THIRD CANADIAN EDITION

Fundamentals of Canadian Nursing
Concepts, Process, and Practice

Barbara Kozier, MN, RN

Glenora Erb, BScN, RN

Audrey Berman, PhD, RN
Professor
Dean, Nursing
Samuel Merritt University
Oakland, California

Shirlee J. Snyder, EdD, RN
Professor
Dean, Nursing
Nevada State College
Henderson, Nevada

Madeleine Buck, RN, BScN, MSc(A)
Assistant Professor
School of Nursing
McGill University
Clinical Associate
McGill University Health Centre

Lucia Yiu, RN, BSc, BA, MScN
Associate Professor
Faculty of Nursing
University of Windsor

Lynnette Leeseberg Stamler, PhD, RN, FAAN
Professor and Associate Dean Graduate Nursing
College of Nursing
South Dakota State University
(formerly of University of Saskatchewan)

WITHDRAWN

SEP 17 2014

PROPERTY OF
SENECA COLLEGE
LIBRARIES
YORKGATE CAMPUS

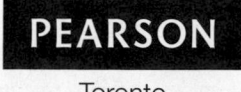
PEARSON

Toronto

Vice-President, Editorial Director: Gary Bennett
Senior Acquisitions Editor: Lisa Rahn
Marketing Manager: Jenna Wulff
Supervising Developmental Editor: Maurice Esses
Senior Developmental Editor: Lise Dupont
Project Manager: Rachel Thompson
Production Editor: Lila Campbell
Copy Editor: Rohini Herbert
Proofreaders: Leanne Rancourt, Tara Tovell
Compositor: Jouve
Photo and Permissions Researcher: Jessica Mifsud, The Editing Company, Toronto
Art Director: Julia Hall
Cover Designer: Anthony Leung
Interior Designer: Anthony Leung
Cover Image: Veer Inc. (Top Left); Corbis Corp. (Top Right); GettyImages (Bottom Left); Masterfile (Bottom Right).

Credits and acknowledgments borrowed from other sources and reproduced, with permission, in this textbook appear on the appropriate page within the text or on page 1675.

Care has been taken to confirm the accuracy of information presented in this book. The authors, editors, and the publisher, however, cannot accept any responsibility for errors or omissions or for consequences from the application of the information in this book and make no warranty, expressed or implied, with respect to its contents.

The authors and publisher have exerted every effort to ensure that drug selections and dosages set forth in this text are in accord with current recommendations and practice at the time of publication. However, in view of ongoing research, changes in government regulations, and the constant flow of information relating to drug therapy and drug reactions, the reader is urged to check the package inserts of all drugs for any change in indications of dosage and for added warnings and precautions. This is particularly important when the recommended agent is a new or infrequently employed drug.

Original edition published by Pearson Education, Inc., Upper Saddle River, New Jersey, USA. Copyright © 2014 Pearson Education, Inc. This edition is authorized for sale only in Canada.

If you purchased this book outside the United States or Canada, you should be aware that it has been imported without the approval of the publisher or the author.

10 9 8 7 6 5 4 3 2 [CKV]

Library and Archives Canada Cataloguing in Publication

Fundamentals of Canadian nursing: concepts, process, and practice / Barbara Kozier ... [et al.]. — 3rd Canadian ed.

Originally publ. under title: Fundamentals of nursing, the nature of nursing practice in Canada.

Includes bibliographical references and index.
ISBN 978-0-13-262761-0

  1. Nursing—Canada—Textbooks. 2. Nursing—Textbooks.
I. Kozier, Barbara

RT41.F86 2013   610.73   C2012-905502-6

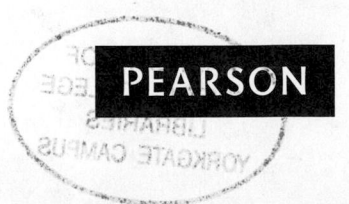

ISBN 978-0-13-262761-0

Contents

Preface *xxi*

Special Features *xxx*

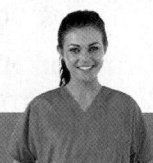

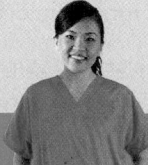

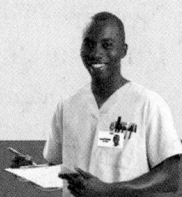

UNIT 3   LIFESPAN AND DEVELOPMENTAL STAGES   323

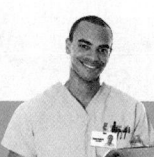

UNIT 4 INTEGRAL ASPECTS OF NURSING 403

UNIT 5 NURSING ASSESSMENT AND CLINICAL STUDIES 591

UNIT 6 PROMOTING PHYSIOLOGICAL HEALTH 1097

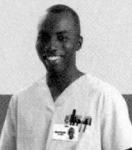

UNIT 7   PROMOTING PSYCHOSOCIAL HEALTH   1473

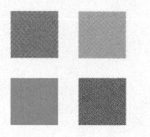

About the Canadian Editors

Madeleine Buck

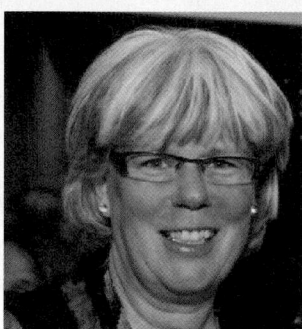

Madeleine Buck is an Assistant Professor and Assistant Director at the McGill University Ingram School of Nursing and a clinical associate at the McGill University Health Centre. Her 35-year career in nursing has provided her with opportunities to work in acute and critical care, community health, and educational settings. She is currently the Program Director of the Bachelor of Science (Nursing) Program at McGill and teaches in the undergraduate and graduate programs, principally in the areas of acute care and illness management. She is active in the Canadian Association of Schools of Nursing (CASN)—as past Chair of the CASN Accreditation Bureau she now sits as co-chair of the CASN Advisory Committee on Accreditation Policies. She is involved in international work and leads McGill Nurses for Highlands Hope, which works with a group of Tanzanian nurses and peer health educators in dealing with the HIV/AIDS pandemic in the Highlands of Tanzania. With her nursing students in the McGill Global Health Masters stream, she works to foster collaboration and development of nursing education and practice relationships, including implementing nursing best practices in low resourced settings in Tanzania. As with previous editions, half of her royalties from the publication of this book will go toward supporting sustainable nursing projects originating from the Tanzanian Highlands Hope Nurse network.

Lucia Yiu

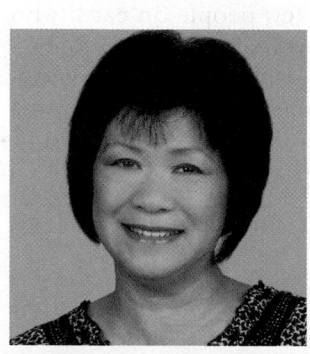

Lucia Yiu, RN, BScN, BA (Psychology, Windsor), BSc (Physiology, Toronto), MScN (Administration, Western Ontario), is an Associate Professor in the Faculty of Nursing, University of Windsor, and an Educational and Training Consultant in community nursing. She has published on family and public health nursing. Her practice and research interests include multicultural health, international health, experiential learning, community development, breast health, and program planning and evaluation. She has worked overseas and served on various community and social services committees involving local and district health planning. Currently, Lucia is board member and committee member with various community organizations related to children's mental health; community health centres; quality assurance; status of women, equity, and diversity; occupational health and employment equity. She is currently president of the World Breast Cancer Organization.

Lynnette Leeseberg Stamler

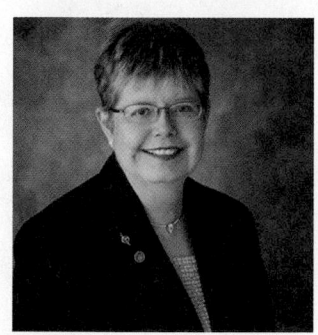

Lynnette Leeseberg Stamler began her nursing career with a BSN from St. Olaf College, Northfield, MN. Her interest in patient teaching began within that program, and inspired her to complete a MEd degree from the University of Manitoba. Although she has worked in many areas of nursing, she has always gravitated to clinical areas where the relationship with patients and families is essential—such as rehabilitation, long-term care, dialysis, and VON (visiting nursing). After teaching in a diploma program at Red River College in Winnipeg, she completed a PhD in nursing from the University of Cincinnati, where she was their third graduate. She has since taught at the University of Windsor, Nipissing University/Canadore College Collaborative BSN program, and the University of Saskatchewan. She has been very active in the Canadian Association of Schools of Nursing (CASN), serving as Treasurer and the first elected President who was not a Dean or Director. She is also active in Sigma Theta Tau International. Her research and international work have focused on aspects of education, from patient to health to nursing. In this spirit, she began work on Canadian nursing textbooks, recognizing that this is one way to influence the next generation of nurses. She has served as an accreditation site visitor. In 2011, her work was recognized when she was inducted as an International Fellow in the American Academy of Nursing, one of eight Canadian nurses to hold that distinction at that time. In the fall of 2012, she embarked on a new adventure, moving to South Dakota to take the position of Associate Dean, Graduate Studies, College of Nursing, South Dakota State University.

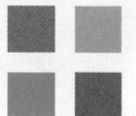

Dedication

Madeleine Buck dedicates this edition to the Highlands Hope Umbrella, an organization that brings together community, professional, and volunteer networks to address the challenge of HIV-AIDS and related social problems in the Njombe region of the Southern Highlands of Tanzania. The knowledge, skill, creativity, and dedication of nurses, nursing students, and other members within the "Umbrella" is truly commendable.

Lucia Yiu dedicates this edition to her family and especially to her students and nursing colleagues who have inspired her to strive for excellence in nursing.

Lynnette Leeseberg Stamler dedicates this edition to her biological sisters, Karen and Marilyn, to her many nonbiological sisters through marriage and friendship, and to her many students and colleagues. Each has contributed to her learning and joy in nursing and teaching. All have supported her in many ways along the journey.

Audrey Berman dedicates this edition to Bo-Gunnar Edvard Dahlström, without whom it would not have been possible. There are few people on earth who can simultaneously challenge and support Audrey—even with all my sharp edges—and he is one. Audrey is grateful for his intellect and English skills, which exceed her own. He loves three nurses unconditionally: his sister, his daughter, and Audrey.

Shirlee Snyder dedicates this edition in loving memory of her late mother, Jean Snyder, and to her husband, Terry J. Schnitter, for his unconditional love and support.

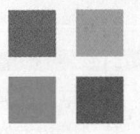

Chapter Features: Walk-Through

We carefully prepared a variety of special features to facilitate learning and to highlight the 5 major themes that form the framework for this edition—namely, *Primary Health Care, Critical Thinking, Clinical Reasoning, Nursing Process,* and *Lifespan Considerations.*

LEARNING OUTCOMES ▶
outline the essential concepts addressed in the chapter

LEARNING OUTCOMES

After studying this chapter, you will be able to:

1. Explain the relationship of individuality and holism to nursing practice.

2. Compare and contrast the elements of physiological and psychological homeostasis.

3. Identify six common factors that can make an individual more vulnerable to some health problems and describe a nursing implication for each.

4. Identify Maslow's five categories in the hierarchy of human needs.

5. Discuss how a nurse might use the three selected types of theories to begin to assess an individual's health needs.

EVIDENCE-INFORMED PRACTICE ▶
boxes highlight relevant Canadian research; systematic reviews and meta-analyses are cited within each box and clinical relevance is carefully described.

EVIDENCE-INFORMED PRACTICE

What Causes Temper Tantrums?

The purpose of the study was to determine how *emotional reactivity* and *emotional competence* of the children contributed to temper tantrums, and 127 families with 3- to 5-year-old children in British Columbia took part in the study. Results showed that children who were more emotionally competent were less likely to display anger and distress. But more importantly, emotionally competent children, while they may be just as emotionally reactive as other children, were less likely to display the full-blown temper tantrum.

NURSING IMPLICATIONS: A child's level of emotional competence, not the tendency to be emotionally reactive, was the key to understanding why some reactive children have tantrums and others do not. Nurses need to understand that two children with similar thresholds for emotional reactivity may display widely different frequencies of temper tantrums and that maturity (i.e., age) and verbal ability had little effect on temper tantrums.

Source: Based on Giesbrecht, G., Miller, M., & Müller, U. (2010). The anger-distress model of temper tantrums: Associations with emotional reactivity and emotional competence. *Infant and Child Development, 19,* 478–497.

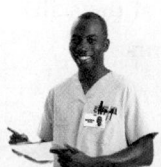

Case Study 18

Billy is a 6-year-old boy entering Grade 1. He is scared and hesitant to let go of his mother's hand. As the nursing student working in this setting, you have the opportunity to work with Billy and other young children as they start school.

CRITICAL THINKING QUESTIONS

1. How would you help Billy's mother reassure him?
2. On the basis of his age, what strategies might you use to teach Billy and his classmates about health promotion?

After working through these questions, visit **www.pearsoncanada.ca/mynursinglab** to check your answers.

◀ CASE STUDIES
present scenarios applicable to Canadian nursing and relevant to the chapter topic at hand.

- *Critical thinking questions* that accompany each Case Study guide students to reflect about the case from different points of view to ensure comprehensive analysis.

- *Suggested answers* to the case-based critical thinking questions can be found in the Instructor's Manual and on the Study on the Go feature.

NURSING AND CANADIAN SOCIETY ▶

boxes summarize relevant facts about issues in Canadian society and their implications for nursing.

Nursing and Canadian Society

Fact	Implications for Nursing Practice
Most older Canadian adults live independently in the community and desire to remain in their homes (PHAC, 2009). In 2008-09, about 0.7% of the Canadian population lived in an institution; of this, about 75% were 65 years and older (Organization for Economic Co-operation and Development, 2011).	Nurses need to be aware of the resources and community services available to their older clients. "Aging in place" interventions can assist older adults to maintain their independence.
Canada has a shortage of health care professionals, including nurses, who specialize in the care of older persons. Numerous Canadian organizations and professional associations actively engage in and disseminate research to better meet the needs of older Canadians (PHAC, 2009).	All nurses need to acquire the requisite knowledge, skills, and expertise to care for the rapidly growing numbers of older adults in Canada—to understand trends that impact health care delivery, plan for evidence-based interventions, and advocate for safe and ethical care.
Although cancer death rate is falling in Canada, cancer incidence and mortality rates continue to be highest among the older adults (Canadian Cancer Society's Steering Committee on Cancer Statistics, 2012).	Nurses are challenged to successfully implement cancer prevention strategies to promote healthy lifestyle changes into the daily lives of older persons (e.g., promoting cancer screening, healthy diet, and active living).

REFLECT ON PRIMARY HEALTH CARE

Nurses apply critical thinking skills as they use a *primary health care approach* to care for their clients. This activity involves knowing *what* are the health-promotion needs of their clients; *how, where,* and *when* to engage their clients and the members of the multidisciplinary team for input regarding their clients' needs, strengths, and barriers; and *what* and *how* to adapt the resources or appropriate technology in order to design services and care that will meet the clients' socioeconomic and cultural needs.

◀ REFLECT ON PRIMARY HEALTH CARE

boxes ask readers to reflect about the clinical application of one or more of the five principles of primary health care (i.e., health promotion, accessibility, public participation, appropriate use of technology, and intersectoral collaboration) in relation to chapter-specific topics.

SKILL BOXES ▶

provide clear step-by-step directions and feature the following:

- Clear purpose statement
- Clinical reasoning questions (for many of the skill instructions).
- Steps to consider during implementation of the skill
- A complete list of equipment required to ensure success
- Patient identification procedures and "infection prevention and control reminders" to promote patient safety

SKILL 39.5 TRANSFERRING BETWEEN BED AND CHAIR

PURPOSE

A client may need to be transferred between the bed and a wheelchair or chair, the bed and the commode, or a wheelchair and the toilet. This technique has numerous variations. Which variation the nurse selects depends on factors related to the client, the environment, and the health care provider, which are assessed before beginning the transfer.

ASSESSMENT

Before transferring a client, assess the following:
- Client's body size
- Client's ability to follow instructions
- Client's activity tolerance
- Client's muscle strength and ability to bear weight
- Client's joint mobility
- Presence of paralysis or paresis
- Client's level of comfort

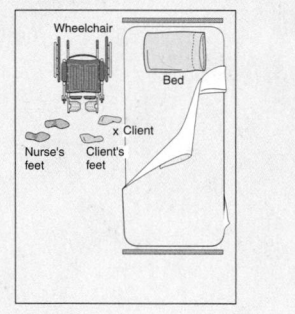

❶ The wheelchair is placed parallel to the bed as close to the bed as possible. Note that placement of the nurse's feet mirrors that of the client's feet.

- Easily identified rationales throughout the skill instructions to ensure complete understanding of each step
- Coloured photos and illustrations provide the visual cues needed to ensure accurate completion of the skill

An evaluation focus at the end of each skill ensures that the relevant assessment and follow-up occurs.

LIFESPAN CONSIDERATIONS ▶

boxes identify clearly when and how nursing care should be adapted for the needs of infants, children, adolescents, and/or older adults.

LIFESPAN CONSIDERATIONS

Positioning, Moving, and Turning Clients

INFANTS
- Position infants on their back for sleep, even after feeding. They have little risk of regurgitation and choking, and the rate of sudden infant death syndrome (SIDS) is significantly lower in infants who sleep on their backs.
- The skin of newborns can be fragile and may be abraded or torn (sheared) if the infant is pulled across a bed.

CHILDREN
- Carefully inspect at least three times in each 24-hour period the dependent skin surfaces of all infants and children confined to bed.

OLDER ADULTS
- Clients who have had cerebrovascular accidents (CVAs, strokes) have a risk of shoulder displacement on the paralyzed side from improper moving or repositioning techniques. Use care when moving, positioning in bed, and transferring. Pillows or foam devices are helpful to support the affected arm and shoulder and prevent injury.
- Decreased subcutaneous fat and thinning of the skin place older adults at risk for skin breakdown. Repositioning approximately every 2 hours (more or less, depending on the unique needs of the individual client) helps reduce pressure on bony prominences and avoid tissue trauma.

CLINICAL ALERTS ▶
focus on patient safety and highlight the potential risks that nurses must watch out for.

CLINICAL ALERT

Take safety measures before faxing confidential information. Consent is needed from the client to fax information. Make sure that personally identifiable information (e.g., client name, social insurance number) has been removed. If needed, confirm that the material is being sent to a confidential fax number or call ahead to ensure the person is present to receive the fax. Check that the fax number is correct before pressing the send button.

HOME CARE CONSIDERATIONS ▶
boxes guide readers to consider the issues that could affect the client's successful home recovery and living.

HOME CARE CONSIDERATIONS

Positioning, Moving, and Turning Clients

- Assess the height of the bed and the person's leg length to ensure that self-movement in and out of the bed are smooth.
- Inspect the client's mattress for support.
- Assess the caregivers' knowledge and application of body mechanics to prevent injury.
- Demonstrate how to turn and position the client in bed. Observe the caregiver performing a return demonstration. Re-evaluate this technique periodically to reinforce correct application of body mechanics.
- Teach caregivers the basic principles of body alignment and how to check for proper alignment after the client has been changed to a new position.

- Warn caregivers of the dangers of lifting and repositioning and encourage the use of assistive devices and a "no solo lift" policy.
- Teach the caregiver to check the client's skin for redness and integrity after repositioning the client. Stress the importance of informing the nurse about the length of time skin redness remains over pressure areas after the person has been repositioned. Emphasize that reddened areas should not be massaged as it may lead to tissue trauma.

CLINICAL MANIFESTATIONS ▶
boxes feature bulleted lists of common signs and symptoms to provide a quick and easy reference to key manifestations of illness situations.

CLINICAL MANIFESTATIONS

Hypothermia

Hypothermia typically manifests in the following ways:

- Decreased body temperature
- Severe shivering (initially)
- Feelings of cold and chills
- Pale, cool, waxy skin
- Hypotension
- Decreased urinary output
- Lack of muscle coordination
- Disorientation
- Drowsiness progressing to coma

PRACTICE GUIDELINES 32.2

Applying Restraints

◀ PRACTICE GUIDELINES
provide clear and succinct summaries of evidence-based clinical actions and their rationales.

Guidelines	Rationales
Ensure that all alternative measures other than restraints have been exhausted and that the least restraint option is being used. Assure the client and the family that the restraint is temporary and protective.	Underlying reasons for restraints must be addressed and corrected, if possible, as their use is associated with psychological (guilt, anger, shame, feeling punished) and physiological (strangulation, skin breakdown, constipation) risks.
Obtain consent from the client or guardian and ensure that necessary collective or physician prescriptions are in order.	Legal and ethical considerations require informed consent, unless in an emergency situation. Health agencies generally have specific protocols and lines of authority to ensure practices are consistent and safe.
If restraints are applied, ensure the following:	
• Apply the restraint so that the client can move as freely as possible without defeating the purpose of the restraint.	Inability to move can cause anxiety and agitation, and enhance the risk of physiological complications, such as aspiration if vomiting.
• Apply a restraint using quick-release buckles or a half-bow (quick-release) knot that does not tighten when pulled and supports the normal anatomy of the body part.	Time is of the essence in emergency situations and tight physical restraints can impede blood circulation and are uncomfortable; contractures and discomfort can arise from poor body alignment.

Sample Care Plan for Amanda Aquilini

Nursing Diagnosis: Ineffective Airway Clearance related to viscous secretions and shallow chest expansion secondary to deficient fluid volume, pain, and fatigue

Goals/Desired Outcomes	Nursing Interventions	Rationale
Demonstrate adequate air exchange (goal), as evidenced by the following: • Absence of pallor and cyanosis (skin and mucous membranes) • Using correct breathing/coughing technique after instruction • Productive cough • Symmetric chest expansion of at least 4 cm	Monitor respiratory status q4h: rate, depth, effort, skin colour, mucous membranes, amount and colour of sputum. Monitor results of blood gases, chest x-ray studies, and incentive spirometer volume, as available. Monitor level of consciousness. Auscultate lungs q4h. Take vital signs q4h (temperature, pulse, respiration [TPR], blood pressure [BP], pulse oximetry, pain).	*This helps identify progress toward or deviations from goal. Ineffective Airway Clearance leads to poor oxygenation, evidenced by pallor, cyanosis, lethargy, and drowsiness.* *Inadequate oxygenation causes increased pulse rate. Respiratory rate may be decreased by narcotic analgesics.*
Within 48–72 hours • Lungs clear to auscultation • Respirations 12–22/min, pulse <100 beats/min	Instruct in breathing and coughing techniques. Remind to perform, and assist q3h.	*This enables the client to cough up secretions. The client may need encouragement and support because of fatigue and pain.*
• Inhaling normal volume of air on incentive spirometer	Administer prescribed expectorant; schedule for maximum effectiveness.	*This helps loosen secretions so they can be coughed up and expelled.*

◀ **SAMPLE CARE PLANS** outline the nursing process relative to specific clinical scenarios; rationales for all nursing actions are provided to help increase the reader's understanding of each component of the plan.

HEALTH-PROMOTION GUIDELINES ▶

provide recommendations for how to promote the health of clients at various stages in the lifespan.

Health-Promotion Guidelines 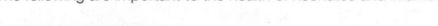 for Neonates and Infants

The following are important to the health of neonates and infants:

HEALTH EXAMINATIONS
• At birth, screening for hearing, congenital hypothyroidism, and phenylketonuria (PKU).
• Physical examination at birth, 2 weeks, and at 2, 4, 6, 9, and 12 months

PROTECTIVE MEASURES
• Routine immunizations: 5-in-1 DTaP-IPV and Hib vaccines protect against diphtheria, tetanus, pertussis, polio, and *Haemophilus influenzae,* type B (Hib) vaccine, hepatitis B vaccine (HepB), varicella vaccine, pneumococcal conjugate vaccine, and meningococcal C conjugate vaccine; influenza vaccine and other vaccines, as recommended. Schedules may vary across provinces and territories. See Table 34.9: Routine Immunization Schedules for Infants and Children (page 988).
• Fluoride supplements, if inadequate water fluoridation (less than 0.7 parts per million [ppm])
• Screening for congenital hypothyroidism, PKU, and other metabolic and congenital disorders, according to jurisdictions
• Prompt attention for illnesses or fever
• Appropriate skin hygiene and clothing
• Assessment of caregiver–infant relationship quality

INFANT SAFETY
• Supervision at all times
• Car seat, crib, playpen, bath, sleeping arrangement, and home environment safety measures
• Feeding measures (e.g., avoid propping the bottle during feeding)

• Toys with no small parts or sharp edges
• Elimination of toxins in the environment (e.g., tobacco, chemicals, radon, lead, mercury)
• Use of smoke and carbon monoxide (CO) detectors in home

NUTRITION
• Exclusive breast-feeding to 6 months
• Proper breast-feeding and bottle-feeding techniques
• Formula preparation
• Feeding schedule
• Introduction of solid foods
• Need for iron supplements at 4 to 6 months; iron-fortified formulas to infants who are not breastfed or for infants receiving formula as well as breast milk; by age 6 months, iron-rich foods
• Continued breast-feeding to age 12 months

ELIMINATION
• Characteristics and frequency of stool and urine elimination
• Diarrhea and dehydration signs

REST AND SLEEP
• Established routine for sleep and rest patterns

SENSORY STIMULATION
• Touch: holding, cuddling, rocking
• Vision: colourful, moving toys
• Hearing: soothing voice tones, music, singing
• Play: toys appropriate for development

TEACHING   CLINICAL

Client Self-Management of Pain by Using a Patient-Controlled Analgesia Pump

Choose a time to teach the client about pain management when the pain is controlled so that the client is able to focus on the teaching.

Teaching the client about self-management of pain can include the following:

• Demonstrate the operation of the patient-controlled analgesia (PCA) pump and explain that the client can safely push the button without fear of overmedicating. Sometimes, it helps clients who are reluctant to repeatedly push the button to know that they must dose themselves (i.e., push the button) 5 to 10 times

to receive the same amount of medication (10 mg morphine equivalent) they would receive in a standard injection.
• Describe the use of the pain scale and encourage the client to respond to demonstrate understanding.
• Explore a variety of nondrug pain relief techniques that the client is willing to learn and use to promote pain relief and optimize functioning.
• Explain to the client the need to notify staff when ambulation is desired (e.g., for bathroom use), if applicable.

◀ **TEACHING: CLINICAL** boxes discuss teaching with regard to the learning needs of the individual client.

TEACHING   HOME CARE

Hygiene

Suggest the client or family do the following:

- Consider purchasing a bath seat that fits in the tub or shower.
- Install a hand shower for use with a bath seat and shampooing.
- Use a nonskid surface on the tub or shower floor.
- Install hand bars on both sides of the tub or shower to facilitate transfers in and out of the tub or shower.
- Carefully monitor the temperature of the bathwater. See Chapter 32 for hot water tank setting recommendations.
- Apply lotion *after* the client is out of the tub or shower since lotions may make the tub surface or shower floor slippery.

◀ **TEACHING: HOME CARE**
boxes describe teaching methods designed to facilitate self-care for clients living at home.

▼ **TEACHING: WELLNESS**
boxes offer teaching methods directed at providing wellness or health-promotion information to help clients live healthier lives.

TEACHING   WELLNESS

Reducing Electrical Hazards

Take the following steps to reduce electrical hazards:

- Check cords for fraying or other signs of damage before using an appliance. Do not use it if the cord is damaged.
- Avoid overloading outlets and fuse boxes with too many appliances; use grounded outlets and plugs.
- Always pull a plug from the wall outlet by firmly grasping the plug and pulling it straight out. Pulling a plug by its cord can damage the cord and plug unit.
- Ensure that ground fault circuit interrupters (GFCIs) have been installed wherever electrical appliances or equipment can inadvertently come in contact with water, such as near sinks, bathtubs, or showers, or outdoors.

- Keep electric cords and appliances out of the reach of children, and place protective covers over wall outlets to protect young children.
- Carefully read instructions before operating electric equipment.
- Always disconnect appliances before cleaning or repairing them.
- Unplug any appliance that has given a tingling sensation or shock and have an electrician evaluate it.
- Keep electric cords coiled or taped to the ground away from areas of traffic to prevent people from damaging the cords or tripping over them.

ASSESSMENT   HOME CARE

- Monitor respiratory rate following the administration of respiratory depressants, such as morphine.
- Assess the home setting for factors that could interfere with breathing, such as exhaust, gas, or cigarette smoke.
- If the client has just come in from another room, allow the client to rest a minute or two before counting respirations.

◀ **ASSESSMENT: HOME CARE**
boxes provide guidelines to assess the needs of clients or families or caregivers and explain how to assess the available community resources for discharge and home care planning.

ASSESSMENT INTERVIEW

Hygiene Practices

The following questions can help the nurse learn about the client's hygiene practices:

SKIN CARE PRACTICES

- What is your usual time to shower or bathe?
- What products, such as soap, shampoo, deodorant, do you prefer to use?
- What products, if any, do you use on your face?
- How frequently do you clean or discard applicators or puffs that you use on your face?
- Are there any products or practices that you avoid because of how they affect your skin?

SELF-CARE ABILITIES

- Do you have any problems managing your own hygiene?
- What assistance can the nurse give you to help you meet your need for hygiene?

SKIN PROBLEMS

- Do you have any tendency toward dry skin, acne, itchiness, rashes, bruising, excessive perspiration, or lack of perspiration?
- Do you have any allergies? If so, to what?

◄ **ASSESSMENT: INTERVIEW** boxes offer examples of interviewing questions that can be used to help elicit relevant assessment data from the client.

ASSESSMENT: DEVELOPMENTAL GUIDELINES ▶

boxes feature critical assessment questions relevant to the growth and developmental needs of the client.

ASSESSMENT DEVELOPMENTAL GUIDELINES

The Young Adult

In these three developmental areas, does the young adult do the following?

1. **PHYSICAL DEVELOPMENT**
   - Exhibit weight and BMI within normal range for age and gender
   - Manifest vital signs (e.g., blood pressure) within normal range for age and gender
   - Demonstrate visual and hearing abilities within normal range
   - Exhibit appropriate knowledge (e.g., STIs) and attitudes about sexuality

2. **PSYCHOSOCIAL DEVELOPMENT**
   - Feel independent from parents
   - Have a realistic self-concept

   - Like self and direction of life
   - Interact well with family
   - Cope with the stresses of change and growth
   - Have well-established bonds with significant others and intimacy with a partner or close friends
   - Have a meaningful social life
   - Demonstrate emotional, social, and economic responsibility for own life
   - Have a set of values that guide behaviour

3. **ACTIVITIES OF DAILY LIVING**
   - Have a healthy lifestyle

CONCEPT MAP Ineffective Airway Clearance (Gas Exchange)

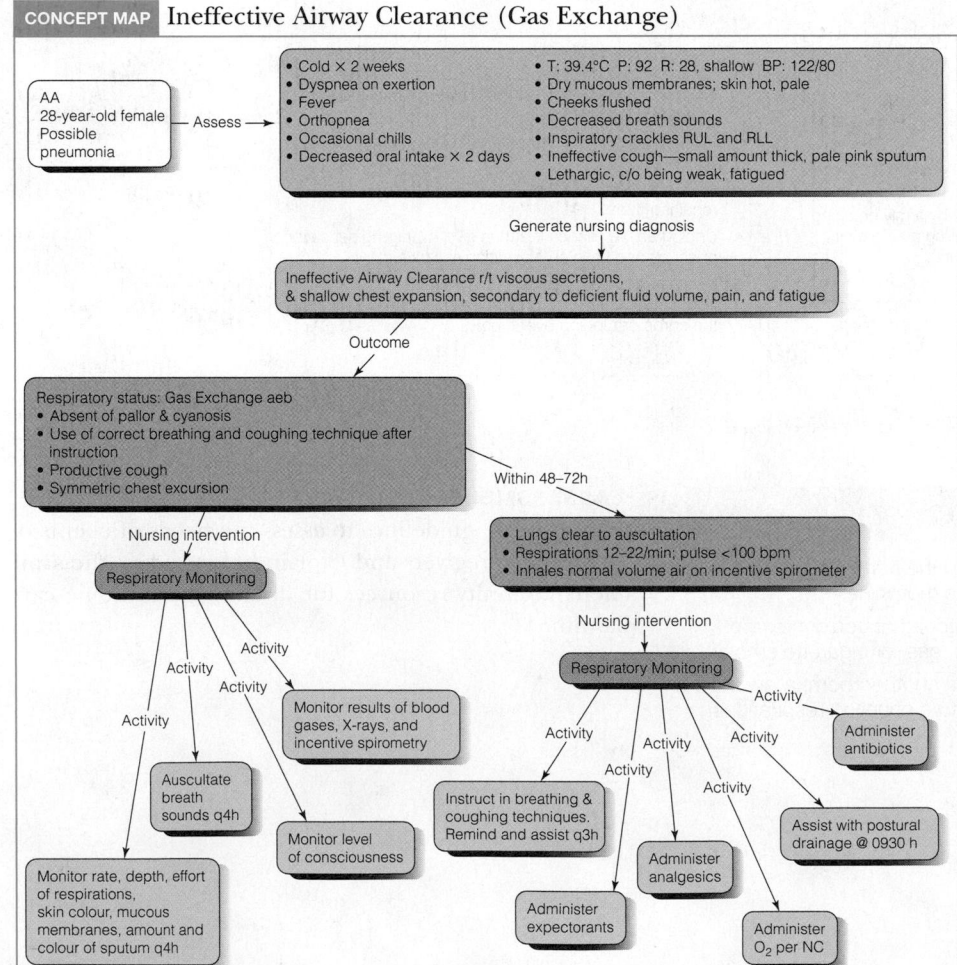

◄ **CONCEPT MAPS** show the schematic relationships of various concepts and elements of both the nursing process and nursing care plans.

KEY TERMS ▶

summarize, in alphabetical order, the essential vocabulary associated with each chapter; the key term is defined and high-lighted in boldface upon first mention in the chapter, and then both the term and the definition appear again in the end-of-book Glossary.

KEY TERMS

capacity building   *p. 189*

climate change   *p. 183*

colonialism   *p. 189*

environmental health factors   *p. 183*

epidemiological transition   *p. 188*

food security   *p. 195*

global health   *p. 187*

Indigenous peoples   *p. 193*

international health   *p. 187*

international nursing   *p. 192*

migration   *p. 193*

Millennium Development Goals (MDGs)   *p. 189*

natural disasters   *p. 195*

pollution   *p. 186*

poverty   *p. 194*

safe water   *p. 186*

sanitation   *p. 186*

social determinants of health   *p. 193*

social justice   *p. 192*

surveillance   *p. 195*

sustainability   *p. 192*

vectors of disease   *p. 185*

ASSESS YOUR LEARNING

1. On the basis of a community needs assessment, a public health nurse develops a program to prevent childhood obesity. Which strategy is most appropriate for successful implementation?
   a. Providing information to the teacher for classroom use
   b. Involving parents, teachers, and children in program development
   c. Asking the school administration to remove all vending machines
   d. Initiating an exercise program during recess for children who are obese

2. In contrast to a home health nurse, the practice of public health nurses is characterized by a focus on what?
   a. Illness and injury prevention
   b. The health of populations
   c. Work in school health, occupational health, and home care

employ which of the following primary health care principles?
   a. Accessibility, health promotion, and public participation
   b. Illness and injury prevention; political action
   c. Social justice and equity
   d. Appropriate use of technology and community organization

5. Planning for discharge from an institutional setting, such as a hospital, can include a referral to a home care nurse. What BEST describes the expectations of the referral?
   a. The home care nurse will deliver all care himself or herself.
   b. The discharge assessment of service needs will be followed exactly.
   c. The home care nurse will coordinate the health care service needs of the client.
   d. The discharge plan is developed solely by the discharge planner and the client.

◀ ASSESS YOUR LEARNING

sections present 10 multiple-choice questions to help reinforce concepts and clinical application. Answers can be found in the Instructor's Manual and in the Study on the Go feature.

WEBLINKS ▶

lists offer readers an annotated list of relevant web-based resources

WEBLINKS

Canadian Interdisciplinary Network for CAM Research (IN-CAM)
http://www.incamresearch.ca
Launched in January 2004, IN-CAM's two primary objectives are to build research capacity and facilitate interdisciplinary CAM research in Canada, particularly from the perspective of health services or social science. It offers a searchable members database, bimonthly e-bulletin, networking opportunities, and an annual research symposium. Membership is free.

the regulating authority for natural health products for sale in Canada.

Canadian Holistic Nurses Association
http://www.chna.ca
This site presents the philosophy and objectives of the Canadian Holistic Nurses Association (CHNA) and information on the levels of training for a holistic nursing specialty.

◀ STUDY ON THE GO—QUICK RESPONSE CODES

align text and mobile learning by providing access to practice assessments, glossary flashcards, and more.

REFERENCES ▶

sections cite the relevant evidence-based sources that appear in each chapter. Readers are encouraged to consult these to further enhance their comprehension of the chapter topics.

REFERENCES

Bowlby, J. (1999). Attachment and loss. Vol. 1. *Attachment* (2nd ed.). New York, NY: Basic Books.

De Pauw, S. S., Mervielde, I., & Van Leeuwen, K. G. (2009). How are traits related to problem behaviour in preschoolers? Similarities and contrasts between temperament and personality. *Journal of Abnormal Child Psychology 37*, 309–325. doi:10.1007/s10802-008-9290-0

Erikson, E. H. (1963). *Childhood and society* (2nd ed.). New York, NY: Norton.

Erikson, E. H. (1964). *Insight and responsibility: Lectures on the ethical implications of psychoanalytic insight.* New York, NY: Norton.

Fowler, J., & Keen, S. (1985). *Life maps: Conversations in the journey of faith.* Waco. TX: Word Books.

Gould, R. L. (1972). The phases of adult life: A study in developmental psychology. *American Journal of Psychiatry, 129,* 33–43.

Havighurst, R. J. (1972). *Developmental tasks and education* (3rd ed.). New York, NY: Longman Publishers.

Kohlberg, L. (1984). *Essays on moral development: Vol. 2. The psychology of moral development.* San Francisco, CA: Harper & Row.

Murray, R. B., Zentner, J. P., & Yakimo, R. (2009). *Health promotion strategies through the life span* (8th ed.). Upper Saddle River, NJ: Prentice Hall.

Peck, R. (1968). *Psychological developments in the second half of life.* In B. L. Neugarten (Ed.), *Middle age and aging* (pp. 88–92). Chicago. IL: University of Chicago Press.

 # Preface

As the scope and pace of nursing and allied health knowledge continues to grow exponentially, one must ask what is truly *"fundamental"* for a nurse to know and understand in order to practice knowledgeably, morally, ethically, accurately, sensitively, and compassionately in both today's and tomorrow's health care delivery system. Within the context of the current and future health-care system, the third Canadian edition of *Fundamentals of Canadian Nursing: Concept, Process, and Practice* provides undergraduate nursing students with the *fundamentals* they will require as they embark on their nursing careers. This textbook aims to provide students with a broad and solid foundation of knowledge about the health of individuals, families, communities, and populations. Also included are the issues that client populations face at varying points in time, as well as the nursing care that is possible in health and illness situations, whether clients are situated at home, in the community, at a clinic, at an extended or palliative care facility, or in an acute care setting. We hope that this text will serve as a "go to" resource for students and practicing nurses working in a wide range of settings.

With the goal of providing a fundamental understanding of what is required for contemporary professional nursing practice in Canada, we built on the first and second editions to ensure that we thoroughly addressed needed *skills,* such as communication, critical thinking, clinical reasoning, decision making, use of the nursing process, development of interpersonal and interprofessional relationships, teaching, leading and managing change, use of technology, and application of primary health-care principles. We placed high importance on such conepts as caring, wellness, health promotion, disease prevention, complementary and alternative health modalities, rural health, environmental and global health, multiculturalism, growth and development, nursing theories, nursing informatics, nursing research and education, ethics, accountability, and advocacy. Furthermore, we highlighted basic nursing care for clients across the lifespan from hospital to community settings in the culturally diverse Canadian health-care system throughout. In all areas, we integrated the most recent literature and clinical best-practice guidelines.

To ensure that our text reflects "pan-Canadian" issues and practices, we enlisted reviewers and contributors from across the country, representing different geographical perspectives. We expended every effort to ensure that the level of specificity and readability is appropriate for beginning nursing students. We believe that this text will also provide a strong foundation for advanced nursing studies. Enjoy!

Organization

For this third Canadian edition, we present 7 units for a total of 49 chapters—one more than our last edition, as we added a new chapter entitled *Environmental and Global Health Nursing* (see page v for a complete list of chapters). The material presented in this publication addresses foundational and fundamental knowledge and skills required for a person entering the nursing profession. Building on the strengths of our first and second editions, we enhanced many features to ensure that our textbook is relevant and informative to nurses across the country.

UNIT 1—THE FOUNDATION OF NURSING IN CANADA (Chapters 1–6) introduces the nature of the nursing profession, from the history of nursing to its current practice, education, and research. Each chapter has been updated since our last edition to reflect evolving trends and emerging issues such as changes to nursing practice standards, the increasing role of nurses as research consumers, the influx of internationally educated nurses, moral distress in the work of nurses, and the role of social media in nursing and health care, among many other topics.

UNIT 2—CONTEMPORARY HEALTH CARE IN CANADA (Chapters 7–16) describes health-care practice in today's multicultural environments. Concepts of health, illness, and wellness are addressed as well as the role nurses can play in health promotion from an individual, family, community and global perspective. This unit addresses foundational concepts related to Canada's health care system and specific issues related to rural and remote health care, including Northern nursing. *Chapter 10: Environmental and Global Health Nursing* is a NEW chapter. Topics addressed include: how the environment influences health; theories related to global development; and major issues in global health such as migration, poverty, inequality, gender, and infectious diseases (to name a few).

UNIT 3—LIFESPAN AND DEVELOPMENTAL STAGES (Chapters 17–20) describes concepts of growth and development and outlines the various developmental stages and their specific health needs throughout the lifespan. Particular attention has been given to the issues facing the very young and older adults.

UNIT 4—INTEGRAL ASPECTS OF NURSING (Chapters 21–27) describes the fundamental nursing tools required for practice, including critical thinking, clinical reasoning and decision making, caring and communicating, the nursing process, documenting and reporting, teaching and learning, and leading and managing change. These tools provide a foundation for competent nursing care.

UNIT 5—NURSING ASSESSMENT AND CLINICAL SKILLS (Chapters 28–36) provides fundamental knowledge to guide comprehensive health assessment, including vital signs, and addresses integral components of care in relation to pain assessment and management, hygiene, safety, medications, infection prevention and control, skin integrity and wound care, and caring for perioperative clients.

UNIT 6—PROMOTING PHYSIOLOGICAL HEALTH (Chapters 37–44) discusses such physiologic concepts as sensory perception; sleep; activity and exercise; nutrition; fecal elimination; urinary elimination; fluid, electrolytes, and acid-base balance; and oxygenation and circulation.

UNIT 7—PROMOTING PSYCHOSOCIAL HEALTH (Chapters 45–49) covers a wide range of areas that affect one's health. Self-concept, sexuality, spirituality, stress and coping, and loss, grieving, and death are all areas that a nurse should consider to care effectively for a client.

Following the book chapters is a **Glossary** in which key terms are defined. Three **Appendices** are provided near the end of the book. They summarize important information about laboratory values, formulae, and vital signs.

What's New in the 3rd Canadian Edition

- NEW approach with adoption of a broader, less prescriptive approach to nursing diagnoses. This new edition encourages students and nurses to use their knowledge, experience, and critical thinking skills to generate diagnoses or analysis.
- NEW focus on "Environmental and Global Health Nursing"—A whole new chapter is devoted to this important and fascinating topic.
- NEW Patient Safety—All national patient safety consensus recommendations from Safer HealthCare NOW!, the Canadian Patient Safety Institute, and Accreditation Canada have been integrated into relevant chapters.

- NEW Community Health Assessment focus—In addition to individual and family assessment features, we have added a community health assessment focus.
- NEW emphasis on Clinical Reasoning—A discussion about the importance of clinical reasoning and the similarities and differences between, and among, clinical reasoning and critical thinking now appear. *Clinical Reasoning* questions appear in several chapters to encourage readers to consider the clinical context as a major factor in determining the specific priorities and approach to nursing care.
- REINSTATED Glossary of Key Terms—Previously, our glossary of key terms was available on-line; based on feedback from users, we have reinstated the glossary as part of the text so that users have ready access to such an important feature.
- UPDATED Reflects the Latest Evidence—A thorough review of the literature was conducted for each chapter. Emphasis was placed on including the results of systematic reviews and meta analyses to ensure the highest level of evidence.
- UPDATED All relevant national consensus guidelines related to nursing care are included in the relevant chapters.
- ENHANCED Rationales for Nursing Care—All Skill instructions and Clinical Guidelines were reviewed and revised to ensure that a rationale is provided for each recommendation to promote clarity and understanding.
- ENHANCED Pan-Canadian Perspective—Reviewers and contributors were selected from across Canada to ensure that the textbook provides a relevant and comprehensive perspective on nursing care and issues facing nurses across the country.
- ENHANCED Level of Foundational Knowledge—We took care to sustain the broad knowledge base provided by this foundational "fundamentals" text; however, the depth and specificity of certain topics were updated and augmented where required throughout the text.
- ENHANCED Images and Photos—Over 50 new colour photos have been added, mostly in the Skill Boxes, to enhance clarity and that the most up-to-date equipment appears.

Resources and Supplements

Student Resources

Clinical Reference Cards

Each copy of the book is accompanied by a series of Clinical Reference Cards, which are intended to serve as a handy reference when engaged in clinical work. The contents include brief summaries of such topics as the normal ranges of vital signs for various age groups, common laboratory values, the Glasgow Coma Scale, and the "10 Rights" of medication administration.

Online Resources

At the end of every chapter, students will find a QR code (also known as a quick response code) that aligns text and mobile learning. Students can access practice quizzes, glossary flashcards, and more text-specific resources through their smartphones, allowing them to study whenever and wherever the wish!

Students can visit one of the sites below to download a free app to their smartphone to gain access to these resources. Once the app is installed, the phone scans the code and links to a website that features Fundamentals of Canadian Nursing's Study on the Go content.

> **ScanLife**
> http://getscanlife.com
> **NeoReader**
> http://get.neoreader.com
> **QuickMark**
> http://www.quickmark.com.tw

MyNursingLab

MyNursingLab engages students in higher level thinking to move beyond knowledge acquisition to true learning through application with its unique, "Review, Remember, Apply" study plan.

Instructor Resources

An **Instructor's Manual** includes answers to all the questions in the book, along with other material to help instructors to design effective classes.

Powerpoint Slides illuminate and build upon key concepts in the text.

An **Image Library** provides electronic files of all the figures, photos, and tables in the book.

Pearson's TestGen computerized **Testbank** is a powerful program that enables professors to view and edit existing questions, create new questions, and generate quizzes, tests, exams, or homework. TestGen also allows for the administration of tests on a local area network, have the tests graded electronically, and have the results prepared in electronic or printed reports.

Acknowledgments

We wish to extend our sincere thanks to the many talented and committed people involved in the development of this third Canadian edition. We are especially grateful to

- The students and colleagues who provided valuable suggestions for developing this edition, in particular users who alerted us to new practices or region-specific variations in practice.
- The Canadian contributors, who worked diligently to provide content in their areas of expertise (listed on pages xxv–xxvii).
- The Canadian reviewers, who provided critical appraisal to strengthen this text (listed on pages xxviii).
- The editors and contributors of the U.S. ninth edition for setting high standards for the book (listed on page xxix).

- The two people who revised the end-of-chapter test questions: Sandy Kostashuk, Grant MacEwan University, and Barbara Thompson, Sault College.
- The expert guidance and ongoing support from the editorial and production teams at Pearson Canada: Lisa Rahn, Lise Dupont, Trish Ciardullo, Rachel Thompson, Avinash Chandra, Lila Campbell, Rohini Herbert, Ben Zaporozan, and many others who worked scrupulously behind the scenes to help realize this project.

Madeleine Buck

Lucia Yiu

Lynnette Leeseberg Stamler

Thank You: Canadian Contributors

We would like to extend our heartfelt thanks to the following instructors, who contributed their knowledge and expertise to the Third Canadian Edition:

Mary-Anne Andrusyszyn, RN, BScN, MScN, EdD
Professor and Director
Arthur Labatt Family School of Nursing
Faculty of Health Sciences
Western University

Yolanda Babenko-Mould, RN, BScN, MScN, PhD
Assistant Professor
Arthur Labatt Family School of Nursing
Faculty of Health Sciences
Western University

Judith Bailey, RN, MN
Associate Professor
Department of Nursing
Cape Breton University

Cynthia Baker, RN, PhD
Executive Director
Canadian Association of Schools of Nursing

Lois E. Berry, RN, PhD
Associate Dean
North & North Western Campus and
Rural & Remote Engagement
College of Nursing
University of Saskatchewan
Northern Campus

Richard Booth, RN, MScN
Doctoral Candidate
Arthur Labatt Family School of Nursing
Faculty of Health Sciences
Western University
Adjunct Professor
Institute of Health Policy, Management, and Evaluation
University of Toronto

Margaret B. Clark, D. Min.
CASC/ACSS Teaching Supervisor, CPE
Associate Faculty
St. Stephen's College

Mary Jane Comiskey, RN, BScN, BEd, MScN
Professor of Nursing
University of Windsor/Lambton Collaborative BScN Program

Jamie Crawley, BA, MBA/HCM, PhD, RN
Assistant Professor
Faculty of Nursing
University of Windsor

Lorie Donelle, RN, PhD
Assistant Professor
Arthur Labatt Family School of Nursing and School of Health Studies
Faculty of Health Sciences
Western University

Elaine Doucette, RN, BScN, MScN
School of Nursing
McGill University

Karen Eisler, RN, BScN, MScN, PhD
Executive Director
Saskatchewan Registered Nurses Association

Linda Ferguson, RN, PhD
Professor
College of Nursing
Director, Centre for the Advancement of the Study of Nursing Education & Interprofessional Education
University of Saskatchewan

Bernie Garrett, PhD, BA (Hons), PGCE, RN
Associate Professor
School of Nursing
University of British Columbia

Céline Gélinas, N, BSc(N), MSc(N), PhD, Post Doc
Assistant Professor
School of Nursing
McGill University
Nurse Scientist, Centre for Nursing Research, Jewish General Hospital
Associate Researcher
McGill University Health Centre

Donna Goodridge, RN, BA, BN, MN, PhD., CHPCN(c)
Professor
College of Nursing
University of Saskatchewan

Holly Graham-Marrs, RN, BA, BScN, MN, PhD, R.D. Psych. (Provisional)
Assistant Professor
College of Nursing
University of Saskatchewan

Jean Hughes, RN, PhD
Professor, School of Nursing
Dalhousie University
and Research Scientist
IWK Health Centre
and Senior Editor-Publications
Canadian Journal of Community Mental Health

Michelle Hughes, RN, BScN, MEd
Professor Nursing
Ryerson, Centennial, George Brown Collaborative
Nursing Degree Program
School of Community & Health Studies
Centennial College

Katharine A. Hungerford, RN, BScN, MEd
Professor of Nursing
University of Windsor/Lambton Collaborative BScN
Program

Joanne Jones, RN, BSN, MSN
School of Nursing
Thompson Rivers University

Oxana Kapoustina, BSc (Physiology), MSc (Biochemistry), MSc(A) (N)
School of Nursing
McGill University

Kristen Knibbs, RN, MN
Lecturer
College of Nursing
University of Saskatchewan

Michael G. Ladouceur, RN, BScN, MPH
Assistant Professor and Co-Chair
Global Health Education Committee
School of Nursing
McMaster University

Sandie Larouche, RN, BSc(N), MSc
School of Nursing
McGill University

Kristen Lethbridge, RN, BScN, MScN, PhD
Research Assistant
Arthur Labatt Family School of Nursing
Faculty of Health Sciences
Western University

Nicole Letourneau, PhD, RN
Norlien/ACHF Chair in Parent-Infant Mental
Health
Alberta Children's Hospital Research Institute for
Child & Maternal Health
Professor
Faculties of Nursing & Medicine (Pediatrics)
University of Calgary
Adjunct Professor
Faculty of Nursing
University of New Brunswick

Caroline Marchionni, N, MSc Admin, MSc A
Knowledge Broker
McGill University Health Centre
Faculty Lecturer
School of Nursing
McGill University

Carol McDonald, PhD, RN
Associate Professor
School of Nursing
University of Victoria

Marjorie McIntyre, RN, PhD
Associate Professor
School of Nursing
University of Victoria

Mitzi G. Mitchell, RN, GNC(C); BScN, BA (Soc), MHSc, MN, DNS, PhD
Professor
Faculty of Applied Health & Community Studies
Sheridan Institute of Technology and Advanced
Learning

Donna Moralejo, BA, BSc, MSc(A), PhD
Professor
School of Nursing
Memorial University of Newfoundland

Glenys Moran, RN, BN, MN
Nurse Educator
Centre for Nursing Studies
St. John's, NL

Nancy Moules, RN, PhD
Professor
Faculty of Nursing
University of Calgary

Iris Mujica, RN, MSc, PhD(s)
Assistant Professor and Co-Chair
Global Health Education Committee
School of Nursing
McMaster University

Ted Naylor, BA (Hons), GDPA, MA
Research Coordinator
School of Social Work
Dalhousie University

Joanne K. Olson, PhD, RN
Professor
Faculty of Nursing
University of Alberta

Kathryn A. Pfaff, RN, MSc, PhD(c)
Level One Coordinator and Lecturer
Faculty of Nursing
University of Windsor

Em M. Pijl Zieber, BScN, MEd, RN
University of Lethbridge

Viola Polomeno, RN, BSc, MSc(A), PhD
Assistant Professor
School of Nursing
University of Ottawa

Joanne Profetto-McGrath, PhD, RN
Professor and Vice Dean
President, Canadian Association of Nursing Research
Faculty of Nursing
University of Alberta

Shelley Raffin Bouchal, RN, PhD
Associate Dean, Graduate Programs
Faculty of Nursing
University of Calgary

Noelle Rohatinsky, RN BSN, MN, PhD(c)
Assistant Professor
College of Nursing
University of Saskatchewan

Robyn Stremler, RN, PhD
Assistant Professor
Lawrence S. Bloomberg Faculty of Nursing
University of Toronto
Adjunct Scientist
The Hospital for Sick Children (SickKids), Toronto

Beth Swart, BScN, MES
School of Nursing
Ryerson University

Olive Wahoush, RN, MSc, PhD
Assistant Professor
School of Nursing,
McMaster University

Donna M. Wilson, RN, PhD
Professor
Faculty of Nursing
University of Alberta

# Canadian Reviewers

Gail Bremer
Langara College
Nursing

Krista Cordell
St. Lawrence College–Cornwall Campus
Health Sciences: Practical Nurse Program

Edward V. Cruz
Centennial College
School of Community and Health Studies

Joanne Folstad
SAIT
Nusring Education Program of Saskatchewan

Sharon Hamilton
University of New Brunswick
Faculty of Nursing

Paul Jeffrey
Sheridan College
School of Community & Liberal Studies

Tracey Jewiss
McMaster University
School of Nursing

Paula Kelly
Memorial University of Newfoundland
School of Nursing

Tania Killian
Seneca College
Health Sciences: Nursing

Sandra Kostashuk
Grant MacEwan
Bachelor of Science in Nursing Program
Faculty of Health and Community Studies

Marion Lougas
Professor of Nursing and Program Coordinator
Georgian College
Health and Wellness Department

Lindsay MacFarlane
Confederation College
Health and Community Services
Practical Nursing Program

Ann MacLeod
Trent/Fleming School of Nursing
Nursing

Joan Martin Saarinen
Northern College
Nursing Department

Carrie Mines
Mohawk College
Nursing Department

Jennifer Miron
Humber College
Health Sciences (Nursing)
Humber College Collaborative Bachelor of Nursing Program

Julie Novakovic
British Columbia Institute of Technology
School of Health Sciences

Andrea Phillips
York University
Nursing Department

Joanna Pierazzo
McMaster University
School of Nursing

Wanda Pierson
Langara College
Nursing

Dawn Prentice
Brock University
Nursing Department

Debbie Rickeard
University of Windsor
Nursing Department

Carolyn Rivard
Fanshawe College
Nursing

Sandra Secord
Sheridan College
Faculty of Health and Community Studies

Lynne Theriault
MacEwan University
Psychiatric Nursing

Margaret Verkuyl
Centennial College
Nursing

 # US Contributors

We would like to extend our heartfelt thanks to more than 90 of our colleagues from schools of nursing across the United States of America who have given their time generously during the past few years. *Kozier & Erb's Fundamentals of Nursing,* Ninth Edition, benefited immeasurably from their efforts, as well as from their vast experience as teachers and nurses.

Aara Amidi-Nouri, PhD, RN
Samuel Merritt University

Betty M. L. Bedner, RN, MSN Ed
Visiting Assistant Professor
University of Pittsburgh, Bradford

Amy Chaffin, PhD, RN, CNS-BC
Associate Professor
Nevada State College

Sherrilyn Coffman, DNS, RN, CPN
Professor, Assistant Dean
Nevada State College

Karen Cuvar, PhD, RN
Assistant Professor
St. Louis University

Pamela Allyn Di Vito-Thomas, PhD, RN, CNE
Director of Nursing
Coffeyville Community College

Ardys Dunn, PhD, PNP
Associate Professor Emeritus
University of Portland

Karen Lee Fontaine, RN, MSN, ASSECT
Purdue University Calumet

Geralyn Frandsen, EdD, RN
Professor
Maryville University

Rebecca E. Swogger-Heyne, RN, MSN, CPNP, CNE
Clinical Assistant Professor
Walsh University Division of Nursing

Lora McDonald McGuire, MS, BSN
Professor
Joliet Junior College

Susan Norwood, EdD, RN
Professor
Gonzaga University

Gail Rattigan
Lecturer
Nevada State College

Melissa Schmidt, PhD, MSN, BSN
Associate Professor
Tompkins Cortland Community College

Elizabeth Johnston Taylor, PhD, RN
Associate Professor, Loma Linda University
Research Director, Mary Potter Hospice
Wellington South, New Zealand

Ruby Wertz, RN, BSN, MHA
Lecturer, Assistant Dean
Nevada State College

Special Features

Health-Promotion Guidelines

Home Care Considerations

Lifespan Considerations

Nursing and Canadian Society

Practice Guidelines

Reflect on Primary Health Care

Sample Care Plan

Teaching: Clinical

Teaching: Home Care

Teaching: Wellness

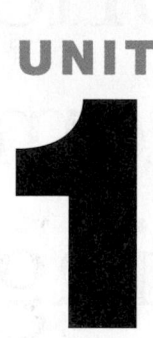

The Foundation of Nursing in Canada

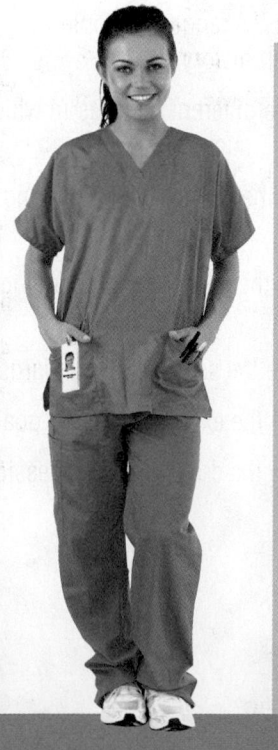

Chapter 1

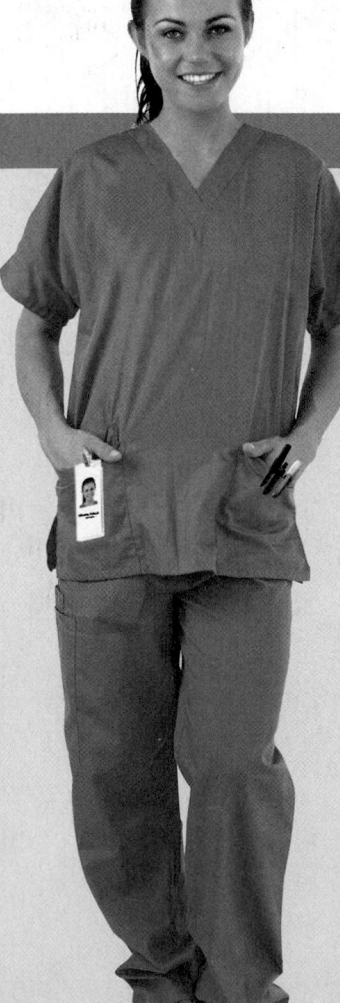

Historical and Contemporary Nursing Practice**

LEARNING OUTCOMES

After studying this chapter, you will be able to:

1. Explain major trends in the writing of nursing history.

2. Discuss the range of people who provided nursing care in different periods in Canadian history.

3. Compare different settings in which nursing care has been provided by Canadian nurses.

4. Explain the usefulness of nursing history for understanding current practice issues.

5. Analyze the influence of changing social, political, and economic conditions over time.

6. Describe the scope and standards of nursing practice.

7. Evaluate the expanded career goals and their functions.

8. Examine the criteria of a profession and the professionalization of nursing.

**The author acknowledges the work of Drs. Jayne Elliott and Cynthia Toman in the historical section.

Nurses have traditionally composed the largest portion of health care workers in Canada. As such, they have enabled and participated in shaping the Canadian health care system and have made a significant impact on the health of individuals, families, and communities. Although public surveys identify nurses as the most trusted of health care providers, gloomy forecasts of massive nursing shortfalls persist. Nurses perceive their work as being undervalued, while others deem it too expensive in the face of persistent cost-cutting measures and concerns over the viability of government-supported health and medical care. At the same time, nurses struggle to articulate what they actually do (Nelson & Gordon, 2006). Nursing policymakers, educators, and union leaders are challenged with defining and defending a unique role for nurses among other health care professionals and within a rapidly changing health care system (Villeneuve & MacDonald, 2006).

Historical Nursing Practice

In the past, Canadian nurses were on the front lines during cholera, influenza, and polio epidemics, as they were for more recent outbreaks of contagious diseases, such as the SARS (severe acute respiratory syndrome) outbreak in 2003 (MacDougall, 2007). They served in military medical units during the South African War, World Wars I and II, the Korean War, and the Gulf War, leaving a rich heritage for Canadian nurses who continue to play important roles in international conflicts. Nurses and their work were critical to the rapid expansion in the number and size of hospitals, and nurses continue to facilitate the spread and acceptance of medical technology both within and outside hospitals. Since the late nineteenth century, public health nurses have provided essential health and medical care to isolated populations in both rural and urban centres, a legacy taken up by street nurses caring for people on new frontiers.

As these situations suggest, nursing takes place within broad cultural, sociopolitical, and economic contexts that also influence both its practitioners and its practice. Nursing evolved similarly in most Western nations, partially shaped by societal events and such changes as industrialization, urbanization, wars, cycles of economic depression and expansion, and the women's movement. Developments in scientific and technological knowledge and the consolidation of Western medicine have changed conceptualizations of health and illness, as well as the meanings associated with them. Historical research contributes to nursing knowledge in two main ways: (a) It develops in-depth analyses of these complex relationships, and (b) it creates enhanced understandings of the past that inform both present and future situations.

Early historians of nursing focused primarily on questions about professionalization, education, and leadership, tending to see their history as a steady march of progress through time. Although indebted to these writers, who have preserved vast amounts of source material, historians since the 1980s have examined the profession more critically—paying closer attention to issues that complicate and add greater complexity to their analyses. It is important, for example, to understand who was considered a "nurse" and what nursing work encompassed in a particular historical period. Answers to these questions are contingent on who was available to work as a nurse, what status or value society attributed to nurses' (and women's) work, and how nurses were compensated for that work within a specific timeframe. Inclusion of gender, race, ethnicity, and class in historical analyses raises important questions about the social arrangements and relationships of power that shaped who was included or excluded as a nurse. Although, for the most part, nurses have worked as subordinates within health care systems, they often held positions of privilege, increased social status, and respect in comparison with other female workers. Analyzing nurses as agents of the state allows us to ask in what ways they did (and do) enable and influence larger social, political, and economic agendas through their participation in systems of health care. Knowledge of how nursing developed in specific contexts or sets of circumstances permits nurses to better understand their present situation and, particularly, to see how contemporary concerns might relate to larger social-structural conditions.

Before the establishment of training schools in Canada, women provided most of the nursing care either for family members and acquaintances or for strangers in their communities. Some took on these roles as charitable acts of kindness; others, self-identifying as nurses in the pretraining era, developed midwifery practices or hired themselves out as "monthly" nurses to care for women in their homes for a month after childbirth (Young, 2004). First Nations women provided much needed help to new, white settler societies as they spread across the frontier—a history too long ignored because the skilled

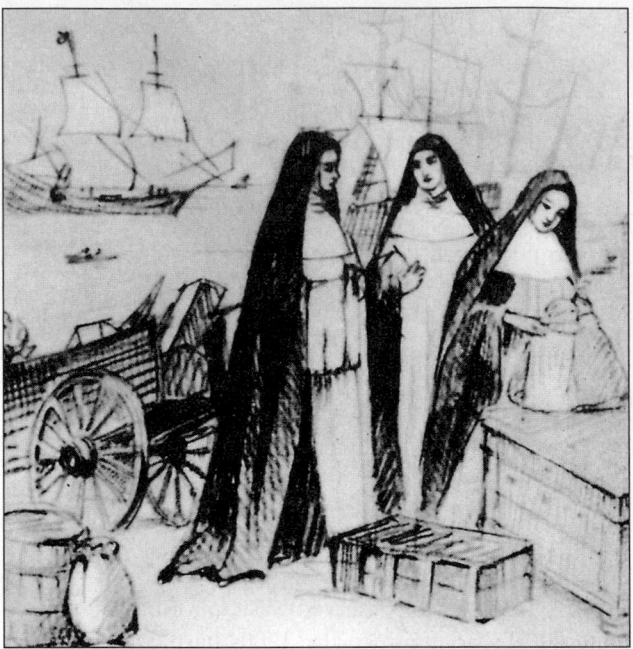

FIGURE 1.1 Arrival of the first three Augustinian sisters in Quebec, 1639

medical care of these women, particularly in midwifery and childhood diseases, was critical to the very survival of these new communities. Women who were members of religious groups were also early skilled caregivers, dating back to the first group of European nuns who arrived (in 1639) in what is now Quebec with a mission to provide care for the bodies and souls of both settlers and native inhabitants. These women cared for the sick and destitute where they landed, but many soon followed the new immigrants west and founded hospitals, some of which have survived into the present (see Figure 1.1).

Immigration, growing urbanization, and changing concepts around the transmission and treatment of diseases contributed to the push for formally trained nurses by the late nineteenth century. Early Canadian towns and cities were plagued by inadequate sanitation and sewage systems. Waves of infectious diseases, such as typhus, influenza, and smallpox, regularly devastated both immigrant and native populations (Cassel, 1994). Wealthy patrons initially established hospitals during the late nineteenth century as philanthropic institutions that served the increasingly visible "sick poor." Measures to improve and protect the delivery of food and water supplies, a gradual acceptance of germ theory in disease transmission, and the availability of anesthesia all helped to increase confidence in the idea of scientific medicine. Although cures for many illnesses often lagged far behind identification of causes, perceptions of increased therapeutic efficacy inclined the better-off classes to choose care in medical institutions over treatments (including surgeries) in their homes. Hospital administrators increasingly relied on these paying patients to offset the costs of caring for the poor (Gagan & Gagan, 2002). Significantly, the advent of

trained nurses lent both efficiency and respectability to this shift toward hospital care.

Two main influences have shaped formally prepared nursing in Canada. The British system, associated primarily with Florence Nightingale during the mid-nineteenth century, has attracted the most historical attention, even if her vision for an independent nursing force complementary to, and not dependent on, hospital administration was never fully realized. French-Canadian religious communities, which also contributed significantly to the development of trained nurses, blended religious and work life to own and manage hospitals and training schools across the country. The Quiet Revolution in Quebec during the 1960s, in reaction to the hegemony of the church over French-Canadian society, brought in a period of rapid secularization with closer government control over institutions, eroding the nuns' authority within their institutions and shifting nursing education into the public sphere (Charles, 2003; Paul, 2005; Violette, 2005) (see Figure 1.2). Both systems built on religious and cultural ideals of respectable femininity that integrated contemporary ideas about scientific thinking with womanly, selfless devotion to duty and service.

The first official training school was established in St. Catharines, Ontario, in 1874 by Dr. Theophilus Mack. Over the next decades, the number of nurses rose dramatically from only 300 at the turn of the twentieth century to 20 000 by the end of World War I (McPherson, 1996). Student nurses formed the major part of the hospital workforce until the 1940s, with the expectation that they would become self-employed as private duty nurses outside the hospital on graduation. The apprenticeship training system was the predominant model of nursing education in both large and small hospitals across the country until the 1970s. Several universities did offer combined programs whereby it was possible to earn a degree in nursing, such as the first degree program established at the University of British Columbia in 1919; the focus of these programs was often on preparing nurses to be supervisors, educators, and public health nurses.

Nursing became one of the few respectable opportunities for paid work available to women in the first half of the twentieth century. The vast majority of student placements in nursing schools were reserved for young, white women whose families could afford to do without their financial contribution, at least for the duration of their training. Two men appear in the 1899 graduating class of Victoria General Hospital in Halifax (Nursing Education in Nova Scotia, n.d.), but men, in general, have remained vastly underrepresented in the ranks of an occupation strongly tied to the concept, promoted sometimes by nurses themselves, that nursing is women's work (McPherson, 1996). Despite the Canadian Nurses Association's official policy of nondiscrimination, in place since the 1940s, few black nurses gained entrance to training programs until the 1970s (McPherson, 1996).

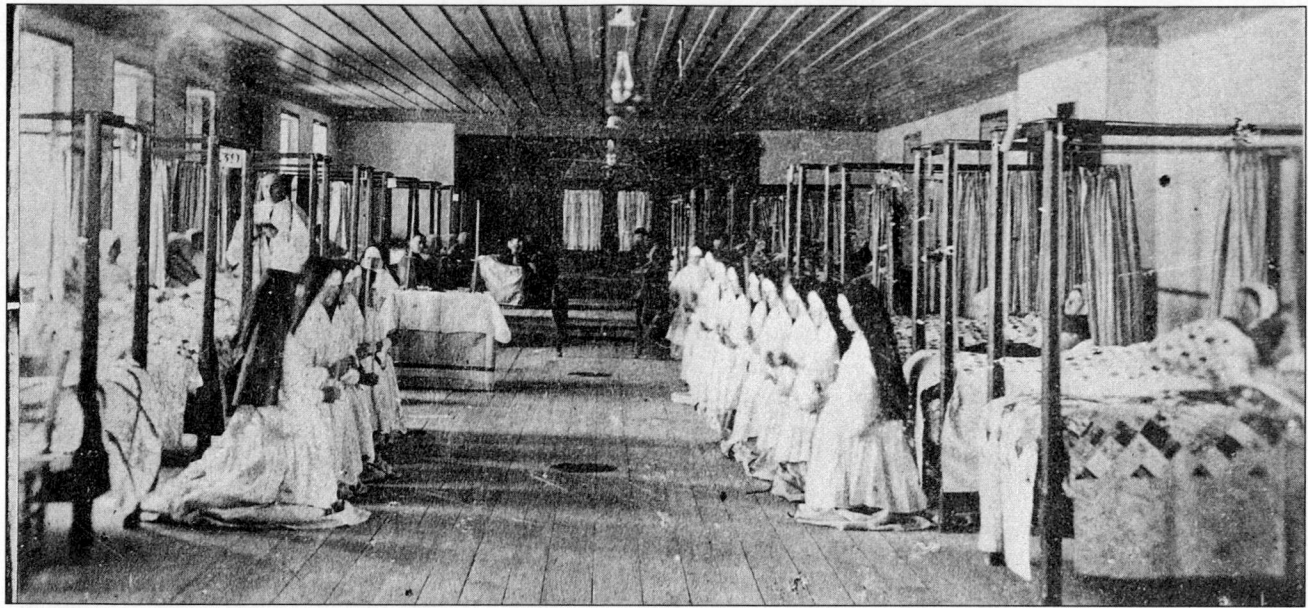

FIGURE 1.2 Nuns at prayer, along with their patients at an early Hotel Dieu hospital

In British Columbia, a few nursing students of Asian background were admitted during the late 1930s for the explicit purpose of nursing among their own ethnic communities. And in 1954, Jean Cuthand Goodwill became the first Aboriginal woman to graduate from nursing school in Saskatchewan, but again, not until the 1970s was a concerted effort made to recruit First Nations and Inuit students into nursing (McBain, 2005) (see Figures 1.3 and 1.4).

Various professionalization movements throughout the twentieth century also intensified debates over who was, or could become, a nurse. In the early decades, nursing leaders attempted to distance skilled nursing work from domestic caregiving and midwifery. Following a successful campaign by physicians to gain control over medical practice, nurses sought to establish control over nursing through the standardization of educational curricula and the legal authority to credential graduates of recognized hospital-based training programs. Most provinces brought in nurse registration between 1910

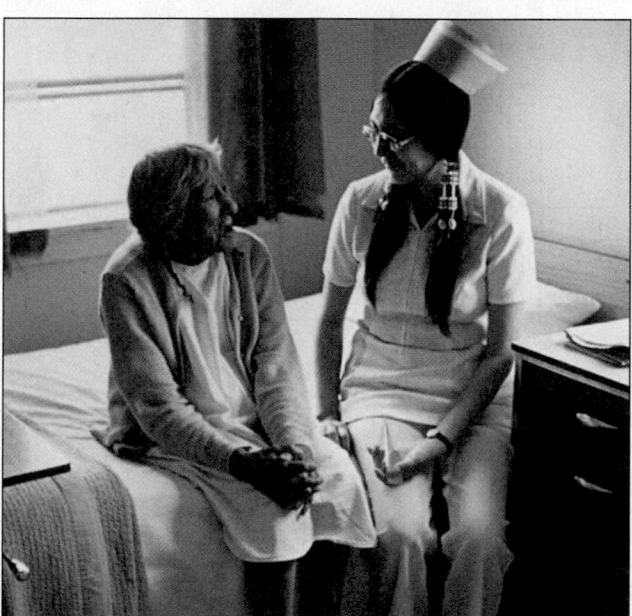

FIGURE 1.3 Ottawa General Hospital graduation 1912

FIGURE 1.4 Aboriginal nurse with a patient at Blood Hospital, Cardston, Alberta

and 1922, thus separating trained nurses from others who used the term *nurse* (Mansell, 2003). Newfoundland and Labrador nurses obtained registration in 1954, Northwest Territories nurses in 1975, and Yukon nurses in 1992.

During the first half of the twentieth century, most nurses worked in private duty after graduation, but changing concepts in public health provided other opportunities. Women's groups were instrumental in pushing for reform, particularly in maternal and child health, and initiated many services that provincial health authorities later took over. Poor health status (and subsequent rejection) of wartime recruits because of preventable and treatable illnesses contracted in childhood, the devastating impact of the influenza epidemic (1917–1918), and a high rate of tuberculosis and venereal diseases among returning World War I soldiers in 1918 fuelled demands for increased government responsibility in matters of health. Specially trained nurses were dispersed into schools and homes across Canada, in both urban and rural districts. Nurses, as women, met gendered expectations that they were the ideal people to bring the new "gospel of good health" to mothers and their families. By helping to spread new scientific theories of health, including those on social and mental hygiene, nurses were responsible for Canadianizing new immigrants through the promotion of white, middle-class, urban-based ideals of health, which they found that their clients sometimes could not, or would not, meet.

The Victorian Order of Nurses was founded in 1897, but other organizations, such as the Margaret Scott Nursing Mission in Winnipeg, the Alberta District Nursing Service, the Newfoundland Outport Nursing and Industrial Association (NONIA), and the Medical Service to Settlers in Quebec, emerged to meet these public health needs. Several provincial divisions of the Canadian Red Cross Society began outpost programs in isolated parts of their territories (Elliott, 2004; McKay, 2007; Penney, 1996; Richardson, 1998; Rousseau & Daigle, 2000). The federal health department did not regularly supply nursing stations and nurses to First Nations and Inuit populations in the sub-Arctic and Arctic regions of the country until after World War II (McPherson, 2003; Meijer-Drees & McBain, 2001). Together, these nurses brought much-needed health care to areas underserved by physicians, and they often found they needed to undertake such tasks as midwifery, stitching of wounds, or teeth pulling, for which they had received little training (see Figures 1.5, 1.6, 1.7, and 1.8).

Several small groups of civilian nurses volunteered with the Canadian militia during the Northwest Rebellion (1885), with the Northwest Mounted Police during the Klondike Gold Rush (1898), and with the

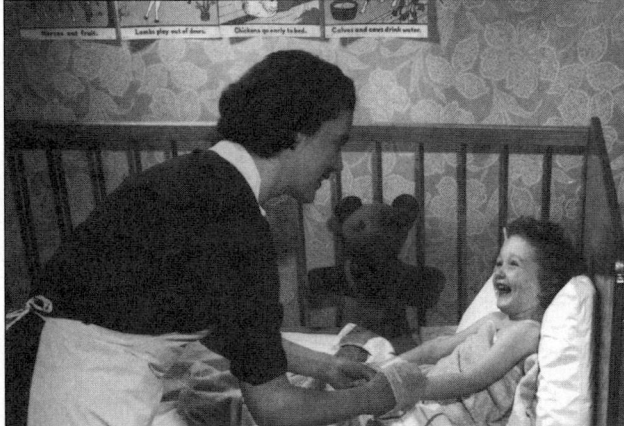

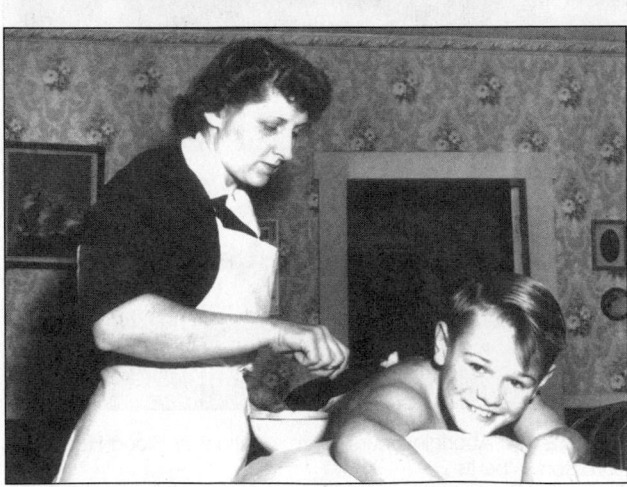

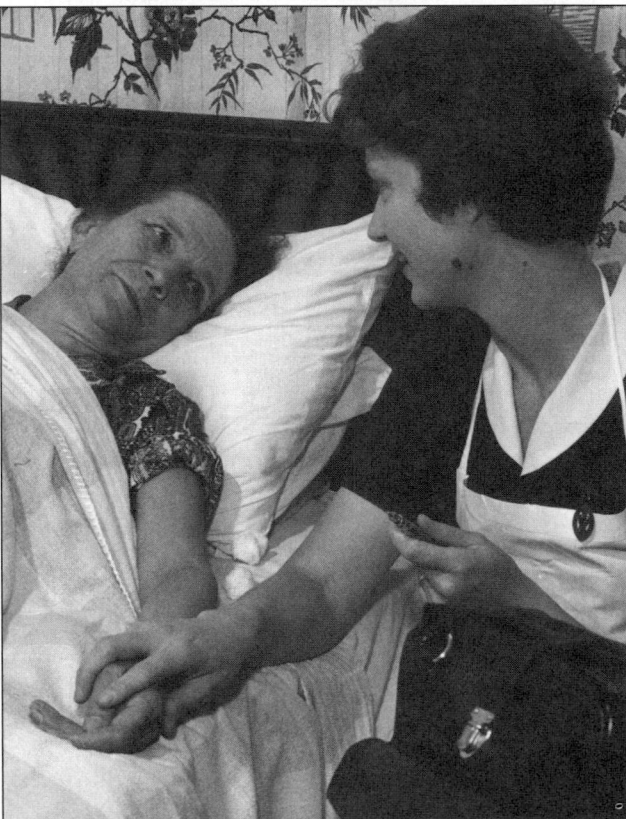

FIGURE 1.5 Three patients of Victorian Order of Nurses (VON) cared for in their own homes. The VON still provides community and home care services across Canada

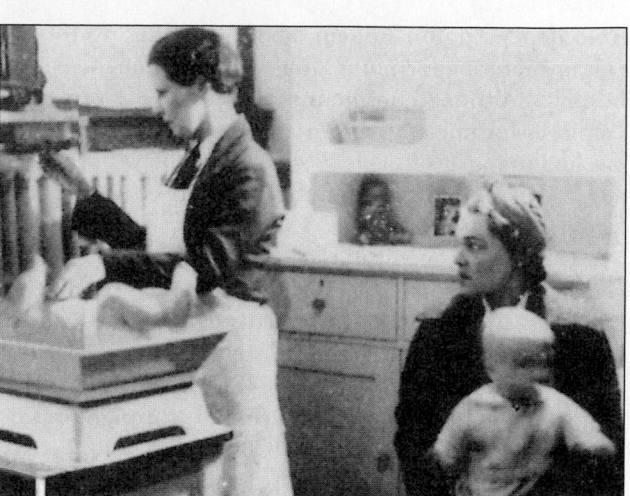

FIGURE 1.6 Well-baby clinic in Manitoba

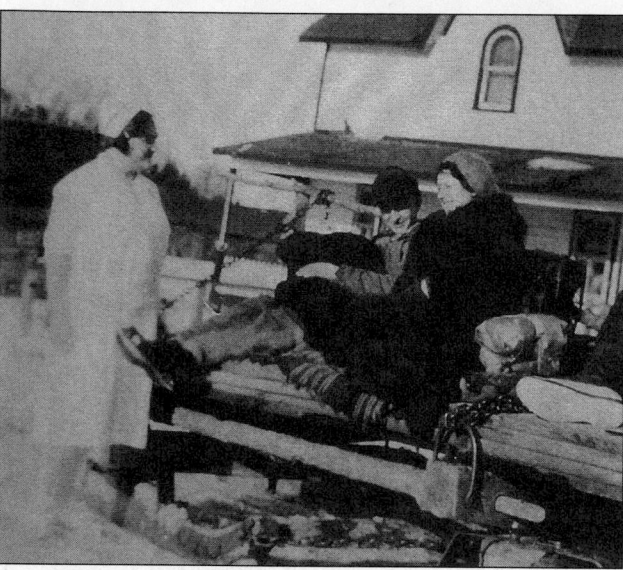

FIGURE 1.8 Red Cross Nurse Gertrude Leroy Miller discharging a patient from the nursing outpost at Wilberforce, Ontario, in the 1930s

British Expeditionary Force during the South African War (1899–1902), but they were not officially part of the Canadian military. With the formation of the first permanent nursing service as part of the Canadian Army Medical Corps (CAMC) in 1904, civilian nurses became fully integrated into the Canadian armed forces as soldiers, enlisting as lieutenants with the specially created officer's rank and title of *nursing sister,* serving under the supervision of higher-ranked matrons. During 1944, Matron-in-Chief Elizabeth Smellie became the first woman in the world to rise to the rank of a full colonel. Initially, nursing sisters were the only women to serve in the military, and they readily filled every available position in the Canadian armed forces throughout both World Wars—even creating long waiting lists to get into the military. Canadian military nurses served with NATO (North Atlantic Treaty Organization) forces in Europe during the 1950s and with the Allied Forces during the

Korean War (1950–1953), as well as with peacekeeping forces during the 1990s and beyond.

At least 3141 nursing sisters served during World War I and 4079 during World War II. They called themselves soldiers and understood their work as winning the war through the salvage of damaged men. They actively sought opportunities to move closer to the front lines, readily accepting increased risk and danger as part of the job. Some died in both wars because of enemy action and military-related illnesses and accidents; two were prisoners of war under the Japanese army in Hong Kong for almost 2 years during World War II; others were torpedoed, bombed, and strafed—and survived to talk about the experiences. Some of them left personal accounts of these experiences; some questioned the contradictory values of caring and saving lives in the midst of organizations designed for the destruction of lives. The armed forces valued the knowledge and skills of nurses highly, reluctantly moving them forward as they demonstrated better outcomes for the soldiers under their care than less-trained personnel could achieve. The military was adamant, however, that nurses were temporary—only for the duration of the war, regardless of what nurses preferred with regard to their military careers (Toman, 2007) (see Figures 1.9, 1.10, and 1.11).

During the 1930s, the private duty market for nurses shrank because of both an oversupply of graduate nurses and the widespread economic depression that left at least 30% of the Canadian population unemployed. But a boom in hospital construction and the growing use of medical technologies, among other factors, increased the need for nurses again, precipitating a nursing shortage that continued into the 1970s. The nursing leadership campaigned to move nurses' training into educational institutions and gradually weaned hospital administrators

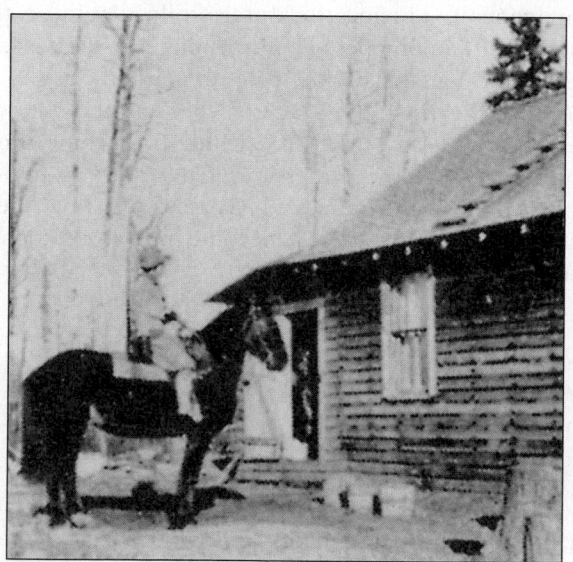

FIGURE 1.7 District nurse at Old Pendryl Cottage, Alberta

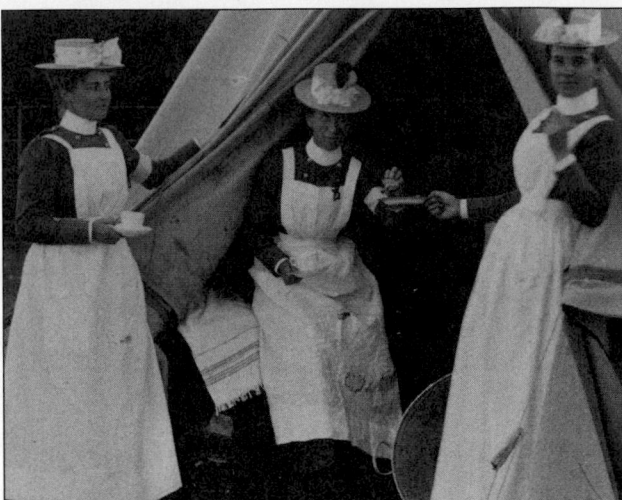

FIGURE 1.9 Canadian civilian nurses with the British Expeditionary Force in South Africa (1899–1902)

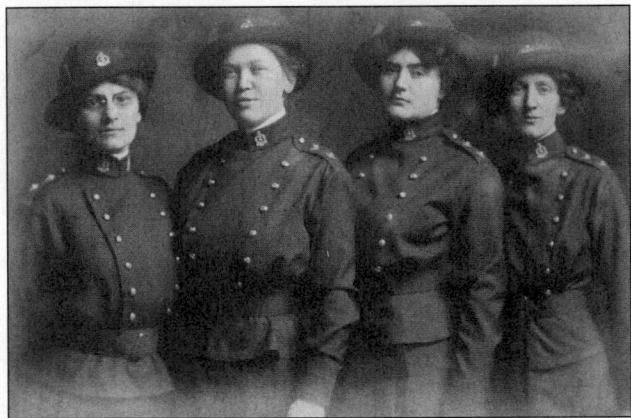

FIGURE 1.10 World War I Nursing Sister Mabel Lucas Rutherford (*left*) and three colleagues in their dress uniforms

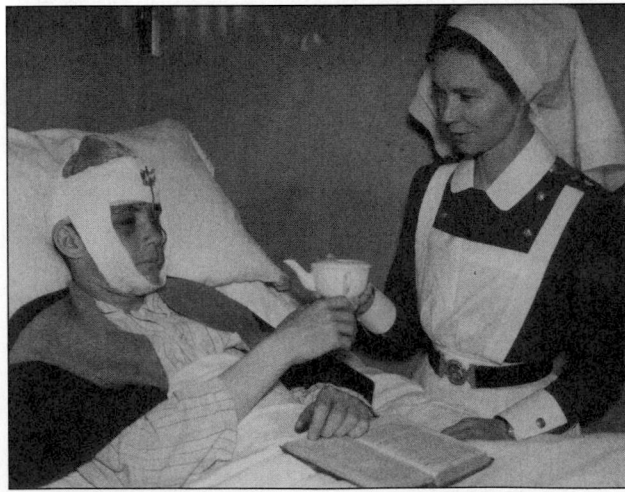

FIGURE 1.11 World War II Nursing Sister Dorothy Macham attending to a wounded soldier

from depending on student labour, opening up further employment opportunities for graduate nurses within hospitals. Although hospitals soon became the preferred employer for nurses, the shortage was so great that hospitals had to make substantial changes in the workplace to attract new students for training and married nurses back into the workforce.

Changes in medical and surgical therapeutics were central forces in defining the nature and scope of nursing practices. By accepting delegated medical tasks, nurses have been instrumental in facilitating the spread and acceptance of many technologies that range from thermometers in the early twentieth century, through routine blood tests in the 1940s and 1950s, to the complex systems of medical monitoring in place today (Sandelowski, 2000; Toman, 2001). An increasingly specialized nursing workforce has resulted in a hierarchical relationship among nurses and between nurses and lesser-skilled auxiliary workers, whose positions emerged initially to help address the shortage of trained nurses.

Each of these issues lies within a body of historical research that offers alternative perspectives through which we can question who and what is determining today's nursing practice. On the one hand, the wider socioeconomic and political milieu has shaped nurses and their work; on the other hand, nurses have participated in shaping the health care system and the role of nursing within it. Curiosity about the roots of the nursing profession has merit in itself, but many would argue that the value of nursing history lies in its relevance to current issues in professional practice. Much more research is needed, for example, on the history of registered psychiatric nursing programs and how the baccalaureate degree as entry to practice has affected perceptions of nursing work among nurses themselves and the wider society. Hospital-based training and work environments tried to standardize nurses, nurses' knowledge, and nursing care, creating the illusion of a homogeneous nursing workforce while devaluing the vast diversity among people performing nursing work. A more critical analysis of the roles of gender, class, race, and ethnicity (including lack of colour), and the way these factors have worked to include or exclude those wanting to enter the profession, is necessary to understand who became nurses in Canada and how these influences still shape who become nurses in today's multicultural health care context.

Contemporary Nursing Practice

An in-depth study of contemporary nursing practice includes a look at selected definitions of nursing, a framework for the Canadian health system, the goals of the nurse within this system, the acts that legislate health care and nursing practice, and the scope and standards of practice. This chapter will concentrate on definitions and the goals and roles of nursing. Currently, four legislated categories of nursing exist in Canada: (a) Licensed (Registered) Practical Nurses, (b) Registered Nurses, (c) Registered Psychiatric Nurses, and (d) Nurse Practitioners (Extended Class). Each has a scope of practice legislated within a province or territory. These acts may be unique for each category of nursing, or together, for example, the Registered Health Professions Act (RPHA) in Ontario. For the Canadian health care system, see Chapter 9, and for legal issues see Chapter 6.

Definitions of Nursing

To understand what nursing is, we must first define the word. Many definitions exist, some of which misrepresent the complex knowledge and skill of professional nursing. Common dictionary definitions, for example, still refer to the nurse as "a person, usually a woman, trained to care for the sick" (Cayne, 1988). Today, however, many men are choosing to become nurses, and nurses also provide preventive and health-promoting care to well clients. This section gives several definitions of nursing, and Chapter 4 provides other definitions created by nursing theorists.

In 1860, Florence Nightingale described nursing as the "use of fresh air, light, warmth, cleanliness, quiet and the proper selection and administration of diet" (Nightingale, 1938, p. 8). She considered a clean, well-ventilated, and quiet environment essential for recovery from illnesses. Often considered the first nurse theorist, Nightingale raised the status of nursing through education. Nurses were no longer untrained housekeepers but persons educated in the care of the sick.

Virginia Henderson was one of the first modern nurses to define *nursing*. In 1960, she wrote, "The unique function of the nurse is to assist the individual, sick or well, in the performance of those activities contributing to health or its recovery (or to peaceful death) that he would perform unaided if he had the necessary strength, will, or knowledge, and to do this in such a way as to help him gain independence as rapidly as possible" (Henderson, 1966, p. 3). Like Nightingale, Henderson described nursing in relation to the client and the client's environment. Unlike Nightingale, Henderson saw the nurse as concerned with both well and ill individuals, acknowledged that nurses interact with clients even when recovery may not be feasible, and mentioned the teaching and advocacy roles of the nurse.

Professional nursing associations have also examined nursing and developed their definitions of it. In 1987, the Canadian Nurses Association (CNA) described nursing practice as a dynamic, caring, helping relationship in which the nurse helps the client to achieve and maintain optimal health (CNA, 1987). Many countries have chosen to use the International Council of Nurses, (2010) definition:

> Nursing encompasses autonomous and collaborative care of individuals of all ages, families, groups and communities, sick or well and in all settings. Nursing includes the promotion of health, prevention of illness, and the care of ill, disabled, and dying people. Advocacy, promotion of a safe environment, research, participation in shaping health policy and in patient and health systems management, and education are also key nursing roles.

In the latter half of the twentieth century, a number of nurse theorists developed their own theoretical definitions of nursing. Theoretical definitions are important because they go beyond simplistic common definitions. They describe what nursing is and the interrelationship among nurses, nursing, the client, and the intended client outcome—health. See Chapters 4 and 23. Several themes are common to all the various definitions of nursing (see Box 1.1).

Caring is described as the "essence of nursing" (Leininger, 1984). It is a complex concept that has multiple aspects: affective, cognitive, and ethical. Research to explore the meaning of caring in nursing has been increasing because nursing, more than any other profession, has "the distinction of being responsible for the caring that clients receive in the health care system" (Miller, 1995, p. 29). Details about caring are discussed in Chapter 22. See also Watson's assumptions of caring in Box 4.2 in Chapter 4 (see page 68).

Recipients of Nursing

Nurses work with many and varied recipients of care. The recipients can be individuals, families, groups, communities, and populations. Even when planning and implementing care to various recipients, it is important for the nurse to recognize that these recipients live within

---

BOX 1.1 THEMES COMMON TO DEFINITIONS

Although several different definitions of nursing have been made over the years, they do share some common themes:

- Nursing is caring.
- Nursing is an art.
- Nursing is a science.
- Nursing is client centred.
- Nursing is holistic.
- Nursing is adaptive.
- Nursing is concerned with health promotion, health maintenance, and health restoration.
- Nursing is a helping profession.

a larger society—for instance, individuals are connected to families, groups live in the community, and multiple communities exist within a given population. Groups are collections of individuals with a shared goal or purpose, and communities may be defined by geography, culture, or other characteristics.

In this book, we have generally identified the recipient of care as the individual (see Chapter 12). We have, however, also provided some beginning information on families and working with families in providing nursing care (see Chapter 13). When referring to individuals who are receiving nursing care, the literature refers to them as consumers, patients, residents, or clients and by other terms. A **consumer** is an individual, a group of people, or a community that uses a service or commodity. People who use health care products or services are consumers of health care.

A **patient** is a person who is waiting for or undergoing medical treatment and care. The word *patient* comes from a Latin word meaning "to suffer" or "to bear." Traditionally, the person receiving health care has been called a *patient*. Usually, people become patients when they seek assistance because of illness or for surgery. Some nurses believe that the word *patient* implies passive acceptance of the decisions and care of health professionals. Additionally, with the emphasis on health promotion and prevention of illness, many recipients of nursing care are not ill. Moreover, in addition to caring for patients, nurses interact with family members and significant others to provide support, information, and comfort.

For these reasons, nurses also refer to recipients of health care as *clients*. A **client** is a person who engages the advice or services of another who is qualified to provide this service. The term *client* presents the receivers of health care as collaborators in the care, that is, as people who are also responsible for their own health. Thus, the health status of a client is the responsibility of the individual in collaboration with health care professionals. In this book, we have generally used the term *patient* to describe the individual admitted to an acute care facility or otherwise seeking care, the term *resident* for an individual cared for in a long-term care facility, and the term *client* to describe recipients of nursing care in other settings. Many times, the topics discussed in this book are equally applicable to clients, patients, and residents. When this is the case, readers may see references to more than one recipient of care in the same paragraph.

Scope of Nursing

Nursing practice involves four areas: (a) promoting health and wellness, (b) preventing illness, (c) restoring health, and (d) caring for the dying. Within each of these areas, nurses seek to articulate and follow best practices in terms of the care they provide. Various chapters of this book relate to each of the areas of nursing practice. The Registered Nurses' Association of Ontario has led the way in developing a series of best practices documents (see the Weblinks section in this chapter). Reference to appropriate best practices documents can be found in the chapters throughout the book.

PROMOTING HEALTH AND WELLNESS "Wellness is a process that engages people in activities and behaviors that enhance quality of life and maximize personal potential" (Anspaugh, Hamrick, & Rosata, 2003, p. 490). Nurses promote wellness in clients who are healthy as well as those who are ill. This promotion may involve individual and community activities to enhance healthy lifestyles, such as improving nutrition and physical fitness, preventing problematic drug and alcohol use, smoking cessation, and preventing accidents and injury in the home and workplace. See Chapters 8 and 14 for further discussion.

PREVENTING ILLNESS The goal of illness-prevention programs is to maintain optimal health by preventing disease. Examples of nursing activities that prevent illness include immunizations, prenatal and infant care, and prevention of sexually transmitted infections.

RESTORING HEALTH Restoring health focuses on the ill client, and it extends from early detection of disease through helping the client during the recovery period. Examples of nursing activities focused on restoring health include the following:

- Providing direct care to the ill person, such as administering medications, baths, and specific procedures and treatments

- Performing diagnostic and assessment procedures, such as measuring blood pressure and examining feces for occult blood

- Consulting and working collaboratively with other health care professionals about client problems

- Teaching clients about recovery activities, such as exercises that will accelerate recovery after a cerebrovascular accident (stroke)

- Rehabilitating clients to their optimal functional level following physical or mental illness, injury, or chemical addiction

CARING FOR THE DYING This area of nursing practice involves comforting and caring for people of all ages who are dying. It includes helping clients live as comfortably as possible until death and helping the support people cope with death. Nurses carrying out these activities work in homes, hospitals, and extended care facilities. Some agencies, called *hospices*, are specifically designed for this purpose. See Chapter 49 for further discussion.

Nursing Settings

Canada has three categories of regulated nurses: (a) registered nurses (RNs), (b) licensed (registered) practical nurses (LPNs/RPNs), and (c) registered psychiatric nurses (RPNs) (see Box 1.2 for definitions of each category of regulated nurses). The Canadian Institute for Health Information reported that Canada had 354 910 employed regulated nurses in 2010. Of these, RNs represented 75.47%, practical nurses 22.9%, and psychiatric nurses 1.5% (Canadian Institute for Health Information [CIHI], 2012). In the past, the acute care hospital was the primary practice setting open to most nurses. In 2010, approximately 63%

of RNs, 45.1% of LPNs/RPNs, and 45.2% of RPNs worked in hospitals, but the rest worked in clients' homes, community agencies, ambulatory clinics, and nursing practice centres (CIHI, 2012). Figure 1.12 shows nurses in a variety of settings.

Nurses have different degrees of nursing autonomy and nursing responsibility in the various settings. They may provide direct care, engage in health teaching for various individuals and groups, serve as nursing advocates and agents of change, and help determine health policies affecting consumers in the community and in hospitals.

The CNA maintains that an individual's health affects the quality of that person's life. Health is influenced not only by the health care system but also by human biology, lifestyle choices, and the environment. With this in mind, the CNA advocates a framework to provide direction for the Canadian health care system that includes (a) the *conditions* of the Canada Health Act and (b) the *principles* of primary health care.

The Canada Health Act (1984) lists the conditions or national standards that provincial and territorial health insurance plans must respect to be able to receive federal cash contributions: public administration, accessibility, comprehensiveness, universality, and portability. The CNA believes that these conditions are essential to Canada's health care system.

1. *Public administration* means that federal, provincial, and territorial health insurance programs should be nonprofit programs operated by public authorities who are appointed by government.

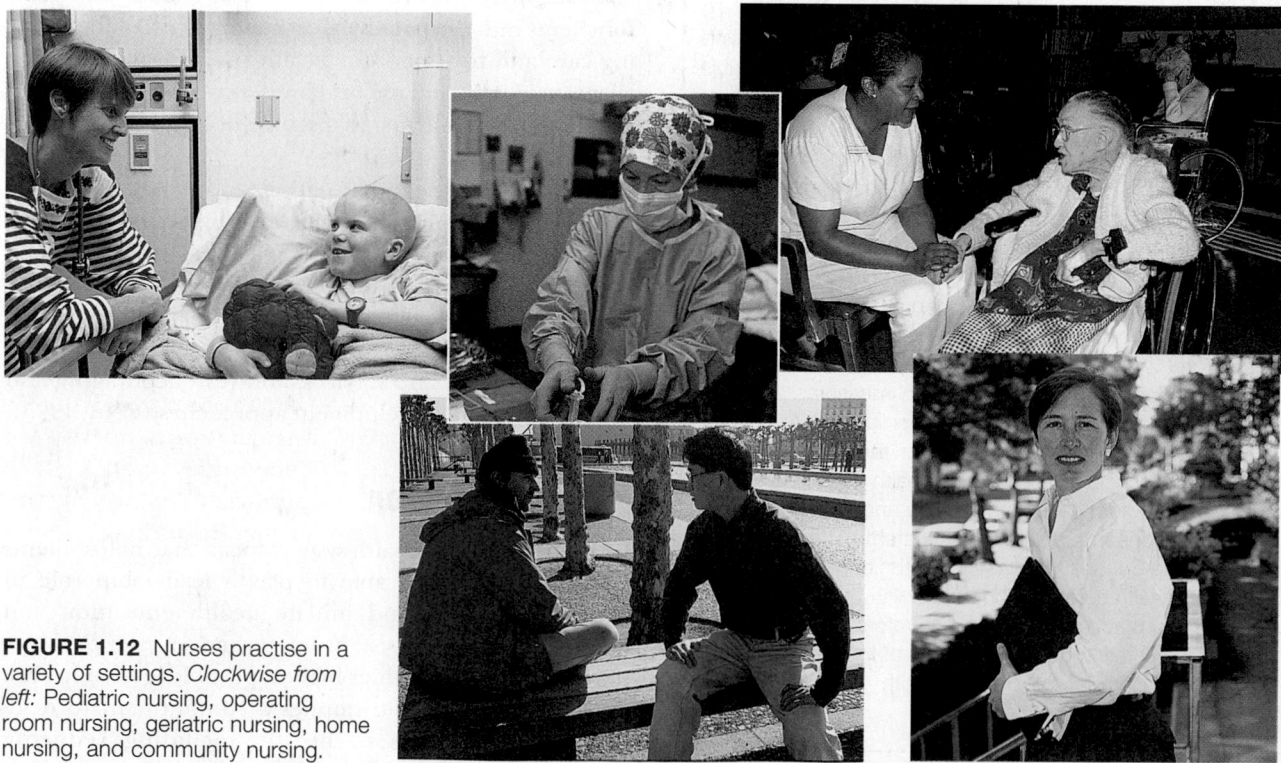

FIGURE 1.12 Nurses practise in a variety of settings. *Clockwise from left:* Pediatric nursing, operating room nursing, geriatric nursing, home nursing, and community nursing.

2. *Accessibility* means that Canadians have reasonable access to essential health care services, with no financial barriers, such as user fees, to impede this access.

3. *Comprehensiveness* means that federal and provincial or territorial health insurance together should cover the full continuum of health care services for all Canadians, including health promotion, the prevention of disease and disability, the treatment of disease and disability, restoration, rehabilitation, and support.

4. *Universal coverage* means that all Canadians are entitled to essential health care services, regardless of gender, culture, income, language, education, marital status, or age.

5. *Portability* means that Canadians should be covered equally for health care services wherever they are in Canada. (Canada, House of Commons, 1984). (See Chapter 9 for more information on Canada's health care system.)

Primary Health Care

Primary health care is essential (promotive, preventive, curative, rehabilitative, and supportive) care that focuses on preventing illness and promoting health. It is both a philosophy of health care and an approach to providing health care services. Primary health care has been adopted by the World Health Organization (WHO) and by Canada as the key to a healthy society. Clients of primary health care can be individuals, families, groups, communities, and populations (CNA, 2005; WHO, 1982).

The principles of primary health care are accessibility, public participation, health promotion, appropriate technology, and intersectoral cooperation. They are outlined in the Reflect on Primary Health Care box.

PRIMARY CARE AND PRIMARY NURSING Primary health care should not be confused with *primary care* or *primary nursing*. Primary care is provider driven and is the entry point to the health care system. Primary nursing is a system of delivering nursing services whereby a nurse is responsible for planning the 24-hour care of a specific patient. Both these concepts are illness-oriented concepts. For more information on primary health care and primary care, see Chapter 14.

The Role of the Nurse

The goal of nursing is to improve the health of clients through partnerships with clients, other health care providers, related community agencies, and government. Nursing practice involves a variety of roles, including direct care provider, educator, administrator, consultant, policy adviser, and researcher. The principles of primary health care apply to nurses in all these roles (CNA, 2005). Nurses are encouraged to examine their own practice and places of work in light of the pillars of the Canada Health Act and the principles of primary health care (CNA, 2005).

To ensure that Canadians have *reasonable access* to essential health care services, nurses provide more options for accessing health care services by (a) acting as an entry point for clients into the health care system; (b) providing nursing care and treatment for health problems; (c) helping clients to identify and use health resources, both formal and informal; and (d) acting as a source of health information for clients (CNA, 1995).

Nurses increase public participation in planning and making decisions about health care by (a) involving clients in decisions about their own health; (b) encouraging clients to take action for their own health; (c) involving clients in identifying their own health care needs; (d) involving clients in planning, using, and evaluating their own health care services; and (e) encouraging and using community development approaches (CNA, 1995).

Health Promotion

In keeping with a health-system focus that helps clients stay well, nurses are able to play a leadership role in health promotion and initiate health education and other activities that assist, promote, and support clients as they strive to achieve their highest possible level of health.

Health promotion implies a commitment to dealing with challenges to health, including reducing

---

REFLECT ON 🔑 **PRIMARY HEALTH CARE**

Principles of Primary Health Care

Accessibility means that essential health care is universally available to all clients in an acceptable and affordable way, "with no unreasonable geographic or financial barrier" (CNA, 2005, p. 1). *Public participation* means clients should be encouraged to participate in making decisions about their own health. *Health promotion* means that the health care system should place more emphasis on helping clients stay well rather than on treating clients when they are ill. *Appropriate technology* means that technology and modes of care should be appropriately adapted to the community's social, economic, and cultural development. *Intersectoral cooperation* recognizes that health activities must be undertaken concurrently with measures aimed at improving economic and social development (CNA, 2005).

Taken together, the conditions of the Canada Health Act and the principles of primary health care serve as a solid framework for health care delivery and the future development of Canada's health care system. The conditions outlined in the Canada Health Act and the principles required for primary health care are congruent with the CNA's beliefs about nursing practice. All nurses, therefore, play a vital role in the implementation of the conditions of the Canada Health Act and the principles of primary health care (CNA, 2005; WHO, 1982).

inequities, extending the scope of prevention, and helping people cope with their circumstances. In keeping with the principles of primary health care outlined above, it means fostering public participation, strengthening community health services, and coordinating public health policy. Moreover, it means creating environments conducive to health, in which people are better able to take care of themselves and to offer one another support in solving and managing collective health problems.

Health status is influenced by social norms, cultural values, economic and environmental conditions and policies, and life practices, such as food and exercise choices, the following of safety precautions, and the problematic use of tobacco, alcohol, and other drugs. Health-promotion initiatives must be widely targeted, beginning with the very young, and extending throughout the lifespan. Nurses must provide leadership for health promotion and addressing the determinants of health (CNA, 2009). This guiding should be done through positive role modelling and personal demonstration of healthy life practices, as well as by assisting, promoting, and supporting clients, individuals, groups, and communities through nursing interventions so that they understand and achieve the highest possible level of health.

In cooperation with clients, with each other, with professionals from other sectors, and with governments, nurses coordinate client care and strive to integrate health care services. Nurses participate with clients in designing public health policies and will continue to do so to achieve health for all. Nurses will continue to work with clients and other health care providers to implement the principles of primary health care (CNA, 2005).

Nurse Practice Acts

Nurse practice acts, or legal acts for professional nursing practice, regulate the practice of nursing in Canada and other countries. Each province and territory in Canada has its own act for each of the regulated nursing groups. Although nurse practice acts differ in various jurisdictions, they all have a common purpose—to protect the public. See Chapter 6 for additional information on scopes of practice and nurse practice acts.

One of the ways that the public is protected is through regulation. The primary purpose of regulation is to "assure the public that they are receiving safe and ethical care from competent, qualified registered nurses" (CNA, 2007b, p. 1). Professions can be regulated in one of two ways: (a) by the government or (b) by the profession itself. In Canada, in all the provinces and territories, self-regulation is in place for registered nurses, licensed or registered practical nurses, and registered psychiatric nurses. In some jurisdictions, it is the professional association that is the self-regulatory body, whereas in other jurisdictions, it is a specific regulatory body. Self-regulation means provincial and territorial governments delegate to professional bodies, through legislative acts, the power to determine who may enter and remain in the profession and under what circumstances. Self-regulation is a privilege granted by governments to professional or regulatory organizations. One way in which nurses in Canada are regulated is through title control. "The use of such titles as 'registered nurse,' 'RN,' and 'nurse' is protected by legislation. Only individuals who are currently registered with a nursing regulatory body may use these titles" (CNA, 2007b, p. 1). Similarly, practical nurses and psychiatric nurses in Canada have title protection. Nurse practitioners are also regulated by the provincial and territorial regulatory bodies.

Nursing regulatory bodies, including the International Council of Nurses (ICN), the CNA, and the provincial and territorial professional organizations, work together to develop frameworks for regulatory matters, such as standards of practice, scope of practice, and continuing competence. *Standards of practice* "reflect the values of the nursing profession, clarify what the profession expects of its members, define the expectations of the public or employers, and provide a benchmark below which performance is unacceptable" (CNA, 2001, p. 6). The *scope of practice* refers to the activities that RNs are educated and authorized to perform as set out in legislation and complemented by standards, guidelines, and policy positions of provincial and territorial nursing regulatory bodies (CNA, 2007a, p. 13). *Continuing competence,* as defined by the CNA and the Canadian Association of Schools of Nursing (CASN), is "the ongoing ability of a nurse to integrate and apply the knowledge, skills, judgment and personal attributes required to practice safely and ethically in a designated role and setting" (CNA, 2004, p. 1).

Differences in the regulation of professionals in Canada can often be traced to the differences in provincial and territorial legislation. Usually, licensed practical nurses (LPNs), who are called registered practical nurses (RPNs) in Ontario, and registered psychiatric nurses are regulated under legislation separate from that for registered nurses. Some provinces regulate more than one profession in a single legislative act. Nonregulated workers also work in the health care system. See Chapter 6 for more information on legislation.

Nursing Practice Standards

Nursing practice standards are mandatory for a self-regulating profession. "A standard is a desired and achievable level of performance against which actual performance can be compared. **Standards for nursing practice** reflect the philosophical values of the profession, clarify what the registered nursing profession expects of its members and inform the public of the minimal level of acceptable practice of registered nurses. These standards apply to every setting and provide a benchmark for the basic level of safe registered nursing practice . . ." (Saskatchewan Registered Nurses' Association [SRNA], 2007, p. 4). Each jurisdiction and regulatory body compiles its own nursing standards in conjunction with the legislation governing nursing practice in that jurisdiction for that group of nurses (e.g., licensed practical nurses, registered practical nurses, registered psychiatric nurses, nurse practitioners) (see Chapter 6).

Roles and Functions of the Nurse

Nurses assume a number of roles when they provide care for clients. Often, nurses carry out these roles concurrently. For example, the nurse may act as a counsellor while providing physical care and the health education aspects of that care. The roles required at a specific time depend on the needs of the client and the aspects of the particular environment. Some of the roles of nurses are described below.

Caregiver

The caregiver role has traditionally included those activities that assist the client physically and psychologically while preserving the client's dignity. The required nursing actions may involve full care for the completely dependent client, partial care for the partially dependent client, and supportive–educative care to assist clients in attaining their highest possible level of health and wellness. Caregiving encompasses the physical, psychosocial, developmental, and spiritual levels. A nurse may provide care directly or delegate it to other caregivers.

Communicator

Communication is integral to all nursing roles. Nurses communicate with clients and their support people, other health care professionals, and people in the community.

Nurses identify client problems and then communicate these verbally or in writing to other members of the health care team. The quality of a nurse's communication is an important factor in nursing care. The nurse must be able to communicate clearly and accurately so that a client's health care needs are met. (See Chapters 6 and 22.)

Educator

As a teacher, the nurse helps clients learn about health and the health care procedures they need to perform to restore or maintain health. In collaboration with the client, the nurse determines the client's learning needs and readiness to learn, sets specific learning goals and teaching strategies, implements teaching strategies, and evaluates learning. Nurses also teach other health care providers to whom they delegate care, and they share their expertise with other nurses and health care professionals. See Chapter 26 for additional details about the teaching and learning processes.

Client Advocate

A client advocate acts to protect the client. In this role, the nurse may represent the client's needs and wishes to other health care professionals, such as relaying the client's request for information to a member of the health care team. They also assist clients in exercising their rights and help them advocate for themselves. See Chapter 5.

Counsellor

Counselling is the process of helping a client recognize and cope with stressful psychological or social problems, develop improved interpersonal relationships, and promote personal growth. It involves providing emotional, intellectual, and psychological support. In contrast to the psychotherapist, who counsels individuals with identified problems, the nurse counsels primarily healthy individuals with normal adjustment difficulties. The nurse focuses on helping the person develop new attitudes, feelings, and behaviours, rather than on promoting intellectual growth. The nurse encourages the client to look at alternative behaviours, recognize the choices, and develop a sense of control.

Change Agent

The nurse acts as a change agent when assisting clients to make modifications in their own behaviour. Nurses also often act to make changes in a system, such as clinical care, if it is not helping a client return to health. Nurses are continually dealing with changes in the health care system. Technological changes, changes in the age of the client population, and changes in medications are just a few of the changes nurses deal with daily. See Chapter 27 for additional information about change.

Leader

The leadership role can be employed at different levels: individual client, family, groups of clients or colleagues, or the community. Effective leadership is a learned process requiring an understanding of the needs and goals that motivate people, the knowledge to apply the leadership skills, and the interpersonal skills to influence others. The leadership role of the nurse is discussed in Chapter 27.

NURSE PRACTITIONER

A nurse practitioner is a registered nurse who has an advanced education and is a graduate of a nurse practitioner program. Nurses can be primary health care nurse practitioners who work with clients of all ages or can specialize in a single area or client age group.

Core Competencies

1. Professional Role, Responsibility, and Accountability
   a. Clinical Practice
   b. Collaboration, Consultation, and Referral
   c. Research
   d. Leadership
2. Health Assessment and Diagnosis
3. Therapeutic Management
4. Health Promotion and Prevention of Illness and Injury (Saskatchewan Registered Nurses' Association, 2010)

CLINICAL NURSE SPECIALIST

The clinical nurse specialist is a registered nurse or registered psychiatric nurse who has an advanced degree or expertise in a specialized area of practice (e.g., gerontology, oncology, mental health, primary health care) and provides direct client care, educates others, consults, conducts research, and manages care.

NURSE MIDWIFE

The nurse midwife is a registered nurse who has completed a program in midwifery and is certified. The nurse gives prenatal and postnatal care and manages deliveries in normal pregnancies. The midwife practises in association with a health care agency and can obtain medical services if complications occur.

NURSE ADMINISTRATOR

The nurse administrator manages client care, including the delivery of nursing services. The administrator may have a middle-management position, such as nurse manager or supervisor, or a more senior management position, such as director of nursing services. The functions of nurse administrators include budgeting, staffing, and planning programs. The educational preparation for nurse administrator positions is at least a baccalaureate degree in nursing and frequently a master's or doctoral degree.

NURSE RESEARCHER

Nurse researchers investigate nursing problems to improve nursing care and to refine and expand nursing knowledge. They are employed in academic institutions, teaching hospitals, and research centres. Nurse researchers usually have advanced education at the doctoral level.

NURSE EDUCATOR

Nurse educators are employed in nursing programs, at educational institutions, and in hospital or institutional (e.g., long-term care) staff education. Many have advanced degrees in nursing or education.

Manager

The nurse manages the nursing care of individuals, families, and communities. The nurse manager also delegates nursing activities to ancillary workers and other nurses, and supervises and evaluates their performance. Managing requires knowledge about organizational structure and dynamics, authority and accountability, leadership, change theory, advocacy, delegation, supervision, and evaluation. See Chapter 27 for additional details.

Case Manager

Nurse case managers work with multidisciplinary health care teams to measure the effectiveness of case management plans and to monitor outcomes. Each agency or unit specifies the role of the case manager.

Research Consumer

Nurses often use research to improve client care. In a clinical area, nurses need to (a) have some awareness of the process and language of research, (b) be sensitive to issues related to protecting the rights of human subjects, (c) participate in the identification of significant researchable problems, and (d) be a discriminating consumer of research findings (see Chapter 3).

Expanded Career Roles

Nurses are fulfilling expanded career roles, such as those of nurse practitioner, clinical nurse specialist, nurse midwife, nurse administrator, nurse educator, and nurse researcher, that allow greater independence and autonomy. See Box 1.3.

Nursing as a Profession

Nursing is gaining recognition as a profession. A **profession** has been defined as an occupation that requires extensive education or a calling that requires special knowledge, skill, and preparation. A profession is generally distinguished from other kinds of occupations by (a) its requirement of prolonged, specialized training to acquire a body of knowledge pertinent to the role to be performed, and (b) an orientation of the individual toward service, either to a community or to an organization. The standards of education and practice for the profession are determined by the members of the profession, rather than by outsiders. The education of the professional involves a complete socialization process, more far-reaching in its social and attitudinal aspects and its technical features than is usually required in other kinds of occupations.

Self-regulation is based on the belief that the profession of nursing has the special knowledge required to set standards of practice and to assess the conduct of its members through peer review. As members of the nursing profession, nurses are bound by the ethical values of the profession to base their practice on relevant and current knowledge. Although not all professional organizations use the same criteria for identifying a profession, most include that a profession has a formal base of knowledge, requires significant educational preparation to be admitted to the profession, maintains control over the standards by which new applicants are evaluated, uses the knowledge for the direct benefit of the public, is self-regulating, and maintains a code of ethics (Ross-Kerr, 2003). See Chapter 5 for more information on the codes of ethics for nursing.

Criteria of a Profession

SPECIALIZED BODY OF KNOWLEDGE As a profession, nursing is establishing a well-defined body of knowledge and expertise. A number of nursing conceptual frameworks (discussed in Chapter 4) contribute to the knowledge base of nursing and give direction to nursing practice, education, and ongoing research.

Increasing research in nursing is contributing to nursing practice and nursing knowledge. In the 1980s, increased federal funding and professional support helped establish centres for nursing research. Most early research was directed to the study of nursing education. In the 1960s, studies were often related to the nature of the knowledge base underlying nursing practice. Since the 1970s, nursing research has focused on practice-related issues. Nursing research as a dimension of the nurse's role is discussed further in Chapter 3.

SPECIALIZED EDUCATION Specialized education is an important aspect of professional status. In modern times, the trend in education for professions has shifted toward programs in colleges and universities. Many nursing educators believe that the undergraduate nursing curriculum should include liberal arts education, in addition to the biological and social sciences and the nursing discipline.

The CNA recommends the baccalaureate degree as the level of education required for entry to practice as a registered nurse. (See Chapter 2 for more information on nursing education at all levels.)

SERVICE ORIENTATION A service orientation differentiates nursing from an occupation pursued primarily for profit. Many consider altruism (selfless concern for others) the hallmark of a profession. Nursing has a tradition of service to others. This service, however, must be guided by certain rules, policies, or codes of ethics. Nursing is an important component of the health care delivery system.

PROFESSIONAL ORGANIZATION Operation under the umbrella of a professional organization differentiates a profession from an occupation. For registered nurses, the CNA, in addition to the provincial and territorial nursing organizations, performs the self-regulatory functions.

AUTONOMY AND SELF-REGULATION A profession is autonomous if it regulates itself and sets standards for its members. Providing autonomy is one of the purposes of a professional association. If nursing is to have professional status, it must function autonomously in the formation of policy and in the control of its activities. To be autonomous, a professional group must be granted legal authority to define the scope of its practice, describe its particular functions and roles, and determine its goals and accountabilities in delivery of its services. See Chapter 6 for additional information on scopes of practice and legislated authority.

CODE OF ETHICS Nurses have traditionally placed a high value on the worth and dignity of others. The nursing profession requires integrity of its members; that is, a member is expected to do what is considered right. Ethical codes change as the needs and values of society change. Nursing has developed its own codes of ethics. It is within the nursing educational program that the nurse develops, clarifies, and internalizes professional values. Specific professional nursing values are stated in nursing codes of ethics (see Chapter 5), in standards of nursing practice (discussed earlier in this chapter), and in the legal system itself (see Chapter 6).

Socialization to Nursing

Socialization can be defined simply as the process by which people (a) learn to become members of groups and society, and (b) learn the social rules defining relationships into which they will enter. Socialization involves learning to behave, feel, and see the world in a manner similar to other persons occupying the same role (Hardy & Conway, 1988). The goal of professional socialization is to instill in individuals the norms, values, attitudes, and behaviours deemed essential for the survival of the profession.

Various models of the socialization process have been developed. Benner's model (1984) describes five levels of proficiency in nursing based on the Dreyfus general model of skill acquisition (Dreyfus & Dreyfus, 1980). The five stages, which have implications for teaching and learning, are novice, advanced beginner,

---

BOX 1.4 BENNER'S STAGES OF NURSING EXPERTISE

STAGE I, NOVICE

No experience (e.g., nursing student). Performance is limited, inflexible, and governed by context-free rules and regulations, rather than experience.

STAGE II, ADVANCED BEGINNER

Demonstrates marginally acceptable performance. Recognizes the meaningful "aspects" of a real situation. Has experienced enough real situations to make judgments about them.

STAGE III, COMPETENT PRACTITIONER

Has 2 or 3 years of experience. Demonstrates organizational and planning abilities. Differentiates important factors from less important aspects of care. Coordinates multiple, complex care demands.

STAGE IV, PROFICIENT PRACTITIONER

Has 3 to 5 years of experience. Perceives a situation as a whole, rather than in terms of parts, as in Stage II. Uses maxims as guides for what to consider in a situation. Has holistic understanding of the client, which improves decision making. Focuses on long-term goals.

STAGE V, EXPERT PRACTITIONER

Performance is fluid, flexible, and highly proficient; no longer requires rules, guidelines, or maxims to connect an understanding of the situation to appropriate action. Demonstrates highly skilled, intuitive, and analytical ability in new situations. Is inclined to take a certain action because "it feels right."

Source: Benner, P. (2001). *From novice to expert: Excellence and power in clinical nursing practice, Commemorative edition,* 1st. Upper Saddle River, NJ: Pearson Education, Inc. Electronically reproduced by permission of Pearson Education, Inc., Upper Saddle River, NJ.

---

competent practitioner, proficient practitioner, and expert practitioner. Benner writes that experience is essential for the development of professional expertise. See Box 1.4.

One of the most powerful mechanisms of professional socialization is interaction with fellow students (Hardy & Conway, 1988). Within this student culture, students collectively set the level and direction of their scholastic efforts. They develop perspectives about the situation in which they are involved, the goals they are trying to achieve, and the kinds of activities that are expedient and proper, and they establish a set of practices congruent with all of these. Students become bound together by feelings of mutual cooperation, support, and solidarity. The Canadian Nursing Students' Association (CNSA) helps link nursing students with nursing leadership groups. This organization exposes student nurses to issues impacting the nursing profession while promoting collegiality and leadership qualities.

Factors Influencing Contemporary Nursing Practice

To understand nursing as it is practised today and as it will be practised tomorrow requires an understanding of some of the social forces influencing this profession. These forces usually affect the entire health care system, and as a major component of that system, nursing cannot avoid the effects.

Economics

Greater financial support provided through public and private health insurance programs has increased the demand for nursing care. While basic health care in Canada is available to all, each provincial and territorial system identifies the services which are covered, and which are not.

Currently, the health care industry is shifting its emphasis from inpatient care to outpatient care with pre-admission testing, increased outpatient same-day surgery, posthospitalization rehabilitation, home health care, health maintenance, physical fitness programs, and community health education programs. As a result, more nurses are being employed in community-based health care settings, such as home health agencies, hospices, and community clinics. As well, advanced practice nurses, such as nurse practitioners or foot care specialists, are practising collaboratively or independently in nontraditional settings. These changes in employment for nurses have implications for nursing education, nursing research, and nursing practice.

Consumer Demands

Consumers of nursing services (the public) have become an increasingly effective force in changing nursing practice. On the whole, people are better educated and have more knowledge about health and illness than in the past. Consumers also have become more aware of others' needs for care. The ethical and moral issues raised by poverty and neglect have made people more vocal about the needs of minority groups and the poor.

Most Canadians strongly believe that health is a right of all Canadians. The media increasingly emphasize the message that individuals must assume responsibility for their own health by obtaining a physical examination regularly, checking for signs of cancer and cardiovascular disease, and maintaining their mental well-being by balancing work and recreation. As more of the population struggles with chronic diseases, expectations of support for self and others continue to rise. Many people now want more than freedom from disease—they want energy, vitality, and a feeling of wellness.

Increasingly, the consumer has become an active participant in making decisions about health and nursing care. Planning committees concerned with providing nursing services to a community usually have an active consumer membership. Recognizing the legitimacy of public input, many federal, provincial, and territorial nursing associations and regulatory agencies have consumer representatives on their governing boards.

Family Structure

Family structures influence the need for and provision of nursing services. More people are living away from the extended nuclear family, and the family breadwinner is no longer necessarily the husband. Many single men and women rear children, and in many two-parent families, both parents work. Thus support, such as daycare or senior assistance, which may have been available historically from family members is sought elsewhere. For additional information about the family, see Chapter 13.

Science and Technology

Advances in science and technology affect nursing practice. For example, people with *acquired immune deficiency syndrome (AIDS)* are receiving new drug therapies to prolong life and delay the onset of AIDS-associated diseases. Nurses must be knowledgeable about the actions of such drugs and the needs of the clients receiving them. Nurses acquire knowledge and skills as they adapt to meet the new needs of clients.

In some settings, technological advances have required that nurses become highly specialized. Nurses frequently have to use sophisticated computerized equipment to provide care for clients. In addition, information technology advances have given the nurse and the client access to much more information. Nurses and clients must view this information with a critical eye. As technologies change, nursing education changes, and nurses require more advanced education to provide effective, safe nursing practice.

The need for long-distance monitoring of astronauts and spacecraft, lighter materials, and miniaturization of equipment in the U.S. space program has given rise to advanced technologies. Health care has benefited as these new technologies have been adapted to health care aids, such as Viewstar (an aid for those with visual impairments), the insulin infusion pump, the voice-controlled wheelchair, magnetic resonance imaging (MRI), laser surgery, filters for intravenous fluid control devices, and monitoring systems for intensive care (see Chapter 25).

Demography

Demography is the study of population, including statistics about distribution by age and place of residence, mortality (death), and morbidity (incidence of disease). From demographic data, the needs of the population for nursing services can be assessed:

- The total population in Canada is increasing. The proportion of older adults has also increased, creating a growing need for nursing services for this group (see the Evidence-Informed Practice box on caring for older adults). This change in demographics has also highlighted differences in generations. For instance, as the baby boomer generation (those born between 1945 and 1964) ages, a variety of social processes, including health care, have been influenced.

- The population is shifting from rural to urban settings. This shift signals increased needs for nursing related to problems caused by pollution and other effects on the environment by concentrations of people. Yet, the rural population still needs access to care.

- Mortality and morbidity studies reveal the presence of risk factors. Many of these risk factors (e.g., smoking) are major causes of death and disease that can be prevented through changes in lifestyle. The nurse's role in assessing risk factors and helping clients make healthy lifestyle changes is discussed in Chapter 8.

EVIDENCE-INFORMED PRACTICE

What Has Influenced Our Care of Older Adults?

Although the historical portion of this chapter has focused on the history of nursing in Canada, these authors have used an historical review to consider the basis for care for older adults. Examining the aging through a philosophical lens, the authors contend that Western society continues to have negative views on aging, which have influenced thinking and actions of all who were exposed to them. As students and teachers we may unconsciously mimic these negative attitudes in our work with older adults, both healthy and those with health challenges.

NURSING IMPLICATIONS: The authors challenge nurse educators and leaders to reassess their thinking and how it affects their practice and their teaching.

Source: Based on Dahlke, S. (2011). Examining nursing practice with older adults through a historical lens. *Journal of Gerontological Nursing, 37*(5), 41–48.

The Women's Movement

The women's movement brought public attention to both women's and human rights. People are seeking equality in all areas, particularly educational, political, economic, and social equality. Because the majority of nurses are women, this movement has altered nursing's perspectives on economic and educational needs. As a result, nurses are increasingly asserting themselves as professional people who have a right to equality with men in health care professions and are demanding more autonomy in client care.

Nursing Organizations

As nursing has developed, an increasing number of nursing organizations have been formed at the local, provincial and territorial, national, and international levels. The organizations that involve most Canadian registered nurses and nursing students are the CNA and the ICN. Psychiatric and practical nurses are also part of nursing organizations, as described shortly. Increasingly, nursing specialty organizations are being formed, for example, the Canadian Association of Nurses in Oncology (CANO). In addition, many nurses are part of unions. Participation in the activities of nursing associations enhances the growth of involved individuals and helps nurses collectively influence policies that affect nursing practice. Nurses advocate

and influence policy at provincial, territorial, and federal levels through professional organizations such as CNA and provincial/territorial professional associations.

Canadian Nurses Association

The CNA is a federation of 11 provincial and territorial nursing associations, representing more than 143 843 registered nurses. The CNA's mission states that it is "the national professional voice of registered nurses . . . advances the practice and profession of nursing to improve health outcomes and strengthen Canada's publicly funded not-for-profit health system" (CNA, 2011). Toward this end, it promotes high standards of practice, education, research, and administration. In many provinces and territories, the regulatory body and the professional association are within the same organization. In other provinces, such as Ontario, these are separate organizations (see Table 1.1).

The CNA is the national nursing association of Canada. Nurses do not join the CNA independently but obtain membership by paying a fee to the provincial or territorial organizations. In November 1985, the Ordre des infirmières et infirmiers du Québec (the Quebec Nurses Association, or OIIQ) withdrew from the CNA. This parallels the history that is noted in the Nursing and Canadian Society box on page 20. The CNA has developed national standards and a code of ethics, and it offers support to all provincial and territorial organizations.

TABLE 1.1   Provincial and Territorial Registered Nursing Associations

Geographical Area	Nursing Association	Website
British Columbia	Association of Registered Nurses of British Columbia	http://www.arnbc.ca
	College of Registered Nurses of British Columbia	http://www.crnbc.ca
Alberta	College and Association of Registered Nurses of Alberta	http://www.nurses.ab.ca
Saskatchewan	Saskatchewan Registered Nurses' Association	http://www.srna.org
Manitoba	College of Registered Nurses of Manitoba	http://www.crnm.mb.ca
Ontario	Registered Nurses' Association of Ontario	http://www.rnao.org
	College of Nurses of Ontario	http://www.cno.org
Quebec	Ordre des infirmières et infirmiers du Québec	http://www.oiiq.org
New Brunswick	Nurses Association of New Brunswick	http://www.nanb.nb.ca
Nova Scotia	College of Registered Nurses of Nova Scotia	http://www.crnns.ca
Newfoundland and Labrador	Association of Registered Nurses of Newfoundland and Labrador	http://www.arnnl.ca
Prince Edward Island	Association of Registered Nurses of Prince Edward Island	http://www.arnpei.ca
Northwest Territories	Registered Nurses Association of Northwest Territories and Nunavut	http://www.rnantnu.ca
Yukon	Yukon Registered Nurses Association	http://www.yrna.ca

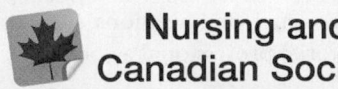

Nursing and Canadian Society

Fact	Implications for Nursing Practice
Canadian nursing history is rooted in the French tradition of nursing sisters and the secular British model.	Understanding history provides registered nurses with an appreciation of present issues, conflicts, and ideologies.
The Canadian Nurses Association (CNA) is a federation of 11 provincial and territorial registered nurses associations. The membership of more than 143 843 registered nurses is broad and diverse, reflecting the face of nursing today.	Strength for changes to health care is often achieved through the large membership of the CNA.
Ordre des infirmières et infirmiers du Québec speaks for registered nurses in that province.	Registration practices differ within Canada, which may influence the employment pattern of nurses.

Through the national testing services, the CNA prepares licensure examinations. These examinations are available to all provinces and territories and provide a national standard for licensure of registered nurses. Certification in specific clinical specialties can also be obtained through the CNA (see Chapter 2). Through the Canadian Nurses Foundation, research grants, fellowships, and scholarships are offered to Canadian nurses. The official journal of the CNA, *Canadian Nurse,* is published monthly and sent to each nurse member.

International Council of Nurses

The ICN was established in 1899. Nurses from Great Britain, the United States, and Canada were among the founding members. The council is a federation of national registered nurses' associations, such as the CNA and the American Nurses Association.

Through the ICN, member national associations can work together for the mission of representing nursing worldwide, advancing the profession, and influencing health care policy. The five core values of the ICN are visionary leadership, inclusiveness, flexibility, partnership, and achievement (ICN, 2011). The official journal of the ICN is *International Nursing Review.*

Canadian Council of Registered Nurse Regulators

As noted earlier in the chapter, as part of self-regulation of registered nurses, there are regulatory bodies within each province and territory, often aligned with the provincial

or territorial nursing association, but sometimes existing as distinct entities. The Canadian Council of Registered Nurse Regulators is a very new national group. The purpose of the council is as follows:

• Promote excellence in professional nursing regulation
• Serve as a national forum and voice regarding interprovincial/territorial, national, and global regulatory matters for nursing regulation (College of Registered Nurses of Nova Scotia, 2012)

Sigma Theta Tau International Honor Society of Nursing

The Sigma Theta Tau International Honor Society of Nursing (STTI) was founded in 1922 and is headquartered in Indianapolis, Indiana. The Greek letters stand for the Greek words *storga, tharos,* and *tima,* meaning "love," "courage," and "honour." The society is a member of the Association of College Honor Societies. The society's purpose is professional, rather than social. Membership is attained through academic achievement. Nursing students in baccalaureate programs and those in master's, doctoral, and postdoctoral programs are eligible to be selected for membership. In addition, community nurses with a "minimum of a baccalaureate degree or equivalent, and demonstrated achievement in nursing" can apply to become members (Sigma Theta Tau International, 2011). STTI became an international organization with the creation of a chapter at the University of Western Ontario. Now chapters span the globe, and there are eight STTI chapters in Canada.

The official journal of STTI, *Journal of Nursing Scholarship,* is published quarterly. The journal publishes scholarly articles of interest to nurses. STTI also organizes at least one international research conference each year, held in a different city each time.

Specialty Organizations

Within Canadian nursing are a large number of specialty organizations. These may be linked to the provincial, territorial, or national (CNA) professional associations. Although some are groups of nurses in specialized practice (e.g., Community Health Nurses Association of Canada [CHNAC]), others are by type of job (e.g., the Provincial Nurse Educator Interest Group [PNEIG], Canadian Association for Nursing Research [CANR], Academy of Canadian Executive Nurses [ACEN], Canadian Association of Practical Nurse Educators [CAPNE]). These organizations further the profession by contributing position statements and group-specific standards of practice, influencing public policy, and participating in knowledge translation and dissemination.

Licensed (Registered) Practical Nurses

Practical nurses are licensed in all provinces and territories except Ontario, where they are registered. Although all provinces have a professional organization (see Table 1.2), the national organization is inactive at this time. Of the territories, only Yukon has a professional association for LPNs, and it is in the beginning stages. In addition, the practical nurse regulatory bodies have a national organization: the Canadian Council for Practical Nurse Regulators (CCPNR). It notes national commonalities, but the organizations are different in all jurisdictions. The CCPNR has contributed to development of national policies for practical nursing. The Canadian Association of Practical Nurse Educators (CAPNE) presents its mission as "to support and enhance the access,

quality, effectiveness and consistency of education for practical nurses to meet the evolving health care needs of Canadians" (CAPNE, 2011). Its membership consists of "practical nursing educators and regulatory bodies from every province/territory with the exception of Quebec" (CAPNE, 2011).

Registered Psychiatric Nurses

In the four Western provinces of Canada, another category of nurses is the registered psychiatric nurse. The Canadian Institute for Health Information's definition of a registered psychiatric nurse is found in Box 1.2 (see page 11). The Registered Psychiatric Nurses of Canada (RPNC) comprises the regulatory bodies or associations from all four provinces. It also liaises with other psychiatric nursing organizations globally. The provincial and national organizations are listed in Table 1.3.

TABLE 1.2 Provincial and Territorial Practical Nurse Professional Organizations

Geographical Area	Organization	Website
British Columbia	College of Licensed Practical Nurses of British Columbia	http://www.clpnbc.org
Alberta	College of Licensed Practical Nurses of Alberta	http://www.clpna.com
Saskatchewan	Saskatchewan Association of Licensed Practical Nurses	http://www.salpn.com
Manitoba	College of Licensed Practical Nurses of Manitoba	http://www.clpnm.ca
Ontario	Registered Practical Nurses Association of Ontario	http://www.rpnao.org
	College of Nurses of Ontario	http://www.cno.org
Quebec	Ordre des infirmières et infirmiers auxiliaires du Québec	http://www.oiiaq.org
New Brunswick	Association of New Brunswick Licensed Practical Nurses	http://www.anblpn.ca
Nova Scotia	College of Licensed Practical Nurses of Nova Scotia	http://www.clpnns.ca
Newfoundland and Labrador	College of Licensed Practical Nurses of Newfoundland and Labrador	http://www.clpnnl.ca
Prince Edward Island	Licensed Practical Nurses Association of Prince Edward Island	http://www.lpna.ca
Yukon	Yukon Practical Nurses Association	Regulatory—Yukon Consumer Services Early stages of development; no website yet
Northwest Territories		Regulatory—Licensed Practical Nurses, Department of Health and Social Services, Government of the Northwest Territories; http://www.hlthss.gov.nt.ca/english/services/professional_licensing/licensed_practical_nurses.htm

TABLE 1.3 Canadian Psychiatric Nursing Professional Organizations

Jurisdiction	Organization	Website
National	Registered Psychiatric Nurses of Canada	http://www.rpnc.ca
British Columbia	College of Registered Psychiatric Nurses of British Columbia	http://www.crpnbc.ca
Alberta	College of Registered Psychiatric Nurses of Alberta	http://www.crpna.ab.ca
Saskatchewan	Registered Psychiatric Nurses Association of Saskatchewan	http://www.rpnas.com
Manitoba	College of Registered Psychiatric Nurses of Manitoba	http://www.crpnm.mb.ca
Yukon	Yukon Consumer Services	http://www.community.gov.yk.ca/rpn/index.html

Unions

The majority of today's nurses are union members by virtue of their employment. The Canadian Federation of Nurses Unions (CFNU) represents nine provincial unions and one students' association and speaks for 176 000 members. Created in 1981 as the National Federation of Nurses Unions, it seeks to "advance solutions to improve patient care, working conditions and our public health care system" (CFNU, 2010). Depending on the worksite and collective agreements, each union may include registered nurses, licensed (registered) practical nurses, and registered psychiatric nurses within the membership.

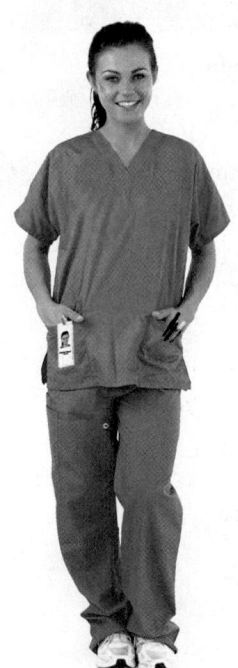

Case Study 1

The supply of nurses in Canada has historically been partially shaped by constraints over who could train as a nurse and who could practise in certain areas, such as pediatrics, obstetrics, psychiatric hospitals, and the military. The following cases illustrate some criteria that have been used in the past to include or exclude people as nurses.

Edith Anderson Monture was a member of the Upper Mohawk band of the Six Nations of the Grand River Reserve near Brantford, Ontario. She was denied entrance to nursing schools in Canada, but she graduated first in her class from the New Rochelle Hospital School of Nursing in New York in 1914. Following volunteer service with the American Expeditionary Force in World War I, she returned to the hospital on the Six Nations Reserve, where she worked as a nurse and midwife until her retirement in 1955 (Moses, 2005).

Estelle Tritt applied for training at the Montreal General Hospital School of Nursing and was told that they did not take Jewish nurses because "they get married too soon" (Toman, 2007, p. 47). She subsequently applied successfully to the Women's General Hospital at Westmount, Quebec, and graduated from training in 1941. After working at the Jewish General Hospital in Montreal to gain the required years of graduate experience, Tritt was accepted as a military nurse (nursing sister) with the Royal Canadian Army Medical Corps and served overseas during World War II.

This memo was sent to Helen Mussallem, CEO of Canadian Nurses Association, January 18, 1966: "The Surgeon General stated today that he has not changed his mind: 'male nurses will not get commissions in the medical services (nursing). . . .' His main objection is that 'the men would stay in nursing and would possibly become Matron in the Armed Services. This would not be good in a male-oriented service'" (Library and Archives Canada, 1966).

CRITICAL THINKING QUESTIONS

1. The preferred candidates for nursing students until the mid-twentieth century were young, white, Canadian-born women. What are the different factors in these examples that have historically determined who could be a nurse?

2. In what ways are these criteria still influencing the composition of the nursing workforce? What has changed regarding the manifestations of such criteria? What additional characteristics are shaping the nursing profession? To what extent is the profession more inclusive now, and how might some people still face barriers?

Check the eText in MyNursingLab for answers and explanations.

KEY TERMS

client *p. 10*

consumer *p. 10*

demography *p. 18*

standards for nursing practice *p. 13*

patient *p. 10*

profession *p. 15*

socialization *p. 16*

CHAPTER HIGHLIGHTS

- Knowledge of how larger and changing sociocultural and political contexts have influenced the development of nurses and their practice in the past is key to understanding the relevance of history to present-day concerns in nursing.

- The term *nursing* has many definitions and descriptions, but the essence of nursing is caring for and caring about people.

- The scope of nursing practice is outlined by the professional associations (or organizations) of each province and territory. It describes what it is that nurses in a particular province or territory have the legislated authority to do.

- Although traditionally the majority of nurses were employed in hospital settings, today the numbers of nurses working in home health care, ambulatory care, and community health settings are increasing.

- Standards of clinical nursing practice reflect the values of the profession and clarify what professional organizations expect of their members.

- Every nurse can function in a variety of roles that are not exclusive; in reality, the functions often occur together and serve to clarify the nurse's activities. These roles include caregiver, communicator, teacher, client advocate, counsellor, change agent, leader, and research consumer.

- A desired goal of nursing is professionalism, which requires specialized education; a unique body of knowledge, including specific skills and abilities; ongoing research; a code of ethics; autonomy; a service orientation; and a professional organization.

- Socialization is a lifelong process by which people become functioning participants of a society or a group. Although several models of the socialization process have been developed, Benner's five stages—novice, advanced beginner, competent practitioner, proficient practitioner, and expert practitioner—can serve as guidelines to establish the phase and extent of an individual's socialization in nursing.

- Participation in the activities of nursing associations and other professional and nonprofessional groups enhances the growth of involved individuals and helps nurses collectively influence policies affecting nursing practice.

ASSESS YOUR LEARNING

1. The primary purpose of historical research on the nursing profession is to do what?

   a. Showcase achievements of nurses in the past

   b. Provide alternative perspectives for understanding nursing issues

   c. Prove that nursing has been a true profession for a long time

   d. Justify nurses' demands for greater respect and improved salaries

2. What is true about the profession of nursing in Canada?

   a. No nurses were practising in Canada prior to the establishment of the first training school.

   b. Nursing has always been an equal opportunity profession, gender blind, and open to all ethnic groups.

   c. Nurses have traditionally relied on hospitals as their main place of work.

   d. The nursing workforce has experienced recurring periods of oversupply and shortages.

3. Which of the following groups had a historically significant influence on the beginnings of formal educational preparation for practicing nurses in Canada?

   a. Federal government

   b. French Canadian religious communities

   c. Victorian Order of Nurses

   d. Canadian Nurses Association

4. The difference between Primary Health Care and Primary Care is BEST explained by which of the following statements?

   a. Primary Health Care is a theoretical approach to health care while Primary Care is a system of delivering services.

   b. Primary Health Care is illness focused while Primary Care is health promotion focused.

   c. Primary Health Care is a set of government standards for Canadian health care while Primary Care provides a set of principles for delivering care.

   d. Primary Health Care is a philosophical approach to providing health care while Primary Care provides an entry point to the health care system.

5. Which activity would be considered in the category of restoring health?

   a. Running a newborn clinic at the local public health facility

   b. Administering medications to a patient in a hospital orthopedic unit

   c. Facilitating a parenting class at the hospital

   d. Starting a seniors' walking program at the local mall

6. What describes the principle of comprehensiveness in the Canada Health Act?

   a. All levels of health care are available to the residents of a particular jurisdiction.

   b. Individuals who move within Canada are covered at all times.

   c. There are no user fees for basic services within the jurisdiction.

   d. The administration of the plan is devolved to the local authorities.

7. What represents the BEST application of nursing practice standards?

   a. A student nurse writes end-of-term examinations.

   b. A physician determines the necessary care for a patient.

   c. Registered nurses receive an increase in salary.

   d. A registered nurse practises in an ethical manner.

8. Benner's stages of nursing expertise were developed primarily to do what?

   a. Assist nursing students to plot their progress to graduation

   b. Ensure performance appraisal forms are measured against practice standards

   c. Describe the characteristics of nurses as they move from novice to expert

   d. Assist nurse managers to ensure they hire only nurses who are experts

9. What does the profession of nursing have that is considered necessary to be called a profession?

   a. Levels of expertise

   b. Payment for services

   c. A code of ethics

   d. Government control

10. Among the many nursing theorists, what is a commonality in the definition of nursing?

    a. Delivery of holistic, adaptive, and client-centred care

    b. Delivery of care to a passive recipient

    c. Assistant to the physician while delivering care

    d. A profession of entrepreneurs delivering independent care

Check the eText in MyNursingLab for answers and explanations.

WEBLINKS

Canadian Association for the History of Nursing (CAHN)

http://cahn-achn.ca

The Canadian Association for the History of Nursing provides a forum for those interested in the history of nursing through annual conferences, biannual newsletters, and financial support of nursing history scholarship. It also promotes the preservation of historical nursing materials through its Guide to Canadian Nursing Archival Resources.

Associated Medical Services Nursing History Research Unit

http://www.health.uottawa.ca/nursinghistory

The Associated Medical Services Nursing History Research Unit is the only funded academic centre in Canada dedicated to the production and dissemination of new knowledge in nursing history. It educates graduate students through academic programs and summer research practicums, publishes new research, hosts conferences and seminars, establishes links with international nursing history units, and maintains a comprehensive bibliography on Canadian nursing history.

Registered Nurses' Association of Ontario

http://www.rnao.org/bestpractices

This group has led the way in developing a series of best practices documents. Thirty-five different publications are available, offering guidelines on such subjects as clinical practice and healthy work environments.

MyNursingLab

MyNursingLab's guided learning path makes reviewing and test preparation straightforward.

- Content summaries, animations, and videos reinforce key concepts and skills
- Practice questions help with test prep by showing gaps in knowledge
- An eText, available online and via the iPad, makes searching, highlighting, and note-taking easy

This QR code appears at the end of every chapter and provides learning resources that you can access with your smartphone to study on the go. Access self-review quizzes, flashcards, and more!

REFERENCES

Anspaugh, D. L., Hamrick, M. H., & Rosata, F. D. (2003). *Wellness: Concepts and applications.* New York, NY: McGraw-Hill.

Benner, P. (1984). *From novice to expert: Excellence and power in clinical nursing practice.* Menlo Park, CA: Addison-Wesley Nursing.

Canada Health Act of 1984, R.S., 1985, c. C-6. Ottawa, ON: Government of Canada.

Canada, House of Commons. (1984). *An Act Relating to Cash Contributions by Canada in Respect of Insured Health Services Provided Under Provincial Health Care Insurance Plans and Amounts Payable by Canada in Respect of Extended Health Care Services and to Amend and Repeal Certain Acts in Consequence Thereof (The Canada Health Act).* Ottawa, ON: Government of Canada.

Canadian Association of Practical Nurse Educators (2011). *About us.* Retrieved from http://www.capne.net/about.php

Canadian Federation of Nurses Unions. (2010). *Home page.* Retrieved from http://www.nursesunions.ca

Canadian Institute for Health Information. (2012). *Regulated nurses: Canadian trends, 2006 to 2010.* Ottawa, ON: Author.

Canadian Nurses Association. (1987). *A definition of nursing practice: Standards for nursing practice.* Ottawa, ON: Author.

Canadian Nurses Association. (1995). *The role of the nurse in primary health care.* Ottawa: Author.

Canadian Nurses Association. (2001). Issues and trends in Canadian nursing. Self-regulation: Safeguarding the privilege. *Nursing Now, 10,* 5–8.

Canadian Nurses Association. (2004). *CNA and CASN Joint Position Statement: Promoting continuing competence for registered nurses.* Ottawa, ON: Author.

Canadian Nurses Association. (2005). *Primary health care: A summary of the issues.* Ottawa, ON: Author.

Canadian Nurses Association. (2007a). *Framework for the practice of registered nurses in Canada.* Ottawa, ON: Author. Retrieved from http://www.cna-aiic.ca/CNA/ documents/pdf/publications/RN_Framework_Practice_2007_e.pdf

Canadian Nurses Association. (2007b). Issues and trends in Canadian nursing. Understanding self-regulation. *Nursing Now, 21,* 1–5.

Canadian Nurses Association. (2009). *Position Statement— Determinants of Health.* Ottawa, ON: Author.

Canadian Nurses Association. (2011). *Who we are.* Retrieved from http://cna-aiic.ca/CNA/about/who/default_e.aspx

Cassel, J. (1994). Public health in Canada. In P. Dorothy (Ed.). *The history of public health and the modern state* (pp. 276–312). London, UK: Wellcome Institute Series in the History of Medicine.

Cayne, B. S. (Ed.). (1988). *New Lexicon Webster's Dictionary of the English Language* (Rev. ed.). New York, NY: Lexicon Publications.

Charles, A. (2003). Women's work in eclipse: Nuns in Quebec hospitals, 1940–1980. In G. Feldberg, M. Ladd-Taylor, A. Li, & K. McPherson (Eds.). *Women, health and nation: Canada and the United States since 1945* (pp. 264–291). Montreal, PQ: McGill-Queen's University Press.

College of Registered Nurses of Nova Scotia. (2012). *Canadian Council of Registered Nurse Regulators.* Retrieved from http://crnns.ca/

Dreyfus, S. E., & Dreyfus, H. L. (1980). *A five-stage model of the mental activities involved in directed skill acquisition.* Unpublished report supported by the Air Force Office of Scientific Research (AFSC), USAF (Contract F49620–79-C-0063), University of California at Berkeley.

Elliott, J. (2004). Blurring the boundaries of space: Shaping nursing lives at the Red Cross outposts in Ontario, 1922–1945. *Canadian Bulletin of Medical History, 21*(2), 303–325.

Gagan, D., & Gagan, R. (2002). *For patients of moderate means: A social history of the voluntary public hospital in Canada, 1890–1950.* Montreal, PQ: McGill-Queen's University Press.

Hardy, M. E., & Conway, M. E. (1988). *Role theory: Perspectives for healthy professionals* (2nd ed.). Norwalk, CT: Appleton & Lange.

Henderson, V. (1966). *The nature of nursing: A definition and its implications for practice, research, and education.* New York, NY: Macmillan.

International Council of Nurses. (2010). *The ICN definition of nursing.* Retrieved from http://www.icn.ch/about-icn/icn-definition-of-nursing

International Council of Nurses. (2011). *Our mission.* Retrieved from http://www.icn.ch/about-icn/icns-mission

Leininger, M. (1984). *Care: The essence of nursing and health.* Thorofare, NJ: Slack.

Library and Archives Canada. (1966). MG 28, I248, Vol. 78, File 30–3-8. Memo to file from Helen Mussallem, January 18, 1966.

MacDougall, H. (2007). Toronto's health department in action: Influenza in 1919 and SARS in 2003. *Journal of the History of Medicine and Allied Sciences, 62,* 56–89.

Mansell, D. (2003). *Forging the future in Canada: A history of nursing in Canada.* Ann Arbor, MI: Thomas Press.

McBain, L. (2005). Jean Cuthand Goodwill. In C. Bates, D. Dodd, & N. Rousseau (Eds.). *On all frontiers: Four centuries of Canadian nursing* (p. 116). Ottawa, ON: University of Ottawa Press & Canadian Museum of Civilization.

McKay, M. (2007). "The tubercular cow must go": Business, politics, and Winnipeg's milk supply, 1894–1922. *Canadian Bulletin of Medical History, 23*(2), 255–380.

McPherson, K. (1996). *Bedside matters: The transformation of Canadian nursing, 1900–1990.* Toronto, ON: Oxford University Press.

McPherson, K. (2003). Nursing and colonization: The work of Indian health service nurses in Manitoba, 1945–1970. In G. Feldberg, M. Ladd-Taylor, A. Li, & K. McPherson (Eds.). *Women, health and nation: Canada and the United States since 1945* (pp. 223–246). Montreal, PQ: McGill-Queen's University Press.

Meijer-Drees, L., & McBain, L. (2001). Nursing and native peoples in northern Saskatchewan: 1930s–1950s. *Canadian Bulletin of Medical History, 18*(1), 43–65.

Miller, K. L. (1995). Keeping the care in nursing care: Our biggest challenge. *Journal of Nursing Administration, 25*(11), 29–32.

Moses, J. (2005). Charlotte Edith Anderson Monture (1890–1996). In C. Bates, D. Dodd, & N. Rousseau (Eds.). *On all frontiers: Four centuries of Canadian nursing* (p. 86). Ottawa, ON: University of Ottawa Press & Canadian Museum of Civilization.

Nelson, S., & Gordon, S. (Eds.). (2006). *The complexities of care: Nursing reconsidered.* Ithaca, NY: Cornell University Press.

Nightingale, F. (1938). *Notes on nursing: What it is, and what it is not.* New York, NY: Appleton-Century Company.

Nursing Education in Nova Scotia. (n.d.). *1899 Graduating class photo.* Retrieved from http://www.msvu.ca/library/archives/nhdp/schools/VGH.htm

Paul, P. (2005). Religious nursing orders of Canada: A presence on all western frontiers. In C. Bates, D. Dodd, & N. Rousseau (Eds.). *On all frontiers: Four centuries of Canadian nursing* (pp. 125–138). Ottawa, ON: University of Ottawa Press & Canadian Museum of Civilization.

Penney, S. M. (1996). *A century of caring: 1897–1997, the history of the Victorian Order of Nurses for Canada.* Ottawa, ON: VON Canada.

Richardson, S. (1998). Frontier health care: Alberta's district and municipal nursing services, 1919 to 1976. *Alberta History, 46,* 2–9.

Ross-Kerr, J. C. (2003). Professionalization in Canadian nursing. In J. C. Ross-Kerr & M. Wood (Eds.). *Canadian nursing: Issues and perspectives* (4th ed.) (pp. 29–38). Toronto, ON: Mosby.

Rousseau, N., & Daigle, J. (2000). Medical service to settlers: The gestation and establishment of a nursing service in Quebec, 1932–1943. *Nursing History Review, 8,* 95–116.

Sandelowski, M. (2000). *Devices and desires: Gender, technology and American nursing.* Chapel Hill, NC: University of North Carolina Press.

Saskatchewan Registered Nurses' Association. (2007). *Standards and foundation competencies for the practice of registered nurses.* Regina, SK: Author.

Saskatchewan Registered Nurses' Association (2010). *Registered Nurse (Nurse Practitioner) RN(NP) Standards and Core Competencies.* Retrieved from http://www.srna.org/images/stories/pdfs/communications/pdf/standards_and_comp_2011.pdf

Sigma Theta Tau International. (2011). *Nurse leader membership criteria.* Retrieved from http://www.nursingsociety.org/Membership/ApplyNow/Pages/nl_memcriteria.aspx

Toman, C. (2001). Blood work: Canadian nursing and blood transfusion, 1942–1990. *Nursing History Review, 9,* 51–78.

Toman, C. (2007). *An officer and a lady: Canadian military nurses and the Second World War.* Vancouver, BC: UBC Press.

Villeneuve, M., & MacDonald, J. (2006). *Towards 2020: Visions for nursing.* Ottawa, ON: Canadian Nurses Association.

Violette, B. (2005). Healing the body and saving the soul: Nursing sisters and the first Catholic hospitals in Quebec (1639–1880). In C. Bates, D. Dodd, & N. Rousseau (Eds.). *On all frontiers: Four centuries of Canadian nursing* (pp. 57–71). Ottawa, ON: University of Ottawa Press & Canadian Museum of Civilization.

World Health Organization (Division of Health Manpower Development). (1982). *Report of a meeting on nursing in support of the goal health for all by the year 2000.* November 16–20, 1981. Geneva, Switzerland: WHO.

Young, J. (2004). "Monthly" nurses, "sick" nurses, and midwives in 19th-century Toronto, 1830–1891. *Canadian Bulletin of Medical History, 21,* 281–302.

Chapter 2

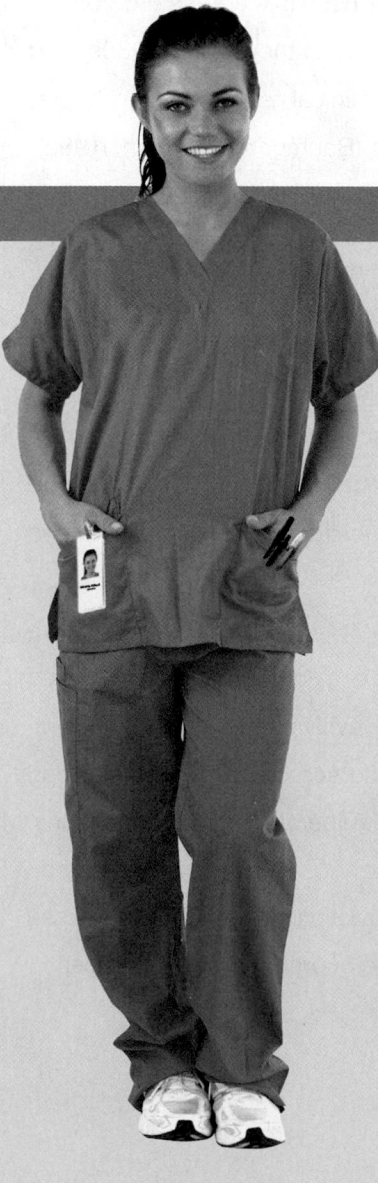

Nursing Education in Canada

LEARNING OUTCOMES

After studying this chapter, you will be able to:

1. Describe the different types of nursing education programs.

2. Identify aspects of the baccalaureate level for entry to professional nursing practice.

3. Explain the importance of continuing nursing education.

4. Describe the role of national nursing associations in shaping nursing education in Canada.

5. Analyze issues influencing nursing education in Canada.

In the early twentieth century in Canada, nursing was viewed in a variety of ways depending on the religion, geographical location, class, status, race, and ethnicity of the people who practised the profession. Schools of nursing focused primarily on teaching students what they needed to know to work in a hospital setting. In fact, the need for student nurses to staff a particular hospital was the major reason for the existence of most nursing schools during this period (Pringle, Green, & Johnson, 2004). Although religious groups were important in developing nursing education in Canada, Cohen (2000) has argued that the Catholic Church, among other agents, also slowed the introduction of sciences into nursing schools. Nursing education has evolved a great deal over the last century and today prepares students to practise in a broad range of areas, to think critically, and to use the best scientific evidence available when providing care. Provincial and territorial nursing organizations and national accrediting bodies provide internal professional control of nursing education.

The General and Marine Hospital in St. Catharines, Ontario, offered the first training program for nurses in Canada in 1874. Following this, it soon became the norm for hospitals across the country to introduce their own schools of nursing. The hospital training programs of the 1920s, 1930s, and 1940s were characterized by limited coordination of classroom and clinical teaching, long hours, night duty without supervision, and numerous housekeeping chores (Baumgart & Larsen, 1992). The medical staff and nursing supervisors provided the instruction and were identified as clinical teachers.

In 1939, the Canadian Nurses Association (CNA) recommended that each province develop educational programs for practical nurses as a solution to a shortage of nurses that had increased as a result of World War II (Mussalem, 1960). In 1941, the Registered Nurses Association of Ontario (RNAO) implemented a demonstration program for Nursing Assistants. The St. Boniface School for Practical Nurses opened its doors in September 1943 with the approval of the Manitoba Association of Registered Nurses. Programs continued to be established for practical nurses as health care services expanded (Pringle, Green, & Johnson, 2004).

Today, as nursing responds to new scientific knowledge and technological innovation and to cultural, political, and socioeconomic changes, nursing education curricula are continually being updated to prepare students for very complex clinical situations and a rapidly evolving health care system. Programs of study for registered nurses and registered psychiatric nurses are based on a broad knowledge of biological, social, and physical sciences, as well as the liberal arts and humanities. There is a strong focus on critical thinking and on health prevention and promotion, as well as on health maintenance and health restoration. Educational programs for practical nurses have increased in length, depth, and breadth in response to an expansion of their scope of practice (Pringle, Green, & Johnson, 2004).

Nursing Education

Today, provincial and territorial laws and union regulations in Canada recognize five distinct groups within the profession of nursing. Not every province or territory, however, recognizes all five of the groups. Each province and territory recognizes the *registered nurse* (*RN*) and the *licensed practical nurse* (*LPN;* called a *registered practical nurse* in Ontario only [*RPN*]). All jurisdictions except the Yukon recognize the *nurse practitioner* (*NP*). Only the four Western provinces recognize the *registered psychiatric nurse* (*RPN*). Quebec distinguishes RNs by type of education: diploma or baccalaureate. Responsibilities differ for the five groups. Definitions and roles for the RN, LPN or RPN, and RPN can be found in Box 1.2 in Chapter 1 (see page 11).

Currently, two *major* educational routes lead to RN licensure: diploma and baccalaureate programs. In most Canadian jurisdictions, however, the baccalaureate degree is required for entry-to-practice. University **baccalaureate nursing degrees** are offered by universities, university colleges, and polytechnic institutes. Many community colleges partner with universities to offer baccalaureate programs. In generic programs, students are admitted directly into the nursing program and graduate with a degree. Programs also exist for students with a previous degree (not in nursing), or credits toward a degree (usually about half the requirement for a degree) in which the nursing content has been reconfigured so that students can graduate with a nursing degree in approximately 24 months. These are variously called *generic master's, second entry, compressed,* or *accelerated programs.* A listing of the programs offered by members of the Canadian Association of Schools of Nursing (CASN) can be found in the Weblinks section of this chapter. In addition, colleges provide diploma education for nurses, although most of these are in Quebec. In some provinces and territories, such as Ontario, polytechnic institutes provide undergraduate degrees. Basic educational programs for practical nurses are generally offered in colleges. No national list exists for practical nursing programs; however, provincial or territorial lists can often be found on the provincial or territorial regulatory websites (see Table 1.1 in Chapter 1 [page 19]). Psychiatric nurses can complete their basic education at the diploma or degree level, depending on the province. A national listing of psychiatric nursing education programs can be found in the Weblinks section of this chapter.

Graduates of all programs take a **licensing examination** for their group (e.g., RN, LPN or RPN, RPN) provided by the appropriate regulatory authority and, if successful, are licensed within their group. The Canadian Registered Nurse Examination (CRNE) is a multiple-choice test that measures the applicant's ability to integrate the competencies expected of a new graduate nurse. The CRNE question format is the basis for the Assess Your Learning questions at the end of each chapter in this book. CRNE results are reported to candidates as pass or fail. National examinations for all the groups of nurses are administered by the provincial or territorial regulatory authority. The successful candidate becomes licensed in that province or territory, even though the examinations are of national origin. To practise nursing in another province or territory, the nurse must receive reciprocal licensure by applying to that province's or territory's regulatory body. Both licensure and registration must be renewed each year to remain valid.

Students in all nursing groups are increasingly more diverse than they were in the past, as many first- and second-generation young Canadian immigrants enrol in nursing education programs. The nursing student body is, therefore, becoming more representative of the cultural diversity in Canadian communities (Anderson et al., 2003). In addition, the trend has been to provide nurses who have been educated in other countries, known as **internationally educated nurses**, or IENs, with educational bridging programs. Bridging programs for IENs include both classroom and clinical experience and are tailored to assist them to meet the educational gaps they may have so that they can obtain licensure in Canada. Bridging programs also provide opportunities to learn about Canadian cultural expectations and health care delivery in this country. IENs first apply to have their credentials assessed and are granted registration after successfully completing the appropriate licensing examinations. Bridging programs are completed before writing the Canadian examination. The legal right to practise within all the nursing groups requires not only a passing grade in licensing examinations but also verification that the graduate has completed a prescribed course of study from an approved program in nursing.

Minimum standards for basic nursing education are established in each province and territory and are monitored by the provincial or territorial nursing regulatory bodies. Schools that meet these minimum standards are granted provincial or territorial approval. In addition to approval in Canada for baccalaureate nursing education, the CASN grants accreditation that is focused on standards of excellence for nursing education.

Types of Educational Programs

Hospital Diploma Programs

Florence Nightingale developed a nursing program based on religious, military, and, what is called today, public health concerns and insisted on the moral superiority of her recruits (Cohen, 2000). After she established the first school of nursing—the Nightingale Training School for Nurses—at St. Thomas's Hospital in England in 1860, the concept travelled quickly to North America. Hospital administrators welcomed the idea of training schools as a source of free or inexpensive staffing for the hospital. Nursing education in the early years largely took the form of apprenticeships. Along with minimal formal classroom instruction, students learned by doing, that is, by providing care to patients in hospitals. The curricula were not standardized and no accreditation was available at that time. Programs were designed to meet the service needs of the hospital, not the educational needs of the students.

Over the years, the curricula in nursing education programs has changed progressively with the development of the health care system, medical care, and knowledge base. New knowledge, new procedures, and new systems of delivery have influenced practice, and in turn, changes in practice have resulted in the development of new knowledge and the creation of new types of nursing groups. The overall goal is the health of Canadians.

In Chapter 1, we discussed the number of regulated nurses in Canada and their distribution by category. In this chapter, we examine the educational background of those nurses. The highest level of education in nursing reported by all regulated nurses in 2009 is given in Table 2.1. These statistics exclude education in disciplines other than nursing. For example, the Canadian Institute for Health Information (2008) lists 482 nurses with a doctoral degree in nursing in Canada in 2008. If doctoral degrees in other disciplines were included, the number would be higher, although still a very small percentage of the total nursing population.

Educational Programs Leading to, or Continuing from, Basic Registered Nursing Education

COLLEGE DIPLOMA PROGRAMS Mussalem (1960) identified problems in hospital-based nursing **diploma programs** caused by the hospital's control over education. Students were used as the primary service providers, and their education was controlled by the hospital. Community college nursing education programs began to appear in the 1960s, also offering diploma preparation, and by the 1970s, most diploma nursing programs had moved into community colleges (Baumgart & Larsen, 1992). Today, the majority of nursing programs for registered nurses in community colleges are offered in a collaborative partnership with university schools which provide a common curriculum leading to a baccalaureate degree in nursing. Some colleges have been granted degree-granting privileges by their provincial legislation and offer a baccalaureate education in nursing independently. In Quebec, the DEC-BACC program (3 years in a *collège d'enseignement général et professionnel,* plus 2 years in a university) was introduced in 2004, with the first cohort graduating in 2006. A DEC-BACC refers to an integrated college diploma and baccalaureate degree program (*diplôme d'études collégiales – baccalauréat*).

BACCALAUREATE DEGREE PROGRAMS In 1919, the first baccalaureate degree program in nursing in English was established at the University of British Columbia in Vancouver, followed by the McGill School (Montreal) of Graduate Nurses in 1920 (Street, 1973). The first baccalaureate program in French was developed by Institut Marguerite d'Youville in 1938. With the establishment of these programs, nursing moved into the university sector.

In 1932, the CNA and the Canadian Medical Association (CMA) commissioned Dr. George Weir to conduct a study of nursing education in Canada. He found that education was secondary to hospital service as a priority in the schools. Weir (1932) recommended, in the *Survey of Nursing Education in Canada,* that nurses be given a liberal education in addition to a technical one and that university training programs award degrees.

The 1950s saw the greatest expansion of university schools of nursing. Students enrolled in the university for 1 year for non-nursing courses and then moved to a hospital-based model for practical experience. A fifth year at the university completed what was labelled a "sandwich" program. It was not until the 1960s that the number of students enrolled in these baccalaureate programs increased markedly. Currently, baccalaureate programs are offered by universities or colleges alone or in collaboration with other postsecondary institutions, depending on the province or territory. The curricula offer courses in the liberal arts, sciences, humanities, and nursing. The degree awarded is usually a bachelor of science in nursing (BScN, BSN) or a bachelor of nursing (BN).

TABLE 2.1 Educational Preparation of the Regulated Nursing Workforce (in percentages)

Education	Registered Nurse	Licensed (Registered) Practical Nurses	Registered Psychiatric Nurses
Diploma	57.7	97.6	88.9
Baccalaureate	38.8	—	10.7
Master's/doctorate	3.5	—	0.4

Source: From Canadian Institute for Health Information. (2012). *Regulated Nurses: Canadian Trends, 2005–2010.* Ottawa, ON: Author. Reprinted with permission.

Most baccalaureate programs also admit registered nurses who have diplomas. Some programs have specifically designed curricula to meet the needs of these students. Some universities offer nursing students the opportunity to pursue a self-paced or independent study program. Many programs offer some distance education and online courses that can be accessed by nursing students. Many accept transfer credits from other accredited colleges and universities and offer students the opportunity for prior learning assessment and recognition (PLAR) when the students believe they have acquired the required competency. These programs are referred to as BScN completion, BN transition, or postdiploma programs. In recent years, however, a downward trend has been seen in the enrollment of diploma nurses in degree programs because of the increase in nurses entering practice with a baccalaureate degree, a requirement in most jurisdictions in Canada.

The newest type of program is one in which the students come with all or part of a university degree in another discipline. These are variously called *second entry, second degree, accelerated,* or *compressed programs.* Usually 2 to 3 years long, they build on the courses already completed and may compress the structure of the nursing curriculum typically by including spring and summer sessions into the program.

Today, universities and colleges have control over all components of education, and nursing students receive a liberal education combined with a professional one. The majority of nursing programs are 4 academic years long, an academic year being approximately 8 calendar months. Many educational institutions offer students the opportunity for accelerated completion of the program. Requirements for university admission include a Grade 12 or a high-school diploma with specific prerequisites, such as chemistry and biology.

GRADUATE NURSING EDUCATION Most graduate programs are conducted by departments within the graduate school or faculty of a university, and the applicant must first meet requirements established by the graduate school. Although graduate schools differ, for Canadian students, common requirements for admission to graduate programs in nursing include the following:

- The applicant must be a registered nurse and licensed or eligible for licensure within the program's province or territory.
- The applicant generally must hold a baccalaureate degree in nursing from a recognized university.
- The applicant must give evidence of scholastic ability.
- Letters of recommendation from supervisors, nursing faculty, or nursing colleagues indicating the applicant's ability to do graduate study are required.

MASTER'S PROGRAMS The growth of university nursing programs encouraged the development of graduate study in nursing. In Canada, the first master's program in nursing was established at the University of Western Ontario in London, Ontario, in 1959. This was followed by a program at McGill University in Montreal in 1961 and a French program at Université de Montréal in 1962. The most recent master's program has been established at Brandon University and is noted in the section on registered psychiatric nurses.

Master's programs may be course based or a combination of course work and thesis research. Programs generally take 1 to 2 years to complete. Degrees most frequently granted are master of nursing (MN), master of science in nursing (MScN), master of science (MS or MSc), and master of psychiatric nursing (MPN). Master's degree programs provide specialized knowledge and skills that enable nurses to assume advanced roles in practice, education, administration, and research.

NURSE PRACTITIONER PROGRAMS "A nurse practitioner (NP) is a registered nurse (RN) with additional education and experience in health assessment, diagnosis and management of illnesses and injuries, including ordering tests and prescribing drugs"(Canadian Nurses Association & Canadian Institute for Health Information [CNA & CIHI], 2005, p. 2). Originally aimed at preparing nurses to work in northern nursing stations, nurse practitioner programs were available as early as 1967 at Dalhousie University. However, these programs did not survive largely because of societal factors, such as a perceived oversupply of physicians, lack of corresponding legislation, and lack of support from policymakers in medicine and in nursing (CNA & CIHI, 2006). Currently, all provinces and territories, with the exception of Yukon, have legislation and regulations regarding NP status in place or in progress. Although NP programs in some provinces are offered at the postdiploma (RN) level, the majority are offered at the master's or post-master's level.

DOCTORAL PROGRAMS Nurses with doctoral and postdoctoral education are needed in both academic and practice settings for advanced clinical practice, administration, education, and research. As of 2011, there are 15 doctoral nursing programs in Canada. A major benefit of doctoral education is that it prepares nurses who are able to develop the nursing knowledge base through research and discover the evidence needed to provide high-quality patient care. As of 2009, approximately 0.2% of registered nurses reported being educated at the doctoral level in the discipline (CNA, 2011) and even fewer at the postdoctoral level. Until recently, nursing programs leading to a doctoral degree in Canada were limited, and many completed a doctor of philosophy (PhD) degree in other disciplines, such as sociology, psychology, or education. Doctoral programs in nursing, which award PhDs, began in the 1960s in the United States. The first formal Canadian program began at the University of Alberta in 1991.

PRACTICAL NURSING PROGRAMS Practical nurses are educated and licensed or registered in all the provinces and territories. Programs for practical nurses were introduced in provinces across the country between 1939 and 1960. The first formal LPN training program was offered in 1945, in Manitoba (CIHI, 2010, p. 81). The last 2 decades has seen an expansion of the scope of practice of practical nurses and a corresponding increase in the length of educational programs. Although LPNs or RPNs have programs of varying lengths, the trend is moving to a 2-year program leading to a diploma in practical nursing. In 2010, 97.6% of practical nurses earned a certificate or diploma as entry to practice (CIHI, 2012). Entrance requirements vary across the provinces and territories but usually include a high-school diploma. Practical nursing educational programs have a tradition of being very innovative in providing education at multiple sites within each jurisdiction. Bridging programs for practical nurses who want to obtain their baccalaureate in nursing are becoming more formalized. One of the leaders in this effort is Ontario, where several programs have recently been initiated.

REGISTERED PSYCHIATRIC NURSING PROGRAMS

RPNs are educated and licensed in the four Western provinces. Educational programs specific to psychiatric nursing began in Canada in the 1920s. Application requirements generally include a high-school diploma. RPNs are educated at the diploma or baccalaureate level. A significant number of RPNs go on to complete graduate-level education. In January 2011, the first students were admitted to the Master of Psychiatric Nursing program at Brandon University, Manitoba, the first graduate program for psychiatric nurses in Canada.

Nursing Associations and Their Influence on Education

Several national nursing associations have influenced nursing education in Canada through their funding of research, pilot education projects, and policy development. These include the CNA, Practical Nurses Canada (although inactive at this time), Registered Psychiatric Nurses of Canada, and the CASN. Although the organizations for practical and psychiatric nurses tend to more strongly influence the education of their own constituents, the CNA and CASN have influenced registered nursing education at all levels. See the Reflect on Primary Health Care box.

REFLECT ON   **PRIMARY HEALTH CARE**

Schools of nursing in Canada generally use a conceptual framework as a guide for their curricula. Some schools of nursing have chosen to use primary health care as one of the foundations for their conceptual framework or their curricula.

Canadian Nurses Association

As early as 1895, a desire was expressed to create a group that would facilitate the integration of francophones and nurses from all provinces and that would represent the nurses of Canada. In 1908, the Canadian National Association of Trained Nurses (Cohen, 2000) became that organization. From this beginning, the CNA has become a federation of 11 provincial and territorial registered nurses' associations, representing more than 146 788 Canadian RNs (see Chapter 1). Quebec nurses do not belong to the CNA.

The CNA has influenced nursing education in Canada in several key areas. Its co-sponsorship of the Weir Report (1932) is one example. In addition, in 1948, the CNA, with financing from the Red Cross, established the Metropolitan School of Nursing in Windsor, Ontario (Jensen, 2007). This demonstration school was Canada's first independent school of nursing, separated financially and physically from the hospital. This pioneer project led to the establishment of the first nursing program in an educational setting in Canada at the Ryerson Institute of Technology in 1963. The growth of similar independent schools of nursing in Canada was delayed until the community college was developed in the 1970s and 1980s. As education is under provincial and territorial jurisdiction, it is through the provincial and territorial registered nurses associations that approval of basic nursing education programs occurs. Approval by the provincial or territorial body ensures that programs meet minimal standards and allows graduates from a specific program, on graduation, to write the CRNE (Canadian Registered Nurse Examination) or the Ordre des infirmières et infirmiers du Québec exams in Quebec. This approval must be renewed on a regular basis. Recently, the CNA, in conjunction with the provincial and territorial bodies, completed a project on entry-level competencies. From this project, each jurisdiction completed and endorsed a set of competencies for new RN graduates. Schools of nursing use these competencies as a basis for their curricula, and the CRNE is based on national competencies.

Another influence of the CNA on nursing education is *certification*, which is a voluntary and periodic process (recertification) by which an organized specialty group verifies that a registered nurse has demonstrated competence in a nursing specialty by having met identified standards of that specialty. Certification was initiated by a CNA membership request in June 1980 through a biennial resolution that directed the board of directors to study the feasibility of developing examinations for certification in major nursing specialties. In 1982, the board of directors adopted a policy of accreditation in nursing as well as a recommendation that the CNA promote the development of certification in nursing specialties (CNA, 1982). The first certification was offered in occupational health nursing. Currently, certification is offered in 19 specialty areas: cardiovascular, community health, critical care, critical care pediatrics, emergency, enterostomal therapy, gastroenterology, gerontology, hospice palliative care, medical-surgical, nephrology, neuroscience, occupational health, oncology, orthopedics, perinatal, perioperative, psychiatric or mental health, and rehabilitation. In Quebec, the first two specialty certifications will be available in mental health and the prevention and control of infections.

The Canadian Association of Schools of Nursing

In 1942, the Provisional Council of University Schools and Departments was formed. The name of the organization was changed in 1971 to the Canadian Association of University Schools of Nursing, with a mandate in 1973 to provide accreditation to university nursing programs in Canada. In 2002, the colleges providing all or part of a baccalaureate degree programs in collaborative partnerships with a university joined the Canadian Association of Schools of Nursing (CASN) (CASN, 2006a). Today, the 91 member schools deliver all or part of a baccalaureate degree, a graduate degree, or both in nursing. The purpose of the CASN is *to lead nursing education and nursing scholarship in the interest of healthier Canadians.* To that end, the CASN (a) speaks for Canadian nursing education and scholarship; (b) establishes and promotes national standards of excellence for nursing education; (c) promotes the advancement of nursing knowledge; (d) facilitates the integration of theory, research, and practice; (e) contributes to public policy; and (f) provides a national forum for issues in nursing education and research (CASN, 2006b).

The CASN baccalaureate accreditation program provides national standards of excellence for programs of baccalaureate nursing education to use in self- and peer evaluation. Although accreditation is voluntary in most jurisdictions, some have mandated that CASN accreditation function as approval in that province or territory. Ontario was the first province to do so. The CASN has also published several position papers on nursing education topics, which schools use to plan curricula and shape new programs. The CASN is a founding member of the Global Alliance for Leadership in Nursing Education and Science (GANES), an organization that provides a global forum to discuss issues of concern for nursing education programs worldwide.

Canadian Nursing Students' Association

The Canadian Nursing Students' Association (CNSA) is a national organization. With more than 20 000 members, the CNSA is an affiliate member of the CNA and Practical Nurses Canada. The CNSA has a close working relationship with the CASN and is a co-chair of the New Health Professionals Network (CNSA, 2004). The CNSA maintains an influence on nursing education through its partnership with other national and international organizations.

Issues Facing Nursing Education

Nursing education is facing a number of complex issues, partly because societal changes in Canada have implications for professional nursing practice. Nurses must have an understanding of the changes themselves and the issues facing education. They must be able to use critical thinking skills to talk about these issues so that they can actively engage in addressing them and in shaping the nursing profession.

Changes in Health Care Needs

Shifts are occurring within health care in Canada today. Whether or not a person agrees with the futuristic pictures painted in such documents as *Toward 2020* (Villeneuve & MacDonald, 2006), it is clear that nursing in the future will be different from what it is today. One anticipated change is the shift away from acute care services toward primary health care. The second is the shift toward community-based care, including home care services, for clients. Clients are being discharged from hospital with higher acuity levels and more complex care needs. Nurses need to work collaboratively and interprofessionally. A third shift is the aging of the Canadian population. Partly because of these shifts, nurses are involved in new roles, such as acting as case manager, program manager, or community developer. Besides new roles, many nurses are performing additional administrative functions, such as participating on boards, chairing committees, and preparing budgets. These shifts influence what is taught in nursing education programs as students require skills to carry out these roles and administrative functions.

Entry to Practice

In 1982, the CNA approved the following policy statement regarding the future educational requirements for RNs: "The Canadian Nurses Association believes that by the year 2000 the minimum educational requirement for entry into the practice of nursing should be the successful completion of a baccalaureate degree in nursing" (CNA, 1982).

The CNA's position was based on an examination of the future health needs of the country and the type of

Nursing and Canadian Society

Fact	Implications for Nursing Practice
The baccalaureate requirement as entry-to-practice for registered nurses has been adopted throughout Canada by the majority of provincial and territorial nurses' associations.	Students and RNs need to be aware that opportunities and graduate study will be open to those with a baccalaureate degree in nursing.
Nurses in Canada can obtain a PhD or a postdoctoral degree within their discipline at a number of Canadian universities.	PhD preparation supports nurses becoming educators and researchers by providing the theoretical knowledge and the practical experience for the roles.
Nursing specialty certification is offered through the CNA certification program.	Employment and personal satisfaction at work may be supported by certification.

nursing services that would be required to meet them. Nurses' associations in every province and territory supported this policy (see the Nursing and Canadian Society box). In 2004, the CASN and the CNA issued a joint statement supporting the baccalaureate degree as the **entry-to-practice** credential in Canada (CASN & CNA, 2004).

In 1991, Premier McKenna of New Brunswick became the first premier to commit his government to support the baccalaureate degree as the entry point into nursing by the year 2000. The following year, 1992, Prince Edward Island became the first province to achieve the goal of a baccalaureate degree as the minimal level of entry into nursing. However, in March 2000, Manitoba's government announced a 23-month diploma program as part of their five-point plan to address the nursing shortage. This move was in direct opposition to the CNA entry-to-practice position. A month earlier, Saskatchewan nurses saw a compromise reached among the provincial government, the Saskatchewan Registered Nurses' Association (SRNA), and the Nursing Education Program of Saskatchewan (NEPS), which protected the nursing degree but offered options regarding accelerated completion of the nursing program. RNs and nursing students had made strong protests over the provincial government's plan to restore diploma education as the entry-level requirement. Manitoba's diploma program admitted its final students in 2010 (CIHI, 2010). In a historic vote in October 2011, the Ordre des infirmières et infirmiers du Québec voted to work with government to ensure that new RNs will get their licence to practise only after a university education. When this is enacted, baccalaureate entry-to-practice will be uniform across Canada.

With the move to the baccalaureate degree as the entry-to-practice requirement for registered nurses, practical nurses have also adjusted their educational requirements in response to the changing skill mix. In Ontario, for example, a fourth semester was added to the diploma program to better prepare the students for the changing skill mix (Baumann et al., 2009).

Educational programs must develop the knowledge, attitudes, and skills a new graduate will need to provide safe and effective care. A National Nursing Competency project involved 26 provincial and territorial bodies that regulate nursing in a collaboration to develop the specific competencies that registered nurses, practical nurses, and psychiatric nurses require on entering the nursing workforce (Black et al., 2008). These competencies are based on a profile of the practice expectations for new graduates and a set of underpinning assumptions. They are used to guide the curricula in nursing education programs. One assumption for entry-to-practice RN competencies is that the new graduate is a beginning practitioner, whose level of practice autonomy and proficiency will grow best through collaboration, mentoring, and support from RN colleagues, managers, other health care team members, and employers. Similarly, an assumption for practical nurses identified in the *Canadian Practical Nurse Registration Examination* (Assessment Strategies Inc., 2012) is that the competencies represent the combined nursing knowledge, skills, behaviours, and clinical judgment that the entry-level practical nurse requires for safe, competent practice.

Ensuring the Appropriate Number of Regulated Nurses

It has proved difficult to accurately project how many new nurses will be needed and align admissions into nursing programs with future demands because of changes in the scope of practice and delivery of care. As a result, there have been both periods of nursing shortages in Canada when the number of graduates have been insufficient to meet the need for new nurses as well as periods of limited employment opportunities for nurses ready to enter the workforce.

After several decades of declining numbers of students enrolled in nursing programs following a peak in the early 1970s, admissions to registered nursing programs began to increase steadily from 8947 in 1999 to 14 010 in 2008–2009 in response to a shortage. As a result, the number of new graduates rose from 4816 in 2003 to 10 074 in 2009–2010 (CNA & CASN, 2012). The numbers enrolled in practical nursing programs have also increased in recent years.

Changing Demographics in Nursing Programs

Student populations in nursing programs are changing. Aboriginal students, mature students, male students, international students, and students with disabilities are enrolling in increasing numbers. In addition, more students work part time while studying to obtain the funds they need for tuition and living expenses. These changes mean that nurse educators must take into account a variety of needs among learners, and nursing programs have changed to accommodate these trends. More options are being explored that permit part-time study and allow students to work while attending school. Many programs are now offering distributed learning courses as an alternative to traditional modes of learning.

Until recently, few Aboriginal people from Northern Canada entered the nursing profession. To provide for Inuit nurses, Nunavut Arctic College in Iqaluit and the School of Nursing at Dalhousie University collaborated on a 4-year baccalaureate program. The program admitted its first class of Inuit students in October 1999. Another solution has been to work within established programs, offering support to Aboriginal students. One such program is the Native Access Program to Nursing (NAPN) at the University of Saskatchewan, begun in 1986. This province has the highest population percentage of Aboriginal persons, and NAPN offered support to more than 500 Aboriginal baccalaureate nursing students (personal communication, Rhonda Goodtrack, October 2011).

The average age of nurse educators in Canada is moving toward retirement age, and active efforts to recruit more nurses are underway. Current initiatives include additional PhD programs in nursing. Where future faculty members will be recruited from and how these members will be prepared to teach are some of the serious questions being asked of nursing programs.

Technological Advancements

The growth of technology is influencing nursing education. Advances in web-based technology and computer-assisted instruction offer the potential for flexible, self-directed, interactive learning activities for students in on-site nursing programs. Computer-mediated distance education also makes it possible for nursing programs to offer courses over a large geographical area through the use of a computer network or the Internet. This method is a relative newcomer to nursing education. By 2004, however, 41 programs were offered in full or part through distance technology (see the Evidence-Informed Practice box). Twenty of these were baccalaureate, 16 were master's programs, and five were PhD programs. Some programs may also include videoconferencing and other means of distance learning. For nurses who already hold a degree, computer-mediated instruction supports continuing education opportunities.

Another technological advance that has been important in nursing education is high-fidelity simulation. Considered an adjunct learning opportunity for students, these highly technical mannequins allow nursing students and graduates to practise specific skills in a safe environment. The use of additional virtual technology offers further opportunities to engage learners in realistic situations where critical thinking and problem-solving skills can be practised.

With the introduction of the electronic record, significant changes in the delivery of health are underway. These changes are having an impact on health care education. Nursing students will need to learn new approaches to information management to provide care in technology-enabled environments (McBride, 2005).

EVIDENCE-INFORMED PRACTICE

How Can Students Overcome Barriers During Their Nursing Programs?

A 3-year study of 10 students was conducted as they moved through a BN online educational program following an LPN program. All students were interviewed at the beginning, middle, and end of their program. They were asked about the barriers they faced and the strategies they used to overcome these barriers. The analysis of the interview data identified three key themes: (a) workplace mentors who helped these students apply their learning; (b) personal learning goals that sustained their motivation; and (c) time-management strategies, which included ending full-time employment to focus on educational activities.

NURSING IMPLICATIONS: While this research was focused on the LPN-to-BN experience, other nursing students may find that some of the same barriers and strategies resonate with them with regard to their personal experience.

Source: Based on Melrose, S. & Gordon, K. (2011). Overcoming barriers to role transition during an online post LPN to BN program. *Nurse Education in Practice, 11*, 31–35.

Interprofessional Education

Nurses have long recognized that they need to work with other health care professionals to deliver quality care to their patients. More recently, however, health care professionals and other stakeholders, such as government, have argued that health care professionals who are educated together will work together more effectively in the health care workplace. Several health care educational programs have already pioneered work in this area, and Health Canada has initiated the Interprofessional Education for Collaborative Patient-Centred Practice (IECPCP) program. The IECPCP program funded 20 research programs at various sites in Canada to pilot, implement, and evaluate strategies to increase **interprofessional education (IPE)** and evaluate its effectiveness (Health Canada, 2007). Interprofessional education is supported by the Accreditation of Interprofessional Health Education (AIPHE) initiative. Eight organizations that accredit prelicensure education for six Canadian health care professions have collaborated in promoting the integration of IPE in their respective accreditation standards. They have developed a framework to assist health care professions to integrate IPE competencies in accreditation standards, and work by each of the accrediting bodies to do this is underway (AIPHE, 2011). With the increase in the scope of practice of LPNs or RPNs, intraprofessional education is important in nursing as is interprofessional education. It is important for nursing students to collaborate with each other for the changing skill mix in the clinical environment.

Continuing Education to Maintain Competency

To provide competent nursing care (see Box 2.1), all nurses, RNs, LPNs/RPNs, RPNs must continually enhance the knowledge, skills, and critical thinking required to meet client needs in a changing health care system. Each jurisdiction and each group of nurses have continuing competency requirements for licence or registration renewal. Continuing education or lifelong learning is a strategy to achieve this goal. The CNA interprets **continuing nursing education** as consisting of planned learning experiences undertaken following a basic nursing education. Acknowledging the need to ensure safe practice, the CNA published *A National Framework for Continuing Competency Programs for Registered Nurses* in September 2000. The framework represents a consensus of nursing regulatory bodies in all provinces and territories, including Quebec.

BOX 2.1   EDUCATIONAL SUPPORT FOR COMPETENT NURSING PRACTICE

The competence of RNs is an essential element of safe and quality nursing practice. Competence is defined as a way to act with the necessary knowledge and skills in a certain context (Le Boterf, 2006; Tardif, 1997).

Competence is one of the main aspects to consider when evaluating quality of care. To practise safely and competently, RNs comply with professional standards, base their practice on relevant knowledge, and, in adherence with the *Code of Ethics for Registered Nurses,* acquire new skills and knowledge in their area of practice on a continuing basis.

Continuing education is the responsibility of each practising nurse and employer. The CNA advocates for the voluntary participation of nurses in continuing education in which they select learning activities based on their own experiences, learning styles, and practice requirements. Constant updating and growth are essential to keep on top of scientific and technological changes, as well as the changes within the nursing profession. A variety of educational and health care institutions conduct continuing education programs. They are usually designed to meet one or more of the following needs: (a) to keep nurses abreast of new techniques and competence; (b) to help nurses attain expertise in a specialized area of practice, such as intensive care nursing or community nursing; and (c) to provide nurses with information essential to nursing practice, for example, knowledge about the legal aspects of nursing.

Mandatory versus voluntary continuing education has been a topic of interest to practising nurses, educators, administrators, professional and regulatory associations, unions, and governments. Most registered, psychiatric, and licensed practical nursing jurisdictions in Canada view continuing education itself as voluntary and a strong link in a mandatory continuing competency or professional development program.

In-Service Education

An **in-service education** program is administered by an employer and is designed to upgrade the knowledge or skills of employees. For example, an employer might offer an in-service program to inform nurses about a new piece of equipment, about specific isolation practices, or about methods of implementing a nurse theorist's conceptual framework for nursing. Some in-service programs are mandatory, such as cardiopulmonary resuscitation (CPR) and fire safety programs.

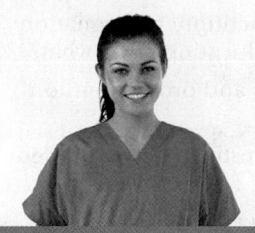

Case Study 2

A friend, who knows that you are a nursing student, tells you that he or she is considering nursing school and wants your advice.

CRITICAL THINKING QUESTIONS

1. What questions would you ask before responding?
2. What did you consider when choosing your nursing educational program?

Check the eText in MyNursingLab for answers and explanations.

KEY TERMS

baccalaureate nursing
degrees *p. 29*

continuing nursing
education *p. 36*

diploma programs
p. 30

entry-to-practice *p. 34*

in-service education *p. 36*

internationally educated
nurses *p. 29*

interprofessional
education (IPE) *p. 36*

licensing examination
p. 29

master's programs
p. 31

CHAPTER HIGHLIGHTS

- Nursing education has changed dramatically since the mid-nineteenth century. Early apprenticeship programs established in the nineteenth century were designed to meet the service needs of hospitals, not the educational needs of students. Today, nursing education is provided primarily in college and university settings independent of hospitals' needs.

- Although baccalaureate programs began in the early twentieth century, baccalaureate education began to take hold only after the release of the Weir Report in 1932. Master's and doctoral programs in nursing grew significantly in the latter part of the

twentieth century. Admission requirements, lengths of programs, curricula, and costs for these programs vary considerably.

- Nursing education curricula are continually being revised in response to new scientific knowledge and technological, cultural, political, and socioeconomic changes in society.

- Continuing education is the responsibility of each practising nurse to keep abreast of scientific and technological changes, as well as changes within the nursing profession.

ASSESS YOUR LEARNING

1. Who is responsible for monitoring minimum standards for basic nursing education in Canada?
   a. Provincial or territorial nursing regulatory bodies
   b. The individual school of nursing
   c. Canadian Association of Schools of Nursing (CASN)
   d. Provincial or territorial governments

2. What was one of the greatest influences on the evolution of Canadian registered nursing education programs?
   a. Requirements of the national regulatory bodies
   b. Introduction of the nursing unions

   c. Recommendations of the Weir Report
   d. Creation of the Mack Training School

3. What would be the best example of continuing nursing education?
   a. A course on leadership offered at a college or university
   b. A course given by the employer on the new electronic charting
   c. CPR (cardiopulmonary resuscitation) recertification offered by a community agency
   d. A course in fitness offered through community services

4. The trend for practical nurse (LPN or RPN) programs to increase program length to a 2-year diploma is largely the result of what?

   a. A shortage of qualified nurses in health care

   b. An expansion in the scope of practice of practical nurses

   c. The increasing cost of baccalaureate education

   d. A decrease in entrance requirements for practical nurse programs

5. The term *entry to practice* refers to what?

   a. The amount of time spent in preparing for professional practice

   b. Courses required by the educational institution

   c. The level of education required to achieve licensure

   d. Curriculum required by the accreditation process

6. What is the purpose of certification?

   a. To achieve advanced standing in a graduate nursing program

   b. A requirement for a nursing leadership position

   c. To acquire new technical skills in nursing practice

   d. To gain competence in a specialized area of nursing

7. What is currently recognized as an important issue that has implications for nursing education in Canada?

   a. The need to establish national competencies

   b. Changing societal health care needs

   c. The increasing cost of nursing education

   d. An oversupply of nurse educators

8. A nurse who has a nurse practitioner designation has completed additional education to do what?

   a. Prescribe common drugs and order common diagnostic tests

   b. Serve as the principal investigator on a funded research project

   c. Teach in graduate nursing programs

   d. Provide high-level leadership in a practice setting

9. Which of the following has responsibility for continuing education?

   a. The college or university

   b. The employing agency

   c. The practising nurse

   d. The provincial or territorial regulating body

10. What was the major impetus for moving nursing education programs away from the hospital setting?

    a. To demonstrate the value of apprenticeship models of education

    b. To force physicians to come to the university to teach

    c. To enable the profession to gain control over the educational process

    d. To remove the influence of religious groups over nursing

Check the eText in MyNursingLab for answers and explanations.

WEBLINKS

Canadian Association of Schools of Nursing

http://www.casn.ca/media.php?mid=200

The Canadian Association of Schools of Nursing is a voluntary association representing all the universities and colleges that offer undergraduate and graduate programs in nursing. This site lists the programs offered by its members.

Canadian Nurses Association

http://www.cna-aiic.ca

This is the website for the national nursing association in Canada.

Canadian Nursing Students' Association

http://www.cnsa.ca

The site is host to the national association for nursing students in Canada.

Registered Psychiatric Nurses of Canada

http://www.rpnc.ca/pages/education

This site of the Registered Psychiatric Nurses of Canada has a national listing of psychiatric nursing education programs.

MyNursingLab

REFERENCES

Accreditation of Interprofessional Health Education. (2011). *Interprofessional health education accreditation standards guide.* Retrieved from http://wwwaiphe.ca

Anderson, J. P, Blue, J. C., Browne, A., Henderson, A., Khan, Koushambhi B., Kirkham, S., . . . Smythe, V. (2003). "Rewriting" cultural safety within the postcolonial and postnational feminist project: Toward new epistemologies of healing. *Advances in Nursing Science, 26*(3), 196–214.

Assessment Strategies Inc. (2012). *Canadian practical nurses registration examination 2012–2016.* Retrieved from http://www.cpnre.ca/documents/Blueprint%20for%20 the%20CPNRE%202012-E.pdf

Baumann, A., Blythe, J., Baxter, P., Alvarado, K., Martin, D. (2009). *Registered practical nurses: An overview of education and practice.* NHSRU: Health Human Resources Series 12. Retrieved from http://www.NHSRU.com

Baumgart, A. J., & Larsen, J. (Eds.). (1992). *Canadian nursing faces the future* (2nd ed.). Toronto, ON: C. V. Mosby.

Black, J., Redern, L., Muzio, L., Rushowick, B., Balishi, B., Martens, P., Crawford, M., . . . Round, B. (2008). Competencies in the context of entry-level registered nurse practice: A collaborative project in Canada. *International Nursing Review, 55*(2), 171–178.

Canadian Association of Schools of Nursing. (2006a). *CASN/ ACESI historical milestones.* Retrieved from http://www.casn .ca/content.php?doc=98

Canadian Association of Schools of Nursing. (2006b). *CASN/ ACESI mission.* Retrieved from http://www.casn.ca/content .php?sec=1

Canadian Association of Schools of Nursing & Canadian Nurses Association. (2004). *Educational preparation for entry to practice.* Retrieved from http://www.casn.ca/media .php?mid=202

Canadian Institute for Health Information. (2008). *Registered Nurses Database.* Ottawa, ON: Author.

Canadian Institute for Health Information. (2012). *Regulated nurses: Canadian trends, 2006 to 2010.* Ottawa, ON: Author.

Canadian Nurses Association. (1982). *The definition and purposes of the CNA certification program.* Ottawa, ON: Author.

Canadian Nurses Association. (2011). *2009 workforce profile of registered nurses in Canada.* Ottawa, ON: Author.

Canadian Nurses Association & Canadian Association of Schools of Nursing. (2012). *Registered nurses education in Canada statistics 2009–10.* Retrieved from http://www.casn.ca

Canadian Nurses Association & Canadian Institute for Health Information. (2005). *The supply and regulation of nurse practitioners in Canada.* Ottawa, ON: Author.

Canadian Nurses Association & Canadian Institute for Health Information. (2006). *The regulation and supply of nurse practitioners in Canada: 2006 Update.* Ottawa, ON: Author.

Canadian Nursing Students' Association. (2004). *The Canadian Nursing Students' Association.* Retrieved from http://www.cnsa.ca

Cohen, Y. (2000). *Profession infirmière: Une histoire des soins dans les hôpitaux du Québec.* Montréal, PQ: Les presses de l'Université de Montréal.

Health Canada. (2007). *Interprofessional education for collaborative patient-centred practice.* Retrieved from http://www.hc-sc.gc.ca/ hcs-sss/hhr-rhs/strateg/interprof/index_ e.htmlHealth

Jensen, P. M. (2007). *Nursing.* Canadian Encyclopedia Historica. Retrieved from http://www.thecanadian encyclopedia.com/ index.cfm?PgNm= TCE&Params=A1SEC825469

Le Boterf, G. (2006). *Contruire les compétences individuelles et collectives* (4e éd.). Paris, France: Éditions d'Organisation.

McBride, A. (2005). Nursing and the informatics revolution. *Nursing Outlook, 53*(4), 183–191.

Mussalem, H. (1960). *Spotlight on nursing education.* Ottawa, ON: Canadian Nurses Association. (1965).

Pringle, D., Green, L., Johnson, L. (2004). *Nursing education in Canada. Historical review and current capacity.* The Nursing Sector Study Corporation, 99 Fifth Avenue, Suite 10, Ottawa K1S 5K4. Retrieved from http://www.cna-nurses.ca/CNA/ documents/ pdf/publications/nursing_education_Canada_e.pdf

Street, M. M. (1973). *Watch-fires on the mountains: The life and writings of Ethel Johns.* Toronto, ON: University of Toronto Press.

Tardif, J. (1997). *Pour un enseignement stratégique: l'apport de la psychologie cognitive.* Montréal, PQ: Éditions Logiques Inc.

Villeneuve, M., & MacDonald, J. (2006). *Toward 2020: Visions for nursing.* Ottawa, ON: Canadian Nurses Association.

Weir, G. M. (1932). *Survey of nursing education in Canada.* Toronto, ON: University of Toronto Press.

Chapter 3

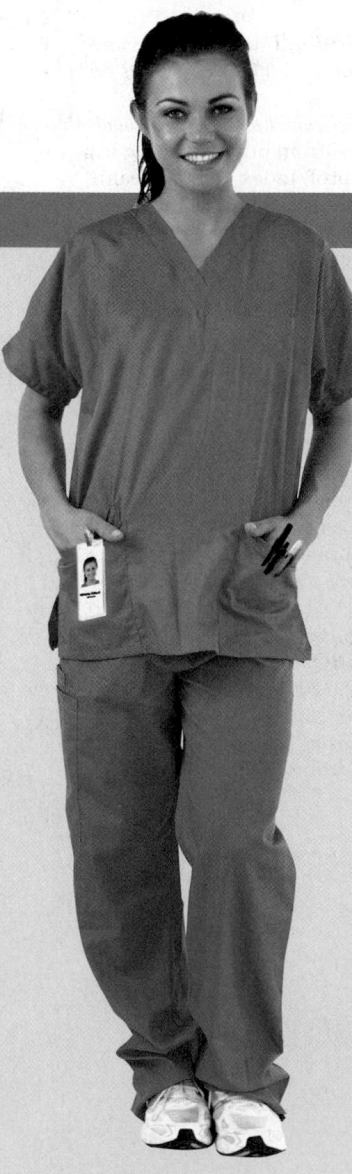

Nursing Research in Canada

LEARNING OUTCOMES

After studying this chapter, you will be able to:

1. Summarize the concepts and language of research.
2. Identify common research methods used in clinical inquiries.
3. Describe the ways that theory, research, and practice interrelate.
4. State the significance of research to the practice of nursing.
5. List seven ways the nurse can participate in research activities in practice.
6. Differentiate the quantitative approach and the qualitative approach in nursing research.
7. Analyze the nurse's role in protecting the rights of human subjects in research.
8. Outline the 11 steps of the research process.

Nurses actively generate, publish, and apply research in practice to improve client care and enhance nursing's scientific knowledge base. The use of research has three main benefits for clients: It helps nurses (a) understand the client's situation more thoroughly, (b) assess more accurately, and (c) intervene more effectively. *Nursing research* findings not only improve client care but also affect the health care system itself. For example, research studies have demonstrated the cost-effectiveness of registered nurses (RNs) as health care providers.

Nursing Research

The Canadian Nurses Association (CNA) is committed to promoting research as the foundation for clinical practice. Reading research, evaluating the results of research studies, and, where appropriate, integrating new findings into practice are necessary competencies of professional nursing practice (see Box 3.1). Nurses who base their clinical decisions on current, scientifically obtained evidence are being professionally accountable. **Research-based nursing practice** simply means nursing practice that is informed by valid and reliable (see page 46 in this chapter) research findings obtained from scientific investigations. The term *evidence-based practice*, or evidence-based decision making, is gaining popularity in nursing and, in some cases, is preferred to research-based practice.

BOX 3.1 COMPETENCIES RELATED TO USE OF EVIDENCE IN PRACTICE

The Canadian Nurses Association's Canadian Registered Nurse Examination (2010–2015) includes the following competencies:

PROFESSIONAL PRACTICE COMPETENCIES:

PP-11 provides rationale for nursing care actions and decisions based on theoretical and evidence-based knowledge from nursing and related disciplines.

PP 15 uses evidence and critical inquiry to challenge, change, enhance, or support nursing practice (e.g., questioning accepted practice, participating in research).

HEALTH AND WELLNESS COMPETENCIES:

HW-26 provides evidence-informed health-related information to clients (e.g., credible electronic sources, relevant and current information).

CHANGES IN HEALTH COMPETENCIES:

CH-12 uses evidence-informed knowledge to assist the client to understand interventions and their relationship to expected outcomes (e.g., possible risks and benefits, discomforts, inconveniences, costs).

Source: From *Canadian Registered Nurse Examination Competences* by Canadian Nurses Association, 2010–2015, Ottawa: Author. © Copyright 2011 Canadian Nurses Association.

Evidence-based practice or **evidence-informed practice** is "broadly defined as the use of the best clinical evidence in making patient care decisions" (Loiselle, Profetto-McGrath, Polit, & Beck, 2011, p. 3). In recent years, more emphasis has been placed on integrating appropriate evidence into practice to inform decisions and policy-making, advance the quality of care, and achieve the best possible outcomes for patients, regardless of setting. Although evidence generated by findings from research studies is of primary importance, it is not the only source of knowledge used by nurses. Carper (1978) identified four patterns of nursing knowledge that are essential to nurses: empirical, aesthetic, personal, and moral.

When nurses have a question they want answered so that they can provide better care to their clients, they can do nursing research. **Nursing research** is the systematic, objective investigation of phenomena (experiences, events, or circumstances) of importance to nursing, with the goal of improving practice. Research can be classified, according to the purpose of the study, as *basic* or *applied*. **Basic research** is concerned with generating knowledge and is sometimes called *pure research*. **Applied research** is concerned with using knowledge to solve immediate problems. Nurse researchers employ a variety of research approaches to substantiate existing knowledge and to discover new knowledge. The two primary approaches are termed *qualitative* and *quantitative*. In quantitative approaches, research problems contain *dependent* and *independent variables*, except for descriptive research, which has no dependent variables. The **dependent variable** is the behaviour, characteristic, or outcome that the researcher wants to explain or predict. The **independent variable** is the presumed cause of, or influence on, the dependent variable. Qualitative studies do not contain variables.

Research is different from problem solving. **Problem solving** is specific to a given situation in which alternatives are explored and chosen and immediate action is taken. Knowledge gained from research is transferable to other situations. The body of knowledge called *nursing science* and the growth and development of professional nursing depend on research undertaken by nurses.

Although the focus for *all* nurses is the use of research findings in practice, the level of participation in research depends on the nurse's educational level, position, experience, and practical environment. Refer to the "Developing Research-Based Practice" section in this chapter for specific examples of ways in which nurses participate in research.

The History

As early as 1854, Florence Nightingale demonstrated the importance of research in the delivery of nursing care. When Nightingale arrived in the Crimea in November 1854, she found the military hospital barracks overcrowded, filthy, rat- and flea-infested, and lacking in food, drugs, and essential medical supplies. As a result of these conditions, men died from starvation and such diseases as dysentery, cholera, and typhus (Woodham-Smith, 1950). By systematically collecting, organizing, and reporting data, Nightingale was able to institute sanitary reforms and significantly reduce the rate of mortality from contagious diseases. Although the Nightingale tradition influenced the establishment of Canadian nursing schools, the research approach did not take hold until the beginning of the twentieth century.

Nursing research has become a significant activity in Canada. The First National Nursing Research Conference was held in 1971 in Ottawa. It was organized by the University of British Columbia School of Nursing and supported by the federal Department of Health and Welfare. Only one of the invited speakers, Dr. Faye Abdellah, was a nurse. This international nursing leader offered a historical perspective of nursing research in the United States. As a result of the conference, the first Centre for Nursing Research in Canada was established at McGill University in Montreal and was funded by the federal government.

Historically, research activity in nursing developed slowly as the result of a gradual increase in the number of nurses with research expertise. Because nurses were not prepared to conduct research, many early studies in nursing were conducted by members of other disciplines. Today, nursing research is developing at a more rapid pace, and most nursing research is initiated in university settings because of faculty members' preparation as researchers.

In 2000, Donaldson reviewed breakthroughs in research over 4 decades and noted that many nurse scientists have played a key role in shaping nursing practice. The breakthroughs have occurred in diverse areas and practice specialties, including personal and family health, child development, dementia care, and pain management.

Linking Theory, Practice, and Research

An interrelationship exists among nursing research, theory, and practice. Research can be used to demonstrate that one nursing practice intervention is more effective than another. Examples of changes in nursing practice motivated by research include the following:

- Incidence and predictors of excess disability in walking among nursing home residents with middle-stage dementia: A prospective cohort study (Slaughter, Eliasziw, Morgan, & Drummond, 2011).
- Storytelling as a communication tool for health consumers: Development of an intervention for parents of children with croup. Stories to communicate health information (Hartling, Scott, Pandya, Johnson, Bishop, & Klassen, 2010).
- Parental decision making regarding treatment of hypoplastic left heart syndrome (Ellinger & Rempel, 2010).

Research ideas, while often born in practice, also come from the nursing literature and nursing theory. Published articles about nursing research may stimulate questions, which lead to interest in further studies. Nursing theorists also generate research questions, since they piece together ideas that explain why something happens. Their explanations are tested, through research, to determine if they are credible enough to be useful in clinical practice.

Hospitals and health care agencies have begun to formally define the link between nursing research and practice. The strategies include the cross-appointment of faculty among hospitals, health care agencies, and universities; the implementation of programs to develop staff nurses as users of research in their practice; the establishment of ethics committees to review research proposals; the appointment of unit research coordinators; the establishment of nursing research committees; the development of strategic plans for nursing research; and the use of evidence-based decision-making models in practice settings. These strategies create an environment to support evidence-informed practice.

Support for Nursing Research

Nursing research costs money. Computer and library services, data collection, statistical consultation, employment of research assistants, and release time for researchers from their regular work responsibilities can be expensive. While funding sources have developed, financial support is still difficult to obtain, especially for new researchers. Collaborative, interdisciplinary studies have a greater chance of receiving financial support than research conducted only by RNs. Insufficient funds to support research are an obstacle for nursing research.

Nursing research funding comes from a variety of sources. At the provincial or territorial level, research funding varies a great deal across the country. A few provincial nursing associations have developed some capacity for the funding of nursing research. Nationally, the Canadian Nurses Foundation funds research. Specialty groups, such as the Canadian Gerontological Nursing Association, also provide financial assistance for their members to conduct research.

Nursing and Canadian Society

Fact	Implications for Nursing Practice
The Canadian Association of Nurse Researchers (CANR) is a national organization with representation from every province and territory.	Nurses need to participate in associations that promote the use of research in practice.
CHSRF works with health services experts across Canada to address challenges facing health decision makers. In collaboration with decision makers, CHSRF tackles questions relevant to the organization, financing, managing and delivery of high-quality, affordable, patient-centred health care for Canadians. CHSRF brings together expert teams who provide the analysis, processes, tools, learning systems and leadership development needed to create breakthroughs with evidence-driven policy and implementation solutions. (http://www.chsrf.ca/AboutUs.aspx)	Nurses interested in research need to be aware of funding opportunities.
In 1969, Moyra Allen of McGill University founded the first Canadian scholarly nursing journal. Initially known as *Nursing Papers*, the journal is now known as the *Canadian Journal of Nursing Research*. Several other Canadian nursing journals have since been established (see Box 3.3).	The reading of research studies promotes Canadian nurses' awareness of available knowledge to meet the health care needs of their clients.

Several non-nursing provincial, territorial, and federal agencies accept proposals that meet their funding guidelines when submitted by qualified nurse researchers. These include the Social Sciences and Humanities Research Council (SSHRC), Canadian Health Services Research Foundation (CHSRF), and the Canadian Institutes of Health Research (CIHR). The SSHRC is a federal agency that promotes and supports university-based research in social sciences and humanities, including health. The CHSRF was founded by Industry Canada under the Canada Corporation Act. The CSHRF is an independent organization dedicated to accelerating healthcare improvement and transformation for Canadians. It collaborates with governments, policymakers, and health system leaders to convert evidence and innovative practices into actionable policies, programs, tools, and leadership development. Its vision is "Timely, appropriate and high-quality services that improve the health of all Canadians." (http://www.chsrf.ca/AboutUs.aspx)

The CIHR was established by an Act of Parliament in 2000 and is Canada's foremost federal agency for health research. Its predecessor was the Medical Research Council. The CIHR provides funding opportunities for biomedical, clinical, health systems services, social, cultural, environmental, and population health research. The CIHR integrates research through a unique interdisciplinary structure made up of 13 "virtual" institutes (e.g., Aboriginal People's Health, Aging, Population & Public Health) that encourage partnership and collaboration across sectors, disciplines, and regions. Each Institute embraces a range of research from fundamental bio-medical and clinical research, to research on health systems, health services, the health of populations, societal and cultural dimensions of health, and environmental influences on health. Other recent funding endeavours include the Canadian Foundation for Innovation (CFI), a nonprofit corporation funded by the federal government, beginning in 1997, to enable Canada's research community to conduct research and develop technology. CIHR unveiled a 10-year plan entitled "Strategy for Patient-Oriented Research" (http://www.cihr-irsc.gc.ca/e/41232.html). One of the major components of this plan is to support best practices in health care.

Foundations and voluntary associations, such as the Canadian Cancer Society and the Kidney Foundation of Canada, are other sources of funds for nurse researchers (see the Nursing and Canadian Society box). The Canadian Nurses Association's current campaign is targeting the federal government to renew a 10-year nursing research fund.

Approaches to Nursing Research

The two predominant research approaches are quantitative and qualitative approaches. *Quantitative research* is generally considered objective and uses data-gathering techniques that can be verified by others. *Qualitative research* is more subjective, which means that qualitative researchers study things in their natural settings, attempting to make sense of phenomena in terms of the meanings people bring to them. Although today both approaches are valued within the nursing research community, in the past, nurse researchers primarily conducted quantitative research.

These approaches originate from different philosophical perspectives and use different methods for the collection and analysis of data.

QUANTITATIVE RESEARCH **Quantitative research** is a systematic, logical approach to studying phenomena that lend themselves to precise measurement by using quantification and statistical analysis (Berman, Snyder, Kozier, & Erb, 2008). The quantitative approach is most frequently associated with **logical positivism**, a philosophical doctrine that asserts that scientific knowledge is the only kind of factual knowledge. Quantitative research is often viewed as hard science and tends to emphasize deductive reasoning and the *measurable* attributes of human experience. Data are usually collected by using structured methods and procedures and are analyzed by using a number of statistical procedures (see the Evidence-Informed Practice box "How Can Employers Promote Empowerment for New Graduate Nurses?").

The following are examples of research questions that lend themselves to a quantitative approach:

- What is the effect of nurse home visits on the parenting ability of teen mothers?

- Does rocking in older adults elicit the physiological changes of the relaxation response?

- What is the effect of social support intervention on coping in nurses working in intensive care units?

QUALITATIVE RESEARCH **Qualitative research** is "associated with naturalistic inquiry, which explores the subjective and complex experiences of human beings" (Berman et al., 2008, p. 32). The collection of rich narrative material and analysis take place simultaneously with the use of an inductive approach to analysis. In the qualitative approach, no formal instruments are used; instead, loosely structured narrative data are collected. Using the inductive method, data are analyzed by identifying themes and patterns that emerge. This approach is most often associated with the **naturalistic paradigm**, which began as a countermovement to positivism. This perspective assumes that multiple perspectives of reality exist, each within a context.

The qualitative approach explores complex human experiences and focuses on the holistic aspects of these experiences from the perspectives of those who are living them (Loiselle et al., 2011). (See the Evidence-Informed Practice box "How Do Health Care Providers Respond to and Empower Adolescent Women's Reproductive Health Concerns through Health Literacy?") The qualitative approach would be appropriate for the following types of research questions:

- What is the nature of the bereavement process in spouses of clients with terminal cancer?

- What is the nature of adjustment after a mastectomy?

- What is the impact of eating disorders on family life?

The Research Process

Loiselle et al. (2011) defined **research** as a "systematic inquiry that uses disciplined methods to answer questions or solve problems" (p. 2). Whether a quantitative or qualitative approach is used, all research must be meticulously planned, systematically implemented, and carefully

---

EVIDENCE-INFORMED PRACTICE

How Can Employers Promote Empowerment for New Graduate Nurses?

The nursing shortage and projected retirement of nurses in the next few years have resulted in the need for enhanced recruitment and retention of nurses. A high priority among health care organizations is the development of strategies to improve working conditions and to provide a supportive environment for new graduate nurses.

A predictive, nonexperimental survey design investigated factors that promote empowerment among new graduate nurses (Cho, Laschinger, & Wong, 2006). This study tested the relationships among structural empowerment, six areas of work life, emotional exhaustion, and organizational commitment. Structural empowerment measured employees' perceptions of access to opportunity, information, support, and resources. The six areas of work life included (a) workload, (b) control, (c) rewards, (d) community, (e) fairness, and (f) values. Emotional exhaustion measured how often an individual experienced feelings of disengagement and burnout in his or her work. Organizational commitment measured the psychological link between the employee and the organization.

The researchers found that structural empowerment had a positive effect on the areas of work life and a negative effect on emotional exhaustion. They concluded that increasing access to job flexibility, strong interpersonal relationships, information, support, and learning opportunities are potential strategies to retain new graduate nurses.

NURSING IMPLICATIONS: **This study suggests the importance of a positive work environment in ensuring the commitment of new graduates and the resulting retention of staff. The following strategies would contribute:**

- Use multiple communication techniques: regular staff meetings, forums, electronic messages, brown bag lunches, and written updates.

- Use support staff to reduce nursing time spent on nonnursing tasks.

- Provide orientation, emotional support, assistance, and collaborative learning opportunities.

- Give new graduates opportunities for leadership roles and involvement in decision making.

- Offer choices and alternatives for flexibility in jobs (e.g., job sharing, innovative scheduling).

- Build strong interpersonal relationships through team building and mentoring programs.

Source: Based on Cho, J., Laschinger, H. K. S., & Wong, C. (2006). Workplace empowerment, work engagement and organizational commitment of new graduate nurses. *Canadian Journal of Nursing Leadership, 19*(3), 43–60.

---

analyzed. To achieve this goal, researchers adhere to a formal course of action known as the research process. This process has 11 steps, beginning with the formulation of the research problem and ending with the communication of the research. However, sometimes variation

EVIDENCE-INFORMED PRACTICE

How Do Health Care Providers Respond to and Empower Adolescent Women's Reproductive Health Concerns through Health Literacy?

According to Banister, Begoray, and Daly (2011), specific health care–related needs of adolescents are frequently unmet. They assert that health care providers, such as nurses, have the ability to overcome barriers that get in the way of adolescents being able to make use of health care services in an effective manner. Specifically, they suggest that developmentally and contextually appropriate health literacy strategies in the active involvement of adolescent women in their learning would be most effective.

The authors provide comprehensive information and research findings about health literacy, adolescent development, barriers to adolescent empowerment, and functional, communicative or interactive, and critical health literacy strategies (e.g., text messaging, writing, visual props and other materials, books). Furthermore, based on their extensive practice and published research experience in Canada with rural and urban high-school adolescent women, they recommend how health care providers can address adolescent women's reproductive health concerns. Banister et al. recommend the following basic approach: (a) Choose a health topic (e.g., use of condoms); (b) integrate functional, communicative or interactive, and critical health literacy; (c) choose one or more learning processes from the list of functional literacy skills; and (d) evaluate outcomes.

NURSING IMPLICATIONS: Consider the developmental stage of the adolescents, determine the knowledge translation strategies available about the topic of interest or need, and collaboratively determine the most appropriate teaching and learning approach.

Source: Based on Banister, E. M., Begoray, D. L., & Daly, L. K. (2011). Responding to adolescent women's reproductive health concerns: Empowering clients through health literacy, *Health Care for Women International, 32*(4), 344–354. Retrieved from http://dx.doi.org/10.1080/07399332.2010.536603.

exists in the terms given to these steps, depending on the nature of the study.

1. STATE A RESEARCH PROBLEM The investigator's initial task is to narrow a broad area of interest to a circumscribed **research problem** that specifies exactly the situation that needs to be described, explained, or predicted. The ideas for research may arise from recurrent problems encountered in practice, questions that are difficult to resolve because of contradictions in the literature, or areas in which minimal or no research has been done.

In formulating a research problem, Loiselle et al. (2011) suggest five important considerations: (a) significance, (b) usefulness, (c) researchability, (d) feasibility, and (e) ethical soundness. A research problem has *significance* if it has the potential to contribute to nursing science by enhancing client care, testing or generating a theory, or resolving a day-to-day clinical problem. The question "So what?" must be answered adequately to determine whether a research problem is significant.

The *usefulness* of a study relates to the potential usefulness in nursing practice of the findings. Not only should the problem be significant, but it must also be relevant and applicable to nursing practice.

Researchability means that the problem can be subjected to scientific investigation by using appropriate and sound methodology. Many significant problems that produce ambiguity and uncertainty in clinical situations are not amenable to research. For instance, "Should nurses support voluntary euthanasia?" is a relevant, timely, and difficult question, but it cannot be answered through research.

Feasibility pertains to practical issues, such as availability of time and the material and human resources needed to investigate a research problem or question. Conducting a study involves the use of space, money, equipment, supplies, computers, subjects, research assistants, and consultants.

A study is *ethically sound* if ethical issues are addressed by adhering to rigorous procedures and appropriate ethical reviews, where needed. See the "Protecting the Rights of Human Subjects" section later in this chapter for details concerning the ethical principles guiding research in Canada.

2. DEFINE THE STUDY'S PURPOSE OR RATIONALE The statement of the study's purpose indicates what the researcher intends to do with the research problem identified. The **study purpose** includes *what* the researcher will do, *who* the subjects will be, and *where* the data will be collected.

3. REVIEW THE LITERATURE Before progressing with the development of the research design, the investigator determines what is known and what is not known about the problem. A thorough **review of the literature** provides the foundation on which to build new knowledge. Through a literature review, a researcher may also acquire information about available techniques, instruments, and methods of data analysis that have been used in prior research, as well as potential flaws or problems and how to avoid them. The literature review helps to determine the best approach for studying the problem (Gillis & Jackson, 2002).

4. FORMULATE THE RESEARCH QUESTION OR HYPOTHESIS Once nurse researchers have identified a research problem and are knowledgeable of the literature, they formulate a **research question**. The question may be stated in one of three ways: (a) a statement, (b) a question, or (c) a hypothesis. If researchers are going to describe something, they may make a statement, such as "The purpose of this study is to identify gender differences in the nursing care of patients admitted to rehabilitation units." They could also ask a question, such as "What are the communication styles of nurses that produce client satisfaction with nursing care?"

If conducting an experiment, researchers must have a **hypothesis** about what the outcome will be so that hypothesis-testing statistics can be applied. For example, "Family members of palliative care patients attending support groups will demonstrate more positive coping strategies compared with those who do not attend" is a testable hypothesis. Whichever way a research question is stated, it must be clearly expressed. Wood and Ross-Kerr (2010) identify three levels of questions: (a) Level one questions relate to topics with little or no prior knowledge, and this leads to an exploration; (b) level two questions are useful when a topic has already been well described and any variables arising from the descriptions prompt the researcher to consider relationships between these variables; and (c) level three questions build on previous research and look for causal relationships.

5. SELECT A RESEARCH DESIGN   A **research design** is the "overall plan for addressing a research question" (Loiselle et al., 2011, p. 422). The choice of design depends on the nature of the problem. Level one questions lend themselves to various qualitative designs, while levels two and three are more appropriate for quantitative designs. Sometimes, a combination of approaches is used. The research design includes the study setting, the sample, and the type of data to be collected, as well as strategies to reduce bias.

Quantitative research design has three categories:

1. **Experimental design**. The investigator manipulates the independent variable by administering an experimental treatment to some subjects while withholding it from others. The conditions are tightly controlled to objectively test the hypothesis to predict cause-and-effect relationships (Potter et al., 2010).

2. **Quasi-experimental design**. The investigator manipulates the independent variable but without either the randomization or the control that characterizes true experiments. This design is common in health care studies because random assignment to treatment and control groups is not always feasible in a clinical setting (Potter et al., 2010).

3. **Nonexperimental design**. The investigator does not manipulate the independent variable. Researchers use nonexperimental designs to measure characteristics and determine relationships or correlations among these variables (Loiselle et al., 2011).

As noted earlier, **qualitative designs** seek to derive meaning and understanding from human experience. In such disciplines as nursing, where it is necessary to know what the participant is experiencing, a qualitative design may be the preferred method of identifying data. A qualitative design differs from a quantitative design in the phenomenon studied, the data collection and analysis procedures, and the interpretation of the data. Often, data collection and analysis are done simultaneously. Qualitative designs do not have identifiable measurable variables and data are not processed through statistical analysis.

Ethnography, grounded theory, and phenomenology are some of the commonly used qualitative methods. **Ethnographic research** is used to describe social behaviours within a particular group or setting. The goal is to understand the culture and norms from the participant's viewpoint (Potter et al., 2010). Studies related to the nursing care or health practices of a particular culture would be examples of ethnographic nursing research. **Grounded theory** research is used to develop nursing theory from collected data. Theory may be generated for relatively new areas, where very little is known, or for more familiar areas where a fresh viewpoint is sought. **Phenomenology** is a philosophical research method that regards each human as having a unique experience. The researcher uses in-depth conversations to attempt to derive meaning from individuals' descriptions of their experiences (Potter et al., 2010).

In selecting the approach, the researcher should try to identify factors that may affect the study's results. Sometimes, these factors are called *limitations*. The researcher should acknowledge the limitations of the study, as much as possible, before the data are collected.

6. SELECT THE POPULATION, SAMPLE, AND SETTING   At this stage, the researcher chooses the study population, selects a sample, and decides on the setting where the sample can be found. The **population** includes all members of the group who meet the criteria for the study. The **sample** is the segment of the population from whom the data will actually be collected.

7. CONDUCT A PILOT STUDY   In quantitative studies, a **pilot study** is a small-scale trial done before the actual study begins. The research procedure is conducted on a few subjects to determine the feasibility of the data collection plan, identify flaws, and refine the proposed plan to strengthen the research methodology (Berman et al., 2008).

8. COLLECT THE DATA   When designing a study, researchers must consider how the data will be collected. The most commonly used methods of collecting data in nursing are questionnaires, rating scales, interviews, observation, and biophysical measures.

In quantitative designs, the validity and reliability of measurement tools need to be established before the start of data collection. **Validity** is the degree to which an instrument measures what it is supposed to measure. If a nurse measures anxiety, how can the nurse be sure that what is being measured is not fear or stress, which are related concepts? **Reliability** is the degree of consistency with which an instrument measures a concept or variable. If an instrument is reliable, repeated measurements of the same variable should yield similar or nearly similar results.

9. ANALYZE THE DATA   In this step, the collected data are organized, coded, and analyzed for the purpose of answering the research question or testing the hypothesis. Even before data collection is initiated, there must be a systematic plan for analyzing the results. Measurement is a critical part of the research process. Measurement is not a feature of qualitative designs; the discussion here is relevant to quantitative designs. Variables are important components of measurement. The identified research question helps the researcher identify the variables and possible relationships among them. The variables must be clearly defined, observable, and measurable to permit the results of a study to be interpretable. Regardless of the method of measurement used, it must have evidence of objectivity. This means that the system of measurement must be so clear that anyone following the prescribed rules will assign the same or similar score to what was observed.

Data analysis can involve descriptive or inferential statistics. **Descriptive statistics**, procedures that summarize large volumes of data, are used to describe and synthesize data, showing patterns and trends. Descriptive statistics include measures of central tendency and measures of variability.

Measures of central tendency describe the centre of a distribution of data, denoting where most of the subjects lie. These include the mean, median, and mode. **Measures of variability** indicate the degree of dispersion, or spread, of the data. These include the range, variance, and standard deviation. See Box 3.2 for definitions of these measures. Typically, in a research report, the mean and the standard deviation are reported together to give the reader an idea of the nature of the data distribution.

The following is an example: systolic blood pressure = 130 ± 30. The two statistics reported are the mean and the standard deviation. The number 130 indicates the mean systolic blood pressure, whereas 30 represents 1 standard deviation (SD) from the mean. Hence, 1 SD from the mean would include blood pressures from 100 mm Hg to 160 mm Hg (1 SD less than the mean to 1 SD more than the mean).

After the data have been analyzed, nurse researchers attempt to determine whether the results are *statistically significant*. Underlying this statement is the notion of *probability*. By convention, a *p* (probability) value less than 0.05 is considered the acceptable level of significance; a *p* value greater than 0.05 is considered statistically insignificant. In research, the desire is to generalize beyond the sample; a need exists to determine the probability that the results were due to chance or a fluke, rather than a true occurrence in the population. Hence, a *p* value of 0.05 means that the probability of the findings being caused by chance alone is 5 in 100 (Berman et al., 2008).

In qualitative studies, data analysis is often done simultaneously with data collection, which enables the researcher to focus and shape the study as it proceeds. The researcher consistently thinks about the data, works to organize it, and tries to discover meaning in it.

10. INTERPRET THE FINDINGS In either quantitative or qualitative research, when interpreting the results of the data analysis, the researcher first reports the findings that are directly related to the research question. Sometimes, the researcher uncovers unexpected findings, and these are also reported. Hirst (2000) articulated a definition of resident abuse as perceived by those living and working within long-term care institutions and unexpectedly found that older adults were devalued in these same facilities.

Conclusions are then drawn: What do these findings mean? At this point, researchers can be subjective and insert some of their own thinking into the research report. The results of the current research are compared with previous studies that investigated the same or similar phenomena. The researcher should discuss any problems encountered in the course of the study or any limitations that may have influenced the findings.

After the findings are interpreted, the researcher should indicate the implications for nursing. **Implications** are suggestions for ways of thinking about the phenomenon in the future. Nursing research may unearth indications for changes to nursing practice, administration, or education. For example, in a review of research literature on the impact of international placements on nursing students, the findings suggested that students become more sensitive to cultural issues and cross-cultural care as a result of these experiences (Button, Green, Tengnah, Johansson, & Baker, 2005). An implication is that nurse educators need to provide culturally diverse opportunities for students. In a study examining what percentage of clients had postoperative pain at home and what impact the pain had on their activity, the findings identified that clients had received no information on how to cope with pain and were not knowledgeable about analgesic use (Collins & MacDonald, 2000). These findings indicate a need for educational resources on the management of postoperative pain following discharge from hospital to be given to clients.

11. COMMUNICATE THE RESEARCH Implicit in conducting research is the requirement to share with others the knowledge generated, primarily through publication in professional journals or by reporting the results orally or in poster format at professional conferences. Interpreting the results, communicating the findings, and suggesting directions for further study conclude the research process.

In Canada, nursing research findings can be communicated in numerous ways. At the local, provincial or territorial, and national levels, nursing associations and special interest groups use their newsletters, publications, annual meetings, and conferences to promote nursing

---

BOX 3.2 DEFINITIONS OF MEASURES OF CENTRAL TENDENCY AND VARIABILITY

CENTRAL TENDENCY

Mean: The sum of all scores divided by the number of subjects; commonly symbolized as X or M

Median: The middle score or value in a distribution of scores; the value above and below which 50% of the scores lie

Mode: The score or value that occurs most frequently in a distribution of scores

VARIABILITY

Range: The difference between the highest and the lowest values in a distribution of scores

Variance: The square of the standard deviation

Standard deviation: The average to which scores deviate from the mean; commonly symbolized as SD or S; the most frequently used measure of variability

---

BOX 3.3 EXAMPLES OF RESEARCH JOURNALS IN NURSING

These are just a few of the nursing journals that are currently available:

Canadian Oncology Nursing Journal

Canadian Journal of Cardiovascular Nursing

Canadian Journal of Nursing Leadership

Canadian Journal of Public Health

Canadian Operating Room Nursing Journal

Canadian Journal of Nursing Research

Canadian Journal of Nursing Informatics

Clinical Nursing Research

Nursing Research

International Journal of Nursing Studies

Nursing Science Quarterly

Qualitative Health Research

Biological Research for Nursing

---

research and disseminate findings. The best method of reaching a large number of nurses is through publication in nursing journals (see Box 3.3 for examples). *Canadian Nurse* (*L'infirmière Canadienne*) publishes news items on research activities, abstracts of Canadian research articles, and articles that report research findings.

Developing Research-Based Practice

The nurse needs to be research minded, that is, aware of and open to nursing research. Nurses should critically read, interpret, and evaluate research evidence for applicability to their nursing practice. When reviewing research articles or reports, consider the philosophical view taken in the study; for example, where does knowledge exist? Does it exist in individuals' experiences (qualitative) or in the logical reasoning of the researcher (quantitative)? Nursing has possibilities for both.

Research-based practice enables nurses to provide high-quality, cost-effective care. Through clinical practice, nurses can identify nursing problems that need to be investigated. Nurses can participate in the implementation of research studies by helping principal researchers collect data in clinical settings. They can also help disseminate research-based knowledge by sharing useful findings with colleagues. Nurses with graduate education also assume the role of clinical experts on clinical practice teams, integrate research findings into practice, design studies, and collaborate with other researchers (Potter et al., 2010).

Research utilization involves a number of activities by nurses to link research findings to practice. To do so, nurses need to access current research findings and critique this literature to determine its appropriateness for a particular clinical setting.

Locating Nursing Research Findings

The journal *Nursing Research* was established in 1952 in the United States to serve as a vehicle to communicate nurses' research and scholarly productivity (Donahue, 1985). The publication of many other nursing research journals followed, some devoted to research and others combining clinical, theory, and research publications. Journals are available in the libraries of academic institutions and large hospitals, and many journals are now published online on the World Wide Web.

The most efficient way to access research articles is to conduct a search on an index of journal articles (Potter et al., 2010). Examples of these indexes include the Cumulative Index to Nursing and Allied Health Literature (CINAHL), International Nursing Index, MEDLINE, and PubMed. Computerized search assistance is available in health care libraries; the trick to finding relevant articles is to identify the key words to be used for the search. It may take several computer searches using different key terms and databases to locate the articles. Increasingly, these searches can be done through the World Wide Web. The Canadian Research Information Database (CRID) is a resource for researchers and others interested in accessing the results of research in Canada on the web. In searching the web, be aware of the credibility of the source and when the site was last updated.

The Cochrane Library is a collection of databases with high-quality evidence obtained through systematic reviews. Results from several similar randomized trials are brought together and combined to produce an overall statistic by using exact methodology. This process facilitates evidence-informed decision making for clinical treatment.

The Virginia Henderson International Nursing Library is sponsored by Sigma Theta Tau International and provides online access to reliable nursing information. It also includes the Registry of Nursing Research Database, with up-to-date study and conference abstracts.

The Canadian Nurses Association (CNA), Health Canada, and the First Nations and Inuit Health Branch of Health Canada have created NurseONE, a secure web-based resource to provide nurses "with access to current and reliable information to support their nursing practice, manage their careers, and connect with colleagues and health care experts" (CNA, n.d., p. 1). It supports an evidence-based approach to care by providing easily accessible digital libraries, online journals, electronic material, and databases that are all approved by the CNA.

Critiquing Research

Critiquing involves intensive scrutiny of a study, including its strengths and weaknesses, its statistical and clinical significance, and the generalizability of the results.

Loiselle et al. (2011) suggest different approaches to critiquing quantitative and qualitative research. For quantitative research, using the IMRAD format (i.e., introduction, method, results, and discussion) will address the study components found in most research reports. See Table 3.1 for relevant questions about each of these components.

TABLE 3.1 Critique of a Quantitative Research Report

Aspect of the Report	Questions to Consider
Title	Does the title inform you of the research problem and study population?
Abstract	Does the abstract summarize the main features of the article?
Introduction	
Problem Statement	Is the problem clear and easy to identify? Does the problem statement identify key concepts and the population? Is the problem significant for nursing? Is a quantitative approach suitable? Does the research problem fit the methods?
Literature Review	Is the literature review current and complete? Is it based mostly on primary sources? Does the literature review summarize what is known about the dependent and independent variables and how they are related? Does it provide a solid framework for the new study?
Conceptual Framework	Are key concepts fully defined from a theoretical perspective? Is a theoretical framework described? Is it appropriate? If no theoretical framework is present, does the report justify the absence?
Hypothesis or Research Questions	Are research questions or hypotheses clear and explicit? If not, is there a rationale for their absence? Is there consistency among the questions and hypotheses, the literature review, and the conceptual framework?
Method	
Research Design	Was a rigorous design used given the study purpose? Were appropriate comparisons made for ease of interpretating the findings? Was there evidence of efforts to minimize threats to internal and external validity?
Population and Sample	Were the population and sample identified and described? Was the sampling design devised to promote a representative sample? Was sample size sufficient? Was a sample size estimate done by using power analysis?
Data Collection and Measurement	Were there congruence between the operational and conceptual definitions? Were key variables defined in an operational manner? Were the instruments well described? Did the report provide evidence of high reliability and validity of data?
Procedures	Was the intervention (if used) described and correctly implemented? Were data collected to minimize bias? Were the staff who collected the data trained in data collection? Were procedures used to safeguard rights of study participants? Was there an ethics review?
Results	
Data Analysis	Did the analysis address each research question or hypothesis? Were statistical methods matched to measurement level of the variables and number of groups being compared?
Findings	Were the findings summarized by using tables and figures? Do findings demonstrate sound evidence about the research questions?

(continued)

TABLE 3.1 *(continued)*

Aspect of the Report	Questions to Consider
Discussion	
Interpretation of Findings	Are major findings interpreted, discussed, and related to prior research and the conceptual framework used?
	Was there consistency among interpretations and results or limitations of the study?
Implications	Does the article provide details about generalizability of the findings?
Overall	
Presentation	Was the report well organized, and did it provide adequate detail for critical analysis?
	Was the study understandable?
	Was the study written in such way as to make the findings accessible to practising nurses?
Summary Assessment	Despite identified limitations, do the findings appear valid?
	Does the study contribute to evidence that can be meaningfully used in nursing practice or the discipline of nursing?

Source: Adapted from Loiselle, C. G., Profetto-McGrath, J., Polit, D. F., & Beck, C. T. (2011). *Canadian essentials of nursing research* (3rd ed.) (pp. 359–361). Philadelphia, PA: Lippincott Williams & Wilkins.

Qualitative research reports are generally less structured and organized according to the themes. However, a similar approach can be used to critique qualitative research (see Table 3.2).

TABLE 3.2 Critique of a Qualitative Research Report

Aspect of the Report	Questions to Consider
Title	Does the title reflect the main phenomenon and the group or community under study?
Abstract	Does the abstract summarize the main features of the article?
Introduction	
Statement of the Problem	Is there a clear identification of the phenomenon of interest?
	Is the problem clearly stated and easy to identify?
	Is the problem significant for nursing?
	Does the research problem fit the methods?
	Is the qualitative approach suitable?
Literature Review	Does the literature review summarize knowledge related to the problem?
	Is the literature review current and complete?
	Does the literature review set down a basis for the new study?
Conceptual Underpinnings	Are key concepts fully defined from a theoretical perspective?
	Does the report identify the philosophical or ideological basis, conceptual framework, and research tradition?
	Is the approach congruent with the research questions?
Research Questions	Are research questions clear and explicit?
	If not, is there a rationale for their absence?
Method	
Research Design and Tradition	Does the research tradition fit with the data collection and analysis methods?
	Was sufficient time spent in the field or with study participants?
	Did the researcher build on early understanding by adapting the design in the field?
	Was there evidence of reflective thought by the researcher?
	Was the number of contacts with participants sufficient?

TABLE 3.2 *(continued)*

Sample and Setting	Were the population, sample, and setting identified and described? Was an appropriate approach used to access participants? Was an optimum sampling method used? Was the sample sufficient? Was there saturation of data?
Data Collection Procedures	Were the data gathered in an appropriate manner? Were two or more methods of data gathering used to achieve triangulation? Were the right questions or observations used? Were these recorded appropriately? Were sufficient data collected for depth and richness? Was there a clear description of data collection and recording procedures? Were steps taken to minimize bias or altered behaviour? Were procedures used to safeguard rights of study participants? Was there an ethics review?
Enhancement of Rigour	Was there a description of methods used to promote trustworthiness of the analysis? Were sufficient methods used to enhance credibility? Were research procedures and decision processes documented to be auditable and confirmable?

Results

Data Analysis	Were methods of data management and analysis clearly described? Did the analysis approach fit with the research tradition, nature, and type of data gathered? Did the analysis produce a tangible output (theory, taxonomy, thematic pattern, etc.)?
Findings	Were the findings summarized with the use of quotes? Do the themes capture the meaning of the data? Did the researcher conceptualize the themes or patterns in the data? Did the analysis identify a thought-provoking and meaningful picture of the phenomenon?
Theoretical Integration	Are there logical connections among the themes or patterns, and do these connect to form a meaningful whole? Were figures, maps, or models effectively used to summarize conceptualization? Are the themes or patterns logically linked to a conceptual framework or ideology (if one was used to guide the study)?

Discussion

Interpretation of Findings	Is the interpretation of the findings situated in an appropriate context (e.g., group, cultural, or social)? Are major findings interpreted, discussed, and related to prior research? Is there consistency between the study's interpretations and limitations? Does the report discuss transferability of findings?
Implications	Are the implications of the study for clinical practice or future study discussed? Are the implications reasonable?

Overall

Presentation	Was the report well organized, and did it provide adequate detail for critical analysis? Were the methods, findings, and interpretations richly described?
Summary Assessment	Do the findings seem trustworthy? Does the study contribute to meaningful evidence that can be used in nursing practice or the discipline of nursing?

Source: Adapted from Loiselle, C. G., Profetto-McGrath, J., Polit, D. F., & Beck, C. T. (2011). *Canadian Essentials of Nursing Research* (3rd ed.) (p. 361). Philadelphia, PA: Lippincott Williams & Wilkins.

In general, the critique should include consideration of the following:

- Amount of detail about the method, ethical considerations, and interpretation of findings
- Clarity of language
- Objectivity and lack of bias in presentation
- Organization and logical presentation of ideas
- Correct use of grammar and rules of good writing
- Sensitivity to gender, race, and ethnicity
- Appropriateness of title to capture key concepts and target population
- Adequacy of summary of research problem, study methods, and key findings (Loiselle et al., 2011)

Protecting the Rights of Human Subjects

When research is conducted with human participants, the researcher and the nurse have a responsibility to protect the research participant from harm that may result from participation in the study. The nurse, as client advocate, must ensure that clients' rights are protected.

All institutions in which research is conducted should have, or have access to, a *research ethics board (REB)*, a committee of qualified individuals to approve the research activity and to ensure that the rights of participants are protected. The principle of protecting rights is enforced, to some extent, by major granting agencies, such as the CIHR and the SSHRC, which make their funding contingent on an REB review. REBs have the authority to require modifications to proposed research and can terminate research that is not conducted according to specific requirements. Also offering guidance to nurse researchers in Canada are the CNA's *Code of Ethics for Registered Nurses* (2008); the Canadian Institutes of Health Research, Natural Sciences, and Engineering Research Council of Canada, and the Social Science and Humanities Research Council of Canada's *Tri-Council Policy Statement on Ethical Conduct for Research Involving Humans* (1998 with 2000, 2002, and 2005 amendments, second edition, 2010).

All nurses who practise in settings in which research is being conducted with human subjects, or who participate in such research as data collectors or collaborators, play an important role in safeguarding the rights of human subjects. The *Tri-Council Policy* is based on the following guiding ethical principles:

RESPECT FOR HUMAN DIGNITY Respect for human **dignity** means protecting the interests of the person in all spheres: physical, psychological, and social/cultural. This cardinal principle forms the basis of ethical obligations in modern research.

RESPECT FOR FREE AND INFORMED CONSENT It is presumed that individuals have the capacity and right to make free and informed decisions. Obtaining **informed consent** is the responsibility of the principal investigator.

It is a contract between the investigator and the participant. All clients must be informed about the consequences of consenting to serve as research participants. The client needs to be able to judge whether a reasonable balance exists between the risks of participating in the study and the potential benefits.

Informed consent may appear to be straightforward and easy to implement, but this is not always true. Sometimes, researchers avoid informed consent, believing that the client's knowledge of being observed could alter behaviour and distort the findings. It is the nurse's responsibility to safeguard participants' human rights and ensure that informed consent takes place before their involvement in any research study.

Informed consent includes written and oral explanations. It should be in the participant's preferred language and at an appropriate educational level. Documenting informed consent by obtaining a participant's consent in writing is important. Participants who can give only oral permission must have their consent witnessed by a third person. If the participant is a minor or is not capable of consenting because of mental or physical disability, a legally authorized representative, such as a parent or guardian, may sign the consent. Consent must be voluntary and informed, and no additional risk, discomfort, or invasion of privacy to that stated in the consent document can take place. In addition, the participant must be guaranteed that refusal to take part in or withdraw from the study will not jeopardize the quality of nursing care.

RESPECT FOR VULNERABLE PERSONS Greater ethical obligations toward vulnerable people and those who have diminished competence or decision-making capacity must be met. Children, people in institutions, and others are entitled to special protection against abuse and exploitation. In research, this often means that special procedures are needed to protect the interests of vulnerable people.

RESPECT FOR PRIVACY AND CONFIDENTIALITY The principle of respect for privacy and confidentiality is considered fundamental to human dignity in many cultures. Standards of privacy and confidentiality protect personal information and enable a client to participate without worrying about later embarrassment. The anonymity of a study participant is ensured if the investigator cannot link a specific subject to the information reported. **Confidentiality** means that any information a subject provides will not be made public or available to others without the subject's consent. Investigators must inform research subjects about the measures that provide for these rights. Such measures may include the use of pseudonyms or code numbers or the reporting of only aggregate or group data in published research.

RESPECT FOR JUSTICE AND INCLUSIVENESS The ethics review process is required to have fair methods and standards for reviewing research protocols so that no segment of the population is unfairly burdened with the harms of research and those who are vulnerable are not exploited for the advancement of knowledge. Conversely, justice also implies a duty to ensure that some individuals and groups are not neglected or discriminated against with respect to inclusion in research studies.

BALANCING HARMS AND BENEFITS Minimizing harm, or **nonmaleficence**, is the duty to avoid, prevent, or minimize harm to others. A research subject should not be exposed to the possibility of injury beyond everyday situations. The risk can be physical, emotional, legal, financial, or social. For instance, withholding standard care from a client in labour for the purpose of studying the course of natural childbirth clearly poses a potential physical danger. Risks can be less overt and involve psychological factors, such as exposure to stress or anxiety, or social factors, such as loss of confidentiality or loss of privacy. This means that research should involve the smallest number of human subjects and smallest number of tests on subjects that will ensure scientifically valid data.

Maximizing benefit, or **beneficence**, is the duty to benefit others and maximize the net benefits. This is particularly relevant in social science disciplines, like social work and nursing, in which the advancement of knowledge can produce benefits for society.

RIGHT TO FULL DISCLOSURE Even though it may be possible to collect data about a client as part of everyday care without the client's particular knowledge or consent, to do so is considered unethical. **Full disclosure** is a basic right. It means that deception, either by withholding information about a client's participation in a study or by giving the client false or misleading information about what participating in the study will involve, will not occur.

RIGHT OF SELF-DETERMINATION Many clients in dependent positions, such as people in nursing homes, feel pressured to participate in studies. They feel that they must please the doctors and nurses who are responsible for their treatment and care. The **right of self-determination** means that subjects should feel free from constraints, coercion, or any undue influence to participate in a study. Masked inducements, for instance, suggesting to potential participants that they might become famous by taking part in the study, make an important contribution to science, or receive special attention, must be strictly avoided. Nurses must be assertive in advocating for this essential right.

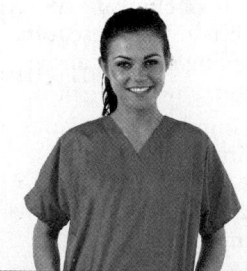

Case Study 3

A research study is being implemented on the unit as Jamie, a third-year baccalaureate nursing student in a large university in Western Canada, starts his adult health course rotation. He participates in the orientation session held by the researchers to inform the staff about their study. The purpose of the study is to understand the presurgical experiences of patients. Jamie is interested in working with the researchers.

CRITICAL THINKING QUESTIONS

1. Identify the responsibilities of beginning nurses in relation to nursing research.

2. What questions might Jamie ask of the researchers as he explores his possible interest in the study?

3. How might Jamie ensure that he protects the rights of his patients, if they decide to participate in the study?

Check the eText in MyNursingLab for answers and explanations.

KEY TERMS

CHAPTER HIGHLIGHTS

- Nurses are now generating new knowledge and applying research in practice to guide and improve client care.

- Nurses at all levels are participating in nursing research activities. All nurses practising in settings in which research is conducted have a role in safeguarding the clients' rights.

- The use of research will help nurses understand the client's situation more thoroughly, assess more accurately, and intervene more effectively.

- The Canadian Nurses Association is a leader in the promotion of evidence-based nursing practice.

- Most nursing research is initiated in university settings because of the preparation of faculty members as researchers; however, many questions are raised by nurses in the practice settings.

- In Canada today, nursing research faces both capabilities and constraints for its ongoing development.

- The nurse has a duty to protect the rights of the research participants.

- There is an ongoing effort to conduct nursing research on a wide range of nursing questions.

- Qualitative and quantitative methods or mixed methods are employed in nursing research.

- Seven ways that nurses can participate in research are by (a) identifying nursing problems that need to be investigated, (b) helping principal researchers collect data in clinical settings, (c) disseminating research-based knowledge by sharing useful findings with colleagues, (d) assuming the role of clinical expert on clinical practice teams, (e) integrating research findings into practice, (f) designing studies, and (g) collaborating with other researchers.

- Research utilization involves a number of activities by nurses to link research findings to practice. To do so, nurses need to access current research findings and critique this literature to determine its appropriateness for a particular clinical setting.

ASSESS YOUR LEARNING

1. Which is an example of a strategy employed to link theory, practice, and research in nursing?

   a. Ensuring that nursing research is exclusively conducted by qualified, university-based scientists

   b. Implementing cross-appointments of faculty among hospitals, health care agencies, and universities

   c. Promoting studies that focus on nursing as a distinct discipline rather than interdisciplinary studies

   d. Establishing concise health information systems containing only essential medical data for ease of use

2. Which of the following research roles is expected of a baccalaureate nurse working as a staff nurse in an acute care hospital?

   a. Designing studies and collaborating with other researchers

   b. Assuming the role of clinical expert on clinical practice teams

   c. Identifying nursing problems that need to be investigated

   d. Submitting research proposals to the hospital ethics board for approval

3. What should you do as a student or staff nurse seeking guidance from published research?

   a. Accept the findings without question, since the study has been published

   b. Compare the study subjects with your clients to determine if the findings are applicable

   c. Look for another study since you need at least two sources to ensure the findings are consistent

   d. Write to the researchers for the raw data so you can analyze the data yourself

4. Which study would best lend itself to a quantitative research approach?

   a. Measuring the effects of preoperative teaching on postoperative wound healing

   b. Examining perceptions of adolescents with type 1 diabetes mellitus

   c. Exploring factors influencing social isolation among seniors living alone in the community

   d. Describing the experience of adjustment following sudden infant death

5. Which study would BEST lend itself to a qualitative research approach?

   a. Measuring nutrition and weight changes in clients with cancer

   b. Examining the relationships between urinary infections and indwelling catheters

   c. Examining the relationships among infant, mother, and contextual factors and mother–low-birth-weight-infant interaction

   d. Exploring the caregiving role adult daughters play when a parent is hospitalized for a cardiac condition

6. The nurse is conducting a research project on differences in long-term psychological functioning in young women following alternative pregnancy resolution decisions (abortion, adoption, keeping the baby). After identifying the problem, what is the next step in the research process?

   a. Select the population and sample

   b. Review the literature

   c. Identify data collection methods

   d. Conduct a pilot study

7. The choice of a research design is determined by what?

   a. Preferences of the researcher conducting the research

   b. Availability of tested measurement instruments for the variables of interest

   c. Availability of potential subjects to participate in the study

   d. The nature of the problem being investigated

8. What should the nurse do to ensure the principle of self-determination related to participation in research studies for residents in a long-term care facility?

   a. Contribute to the research process by offering staff assistance to gather all the data from the residents

   b. Insist on personally gathering the informed consent from the residents

   c. Recognize that the residents are in a dependent position and should not be coerced into participating

   d. Refuse to allow researchers into the facility, since the residents are in no condition to consent

9. You work as a nurse on a special assessment unit in a rehabilitation hospital with children who have developmental disorders. You have been asked to help identify potential participants for an institutionally approved research study on independent community living options for adolescents with Down syndrome. One of your clients is an 18 year old, who has told you previously that he wants to move out of his parents' home and live independently, but his parents are against such a move. How would you protect the rights of the client in this case?

   a. Discuss your dilemma with the client and his family together

   b. Refer the client's name to the researcher and leave the decision up to her

   c. Talk to your nursing manager and seek her advice in this matter

   d. Talk to the client alone and ask him what he would like to do about participation in the study

10. The nurse is developing a workshop on teenage pregnancy for school children from 12 to 14 years of age. What is the BEST way to gather information for the presentation?

    a. Ask parents what they think teenagers should know about pregnancy

    b. Do an Internet search of websites for pregnant teenagers

    c. Conduct a literature review of research on teenage pregnancy

    d. Consult other nurses who work with pregnant teenagers

Check the eText in MyNursingLab for answers and explanations.

WEBLINKS

Canadian Association of Nursing Research (CANR)

http://www.canr.ca

CANR is a national organization with representation from every province and territory. It fosters research-based nursing practice and practice-based nursing research.

Canadian Nurses Association (CNA)

http://www.cna-aiic.ca

Through its search mechanism, the CNA provides access to research initiatives specific to the practice of nursing.

Canadian Institutes of Health Research (CIHR)

http://www.cihr-irsc.gc.ca

The CIHR is a primary funding source for Canadian nurse researchers.

Canadian Consortium for Health Promotion Research

http://www.utoronto.ca/chp/CCHPR/introe.htm

The focus of the consortium is to improve health-promotion research, policy, and practice in Canada by linking research, capacity development, and information dissemination.

Canadian Nursing Informatics Association (CNIA)

http://www.cnia.ca

The CNIA exists to help nurses across Canada to learn, share, research, and create informatics-related projects and experiences that can help to boost the competencies, theory, and practice of informatics on a national level.

Canadian Cochrane Centre (CCNC)

http://www.ccnc.cochrane.org

The centre's mandate is to promote health care decisions based on accurate knowledge (evidence-based health care) through the dissemination and application of systematic reviews of health care interventions. This site provides evidence-based resources.

Queen's Joanna Briggs Collaboration for Patient Safety

http://meds.queensu.ca/qjbc/index.php?id_mnu=1

It involves a pan-Canadian collaboration for synthesis of evidence in patient safety. Its mission is to improve the quality and reliability of practice, and ultimately health outcomes by enabling the use of best available evidence on patient safety.

Social Sciences and Humanities Research Council of Canada (SSHRC)

http://www.sshrc.ca

This council is an arm's-length federal agency that promotes and supports university-based research and training in the social sciences and humanities.

NurseONE Portal

http://www.nurseone-inf-fusion.ca

This web-based resource was developed by the CNA, Health Canada, and the First Nations and Inuit Health Branch of Health Canada. It provides a variety of resources to support evidence-based clinical practice for Canadian nurses.

MyNursingLab

REFERENCES

Banister, E.M., Begoray, D. L., & Daly, K. (2011). Responding to adolescent women's reproductive health concerns: Empowering clients through health literacy. *Health Care for Women International, 32*(4), 344–354.

Berman, A., Snyder, S. J., Kozier, B., & Erb, G. (2008). *Kozier and Erb's fundamentals of nursing* (8th ed.). Upper Saddle River, NJ: Pearson/Prentice Hall.

Button, L., Green, B., Tengnah, C., Johansson, I., & Baker, C. (2005). The impact of international placements on nurses' personal and professional lives: Literature review. *Journal of Advanced Nursing, 50*(3), 315–324.

Canadian Institutes of Health Research, Natural Sciences, and Engineering Research Council of Canada, & The Social Science and Humanities Research Council of Canada. (1998 with 2000, 2002, and 2005 amendments, second edition, 2010).

Tri-council policy statement: Ethical conduct for research involving humans. Ottawa, ON: Author.

Canadian Nurses Association. (n.d.). *NurseONE: The Canadian nurse's portal.* Ottawa, ON: Author. Retrieved from http://www.cna-aiic.ca/CNA/documents/pdf/publications/Portal_Overview_2_e.pdf

Canadian Nurses Association. (2008). *Code of ethics for registered nurses.* Ottawa, ON: Author.

Canadian Nurses Association. (2010–2015). *Canadian registered nurse examination competences.* Ottawa, ON: Author.

Carper, B. (1978). Fundamental patterns of knowing in nursing. *Advances in Nursing Science, 1*(1), 13–23.

Collins, M., & MacDonald, V. (2000). Managing postoperative pain at home. *Canadian Nurse, 96*(7), 26–29.

Donahue, M. P. (1985). *Nursing: The finest art.* St. Louis, MO: Mosby.

Donaldson, S. K. (2000). Breakthroughs in scientific research: The discipline of nursing, 1960–1999. *Annual Review of Nursing Research, 18,* 247–311.

Ellinger, M. K. & Rempel, G. R. (2010). Parental decision making regarding treatment of hypoplastic left heart syndrome. *Advanced Neonatal Care, 10*(6), 323–324.

Gillis, A., & Jackson, W. (2002). *Research for nurses: Methods and interpretation.* Philadelphia, PA: Davis.

Hartling, L., Scott, S., Pandya, R., Johnson D., Bishop T., Klassen T. P. (2010). Storytelling as a communication tool for health consumers: Development of an intervention for parents of children with croup. Stories to communicate health information. *BMC Pediatrics, 10,* 64.

Hirst, S. (2000). Resident abuse: An insider's perspective. *Geriatric Nursing, 21,* 38–42.

Loiselle, C. G., Profetto-McGrath, J., Polit, D. F., & Beck, C. T. (2011). *Canadian essentials of nursing research* (3rd ed.). Philadelphia, PA: Lippincott Williams & Wilkins.

Potter, P., Perry, A., Ross-Kerr, J., & Wood, M. (2010). *Canadian fundamentals of nursing* (4th ed.). Toronto, ON: Elsevier Canada.

Slaughter, S. E., Eliasziw, M., Morgan, D., & Drummond, N. (2011). Incidence and predictors of excess disability in walking among nursing home residents with middle-stage dementia: A prospective cohort study. *International Psychogeriatrics, 23*(1), 54–64. doi:10.1017/S1041610210000116

Wood, M. J., & Ross-Kerr, J. C. (2010). *Basic steps in planning nursing research: From question to proposal* (7th ed.). Sudbury, MA: Jones and Bartlett.

Woodham-Smith, C. (1950). *Florence Nightingale.* London, UK: Constable & Co.

Chapter 4

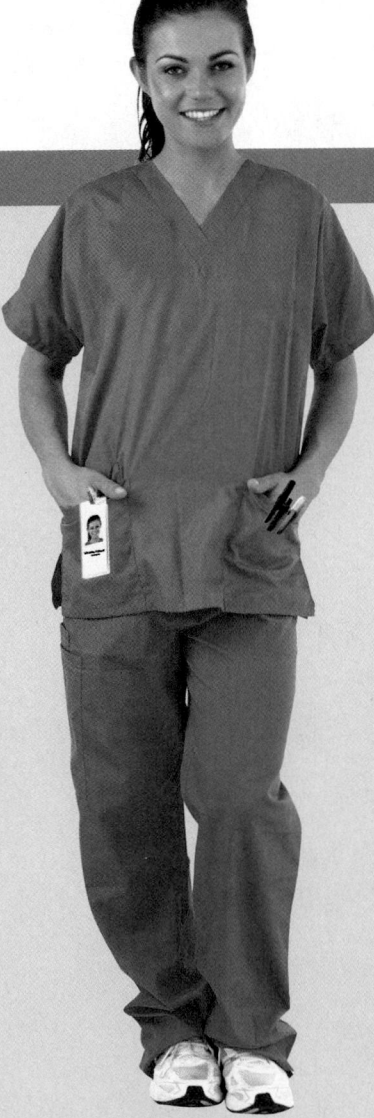

Nursing Philosophies, Theories, Concepts, Frameworks, and Models

LEARNING OUTCOMES

After studying this chapter, you will be able to:

1. Identify the purposes and essential elements of theories in nursing.

2. Examine the purposes and benefits of philosophies in nursing.

3. Describe three main areas of philosophical inquiry and two research traditions.

4. Compare selected philosophical approaches in relation to the questions they pose for nursing.

5. Identify selected theoretical works in terms of how nursing is conceptualized and the assumptions underpinning these conceptualizations.

6. Define the terms *philosophy, paradigm, assumption, concept, conceptual framework, conceptual model,* and *theory.*

Philosophical thinking is an indispensable feature of our everyday lives. When people reflect on the meaning of their experiences, consider how they might evaluate the *truth* of an observation, or try to determine the *best* course of action in a particular situation, they are engaging in philosophical thought. The word *philosophy*, translated from its original Greek, means simply "love of wisdom." Philosophical thinking is also what people draw on to make their way, as wisely as they can, through their lives. To be wise means, in part, to use knowledge well. Therefore, nurses should be committed to using philosophical thinking to improve their understanding of the particular values, beliefs, and assumptions that inform their thinking and influence what they say and do.

Philosophical thinking provides the foundation for the development and analysis of the concepts (including conceptual models and conceptual frameworks) and theories used to articulate knowledge of the discipline. **Concept** is another word for idea. Nurses make use of concepts to highlight the ideas that are important to the discipline. A **conceptual framework**, viewed simply, is a cluster of related concepts around a particular topic. A **conceptual model** is a diagram or illustration showing graphically how concepts within a particular cluster are positioned in relation to each other. A **theory** goes beyond conceptual models and frameworks to show the nature and significance of relationships among concepts. Theories offer ways of looking at (conceptualizing) a discipline—such as nursing—in clear, explicit terms that can be communicated to others.

Philosophical and theoretical thinking support the discipline's professionalism and collegial status with other health care professionals. Nurses must communicate clearly what makes their place in the interdisciplinary team important. To achieve this clarity, concepts and theories are used to organize and analyze nursing knowledge. To use this knowledge wisely, the philosophical beliefs and assumptions that are the foundation for its creation and use must be made clear.

What Is Philosophy?

Although the word *philosophy* has an ordinary, everyday meaning—in the sense that people say they each have their own philosophy, or set of beliefs and assumptions, about the world and their place in it—philosophy is also a scientific discipline. *Science* here means the systematic formulation of a body of knowledge. In a formal sense, philosophy is a scientific discipline that raises, explores, and attempts to answer questions bearing on "our ideas about our experience, the universe, and human affairs" (Fry, 1992, p. 87). In philosophy, people use critical analysis in pursuit of goals.

Philosophical thinking can assist with the following:

- Identifying and questioning assumptions
- Clarifying how concepts are used and how they have meaning
- Assessing arguments made to defend or critique particular ways of thinking

Philosophy's Three Primary Areas of Inquiry

Philosophy's three primary areas of inquiry are *ontology*, *epistemology*, and *ethics*. These terms refer to areas of inquiry somewhat familiar to most people. **Ontology** investigates the nature of being. It asks such questions as: What is the nature of reality? What is the meaning and purpose of our existence? What does it mean to be a person? **Epistemology** investigates the nature of knowledge: How do we know something? What are the limits of knowledge? On what grounds can we say something is true? What is the difference between what is believed to constitute knowledge and what is described as opinion? **Ethics** explores the nature of moral conduct and judgment: What is good? How should people behave or react in particular circumstances? How should people judge the actions of others? The ways in which we answer these kinds of ontological, epistemological, and ethical questions reflect our basic assumptions and beliefs about the world.

Paradigms or World Views

A **paradigm** (or world view) is a particular way of thinking based on a specific set of beliefs, values, and assumptions. Each person's world view influences how he or she perceives, comprehends, and interprets the world. It shapes people's understanding of events and the means used to seek knowledge. Nevertheless, people are often unaware of their underlying beliefs, values, and assumptions. In particular, **assumptions** often operate unconsciously and are beliefs that are taken for granted, without evidence that has been systematically generated.

Many social arrangements rest solely on assumptions. For example, the idea that nursing is "women's work" relies on an assumption that particular kinds of work are best suited for women and other kinds of work are more appropriate for men. This assumption is often based on other unexamined beliefs about what is sometimes described as women's natural capacity for caring and nurturing. To critique this assumption requires examining particular beliefs and values: such notions as caring, men's and women's "proper" positions in society, the difference between men and women, and the social value attributed to various kinds of work. This kind of inquiry might suggest that women's historical association with activities of care is a reflection not so much of women's essential nature but rather of the ways in which social roles and responsibilities have been allocated throughout history. Philosophical inquiry helps to make explicit what underlies the assumption that nursing is women's work.

Empiricist and Interpretive Traditions

Though many world views or paradigms exist, two ways of understanding the world have been particularly influential in nursing: the empiricist and the interpretive traditions. According to the **empiricist tradition**, a single reality exists independently of our knowledge of it. The world exists separate from human knowers. Knowledge can be obtained by observation and experiment—in other words, by means of the **scientific method**. Truth can be determined by comparing knowledge claims against this independently existing reality. In making discoveries about this world as it really is, scientists can and should prevent subjective biases and beliefs from influencing their perceptions. According to this tradition, it is possible to produce objective knowledge of the world.

By contrast, according to the **interpretive tradition**, no single fixed reality exists against which knowledge can be measured. Knowledge of the world independent of theorizing about it is not possible. Knowledge of the world is always mediated through assumptions. In fact, some scholars in the interpretive tradition argue that the nature of human understanding is itself interpretive and that it is our nature as human beings to create meaning from our experiences.

Each of these two philosophical traditions includes many variations. People who work in one of these traditions often express their beliefs and assumptions somewhat differently. Therefore, simply labelling a work as empiricist or interpretive is of limited use. It is much more fruitful to consider the specific beliefs and assumptions that underlie a particular work.

Both the empiricist and the interpretive traditions have strong adherents, but the point here is not to suggest the rightness or wrongness of either tradition. Rather, it is to recognize that world views provide a general orientation to the world, a way to organize perceptions and experience. In knowledge-generating activities, paradigmatic views influence directions for research and study, problem identification, and guidelines for inquiry and action. Because writers often do not make their world views explicit, readers of nursing research and theory should carefully consider exactly what assumptions are in play.

Philosophy in Nursing

Philosophy is an essential feature of all scientific disciplines, and nursing is no exception. The study of philosophy in nursing enables nurses to further their understanding of the values, beliefs, assumptions, and knowledge that constitute the discipline. Generally speaking, the study of philosophy in nursing can be understood as the "philosophical inquiry about nursing's social and humanitarian roles, its form of thought, nature, scope, purpose, methods, language, moral presuppositions, and knowledge claims" (Fry, 1999, p. 6). Philosophy in nursing involves consideration of the same sorts of ontological, epistemological, and ethical questions mentioned earlier in the chapter. Here, we formulate how these questions are studied in relation to the art, science, and practice of nursing. Thus, an ontological inquiry will consider the nature of nursing; an epistemological inquiry will consider nursing knowledge; and an ethical inquiry will consider the moral questions that arise in nursing. Nurses use philosophy to think, to examine assumptions, to analyze concepts, and to carefully consider arguments. In this sense, philosophical inquiry in nursing is an invaluable practical activity in which all nurses should participate.

Developing a particular philosophy of nursing involves careful clarification and reflection on what nurses are trying to do, why they do it, and what knowledge they use. A useful philosophy of nursing will help accomplish these goals. First, it will identify the central phenomena of the discipline. Second, it will relate nursing to a particular world view or philosophical tradition. Third, it will offer some criteria concerning knowledge development in the discipline (Salsberry, 1994). Formulating a philosophy of nursing is about making nurses' frame of reference for being in the world explicit (Smith, 1994).

Nursing and Canadian Society

Fact	Implications for Nursing Practice
In 1988, the Institute for Philosophical Nursing Research was founded at the University of Alberta.	The aim of the institute is to provide leadership in the pursuit of philosophical nursing knowledge that underlies the advancement of the nursing practice.
Philosophical methods raise certain kinds of questions about the discipline of nursing.	Nurses can appreciate the necessity to support within nursing a number of different approaches to philosophy.
Techniques of science cannot answer some questions concerning the nature of nursing, the moral ground of nursing practice, or the particular meanings of nurse–client relationships.	The position statement of the Canadian Nurses Association (CNA, 2002), *Evidence-Based Decision-Making and Nursing Practice,* provides directives to nurses concerning the need for scientific evidence to underlie practice.

Scientific inquiry is still the predominant mode of inquiry in nursing. However, science cannot answer some nursing questions (Kikuchi, 1992). Scientific inquiry is directed toward the material world, to what can be measured or is observable through the senses. Thus, techniques of science cannot answer some questions concerning the nature of nursing, the moral ground of nursing practice, or the particular meanings of nurse–client relationships. Interpretive approaches as well as empiricist approaches are important in nursing philosophy.

Philosophical thinking in nursing has developed on many fronts, and nurses have used philosophy in many different ways (see the Nursing and Canadian Society box). Since the 1980s, nurses have published many articles and books about nursing philosophy, and they have organized many conferences around philosophical themes. In 1988, the Institute for Philosophical Nursing Research was founded at the University of Alberta. If the philosophy of nursing is understood as simply an activity that uses philosophical methods and raises certain kinds of questions about the discipline of nursing, it is possible to appreciate the necessity to support within nursing a number of different approaches to philosophy.

Overview of Selected Nursing Philosophies

The work of selected nurse philosophers demonstrates the ways in which philosophy can be used in nursing and the kinds of questions a philosophical perspective can address. In the survey that follows, selected nurse philosophers are organized into four groups, according to the types of topics they might address (see Table 4.1). This survey is, of necessity, a partial one, but a range of philosophical positions are included.

Some nurse philosophers directly address nursing philosophy itself as a topic for discussion. For example, Kikuchi (1992) argued for a place for philosophical inquiry in nursing by reasoning that science cannot answer all of nursing's questions. In a later paper, Kikuchi and Simmons

TABLE 4.1 Selected Nurse Philosophers

Topics They Might Address	Nurse Philosophers	Approach to Inquiry
Argument	Kikuchi, J., & Simmons, H.	Philosophical Analysis
	Johnson, J.	Philosophical Analysis
Values and Ethics	Sellman, D.	Philosophical Analysis
Epistemology	Edwards, S.	Philosophical Analysis
	Purkis, M. E.	Critical Philosophical Analysis
	Ceci, C.	Critical Philosophical Analysis
	Holmes, D.	Critical Philosophical Analysis
	Nelson, S.	Philosophical/ Historical Analysis
	McIntyre, M.	Philosophical Hermeneutics
	McDonald, C.	Philosophical Hermeneutics
Research	Cameron, B.	Interpretive Phenomenology
Ethics	Gadow, S.	Relational Ethics
	Bergum, V.	Relational Ethics
	Storch, J.	Bioethics

(1994) presented a philosophical argument against the appropriateness of particular philosophies for nursing. Salsberry (1994) claimed that a philosophy of nursing will identify the central phenomena of the discipline and relate nursing to a particular world view or philosophical tradition. Smith (1994) asserted that arriving at a philosophy of nursing makes explicit our frame of reference for being in the world. Edwards (1997) explored what constitutes a philosophy of nursing, considering not only *what* should be included under this heading but also *how* it should be included. For Edwards, a philosophy of nursing should include an analysis of the concepts deemed to be central to the discipline. Such analysis would include ontological and epistemological values and logic. Johnson (1994) took up the question regarding what is meant by the art of nursing by using a philosophical method of argument to arrive at a definition of nursing as an art associated with expressive, creative, and intuitive abilities.

Beginning from a different philosophical perspective, Bishop and Scudder (1999) used an interpretive approach to articulate a meaning of nursing from the point of view of practising nurses. Their interpretation focused on nursing as the practice of caring, as a way of being for others, and as a relationship. In all these papers, the authors did not insist that they were offering correct knowledge as found in a scientific paper. Rather, they presented arguments, defended positions, and invited readers to consider the persuasiveness of their analyses and conclusions.

A second group of nurse philosophers used philosophy to address nursing research questions. Often, these inquiries took a phenomenological approach, which means that the researcher investigated and described particular phenomena as they are consciously experienced in nursing practice. Topics of this kind of research range from experiences of illness or grief to experiences of homelessness. For example, Cameron (1992) considered the meanings that the question "How are you?" can have in the context of a nurse–client relationship, showing that nurses should not take their understanding of these words for granted. Bergum (1989) philosophically explored a woman's experience of becoming a mother. These kinds of philosophical writings stimulate nurses to reflect on the meanings of experiences and phenomena that they sometimes assume they already understand. In other words, these types of philosophical inquiries expand thinking by giving us more to *think about*.

A third group of nurse philosophers asked epistemological questions about the practice of nursing. Some of these writers explicitly drew on other philosophers or philosophical traditions to explicate nursing practice. Purkis (1997) used ideas from the writings of the French philosopher Michel Foucault (1926–1984), such as the disciplined and disciplining gaze of the nurse (how nurses communicate what counts as health and its promotion), to reflect on the implications of health-promotion discourses and practice. Lawler (1997) also drew on Foucault's writings to suggest that the disciplines of science and economics have influenced how people speak and think about nursing. In particular, the world views that prevail in science and economics do not recognize the importance of relationship and contexts, concepts that nurses consider central to the practice of nursing.

In the area of ethics, a fourth group of nurse philosophers addressed ethical questions about the practice of nursing. Gadow (1994) suggested that the inability of patients to determine the meaning of their own experiences is a moral issue for nursing. Liaschenko (1997) suggested that serious ethical dilemmas can arise for nurses because of the systems and structures that contribute to the powerlessness that some nurses experience in practice.

Even this abbreviated discussion of nurse philosophers reveals that nursing philosophy can be approached in many ways. Note, however, that although they are often not stated, philosophical ideas are an integral component of nursing practice, research, and theory development. Foregrounding, or making explicit philosophical thinking, furthers our understanding of current nursing practices and develops the profession more effectively for the future.

Concepts and Theories

Philosophical thinking provides the foundation for the development and critical analysis of nursing knowledge. Nursing knowledge is organized and communicated by using concepts, models, frameworks, and theories. A theory of nursing will address the subject matter of the discipline of nursing in accordance with a particular philosophical world view. For example, a theory of nursing will include some conceptualization of the nature of nursing, its scope, and purpose. It will identify and describe the central nursing concepts, such as person, health, nursing, and environment (see Table 4.2), and also propose how these phenomena can be known. It may also address ethical concerns by specifying how to understand moral phenomena encountered in nursing practice. The building blocks of theories are concepts.

Concepts are abstract ideas or mental images of phenomena. They are words that bring forth mental pictures of the properties and meanings of objects, events, or things. Concepts can be (a) readily observable, or *concrete*, ideas, such as thermometer, rash, and lesion; (b) indirectly observable, or *inferential*, ideas, such as pain and temperature; or (c) nonobservable, or *abstract*, ideas, such as equilibrium, adaptation, stress, and powerlessness. Many concepts apply to nursing: concepts about human beings, health, helping relationships, and communication. Nursing theories address and specify relationships among four major abstract concepts referred to as the **metaparadigm** of nursing—the most global philosophical or conceptual framework of a profession. A metaparadigm is a higher level of abstraction than a paradigm. It identifies the concepts central to the discipline without relating them to the assumptions of a particular world view. Although consensus exists that the following four concepts make up nursing's metaparadigm (Fawcett, 2005), others have proposed an alternative metaparadigm (Newman, Sime, & Corcoran-Perry, 1991; Parse, 1987):

1. *Person or Client:* the recipient of nursing care (includes individuals, families, groups, and communities)

2. *Environment:* the internal and external surroundings that affect the client, which includes people in the physical environment, such as families, friends, and significant others

3. *Health:* the degree of wellness or well-being that the client experiences

4. *Nursing:* the attributes, characteristics, and actions of the nurse providing care on behalf of, or in conjunction with, the client

Nurse theorists' definitions of nursing's major concepts vary in accordance with their world view, their philosophy, and their experience in nursing. Nursing theories serve several purposes (see Box 4.1).

BOX 4.1 PURPOSES OF NURSING THEORIES AND CONCEPTUAL FRAMEWORKS

Nursing theories and conceptual frameworks provide direction and guidance for (a) structuring professional nursing practice, education, and research, and (b) differentiating the focus of nursing from other professions.

IN PRACTICE

- Help nurses to describe, explain, and predict everyday experiences

- Guide assessment, intervention, and evaluation of nursing care

- Provide a rationale for collecting reliable and valid data about the health status of clients, which are essential for effective decision making and implementation

- Help establish criteria to measure the quality of nursing care

- Help build a common nursing terminology to use in communicating with other health care professionals: ideas are developed and words defined

- Enhance the autonomy (independence and self-governance) of nursing by defining its own independent functions

IN EDUCATION

- Provide a general focus for curriculum design

- Guide curricular decision making

IN RESEARCH

- Offer a framework for generating knowledge and new ideas

- Assist in discovering knowledge gaps in the specific field of study

- Offer a systematic approach to identify questions for study, select variables, interpret findings, and validate nursing interventions

---

The terms *theory* and *conceptual framework* are often used interchangeably in the nursing literature. Strictly speaking, they differ in their levels of abstraction; a conceptual framework is more abstract than a theory. As noted earlier, a *conceptual framework* is a group of related concepts. It provides an overall view or orientation to focus thoughts. A conceptual framework can be visualized as an umbrella under which many concepts can exist. A *theory* is a supposition or system of ideas that is proposed to explain a given phenomenon. For example, Newton proposed his theory of gravity to explain why objects always fall to the ground. A theory goes one step beyond a conceptual framework by relating concepts through definitions that state significant relationships between concepts.

Frameworks, Concepts, and Theories: Direction for Nursing Practice

The major purpose of a conceptual framework is to give clear and explicit direction to the three areas of nursing: (a) practice, (b) education, and (c) research. A conceptual framework makes explicit the concepts important to the discipline and the professional practice of nursing. Theories are constructed by making explicit the relationships between and among these identified concepts. Most, if not all, nursing theories include either implicitly or explicitly the concepts of health, persons, environment, and nursing. What distinguishes one theory from another is the way in which the relationships among them are conceptualized. We speak of this process of theorizing as the making explicit the relationships between and among those concepts. The product of the theorizing—that is, the theory—provides direction for nursing practice. The nature of the direction provided for nursing practice can be traced back to the philosophical views underpinning each of the concepts. An example might be useful here. Select any one of the theorists discussed in this chapter. Ask yourself which of his or her concepts are highlighted as important and what the nature of the relationship between these concepts is. The final question for you will be whether you can see the direction this relationship provides for professional nursing practice.

Because the purpose of nursing theory is to generate knowledge to direct nursing practice, nursing theory and nursing research are closely related (see the Evidence-Informed Practice box on the next page). Nursing knowledge is generated within empiricist and interpretive research traditions. Empiricist approaches can be theory generating or theory testing, whereas interpretive approaches expose the understandings of experiences.

Empirical knowledge is derived from testing hypotheses (assumptions). In the research process, comparisons are made between the observed outcomes of research and the relationship predicted by the hypotheses. Research findings may be developed into theories to provide direction for nursing practice or education.

EVIDENCE-INFORMED PRACTICE

How Important Is Patient Involvement in Planning Complex Medication Regimes?

Using a case study approach, researchers Leslie Paldry and Alice March examined how experienced registered nurses can engage the circle of caring model to improve a patient's adherence to complicated medication regimens following cardiac transplantation. The model incorporates nursing and medical information alongside an assessment of the patient's readiness to learn, learning style, and perceptions of the meaning of his or her illness and need for medication.

The use of the theoretical circle of caring model resulted in increased ownership of health outcomes by patients and an understanding of the importance of following the agreed-upon plan for medication administration. The advantage of the circle of caring model is that it takes into account the patient's needs and desires, ensuring participation in the plan and thus improving the long-term quality of life and survival for people receiving cardiac transplants.

NURSING IMPLICATIONS: Theoretical models such as the circle of caring, where the planning and implementation of medication administration takes into account not only nursing and medical information but also the individual life of the patient, can lead to increased patient commitment to long-term medication regimes.

Source: Based on Paldry, I., & March, A. (2011). Circle of caring model: Medication adherence in cardiac transplant patients. *Nursing Science Quarterly, 24*(2). 120–125.

The Influence of Ways of Knowing on Theory Development and Direction for Practice

In addition to conceptual frameworks already discussed, writers have also proposed ways of knowing as influencing the generation of nursing theory. One such framework, originally developed by Barbara Carper (1978) is commonly referred to as *Carper's ways of knowing* and includes personal, empirical, aesthetic, and ethical ways of knowing. *Personal knowing* is about the nurse's knowledge of himself or herself, and the way in which that knowledge is used to authentically engage in relationships with others. Empirical knowing addresses the knowledge of nursing science needed for professional practice. *Empirical knowing* includes knowledge generated through research and theory from within and beyond the discipline of nursing. *Aesthetic knowing,* sometimes described as the art of nursing, is the unique interpretation and particularizing of nursing science in the momentary encounter experienced by the nurse in relationship with others. *Ethical knowing,* which is essential in decision making, is central to nursing practice. This form of knowledge underpins daily decisions about what one ought to know and how this knowledge obligates the nurse to act in particular ways in professional practice.

Building on Carper's four ways of knowing, Chinn and Kramer introduced the additional pattern of *emancipatory knowing.* Emancipatory knowing supports nurses to engage with issues of justice and equity in nursing practice. This knowing "cultivates awareness of how problematic conditions converge, reproduce, and remain in place to sustain a status quo that is unfair for some groups within society" (Chinn & Kramer, 2011, p. 64).

Overview of Selected Nursing Theories

Theory development gained momentum in the 1960s and has progressed markedly since then. Because opinions on the nature and structure of nursing vary, theories continue to be developed. Each theory bears the name of the person or group that developed it and reflects the beliefs of the developer.

The following nursing theories vary considerably in their (a) level of abstraction; (b) conceptualization of the client, health or illness, and nursing; and (c) ability to describe, explain, or predict. Some theories are broad in scope; others are limited. See Table 4.2 for a summary.

Only brief summaries of the theorists' central theme and basic assumptions are included here. For more detailed information on how specific theories are used in current nursing practice, refer to Alligood and Tomey (2010) and Alligood (2010) listed in the references of this chapter.

Nightingale's Environmental Theory

Florence Nightingale, often considered the first nurse theorist, defined nursing more than 100 years ago as "the act of utilizing the environment of the patient to assist him in his recovery" (Nightingale, 1860/1957). She linked health with five environmental factors: (a) pure or fresh air, (b) pure water, (c) efficient drainage, (d) cleanliness, and (e) light, especially direct sunlight. Deficiencies in these five factors caused lack of health, or illness.

These environmental factors attain significance when we consider that sanitation conditions in the hospitals of the mid-nineteenth century were extremely poor and that women working in the hospitals were often unreliable, uneducated, and incompetent.

In addition to those factors, Nightingale also stressed the importance of keeping the client warm, maintaining a noise-free environment, and attending to the client's diet in terms of assessing intake, timeliness of the meal, and its effect on the person.

Nightingale set the stage for further work in the development of nursing theories. Her general concepts about ventilation, cleanliness, quiet, warmth, and diet remain integral parts of nursing and health care today. Dunphy (2010) reminds us that in addition to manifesting these core ideals of health, Nightingale, as an original

TABLE 4.2 Selected Nurse Theorists' Conceptualization of Nursing, Health, Environment, and Human Beings

Nightingale	• *Nursing* is the act of using the environment of the patient to assist in recovery. • *Health* is linked to five *environmental* factors: fresh air, pure water, efficient drainage, cleanliness, and light. A deficiency in any of these factors is linked to illness. • *Human beings* are described as recipients of compassionate care.
Peplau	• *Nursing* is a therapeutic relationship between the nurse and the client. • *Health* includes interpersonal and intrapersonal experiences. • *Environment* includes the client's internal experiences and the relational environment in which he or she lives. • *Human beings* are conceptualized as subjects of their own experience rather than as objects of professional care.
Henderson	• *Nursing* is assisting sick or well individuals to gain independence in meeting their fundamental needs, or accompanying the client to a peaceful death. • *Health* is linked to the 14 fundamental needs identified by Henderson. • *Environment* is understood as the physicality of the client and his or her immediate physical surroundings. *Nurses* manage the environment as a way of moving the client toward performing activities unaided. • *Human beings* are physical beings who experience a variety of needs and are in relation with others for the purpose of meeting those needs.
Roy	• *Nursing* is the promotion of client adaptation in experiences of health, quality of life, and death with dignity. • *Health* is the way in which human beings interact with and adapt to environmental stimuli. • *Environment* is understood as the variable and constantly changing stimuli to which a person must adapt. • *Human beings* are seen as interacting with their physical and social environments and in relationship with the world and with God: "Persons are seen as adapting to those stimuli present as a result of his or her position on the health–illness continuum" (Roy & Andrews, in Fawcett, 2005, p. 367).
Watson	• *Nursing* is an intentional consciousness of caring enacted between a nurse and another, transcending the boundaries of time, space, and physicality. • *Health* "refers to unity and harmony within the mind, body and soul. Health is also associated with the degree of congruence between the self as perceived and the self as experienced" (Watson, 1988, p. 48). • *Environment*, both internal and external, is interdependent and strongly influence health and illness. Healing environments comprise physical and nonphysical energies and consciousness whereby wholeness, comfort, beauty, dignity, and peace are potentiated. • *Human beings* physically are confined in space and time, whereas the mind and soul are not.
Parse	• *Nursing* is co-creating a situation in which clients choose and bear responsibility for patterns of health. • *Health* is a continuously changing process, the quality of life co-created by human beings in relation with the universe. • *Environment* is understood as the world in which lived experiences unfold. • *Human beings* are open, indivisible, freely choosing beings who co-create patterns of relating.
Leininger	• *Nursing* is "a learned humanistic and scientific profession and discipline which is focused on human care phenomenon and activities to help people maintain or regain their well-being or health in culturally meaningful ways" (Leininger & McFarland, 2006, p. 7). • *Health* is a culturally defined, valued, and practised state of well-being that reflects people's abilities to perform their daily activities.

(continued)

TABLE 4.2 *(continued)*

	• *Environment* is the physical, ecological, sociopolitical, and cultural context of events or experiences. • *Human beings,* families, clans, and collective groups are constituted within cultural contexts, including values, beliefs, and life ways.
Newman	• *Nursing* is the study of caring in the human health experience. • *Health* is conceptualized as expanding consciousness that occurs when a person gains insight from a disturbance in the flow of daily living. The process of evolution of consciousness is also the process of health. • *Environment* is unbroken wholeness in which health and illness are viewed as a single process. • *Human beings* are continuous with the undivided wholeness of the universe and can be identified by their patterns of consciousness: "The person does not *possess* consciousness, the person *is* consciousness" (Newman, in Fawcett, 2005, p. 452).
Campbell (UBC [University of British Columbia] Model)	• *Nursing* is the activities that help patients to learn and maximize their coping abilities to manage critical situations within their life cycle. • *Health* is stability—preferably at the most optimum level possible within the situation. • *Environment* is anything that is outside the individual's system. • *Person* refers to individuals, each of whom shares nine basic needs. The individual meets those needs through coping mechanisms.
Allen (McGill Model)	• *Nursing* is the response of the profession to individuals' search for healthy living. • *Health* is a social process. Health can be described, measured, and modified. • *Environment* is the social context in which learning takes place. • *Person* in this model refers to the family or other social group.

nurse-activist, demonstrated the ways in which the values of caring can be transformed into an activism capable of transforming "our current health care system into a more humanistic and just one" (p. 51). In this way, Nightingale was a role model for showing through practice that actions driven by caring and compassion bring about justice.

Peplau's Interpersonal Relations Model

Hildegard Peplau, a psychiatric nurse, introduced her interpersonal concepts in 1952. Central to Peplau's theory is the use of a therapeutic relationship between the nurse and the client. Though now a taken-for-granted practice in nursing, in the early 1950s, the idea of engaging with clients as subjects, rather than treating them as objects, was a revolutionary one. Despite the early resistance to her approach, Peplau's work is responsible for the integration of the therapeutic relationship, the nurse–client relationship, into nursing theory. Traces of Peplau's emphasis on the nurse–client relationship can be found in all the major theoretical works today.

Nurses enter into a personal relationship with an individual when the need is present. The nurse–client relationship evolves in four phases:

1. *Orientation.* During this phase, the client seeks help, and the nurse establishes trust and helps the client understand the problem and the extent of the need for help.

2. *Working Phase: Identification.* During this phase, the client may assume a posture of dependence, interdependence,

or independence in relation to the nurse (relatedness); the nurse uses her or his professional knowledge "to aid the patience [*sic*] to make full use of the relationship, in order to solve the health problem" (Fawcett, 2005, p. 535). The nurse's focus is on helping the client understand the interpersonal meaning of their situation or behaviour (Peplau, 1952).

3. *Working Phase: Exploitation.* In this phase, the client derives full value from what the nurse offers through the relationship. The client uses available services on the basis of self-interest and needs. Power shifts from the nurse to the client.

4. *Termination.* In this final phase, the nurse–client relationship has closure (Peplau, 1952). Termination is seen as the end point of a time-limited relationship and calls for a marking of the end of the relationship.

To help clients fulfill their needs, nurses assume many roles: stranger, teacher, resource person, surrogate, leader, and counsellor. Peplau's model continues to be used by clinicians and has contributed significantly to the use of therapeutic relationships and the nurse as a therapeutic tool in many areas of nursing practice.

Henderson's Definition of Nursing

In 1966, Virginia Henderson formulated a definition of the unique function of nursing. This definition was a major stepping stone in the emergence of nursing as a discipline separate from medicine. Like Nightingale,

Henderson described nursing in relation to the client and the client's environment. Unlike Nightingale, Henderson saw the nurse as being concerned with both well and ill individuals, acknowledged that nurses interact with clients even when recovery may not be feasible, and described the teaching and advocacy roles of the nurse.

Henderson conceptualized the nurse's role as helping sick or well individuals to gain independence in meeting these 14 fundamental needs (1966; 1991, p. 22–23):

1. Breathe normally
2. Eat and drink adequately
3. Eliminate body wastes
4. Move and maintain desirable positions
5. Sleep and rest
6. Select suitable clothes, dress and undress
7. Maintain body temperature within a normal range by adjusting clothing and modifying the environment
8. Keep the body clean and well groomed and protect the integument
9. Avoid dangers in the environment and avoid injuring others
10. Communicate with others in expressing emotions, needs, fears, or opinions
11. Worship according to one's faith
12. Work in such a way that there is a sense of accomplishment
13. Play or participate in various forms of recreation
14. Learn, discover, or satisfy the curiosity that leads to normal development and health, and use the available health facilities

Henderson published many works and continues to be cited in current nursing literature. Her emphasis on the importance of nursing's independence from, and interdependence with, other health care disciplines is well recognized. In Henderson's later work (1991), she questioned whether nurses continue to value engagement with clients in the *palliative* (relieving suffering and providing comfort) experience or if the profession has shifted toward a medical approach in which the focus is prolonging life, even when death is inevitable.

Roy's Adaptation Model

Sister Callista Roy's adaptation model was first published in book form in 1976. She defined *adaptation* as "the process and outcome whereby the thinking and feeling person uses conscious awareness and choice to create human and environmental integration" (Roy, 1997, p. 44).

Roy later restated her scientific and philosophical assumptions for the twenty-first century. These assumptions focused on the increasing complexity of person and environment, self-organization, and the relationship among human beings, the universe, and God, or what can be considered a supreme being. Her philosophical

assumptions were refined by using major characteristics of "creation spirituality"—a view that "persons and the earth are one and that they are in God and of God" (Roy, 1997, p. 46). "Roy also uses the idea of cosmic unity that stresses her vision for the future and emphasizes the principle that people and Earth have common patterns and integral relationships" (Roy & Zhan, 2010, p. 171). In this way, Roy moved past her earlier supposition that the system acts to maintain itself, shifting the emphasis to the "purposefulness of human existence in a creative universe" (p. 171).

Roy focused on the individual as a biopsychosocial adaptive system that employs a feedback cycle of input (stimuli), throughput (control processes), and output (behaviours or adaptive responses). Both the individual and the environment are sources of stimuli that require modification to promote adaptation, an ongoing purposive response. Central to Roy's theoretical model is the belief that "health is defined as (a) a process, (b) a state of being, and (c) becoming whole and integrated in a way that reflects individual and environment mutuality" (Roy & Zahn, 2010, p. 174). Although Roy originally conceptualized her model with regard to the health of the individual, more recently, the modes of the model have been expanded to speak to groups as well as individuals. Each person's or group's adaptation level is unique and constantly changing.

Individuals and groups respond to needs (stimuli) in one of four modes:

1. The *physiological mode* involves the body's basic physiological needs and ways of adapting to fluid and electrolytes, activity and rest, circulation and oxygen, nutrition and elimination, protection, the senses, and neurological and endocrine functions.
2. The *self-concept mode* includes two components: (a) the *physical* self, which involves sensation and body image, and (b) the *personal* self, which involves self-ideal, self-consistency, and the moral–ethical self.
3. The *role function mode* is determined by the need for social integrity and refers to the performance of duties based on given positions within society.
4. The *interdependence mode* involves a person's relations with significant others and support systems that provide help, affection, and attention.

The goal of Sister Callista Roy's model is to enhance life processes through adaptation in these four adaptive modes.

Watson's Human Caring Theory

Jean Watson (1979) believed the practice of caring is central to nursing; it is the unifying focus for practice. Her major assumptions about caring are shown in Box 4.2 on the next page. Watson originally referred to the nursing interventions related to human care as *carative factors,* a guide Watson refers to as the "core of nursing." Watson later expanded each of the carative factors to become *clinical caritas processes.* Watson explains: "What differs in the

BOX 4.2 WATSON'S ASSUMPTIONS OF CARING

- Human caring in nursing is not just an emotion, concern, attitude, or benevolent desire. Caring connotes a personal response.
- Caring is an intersubjective (between human subjects) human process and is the moral ideal of nursing.
- Caring can be effectively demonstrated only interpersonally.
- Effective caring promotes health and individual or family growth.
- Caring promotes health more than does curing.
- Caring responses accept people not only as they are now but also for what they may become.
- A caring environment offers the development of potential while allowing the person to choose the best action at a given time.
- Caring occasions involve action and choice by nurse and client. If the caring occasion is transpersonal, the limits of openness expand, as do human capacities.
- The most abstract characteristic of a caring person is that the person is somehow responsive to another person as a unique individual, perceives the other's feelings, and sets one person apart from another.
- Human caring involves values, a will and a commitment to care, knowledge, caring actions, and consequences.
- The ideal and value of caring is a starting point, a stance, and an attitude that has to become a will, an intention, a commitment, and a conscious judgment that manifests itself in concrete acts.

clinical caritas framework is that a decidedly spiritual dimension and an overt evocation of love and caring are merged for a new paradigm for this millennium" (Watson & Woodward, 2010, p. 355). The term *caritas* originates from a Greek word meaning "to cherish or appreciate."

Watson (1979) outlined the original carative factors with the addition of the clinical caritas processes in 2005 (Watson, 2005):

1. Formation of humanistic–altruistic system of values becomes a practice of living kindness and equanimity within the context of caring consciousness.

2. Instillation of faith–hope becomes being authentically present and enabling and sustaining the deep belief system and subjective life world of self and one being cared for.

3. Cultivation of sensitivity to one's self and to others becomes cultivation of one's own spiritual practices and transpersonal self, going beyond ego self, opening to others with sensitivity and compassion.

4. Development of a helping–trusting, human caring relationship becomes developing and sustaining a helping–trusting, authentic caring relationship.

5. Promotion and acceptance of the expression of positive and negative feelings becomes being present to, and supportive of, the expression of positive and negative feelings as a connection with deeper spirit of self and the one being cared for.

6. Systematic use of a creative problem-solving caring process becomes creative use of self and all ways of knowing as part of the caring process; to engage in artistry of caring–healing practices.

7. Promotion of transpersonal teaching–learning becomes engaging in genuine teaching–learning experience that attends to unity of being and meaning, attempting to stay within others' frames of reference.

8. Provision for a supportive, protective, and/or corrective mental, physical, societal, and spiritual environment becomes creating a healing environment at all levels (a physical and nonphysical, subtle environment of energy and consciousness, whereby wholeness, beauty, comfort, dignity, and peace are potentiated).

9. Assistance with gratification of human needs becomes assisting with basic needs, with an intentional caring consciousness, administering "human care essentials," which potentiate alignment of mind–body–spirit, wholeness, and unity of being in all aspects of care, tending to both embodied spirit and evolving spiritual emergence.

10. Allowance for existential–phenomenological–spiritual forces becomes opening and attending to spiritual–mysterious and existential dimensions of one's own life–death; soul care for self and the one being cared for.

In addition to the carative factors or caritas processes, three major ideas underpin all of Watson's work: (a) the transpersonal caring relationship, (b) the caring moment, or caring occasion, and (c) the caring (healing) consciousness.

Although numerous theorists include the idea of caring in their work, Watson's work spoke particularly of *transpersonal caring*, in which the nurse seeks to "connect with and embrace the spirit or soul of the other" through genuine and authentic engagement (Watson & Woodward, 2010, p. 356). The *caring moment* is understood to be "the moment of coming together" of the nurse and the client in which each person brings all of his or her experiential history with an intention of care and a possibility of connection. "If the caring moment is transpersonal, each feels a connection with the other at the spirit level; thus, the moment transcends time and space, opening up new possibilities for healing and human connection at a deeper level than physical interaction" (p. 358). The relationship between the nurse and the client is affected by the nurse's consciousness in the moment, and thus, transpersonal caring within a caring moment is manifested in an intentional *consciousness of caring or healing* by the nurse. For Watson, the process of an intentional (conscious) transpersonal caring occasion transcends time, space, and physicality: the effect of a caring interaction can go beyond the time and space boundaries of a given caring moment.

Watson's theory of human caring has received worldwide recognition and is a major force in redefining nursing as a *caring–healing health* model. Watson described her theory as building on nursing's disciplinary heritage, while also challenging nursing to mature in its own discipline and to affect health care providers beyond disciplinary boundaries in a caring model of health (Watson & Woodward, 2010).

Parse's Theory of Humanbecoming

Parse first published her theory in 1981 in *Man-Living-Health: A Theory for Nursing* and later retitled her work as *A Theory of Humanbecoming*, substituting the term *human* for *man*. Parse proposed three assumptions about "humanbecoming" (1995):

1. Humanbecoming is freely choosing personal *meaning* in situations in the intersubjective process of relating value priorities.
2. Humanbecoming is co-creating *rhythmic patterns* or relating in a mutual process with the universe.
3. Humanbecoming is *co-transcending* multidimensionally with the emerging possibilities.

These three assumptions focus on the concepts of meaning, rhythmicity, and co-transcendence:

- Meaning arises from a person's interrelationship with the world and refers to happenings to which the person attaches varying degrees of significance.
- Rhythmicity is the movement toward greater diversity.
- Co-transcendence is the process of reaching out beyond the self.

Parse's theory of humanbecoming emphasizes how individuals choose and bear responsibility for patterns of personal health. Parse contends that the client, not the nurse, is the authority figure and decision maker. The nurse's role involves helping individuals and families in choosing the possibilities for changing the health process. Specifically, the nurse's role consists of illuminating meaning (uncovering what was and what will be), synchronizing rhythms (leading through discussion to recognize harmony), and mobilizing transcendence (dreaming of possibilities and planning to reach them).

The Parse nurse uses "true presence" in the nurse–client process. "In true presence, the nurse's whole being is immersed with the client as the other illuminates the meanings of his or her situation and moves beyond the moment" (Parse, 1994, p. 18).

Leininger's Cultural Care Diversity and Universality Theory

Madeleine Leininger, a well-known nurse anthropologist, first published her cultural care diversity and universality theory in 1985 in the journal *Nursing and Health*

Care and explained it further in 1988 and then in 1991 in her book *Culture Care Diversity and Universality: A Theory of Nursing*.

Leininger stated that *care* is the essence of nursing and the dominant, distinctive, and unifying feature of nursing. She emphasized that human caring, although a universal phenomenon, varies among cultures in its expressions, processes, and patterns; it is largely culturally derived. Leininger's work draws on the premise that people of different cultures are capable of informing caregivers of the kind of care they need. McFarland points out that Leininger's theory was the first nursing theory "explicitly focused on care and culture in nursing environments" (2010, p. 320). Leininger defined culture, culture care, culture care diversity, culture care universality, generic care, and professional care. Her sunrise model, which depicts her theory, is presented in the MyNursingLab. For nurses to assist people of diverse cultures, Leininger also presented three intervention modes:

- Culture care preservation and maintenance
- Culture care accommodation, negotiation, or both
- Culture care restructuring and repatterning

Margaret Newman and Expansion of Consciousness

Margaret Newman's theory was influenced by her early life experiences in caring for her mother, when she began to think of health as other than the absence of disease. Following her undergraduate and graduate nursing education, informed by Martha Rogers, Newman proposed that illness reflects the life pattern of the person and that illness and health are part of a unitary life process, one no more important than the other. As she continued to develop her theory in the 1970s, Newman articulated the central thesis of her work that health is the expansion of consciousness (Newman, 1986).

When challenged about the scientific basis for her theory, Newman interestingly sidestepped the controversy of the scientification of nursing theory and instead claimed that her work "is not necessarily about science but rather about *meaning*: the meaning of life and health . . . found in the evolving process of expanding consciousness" (Newman, 1986, p. 4). Newman suggested that the use of the theory of health as expanded consciousness requires education in a curriculum that disrupts a view of health and illness as dichotomous or even as disparate ends of a continuum and instead has a "view of disease as a meaningful aspect of health. Furthermore the nurse has to let go of wanting to control the situation. The client's choices have to be respected and supported, even when those choices conflict with the nurse's personal values" (Fawcett, 2005, p. 462).

Campbell's UBC (University of British Columbia) Model of Nursing

Margaret Campbell (1987) developed the UBC model of nursing. Campbell guided nurse practitioners, researchers, and educators to look to the following elements of a model to guide their practice: "the view of the client" or "the recipient of care" and "the role and function of nursing in relation to the recipient of care and as a distinct and separate member of the team of health care professionals" (p. 5). In the UBC model, the major theme is a behavioural system with interacting and interdependent subsystems, each representing a basic human need. Campbell viewed human beings as having nine basic human needs, constantly striving to satisfy these needs by using a range of coping behaviours, both innate and acquired. According to this model, environment is that which lies outside the boundary of the system. The nurse is seen as nurturing "individuals experiencing critical periods so that they may develop and use a range of coping behaviours that will permit them to satisfy their basic human needs, to achieve stability and to reach optimum health" (Campbell, 1987, p. 10).

Campbell developed this model on the basis of several assumptions about Canadian society. She assumed that society views optimal health as a desirable goal for all of its members and that members of society would assume responsibility for utilizing behaviours that promote and maintain positive health. She further assumed that society expects its members will behave in ways that will not be harmful to themselves or others in the satisfaction of their needs. She assumed that society expects health care professionals to function competently and ethically. Lastly, Campbell assumed that society expects the UBC model for nursing, or any model for nursing, to be congruent with the values of that society. These assumptions about the values that Canadians hold and the beliefs about nursing that Campbell identified then guided her to conceptualize the UBC model in a particular way.

The UBC model in Figure 4.1 shows the nine subsystems that make up the behavioural system, with each subsystem representing one basic need. This illustration also shows how each of these subsystems relates to the others and how they interrelate to the system as a whole, a feature of significance to nursing. For example, whatever happens to one subsystem (including nursing interventions) can influence the system as a whole. Figure 4.2 shows the structure of each of the subsystems. Each subsystem is responsible for the satisfaction of one of the basic needs. Each subsystem consists of (a) an inner region that includes the need and the abilities to meet that need, and (b) an outer region that includes the need-related goal and the forces influencing attainment of that goal. Figure 4.3 shows how the parts of a subsystem relate to one another. The determinants of coping behaviours are both cognitive (knowing what

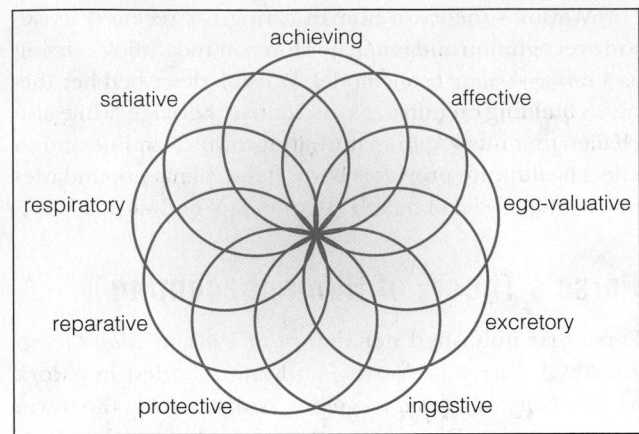

FIGURE 4.1 The nine basic needs of the individual

Source: From Campbell, M. (1987). *The UBC model for nursing: Directions for practice* (p. 32). Vancouver, BC: University of British Columbia School of Nursing.

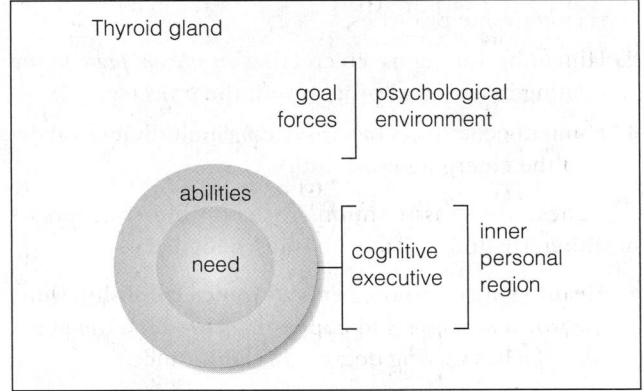

FIGURE 4.2 Structure of a subsystem: The parts

Source: From Campbell, M. (1987). *The UBC model for nursing: Directions for practice* (p. 33). Vancouver, BC: University of British Columbia School of Nursing.

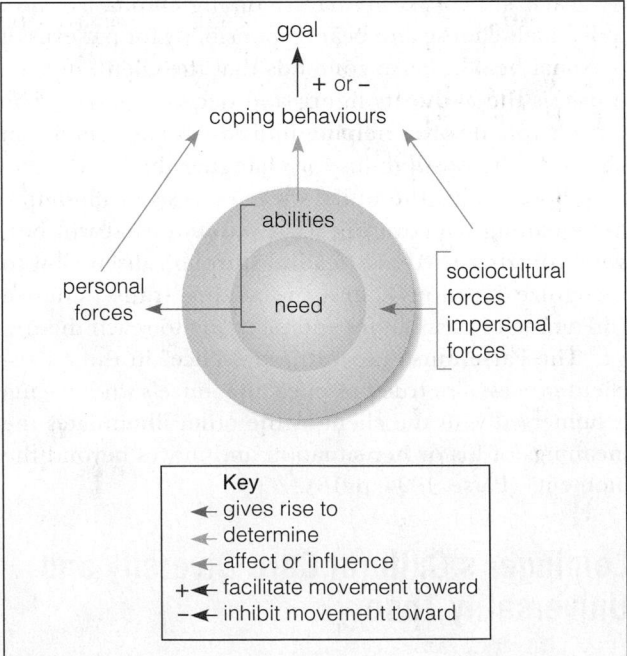

FIGURE 4.3 Structure of a subsystem: Interrelationship of the parts

Source: From Campbell, M. (1987). *The UBC model for nursing: Directions for practice* (p. 34). Vancouver, BC: University of British Columbia School of Nursing.

to do) and executive (carrying out the needed action). These forces influence movement toward or away from desired goals. It is the understanding of the detailed structure and function of a particular subsystem, and its interrelation with other subsystems and with the behavioural system as a whole, that guides the nurse in making decisions relative to providing care.

Allen's McGill Model of Nursing

Another example of a nursing model is the McGill model developed by Moyra Allen (1986). The McGill Model of Nursing espouses a collaborative, family-centred approach to care. Health is the central element of the model and the goal of nursing is to engage the individual, family, and community in the process of learning about and acquiring healthier ways of living. Health is a complex phenomenon and has multiple determinants that include income and social status, social support networks, education and literacy, employment or working conditions, social environments, physical environments, personal health practices and coping skills, healthy child development, biology and genetic endowment, health services, gender, and culture (Public Health Agency of Canada, 2010). Health is a process rather than an end point and it develops throughout the lifespan. It involves setting and achieving goals and developing competencies to manage normative and non-normative life events. Competencies include such skills as regulating and expressing emotion, problem solving, developing supportive relationships, and carrying out roles and responsibilities (Gottlieb, 1998). *Coping*, a component of health, refers to efforts made to deal with some problematic situation—it is aimed at mastery or problem solving, rather than at simply reducing tension. *Development,* another dimension of health, relates to the achievement of life goals. This broad concept of health means that the nurse focuses on strengths and potential rather than only on weaknesses or deficits. Within the McGill model, health is conceptualized as a distinct entity that exists alone or co-exists with illness (Gottlieb, 1998). The *optimal* state exists when the individual is free of disease and displays positive and constructive health behaviour; the *least satisfactory* state is when an individual has a disease and, at the same time, his health behaviours fail to permit him to cope with it and to learn further (Allen, 1981).

The McGill Model of Nursing directs the nurse to focus on the family as the unit of concern; when working with individuals, the nurse understands the person through a "family filter" (Gottlieb & Rowat, 1987). "The family influences healthy development and coping and is where people learn healthy ways of living. The nature of the nurse–person relationship is a collaborative partnership. The person is active and shares responsibility for his care. The person has knowledge and capabilities

that he can use to understand and manage his illness or problems or work toward his goals in ways that are meaningful to him; the nurse is a facilitator who encourages people to share their perceptions and expertise, to participate in joint decision making, and to develop the person's autonomy and self-efficacy. The nurse helps people more fully use their strengths and resources and has knowledge of their illnesses and themselves. . . . The nature of the nurse–person relationship is reciprocal and mutual; each partner gives and receives and, thus, the relationship is balanced. It involves the continual negotiation of goals, roles, and responsibilities. Both partners give up some autonomy as they value and trust the other's expertise. Both partners gain and grow" (Gottlieb & Feeley, 2006, p. 6). "Collaboration is not coercion, cooperation, or co-opting." (Buck, 2011).

Sister Simone Roach's Attributes of Professional Caring

In her book *The Human Act of Caring*, first published in 1992, Dr. Simone Roach put forth the notion that "caring is an essential ingredient in human development and survival" (p. 2). Roach claimed that nurses' professional caring has five important attributes: (a) *compassion*, (b) *competence*, (c) *confidence*, (d) *conscience*, and (e) *commitment*. In the 2002 edition of the book, she added the sixth attribute, *comportment* (see Box 4.3 for a description of each).

BOX 4.3 ROACH'S ATTRIBUTES OF PROFESSIONAL CARING

Roach claims that nurses' professional caring has six important attributes:

1. *Compassion:* a sensitivity to the pain and brokenness of the other; a quality of presence that allows one to share with and make room for the other

2. *Competence:* having the knowledge, judgment, skills, energy, experience, and motivation required to respond adequately to the demands of the professional responsibilities

3. *Confidence:* the self-belief that fosters trusting relationships

4. *Conscience:* a state of moral awareness that grows with experience

5. *Commitment:* a complex, affective response characterized by convergence between desires and obligations and by the deliberate choice to act in accordance with them

6. *Comportment:* use of dress, language, and personal bearing to communicate caring and respect for the dignity of both the patient and the nurse

Source: Adapted from M.S. Roach (2002). *The Human Act of Caring: A Blueprint for the Health Professions* (2nd revised edition). Ottawa, ON: CHA Press.

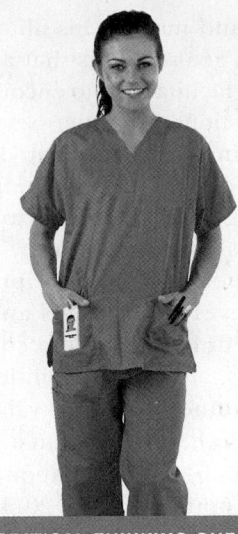

Case Study 4

Kaili is a 32-year-old man with human immunodeficiency virus (HIV) infection. His first acquired immuno-deficiency syndrome (AIDS)–defining illness caused his weight to drop from 80 kg to 54 kg because of intractable diarrhea. The physician thought caloric intake was of primary importance and urged Kaili to eat whatever he desired. Medications for the diarrhea were also prescribed, but Kaili was not happy because of the adverse effects of these medications. Since Kaili was getting worse, the nurse argued that he needed intravenous feedings and that his oral intake should be restricted to bland foods until the diarrhea stopped. The nurse suggested further that additional foods could be added one at a time, based on Kaili's tolerance of them. Kaili's family and friends offered to manage his intake.

The physician's stance was that AIDS was similar to advanced cancer in terms of quality of life, so he would not order intravenous feedings, just as he would not for someone with advanced cancer. The nurse argued that this was Kaili's first AIDS infection and that his prognosis was better than that for an individual with advanced cancer. The nurse wanted to stop the diarrhea and supplement nutrition in the meantime. Kaili's friends and family were pleased with the nurse's approach, but Kaili was not as easily convinced.

CRITICAL THINKING QUESTIONS

1. What concepts are present in this case?

2. How are the nurse and the physician defining the paradigm? What are their main perspectives?

3. How might Florence Nightingale analyze this situation?

4. Which of the nursing models in this chapter best supports the nurse's plan of care?

Check the eText in MyNursingLab for answers and explanations.

KEY TERMS

assumptions *p. 60*

concept *p. 59*

conceptual framework
  p. 59

conceptual model
  p. 59

empiricist tradition
  p. 60

epistemology *p. 59*

ethics *p. 59*

interpretive tradition
  p. 60

metaparadigm *p. 62*

ontology *p. 59*

paradigm *p. 60*

scientific method *p. 60*

theory *p. 59*

CHAPTER HIGHLIGHTS

- Nursing is now deeply involved in identifying its own unique knowledge base—that is, the body of knowledge essential to nursing practice, or a nursing science.

- Nurses must communicate exactly what makes their place in the interdisciplinary team unique and important.

- Theories offer ways of conceptualizing a discipline in clear, explicit terms that can be communicated to others.

- Because opinions about the nature and structure of nursing vary, theories continue to be developed. Each nursing theory bears the name of the person or group who developed it and reflects the beliefs of the developer.

- The theories vary considerably in (a) their level of abstraction; (b) their conceptualization of the client, health and illness, and nursing; and (c) their ability to describe, explain, or predict. Some theories are broad in scope; others are limited.

- Nursing theories serve several essential purposes, some of which are to differentiate the focus of nursing from those of other professions; to structure professional nursing practice, education, and research; to help build a common nursing terminology to use in communicating with other health care professionals; and to enhance the autonomy of nursing by defining its own independent functions.

- Because the primary purpose of nursing theory is to generate scientific knowledge, nursing theory and nursing research are closely related. Scientific knowledge is derived from testing hypotheses generated by theories for nursing. Research determines the utility of those hypotheses, and research findings may be developed into theories for nursing.

- The major distinction between a theory and a conceptual framework or model is the level of abstraction, with the conceptual framework being more abstract than theory. A conceptual model is a system of related concepts or a conceptual diagram. Its major purpose is to give clear and explicit direction to the three areas of nursing: practice, education, and research. A theory generates knowledge in a field.

- Nursing theories address and specify relationships among four major concepts, the building blocks of theory: nursing, health and illness, environment, and the person or client.

- Each nurse theorist's definitions of these four major concepts vary in accordance with personal

philosophy, scientific orientation, experience in nursing, and how that experience has affected the theorist's view of nursing.

- Conceptual models for nursing relate to the nursing process in that they are operationalized or made real by the use of the nursing process. How nurses view human beings influences how they assess and intervene.

- Today, models for nursing are being refined in accordance with societal needs and with their tested usefulness.

ASSESS YOUR LEARNING

1. What is true about philosophical thinking in nursing?

   a. It provides a graphical illustration of how concepts within the profession are related to one another.

   b. Nursing philosophy offers a way of conceptualizing the discipline in clear, explicit terms that can be communicated to others.

   c. There is only one philosophical perspective that is appropriate for nursing practice.

   d. It provides a foundation for the development and analysis of concepts and theories used to articulate nursing knowledge.

2. Nursing theory is important to the development of the nursing discipline for what reason?

   a. It specifies the direction of research efforts in the profession.

   b. It tells us exactly how to act in various situations.

   c. It articulates the role of nurses and differentiates nursing from other professions.

   d. It helps us to question our assumptions.

3. Which of the following describes the concept of caring?

   a. Concrete

   b. Objective

   c. Empirical

   d. Abstract

4. While Jane and Marcy are studying for a nursing exam, Marcy asks what the difference is between a theory and a conceptual framework. Which statement made by Jane would reflect an accurate understanding of the two terms?

   a. "A theory explicitly states the relationship between concepts, whereas a conceptual framework is a group of related concepts."

   b. "A theory is more abstract than a conceptual framework."

   c. "There is absolutely no difference between the terms *theory* and *conceptual framework;* the terms are used interchangeably."

   d. "A theory is limited in scope, and its purpose is to give direction to nursing research, practice, and education, whereas a conceptual framework is broad in scope, and its purpose is to relate concepts through definitions."

5. A nurse is taking care of a pediatric client who has undergone surgery for a ruptured appendix. Postoperatively, the nurse is reluctant to administer any analgesics to her client because she believes children experience pain less than adults do. Her belief exemplifies what?

   a. A philosophical inquiry

   b. An ethical opinion

   c. An assumption

   d. A physiological fact

6. In 1978, the nursing scholar Carper identified four patterns of nursing knowledge, including empirics, aesthetics, personal knowledge, and ethics. What area of philosophical inquiry does this represent?

   a. Ontology

   b. Epistemology

   c. Paradigm

   d. Scientific method

7. Nurse John has been working with Lana, an inpatient with a history of depression and suicide ideation, for the past 2 weeks. In conversation, Lana has demonstrated readiness for discharge and has asked John to help her access services in the community to help her cope when she goes home. According to Peplau's interpersonal relations model, John and Lana are demonstrating which phase of the nurse–client relationship?

   a. Orientation

   b. Identification

   c. Exploitation

   d. Termination

8. Which abstract concept is generally included in the metaparadigm of nursing, the global framework of the profession?

    a. Caring

    b. Research

    c. Client

    d. Practice

9. Many of the nursing theorists use the concept of caring as a strong element within their theory. Which of the following theorists is BEST known for her theory on caring?

    a. Florence Nightingale

    b. Jean Watson

    c. Virginia Henderson

    d. Madeleine Leininger

10. The UBC (University of British Columbia) model of nursing could be considered which type of theory?

    a. Systems

    b. Interpersonal

    c. Caring

    d. Developmental

Check the eText in MyNursingLab for answers and explanations.

WEBLINKS

Hahn School of Nursing and Health Science: Nursing Theory and Research

http://www.sandiego.edu/academics/nursing/theory

This site was developed by the Faculty of Nursing, University of Alberta, and provides an overview of a number of nursing theorists. It is now hosted by the Hahn School of Nursing and Health Sciences at the University of San Diego, California.

Clayton State University Department of Nursing: Nursing Theory Link Page

http://www.clayton.edu/health/nursing/nursingtheory

This site provides access to the writings of a number of nursing theorists.

Information and Resources for Nurses Worldwide

http://www.nurses.info/nursing_theory_accepted_theories. htm

This website has links to numerous sites for nursing theory and nurse theorists.

International Consortium of Parse Scholars' Home Page

http://www.humanbecoming.org

This is a website for Dr. Rosemarie Parse, author of Illumination: The Humanbecoming Theory in Practice and Research.

Health as Expanding Consciousness

http://www.healthasexpandingconsciousness.org

This website features Dr. Margaret Newman's theory of nursing health as expanding consciousness.

MyNursingLab

REFERENCES

Allen, F. M. (1981). The health dimension in nursing practice: Notes on nursing in primary health care. *Journal of Advanced Nursing 6*, 153–154.

Allen, M. (1986). A developmental health model: Nursing as continuous inquiry (audio tape). In series *Nursing Theory Congress. Theoretical pluralism: Direction for a practice discipline.* Markham, ON: Audio Archives of Canada.

Alligood, M. (2010). *Nursing theory: Utilization and application* (4th ed.). St. Louis, MO: Mosby.

Alligood, M. & Tomey, A. (2010). *Nursing theorists and their work* (7th ed.). St. Louis, MO: Mosby.

Bergum, V. (1989). *Woman to mother: A transformation.* Granby, MA: Bergin & Garvey.

Bishop, A., & Scudder, J. (1999). A philosophical interpretation of nursing. *Scholarly Inquiry for Nursing Practice, 13*(1), 17–27.

Buck, M. (2011). *Excerpts from undergraduate nursing student handbook.* Montreal, PQ: McGill University.

Cameron, B. (1992). The nursing "how are you?" *Phenomenology & Pedagogy, 10,* 173–185.

Campbell, M. (1987). *The UBC model for nursing: Directions for practice.* Vancouver, BC: University of British Columbia School of Nursing.

Canadian Nurses Association. (2002). *Evidence-based decision-making and nursing practice.* Ottawa, ON: Author.

Carper, B. (1978). Fundamental patterns of knowing in nursing. *Advances in Nursing Science, 1*(1), 13-23.

Chinn, P., & Kramer, M. (2011). *Integrated theory and knowledge development in nursing* (8th ed.) St. Louis, MO: Mosby.

Dunphy, L. (2010). Florence Nightingale's legacy of caring and its applications. In M. E. Parker & M. Smith (Eds.), *Nursing theories and nursing practice* (3rd ed.) (pp. 35–53). Philadelphia, PA: Davis.

Edwards, S. (1997). What is philosophy of nursing? *Journal of Advanced Nursing, 25,* 1089–1093.

Fawcett, J. (2005). *Contemporary nursing knowledge: Analysis and evaluation of nursing models and theories.* Philadelphia, PA: Davis.

Fry, S. (1992). Neglect of philosophical inquiry in nursing: Cause and effect. In J. Kikuchi & H. Simmons (Eds.), *Philosophic inquiry in nursing* (pp. 85–96). Newbury Park, CA: Sage.

Fry, S. (1999). The philosophy of nursing. *Scholarly Inquiry for Nursing Practice, 13*(1), 5–15.

Gadow, S. (1994). Whose body? Whose story? The question about narrative in women's health care. *Soundings, 77*(3/4), 295–307.

Gottlieb, L. N. (1998). Evolutionary principles can guide nursing's future development. *Journal of Advanced Nursing, 28*(5), 1099–1105.

Gottlieb, L. N., & Feeley, N. (2006). *The collaborative partnership approach to care: A delicate balance.* Toronto, ON: Elsevier Canada.

Gottlieb, L. N., & Rowat, K. (1987). The McGill Model of Nursing: A practice-derived mode. *Advances in Nursing Scholarship, 9*(4), 51–61.

Henderson, V. (1966). *The nature of nursing: A definition and its implications for practice, research, and education.* Riverside, NJ: Macmillan.

Henderson, V. A. (1991). *The nature of nursing: Reflections after 25 years.* New York, NY: National League for Nursing Press. Pub. No. 15–2346.

Johnson, J. A. (1994). Dialectical examination of nursing art. *Advances in Nursing Science, 17*(1), 1–14.

Kikuchi, J. (1992). Nursing questions that science cannot answer. In J. Kikuchi & H. Simmons (Eds.), *Philosophic inquiry in nursing* (pp. 26–37). Newbury Park, CA: Sage.

Kikuchi, J. & Simmons, H. (1994). A pragmatic philosophy of nursing: Threat or promise? In J. Kikuchi & H. Simmons (Eds.), *Developing a philosophy of nursing* (pp. 79–94). Thousand Oaks, CA: Sage.

Lawler, J. (1997). *The body in nursing.* Melbourne, Australia: Churchill Livingstone.

Leininger, M. M. (1985). Transcultural care diversity and universality: A theory of nursing. *Nursing and Health Care, 6,* 208–212.

Leininger, M. M. (1988). Leininger's theory of nursing: Cultural care, diversity and universality. *Nursing Science Quarterly, 1*(4), 152–160.

Leininger, M. M. (Ed.). (1991). *Culture care diversity and universality: A theory of nursing.* New York, NY: National League for Nursing Press. Pub. No. 15–2402.

Leininger, M., & McFarland, M. (2006) *Cultural care, diversity and universality: A worldwide nursing theory.* Sudbury, ON: Jones and Bartlett.

Liaschenko, J. (1997). Ethics and the geography of nurse–patient relationship: Spatial vulnerabilities and gendered space. *Scholarly Inquiry for Nursing Practice, 11*(1), 45–59.

McFarland, M. (2010). Part two: Application of Leininger's theory of culture care diversity and universality. In M. E. Parker & M. Smith (Eds.), *Nursing theories and nursing practice* (3rd ed.) (pp. 329–336). Philadelphia, PA: Davis.

Newman, M. (1986). *Health as expanding consciousness.* St. Louis, MO: Mosby.

Newman, M., Sime, A., & Corcoran-Perry, S. (1991). The focus of the discipline of nursing. *Advances in Nursing Science, 14*(1), 1–6.

Nightingale, F. (1957). *Notes on nursing.* Philadelphia, PA: Lippincott. (Original work published 1860).

Parse, R. R. (1981). *Man-living-health: A theory of nursing.* New York, NY: Wiley.

Parse, R. R. (1987). *Nursing science: Major paradigms, theories, and critiques.* Philadelphia, PA: Saunders.

Parse, R. R. (1994). Quality of life: Sciencing and living the art of humanbecoming. *Nursing Science Quarterly, 7*(1), 16–21.

Parse, R. R. (Ed.). (1995). *Illumination: The humanbecoming theory in practice and research.* New York, NY: National League for Nursing Press. Pub. No. 15–2670.

Peplau, H. E. (1952). *Interpersonal relations in nursing.* New York, NY: Putnam.

Public Health Agency of Canada. (2010). *Determinants of health: What makes Canadians healthy.* Retrieved from http://www.phac-aspc.gc.ca/ph-sp/determinants/index-eng.php#determinants

Purkis, M. E. (1997). The "social determinants" of practice: A critical analysis of the discourse of health promotion. *Canadian Journal of Nursing Research, 29*(1), 47–62.

Roach, Sr. S. (2002). *The human act of caring: A blueprint for the health professions* (2nd Rev. Ed.). Ottawa, ON: Canadian Hospital Association Press.

Roy, C. (1976). *Introduction to nursing: An adaptation model.* Englewood Cliffs, NJ: Prentice-Hall.

Roy, C. (1997). Future of the Roy model: Challenge to redefine adaptation. *Nursing Science Quarterly, 10*(1), 42–48.

Roy, C., & Zahn, L. (2010). Sister Callista Roy's adaptation model. In M. E. Parker & M. Smith (Eds.), *Nursing theories and nursing practice* (3rd ed.) (pp. 167–181). Philadelphia, PA: Davis.

Salsberry, P. (1994). A philosophy of nursing: What it is? What it is not? In J. Kikuchi & H. Simmons (Eds.), *Developing a philosophy of nursing* (pp. 11–19). Thousand Oaks, CA: Sage.

Smith, M. (1994). Arriving at a philosophy of nursing: Discovering? Constructing? Evolving? In J. Kikuchi & H. Simmons (Eds.), *Developing a philosophy of nursing* (pp. 43–59). Thousand Oaks, CA: Sage.

Watson, J. (1979). *Nursing: The philosophy and science of caring.* Boston, MA: Little, Brown.

Watson, J. (1988). *Nursing: Human science and human care: A theory of nursing.* New York, NY: National League for Nursing Press. Pub. No. 15–2236.

Watson, J. (2005) Jean Watson: Theory of human caring. In M. E. Parker (Ed.), *Nursing theories and nursing practice* (2nd ed.) (pp. 295–301). Philadelphia, PA: Davis.

Watson, J., & Woodward, T. (2010). Jean Watson's theory of human caring. In M. E. Parker & M. Smith (Eds.), *Nursing theories and nursing practice* (3rd ed.) (pp. 351–369). Philadelphia, PA: Davis.

Chapter 5

Values, Ethics, and Advocacy

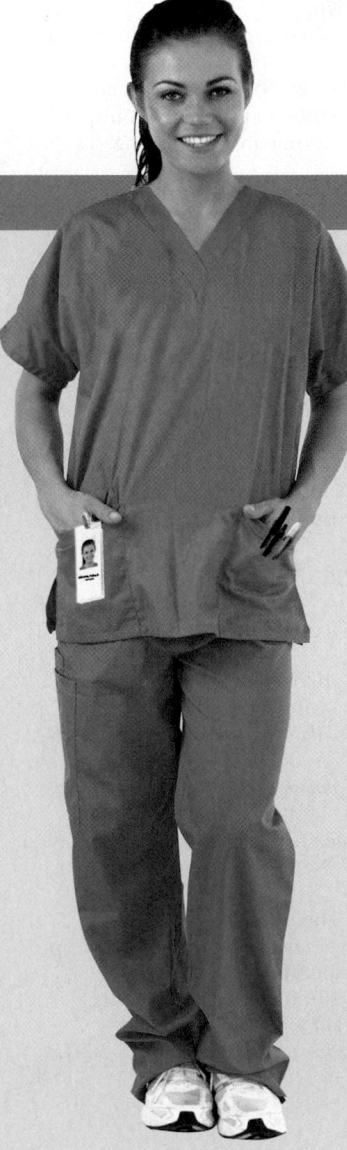

LEARNING OUTCOMES

After studying this chapter, you will be able to:

1. Explain how values, moral frameworks, and codes of ethics affect moral decisions.

2. Explain how nurses can use their knowledge of values and values clarification to facilitate ethical decision making by clients.

3. Identify the moral issues and principles involved when presented with an ethical situation.

4. Explain the uses and limitations of professional codes of ethics.

5. Describe reflective practice in nursing.

6. Describe common ethical problems facing health care professionals, including moral distress, moral residue, and integrity.

7. Describe ways in which nurses can enhance their ethical decision making and practice.

8. Discuss the advocacy role of the nurse.

I n their daily work, nurses deal with intimate and fundamental human events, such as birth, death, and suffering. They must evaluate the morality of their own actions when they face the many ethical issues that surround such sensitive areas. Because of the special nature of the nurse–client relationship, nurses are the ones who support and advocate for clients and families who are facing difficult choices and for those who are living with the results of choices that others make for and about them. The nurse is frequently confronted with decisions about the rightness or wrongness of particular actions within a given context. It is essential, therefore, that nurses have a strong grounding in ethics and a sound approach to ethical decision making.

Ethical issues in nursing evolve to reflect the challenges facing society. Although numerous ethical challenges affect patients and families in health care settings, a panel of Canadian clinical bioethicists identified 10 that they felt were the most pressing (Breslin, MacRae, Bell, & Singer, 2005). The Nursing and Canadian Society box lists these by rank. Nurses face many of these challenges on a daily basis.

According to the Canadian Nurses Association (CNA, 2004), nurses have increasingly expressed concern about their ability to deliver safe care in today's health care system. The potential for compromised safety creates new moral problems and intensifies old ones, making it critical for nurses to make sound moral decisions. Therefore, nurses need to (a) develop sensitivity to the ethical dimensions of nursing practice, (b) examine their own and their clients' values, (c) understand how values influence their decisions, and (d) think ahead to the kinds of moral problems they are likely to face. This chapter explores the influences of values and moral frameworks on the ethical dimensions of nursing practice and on the nurse's role as a client advocate.

Values

Values are enduring beliefs or attitudes about the worth of a person, an object, an idea, or an action. Values are important because they influence decisions and actions, including nurses' ethical decision making. Even though they may be unspoken and perhaps even unconsciously held, values underlie all moral dilemmas. Of course, not all values are moral values. For example, people hold values about work, family, religion, politics, money, and relationships, to name just a few. Values are often taken for granted. In the same way that people are not constantly aware of their breathing, they usually do not think about their values; they simply accept them and act on them.

A **value set** is the small group of values held by an individual. People organize their sets of values internally along a continuum from most important to least important, forming a **value system**. Value systems are basic to

a way of life, give direction to life, and form the basis of behaviour—especially behaviour that is based on decisions or choices.

Values consist of beliefs and attitudes, which are related, but not identical, to values. People have many different beliefs and attitudes but only a small number of values. **Beliefs** (or opinions) are interpretations or conclusions that people accept as true. They are based more on faith than on fact and may or may not be true. Beliefs do not necessarily involve values. For example, the statement "If I study hard I will get a good grade" expresses a belief that does not involve a value. By contrast, the statement "Good grades are really important to me, and I must study hard to obtain good grades" involves both a value and a belief.

Attitudes are mental positions or feelings toward a person, an object, or an idea (e.g., acceptance, compassion, openness). Typically, an attitude lasts over time, whereas a belief may last only briefly. Attitudes are often judged as bad or good, positive or negative, whereas beliefs are judged as correct or incorrect. Attitudes have thinking and behavioural aspects. Attitudes vary greatly among individuals. For example, some clients may feel strongly about their need for privacy, whereas others may dismiss it as unimportant.

Values Transmission

Values are learned through observation and experience. As a result, they are heavily influenced by a person's sociocultural environment—that is, by societal traditions; by cultural, ethnic, and religious groups; and by family and peer groups. For example, if a parent consistently demonstrates honesty in dealing with others, his or her child will probably begin to value honesty. Nurses should keep

Nursing and Canadian Society

Top 10 Health Care Ethics Challenges Facing the Canadian Public

Rank	Scenario	Implications for Nursing Practice
1	"Disagreement between patients/families and health care professionals about treatment decisions" (Breslin et al., 2005)	Ongoing dialogue about treatment between patients or families and providers is a key component of nursing care.
2	"Waiting lists" (Breslin et al., 2005)	Demand for nurses specializing in perioperative, rehabilitation, and surgical nursing will continue to increase.
3	"Access to needed health care resources for the aged, chronically ill and mentally ill" (Breslin et al., 2005)	Nurses with the skills and abilities to provide care to these vulnerable populations across diverse settings is essential.
4	"Shortage of family physicians or primary care teams in both rural and urban settings" (Breslin et al., 2005)	Expanded nursing practice and roles, such as the nurse practitioner, will form a cornerstone of our health care system.
5	"Medical error" (Breslin et al., 2005)	Accountability for individual nursing practice and the recognition of systemic causes of medical error will gain importance.
6	"Withholding/withdrawing life-sustaining treatment in the context of terminal or serious illness" (Breslin et al., 2005)	Earlier and improved communication between health care providers and patients or families can prevent the use of unwanted and inappropriate therapies. Nurses are key players in discussions with families and other providers about withholding or withdrawing therapies.
7	"Achieving informed consent" (Breslin et al., 2005)	Nurses are in a position to assess whether the patient and family have fully understood the procedure for which they gave consent, and nurses can advocate for additional discussion.
8	"Ethical issues related to subject participation in research" (Breslin et al., 2005)	Nursing research often deals with vulnerable populations, such as children, those with dementia, or those who are incarcerated. Nursing researchers abide by guidelines for ethical conduct of research.
9	"Substitute decision making" (Breslin et al., 2005)	When patients are physically or cognitively compromised and unable to consent to medical interventions, nurses work with substitute decision makers, such as family members, to promote sound ethical decisions.
10	"The ethics of surgical innovation and incorporating new technologies for patient care" (Breslin et al., 2005)	Nurses should engage in dialogue with other health care providers to consider the implications of new technologies from an ethical perspective.

Source: Based on Breslen, J. M., MacRae, S. K., Bell, J., & Singer, P. A. (2005). *Top 10 health care ethics challenges facing the public: Views of Toronto bioethicists* (table 1). *BMC Medical Ethics, 6*, 5.

in mind the influence of values on health. For example, some cultures value treatment by a folk healer over that by a health care provider. For additional information about cultural values related to health and illness, see Chapter 11.

PERSONAL VALUES Although people derive values from society and their individual subgroups, they internalize some or all of these values and perceive them as **personal values**. People need societal values to feel accepted, and they need personal values to have a sense of individuality.

PROFESSIONAL VALUES Nurses' **professional values** are acquired during socialization into nursing from codes of ethics, nursing experiences, teachers, and peers. The College of Nurses of Ontario (2005) identifies the following values as being most important to nursing care: client well-being, client choice, privacy and confidentiality, respect for life, the maintaining of commitments, truthfulness, and fairness. The Registered Nurses' Association of Ontario (RNAO, 2006) has framed its *Client-Centred Care Best Practice Guidelines* program around a widely accepted set of professional values (see Box 5.1). In client-centred care, the client is viewed as a whole person

BOX 5.1 CLIENT-CENTRED BEST PRACTICE RECOMMENDATION

Nurses embrace as foundational to client-centred care the following values and beliefs:

- Respect
- Human dignity
- Clients are experts for their own lives
- Clients as leaders
- Clients' goals coordinate care of the health care team
- Continuity and consistency of care and caregiver
- Timeliness
- Responsiveness
- Universal access to care

These values and beliefs must be incorporated into, and demonstrated throughout, every aspect of client care and service.

Source: Registered Nurses' Association of Ontario. (2006). *Client centred care* (rev. suppl.). Toronto, ON: Author.

and the approach involves advocacy, empowerment, and respect for the client's autonomy, voice, self-determination, and participation in decision making. Table 5.1 lists the values and professional behaviours associated with these values.

Values Clarification

Values clarification is a process by which people identify, examine, and develop their own individual values. A principle of values clarification is that no one set of values is right for everyone. When people can identify their values, they can retain or change them and thus act based on freely chosen, rather than unconscious, values. Values clarification promotes personal growth by fostering awareness, empathy, and insight. Therefore, it is an important step that nurses must take in dealing with ethical problems.

Often, values clarification is an internal process not apparent to the person. In some cases, a values clarification

TABLE 5.1 Essential Nursing Values and Behaviours

Values	Professional Behaviours
Altruism is a concern for the welfare and well-being of others. In professional practice, altruism is reflected by the nurse's concern for the welfare of patients, other nurses, and other health care providers. *Autonomy* is the right to self-determination. Professional practice reflects autonomy when the nurse respects patients' rights to make decisions about their health care. *Human dignity* is respect for the inherent worth and uniqueness of individuals and populations. In professional practice, human dignity is reflected when the nurse values and respects all patients and colleagues. *Integrity* is acting in accordance with an appropriate code of ethics and accepted standards of practice. Integrity is reflected in professional practice when the nurse is honest and provides care based on an ethical framework that is accepted within the profession. *Social justice* is upholding moral, legal, and humanistic principles. This value is reflected in professional practice when the nurse works to ensure equal treatment under the law and equal access to quality health care.	1. Demonstrate the professional standards of moral, ethical, and legal conduct. 2. Assume accountability for personal and professional behaviours. 3. Promote the image of nursing by modelling the values and articulating the knowledge, skills, and attitudes of the nursing profession. 4. Demonstrate professionalism, including attention to appearance, demeanour, respect for self and others, and attention to professional boundaries with patients and families as well as among caregivers. 5. Demonstrate an appreciation of the history of and contemporary issues in nursing and their impact on current nursing practice. 6. Reflect on one's own beliefs and values as they relate to professional practice. 7. Identify personal, professional, and environmental risks that impact personal and professional choices and behaviours. 8. Communicate to the health care team one's personal bias on difficult health care decisions that impact one's ability to provide care. 9. Recognize the impact of attitudes, values, and expectations on the care of the very young, frail older adults, and other vulnerable populations. 10. Protect patient privacy and confidentiality of patient records and other privileged communications. 11. Access interprofessional and intraprofessional resources to resolve ethical and other practice dilemmas. 12. Act to prevent unsafe, illegal, or unethical care practices. 13. Articulate the value of pursuing practice excellence, lifelong learning, and professional engagement to foster professional growth and development. 14. Recognize the relationship between personal health, self-renewal, and the ability to deliver sustained quality care

Source: From American Association of Colleges of Nursing. (2008). *The essentials of baccalaureate education for professional nursing practice* (pp. 8–9). Washington, DC: Author. Reprinted with permission.

exercise can be useful in helping individuals or groups to become more aware of their values and how they may influence their actions. For example, asking a client to agree or disagree with a list of statements or to rank in order of importance a list of beliefs can assist the nurse and client to make the client's values more open so they can be considered in planning the client's care. See Table 5.2 for an example of a general values clarification exercise.

TABLE 5.2 Questionnaire for Personal Values Clarification

Rating on a Scale of 1 to 3*	Personal Value	Example of Activity That Demonstrates That Value
	Help Society	Do something which contributes to improving the world we live in
	Help Others	Be directly included in helping other people, either individually or in small groups
	Work Ethics	Feeling satisfied from a job well done
	Enjoyment of Life	Enjoying life, having fun in life
	Honesty	Being able to tell people what I really think and believe; having them be honest with me
	Approval	Having other people like me
	Competition	Engage in activities which pit my abilities against others
	Make Decisions	Have the power to decide courses of action
	Respect	Having other people think highly of me and hold me in good esteem
	Leadership	Be in a position to influence the attitudes or opinions of other people
	Knowledge	Understanding gained through study, and/or experience
	Work Mastery	Become an expert in whatever work I do
	Peace	Living in a peaceful, harmonious society and environment
	Creativity	Have the opportunity to create new things, ideas, products, works of art
	Freedom	Being able to do or say what I want
	Good Character	Knowing inside that I do the right, moral, just thing
	Loyalty	Sticking with people who are close to me and/or believe in what I do
	Justice	Being fair and just and having others treat me fairly and justly
	Stability	Have a routine and duties that are largely predictable
	Safety	Be assured of being safe and free from harm
	Recognition	Be publicly recognized
	Children	Having happy, healthy children
	Excitement	Experience a high degree of (or frequent) excitement
	Adventure	Have duties which require frequent risk-taking
	Power	Having authority over others
	Economic Security	Having enough money to buy whatever I want

TABLE 5.2 (*continued*)

Rating on a Scale of 1 to 3*	Personal Value	Example of Activity That Demonstrates That Value
	Leisure	Having time for hobbies, sports, other activities
	Inner Harmony	Being at peace with one's self
	Wealth	Profit, gain, making a lot of money
	Trustworthiness	Having people trust me and being able to trust them
	Challenge	Do activities that use my physical and/or mental capabilities
	Independence	Be able to determine the nature of my day without significant direction from others
	Change and Variety	Varied, frequently changing responsibilities and settings
	Moral Fulfillment	Feel that whatever I do contributes to a set of moral standards that I feel are very important
	Community	Being a part of a close and supportive community
	Caring	Experiencing love and affection daily
	Health	Being free from disease or sickness, feeling good physically
	Religion/Spirituality	Doing what's right according to my religious and/or spiritual beliefs
	Family	Making sure my family members are healthy and safe
	Friendship	Having good, reliable friends I can count on

*1 = Things I value very much; 2 = Things I value; 3 = Things I don't value very much.

Now, list your top five essential values (from those rated 1 above).
MY FIVE MOST ESSENTIAL VALUES
1.   4.
2.   5.
3.

Source: From Johns Hopkins Bloomberg School of Public Centre for Communication Programs. (2002). *Questionnaire for values clarification.* Copyright 2002. Retrieved from http://www. jhuccp.org/research/download/Valuesinstrument.pdf

CLARIFYING THE NURSE'S VALUES Nurses and nursing students need to examine the values they hold about life, death, health, and illness (College of Nurses of Ontario, 2005). One strategy for gaining awareness of personal values is to consider your own attitudes about specific issues, such as abortion or euthanasia, by asking the following questions: Can I accept this, or live with this? Why does this bother me? What would I do or want done in this situation? Nurses use critical thinking (see Chapter 21) to reflect on various viewpoints and previous experiences that may have influenced their own values.

CLARIFYING CLIENT VALUES To plan effective care, nurses need to identify clients' values as they influence and relate to a particular health problem. For example, a client with failing eyesight will probably place a high value on the ability to see, and a client with chronic pain will value comfort. Normally, people take such things for granted. The nurse needs to ask such questions as these: "What really matters to you in this situation?" "What would have to happen to make this seem like a good experience for you?" "What do you think you want to have happen here?" "Who do you want to make decisions for you?" "What do you want from me as a nurse?" The reflective nurse will soon recognize that without an understanding of a client's values, it is impossible to answer the questions. Therefore, this understanding is foundational for ethical practice. For information about health beliefs and values, see Chapter 7.

When clients hold unclear or conflicting values that are detrimental to their health, the nurse should use values clarification as an intervention. Examples of behaviours that may indicate the need for clarification of health values are listed in Table 5.3 on the next page.

TABLE 5.3 Client Behaviours That May Indicate Unclear/Conflicting Values

Behaviour	Example
Ignoring a health care professional's advice	A client with heart disease who values hard work ignores advice to exercise regularly.
Inconsistent communication or behaviour	A pregnant woman says she wants a healthy baby but continues to drink alcohol and smoke tobacco.
Numerous admissions to a health care agency for the same problem	A middle-aged, obese woman repeatedly seeks help for back pain but does not lose weight.
Confusion or uncertainty about which course of action to take	A woman wants to obtain a job to meet financial obligations but also wants to stay at home to care for her ailing husband.

The following process may help clients clarify their values:

1. *List alternatives.* Make sure that the client is aware of all alternative actions. Ask, "Are you considering other courses of action?" "Tell me about them."

2. *Examine possible consequences of choices.* Make sure the client has thought about the possible results of each action. Ask, "What do you think you will gain from doing that?" "What benefits do you foresee?"

3. *Choose freely.* To determine whether the client chose freely, ask, "Did you have any say in that decision?" "Do you have a choice?"

4. *Feel good about the choice.* To determine how the client feels, ask, "How do you feel about that decision (or action)?" Because some clients may not feel satisfied with their decision, a more sensitive question may be "Some people feel good after a decision is made; others feel bad. How do you feel?"

5. *Affirm the choice.* Ask, "How will you discuss this with others (family, friends)?"

6. *Act on the choice.* To determine whether the client is prepared to act on the decision, ask, for example, "Will it be difficult to tell your partner about this?"

7. *Act with a pattern.* To determine whether the client consistently behaves in a certain way, ask, "How many times have you done that before?" or "Would you act that way again?"

When implementing these seven steps to clarify values, the nurse helps the client think through each question but does not impose personal values. The nurse rarely, if ever, offers an opinion when the client asks for it—and then only with great care or when the nurse is an expert in the content area. Because each situation is different, what the nurse would choose in his or her own life may not be relevant to the client's circumstances.

Thus, if the client asks the nurse, "What would you have done in my situation?" it is best to redirect the question back to the client rather than answering from a personal point of view.

CLARIFYING VALUES AND OBLIGATIONS IN CARE SITUATIONS Nurses need to understand their own values in the broader sense, but they also need to identify values that are relevant in individual care situations. They need to ask themselves the following: What factors in this situation might affect how I think about "right" action? Are there particular contextual features that might change my views? For example, the nurse might value autonomy as a general rule but might question this value if it means supporting a client's decision to commit suicide.

Because of their unique position in the health care hierarchy, nurses often experience conflicts among their loyalties and obligations to clients, families, other health care providers, employing institutions, and licensing bodies. Client needs may conflict with institutional policies, physician preferences, needs of the client's family, or even laws. According to the CNA's code of ethics, the nurse's first loyalty is to the client. However, it is not always easy to determine which action best serves the client's needs. For instance, a nurse may think that a client needs to be provided with the most current evidence-based information, but that information may conflict with the physician's advice; if the client goes against that advice, it may damage the physician–client relationship. The nurse will then have to decide what the greater good is in the situation.

Ethical Obligations

Making a commitment to treat others with respect and to uphold the values of well-being, choice, and dignity are fundamental to nursing. Nurses have an obligation to maintain commitments that they assume as regulated health care professionals, such as keeping promises, being honest, and meeting implicit or explicit obligations toward their clients, themselves, one another, the nursing profession, other members of the health care team, and quality practice settings (College of Nurses of Ontario, 2005). However, despite such clear moral commitments, nurses may still face situations in which the right action is not easily identified (Davis, Fowler & Aroskar, 2009). A good decision is one that is in the client's best interests and at the same time preserves the integrity of all involved. Nurses have **ethical obligations**, or responsibilities imposed as a result of ethical imperatives, to their clients, to the agency that employs them, and to other health care professionals. Unfortunately, there will be times when some of these obligations appear to be in conflict, as when the nurse feels a strong duty to follow institutional policy but at the same time feels that the policy does not serve the best interests of the client.

Ethics

The term **ethics** has several meanings in common use. It refers to (a) a method of inquiry that helps people understand the morality of human behaviour (i.e., it is the study of morality), (b) the practices or beliefs of a certain group (e.g., medical ethics, nursing ethics), and (c) formal statements about expected standards of moral behaviour of a particular group. Thus, it is generally used to refer to a broader understanding of moral life through the application of theories and sets of principles that give structure to morality (Yeo & Moorhouse, 1996).

Nurses are often faced with moral quandaries in practice, that is, with decisions about *ought, should, good,* and *bad*. For example, the nurse might have to decide about whether or not to use physical restraints on clients who are confused and in danger of hurting themselves. The question is whether taking away a person's free choice is truly in that person's best interests and, therefore, whether the nurse *ought* or *ought not* to do it. The nurse's action will be guided by his or her individual belief system (morality) and by the broadly accepted standards of the society and the profession (as articulated in ethics theory and codes of ethics). A **code of ethics** is a formalized statement of a group's beliefs.

When faced with difficult decisions, it is important that the nurse be able to distinguish between *ethics* and *law*. Laws do reflect the moral values of a society, and they offer guidance in determining what is moral. However, an action can be legal but not moral. For example, an order for full resuscitation of a dying client is legal, but the nurse could question whether the act is moral. Conversely, an action can be moral but illegal. If a child at home stops breathing, it is moral but not legal to exceed the speed limit when driving to the hospital. The legal aspects of nursing practice are covered in Chapter 6.

Moral Theories

Moral theories, which are a set of abstract principles, provide different lenses through which nurses can view and clarify disturbing client care situations. Nurses can use moral theories in developing explanations for their ethical decisions and actions and in discussing problem situations with others. Three types of moral theories are widely used, and they can be differentiated by their emphasis on (a) consequences, (b) principles and duties, or (c) relationships.

Consequence-based (teleological) theories look to an action's outcomes (consequences) in judging whether that action is right or wrong. **Utilitarianism**, one form of consequentialist theory, views a good act as one that brings the most good and the least harm for the greatest number of people. This is called the **principle of utility**. This approach is often used in making decisions about the funding and delivery of health care. Teleological theories focus on issues of fairness.

Principles-based (deontological) theories involve logical and formal processes and emphasize individual rights, duties, and obligations. The morality of an action is determined not by its consequences but by whether it is done according to an impartial, objective principle. For example, while following the rule "Do not lie," a nurse might believe he or she should tell the truth to a dying client, even though the physician has given instruction not to do so. There are many deontological theories; each justifies the rules of acceptable behaviour differently.

Relationships-based (caring) theories stress courage, generosity, commitment, and the need to nurture and maintain relationships (Figure 5.1). Unlike the two preceding theories, which frame problems in terms of justice

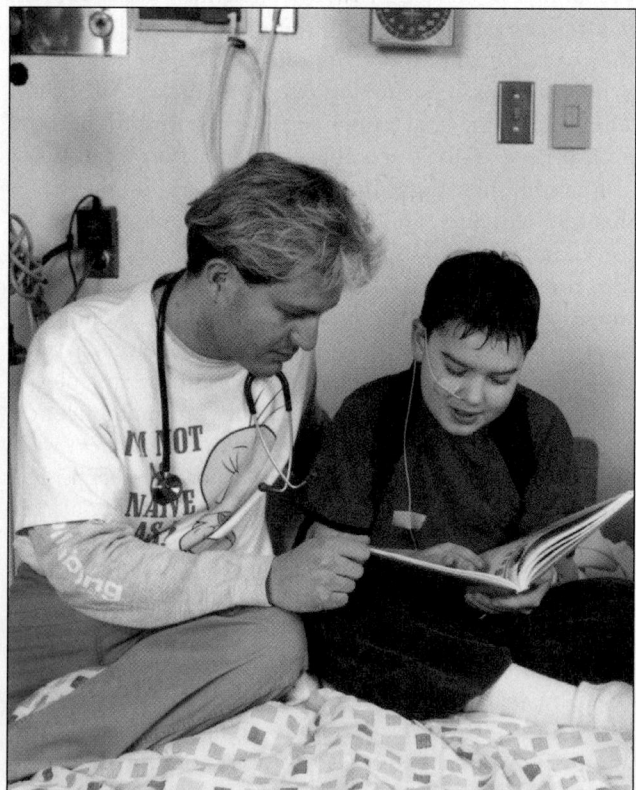

FIGURE 5.1 Relational caring is a professional relationship.

(fairness) and formal reasoning, caring theories (see Chapter 4) judge actions according to a perspective of caring and responsibility. Principles-based theories stress individual rights, but caring theories promote the common good or the welfare of the group.

A moral theory guides moral decisions, but it does not determine the outcome. Imagine a situation in which a frail older client has made it clear that he does not want further surgery, but the family and surgeon insist. Three nurses have each decided that they will not help with preparations for surgery and that they will work through proper channels to try to prevent it. Using consequence-based reasoning, Nurse A thinks, "Surgery will cause him more suffering; he probably will not survive it anyway, and the family may even feel guilty later." Using principles-based reasoning, Nurse B thinks, "This violates the principle of autonomy. This man has a right to decide what happens to his body." Using caring-based reasoning, Nurse C thinks, "My relationship to this client commits me to protecting him and meeting his needs, and I feel such compassion for him. I must try to help the family understand that he needs their support." Each perspective is based on the nurse's moral framework.

Principle-Based Ethics

Principle-based ethics is the most widely known approach to health care ethics. This approach was first described in Beauchamp and Childress's *Principles of Biomedical Ethics* (2009, first published in 1979). Their idea was that when health care providers encountered an ethical problem, they would examine the situation, decide which ethical principles applied, and use them to make a decision. Their belief was that principles would be useful because even if people disagreed about which action was right in a situation, they might be able to agree on the principles that applied. Such an agreement could serve as the basis for a solution that was acceptable to all parties. For example, most people would agree with the principle that nurses are obligated to respect their clients, even if they disagree as to whether the nurse should deceive a particular client about the prognosis. The original principles of bioethics were *autonomy*, beneficence, nonmaleficence, and *justice*. Later, principles of *fidelity* and *veracity* were added, and autonomy was expanded to *respect for persons*. These principles are very useful in discussions about ethical dimensions of particular care situations in nursing, although it is increasingly being realized that the biomedical ethics paradigm falls short of recognizing concepts important to nursing, such as nurturance, compassion, and communication (Ferrell, 2006).

The principle of **autonomy (respect for persons)** states that individuals have the right to make choices about their own lives. It also means showing respect for others and accepting them as unique individuals with personal histories that influence their decision making.

In health care, this means that health care providers must honour the person's right to choose methods or approaches to diagnosis and treatment. Choices must be free and informed, that is, made without coercion and with the benefit of all necessary information (see Chapter 6). Some clients are unable to make their own decisions (e.g., cognitively impaired older persons, young children, or comatose patients); health care professionals are obligated to try to make decisions that, to the best of their knowledge, the persons would make for themselves. Usually, the nurse gains information about the person's preferences from that person's family.

Nonmaleficence is the duty to do no harm. Although this would seem to be a simple principle to follow, in reality, it is complex. Harm can mean intentional harm, risk of harm, and unintentional harm. In nursing, intentional harm is never acceptable; nurses must not deliberately harm patients. However, nurses sometimes inflict harm during a nursing intervention that is intended to be helpful. Causing such harm would not be unethical as such. For example, a nurse may be required to carry out treatments that cause pain or discomfort, such as administering chemotherapy that has the side effects of severe nausea and vomiting. If the principle of nonmaleficence were taken on the surface, it would appear to dictate that the nurse should not carry out such actions. On reflection, however, the nurse would realize that failure to administer the drugs would cause the patient greater harm by allowing the cancer to progress unchecked. Similarly, nurses are often in the position of trying to mobilize patients after surgery, even when they are in pain and resist movement. Again, the nurse must realize that the effects of immobility are potentially more harmful than the increased discomfort. The nurse must consider the risk of harm from various sources and consider which action would be the most beneficial to the patient. Thus, the nurse must examine potential harms *and* benefits in considering whether the acts of harm were unethical. Unintentional harm is often unpredictable and could result from a lack of specific knowledge about a patient or from unexpected consequences of certain actions. Harm of that nature would be an error but would not necessarily have ethical implications, as the intent was positive.

Beneficence is the obligation to "do good." Nurses have a duty to implement actions that benefit their clients, that is, to act in the client's best interests. However, what is considered "good" in any situation is not always clear. Is it better, for instance, to tell a patient the truth about the diagnosis of a terminal disease or withhold the information? Which would be of greater benefit? An important question that arises in discussions of benefit is: Who defines "good"? Should it be the health care professional or the patient and family? For example, a nurse might believe that it is in a patient's best interests to get up and walk, whereas the patient might believe otherwise. The nurse must then consider whose beliefs should prevail in this instance. When health care providers make decisions for clients without seeking their input, it is called **paternalism**. In the past, a paternalistic attitude was accepted; people expected doctors and nurses to make decisions for them. Today, clients are respected as having the ability to make decisions for themselves, and paternalism is not considered ethical. Nurses who want to make decisions for patients "in their best interests" must question whether they are being paternalistic.

Justice is often referred to as fairness. In health care, justice issues arise most often in deciding how scarce resources should be used. Such questions as who should get a heart for transplantation, whether a patient should be discharged to make room for another patient who seems more ill, or whether funding should be directed to heart-health programs or home care for the seniors require justice-based decisions. Nurses make justice decisions all the time in prioritizing care. For example, a nurse making home visits finds one client tearful and depressed and knows that staying for 30 minutes more to talk would help. However, that would take time from another client, who has diabetes and needs a great deal of teaching and observation. Many factors must be weighed in the decision, and a nurse must be prepared to do some hard thinking.

Fidelity means to be faithful to agreements and promises. Nurses often make promises to patients, such as "I'll be right back with a medication for your pain," or "I'll find out for you." Clients take such promises seriously. As professional caregivers, nurses have responsibilities to clients, employers, government, and society, as well as to themselves. Sometimes, these responsibilities are in conflict, as when institutional policy suggests one thing, and the nurse believes the patient would benefit from something else. Nurses need to be prepared to make decisions about where their primary responsibilities lie.

Veracity refers to telling the truth. Although this seems straightforward, in practice, choices are not always clear. Should a nurse tell the truth when it is known that it will cause harm? Does a nurse tell a lie if the lie will relieve anxiety and fear? These kinds of decisions form the basis for many moral dilemmas in nursing.

Although bioethics principles are meant to help the health care provider make decisions, it is never quite as simple as deciding which principle applies in any one case. Often, several principles apply, and the principles may conflict with each other. If a nurse working in community health observes a young mother exhibiting inappropriate parenting practices, does the nurse respect the mother's autonomy and right to care for her child as she sees fit (respecting autonomy), or does the nurse intervene and insist that changes be made (beneficence)? Does a nurse restrain confused senior patients to keep them from hurting themselves (nonmaleficence) or let them wander and risk a serious fall (respecting autonomy)? Such questions are very difficult and require active reflection. The nurse who is insensitive to or unaware of the ethical dimensions of such practice decisions is less likely to choose the most ethically sound course of action.

Nursing Ethics and Relational Ethics

Some authors believe that nursing's ethical foundation must be based on caring and, therefore, nursing is better served by an approach that takes into account the relationship between nurse and patient (Gastmans, 2006). Some also suggest that caring is a **virtue**, that is, an "excellence of character" (Begley, 2005) or a highly valued personality characteristic that predisposes a person to act in a certain way, and that nurses must possess the virtue of caring if they are to make ethical decisions in practice (Armstrong, 2006).

Ethical theories coming from these perspectives are called **relational ethics theories** or **ethics of care**. These theories suggest that we all have a moral obligation to others simply because we are human and that we ought to act in others' best interests. Actions are judged according to whether they demonstrate caring and responsibility. Bioethics theory tends to consider situations more in the abstract, whereas relational theories take into account the individual's personal story or *narrative*. Thus, they are more concrete and rooted in the client's own reality.

Relational ethics theory seems to fit well with the caring concepts that are central to nursing, as it demands that clients be affirmed as persons, not objects (Marck, 2000a, 2000b). However, it is important to remember that caring is not unique to nursing and that some have criticized the caring perspective for (a) reinforcing the stereotype of women as caretakers and (b) overlooking other important moral principles, such as fairness and autonomy (Bowden, 1995). Nonetheless, nursing scholars seem to be in agreement that the commitment to others that is reflected in an attitude of caring is the basis, if not the whole, of nursing ethics (Marck, 2000b).

Nursing Codes of Ethics

No single theory of ethical decision making is universally applicable to nursing. However, within the profession, norms of practice can be used to help the nurse make moral decisions. These norms are reflected in a professional code of ethics, which is a set of ethical principles that (a) is shared by members of the group, (b) reflects their moral judgments over time, and (c) serves as a standard for their professional actions. Codes of ethics usually have higher requirements than do legal standards. Nursing codes of ethics have the following purposes:

- To inform the public about the minimum standards of the profession and help them understand professional nursing conduct
- To provide a sign of the profession's commitment to the public it serves
- To outline the major ethical considerations of the profession
- To provide general guidelines for professional behaviour
- To guide the profession in self-regulation

- To remind nurses of the special responsibility they assume when caring for clients

Codes of ethics for nursing have been developed at the international level by the International Council of Nurses (ICN), and at the national level by different countries. The ICN (2006) *Code of Ethics for Nurses* notes that nurses have four fundamental responsibilities: to promote health, to prevent illness, to restore health, and to alleviate suffering. The CNA *Code of Ethics for Registered Nurses* (2008) articulates the value system held by the nursing profession in Canada and, as such, serves as a blueprint for ethical practice by Canadian nurses [RNs, LPNs/RPNs, RPNs]. However, the code cannot provide answers to particular care decisions. Instead, the code reflects the mandate of professional nursing and the elements that must be considered in making ethical practice decisions. Nurses are responsible for being familiar with the code that governs their practice. Box 5.2 describes the nursing values that are the foundation for the CNA's *Code of Ethics*. See the Weblinks section of this chapter for a link to the complete *Code of Ethics*.

! CLINICAL ALERT

Ethical behaviour is contextual; what is an ethical action or decision in one situation may not be so in a different situation.

BOX 5.2 CANADIAN NURSES ASSOCIATION'S *CODE OF ETHICS FOR REGISTERED NURSES*

The CNA's *Code of Ethics for Registered Nurses* (2008) outlines the values that should guide Canadian nursing practice. Each value is accompanied by an itemized list of ethical responsibilities:

1. *Providing safe, compassionate, competent, and ethical care:* Nurses provide safe, compassionate, competent, and ethical care.

2. *Promoting health and well-being:* Nurses work with people to enable them to attain their highest possible level of health and well-being.

3. *Promoting and respecting informed decision making:* Nurses recognize, respect, and promote a person's right to be informed and make decisions.

4. *Preserving dignity:* Nurses recognize and respect the intrinsic worth of each person.

5. *Maintaining privacy and confidentiality:* Nurses recognize the importance of privacy and confidentiality and safeguard personal, family, and community information obtained in the context of a professional relationship.

6. *Promoting justice:* Nurses uphold principles of justice by safeguarding human rights, equity, and fairness and by promoting the public good.

7. *Being accountable:* Nurses are accountable for their actions and answerable for their practice.

Source: Canadian Nurses Association. (2008). *Code of ethics for registered nurses.* Ottawa, ON: Author. Reprinted with permission.

Ethical Decision Making

In this chapter, we have discussed several types of ethics theory (teleological, deontological, and relational ethics). In addition, we have discussed codes of ethics and the impact of personal and professional values on decision making. How can these various parts be brought together to help a nurse develop a plan to enhance ethical practice? Providing ethical care requires considerable thought and reflection, and ethical decision making can be enhanced if nurses have an understanding of the values that drive their practice.

Making Ethical Decisions

Responsible ethical reasoning is rational and systematic. It should be based on ethical principles and codes rather than solely on emotions, intuition, fixed policies, or precedent (that is, an earlier similar occurrence). One decision-making model is shown in Box 5.3.

A good decision is one that is in the client's best interests and also preserves the integrity of all involved. Nurses have ethical obligations to their clients, to the agency that employs them, and to health care providers. Therefore, nurses must weigh competing factors when making ethical decisions. See Box 5.4 for examples. Although ethical reasoning is principle based and has the client's well-being at its centre, being involved in ethical problems and dilemmas is stressful for a client who has not responded to mainstream therapies. Although legal issues are involved, the nurse must determine if, ethically, the client should be made aware of a potentially effective alternative. Another example is individual nurses' decisions regarding honouring picket lines during employee strikes. The nurse may experience conflict, feeling the need to support coworkers in their efforts to improve working conditions, feeling the need to ensure clients receive care and are not abandoned, and feeling loyalty to the hospital employer.

BOX 5.3 AN ETHICAL DECISION-MAKING MODEL

This is an example of an ethical decision-making model (Toren & Wagner, 2010) that can be used in clinical practice to facilitate ethical choices.

- Define the ethical dilemma.
- Clarify the personal and professional values, ethical principles, and laws involved.
- Identify the alternatives for actions.
- Choose an action.
- Generalize the solution to other similar cases.

Source: Based on Toren, O. & Wagner, N. (2010). Applying an ethical decision-making tool for a nurse management dilemma. *Nursing Ethics, 17,* 393–402.

BOX 5.4 EXAMPLES OF NURSES' OBLIGATIONS IN ETHICAL DECISIONS

Nurses must meet a variety of obligations in making ethical decisions:

- Maximize the client's well-being.
- Balance the client's need for autonomy with family members' responsibilities for the client's well-being.
- Support each family member, and enhance the family support system.
- Carry out agency policies.
- Protect other clients' well-being.
- Protect the nurse's own standards of care.

Reflective Practice

Reflection is a method of accessing, making sense of, and learning through experience (Johns, 1995). As a key competency of self-directed learners, evidence of reflective practice is a mandated element of the continuing competency requirements for most nursing jurisdictions. Schon (1983) described reflective practice several years ago, but it has become part of nursing's professional requirements more recently. Schon described two components: reflection in action and reflection on action. *Reflection in action* outlines the thinking processes in the midst of practice—what contributes to the actions of the novice and experienced nurse. *Reflection on action* is the process of reflecting after the fact and thinking about how one might improve on one's performance when faced with a similar situation in the future. It is this component that has often been termed **reflective practice** in nursing circles today. There are several structures that can assist nursing students and nurses to engage in reflective practice; one that has been quite popular is the

BOX 5.5 EXAMPLES OF REFLECTIVE QUESTIONS

WHAT?

– How did the situation begin?

– What did you observe or hear?

– How did the situation end?

SO WHAT?

– Did you learn something new?

– How might someone else in the situation view the same situation?

– Did anything about the situation surprise you?

– Are you pleased with the outcome?

– Are others in the situation pleased with the outcome? How do you know?

NOW WHAT?

– What learning did you take from this experience?

– Would you engage in the same actions another time? Different actions?

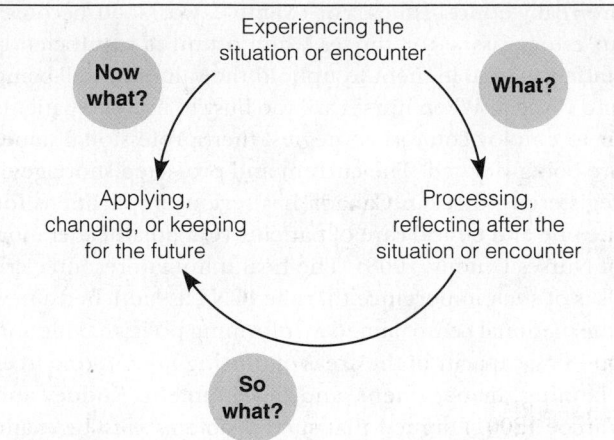

What? The "what" consists of observations and/or information that can be the result of your personal reflections about a specific situation or the results of a broader self, and/or other, assessment.

So What? The "so what" is what you make of the information after thinking about it or reflecting on it, or what it means to you.

Now What? The "now what" is what you will do with the information to reinforce what you feel good about and/or to change knowledge and skills for the future where necessary. "What, so what, and now what" thinking is a critical part of self-reflection.

FIGURE 5.2 "What? So What, and Now What?" Model.

"What—So What—Now What" model. The "What" refers to observations and/or information that can be the result of your personal reflections about a specific situation or the results of an assessment. The "So What" refers to what you make of the information after reflection. The "Now What" is what you will do with the information to reinforce what you feel good about or what changes in knowledge or skills will be made in the future. Figure 5.2 illustrates the process, while Box 5.5 outlines questions that can be asked as part of the process.

Decision Making in Practice

A decision-making framework can help the nurse in making ethical decisions. Frameworks must take into account the facts, beliefs, and values inherent in the situation. Knowing the kinds of questions to ask in a situation is essential if the nurse is to get the necessary information.

Selected Ethical Issues in Nursing

In the past, nurses did not consider themselves to be **moral agents**. Moral agents have the capacity for making moral judgments and for taking actions that are consistent with morality. With changes in the profession, nurses' awareness of ethical issues in practice is growing. Nurses are beginning to realize that many problems at the institutional level are really ethical issues. For example, workload becomes an ethical issue for nurses when a unit is insufficiently staffed to enable them to uphold the values of well-being and respect. When nurses are too busy to listen to patients or to employ comfort strategies, then professional values are being violated. The current and projected shortage of registered nurses in Canada has serious implications for the safe and ethical care of patients (Canadian Federation of Nurses Unions, 2008). The health human resource crisis is of such importance that the ICN has launched a new international centre aimed at informing policymaking and building capacity in the areas of nursing human resources planning, management, and development. Rodney and Varcoe (2001) argued that such problems *must* be examined from an ethics perspective and that nurses must begin to understand that striving for better working conditions is part of nursing's moral imperative. If the quality of work life is unsatisfactory, and the standard of care is compromised, nurses' moral base is eroded.

Developing and maintaining a trusting, caring, and supportive relationship with a client is the foundation of nursing ethics (Gastmans, Dierckx de Casterle, & Schotsmans, 1998). The CNA's *Code of Ethics for Registered Nurses* (2008) indicates the values held by the profession. However, the code acknowledges that "given the complexity of ethical situations, the code can only outline nurses' ethical responsibilities and guide nurses in their reflection and decision-making. It cannot ensure ethical practice" (p. 4). Thus, it points again to the need for nurses to have a clear understanding of their own values.

Nurses must consider how their values might affect the care they give to clients. Certainly, every caregiving situation has moral components and will be affected by the values, beliefs, and attitudes of all those involved. However, some kinds of care situations cause nurses to pay particular attention to their own values. **Moral integrity** refers to the quality of one's character and has integrated virtues including honesty and truthfulness (Butts & Rich, 2005). **Moral dilemmas** are situations involving conflicting ethical claims and often create such questions as these: "What ought I to do?" "What harm and benefit will result from this decision or action?" (Davis, Fowler, & Aroskar, 2009). **Moral distress** occurs when the individual knows the ethically correct action to take but is unable to take the action because of internal or external barriers (Jameton, 1992). As seen in the Evidence-Informed Practice box, situations causing moral distress can occur during the practice of nursing. To address moral distress, the American Association of Critical Care Nurses (McCue, 2010) advises that nurses consider "four A's: Ask, Affirm, Assess, and Act." This framework is depicted in Figure 5.3.

The unprecedented advances in medical technology over the past 4 decades have engendered significant changes in professional, social, and legal expectations about care outcomes (Ferrell, 2006). Ethical issues related to **medical futility**, defined as life-sustaining care that is unlikely to result in meaningful survival, continue

EVIDENCE-INFORMED PRACTICE

Encountering Situations of Moral Conflict and Distress in Practice

This study examined moral distress experienced by professionals who provided home palliative care. Using a critical incident approach, qualitative interviews were used to elicit the experiences of 18 providers from five home visiting organizations in Ontario. A total of 47 critical incidents were described and revealed 11 issues that triggered moral distress.

Primary themes included: (1) the role of informal caregivers, (2) challenging clinical situations, and (3) service delivery issues. Informal caregiver issues were described in terms of caregiver burden, neglect or abuse of the patient, and competency of informal caregivers to provide care. Challenging clinical situations were found to include issues related to respect for patient decision making, appropriateness of treatment, inability to have an impact, unexpected death, and communication. Service delivery issues included access to appropriate care, inadequately trained staff, and lack of information.

NURSING IMPLICATIONS: While nurses frequently have experiences that cause emotional distress, moral distress involves the added dimension that personal or professional values are being violated. The caregiving experience at the end of life is complex, and there are often no clear decision-making guidelines. Collaborative, respectful relationships, attention to norms for behaviour, support, and communication, as well as resolution of moral conflicts are essential.

Source: Based on Brazil, K., Kassalainen, S., Ploeg, J., & Marshall, D. (2010). Moral distress experienced by health care professionals who provide home-based palliative care. *Social Science and Medicine, 71,* 1687–1691.

to present challenges in nursing practice. Euthanasia and the withholding or withdrawal of life-sustaining treatment are frequently cited by Canadian nurses as ethical issues (Oberle & Hughes, 2001). Often, the problem is that the family or the physician wants aggressive care to continue, whereas nurses believe that the client's dignity is being eroded by continued treatment. Sometimes, the opposite applies; nurses believe that treatment should continue, and others want it to be terminated. Either way, the situation can cause the nurse moral distress, particularly if he or she feels powerless to affect the decision making.

Redman and Fry (2000) analyzed numerous published reports of studies of ethical conflict in nursing and determined that the most common disagreements centre on decisions about the medical treatment of patients. When such disagreement exists, communication and problem-solving skills are particularly important. The nurse can use a framework to analyze the problem on the basis of understanding the patient's and family's wishes

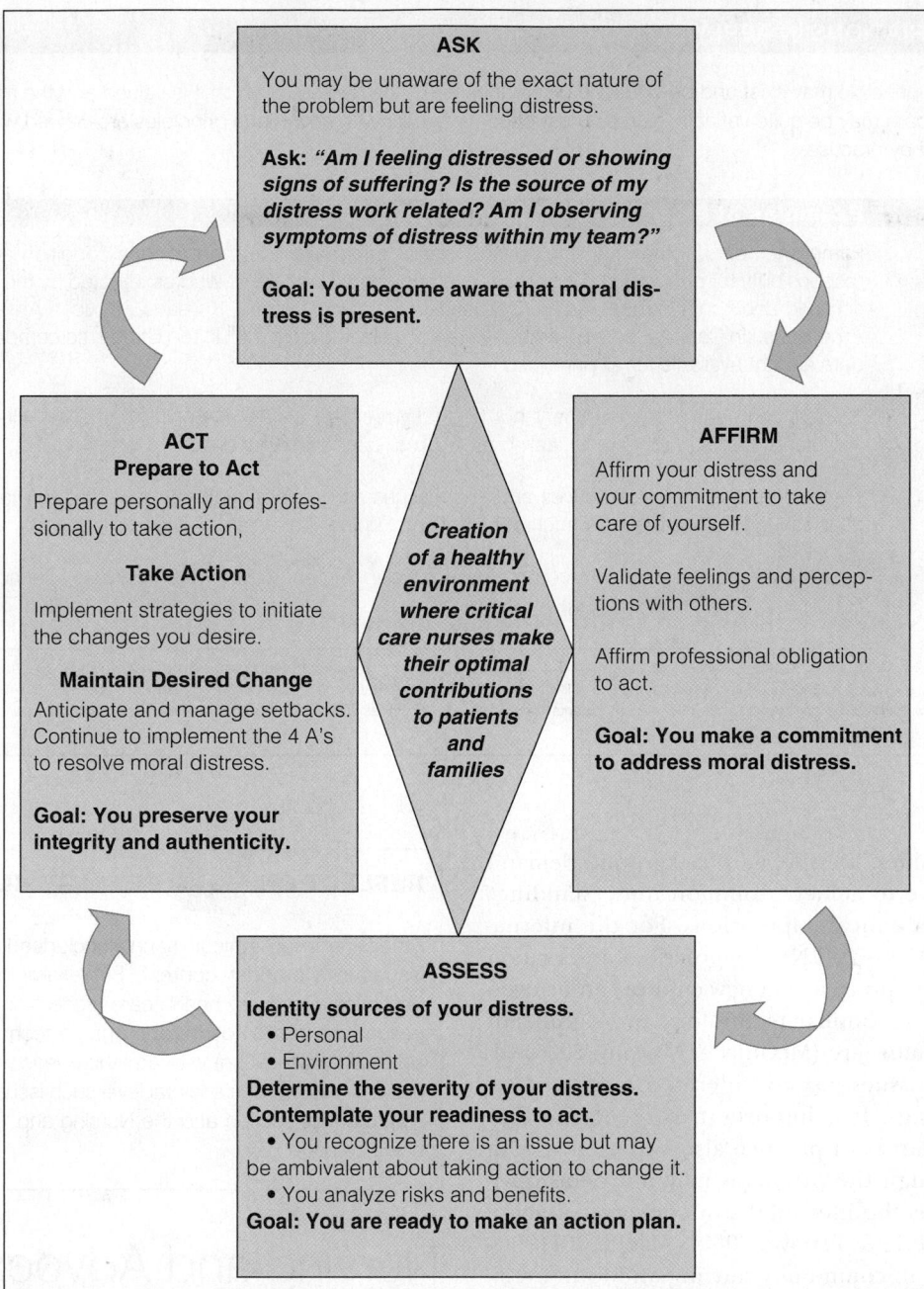

ASK

You may be unaware of the exact nature of the problem but are feeling distress.

Ask: "Am I feeling distressed or showing signs of suffering? Is the source of my distress work related? Am I observing symptoms of distress within my team?"

Goal: You become aware that moral distress is present.

ACT
Prepare to Act

Prepare personally and professionally to take action,

Take Action

Implement strategies to initiate the changes you desire.

Maintain Desired Change

Anticipate and manage setbacks. Continue to implement the 4 A's to resolve moral distress.

Goal: You preserve your integrity and authenticity.

Creation of a healthy environment where critical care nurses make their optimal contributions to patients and families

AFFIRM

Affirm your distress and your commitment to take care of yourself.

Validate feelings and perceptions with others.

Affirm professional obligation to act.

Goal: You make a commitment to address moral distress.

ASSESS

Identity sources of your distress.
- Personal
- Environment

Determine the severity of your distress.
Contemplate your readiness to act.
- You recognize there is an issue but may be ambivalent about taking action to change it.
- You analyze risks and benefits.

Goal: You are ready to make an action plan.

FIGURE 5.3 The four A's to rise above moral distress.

Source: American Association of Critical Care Nurses (AACN) from AACN Ethics Work Group. (2004). The 4 A's to Rise above moral distress. Aliso Viejo, CA: AACN.

and can use values cited in the CNA *Code of Ethics* (2008) to develop an argument for approaching the problem from a nursing ethics perspective. Nurses need to be prepared to explore, with the physician, patient, and family, why they each believe that a particular pathway should be followed and work with them to come to a common understanding that is acceptable to all. Sometimes, agreement is not possible, and nurses must look carefully at their own frame of reference and why they believe the treatment decisions are incorrect. See Box 5.6 on the next page for additional discussion. The question that must be asked in every instance is this: Whose needs are

being met? If the nurses place priority on their own values above those of the patients (which may be contrary to the CNA *Code of Ethics for Registered Nurses*), they may be unable to resolve the dilemma and may continue to experience moral distress. Thus, the importance of values clarification again becomes evident. Discussion with clients and other health care providers about differences in values can help ease the tension that such situations produce (CNA, 2008).

The increasing cultural diversity evident in both patients and their families and in the nursing population in Canada can create ethically charged situations.

BOX 5.6 VARIATIONS IN APPLYING MORAL PRINCIPLES

Although a moral principle may exist and be valued in different cultures, the degree to which it is valued and the manner in which it is used in health care may be quite variable. Nurses must become familiar with how moral principles are viewed within the cultural groups in which they practise.

Principle	Examples of Ethnic and Cultural Variations
Autonomy	Family members, rather than the patient, receive information on the patient's condition and take primary responsibility for decision making. The family and community are viewed as affected by the patient's condition and decisions as much as the individual is affected: Chinese, Koreans, Mexican Americans, Bosnian Americans. (In Canada, data on ethnicity are not collected as in the United States, so comparable Canadian data are not available for all principles.)
Veracity	The preference is that the patient not be told directly of a life-threatening condition: Hispanics, Asians, Pakistanis, Bosnian Americans, Italian Americans, Canadian Aboriginals.
Nonmaleficence	Discussion of advance directives and such issues as cardiopulmonary resuscitation may be viewed as physically and emotionally harmful to the patient: Filipino, Canadian Aboriginals, Chinese.
Beneficence	Health care providers should promote patient well-being and hope: Asian cultures, Canadian Aboriginals, Russians.

Sources: From Ellerby, J. H., McKenzie, J., McKay, S., Gariepy, G. J., & Kaufert, J. M. (2000). Bioethics for clinicians: 18. Aboriginal cultures., *Canadian Medical Association Journal, 163,* 845–850; Searight, H. R., & Gafford, J. (2005). Cultural diversity at the end of life: Issues and guidelines for family physicians. *American Family Physician, 71,* 515–522; and Searight, H. R., & Gafford, J. (2005). It's like playing with your destiny: Bosnian immigrants' views of advance directives and end-of-life decision-making. *Journal of Immigrant Health, 7*(3),195–203.

Differences in values, lifestyle, and background demand ongoing dialogue to achieve common understandings about issues with ethical implications. For the internationally educated nurse (IEN), the process of integration and transition into practice in a new culture can be overwhelming, given unfamiliar technology and significant differences in health care (McGuire & Murphy, 2005).

Most of the issues just considered are centred on acute care settings. It is important to recognize that nurses in other areas of practice also experience ethical issues, although the problems may not be as obviously dramatic as the life-and-death concerns of acute care nurses (Oberle & Tenove, 2000). MacPhail (1996) examined ethics in community nursing and found relationship, trust, and advocacy to be central to community health nursing practice. For example, nurses in the study talked about difficulties in working with individuals who had chosen to adopt at-risk lifestyles, such as problematic drug use and prostitution. How could they provide support for the person without appearing to condone or support the lifestyle? How could they honour autonomy and at the same time try to change the individuals' behaviours? How could they maintain trust while adhering to legal requirements to report certain practices, such as child abuse? This study demonstrated that community health nursing is rooted in relationships and that the nurses who fail to attend to the ethical dimensions of relationships will be unable to provide effective care. These issues must be considered within the context of the broader society (see the Reflect on Primary Health Care box).

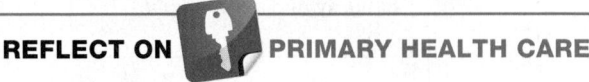

REFLECT ON PRIMARY HEALTH CARE

Practising in an ethical manner includes looking at ethical issues in a broader context. For example, examining the principles of primary health care (accessibility, public participation, health promotion, appropriate technology, and intersectoral collaboration) with an ethical lens will encourage the nurse to explore at a societal level such issues as those mentioned in this section and the Nursing and Canadian Society box (see page 78).

Nursing and Advocacy

Within the powerful institutional machinery of the health care system is the significant potential for the client to be a relatively powerless player in his or her own care (Hewitt, 2002). The notion of **advocacy** in nursing is closely tied to empowering clients through the provision of information, support, and intervention. One definition of advocacy is "acting to the limit of professional ability to provide for the client's interests and needs as the patient defines them" (Dubler, 1992). Curtin (1979) defined advocacy as the moral art in nursing that evolves from shared vulnerability, past experiences, and humanity in the nurse–patient relationship. The overall goal of a client advocate is to protect clients' rights.

An advocate is one who expresses and defends the cause of another. Three primary elements constitute advocacy by the nurse, according to Tschudin and Hunt (1994).

The first is that the nurse's position is proactive, rather than passive and subordinate. Second, the nurse speaks up and acts on behalf of the patient. Finally, some kind of difficulty or conflict exists that necessitates the need for advocacy.

Nurses are frequently placed in an advocacy role when clients and families are unable, or unwilling, to speak up for themselves. Nurses must ensure that clients and families have the necessary information to enable them to consider options and must provide them with support when they make decisions. Sometimes, the nurse must defend the client's or family's views when others are trying to coerce them into making a different decision. This is often a difficult role for the nurse because it may pit the nurse against other members of the health care team. However, the nurse must be guided by the professional code, which places choice, dignity, and well-being as the highest values. To be an effective advocate involves the following:

- Recognizing that the rights and values of clients and families must take precedence when they conflict with those of health care providers

- Being aware that conflicts may arise over issues that require consultation, confrontation, or negotiation

- Being assertive and using excellent communication techniques

Advocacy may be required at the broader, systems level as well. For example, the CNA *Code of Ethics* (2008) articulates a value of **quality practice environments**, that is, environments conducive to safe, competent, and ethical care. Nurses may have to be involved in political action when underfunding threatens the integrity of the health care system. It is a nurse's moral obligation to work to ensure that the best possible conditions exist for the clients' health care needs to be met. This is another demanding role for nurses, one with which many nurses are unfamiliar. Nurses may choose not to act because it is too much trouble or they are reluctant to engage with unfamiliar administrative personnel or agencies. However, providing ethical care for clients is not an easy task, and nurses must be prepared to take action to ensure quality care.

Advocacy is an important role for nurses. Nonetheless, nurses must be careful not to suggest (or believe) that they are the only advocates for the client. The term *advocacy* is potentially divisive; that is, it could cause conflict in itself because it suggests that the client needs to be protected. Not all clients feel the need for protection, and the nurse must honour their right to self-determination. As well, other health care providers, such as physicians, may resent the implication that clients need to be protected from them. Physicians, too, consider themselves to be client advocates, as do many other concerned professionals, such as social workers and physiotherapists. The nurse has a moral obligation to the client but also an obligation to keep the health care team functioning cohesively. Therefore, the nurse must be sensitive to the implications of such terms as *advocacy* and use them carefully. The basic values in client advocacy are shown in Box 5.7.

BOX 5.7 BASIC VALUES IN CLIENT ADVOCACY

The basic values in client advocacy are the following:

- The client is a holistic, autonomous being who has the right to make choices and decisions.

- Clients have the right to expect a nurse–client relationship that is based on shared respect, trust, collaboration in solving problems related to health and health care needs, and consideration of their thoughts and feelings.

- It is the nurse's responsibility to ensure the client has access to health care services that meet health needs.

Enhancing Ethical Practice

It should be noted that decisions about a client's care are not made by nurses alone. Although the nurse's input is important, in reality, several people are usually involved in making an ethical decision. Therefore, collaboration, communication, and compromise are important skills for health care professionals. When nurses do not have the autonomy to act on their moral or ethical choices, compromise becomes essential. Integrity-preserving compromises are most likely to be produced by collaborative decision making. The mnemonic device LEARN can remind nurses to work toward collaboration in ethical decisions (Berlin & Fowkes, 1983):

> **L**isten to others.
> **E**xplain your perceptions.
> **A**cknowledge and discuss differences.
> **R**ecommend alternatives.
> **N**egotiate agreement.

As should be evident from the preceding discussion, excellent ethical decision-making skills require considerable reflection and practice. Davis and Aroskar (1991), Rodney and Starzomski (1993), and Wilkinson (1996) described a number of strategies to help nurses overcome possible organizational and social constraints that may hinder the ethical practice of nursing:

- Become aware of your own values and the ethical aspects of nursing.

- Be familiar with the code of ethics that is to guide your practice.

- Learn about and respect the values, opinions, and responsibilities of other health care professionals.

- Participate in or establish ethics rounds. Ethics rounds, using hypothetical or real cases, incorporate the traditional teaching approach for clinical rounds but focus on the ethical dimensions of client care, rather than clinical diagnosis and treatment.

- Serve on institutional ethics committees.

In addition, the researchers stressed the importance of striving for collaborative practice in which nurses function effectively in cooperation with clients and other health care professionals. Ethical practice does not just happen—it takes a great deal of work. Every nurse has an obligation to understand the ethical foundations of practice and to make a conscious effort to examine and reflect on the ethical dimensions of each caregiving encounter. It is only with an understanding of the ethical components of a situation that nurses can meet their obligation to act in the best interests of their clients.

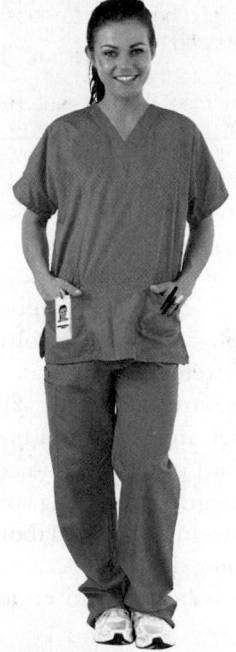

Case Study 5

At a Canadian acute care hospital, nurses expressed concern with the plan of care for a 98-year-old Asian woman. She had been in a nursing home for several years and had been bedridden because of severe arthritis. As a result, she had numerous contractures that made it difficult to position her, and her skin had broken down in several areas. She was responding only to painful stimuli, and the nurses observed indications of considerable pain whenever she was moved. She had a pulmonary infection and was receiving triple-antibiotic therapy. The antibiotics gave her severe diarrhea, which necessitated more frequent moving and bathing. The antibiotics had not been effective, and the order was due for renewal. The nurses expressed the view that the antibiotics ought to be discontinued and that further aggressive care should be terminated. In their view, continuing treatment was robbing the patient of the possibility of a dignified death. Nurses wanted a DNR (do not resuscitate) order instituted. The patient's daughter adamantly disagreed, saying that it was her obligation to see that her mother got every possible treatment. In their culture, she argued, it was a demonstration of respect to try to preserve life at all costs.

What could the nurses do? They wanted to respect the daughter's wishes, but they believed that treatment was causing harm to the patient and that it was wrong to continue to use scarce resources trying to preserve life in this futile situation. They felt constrained by the desire to respect cultural differences but also felt strongly that the patient was being harmed, even tortured, by nursing actions. Because of their distress, they put pressure on the physician to have the DNR order instituted and discontinue therapy. The physician was reluctant. A consultation with the clinical ethics committee was called by the unit manager.

CRITICAL THINKING QUESTIONS

1. How can this situation be explored by applying ethical principles?

2. What are the goals of care? Are these goals shared by the patient? the nurses? other health care professionals?

3. How does a focus on relationships improve your ethical understanding of the situation?

4. How would everyone (client, family, caregivers, institutions, organization, society) be affected by the decision?

5. What external conditions must be considered?

6. What (and whose) values must be considered?

7. Discuss the features of this case that make the experience of moral distress likely for the providers involved. What could be done to mitigate moral distress in this case?

Check the eText in MyNursingLab for answers and explanations.

KEY TERMS

advocacy *p. 90*

attitudes *p. 77*

autonomy (respect for persons) *p. 84*

beliefs *p. 77*

beneficence *p. 84*

code of ethics *p. 83*

consequence-based (teleological) theories *p. 83*

ethical obligations *p. 83*

ethics *p. 83*

ethics of care *p. 85*

fidelity *p. 85*

justice *p. 85*

medical futility *p. 88*

moral agents *p. 87*

moral dilemmas *p. 88*

moral distress *p. 88*

moral integrity *p. 88*

moral theories *p. 83*

nonmaleficence *p. 84*

paternalism *p. 85*

personal values *p. 78*

principle of utility *p. 83*

principles-based (deontological) theories *p. 83*

professional values *p. 78*

quality practice environments *p. 91*

reflective practice *p. 87*

relational ethics theories *p. 85*

relationships-based (caring) theories *p. 83*

utilitarianism *p. 83*

value set *p. 77*

value system *p. 77*

values *p. 77*

values clarification *p. 79*

veracity *p. 85*

virtue *p. 85*

CHAPTER HIGHLIGHTS

- Values are enduring beliefs that give direction and meaning to life and guide a person's behaviour.
- Values clarification is a process in which people identify, examine, and develop their own values.
- Nursing ethics refers to the moral problems that arise in nursing practice and to ethical decisions that nurses make.
- Morality refers to what is right and wrong in conduct, character, or attitude.
- Moral issues are those that arouse conscience, are concerned with important values and norms, and evoke such words as *good, bad, right, wrong, should,* and *ought.*
- Three common moral frameworks (approaches) are consequence-based (teleological), principles-based (deontological), and relationships-based (caring) theories.
- Moral principles (e.g., autonomy, beneficence, nonmaleficence, justice, fidelity, and veracity) are broad, general philosophical concepts that can be used to make and explain moral choices.
- A professional code of ethics is a formal statement of a group's ideals and values that serves as a standard and guideline for the group's professional actions and informs the public of its commitment.
- Moral distress occurs when the individual knows the ethically correct action to take, but is unable to take the action because of internal or external barriers.

- Nurses' ethical decisions are influenced by their moral theories and principles, personal and professional values, and nursing codes of ethics.
- The goal of ethical reasoning, in the context of nursing, is to reach a mutual, peaceful agreement that is in the best interests of the client; reaching the agreement may require compromise.
- Reflective practice refers to the ability to take information about experience, knowledge, or skills levels based on assessments (by the nurse herself or by others), analyze this information, and determine how to act on this information in the future.
- Nurses are responsible for determining their own actions and for supporting clients who are making moral decisions or for whom decisions are being made by others.
- Nurses can enhance their ethical practice and client advocacy by clarifying their own values, understanding the values of other health care professionals, becoming familiar with nursing codes of ethics, and participating in ethics committees and rounds.
- Client advocacy involves concern for and actions on behalf of another person or organization to bring about change.
- The functions of the advocacy role are to inform, support, and mediate.

ASSESS YOUR LEARNING

1. When an ethical issue arises, what is one of the most important nursing responsibilities in managing client-care situations?

   a. Being able to defend the morality of your own actions

   b. Remaining neutral and detached when making ethical decisions

   c. Ensuring that a team is responsible for deciding ethical questions

   d. Following the client's and family's wishes exactly

2. Which situation is most clearly a violation of the underlying principles associated with professional nursing ethics?

   a. The hospital policy permits use of internal fetal monitoring during labour. However, literature both supports and refutes the value of this practice.

   b. When asked about the purpose of a medication, a nurse colleague responds, "Oh, I never look them up. I just give what is prescribed."

   c. The nurses on the unit agree to sponsor a fundraising event to support a labour strike proposed by fellow nurses at another facility.

   d. A client reports that he did not quite tell the doctor the truth when asked if he was following his therapeutic diet at home.

3. Following a motor vehicle collision, the parents refuse to permit withdrawal of life support from their child, who has no apparent brain function. Although the nurse believes the child should be allowed to die and organ donation considered, the nurse supports the parents' decision. Which moral principle provides the basis for the nurse's actions?

   a. Respect for autonomy

   b. Nonmaleficence

   c. Beneficence

   d. Justice

4. Which statement would be MOST helpful when a nurse is assisting clients in clarifying their values?

   a. "That was not a good decision. Why did you think it would work?"

   b. "The most important thing is to follow the plan of care. Did you follow all your doctor's orders?"

   c. "Some people might have made a different decision. What led you to make your decision?"

   d. "If you had asked me, I would have given you my opinion about what to do. Now, how do you feel about your choice?"

5. After recovering from her hip replacement, an older client wants to go home. The family wants the client to go to a nursing home. If the nurse were acting as a client advocate, what should the nurse do?

   a. Inform the family that the client has a right to decide on her own

   b. Ask the primary care provider to discharge the client to her home

   c. Suggest the client hire a lawyer to protect her rights

   d. Help the client and family communicate their views to each other

6. Mr. Goldman, 78 years old, was admitted with congestive heart failure. His wife tells the nurse that she is afraid her husband's condition is deteriorating, and despite several requests, the physician has not been in to see him. Which of the following is the most appropriate nursing action?

   a. Assess Mr. Goldman and inform the couple that the physician will be contacted to convey their concerns

   b. Explain to Mrs. Goldman that she may speak with the physician later during rounds

   c. Reassure Mrs. Goldman that her husband is receiving appropriate care

   d. Inform Mrs. Goldman that the nurse-in-charge will be notified of her concerns

7. Which is an example of a nurse engaging in reflective practice?

   a. Contributing to decision making about a client within an interprofessional team

   b. Asking for feedback and engaging in discussion with a colleague about the nurse's own performance.

   c. Giving advice to a student nurse regarding his performance

   d. Documenting care the nurse gave to a client in the client's record

8. A daughter does not want her mother to learn of the mother's diagnosis of advanced cancer. She asks you to tell her mother that you do not know why she is in the hospital if her mother asks you. In this situation, you are being asked to compromise which ethical principle?

   a. Beneficence

   b. Nonmaleficence

   c. Veracity

   d. Fidelity

9. Which is defined as the professional obligation of a nurse to assume responsibility for his or her own actions?

   a. Individuality

   b. Accountability

   c. Bioethics

   d. Utilitarianism

10. Which activity reflects the nurse's role as advocate?

   a. Conducting a research study into the benefits of exercise

   b. Notifying the supervisor about a client's adverse drug reaction

   c. Teaching clients how to care for themselves after surgery

   d. Assessing changes in blood pressure

Check the eText in MyNursingLab for answers and explanations.

WEBLINKS

NursingEthics.ca

http://www.nursingethics.ca

This site lists Canadian resources related to ethical practice.

Canadian Nurses Association's Code of Ethics

http://www.cna-aiic.ca/en/improve-your-workplace/ nursing-ethics/

This site provides access to the Code of Ethics for the Canadian Nurses Association (CNA) and links to provincial and territorial websites for related documentation.

The W. Maurice Young Centre for Applied Ethics

http://www.ethics.ubc.ca/

Established in 1993 by the University of British Columbia, the Centre for Applied Ethics is an interdisciplinary research centre

that studies a variety of topics, including health care practices. Its newsletter is available on the site.

Canadian Bioethics Society

http://www.bioethics.ca

The Canadian Bioethics Society was established in 1988 by the union of the Canadian Society of Bioethics and the Canadian Society for Medical Bioethics. Its members include health care administrators, lawyers, nurses, philosophers, physicians, theologians, and others interested in the ethical dimensions of health care.

MyNursingLab

REFERENCES

Armstrong, A.E. (2006). Towards a strong virtue ethics for nursing practice. *Nursing Philosophy 7*, 110–124.

Beauchamp, T. L., & Childress, J. F. (2009). *Principles of biomedical ethics* (6th ed.). New York, NY: Oxford University Press.

Begley, A. M. (2005). Practising virtue: A challenge to the view that a virtue centred approach to ethics lacks practical content. *Nursing Ethics, 12*(6), 622–637.

Berlin, E. A., & Fowkes, W. C. (1983). Teaching framework for cross-cultural care: Application in family practice. *Western Journal of Medicine, 139*(6), 934–938.

Bowden, P. L. (1995). The ethics of nursing care and "the ethic of care." *Nursing Inquiry, 2*(1), 10–21.

Breslin, J. M., MacRae, S. K., Bell, J., & Singer, P. A. (2005). Top 10 health care ethics challenges facing the public: Views of Toronto bioethicists. *BMC Medical Ethics, 6*, 5.

Butts, J.B. & Rich, K. (2005) *Nursing ethics: Across the curriculum and into practice.* Sudbury, MA: Jones & Bartlett Learning.

Canadian Federation of Nurses Unions. (2008). *Nursing health human resources in Canada: The time for action was yesterday!* Retrieved from http://www.nursesunions.ca/content.php?doc=90

Canadian Nurses Association. (2004). *Everyday ethics: Putting the code into practice* (2nd ed.). Ottawa, ON: Author.

Canadian Nurses Association. (2008). *Code of ethics for registered nurses.* Ottawa, ON: Author.

College of Nurses of Ontario. (2005). *Practice standard: Ethics.* Retrieved from http://www.cno.org/docs/prac/41034_Ethics.pdf

Curtin, L. L. (1979). The nurse as advocate: A philosophical foundation for nursing. *Advances in Nursing Science, 1*(3), 1–10.

Davis, A. J., & Aroskar, M. A. (1991). *Ethical dillemas and nursing practice* (3rd ed.). East Norwalk, CT: Appleton & Lange.

Davis, A., Fowler, M, & Aroskar, M. (2009). *Ethical dilemmas and nursing practice* (5th ed.). Toronto, ON: Pearson Education.

Dubler N. (1992). Individual advocacy as a governing principle. *Journal of Case Management, 1*(3), 82–86.

Ferrell, B. R. (2006). Understanding the moral distress of nurses witnessing medically futile care. *Oncology Nursing Forum, 33*(5), 922–930.

Gastmans, C. (2006). The care perspective in healthcare ethics. In A. J. Davis, V. Tschudin, & L. Raeve (Eds.), *Essentials of teaching and learning in nursing ethics: Perspectives and methods* (pp. 76–89). Toronto, ON: Churchill Livingstone Elsevier.

Gastmans, C., Dierckx de Casterle, B., & Schotsmans, P. (1998). Nursing considered as moral practice: A philosophical-ethical interpretation on nursing. *Kennedy Institute of Ethics, 8*, 43–69.

Hewitt, J. (2002). A critical review of the arguments debating the role of the nurse advocate. *Journal of Advanced Nursing, 37*(5), 439–455.

International Council of Nurses. (2006). *Code of ethics for nurses.* Geneva, Switzerland: Imprimerie Fornara.

Jameton, A. (1992). Nursing ethics and the moral situation of the nurse. In E. Friedman (Ed.). *Choices and conflict* (pp. 101–109). Chicago, IL: American Hospital Association.

Johns, C. (1995). The value of reflective practice for nursing. *Journal of Clinical Nursing, 4*(1), 23–30.

MacPhail, S. (1996). *Ethical issues in community nursing.* Unpublished doctoral dissertation, University of Alberta.

Marck, P. (2000a). Recovering ethics after "technics": Developing critical text on technology. *Nursing Ethics, 7*(1), 5–14.

Marck, P. (2000b). Nursing in a technological world: Searching for healing communities. *Advances in Nursing Science, 23,* 63–81.

McCue, C. (November 9, 2010). Using the American Association of Critical Care Nurses framework to alleviate moral distress: The 4 A's to rise above moral distress. *OJIN: The Online Journal of Issues in Nursing, 16*(1). DOI: 10.3912/OJIN.Vol16No01PPT02. Retrieved from http://nursingworld.org/MainMenuCategories/ANAMarketplace/ANAPeriodicals/OJIN/TableofContents/Vol-16-2011/No1-Jan-2011/Articles-Previous-Topics/AACN-Framework-and-Moral-Distress.html

McGuire, M., & Murphy, S. (2005). The internationally educated nurse. *Canadian Nurse, 101,* 25–29.

Oberle, K., & Hughes, D. (2001). Doctors' and nurses' perceptions of ethical problems in end-of-life decisions. *Journal of Advanced Nursing, 33,* 707–715.

Oberle, K., & Tenove, S. (2000). Ethical issues in public health nursing. *Nursing Ethics, 7,* 425–438.

Redman, B. K., & Fry, S. (2000). Nurses' ethical conflicts: What is really known about them? *Nursing Ethics, 7,* 360–366.

Registered Nurses' Association of Ontario. (2006). *Client centred care best practice guidelines.* Toronto, ON: Author.

Rodney, P., & Starzomski, R. (1993, October). Constraints on the moral agency of nurses. *Canadian Nurse, 89,* 23–26.

Rodney, P., & Varcoe, C. (2001). Towards ethical inquiry in the economic evaluation of nursing practice. *Canadian Journal of Nursing Research, 33*(1), 35–57.

Schon, D. A. (1983). *The reflective practitioner.* New York, NY: Basic Books.

Toren, O. & Wagner, N. (2010). Applying an ethical decision-making tool for a nurse management dilemma. *Nursing Ethics, 17,* 393–402.

Tschudin, V., & Hunt, G. (1994). Dissatisfaction: With professional relationships, with the status quo and with health care in general. *Nursing Ethics: An International Journal for Health Care Professionals, 1*(2), 69–70.

Wilkinson, J. M. (1996). *Toward a context-sensitive theory of nursing ethics: Classification and comparison of nurses' narratives from four time periods (1934, 1979, 1989 and 1995).* Doctoral dissertation, University of Kansas.

Yeo, M., & Moorhouse, A. (Eds.). (1996). *Concepts and cases in nursing ethics* (2nd ed.). Peterborough, ON: Broadview Press.

Chapter 6

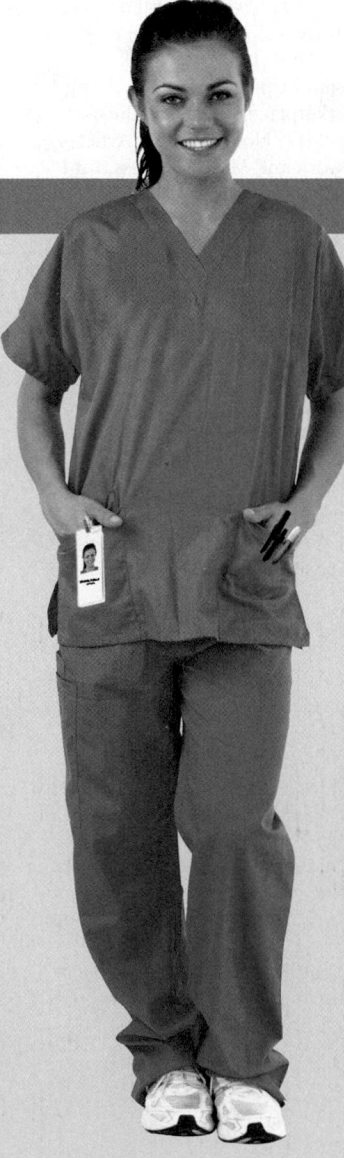

Accountability and Legal Aspects of Nursing

LEARNING OUTCOMES

After studying this chapter, you will be able to:

1. Describe the history and sources of Canadian law.

2. Identify regulatory considerations in nursing and their impact on the practice of nursing in Canada.

3. Identify selected aspects of professional regulation and their role in governing the practice of nursing, including expanding the scope of nursing practice.

4. Discuss measures of accountability and discipline in nursing practice.

5. Identify the two interdependent legal roles of provider of service and employer or contractor for service in nursing.

6. Discuss areas of potential tort liability in nursing.

7. Discuss informed consent, confidentiality, problematic substance use, and chemical dependency.

8. Discuss legal issues and safe practices in documentation, telephone advice, incident reports, and reports of unsafe practices.

9. Identify ways nurses and nursing students can minimize their chances of liability.

10. Discuss legal protection of nurses in practice.

Nursing practice is governed by many legal concepts. It is important for nurses to know the basics of the Canadian legal system and its relationship to the profession of nursing. Accountability is an essential concept of professional nursing practice and the law. Knowledge of laws that regulate and affect nursing practice is needed for the following reasons:

- To ensure that the nurse's decisions and actions are consistent with current legal principles
- To protect the nurse from liability
- To protect the public

Relationship between Nurses and the Law

Law can be defined as "the sum total of rules and regulations by which a society is governed. As such, law is created by people and exists to regulate all persons" (Guido, 2006, p. 31).

Functions of the Law in Nursing

The law serves a number of functions in nursing:

- It provides a framework for establishing which nursing actions in the care of clients are legal.
- It outlines the responsibilities that govern nursing practice and nurses' relationships with physicians, other health care practitioners, and the health care system.
- It helps establish the boundaries of independent nursing action.
- It assists nurses in ensuring that they are consistent, competent, and safe in providing quality care that serves society while preserving individual rights and human dignity.

History and Source of Canada's Laws

Historically, Canadian law is derived from two distinct European systems, namely, English common law and French civil law. Quebec follows the civil law system, whereas the other Canadian provinces and territories follow the common law legal tradition.

THE COMMON LAW TRADITION In the English **common law** tradition, legal principles and rules evolve through the courts. Judges interpret and apply principles from similar decisions in previous cases (*precedents*) to the particular case before them to reach a decision. For this reason, common law is sometimes called *case law* or *judge-made law*. In reality, no two cases are identical, and common law develops through judges making distinctions between cases and determining when an earlier case is not applicable to the case being considered. In this way,

common law at once provides some consistency and predictability regarding what legal solution will be appropriate in a given instance and is flexible enough to allow for the particulars of a specific situation to be considered (Keatings & Smith, 2009).

The hierarchy within the courts has important implications for how common law develops. Each province and territory has a lower-level trial court and a higher-level appeal court. The decisions of higher courts are binding on the lower courts in the same jurisdiction. Decisions in one jurisdiction, province, or territory are not binding in another jurisdiction, province, or territory, but such decisions are often treated as a persuasive source of law. This is particularly true when lower courts in one jurisdiction are considering a judgment from a higher-level court in a different jurisdiction. In contrast, a decision from the Supreme Court of Canada is binding on all other courts in the country (Keatings & Smith, 2009).

THE CIVIL LAW TRADITION The tradition of **civil law**, with its Roman roots, is quite different. A key distinguishing feature is that instead of emerging through the courts, laws are written down in what is referred to as a *code*. This code provides all citizens with an accessible and written collection of the laws that apply to them and that judges must follow. Quebec's Civil Code, first enacted in 1866 just before Confederation, is amended periodically and underwent a major revision in 1994. Like other civil codes, it contains a comprehensive statement of rules and general principles. Unlike common law courts, courts in a civil law system first look to the code, and then refer to previous decisions for consistency.

STATUTORY LAW The distinction between the common and civil law traditions reveals two different sources of legal authority: (a) case law or judge-made law and (b) the Civil Code. Parliament and the provincial or territorial legislatures are another key source of Canadian law. Parliament has the power to pass laws for all of Canada, whereas the legislatures of each province and territory pass laws of a more local nature. Laws enacted by either of these legislative bodies are called *statutes, legislation,* or *acts.* When Parliament or one of the legislatures enacts legislation, that legislation then supersedes any case law dealing with the same subject. In Quebec, much legislation exists to cover areas not dealt with in the Civil Code.

Responsibility for the Canadian health care system is shared between the federal and provincial or territorial governments, according to the division of powers set out in the Constitution Act, 1867. As a leading constitutional scholar notes, "health is an 'amorphous topic' which is distributed to the federal parliament or provincial legislatures depending on the purpose and effect of the particular health matter at issue" (Hogg, 1997, p. 445). However, despite the federal government having some jurisdiction in this area, health care delivery is interpreted as being largely within provincial and territorial authority. For example, regulation of health care professionals is a responsibility of the provinces and territories and is one that, as will be discussed here, has, in many instances, been delegated by the provinces and territories to the provincial and territorial professional organizations.

Tort law refers to that body of the law through which a person who suffers injury caused by another person is able to claim compensation for that injury. Tort law is divided into two main categories: (a) intentional torts and (b) negligence. When a person proves that he or she has suffered harm caused by another, either through intentional action or through negligence, that person will have a claim for damages (*compensation*) against the person who caused the harm (called the *tortfeasor*). The goal of compensation in tort law is to put the person who suffered the harm back in the position he or she would have been in had the tortfeasor not acted. This is a guiding principle and is clearly more feasible in some cases than in others. Negligence and those intentional torts most applicable to the nursing context are discussed in greater detail later in this chapter. See Table 6.1 for examples of laws that affect nurses and nursing practice.

TABLE 6.1 Selected Categories of Laws Affecting Nurses

Category	Examples
Constitutional	Due process, equality protection
Statutory (legislative)	Nursing legislation; Good Samaritan/ Emergency Medical Aid acts; child protection legislation; vulnerable persons legislation, such as Protection for Persons in Care acts; laws regarding advance directives or power of attorney for personal care; laws regarding privacy and protection of health information; human rights acts
Criminal (public)	Murder, manslaughter, theft, assault, active euthanasia, illegal possession of controlled drug or substance
Contracts (private or civil)	Nurse and client, nurse and employer, nurse and insurance, client and agency, employer and union (collective agreement)
Torts (private or civil)	Negligence, defamation, invasion of privacy, assault and battery, false imprisonment

Regulatory Considerations in Nursing

In Canada, provincial and territorial governments give the nursing profession the legislation to regulate the profession in the public interest. Although it gets its authority from provincial and territorial governments, the profession itself is self-governing (see the Nursing and Canadian Society box). Each province and territory has a professional regulatory body that, depending on the jurisdiction, is called a *college* or an *association* or both. The following section reviews the roles and responsibilities of these provincial and territorial professional bodies and their impact on the practice of nursing in Canada.

 Nursing and Canadian Society

Fact	Implications for Nursing Practice
Profession-led regulation is a privilege that is granted by government through legislation that gives the nursing profession the power to regulate its peers in the public interest.	This regulation assures the public that they are receiving safe and ethical care from competent, qualified practitioners.
This is based on the belief that the profession has the knowledge required to set standards of practice and assess the conduct of its members through peer review.	One part of the nursing regulations is protection of title. Registered nurse (RN) and nurse practitioner (NP), registered (licensed) practical nurse (RPN/LPN), and registered psychiatric nurse (RPN) are protected in provincial legislation. Only nurses currently registered with a nursing regulatory body can use these titles.
Canadian public interest is best served when regulatory bodies adopt a framework that strengthens clinical nursing practice and leadership and promotes public safety.	A regulatory framework used by many of the provincial or territorial nursing regulatory bodies embodies such principles as promoting good practice, preventing poor practice, and intervening in unacceptable practice.

Source: Adapted from Canadian Nurses Association. (2007). Understanding self-regulation. *Nursing Now: Issues and Trends in Canadian Nursing, 21,* 1–5.

PROVINCIAL AND TERRITORIAL REGULATORY BODIES

In Canada, the regulation of nursing is a function of provincial and territorial law. Nurses have been granted an exclusivity of practice (a right of self-government or self-regulation) and an obligation to monitor and discipline their own membership (Canadian Nurses Association [CNA], 2007). The provincial and territorial nursing **regulatory bodies**, such as the College of Registered Nurses of British Columbia (CRNBC), the College and Association of Registered Nurses of Alberta (CARNA), the Saskatchewan Registered Nurses' Association (SRNA), or the College of Nurses of Ontario (CNO), are given their authority by provincial and territorial governments through legislation. Through such legislation and the associated regulations, these bodies are charged with regulating entry into the profession, approving entry-level nursing education programs, setting standards of competent practice, establishing continuing competence or education and quality assurance improvement programs, and drafting bylaws for the general and day-to-day governance of the profession. (See the Nursing and Canadian Society box for additional information.)

All entry-level nursing education programs must receive approval from their regulatory body in order for their graduates to write the registration examination and apply for registration. Approval is based on the nursing education programs meeting the standards and competencies set by the regulatory bodies.

Accreditation for baccalaureate programs is completed by the Canadian Association of Schools of Nursing (CASN). See Chapter 2 for additional information.

The laws regulating nursing in the provinces and territories (other than Ontario and Quebec) are fairly uniform. Several provinces have umbrella legislation containing general provisions regarding all recognized health care professionals within the province, as well as companion legislation relating specifically to nursing (see examples of the legislation for each province and territory listed in Table 6.2). In Ontario, the Regulated Health Professions Act and the Nursing Act govern the nursing profession (Keatings & Smith, 2009). This legislation makes the CNO the governing body responsible for the regulation of nursing in the province. Section 11 of the Nursing Act prohibits anyone from declaring himself

TABLE 6.2 Nursing Legislation in Canadian Provinces and Territories

Province or Territory	Health Care and Nursing Legislation for *Registered Nurses (RN)*
British Columbia	Health Professions Act
Alberta	Health Professions Act and Nursing Professions Act
Northwest Territories and Nunavut	Nursing Profession Act and Nunavut Nursing Professions Act
Saskatchewan	The Registered Nurses Act
Manitoba	Regulated Health Professions Act
New Brunswick	Nurses Act
Nova Scotia	Registered Nurses Act
Prince Edward Island	Registered Nurses Act
Newfoundland and Labrador	Registered Nurses Act
Ontario	Regulated Health Professions Act, Nursing Act, and Health Professions Procedural Code
Quebec	Professional Code of Quebec and Nurses Act
Yukon	Registered Nurses Profession Act

Province or Territory	Health Care and Nursing Legislation for *Licensed Practical Nurses (LPN)*
British Columbia	Health Professions Act and CLPNBC bylaws
Alberta	Health Professions Act and Health Disciplines Act
Northwest Territories and Nunavut	Licensed Practical Nurses Act
Saskatchewan	Licensed Practical Nurses Act
Manitoba	Regulated Health Professions Act
New Brunswick	Licensed Practical Nurses Act
Nova Scotia	Licensed Practical Nurses Act
Prince Edward Island	Licensed Practical Nurses Act
Newfoundland and Labrador	Licensed Practical Nurses Act
Ontario (Registered Practical Nurse)	Regulated Health Professions Act, Nursing Act, and Health Professions Procedural Code
Quebec	Professional Code of Quebec, Nurses Act, and Licensed Practical Nurses Act

Province or Territory	Health Care and Nursing Legislation for *Registered Psychiatric Nurses*
British Columbia	Health Professions Act and Registered Psychiatric Nurses Act
Alberta	Health Professions Act and Health Disciplines Act
Saskatchewan	Registered Psychiatric Nurses Act
Manitoba	Regulated Health Professions Act and Registered Psychiatric Nurses Act

Source: Updated and adapted from Keatings, M., & Smith, O. (2009). The Canadian legal system. In M. Keatings and O. Smith (Eds.), *Ethical and Legal Issues in Canadian Nursing* (pp. 51–94). Toronto, ON: W.B. Saunders.

or herself as competent to practise as a registered nurse unless the CNO has licensed that person.

As further examples, Manitoba, Alberta, and British Columbia have legislation called the Health Professions Act. These acts provide a common regulatory structure for the governance of health care professions within the provinces. Regulations (or subordinate legislation) are enacted under the Health Professions Act that designate nursing as a regulated profession under the act with its own self-governing body. In British Columbia, for example, the Nurses (Registered) and Nurse Practitioner Regulation was approved by Cabinet in 2005. This regulation not only governs registered nurses but also establishes nurse practitioners as a recognized category of registered nurse under CRNBC. The Nurses (Registered) and Nurse Practitioner Regulation sets out reserved titles and the scope of practice for CRNBC registrants, including reserved actions for general and certified registered nurse practice as well as nurse practitioner practice. As explained on the CRNBC website, under the province's Health Professions Act, the CRNBC is responsible for serving and protecting the public, and for exercising its powers in the public interest. To fulfill that role, the act empowers the CRNBC to make bylaws to govern registrants, though most of the bylaws still do require government approval.

Licensure and registration together are a way to protect the public from unsafe practitioners and to assure employers that the nurse has met minimum requirements for entry to practice. The term **registration** means the listing of an individual's name on an official roster. In Canada, practising nurses in all provinces and territories are required by law to be registered or to hold a valid permit or licence with their provincial or territorial nursing association. Registration usually occurs every year. Only those who are registered are entitled to call themselves registered nurses, licensed (registered) practical nurses, or registered psychiatric nurses, or to use the initials RN, LPN, or RPN. To be registered, the regulated nurse must have completed a basic course of nursing studies in an approved program of the registering body and have passed the national qualifying exams.

The Agreement on Internal Trade (AIT) came into effect in 2009. It reads as follows:

> *AIT promotes harmonization of standards across provinces such that a qualified practitioner in one province would ultimately be able to move to another province and practice without going through an entirely new application/examination/supervision process. AIT is not aimed at creating a uniform standard for practice across the country, although that may be the intent of some of its proponents. Rather, the Agreement is directed at facilitating the movement of capable professional workers across provincial boundaries by reducing those barriers that appear to have nothing to do with a professional's competence to provide services.* (King, 2011, p.4)

Certification is a voluntary practice that proves that a nurse has met minimum standards of nursing competence in specialty areas, such as perinatal nursing, pediatrics, mental health, gerontology, or critical care nursing. Certification enhances a nurse's confidence and proficiency in a specialty area. Certification is a commitment to the leading edge in national health care standards. It gives national scope to the principle of continued competence encouraged by provincial and territorial quality assurance programs. The CNA offers certification in many areas.

EXPANDING THE ROLE OF REGISTERED NURSES   The various acts and regulations that govern the practice of nursing in Canada means they are responsible for setting the scope and nature of nursing in Canada. Recently, the development of policy and legislation to expand the scope of RNs' practice has become a prominent issue across the country. Diverse models have been used to provide authority to RNs performing extended or expanded roles. Diagnostic and treatment functions have been delegated by government to the medical profession through legislation (CNA, 2002). The CNA formed a committee of provincial and territorial representatives to establish a framework to guide the development and implementation of legislation dealing with nursing roles that require additional regulation (i.e., primary care functions). In 2008, the CNA published *Advanced Nursing Practice: A National Framework*, which includes information about various aspects of advanced nursing practice (ANP), such as competencies, educational preparation, and regulation (CNA, 2008a).

STANDARDS   The establishment of nursing practice standards is essential for a self-regulating profession. In assessing the quality of care provided by nurses, it is crucial to have objective criteria by which to judge whether the care given is good, adequate, or unsafe. Nursing practice standards are generally broad in nature to capture the varied roles and practice settings in which nurses practise. Each regulatory body will have a document regarding Standards of Practice for their members. Standards are also used as a template for nurses to assess their own nursing practice annually to determine their professional development goals and meet continuing competence requirements set out by the provincial or territorial body. It is the responsibility of all regulated members to understand their practice standards and apply them to their nursing practices, specific to their areas of practice and roles.

Best practice guidelines are a general form of nursing practice standards, for example, the Registered Nurses' Association of Ontario (RNAO) has produced a variety of documents that explain nursing practices that are research based, such as *Therapeutic Nurse–Client Relationship, Culturally Sensitive Care,* and *Documentation*.

Accountability and Discipline in Nursing

In addition to the elements just outlined, the nursing regulatory bodies are also responsible for ensuring that standards are established and maintained. This task includes investigating complaints regarding the level of practice or other competency issues of individual registrants and, where appropriate, addressing them through disciplinary action.

COMPLAINT PROCESS Each provincial and territorial nursing body has a mechanism in place to review the conduct of its members to ensure safe and ethical nursing practice. They are required to investigate complaints against members and discipline those who fail to meet the standards of the profession. The regulatory body may receive complaints about regulated nurses from a variety of sources, including the public, hospitals or other employers, and other nurses or health care providers. Occasionally, nurses may decide to self-report if they are concerned that they are not able to practise safely. The complaint process comprises a number of steps, including the complaint intake or receipt and initial assessment, the investigation process, the review process, and possibly a hearing and an appeal. Although variations exist across jurisdictions, so, too, do many similarities. Nurses are encouraged to check with their provincial or territorial association to determine the process to follow. The disciplinary role is central to the regulatory body's duty to protect the public, is taken very seriously, and can have significant consequences for the registrant. When a case involves either civil or criminal wrongs, further legal consequences may follow, separate and apart from the provincial and territorial regulatory body discipline process.

Contractual Arrangements in Nursing

Legal Roles of Nurses

Nurses have two separate but interdependent legal roles, each with rights and associated responsibilities: (a) provider of service and (b) employee or contractor for service.

PROVIDER OF SERVICE The nurse is expected to provide safe and **competent care** so that no harm (physical, psychological, or material) comes to the recipient of the service. A nurse, for example, has an obligation to practise and direct the practice of others under the nurse's supervision so that harm or injury to the client is prevented and standards of care are maintained. When **delegating care** to others, the nurse is responsible for ensuring that this delegation is appropriate and that those delegated to (e.g., family, other health care members, students) have

the skills to fulfill the functions (CNA, 2002). Nurses are obligated to follow physicians' orders, unless they believe that these orders have the potential to harm or injure the patient. The nurse must then carefully assess the situation and obtain clarification from the physician, if necessary. If the physician confirms the order and the nurse still believes the order to be unsafe, informing the supervisor is the next responsibility. The nurse also needs to carefully document, in chronological order, the steps taken. At this point, resolving the problem of the questionable order should be the supervisor's responsibility. It is imperative that a nurse speak out and investigate orders that are believed to be unsafe, as the nurse who carries out the order could be held legally responsible for any harm suffered by the patient.

The **standards of care** by which a nurse acts or fails to act are legally defined by nurse practice acts and by the rule of reasonable and prudent action—what a sensible and careful professional with similar preparation and experience would do in similar circumstances. The **contractual obligations** of a nurse toward the patient may be either implied, such as to render safe and competent care, or be more specifically stated, such as they might be within a contract for private employment, specifying what types of services will be provided, when, and for what payment. Employment contracts are discussed further in the following section.

EMPLOYEE OR CONTRACTOR FOR SERVICE Nurses, whether in independent practice or as employees, have employment contracts. A **contract** is an agreement between two or more persons that creates an obligation to do or not do a particular thing (*Black's Law Dictionary*, 2004). For a contract to exist (Parisi, 1999), the following conditions must be met:

* Each contract must have a lawful purpose.
* Each party entering the contract must be competent and understand the subject matter.
* Each party must understand the obligations of the contract.
* Each party must have obligations and benefits derived from the contract.
* At minimum, all employment contracts must meet the standards set forth in provincial, territorial, and federal labour standards and codes.

Employment contracts can be oral, written, or implied. If a union is not involved, the nurse and the employer can negotiate an individual employment contract that sets forth the rights and obligations of each party. A nurse who is employed directly by a client (a nurse in private practice) usually has a written contract with that client in which the nurse agrees to provide professional services for a certain fee. In a unionized organization, the terms and conditions of employment are those of the union contract with the employer. Verbal employment contracts can be problematic because they lack proof of the terms negotiated.

Contractual relationships vary among practice settings. The nurse employed by a hospital typically functions within an employer–employee relationship, in which the hospital is responsible for the workplace, and the nurse provides nursing care on behalf of the hospital. As an employee, a nurse must abide by the employer's policies. A nurse in independent practice is a contractor for service, whose contractual relationship with the client is an independent one. No matter what the practice setting, the parties involved should have a common understanding of the nurses' status as employee or independent contractor. It will have an impact on their daily working relationship and will be relevant should the nurse be the subject of an allegation of negligence.

If a nurse is found negligent, a court may order that nurse to pay damages to the plaintiff. This form of liability is called direct liability. The Canadian Nurses Protective Society (CNPS) professional liability protection is designed to assist nurses with this kind of damage award. A health care facility may also be found negligent and held directly liable for breaching duties it owed to the patient. These could include, for example, the duty to select professional staff using reasonable care, adopt and enforce appropriate policies and procedures, provide reasonable supervision of staff, and provide adequate staffing, equipment or resources.

If a nurse working as an employee is found negligent, the court may order that damages be paid by the nurse's employer pursuant to the doctrine of **vicarious liability**. This legal doctrine provides that an employer, which may be an individual or an institution, is held financially responsible for the negligence of its employees to an individual harmed by this negligence. This is in recognition of the control an employer has in the workplace and to ensure a remedy for successful plaintiffs. An employment relationship must have existed at the time of the incident and the defendant employee must have been sued for work done within the scope of his or her employment. Consequently, it is very common for the employer's liability insurance to cover the legal defence costs (legal fees, related disbursements, and damages) of nurses who are sued in connection with the work they are employed to do (CNPS, 1998). The doctrine of vicarious liability does not imply that the nurse cannot be held liable as an individual. Employees should verify whether they are covered by their employer or their employer's insurance in the event of claims arising out of their employment. An employer generally cannot be held liable under the doctrine of vicarious liability for conduct falling outside the scope of employment, such as theft of narcotics or assault.

The doctrine of vicarious liability does not generally apply to nurses who are independent contractors or self-employed. Independent contractors must

---

BOX 6.1 LEGAL PROTECTION IN AN EMPLOYEE–EMPLOYER RELATIONSHIP

Nurses should be aware of the liability protection they have:

- Nurses should seek written confirmation of their employment status and professional liability coverage.
- Nurses should ensure that the employer is notified immediately if they are sued or involved in a potential liability situation.
- Nurses should be aware of the process and cooperate with the employer's insurer and lawyer representing (defending) them in a legal suit.
- Nurses who practise as independent practitioners should contact their insurer, if they have one, and CNPS to discuss their existing liability protection.

Source: Based on Canadian Nurses Protective Society. (1998). Vicarious liability. *infoLAW, 7*(1).

---

decide on the type and amount of liability protection they require, which will respond to the types of liability they may incur. Seeking advice from a business advisor is recommended (CNPS Briefing Note, Collaborative Practice: Are Nurses Employees or Self-employed? 2006). See Box 6.1 for information on legal protection for nurses.

The nurse is expected to respect the rights and responsibilities of other health care participants. For example, although the nurse has a responsibility to explain nursing activities to a patient, the nurse does not have the right to comment on medical practice in a way that disturbs the client or denounces the physician. At the same time, the nurse has the right to expect reasonable and prudent conduct from other health care professionals. See Table 6.3 for examples of roles, responsibilities, and rights of nurses.

Areas of Potential Tort Liability in Nursing

Tort Law

A **tort** is a civil wrong committed against a person or a person's property. Battery and the failure to obtain informed consent, discussed later in this chapter, are examples of torts. Torts are usually litigated in court by civil action between individuals. In other words, the person claimed to be responsible for the tort is sued for damages. Tort liability is based on fault, that is, something that was done incorrectly (an unreasonable act of commission) or something that should have been done but was not (omission). Torts can be broadly categorized as either negligence or intentional.

TABLE 6.3 Legal Roles, Responsibilities, and Rights

Role	Responsibilities (Obligations)	Rights
Provider of service	To provide safe and competent care commensurate with the nurse's preparation, experience, and circumstances To inform clients of the consequences of various alternatives and outcomes of care To provide adequate supervision and evaluation of others for whom the nurse is responsible	The right to reasonable and prudent conduct from clients (e.g., provision of accurate information, as required)
Employee or contractor for service	To fulfill the obligations of contracted service with the employer To respect the employer To respect the rights and responsibilities of other health care providers	The right to adequate working conditions (e.g., safe equipment and facilities) The right to compensation for services rendered The right to reasonable and prudent conduct by other health care providers
Citizen	To protect the rights of the recipients of care	The right to respect of the nurse's own rights and responsibilities by others Right to physical safety

NEGLIGENCE In the nursing context, **negligence** consists of conduct and behaviour that falls below the standard expected of an ordinary, reasonable, and prudent nurse. Such conduct places another person at risk for harm. Failing to obtain informed consent, failing to follow proper procedure in moving a patient, or administering the wrong dosage of medication all constitute examples of negligence in nursing. Four elements must be present in a negligence lawsuit against a nurse:

1. *Duty.* The nurse must have a relationship with the client that involves providing care. Such duty is evident when the nurse has been assigned to care for a client in the home, hospital, or community by virtue of employment. In contrast, a nurse in private practice may have the option of deciding whether to accept a patient for care; as such, the duty is established when the nurse takes on an individual as a patient.

2. *Breach.* A standard of care must be expected in the specific situation that the nurse did not observe. This is the failure to act as a reasonable, prudent nurse under the circumstances. The practice is measured against that of similar nurses, unless the nurse undertakes a practice outside the usual nursing role. In such an instance, the nurse may be held to a higher standard based on advanced training. The standard can come from documents published by national or professional organizations, provincial or territorial nursing practice standards, institutional policies and procedures, or textbooks or journals, or it may be stated by expert witnesses.

3. *Harm.* The client must have sustained injury, damage, or harm. The plaintiff will be asked to document physical injury, medical costs, loss of wages, pain and suffering, and any other damages.

4. *Causation.* It must be proved that the harm occurred as a *direct result* of the nurse's failure to follow the standard, and the nurse could have (or should have) known that failure to follow the standard could result in such harm.

To avoid charges of negligence, nurses need to recognize those nursing situations in which negligent actions are most likely to occur and to take measures to prevent them (see Box 6.2). A common situation is *medication error*. Because of the large number of medications taken by patients, and the numerous commercial names commonly used for the various drugs, safety precautions assume greater importance to ensure that the patient receives the right drug, in the proper dose, at the right time, for the right reason, and in the proper manner. Medication errors include failing to read the medication label, misreading or incorrectly calculating the dosage, failing to identify the client correctly, preparing the wrong concentration, or administering a medication by the wrong route (e.g., intravenously instead of intramuscularly). Nurses always need to check medications very carefully (see Chapter 33). Even after checking, the nurse should recheck the medication order and the medication before administering it if, for example, the client states, "I did not have a green pill before."

A nurse's responsibility for adverse effects and critical incidents (National Steering Committee on Patient Safety, 2002) will be weighed in accordance with the provincial or territorial professional nursing standard. Health care employers often have policies and procedures for

---

BOX 6.2 BASIC NURSING CARE ERRORS RESULTING IN NEGLIGENCE

Three kinds of nursing errors can result in negligence. Examples of each kind of error are listed below.

ASSESSMENT ERRORS

- Failing to gather and chart client information adequately
- Failing to recognize the significance of certain information (e.g., laboratory values, vital signs)

PLANNING ERRORS

- Failing to chart each identified problem
- Failing to use language in the care plan that other caregivers understand
- Failing to ensure continuity of care by ignoring the care plan
- Failing to give discharge instructions that the client understands

INTERVENTION AND EVALUATION ERRORS

- Failing to interpret and carry out a doctor's orders
- Failing to perform nursing tasks correctly
- Failing to pursue the physician if the physician does not respond to calls or failing to notify the nurse manager if the physician is unavailable
- Failing to report unsafe working conditions

---

medication administration and standards for documentation that include the steps to follow once an error has been discovered. Such standards also include the requirement to keep up to date with the latest professional and technological developments, such as new intravenous tubing or intravenous pumps. Additional education should be taken as required to maintain expertise to the appropriate standard.

A nurse must administer medications according to the 10 *rights* of medication administration (see Chapter 33). Nurses must take action to ensure that they do not misread, mishear, or misunderstand the drug that they are giving. For example, such a drug as hydromorphone can easily be mistaken for morphine. This error is known as *confirmation bias*: seeing what you expect to see (Borg, 2008).

Despite this diligence, medication errors still occur. Such was the case in which a 67-year-old man in the emergency department was given 10 mg of hydromorphone intramuscularly (IM) instead of 10 mg of morphine. He was given this drug just before discharge as the patient declined to stay for observation. Hydromorphone that was packaged in a similar way to morphine was mistakenly selected from the opioid cupboard. The dose given to the patient (who was opioid naive) was equivalent to about 60 mg to 70 mg of morphine. Within 1 hour of the patient's discharge, the opioid count revealed the error. The hospital took immediate action to find the

patient; unfortunately, he had experienced cardiac arrest and died in another rural hospital. Possible legal investigations in such a case may or may not lead to legal proceedings and penalties. In 2004, the Institute for Safe Medication Practices Canada generated a detailed report with recommendations for practitioners and institutions; "unfortunately in the years since the report morphine/hydromorphone substitution errors continue to be made" (Borg, 2008, p. 35).

Patients can fall accidentally, sometimes with resultant injury. Some falls can be prevented by elevating the side rails on the cribs, beds, and stretchers for babies, small children, and, when necessary, adults. If a nurse leaves the rails down, or leaves a baby unattended on a bath table, that nurse may be found liable in negligence if the patient falls and is injured as a direct result. Most hospitals and nursing homes have policies regarding the use of safety devices, such as side rails and restraints. The nurse needs to be familiar with these policies and to take precautions to prevent accidents. Information about providing a safe environment for patients can be found in Chapter 32.

In some instances, ignoring a patient's complaints can constitute negligence. The nurse who does not report a client's complaint of acute abdominal pain is negligent and may be found liable for the ensuing appendix rupture and death. By failing to take vital signs and to check the dressing of a patient who has just had abdominal surgery, a nurse omits important assessments. If the patient has a hemorrhage and dies, the nurse may be found liable for negligence.

The case of *Downey v. Rothwell* (1974) is a clear, often cited example of negligence in the nursing context. In this case, a 35-year-old plaintiff, who had a history of grand mal epileptic seizures and recently had discontinued her anticonvulsant prescription for phenobarbital, suffered a severe arm injury after falling off an examining room table. Mrs. Downey was under the care of an RN (of 40 years' experience) who had worked in this doctor's clinic for the past 22 years. The client informed the nurse that she was experiencing the sensation (called an *aura*) that precedes an epileptic seizure. The nurse remained in the room with the client for about a half an hour. When nothing happened, however, the nurse left the room to locate Mrs. Downey's file, leaving her unattended. During this time, the client experienced a severe seizure, fell onto the floor, and broke her arm. The nurse, having knowledge about epileptic seizures, should have recognized an aura and remained with the client, ensuring her safety on the examination table.

In this case, the judge concluded that leaving the client unattended constituted a breach of the standard of care expected of an RN. A nursing instructor who testified as an expert witness and textbook materials were both presented to establish the appropriate standard of care. These sources were unanimous in stating that the nurse in this situation should have remained with the client. The nurse was found to be negligent, and for that negligence, her employers were made vicariously liable.

INTENTIONAL TORTS Negligence is different from **intentional torts**. The main difference is that negligent acts are unintentional, and intentional torts are committed on purpose by the tortfeasor. Another difference is that harm is a required element in negligence, whereas no harm need be suffered by the plaintiff for a defendant to be found liable of an intentional tort. Also, because no standard of care is involved, no expert witnesses are needed. Assault, battery, false imprisonment, and invasion of privacy are some of the intentional torts most likely to be relevant in the nursing context.

Assault can be described as an attempt or threat to touch another person unjustifiably. Assault precedes battery; it is the act that causes the person to believe a battery is about to occur. For example, the person who threatens someone by making a menacing gesture with a club or a closed fist is guilty of assault. A nurse who threatens a client with an injection after the client refuses to take the medication orally would be committing assault.

Battery is intentional harmful or offensive contact with another person (or the person's clothes or even something the person is carrying), without that person's consent. It is not necessary that a battery actually result in harm to the plaintiff; instead, "offensive contact is enough, however trivial it may seem, for it may trigger retaliatory measures by persons whose dignity and self-respect are threatened" by the contact (Linden & Feldthusen, 2006, p. 44). "[B]attery is . . . a tort or legal wrong which protects people's 'dignitary interests,' their rights to personal autonomy and to freedom from wanton, humiliating or otherwise unwelcome interference" (Sneiderman et al., 2003, p. 160). In the previous example, if the nurse followed through on the threat and gave the injection without the client's consent, the nurse would be committing battery. Liability applies even though the physician ordered the medication or the activity and even if the client benefits from the nurse's action. Case law also indicates that it is battery "where a nurse in good faith administers a vaccination believing wrongly that there has been consent" (*Toews v. Weisner*, [2001, BCSC] as cited by Linden & Feldthusen, 2006).

A good example of a case involving battery is *Malette v. Shulman* (1990), from the Ontario Court of Appeal. In this case, an unconscious patient arrived in the emergency department following a car accident. The physician determined that the patient required a blood transfusion to survive and proceeded to transfuse her even after being advised that she carried a card in her wallet that identified her as a Jehovah's Witness. The card indicated that on the basis of her religious convictions, she did not want

to be given blood under any circumstances. The card was neither dated nor witnessed. The patient survived and successfully sued the physician for battery. Although this case did not involve nurses, it serves to highlight the fact that even though consent is often deemed to be implied in emergency situations, such consent may in some circumstances be set aside when a strong indication exists that the patient would not have consented to the treatment.

Battery clearly exists when consent is not obtained for treatment. However, the courts will also consider as battery treatments given that either go beyond or are different from that for which consent was obtained (such as when the wrong spinal disc is operated on), or when consent is obtained through fraud or misrepresentation (Linden & Feldthusen, 2006). In contrast, when a patient has consented to treatment but then complains that he or she was not given adequate information, for example, as to the risks associated with the procedure, the plaintiff would properly bring the claim of negligence. For consent to be valid, the patient must be competent to give consent. It can be very difficult to determine whether clients who are very old, who have specific mental disorders, or who take particular medications are competent to agree to treatments. If the nurse is uncertain whether a client refusing a treatment is competent, the supervisor and physician should be consulted to ensure that the treatment is ethically and legally permissible.

False imprisonment is the intentional confining of a person within fixed boundaries, without that person's consent. As others have explained, the name is somewhat misleading. Linden and Feldthusen (2006) explain as follows:

Firstly, there is no need for any prison to be involved. Although one can certainly imprison someone by incarceration behind prison walls, it can also be accomplished in other ways [for example, one can imprison someone in a psychiatric hospital, room, car, or boat]. Secondly, the confinement cannot be "false" in the sense of being unreal. The word "false" is intended to impart the notion of unauthorized or wrongful detention. (p. 50)

The plaintiff does not need to prove damages to successfully bring a false imprisonment action but must show that he or she "was intentionally restrained and that no reasonable avenue of escape was available. [Moreover], the plaintiff need not be conscious of the confinement" at the time it occurred (Picard & Robertson, 1996, p. 338).

The 1994 case *Lebel v. Roe* in the Yukon provides a clear example of false imprisonment in the nursing context. In that case, a patient agreed to be admitted to a psychiatric facility after being advised (incorrectly) by a mental health nurse that she would be apprehended by the Royal Canadian Mounted Police (RCMP) if she refused to come voluntarily. The court awarded the patient $5000, holding that the nurse ought to have known her statement was incorrect, that her statement resulted in the patient believing that her freedom was restricted, and that her admission to the facility constituted false imprisonment (as discussed by Picard & Robertson, 1996, p. 339). Although nurses may suggest under certain circumstances that a patient remain in the hospital room or in bed, the patient must not be detained against his or her will. The patient has the right to leave, even though it may be detrimental to his or her health.

If the patient insists on leaving, most institutions require that he or she sign a release stating that the agency will not be held responsible for any resulting harm. As with all situations, the nurse should try to inform the patient of potential risks and alternative courses of action. The use of force to detain someone against his or her will can constitute battery, and even the threat of restraint made to detain the patient can be considered assault. The nurse must be cautious with the use of restraints (see Chapter 32).

Invasion of privacy is a developing area of Canadian law: "Although the right to privacy is well-entrenched in American tort law, the Canadian and English courts have been reluctant to recognize a separate common law right to privacy . . . [however,] we seem to be drifting closer to the American model" (Linden & Feldthusen, 2006, p. 59). The American model outlines four distinct privacy torts: (a) intrusion on the plaintiff's seclusion or private affairs, (b) public disclosure of embarrassing private facts about the plaintiff, (c) publicity that places the plaintiff in a false light in the public eye, and (d) appropriation of the plaintiff's name or likeness for the defendant's advantage (Linden & Feldthusen, 2006, p. 59).

Canadian courts have generally recognized invasions of privacy that fall under the fourth category only; however, an Ontario case, *Somwar v. McDonald's Restaurants of Canada* (2006), suggested that in light of technological advancements that allow for easy (proper and improper) collection, access, and dissemination of personal information, the courts may well be more willing to recognize invasion of privacy as a distinct tort. This case was not in the medical context, but it does demonstrate that the longstanding position of the courts in this area might be changing. The case involved an action for invasion of privacy as a result of an unauthorized credit check by the plaintiff's employer. The defendant employer sought to have the claim dismissed on the ground that Ontario law did not recognize such a cause of action. However, the judge found that "it is not settled law in Ontario that there is no tort of invasion of privacy" (*Somwar v. McDonald's Restaurants of Canada*, 2006) and refused to strike the claim.

A number of Canadian provinces have also implemented privacy legislation that make it a "tort, actionable without proof of damage, for a person, willfully and without a claim of right, to violate the privacy of another" (Privacy Act, RSBC, 1996, as cited by Linden & Feldthusen, 2006). Despite these legislative advances, in most cases, although the possibility of pursuing a civil claim for breach of privacy exists, it seems that "professional disciplinary proceedings remain by far the more realistic deterrent to this variety of nursing malpractice" (Sneiderman et al., 2003, p. 179).

One important exception exists to the courts' hesitation in awarding liability for invasions of privacy: Breach of confidentiality will give rise to legal remedy against, for example, a nurse or other health care provider who divulges confidential patient information (Sneiderman et al., 2003). In nursing, liability can result if the nurse breaches confidentiality by passing along confidential patient information to others who are not directly involved in the care of that patient or by intruding into the patient's private domain. In this context, a delicate balance must be maintained between the need for a number of people to contribute to the diagnosis and treatment of a client and the client's right to confidentiality. In most situations, necessary discussion about a client's medical condition is considered appropriate, but unnecessary discussions and gossip are considered a breach of confidentiality. Necessary discussion involves only those engaged in the client's care. In some instances, however, a statutorily imposed duty exists to report what would normally constitute confidential information. Most provinces and territories have a variety of statutes that impose a duty to report some confidential patient information. Four major categories are (a) vital statistics, such as births and deaths, (b) infections and communicable diseases, such as diphtheria, syphilis, and typhoid fever, (c) child or elder abuse, and (d) violent incidents, such as gunshot wounds and knife wounds.

Consent Issues

Patients are entitled to make decisions about their health care and have the right to be given all available information relevant to such decisions. Obtaining consent is not a discrete event; rather, it is a process that should occur throughout the relationship between the patient and all health care providers.

Consent has three components: (a) disclosure, (b) capacity, and (c) voluntariness. **Disclosure** refers to the provision of information, including the risks of treatment, alternative treatment and its associated facts and risks, and the effects and risks of no treatment. **Capacity** refers to the patient's ability to understand the relevant information and appreciate the consequences of the decision. **Voluntariness** refers to the patient's right to come to a decision without force, coercion, or manipulation from others (Etchells, Sharpe, Elliott & Singer, 1999). When these three requirements are met—that is, when a patient has received all the information, when the patient has the capacity to make the decision, and when the patient is free from coercion—the patient is then in a position to provide what is called **informed consent** to the medical treatment.

Consent is of two types: *express* and *implied.* **Express consent** is a clear statement by the patient and can be either oral or written. "It is important to remember that the patient has the right to withdraw consent or revoke a previously given consent at any time, even orally, provided he/she is mentally competent to do so" (Keatings & Smith, 2009, p. 186). **Implied consent** exists when the individual's nonverbal behaviour indicates willingness. Examples of implied consent include the following:

- In emergency situations, when the individual cannot provide express consent

- During surgery, when additional procedures are needed that are consistent with the procedure already consented to

- In therapy, when the person continues to participate without withdrawing previously provided consent

In such situations, the CNPS (1994) suggests that provincial and territorial legislation, including hospital or institutional policies and procedures, be followed.

OBTAINING CONSENT AND DISCLOSING INFORMATION
Obtaining consent to medical or nursing care is a legal requirement. Under common law, treating a competent patient without obtaining any consent, or treating a patient who is refusing treatment, constitutes battery, whereas treating a patient without obtaining fully informed consent constitutes negligence (Parisi, 1999).

Obtaining informed consent for specific *medical* and *surgical* treatments is the responsibility of a physician. Although this responsibility is delegated to nurses in some agencies and no laws prohibit the nurse from being part of the information-giving process, the practice, nevertheless, is highly undesirable. The nurse does not perform direct medical procedures and may not have the detailed medical knowledge of the physician performing the procedure. Also, it is not the nurse's responsibility to "supply the gaps or deficiencies in the physician's dialogue with the patient"; however, it is the responsibility of the nurse to "respond appropriately and ensure that when information gaps occur the physician is alerted in time to put things right" (Sneiderman et al., 2003, p. 164). Often, the nurse's responsibility is to witness the giving

of informed consent for medical procedures, which involves the following:

- Witnessing the exchange between the client and the physician

- Establishing that the client really did understand, that is, was truly informed

Obtaining informed consent for *nursing* procedures is the responsibility of the nurse. This applies, in particular, to nurse midwives and nurse practitioners in performing procedures in their advanced practices. However, it also applies to other nurses performing direct care, such as inserting nasogastric tubes or starting an intravenous infusion. It can be a challenge to determine the amount and type of information required for the client to make an informed decision. The client should have the following general information:

- The purposes of the treatment

- What he or she can expect to feel or experience

- The intended benefits of the treatment

- The possible risks or negative outcomes of the treatment

- The advantages and disadvantages of possible alternatives to the treatment (including no treatment)

Informed consent regulations were originally written with acute care settings in mind. Nonetheless, ensuring informed consent is equally important in providing nursing care in the home and community. Because the provision of home care often occurs over an extended period, the nurse has multiple opportunities to ensure that the client agrees to the plan of treatment. A challenge to informed consent in the home, however, is that the plan may affect other members of the family, and, if so, they need to be consulted.

In many areas of health care law and capacity, consent remains a confusing issue. The first is related to minors. Canadian common law does not specify an age below which a person is not presumed capable (Etchells, Sharpe, Elliott, & Singer, 1999). Some provinces have legislation that lowers the age of consent below 18 years. A minor can give consent if it is determined that the person has adequate knowledge and judgment (is able to reasonably foresee consequences of a decision or lack of a decision) (Sharpe, 1993). Some provinces have legislation that establishes the age of consent to treatment; health care providers should be aware of the legislative requirements of their own province or territory.

It is also important to remember that capacity can change over time. A patient who is confused, disoriented, or sedated is not considered functionally competent; however, this state may be temporary and requires careful, skilled assessment. Individuals who are unconscious or injured in such a way that they are unable to give consent require substitute consent from another individual.

Statutes tend to provide a hierarchy of **substitute decision makers**. Priority is given to a court-appointed substitute decision maker or person with power of attorney for personal care or proxy. If these do not exist, authority falls to a spouse, and then to various family members in accordance with the statutory list (CNPS, 2009, p. 2). The substitute decision maker should be the person with the best knowledge of the patient's specific wishes or of the patient's values and beliefs. In general, close relatives are preferred as substitute decision makers as they "know the patient best" and are able to make a decision that would be as close to the patient's as possible.

In the case of a patient with a mental illness, capacity to consent may or may not be valid, depending on whether the mental illness makes that patient unable to appreciate the nature, quality, and consequences of the proposed treatment. In this case, patients who refuse treatment can have their capacity questioned by the clinician. Provincial and territorial mental health acts or similar statutes generally provide direction and specify the rights of people with mental illness under the law, as well as the rights of the professionals caring for such patients.

Patient Safety

Significant attention has been focused on issues related to patient safety in Canada's health care system because "the costs of unsafe health care—both personal and fiscal—to individuals, their families and their communities and to the state are massive" (Downie, Lahey, Ford, Gibson, Thomson, Ward, et al., 2006). In 2006, a report entitled *Patient Safety Law: From Silos to Systems*, funded by Health Canada, "explored the use of legal instruments by governments to improve patient safety" (Downie et al., 2006, p. 1). The report provides an overview of the various legal tools in Canada that, in patchwork fashion, address issues of patient safety. It also identifies strengths and weaknesses for each area as well as for the system as a whole. Some of the elements reviewed include approaches to institutional, professional, and products regulation in Canada, as well as adverse event reporting frameworks and relevant aspects of the complaint and inquiry processes and available compensation systems. The authors' comments provide some helpful insights into some of the problems and suggest some possible solutions:

> *Having taken a system governance perspective, we identified a body of law that can be described as patient safety law, in that it functions to protect the patient by reducing unsafe acts within the health care system. The different areas of law that affect patient safety (e.g., tort law, professional regulation, institutional regulation) are not usually conceived of as an integrated system of law. However, conceiving of patient safety law as an integrated entity has value since it allows the discussion to move away from thinking in terms of narrow siloed categories of law to thinking of the larger systemic objectives the legal framework should enable regarding the governance of patient safety. (Downie et al., 2006, p. 2)*

EVIDENCE-INFORMED PRACTICE

What Are the Clinical Ethical Conflicts that Hospital Nurses and Physicians Experience in Their Practice Today?

In a qualitative descriptive study, part of a larger investigation of four hospital clinical ethics committees in Atlantic Canada, nurses and physicians were interviewed about their ethical conflicts in clinical situations. The results were nine themes of clinical ethical conflict common to both nurses and physicians:

- Disagreement about care decisions or treatment options
- Others not respecting a patient's wishes
- Patient not receiving quality end-of-life care
- Patient's or family's behaviour preventing safe or quality care for self or others
- Patient and/or family not having informed consent or full disclosure
- Not knowing the "right thing to do"
- System deficit or deficiency preventing quality care
- Nurse or physician values conflict with patient values or lifestyle choices
- Possible or perceived deficiencies in care owing to nurse or physician competency

Three additional themes were specific to physicians:

- Disagreement with national clinical practice guidelines
- Estimating the odds of survival and futility of treatment
- Balancing merit of survival with disability in an infant or child

NURSING IMPLICATIONS: All themes relate to the nurse's and physician's desire to do the right thing for a patient and/or family. The core theme "striving to do what is best for the patient" underpins all the clinical ethical conflict themes described in this study.

Source: Based on Gaudine, A., Lefort, S., Lamb, M., & Thorne, L. (2011). Clinical ethical conflicts of nurses and physicians. *Nursing Ethics, 18*(1), 9–19.

The report clearly highlights that a more holistic, system-wide approach to patient safety is in line with international trends and would address some of the gaps identified in our current approach.

See the Evidence-Informed Practice box on the clinical ethical conflicts that hospital nurses and physicians experience in their practice today.

Adverse Event Reporting

One of the key areas addressed in the report on patient safety was **adverse event reporting**. Although "adverse events reporting systems are a structural facet of safety regulation in other sectors . . . they are a relatively recent innovation in the health care system" (Downie et al., 2006, p. 56). In some provinces (including Saskatchewan, Manitoba, and Quebec), adverse event reporting frameworks have been established through legislative initiatives. The first example of this was Saskatchewan's Regional Health Services Act, passed in 2002, which gave rise to mandatory reporting of adverse events to the provincial health department. In 2004, with the addition of the Critical Incident Regulation under the act, the requirements and details of the reporting structure were made clearer and more complete. Under this framework, for example, health care organizations and the regional health authorities to which they report "are required to give notice of critical incidents arising from their operations within 3 business days, or as soon as possible thereafter" to the Department of Health (Downie et al., 2006, p. 56). Notification must be followed up by a detailed written report. The *Saskatchewan Critical Incident Reporting Guideline* (Government of Saskatchewan, 2004) offers some additional insight into what is required under the framework. The guideline defines a **critical incident** as "a serious adverse health event including, but not limited to, the actual or potential loss of life, limb or function related to a health service provided by, or a program operated by, a regional health authority (RHA) or health care organization (HCO)" (p. 1). Some of the categories under which a reportable incident can arise include "surgical events, product or device events, patient protection events, care management events, environmental events and criminal events" (Downie et al., 2006, p. 56).

Although developments and initiatives, such as those in Saskatchewan, Manitoba, and Quebec, suggest that improvements are underway, the concern expressed in the report of the National Steering Committee on Patient Safety (2002) that Canada is behind several other countries in the development of such mechanisms has not yet been fully addressed. Some of the recommendations made in the committee's report specifically address the issue of how to improve the reporting of adverse events:

- The adoption of nonpunitive reporting policies within a quality improvement framework across the system that encourage and reward reporting, with limited exceptions

- The review and revision of legislation across all Canadian jurisdictions to protect patient safety data and reports from disclosure in legal proceedings. Facts relating to the event should be recorded on the patient's health record and should not be privileged. Deidentified information could be entered into a provincial or territorial or national database to facilitate the sharing of lessons learned across jurisdictions (Downie et al., 2006, p. 59).

The recommendations indicate a tension between litigation and quality assurance or improvement systems. The former does not encourage openness or

---

BOX 6.3 CANADIAN DISCLOSURE GUIDELINES

The *Canadian Disclosure Guidelines* focus on disclosure of adverse events and were developed by the Canadian Patient Safety Institute (CPSI), a nonprofit organization that raises awareness and facilitates the implementation of ideas and best practices to achieve a transformation in patient safety.

"Healthcare providers have ethical and professional obligations to be open and honest when communicating with patients" (p. 10). The guideline outlines a process for health care providers that promotes a clear and consistent approach to disclosure.

Source: Based on information obtained from The Canadian Patient Safety Institute. (2008). *Canadian disclosure guidelines: Being open with patients and families.* Retrieved from http://www.patientsafetyinstitute.ca/English/toolsResources/disclosure/Documents/CPSI%20Canadian%20Disclosure%20Guidelines.pdf. Edmonton, AB: Author.

---

transparency in the wake of an adverse event, as this has the potential to expose those health care providers and institutions involved to liability; in contrast, to fully identify, understand, learn from, and thereby reduce future likelihood of adverse events, mechanisms that will encourage reporting and open discussion of such events are needed. Ultimately, such a system will help increase patient safety, as well as the accountability of both individuals and organizations within the health care system. See Box 6.3 on Canadian disclosure guidelines.

Selected Legal Aspects of Nursing Practice

Confidentiality and Privacy

As discussed earlier, fundamental to the nurse–patient relationship is the professional obligation to respect patient confidentiality. Confidentiality brings with it both moral and legal obligations for nurses. Whenever possible, nurses uphold confidentiality, except when harm might result to the patient or others or when statute law or legislation requires disclosure (i.e., suspected child abuse, infectious disease, information for workers' compensation boards, or a court order). The CNA *Code of Ethics* (2008) states: "When nurses are required to disclose information for a particular purpose, they disclose only the amount of information necessary for that purpose and inform only those necessary. The attempt is to do so in ways that minimize any potential harm to the individual, family or community" (p. 15). Legally, the betrayal of a patient's confidence is covered under the area of professional misconduct and may result in discipline by the provincial or territorial conduct committee of the professional nursing regulatory body.

Confidential information is "intimate or private knowledge" protected under a duty of confidentiality.

Confidentiality can be summarized as the duty of someone (a professional) who has received confidential information in trust to protect that information and disclose it to others only with permission, or when rules or laws authorize its disclosure. Confidential information can come directly from the patient, received through written documents or electronic data, or come from a third party. A common rule frequently noted in policy is that all knowledge is considered confidential unless otherwise stated by the patient.

Often, the notion of confidential information is discussed within the framework of the legal right to *privacy*. In simple terms, **privacy** is about people, while confidentiality is about duty to protect information. Privacy is about a person's right to control the intrusion of others into his or her life. In other words it concerns what information a health care provider can have. A patient's right to privacy means that he or she has the right to disclose details of his or her life, illness, feelings, finances, and family interactions, or *not* to disclose them. Confidentiality is about what a nurse does with the information. When patients give their personal information to nurses, they trust that the nurses will disclose it only to appropriate members of the health care team. Maintaining patient confidentiality is an important element of trust and as such is a moral obligation of nurses.

Many key documents have been written in the development and evolution of public policy concerning informational privacy. The Office of the Privacy Commissioner of Canada (2004) offers information to help individuals learn about their rights under the Personal Information Protection and Electronic Documents Act (PIPEDA), Canada's private sector privacy law (http://www.priv.gc.ca).

The primary legal consideration with respect to any information that the nurse obtains from a patient during the course of the professional relationship is that such information is confidential and cannot be disclosed to anyone who has no valid purpose for requesting it. The rule has some exceptions, both in the common law and as provided by statute. But in many provinces, if an unauthorized person accesses a patient's health record, or if health information is inappropriately released, a breach of patient's privacy rights can result in legal liability for the custodian of the records and the individuals involved in the incident. Because of that risk, it is important for all nurses, health care professionals, and employees to be aware of current developments in and comply with the legislated requirements of Canadian privacy law.

Confidentiality and Social Media

All health care professionals, are held to a high standard of confidentiality with respect to all patient information. "Professional practice standards may also be applicable when nurses use social media in connection with their professional activities and require nurses to display professional conduct towards both patients and colleagues. Failure to abide by these standards can lead to serious legal consequences. For example, a nurse was found guilty of unprofessional conduct by her professional licensing body because she posted a patient's first name and the patient's personal health information on a coworker's Facebook page" (CNPS, 2010).

Risk management for nurses using social media (CNPS, 2010) involves the following:

- Avoid posting/sharing confidential information: an unnamed patient or person may be identifiable from posted information.

- Avoid using social media to vent or discuss work-related events or to comment on similar postings by others.

- Avoid posting negative comments about your colleagues, supervisors, and other health care professionals; disclosing information obtained at work could be considered unprofessional and, if erroneous, could lead to a defamation claim.

- Respect and enforce professional boundaries: becoming a patient's electronic "friend" or communicating with him or her through social media sites may extend the scope of professional responsibility.

- Be aware that it is difficult to ascertain whether individuals providing or seeking information through a social media account are who they say they are.

- Avoid offering health-related advice in response to comments or questions posted on social media sites; if relied upon, such advice could trigger professional liability.

- Make your personal profile private and accessible only by people you know and trust.

- Create strong passwords, change them frequently, and keep them private.

- Present yourself in a professional manner in photos, videos, and postings.

Problematic Substance Use and Chemical Dependency

"It is thought that between 10 and 20 percent of nurses will have a substance abuse problem at some point in their lives" (CNA, 2011, p. 24). Problematic substance use and chemical dependency are serious problems, endangering the safety of the public and the health of nurses. Many factors in the workplace are linked to nurses' problematic substance use: shift work, stress, long working hours, and access to a large variety of pharmacological substances all contribute to the risk (Adlersberg & Mackinnon, 2004). Prevention, early recognition, and effective treatment programs are essential to promote the health of nurses and ensure public safety.

Nurses have a professional responsibility to protect patients from harm. Education and prevention of problematic substance use must begin in schools of nursing and nurses' workplaces to heighten awareness and

BOX 6.4 BEHAVIOURAL INDICATORS OF CHEMICAL MISUSE

Nurses need to be aware of the signs of problematic drug or alcohol use:

- Increased isolation from colleagues, friends, and family
- Frequent reports of illness, minor accidents, and emergencies
- Complaints about poor work performance
- Inability to meet schedules and deadlines
- Tendency to avoid new and challenging assignments
- Mood swings, irritability, and depression
- Request for night shifts
- Social avoidance of staff
- Illogical and sloppy charting
- Excessive errors
- Increasing carelessness about personal appearance
- Medication errors that require many changes in charting
- Arriving early or staying late for no reason
- Volunteering to administer client medications, especially pain medications

Source: Adapted from Springhouse Corporation. (2004). *Nurse's legal handbook* (5th ed.) Springhouse, PA: Springhouse.

promote early detection. Denying that a problem exists is a common first sign of problematic substance use. Admitting there is a problem may be the hardest step. It is not uncommon for coworkers to explain or excuse unacceptable behaviour rather than consider the possibility of problematic drug or alcohol use (CNA, 2009). Nurses need to be aware of signs of a potential problem (see Box 6.4). Consultation with licensing bodies is available to help deal with suspected problems. Guidance for nurses is also provided by the CNA *Code of Ethics* and CNA Position Statement on Problematic Substance Use by Nurses (2009). Nurses must adhere to the reporting requirements of the licensing bodies.

Employers must have sound policies and procedures for identifying and intervening in situations involving a possibly impaired nurse. The primary concern is for the protection of clients, but it is also critically important that the nurse's problem be identified quickly so that appropriate treatment may be instituted. The signs presented in Box 6.4 can be used to report the nurse suspected of chemical impairment.

A variety of programs have been developed to help nurses recover from problematic substance use. Nurses need the same caring attitude from peers as that shown to patients. The goal is to have nurses enter rehabilitative treatment. Employee and family assistance programs can provide support and direction for nurses who require assistance to deal with their substance involvement. Rehabilitation is a complex process. A work re-entry plan can assist nurses to return to their job and provide safe and competent care.

Legal Protections in Nursing Practice

Professional Liability Insurance

All nurses are advised to have professional liability insurance. Despite the high level of competence promoted and maintained, excellent communication with clients, and increasing awareness of the risks involved in giving care, a lawsuit can still be initiated by a client. "Nurses who are employees are covered by their employer's insurance through the operation of vicarious liability" (CNPS, 2004a, p. 2). An employment relationship must have existed at the time of the incident and the defendant employee must have been sued for work done within the scope of his or her employment. The determination regarding whether an employer–employee relationship existed will be identified by the courts (CNPS, 2006). Nurses in independent practice do not have this protection; they are held directly accountable for their practice and thus require their own insurance (CNPS, 2004b).

In Canada, legal support and liability protection insurance can be obtained through the CNPS, a nonprofit society established in 1988. As a member in good standing in most provincial and territorial associations, nurses are able to obtain the services of the CNPS free of charge. Nurses in British Columbia and Quebec are not included in the CNPS and are covered by other insurance agents. CNPS Plus offers additional insurance to all registered nurses at an annual premium. This added insurance, originally designed for independent practitioners, nurse practitioners, and independent contractors, offers insurance for malpractice coverage, business protection, professional discipline costs, and directors' and officers' liability coverage (CNPS, 2008).

Nurses often provide nursing services outside of employment-related activities, such as being available for first aid at children's sport or social activities or providing health screening and education at health fairs. Neighbours or friends may seek advice about illnesses or treatment for themselves or family members. In the latter situation, the nurse may be tempted to give advice; however, it is always advisable for the nurse to refer the friend or neighbour to the family physician.

Nurses may also act as **good Samaritans** by providing emergency assistance at an accident scene. This type of professional activity is not covered by an employer's insurance policy because the care given was not the responsibility of the employer. The good Samaritan or emergency medical aid acts are designed to protect those acting reasonably, without gross negligence. Although the *Code of Ethics for Registered Nurses* (CNA, 2008) no longer specifically mentions emergency care, it does note that "during a natural or human-made disaster, including a communicable disease outbreak, nurses have a duty to provide care, using appropriate safety measures" (p. 9).

To encourage citizens to be good Samaritans, most provinces and territories have now enacted legislation releasing a good Samaritan from legal liability for injuries caused in such circumstances, even if the injuries resulted from negligence of the person offering emergency aid. The Alberta Emergency Medical Act, established in 1980, protects physicians and other registered health-discipline members, including nurses, unless gross negligence is involved. The act covers people who give help in an emergency, at a level that would be provided by a reasonably careful person under similar circumstances (Phillips, 2006). Manitoba, Ontario, New Brunswick, and Nunavut do not have good Samaritan legislation, although New Brunswick does protect physicians who voluntary give first aid or emergency treatment outside of a hospital or doctor's office from liability, under the Medical Act of 1981 (Phillips, 2006).

It is vital for the good Samaritan to consider that once he or she has begun to help the victim, he or she has entered into a nurse–client relationship with that person and is bound by a duty of care to that person. "You now have a duty, in law, to the injured person to continue to treat that person until you are relieved by another competent professional, the preference being one with medical training, or until the person is out of immediate danger" (Phillips, 2006, p. 2).

Carrying out a Physician's Orders

Nurses are expected to analyze the procedures and medications ordered by physicians. It is the nurse's responsibility to seek clarification of ambiguous or seemingly erroneous orders from the prescribing physician or covering on-call physician.

Nurses are not absolved of responsibility for their actions simply because they are following a physician's order. The law states that nurses must understand the cause and effect of the treatment. If nurses carry out treatment they know is wrong, they are guilty of negligence.

If the order is neither ambiguous nor erroneous, the nurse is responsible for carrying it out. For example, if the physician orders oxygen to be administered at 4 L per minute, the nurse must administer oxygen at that rate, and not at 2 L or 6 L per minute. If the orders state that the client is not to have solid food after a bowel resection, the nurse must ensure that no solid food is given to the client.

To protect themselves legally, nurses must question several categories of orders:

1. *Question any order a client questions.* For example, if a client who has been receiving intramuscular injections tells the nurse that the doctor changed the order from an injectable medication to an oral medication, the nurse should recheck the order before giving the medication.

2. *Question any order if the patient's condition has changed.* The nurse is considered responsible for notifying the physician of any significant changes in the patient's condition, whether the physician requests notification or not. For example, if a client who is receiving an intravenous infusion suddenly develops a rapid pulse, chest pain, and a cough, the nurse must notify the physician immediately and question continuance of the ordered rate of infusion. If a patient who is receiving morphine for pain develops severely depressed respirations, the nurse must withhold the medication and notify the physician.

3. *Question and record verbal orders to avoid miscommunications.* In addition to recording the time, the date, the physician's name, and the orders, the nurse documents the circumstances that occasioned the call to the physician, reads the orders back to the physician, and documents that the physician confirmed the orders as the nurse read them back. To avoid miscommunication there should be limited verbal orders.

4. *Question any order that is illegible, unclear, or incomplete.* Misinterpretations in the name of a drug or in dose, for example, can easily occur with handwritten orders. The nurse is responsible for ensuring that the order is interpreted the way it was intended and that it is a safe and appropriate order.

Providing Safe, Competent Nursing Care

Competent practice is a major legal safeguard for nurses. Nurses need to provide care that is within the legal scope of their practice and within the boundaries of agency policies and procedures. Nurses, therefore, must be familiar with their legislated scope of practice and the various job descriptions, which may be different across agencies. All nurses are responsible for ensuring that their educational qualifications and experiences are adequate to meet the responsibilities delineated in their job description.

Competency also involves care that protects clients from harm. Nurses need to anticipate sources of client injury, educate clients about hazards, and implement measures to prevent injury. Nursing competency is one measure of accountability that allows the nurse to uphold the special knowledge, skill, and ability associated with nursing. Because of this knowledge, patients rely on the nurse to provide the standard of care a reasonable, prudent nurse with similar training would in similar circumstances. If the nurse breaches this knowledge, he or she could injure the client and incur liability.

Application of the nursing process is another essential aspect of providing safe and effective client care. All assessments and care must be documented accurately. Effective communication can also protect the nurse from

BOX 6.5 LEGAL PRECAUTIONS FOR NURSES

Nurses can do several things to protect themselves legally:

- Function within the legislated scope of nursing practice (set by regulatory bodies), your education, and job description.
- Follow the procedures and policies of the employing agency.
- Build and maintain good rapport with clients. Keeping clients informed about diagnostic and treatment plans, giving feedback on their progress, and showing concern for the outcome of their care can prevent a sense of powerlessness and a buildup of hostility in the client.
- Always identify clients, particularly before initiating major interventions (e.g., surgical or other invasive procedures, or when administering medications or blood transfusions).
- Observe and monitor the client accurately. Record and communicate to the physician any significant changes in the client's condition.
- Promptly and accurately document all assessments and care given. Records must show that the nurse provided and supervised the client's care at regular intervals (the frequency of required reporting varies with the agency).
- Be alert when implementing nursing interventions and give each task your full attention and skill.
- Perform procedures appropriately. Negligent incidents during procedures generally relate to equipment failure, improper technique, and improper performance of the procedure. For instance, the nurse must know how to safeguard the client in the event that a respirator or other equipment fails.

- Make sure the correct medications are given in the correct dose, by the right route, at the scheduled time, and to the right client. See Chapter 33 for more detailed information about the administration of medications.
- When delegating nursing responsibilities, make sure that the person who is delegated a task understands what to do and that the person has the required knowledge and skill. As the delegating nurse, you can be held liable for harm caused by the person to whom the care was delegated.
- Protect clients from injury. Inform clients of hazards and use appropriate safety devices and measures to prevent falls, burns, or other injuries.
- Report all incidents involving clients. Prompt reports enable those responsible to attend to the client's well-being, to analyze why the incident occurred, and to prevent recurrences.
- Always check any order that a client questions and ensure that verbal orders are accurate and documented appropriately. Question and confirm standing orders if you are inexperienced in a particular area.
- Know your own strengths and weaknesses. Ask for assistance and supervision in situations for which you feel inadequately prepared.
- Maintain your clinical competence. For students, this demands study and practice before caring for clients. For graduate nurses, it means continued study, including maintaining and updating clinical knowledge and skills.

negligence claims. Nurses need to approach every client with sincere concern and include the client in conversations. In addition, nurses should always acknowledge when they do not know the answer to a client's questions, telling the client they will find out the answer and then following through. Ways to take legal precautions are summarized in Box 6.5.

Quality Documentation

The client's medical record is a legal document and can be produced in court as evidence. Licensing bodies have documentation standards in place to which nurses are held accountable. Failure to meet these standards can result in disciplinary action against the nurse (CNPS, 2007). The courts look to the chart as a chronological record of all aspects of care from admission until discharge. Nursing documentation is often used as a means of reconstructing events surrounding the care given and dates and times, as a way of refreshing the memory of a witness, because often several months or years elapse before the lawsuit goes to trial. The effectiveness of a witness's testimony can depend on the accuracy of such records. Nurses, therefore, need

to keep accurate and complete records of nursing care provided to clients.

Nurses have obligations to perform certain nursing acts, such as taking vital signs. In the eyes of the court, failure to document these acts may suggest that the act was not performed. Omissions can constitute negligence and be the basis for tort liability. Insufficient or inaccurate assessments and documentation can hinder proper diagnosis and treatment and result in injury to the client.

Privacy and confidentiality are also important considerations if e-mail is being considered as a method of transferring patient health records or health information. Because the security and confidentiality of e-mail systems are not guaranteed, it is not the recommended method for transmission of health information. If this method of transmission is used, legal writers recommend that any e-mail messages containing confidential health information be encrypted. Additionally, the patient should be informed of the risks of disclosure and presented with alternative methods of communication; if the patient agrees to the transmission of the health information by e-mail, it is prudent to obtain written consent from the patient for the transmission (Tapp, 2001). See Chapter 24 for types of records and facts about recording.

Reporting Crimes, Torts, and Unsafe Practices

Nurses may need to report nursing colleagues or other health care professionals for practices that endanger the health and safety of clients. For instance, problematic alcohol and drug use, theft from a client or agency, and unsafe nursing practice should be reported. Reporting a colleague is not easy. The person reporting may feel disloyal, incur the disapproval of others, or feel that chances for promotion are endangered. When reporting an incident or series of incidents, the nurse must be careful to describe observed behaviour only and not make inferences as to what might be happening. Box 6.6 outlines guidelines for reporting a crime, tort, or unsafe practice. Reporting these events is referred to as *whistle-blowing*.

"**Whistle-blowers** are people who expose negligence, abuses, [and] dangers, such as professional misconduct or incompetence in the organization in which they work" (Hardingham, 1999, p. 1). The decision to be a whistle-blower is never an easy one, unless there is a legal obligation (such as in the cases of child abuse or the abuse of vulnerable adults). Reporting it should be considered as the step to take when all else has failed. Nurses may be the first to come upon unsafe practice or to identify actual or potential hazards. It can be a difficult situation, where the nurse is caught between the values and standards of the profession and the values and norms of the employing organization. The CNA's *Code of Ethics* (CNA, 2008) can be used as a guideline. Four values in the code are especially relevant to nurses deciding whether to report:

1. Promoting health and well-being
2. Preserving dignity
3. Maintaining privacy and confidentiality
4. Being accountable

BOX 6.6 GUIDELINES FOR REPORTING A CRIME, TORT, OR UNSAFE PRACTICE

Nurses should follow these guidelines when reporting a crime, tort, or unsafe practice:
- Write a clear description of the situation you believe you should report.
- Make sure that your statements are accurate.
- Make sure you are credible. Obtain support from at least one trustworthy person before filing the report.
- Report the matter by starting at the lowest possible level in the agency hierarchy.
- Assume responsibility for reporting the individual by being open about it. Sign your name to the letter.
- See the problem through once you have reported it.

Legal Responsibilities of Nursing Students

Nursing students are responsible for their own actions and liable for their own acts of negligence committed during the course of clinical experiences. When they perform duties that are within the scope of professional nursing, such as administering an injection, they generally share the responsibility with the instructor, health care facility, and educational institution. Communication among all individuals must be clear and unambiguous in relation to goals and objectives to be achieved to meet the students' needs during the clinical experience. "Student nurses are not held to a standard of perfection; rather, they are held to the standard of their peers" (Phillips, 2007, p. 2).

In the past, in cases arising from negligent acts by nursing students, the student was traditionally treated as an employee of the hospital, which was held liable under the doctrine of *respondent superior*. Today, nursing students are not usually considered employees of the agencies in which they receive clinical experience because nursing programs usually contract with agencies to provide clinical experiences for students.

Managing legal risks means considering first the competence of the student. The responsibility for ensuring that the clinical experience is safe is shared by the student, the educational institution, the health care agency, and the instructor or preceptor accompanying the student. Before the student enters clinical practice, the educator must be aware of the student's capabilities and whether the curriculum is current and relevant.

Students in clinical situations must be assigned activity within their capabilities and be given reasonable guidance and supervision. Nursing instructors are responsible for assigning students to the care of clients and for providing reasonable supervision. Failure to provide reasonable supervision or the assignment of a client to a student who is not prepared and competent can be a basis for liability.

To fulfill responsibilities to clients and to minimize chances for liability, nursing students need to do the following:

- Make sure they are prepared to carry out the necessary care for assigned clients.
- Ask for additional help or supervision in situations for which they feel inadequately prepared.
- Comply with the policies of the agency in which they obtain their clinical experience.
- Comply with the policies and definitions of responsibility supplied by the school of nursing.

Students who work as part-time or temporary nursing assistants or aides must also remember that legally they can perform only those tasks that appear in the job description of a nurse's aide or assistant. Even though a student may have received instruction and acquired competence in administering injections or suctioning a tracheostomy tube, the student cannot legally perform these tasks while employed as an aide or assistant. While acting as a paid worker, the student is covered for negligent acts by the employer, not by the school of nursing.

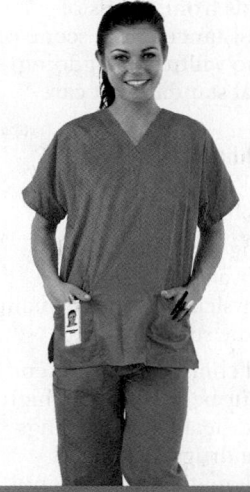

Case Study 6

Mrs. Jiminez in the Royal Victoria Hospital in Montreal is not progressing well following extensive surgery for gastrointestinal cancer. She has experienced severe weight loss and has little desire to eat. Dr. Jones, the physician, has elected to place a subclavian catheter to administer total parenteral nutrition. Dr. Jones telephones the nursing unit and requests that the nurse obtain the patient's informed consent for this invasive procedure. The nurse completes the procedural consent form according to the physician's orders and goes to Mrs. Jiminez's room.

  The nurse informs Mrs. Jiminez that the physician plans to place a catheter into her subclavian vein so that additional nutrients can be administered to her. The nurse further explains that these nutrients will help Mrs. Jiminez heal and regain her strength. In making decisions, Mrs. Jiminez often relies on her eldest son because "he knows best." Mrs. Jiminez asks, "Will it hurt? I'm so tired of all this pain, I'm not sure I want anything else done." The nurse replies, "Oh, don't worry, we'll make sure you don't feel a thing. Your doctor will be here shortly, and he is expecting this permit to be signed, so will you please sign it now?"

CRITICAL THINKING QUESTIONS

1. When the nurse takes the consent form into Mrs. Jiminez's room for her to sign, is the patient actually signing a valid consent?

2. What is the difference between informed consent and signing a consent form?

3. Evaluate the nurse's approach to Mrs. Jiminez regarding this invasive procedure.

4. Who is responsible for obtaining the consent?

Check the eText in MyNursingLab for answers and explanations.

KEY TERMS

adverse event reporting *p. 108*	confidentiality *p. 110*	false imprisonment *p. 105*	privacy *p. 110*
assault *p. 105*	contract *p. 101*	good Samaritan *p. 111*	registration *p. 100*
battery *p. 105*	contractual obligations *p. 101*	implied consent *p. 107*	regulatory bodies *p. 99*
capacity *p. 106*	contractual relationships *p. 102*	informed consent *p. 107*	standards of care *p. 101*
certification *p. 100*	critical incident *p. 109*	intentional torts *p. 105*	substitute decision makers *p. 107*
civil law *p. 97*	delegating care *p. 101*	invasion of privacy *p. 106*	tort *p. 102*
common law *p. 97*	disclosure *p. 106*	law *p. 97*	tort law *p. 98*
competent care *p. 101*	express consent *p. 107*	licensure *p. 100*	vicarious liability *p. 102*
confidential information *p. 109*		negligence *p. 103*	voluntariness *p. 107*
			whistle-blowers *p. 114*

CHAPTER HIGHLIGHTS

- Accountability is an essential concept of professional nursing practice.
- Nurses need to understand laws that regulate and affect nursing practice to ensure that their actions are consistent with current legal principles and to protect themselves from liability.

- In Canada, the regulation of nursing is a function of the provinces and territories.
- Nursing has been granted an exclusivity of practice (a right of self-government or self-regulation).
- Professional regulation in nursing practice is determined and maintained by licensure and

registration, continuing competence programs, discipline and certification, in the public interest.

- Scope of practice and standards of practice are developed and published by provincial and territorial nursing regulatory bodies.

- Agency policies, procedures, and job descriptions further delineate a nurse's practice, but they cannot increase the scope of practice.

- The nurse has specific legal obligations and responsibilities to clients, employers, and the profession. As a citizen, the nurse has the rights and responsibilities shared by all individuals in the society.

- Nursing regulatory bodies are also responsible for accountability and discipline in nursing.

- Legal roles in nursing vary according to nurses' roles as provider of service and employee or contractor for service.

- Nurses can be held liable for unintentional torts, such as negligence, and for intentional torts, such as invasion of privacy, assault, and battery.

- Negligence of nurses can be established when (a) the nurse (defendant) owed a duty to the client, (b) the nurse failed to carry out that duty according to standards, (c) the client (plaintiff) was injured, and (d) the client's injury was caused by the nurse's failure to follow the standard.

- The nurse is responsible for ensuring that the informed consent of a client is complete before nursing treatment regimens and procedures begin.

- Informed consent implies that (a) the consent was given voluntarily, (b) the client had the capacity and competency to understand, and (c) the client was given enough information with which to make an informed decision.

- Good Samaritan and emergency medical aid acts protect health care professionals from claims of malpractice when they offer assistance at the scene of an emergency, provided that no willful wrongdoing or gross departure from normal standards of care take place.

- Nurses can obtain professional liability insurance through the Canadian Nurses Protective Society except in Quebec or British Columbia.

- Selected legal aspects of nursing practice include issues of confidentiality and privacy, informed consent, the carrying out of physicians' orders, quality documentation, and problematic substance use.

- Problematic substance use and chemical dependency in health care workers can occur because of the high levels of stress involved in many health care settings and the easy access to addictive drugs. Chemical impairment includes the problematic use of alcohol and addictive drugs. The nurse needs to know the proper methods for reporting nursing colleagues who are chemically impaired.

- Nursing students need to make certain that they are prepared to provide the necessary care to assigned clients and to ask for help or supervision in situations for which they feel inadequately prepared.

ASSESS YOUR LEARNING

1. What is an unintentional tort?
   a. Commonly regarded as an act of battery
   b. The least common of the torts committed by nurses
   c. Commonly regarded as an act of negligence
   d. A wrongful act, but one that cannot lead to a client lawsuit

2. Which is an example of application of common law?
   a. The provincial government legislates tougher laws with regard to drinking and driving.
   b. A court judge rules against a nurse named in a lawsuit based on similar decisions in previous cases.
   c. The federal government establishes new tax legislation.
   d. Provincial/territorial nursing regulatory bodies establish new practice standards.

3. Which is true about licensure in Canadian nursing?
   a. It is a legal method to control the standards of the nursing profession.
   b. Standards for licensure are established and regulated by the Canadian Nurses Association.

   c. It applies only to those nurses returning to the profession who have completed a refresher course.
   d. Membership in each provincial or territorial nursing association does not require licensure.

4. Which is MOST accurate regarding nursing liability?
   a. Nursing liability refers to not accepting responsibility for your own actions.
   b. A nurse can be held legally liable even though the client did not sustain injury, damage, or harm.
   c. Nurses can deny responsibility for a harmful act or inaction on the grounds that someone else was also involved.
   d. Nurses are legally responsible for harm caused to a client by an inappropriate nursing action or by a failure to perform a required nursing action.

5. Mrs. Jack, who is alert and oriented, refuses to take an antipsychotic medication that you, the nurse, bring to her. She states, "I don't like the way it makes me feel." What would be the MOST legally prudent action that you could take?
   a. Tell Mrs. Jack that the medication is prescribed for her and she should take it.

b. Crush her medication and administer it in her food.

c. Ask her son to convince her to take the medication.

d. Withhold the medication, talk to Mrs. Jack about the importance of taking the medication, document the incident, and notify the physician.

6. Which of the following is an accurate reflection of provincial or territorial documentation standards?

a. Failure to meet these standards would not destroy the nurse's defence in a lawsuit as he or she would be protected by the professional association.

b. The courts look only at the documentation done by the physician.

c. Failure to meet these standards could result in disciplinary action against individual nurses.

d. Documentation is used strictly as a means of communication between health care professionals and is not used by the courts in a lawsuit.

7. What is true regarding the clinical practice of student nurses?

a. Student nurses are legally considered employees of the clinical agency.

b. The nursing instructor and school of nursing are solely accountable for client care administered by students.

c. The school of nursing has sole responsibility for ensuring students are competent to practise.

d. Student nurses are responsible for their own actions and liable for their own acts of negligence committed during the course of clinical experiences.

8. *Capacity* in informed consent is MOST accurately defined as what?

a. A clear statement of consent by the client that can be either oral or written

b. The provision of information, including the risks of treatment, alternative treatment, and its associated facts and risks

c. An understanding of the nature of the decision to be made and the consequences of the decision, including the decision to decline the treatment

d. The client's right to come to a decision without force, coercion, or manipulation from others

9. Which of the following would suggest a situation of potential liability for you, the nurse?

a. A child admitted to your unit is too weak to be weighed. The nurse obtains a verbal estimate from the mother, documents the situation and the child's estimated weight, and ensures that the procedure is done when safe to do so.

b. Your client Mr. Jones, who is very obese, has come to your unit after abdominal surgery. As you care for him the next day, he continues to refuse to move out of bed and walk. You document the situation, inform the charge nurse, and continue to encourage Mr. Jones by exploring other related range-of-motion exercises and teaching related to the importance of walking after surgery.

c. While admitting Mrs. White, 78 years old, to your unit, the daughter informs you that her mother sometimes coughs and even chokes when she is eating. At dinner you inform the care aide that Mrs. White can feed herself and can be left alone as long as she sits up to eat.

d. You question the physician about an order for an antihypertensive medication dose that seems rather high to you. After checking with the pharmacist, who feels the dose is high but safe, you give the medication, document the client's response to the medication (low blood pressure), and ensure that the risk for falls is noted on the client's care plan.

10. A personal care attendant introduces herself to Rita, 18 years old, by saying, "I am the nurse who will give you a bath today." The nurse provides feedback to the attendant based on which of the following principles?

a. Clients should be able to address by name those caring for them.

b. Young people do not understand the various levels of nursing staff.

c. All health care workers giving basic care to clients may introduce themselves as a member of the care team.

d. Clients should know the title and responsibilities of those providing their care.

Check the eText in MyNursingLab for answers and explanations.

WEBLINKS

Canadian Nurses Protective Society
http://www.cnps.ca
The Canadian Nurses Protective Society website offers information about several legal issues and liability protection for nurses who are members in a provincial or territorial nursing association in Canada.

Canadian Nurses Association: Certification
http://www.cna-aiic.ca
Go to the Professional Development section of the Canadian Nurses Association website, and click on Specialty Certification to learn more about how to become certified.

CASN Accreditation Program

http://www.casn.ca/en/21

This website offers information about the accreditation standards and policies of the Canadian Association of Schools of Nursing.

University of Toronto Joint Centre for Bioethics

http://www.jointcentreforbioethics.ca/tools/livingwill.shtml

This website allows you to download a blank living will (which includes legal information specific to each province and territory, as well as further information on personal care decisions).

Canadian Bioethics Society

www.bioethics.ca

This society is a nonprofit organization. The website is designed to provide a forum for professionals interested in sharing ideas relating to bioethics and in finding solutions to bioethical problems.

MyNursingLab

REFERENCES

Adlersberg, M. & MacKinnon, J. (2004). Registered nurses and substance misuse or abuse: RNABC's role. *Nursing BC, 36*(2), 13–15.

Black's law dictionary (8th ed.). (2004). St. Paul, MN: Thomson West Publishing.

Borg, E. (2008). Hydromorphone: Handle with care. *Canadian Nurse, 104*(1), 35.

Canadian Nurses Association. (2002). *Position statement on advanced nursing practice.* Ottawa, ON: Author.

Canadian Nurses Association. (2007). Understanding self-regulation. *Nursing Now: Issues and Trends in Canadian Nursing, 21,* 1–5.

Canadian Nurses Association. (2008a). *Advanced nursing practice: A national framework.* Ottawa, ON: Author.

Canadian Nurses Association. (2008b). *Code of ethics for registered nurses.* Centennial Edition. Ottawa, ON: Author.

Canadian Nurses Association. (2009). *Problematic substance use by nurses.* Ottawa, ON: Author

Canadian Nurses Association. (2011). I think my colleague has a problem. *Canadian nurse.* Ottawa, ON: Author.

Canadian Nurses Protective Society. (1994). Consent to treatment: The role of the nurse. *InfoLAW, 3*(2). Ottawa, ON: Author.

Canadian Nurses Protective Society. (1998). Vicarious liability. *InfoLAW, 7*(1). Ottawa, ON: Author.

Canadian Nurses Protective Society (2004a). Negligence. *InfoLAW 4*(1). Ottawa, ON: Author.

Canadian Nurses Protective Society. (2004b). Independent practice: Legal considerations. *InfoLAW 4*(1). Ottawa, ON: Author.

Canadian Nurses Protective Society. (2006). *Collaborative practice: Are nurses employees or self-employed?* Ottawa, ON: Author.

Canadian Nurses Protective Society. (2007). *Quality documentation: Your best defence. InfoLAW, 1*(1). Ottawa, ON: Author.

Canadian Nurses Protective Society. (2008). *CNPS Plus: An optional extended protection plan for Canadian nurses.* Retrieved from http:// www.cnps.ca/cnps_plus/index_e.html

Canadian Nurses Protective Society. (2009). *Consent for the incapable adult. 13*(3). Ottawa, ON: Author.

Canadian Nurses Protective Society. (2010). Social Media. *InfoLAW, 19*(3). Ottawa, ON: Author.

Canadian Patient Safety Institute. (2008). *Canadian disclosure guidelines.* http://www.patientsafetyinstitute.ca/English/toolsResources/disclosure/Documents/CPSI%20Canadian%20Disclosure%20Guidelines.pdf. Edmonton, AB: Author.

Downey v. Rothwell (1974). 5W.W.R. 311, 49 D.L.R. (3d) 82 (Alta, S.C.)

Downie, J., Lahey, W., Ford, D., Gibson, E., Thomson, M., Ward, T., . . . Shea, A. (2006). *Patient safety law: From silos to systems (final report), country report: Canada.* Ottawa, ON: Health Canada (Project number: HPRP 6795–15–5760009).

Etchells, E., Sharpe, G., Elliott, C., & Singer, P. (1999). Capacity. In P. Singer (Ed.), *Bioethics at the bedside: A clinician's guide* (pp. 17–24). Ottawa, ON: Canadian Medical Association.

Gaudine, A., Lefort, S., Lamb, M., & Thorne, L. (2011). Clinical ethical conflicts of nurses and physicians. *Nursing Ethics, 18*(1), 9–19.

Guido, G. W. (2006). *Legal and ethical issues in nursing* (4th ed.). Upper Saddle River, NJ: Prentice Hall.

Government of Saskatchewan. (2004). *Saskatchewan critical incident reporting guideline.* Regina, SK: Author.

Hardingham, L. (1999). I see and am silent/I see and speak out: The ethical dilemma of whistle-blowing. In *Ethics in Practice* (pp. 1–4). Ottawa, ON: Canadian Nurses Association.

Hogg, P. W. (1997). *Constitutional law of Canada* (4th ed.). Scarborough, ON: Carswell.

Institute for Safe Medication Practices Canada. (2004). *Event analysis report: Hydromorphone/morphine event Red Deer Regional Hospital.* Red Deer, AB: Author.

Joseph Brant Memorial Hospital v. Koziol, [1978] 1 SCR 491.

Keatings, M., & Smith, O. (2009). The Canadian legal system. In M. Keatings & O. Smith (Eds.), *Ethical and legal issues in Canadian nursing* (3rd ed.), (pp. 51–94). Toronto, ON: W.B. Saunders.

King, M. C. (2011). *An introduction to the Health Professions Act.* Calgary, AB: Calgary Regional Health Authority.

Lebel v. Roe, [1994] Y.J. No. 62.

Linden, A. M., & Feldthusen, B. (2006). *Canadian tort law* (8th ed.). Toronto, ON: LexisNexis Canada.

Malette v. Shulman (1990), 67 D.L.R. (4th) 321 (Ont. C.A.).

National Steering Committee on Patient Safety. (2002). *Building a safer system: A national integrated strategy for improving patient safety in Canadian health care.* Ottawa, ON: Author.

Office of the Privacy Commissioner of Canada. (2004). *Fact sheet: Questions and answers regarding the application of PIPEDA, Alberta and British Columbia's Personal Information Protection Act (PIPAs).* Retrieved from http://www.privcom.gc.ca

Parisi, L. (1999). Legal framework for health-care services. In J. Hibbard & D. Smith (Eds.), *Nursing management in Canada* (2nd ed.) (pp. 43–64). Toronto, ON: W.B. Saunders.

Phillips, E. (2006). *Is there a risk in being a good Samaritan?* Retrieved from http://www.cnps.ca/members/publications/articles/good_sam/good_sam_e.html

Phillips, E. (2007). *Managing legal risks in preceptorships.* Retrieved from http://www.cnps.ca/members/publications/articles/preceptor/preceptor_e.html

Picard, E., & Robertson, G. (1996). *Legal liability of doctors and hospitals in Canada* (3rd ed.). Toronto, ON: Carswell.

Sharpe, G. (1993). Consent and minors. *Health Law Canada, 13,* 197–207.

Sneiderman, B., Irvine, J. C., & Osborne, P. (2003). *Canadian medical law: An introduction for physicians, nurses and other health care professionals* (3rd ed.). Scarborough, ON: Thomson Canada.

Somwar v. McDonald's Restaurants of Canada Ltd., [2006] O.J. No. 64 (Ont. S.C.J.).

Tapp, A. (2001). *The legal risks of email.* Retrieved from http://www.cnps.ca/index.php?page=122

UNIT 2

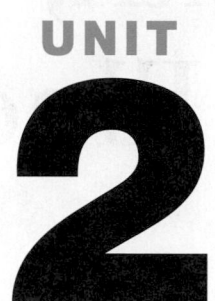

Contemporary Health Care in Canada

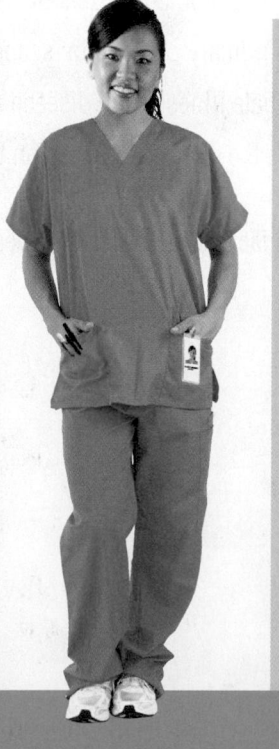

Chapter 7

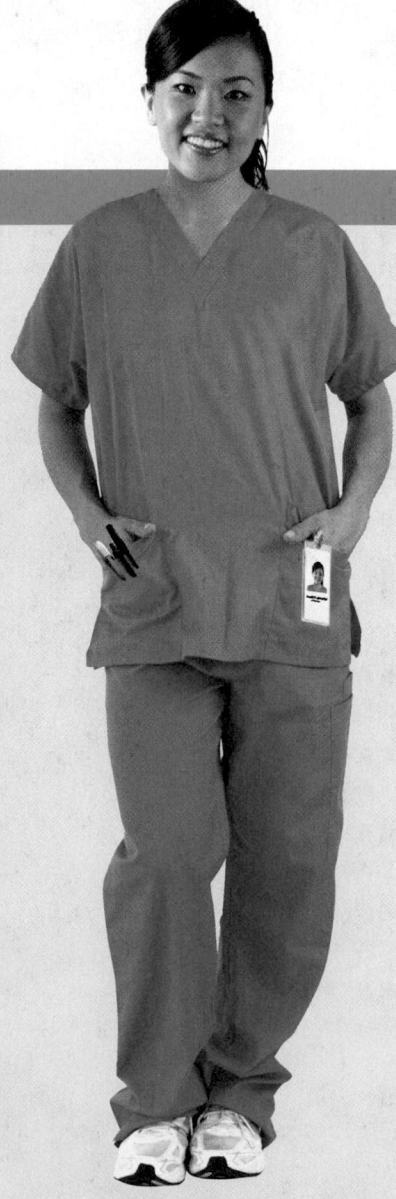

Health, Wellness, and Illness

LEARNING OUTCOMES

After studying this chapter, you will be able to:

1. Explain the concepts of health, wellness, and well-being.

2. Explain the common models of health and wellness.

3. Discuss primary prevention, secondary prevention, and tertiary prevention.

4. Differentiate illness from disease and acute illness from chronic illness.

5. Describe the effects of illness on the roles and functions of individuals and families.

6. Discuss factors that determine health.

For many years, the focus for health was on treatments and cures for diseases. Today, the emphasis is on promoting health and wellness in individuals, families, and communities. People's health beliefs influence their health practices. Similarly, nurses' understanding of health and wellness will determine the scope and nature of their nursing practice. Throughout this chapter, the word *clients* refers to patients in hospitals as well as those in community settings.

Concepts of Health, Wellness, and Well-Being

Health, wellness, and well-being have many definitions and interpretations. Nurses must be familiar with their conceptual commonalities and consider how each term is individualized with specific clients.

Health

Health is a state of being well and using every power individuals' possess to the fullest extent (Nightingale, 1960/1969). The World Health Organization (WHO) defines health as "a state of complete physical, mental, and social well-being, and not merely the absence of disease or infirmity" (WHO, 1948). This definition reflects a concern for the functioning of individuals physically, psychologically, and socially within their environments. Peoples' lives and health are affected by all interactions with their environments. These environmental interactions may include such elements as climate, food, shelter, clean air, and water, as well as interactions with family, employers, coworkers, friends, and associates (see the Reflect on Primary Health Care box).

Health has also been defined in terms of roles and performance. Talcott Parsons (1951) conceptualized health as the ability to maintain roles. Marc Lalonde (1974), in his report *A New Perspective on the Health of Canadians*, presented the *health field concept*, which included human biology, environment, lifestyle, and health care organizations. This landmark document shifted the focus of care from treatment to the importance of lifestyle and environmental factors for health (see Figure 8.1 on page 139, Lalonde's health field concept).

PERSONAL DEFINITION OF HEALTH   Health is a highly individualized experience. People may say they feel healthy, even though they have physical challenges that some would consider illnesses. A person can view health as having fewer symptoms of disease and pain, being active, or remaining in good spirits. It is a way of life through which the body, mind, and emotions interrelate harmoniously.

Many factors affect individual definitions of health, including an individual's previous experiences, expectations of self, age, and sociocultural influences. How people define health influences their behaviours. By understanding clients' perceptions of health and illness, nurses can provide more meaningful assistance to help them regain or attain a state of health. Nurses should be aware of their own personal definitions of health and appreciate that other people will have their unique definitions. See Box 7.1 on developing a personal definition of health.

REFLECT ON **PRIMARY HEALTH CARE**

Many Canadians view having access to clean air and water, balancing personal life and school or work to avoid stress, being physically active to prevent disease, and so on as measures of good health, wellness, and quality of life. People living in poverty, here as well as in developing countries, think that being healthy includes having adequate food supplies, proper nutrition, safe water, basic sanitation, education, basic health care for maternal and child health, immunizations, and the treatment of injuries and communicable diseases. The WHO (1978) articulated these as essential *elements of primary health care* for program planning and policy development. Consider how they are related to the determinants of health outlined in Table 7.2 (on page 132).

Source: Based on World Health Organization. (1978). *The Declaration of Alma-Ata.* Geneva, Switzerland: Author.

BOX 7.1   DEVELOPING A PERSONAL DEFINITION OF HEALTH

The following questions can help nurses develop a personal definition of health:

- Is health more than the absence of disease symptoms?
- Are health and wellness the same?
- Are disease and illness different?
- Is health static or changing?
- Are wellness, health, and illness separate entities or points along a continuum?
- Is health the ability of an individual to adapt to the environment?
- Is health a condition of a person's actualization?
- Is health the effective functioning of self-care activities?
- Is health socially determined?
- How do you rate your health, and why?

Wellness and Well-Being

Wellness is a state of well-being, which is also a component of health. The basic concept of wellness includes developing self-awareness or self-responsibility to reach an ultimate goal of optimal health and happiness. Wellness is a dynamic and growing process that involves daily decision making in the areas of nutrition, stress management, physical fitness, preventive health care, and emotional health.

According to Human Resources and Skills Development Canada (HRSDC, 2012), **well-being** refers to quality of life and individual and societal well-being. Ten indicators influence individual and societal well-being (see Figure 7.1). *Individual well-being* includes such factors as personal values, relationships with family and friends, work, health, and so on. *Societal well-being* includes the collective well-being of people and the quality of interactions between and among people and their social institutions, for example, communities, the health care system, and so on.

Areas of Well-Being

The following summarizes the 10 indicators of well-being, with selected indicators highlighted in the Nursing and Canadian Society box (HRSDC, 2012):

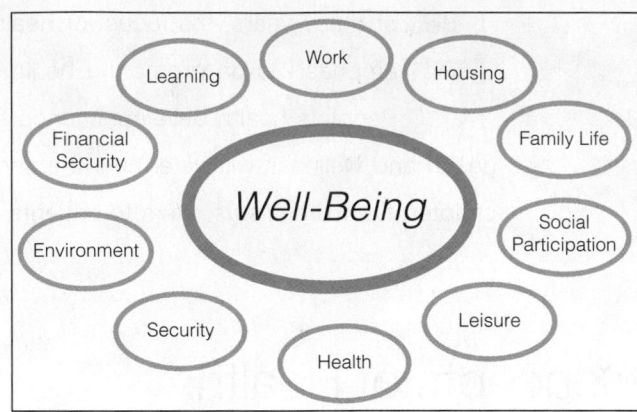

FIGURE 7.1 The 10 indicators of well-being.

Source: Indicators of Well-Being in Canada, 2011. Reproduced with the permission of the Minister of Public Works and Government Services Canada, 2012.

1. *Work:* Individuals may obtain their purpose in life through their work accomplishments, and monetarily meet their basic and other needs through work. The Canadian economy remains competitive when people are employed, which promotes societal well-being.

 Nursing and Canadian Society

Facts	Implications for Nursing Practice
Single parents, unattached individuals, new immigrants, people with disabilities, and Aboriginal people were more at risk of experiencing low income than other Canadians in 2007.	Nurse must understand that individual well-being and societal well-being are interrelated and that *financial security* depends on how incomes are distributed among the priority populations across society and primarily on the level of income of individual Canadians.
In 2003, half of Canadians (52%), age 16 and older, had literacy levels sufficient for them to function well in today's society. In 2008, about one-third of Canadian adult workers participated in formal job-related training.	Nurses can identify the needed learning opportunities and training and refer individuals to pursue them. These individuals can then acquire the necessary knowledge, skills, and competencies to enter the job market and make effective economic contributions to society. *Learning* can bring personal pleasure and pride and can improve one's standard of living and quality of life.
Although the homicide rate in Canada has been decreasing since 1975, it rose by about 18% from 2003 to 2005. Also, between 1999 and 2004, the reported rate of incidents of violent crime (assault, sexual assault, or robbery) declined by about 5%. More women than men report being victims of sexual assault. More men than women report being victims of robbery and physical assault. Victims of robbery or physical assault were more likely to report the crime to police than the sexually assaulted victims.	*Security* involves safety and protection from harm. Nurses must assess individual and community perceptions of safety in relation to clients' experiences of harm or threats of harm. They can provide primary prevention activities, such as education on workplace safety, family violence, equity, individual rights, and organizational and society obligations. When working with victims, nurses can provide secondary and tertiary prevention activities focusing on counselling, referring, and treatment.
Between 1998 and 2005, average leisure time for Canadians decreased from 5.8 to 5.5 hours (18 minutes) per day. Time spent on socializing decreased by about 1.5 hours per week on average between 1998 and 2005. Older Canadians (those 65 and older) spent nearly 1.5 hours more per day on passive leisure (e.g., watching TV) compared with other Canadians. Older Canadians also spent more time (~0.5 hours/day) on hobbies, reading, and other activities that stimulate thinking.	*Leisure* offers personal and social benefits. It promotes relaxation, reduces stress, and improves mental health and physical fitness. Nurses must recognize the importance of physical and mental stimulation to healthy growth and development and aging. They can design leisure-focused health-promotion activities to take place between stimulating and relaxing forms of recreation in the areas of social connection, cognitive stimulation, and physical exercise.

2. *Housing:* Individual and societal well-being may suffer when safe and affordable housing is inadequate or unavailable.

3. *Family Life:* Families influence individual and societal well-being through their participation in the community and the provision of social, physical, and emotional supports.

4. *Social Participation:* Trust and a sense of belonging promote the level of participation of individuals within their communities. Social networks are strengthened through volunteerism, recreational and sports participation, and political activism.

5. *Leisure:* Participating in enjoyable activities that reduce stress and promote growth and well-being are beneficial to health, aging, and development.

6. *Health:* Mental and physical well-being may be enhanced in those individuals who are in good health, thus enabling individuals to participate in the growth of the community's health and well-being.

7. *Security:* Actual or perceived threats to safety will influence individual and community well-being.

8. *Environment:* Balancing the use and protection of the surrounding physical environment is important for the well-being of all.

9. *Financial Security:* The ways in which income is equitably distributed across society will influence individual and societal well-being.

10. *Learning:* Training and education may improve quality of life through the enhancement of skills and knowledge, thus offering new opportunities for individuals within their communities.

ABORIGINAL VIEWS OF WELLNESS The Canadian Population Health Initiative (CPHI) (Canadian Institute for Health Information [CIHI], 2009) acknowledges the diversity within First Nations, Inuit, and Métis groups. In all groups, however, there exists a belief of the interconnectedness of Aboriginal people with all creation. This includes family, community, nation, plants, animals, and the spirit people, as well as those who have died and those not yet born. In addition, Aboriginal people have a strong sense to use mutual decision making to plan for future generations, to believe that they have the duty to family and to all creation, to be observant of their surroundings, and to believe that all members have special gifts that can benefit the community.

Hales and Lauzon (2010) describe the holistic world view of health and wellness of Aboriginal people by using the medicine wheel. The **medicine wheel** has many variations, but they all emphasize "the way of good life" or "everyday good living" in the context of human behaviour and interaction. The term *medicine* refers to spiritual energy and healing or enlightened experience. Aboriginal people see the interconnectedness between the physical and spiritual world, and the mind, body, and spirit, and healing is created when balance and harmony are attained in one's decisions and actions. The medicine wheel has

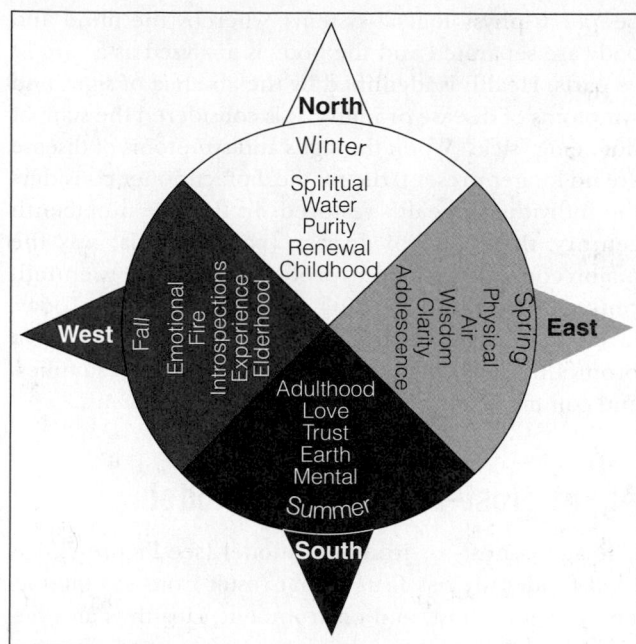

FIGURE 7.2 Aboriginal medicine wheel.

four colours representing north, south, east, and west (see Figure 7.2). These coloured directions refer to seeking healthy minds (East), strong inner spirits (South), inner peace (West), and strong, healthy bodies (North). A medicine wheel encourages reflection on one's life.

The conceptualization of the medicine wheel helps understand human development as following four sequential life cycles associated with specific developmental tasks, including (a) learning of belonging; (b) learning new skills and behaviours; (c) service for the benefit of family, community, and nation; and (d) the giving away of wisdom. Traditional healing practices focus on restoring balance when a disruption of developmental tasks occurs during one of these life cycles. In the words of one Inuit elder, "The living person and the land are tied up together because without one the other doesn't survive. . . . The land is so important for us . . . that's why we treat it as part of ourselves"(CIHI, 2009, p. 10). When working with Aboriginal people, it is important to remember that health care providers also bring their own culture and attitudes to the relationship; therefore, it is important to provide care that is culturally safe. Cultural safety requires that health care providers be "respectful of nationality, culture, age, sex, political and religious beliefs, and sexual orientation" (p. 11).

Models of Health and Wellness

Medical Model of Health

The *medical model* of health has the narrowest interpretation of health. This mechanistic concept presented by Descartes in the seventeenth century (Curtis, 2000) views people as physiological systems, whereby the mind and body are separated and the body is analyzed as a sum of its parts. Health is identified by the absence of signs and symptoms of disease or injury. It is considered the state of not being "sick." When the signs and symptoms of disease are no longer present, the medical practitioner considers the individual's health restored. In the late nineteenth century, the "how" of disease (pathogenesis) was the major concern of health professionals. The twentieth century focused on finding cures for diseases. Today, health care providers are placing increased emphasis on promoting health and wellness in individuals, families, and communities.

Agent–Host–Environment Model

The agent–host–environment model (see Figure 7.3) is used to identify risk factors that result from the interaction of agent, host, and environment. Health is an ever-changing state, and the goal is to promote and maintain health. When the variables are in balance, health is maintained; when variables are not in balance, disease occurs. The model has three dynamic, interactive elements:

1. *Agent.* Any environmental factor or stressor (biological, chemical, mechanical, physical, or psychosocial) that by its presence or absence (e.g., lack of essential nutrients) can lead to illness or disease.

2. *Host.* A person or people who may or may not be at risk of acquiring a disease. Family history, age, and lifestyle habits influence the host's reaction to an agent.

3. *Environment.* Includes all factors external to the host that may or may not predispose the person to the development of the disease. The physical environment includes climate, living conditions, sound (noise) levels, and economic level. The social environment can include interactions with others and life events, such as the death of a spouse.

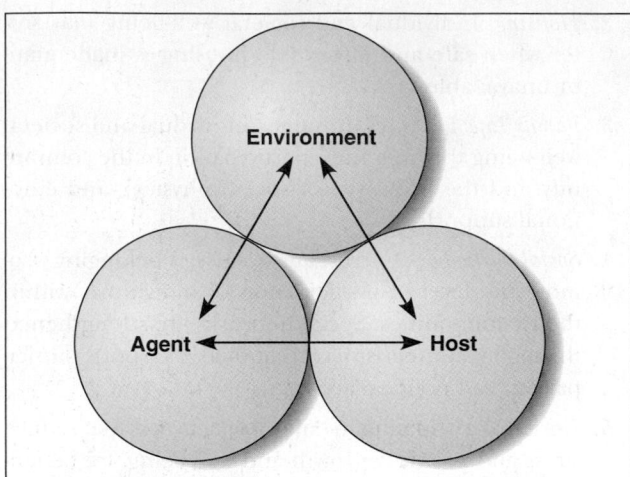

FIGURE 7.3 The agent–host–environment triangle.

Travis's Illness–Wellness Continuum

Travis's illness–wellness continuum (see Figure 7.4) ranges from high-level wellness to premature death (Travis & Ryan, 2004), shown by two arrows pointing in opposite directions and joined at a neutral point. People move back and forth within the continuum. Movement to the right of the neutral point indicates increasing levels of health and well-being. This improvement is achieved in three steps: (a) awareness, (b) education, and (c) growth. In contrast, movement to the left of the neutral point indicates decreasing levels of health. One may be physically ill and at the same time oriented toward wellness, or be physically healthy and at the same time function from an illness perspective.

Levels of Prevention

Prevention refers to avoiding the development of disease and occurs in three levels: primary, secondary, and tertiary (Leavell & Clark, 1965). Table 7.1 summarizes

TABLE 7.1 Levels of Prevention, Foci, and Activities

Level	Focus	Examples of Activities
Primary prevention	Focuses on health promotion and protection against specific health problems or disease. Precedes disease or dysfunction and is applied to generally healthy individuals or groups.	• Teaching accident and poisoning prevention, immunizations, family planning, nutrition, exercise, stress management, home and occupational safety; lifestyle and nutrition to prevent cancer or heart disease
Secondary prevention	Focuses on early identification or detection of health problems and prompts intervention to alleviate health problems and limit future disability.	• Screening for developmental delays and hypertension; tuberculosis skin test; clinical breast examination and testicular examination; annual physical and dental examinations
Tertiary prevention	Focuses on restoration and rehabilitation to an optimal level of functioning. Begins after an illness, when a defect or disability is stabilized or determined to be irreversible.	• Teaching foot care to diabetic clients • Teaching range-of-motion exercises to patients who have suffered a cerebrovascular accident

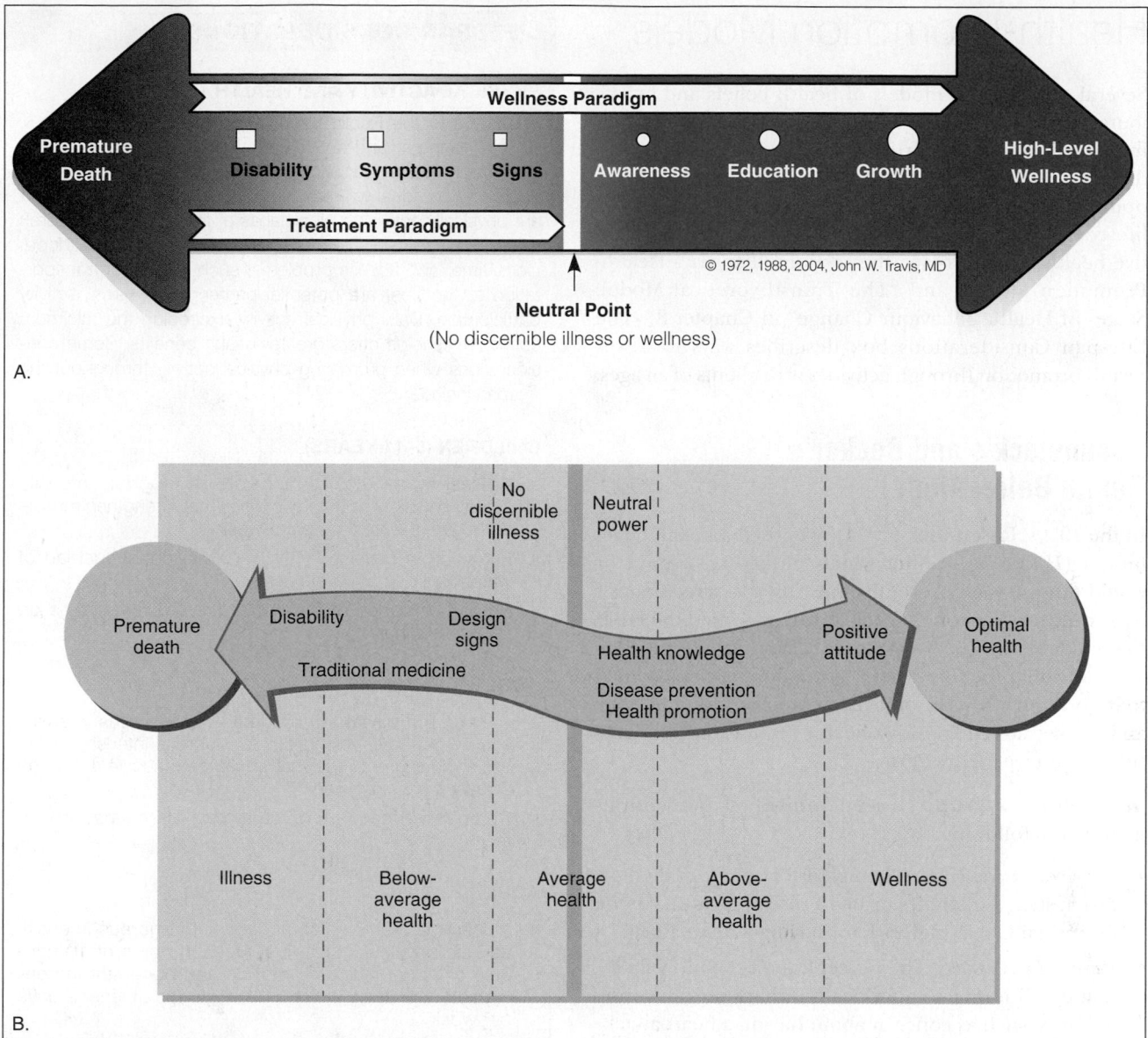

FIGURE 7.4 Illness–wellness continuum.

Source: From Travis, J. W., & Ryan, R. S. (2004). *Wellness workbook: How to achieve enduring health and vitality* (3rd ed.)., Berkeley, CA: Celestial Arts. Retrieved from http://www. thewellspring.com/wellspring/introduction-to-wellness/357/key-concept-1-the-illnesswellness-continuum.cfm. Used by permission of the author.

the levels and their foci and provides examples of prevention activities. The levels can occur at various points during the course of a disease and can overlap in practice. For example, a client may have experienced a heart attack, and a goal of secondary prevention is to give cardiac medications immediately to limit disability. The teaching (e.g., lifestyle changes) given to the client to prevent new complications will be similar to the health-education activities in primary prevention, and the goal of the client to return home with follow-up appointments, such as for cardiac rehabilitation, is tertiary prevention.

See Box 7.2 on examples of healthy lifestyle choices.

BOX 7.2 EXAMPLES OF HEALTHY LIFESTYLE CHOICES

- Regular exercise
- Weight control
- Avoidance of saturated fats
- Responsible use of alcohol and tobacco avoidance
- Seat belt use
- Bike helmet use
- Immunization updates
- Regular dental checkups
- Regular health maintenance visits for screening examinations or tests

Health-Promotion Models

Several theories and models of health beliefs and behaviours have been developed to help determine whether an individual is likely to participate in health-promotion or disease-prevention activities. They are useful tools in developing programs for helping people change to healthier lifestyles and develop positive attitudes toward preventive health measures (see the sections "Pender's Health-Promotion Model" and "The Transtheoretical Model: Stages of Health Behaviour Change" in Chapter 8). The Lifespan Considerations box describes ways to foster health promotion through activities with clients of all ages.

Rosenstock's and Becker's Health Belief Model

In the 1950s, Rosenstock (1974) proposed a health belief model (HBM) to predict which individuals would or would not use such preventive measures as screening for early cancer detection. Becker (1974) modified the HBM to include *individual perceptions, modifying factors,* and variables affecting the *likelihood of action.* Rosenstock assumed that good health is an objective common to all people; and Becker added "positive health motivation" as a consideration (see Figure 7.5).

INDIVIDUAL PERCEPTIONS Individual perceptions include the following:

- *Perceived susceptibility.* A family history of a certain disorder, such as diabetes or heart disease, may make the individual feel at high risk for having a heart attack.
- *Perceived seriousness.* The perception of the individual that the illness may cause death or have serious consequences, such as concern about having a heart attack and the subsequent financial and lifestyle challenges.
- *Perceived threat.* Perceived susceptibility and perceived seriousness combine to determine the total perceived threat of an illness to a specific individual. For example, a person who has high cholesterol, does not exercise, and is the sole financial provider for the family may have an increased perceived threat of having a heart attack.

MODIFYING FACTORS Factors that modify a person's perceptions include the following:

- *Demographic variables.* Demographic variables include age, gender, race, and ethnicity. An infant, for example, does not perceive the importance of a healthy diet. An adolescent may perceive peer approval as more important than family approval and, subsequently, participate in risk-taking activities or adopt unhealthy eating and sleeping patterns.
- *Sociopsychological variables.* Social pressure or influence from peers or other reference groups (e.g., self-help or vocational groups) may encourage preventive

---

LIFESPAN CONSIDERATIONS

PHYSICAL ACTIVITY AND HEALTH

According to the Public Health Agency of Canada (PHAC, 2011), staying fit and active early in life can positively influence future health behaviours and the likelihood that, as an adult, the individual will remain physically active. Families that are physically active develop habits of fitness in their children that typically remain with them as they mature into adulthood. Cost, time, and access problems, such as lack of transportation to facilities, are potential barriers to physical activity participation. Daily physical activity exceeding the minimum activity thresholds offers greater health benefits. Some considerations when promoting physical activity throughout the lifespan include:

CHILDREN (5–11 YEARS)

- At least 60 minutes of moderate- to vigorous-intensity activity per day, including activities that strengthen muscle and bone at least 3 days per week
- Engaging in physical activities after school, instead of watching TV or using the computer
- Positive influence of physically active older siblings on younger siblings

ADOLESCENTS

- At least 60 minutes of moderate- to vigorous-intensity activity per day, which includes vigorous-intensity activities, including activities that strengthen muscle and bone at least 3 days per week
- Competitive team sports as a form of socialization for teens

ADULTS

- At least 150 minutes of moderate- to vigorous-intensity aerobic physical activity per week in bouts of 10 minutes or more, including muscle and bone strengthening activities using major muscle groups at least 2 days per week
- Previous levels of exercise, which predict continued and future participation in physical activity
- Family obligations and work stressors, which influence the ability to remain fit
- Improvement of well-being and self-esteem, increased energy, reduced stress and positive mental health
- Reduction in the risk of premature death and chronic diseases, such as osteoporosis, coronary heart disease, breast and colon cancers, and type 2 diabetes

OLDER ADULTS

- At least 150 minutes of moderate- to vigorous-intensity physical activity per week, in bouts of 10 minutes or more, including muscle and bone strengthening activities using major muscle groups at least 2 days per week
- Physical activities that can enhance balance, prevent falls, and improve mental alertness
- Participating in personally enjoyable activities (e.g., walking, golfing, or swimming) that will improve overall health
- Physical group activities, including social time with friends and family, which reduce feelings of social isolation

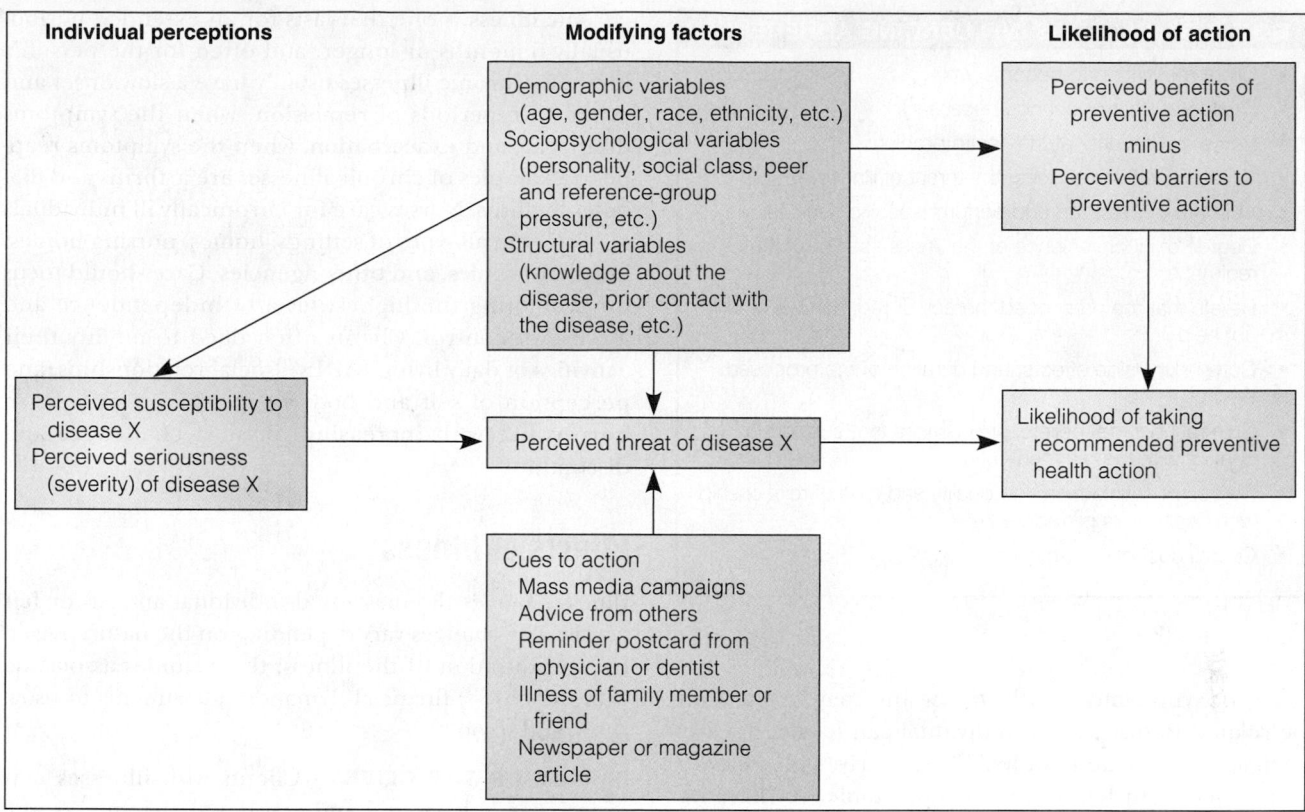

FIGURE 7.5 The health belief model.

Source: From Becker, M. H., Haefner, D. P., Kasl, S. V., et al. (1977). Selected psychosocial models and correlates of individual health-related behaviours. *Medical Care, 15*(5 Suppl), pp. 27–46. Medical care by AMERICAN PUBLIC HEALTH ASSOCIATION. Reproduced with permission of LIPPINCOTT WILLIAMS & WILKINS in the format Journal via Copyright Clearance Center.

health behaviours, even when individual motivation is low. The expectations of others may motivate people, for example, not to drive after drinking alcohol.

- *Structural variables.* Knowledge about the target disease and prior contact with it are structural variables that are presumed to influence preventive behaviours. For example, people who have had skin cancer may use sunscreen with a high sun protection factor (SPF) before going outside.

- *Cues to action.* Cues can be either internal or external. Internal cues include thoughts about an ill family member. External cues include Internet and television advertisements.

LIKELIHOOD OF ACTION The likelihood of a person taking recommended preventive health action depends on the perceived benefits of the action minus the perceived barriers to the action.

- *Perceived benefits of the action.* Examples include refraining from smoking to prevent lung cancer, and eating nutritious foods and avoiding snacks to maintain weight control.

- *Perceived barriers to action.* Examples include cost, inconvenience, unpleasantness, and lifestyle changes.

Pender, Murdaugh, and Parsons (2011) modified the HBM to develop a health-promotion model. According to Pender, the HBM explains health-protecting or preventive

behaviours but does not emphasize health-promoting behaviours (see the section "Pender's Health-Promotion Model" in Chapter 8).

Health Care Adherence

Adherence is the extent to which an individual's behaviour (e.g., taking medications as prescribed, following a diet plan, or making lifestyle changes) coincides with medical or health advice. Degree of adherence may range from disregarding every aspect of the recommendations to following the total therapeutic plan. There are many reasons why some people adhere and others do not (see Box 7.3 on the next page). The nurse must be aware that knowledge of health behaviours does not always translate into action. To enhance adherence, nurses need to ensure that the client is able to perform the activities, understands the necessary instructions, is a willing participant in establishing goals of therapy, and values the planned outcomes of behaviour changes.

Illness and Disease

Illness is a highly personal state in which the person's physical, emotional, intellectual, social, developmental, or spiritual functioning is thought to be diminished.

It is not synonymous with *disease* and may or may not be related to disease. An individual can have a disease, such as diabetes, and not feel ill. Similarly, a person with a headache can feel ill or uncomfortable, yet have no discernible disease. Illness is highly subjective; only the person experiencing it can say that he or she is ill.

Disease can be described as an alteration in bodily functions resulting in a reduction of capacities or a shortening of the normal lifespan. People once thought disease was caused by "forces" or spirits. This belief was replaced by causation theory, in which multiple factors interact to cause disease and determine an individual's response to treatment.

The causation of a disease is called its **etiology**. For example, a virus is the biological agent of severe acute respiratory syndrome (SARS). However, other etiological factors, such as age, nutritional status, and occupation, are involved in the development of SARS and the course of infection.

Illness can be acute or chronic. **Acute illness** is typically characterized by severe symptoms of relatively short duration. The symptoms appear abruptly and subside quickly and, depending on the cause, may or may not require intervention by health care providers. Some acute illnesses are serious (e.g., appendicitis may require immediate surgical intervention), but many acute illnesses, such as colds, subside without medical intervention or after using over-the-counter (OTC) medications. Following an acute illness, most people return to their prior level of wellness.

Canadians living with a chronic illness often require the use of multiple resources to maintain self-management. Chronic illness is a health priority due to increased health care costs, and the incidence of older Canadians living with chronic illnesses is on the rise (Registered Nurses' Association of Ontario, 2010). A **chronic illness** is one that lasts for an extended period, usually 6 months or longer, and often for the person's lifetime. Chronic illnesses usually have a slow onset and often have periods of **remission**, when the symptoms disappear, and **exacerbation**, when the symptoms reappear. Examples of chronic illnesses are arthritis and diabetes mellitus. Nurses care for chronically ill individuals of all ages in all types of settings: homes, nursing homes, hospitals, clinics, and other agencies. Care should focus on promoting the highest level of independence and a sense of control. Clients often need to modify their activities of daily living (ADLs), social relationships, and perception of self and body image. Many must learn how to live with increasing physical challenges and discomfort.

Effects of Illness

Illness changes the diagnosed individual and his or her family. The changes vary depending on the nature, severity, and duration of the illness; the attitudes associated with the illness; financial demands; adjustments to usual roles; and so on.

IMPACT ON THE CLIENT Clients with illnesses may experience behavioural and emotional changes, as well as changes in lifestyle, self-concept, and body image. Behavioural and emotional changes associated with short-term illness are generally mild and short lived. The individual, for example, may become irritable and lack the energy or desire to interact in the usual fashion with family members or friends. Heightened responses are likely with severe, life-threatening, chronic, or disabling illnesses. Anxiety, fear, anger, withdrawal, denial, a sense of hopelessness, and powerlessness are all common responses to severe or disabling illnesses.

Certain illnesses can also change the client's body image or physical appearance, especially if it entails severe scarring or the loss of a limb. The client's self-esteem and self-concept may also be affected (e.g., loss of bodily function, increased dependence on others, unemployment, and strained relationships with others). (See Chapter 45.) Besides participating in treatments and taking medications, the person with illness may need to change his or her diet and activity, exercise, rest, and sleep patterns. See the Evidence-Informed Practice box.

Individuals with illness are vulnerable to loss of **autonomy**, which is the state of being independent and self-directed without outside control. Nurses need to support clients' right to self-determination and autonomy by providing them with sufficient information to participate in decision making and maintain feelings of control. Nurses can help their clients express their thoughts and provide care to help them effectively cope with change by doing the following:

- Providing explanations about any necessary adjustments to the client and their significant others

EVIDENCE-INFORMED PRACTICE

How Can Nurses Help Improve the Physical Activity of Older Adults?

A systematic review of 66 articles were examined to determine the relationships of healthy community-dwelling older adults (age >65 years) participating in physical activity and the effects of this activity on disability, functional limitations, or loss of independence. The authors found that greater physical activity, particularly if the activity was moderate to vigorous and aerobic in nature, was associated with overall greater functional independence and higher functional status for older adults, thus conferring a reduced risk (odds ratio ~0.5) of disability or functional limitation. Resistance training and aerobic exercises performed by older adults showed reductions with the incidence of mobility disabilities and improvements in functional and physiological measures. The risk of developing dementia was reduced and cognitive function was improved when older adults participated in relatively high levels of physical activity.

NURSING IMPLICATIONS: The findings suggest that regular aerobic activities and exercise programs for older adults do reduce functional limitations and disability and improve cognitive function. Improved cognitive function and improved mobility may help keep older adults independent in their homes. Nurses can assist with health teaching that reinforces physical activities that are appropriate and enjoyable for community-dwelling older adults.

Source: Based on Paterson, D. H., & Warburton, D. (2010). Physical activity and functional limitations in older adults: A systematic review related to Canada's physical activity guidelines. *International Journal of Behavioral Nutrition and Physical Activity, 7*, 38. Retrieved from http://www.ijbnpa.org/content/pdf/1479-5868-7-38.pdf

- Making arrangements, wherever possible, to accommodate the client's lifestyle
- Actively listening to clients as they share their feelings about various changes
- Reinforcing and incorporating desirable changes as a permanent part of the client's lifestyle

IMPACT ON THE FAMILY A person's illness affects not only the person who is ill but also the family or significant others. The kind of effect and its extent depend chiefly on three factors: (a) the member of the family who is ill, (b) the seriousness and length of the illness, and (c) the cultural and social customs the family follows.

The changes that can occur in the family include the following:

- Role changes
- Task reassignments and increased demands on time
- Increased stress because of anxiety about the outcome of the illness for the client and conflict about new responsibilities
- Financial problems

- Loneliness as a result of separation and pending loss
- Change in social customs

What Makes Canadians Healthy?

Everything in the environment and society affects the health of individuals, families, and communities. Nurses must maintain a spirit of inquiry and inquisitiveness about the world and the root causes of what determines health. Box 7.4 describes a simple story that speaks to the complex set of factors that determines the health conditions surrounding individuals, families, communities, and nations.

Upstream and Downstream Views

Imagine you are the nurse caring for Jason's infected leg as described in Box 7.4. How many more children with infected legs from this neighbourhood would you need to take care of if the roots of the problems were not eliminated?

This metaphor speaks about the importance of looking beyond the immediate event when studying health. Nurses can make a difference every day in the lives of patients or clients. As *downstream thinkers*, nurses act on the immediate problem at hand and provide only

---

BOX 7.4 **WHAT MAKES CANADIANS HEALTHY?**

This story speaks to the complex set of factors that determine health conditions.

Why is Jason in the hospital? Because he has a bad infection in his leg.

But why does he have an infection? Because he has a cut on his leg, and it got infected.

But why does he have a cut on his leg? Because he was playing in the junk yard next to his apartment building, and there was some sharp, jagged steel there that he fell on.

But why was he playing in a junk yard? Because his neighbourhood is kind of rundown. A lot of kids play there, and there is no one to supervise them.

But why does he live in that neighbourhood? Because his parents can't afford a nicer place to live.

But why can't his parents afford a nicer place to live? Because his Dad is unemployed and his Mom is sick.

But why is his Dad unemployed? Because he doesn't have much education and he can't find a job.

But why . . . ?

Source: Toward a Healthy Future—Second Report on the Health of Canadians. Public Health Agency of Canada, 2009. Reproduced with the permission of the Minister of Health, 2012.

episodic care. Nurses who examine problems as *upstream thinkers* promote and advocate for their clients' health. They invest not only in the biological factors but also in the physical, psychological, cultural, spiritual, and socio-economic factors associated with health.

Social Determinants of Health

"A health care system—even the best health care system in the world—will be only one of the ingredients that determine whether your life will be long or short, healthy or sick, full of fulfillment, or empty with despair."

—The Honourable Roy Romanow, 2004
(*from Mikkonen & Raphael, 2010, p. 7*)

It is not lifestyle choices or medical treatments that are the primary factors shaping Canadians' health; instead, it is their experiences within their living environments. These conditions are called the *social determinants of health* (Mikkonen & Raphael, 2010). The health of Canadians is largely shaped by access to quality housing and nutrition, living conditions, and how wealth is distributed, and so on; and these factors, among others, influence the range of health inequities that exist.

The Public Health Agency of Canada (2003) uses a population health approach when examining the health of Canadians. It is individuals' interactions with their environments that have greater impacts on their health than do individual lifestyle choices and behaviours. Originating from the Lalonde Report (1974), the 12 determinants of health have been modified to include the 15 social determinants of health listed below (see Table 7.2). Advocating for public policies that strengthen the health of Canadians, educating Canadians about the influence of the determinants of health on health, and lobbying political offices and agencies to allocate resources that support a broader view of health will improve the health of individuals and the overall health of Canadian society.

TABLE 7.2 Social Determinants of Health

Stress, Bodies, and Illness
Individuals living in adverse conditions experience excess psychological and physiological stress. When one experiences prolonged stress, excess strain is placed on the body, which alters the metabolic, hormonal, and immune systems within the body. Prolonged stress makes one more vulnerable to disease, illness, and coping choices that may be unhealthy.

Income and Income Distribution
The most important social determinant of health is income. Income influences the ability to purchase food, housing, and other basic health prerequisites, and this affects psychological functioning. The health of a society can be predicted by examining the income distribution within that society; equal distribution equates to a healthier society. Families with higher incomes were more likely to save for their retirement and their children's postsecondary education. Families with lower incomes placed greater emphasis on saving for education (Statistics Canada, 2011).

Education
Literacy and education provide greater access to resources that bring about changes in society. Movement up the socioeconomic ladder may also be attributed to education. As with the other determinants, this greater access is not gained in isolation and influences other social determinants of health.

Unemployment and Job Security
Psychological stress, including depression and anxiety, social and material deprivation and adapting unhealthy coping behaviours may be the results of unemployment or lack of job security. Employment influences one's daily life and provides a sense of identity. Forcing one into part-time work and needing to seek employment with multiple jobs can lead to reduced health.

Employment and Working Conditions
Adverse working conditions, including long hours of work and not feeling valued, may lead to excess stress. This excess stress may lead to the development of psychological and physical illnesses. Women, in particular, have reported that they are exposed to too many daily demands and reduced time.

Early Childhood Development
The social and economic resources available to one's family influence early childhood development. Latent and cumulative effects of deprivation and loss may lead to lasting psychological, social, and physical influences on health well into adulthood.

Food Insecurity
Inadequate diet in terms of the quantity or quality of food may lead to dietary deficiencies. These deficiencies are associated with the development of illnesses and difficulty with the management of those illnesses. Academic problems may develop in children living in food-insecure households.

Housing
Homelessness, overcrowding, and inadequately maintained homes allow for the transmission of illnesses and may lead to poor health and academic outcomes. Some Aboriginal people live in homes lacking even basic sanitation and clean water.

TABLE 7.2 *(continued)*

Social Exclusion

Chronic illness, crime, and a lack of educational attainment may be exacerbated due to social exclusion. Canadians who are socially excluded, such as women, people with disabilities, new immigrants, and Aboriginal people, have reduced access to cultural, economic, and social resources, and this leads to reduced health.

Social Safety Net

Services, such as employment training, counselling, and community services, lead to increased social cohesion. These supportive social and financial services particularly help protect people's health during unexpected life events.

Health Services

Many Canadians do not have private health insurance; therefore, the amount of out-of-pocket spending by individuals influences other determinants of health. While Canadian citizens should enjoy the universality of health care, but many treatments are not completed, dental appointments are not kept, or prescriptions are not filled due to cost.

Aboriginal Status

Colonization, relocation of families, and residential schools have led to adverse health outcomes for many of Canada's Aboriginal peoples. Overcrowding in homes, food insecurity, and low income have caused increased rates of chronic illness and reduced life expectancy.

Gender

Women most often do not have secure employment and earn lower wages compared with men. Men experience more violence, homelessness, and reduced life expectancy during their lifetimes. Lesbian, gay, and transgendered Canadians experience discrimination, which leads to adverse health outcomes.

Race

Racism negatively influences the health outcomes of individuals and society. Devaluing, government inaction, and segregation influence health outcomes. Newcomers to Canada experience worsening health over time.

Disability

People with disabilities are more unemployed or are earning lower wages compared with those without any disability. Social benefits provided to Canadians with disabilities are some of the lowest in the developing world, lessening their ability to participate in society and meet the basic requirements of life.

Source: Copyright © 2010 Juha Mikkonen and Dennis Raphael.

Summary

Nurses play an important role in helping their clients attain optimal health. Future health care will need to be client centred, respect people's values, avoid fragmentation of care, and ensure equitable access to services, while maximizing financial, human, and structural resources (South West Local Health Integration Network, 2009). The future includes enhancing capacity for community-based care, increasing access and sustainability for hospital-based care, integrating information technology systems, and improving accountability and leadership for health care and human resources. It will be the norm for health care providers and clients to share the responsibility for health and wellness. An understanding of various approaches to health will enhance health care providers' ability to impart knowledge on health, identify the root causes of problems, reduce barriers, and support positive actions toward good health (see Case Study 7).

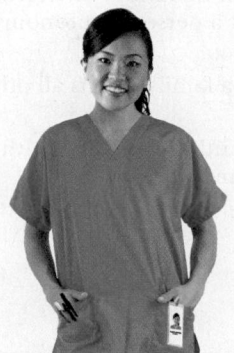

Case Study 7

Russel and Rayne have both suffered heart attacks; they live near downtown Toronto and are members of the Anishnawbe First Nation people. Russel, on advice from his traditional healer and physician, requested a healing ceremony, started exercising, reduced his salt and fat intake, entered stress-reduction classes, and with the support of his partner returned to work 6 weeks after his heart attack. He has a positive outlook, is doing well, and talks about "feeling well." Rayne has also changed his dietary habits and has started exercising; however, he has been unable to quit smoking, even though he wants to and has been advised to do so. Rayne is frequently despondent, very fearful of having another heart attack, has not yet returned to work, and frequently talks about "feeling ill."

(continued)

1. How does Russel's psychological dimension of health status differ from Rayne's?

2. Both Russel and Rayne have heart disease. Russel considers himself to be well, whereas Rayne considers himself to be ill. Explain this phenomenon on the basis of the social determinants of health.

3. What external factors may have influenced Russel's decision to implement positive health behaviours?

4. What factors may have prevented Rayne from developing the same positive outlook and taking the same actions as Russel did to manage his illness?

5. What nursing interventions would be most beneficial to Rayne with regard to his smoking problem?

6. What would be some cultural considerations when teaching Russel and Rayne?

Check the eText in MyNursingLab for answers and explanations.

KEY TERMS

acute illness *p. 130*

adherence *p. 129*

autonomy *p. 130*

chronic illness *p. 130*

disease *p. 130*

etiology *p. 130*

exacerbation *p. 130*

health *p. 123*

illness *p. 129*

medicine wheel *p. 125*

remission *p. 130*

well-being *p. 124*

wellness *p. 124*

CHAPTER HIGHLIGHTS

- Nurses need to understand the concept of *health* because their personal definitions of health largely determine the scope and nature of their nursing practice.

- Perspectives on health have changed; instead of being the absence of disease, *health* has come to mean the fulfillment of a person's maximum potential for physical, psychosocial, and spiritual functioning.

- Notions of health are highly individualized; the nurse works with the client and the client's perception of health to provide meaningful assistance.

- Well-being is composed of 10 indicators and refers to quality of life and individual and societal well-being. Individual well-being includes personal values, relationships with family and friends, and so on. Societal well-being includes the quality of interactions between and among people and their social institutions, for example, interactions with the health care system, and so on.

- Most people describe health as freedom from symptoms of disease, the ability to be active, and a state of being in good spirits.

- Health belief and behaviour models, such as Rosenstock's and Becker's health belief models (HBMs), have been developed to help determine whether an individual is likely to participate in disease-prevention and health-promotion activities.

- Nurses can enhance health care adherence by identifying the reasons for nonadherence if it occurs, demonstrating caring, and using positive reinforcement to encourage healthy behaviours.

- Illness is usually associated with disease but may occur independently. Illness is a personal experience in which the person feels unhealthy or ill. Disease alters bodily functions and results in a reduction of capacities or a shortened lifespan.

- An individual's usual pattern of behaviour changes with illness, which may disrupt a person's autonomy, lifestyle, roles, and finances.

- The illness of one member of a family affects all other members.

- Various determinants significantly affect the health of individuals, families, and communities.

ASSESS YOUR LEARNING

1. Mr. Smith is a 72-year-old man who lives alone in an apartment in an urban setting in Canada. He describes himself as healthy, self-sufficient, and financially secure. Mr. Smith has no living relatives and states that he often feels sad and lonely. He does his shopping at a grocery store across the street and eats a well-balanced diet. Which health determinant may have the most influence on Mr. Smith's ability to maintain his health over the next few years?

   a. Income and income distribution

   b. Social exclusion

   c. Housing

   d. Gender

2. Modified social relationships, change in body image, and feelings of hopelessness are best associated with what?

   a. Disability

   b. Disease

   c. Chronic illness

   d. Acute illness

3. A person who is worried about her own health because her mother and grandmother both developed breast cancer has individual perceptions about which of the following, which may subsequently influence her future prevention activities?

   a. Perceived susceptibility

   b. Perceived seriousness

   c. Sociopsychological variables

   d. Demographic variables

4. Which of the following is defined as a "subjective perception of vitality and feeling well; it can be described objectively, experienced, and measured, and can be plotted on a continuum"?

   a. Health

   b. Perception

   c. Wellness

   d. Well-being

5. Mr. Street is a middle-aged homeless man who has come into the clinic with a generalized body rash. Mr. Street has strong body odour and appears very dirty. Which concept is most important for the nurse to understand?

   a. Mr. Street needs education on proper bathing and hygiene practices.

   b. Education regarding self-care hygiene practices is not going to be enough to change Mr. Street's behaviours.

   c. Homeless people are always very dirty, and nothing can be done to change that.

   d. Homeless people often do not care as much about their hygiene as do the rest of the population.

6. Ms. Run, age 52 years, has an annual mammography for breast cancer. She does not have a diagnosis of breast cancer or a family history of this type of cancer. This screening is BEST described as what?

   a. Primary prevention

   b. Secondary prevention

   c. Tertiary prevention

   d. Health promotion

7. A new mother brings her newborn daughter to your wellness clinic for a checkup. In the course of the assessment, you notice that the mother holds the baby only when necessary and does not communicate with or look at her new baby. Believing this new family to be at risk, you offer support services of home care visits and counselling. Which determinant of health is most at risk in this situation?

   a. Social safety net

   b. Early child development

   c. Gender

   d. Income and income distribution

8. Mrs. Jog has been exercising and calorie counting ever since her diagnosis of hypertension last fall. She has set a goal of reducing her blood pressure over the next 6 months. Her strategy is BEST described as what?

   a. Primary prevention

   b. Secondary prevention

   c. Tertiary prevention

   d. Disease prevention

9. Mr. Chan was recently diagnosed with diabetes mellitus. He is confident that he can control his blood sugar with diet and exercise alone. He recently checked out a video on the management of diabetes at a community diabetes education centre. Mr. Chan's actions are most representative of which one of the following models?

   a. Health belief model

   b. Clinical model

   c. Role-performance model

   d. Health and wellness model

10. Mrs. Jones sees a nurse at the local diabetes centre. She states, "I feel healthy, even though I have diabetes." Which of the following responses by the nurse is consistent with the generally recognized definition of health?

    a. "Health is influenced mainly by biology."

    b. "The definition of health is a personal belief."

    c. "Health is a state of complete physical, mental, and social well-being."

    d. "Health is defined as the absence of disease."

Check the eText in MyNursingLab for answers and explanations.

WEBLINKS

Public Health Agency of Canada (PHAC)

http://www.phac-aspc.gc.ca/chn-rcs/index-eng.php

This website provides information related to diseases and conditions, health and safety, research and statistics, and health indicators for age groups across the lifespan, including a section dedicated to Aboriginal peoples' health.

Canadian Holistic Nurses Association (CHNA)

http://www.chna.ca

This site presents the philosophy and objectives of the CHNA and information on the levels of training for a Holistic Nursing Specialty.

Health Canada

http://www.hc-sc.gc.ca/index-eng.php

This client-centred government website provides a collection of health-related resources and services.

MyNursingLab

MyNursingLab's guided learning path makes reviewing and test preparation straightforward.

– Content summaries, animations, and videos reinforce key concepts and skills

– Practice questions help with test prep by showing gaps in knowledge

– An eText, available online and via the iPad, makes searching, highlighting, and note-taking easy

---

This QR code appears at the end of every chapter and provides learning resources that you can access with your smartphone to study on the go. Access self-review quizzes, flashcards, and more!

REFERENCES

Becker, M. (Ed.). (1974). *The health belief model and personal health behavior.* Thorofare, NJ: Charles B. Slack.

Canadian Institute for Health Information. (2009). *Mentally healthy communities: Aboriginal perspectives.* Ottawa, ON: CIHL. Retrieved from http://secure.cihi.ca/cihiweb/products/ mentally_healthy_communities_aboriginal_perspectives_e.pdf

Curtis, A. J. (2000). *Health psychology.* New York, NY: Routledge.

Hales, D. R., & Lauzon, L. (2010). *An invitation to health* (Canadian 2nd ed.). Toronto, ON: Thomson Canada Ltd., Nelson Division.

Human Resources and Skills Development Canada. (2012). *Indicators of well-being in Canada.* Retrieved from http://www4. hrsdc.gc.ca/c.4nt.2nt@-eng.jsp?cid=14

Lalonde, M. (1974). *A new perspective on the health of Canadians.* Ottawa: Government of Canada.

Leavell, H. R., & Clark, E. G. (1965). *Preventive medicine for the doctor in his community* (3rd ed.). New York, NY: McGraw-Hill.

Mikkonen, J., & Raphael, D. (2010*). Social determinants of health: The Canadian facts.* Toronto, ON: York University School of Health Policy and Management. Retrieved from http://www. thecanadianfacts.org/

Nightingale, F. (1960/1969). *Notes on nursing: What it is, and what it is not.* New York, NY: Dover Books. (Original work published in 1860).

Parsons, T. (1951). *The social system.* Glencoe, IL: Free Press.

Paterson, D. H., & Warburton, D. (2010). Physical activity and functional limitations in older adults: A systematic review related to Canada's physical activity guidelines. *International Journal of Behavioral Nutrition and Physical Activity, 7*, 38. Retrieved from http://www.ijbnpa.org/content/pdf/1479-5868-7-38.pdf

Pender, N. J., Murdaugh, C. L., & Parsons, M. J. (2011). *Health promotion in nursing practice* (6th ed.). Upper Saddle River, NJ: Prentice Hall.

Public Health Agency of Canada. (2003). *What makes Canadians healthy or unhealthy—key determinant.* Retrieved from http://www.phac-aspc.gc.ca/ph-sp/determinants/determinants-eng.php#income

Public Health Agency of Canada. (2011). *Physical activity, tips to get active: Adding physical activity to your day.* Retrieved from http://www.phac-aspc.gc.ca/hp-ps/hl-mvs/pa-ap/04paap-eng.php

Registered Nurses' Association of Ontario. (2010). *Strategies to support self-management in chronic conditions: Collaboration with clients.* Toronto, ON. Registered Nurses' Association of Ontario. Retrieved from http://www.rnao.org/Storage/72/6710_SMS_Brochure.pdf

Rosenstock, I. M. (1974). Historical origins of the health belief model. In M. H. Becker, (Ed.), *The health belief model and personal health behavior* (pp. 27–59). Thorofare, NJ: Charles B. Slack.

South West Local Health Integration Network. (2009). *A healthier tomorrow: Integrated health service plan 2010–2013.* Chatam, ON: Author.

Statistics Canada. (May, 2011). *Competing priorities—Education and retirement saving behaviours of Canadian families.* Retrieved from http://www.statcan.gc.ca/pub/81-004-x/2011001/article/11432-eng.htm

Travis, J. W., & Ryan, R. S. (2004). *Wellness workbook: How to achieve enduring health and vitality* (3rd ed.). Berkeley, CA: Celestial Arts. Retrieved from http://www.thewellspring.com/wellspring/introduction-to-wellness/357/key-concept-1-the-illnesswellness-continuum.cfm

World Health Organization. (1948). *Preamble to the constitution of the World Health Organization as adopted by the International Health Conference.* New York, June 19–22, 1946; signed on July 22, 1946, by the representatives of 61 States (Official Records of the World Health Organization, no. 2, p. 100) and entered into force on April 7, 1948.

World Health Organization. (1978). *The Declaration of Alma-Ata.* Geneva, Switzerland: Author.

Chapter 8

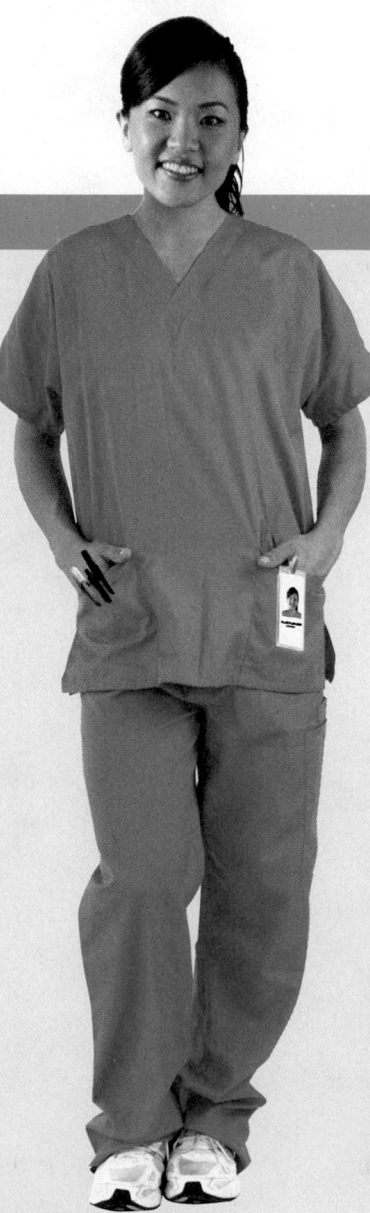

Health Promotion

LEARNING OUTCOMES

After studying this chapter, you will be able to:

1. Describe the development of health-promotion initiatives in Canada.

2. Discuss the essential components of the following health-promotion models and documents: *Lalonde Report*, *Ottawa Charter for Health Promotion*, Epp's health-promotion framework, population health-promotion model, the *Jakarta Declaration*, and Pender's health-promotion model.

3. Describe the national health goals and the development process specific to improve the health of Canadians.

4. Differentiate health promotion from health protection and health education.

5. Identify various sites of health-promotion programs.

6. Explain the six stages of change in Prochaska's transtheoretical model.

7. Discuss the nurse's role in health promotion.

8. Discuss how nursing process is applied to health promotion.

Health promotion is a cornerstone of professional nursing practice (Community Health Nurses of Canada, 2003, revised 2011). In the past 3 decades, the public has become increasingly aware of the relationship between lifestyle and illness and has begun to adopt health-promoting habits, such as being more physically active, balancing stress and relaxation, maintaining good nutrition, achieving healthy weight, and controlling the use of tobacco, alcohol, and other drugs. Nurses must understand what health promotion is to effectively prevent illness and promote individual and community health.

Development of Health-Promotion Initiatives in Canada

Health promotion has been a practice dating back to 4000 B.C.E. with the Egyptians' sewage disposal system, feeding of the poor, and warnings about excessive alcohol consumption. Florence Nightingale was the very first nurse to promote clean air and hygiene during the Crimean War in the 1800s. In the early 1900s, public health movements in Canada focused on the control of communicable diseases. At the turn of the twentieth century, this work was exemplified by the Victorian Order of Nurses (VON) and by public health nurses promoting nutrition and maternal and child health among the poor (Stamler & Yiu, 2012). See Chapter 1.

Changing Focus in Public Health (Post–World War II)

Since World War II, continued advances in scientific medicine and technology have led to marked improvement in health and mandatory public health measures, such as immunization, sanitation, water purification, and the pasteurization of milk, to control communicable diseases have prevented many illnesses and deaths. Union movements helped improve working conditions and income. Economic improvement also led to better housing and living conditions and improved nutrition. As Canadians enjoyed longer life expectancy, chronic diseases (e.g., diabetes and heart disease), cancer, and accidents gradually replaced tuberculosis, diarrhea, and influenza as the leading causes of death. Public health practice began shifting its emphasis from infection control to health-promotion activities by addressing risk factors, such as tobacco use, lack of physical activity, and poor eating habits, which contribute to various diseases (Stamler & Yiu, 2012).

Lalonde Report (1974)

With the passing of the Medical Care Act of 1966, governments became responsible for financing a universal health care system with services that are accessible to all Canadians. In an effort to control the escalating health care costs, governments began to explore factors that influenced the health of Canadians and evidence that supported health outcomes. This led to the first landmark health-promotion document in Canada, *A New Perspective on the Health of Canadians* (Lalonde, 1974), known as the *Lalonde Report*.

Lalonde conceptualized the **health field concept**, which listed the four elements that determine health: (a) biology, (b) lifestyle, (c) environment, and (d) health care organizations (see Figure 8.1). The concept marked a shift from a medical approach to a behavioural approach to health and put the emphasis on individuals' responsibility for their own health. Nevertheless, this approach was heavily criticized for blaming people for their poor health

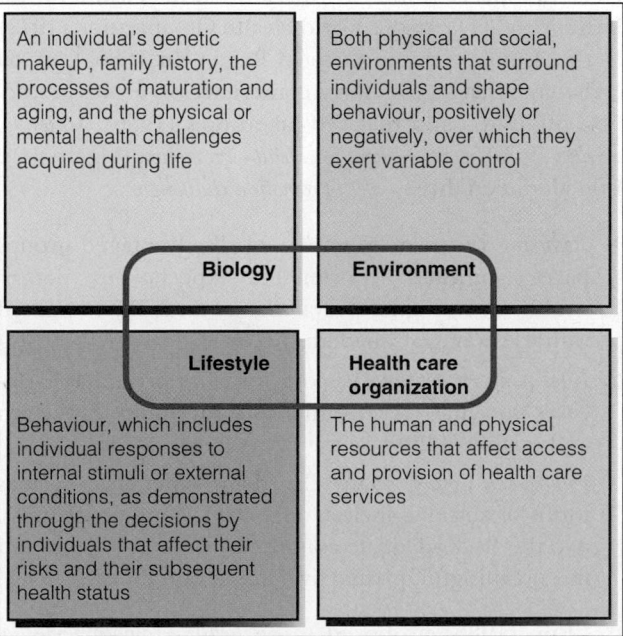

An individual's genetic makeup, family history, the processes of maturation and aging, and the physical or mental health challenges acquired during life	Both physical and social, environments that surround individuals and shape behaviour, positively or negatively, over which they exert variable control
Biology	**Environment**
Lifestyle	**Health care organization**
Behaviour, which includes individual responses to internal stimuli or external conditions, as demonstrated through the decisions by individuals that affect their risks and their subsequent health status	The human and physical resources that affect access and provision of health care services

FIGURE 8.1 Lalonde's health field concept.

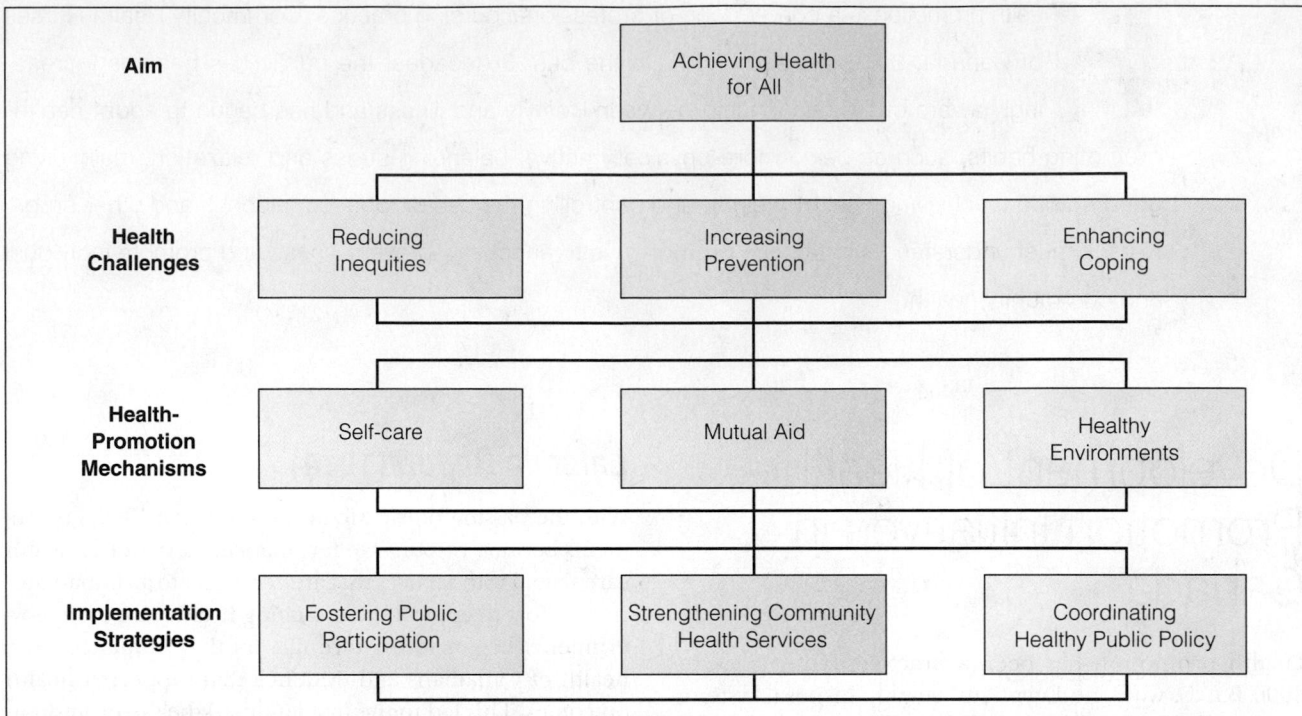

FIGURE 8.2 A framework for health promotion.

Source: From Achieving health for all: A framework for health promotion. Health Canada, 1986. Reproduced with permission from the Minister of Health, 2012.

and failing to recognize the socioeconomic barriers to making healthy lifestyle choices.

Epp Report (1986)

By the mid-1980s, health promotion became a global discussion, especially after the declaration of "Health for All by the Year 2000" by the World Health Organization (1978) at the Alma-Ata conference in Russia. In 1986, Canada hosted the first international conference on health promotion in Ottawa and released Jake Epp's (1986) *Achieving Health for All: A Framework for Health Promotion* (Figure 8.2). Epp identified three *health-promotion challenges*:

1. *Reducing Inequities.* Members of disadvantaged groups have significantly shorter life expectancies, poorer health, and a higher prevalence of disability compared with the average Canadian.
2. *Increasing Prevention.* Various forms of preventable diseases and injuries continue to undermine the health and quality of life of many Canadians.
3. *Enhancing Coping.* Many Canadians suffer from various forms of chronic disease, disability, or emotional stress, and they lack adequate community support to cope and live meaningful, productive, and dignified lives.

Epp (1986) proposed three *health-promotion mechanisms* to overcome these challenges:

1. Self-care, or the decisions and actions individuals take in the interest of their own health

2. Mutual aid, or the actions people take to help one another cope
3. Healthy environments, or the creation of conditions and surroundings conducive to health

Epp also suggested three key *health-promotion implementation strategies*:

1. Fostering public participation
2. Strengthening community health services
3. Coordinating healthy public policy

Epp (1986) believed that decisions about health should not belong exclusively to experts or governments. He stressed the need for *partnerships in health* with all stakeholders and the importance of *public participation* in implementing health-promotion programs. As communities began to see health as their prerogative, they took collective action on what they saw as priorities for their well-being. This led to the *healthy communities* movement to improve social and working environments; it was initiated in Toronto in 1984 and later spread worldwide (Raeburn & Rootman, 1998).

Ottawa Charter for Health Promotion (1986)

The *Ottawa Charter for Health Promotion* (World Health Organization, Health and Welfare Canada, & Canadian Public Health Association, 1986), shown in Figure 8.3 on the next page, was conceived and signed by delegates from 38 countries at the end of the 1986 First

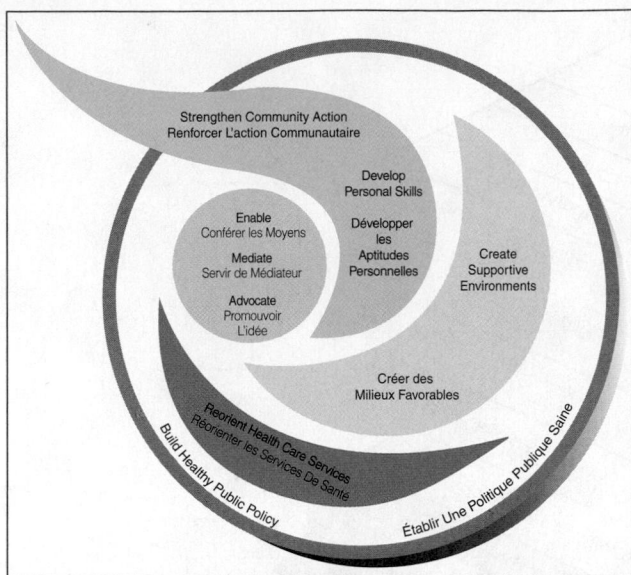

FIGURE 8.3 The *Ottawa Charter for Health Promotion.*

Source: From World Health Organization, Health and Welfare Canada, and Canadian Public Health Association. (1986). *The Ottawa Charter for Health Promotion.* Geneva, Switzerland: World Health Organization. Retrieved from http://www.who.int/ healthpromotion/conferences/previous/ottawa/en/index4.html

International Conference on Health Promotion in Ottawa. This charter addresses the importance of a socioenvironmental approach to achieving equity in health. It viewed health as a "resource for everyday living" and identified the fundamental conditions or *prerequisites for health* as peace, shelter, education, food, income, social justice, equity, sustainable resources, and a stable ecosystem. The charter also stressed that individuals, government, and nongovernment sectors must work in partnership for health. It outlined five health-promotion strategies and aims:

1. Build healthy public policy—aim to make healthier choices by adopting healthy public policy.

2. Create supportive environments—aim to generate safe, stimulating, satisfying, and enjoyable living and working conditions.

3. Strengthen community action—aim to empower communities to take ownership and control of their own endeavours and destinies.

4. Develop personal skills—aim to assist people to make informed choices so that they can have control over their own health.

5. Reorient health services—aim to organize health, social, political, economic, and physical sectors by focusing on the total needs of the individual.

Strategies for Population Health (1994)

The progress of health promotion was set back by the severe global economic recession in the early 1990s. The need for all health services to demonstrate evidence

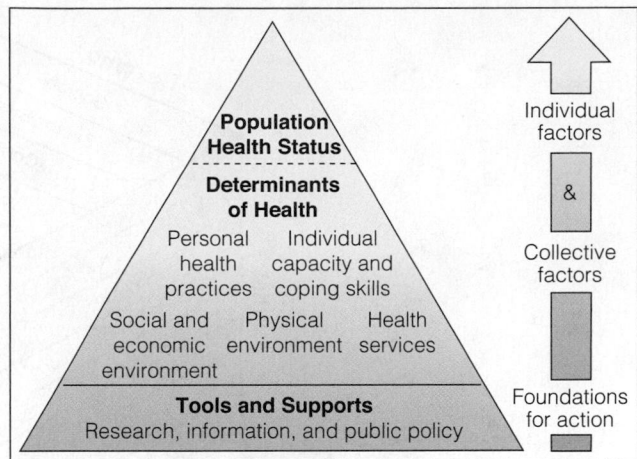

FIGURE 8.4 Framework for population health.

Source: From *Achieving Health for All: A Framework for Health Promotion.* Health Canada, 1986. Reproduced with the permission of the Minister of Health, 2012.

of health outcomes, accountability, cost-effectiveness, and efficiency became more important than ever. The Canadian Institute of Advanced Research released a report, *Strategies for Population Health: Investing in Health of Canadians* (Federal, Provincial, and Territorial Advisory Committee on Population Health, 1994), which set the *determinants of health* at the centre of the *framework for population health* (Figure 8.4). In this framework, all known determinants of health must be considered in planning action to improve health. Evidence-based health outcomes through research will be tracked and used to formulate public policy. The 15 determinants of health (see Chapter 7) were divided into five groups of population health initiatives as follows:

1. *Social and economic environments:* education, employment and working conditions, income and social status, social support networks, and social environments

2. *Individual capacity and coping skills:* healthy child development, biology and genetic endowment, gender

3. *Health services:* health services

4. *Physical environments:* physical environments

5. *Personal health practices:* personal health practices and coping skills, culture

Population Health-Promotion Model (1996)

Hamilton and Bhatti (1996) developed a population health-promotion model, shown in Figure 8.5, to improve population health. The model *integrated* the concepts of health-promotion strategies from the *Ottawa Charter for Health Promotion*, the determinants of health from the *Strategies for Population Health*, and the levels of potential clients for intervention. These clients may be individuals, families, communities, groups, or societies. This

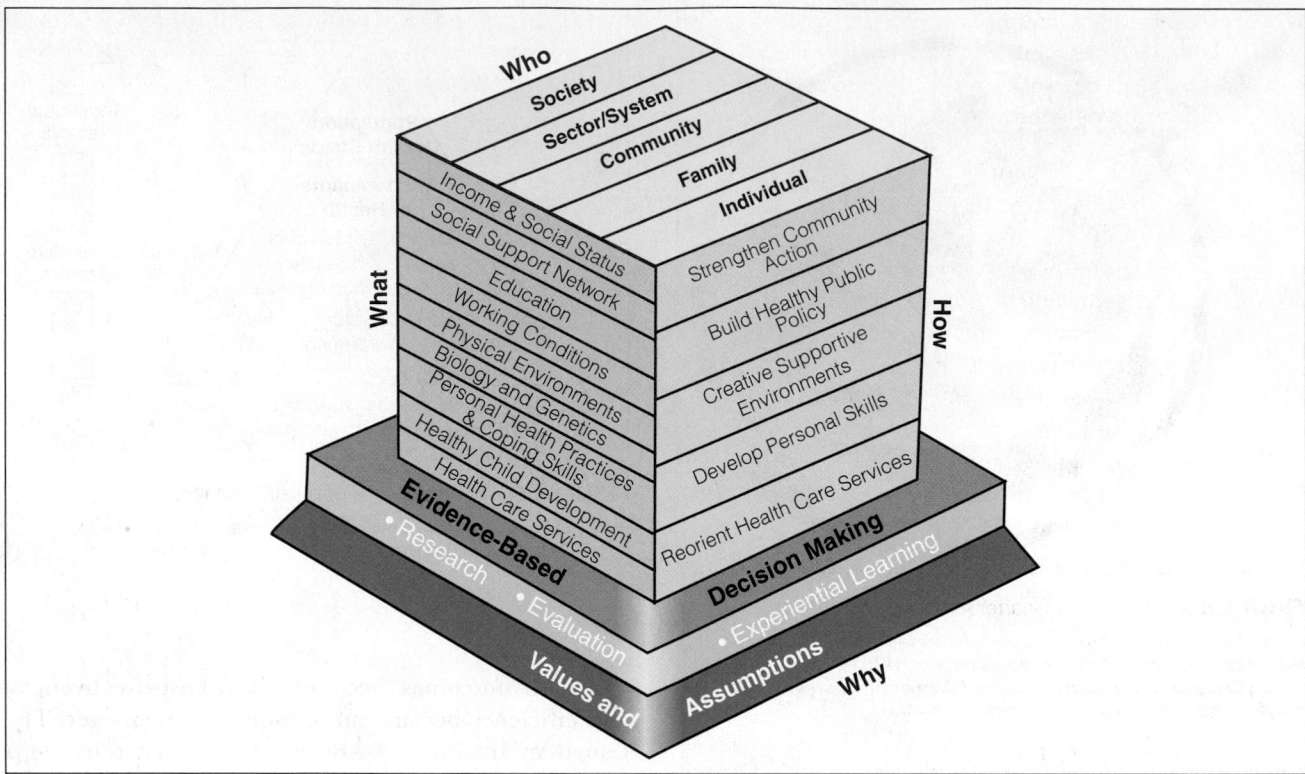

FIGURE 8.5 An integrated model of population health and health promotion.

Source: From *Population health promotion: An integrated model of population health and health promotion.* Public Health Agency of Canada, 2001. Reproduced with the permission of the Minister of Health, 2012.

model presented four key questions for examination when implementing health-promotion actions: (a) *what* actions are being taken, (b) *how* these actions can be implemented, (c) *with whom* the actions can be taken, and (d) *why* such actions are taken. It also emphasized the importance of research and evidence-based decision making.

Jakarta Declaration and Toronto Charter for a Healthy Canada (1997–2002)

In the late 1990s, poverty, social and economic inequities, globalization, and environmental degradation gained increasing recognition as threats to health. Social determinants of health became the key themes in health-promotion discussions and resulted in the adoption of the 1997 *Jakarta Declaration on Health Promotion* (WHO, 1997). Canada, together with other nations, affirmed social justice, equity, and sustainability as new commitments for health promotion at the local, national, and international levels. The *Jakarta Declaration* endorsed the *Ottawa Charter for Health Promotion*, as its principles were grounded in primary health care, social justice, and community empowerment. It identified five priorities for health promotion in the twenty-first century:

1. Promoting social responsibility for health
2. Increasing investment for health development

3. Consolidating and expanding partnerships for health
4. Increasing community capacity and empowering the individual
5. Securing an infrastructure for health promotion

The 2002 *Toronto Charter for a Healthy Canada* (Raphael, Bryant, & Curry-Stevens, 2004) further addressed the social determinants of health, their implications, and policy development in such areas as early childhood development, education, employment and working conditions, food security, health care services, housing shortages, income and its equitable distribution, social safety nets, social exclusion, unemployment, and job security.

A Population Health Approach: The Organizing Framework (2006)

In 2006, the Public Health Agency of Canada (2010) launched *A Population Health Approach: The Organizing Framework,* which focuses on eight elements essential to improve the health of the population and reduce health disparities: (a) focusing on the health of the population, (b) addressing the determinants of health and their interactions, (c) basing decisions on evidence, (d) increasing upstream investments to examine the root causes of a problem or a benefit, (e) applying multiple interventions and strategies, (f) collaborating across sectors and levels, (g) employing mechanisms for public involvement, and

(h) demonstrating accountability for health outcomes. These elements cover a broad context of diseases and risk factors, and the framework supports decision making for the desired health outcomes.

Public Health Goals for Canada

Between 1989 and 1998, attempts by each province to develop health goals failed to address ways to integrate planning, policy formulation and decision making, and accountability to measure performance on the goals. In 2004, the newly established Public Health Agency of Canada (PHAC) led extensive consultations with experts, stakeholders, and Canadians from all regions to articulate their priorities and vision for the health goals for the nation, and benchmarks were set to improve the health status of Canadians (see Table 8.1). These health goals are framed as public health goals to achieve population health and not just individual health. The goals are broad and take an upstream approach to look beyond health care but focus on the social determinants of health (Clement, 2005).

Canada was once a world leader in health promotion. However, inequities in health have been largely ignored due to various funding priorities. There needs to be political and health care system leadership to invest adequately in disease prevention and health promotion (Handcock, 2011). Ongoing collaborative research in health promotion and translating knowledge to practice must be fostered, and policies must be established to address major health issues, such as tobacco and drug use, obesity, mental health, poverty, early childhood development, diabetes, heart disease, and Aboriginal health. Nurses must understand the implications of various health-promotion initiatives for their practice, as shown in the Nursing and Canadian Society box on the next page.

Defining Health Promotion

What, then, is health promotion? **Health promotion** is "a *strategy* that aims at informing, influencing, and assisting both individuals and organizations so that they will accept more responsibility and be more active in matters affecting mental and physical health" (Lalonde, 1974, p. 66). It involves any *activity* or *program* designed to improve the social and environmental living conditions that enhance people's well-being (Labonte, 1992). Health promotion is also a *process* of enabling or empowering people to increase control over their health and to improve their health by maximizing positive changes to their physical, economic, social, and political environments (Epp 1986; Health Canada, 2005; WHO, 1984). **Empowerment** is a social action process "through which people gain greater control over decisions and actions affecting their health" (WHO, 1998, p. 16). Health promotion, therefore, is a philosophy, a process, and a multisectoral and sociocultural approach that aims to enhance the health and well-being of individuals

TABLE 8.1 Health Goals for Canada

Overarching Goal: As a nation, we aspire to a Canada in which every person is as healthy as they can be—physically, mentally, emotionally, and spiritually.

Health Goals	Canada is a country where:
Basic Needs (Social and Physical Environments)	Our children reach their full potential, growing up happy, healthy, confident, and secure.
	The air we breathe, the water we drink, the food we eat, and the places we live, work, and play are safe and healthy—now and for generations to come.
Belonging and Engagement	Each and every person has dignity and a sense of belonging and contributes to supportive families, friendships, and diverse communities.
	We keep learning throughout our lives through formal and informal education, relationships with others, and the land.
	We participate in and influence the decisions that affect our personal and collective health and well-being.
	We work to make the world a healthy place for all people, through leadership, collaboration, and knowledge.
Healthy Living	Every person receives the support and information they need to make healthy choices.
A System for Health	We work to prevent, and are prepared to respond to, threats to our health and safety through coordinated efforts across the country and around the world.
	A strong system for health and social well-being responds to disparities in health status and offers timely, appropriate care.

Source: Adapted from *Health goals for Canada: A federal, provincial and territorial commitment to Canadians.* Public Health Agency of Canada, 2005. Reproduced with permission from the Minister of Health, 2012.

Nursing and Canadian Society

Fact	Implications for Nursing Practice
The 1974 *New Perspective on the Health of Canadians*, also known as the *Lalonde Report*, is often cited as the beginning of health promotion.	Nurses must appreciate and understand the historical development and achievements of health promotion and continue to explore what determines Canadians' health.
Jake Epp's *Achieving Health for All: A Framework for Health Promotion* reinforced the WHO's goal of health for all by 2000.	Nurses must continue to investigate ongoing health-promotion challenges and mechanisms to plan and implement participatory actions to achieve equity in health.
The 1986 *Ottawa Charter for Health Promotion* marked the shift from traditional treatment and preventive health care to health-promotion strategies that feature empowerment.	Nurses must focus on the broader definitions of health, go beyond health education, and work with intersectoral partners to empower clients to take control of their lives through policy changes and supportive environments.
Hamilton and Bhatti's 1996 population health-promotion model outlined the *who*, *what*, *where*, and *how* of population health promotion and stressed the importance of evidence-based practice.	Nurses must integrate the needed knowledge and skills to promote health for individuals, families, groups, and communities in various settings. Accountable actions and ongoing monitoring and evaluation while striving for evidence-based outcomes must be emphasized.
The 2002 *Toronto Charter for a Healthy Canada* expanded on the 1997 *Jakarta Declaration on Health Promotion* to address the importance of the social determinants of health, their implications, and policy development.	Nurses must advocate and be politically active from local to international levels to address the broader determinants of health and work and move toward sustainability, social justice, and equity in health.
Health goals for Canadians are developed through extensive consultations with Canadians and stakeholders across the nation and all government levels.	Nurses must implement evidence-based outcome oriented programs to address the interacting social determinants of health.

and communities through policy formulation, supportive environments, and health education. Alternatively, some viewed health promotion as "marginal in health care and was more of a professional movement than a social movement"(Rootman, Dupéré, Penderson, & O'Neill, 2012, p. ix) (see the Reflect on Primary Health Care box).

 REFLECT ON PRIMARY HEALTH CARE

Health promotion is a principle of primary health care. Nurses adopt the primary health care approach to provide promotive, preventive, curative, rehabilitative, and supportive or palliative care to their clients. The focus of their care is on preventing illness and promoting health and well-being. In promoting the health of individuals, families, groups, and communities, nurses must help their clients understand factors that determine their health and develop effective skills to improve and maintain their own health and well-being. Consider how you can work with your clients and interdisciplinary health care providers to provide health-promotion services that are culturally sensitive and accessible to your clients. Also, examine whether the educational material is written in a language and at a level that can be understood by clients from another culture.

Health promotion is not synonymous with health education. WHO (1998) defined **health education** as "consciously constructed opportunities for learning designed to facilitate changes in behaviour towards a predetermined goal, and involving some form of communication designed to improve health literacy, knowledge, and life skills conducive to individual and community health" (p. 14). Health education, therefore, is a strategy of health promotion; it is concerned with the communication of information and the fostering of motivation, skills, and confidence to take action to improve health.

Central to health promotion is prevention. Leavell and Clark (1965) described *three levels of prevention* during a course of disease progression (see Chapter 7 for primary, secondary, and tertiary levels of prevention). The notions of *health promotion, health protection,* and *disease prevention* are significantly different. Pender, Murdaugh, and Parsons (2011) define health promotion as "behaviour motivated by the desire to increase well-being and actualize human health potential." **Health protection** involves activities focused on preventing, avoiding, or minimizing injuries that individuals have little or no control over and preventable illnesses. **Disease prevention** is concerned with taking measures to prevent and control common risk factors for diseases.

TABLE 8.2   Differences between Health Promotion, Health Protection, and Disease Prevention

	Health Promotion	Health Protection and Disease Prevention
Aim	To attain a higher level of wellness by modifying own behaviours and improving social, environmental, and economic conditions	To increase resistance to harm by modifying the environment to minimize preventable illness or injury
Motivation	Motivated by personal, positive desire for wellness	Motivated by avoidance of harm or illness
Examples of Activity Focus	• Stress management • Active living • Nutrition • Sexual health • Injury prevention • Smoking cessation • Substance use and abuse • Responsible alcohol use	• Emergency responses • Vehicle, water, food, and drug safety • Infectious disease control • Occupational health safety • Early detection of cancer (e.g., breast health) • Health hazard investigation (e.g., chemical, radiation, and water)

Behaviours in both *health protection* and *disease prevention* are "motivated by a desire to actively avoid illness, detect it early, or maintain functioning within the constraints of illness" (p. 5). The major difference in these terms lies with the underlying *motivation* for the individual behaviour (see Table 8.2).

Activities for health promotion, health protection, and disease prevention are complementary processes and are carried out for numerous reasons. For example, suppose a 40-year-old male begins a program of walking 5 kilometres each day. If the goal of his program is to decrease his risk of cardiovascular disease, then the activity is considered disease prevention. By contrast, if the motivation for walking is to increase his overall health and feeling of well-being, then it is considered health-promotion behaviour. Health promotion can be offered to all clients regardless of their age or state of health. Age-specific health-promotion activities are discussed in Chapters 17 to 20. (See Lifespan Considerations on the next page for examples of health-promotion topics).

Sites for Health-Promotion Activities

Health-promotion programs and activities can be offered to individuals and families in the home or in the community setting, such as in schools, hospitals, or worksites. Individual teaching or home visits can be costly, while group teaching is more cost-effective and can offer a setting for socialization and peer support.

Community health-promotion programs are frequently offered by health units, community health centres, and nonprofit health agencies. They may include immunization programs or blood pressure screenings, fire prevention information, bicycle safety programs for children, or a safe-driving campaign for young adults.

School health-promotion programs form a foundation of good health practices for children of all ages. They are cost-effective and offer a convenient setting for health-promotion programs. The school nurse works with teachers to plan and deliver information on various health topics, such as basic nutrition, dental care, activity and play, drug and alcohol use, domestic violence, child abuse, and issues related to sexuality and pregnancy.

Worksite programs may include programs that address air quality, accident prevention, back safety programs, blood pressure screening, fitness information, and relaxation techniques. Benefits to the employees can include an increased feeling of well-being, fitness, weight control, and decreased stress. Benefits to the employers can include an increase in productivity and morale, a decrease in absenteeism, and a lower rate of employee turnover, all of which can help decrease business and health care costs.

Effective health-promotion activities must be guided by models or conceptual frameworks for practice. The rest of this chapter presents two common practice models in health promotion, as well as the use of the nursing process in health promotion. See the Evidence-Informed Practice box on the next page.

Pender's Health-Promotion Model

Nola Pender's revised health-promotion model (HPM), shown in Figure 8.6 on page 147, considers the motivational source for behaviour change that is based on how the client perceives the benefits of changing the given health behaviour. Unlike the health belief model (see Chapter 7 for Rosenstock and Becker's health belief model), the HPM does not include "fear" or "threat" as a motivating

LIFESPAN CONSIDERATIONS

Health-Promotion Topics

INFANTS

Infant–parent attachment/bonding

Breast-feeding

Sleep patterns

Playful activity to stimulate development

Immunizations

Safety promotion and injury control

CHILDREN

Nutrition

Dental checkups

Rest and exercise

Immunizations

Safety promotion and injury control

ADOLESCENTS

Communicating with the teen

Hormonal changes

Nutrition

Exercise and rest

Peer group influences

Self-concept and body image

Sexuality

Safety promotion and accident prevention

ADULTS

Adequate sleep

Appropriate use of alcohol

Mental health

Stress and coping

Exercise

Weight control

Health screening recommendations

Preventive health services

OLDER ADULTS

Mental health

Physical fitness

Dental/oral health

Drug management

Nutrition

Safety precautions

Foot health

Hearing aid use

Immunizations

Medication management

Coping with loss

EVIDENCE-INFORMED PRACTICE

How Many Canadians Will Be Diagnosed with Diabetes over the Next Decade?

Based on the data on diabetes risk factors and the current levels of obesity from the 2007 Canadian Community Health Survey (CCHS cycle 4.1), the *Diabetes Population Risk Tool* (DPoRT) was used to estimate Canadians' future risk of developing diabetes in the following 10 years. The findings revealed that between 2007 and 2017, 1.9 million (or 9 of 100) Canadians will develop diabetes during the 10-year period. In 2007, Quebec, British Columbia, and Canada's urban regions had the lowest 10-year risk of diabetes. Individuals who are obese, with obesity defined as a body mass index (BMI) of >35, and overweight (BMI of 25–30) have an increased risk for developing diabetes. In total, 712,000 cases are predicted to develop among people who are overweight, compared with 247,000 cases among people who are very obese.

NURSING IMPLICATIONS: **Understanding the population at risk for developing diabetes is a cornerstone in health planning. With this information, the nurse can determine the target population and where to implement preventive activities. One of the diabetes intervention strategies may include targeting overweight individuals and achieving weight reduction in the overall population through public policy, such as controlling the sale of junk food in the community and providing individual pharmacotherapy or lifestyle counselling to high-risk obese individuals.**

Source: Based on Manuel, D. G., Rosella, L. C. A., & Tuna, M. (2010). *How many Canadians will be diagnosed with diabetes between 2007 and 2017? Assessing population risk.* Toronto, ON: Institute for Clinical Evaluative Sciences.

source for changing health behaviour (Pender et al., 2011, p. 44). The variables in the revised HPM are described below.

Individual Characteristics and Experiences

The importance of an individual's unique personal factors or characteristics and experiences depends on the target behaviour for health promotion. Personal factors are categorized as biological (e.g., age, strength, balance), psychological (e.g., self-esteem, self-motivation), and sociocultural (e.g., race, ethnicity, education, socioeconomic status). Some personal factors can influence health behaviours, while others, such as age, cannot be changed. Prior related behaviour includes previous experience, knowledge, and skill in health-promoting actions. Individuals who received benefits from previous health-promoting behaviours will engage in future health-promoting behaviours. In contrast, a person with a history of barriers to

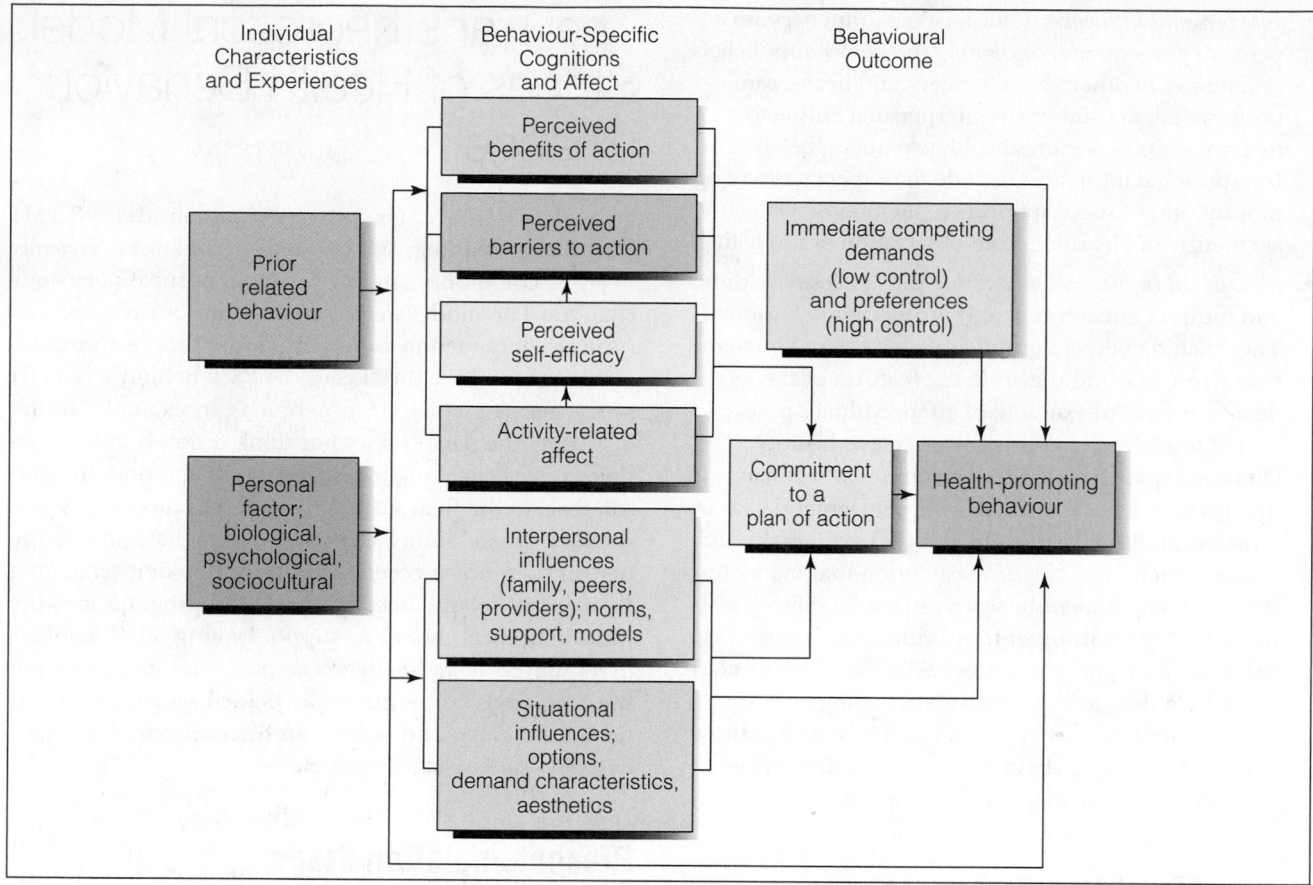

FIGURE 8.6 The health-promotion model (revised).

Source: From Pender, N. J., Murdaugh, C. L., & Parsons, M. A. (2011). *Health promotion in nursing practice* (6th ed.) (p. 45). Upper Saddle River, NJ: Prentice Hall. Copyright 2006 by Prentice Hall. Reprinted with permission.

achieving the behaviour remembers the "hurdles" and will avoid making changes.

Nurses can assist by focusing on the positive benefits of the behaviour, teaching how to overcome the barriers, and providing positive feedback for the client's successes. Nursing interventions usually focus on factors that can be modified, as well as those that cannot be changed, such as family history. For instance, nurses could direct more support and information to women with a strong family history of breast cancer by emphasizing the importance of early detection and treatment and offering more hope for a cure. Helping to transform fear into hope through early detection can make a difference in health attitudes and behaviours.

Behaviour-Specific Cognitions and Affect

Behaviour-specific cognitions and affect have major motivational significance for acquiring and maintaining health-promoting behaviours, which can be modified through nursing interventions. They include the following:

• *Perceived Benefits of Action:* Anticipated benefits or outcomes (e.g., physical fitness, stress reduction) affect the person's plan to participate in health-promoting behaviours and may facilitate continued practice. Prior positive experience with the behaviour or observations of others engaged in the behaviour is a motivational factor.

• *Perceived Barriers to Action:* A person's perceptions about available time, inconvenience, expense, and difficulty performing the activity can act as barriers (imagined or real) to the individual's commitment to a plan of action.

• *Perceived Self-Efficacy:* This concept refers to the person's competencies in successfully carrying out the behaviour needed to achieve a desired outcome, such as maintaining an exercise program to lose weight. Often, people who have serious doubts about their capabilities decrease their efforts and give up, whereas those with a strong sense of efficacy exert greater effort to master problems or challenges.

• *Activity-Related Affect:* The subjective feelings, such as reaction to the thought of the behaviour, perceived enjoyment, or unpleasant activities, that occur before, during, and following an activity can influence whether a person will repeat the behaviour or maintain the behaviour. A positive affect or emotional response to a behaviour is likely to be repeated, and behaviours associated with a negative affect are usually avoided.

- *Interpersonal Influences:* Interpersonal influences are a person's perceptions concerning the behaviours, beliefs, or attitudes of others. Family, peers, and health care professionals are sources of interpersonal influences that can shape a person's health-promoting behaviours. Interpersonal influences include the expectations of significant others, social support (e.g., emotional encouragement), and learning from observation or modelling.

- *Situational Influences:* Situational influences have direct and indirect effects on health-promoting behaviours. They include perceptions of available options, demand characteristics, and the aesthetic features of the environment. An example of an individual's perception of available options is easy access to healthy alternatives, such as vending machines and restaurants that provide healthful menu options. Demand characteristics can directly affect healthy behaviours through policies, such as a company regulation that mandates that safety equipment be worn or that establishes a nonsmoking environment. Individuals are more apt to adopt health-promotion behaviours if they are comfortable in the environment versus feeling alienated. Environments that are considered safe as well as those that are interesting are also desirable aesthetic features that facilitate health-promotion behaviours.

Commitment to a Plan of Action

Commitment to a plan of action involves dedication and the identification of specific strategies for carrying out and reinforcing a behaviour. Strategies are important because commitment alone often results in good intentions but not in the actual performance of the behaviour.

Immediate Competing Demands and Preferences

Competing demands are those behaviours over which an individual has a low level of control. For example, an unexpected work or family responsibility may compete with a planned visit to the health club, and not responding to this responsibility may cause a more negative outcome than missing the exercise routine. *Competing preferences* are behaviours over which an individual has a high level of control; however, this control depends on the individual's ability to be self-regulating or not give in. For example, a person who chooses a better-tasting high-fat food over a low-fat food has given in to an urge based on a competing preference.

Behavioural Outcome

Health-promoting behaviour, the outcome of the health-promotion model, is directed toward the client attaining positive health outcomes, such as improved health, enhanced functional ability, and better quality of life at all stages of development (Pender et al., 2011).

The Transtheoretical Model: Stages of Health Behaviour Change

The Prochaska's transtheoretical model (TTM) (Prochaska, Redding, & Evers, 2009), also known as *change theory*, is commonly used to promote positive behaviour changes. The model views health behaviour change as a cyclical phenomenon in which people progress through several stages. Take the "Leave the Pack Behind" ([LTPB] 2012) smoking cessation program as an example. In the first stage, the person does not think seriously about quitting smoke (changing a behaviour); by the time the person reaches the final stage, he or she has successfully quit smoking (maintaining the change in behaviour). If the person does not succeed in quitting smoking (changing behaviour), relapse occurs. The LTPB program uses the transtheoretical model to support young adult smokers in 44 university and college campuses in Ontario to quit smoking, and the program has yielded significant reductions in smoking and at least an 8% quit rate. Figure 8.7 describes the six stages of change.

Precontemplation Stage

In the precontemplation stage, the person does not think about changing his or her behaviour in the future 6 months. They may be uninformed or underinformed about the consequences of the risk behaviours; or the person may have tried changing and been unsuccessful and now sees the behaviour as "fate" or feels that change is hopeless. Individuals in this stage tend to avoid reading, talking, or thinking about their high-risk behaviours (Prochaska, Redding, & Evers, 2009).

Contemplation Stage

During the contemplation stage, the person acknowledges having a problem, seriously considers changing a specific behaviour, actively gathers information, and verbalizes plans to change the behaviour in the near future (e.g., the next 6 months). The person, however, may not be ready to commit to action. Some people may stay in the contemplative stage for months or years before taking action. Their thinking is clearly focused on the solution rather than the problem, and they are thinking more about the future than the past.

Preparation Stage

The preparation stage occurs when the person intends to take action in the immediate future (e.g., within the next month). Some people in this stage may have already started making small behavioural changes, such as buying

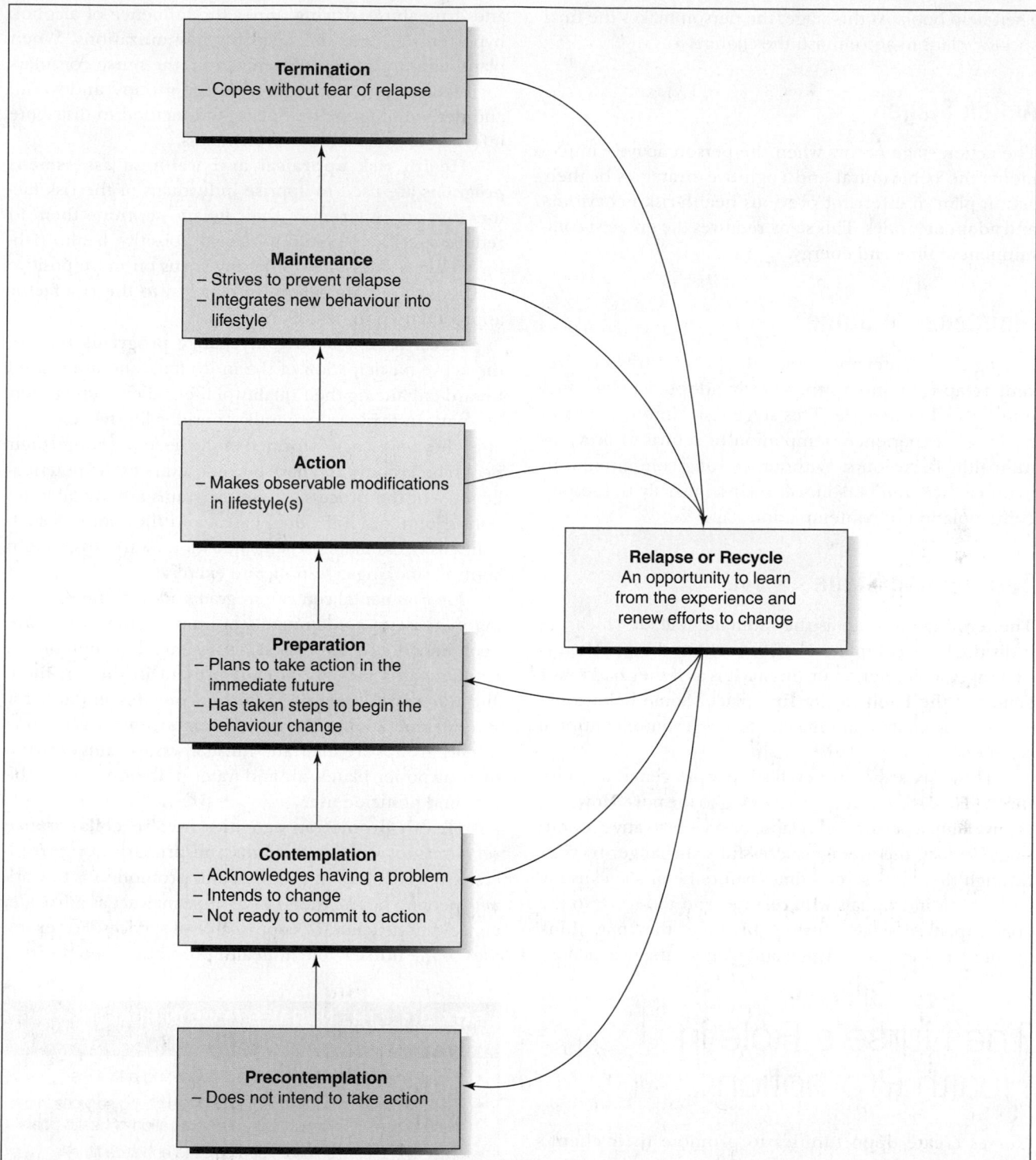

FIGURE 8.7 The transtheorectical model: Stages of change. The stages of change are rarely linear. It is more common for people to recycle several times through the stages. The person who takes action and has a relapse (recycles through some or all of the stages) is more apt to be successful the next time than the individual who never takes action.

Sources: Based on content from Prochaska, J. O., Norcross, J. C., & DiClimente, C. C. (1994). *Changing for good.* New York, NY: HarperCollins Publishers. Copyright 1994 by James O. Prochaska, John C. Norcross, and Carlo C. DiClimente; Prochaska, J. O., Redding, C. A., & Evers, K. E. (2009). The transtheoretical model and stages of change. In Glanz, K., Rimer, B. K., & Lewis, F. M., (Eds.). *Health behaviors and health education: Theory, research, and practice* (4th ed.). (2009). San Francisco, CA: Jossey-Bass.

a self-help book. At this stage, the person makes the final specific plans to accomplish the change.

Action Stage

The action stage occurs when the person actively implements the behavioural and cognitive strategies of their action plan to interrupt previous health-risk behaviours and adopt new ones. This stage requires the greatest commitment of time and energy.

Maintenance Stage

During the maintenance stage, the person strives to prevent relapse by integrating newly adopted behaviours into his or her lifestyle. This stage lasts until the person no longer experiences temptation to return to previous unhealthy behaviours. Without a strong commitment to maintenance, the person will relapse, usually to the precontemplation or contemplation stage.

Termination Stage

The termination stage is the ultimate goal, at which the individual has complete confidence that the problem is no longer a temptation or threat. It is as if they had never acquired the habit in the first place. Some behaviours may be terminated and may no longer require continual maintenance.

These six stages are cyclical; people generally move through one stage before progressing to the next. However, at any point, a person can relapse or recycle to any previous stage. In fact, the average successful self-changer recycles through the stages several times before he or she exits the cycle. Most individuals who relapse tend to return to the contemplation stage. During this time, they may think about what they have learned and plan for the next action.

The Nurse's Role in Health Promotion

Nurses create opportunities to promote their client's health. They can use a variety of programs (described below) to assist individuals and communities to adopt healthy behaviours.

Information dissemination is used to raise the level of knowledge and awareness of individuals and groups about health habits. It uses a variety of media to educate the public and raise their awareness about the risks of particular lifestyle choices and about changing personal behaviours to improve the quality of life. Billboards, posters, brochures, newspaper features, books, health fairs, and community forums all offer opportunities for information dissemination on health promotion topics, such as alcohol

and drug abuse, driving under the influence of alcohol, hypertension, and the need for immunizations. When planning information dissemination, the nurse considers such factors as culture, different age groups, and so on, and determining the best place and method to distribute information will increase effectiveness.

Health risk appraisal and **wellness assessment programs** are used to apprise individuals of the risk factors that are inherent in their lives to motivate them to reduce specific risks and to develop positive health habits. Wellness assessment programs focus on more positive methods of enhancement, in contrast to the risk-factor approach used in health appraisal.

Lifestyle and behaviour change programs require the active participation of the individuals and are geared toward enhancing their quality of life and extending their lifespan. Individuals generally consider lifestyle changes after they have been informed of the need to change their health behaviours and have become aware of the potential benefits of the process. These programs are available on both group and individual bases, and they address such issues as stress management, nutrition awareness, weight control, smoking cessation, and exercise.

Environmental control programs address the continuing increase of contaminants of human origin that have been introduced into our environment. The amounts of contaminants that are already present in the air, food, and water will affect the health of our descendants for several generations. The most common concerns of community groups are toxic and nuclear wastes, dangers from nuclear power plants, air and water pollution, and herbicide and pesticide use.

Health promotion activities involve collaborative relationships with both clients and primary care providers. The role of the nurse in health promotion is to work *with* people, not *for* them. The nurse may act as advocate, consultant, teacher, or coordinator of services. For examples of the nurse's role in health promotion, see Box 8.1.

BOX 8.1 THE NURSE'S ROLE IN HEALTH PROMOTION

- Modelling healthy lifestyle behaviours and attitudes
- Facilitating client involvement and coordinating services in the assessment, implementation, and evaluation of health goals
- Teaching clients self-care strategies to enhance fitness, improve nutrition, manage stress, and enhance relationships
- Educating clients to be effective health care consumers
- Guiding clients' development in effective problem solving and decision making
- Reinforcing clients' personal and family health-promoting behaviours
- Advocating in the community for changes that promote a healthy environment
- Empowering individuals, families, and communities to increase their levels of health by developing and choosing health-promoting options

The Nursing Process and Health Promotion

Nurses work with individuals, families, groups, and communities in diverse settings; they apply the nursing process to assess clients' health and assist them in setting goals and plans and to take responsibility for positive health changes. Refer to the section "Overview of the Nursing Process" in Chapter 23.

Assessing

Components of this assessment are the health history and physical examination, lifestyle assessment, spiritual health assessment, social support systems review, health-risk appraisal, health beliefs review, and life stress review.

HEALTH HISTORY AND PHYSICAL EXAMINATION
Health history and physical examination (discussed in Chapter 28) provide guidelines for detecting any existing problems. Medical history, age, gender, race, ethnicity, and culture of the individual must be considered when collecting data. For example, an environmental safety assessment and immunization history must be appropriate to the person's age and gender. Also, when doing a nutritional assessment, the nurse must consider how age, lifestyle, and cultural practices influence the dietary patterns of a client (see Chapter 40 for more information on nutrition assessment).

PHYSICAL FITNESS ASSESSMENT   The nurse assesses several components of the body's physical functioning: muscle endurance, flexibility, body composition, and cardiorespiratory endurance. There are specific guidelines for obtaining measurements and the optimal values for men, women, and children. Older adults need to be monitored carefully for fatigue during strength and endurance tests.

LIFESTYLE ASSESSMENT   **Lifestyle assessment** focuses on the personal lifestyle of the client, such as physical activity, nutritional practices, and stress management, and such habits as smoking, alcohol consumption, and drug use as they affect health. Lifestyle assessment provides a basis for decisions related to desired behaviour and lifestyle changes.

SPIRITUAL HEALTH ASSESSMENT   **Spiritual health** is the ability to develop our inner nature to its fullest potential, including the ability to discover and articulate a basic purpose in life, to learn how to experience love, joy, peace, and fulfillment, and how to help ourselves and others achieve their fullest potential (Pender et al., 2011). Individuals' spiritual beliefs can affect their interpretation of events in their life, and therefore, an assessment of spiritual well-being is a part of evaluating overall health (see Chapter 47).

SOCIAL SUPPORT SYSTEMS REVIEW   Through interpersonal relationships, individuals and groups can provide comfort, assistance, encouragement, and information. **Social support** fosters successful coping and promotes satisfying and effective living. **Social support systems** create an environment that encourages healthy behaviours, promotes self-esteem and wellness, and provides feedback that the person's actions will lead to desirable outcomes. Examples of social support systems include family, peer support groups, computer-based support groups, community organized religious support systems (e.g., churches), and self-help groups (e.g., Alcoholics Anonymous, Weight Watchers). The nurse can evaluate the adequacy of the client's social support systems by asking if clients have a source of support in the last 5 years or more, and, if necessary, make a plan *with* them for exploring other options for enhancing the support system.

HEALTH-RISK ASSESSMENT (HRA)   A health risk assessment (HRA) is an assessment and educational tool that indicates a client's risk for disease or injury during the next 10 years by comparing the client's risk with the mortality risk of the corresponding age, gender, and racial group. The objectives of most HRAs are twofold:

1. To assess risk factors that may lead to health problems
2. To change the health behaviours that place the client at risk of developing an illness

The HRA includes a summary of the person's health risks and lifestyle behaviours with educational suggestions on how to reduce the risk. **Risk factors** are features that can cause a client to be vulnerable to developing a specific health problem, such as cancer. An **at-risk aggregate** refers to a subgroup within the community or population that is at greater risk of illness or poor recovery. Occupational health nurses often use HRA to identify risk factors and subsequently plan interventions aimed to decrease illness, absenteeism, and disability.

HEALTH BELIEFS REVIEW   Assessment of clients' health care beliefs reveals how much the clients believe or perceive they can influence or control health through personal behaviours. **Locus of control** is a measurable concept that can be used to predict which people are most likely to change their behaviour. Some cultures have a strong belief in fate: "Whatever will be, will be." An example is teaching about diabetes control, which often requires many lifestyle changes in diet and exercise, and close control of blood glucose levels to prevent complications. If the person believes he or she has no control over the outcome, it is difficult to motivate the client to make the necessary changes. Awareness of these differences in beliefs can provide a better indication of readiness and motivation on the part of the client to engage in healthy behaviours.

LIFE STRESS REVIEW   Abundant literature and a variety of stress-related tools are available to measure the impact of stress on mental and physical well-being. High levels of stress are associated with an increased possibility of illness (see the section "Concept of Stress" in Chapter 48). Thomas Holmes's Life Change Index Scale rates 43 life events on the degree of stress each produces. This life stress scale can be accessed online at http://www.psychbytes.com/Quizzes/Life%20Changing%20Index/Life%20Changing%20Index%20Scale.htm.

VALIDATING ASSESSMENT DATA   Following the collection of assessment data, the nurse and client jointly review the client's current health practices and attitudes. This allows for validation of the information by the client and may increase awareness of the need to change behaviour. The nurse and client should consider the following:

- Any existing health problems
- Perceived degree of control over health status
- Level of physical fitness and nutritional status
- Illnesses for which the client is at risk
- Health beliefs, cultural and spiritual practices
- Current health practices and coping skills
- Sources of stress and ability to handle stress
- Social support systems
- Client's strengths and needs

Analyzing

Wellness nursing diagnoses, or *strength-oriented diagnoses,* provide a clear focus for planning interventions and can be applied at all levels of prevention. Wellness diagnoses are particularly useful for healthy clients who require teaching on health promotion, illness or disease prevention, and personal growth. When the nurse and client conclude that the client has positive health functioning, such as adequate nutrition or effective coping, the nurse can use this information to help the client reach a higher level of functioning. Some examples of wellness diagnoses are as follows:

- Health-seeking behaviours
- Effective breast-feeding
- Anticipatory grieving
- Readiness for enhanced parenting

Planning

Health-promotion plans should be mutually developed according to the needs, desires, and priorities of the client. The client chooses the health-promotion goals; the frequency, duration, and course of actions; and the method of evaluation. As a resource person, an adviser, and a counsellor, the nurse provides information, emphasizes the importance of small steps in making behavioural changes, and helps the client set realistic and measurable goals.

STEPS IN PLANNING   Pender et al. (2011) outline several steps in the process of planning health promotion, which are carried out jointly by the nurse and the client (see Box 8.2 for an example of an individualized health-promotion plan):

1. *Review and summarize the data from the assessment.* The nurse discusses with the client a summary of the data collected from the various assessments (e.g., physical health and fitness, nutrition, sources of stress, spirituality, health practices).

2. *Reinforce strengths and competencies.* The nurse and the client come to a consensus about areas in which the client is doing well and areas that need work.

3. *Identify health care goals.* The client selects two or three top-priority short-time and long-term goals and reviews the behaviour change options. These goals are formulated during the planning phase, and a date is determined for attaining them.

4. *Identify behavioural or health outcomes.* For each of the selected goals or areas in step 3, the nurse and client determine what specific behavioural changes are needed to bring about the desired outcome. For example, to reduce the risk of cardiovascular disease, the client may need to change behaviours, such as stopping smoking, losing weight, and increasing his or her activity level.

5. *Develop a behaviour change plan.* A successful program of change is based on client *ownership* of the behaviour changed (Pender et al., 2011). Clients may need help in examining value–behaviour inconsistencies and in selecting behavioural options that are most appealing and that they are most willing to try. The client's priorities will reflect personal values, activity preferences, and expectations of success.

6. *Reiterate the benefits of change.* The benefits will probably need to be reiterated even though the client is committed to the change. The health-related and non–health-related benefits should be discussed with the client as central motivating factors.

7. *Address environmental and interpersonal facilitators and barriers to change.* Environmental and interpersonal factors and available resources that support positive change should be explored and used to reinforce the client's efforts to change his or her lifestyle. All people experience barriers, some of which can be anticipated and planned for, thereby increasing the chances for the change to occur.

8. *Determine a time frame for implementation.* Setting a time frame helps the client target when to develop the

BOX 8.2 EXAMPLE OF AN INDIVIDUAL DISEASE-PREVENTION AND HEALTH-PROMOTION PLAN

Designed for: James Moore
Home Address: 714 George Street
Home Telephone Number: 222-3333
Occupation (if employed): Building services supervisor
Work Telephone Number: 445-6666
Cultural Identification: African Canadian
Birth Date: 3/14/59   Date of Initial Plan: 1/15/2010

Client strengths	Satisfactory peer relationships, spiritual strength, adequate sleep pattern
Major risk factors	Elevated cholesterol, mild obesity, sedentary lifestyle, moderate life change, multiple daily hassles
Nursing analysis	Deficient Diversional Activity
(derived from assessment of functional health patterns)	Imbalanced Nutrition: More than Body Requirements
	Caregiver Role Strain (elderly mother)
Medical diagnoses (if any)	Mild hypertension
Age-specific screening recommendations	Blood pressure, cholesterol, fecal occult blood, malignant skin lesions, depression
Desired behavioural and health outcomes	Become a regular exerciser (3×/week), lower my blood pressure, reduce weight to 75 kg

Personal Health Goals (1 = highest priority)	Selected Behaviours to Accomplish Goals	Stage of Change	Strategies/Interventions for Change
1. Achieve desired body weight	• Begin a progressive walking program • Decrease caloric intake while maintaining good nutrition	• Planning • Action (eating 4 fruits and 4 vegetables daily; using low-fat dairy products for last 2 months)	• Counterconditioning • Reinforcement management • Client contracting • Stimulus control • Cognitive restructuring
2. Decrease risk for hypertension-related disorders	Change from high- to low-sodium snacks	Contemplation	• Consciousness raising • Learning facilitation
3. Learn to manage stress effectively	Attend relaxation classes and use home relaxation tapes	Contemplation	• Contemplation • Consciousness raising • Self-revaluation • Simple relaxation therapy
4. Increase leisure-time activities	Join a local bowling league	Contemplation	• Support system enhancement

Source: From Pender, N. J., Murdaugh, C. L., & Parsons, M. A. *Health promotion in nursing practice* (6th ed.) © 2011 (pp. 124–125). Reprinted and electronically reproduced by permission of Pearson Education, Inc., Upper Saddle River, New Jersey.

needed knowledge and skills for implementation of a new behaviour. The time frame may be several weeks or months. Scheduling short-term goals and rewards can offer encouragement to achieve long-term objectives. Clients may need help to be realistic and to deal with one behaviour at a time.

9. *Formalize commitment to behaviour change.* Commitments to changing behaviours are usually verbal, but increasingly a formal, written behavioural contract is being used to motivate the client to follow through with selected actions. Motivation to follow through is provided by a positive reinforcement or reward stated in the contract. *Contracting* is based on the belief that all people have the potential for growth and the right of self-determination, even though their choices may be different from the norm.

Implementing

Self-responsibility is emphasized in making plans to change the behaviour. Depending on the client's needs, the nursing strategies may include supporting, teaching, consulting, coordinating, facilitating, counselling, and modelling to enhance behaviour change.

PROVIDING AND FACILITATING SUPPORT The focus of providing support is on the desired behaviour change. The nurse must be nonjudgmental when offering support, whether on an individual basis or in a group setting. The nurse may also facilitate the development of support networks for the client, such as family members and friends.

Individual Counselling Sessions Counselling sessions may be routinely scheduled as part of the plan to support the client's decision making in regard to the health-promotion plan. They may be provided if the client encounters difficulty in carrying out interventions or meets insurmountable barriers to change.

Telephone or Computer Counselling Telephone or computer counselling may be provided to the client to answer questions, review goals and strategies, and reinforce progress. This form of support can be useful and convenient for the busy client who may not have the time for regular in-person sessions.

Group Support Group sessions provide an opportunity for participants to learn the experiences of others in changing behaviour. Regular group contacts give individuals a renewed commitment to their goals.

Facilitating Social Support Social networks, such as family and friends, can facilitate or impede the efforts directed toward prevention and health promotion. The nurse's role is to communicate the client's needs and goals, and assist the client to assess, modify, and develop the social support necessary to achieve the desired change.

PROVIDING HEALTH EDUCATION Health education programs on a variety of health-promotion topics can be provided to groups, individuals, or communities. The health-promotion topics must be based on the health needs of the people. Specific health-promotion goals must be set and outcomes evaluated after the program implementation.

ENHANCING BEHAVIOUR CHANGE To help clients succeed in implementing behaviour changes, the nurse needs to understand the stages of change and effective

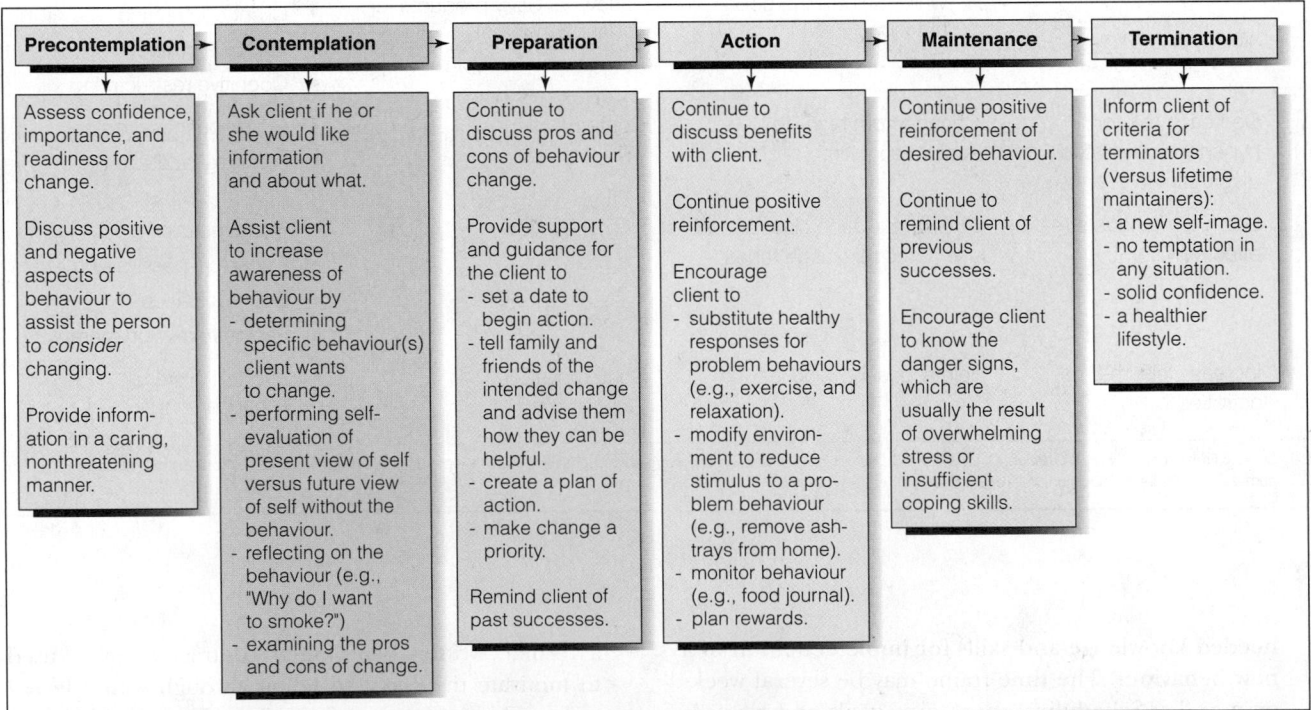

FIGURE 8.8 Strategies to promote behavioural change for each stage of change.

Sources: Data are from Prochaska, J. O., Colleen A., Redding, C. A., & Evers, K. E. (2002). The transtheoretical model and stages of change. In K. Glanz, B. K. Rimer, & F. M. Lewis, (Eds.). *Health behaviors and health education: Theory, research, and practice* (3rd ed.). San Francisco, CA: Jossey-Bass; Prochaska, J. O., Norcross, J. C., & DiClimente, C. C. (1994). *Changing for good.* New York, NY: HarperCollins Publishers. Copyright 1994 by James O. Prochaska, John C. Norcross, and Carlo C. DiClimente; Rollnick, S., Mason, P., & Butler, C. (1999). *Health behavior change: A guide for practitioners.*, Edinburgh, UK: Churchill Livingstone; Saarmann, L., Daugherty, J., & Riegel, B. (2000). Patient teaching to promote behavioral change. Nursing Outlook, *48*(6), 281–287.

BOX 8.3 GUIDELINES FOR MOTIVATING BEHAVIOURAL CHANGE

The following are guidelines for nurses to motivate their clients to achieve the desired behaviour change:

- Establish a trusting relationship with the clients.
- Assess the clients' perception of their presenting problems or concerns.
- Explain the importance of behaviour change can benefit clients' health and explore the clients' feelings, values, and beliefs as well as readiness and motivation to change.
- Encourage the clients to consider the pros and cons of behaviour change; guide them to formulate their own action plan that will be realistic and can be easily integrated by the clients into their current lifestyle.
- Be supportive and nonjudgmental when assisting the clients to select priority behaviour for change.
- Provide information and other resources including follow-up contact that will support the clients to act on behavioural change.
- Encourage the clients to monitor own progress of change, emphasizing they have control over the change process.
- Reassure the clients that relapse may occur and is common. Encourage the clients to reflect on the importance of and confidence in making the specific change. Discuss alternatives when the intended behaviour change is unmet.

interventions that focus on moving the individual through the stages of change. Figure 8.8 provides suggested strategies for helping clients, depending on their individual stage of change. Guidelines for assisting the client toward behaviour change are provided in Box 8.3. The nursing goal is not necessarily to change behaviour but to advance the client to the next stage of change.

HARM REDUCTION **Harm reduction** is a health-promotion approach that aims to minimize harm or reduce the negative consequences of risk behaviour by keeping people as safe and healthy as possible in their current lifestyle realities (Canadian Nurses Association [CNA], 2011). The nurse provides the needed knowledge, skills, resources, and support to those who are at risk, to reduce the harm done to those engaging in these behaviours and to the overall community. Examples of harm reduction are the Prevent Alcohol and Risk-related Trauma in Youth (PARTY) programs to promote responsible drinking and the needle exchange program to prevent the spread of acquired immunodeficiency syndrome (AIDS) or hepatitis C.

Some nurses may experience value conflicts and be concerned that they are not providing health-promoting behaviours with this approach. Regardless, they need to recognize that clients have rights to accessible,

nonjudgmental, and noncoercive treatments (see the section "Ethical Decision Making" in Chapter 5), and that prevention activities are best aimed at people engaging in high-risk behaviours (CNA, 2011).

ROLE MODELLING Through observing a role model during the early stages of learning and change, the client acquires ideas for behaviour and coping strategies for specific problems. The nurse and client should mutually select role models with whom the client can identify and whom he or she respects. Nurses need to have a philosophy and lifestyle that demonstrate good health habits and serve as models of wellness for their clients.

Evaluating

Evaluation of the plan is an ongoing, collaborative effort between the nurse and the client, both during the attainment of short-term goals and after the completion of long-term goals. During evaluation, the client may decide to continue with the plan, reorder priorities, change strategies, or revise the health-promotion contract.

Promoting Canadians' Health

Canada has been at the forefront of influencing health promotion. Canadian nurses must understand the historical development of health promotion and its significant contributions nationally and internationally. While health promotion has shown effectiveness from local to international levels, broader challenges remain and better effort must be made in the following: (a) building capacity for health promotion, (b) strengthening health systems, (c) partnerships and intersectoral action, (d) community empowerment, and (e) health literacy and health behaviours (7th Global Conference, 2009). The goal of nursing is to promote clients' health and to reduce inequities in health. Canadian nurses must, therefore, possess the necessary knowledge and skills in health promotion to address the social determinants of health, to promote positive behaviour change in their clients, and to develop healthy public policies at the community level. Through the use of the nursing process (see the section "Overview of the Nursing Process" in Chapter 23), nurses work with individual clients of all ages, families, groups, and communities and help them attain the highest level of functioning (see the section "Health" in Chapter 7; the section "Overview of the Nursing Process" in Chapter 23; and the Lifespan Considerations box on the next page).

LIFESPAN CONSIDERATIONS

Factors Affecting Health Promotion and Illness Prevention

CHILDREN

In Canada, national obesity rates continue to rise. Between 1981 and 2009, more than 1 in 4 adults and less than 1 in 11 children in Canada were found to be obese. The obesity rate is now roughly doubled across all age groups and tripled for youth, aged 12 to 17 (Canadian Institute for Health Information, 2011).

Obesity and overweight in children contribute to long-term health problems, such as heart disease and diabetes mellitus. Healthy eating habits and adequate exercise patterns form the basis for healthy growth and prevention of excessive weight gain in children. It is the responsibility of parents and caregivers to provide children with healthy food choices and an environment that makes eating a pleasure. Adults must be role models for their children, eating well and exercising regularly themselves.

OLDER ADULTS

In older adults, health promotion and illness prevention are important, but often the focus is on learning to adapt to and live with increasing changes and limitations. Maximizing strengths continues to be of prime importance in maintaining optimal function and quality of life. Factors to be aware of that might indicate a need for additional information or resources include the following:

- An increase in physical limitations
- Presence of one or more chronic illnesses
- Change in cognitive status
- Difficulty in accessing health care services because of transportation problems
- Poor support system
- Need for environmental modifications for safety and to maintain independence
- Attitude of hopelessness and depression, which decreases the motivation to use resources or learn new information

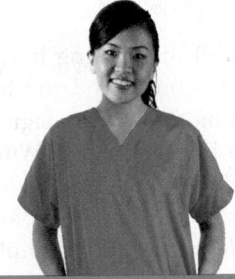

Case Study 8

Mr. W., a 50-year-old professional, has pneumonia and is currently being treated with antibiotics. He smokes two packs of cigarettes a day. Following this bout of pneumonia, he voices his concern about his smoking and wonders if he should try to quit again. He states, "I've tried everything and nothing works. The longest I last is about one month." He admits to being 13 kg overweight and states that he and his wife have started walking for 30 minutes every evening. His wife has also started making low-fat meals. He is concerned that if he quits smoking, he will gain more weight.

CRITICAL THINKING QUESTIONS

1. What information or knowledge is important for the nurse to remember when assisting a client to advance to the next stage of change?

2. Each contact between a nurse and a client is an opportunity for health promotion. On the basis of the knowledge or key concepts listed above, what question(s) would you ask Mr. W.?

3. In which stage of change relating to his cigarette smoking would you place Mr. W.? What strategies could you, as the nurse, consider?

Check the eText in MyNursingLab for answers and explanations.

KEY TERMS

locus of control   *p. 151*
risk factors   *p. 151*
social support   *p. 151*

social support
systems   *p. 151*

spiritual health   *p. 151*
wellness assessment
programs   *p. 150*

wellness nursing
diagnoses   *p. 152*

CHAPTER HIGHLIGHTS

- Canada is a world leader in health promotion and has taken a sociocultural approach to examining what determines health.

- Key documents have influenced health promotion in Canada: the *Lalonde Report*, the *Ottawa Charter for Health Promotion*, *Achieving Health for All*, the *Jakarta Declaration on Health Promotion*, the *Toronto Charter for a Healthy Canada*, and *Health Goals for Canada*.

- Health promotion is defined as client behaviour directed toward developing well-being and actualizing human health potential. Health protection is client behaviour geared toward preventing illness, detecting it early, or maintaining function.

- Health-promotion activities are directed toward developing client resources that maintain or enhance well-being. Health-protection activities are geared toward preventing specific diseases, for example, immunization to prevent poliomyelitis.

- Nurses play a critical role in promoting health through programs that focus on (a) information dissemination, (b) health appraisal and wellness assessment, (c) lifestyle and behaviour change, and (d) environmental control programs. These programs can be carried out in the home, schools, community centres, hospitals, and worksites.

- Pender's health-promotion model depicts the multidimensional nature of persons interacting with their interpersonal and physical environments as they pursue their health goals. The major motivational variables that are modifiable through nursing interventions include perceived benefits of action, perceived barriers to action, perceived self-efficacy, activity-related affect, interpersonal influences, and situational influences.

- Prochaska et al. proposed a six-stage model for health behaviour change: (a) precontemplation, (b) contemplation, (c) preparation, (d) action, (e) maintenance, and (f) termination. If a person is not successful in changing behaviour, relapse occurs. At any point in these stages, people can move to any previous stage. An understanding of these stages enables the nurse to provide appropriate nursing interventions.

- The nurse's role in health promotion is to act as a facilitator of the process of assessing, planning, implementing, evaluating, and understanding health. Nurses seek opportunities to strengthen the profession's influence on health promotion, disseminate information that promotes an educated public, and help individuals and communities to change long-standing adverse health behaviours.

- A complete and accurate assessment of the individual's health status is basic to health promotion. Assessments or reviews of a client's spiritual health, social support, health beliefs, and life stress are also important because they affect a person's health.

- Organizing assessment data from individual and family assessments enables the nurse to identify client strengths, recognize self-care abilities, and enhance health-promotion goals to help the client reach a higher level of functioning.

- Health-promotion activities are mutually planned and directed according to the client's needs, desires, and priorities.

- The nurse provides ongoing support and supplies additional information and education to help individuals change their lifestyles or health behaviours.

- During the evaluation phase of the health-promotion process, the nurse assists clients in determining whether they will continue with the plan, reorder priorities, or revise the plan.

- As role models for their clients, nurses should develop attitudes and behaviours that reflect healthy lifestyles.

ASSESS YOUR LEARNING

1. What is the aim of health promotion?
   a. Reduce premature death
   b. Empower and expand positive potential for health
   c. Minimize the occurrence of harms to health and well-being
   d. Avoid illness and maintain health functioning

2. According to the Public Health Agency of Canada (PHAC), what is a current health-promotion priority for Canadians?
   a. Securing an infrastructure for health promotion and consolidating and expanding partnerships
   b. Developing personal skills and orienting health care services
   c. Developing population health models
   d. Creating new determinants of health

3. Using a condom during sexual activity is an example of what?

    a. Health promotion

    b. Health protection

    c. Disease prevention

    d. Harm reduction

4. What is the best way for the nurse to promote safe sexual practices in a group of adolescents?

    a. Provide condoms

    b. Encourage abstinence

    c. Teach ways to prevent pregnancy

    d. Teach safe sex practices

5. Which statement reflects the contemplation stage of behaviour change?

    a. "I currently do not exercise 30 minutes three times a week and do not intend to start in the next 6 months."

    b. "I have tried several times to exercise 30 minutes three times a week but am seriously thinking of trying again in the next month."

    c. "I currently do not exercise 30 minutes three times a week, but I am thinking about starting to do so in the next 6 months."

    d. "I have exercised 30 minutes three times a week regularly for more than 6 months."

6. A female client is 20 kg overweight. She previously attended two programs that guaranteed weight loss. Although she lost some weight, she gained it back and more after each program. She tells you, "I was just born to be fat. I don't have the willpower." According to Pender's health-promotion model, the nurse should focus on which behaviour-specific cognition and affect variables for this client?

    a. Perceived barriers to action

    b. Perceived self-efficacy

    c. Interpersonal influences

    d. Situational influences

7. If a client fails to follow the information or teaching provided, how should the nurse respond?

    a. Give up, since the client does not want to change his behaviour

    b. Tell the client that he must follow your instructions

    c. Act as the role model for the client so that he can imitate the expected behaviour

    d. Assess what the barriers are and allow the client to determine what he can or will do

8. Which individual would have an increased possibility of illness in the near future?

    a. A 25-year-old man who recently married his high school sweetheart

    b. A 35-year-old man who was fired from his job

    c. A 40-year-old woman who started a nursing program

    d. A 50-year-old woman whose husband died a month ago

9. A client is very worried about how his business is doing while he is hospitalized. He spends much time on the phone and with colleagues instead of resting. To promote the client's health, what should the nurse do first?

    a. Assess the client's physiological needs

    b. Assess the client's perception of his health status

    c. Discuss with the client plans for the needed behavioural change

    d. Eliminate stress and distraction by offering the client a private room

10. Which provides data that indicate whether the person has an increased chance of acquiring a specific disease?

    a. Lifestyle assessment

    b. Health risk appraisal

    c. Health beliefs review

    d. Health education

Check the eText in MyNursingLab for answers and explanations.

WEBLINKS

Global Health Promotion Consortium

http://global-health-promotion-consortium.spruz.com

This global health-promotion consortium is internationally recognized for leading and linking community and academia into partnership in education, evaluation, and research. It focuses on strengthening the capacity for effective delivery of health promotion and health education, support theory and practice of evaluation, and conduct research and disseminate scientific and technical information for global development.

Public Health Agency of Canada: Canadian Best Practices Portal

http://cbpp-pcpe.phac-aspc.gc.ca

This portal is a virtual entry point to organizing framework and evidenced-based interventions and resources related to chronic disease prevention and health promotion for community and population health program planning.

MyNursingLab

REFERENCES

7th Global Conference. (2009). *The Nairobi call to action for closing the implementation gap in health promotion.* Retrieved from http://www.iuhpeconference.net/downloads/en/Thematisches/0910_WHO_Conference_Health_Promotion.pdf

Canadian Institute for Health Information. (2011). Increased activity and healthier eating can improve obesity rates, but aren't the only factors at play. Retrieved from http://www.cihi.ca/CIHI-ext-portal/internet/en/Document/factors+influencing+health/RELEASE_20JUNE11

Canadian Nurses Association. (2011). *Harm reduction and currently illegal drugs: Implications for nursing policy, practice, education and research: Discussion paper.* Ottawa, ON: Author.

Clement, C. (2005). *Health goals: Coming soon to a Canada near you.* Ontario Prevention Clearinghouse. OHPE Bulletin 408, 2005 (408). Retrieved from http://www.ohpe.ca/node/284

Community Health Nurses of Canada. (2003, revised 2011). *Canadian community health nursing: Professional practice model and standards of practice.* Retrieved from http://www.chnc.ca/documents/CHNC-ProfessionalPracticeModel-EN/index.html

Epp, J. (1986). *Achieving health for all: A framework for health promotion.* Ottawa, ON: Health and Welfare Canada.

Federal, Provincial, and Territorial Advisory Committee on Population Health. (1994). *Toward a healthy future: Second report on the health of Canadians.* Ottawa, ON: Minister of Public Works and Government Services Canada.

Hamilton, N., & Bhatti, T. (1996). *Population health promotion: An integrated model of population health and health promotion.* Ottawa, ON: Health Canada, Health Promotion and Development Division.

Handcock, T. (2011). Health promotion in Canada: 25 years of unfulfilled promise. *Health Promotion International, 26*(S2), doi:10.1093/heapro/dar061

Health Canada. (2005). *Health protection and promotion.* Retrieved from http://www.hc-sc.gc.ca/sr-sr/activ/protection/index_e.html

Health Goals for Canada. (2011). *Health goals for Canada: A federal, provincial and territorial commitment to Canadians. October 2005.* Retrieved from http://www.phac-aspc.gc.ca/hgc-osc/new-1-eng.html

Labonte, R. (1992). *Determinants of health: Empowering strategies for nursing practice.* Vancouver, BC: Registered Nurses Association of British Columbia.

Lalonde, M. (1974). *A new perspective on the health of Canadians.* Ottawa, ON: Government of Canada.

Leave the Pack Behind. (2011). *LTPB final report: Working together to achieve smoke-free campuses, 2011–2012.* Retrieved from http://www.leavethepackbehind.org/pdf/11-12%20LTPB%20Final%20Activity%20Report_final.pdf

Leavell, H. R., & Clark, E. G. (1965). *Preventive medicine for the doctor in the community* (3rd ed.). New York, NY: McGraw-Hill.

Pender, N. J., Murdaugh, C. L., & Parsons, M. A. (2011). *Health promotion in nursing practice* (6th ed.). Upper Saddle River, NJ: Prentice Hall.

Prochaska, J. O., Redding, C. A., & Evers, K. E. (2009). The transtheoretical model and stages of change. In K. Glanz, B. K. Rimer, & F. M. Lewis (Eds.), *Health behavior and health education: Theory, research, and practice* (4th ed., pp. 97–121). San Francisco, CA: Jossey-Bass.

Public Health Agency of Canada. (2010). *A population health approach: The organizing framework.* The Canadian Best Practices Portal. Retrieved from http://66.240.150.14/population_health/index-eng.html

Raeburn J., & Rootman, I. (1998). *People-centered health promotion.* Chichester, UK: John Wiley & Sons.

Raphael, D., Bryant, T., & Curry-Stevens, A. (2004). Toronto charter outlines future health policy directions for Canada and elsewhere. *Health Promotion International, 19*(2), 269–273.

Rootman, I., Dupéré, S., Penderson, A., & O'Neill, M. (2012). *Health promotion in Canada: Critical perspective on practice* (3rd ed.). Toronto, ON: Canadian Scholars Press.

Stamler, L., & Yiu, L. (2012). *Community health nursing: A Canadian perspective* (3rd ed.). Toronto, ON: Pearson Canada.

World Health Organization. (1978). *The declaration of Alma-Ata.* Geneva, Switzerland: Author.

World Health Organization. (1984). *Health promotion: A discussion document on the concepts and principles.* Copenhagen, Denmark: WHO Regional Office for Europe.

World Health Organization. (1997). *The Jakarta declaration on health promotion.* Geneva, Switzerland: Author.

World Health Organization. (1998). *Health promotion glossary.* Geneva, Switzerland: Author. Retrieved from http://www.who.int/hpr/NPH/docs/hp_glossary_en.pdf

World Health Organization, Health and Welfare Canada, & Canadian Public Health Association. (1986). *Ottawa Charter for Health Promotion.* Geneva, Switzerland: WHO.

Chapter 9

The Canadian Health Care System

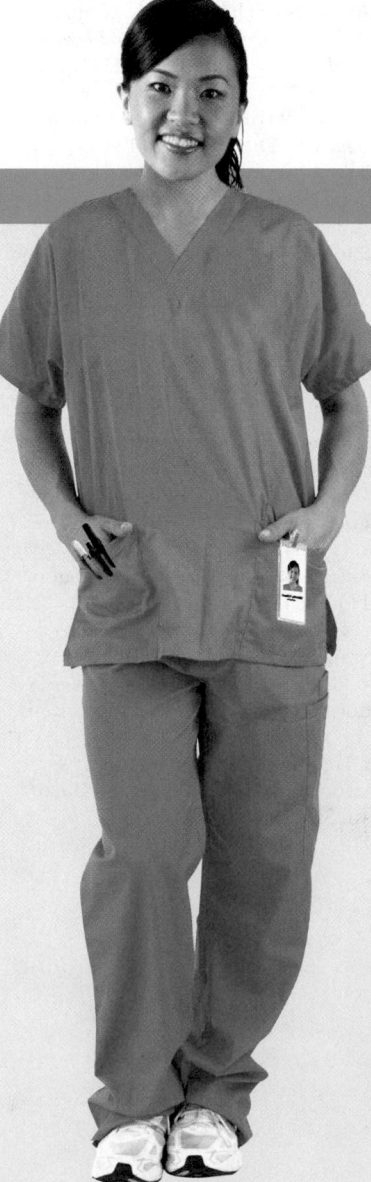

After studying this chapter, you will be able to:

1. Outline the history of the Canadian health care system as a major component of Canada's social safety network.

2. Describe the five criteria or principles of the Canada Health Act (1984).

3. List the four essential elements of the patient's Bill of Rights and the social values underpinning both it and a universal publicly funded health care system.

4. Define the impact and value of urgency-of-need determinations for gaining access to health care services.

5. Describe the functions and purposes of the health care sectors outlined in this chapter.

6. Differentiate primary, secondary, tertiary, and quaternary health care services.

7. Report on the social, political, technological, and other main factors that impact health care delivery and that influence health care system reform.

8. Identify the complementary but distinct roles and functions of other health care professionals and para-professionals, and the significance of interdisciplinary health care teams.

9. Describe contemporary models of nursing care.

10. Outline the contributions of nurse practitioners, nurse managers, nurse researchers, and nursing sociopolitical action for engendering beneficial health care and health care system changes.

A **health care system** is the sum of health care services provided by all individuals and organizations that aim to meet the health care needs of target populations. In Canada, the health care system is a major contributor to the well-being of its citizens and Canada as a whole. Although other comparisons can be made, the Canadian health care system is often used to define Canada against other countries where health care is neither as advanced nor as accessible to their citizens. Even though health care in Canada is normally considered an essential public service, it is also "big business." It is a major source of direct and indirect employment and a major component of government spending, as Canada's large health care system is primarily publicly funded. Traditionally, this health care system is expected to provide care for acutely ill and injured persons. However, health promotion, illness prevention, wellness initiatives, and technological advancements that permit earlier detection of and intervention for health problems, as well as many other developments, including an increase in chronic or incurable illnesses and an aging population, are changing the health care system. The roles of nurses are also changing in response to changes in health care, the health care system, and population health and because nurses have formulated and implemented beneficial nursing, health care, and health care system reforms.

History

Canada's large system of health care services did not emerge suddenly or without precedent. The British North America Act (1867) established Canada as a country and laid out the respective jurisdictions of the federal and provincial governments. Responsibility for health, education, and social services was delegated to the provinces. As Canada grew through immigration, high birthrates, and industrialization, the population became urbanized. Poor housing and sanitation, crowded living conditions, poverty, and a volatile economy contributed to the already high rates of morbidity and mortality. In response to this, public health legislation was enacted to deal with infectious diseases, maternal and child health, workplace safety, and environmental sanitation. Churches and charities continued to provide hospital care (as they did before Confederation), and voluntary organizations emerged. Some of these organizations continue to serve the Canadian public today (e.g., Victorian Order of Nurses, Children's Aid Societies, Canadian Mental Health Association). Municipal governments also became involved, often to assist those who were poverty stricken or ill. The union movement and fraternal brotherhoods established benevolent funds, which members contributed to and could access in the event they were unable to work. These funds were the precursors to today's employment insurance program and workers' compensation.

The two World Wars (1914–1918 and 1939–1945) were instrumental in highlighting the importance of a social safety network. Many injured soldiers returned with permanent disabilities, needing health care and other assistance. These wars also created a demand for services by the soldiers' widows, children, and parents, all of whom had lost their main source of support. Rural municipalities were given power by the Government of Canada to levy taxes to pay for local physician services (through the Municipality Act, 1916) and then hospital services (through the Municipal Medical and Hospital Services Act, 1939). In 1927, the federal government implemented a cost-sharing pension program for older persons in need. The Family Allowance Act (1945), however, was the first universal social program in Canada. It provided every Canadian family with a stipend for each child regardless of family income. Other universal programs that formed the Canadian social safety network include Old Age Security (through the Old Age Security Act, 1952, 1975) and the Canada Pension Plan (which came into force in 1966). Today, a comprehensive range of programs are in place, although many are no longer universal. The Canadian health care system is one exception. It was designed as a universal program through the federal Hospital Insurance and Diagnostic Services Act (1957), which brought uniform coverage for these services across Canada, with the 1966 Medical Care Act extending this coverage to include physician services. In 1984, the Canada Health Act was passed, in large part to assure universal health care accessibility for all citizens through outlawing extra-billing and other co-payments or user charges for insured health care services. Each province and territory today has a health care insurance plan that continues to be governed by the Canada Health Act (1984). This Act provides for federal cost sharing, whereby the Government of Canada pays a proportion of the provincial or territorial costs of provided health care, on the condition that five criteria are met: **public administration**, **comprehensiveness**, **universality**, **portability**, and **accessibility** (Table 9.1).

Even though Canada's social safety network was developed to meet the needs of individuals requiring assistance and to address societal values of compassion and equity, many social, economic, and other developments, including rising costs and demands for services, have challenged each program. In response to these developments, the provinces and territories have been restructuring their programs, including their health care systems, although much of this redevelopment has been done to accommodate evidence-based practice and technological developments, allowing health care to be delivered in new ways with better outcomes. For instance, surgical and diagnostic developments have resulted in most people receiving ambulatory care in day surgery or outpatient clinics, when only a few short years ago, they would have been admitted to hospital for a few days or even weeks. Over 90% of all surgeries now are done in day surgery clinics and well over 90% of all diagnostic

TABLE 9.1 Canada Health Act

1. **Public administration**	The public administration criterion applies to provincial and territorial health care insurance plans. The act specifically states that to satisfy the criterion respecting public administration, the health care insurance plan of each province or territory "must be administered and operated on a non-profit basis by a public authority appointed or designated by the government of the province; the public authority must be responsible to the provincial government for that administration and operation; and the public authority must be subject to audit of its accounts and financial transactions by such authority as is charged by law with the audit of the accounts of the province."
2. **Comprehensiveness**	The comprehensiveness criterion requires that to be eligible for federal cash transfer payments, the health care insurance plan of each province or territory "must insure all insured health services provided by hospitals, medical practitioners or dentists (i.e., such as in the case of surgical-dental services that require a hospital setting) and, where the law of the province so permits, similar or additional services rendered by other health care practitioners."
3. **Universality**	Under the universality criterion, "the health care insurance plan of a province must entitle one hundred percent of the insured persons of the province to the insured health services provided for by the plan on uniform terms and conditions."
4. **Portability**	To satisfy the criterion of portability, "the health care insurance plan of a province must not impose any minimum period of residence in the province, or waiting period, in excess of three months before residents of the province are eligible for or entitled to insured health services; must provide for and be administered and operated so as to provide for the payment of amounts for the cost of insured health services provided to insured persons while temporarily absent from the province on the basis that (i) where the insured services are provided in Canada, payment of health services is at the rate that is approved by the health care insurance plan of the province in which the services are provided, unless the provinces concerned agree to apportion the cost between them in a different manner, or (ii) where the insured health services are provided out of Canada, payment is made on the basis of the amount that would have been paid by the province for similar services rendered in the province, with due regard, in the case of hospital services, to the size of the hospital, standards of service and other relevant factors; and must provide for and be administered and operated so as to provide for the payment, during any minimum period of residence, or any waiting period, imposed by the health care insurance plan of another province, of the cost of insured health services provided to persons who have ceased to be insured persons by reason of having become residents of that other province, on the same basis as though they had not ceased to be residents of the province."
5. **Accessibility**	The intent of the accessibility criterion is to ensure that residents of a province or territory have reasonable access to insured hospital, medical, and surgical–dental services on uniform terms and conditions, unprecluded or unimpeded, either directly or indirectly, by charges (user charges or extra-billing) or other means (e.g., discrimination on the basis of age, health status, or financial circumstances). In addition, the health care insurance plans of the province or territory must provide reasonable compensation to physicians and dentists for all the insured health care services they provide; and payment to hospitals to cover the cost of insured health care services.

Note: Since 1984, slight changes through reinterpretation of the act have occurred. These changes and health care system changes are outlined each year in Health Canada's Canada Health Act Annual Report.

Source: © Adapted and reproduced with the permission of the Minister of Public Works and Government Services Canada, 2003. Health Canada assumes no responsibility for any errors or omissions which may have occurred in the adaptation of its material. Canada Health Act available at http://laws-lois.justice.gc.ca/eng/acts/C-6

tests are done on an ambulatory or outpatient basis. More accurate diagnostic tests and new medicines are also reducing the need for surgery, and complication rates and recovery times are much better with the newer laparoscopic and laser surgery methods. Another major development factor has been changing views of health, with 12 determinants of health considered highly important for preventing illnesses and injuries, and maintaining or improving health. Intersectoral collaboration, strategic long-range planning, and public participation are strategies being used to create more equitable distribution of scarce and costly resources and services. Efforts are being made to curb costs and make more effective use of health care personnel and infrastructure through such initiatives as regionalization, integration, and the continued shift of what was hospital-based care to families and community agencies, such as extended care facilities, hospices, and seniors' daycare centres.

Increasingly, Canadians are paying out of pocket or contributing to supplementary insurance plans that cover uninsured or extra health care services such as physiotherapy; prescription drugs and home care supplies; vision, hearing, and dental care; care in assisted-living facilities; and complementary or alternative therapies. These costs can be considerable, with low-income Canadians disproportionately disadvantaged by this shift from public funding to private funding. The corresponding shift from public control and public delivery of services to private for-profit and private not-for-profit providers affects all Canadians.

Rights and Health Care

Although health care is widely considered a right by citizens of Canada, an important patients' rights, or **clients' rights** (which includes patients and residents), movement began in the late 1960s. Its broad goal was to improve the quality of health care, largely by making the health care system and health care professionals more aware of and responsive to client needs and interests. At that time, individuals wanted self-determination and control over their own bodies when ill. Informed consent, confidentiality of information, and the right of the patient to accept or refuse treatment are all accepted and influential aspects of self-determination now. The need for concern about rights continues, however, because of their vulnerability and the ongoing uncertainty, coupled with differing judgments, over the expected or probable outcomes of health care. More recently, timely access to health care has become a clients' rights concern. Although legal opinions have indicated that Canadians do not actually have a "right" to health care, Section 7 of the 1982 Canadian Charter of Rights and Freedoms could be interpreted as outlining the rights or entitlements of persons waiting for health care. At the heart of clients'

rights is the need for clients and care providers to respect each other. Although nurses have the Canadian Nurses Association (CNA, 2008) *Code of Ethics* mandating and supporting their respect for clients, many governments across Canada are developing legislation or policy documents to demonstrate that their citizens should be able to expect timely access to health care and other assurances, such as to safe high-quality health care.

Although many comparisons reveal Canada has a top performing health care system, Canada's performance in relation to rights and information for clients, patients, and residents has been judged as below that of many European countries (Eisen & Bjornberg, 2010). When people are ill, they are frequently unable to assert their rights as they would if they were healthy. Asserting rights requires energy, mental competency, knowledge about their health problem and care options, an underlying awareness of their rights in the situation, and organizational support for them to exercise their rights. In 1972 (revised in 1989), the Consumers' Association of Canada published the *Consumer Rights to Health Care.* Their current 2011 version are outlined in Table 9.2. The consumer movement was also important for helping initiate legislation on advance directives. All adults in Canada now have the legislated right to make a statement about their care preferences, such as through a living will or a personal directive, preferences that should be adhered to by all health care organizations and health care professionals, if permitted by law. Client requests for assisted suicide and other illegal or criminal acts, however, cannot be carried out.

It is widely understood now that adults have the right to verbally or in writing refuse treatment, even when it is life saving; the right to review their health care records and have them explained; the right to receive publicly funded health care when it is appropriate for them; and the right to be informed of any business or other arrangements among institutions or people involved in their care. In addition, they have the right to be informed of resources that can be used to resolve a dispute or grievance and of health care agency policies and practices that relate to their care, treatment, and responsibilities, including any extra charges or out-of-pocket costs associated with these care options. Furthermore, they have the

TABLE 9.2 Consumer Rights

- The right to choice
- The right to be informed
- The right to safety
- The right to be heard
- The right to amends
- The right to participate in marketplace decision making
- The right to basic services
- The right to a sustainable environment

Source: Consumers' Association of Canada. (2011). *Consumer rights.* Retrieved from http://www.consumer.ca/1625

right to have options explained when hospital care is no longer appropriate and to expect a reasonable continuity of care both within and across health care settings when moved. Clients can also refuse to participate in research studies.

Nurses and other health care professionals are also obliged to advise patients of their rights to make informed choices about their health and health care. Every patient or resident should be asked about advance directives (i.e., such instructions as DNR [Do Not Resuscitate] in the event of a cardiac or respiratory arrest), and this information must be placed on their health care record. Details about advance directives are provided in Chapter 49.

If a person lacks decision-making capacity, such as in the case of being a minor, very ill, and temporarily or permanently mentally incompetent, his or her rights can be exercised by a designated surrogate or proxy decision maker. Nurses are often advocates for clients in these and other situations. Nursing organizations, such as the Canadian Nurses Association (CNA), have also been advocates for the rights of individuals and for the good of Canadian society through lobbying governments and through the development of documents to unite nurses and influence public policy, such as their 2009 *Position Statement: Financing Canada's Health System.*

Categories of Health Care

Health care services are commonly categorized according to type and level. In Canada, health care services are also categorized on the basis of urgency of need.

Types of Health Care

Four types of health care services are often described: (a) health promotion and illness prevention, (b) diagnosis and treatment, (c) rehabilitation and health restoration, and (d) hospice–palliative, or end-of-life, care. These types can be linked to the levels of prevention discussed in Chapter 7.

HEALTH PROMOTION AND ILLNESS PREVENTION In 1979, one of the most influential organizations globally, the World Health Organization (WHO), "reaffirmed that health is a basic human right and a worldwide social goal; that it is essential to the satisfaction of basic human needs and the quality of life; and that it is to be attained by all people," and emphasized their 1977 resolution that the main target of governments and the WHO should be "the attainment by all citizens of the world by the year 2000 of a level of health that will permit them to lead a socially and economically productive life" (WHO, 1979, p. 7). The overall goal then and in subsequent WHO (1981) documents was to ensure health for all individuals globally in part by increased access to and distribution of health care

services. This goal was developed and has been maintained in keeping with a series of Canadian documents that emphasize health and wellness, as opposed to illness care. These documents illustrate Canadian interest in and awareness of the importance of health promotion; including Marc Lalonde's (1974) *A New Perspective on the Health of Canadians*, the *Ottawa Charter for Health Promotion* (World Health Organization, Health and Welfare Canada, & Canadian Public Health Association, 1986), and Jake Epp's (1986) *Achieving Health for All: A Framework for Health Promotion* (see Chapter 8 for additional discussion on health promotion).

Since the 1980s, more and more individual Canadians and Canadian groups have been recognizing the advantages of staying healthy and avoiding illness. Health-promotion programs address determinants of health, such as physical, psychological, and social environments. Activities for **health promotion** emphasize the important role that clients have in actively maintaining or improving their own health. Health care services are increasingly emphasizing health promotion, such as in public health clinics, where community health nurses offer a wide range of health-promotion programs; home care programs, where nurses work to maintain or improve the health of older and younger persons who have disabilities and are at risk; and primary care clinics or primary care networks, where interdisciplinary health care teams emphasize health promotion.

The health care system similarly offers programs for **illness and injury prevention**. These may be directed at the client or the community and involve such practices as providing immunizations, identifying risk factors for illnesses and injuries (e.g., dietary habits or blood lipid levels for cardiovascular disease), and helping people take measures to prevent both acute and chronic health problems. Illness prevention also includes programs to reduce the incidence of illness, injury, or disability, such as through mandating helmets for children riding bicycles. Environmental protective measures are often legislated by governments after they have been lobbied by citizens' or health care provider groups (for a discussion on further issues of safety, see Chapter 32).

DIAGNOSIS AND TREATMENT Traditionally, the greatest emphasis of Canada's health care system has been on the **diagnosis** and **treatment** of illnesses and injuries. Physicians' offices and hospitals, on an inpatient or, increasingly, an ambulatory basis, are the major settings for these services. However, community-based organizations are increasingly providing these services. For example, community health centres provide a wide range of services for clients with chronic illnesses (e.g., diabetes mellitus or schizophrenia). Limited diagnostic technology may be available in these places, but referrals are made for laboratory or diagnostic imaging services elsewhere. Some shopping malls and high-density commercial or residential areas have walk-in clinics that provide a wide range of services, usually without appointment.

REHABILITATION AND HEALTH RESTORATION

Rehabilitation and **health restoration** involve a process of restoring people with illnesses and injuries to more optimal levels of health and functioning. Rehabilitative care emphasizes the importance of assisting clients to function adequately in the physical, cognitive, social, and perhaps vocational areas of their lives. The goal of rehabilitation is to help people return to their previous level of health and self-care capabilities or to the highest level they are capable of given their current health status. Often, the aim is for the person to become independent, although this aim is impossible for some. If the person is hospitalized, rehabilitation will begin in the hospital and may continue in a subacute care unit, rehabilitative hospital, or nursing home. Increasingly, with hospital stays that typically last less than 7 days and the majority of surgeries and other treatments done on an ambulatory basis, rehabilitation is taking place at home. Rehabilitation can occur through such simple means as having the client resume self-care activities, but some clients will need extensive rehabilitative treatment, such as occupational therapy and ongoing physiotherapy.

HOSPICE–PALLIATIVE AND END-OF-LIFE CARE The term **hospice–palliative care** refers to the provision of compassionate care to the dying (see Chapter 49). Some nurses and other professionals specialize in hospice–palliative care, with this care often limited to persons experiencing difficult dying processes, typically younger people with incurable cancers. Nurses who specialize in hospice–palliative care may become credentialed; these specialists are recognized as having advanced competencies in hospice–palliative care nursing through the CNA designation of CHPCN(C): Certified in Hospice and Palliative Care Nursing (Canada).

Currently, fewer than 30% of decedents in Canada received specialized hospice–palliative care services in hospital palliative care units or other places following a referral for specialist palliative care. The remaining decedents typically would have received some assistance while terminally ill from nurses and others who are not hospice–palliative care specialists. Increasingly, family members are providing **end-of-life care** in the home, with some receiving assistance from home care nurses. Some dying processes, however, such as those associated with a long decline in health through advanced aging and/or serious progressive chronic illnesses, require much more support in a free-standing hospice or extended care facility (i.e., a nursing home or long-term care facility). Nurses are a major provider of both specialized hospice–palliative care and basic end-of-life care as they help dying people and family members in all care settings.

Levels of Health Care

Health care services can also be categorized according to the complexity or level of the services provided: primary, secondary, tertiary, or quaternary. Table 9.3 outlines the

TABLE 9.3 Levels of Health Care Classified According to Increasing Complexity

Primary care (first point of contact)	Health promotion
	Preventive care
	  (e.g., immunizations,
	  prenatal or well-baby clinics)
	Health education
	Environmental protection and
	  risk assessment
	Early detection and treatment
	  (e.g., physician office nursing
	  and telehealth nursing)
	Long-term care
	Emergency room care

Secondary care (care from specialist following referral)	Diagnosis and treatment (complex)

Tertiary (settings of highly specialized skills, technology, supports)	Acute care
	Care of the dying in hospital
	  palliative care units or
	  hospices
	Rehabilitation

Quaternary (centres of highly specialized care)	Transplantation perioperative and postsurgical nursing

levels of care and the kinds of services that may be provided by nurses at these levels. Services provided within one level of care can often be coordinated and implemented in many different health care settings besides hospitals. Nurses have a key role in health-promotion activities and in providing health care, whether in the hospital or the community. Planning for nursing services in an institution or community must be approached with the four levels of care in mind.

Categories of Need for Health Care

Although all Canadians can access the health care system if they require any of the many insured services available, an assessment of their urgency of need for health care is the major defining criterion in Canada affecting the speed at which health care is provided. Physicians and nurse practitioners, as well as triage nurses in emergency departments, are charged with the responsibility of determining how urgent each presenting person's need for health care is. Different systems of classifying the nature of illnesses exist, but most are oriented to identifying whether the person has one of three categories of need:

1. *Urgent:* An urgent health problem is one that requires immediate treatment to save a life or prevent serious complications, such as in cases of myocardial infarction (heart attack) or a cardiovascular accident (stroke).

2. *Emergent:* An emergent health problem is one where diagnostic and often treatment services are required in the next few days or weeks, such as when there is a possibility of cancer or any other condition that could become serious in the near future.

3. *Elective:* An elective or nonurgent health problem is one that will progress slowly, if at all, or may resolve without health care intervention. Knee and hip replacements for arthritic joints are common elective procedures. It normally takes many years for arthritis to progress to a state where a joint replacement requiring major surgery is indicated. Waiting for this surgery for a few weeks is not normally a health hazard, as the disease continues to progress slowly, if at all. In addition, waiting for this surgery allows time for the person to make living or other arrangements, as their postoperative recovery will be many weeks or months in length. A high proportion, as many as 50%, of all persons who are booked for elective surgeries and elective diagnostic tests do not choose to have these procedures performed. Unfortunately, many of these people do not call to cancel their booked appointments, leaving gaps in operating room and diagnostic imaging schedules, unless someone else can quickly fill in.

This determination of need, a resource-allocation and planning process, although difficult to understand for clients who want to have their health problem immediately diagnosed and addressed, is important for ensuring health care system efficiency and for containing health care costs. People who have emergent and elective health care needs have their names added to a wait list, with their urgency of need clearly listed. These people have booked tests or treatments, compared with over half of all hospital inpatients who are admitted through the emergency department. People who have urgent health problems are sent directly to the emergency department, diagnostic imaging clinic, or operating room, with arrangements being made while they are in transit for immediate care.

One example of a system for classifying the severity of illnesses is the Canadian Triage and Acuity Scale, widely used across Canada to ensure people of all ages receive health care that is appropriate to their needs (Warren, Jarvis, LeBlanc, Gravel, & the CTAS National Working Group, 2008). At times, this scale is used to illustrate the inappropriate use of emergency departments. For example, the Canadian Institute for Health Information (CIHI, 2005) reported that more than one-half of all visits to Canadian emergency rooms in 2004 were for health problems of a nonurgent nature, with almost 20% of adults indicating they could have received treatment for their condition at a physician's office.

Wait lists have been a longstanding method in Canada of ensuring appropriate access to health care and the effective use of expensive and sometimes scarce health care resources, which typically is the newest diagnostic machinery. Although quality of life may be influenced while waiting for emergent or elective diagnostic tests, surgery, or other treatments, the health of the individual is not normally impacted. However, considerable concern over waiting too long for health care has arisen in recent years. This concern is valid when the health of an individual is negatively impacted by the wait. For instance, if the delay is too long in obtaining a joint replacement and the affected person develops a secondary health problem because of that delay, such as depression or a bed sore, then the wait clearly was too long. A growing number of research investigations and other attempts at tracking wait times and identifying appropriate waits for select health care services have been conducted. This work is ongoing, with many different approaches in use now to reduce wait times for health care. The 2003 First Ministers' Accord on Health Care Renewal and their subsequent 10-year plan in 2004 to improve health care have had some impact across Canada in reducing wait lists and wait times (Health Canada, 2006a, 2006b). A recent CIHI (2011) report revealed that 8 of every 10 patients across Canada received care within benchmarked timelines.

Despite wait lists, the vast majority of Canadians needing health care get same-day service, as they can call a telehealth line to talk to a nurse for health care advice or see a health care provider in a physician's or nurse practitioner's office, medi-clinic, community care centre, primary care clinic, or hospital emergency department. Blood work and x-rays or other common diagnostic tests will often be done that same day. Furthermore, same-day service is provided if the health problem is urgent and also, in many cases, when it is emergent.

Types of Health Care Organizations and Care Settings

In Canada, health care organizations are numerous and care settings varied. Some organizations provide many services; for example, a hospital provides a wide range of inpatient and outpatient or ambulatory care services, including emergency room services. Some of these services can also be obtained through community-based agencies. For example, specialized hospice–palliative care can be provided in a hospital, the home, or another community setting, such as a hospice or long-term care facility. The **continuum of care** refers to care given in a variety of settings from the onset of the health challenge to the point where the recipient no longer requires care.

A client can be categorized as either an inpatient or an outpatient. An *inpatient* is admitted to hospital and is expected to remain for 1 or more days of care. With technological and other advances, most hospital stays now are shorter than 7 days. A client who is an *outpatient* similarly requires health care but does not stay more than a few hours in the hospital or clinic. The majority of diagnostic tests and treatments, including around 90% of surgical procedures, are done on an outpatient basis now. Although this shift to ambulatory care has greatly increased the efficiency of the health care system, this shift has major implications for clients and their families. For instance, a person can become ill, undergo a number of diagnostic tests that diagnose a type and stage of cancer, have ongoing blood work and other cancer clinic examinations, receive monthly chemotherapy treatments, and then have 2 weeks of daily radiation for palliative pain reduction and never once be a hospital inpatient. Traditional nursing roles and responsibilities have changed and are continuing to change in response to this considerable shift of client care out of inpatient hospital beds.

Clients, particularly those with severe or chronic and incurable health conditions requiring various forms of care over an extended time, often receive their care through a number of health care organizations. This care and the location of this care will depend on the care needs, availability of family or friends to assist them, number and type of services or care agencies within their community, supplementary insurance coverage, and many other potential factors. To address the health and health care needs of an entire population, a wide range of health care organizations have developed in Canada.

Public Health

Public health, a subset of community health, includes services that focus on promoting health and preventing illness. Depending on the needs of people in the immediate or larger community, public health offices may offer immunization programs; well-baby clinics and prenatal health programs; cancer screening and screening for other conditions, such as communicable and genetic diseases; education and support for persons living with chronic mental or physical illnesses; school health education programs to prevent teenage pregnancy and other common age-based health issues, such as sports injuries; alcohol, drug, and gambling addiction detection and abuse services; water and air testing services; restaurant inspections; and so on. In some areas, the local public health office is also the site where people can request home care services for people who need assistance in the home and where home care employees report to work.

Public health services are provided through government departments established at the local, regional (in provinces with regionalization), provincial or territorial, and federal levels. Although their aims have considerable similarity, the health programs and services at the federal, provincial or territorial, regional, and local rural or urban levels vary according to the public health needs of the people over whom they have jurisdiction.

At the federal level, Health Canada (2011) is responsible for "helping Canadians maintain and improve their health, while respecting individual choices and circumstances," with the goal "for Canada to be among the countries with the healthiest people in the world." Public health is a primary focus of its various branches and agencies. Health Canada is also charged with providing health care services directly to First Nations and Inuit peoples. The federal government also administers a number of veterans' health services in Canada and has other departments that directly or indirectly support the health and well-being of Canadians.

In 2004, the increasingly influential Public Health Agency of Canada (PHAC) was created by the federal government with the goal to "strengthen Canada's capacity to protect and improve the health of Canadians and to help reduce pressures on the health care system" (PHAC, 2011). This agency is expected to promote health, prevent and control chronic diseases and injuries, prevent and control infectious diseases, prepare for and respond to public health emergencies, and strength public health capacity through focusing on the determinants of health and common factors that maintain or reduce health (PHAC, 2011). It is responsible for the Centre for Immunization and Respiratory Infectious Diseases, the Centre for Communicable Diseases and Infection Control, the Centre for Emergency Preparedness and Response, the National Microbiology Laboratory, and the Centre for Food-borne, Environmental, and Zoonotic Infectious Diseases.

The federal minister of health is also responsible for the Canadian Institutes of Health Research (2007), Canada's major agency for funding and directing health research. Thirteen institutes are charged with fostering needed research. One of these is the Institute of Population and Public Health. The research that is conducted through this institute is commonly oriented to health promotion and illness prevention. Nurses are often principal investigators and research team members, as well as institute board members and members of the scientific teams that judge the quality and importance of the many research proposals that are submitted in competition for funding. Much intergovernmental communication and program coordination occurs among Health Canada, the Public Health Agency of Canada, and provincial or territorial health departments. Contact is at the political or top level through the elected and appointed federal and provincial or territorial ministers of health and chief public health officer as well as at the front lines through the ongoing work of the many nurses and other personnel hired to support their organization's mandate.

Provincial and territorial health departments are as broadly oriented as the federal health department is to public health and thus to supporting both health and wellness through health promotion and effective health care, although their mandates are confined to policies and programs or services on a provincial or territorial basis. Although all provinces and territories have similar public health and other health care services, some differences exist. Some provinces, for instance, have established agencies specifically for drug, alcohol, and gambling abuse.

Regional health departments and local agencies traditionally have responsibility for developing programs and providing the services that meet the health needs of people living in or travelling through a defined geographical area, by providing the necessary staff and facilities to carry out these programs, continually evaluating the need for and effectiveness of their programs, and monitoring changing health needs. Client and service utilization information collected at this level is crucial for provincial or territorial and federal monitoring of public health and the efficacy of services.

Nurses work at all levels of public health service, as direct care providers, care coordinators, department or office managers, and policymakers. Nurses who are certified in community health nursing have met specific eligibility requirements, passed a written examination, and met a national standard of competency in community health nursing. In Canada, expertise in this specialty is recognized with the initials CCHN(C)—Certified in Community Health Nursing (Canada)—granted by the CNA. (See Chapters 1 and 2 for more information on certification and competency, and Chapter 14 for more information on public health nursing.)

Home Care

Home care services are provided to people outside hospitals and long-term care facilities who need temporary or permanent assistance with health care needs, such as complex dressing changes, or with activities of daily living, such as bathing. Home care is traditionally provided to seniors and younger persons with disabilities. Earlier discharge of clients from hospital has made home care an important aspect of the health care delivery system. The home is now a common health care delivery site, with expectations that care at this site will increase. In addition, the scope of services offered in the home has broadened. Home care organizations now provide a wide range of education and comprehensive care to clients with acute, chronic, and terminal illnesses. Nurses and nursing aides or assistants are the most common home care employees (Wilson, Birch, Cohen, MacLeod, Mohankumar, & Williams, 2011). See Chapter 14.

Community Health Centres and Primary Care Clinics

Community health centres or primary care clinics are found in many Canadian communities. Most of these ambulatory care centres have a wide range of health-promotion,

diagnostic, and treatment services. These facilities normally provide medical, nursing, nutrition, social work, and basic laboratory and radiological services. Some provide services to people who require minor surgical procedures that can be performed outside hospitals. These centres offer three main advantages: (a) They are more accessible to clients and thus help them obtain necessary and timely health care; (b) they are more holistic in their approach to health and illness, as they typically focus on more than just the single presenting health problem and symptoms; and (c) they free up costly and scarce hospital services for clients who are more seriously ill. Nurses working here may have basic or advanced education. Nurse practitioners and clinical nurse specialists are often needed for their specialized knowledge and skills.

Physician Offices

In Canada, the family physician's office was the traditional setting where first contact between clients and the health care system occurred. Although the majority of family and specialist physicians have their own offices or work with several other physicians in a group practice, the trend now is toward community health centres and primary care clinics in which physicians work with an interdisciplinary team comprising nurse practitioners, nurses, and other health care or social service professionals. Community health centres and primary care clinics are expected to provide a holistic range of health services, compared with the more limited set of medical services that are provided by physicians in their offices, usually in keeping with the fee-for-service schedule of payments that is negotiated by medical groups with their provincial or territorial health departments.

Clients most often go to physician offices for illness diagnosis and treatment, and for routine health monitoring and ongoing chronic illness management. Medication prescriptions, either new or refills, are a common outcome of visits to physician offices, along with referrals for laboratory and other diagnostic tests, and referrals to medical or other specialists. An increasing criticism of physician offices is that they are reactive to health problems and do not address the broader aim of health care, which is to prevent illnesses through improving health and through better management of health problems to prevent acute episodes of illness and chronic disease progression.

Nurses employed in physician offices have many roles and responsibilities. Some nurses carry out traditional functions, including client registration, preparing clients for examination, obtaining information, and providing information to clients and other persons or organizations. Other functions may include obtaining specimens, assisting with procedures, and providing some treatments. Nurse practitioners and clinical nurse specialists may be employed to provide primary care to clients in stable health or to those in unstable health. Nurse practitioners diagnose health conditions that require intervention, plan and provide this intervention or make referrals to other professionals (CNA, 2002), and typically prescribe medications. Nurse practitioners and clinical nurse specialists (although their scope of practice is more limited) are expected to have a holistic and wellness orientation to their care.

Nurse Practitioner Offices

Nurse practitioner offices are opening in Canada as places for first contact between clients and the health care system (NP-led clinics, 2010). As in physician offices, a wide range of diagnostic and treatment services are normally offered. Health promotion is a key difference, as nurse practitioners focus on wellness. Some nurse practitioners specialize, such as those who offer health promotion and other services to seniors. These offices tend to be situated in regions where health care needs are not being met, such as in areas with sparse populations and chronic shortages of family physicians.

Specialist Clinics

The term *specialist clinic* refers to a health care organization that is managed by physicians, nurses, or physiotherapists, with these situated either in a hospital or community setting. Most provide a distinct or specialized set of health services, such as physiotherapy, breast-feeding support, midwifery, or diabetes mellitus education and ongoing care. If based in a hospital, these clinics are also called *outpatient or ambulatory care clinics,* normally serving people not currently admitted to hospital as inpatients. Nurses in these clinics have a wide range of functions, in keeping with their education and their specific level of needed skills and knowledge.

Occupational Health Clinics

The occupational health clinic or office is gaining importance as a common setting for employee health care. Employee health has long been recognized as significant to workplace productivity. Today, more companies encourage workplace wellness by providing on-site exercise facilities and through the coordination or provision of a wide range of health-promotion activities.

Community nurses in occupational health settings have a variety of roles. Worker safety has been a traditional concern of occupational health nurses. Today, nursing functions in occupational health may include work safety and health education; immunizations; and pre-employment and annual employee health screening for tuberculosis, hearing loss, and vision or eye problems.

Other functions may include screening for health problems, such as hypertension and obesity; assessing disability and readiness to return to work; providing workplace discord counselling and crisis intervention; and planning preretirement or retirement programs. Managers are realizing that occupational health clinics can be a significant factor in staff attraction and retention.

In Canada, occupational health nurses are typically registered nurses. They may also have a certificate, diploma, or degree in occupational health and safety from a college or university. Nurses certified in occupational health nursing have met specific eligibility requirements, passed a written examination, and met a national standard of competency in occupational health. In Canada, expertise unique to this specialty is recognized with the initials COHN(C)—Certified in Occupational Health Nursing (Canada)—granted by the CNA. (See Chapters 1 and 2 for more information on certification and competency.)

Hospitals

Hospitals traditionally have provided a broad range of services for persons who are ill, injured, or dying. Most hospitals are open to any person needing health care. However, military hospitals provide care only to military personnel and their dependants. Although hospitals are chiefly viewed as institutions that provide health care, they have other functions, such as being a resource for research and for nursing education.

Hospitals can be classified by the services they provide. General hospitals admit clients requiring a variety of services; most often these are emergency, medical, surgical, obstetric, pediatric, and psychiatric or mental health services. Hospitals are becoming more specialized, however, such as when one hospital in a region becomes the maternal or child centre, with no other hospitals in that region offering these services. Some hospitals only offer a specialty service, such as psychiatric or pediatric care.

Hospitals are usually described as acute care or chronic care (i.e., auxiliary) facilities. An acute care hospital provides assistance to clients who are acutely ill and who need short-term hospitalization, for example, a few hours or days. Increasingly, with health care advances, acute care clients are requiring only a few hours of observation following surgery, other treatments, and major diagnostic procedures. Chronic care or auxiliary hospitals provide care for extended periods, sometimes for the remainder of a person's life.

The variety of health care services that each hospital provides usually depends on their expected duties, as well as their size and location. Hospitals vary considerably in size, from small rural hospitals with only a few inpatient beds to large urban hospitals that may have as many as 1000 beds. Large urban hospitals typically have a wide range of inpatient services, a large capacity emergency department, advanced diagnostic equipment and laboratories, day surgery units, pharmacy services, intensive care and coronary care services, and different outpatient clinics. Some large hospitals also have ultra-specialized or quaternary services, such as spinal cord injury or burn units, organ transplantation programs, oncology services, and kidney dialysis units. Small rural hospitals are often limited to some inpatient beds, basic radiological and laboratory services, and first-response emergency services. The number of services that a rural hospital provides is related to the educational and practice qualifications of the hospital's staff and physicians, the number of people who rely on it for health care, and its distance from an urban centre.

Hospitals in Canada have undergone massive changes over time. One of the most common changes since the mid-1990s has been a reduction in the number of inpatient beds, offset by an increase in outpatient and day surgery services. Some hospitals began providing innovative services, such as daycare for older persons or those who are terminally ill and nutrition classes. Some established alternative birth centres to make birthing a more normal and natural life event. Within some provinces and territories, regional health authorities have been given the responsibility for needed changes and for the overall planning and provision of health care services in their region. In others, the provincial or territorial government and local hospital or health care boards are responsible for operating, planning, and policymaking for hospitals.

Another change relates to clientele. Most patients admitted to hospitals today are seriously ill and require complex nursing and other care on an inpatient basis; others are less ill and can be treated on an outpatient or ambulatory basis. With the increasing acuity (or severity) of illness among hospital inpatients, hospitals have become complex care centres. Hospital nurses consequently need to have advanced assessment and other skills and knowledge.

Nurses in hospitals have multiple responsibilities, including coordinating patient care, assessing and monitoring client health, providing a wide range of direct care services, conducting research studies, orienting new staff, and educating staff for continuing competency. Management roles are often fulfilled by nurses, with nurses having responsibility for a hospital or a hospital unit or department, increasingly as top-level executives.

Rural Primary Care Hospitals

Rural primary care hospitals were created in some provinces during the 1990s process of health system reform. They provide emergency care to patient in rural areas who require stabilization before transfer to a larger hospital. Usually, basic laboratory and radiological services are also available.

Telehealth

Telephone health care advice is now common across Canada. Telehealth nurses are often seasoned nurses who can ask key questions to elicit needed information and can supply appropriate answers to the wide range of persons calling in with health concerns. These nurses also advise callers how to manage nonurgent situations at home and, in some instances, how and when to seek appropriate medical or hospital care. Telehealth services are typically available 24 hours a day, 7 days a week. Telehealth services greatly assist people at home who have a health concern and little or no knowledge about it. The number of visits to hospital emergency departments is greatly reduced in areas with telehealth, a benefit for both those who do not need to travel to the emergency department as well as those who need care in emergency departments.

Rehabilitation Centres

Rehabilitation centres include half-way houses, entire hospitals, or special units in hospitals and other sites such as extended care facilities. Because rehabilitation ideally starts the moment a patient enters hospital, hospital nurses help rehabilitate patients. Rehabilitation centres have an important role in helping clients recuperate. Drug and alcohol rehabilitation centres, for example, help clients free themselves from chemical dependence and assist them to return home and function to the best of their abilities. Today, the concept of rehabilitation is applied to all injuries, illnesses (physical and mental), and addictions. Nurses in rehabilitation centres generally plan and coordinate client activities and treatments. This type of nursing often requires specialized skills and knowledge.

Extended Care Facilities

Extended care facilities have more traditionally been called *nursing homes* or *long-term care facilities*, although they are also called *continuing care facilities* and, in British Columbia, *complex care facilities*. Extended care facilities include skilled nursing homes (for intermediate- to top-level care) and extended care facilities (for long-term or permanent care); typically these provide personal care for those with chronic illnesses or disabilities who are unable to care for themselves. These facilities often become home, with clients living there being referred to as *residents*. A new type of extended care facility is one offering subacute care. Subacute care helps acute care hospital clients who no longer need acute care but require additional rehabilitation before they return home.

Because long-term disability occurs most often among seniors, extended care facilities have programs that are largely oriented to the needs of this age group. Typically, these facilities are intended for people who require not only basic personal services (i.e., bathing, hygiene, assistance with daily activities, and so on) but also some regular nursing care and periodic medical or nurse practitioner attention.

Nurses working in extended care facilities have a wide range of possible responsibilities. Some assist clients with their daily activities and provide care when necessary, whereas others plan and coordinate daily care and rehabilitation activities or manage part or all of the facility.

Retirement Homes, Lodges, and Assisted-Living Facilities

Many forms of housing exist for seniors and those with disabilities who require little, if any, assistance. Residents in these housing, condominium, or apartment complexes live relatively independently; however, many of these facilities offer meals, laundry services, transportation, and social activities. Some have additional capacity to care for residents experiencing short-term or long-term illnesses through visiting home care nurses or employed on-site nurses. However, lodges and some other facilities admit and retain only residents who are ambulatory and able to dress and bathe themselves. Nurses working in these facilities provide limited care directly to residents; usually their work is related to medication monitoring, minor treatments, resident or staff supervision, and the administration or management of the facility.

Daycare Centres

Daycare centres serve many functions and many age groups. Some provide care for children with disabilities while their parents work. Others similarly provide care for adults who cannot be left at home alone. Eldercare centres generally provide care involving meals, socializing, exercise programs, and stimulation. Some centres provide counselling and physical therapy. Others provide hospice–palliative care. Nurses who are employed in daycare centres typically provide medications, treatments, and counselling; or perform other functions, such as education and management.

Hospice–Palliative Care Services

Long ago, a *hospice* was a place for travellers to rest. This term has currently come to mean a home-like health care facility specifically for dying people (see Chapter 49 for more information on hospice care). Hospice–palliative care, more broadly, is a type of end-of-life care that may be offered in any setting, such as a home, nursing home, or hospital. Its central concept is not saving life but improving or maintaining quality of life until death. Cicely Saunders, a nurse who later became a physician and the founder of

EVIDENCE-INFORMED PRACTICE

What Are the Concerns of Rural Persons with Advanced Cancer and of Their Families?

In this study, the researchers were trying to understand how older rural patients with advanced cancer manage transitions during their care. Based on individual interviews with six rural patients, 10 bereaved family members, 12 rural health care professionals, and four focus groups, four themes were identified. The first was community connectedness and isolation— where participants noted that they did feel connected to their community and supported by it, but also felt isolated, especially during certain parts of the illness process. This was increased if the participant was geographically distant from others. The second theme was lack of accessibility to care—especially if care was required after hours or if they lived long distances from treatment centres. The third identified theme was communication and information issues—where participants identified not knowing what was going to happen as the disease progressed, and health care workers expressed that sometimes patients and families were struggling, and the health care worker had not been notified that they needed help. The fourth theme, independence and dependence, reflected the patients' desire to remain independent as well as their realization that they needed help as more care was required.

NURSING IMPLICATIONS: Although independence and community support are valued by patients and their families, nurses need to be alert to changing needs during the progression of a terminal disease.

Source: Based on Duggleby, W. D., Penz, K., Liepert, B. D., Wilson, D. M., Goodridge, D., & Williams, A. (2011)."I am part of the community but. . . ." The changing context of rural living for persons with advanced cancer and their families. *Rural and Remote Health, 11,* 1733. (online) PMID21787109

St. Christopher's Hospice in London, England, believed that the physical and social environments of dying people are as important as medical interventions on their behalf. Nurses who work in hospice–palliative care may or may not have advanced education and preparation for this important work. A growing number of nurses are obtaining CHPCN(C) designation. (See the Evidence-Informed Practice box on the concerns of rural persons with advanced cancer and of their families.)

Crisis Centres

Crisis centres provide emergency support to clients. These centres operate out of a community organization or hospital, and most provide 24-hour telephone service. Some also provide direct counselling to people at the centre or in their homes. The primary purpose of a crisis centre is to help people cope with an immediate crisis and provide guidance and support to prevent further crises.

Nurses working in crisis centres need crisis communication and counselling skills. These nurses must immediately identify the person's problem, offer assistance to help the person cope or obtain needed help, and perhaps later direct the person to resources for ongoing support.

Mutual Support and Self-Help Groups

Canada has hundreds of support or self-help groups that focus on nearly every health problem or life crisis that people may experience. Such groups arose largely because people felt their needs were not being met by the health care system. Alcoholics Anonymous, which was formed in 1935, served as the model for many of these groups.

Providers of Health Care

The providers of health care, collectively referred to as the *health care team,* are health care personnel from a variety of disciplines who coordinate their knowledge and skills to assist patients (clients or residents), families, select population groups, and whole communities. Their broad mutual goal is to restore patient health and promote wellness. The choice of personnel for a particular individual or group client depends on the needs of the client or patient. The roles of the categories of nurses are found in Chapter 1; Table 9.4 defines the roles of other needed health care providers. **Alternative care providers**, such as chiropractors, herbalists, naturopaths, acupuncturists, and many others, offer services that are not typically listed as medically necessary for provincial and territorial health care insurance coverage, although it could be argued that they are also health care team members.

Factors Impacting the Health Care System

People now have greater knowledge about their health and health care than in previous years. In the past, physicians and nurses made all the necessary health care decisions; today, people usually want to be involved in these decisions, if not be solely responsible for them. People also have higher expectations about health care. Canadians want up-to-date, appropriate, effective, and mistake-free health care. Most citizens have also become

TABLE 9.4 Roles of Select Health Care Team Members

Dentists	Dentists diagnose and treat diseases, conditions, and disorders of teeth, the mouth, and surrounding tissues and structures.
Dietitians or **nutritionists**	Dietitians plan, implement, and manage individual nutritional support and food service programs.
Laboratory or **radiologic technologist**	These health care workers assist or complete diagnostic tests—often laboratory or radiology tests.
Nurse practitioners	Nurse practitioners diagnose and treat human illness and assist in rehabilitation, with their role also expected to be holistic and health promotive.
Occupational therapists	The primary goal of occupational therapists is to enable people to participate in activities of daily living.
Paramedical technologist; emergency medical and ambulance attendants	These first-response health care personnel deliver on-site first-aid to ill or injured persons and transport them to hospitals.
Pharmacists	Pharmacists dispense medications and help people understand and use their medications safely to achieve desired health outcomes. In some provinces, they can renew and alter prescriptions.
Physicians	Physicians diagnose and treat human illnesses and assist rehabilitation after the onset of disease or injury.
Physiotherapists	Physiotherapists or physical therapists are professionals who analyze and address the impact of injuries, diseases, or disorders on movement and physical functioning.
Respiratory therapists	Respiratory therapists assist the diagnosis and treatment of lung disorders.
Social workers	Social workers seek to improve the social health and well-being of individuals or families.

Source: Adapted from the Canadian Institute for Health Information. (2006). *Health Personnel Trends in Canada, 1995 to 2004.* Ottawa: Author. Reprinted by permission of CIHI.

aware that their lifestyle and their home or work environments impact their health. As a result, they desire more information and services related to health promotion and illness prevention. These factors and many others are affecting the health care system.

Advancements in Technology and Evidence-Based Care

With more research being done and more effective knowledge translation, scientific knowledge is rapidly increasing. Improved diagnostic and treatment procedures, more highly sophisticated equipment, and very knowledgeable health care professionals create better outcomes for those who are seriously ill and allow for earlier diagnosis of health problems that might otherwise have remained undetected until late in the illness, when death was inevitable or major surgery and long hospitalizations were needed. New medications are continually being developed to treat and prevent both chronic and acute health problems. The higher prevention, cure, and remission rates with cancer are but one example of the life-saving impact of these advancements.

Surgical procedures involving the heart, lungs, brain, and other organs that were nonexistent as recently as 10 years ago are possible today. Recovery following major surgery has also improved in terms of health outcomes and speed of recovery. Laser, laparoscopic, and microscopic procedures have streamlined the treatment of illnesses that required major surgery not long ago. Nonsurgical techniques and medications have made some surgeries unnecessary. A prime example is gallbladder removal, which used to be a major surgical procedure involving a 10-day hospital stay and a high probability of wound infections and pneumonia. Although gallbladder disease is still very common in Canada, it can now be treated either with medications to dissolve gallbladder stones or through laparoscopic gallbladder removal, which is a day surgery procedure. Day surgery has many advantages; even when the person is hospitalized, the hospital stays are much shorter; recovery at home is improved; and hospital-acquired, or nosocomial, infections are avoided.

People are now more likely to be treated in the community or to recover at home after receiving care in hospital. A person having cataract surgery used to have to remain in bed in hospital for 10 days; today, cataract surgeries are performed on an outpatient basis, with the person returning home with instructions for immediate and follow-up postsurgical care. As a result of this shift out of hospital, some direct and indirect costs have been passed to the individual or family. These include the cost of medications and supplies that would be provided at no charge if hospitalized. Lost time from work and interrupted careers are indirect costs, as family members normally are needed for transportation purposes and for providing both pretreatment and post-treatment care in the home.

Family caregiving may be long term, with informal caregiver burden increasingly linked to health issues for family members who provide ongoing 24-hour 7-day-a-week care for loved ones who are chronically ill or dying.

Computers, which have improved client care and can store and retrieve large volumes of information in databases, are commonplace in health care organizations now. Health care research is also greatly advanced, with the knowledge gained important for evidence-informed practice improvements by current health care professionals and in the education of new health care professionals.

Technological advances and specialized treatments or procedures come with a high price tag for the health care system. This cost is offset, however, by the cost savings that result from health care advancements. Unfortunately, it is much easier to cost out the price of a new diagnostic machine than calculate the savings that arise from preventing some illnesses and successfully treating others earlier.

Economics

Paying for health care has been an issue for governments and, particularly since 1966 when the Medical Care Act (the precursor of the 1984 Canada Health Act) was passed, containing a promise of 50/50 cost sharing between the federal and provincial governments. The health care system, then and now, is very much affected by the country's overall economic status. The economic recessions of the 1970s, 1990s, and the current period after 2008 increased concern about escalating health care costs. Canada's health care costs have increased considerably since 1966, and they continue to increase above inflation. Many factors contribute to this, including the cost of not doing more to prevent illnesses and injuries, and the high cost of delivering health care across Canada. Although 80% of citizens live in or near urban centres, 20% live in rural and remote areas across 95% of Canada's land surface.

Other reasons for this cost increase include the following:

- The cost of drugs and health care supplies have risen substantially.

- Inflation continually increases all costs, including wages of health care providers.

- Existing equipment and facilities become obsolete or in need of repair and replacement.

- Additional space, sophisticated equipment, and specially trained personnel to use and maintain this new equipment are required to provide modern evidence-informed care.

- The number of people working within the health care system has increased.

- The total population has grown, and the number of people needing health care services has also increased.

- Health care system inefficiency, with only minimal home care and extended care services to permit more care out of hospitals, although increases in this area are becoming more common.
- Changes in illnesses have occurred; more clients have multiple chronic or incurable illnesses that need ongoing care, and more are acquiring infections that delay hospital discharge.

Growth and Demographic Changes

In 1966 and 1984, when the two acts that sequentially formed the current health care system were passed, the population of Canada was 20 million and 26 million, respectively. Today, there are 34 million Canadians, each of whom can be expected to see a physician or nurse practitioner at least once a year. Approximately 9% of Canadian citizens of all ages will be admitted to hospital for inpatient care, and 40% to 50% will require ambulatory care in emergency departments or other outpatient settings.

The characteristics of the Canadian family have also changed considerably in the last few decades. The numbers of single-parent families and alternative family structures have increased markedly. Most single-parent families are headed by women, many of whom work in low-paying jobs; they typically require assistance with childcare or when a child is sick at home. Divorce continues to be common, with more divorced or never-married persons entering old age without the assurance of assistance from spouses or children. Considerable geographical mobility also means that family members may not be available to help. The birthrate continues to be low, with immigration needed to maintain the population levels of the youth and working-age persons.

Recognition of the cultural and ethnic diversity of Canada is also increasing. In 2000, the CNA published *Cultural Diversity: Changes and Challenges* and, in 2004, a position statement entitled *Promoting Culturally Competent Care*, which acknowledges the increasingly diverse clients that nurses work with. Health care professionals and organizations are aware of this diversity and are meeting the challenges presented by persons who have different languages, social customs, illnesses, diets, and health care practices and beliefs. For example, more organizations are ensuring translators are available, and many are hosting opportunities for staff to increase their cultural knowledge and respect.

Uneven Distribution of Services

Some problems in the distribution of health care services across Canada exist. Two main considerations are (a) uneven distribution and (b) increased specialization. In some areas, particularly the inner city and remote or rural locations, the numbers of health care professionals and services available locally are insufficient to meet the health care needs of individuals, families, and communities. Rural and remote clients, such as Inuit and other northern residents, often need to travel long distances to obtain the services they require. Even if there is a local hospital, small hospitals usually do not offer surgical, childbirthing, and many other services; this may be because of personnel and equipment shortages or increased health care specialization.

Health care is continually becoming more specialized, with cancer care and many other health care services only provided in a few larger organizations where economies of scale can reduce costs and where the frequency of care delivery helps to ensure current knowledge and competent practice. Because of the highly specialized techniques and new knowledge that have emerged with research, an increasing number of health care personnel provide only specialized services. They may be highly specialized technicians or technologists with narrow and exacting jobs, such as orthotic technologists, biomedical electronic technologists, and nuclear medicine technologists. Increased specialization is evident also among nurses, physicians, and other health care professionals. This specialization, although beneficial, contributes to fragmentation of care and to other concerns. To a client, it may mean receiving care from 5 to 30 different health care professionals in the hospital and many more over the course of a terminal illness or a treatable illness. Having to deal with this seemingly endless stream of personnel can cause confusion and fear. It can also lead to errors.

Providing safe care is very important. The Canadian Patient Safety Institute was established by Health Canada in 2003 as an independent nonprofit corporation, operating collaboratively with health care professionals and organizations, regulatory bodies, and governments to build and advance a safer health care system for Canadians (Canadian Patient Safety Institute, 2010). Nursing has contributed to these efforts, such as through the position statement by the CNA (2009) entitled *Patient Safety*. The Canadian Council on Health Services Accreditation is another key national nongovernmental organization that assesses health care organizations for their ability to meet expected health care and workplace standards. This organization has health care excellence as its aim. Clients are also more aware of patient safety issues because of media attention, with health care organizations expected to have safety policies and safe workplace practices. While patient safety has been an increasing focus of attention, health care worker safety is lagging behind.

Access to Health Care

Not all population groups in Canada have equitable access to health care. Rural and remote residency has been associated with higher rates of risk factors, illnesses, and death; and reduced access to health care for people living in rural and remote communities compared with urban Canadians has been identified as a factor (CIHI, 2006). Low education and income are other major factors associated with greater health care needs and with poorer health care outcomes (CIHI, 2004). Access to, and thus use of, available health care services is adversely affected by poverty. Although Canadians do not have to pay to see a physician or to receive hospital care, taking a day off from work for health care could mean a day without pay for someone in a low-paying job. The transportation costs to access health care and the costs of out-of-hospital care are also disproportionately higher for persons with low incomes. Limited government assistance may be available, but the eligibility for programs and benefits varies considerably across provinces and territories. (See Chapter 15 for more information on rural health care.)

Population Aging and Aging among Older Adults

An increase is anticipated in the number of older Canadians: from 4.8 million in 2010 to 10.4 million by 2036 (Statistics Canada, 2009). Seniors aged 85 years and older are the fastest-growing population group; seniors in this age group are more likely to need assistance to remain in their own homes or to accomplish activities of daily living. Most seniors live independently; only 7% live in extended care or other seniors' facilities. Chronic illnesses are more prevalent among seniors and with aging, although three of every four seniors aged 65 to 74 years and two of every three seniors aged 75 years and older rate their health as good, very good, or excellent (Public Health Agency of Canada, 2005). Considerable concern exists over the use of health services by seniors, despite 86% of the Canadian population being younger and potentially as likely to need health care. Some age-based differences in health care needs are becoming evident, as 90% of the persons living in extended care facilities and 80% of all persons who require end-of-life care are seniors. Some differences in health care services use are also becoming more evident, such as seniors having higher rates of home care and longer hospital stays if admitted to hospital.

Older people are increasingly healthy and active into advanced old age. They fulfill many important responsibilities through volunteering, holding political office, heading boards or corporations, caring for grandchildren or family members or friends who are ill, and, increasingly, maintaining paid employment (Health Canada, 2002). The feeling of being a useful person is important for health. Special programs are being designed in communities so that the talents and skills of this group are not lost to society. Other programs, such as seniors' daycare, are being designed for

health-promotion purposes and earlier detection and proactive management of health problems. These programs are often used by women, as they are more likely to live longer and to live alone in old age.

Women's Health

The women's movement has been instrumental in changing health care practices. Examples are the provision of childbirth services in more relaxed settings, such as birthing centres, and the provision of overnight facilities for parents of children who are in hospitals. Traditionally, many health care concerns that are unique to women, both young and old, have been overlooked, with rising concern, for instance, that heart disease among women is often not detected. One of Health Canada's responses in this area is the Gender-Based Analysis initiative, which recognizes the variety of factors that contribute to gender differences in health and health care needs, as well as providing evidence of the effects of gender on the determinants of health (Health Canada, 2010).

Homeless Populations

The growing number of homeless individuals and families is a health problem, too. The homeless differ from people who are poor. The homeless are socially isolated, lack any type of permanent residence, and are often disaffiliated from family or friends. Because of the conditions in which homeless people live (e.g., in temporary shelters, tents, or cars or on the street), existing health challenges are often exacerbated and new health challenges, such as frost bite, malnutrition, and injuries, often emerge.

Factors contributing to homelessness include the high cost of housing and the change from inpatient to outpatient mental care services. Some homeless people have mental as well as physical, social, and emotional health challenges. Limited access to health care services is another significant contributor to poor health. Tuberculosis, for instance, is more common among homeless people.

Evidence-Informed Practice

It is sometimes said that over half of all health care practices are not research based and that, instead, practices that have developed in response to needs have been refined over time. Nurses are rapidly addressing this issue, with many nurse researchers seeking to prove that current nursing or health care practices are safe and effective or that alternatives are better.

Climate Change

Evidence of climate change, broadly referred to as global warming, is also growing, including information on the varied impacts of climate change. Although distinct weather-related emergencies, such as Hurricane Katrina in 2005 and the 2011 tsunami in Japan, cause considerable health impacts to those directly and indirectly affected, global health is being affected by the daily effects of increased greenhouse gases. Unfortunately, we can expect to see more pandemics, heat waves, and violent weather because of unchecked climate change. Other less visible, but serious, impacts from increased greenhouse gases should also be of concern, such as rising rates of asthma and chronic obstructive lung disease.

Leadership

Another important influence on the health care system is leadership by elected and appointed persons, as well as nurses and others who advocate for beneficial reforms. A change in or threat to a political party at the provincial, territorial, and federal levels often leads to reforms through task forces or commission reports (see the Nursing and Canadian Society box). Increasingly, leaders are using visions of health promotion and sustainable health care coupled with evidence from research to plan policy and programs that incrementally change the Canadian health care system.

Contemporary Frameworks for Care

A number of newer approaches to client care support continuity of care and cost-effectiveness. Continuity of care across organizations and care providers is increasingly important, as is cost-effectiveness.

Case Management

Case management describes a range of models of integrated health care services. Case managers may also be referred to as patient navigators or care managers. Nurses are commonly hired for this type of work. Case managers typically assume responsibility for assessing needs, planning, coordinating, implementing, and evaluating care for individuals after hospital discharge over their lifetimes.

Nurse **case managers** may be hired by a hospital or another health care organization, such as a home care agency. They may coordinate care for a specific client population, such as clients with chronic obstructive lung disease or mental health problems, or for all persons receiving long-term home care. A critical component of their role is communication and collaboration with other health care professionals and the client to achieve optimal immediate and long-term outcomes.

 Nursing and Canadian Society

Fact	Implications for Nursing Practice
The five criteria of the Canada Health Act (CHA) are the cornerstone of the Canadian health care system.	Nurses need to understand the criteria of the Canada Health Act and the health care system to deliver effective quality care within and outside of this act.
The Canadian health care system has evolved into its present form over many years. Saskatchewan, in 1947, was the first province to establish public, universal hospital insurance. Ten years later, the Canadian government passed legislation to permit the federal government to share in the cost of provincial hospital insurance plans. By 1961, all provinces and territories had public insurance plans that provided comprehensive coverage for in-hospital care.	Then and now, nurses have been system and client advocates to ensure that the health care needs of people are served.
Canada's health expenditures stand fifth of all industrialized nations and Canada's system is the highest in per capita (or per person) costs among all publicly funded universal health care systems worldwide.	Nurses consequently have a responsibility to be fiscally accountable and to advocate for economic accountability.
Recent federal initiatives have included the Commission on the Future of Health Care, chaired by Roy Romanow, and the Standing Senate Committee on Social Affairs, Science and Technology (the Health of Canadians–the Federal Role), chaired by the Honourable Michael Kirby.	Nurses need to lead, participate in, and understand government initiatives that will affect health care.

Case management can be used as a cost-containment strategy, as hospital avoidance and earlier discharge from hospital reduce health care costs. Case managers often use **critical pathways** to track each client's progress. A critical pathway is a plan or tool for the managed care of a client that specifies assessments, interventions, treatments, and outcomes for specific health-related conditions across time. Critical pathways are also called *interdisciplinary care plans*, *anticipated recovery plans*, and *action plans*. These plans can be developed for most surgical procedures, and for other emergency care, trauma care, and additional health-related interventions. They are usually used for high-volume case types or situations with relatively predictable outcomes. The pathways are designed in collaboration with members of the health care team who are involved in managing each case type, and the pathways are considered best practices as they are based on a body of evidence in that field. It is important to exercise clinical judgment, however, when applying standard protocols and to refrain from using them as a checklist for all clients. Critical pathways are presented in later chapters.

Patient-Focused Care

Patient-focused care (also called client-centred care) is a delivery model that emphasizes the importance of the client and his or her needs. The supposition is that if health care is more directly aimed at determining and meeting client needs there will be cost-savings through earlier diagnosis and more successful treatment. For instance, breast screening vans go out to rural areas to increase the likelihood of screening and thus early detection of breast cancer, and health care teams develop satellite centres for kidney dialysis, cancer care, or hospice–palliative care so that people needing these services do not have to travel to large urban hospitals for their ongoing health care.

Cross-training, the development of multiskilled workers who can perform tasks or functions normally done by more than one discipline, can also illustrate patient-focused care. For example, an unlicensed health care worker may be taught to obtain a 12-lead electrocardiogram (ECG) and perform phlebotomy, or individuals who are already certified in one occupation can take on a second certification, such as nurses also providing medical laboratory and x-ray technology, respiratory therapy, and physical or occupational therapy. Because patient-focused care can result in the blurring of role boundaries, collaboration is vital during the design and implementation process.

Another initiative to foster patient-focused care is **interprofessional collaboration**, which has long been a topic in practice and educational arenas. In light of the need for interdisciplinary teamwork, Health Canada developed the *Interprofessional Education for Collaborative Patient-Centred Practice* (IECPCP) initiative in 2005.

"Collaborative patient-centred practice is designed to promote the active participation of several health care disciplines and professions. It enhances patient-, family-, and community-centred goals and values, provides mechanisms for continuous communication among health care providers, optimizes staff participation in clinical decision making (within and across disciplines), and fosters respect for the contributions of all providers" (Health Canada, 2007, p. 1).

Models for the Delivery of Nursing

Contemporary configurations for the delivery of nursing include collaborative arrangements, such as managed care, case management, and patient-focused care discussed earlier. Frequently, delivery methods comprise components of more than one configuration. Box 9.1 describes the most common nursing care delivery methods used in acute care and other settings: **case method**, **functional method**, **team nursing**, and **primary nursing**.

BOX 9.1 NURSING DELIVERY METHODS USED IN HEALTH CARE SETTINGS	
Case method	• One nurse is assigned to and is responsible for the comprehensive care of one or more assigned clients over the course of a shift.
Functional method	• This method focuses on the jobs to be completed (e.g., vital signs, medication administration).
	• Personnel with less preparation than the professional nurse perform less complex care.
	• It gives authority and responsibility to the person assigning the work, for example, the charge nurse or team leader.
Team nursing	• The collective delivery of individualized nursing care to clients through a nursing team that is led by a professional nurse.
	• The team consists of registered nurses, often working with licensed (or registered) practical nurses, unlicensed assistive personnel, such as nurse aides, and possibly psychiatric nurses and others.
Primary nursing	• One nurse is responsible for the total care of clients, 24 hours a day, 7 days a week.
	• Associates provide care when the primary nurse is not available.

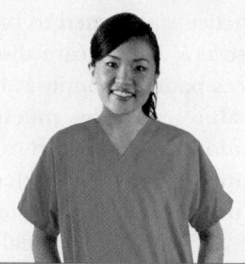

Case Study 9

Rebecca Konapinksi is leaving the hospital after major surgery. She is leaving with a drain that will stay in place for about 10 days. It is obvious in talking to her that she is apprehensive and worried about who will change her dressing when she gets home. Her two children are young and her husband travels a great deal.

CRITICAL THINKING QUESTIONS

1. What is meant by continuum of health care service delivery?

2. How might Rebecca's family and friends provide health care services to her?

3. How would a nurse provide health care to her?

Check the eText in MyNursingLab for answers and explanations.

KEY TERMS

accessibility *p. 162*

alternative care
  providers *p. 172*

case management *p. 176*

case managers *p. 176*

case method *p. 177*

clients' rights *p. 163*

comprehensiveness *p. 162*

continuum of care *p. 166*

critical pathways *p. 177*

dentist *p. 172*

diagnosis *p. 164*

dietitian *p. 172*

end-of-life care *p. 165*

functional
  method *p. 177*

health promotion
  p. 164

health restoration *p. 165*

health-care system *p. 161*

hospice–palliative
  care *p. 165*

illness and injury
  prevention *p. 164*

interprofessional
  collaboration *p. 177*

laboratory/radiologic
  technologist *p. 172*

nurse practitioner
  p. 172

nutritionist *p. 172*

occupational
  therapist *p. 172*

paramedical
  technologist *p. 172*

patient-focused
  care *p. 177*

pharmacist *p. 172*

physician *p. 172*

physiotherapist *p. 172*

portability *p. 162*

primary nursing *p. 177*

public administration
  p. 162

rehabilitation *p. 165*

respiratory
  therapist *p. 172*

social worker *p. 172*

team nursing *p. 177*

treatment *p. 164*

universality *p. 162*

CHAPTER HIGHLIGHTS

- The health care system has developed into a large, complex organization comprising a wide variety of organizations, services, and health care providers. At the heart of this system is the client.

- Health care should be considered a right of citizens of Canada.

- Health care services can be categorized as primary, secondary, tertiary, or quaternary and grouped by type of service: (a) health promotion and illness prevention, (b) diagnosis and treatment, (c) rehabilitation, and (d) hospice–palliative and end-of-life care.

- Hospitals provide a wide variety of services on inpatient and outpatient bases. Hospitals can be categorized as acute care or extended care. Many other settings, such as clinics, offices, and daycare centres, also provide health care.

- Various providers of health care coordinate their skills to assist clients. Their mutual goal is to restore a client's health and promote wellness. This coordination can occur even when hospice–palliative care is provided.

- The many factors affecting health care delivery include consumers' rights, women's health, an increasing population, advances in knowledge and technology, economic factors, fragmentation of care, increased costs, health care of the homeless, uneven distribution of health services, demographic changes, and access barriers to health care.

- A number of different nursing care delivery models are used, often the case method, functional method, team nursing, and primary nursing.

ASSESS YOUR LEARNING

1. Alicia, a 24-year-old from Ontario was vacationing in British Columbia when she injured herself. She was given immediate treatment at the nearest hospital and was not charged any additional cost for her treatment though she lives out of province. This example best demonstrates which of the five principles of the Canada Health Act?

   a. Comprehensiveness

   b. Universality

   c. Public Administration

   d. Portability

2. John is diagnosed with a condition requiring a blood transfusion. John declines the transfusion because of his religious beliefs. This exemplifies which right of health-care consumers?

   a. To be informed

   b. The right to choice

   c. Right to consumer education

   d. Access to basic services

3. Which types of health-care services have traditionally been emphasized within the Canadian health-care system?

   a. Diagnosis and treatment

   b. Rehabilitation and health restoration

   c. Health promotion and illness prevention

   d. Hospice palliative and end-of-life care

4. Which of these examples is considered a primary health-care service?

   a. A visit to an orthopedic specialist

   b. Screening for scoliosis

   c. Emergency room care

   d. Diagnostic imaging

5. Part of the responsibility of a registered nurse is to understand the role of health-care personnel involved in the different dimensions of client care. Wendy, an experienced RN, is working on a busy cardiology ward. One of her patients is being discharged home with a prescription for eight new cardiac drugs to add to his health-care regime. Which health-care provider might best be suited for the role of complex medication education?

   a. Registered nurse

   b. Pharmacist

   c. Social worker

   d. Physician

6. Which statement is *true* regarding societal and demographic factors affecting the Canadian health-care system?

   a. Most older people in Canada are no longer independent, with the majority living in extended-care facilities.

   b. Reduced access to health care by the rural populations in Canada may be a factor associated with higher rates of rural illness and death.

   c. Canadians are realizing the health-care system may not meet all their needs and therefore have lower expectations regarding the care and delivery of health services.

   d. Advancements in technology have decreased the amount of time spent in hospital and concurrently decreased care requirements from community health agencies and individual clients.

7. What best describes team nursing?

   a. Delegation of tasks to other members of the health-care team

   b. Planning and delivery of care for a group of patients on a 24/7 basis

   c. Fragmentation of nursing care

   d. First point of contact for most patients within the health-care system

8. Mrs. Mack, 70 years old, requires a surgical procedure and has been placed on a waiting list. What describes the category of urgency for need in which she has been placed?

   a. Urgent

   b. Emergent

   c. Elective

   d. Diagnostic

9. There has been a shift from inpatient hospital care to care in the ambulatory or community arena. This change has also resulted in what?

   a. An increase in out-of-pocket expenses for individuals and families

   b. A decrease in the availability of treatments requiring sophisticated equipment

   c. A decreased requirement for professional nurses to work in hospitals

   d. A decrease in the number of extended-care facilities required for the population

10. Which is an example of an illness- and injury-prevention program?

    a. Analysis of motor vehicle collisions

    b. Use of occupational protective equipment

    c. Teaching crutch walking in an ambulatory care clinic

    d. Support group for women with breast cancer

Check the eText in MyNursingLab for answers and explanations.

WEBLINKS

Accreditation Canada

http://www.accreditation.ca

Accreditation Canada (formerly the Canadian Council on Health Services Accreditation) is a national nongovernmental body that assesses health care organizations' ability to meet or exceed expected standards.

Canadian Healthcare Association

http://www.cha.ca

The Canadian Healthcare Association is a federation of provincial and territorial hospital and health care organizations.

Canadian Nurses Association

http://www.cna-aiic.ca

This site provides access to the position statements and other publications of this national nursing organization.

Canadian Occupational Health Nurses Association

http://www.cohna-aciist.ca

The site is sponsored by and speaks for occupational health nurses in Canada.

Canadian Public Health Association

http://www.cpha.ca

The Canadian Public Health Association advocates for improvements to health care according to the principles of disease prevention, health promotion and protection, and healthy public policy.

Commission on the Future of Health Care in Canada

http://www.hc-sc.gc.ca/hcs-sss/com/fed/romanow/index-eng.php

Chaired by Roy Romanow, the mandate of the Commission on the Future of Health Care in Canada was "to ensure that our health system meets the challenges of the 21st century." The site provides access to the work of the Commission.

Health Canada

http://www.hc-sc.gc.ca

This is a site of the federal government and provides access to national legislation, policy statements, and related health care information.

Public Health Agency of Canada

http://www.phac-aspc.gc.ca

Since 2004, this has been the main Government of Canada agency responsible for public health in Canada.

MyNursingLab

REFERENCES

Canada Health Act. R.S., 1984, c. C-6.

Canadian Institute for Health Information. (2004). *Improving the health of Canadians.* Ottawa, ON: Author.

Canadian Institute for Health Information. (2005). *Understanding emergency department wait time.* Ottawa, ON: Author.

Canadian Institute for Health Information. (2006). *How healthy are rural Canadians? An assessment of their health status and health determinants.* Ottawa, ON: Author.

Canadian Institute for Health Information. (2011). *Wait times in Canada—A comparison by province, 2011.* Retrieved from http://secure.cihi.ca/cihiweb/products/Wait_times_tables_2011_en.pdf

Canadian Institutes of Health Research. (2007). *CIHR institutes.* Retrieved from http://www.cihr-irsc.gc.ca/e/9466.html

Canadian Nurses Association. (2000). *Cultural diversity: Challenges and changes. NursingNow,* 7. Retrieved from http://www.cna-aiic. ca/CNA/documents/pdf/publications/CulturalDiversity_February2000_e.pdf

Canadian Nurses Association. (2002). *Fact sheet: Role of the nurse practitioner around the world.* Ottawa, ON: Author.

Canadian Nurses Association. (2004). *Position statement: Promoting culturally competent care.* Ottawa, ON: Author.

Canadian Nurses Association. (2008). *Code of ethics.* Ottawa, ON: Author.

Canadian Nurses Association. (2009). *Position Statement: Patient safety.* Retrieved from http://www.cna-nurses.ca/CNA/documents/pdf/publications/PS102_Patient_Safety_e.pdf

Canadian Nurses Association. (2009). *Position statement. Financing Canada's health system.* Retrieved from http://www.cna-aiic.ca/CNA/documents/pdf/publications/PS108_Financing_2009_e.pdf

Canadian Patient Safety Institute. (2010). Retrieved from http://www.hc-sc.gc.ca/hcs-sss/qual/patient_securit/cpsi-icsp-eng.php

Consumers' Association of Canada. (1989). *Consumer rights to health care.* Ottawa, ON: Author.

Eisen, B., & Bjornberg, A. (2010, May). *Euro-Canada health consumer index 2010.* Retrieved from http://www.fcpp.org/files/1/10-05-10-Euro-Canada_Index_2010_FINAL.pdf

Epp, J. (1986). *Achieving health for all: A framework for health promotion.* Ottawa, ON: Health and Welfare Canada.

Health Canada. (2002). *Canada's aging population.* Ottawa, ON: Author.

Health Canada. (2005). *Interprofessional education for collaborative patient-centred practice.* Retrieved from http://www.hc-sc.gc.ca/hcs-sss/hhr-rhs/strateg/interprof/index-eng.php

Health Canada. (2006a). *2003 First Ministers' Accord on Health Care Renewal.* Retrieved from http://www.hc-sc.gc.ca/hcs-sss/delivery-prestation/fptcollab/2003accord/index-eng.php

Health Canada. (2006b). *First Minister's Meeting on the Future of Health Care 2004. A 10-year plan to strengthen health care.* Retrieved from http://www.hc-sc.gc.ca/hcs-sss/delivery-prestation/fptcollab/2004-fmm-rpm/index-eng.php

Health Canada. (2010). *Health portfolio sex and gender-based analysis policy.* Retrieved from http://www.hc-sc.gc.ca/hl-vs/pubs/women-femmes/sgba-policy-politique-ags-eng.php

Health Canada. (2011). *About Health Canada.* Retrieved from http://www.hc-sc.gc.ca/ahc-asc/index-eng.php

Lalonde, M. (1974). *A new perspective on the health of Canadians.* Ottawa, ON: Government of Canada.

NP-led clinics: Ontario leads the way. (2010). *Canadian Nurse Journal, 106*(9), 30–35.

Public Health Agency of Canada. (2005). *Canada's seniors at a glance.* Retrieved from http://www.phac-aspc.gc.ca/seniors-aines/pubs/seniors_at_glance/poster2_e.html

Public Health Agency of Canada. (2011). *About the agency.* Retrieved from http://www.phac-aspc.gc.ca/about_apropos/index-eng.php

Statistics Canada. (2009). *2006 census: Portrait of the Canadian population in 2006, by age and sex: Findings.* Retrieved from http://www12.statcan.ca/census-recensement/2006/as-sa/97-551/index-eng.cfm

Warren, D. W., Jarvis, A., LeBlanc, L, Gravel, J., & the CTAS National Working Group. (2008). Revisions to the Canadian Triage and Acuity Scale Paediatric Guidelines (PaedCTAS). *Canadian Journal of Emergency Medicine, 19*(3), 224–232.

Wilson, D. M., Birch, S., Cohen, J., MacLeod, R., Mohankumar, D., & Williams, A. (2011). Home care developments in the Canadian province of Alberta with regionalization. *Global Journal of Health Science, 3*(1), 3–9.

World Health Organization. (1979). *Formulating strategies for health for all by the year 2000.* Geneva, Switzerland: Author.

World Health Organization. (1981). *Global strategy for health for all by the year 2000.* Geneva, Switzerland: Author.

World Health Organization, Health and Welfare Canada, & Canadian Public Health Association. (1986). *Ottawa charter for health promotion.* Ottawa, ON: Canadian Public Health Association.

Chapter 10

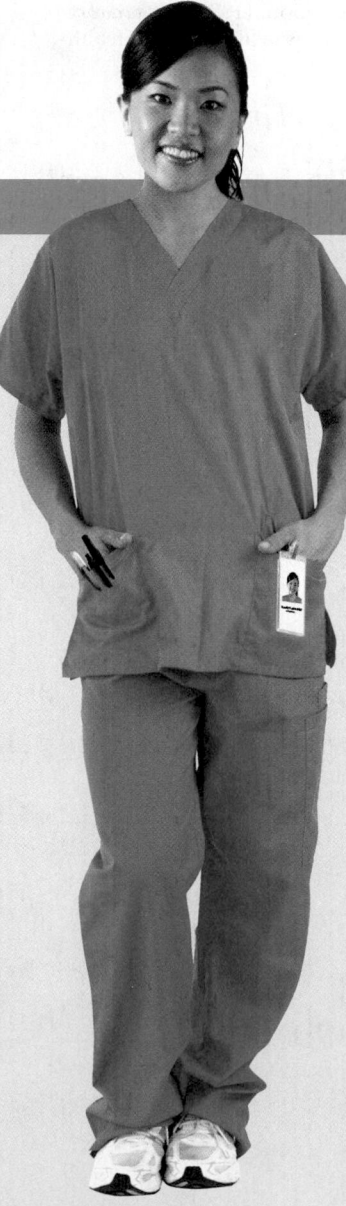

Environmental and Global Health Nursing

LEARNING OUTCOMES

After studying this chapter, you will be able to:

1. Describe the main factors related to environmental health: climate change, global warming, air pollution, water, and sanitation

2. Describe how environmental health factors affect health in Canada.

3. Examine the changes in population health over time and between countries, including lifespan differences and epidemiologic transition.

4. Distinguish between global health and international health.

5. Summarize the ways in which countries are organized and current theories of development in relation to global health.

6. Discuss the relevance of the Millennium Development Goals in reducing poverty and fostering development.

7. Describe the features of four main issues of global health and explain how they relate to life in Canada.

8. Describe the role of nursing in global health and the importance of educating nurses in global health issues.

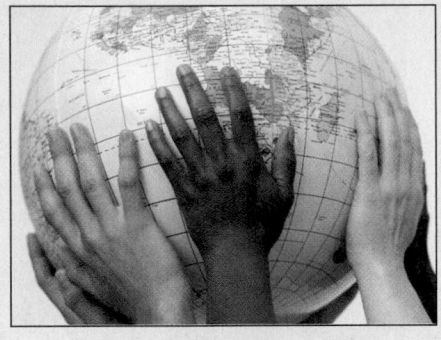

his chapter will help you understand the evolution and characteristics of environmental and global health. **Environmental health** and global health are both important and relevant to nurses in Canada, even if they never travel out of Canada. It is already clear that climate change and changes in the global economy exert powerful effects on Canadians and Canada. Environmental and global health are not static fields; each is a rapidly changing and dynamic interface of many factors that impact how we live and work now and in the future. We present definitions of key terms, history, and development of these broad fields of health and introduce the idea of transitions for nations and populations in each section.

Environment and Health

Environmental factors exert significant influence on human health in all countries, including Canada. Climate change, access to safe water, sanitation, and indoor and outdoor pollution are perhaps most important as they are major factors in the deaths and burden of illness for millions of adults and children annually.

Almost 25% of all diseases and 23% of all deaths are caused by environmental factors. The most vulnerable are those who experience unequal access to health care resources or have specific vulnerabilities, for example, children, Indigenous peoples, people who live in poverty, and those who live on small islands and in rural or isolated communities (Griffiths, & Winant, 2007; United Nations Environment Programme [UNEP], 2010; World Health Organization [WHO], 2009a).

Young children are particularly vulnerable to illnesses and death related to environmental factors because children breathe, eat, and drink more in proportion to body size compared with adults (Prüss-Üstün & Corvalán, 2006). Globally, a third of illnesses and death in childhood are caused by environmental factors and from toxins, sometimes resulting in permanent developmental damage.

Climate Change

Climate change and its effects are now well documented (Balbus, 2010; Pachauri, & Reisinger, 2007; UNEP, 2010) and reasonable estimates of future effects are possible (Prüss-Üstün & Corvalán, 2006). **Climate change** occurs when long-term weather patterns change. Changes noted in weather patterns over the last few decades include global warming, increased rainfall in some regions,

prolonged periods of no rainfall in others, extreme storm systems, and rising sea levels. Possible effects of climate change are presented in Table 10.1 on the next page.

Global warming is caused by increases of "greenhouse gases," primarily carbon dioxide, methane, and nitrous oxide. Their emissions vary widely by country (see Table 10.2 on page 185). It is important to understand that some countries with lower per capita rates of carbon production have, in fact, the largest total rate because they have very large populations. Others with very high per capita rates have a low total rate, as their national population is quite small in global terms (see Table 10.3 on page 185). Both measures provide direction for carbon reduction activities.

The greenhouse gases are produced from human activity in industry, power generation, vehicle use, agriculture, and deforestation (Birn, Pillay, & Holtz, 2009a). Burning fossil fuels is the principal source of greenhouse gases, and deforestation adds to this, as trees are essential for absorption. Greenhouse gases cause global warming as they form a layer above the earth's atmosphere. Radiation from the sun penetrates these gases and warms the earth. The greenhouse gas layer, however, limits the normal reflection of the sun's rays back into the upper atmosphere, which is necessary to maintain normal cycles of the earth's temperature. Global warming has been increasing more rapidly since the 1970s. Patterns of change may last a decade or two, while others may persist and become permanent without interventions for change (Birn, Pillay, & Holtz, 2009b).

Global warming effects vary. For instance, warming is greatest over land, highest over high northern latitudes, and least over the Southern Ocean and northern part of the North Atlantic (Pachauri & Reisinger, 2007). Predicted changes include increased frequency of tropical storms and heat waves, with precipitation increasing in some regions and decreasing in others. These changes will impact how and where people live and ultimately their health.

TABLE 10.1 Examples of Possible Impacts of Climate Change Due to Changes in Extreme Weather and Climate Events

Phenomenon and Direction of Trend	Likelihood of Future Trends for Twenty-First Century Using SRES Scenarios	Examples of Major Projected Impacts by Sector*			
		Agriculture, Forestry	Water Resources	Human Health	Industry, Settlement Projections, Ecosystems, and Society
Land areas, warmer; ↓ Cold days and nights; ↑ Hot days and nights	Virtually certain	↑ Crops in colder environments; ↓ Crops in warmer environments; ↑ Insect outbreaks	Effects on water resources relying on snowmelt; effects on some water supplies	↓ Human mortality from less cold exposure	↓ Energy demand for heating; ↑ Demand for cooling; Poor air quality in cities; ↓ Disruption to transport due to snow; ice effects on winter tourism
Warm spells/heat waves; more often over land areas	Very likely	↓ Crops in warmer regions due to heat stress; ↑ Danger of wild fire	↑ Water demand; water quality problems (e.g., algal blooms)	↑ Risk of heat-related mortality, especially for older adults, chronically sick, very young, and socially isolated	↓ Quality of life for people in warm areas without appropriate housing; impacts on the very young and poor
Heavy precipitation events ↑ frequency over most areas	Very likely	Damage to crops, soil erosion, inability to cultivate land due to waterlogged of soils	↓ Quality of surface and groundwater; contamination of water supply; water scarcity may be relieved	↑ Risk of deaths, injuries; ↑ Infectious, respiratory, and skin diseases	Disruption of settlements, commerce, transport, and societies due to flooding; pressures on urban and rural infrastructures, and loss of property
↑ Area affected by drought	Likely	Land degradation; ↓ Yields due to crop damage and failure; ↑ Livestock deaths; ↑ Risk of wild fire	More widespread water stress	↓ Risk of food and water shortages; ↑ Risk of malnutrition; ↑ Risk of water- and food-borne diseases	Water shortage for settlements, industry, and societies; ↓ Hydropower generation potential; ↑ Possibility for population migration
↑ Intense tropical cyclone activity	Likely	Damage to crops; windthrow (uprooting) of trees; damage to coral reefs	Power outages causing disruption to public water supply	↑ Risk of deaths, injuries, water- and food-borne diseases; post-traumatic stress disorder	Disruption by flood and high winds; Loss of risk coverage in vulnerable areas by private insurers; ↑ Potential for population migrations and loss of property
↑ Incidence of extreme high sea level (excludes tsunamis)	Likely	Salinization of irrigation water, estuaries, and freshwater systems	↓ Freshwater availability due to saltwater intrusion	↑ Risk of deaths and injuries by drowning in floods; ↑ Migration-related health effects	Similar to tropical cyclones above

Note: These projections do not take into account any changes or developments in adaptive capacity. SRES, Special Report on Emissions Scenarios.

Source: Adapted from Pachauri, R. K., & Reisinger, A. (2007). Climate change: Synthesis report, fourth assessment report of the Intergovernmental Panel on Climate Change. (Fourth Assessment of the Intergovernmental Report on Climate Change No. 2011). Geneva, Switzerland: IPCC.

TABLE 10.2 Top 10 Countries in Total Carbon Emissions in Metric Tonnes, 2008

Country	Metric Tonnes (Thousands)
China	7 031 916
United States	5 461 014
India	1 742 698
Russian Federation	1 708 653
Japan	1 208 163
Germany	786 660
Canada	544 091
Iran	538 404
United Kingdom	522 856
Korea (South)	509 170

Source: World Bank (2012),CO2 emissions (metric tons per capita). Available from http://data.worldbank.org/indicator/EN.ATM.CO2E.PC

TABLE 10.3 Top 10 Countries Based on Per Capita Rates of Carbon Emissions, 2008

Country	Tonnes Per Capita
Qatar	49.1
Trinidad & Tobago	37.4
Kuwait	30.1
Brunei Darussalam	27.5
United Arab Emirates	25.0
Aruba	21.7
Luxemburg	21.5
Bahrain	21.4
Australia	18.6
United States	18.0

Source: World Bank (2012),CO2 emissions (metric tons per capita). Available from http://data.worldbank.org/indicator/EN.ATM.CO2E.PC

Over time, changes in temperature and weather patterns will change land use; rising seas levels will cause loss of coastal plains and small islands; and populations will be displaced and forced to migrate. Forest clearance, accompanied by changing weather patterns, will cause **vectors of diseases**, such as rats, ticks, flies, and mosquitoes, to migrate, bringing old diseases to new areas and giving rise to new diseases. West Nile virus infection is an example of a new disease in Canada.

Health Effects of Climate Change

Climate change is implicated in 13 million deaths worldwide annually and is a significant portion of disease burden. Globally, increasing millions will suffer malnutrition, death, and injuries related to extreme weather. In 2003, an extreme heat wave in Europe caused an estimated 70 000 deaths; such events are expected to be the norm by 2050. Diarrheal diseases associated with warmer temperatures and cardiorespiratory problems related to poor air quality will increase, and other diseases will emerge in new regions; malaria and Dengue fever have already extended into new regions and higher altitudes (WHO, 2009a). Changes in disease patterns require vigilance from public health systems so that early identification can lead to effective management for population health.

Although deaths from such causes as extreme cold may be reduced, benefits from climate change are believed to be far outweighed by its negative consequences, especially where resources are limited and in vulnerable populations (Pachauri & Reisinger, 2007). Knowledge and access to such resources as safe water will, in part, determine who survives and who does not.

Solutions for Climate Change

Three potential solutions for climate change are proposed: (a) adaptation, (b) mitigation, and (c) reducing emissions from deforestation and forest degradations (REDD); these solutions will be effective if widely adopted and implemented (McMullen & Jabbour, 2009).

Adaptation includes actions to live with climate changes and to identify shifts in disease patterns. Examples of adjusting to climate change include changing the timing of the planting season, matching types of crops planted regionally to suit new temperature and rainfall patterns, and new standards for insulation of buildings to protect against extreme cold or heat. Health care system adaptations include implementing heat and cold alert protocols and early identification of new patterns in disease. Successful adaptation results in reduced vulnerability to climate change.

Mitigation focuses on reducing greenhouse gas emissions. Actions include switching to cleaner, renewable energy sources, such as solar power and wind power. Reducing deforestation will decrease emissions from wood burning and help maintain the earth's capacity to absorb greenhouse gases, particularly carbon dioxide. Deforestation is an ongoing challenge, as national and corporate interests are heavily invested in clearing forests to access mineral and other resources. Climate change is created locally but acts globally, so remediation efforts must start locally but extend globally to halt or reverse climate change. Successful actions will require intersectoral and intergovernmental collaborations and sharing of information and resources. Future health care needs will include managing heat exposure, old infectious diseases in new locations, and malnutrition, as well as disaster planning.

Water and Sanitation

Safe and clean drinking water and sanitation, a human right essential to the full enjoyment of life and all other human rights (WHO, 2010), are important for health and are closely linked. Water supplies are often contaminated when effective sanitation measures are not used to dispose of human waste. Sanitation systems can be compromised by flooding that overruns pit latrines, septic tanks, or piped sewage systems.

Safe water is essential for health, yet globally 884 million people do not have access to safe drinking water. Most live in rural areas and in Sub-Saharan Africa and East and Southeast Asia. Almost 94% of diarrheal diseases are related to unsafe drinking water. Access to safe drinking water is a key target of Millennium Development Goal 7 (MDG 7) (Prüss-Üstün & Corvalán, 2006).

Water comes from two main sources: (a) surface sources, such as pools and rivers, and (b) groundwater sources, such as wells. Surface water sources are easily contaminated by animal and human activities and should not be used without treatment. Groundwater sources are more protected, as water is filtered by soil and other layers until it is trapped by impervious bedrock. Groundwater may be accessed through springs or wells, which are often susceptible to contamination. Deep or bore wells are much safer sources of water; however, specialized equipment is required to construct them.

Contamination of water may also involve toxic substances, such as fertilizers, pesticides, dioxins, or polycyclic aromatic hydrocarbons (PAHs), which are a result of fires or petroleum production. All have been associated with risks to health and to diseases, such as cancer; these substances have been found in the breast milk of women living near a contaminated water source (Courter, Pereira, & Baird, 2007; Sudaryanto et al., 2006). Water is vulnerable to contamination at many points through animal or human feces at the source (surface water), chemical runoff from nearby industries and farms (groundwater), and improper purification procedures. Contaminated water supply results in death, as occurred in the United States (Milwaukee, 1993) and Canada (Walkerton, 2000).

The principles of safe drinking water are prevention of contamination, water treatment, and clean storage for use. The best source of water for drinking is piped from a central clean supply either to individual households or to community centres where people can easily access water for their use.

Sanitation is the treatment and disposal of waste products making them safe for public health. Sanitation is divided into two main activities: (a) wastewater treatment and (b) solid waste disposal. Wastewater treatment is the management of human sewage; solid waste management includes garbage collection and disposal.

The safe disposal of human feces to prevent contamination of soil is important to reduce the spread of diarrheal disease, intestinal nematodes, and hookworms. These parasites cause malnutrition and anemia in infected individuals. Parasites may be ingested in soil or in uncooked food that is contaminated. Sanitation of human waste is achieved using a latrine, septic tank, or piped system to a sewage treatment plant. The simplest is storage, usually in a pit latrine or outhouse; the mostly solid waste is stored until the pit is full, at which time the solids must be removed or a new pit must be prepared. Improvements have been made to improve privacy and ventilation (Markle, Fisher, & Smego, 2007). Septic tanks are often used around the world in rural communities; they handle larger quantities of human waste and are efficient and effective over longer periods. They work well in low-density housing locations, such as rural areas, and require little maintenance (Markle et al., 2007). The most efficient method of managing human waste comprises collection systems that use large sewer pipes conveying the waste material to a treatment plant. The raw sewage is processed through a number of phases enhanced with disinfection procedures, which allows the fluid content to be returned to surface water supplies and the separated solids to be further processed for soil enrichment or as crop fertilizer.

Solid waste management (garbage removal and disposal) is also important, and in many communities across the developing world, this means collecting these materials and burning them, even when they include materials that create toxic fumes and smoke. In many countries, sorting garbage into various components for recycling is an important diversion strategy to reduce landfills. Landfills have generated public resistance, as they pose a risk for harmful substances leaking into surrounding soil and water tables.

Access to safe drinking water and sanitation systems is important in promoting human health. Globally, children, Indigenous peoples, and those living in rural and remote areas or in urban slums are most at risk of living with inadequate access to safe drinking water or sanitation.

Air Pollution

Indoor and outdoor air **pollution** each cause respiratory illnesses, particularly among children, older adults, and those with compromised health.

Globally, indoor pollution is primarily caused by the use of biofuels for cooking and heating with inadequate ventilation in homes (Birn et al., 2009b; UNEP, 2010). Biofuels include wood, coal, and dried animal dung. Women and young children are the most commonly affected and have high rates of acute and chronic respiratory illnesses. Other causes of indoor pollution include tobacco smoke, industrial processes, and toxic chemicals in paint, wood finishes, and cleaning chemicals.

A few approaches are already bringing about reductions in indoor pollution. Simple, inexpensive, improved cooking stoves are being distributed in many developing countries to reduce indoor pollution among most of the affected population. Smoking is prohibited in public settings in many developed and developing countries. Paints and wood finishes are produced without noxious chemicals, and safety filtration masks are readily available for those who must use paints and wood finishes.

Outdoor pollution is more pervasive and causes chronic obstructive pulmonary disease (COPD). Outdoor pollution is produced largely by industry, emissions from vehicles, power generation, new allergens following forest clearing, and such natural events as volcanic eruptions. Some of the worst air quality is found in Linfen, China (Birn et al., 2009a, 2009b), mainly from coal-based industry, which is associated with acute respiratory infections and lung cancer. Plans to remediate this situation include the replacement of 200 industrial plants in the region.

Controls on car emissions, garbage burning, and industrial exhausts are important strategies for improving air quality. However, with a rapidly expanding airline industry, aircraft exhaust is a growing concern as is the expanding automobile markets in India and China. Cleaner fuels are more important than ever if outdoor air quality is to be improved and sustained.

Environmental factors are interactive and difficult to separate for independent actions. Their effects are pervasive and affect many millions of people globally, usually those who are already vulnerable because of age, location, or income. Successful resolution of these problems requires intersectoral and intergovernmental cooperation and collaboration. Nurses and other health care professionals have roles and responsibilities as citizens and professionals working for global health in health promotion, illness prevention, and public health.

Global Health versus International Health: What Is the Difference?

For many decades the terms "international health," "health geography," and "tropical medicine" were used to describe this growing field (Brown, Cueto, & Fee, 2006).

While "international health" is still very much in use, those who work internationally are increasingly using the term "global health" to characterize their field of activity.

The term "**international health**" literally means "health status among nations" and has emphasized differences among countries rather than their commonalities. It is historically a concept more focused on the control of epidemics in developing countries that require nation-to-nation solutions, such as foreign aid and medical missionary work, rather than on collective action (Global Health Education Consortium, 2011).

The term "**global health**" refers to health issues and concerns that typically transcend national borders (Brown et al., 2006), class, race, ethnicity, and culture. The term acknowledges the ongoing process of the integration of national economies, societies, and cultures and emphasizes the commonality of health issues that require collective action. It has been defined as "the area of study, research and practice that places a priority on improving health and achieving equity in health for all people worldwide" (Koplan, Bond, Merson, Reddy, Rodriguez, Sewankambo, & Wasserheit, 2009, p. 1995). The term "global" is also associated with the growing importance of actors beyond governmental or intergovernmental organizations and such agencies as the media, internationally influential foundations, nongovernmental organizations, and transnational corporations (Macfarlane, Jacobs, & Kaaya, 2008).

The major international agency for health is the World Health Organization (WHO). Other important agencies are the United Nations Development Program (UNDP, 1992) and the World Bank, which are introduced later. A major initiative for improved global health is the United Nations Millennium Declaration, which includes the globally endorsed *Millennium Development Goals* (Patel & Prince, 2010). (See Weblinks for Canadian Nurses Association position statement.)

Global Health: Historical Perspective

The collective personal health of a population is defined as *public health*. At the turn of the twentieth century, the life expectancy for a citizen living in Canada was 47 years for a male and 50 years for a female, and the five leading causes of death were (a) influenza and pneumonia, (b) tuberculosis, (c) diarrhea and enteritis, (d) heart disease, and (e) stroke (Norris & Williams, 2000). The median lifespan for persons residing in the less developed regions of the world was even lower, and most public health problems largely were infections. Now, more than 100 years later, the health of populations globally has dramatically improved. In 2011, the average Japanese is living as long as 82 years, the average Canadian 80 years, and the average Costa Rican 77 years. Even in impoverished parts of Africa, Asia, and

Latin America, tremendous public health gains were seen in the twentieth century. Unfortunately, poverty and political strife have resulted in undermining these improvements. As of 2011, the average life expectancy of a person in Afghanistan is 45 years, in Zimbabwe 47.5 years, and in Guatemala 68 years. Longevity in Africa has been severely limited by the ongoing human immuno-deficiency virus/acquired immunodeficiency syndrome (HIV/AIDS) pandemic. For example, the life expec-tancy for a Ugandan man has decreased from 47.4 years (1980–1985) to 39.7 years (1985–1990) to 38.9 years (1995–2000) (Watkins, 2005).

Globally, populations seem to be trading one set of diseases for another. In many countries, improved socioeconomic and public health conditions that led to a reduction in infectious disease-related morbidity and mortality have, however, resulted in the introduction of lifestyle-related diseases, such as obesity, coronary artery disease, hypertension, and other diseases related to excessive eating, smoking, alcohol consumption, and illicit drug use. Scientific, social, cultural, economic, and political factors all contribute to the overall wellness of a community, whether local or international. The impact of disease-oriented medical care on the overall health status of a country is relatively small compared with the collective contributions made by improved living condi-tions, including better nutrition, sanitation, housing, education, and income.

Epidemiological Transition

According to the theory postulated by Omran in 1971, an **epidemiological transition** occurs as a country under-goes the process of modernization from third-world status to first-world status (Omran, 2005). The develop-ment of cleaner water and better nutrition drastically reduces infant mortality rates and extends the average life expectancy, which, coupled with subsequent declines in fertility rates, reflects a shift from infectious diseases to chronic and degenerative diseases as more important causes of death.

Classification of Countries

For purposes of thinking in a global context, there are approximately 200 countries in the world. There are many ways of organizing or classifying these countries; by income, by level of development, and by geogra-phy. Such terms as "Western World," "First World" and "Third World" are well known. The term "developing country" is generally used to describe a nation with a low level of material well-being. There is no international definition of the term "developed country," and levels of development may vary widely within the so-called devel-oped countries (e.g., certain population groups that do not share in the prosperity of the mainstream). In

addition, some so-called developing countries have high average standards of living (e.g., South Korea, Brazil). All of these terms may be perceived as negative stereo-typing, so some have suggested that classification on a North–South axis would be more accurate. The North is home to all members of the G8 wealthiest democra-cies. "The North" mostly covers the West and the so-called First World as well as much of the Second World (former Communist countries). Although the terms "North" and "South" are in common use, they lack pre-cision as a method of classifying countries. As nations become more economically developed and integrated, they become part of the global economy regardless of geographical location.

Nation States Classified by Income

For analytical purposes, the World Bank's main criterion for classifying its 187 member countries is gross national income (GNI) per person per year. On the basis of GNI, every country is classified as high-income, middle-income (subdivided into lower-middle and upper-middle), or low-income (World Bank, 2011) countries. In addition, there are two elite groups classified as major industrial-ized democracies (the G8) and the world's top major economies (the G20). Canada belongs to both groups. (See http://data.worldbank.org/about/country. classifications.)

In 2008, the richest fifth of the world's popula-tion received 82.7% of the total world income, whereas the poorest fifth received merely 1.4%. Just 1% of the world's adults owned 40% of the wealth, whereas 50% of the world's adults owned just 1% of the wealth (Davies, Sandström, Shorrocks, & Wolff, 2008). Almost half the world (>3 billion people) lived on less than $2.50 a day (Chen & Ravallion, 2008). Nearly one in four people (1.3 billion) lived on less than $1 per day, whereas, in 2007, the world's 358 billionaires had assets exceeding the combined annual incomes of countries with 45% of the world's people (UNDP, 2007). Figure 10.1 provides a dramatic illustration of "the champagne glass distribu-tion" of the world's population by income divided into 20% increments (quintiles) (Conley, 2008).

Countries Organized by Religion

When one thinks of "culture," one can think of language groupings, nationality, religious traditions, and ethni-city. The world's principal religions and spiritual tra-ditions may be classified into a small number of major groups, arranged by historical origin and mutual influ-ence. Abrahamic religions originated in the Middle East, Indian religions in India, and Far Eastern religions in East Asia. Another group with supraregional influence are African diasporic religions, which have their origins in Central and West Africa.

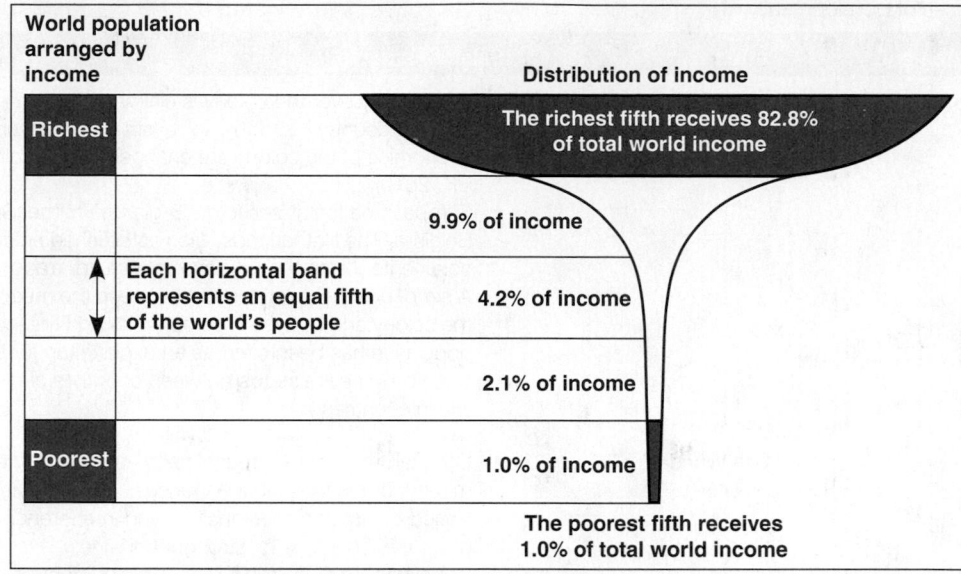

FIGURE 10.1 Champagne glass distribution of income for world populations

Source: Ortiz, I. & Cummins M. (2011). Global inequality: Beyond the bottom billion - a rapid review of income distribution in 141 countries. *UNICEF Social and Economic Policy Working Paper* (p. 6). New York, NY: UNICEF

Countries Organized by Language

There are more than 2700 languages in the world. Some of the top languages by population are the six official languages of the United Nations: Arabic, Chinese (Mandarin), English, French, Russian, and Spanish. English is currently one of the most widely spoken and written languages worldwide. The impact of **colonialism** and the continued influence of Western power have contributed to making European languages dominant in many parts of the world.

Theories of Development

The observation that some countries are wealthier (and healthier) than others has spawned a host of theories to explain such differences, a few of the better known ones are presented in Table 10.4 on the next page.

Regardless of which theories are used to describe or explain why some countries are wealthier and healthier than others, the inevitable fact is that the world is becoming increasingly more integrated, there has been an increase in overall life expectancy (Markle et al., 2007), and calls for social justice and equity are rising in every corner of the world. It can be argued that only when humanity tackles issues that confront all people globally will global solutions become possible.

Millennium Development Goals

During the 2000 Millennium Summit, all state members of the United Nations approved the United Nations Millennium Declaration, which asserts that all individuals have the right to dignity, equality, freedom, a basic standard of living that includes freedom from hunger and violence, and encourages tolerance and solidarity (United Nations, 2001). Among the several commitments stated in the declaration was the commitment to significantly reduce poverty and promote development by reducing economic and social conditions in the world's poorest countries. Eight **Millennium Development Goals (MDGs)** were identified to operationalize this priority area between 1990 and 2015. See Table 10.5 on page 191.

The government of Canada, along with other nations, has demonstrated commitment to achieving these goals, particularly in the areas of maternal, newborn, and child health; education; gender equality; and food security (Canadian International Development Agency [CIDA], 2010).

CAPACITY BUILDING In health, capacity building aims at developing new structures, approaches, or values to address the health challenges of the population (Crisp, Swerissen, & Duckett, 2000). **Capacity building** is a long-term, continual process of development that involves all stakeholders in a population, and uses a country's human, scientific, technological, and organizational resources and capabilities (United Nations, 2006). For capacity building to be successful, the interventions must be addressed at the individual, institutional, and societal levels and at both the local and international levels. Individually, people build capacity by enhancing existing knowledge and skills. Education and health are closely related in development; as people become more knowledgeable about their health, they are more able to care for themselves, and thus the burden of disease is reduced (Todaro & Smith, 2009c). At institutional and societal levels, capacity building can be achieved by strengthening existing organizations, through supporting the development of sound policies, organizational structures, and

TABLE 10.4 Theories of Development

Theory of Development	Period	Salient Features
Colonialism	15th–20th centuries	• Sovereignty over the colony is claimed by the metropole or "mother country," and the social structure, government, and economics of the colony are changed by the colonists (Collins UK, 2010). • European nation states (e.g., England, France, Spain, Portugal, Belgium, The Netherlands, etc.) established colonies on other continents (Africa, Asia, Latin America) for trade. • A set of unequal relationships between the metropole and the colony and between the colonists and the Indigenous population has been cited as an explanation for extreme variation in health status between countries and certain groups within countries.
Neocolonialism	Post–World War II (1945–1960)	• Colonialism by other means, such as economic arrangements, military, or technological influences. • Based on unequal relationships and interference in the politics of weaker countries by stronger countries. • Certain forms of foreign aid or "development assistance" have amounted to neocolonialism. • Has also been used as a label to describe governmental social policy or attitude toward certain groups within countries.
Modernization Theory	18th century–present day	• Used to explain the process of improvements made within societies. • Looks at internal dynamics while referring to social and cultural structures and the adaptation of new technologies. • Assumes that with assistance, "traditional" countries and societies can be brought to "development" in the same manner that wealthier countries have (e.g., from hunting and gathering, to subsistence farming, to an industrial revolution, to the knowledge economy). • Criticized by communist ideologies, world systems theorists, globalization theorists, and dependency theorists, among others.
Linear Stages of Growth (also called Rostow's Stages of Growth) Model (Rostow, 1960)	1960s–1980s	• Developed by Walt W. Rostow, an American economist. • Economic modernization occurs in five fairly linear stages of varying lengths: (a) traditional society, (b) preconditions for takeoff, (c) takeoff, (d) drive to maturity, and (e) age of high mass consumption (Todaro & Smith, 2009a). • Economic "takeoff" must initially be led by a few individual sectors, such as agriculture, transportation, and manufacturing. • Criticized by Marxists, who push for economic self-reliance and development of all sectors equally, including the education and health sectors.
Dependency Theory	1970s–present day	• Resources flow from a "periphery" of poor and underdeveloped states to a "core" of wealthy states, enriching the latter at the expense of the former (Dos Santos, 1971). • Poor states are impoverished and rich ones enriched by the way poor states are integrated into the "world system." • The task in helping underdeveloped areas out of poverty is to accelerate them along a supposed common path of development, by such means as investment, technology transfers, and closer integration into the world market. • Opposes free market economists and modernization theorists. • "Underdeveloped" countries need to reduce their connectedness with the world market so that they can pursue a path more in keeping with their own needs, less dictated by external pressures (Todaro & Smith, 2009b).

TABLE 10.5 Millennium Development Goals

1. Eradicate extreme poverty and hunger 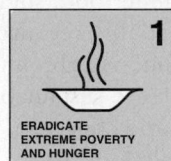	Reducing by half the proportion of the world's population suffering from hunger and those whose income is less than 1 dollar a day and achieving full and productive employment for all, including women and young people.
2. Achieve universal primary education 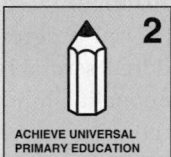	Ensuring that children in the world, girls and boys alike, will be able to complete a full course of primary schooling and will have equal access to all levels of education.
3. Promote gender equality and empower women 	Eliminating gender disparity in primary and secondary education as an effective way to stimulate sustainable development as women are still the poorest of the world's poor (United Nations, 2006).
4. Reduce child mortality 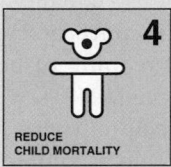	Reducing by two-thirds the under-5 mortality rate, a 4% reduction per year (You, Jones, & Wardlaw, 2010) and increasing the proportion of 1-year-old children immunized against measles.
5. Improve maternal health 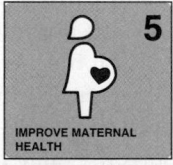	Reducing by three-quarters the maternal mortality ratio and achieving universal access to reproductive health.
6. Combat HIV/AIDS, malaria, and other diseases 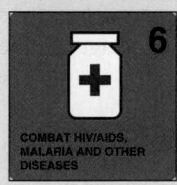	Halting and beginning to reverse the spread of HIV/AIDS, the incidence of malaria, and other major diseases. This will be achieved through universal access to treatment for these diseases.
7. Ensure environmental sustainability 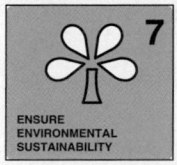	Reducing the loss of biodiversity and environmental resources, reducing by half the proportion of people without sustainable access to safe drinking water and basic sanitation, and achieving a significant improvement in the levels of at least 100 million slum dwellers.
8. Global partnership for development 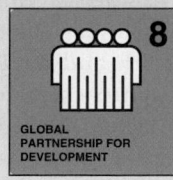	Identifying targets for aid, trade, and debt relief.

Source: Adapted from United Nations. (2011). *The Millennium Development Goals report (United Nations, 2006) and a gateway to the UN System's work on the MDGs.* Geneva, Switzerland: United Nations.

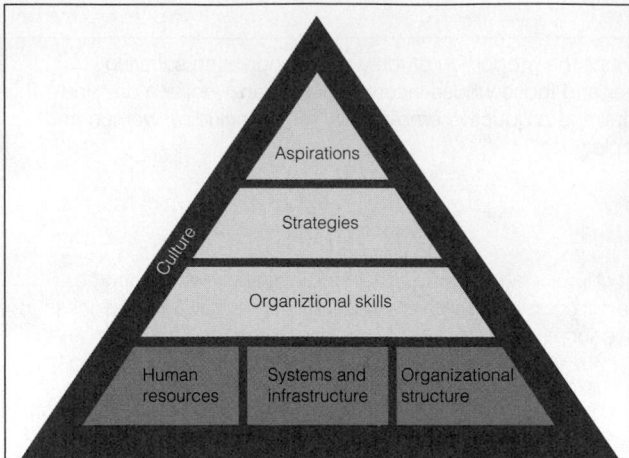

Aspirations: An organization's mission, vision, and overarching goals, which collectively articulate its common sense of purpose and direction

Strategy: The coherent set of actions and programs aimed at fulfilling the organization's overarching goals

Organizational Skills: The sum of the organization's capabilities, including performance measurement, planning, resource management, and external relationship building

Human Resources: The collective capabilities, experiences, potential and commitment of the organization's board, management team, staff, and volunteers

Systems and Infrastructure: The organization's planning, decision making, knowledge management, and administrative systems, as well as the physical and technological assets that support the organization

Organizational Structure: The combination of governance, organizational design, interfunctional coordination, and individual job descriptions that shapes the organization's legal and management structure

Culture: The connective tissue that binds together the organization, including shared values and practices, behaviour norms, and, most important, the organization's orientation toward performance.

FIGURE 10.2 Capacity building framework

effective methods of management. Both governmental and nongovernmental organizations (NGOs) have active roles in global capacity building. The key is that people, organizations, and societies develop partnerships in pursuit of the same goal and use a framework to aid their success (see Figure 10.2).

SUSTAINABILITY Similar to capacity building, the concept of **sustainability** in global health refers to the long-term maintenance of developed programs in a society. Sustainable development, as described by the United Nations World Commission on Environment and Development (WCED) (also known as the Brundtland Commission), is "development that meets the needs of the present without compromising the ability of future generations to meet their own needs" (WCED, 1987). People's basic needs include food, shelter, health, and protection, and when available resources cannot meet any of these needs, a condition of absolute underdevelopment occurs. Thus, to achieve sustainable development, a process of change must be consistent with future and present needs of the population.

The main indicators of sustainable development are environmental (water, land, atmosphere, and waste), economic, institutional, and social progress (Bell & Morse, 2008). These indicators address several interrelated global issues, such as poverty, inequality, hunger, and environmental degradation. Alleviation of poverty is a major hurdle to achieve sustainability and is considered a major cause of global health problems (Lusigi, 2008). Sustainability of health is important for reducing mortality, morbidity, and disability, especially in poor and marginalized populations, and is achieved through specific strategies that target health issues and create health systems that unfold over time (Yang, Farmer, & McGahan, 2010).

SOCIAL JUSTICE The concept of **social justice** is based on the principles of equity, equality, and respect for human rights. It is broadly concerned with the equitable bearing of burdens and reaping of benefits in society (Drevdahl, Dorcy, & Grevstad, 2001).

In health care, the focus of social justice is the allocation of health care resources and equitable access to these resources, as well as the broader determinants of health. The disparity in health status of virtually all populations in terms of their socioeconomic status, gender, race or ethnicity, and geographical location makes it necessary to identify and intervene within these determinants (Canadian Institutes of Health Research, 2005).

Nursing actively supports the value of social justice in health through national and **international nursing** associations' mandates. The Canadian Nurses Association (CNA) *Code of Ethics* states the following: "Nurses uphold principles of equity and fairness to assist persons in receiving a share of health services and resources proportionate to their needs and in promoting social justice" (CNA, 2008).

Major Issues in Global Health

Major issues in global health are related to the circumstances in which people live, their behaviour, and the environment. These factors, the determinants of health, were described more than 30 years ago, when the need for a focus on public health and primary health care was identified as the best approach to improve health in Canada (Lalonde, 1974). These ideas were reaffirmed by the declaration of Alma Ata a few years later (1978), which added that health is a fundamental human right and called on governments, the WHO, and others to act (WHO, 1978). The Commission on Social Determinants of Health (CSDH) described the impact of **the social determinants of health** and the link to health inequities within and between nations (CSDH, 2008).

> *The poor health of the poor, the social gradient in health within countries, and the marked health inequities between countries are caused by the unequal distribution of power, income, goods, and services, globally and nationally, the consequent unfairness in the immediate, visible circumstances of people's lives—their access to health care, schools, and education, their conditions of work and leisure, their homes, communities, towns, or cities—and their chances of leading a flourishing life.*

These differences in health status of populations are areas for action; many examples of successful change and ongoing problems are presented in the report of the Commission for the Social Determinants of Health (Marmot & Friel, 2008).

Migration

In global terms, **migration** means the movement of people, usually from one country to another. It is increasing, and at present, there are an estimated 214 million international migrants worldwide (International Office of Migration, 2011). Migration brings many benefits to the receiving countries, such as new ideas, skills, and resilience. Migrants stimulate local economies as they establish themselves in their community.

There are a few important distinctions among migrants. Voluntary migrants move for many reasons, primarily to improve their circumstances. Significant numbers of business class or skilled workers, including health care professionals, migrate to other countries to improve their opportunities (Dumont & Widmaier, 2010). Forced migrants include refugees and asylum seekers, who are unable to remain in their country of origin because they are at risk from war, persecution, or natural disasters. They are usually not able to return to their homeland until significant changes occur.

The 1951 Refugee Convention establishing the United Nations High Commission for Refugees (UNHCR) states that a refugee is someone who:

> *owing to a well-founded fear of being persecuted for reasons of race, religion, nationality, membership of a particular social group or political opinion, is outside the country of his nationality, and is unable to, or owing to such fear, is unwilling to avail himself of the protection of that country.* (UNHCR, 2012)

The majority of refugees (approximately 80%) live in neighbouring countries to their country of origin

(Baba Fall, Das, Kintu, Wilkinson, Zhdanov, & Zuefle, 2009; UNHCR, 2012). Canada is a destination or receiving country for immigrants and refugees. This means that nurses and health care professionals will care for people with different beliefs and expectations and whose needs will relate to their migration history. Evidence suggests that access to health care (Gagnon, 2004; Wahoush, 2009) and health vary by immigration status (Gagnon et al., 2007; Newbold, 2005; Newbold, 2009). Nurses in Canada must be proficient in caring for culturally diverse populations (see Chapter 11) and understand the additional impact of migration on expectations for health.

Indigenous Peoples

Indigenous peoples, or Aboriginal populations, are described by the WHO as:

> *. . . communities that live within, or are attached to, geographically distinct traditional habitats or ancestral territories, and who identify themselves as being part of a distinct cultural group, descended from groups present in the area before colonists arrived, modern states were created and current borders defined. They generally maintain cultural and social identities, and social, economic, cultural and political institutions, separate from the mainstream or dominant society or culture* (WHO, 2011a)

This description does not mention the forcible displacement that is characteristic of many Indigenous populations with loss of land and sometimes catastrophic lifestyle changes. Globally, there are approximately 350 million Indigenous people living in more than 70 countries. They are often marginalized and experience poorer health than the general population. For example, infant mortality is almost always higher among Indigenous populations (see Figure 10.3 on the next page) (Stephens, Porter, Nettleton, & Willis, 2006). Although Indigenous populations around the world are diverse, they experience similar health issues and determinants of health (Gracey & King, 2009; King, Smith, & Gracey, 2009). Many live in isolated communities with limited access to services, water, and sanitation and experience inadequate nutrition and poverty.

In Canada, Indigenous peoples include First Nations, Inuit, and Métis. Like many other Indigenous populations, they experience poorer health compared with the general population. Suicide, diabetes, and premature deaths occur more frequently than in the general population (Gracey & King, 2009; WHO, 2011a). Health Canada has targeted improved health outcomes and reduction in health inequalities between First Nations, Inuit, and other Canadians as a priority (see Chapter 11). A global perspective of Indigenous health can be found in the *Lancet* series (Gracey & King, 2009; King et al., 2009).

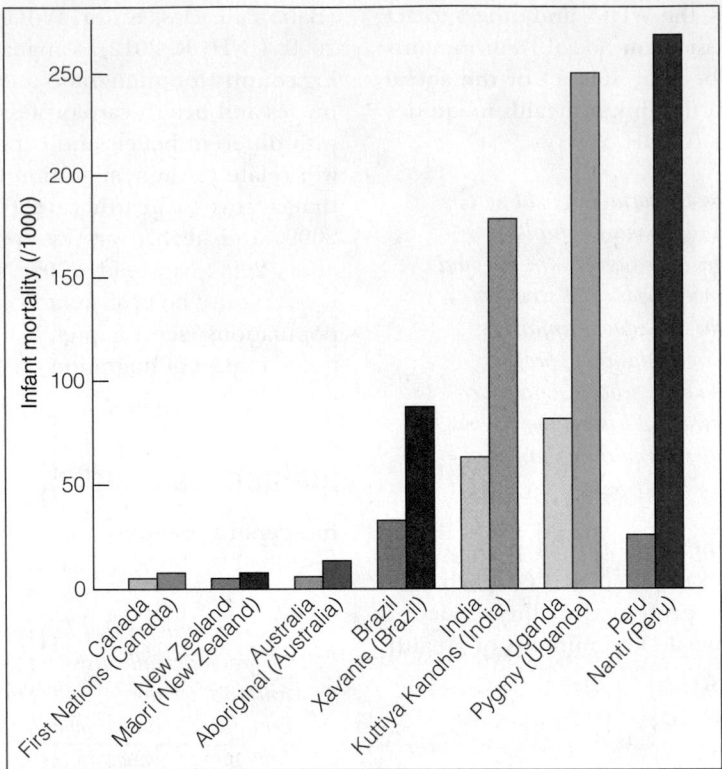

FIGURE 10.3 Infant mortality among Indigenous populations across the globe

Source: Reprinted from *The Lancet*, 367.9527, C. Stephens, J. Porter, C. Nettleton, & R. Willis, "Disappearing, displaced, and undervalued: A call to action for indigenous health worldwide," pp. 2019–2028, Copyright © 2006 with permission from Elsevier.

Poverty and Inequality

Poverty is a complex concept with many definitions; in this chapter, poverty means more than low income. Our definition includes the limited choices and opportunities that are often associated with low income, that is, limited choices with regard to where people live, food, and recreational activities. Measuring poverty is also challenging but is necessary to evaluate changes over time and differences between groups or populations. Comparisons between countries are possible using a purchasing power parity (PPP) estimate in dollars. This estimate is calculated such that differences in currency values are accounted for and the measure focuses on what it takes to buy the same bundle of goods in different countries.

The World Bank defines extreme poverty as having an average daily consumption of $1.25 or less; this means living on the edge of subsistence (World Bank, 2010). Globally, poverty rates are declining, but the improvements are not universal, and the proportion of those living in deep poverty remains largely unchanged (Chen & Ravallion, 2008). Between 1980 and 2005, almost half of the population in Sub-Saharan Africa lived in extreme poverty, and in Southeast Asia, extreme poverty was significantly reduced from 80% to 20%. Poverty is implicated in the death of more than 10 million children annually. Children growing up poor face many challenges that

have negative consequences for their health in adulthood and their future earning power, which affects their living standard, health, and well-being and the material circumstances of their future children.

In developed countries, income inequality is more damaging to health and well-being than low income alone (Marmot, Friel, Bell, Houweling, & Taylor, 2008). Income inequality, which was reduced in many countries during the mid-1990s, is increasing again, and in Canada, it is now above the OECD (Organisation for Economic Co-operation and Development) average (Gurria, 2008). Globally, Indigenous peoples, recent immigrants, and women, especially those in single-parent households, are most at risk of low income and the associated risks of poor living conditions and homelessness. They are also less likely to move out of poverty.

The current global economic downturn is a concern for everyone; as countries are forced to reorganize their financial systems, trade and the prices of goods will be negatively affected. Social programs and other supports for families and those living in poverty may be cut or reduced or may fail to keep up with the growing needs that are anticipated during a recession. Many countries across Europe and the United States currently facing these challenges are also major trading partners with Canada. The consequences of economically restrained economies will likely affect everyone, in particular those living in poverty and many working families within the affected countries and within their trading partner countries.

Food Security

The WHO (2011b) considers that **food security** exists "when all people at all times have access to sufficient, safe, nutritious food to maintain a healthy and active life." Food security is based on three pillars: (a) *food availability,* or having sufficient amount of food available on a consistent basis; (b) *food access,* or having sufficient amount of resources, both physical and economic, to obtain appropriate and nutritious food; and (c) *food use,* or the appropriate use of available food based on knowledge of basic nutrition and adequate water and sanitation. If one of these three pillars is affected, then food security is at risk. There are many factors that jeopardize food security in the world; however, poverty is the major contributor to food insecurity, leading to hunger and malnutrition. Around 1.2 billion people in the world are chronically hungry due to extreme poverty, and up to 2 billion people lack food security intermittently due to varying degrees of poverty (Food and Agriculture Organization [FAO], 2009).

Food safety is also important in maintaining health. Food can become contaminated with biological and chemical agents, causing adverse effects on health. Currently, the most common threats to food safety are pesticides, industrial chemicals and metals, allergens, bacteria, viruses and parasites, natural toxins, veterinary drugs, and food additives. That is why it is important that food safety regulatory agencies such as the Canadian Food Inspection Agency (CFIA) in Canada ensure that food is safe for consumption (Chassy, 2010).

Disasters

Disasters are situations where the normal infrastructure is severely disrupted on a large scale, necessitating external help to enable people to live their lives in safety and health. Many die at the time of the disaster and others continue to die later because of longer-term impacts of disease and contamination from the event. **Natural disasters** are often climate related. They include storm systems, such as typhoons that cause severe and extensive floods; extreme weather conditions, such as heat waves or extreme cold; earthquakes; and drought. The March 2011 earthquake in Japan is an example of how a natural disaster can have significant impact well beyond national borders, as the resulting tsunami damaged a nuclear power plant, causing radiation leakage into the air and seawater.

Disasters generally include the disruption of normal services, including access to clean water, sanitation, school or work, and health care services. Organizations providing help on the large scale needed include national governments, International Red Cross, Save

the Children, Oxfam International, and Médecins Sans Frontières. Initial activities focus on providing temporary shelter, clean water, and latrines and on assessment of the extent of damage and need for help in the immediate as well as longer term. Disaster relief teams are multidisciplinary and often include nurses along with other health care professionals, logistics support personnel, engineers, skilled workers, and volunteers. The Disaster Assistance Response Team (DART) includes 200 members of the Canadian forces, who arrive quickly and establish mechanisms for safe drinking water, shelter, safety, and urgent health care and eventually leave to allow space for other personnel engaged in longer-term relief activities.

Infectious Diseases and Surveillance

In global health terms, monitoring disease outbreaks and threats to public health is a priority for the global community; 194 countries have committed to implementing global rules to improve global health security. This monitoring is called **surveillance**. The International Health Regulations (IHRs) developed these rules after the severe acute respiratory syndrome (SARS) outbreak in Canada. An international example is the global monitoring of the H1N1 virus (WHO, 2008). The Public Health Agency of Canada (PHAC) is responsible for the implementation of the IHRs and leads the Emergency Preparedness Response in Canada (PHAC, 2008).

Gender

Gender may not relate to the biological sex distinction of the individual alone but refers to the socially constructed roles, behaviour, activities, and attributes that a particular society considers appropriate for men and women (WHO, 2009b). Inequities between men and women exist in many societies, often with men enjoying better health compared with women. Yet women live longer than men in almost every country; this means that life expectancy is not the best measure of health when exploring gender issues. Measuring gender inequalities is difficult, but two measures that assess different but complementary aspects of gender are widely used: (a) the Gender Inequalities Index and (b) the Social Institutions and Gender Index.

The Gender Inequalities Index (GII) compares outcomes for women against those for men within a nation (Klugman, 2010); the score represents women's loss of potential for human development in comparison with men within the same country. This new experimental measure includes features of reproductive health, empowerment, and labour market participation at national levels, comparing men and women on these aspects of life. The world average GII score is 0.56, which means that 56% of potential human development is lost because of discrimination against women; the score for Canada is 0.289 (Klugman, 2010; Varkey & Gupta, 2005).

In contrast, the Social Institutions and Gender Index (SIGI) is a measure of gender equality. Developed by the OECD (Branisa, Klasen, & Zeigler, 2009), SIGI employs different indicators or factors at the root of gender inequity. Factors include measures of civil liberty, decision-making power, exposure to violence, male offspring preference, and ownership rights. Scores range from 0 to 1; a lower number indicates less discrimination against women compared with higher scores. In 2009, using this scale, the OECD reported that Paraquay (0.00248) had the lowest and that Sudan (0.67781) had the highest level of discrimination against women (OECD, 2010).

These measurements are significant, as they provide a mechanism to evaluate changes over time and to compare countries. Most important, readers need to understand what each measure includes and to use more than one to get a clearer picture of gender equity and inequality.

Women's Health

Women in low-income countries face high levels of mortality, associated with poor nutrition, unsafe water, poor sanitation, smoke from solid-fuel stoves, and lack of care during pregnancy and childbearing. This section will focus on reproductive health, as reproductive health is the most significant factor in gender inequality.

Many of the causes of death and illness in the childbearing years, such as HIV/AIDs, complications of pregnancy and childbirth, and vesicovaginal fistula, are preventable with simple improvements in care during and after pregnancy (Lester, Benfield, & Fathalla, 2010). Risks to women's health in the childbearing years impact more than the health of women; they have negative consequences for their children, families, and communities. Poor nutrition, infectious diseases, and limited access to health care are associated with low-birth-weight infants, and women in low-income countries often experience all three. Low-birth-weight infants have increased risk of death or poor health in the long term.

Maternal Health Guideline 5 (MDG 5) is now part of a global strategy to improve women's and children's health. Almost all (98%) of the more than a half million maternal deaths occur in 68 priority countries, with little progress on improvements to date. The most common causes of maternal death include hypertension, hemorrhage, sepsis, and other direct causes (e.g., those related to cesarean section and anesthesia). Improvement in the ratio of maternal deaths globally has been slow, going from 430 down to 400 per 1 000 000 births from 1990 to 2005 (Lester et al., 2010). Interventions to achieve sustainable reduced rates of maternal mortality are similar to those in Box 10.1, along with four prenatal checks. In low-income and middle-income countries, almost three-quarters of pregnant women had at least one antenatal check, but this rate drops to less than half for pregnant women in Sub-Saharan Africa. Births attended by a skilled

---

BOX 10.1 WHY INVESTING IN WOMEN'S AND CHILDREN'S HEALTH MAKES SENSE

To reduce poverty and improve a country's overall well-being:

- Research confirms that a health system that delivers reproductive health care is a strong system that delivers for everyone.
- A woman's poor health often pushes her family further into poverty.
- Children born to women who have had at least 5 years of education are 40% more likely to live past age 5 years.

To enable families to thrive:

- A mother's death or disability greatly raises the chances her newborn and her other children will die before age 5 years.
- Women connect their families and communities, instilling cultural and social values.
- It helps women and children to realize their fundamental human rights.
- Women's health and children's health are inextricably linked to meeting the other Millennium Development Goals (MDGs).

The principal strategies to reduce maternal mortality include the following:

- Improved nutrition and education of girls—improved physical health; growth and development
- Gender equality and women's empowerment—enables choices by women
- Reducing adolescent pregnancies—deferred age of marriage and access to contraception
- Promoting access to contraception—enables birth spacing, reduces unwanted pregnancies, and limits unsafe abortions
- Skilled birth attendants—evidence-based practice promoted via the Integrated Management of Pregnancy and Childbirth (IMPAC)
- Postbirth care for mother and infant

Source: Ki-Moon, B. (2010). Investing in our common future: Global strategy for women's and children's health. Retrieved from http://www.who.int/pmnch/topics/maternal/201009_globalstrategy_wch/en/index.html

---

birth attendant increased from 41% to 65.7% from 1996 to 2008, but varied with the much lower rates in Eastern Africa (33.7%), Western Africa (41.2%), and South Central Asia (46.9%) (WHO, 2009b; WHO, 2009c).

Progress is also hampered by the shortage of skilled health care providers (doctors, nurses, and midwives). See the Evidence-Informed Practice box on the provision of essential newborn care (ENC) training to midwives (on the next page). The WHO estimates that approximately 700,000 midwives are needed to achieve the goal of skilled care at every birth. Migration of skilled health care providers to urban settings, the private sector, or out of the country further hampers progress. Improvements that have been achieved in some countries demonstrate that improvements are possible.

EVIDENCE-INFORMED PRACTICE

Is the Provision of Essential Newborn Care (ENC) Training to Midwives a Cost-Effective Intervention to Reduce Neonatal Mortality in Zambia?

Manasyan, Chomba, McClure, Krzywanski, and Carlo (2011) conducted a cost-effectiveness analysis to evaluate whether the training of midwives who worked in first-level (primary care, low-risk) health facilities in Zambia and participated in the WHO ENC (essential newborn care) course on 7-day neonatal mortality was effective in reducing early neonatal mortality (ENM) rates. Eighteen college-trained midwives were certified as ENC instructors after a 5-day ENC training-of-trainer course. The course included universal precautions, routine neonatal care, resuscitation, prevention of hypothermia, early and exclusive breast-feeding, "kangaroo care," small infant management, danger signs, and recognition of illness. These instructors were responsible for training a total of 123 midwives in each of the 18 delivery clinics in two urban areas. The effect of training was calculated by comparing ENM rates before and after ENC training. It was found that all-cause 7-day neonatal mortality decreased from 11.5/1000 to 6.8/1000 live births after ENC training. This was indicative of 97 lives being saved. With Zambia's gross domestic product (GDP) of $1500, the intervention cost was calculated to be $208 per life saved.

NURSING IMPLICATIONS: The WHO developed the ENC course, as neonatal deaths in the first 7 days are significantly higher in developing countries than in the industrialized world. Nurses in developing countries benefit from this type of training, as they are often the first health care team member that expecting mothers would see in a care facility and as they also work closely with midwives or receive midwifery training. In addition, this training-the-trainer approach allows for knowledge transfer to occur between nurses and nursing students. Having knowledge of the different topics offered by this course would be an empowering asset for nursing students. In Canada, the low cost of this intervention would make it possible to use it in limited resource settings.

Source: Based on Manasyan, A., Chomba, E., McClure, E. M., Krzywanski, S., & Carlo, W. A. (2011). Cost-effectiveness of essential newborn care training in urban first-level facilities. *Pediatrics, 127*(5), e1176–e1181.

Child Health

Risks to newborn health are highest during the first month after birth; deaths during this time occur most often when mothers have limited access to skilled health care during pregnancy, during birth, and after birth. Improved maternal care improves outcomes for newborns. Globally, most deaths among children less than

5 years old are caused by infections and malnutrition (see Box 10.2). Children in this age group are particularly vulnerable because of their immaturity.

Worldwide, improvements reduced mortality rates in this age group from 89 to 60 per 1000 live births in 2009. Almost two-thirds of these 8 million deaths in 2008 were caused by infectious diseases (WHO, 2011c). In the period 1990 to 2009, only three regions—Sub-Saharan Africa, Southeast Asia, and Oceania—failed to achieve reductions of more than 50% in child mortality (You et al., 2010).

Data on infants or children in marginalized groups, such as refugees and Indigenous or Aboriginal populations, are limited. Evidence suggests that children in these groups are at additional risk of poor health and premature death (see Box 10.3).

BOX 10.2 SUMMARY FACTS ABOUT MORTALITY IN CHILDREN UNDER 5 YEARS

- Approximately half of all deaths in children under 5 years occur in five countries: India, Nigeria, Democratic Republic of Congo, Pakistan, and China.
- Girls are more at risk of early death compared with boys (due to selective abortion and infanticide).
- One-third of deaths are caused by pneumonia (18%) and diarrhea (15%).
- Almost half of mortality (40%) in those under age 5 years occurs within the first month after birth.
- The majority of deaths (70%) in those under age 5 years occurs within the first year of life.

BOX 10.3 SUMMARY OF INTERVENTIONS KNOWN TO REDUCE CHILD MORTALITY IN CHILDREN UNDER 5 YEARS

- Care during pregnancy, during birth, and after birth by a skilled health care provider
- Early initiation of breast-feeding, that is, within 1 hour of birth
- Exclusive breast-feeding for the first 6 months of life
- The introduction of nutritionally adequate and safe complementary foods at 6 months, together with continued breast-feeding for up to 2 years and beyond
- Immunization programs
- Sleeping under mosquito nets treated with insecticide
- Use of oral rehydration salts and zinc supplements for diarrheal diseases
- Hand washing and hygiene (safe disposal of feces)
- Reduction of indoor pollution (see environmental health)
- Prompt care by a skilled health care provider
- Improved standards and delivery of care through the Integrated Management of Childhood Illness (IMCI) available to children under 5 years, with specific emphasis on common diseases in the region (WHO, 2001)

The Integrated Management of Childhood Illness (IMCI) program, now operational in more than 70 countries, strengthens the capacity of health care providers, families, and communities to support child health and development and reduce child mortality, illness, and disability (Rowe, Rowe, Holloway, Ivanovska, Muhe, & Lambrechts, 2008).

Child health and deaths among children under 5 years old represents a significant loss of potential for human development. Effective low-cost interventions have reduced child mortality rates in some countries, but some others lag behind. Success in reducing child mortality to meet MDG 4 requires additional efforts to accelerate progress (Ki-Moon, 2010). A collaborative global partnership is now in place to achieve accelerated improvements in the least improved countries.

Nurses and Global Health

Nurses have many roles in global health. Information in this section describes such changes as the inclusion of global health into nursing curriculae, the relevance of nursing and nursing organizations to global health, and finally suggestions from our collective knowledge and experience as practitioners, educators, researchers, and nursing leaders in global and international health settings.

Global Health Nursing Education

Global health issues are now an important part of nursing education, health policy, research, and practice. As societies interact, share common concerns, and face similar health challenges, nurses in Canada and around the world are becoming more aware of global health issues. Nurses need to understand cultural, social, political, economic, environmental, and ethical issues that affect health. Nursing curriculae now often include these topics and may offer opportunities for students to gain experience in international settings.

Globally, increased migration, international travel, and commerce are associated with new patterns of diseases and risks, such as SARS, tuberculosis, and avian flu. Also, the impact of global warming, environmental pollution, and natural disasters affect the entire world (Carlton, Ryan, Ali, & Kelsey, 2007; Dickenson-Hazard, 2004; Tanner, 2002).

According to the 2009 annual report to parliament on immigration, Canada has the highest per capita immigration rate in the world (Citizenship and Immigration Canada, 2009). Statistics Canada predicts that by 2031, an unprecedented 25% to 28% of the country's population could be foreign-born persons (Statistics Canada, 2010). The implication of these immigration trends for nurses

is clear: At some point in their careers, nurses will be responsible for patients from diverse cultures and areas in the world. This idea is supported by professional nursing organizations, who maintain that nurses should be able to provide safe, culturally congruent, and ethical care to their patients (American Association of Colleges of Nursing [AACN], 2008; CNA, 2009; College of Nurses of Ontario [CNO], 2009; Registered Nurses, Association of Ontario [RNAO], 2007).

Schools of nursing have addressed education in global health in their curricula in a variety of ways. Some have integrated theoretical concepts, such as principles of primary care, health promotion, environmental aspects of global health, population and development, prevention of infectious diseases, health systems, social justice, and so on (Hegyvary, 2004; Messias, 2001; Mill, Astle, Ogilvie, & Gastaldo, 2010; Mill, Astle, Ogilvie, & Opare, 2005). Others provide international cultural immersion opportunities to increase students' understanding of culture on health (Mill et al., 2010). These exposures to different global health concepts enable nursing students to become competent caregivers, educators, and global citizens.

Nursing and Global Health

National and international nursing organizations have emphasized the importance of addressing global health issues in clinical practice (AACN, 2008; CNA, 2008; International Council of Nursing [ICN], 2007). The CNA (2009) endorses the principles of primary health care, whereby essential health care in the form of health promotion and illness prevention is universally accessible to the entire population. The CNA also considers global health a fundamental right; therefore, nurses have the right and responsibility to learn about the root causes of inequity in global health and be actively involved in developing solutions. Furthermore, although there is no defined set of competencies needed for nurses to practise safely and ethically in the global health context, there has been an emphasis on cultural competence as a key component of global health (CNA, 2008; RNAO, 2007).

Currently, nurse migration is a growing phenomenon in the world, and there is a need to ensure the availability of well-trained nurses in all health care settings to meet patients' needs in diverse cultural and geographical areas (WHO, 2006). Nurses should be active participants in the development of clinical practice guidelines that ensure comprehensive global health care.

Preparing to Work in Global Health

Nurses interested in working in global health need to consider their motivation and the assets that they may bring to the job and share with others. Skills and knowledge in nursing and the ability to prioritize, make decisions, and work with limited technologies are all important, as are general abilities, such as being able to drive and speak or understand languages other than one's own. Such attributes as personal interest, sense of adventure, and willingness to learn from and with others in the local setting are important for success. Many education programs for health care professionals now include specifically relevant courses to help prepare them for work in international settings (Markle et al., 2007). Nurses work overseas as volunteers, nurses, or support staff in some projects. Roles are often flexible and multitasked. Before applying for or accepting any offer, you should review information about the mission and values of the proposed receiving organization, conditions of employment and living arrangements, expectations of duration on site, expenses, and security. Consider the ethical perspectives of the role you will fill and the code of ethics and practice from your jurisdiction in Canada in comparison with those of the organization you will be working with and the setting in which you will work. Country reports are available from the Department of Foreign Affairs and International Trade Canada (DFAIT, 2011) and the Central Intelligence Agency (CIA) *World Fact Book* (CIA, 2011). A sample of organizations that hire, place, or support nurses and undergraduate students who work abroad is presented in Table 10.6.

TABLE 10.6 Organizations of Interest to Nurses and Students Interested in Working Overseas

Organization	Role	Weblink
Global Health Council	The Global Health Council is a membership organization with an extensive list of NGOs, faith-based foundations, academic institutions, and government agencies.	http://www.globalhealth.org
Canadian International Development Agency (CIDA)	Three priority themes are food security, securing the future of children and youth, and supporting sustainable economic growth.	http://www.cida.gc.ca
Canadian Red Cross	The Canadian Red Cross Society is linked to the International Red Cross and Red Crescent Society providing relief during crises.	http://www.redcross.ca
Canadian Institutes of Health Research (CIHR)	Health care professional student grants are provided for study or research abroad. Global health research is a priority interest.	http://www.cihr-irsc.gc.ca
Médecins Sans Frontières (MSF)	MSF is an international, independent medical humanitarian organization. Medical staff include nurses, midwives, dieticians and doctors. Support staff are also hired.	http://www.msf.org
FHI 360	FHI 360 is a global health and development organization, with programs that aim to bring lasting change to the world's most vulnerable people.	http://www.fhi.org
Save the Children	Save the Children is the world's leading independent organization for children.	http://www.savethechildren.net http://www.savethechildren.ca
The Canadian Nurses Association (CNA)	The Canadian Nurses Association (CNA) is a federation of 11 provincial and territorial registered nurses' associations and colleges.	http://www.cna-aiic.ca
Provincial Nurses Associations, for example, Registered Nurses, Association of Ontario (RNAO)	These associations provide information that helps with career planning and provides a link to interest groups, such as the International Nurses' Interest Group, which has information about working overseas and in global health.	http://www.rnao.org

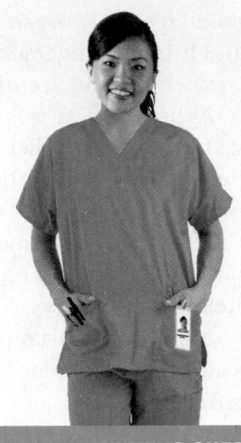

Case Study 10

Following the civil war in Somalia in the1990s, Canada accepted large numbers of Somali refugees. The first wave of families were settled in two large urban cities (Toronto and Vancouver), and these families tended to group together socially and geographically. Some administrators in charge of resettlement felt this was hindering their assimilation into Canadian society by allowing small ghettos of refugees to develop. Consequently, the next wave of Somali refugees were dispersed throughout the country to small towns—in many cases, only one or two families per town. However, when an evaluation of the resettlement program was carried out a year later by qualified, independent evaluators, it was found that the separated families had poorer scores in English skills and had higher rates of health and adjustment problems and work absenteeism, compared with the concentrated families. The administrators were puzzled by these results.

CRITICAL THINKING QUESTIONS

1. How would you satisfactorily explain the results to the administrators?

2. What are some of the barriers that you would expect Somali refugees would have to face in Canada?

3. What sorts of health problems would you expect to find in a cluster of Somali refugee families?

4. Which level(s) of government is/are responsible for the health and well-being of refugees and asylum seekers in Canada?

Check the eText in MyNursingLab for answers and explanations.

KEY TERMS

capacity building *p. 189*

climate change *p. 183*

colonialism *p. 189*

environmental health factors *p. 183*

epidemiological transition *p. 188*

food security *p. 195*

global health *p. 187*

Indigenous peoples *p. 193*

international health *p. 187*

international nursing *p. 192*

migration *p. 193*

Millennium Development Goals (MDGs) *p. 189*

natural disasters *p. 195*

pollution *p. 186*

poverty *p. 194*

safe water *p. 186*

sanitation *p. 186*

social determinants of health *p. 193*

social justice *p. 192*

surveillance *p. 195*

sustainability *p. 192*

vectors of disease *p. 185*

CHAPTER HIGHLIGHTS

- International organizations agree that climate change is the most significant environmental challenge and that multiple actions are needed to cope with climate change already in progress and to reduce carbon emissions now and in the future.

- Access to clean water and sanitation, which is important for human health, has improved globally. However, people living in rural and remote areas or in urban slums face increased risks to their health in many regions of the world because they continue to have limited or no access to safe drinking water or appropriate sanitation.

- Pollution continues to reduce indoor and outdoor air quality and is associated with increased risks of respiratory and other illnesses.

- There is a difference between international health and global health. International health is health status among nations, and global health relates to worldwide improvement of health, reduction of disparities, and protection against global threats that disregard national borders.

- The United Nations Millennium Declaration asserts that all individuals in the world have the right to dignity, equality, freedom, a basic standard of living that includes freedom from hunger and violence, and encourages tolerance and solidarity.

- Eight Millennium Development Goals (MDGs) have been identified to significantly reduce poverty and promote development by reducing economic and social conditions in the world's poorest countries by the year 2015.

- Capacity building, sustainability, and social justice are important for development to occur.
- Theories of development, such as colonialism, neocolonialism, modernization, and linear stages of growth, attempt to explain the economic growth of countries around the world.
- Globally, major issues include the health of migrants and Indigenous peoples, and issues of poverty and inequality.
- Women's and children's health and mortality have improved globally, but some regions have not realized

these improvements. Unacceptable mortality rates in some regions require focused efforts to accelerate the rate of improvement.

- National and international nursing organizations have emphasized the importance of addressing global health issues in clinical practice.
- Global health education in nursing has become important in the Canadian undergraduate nursing curriculum.

ASSESS YOUR LEARNING

1. The Millennium Development Goals (MDGs) are expected to be achieved by:
   a. 2015
   b. 2018
   c. 2020
   d. 2025

2. Which of the following BEST describes the process of economic development from traditional society, through economic "takeoff," initially led by a few individual sectors such as agriculture, transportation, and manufacturing, and ending in mass consumption?
   a. The neocolonial theory
   b. The only reasonable development path for poor countries
   c. Rostow's linear stages of growth theory
   d. How "underdeveloped" countries can reduce their connectedness to world markets

3. Which of the following is an example of a new disease in Canada believed to be caused by changes in temperature and weather?
   a. Dengue fever
   b. Tuberculosis
   c. Malaria
   d. West Nile virus

4. Food insecurity is the lack of access to nutritious food to support a healthy life. Which of the following is the greatest contributor to food insecurity?
   a. Plant diseases
   b. Poverty
   c. Population overcrowding
   d. Lack of proper food storage

5. The six official languages of the United Nations include:
   a. English, French, Spanish, Arabic, Russian, Chinese (Mandarin)
   b. English, French, German, Arabic, Russian, Chinese (Mandarin)

   c. English, Spanish, Arabic, Russian, Chinese (Mandarin), Hindi
   d. English, French, German, Dutch, Spanish, Russian

6. Which of the following BEST describes the distribution of the world's income per capita?
   a. Equal among the 20% quintiles (5ths)
   b. Half are rich and half are poor
   c. The richest 20% own more than 80% of the wealth
   d. The poorest 60% own less than 10% of the wealth

7. What has sometimes caused catastrophic lifestyle changes in Indigenous (Aboriginal) populations?
   a. Education
   b. Economic assistance
   c. Migration
   d. Forcible displacement

8. You are a student nurse working with a nongovernmental organization (NGO) on a community development project with women and children in Indonesia. Which would be a key capacity building intervention?
   a. Sitting with families at a community feast upon arrival
   b. Leading a consultation with prominent community members
   c. Reflecting on your motivation for undertaking this opportunity
   d. Relying on the expertise of professional occupational trainers in Canada prior to departure

9. An unnamed country has a Gender Inequality Index score of 0.446. What does this mean?
   a. Women are almost 45% less powerful than women in other countries.
   b. Women earn almost 45% less than men.
   c. Almost 45% of human development potential is lost.
   d. Women have almost 45% more power than men.

10. Which is the safest source of clean drinking water?
    a. A natural spring
    b. A deep and covered well
    c. Piped water at a community centre
    d. A clear stream with a rocky riverbed

Check the eText in MyNursingLab for answers and explanations.

WEBLINKS

Global Health Council

http://www.globalhealth.org

The official website of the Global Health Council, this site, funded by the Bill and Melinda Gates Foundation, hosts current information about global health issues. The Global Health Council informs and supports those working to improve global health and equity.

David Suzuki Foundation

http://www.davidsuzuki.org/issues

This website presents information and updates on climate, health, oceans, wildlife and habitat, and freshwater. Information about what a single individual or groups of individuals can do to improve the present and the future in relation to these five topic areas is also presented.

Canadian Nurses Association

www.cna-aiic.ca

This group revised their position statement on Global Health and Equity in 2009. They also have other position statement relevant to global health.

Measure DHS (Demographic and Health Surveys)

http://measuredhs.com

This website presents information and data on many health topics collected from more than 75 countries across the world. Topics include HIV/AIDS, women's and children's health, and many more. Data that are available are current.

Futures Institute

http://www.futuresinstitute.org

The Futures Institute started in 2006 in the United States, and its work focuses on longer-term improvements achieved through policy and long-range planning projects. Maternal and child health and HIV/AIDS and other infectious diseases are featured in their work to date. Information on this website includes details of current and past projects.

MyNursingLab

REFERENCES

American Association of Colleges of Nursing. (2008). *The essentials of baccalaureate education for professional nursing practice.* Washington, DC: AACN. Retrieved from http://www.aacn.nche.edu/Education/pdf/BaccEssentials08.pdf

Baba Fall, A., Das, S., Kintu, P., Wilkinson, C., Zhdanov, O., & Zuefle, J. (2009). *Statistical yearbook 2008: Trends in displacement, protection and solutions.* Geneva, Switzerland: United Nations High Commissioner for Refugees.

Balbus, J. A. (2010). *Fact sheet—health effects of climate change.* Bethesda, MD: National Institutes of Health. Retrieved from http://report.nih.gov/nihfactsheets/ViewFactSheet.aspx?csid=44&key=H

Bell, S., & Morse, S. (2008). *Sustainability indicators: Measuring the immeasurable.* London, UK, & Philadelphia, PA: Earthscan.

Birn, A., Pillay, Y., & Holtz, T. (2009a). Globalization, trade, work and health. In *Textbook of international health: Global health in a dynamic world* (3rd ed.) (pp. 417–463). New York, NY: Oxford University Press.

Birn, A., Pillay, Y., & Holtz, T. (2009b). Health and the environment. In *Textbook of international health: Global health in a dynamic world* (3rd ed.) (pp. 470–529). New York, NY: Oxford University Press.

Branisa, B., Klasen, S., & Zeigler, M. (2009). *Background paper: The construction of the Social Institutions and Gender Index.* (Background paper No. 2011). Goettingen, Germany: OECD. Retrieved from http://www.oecd.org/dataoecd/49/19/42295804.pdf

Brown, T. M., Cueto, M., & Fee, E. (2006). The World Health Organization and the transition from "international" to "global" public health. *American Journal of Public Health, 96*(1), 62–72. doi:10.2105/AJPH.2004.050831

Canadian Institutes of Health Research. (2005). *Reducing health disparities and promoting equity for vulnerable populations.* Retrieved from http://www.cihr-irsc.gc.ca/e/25703.html

Canadian International Development Agency. (2010). *Canada's contribution to the global effort to reach the Millennium Development Goals.* Ottawa, ON: CIDA.

Canadian Nurses Association. (2008). *Code of ethics for registered nurses*. Ottawa, ON: Author.

Canadian Nurses Association. (2009). *Global health equity*. Ottawa, ON: Author.

Carlton, K. H., Ryan, M., Ali, N. S., & Kelsey, B. (2007). Integration of global health concepts in nursing curricula: A national study. *Nursing Education Perspectives, 28*(3), 124–129.

Central Intelligence Agency. (2011). *The World Factbook 2009.* Retrieved from https://www-cia-gov/library/publications/the-world-factbook/index.html

Chassy, B. M. (2010). Food safety risks and consumer health. *New Biotechnology, 27*(5), 534–544. doi:10.1016/j.nbt.2010.05.018

Chen, S., & Ravallion, M. (2008). *The developing world is poorer than we thought, but no less successful in the fight against poverty.* Retrieved from http://www-wds.worldbank.org/external/default/WDSContentServer/IW3P/IB/2010/01/21/0001583 49_20100121133109/Rendered/INDEX/WPS4703.txt

Citizenship and Immigration Canada. (2009). Section 1: Making immigration work for Canada. In *Annual report to parliament on immigration, 2009*. Ottawa, ON: Author. Retrieved from http://www.cic.gc.ca/english/resources/publications/annual-report2009/section1.asp

College of Nurses of Ontario. (2009). *Practice guideline: Culturally sensitive care*. Ottawa, ON: Author. Retrieved from http://www.cno.org/Global/docs/prac/41040_CulturallySens.pdf

Commission on Social Determinants of Health. (2008). *Closing the gap in a generation: Health equity through action on the social determinants of health. Final report of the Commission on Social Determinants of Health*. Geneva, Switzerland: World Health Organization.

Conley, D. (2008). Champagne glass distribution. In *You may ask yourself: An introduction to thinking like a sociologist*. (1st ed.), (p. 392). New York, NY: WW Norton and Company.

Courter, L. A., Pereira, C., & Baird, W. M. (2007). Diesel exhaust influences carcinogenic PAH-induced genotoxicity and gene expression in human breast epithelial cells in culture. *Mutation Research/Fundamental and Molecular Mechanisms of Mutagenesis, 625*(1–2), 72–82.

Crisp, B., Swerissen, H., Duckett, S.J. (2000). Four approaches to capacity building in health: Consequences for measurement and accountability. *Health Promotion International, 15*(2), 99–107.

Davies, J.B., Sandström, S., Shorrocks, A., & Wolff, E.N. (2008). *The world distribution of household wealth* (Discussion Paper No. 2008/0.). Geneva, Switzerland: United Nations University, World Institute for Development Economics Research of the United Nations.

Department of Foreign Affairs and International Trade. (2011). *Voyage.gc.ca—essential information for Canadians abroad*. Retrieved from http://www.voyage.gc.ca/index-eng.asp

Dickenson-Hazard, N. (2004). Global health issues and challenges. *Journal of Nursing Scholarship: An Official Publication of Sigma Theta Tau International Honor Society of Nursing/Sigma Theta Tau, 36*(1), 6–10.

Dos Santos, T. (1971). The structure of dependence. In K. T. Fann, & D. C. Hodges (Eds.), *Readings in U.S. Imperialism* (p. 226). Boston, MA: Porter Sargent.

Drevdahl, D., Dorcy, K. S., & Grevstad, L. (2001). Integrating principles of community-centered practice in a community health nursing practicum. *Nurse Educator, 26*(5), 234–239.

Dumont, J., & Widmaier, S. (2010). *Database on immigrants in OECD and non-OECD countries (DIOC-E)*. Retrieved from http://www.oecd.org/document/33/0,3746,en_2649_37415_46561249_1_1_1_37415,00.html

Food and Agriculture Organization. (2009). *The state of food insecurity in the world 2009*. Retrieved from http://www.fao.org/docrep/012/i0876e/i0876e00.htm

Gagnon, A. (2004). *Health insurance coverage in Canada.* Unpublished manuscript.

Gagnon, A. J., Dougherty, G., Platt, R. W., Wahoush, E. O., George, A., Stanger, E., . . . Stewart, D. E. (2007). Refugee and refugee-claimant women and infants post-birth: Migration histories as a predictor of Canadian health system response to needs. *Canadian Journal of Public Health, 98*(4), 287–291

Global Health Education Consortium. (2011). *Global health vs. international health: What is the difference?* Retrieved from http://globalhealtheducation.org/Pages/GlobalvsInt.aspx

Gracey, M., & King, M. (2009). Indigenous health part 1: Determinants and disease patterns. *Lancet, 374*(9683), 65–75.

Griffiths, J. K., & Winant, E. (2007). Environmental heath in the global context. In W. H. Markle, M. A. Fisher & R. A. Smego (Eds.), *Understanding global health* (pp. 86–103). New York, NY: McGraw-Hill.

Gurria, A. (2008). In Organization for Economic Development: Secretary General (Ed.), *Growing unequal? Income distribution and poverty in OECD countries* (http://www.oecd.org/document/4/0,3343,en_2649_33933_41460917_1_1_1_1,00.html). Paris, France: OECD Publishing. Retrieved from http://www.oecdbookshop.org/oecd/display.asp?sf1=identifiers&st1=9264044183

Hegyvary, S. T. (2004). Working paper on grand challenges in improving global health. *Journal of Nursing Scholarship: An Official Publication of Sigma Theta Tau International Honor Society of Nursing/Sigma Theta Tau, 36*(2), 96–101.

International Council of Nursing. (2007). *Cultural and linguistic competence*. Geneva, Switzerland: Author.

International Office of Migration. (2011). *IOM—facts & figures*. Retrieved from http://www.iom.int/jahia/Jahia/about-migration/facts-and-figures/lang/en

Ki-Moon, B. (2010). *Investing in our common future: Global strategy for women's and children's health* (Paper presented at the 2010 conference). Retrieved from http://www.who.int/pmnch/topics/maternal/201009_globalstrategy_wch/en/index.html

King, M., Smith, A., & Gracey, M. (2009). Indigenous health, part 2: The underlying causes of the health gap. *Lancet, 374*(9683), 76–85.

Klugman, J. (2010). *Human Development Reports (HDR), 2010: The real wealth of nations: Pathways to human development*. (20th Anniversary Edition No. 2011). New York, NY: Palgrave McMillan. Retrieved from http://hdr.undp.org/en/reports/global/hdr2010/ (Gender Inequality Index)

Koplan, J., Bond, T., Merson, M., Reddy, K., Rodriguez, M., Sewankambo, N., & Wasserheit, J. (2009). Towards a common definition of global health. *Lancet, 373*(June 6), 1993–1995.

Lalonde, M. (1974). *A new perspective on the health of Canadians a working document*. Ottawa, ON: Minister of Supply and Services Canada.

Lester, F., Benfield, N., & Fathalla, M. M. (2010). Global women's health in 2010: Facing the challenges. *Journal of Women's Health, 19*(11), 2081–2089.

Lusigi, A. (2008). *Linking poverty to environmental sustainability*. (UNDP-UNEP Poverty-Environment Initiative. Retrieved from http://www.povertyandconservation.info/docs/20080524-UNDP-UNEP_Poverty_Environment_Initiative.pdf

Macfarlane, S. B., Jacobs, M., & Kaaya, E. E. (2008). In the name of global health: Trends in academic institutions. *Journal of Public Health Policy, 29*(4), 383–401. doi:10.1057/jphp.2008.25

Manasyan, A., Chomba, E., McClure, E. M., Krzywanski, S., & Carlo, W. A. (2011). Cost-effectiveness of essential newborn care training in urban first-level facilities. *Pediatrics 127*(5), pp. e1176–e1181.

Markle, W. H., Fisher, M. A., & Smego, R. A. (2007). *Understanding global health*. New York, NY: McGraw-Hill.

Marmot, M., & Friel, S. (2008). Global health equity: Evidence for action on the social determinants of health. *Journal of Epidemiology & Community Health, 62*(12), 1095–1097. doi: http://dx.doi.org/10.1136/jech.2008.081695

Marmot, M., Friel, S., Bell, R., Houweling, T. A. J., & Taylor, S. (2008). Closing the gap in a generation: Health equity through action on the social determinants of health. *Lancet (British Edition), 372*(9650), 1661–1669. doi: http://dx.doi.org/10.1016/S0140-6736(08)61690-6

McKinsey & Company. (2001). *Effective capacity building in nonprofit organizations*. In Venture Philanthropy Partners (Eds.). *The capacity framework*. Washington, DC: McKinsey & Company. Retrieved from http://www.vppartners.org/sites/default/files/reports/full_rpt.pdf

McMullen, C., & Jabbour, J. (2009). *Climate change science compendium 2009*. New York, NY: United Nations Environment Programme. Retrieved from http://www.unep.org/pdf/ccScienceCompendium2009/cc_ScienceCompendium2009_full_en.pdf

Messias, D. K. (2001). Globalization, nursing, and health for all. *Journal of Nursing Scholarship: An Official Publication of Sigma Theta Tau International Honor Society of Nursing/Sigma Theta Tau, 33*(1), 9–11.

Mill, J., Astle, B., Ogilvie, L., & Gastaldo, D. (2010). Linking global citizenship, undergraduate nursing education and professional nursing: Curricular innovation in the 21st century. *Advances in Nursing Science, 33*(3), E1–E11.

Mill, J., Astle, B., Ogilvie, L., & Opare, M. (2005). Global health and equity, part 1: Setting the context. *Canadian Nurse, 101*(5), 22–24.

Newbold, B. (2005). Health status and health care of immigrants in Canada: A longitudinal analysis. *Journal of Health Services & Research Policy, 10*(2), 77–83.

Newbold, B. (2009). The short-term health of Canada's new immigrant arrivals: Evidence from LSIC. *Ethnicity & Health, 14*(3), 315–336.

Norris, S., & Williams, T. (2000). *Healthy aging: Adding life to years and years to life*. (No. PRB 00-23E). Ottawa, ON: Health Canada: Science and Technology Division. Retrieved from http://dsp-psd.pwgsc.gc.ca/Collection-R/LoPBdP/BP/prb0023-e.htm

Omran, A. R. (2005). The epidemiologic transition: A theory of the epidemiology of population change. 1971. *The Milbank Quarterly, 83*(4), 731–757. doi:10.1111/j.1468-0009.2005.00398.x

Organisation of Economic Co-operation and Development. (2010). *The OECD Social Institutions and Gender Index: Results 2009*. Retrieved from http://www.oecd.org/document/39/0,3746,en_21571361_38039199_42274663_1_1_1_1,00.html#results

Pachauri, R. K., & Reisinger, A. (2007). *Climate change: Synthesis report fourth assessment report of the Intergovernmental Panel on Climate Change*. (Fourth Assessment of the Intergovernmental Report on Climate Change No. 2011). Geneva, Switzerland: IPCC.

Patel, V., & Prince, M. (2010). Global mental health: A new global health field comes of age. *JAMA: The Journal of the American Medical Association, 303*(19), 1976–1977. doi:10.1001/jama.2010.616

Prüss-Üstün, A., & Corvalán, C. (2006). *Preventing disease through healthy environments: Towards an estimate of the environmental burden of disease*. Geneva, Switzerland: World Health Organization.

Public Health Agency of Canada. (2008). *Revising the International Health Regulations*. Retrieved from http://www.phac-aspc.gc.ca/cepr-cmiu/ihr-eng.php

Registered Nurses' Association of Ontario. (2007). *Healthy work environments best practice guidelines: Embracing cultural diversity in health care: Developing cultural competence*. Ottawa, ON: Author.

Rostow, W. W. (1960). The stages of economic growth: A non-communist manifesto (pp. 4–16). Cambridge, MA: Cambridge University Press.

Rowe, A. K., Rowe, S. Y., Holloway, K. A., Ivanovska, V., Muhe, L., & Lambrechts, T. (2008). *A systematic review of the effectiveness of shortening Integrated Management of Childhood Illness guidelines training*. Geneva, Switzerland: WHO.

Statistics Canada. (2010). *Study: Projections of the diversity of the Canadian population*. Ottawa, ON: Author.

Stephens, C., Porter, J., Nettleton, C., & Willis, R. (2006). Disappearing, displaced, and undervalued: A call to action for indigenous health worldwide. *Lancet, 367*(9527), 2019–2028.

Sudaryanto, A., Kunisue, T., Kajiwara, N., Iwata, H., Adibroto, T. A., Hartono, P., & Tanabe, S. (2006). Specific accumulation of organochlorines in human breast milk from Indonesia: Levels, distribution, accumulation kinetics and infant health risk. *Environmental Pollution, 139*(1), 107–117.

Tanner, C. A. (2002). Global perspectives in nursing education. *The Journal of Nursing Education, 41*(7), 287–288.

Todaro, M. P., & Smith, S. C. (2009a). Classic theories of economic growth and development. In M. P. Todaro & S. C. Smith, (Eds.), *Economic development* (10th ed.) (pp. 109–111). Toronto, ON: Addison-Wesley.

Todaro, M. P., & Smith, S. C. (2009b). The neocolonial dependence model. In M. P. Todaro & S. C. Smith (Eds.), *Economic development* (10th ed.) (pp. 122–124). Toronto, ON: Addison-Wesley.

Todaro, M. P., & Smith, S. C. (2009c). Human capital: Education and health in economic development. In M. P. Todaro, & S. C. Smith (Eds.), *Economic development* (10th ed.) (pp. 369–430). Toronto, ON: Addison-Wesley.

United Nations. (2001). *Road map towards the implementation of the United Nations Millennium Declaration*. (Report of the secretary-general). Geneva, Switzerland: UN.

United Nations. (2006). *The Millennium Development Goals report: 2006*. (United Nations Development Programme). Geneva, Switzerland: UN.

United Nations. (2011). *A gateway to the UN system's work on the MDGs*. http://www.un.org/millenniumgoals

United Nations Development Programme. (1992). The widening gap in global opportunities. In *UNDP Human Development Report* (p. 34). New York, NY: Oxford University Press.

United Nations Development Programme. (2007). *Human Development Report 2007*. Geneva, Switzerland: UNDP.

United Nations Environment Programme. (2010). *United Nations Environment Programme (UNEP)— six priority areas Factsheets—harmful substances and Hazardous waste*. Geneva, Switzerland: UN. Retrieved from http://www.unep.org/publications/contents/pub_details_search.asp?ID=4193

United Nations High Commission for Refugees. (2012). *UNHCR—statistics*. Geneva, Switzerland: UN. Retrieved from http://www.unhcr.org/pages/49c3646c125.html

Varkey, S., & Gupta, S. S. (2005). How gender (in)sensitive are the gender-related indices? *Bulletin of the World Health Organization, 83*(12), 954–956.

Wahoush, E. O. (2009). Equitable health-care access: The experiences of refugee and refugee claimant mothers with an ill preschooler. *Canadian Journal of Nursing Research, 41*(3), 186–206.

Watkins, K. (2005). *Human Development Report 2005: International cooperation at a crossroads, air, trade and security in an unequal world*. New York, NY: UNDP. Retrieved from http://hdr.undp.org/en/media/HDR05_complete.pdf

World Bank. (2010). *Extreme poverty rates continue to fall*. Retrieved from http://data.worldbank.org/news/extreme-poverty-rates-continue-to-fall

World Bank. (2011). *How we classify countries*. Retrieved from http://data.worldbank.org/about/country-classifications

World Commission on Environment and Development. (1987). *Our common future, report of the World Commission on*

Environment and Development. (Published as Annex to General Assembly document A/42/427). Geneva, Switzerland: WCED: Environment.

World Health Organization. (1978). *Declaration of Alma Ata.* Geneva, Switzerland: UN. Retrieved from http://www.who.int/publications/almaata_declaration_en.pdf

World Health Organization. (2001). Integrated Management of Childhood Illness: Model chapter for textbooks. In World Health Organization Department of Child and Adolescent Health and Development. WHO/CAH/01.01 Paris, France: WHO. Retrieved from whqlibdoc.who.int/hq/2001/WHO_CAH_01.01.pdf

World Health Organization. (2006). *The World Health Report 2006—working together for health.* Geneva, Switzerland: World Health Organization. Retrieved from http://www.who.int/hrh/whr06/en/index.html

World Health Organization. (2008). In World Health Organization (Ed.), *International Health Regulations 2005* (http://www.who.int/ihr/about/en/ed.). Geneva, Switzerland: WHO.

World Health Organization. (2009a). *Protecting health from climate change: Connecting science, policy and people.* Geneva, Switzerland: WHO. Retrieved from http://whqlibdoc.who.int/publications/2009/9789241598880_eng.pdf

World Health Organization. (2009b). *Women and health: Today's evidence, tomorrow's agenda.* (No. 2011). Geneva, Switzerland: WHO.

World Health Organization. (2009c). *Proportion of births attended by a skilled health worker: 2008 updates.* Department of Reproductive Health and Research. Retrieved from http://www.who.int/reproductivehealth/publications/maternal_perinatal_health/2008_skilled_attendants/en/index.html

World Health Organization. (2010). *Water, sanitation and health: Recent developments on the recognition of safe and clean water and sanitation as a human right.* Geneva, Switzerland: WHO. Retrieved from http://www.who.int/water_sanitation_health/recognition_safe_clean_water/en

World Health Organization. (2011a). *WHO: Health of indigenous peoples.* Retrieved from http://www.who.int/topics/health_services_indigenous/en

World Health Organization. (2011b). *Trade, foreign policy, diplomacy and health: Food security.* Retrieved from http://www.who.int/trade/glossary/story028/en

World Health Organization. (2011c). World Health Statistics 2011 (pp. 12–14). *Health statistics and informatics of the innovation, information, evidence and research cluster.* Retrieved from http://www.who.int/gho/publications/world_health_statistics/en/index.html

Yang, A., Farmer, P. E., & McGahan, A. M. (2010). "Sustainability" in global health. *Global Public Health, 5*(2), 129–135. doi:10.1080/17441690903418977

You, D., Jones, G., & Wardlaw, T. (2010). *Levels and trends in child mortality, report 2010: Estimates developed by the UN inter-agency group for child mortality estimation.* New York, NY: United Nations Children's Fund.

Chapter **11**

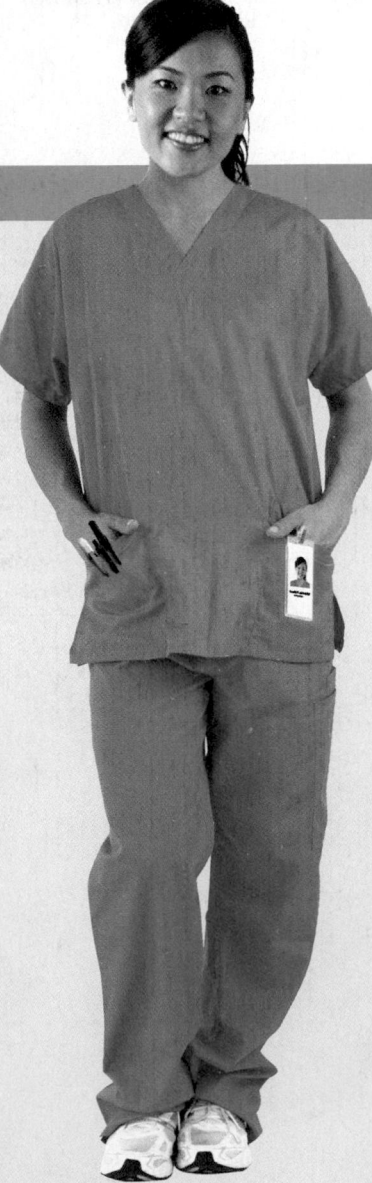

Cultural Caring

After studying this chapter, you will be able to:

1. Describe the concept of culture and its impact on the nursing process.

2. Describe the unique world views/perspectives that all peoples (i.e., Indigenous, non-Indigenous, immigrants) in Canada have that impact their health practices.

3. Differentiate among *cultural awareness*, *cultural sensitivity*, and *cultural competence*, and describe the process of working toward cultural safety.

4. Identify seven characteristics of culture and describe how they pertain to nursing.

5. Discuss Srivastava's (2008) ABCDE model of cultural competence.

6. Describe and apply guidelines for culturally sensitive, competent, and safe health care.

7. Describe four cultural barriers to cultural sensitivity and safety and identify ways to overcome them.

8. Analyze the different health views of culturally diverse clients: traditional healing, biomedical, and holistic.

9. List the determinants of health and understand that they influence the health and well-being of an individual.

10. Assess clients from a holistic perspective and individualize their care to facilitate culturally sensitive, competent, and safe client care, thus recognizing that all clients require a cultural assessment.

n this chapter, we explore the diverse elements of Canadian culture. We examine culture as a concept and discuss using a cultural safety lens to guide nursing practice. Cultural awareness, sensitivity, competence, and safety are then applied to primary care and health promotion. Cultural competence is linked increasingly to reducing health disparities among racial, ethnic, and underserved populations (Lipson & Desantis, 2007). Thus, it is imperative that Canadian nurses be informed, become culturally sensitive, and work toward cultural competence to safely care for the diverse ethnic and Indigenous populations in Canada.

The demographic profile of Canada has been changing over the last several decades, creating a greater racial and ethnic diversity. All health care providers must understand the intricate relationship between cultural and ethnic beliefs and values and the ways in which these concepts impact the context of health care services both delivered (by providers) and received (by those in need of care) (Escallier, Fullerton, & Messina, 2011). Initially, cultural competence was perceived as a moral and ethical imperative; however, there is increasing evidence stressing the importance of cultural competence when addressing disparities in health care quality and outcomes (Srivastava, 2008). Thus, nurses can directly impact health disparities by improving health care services.

Canada's Cultural Mosaic

It is important to understand the history of the peoples in Canada to truly comprehend and appreciate their diverse ethnic and cultural origins. Examining the historical context and national policies of Canada that affect immigrants, refugees, and Indigenous peoples provides nurses with insight into the evolution of Canada's cultural mosaic, and ultimately lays the foundation to think critically about providing culturally competent and culturally safe care.

Indigenous communities, peoples and nations are those which, having a historical continuity with pre-invasion and pre-colonial societies that developed on their territories, consider themselves distinct from other sectors of the societies now prevailing in those territories, or parts of them. They form at present non-dominant sectors of society and are determined to preserve, develop and transmit to future generations their ancestral territories, and their ethnic identity, as the basis of their continued existence as peoples, in accordance with their own cultural patterns, social institutions and legal systems. (M. Cobo, as cited in United Nations Permanent Forum on Indigenous Issues, 2007. p 12)

In this chapter, the use of the term *Indigenous* will be used to refer to the three groups of Aboriginal peoples who are recognized by the Canadian Constitution: Indians (First Nations), Métis, and Inuit (Health Canada, 2009). In general, the Government of Canada and some organizations use the term *Aboriginal*, whereas other organizations use *Indigenous* (e.g., Indigenous Peoples Health Research Centre).

Canada has a long history of emigration and immigration; individuals from diverse backgrounds and cultures have come to Canada and called it home. The Indigenous peoples were the original inhabitants of North America. Theories conflict about when and how Indigenous peoples arrived in this part of North America. One theory is the Bering land bridge theory, which speculates that the Indigenous peoples crossed a land bridge between what is now Alaska and Asia. However, the Indigenous peoples and their traditional teachings maintain that they are the first peoples of Canada and have existed here from the very beginning. Despite colonization and numerous attempts to totally assimilate Indigenous peoples, they remain as distinct in language, culture, and ethnicity as more recent immigrants to Canada.

Early in the seventeenth century, Europeans established settlements primarily in Quebec, New Brunswick, and Nova Scotia. They also moved westward into Ontario, the Prairie provinces, and British Columbia. With the defeat of French General Montcalm by British General Wolfe in 1769, Canada became a British colony. By 1891, Canada's population growth was small compared with that in the United States. Canada's population of 4.8 million persons was distributed unevenly across its vast territory, with the majority concentrated in Ontario, Quebec, and the Atlantic region. With the completion of the transcontinental railway in 1885, all of Canada became accessible, from the east coast to the west coast. This allowed settlers to travel more easily and provided a means for farmers to export their grain. In addition, the dispossession of Indigenous land rights through the signing of the seven numbered treaties in the 1870s enabled the federal government to open up the west to agricultural settlement. The closing of the American frontier meant that Canada could attract immigrants from the United States, Britain, and Europe.

During the twentieth century, three major migrations helped shape the present composition of the Canadian population. The first occurred between 1901 and 1912, when almost 3 million people arrived, mainly from Britain and northern European countries. By 1911, immigrants accounted for 22% of the population, compared with 13% in 1901. Between 1919 and 1931, only 1.2 million immigrants arrived in Canada. This decline occurred for several reasons: Canadians were involved in social policies that influenced the character of the country, including its immigration policy; the years between World War I and II was a period of immigration restriction and reduction; the Canadian government increased sanctions with regard to certain immigrant groups; and the war-torn conditions of Europe left many individuals without the means to immigrate to other countries.

The second group of immigrants came after World War II, when hundreds of thousands of people in Europe were displaced from their homelands or were refugees. More than 1 million immigrants arrived in Canada between 1946 and 1955, with most of them still coming from Britain and other European countries. The third major migration began in 1977 and continues today. Between 2001 and 2006, more than 1 million immigrants were accepted into Canada.

In proportion to its population, Canada permits about twice as many people as does the United States. Consequently, the proportion of foreign-born individuals in Canada is more than 20%, whereas the proportion in the United States is 12.5%. Only Australia rivals Canada in its proportion of first-generation immigrants: 22.2% (Chui, Tran, & Maheux, 2007). The Atlantic provinces are the only areas in which people of British origin are the majority ethnic group, while Quebec retains French as the most common ethnic origin of its population. Statistics Canada projects that by 2030, immigration may be the only source of population growth in Canada (Chui, Tran, & Maheux, 2007).

New immigrants tend to settle in geographical areas that have individuals from their homeland; in a new country, the presence of others from a familiar linguistic, religious, and cultural background makes the transition to a new way of life easier. The vast majority, 97.2%, of immigrants entering Canada between 2001 and 2006 (Chui, Tran, & Maheux, 2007) settled in urban areas, with more than half in the large cities of Toronto, Montreal, and Vancouver.

Historical events and immigration patterns and policies have shaped the ethnocultural composition of Canada. In the beginning, Canada was dominated by French and British cultures, as a consequence of colonization. These two groups remain unassimilated by each other. Indigenous peoples were also not completely assimilated, even though numerous government policies attempted to do that. Today, Canada is a multicultural nation in which a plethora of languages, religions, belief systems, values, and life patterns prevail.

Demographic Profile

A demographic profile of Canada includes statistical descriptions and analyses of its population; for example, the number of people in the country or in a region, or the number of people who speak both official languages. See Table 11.1 for information about the Aboriginal population.

In terms of the whole population, the results of the 2006 census (Chui, Tran, & Maheux, 2007; Martel & Caron-Malenfant, 2007a, 2007b; Statistics Canada, 2008a, 2008c, 2008d) identify the following points:

- Canada's population has more than doubled in the past 50 years, from just over 14 million in 1951 to just over 31 million in 2006.
- The People's Republic of China was the main source country of immigrants to Canada in 2001 and again in 2006. In 2006, 14% of recent immigrants came from China, and India counted for 11.6%, followed by the Philippines (7%) and Pakistan (5.2%). Six of the top 10 countries of birth of all newcomers in the 2006 census were in Asia and the Middle East.
- Canada's national median age reached an all-time high of 39.5 years in 2006, rising steadily since 1966. Statistics Canada's demographic projection is that by 2031 the median age of the population will be 44 years.
- In 2006, the median age of Canada's workforce increased to 41.2 from 39.5 in 2001. This rise is especially strong in the percentage of workers that are more than 55 years of age, which increased to 15.3% from 11.7% in 2001.
- Chinese is the most common language spoken at home, after English and French.
- Aboriginal people are a young and urban population. The median age of the Aboriginal population is 24.7 years, 14 years younger than the non-Aboriginal population.
- Older Canadians are shaping national demographics. Between 2001 and 2006, the population older than 80 years increased by 25%. Statistics Canada projects that the number of seniors (65 years of age and older) could outpace the number of children younger than 15 years of age within the next 10 years.
- The increase in visible minority populations has outpaced the natural population increase, increasing by 27.2% compared with the total population increase of 5.4%. In 2006, visible minorities accounted for 16.2% of the population, compared with 11.2% in 1996.

TABLE 11.1 Population by Aboriginal Group, 2006 Census

| Region | Total Population | Aboriginal Population | | | | Non-Aboriginal Identity Population |
		Aboriginal Identity Population*	North American Indian	Métis	Inuit	
Canada	**31 241 030**	**1 172 785**	**698 025**	**389 780**	**50 480**	**30 068 240**
Newfoundland and Labrador	500 610	23 455	7 765	6 470	4 715	477 160
Prince Edward Island	134 205	1 730	1 225	385	30	132 475
Nova Scotia	903 090	24 175	15 240	7 680	325	878 920
New Brunswick	19 650	17 650	12 385	4 270	185	701 995
Quebec	7 435 905	108 425	65 085	27 980	10 950	7 327 475
Ontario	12 028 895	242 495	158 395	73 605	2 035	11 786 405
Manitoba	1 133 515	175 395	1 006 407	1 805	565	958 115
Saskatchewan	953 850	141 890	91 400	48 120	215	811 960
Alberta	3 256 355	188 365	97 275	85 495	1 610	3 067 990
British Columbia	4 074 385	196 075	129 580	59 445	795	3 878 310
Yukon	30 190	7 580	6 280	800	255	22 615
Northwest Territories	41 060	20 635	12 640	3 580	4 160	20 420
Nunavut	29 325	24 915	100	130	24 635	4 405

*Includes Aboriginal groups (North American Indian, Métis, and Inuit), multiple Aboriginal responses, and Aboriginal responses not included elsewhere.

Source: Adapted from Statistics Canada. (2010b). *Aboriginal identity population by age groups, median age and sex, 2006 counts, for Canada, Provinces and Territories and Census Metropolitan Areas and Census Agglomerations—20% sample data.* Retrieved from http://www12.statcan.ca/census-recensement/2006/dp-pd/hlt/97-558/pages/page.cfm?Lang=E&Geo=PR&Code=01&Table=1&Data=Count&Sex=1&Age=1&StartRec=1&Sort=2&Display=Page

- Since the end of World War II, a substantial proportion of immigrants, in excess of 500 000 in total, have been refugees, coming from Hungary in 1956; Czechoslovakia in 1968; Southeast Asia, the Middle East, South and Central America, Africa, and, more recently, from Bosnia and Somalia.

- Discerning whether an individual is an immigrant or a refugee—that is, whether or not the move to Canada was a choice or forced—is a consideration in providing culturally safe care.

Language

During each of the census periods, Canadians were asked to identify their mother tongue, which was defined as "the first language that a person learned at home in childhood and still understands" (Statistics Canada, 2012a). In 2011, for the first time, language questions were asked of the total population, and more than 200 languages were reported, including Aboriginal languages. English was most commonly spoken at home by 66%, whereas 21% of the population reported that French was most commonly spoken at home (Statistics Canada, 2012b). One in five of the population in 2006 was an allophone (i.e., mother tongue other than English or French). Asian languages are identified as mother tongue by 56% of the allophone population, with Tagalog (from the Philippines) having the greatest increase since 2006 (Statistics Canada, 2012b). Also, in 2011, over 200 000 Canadians reported an Aboriginal mother tongue. These persons were most often living in Quebec, Manitoba, and Saskatchewan (Statistics Canada, 2012c).

According to the 2006 census, 81% of the new immigrants who had arrived in the previous 5 years were unable to speak either one of the two official languages (Corbeil & Blaser, 2007). This situation puts a strain on certain services, such as English or French language training and translation services, and posed challenges in the delivery of health care. Statistics Canada (Schellenberg & Maheux, 2007) conducted a longitudinal survey of immigrants to Canada, and 32% of immigrants who sought employment in Canada identified language as a major barrier to employment.

Indigenous Peoples

It is important to understand how contact with colonizers changed every aspect of life for the Indigenous peoples. As a result of colonization the Indigenous peoples of Canada lost their autonomy, self-determination, ability to practise their cultural and spiritual beliefs, and most importantly, they were disconnected from their identity. With the occurrence of epidemics, social, economic, political, cultural, and community structures were severely disrupted and, in some cases, annihilated. Within the residential school system Indigenous children were exposed to physical, mental, emotional, religious, and sexual abuses. These practices that were legally enforced by non-Indigenous peoples have contributed to the current health disparities between the Indigenous and non-Indigenous peoples in Canada (Chansonneuve, 2005; Chartrand & McKay, 2006; Wesley-Esquimaux & Smolewski, 2004).

The negative consequences of colonization, specifically the epidemics and the residential school experiences, led to cultural discontinuity, which has been linked to high rates of depression, alcoholism, suicide, and violence in many communities (Kiramayer, Brass, & Tait, 2000). The First Nations adults who were surveyed by the Regional Health Survey (2002–2003) believed that their parents' attendance at residential school had negatively affected the parenting they received as children. Also, even if only one of the parents had attended a residential school, the chances of the children thinking about committing suicide in their lifetime were higher. At a 5-day retreat for those who had experienced residential abuse in eastern Ontario, participants reported the continued negative impact of attending residential schools on themselves, their families, their communities, and their clients (Chansonneuve, 2005). These participants attributed to the residential school legacy the high rates of suicide; family violence; addictive and self-destructive behaviours; mental illness and emotional disorders; histories of intergenerational family violence and abuse; histories of involvement with foster care; unhealthy coping, social, and life skills; emotional numbness, with anger toward authority figures; low self-esteem from deep-rooted feelings of humiliation, shame, and abandonment; and disconnection from family and culture (Chansonneuve, 2005). There are unequivocal disparities between Indigenous and non-Indigenous peoples in Canada related to income, employment, education, housing, health, and mental health (Health Canada, 2005; Statistics Canada, 2010). Ermine, Sinclair, and Jeffery

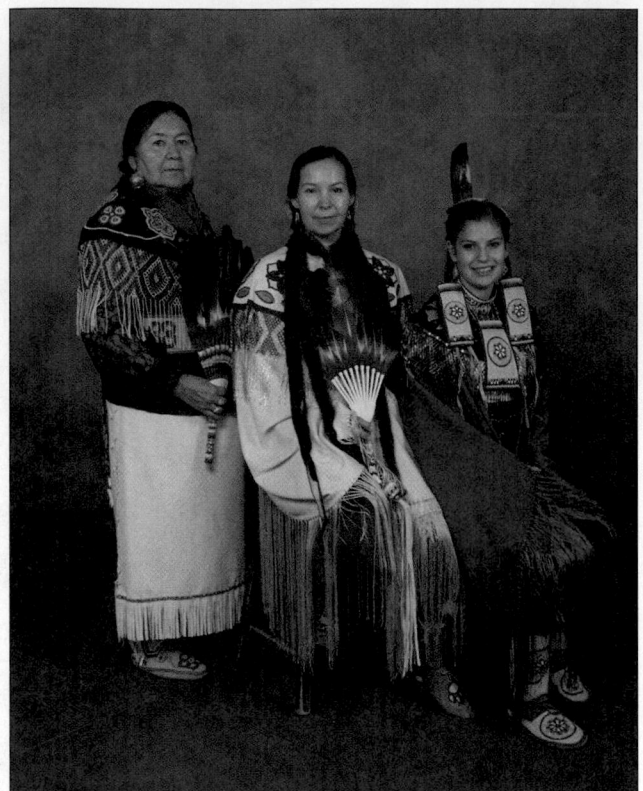

FIGURE 11.1 This photograph represents three generations of Plains Cree people from the Thunderchild First Nation, Saskatchewan: grandmother, mother, and granddaughter.

(2004) asserted that "despite the unpalatable nature of colonial history . . . Indigenous people experience those realities daily. While it may be difficult to read about the realities of Indigenous peoples, it is without a doubt more difficult to live those realities" (p. 9). This the changing face of Indigenous peoples as illustrated by Figure 11.1.

Visible Minorities

In Canada, non-British and non-French immigrants remained on the fringes of mainstream society until the middle of the twentieth century. The 2006 census collected information on members of visible minority groups in Canada, defined by the Employment Equity Act as "persons, other than aboriginal people, who are non-Caucasian in race, or non-white in colour" (Statistics Canada, 2008b). In 2006, over 5 million persons identified themselves as members of visible minority groups, representing 16.2% of the Canadian population. The numbers of visible minorities have steadily increased over the past 25 years. Indeed, visible minorities represented 4.7% of Canadians in 1981, 9.4% in 1991, 11.2% in 1996, 13.4% in 2001, and 16.2% in 2006. Ontario is home to more than half of the visible minority population (Statistics Canada, 2008c).

The rise of the visible minority population was five times the increase in the general population since 2001

TABLE 11.2 Visible Minority Population, by Place of Origin, 1996 Census and 2006 Census

	1996 Census	2006 Census
Total population	28 528 125	31 241 030
Visible minority population	3 197 480	5 068 095
South Asian	670 590	1 262 865
Chinese	860 150	1 216 565
Black	573 860	783 795
Filipino	234 195	410 700
Latin American	176 970	304 245
Arab/West Asian	244 665	422 245
Southeast Asian	172 765	239 935
Korean	64 835	141 890
Japanese	68 135	81 300
Multiple visible minority	61 575	133 120
Visible minority (not included elsewhere)	69 745	71 420

Source: Adapted from Statistics Canada. (2001). Total population by visible minority population for Canada, 1996. Retrieved from http://www.statcan.ca/english/census96/feb17/vmcan.htm; and Statistics Canada. (2009). 2006 Census of Population. Retrieved from http://www40.statcan.gc.ca/l01/cst01/demo50a-eng.htm

(Statistics Canada, 2008c). The largest visible minority population is the South Asian group (4% of total population), followed by the Chinese (3.9%) and blacks (2.5%). Other visible minority groups included Filipinos, who represented 8.1% of the visible minority population, Latin Americans (6.0%), Arabs (5.2%), Southeast Asians (4.7%), West Asians (3.1%), Koreans (2.8%), and Japanese (1.6%) (see Table 11.2).

The Toronto, Montreal, and Vancouver census metropolitan areas (CMAs) were home to 68.9% of recent immigrants in 2006. Between 2001 and 2006, higher proportions of recent immigrants chose to settle in smaller CMAs. Fully 16.6% of newcomers in 2006 settled in the CMAs of Calgary, Ottawa-Gatineau, Edmonton, Winnipeg, Hamilton, and London. In 2001, by comparison, 14.3% of newcomers lived in these CMAs (Statistics Canada, 2008c).

Canada's Multicultural Policy

The multicultural policy in Canada was initiated in 1971 as a guideline for federal government policy and reflects the evolving nature of Canadian society. However, it is important to note that Canada did have previous policies of assimilation and/or **colonization** that focused on the absorption of people into a dominant culture. In Canada, an example of assimilation would be the forced integration of Indigenous peoples into the European-Canadian culture. **Assimilation** was an explicit policy of the Canadian government that led to the removal of Indigenous children from their homes and families and their subsequent institutionalization in residential schools. Colonization has shaped and continues to influence families around the globe. The purpose of assimilation or colonization is to impose the values, attitudes, beliefs, or practices of a dominant group in society on a minority group. Through colonial rule, many cultures have had to cope with the imposition of Christian-European family norms and with the values of their colonizers.

In 1988, the Multiculturalism Act was passed, guaranteeing multiculturalism as a legal entity and affirming its importance to Canada. As a policy promoting tolerance and diversity, multiculturalism was to be the opposite of assimilation, for to assimilate is to lose those characteristics that distinguish a group from the culture that surrounds it. Canada has been called a *mosaic* or an *ethnically plural society* because of the way it has absorbed immigrants. It has supported people in retaining a distinct sense of cultural identity. This is in contrast to the melting pot of the United States, where immigrants are assimilated into the mainstream of that culture. (See the Nursing and Canadian Society box on the next page for a summary of Canadian legislation and important facts on multiculturalism in Canada.)

An ethnocultural profile of Canada today shows a nation that has become increasingly multiethnic and multicultural. This portrait is diverse and varies from province to territory, city to city, and community to community. Immigration over the past 100 years has shaped Canada, with each new wave of immigrants adding to the nation's ethnic and cultural composition. Half a century ago, most immigrants came from Europe; now most are from several parts of Asia. The number of visible minority groups in Canada is growing. Canadians listed more than 200 ethnic groups in answering the 2006 census question on ethnic ancestry, thus reflecting a varied and rich cultural mosaic (Statistics Canada, 2008c).

Culture as a Concept

COMPONENTS OF CULTURE Cultures are complex. Their facets relate to all aspects of life: language, art, music, values systems (beliefs, morals, rules), spirituality and religion, philosophy, family roles and organization, patterns of behaviour, childrearing practices, rituals or ceremonies, recreation and leisure activities, festivals and holidays, nutrition, food preferences, and health practices. Many parts of culture (e.g., health and illness practices; attitudes about touch, territory, and privacy; childbirth; and death and dying practices) affect nursing practice.

Nursing and Canadian Society

Fact	Implications of Legislation for Nursing Practice
1960: The Canadian Bill of Rights barred discrimination by federal agencies on the grounds of race, national origin, colour, religion, or gender. 1961: Changes to Canada's Immigration Act meant that fewer immigrants were European and the mix of source countries shifted to nations in southern Europe, Asia, and the West Indies.	These rights are legally protected. Nurses must have knowledge of the ethnic and cultural makeup of the Canadian population and use that knowledge to provide culturally competent and safe care.
1969: The Official Languages Act was enacted to protect minority language rights.	Clients have the right to have health care services provided in either official language in any part of Canada.
1971: The federal government announced its policy of multiculturalism.	People are encouraged to retain their cultural beliefs and practices, rather than being assimilated into the mainstream culture. This means that nurses need to be culturally sensitive and incorporate appropriate measures into health care assessment and delivery.
1982: The Canadian Charter of Rights and Freedoms considered multiculturalism to be constitutional and protected equality rights without discrimination (in particular based on race, national or ethnic origin, colour, religion, gender, age, or mental or physical disability). Section 27 explicitly states that the Charter will be interpreted in a manner consistent with the preservation and enhancement of the multicultural heritage of Canadians; by virtue of this section of the Charter, Canada became a constitutional multicultural stage.	The Charter entrenches equality rights without discrimination, again obligating nurses to provide culturally competent and safe care grounded in respect for the self and the client.
1982: The Canada Act replaced the British North America Act as Canada's constitution and also recognized the three main groups of Indigenous peoples in Canada: First Nations, Métis, and Inuit.	This policy acknowledged the rights of the Indigenous peoples in Canada. Nurses must have knowledge of and respect for the customs and beliefs of First Nations, Métis, and Inuit and integrate that knowledge into the provision of culturally safe care.
1986: The Employment Equity Act was established to achieve equality in the workplace so that no persons would be denied employment opportunities or benefits for reasons unrelated to ability; it established the principle that employment equity means more than treating persons in the same way but also requires special measures and the accommodation of differences; it identified four groups thought to experience disadvantage in employment: women, Aboriginal peoples, persons with disability, and persons in a visible minority (Canadian Human Rights Commission, n.d.).	This policy recognizes the challenges faced by Indigenous peoples and other groups in seeking and maintaining employment, and hence the impact of unemployment on poverty and self-esteem. In assessing, planning, and providing care, it is the nurse's responsibility to consider the impact of poverty and self-esteem on the health and well-being of all peoples, especially those identified in the act.
Previous censuses have shown that the Indigenous population is growing much faster than the total population. Given the younger age of the Indigenous population, this trend is expected to continue (Statistics Canada, 2008d).	This rapid increase in the Indigenous populations will have an impact on health care services for both young and older adults.
Approximately two-fifths of the Canadian population have one origin other than British, French, or Indigenous.	The fact that the Canadian population is increasing in diversity has implications for how nurses incorporate the changes in practice needed to address this diversity. The importance of culture is highlighted in the fact that this topic is listed in the Canadian Nurses Association (CNA, 2006) *Blueprint for the Registered Nurse Examination*, which parallels nursing competencies and standards of practice. The CNA (2010) now has a position statement *promoting cultural competence in nursing*.

Religious and spiritual beliefs are part of cultural values, and they can influence dietary restrictions, family planning, the use of blood transfusions, and death-related practices, such as autopsy, organ donation, cremation, and prolonging life. Understanding the unique values and belief systems of particular religious groups is important in providing culturally safe care. For example, many Orthodox Jews believe in prolonging life as much as possible and do not believe in cremation; some Indigenous peoples practise traditional healing methods, such as use of the sweat lodge; many Jehovah's Witnesses will not accept blood transfusions; and many Jewish and Muslim dietary practices prohibit eating pork or pork products. These are just a few examples; however, in providing culturally safe care, the important nursing action is to conduct a cultural assessment on all clients (Indigenous, non-Indigenous, immigrants) and ask the client about his or her preferences.

CHARACTERISTICS OF CULTURE Culture exhibits the following characteristics:

- *Culture is learned.* It is neither instinctive nor innate. It is learned through life experiences from birth.

- *Culture is taught.* It is transmitted from parents, extended family, and peers to children over successive generations. Verbal and nonverbal communication patterns transmit culture.

- *Culture is social.* It originates and develops through people's interactions: families, groups, and communities.

- *Culture is adaptive.* Customs, beliefs, and practices change as people adapt to the social environment and as people's biological and psychological needs change. For example, the idea of the extended family still exists; however, the means by which families interact and communicate has been transformed, despite large geographical distances, by the World Wide Web, which facilitates instant visual and verbal communication. Messages can now be transmitted instantaneously around the world to children, grandchildren, brothers, sisters, mothers, fathers, grandmothers, grandfathers, aunts, and uncles.

- *Culture is shared.* This is true to varying degrees. Even though values, beliefs, and traditions may be shared, unique differences still exist for each individual within a cultural group.

- *Culture is difficult to articulate.* Members of a specific cultural group often find it difficult to explain their own culture. Many of the values and behaviours are habitual and are carried out subconsciously.

- *Culture exists at many levels.* Culture is most easily identified at a visible level. Rituals (e.g., funerals), dress, and celebrations are visual cues to culture that are easily revealed. Often, it is more difficult to find out about the more abstract concepts, such as values, beliefs, and traditions.

Definitions and Concepts Related to Culture

Culture is a universal experience, but no two cultures are exactly alike. Two important terms identify the differences and similarities among peoples of different cultures. **Culture-universals** are the commonalities of values, norms of behaviour, and life patterns among different cultures. **Culture-specifics** are those values, beliefs, and patterns of behaviour that tend to be unique to a designated culture, rather than shared with members of other cultures. For example, Aboriginal peoples' pow-wows, the date on and the way in which Chinese New Year is celebrated, East Indian Diwali celebrations, Robbie Burns Day for the Scottish, and Saint-Jean-Baptiste Day for the Québécois are all culture-specifics.

The terms *culture, diversity, ethnicity,* and *race* are often used interchangeably, but they are not synonymous. **Culture** is defined as "the learned, shared, and transmitted values, beliefs, norms, and lifeway practices of a particular group that guide thinking, decisions, and actions in patterned ways" (Leininger, 1988, p. 158). Because cultural patterns are learned, it is important for nurses to note that all members of a particular group may not share identical cultural experiences. Thus, individual members of a cultural group will be somewhat different from their own cultural counterparts. For example, generations have different appreciations of music according to exposure within their peer group—swing from the 1940s, jive from the 1950s, rock and roll from the 1960s, and so on. Large cultural groups often have cultural subgroups or subsystems. A **subculture** usually comprises people who have a distinct identity and yet are also related to a larger cultural group.

Bicultural "is used to describe a person who crosses two cultures, lifestyles, and sets of values" (Giger & Davidhizar, 2004, p. 67). For example, a young man whose father is Cree and whose mother is European Canadian may maintain his traditional Cree heritage while also being influenced by his mother's cultural values.

Diversity refers to the fact or state of being different. Many factors account for differences: race, gender, sexual orientation, culture, ethnicity, socioeconomic status, educational attainment, religious affiliation, ability, marital status, age, and so on. Diversity, therefore, occurs not only between cultural groups but also within a cultural group.

The term **ethnic** refers to a group of people who share a common and distinctive culture and who are members of a specific group. Although ethnicity has sometimes been used to identify race, Giger and Davidhizar (2004) suggest that it is "a common social and cultural heritage that is passed on to successive generations" (p. 67). The characteristics of the group give an individual a sense of **cultural identity**. Other factors that help define ethnicity may include religion and the geographical background of the family.

Race is a controversial term. For some people, the definition of race includes having common characteristics, such as skin colour, bone structure, facial features, hair texture, and blood type. The American Anthropological Association (AAA) statement on race defines it as an idea created by Western Europeans following exploration across the world to account for differences among people and justify colonization, conquest, enslavement, and social hierarchy among humans. It has been used to refer to groupings of people according to common origin or background and associated with perceived biological markers. Among humans, there are no races except the human race. Ideas about race are culturally and socially transmitted and form the basis of racism, racial classification, and often complex racial identities (AAA, 1998). The Human Genome Project has discovered that humans are 99.9% genetically alike and that the genetic variations related to geography or ancestry do not correlate with the socially constructed racial classifications; that is, there are no genetically discrete races. In fact, there is greater genetic variability within the racial categories than among them. Although it is now recognized that there is no scientific merit to the concept of race, race remains an important social construct, whereby social meanings are attached to perceived physical differences, resulting in inequality among racial groups. Thus, the term *race* becomes problematic when it leads to negative stereotyping. *Culture* should not be confused with either *race* or *ethnic group*. *Race, culture,* and *ethnic origin* are three different terms that are often used interchangeably; however, it is inappropriate to do so.

Considerations for Culturally Safe Nursing Practice

Similar to giving ethical care, nurses must consider cultural and ethnic factors in themselves and others in providing quality nursing care. A group's world views shape its health culture—the values, beliefs, and practices it holds about health promotion, disease prevention, illness treatment, and the expectations that guide the nurse–client encounter.

People who belong to the same ethnic group may have little in common in their lifestyles, beliefs, and values. For example, a Canadian of East Indian ancestry could be a third-generation Canadian who cannot speak a word of Hindi, a recently arrived lawyer from New Delhi, or an ethnic refugee from a small mountain village in northern India.

Health care providers must understand the overarching influence of the determinants of health that also influence health inequities and disparities (Public Health Agency of Canada [PHAC], 2010; Raphael, 2006). For example, socioeconomic status, length of time in Canada, educational level, age, sex, and country of origin will influence the perspectives of health and health behaviours. However, some genetically acquired biological traits, such as differences in skin pigmentation, body build, and

metabolism, can have a bearing on a person's health. For example, individuals who trace their ancestry to black racial groups of Africa, among others, are predisposed to a genetic blood condition known as sickle-cell anemia.

It is important for nurses to explore the cultural and ethnic beliefs and the health care practices of *all* Canadians (see the Evidence-Informed Practice box). The Canadian health care system is rooted in Western biomedical principles, in which outcome is oriented toward the effective diagnosis and treatment of disease. Clients from a nondominant culture may view nurses of the predominant culture as a threat to their traditional ways of dealing with health care concerns. For example, ethnic minority immigrants may not be able to read and write in either official language of Canada. Written instructions from a nurse may be misunderstood or not fully understood.

Escallier, Fullerton, and Messina (2011) contended that cultural competence is really nursing competence. The "real issue in a clinical event is individualized patient care—which is the signature of contemporary nursing—which has been repackaged by the medical profession as 'culturally competent' care" (p. 185). Essentially, the various cultural assessments are simply strategies for eliciting the patient's understanding of his or her illness, individualizing his or her care, and improving communication.

Before presenting a cultural safety lens, it is necessary to elaborate on the diversity of the health beliefs and practices, family patterns, communications styles,

---

EVIDENCE-INFORMED PRACTICE

How Do Contemporary néhiyawak (Plains Cree) Describe miyo-mahcihoyān (Well-Being)?

Given the negative history of research with Indigenous peoples, there has been a shift to new research paradigms as a result of the "decolonizing agenda that has a principal goal, the amelioration of disease and the recovery of health and wellness for Indigenous populations" (Ermine, Sinclair & Jeffery, 2004, p. 9). Research guidelines and policies now reflect a greater sensitivity to Indigenous knowledge and to the rights of Indigenous peoples and their communities. Graham-Marrs (2011) explored what improved the mental health and well-being of the Plains Cree people from Thunderchild First Nation and what they perceived as necessary to attain optimal mental health and well-being. Each step of the research process was intended to benefit the participants, the same way the nursing process is expected to benefit clients.

NURSING IMPLICATIONS: Through research such as this, nurses can begin to understand how cultural perspectives influence clients' views of health and health challenges.

Source: Based on Graham-Marrs, H. A. (2011). *Narrative descriptions of miyo-mahcihoyān (well-being) from a contemporary néhiyawak (Plains Cree) perspective* (Doctoral dissertation). Saskatoon, SK: University of Saskatchewan.

space and time orientation, nutritional patterns, pain responses, and death and dying practices of Canadians.

Health Beliefs and Practices

The **scientific or biomedical health belief** is based on the belief that life and life processes are controlled by physical and biochemical processes that can be manipulated (Andrews & Boyle, 2003). The client with this view will believe that illness is caused by germs, viruses, bacteria, or a breakdown of the human machine, the body. This client will expect a pill, treatment, or surgery to cure health problems.

From an Indigenous perspective, the **holistic health belief** approaches health and well-being from a perspective that takes into consideration interconnectedness, interrelatedness, balance, and harmony within an individual and extends outward into the community (Hart, 2002). Many Indigenous peoples of North America and South America use the medicine wheel to symbolize these concepts. For example, the medicine wheel teaches that there are four aspects to an individual's well-being—the physical, the mental or intellectual, the emotional, and the spiritual (Mussell, 2005). See Figure 11.2.

The concept of yin and yang in the Chinese culture and the hot–cold theory of illness in many Spanish cultures are examples of holistic health beliefs. When a Chinese client has a yin illness or a cold illness, the treatment may include a yang or hot food (e.g., hot tea). For example, a Chinese client who has been diagnosed with cancer, a yin disease, will want to eat foods considered to have yang properties.

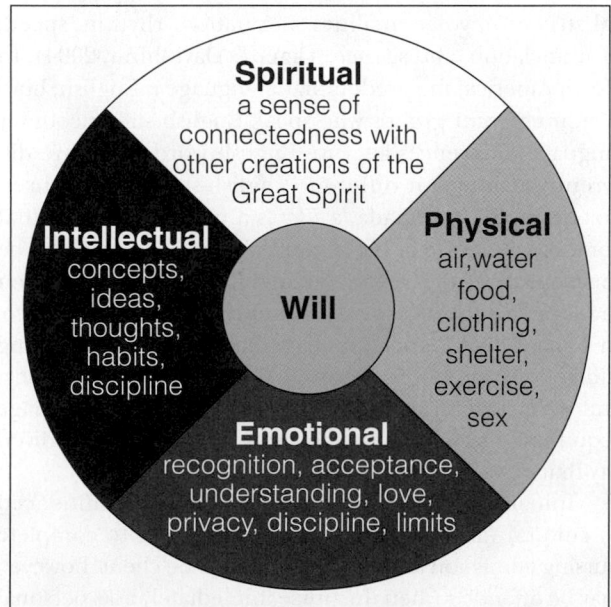

FIGURE 11.2 Medicine Wheel.

Source: Mussel, W. J. (2005). *Warrior-caregivers: Understanding the challenges and healing of First Nations men* (p. 115). Ottawa, ON: Aboriginal Healing Foundation. Photo courtesy of the Aboriginal Healing Foundation, www.ahf.ca

What is considered hot or cold varies considerably across cultures. In many cultures, the mother who has just delivered a baby should be offered warm or hot foods and kept warm with blankets because childbirth is seen as a cold condition. Conventional scientific thought recommends cooling the body to reduce a fever. The physician may order liquids for the client and cool compresses to be applied to the forehead, the axillae, or the groin. Galanti (2004) stated that many cultures believe that the best way to treat a fever is to "sweat it out." Clients from these cultures may want to cover up with several blankets, take hot baths, and drink hot beverages. Giger and Davidhizar (2004) stated that the nurse must keep in mind that a treatment strategy that is consistent with the client's beliefs may have a better chance of being successful. For example, the Latin American client who avoids spicy foods when experiencing a stomach disturbance may be eating foods consistent with the bland diet that is normally prescribed by physicians.

People who have limited access to scientific health care or strong cultural beliefs may turn to traditional medicine or healing. **Traditional medicine** is defined as those beliefs and practices relating to illness prevention and healing that are derived from cultural traditions, rather than from modern medicine's scientific base. Many students might recall special teas or cures used by older family members to prevent or treat colds, fevers, indigestion, and other common health problems. People continue to use chicken soup as a treatment for the flu.

Why do individuals use these traditional healing methods? Traditional medicine, in contrast to biomedical health care, is thought to be more humanistic. The consultation and treatment often takes place in the community of the recipient, frequently in the home of the healer. The healer often prepares the treatments, for example, teas to be ingested, poultices to be applied, or charms or amulets to be worn. It is important for the nurse to be mindful that these amulets or culture-specific items may be placed under their pillow to assist with the healing process; thus, it is essential to ensure that these items are kept intact and remain in place throughout the person's hospitalization. A frequent component of treatment is some ritual practice on the part of the healer or the client to cause healing to occur. For example, Indigenous peoples may participate in a sundance as part of their healing process. Because traditional healing practices are culturally based, they are often more comfortable and less frightening for the client.

It is important for the nurse to obtain information about traditional healing practices that may have been used before and currently in use when the client is seeking Western medical treatment. Often, clients are reluctant to share home remedies with health care professionals for fear of being laughed at or rebuked. The nurse should remember that treatments once considered to be traditional treatments, including acupuncture, therapeutic touch, and massage, are now being investigated for their therapeutic effect. However, herbal remedies sometimes interact with cardiac medications, for example, with deleterious effects on a person's health, ranging from discomfort to death.

Family Patterns

The family is the basic unit of society. Cultural values can determine communication within the family group, the norm for family size, and the roles of specific family members. In some families, the man is considered the provider and decision maker. The woman may need to consult her family before making decisions about her medical treatment or the treatment of her children. Some families are matriarchal; that is, the mother or grandmother is viewed as the leader of the family and is usually the decision maker. The nurse needs to identify who has the authority to make decisions in a client's family. If the decision maker is someone other than the client, the nurse needs to include that person in health care discussions.

The value placed on children and older people within a society is culturally derived. In some cultures, older people are considered the holders of the culture's wisdom and are, therefore, highly respected. Responsibility for caring for older relatives is determined by cultural practices. In many cultures, older relatives who cannot live independently often live with a married son or daughter and his or her family.

Cultural gender-role behaviour may also affect nurse–client interaction. In some countries, men dominate, and women have little status. Men from these countries may not accept instruction from a female nurse or physician but are receptive to the same instruction given by a male physician or nurse. Some cultures have a prevailing concept of *machismo,* or male superiority. Machismo requires that the adult man provide for and protect his family, including extended family members. The woman is expected to maintain the home and raise the children.

Cultural family values may also dictate the extent of the family's involvement in the hospitalized client's care. In some cultures, the nuclear and the extended family will want to visit for long periods and participate in care. In other cultures, the entire clan may want to visit and participate in the client's care. This can cause concern on nursing units with strict visiting policies. The nurse should evaluate the positive benefits of family participation in the client's care and modify visiting policies, as appropriate.

Cultures that value the needs of the extended family as much as those of the individual may hold the belief that personal and family information must stay within the family. Some cultural groups are very reluctant to disclose family information to outsiders, including health care professionals. This attitude can present difficulties for health care professionals who require knowledge of family interaction patterns to help clients with emotional problems.

Naming systems in many cultures differ from those in North America. In some cultures (e.g., Japanese and Vietnamese), the family name comes first and the given name second. One or two names may or may not be added between the family and given names. Other nomenclature may be used to delineate sex and child or adult status. For example, in traditional Japanese culture, adults address other adults by their surname followed by *san,* meaning *Mr., Mrs.,* or *Miss.* An example is "Maurakami san." The children are referred to by their first names followed by *kun* for boys and *chan* for girls. Sikhs and Hindus traditionally have three names. Hindus have a personal name, a complementary name (such as the father's first name), and then a family name. Sikhs have a personal name, the title *Singh* for men and *Kaur* for women, and then the family name. Names by marriage also vary. In Central America, a woman who marries retains her father's name and takes her husband's. For example, if Louisa Viccario marries Carlos Gonzales, she becomes Louisa Viccario de Gonzales. The connecting *de* means "belonging to." Nurses need to become familiar with appropriate ways to address clients.

Communication Style

Communication and culture are closely interconnected. Through communication, culture is transmitted from one generation to the next, and knowledge about the culture is transmitted within the group and to those outside the group. Effective communication with clients of various ethnic and cultural backgrounds is critical to providing culturally competent, safe nursing care. A therapeutic nurse–client relationship is grounded in meaningful communication between the nurse and the client. Cultural variations in both verbal and nonverbal communication can require the development of a communication plan that incorporates the client as an informed partner in care.

VERBAL COMMUNICATION The most obvious cultural difference is in verbal communication: vocabulary, grammatical structure, voice qualities, intonation, rhythm, speed, pronunciation, and silence (Giger & Davidhizar, 2004). In North America, the predominant language is English; however, immigrant groups who speak English still encounter language differences because English words can have different meanings in different English-speaking cultures. For example, in Canada, a *boot* is a type of footwear that comes to the ankle or higher; in England, a *boot* can also be the trunk of a car. Similarly, great differences exist between the French spoken in Canada and that spoken in France. In Canada, the French language has evolved, assimilating Indigenous and English terms. In Quebec, New Brunswick, and other places, nurses must meet the French-language requirements and need to be aware of the language diversity that exists within the province.

Initiating verbal communication may be influenced by cultural values. The busy nurse may want to complete nursing admission assessments quickly. The client, however, may be offended when the nurse immediately asks personal questions. In some cultures, it is believed that social courtesies should be established before business or personal topics are discussed. Discussing general topics can convey that the nurse is interested in the client and has time for the client. This enables the nurse to develop a rapport with the client before progressing to more personal discussion.

Verbal communication becomes even more difficult when an interaction involves people who speak different languages. Both clients and health care professionals experience frustration when they are unable to communicate verbally with each other. For clients who have limited knowledge of English, the nurse should avoid slang words, medical terminology, and abbreviations. Augmenting spoken conversation with gestures or pictures can increase the client's understanding. The nurse should speak slowly, in a respectful manner, and at a normal volume. Speaking loudly does not help the client understand and may be offensive. The nurse must also frequently validate the client's understanding of what is being communicated. The nurse must be wary of interpreting a client's smiling and nodding to mean that the client understands; the client may only be trying to please the nurse while not understanding what is being said.

For the client who speaks a different language, an interpreter may be necessary. Galanti (2004) noted that cultural rules often dictate who can discuss what with whom. Guidelines for using an interpreter are shown in Box 11.1. Whenever possible, professional health care interpreters should be used.

Interpreters should be objective individuals who can provide accurate interpretation of the client's information and of the health care professional's questions, information, and instruction. Many institutions that are located in culturally diverse communities have interpreters available on staff or maintain a list of employees who are fluent in other languages. Embassies, consulates, ethnic churches, ethnic clubs, or telephone companies may also be able to provide interpretation services. Nurses and other health care personnel can use pictures and gestures to augment verbal communication.

Nurses who speak a second language may be asked to interpret for others. Some nursing schools and health care institutions do not permit nursing students to interpret for a procedure consent because a lack of knowledge about the procedure may lead the student to give inaccurate information. The student should check the institution's policy before agreeing to interpret for institutional staff and physicians.

Nurses and other health care providers must remember that clients for whom English is a second language may lose command of their English when they are in stressful situations. Clients who have used English comfortably for years in social and business communication may forget and revert back to their primary language when they are ill or distressed. It is important for the nurse to assure the client that this is normal and to promote behaviours to facilitate verbal communication.

NONVERBAL COMMUNICATION To communicate effectively with culturally diverse clients, the nurse needs to be aware of two aspects of nonverbal communication behaviours: (a) what nonverbal behaviours mean to the

---

BOX 11.1 USING AN INTERPRETER

When using an interpreter, nurses should use the following guidelines:

- Avoid asking a member of the client's family, especially a child or spouse, to act as interpreter. Some clients, not wanting family members to know about their problems, may not provide complete or accurate information.

- Be sure to obtain client consent to use an interpreter or for any other arrangement for communication.

- Avoid complex language, as the client may have limited understanding of vocabulary in English related to health problems.

- Be aware of sex, age, dialect, and religious differences; it is preferable to use an interpreter of the same sex as the client to avoid embarrassment and faulty translation of sexual matters.

- Avoid an interpreter who is politically or socially incompatible with the client. For example, a Bosnian Serb may not be the best interpreter for a Muslim, even if he speaks the language.

- Address the questions to the client, *not* to the interpreter.

- Ask the interpreter to interpret as closely as possible the words used—the interpreter's role is to be the voice of the client.

- Speak slowly and distinctly. Do *not* use metaphors—for example, "Does it swell like a grapefruit?" or "Is the pain stabbing like a knife stab?"

- Observe the facial expressions and body language that the client assumes when listening and talking to the interpreter.

- Ask the interpreter to share any insights about the client; however, be sure these are perceived to be insights and not facts or the client's actual beliefs.

- Explain to the client and the interpreter that all communication is confidential—no client information will be disclosed to anyone.

- Write down key points, directions, and/or appointment times so they are not confused or forgotten.

- Ask the client to repeat in his or her own words all instructions and information.

- Determine from the interpreter whether or not any aspects of the interaction were difficult.

---

client, and (b) what specific nonverbal behaviours mean in the client's culture. It is not required that the nurse be knowledgeable about the nonverbal behaviour patterns of all cultures; however, before assigning meaning to nonverbal behaviour, the nurse must consider the possibility that the behaviour may have a different meaning for the client and the family. Furthermore, to provide safe and effective care, nurses who work with specific cultural groups should learn more about cultural behaviour and communication patterns within these cultures.

Nonverbal communication can include the use of silence, touch, eye movement, facial expressions, and body posture. Some cultures are quite comfortable with long periods of silence, whereas others consider it appropriate to speak before the other person has finished talking. Many people value silence and view it as essential to understanding a person's needs or use silence to preserve privacy. Some cultures view silence as a sign of respect, whereas to other people, silence may indicate agreement (Giger & Davidhizar, 2004).

Touching involves learned behaviours that can have both positive and negative meanings. In the North American culture, a firm handshake is a recognized form of greeting that reflects cordiality (Giger & Davidhizar, 2004). In some European cultures, greetings may include a kiss on one or both cheeks along with the handshake. In some societies, touch is considered magical, and because of the belief that the soul can leave the body on physical contact, casual touching is forbidden. Vietnamese Canadians may find touching of the head or shoulders to be anxiety producing because of such a belief (Giger & Davidhizar, 2004). Nurses should, therefore, touch a client's head only with permission. The sex of the person touching and being touched often has cultural significance.

Cultures dictate what forms of touch are appropriate for individuals of the same sex and opposite sex. In many cultures, for example, a kiss is not appropriate for a public greeting between persons of the opposite sex, even those who are family members; however, a kiss on the cheek is acceptable as a greeting among individuals of the same sex. The nurse should watch interaction among clients and families for cues to the appropriate degree of touch in that culture. The nurse can also assess the client's response to touch when providing nursing care, for example, by noting the client's reaction to the physical examination or a bath.

Facial expression can vary among cultures. Giger and Davidhizar (2004) stated that Italian, Jewish, black, and Spanish-speaking persons are more likely to smile readily and use facial expression to communicate feelings, whereas Irish, English, and northern European people tend to have less facial expression and are less open in their response, especially to strangers. Facial expressions can also convey a meaning opposite to what is felt or understood.

Eye movement during communication has cultural foundations. In Western cultures, direct eye contact is regarded as important and generally shows that the other is attentive and listening. It conveys self-confidence, openness, interest, and honesty. Lack of eye contact may be interpreted as secretiveness, shyness, guilt, lack of interest, or even a sign of a mental health problem. However, other cultures view eye contact as impolite or an invasion of privacy.

Body posture and gesture are also culturally learned. Finger pointing, the "V" sign with the index and middle fingers, and the thumbs-up sign have different meanings. For example, the "V" sign means victory in some cultures, but it is an offensive gesture in other cultures (Galanti, 2004). In the Hmong culture, bowing the head slightly when entering the room where an older person is present and using both hands to give something to someone are considered signs of respect (Rairdan & Higgs, 1992).

Communication is an essential part of establishing a relationship with clients and their families. It is also important for developing effective working relationships with health care colleagues. To enhance their practice, nurses can observe the communication patterns of clients

and colleagues and be aware of their own communication behaviours.

Space Orientation

Space is a relative concept that includes the individual, the body, the surrounding environment, and objects within that environment. The relationship between the individual's own body and objects and persons within a space is learned and is influenced by culture. For example, in nomadic societies space is not owned; it is occupied temporarily until the tribe moves on. In Western societies, people tend to be more territorial, as reflected in such phrases as "This is my space" or "Get out of my space." In Western cultures, spatial distances are defined as the intimate zone, the personal zone, and the social and public zones. The size of these areas may vary with the specific culture. Nurses move through all three zones as they provide care for clients. The nurse needs to be aware of the client's response to movement toward him or her. The client may physically withdraw or back away if the nurse is perceived as being too close. The nurse will need to explain to the client why there is a need to be close. To assess the lungs with a stethoscope, for example, the nurse needs to move into the client's intimate space. The nurse should first explain the procedure and await permission to continue.

Residents in long-term care facilities or patients who are hospitalized for an extended time may want to personalize their space. They may want to arrange their room differently or control the placement of objects on their bedside cabinet or overbed table. The nurse should be responsive to clients' needs to have some control over their space. When there are no medical contraindications, clients should be permitted and encouraged to wear their own clothing and have objects of personal significance. Wearing cultural dress or having personal and cultural items in the environment can increase self-esteem by promoting not only the client's individuality but also his or her cultural identity. Of course, the nurse should caution the client about responsibility for loss of personal items.

Time Orientation

Time orientation refers to an individual's focus on the past, the present, or the future. Most cultures combine all three time orientations, but one orientation is more likely to dominate. The North American focus on time tends to be directed to the future, emphasizing time and schedules (Galanti, 2004). Nursing students know what times they must be in class or clinical. They know what courses they will take in future semesters. European Canadians often plan for next week, their vacation, or their retirement. Other cultures may have a different concept of time. Members of First Nations communities may be perceived as being present oriented and not being concerned with the future. Other values, such as family and community, may override or come into conflict with European views or orientations with regard to time. For example, going to class or to a medical appointment may take a backseat if a family member becomes ill. The first obligation is always to family and community. Often, no explanations are given, perhaps because none are expected within the Indigenous culture.

The culture of nursing and health care values time. Appointments are scheduled, and treatments are prescribed with time parameters (e.g., changing a dressing once a day). Medication orders include how often the medicine is to be taken and when (e.g., digoxin 0.25 mg, once a day, in the morning). Nurses need to be aware of the meaning of time for clients. Giger and Davidhizar (2004) stated that when caring for clients who are "present-oriented," it is important to avoid fixed schedules. The nurse can offer a time range for activities and treatments. For example, instead of telling the client to take digoxin every day at 10 a.m., the nurse might tell the client to take it every day in the morning, or every day after getting out of bed.

Nutritional Patterns

Most cultures have staple foods, that is, foods that are plentiful or readily accessible in the environment. For example, the staple food of most Asians is rice; of Italians, pasta; and of Eastern Europeans, wheat. Even clients who have been in Canada for several generations often continue to eat the foods of their cultural homelands.

The way food is prepared and served is also related to cultural practices. For example, in Canada, a traditional food served for the Thanksgiving holiday is stuffed turkey; however, in different regions of the country, the contents of the stuffing may vary. The variation may be influenced by ethnic preference or by regional tradition, such as including oysters, fruits, or nuts, or using rice instead of bread.

Food-related cultural behaviours can include whether to breast-feed or bottle-feed infants and when to introduce solid foods to them. Food can also be considered part of the remedy for illness. Foods classified as hot foods or foods that are hot in temperature may be used to treat illnesses that are classified as cold illnesses, as noted earlier. For example, corn meal (a hot food) may be used to treat arthritis (a cold illness). Each cultural group defines what it considers to be hot and cold entities.

Religious practice associated with specific cultures also affects diet. Some Roman Catholics avoid meat on certain days, such as Ash Wednesday and Good Friday, and some Protestant denominations prohibit meat, tea, coffee, or alcohol. Both Orthodox Judaism and Islam prohibit the ingestion of pork or pork products. Orthodox Jews observe kosher customs, eating certain foods only if they are inspected by a rabbi and prepared according to dietary laws. For example, the eating of milk products and meat products at the same meal is prohibited. Some Buddhists, Hindus, and Sikhs are strict vegetarians. The nurse must be sensitive to such religious dietary practices.

Pain Responses

It has been demonstrated that beliefs about and responses to pain vary among ethnic and racial groups. Cultural response to pain must be viewed in relation to both the actual perception of pain and the meaning or significance of pain to the client and family. In some cultures, pain is considered a punishment for bad deeds; the individual is, therefore, to tolerate pain without complaint to atone for sins. In other cultures, self-infliction of pain is a sign of mourning or grief. In other groups, pain is anticipated as a part of the ritualistic practices of passage ceremonies and, therefore, tolerance of pain signifies strength and endurance. In some cultures, boys especially are taught "to take pain like a man" and that "big boys don't cry," but in other cultures, the expression of pain elicits attention and sympathy.

Galanti (2004) noted that nurses and clients may assess pain differently. Nurses and physicians may underestimate or overestimate (and treat accordingly) their client's pain in relation to the client's expression of pain and their own cultural context. Client responses to pain should be assessed within the context of their culture. If the client does not complain of pain, it should not be assumed that the client is not experiencing pain. The nurse must be aware of what conditions are likely to cause pain and offer clients pain relief, as appropriate.

Treatment for pain may also vary with culture. In European Canadian cultures, medication is typically used for pain relief. In other cultures, heat, cold, relaxation, or other techniques and treatments may be used.

Death and Dying Practices

Death is a universal experience, and people want to die with dignity. Various cultural and religious traditions and practices associated with death, dying, and the grieving process help people cope with these experiences. Nurses are often present through the client's dying process and at the moment of death, especially when it occurs in a health care facility. Knowledge of the client's religious and cultural heritage helps nurses provide individualized care to the client and the family, even though the nurses themselves may not participate in the family's rituals associated with death. It is important for the nurse to ask the family if any special customs or practices are required prior to and after the death of the client.

Dying in solitude is unacceptable in most cultures. In many cultures, people prefer a peaceful death at home rather than in the hospital. Some ethnic groups may request that health care professionals not reveal the prognosis to dying clients. They believe the person's last days should be free of worry and pain. People in other cultures prefer that a family member (preferably a male in some cultures) be told the diagnosis so that the client can be tactfully informed by a family member in gradual stages or not told at all. Nurses also need to determine whom to call and when as the client's death draws near.

Beliefs and attitudes about death, its cause, and the soul also vary among cultures. Unnatural deaths, or "bad deaths," are sometimes distinguished from "good deaths." In some cultures, the death of a person who has behaved well in life is considered less threatening because that person will be reincarnated into a good life next time.

Beliefs about preparation of the body, autopsy, organ donation, cremation, and prolonging life can be closely allied to the person's religion. *Autopsy,* for example, may be prohibited, opposed, or discouraged by Eastern Orthodox religions, Muslims, Jehovah's Witnesses, and Orthodox Jews. Some religions prohibit the removal of body parts and dictate that all body parts be given appropriate burial. *Organ donation* is prohibited for Jehovah's Witnesses and Muslims, whereas Buddhists in North America consider it an act of mercy and encourage it. *Cremation* is discouraged, opposed, or prohibited by the Mormon, Eastern Orthodox, Islamic, and Jewish faiths. Hindus, in contrast, prefer cremation and cast the ashes into what they consider a holy river. *Prolongation of life* is generally encouraged; however, some religions, such as Christian Science, are unlikely to use medical means to prolong life, and the Jewish faith generally opposes prolonging life after irreversible brain damage. In terminal illness, Buddhists may permit euthanasia.

Nurses also need to be knowledgeable about the client's death-related rituals, such as last rites and administration of Holy Communion, chanting at the bedside, and other rituals, such as special procedures for washing, dressing, positioning, and shrouding the dead. For example, certain people may want to retain their native customs, in which family members of the same sex wash and prepare the body for burial and cremation. Muslims customarily turn the body to face Mecca. Nurses need to ask family members about their preferences and verify who will carry out these activities. Burial clothes and other cultural or religious items are often important symbols for the funeral. For example, those of the Mormon faith are often dressed in their temple clothes. The nurse must ensure that any ritual items present in the health care agency are given to the family or to the funeral home.

Providing Culturally Safe Care

Leininger (1991) produced one of the first models of cultural care diversity and universality (see MyNursingLab for the model). Since the development of Leininger's sunrise model, several other models have been developed. All of these models address similar elements of culture pertinent to nursing care. Some focused on broad concepts, such as an emphasis on understanding of personal biases, prejudices, values, and beliefs,

combined with an understanding of power, trust, and equity (Srivastava, 2007); and others emphasized learning the practices and beliefs that are attributed to particular cultures (Purnell & Paulanka, 2005). Some others introduced notions of time, space (Giger & Davidhizar, 2004; Spector, 2004), and communication (Andrews & Boyle, 2003). Although these models have elements in common, each model emphasizes slightly different attributes that can guide the nurse to assess patient, family, or community culture. However, health care providers should use these models in conjunction with a cultural safety lens to avoid a checklist approach. The assumption that checklists and learning about rituals and practices in general will provide insight into the complexity of social human behaviour is risky. **Cultural safety** takes into consideration power relations and the uniqueness of human beings and avoids stereotyping.

Cultural competence requires acknowledging the fundamental ethnocentrism of contemporary Western health care and the differences in the way patients and families respond to illness and treatment (Escallier, Fullerton, & Messina, 2011). Cultural competence is "the process in which the health care provider continuously strives to achieve the ability to effectively work within the cultural context of a client, individual, family, or community (Campinha-Bacote, 1998, p. 6). Srivastava's (2008) ABC (and DE) model of cultural competence (see Figure 11.3) provides a comprehensive context to guide safe nursing care for the diverse populations in Canada. Srivastava's (2008) ABCDE approach to cultural competence is based on assumptions and concepts that provide a way of viewing a complex issue:

A = Affective domain
B = Behavioural domain
C = Cognitive domain
D = Dynamics of difference
E = Equity and Environment

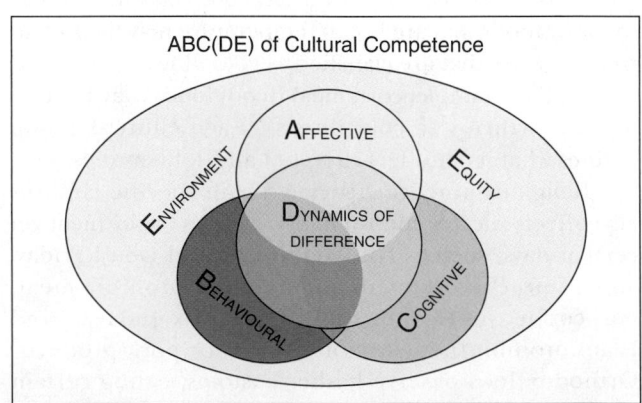

FIGURE 11.3 Srivastava's (2008) ABC (and DE) Model of Cultural Competence.

Source: Srivastava, R. (2008). PowerPoint slide from the Canadian Federation of Mental Health Nurses Conference Presentation. Toronto, ON: Author. Reprinted by permission of Rani Srivastava.

The first three domains have been described extensively in the literature. The **affective domain** of cultural competence is demonstrated by cultural awareness and sensitivity and is viewed as a vital first step in the cultural competence journey. **Cultural awareness** is the self-examination and in-depth exploration of one's own cultural and professional backgrounds. This process involves the recognition of one's biases, prejudices, and assumptions about individuals who are different (Campinha-Bacote, 2002). Without being aware of the influence of one's own culture or professional values, there is a risk that the health care provider may engage in cultural imposition. Cultural imposition is the tendency of an individual to impose their beliefs, values, and patterns of behaviour on another culture (Leininger, 1978). **Cultural sensitivity** is the respect and appreciation for cultural behaviours based on an understanding of the other person's experience and perspective. This domain reflects an intentional respect for cultural differences and having an accepting attitude. To develop this awareness and sensitivity requires openness, critical self-reflection, and experience (Srivastava, 2008). In addition, the Registered Nurses' Association of Ontario (RNAO, 2007) reminds health care providers that exposure to different cultures does not necessarily lead to cultural sensitivity; it is a focused commitment to learning from and about others alongside critical self-reflection that will develop one's cultural sensitivity.

The **behavioural domain** of cultural competence is typically described as the cultural skill that enables the health care provider to learn about client's cultural values, beliefs, and practices to determine the most appropriate goals and interventions (Srivastava, 2008).

The **cognitive domain** addresses the need for knowledge-based care. The nature of knowledge required for cultural competence is not clear (Srivastava, 2008). She suggests health care providers assess the extent to which the issues involved can be categorized as (a) unique to the individual, (b) reflective of the broader culture, and (c) reflective of cultural processes in general. Ideally, health care providers would learn the rituals, customs, and practices of the major cultural groups within the geographical location where they practice.

Understanding the **dynamics of difference** is a key attribute of cultural competence. Given the "significant influence that minority group or marginalized status can have on healthcare quality and outcomes, there is merit in highlighting this attribute as a separate domain" (Srivastava, 2008, p. 31). Cultural competence in this domain requires health care providers to acknowledge and understand the impact of systemic oppression, discrimination, and racism. In addition, these dynamics of difference occur at multiple levels: (a) client–clinician, (b) client–system, (c) clinician–colleagues, and (d) clinician–system. Dynamics of difference recognize the impact of both marginalization and privilege (Srivastava, 2008).

"E" represents **equity** and **environment**. Equity focuses on "equality of outcomes and means that people with unequal need require different or differential treatment to achieve identical results" (Srivastava, 2008, p. 32). By keeping the concept of equity as a desired goal for cultural competence, health care providers are reminded to "identify and address the unique needs and barriers for each patient" (Srivastava, 2008, p. 32). The environment— that is, the practice setting—also plays an important role in promoting and supporting client care. Health care providers require the support of their practice setting to effectively deliver culturally competent care to their clients. For example, interpreter services may need to be accessed for care in the home.

Guidelines for Best Practices

Several national and provincial nursing groups have developed position statements and best practices for delivery of appropriate cultural care. Examples are the Canadian Nurses Association (CNA, 2010) *Position Statement: Promoting Cultural Competence in Nursing*; the RNAO (2007) *Embracing Cultural Diversity in Health Care: Developing Cultural Competence*; and the Aboriginal Nurses Association of Canada (2009) *Cultural Competence and Cultural Safety in Nursing Education: A Framework for First Nation, Inuit and Métis Nursing*. The College of Nurses of Ontario's *Practice Guideline for Culturally Sensitive Care* (2008) emphasizes the following elements for providing culturally sensitive care:

1. *Being culturally knowledgeable:* It is impossible to possess in-depth knowledge about all cultures; however, it is possible to have a general understanding of how cultures can affect health practices and beliefs.

2. *Being client centred:* Client-centred care requires that nurses recognize the client's culture, the nurse's own culture, and how both affect the nurse–client relationship—the focus of care is always the client's needs. Each client and each situation is unique and requires individual assessment and planning.

3. *Being self-reflective:* Self-reflection is a fundamental element of providing culturally sensitive, competent, and safe care. Nurses may fall into the trap of thinking they know a culture and therefore know what is best for the client, or nurses might impose their beliefs and values on the client or presuppose that their own values are the same as the clients'. Understanding the self as distinct from others in the broadest sense is critical in the provision of culturally safe care.

4. *Recognizing potential conflict between the culture of the nursing profession's values and beliefs and client cultural values and beliefs:* The nursing profession itself has a culture that can come into conflict with the cultural values and beliefs of clients. When beliefs and values come into conflict, it is the nurse's role to reflect on her professional beliefs and values and to explore and reframe the treatment or therapy in a culturally appropriate way that meets the client's goal of care.

5. *Facilitating client choice:* This is part of the nurse's role in providing quality care. A client's choice could place other clients at risk or be threatening to their care. In such situations, it is the nurse's responsibility to balance these demands. The nurse attempts to meet some of the client's wishes while at the same time protecting other clients.

6. *Incorporating client's cultural preferences:* Adding these into the client's nursing care plan can facilitate the client's physical, emotional, or spiritual health, taking into consideration whether or not the practices are harmful to the client or other clients. Endorsement of one client's cultural beliefs, practices, or values does not mean the nurse adopts these views or requires other clients to do so.

7. *Accommodating client cultural beliefs and practices:* This can be done by finding ways to minimize risks or remove obstacles.

It is interesting to note that the study by Purnell (2002) on the perceptions of preferred care of patients in a Guatemalan clinic indicated little concern for sensitivity to cultural traditions. Rather, they looked for behaviours such as greeting the patient with a handshake, calling the person by name, explaining procedures at every opportunity, asking permission for and explaining the necessity of examination, informing the patient ahead of time whether procedures were painful, and maintaining a professional demeanour. Similar conclusions were reached by McGee (2001), who stated that caring, respect, compassion, and sincerity were central to cultural competence.

Barriers to Cultural Sensitivity and Safety

Many factors can be barriers to providing culturally sensitive or culturally safe care to clients and their support people. These issues can also affect communication and working relationships with other health care personnel. Ethnocentrism, stereotyping, prejudice, and discrimination are some of these elements.

Ethnocentrism refers to the view that the beliefs and values of one person's own culture are superior to those of other cultures. In health care, ethnocentrism can include the view that the only valid health care beliefs and practices are those held by the professionals in the health care system. Nurses who take a transcultural view, however, value their own beliefs and practices while respecting the beliefs and practices of others. It is important for nurses to realize that although many people of diverse racial and religious backgrounds have combined their traditional health practices with Western health practices, other people may be unable or unwilling to do so.

Most people are gradually exposed to their culture's beliefs, values, and practices over a period of years, starting at birth. Ethnocentrism is thought to result from lack of exposure or knowledge of other cultures. **Ethnorelativity** is the ability to appreciate and respect the viewpoints of other cultures.

Stereotyping occurs when the assumption is made that all members of a culture or ethnic group are alike. For example, a nurse may assume that all Italians express pain volubly or that all Chinese people like rice. Stereotyping may be based on generalizations founded in research, or it may be unrelated to reality. For example, research indicates that Italians are likely to express pain verbally; however, a particular Italian client may not verbalize pain. Stereotyping that is unrelated to reality can be either positive or negative and is frequently an outcome of racism or discrimination. Nurses need to realize that not all people of a specific group have the same health beliefs, practices, and values. It is, therefore, essential to identify a specific client's beliefs, needs, and values, rather than assuming they are the same as those attributable to the larger group.

Prejudice is a strongly held opinion about some topic or group of people. A prejudice may be positive or negative. A positive prejudice often stems from a strong sense of ethnocentrism (Eliason, 1993). Prejudice may also derive from ignorance, misinformation, past experience, or fear. Types of negative prejudice include ageism, which is negative attitudes toward older adults; sexism, meaning negative attitudes toward women; and homophobia, which is negativism toward lesbian women and gay men.

Discrimination refers to the differential and negative treatment of individuals on the basis of their race, ethnicity, gender, or other group membership. **Institutional discrimination** refers to the uneven access by group membership to resources, status, and power resulting from policies and practices of organizations and institutions. Deliberate discrimination in Canadian history has created inequalities between racial groups, specifically, within the Indigenous peoples of Canada (Office of the Treaty Commissioner, 2008). **Racism** is a form of discrimination related to ethnocentrism in which a person believes that race is the primary determinant of human traits and capacities and that racial differences result in an inherent superiority of a particular race.

Implementing Best Practices for Safe Cultural Caring

It is important for nurses to be culturally sensitive and to convey this sensitivity to clients, support people, and other health care personnel. Some ways to do so include the following:

- Always address clients by their last names (e.g., Mrs. Aylia, Dr. Rush) until they give you permission to use other names. In some cultures, the more formal style of address is a sign of respect, whereas the use of first names may be considered disrespectful. It is important to ask clients how they want to be addressed.

- When meeting a person for the first time, introduce yourself by your full name and explain your role in the person's health care. This helps establish a relationship and provides an opportunity for clients and nurses to learn the pronunciation of one another's names.

- Be genuine with people, and be honest about the knowledge you lack about their culture.

- Use language that is culturally sensitive; for example, use terms such as *gay, lesbian, bisexual, transgendered,* or *two-spirited* rather than *homosexual;* do not use *man* or *mankind* when referring to a woman; *African Canadian* is preferred by some over *black,* and *Latin American* is preferred over *Hispanic. Asian* is more acceptable than *Oriental* (Eliason, 1993). In Canada, use the term *Aboriginal* or *Indigenous* to refer to First Nations, Inuit, and Métis. Even better, ask the person what term they prefer. Members of some ethnic groups may prefer the appellation of *Hispanic* or *Oriental,* for example.

- Find out what the clients know about their health problems, illnesses, and treatments. Assess whether this information is congruent with the predominant health care culture. If the beliefs and practices are incongruent, establish whether this will have a negative effect on the client's health.

- Do not make any assumptions about the client, and always ask about anything you do not understand.

- Respect the client's values, beliefs, and practices, even if they differ from your own or from those of the predominant culture. If you don't agree with them, it is important to respect the client's rights to hold these beliefs. It is important for the client to feel safe in the nurse–client relationship.

- Show respect for the client's support people. In some cultures, men in the family make decisions affecting the client, while in other cultures, women make the decisions.

- Make a concerted effort to earn the client's trust, but do not be surprised if it develops slowly or not at all.

Remember, "it is impossible to become an authority on your own culture(s), let alone someone else's and it is counter to the concept of cultural safety, where differences within cultures, not just between them is acknowledged and respected. What cultural safety asks us to do when we face a nursing situation outside of our sphere of cultural experience is to 'ask'" (Hughes & Farrow, 2006, p. 13).

Cultural Assessment

Students in Canadian nursing programs are expected to learn about cultural diversity, and all nurses are expected to provide safe care, regardless of the culture of the client. The CNA (2010) believes that cultural competence is the application of knowledge, skills, attitudes, or personal attributes required by nurses to maximize respectful relationships with diverse populations. The underlying values for cultural competence are inclusivity, respect, valuing differences, equity, and commitment (CNA, 2010).

All phases of the nursing process are affected by the client's and the nurse's cultural values, beliefs, and behaviours. As the client's culture and the nurse's culture come together in the nurse–client relationship, a unique cultural environment is created that can improve or impair the client's outcome. Self-awareness of personal biases can enable nurses to develop modifying behaviours or (if they are unable to do so) to remove themselves from situations where care may be compromised. Nurses can become more aware of their own culture through a values clarification (see Chapter 5). As an example, see Box 11.2 for recommendations for working with Indigenous clients.

A thorough cultural assessment provides a nurse with the necessary information and understanding of how a client's cultural beliefs and practices will impact the nursing process and ultimately the client's health outcome. A cultural assessment takes time and usually needs to extend over several sessions. The process of assessment is important; how and when questions are asked require sensitivity and clinical judgment. Trust must be established before clients can be expected to volunteer and share sensitive information. The nurse, therefore, needs to spend time with clients, introduce some social

---

BOX 11.2 GUIDE FOR HEALTH CARE PROFESSIONALS WORKING WITH INDIGENOUS PEOPLES

According to the Society of Obstetricians and Gynaecologists of Canada (2000) and the Indigenous Physicians Association of Canada (2011), health care professionals should do the following:

1. Have a basic understanding of the appropriate names with which to refer to the various groups of Indigenous peoples in Canada;

2. Have a basic understanding of the current sociodemographics of Indigenous peoples in Canada;

3. Familiarize themselves with the traditional geographical territories and language groups of Indigenous peoples;

4. Understand the connection between historical and current government practices toward First Nations/Inuit/Métis peoples (including, but not limited to, colonization, residential schools, treaties, and land claims), and the resultant intergenerational health outcomes;

5. Recognize that the current sociodemographic challenges facing many Indigenous individuals and communities have a significant impact on health status;

6. Recognize the need to provide health care services for Indigenous peoples as close to home as possible;

7. Have a basic understanding of governmental obligations and policies regarding the health of Indigenous peoples in Canada;

8. Recognize the need to support Indigenous individuals and communities in the process of self-determination.

Source: Adapted from Smylie, J. Policy statement: A guide for health professionals working with Aboriginal peoples, *J Soc Obstet Gynaecol Can 2000,* 22(12): 1056–61.

conversation, and convey a genuine desire to understand their values and beliefs.

Before a cultural assessment begins, the nurse determines what language the client speaks and the client's degree of fluency in English. The nurse can also learn about the client's communication patterns and space orientation by observing both verbal and nonverbal communication. For example, does the client do the speaking or defer to another? What nonverbal communication behaviours does the client exhibit (e.g., touching, eye contact)? What significance do these behaviours have for the nurse–client interaction? What is the client's proximity to other people and objects within the environment? How does the client react to the nurse's movement toward him or her? What cultural objects within the environment have importance for health promotion or health maintenance?

To obtain cultural assessment data, the nurse uses broad statements and open-ended questions that encourage clients to express themselves fully (see Box 11.3 for examples). The important principle to remember when conducting an assessment is that "the client is the teacher and expert regarding his or her culture, and the nurse is the learner" (Rosenbaum, 1995, p. 188). At this stage, the nurse draws no conclusions but obtains information from the client.

Many cultural assessment tools are available. The nurse needs to use a tool appropriate to the situation and adapt it, as required. For example, a nurse in an emergency department of an urban hospital may need a different format from a nurse working in a home care setting. Nurses need to ensure they collect enough basic cultural data to identify patterns of behaviour that may either facilitate or interfere with a nursing strategy or treatment plan.

When a client chooses to follow only cultural practices and refuses all prescribed medical or nursing interventions, nursing goals for the client need to be adjusted. Anderson, Waxler-Morrison, Richardson, Herbert, & Murphy (1990) pointed out that monitoring the client's condition to identify changes in health state and to recognize impending crises before they become irreversible may be all that is realistically achievable. At a time of crisis,

---

BOX 11.3 EXAMPLES OF OPEN-ENDED QUESTIONS FOR A CULTURAL ASSESSMENT

CULTURAL AFFILIATION

I am interested in learning about your cultural heritage. Can you tell me about your cultural group, where you were born, and how long you have lived in this country?

BELIEFS ABOUT CURRENT ILLNESS

What do you call your problem? What name do you give it? What do you think has caused it? Why did it start when it did? What does your sickness do to your body? How severe is it? What do you fear most about your sickness? What are the chief problems your sickness has caused for you personally, for your family, and at work?

COMMUNICATION

What languages do you speak at home? What languages are you most comfortable speaking? In what language(s) can you read and write? How would you like us to address you? by your first name? by your last name? Would you like an interpreter?

HEALTH CARE PRACTICES

What kinds of things do you do to maintain health? For example, what types of food do you eat to maintain health? What foods do you eat during illness, and how is food prepared? What other activities do you or your family do to keep people healthy (e.g., wearing amulets, religious or spiritual practices)? How do you know when you are healthy?

ILLNESS BELIEFS AND CARE PRACTICES

What kinds of things do you do to treat illness? Do you use traditional healers (shaman, curandero, priest, spiritualist, minister, monk)? Who determines when a person is sick? How would you describe your past experiences with cultural healers and Western health care professionals? What special remedies are generally used for the illness you have? What remedies are you currently using (e.g., herbal remedies, potions, massage, wearing of talismans, copper bracelets, or charms)? What remedies have you used in the past, and which did you find helpful? What remedies or treatments are you considering now, and how can we help? Is the care we are giving you what you think it should be? How would you like us to care for you?

FAMILY LIFE AND SUPPORT SYSTEM

I would like to learn about your family. Who are the members of your family? What family duties do women and men usually perform in your culture? Whom do you consult when making health care decisions (e.g., another family member, cultural or religious leader)? Who will be able to help you during and after treatment? Do you need help to contact these people?

Sources: Based on Andrews, M. M. & Boyle, J. S. (2003). *Transcultural concepts in nursing care* (4th ed.). Philadelphia, PA: Lippincott; Kleinman, A., Eisenberg, L., & Good, B. (1978). Culture, illness and care. *Annals of Internal Medicine, 88,* 251–258; Rosenbaum, J. N. (1991). A cultural assessment guide: Learning cultural sensitivity. *Canadian Nurse, 88,* 32–33; and Waxler-Morrison, N., Anderson, J., & Richardson, E. (Eds.). (1990). *Cross-cultural caring: A handbook for health professionals in Western Canada.* Vancouver, BC: University of British Columbia (UBC) Press.

the nurse may then have the opportunity to renegotiate the original care approach.

Safe cultural caring is challenging. It requires discovery of the meaning of the client's behaviour, flexibility, creativity, and knowledge to adapt nursing interventions. For example, a culturally sensitive nurse knows that a Chinese woman who has just given birth and refuses to eat fruits and vegetables, refuses to drink the cold water at her bedside, stays in bed, and refuses to take sitz baths, baths, or showers needs to increase her yang forces. The nurse will make plans to adapt nursing interventions accordingly, recognizing that it is the client's (or family's) right to make his or her own health care choices. Nurses also need to identify community resources that are available to assist clients of diverse cultures. Cultural competence is an ongoing process, multifaceted, and requires a personal and organizational commitment to enhance the health outcomes for all Canadians (Srivastava, 2008).

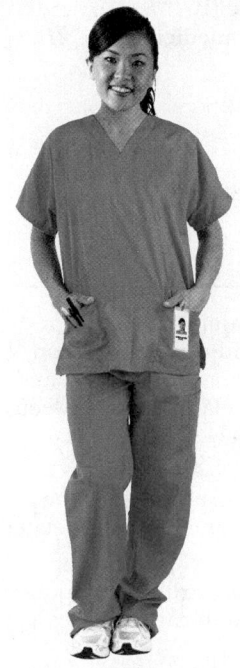

Case Study 11

Rose Maniwaki is a 65-year-old Indigenous person with a history of diabetes. She was diagnosed with gestational diabetes during her first pregnancy in her early twenties. She has had six pregnancies and, during each, her diabetes was significantly aggravated. She is now fully insulin dependent with type II diabetes and is clinically obese (175 cm tall and weighs 110 kg). Her diabetes is extremely difficult to control. She has had her right foot amputated below the knee and has had a prosthesis since age 60 She has osteoarthritis, osteoporosis, and high blood pressure.

Rose is a widow. Her husband died in his forties of uncontrolled diabetes combined with alcoholism. She lives in a small, poorly insulated, mouldy, overcrowded, two-bedroom house in a First Nations community in northern Ontario. After her husband's death, she raised her children alone on social assistance and is now raising five grandchildren so that her daughter can attend nursing school in a community 400 km away. Two of Rose's other children are dead—one from suicide, the other from a car accident caused by drunk driving. Her other surviving children have left northern Ontario, and she has had little or no contact with them. Rose is also struggling with alcoholism.

Rose experiences depression and takes Prozac to help with her health problems and sense of loss. The Prozac does not help very much. Rose uses sleeping pills to assist with sleep. Rose attended residential school from age 6 to 13 years and, therefore, is not as connected to her family and community as she might otherwise be. She has had trouble connecting with her culture and its values. However, there is a new community health centre with a traditional circular healing room, where traditional healers are available alongside a nurse practitioner, nurses, community health representatives, a nutritionist, and a social worker. Rose has been coming to the health centre on a more or less regular basis and has found herself drawn to the traditional healers.

Rose has come to the health centre because she is experiencing breakdown of her stump, which is cracked and painful, as well as draining pus. The nurse practitioner advises her that she may need to travel south to the hospital if the infection persists. Rose has no other family members in the community and worries about who would care for her grandchildren if she has to fly out for hospital care. Rose has brought one of her granddaughters with her to the clinic. Rose's granddaughter is extremely overweight—and, given her family history, at high risk for diabetes.

Through her involvement at the community health centre and interactions with the traditional healers, Rose has begun to become more active in the community and has joined a women's drumming group. She has found the regular gatherings of her drumming group, comprising women of varying ages, to be very helpful in her struggle with alcoholism and depression. Her drumming group gave the opening welcome to an evening heart health talk held in her community for First Nations women and Rose discovered that diabetes is a major risk factor.

As a result of her experiences at the community health centre and in her drumming group, Rose has become involved in self-governance and has joined a group in the local band office, particularly focusing on health issues, such as diabetes, alcoholism, and depression.

CRITICAL THINKING QUESTIONS

1. Using the nursing process, develop a plan of care for Rose and her family (assessment, nursing diagnosis, planning, intervention, and evaluation; see Chapter 23).

   a. How would you integrate holistic health beliefs into your nursing care plan for Rose and her family?

   b. How would you integrate knowledge of colonization and residential schools into Rose and her family's care?

   c. How would you integrate Rose's newly discovered appreciation of traditional healing to her plan of care?

   d. As a health care provider, what questions would you ask Rose about her family, her community, and her diabetes?

   e. How would you integrate your knowledge of the determinants of health into her plan of care?

   Check the eText in MyNursingLab for answers and explanations.

KEY TERMS

affective domain *p. 221*	cultural identity *p. 213*	environment *p. 221*	race *p. 213*
assimilation *p. 211*	cultural safety *p. 220*	equity *p. 221*	racism *p. 222*
behavioural	cultural sensitivity *p. 221*	ethnic *p. 213*	scientific or biomedical
domain *p. 221*	culture *p. 213*	ethnocentrism *p. 222*	health belief *p. 215*
bicultural *p. 213*	culture-specifics *p. 213*	ethnorelativity *p. 222*	stereotyping *p. 222*
cognitive domain *p. 221*	culture-universals *p. 213*	holistic health	subculture *p. 213*
colonization *p. 211*	discrimination *p. 222*	belief *p. 215*	traditional
cultural awareness *p. 221*	diversity *p. 213*	institutional	medicine *p. 215*
cultural	dynamics of	discrimination *p. 222*	
competence *p. 220*	difference *p. 221*	prejudice *p. 222*	

CHAPTER HIGHLIGHTS

- Canadians come from a variety of ethnic and cultural backgrounds, and many Canadians retain at least some of their traditional values, beliefs, and practices.

- Many groups in Canada are bicultural; that is, they embrace two cultures: their original ethnic culture and a Canadian culture.

- An individual's ethnic and cultural background can influence beliefs, values, and practices.

- Through acculturation, most ethnic and cultural groups in Canada modify some of their traditional cultural characteristics.

- Personal characteristics also modify an individual's cultural values, beliefs, and practices.

- Health beliefs and practices, family patterns, communication style, space and time orientation, nutritional patterns, pain response, and death and dying practices influence the relationship between the nurse and the client who have individual cultural backgrounds.

- When assessing a client, the nurse considers the client's cultural values, beliefs, and practices related to health and health care.

- Self-reflection and awareness is a critical component of providing culturally safe health care.

ASSESS YOUR LEARNING

1. Canada's population has more than doubled in the past 50 years as a result of what?
   a. Immigration
   b. Longer life expectancy
   c. Higher birthrates
   d. Immunization

2. A nurse is starting a new job in a community health setting where many of the clients have a different culture than her own. According to Srivastava's ABCDE model of cultural competence (2008), which action by the nurse would BEST satisfy the affective domain of the model?
   a. Set goals for nursing interventions
   b. Discuss the impact of discrimination with the clients
   c. Ensure an interpreter is available for all client interactions
   d. Reflect on her (the nurse's) own values and beliefs about culture

3. What is the focus of cultural safety?
   a. Transcultural nursing theories
   b. Cultural awareness
   c. Cultural competence
   d. Self-reflection and power

4. Which of the following is an example of stereotyping?
   a. Holding a strong opinion against an individual or group of individuals
   b. Giving preferential treatment based on gender, social class, or ethnicity
   c. Assuming that all members of a group are alike
   d. Seeing your one own group as superior to another

5. You are about to begin assisting a young woman from a Middle Eastern country with her morning care; she suddenly appears to be very uncomfortable and asks if she can do it later. In keeping with

the College of Nurses of Ontario's *Guidelines for Culturally Sensitive Care*, what should you do?

a. Immediately pack up your equipment and tell her you will be back later

b. Explain that you are very busy and that this is the only time that her morning care can be done

c. Discuss with the client when she would like to do her morning care and plan to do it then

d. Tell the client that if she does not do it now, she will have to wait until tomorrow

6. You are assigned to care for an older Aboriginal man. In keeping with his traditions, he would like to do a "smudge," that is, ignite a very small quantity of tobacco that he keeps in a pouch with him at all times. What should you do?

a. Explain that there is a no smoking bylaw and that he cannot smoke at any time

b. Inform him that lighting fires in the hospital is against the law

c. Insist that he give you his tobacco, since smoking is bad for him

d. Ask him what a "smudge" is and why he wants to do it

7. What is the most important aspect of providing culturally competent nursing care demonstrated in the scenarios in questions 5 and 6?

a. The client feels safe in the nurse–client relationship.

b. You feel that you have done everything to make the client like you.

c. You have learned something about a new culture.

d. Your clients' preferences are as important as your own.

8. You are assigned to care for a client who does not speak or understand English, the only language that you speak and understand. The client is accompanied by his young grandson, who appears to be about 8 years of age. What would be the BEST course of action?

a. Find an older member of the family to act as an interpreter

b. Request a professional health care interpreter

c. No additional help is necessary—the grandson will be a sufficient interpreter

d. Use nonverbal methods of communication, such as drawing pictures or gesturing

9. You are working in a community agency and one of your clients is consistently late for appointments. This is very distressing to you, since you are very busy and cannot always accommodate the client when she does eventually turn up. You are aware that not all cultures have the same time orientation as Western cultures, that is, to be on time and to keep their scheduled appointments. However, you are not sure whether that is the only reason for the lateness. What should you do?

a. Tell the client that you are very busy and that she should let you know in advance if she is going to be late for the appointment

b. Ask the client why she is late for appointments and ask if you can assist her to keep the scheduled appointments

c. Explain to the client that time is very important in Western or Canadian culture

d. Offer to get her a watch so she can keep track of the time

10. You are assigned two patients who have had abdominal surgery; one patient is constantly complaining about pain, and the other patient does not tell you he is experiencing pain, but you can tell by his facial expressions and body language that he is. What should you do?

a. Assess the patient's pain within the context of the patient's culture.

b. Treat each patient equally and according to Western beliefs and values.

c. Insist that the patient who is more vocal about his pain express his discomfort in more acceptable ways.

d. Ask their physicians to increase their doses of analgesic.

Check the eText in MyNursingLab for answers and explanations.

WEBLINKS

Citizenship and Immigration Canada, Multiculturalism

http://www.cic.gc.ca/english/multiculturalism/index.asp

This site has multiple links to governmental, nongovernmental, Canadian, and international organizations.

Virtual Museum Canada

http://www.museevirtuel-virtualmuseum.ca

This site is the result of a partnership between Canada's museum community and the Department of Canadian Heritage. Through this site, the user can celebrate the stories and treasures that have helped to define Canada.

Aboriginal Affairs and Northern Development Canada

http://www.aadnc-aandc.gc.ca

This site describes the First Nations peoples and their cultures. The Indian Act, the Oka Crisis, and the Royal Commission on Aboriginal Peoples are among some of the topics addressed through the publications available on the site.

Aboriginal Nurses Association of Canada

http://www.anac.on.ca

This is the website of the only professional Aboriginal nursing organization in Canada. It contains information on history, statistics, and current events and initiatives.

First Nations and Inuit Branch of Health Canada

http://www.hc-sc.gc.ca/fnih-spni/index_e.html

This government site gives information on history, health challenges, funding, and programming focused on Canada's Aboriginal groups.

Canada's Food Guide

http://www.hc-sc.gc.ca/fn-an/food-guide-aliment/ fnim-pnim/index-eng.php

http://www.hc-sc.gc.ca/fn-an/food-guide-aliment/ index-eng.php

At the first site, you will find culturally appropriate information for using Canada's Food Guide with Aboriginal groups, in a publication called Eating Well with Canada's Food Guide: First Nations, Inuit and Métis. *The second link is to the original Canada's Food Guide.*

MyNursingLab

REFERENCES

Aboriginal Nurses Association of Canada. (2009). *Cultural competence and cultural safety in First Nations, Inuit and Métis nursing education: An integrated review of the literature*. Ottawa, ON: Author.

American Anthropological Association. (1998). *Statement on "race."* Retrieved from http://www.aaanet.org/stmts/racepp.htm

Anderson, J. M., Waxler-Morrison, N., Richardson, E., Herbert, C., & Murphy, M. (1990). Delivering culturally sensitive health care. In N. Waxler-Morrison, J. Anderson, & E. Richardson (Eds.), *Cross-cultural caring: A handbook for health professionals in Western Canada* (pp. 245–267). Vancouver, BC: UBC Press.

Andrews, M. M., & Boyle, J. S. (2003). *Transcultural concepts in nursing care* (4th ed.). Philadelphia, PA: Lippincott.

Campinha-Bacote, J. (1998). *The process of cultural competence in the delivery of healthcare services* (3rd ed.). Cinacinnati, OH: Transcultural C.A.R.E Associates

Campinha-Bacote, J. (2002). The process of cultural competence in the delivery of healthcare services: A model of care. *Journal of Transcultural Nursing, 13*(3), 181–184.

Canadian Human Rights Commission. (n.d.). *Human rights in Canada: A historical perspective*. Retrieved from http://www.chrc-ccdp.ca/en/timePortals/milestones/118mile.asp

Canadian Multiculturalism Act. RS 1985, c.24 (4th Suppl.). *Statutes of Canada*. Ottawa, ON: Queen's Printer. pp. 835–841.

Canadian Nurses Association. (2006). *Blueprint for the Canadian Registered Nurse Examination*. Ottawa, ON: Author.

Canadian Nurses Association. (2010). *Promoting cultural competence in nursing: CNA position*. Ottawa, ON: Author.

Chansonneuve, D. (2005). *Reclaiming connections: Understanding residential school trauma among Aboriginal people*. Ottawa, ON: Aboriginal Healing Foundation.

Chartrand, L., & McKay, C. (2006). *A review of research on criminal victimization and First Nations, Métis and Inuit peoples 1990 to 2001*. Ottawa, ON: Policy Centre for Victim Issues and the Research and Statistics Division, Department of Justice, Canada.

Chui, T., Tran, K., & Maheux, H. (2007). *Immigration in Canada: A portrait of the foreign-born population, 2006 census: Findings*. Retrieved from http://www12.statcan.ca/english/census06/analysis/immcit/index.cfm

College of Nurses of Ontario. (2008). *Practice guideline for culturally sensitive care*. Retrieved from http://www.cno.org/docs/prac/41040_CulturallySens.pdf

Corbeil, J.-P., & Blaser, C. (2007). *The evolving linguistic portrait, 2006 census: Findings*. Retrieved from http://www12.statcan.ca/english/census06/analysis/language/index.cfm

Eliason, M. J. (1993). Ethics and transcultural nursing care. *Nursing Outlook, 4,* 225–228.

Ermine, W., Sinclair, R., & Jeffery, B. (2004). *The ethics of research involving Indigenous peoples: Report of the Indigenous Peoples' Health Research Centre to the interagency advisory panel on research ethics (PRE)*. Regina, SK: Indigenous Peoples' Health Research Centre.

Escallier, L. A., Fullerton, J. T. & Messina, B. A. M. (2011). Cultural competence outcomes assessment: A strategy and model. *International Journal of Nursing and Midwifery, 3*(3), 35–42.

Galanti, G. (2004). *Caring for patients from different cultures* (3rd ed.). Philadelphia, PA: University of Pennsylvania Press.

Giger, J. N., & Davidhizar, R. (2004). *Transcultural nursing: Assessment and interventions* (4th ed.). St. Louis, MO: Mosby.

Graham-Marrs, H. A. (2011). *Narrative descriptions of miyo-mahcihoyān (well-being) from a contemporary néhiyawak (Plains Cree) perspective* (Doctoral dissertation). Saskatoon, SK: University of Saskatchewan.

Hart, M. A. (2002). *Seeking mino-pimatisiwin: An Aboriginal approach to helping.* Halifax, NS: Fernwood Publishing.

Health Canada. (2005). A statistical profile on the health of First Nations in Canada. Ottawa, ON: Health Canada.

Health Canada (2009). *Closing the gaps in Aboriginal health.* Retrieved from http://www.hc-sc.gc.ca/sr-sr/pubs/hpr-rpms/bull/2003-5-aboriginal-autochtone/index-eng.php

Hughes, M., & Farrow, T. (2006). Preparing for cultural safety assessment. *Kai Tiaki Nursing New Zealand, February 2006,* 12–14.

Kiramayer, L. J., Brass, G. M., & Tait, C. L. (2000). The mental health of Aboriginal peoples. In L. J. Kiramayer, M. E. Macdonald, & G. M. Brass (Eds.). *Proceedings of the Advanced Study Institute: The mental health of indigenous peoples. McGill Summer Program in Social & Cultural Psychiatry and the Aboriginal Mental Health Research Team, May 29–31, 2000.* Montreal, PQ: McGill University.

Leininger, M. M. (1978). *Transcultural nursing: Concepts, theories, and practices.* New York, NY: Wiley.

Leininger, M. M. (1988). Leininger's theory of nursing: Cultural care diversity and universality. *Nursing Science Quarterly, 14,* 152–160.

Leininger, M. M. (Ed.). (1991). *Culture care diversity and universality: A theory of nursing.* New York, NY: National League for Nursing Press. Pub. No. 15–2402.

Lipson, J. G. & Desantis, L. A. (2007). Current approaches to integrating elements of cultural competence in nursing education. *Journal of Transcultural Nursing, 18*(1), 10S–20S.

Martel, L., & Caron-Malenfant. (2007a). *Portrait of the Canadian population in 2006, Findings.* Retrieved from http://www12.statcan.ca/english/census06/analysis/popdwell/index.cfm

Martel, L., & Caron-Malenfant. (2007b). *Portrait of the Canadian population in 2006, age and sex: Findings.* Retrieved from http://www12.statcan.ca/english/census06/analysis/agesex/index.cfm

McGee, C. (2001). When the golden rule does not apply: Starting nurses on the journey toward cultural competence. *Journal for Nurses in Staff Development, 17*(3), 105–112.

Mussel, W. J. (2005). *Warrior-caregivers: Understanding the challenges and healing of First Nations men.* Ottawa, ON: Aboriginal Healing Foundation.

Office of the Treaty Commissioner. (2008). *Treaty essential learnings: We are all treaty people.* Saskatoon, SK: Author.

Public Health Agency of Canada. (2010). *What determines health?* Retrieved from http://www.phac-aspc.gc.ca/ph-sp/determinants/index-eng.php

Purnell, L. (2002). The Purnell model for cultural competence. *Journal of Transcultural Nursing, 13,* 193–196.

Purnell, L., & Paulanka, B. (2005). *Transcultural health care: A culturally competent approach.* Philadelphia, PA: Davis.

Rairdan, B., & Higgs, Z. R. (1992). When your patient is a Hmong refugee. *American Journal of Nursing, 92,* 52–55.

Raphael, D. (2006). Social determinants of health: An overview of concepts and issues. In D. Raphael, T. Bryant, & M. Rioux (eds.), *Critical perspectives on health, illness, and health care: Staying alive* (pp. 115–138). Toronto, ON: Canadian Scholars' Press Inc.

Registered Nurses' Association of Ontario. (2007). *Best practice guideline: Embracing cultural diversity in health care: Developing cultural competence.* Toronto, ON: Author.

Rosenbaum, J. N. (1995). Teaching cultural sensitivity. *Journal of Nursing Education, 34,* 188–189.

Schellenberg, G., & Maheux, H. (2007). *Immigrants' perspectives on their first four years in Canada: Highlights from three waves of the longitudinal survey of immigrants to Canada.* Retrieved from http://www.statcan.ca/english/freepub/11-008-XIE/2007000/11-008-XIE20070009627.htm

Spector, R. E. (2004). *Cultural diversity in health and illness* (6th ed.). Upper Saddle River, NJ: Pearson Prentice Hall.

Srivastava, R. H. (2007). *The healthcare professional's guide to clinical cultural competence.* Toronto, ON: Mosby Elsevier Canada.

Srivastava, R. H. (2008). The ABC (and DE) of cultural competence in clinical care. *Ethnicity and Inequalities in Health and Social Care, 1*(1), 27–33.

Statistics Canada. (2008a). *Canada's changing labour force, 2006 census: Findings.* Retrieved from http://www12.statcan.ca/english/census06/analysis/labour/index.cfm

Statistics Canada. (2008b). *Visible minority population and population group reference guide, 2006 census.* Retrieved from http://www12.statcan.ca/english/census06/reference/reportsandguides/visible-minorities.cfm

Statistics Canada. (2008c). *Canada's ethnocultural mosaic, 2006 census: Findings.* Retrieved from http://www12.statcan.ca/english/census06/analysis/ethnicorigin/index.cfm

Statistics Canada. (2008d). Aboriginal peoples in Canada in 2006: Inuit, Métis and First Nations, 2006 census. *The Daily,* January 15. Retrieved from http://www.statcan.ca/Daily/English/080115/d080115a.htm

Statistics Canada. (2010). *Aboriginal statistics at a glance.* Retrieved from http://www.statcan.gc.ca/pub/89-645-x/89-645-x2010001-eng.htm

Statistics Canada. (2012a). Immigrant languages in Canada. Retrieved from http://www12.statcan.gc.ca/census-recensement/2011/as-sa/98-314-x/98-314-x2011003_2-eng.cfm

Statistics Canada. (2012b). Linguistic characteristics of Canadians. Retrieved from http://www12.statcan.gc.ca/census-recensement/2011/as-sa/98-314-x/98-314-x2011001-eng.cfm

Statistics Canada. (2012c). Aboriginal languages in Canada. Retrieved from http://www12.statcan.gc.ca/census-recensement/2011/as-sa/98-314-x/98-314-x2011003_3-eng.cfm

United Nations Permanent Forum on Indigenous Issues, (2007). *Indigenous peoples, Indigenous voices.* Retrieved from www.un.org/esa/socdev/unpfii/documents/unpfiibrochure_en07.pdf

Wesley-Esquimaux, C. C., & Smolewski, M. (2004). *Historic trauma and Aboriginal healing.* Ottawa, ON: Aboriginal Healing Foundation.

Chapter 12

Individual Care

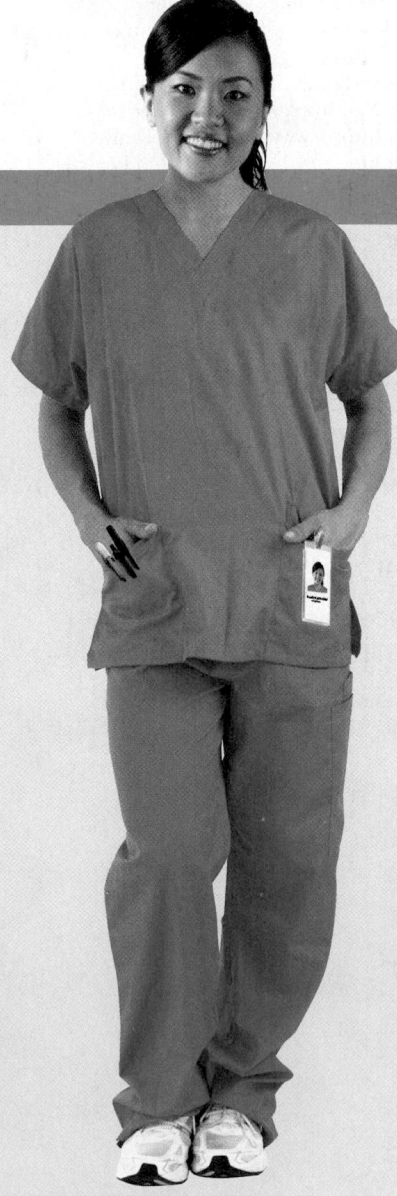

After studying this chapter, you will be able to:

1. Explain the relationship of individuality and holism to nursing practice.

2. Compare and contrast the elements of physiological and psychological homeostasis.

3. Identify six common factors that can make an individual more vulnerable to some health problems and describe a nursing implication for each.

4. Identify Maslow's five categories in the hierarchy of human needs.

5. Discuss how a nurse might use the three selected types of theories to begin to assess an individual's health needs.

Nurses assess and plan health care for individuals. Care of the individual is enhanced when the nurse understands the concepts of individuality, holism, homeostasis, human needs, and systems theory. The beliefs and values of clients and the support they receive come, in large part, from the family and are reinforced by the community. Thus, an understanding of family dynamics and the context of the community assists the nurse in planning care. For additional information on the family and community, see Chapters 13 and 14. To assist clients toward health, nurses must understand them as individuals. The nurse uses knowledge of individuality, holism, homeostasis, human needs, and systems theory in the context of the client's situation, whomever the client may be (individual, family, group, community, population).

Individual application of knowledge is known as client-centred care and is the centrepiece of the profession and of this text. As outlined in Chapter 1, the individual recipient of care may be called a *patient*, *resident*, or *client*. This terminology has been a topic of some controversy, with several organizations using both *patient* and *client* in their published documents. For example, we might talk about patient safety, or client-centred care. Wing (1997) surveyed individuals attending a back pain clinic and contended that the majority of individuals seeking care prefer to be called *patients*. He made the point that the health care professional should follow the person's lead and use the terminology preferred by the individual. In this text, we have chosen to refer to the individual seeking care, especially within an acute care setting as a *patient*, and the person living in a long-term care setting as a *resident*. We have referred to individuals receiving care in community settings as *clients*. Sometimes, concepts that are developed for individuals can be applied to communities, and vice versa (see the Reflect on Primary Health Care box).

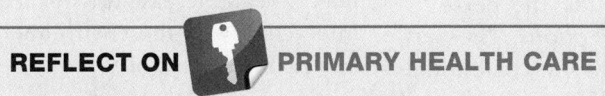

REFLECT ON PRIMARY HEALTH CARE

Often, the principles of primary health are considered in light of the health of communities and populations. However, each of the principles can be applied to the individual seeking care. For instance, accessibility may be difficult even when the service is present if it has limited hours or affordable public transportation to get to the service is lacking. Public participation may refer to the individual's contributions to decisions about his or her health care.

It is important to remember, as you read this chapter, that you are an individual and are influenced by the same factors as are your clients. For example, when reading the Nursing and Canadian Society box, do you identify in your home community with the nursing implications presented?

Nursing and Canadian Society	
Fact	**Implications for Nursing Practice**
In a list of Organisation for Economic Co-operation and Development (OECD) countries, only Iceland and Australia have a smaller population density per square kilometre than Canada (OECD, 2010).	Access to health care may be difficult for some people in Canada.
The trend was to see higher levels of education in the population from 1986 to 2006. For example, persons with a high-school diploma rose from 20% to 24%. In the same population, persons with a college certificate or degree went from 10.4% to 32%, and those with a completed bachelor's degree went from 6% to 23% (Statistics Canada, 2004, 2008).	Nurses may expect that patients come with higher levels of health care knowledge and also expect to be provided with more information about health and health care.
In 2011, the total population had increased by 5.9% since 2006. In 2011, one person households had increased to 27.6%, a rise of 2.1% since 2001. For the first time, there were more one person households than households of couples with children (Statistics Canada 2012a, b).	More people are living alone in Canada and may not have readily available assistance from family members.

Individual Health

Concept of Individuality

To help clients attain, maintain, or regain an optimal level of health, nurses need to understand clients as individuals. Each individual is a unique being who is different from every other human being, with a different genetic makeup, life experiences, and environmental interactions.

Dimensions of individuality include the person's total character, self-identity, and perceptions. The person's *total character* encompasses behaviours, emotional states, attitudes, values, motives, abilities, habits, and appearances. The person's *self-identity* encompasses perception of self as a separate and distinct entity, alone and in interactions with others. Identity is often threatened by actual or perceived alterations in wellness. Some changes are minor and may be considered merely inconveniences; others can compromise existence in profound ways. The person's *perceptions* encompass the way the person interprets the environment or situation, directly affecting how the person thinks, feels, and acts in any given situation.

Nurses' and clients' perceptions determine their subjective realities at the time of their interaction. Differences can exist in the two views of reality that will influence communication, acceptance of each other, and whether the client's health care needs are being met. Sometimes, the views of nurses and clients differ because of their own unique experiences.

When providing care, nurses need to focus on the client within both a total care and an individualized care context. In the total care context, the nurse considers all the principles and areas that apply when taking care of any client of that age and condition. In the individualized care context, the nurse becomes acquainted with the client as an individual, referring to the total care principles and using the principles that apply to this person at this time. For example, a nurse who is advising the mother of a preschooler understands that the child's desire to explore the world is a developmental stage that all preschoolers experience. However, the preschooler diagnosed with attention deficit disorder with hyperactivity may have an increased risk of accidents and injuries when interacting with the environment because of impulsivity and poor self-control.

Concept of Holism

Nurses are concerned with the individual as a whole, that is, with the complete, or holistic, person, not as an assembly of parts and processes. The terms **holistic** and **holism** are derived from the Greek word meaning "whole." The term *holism* itself was coined by Jan Smuts, a South African scholar and political leader, in his book *Holism and Evolution* (1926). In holistic theory, a living organism is seen as an interacting, unified whole that is more than the mere sum of its parts. Viewed in this light, any disturbance in one part is a disturbance of the whole system or being (see Box 12.1).

When applied in nursing, the concept of holism emphasizes that nurses must keep the whole person in mind and strive to understand how one area of concern relates to the whole person. The nurse must also consider the relationship of the individual to the external environment and to others. For example, in helping a man who is grieving over the death of his spouse, the nurse explores the impact of the loss on the whole person (i.e., on the man's appetite, rest and sleep patterns, energy level, sense of well-being, mood, usual activities, family relationships, and relationships with others). Nursing interventions are directed toward restoring overall harmony, so they depend on the man's sense of purpose and meaning of his life. Nursing theorists, such as Parse and Newman (see Chapter 4 for additional information), based their theories on looking at the whole person.

Concept of Homeostasis

The concept of homeostasis was first introduced by Cannon (1939) to describe the relative constancy of the internal processes of the body, such as blood oxygen and carbon dioxide levels, blood pressure, body temperature, blood glucose, and fluid and electrolyte balance. To Cannon, the word *homeostasis* did not imply something stagnant, set, or immobile; it meant a condition that might vary but remained relatively constant. Cannon viewed the human being as separate from the external environment and constantly endeavouring to maintain physiological **equilibrium**, or balance, through adaptation to that environment. **Homeostasis**, then, is the tendency of the body to maintain a state of balance or equilibrium while continually changing.

PHYSIOLOGICAL HOMEOSTASIS   Physiological homeostasis means that the internal environment of the body is relatively stable and constant. All cells of the body require a relatively constant environment to function; thus, the body's internal environment must be maintained within narrow limits. Homeostatic mechanisms have four main characteristics:

1. They are self-regulating.
2. They are compensatory.
3. They tend to be regulated by negative feedback systems.

4. They can require several feedback mechanisms to correct only one physiological imbalance.

Self-regulation means that homeostatic mechanisms come into play automatically in the healthy person. However, if a person is ill or if an organ, such as a lung, is injured, the homeostatic mechanisms may not be able to respond to the stimulus as they would normally. Homeostatic mechanisms are **compensatory** (counterbalancing) because they tend to counteract conditions that are abnormal for the person. An example is a sudden drop in temperature. The compensatory mechanisms are that the peripheral blood vessels constrict, thereby diverting most of the blood internally, muscular activity increases and shivering occurs to create heat. Through these mechanisms the body temperature remains stable, despite the cold.

Feedback is the mechanism by which some of the output of a system is fed back into the system as input. This input influences the behaviour of the system and its future output. **Negative feedback** inhibits change; **positive feedback** stimulates change. Most biological systems are controlled by negative feedback to bring the system back to stability. This type of feedback system senses and counteracts any deviations from normal. Negative feedback is a common control mechanism for hormone levels. For example, an increase in the production of parathyroid hormone is stimulated by a drop in blood calcium, but when additional parathyroid hormone raises the level of blood calcium, the hormone's production is then inhibited. As noted, several negative feedback systems can be required to correct one physiological imbalance. For example, with hypoxia (shortage of oxygen), the concentration of red blood cells increases and the heart rate becomes faster to transport the blood and available oxygen around the body adequately.

The two major homeostatic regulators are the autonomic nervous system and the endocrine system. In addition, the cardiovascular system, the renal system, the respiratory system, and the gastrointestinal system are important in maintaining homeostasis. See Figure 12.1 on the next page.

PSYCHOLOGICAL HOMEOSTASIS   The term *psychological homeostasis* refers to emotional or psychological balance or a state of mental well-being. Each person has certain psychological needs, such as the need for love, security, and self-esteem, that must be met to maintain psychological homeostasis. When one or more of these needs is not met or is threatened, certain coping mechanisms are activated to protect the person and return him or her to psychological homeostasis (see Chapter 48 for additional information on stress and coping).

Psychological homeostasis is acquired or learned through the experience of living and interacting with others. In addition, societal norms and culture influence individual expectations and the behaviour or actions used to meet those expectations. Some prerequisites for a

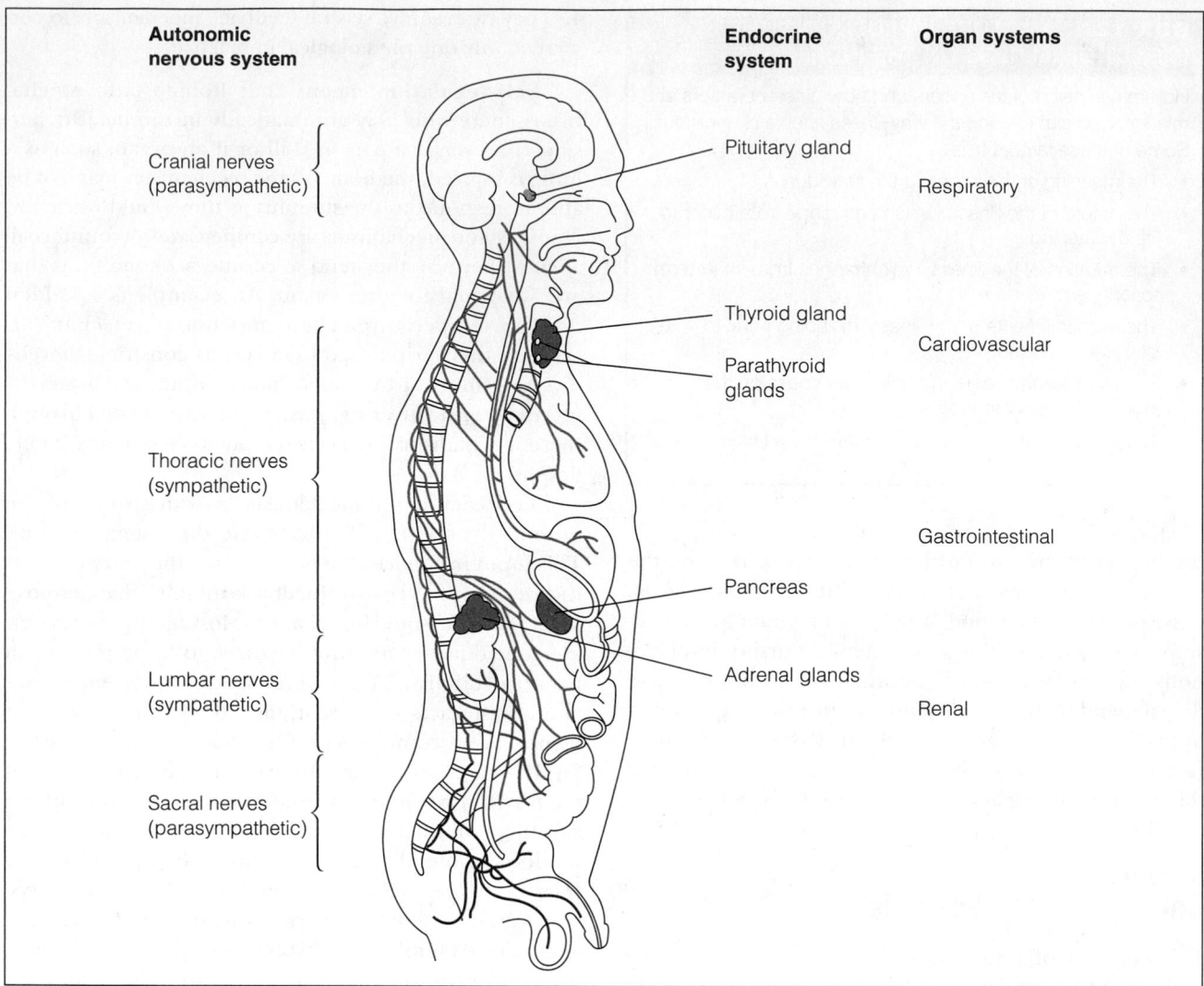

Autonomic nervous system

Cranial nerves (parasympathetic)

Thoracic nerves (sympathetic)

Lumbar nerves (sympathetic)

Sacral nerves (parasympathetic)

Endocrine system

Pituitary gland

Thyroid gland

Parathyroid glands

Pancreas

Adrenal glands

Organ systems

Respiratory

Cardiovascular

Gastrointestinal

Renal

FIGURE 12.1 The homeostatic regulators of the body: autonomic nervous system, endocrine system, and specific organ systems.

person to develop psychological homeostasis can be summarized as follows:

- *A stable physical environment in which the person feels safe and secure.* For example, the basic needs for food, shelter, and clothing must be met consistently from birth onward.

- *A stable psychological environment from infancy onward, so that feelings of trust and love develop.* Growing children and adolescents also need kind but firm and consistent discipline, encouragement, and support to be their own unique selves.

- *A social environment that includes adults who are healthy role models.* Children learn the customs and values of society from these individuals.

- *A life experience that provides satisfaction.* Throughout life, people encounter many frustrations. They deal with these better if enough satisfying experiences have occurred to counterbalance the frustrating ones.

It is interesting to note that these prerequisites are embedded within the social determinants of health, described in Chapter 7. An example of the importance of psychological homeostasis is the training of athletes. A winning attitude and feeling supported by coaches, family, and friends may be as important as strength and speed training.

Assessing the Health of Individuals

A thorough assessment of the individual's health status is basic to health promotion (see Figure 12.2). Components of this system may include the health history and physical examination, physical fitness assessment, lifestyle assessment, health-risk appraisal, health beliefs review, spiritual health assessment, social support systems review, and life-stress review. Details about selected assessments are discussed in Chapters 8, 28, 47, and 48.

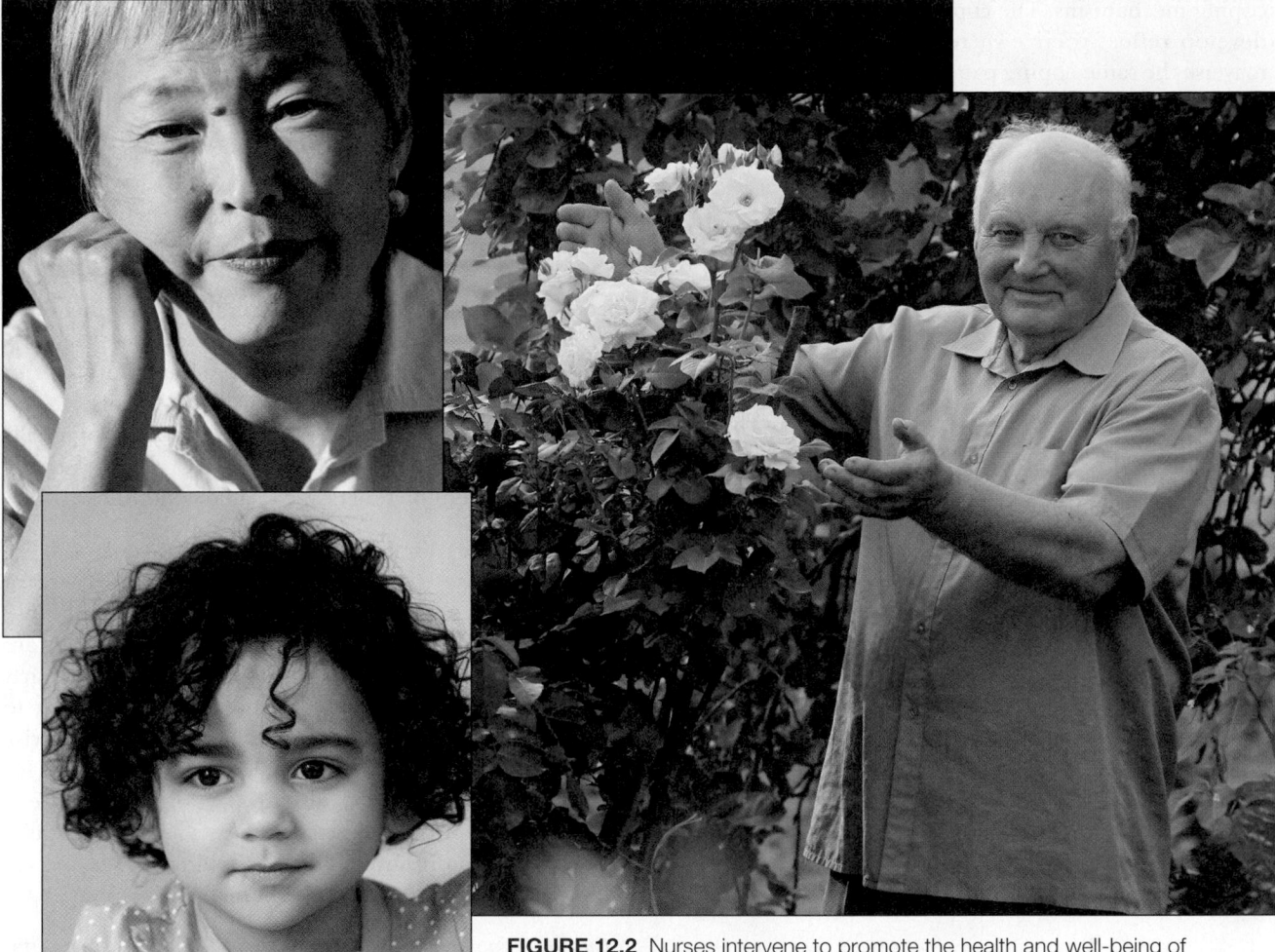

FIGURE 12.2 Nurses intervene to promote the health and well-being of individuals of diverse ages and backgrounds.

HEALTH APPRAISAL The *health appraisal* begins with a complete health history. The health history is one of the most effective ways of identifying existing or potential health problems (see Chapter 28). If further evaluation is indicated, a referral is made to the appropriate health care professional. When the focus is on health, the appraisal includes information on lifestyle behaviours and health beliefs. The nurse uses data from the health appraisal to formulate a health profile. The health profile provides the data necessary to determine wellness or to establish a nursing diagnosis and to plan appropriate nursing interventions to promote optimal health through lifestyle modification.

HEALTH BELIEFS To promote health, the nurse must understand the health beliefs of individuals. Health beliefs may reflect a lack of information or misinformation about health or disease. They may also include folklore and practices from different cultures. Many clients may have outdated information about health, illness, treatment, and prevention. The nurse is frequently in a position to give the latest information or to correct misconceptions. For additional information on health beliefs, see Chapters 7, 8, and 11.

COPING MECHANISMS Individual coping mechanisms are the behaviours individuals use to deal with stress or changes. Coping mechanisms can be viewed as an active method of problem solving developed to meet life's challenges. See Box 12.2 for some health-promoting

---

BOX 12.2 HEALTH-PROMOTING COPING MECHANISMS

The following coping mechanisms can be beneficial when they promote health:

- Problem solving
- Positive thinking
- A sense of personal control over own life
- Delayed gratification
- Healthy behaviours (e.g., exercise, good nutrition)
- Social support relationships

coping mechanisms. The coping mechanisms individuals develop reflect their own resourcefulness. Individuals may use the same coping patterns rather consistently over time or may change their coping strategies when new demands are made on them. See Chapter 48 for a more detailed discussion on coping mechanisms.

Nurses working with individuals realize the importance of assessing coping mechanisms as a way of determining how individuals relate to stress. Also important are the resources available to the individual (see the Evidence-Informed Practice box). Internal resources, such as knowledge, skills, effective communication patterns, and a sense of purpose, assist in the problem-solving process. Age and the individual's developmental stage often bring with them experiences that may or may not support positive coping strategies. In addition, external support systems promote coping and adaptation. For additional information on coping, see Chapter 48.

RISK FOR HEALTH PROBLEMS Risk assessment helps the nurse identify individuals at higher risk than the general population of developing specific health problems, such as a cerebrovascular accident, diabetes, and lung cancer. The vulnerability of individuals to health problems may be based on age, hereditary or genetic factors, gender or race, cultural factors, sociological factors, and lifestyle practices.

Developmental Factors Individuals at both ends of the age continuum are at risk of developing health problems.

Young children lack the knowledge, skills, and experience to establish a repertoire of coping strategies. Many older adults feel a lack of purpose and decreased self-esteem. These feelings, in turn, reduce their motivation to engage in health-promoting behaviours, such as exercise or community and family involvement.

Hereditary Factors Individuals born into families with a history of certain diseases, such as diabetes or cardiovascular disease, are at greater risk of developing these conditions. A detailed individual and family history, including genetically transmitted disorders, is essential to the identification of individuals at risk. These data are used not only to monitor the health of individuals but also to recommend modifications in health practices that potentially reduce the risk, minimize the consequences, or postpone the development of genetically related conditions.

Gender or Race Some individuals may be at risk of developing a disease by reason of gender or race. Males, for example, are at greater risk of having cardiovascular disease at an earlier age than are females, and females are at greater risk of developing osteoporosis, particularly after menopause. Although it is sometimes difficult to separate genetic factors from cultural ones, certain risk factors seem to be related to race. Sickle-cell anemia, for example, is a hereditary disease predominantly affecting people of African descent. Indigenous or Aboriginal people seem more susceptible to certain diseases, such as diabetes, compared with the general population.

Cultural Factors Culture creates an atmosphere that influences the health beliefs and practices of an individual. To provide culturally sensitive care, nurses need to recognize and understand a broad spectrum of cultural values, beliefs, and practices (see Chapter 11).

Sociological Factors The individual's health is influenced by a variety of sociological factors. One of the most noteworthy is poverty. Poverty is a major problem that affects the health of the individual. If an individual is born into or grows up in a single-parent family headed by a female, then the risk of poverty increases. Other factors include the person's roles within society, at work, and in the community, and personal interests and activities.

Lifestyle Factors It has become clear that many diseases are preventable, that the effects of some diseases can be minimized, and that the onset of disease can be delayed through lifestyle modifications. Cancer, cardiovascular disease, Type 2 diabetes, and tooth decay are among lifestyle diseases. The incidence of lung cancer, for example, would be greatly reduced if people stopped smoking. Good nutrition, dental hygiene, and use of fluoride—in the water supply, in toothpaste, as topical supplements—have been shown to reduce caries (dental decay).

One of the most important lifestyle issues today is obesity. Obesity has become pandemic in Canada, and

---

EVIDENCE-INFORMED PRACTICE

What Needs Do Men with Advanced Prostate Cancer Identify?

In this research study, the authors met with 29 men in focus groups or individual interviews. All the men had advanced prostate cancer, and the researchers were seeking greater understanding of the priority supportive needs for these men. After analyzing the taped interview data, they found that there were three primary needs. The first was support to "maintain their ability 'to do what they want to do,'" (p. 189), or preserve their functional abilities. The second was greater disease-specific information to understand what was happening to them and their treatment options. Finally, the participants noted that assistance with emotional distress, including such emotions as sadness, anger, and frustration, was important.

NURSING IMPLICATIONS: It is important for nurses to address each of these areas with patients who have complex physical care needs. By asking questions, the nurse can assist the patient to express his needs and then plan a strategy for meeting the needs.

Source: Based on Carter, N., Bryant-Lukosius, D., DiCenso, A., Blythe, J., & Neville A. J. (2011). The supportive care needs of men with advanced prostate cancer. *Oncology Nursing Forum, 38*(2), 189–197.

the negative health effects of obesity are many and varied. Other important lifestyle considerations are exercise, stress management, and rest. Today, nurses have the knowledge to prevent or minimize the effects of some of the main causes of disease, disability, and death. The challenge is to disseminate information about prevention and to motivate individuals to make lifestyle changes before the onset of illness.

Nursing Process

Nurses committed to individualized care involve the client in the nursing process. The process is discussed in Chapter 23. Data gathered during an individual assessment can lead to different nursing diagnoses. Planned nursing interventions that are needed to assist the individual to health and that enhance personal well-being are identified on the basis of a diagnosis. Evaluation determines whether the planned interventions have led to the achievement of the established goals and outcomes.

Applying Theoretical Frameworks to Individuals

A variety of theoretical frameworks provide the nurse with a holistic overview of health promotion for the individual across the lifespan. Major theoretical frameworks that nurses use in promoting the health of the *individual* are needs theories, developmental stage theories, and systems theories.

Needs Theories

In needs theories, human needs are ranked on an ascending scale according to how essential the needs are for survival. Abraham Maslow, perhaps the most renowned needs theorist, ranks human needs on five levels in ascending order (1970):

1. *Physiological Needs.* Such needs as air, food, water, shelter, rest, sleep, activity, and temperature maintenance are crucial for survival.

2. *Safety and Security Needs.* The need for safety has both physical and psychological aspects. The person needs to feel safe, both in the physical environment and in relationships.

3. *Love and Belonging Needs.* The third level of needs includes giving and receiving affection, attaining a place in a group, and maintaining the feeling of belonging.

4. *Self-Esteem Needs.* The individual needs both self-esteem (i.e., feelings of independence, competence, and self-respect) and esteem from others (i.e., recognition, respect, and appreciation).

5. *Self-Actualization.* When the need for self-esteem is satisfied, the individual strives for self-actualization, the innate need for a person to develop his or her maximum potential and realize abilities and qualities. (See Box 12.3.)

KALISH'S HIERARCHY OF NEEDS Richard Kalish (1983) adapted Maslow's hierarchy of needs into six levels, rather than five. He suggests an additional category of needs between the physiological needs and the safety and security needs. This category, referred to as *stimulation needs*, includes sex, activity, exploration, manipulation, and novelty. See Figure 12.3 on the next page. Kalish emphasizes that children need to explore and manipulate their environments to achieve optimal growth and development. He notes that adults, too, often seek novel adventures or stimulating experiences before considering their safety or security needs. Maslow, by contrast, includes the pursuit of knowledge and aesthetic needs in the category of self-actualization needs.

BOX 12.3 MASLOW'S CHARACTERISTICS OF A SELF-ACTUALIZED PERSON

According to Maslow, a self-actualized person has the following characteristics:

- Is realistic and objective about life
- Judges people correctly
- Is perceptive and decisive
- Has a clear notion of right and wrong
- Is usually accurate in predicting future events
- Understands art, music, politics, and philosophy
- Possesses humility and listens to others carefully
- Is dedicated to some work, task, duty, or vocation
- Is highly creative, flexible, spontaneous, courageous, and willing to make mistakes
- Is open to new ideas
- Is self-confident, has self-respect and self-control
- Has low degree of self-conflict; personality is integrated
- Does not need fame
- Is highly independent and desires privacy
- Can appear remote and detached
- Is governed more by inner directives than by society
- Can make decisions contrary to popular opinion
- Is problem centred rather than self-centred
- Accepts the world for what it is

Source: Based on Chapter 3, "The study of self-actualization," from *The third force: The psychology of Abraham Maslow,* by Frank Goble. Copyright © 1970 by Thomas Jefferson Research Center.

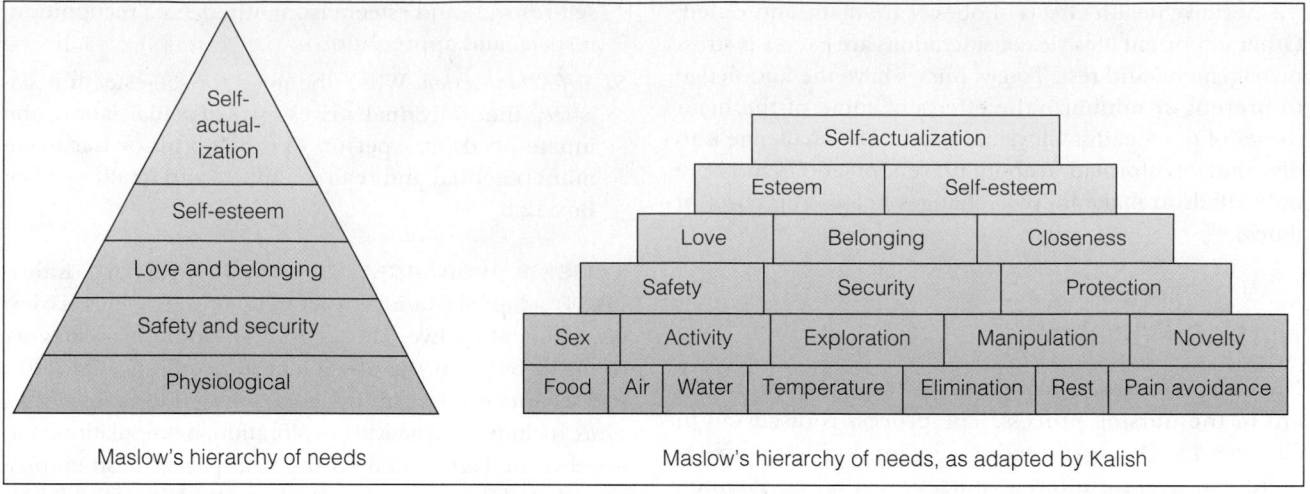

FIGURE 12.3 Maslow's needs and Kalish's adaptation.

Source: From KALISH. *Psychology of Human Behavior*, 5E. © 1983 Wadsworth, a part of Cengage Learning, Inc. Reproduced by permission. www.cengage.com/permissions

CHARACTERISTICS OF BASIC NEEDS   All people have the same basic needs; however, a person's perception of a need varies according to learning and the standards of his or her culture. For example, professional achievement may be important in one culture or subculture and unimportant in another. People's needs have the following characteristics:

- People meet their own needs relative to their own priorities. For example, during a drought, a mother might give up her share of water or food and risk starvation or die so that her child can live.

- Although basic needs generally must be met, some needs can be deferred. An example is the need for independence. During an acute illness, the individual may prefer to be somewhat dependent on health care professionals and other caregivers, and then resume the desire for independence after recovery.

- Failure to meet needs results in one or more homeostatic imbalances, which can eventually result in illness.

- A need can make itself felt by either external or internal stimuli. An example is the need for food. A person may experience hunger as a result of thinking about food (internal stimulation) or as a result of seeing a beautifully decorated cake (external stimulation).

- A person who perceives a need can respond in several ways to meet it. The choice of response is largely a result of learned experiences, lifestyle, and the values of the culture. For example, the professional woman who comes home from work feeling tired may meet the need for relaxation by walking around the park after dinner. Many people's food choices at mealtimes and snack times are based on past experiences, lifestyle, and culture.

- Needs are interrelated. Some needs cannot be met unless related needs are also met. The need for

hydration can be seriously altered if the need for elimination of urine is not also met. Likewise, the need for security can be markedly altered if the need for oxygen is threatened by a respiratory obstruction.

Needs can be satisfied in healthy and unhealthy ways. Ways of meeting basic needs are considered healthy when they are not harmful to others or to the self, conform to the individual's sociocultural values, and are within the law. Conversely, unhealthy behaviour may be harmful to others or to the self, does not conform to the individual's sociocultural values, or is not within the law. People who satisfy their basic needs appropriately are healthier, happier, and more effective than those whose needs are frustrated.

Throughout their lifetime, individuals strive to meet needs. A person's perception of a need and his or her response to satisfy a need can be influenced by ethnocultural standards, by external and internal stimuli (e.g., hunger), and by self-determined priorities (e.g., stopping smoking). Positive factors that affect the satisfying of needs are the presence of supportive relationships, a strong self-concept, and the satisfactory achievement of developmental stages. For example, if an infant achieves the developmental task of learning to trust, then the basic needs of feeling loved and secure are readily resolved.

Knowledge of the theoretical bases of human needs assists nurses in responding therapeutically to a client's behaviours and in understanding themselves and their own responses to needs. Human needs serve as a framework for assessing behaviours, assigning priorities to desired outcomes, and planning nursing interventions. For example, an adult with poor self-esteem would have difficulty becoming self-actualized. Therefore, nursing interventions would focus on increasing the client's self-esteem.

Developmental Stage Theories

Developmental stage theories related to individuals categorize a person's behaviours or tasks into approximate age ranges or in terms that describe the features of an age group. The age ranges of the stages do not take into account individual differences; however, the categories do describe characteristics associated with the majority of individuals at periods when distinctive developmental changes occur and with the specific tasks that must be accomplished. Because human development is highly complex and multifaceted, developmental stage theories describe only one aspect of development, such as cognitive, psychosexual, psychosocial, moral, or faith development. Stage theories emphasize a definite, predictable sequence of development that is orderly and continuous. Each stage is affected by those stages preceding it and affects those stages that follow. For example, an adolescent who is unable to establish a stable sense of personal identity may have difficulty in later developmental stages with adult roles and career aspirations. See Chapter 17 for further information about developmental stages.

Developmental stage theories allow nurses to describe the typical behaviours of an individual within a certain age group, explain the significance of those behaviours, predict behaviours that might occur in a given situation, and provide a rationale to control behavioural manifestations. Individuals can be compared with a representative group of people at the same time or be compared at different times. During care, the nurse's knowledge of stage theories can be used in parental and client education, counselling, and anticipatory guidance.

Systems Theories

General systems theory explains the breaking of whole things into parts and the working together of those parts in systems. The theory explains the relationship between wholes and parts, describes concepts about them, and predicts how the parts will behave and react.

The basic concepts of systems theory were proposed in the 1950s. One of its major proponents, Ludwig von Bertalanffy (1968) introduced systems theory as a universal theory that could be applied to many fields of study. Systems theory is applied in health professions when curricula are focused on body systems, such as the respiratory, cardiac, or gastrointestinal system. Nurses are increasingly using systems theory to understand not only biological systems but also systems in families, communities, and nursing and health care. General systems theory provides a way of examining interrelationships and deriving principles. Systems theory can also be used in nursing theories and curricula, such as Campbell's UBC (University of British Columbia) model (see Chapter 4).

A **system** is a set of interacting identifiable parts or components. A system can be an individual, a family, or a community. The fundamental components of a system are matter, energy, and communication. Without any one of these, a system does not exist. The individual is a human system with matter (the body), energy (chemical or thermal), and communication (e.g., the nervous system). The **boundary** of a system, such as skin in the integumentary system in humans, is a real or imaginary line that differentiates one system from another system or a system from its environment.

Systems can be complex and, therefore, are often studied as *subsystems*. Each subsystem belongs to a higher system. In the individual or human system, the subsystems (or lower-level systems) are the organ systems, such as the respiratory system and the digestive system; the *suprasystems* are the family systems. See Figure 12.4 for a hierarchy of the human system.

Because all the parts of a system are interrelated, the whole system responds to changes in one of its parts. This interrelatedness is the basis for nursing's holistic view of the client. For example, a tumour of the liver affects the whole individual, that is, the person may be nauseated, tired, anxious, and so on. A psychological problem, such as stress or anxiety, can also manifest itself in physiological symptoms, such as sleeplessness, nausea, or changes in cardiac function.

Systems come in two general types: *closed* and *open*. A **closed system** does not exchange energy, matter, or information with its environment. An example of a closed system is a chemical reaction that takes place in a test tube. In reality, outside the laboratory, no closed systems exist. In an **open system**, energy, matter, and information move into and out of the system through

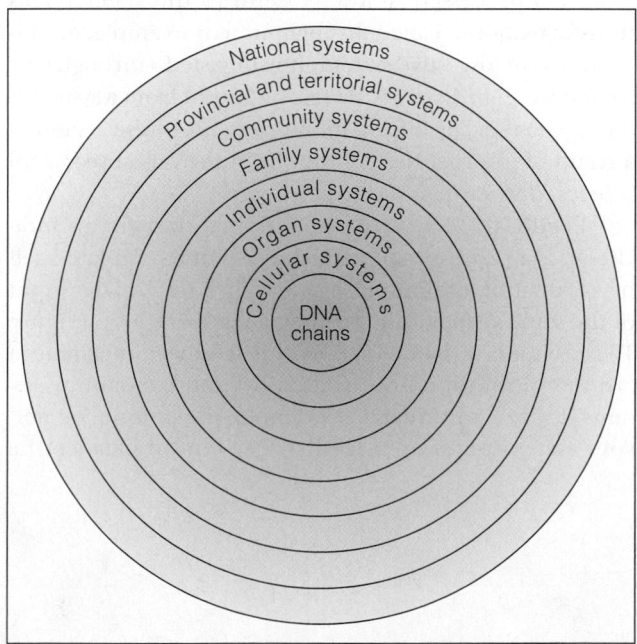

FIGURE 12.4 A common system hierarchy.

the system boundary. All living systems, such as plants, animals, people, families, and communities, are open systems, since their survival depends on a continuous exchange of energy. They are, therefore, in a constant state of change.

Because humans are biopsychosocial beings, their biological, psychological, social, and spiritual components can be regarded as systems with hierarchical, interrelated subsystems.

The *biological system* can be subdivided into the neurological, musculoskeletal, respiratory, circulatory, gastrointestinal, and urinary subsystems, among others. Each subsystem can, in turn, be subdivided. For example, the urinary system consists of the kidneys, the ureters, and the bladder; the circulatory system consists of the heart and blood vessels. The biological system can also be subdivided into categories of needs or functional health patterns or activities of daily living, such as nutrition and hydration, sleep or rest, activity or exercise, elimination, and so on.

The *psychological, social,* and *spiritual systems* are a focus of research in several disciplines. Although the interrelatedness of the systems is clearly evident, the explicit delineation of specific subsystems, the exact relationships among them, and their influence on health are still not well understood (Belar, 2003). Topics within these systems include thinking, feeling, faith, empathy, coping, hardiness, quality of life, self-efficacy, power, and social support. Nurse researchers and theorists have used research results on these topics as a basis for theory development and improving practice.

For its functioning, an open system depends on the quality and quantity of its input, output, and feedback. **Input** consists of information, material, or energy that enters the system. After the input is absorbed by the system, it is processed in a way useful to the system. This transformation is called **throughput**. For example, food is input to the digestive system; it is digested (throughput) so that it can be used by the body. **Output** from a system is energy, matter, or information given out by the system as a result of its processes. Output from the digestive system is feces, nutrients, and caloric energy.

Feedback, as discussed for homeostasis in an individual, is a process that enables a system to regulate itself by redirecting the output of a system to affect the input of the same system, thus forming a feedback loop (Figure 12.5). Numerous examples of this feedback mechanism are found within individual, family, and community systems. In the individual, for example, the autonomic nervous system relies on a feedback system to balance the

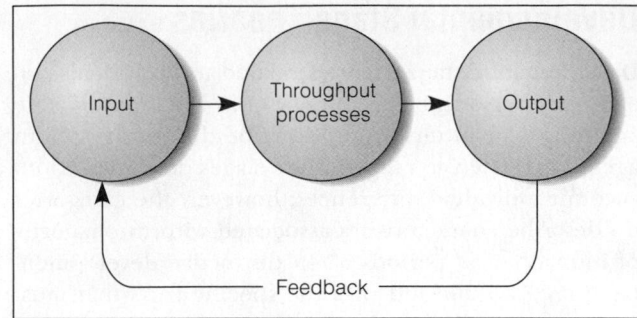

FIGURE 12.5 An open system with a feedback mechanism.

effects of the sympathetic and parasympathetic centres, which modify heart and respiratory rates. In the family system, parents provide feedback to children to modify behaviour. In the community, laws, rules, and regulations guide the behaviour of citizens.

Human systems theories assert that the individual is an open system in constant interaction with a changing environment. People interact with the environment by adjusting themselves to it or adjusting it to themselves. For instance, increasing environmental (societal) emphasis on physical activity has caused many Canadians to increase their own activity levels and to encourage family members to do so as well. Constant input into the system and feedback to it maintain the system in a state of dynamic equilibrium (homeostasis). This premise directs the nurse to look at environmental factors influencing the system and to plan nursing interventions to help the client maintain homeostasis. For example, the individual who is experiencing severe anxiety may be taught a variety of stress-management techniques.

The family unit can also be viewed as a system. Its members are interdependent, working toward specific purposes and goals. Many families are described as *open systems,* for they are continually interacting with and influenced by other systems in the community. Boundaries regulate the input from other systems that interact with the family system; they also regulate output from the family system to the community or to society. Boundaries protect the family from the demands and influences of other systems. Open families are likely to welcome input from without, encouraging individual members to adapt beliefs and practices to meet the changing demands of society. Such families are more likely to seek out health care information and use community resources. These families are adaptable and, therefore, better prepared to cope with changes in lifestyle needed to restore, maintain, or promote health.

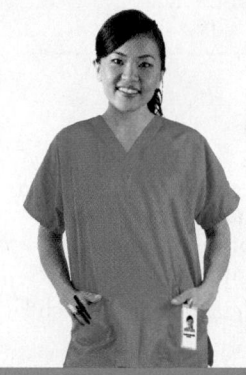

Case Study 12

Aliyah is a young mother of three children who lives in Windsor, Ontario. She has developed a severe arthritic condition that has affected her ability to work and adequately care for her family. Her illness has created a financial hardship for the family and has strained their roles. She has given up her position as a secretary at an automotive plant. Aliyah and her husband have custody of their children from previous marriages, as well as a daughter together. She is reluctant to seek assistance from outside sources because she fears interference from her ex-husband concerning her children.

CRITICAL THINKING SKILLS

1. What type of assessment data might you collect?

2. When dealing with Aliyah's physical problem, what other issues occurring in Aliyah's life might the nurse consider?

3. Explore Aliyah's situation from the perspective of Maslow.

4. What class of theories might you use to understand Aliyah's situation?

Check the eText in MyNursingLab for answers and explanations.

KEY TERMS

boundary *p. 239*	**feedback** *p. 233*	**input** *p. 240*	**positive feedback** *p. 233*
closed system *p. 239*	**holism** *p. 232*	**negative feedback** *p. 233*	**self-regulation** *p. 233*
compensatory *p. 233*	**holistic** *p. 232*	**open system** *p. 239*	**system** *p. 239*
equilibrium *p. 233*	**homeostasis** *p. 233*	**output** *p. 240*	**throughput** *p. 240*

CHAPTER HIGHLIGHTS

- Nursing involves viewing the client as an individual and in a holistic way.

- To ensure holistic health care, the nurse considers all the components of health (health promotion, health maintenance, health education and illness prevention, and restorative–rehabilitative care) and recognizes that disturbance in one part of a person affects the whole being.

- Homeostasis is the tendency of the body to maintain a state of relative balance or constancy in response to changing internal and external environments.

- Physiological homeostasis is maintained by coordinated functioning of the autonomic, nervous, endocrine, respiratory, cardiovascular, renal, and gastrointestinal systems.

- Homeostatic mechanisms regulate hormone secretion, fluid and electrolyte levels, the functions of body viscera, and metabolic processes that provide energy for the body.

- Psychological homeostasis, or emotional well-being, is acquired or learned through the experience of living and interacting with others.

- Although each individual has unique characteristics, certain needs are common to all people.

- A variety of social, psychological, and nursing theoretical frameworks provide the nurse with a holistic overview of the health promotion of individuals and families across the lifespan.

- Maslow's hierarchy of human needs consists of five categories: physiological (survival) needs, safety needs, love and belonging needs, self-esteem needs, and self-actualization needs.

- People vary in how they rank their needs at any given moment.

- Needs satisfaction can be altered by illness, significant relationships, self-concept, and developmental levels.

ASSESS YOUR LEARNING

1. In her health history, Sally, age 46 years, reveals that both her sister and her mother have diabetes. The interviewing nurse should inform Sally that this puts her at higher risk for developing this disease because of what factors?

    a. Developmental

    b. Sociological

    c. Lifestyle

    d. Hereditary

2. The way an individual interprets the environment can be considered part of which of the following dimensions of individuality?

    a. Self-identity

    b. Total character

    c. Perceptions

    d. Values

3. Mr. Greer, who has metastatic cancer of the liver and is severely jaundiced, asks you to assist him in planning a cruise 9 months in the future. You assess that he is using a coping mechanism. You remember that one purpose of coping mechanisms is to do which of the following?

    a. Protect the person

    b. Provide feedback

    c. Stimulate the endocrine system

    d. Change reality

4. Developmental theories are useful because they do which of the following?

    a. Provide a basis for comparison with the individual characteristics

    b. Provide a set of rules for structuring individual care

    c. Focus on year-by-year changes in the individual

    d. Are not affected by the situation the individual is experiencing

5. When a father prepares to leave for work in the morning, his 3-year-old son starts to cry and scream. The father picks him up and delays leaving for a while. The child's behaviour most reflects which part of the family system?

    a. Input

    b. Throughput

    c. Output

    d. Feedback

6. Maslow would identify which of the following as belonging on the first (lowest, bottom) level of his hierarchy of needs?

    a. Ability to move around

    b. Recognition as a member of a peer group

    c. Feelings of independence

    d. Safety from physical harm

7. Baljit, a student nurse, has recently learned about the use of holistic thinking in nursing. When interviewing a client, which of the following rationales will he use in planning his questions?

    a. Individual processes are detached from each other.

    b. The reason for consulting the health care professional is of primary importance.

    c. Each individual is more than the sum of his or her parts.

    d. The individual and the immediate environment are the focus of care.

8. Mr. Hannah, 28 years old, has been positive for human immunodeficiency virus (HIV) for 5 years. Recently, he has been admitted to the hospital with a confirmed diagnosis of *Pneumocystis carinii* [now known as *Pneumocystis jiroveci*]. Mr. Hannah tells the nurse that he notices people seem to avoid coming into his room and that he is lonely. What strategy should the nurse use to provide support to the client?

    a. Explain to him the reason he is isolated is due to his susceptibility to infections.

    b. Explain to him that people do not come in to his room because they are afraid of getting HIV infection.

    c. Ask him if any of his family can come to the hospital to keep him company.

    d. Spend time talking with him during and between care activities.

9. Sarah, your friend, is trying to make some changes to her lifestyle. You support her by giving positive feedback because positive feedback does what?

    a. Inhibits change

    b. Stimulates change

    c. Maintains homeostasis

    d. Regulates change

10. Psychological homeostasis, or emotional well-being, can be described as what?

    a. Inherited from parents

    b. Dependent on a person's role in family life

    c. Acquired or learned from living and interacting with others

    d. Totally independent from a person's culture

Check the eText in MyNursingLab for answers and explanations.

WEBLINKS

Public Health Agency of Canada
http://www.phac-aspc.gc.ca
This site provides current Canadian-specific information about many health topics.

Statistics Canada
http://www.statcan.gc.ca
This site provides a variety of federal government statistics related to Canadian life and health.

MyNursingLab

REFERENCES

Belar, C. (2003). Concepts and models. In S. Llewelyn & P. Kennedy (Eds.), *Handbook of clinical health psychology* (pp. 7–19). Chichester, UK: John Wiley & Sons.

Cannon, W. B. (1939). *The wisdom of the body* (2nd ed.). New York, NY: Norton.

Kalish, R. A. (1983). *The psychology of human behaviour* (5th ed.). Montery, CA: Brooks/Cole.

Maslow, A. H. (1970). *Motivation and personality* (2nd ed.). New York, NY: Harper & Row.

Organisation for Economic Co-operation and Development (OECD) (2010). *Broadband penetration and population density.* Retrieved from http://www.oecd.org/21/60/39574903.xls

Smuts, J. (1926). *Holism and evolution.* New York, NY: Macmillan.

Statistics Canada. (2004). *Population 15 years and over by highest degree, certificate or diploma (1986–2001).* Retrieved from http://www40.statcan.ca/101/cst01. educ42.htm

Statistics Canada. (2008). *Number and proportion of persons aged 25 to 64 by level of educational attainment and age groups, Canada, 2006.* Retrieved from http://www12.statcan.ca/english/census06/analysis/education/tables/table2.htm

Statistics Canada (2012a). *The Canadian population in 2011: Population counts and growth.* Retrieved from http://www12.statcan.gc.ca/census-recensement/2011/as-sa/98-310-x/98-310-x2011001-eng.cfm

Statistics Canada (2012b). *Canadian households in 2011: Type and growth.* Retrieved from: http://www12.statcan.gc.ca/census-recensement/2011/as-sa/98-312-x/98-312-x2011003_2-eng.cfm

von Bertalanffy, L. (1968). *General systems theory: Foundation, development, applications.* New York, NY: Braziller.

Wing, P. (1997). Patient or client? If in doubt, ask. *Canadian Medical Association Journal, 157*(3), 287–289.

Chapter **13**

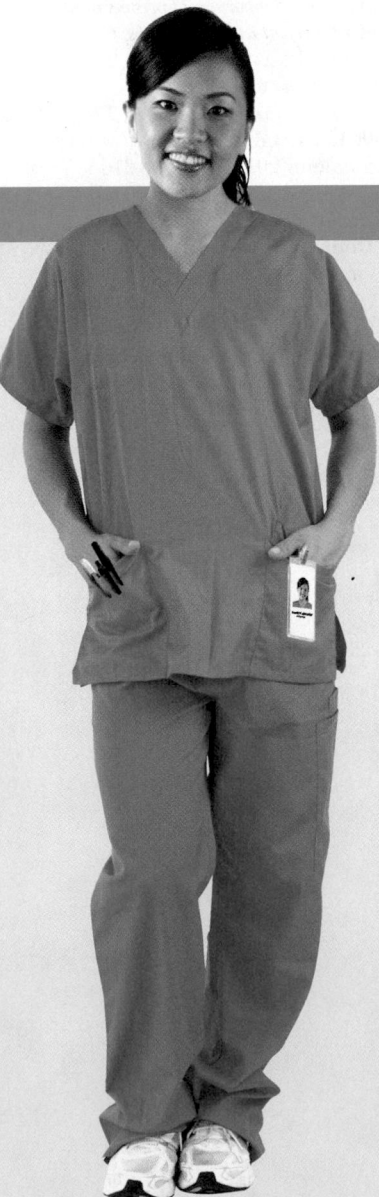

Nursing Care of Families

After completing this chapter, you will be able to:

1. Define "family" in a way that accounts for diverse forms of structure and relationship.

2. Describe factors influencing a shift in nursing perspective from the individual to the person in the context of the family.

3. Outline historical developments in the history of family nursing.

4. Discuss the impact of trends in health care services on family involvement.

5. Propose possible family member expectations for their involvement in care.

6. Analyze demographic trends in Canadian families that influence health and family structure.

7. Identify questions to be posed during a genogram and ecomap inquiry.

8. Formulate questions aimed at exploring reciprocal influences between health or illness and the family.

9. Describe relational practices that foster a collaborative stance with family members.

10. Explain five relational practices that can be integrated when providing nursing care with families.

Whenever concerns related to health and illness arise, both individual persons and those who are involved in their lives are affected. Usually these are family members. Nurses encounter family members in every practice setting, including home care, community clinics, and hospitals. As health care services have shifted away from institutional care with shorter hospital stays, family members are increasingly called upon to provide care at home. Care can involve emotional support, symptom monitoring, and such technical procedures, such as dressing changes or dialysis and intravenous therapies. Family members can be a tremendous resource to nurses through their knowledge of patient preferences and usual patterns of response to difficulties. However, family members do not always hold similar views about caregiving roles. Nurses are challenged to invite and respect all views of family members and provide them with information and emotional support. Nurses are also challenged to involve family members in decision making, in ways that respect the rights and wishes of patients, and to prepare family members with appropriate knowledge, skills, and supports for caregiving roles.

What Is "Family?"

Standards of family structure have shifted dramatically over the past three decades. Couples now often postpone childbearing for prolonged periods of education or establishment of careers. Rising rates of divorce and remarriage have resulted in more blended and lone-parent families. Increased family mobility has also shifted the roles of extended family members (see Box 13.1). These changes challenge definitions of family based on long-held assumptions. Persons choosing to define themselves as family may or may not be bound by blood or legal status. The following definition attempts to be open and respectful of the many different ways families may organize themselves:

> *The Vanier Institute of the Family* (n.d.) *defines family as any combination of two or more persons who are bound together over time by ties of mutual consent, birth and/or adoption, or placement and who, together, assume responsibilities for variant combinations of some of the following:*

- *Physical maintenance and care of group members*
- *Addition of new members through procreation or adoption*
- *Socialization of children*
- *Social control of members*
- *Production, consumption, distribution of goods and services*
- *Affective nurturance—love*

In clinical practice, it is helpful to the nurse to understand how members of a particular family identify themselves in relation to each other. Who is in *this* family? How do *these* family members view their relationships, priorities, concerns, responsibilities, and preferences? To establish a therapeutic relationship with a family, nurses need to be respectful of the ways that families define and describe themselves.

BOX 13.1 TYPES OF FAMILIES IN TODAY'S SOCIETY

Family may be described in different ways according to characteristics of the members (e.g., age, ethnicity, number, sexual orientation, employment), their relationship (e.g., marital, cohabitation, biological, blended, adoptive), or their generation (*nuclear*: parents and child(ren); *extended*: aunts, uncles, cousins; *intergenerational*: grandparents, great grandparents).

- Traditional—both parents reside in the home with children; mother assumes nurturing role and father provides economic necessities
- Two career—both husband and wife are employed
- Lone parent—one parent with child(ren)
- Adolescent—an infant is born to adolescent parents
- Blended—existing families that join together to form a new one
- Cohabiting—unrelated individuals or families who live under one roof
- Adoptive—children are adopted by parent(s)
- Mixed race—parents and/or children of different ethnicities
- Nuclear—parent(s) and child(ren) from same generation
- Mixed generation—parent(s) and child(ren) from several generations
- Gay or lesbian—same-sex couple

Family Nursing

Family nursing refers to relational practices that involve family members in care, respond to their concerns, or provide information and emotional support. Care of family members calls for nursing practices that occur within conversation and relationship, across every health care setting. You will notice that the terms *patient* and *client* are used in this chapter, as nursing care of families can occur in inpatient and community settings.

When nurses encounter families in their day-to-day practice, each encounter affords a possibility for nursing of families. Family members may be present when the home care nurse visits. They may be maintaining a rotating vigil at the bedside of an ill family member, and the nurse may have several brief conversations with them over a particular shift. The nurse may conduct a more formal family assessment interview upon the patient's admission to an outpatient or inpatient facility. The nurse may be involved in a family conference with family and other health care team members to facilitate decision making, treatment planning, or discharge. In some situations, the nurse has little or no direct contact with family members of the individual client, yet the needs and concerns of family members may still be addressed in their absence.

Frequently in nursing, the individual is the focus of care and the extent to which family members are encouraged to be involved in health care encounters varies. Many agencies now provide structural supports to include family members and value their presence and contribution to care. These supports include open or flexible visiting policies; comfortable waiting rooms and access to overnight facilities, refreshments, telephones; and increased access to information from health care professionals.

Nursing of families challenges nurses to shift their perspective from thinking of the client as an individual to "thinking family" or "thinking interactionally." This means that the nurse must forge a collaborative relationship not only with the patient but also with persons who are involved with the patient during the health care encounter. Involvement of family members helps the nurse better understand the meaning of illness to the patient and family, and the possibilities for support during recovery, health maintenance, or health promotion. Unfortunately, despite the growing recognition of the importance of family in health care, there has been limited transfer of family theory to nursing practice (e.g., Segaric & Hall, 2005). This may, in part, be due to conceptual confusion. Few practice areas view the family as context for the patient or view the family as the unit of care. However, nurses need family theory to provide truly relevant care, given that the family is the fundamental unit of society with norms, values, and roles distinct from that of the individual (Dwairy, 2002). Wright and Leahey (2009) described four theoretical frameworks that have contributed to their family nursing work: (a) systems theories, (b) cybernetics theory, (c) communications theory, and (d) change theory. Systems theories help nurses understand the family as a group of interconnected individuals (see Chapter 12). Cybernetics theory looks at communication and control—that the family can be self-regulating, as the body is self-regulating, at differing levels at the same time. In family nursing, communications theory focuses on how family members interact with each other, and change theory examines how changes happen within individuals and groups such as families (Wright & Leahey, 2009). Wright and Leahey (2009) also posited that postmodernism and the biology of cognition have influenced their work, particularly the understanding of multiple realities, perceptions, and possible interventions to achieve family goals.

In some practice settings, the "patient" or "client" is conceptualized as the **person in the context of the family**. Here, the individual is viewed as the primary focus of nursing concern and the family as a significant contextual influence in health, illness, and recovery. Family nursing focuses on *both* individuals (foreground) and families (background). Family members are viewed as connected to the person, relevant to the health concerns of the individual and his or her environment. For example, participation of family members in decisions related to discharge planning is desirable as they can provide emotional support and instrumental assistance to the individual upon returning home. Likewise, family members can be a valuable resource to both the patient and the health care team for decision making around serious illness (Heyland, Tranmer, O'Callaghan, & Gafni, 2003). Though the individual is the focus of care, evidence shows there should also be varying degrees of intent to nurse family members by attending to the impact of the health situation on the family. For example, nurses can *reduce family stress* by providing education to parents of neonatal or pediatric patients around their children's painful procedures, or changes in appearance, behaviour or emotions (Board & Ryan-Wegner, 2003; Davidson et al., 2007). Similarly, nurses can lessen the anxiety of an ICU patient's children by helping them to visit their parent in hospital (Davidson et al., 2007).

Nurses can also *improve the health* of family members caring for loved ones with dementia by teaching them personal coping strategies (Selwood, Johnston, Katona, Lyketsos, & Livingston, 2006). Likewise, nurses can *acknowledge families* by including them in discharge planning discussions and showing concern for its impact on the demands of the family caregiver (their time, energy, and health) when the patient returns home (Davidson et al., 2007). As Friedemann (1995) argued, "all nursing is family nursing and is practised in all clinical settings" (p. 34). She proposed that nurses cannot contribute to the healing of persons without attention to the contexts and relationships in which they live.

Nursing practice may also focus on the **family unit as the client of care**. Attention is simultaneously directed toward the individual *and* family—with the family in the foreground. The family unit is assisted to make change in family *relationships* and *processes* around the difficulties they encounter (Wright, Watson, & Bell, 1996). Heightened attention is given to reciprocity within relationships between family members, between the family and the nurse, and between illness and the family. This work typically requires advanced practice skills.

Development of Family Nursing

Historically, nurses have encountered family members by virtue of their shared presence in homes, communities, and hospitals. However, while the interest in the family as a focus of nursing care extends back to the earliest traditions of modern nursing (Whall & Fawcett, 1991), it is important to note that the family unit, and its activities (including childrearing), were considered a private matter rather than a public societal concern until very recently (Hart, 1991; Bell, Moules, & Wright, 2009).

During the early decades of the twentieth century, there was interest, in both clinical practice and nursing curricula, on nurses (public health nurses and private duty) providing care to families at home or assisting families to care for loved ones and providing them with respite from caregiving activities. Public health nurses have a longstanding tradition of educating families to address the health needs of all family members. In Canada, by the 1920s, there was a growing reliance on hospital services and reduced demand for health care provided at home by private duty nurses (McPherson, 2003). By the 1940s and 1950s, private duty nursing declined dramatically and was coupled with federal and provincial legislation that increased construction of public hospitals across the country. This was followed by the advent of the Canadian system of Medicare, which provided public health care insurance for medical and hospital services. Illness care became increasingly entrenched within hospitals.

Focus on Individuals in Hospital Care

The rise of scientific biomedicine and the organizational efficiencies of hospital care contributed to a focus on the individual. The client was viewed as the individual patient, with a particular pathology, requiring diagnosis and treatment. As medicine focused on curing disease, nurses contributed greatly to the achievement of organizational efficiencies that supported these activities (McPherson, 2003). Families were overlooked as less relevant, with little entitlement to involvement in hospital care. In recent years, there has been renewed attention to the psychosocial aspects of health and illness, including recognition of the influence of family (Firth, 2006). As health care services have been challenged to reconsider the importance of family, many changes in practice and policy have been guided by nurses' responsiveness to the needs, requests, and expectations of families.

Family Care Traditions in Public Health, Maternal–Child, Pediatric, and Mental Health Nursing

Throughout these developments, public health nurses, maternal–child nurses, and pediatric nurses maintained an enduring interest in family care. Hospitals were challenged to provide structural support for family involvement. In maternity settings, couples demanded the presence of fathers in the delivery room. Mothers objected to postpartum separation from their newborns, leading to "rooming-in" practices, with infants cared for at the mother's bedside. In pediatric settings, parents desired round the clock access to their children through flexible visiting policies. Nursing research in the 1970s and 1980s addressed such topics as parent–infant attachment, maternal role attainment, and childbearing or childrearing transitions in the family life cycle with little emphasis on parenting (Gage, Everett, & Bullock, 2006) and the impact of pediatric illness on family members. While much of this early work focused on mother–child relationships, current emphasis on the roles of fathers and husbands has increased (e.g., role of fathers with children who have life-threatening illnesses [Wolff, Pak, Meeske, Worden, & Katz, 2011]). Family nursing research has broadened its focus to include more theory development (e.g., enacting nursing obligations and high family priorities in practice [Doane, Brown, Reimer, MacLeod, & McLellan, 2009]), best practices or standards (e.g., meeting families' needs of patients with parenteral nutrition [Federico & Forbes, 2009], cancer care [Copeland, Pimiento, & Dudrick, 2011], and an examination of best ways to work with families through family- and patient-centred care [Hundon, Fortin, Haggerty, Lambert, & Poitras, 2011; and DiGioia, Lorenz, Greenhouse, Bertoty, & Rocks, 2010]).

Interestingly, the importance of family in mental health nursing is a relatively recent phenomenon. Families often feel rejection or stigma when their loved one is diagnosed with a mental illness and try to conceal the diagnosis and avoid involvement in care (Phelan, Bromet, & Link, 1998). Even when families try to contact care providers for information and emotional support (Doornbos, 2001, 2002), they are sometimes unsuccessful as staff often place their loyalty with the patient (Sjobloom, Pejlert, & Asplund, 2005). Only recently has nursing research begun to understand the experience (Wade, 2006) and needs (Clarke, 2006) of families whose loved ones have a mental illness and begun to explore the effects of different models of family nursing care delivery (Goudreau, Duhamel, & Ricard, 2006).

Family Nursing in Critical Care Settings

During the last 4 decades of the twentieth century, acute care hospitals introduced specialized critical care units. Nurses recognized the impact on family members of implementing highly invasive and technological procedures under tenuous life-and-death circumstances. Nursing research reflected a desire to understand and assist with the emotional distress, uncertainty, and informational needs of family members under these extraordinary circumstances (Myers, Eichhorn, & Guzzetta, 2000). Again, nurses were challenged to humanize these environments by finding ways to enable family access to patients and information and to facilitate family involvement in decision making (Davidson, et al., 2007; Hudson & Payne, 2011).

Shifting Focus to Family Involvement in Health Care

During the 1990s, Canadian hospitals changed dramatically with increasing political pressure for fiscal restraint within the public health care system. Length of hospital stays was considerably reduced, reserved for management of acute episodic events, urgent diagnostic assessment, and treatment requiring intensive physiological monitoring. Outpatient services, home care, and community service increased as an alternative. These changes were coupled with the shifting demographics of the Canadian population. Average life expectancy is increasing, and key causes of death and disability have shifted to chronic illnesses (heart disease, cancer, and respiratory diseases) prompting a shift in direction of care—from one that focuses on hospitals and professionals to a focus on home and family.

More than at any time in the past, family members are implicitly expected to be involved in the complex ongoing medical management of an ill family member at home (Mayer, 2001). Health care providers rely on family members to assist with administration of medication regimes, symptom management, dressing changes, and even technical procedures, such as intravenous therapies, feeding systems, respiratory ventilators, and home dialysis. To be effective, the relationship between health care providers and family members must be collaborative and reciprocal—each needs the support of the other (Ting, 2007).

Family Expectations for Involvement in Care

Clinical practice guidelines (e.g., American College of Critical Care Medicine; Davidson et al., 2007) offer examples of family's hopes and expectations for involvement in care. Family members want to be able to *communicate* with health care professionals about the ill person's condition. They want *access to information* about test results, diagnosis,

treatment plans, and prognosis. Family members want to be able to *trust* that the ill person will be given good care and treated compassionately. They may feel compelled to be vigilant to protect the ill family member at a time of vulnerability. Family members want *recognition* that they are included and valued. Emotional attachment to the ill person may be a powerful motive for their involvement in providing care, but they also seek recognition of their own emotional distress. Finally, family members want *information and preparation* for their roles so they can confidently provide ongoing physical and emotional care. Unfortunately, evidence shows that regardless of culture, most caregivers provide ongoing care without support from any formal caregivers (Navaie-Waliser, Feldman, Gould, Levine, Kuerbis, & Donelan, 2001, 2002).

Canadian Contributions to the Field of Family Nursing

Canadian nurses have made significant contributions to the field of family nursing (Bell, 1996). The "Calgary Family Assessment Model" was first published in 1984, updated, and then enhanced with "The Calgary Family Intervention Model" in subsequent editions of the landmark text *Nurses and Families: A Guide to Family Assessment and Intervention* (Wright & Leahey, 2009). The first International Family Nursing Conference, held in Calgary, Alberta, in 1989, continues to meet regularly. The *Journal of Family Nursing* was first published in 1995 under the editorship of Dr. Janice Bell, University of Calgary. Nursing education programs increasingly offer family nursing in both undergraduate and specialized graduate programs in Canadian universities.

Canadian Families: A Demographic Snapshot

Canada has a growing population of about 34 million people (Statistics Canada, 2011). However, its growth is not sustained from within. Indeed, Canada has a declining fertility rate (1.5 children per woman compared with a replacement rate of 2.1 children) and a population of seniors whose numbers will surpass those of the child population (under 15 years) by 2027. Canada's growth is largely due to immigration (roughly twice the rate of that of the United States and second largest among the G8 countries) (Chui, Tran, & Maheux, 2007). More than one in five Canadians was born in another country and about 43% of Canada's population has origins other than Aboriginal, French, or English. The following depiction of Canadian demographics is based on an analysis of data from Statistics Canada and by The Vanier Institute of the Family (VIF). Some of these trends and implications are summarized in the Nursing and Canadian Society box.

Nursing and Canadian Society

Fact	Implications for Nursing Practice
The average age of first marriages has been rising but seems to have stabilized (28.5 years for women, 30.6 years for men).	Assess impact of family developmental tasks on health maintenance routines and practices.
Changes to the Divorce Act in 1985 resulted in a peak in divorce rates in the decade that followed.	Genogram inquiries should routinely include consideration of step-parenting and blended family arrangements.
Divorce rates are currently declining (38% in 2001 data from Statistics Canada; 40% of first marriages end in divorce according to the Vanier Institute of the Family [2010]) due to lower marriage rates and increasing common-law partnerships.	
More than 9 of 10 individuals with special needs or disabilities live with their families.	Nurses should routinely assess the need for respite care and home care support for family members who are willing and able to fulfill ongoing caregiving responsibilities.
Canadian families are highly mobile—between 1996 and 2000, about 40% of all Canadian residents moved to a different location, though there has been a decline in mobility since 2001.	Explore accessibility of family members to provide emotional and instrumental assistance during health difficulties.

Source: Adapted from The Vanier Institute of the Family. (2010). *Families Count: Profiling Canada's Families IV*. Ottawa, ON: Author.

Cultural Diversity

Canada is heavily influenced by diverse ethnic, religious, and cultural traditions. In 2006, just over 1.2 million Canadians (3.8% of the Canadian population) reported some Aboriginal ancestry (including Indian, Inuit, and Métis) (Statistics Canada, 2008a). The Aboriginal community is generally younger than their counterparts in the general population, with one-third of its population under the age of 24 years. Although some Aboriginal people live on designated reserves, many are integrated into the general communities, and about half live in urban areas located in the Northern and Prairie communities west of Ontario.

Immigrants represent a large composition of the Canadian population. In 2006, the total number of immigrants in Canada was estimated at 6.1 million, representing approximately 19.8% of Canada's total population (Chui, Tran, & Maheux, 2007). Each year, Canada welcomes between 200 000 to 300 000 immigrants and refugees into the country. Before 1970, Canadian culture was powerfully shaped by European immigration. However, post-1970 statistics reveal that the majority of immigrants now come from Asia (Chui, Tran, & Maheux, 2007). Canada's foreign-born population, representing more than 200 countries of origin, increased by 13.6% between 2001 and 2006, which is four times faster than the Canadian-born population (which saw an increase of just 3.3% in comparison) (Chui, Tran, & Maheux, 2007).

Mobility

Canadian families are characterized by high mobility. In the 2006 census, over 40% of Canadian residents moved within the past 5 years (VIF, 2010). About 37% moved to another location within their municipality, whereas more than 3% moved to another province. This is noteworthy since mobility occurred most often among those 15 to 44 years old, in which group families tend to be young and vulnerable. Mobility can trigger family stress, as families join new communities, establish friendships, schools, employment, or handle a long-distance relationship (e.g., with an older parent or a spouse who works away from home). Many young families also experience difficulty with regard to coping with their jobs as they are unable to call on their usual supports (e.g., parents, grandparents, friends) for childcare.

Family: Trends in Marriage, Divorce, Common-Law Relationships, and Parenting

As with other social structures, the family (more than 9 million in Canada) is experiencing a number of significant changes. Although married couple families accounted for nearly 67% of families in 2011, their numbers are falling (down from 69% in 2006, 71% in 2001, and 80% in 1986) (Statistics Canada, 2012). According to Statistics Canada (2012), the number of common-law families increased 13.9% between 2006 and 2011, which is more than four times the gains observed for married-couple families (3.1%). Lone-parent families increased by 8% for a total of 16.3% with higher growth for lone-parent families headed by males. For the first time in the history of Canadian census, common-law couple families were a higher proportion (16.7%) than lone-parent families. Same-sex couples rose 42.4% between 2006 and 2011, with a tripling of married same-sex couples, recognizing the legality of same-sex marriage.

While almost 41% of marriages end in divorce (VIF, 2010), divorce rates are declining—reflecting lower rates of marriage, increasing common-law partnerships, and the drop that followed a peak subsequent to the 1986 amendments to the Divorce Act. The 2011 Census recorded a higher percentage of census families without children (44.5%) than with children (39.2%), a phenomenon first noted in 2006 (Statistics Canada, 2012). In 2011, just over one-fifth of Canadians lived alone. This was a small percentage until the fifth decade or so, 40.1% of persons over 80 who were not institutionalized lived alone (Statistics Canada, 2012).

In 2011, over 3.5 million step-couples with children were counted and stratified as simple or complex families. Eighty-seven point four percent of the step-families were simple step-families, comprised of two parents and their children (Statistics Canada 2012). In 2011, 10% of children 14 and younger lived in step-families. Almost 5% of this age group lived with one or more grandparents, an increase from 2006. These families are frequently intergenerational, including three generations (Statistics Canada, 2012). See Box 13.2 on the top trends for Canadian families.

Income

Seven out of ten couples with children in Canada are dual-income families. Working couples with children are the highest average earners of all family types (Statistics Canada, 2008b). Although the after-tax income for families decreased slightly between 1976 and 1997, the decade ending in 2007 saw a 27.5% rise in family income

after taxes (VIF, 2010), albeit before the latest recession. However, Canadian families are spending faster than they are earning. In 1990, the typical household was able to put aside 13% of its disposable income, but by 2008, this was down to only 3% (VIF, 2010). In 2011, personal debt continued to climb; if household debt were spread evenly across all Canadian families, a family with two children would owe approximately $176 461 (Certified General Accountants of Canada [CGA], 2011). More than 73% of females with school-aged children were employed in 2008 (VIF, 2010). However, employment does not guarantee prosperity, especially in lone-parent families. Even though the picture has improved over time, more than half (56%) of female lone-parent families lived in poverty, more than double the number for all other groups—male lone parents (24%), two-parent families (12%), couples without children (11%), and older adults (7%). For example, earnings for working couples are an estimated $75 997, up 20.6% from 1980. Yet, for lone-parent families headed by women, median earnings rose just 10.9% to $30 958 (Statistics Canada, 2008b). Nearly one in ten Canadians receives social assistance or welfare and has an income well below the poverty line. Reduced access to employment insurance and the lack of affordable housing and dependable childcare force many families to rely on social assistance at some time (Morissette & Ostrovsky, 2007). Thus, almost 13% of all Canadian households were living in poverty in 2007 (VIF, 2010). Nobody knows how many homeless people live in Canada, but it is estimated that from 150 000 to 300 000 are on the streets or in shelters (Human Resources and Skills Development Canada, 2010). However, as many homeless families do not go to shelters or facilities, their numbers are not reflected in homeless counts, and they thus remain almost invisible. Instead, they live in unsafe, overcrowded housing, with friends and family, or in cheap motels. These families are often headed by lone-parent mothers who are struggling with mental health issues, addiction problems, or abuse. Families who do access shelters are often forced to split up.

Families Providing Care

More than 8 of 10 Canadians over the age of 85 years have some form of disability and more than 9 of 10 individuals with special needs or disabilities live with their families in their own, their parents', or their children's home. Although many persons with disabilities are capable of caring for themselves, when they do require assistance, they most often turn to their families. Families continue to provide much of the care required for family members who are aging or disabled. Although many do not identify themselves as such, this is a very large population. About 21% of women and 19% of men provide care to seniors, but it is not known how many

---

BOX 13.2 THE TOP 10 TRENDS FOR CANADIAN FAMILIES

Although these were written several years ago, current statistics attest that the top 10 trends for Canadian families are still relevant:

- Fewer couples are getting legally married.
- More couples are breaking up.
- Families are getting smaller.
- Children experience more transitions as parents change their marital status.
- Canadians are generally satisfied with life.
- Family violence is underreported.
- Multiple-earner families are now the norm.
- Women still do most of the juggling involved in balancing work and home.
- Inequality is worsening.
- The future will have more aging families.

Source: From Sauvé, R. (2004). *Profiling Canada's families III.* Ottawa, ON: The Vanier Institute of the Family. Retrieved from http://www.vifamily.ca. © 2007. Reproduced with permission from The Vanier Institute of the Family.

families care for a child or family member with a disability (VIF, 2010). Caregivers make a significant contribution to the health and well-being of the country; indeed, they are the very foundation to the nation's long-term care system (Gibson & Houser, 2007). It is estimated that Canadian caregivers contribute more than $5 billion worth of free services annually (Fast, Eales, & Keating, 2001).

Older adults often serve as caregivers for their partners, but women between the ages of 35 and 54 years are most likely to provide unpaid care to seniors, and they do so while maintaining other career and family responsibilities. Little is known about children who serve as caregivers, for example, to a lone parent with a debilitating mental illness, out of fear of having the family separated if authorities are informed.

Caregiving affords many personal rewards. However, there are numerous physical, psychological, social, and financial risks assumed by family and friends providing care (Gibson & Houser, 2007; VIF, 2010). Unfortunately, limited health care resources or government financial supports and lack of employment flexibility or respite alternatives isolate caregivers and can increase their distress and burnout (VIF, 2010). The current health care system would not function without caregivers. Nurses are in a position to afford them much needed support.

Understanding Families

Nursing care of families begins with understanding the family at a particular point in time, that is, *who* is involved and *how*. It is not realistic to expect that the nurse will "fix" all the past, present, or future problems confronting the family. However, it is reasonable to expect the nurse to assist the family to navigate through a particular difficulty with a health problem or life transition. The focus of these encounters is the family's hopes and expectations for the present situation and ways the nurse can assist with reciprocal influences between the health or illness concern and the family members.

Illness affects the family, and the family affects the illness (see Figure 13.1 on the next page). By exploring both segments of this reciprocal loop in clinical conversation, the nurse can uncover many areas of inquiry that inform the nurse and create openings for addressing concerns of family members.

Who Is Involved in the Situation?

Family supports may assist the patient at the clinic, at the bedside, or in the home. However, the nurse may not actually see them because of work commitments, transportation difficulties, childcare responsibilities,

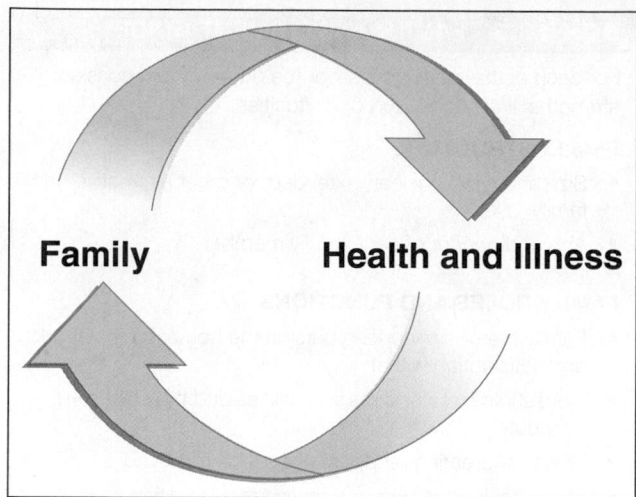

FIGURE 13.1 Reciprocal influence between family and health or illness.

economic constraints, or their own poor health. In addition, family members may not wish to be involved or the patient may not wish to have them involved. If the nurse does not engage family members in conversation when encountering them, or does not ask about them in their absence, it becomes impossible to understand the possibilities for family support or the constraints and limits for family involvement. See Box 13.3 on the family assessment guide for nurses (on the next page).

At a minimum, the nurse must acknowledge the presence of family members, inviting their questions and concerns, explaining the value of family to patient health, and welcoming their participation. More specifically, the nurse can ask what family members understand of the health situation; provide clear, honest information; answer questions; and strive for consensus (Davidson et al., 2007).

Unfortunately, much of this information is lost because it is not documented or communicated. More structured documentation about the family can be facilitated by a genogram inquiry (Hanson, Kaakinen, & Gedaly-Duff, 2005; Wright & Leahey, 2009). The **genogram** is a concise visual depiction of the family structure and relevant situational information that can be sketched on nursing admission forms, progress notes, or Kardex® cards and used with numerous areas of nursing such as postpartum families (Holtslander, 2005) or in pediatrics (Martinez, D'Artois, & Rennick, 2007).

Mapping out a genogram can be brief (minutes) or the focus of an entire family assessment interview. The nurse can introduce the genogram by explaining that it helps the health care team understand the family situation and provide more effective care, for example, by identifying others who might be involved in the care, have access to information, or assist with discharge planning.

For each of the areas assessed, the nurse should consider strengths, limitations, and opportunities.

FAMILY STRUCTURE

- Size and type: nuclear, extended, or other alternative family
- Age and gender of each family member

FAMILY ROLES AND FUNCTIONS

- Family members working outside the home; type of work and satisfaction with it
- Household roles and responsibilities and how tasks are distributed
- Ways childrearing responsibilities are shared
- Major decision maker and methods of decision making
- Family members' satisfaction with roles, the way tasks are divided, and the way decisions are made

PHYSICAL HEALTH STATUS

- Current physical health status of each member
- Perceptions of own health and other family members' health
- Preventive health practices (e.g., status of immunizations, oral hygiene practices, regularity and frequency of visits to the dentist, regularity of visual examinations)
- Routine health care, when and why physician last seen

INTERACTION PATTERNS

- Ways of expressing affection, love, sorrow, anger, and so on
- Most significant family member in person's life
- Openness of communication with all family members

FAMILY VALUES

- Cultural and religious orientations; degree to which cultural practices are followed
- Use of leisure time and whether leisure time is shared with total family unit
- Family's view of education, teachers, and the school system
- Health values: how much emphasis is put on exercise, diet, preventive health care

COPING RESOURCES

- Degree of emotional support offered to one another
- Availability of support persons and affiliations outside the family (e.g., friends, church memberships)
- Methods of handling stressful situations and conflicting goals of family members
- Financial ability to meet current and future needs

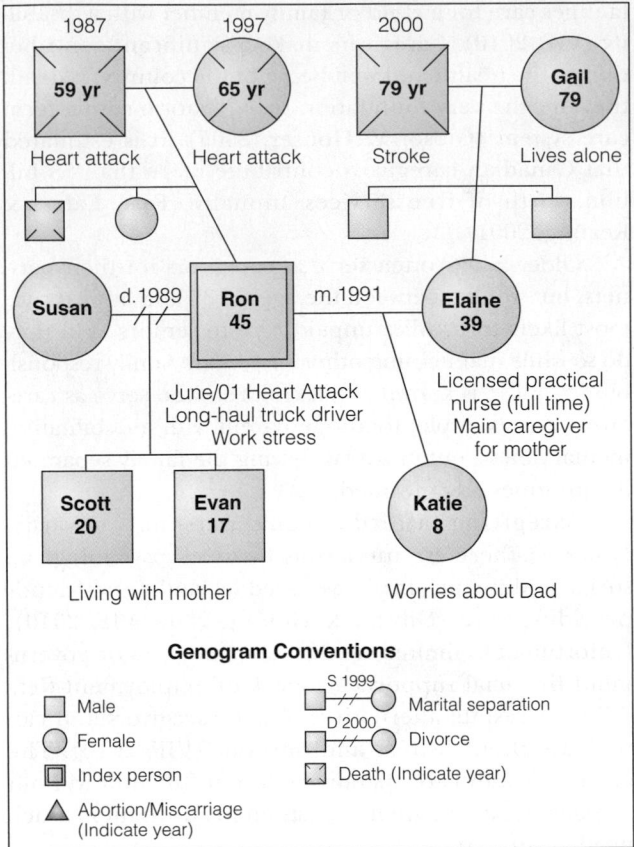

FIGURE 13.2 Family genogram.

Figure 13.2 illustrates an example of a detailed genogram and common conventions for constructing these diagrams. The situation involves a family in which the father, Ron, is hospitalized following a heart attack. He is a long haul truck driver and divorced from Susan, with whom he had two children (Scott and Evan). Ron is now married to Elaine, a licensed practical nurse. Together, they have a daughter, Katie. Elaine is the main caregiver for her mother, the only living grandparent in the family, who lives a 45-minute drive away. The family resides in a small city in which one of the main industries is closing. Ron does most of his driving for this company.

The nurse can introduce the genogram with basic questions about individuals' ages, interests, and occupations. Age-appropriate questions can also be directed to young children about school, friends, and favourite games or toys. Beginning questions usually focus on the family members currently residing together or who are involved in some way in the health care situation. However, inquiry should also explore other family relationships that seem to be relevant to the current situation. For example, in Figure 13.2, the genogram inquiry uncovered the 8-year-old daughter's worries about her father's health, Ron's significant family history with heart disease, and Elaine's caregiving responsibilities for her aging mother. The genogram inquiry may reveal recent losses in the family or significant family events that may contribute to concurrent stress or difficulties confronted by the family. Asking questions about relationships with previous marital partners who are involved in ongoing coparenting responsibilities may also be important. For example, the nurse could ask Ron how his ex-wife, Susan, believes that Scott and Evan have been reacting to the news of his heart attack. This discussion not only builds an understanding of Ron's relationship with the two sons but also the nature of his relationship with his ex-wife. It is important that the genogram questions explore and focus on family concerns and the impact of the health problem on family members and their relationships. As they explore the genogram information together, the nurse and family members can become more engaged and committed to working together. Initiating a genogram inquiry can be an intervention that encourages the nurse *and* family to "think family" and to consider the impact of the situation on all family members.

The context and external environment of the family can similarly be explored by sketching an **ecomap** (Figure 13.3). This diagram uses symbols to depict the family's connections to larger systems, including community agencies, health care providers, work, church, friends, and other meaningful activities in their lives (Bomar, 1996; Kaakinen, Gedaly-Duff, Hanson, & Coehlo 2011; Wright & Leahey, 2009). The symbols are able to express relationships in ways that may be inadequately portrayed in words (Ray & Street, 2005). The genogram of family members sharing a household is sketched at the

centre of the diagram. Ecomap questions could include the following examples:

- *To understand how connected the family is with other resources:* Are there any other clinics, health care professionals, or community agencies that are involved with your family regarding this health concern?
- *To understand the family's level of satisfaction:* Which of these contacts have been most or least helpful to you?
- *To understand the family's support network:* Are there any other religious groups, self-help groups, or personal relationships outside your family that either have been supportive to you or have contributed to your stress?

The ecomap can also depict the dynamic nature of the relationships and stressors with extended family members, work colleagues, or friends. For example, Figure 13.3 helps highlight many external demands on Elaine. In addition to coping with her husband's heart attack, she does shift-work and is a caregiver for her mother. She is dealing with the often difficult transition of placing her mother in a nursing home, with little apparent support from her brothers.

Each circle on the ecomap represents an outside contact with either an individual or the entire family. Straight lines are drawn to indicate the intensity of helpful relationships (for either party); dotted lines indicate ambivalent relationships; and slashed (or jagged) lines indicate difficult or stressful relationships. The ecomap can heighten the nurse's awareness of the possibility of social isolation or of family overload with multiple overlapping connections with health care professionals or agencies. The number of identified contacts in the social network should not be assumed to indicate that support is provided or received or that such contacts are easily accessible (Bomar, 1996). The ecomap inquiry provides an opportunity to explore the nature and quality of these networks.

How Does Illness Affect the Family?

Exploring the impact of illness on the family increases the nurse's appreciation of the distress and suffering of all family members, including the person who is experiencing the health problem (Wright & Leahey, 2005b). The long-term impact of illness demands will differ when the family is confronted with recovery from an acute illness episode, compared with those who face these responsibilities on an ongoing basis, as with a chronic or debilitating illness (Hopkins & Brett, 2005). Instrumental functioning of the family (i.e., activities of daily living [ADLs]) may be affected. If caring for a person who is ill or recovering at home, family members may need to assist with hygiene or mobilization, medication administration, changes in meal preparation, or follow-up visits to doctors and clinics.

Illness may also impact on expressive functioning and communication within the family (Gjerberg, Førde, & Bjørndal, 2011). Anxiety, depression, and uncertainty

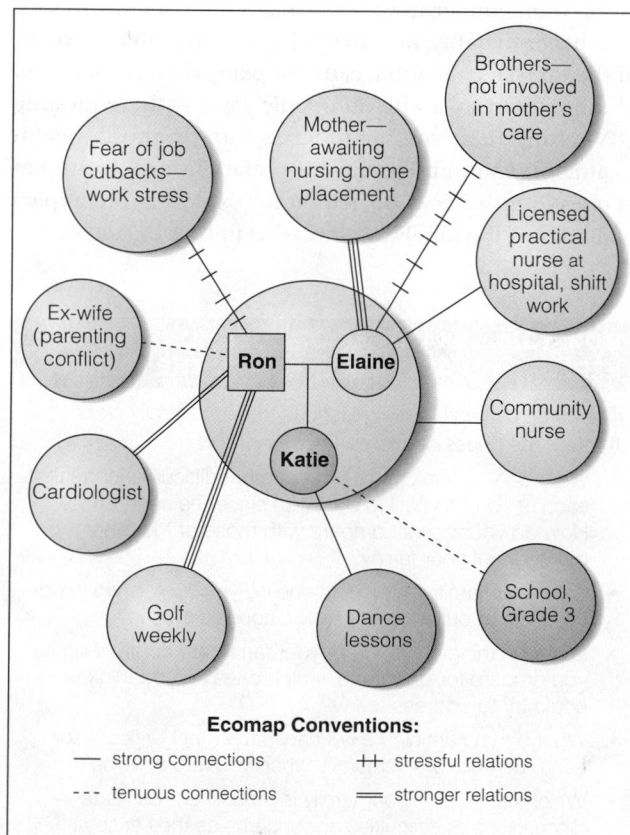

Ecomap Conventions:

— strong connections   ++ stressful relations

--- tenuous connections   = stronger relations

FIGURE 13.3 Family ecomap.

not only can cause distress for the person who is ill but may be an even greater difficulty for others in the family. There may be concern regarding the loss of physical functioning, the implications of a poor prognosis, or the possibility of premature death. It may be difficult for family members to discuss their distress and worries. Communication patterns may shift as family members either address these concerns together or conceal these worries from each other. Family members often feel compelled to maintain an optimistic attitude regarding the future and family roles may shift dramatically. If one partner is unable to work and struggling with physical limitations, the other partner may be pressed to take on new responsibilities for childcare, household maintenance, or employment. Every new diagnosis, change in treatment plan, or contact with a new health care setting potentially has an impact on family members, including heightened vulnerability to illness in other members (e.g., Goodwin, Wickramaratne, Nomura, & Weissman, 2007) (see the Evidence-Informed Practice box on the consequences for nurse–daughters who are caring for older parents).

Nurses need to encourage productive conversations that explore family understandings of the impact of illness. Such conversations can help reveal family values (e.g., family beliefs about appropriate roles and responsibilities for different members, family beliefs about why people get ill and strategies for healing) which, in turn,

can assist in understanding their decisions. The nurse who initiates these conversations in the combined presence of several family members creates an opportunity for each to listen to the others' concerns. Such discussions can help family members become mutually supportive.

The nurse may help a family who is hesitant to raise sensitive matters by asking members to *meet together*, introducing topics and helping them explore the issues. Alternatively, the nurse may *meet privately* with individual members with an understanding that some highly stigmatized behaviour and health conditions are disclosed at considerable risk to those affected. For example, the nurse may meet alone with a mother who has brought her child to the pediatric emergency room, to initiate a discussion of interpersonal partner violence. In this case, the nurse needs to first wait until the child's health problem has been addressed and then, when raising the possibility of abuse, reassure the mother that immediate assistance is available if needed (Dowd, Kennedy, Knapp, & Stallbaumer-Rouyer, 2002). In the case of sexually transmitted infections (STIs), such as human immunodeficiency virus/acquired immunodeficiency syndrome (HIV/AIDS), nurses need to be sensitive to the fact that making a disclosure to family is not only a difficult task but may require different approaches according to gender, sexual orientation, and cultural background (Korner, 2007). For example, a discussion of positive HIV test results with an undeclared bisexual married man attending an infertility clinic will address very different issues (e.g., coming to terms with the diagnosis, coming to terms with his bisexuality, how to tell his wife, possible breakup of the marriage, health treatment plan) than a discussion of the same results with an openly gay couple requesting HIV testing (e.g., coming to terms with diagnosis, health treatment plans, implications for relationship). Examples of questions that may be helpful for exploring the impact of illness on the family are provided in Box 13.4.

EVIDENCE-INFORMED PRACTICE

What Are the Consequences for Nurse–Daughters Who Are Caring for Elderly Parents?

These authors have been examining the experiences of registered nurses who were also daughters of older parents. For this study, they interviewed 20 nurses who care for their older relatives. Qualitative analysis revealed themes (context, characteristics, and consequences) from the interview data. The nurses described situations where the boundaries between professional identity and work was blurred with personal identity and work. These nurses were often so caught up in their relatives' health care needs, in addition to their professional work, that they developed what is described as compassion fatigue. In fact, some of the participants noted that the continuous balancing between work and family could and did result in the nurses experiencing adverse health themselves.

NURSING IMPLICATIONS: With an aging nursing profession caring for older relatives, society needs to re-examine its expectations of care from professional family members, and the support available for families to ensure that all needs are met.

Source: Based on Ward-Griffin, C., St-Amant. O., & Brown, J. B. (2011). Compassion fatigue within double duty caregiving: Nurse-daughters caring for elderly parents. *The Online Journal of Issues in Nursing, 16*(1), 4.

BOX 13.4 EXAMPLES OF QUESTIONS THAT EXPLORE IMPACT OF ILLNESS ON THE FAMILY

The nurse can ask these questions to help a family work through the illness of a family member:

- What do you think has been the most difficult change that each of you has had to deal with since the heart attack? How do your views compare with those of the other members of your family?

- Of all your family members, who do you think is worrying the most about what this new diagnosis means?

- Of all the things that you or your family are confronting as you prepare for discharge, which ones do you think we could try to address today?

- What do you anticipate will cause the most difficulty for each member of your family when you return home?

- Which member of your family is most likely to initiate discussions of difficulties or concerns as they arise at home?

How Does the Family Affect the Illness?

Just as the illness has an influence on each family member, each family member also has an influence on the illness (Firth, 2006). This does not mean that they can control the illness or determine health outcomes. Family members cope with and respond to the illness in many different ways—each journey is unique and different from that of the patient. However, the need for support, information, valuing, and respect is the same. Therapeutic conversation in this domain helps uncover ways family members have found to manage the demands of the illness in their daily lives. They may view a health concern as a challenge and embrace changes necessitated by health maintenance or illness management. They may be overwhelmed by illness demands that compound other concurrent life stressors. A new diagnosis may challenge family members to seek new information and to figure out what this means for their lives. Family members may develop expertise in their vigilance for the return of troublesome symptoms or potential complications.

Family members typically attempt to offer help and encouragement to the person who is ill or recovering while also attempting to manage their own distress. On occasion, family offers of support are seen by the person who is ill as intrusive or as a limitation to their independence. Conversations about these attempts to influence illness can help family members understand their sense of helplessness and explore how they would most prefer to be involved, to limit the caregiving burden, and to enable family members to show their caring in a manner that is experienced as supportive. In some instances, the illness may compound other life stressors. Marital discord, difficulties with parenting of teenagers, unemployment, and conflict within the extended family are examples of adverse circumstances that can interfere with family coping and increase the complexity of family involvement during health care encounters. In such circumstances, the nurse might have a discussion with the family about strengths observed and ways they might be used to overcome the family's sense of helplessness.

Conversely, conversations that explore family responses to illness can reveal incredible capability and competency on the part of family members. Learning about the family's resourcefulness provides the nurse with opportunities to help the family recognize their own capability and explore other possible ways of coping based on the family's knowledge. These conversations help the nurse understand the family's usual ways of coping with difficulties and introduce ideas that may be different from those that the family has already attempted. Exploration of family strengths in illness management is an often-neglected domain of inquiry. Some examples of questions that explore family influence on the illness are provided in Box 13.5.

BOX 13.5 EXAMPLES OF QUESTIONS THAT EXPLORE THE IMPACT OF THE FAMILY ON ILLNESS

These questions can help debrief families when someone experiences an illness:

- What has been the most helpful thing that your family has done for you that has made a difference to this hospitalization?
- What have each of you learned about limiting stress that will be most useful to you when you return home?
- How have each of your family members been most helpful to you as you have been preparing for discharge?
- Of all of the lifestyle changes that have been recommended to you, which ones do you believe each of your family members will be able to implement most successfully?
- How would you like each of your family members to be involved in your recovery at home?

Nursing Care of Families

As stated earlier, nursing care of families is exercised almost exclusively through relational practices. Even if there are only one or two family members directly involved in the health care encounter, the nurse–family relationship is more complex than when working with individual clients. The nurse needs to engage and understand each family member to elicit concerns and invite questions. Family members and patients may hold similar or different perspectives and may require different supports. The nurse needs to not only appreciate these multiple perspectives but also attempt to respond in ways that account for these similarities or differences. Nurses can enhance their family nursing practice by using the guidelines in Box 13.6.

BOX 13.6 FAMILY NURSING PRACTICES

Effective family nursing practices include the following:

- Engaging in a collaborative relational stance
- Asking reflective questions
- Enabling access to the patient
- Eliciting illness narratives
- Commending family and individual strengths
- Offering information
- Creating and encouraging family support
- Suggesting respite from caregiving

Engaging in a Collaborative Relational Stance

Relational practices are influenced by nurses' beliefs about the kinds of obligations we have toward family members, about our expectations of family members, and about the skills and knowledge that nurses bring to family encounters. Many of these ideas presupposed in nursing practice, for example, the idea that recovery from an acute episode of illness will affect family members. However, ideas about whether nurses are responsible to care for family members and what ought to be done may be less clear. The nurse's stance toward the family is influenced by the habits, practices, concerns, and skills the nurse brings to the situation (Browning & Warren, 2006). In family nursing, **relational stance** refers to the thoughtful and purposeful choices that nurses make in clinical practice about the ways that they will engage and involve families and respond to their concerns (Tapp, 2000; Walker, & Dewar 2001). Families feel engaged when information is shared and they are included in decision making—when there is someone to contact when needed and when services are responsive to their needs (Walker, & Dewar, 2001). Nurses can evaluate their relational practice by asking themselves questions, such as those summarized in Box 13.7.

It is often assumed that having a good nursing relationship with the patient and family will increase the effectiveness of their work together. Robinson's (1996) research challenged nurses to reconsider relational practices—to see that they not only create a context or climate in which "interventions" can be more effective but that these relational practices in themselves *are* interventional. This research described examples of relational practices that were noticed by family members in this study of women and families experiencing chronic illnesses. They described the nurse as a *curious listener,* who found a balance between listening and asking good questions that focused conversation and brought out in the open significant differences in family perspectives. They viewed the nurse as a *compassionate stranger,* someone who was deeply interested in the family's situation and yet had some objectivity and could offer a new point of view that was impartial to various family members. Families valued

the nurse as a *nonjudgmental collaborator* whose avoidance of blaming and criticism helped family members speak with less reservation. This collaborative stance helped families realize what they needed to do and then to do it together. Families appreciated the nurse as a *mirror for family strengths,* whose positive orientation toward strengths, resources, and possibilities fostered family confidence and capability. Collaboration entails working with the family to co-evolve shared understandings of the difficulties they are encountering. Together, the family and the nurse generate other possibilities for dealing with health concerns or illness. A **collaborative relational stance** is one that values the multiple ideas and perspectives that are inevitably encountered within the family and demonstrates respect for family strengths and capabilities in addressing health concerns and living with illness. It is through the process of "shaping mutuality" that a nurse and family caregiver learn to collaborate and achieve their individual goals and desired outcomes, both for the patient and for themselves (Jeon, 2004).

Asking Reflective Questions

A series of studies have consistently shown that families find nurses to be particularly helpful when they ask good questions (Tapp, 1997; Wright, Watson, & Bell, 1996). The best questions enable them to think differently about themselves, about other family members, and about health and illness—both in the present and future (Firth, 2006). Wright et al. (1996) describe this practice as "asking questions that invite reflection" (p. 116) to promote understanding of events and relationships of everyday life. Wright and Leahey (2005b) describe **reflective questions** as interventional because they not only *provide information* to the nurse but they also *facilitate changes in the family* as new information emerges in conversations. Family members come to understand each other, their difficulties, and possible solutions differently as they listen to each other's responses to reflective questions. Table 13.1 summarizes examples of reflective questions, including **difference questions**, **behavioural effect questions**, and **hypothetical/future-oriented questions** (Wright & Leahey, 2009). In addition, the three most common errors in family nursing are also included along with strategies for avoiding such mistakes (Wright & Leahey, 2009).

Enabling Access to the Hospitalized Patient

Within inpatient practice settings, an issue commonly encountered by families is that of visiting hours (Farrell, Joseph, & Schwartz-Barcott, 2005). Hospital policies regarding visiting hours may impose constraints for family members who want to be present at the patient's bedside.

BOX 13.7 QUESTIONS INVITING NURSING REFLECTION ON RELATIONAL STANCE

A collaborative relational stance is important in the nurse–family relationship. Use the questions that follow to evaluate your own relational stance:

- To what extent am I imposing my beliefs on the family?
- To what extent did I elicit the patient's and family members' expectations, hopes, questions, and ideas?
- How frequently are decisions about the patient's health care made mutually by the patient, family, and myself?
- Do my actions and comments acknowledge the strengths and abilities of this family?
- What can I learn from this family about their experiences in living with this health problem?

Source: Leahey, M., & Harper-Jaques, S. "Family-nurse relationships: Core assumptions and clinical implications." *Journal of Family Nursing, 2*(2), 133–151. Copyright © 1996 by SAGE. Reprinted by Permission of SAGE Publications.

TABLE 13.1 Types of Reflective Questions

Types of Question	Examples
Difference Question	
Explores differences among people, relationships, time, ideas, or beliefs	Who do you think will be most affected by this new diagnosis of heart disease as you return home? What impact has this experience with heart attack had on your relationship as a couple?
Behavioural Effect Question	
Explores the effect of one family member's behaviour on another	When your daughter Katie is worried about her dad's health, what do you tell her? How does Ron show his stress when his work is demanding? What impact does this have on you, Elaine? What impact does it have on Katie?
Hypothetical/Future-Oriented Question	
Explores family options and alternative actions or implications in the future	What do you predict will be the most difficult change for you as you try to implement lifestyle changes? How do you anticipate your family's daily routine to be different when you are discharged home?
Most Common Errors	**How to Avoid**
Failing to create a context for change (being curious about the problem)—the foundation of the therapeutic relationship	• Show interest. • Obtain a clear understanding of the most pressing concern. • Validate each family member's experience. • Acknowledge suffering and the sufferer.
Taking sides	• Maintain curiosity. • Identify all the perspectives (identifying does not equate with condoning). • Remember that all members experience some suffering during a family illness/problem. • Give equal time to each concern and each member. • Treat all information as a new discovery. • Avoid having private conversations with one family member reporting on another.
Giving too much advice	• Give advice, opinions, recommendations only after a thorough assessment. • Offer advice without believing that the nurse's ideas are the best or better. • Focus more on asking questions than giving statements during initial conversations.

Source: Wright, L. M. & Leahey, M. (2013). *Nurses and families: A guide to family assessment and intervention*, 6th edition. Philadelphia, PA: F.A. Davis and Wright, L. M. & Leahey, M. (2013). The three most common errors in family nursing: How to avoid or sidestep. *Journal of Family Nursing, 11*, 90. Copyright © 2005 SAGE. Reprinted by Permission of SAGE Publications.

Reasons for limiting family access may include concerns for patient rest and privacy, infection control, limited space at the bedside, patient instability, and the possible impact of viewing procedures on family members. Nurses may not be comfortable when family members observe their performance of bedside care or technical procedures. Nurses may believe that the impact of an emotionally distraught family member at the bedside can upset the patient. Sometimes, the patient may request limitations to family visiting.

Family members may want to be present to provide emotional support to the person who is ill, to protect him or her from harm through possible mistakes or careless treatment by health care providers, or to quell their own emotional distress (Mitchell, Courtney, & Coyer, 2003). Access to the patient often means access to information. Family members who are present at the bedside may have more opportunities to consult directly with the health care team. When family members are able to access the patient, they also have more opportunity to understand their loved one's condition, which, in turn, can help them gain confidence as they see the patient progress in strength and recovery or assist them to prepare for difficulties and loss. Nurses have a responsibility to facilitate that understanding. Families want different kinds of information in different situations. For example, when removing life supports from a patient, families want (a) assurances that the patient will not be abandoned before death, (b) assurances that the patient will be comfortable and will not suffer, and (c) support for family's decisions about end-of-life care, including support for family's decision to withdraw or not to withdraw life support (Stapleton, Engelberg, Wenrich, Goss, & Curtis, 2006).

Nurses interpret hospital policy and unit guidelines and often have discretion to be flexible with visiting rules when warranted in particular situations or to collectively generate a unit culture that is more family friendly. Many nurses argue that visiting hours require balancing the visitors' needs for information and access to a loved one with the nurse's need to safely manage the care of a critically ill individual (Farrell et al., 2005). Studies of the effects of visiting on mental status and various physiological systems have shown no physiological rationale for restricting visitors and some reasons for making visiting hours more flexible, even in the intensive care unit (ICU) (e.g., Griffin, 2003; Lee et al., 2007). Many pediatric settings and, increasingly, adult ICU or emergency settings show positive effects on the family when they have open, unrestricted visiting policies, even during resuscitation (e.g., Myers et al., 2000). However, these situations require adequate preparation of the family, availability of support personnel to help the family through a crisis situation, and family debriefing and support following a crisis (Benner, Hooper-Kyriakidis, & Stannard, 1999). In addition, patients, families, and staff do not always share the same views around visiting hours (Tanner, 2005), so it is important to check with the patient, where possible, when discussing visitation.

Eliciting Illness Narratives

Nurses access the beliefs and meanings that people hold about their day-to-day experience of illness through illness narratives, rather than medical narratives (Morris, 1998). **Medical narratives** provide clinicians with information relevant to the nature and course of physical symptoms, diagnosis and treatment of a disease process, and concurrent or past illness problems for the person or other family members. In contrast, **illness narratives** seek understanding of the person's or family's experience of illness in the ordinary acts of everyday living; the influence of illness on relationships with family, friends, and workmates; the persons' ability to gain influence over the impact of illness in their lives; and the stories told of encounters with the health care system. Both medical and illness narratives are important and useful, and nurses must be able to conduct both forms of inquiry. Table 13.2 offers examples of questions that illustrate differences between medical and illness narratives.

Eliciting illness narratives with families is an important relational practice. These stories help the nurse understand family strengths and difficulties and also help patients and their families come to terms with their own experiences. In the telling of these stories, people reach a new understanding of their experiences with illness. Family members are better able to appreciate what is happening and to realize that their experiences are both similar and different. Family members may describe the telling of illness stories as therapeutic in itself (e.g., Berg, 2006). However, there are many constraints against having illness conversations. Family members may want to maintain privacy or may not want to burden friends or other family members. People expect to tell health care professionals their medical story. They are often surprised that health care professionals are interested

TABLE 13.2 Examples of Questions to Elicit Medical and Illness Narratives

Medical Narrative	Illness Narrative
Could you describe the onset of the chest pain?	What does it mean to you when the chest pains come and are very unpredictable?
Have you had any acute health problems or chronic illnesses in the past?	Of all of the health problems that you have encountered in the past, what has been the most difficult thing you have had to deal with?
Does your extended family have any previous history of heart disease?	What have you learned from your parents' experiences with heart disease that might be helpful during your own recovery?
Have you had any cardiac diagnostic tests done in the past?	Based on the diagnostic tests that you have had done, what are your predictions about your health in the future?
Which of the following cardiac risk factors would apply to you? (e.g., smoker, sedentary lifestyle, high-fat diet)	Tell me how it has been for you and your family as you have tried to incorporate the lifestyle changes that have been recommended.

in illness stories, and they often tell of encounters with health care systems that contributed to difficult illness experiences.

When nurses elicit illness stories, they are drawn into the richly contextualized lives of the people they encounter. It becomes much more difficult to objectify or depersonalize people and easier to recognize the strengths, resourcefulness, and capabilities of the family members. It is through illness stories that nurses will be able to offer family commendations to acknowledge their efforts to maintain health or manage illness.

Commending Family and Individual Strengths

Nurses may adopt the stance that patients and families have strengths and capabilities, that they have solved problems before and are resourceful and only temporarily in need of assistance from health care professionals (McElheran & Harper-Jaques, 1994). This stance heightens the nurse's ability to recognize and elicit examples of the family's resourcefulness throughout their work together. Examples of strength and capability appear in the illness narratives as persons and families tell of ways they have been able to manage or live with a health problem or illness. Other examples may be evident in the day-to-day situations and conversations that occur as nurses and families work together. When nurses acknowledge strengths directly to the family, the practice of offering commendations emerges. This practice can help families recognize their own strengths and realize that these can be transferred to other situations and are valued by other health care professionals. Commendations are not always experienced as warm and gentle. Indeed, while considered constructive, they may also be experienced as provocative, potent, and powerful (Limacher & Wright, 2006).

Commendations are statements of praise that "highlight strengths, support movement of the nurse–patient–family system in ways that meet the family's needs and assist the nurse in engaging the patient and family at levels of interaction that are not problem saturated, but are resource focused" (McElheran & Harper-Jaques, 1994, p. 7). When health problems occur, families may be overwhelmed by difficulties and feel unable to cope with the uncertainty or transitions they are facing. Commendations can help change the view that families have of themselves or their situations and support their confidence in each other. Commendations support the idea that the patient and the family are active participants who are in charge of their health or life situation and can offer hope for the future (McElheran & Harper-Jaques, 1994). This practice can encourage families to continue seeking further options to discover their own solutions to problems (Wright & Leahey, 2009). Commendations can also enhance connection in the family–nurse relationship as the nurse conveys

respect and appreciation for the family's contributions and efforts within difficult situations.

Commendations should echo the family's own language and fit with their values and perceptions of their experiences. When the nurse does not know the family well, commendations can be offered as "beginning impressions" of what they have been doing well. Commendations can be introduced by comments such as the following:

> "What I've noticed about your family (or about what you've told me) is that . . ."
> "I'm really impressed by the way that . . ."
> "I appreciate how you have been able to . . ."
> "I'm wondering if your talent in this situation is the way that you . . ."

It may be helpful to offer a commendation prior to offering an opinion or idea that might be difficult for family members to accept, with comments such as the following:

> "You have all really pulled together in wonderful ways to understand your son's illness. Unfortunately, as there is no cure for his illness, he will need increasing amounts of care . . . care that is often painful."

Commendations offered at the end of a conversation can highlight change or support family choices that have emerged within the discussion through comments such as:

> "It is quite remarkable how many decisions you have made today, given that, when we started our discussion today, you each said that you were in no position to make any decisions."

Offering Information

Families indicate that obtaining information about the health situation greatly assists them to make decisions, to cope more effectively, and to be able to support their ill family member appropriately (Davidson et al., 2007). Nurses play an important role in providing information for health promotion, recovery, and health maintenance, or during acute episodes of illness. Health-promotion messages within the media and public domain are often confusing or contradictory. Illness care operates within an increasingly technical biomedical domain with a specialized jargon. Nurses are positioned in the middle of these public and biotechnical discourses and can help families interpret this information. Also, nurses typically know the health care system well and can offer information to help people access appropriate services effectively. They can, for example, provide handouts of resource lists, teach steps for navigating bureaucratic systems, make advance contact to services when referring, and make follow-up phone calls to families. These actions foster a sense of partnership with families and facilitate service access.

Family members other than the ill individual may play an important role in garnering information about diagnosis, treatment, and health maintenance. The ill person may be less able to seek out or comprehend new information because of illness, effects of medications, or invasive diagnostics and treatment. By informing and educating family members, the nurse helps them understand illness events, anticipate likely events on a trajectory of illness, and prepare for their caregiving roles (Levine, 1998).

Nurses often make assumptions about the kind of information that would be most helpful to particular persons or families. Often, these assumed essentials concern the details of the disease process, medication management, and activity guidelines. However, it is important to discuss with the family the kind of information they believe would be most helpful. Other concerns may be far more pressing, such as how to provide emotional support at home or how to arrange for transportation to a follow-up appointment and how to pay for it—concerns that families may be hesitant to raise on their own. Nurses often believe that more information will result in decreased anxiety, but it is not always so. Nurses can be very helpful to families by assisting them to locate other sources of information, such as availability of self-help or support groups, public service groups, websites, or community resource centres. The challenge is to offer resources (information and support) that address family questions or needs in a timely fashion (as needed) and in suitable ways (e.g., plain language).

Creating and Encouraging Family Support

When nurses are thinking in a family context, they are more likely to be aware that all family members may be in need of various degrees of support. The health care literature often conceptualizes **family support** as a form of social support—the provision of emotional, instrumental, informational, and appraisal assistance that helps to buffer stress. It is not unidirectional, but rather **reciprocal** and **mutual** as individuals attempt to be supportive of each other. Therefore, in health care, the focus remains not solely on the patient but, instead, on identified caregiver(s) and other family members as well.

Social support is not simply "nice to have"; it actually plays a critical role in psychological health (Deci, La Guardia, Moller, Scheiner, & Ryan, 2006). In addition, *giving* support has been found to be a stronger predictor of psychological health than the act of *receiving* support (Deci et al., 2006). Further, the number of contacts within a social network is less important

than the perceived quality of social relationships and the extent to which they are experienced as supportive (Bomar, 1996).

Nurses provide family support as they involve family members in care and respond to their concerns and questions. Nurses can assist family members to listen to each other's concerns, feelings, and stories and make meaning of illness and health care encounters, thus increasing the possibility for them to be supportive of each other.

Family members may seek guidance about how they can be supportive of the ill person. These needs typically arise at times when family members are also experiencing distress, concern, and need for emotional support. Nurses can help family members discuss their preferences about the kind of assistance or support they desire from each other (Tapp, 1997). For example, following an acute episode of illness, the patient may want to regain a sense of independence. Family members may have difficulty gauging how much assistance is desired or appropriate. If the ill person views needing help as a sign of weakness, offers of assistance from family members may be unwelcome.

As another example, following diagnosis of diabetes, family members frequently attempt to be helpful through watchful monitoring of medications, activity, or diet while the person who is ill may find these reminders unhelpful or intrusive. At the same time, it can be hurtful to family members when their well-intended efforts are rebuffed, especially if they view the ill person as not attending "responsibly" to health maintenance activities.

The person who is ill may be self-absorbed with the experience of illness and recovery and may be less aware of impacts on other family members. Illness conversations may be constrained by a desire to maintain a positive attitude. Family members may be reluctant to discuss their own needs or frustrations, especially if their distress is motivated by worries about the future or prognosis. These difficulties can contribute to significant family conflict. Using reflective questions, the nurse can assist family members to explore their perceptions and concerns, come to appreciate the perspective of other members, and discuss how each person would prefer to both receive and offer assistance.

Suggesting Respite from Caregiving

Families differ in their desire to be directly involved in caregiving. For example, Benner and colleagues (1999) suggested that family members of patients who are chronically ill and hospitalized may wish to participate in familiar caregiving rituals (such as grooming, assisting with meals, comfort measures) to maintain connection.

Others may be exhausted from caregiving at home and welcome respite from these demands. It is important to encourage family participation in caregiving to the extent that they desire, but this should be facilitated following careful exploration of both patient and family preferences. Such discussions are not always easy. Indeed, evidence suggests that nurses and families have difficulty discussing family participation in caretaking activities (e.g., Roden, 2005).

A study by Ward-Griffin (1999) explored transitions in caregiving between community nurses and family members caring for an older person at home. Initially, family members were encouraged to be involved and were grateful to be of assistance. They became knowledgeable and skillful in these activities as the nurse shifted care to the family caregiver at a comfortable pace. However, family members gradually reported feeling overwhelmed as nurses reduced their time and involvement. Eventually, many family caregivers reported that the amount of care they were expected to provide led to physical and emotional exhaustion, social isolation, and strained family relationships. This report heightens sensitivity to the potential for caregiver burden. Another study by Leenerts and Teel (2006) explored communication skills used by nurses to create partnerships with the older spouses of persons with dementia who are their caregivers. Conversations that resulted in partnerships depended on one theme only: relational conversation—that is, conversation that included listening with intent, affirming emotions, creating relational images, and planning enactment.

Financial constraints may make it difficult for families to secure respite from caregiving. Research shows that caregivers who are poor, married, have a poor health status, provide care for a long time, care for patients with poor performance status, and pay high medical expenses are more likely to lose their family savings (Yun et al., 2005). Household income may be reduced due to the person's inability to work, or family members may be forfeiting income to be available to the family member who is ill. Finances may limit options to compensate a replacement caregiver or to allow for a vacation. Additionally, it may be difficult for family members to allow themselves to take respite from caregiving without guilt (Wright & Leahey, 2005b). The person who is ill may be reluctant to accept an alternative caregiver. A primary caregiver may be reluctant to request assistance from, or disagree with, extended family members. Possible constraints should be explored with the family, perhaps by discussing the implications should the caregiver get rundown or ill without a break, or measures that would give the caregiver comfort if respite care were provided.

Many possible options are available for **respite care**. Regularly obtaining a few hours away from home may be sufficient in some instances. Others may prefer an extended vacation for several weeks. Some may desire respite for brief 1- or 2-day periods. Respite programs may be available either to provide care in home or for temporary inpatient placement. Unfortunately, respite care is not available in all provinces and territories or in many rural areas. Hence, for many families, respite care must be provided by other family members or friends.

Evaluating Nursing Care of Families

Relational practices are inherent in nurses' efforts to evaluate their clinical practice with families. Every encounter with patients and families provides opportunities for the nurse to invite their viewpoint. The nurse can reflect on the extent to which information was communicated to families, how families were involved in decision making, and the ways that patient and family expectations, hopes, questions, and ideas were discussed (Leahey & Harper-Jaques, 1996) and met, or not, and barriers that might have surfaced. The nurse can also solicit feedback from the patient and family about their experience of the family–nurse relationship (see Box 13.8). Their comments and suggestions may provide useful opportunities for fostering ongoing development in clinical skills that enable nursing care of families to be provided in a respectful and healing manner.

BOX 13.8 EVALUATING THE NURSING CARE OF FAMILIES

Gaining feedback from the patient and family about their experience of the family–nurse relationship is important for professional development. These questions can assist in getting started:

- Of all the things that we have talked about today, which of these ideas, if any, seemed most useful to you? In what way is it useful?

- What else could we have talked about that would be more helpful?

- Which family member do you think has benefited most from our conversation? How?

- If I were to encounter another family in a similar situation tomorrow, what do you think I should be sure to talk with them about?

- What advice would you give to me about working with other families who might run into this situation?

- Is there anything in our work together that supported your confidence in dealing with this difficulty?

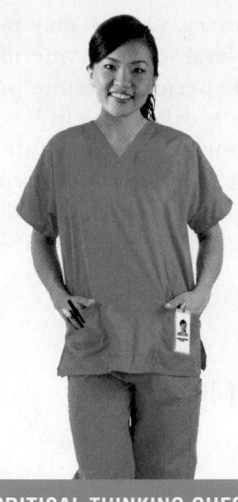

Case Study 13

At the morning change of shift report on the medical unit of a large city hospital where you work, you are warned about John's "demanding family." The family has recently immigrated to Canada looking for a safer country to call home. They speak English as a second language. The father, although a teacher in his home country, has been working as a dishwasher or cleaner on nightshift when he can find a job. John, his Canadian name, is a 1-year-old boy who has been hospitalized for the past week for diagnostic tests that have attempted to locate the cause for his progressive neurological deficits. Test results have been inconclusive. The mother has not left John's side since his admission. Each morning, when the father arrives, with limited English, he interrogates the nurse about John's progress overnight and the plan of action for the day. The nurses are concerned by what they describe as "overly strict" parenting practices with John, and the wife's overly subservient attitude toward her husband. The father approaches you as you begin your shift.

CRITICAL THINKING QUESTIONS

1. How might the family's cultural background be affecting their response to this health situation?

2. How would you engage this family to foster a more productive and collaborative relationship?

3. How would you attempt to address their concerns?

4. What is the relationship between the health problem and the family members?

5. How might the family's cultural background be affecting the parenting practices? How would you engage the family in a discussion about this matter?

Check the eText in MyNursingLab for answers and explanations.

KEY TERMS

behavioural effect questions *p. 256*

collaborative relational stance *p. 256*

commendations *p. 259*

difference questions *p. 256*

ecomap *p. 253*

family *p. 245*

family nursing *p. 246*

family support *p. 260*

family unit as the client of care *p. 246*

genogram *p. 251*

hypothetical/ future-oriented questions *p. 256*

illness narratives *p. 258*

medical narratives *p. 258*

mutual *p. 260*

person in the context of the family *p. 246*

reciprocal *p. 260*

reflective questions *p. 256*

relational stance *p. 256*

respite care *p. 261*

CHAPTER HIGHLIGHTS

- Definitions of "family" should include shifting social norms in family structure and each family's mode of describing themselves.

- Nursing care of families is based on relational practices that involve family members in care, respond to their concerns, provide them with information, and/or offer emotional support.

- Family expectations of health care providers may include a desire for access to information about diagnosis and treatment, ability to trust that their ill family member will receive good care and be treated compassionately, recognition for their own involvement in care, and preparation for their roles at home.

- The genogram inquiry helps the nurse demonstrate a concern for all family members, to document relevant information about those involved in the health situation, to appreciate developmental transitions in the family, and to begin to understand family relationships.

- The ecomap inquiry helps the nurse understand sources of family support or stress by tracing external connections to employment, health care services, and recreational and religious communities.

- Reflective questions invite family members to think differently about themselves, health and illness concerns, and options for addressing concerns.

- Illness narratives help nurses more fully understand the reciprocal influences between health and the family and can assist families to make sense of the illness experience.
- Commendations acknowledge and convey respect for family capabilities and strengths.
- Families vary in their desire to be directly involved in caregiving activities and may need encouragement to take a respite from prolonged caregiving.
- Nurses can evaluate nursing care of families by reflecting on their efforts to invite family questions and concerns, by involving family members in decision making, and by asking the family directly about their experience of the family–nurse relationship.

ASSESS YOUR LEARNING

1. Chris is a 42-year-old father who is terminally ill. He continues to want to drive his children to school, but his wife, Susan, fears that his illness makes him an unsafe driver. Susan asks the nurse to reinforce her view. Which response by the nurse BEST reflects a family nursing approach?

   a. "You have raised an important issue. However, this is a family matter and not really any of my business."

   b. "You both have very legitimate concerns. Can we talk about some ways for you, Chris, to maintain independence despite your illness and for you, Susan, to ensure that everyone is safe?"

   c. "Chris, your wife is only looking out for your best interests. I know it is a painful reality, but you are too ill to be driving."

   d. "Susan, I think driving is only one of many issues that you and Chris are going to have to address around your husband's illness. I'd like to refer you for counselling."

2. Skyla is a 35-year-old Aboriginal woman with rapidly advancing cancer. She has the choice of following the usual course of treatment, known to have mixed outcomes, or trying an experimental treatment with little or no clear outcome data. The client asks the nurse to help her plan for a discussion of the dilemma with her family. Which response by the nurse BEST indicates the use of a difference question?

   a. "Who do you think will be most affected by these treatment choices?"

   b. "Are you nervous about your family's reaction?"

   c. "Your decision is very personal—no one but you can decide."

   d. "What effect do you think your cultural beliefs will have on your decision?"

3. Eight-year-old Darren was diagnosed with kidney disease 2 years ago. He lives with his parents and 5-year-old sister in a small rural community 4 hours away from the closest tertiary health centre. Since his diagnosis, Darren and his mother have travelled to the city eight times—three times for admission. At first, the entire family came to the hospital, but now his father and sister stay home for work and school. Darren has been hospitalized this admission for 3 weeks. The nurse notices that Darren's mother is becoming exhausted; but when invited to take breaks, she politely, but firmly, refuses. What BEST explains the mother's reaction as a family caregiver?

   a. Darren's mother fears that Darren will not receive good care or be treated compassionately.

   b. She has become overly possessive of Darren since his hospitalization.

   c. She would actually be relieved if the nurse "ordered" her to take a break.

   d. She wants to ensure that hospital staff consider her a "good" mother.

4. Tracy, an 8-year-old girl with cystic fibrosis, is hospitalized with a respiratory infection. Even though she is very ill, the nurse notices that Tracy tries to help her mother, who has been at her bedside night and day, by doing simple tasks. What BEST explains Tracy's demonstration of social support?

   a. Tracy's psychological development will be compromised if she continues to take on caregiving responsibilities at such a young age.

   b. The nurse knows that she will have to explain to Tracy that although her gestures are very thoughtful, she should call the nurse when she thinks her mother needs help as Tracy is too ill.

   c. Relationships are reciprocal, and even though Tracy is young and ill, both she and her mother gain strength when they each give and receive support.

   d. Tracy is a born helper, and she should be encouraged to help out on the unit, whenever possible.

5. The nurse expresses her concerns about a patient's wife who has been at her husband's bedside round the clock over the past 2 months to other team members. Misha, the husband, has a terminal illness and is not expected to live more than a few weeks. He is a 36-year-old father of three young children who immigrated to Canada 4 years ago

with his family and parents. He had high hopes of setting up his own engineering business but found himself driving a taxi. Misha has been the sole breadwinner for the family. The nurse notes that the family is in need of additional supports. Which approach by the nurse BEST reflects family-centred nursing?

a. Demonstrating sympathy and making the hospital environment as comfortable as possible for his wife

b. Working with Misha's wife to connect her with support services for the family situation

c. Calling regular family meetings and ensuring that together, they plan and carry out a family plan of care

d. Introducing Misha's wife to another family on the unit with a family member with a similar terminal illness

6. Ashley Jackson recently lost her job when the candy factory where she had been a line worker for 6 years closed. Her oldest son, Tremaine, aged 4 years, has asthma and needs weekly visits to the community health clinic to get established on a new treatment regime. The family has missed the last three appointments because of the cost of transportation, but Ashley denies any financial difficulty when asked directly. What information would an ecomap inquiry regarding Ashley and her family provide for the nurse?

a. Family financial information

b. Developmental transitions in the family

c. An understanding of family relationships

d. Sources of family stress and supports

7. Grandparents Hester and Randy Bishop have had custody of their grandchildren (ages 10, 12, and 14 years) for 13 months. The mother, who has been getting treatment for a drug addiction, comes to visit her 12-year-old daughter, Sarah, who has been hospitalized for minor surgery. Which response by the nurse BEST reflects a family nursing perspective to the mother?

a. "I can see that you care about your daughter, but as you do not have custody, I'll have to ask you to leave."

b. "I can see that you have made good progress with your addiction, so I think it is important that you visit your daughter. If your parents do not want to meet with you, then I will stay with your daughter during the visit."

c. "I can see that it is very important to you that your daughter and family see that you care about Sarah and are making a real effort to address your addiction. However, this may not be an easy visit for your family. What challenges do you think your daughter and parents might have around accepting your visit?"

d. "I'll have to ask your daughter and, if she agrees to see you, then you are welcome to visit."

8. The community health nurse is doing a hospital discharge follow-up visit with 74-year-old Mrs. Pineau. She recently suffered a cerebrovascular accident that has caused some cognitive impairment with short-term memory loss. She can still carry out many activities of daily living (e.g., shopping, cooking, and going to the bank) with minimal assistance. In discussion with Mrs. Pineau, the nurse learns that she has one son, who rarely visits and does not appear to be very supportive. Mrs. Pineau mentions that she is going to give her life savings to her son so that he can buy a house. Which immediate actions by the nurse BEST reflects a family nursing approach?

a. Calling for a thorough assessment of Mrs. Pineau's mental competence

b. Telling Mrs. Pineau that her intentions may not be a good idea and that she should call her lawyer to discuss the matter

c. Inviting Mrs. Pineau to discuss her intentions more fully and how she thinks family members, including her son, might view the decision

d. Calling individual family members to tell them of Mrs. Pineau's intentions

9. Mabel, 70 years old, was diagnosed with Alzheimer's dementia 2 years ago. She and her husband, Harold, were adamant that they would stay in their home, even though their two children lived a 5-hour drive away and could visit only once a month. Mabel has been cared for by her husband with the help of home care services (personal care workers under the direction of community health nurses). Mabel's memory loss has now progressed to the point that her husband is exhausted with the caregiving responsibilities. Yet, he fiercely denies that the care is a burden. Which statements by the community health nurse BEST demonstrates a reflective response?

a. "I know that you love your wife very much, but her care is wearing you out."

b. "Maybe it is time for your children to move closer so that they could help you care for your wife?"

c. "I think your wife would be best cared for in a nursing home."

d. "If she could talk, what do you think your wife would be telling your children?"

10. Eric is a 14-year-old boy who was diagnosed with cystic fibrosis during infancy. His parents appear to be coping well, but they state that there are times when they feel very alone when dealing with the chronic aspects of Eric's condition. Which response by the nurse BEST reflects a family nursing approach?

a. "You seem lonely and depressed; talking to a counsellor may relieve some of your concerns."

b. "You appear to be coping well. Although things may seem difficult now, they will improve."

c. "Would you like me to arrange for you to talk with another family experiencing cystic fibrosis?"

d. "You should join the Cystic Fibrosis Association. It always needs volunteers, and it can help you meet people."

Check the eText in MyNursingLab for answers and explanations.

WEBLINKS

The Vanier Institute of the Family

http://www.vanierinstitute.ca

The Vanier Institute is a national charitable organization dedicated to promoting the well-being of Canadian families through research, consultation, and policy development. The website accesses online publications related to contemporary family trends and such issues as aging, divorce, employment, and family income.

Department of Justice Canada

http://www.justice.gc.ca/eng/pi/fcy-fea/lib-bib/pub/index.html

This Government of Canada website provides information about legal issues, programs, and services of interest to families (such as child custody, access, and support), fact sheets on family violence and child abuse, and links to research publications on these topics.

Canadian Council on Social Development

http://www.ccsd.ca

The website of this national nonprofit organization provides information and publications relevant to the social and economic security of Canadian families.

Family Nursing Resources

http://www.eFamilyNursing.com

This website markets educational products (books and videotapes) to family nursing educators and students.

MyNursingLab

REFERENCES

Bell, J. M. (1996). Signal events in family nursing. *Journal of Family Nursing, 2*(4), 347–349.

Bell, J. M., Moules, N. J., & Wright, L. M. (2009). Therapeutic letters and the family nursing unit: A legacy of advanced nursing practice. *Journal of Family Nursing, 15*(1), 6–30.

Benner, P., Hooper-Kyriakidis, P., & Stannard, D. (1999). *Clinical wisdom and interventions in critical care: A thinking-in-action approach.* Philadelphia, PA: W. B. Saunders.

Berg, S. (2006). In their own voices: Families discuss end-of-life decision making—part 2. *Pediatric Nursing, 32*(3), 237–242.

Board, R. & Ryan-Wenger, N. (2003). Stressors and stress symptoms of mothers with children in the PICU. *Journal of Pediatric Nursing, 18*(3), 195–202.

Bomar, P. J. (Ed.). (1996). *Nurses and family health promotion.* Philadelphia, PA: Saunders.

Browning, G., & Warren, N. A. (2006). Unmet needs of family members in the medical intensive care waiting room. *Critical Care Nursing Quarterly, 29*(1), 86–95.

Certified General Accountants of Canada. (2011). *A driving force no more: Have Canadians consumers reached their limits?* Retrieved from http://www.cga-canada.org/en-ca/ResearchAndAdvocacy/AreasofInterest/DebtandConsumption/Pages/ca_debt_default.aspx

Chui, T., Tran, K., & Maheux, H. (2007). *Immigration in Canada: A portrait of the foreign-born population 2006 census: Findings.* Retrieved from http://ww12.statcan.ca/english/census06/analysis/immcit/index.cfm

Clarke, C. (2006). Relating with professionals. *Journal of Psychiatric Mental Health Nursing, 13*(5), 522–526.

Copeland, E. M., Pimiento, J. M., & Dudrick, S. J. (2011). Total parenteral nutrition and cancer: From the beginning. *Surgical Clinics of North America, 91*(4), 727–736.

Davidson, J. E., Powers, K., Hedayat, K. M., Tieszenm M., Kon, A. A., Shepard, E., ... Armstrong, D. (2007). American College of Critical Care Medicine Task Force 2004–2005, Society of Critical Care Medicine. Clinical practice guidelines for support of the family in the patient-centered intensive care unit: American College of Critical Care Medicine Task Force 2004–2005. *Critical Care Medicine, 35*(2), 605–622.

Deci, E. L., La Guardia, J. G., Moller, A. C., Scheiner, M. J., & Ryan, R. M. (2006). On the benefits of giving as well as receiving autonomy support: Mutuality in close friendships. *Personal and Social Psychology Bulletin, 32*(3), 313–327.

DiGioia, A., Lorenz, H., Greenhouse, P. K., Bertoty, D. A., & Rocks, S. D. (2010). A patient-centered model to improve metrics without cost increase: Viewing all care through the eyes of patients and families. *Journal of Nursing Administration, 40*(12), 540–546.

Doane, G. H., Browne, A. J., Reimer, J., MacLeod, J., & McLellan, E. (2009). Enacting nursing obligations: Public health nurses' theorizing in practice. *Research and Theory for Nursing Practice, 23*(2), 88–106.

Doornbos, M. M. (2001). Professional support for family caregivers of people with serious and persistent mental illnesses. *Journal of Psychosocial Nursing and Mental Health Service, 39*(12), 38–45.

Doornbos, M. M. (2002). Family caregivers and the mental health care system: Reality and dreams. *Archives of Psychiatric Nursing, 16*(1), 39–46.

Dowd, M. D., Kennedy, C., Knapp, J. F., & Stallbaumer-Rouyer, J. (2002). Mothers' and health care providers' perspectives on screening for intimate partner violence in a pediatric emergency department. *Archives of Pediatric and Adolescent Medicine, 156*(8), 794–799.

Dwairy, M. (2002). Foundations of psychosocial dynamic personality theory of collective people. *Clinical Psychology Review, 22*(3), 345–362.

Farrell, M. E., Joseph, D. H., & Schwartz-Barcott, D. (2005). Visiting hours in the ICU: Finding the balance among patient, visitor and staff needs. *Nursing Forum, 40*(1), 18–28.

Fast, J., Eales, J., & Keating, N. (2001). *Economic impact of health, income security, and labour policies on informal caregivers of frail seniors. Status of women.* Ottawa, ON: Author. Retrieved from http://dsp-psd.pwgsc.gc.ca/Collection/SW21-67-2001E.pdf

Federico, B., & Forbes, A. (2009). The ESPEN clinical practice guidelines on parenteral nutrition: Present status and perspectives for future research. *Clinical Nutrition, 28,* 359–364.

Firth, P. (2006). Patients and their families. *Recent Results in Cancer Research, 168,* 61–71.

Friedemann, M. (1995). *The framework of systemic organization: A conceptual approach to families and nursing.* Thousand Oaks, CA: Sage.

Gage, J. D., Everett, K. D., & Bullock, L. (2006). Integrative review of parenting in nursing research. *Journal of Nursing Scholarship, 38*(1), 56–62.

Gibson, M. J, & Houser, A. (2007). Valuing the invaluable: A new look at the economic value of family caregiving. *Issue Brief* (Public Policy Institute [American Association of Retired Peers]). *IB82,* 1–12.

Gjerberg, E., Førde, R., & Bjørndal, A. (2011). Staff and family relationships in end-of-life nursing home care. *Nursing Ethics, 18*(1), 42–53.

Goodwin, R. D., Wickramaratne, P., Nomura, Y., & Weissman, M. M. (2007). Familial depression and respiratory illness in children. *Archives of Pediatric and Adolescent Medicine, 161*(5), 487–494.

Goudreau, J., Duhamel, F., & Ricard, N. (2006). The impact of a family systems nursing educational program on the practice of psychiatric nurses: A pilot study. *Journal of Family Nursing, 12*(3), 292–306.

Griffin, T. (2003). Facing challenges to family-centered care: Conflicts over visitation. *Pediatric Nursing, 29*(2):135–137.

Hanson, S. M. H., Kaakinen, J., & Gedaly-Duff, V. (2005). *Family health care nursing: Theory, practice, and research* (3rd ed.). Philadelphia, PA: F.A. Davis.

Hart, S. N. (1991). From property to person status. *American Psychologist, 46,* 53–59.

Heyland, D. K., Tranmer, J., O'Callaghan, C. J., & Gafni, A. (2003). The seriously ill hospitalized patient: Preferred role in end-of-life decision making? *Journal of Critical Care, 18*(1), 3–10.

Holtslander, L. (2005). Clinical application of the 15-minute family interview: Addressing the needs of postpartum families. *Journal of Family Nursing, 11*(1):5–18.

Hopkins, R. O., & Brett, S. (2005). Chronic neurocognitive effects of critical illness. *Current Opinions in Critical Care, 11*(4), 369–375.

Hudson, P., & Payne, S. (2011). Family caregivers and palliative care: Current status and agenda for the future. *Journal of Palliative Medicine, 14*(7), 864–869.

Human Resources and Skills Development Canada. (2010). *The homeless partnering strategy.* Retrieved from http://www.hrsdc.gc.ca/eng/homelessness/index/shtml

Hundon, C., Fortin, M., Haggerty, J. L., Lambert, M., & Poitras, M. E. (2011). Measuring patients' perceptions of patient-centered care: A systematic review of tools for family medicine. *Annals of Family Medicine, 9*(2), 155–164.

Jeon, Y. H. (2004). Shaping mutuality: Nurse-family caregiver interactions in caring for older people with depression. *International Journal of Mental Health Nursing, 13*(2), 126–134.

Kaakinen, J., Gedaly-Duff, V., Hanson, S., & Coehlo, D. (2011). *Family health care nursing: Theory, practice and research* (4th ed.). Philadelphia, PA: F.A Davis Publishing.

Korner, H. (2007). Negotiating cultures: Disclosure of HIV-positive status among people from minority ethnic communities in Sydney. *Cultural Health and Sexuality, 9*(2), 137–152.

Leahey, M., & Harper-Jaques, S. (1996). Family-nurse relationships: Core assumptions and clinical implications. *Journal of Family Nursing, 2*(2), 133–151.

Lee, M. D., Friedenberg, A. S., Mukpo, D. H., Conray, K., Palmisciano, A., Levy, M. M. (2007). Visiting hours policies in New England intensive care units: Strategies for improvement. *Critical Care Medicine, 35*(2), 497–501.

Leenerts, M. H., & Teel, C. S. (2006). Relational conversation as method for creating partnerships: Pilot study. *Journal of Advanced Nursing, 54*(4), 467–476.

Levine, C. (1998). *Rough crossings: Family caregivers' odysseys through the health care system.* New York, NY: United Hospital Fund of New York.

Limacher, L. H., & Wright, L. M. (2006). Exploring the therapeutic family intervention of commendations: Insights from research. *Journal of Family Nursing, 12*(3), 307–331.

Martinez, A. M., D'Artois, D., Rennick, J. E. (2007). Does the 15-minute (or less) family interview influence family nursing practice? *Journal of Family Nursing, 13*(2), 157–178.

Mayer, G. G. (2001). Families as hospital care givers: A self-service approach to the nursing shortage. *Journal of Nursing Administration, 31*(10), 457–458.

McElheran, N., & Harper-Jaques, S. (1994). Commendations: A resource intervention for clinical practice. *Clinical Nurse Specialist, 8*(1), 7–10.

McPherson, K. (2003). *Bedside matters: The transformation of Canadian nursing, 1900–1990.* Toronto, ON: Oxford University Press.

Mitchell, M. L., Courtney, M., & Coyer, F. (2003). Understanding uncertainty and minimizing families' anxiety at the time of transfer from intensive care. *Nursing Health Science, 5*(3), 207–217.

Morissette, R., & Ostrovsky, Y. (2007). *Income instability of lone parents, singles and two-parent families in Canada, 1984–2004.* Retrieved from http://www.statcan.ca/english/research/11F0019MIE/11F0019MIE2007297.pdf

Morris, D. B. (1998). *Illness and culture in the postmodern age.* Berkeley, CA: University of California Press.

Myers, T. A., Eichhorn, D. J., Guzzetta, C. E. (2000). Family presence during invasive procedures and resuscitation. *American Journal of Nursing, 100,* 32–43.

Navaie-Waliser, M., Feldman, P. H., Gould, D. A., Levine, C., Kuerbis, A. N., & Donelan, K. (2001). The experiences and challenges of informal caregivers: Common themes and differences among whites, blacks, and Hispanics. *Gerontologist, 41*(6), 733–741.

Navaie-Waliser, M., Feldman, P. H., Gould, D. A., Levine, C., Kuerbis, A. N., & Donelan, K. (2002). When the caregiver needs care: The plight of vulnerable caregivers. *American Journal of Public Health, 92*(3), 409–413.

Phelan, J. C., Bromet, E. J., & Link, B. G. (1998). Psychiatric illness and family stigma. *Schizophrenia Bulletin, 24*(1), 115–126.

Ray, R. A., & Street, A. F. (2005). Ecomapping: An innovative research tool for nurses. *Journal of Advanced Nursing, 50*(5), 545–552.

Robinson, C. A. (1996). Health care relationships revisited. *Journal of Family Nursing, 2*(2), 152–173.

Roden, J. (2005). The involvement of parents and nurses in the care of acutely-ill children in a non-specialist paediatric setting. *Journal of Child Health Care, 9*(3), 222–240.

Segaric, C. A., & Hall, W. A. (2005). The family theory-practice gap: A matter of clarity? *Nursing Inquiry, 12*(3), 210–218.

Selwood, A., Johnston, K., Katona, C., Lyketsos, C., & Livingston, G. (2007). Systematic review of the effect of psychological interventions on family caregivers of people with dementia. *Journal of Affective Disorders, 101*(1–3): 75–89.

Sjöblom, L. M., Pejlert, A., & Asplund, K. (2005). Nurses' view of the family in psychiatric care. *Journal of Clinical Nursing, 14*(5), 562–569.

Stapleton, R. D., Engelberg, R. A., Wenrich, M. D., Goss, C. H., & Curtis, J. R. (2006). Clinician statements and family satisfaction with family conferences in the intensive care unit. *Critical Care Medicine, 34*(6), 1679–1685.

Statistics Canada. (2008a). *Aboriginal Peoples in Canada in 2006: Inuit, Métis, and First Nations, 2006 Census.* Ottawa, ON: *The Daily.* Retrieved from http://www.statcan.gc.ca/daily-quotidien/080115/dq080115a-eng.htm

Statistics Canada. (2008b). *2006 Census: Earnings, income and shelter costs.* Ottawa, ON: *The Daily.* Retrieved from http://www.statcan.gc.ca/daily-quotidien/080501/dq080501a-eng.htm

Statistics Canada. (2011). *Canada's population clock.* Ottawa, ON: Author. Retrieved from http://www.statcan.gc.ca/ig-gi/pop-ca-eng.htm

Statistics Canada. (2012). *Portrait of families and living arrangements in Canada.* Retrieved from http://www12.statcan.gc.ca/cencus-recensement/2011/as-sa/98-312-x/98-312-x2011001-eng.cfm a4.

Tanner, J. (2005). Visiting time preferences of patients, visitors and staff. *Nursing Times, 101*(27), 38–42.

Tapp, D. M. (1997). *Exploring therapeutic conversations between nurses and families experiencing ischemic heart disease* (Unpublished doctoral dissertation). Calgary, AB: University of Calgary.

Tapp, D. M. (2000). The ethics of relational stance in family nursing: Resisting the view of "nurse as expert." *Journal of Family Nursing, 6*(1), 69–91.

The Vanier Institute of the Family (n.d.) *Definition of family.* Retrieved from http://www.vanierinstitute.ca/definition_of_family.

The Vanier Institute of the Family & Roger Sauvé. (2004). *Profiling Canada's families III.* Ottawa, ON: Author.

The Vanier Institute of the Family. (2010). *Families count—Profiling Canada's families IV.* Ottawa, ON: Author.

Ting, J. (2007). Family orientated delivery of routine nursing care in hospital. *Australian Nursing Journal, 14*(10), 27.

Wade, J. (2006). "Crying alone with my child": Parenting a school age child diagnosed with bipolar disorder. *Issues in Mental Health Nursing, 27*(8), 885–903.

Walker, E., & Dewar, B. J. (2001). How do we facilitate carers' involvement in decision making? *Journal of Advanced Nursing, 34*(3), 329–337.

Ward-Griffin, C. (1999, Nov/Dec). Nurse–family caregiver relationships: Moving beyond the rhetoric of shared care. *Registered Nurse,* 8–10.

Whall, A. L., & Fawcett, J. (1991). The family as a focal phenomenon in nursing. In A. L. Whall & J. Fawcett (Eds.), *Family theory development in nursing: State of the science and art* (pp. 7–29). Philadelphia, PA: F.A. Davis.

Wolff, J. R., Pak, J., Meeske, K., Worden, J., & Katz, E. (2011). Understanding why fathers assume primary medical caretaker responsibilities of children with life-threatening illnesses. *Psychology of Men and Masculinity,* April 12(2): 144–157.

Wright, L. M., & Leahey, M. (2005a). *Nurses and Families: A Guide to Family Assessment and Intervention* (4th ed.). Philadelphia, PA: F. A. Davis.

Wright, L. M., & Leahey, M. (2005b). The three most common errors in family nursing: How to avoid or sidestep. *Journal of Family Nursing, 11,* 90.

Wright, L. M., & Leahey, M, (2009). *Nurses and families: A guide to family assessment and intervention* (5th ed.). Philadelphia, PA: F. A. Davis.

Wright, L. M., Watson, W. L., & Bell, J. M. (1996). *Beliefs: The heart of healing in families and illness.* New York, NY: Basic Books.

Yun, Y. H., Rhee, Y. S., Kang, I. O., Lee, J. S., Bang, S. M., Lee, W. S. . . . Hong, Y. S.. (2005). Economic burdens and quality of life of family caregivers of cancer patients. *Oncology, (2–3),* 107–114.

Chapter 14

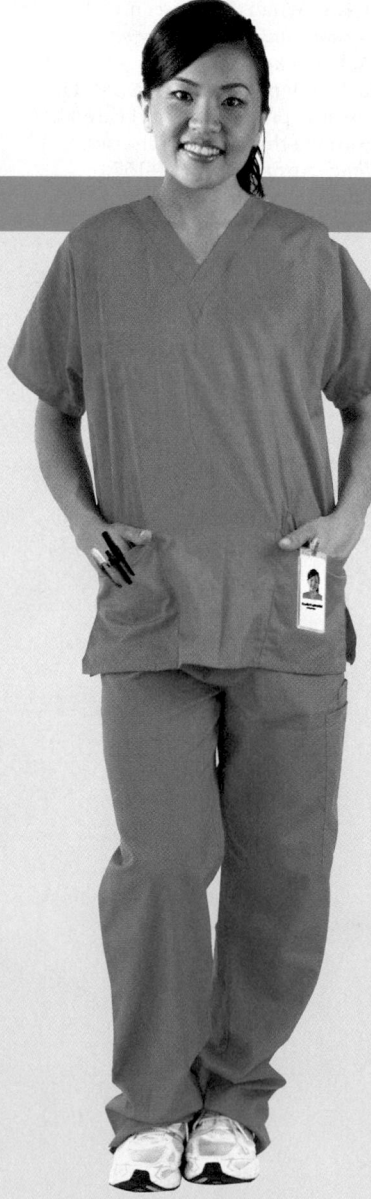

Community-Based Nursing

LEARNING OUTCOMES

After studying this chapter, you will be able to:

1. Discuss factors influencing community-based health care.

2. Identify the five essential aspects of the Alma-Ata Declaration, particularly primary health care and its impact on community health nursing.

3. Describe community-based health care.

4. List and describe the following:

   • The Community Health Nurses Association of Canada's *community health nursing standards of practice*

   • The Canadian Public Health Association's *roles and activities of the public/ community health nurse*

   • The Community Health Nurses Association's *discipline specific competencies for public health and home care nursing*

5. Explain essential aspects of cooperative partnerships in health care: definitions, objectives, benefits, and the nurse's role.

6. Describe the role of a community health nurse, a home health nurse, and a public health nurse (PHN), and describe the environments in which they practise.

7. Delineate the role of the nurse in providing continuity of care.

8. Compare and contrast community-based nursing and traditional institution-based nursing.

The Canadian health care system is evolving. Escalating health care costs, expanding technology, changing demographics, shorter hospital stays, and recent public health emergencies are just some of the factors motivating these changes. One of the most significant changes has been the shift of health care delivery from institutions to the community and home environments. Health care, once delivered predominantly in hospital settings, is now routinely provided in the home and other community-based environments. Though acute care institutions will undoubtedly remain a vital component of the health care system, their prominence may be lessened in the future. The trend toward community-based care will play a significant role in the future of Canada's health care system.

According to the Canadian Institute for Health Information (CIHI), between 2006 and 2010, the number of regulated nurses continued to rise, with a small increase in the proportion of those in community-based settings (CIHI, 2012).

Canada continues to move toward an integrated health care system—one that is community based, multidisciplinary, and collaborative. However, with the shift from institutional to community-based care comes changes in the roles and responsibilities of nurses and other health care professionals.

Shifts in the Canadian Health Care System

The Canadian health care system is continually adapting to meet the changing needs of health care consumers. In the report *An Ounce of Prevention: Strengthening the Balance in Health Care Reform*, the Canadian Public Health Association (CPHA) suggested that though developments in health over the past century have been remarkable, if Medicare is to remain sustainable, we must "build on the opportunities afforded by past successes, improved information, knowledge and research capacities, and technological advances" (Canadian Public Health Association Board of Directors, 2000, p. vii) (see Chapter 9 for more details). Many of these system changes have been precipitated by recent world events such as the severe acute respiratory syndrome (SARS) epidemic, the terrorist attacks in the United States on September 11, 2001, and the H1N1 virus outbreak. In each of these events, and many others, nursing played an invaluable role in the promotion and protection of the public's health. Knowledge gained from recent world health crises and an increasing body of evidence supporting the impact of social determinants on health have heightened the government's focus on public health capacity (Underwood et al., 2009). In 2010, the Ministers of Health and Health Promotion/ Healthy Living made a declaration in *Creating a Healthier Canada: Making Prevention a Priority* that " . . . the promotion of health and the prevention of disease, disability

and injury are a priority and necessary to the sustainability of the health system" (2010, p. 1).

Whatever the approach, agreement exists that care must continue to shift from a strict illness focus to one that includes the promotion of health, a strong focus on the social determinants of health (see Chapter 7), and features service in a community-based environment. This systemic shift is occurring. According to Health Canada (2010), as a result of the above policy and societal shifts away from institutional care, an increasing number of Canadians are being cared for in their home communities, and much of this community-based care is being facilitated by nurses. In 2010, 45 067 (12.7%) of the 354 910 regulated nurses in Canada were community health nurses, most of whom worked in community health clinics or home health care agencies (CIHI, 2012). The Canadian Nurses Association (CNA) predicts that by the year 2020, 60% of all nurses will be practising in the community (Villeneuve & MacDonald, 2006).

The CNA (2005a) endorsed a restructured health care system based on the principles of primary health care as the most effective way to achieve optimal health care for the population. Specifically, the CNA recommended that governments commit to a strong publicly funded health care system that permits accessibility to essential health services, allows for public participation in health decisions, and emphasizes health promotion and the adoption of a community health approach.

The precursor of much of Canada's focus on health promotion and illness prevention was the 1978

BOX 14.1 FIVE PRINCIPLES OF PRIMARY HEALTH CARE

The following five principles of primary health care are endorsed by the Canadian Nurses Association:

1. *Accessibility:* A continuing and organized supply of essential health services is available to all people with no unreasonable geographic or financial barriers

2. *Public Participation:* Individuals and communities have the right and responsibility to be active partners in making decisions about their health care and the health of their communities

3. *Health Promotion:* The process of enabling people to increase control over and to improve their health

4. *Appropriate Technology:* This includes methods of care, service delivery, procedures, and equipment that are socially acceptable and affordable

5. *Intersectoral Cooperation:* Commitment from all sectors (government, community, and health care professionals) is essential for meaningful action on health determinants

Source: From Canadian Nurses Association. (2005). *Primary health care: A summary of the issues.* Ottawa, ON: Author. Reprinted with permission.

International Conference on Primary Health Care. This meeting of the World Health Assembly resulted in a report known as the Declaration of Alma-Ata (so named for the geographical location in which the conference was held). In this report, the term *primary health care* was coined by the World Health Organization (WHO) and the United Nations International Children's Emergency Fund (UNICEF). Subsequently, five principles central to the care delivery philosophy were outlined (see Box 14.1). These principles are still commonly referred to today.

Primary health care (PHC) is defined as:

essential health care based on practical, scientifically sound, and socially acceptable methods and technology made universally accessible to individuals and families in the community through their full participation and at a cost that the community and country can afford to maintain at every stage of their development in the spirit of self-reliance and self-determinations.
(World Health Organization [WHO] & United Nations International Children's Emergency Fund [UNICEF], 1978, para. 7)

Deep concern for the health of the world's population, specifically short life expectancies and high mortality rates among children, led to the formation of the global health strategy of primary health care. All members of the WHO were encouraged to take actions toward the attainment of "health for all by the year 2000" through an adequate food supply, safe water, adequate sanitation, maternal and child health care, immunization, the prevention and control of endemic diseases, the provision of essential drugs, health education, and the treatment of common diseases and injuries. Despite strong efforts, there is little argument that health

disparities continue to exist worldwide. "Moving towards health for all requires that health systems respond to the challenges of a changing world and growing expectations for better performance" (WHO, 2008). These continued systemic changes constitute the agenda of the renewal of PHC made by the WHO in response to the continued need for health care mobilization toward the decades old principles of PHC.

The Declaration of Alma-Ata (WHO & UNICEF, 1978) emphasized health, or well-being, as a fundamental right and a worldwide social goal. It was an attempt to address inequality in the health status of persons in all countries and to target governments that needed to be responsible for policies that would promote economic, social, and health development, which were considered basic to the achievement of "health for all." PHC extends beyond traditional health care services. It involves issues of the environment, agriculture, housing, and other social, economic, and political issues, such as poverty, transportation, unemployment, and economic development. A major feature of PHC is that consumers, governments at all levels, and public institutions are involved in the planning and delivery of health care. As a result, the roles of physicians and nurses must change. For PHC to be realized, and health care reform to be successful, health care needs to be organized in such a way that it spans geographical boundaries, bridges service sectors, and creates seamless linkages within and across disciplines serving the public. Additionally, it requires health care providers, nurses included, to develop specialized skills in working with individuals, families, and communities that enable them to collaborate with, rather than merely provide care to, clients.

In *Building on Values: The Future of Health Care in Canada*, Roy Romanow stressed "the need to change the scopes and patterns of practice of health care providers to reflect changes in how health care services are delivered, particularly through new approaches to primary health care" (Romanow, 2002, p. xxvii). This focus on population health and primary health care was echoed by the CPHA Campaign 2008, which identified the following three priority public health issues that warrant national political attention: (a) reinforced national leadership on public health, (b) enhanced public health capacity, and (c) increased investment in public health (CPHA, 2008).

As highly educated, caring professionals, nurses have a responsibility to influence change by attending to the history, current status, and future projections of health care. By taking action individually and collectively, the nursing profession has the power to bring greater attention to the social determinants of health and to ensure more effective delivery of care under the primary health care philosophy.

The distinction between primary health care (PHC) and primary care (PC) is an important one. PHC differs from PC in that although PC includes the need to

TABLE 14.1 Differences between Primary Care and Primary Health Care

Primary Care	Primary Health Care
• Community participation is provider directed.	• Community participation is client directed.
• The professional's role is as expert, provider, authority, team leader.	• The professional's role is as facilitator, consultant, and resource.
• Collaboration occurs among members of the health care team.	• Collaboration goes beyond the health care sector.
• The individual or family is the focus.	• The community or some aggregate is the focus.
• Access is limited.	• Access is universal.
• Health care is available within given health care institutions.	• Health care is available where people live and work.
• Empowerment is a provider-assisted process.	• Empowerment is a collaborative, enabling process.

Source: Reprinted from *Nursing Outlook*, 43/1, Barnes et al., "Primary Health Care and Primary Care: A Confusion of Philosophies," pp. 7–16, Copyright (1995), with permission from Elsevier.

practise in the context of family and community, the emphasis is on the delivery of personal health services by clinicians. PC addresses personal health services and not population-focused public health services.

Barnes et al. (1995) stated that PHC is community driven and involves a "bottom-up" approach that requires active community involvement in decision making to improve health. PC, conversely, is expert driven and involves a "top-down" approach by health care professionals who advise individuals and communities about what is best for their health. Other differences are shown in Table 14.1.

PHC and PC also have similarities. Both systems acknowledge the prevention and promotion components of health and well-being. Both systems strive for universal access to and affordability of health care, support empowerment of the client, and target those at risk for preventable health problems.

Over the past 30 years, Canadians have embraced the notions of PHC and the resulting strategies for health promotion that have arisen from them. (See Chapter 8 for more details.) Canadian consumers also effect major changes in the delivery of health care as they increase their knowledge of health promotion, illness prevention, and treatment options. The resulting expectation of collaboration in decision making about their own, their families, and, to some extent, their communities' health has changed the role of the health care consumer and, as a result, that of the health care professional.

Community-Based Health Care

Community-based health care (CBHC) is a system that provides health-related services within the context of people's daily lives—that is, in places where people spend their time in the community. Care can be delivered in a variety of settings, including, but not limited to, homes, shelters, workplaces, schools, and seniors' centres. In contrast to the traditional health care system that focused primarily on the ill and the injured, community-based care is holistic. It involves a broad range of services designed not only to restore health but also to promote health and prevent illness in the public.

In the past two decades, the delivery of nursing services in the community has increased dramatically. A number of factors have contributed to this trend, among them rising health care costs, an aging population, and a growing emphasis on preventing illness and enhancing quality of life. CBHC is not simply an adjunct to acute care; in fact, many individuals seek community health care services in an effort to avoid hospitalization altogether.

In the context of CBHC, the term *client* is often defined more broadly than in acute care. Community-based care can be delivered to an individual, a family, a group, or an entire population. In each case, the individual or group of people with whom the nurse is working is considered the client.

In Canada, health care delivery is a provincial and territorial responsibility, and the manner in which health regions finance and deliver CBHC differs widely across the provinces and territories. However, to ensure its effectiveness, key features are common to CBHC in all regions:

• A focus on health promotion and prevention whether at the primary, secondary, or tertiary level

• Flexibility in responding to the health care needs of individuals, families, and communities, with these clients assuming primary decision making for their health care

• A realization that care must be provided within the context of the community; that health and the social environment are interactive and must take into account the determinants of health and resources of the individual, family, and community

• Promotion of communication and collaboration and continuity of care among health care agencies

Approaches in Community-Based Health Care

A community may be defined as a group of people who live, learn, work, and/or play in an environment at a given time. They function in a social system such as an organization or region, based on shared characteristics and interests. A population can be thought of as a community on a larger scale, for instance, a city, province, or nation (Yiu, 2012).

As greater emphasis is placed on the general health of the community and population, in contrast to the traditional system that focused on care of ill and injured individuals, alternative approaches to health care delivery become integral. Some of these include an integrated health care system, community initiatives and coalitions, population health promotion programs, and outreach programs:

- An *integrated health care system* is one that makes all levels of prevention—primary, secondary, and tertiary—available in an integrated form. (See Chapter 7 for descriptions of these levels.) The goals are to facilitate continuity of care, recovery, positive health outcomes, and the long-term benefits of modifying harmful lifestyles through health promotion and disease prevention. Community-based clinics, mobile services, home visiting programs, and public health programs are important components of this integrated system.

- *Community initiatives and coalitions* rely on community-based interest groups or individual members of the community to establish health priorities, set measurable goals, and determine actions required to attain these goals. Nurses are major participants and contributors in these coalitions and often assume leadership roles. However, the nurse and community members assume a shared responsibility for the direction, coordination, and implementation of health care initiatives. These initiatives may focus on a single or multifaceted problem and can be health promotive, illness and injury preventive, or restorative in nature. Examples include the establishment of an abuse prevention program, a gang prevention program, an older adult assessment program, and an immunization program for a high-risk group.

- *Population health-promotion programs* focus on the health needs of larger groups. Nurses employ research, epidemiology, and community assessment data in the development and delivery of population-based initiatives. These include, but are not limited to, immunization, social marketing, program planning or evaluation, policy development, and media advocacy.

- *Outreach programs* that use lay health workers are a method of linking underserved or high-risk populations (such as immigrant populations, homeless people, or single parents) with the formal health care system. They can minimize or reduce barriers to health care, increase access to services, and thus improve the health status of the community. They involve partnerships among nurses, community members, and lay health workers who assist their neighbours through outreach networks. Nurses often

provide training, consultation, and support to these individuals, who then assume responsibility for contact with marginalized individuals and groups in their community.

Community Health Nursing

As CBHC becomes more widespread, the requirement for nursing care delivered in the community also increases. Across Canada, there are many nurses with varying educational backgrounds providing community health care. Each province and territory, and even health regions within these, employs nurses with varying scopes of practice in the delivery of health education, health promotion, and primary care in the community. The Evidence-Informed Practice box illustrates the variety of CHNs and the attributes of their workplaces. These nurses, include registered nurses (RNs), registered psychiatric nurses (RPNs), registered practical nurses (RPNs), licensed practical nurses (LPNs), nurse care aids (NCAs), nurse practitioners (NPs), and advanced practice nurses (APNs). As a result, it is important that the practice of community health nurses be distinguished and their practice competencies defined.

The Community Health Nurses of Canada (CHNC) is a national association of community health nurses and community health nursing interest groups that promotes community health nursing and the health of communities. As such, they have defined the scope of and established standards of practice for community health nurses. These standards of (a) promoting health, (b) building individual and community capacity, (c) building relationships, (d) facilitating access and equity, and (e) demonstrating professional responsibility and accountability form the basis of CHNs' and public health nurses' (PHN) practice in Canada (CHNC, 2008).

According to the CHNC, **community health nurses (CHNs)** "are registered nurses whose practice specialty promotes the health of individuals, families, communities, and populations, and an environment that supports health. . . . The practice of community health nurses combines nursing theory and knowledge, social sciences and public health science with primary health care" (CHNC, 2008, p. 6).

It is under this broad umbrella of CHNs that home health nurses (HHNs) and PHNs practice. A **home health nurse (HHN)** "is a community health nurse who combines knowledge from primary health care (including determinants of health), nursing science, and theory and knowledge of the social sciences" to focus on "prevention, health restoration, maintenance, or palliation" (CHNC, 2008, p. 8). Home health nurses provide care in the client's home, school, or workplace.

In contrast, a **public health nurse (PHN)** "is a community health nurse who combines knowledge from public health science, primary health care (including

EVIDENCE-INFORMED PRACTICE

Demographic Profile of Community Health Nurses in Canada and the Organizational Attributes That Support Their Unique Practice

According to a recent national study, as health care shifts from hospital care to in-home and community care, "it is essential that adequate numbers of skilled staff are available to meet the community health care needs" (Underwood et al., 2009, p.10). From 1996 to 2007, the distribution of community health nurses across Canada has evolved.

- The vast majority of community health nurses are registered nurses (RNs), with 17% of the total number of RNs practising in community health (46 273 in 2007). Most of these nurses (81%) have baccalaureate preparation.

- 50% of nurse practitioners practise in community health, largely in clinics and physicians' offices.

- Licensed practical nurses (LPNs/RPNs) practising in community health is rising (7131 in 2007).

- Most RNs work in community health clinics, public health offices, and home care agencies. Most LPNs (also known as registered practical nurses in Ontario) work solely in home care agencies.

Just as the areas of nursing are specialized, so, too, are the organizational attributes that support the unique practices of these specialties. To gain insight into which factors promote the most effective practice of PHNs in Canada, 23 focus groups were conducted with PHNs, managers, and policymakers in diverse regions and urban and rural or remote settings across the country. Attributes at all levels of the public health system were identified, including (a) government and system level action, (b) local organizational culture of employers, (c) supportive management practices, (d) effective leadership, (e) valuing of PHNs, (f) shared vision, (g) collaborative partnerships, (h) flexibility and creativity, and (i) support for ongoing learning.

NURSING IMPLICATIONS: Community health nurses thrive in workplaces where they share the vision and goals of their organization and have flexibility to work collaboratively, creatively, and autonomously. Given the complexity of their practice, they require the time, flexible funding, and management support to develop the relationships necessary for effective community health nursing interventions. Their specialty knowledge and competencies necessitate access to continued education and policies that support evidence-informed practice.

Sources: Underwood, J. et al. (2009). Building community and public health nursing capacity: A synthesis report of the national community health nursing study. *Canadian Public Health Association, 100*(5), 1-1 to 1-12; Underwood , J., Deber, R., Baumann, A., Dragan, A., Laporte, A., Alameddine, M., Wall, R. (2009). *Demographic profile of community health nurses in Canada 1996–2007*. Hamilton, ON: Nursing Health Services Research Unit; and Meagher-Stewart, D. (2010). Organizational attributes that assure optimal utilization of public health nurses. *Public Health Nursing, 27*(5), 443–441.

determinants of health), nursing science, and theory and knowledge from the social sciences" and "focuses on promoting, protecting, and preserving the health of populations" (CHNC, 2008, p. 8). PHNs practise in a variety of settings, including but not limited to, "community health centres, schools, street clinics, youth centres, and nursing outposts" (p. 8). However, it is their focus on the health promotion of populations that distinguishes their practice. In contrast to HHNs, who work mainly with individuals and families, the focus of PHNs' practice is at the larger population level. PHNs do recognize that the health of a population is inextricably linked to that of its constituent members, and as a result, PHNs may work with individuals and families to realize the ultimate goal of population health.

Based on the Canadian Nurses Association's *Code of Ethics for Registered Nurses* (2008), CHNC (2008) developed a list of values and beliefs common to CHNs. These values and beliefs include caring, the principles of PHC, multiple ways of knowing, individual and community partnership, and empowerment. On the basis of these values and beliefs, as well as nursing knowledge and community partnerships, the five interrelated standards of practice (listed earlier) were defined. The Canadian community health nursing practice model was first developed in 2008 and illustrates the dynamic nature of community health nursing practice. It demonstrates the interrelatedness of the practice standards, client groups, values and beliefs, and CHN process. It is currently being revised. The CNA has also acknowledged the specialized knowledge and skill inherent in working with communities. It now offers a certification exam in community health nursing (CNA, 2011).

Public Health Nursing Competencies

The CNA (1998) in its document *Nursing with Communities—Making the Transition* suggested that the knowledge and skills required of CHNs has steadily grown since public health certificates were first offered in Canadian universities in 1920. Today, nurses practising in community-based integrated health care systems require highly specialized knowledge and skills. Over the past 5 years, several foundational documents have been released describing the functions and competencies of this nursing specialty.

In 2008, the Public Health Agency of Canada (PHAC) released a set of core competencies that reflect "essential knowledge, skills and attitudes necessary for the practice of public health. They transcend boundaries of specific disciplines . . . and provide the building blocks for effective public health practice . . . " (PHAC, 2008, p. 1). These generic competencies describe a baseline required to address public health system core functions, including population health assessment, surveillance, disease and injury prevention, health promotion, and health protection. In all, there are 36 core competencies divided among seven categories, including (a) public health science, (b) assessment and analysis, (c) policy and program planning, implementation, and evaluation, (d) partnerships, collaboration, and advocacy, (e) diversity and inclusiveness, (f) communication, and (g) leadership.

The CHNC built on the PHAC Core Competencies in developing the *Public Health Nursing Discipline Specific Competencies*, which was released in 2009. These competencies ". . . are the integrated knowledge skills, judgement and attributes required of a public health nurse to practice safely and ethically" (CHNC, 2009, p. 2).

The CHNC (2009) PHN discipline specific competencies include the following:

1. Public health and nursing science

2. Assessment and analysis

3. Policy and program planning, implementation, and evaluation

   a. Policy development

   b. Program planning

   c. Implementation and intervention

   d. Evaluation

4. Partnerships, collaboration, and advocacy

5. Diversity and inclusiveness

6. Communication

7. Leadership

8. Professional responsibility and accountability

These public health nursing competencies do not replace the *CHNC Standards of Practice* described earlier in this chapter. Rather, the CHNC standards define the scope of practice, whereas the PHN competencies define essential skills, knowledge, and abilities required of PHNs. Underwood (2007) described competencies as "behaviours" and standards as "outcome," competencies being the activities that PHNs engage in to meet the standards of practice.

The PHAC has also described expectations of practice of PHNs in *Public Health—Community Health Nursing Practice in Canada: Roles and Activities*. Table 14.2 identifies these roles and activities, as well as the practice foundations on which they were based.

Home Health Nursing Competencies

"Home health nursing encompasses disease prevention, rehabilitation, restoration of health, health protection, and health promotion with the goal of managing existing problems and preventing potential problems" (CHNC, 2010, p. 7). The *Home Health Nursing Competencies* (CHNC, 2010) were developed to describe the nursing standards in this specialty area of practice. Table 14.3 identifies these elements, foundations, and areas of responsibility.

Community-Based Roles and Settings

Traditionally, community nursing services have been provided by regional and provincial or territorial health departments. Over the years, many community settings have been established, including schools (school health

---

TABLE 14.2 Public Health: Community Health Nursing Practice in Canada: Roles and Activities

Foundations of Public Health Practice	Roles of the PHN	Activities of the PHN
I. Focuses on entire populations and subpopulations that have similar health concerns and characteristics II. Is guided by an assessment of population health status that is determined through a community health assessment process III. Considers the broad determinants of health IV. Considers all levels of prevention, with a focus on primary prevention V. Considers all levels of practice by including a community focus, a system focus, and an individual and family focus	I. Health promotion II. Disease and injury prevention III. Health protection IV. Health surveillance V. Health assessment VI. Emergency preparedness and response	• Advocacy • Building capacity • Building coalitions and networks • Care and counselling • Case management • Communication • Community development • Consultation • Facilitation • Health education • Health threat response • Leadership • Outreach • Policy development and implementation • Referral and follow-up • Research and evaluation • Resource management, planning, coordination • Screening • Surveillance • Team building and collaboration

Source: Adapted from Canadian Public Health Association. (2010). *Public Health—Community health nursing practice in Canada: Roles and activities*. Ottawa, ON: Author.

TABLE 14.3 Home Health Nursing Competencies

Elements of Home Health Nursing	Foundations of Home Health Nursing	Quality and Professional Responsibility
- Assessment monitoring and clinical decision making - Care planning and care coordination - Maintenance, restoration, and palliation - Teaching and evaluation - Communication - Relationships - Access and equity building capacity	- Health promotion - Illness prevention and health protection	- Quality care - Professional responsibility

Source: Adapted from Community Health Nurses of Canada. (2010). Home health nursing competencies. Toronto, ON: Author.

nursing), workplaces (occupational health nursing), homes (home care nursing), clinics (public health nursing), churches (parish nursing), and correctional facilities (forensic nursing). Nurses access clients through these as well as countless other community agencies (such as homeless shelters, mental health shelters, drug and alcohol rehabilitation centres, and harm reduction programs).

Regardless of the practice setting, several overreaching roles are shared by all CHNs:

- *Advocate:* Advocacy involves supporting the client's choices in health care and includes discussion about client rights and the provision of assistance in accessing community resources. The role of advocate can be particularly challenging when family members' or other caregivers' views differ from those of the client. In the event of conflict, it is the nurse's responsibility to ensure the client's rights and desires are upheld. CHNs also advocate in terms of pubic policy.

- *Caregiver:* The role of caregiver is one common to every nursing specialty. In community health, this role may or may not include the provision of direct client care. The CHN may provide direct care, such as sexual health services, intravenous therapy, medication administration, or complex dressing changes. However, much of the CHNs time can also be spent teaching the client or family and friends to provide required care. In home care, additional nursing care, such as bathing, feeding, and maintaining a clean and safe environment, may be provided by care aides or practical nurses.

- *Educator:* In the role of educator, a CHN focuses on illness care, prevention of health problems, and the promotion of optimal wellness. The context of health education will vary, depending largely on the practice setting and client population with which the CHN works. Teaching can take the form of group presentations (as seen in public health or occupational health) or individual client teaching (as seen in home care). The role of educator is critical to community health nursing; informing clients enables them to

become active participants in their own health care. As such, it is imperative that every CHN have knowledge of teaching and learning principles and be skilled in the use of strategies that facilitate learning (see Chapter 26 for additional information).

- *Case Manager or Coordinator:* Ultimately, it is often the CHN who is responsible for the assessment of actual and potential health problems, the coordination of care plans, and the evaluation of client outcomes. When multiple professions are involved in the delivery of care, the role of case manager can shift among the professions, depending on the needs of the client. Some of the professions with which CHNs routinely collaborate include occupational therapy, physical therapy, medicine, pharmacy, nutrition, education, and social work.

- *Health Promoter:* Health promotion is certainly within the scope of every nurse. However, for many CHNs, health promotion constitutes the majority of their practice. For some, health promotion occurs at the population level through such activities as policy development or social marketing, immunization or disaster planning; for others, it occurs at the individual or small group level through such activities as prenatal classes. CHNs function highly independently in the community, often visiting clients in their home or workplace. Because these nurses interact with clients in their territory, their approach often differs from a hospital setting. For example, entry into a home is granted, not assumed; therefore, the development of trust and rapport are crucial. As well, unlike in hospital settings, the family and client set their own priorities and schedules. Engaging with clients in their own environment fosters rapport and trust. As a result, behaviours are more natural, cultural beliefs and practices are more visible, and multigenerational interactions are more readily displayed. Home care nurses and PHNs are able to complete more in-depth individual or community assessments and deliver care that meets the client's needs (whether the client is an individual, a family, or a community).

COMMUNITY HEALTH CENTRE NURSING Community health nursing centres provide patient care (PC) to specific populations and are generally managed by advance practice nurses, such as nurse practitioners. These nurses provide services from community outreach, to health promotion, to screening, to PC. Although the nurses are the primary providers of care to clients visiting the centre, consultation with other health care professionals, including physicians, is available, as needed. Nursing centres are located in both urban and rural communities (see the Nursing and Canadian Society box for nursing resources).

Telehealth projects use communication and information technology to provide health information and health care services to people in rural, remote, or underserved areas, or clients with mobility challenges. Video conferences or video clinics enable health care workers to provide remote assessment, treatment, and monitoring for clients with a variety of health care needs. These video conferences are similar to any outpatient clinic visit, except that the client and health care specialist are kilometres apart. With every changing technology at their disposal, it is critical that nurses must learn to use technology in a manner that can enhance the quality of care, while making every attempt to ensure that the essence of nursing, the relationship between nurse and client, is not disrupted.

PUBLIC HEALTH NURSING Public health nurses practise in a variety of settings including, but not limited to, immunization and well-baby clinics, postnatal visiting programs, and population health-promotion programs. Some PHNs spend much of their time with individual clients, whereas others are involved predominantly with population level interventions such as social marketing, media advocacy, policy planning, program development, disaster planning, community health assessment and more.

PARISH NURSING Parish nursing was first established in Canada in 1992. Since then, the specialty has become more common as faith communities seek to sustain and improve the health of their members. "A parish nurse is a registered nurse with specialized knowledge, who is called to ministry and affirmed by a faith community to promote health, healing and wholeness" through health advocacy, health counselling, health education, and resource referral (Canadian Association for Parish Nursing Ministry, 2011). Though a parish nurse is, by definition, a holistic practitioner, the focus is on the spiritual component of health promotion, not necessarily hands-on care. Initially, parish nurses were volunteers, but now, many are employees paid by the congregation or an affiliated institution, such as a health system or community agency.

SCHOOL HEALTH NURSING School health services are provided at the individual, family, and community levels in an effort to ensure an optimal level of health within the school community. A school health nurse will work within the school and surrounding community by using primarily health-promotion and illness-prevention strategies. As a part of an interprofessional team, he or she is responsible for the assessment, planning, implementation, and evaluation of school health programs. Within this context, a school health nurse provides direct care to students, provides leadership in the development and implementation of health policy and services, promotes a healthy school environment, and acts as a liaison among the school, family, community, and health care system (see Figure 14.1).

OCCUPATIONAL HEALTH NURSING Employers of all sizes are increasingly concerned with the health and safety of their employees. As a result, the need for health services in the workplace is greater than ever before.

Nursing and Canadian Society

Facts	Implications for Nursing
Every year, the Victorian Order of Nurses Canada delivers more than 50 different home nursing, health-promotion, support, and other services to 1 million Canadians and their families in 1300 communities, coast to coast.	Nurses need to be aware of resources that are available to clients under their care so that supplied services meet identified needs.
A World Health Organization (WHO) meeting in Canada in 1986 produced the *Ottawa Charter for Health Promotion*. The *Charter* highlighted the importance of strengthening community action, reorienting health services to place greater emphasis on health promotion, and the necessity for intersectoral action for health. In 2008, the WHO reaffirmed the need for a commitment to health promotion in *Primary Health Care: Now More Than Ever*.	The nurse will need to involve individual and community-focused strategies to ensure health for all. An individual action may be referring a client to a weight-loss program; a community-focused strategy may be providing improved access to immunization services for new parents.
The Community Health Nurses of Canada (CHNC), the Public Health Agency of Canada (PHAC), and the Canadian Public Health Association (CPHA) have all recently released foundational documents that describe the standards, competencies, roles, and activities of community health nurses.	Community health nurses must be aware of these documents that outline the scope of this nursing.

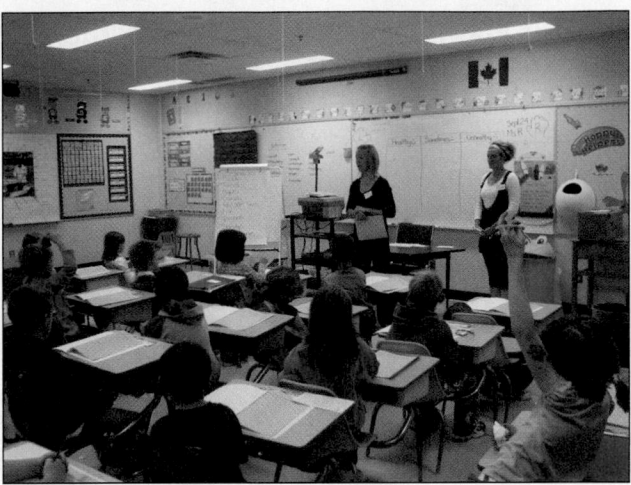

FIGURE 14.1 A school health nurse provides health-promotion teaching in the classroom.

According to the Canadian Occupational Health Nurses Association, "the primary role of the occupational health nurse is to coordinate the delivery of comprehensive, equitable, quality occupational health services for workers and worker groups" (2003, p. 2). Within this role, nurses may be charged with the development of programs that promote safety and accident prevention, and prevention and control of contagious diseases, as well as providing acute emergency care. Typically, the work of an occupational health nurse (OHN) also includes multidisciplinary teamwork; workplace health services often involve the collaboration of OHNs, physicians, human resource members, and specialized physical and occupational therapists.

FORENSIC NURSING   Forensic nurses specialize in the care of both victims and perpetrators of violence. These nurses form an important link between the medical and legal systems in Canada through direct care, legal consultation, and evidence collection. The forensic nurses deliver comprehensive, equitable treatment to victims of crime (such as sexual assault nurse examiners or nurse coroners) and to perpetrators of crime (such as nurses in custody environments). In either case, it is their focus on the health of those affected by crime that distinguishes their practice (Forensic Nurses Society of Canada, n.d.).

HOME CARE NURSING   Home care nursing is the delivery of health care services in the client's home environment, often with the effect of delaying or alleviating the need for long-term care or acute care alternatives (see Figure 14.2). These services are delivered by a variety of agencies (see Box 14.2) and focus on health promotion (such as diabetic nutrition counselling), acute health care (such as central venous or intravenous line management), chronic health care (medication management), or palliative care at the end of life.

Home care is not included in the Canada Health Act. Therefore, its services are not insured in the same way as

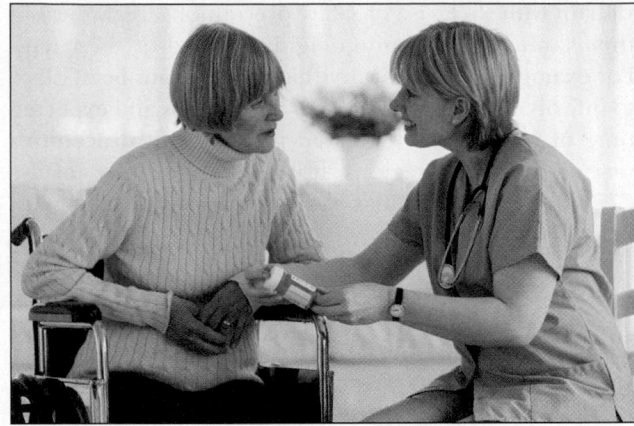

FIGURE 14.2 A home care nurse provides direct client care in the home.

are other basic services. Home care is delivered by public, private nonprofit, and private for-profit agencies in Canada, with the proportion of private versus public services varying by province and territory. Home care services are reimbursed by three mechanisms: (a) provincial or territorial and municipal government funds, (b) private insurance, and (c) private payment by home care recipients. Within public home care agencies, professional services (e.g., nursing, therapies) are generally provided free up to an identified figure per month, whereas user fees may apply to support services (personal care, house cleaning, and transportation). User fees are generally allocated on a sliding scale based on income, as determined by income tax returns. Clients may or may not be responsible for the cost of supplies, equipment, and medications.

Safety Concerns in Community Health Nursing

Any time a nurse visits the home of a client, whether the client is known to the nurse or not, precautions should be taken to ensure nurse safety. Many clients live in neighbourhoods that may present safety concerns for a visiting or street health nurse. It is important that CHNs are

---

BOX 14.2   HOME CARE AGENCIES

A variety of agencies can provide home care services:

- *Public or government agencies* are operated by provincial and territorial or local governments and financed primarily by public funds.
- *Voluntary or private nonprofit agencies,* such as the Victorian Order of Nurses, are supported by donations, endowments, charities, and third-party reimbursement.
- *Private, proprietary agencies,* are for-profit organizations that are governed by either individual owners or national corporations. Some of these agencies participate in third-party reimbursement; others rely on private payment for service.

vigilant with their use of safety precautions, regardless of their familiarity with the neighbourhood or the client. For example, it is important that mechanisms be in place to inform colleagues of the visit destination and expected time of return. Safety-related policies and procedures vary across health regions. It is the responsibility of the CHN to become familiar with regulations in his or her place of work.

The Community Health Nurse as a Collaborator

CHNs routinely collaborate with clients, peers, and other health care professionals. They frequently collaborate about client care but can also be involved in collaboration on bioethical issues, legislation, and health-related research with other professional organizations. Box 14.3 outlines selected aspects of the nurse's role as a collaborator.

COLLABORATIVE PARTNERSHIP IN HEALTH CARE
The traditional hierarchical relationship that has dominated health care delivery emerged from an illness focus in which the health care professional assumed the role of expert. This model of care delivery is no longer functional in our changing health care system. As the boundaries of each health care profession change and as consumers play an increasingly active role in care delivery, a collaborative approach is required. Collaborative partnership is defined as "the pursuit of person-centred goals through a dynamic process that requires the active participation and agreement of all partners. The relationship is one of partnership and the way of working together is collaborative, hence the term *collaborative partnership*" (Gottlieb & Feeley, 2006, p. 8).

In the collaborative partnership model of health care, the client shares responsibility for his or her health, and the nurse acknowledges that clients have knowledge and capabilities that can be used to understand and manage their illness in a meaningful way. The relationship between the nurse and client is reciprocal and mutual: goals and plans of care are jointly determined. Within this context, the role of the nurse is one of facilitator. He or she encourages clients to share their perceptions and expertise. Joint decisions are made in an effort to develop the client's autonomy and self-efficacy. In the end, the health problem may or may not be resolved, but more importantly, the client's capacity to manage current and future problems is enhanced (Gottlieb & Feeley, 2006). Six key forces have contributed to the development of a collaborative partnership approach within health care systems in many countries, including, but not limited to, Australia, Canada, the United Kingdom, and the United States: (a) consumerism and patient rights, (b) PHC and health promotion, (c) accessibility of health information, (d) changes in thinking about nursing and ethical care, (e) the shift from hospital-based to home-based care, and (f) knowledge about how people change (Gottlieb & Feeley, 2006).

BOX 14.3 THE COMMUNITY HEALTH NURSE AS A COLLABORATOR

The community health nurse's role as a collaborator covers many different aspects:

WITH CLIENTS
- Acknowledges, supports, and encourages clients' active involvement in health care decisions
- Encourages a sense of client autonomy and an equal position with other members of the health care team
- Helps clients set goals and objectives for health care that are mutually agreed upon
- Provides client consultation in a collaborative fashion

WITH PEERS
- Shares personal expertise with other nurses and elicits the expertise of others to ensure quality client care
- Develops a sense of trust and mutual respect with peers that recognizes their unique contributions

WITH OTHER HEALTH CARE PROFESSIONALS
- Recognizes the contribution that individual members of the interdisciplinary team can make by virtue of their expertise and view of the situation
- Listens to each individual's views
- Shares health care responsibilities in exploring options, setting goals, and making decisions with clients and families
- Participates in collaborative interdisciplinary research to increase knowledge of a practice problem or situation

WITH PROFESSIONAL NURSING ORGANIZATIONS
- Seeks out opportunities to collaborate with and within professional organizations
- Serves on committees in local, provincial or territorial, and national nursing organizations or specialty groups
- Supports professional organizations in political action to create solutions for professional and health care concerns

WITH LEGISLATORS
- Offers expert opinions on legislative initiatives related to health care
- Collaborates with other health care providers and consumers on health care legislation to best serve the needs of the public

---

INTERPROFESSIONAL COOPERATION IN HEALTH CARE It is the position of the CNA (2005b) that every Canadian is entitled to health care within a system that has the capacity to help them meet their needs. The responsiveness of the health care system is directly related to the effectiveness of cooperation among health care professionals. This **interprofessional cooperation** is a hallmark of PHC and involves the development of a common purpose or care outcome, the acceptance and recognition of complementary skills and expertise among different providers, and the effective coordination and ongoing communication among professionals.

COMPETENCIES BASIC TO COLLABORATION Key elements necessary for collaboration include effective communication skills, mutual respect and trust, and a decision-making process.

Communication Collaborating to solve complex problems requires effective communication skills. Effective *communication* can occur only if the involved parties are committed to understanding one another's professional roles and appreciating one another as individuals. Instead of focusing on distinctions, health care professionals must concentrate on their common ground—the client's needs.

Mutual Respect and Trust *Mutual respect* occurs when two or more people show or feel honour or esteem toward one another. *Trust* occurs when a person is confident in the actions of another person. Both mutual respect and trust imply a mutual process and outcome. They must be expressed both verbally and nonverbally.

Decision Making The *decision-making* process at the team level involves shared responsibility for the outcome. Obviously, to create a solution the team must follow each step of the decision-making process, beginning with a clear definition of the problem. Team decision making must be directed at the objectives of the specific effort. It requires full consideration and respect of diverse viewpoints. Members must be able to verbalize their perspectives in a nonthreatening environment. An important aspect of decision making is the interdisciplinary team focus on the client's priority needs and the organization of interventions accordingly. The discipline best able to address the client's needs is given priority in planning. Nurses, by the nature of their holistic practice, are well suited for interprofessional cooperation.

Continuity of Care

A major responsibility of the CHN is to ensure continuity of care. **Continuity of care** is the coordination of health care services by health care providers for clients moving from one health care setting to another and among health care professionals. Continuity ensures uninterrupted health care services as the client moves from one level of care to another, for example, from an acute care hospital to home, or from home to a long-term care facility. This link is of increasing importance as changes in the health care system, nursing roles, interprofessional relationships, and client populations continue. In an integrated review of continuity of care, Sparbel and Anderson found that although the concept was not consistently or well defined, it was "strongly affected by a variety of communication and systems factors" (2000, p. 22). To provide continuity of care, nurses need to do the following:

- Initiate discharge planning for all clients when they are admitted to any health care setting or program

- Involve the client and family or support persons in all phases (assessing, planning, implementing, and evaluating care) of the planning process

- Collaborate and communicate with other health care professionals, as needed, to ensure the highest quality of care possible

- Ensure accessibility to required services to facilitate seamless care

Case management is an integrative health care model that tracks a client through a variety of care settings to ensure care continuity. The following are the three models of case management used in Canada:

1. *The brokerage or service management model*, wherein health care professionals are designated to assess client needs, implement service, and evaluate client progress while ensuring cost-effectiveness and, ideally, cost reduction

2. *Integrated team or provider-driven model*, wherein one professional provider is designated as primary caregiver to provide the leadership for care, and a team delivers services with the goal of achieving care continuity

3. *Self-managed care or client-centred model*, wherein clients assume, with caregiver support, personal control over care decisions

Discharge Planning

Discharge planning is frequently viewed as synonymous with continuity of care. Traditional discharge planning has referred to discharge from the hospital to home. However, discharges occur from many other settings. Discharge planning can be viewed as the process of preparing a client to transition between care environments in the same facility. For example, a client with a cerebrovascular accident may move from a medical unit to a community-based rehabilitation unit, or a client with multiple traumas may move from an intensive care unit, to a medical or surgical unit, to home care. The term *discharge planning* can also refer to the movement of a client from one care environment to another entirely. For example, an older adult client may transition to long-term care when he or she is no longer able to live at home. The focus of discharge planning is always at the individual client and family level, but each agency generally has its own policies and procedures to guide the process. Many agencies have *discharge planners,* a health or social services professional who coordinates the transition and acts as a link between the discharging and the receiving facilities. Often, a nurse assumes the responsibility of providing continuity of care.

Discharge planning needs to begin when a client is admitted to an agency, especially in hospitals where the lengths of stays are considerably shortened and care is often continued through public health (as with postnatal care) or home care services. Effective discharge planning involves (a) ongoing assessment to obtain comprehensive information about the client's ongoing needs, (b) statements of nursing care, and (c) plans to ensure the client's and caregivers' needs are met. In some situations, discharge planning necessitates health care team and family conferences. At a health care team conference, health care professionals focus on ways to individualize care for the client. At a family conference, both health care professionals and the family discuss family issues related to the client. Both types of conferences give the client, family, and health care professionals the opportunity to mutually plan care and set goals. See Box 14.4 for a description of home assessment parameters.

It is important that assessment focus equally on the client's strengths and deficits, as well as his or her home, family, and community environments. Since all these factors play a part in the optimal care of the client, the nurse must build on strengths while attending to the deficits that currently impede optimal health. The diagnoses and plan of care establish nursing activities necessary before the client is discharged. These activities most often include (a) teaching the client (and family) to cope with continuing self-care at home, and (b) a home care referral. Clients need help to

---

BOX 14.4 DISCHARGE PLANNING: HOME ASSESSMENT PARAMETERS

When planning the discharge of a client, the nurse needs to assess the client's strengths and deficits.

PERSONAL AND HEALTH DATABASE

Age; gender; height and weight; cultural data; medical history; current health status; surgery

ABILITIES TO PERFORM ACTIVITIES OF DAILY LIVING (ADLs)

Abilities for dressing; eating; toileting; hygienic care (tub, shower, or sponge bathing, oral care); ambulating (with or without aids, such as a cane, crutches, walker, wheelchair); transferring (from bed to chair, in and out of a bath, in and out of a car); preparing meals; using transportation; and shopping

DISABILITIES AND LIMITATIONS

Sensory losses (auditory, visual); motor losses (paralysis, amputation); communication disorders; mental confusion or depression; incontinence; and so on

CAREGIVERS' RESPONSES AND ABILITIES

Principal caregiver's relationship to client; thoughts and feelings about client's discharge; expectations for recovery; health and coping abilities; comfort with performing needed care

FINANCIAL RESOURCES

Financial resources and needs (note equipment, supplies, medications, special foods required)

COMMUNITY SUPPORTS

Family members, friends, neighbours, volunteers; resources, such as the Victorian Order of Nurses and Meals on Wheels; nutrition services; health centres; CHNs; day programs; legal assistance; home care; respite care

HOME HAZARD APPRAISAL

Safety precautions, self-care barriers, and home hazards. Assess the following:

- *Walkways and Stairways (inside and outside).* Note uneven sidewalks or paths, broken or loose steps, absence of handrails or placement on only one side of stairways, insecure handrails, congested hallways or other traffic areas, and adequacy of lighting at night.
- *Floors.* Note uneven and highly polished or slippery floors and any unanchored rugs or mats.

- *Furniture.* Note hazardous placement of furniture with sharp corners. Note chairs or stools that are too low to get into and out of or that provide inadequate support.
- *Bathrooms.* Note presence of grab bars around tubs and toilets, nonslip surfaces in tubs and shower stalls, handheld showerhead, adequacy of night lighting, need for raised toilet seat or bath chair in tub or shower, ease of access to shelves, and water temperature regulated at a maximum of 48°C.
- *Kitchen.* Note pilot lights (gas stove) in need of repair, inaccessible storage areas, and hazardous furniture.
- *Bedrooms.* Note adequacy of lighting, in particular the availability of night lights and accessibility of light switches; ease of access to commode, urinal, or bedpan; and need for hospital bed or bed rails.
- *Electrical.* Note unanchored or frayed electrical cords and outlets that are overloaded and/or near water.
- *Fire Protection.* Note the presence or absence of smoke detectors, fire extinguisher, and fire escape plan, improper storage of combustibles (e.g., gasoline) or corrosives (e.g., rust remover, phosphoric acid), and accessibility of emergency telephone numbers (fire, police).
- *Toxic Substances.* Note improperly labelled cleaning solutions.
- *Communication Devices.* Note presence of methods to call for help, such as a telephone or internal intercom in the bedroom and elsewhere (e.g., kitchen), and access to emergency telephone numbers.
- *Medications.* Note medications kept beyond date of expiry, adequacy of lighting for medication cabinet or storage, and method of disposal of sharp objects, such as needles used for injections.
- *Pets.* Note the presence of any pets, whether the pet supports the client (such as a dog that barks when someone knocks on the door) or is often in the way, the safety for home care workers entering the home, and food supplies for pet and owner.

NEED FOR HEALTH CARE ASSISTANCE

Home-delivered meals; special dietary needs; volunteers for telephone reassurance, friendly visiting, transportation, shopping; assistance with bathing; assistance with housekeeping; assistance with wound care, ostomies, tubes, intravenous medications, and so on.

understand their situation, to make health care decisions, and to learn new health behaviours. As a result of shortened hospital stays, it is often unrealistic to try to teach clients everything they need to know. Referral to a home health agency for follow-up teaching may be necessary (see Chapter 26 for details about effective teaching strategies).

Referrals

Regardless of the setting from and to which clients are moving, the referral process is a systematic problem-solving approach that ensures appropriate and timely information is communicated to assist the client in accessing resources that meet his or her health care needs. During the referral, pertinent information about the client's health, care needs, and social environment is communicated between discharging and care-providing agencies. An effective referral involves all of the following: the information is reliable and up to date, the referral is practical and timely, the referral is individualized to the client, and the referral is coordinated and mutually agreed upon by health care practitioners, caregivers, and, of course, the client him- or herself.

Referrals need to present as much information as possible about the client and the hospitalization. Most agencies have well-established protocols and detailed referral forms for this purpose. The assessment guide in Box 14.4 can also be used, but increasingly, nurses must learn to both assess and clearly articulate those assessments to multiple audiences, including families and health care providers. Beyond this, nurses are often called on to examine client and family needs at a larger systems level to assist in the deliberations around the provision of health care services in a community to ensure that the full spectrum of client needs can be addressed and met in the spirit of PHC. Education in public health policy and strategies to influence and effect change is essential.

Community Health Promotion

Though assessment and intervention at the individual and family level is a major component of the scope of community health nursing (as described above), there is also a significant community and public level component to the health promotion work of CHNs.

These community-level assessments and interventions are based on the principles of PHC, health promotion, and behaviour change theory. **Community health assessment**

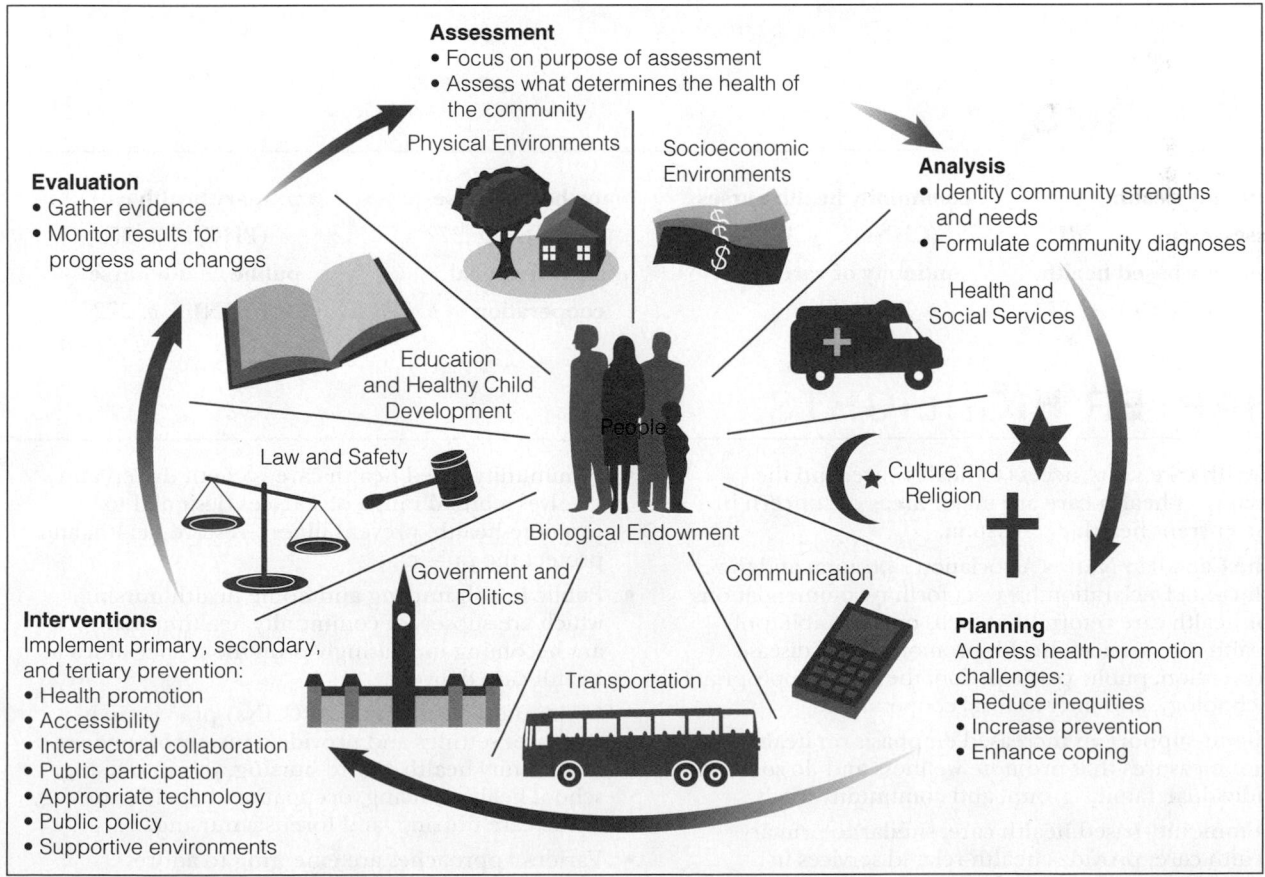

FIGURE 14.3 Community health-promotion model.

Source: From Stamler, L. L., & Yiu, L. (2012). *Community health nursing: A Canadian perspective* (Figure 13-1, p. 216). Toronto, ON: Pearson Canada Inc. Reprinted with permission from the illustrator, Camillia Matuk.

involves many areas including community members, physical environments, socioeconomic environments, health and social services, culture and religion, communication, transportation, government and politics, law and safety, and education and healthy childhood development. The community health-promotion process begins with this holistic assessment, moves through analysis, planning, intervention, and evaluation and ends with assessment again (see Figure 14.3 on the previous page for more detail). This model of care illustrates the complexity of community health nursing. With firm grounding in primary health care, health promotion, health education, and the determinants of health, community health nurses are especially qualified to effect positive health behaviour change within the community.

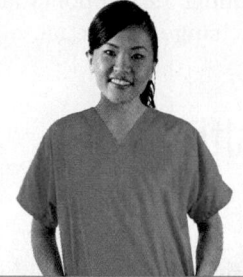

Case Study 14

Mrs. Smith is a 21-year-old new mother who recently gave birth to her first child in hospital. Her labour and delivery were without complications, but she is apprehensive about breast-feeding, bathing, and caring for her infant once home. Today is Mrs. Smith's postpartum day 2, and she is being discharged. She has been referred to the public health postpartum home-visiting program; she will be assigned a nurse to visit her in her home for follow-up physical assessment of mother and baby as well as for health teaching.

CRITICAL THINKING QUESTIONS

1. How will the nurse's role differ when delivering care in the client's home instead of the hospital?

2. What factors within the home environment might affect Mrs. Smith's care?

3. What financial and health benefits might be derived from caring for a client at home rather than in a hospital or other institution?

Check the eText in MyNursingLab for answers and explanations.

KEY TERMS

community health
   assessment *p. 281*

community-based health
   care (CBHC) *p. 271*

community health nurses
   (CHNs) *p. 272*

continuity of care
   p. 279

home health nurse
   (HHN) *p. 272*

interprofessional
   cooperation *p. 278*

primary health care
   (PHC) *p. 270*

public health nurse
   (PHN) *p. 272*

CHAPTER HIGHLIGHTS

- Health care costs, access to health care, and the quality of health care are major areas of concern in the current health care system.

- The Canadian Nurses Association's position and the Alma-Ata Declaration have set forth recommendations for health care reform that focus on accessibility of health care services, health promotion and disease prevention, public participation, the use of appropriate technology, and intersectoral cooperation.

- Clients support an increased emphasis on health care measures that promote wellness and do so at individual, family, group, and community levels.

- Community-based health care, similar to primary health care, provides health-related services in places where people spend their time—in homes, in shelters, in long-term care residences, at work, in schools, in seniors' centres, and so on.

- Community-based health care is client driven and involves a broad range of services designed to promote health, prevent illness, restore health, and protect the public.

- Public health nursing and home health nursing, which are subsets of community health nursing, are becoming increasingly prominent specialties in health care delivery.

- Community health nurses (CHNs) practise in a variety of settings and provide a variety of services: community health centre nursing, parish nursing, school health nursing, occupational health nursing, home care nursing, and forensic nursing.

- Various approaches are emerging to address community-based care: an integrated health care system, community initiatives, community coalitions, and outreach programs using lay health workers.

- Community-based nursing directs nursing care toward a specific population or group. It is not confined to one practice setting; it extends beyond institutional boundaries to involve a network of nursing services: nursing wellness centres, ambulatory care, long-term care, home health, and hospice care.

- To practise in community-based health care systems, nurses will need to learn new knowledge and competencies, such as determinants of a healthy community, primary and secondary preventive strategies, health-promotion strategies, collaborative and interdisciplinary teamwork, information management, and so on. Education in public health policy and strategies to influence and effect change is also essential.

- Intrasectoral and intersectoral cooperation are essential components of community-based care. Key elements of cooperation include effective communication skills, mutual respect and trust, and a good decision-making process.

- It is predicted that nurses will emerge as community health care leaders. Because primary health care is directed toward the community and client, nurses' roles will change to those of facilitator, consultant, and resource, rather than those of expert provider and team leader.

- A major responsibility of the nurse is to ensure continuity of care as clients move from one level of care to another.

- Continuity of care extends beyond the individual and includes a series of actions both within and outside an individual agency, which involve (a) discharge planning that begins when clients are admitted to an agency, (b) collaboration with the client and support persons, and (c) interdisciplinary cooperation.

ASSESS YOUR LEARNING

1. On the basis of a community needs assessment, a public health nurse develops a program to prevent childhood obesity. Which strategy is most appropriate for successful implementation?

   a. Providing information to the teacher for classroom use

   b. Involving parents, teachers, and children in program development

   c. Asking the school administration to remove all vending machines

   d. Initiating an exercise program during recess for children who are obese

2. In contrast to a home health nurse, the practice of public health nurses is characterized by a focus on what?

   a. Illness and injury prevention

   b. The health of populations

   c. Work in school health, occupational health, and home care

   d. Work with marginalized groups

3. The concept of primary health care can BEST be described as what?

   a. Medical care provided at the initial point of contact within the health care system

   b. Synonymous with community-based nursing

   c. More relevant for developing countries than for industrialized nations

   d. A philosophy of care delivery that can be applied in any sector

4. A community health nurse involved in political action to reduce homelessness through increased availability of affordable housing would MOST likely employ which of the following primary health care principles?

   a. Accessibility, health promotion, and public participation

   b. Illness and injury prevention; political action

   c. Social justice and equity

   d. Appropriate use of technology and community organization

5. Planning for discharge from an institutional setting, such as a hospital, can include a referral to a home care nurse. What BEST describes the expectations of the referral?

   a. The home care nurse will deliver all care himself or herself.

   b. The discharge assessment of service needs will be followed exactly.

   c. The home care nurse will coordinate the health care service needs of the client.

   d. The discharge plan is developed solely by the discharge planner and the client.

6. The Victorian Order of Nurses exemplifies which type of home care agency?

   a. Public or government agency

   b. Voluntary or private nonprofit agency

   c. Private proprietary agency

   d. Private cooperative agency

7. An older adult client is being discharged from the home care services program. Which of the following strategies is most appropriate to ensure a successful transition?

   a. Making one last home visit to review client teaching

b. Calling the client's family physician to advise him or her of the change

c. Scheduling a case conference with the client, his or her family, and relevant health care professionals

d. Providing the client with a list of applicable community resources

8. At the end of the postpartum home visiting period with a first-time mother, which of the following is MOST important for the nurse to assess?

a. The new mother has been given the answers to all of her questions about breast-feeding.

b. Mother and baby are no longer experiencing difficulty with breast-feeding.

c. The mother feels confident that she can access the necessary resources to deal with current and future difficulties with breast-feeding.

d. Baby is gaining weight appropriately.

9. Which of the following BEST exemplifies the three competencies basic to collaboration in the care of a home care client by a home care nurse?

a. Questioning the appropriateness of a prescription from the client's attending physician

b. Involving physical therapy and occupational therapy in the client's plan of care

c. Informing the client's family of changes made to the client's plan of care

d. Calling a case planning meeting for the client, the family, and the involved health care professionals

10. A young woman receiving services from an occupational health nurse for an injury sustained at work has assumed personal control over her plan of care in consultation with the occupational health nurse and other health care providers. Which of the following BEST describes the model of case management being employed?

a. Self-managed care or client-centred model

b. Integrated team model

c. Brokerage or service management model

d. Collaborative care model

Check the eText in MyNursingLab for answers and explanations.

WEBLINKS

Health Canada
http://www.hc-sc.gc.ca/

Health Canada is a national government agency. Its website provides links to current health-related programs and documents.

Department of Justice Canada: Canada Health Act
http://laws.justice.gc.ca/en/C-6/index.html

This Department of Justice site provides access to federal legislation, including the Canada Health Act and regulations concerning billing.

Canadian Public Health Association
http://www.cpha.ca

The Canadian Public Health Association (CPHA) is a national, independent, nonprofit association representing public health interests in Canada.

Canadian Home Care Association
http://www.cdnhomecare.ca

The Canadian Home Care Association represents more than 600 Canadian organizations that are involved in home care and community care.

MyNursingLab

REFERENCES

Barnes, D., Eribes, C., Juarbe, T., Nelson, M., Proctor, S., Sawyer, L., . . . Meleis, A. I. (1995). Primary health care and primary care: A confusion of philosophies. *Nursing Outlook, 43*(1), 7–16.

Canadian Association for Parish Nursing Ministry. (2011). *The Canadian Association for Parish Nursing Ministry.* Retrieved from http://www.capnm.ca.

Canadian Institute for Health Information. (2012). *Regulated nurses: Canadian trends, 2006 to 2010.* Ottawa, ON: Author.

Canadian Nurses Association. (1998). *Nursing with communities: Making the transition.* Ottawa, ON: Author.

Canadian Nurses Association. (2005a). *Primary health care: A summary of the issues.* Ottawa, ON: Author.

Canadian Nurses Association. (2005b). *Interprofessional collaboration.* Ottawa, ON: Author.

Canadian Nurses Association. (2011). *CNA certification.* Ottawa, ON: Author. Retrieved from http://www.cna-aiic.ca/CNA/nursing/certification/default_e.aspx

Canadian Occupational Health Nurses Association. (2003). *Occupational health nursing practice standards.* Ottawa, ON: Author. Retrieved from http://www.cohna-aciist.ca/english

Canadian Public Health Association. (2008). *Campaign 2008: CPHA's priority issues for public health.* Ottawa, ON: Author. Retrieved from http://www.cpha.ca/en/programs/briefs/election2008/election2008-5.aspx

Canadian Public Health Association. (2010). *Public health—community health nursing practice in Canada: Roles and activities.* Ottawa, ON: Author. Retrieved from http://www.cpha.ca/uploads/pubs/3-1bk04214.pdf

Canadian Public Health Association Board of Directors. (2000). *An ounce of prevention: Strengthening the balance in health care reform.* Ottawa, ON: Author.

Community Health Nurses of Canada. (2008). *Canadian community health nursing standards of practice.* Toronto, ON: Author. Retrieved from http://www.chnac.ca/images/downloads/standards/ chn_standards_of_practice_mar08_english.pdf

Community Health Nurses of Canada. (2009). *Public health nursing discipline specific competencies version 1.0.* Toronto, ON: Author. Retrieved from http://www.chnc.ca/documents/competencies_june_2009_english.pdf

Community Health Nurses of Canada. (2010). *Home health nursing competencies version 1.0.* Toronto, ON: Author. Retrieved from http://chnc.ca/documents/HomeHealth NursingCompetenciesVersion1.0March2010.pdf

Forensic Nurses Society of Canada. (n.d.). *Forensic nursing in Canada.* Retrieved from http://www.forensicnurse.ca

Gottlieb, L., & Feeley, N. (2006). *The collaborative partnership approach to care: A delicate balance.* Toronto, ON: Mosby Elsevier.

Health Canada. (2010). *Health care system.* Ottawa, ON: Author.

Stamler, L.& Yiu, L. (2012). *Community health nursing: A Canadian perspective.* Toronto, ON: Pearson Canada Inc.

Ministers of Health and Health Promotion/Healthy Living. (2010). *Creating a healthier Canada: Making prevention a priority.* Retrieved from http://www.phac-aspc.gc.ca/hp-ps/hl-mvs/declaration/pdf/dpp-eng.pdf

Public Health Agency of Canada. (2008). *Core competencies for public health in Canada, Release 1.0.* Ottawa, ON: Author.

Romanow, R. (2002). *Building on values: The future of health care in Canada.* Ottawa, ON: Commission on the Future of Health Care in Canada.

Sparbel, K., & Anderson, M. (2000). Clinical scholarship. Integrated literature review of continuity of care: Part 1, conceptual issues. *Journal of Nursing Scholarship, 32*(1), 17–24.

Underwood, J. (2007). *Competencies and standards: In a public health context, what is the difference?* Retrieved from info@chnc.ca

Underwood, J., Mowat, D., Meagher-Stewart, D., Deber, R., Baumann, A., MacDonald, M., . . . Munroe, V. (2009). Building community and public health nursing capacity: A synthesis report of the national community health nursing study. *Canadian Public Health Association, 100*(5), 1-1–1-12.

Villeneuve M., & Macdonald, J. (2006). *Towards 2020: Visions for nursing.* Ottawa, ON: Canadian Nurses Association. Retrieved from http://www.cna-nurses.ca/CNA/documents/pdf/publications/Toward-2020-e.pdf

World Health Organization & United Nations International Children's Emergency Fund. (1978). *Declaration of Alma-Ata: Health for all by the year 2000.* Geneva, Switzerland: Author.

World Health Organization. (2008). *The world health report: Primary health care (now more than ever).* Geneva, Switzerland. Retrieved from http://www.who.int/whr/2008/en

Yiu, L. (2012). Community care. In L. L. Stamler & L. Yiu (Eds.). *Community health nursing: A Canadian perspective* (3rd ed.) (pp. 213–235). Toronto, ON: Pearson Education Canada.

Chapter 15

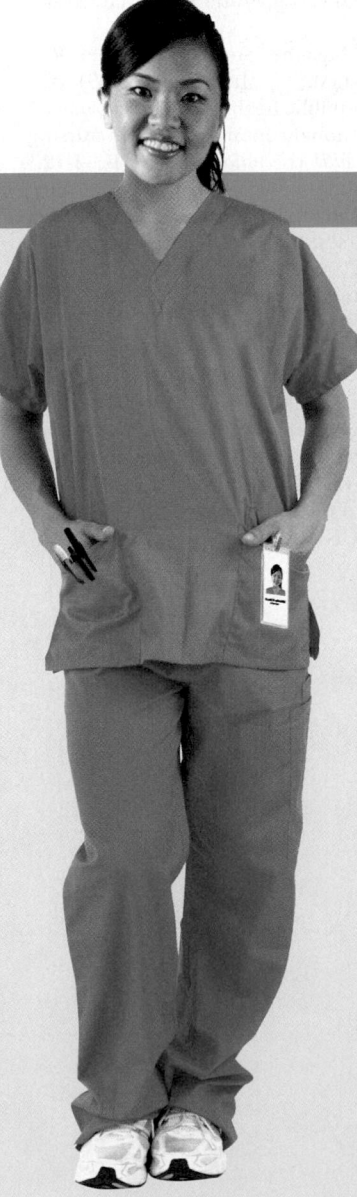

Rural and Remote Health Care

LEARNING OUTCOMES

After studying this chapter, you will be able to:

1. Describe the issues related to establishing universal definitions of rural, remote, and isolated communities.

2. Describe the geographical characteristics of rural, remote, and isolated communities and associated health care issues.

3. Describe the predominant occupational trends in rural, remote, and isolated communities and the associated health care issues.

4. Summarize the health concerns of individuals, families, and communities within rural, remote, and isolated contexts, including a specific focus on Aboriginal people on and off reserve.

5. Identify existing and emerging health care delivery issues within rural, remote, and isolated contexts.

6. Analyze the broad scope of rural, remote, and isolated nursing practice.

7. Examine topics of concern to nurses in rural, remote, and isolated practice.

Canada was originally a predominantly **rural** (a word to describe places like the countryside, towns, and small cities outside urban centres), agrarian-based nation, and it remained so until societal changes following World Wars I and II resulted in the growth of industry in urban centres. This growth led to the migration of rural residents to find employment in these industrial centres. In 1901, 37% of the population lived in urban centres, compared with over 80% in 2011 (Statistics Canada, 2012a). Urban populations surpassed rural ones in the period between 1921 and 1931; before that time, agriculture and natural resources were dominant industries. In **agriculture**, assets come from cultivating soil, producing crops, and raising livestock. **Natural resources** are assets supplied by nature, such as oil, coal, water, and timber, that can be used to create wealth. Since that time, the number of census farms has steadily declined, most recently with a 10.3% drop from 2006 to 2011 (Statistics Canada, 2012b).

Although approximately 19% of Canadians continue to live in rural and **remote** regions, those areas located far from urban and even rural centres, the realities of rural life belie the myth of a tranquil, healthy existence. Many rural communities in Canada are confronted by demographic, ecological, economic, and social challenges related to geographical **isolation** (a state of complete physical separation from other regions), boom–bust cycles, a reliance on nonrenewable natural resources, chronic high unemployment, the vulnerability of single-industry communities, aging populations, and so on (Pong, 2007). Correspondingly, nursing practice is affected by the diversity found within this huge geographical region of Canada. Health care delivery is further complicated by incomplete and sometimes conflicting data on the health status of residents in these regions.

Definition of *Rural*

One obstacle identified by researchers is the lack of consensus regarding the definition of the term *rural* (MacLeod, Martin–Meisner, Banks, Morton, Vogt, & Bentham, 2008). A common definition could facilitate comparison of study findings and experiences by researchers, clinicians, health policymakers, and health care delivery agencies (Ali, Rose Olfert, & Partridge, 2007; Thomlinson, McDonagh, Crooks, & Lees, 2004).

Statistics Canada and the Rural Secretariat used six definitions to outline how *rural* could be defined (du Plessis, Beshiri, Bollman, & Clemenson, 2001) and suggested that the appropriate definition be chosen based on the particular question being asked. How *rural* is defined can profoundly affect research results, policy development and use, program administration, and even how funding is distributed by governments at all levels (a **policy** is a plan or a course of action that the government follows). So, understanding the limitations and benefits of definitions based on geographical scale

(local, community, or regional), a geographical dimension (population size, density, labour market), a rural small town, or degrees of rurality, and whether more than one definition is used is important. Du Plessis and her colleagues (2001) identified some limitations of geographical definitions: the use of only one definition cannot capture the complexity of rurality, a common definition is lacking, qualitative data is disregarded, and definitions are preset. Du Plessis et al. (2001) indicated that the proportion of the population considered rural varies from 22% to 38%, depending on which definition is used.

In discussing rural demography, Statistics Canada uses a definition referring to *rural and small town Canada,* which it defines as labour market areas that are outside of the commuting areas of larger urban centres with core populations of 10 000 or more (Beshiri & He, 2009). This definition was used by the largest national research project to date on nursing in rural Canada, *The Nature of Nursing Practice in Rural and Remote Canada* (MacLeod et al., 2004).

Rural Health: Place, Space, and Time

Health geography examines the interaction of spatial factors and health, or the relationship between health and "place." Evidence has shown that place can affect health both directly and indirectly (Rainham, McDowell, Krewski, & Sawada, 2010). Examples of how geography can affect rural health include such issues as environmental factors that affect residents of a certain area, the type of employment associated with a particular geographical area, or the distances required to travel to obtain health care. Health geographers in Canada have traditionally looked at two issues in particular: using geographical techniques to map disease and epidemics, and looking at the geography of access to health care services (Luginaah, 2009.)

Carolan, Andrews, and Hodnett (2006) described some of the elements of place from a health geography perspective and debated the fit with nursing. These authors described *place* in several ways in relation to nursing, including as "situatedness," or being in and feeling place; creating a healing place; place in terms of disembodiment or displacement and the nurse's "place" involving issues of workplace, power, and gender (p. 203).

The characteristics or attributes of *rural place* can contribute to the uniqueness and peculiarities of being rural, and a framework to guide the assessment, planning, implementation, and evaluation of rural health care for individuals, families, and communities is critical. In particular, such a framework helps us understand and provide the optimal care possible to rural residents in relation to research, policy, and practice. Health Canada, working with the Canadian Nurses Association (CNA), the Canadian Medical Association (CMA), and other stakeholders, developed a rural health framework that can be found at the CNA website (see the Weblinks section at the end of this chapter).

Elements of a Rural Health Framework

The Canada Health Act provides for the "right to health care for all." The five federally defined principles that comprise the core of this act are universality, accessibility, portability, comprehensiveness, and public administration. Rural, remote, and isolated communities are confronted by challenges in gaining access to **equitable health care**, that is, the same or comparable health care as is provided elsewhere (Smith, Humphreys, & Wilson, 2008). It is a balancing act to maintain high-quality health care systems and manage the conflicting demands of the public.

Acury, Gesler, Preisser, Sherman, Spencer, and Perrin (2005) put forth a framework that incorporated geography and spatial behaviour as enabling factors in rural health care utilization, controlling for demographic, social, cultural, and health status factors. These authors, in a survey of 1059 adults in 12 rural communities, found that several factors, including having a driver's licence, using provided rides, and being within a reasonable distance for regular care, were significantly related to health care utilization for regular health care appointments and chronic care. Geographical and spatial behaviour are important to consider as factors in rural health care utilization.

Geography

Even though Canada is the second-largest country in the world in size of landmass, it has a relatively small population, the majority of which is concentrated close to the Canada–United States border. According to Statistics Canada (2011), in 2011, Canada's population was more than 34.4 million, an increase of 5.7% since the 2006 census. In 2011, 6.3 million people lived in rural areas, a number that has remained relatively constant since 1991 (Statistics Canada, 2012a). While the numbers in rural Canada remain relatively stable, the population in urban areas continues to increase, resulting in a decrease in the proportion of the Canadian population that lives in rural areas. In 2011, 18.9% of the Canadian population lived in rural areas (Statistics Canada, 2012a). Between 2006 and 2011, Canada's rural population increased by 1.1%, compared with Canada's overall population increase of 5.9%.

Regional variations in Canada's rural population exist. For example, rural areas in the Atlantic provinces and Saskatchewan declined in population, while the Northwest Territories, Nunavut, and Alberta had the fastest-growing rural populations (Statistics Canada, 2007a). For the first time, the population of the territories in the 2006 census surpassed 100 000 people, nearly half of whom live in the three capital cities. Small rural towns and hamlets increased in some cases by as much as 20% over the previous census. The population increase in Nunavut was due to natural increase from 2001 to 2006, when the fertility rate was twice the national average (3.1 versus 1.5 children per woman). Indeed, the **Aboriginal population**, those who can trace their origins to First Nations, Inuit, or Métis, had the fastest-growing natural increase (Aboriginal Affairs and Northern Development Canada, 2010).

These regional variations, combined with the concentration of population in major urban regions, contribute to issues for the delivery of health care to rural residents (see the Nursing and Canadian Society box).

Nursing and Canadian Society

Fact	Implications for Nursing
Over 6 million Canadians live in rural and remote areas of the country.	Particular geographical factors influence access to health care services. For example, distance and lack of resources affect emergency care for persons involved in farming and resource industry accidents.
Various governments have indicated a need to work with rural communities to develop successful solutions to the challenges they face.	Nurses working in rural areas need to participate in policy and program development initiatives of various governmental departments, recognizing how these actions affect health and health care delivery within their communities.
The Aboriginal population is the fastest-growing population in Canada, with most being youth and children living in underserviced Northern, rural, and remote communities.	Nurses working in Northern, rural, and remote communities need to participate in policy and program initiatives to address health care inequities.

It is difficult to specifically locate where the North begins. General agreement exists that great distances and difficult terrain often separate the communities in Northern Canada. With relatively few roads through a large geographical area, travel is still often dependent on weather. For example, winter roads built on the ice and snow can only be built when the weather is cold enough to permit travel across the frozen expanses of northern lakes and rivers. This, in turn, affects the type of goods transported into Northern communities. These factors are not as important in areas of Canada with an integrated highway system.

Enormous diversity exists within Canada in rural and Northern communities. Some rural communities remain relatively self-contained with limited impact from and relationship to urban areas. However, with the advent of improved transportation, the decline in farm income and income from other commodities, increasing numbers of rural and small town residents commute to work in urban centres on a daily basis, or to remote mining and resource jobs on a weekly or biweekly basis (Ali et al., 2007). This lack of geographical homogeneity adds to the complexity of health care issues and delivery systems across the country.

Demography

The ethnic composition of rural areas differs from urban areas. Rural Canada has the lowest proportion of immigrants, including new immigrants and visible minorities; 95.9% live in urban regions (Statistics Canada, 2008a). However, immigration settlement patterns are changing with the growth in the economies of some provinces, such as Saskatchewan and Manitoba, reversing traditional patterns of population decline (Beshiri & He, 2009). Smaller centres are increasingly developing strategies to recruit and retain immigrants to fill jobs in their growing manufacturing and processing industries (Beshiri & He, 2009).

Economic conditions vary by region and the degree of reliance on single industries, such as agriculture and natural resources. Population growth rates in rural and small town areas vary depending on the nature of the community. Given the recent slump in profits and sales of primary commodities (agriculture, forestry, fishing, and mining), communities dependent on such production have declined in population (Bollman & Reimer, 2009). Communities dependent on production of commodities that are growing in value, such as oil and potash, are growing rapidly, with resulting challenges of housing, service availability, and such infrastructure as servicing of building lots and provision of sewer and water services. Populations are growing in rural and small town areas within commuting distance of large urban centres. Populations are also growing in areas around lakes and mountains—preferred areas for many retiring "baby boomers."

Over time, a significant reduction in the number of family farms has been associated with a decrease in rural population. The majority of these larger farms are family corporations. Despite overall recent improvements in the farming economy, the countrywide trend has been for older farm operators to retire but for fewer of their children to continue with the family farm. The consequent decrease in population has a significant economic and sociocultural impact on the residents and communities in rural areas.

Many (46%) (Statistics Canada, 2008b) Canadians who identify themselves as First Nations, Inuit, and Métis live in remote, Northern, and rural areas of the country. Thirty-five percent of Canada's rural Northern population report Aboriginal identity. The majority of Aboriginal communities (64%) are non-isolated; 14% are semi-isolated; and 22% are isolated or remote isolated.

Most rural communities have large populations of children and youth (0 to 19 years) and seniors (older than 60 years), in comparison with a somewhat smaller population of working-age people (20 to 59 years). Overall they are, for the most part, older than urban populations. Factors that contribute to the bimodal population age pattern include the aging of the rural population, out-migration of rural youth for education and employment, and in-migration of retirees (Pong, 2007).

Rural communities support many different occupations. The following are a few of the major ones:

Agriculture	Mining
Logging	Fishing
Oil and potash extraction	Tourism
Merchants	Service sector

Occupations

Although the term *rural* is often equated with agriculture, other major industries in rural regions include mining, fishing, logging and forestry, and resource extraction, such as for oil and potash. In addition, rural communities have a variety of merchants, service dealers, and support services (see Box 15.1). The concentration of unskilled occupations is sizeably higher in predominantly rural regions (Bollman & Reimer, 2009).

Bollman and Reimer (2009) described a significant shift from farming to nonfarming activities in rural Canada. They noted: "The landscape may still be agricultural. The rural people-scape is decidedly non-agricultural" (p. 135). Less than 10% of Canadians live on farms, a decrease from two-thirds of the population prior to World War II. Only in Manitoba and Saskatchewan is agriculture a major employment sector in rural areas. Economists predict that economic growth in rural communities will be dependent on manufacturing growth in the future.

Although traditionally rural and small town families had lower per capita incomes compared with urban families, currently, the rural incidence of low income is similar to that of those living in urban areas (Bollman & Reimer, 2009). Rural employment has matched that in urban areas since 2001, after lagging throughout the previous decade. The biggest employment increases occurred in northern Manitoba, followed by Athabasca, Alberta, driven by the development of the oil sands. Rural areas that are reliant on such commodities as agriculture, forestry, or mineral extraction for their economic welfare are subject to "boom and bust" economic changes that result in a lack of predictable income. This lack of security can act as a major source of stress in rural areas (Brannen, Johnson Emberly, & McGrath, 2009).

Health of Rural Residents

Health Issues

Although there is a perception that rural residents are healthier than their urban counterparts, statistics demonstrate that, for the majority, this is not the case

(DesMeules et al., 2006). DesMeules et al. (2006) completed the first report produced at the pan-Canadian level that provides a broad picture of the health of rural populations. They did so by analyzing data from three different sources: (a) the Canadian annual mortality database, (b) the Canadian Community Health Survey, and (c) the Cancer Registry (see Box 15.2). Some of the findings affirmed previously identified health-related factors, such as the prevalence of smoking and obesity, compared with urbanites (Mitura & Bollman, 2004). Other health influences, such as eating habits and physical activity, showed lower practice levels in rural communities. These statistics are supported by research examining the perceptions of rural women, who identified that they felt more vulnerable because of living in the rural North (Leipert & Reutter, 2005). Smith et al. (2008) reported lower life expectancy for men in rural Canada than for urban men.

Higher overall rural mortality risks were attributed to such causes as **circulatory diseases** (those that affect the heart, arteries, capillaries, or veins), **respiratory diseases** (those that affect the nose, throat, larynx, trachea, bronchi, or lungs), **injuries** (harm, hurt, trauma, or a wound that is caused accidentally or deliberately), and **suicide** (the act of a person deliberately causing his or her own death). Indeed, people living in rural areas farthest from urban centres were at the greatest risk for all causes. Respiratory disease risks were, for the most part, significantly higher in rural areas, except for women

Rural residents face a number of health concerns:
- Respiratory problems
- Circulatory diseases
- Stress related to farm production and declining income
- Pesticide use
- Chemical contaminants
- Skin diseases
- Zoonoses
- Mental health issues
- Water safety around dugouts and ponds
- Machinery injuries
- Injuries from livestock
- Safe play spaces for children
- Water supply safety
- Hearing protection
- Eyesight protection
- Suicide
- Injuries
- Motor vehicle collisions
- Problematic substance use

living in more rural areas, who reported a prevalence of asthma significantly lower than that among their urban counterparts. Interestingly, the incidence rates of most cause-specific cancers were lower in rural areas than in urban areas. A full report by DesMeules et al. (2006) can be found at a link listed in the Weblinks at the end of the chapter.

Pampalon, Martinez, and Hamel (2006) conducted a study that looked at the health status of rural populations and the major determinants of health in Quebec. Similar to Pong et al. (2006), these researchers found that health varied within rural areas; generally, the closer the residents lived to urban centres, the better was their health. They further stated that what really discriminates urban from rural and areas within rural regions are health determinants (socioeconomic) and the presence of specific health conditions, such as respiratory disease, trauma (motor vehicle accidents and suicide), breast cancer, heart disease, infant mortality, smoking, and obesity.

RESPIRATORY PROBLEMS

Respiratory disease is a common health problem among agrarian rural dwellers, and rates of respiratory diseases are significantly higher across the board in rural communities, compared with urban centres, according to DesMeules et al. (2006). Exposure to grain dust, wood smoke, agricultural chemicals for crop production, and noxious gases emitted from silos or oil and gas wells have all been implicated as having immediate or long-term adverse effects on the health of this population. Depending on the specific chemical and length of exposure, ill effects resulting from inhalation of toxic substances can result in systemic problems, such as headaches, blurred vision, or possibly convulsions. Asthma is particularly prevalent in southern Alberta, an area noted for its wind and cattle feedlots; however, in the pan-Canadian health report, this regional rural difference does not show up in the overall health of rural residents, highlighting the need for both pan-Canadian and regional health and illness data.

CHEMICALS

Chemical contaminants can cause a variety of clinical manifestations, depending on the agent, source, amount, and route of absorption. Skin disorders, such as dermatitis, are a common problem for those working with chemicals without the use of personal protective equipment, such as gloves and coveralls. Canadian studies of pesticide use among farmers have found an increased risk of cancers among those exposed (Bushy, 2000). Gastrointestinal problems from acute or insidious poisoning through ingestion of contaminated food or water supplies are also concerns encountered, particularly after crop spraying. Arbuckle, Bruce, Ritter, and Hall (2006) recommended that people who apply pesticides and their families be counselled on hygienic practices (e.g., removing footwear and washing soiled hands before entering the home) to reduce indirect sources of exposure to herbicides.

CANCER

Differences in incidence of cancers between rural and urban areas in Canada vary widely. Cervical, prostate, melanoma, lip, and eye cancers are more common in rural areas, whereas the incidence of breast, lung, stomach, and lymph cancers are more often found in urban areas (Smith et al., 2008). Lip cancer is linked to increased exposure to the sun and its ultraviolet (UV) radiation among farmers and others who work in the sun without adequate UVB protection. Pong (2007) found that cervical cancer rates were significantly higher for women in the two most rural categories, compared with urban areas, in the 20- to 44-year age group, and the rate of having a Papanicolaou (Pap) test was lower. As well, cancer was more prevalent in the Aboriginal population. However, according to DesMeules et al. (2006) in the pan-Canadian study of rural health, in general, no significant differences exist between rural and urban residents in terms of cause-specific cancers.

WATER SAFETY

Water safety is a twofold concern: first, irrigation ditches, dugouts, and northern lakes and rivers are common sites of drowning; second, contaminated wells and creeks that supply drinking water for rural residents pose health risks.

The events in Walkerton, Ontario; North Battleford, Saskatchewan (Eggertson, 2008; Hrudey, 2008); and Kashechewan in Northern Ontario serve as examples of the enormous challenges Canadian rural society faces in terms of potable drinking water. Infrastructure to support potable water is either deteriorating or has never met rigorous health standards. In Walkerton, *Escherichia coli* bacterial contamination of the water transportation system caused seven deaths and made 2300 other residents ill. Vicente and Christoffersen (2006) examined the sequence of events in Walkerton and revealed an interaction among all levels in a complex community system, including "physical factors, unsafe practices of individual workers, inadequate oversight and enforcement by local government and a provincial regulatory agency and budget reductions imposed by the provincial government" (p. 93). Many remote and Northern residents continue to obtain their drinking water from sources that are not treated to remove bacteria and parasites. This fact, coupled with inadequate sewage disposal and contamination from livestock, has resulted in outbreaks of infection that are most harmful to infants, children, older adults, and persons who are immunocompromised. The development of water and sewage treatment plants, the education of communities with respect to their maintenance, and the creation and enforcement of stringent regulatory standards for water quality at a national level are significant requirements for health in rural and Northern areas (Eggertson, 2008; Hrudey, 2008).

ZOONOSES

Other risks for rural and remote residents are zoonoses (LeJeune & Kersting, 2010). These are diseases that are communicated from animals to humans. One of the more common zoonoses is brucellosis, which is contracted from cattle, swine, and goats. Humans acquire this disease, known as *undulant fever*, from ingestion of unpasteurized dairy products. Agricultural employees are especially at risk for transmission of zoonoses (Smith et al., 2008).

Bovine spongiform encephalopathy (BSE) is a progressive, fatal disease of the nervous system of cattle. It is one member of a family of diseases known as *transmissible spongiform encephalopathies* (TSEs). Other TSEs include scrapie in sheep, chronic wasting disease (CWD) in deer and elk, and Creutzfeldt-Jakob disease (CJD) in humans. Although the exact cause of BSE is unknown, it is associated with the accumulation of abnormal proteins, or BSE prions, in the brain. No treatment or vaccine is currently available for the disease (Agriculture and Food, Alberta, 2007; Canadian Food Inspection Agency, 2005).

Another zoonosis seen in rural and Northern areas is rabies, which is often transmitted from foxes, raccoons, and skunks. Diseases such as tularaemia, which produces lung, skin, and eye problems, are transmitted from muskrats, rabbits, and ticks. Leptospirosis, which produces flu-like symptoms from kidney, liver, and brain involvement, can be contracted from wildlife or contact with contaminated water. Hunters should be taught the proper handling of wild meat (Campagna, 2009).

In Northern and Arctic regions, trichinosis is a parasitic infection that is commonly found in wild game, such as bears, cougars, and walruses. From 1970 to 1997, Labrador, Quebec, the Northwest Territories (including present-day Nunavut), and Yukon had the highest number of reported cases of trichinosis, numbering more than 100 (Appleyard & Gajadhar, 2000). Hantavirus is a recent health concern that is prevalent in arid rural areas. This pathogen is spread through droppings from deer mice.

BLASTOMYCOSIS Though rare and nonreportable in most Canadian provinces, blastomycosis is a serious infectious disease that is endemic to much of central Canada and the United States (Saccente & Woods, 2010). Infection is caused by inhalation of the soil-dwelling fungal spores of *Blastomyces dermatitidis*, usually around river banks and other moist areas. Rural residents are particularly susceptible because of opportunity for exposure, whereas some urban dwellers have become infected after a vacation in the lake country (Parman, 2005). The Kenora region of northwestern Ontario has been identified as a region of high infection rate, particularly in Aboriginal populations (Saccente & Woods, 2010). Blastomycosis presents a particular challenge for health care providers because there is no simple test for detection and patients' symptoms are often mistaken for community-acquired bacterial pneumonia or chronic respiratory diseases, such as tuberculosis (Saccente & Woods, 2010).

AGRICULTURAL INJURIES In the 2006 census, 13 801 farms reported farm-related injuries in the previous 12 months. This represents 6.0% of all Canadian farms (Statistics Canada, 2007b). In the 16 years from 1990 to 2005, 1769 people were killed in agricultural injury events in Canada (Canadian Agricultural Injury Surveillance Program [CAISP], 2009). Comparisons by farm type of all farms reporting injuries show that livestock operations have a higher proportion of injuries than crop operations. Other than poultry and egg operations, all livestock operations had a higher incidence of injury than their overall share of operations by farm type.

Maltais (2007) determined that nearly two agricultural injuries in five are fractures (20.70%) or open wounds (19.79%), as reported by farm operators in Canada in 2001. The majority of farm injuries (51.95%) are musculoskeletal (fractures, dislocations, sprains or strains, and back injuries). Reported injury cases are more frequent among men (4.04%) than among women (1.89%). When injuries occur, farm income is jeopardized because operators of small family farms are not usually covered by workers' compensation. Farm injury-prevention programs should stress gender sensitivity (e.g., women completing tasks by using machinery designed for men's generally larger bodies) by using education, regulation, or engineering approaches (Dimich-Ward, Guernsey, Pickett, Rennie, Hartling, & Brison, 2007).

PRIMARY INDUSTRY INJURIES The most dangerous industries to work in from 1996 to 2005 were mining, quarrying, and oil wells (49.9 fatalities per 100 000 workers); followed by logging and forestry (42.9 fatalities per 100 000 workers); fishing and trapping (35.6 fatalities per 100 000 workers); agriculture (28.1 fatalities per 100 000 workers); and construction (20.6 fatalities per 100 000 workers) (Sharpe & Hardt, 2006). From 1996 to 2005, primary industry occupations had the highest fatality rate at 19.5 per 100 000 workers. Occupational health and safety programs should ensure that appropriate safety equipment is available, properly maintained, and used correctly. Such programs have done much to reduce the incidence of occupational injuries and fatalities in these primary industries.

SAFE PLAY AREAS FOR CHILDREN Agricultural injuries and fatalities are an important health issue for preschool children. From 1990 to 2005, there were 217 agricultural fatalities among children and youth in Canada aged 14 and under, an average of 13.6 per year (CAISP, 2009). Brison, Pickett, Berg, Linneman, Zentner, and Marlenga (2006) analyzed pan-Canadian data related to fatal injuries in children aged 1 to 6 years and found that death caused by fatal farm injuries was almost double all-cause unintentional fatal injury. Three major causes were identified: (a) being run over as a bystander, (b) being run over as an extra rider, and (c) drowning. The implications for providing health care include restricting preschool-age children's access to agricultural work sites and developing and delivering communication strategies to educate families as to the lethal danger exposure the work site engenders. Designated safe play areas for small children living on farms are rare but needed. Once children reach school age, statistics show a decrease in agriculture-related injuries and fatalities, until children are 10 years of age or older. At that age, many farm children begin to help with work. Schools not only provide farm children with an education but also serve to protect them from farm hazards for several hours a day. The CAISP (2009) reported a decline in the rate of injury from 17 injuries per year from 1900 to 1998, compared with 10.1 from 1999 to 2005. It is thought that this decline may be due, in part, to safety education and better safety practices (CAISP, 2009).

MOTOR VEHICLE COLLISIONS When discussing motor vehicles, the ones most commonly considered are cars, trucks, and motorcycles. However, farm vehicles, such as tractors, all-terrain vehicles (ATVs), dirt bikes, and snow-mobiles, are also included in this category, even though they are primarily used for off-road activities. Close to 40% of all motor vehicle collisions (MVCs) occur in rural areas and small towns, and they are the most important cause of injury mortality (DesMeules et al., 2006). Conditions thought to affect the mortality rate of rural and Northern regions include the following:

- Road conditions: narrow gravel roads, rock cuts, winter ice and snow
- High traffic speeds
- Wildlife or livestock on the roads
- Lower rates of seat belt and child restraint use
- The practice of riding in the back of open pick-up trucks
- Limited emergency medical personnel
- Greater distances to emergency medical services

In addition to the majority of collisions involving more than one vehicle, single-vehicle rollovers are common. These may be the result of high speed and loose gravel on country roads. ATV rollovers occur in the process of carrying out farm or ranch work. Numerous injuries are incurred when ATV, dirt bike, and snowmobile riders encounter barbed-wire fences, especially while travelling at high speeds. In Northern areas, snowmobile mishaps are the leading cause of injury and death.

Another factor related to the increased mortality in MVCs in rural areas is the distance that must be travelled to get either the necessary resources to the person in need or the injured individual to the appropriate level of care. In trauma care, the first hour following a traumatic event is commonly referred to as the "golden hour," since the care delivered to the victim during this initial phase strongly influences patient outcome.

MVCs caused 2578 deaths in Canada in 2005, and 1606 of these were in rural areas (Transport Canada, 2005). In 2004, 62% of collisions resulting in a fatality were in rural areas (Statistics Canada, 2008c). Of those drivers who were fatally injured, most had been drinking and driving and had an average blood alcohol level

of twice the legal limit. Compared with the 2578 deaths in 2005, some 4063 fatalities occurred in 1986. This decrease can be attributed to a combination of factors: better engineering of vehicles and roads, advances in medical care, increased public awareness campaigns, and education regarding traffic safety through such initiatives as Mission Possible, supported by the Canadian Automobile Association; the Heroes program from the Canadian Injury Prevention Foundation; and the Prevent Alcohol and Risk-Related Trauma in Youth (PARTY) program in Alberta and Ontario.

HEARING LOSS Many rural residents are at increased risk for noise-induced hearing loss. Working with heavy equipment, such as grain dryers, tractors, combines, and augers, can lead to intense exposure to loud noises for long periods. Pig farmers are especially at risk during feeding time when they are exposed to high-pitched squeals (Winters, MacIntyre, Peters, Thom, Teschke, & Davies, 2005).

Prevention of hearing loss and preservation of residual hearing may be accomplished through occupational health and safety education regarding these issues:

- Reducing the length of exposure to harmful noise
- Surrounding the sound with a sound-dampening enclosure
- Isolating the sound by placing a barrier around the driver, such as a tightly enclosed tractor or heavy machinery cab
- Wearing proper hearing-protection equipment (Winters et al., 2005)

Otitis media (middle-ear infection) and resultant hearing loss are endemic in Aboriginal children in Northern Canada, with the prevalence in some communities as much as 40 times greater than in urban southern communities (Bowd, 2005). Causes include increased susceptibility to infection because of immunity deficits, a decline in breast-feeding, cigarette smoke exposure, and poor diet. Hearing impairment can affect learning and literacy and have profound economic and social costs. Public health care providers need to be informed and provide care that includes traditional knowledge and practices.

LOSS OF EYESIGHT Loss of sight and eye injuries are health concerns for both rural and urban populations. However, because of the very nature of the work performed by rural residents, more eye injuries are treated in rural acute care facilities. Farmers, ranchers, loggers, and sawmill workers often have foreign bodies, such as gravel and wood chips, lodged in their eyes. Farmers are at increased risk of getting chemical spray in their eyes when applying a variety of fertilizers, herbicides, and pesticides. Those who work in the oil industry on the rigs or as heavy-duty mechanics require medical attention regularly for a variety of chemicals splashed into their eyes. For example, one particularly caustic substance known as "big orange" is a powerful engine degreaser that quickly causes sloughing of delicate ophthalmic tissues if it is not vigorously and immediately flushed.

Flash burns are one of the more common injuries seen among welders. A similar type of burn also occurs when persons are in the sun for long periods without proper eye protection from UV rays. This injury can manifest as snow blindness in trappers or outfitters, especially in springtime, or in any other rural or remote area resident who is not wearing protective eye lenses.

MENTAL HEALTH ISSUES   Mental health issues are those that affect an individual's mood, behaviour, thinking, and perceptions. The problem may be the result of an organic process, such as Alzheimer's disease, or be of a functional nature, such as depression.

Mental health problems affect more people than does breast cancer, Alzheimer's disease, or diabetes (Alberta Health and Wellness, 1999). There is conflicting evidence regarding whether rural individuals experience greater mental health issues than urban dwellers (Brannen et al., 2009). A recent study showed that rural residents experienced stress as a result of a variety of stressors related to individual factors, relationships issues, health work and education, community, finances and the environment (Brannen et al., 2009).

Several factors differentiate rural mental health issues and care from urban ones and may affect whether or not residents seek care:

- The lack of infrastructure to support and mobilize resources
- Different situational variables precipitating a mental health event or crisis, such as drought conditions during which farmers are unable to produce crops
- The lack of anonymity in rural communities
- The stigma still associated with mental health problems
- Concern regarding confidentiality

PROBLEMATIC SUBSTANCE USE   The onset of problematic substance use can be inadvertent and insidious. Commonly misused substances include tobacco, alcohol, opioids, and a wide range of illicit drugs, such as cannabis and hallucinogens. In addition, the inhalation of various aerosol products, glues, and gasoline is a growing problem among Canadian youth, especially in the more remote regions.

Substance use may begin in response to curiosity, in an attempt to achieve peer approval, as is often the case with tobacco and alcohol use among youth, or as a means of achieving an altered mental state in an attempt to escape situations or events. Problematic substance use refers to the inappropriate use of prescription drugs and nonprescription drugs (including alcohol) and the use of illicit drugs.

Alcohol continues to be the primary drug leading to health-related problems (Centre for Addiction and Mental Health, 2002). Problematic alcohol use causes chronic disease, permanent disabilities, and fatalities that result from sensory and motor impairment. This, in turn, leads to a variety of traumatic injuries and deaths as a result of falls, drowning, and MVCs. Multiple social and economic factors contribute to the fact that the Canadian Aboriginal population is at increased risk of death through alcohol and suicide (Health Canada, 2001).

SUICIDE   Even though DesMeules et al. (2006) reported that across Canada, suicide continues to be a major risk for rural and remote residents, their study did not find a high prevalence of depression, compared with their urban counterparts. DesMeules and colleagues suggested that this finding can be explained methodologically as the data for suicide and depression were obtained from two different sources at two different times. As well, factors such as personal stigma, visibility, and confidentiality may have affected self-reported responses to questions regarding depression.

In recent years, the incidence of suicide among rural youth has increased, with the highest rate occurring among the Canadian Aboriginal population. The national suicide rates for 2000–2004 ranged from 11.3 to 11.9 per 100 000 (Statistics Canada, 2008d). Smith et al. (2008) report higher male suicide in rural and remote populations, while female suicide rates were similar in both rural or remote and urban populations. Pong et al. (2006) reported that low-income single men and women in the 15 to 24 age group living in the most rural and remote communities are at greatest risk of dying from suicide, with rates four times as high for men as for women.

Factors that are believed to contribute to a high incidence of suicide are depression; problematic substance use; changing family, community, and economic dynamics; cultural changes that emphasize the valuing of increased personal freedom and heterogeneity; declining religious affiliations; and Western society's tendency to view suicide as a terminal means of problem solving. Although these factors are also influential in urban settings, rural communities tend to be more isolated from formalized health and social services. The lack of anonymity within small communities and the fear of being stigmatized with a mental health problem pressure some rural and Northern residents to keep their problems to themselves.

Special Concerns in Aboriginal Communities

The problems that exist for rural residents are magnified for those who live in First Nations communities. Aboriginal Canadians have been found to have significantly greater health challenges than people in the general population. Lower income and education levels for Aboriginal people account for some but not all of these differences (Garner, Carriére, & Sanmartin, 2010). Infant mortality rates for First Nations people, both on and off reserve, are reported to be two times that of the general population (Smylie, Fell, & Ohlsson, 2010). These rates, coupled with significantly higher accident and injury rates among all ages, contribute to lowered life expectancies. Lack of clean water and sewage systems, inadequate housing, and high unemployment are contributing factors. Despite the fact that the 2007 federal budget speech stated unequivocally that "all Canadians deserve clean drinking water," in February 2008, there were 93 First Nations communities in Canada living under boil-water or "Do not consume" orders. One of those communities had been living under the order issued in 1995 (Eggertson, 2008).

Diabetes is a major health issue—the prevalence being two times higher for the Métis population as the general population, and 3.5 times higher for First Nations people as compared with people in the general population (Tjepkema, Wilkins, Senecal, Guimond, & Penney, 2009). **Diabetes** is a metabolic disease in which high blood glucose levels are caused by defects in insulin secretion, action, or both.

The most common causes of death for First Nations people aged 1 to 44 years were poisoning and injury. Children under 10 years died predominantly from unintentional injuries. In a study of unintentional injuries in children and adolescents in Newfoundland and Labrador, Alaghehbandan, Sikdar, MacDonald, Collins, and Rossignol (2010) found the mortality rate due to unintentional injury to be eight times higher in Aboriginal children than that of children in the general population.

As previously noted, suicide rates in the Aboriginal population are dramatically higher than in the general population, with the First Nation suicide rate twice that of people in the general population, and the Inuit suicide rate over 10 times that of others (Kirmayer, Brass, Holton, Paul, Simpson, & Tait, 2007). Suicide and self-injury were the leading cause of death for youth and adults up to 44 years. Suicide accounted for 22% of deaths in youth and 16% in early adulthood. Social disruption, lack of hope for the future, problematic substance use, and family violence have all been suggested as underlying or related factors for suicide. Efforts to combat these problems include community mobilization and awareness campaigns (Kirmayer et al., 2007).

Kirmayer et al. (2007) suggested that even though direct causal links are a challenge to show quantitatively, obvious and convincing evidence shows that a long history of cultural oppression and marginalization has played a role in the high levels of mental health problems found in many Aboriginal communities. On the positive side, evidence also shows that fortifying an ethnocultural sense of identity, community unity, and political empowerment can assist in improving mental health in Aboriginal communities. Mental health promotion

that emphasizes youth and community empowerment through individual and community-based initiatives, as well as larger political and cultural processes, is likely to have broad effects on mental health and general well-being in these communities.

Tradition and healing are central to current efforts by Aboriginal peoples to confront historical injustices and suffering brought on by **colonialism**, when European settlers arrived in Canada and assumed control of the land and its resources. Aboriginal peoples in Canada are involved in healing their own traditions, repairing the ruptures and discontinuity in the sharing of traditional knowledge and values, and asserting their collective identity and power (Kirmayer et al., 2007).

According to Llewellyn (2002), residential schools were established by the Canadian government in the late nineteenth century and were in operation until the 1980s to provide education to First Nations children. They were administered by Christian churches: Methodist (United Church of Canada), Presbyterian, Anglican, and several Roman Catholic orders. The policies by which the schools were run came from the Canadian government; however, day-to-day management lay with the religious organizations. The government used these schools to implement its policy of assimilation. "Settlers demanded that the colonial government respond to the so-called Indian problem," which arose with the arrival and spread of British settlers into First Nations lands (p. 256). These schools created and enforced situations of shame, humiliation, and physical, mental, emotional, and spiritual disconnectedness that led to feelings of helplessness and powerlessness (Chansonneuve, 2005). The removal of children from their families; the destruction of First Nations languages, culture, and spirituality; and the physical and emotional abuse the children endured are at the core of many of the health and social challenges that face First Nations and their communities today.

Llewellyn (2002) presented arguments in support of and against the use of litigation to resolve the more than 100 years of abuse perpetrated by the policies and practices of residential schools. Llewellyn introduced and made a case for **restorative justice**, an approach to justice that involves righting the wrong, as much as possible, through reconciliation, healing, and building peace within communities, which builds on and learns from the successes and failures of the South African Truth and Reconciliation Commission. "The idea of such a process has been supported by a variety of groups, including the Royal Commission on Aboriginal Peoples, the Assembly of First Nations, the Law Commission of Canada and several of the church organizations implicated in residential school cases" (p. 289). On June 11, 2008, the Prime Minister of Canada, Stephen Harper, officially apologized to Aboriginal people on behalf of the people of Canada for the abuses suffered in residential schools. Also in June 2008, the Indian Residential Schools Truth and Reconciliation Commission began its national work to understand how Aboriginal people were affected by the residential school experience (Truth and Reconciliation Commission, 2011). Health care providers working in rural, remote, and isolated communities must be knowledgeable about this issue and the impact it has had on the culture, spirituality, health, and well-being of Aboriginal people. Health care workers must also be able to provide culturally safe care.

Health Care Delivery

Health Care Delivery Issues

Many factors contribute to making the delivery of appropriate and cost-effective health services to rural, remote, and Northern populations a challenge (see Box 15.3). Accessibility to equitable health care services is at the heart of health care delivery issues. A major factor is the need to deliver a variety of health services to a population that is sparsely distributed over a large geographical area, with a limited number of health care professionals. Current and impending shortages of health care professionals will only exacerbate an already challenging health human resources problem (Rukholm, 2006). In addition, the current practice of educating health care professionals in urban settings with limited clinical exposure to rural settings results in health professionals being less inclined to practise in rural settings on completion of their programs (Blankenau, 2010).

The inclusion of health issues of rural, remote, and Northern residents within general statistics contributes to difficulties in being able to focus on specific concerns affecting these populations. The work of DesMeules et al. (2006) was a beginning step in addressing the challenge of adequate and useful statistical data to affect health care policy and practice in rural, remote, and isolated

---

BOX 15.3 NURSING AND HEALTH CARE DELIVERY ISSUES

Nursing in rural and remote areas can be affected by a number of delivery issues:

- Data gaps and inadequate information about the health status of rural residents
- Distance
- Sparse population
- Limited infrastructure, including transportation and communication
- Limited health care resources and access to technology
- Educational preparation for generalist-specialist practice
- Recruitment and retention of professionals
- Ethical issues (lack of anonymity, confidentiality, resources)
- Changing demographics and care requirements of the community

---

communities across Canada. Smaller independent studies have added to our understanding of rural health issues in specific areas, including the health issues of rural and remote black women in Nova Scotia (Etowa, Wiens, Thomas Bernard, & Clow, 2007) and determinants of women's health in southwest Ontario (Leipert & George, 2008). However, a comprehensive review of the literature of rural–urban health differences notes that although rurality plays a major role in the nature of services and level of access available, rurality itself does not lead to health disparities. "Much of the variation between rural and urban health status [can] be explained by socioeconomic factors affecting the use of health services" (Smith, Humphreys, & Wilson, 2008, p. 59).

Health care providers in rural, remote, and Northern areas must possess a broad generalized knowledge base to meet the diverse health care needs of the residents. **Interdisciplinary or interprofessional approaches**, in which nurses interact with many other health care professionals from all areas, have been suggested as one way to increase the effectiveness of health care delivery (MacLeod et al., 2004; MacLeod et al., 2008). MacLeod et al. (2004) suggested that nurses working in rural, remote, and Northern communities often interact with other health care professionals at a distance. These researchers further stated that "new models of interprofessional practice can be developed that are supportive of the varied strengths of and resources available to rural and remote communities" (MacLeod et al., 2004, p. 4). Hayward (2005) described the facilitation of interdisciplinary practice through the provision of a mobile service to older adults in rural seniors' centres and in the home by students and faculty in nursing, physical therapy, occupational therapy, pharmacy, and dietetics, as well as other disciplines.

RURAL, REMOTE, AND NORTHERN NURSING PRACTICE
Nurses practise in multiple settings in rural, remote, and Northern sites; they provide acute and extended care, community health services, home care, occupational health services, and mental health services, and, in some provinces and territories, they are taking on **expanded practice** roles, in which nursing goes beyond the traditional nursing roles. Often, these nurses, especially in remote communities, work alone (MacLeod et al., 2008).

Nursing Practice Issues

In the past, the majority of research regarding rural and remote nursing has come from Australia and the United States. During the last few years, there has been an explosion of Canadian research focusing on rural nursing practice (e.g., Jackman, Myrick, & Yonge, 2010; Martin Meisner, MacLeod, Banks, Morton, Vogt, & Bentham, 2008; Montour, Baumann, Blythe, & Hunsberger, 2009; Penz, Stewart, D'Arcy, & Morgan, 2008; Thomlinson et al., 2004), nurses (e.g., Andrews, Stewart, Morgan, &

D'Arcy, 2011; Kulig, Stewart, Penz, Forbes, Morgan, & Emerson, 2009; MacLeod et al., 2004), nurse practitioners (Way, Jones, Baskerville, & Busing, 2001), and nursing education and professional development (Kosteniuk, D'Arcy, Stewart, & Smith, 2006; Rukholm, 2004). Issues that were identified in the MacLeod et al. (2004) pan-Canadian study of rural nursing practice and rural nurses included the following:

- Managers and policymakers need to better understand the realities of rural and remote practice to develop a "rural lens" that could be used as part of a pan-Canadian rural and remote nursing strategy.
- Nurses' personal and professional roles are inseparable in small communities.
- Many rural nurses work alone, indicating a need for at-a-distance, face-to-face, and technological supports.
- Understanding of nurses and their partnerships with their communities could aid recruitment and retention.
- Support for new ways of interprofessional practice is essential.
- Particular attention must be paid to and support given to nurses in Aboriginal communities to provide culturally competent, appropriate care.
- Retirement and migration need to be addressed by providing relevant continuing education.
- The distinctiveness of rural and remote nursing practice cannot be captured until unique personal identifiers are created along with relevant urban rural indicators (MacLeod et al., 2004, p. v).

Rural nursing in Canada has lacked a consistent definition and has not yet been formally recognized as a distinct specialized area of nursing practice (Crooks, 2004). Although some claim that the only difference between rural and urban nursing is the environment in which nursing is practised, others disagree. Crooks (2004) maintained that it is the development of deep, meaningful professional relationships that is the heart of rural nursing practice. Developing multiple relationships with other health care professionals, addressing the vulnerability of their clients due to lack of anonymity, difficulty stepping out of the nursing role in nonwork situations—all of these things challenge the rural nurse to develop a clear sense of the nurse's role and how that role plays out in a rural setting. See the Evidence-Informed Practice box on the working relationships of public health nurses and high-priority families in Northern Canadian communities. The caring that emerges in rural nursing is based on interpersonal knowledge of the patients and clients, their families, and their communities, as well as the relationship that exists between the nurses and their coworkers.

Rural nurses in Canada, the United States, and Australia share many common characteristics. Nurses are often described as highly visible members of the community, resourceful, flexible, autonomous, self-reliant, and

---

EVIDENCE-INFORMED PRACTICE

"And Then You'll See Her in the Grocery Store:" The Working Relationships of Public Health Nurses and High Priority Families in Northern Canadian Communities

Moules, MacLeod, & Hanlon (2010) completed a qualitative study exploring the nature of working relationships between health care professionals and high needs families in small rural, Northern communities. The researchers interviewed 32 public health nurses, 25 families, and 3 lay home visitors from 14 communities across northern British Columbia to determine the unique experiences and challenges faced. The study found that the relationships established were multifaceted and that the nature of small communities increased the complexity of the health care professional–client relationship. The multiple roles played by nurses in small communities and the negotiation of relationship boundaries were major issues. The nurses described the issues that arose from knowing clients in multiple contexts and being known to them. They spoke of the pressure to bend the rules because of the complexity of these relationships. Confidentiality, anonymity, role confusion, and proximity all posed challenges. The study provided insights into the day-to-day issues that arise when working with vulnerable, marginalized families in small community settings and the challenges faced by nurses when living and working in small communities.

NURSING IMPLICATIONS: Nurses working in small communities must be aware of the unique demands that this work situation creates. Relationships may not begin or end at the clinic door or in the home visit. They simply change. Nurses working in rural communities must have a clear understanding of their professional role, an ability to negotiate shifting boundaries, and supports to assist them in this complex work.

Source: Based on Moules, N., MacLeod, M., & Hanlon, N. (2010). "And then you'll see her in the grocery store": The working relationships of public health nurses and high priority families in northern Canadian communities. *Journal of Pediatric Nursing, 25,* 327–334.

---

effective team members (MacLeod et al., 2008). Above all else, rural nurses are described as *generalists* and *specialist-generalists.* The need to maintain general practice skills covering all ages and all the conditions that clients or patients can present with is a major challenge for rural nurses.

Nurses working in rural and remote areas face occupational risks that differ from those in metropolitan areas. An Australian study comparing the risks faced by rural nurses with those of their urban counterparts found that rural nurses lifted and transferred patients more often than their urban colleagues. Rural nurses reported less risk of blood-borne pathogens and excessive noise but more risk for temperature extremes than metropolitan nurses (Timmins, Hogan, Duong, & Miller, 2008). Rural nurses are exposed to weather extremes more frequently than their urban counterparts. The impact of extreme weather challenges is rarely identified in the literature as a concern in the provision of home, community, and emergency care, and even more rarely reflected in health policy (Skinner, Yantzi, & Rosenberg, 2009). Distance and geography also pose significant challenges and potential risks (Skinner et al., 2009).

A Canadian study published in 2010 found that rates of workplace injury for rural health care workers, particularly musculoskeletal injury, were remarkably high. This study found that risk factors for poor work disability prevention outcomes were different for rural health care workers due to older age, lower education levels, high workloads (long hours, extensive on-call demands, complex patient needs), low staff support, exposure to violence, lack of replacement staff, and inadequate safety features in buildings (Franche, Murray, Ostry, Ratner, Wagner, & Harder, 2010).

Despite these risks, rural nursing practice provides many rewards, including the following:

- Greater autonomy because there are fewer nurses and other health care professionals
- Greater knowledge of the client's or patient's home and family conditions
- Closer interface with other health care professionals
- Greater opportunity to affect health care planning and policy at the local level because of the recognized role as a resource on health care and the prominence in the community

EDUCATION FOR RURAL AND REMOTE PRACTICE

As early as 1975, a course in rural hospital nursing was offered at the Foothills Hospital School of Nursing in Calgary (Reimer & Mills, 1988). Across the country, some undergraduate nursing programs are beginning to include theory and clinical practice specific to rural nursing in their curricula. Other programs continue to use rural placements as practicum sites, with a lesser emphasis placed on the setting itself. The recruitment and retention of nurses for practise in rural, remote, and Northern regions of Canada have been persistent problems, and these continue to grow in importance (MacLeod et al., 2008; Rukholm, 2006). Nursing leaders and educators have a role in the education and psychological preparation of nurses to work in these diverse settings. It is essential that more nursing students be educated to practise in rural and remote acute care and community settings. Programs based at Lakehead University in Thunder Bay, Ontario, the University of Northern British Columbia in Prince George, British Columbia, the University of the North in The Pas/Thompson, Manitoba, and the University of Saskatchewan are delivering baccalaureate nursing programs in smaller rural centres in an attempt to address rural and remote health care needs.

Although the number of programs being offered across the country for nurses working in rural, remote, and Aboriginal communities has increased, not enough nurses are graduating from nursing programs to fill the gaps left by retirements and migration (Rukholm, 2006). New programs have recently emerged from many universities. One example is the University of Northern British Columbia, which is offering a 1-year certificate program in rural and Northern nursing for experienced registered nurses, with an option to complete an undergraduate degree in nursing. As well, a graduate program with a focus on rural and Northern nursing is offered through a blended-mode (face-to-face and online) delivery at Laurentian University in Northern Ontario. Laurentian also offers a unique interdisciplinary program at the doctoral level in rural and Northern health, focusing on health services and health policy. Aboriginal nursing–specific programs are reported by 8 of the 91 Canadian Association of Schools of Nursing members (Gregory, 2007).

TELEHEALTH AND RURAL AND REMOTE PRACTICE

Telehealth (the sharing of nursing information by using electronic means, such as a telephone or the Internet, to answer consumers' questions), **telemedicine** (the use of technology to transmit electronic medical data about clients to persons at distant locations), and blended-mode learning (a combination of face to face, videoconferencing, Internet, paper-based, and web casting) have mushroomed with technological advances and increased access to high-speed Internet connections and videoconferencing capacity (Atack, 2003; Carter, Rukholm, Mossey, Viverais-Dresler, Bakker, & Sheehan, 2006). In Alberta, a provincial early intervention stroke protocol allows diagnostic test results to be transmitted immediately from rural hospitals to specialists in urban centres, who review the results and view the patient on a bedside video monitor to determine treatment to be carried out locally. In remote Labrador, Rosie the Robot moves throughout the health centre, allowing the patients to talk with physicians 350 km away. Physicians perform visual assessments and have access to all diagnostic data while they interact with each patient (Canadian Broadcasting Corporation, 2010).

Gibson, Kakepetum-Shultz, Coulson, and O'Donnell (2009) explored the use of telehealth in mental health services in Northern Ontario. Telemental health, using primarily videoconferencing, was used in mental health services provided to First Nations people. Telehealth was seen as useful by clients in providing greater access to and better continuity of service. Community members reported a degree of comfort with the process, indicating that having the counsellor at a distance actually facilitated disclosure. There was concern expressed by some individuals about the challenge of building trust using these methods. Privacy and security were concerns for some community members, who indicated that they felt that the staff in the rest of the health centre might overhear their interactions. Others noted concerns about the therapist not being in the community, both from the perspective of developing an understanding of the context of people's lives, and also in relation to the lack of contribution to community capacity building if the therapist does not participate in the fabric of the community.

Technological approaches are not only seen in service delivery. Russell and Perris (2003) reported on a 6-month telementoring staff development initiative in a Canadian community nursing agency. The online discussions focused on collaborative learning and professional development that showed improved asynchronous communication and problem-solving skills as a result of online discussions and fostered "communal opportunistic learning and professional development" (p. 227).

Technology has the potential to support service provision, accessing health information for clients, nursing education, and staff development in rural and remote settings. Given the distances required for travel, technology is an important aspect of rural and remote health care now and in the future.

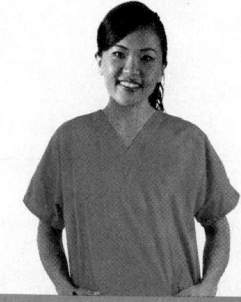

Case Study 15

Mr. Donaldson is a 45-year-old farmer living in rural Saskatchewan who presented to the emergency department with cellulitis in his right leg, secondary to a puncture wound from the tine of a pitchfork. He runs a family grain-and-cattle operation about 50 km from town and the nearest hospital. He is given the choice of being admitted to hospital or returning to hospital every 8 hours for a one-hour antibiotic treatment and for a daily dressing change. He is told he must limit his activity and keep his leg elevated as much as possible.

CRITICAL THINKING QUESTIONS

1. What issues should the nurse discuss with Mr. Donaldson to assist him in choosing his treatment options?

2. How might the patient's regime vary from that in an urban setting?

3. How might Mr. Donaldson's occupation influence his recovery?

4. What health care delivery issues common to rural and remote residents affect Mr. Donaldson's treatment?

Check the eText in MyNursingLab for answers and explanations.

KEY TERMS

Aboriginal population   *p. 288*

agriculture   *p. 287*

circulatory diseases   *p. 290*

colonialism   *p. 295*

diabetes   *p. 295*

equitable health care   *p. 288*

expanded practice   *p. 296*

injuries   *p. 290*

interdisciplinary or interprofessional approaches   *p. 296*

isolation   *p. 287*

natural resources   *p. 287*

policy   *p. 287*

remote   *p. 287*

respiratory diseases   *p. 290*

restorative justice   *p. 295*

rural   *p. 287*

suicide   *p. 290*

telehealth   *p. 298*

telemedicine   *p. 298*

CHAPTER HIGHLIGHTS

- Consensus on clear, comprehensive definitions for *rural* and *remote* areas is required to allow for data collection on health care information of residents in these regions of the country.

- Rural communities are diverse. Issues vary depending on rurality, demography, and economic base.

- Great diversity in the geography of Canada contributes to particular regional issues.

- Rural and remote residents have higher infant mortality, lower life expectancy, and higher rates of injuries and death than urban residents.

- Common health concerns include respiratory illnesses, chemical exposures, circulatory diseases, hearing and sight problems, and zoonoses.

- Water safety concerns include the contamination of drinking water supplies and drowning in ditches, dugouts, rivers, and lakes.

- Injuries and deaths within rural and remote primary industries are a significant factor in the health care of rural populations.
- Children are at particular risk for injury or death because of the lack of designated safe play areas for young children.
- Numerous factors contribute to high mortality rates from motor vehicle collisions.
- Social and economic factors contribute to increased mortality and morbidity within the Aboriginal population in Canada.
- Challenges to health care delivery are sparse population, distance, and difficulties in recruiting and retaining health care professionals.

- Knowledge about the impact of residential schools on the culture, spirituality, health, and well-being of Aboriginal people must be considered in the delivery of culturally safe health care.
- A major challenge for rural nurses is to attain and maintain practice skills for providing care for all ages and health conditions.
- Nurses in rural areas face issues of confidentiality, anonymity, proximity, and boundary definition in working with clients from their home communities.
- Key characteristics of rural and remote practice are lack of anonymity, greater autonomy, and broad generalist practice.

ASSESS YOUR LEARNING

1. Which term BEST describes a significant challenge confronting delivery of rural health care in Canada?
   a. Universality
   b. Portability
   c. Public administration
   d. Equitability

2. Originally, the Canadian economy was mainly based on what?
   a. Agrarian, natural-resource based, and rural
   b. An even blend of rural agrarian and urban industry
   c. Urban with some agriculture and industry
   d. Urban based on a skilled knowledge industry

3. What is the primary reason rural populations have declined in relation to urban populations in the past century?
   a. Few new immigrants choose to live in rural areas.
   b. Rural Aboriginal populations are not increasing.
   c. Urban residents have a higher birth rate than rural residents.
   d. An increase in farming technology means there is less rural opportunity.

4. What are the main causes of mortality in rural and Northern Canadian communities?
   a. Motor vehicle collisions, respiratory diseases, homicide, and circulatory diseases
   b. Injuries, poisonings, arthritis, and cancer
   c. Cardiovascular disease, cancer, and arthritis
   d. Injuries, suicide, and circulatory and respiratory diseases

5. You are the nurse in a rural First Nations community in Northern Ontario. Lately, there have been a number of serious motor vehicle collisions, including one that killed four local teenagers. Problematic substance use was part of the causes of the accidents. What should be your next step?
   a. Approach the local high school about doing a lecture on the dangers of alcohol and substance use
   b. Approach the local high school and invite students to participate in a stop drinking and driving contest you have designed
   c. Meet with a group of local teenagers and community elders and work with them to develop a video game they created on stopping drinking and driving
   d. Meet with the high school principal to tell him or her about the dangers of substance use, drinking, and fatal accidents

6. As a nurse working in a rural and remote community in Saskatchewan, you know that farm injuries are a major health issue. Preschool children are at particularly high risk of fatal injuries. You have been approached by the wife of a local farmer who wants you to help her organize a safe play area for preschool children. What should be your next step?
   a. Arrange to meet with the farmers at a local fall fair to talk with them about the hazards of farming
   b. Post signs in the community about farm hazards
   c. Talk to the town mayor, the school principal, and other civic leaders, along with parents, and tell them they must recognize farm hazards for children
   d. Invite parents, teachers, the school principal, the mayor, and other civic leaders to a meeting to talk about safe play areas for preschool children

7. After suffering a detached retina, Mr. Boucher, 78 years old and a retired farmer, must adapt to his blindness while continuing to live in the rural area with his wife. What is the most important factor that

the nurse should consider to help them rearrange the inside of their house?

  a. The distance separating the couple from their neighbours

  b. The family's beliefs

  c. The availability of resources

  d. Mrs. Boucher's level of literacy

8. What has research shown about the health practices of individuals living in Canadian rural communities in comparison with those in urban communities?

  a. A lower incidence of smoking

  b. Better eating habits

  c. A higher rate of physical activity

  d. A higher incidence of obesity

9. Why is providing health care to inhabitants of rural and remote communities experiencing motor vehicle collisions particularly challenging?

  a. So many new immigrants live in rural communities.

  b. The primary industries are fishing, farming, mining, and forestry.

  c. The population is sparsely distributed over a wide geographical area.

  d. The nurse must be flexible and friendly with local inhabitants.

10. Children in Northern Aboriginal communities are at increased risk for type 2 diabetes. As the nurse in the community, you want to raise awareness about this health risk. What should be your next step?

  a. Talk with the teenagers in the community because they may have younger siblings

  b. Meet with the school principal and launch a poster contest featuring student-drawn pictures of healthy foods

  c. Ask the children to draw pictures of their healthy community and post these on the walls

  d. Ask the children to draw and post pictures of healthy foods that come from their community

Check the eText in MyNursingLab for answers and explanations.

WEBLINKS

Canadian Association for Rural and Remote Nursing

http://www.carrn.com

This site provides access to the Canadian Association for Rural and Remote Nursing. The association is meant to be a voice for rural and remote nursing and to promote the speciality.

Canadian Rural Health Research Society

http://crhrs-scrsr.usask.ca

The Canadian Rural Health Research Society offers the opportunity for researchers engaged in rural, remote, and Northern health research to network with researchers of many disciplines.

Canadian Institute for Health Information

https://www.cihi.ca

Source of many health related reports including DesMeules et al. (2006).

Government of Canada: Canada's Rural Partnership

http://www.rural.gc.ca/home_e.phtml

This site provides access to knowledge, information, programs, and services for and about rural and remote Canada.

International Council of Nurses, Rural and Remote Nursing Network

http://www.icn.ch/networks/rural-and-remote-nursing-network

This site provides a global forum for discussing issues related to rural and remote nursing.

Health Canada: Office of Nursing Services

http://www.hc-sc.gc.ca/ahc-asc/branch-dirgen/fnihb-dgspni/ons-bsi/index_e.html

This office provides support to the First Nations and Inuit Health Branch of Health Canada.

The Development of a Multistakeholder Framework/Index of Rurality

http://www2.cna-aiic.ca/CNA/documents/pdf/publications/Final_Report_e.pdf

This report describes the rural health framework developed by Health Canada, the Canadian Nurses Association (CNA), and the Canadian Medical Association (CMA).

MyNursingLab

REFERENCES

Aboriginal Affairs and Northern Development Canada (2010, September 15). *Fact sheet: Urban Aboriginal population in Canada*. Ottawa, ON: Author. Retrieved from http://www.aadnc-aadnc.gc.ca/eng/1100100014298/1100100014302

Acury, T., Gesler, W., Preisser, J. L., Sherman, J., Spencer, J., & Perrin, J. (2005). The effects of geography and spatial behavior on health care utilization among the residents of a rural region. *Health Services Research, 40*(1), 135–155.

Agriculture and Food, Alberta. (2007). *Bovine spongiform encephalopathy (BSE) fact sheet*. Retrieved from http://www1.agric.gov.ab.ca/$department/deptdocs.nsf/all/cpv8104?opendocument

Alaghehbandan, R., Sikdar, K., MacDonald, D., Collins, K., & Rossignol, A. (2010). Unintentional injuries in children and adolescents in Aboriginal and non-Aboriginal communities, Newfoundland and Labrador, Canada. *International Journal of Circumpolar Health, 69*(1), 61–71.

Alberta Health and Wellness. (1999). *Report on the health of Albertans: Looking through a wider lens*. Edmonton, AB: Government of Alberta, Alberta Health and Wellness.

Ali, K., Rose Olfert, M. R., & Partridge, M. D. (2007). Urban footprints in rural Canada: Employment spillovers by city size. *Regional Studies, 45*(2), 245–260.

Andrews, M. E., Stewart, N., Morgan, D., & D'Arcy, C. (2011). More alike than different: A comparison of male and female RNs in rural and remote Canada. *Journal of Nursing Management, 20*(4), 1–10.

Appleyard, G. D., & Gajadhar, A. A. (2000). A review of trichinellosis in people and wildlife in Canada. *Canadian Journal of Public Health, 91*, 293–297.

Arbuckle, T. E., Bruce, D., Ritter, L., & Hall, J. C. (2006). Indirect sources of herbicide exposure for families on Ontario farms. *Journal of Exposure Science and Environmental Epidemiology, 16*, 98–104.

Atack, L. (2003). Becoming a web-based learner: Registered nurses experiences. *Journal of Advanced Nursing, 44*(3), 289–297.

Beshiri, R., & He, (2009). Immigrants in rural Canada: 2006. *Rural and Small Town Analysis Bulletin, 8*(2), 1–28. Retrieved from http://www.statcan.gc.ca/pub/21-006-x/21-006-x2008002-eng.htm

Blankenau, J. (2010). Comparing rural health and health care in Canada and the United States: The influence of federalism. *The Journal of Federalism, 40*(2), 332–349.

Bollman, W., & Reimer, W. (2009). Demographics, employment, income, and networks: Differential characteristics of rural populations. *Rural and Small Town Analysis Bulletin, 14*(2), 131–142.

Bowd, A. D. (2005). Otitis media: Health and social consequences for Aboriginal youth in Canada's North. *International Journal of Circumpolar Health, 64*(1), 5–15.

Brannen, C., Johnson Emberly, D. J., & McGrath, P. (2009). Stress in rural Canada: A structured review of context stress levels, and sources of stress. *Health & Place, 15*, 219–227.

Brison, R., Pickett, W., Berg, W., Linneman, J., Zentner, J., & Marlenga, B. (2006). Fatal agricultural injuries in preschool children: Risks, injury patterns and strategies for prevention. *Canadian Medical Association Journal, 174*(12), 1723–1726.

Bushy, A. (2000). Behavioral health care: Rural issues and strategies. In A. Bushy (Ed.), *Orientation to nursing in the rural community* (pp. 107–123). Thousand Oaks, CA: Sage Publications.

Campagna, S. (2009). *Prevalence and environmental risk for ten zoonoses in two Cree communities of James Bay (Canada)*. Retrieved from https://www.usherbrooke.ca/environnement/fileadmin/sites/environnement/documents/Essais2009/Campagna_S.pdf

Canadian Agricultural Injury Surveillance Program. (2009). *Agricultural fatal injuries in Canada 1990–2005*. Retrieved from http://cair-sbac.ca/natfull.pdf

Canadian Broadcasting Corporation. (2010). *Robot helps connect Labrador patients, doctors*. Retrieved from http://www.cbc.ca/news/health/story/2010/07/09/nl-rosie-robot-709.html

Canadian Food Inspection Agency. (2005). *Technical overview of BSE in Canada—March 2005*. Retrieved from http://www.inspection.gc.ca/english/anima/heasan/disemala/bseesb/200503canadae.shtml

Carolan, M., Andrews, G., & Hodnett, E. (2006). Writing place: A comparison of nursing research and health geography. *Nursing Inquiry, 13*(3), 203–219.

Carter, L., Rukholm, E., Mossey, S., Viverais-Dresler, G., Bakker, D., & Sheehan, C. (2006). Critical thinking in the online nursing educational setting: Raising the bar. *Canadian Journal of University Continuing Education, 32*(1), 27–46.

Centre for Addiction and Mental Health. (2002). *Alcohol, tobacco and other drug use among Ontario students*. Sheet #2. Toronto, ON: Author.

Chansonneuve, D. (2005), Reclaiming connections: Understanding residential school trauma among Aboriginal people. Retrieved from http://www.ahf.ca/publications/research-series

Crooks, C. (2004). Is rural nursing a speciality? *Online Journal of Rural Nursing and Health Care, 4*(1), 1–4.

DesMeules, M., Pong, R., Legacé, C., Heng, D., Manuel, D., Pitblado, R., ... & Koren, I. (2006). *How healthy are rural Canadians? An assessment of their health status and health determinants*. Ottawa, ON: Canadian Institutes for Health Information.

Dimich-Ward, H., Guernsey, J. R., Pickett, W., Rennie, D., Hartling, L., & Brison, R. J. (2007). Gender differences in the occurrence of farm related injuries. *Occupational and Environmental Medicine, 61*, 52–56.

du Plessis, V., Beshiri, R., Bollman, R. D., & Clemenson, H. (2001). Definitions of rural. *Rural and Small Town Canada Analysis Bulletin, 3*(3).

Eggertson, L. (2008). Despite federal promises, First Nations' water problems persist. *Canadian Medical Association Journal, 178*(8), 985.

Etowa, J., Wiens, J., Thomas Bernard, W., & Clow, B. (2007). Determinants of black women's health in rural and remote communities. *Canadian Journal of Nursing Research, 39*(3), 56–76.

Franche, R. L., Murray, E., Ostry, A., Ratner, P., Wagner, S., & Harder, H. (2010). Work disability prevention in rural health care workers. *The International Electronic Journal of Rural and Remote Health, Education, Practice and Policy, 10*, 1502 (Online).

Garner, R., Carrière, G., & Sanmartin, C. (2010). *The health of First Nations living off-reserve, Inuit, and Métis adults in Canada: The impact of socio-economic status on inequalities in health*. Retrieved from http://www.statcan.gc.ca/pub/82-622-x/82-622-x2010004-eng.htm

Gibson, K., Kakepetum-Schultz, T., Coulson, H., & O'Donnell, S. (2009) Telemental health with remote and rural First Nations: Advantages, disadvantages, and ways forward. Retrieved from National Aboriginal Health Organization: http://nparc.cisti-icist.nrc-cnrc.gc.ca/npsi/ctrl?action=rtdoc&an=15084644

Gregory, D. (2007). *Against the odds: An update on Aboriginal nursing in Canada. Report funded by Canadian Association of Schools of Nursing under the auspices of Health Canada* (First Nations and Inuit Health Branch). Lethbridge, AB: University of Lethbridge.

Hayward, K. (2005). Facilitating interdisciplinary practice through mobile service provision to the rural older adult. *Geriatric Nursing, 26*(1), 29–33.

Health Canada. (2001). *Preventing substance use problems among young people—A compendium of best practices.* Retrieved http://www.hc-sc.gc.ca/hl-vs/pubs/adp-apd/prevent/pattern-tendance_e.html

Hrudey, S. (2008). Safe water? Depends on where you live. *Canadian Medical Association Journal, 178*(8), 975.

Jackman, D., Myrick, F., & Yonge, O. (2010). Rural nursing in Canada: A voice unheard. *Online Journal of Rural Nursing and Health Care, 10*(1), 60–69.

Kirmayer, L., Brass, G., Holton, T., Paul, K., Simpson, C., & Tait, C. (2007). *Suicide among Aboriginal people in Canada.* Retrieved from http://www.ahf.ca/downloads/suicide.pdf 2, or.r_gc.r_pw.&fp=ebd2c2647c16acfc&biw=1073&bih=407

Kosteniuk, J., D'Arcy, C., Stewart, N., & Smith, B. (2006). Central and peripheral information source use among rural and remote registered nurses. *Journal of Advanced Nursing, 55*(1), 100–114.

Kulig, J., Stewart, N., Penz, K., Forbes, D., Morgan, D., & Emerson, P. (2009). Work setting, community attachment, and satisfaction among rural and remote nurses. *Public Health Nursing, 26*(5), 430–439.

Leipert, B., & George, J. (2008). Determinants of rural women's health: A qualitative study in southwest Ontario. *Journal of Rural Health, 24*(2), 210–218.

Leipert, B., & Reutter, L. (2005). Developing resilience: How women maintain their health in northern geographically isolated settings. *Qualitative Health Research, 15*(1), 49–65.

LeJeune, J., & Kersting, A. (2010). Zoonoses: An occupational hazard for livestock workers and a public health concern for rural communities. *Journal of Agricultural Safety and Health, 16*(3), 161–179.

Llewellyn, J. (2002). Dealing with the legacy of native residential school abuse in Canada: Litigation, ADR, and restorative justice. *University of Toronto Law Journal, 52,* 253–300.

Luginaah, I. (2009). Health geography in Canada: Where are we headed? *The Canadian Geographer, 53*(1), 91–99.

MacLeod, M., Kulig, J., Stewart, N., Pitblado, R., Banks, K., D'Arcy, C., & ... Bentham, D. (2004). *The nature of nursing practice in rural and remote Canada.* Ottawa, ON: Canadian Health Services Research Foundation.

Macleod, M., Martin-Meisner, R., Banks, K., Morton, A. M., Vogt, C. & Bentham, D. (2008). "I'm a different kind of nurse": Advice from nurses in rural and remote Canada. *Nursing Leadership, 21*(3), 40–53.

Maltais, V. (2007). Risk factors associated with farm injuries in Canada 1991 to 2001. *Agriculture and Rural Working Paper Series.* Ottawa, ON: Agriculture Division, Statistics Canada.

Martin-Meisner, R., MacLeod, M., Banks, K., Morton, A. M., Vogt, C., & Bentham, D. (2008). "There's rural and then there's rural": Advice from nurses providing health care in rural and remote Canada. *Nursing Leadership, 21*(3), 54–63.

Mitura, V., & Bollman, R. (2004). Health status and behaviours of Canada's youth: A rural-urban comparison. *Rural and Small Town Canada Analysis Bulletin, 5*(3), 1–22.

Montour, A., Baumann, A., Blythe, J., & Hunsberger, M. (2009). The changing nature of nursing work in rural and small community hospitals. *Rural and Remote Health, 9*(1), 1–13.

Pampalon, R., Martinez, J., & Hamel, D. (2006). Does living in rural areas make a difference for health in Quebec? *Health & Place, 12,* 421–435.

Parman, M.S. (2005). Paradise—not without its plagues: Overwhelming blastomycosis pneumonia after visit to lakeside cottages in Northeastern Ontario. *BMC Infectious Diseases, 5*(30). doi:|10.1186/1471-2334-5-30

Penz, K., Stewart, N., D'Arcy, C., & Morgan, D. (2008). Predictors of job satisfaction for rural acute care registered nurses in Canada. *Western Journal of Nursing Research, 30*(7), 785–800.

Pong, R. (2007). *Rural poverty and health: What do we know?* Paper presented to the Standing Senate Committee on Agriculture and Forestry. Ottawa, ON.

Pong, R., DesMeules, M., Legace, C., Heng, D., Manuel, D., Pitblado, R., et al. (2006). *How healthy are rural Canadians? An assessment of their health status and health determinants.* Ottawa: Canadian Institutes for Health Information.

Rainham, D., McDowell, I., Krewski, D., & Sawada, M. (2010). Conceptualizing the healthscape: Contributions of time geography, location technologies and spatial ecology to place and health research. *Social Science & Medicine, 70,* 668–676.

Reimer, M., & Mills, C. (1988). Rural hospital nursing as an elective. *Journal of Rural Health, 4*(2), 5–8. Retrieved from http://www12.statcan.ca/english/ census06/analysis/ aboriginal/ index.cfm

Rukholm, E. (2004). Professional development opportunities. In L. McGillis Hall (Ed.), *Quality work environments for nurse and patient safety* (pp. 163–180). Sudbury, MA: Jones & Bartlett.

Rukholm, E. (2006). *Recruitment and retention of RNs and RPNs in Northeastern Ontario.* A report for the Nursing Secretariat, Ontario Ministry of Health and Long-Term Care. Toronto, ON: Ministry of Health and Long-Term Care. Retrieved from http://www.cranhr.ca/

Russell, A., & Perris, K. (2003). Telementoring in community nursing: A shift from dyadic to communal models of learning and professional development. *Mentoring and Tutoring, 11*(2), 227–237.

Saccente, M., & Woods, G. L. (2010). Clinical and laboratory update on Blastomycosis. *Clinical Microbiology Reviews, 23*(2): 367–381.

Sharpe, A., & Hardt, J. (2006). *Five deaths a day: Workplace fatalities in Canada, 1993–2005.* Ottawa, ON: Center for the Study of Living Standards.

Skinner, M. W., Yantzi, N. M., & Rosenberg, M. W. (2009). Neither rain nor hail nor sleet nor snow: Provider perspectives on the challenges of weather for home and community care. *Social Science & Medicine, 68,* 682–688.

Smith, K., Humphreys, J., & Wilson, M. (2008) Addressing the health disadvantage of rural populations: How does epidemiological evidence inform rural health policies and research? *Australian Journal of Rural Medicine, 16,* 56–66.

Smylie, J., Fell, D., & Ohlsson, A. (2010). A review of Aboriginal infant mortality rates in Canada: Striking and persistent Aboriginal/non-Aboriginal inequities. *Canadian Journal of Public Health 101*(2), 143–148.

Statistics Canada. (2007a). Portrait of the Canadian population in 2006. *Population and dwelling counts, 2006 census.* Ottawa, ON: Author.

Statistics Canada. (2007b). *2006 census of agriculture.* Retrieved from http://www.statcan.ca/ english/agcensus2006/index.htm

Statistics Canada. (2008a). *Canada's ethnocultural mosaic, 2006 census: Findings.* Retrieved from http://www12.statcan.ca/ english/census06/analysis/ethnicorigin/index.cfm

Statistics Canada. (2008b). *Aboriginal peoples in Canada in 2008, Inuit, Métis and First Nations, 2006 census: Findings.* Retrieved from http://www12.statcan.ca/english/census06/analysis/ aboriginal/index.cfm

Statistics Canada. (2008c). *Motor vehicle accident deaths 1979 to 2004.* Retrieved from http://www.statcan.gc.ca/pub/ 82-003-x/2008003/article/10648-eng.htm

Statistics Canada. (2008d). *Suicide and suicide rate, by sex and age group*. Retrieved from http://www40.statcan.ca/l01/cst01/perhlth66a.htm

Statistics Canada (2011, September). *Population by year, by province and territory*. Ottawa, ON: Author. Retrieved from http://www.statcan.gc.ca/tables-tableaux/sum-som/l01/cst01/demo02a-eng.htm

Statistics Canada (2012a). *Canada's rural population since 1851*. Ottawa, ON: Author. Retrieved from http://www12.statcan.gc.ca/census-recensement/2011/as-sa/98-310-x/98-310-x2011003_2-eng.cfm

Statistics Canada (2012b). *2011 Census of agriculture*. Ottawa, ON: Author. Retrieved from http://www.statcan.gc.ca/daily-quotidien/120510/dq120510a-eng.htm

Thomlinson, E., McDonagh, M., Crooks, K., & Lees, M. (2004). Health beliefs of rural Canadians: Implications for practice. *Australian Journal of Rural Health, 12*, 258–263.

Timmins, P., Hogan, A., Duong, L., & Miller, P. (2008). *Occupational health and safety risk factors for rural and metropolitan nurses*. Retrieved from Safe Work Australia: http://www.safeworkaustralia.gov.au/ABOUTSAFEWORKAUSTALIA/WHATWEDO/PUBLICATIONS/pages/RR200811OHSRiskFactorsForRuralAndMetropolitanNurses.aspx

Tjepkema, M., Wilkins, R., Senécal, S.I, Guimond, E., & Penney, C. (2009). Mortality of Métis and Registered Indian adults in Canada: An 11-year follow-up study. *Health Reports, 20*(4), 31–51.

Transport Canada. (2005). *Canadian motor vehicle traffic collision statistics*. Ottawa, ON: Author. Retrieved from http://www.tc.gc.ca/pol/en/t-facts_e/Highways_ Data_Menu.htm

Truth and Reconciliation Commission. (2011). *Mandate of the Truth and Reconciliation Commission*. Retrieved from http://www.trc.ca/websites/trcinstitution/index.php?p=3

Vicente, K., & Christoffersen, K. (2006). The Walkerton *E. coli* outbreak: A test of Rasmussen's framework for risk management in a dynamic society. *Theoretical Issues in Ergonomics Science, 7*(2), 93–112.

Way, D., Jones, L., Baskerville, B., & Busing, N. (2001). Primary health care services provided by nurse practitioners and family physicians in shared practice. *Canadian Medical Association Journal, 165*(9), 1210–1214.

Winters, M., MacIntyre, E., Peters, C., Thom, J., Teschke, K., & Davies, H. (2005). *Noise and hearing loss in farming*. Retrieved from http://www.cher.ubc.ca/PDFs/FARSHAFinalRevised.pdf

Chapter 16

Complementary and Alternative Health Modalities

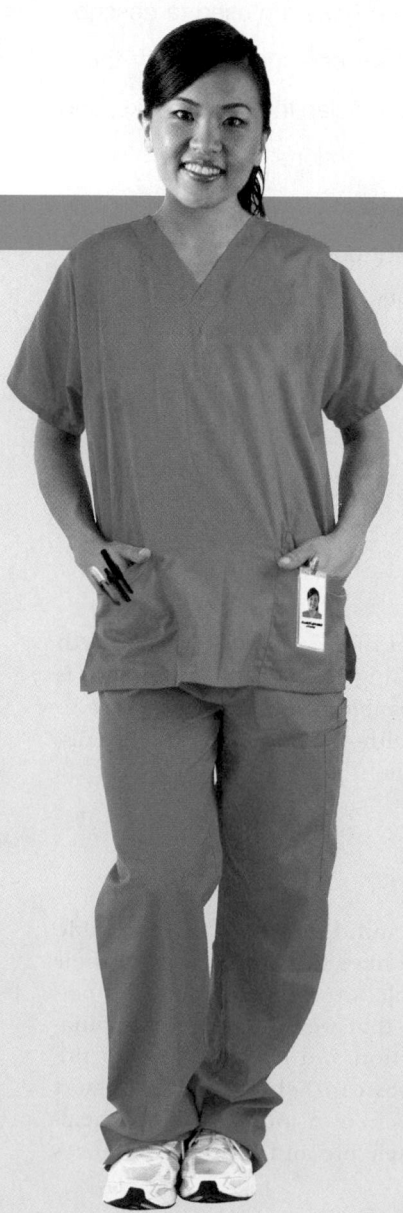

LEARNING OUTCOMES

After studying this chapter, you will be able to:

1. Describe the terms *complementary medicine, alternative medicine*, and *integrative medicine*.

2. Explain the basic concepts of complementary and alternative health modalities: holism, humanism, balance, spirituality, energy, and healing environments.

3. Describe the key principles and clinical application used in complementary and alternative health modalities: whole medical systems, biological-based treatment, nutritional therapy, manual healing methods, mind–body therapies, and spiritual therapy.

4. Describe the role of Health Canada in complementary and alternative medicine.

5. Explain why natural health products should be used with care.

6. Discuss the role of the nurse in teaching clients the uses and safety precautions regarding complementary health modalities.

As our Canadian population becomes increasingly older and more ethnically diverse, more and more Canadians are using complementary and alternative health modalities (CAHM). Some of the reasons for clients to use CAHM are an increase in chronic illnesses, better access to information, and personal and cultural beliefs to control one's own health (Boon, Verhoef, Vanderheyden, & Westlake, 2006; McFarland, Bigelow, Zani, Newsom, & Kaplan, 2002). Yet, not many nurses are prepared to assist clients to obtain alternative medical therapies and, as a result, may lack information or even harbour misinformation (Canadian Nurses' Association [CNA], 2008a). In response to this trend, Health Canada (2011) has been raising awareness among Canadians about natural health products (NHPs) and regulating the safety and efficacy of these products. Most provincial and territorial nursing associations also have developed position statements on the provision of holistic therapies. Thus, nurses must understand the different interventions that complement Western medicine and their potential risks and benefits. They must also practise within their professional guidelines to provide safe and effective nursing care.

In this chapter, the terms *complementary medicine* and *alternative medicine* are used to describe as many as 1800 therapies that have been practised around the world for centuries. Many of these modalities originated from ancient medical systems of Egyptians, Chinese, Asian Indians, Greeks, and Aboriginal peoples. **Complementary medicine** is used *together with* conventional or Western medicine. For example, the scent of essential oils from flowers or herbs used in aromatherapy can help promote relaxation and well-being. **Alternative medicine** is used *in place of* conventional medicine. An example of an alternative therapy is the use of acupuncture for back pain relief instead of surgery, as recommended by the health care provider. **Integrative medicine** combines treatments from Western medicine and complementary and alternative medicine (CAM) to achieve maximum safety and effectiveness of care (National Institutes of Health, 2010).

Basic Concepts

Several concepts are common to most alternative health practices. These are holism, humanism, balance, spirituality, energy, and healing environments.

Holism

Holism refers to the combining of mental, emotional, spiritual, relationship, and environmental components, and individuals are central to their own healing. **Holistic health** involves the whole of the person's being and the overall quality of life. **Holistic health care** considers all the components of health: health promotion, health maintenance, health education, illness prevention, restorative care, and palliation. The focus of interventions is to enhance the healing of the whole person from birth to death. Florence Nightingale noted, ". . . nursing is putting us in the best possible conditions for nature to restore or to preserve health—to prevent or to cure disease or injury" (Nightingale, 1954/1982, p. 334).

Humanism

The **humanist** views the mind and body as indivisible and believes that people have the power to solve their own problems, that people are responsible for the patterns of their lives, and that well-being is a combination of personal satisfaction and contributions to the larger community. Nurses can help consumers assert their right to choose their own journey toward healing and the quality of their life and death experiences (Fontaine, 2010).

Balance

The concept of **balance** consists of mental, physical, emotional, spiritual, and environmental components. Balance is attained when each component reaches a state of equilibrium. *Physical* aspects include optimal functioning of all body systems. *Emotional* aspects include the ability to feel and express the entire range of human emotions. *Mental* aspects include feelings of self-worth, a positive identity, a sense of accomplishment, and the ability to appreciate and create. *Spiritual* aspects involve moral values, a meaningful purpose in life, and a feeling of connectedness to others and to a divine source. *Environmental* aspects include physical, biological, economic, social, and political conditions. Being in balance is a learned skill and must be practised regularly to engage in the process of healthful living.

Spirituality

Spiritual healing techniques and spirituality-based health care systems are among the most ancient healing practices. Spirit is the liveliness and richness of one's life. **Spirituality** includes the drive to become all that we can be, and it is bound to intuition, creativity, and motivation. It is the dimension that involves relationship with the self, with others, and with a higher power. Spirituality gives people meaning and purpose in their lives. It involves finding significant meaning in the entirety of life, including illness and death (see Chapter 47).

Energy

For centuries, in most cultures, **energy** has been viewed as the force that integrates and connects body, mind, and spirit. Chinese Taoist scholars believed that energy was the basic building material of the universe. Albert Einstein and other physicists proved that matter and energy are the same and that energy is not only the raw material of the cosmos but also the glue that holds it together. People are beings of energy, living in a universe composed of energy.

Grounding and *centring* are common terms used in various healing practices. *Grounding* relates to a person's connection with the ground and, in a broader sense, to that person's whole contact with reality. The phrase "being grounded" suggests stability, security, independence, the presence of a solid foundation, and the ability to live in the present rather than escape into dreams. *Centring* refers to the process of focusing the mind on the centre of energy, allowing the person to operate intuitively, with awareness, and to channel energy throughout the body. When people are centred, they are fully connected to the part of their bodies where all their energies meet.

Healing Environments

Nursing has always focused on creating healing environments for clients. Nurses create these environments by providing compassionate and holistic care through the use of their hands, hearts, and minds. Nurses must also create healing environments for themselves. Working with people can be draining work. Nurses need to learn how to restore their energy and replenish themselves to avoid burnout. (See Box 16.1.)

BOX 16.1 SELF-HEALING METHODS FOR NURSES

- Check your posture. Sit up, or stand straight. Imagine that a cord is attached to the top of your head, pulling it gently toward the sky. This image helps readjust your posture.

- Boost your energy. Take your shoes off; sit on the floor with your legs stretched out in front of you and your palms facing down at your sides. Point your toes as hard as you can and hold for 5 seconds, then dorsiflex your feet as hard as you can and hold for 5 seconds. Repeat 10 times.

- Check your breathing. Sit comfortably and close your eyes. Note your breathing without trying to change it. Breathe in, and breathe out. Feel your breath flowing in and out of your heart. Do this for 5 to 10 minutes.

Complementary and Alternative Health Modalities

Ethnocentrism, the assumption that one's own cultural or ethnic group is superior to others, has often prevented Western health care practitioners from learning new ways to promote health and prevent chronic illness. With consumers demanding a broader range of health options, health care providers must be open and learn about various complementary health modalities being practised in other cultures and countries for disease prevention and treatment. The World Health Organization (WHO, 2010) endorses traditional healing practices that have been used in various cultures in many communities for thousands of years; however, there are challenges (see Box 16.2 on the next page). The Nursing and Canadian Society box on the next page outlines some of the nursing implications with the increasing use of NHPs among Canadians.

The National Center for Complementary and Alternative Medicine (NCCAM) of the National Institutes of Health (NIH) in the United States has grouped complementary and alternative health modalities into five major categories: (a) whole medical systems, (b) biologically based treatments, (c) manipulative and body-based therapies, (d) energy therapies, and (e) mind–body interventions.

BOX 16.2   TRADITIONAL MEDICINE: KEY FACTS AND WHO RESPONSE

The WHO outlined some key facts of traditional medicine around the world and WHO's response.

KEY FACTS

- In some Asian and African countries, 80% of the population depend on traditional medicine for primary health care.

- In many developed countries, 70% to 80% of the population has used some form of alternative or complementary medicine (e.g., acupuncture).

- Herbal treatments are the most popular form of traditional medicine and are highly lucrative in the international marketplace. Annual revenues in Western Europe reached US$5 billion in 2003–2004. In China, sales of products totalled US$14 billion in 2005. Herbal medicine revenue in Brazil was US$160 million in 2007.

- Counterfeit, poor-quality, or adulterated herbal products in international markets are serious threats to patient safety.

- More than 100 countries have regulations for herbal medicines.

WHO RESPONSE

Traditional medicine has been used in some communities for thousands of years. As traditional medicine practices are adopted by new populations, there are challenges concerning international diversity; national policy and regulation; safety, effectiveness, and quality; knowledge and sustainability; and patient safety and use. The WHO aims to do the following:

- Support and integrate traditional medicine into national health systems in combination with national policy and regulation for products, practices, and providers to ensure safety and quality.

- Ensure the use of safe, effective, and good-quality products and practices, based on available evidence.

- Acknowledge traditional medicine as part of primary health care, to increase access to care and preserve knowledge and resources.

- Ensure patient safety by upgrading the skills and knowledge of traditional medicine providers.

Source: Excerpts based on World Health Organization. (2010). Traditional medicine. *Fact sheet No. 134, December 2008.* Copyright by the World Health Organization. Retrieved from http://www.who.int/mediacentre/factsheets/fs134/en

Nursing and Canadian Society

Fact	Implications for Nursing Practice
Nearly 71% of Canadians consume NHPs, such as vitamins and minerals, herbal remedies, and other complementary or alternative therapies, for disease prevention, health maintenance, and treatment of illnesses; 12% reported experiencing unwanted side effects, and only 41% of these reported them (Health Canada, 2011).	By understanding the interaction between natural and pharmaceutical products, nurses can offer informed advice to clients about self-care decisions. Nurses must also be culturally sensitive to the unique health care beliefs and practices with regard to CAHM among cultural groups.
A majority of Canadians (81%) think that the use of NHPs will increase over the next 10 years, and 7 in 10 (72%) believe that Canadians have the right to use any NHP they choose (Health Canada, 2011).	Nurses need to be aware of their provincial or territorial nursing guidelines regarding alternative and complementary therapies to ensure that their advice is ethically sound and that their services fall within their scope of practice.
The costs of complementary and alternative therapies are rarely covered by provincial, territorial, or private health insurance plans.	Nurses need to know how to access information on the credentials of therapists and the costs of these therapies.
The most commonly used manual therapies in Canada are chiropractic and massage therapy, but physicians know very little about these therapies (Verhoef, 2005).	Manual therapies have clinical importance in treating clients. Health care providers can advance integrative health care through developing interprofessional education, and interdisciplinary practice, research, and education (Verhoef, 2005; Willison, 2008).

Whole Medical Systems

A number of health care practices have been systematized throughout the centuries and throughout the world. These typically include an entire set of values, attitudes, and beliefs that generate a philosophy of life, not simply a group of remedies.

AYURVEDA   The Indian system of medicine, Ayurveda, is at least 2500 years old. **Ayurveda** views illness as a state of imbalance among the body's systems. The individual aims to minimize stress by achieving an optimal balance of emotional health, physical health, spiritual health, mental health, and environmental health. Specific lifestyle interventions are a major preventive and therapeutic approach in Ayurveda. Each person is prescribed an individualized diet and exercise program depending on *dosha* (body) type and the nature of the underlying dosha imbalance. Herbal preparations are added to the diet for preventive or regenerative purposes as well as for the treatment of specific disorders. Yoga, breathing exercises, and meditative techniques are also prescribed by the practitioner.

TRADITIONAL CHINESE MEDICINE   **Traditional Chinese medicine (TCM)** has been practised in China for more than 3000 years. TCM sees the body as a delicate balance of *yin* and *yang*: two opposing but inseparable forces. *Yin* represents the cold, slow, or passive principle, while *yang* represents the hot, excited, or active principle. Health is achieved by maintaining the body in a balanced state, and disease is caused by an internal imbalance of yin and yang. This imbalance leads to blockage in the flow of *qi* (pronounced *chee*), or vital energy, and of blood along pathways known as *meridians*.

TCM views a person's mind, body, spirit, and emotions as inseparable. The heart is not just a blood pump; it also influences a person's capacity for joy, a sense of purpose in life, and connectedness with others. Kidneys filter fluids, but they also manage the capacity for fear, will and motivation, and faith in life. Lungs breathe in air and breathe out waste products, but they also regulate the capacity to grieve, as well as a person's acknowledgment of the self and of others. The liver cleanses the body, and it also influences feelings of anger, vision, and creativity. The stomach has a part in the digestion of food and influences the ability to be thoughtful, kind, and nurturing as well. These are just a few of the mind–body connections that TCM practitioners recognize.

TCM practitioners use a variety of ancient and modern therapeutic methods, including acupuncture, acupressure, herbal medicine, massage, heat therapy, qigong, Tai Chi, and nutritional lifestyle counselling. Multiple herbs in combinations may be used to treat individual clients.

TRADITIONAL ABORIGINAL HEALING Spirituality and medicine are inseparable in Aboriginal healing. Medicine women and men see themselves as channels through which the Great Power helps others achieve well-being in mind, body, and spirit. The only healer is the One, who created all things. Medicine people consider that they have certain knowledge to put things together to help the sick person heal and that knowledge has to be dispensed in a certain way, often through ritual or ceremony. Healers use medicine objects to assist them and ceremony treatments, such as the sweat lodge, singing, the pipe ceremony, the sun dance, and the vision quest. Other treatments include smudging, drumming and chanting, healing lodges, healing touch, acupressure, and herbs.

Health is viewed as a balance or harmony of mind and body. The goal is to be in harmony with all things, which means first being in harmony with oneself. If the mind is negative, the body will be drained, making it more vulnerable. When people open up to the universe, learn what is good for them, and find ways to be happier, they can begin to work toward a longer and healthier life (see the section "Aboriginal Views of Wellness" in Chapter 7).

HOMEOPATHY Homeopathy is a self-healing system, assisted by small doses of remedies or medicines, which is useful in treating a variety of acute and chronic disorders. It is based on the premises of the *law of similar*, which claims that a natural substance that produces a given symptom in a healthy person cures it in a sick person.

If taken in large amounts, these natural compounds will produce symptoms of disease.

Natural healing compounds are prepared through a process of serial dilution. The compound is first dissolved in a water–alcohol mixture called the *mother tincture*. One drop of the tincture is then mixed with 10 drops of the water–alcohol mixture, and this process is repeated hundreds or thousands of times, depending on the potency of the compound being prepared. The homeopathic belief is that the more the substance is diluted, the more potent it becomes as a remedy. It is not currently understood how homeopathic remedies work.

NATUROPATHY Naturopathic medicine "blends modern scientific knowledge with traditional and natural forms of medicine. It is based on the healing power of nature and it supports and stimulates the body's ability to heal itself" (Canadian Association of Naturopathic Doctors, 2011, para.1). Based on the individual clients' physiological, structural, psychological, social, spiritual, environmental, and lifestyle factors, the treatment goal is to promote health through diet and exercise rather than through the application of a particular therapy. This may involve botanical medicine, homeopathy, clinical nutrition, hydrotherapy, naturopathic manipulation, TCM and acupuncture, and prevention and lifestyle counselling. Clients are given the responsibility for their own health and well-being, and traditional pharmaceuticals and surgical interventions are rarely used. In Canada, practitioners of naturopathic medicine are primary health care providers trained at an accredited school of naturopathic medical in a four-year, full-time program; they are required to pass licensing board exams to practise.

Biologically Based Treatments

Botanical (plant) healings are used by 80% of the world's population. These include herbs, aromatherapy, homeopathy, and naturopathy. **Herbal medicine** refers to the use of herbs to treat disease and supplement other treatments. **Herbal therapy** is used to prevent disease or promote health through the routine use of herbs.

HERBAL MEDICINE Herbs have been used by humans since antiquity for the prevention and treatment of illness. Herbs or botanicals are plants that are valued for their medicinal properties, flavour, scent, and so on. Herbs contain dozens of bioactive compounds. It is often not clear which of these compounds underlie an herb's medical use. More than 10 000 herbs have been identified as useful for medicinal purposes. Over 30% of all prescription drugs sold in North America are derived from plants.

Health Canada (2011) plays a key role in ensuring that Canadians have access to high-quality, safe, and effective NHPs while respecting culturally oriented health care practices. Under the 2004 Natural Health Products Regulations, **natural health products (NHPs)** include vitamins and minerals, herbal remedies, homeopathic medicines, traditional medicines, probiotics, and other products such as amino acids and essential fatty acids.

The determination of the safety and efficacy of herbal products presents a challenge, as herbal experts often disagree on how to interpret the varying evidence available for many types of herbal remedies (WHO, 2010). Most herbs are consumed without untoward reactions when they are taken in small amounts. It is when the product is consumed in excessive amounts that problems arise.

With the current proliferation of lay literature on herbal remedies and the wide availability of such products in health food stores, more people are relying on herbal and other less conventional therapies for a wide variety of problems. Health care professionals must become aware of their clients' use of herbs and be knowledgeable, using evidence-based practice by referring to resources such as Health Canada (2009), the Canadian Adverse Reaction Newsletter, and MedEffect Canada. See Table 16.1 for some of the more commonly used herbs.

AROMATHERAPY **Aromatherapy** is the therapeutic use of plant essential oils, in which the odour or fragrance plays an important part. The essential oils that are used in aromatherapy are plant oils extracted from flowers, roots, bark, leaves, wood resins, and lemon or orange rinds. The oils are massaged into skin, inhaled, placed in baths, used as compresses, or mixed into ointments. The chemicals in the essential oils are absorbed into the body, resulting in physiological or psychological benefit. Different oils calm, stimulate, improve sleep, change eating habits, or boost the immune system.

Nurses should be aware of the potential complications from using certain oils and caution clients about their use and storage. Essential oils, other than lavender and tea tree oil, are quite potent and can irritate skin. They should be diluted with a carrier oil before being used on skin. Carrier oils, such as sunflower oil, grapeseed oil, and soy oil, contain vitamins, proteins, and minerals that provide added nutrients to the body. Essential oils should not be ingested because even modest amounts can be fatal. Pregnant women and people with epilepsy should consult a knowledgeable health care practitioner or qualified aromatherapist before using essential oils. Some oils can trigger bronchial spasms, so people with asthma should consult their primary health care provider before using oils. Table 16.2 describes oils that may be used at home.

DIETARY THERAPY **Dietary therapy**, or nutritional therapy, consists of the consumption of specific types of diets (see Chapter 40) or supplements—including vitamins, minerals, amino acids, herbs and other botanicals, and miscellaneous substances, such as enzymes and fish oils—to prevent or treat illness. The therapy focuses on

TABLE 16.1 Uses, Cautions, and Contraindications for Popular Herbal Preparations

Herb	Traditional Uses	Selected Warnings
Feverfew	Prevents migraine headaches, arthritis; stimulates digestion	May increase the anticoagulant effects of aspirin and anticoagulant medications
Garlic	Reduces high blood pressure and cholesterol; antibiotic/antifungal; anticlotting	May increase the anticoagulant effects of aspirin and anticoagulant medications
Ginger	For digestion; relieves motion sickness, dizziness, and nausea	May increase the anticoagulant effects of aspirin and anticoagulant medications
Ginkgo	May improve memory function, relieve stress, treat dizziness	May increase the anticoagulant effects of aspirin and anticoagulant medications
Echinacea	May boost the immune system, enhance wound healing	May reduce the effectiveness of immunosuppressants; has not been found effective in treating colds in children ages 2 to 11 years
Ginseng	Stimulates mental activity; enhances immune system and appetite	May interact with caffeine and cause irritability; may decrease the effectiveness of glaucoma medications
Milk thistle	Enhances flow in gallbladder, liver, spleen, and stomach	Reduces the effectiveness of oral contraceptives
St. John's wort	Acts as antidepressant, antiinflammatory; is antiviral	May potentiate antidepressant medications, causing severe agitation, nausea, confusion, and possible cardiac problems
Saw palmetto	Treats prostate hypertrophy; antiinflammatory	May give false low prostate-specific antigen (PSA) levels, thereby delaying diagnosis of prostate cancer
Valerian	Sedative, tranquilizer; lowers blood pressure; helps menstrual cramps	May increase the sedative effects of antianxiety medication

TABLE 16.2 Oils That May Be Useful to Have at Home

Oil	Use
Chamomile	Soothes muscle aches, sprains, swollen joints; acts as gastrointestinal (GI) antispasmodic; can be rubbed on abdomen for colic, indigestion, gas; decreases anxiety, stress-related headaches; decreases insomnia; can be used in children
Eucalyptus	Feels cool to skin and warm to muscles; decreases fever; relieves pain; antiinflammatory; antiseptic, antiviral, and expectorant to respiratory system in steam inhalation; boosts immune system
Ginger	Helps ward off colds; calms upset stomach, decreases nausea; soothes sprains and muscle spasms
Jasmine	Is uplifting and stimulating, antidepressant; can be used to massage abdomen and lower back to treat menstrual cramps
Lavender	Is calming, sedative for insomnia; can be used to massage around temples for headache; can be inhaled to speed recovery from colds, flu; can be used to massage chest to decrease congestion; heals burns
Tea Tree	Works as an antifungal agent for athlete's foot; soothes insect bites, stings, cuts, wounds; can be used in baths for yeast infection; is used as drops on handkerchief for relief from coughs, congestion

eating more fresh vegetables, fruits, and whole grains. A variety of diets are offered for treating cancer, cardiovascular disease, and food allergies. In many cases, diet therapy mirrors traditional dietary and medical advice: reducing excessive use of sugar and salt, reducing excess fat, increasing the intake of fruit and vegetables, and stressing the need for a well-balanced diet.

Not all nutritional supplements are harmless. Three major concerns regarding the use of nutritional supplements by clients are (a) efficacy, (b) consistency, and (c) safety (Health Canada, 2011; WHO, 2010). Evidence to determine the effectiveness of supplements remains inconclusive. Supplements manufactured by different companies often contain a variety of substances in varying amounts; and there are no legal definitions for the words *standardized*, *certified*, or *verified* for supplements. Some supplements cause adverse effects, such as diarrhea or high blood pressure, and some others become dangerous when taken in combination with certain medications. Another safety concern with supplements is that they may be contaminated with dangerous substances, such as mould, bacteria, pesticides, and metals (Rolfes, Pinna, & Whitney, 2009). Nurses must assess clients for use of dietary supplements and include teaching about the supplements, their known benefits, and risks of supplements in the care planning.

Manipulative and Body-Based Therapies

Some manual healing methods come from ancient times, and some were developed in the latter half of the twentieth century. These healing practices include chiropractic; massage; acupuncture, acupressure, and reflexology; and hand-mediated biofield therapies.

CHIROPRACTIC THERAPY **Chiropractic therapy** is the third-largest independent health profession in the Western world, after conventional medicine and dentistry. Chiropractic doctors focus on the spine and its relationship to the component bone structures, muscles, and nerves. Chiropractors believe that displacements of the spine can result in a variety of symptoms that can be treated by spinal manipulation or adjustment. Three primary goals guide chiropractic intervention. The *first* goal is to reduce or eliminate pain. The *second* goal is to correct the spinal dysfunction thereby restoring biomechanical balance to re-establish shock absorption, leverage, and range of motion. In addition, muscles and ligaments are strengthened by spinal rehabilitative exercises to increase resistance to further injury. The *third* goal is preventive maintenance to ensure the problem does not recur.

Clients need to be aware of the benefits and limitations of chiropractic care. Chiropractors work with many facets of clients' lifestyles. Exercise programs are designed, rehabilitation measures are planned, correct posture and lifting techniques are explained, and activities of daily living are assessed and improved.

MASSAGE Healing through touch, or massage, goes back to early civilization. Touch is an important part of healing. One possible explanation is that touch stimulates the production of certain chemicals in the immune system that promote healing.

Therapeutic Massage Physically, **massage** relaxes muscles and releases the buildup of lactic acid that accumulates during exercise (see Figure 16.1). It can also improve

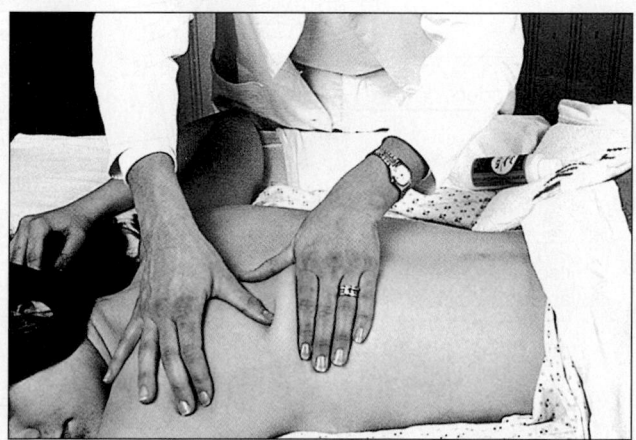

FIGURE 16.1 Massage over the shoulder and back.

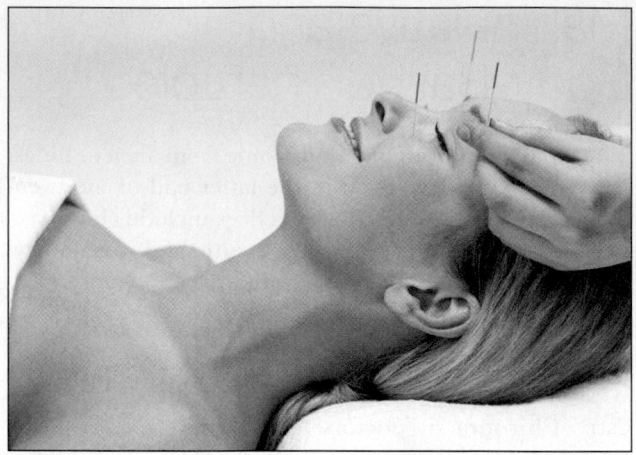

FIGURE 16.2 Acupuncture involves the insertion of thin, sterile needles.

blood and lymph circulation, stretch joints, and relieve pain and congestion. On the emotional level, massage can relieve anxiety and provide a sense of relaxation and well-being (Fontaine, 2010). Spiritually, it provides a sense of harmony and balance. Individuals receiving a massage may enter a meditative state, which relaxes their minds and expands their awareness. A variety of massage strokes or movements can be used singly or in combination, depending on the outcome desired. These include *effleurage* (stroking), friction, pressure, *petrissage* (kneading, or large, quick pinches of the skin, subcutaneous tissue, and muscle), and **Tui Na** (an oriental massage using a series of pressing, tapping, and kneading with palms, fingertips, knuckles, or implements that help remove blockages along the meridians of the body and stimulate

the flow of qi and blood to promote healing). Almost anyone can benefit from massage (see the Lifespan Considerations box).

ACUPUNCTURE, ACUPRESSURE, AND REFLEXOLOGY

Acupuncture and **acupressure** are techniques of applying pressure or stimulation to specific points on the body, known as *acupuncture points*, to relieve pain, cure certain illnesses, and promote wellness. Acupuncture uses needles (see Figure 16.2), whereas acupressure uses finger pressure. **Reflexology** is a form of acupressure most commonly performed on feet, but hands or ears may also be manipulated. See Figure 16.3 for foot reflex areas.

Acupuncture, acupressure, and reflexology are treatments rooted in the traditional Eastern philosophy that qi flows through the body along the meridians. This leads to the formation of tiny whirlpools close to the skin's surface at the acupuncture points, which function somewhat like gates to moderate the flow of qi.

When the flow of energy becomes blocked or congested, people experience discomfort or pain on the physical level, may feel frustrated or irritable on the emotional level, and may experience a sense of vulnerability or lack of purpose in life on the spiritual level. The goal of care in wellness acupuncture is to recognize and manage the disruption before illness or disease occurs. Practitioners bring balance to the body's energies, which promotes optimal health and well-being, and facilitates people's own healing capacity (Dale, 2009). A systemic review and a number of clinical trials have reported that acupuncture increases the chance of pregnancy in women undergoing in vitro fertilization (Manheimer et al., 2008), improves symptoms of dyspnea (Suzuki et al., 2008),

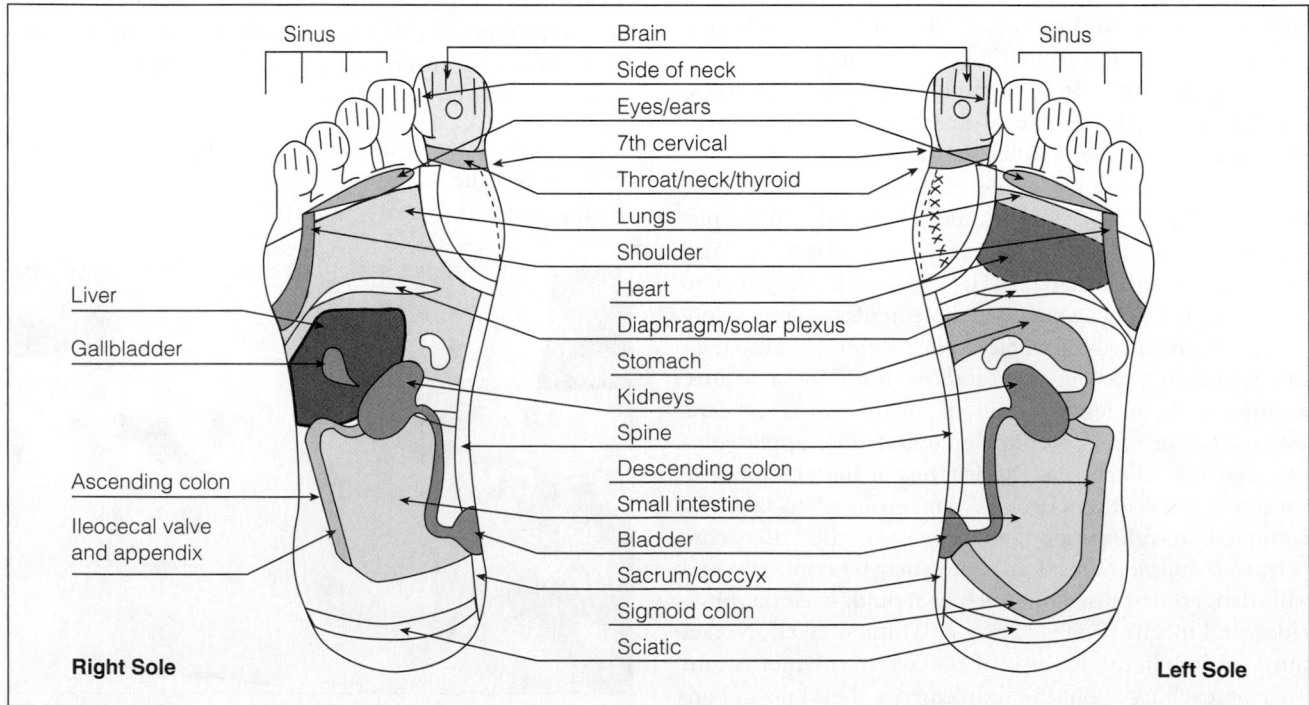

FIGURE 16.3 Foot reflex areas.

Examples of the Uses of Massage

Following are a few of the many examples illustrating the uses of massage in children, adults, and older adults.

CHILDREN

Infant massage is gaining in popularity in Canada. Infant massage stimulates weight gain in premature infants, reduces complications in "cocaine babies" (infants born to mothers addicted to cocaine), and helps mothers soothe their babies. It improves parent–infant bonding; eases painful procedures, such as immunizations; reduces pain from teething and constipation; reduces colic; induces sleep; and makes parents feel they are doing something good for their baby.

ADULTS

- Although massage relaxes the prenatal woman, it is usually contraindicated until after the first trimester of pregnancy because of the danger of miscarriage during that time. During the second and third trimesters, massage can ease pain and provide comfort to the pregnant woman. Pregnancy massage is usually done with the client in the side-lying position, with plenty of pillows or cushions for support. The massage usually is done to the neck, arms and hands, back, pelvis, legs, and feet. Since not all massage therapists are trained in pregnancy massage, consumers must ask about the experience and credentials of a particular therapist.

- Massage has become popular among athletes. Prior to an athletic event, massage loosens, warms, and readies the athlete's muscle for intensive use, especially when combined with stretching. Besides helping prevent injury, it can improve performance and endurance. Postevent massage relieves pain, prevents stiffness, and returns the muscles to their normal state more rapidly. The use of massage in sports health care is increasing rapidly in both training and competition. Recreational athletes have also discovered the benefits of sports massage as a regular part of their workouts.

OLDER ADULTS

A randomized study of the effects of massage on well-being and stress perception among older adults found that there was significant improvement in the massage group (50-minute massages twice a week for four weeks) compared with the control group (guided relaxation sessions for the same frequency). The massage group demonstrated improvement in anxiety, depression, vitality, general health, and positive well-being on the General Well-being Schedule and the Perceived Stress Scale (Sharpe, Williams, Granner, & Hussey, 2007).

decreases pain (Singh et al., 2006), and improves memory, orientation, and the ability to perform the activities of daily living (Yu, Zhang, Liu, Meng, & Han, 2006). (See the Evidence-Informed Practice box.)

QIGONG AND TAI CHI A number of therapies focus on movement, body awareness, and breathing, and their purpose is to maintain health as well as to correct specific problems. **Qigong** (pronounced *chee goong*) is a Chinese discipline consisting of breathing and mental exercises combined with body movements. **Tai Chi** (pronounced

What Is the State of Research on Complementary and Alternative Medicine in Pediatric Rheumatology?

The authors conducted a comprehensive literature review on the use of complementary and alternative medicine in pediatric rheumatology. Between 1994 and 2003, pediatric CAHM use increased from 10% to 35%, depending on the study and country (e.g., about 2% of children in the United States, 11% in Canada, 18% in the United Kingdom, and 31% in Australia). Children with chronic illnesses and adolescents (with or without chronic disease) were frequent users. Overall, evidence suggests between 34% to 92% use pediatric CAHM. However, the results seem only promising in such treatments as massage, acupuncture, mind–body interventions (e.g., guided imagery and meditative breathing) and in some natural health products. The efficacy and safety of CAHM are still inconclusive.

NURSING IMPLICATIONS: Further research is needed for high-quality trials to investigate the long-term effects and underlying mechanisms of these CAHM therapies and their use in this population. Nurses must be knowledgeable about the potential benefits and harms of natural and pharmaceutical products and adhere to their practice guidelines when assisting their clients to make decisions regarding the safe use of CAHM.

Source: Based on April, K. T. & Walji, R. (2011). The state of research on complementary and alternative medicine in pediatric rheumatology. *Rheumatic Diseases Clinics of North America, 37*(1), 85–94. doi:10.1016/j.rdc.2010.11.011

teye chee) arose out of qigong and is a discipline that combines physical fitness, meditation, and self-defence. Both disciplines consist of soft, slow, continuous movements that are circular in nature. The slowness of movements requires attentive control that quiets the mind and develops the person's powers of awareness and concentration. The continuous circular nature of the movements develops strength, balance, and endurance. Almost anyone can participate in movement-oriented therapies.

These movement-oriented therapies can be learned by the young and by seniors, by people with physical challenges or who are physically fit, and by those in good health and those recovering from long-term injury or illness. These Eastern practices can be done alone, in pairs, or in large groups.

Energy Therapies

The three most prominent therapies that use the hands to alter the biofield, or energy field, are (a) therapeutic touch (TT), (b) healing touch, and (c) reiki. The goals are to accelerate the person's own healing process and to facilitate healing at all levels of body, mind, emotions, and spirit. These treatments are designed neither to diagnose physical conditions nor to replace conventional surgery, medicine, or drugs in treating organic or pathological disease.

THERAPEUTIC TOUCH Noncontact **therapeutic touch (TT)** is a process by which practitioners believe they can transmit energy to a person who is ill or injured to potentiate the healing process. TT involves four steps:

1. *Centring* to achieve a sense of detachment, sensitivity, and balance
2. *Assessing* the client's energy field from head to toe by moving the palms of both hands 5 to 15 cm above the client's skin surface
3. *Mobilizing* or unruffling the client's congestive energy field by moving the hands in sweeping motion from the pressure field down along the long bones of the body
4. *Transferring energy* from the practitioner to the client over the identified area of congestion to help the client regain balance in the energy field and to promote healing

HEALING TOUCH **Healing touch** is a group of noninvasive energy-based techniques that incorporate TT. Healing touch can be helpful in promoting relaxation, reducing pain, and managing stress.

REIKI Reiki (*ray-key*), a Japanese word for "universal life force," is a healing technique that channels life energy to someone through the hands. It is a stress-reduction and relaxation technique that taps into the client's own life-force energy to improve health and enhance quality of life.

BIOELECTROMAGNETIC THERAPIES **Bioelectromagnetic therapies** involve the use of electromagnetic fields, such as pulsed fields, magnetic fields, or alternating current or direct current fields, in people with diseases ranging from asthma and arthritis, to poisoning and tubal pregnancy, to wrinkles. It is thought that some types of illness and pain are associated with imbalances in biological electric and magnetic fields. Bioelectromagnetic therapy realigns the fields to correct imbalances through the application of magnets, the use of lasers or direct electrical stimulation, and even the ingestion of magnetized liquids.

Magnetic therapy is one of the most common of the bioelectromagnetic therapies, and it involves the application of magnets to the body to stimulate the nerves to create a better blood flow to various parts of the body. Common magnetic therapies involve the use of bracelets, mattress pads, necklaces, bands, and so on, with magnets placed in them, which are then worn on the body or, in the case of mattress pads, slept on. Currently, there is no scientific evidence that supports the use of magnets for pain relief. However, some argue that the effects may depend on the type and strength of the magnets used, and the frequency and duration the magnet was applied (National Centre for Complementary and Alternative Medicine, 2010).

Mind–Body Interventions

The following mind–body interventions guide the individuals to focus on realigning or creating balance in mental processes to bring about healing.

YOGA The word **yoga** refers to the uniting of all the powers of the body, mind, and spirit. Yoga has been practised for thousands of years in India. It is an approach to living a balanced life that includes mental and physical exercises aimed at producing spiritual enlightenment. Yoga has many different schools. Each school stresses a different technique, but all have as their goal the mastery of self. Yoga can be a series of gentle stretching exercises to breathing techniques, hot yoga, or antigravity yoga. The Western approach to yoga tends to be more fitness oriented, with the goal of managing stress, learning to relax, and increasing vitality and well-being. Individuals interested in beginning yoga are advised to explore the specific program offered to ensure that it includes the techniques most suited to their needs. Clinical studies have found that yoga can improve cardiovascular fitness and psychological well-being in older adults (Buranruk et al., 2010), as well as improve sleep quality, alleviate depression, and enhance self-perception of health status (Chen et al., 2009).

HYPNOSIS **Hypnosis** is a trance state, or an altered state of consciousness, in which an individual's concentration is focused and distraction is minimized. People in trances are aware of what is going on around them but choose not to focus on it. They can return to normal awareness whenever they choose. Hypnosis is not a surrender of control; it is only an advanced form of relaxation. It can be used to help people gain self-control, improve self-esteem, and become more autonomous. Hypnosis is routinely used with a variety of clients with different medical problems, usually in conjunction with other forms of medical, surgical, psychiatric, or psychological treatment. It can be used with clients with nonmedical problems as well for the management of such problems as performance anxiety or for changing bad habits, such as smoking. Depending on the complexity and seriousness of the complaint, treatment typically runs from 2 to 10 sessions.

MEDITATION **Meditation** is a technique used to relax the body and calm the mind. It produces a state of deep peace and rest combined with mental alertness, and it involves both relaxation and focused attention. Anyone can meditate to feel calm, cope with stress, and, for those with spiritual inclinations, feel as one with a higher power or the universe. Meditation can be practised individually or in groups and is easy to learn.

If practised regularly, such as 20 minutes twice a day, meditation produces widespread positive effects on physical and psychological functioning. The autonomic nervous system responds with a decrease in heart rate, lower blood pressure, decreased respiratory rate and oxygen consumption, and a lower arousal threshold. People who meditate say that they have clearer minds and sharper thoughts. Meditation's residual effects—improved stress-coping abilities—are a protection against daily stress and anxiety. All other self-healing methods are improved with the practice of meditation. Skill in meditation is enhanced when the person first masters the skills of breathing, progressive relaxation, and imagery. See Box 16.3 for some of the guidelines for meditation.

> **BOX 16.3 GUIDELINES FOR MEDITATION**
>
> Practise this process daily for 10- to 20-minute periods:
>
> 1. Create a special time and place for meditation. Ideally, choose the early morning or evening, and wait at least two hours after eating so that complete energy is devoted to meditation, rather than to digestive demands. A quiet, comfortable place, devoid of distractions, is essential.
> 2. Sit either cross-legged on the floor or upright in a straight-backed chair, keeping the spine straight and the body relaxed. Avoid the side-lying position; this increases the tendency to fall asleep.
> 3. Support your palms on the thighs, and close your eyes.
> 4. Follow deep-breathing or progressive relaxation exercises.
> 5. Focus your attention completely on either breathing or a chosen mental image. If using a mantra, repeat the word or phrase either aloud or silently while exhaling. When distracting thoughts appear, allow them to drift into and out of your mind without giving them undue attention; then refocus on your breathing or your mantra.

PROGRESSIVE RELAXATION Relaxation techniques are commonly used to reduce high levels of stress and chronic pain. **Progressive relaxation** requires that the client (a) tense and then relax successive muscle groups, and (b) focus attention on discriminating between the feelings experienced when the muscle group was relaxed and when it was tense. Such techniques enable the client to exert control over the body's responses to tension and anxiety by creating a second centre of concentration.

Three requisites to relaxation are (a) correct posture, (b) a mind at rest, and (c) a quiet environment. Procedures for teaching progressive relaxation vary. The method for relaxing muscle groups, the specific muscle groups to be relaxed, the number of sessions involved, and the role of the instructor (taped versus live instructions) can differ. Tensing of muscle groups is often maintained for five to seven seconds and is followed by relaxation of the muscle group at a predetermined cue. To achieve maximum relaxation, various positive and affirmative phrases are used, such as "Let all the tension go" and "Enjoy the feelings as your muscles become relaxed and loose." Guidelines for progressive relaxation are outlined in Box 16.4.

GUIDED IMAGERY Imagery is a two-way communication between the conscious and unconscious mind and involves the whole body and all of its senses. Imagery enables people to open their minds to mental ideas of positive creative

> **BOX 16.4 GUIDELINES FOR PROGRESSIVE RELAXATION**
>
> Relaxation techniques have been used extensively to reduce high levels of stress and chronic pain. The steps in progressive relaxation are as follows:
>
> - Sit comfortably in a chair, with your feet flat on the ground.
> - Tense and tighten your right fist. Focus on the feeling of tension as you do so.
> - Allow the muscles in your right fist to relax. Contrast the difference in feeling from tension to relaxation.
> - Repeat the preceding two steps for the left fist.
> - Tense and relax both your left and right fists.
> - Focus on and relish the feeling of relaxation.
> - Tighten the muscles in both fists and both arms. Feel the tension, fully relax the muscles, and again focus on the sensation of relaxation.
> - Progressively tighten and relax each muscle group in the body: toes, ankles, knees, buttocks and groin, stomach and lower back muscles, chest and upper back muscles, shoulders, forehead, and jaw muscles.
> - Couple deep breathing with progressive relaxation. While relaxing your muscles, inhale deeply, send the breath to the fist (or other muscle group), and exhale.
>
> The entire exercise should last a minimum of 10 minutes.

images that can foster self-healing and bring about desired achievements. Worry is the most common form of imagery that affects our health. In our imagination, we react to current stressors and anticipated dangers. Our bodies become aroused and tense and we activate the fight-or-flight mechanism. **Guided imagery** is a state of focused attention, much like hypnosis, that encourages changes in attitudes, behaviour, and physiological reactions. Guided imagery can help people learn how to stop troublesome thoughts and focus on images that help them relax and decrease the negative impact of stressors.

In guided imagery, the images may be created by the therapist based on the needs and desires of the client. Clients can also create the images as a way to understand the meaning of symptoms or to access inner resources. Imagery stimulates changes in many body functions, such as heart rate, blood pressure, respiratory patterns, brain-wave rhythms and patterns, electrical characteristics of the skin, local blood flow and temperature, GI motility and secretions, sexual arousal, and levels of various hormones and neurotransmitters. Table 16.3 describes several types of imagery.

BIOFEEDBACK **Biofeedback** is a method by which a person can learn to control certain physiological responses of the body. The technique uses electronic equipment to provide clients with visible or audible evidence that they are controlling their body in the desired manner. For example, a sensor attached from a person to a computer screen shows a wave pattern changing as the

TABLE 16.3 Types of Imagery

Type	Description	Example
Feeling state	Move from a feeling state of tension to one of peace	Imagine self at a beach or floating gently on water
End state	Imagine self in the situation wanted	See self as strong and healthy
Energetic	Imagine free-flowing energy	Feel self by pulling up energy from the earth through the soles of the feet
Cellular	Imagine events at cellular level	Imagine natural killer cells surrounding and attacking cancer cells
Physiological	Imagine events at the bodily level	Imagine all blood vessels relaxed and wider in order to lower blood pressure
Psychological	Change perception of self	Imagine a dialogue with a person with whom you are in conflict in an effort to find a new solution to the problem
Spiritual	Make contact with God, or the Divine	Imagine being held in the hands of God where you are perfectly safe

person concentrates on such processes as increasing blood flow in the hands, decreasing sweat gland activity, lowering blood pressure, and controlling incontinence. Biofeedback teaches clients to achieve a generalized state of relaxation, which is characterized by parasympathetic dominance, in opposition to the pattern of physiological arousal manifested in stress-related disorders.

PILATES **Pilates** is a method of physical movement and exercise designed to stretch, strengthen, and balance the body, in particular the core or centre, including the abdominal region. It is based on the principles of yoga, Zen meditation, and ancient Greek and Roman physical regimens. Exercises, coupled with focused breathing patterns, are done on the floor or with simple types of equipment. Benefits include increased lung capacity, improved flexibility and joint health, muscular coordination, increased bone density, and better posture and balance. Pilates can help rehabilitate back, knee, hip, shoulder, and stress injuries, and relieve muscle aches.

Spiritual Therapy

Health care sciences have begun to demonstrate that spirituality, faith, and religious commitment may play a role in promoting health and reducing illness. For more information about spirituality, see Chapter 47.

FAITH **Faith** refers to our beliefs and expectations about life, ourselves, and others. In a religious context, faith refers to a belief in a Supreme Being who listens and responds to people and who cares about their well-being. In a spiritual context, faith is thought of as the power to accept the nature of life as it is and live in the present moment. It is a sense of letting go of the need to control while trusting and waiting for the moment when answers come.

PRAYER **Prayer** is an active process of communication with God, a saint, or any kind of higher power that answers the prayer. Prayer can be conducted individually or in groups and may even be conducted at a distance by individuals unknown to the person for whom the prayers of healing are made. The universality of prayer is evidenced in all cultures having some form of prayer. Prayer has been, and continues to be, used in times of difficulty and illness, even in the most secular societies.

Prayer can also be described according to form. *Colloquial prayer* is an informal talk with God, as if talking to a good friend. *Intercessory prayer* is asking God for things for yourself or others. The focus is on what God can provide. Intercessory prayer for others may be called *distant prayer*, if the person being prayed for is in a remote place from the person who is praying. This form of prayer is of interest to researchers, but at the present time, scientific evidence is not conclusive (Roberts, Ahmed, Hall, & Davison, 2009). *Ritual prayer* is the use of formal prayers or rituals, such as prayers from a prayer book or the Jewish siddur, or the Catholic practice of saying the rosary. *Meditative prayer*, also known as *contemplative prayer*, is similar to meditation and is a process of focusing the mind on an aspect of God for a period. Prayer is a self-care strategy that provides comfort, increases hope, and promotes healing and psychological well-being (Masters & Spielmans, 2007).

Miscellaneous Therapies

These include music therapy, humour and laughter, bio-electromagnetics, detoxifying therapies, animal-assisted therapy, and horticultural therapy.

MUSIC THERAPY **Music therapy** consists of listening, rhythm, body movement, and singing. It is used for a variety of reasons in practice settings (e.g., perioperative holding areas, cardiac care units, birthing rooms, counselling rooms, rehabilitation and physical therapy units, and sleep induction units). Music can alter ordinary levels of consciousness to achieve the mind's fullest potential. Quiet, soothing music without words is often used to induce relaxation and promote self-expression. To select the appropriate music, the nurse needs to consider the client's preferences as well as the goals of therapy. The usual duration of a session is about 20 minutes. Clients are encouraged to let the body respond to the music as it wants to, that is, to relax the muscles, lie down, hum, clap, or dance.

HUMOUR AND LAUGHTER   **Humour** involves the ability to discover, express, or appreciate the comical or absurdly incongruous, to be amused by our own imperfections or the whimsical aspects of life, and to see the funny side of an otherwise serious situation. The use of humour in nursing is defined as assisting the client "to perceive, appreciate, and express what is funny, amusing, or ludicrous in order to establish relationships, relieve tension, release anger, facilitate learning, or cope with painful feeling" (Bulechek, Butcher, & Dochterman, 2008, p. 409). Elaboration of these functions of humour in nursing situations is described as follows:

- *Establishing relationships.* Humour decreases the social distance between persons and helps put people at ease. When tension is decreased, people can focus on the message and on other people rather than on their own feelings. The use of humour helps the nurse establish rapport with clients, an important factor in achieving success in nursing interventions.

- *Relieving tension and anxiety.* The effective use of humour relieves the tension of emotionally charged events. The personal nature of humour, for example, helps clients deal with the impersonal nature of wearing a hospital gown and a numbered identity (ID) band and with answering embarrassing questions and undergoing uncomfortable tests. People can also use humour prophylactically to decrease stress.

- *Releasing anger and aggression.* Humour helps individuals act out impulses or feelings in a safe and nonthreatening manner. It dissipates feelings of anger and aggression by focusing on the comic elements of a situation.

- *Facilitating learning.* Many lectures and presentations begin with a joke or cartoon. Humour not only reduces the presenter's anxiety but also gains the audience's attention. People learn more when humour is used and anxiety levels are reduced. People also recall more information when they associate information with a joke. Use of humour in instruction, however, needs to be carefully planned so that it will contribute to learning.

- *Coping with painful feelings.* People may use humour to blunt the immediate effect of situations that are too painful, such as the effect of a threatening diagnosis or treatment. Humour diminishes anxiety and fear and reduces tension, thus enabling the person to confront and deal with the situation.

Humour also has physiological benefits that involve alternating states of stimulation and relaxation. Humour stimulates the production of catecholamines and hormones. It also releases endorphins, thereby increasing pain tolerance. Laughter, for example, helps relieve tension. It stimulates increases in respiratory rate, heart rate, muscular tension, and oxygen exchange. A state of relaxation follows laughter, during which heart rate, blood pressure, respiration, and muscle tension decrease.

Many health care settings are now interested in providing humour as a caring skill and have recognized that "laughter is the best medicine." The nurse needs to use humour effectively and cautiously by considering the feelings of others and cultural variations in what people consider humorous. "Humour rooms," which are supplied with games, funny audiotapes and videotapes, humorous books, collections of cartoons, and so on, are being created for clients and staff.

ANIMAL-ASSISTED THERAPY   **Animal-assisted therapy** is the use of specifically selected animals as a treatment modality in health and human service settings. It has been shown to be a successful intervention for people with a variety of physical or psychological conditions. Throwing an object for a dog to retrieve or brushing the animal increases upper extremity range of motion. Reaching for the object the dog has retrieved improves coordination. Ambulating with a dog improves mobility. Giving simple commands to the animal increases language production. Attending to the animal and the situation increases attention and concentration. Therapeutic horseback riding, or *hippotherapy*, uses the rhythmic movement of the horse to increase sensory processing and improve posture, balance, and mobility in people with movement dysfunctions.

Long-term health care facilities may have animals such as fish, birds, hamsters, gerbils, guinea pigs, rabbits, cats, and dogs. Some staff report that some pets become so perceptive that they gravitate to people who are the most isolated or depressed. The contributions pet animals make to the emotional well-being of people include unconditional love and opportunities for affection; achievement of trust, responsibility, and empathy toward others; hope and motivation; and a source of reassurance.

DETOXIFYING THERAPIES   Many cultures and religions have rituals of purification. **Detoxification** is a practice to clear the physical impurities and toxins from the body to achieve better health. The use of water as a healing treatment is known as *hydrotherapy*. The use of hot and cold moisture in the form of solid, liquid, or gas makes use of the body's response to heat and cold. Hydrotherapy is used to decrease pain, fever, swelling, and cramps; induce sleep; and improve physical and mental tone. It must be used with great care in the very young or old, who have poor heat regulation, and also with people experiencing any prolonged illness or fatigue. *Colonics*, or colon therapy, is the procedure for cleansing the fat accumulated on the inner wall of the colon by filling it with water or herbal solutions and then draining it. *Colon cleansing* is a controversial method of detoxification. Contraindications include people in a weakened state and those having ulcerative colitis, diverticulitis, Crohn's disease, severe hemorrhoids, or tumours of the large intestine or rectum.

HORTICULTURAL THERAPY **Horticultural therapy**, also called *gardening* or a *healing garden*, is an adjunct therapy to occupational and physical therapy. People may view nature, visit a healing garden or a wander garden, or actually participate in gardening. When it is a communal activity, gardening decreases social isolation by fostering interactions with others. Horticultural therapy stimulates the five senses, provides leisure activities, improves motor function, provides a sense of achievement, and improves self-esteem (Smilski, 2008). Nurses must also be aware, however, that clients who are prone to infection should not come into contact with garden soil, perform activities that can cause skin punctures or scratches, or come in proximity to stagnant water that can contain insects or infectious organisms.

Nursing Role in Complementary and Alternative Health Modalities

Every year, billions of dollars are spent on unproven, fraudulently marketed, and potentially dangerous health products. The nurse must ask the obvious questions: Is there any supportive evidence? Does it sound too good to be true? Do the claims for the product seem exaggerated or unrealistic for the purpose of selling a product? Remember that the only way to know if a drug is working or is harmful is through large, preferably placebo-controlled, double-blind studies. See the Assessment: Interview box for more questions.

The Internet can be a valuable source of accurate, reliable information. However, it also has a wealth of misinformation that may not be obvious to distinguish hype from evidence-based science (see Chapter 25). In today's health care environment, health care consumers are more knowledgeable than ever and are demanding a broader range of health options. Additionally, the Canadian population is getting more culturally diverse and older. The CNA (1999, 2008a) expects nurses to demonstrate safe, competent, and ethical care (see the Reflect on Primary Health Care box). It requires nurses to *competently* "facilitate and respect the client's informed choice to use alternative or complementary therapies

---

ASSESSMENT	INTERVIEW

Complementary and Alternative Health Modalities

Nurses can use these questions to ask their clients about their use of CAHM:

- Tell me about your use of teas, herbs, vitamins, or other natural products to improve your health.
- What traditional or folk remedies are used in your family?
- Do you meditate, pray, or use relaxation techniques, music, or yoga for healing purposes?
- What alternative therapies have you used (acupuncture, touch therapies, magnets, hypnosis, etc.)?
- Tell me what you know about the benefits and risks of the CAHM you are using.
- Have you discussed your use of CAHM with your health care provider?

(e.g., aromatherapy, acupressure, therapeutic touch, nutritional supplements, diets)" (CNA, 2008b). Nurses must inquire about healing practices the client may have used previously (see the Assessment: Interview box). In relation to CAHM, nurses must develop the following healing attitudes and behaviours:

1. Have a strong fundamental, evidence-based knowledge of the human body and various CAHM

2. Demonstrate practice competencies in teaching clients related to the safe and appropriate use of complementary medicine

3. Be nonjudgmental and respectful regarding clients' choices to use any of the CAHM within his or her own cultural context

4. Act as an advocate and facilitator by providing accurate information on CAHM modalities, NHPs, and the risks and benefits as opposed to conventional health care practices to help clients make informed decisions

5. Encourage clients to discuss their use of CAHM with their health care provider

---

REFLECT ON 🔑 **PRIMARY HEALTH CARE**

To improve the health of clients, nurses act by working in partnerships with clients, other health care providers, and related community partners. They are the entry point for clients to access the health care system. They assess the client's health problems, provide accurate information, from conventional Western medicine to available CAHM, and assist the client in making the choice of treatment as desired. Consider how these nursing roles reflect the primary health care principles of accessibility, intersectoral collaboration, and health promotion.

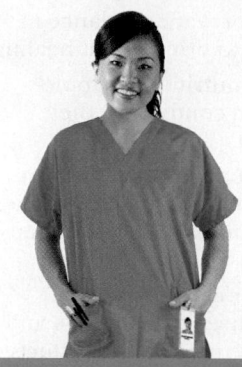

Case Study 16

Tim Le is a 68-year-old accountant who has been diagnosed with gastric cancer. He had lost a great deal of weight before the diagnosis and during chemotherapy and radiotherapy. He is now admitted to the hospital with pain and weakness, which are preventing him from working or performing many activities of daily living. His wife, Susan, stays with him most of the day. His elderly parents visit often and bring him homemade food and drink. They do not speak English. In the process of placing bathing items on Tim's bedside stand, the nurse notices several plastic bags of a tea-like product in the drawer.

CRITICAL THINKING QUESTIONS

1. What aspects of this case suggest that it would be appropriate for the nurse to discuss the use of alternative therapies with the client or his family?

2. Which alternative therapies might be most useful for this client and are in keeping with the principle of "do no harm"?

3. How should the nurse respond to finding the bags in the client's drawer? What options should be considered, and what are the likely results of each?

4. How might the nurse's own belief system influence his or her interactions with the client and family regarding CAHM?

Check the eText in MyNursingLab for answers and explanations.

KEY TERMS

CHAPTER HIGHLIGHTS

- Complementary health modalities are practised by a majority of Canadians. Therefore, nurses need to be aware of the different types of therapies and their potential benefits and harms.

- The concepts common to most alternative practices include holism, humanism, balance, spirituality, energy, and healing environments.

- Ancient health care practices typically include an entire set of values, attitudes, and beliefs that generate a philosophy of life, not simply a group of remedies. Harmony or balance in energy is the emphasis.

- Complementary and alternative health modalities are generally classified into these categories: total medical systems, biologically based therapies, manipulative and body-based methods, energy therapy, mind–body interventions, and spiritual therapy.

- Total medical systems include Ayurveda, traditional Chinese medicine, traditional Aboriginal medicine, homeopathy, and naturopathy.
- Biologically based treatments include herbal medicine, aromatherapy, and dietary therapy.
- Manipulative and body-based treatments include chiropractic therapy; massage therapy; acupuncture, acupressure, and reflexology; qigong and Tai Chi.
- Energy therapies include therapeutic touch, healing touch, reiki, and bioelectromagnetic therapies.
- Mind–body interventions include yoga, hypnosis, meditation, progressive relaxation, guided imagery, biofeedback, Pilates, prayer, music therapy, humour, animal-assisted therapy, and horticultural therapy.

They all focus on realigning or creating balance in mental and physical processes to bring about healing.

- Although many botanical and nutritional supplements can be helpful in certain conditions, their effectiveness and safety are not all well studied.
- Other CAHM approaches include faith and prayer, music therapy, humour and laughter, bioelectromagnetics, detoxifying therapies, animal-assisted therapy, and horticultural therapy.
- Nurses act as the entry point for clients to access various health care services. Nurses can advocate and facilitate their clients' use of natural health products and complementary and alternative health modalities within their cultural context as an integral part of care.

ASSESS YOUR LEARNING

1. A nurse is teaching a prenatal class to a group of women about pain relief measures during labour. A young woman states, "I prefer not to use any medication during labour; aromatherapy oils have a calming effect on me." What is the nurse's most appropriate response?
   a. "Aromatherapy oils may work for mild pain but will not reduce labour pain."
   b. "Keep your options open at this point, since aromatherapy may not be sufficient to manage labour pain."
   c. "Aromatherapy oils are a good choice to use with medication for labour pain."
   d. "You need to determine if aromatherapy oils are safe to use during pregnancy."

2. What is true about the differences between traditional therapies and alternative therapies?
   a. Alternative therapies cost less compared with traditional therapies.
   b. Alternative therapies are used if traditional therapies are ineffective.
   c. Alternative therapies can be as effective as traditional therapies for some conditions.
   d. Alternative therapies use products from nature but traditional therapies do not.

3. Which of the following is the BEST explanation of spirituality?
   a. Something that gives people purpose and meaning in their lives
   b. A formalized religious dogma
   c. A non-denominational community service
   d. People being responsible for their life patterns

4. In what ways do nurses create healing environments?
   a. Using technology to prevent hospital-acquired infections

   b. Empowering clients to make healthy decisions for themselves
   c. Placing aquariums in day rooms of nursing homes
   d. Ensuring that physicians' orders are carried out

5. A client asks the nurse to state one of the primary principles associated with naturopathy. Which is the BEST response?
   a. "A higher being guides the learning needed to treat disease."
   b. "It focuses on environmental causes when treating illnesses."
   c. "It focuses on early detection and treatment of disease."
   d. "It is a way of life to maintain health and prevent disease."

6. From the perspective of traditional Chinese medicine (TCM), which is the BEST definition of disease?
   a. Imbalance or disruption in food digestion
   b. Imbalance or interruption in the flow of qi
   c. Imbalance or disruption in key social relationships
   d. Imbalance or disruption in thoughts or emotions

7. A hospitalized client is due for surgery tomorrow. You learn that he had not told his physician that he was taking natural health products (NHPs) in addition to his other prescribed medication. What should you do?
   a. Encourage the client to continue taking the NHPs as they are harmless.
   b. Tell the client to stop taking the NHPs immediately.
   c. You would report all medications and NHPs the client is taking to the attending physician.
   d. You would offer some additional herbal medicine to the client before the surgery.

8. You are caring for James, who has colon cancer and has undergone chemotherapy. His prognosis is unknown. James has experienced much pain. He is depressed and anxious. He asks you for advice regarding the use of therapeutic touch to ease his pain. Which is the most appropriate nursing action?

   a. You cannot endorse the use of any complementary and alternative health modalities.

   b. You first ensure that James understands what therapeutic touch is.

   c. You encourage James to consider music therapy to relieve his pain.

   d. You encourage James to pray so that he will be protected from harm.

9. A two-month pregnant woman has told you that she wants to take ginseng to avoid stretch marks. Which is the MOST appropriate nursing action?

   a. Advise the mother not to take ginseng, as it may be toxic if taken in very large quantities.

   b. Advise against using ginseng, as it is not recommended for pregnant and nursing mothers.

   c. Endorse the use of ginseng, as it is a well-known and popular Chinese medicine.

   d. Advise the mother on other ways to reduce stretch marks, such as aiming for gradual weight gain during pregnancy.

10. Which would be the most appropriate form of mind–body interventions for older clients who are at risk for falls?

    a. Music therapy

    b. Tai Chi

    c. Diet therapy

    d. Guided imagery

> *Check the eText in MyNursingLab for answers and explanations.*

WEBLINKS

Canadian Interdisciplinary Network for CAM Research (IN-CAM)

http://www.incamresearch.ca

Launched in January 2004, IN-CAM's two primary objectives are to build research capacity and facilitate interdisciplinary CAM research in Canada, particularly from the perspective of health services or social science. It offers a searchable members database, bimonthly e-bulletin, networking opportunities, and an annual research symposium. Membership is free.

Canadian Pediatric Complementary and Alternative Medicine Network (PedCAM)

http://www.pedcam.ca

A new network to link pediatric CAM researchers and educators. Free membership provides access to an online, searchable database of members, bimonthly bulletin, and an annual research forum.

Health Canada

http://www.hc-sc.gc.ca/dhp-mps/prodnatur/index_e.html

As part of the Drugs and Health Products branch of Health Canada, the Natural Health Products Directorate (NHPD) is the regulating authority for natural health products for sale in Canada.

Canadian Holistic Nurses Association

http://www.chna.ca

This site presents the philosophy and objectives of the Canadian Holistic Nurses Association (CHNA) and information on the levels of training for a holistic nursing specialty.

Videos

Health Canada. (n.d.). Natural Health Product Regulations in Canada.

http://www.howtodothings.com/video/natural-health-product-regulations-in-canada

Johnson, E. (2011, January 14). Marketplace investigates homeopathy. *CBC News.*

http://www.cbc.ca/video/player.html?category=News&zone=health&site=cbc.health.ca&clipid=1742776936

MyNursingLab

REFERENCES

Boon, H. S, Verhoef, M. J., Vanderheyden, L. C., & Westlake, K. P. (2006). Complementary and alternative medicine: A rising healthcare issue. *Healthcare Policy, 1*(3), 19–30.

Bulechek, G. B., Butcher, H. K., & Dochterman, J., (Eds.). (2008). *Nursing interventions classification (NIC)* (5th ed.). St. Louis, MO: Mosby.

Buranruk, O., La Grow, S., Ladawan, S., Makarawate, P., Suwanich, T., & Leelayuwat, N. (2010). Thai Yoga as an appropriate alternative physical activity for older adults. *Journal of Complementary and Integrative Medicine, 7*(1). Article 6. doi: 10.2202/1553-3840.1290

Canadian Association of Naturopathic Doctors. (2011). *What is naturopathic medicine?* Retrieved from http://www.cand.ca/index.php?36

Canadian Nurses Association. (1999). Complementary therapies—Finding the right balance. *Nursing Now: Issues and Trends in Canadian Nursing, 6.*

Canadian Nurses' Association. (2008a). *Code of ethics for registered nurses* (Centennial edition). Ottawa, ON: Author.

Canadian Nurses Association. (2008b). *Nursing in Canada: Canadian registered nurse examination—Competencies.* Retrieved from http://www.cna-aiic.ca/CNA/nursing/rnexam/competencies/default_e.aspx

Chen, K. M., Chen, M. H., Chao, H. C., Hung, H. M., Lin, H. S., & Li, C. H. (2009). Sleep quality, depression state, and health status of older adults after silver yoga exercises: Cluster randomized trial. *International Journal of Nursing Studies, 46,* 154–163. doi:10.1016/j.ijnurstu.2008.09.005

Dale, C. (2009). *The subtle body.* Louisville, CO: Sounds True.

Fontaine, K. L. (2010). *Complementary & alternative therapies for nursing practice* (3rd ed.). Upper Saddle River, NJ: Prentice Hall.

Health Canada. (2009). *Advisories, warnings and recalls for health professionals.* Retrieved from http://www.hc-sc.gc.ca/dhp-mps/medeff/advisories-avis/prof/_2008/index-eng.php.

Health Canada. (2011). *Natural health products, drug and health products.* Retrieved from http://www.hc-sc.gc.ca/dhp-mps/prodnatur/about-apropos/cons-eng.php

Manheimer, E., Zhang, G., Udoff, L., Haramati, A., Langenberg, P., Berman, B. M., & Bouter, L. M. (2008). Effects of acupuncture on rates of pregnancy and live birth among women undergoing in vitro fertilization: Systematic review and meta-analysis. *British Medical Journal, 336,* 545–549. doi:10.1136/bmj.39471.430451.BE

McFarland,B., Bigelow, D., Zani, B., Newsom, J., & Kaplan, M. (2002). Complementary and alternative medicine use in Canada and the United States. *American Journal of Public Health, 92*(10), 1616–1618. PMCID:1447296.

Masters, K. S., & Spielmans, G. I. (2007). Prayer and health: Review, meta-analysis, and research agenda. *Journal of Behavioral Medicine, 30,* 329–338. doi:10.1007/s10865-007-9106-7

National Centre for Complementary and Alternative Medicine. (2010). *Magnets for pain.* Retrieved from http://nccam.nih.gov/health/magnet/magnetsforpain.htm

National Institutes of Health. (2010). *CMA basics: National Centre for Complementary and Alternative Medicine.* Retrieved from http://nccam.nih.gov/health/whatiscam

Nightingale, F. (1954, originally published 1882). Nurses, training of and nursing the sick. In L.R. Seymer (Ed.), *Selected writings of Florence Nightingale* (pp. 319–351). New York, NY: MacMillan.

Roberts, L., Ahmed, I., Hall, S., & Davison, A. (2009). Intercessory prayer for the alleviation of ill health. *Cochrane Database of Systematic Reviews,* Issue 2, Art. No.: CD000368. doi:10.1002/14651858.CD000368.pub3

Rolfes, S. R., Pinna, K., & Whitney, E. (2009). *Understanding normal and clinical nutrition* (8th ed.). Belmont, CA: Wadsworth Cengage Learning. doi: 10.1002/14651858. CD000368.pub3

Sharpe, P. A., Williams, H. G., Granner, M. L., & Hussey, J. R. (2007). A randomized study of the effects of massage therapy compared to guided relaxation on well-being and stress perception among older adults. *Complementary Therapies in Medicine, 15,* 157–163. doi:10.1016/j.ctim.2007.01.004

Singh, B. B., Wu, W. S., Hwang, S. H., Khorsan, R., Der-Martirosian, C., Vinjamury, S. P., . . . Lin, S. Y. (2006). Effectiveness of acupuncture in the treatment of fibromyalgia. *Alternative Therapies in Health and Medicine, 12*(2), 34–41.

Smilski, A. (2008). Cultivations . . . and potting on a strategic plan for a social and horticultural therapy program. *Perspectives, 32*(2), 5–14.

Suzuki, M., Namura, K., Ohno, Y., Tanaka, H., Egawa, M., Yokoyama, Y., . . . , & Tadashi, Y. (2008). The effect of acupuncture in the treatment of chronic obstructive pulmonary disease. *Journal of Alternative and Complementary Medicine, 14,* 1097–1105. doi:10.1089/acm.2007.0786

Verhoef, M. (2005). Overview of manual therapy use in Canada. Natcher Conference Center, National Institutes of Health, June 9–10, 2005. Retrieved from http://nccam.nih.gov/news/events/Manual-Therapy/overview_canada.htm

Willison, K. D. (2008). Advancing integrative medicine through interprofessional education. *The International Journal of Health Sociology, 17*(4), 342–352.

World Health Organization. (2010). *Traditional medicine.* Fact sheet, #134, December 2008. Retrieved from http://www.who.int/mediacentre/factsheets/fs134/en

Yu, J., Zhang, X., Liu, C., Meng, Y., & Han, J. (2006). Effect of acupuncture treatment on vascular dementia. *Neurological Research, 28,* 97–103.

UNIT
3

Lifespan and Developmental Stages

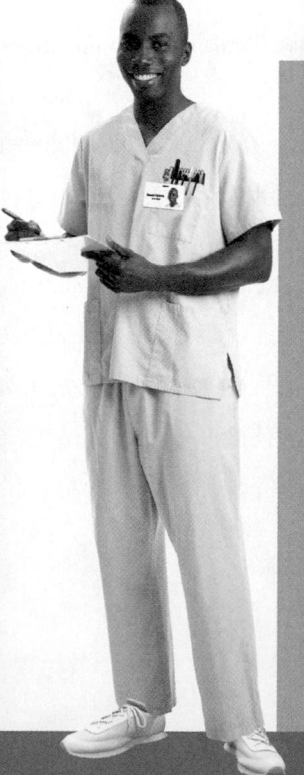

Chapter 17

Concepts of Growth and Development

LEARNING OUTCOMES

After studying this chapter, you will be able to:

1. Differentiate between the terms *growth* and *development*.

2. Describe the factors that influence human growth and development.

3. Discuss the principles and stages of human growth and task development.

4. Describe Havighurst's developmental tasks theory.

5. Describe the characteristics and implications of Freud's theory of psychosexual development.

6. Describe Erikson's eight stages of psychosocial development.

7. Compare Peck's and Gould's stages of adult development.

8. Explain Piaget's theory of cognitive development.

9. Compare Kohlberg's and Gilligan's theories of moral development.

10. Compare Fowler's and Westerhoff's stages of spiritual development.

We live through various stages of growth and development, from the moment of conception through to the end of life. Understanding normal growth and development provides a framework for age-specific health assessment and health promotion throughout a person's lifespan. The terms *growth* and *development* are often used interchangeably, but they have different meanings. **Growth** is physical change and increase in size. Indicators of growth include height, weight, bone size, and dentition. Growth rates vary during different stages; for example, growth rate is rapid during the prenatal, neonatal, infancy, and adolescent stages. **Development** is an increase in the complexity of function and skill progression. It is the capacity and skill of a person to adapt to the environment. Development is the behavioural aspect of growth; for example, a person develops the ability to walk, to talk, and to run. **Developmental milestones** are the developmental sequences and patterns that are predictable in a child's growth. These milestones may vary from one culture to another; they are the benchmarks for determining when to expect developmental tasks to take place.

Growth and development are independent but interrelated processes. For example, an infant's muscles, bones, and nervous system must grow to a certain point before the infant can sit up or walk. Growth generally takes place during the first 20 years of life; development continues after that. Principles of growth and development are shown in Box 17.1.

BOX 17.1 PRINCIPLES OF GROWTH AND DEVELOPMENT

All humans follow the same pattern of growth and development. The process is independent, interactive, and governed by the following general principles:

- The sequence of each stage is predictable, although the time of onset, the length of the stage, and the effects of each stage vary from person to person.

- Each developmental stage has its own characteristics. For example, Piaget suggests that in the sensorimotor stage (birth to two years), children learn to coordinate simple motor tasks.

- Growth and development occur as follows:

  - In a *cephalocaudal direction*, that is, starting at the head and moving to the trunk, legs, and feet. This pattern is particularly obvious at birth, when the head of the infant is disproportionately large.

  - In a *proximodistal direction*, that is, from the centre of the body outward (see Figure 17.1). For example, infants can roll over before they can grasp an object with the thumb and the second finger.

  - In *continuous, orderly, sequential processes* influenced by maturational, environmental, and genetic factors.

- Development proceeds from simple to complex or from single acts to integrated acts. To accomplish the integrated act of drinking and swallowing a liquid from a cup, for example, the child must first learn a series of single acts: eye–hand coordination, grasping, hand–mouth coordination, controlled tipping of the cup, and then mouth, lip, and tongue movements to drink and swallow.

- Development becomes increasingly differentiated. *Differentiated development* begins with a generalized response and progresses to a skilled specific response. For example, an infant's initial response to a stimulus

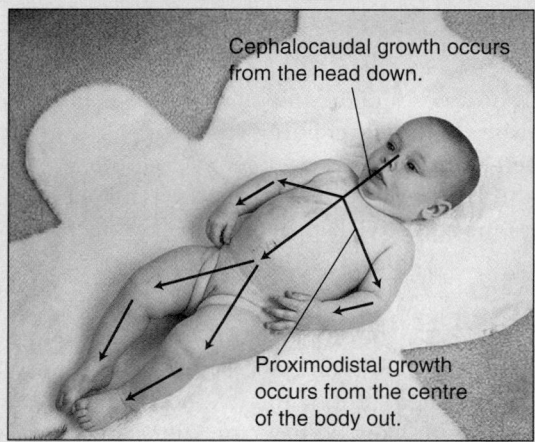

FIGURE 17.1 Cephalocaudal and proximodistal growth.

involves the total body; a 5-year-old child can respond more specifically with laughter or fear.

- Certain stages of growth and development are more critical than others. For example, the first 10 to 12 weeks after conception are critical. The incidence of congenital anomalies as a result of exposure to certain viruses, chemicals, or drugs is greater during this stage than in others.

- The pace of growth and development is uneven. It is known that growth is greater during infancy than during childhood. Asynchronous development is demonstrated by rapid growth of the head during infancy and of the extremities at puberty.

Factors Influencing Growth and Development

Many factors can influence growth and development. Knowledge of these factors helps the nurse provide anticipatory guidance to promote optimal growth and development of an individual.

Genetic

The genetic inheritance of an individual is established at conception. It remains unchanged throughout life and determines such characteristics as gender, physical characteristics (e.g., eye colour, potential height), and, to some extent, temperament.

Temperament

Temperament (i.e., the way individuals respond to their external and internal environments) sets the stage for the interactive dynamics of growth and development. Temperament may persist throughout the lifespan, though caution must be taken not to label or categorize infants and children.

Family

Family provides support and safety for the child. Families are involved in their children's physical and psychological well-being and development. Children are socialized through family dynamics. The parents set expected behaviours and model appropriate behaviour.

Nutrition

Adequate nutrition is an essential component of growth and development. For example, poorly nourished children are more likely to have infections compared with well-nourished children. In addition, poorly nourished children may not attain their full height potential.

Environment

A few environmental factors that can influence growth and development are the child's living conditions (e.g., homelessness), socioeconomic status (e.g., poverty versus financial stability), climate, and community (e.g., one that provides developmental support versus one that exposes the child to hazards).

Health

Illness or injury can affect growth and development. Hospitalization is stressful for a child and can affect his or her coping mechanisms. Prolonged or chronic illness may affect normal developmental processes.

Culture

Cultural customs, nutritional practices, and childrearing practices may all influence growth and development in infants and children.

Stages of Growth and Development

The *rate* of a person's growth and development is highly individual. However, the *sequence* of growth and development is predictable. Stages of growth usually correspond to certain developmental changes (see Table 17.1).

Growth and development are commonly thought of as having eight major components: (a) biophysical, (b) psychosocial, (c) cognitive, (d) behavioural, (e) social, (f) ecological, (g) moral, and (h) spiritual. A discussion of some of the major theories relating to these components follows.

TABLE 17.1 Stages of Growth and Development

Stage	Age	Significant Characteristics	Nursing Implications
Neonatal	Birth to 28 days	Behaviour is largely reflexive and develops to more purposeful behaviour.	Assist parents to identify and meet unmet needs.
Infancy	1 month to 1 year	Physical growth is rapid.	Control the infant's environment so that physical and psychological needs are met.
Toddlerhood	1 to 3 years	Motor development permits increased physical autonomy. Psychosocial skills increase.	Safety and risk-taking strategies must be balanced to permit growth.
Preschool	4 to 6 years	The preschooler's world is expanding. New experiences and the preschooler's social role are tried during play. Physical growth is slower.	Provide opportunities for play and social activity.

Stage	Age	Significant Characteristics	Nursing Implications
School age	6 to 12 years	This stage includes the preadolescent period (10 to 12 years). The peer group increasingly influences behaviour. Physical, cognitive, and social development increase, and communication skills improve.	Allow time and energy for the school-age child to pursue hobbies and school activities. Recognize and support the child's achievements.
Adolescence	13 to 19 years	The self-concept changes with biological development. Values are tested. Physical growth accelerates. Stress increases, especially in the face of conflicts.	Assist adolescents to develop coping behaviours. Help adolescents develop strategies for resolving conflicts.
Young adulthood	20 to 39 years	A personal lifestyle develops. The person usually establishes a relationship with a significant other and a commitment to something.	Accept the adult's chosen lifestyle and assist with necessary adjustments relating to health. Recognize the person's commitments. Support change, as necessary, for health.
Middle adulthood	40 to 64 years	Lifestyle changes because of other changes; for example, children leave home, occupational goals change.	Assist clients to plan for anticipated changes in life, to recognize the risk factors related to health, and to focus on strengths rather than weaknesses.
Older adulthood			
Young-old	65 to 74 years	Adaptation to retirement and changing physical abilities is often necessary. Chronic illness may develop.	Assist clients to keep physically and socially active and to maintain peer group interactions.
Middle-old	75 to 84 years	Adaptation to decline in speed of movement, reaction time, and sensory abilities, and increasing dependence on others may be necessary.	Assist clients to cope with loss (e.g., hearing, sensory abilities, eyesight, death of loved one). Provide necessary safety measures.
Old-old	85 and over	Physical problems may increase.	Assist clients with self-care, as required, and with maintaining as much independence as possible.

Growth and Development Theories

Biophysical Theory

Biophysical development theories describe the development and physical changes of the body compared against established norms. Arnold Gesell's (1880–1961) theory states that development is directed by genetics. He asserts that child development is a maturational process based on an inborn timetable. For example, children achieve maturational milestones, such as rolling over, sitting, and walking, at specific times.

Psychosocial Theories

Psychosocial development refers to the development of personality. **Personality** is a complex concept that is difficult to define. It can be considered as the outward (interpersonal) expression of the inner (intrapersonal) self. It encompasses a person's temperament, feelings, character traits, independence, self-esteem, self-concept, behaviour, ability to interact with others, and ability to adapt to life changes.

ROBERT HAVIGHURST (1900–1991) Robert Havighurst believed that learning is basic to life and that people continue to learn throughout life. He described growth and development as occurring during six stages, with tasks to be learned in each (see Table 17.2). A **developmental task** is "a task which arises at or about a certain period in the life of an individual, successful achievement of which leads to his happiness and to success with later tasks, while failure leads to unhappiness in the individual, disapproval by society, and difficulty with later tasks" (Havighurst, 1972, p. 2).

Havighurst's developmental tasks provide a framework to evaluate a person's general accomplishments. However, the broad categories limit its usefulness as a tool in assessing specific accomplishments, particularly

TABLE 17.2 Havighurst's Age Periods and Developmental Tasks

Infancy and Early Childhood

1. Learning to walk
2. Learning to take solid foods
3. Learning to talk
4. Learning to control the elimination of body wastes
5. Learning sex differences and sexual modesty
6. Achieving psychological stability
7. Forming simple concepts of social and physical reality
8. Learning to relate emotionally to parents, siblings, and other people
9. Learning to distinguish right from wrong and developing a conscience

Middle Childhood

1. Learning physical skills necessary for ordinary games
2. Building wholesome attitudes toward oneself as a growing organism
3. Learning to get along with age-mates
4. Learning an appropriate masculine or feminine social role
5. Developing fundamental skills in reading, writing, and arithmetic
6. Developing concepts necessary for everyday living
7. Developing conscience, morality, and a scale of values
8. Achieving personal independence
9. Developing attitudes toward social groups and institutions

Adolescence

1. Achieving new and more mature relations with age-mates of both genders
2. Achieving a masculine or feminine social role
3. Accepting one's physique and using the body effectively
4. Achieving emotional independence from parents and other adults
5. Achieving assurance of economic independence
6. Selecting and preparing for an occupation

7. Preparing for marriage and family life
8. Developing intellectual skills and concepts necessary for civic competence
9. Desiring and achieving socially responsible behaviour
10. Acquiring a set of values and an ethical system as a guide to behaviour

Early Adulthood

1. Selecting a mate
2. Learning to live with a partner
3. Starting a family
4. Rearing children
5. Managing a home
6. Getting started in an occupation
7. Taking on civic responsibility
8. Finding a congenial social group

Middle Age

1. Achieving adult civic and social responsibility
2. Establishing and maintaining an economic standard of living
3. Assisting teenage children to become responsible and happy adults
4. Developing adult leisure-time activities
5. Relating oneself to one's spouse as a person
6. Accepting and adjusting to the physiological changes of middle age
7. Adjusting to aging parents

Later Maturity

1. Adjusting to decreasing physical strength and health
2. Adjusting to retirement and reduced income
3. Adjusting to death of spouse
4. Establishing an explicit affiliation with one's age group
5. Meeting social and civic obligations
6. Establishing satisfactory physical living arrangements

Source: Havighurst, Robert J. *Developmental Tasks,* 1st Ed., © 1930. Reprinted and Electronically reproduced by permission of Pearson Education, Inc., Upper Saddle River, New Jersey.

those of infancy and childhood. In a multicultural society, the definition of success of tasks may vary with values and belief systems (e.g., not all individuals may wish to marry or bear children), making these tasks less relevant for some.

SIGMUND FREUD (1856–1939) Sigmund Freud (1923) introduced the following concepts about development: the unconscious mind; defence mechanisms; and the id, the ego, and the superego. The **unconscious mind** is the part of a person's mental life that the person is unaware of. This concept of the unconscious is one of Freud's major contributions to the field of psychiatry. **Defence mechanisms**, or **adaptive mechanisms**, are the result of

conflicts because of environmental and social restrictions. The id is the source of instinctive and unconscious urges, which Freud considered chiefly sexual in nature. The **id** is also the source of all pleasure and gratification. The **ego** is formed by the person to make effective contact with social and physical needs. Through the ego, the id impulses are satisfied. The **superego** contains the conscience and the ego ideal. The conscience consists of society's "do not's," usually as a result of parental and cultural expectations. The ego ideal comprises the standards of perfection toward which the individual strives. Freud proposed that the underlying motivation to human development is an energy form or life instinct, which he called **libido**.

According to Freud's theory of psychosexual development, the personality develops in five overlapping stages from birth to adulthood. The libido changes its location of emphasis within the body from one stage to another. Therefore, a particular body area has special significance to a client at a particular stage. The first three stages (oral, anal, and phallic) are called *pregenital stages.* The next stage is the *latency stage.* The culminating stage is the *genital stage.* Table 17.3 indicates the characteristics for each stage.

If the individual does not achieve a satisfactory resolution at each stage, the personality becomes fixated at that stage. **Fixation** is immobilization or the inability of the personality to proceed to the next stage because of anxiety. For example, nurses can assist an infant's development by making feeding a pleasurable experience and by making toilet training a positive experience, thereby enhancing the child's feeling of self-control. If, however, the toilet training has been a negative experience, the resulting conflict or stress could delay or prolong progression through a stage or cause a person to regress to a previous stage. Ideally, an individual progresses through each stage with balance among the id, the ego, and the superego.

ERIK ERIKSON (1902–1994) Erik H. Erikson (1963, 1964) expanded Freud's theory of development to include the entire lifespan, believing that people continue to develop throughout life. He described eight stages of development. In contrast to Freud, Erikson believed the ego to be the conscious core of the personality (see Table 17.4 on the next page).

Erikson envisioned life as a sequence of developmental stages or levels of achievement. Each stage signals a task that must be achieved. The resolution of the task may be complete, partial, or unsuccessful. The greater the task achievement, the healthier is the personality of the person; failure to achieve a task influences the person's ability to achieve the next task. These developmental tasks can be viewed as a series of crises, and successful resolution of these crises is supportive to the person's ego. Failure to resolve the crises is damaging to the ego.

TABLE 17.3 Freud's Five Stages of Development

Stage	Age	Characteristics	Implications
Oral	Birth to 1.5 years	The mouth is the centre of pleasure (major source of gratification and exploration). Security is a primary need. *Major conflict*: weaning	Feeding produces pleasure and a sense of comfort and safety. Feeding should be pleasurable and provided when required.
Anal	1.5 to 3 years	The anus and the bladder are the sources of pleasure (sensual satisfaction, self-control). *Major conflict*: toilet training	Controlling and expelling feces provide pleasure and sense of control. Toilet training should be a pleasurable experience.
Phallic	4 to 6 years	The child's genitals are the centre of pleasure. Masturbation offers pleasure. Other activities can include fantasy, experimentation with peers, and questioning of adults about sexual topics. *Major conflict*: the Oedipus or Electra complex, which resolves when the child identifies with parent of same sex. (The *Oedipus complex* refers to the male child's attraction for his mother and hostile attitudes toward his father. The *Electra complex* refers to the female's attraction for her father and hostile attitudes toward her mother.)	The child identifies with the parent of the opposite sex and later takes on a love relationship outside the family. Encourage identity.
Latency	6 years to puberty	Energy is directed to physical and intellectual activities. Sexual impulses tend to be repressed. Relationships with peers of the same sex develop.	Encourage the child with physical and intellectual pursuits. Encourage sports and other activities with same-sex peers.
Genital	Puberty and after	Energy is directed toward full sexual maturity and function and the development of skills needed to cope with the environment.	Encourage separation from parents, achievement of independence, and decision making.

Source: From Murray, R. B., Zentner, J. P., & Yakimo, R. (2009). *Health promotion strategies through the life span* (8th ed.) (p. 19). Upper Saddle River, NJ: Merrill/Prentice Hall. Adapted with permission. Electronically reproduced by permission of Pearson Education, Inc., Upper Saddle River, New Jersey.

TABLE 17.4 Erikson's Eight Stages of Development

Stage	Age	Central Task	Indicators of Positive Resolution	Indicators of Negative Resolution
Infancy	Birth to 18 months	Trust versus mistrust	Learning to trust others	Mistrust, withdrawal, estrangement
Early childhood	18 months to 3 years	Autonomy versus shame and doubt	Self-control without loss of self-esteem Ability to cooperate and to express oneself	Compulsive self-restraint or compliance Willfulness and defiance
Late childhood	3 to 5 years	Initiative versus guilt	Learning the degree to which assertiveness and purpose influence the environment Beginning ability to evaluate one's own behaviour	Lack of self-confidence Pessimism, fear of wrongdoing Overcontrol and overrestriction of own activity
School age	6 to 12 years	Industry versus inferiority	Beginning to create, develop, and manipulate Developing sense of competence and perseverance	Loss of hope, sense of being mediocre Withdrawal from school and peers
Adolescence	12 to 20 years	Identity versus role confusion	Coherent sense of self Plans to actualize one's abilities	Feelings of confusion, indecisiveness, and possible antisocial behaviour
Young adulthood	18 to 25 years	Intimacy versus isolation	Intimate relationship with another person Commitment to work and relationships Impersonal relationships	Avoidance of relationship, career, or lifestyle commitments
Adulthood	25 to 65 years	Generativity versus stagnation	Creativity, productivity, concern for others	Self-indulgence, self-concern, lack of interests and commitments
Maturity	65 years to death	Integrity versus despair	Acceptance of the worth and uniqueness of one's own life	Acceptance of death Sense of loss, contempt for others

Source: Adapted from Erikson, E. H. (1991). *Childhood and society.* New York, NY: W. W. Norton. Copyright 1950, 1963 by W. W. Norton & Company, Inc., renewed 1978, 1991 by Erik H. Erikson. Reprinted by permission of W. W. Norton & Company, Inc.

After attaining one developmental stage, the person may fall back and need to approach it again.

Erikson's eight stages reflect both positive and negative aspects of the critical life periods. The resolution of the conflicts at each stage enables the person to function effectively in society. Each stage has its developmental task, and the individual must find a balance between, for example, trust versus mistrust (stage 1) or integrity versus despair (stage 8) (see Figures 17.2 and 17.3).

When using Erikson's developmental framework, nurses should be aware of indicators of positive and negative resolutions of each stage and note that the environment is highly influential in development. Nurses can enhance a client's development by being aware of the person's developmental stage and by helping the person develop coping skills relative to stressors experienced at that level and by providing the individual with appropriate opportunities and encouragement. For example, a 10-year-old child with an illness can be encouraged to

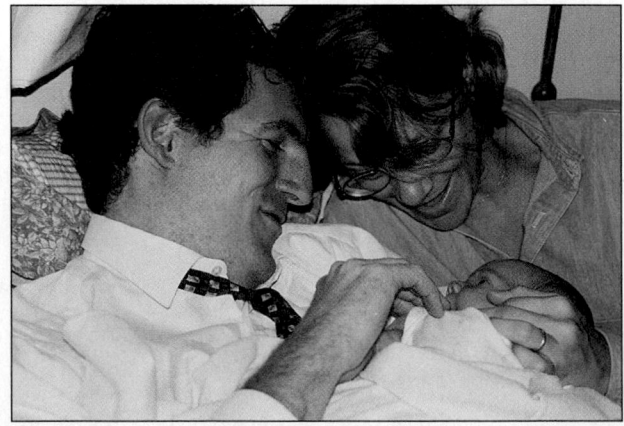

FIGURE 17.2 Trust is established when the infant's basic needs are met.

be creative, to finish schoolwork, and to learn how to accomplish these tasks within the limitations imposed by his or her illness.

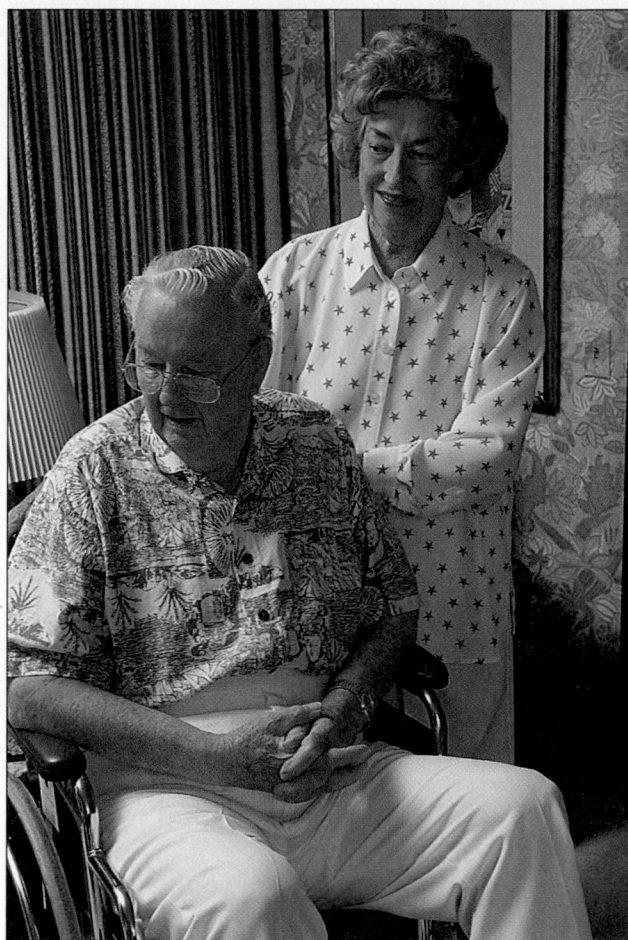

FIGURE 17.3 Assistive devices help maintain independence and self-esteem, which also helps the older adult's ego integrity to adapt and cope with the reality of aging.

Erikson emphasized that people must change and adapt their behaviour to maintain control over their lives. No stage in personality development can be bypassed, but people can become fixated at one stage or regress to a previous stage. For example, a middle-aged woman who has never satisfactorily accomplished the task of resolving identity versus role confusion might regress to an earlier stage when stressed by an illness she cannot cope with.

ROBERT PECK (1919–2002) Robert Peck believed that physical capabilities and functions decrease with old age but that mental and social capacities tend to increase in the latter part of life (Peck, 1968). He proposed three developmental tasks during old age, in contrast to Erikson's stage of maturity (integrity versus despair):

1. *Ego differentiation versus work-role preoccupation.* An adult's identity and feelings of worth are highly dependent on that person's work role. On retirement, people may experience feelings of worthlessness unless they derive their sense of identity from a number of roles so that one such role can replace the work role or occupation as a source of self-esteem. For example, a man who likes to garden or golf can obtain ego rewards from those activities, replacing rewards formerly obtained from his occupation.

2. *Body transcendence versus body preoccupation.* This task calls for the individual to adjust to decreasing physical capacities and, at the same time, maintain feelings of well-being. Preoccupation with declining body functions reduces happiness and satisfaction with life.

3. *Ego transcendence versus ego preoccupation.* Ego transcendence is the acceptance, without fear, of death as inevitable. This acceptance includes being actively involved in our own future beyond death. Ego preoccupation, in contrast, results in holding onto life and a preoccupation with self-gratification.

ROGER GOULD (B. 1935) Roger Gould (1972) believed that transformation is a central theme during adulthood. (See the Evidence-Informed Practice box.) He described seven stages of adult development:

1. *Stage 1 (ages 16–18).* Individuals consider themselves part of the family, rather than individuals, and want to separate from their parents.

2. *Stage 2 (ages 18–22).* Although the individuals have established autonomy, they feel it is in jeopardy; they feel they could be pulled back into their families.

EVIDENCE-INFORMED PRACTICE

Does Masculinity Have Anything to Do with Men's Depression?

Depression affects between 3% and 16.9% of individuals worldwide. International university male students are particularly vulnerable to depression because of social isolation in addition to academic pressures while transitioning into adulthood. The purpose of this study was to explore their perceptions about the cause, implications, and management of their depression. Fifteen international male students at a Canadian university who suffered from depression were interviewed after they completed a 21-item Beck Depression Inventory. The findings revealed three intricately connected themes as the cause of depression: (a) sex and gender, (b) the limits of self-disclosure, and (c) self-managed men. These male students denied illness, treated their own symptoms, and avoided professional services so as to maintain their masculinity.

NURSING IMPLICATIONS: Life circumstances can exacerbate depression. Any university students, including international university students, may experience isolation amid academic pressures. Nurses must assess the gender and role ideals as well as cultural expectations of their adult clients, determine if their perceptions are congruent with the society norms, and encourage their client to seek the needed care for depression.

Source: Based on Oliffe, J. L., Robertson, S., Kelly, M. T., Roy, P., & Ogrodniczuk, J. S. (2010). Connecting masculinity and depression among international male university students. *Quality Health Research, 20*(7), 987–998. doi: 20360568.

3. *Stage 3 (ages 22–28).* Individuals feel established as adults and autonomous from their families. They see themselves as well defined but still feel the need to prove themselves to their parents. They see this as the time for growing and building for the future.

4. *Stage 4 (ages 28–34).* Marriage and careers are well established. Individuals question what life is all about and want to be accepted as they are, no longer finding it necessary to prove themselves.

5. *Stage 5 (ages 34–43).* Through self-reflection, individuals question values and life itself. They see time as finite, with little time left to shape the lives of adolescent children.

6. *Stage 6 (ages 43–50).* Personalities are seen as set. Time is accepted as finite. Individuals are interested in social activities with friends and spouse and desire both sympathy and affection from spouse.

7. *Stage 7 (ages 50–60).* This is a period of transformation, with a realization of mortality and a concern for health. There is an increase in warmth and a decrease in negativism. The spouse is seen as a valuable companion (Gould, 1972).

The concept map below provides an overview of growth and development theories and theorists.

CONCEPT MAP Overview of Growth and Development Theories and Theorists

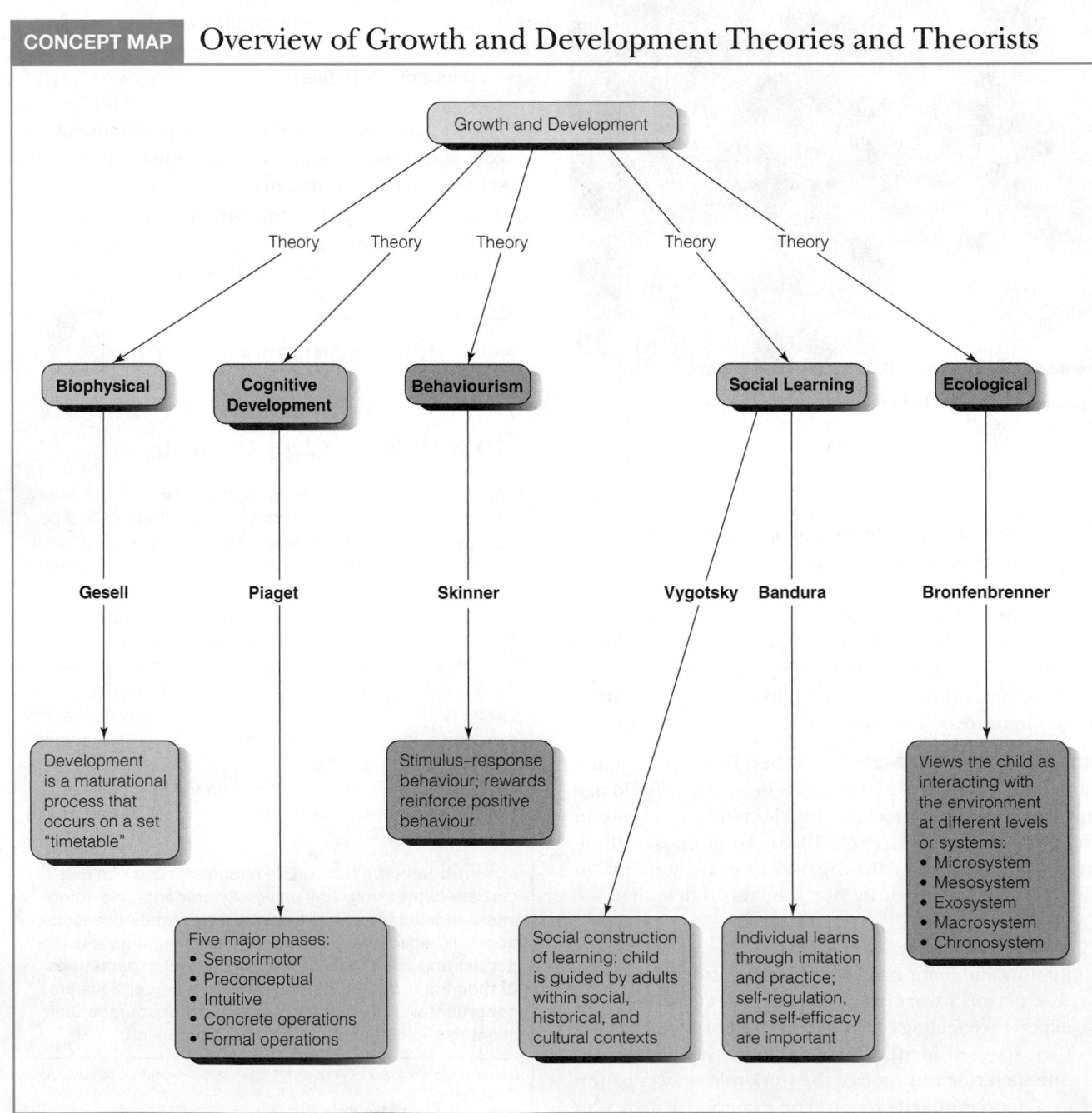

Temperament Theories

STELLA CHESS (1914–2007) AND ALEXANDER THOMAS (1914–2003) Stella Chess and Alexander Thomas identified nine temperamental qualities seen in children's behaviour (see Table 17.5). The "goodness of fit" between children's temperamental qualities and the demands of their environment contributes to positive interaction and positive growth and development (De Pauw, Mervielde, & Van Leeuwen, 2009). **Goodness of fit** refers to whether parents' expectations of their child's behaviour are consistent with the child's temperament type. When parents understand a child's temperament characteristics, they are better able to shape the environment to meet the child's needs.

Attachment Theory

JOHN BOWLBY (1907–1990) British psychologist and physician John Bowlby's attachment theory shares a common belief with Freud's psychoanalytic theories that early childhood experiences have a strong influence on the child's development and later behaviour. He hypothesized that humans have an essential need for **attachment**—or lasting, strong emotional bonds—to others and that the infant–caregiver relationship is the first such attachment. Attachment served as a protective or survival mechanism for the infant. For example, the infant experiences separation anxiety when the attachment figure is absent (Bowlby, 1999).

TABLE 17.5 Characteristics of Temperament

Characteristic	Examples of Behaviour Style
Activity level	Active, restless, always on the move versus quiet, inactive
Sensitivity	Apparently oblivious to stimuli versus reacts to minimal stimuli
Intensity	Minimal reaction to stimuli versus strong and intense reaction
Adaptability	Responds smoothly to unexpected events versus resists change
Distractibility	Focuses on tasks versus easily distracted by minimal stimuli
Approach/ Withdrawal	Jumps right into activities versus hesitant to engage, slow to warm up
Mood	Cheerful, happy versus serious, sombre
Persistence	Sticks to tasks versus easily gives up
Regularity	Demonstrates patterns of behaviour versus random activity

Cognitive Theory

JEAN PIAGET (1896–1980) **Cognitive development** refers to the manner in which people learn to think, reason, and use language. It involves a person's intelligence, perceptual ability, and ability to process information. Cognitive development represents a progression of mental abilities from illogical thinking to logical thinking, from simple problem solving to complex problem solving, and from understanding concrete ideas to understanding abstract concepts.

According to Piaget (1966), the most widely known cognitive theorist, cognitive development is an orderly, sequential process in which a variety of new experiences (stimuli) must exist before intellectual abilities can develop. Piaget's cognitive developmental process is divided into five major phases: (a) the sensorimotor phase, (b) the preconceptual phase, (c) the intuitive thought phase, (d) the concrete operations phase, and (e) the formal operations phase. A person develops through each of these phases, and each phase has its own unique characteristics. See Table 17.6.

In each phase, the person uses three primary abilities: (a) assimilation, (b) accommodation, and (c) adaptation. **Assimilation** is the process through which humans encounter and react to new situations by using the mechanisms they already possess. In this way, people acquire knowledge and skills as well as insights into the world around them. **Accommodation** is a process of change whereby cognitive processes mature sufficiently to allow the person to solve problems that were unsolvable before. This adjustment is possible chiefly because new knowledge has been assimilated. **Adaptation**, or coping behaviour, is the ability to handle the demands made by the environment.

Nurses can employ Piaget's theory of cognitive development when developing teaching strategies. For example, a nurse can expect a toddler to be egocentric and literal; therefore, explanations to the toddler should focus on the needs of the toddler, rather than on the needs of others. When teaching adults, nurses may become aware that some adults are more comfortable with concrete thought and are slower to acquire and apply new information than are other adults.

Behaviourist Theory

B. F. SKINNER (1904–1990) Behaviourist theory, or behaviourism, states that learning takes place when an individual's reaction to a stimulus is either positively or negatively reinforced. The more rapid, consistent, and positive the reinforcement is, the more likely it is that a behaviour will be learned and retained. Skinner believed that organisms learn as they respond to or operate in their environment. He maintained that rewarded or reinforced behaviour will be repeated; behaviour that is punished will be suppressed.

TABLE 17.6 Piaget's Phases of Cognitive Development

Phases and Stages	Age	Significant Behaviour
Sensorimotor phase	**Birth to 2 years**	
Stage 1 Use of reflexes	Birth to 1 month	Most actions are reflexive.
Stage 2 Primary circular reaction	1 to 4 months	Perception of events is centred on the body; objects are extension of self
Stage 3 Secondary circular reaction	4 to 8 months	Acknowledges the external environment; actively makes changes in the environment
Stage 4 Coordination of secondary schemata	8 to 12 months	Can distinguish a goal from the means of attaining it
Stage 5 Tertiary circular reaction	12 to 18 months	Tries and discovers new goals and ways to attain them; rituals are important
Stage 6 Inventions of new means	18 to 24 months	Interprets the environment by mental image; uses make-believe and pretend play
Preconceptual phase	**2 to 4 years**	Uses an egocentric approach to accommodate the demands of an environment Everything is significant and relates to "me" Explores the environment; language development is rapid Associates words with objects
Intuitive thought phase	**4 to 7 years**	Egocentric thinking diminishes; thinks of one idea at a time Includes others in the environment; words express thoughts
Concrete operations phase	**7 to 11 years**	Solves concrete problems; begins to understand relationships such as size; understands right and left; cognizant of viewpoints
Formal operations phase	**11 to 15 years**	Uses rational thinking; reasoning is deductive and futuristic

Sources: Based on Piaget, J. (1966). *The origins of intelligence in children.* New York, NY: W. W. Norton and Company, Inc.; and Murray, R. B., Zentner, J. P., & Yakimo, R. (2009). *Health promotion strategies through the life span.* (8th ed.) (pp. 32–33). Upper Saddle River, NJ: Prentice Hall.

Social Learning Theory

Social learning theory is based on the principle that individuals learn by observing and thinking about the behaviour of the self and others and can be seen as spanning both behaviourist and cognitive learning theories.

ALBERT BANDURA (B. 1925) Albert Bandura believes that learning occurs through imitation and practice; that it requires more awareness, self-motivation, and self-regulation of the individual; and that the individual actively interacts with the environment to learn new skills and behaviours.

LEV VYGOTSKY (1896–1934) Lev Vygotsky explored the concept of cognitive development within social, historical, and cultural contexts. His view was that adults guide children to learn and that development depends on the use of language, play, and extensive social interaction. His ideas have been used in the treatment of children with learning disorders, autism, mental challenges, and other disabilities. His work also supports the benefit of

adult social learning opportunities via group interaction and observation.

Ecological Systems Theory

URIE BRONFENBRENNER (1917–2005) Urie Bronfenbrenner viewed the child as interacting with the environment at different levels, or systems. He believed each child brings a unique set of genes—and specific attributes, such as age, gender, health, and other characteristics—to his or her interactions with the environment.

There are five levels or systems in the ecological systems theory. (a) The *microsystem* includes close relationships the child has on a daily basis (e.g., home, school, friends). (b) The *mesosystem* level includes relationships of microsystems with one another. For example, two common microsystems for children are home and school. (c) The *exosystem* includes those settings that may influence the child but with which the child does not have daily contact (e.g., parent's job, local school board). (d) The *macrosystem* includes attitudes and beliefs of the child's culture. (e) The *chronosystem* involves the period in which the child is growing up as it influences views of health and illness.

Theories of Moral Development

Moral development, a complex process not fully understood, involves learning what ought to be and what ought not to be done. It is more than imprinting parents' rules and virtues or values on children. The term **moral** means "relating to right and wrong." The terms *morality, moral behaviour,* and *moral development* need to be distinguished. **Morality** refers to the requirements necessary for people to live together in society; **moral behaviour** is the way a person perceives those requirements and responds to them; **moral development** is the pattern of change in moral behaviour with age (see Chapter 5).

LAWRENCE KOHLBERG (1927–1987) Lawrence Kohlberg's theory specifically addressed moral development in children and adults (Kohlberg, 1984). Kohlberg focused on the reasons an individual makes a decision. He viewed moral development as progressing through three levels and six stages. These levels and stages are not always linked to a certain developmental stage because some people progress to a higher level of moral development than others do.

At Kohlberg's first level, called the *premoral* or *preconventional level,* children are responsive to cultural rules and labels of good and bad, right and wrong. However, children interpret these in terms of the physical consequences of their actions, that is, punishment or reward. At the second level, the *conventional level,* the individual is concerned about maintaining the expectations of the family, group, or nation and sees this as right. The emphasis at this level is on conformity and loyalty to his or her own expectations as well as society's. (See Evidence-Informed Practice Box on page 329.) Level three is called the *postconventional, autonomous,* or *principled level.* At this level, people make an effort to define valid values and principles without regard to outside authority or to the expectations of others. (See Table 17.7.)

TABLE 17.7 Kohlberg's Stages of Moral Development

Level	Stage	Average Age
I. Preconventional The person is responsive to cultural rules and labels of good and bad, right or wrong. Externally established rules determine right or wrong actions. The person reasons in terms of punishment, reward, or exchange of favours.	**1. Punishment and Obedient Orientation** Fear of punishment, not respect for authority, is the reason for decisions, behaviour, and conformity.	Toddler to 7 years
Egocentric focus	**2. Instrumental Relativist Orientation** Conformity is based on egocentricity and narcissistic needs. There is no feeling of justice, loyalty, or gratitude. "I'll do something if I get something for it or because it pleases you."	Preschool age through school age
II. Conventional The person is concerned with maintaining the expectations and rules of the family, group, nation, or society. A sense of guilt has developed and affects behaviour. The person values conformity, loyalty, and active maintenance of social order and control. Conformity means good behaviour or what pleases or helps another and is approved.	**3. Interpersonal Concordance Orientation** Decisions and behaviour are based on concerns about others' reactions; the person wants others' approval or a reward. An empathic response, based on understanding of how another person feels, is a determinant for decisions and behaviour. ("I can put myself in your shoes.")	School age through adulthood Most Canadian women are in this stage.
Societal focus	**4. Law-and-Order Orientation** The person wants established rules from authorities, and the reason for decisions and behaviour is that social and sexual rules and traditions demand the response. ("I'll do something because it's the law and my duty.")	Adolescence and adulthood Most Canadian men are in this stage.

(continued)

TABLE 17.7 *(continued)*

Level	Stage	Average Age
III. Postconventional The person lives autonomously and defines moral values and principles that are distinct from personal identification with group values. He or she lives according to the principles that are universally agreed on and that the person considers appropriate for life.	**5. Social Contract Legalistic Orientation** The social rules are not the sole basis for decisions and behaviour because the person believes a higher moral principle applies, such as equality, justice, or due process.	Middle-age or older adult. (Only 20% or less of Canadians achieve this stage.)
Universal focus	**6. Universal Ethical Principle Orientation** Decisions and behaviours are based on internalized rules, on conscience rather than social laws, and on self-chosen ethical and abstract principles that are universal, comprehensive, and consistent.	Middle-age or older adult. Few people attain or maintain this stage. Examples of this stage are seen in times of crisis or extreme situations.

Source: Adapted from Murray, R. B., Zentner, J. P., & Yakimo, R. (2009). *Health promotion strategies through the life span* (8th ed.) (pp. 32–33). Upper Saddle River, NJ: Merrill/ Prentice Hall. Adapted with permission.

CAROL GILLIGAN (B. 1936) Carol Gilligan (1982) believes that moral development needs to include the concepts of caring and responsibility. She views moral development as proceeding through three levels and two transitions, with each level representing a more complex understanding of the relationship of the self and others and each transition resulting in a crucial reevaluation of the conflict between selfishness and responsibility (Murray, Zentner, & Yakimo, 2009, p. 251).

- *Stage 1, caring for the self.* In this stage, the person is concerned only with caring for the self. The individual feels isolated, alone, and unconnected to others and has no concern or conflict with the needs of others because the self is most important. The focus of this stage is survival. The end of this stage occurs when the individual begins to view this approach as selfish. At this time, the person also begins to see a need for relationships and connections with other people.

- *Stage 2, caring for others.* The individual recognizes the selfishness of earlier behaviour and begins to understand the need for caring relationships with others. Caring relationships bring with them responsibility. The definition of *responsibility* includes self-sacrifice, where "good" is considered to be "caring for others." The individual now approaches relationships with a focus of not hurting others. This approach causes the individual to be more responsive and submissive to others' needs, excluding any thoughts of meeting his or her own. A transition occurs when the individual recognizes that this approach can cause difficulties with relationships because of the lack of balance between caring for the self and caring for others.

- *Stage 3, caring for the self and others.* A person sees the need for a balance between caring for others and caring for the self. The concept of responsibility now includes responsibility for the self and for other people. Care remains the focus by which decisions are made.

However, the person recognizes the interconnections between the self and others and realizes that if his or her own needs are not met, other people may also suffer.

Gilligan believes women often see morality in the integrity of relationships and caring so that the moral problems they encounter are different from those of men. Men tend to consider what is right to be what is just, whereas for women, what is right is taking responsibility for others as a self-chosen decision (Gilligan, 1982). The ethic of justice, or fairness, is based on the idea of equality and equal treatment.

Theories of Spiritual Development

The spiritual component of growth and development refers to individuals' understanding of their relationship with the universe and their perceptions about the direction and meaning of life.

JAMES FOWLER (B. 1940) James Fowler describes **faith** as a force that gives meaning to a person's life. *Faith* is a form of knowing, a way of being in relation to "an ultimate environment"; it is a relational phenomenon and is "an active 'mode-of-being-in-relation' to another or others in which we invest commitment, belief, love, risk and hope" (Fowler & Keen, 1985, p. 18). (See Table 17.8.)

Fowler believes that the development of faith is an interactive process between the person and the environment. In each of Fowler's stages, new patterns of thought, values, and beliefs are added to those already held by the individual; therefore, the stages must follow in sequence.

JOHN WESTERHOFF (B. 1933) Westerhoff (2000) described faith as a way of being and behaving that evolves from an experienced faith guided by parents and others during a person's infancy and childhood to an

TABLE 17.8 Fowler's Stages of Spiritual Development

Stage	Age	Description
0. Undifferentiated	0 to 3 years	Infant unable to formulate concepts about self or the environment
1. Intuitive–projective	4 to 6 years	A combination of images and beliefs given by trusted others, mixed with the child's own experience and imagination
2. Mythical–literal	7 to 12 years	Private world of fantasy and wonder; symbols refer to something specific; dramatic stories and myths used to communicate spiritual meanings
3. Synthetic–conventional	Adolescent or adult	World and ultimate environment structured by the expectations and judgments of others; interpersonal focus
4. Individuating–reflective	After 18 years	Constructing one's own explicit system; high degree of self-consciousness
5. Paradoxical–consolidative	After 30 years	Awareness of truth from a variety of viewpoints
6. Universalizing	Maybe never	Becoming an incarnation of the principles of love and justice

Sources: Adapted from Fowler, J. & Keen, S. (1985). *Life maps: Conversations in the journey of faith.* Waco, TX: Word Books; and Hollander, A. (1980). *How to help your child have a spiritual life: A parents' guide to inner development.* New York, NY: A and W Publishers. Used with permission.

TABLE 17.9 Westerhoff's Four Stages of Faith

Stage	Age	Behaviour
Experienced faith	Infancy/early adolescence	Experiences faith through interaction with others living a particular faith tradition
Affiliative faith	Late adolescence	Actively participates in activities that characterize a particular faith tradition; experiences awe, wonderment, and a sense of belonging
Searching faith	Young adulthood	Through a process of questioning and doubting own faith; acquires a cognitive as well as an affective faith
Owned faith	Middle adulthood/old age	Puts faith into personal and social action and is willing to stand up for beliefs, even against a nurturing community

Source: Based on Westerhoff, J. (2000). *Will our children have faith?* New York, NY: Morehouse Publishing.

owned faith that is internalized in adulthood and serves as a directive for personal action (see Table 17.9). For the client who is ill, faith—whether in a higher authority (e.g., God, Allah, Jehovah), in the client's own self, in the health care team, or in a combination of all—provides strength and trust.

Applying Growth and Development Concepts to Nursing Practice

Different theories explain one or more aspects of an individual's growth and development. The nurse may find it necessary to apply several theories for an adequate understanding of the growth and development of a client (see the Reflect on Primary Health Care box). Developmental theories can be useful in guiding assessment, explaining behaviour, and providing a direction for nursing interventions. An understanding of a child's intellectual ability helps a nurse anticipate and explain certain reactions, responses, and needs. Nurses can then encourage client behaviour that is appropriate for that particular developmental stage. In adult care, knowledge about the physical, cognitive, and psychological aspects of the aging process is a fundamental aspect of administering sensitive nursing care.

REFLECT ON 🔑 **PRIMARY HEALTH CARE**

By understanding human growth and development, nurses can provide anticipatory *health-promotion* teaching to help clients reach their optimal health. Consider this example: Pregnant adolescents tend to make egocentric and lifestyle choices without regard for the future health consequences of the unborn child; nurses can teach pregnant teens that maternal alcohol consumption during pregnancy can negatively alter the growth and developmental potential of the fetus. Find out if pregnant teens have *access* to early prenatal care in your community.

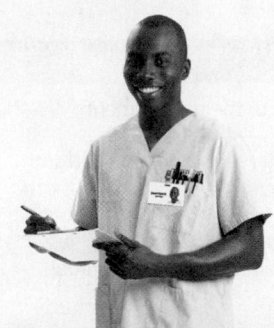

Case Study 17

Finnegan, an inquisitive, energetic 2-year-old, is diagnosed with amblyopia (lazy eye) and far-sightedness in his stronger eye. Untreated, this condition will lead to blindness in the affected eye. Treatment includes wearing an eye patch over his stronger eye for two hours a day and wearing glasses with a corrective lens at all times when he is awake. Finnegan's mother says he resists actively when she or his father places the patch and that it is "almost impossible" to get him to leave his glasses on.

CRITICAL THINKING QUESTIONS

1. According to Erikson, at what stage of development is Finnegan?

2. What strategies could you suggest Finnegan's parents use to increase his cooperation with treatment?

3. Specifically describe strategies based on Piaget's theory of cognitive development and the theory of social learning.

Check the eText in MyNursingLab for answers and explanations.

KEY TERMS

accommodation *p. 333*

adaptation *p. 333*

adaptive mechanisms *p. 328*

assimilation *p. 333*

attachment *p. 333*

cognitive development *p. 333*

defence mechanisms *p. 328*

development *p. 325*

developmental milestones *p. 325*

developmental task *p. 327*

ego *p. 328*

faith *p. 336*

fixation *p. 329*

goodness of fit *p. 333*

growth *p. 325*

id *p. 328*

libido *p. 328*

moral *p. 335*

moral behaviour *p. 335*

moral development *p. 335*

morality *p. 335*

personality *p. 327*

superego *p. 328*

temperament *p. 326*

unconscious mind *p. 328*

CHAPTER HIGHLIGHTS

- Growth is physical change and an increase in size. The pattern of physiological growth is similar for all people.

- Development is an increase in the complexity of function and skill progression. It is the capacity and skill of the individual to adapt to the environment.

- The rate of a person's growth and development is highly individual, but the sequence of growth and development is predictable.

- Heredity and environment are the primary factors influencing growth and development.

- Components of growth and development are generally categorized as biophysical, psychosocial, cognitive, behavioural, social, ecological, moral, and spiritual.

- Temperament, the way in which individuals respond to their external and internal environments, influences the interactive dynamics of growth and development.

- Gesell's biophysical development theory stated that development is directed by genetics.

- Psychosocial development refers to the development of personality. Psychosocial theorists include Havighurst, Freud, Erikson, Peck, and Gould.

- Attachment theory states that humans have a need for strong emotional bonds to others.

- Havighurst believed that learning is basic to life and that people continue to learn throughout life. His theory describes six age periods, with developmental tasks for each period.

- Cognitive development refers to the manner in which people learn to think, reason, and use language. The most widely known cognitive theorist is Piaget.

- Behaviourist learning theory emphasizes stimulus response and either positive or negative reinforcement as the basis for learning and behaviour change.

- Social learning theory states that learning can occur by observation. Role modelling and learning from watching role models are a part of social learning theory.
- Ecologic systems theory sees the child as interacting with the environment at different levels, or systems. Bronfenbrenner described five levels or systems of interaction.
- Moral development, a complex process not fully understood, involves learning what ought to be and what ought not to be done. Kohlberg's theory focuses on the reasons an individual makes a decision.

- Gilligan's theory included the concepts of caring and responsibility.
- The spiritual component of growth and development refers to individuals' understanding of their relationship with the universe and their perceptions about the direction and meaning of life. Fowler and Westerhoff are two theorists who describe stages of spiritual development or faith.
- The nurse uses developmental theories in guiding assessment, explaining behaviour, and providing a direction for interventions to promote the client's health.

ASSESS YOUR LEARNING

1. Which of the following is true about human growth and development?

   a. The time of onset, length, and pace of developmental stages is predictable.

   b. Some stages are more critical than others.

   c. Growth and development occur in a proximal to distal direction.

   d. It proceeds from a specific response to a more generalized one.

2. Which is one example of how to integrate Piaget's theory to nursing practice?

   a. Giving a thorough explanation of why taking medication is important to a 3-year-old

   b. Providing a choice of two methods of medicine administration, by glass or spoon, to a 5-year-old.

   c. Assimilating family members into the care plan to promote positive outcomes

   d. Providing a structured daily routine for a hospitalized adolescent

3. Constance, age 12 years, is crying by her locker at school. Her friends are gathered around, trying to "give her some protection." You are the school nurse who is called by the physical education teacher to come and help out. On the way, you reflect on the most likely scenario you will find. Based on the norms of growth and development, you would most likely find which situation?

   a. Constance has begun her menstrual cycle, was unprepared, and is embarrassed and frightened.

   b. Students want to focus on Constance's need for peer pressure.

   c. Constance has fallen or been injured and has collapsed by her locker in pain.

   d. Her friends have been trying to protect her from bullies in the school.

4. The parents of a 5-month-old infant and a 3-year-old child ask the nurse about the sequence and timing of developmental milestones. Which of the following is the MOST appropriate response?

   a. "This infant should reach the milestones at the same time as your older child did."

   b. "The infant may reach the milestones in a different order from your older child."

   c. "The sequence of milestones should follow the same pattern.

   d. "There are no predictable patterns. Try to enjoy the uniqueness of each child."

5. Fred, a university student, is invited by a group of students to cheat on an exam. He declines and reports the situation to university officials as he believes the behaviour is unethical. Which of Kohlberg's stages of moral development does this exemplify?

   a. Conventional

   b. Societal focus

   c. Postconventional

   d. Universal

6. A 14-year-old is scheduled to have surgical repair of a spinal curvature (scoliosis). The adolescent will be hospitalized for about 2 weeks. What nursing intervention will be MOST helpful during the hospital stay?

   a. Having peers visit frequently during the day

   b. Instructing parents to room-in with her

   c. Encouraging her to go to the recreation room

   d. Encouraging her to arrange for her teachers to provide her with homework

7. A 70-year-old man who recently retired after 40 years of work as an independent contractor is scheduled for a physical examination. Using Erikson's stages of social development the nurse should be concerned about which of the following comments?

   a. "My wife and I are planning to drive to Halifax in June to visit our grandkids."

   b. "Every day, when I wake up, it's hard to find a reason to get out of bed."

   c. "I often take ibuprofen for the pain in my knees."

   d. "People still call me for advice on building projects. I may never get to retire!"

8. An 11-year-old child is scheduled for a yearly physical examination. The accompanying parent expresses concern because the child "seems all wrapped up in the soccer teammates and other peers, leaving very little time for the family." Using Havighurst's developmental tasks, what would be the nurse's BEST response?

   a. "This is somewhat unusual. Are there problems that we need to discuss?"

   b. "Although this is normal for 11-year-olds, this transition can be difficult for families."

   c. "Become involved in her life and insist that she set aside time for the family."

   d. "This is normal development. You need to let her grow up."

9. A 5-year-old boy arrives for the pre-admission work-up for a surgical procedure. When the nurse brings in the intravenous (IV) control pump the child states, "I am afraid that it will bite me because I have been bad." Using knowledge of Piaget, Erikson, and Fowler, which of the following is the BEST nursing intervention?

   a. Reassure the child by providing opportunities for touching and exploring the machine, as well as explaining how it works.

   b. Understand that his imagination is out of control. Tell him that his fears are unfounded and that he should act like a "big boy."

   c. Recognize that he is too young to understand and that he needs to be quickly distracted.

   d. Acknowledge his need for fantasy by reassuring him that if he is a "good boy" the bad machine will not bite him.

10. Nursing implications associated with the care of people in middle adulthood must consider which of the following?

   a. Clients' stage of development encourages them to be self-centred and actively changing.

   b. Individuals will be focused on their increasing age and physical limits.

   c. Personal lifestyle changes result from physical changes in the self and others.

   d. The peer group is vitally important to the accomplishment of developmental tasks.

> *Check the eText in MyNursingLab for answers and explanations.*

WEBLINKS

Ontario Ministry of Education. (2010). Health and physical education: The Ontario curriculum for grades 1-8 students.

http://www.canadianvalues.ca/SCC/health18curr2010.pdf

This document outlines physical education programs standards, goals, and activities for grades 1-8 students to promote healthy growth and development.

Canadian Institute of Child Health

http://www.cich.ca

The site provides information on children's policies, research, and programs pertaining to nurturing, protecting, educating, and empowering children.

Public Health Agency of Canada—Division of Childhood and Adolescence

http://www.phac-aspc.gc.ca/dca-dea/main_e.html

The Division of Childhood and Adolescence serves as a centre of expertise, leadership, and coordination within the federal government and Health Canada for issues, activities, and programs concerning children and youth.

MyNursingLab

MyNursingLab's guided learning path makes reviewing and test preparation straightforward.

– Content summaries, animations, and videos reinforce key concepts and skills

– Practice questions help with test prep by showing gaps in knowledge

– An eText, available online and via the iPad, makes searching, highlighting, and note-taking easy

This QR code appears at the end of every chapter and provides learning resources that you can access with your smartphone to study on the go. Access self-review quizzes, flashcards, and more!

REFERENCES

Bowlby, J. (1999). Attachment and loss. Vol. 1. *Attachment* (2nd ed.). New York, NY: Basic Books.

De Pauw, S. S., Mervielde, I., & Van Leeuwen, K. G. (2009). How are traits related to problem behaviour in preschoolers? Similarities and contrasts between temperament and personality. *Journal of Abnormal Child Psychology 37*, 309–325. doi:10.1007/s10802-008-9290-0

Erikson, E. H. (1963). *Childhood and society* (2nd ed.). New York, NY: Norton.

Erikson, E. H. (1964). *Insight and responsibility: Lectures on the ethical implications of psychoanalytic insight.* New York, NY: Norton.

Fowler, J., & Keen, S. (1985). *Life maps: Conversations in the journey of faith.* Waco, TX: Word Books.

Freud, S. (1923). *The ego and the id.* London, UK: Hogarth Press.

Gilligan, C. (1982). *In a different voice: Psychological theory and women's development.* Cambridge, MA: Harvard University Press.

Gould, R. L. (1972). The phases of adult life: A study in developmental psychology. *American Journal of Psychiatry, 129,* 33–43.

Havighurst, R. J. (1972). *Developmental tasks and education* (3rd ed.). New York, NY: Longman Publishers.

Kohlberg, L. (1984). *Essays on moral development: Vol. 2. The psychology of moral development.* San Francisco, CA: Harper & Row.

Murray, R. B., Zentner, J. P., & Yakimo, R. (2009). *Health promotion strategies through the life span* (8th ed.). Upper Saddle River, NJ: Prentice Hall.

Peck, R. (1968). *Psychological developments in the second half of life.* In B. L. Neugarten (Ed.), *Middle age and aging* (pp. 88–92). Chicago, IL: University of Chicago Press.

Piaget, J. (1966). *Origins of intelligence in children.* New York, NY: Norton.

Westerhoff, J. (2000). *Will our children have faith?* (Rev. Ed.). New York, NY: Seabury Press.

Chapter 18

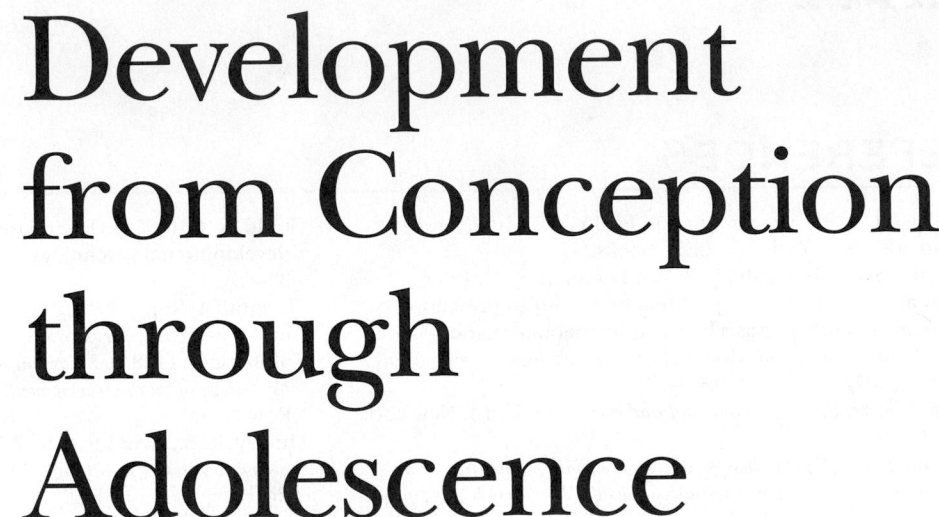

Development from Conception through Adolescence

After studying this chapter, you will be able to:

1. Identify the characteristics and tasks at different stages of development, from infancy through adolescence.

2. Describe expected physical development from infancy through adolescence.

3. Trace psychosocial development according to Erikson, from infancy through adolescence.

4. Explain cognitive development according to Piaget, from infancy through adolescence.

5. Describe the influence of relationships on mental health, from infancy through adolescence.

6. Describe spiritual development according to Fowler and moral development according to Kohlberg throughout childhood and adolescence.

7. Discuss assessment activities and expected characteristics from birth through late childhood.

8. List essential nursing activities to promote and protect the health of infants, toddlers, preschoolers, school-age children, and adolescents.

Knowledge of growth and development is essential for nurses to provide clients with antici-pated guidance for optimal developmental milestones. On the basis of the concepts of growth and development introduced in Chapter 17, this chapter will emphasize health assessment, including health-promotion and health-protection activities to meet physical, psycho-social, cognitive, moral, and spiritual developmental needs from infancy through adolescence.

Conception and Prenatal Development

Conception and prenatal, or intrauterine, develop-ment lasts approximately 9 calendar months (10 lunar months) or 38 to 40 weeks, depending on the method of calculation. A lunar month of pregnancy comprises 28 days. Pregnancy is divided into three periods called **trimesters**, each of which lasts about 3 months. The two phases of intrauterine life are the *embryonic phase* in the first trimester and the *fetal phase* in the second and third trimesters.

The fertilized ovum develops into an organism with most of the human features in the *embryonic phase*. The embryo is implanted in the endometrium of the uterus. The *placenta* is a flat, disc-shaped organ that is highly vascular. It normally forms in the upper segment of the endometrium of the uterus. Its functions are to exchange nutrients and gases between the embryo or fetus and the mother to sustain growth in utero.

Within the first three weeks of life, tissues differenti-ate into three layers—the *ectoderm* (outer layer), the *meso-derm* (middle layer), and the *endoderm* or *entoderm* (inner layer). The ectoderm and endoderm are formed in the second week; the mesoderm forms in the third week. These layers form all of the body's complex organs and systems as a series of outpouchings, inpouchings, fold-ings, and tubular formations. Organs are developed between 8 to 12 weeks during this *embryonic phase*. The *fetal phase* is characterized by a period of rapid growth in the size of the fetus. Both genetic and environmen-tal factors affect its growth (Murray, Zentner, & Yakimo, 2009).

At the end of the second trimester, the fetus resem-bles a small baby. Because very little fat is present beneath the skin of the fetus, skin appears wrinkled, red, and transparent. The underlying blood vessels are visible. A protective covering, called **vernix caseosa**, begins to develop over the fetus's skin. This is a white, cheese-like substance that adheres to skin and may become 3 mm thick by birth. **Lanugo**, fine, downy hair, covers the body. At about 5 months, the mother begins to feel fetal move-ment, and the fetal heartbeat is audible.

At the end of the third trimester, the fetus is approxi-mately 50 cm long and weighs 3.2 to 3.8 kg (Public Health Agency of Canada, 2012). Lanugo has disappeared, and skin has a normal colour and appears less wrinkled. More subcutaneous fat makes the fetus look more rotund. The fetus gains most of its weight during the last 2 months in utero. Box 18.1 lists maternal factors that can lead to a higher risk of a low-birth-weight baby (<2.5 kg).

Health Promotion

During the intrauterine stage of fetal development, the embryo or fetus relies on the maternal blood flow through the placenta to meet its basic survival needs. The health of the mother is essential for optimal fetal growth and development.

OXYGEN To meet the fetal demands for oxygen, the pregnant mother gradually increases her normal blood flow by about one-third, peaking at about 8 months;

BOX 18.1 MATERNAL FACTORS THAT CONTRIBUTE TO A HIGHER RISK OF LOW-BIRTH-WEIGHT BABIES

The following factors can contribute to mothers having low-birth-weight babies:

- Underweight before pregnancy
- Less than 9 kg weight gain during pregnancy
- Inadequate prenatal care
- Age 17 years or younger, or 49 years or older
- History of hypertension
- Low socioeconomic level
- Exposure to toxic substances or chemicals
- Smoking cigarettes during pregnancy
- Use of addictive drugs or alcohol during pregnancy
- Complications during pregnancy, poor health status, exposure to infections
- High stress levels, including physical or emotional abuse
- Previous low-birth-weight infants or multiple miscarriages
- Having given birth less than 6 months or 10 or more years ago

Source: Adapted from R. B. Murray, & J. P. Zentner, & R. Yakimo. (2009). *Health promotion strategies through the life span* (8th ed.) (p. 233)., Upper Saddle River, NJ: Prentice Hall. Reprinted with permission.

increases tidal volume by about 40% with associated increased respiration; and increases her cardiac output significantly. Fetal circulation travels from the placenta through two umbilical arteries, which carry deoxygenated blood away from the fetus. By 20 weeks, the fetal heartbeat is audible through a fetoscope, or as early as the tenth week if a Doppler stethoscope with ultrasound is used.

NUTRITION AND FLUIDS The fetus obtains nourishment from the placental circulation and by swallowing amniotic fluid. Nutritional needs are met when the mother eats a well-balanced diet containing sufficient calories to meet both her needs and those of the fetus. Adequate folic acid, which is one of the B vitamins, is important to prevent neural tube defects (e.g., spina bifida) in the fetus.

REST AND ACTIVITY The fetus sleeps most of the time but develops a pattern of sleep and wakefulness that can persist after birth. Fetal activity begins about the fifth lunar month of pregnancy.

ELIMINATION Throughout pregnancy, fetal feces are formed from swallowed amniotic fluid, but normally no stool is passed until after birth. Inadequate oxygenation of the fetus during the third trimester can result in relaxation of the anal sphincter and passage of feces into the amniotic fluid. Urine normally is excreted into the amniotic fluid when the kidneys mature (16 to 20 weeks).

TEMPERATURE MAINTENANCE Although amniotic fluid provides a constant temperature for the fetus, significant increases in temperature caused by maternal fever or the use of hot whirlpool baths or saunas can alter the temperature of the amniotic fluid and that of the fetus and may result in birth defects. In the last weeks of gestation, the fetus develops subcutaneous fatty tissue stores that will help maintain body temperature at birth.

SAFETY The embryo is particularly vulnerable to damage or harm from a **teratogen**—anything that adversely affects normal cellular development in the embryo or fetus. Expectant mothers must avoid radiography (x-ray) and medications that are known teratogens.

Exposure to environmental tobacco smoke has been associated with preterm labour, spontaneous abortion, low-birth-weight infants, sudden infant death syndrome, and learning disorders (Pogodina, Brunner Huber, Racine, & Platanova, 2009). Maternal, neonatal, and infant mortality are significantly increased with maternal use of drugs or alcohol and exposure to other chemicals (Wigle et al., 2008). **Fetal alcohol spectrum disorder** (FASD), a result of alcohol use by the pregnant woman, is defined as impaired mitochondrial development in the fetus that leads to microcephaly, intellectual disability (also known as mental retardation), learning disorders, and other central nervous system defects (Rasmussen, Andrew, Zwaigenbaum, & Tough, 2008). All women of childbearing age should abstain from alcohol and drug use. Those who engage in unprotected sex are at significant risk for sexually transmitted infections (STIs).

Neonates and Infants (Birth to One Year)

Physical Development

The neonate's basic task is survival, which requires breathing, sleeping, sucking, eating, swallowing, digesting, and eliminating. Newborns and infants undergo significant physiological change in weight, length, head growth, vision, and motor development. Because many of the infant's activities and pleasures are mouth centred, this stage in development is often referred to as the *oral stage* (see Chapter 17, the section on Freud).

WEIGHT At birth, most babies weigh about 3.2 to 3.8 kg. Just after birth, most newborns lose 5% to 10% of their birth weight because of fluid loss and regain that weight in about 1 week. After several days, they gain weight at the rate of 150 g to 210 g weekly for 6 months. By 5 months of age, infants usually double their birth weight, and by 12 months, triple their birth weight. Rapid weight gain in the first year of life, especially in the first 5 to 6 months, is related to obesity in children and adults (Goodell, Wakefield, & Ferris, 2009). Exclusive breast-feeding in the first 4 to 6 months may be helpful in preventing excessive weight gain. (See the Reflect on Primary Health Care box.)

LENGTH The average length of a Canadian newborn is about 50 cm to 52 cm. At birth, black Canadian infants tend to be shorter. Female babies, on average, are smaller

---

REFLECT ON 🔑 **PRIMARY HEALTH CARE**

Growth monitoring is an integral part of physical assessment of children. Aboriginal children tend to be heavier at birth and in early life compared with children from other ethnic groups. The Canadian Paediatric Society (CPS) (Marchand, 2010) saw little purpose in devising a special growth curve for each ethnic group. It adapted the World Health Organization's growth charts (see the Weblinks section of this chapter) for *all* Canadian children, from birth to age 19 years, regardless of their race and ethnicity. The CPS emphasized the importance of assessing growth patterns over time to detect deviations, addressing the nature of the problem early, and not focusing on race and ethnicity. Growth charts are useful health assessment tools for children. Consider how using growth charts is a reflection of the primary health care principles of *appropriate technology* and *health promotion*.

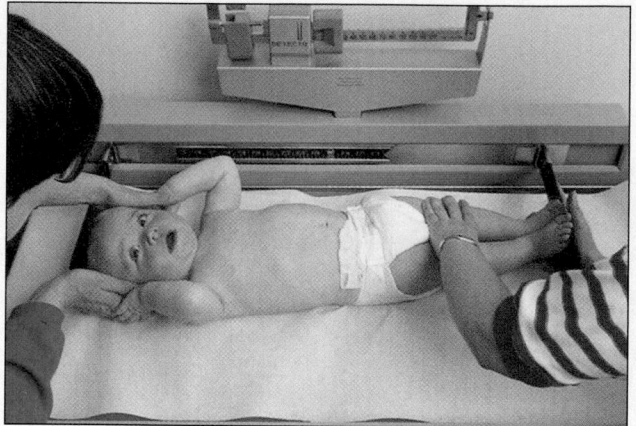

FIGURE 18.1 Measuring an infant head to heel, from the top of the head to the base of the heels.

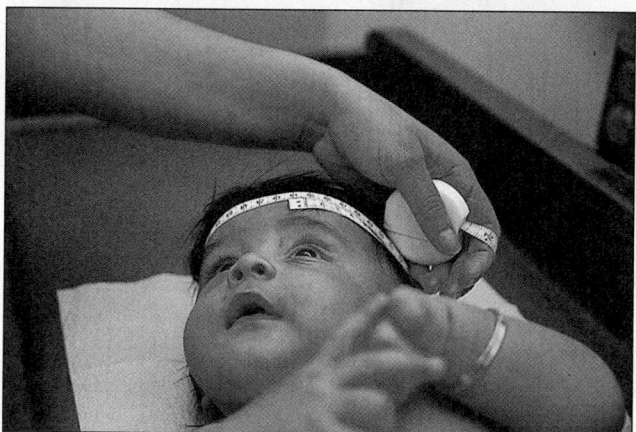

FIGURE 18.2 An infant's head circumference is measured around the skull, above the eyebrows.

than male babies. Two lengths measured are (a) the crown-to-rump length (the sitting length) and (b) the recumbent head-to-heel length (from the top of the head to the base of the heels). See Figure 18.1. Normally, the crown-to-rump length is approximately the same as the head circumference. By 6 months, infants gain another 13.75 cm of length. By 12 months, they add another 7.5 cm. The rate of increase in length is largely influenced by the baby's size at birth and by nutrition.

HEAD AND CHEST CIRCUMFERENCE Assessment of head circumference is of particular importance in infants and children to determine the growth rate of the skull and the brain. An infant's head should be measured at every checkup until the child is 2 years old (Figure 18.2). Normal head circumference (**normocephaly**) is often related to chest circumference. At birth, the average head circumference is 33 cm to 35 cm and generally varies only by 1 cm or 2 cm. The chest circumference is usually less than the head circumference by about 2.5 cm. As the infant grows, the chest circumference becomes larger than the head circumference. At about 9 or 10 months,

both circumferences are about the same, and after 1 year of age, the chest circumference is larger.

HEAD MOULDING Moulding of the heads in newborn babies can occur during vaginal deliveries. Moulding of the head is made possible by *fontanelles* (unossified membranous gaps) in the bone structure of the skull and by overriding of the *sutures* (junction lines of the skull bones). Within a week, a newborn's head usually regains its symmetry. The larger anterior fontanelle (4 cm to 6 cm in diameter and diamond shaped) can increase in size for several months after birth. After 6 months, the size gradually decreases until closure occurs between 9 and 18 months. The posterior fontanelle, between the parietal bones and the occipital bone, closes from 4 to 8 weeks after birth (Figure 18.3).

VISION Newborns can follow large moving objects and blink in response to bright light and sound. A newborn's pupils respond slowly, and the eyes cannot focus on close objects. By 1 month, infants can focus their gaze on objects 18–25 cm from their face and follow moving ones. At 4 months, the infant recognizes a parent's smile, although social smiles may appear as early as 2 months. The 4-month-old has almost complete colour vision and follows objects through a 180-degree arc. A 5-month-old infant reaches for objects. Between 6 and 10 months, the infant can fix on an object and follow it in all directions. By 12 months, the infant will have depth perception and recognize drop-offs, such as steps or the edge of the bed.

HEARING Newborns with normal hearing will react with a startle to a loud noise, a reaction called the *Moro reflex.* Within a few days, they are able to distinguish different sounds and may distinguish between the mother's voice and that of another woman. Between 3 and 6 months, the infant will look for sounds, stop an activity to listen, and respond with distress or pleasure to angry or happy voices.

SPEECH Between 6 and 9 months, individual words begin to take on meaning, and the infant may look at named objects or people. The 9- to 12-month-old infant understands many words (e.g., "no," "hot," "dog"), uses gestures (e.g., waves "bye-bye"), may articulate one or two words with a specific reference (e.g., "mama," "dada"), and may respond to simple commands.

SMELL AND TASTE The senses of smell and taste are functional shortly after birth. Newborns can recognize the smell of their mother's milk and respond to this smell by turning toward their mother.

TOUCH The sense of touch is well developed at birth. Skin-to-skin touching (also known as "kangaroo care")

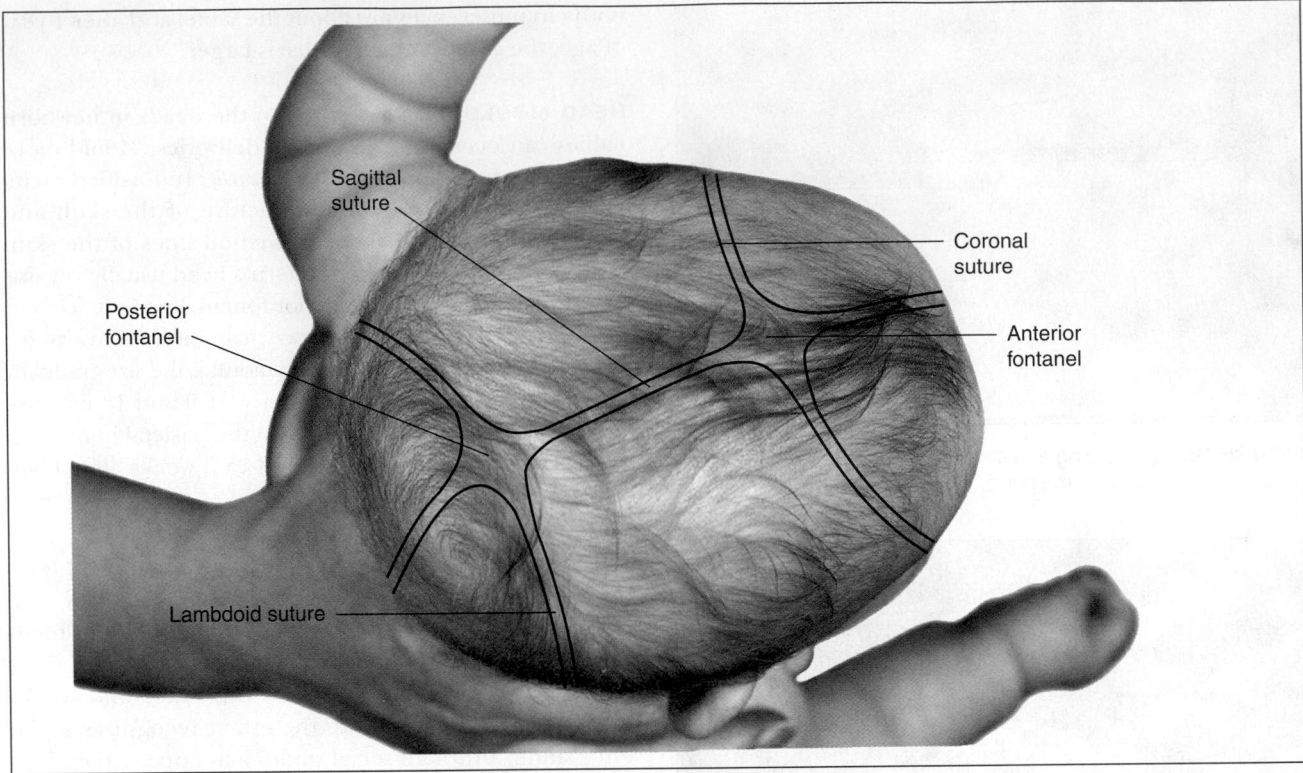

FIGURE 18.3 The bones of the skull, showing the fontanelles and the suture lines.

BOX 18.2 INFANT REFLEXES

From the moment of birth, newborns display the following reflexes of the involuntary nervous system:

- *Sucking Reflex:* A feeding reflex occurs when the infant's lips are touched; it lasts throughout infancy.

- *Rooting Reflex:* A feeding reflex is elicited by touching the baby's cheek, causing the baby's head to turn to the side that was touched; it usually disappears after 4 months.

- *Moro Reflex:* This reflex is often assessed to estimate the maturity of the central nervous system. A loud noise or a sudden change in position elicits this startle reflex. The infant reacts by extending both arms and legs outward with the fingers spread, then suddenly retracting the limbs. The infant may cry at the same time. This reflex disappears after 4 months.

- *Palmar Grasp Reflex:* This reflex occurs when a small object is placed against the palm of the hand, causing the fingers to curl around it. This reflex disappears after 3 months.

- *Plantar Reflex:* When an object is placed just beneath the toes, they curl around it. This reflex disappears after 8 months.

- *Tonic Neck Reflex (TNR) or Fencing Reflex:* When a baby lying on its back turns its head to the right side, for example, the left side of the body shows a flexing of the left arm and the left leg. This postural reflex disappears after 4 months.

- *Stepping Reflex (Walking or Dancing Reflex):* This reflex can be elicited by holding the baby upright so that the feet touch a flat surface. The legs then move up and down as if the baby were walking. This reflex usually disappears at about 2 months.

- *Babinski Reflex:* A newborn baby has a positive Babinski if when the sole of the foot is stroked, the big toe rises and the other toes fan out. After age 1 year, the infant exhibits a negative Babinski; that is, the toes curl downward. A positive Babinski after age 1 year indicates brain damage.

---

is important for an infant's development. The newborn responds positively to warmth, love, and comfort when touched, held, and cuddled and is also sensitive to temperature extremes and pain.

REFLEXES The reflexes of the newborn are involuntary nervous system responses to stimuli. They are neither learned nor consciously carried out. Reflexes normally present at birth are the rooting, sucking, Moro, palmar grasp, plantar, tonic neck, stepping, and Babinski reflexes. See Box 18.2 for a description of these reflexes. Infant reflexes disappear during the first year of life. In addition, the abilities to yawn, stretch, sneeze, burp, and hiccup are all present at birth.

MOTOR DEVELOPMENT Motor development increases with the infants' abilities to move and to control the body. Initially, body movement is uncoordinated. At 1 month,

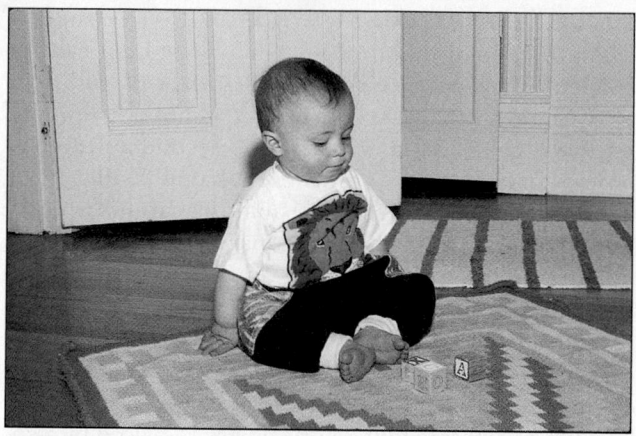

FIGURE 18.4 An infant sits without support at 6 months of age.

they lift their head momentarily when prone, turn their head, and have a head lag when pulled to a sitting position. After 6 months, they can sit without support (Figure 18.4). At 9 months, they can sit, reach, grasp a rattle, and transfer it from hand to hand. At 12 months, they can turn the pages of a book, put objects into a container, and walk and dress themselves with some assistance.

Psychosocial Development

According to Erikson (1963), the central crisis at this stage is *trust versus mistrust* (see Table 17.4 on page 328). Fulfillment of needs is required for the infant to develop a basic sense of trust. Parents can enhance this sense of trust by (a) responding consistently to an infant's needs, (b) providing a predictable environment in which routines are established, and (c) being sensitive to the infant's needs and meeting these needs skillfully and promptly.

Newborns are helpless to care for themselves; they cry to elicit care from their caregivers (Crittenden, 2008). Infants react socially to caregivers by paying attention to the face or voice and by cuddling when held. See Table 18.1

for examples of motor and social development. Mothering behaviour, such as consistent care, handling, stroking, and cuddling, is essential for healthy psychosocial development. By 8 months, most infants tend to attach to their parents and may show displeasure when left with strangers.

Cognitive Development

Piaget (1966) viewed cognitive development as a result of interaction between an individual and the environment. The initial period of cognitive development is the *sensorimotor phase* (see Table 17.6 on page 332). This phase has six stages, three of which take place during the first year. From 4 to 8 months, infants begin to have perceptual recognition. By 6 months, they attend to new stimuli, while familiar objects are looked at for a short time. By 12 months, infants have a concept of both space and time. They experiment to reach a goal, such as a toy on a chair.

Moral Development

Infants associate right and wrong with pleasure and pain. What gives them pleasure is right, since they are too young to reason otherwise. Positive responses from the parents, such as smiles, caresses, and voice tones of approval, in these early months teach that certain behaviours are "good." Pain or harsh voices are associated with "bad" behaviour. In later months and years, children can tell easily and quickly by changes in parental facial expressions and voice tones whether their behaviour is approved or disapproved.

Health Risks

A number of health problems of neonates and infants require interventions from health care providers. Safety concerns are of particular importance.

TABLE 18.1 Examples of Motor and Social Development in Infancy

Age	Motor Development	Social Development
Newborn	Turns head from side to side when in a prone position; grasps by reflex when object is placed in palm of hand	Displays displeasure by crying and satisfaction by soft vocalizations; attends to adult face and voice by eye contact and quieting
4 months	Rolls over; sits with support, holds head steady when sitting	Babbles, laughs, and exhibits increased response to verbal play
6 months	Lifts chest and shoulders off table when prone, bearing weight on hands; manipulates small objects	Starts to imitate sounds; vocalizes one-syllable sounds: "ma ma," "da da"
9 months	Creeps and crawls; uses pincer grasp with thumb and forefinger	Complies with simple verbal commands; displays fear of being left alone (e.g., going to bed); waves "bye-bye"
12 months	Walks alone with help; uses spoon to feed self	Clings to caregiver in unfamiliar situations; demonstrates emotions, such as anger and affection

FAILURE-TO-THRIVE SYNDROME **Failure to thrive** (FTT) is a condition in which an infant falls below the fifth percentile for weight and height or whose growth declines across two percentiles on a standard growth chart over time (Emond, Drewett, Blair, & Emmett, 2007). Weight is altered initially, followed by length and head circumference.

FTT may have *organic* causes (e.g., causes associated with physiological or genetic disorders, such as cardiac disease) or *inorganic* causes, which usually involve the parent–child relationship. Infants deprived of mothering, especially from months 3 to 15, will not learn to form significant relationships or to trust others. These infants show delayed physical and emotional development without any physical cause. They are often malnourished; they fail to gain weight or grow normally.

INFANT COLIC **Colic** is acute abdominal pain caused by periodic contractions of the intestines during the first 3 months of life. The peak colicky period usually is between 3 and 8 weeks. Infants who cry up to 10 to 12 hours a day are described as being *colicky*. A crying or fussy period lasting 1 to 2 hours a day is not uncommon but is a concern and is stressful for the parents or caregivers. Although the direct cause is not known, temperament, swallowing air, feeding too rapidly, having allergies, infant taking in excessive amounts of carbohydrates, or experiencing emotional distress, and feeling the anxiety of the caregiver may be associated with colic.

The nurse can help relieve colic by assessing the infant during feeding and suggesting possible changes, such as cuddling the infant and finding the position that provides the infant with the most comfort (e.g., wearing the baby in a front pack, placing the infant in a swinging or vibrating chair, playing soft music, dimming the light, giving the baby a warm bath) (Canadian Paediatric Society, 2011). Providing parental respite care or support is essential.

CHILD ABUSE Abuse can take various forms, including physical abuse and neglect, sexual abuse, and emotional abuse and neglect. Child abuse may be associated with parental mental illness, substance abuse, or exposure to violence. Deliberate whiplash shaking can lead to **shaken baby syndrome (SBS)**, a constellation of severe injuries, such as cerebral damage, neurological defects, blindness, and intellectual disability, in infants. These injuries often occur without external evidence of head injury. Nurses should suspect SBS in infants less than 1 year old who have apnea (a pause in or stoppage of breathing), seizures, lethargy or drowsiness, bradycardia (a slow heart rate), or respiratory difficulty, who are in coma, or who die. Subdural and retinal hemorrhages with the absence of external signs of trauma are hallmarks of the syndrome (Altimier, 2008). Parents need to be aware of the dangers in shaking infants and ask for assistance if they feel they could harm their baby (Canadian Paediatric Society, 2009).

SUDDEN INFANT DEATH SYNDROME The sudden and unexpected death of an infant may be a case of **sudden infant death syndrome (SIDS)**. A postmortem examination usually fails to reveal a cause. The highest incidence of SIDS occurs in the second and fourth months of life, and boys are more susceptible than girls. SIDS is less common among babies of parents who do not smoke, when infants do not share the same bed with adults, and when infants sleep on their back. Sleeping on the back is preferred as infants may roll onto their stomach from the side-lying position, blocking their breathing. Infants are at risk for asphyxia when sharing the bed with adults who cannot be easily aroused because of extreme fatigue or who are impaired by alcohol or drug use. Nurses must assess the cultural practice for sleeping arrangements in the home, discuss the dangers of bed-sharing practices with the parents, and suggest alternatives for a safe sleeping environment for infants (Canadian Paediatric Society, 2004, 2010). (See Figure 18.5.)

Health Assessment and Promotion

APGAR SCORING **Apgar scores** are usually assessed in neonates 60 seconds after birth and repeated 5 and 10 minutes later. These scores provide a numeric indicator of the baby's physiological capacities to adapt to

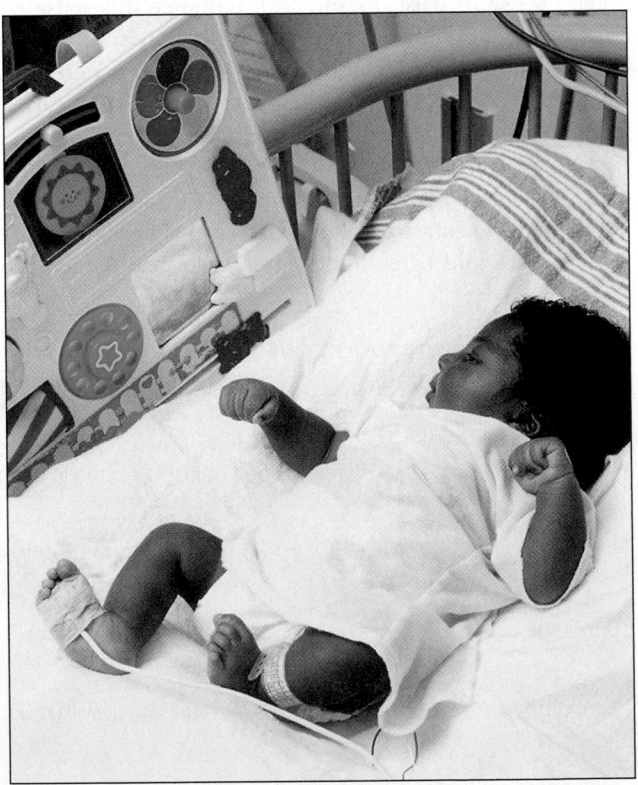

FIGURE 18.5 Place an infant on his or her back for sleeping. Note the infant's tonic neck reflex.

TABLE 18.2 Apgar Scoring System to Assess the Newborn

Sign	Score 0	1	2
1. Heart rate	Absent	Slow (fewer than 100 beats per minute)	Above 100 beats per minute
2. Respirations	Absent	Slow, irregular	Regular rate, crying
3. Muscle tone	Flaccid	Some flexion of extremities	Active movements
4. Reflex irritability	None	Grimace	Cries
5. Colour	Body pale or cyanotic	Body pink; in babies with dark skin (e.g., black Canadian, some East Indian, Hispanic), check mucous membranes, extremities	Body completely pink; pink mucous membranes in babies with dark skin

---

ASSESSMENT DEVELOPMENTAL GUIDELINES

The Infant

In these five developmental areas, does the infant do the following?

1. PHYSICAL DEVELOPMENT

- Demonstrate physical growth (weight, length, head and chest circumference) within the normal range
- Manifest appropriately sized fontanelles for age
- Exhibit vital signs within normal range for age

2. MOTOR DEVELOPMENT

- Perform gross and fine motor milestones within the normal range for age
- Exhibit reflexes appropriate for age

3. SENSORY DEVELOPMENT

- Follow a moving object within normal range for age
- Respond to sounds, such as talking or clapping hands

4. PSYCHOSOCIAL DEVELOPMENT

- Interact appropriately with caregiver through body movements and vocalizations
- Respond to caregiver and provide clear infant cues

5. DEVELOPMENT IN ACTIVITIES OF DAILY LIVING

- Eat and drink appropriate amounts of breast milk, formula, or solid foods
- Exhibit an elimination pattern within normal range for age
- Exhibit rest and sleep patterns appropriate for age

---

extrauterine life. Each of five signs is assigned a maximum score of 2, with a total achievable score of 10. A score less than 7 suggests that the baby is having difficulty, and a score less than 4 indicates that the baby's condition is critical. Those with very low scores require special resuscitative measures and care. See Table 18.2.

DEVELOPMENTAL SCREENING TESTS The development of infants can be assessed by observing the infant's behaviour and by using standardized tests, such as the **Denver Developmental Screening Test (DDST-II)**. The DDST-II is used to screen children from birth to age 6 years. Four main areas are screened: *personal–social, fine motor–adaptive, language,* and *gross motor* skills.

ONGOING NURSING ASSESSMENTS The nurse assesses the infant while noting the variations that occur with developmental age and activity. The nurse listens to the parents

for possible problems or areas of concern and reviews with the parents the expected behaviours or characteristics for the particular age group, reinforcing certain behaviours, responses, and activities of the infant as normal and expected, given individual differences that occur. The nurse assesses maternal bonding and infant attachment and provides anticipatory parental support and guidance as needed. See the Assessment: Developmental Guidelines box.

The first month of life is critical for physical adjustments to extrauterine life and for the psychosocial adjustment of the parents or caregivers. From 1 to 12 months, infants experience rapid change, with advances in growth and psychosocial development. For a summary of health and wellness promotion, see the Health-Promotion Guidelines box for Neonates and Infants. (See the section titled "Promoting Safety across the Lifespan" in Chapter 32.)

Health-Promotion Guidelines for Neonates and Infants

The following are important to the health of neonates and infants:

HEALTH EXAMINATIONS
- At birth, screening for hearing, congenital hypothyroidism, and phenylketonuria (PKU).
- Physical examination at birth, 2 weeks, and at 2, 4, 6, 9, and 12 months

PROTECTIVE MEASURES
- Routine immunizations: 5-in-1 DTaP-IPV and Hib vaccines protect against diphtheria, tetanus, pertussis, polio, and *Haemophilus influenzae,* type B (Hib) vaccine, hepatitis B vaccine (HepB), varicella vaccine, pneumococcal conjugate vaccine, and meningococcal C conjugate vaccine; influenza vaccine and other vaccines, as recommended. Schedules may vary across provinces and territories. See Table 34.9: Routine Immunization Schedules for Infants and Children (page 988).
- Fluoride supplements, if inadequate water fluoridation (less than 0.7 parts per million [ppm])
- Screening for congenital hypothyroidism, PKU, and other metabolic and congenital disorders, according to jurisdictions
- Prompt attention for illnesses or fever
- Appropriate skin hygiene and clothing
- Assessment of caregiver–infant relationship quality

INFANT SAFETY
- Supervision at all times
- Car seat, crib, playpen, bath, sleeping arrangement, and home environment safety measures
- Feeding measures (e.g., avoid propping the bottle during feeding)

- Toys with no small parts or sharp edges
- Elimination of toxins in the environment (e.g., tobacco, chemicals, radon, lead, mercury)
- Use of smoke and carbon monoxide (CO) detectors in home

NUTRITION
- Exclusive breast-feeding to 6 months
- Proper breast-feeding and bottle-feeding techniques
- Formula preparation
- Feeding schedule
- Introduction of solid foods
- Need for iron supplements at 4 to 6 months; iron-fortified formulas to infants who are not breastfed or for infants receiving formula as well as breast milk; by age 6 months, iron-rich foods
- Continued breast-feeding to age 12 months

ELIMINATION
- Characteristics and frequency of stool and urine elimination
- Diarrhea and dehydration signs

REST AND SLEEP
- Established routine for sleep and rest patterns

SENSORY STIMULATION
- Touch: holding, cuddling, rocking
- Vision: colourful, moving toys
- Hearing: soothing voice tones, music, singing
- Play: toys appropriate for development

Toddlers (1 to 3 Years)

Toddlers develop from having no voluntary control to learning to walk, speak, and control their bladder and bowels, and acquiring all kinds of information about their environment.

Physical Development

Two-year-old toddlers are usually chubby, with relatively short legs and large heads. Their face appears small when compared with the skull. As the toddler grows, the face seems to grow from under the skull and appears better proportioned. Toddlers have a pronounced lumbar lordosis and a protruding abdomen. The abdominal muscles grow and strengthen gradually and the abdomen flattens.

WEIGHT   Two-year-olds can be expected to weigh approximately four times their birth weight, gaining about 2 kg between 1 year and 2 years and about 1 to 2 kg between 2 and 3 years. The 3-year-old weighs about 13.6 kg.

HEIGHT   *Height* is measured while the toddler stands. *Length* is measured while the toddler is in a recumbent position. The measurements differ slightly, so nurses must specify which measurement is used. Between 1 and 2 years, the average growth in height is 10 cm to 12 cm, and between 2 and 3 years, it slows to 6 cm to 8 cm.

HEAD CIRCUMFERENCE   The head circumference of the toddler increases about 2.5 cm on average during this period. By 24 months, the head is 80% of the average adult size and the brain is 70% of its adult size.

SENSORY ABILITIES   Visual acuity is fairly well established at age 1 year. Estimates of visual acuity for toddlers are 20/70 at 18 months and 20/40 at age 2 years. Accommodation to near and far objects is fairly well developed by 18 months and continues to mature with age. At age 3 years, the toddler can look away from a toy before reaching out and picking it up. This ability requires the integration of visual and neuromuscular mechanisms.

The senses of hearing, taste, smell, and touch become increasingly developed and associated with one another. Hearing in the 3-year-old is at adult levels. The taste buds of the toddler are sensitive to the natural flavours of food, and the 3-year-old prefers familiar odours and tastes. A distressed toddler is often soothed by tactile sensations.

MOTOR ABILITIES *Fine muscle coordination* and *gross motor skills* improve during toddlerhood. At the age of 18 months, toddlers can pick up small beads and place them in a receptacle. They can also hold a spoon and a cup and can walk upstairs with assistance. They will probably crawl down the stairs.

At age 2 years, toddlers can hold a spoon and put it into their mouths correctly. They are able to run; their gait is steady; and they can balance on one foot and ride a tricycle. By age 3 years, most children are toilet trained, although they still may have the occasional accident when playing or during the night.

Psychosocial Development

According to Freud (1923), the ages of 2 and 3 years represent the *anal phase,* when the rectum and anus are particularly significant areas of the body (see Table 17.3 on page 327). Erikson sees the period from 18 months to 3 years as the time when the central developmental task is autonomy versus shame and doubt (see Table 17.4 on page 328).

Toddlers begin to develop their *sense of autonomy* by asserting themselves with the frequent use of the word "no." They are often frustrated by restraints on their behaviour and may have temper tantrums and act out to elicit a response from their caregivers (see the Evidence-Informed Practice box on what causes temper tantrums). Toddlers learn to gain control over their emotions with guidance from their caregivers. Parents need to be patient and understand the importance of this developmental milestone. They need to give the child some measure of control and, at the same time, be consistent in setting limits so that the child learns the results of misbehaviour. The nurse can also assist the parents and caregivers in promoting the toddler's development by suggesting the activities summarized in Box 18.3.

Self-concept is made up of body image, feelings about the self, adaptive and defensive mechanisms, reactions from others, and our own perceptions of these reactions, attitudes, values, and many of life's experiences (Burns, Dunn, Brady, Starr, & Blosser, 2008). Children learn to develop a sense of self through their immediate social environment, in which their parents play a significant role. If the children's social interactions with their parents are negative (e.g., constant disapproval regarding eating, toilet training, or other behaviour), they may begin to see themselves as bad. Parents need to give toddlers positive input so that they can develop a positive and healthy self-concept. Children with a strong self-concept and security are able to deal with periodic failures later in life without damage to their self-esteem. (See Chapter 45.)

EVIDENCE-INFORMED PRACTICE

What Causes Temper Tantrums?

The purpose of the study was to determine how *emotional reactivity* and *emotional competence* of the children contributed to temper tantrums, and 127 families with 3- to 5-year-old children in British Columbia took part in the study. Results showed that children who were more emotionally competent were less likely to display anger and distress. But more importantly, emotionally competent children, while they may be just as emotionally reactive as other children, were less likely to display the full-blown temper tantrum.

NURSING IMPLICATIONS: A child's level of emotional competence, not the tendency to be emotionally reactive, was the key to understanding why some reactive children have tantrums and others do not. Nurses need to understand that two children with similar thresholds for emotional reactivity may display widely different frequencies of temper tantrums and that maturity (i.e., age) and verbal ability had little effect on temper tantrums.

Source: Based on Giesbrecht, G., Miller, M., & Müller, U. (2010). The anger-distress model of temper tantrums: Associations with emotional reactivity and emotional competence. *Infant and Child Development, 19,* 478–497.

BOX 18.3 FOSTERING THE TODDLER'S PSYCHOSOCIAL DEVELOPMENT

Parents and caregivers can do many things to stimulate a toddler's psychosocial development:

- Provide toys suitable for the toddler, including some toys challenging enough to motivate but not so difficult that the toddler will fail. (Failure will intensify feelings of self-doubt and shame.)

- Make positive suggestions rather than giving commands. Avoid an emotional climate of negativism, blame, and punishment.

- Give the toddler two or three options, all of which are safe.

- When the toddler has a temper tantrum, make sure he or she is safe, and then leave.

- Help the toddler develop inner control by setting and enforcing consistent, reasonable limits.

- Praise the toddler's accomplishments; give spontaneous feedback for positive behaviour.

Young children can experience acute **separation anxiety**—the fear and frustration that come with parental absences—peaking around 8–9 months. At this age, abandonment is their greatest fear. The child may also have difficulty accepting a babysitter or strongly resist being left by the parents at a daycare centre or when separated from their parents or admitted to hospital.

Toddlers need room for exploration and interaction with other children and adults. At the same time, they need to know that they are loved, safe, and secure. They assert their independence by saying "no." Toddlers acquire receptive and expressive language skills quickly. They can understand words and follow directions long before they can actually speak them.

Regression, or reverting to an earlier development stage, can take the form of bedwetting or using baby talk. Nurses can help parents to understand that this behaviour is normal and indicates that the toddler is trying to establish his or her position in the family.

Cognitive Development

According to Piaget (1966), the toddler completes the fifth and sixth stages of the *sensorimotor phase* and starts the *preconceptual phase* at about age 2 years. In the fifth stage, the toddler solves problems by a trial-and-error process. By stage 6, toddlers can solve problems mentally. During Piaget's preconceptual phase, toddlers have some symbolic thought; for example, a chair may represent a place of safety, and a blanket may symbolize comfort. Concepts develop in late toddlerhood when the child learns words to represent classes of objects or thoughts. An example of a concrete concept is *table*, representing a number of articles of furniture that may look different but match the characteristics of a table.

Moral Development

According to Kohlberg (1977), the first level of moral development is *preconventional,* when children respond to punishment and reward. During the second year, children begin to know that some activities elicit affection and approval and recognize that certain rituals create feelings of security. Children also sense what attitudes their parents hold about moral matters.

Spiritual Development

Fowler (1981) believed the toddler may be aware of some religious practices, but they are primarily involved in acquiring knowledge and learning emotional reactions. For example, a toddler may repeat short prayers at bedtime, conforming to a ritual for praise and affection.

Health Risks

ACCIDENTS   Accidents are the leading cause of death for toddlers (Health Council of Canada, 2006), as they are curious and like to feel and taste everything. The most common causes of fatal injuries are automobile accidents, drowning, burns, poisoning, and falls. Parents or other caregivers need to take measures to prevent accidents (see Figure 18.6).

VISION PROBLEMS   Early screening to detect amblyopia and strabismus can correct common problems in toddlers. **Amblyopia** (lazy-eye) is reduced visual acuity in one eye without obvious defect or change in the eye; the brain favours the images from the stronger eye over those from the affected eye. **Strabismus** (cross-eye) is unequally

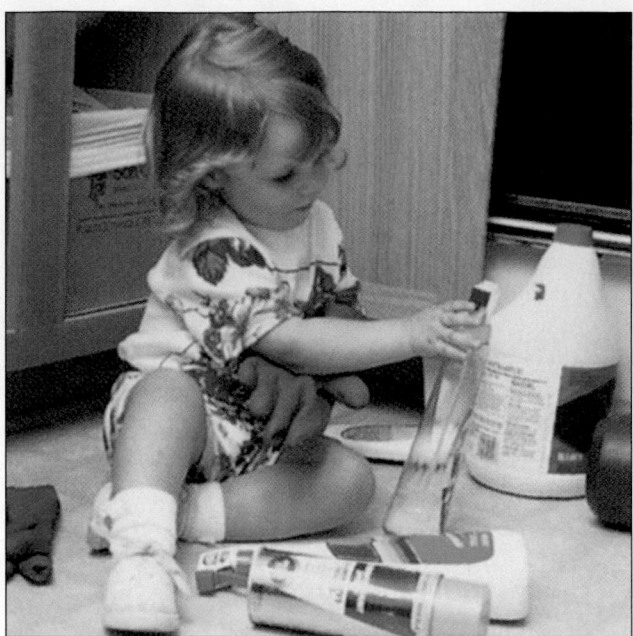

FIGURE 18.6 Keep medicines and other poisonous material locked away.

aligned eyes, which distorts vision so that the child's brain suppresses vision in one eye.

DENTAL CARIES   Dental caries are common and often a result of the excessive ingestion of sweets or a prolonged exposure of teeth to carbohydrates, such as through the use of the bottle during naps and at bedtime. Good dental hygiene can prevent dental caries and hence promote proper speech development and nutrition.

RESPIRATORY TRACT AND EAR INFECTIONS   Respiratory and middle ear infections are common during toddlerhood and contribute significantly to visits to health care providers. The incidence increases with exposure to other children and the use of a bottle during naps or at bedtime or if bottles are propped for feedings.

Health Assessment and Promotion

Growth and development in the toddler and preschool years provide the basis for a child's future health and well-being. It is essential that nurses provide anticipatory guidance and accurate assessments to promote health and detect problems for early interventions.

Guidelines for growth and development of the toddler are shown in the Assessment: Developmental Guidelines box.

Promoting health and wellness includes such areas as accident prevention, toilet training, and good dental hygiene. See the Health-Promotion Guidelines box for Toddlers.

ASSESSMENT   DEVELOPMENTAL GUIDELINES

The Toddler

In these four developmental areas, does the toddler do the following?

1. PHYSICAL DEVELOPMENT

- Demonstrate physical growth (weight, height, and head circumference) within normal range
- Manifest vital signs within normal range for age
- Exhibit vision and hearing abilities within normal range

2. MOTOR DEVELOPMENT

- Perform gross and fine motor milestones within the normal range for age. For example, by age 3 years, is the toddler able to do the following?
  - Walk up steps without assistance
  - Balance on one foot, jump, and walk on toes
  - Copy a circle
  - Build a bridge from blocks
  - Ride a tricycle

3. PSYCHOSOCIAL DEVELOPMENT

- Perform psychosocial developmental milestones for their age. For example, by age 3 years, is the toddler able to do the following?

- Express likes and dislikes
- Display curiosity and ask questions
- Accept separation from mother for short periods
- Begin to play and communicate with children and others outside the immediate family
- Understand such words as *up, down, cold,* and *hungry*
- Speak in sentences of three to four words
- Imitate religious rituals of the family

4. DEVELOPMENT IN ACTIVITIES OF DAILY LIVING

- Feed self
- Eat and drink a variety of foods
- Begin to develop bowel and bladder control
- Exhibit a sleep pattern appropriate for age
- Dress self

Health-Promotion Guidelines for Toddlers

The following are important to the health of toddlers:

HEALTH EXAMINATIONS

- At 15 and 18 months and then as recommended by the health care provider
- Supervise tooth brushing and start regular dental visits at age 3 years or earlier
- Hearing tests by 18 months or earlier

PROTECTIVE MEASURES

- Routine immunizations: continuing 5-in-1 DTaP-IPV and Hib series, measles-mumps-rubella vaccine (MMR), pneumococcal conjugate vaccine, influenza vaccine, varicella vaccine, flu vaccine, and other vaccines, as recommended by jurisdiction
- Screenings for tuberculosis (TB) and lead poisoning, as recommended
- Fluoride supplements, if inadequate water fluoridation (less than 0.7 ppm)

TODDLER SAFETY

- Importance of supervision and teaching child to obey instructions
- Home environment safety measures (e.g., lock medicine cabinet)

- Outdoor safety measures (e.g., close supervision near water, use of car seat)
- Appropriate toys with lift locks on toy boxes
- Elimination of toxins in environment (e.g., pesticides, herbicides, mercury, lead, arsenic in playground materials)
- Use of smoke and carbon monoxide detectors in home

NUTRITION

- Importance of nutritious meals and snacks
- Teaching of simple mealtime manners
- Dental care

ELIMINATION

- Toilet training techniques

REST AND SLEEP

- Dealing with sleep disturbances

PLAY

- Provision of adequate space and a variety of activities
- Encouraging regular, vigorous physical activity
- Toys that allow "acting out" behaviours and provide motor and sensory stimulation safety

Preschoolers (4 to 5 Years)

During the preschool period, physical growth slows, but control of the body and coordination increase greatly. Preschoolers' worlds expand as they meet relatives, friends, and neighbours.

Physical Development

By age 4 or 5 years, preschool children appear taller and thinner than toddlers because they tend to grow more in height than in weight. The preschooler's brain reaches almost adult size by age 5 years. The extremities grow more quickly than the body trunk, making the child's body appear somewhat out of proportion. The preschooler appears slender with erect posture as their pelvis is straightened and the abdominal muscles become stronger.

WEIGHT Weight gain in preschool children is generally slow. By age 5 years, they gain about 3 kg to 5 kg and reach between 18 kg and 20 kg.

HEIGHT Preschool children grow about 5 cm to 6.25 cm each year. By age 5 years, they double their birth length and measure 102 cm.

VISION Preschool children are generally **hyperopic** (farsighted), that is, unable to focus on near objects. As the eye grows in length, it becomes **emmetropic** (it refracts light normally). If the eyes become too long, the child becomes **myopic** (nearsighted), that is, unable to focus on objects that are far away. In severe cases of hyperopia or myopia, glasses may be prescribed. Visual acuity generally improves by the end of the preschool years. Normal vision for the 5-year-old is approximately 20/30. The Snellen E chart can be used to assess the preschooler's vision (see the section titled "Eyes and Vision" in Chapter 28).

HEARING AND TASTE The hearing of the preschool child has reached optimal levels, and the ability to listen (attending to and comprehending what is said) has matured since the toddler age. Preschoolers show their taste preferences by asking for something "yummy," and they may refuse to eat a few particular foods. Parents should not "nag" the child to eat certain foods. The child will eat what is needed if there is a pleasant environment and a variety of healthful foods that is pleasing for eating.

MOTOR ABILITIES By age 5 years, children can wash hands and face and brush teeth by themselves. They are self-conscious about exposing their bodies and go to the bathroom without telling others. Typically, preschool children run with increasing skill each year. They can jump three steps and can balance on their toes and dress themselves without assistance.

Psychosocial Development

Erikson (1963) writes that the major developmental crisis of the preschooler is *initiative versus guilt* (see Table 17.4 on page 328). Preschoolers begin to solve problems in accordance with their consciences as their personalities and self-concepts develop. Parents can enhance the self-concept of the preschooler by providing opportunities for new achievements where the child can learn, repeat, and master. For example, a child obtains a two-wheel bike with safety wheels and quickly learns coordination, balance, use of the brakes, and bicycle safety. Mastery of these tasks provides children with a sense of accomplishment and prepares them for new challenges.

The self-concept of the preschooler is also based on gender identification. Preschoolers often imitate sexual stereotypes and usually begin by identifying with the parent of the same sex. They may mimic the parent's behaviour, attitudes, and appearance (Figure 18.7). Preschoolers will be curious about their own bodies and sexual functions as well as those of others, and they will often ask questions.

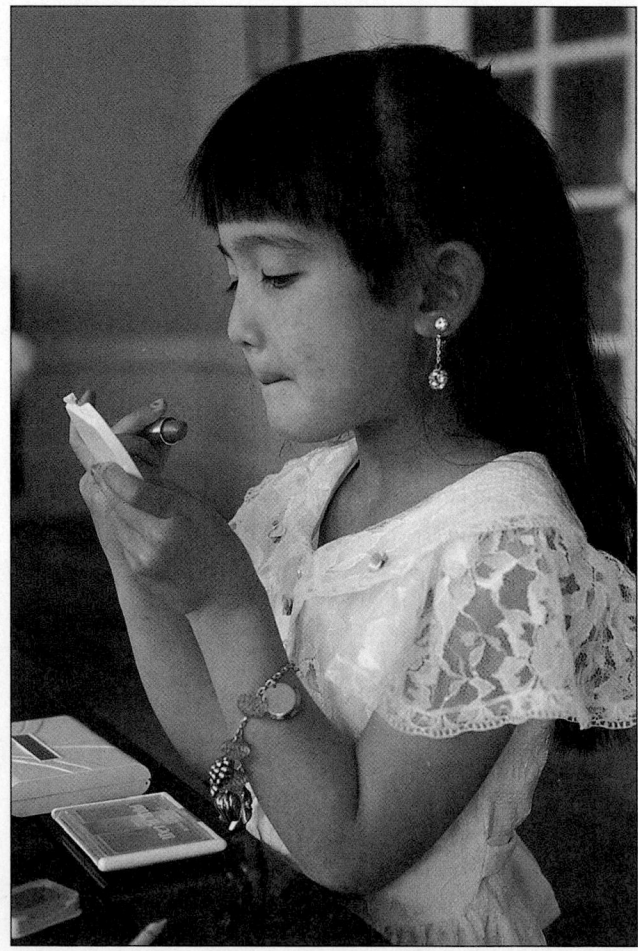

FIGURE 18.7 Preschoolers often identify with the parent of the same sex and like to mimic behaviour.

Freud (1923) theorized that the preschooler is in the *phallic stage* of development (see Table 17.3 on page 327). The focus during this stage is the genital area. In the Electra or Oedipus complex, the child focuses feelings of love chiefly on the parent of the opposite sex, and the parent of the same sex may receive some hostile feelings. The child begins to develop sexual interests and becomes interested in clothes and hair styles.

Four *adaptive mechanisms* are learned: identification, introjection, imagination, and repression. **Identification** occurs when the child perceives the self as similar to another person and behaves like that person. For example, a boy may internalize the attitudes and gender behaviour of his father. **Introjection** is the assimilation of the attributes of others. When preschoolers observe their parents, they assimilate many of their values and attitudes. **Imagination**, or make-believe, is an important part of preschoolers' lives and is culturally and socially dependent. For example, boys may fantasize that a stool becomes a robot warrior and girls may imagine it as a beautiful swan. **Repression** is removing experiences, thoughts, and impulses from awareness. Preschoolers learn to play with their peers, and socialize and participate more in the family. Associations with neighbours, family guests, and babysitters reinforce social relationships.

In their *speech,* 4-year-old children are often dogmatic; they tend to believe that what they know is right. They can speak and understand 1500 or more words. They love making up their own words and mixing fact and fiction. Exaggeration is common. Their language skills are well developed by age 5 years. They use words purposefully, ask questions to acquire information, speak as a means of social interaction, and are capable of long conversations.

Preschoolers become increasingly aware of themselves, and they play with their bodies largely out of curiosity. By age 5 years, they know the correct names for the different body parts and can draw various features of a person. Preschoolers can also describe their feelings, such as *sad, happy,* or *angry.* The preschooler begins to learn how to control his or her feelings and behaviour, and uses the same types of *coping mechanisms* in response to stress as the toddler does, although protest behaviour (kicking, screaming) is less likely to occur.

Preschoolers need to feel that they are loved and are an important part of the family. The child who has to compete with siblings for parental attention will often display jealousy or sibling rivalry. Parents and caregivers should be aware that preschoolers need time to adjust to a new baby and may need additional attention or special activities to go through this adjustment period.

Guidance and discipline are important parts of the parental role. As children seek independence from adults, they often test limits by refusing to cooperate and by ignoring parental requests. Such power struggles can be controlled by encouraging children to be responsible for their own behaviour and setting reasonable expectations and consistent limits.

Cognitive Development

According to Piaget (1966), preschoolers gain *intuitive thought* and form concepts by learning through trial and error (see Table 17.6 on page 332). Children are still egocentric, but egocentrism gradually subsides as they encounter wider experiences. Preschoolers learn through trial and error, observation, imitation, and practice in play and make-believe. Preschoolers can become concerned about death as something inevitable and they also associate death with others rather than themselves. Death may still be confused with sleep and "going away" for prolonged periods. Reading and mathematical skills (e.g., recognizing and naming letters and numbers, counting, and "reading" age appropriate books) begin to develop at this age. Young children like fairy tales and books about animals and other children and should be read to often.

Moral Development

Moral behaviour to a preschooler may mean taking turns at play or sharing. Preschoolers enjoy sharing, helping, protecting, befriending, showing affection, and giving encouragement to others. Children who perceive their parents as strict may become resentful or overly obedient. Preschoolers usually control their behaviour because they want love and approval from their parents. It is also important for parents to answer preschoolers' "why" questions and discuss values with them.

Spiritual Development

According to Fowler (1981), children from ages 4 to 6 years are at the *intuitive–projective stage* of spiritual development (see Table 17.8 on page 335). At this stage, faith is primarily taught by parents and teachers through picture books or simple explanations of spiritual matters. Preschoolers' imaginations can envision such ideas as angels or the devil. Children imitate religious behaviour, for example, by bowing their heads in prayer, although they do not understand the meaning of the behaviour.

Health Risks

Respiratory tract problems and communicable diseases, such as *fifth disease* (a viral disease that causes a distinctive rash on the face, arms, and body), meningitis, and head lice, are common as the preschooler interacts with other children. Accidents and dental caries continue to be problems. Congenital abnormalities, such as cardiac disorders and hernias, are often corrected by this age.

Health Assessment and Promotion

During assessment, the preschooler can often participate in answering questions with assistance from parents or caregivers. They are fairly independent but still need supervision and guidance (see the Assessment: Developmental Guidelines box for preschoolers). Promoting health and wellness includes such areas as preventing accidents and ensuring dental health, good nutrition, cognitive stimulation, and sufficient sleep. See the Health-Promotion Guidelines box for Preschoolers.

ASSESSMENT | **DEVELOPMENTAL GUIDELINES**

The Preschooler

In these four developmental areas, does the preschooler do the following by age 5 years?

1. **PHYSICAL DEVELOPMENT**
   - Demonstrate physical growth (weight, height) within normal range
   - Manifest vital signs within normal range for age
   - Exhibit vision and hearing abilities within normal range

2. **MOTOR DEVELOPMENT**
   - Perform gross and fine motor milestones within the normal range for age:
     - Jump rope and skip
     - Climb playground equipment
     - Ride a bicycle with training wheels
     - Print letters and numbers

3. **PSYCHOSOCIAL DEVELOPMENT**
   - Perform psychosocial developmental milestones for age:
     - Separate easily from parents
   - Display imagination and creativity
   - Enjoy playing with peers in cooperative activities
   - Understand right from wrong and respond to others' expectations of behaviour
   - Identify four colours
   - Exhibit increasing vocabulary using complete sentences and all parts of speech
   - Cooperate in doing simple chores (e.g., putting away toys)
   - Demonstrate awareness of sexual differences

4. **DEVELOPMENT IN ACTIVITIES OF DAILY LIVING**
   - Demonstrate development of toilet training
   - Perform simple hygiene measures
   - Dress and undress self
   - Engage in bedtime rituals and demonstrate ability to put self to sleep

---

Health-Promotion Guidelines for Preschoolers

The following are important to the health of preschoolers:

HEALTH EXAMINATIONS
- Every 1 to 2 years

PROTECTIVE MEASURES
- Routine immunizations: DTaP-IPV, IPV series, MMR, and other immunizations, as recommended
- Tuberculin skin test, as recommended
- Vision and hearing screening
- Regular dental screenings and fluoride treatment

PRESCHOOLER SAFETY
- Education about simple safety rules (e.g., crossing the street, use of car seat, avoid strangers)
- Teaching of ways to play safely (e.g., bicycle and playground safety, use of helmets)
- Education to prevent poisoning, exposure to toxic materials

NUTRITION
- Importance of nutritious meals and snacks

ELIMINATION
- Teaching of proper hygiene (e.g., washing hands after using bathroom)

REST AND SLEEP
- Ways to deal with sleep disturbances (e.g., nightmares, sleepwalking)

PLAY
- Encouraging regular, vigorous physical activity
- Provision of times for group play activities
- Teaching of simple games that require cooperation and interaction
- Provision of toys and dress-ups for role playing

School-Age Children (6 to 12 Years)

The school-age period starts at about age 6 years, when the deciduous teeth are shed, and ends with the pre-adolescent (prepuberty) period at about age 12 years with the onset of puberty. **Puberty** is the age at which the reproductive organs become functional and secondary sex characteristics develop. The average age of onset of puberty is 10 years for girls and 12 years for boys. Skills learned and willingness to try new tasks during this stage are particularly important for later life.

Physical Development

The school-age child gains weight rapidly and thus appears less thin than previously. Individual differences because of both genetic and environmental factors are obvious at this time.

WEIGHT At age 6 years, boys tend to weigh about 21 kg, about 1 kg more than girls. The weight gain from ages 6 to 12 years averages about 3.2 kg per year, but the major weight gains occur from ages 10 to 12 for boys and from ages 9 to 12 for girls. By age 12 years, boys and girls weigh 40 kg to 42 kg on average; girls are usually heavier. Overweight and obesity is unlikely at this age if the child has demonstrated a pattern of good nutrition and regular, vigorous exercise in the infant, toddler, and preschool years.

HEIGHT At age 6 years, both boys and girls are about the same height, 115 cm. They are about 150 cm by age 12 years. Before puberty, children of both sexes have a growth spurt—girls between ages 10 and 12 years and boys between ages 12 and 14 years. Thus, girls may well be taller than boys at age 12 years, but boys are usually stronger.

The extremities tend to grow more quickly compared with the trunk; thus, school-age children's bodies appear somewhat ill-proportioned. By age 6 years, the thoracic curvature starts to develop, and the lordosis disappears. Full adult posture is not assumed until after the complete development of the skeletal musculature during the adolescent period.

VISION The depth and distance perception of 6- to 8-year-olds is accurate. By age 6 years, the eye muscles are well developed and coordinated. Because the shape of the eye changes during growth, the farsightedness of the preschool years gradually changes to 20/20 vision during the school-age years; 20/20 vision is usually well established between ages 9 and 11 years.

HEARING AND TOUCH Auditory perception is fully developed in school-age children. They are able to identify fine differences in voices, both in sound and in pitch. They have a well-developed sense of touch for heat and cold on all body surfaces; they are also able to identify an unseen object, such as a pencil or a book, simply by touch. This ability is called **stereognosis**.

PREPUBERTAL CHANGES Little change takes place in the reproductive and endocrine systems until the prepuberty period. At about ages 9 to 13 years, endocrine functions slowly increase, which can result in increased perspiration and more active sebaceous glands. Girls may have sticky vaginal discharge prior to puberty. Early-onset menses should be followed up with a health care practitioner.

MOTOR ABILITIES Between ages 6 and 10 years, children perfect their muscular skills and coordination. By age 9 years, most are becoming skilled in games of interest or school sports, such as football or baseball. Most have sufficient fine motor control for such activities as building models, sewing, or playing musical instruments.

Psychosocial Development

The central task of school-age children is *industry versus inferiority* (Erikson, 1963). At this time, children begin to create and develop a sense of competence and perseverance. They are motivated by activities that provide a sense of self-worth. They concentrate on mastering skills that will help them function in the adult world. Children who are successful and receive recognition for their efforts feel competent and confident. Children who feel unaccepted by their peers, or who receive negative feedback and little recognition, may feel inferior and worthless (see Table 17.4 on page 328).

Freud (1923) describes a *latency stage* in school-age children. Their focus is on physical and intellectual activities, while sexual tendencies seem to be repressed (see Table 17.3 on page 327). Curiosity about sexual matters is present, however, and children are aware of the messages related to sex in popular media, films, and on the Internet; parents need to set limits, answer questions, and provide guidance to help their children understand and cope with information and feelings. Although the focus of interest for this age group has moved to school, peers, and other activities, the home remains the crucial place for the child's development of high self-esteem.

Cognitive Development

The ages 7 to 11 years mark Piaget's (1966) *concrete operations phase* (see Table 17.6 on page 332). These children change from egocentric interactions to cooperative interactions. They also develop an increased understanding of concepts that are associated with specific objects, for example, associating "conservation" with "wildlife." Logical reasoning develops from intuitive reasoning (e.g., adding and subtracting to obtain an answer to a problem). Children also learn about cause-and-effect relationships (e.g., knowing that a stone will not float because it is heavier than water).

By age 6 years, children learn the concept of time and can read both digital and numerical clocks. The schedule in school helps them learn the time periods. By age 7 or 8 years, children usually know the value of money.

Reading skills are usually well developed. What a child reads is largely influenced by the family. By age 9 years, most children are self-motivated. They may compete with themselves; they like discussion and debate and like to plan ahead. By age 12 years, they are motivated by inner drive rather than by competition with peers.

Moral Development

In Kohlberg's (1977) stage 1 of the *preconventional* level (punishment and obedience), school-age children act to avoid being punished. Some, however, are at stage 2 (*instrumental-relativist orientation*): they do things to benefit themselves, but getting a fair share or chance for everyone is important. Between ages 10 and 13 years, most children progress to the *conventional* level. This level has two stages: stage 3 is the *interpersonal concordance* (good boy or nice girl) stage, and stage 4 is the *law and order orientation*. The child shifts from the concrete interests of individuals to the interests of groups. They are motivated to living up to what significant others think of them (see Table 17.7 on page 333).

Spiritual Development

According to Fowler (1981), the school-age child is at stage 2 in spiritual development, the *mythical–literal* stage. Children learn to distinguish fantasy from fact. *Spiritual facts* are those beliefs that are accepted by a religious group, whereas *fantasy* is thoughts and images formed in the child's mind. School-age children may ask many questions about God and religion in these years. Parents and religious leaders still influence the child more than peers do in spiritual matters (see Table 17.8 on page 335).

Health Risks

Communicable diseases, dental caries, accidents, and the achievement of a healthy weight are health risks for school-agers. The most common nutritional problem among children is obesity, which contributes to breathing difficulties, increased risk of fractures, increased incidence of hypertension, and type 2 diabetes in childhood and increases the risk for diabetes, hypertension, and cardiovascular disease in adulthood (DeCorby, Graham, & Dobbins, 2012).

Health Assessment and Promotion

Comprehensive assessment relies on the nurse's ability to respond to questions from the child, parent, or other caregiver, and provide feedback, encouragement, and support, and build on the child's strengths. See the Assessment: Developmental Guidelines box for the school-age child.

ASSESSMENT | DEVELOPMENTAL GUIDELINES

The School-Age Child

In these four developmental areas, does the school-age child do the following?

1. **PHYSICAL DEVELOPMENT**
   - Demonstrate physical growth (weight, height) within normal range
   - Manifest vital signs within normal range for age
   - Exhibit vision and hearing abilities within normal range
   - Demonstrate male or female prepubertal changes within normal range
2. **MOTOR DEVELOPMENT**
   - Possess coordinated motor skills for age
   - Do tricks on a bike or climb a tree
   - Throw and catch a small ball
   - Play a musical instrument
3. **PSYCHOSOCIAL DEVELOPMENT**
   - Meet psychosocial developmental milestones for age
   - Make friends of the same sex and establish a peer group
   - Become less dependent on family and venture away from them

- Interact well with parents
- Control strong and impulsive feelings
- Participate in organized competitions
- Read, print, and manipulate numbers and letters easily
- Exhibit a concept of money and make change for small amounts of money
- Express self in a logical manner and talk through problems
- Enjoy riddles and read and understand comics
- Invest in a hobby or collection
- Like to help others
- Think of self as likable and healthy

4. **DEVELOPMENT IN ACTIVITIES OF DAILY LIVING**
   - Demonstrate concern for personal cleanliness and appearance
   - Express need for privacy

Health-Promotion Guidelines for School-Age Children

The following are important to the health of school-age children:

HEALTH EXAMINATIONS

- Annual physical examination or as recommended

PROTECTIVE MEASURES

- Immunizations as recommended. Human papillomavirus (HPV) vaccination is given only to females age 9 to 26 years at a three-dose schedule (0, 2, and 6 months)
- Tuberculin skin test, as recommended
- Periodic vision, speech, and hearing screenings
- Regular dental screenings and fluoride treatment
- Provision of accurate information about sexual health (e.g., reproduction, acquired immunodeficiency syndrome [AIDS], chlamydiasis)
- Using the right gear for the sport: helmets, pads, face and mouth guards

SCHOOL-AGE CHILD SAFETY

- Use of proper sport equipment (e.g., helmets, pads) and booster seat in car, as applicable
- Taking responsibility for own safety (e.g., participating in bicycle and water safety courses)

NUTRITION

- Importance of eating a balanced diet and not skipping meals
- Minimization of food related to obesity

ELIMINATION

- Using positive approaches for elimination problems (e.g., enuresis)

PLAY AND SOCIAL INTERACTIONS

- Provision of opportunities for a variety of organized group activities
- Acceptance of realistic expectations of child's abilities
- Being a role model for acceptance of other persons who may be different
- Provision of a home environment that limits television viewing and video games and encourages completion of homework

---

Promoting health and wellness includes dental examinations and hygiene, immunization, safety measures to prevent accidents, physical fitness, supporting autonomy, self-esteem, and infection control. See the Health-Promotion Guidelines box for School-Age Children.

Adolescence (12 to 18 Years)

Adolescence is the period during which the person becomes physically and psychologically mature and acquires a personal identity. At the end of this period, the teen is ready to enter adulthood and assume responsibilities. The length of adolescence is culturally determined to some extent and may extend to ages 18 or 20 years in North America.

Puberty is the first stage of adolescence, in which the sexual organs begin to grow and mature. **Menarche** (onset of menstruation) occurs in girls and **ejaculation** (expulsion of semen) in boys. For girls, puberty normally starts between ages 10 and 14 years and for boys between ages 12 and 16 years. The adolescent period is often subdivided into three stages: early adolescence (ages 12 to 13), middle adolescence (14 to 16 years), and late adolescence (from 17 to 18 or 20 years). Late adolescence is a more stable stage, when adolescents are involved with planning their future and economic independence.

Physical Development

During puberty, growth is accelerated through an *adolescent growth spurt*. In males, it begins between ages 12 and 16 years; in females, it begins between ages 10 and 14 years. Because the growth spurt begins earlier in girls, many girls surpass boys in height at this time. Boys will catch up and often surpass the girls by the end of this period.

PHYSICAL GROWTH Physical growth continues throughout adolescence. Growth is fastest for boys at about age 14 years, and the maximum height is often reached at about age 18 or 19 years. Some males add another 1 cm or 2 cm to their height during their 20s. From ages 10 to 18 years, the average Canadian male doubles his weight, gaining about 32 kg, and grows about 41 cm. The fastest rate of growth in girls occurs at about age 12 years; they reach their maximum height at about ages 15 to 16 years. From ages 10 to 18 years, the average Canadian female gains about 25 kg and grows about 24 cm.

Physical growth is largely influenced by heredity, nutrition, medical care, illness, physical and emotional environment, family size, race, and culture. Growth is noted first in the musculoskeletal system, which follows a sequential pattern: the head, hands, and feet are the first to grow to adult status, followed by the extremities. Because the extremities grow before the trunk, the adolescent looks "leggy." After the trunk grows to full size, the shoulders, chest, and hips grow. Skull and facial bones also change proportions—the forehead becomes more prominent, and the jawbones develop.

GLANDULAR CHANGES The eccrine and apocrine glands increase their secretions and become fully functional during puberty. The **eccrine glands**, found over most of the body, produce sweat. The **apocrine glands** develop in the axillae, anal, and genital areas; external auditory canals; and around the umbilicus and areolae of the breasts. Apocrine sweat is released onto the skin in response to emotional stimuli only. **Sebaceous glands** also become active under the influence of androgens in both males and females. The sebaceous glands, which secrete *sebum*, become most active on the face, neck, shoulder, upper back, chest, and genitals.

SEXUAL CHARACTERISTICS **Primary sexual characteristics** relate to the organs necessary for reproduction, such as the testes, penis, vagina, and uterus. **Secondary sexual characteristics** differentiate the male from the female but do not relate directly to reproduction. Examples are pubic hair growth, breast development, and voice changes.

Both primary and secondary sex characteristics develop during puberty. The first noticeable sign that puberty has begun in males is the appearance of pubic hair. The milestone of male puberty is considered to be the first ejaculation, which commonly occurs at about age 14 years. Fertility follows several months later. Sexual maturity is achieved by age 18 years. Often, the first noticeable sign of puberty in females is the appearance of the *breast bud*, although the appearance of hair along the labia may precede this. The milestone of female puberty is the menarche, which occurs about 2 years after the breast bud appears. At first, menstrual periods are scanty and irregular and may occur without ovulation. Ovulation is usually established 1 to 2 years after menarche. Female internal reproductive organs reach adult size about ages 18 to 20 years.

Psychosocial Development

According to Erikson (1963), the psychosocial task of the adolescent is the *establishment of identity*. The danger of this stage is *role confusion* (see Table 17.4 on page 328). The inability to settle on a career path commonly disturbs the adolescent. Less commonly, doubts about sexual identity arise. Adolescents help one another through this identity crisis by forming cliques and a separate youth culture, often excluding all those who are "different" in cultural background and lifestyles. Hair styling, skin care, and clothes become very important. In-groupers of an adolescent clique can be excessively clannish and cruel in excluding out-groupers; this intolerance is a temporary defence against identity confusion.

The adolescent has unlimited imagination and ambition and aspires to great accomplishments. The sense of industry is reenacted when the adolescent chooses a career. The extent to which these tasks were achieved earlier influences the adolescent's ability to achieve a healthy self-concept and self-identity.

The adolescent needs to establish a self-concept that accepts both personal strengths and personal weaknesses. Faced with dramatic changes in body structure and function, and greater expectations to assume responsibilities, many adolescents experience temporary difficulty in developing a positive self-image (e.g., preoccupation with acne problem). Adolescents with physical challenges or illnesses are particularly vulnerable to peer rejection or bullying. Those who are accepted, loved, and valued by family and peers generally tend to gain confidence and feel good about themselves. Those who have difficulty forming relationships, or who are perceived by peers as too different and who are not included in adolescent cliques, may develop less favourable self-images and have low self-esteem.

Because sex roles are becoming less defined in Canadian society, adopting the masculine or feminine role is increasingly confusing for today's adolescent. In forming a sexual identity, adolescents first fantasize the male or female role and then enact various aspects of that imagined role. Later, adolescents begin to establish intimacy with a partner or partners. This intimacy lays the groundwork for the commitments of adulthood. Sexual experimentation is not part of true intimacy, but once intimacy is realized, sexual activity follows. Gay and lesbian youth can experience a great deal of confusion during this period as their questions about self and identity may go unanswered.

Many adolescents may engage in masturbation as well as sexual activity with those of the same or opposite sex. Frappier and colleagues (2008) reported that 27% of teens were sexually active, with a mean age of 15 years and a lifetime average of 2.5 partners. The last time they had sex, 76% reported using a condom. Most valuable sources of information about sexual relations and contraception were school, parents, friends, and doctors. In general, teens lacked knowledge of STIs and their consequences. Most teens trusted the information given to them by health care professionals. (See Chapter 46.)

At about age 15 years, the *need for independence*, combined with the need for family support, sometimes creates conflict within the adolescent and between the adolescent and the family. The young person may appear hostile or depressed at times during this crisis. Adolescents prefer to be with their peers and may seek advice from adults other than parents. Parents sometimes are bewildered by this stage, and instead of reducing controls, they increase them, which causes the adolescent to rebel.

Adolescents may develop brief crushes on adults outside the family. They sometimes adopt some of the attributes of the adults with whom they are infatuated. This modelling can be helpful in the maturing process.

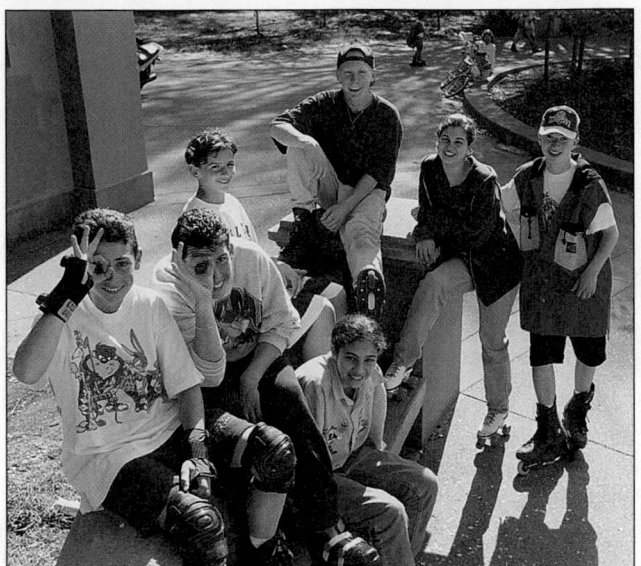

FIGURE 18.8 Adolescent peer group relationships enhance a sense of belonging, self-esteem, and self-identity.

Some of the discord in the family at this time is caused by the generation gap. Adolescents' values may differ from those of their parents and be difficult for the parents to understand and to accept. Restrictions and guidance need to be presented in a manner that makes adolescents feel loved. They need consistency in guidance, fewer restrictions, and as much independence as they can handle, but they need to know that their parents will assist them when necessary.

Peer groups are defined by like-minded, loosely bonded, and self-identified cohorts who influence one another's ideas, values, behaviours, and lifestyle choices and provide one another with a sense of belonging, pride, social learning, and gender roles (Figure 18.8). Most peer groups have well-defined, gender-specific modes of acceptable behaviour. Peer groups change with age, starting as same-sex groups, evolving into mixed groups, and finally narrowing to couples who share activities.

For gay and lesbian youth, adolescence is a difficult time. Because peer acceptance is crucial to self-acceptance, lesbian and gay adolescents usually conform to the heterosexual codes and behaviours, even though these do not feel natural or correct. Adolescents who are openly gay or lesbian may face not only the ostracism of their peers but also the misunderstanding and hostility of parents, teachers, and other important adults.

Cognitive Development

Adolescents begin Piaget's *formal operations phase* of cognitive development (see Table 17.6 on page 332), with cognitive abilities maturing between age 11 and 15 years. At this stage, adolescents can think beyond the present and are highly idealistic. They become more informed about the world and environment. They use new information to solve everyday problems and communicate with adults on most subjects, such as interest areas and career plans.

Moral Development

According to Kohlberg (1977), the young adolescent is usually at the *conventional level* of moral development. Although most still want to abide by social order and existing laws, many discard the values they have adopted from parents in favour of those they consider more suitable. In the *postconventional* or *principled level*, they start to question the rules and laws of society, especially if their personal views are in conflict with societal laws and what they perceive as individual rights. Not all adolescents, or even adults, proceed to this postconventional level. See Kohlberg's stages of moral development in Table 17.7 on page 333.

Spiritual Development

According to Fowler (1981), the adolescent reaches the *synthetic–conventional* stage of spiritual development. As they encounter different groups in society, they are exposed to a wide variety of opinions, beliefs, and behaviours regarding religious matters; some may seek advice from a significant other, such as a parent or a minister. Often, the adolescent believes that various religious beliefs and practices have more similarities than differences. At this stage, the adolescent's focus is on interpersonal, rather than conceptual matters.

Health Risks

Adolescents can be at risk for unintentional injuries, STIs, inactivity, unhealthy eating, mental health problems, teen pregnancy, and problematic tobacco, alcohol, and other drug use (Canadian Institute for Health Information, 2005). Common problems related to nutrition and self-esteem among adolescents include obesity, anorexia nervosa, and bulimia (see the Nursing and Canadian Society box). Psychological and emotional challenges may lead to mental health problems, and the first manifestation of schizophrenia can appear in late adolescence (Toga, Thompson, & Sowell, 2006). Adolescents in communal living, such as in college or university dormitories, may have increased risk for infectious diseases, such as measles, mumps, mononucleosis, and meningitis. Other health problems include acne, cardiovascular disease, tooth decay, gingivitis, misalignment of teeth, neglect, and abuse.

Three leading causes of death in the 10-to-24 age group are unintentional injuries (e.g., motor vehicle collisions, falls, drowning, poisoning,), suicide, and cancer (Public Health Agency of Canada, 2008). The Health Council of Canada (2006) estimated about "1.1 million—or 14%—of

Nursing and Canadian Society

Fact	Implications for Nursing Practice
Six percent of Canadian babies are born underweight (<2500 g) because of poor maternal diet, lifestyle, poverty, smoking, and dieting (Statistics Canada, 2006).	Preconceptual health and prenatal care are important for healthy pregnancy outcomes.
Cancer is the second-leading cause of death in Canada; mortality rates have continued to decline (Canadian Cancer Society's Steering Committee on Cancer Statistics, 2012).	Nursing health assessment needs to include screening for early detection of cancer among children. The importance of regular physical examination and harm reduction to provide a safe environment must be emphasized.
Rates of overweight and obesity among Canadian youth have more than doubled in the last 25 years. One million young Canadians are overweight, and half a million are obese (Health Council of Canada, 2006). Overweight and obesity is the fifth highest global risk for mortality. The prevalence of overweight and obesity in Canadian children ages 2–5 is estimated at 15.2% and 6.3%, respectively (DeCorby et al., 2012).	Obesity is a result of the lack of physical activity and poor food choices. Nurses can prevent childhood obesity at both family and societal levels by creating a supportive environment for healthy eating and active lifestyle.
Rates of adolescent pregnancy continue to be high, though pregnancy rates in Canada among 15- to 19-year-olds declined from 68.9 per 1000 in 1997 to 27.9 in 2006 (McKay & Barrett, 2010).	Nurses can help prevent unintended pregnancy by promoting the use of birth control methods and teaching or counselling teens about themselves (roles, self-concepts, etc.).

Canada's children under age 20 years have mental health conditions that affect their lives at home, at school, and in the community."

Suicide accounts for 24% of all deaths among 15- to 24-year-olds and is the second-leading cause of death for Canadians between 10 and 24 years (Canadian Mental Health Association [CMHA], 2006). Females experience more depression and suicidal ideas compared with males, whereas males act on their thoughts four times more often than females do (Cheung & Renaud, 2007). The rate of suicide among Aboriginal Canadians is twice the national average and shows no sign of decreasing. Some communities have epidemics of youth suicides. The Canadian average is around 4% for females, and 2% of males report a suicide attempt; among Aboriginals, the rate of attempts are 19% and 13% among males and females, respectively (Government of Canada, 2006). In general, suicide rates increase with age, poverty, Aboriginal heritage, seasonal darkness, untreated mental disorders, a history of sexual abuse, and location (CMHA, 2006). Motor vehicle collisions, drug and alcohol overdoses, firearm accidents, and even homicides can be disguised suicides.

Violence

School bullying among adolescents affects the school achievement and psychological well-being of both victims and perpetrators. Bullying is generally defined as a specific type of aggression that is intended to harm and occurs repeatedly over time with a more powerful person or group attacking someone less powerful (Reuter-Rice, 2008). Adolescent bullying can take different forms: physical (e.g., hitting, pushing, and kicking), verbal (e.g., name calling), relational or social (e.g., social exclusion, spreading rumours), and the emerging new form cyber bullying or electronic bullying. Studies show that boys are more involved in direct bullying (physical and verbal), whereas girls are more involved in indirect bullying (social) (Wang, Iannotti, & Nansel, 2009, p. 368).

Eating Disorders

Many adolescents engage in unhealthy dietary practices, and eating disorders are a serious health problem (Sigel, 2008). Increasing obesity rates are making type 2 diabetes more common among teens, whereas previously it occurred mostly in adults (Edelman & Mandle, 2010). As discussed in Chapter 40, common problems related to nutrition and self-esteem among adolescents include obesity, anorexia nervosa, and bulimia. Nurses need to help adolescents create a wellness plan that addresses body image, diet, weight concerns, and exercise.

Nonsuicidal Self-Injury

The number of adolescents who engage in nonsuicidal self-injury appears to be increasing internationally, with self-cutting as a primary form of self-harm. Adolescents who harm themselves have a wide range of psychosocial problems, including anxiety disorder, which may contribute to the behaviour. Eating disorders and self-injury are often related. Further investigation of this problem is needed to clarify its causes and guide treatment (Hintikka et al., 2009; Ross, Heath, & Toste, 2009).

Health Assessment and Promotion

Guidelines for growth and development of the adolescent are shown in the Assessment: Developmental Guidelines box below.

Adolescents are usually self-directed in meeting their health needs. Because of maturational changes, however, they need teaching and guidance, such as screening for hearing and vision; information on avoiding tobacco, alcohol, and drug use; and facts about healthy sexual practices, blood pressure maintenance, healthy weights, and immunizations. See the Health-Promotion Guidelines box for Adolescents.

ASSESSMENT **DEVELOPMENTAL GUIDELINES**

The Adolescent

In these three developmental areas, does the adolescent do the following?

1. **PHYSICAL DEVELOPMENT**
   - Exhibit physical growth (weight, height) within normal range for age and gender
   - Demonstrate male or female sexual development consistent with standards
   - Manifest vital signs within normal range for age and gender
   - Exhibit vision and hearing abilities within normal range

2. **PSYCHOSOCIAL DEVELOPMENT**
   - Interact well with parents, teachers, peers, siblings, and persons in authority
   - Like self
   - Think and plan for the future, such as university, a relationship, or a career
   - Choose a lifestyle and interests that fit own identity

   - Determine own beliefs and values
   - Begin to establish a sense of identity in the family
   - Seek help from appropriate persons about problems

3. **DEVELOPMENT IN ACTIVITIES OF DAILY LIVING**
   - Demonstrate knowledge of physical development, menstruation, reproduction, birth control, and methods for the prevention of STIs
   - Exhibit healthy lifestyle practices in nutrition, exercise, recreation, sleep patterns, and personal habits
   - Demonstrate concern for personal cleanliness and appearance
   - Reach out to members of their religious faith, peer group for support
   - Have a comfortable environment to practise the rituals of their faith

---

Health-Promotion Guidelines for Adolescents

The following are important to the health of adolescents:

HEALTH EXAMINATIONS
- Yearly or as recommended by the health care provider

PROTECTIVE MEASURES
- Immunizations, such as adult diphtheria-tetanus and pertussis (DTap) vaccine, as recommended; and hepatitis B vaccine, meningococcal vaccine, and human papillomavirus vaccine (HPV), if not yet immunized
- Screening for tuberculosis (TB) and STIs, as recommended
- Periodic vision and hearing screenings
- Regular dental assessments
- Provision of accurate information about sexuality and safe sex practices
- Mental health status assessment
- No salon tanning if under age 16

ADOLESCENT SAFETY
- Motor vehicle safety (e.g., driver's education course, seat belts, motorcycle helmets)
- Implementation of proper precautions during all athletic activities (e.g., medical supervision, proper equipment, hydration, and nutrients)
- Open lines of communication and being alert to signs of bullying or harassment, problematic substance use, emotional disturbances, and depression

NUTRITION AND EXERCISE
- Importance of healthy snacks and appropriate patterns of food intake and exercise
- Control of factors that may lead to nutritional problems (e.g., obesity, anorexia nervosa, bulimia, orthorexia)
- Balance of sedentary activities with regular vigorous exercise, at least three times a week for one hour each time

SOCIAL INTERACTIONS
- Parents are emotionally available and physically proximal to adolescents
- Encouragement of relationships that respect feelings, concerns, and fears
- Parental encouragement of peer group activities promoting moral and spiritual values
- Parents acting as role models for appropriate social interactions
- Parents provision of a comfortable home environment for appropriate adolescent peer group activities
- Encouragement of adolescents to participate in and contribute to family and community activities

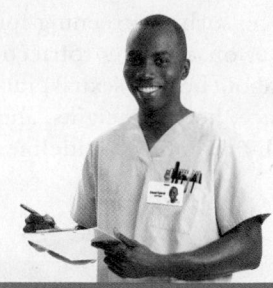

Case Study 18

Billy is a 6-year-old boy entering Grade 1. He is scared and hesitant to let go of his mother's hand. As the nursing student working in this setting, you have the opportunity to work with Billy and other young children as they start school.

CRITICAL THINKING QUESTIONS

1. How would you help Billy's mother reassure him?
2. On the basis of his age, what strategies might you use to teach Billy and his classmates about health promotion?

Check the eText in MyNursingLab for answers and explanations.

KEY TERMS

adolescence *p. 359*
amblyopia *p. 352*
Apgar scores *p. 348*
apocrine glands *p. 360*
colic *p. 348*
Denver Developmental
 Screening Test
 (DDST-II) *p. 349*
eccrine glands *p. 360*
ejaculation *p. 359*
emmetropic *p. 354*

failure to thrive *p. 348*
fetal alcohol spectrum
 disorder *p. 344*
hyperopic *p. 354*
identification *p. 355*
imagination *p. 355*
introjection *p. 355*
lanugo *p. 343*
menarche *p. 359*
myopic *p. 354*
normocephaly *p. 345*

peer groups *p. 361*
primary sexual
 characteristics *p. 360*
puberty *p. 357*
regression *p. 352*
repression *p. 355*
sebaceous glands *p. 360*
secondary sexual
 characteristics *p. 360*
self-concept *p. 351*
separation anxiety *p. 351*

shaken baby syndrome
 (SBS) *p. 348*
stereognosis *p. 357*
strabismus *p. 352*
sudden infant death
 syndrome (SIDS)
 p. 348
teratogen *p. 344*
trimesters *p. 343*
vernix caseosa *p. 343*

CHAPTER HIGHLIGHTS

- Intrauterine development lasts about nine months.
- Genetic and environmental factors affect the development of the fetus.
- A sense of trust and security in the newborn is essential for subsequent development; the infant derives this sense from parental love, warmth, and prompt attention to physical needs.
- Measurements of length, weight, head and chest circumferences, fontanelle size and status, reflex abilities, and motor development are important indicators of the newborn's growth and health.
- Infants from ages 1 month to 1 year reveal marked growth in size and stature with appropriate nutrition and care: birth weight doubles by age 6 months and triples by age 12 months.
- During infancy, motor development is notable: at age 3 months, infants can raise their heads from the prone position; at age 6 months, they can sit unsupported; and at age 12 months, they can stand momentarily and walk with help.
- To develop cognitively, the infant needs a variety of sensory and motor stimuli.

- Early childhood spans the period from ages 1 to 6 years and is subdivided into the toddler group, ages 1 to 3 years, and the preschool group, ages 4 and 5 years.
- During childhood, dramatic changes occur as the child moves from being a dependent person to becoming an independent person entering school.
- As the nervous system develops, body systems mature to the point at which the child can control his or her body, achieve finer muscle control, and perform all the activities of daily living, such as washing and dressing.
- Critical to psychosocial development during childhood is the development of a sense of autonomy and initiative.
- By the end of early childhood, the child has reached the phase of intuitive thought, has developed some internal moral controls, and is at the undifferentiated level of spiritual development.
- School-age children perfect their muscular skills and coordination and develop a sense of competence, perseverance, and self-worth.
- During emotional development, school-age children face Erikson's conflict of industry versus inferiority.

- School-age children begin to understand relationships and change from being egocentric to having cooperative interactions; according to Piaget, they are in the concrete operations phase of cognitive development.

- Most school-age children progress to the conventional level of moral development and to the mythical–literal stage of spiritual development.

- Rapid growth in height, secondary sexual characteristics, sexual maturity, and increasing independence from the family are major landmarks of adolescence.

- Peer groups assume great importance during adolescence; they provide a sense of belonging and self-esteem and facilitate the development of a positive self-concept.

- Adolescents are at Fowler's synthetic–conventional stage of spiritual development.

- Adolescents between ages 11 and 15 years begin the formal operations stage of cognitive development; they are able to think logically, rationally, and futuristically and can conceptualize things as they could be, rather than as they are.

- The adolescent is at Kohlberg's conventional level of moral development, and some proceed to the postconventional, or principled, level.

- The three leading causes of adolescent death are unintentional injuries, suicide, and cancer.

- Adolescents can be at risk for unintentional injuries, STIs, inactivity, unhealthy eating, mental health problems, teen pregnancy, and problematic tobacco, alcohol, and other drug use.

- The four leading causes of adolescent death are motor vehicle crashes, other unintentional injuries, homicide, and suicide.

ASSESS YOUR LEARNING

1. What is the most appropriate strategy for teaching kindergarten children effective hand hygiene techniques?

   a. Explaining and demonstrating the proper procedure for hand hygiene

   b. Involving the children in initiative and imaginative techniques on hand hygiene

   c. Developing a poster showing colourful bacteria growing on hands

   d. Providing a video for the children to watch at home

2. A nurse is involved with a new Family Health Network in a community that has many young families and many new babies. The nurse's responsibility is to complete the neonatal assessments of the new babies of the families in the clinic. Newborn health can be appraised through measuring which of the following?

   a. Muscular skills, vocalization, and feeding

   b. Weight, height, fontanelle size, and head circumference

   c. Tolerance for separation, sleep, and number of wet diapers

   d. Assessment of the levels of formal operations and responses to parental smiles

3. A nurse working with teens in a local high school should know the healthy indicators of developmental maturation. Which of the following is a landmark of adolescent development into adulthood?

   a. Increased self-care activities, sexually mature behaviours, close interpersonal relationships outside the family

   b. Peer pressure, a successful part-time job, graduation from secondary school

   c. Successful family dynamics, peer cohesion, and increased size

   d. Cooperative interactions, peer-focused language, and concern about personal health

4. Nurses can meet the health care needs of adolescents through which of the following?

   a. Encouraging teens to take responsibility for their behaviours and actions based on correct knowledge of health care measures

   b. Promoting parental accountability for yearly physicals, dental exams, and dietary requirements

   c. Providing many free clinics and numerous pamphlets to teach families about proper health activities

   d. Creating injury-proof strategies and requiring the use of helmets and pads during all sports

5. A parent is worried about his 1-year-old child's vision as the child seems to be unable to put his toys into the correct shapes into the holder held right on his lap. The parent indicates that the child wants to sit close to the TV screen to watch his favourite cartoon characters and does not seem to respond to smiles on other people's faces. Which of the following is the correct age and characteristic match regarding vision?

   a. At 4 months, infants still have problems focusing on close objects.

   b. At 9 months, infants begin to recognize and stare at colours.

   c. By 12 months, depth perception is developed.

   d. Rooting and Babinski reflexes mature as infants gain visual coordination.

6. Knowing what you do about new parents and their transition to baby care at home, which is the best choice from the titles below for a presentation you,

as the nurse, would give just before the mother is discharged?

a. *Apgar Scoring: The Way to Help Baby Learn*

b. *Safety Proofing Baby: Tips from A to Z*

c. *For Crying Out Loud! Keep That Baby Quiet!*

d. *Better Not Spoil That Baby: Cleaning Up after Baby*

7. An 18-month-old is rushed to the emergency room by ambulance with a pulse but absent respirations. The nurse performs an assessment. When should shaken baby syndrome (SBS) be suspected?

a. The child is 3 months old.

b. The parents claim the child is a good baby most of the time.

c. Assessment reveals injury, apnea, lethargy, and retinal hemorrhage.

d. An Apgar score of 10 is obtained.

8. Toddlers are prone to fatal injuries for which one of the following reasons?

a. Care is often provided in daycares and other settings outside the home.

b. Recurrent respiratory and ear infections create increased risk for health problems.

c. They are able to walk up and down stairs easily without assistance.

d. Most are curious about the tastes of everything and often copy others' actions.

9. Immunization for all children up to age 6 years should include which of the following?

a. One-time injections to combat measles, tetanus, and polio

b. Sequential injections at specific ages for DPT-Polio, MMR, Hib, HepB

c. Yearly tuberculosis (TB) immunizations in any province or territory

d. Examination of the child for allergies after administering the vaccines

10. School-age children enjoy group activities. These may lead to which of the following health problems?

a. Motor vehicle accidents (MVAs), broken legs, and concussions

b. Head injuries, bullying, and poisoning

c. Lost teeth, eye injuries, and abrasions

d. Communicable diseases, such as scabies, head lice, chickenpox

Check the eText in MyNursingLab for answers and explanations.

WEBLINKS

Canadian Paediatric Society

http://www.caringforkids.cps.ca

This site provides information about children from Canadian pediatric experts.

Dietitians of Canada

http://www.dietitians.ca/Secondary-Pages/Public/Who-Growth-Charts.aspx

This website has a series of World Health Organization (WHO) growth charts adapted for boys and girls (ages birth to 19 years) in Canada.

NCAST Programs: Promoting Nurturing Environments for Young Children

http://www.ncast.org

This website provides professionals, parents, and other caregivers with the knowledge and skills to provide nurturing environments for young children by developing and disseminating research-based products and training programs.

Public Health Agency of Canada: Division of Childhood and Adolescence

http://www.phac-aspc.gc.ca/dca-dea/yjc/summ-eng.php

This cross-national research study is Canada's only national database for health behaviour in school-age children. It aims to explore the health, well-being, and health behaviours of young people (ages 11 to 15 years) and their social settings, specifically, their school environment.

MyNursingLab

REFERENCES

Altimier, L. (2008). Shaken baby syndrome. *Journal of Perinatal & Neonatal Nursing, 22,* 68–76.

Burns, C. E., Dunn, A. M., Brady, M. A., Starr, N. B., & Blosser, C. (2008). *Pediatric primary care: A handbook for nurse practitioners.* Philadelphia, PA: W. B. Saunders.

Canadian Cancer Society's Steering Committee on Cancer Statistics. (2012). *Canadian cancer statistics 2012.* Toronto, ON: Canadian Cancer Society.

Canadian Institute for Health Information. (2005). *Improving the health of young Canadians.* Ottawa, ON: Author.

Canadian Mental Health Association. (2006). *Suicide.* Retrieved from http://www.ontario.cmha.ca/about_mental_health.asp?cID=7608

Canadian Paediatric Society. (2004). Recommendations for safe sleeping environments for infants and children. *Paediatrics & Child Health, 9*(9), 659–663.

Canadian Paediatric Society. (2009). *Shake a baby.* Retrieved from http://www.caringforkids.cps.ca/pregnancybabies/SBS.htm

Canadian Paediatric Society. (2010). *Safe sleep for babies.* Retrieved from http://www.caringforkids.cps.ca/pregnancybabies/safesleepforbaby.htm

Canadian Paediatric Society. (2011). *Colic and crying.* Retrieved from http://www.caringforkids.cps.ca/pregnancybabies/Colic.htm

Cheung, A., & Renaud, C. (2007). *Teen suicide rates in Canada similar to US despite universal health care. Insight Wellness News Article.* Retrieved from http://www.anxiety-and-depression-solutions.com/articles/news/Teen_suicide_rates_in_Canada_similar_to_US_despite_universal_health_care.php

Crittenden, P. (2008). *Raising parents: Attachment, parenting and child safety.* Portland, OR: Willan Publishing.

DeCorby, K., Graham, K., & Dobbins, M. (2012). Interventions to prevent obesity in 0–5 year olds: Evidence and implications for public health. Hamilton, ON: McMaster University. Retrieved from http://health-evidence.ca/documents/20391/Hesketh__2010__Summary_Statement_-_English.pdf

Edelman, C. L., & Mandle, C. L. (2010). *Health promotion throughout the life span* (7th ed.). St. Louis, MO: Mosby Elsevier.

Emond, A., Drewett, R., Blair, P., & Emmett, P. (2007). Postnatal factors associated with failure to thrive in term infants in the Avon Longitudinal Study of Parents and Children. *Child: Care, Health and Development, 33*(3), 351.

Erikson, E. H. (1963). *Childhood and society* (2nd ed.). New York, NY: Norton.

Fowler, J. W. (1981). *Stages of faith: The psychology of human development and the quest for meaning.* New York, NY: Harper & Row.

Frappier, J-Y, Kaufman, M., Baltzer, F., Elliott, A., Lane, M., Pinzon, J., & McDuff, P. (2008). Sex and sexual health: A survey of Canadian youth and mothers. *Pediatrics and Child Health, 13*(1), 25–30.

Freud, S. (1923). *The ego and the id.* London, UK: Hogarth Press.

Goodell, L. S., Wakefield, D. B., & Ferris, A. M. (2009). Rapid weight gain during the first year of life predicts obesity in 2–3 year olds from a low-income minority population. *Journal of Community Health.* Advance online publication. doi: 10.1007/s10900-009-9164-6

Government of Canada. (2006). *Aboriginal mental health and well-being. In the human face of mental health and mental illness in Canada.* Ottawa, ON: Minister of Public Works and Government Services Canada.

Health Council of Canada. (2006). *Their future is now: Healthy choices for Canada's children & youth.* Retrieved from http://www.healthcouncilcanada.ca/docs/rpts/2006/HCC_ChildHealth_EN.pdf

Hintikka, J., Tolmunen, T., Rissanen, M. L., Honkalampi, K., Kylma, J., & Laukkanen, E. (2009). Mental disorders in self-cutting adolescents. *Journal of Adolescent Health, 44,* 464–467. doi: 10.1016/j.jadohealth.2008.10.003

Kohlberg, L. (1977). *Recent research in moral development.* New York, NY: Holt, Rinehart, Winston.

Marchand, V. (2010). *Promoting optimal monitoring of child growth in Canada: Using the new World Health Organization growth charts.* Ottawa, ON: Canadian Paediatric Society.

McKay, A., & Barrett, M. (2010). Trends in teen pregnancy rates from 1996–2006: A comparison of Canada, Sweden, USA and England/Wales. *Canadian Journal of Human Sexuality.* http://www.highbeam.com/doc/1G1-229542649.html

Murray, R. B., Zentner, J. P., & Yakimo, R. (2009). *Health promotion strategies through the life span* (8th ed.). Upper Saddle River, NJ: Prentice Hall.

Piaget, J. (1966). *Origins of intelligence in children.* New York, NY: Norton.

Pogodina, C., Brunner Huber, L. R., Racine, E. F., & Platonova, E. (2009). Smoke-free homes for smoke-free babies: The role of residential environmental tobacco smoke on low birth weight. *Journal of Community Health, 34,* 376–382.

Public Health Agency of Canada. (2012). *Canadian perinatal health report—2008 edition.* Retrieved from http://www.phac-aspc.gc.ca/publicat/2008/cphr-rspc/index-eng.php

Public Health Agency of Canada. (2008). *Leading causes of death and hospitalization in Canada.* Retrieved from http://www.phac-aspc.gc.ca/publicat/lcd-pcd97/index-eng.php

Rasmussen, C., Andrew, G., Zwaigenbaum, L., & Tough, S. (2008). Neurobehavioural outcomes of children with fetal alcohol spectrum disorders: A Canadian perspective. *Paediatric Child Health, 13*(3), 185–191.

Reuter-Rice, K. (2008). Male adolescent bullying and the school shooter. *Journal of School Nursing, 24,* 350–359. doi: 10.1177/1059840508324577

Ross, S., Heath, N. L., & Toste, J. R. (2009). Eating disorders related to non-suicidal self-injury (cutting). *American Journal of Orthopsychiatry, 79*(1), 83–92. doi: 10.1037/a0014826

Sigel, E. (2008). Eating disorders. *Adolescent Medicine State of the Art Review, 19*(3), 547–572.

Statistics Canada. (2006). *Pregnancy outcomes by age group, 2004.* Retrieved from http://www40.statcan.ca/l01/cst01/hlth65a.htm

Toga, A. W., Thompson, P. M., & Sowell, E. R. (2006). Mapping brain maturation. *Trends in Neurosciences, 29*(3), 148–159.

Wang, J. Iannotti, R. J., & Nansel, T. R. (2009). School bullying among adolescents in the United States: Physical, verbal, relational, and cyber. *Journal of Adolescent Health, 45*(4), 368–375.

Wigle, D. T., Arbuckle, T. E., Turner, M. C., Berube, A., Yang, Q., Liu, S., & Krewski, D. (2008). Epidemiologic evidence of relationships between reproductive and child health outcomes and environmental chemical contaminants. *Journal of Toxicology and Environmental Health. Part B, Critical Reviews, 11*(5–6), 373–517. doi: 10.1080/10937400801921320

Chapter 19

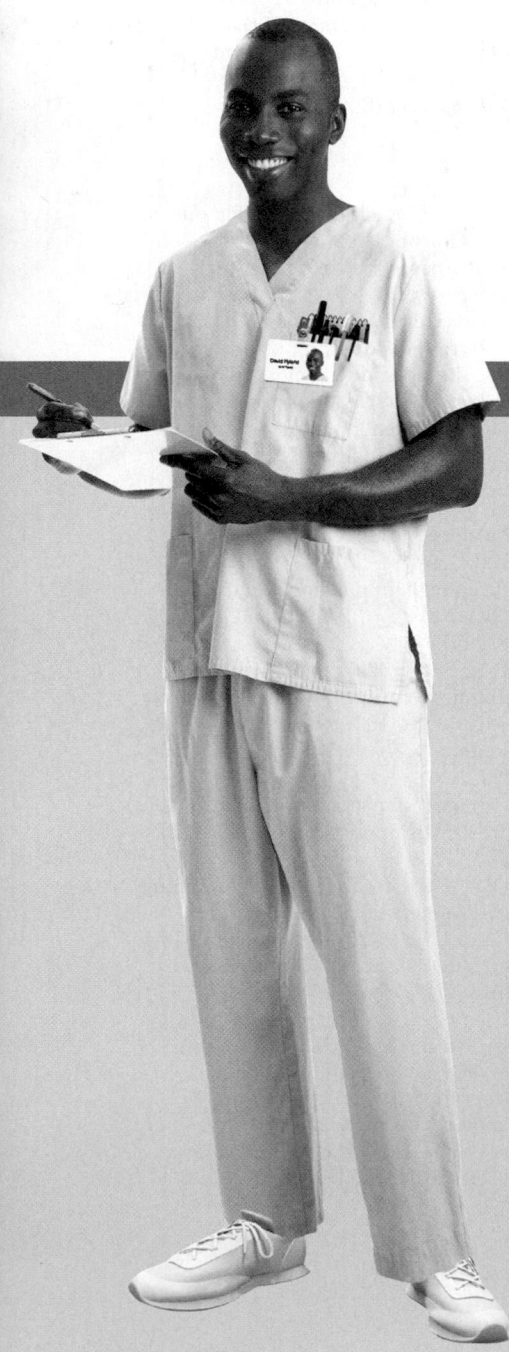

Young and Middle Adulthood

After completing this chapter, you will be able to:

1. Compare and contrast attributes that differentiate baby boomers, Generation X, and Generation Y.

2. Describe the normal physical development during young and middle adulthood.

3. Identify characteristic tasks of psychosocial development during young and middle adulthood.

4. Identify changes in cognitive development, according to Piaget, throughout adulthood.

5. Differentiate moral development, according to Gilligan and Kohlberg, throughout adulthood.

6. Examine spiritual development, according to Fowler, throughout adulthood.

7. Identify developmental assessment guidelines for young and middle-aged adults.

8. Identify selected health risks for young and middle-aged adults.

9. List examples of health-promotion strategies for young and middle adulthood.

The adult phase of development encompasses the years from the end of adolescence to death. Adulthood is often divided into three phases: young adulthood (20–40 years), middle adulthood (40–65 years), and late adulthood (65 years and older).

The adult period spans three different generations: the **baby boomers** (those born between 1945 and 1964), **Generation X** (those born between 1965 and 1978), and **Generation Y** (the *Millennials,* born between 1979 and 2000). Baby boomers are characterized by an individualistic outlook, tend toward a "workaholic" orientation, want to be respected at work, and are loyal and dedicated (Sudheimer, 2009). Many Generation Xers (Gen Xers) were raised by parents who were employed in full-time jobs outside the household. Watching their parents work long hours made Gen Xers less impressed with corporate values, more skeptical, and resistant to authority, but they enjoy challenges and opportunities to creatively solve problems. Generation Y, or Millennials, face an increasingly multicultural and technologically sophisticated society, and they enjoy public affirmation of their efforts.

Across the life continuum, individuals display differing degrees of physiological, cognitive, psychological, moral, emotional, and spiritual development. Nurses need to recognize individual variations when applying theories to meet caregiving.

Young Adults (20–40 Years)

The age at which a person is considered an adult depends on how the term *adulthood* is defined. In Canada, 18 years is the legal age for voting in government elections. Some mark the passage into adulthood with the legal smoking and drinking age, which varies from 18 to 21 years among the Canadian provinces and territories. Others consider adulthood has been reached when financial independence has been obtained. However, some adolescents support themselves as early as 16 years of age, whereas some persons remain financially dependent on their families for many years.

One may be considered an adult upon moving away from home and establishing one's own living arrangements. According to Statistics Canada (2012), an increasing number of young adults in their 20s (42% or 4.3 million, as compared to 32% in 1991) had either never left home or moved back to their parents' home. A relatively new term, "**boomerang kids**" describes young adults who move back into their parents' homes after an initial period of independent living. Returning home is often attributed to such reasons as increasing housing costs, divorce, high unemployment rates, and to some extent, cultural expectations. Many employed in minimum wage jobs do not earn enough money to be totally independent.

Young adults lead busy lives as they acclimatize to new roles at work, at home, and in the community. According to Erikson's developmental stages, this is a time of intimacy versus isolation and is a time for choosing a partner and becoming active in the community. The individual who has progressed through the first five stages should exhibit a strong sense of personal identity at this stage (Erikson, 1963).

Physical Development

People in their early 20s are in their prime physical years. The human body is at its most efficient functioning at about age 25 years. The musculoskeletal system is well developed and coordinated. This is the period when athletic endeavours reach their peak. All other systems of the body (e.g., cardiovascular, visual, auditory, and reproductive) are also functioning at peak efficiency. Young adults tend to be high risk takers, placing their high-functioning bodies at substantial risk of serious injury.

Although physical changes are minimal during this stage, weight and muscle mass may change as a result of diet and exercise. Additionally, extensive physical and psychosocial changes occur in pregnant and lactating women. Health outcomes in middle and older adulthood are somewhat dependent on behaviours during the younger adult stage.

Psychosocial Development

The psychosocial development milestones of the young adult are outlined in Box 19.1 on the next page, which highlights theorists Freud, Erikson, and Havighurst.

BOX 19.1 PSYCHOSOCIAL DEVELOPMENT: YOUNG ADULT

Young adults' psychosocial development is contingent on fulfilling the tasks listed in various stages of development:

- According to Freud's theory (1923), the young adult is in the genital stage, where one's energy is directed toward attaining a mature sexual relationship.
- According to Erikson's stages of development (1963), the young adult is in the intimacy versus isolation phase.
- According to Havighurst (1972), the young adult has the following developmental tasks:

  - Selecting a mate
  - Learning to live with a partner
  - Starting a family
  - Rearing children
  - Managing a home
  - Establishing a career
  - Taking on civic responsibility
  - Finding a congenial social group

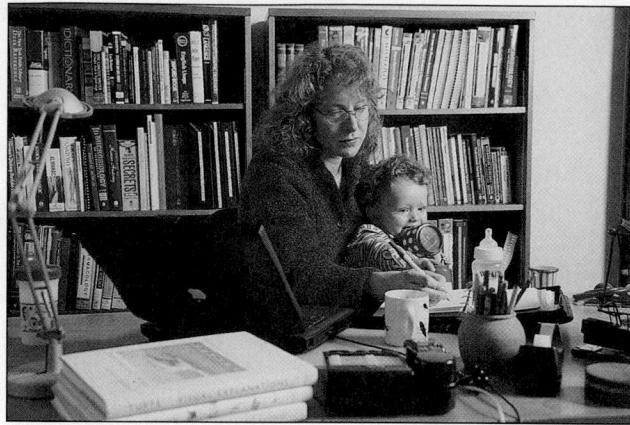

FIGURE 19.1 Many young women combine active careers with motherhood.

Young adults face new experiences and changes in lifestyle as they mature. It is the time in their lives when they are expected to make choices with regard to education and employment; sexual orientation; choosing a life partner and deciding whether to marry, to have a common law relationship, or to remain single; purchasing a home; and having children. Socially, their activities may include forming new friendships and taking on roles to establish themselves as responsible members of a community.

Many young adults have experienced stress related to the divorce of their parents and have experienced life in blended families or stepfamilies. Feelings of divided loyalties for divorced parents can create added stress. Their concerns may be about adequate financial resources, privacy and personal issues, and worries about loyalty and disloyalty to others. These childhood experiences can impact the development of intimate relationships in young adults (Mustonen, Huurre, Kiviruusu, Haukkala, & Aro, 2011). **Intimacy**, according to Erikson (1963), concerns developing affectionate relationships and lengthy attachments and making personal commitments to another that may include marriage or sexual relations.

A career choice may determine the educational requirements for a chosen path, or inversely, one's education may determine where one can obtain employment. Usually, the higher the level of education completed, the greater the opportunities for employment and increased socioeconomic status (SES). The traditional roles of women have evolved from that of wife and mother to one that includes employment outside the home (Figure 19.1).

Remaining single is becoming a chosen lifestyle among young adults, perhaps to pursue an education and then to have the freedom to pursue a chosen vocation. Some unmarried individuals choose to live with another person of the opposite or same sex and share living arrangements and expenses. They do not consider themselves to be single. The traditional definition of marriage has been forever altered with the Canadian government passing Bill C-38, The Civil Marriage Act, on July 20, 2005 (Department of Justice, 2006). The act extends equal access to civil marriage to same-sex couples while respecting religious freedom.

Although nontraditional lifestyles are becoming widely acceptable in society, traditional attitudes can contribute social pressures that lead to stress. The multiple roles of adulthood (citizen, worker, taxpayer, homeowner, spouse, grown child, sibling, parent, and friend) can create stress as a result of role conflict, role ambiguity, and role confusion.

Cognitive Development

Young adults in the *formal operations stage* think abstractly and employ logic (Piaget, 1966). These young adults relate strongly to the values and norms of their social group and will conduct themselves according to those norms.

Postformal thought is defined as a concept that includes creativity, intuition, and the ability to consider information related to other ideas. Postformal thinkers can comprehend and balance arguments created by both logic and emotion and proceed from abstract reasoning to practical considerations. They are aware that most problems have more than one cause and more than one answer and some solutions will work better than others. They are able to comprehend and balance arguments created by both logic and emotion (Beckmann Murray, Zentner, Pangman, & Pangman, 2008).

Moral Development

Young adults who have mastered the first two stages of Kohlberg's theory of moral development enter level III, the *postconventional level*. At this stage, the person understands human rights and what is acceptable as determined by societal norms, rules, and obligations. However, when one has a perceived conflict with society's rules or laws, there is a realization that laws can be changed if it means improving society or righting what they have determined is a wrongful act. For example, consider the media attention around the seal hunt in Newfoundland. A person may intentionally break the law and join a protest group to stop hunters from killing wild animals, believing that the principle of conservation of wildlife justifies the protest action. This type of reasoning is called *principled reasoning*. Gilligan (1982) argued that as individuals approach young adulthood, each gender tends to define moral problems somewhat differently (see the section on Gilligan in Chapter 17). Men often use an ethic of justice and define moral problems in terms of rules and rights. Women, by contrast, often define moral problems in terms of obligations to care and to avoid hurt.

Spiritual Development

According to Fowler (1981), the individual enters the individuating–reflective period sometime after 18 years of age. During this period, the individual focuses on reality. The religious teaching that the young adult had as a child may now be accepted or redefined. Murray, Zentner, & Yakimo (2009) state that the young adult searches for a new connectedness with others, nature, the universe, or a higher being. The mysteries of life, faith, and belief in God are explored actively by some young adults.

Health Risks

Young adulthood is generally a healthy time in life. Health risks that do occur and are common in this age group include accidents, suicide attempts, substance misuse, hypertension, sexually transmitted infections (STIs), eating disorders, interpersonal violence (bullying), and certain malignancies. Some of the problems such as injuries, substance abuse, and STIs are related to behaviours that could possibly be prevented through primary prevention strategies.

INJURY AND VIOLENCE In Canada, injury is the leading cause of death and hospitalization of children and young adults. It is also a major cause of long- and short-term impairment and disability for Canadians. The leading causes of injury were motor vehicle collisions for all age groups except those 65 years and older, followed by falls, gunshot wounds, and stab wounds (Health Canada, 2003).

Violence is a growing concern among Canadians. No one is immune regardless of age, gender, sexual orientation, class, ethnic background, religious or spiritual group membership, physical and mental ability, or place of residence. The problem of battering, or abuse, affects families at all socioeconomic levels. Stresses that predispose

families to abuse may include financial problems, lack of family and community supports, and physical as well as social isolation. Females and children continue to be targets of both physical and sexual assaults (Edelman & Mandle, 2010). Other examples of violence include workplace violence, random shootings, and a phenomenon known as homicide–suicide (H-S). Most H-S offenders are men who kill their partners and sometimes also their children, and a close relationship with the homicide victim predicts subsequent suicide risk by the H-S offender (Large, Smith, & Neilssen, 2009).

INTIMATE PARTNER VIOLENCE (IPV) **Intimate partner violence** refers to dating and cohabiting violence, same-sex violence, and violence by heterosexual women (Hamel, 2009). IPV can include physical violence and nonphysical abuses, including emotional, psychological, economic, and social abuse. Factors such as secondary education, high SES, and formal marriage decrease the incidence of IPV, while alcohol abuse, cohabitation, young age, attitudes supportive of wife beating, having outside sexual partners, experiencing childhood abuse, growing up with domestic violence, and experiencing or perpetrating other forms of violence in adulthood increased the risk of IPV (Abramsky, et al., 2011). Violence between genders is equal; that is, women initiate violence as often as men; and male abuse victims may not report being victimized for fear of being ridiculed or discriminated against by health care professionals (Hamel, 2009; Outlaw, 2009; Wigman, 2009).

Aboriginal men reported two to three times the risk of experiencing partner violence in comparison to men in the general Canadian population. Reports of violence included severe forms of physical assault, being choked, being threatened with or having a knife or gun used against them, and being beaten (Brownridge, 2010).

Lesbian mothers are another vulnerable group for IPV. Education, awareness, and understanding of the lesbian community can assist providers to work with these victims (see Chapter 46). Health care providers need to be able to establish a therapeutic relationship with members of this group; they can be instrumental in spreading cultural awareness and lobbying for policy or institutional changes to include same-sex IPV (Oswald, Fonseca, & Hardesty, 2010).

Efforts to prevent injury and violence can occur at primary, secondary, or tertiary levels of prevention. Education about safety precautions and accident prevention is a major role of the nurse who is promoting the health of Canadians (see the section "Promoting Safety across the Lifespan" in Chapter 32). Nurses who are familiar with community resources can provide valuable safety information for health care professionals, parents, and caregivers on how to keep children and the community safe. Culturally sensitive communication on the part of the nurse is imperative in gathering information from both female and male victims of IPV.

SUICIDE   Suicide is a leading cause of death in the young adult age group (Edelman & Mandle, 2010). Many suicides may be mistaken for accidental death (motor vehicle crashes, combining alcohol and barbiturates, or discharging a gun while cleaning it). Suicide may result from problems with close relationships (marriage partners or parents) or from depression related to perceived occupational, academic, or financial failure. In general, suicide results from the young adult's inability to cope with the pressures, responsibilities, and expectations of adulthood.

The nurse's role in the prevention of suicide includes identifying behaviours that may indicate potential problems: depression; a variety of physical complaints, including weight loss, sleep disturbances, and digestive disorders; and decreased interest in social and work roles along with an increase in isolation. A young adult identified as at risk for suicide must be referred to a mental health specialist or a crisis centre. A suicide threat should never be ignored. Nurses can reduce the incidence of suicide by participating in educational programs that provide information about the early signs of suicide. See the Reflect on Primary Health Care box on depressed young adults in Canada.

SUBSTANCE ABUSE (SA)   The use of alcohol, marijuana, amphetamines, and cocaine, to name just a few, is on the rise, and it is a major threat to the health of young adults. The transient feelings of well-being resulting from substance use may seem to help one escape from reality when problems are overwhelming. Prolonged use can lead to physical and psychological dependency, and deterioration of one's physical and mental health. Health care providers and educators need to understand SA and work collaboratively and pedagogically to eliminate SA in schools (Salm, Sevigny, Mulholland, & Greenberg, 2011). Substance abuse and addiction are at epidemic proportions in Aboriginal communities. Health Canada (2006a) established the National Native Alcohol and Drug Abuse Program (NNADAP) to assist First Nations and Inuit communities to reduce alcohol, drug, and solvent abuse among on-reserve populations.

Nursing strategies related to problematic substance use include teaching about the complications of substance use, changing individual attitudes toward problematic substance use, and counselling clients to learn effective coping strategies.

Smoking can lead to lung cancer and cardiovascular disease. The nurse's role regarding smoking is to (a) serve as a role model by not smoking; (b) provide educational information regarding the dangers of smoking and second-hand smoke; (c) help make smoking socially unacceptable; (d) suggest resources, such as hypnosis, lifestyle training, and behaviour modification, to clients who want to stop smoking; and (e) lobby for antismoking legislation.

SEXUALLY TRANSMITTED INFECTIONS   Sexually transmitted infections (STIs), such as genital herpes, acquired immune deficiency syndrome (AIDS), syphilis, and gonorrhea, are common infections in young adults. Chlamydia is the most prevalent STI (Public Health Agency of Canada, 2010). However, human papilloma virus (HPV) infection is of growing concern in Canada and worldwide. There is no cure for HPV infection, which can lead to skin lesions (i.e., genital warts) or cancer (Health Canada, 2010). In 2007, the National Advisory Committee on Immunization (NACI) recommended the use of Gardasil vaccination for immunization against HPV in females between 9 and 26 years of age. Specifically, Gardasil is recommended for females between 9 and 13 years of age, before they become sexually active, and for females between 14 and 26 years of age, even if they are already sexually active, have had previous Pap test abnormalities, or have had a previous HPV infection.

The nurse's role is to prevent the incidence of STIs by promoting safe sex practices, such as the use of condoms, and to educate individuals about the risks attached to multiple sexual relationships. The nurse must be nonjudgmental and accepting of the client's lifestyle and treat any information obtained as confidential (see Chapter 46).

EATING DISORDERS   Statistics Canada (2011) reported that obesity is a growing health concern in Canada. Both obesity (body mass index [BMI] >30 kg/m²) and overweight (BMI between 25 and 30) affect the health of individuals and populations, as they are contributors to a wide variety of chronic diseases, such as diabetes, cardiovascular disease, hypertension, and liver disease, as well as to breast, colon, and prostate cancers. Approximately 5.5 million, or 23%, of Canadian adults were obese. Obesity rates are rising among 25- to 34-year-olds, and 23% of Canadian women of childbearing age are obese. Nutrition assessment, diet teaching, and exercise are important elements in developing an individualized wellness plan for clients. Individuals who have anorexia nervosa, orthorexia nervosa, and bulimia, as well as vegetarians, are at an increased risk of nutritional deficiencies. Young women require more calcium and proper nutrition during their childbearing years. The nurse assesses nutritional concerns and discusses diet and exercise patterns with the client for the subsequent development of an individualized wellness plan.

REFLECT ON **PRIMARY HEALTH CARE**

Because of the stigma and inadequate support services, almost half of depressed young adults in Canada do not seek or have access to mental health services. Teenagers and young adults age 15 to 24 years' experience the highest incidence of mental disorders of any age group in Canada (Canadian Mental Health Association, 2012). Nurses educate the public, service providers, and politicians about mental health and lobby for accessible and timely services to meet the needs of the clients and their families. Through these activities, consider how nurses use the primary health care principles of *health promotion, accessibility, intersectoral cooperation,* and *public participation* to make this happen.

MALIGNANCIES The Canadian cancer statistics (Canadian Cancer Society's Steering Committee on Cancer Statistics, 2012) showed that the leading cause of cancer morbidity and mortality for both men and women is lung cancer, followed by colorectal cancer (see the Evidence-Informed Practice box on colorectal cancer screening among young women in Canada). Close to 30% of the newly diagnosed cancers and 17% of deaths occurred in young and middle-aged adults. Testicular cancer is the most common neoplasm in men 20 to 34 years of age. *Monthly testicular self-examination* (TSE) is recommended as a health screening strategy (see the Teaching: Wellness box on testicular self-examination in Chapter 46, page 1508). Breast cancer is the most common cancer in women worldwide. Young women are encouraged to be breast aware (Canadian Cancer Society [CCS], 2010). Average-risk women do not need to have routine mammography screening, clinical breast exams, and do breast self-examinations. Women between 50 and 74 years of age should have a mammogram every two to three years. After age 74 years, the woman's health care provider will determine the need for any further mammograms (Canadian Task Force on Preventive Health Care, 2011) (see Chapter 46).

Young adult females should have a routine **Pap (Papanicolaou) test** starting at age 18 years or sooner if they are sexually active. A second test should be taken after one year. If results are normal a repeat Pap test should be done every three years to age 69 years. No rescreening is necessary if the female has never had sexual intercourse or if the woman had a hysterectomy and her previous tests were normal. A female over age 69 years who has had at least two clear Pap tests, no cervical abnormalities for nine years, and no history of cancer, does not need regular screening (Health Canada, 2006b).

Many young adults are reluctant to have these examinations and screenings. It is important for nurses to explain the purpose of these tests and to encourage all young women to take preventive measures, such as undergoing regular screening for early detection of cancer.

EVIDENCE-INFORMED PRACTICE

Prevalence of and Factors Associated with Colorectal Cancer Screening in Canadian Women

This study compared women ages 50 to 74 years from Ontario who had never been screened for colorectal cancer (CRC) (*n* = 3676) with women who had CRC screening (*n* = 2105). Despite vigorous campaigns by Canadian health organizations for CRC screening, <40% of women reported ever having CRC screening in 2005. Higher rates of screening were noted in the group comprising women who were older, had higher levels of education, were Caucasian, or had had a cancer diagnosis other than colorectal cancer. This group was also more likely to engage in a healthy lifestyle and had easier access to health care resources. Lower socioeconomic status (SES) was a common factor in women who never had CRC screening.

NURSING IMPLICATIONS: Nurses need to develop effective ways to increase CRC screening. Education of the public regarding early detection of colorectal cancer is lifesaving. Providing easier access to CRC screening is essential through community health centres and walk-in clinics.

Source: Based on Brennenstuhl, S., Fuller-Thomson, E., & Popova, S. (2010). Prevalence and factors associated with colorectal cancer screening in Canadian women. *Journal of Women's Health, 19*(4), 775–784. doi:10.1089/jwh.2009.1477

Health Assessment and Promotion

Assessment guidelines for the growth and development of the young adult are shown in the Assessment: Developmental Guidelines box.

ASSESSMENT	**DEVELOPMENTAL GUIDELINES**

The Young Adult

In these three developmental areas, does the young adult do the following?

1. **PHYSICAL DEVELOPMENT**
   - Exhibit weight and BMI within normal range for age and gender
   - Manifest vital signs (e.g., blood pressure) within normal range for age and gender
   - Demonstrate visual and hearing abilities within normal range
   - Exhibit appropriate knowledge (e.g., STIs) and attitudes about sexuality

2. **PSYCHOSOCIAL DEVELOPMENT**
   - Feel independent from parents
   - Have a realistic self-concept

- Like self and direction of life
- Interact well with family
- Cope with the stresses of change and growth
- Have well-established bonds with significant others and intimacy with a partner or close friends
- Have a meaningful social life
- Demonstrate emotional, social, and economic responsibility for own life
- Have a set of values that guide behaviour

3. **ACTIVITIES OF DAILY LIVING**
   - Have a healthy lifestyle

Health-Promotion Guidelines for Young Adults

HEALTH TESTS AND SCREENINGS

Young adults should engage in the following health-promotion activities:

- Routine physical examination (every one to three years for females; every five years for males)
- Immunizations, such as tetanus and diphtheria boosters every 10 years, as recommended; meningococcal vaccine, if not given in early adolescence; hepatitis B vaccine
- HPV vaccine for males and females 9 to 26 years of age who have not yet received or completed the vaccine series
- Regular dental assessments (every 6 to 9 months)
- Periodic vision and hearing screenings
- Being breast aware
- Pap test annually within three years of onset of sexual activity and every three years if normal results
- Testicular examination every year
- Screening for cardiovascular disease (e.g., cholesterol test every five years if results are normal; blood pressure to detect hypertension; baseline electrocardiogram at age 35 years or as needed)
- Tuberculosis skin test every two years or as needed
- Smoking: history taking and counselling, if needed

SAFETY

- Motor vehicle safety reinforcement (e.g., using designated drivers when drinking, not texting or using cell phones when driving a car)
- Sun protection measures
- Workplace safety measures
- Water safety reinforcement (e.g., no diving in shallow water)

NUTRITION AND EXERCISE

- Importance of adequate iron intake in diet
- Nutritional and exercise factors that may lead to cardiovascular disease (e.g., obesity, cholesterol and fat intake, lack of vigorous exercise)

SOCIAL INTERACTIONS

- Encouraging personal relationships that promote discussion of feelings, concerns, and fears
- Setting short-term and long-term goals for work and career choices

Young adults are usually interested in meeting their health needs. However, because of the many stresses and changes that occur throughout this 20-year period, the nurse's role is to engage the young adult in health promotion by disseminating information regarding health tests and screening (see the Health-Promotion Guidelines box for Young Adults).

Middle-Aged Adults (40 to 65 Years)

Middle-aged adults (40 to 65 years) enter a time referred to as "generativity versus self-absorption and stagnation" in Erikson's eight developmental stages of life. Children have grown up, and parents may be experiencing the "empty nest syndrome." The partners generally have more time for each other and to pursue interests they may have deferred for years (Figure 19.2).

Maturity is the state of maximal function and integration, or the state of being fully developed. Mature individuals generally have a broader world view of issues; they demonstrate self-acceptance, are able to be reflective and insightful about life, and see themselves as others see them. Mature adults assume responsibility for themselves and expect others to do the same. They confront

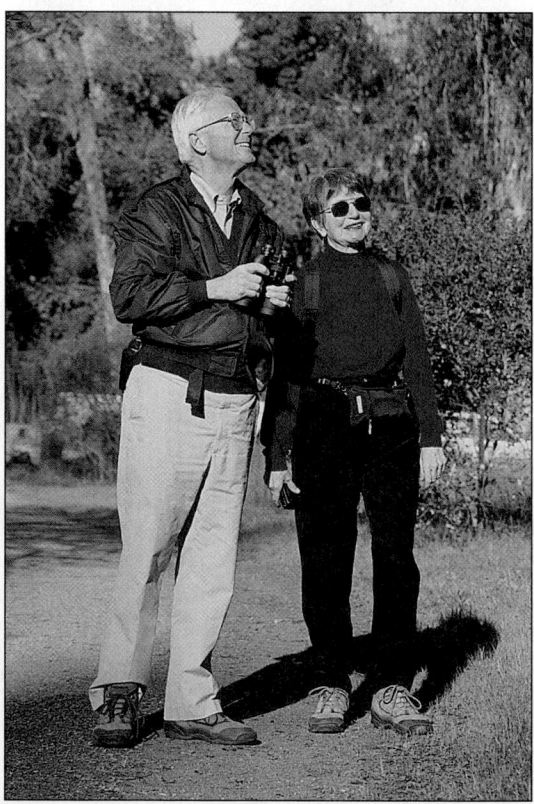

FIGURE 19.2 Middle-aged adults have time to pursue interests that may have been put aside for childcare.

the tasks of life in a realistic manner, make decisions, and accept responsibility for those decisions.

Physical Development

A number of changes take place during the middle years. At age 40 years, most adults function as effectively as they did in their 20s. Between ages 40 to 65 years, many physical changes take place. See Table 19.1 for a summary of these changes.

Both men and women experience decreasing hormonal production during the middle years. **Menopause** refers to the change of life in women and is defined as not having had a menstrual period for 1 year. Menopause usually occurs between ages 45 and 55 years. The average age is about 47 years. At this time, ovarian secretion of estrogen and progesterone decreases. Common symptoms are hot flashes, chills, decrease in breast size and loss of elasticity causing breasts to droop, and weight gain. Insomnia and headaches also occur with relative frequency. Psychologically, menopause can be an anxiety-producing time, especially if the ability to bear children is an integral part of the woman's self-concept.

Climacteric (andropause) refers to the change of life in men, when sexual activity decreases. Androgen levels decrease very slowly; however, men can father children even in late life. Some men may have difficulty achieving sexual arousal for psychological reasons (e.g., financial worries, fear of aging, concerns about retirement, and boredom). (See the section on "Development of Sexuality: Adulthood" in Chapter 46.)

Psychosocial Development

Havighurst (1972) outlined eight tasks for the middle-aged adult (see Box 19.2). Erikson (1963) viewed the developmental choice of the middle-aged adult as *generativity versus stagnation*. **Generativity** is defined as the concern for establishing and guiding the next generation. Couples have more time for companionship and recreation, and relationships can be more satisfying. In middle adulthood, the self seems more altruistic, and concepts of service to others and love and compassion gain prominence. These concepts motivate charitable actions, such as volunteering at church or fundraising

---

BOX 19.2 PSYCHOSOCIAL DEVELOPMENT: MIDDLE-AGED ADULT

According to Havighurst (1972), the middle-aged adult has the following developmental tasks:

- Achieving adult civic and social responsibilities
- Establishing and maintaining an economic standard of living
- Assisting teenage children to become responsible and happy adults
- Developing adult leisure-time activities
- Relating to his or her spouse as a person
- Accepting and adjusting to the physiological changes of middle age
- Adjusting to aging parents
- Balancing the needs of children, parents, work, and so on

TABLE 19.1 Physical Changes in the Middle-Aged Adult

Category	Description
Appearance	Hair begins to thin, and grey hair appears. Skin turgor and moisture decrease, subcutaneous fat decreases, and wrinkling occurs. Fatty tissue is redistributed, resulting in fat deposits in the abdominal area.
Musculoskeletal system	Skeletal muscle bulk decreases at about age 60 years. Thinning of the intervertebral discs causes a decrease in height of about 2 cm or 3 cm. Calcium loss from bone tissue is more common among postmenopausal women. Muscle growth continues in proportion to use.
Cardiovascular system	Blood vessels lose elasticity and become thicker; and the heart has to work harder to pump blood through these blood vessels.
Sensory perception	Visual acuity declines, often by the late 40s, especially for near vision (presbyopia). Auditory acuity for high-frequency sounds also decreases (presbycusis), particularly in men. Taste sensations also diminish.
Metabolism	Metabolism slows, resulting in weight gain.
Gastrointestinal system	Gradual decrease in tone of the large intestine may predispose the individual to constipation.
Urinary system	Nephron units of the kidneys are lost during this time, and the glomerular filtration rate decreases.
Sexuality	Hormonal changes take place in both men and women resulting in decline in sexual function with increasing age.

for charitable causes. Generative middle-aged persons have attained a sense of comfort and satisfaction with their lives.

Erikson (1963) believed that people who are unable to expand their interests at this time and who do not assume the responsibilities of middle age suffer a sense of boredom and impoverishment known as **stagnation**. These individuals have difficulty accepting their aging bodies and become withdrawn and isolated. They are preoccupied with the self and unable to give to others. Some may regress to younger patterns of behaviour. The "midlife crisis" occurs when individuals recognize that they have reached the halfway mark of life and that life is finite. Midlife crisis is *not* universal but is more common in men (Beckmann Murray et al., 2008).

The term **sandwich generation** refers to individuals who are providing for the needs of both their children and their aging parents. They are facing two competing sets of demands. Many employed middle-aged adults have to adjust their work schedules to care for their aging parents. The financial implications and the psychological stresses for this group can be overwhelming and can affect their general health (Chassin, Macy, Seo, Presson, & Sherman, 2010). Caregiving responsibility tends to lie with the female in the family.

Cognitive Development

The middle-aged adult's cognitive and intellectual abilities change very little. Cognitive processes include reaction time, memory, perception, learning, problem solving, and creativity. Reaction time during the middle years stays much the same or diminishes during the latter part of the middle years. Memory and problem solving are maintained through middle adulthood. Learning continues and can be enhanced by increased motivation at this time in life.

Genetic, environmental, social, and personality factors in early and middle adulthood account for the large difference in the ways in which individuals maintain mental abilities (Edelman & Mandle, 2010). Thus, approaches to problem solving and task completion will vary considerably in the middle-aged group.

Moral Development

According to Kohlberg (1971, 1981), most adults move beyond the *conventional level* to the *postconventional level*. Extensive experience of personal moral choice and responsibility is required before people can reach the postconventional level. To move from stage 4, a *law and order orientation,* to stage 5, a *social contract orientation,* requires that the individual move to a stage in which the rights of others take precedence. Moral development continues through adulthood and few individuals attain stage 5 before age 40 years.

Spiritual Development

Not all adults progress through Fowler's stages (1981) to the fifth, called the *paradoxical-consolidative stage.* At this stage, the individual can view *truth* from a number of viewpoints. Fowler's fifth stage corresponds to Kohlberg's fifth stage. Fowler believed that only some individuals after age 30 years reach these levels.

In middle adulthood, people tend to be less dogmatic about religious beliefs, and religion often offers more comfort to these individuals than it did previously. They become more in touch with their own mortality and often rely on spiritual beliefs to help them deal with illness, death, and tragedy.

Health Risks

Many middle-aged adults remain healthy; however, the risk of developing a health problem is greater than that in the young adult. Leading causes of death in this age group include motor vehicle and occupational accidents; chronic diseases, such as cancer; and cardiovascular disease. Lifestyle patterns, in combination with aging, family history, developmental stressors (e.g., menopause, climacteric), and situational stressors (e.g., divorce), often trigger health problems. Smoking and excessive alcohol consumption place an individual at greater risk of developing chronic respiratory problems, lung cancer, and liver disease. Overeating can result in obesity, diabetes mellitus, atherosclerosis, and associated risks for hypertension and coronary artery disease. The role of the nurse in health promotion and illness prevention is to enhance the quality of life and longevity in older adulthood.

INJURIES Changing physiological factors, such as decreased visual acuity and reaction times, increase the risk of injury in middle-aged people. Occupational accident is a significant safety hazard during the middle years. Motor vehicle collisions are the most common cause of accidental death. Other causes of death include falls, fires, burns, poisonings, and drowning.

CANCER In Canada, cancer is the second leading cause of death among people between ages 25 and 64 years. Men have a high incidence of lung and prostate cancers. In women, breast cancer is highest in incidence, followed by lung and colon cancers. About 40% of Canadian females and 45% of men will develop cancer in their lifetime, and one in five Canadians will be diagnosed with some type of cancer and nine people will die from cancer (Canadian Cancer Society's Steering Committee on Cancer Statistics. 2012). The nurse's role is to emphasize the importance of a healthy lifestyle, regular medical examination, and early screening for detection of cancer.

CARDIOVASCULAR DISEASE Coronary artery disease (CAD) is the second leading cause of death in Canada. Several factors contribute to the risk of CAD: smoking, obesity, hypertension, hyperlipidemia, diabetes mellitus, and a sedentary lifestyle. A family history of myocardial infarction, such as the sudden death of a father younger than age 55 years or a mother younger than age 65 years, is of significance. Men over 45 years of age and women over 55 years of age are at a greater risk of developing CAD than are younger adults. Physical inactivity is the greatest risk factor for developing CAD (Edelman & Mandle, 2010).

OBESITY Middle-aged adults who gain weight may not be aware of some common facts about this age period. Decreased metabolic activity and decreased physical activity mean a decrease in caloric need. The nurse can counsel clients to prevent obesity by reducing caloric intake and participating in regular exercise. Clients should be educated that being overweight is a risk factor for many chronic diseases, such as diabetes and hypertension, and for problems of mobility, such as arthritis. (See the Lifespan Considerations box on age-specific physical activity guidelines for Canadians in Chapter 7).

ALCOHOLISM The excessive use of alcohol can lead to unemployment, disrupted families, accidents, and diseases. Nearly 1 in 10 Canadians report problems with alcoholism. Nurses can educate clients about the risks related to excessive alcohol use, examine the individual causes of abuse, and refer the client to a support group, such as Alcoholics Anonymous.

MENTAL HEALTH ALTERATIONS Failure to adapt to the physiological and developmental changes of middle age can have a negative impact on an individual's mental health. Developmental stressors, such as menopause, climacteric, aging, and impending retirement, as well as situational stressors, such as divorce, unemployment, and the death of a spouse, can precipitate increased anxiety and depression. A nurse can help individual clients develop coping strategies to get through difficult times.

BOX 19.3 THE NINE CHOICES OF HAPPINESS

Intention:	Committing to a positive attitude and behaviours that lead to happiness
Accountability:	Assuming personal responsibility for your actions, thoughts, and feelings, and refusing to view yourself as a victim
Identification:	Assessing what makes you uniquely happy and not what others want to do
Centrality:	Focusing on what is central to your life that will bring you happiness
Recasting:	Transforming stressful problems into something meaningful, important, and a source of emotional energy
Options:	Opening to new possibilities and adopting a flexible approach to life's journeys
Appreciation:	Appreciating your life and the people in the present and turning each experience into something precious
Giving:	Sharing yourself with friends and community without the expectation of a return
Truthfulness:	Choosing to be honest with yourself and others.

Source: Based on Foster, R., & Hicks, G. (1999). *How we choose to be happy.* New York, NY: Perigree. pp. 9–10.

SUSTAINABLE HAPPINESS Sustainable happiness is a relatively new paradigm in happiness studies. **Sustainable happiness** is "happiness that contributes to individual, community and/or global well-being and does not exploit other people, the environment or future generations" (O'Brien, 2011, para 1). "True happiness is a profound, enduring feeling of contentment, capability, and centeredness" (Foster & Hicks, 1999, p. 6). Happiness is a life choice. There are nine choices to help one get through tough times (see Box 19.3). Happy

---

ASSESSMENT DEVELOPMENTAL GUIDELINES

The Middle-Aged Adult

In these three developmental areas, does the middle-aged adult do the following?

1. PHYSICAL DEVELOPMENT
- Exhibit weight within normal range for age and gender
- Manifest vital signs (e.g., blood pressure) within normal range for age and gender
- Manifest visual and hearing abilities within normal range
- Exhibit appropriate knowledge and attitudes about sexuality (e.g., about menopause)
- Verbalize any changes in eating, elimination, sleep, or exercise

2. PSYCHOSOCIAL DEVELOPMENT
- Accept the aging body
- Feel comfortable and respect self
- Enjoy new freedom to be independent
- Accept changes in family roles (e.g., having teenage children and aging parents)
- Interact well and share companionable activities with life partner
- Expand and renew previous interests
- Pursue charitable and altruistic activities
- Have a meaningful philosophy of life

3. DEVELOPMENT IN ACTIVITIES OF DAILY LIVING
- Follow preventive health practices

Health-Promotion Guidelines for Middle-Aged Adults

The following are important to the health of middle-aged adults:

HEALTH TESTS AND SCREENING

- Routine physical examination (annually for females; every two to three years or as directed by health-care provider for males)
- Immunizations, such as a tetanus booster every 10 years and influenza and pneumococcal vaccinations, as recommended
- Regular dental assessments (e.g., yearly), daily brushing, flossing, gum massage
- Tonometry (to test pressure in the eye) for signs of glaucoma and eye exams for other eye diseases (e.g., macular degeneration) every two to three years or annually, if indicated
- Screening for breast cancer: mammography every two to three years between ages 50 and 74 years
- Testicular self-examination monthly
- Screenings for cardiovascular disease (e.g., blood pressure measurement; electrocardiographic and cholesterol tests, as directed by health care provider)
- Screenings for colorectal, cervical, uterine, and prostate cancers
- Screening for tuberculosis every two years

SAFETY

- Motor vehicle safety reinforcement, especially when driving at night
- Workplace safety measures (e.g., avoid repetitive strain)
- Home safety measures: keeping hallways and stairways lighted and uncluttered, using smoke and carbon monoxide detectors, using nonskid mats and hand rails in the bathrooms
- The practice of safe sex

NUTRITION AND EXERCISE

- Importance of adequate fibre, protein, calcium, and vitamin D in diet
- Avoidance of excessive intake of caffeine
- Avoidance of nutritional and exercise factors that may lead to cardiovascular disease (e.g., obesity, sedentary lifestyle); monitoring of cholesterol and lipid levels; avoidance of saturated and trans fat intake
- Vigorous exercise program that emphasizes skill and coordination; daily exercise for a minimum of 30 minutes

SOCIAL INTERACTIONS

- Recognition of the possibility of midlife crisis; need for discussion of feelings, concerns, depression, and fears
- Time to expand and review previous interests
- Retirement planning (financial and possible diversional activities), with partner, if appropriate

people are known to be healthier people. Depression increases the risk of cardiovascular disease 1.5 to 2 times, while a positive affect can decrease the risks of disease onset (Davidson, Mostofsky, & Whang, 2010; Pitt & Deldin, 2010).

Assessment guidelines for the growth and development of the middle-aged adult are shown in the Assessment: Developmental Guidelines box on the previous page. The nurse can choose to discuss some or all of the health-promotion topics outlined in the Health-Promotion Guidelines box for Middle-Aged Adults.

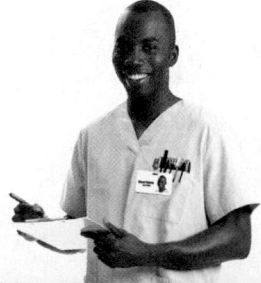

Case Study 19

Mark Jones, a 22-year-old construction worker, comes into the health centre for a "physical." He states that the last time he saw a health care provider was during high school, and he is only here today because his employer required that he be examined prior to returning to work. Mr. Jones has been off the job for two weeks following an accident in which he had fallen off a ladder, sustaining multiple contusions and a concussion. He mentions that he and "his buddies" have enjoyed his two weeks off from work and have used the time to "drink beer and chase women."

CRITICAL THINKING QUESTIONS

1. What questions would you ask Mr. Jones about his usual health-promotion activities?
2. How would you ask Mr. Jones about his risk for sexually transmitted infections?
3. What health conditions are young adults at risk for, and how would you explain these to Mr. Jones?
4. What health screening activities would you suggest to Mr. Jones? How would you explain the rationale to him?

5. How would you assess Mr. Jones's psychosocial development?

Check the eText in MyNursingLab for answers and explanations.

KEY TERMS

baby boomers *p. 369*   generativity *p. 375*   menopause *p. 375*   sandwich generation
boomerang kids *p. 369*   intimacy *p. 370*   Pap (Papanicolaou)   *p. 376*
climacteric *p. 375*   intimate partner violence   test *p. 373*   stagnation *p. 376*
Generation X *p. 369*   (IPV) *p. 371*   postformal thought   sustainable happiness
Generation Y *p. 369*   maturity *p. 374*   *p. 370*   *p. 377*

CHAPTER HIGHLIGHTS

- Distinct characteristics are associated with the three generations which comprise adulthood: baby boomers, Generation Xers, and Generation Yers.
- Physical growth and development peaks in the mid-20s.
- Emerging and young adults develop a self-identity and prepare for intimate relationships with others.
- Moral development continues throughout adulthood.
- Spirituality may be important to young adults but is considered a private matter.
- Health problems for young adults are primarily related to lifestyle and behaviour.
- Middle-aged adults begin to notice physical changes associated with aging.

- The developmental choice for middle-aged adults is generativity versus stagnation.
- Adults in midlife must balance the needs of many, including their own parents and children.
- Health decisions made by middle-aged adults may affect their health in later life.
- Health risks, including cancer and heart disease, become a real threat to individuals categorized as middle-aged. Physical activity, healthy nutrition choices, and routine care by a health care provider are important throughout the adult years.
- The concept of sustainable happiness and its positive effects are related to health outcomes.

ASSESS YOUR LEARNING

1. Mrs. Kelly, 52 years old, is experiencing symptoms of menopause, including frequent hot flashes and insomnia. She states that she exercises daily, meditates, and has consulted a naturopath. She asks the nurse what else she could do to handle these life changes. How should the nurse respond?

   a. Refer Mrs. Kelly for a medical checkup
   b. Advise Mrs. Kelly to take estrogen
   c. Ask Mrs. Kelly to keep an exercise diary
   d. Encourage Mrs. Kelly to continue what she has been doing

2. The adult children of a couple have just helped them celebrate retirement after 35 years of employment. The parents are not concerned and seem ready to make the changes necessary, but their children are worried. To help this family adapt to the parents' retirement, you must understand which of the following?

   a. Young adults are concerned about future caregiver roles in relation to their parents' ages.
   b. Seniors become worried about their health status, ability to travel, and cognitive ability.
   c. Middle-aged adults can adjust to altered schedules, roles, physical strength, and economic changes.
   d. Retired persons focus on themselves, avoiding relationships with peers of bygone days.

3. You are the occupational health nurse (OHN) in a large manufacturing company in Eastern

Canada. You promote health and injury and illness prevention with many employees through the year. Given your mandate, you would be most concerned about which of the following issues for the middle-aged cohort in your workplace?

   a. The promotion of workplace safety
   b. Productivity deadlines
   c. Workplace benefits, including vacations
   d. Work contract performance

4. As a parish nurse, you have the opportunity to provide nursing outreach to many individuals from a variety of cultures and from across all age groups. You are struck by the common traits you are seeing in the healthy and contented adults. What stage of development describes this group?

   a. Trust versus mistrust
   b. Industry versus guilt
   c. Autonomy versus dependence
   d. Generativity versus stagnation

5. Mrs. T. has come to the clinic with her husband for a checkup. She has shared with the nurse that she is afraid her husband may not be able to drive anymore. She became worried the previous week when he did not come home from curling at the usual time. Since then, on two subsequent outings by himself, he was brought home by a good Samaritan. As a nurse in the clinic, taking the

history of Mr. and Mrs. T., what would be your next steps?

  a. Ask Mr. T. if he and Mrs. T. have had a fight recently.

  b. Ask Mr. T. about any headaches, visual problems, or unusual symptoms.

  c. Ask each, separately, about what they did in the past 10 days.

  d. Listen to each person's story, take blood pressures for both, and ask about time, date, persons, and places.

6. The community health nurse at the Halifax Metro Family Wellness Centre has been asked to create a weekly Wellness Program for Working Mothers. Based on the needs of working mothers, which of the following would be the best focus for the program?

  a. Health problems of aging

  b. Immunizations and smoking cessation

  c. Personal changes and home safety

  d. Planning for retirement

7. The home health nurse is visiting Mr. P. (56 years old) in his home for a wound dressing to a chronic leg ulcer. The ulcer is related to varicose veins caused by the many hours he was required to stand in his job from which he is now retired after 30 years. He lives alone with his two cats. He complains of having to get up to go to the bathroom several times during the night to urinate, so he still feels tired in the morning. He is 26 kg overweight and eats packaged frozen foods. In addition to updating his history and caring for the wound, the nurse should assess for which of the following?

  a. Personal neglect

  b. Chronic disability criterion

  c. Measures to prevent constipation

  d. Health concerns, individual strengths, and safety risks

8. Integration of developmental transitions experienced by middle-aged adults is necessary for meaningful health teaching. Most relevant topics would include which of the following?

  a. Accepting an aging body, handling dependent parents, and handling departing children

  b. Wear and tear, interpersonal stress, and sleep deprivation as new parents

  c. Education and career preparation, childbearing roles, and increasing free time

  d. Formal operations and the law and order orientation of Havighurst's theory

9. You are a school nurse helping parents to create health learning resources for their teen children. Which of the following subjects would be the BEST choice of mutual interest for both parents and teens?

  a. Sexually transmitted infections

  b. Internet crime

  c. Eating disorders

  d. Rules of the road and drivers' training

10. Motor vehicle safety is an ongoing safety concern. When promoting motor vehicle safety, nurses should suggest which of the following to young adults?

  a. "Use designated drivers, day or night, as needed."

  b. "Text a cell message only while driving on residential streets."

  c. "Just read and do the computer-simulated games in drivers' ed."

  d. "Keep the car clean, waxed, filled up, and environmentally friendly."

Check the eText in MyNursingLab for answers and explanations.

WEBLINKS

Canadian Public Health Agency, Adult Health

http://www.phac-aspc.gc.ca/ah-sa-eng.php

This site provides various topics related to adult health, from chronic diseases and infectious diseases, to health promotion, travel health, and adult health projects.

The Jack Project at Kids Help Phone

http://www.thejackproject.org

The Jack Project at Kids Help Phone is an outreach pilot project that promotes mental health and well-being among Canadian youth aged 15–20 by providing mental health information and support.

The Health and Well-Being of Canadian Youth and Young Adults

http://www.phac-aspc.gc.ca/cphorsphc-respcacsp/2011/cphorsphc-respcacsp-06-eng.php

This website presents a demographic profile and physical and mental health status of youth and young adults, including their health risk behaviours and what determines their well-being.

MyNursingLab

REFERENCES

Abramsky, T., Watts, C. H., Garcia-Moreno, C., Devries, K., Kiss, L., Ellsberg, M., & Heise, L. (2011). What factors are associated with recent intimate partner violence? Findings from the WHO multi-country study on women's health and domestic violence. *BMC Public Health, 11*(1), 109–125. doi:10.1186/1471-2458-11-109

Beckmann Murray, R., Zentner, J., Pangman, V., & Pangman, C. (2008). *Health promotion strategies through the lifespan* (2nd Canadian ed.). Toronto, ON: Pearson Canada.

Brownridge, D. (2010). Intimate partner violence against Aboriginal men in Canada. *Australian & New Zealand Journal of Criminology (Australian Academic Press), 43*(2), 223–237. doi:10.1375/acri.43.2.223

Canadian Cancer Society. (2010). *Early detection and screening for breast cancer.* Retrieved from http://www.cancer.ca/Saskatchewan/Prevention/Get%20screened/Early%20detection%20and%20screening%20for%20breast%20cancer.aspx?sc_lang=en&r=1

Canadian Cancer Society's Steering Committee on Cancer Statistics. (2012). *Canadian Cancer Statistics 2012.* Toronto, ON: Canadian Cancer Society.

Canadian Mental Health Association. (2012). *Education and mental health.* Retrieved from http://www.cmha.ca/bins/content_page.asp?cid=3-110

Canadian Task Force on Preventive Health Care. (2011). Screening for breast cancer: Summary of recommendations for clinicians and policy-makers. Retrieved from http://www.canadiantaskforce.ca/recommendations/2011_01_eng.html

Chassin, L., Macy, J. T., Seo, D., Presson, C. C., & Sherman, S. J. (2010). The association between membership in the sandwich generation and health behaviors: A longitudinal study. *Journal of Applied Developmental Psychology, 31*(1), 38–46. doi:10.1016/j.appdev.2009.06.001

Davidson, K., Mostofsky, E., & Whang, W. (2010). Don't worry, be happy: Positive affect and reduced 10-year incident coronary heart disease: The Canadian Nova Scotia Health Survey. *European Heart Journal 31*(9), 1065–1070.

Department of Justice. (2006). *Bill C-38 – The Civil Marriage Act.* Retrieved from http://www.justice.gc.ca/eng/news-nouv/nr-cp/2005/doc_31578.htmlEdelman, C. L., & Mandle, C. L. (2010). *Health promotion throughout the life span* (7th ed.). St. Louis, MO: Mosby Elsevier.

Erikson, E. H. (1963). *Childhood and society* (2nd ed.). New York, NY: Norton.

Foster, R., & Hicks, G. (1999). *How we choose to be happy.* New York, NY: Perigree.

Fowler, J. W. (1981). *Stages of faith: The psychology of human development and the quest for meaning.* New York, NY: Harper & Row.

Freud, S. (1923). *The ego and the id.* London, UK: Hogarth Press.

Gilligan, C. (1982). *In a different voice: Psychological theory and women's development.* Cambridge, MA: Harvard University Press.

Hamel, H. (2009). Toward a gender-inclusive conception of intimate partner violence research and theory: Part 2—New directions. *International Journal of Men's Health, 8,* 41–59. doi:10.3149/jmh.0801.41

Havighurst, R. J. (1972). *Developmental tasks and education* (3rd ed.). New York, NY: Longman.

Health Canada. (2003). *Injury surveillance in Canada: Current realities and challenges.* Ottawa, ON: Author. Retrieved from http://www.injurypreventionstrategy.ca/downloads/InjurySurveillanceinCanada.pdf

Health Canada. (2006a). *First Nations, Inuit and Aboriginal Health: National native alcohol and drug abuse program.* Retrieved from http://www.hc-sc.gc.ca/fniah-spnia/substan/ads/nnadap-pnlaada-eng.php

Health Canada. (2006b). Healthy living: Screening for cervical cancer. Retrieved from http://www.hc-sc.gc.ca/hl-vs/iyh-vsv/diseases-maladies/cervical-uterus-eng.php

Health Canada. (2010). Healthy living: Human papillomavirus (HPV). Retrieved from http://www.hc-sc.gc.ca/hl-vs/iyh-vsv/diseases-maladies/hpv-vph-eng.php

Kohlberg, L. (1971). *Recent research in moral development.* New York, NY: Holt, Rinehart & Winston.

Kohlberg, L. (1981). *The psychology of moral development: Moral stages and the idea of justice.* San Francisco, CA: Harper & Row.

Large, M., Smith, G., & Nielssen, O. (2009). The epidemiology of homicide followed by suicide: A systematic and quantitative review. *Suicide and Life-Threatening Behavior, 39*(3), 294–306.

Murray, R. B., Zentner, J. P., & Yakimo, R. (2009). *Health promotion strategies through the life span* (8th ed.). Upper Saddle River, NJ: Prentice Hall.

Mustonen, U., Huurre, T., Kiviruusu, O., Haukkala, A., & Aro, H. (2011). Long-term impact of parental divorce on intimate relationship quality in adulthood and the mediating role of psychosocial resources. *Journal of Family Psychology, 25*(4), 615–619. doi:10.1037/a0023996

O'Brien, C. (2011). *What is sustainable happiness?* Retrieved from www.sustainablehappiness.ca

Oswald, R. F., Fonseca, C. A., & Hardesty, J. L. (2010). Lesbian mothers' counseling experiences in the context of intimate partner violence. *Psychology of Women Quarterly, 34*(3), 286–296. doi:10.1111/j.1471-6402.2010.01575.x

Outlaw, M. (2009). No one type of intimate partner abuse: Exploring physical and non-physical abuse among intimate partners. *Journal of Family Violence, 24,* 263–272. doi:10.107/s10896-009-9228-5

Piaget, J. (1966). *Origins of intelligence in children.* New York, NY: Norton.

Pitt, B. & Deldin, P. (2010). Depression and cardiovascular disease: Have a happy day—just smile! *European Heart Journal 31*(9), 1036–1037. doi; 10.1093/eurheart/ehq031

Public Health Agency of Canada. (2010). *Report on sexually transmitted infections in Canada: 2008. Chlamydia (Chlamydia trachomatis).* Retrieved from http://www.phac-aspc.gc.ca/std-mts/report/sti-its2008/03-eng.php#Fig1

Salm, T., Sevigny, P., Mulholland, V., & Greenberg, H. (2011). Prevalence and pedagogy: Understanding substance abuse in schools. *Journal of Alcohol and Drug Education, 55*(1), 70–93.

Statistics Canada. (2011, March 2). Canadian health measures survey: Adult obesity prevalence in Canada and the United States . *The Daily.* Retrieved from http://www.statcan.gc.ca/daily-quotidien/110302/dq110302c-eng.htm

Statistics Canada. (2012). *2011 Census of Population: Families, households, marital status, structural type of dwelling, collectives.* Retrieved from http://www.statcan.gc.ca/daily-quotidien/120919/dq120919a-eng.htm

Sudheimer, E. E. (2009). Appreciating both sides of the generation gap: Baby boomer and Generation X nurses working together. *Nursing Forum, 44,* 57–63. doi:10.1111/j.1744-6198.2009.00127.x

Wigman, S. A. (2009). Male victims of former-intimate stalking: A selected review. *International Journal of Men's Health, 8*(2), 101–115. doi:10.3149/jmh.0802.101

Chapter 20

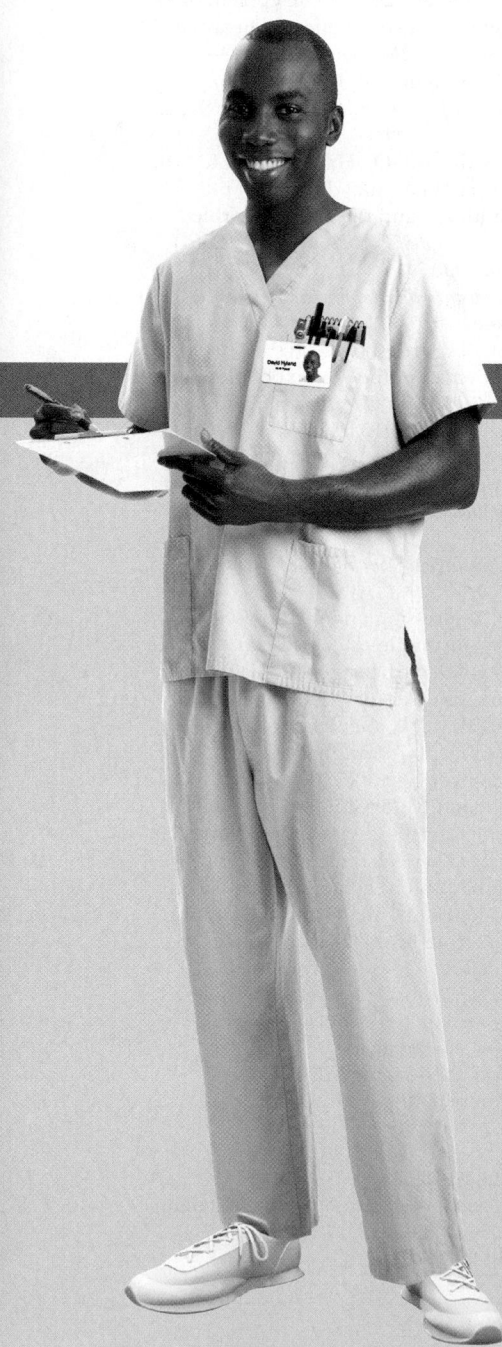

Older Adults

After studying this chapter, you will be able to:

1. Describe the demographic characteristics and the social determinants of health of older adults in Canada.

2. Describe ageism and its contribution to the development of negative stereotypes about older adults.

3. Describe the development of gerontological nursing and the roles of gerontological nurses in Canada.

4. Describe the different care settings for older adults.

5. Explain the common biological theories of aging and related developmental tasks of the older adult.

6. Describe cognitive, physical, and psychosocial changes to which the older adult adjusts.

7. Compare and contrast Kohlberg's and Gilligan's theories of moral reasoning in older adults.

8. Discuss selected health problems associated with older adults.

9. Discuss the role of the nurse in promoting the health and well-being of older adults.

Older adults are the fastest growing segment in the world. The population of people age 65 years and older is projected to triple from 516 million in 2009 to 1.53 billion in 2050 (World Health Organization [WHO], 2012). In Canada, the number of seniors or older adults is expected to reach 10 million by 2036, more than double the 4.7 million in 2009. If this occurs, the number of older adults will surpass the number of children for the first time in Canadian history (Statistics Canada, 2010a).

Characteristics of Older Adults in Canada

Older adults represent an increasingly diverse Canadian population. At one time, all individuals over the age of 65 years were considered old. With advancements in disease control and health technology, the life expectancies of Canadians continue to increase. In 2009, there were roughly 1.3 million people aged 80 years or over. By the year 2036, this number is projected to triple, with 25% of the Canadian population being 65 years and older. In Canada, women outnumber men because of longer life expectancies. About one-third of older women are widowed (Government of Canada, 2010).

Because the chronological age of older adults can span 40 years or more, some authors have expanded the older adult category from one to four, with each having a distinct set of interests and health care needs (Box 20.1). It is important to note that *functional age* is often more useful than chronological age or categorized age groups. **Functional age** refers to the individuals' functional fitness level when compared with others of the same gender and of similar chronological, physiological, mental, and emotional ages (*Mosby's Medical Dictionary*, 2009).

The term **baby boomer** is used to describe a person born between 1946 and 1964. Between these years, there was a large increase in Canadian birthrates. Although not all Canadians report healthy aging, many are entering their senior years with better education, higher household incomes, and very active lifestyles compared with previous generations of seniors. The term "**zoomers**," coined by Demko (1998), refers to older adults who tend to be informed consumers of health care. In fact, seniors

are the fastest growing age group using the Internet (Madden, 2010). Researchers have found that Internet use by older adults can result in enhancements to self-esteem, perceived productivity and accomplishment, social interaction, and mental stimulation (Mauk, 2010) (see Figure 20.1).

Chronic disease and disability increases with age; however, disease is *not* a normal outcome of aging. In fact, aging Canadians report their health as excellent or very good (Touhy, Jett, Boscart, & McCleary, 2011). Nurses need to be aware that promoting health continues to be important for older adults, regardless of chronological age.

Frailty is also not a normal outcome of aging. **Frailty** is a general decline in an older adult's physical functioning that can result in increased vulnerability to illness and disability. The term, *frailty*, is often misinterpreted by health care providers. The most accepted definition classifies someone as "frail" if he or she has three or more of the following: muscle weakness, slow walking speed,

BOX 20.1 CATEGORIZING THE AGING POPULATION	
Young-old	60 to 74 years
Old	75 to 84 years
Old-old	85 to 100 years
Centenarians	Over 100 years

Source: From Eliopoulos, C. (2010). *Gerontological nursing* (7th ed.). Philadelphia, PA: Lippincott Williams & Wilkins.

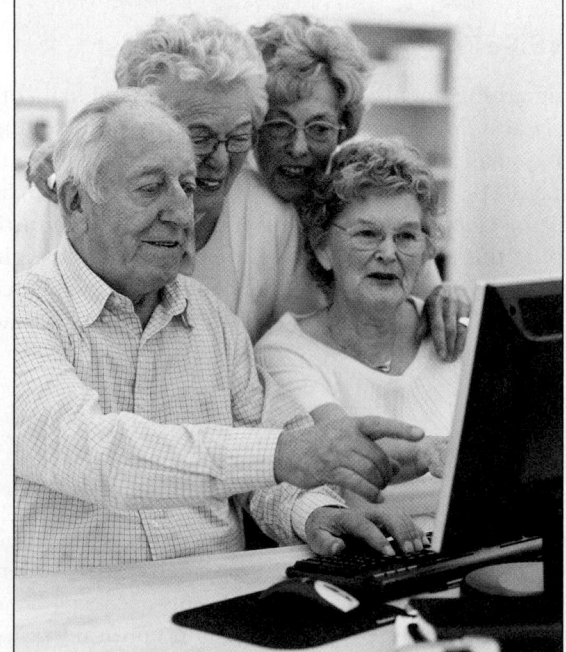

FIGURE 20.1 Older adults are the fastest growing group of computer users.

exhaustion, low physical activity levels, or unintentional weight loss (Woods et al., 2005).

The characteristics of these older adults can be better understood by examining several determinants of health, including socioeconomic status, education, physical environment, culture, and ethnicity.

Socioeconomic Status

Socioeconomic characteristics, such as gender, marital status, education, income, and living arrangements, vary among older adults. Overall, today's seniors are financially secure (Government of Canada, 2008). Older adults who are at highest risk of low income are those who are unattached (living alone, widowed, or never married), those who have worked less than 10 years, new immigrants, and Aboriginal peoples. Although more women now work outside the home, they are still more likely than men to work part time or interrupt employment for caregiving responsibilities.

Education

Educational level can affect the socioeconomic status of the older adult. Generally, higher education is associated with higher income, stronger literacy skills, and better overall health. The number of older adults with completed high school diplomas is gradually increasing. Despite increasing educational levels, many Canadian seniors have literacy skills below the desired threshold for coping well in a complex society.

Physical Environment

Living arrangements of older adults are linked to income and health. Most live in a variety of community settings, with a small minority living in nursing homes (Touhy et al., 2011). Nationally, there is increasing support for *aging in place* initiatives. Senior-friendly communities support the accessibility needs of those with changing physical abilities and provide opportunities for enhanced social interaction (Public Health Agency of Canada [PHAC], 2009).

Culture and Ethnicity

The Canadian population continues to be increasingly diverse. Currently, Asian Canadians comprise the largest ethnic group in Canada (Statistics Canada, 2010a). Some ethnic older adults experience difficulty accessing health care services because of language and cultural barriers, inadequate knowledge of resources, and lack of culturally competent care. Older adults who are newer immigrants

are more likely to suffer from low income. This is because recent arrivals have fewer years to accumulate wealth through home ownership and savings; many may not qualify for government pensions. (See Chapter 11.)

In Canada, Aboriginal older adults are divided into three groups: (a) First Nations, (b) Inuit, and (c) Metis. When compared with the overall Canadian population, Aboriginal older adults tend to have lower income, increased rates of chronic disease, lower educational levels, and shorter life expectancies (Statistics Canada, 2010b). Although the life expectancy of Aboriginals is slowly increasing, it remains lower than other Canadians. The Inuit population has the lowest life expectancy. Lack of quality, affordable housing is a significant challenge to Aboriginal seniors (Special Senate Committee on Aging [SSCA], 2009). Literacy and cultural identity should be considered when working with these older adults. (See Chapter 15.)

Attitudes toward Aging

The Western world values youth. The term **ageism** describes negative societal attitudes toward aging or older adults (Butler, 1963). Unfortunately, these attitudes exist even among some health care professionals (Phelan, 2008). These ideas can be influenced by cultural and societal expectations, family, colleagues, and work experiences, and they can contribute to negative stereotypes about older adults.

Stereotyping can occur when people do not understand or identify with older adults as unique human beings. Instead, undesirable characteristics (e.g., senile, old-fashioned) are generalized to all older adults. Negative attitudes about aging are often based on incorrect information (Table 20.1). It is essential that nurses develop awareness of their own values and attitudes toward aging and examine whether myths or stereotypes influence those attitudes. It is also important for nurses to provide accurate information about aging to reduce stereotypes about aging.

Gerontological Nursing in Canada

Older adults are unique individuals who may require a variety of health care professionals to meet their health care needs. **Gerontology** is a term used to define the study of aging and older adults. Gerontology is multidisciplinary and is a specialized area within such disciplines as nursing, psychology, and social work. **Geriatrics** is associated with the medical care (e.g., diseases and disabilities) of older adults.

TABLE 20.1 Myths and Realities of Aging

Myth	Reality
People consider themselves to be old at 65 years.	People feel old on the basis of their health and functional ability, rather than their chronological age.
In old age, there is an inevitable decline in all intellectual abilities.	A few areas of cognitive ability decline in older adulthood, but others may improve.
Older adults cannot learn complex new skills.	Older adults are capable of learning new things, but the speed with which information is processed slows with age.
Older people have decreased levels of sexual activity because they are less able to perform sexually.	If sexual activity in older people declines, it is because of social reasons or other factors, such as disease and medication effects.
Most older people are depressed and should be allowed to withdraw from society.	Although many older people exhibit depression, particularly with chronic disease, it is a treatable condition at any age.

Source: From Miller, C.A. (2012). *Nursing for wellness in older adults* (6th ed.). Copyright © Lippincott, Williams & Wilkins.. Reprinted with permission.

Gerontological nursing is a separate branch of professional nursing practice. It involves advocating for the health of older persons at all levels of prevention. Although the first North American gerontological nursing textbook was published in 1950, it took more than a decade before gerontological nursing was officially recognized as a specialty. In the 1980s, nursing leaders recognized that practising nurses had insufficient knowledge about gerontology. This prompted the need to prepare all nurses in basic gerontological practice.

In 1985, the Canadian Gerontological Nursing Association was formed. The Hartford Institute for Geriatric Nursing (2011) was later established at New York University in 1996. In Canada, gerontological nursing certification is available through the Canadian Nurses Association (CNA). The National Institute for the Care of the Elderly (NICE) is a champion for improving evidence-based gerontological health care in Canada.

Care Settings for Older Adults

Any nurse who works with older adults might be called a *gerontological nurse*. Gerontological nurses practise in many settings and have many roles: provider of care, teacher, manager, and advocate. Regardless of the setting, nurses can assess and promote the health of older adults.

Acute Care Facilities

Older adults represent the majority of clients cared for in acute care. They use emergency departments at a higher rate than other age groups and are most likely to be admitted to the hospital (Canadian Institute for

Health Information [CIHI], 2010). Nurses in acute care settings focus on protecting the health of older adults, with the goal of returning them to their prior level of independence.

Long-Term Care Facilities

In Canada, long-term care is not publicly insured under the Canada Health Act; it is governed by provincial and territorial legislation. Therefore, there is great variation in the range of services and costs across the country (Health Canada, 2004). Levels of care may include assisted living, long-term care, and chronic continuing care.

Older adults who do not feel safe living alone or require additional help with activities of daily living (ADLs) may desire to reside in *assisted living* facilities. Also known as *retirement settings*, these facilities meet the functional, safety, and socialization needs of older persons. *Long-term care* clients are those who can no longer live independently and require 24-hour direct nursing contact. Many long-term care facilities offer specialized units for clients with dementia. Gerontological nurses working in these units have expertise in family-centred dementia care. *Complex continuing care units* are designed to provide for the needs of clients whose acuity levels require a higher level of nursing care. Specialized care may include tube feedings, intravenous therapy, and mechanical ventilation.

Hospice

Gerontological nurses may also care for older dying persons and their families. These nurses must possess specialized end-of-life knowledge, expert clinical skills, and compassion.

Rehabilitation

Gerontological rehabilitation nursing combines expertise in gerontological nursing with rehabilitation practice. Working as a member of a team, gerontological nurses often care for older adults with functional limitations (e.g., orthopedic surgery, stroke, or amputation).

Community

Gerontological nurses provide nursing care in many types of community settings. Community practice areas may include home health care, adult daycare programs, and primary health care clinics.

Theories of Aging

There are many different theories of aging proposed by scientists in the biological, psychological, and social disciplines. Biological theories of aging are either intrinsic

or extrinsic. *Intrinsic* theory addresses factors within the body; *extrinsic* theory encompasses factors in the environment. Table 20.2 describes the various biological theories of aging.

Physiological Aging

Although people age differently, many changes occur in almost everyone and are considered normal. A more accurate description of these changes is *usual. Usual aging* refers to what happens to most people, including disorders that are common in the aging process. Usual aging does not mean that the changes are unavoidable or desirable. Unfortunately, it is often difficult to determine usual aging when the majority of older Canadians have one or more chronic health conditions (PHAC, 2009).

As a person ages, many physical changes occur; some are visible, and some are not. Table 20.3 provides a summary of the normal physical changes associated with aging.

TABLE 20.2 Common Biological Theories of Aging

Theory Type	Hypotheses
Wear-and-tear theories	• Humans, like automobiles, have vital parts that run down with time, leading to aging and death. • The faster an organism lives, the quicker it dies. • Cells wear out through exposure to internal and external stressors, including trauma, chemicals, and buildup of natural wastes.
Endocrine theory	• Events occurring in the hypothalamus and pituitary are responsible for changes in hormone production and response that result in the organism's decline.
Free radical theory	• Unstable free radicals (groups of atoms) result from the oxidation of organic materials, such as carbohydrates and proteins; these radicals cause biochemical changes in the cells, preventing cellular regeneration.
Genetic theories	• The organism is genetically programmed for a predetermined number of cell divisions, after which the cells/organism dies. • When damage to the protein synthesis occurs, faulty proteins will be synthesized and will gradually accumulate, causing a progressive decline in the organism.
Cross-linking theories	• The irreversible aging of proteins, such as collagen, is responsible for the ultimate failure of tissues and organs. • As cells age, chemical reactions create strong bonds, or cross-linkages, between proteins; these bonds cause loss of elasticity, stiffness, and eventual loss of function.
Immune theories	• The immune system becomes less effective with age, resulting in reduced resistance to infectious disease. • A decrease in immune function may result in an increase in autoimmune responses, causing the body to produce antibodies that attack the body itself.

TABLE 20.3   Normal Physical Changes Associated with Aging

Physical Changes	Rationale
Integumentary	
Increased skin dryness	Decreased sebaceous gland activity and tissue fluid
Increased skin pallor	Decreased vascularity
Increased skin fragility	Reduced thickness and vascularity of the dermis; loss of subcutaneous fat
Progressive wrinkling and sagging of skin	Loss of skin elasticity, increased dryness, and decreased subcutaneous fat
Lentigo senilis (brown age spots) on exposed body parts (e.g., face, hands, arms)	Clustering of melanocytes (pigment-producing cells)
Decreased perspiration	Reduced number and function of sweat glands
Thinning and greying of scalp, pubic, and axillary hairs	Progressive loss of pigment cells from the hair bulbs
Slower nail growth and increased thickening with ridges	Increased calcium deposition
Neuromuscular	
Decreased speed and power of skeletal muscle contractions	Decrease in muscle fibres
Slowed reaction time	Diminished conduction speed of nerve fibres and decreased muscle tone
Loss of height (stature)	Atrophy of intervertebral discs, increased flexion at hips and knees
Loss of bone mass	Bone reabsorption outpaces bone reformation
Joint stiffness	Drying and loss of elasticity in joint cartilage
Impaired balance	Decreased muscle strength, reaction time, and coordination, change in centre of gravity
Greater difficulty in complex learning and abstraction	Fewer cells in cerebral cortex
Sensory and Perceptual	
Loss of visual acuity	Degeneration leading to lens opacity (cataracts), thickening, and inelasticity (presbyopia)
Increased sensitivity to glare and decreased ability to adjust to darkness	Changes in the ciliary muscles; rigid pupil sphincter; decrease in pupil size
Arcus senilis (partial or complete glossy white circle around the periphery of the cornea)	Fatty deposits
Presbycusis (progressive loss of hearing)	Changes in the structures and nerve tissues in the inner ear; thickening of the eardrum
Decreased sense of taste, especially the sweet sensations at the tip of the tongue	Decreased number of taste buds in the tongue because of tongue atrophy
Decreased sense of smell	Atrophy of the olfactory bulb at the base of the brain (responsible for smell perception)
Increased threshold for sensations of pain, touch, and temperature	Possible nerve conduction and neuron changes

(continued)

TABLE 20.3 Normal Physical Changes Associated with Aging *(continued)*

Physical Changes	Rationale
Pulmonary	
Decreased ability to expel foreign or accumulated matter	Decreased elasticity and ciliary activity
Decreased lung expansion, less effective exhalation, reduced vital capacity, and increased residual volume	Weakened thoracic muscles; calcification of costal cartilage, making the rib cage more rigid with increased anteroposterior diameter; dilation from inelasticity of alveoli
Dyspnea (difficulty breathing) following intense exercise	Diminished delivery and diffusion of oxygen to the tissues to repay the normal oxygen debt because of exertion or changes in both respiratory and vascular tissues
Cardiovascular	
Reduced cardiac output and stroke volume, particularly during increased activity or unusual demands; may result in shortness of breath on exertion and pooling of blood in the extremities	Increased rigidity and thickness of heart valves (hence decreased filling and emptying abilities); decreased contractile strength
Reduced elasticity and increased rigidity of arteries	Increased calcium deposits in the muscular layer
Increase in diastolic and systolic blood pressure	Inelasticity of systemic arteries and increased peripheral resistance
Orthostatic hypotension	Reduced sensitivity of the blood pressure–regulating baroreceptors
Gastrointestinal	
Delayed swallowing time	Alterations in the swallowing mechanism
Increased tendency for indigestion	Gradual decrease in digestive enzymes, reduction in gastric pH, and slower absorption rate
Increased tendency for constipation	Decreased muscle tone of the intestines; decreased peristalsis; decreased free body fluid
Urinary	
Reduced filtering ability of the kidney and impaired renal function	Decreased number of functioning nephrons (basic functional units of the kidney) and arteriosclerotic changes in blood flow
Less effective concentration of urine	Decreased tubular function
Urinary urgency and urinary frequency	Enlarged prostate gland in men; weakened muscles supporting the bladder or weakness of the urinary sphincter in women
Tendency for nocturnal frequency and retention of residual urine	Decreased bladder capacity and tone
Genitals and Reproduction	
Prostate enlargement (benign) in men	Exact mechanism is unclear; possible endocrine changes
Multiple changes in women (shrinkage and atrophy of the vulva, cervix, uterus, fallopian tubes, and ovaries; reduction in secretions; and changes in vaginal flora)	Diminished secretion of female hormones and more alkaline vaginal pH
Increased time to sexual arousal	Changes in blood supply to penis, clitoris

TABLE 20.3 Normal Physical Changes Associated with Aging *(continued)*

Physical Changes	Rationale
Decreased firmness of erection, increased refractory period (men)	Changes in blood supply
Decreased vaginal lubrication and elasticity (women)	Loss of estrogen effects
Immunological	
Decreased immune response; lowered resistance to infections	T cells less responsive to antigens; B cells produce fewer antibodies
Poor response to immunization	Immune system changes may precipitate insulin resistance
Decreased stress response	Cortisol (a stress hormone) increases with age and can impair the immune system's ability to fight against diseases
Endocrine	
Increased insulin resistance	Immune system changes may precipitate insulin resistance
Decreased thyroid function	Unclear mechanism

Integument

As chronological age increases, the skin becomes drier, less elastic, and more fragile, making the older person more susceptible to skin tears and shearing injuries. The hair loses colour and becomes thinner, the fingernails and toenails become thickened and brittle, and in women over 60 years, facial hair increases.

These integumentary changes accompany progressive losses of subcutaneous fat and muscle tissue, muscle atrophy, and loss of elastic fibre. This results in a double chin, sagging of eyelids and earlobes, and wrinkling of skin. Bony prominences become visible. In older women, the breasts become smaller and may sag; if large and pendulous, they may cause chafing where the skin surfaces touch. Loss of subcutaneous fat decreases the older adult's tolerance of the cold.

Health-promotion teaching about skin care for older adults can include information about maintaining healthy skin, avoiding sun damage, and preventing injury to the skin.

Neuromusculoskeletal

With aging comes gradual reduction in the speed and power of skeletal or voluntary muscle contractions and sustained muscular effort. Despite regular exercise, a steady decrease in muscle fibres occurs (**sarcopenia**) after the age of 50 years. Age-related sarcopenia appears to be related to denervation of the muscle. Thus, older adults often report lack of strength and early fatigue. Activities can still be carried out but at a slower pace. Often, balance is impaired with age and is related to a loss of muscle strength. Muscle endurance also diminishes, resulting in muscle fatigue after short periods of exercise.

Reaction time slows with age. As a result of diminished physical activity, it can be further delayed by decreased muscle tone. A slight loss in overall stature occurs with age. This can be exaggerated by muscular weakness, resulting in a stooping posture and **kyphosis**. Imbalance in the rates of absorption and formation of bone tissue also occurs. The result is **osteoporosis**, a pathological decrease in bone density that makes the older adult prone to serious fractures, some of which may be spontaneous (**pathological fractures**). Osteoporosis occurs more frequently in people with insufficient intake of dietary calcium and vitamin D, in postmenopausal women, in Caucasians and Asians, and in individuals who are immobilized or physically inactive. It is important to remember that osteoporosis affects both men and women.

Joints and their supporting structures change with age. Decreased elasticity, strength, and hydration of the tendons and ligaments make movement stiffer and more restricted. Stiffness is aggravated by inactivity; for example, if a person sits too long, the joints become stiff, and the person has difficulty initiating activity (see Figure 20.2 on the next page).

As indicated, these age-related changes may affect the mobility and safety of the older adult. The nurse should identify any risk factors that may contribute to decreased functional ability and falls.

Health-promotion interventions include the following:

- Encouraging adequate intake of calcium and vitamin D
- Promoting physical activity and proper nutrition to slow bone density loss and decrease muscle atrophy
- Suggesting rest pauses and avoidance of peak performance to promote safety and prolonged exercise

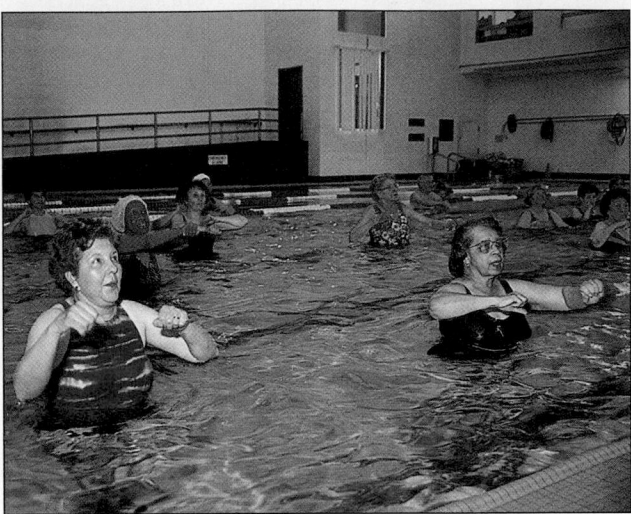

FIGURE 20.2 A regular program of exercise is important for maintenance of joint mobility and muscle tone and can promote socialization.

Sensory and Perceptual

Each of the five senses becomes less efficient in older adulthood. Changes in the eye include a shrunken appearance, a slowed blink reflex, and diminished eyelid muscle tone. Other changes result in loss of visual acuity, less power of adaptation to darkness and dim light, and decrease in accommodation to near and far objects. Loss of peripheral vision, atrophy of lacrimal glands resulting in dry eyes, and difficulty in discriminating similar colours, especially blues, greens, and purples, also occur.

Presbyopia, the inability of the eye to focus or accommodate because of a loss of flexibility of the lens, causes a decrease in near vision. This generally starts around age 40 years. Visual acuity lessens gradually after age 50 years, and more rapidly after age 70 years (Touhy et al., 2011). By the age of 80 years, adults have some lens opacity (**cataracts**) that reduces visual acuity and causes glare to be a problem. Changes in the ciliary muscles reduce the power of the lens to adjust to near and far vision. The pupil's diameter is reduced, and the amount of light entering the eye is thereby restricted. This slows the reaction time to decreases in light, a problem compounded with night driving. Other diseases of the eye that can result in visual impairment and blindness include age-related macular degeneration, glaucoma, and diabetic retinopathy.

Age-related hearing loss, called **presbycusis**, affects people over age 65 years. Gradual loss of hearing is more common among men than among women. Hearing loss is greater in the higher frequencies than the lower frequencies. Thus, older adults with hearing loss usually hear speakers with low, distinct voices best. Hard consonants (e.g., *k, d, t*) and long vowel sounds (e.g. *ay, ee*) are more easily recognized. Sibilant sounds (e.g. *s, th, f*) are the most difficult to hear. If communication problems or social withdrawal is noted, the nurse should suggest a referral for hearing screening. Ears should also be checked for impacted earwax. If hearing has diminished, assistive listening devices are available.

The taste and smell senses are often reduced with aging. These changes significantly affect appetite, contributing to poor nutrition. Decreased or absent sense of smell and taste can also lead to nutrition and safety issues, such as being unable to smell a gas leak. It is important for the nurse to teach the older client with alterations in taste and smell about health and safety strategies (e.g., no added salt, using smoke and carbon monoxide alarms).

Loss of skin receptors takes place gradually, producing an increased threshold for sensations of pain, touch, and temperature. The older person may not be able to distinguish hot from cold, or sense the intensity of heat. This places the older adult at higher risk for burns and other injuries. Again, it is important for the nurse to teach about safety risks and subsequent interventions. For example, water heaters should be set to no more than 49°C to prevent scalding (PHAC, 2009).

Pulmonary

Respiratory efficiency is reduced with age. The respiratory muscles weaken and the chest wall becomes less compliant. The muscles used in breathing also tend to weaken. Tidal volume (the measurement of air moved in and out during normal respiration) remains the same; however, the older adult has a decreased vital capacity. This means the older adult inhales a smaller volume of air and is unable to compensate for increased oxygen need by significantly increasing the amount of air inspired.

Dyspnea (difficulty breathing) occurs frequently with physically demanding activities, such as carrying heavy items upstairs. A greater volume of residual air is left in the lungs after expiration, and the capacity to cough efficiently decreases because of weaker expiratory muscles. Mucous secretions tend to collect more readily in the respiratory tree, increasing the risk of respiratory infection.

Older adults are at great risk of influenza infections and many die as a result of complications. Evidence showed that influenza vaccination could prevent influenza-related illness by 20–40% and influenza-related death by 80% (Thomas, Jefferson, & Lasserson, 2010). Health-promotion teaching includes information about the following:

- Cessation of smoking
- Hand hygiene to prevent respiratory infections
- Influenza and pneumonia vaccinations

Cardiovascular

The working capacity of the heart diminishes with age. This is particularly evident when increased demands are made on the heart muscles, such as during exercise or emotional stress. The resting heart rate does not change with age; however, the heart rate can be slow to respond to stress and slow to return to normal after periods of physical activity.

Changes in the arteries occur concurrently. Reduced arterial elasticity may result in diminished blood circulation to such areas as the legs, resulting in calf muscle pain on exertion (**claudication**). In addition, there may be a delay in the circulatory adjustments required when a person stands up from a lying or sitting position. The delay results in an abrupt drop in systolic blood pressure known as **orthostatic hypotension**.

Systolic hypertension was previously considered "normal" in older adults. A target blood pressure of less than 140/90 mm Hg is now recommended, with a further reduction of less than 130/80 mm Hg for people with diabetes or chronic kidney disease (Campbell, Grover, Hill, & Padwal, 2011).

Health-promotion activities are aimed at detecting and reducing risks for cardiovascular disease. The nurse should inform the older adult about the importance of smoking cessation, maintaining a healthy body weight, exercising daily, reducing sodium and fat intake, and consuming a diet rich in fruits and vegetables.

Gastrointestinal

Age-related changes in the gastrointestinal system are summarized below:

- Periodontal disease, which can lead to tooth loss, which, in turn, affects proper diet intake
- Reduced production of saliva, which may lead to **xerostomia** (dry mouth), making the oral mucosa more susceptible to infection
- Decreased esophageal and gastric motility and emptying time including liver and pancreas functions
- Gradual decrease in digestive enzymes and intrinsic factor (protein needed to make vitamin B_{12})
- Decreased intestinal absorption, motility, and blood flow

Health-promotion teaching for the gastrointestinal health of older adults includes food safety, effective oral hygiene, and regular preventive dental care. Nutrition is also important, including healthy diet and sufficient fluid intake. Maintenance of a regular bowel routine and screening for colorectal cancer is vital.

Urinary

The excretory function of the kidney diminishes with age, but usually not significantly below normal levels. The kidney's filtering abilities may also be impaired; thus, waste products may be excreted more slowly. Drugs that are metabolized predominantly in the kidney may accumulate in the older adult, and the nurse should watch for signs of toxicity.

The capacity of the bladder, and its ability to completely empty, noticeably diminish with age. Many older adults need to get up during the night to void (**nocturia**), and may experience retention of urine, predisposing them to bladder infections. Although older adults are susceptible to urinary incontinence (UI), UI is *never* normal, and it can contribute to falls (caused by rushing to the washroom), skin breakdown in the genital area (due to constant irritation by leaking urine), and social isolation (due to the embarrassing problem).

As the thirst mechanism in aging adults is diminished, the nurse should encourage regular fluid intake. The nurse can also teach pelvic muscle exercises to control stress incontinence.

Genitals and Reproduction

Degenerative changes in the gonads (reproductive glands that produce germ cells) are gradual in men. Production of testosterone and sperm continues well into old age, although sperm production gradually decreases. Older men will notice several age-related changes in their sexual response and performance. In general, the older man's libido may decrease but does not disappear.

Older men achieve an erection that is less firm than in younger men but still capable of penetration. Ejaculation may take longer to occur, and the older man may have difficulty anticipating or delaying ejaculation.

The risk of erectile dysfunction (ED) increases with each decade of age (Tabloski, 2010). ED is the subjective complaint of an inability to achieve or maintain an erection that is satisfactory for the completion of sexual activity (Ellsworth & Kirshenbaum, 2008). There are many possible causes of ED, including atherosclerosis, diabetes, medications, and psychological factors.

In women, the degenerative changes in the ovaries are noticed by the abrupt cessation of menses in middle age. Changes in the gonads of older women result from diminished secretion of the ovarian hormones. Some changes, such as the shrinking of the uterus and ovaries, go unnoticed. Other changes are obvious. The breasts atrophy, and lubricating vaginal secretions are reduced.

Older women also experience changes in their sexual responses. It takes longer for the woman to become sexually aroused and produce vaginal lubrication, making penetration slightly more difficult and uncomfortable (Wallace, 2008). During orgasm, the uterus will contract less frequently, but contractions remain vigorous, and orgasm is as intense as in younger women.

The nurse needs excellent communication skills when providing sexual health education. The process must be open, respectful, and nonjudgmental (Touhy et al., 2011). Older men and women are fully capable of enjoying sexual activity. If they experience problems with sexual function, they should be encouraged to seek advice from their health care provider (see Chapter 46).

Psychosocial Aging

A number of theories explain psychosocial aging. These theories focus on behaviour and attitude changes during the aging process. Developed in the early 1960s, **disengagement theory** proposed that aging involves mutual withdrawal (disengagement) between the older person and others in the older person's environment (Tabloski, 2010). This withdrawal relieves the older person of societal pressures and gradually reduces the number of people with whom the older person interacts. It has been widely criticized for the assumption that disengagement is appropriate for the older adult.

According to Havighurst's **activity theory** (1972), the best way to age is to stay physically and mentally active. **Continuity theory** proposes that people maintain their values, habits, and behaviours in old age. A person who is accustomed to socializing will continue to do so, and the person who prefers not to be involved with others will more likely disengage (Tabloski, 2010).

Erikson (1982) views the developmental task of late adulthood to be integrity versus despair. People who attain ego integrity view life with a sense of wholeness, derive satisfaction from past accomplishments, and accept events, such as death, as part of the life cycle. Acknowledging that the "young-old" and the "old-old" differ in both physical characteristics and psychosocial responses, many people have difficulty with Erikson's singular developmental task. Peck (1968) proposes three developmental tasks of the older adult:

1. Ego differentiation versus work-role preoccupation
2. Body transcendence versus body preoccupation
3. Ego transcendence versus ego preoccupation

For details about these tasks, see Chapter 17. See Box 20.2 for the developmental tasks of the older adult.

Retirement

Retirement is a period of adjustment for most older adults. Although retirement is a challenging transition for many older adults, people who live well-balanced and fulfilling lives may adjust more easily. In fact, some continue to work on a full-time or part-time basis; working can provide a sense of self-worth and continued income. Retirement can also be a time when recreational activities can be pursued. Older adults find outlets in travelling, volunteering, physical fitness, intellectual pursuits, and hobbies (Figure 20.3).

Economic Change

The financial needs of older adults vary considerably. Although many older adults are mortgage-free and require less money for living expenses, rising costs can make it difficult for some to manage. Food and medical

---

BOX 20.2   DEVELOPMENTAL TASKS OF THE OLDER ADULT

65 TO 75 YEARS

- Adjusting to decreasing physical strength and health
- Adjusting to retirement and lower and fixed income
- Adjusting to the death of parents, spouses, and friends
- Adjusting to new relationships with adult children
- Adjusting to leisure time
- Adjusting to slower physical and cognitive responses
- Keeping active and involved
- Making satisfying living arrangements as aging progresses

75 YEARS AND OLDER

- Adapting to living alone
- Safeguarding physical and mental health
- Adjusting to the possibility of moving into a nursing home
- Remaining in touch with other family members
- Finding meaning in life
- Adjusting to the prospect of one's own death

Source: From Murray, R. B., Zentner, J. P., & Yakimo, R. (2008). *Health promotion strategies through the life span* (8th ed.). Upper Saddle River, NJ: Pearson Education, Inc. © 2008. Printed and electronically reproduced by permission of Pearson Education, Inc., Upper Saddle River, New Jersey.

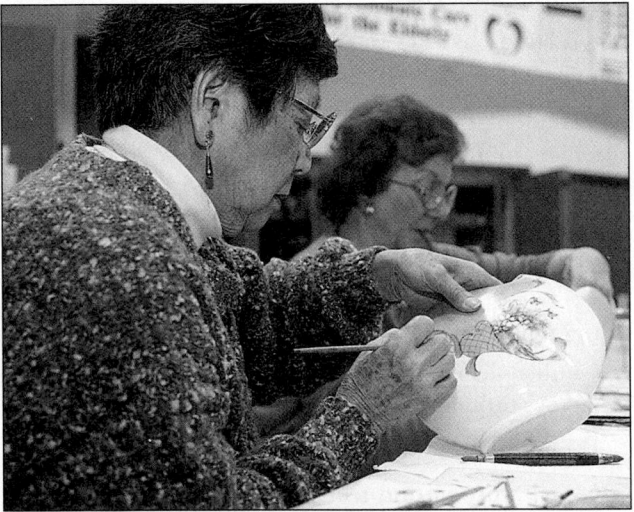

FIGURE 20.3 Many older adults find creative outlets during retirement.

---

costs are a significant financial burden for older adults (Government of Canada, 2009). Challenges are often related to low retirement benefits, lack of pension and health insurance plans, and the increased length of the retirement years. Older women and senior members of minority groups often experience financial difficulty (Touhy et al., 2011). In Canada, the oldest women tend to be the poorest.

Nurses should be aware of health care costs. For example, supplies used in an older adult's care should be as economical as possible. The nurse should also refer the client to social assistance programs that can help with financing health care–related supplies.

Relocation

During late adulthood, a variety of factors can lead to the decision to relocate. The house may be too large, too expensive, or inaccessible. The ongoing maintenance may become burdensome. Some older adults move nearer to their children for support; others may seek a more moderate climate geared to an active lifestyle.

Unfortunately, relocation is often stressful for many older adults and their families, especially if the move is not voluntary. The decision to relocate to a long-term care facility is frequently made when older adults can no longer care for themselves because of mobility problems or memory impairment. It is important for nurses to assist in facilitating the older adult's decision making. During transition, the older adult may require professional services, such as nursing and occupational therapy.

Maintaining Independence and Self-Esteem

Most older Canadians thrive on independence. **Aging in place** describes a process that enables older adults to age within the comfort and familiarity of their own homes. It is important that older adults care for themselves, even if this is challenging. To maintain the older adult's sense of self-respect, the nurse and caregivers need to encourage independence and acknowledge the older adult's ability to think, reason, and make decisions. The values and decisions held by older people need to be accepted whether they are related to ethical, religious, or household matters. For example, the nurse should respect an older person's decision to bathe rather than shower.

Some older adults experience discomfort when doing activities they enjoyed in their younger years. Assistive devices can ease the strains of daily activities. They include medical equipment and mobility aids. These devices can help older adults improve their quality of life and maintain their independence.

Social Relationships

Older adults with increased social contacts tend to receive more support and usually demonstrate health-promoting behaviours.

Grandparenting provides a unique opportunity to form special relationships with grandchildren. This role is now changing, and grandparents are increasingly functioning as the primary caregivers for their grandchildren. This is occurring for a variety of reasons, including teen pregnancy, parental mental health issues, and parental death. While grandparenting, older adults can experience stress related to personal health challenges and parental caregiving. Older adults may also feel family pressure to care for their grandchildren. In some cases, external pressure from family members may become a form of emotional abuse (SSCA, 2009). See the section titled "Mistreatment of Older Adults" in this chapter.

Relatively little is known about the social relationships of lesbian, gay, transgender, and bisexual older adults. As rates of HIV infections increase in Canada, many face unique challenges, such as the loss of a partner and social isolation. When these older adults relocate to assisted living facilities, they may encounter stigmatization, even from some health care practitioners.

It is important for nurses to promote the social relationships of all older adults, regardless of care setting. See the Nursing and Canadian Society box.

Facing Death and Grieving

Well-adjusted aging couples usually thrive on each other's companionship. When a mate dies, the partner often experiences loss, emptiness, and loneliness. Many are capable of living alone; however, reliance on family members may increase with advancing age. Older people are often reminded of their own mortality by the death of friends. A person who has successful relationships with family, meaningful friendships, economic security,

 Nursing and Canadian Society

Fact	Implications for Nursing Practice
Most older Canadian adults live independently in the community and desire to remain in their homes (PHAC, 2009). In 2008-09, about 0.7% of the Canadian population lived in an institution; of this, about 75% were 65 years and older (Organization for Economic Co-operation and Development, 2011).	Nurses need to be aware of the resources and community services available to their older clients. "*Aging in place*" interventions can assist older adults to maintain their independence.
Canada has a shortage of health care professionals, including nurses, who specialize in the care of older persons. Numerous Canadian organizations and professional associations actively engage in and disseminate research to better meet the needs of older Canadians (PHAC, 2009).	All nurses need to acquire the requisite knowledge, skills, and expertise to care for the rapidly growing numbers of older adults in Canada—to understand trends that impact health care delivery, plan for evidence-based interventions, and advocate for safe and ethical care.
Although cancer death rate is falling in Canada, cancer incidence and mortality rates continue to be highest among the older adults (Canadian Cancer Society's Steering Committee on Cancer Statistics, 2012).	Nurses are challenged to successfully implement cancer prevention strategies to promote healthy lifestyle changes into the daily lives of older persons (e.g., promoting cancer screening, healthy diet, and active living).

ongoing interests, and a peaceful philosophy of life generally copes more easily with bereavement. See Chapter 49.

It is the role of every nurse to support those who are grieving. There are support programs in many communities that assist older adults to cope with bereavement. Nurses need to be aware of these programs, and refer their clients to appropriate support services.

Cognitive Abilities and Aging

Piaget's phases of cognitive development end with the formal operations phase (1981); however, considerable research on cognitive abilities and aging is currently being conducted. Intellectual capacity includes perception, cognitive agility, memory, and learning.

Perception

Perception, or the ability to interpret the environment, depends on the acuteness of the senses. If the aging person's senses are impaired, the ability to perceive the environment and react appropriately is diminished. Changes in the nervous system can also affect perceptual capacity. Changes in the cognitive structures occur with age: Neurons are progressively lost; blood flow to the brain decreases; the meninges appear to thicken; and brain metabolism slows.

Cognitive Agility

Changes in cognitive abilities are more often a difference in speed than ability. Overall, the older adult maintains problem-solving, judgment, creativity, and other well-practised cognitive skills. Intellectual loss generally reflects a disease process, such as atherosclerosis, which causes the blood vessels to narrow and diminishes perfusion of nutrients to the brain. Most older adults do not experience cognitive impairments. A cognitive impairment that interferes with social or occupational functions is not considered part of normal aging and should always be regarded as abnormal. Prompt medical evaluation is needed. Lifelong mental activities, particularly verbal activity, help the older adult retain a high level of cognitive function.

Memory

Memory is also a component of intellectual capacity that involves the following steps:

1. The first step is momentary perception of stimuli from the environment, referred to as **sensory memory**.

2. The second step involves storage in **short-term memory** (information held in the brain for immediate use or what a person has in mind at a given moment). An example of this type of memory is calling information for a telephone number and remembering the number for only the brief time needed to dial it. Short-term memory that deals with activities or the recent past (minutes to a few hours) is often referred to as **recent memory**.

3. The final stage is encoding, by which information leaves short-term memory and enters **long-term memory**, the repository for information stored for periods longer than 72 hours and usually weeks and years. Memories of childhood friends and events are stored in long-term memory. Older people who remember the names of their childhood pets are drawing from long-term memory.

In older adults, retrieval of information from long-term memory can be slower, especially if the information is not frequently used. Most age-related differences occur in short-term memory. Older adults tend to forget the recent past. This forgetfulness can be improved by the use of memory aids, making lists, and placing objects in consistent locations.

Learning

Older adults need additional time for learning, largely because of difficulty retrieving information. Active participation and motivation are also important. Older adults can have difficulty learning information they do not consider meaningful; therefore, the nurse should discover what is meaningful to the older adult, including their learning needs and experiences, before attempting client education. Refer to Chapter 26 for strategies to enhance learning among seniors.

Moral Development

According to Kohlberg (1984), moral development is completed in the early adult years. Kohlberg hypothesized that an older person at the preconventional level obeys rules to avoid pain and the displeasure of others. At stage 1, a person defines good and bad in relation to self, whereas older people at stage 2 may act to meet another's needs as well as their own. Older adults at the conventional level follow society's rules of conduct in response to the expectations of others.

Gilligan (1982) developed a theory of moral reasoning based on the concept of caring, whereas Kohlberg based his stages on concepts of justice, objectivity, and preservation of rights. She believed that women base moral judgments on connectedness to others and the value of relationships. Research has demonstrated that men and women make moral decisions differently. Older adults make moral decisions that are consistent with *both*

Kohlberg and Gilligan (Pinch & Parsons, 1997). Older men consider relationships as well as justice in moral decisions, and older women add justice to the factors they consider in moral situations.

Factors such as cultural background, life experiences, and religion influence people's values. Therefore, the values and beliefs that are important to older adults may be different than those held by younger people. The nurse must identify and consider the specific values of the older client when nursing care is planned.

Spirituality

Many older adults take their faith and religious practice very seriously, and display a high level of spirituality. It would be a mistake, however, to assume that religiosity increases with age. Today's older adults grew up in a time when religion held greater importance in society than it does today. The participation of older adults in religious organizations, therefore, is more likely a continuation of lifelong habits than a result of aging (Lawlor-Row & Elliott, 2009).

Involvement in religion often helps the older adult to resolve issues related to the meaning of life, adversity, or good fortune. The older person may derive a sense of worth by sharing spiritual views. Religion may also be an important coping resource, leading to enhanced well-being. Assisting the older person to participate in religious and spiritual practices is an important nursing responsibility.

Promoting Healthy Aging

A primary role of nurses is to promote healthy aging, the goals of which are to maintain physical and emotional health, avoid disease and injury, and remain active and independent. Health-promoting behaviours, such as healthy nutrition and regular physical exercise have been shown to reduce the risk of developing several disorders that commonly occur with age.

Health Assessment

The initial step in promoting health is a detailed assessment of the older adult. The accompanying Developmental Assessment Guidelines box provides the types of information that should be gathered. Because of the increased complexity of an older client, the assessment of an older adult is often more comprehensive than one conducted on a younger adult. It may address other areas such as chronic illness, drug use, and mental health.

A number of guidelines and screening tools have been developed to promote valid and reliable assessment of the older adult. Exactly what tools are used depends on the purpose and the setting. Assessment by the nurse also requires an ability to listen, ask questions, obtain data from multiple sources, and differentiate normal aging changes from abnormal ones. Assessment includes a relevant physical examination, including height, weight, and vital signs (see Chapter 28). A health history should include questions about the following:

- Usual dietary pattern
- Bowel or urinary elimination problems
- Activity, exercise, sleep, and rest patterns
- Family and social activities and interest
- Reading, writing, and problem solving
- Adjustment to retirement or loss of partner
- Economic situation
- Mental and emotional status

ASSESSMENT | **DEVELOPMENTAL GUIDELINES**

The Older Adult

In these developmental areas, does the older adult do the following?

1. PHYSICAL DEVELOPMENT
- Adjust to physiological changes (e.g., appearance, sensory and perceptual, musculoskeletal)
- Adapt lifestyle to diminishing energy and ability
- Maintain vital signs (especially blood pressure) within the recommended target range

2. PSYCHOSOCIAL DEVELOPMENT
- Manage retirement years in a satisfying manner
- Participate in social and leisure activities
- Have a social network of friends and support persons
- View life as worthwhile

- Have high self-esteem
- Gain support from value system or spiritual philosophy
- Accept and adjust to the death of significant others

3. DEVELOPMENT IN ACTIVITIES OF DAILY LIVING
- Exhibit healthy practices in nutrition, exercise, recreation, sleep patterns, and personal habits
- Have the ability to care for self or to secure appropriate help with activities of daily living
- Have satisfactory living arrangements and income to meet changing needs

Health Problems and Chronic Disabling Illnesses

Many Canadian older adults are afflicted with one or more health problems or chronic illnesses that may seriously impair their functioning. Examples of these are arthritis, osteoporosis, cardiovascular disease, chronic obstructive pulmonary disease, diabetes, hypertension, and cognitive dysfunctions. Acute illnesses, such as pneumonia and fractures, may create chronic health problems. Frequently, pain accompanies chronic disease and acute illnesses. Chapter 30 provides a description of pain management. Older adults with cognitive impairment require a specialized approach to pain assessment and management.

In Canada, the presence of chronic conditions varies regionally; for example, rates of chronic disease are higher in the Atlantic region and lower in Western Canada (Touhy et al., 2011). Chronic illness often impacts adaptation and role performance. For example, the client may need increasing help with ADLs, such as ambulation and hygiene. Health care expenses may become an economic concern. Family roles may need to be altered, and family members may need to change their lifestyle to achieve caregiving needs and optimal family functioning.

INJURIES Injury prevention is a major concern for older people. Many accidents are preventable and are directly related to the physiological changes that accompany normal aging. Falls are a leading cause of morbidity and mortality among older adults (Scott, Wagar, Sum, Metcalfe, & Wager, 2010). Carefulness is required in everyday activities, particularly night driving. Older persons should not rely on side vision when crossing a street or changing lanes when driving. Walking and driving in inclement weather conditions should be avoided.

Fires are a hazard for the older adult. The older person may forget that the stove is on or fail to extinguish a candle completely. Because of reduced sensitivity to pain and heat, care must be taken to prevent burns when the person bathes or uses heating devices.

Each year, many older adults die from hypothermia. **Hypothermia** occurs when the body temperature goes below normal. A lowered metabolism and loss of subcutaneous tissue decrease the older client's ability to retain heat. The older adult who spends time outdoors in cold weather or does not turn on the heat in the home is at significant risk for hypothermia.

Older clients who take analgesics or sedatives are at an increased risk for falls. Use of narcotic analgesics and sedatives by older adults should be avoided. Nonpharmaceutical measures to reduce pain and induce sleep should be used whenever possible.

Individuals with dementia experience increased risk for injury as their conditions deteriorate. Judgment becomes impaired as the disease progresses, and some environmental modification is needed to maintain safety. These may include taking knobs off kitchen stoves to prevent burns and fire and installing warning devices on doors for older adults who tend to wander off. Attention should be given to these safety risks, whether the person lives at home or in a health facility.

Nurses can promote environmental safety by identifying and eliminating specific hazards. Injury prevention is detailed in Chapter 32.

CANCER According to the Canadian Cancer Society's Steering Committee on Cancer Statistics (2012), cancer affects Canadians of all ages, and age is a risk factor for cancer. The highest number of new cancer cases (incidence) will occur in the 60–69 age group, while the highest number of cancer deaths (mortality) will be in those 80 and older. More than one-half (53%) of the newly diagnosed cancers are lung, colorectal, prostate, and breast cancers. The most common cancer is prostate cancer in men (27%) and breast cancer in women (26%).

The burden of cancer in older Canadians has serious implications for cancer prevention and cancer care. The aging Canadian population is expected to double by 2030, and 14% of the Canadian population are aged 65 and older. While older adults live longer, many also live with pre-existing health problems, such as chronic conditions, frailty, and physical limitations. As this situation is coupled with an aging population and increased cancer survival rates because of improved cancer treatments, nurses are challenged to develop and implement cancer prevention strategies into the daily lives of older persons to promote healthy aging. For older adults with cancer, nurses play a key role in providing palliative and hospice care to promote end of life quality care.

DRUG USE AND MISUSE Polypharmacy is a significant concern among older Canadian adults, who consume 25% of all medications that are prescribed by health care practitioners (PHAC, 2009) and also purchase over-the-counter (OTC) drugs to remedy discomforts, such as constipation and pain. The use of vitamins, food supplements, and herbal remedies has also increased.

The complexities involved in the self-administration of medication may lead to misuse, including taking too much or too little medication, combining prescribed medications with alcohol or OTC drugs, taking medications at the wrong time, or taking someone else's medication. Misuse can also occur when more than one care provider prescribes medications, and each care provider is not aware of what the other has prescribed. Additionally, because the pharmacodynamics of drugs is altered in older adults, variations in absorption, distribution, metabolism, and excretion of drugs can occur. These variations are discussed in Chapter 33.

Nurses should complete an accurate medication history, including an assessment of all prescription and OTC drugs, many of which can interact with other medications.

MENTAL HEALTH AND ADDICTION PROBLEMS

Although older Canadians report a high level of life satisfaction, factors such as retirement, disability, and relocation can result in mental health challenges (Canadian Mental Health Association [CMHA], 2011). Depression is common in the older adult population, especially among those with a chronic disease. In long-term care settings, the majority of residents have a mental health diagnosis, including dementia and depression (Canadian Coalition for Seniors' Mental Health, 2009). It is difficult to determine the prevalence of mental health among older adults, as many are hesitant to disclose their illness because of fear of stigmatization. In addition, mental health conditions are often masked or confused by physiological aging.

All older individuals with a chronic disease should be screened regularly for depression. Signs and symptoms include a lack of interest in people and things, trouble sleeping, significant changes in appetite, visible sadness, withdrawal from social activities, and feelings of worthlessness. Depression may also be triggered by personal losses, such as the loss of a spouse (CMHA, 2011). In some cases, depression can lead to suicide. Caregivers and health care professionals should be alert to the warning signs of suicide and access mental health services immediately.

Some older adults may use alcohol to cope with the changes of aging. Chronic drinking has negative effects on all body systems and can lead to injuries and death. Risk factors include living alone, having experienced multiple losses, a history of alcohol abuse, a debilitating disease, or all of these factors. Alcohol interacts with various drugs, altering the effect of the medication on the body. Some medications have an increased effect when taken with alcohol (e.g., anticoagulants and narcotics), whereas the action of other medications (e.g., antibiotics) is inhibited. The combination of drugs and alcohol can lead to a serious drug overdose.

Clients who have an alcohol addiction should not be stereotyped; rather, the nurse should support the older adult and advocate for appropriate treatment. The nurse should assess the number and type of alcoholic beverages consumed, as well as the pattern and frequency of consumption. It is also important for the nurse to review the interaction effects of alcohol with the older adults' medications. Referral to community support services is appropriate.

DEMENTIA   **Dementia** is a progressive loss of cognitive function. The most common type of dementia is **Alzheimer's disease** (AD). Identified by Dr. Alois Alzheimer in 1906, the two hallmarks of the disease are (a) plaques, numerous tiny dense and toxic deposits scattered throughout the brain, and (b) tangles, which interfere with vital processes, eventually choking off the living cells. The course of this disease is slow and insidious, affecting half a million people in Canada (Alzheimer's Society of Canada, 2010). In 2008, the incidence of Alzheimer's disease was 103 700 cases per year. Unless a prevention or cure is found, it is estimated that the incidence will increase by 2.5 times the current rate by the year 2038.

The symptoms of AD vary from person to person. The most prominent symptoms are cognitive dysfunctions, including decline in memory, learning, attention, judgment, orientation, and language skills. The symptoms are progressive, leading to a steady decline in cognitive and physical abilities, lasting between 7 and 15 years, and ending in death.

There is no cure for AD. Although several drugs have been developed, none reverse the progression of the disease. AD is devastating for clients, families, and caregivers. Depression and social isolation is common among those who are diagnosed with AD. The nurse's responsibility is to monitor the older adult's cognitive functioning. Nurses use structured tools, such as the mini-mental status exam to assess the older adult's cognition. The nurse also provides supportive nursing care, accurate information, and referral assistance from diagnosis through the various adjustment periods. Referral to home care and respite services is helpful for the caregiver. Canada is one of only a few countries that offer financial support for individuals who leave work to care for an aging family member (Government of Canada, 2008). See the Evidence-Informed Practice box about caring for a family member with dementia.

EVIDENCE-INFORMED PRACTICE

Is Caring for a Family Member with Dementia a Burden?

Caring for a family member with dementia is often perceived as a burdensome responsibility. Using a strengths-based approach, Peacock and colleagues conducted a qualitative exploration of the positive aspects of the caregiving journey. Analysis was conducted of the transcripts from six focus groups and three personal interviews of family members who care for individuals with dementia. The findings suggested that family caregivers perceived their role as an opportunity to give back, to discover personal strengths, and to become closer to the care receiver. The researchers concluded that identifying and mobilizing caregiver strengths may help support family caregivers.

NURSING IMPLICATIONS: With the increasing prevalence of dementia in older adults, more and more caregiving responsibilities will fall on their family members. Nurses must have a sound knowledge in family nursing when working with these families. They can assist the family members to discover their strengths and to positively reframe their family situation as they carry out their roles and functions in caregiving.

Source: Based on Peacock, S., Forbes, D., Markle-Reid, M., Hawranik, P., Morgan, D., Jansen, L., Henderson, S. R. (2010). The positive aspects of the caregiving journey with dementia: Using a strengths-based perspective to reveal opportunities, *Journal of Applied Gerontology, 29*(5), pp. 640–659. doi: 10.1177/0733464809341471

It is critical that dementia be differentiated from **delirium** (see Chapter 37). In contrast to dementia, delirium is an acute and reversible syndrome characterized by a new or different onset of disorientation. The most common causes of delirium are infection, medications, and dehydration. Nurses need to identify when delirium is superimposed on dementia and intervene immediately (Registered Nurses' Association of Ontario [RNAO], 2004, revised 2010).

Although there is no cure for dementia, there is increasing evidence that increased physical activity and diets low in saturated fat can prevent or delay the progression of AD (Alzheimer's Society, 2010; Bayer-Carter et al., 2011).

MISTREATMENT OF OLDER ADULTS One in five Canadians reports knowing a senior who might be experiencing some form of abuse. Elder abuse is defined as "any action by someone in a relationship of trust that results in harm or distress to an older person" (Government of Canada, 2009, para 3). Neglect is as serious as abuse and is defined as lack of action by a person in a trusting relationship, which results in harm or distress. All seniors are vulnerable to elder abuse.

Mistreatment can be classified as physical, psychological, financial, or neglect. Sexual abuse has also been documented. Abuse can be a single incident or a repeated pattern of behaviour. Often, more than one type of abuse occurs simultaneously. Financial abuse is the most commonly reported form of abuse. Abuse or neglect of older adults may occur in all care settings. Abusers can be family members, a friend, someone who provides assistance with basic needs, or health care providers. In many situations, the abuser is dependent on the older adult for money, food, or housing.

The following are some signs and symptoms that may indicate that an older adult is being mistreated:

- Fear, anxiety, depression, agitation, or passivity
- Unexplained physical injuries
- Poor nutrition, dehydration, or poor hygiene
- Confusion about legal documents, such as a will

Older adults at home may fail to report abuse or neglect for many reasons. They may be ashamed or fear retaliation, including institutionalization, if they seek help. Some older adults lack the mental capacity to be aware of the situation.

Nurses should also be familiar with governmental laws regarding the reporting of suspected or known abuse. They can intervene by educating caregivers about the needs of older adults and about available resources to increase home support. Three elements compose the assessment process: (a) the older client, (b) the health care provider, and (c) the context in which abuse or neglect may occur. The nurse also needs to ask about family structure and relationships, caregiving, and lifestyle practices. Screening tools are available to assist in detecting and intervening in elder abuse (NICE, 2011).

Planning for Health Promotion

It is important that older adults take an active role in the care planning process. Most older adults want to be involved in decision making about their health (see the Reflect on Primary Health Care box). It is important to set goals that are mutually agreed upon and realistic for the older adult to achieve. Smaller goals that can be accomplished in shorter time frames may enhance motivation and success.

Nursing Interventions for Health Promotion

A variety of nursing interventions and health-promotion guidelines for older adults (see the Health-Promotion Guidelines box) have been provided throughout this chapter. Communicating with older adults can also be challenging (see Chapter 22 for the box Lifespan Considerations: Communication with Older Adults). To support nurses in their work with older adults, the RNAO has published a number of guidelines related to the care of older clients. These guidelines are intended to help nurses make evidence-informed decisions specific to their practice circumstances. The following selected guidelines are available on the RNAO website:

- Prevention of falls and injuries in the older adult
- Prevention of constipation in the older adult population
- Screening for delirium, dementia, and depression in older adults

Other guidelines are available through a variety of professional organizations. See the Weblinks section at the end of this chapter for two information-rich sources.

REFLECT ON **PRIMARY HEALTH CARE**

As older Canadians enjoy longer lives, they are faced with the potential burden of chronic illness and disability. Nurses use *health-promotion* strategies to engage older adults so that their clients will learn about healthy aging and how to reduce the risks of illness and injury. The emergence of community health centres and use of health-focused Internet sites (*technology*) can increase *accessibility* to health services for older adults living in the community. In providing seamless, quality care for older adults and their caregivers, nurses can invite interprofessional and family input in the planning process. Reflect on how *public participation* and *intersectoral cooperation* can lead to one-stop shopping or multiservice agencies in many communities (e.g., Community Health Centres).

Health-Promotion Guidelines for Older Adults

The following are important to the health of older adults:

HEALTH TESTS AND SCREENING

- Annual health examination, including height and weight
- Total cholesterol and lipid profile every 1 to 3 years, or as recommended by health care provider (Canadian Cardiovascular Society, 2006)
- Screening for type 2 diabetes using a fasting plasma glucose every 3 years (Canadian Diabetes Association, 2008)
- Smoking cessation
- Immunizations, as recommended, including tetanus and diphtheria booster every 10 years; pneumococcal vaccination at age 65 years and every 10 years; annual influenza vaccine
- Dental assessments every 9 months
- Annual eye examination
- Regular testicular self-examination (for men)
- Routine prostate screening for men beginning at the age of 50 years, or earlier with symptoms, a family history of prostate cancer, or of African descent (Canadian Cancer Society, 2011)
- Colorectal screening, including a fecal occult blood test, every 2 years after the age of 50 years (Canadian Cancer Society, 2011)
- Breast awareness, including mammograms every 2 to 3 years between the ages of 50 and 74 years for those who are at average risk for cancer (Canadian Task Force on Preventive Health Care, 2011)
- Cervical cancer screening every 2 to 3 years after three annual negative Pap tests. Screening may be discontinued after the age of 70 years if there is an adequate negative screening history in the previous 10 years.
- Annual screening for immunocompromised or HIV-positive women (National Guideline Clearinghouse, 2005).
- Depression screening periodically

- Family violence screening periodically
- Sexually transmitted infections (STIs) testing, if in high-risk group

SAFETY

- Home injury prevention measures (e.g. falls, burns, poisoning)
- Working smoke detectors and carbon monoxide detectors in the home
- Motor vehicle safety reinforcement
- Precautions to prevent pedestrian accidents
- Older-driver skills evaluations
- Education about safe medication use

NUTRITION AND EXERCISE

- A well-balanced diet using *Canada's Food Guide*, with fewer calories to accommodate lower metabolic rate and decreased physical activity
- Sufficient amounts of vitamin D and calcium to prevent osteoporosis
- Low sodium or no-added-salt diet
- Moderate, daily physical exercise

ELIMINATION

- Adequate roughage in the diet, adequate exercise, and adequate fluids to prevent constipation

SOCIAL INTERACTIONS

- Intellectual and recreational pursuits
- Personal relationships that promote discussion of feelings, concerns, and fears
- Assessment of risk factors for abuse and neglect
- Availability of community centres, programs, and support groups for older adults

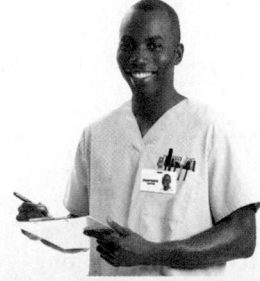

Case Study 20

Mrs. Alice Green, a 78-year-old female, has had a bone density scan as part of a regular physical exam and has been told that she has severe osteoporosis. Her primary care health practitioner has ordered a new medication that is supposed to maintain bone mass in clients with osteoporosis. Mrs. Green lives alone in her own home and is able to perform her activities of daily living (ADLs) independently.

CRITICAL THINKING QUESTIONS

1. How would you define osteoporosis to Mrs. Green?
2. What risk factors related to osteoporosis should be included in an assessment of Mrs. Green?
3. Which of the risk factors are modifiable or can be altered by a change in lifestyle?
4. What medication teaching is essential when a client is taking medications to increase or maintain bone mass in osteoporosis?

5. What preventive measures should be taught to decrease risks of fractures and to maintain bone mass?

Check the eText in MyNursingLab for answers and explanations.

KEY TERMS

activity theory   *p. 392*

ageism   *p. 384*

aging in place   *p. 393*

Alzheimer's disease   *p. 397*

baby boomer   *p. 383*

cataracts   *p. 390*

claudication   *p. 391*

continuity theory   *p. 392*

delirium   *p. 398*

dementia   *p. 397*

disengagement theory   *p. 392*

dyspnea   *p. 390*

frailty   *p. 383*

functional age   *p. 383*

geriatrics   *p. 384*

gerontology   *p. 384*

hypothermia   *p. 396*

kyphosis   *p. 389*

long-term memory   *p. 394*

nocturia   *p. 391*

orthostatic hypotension   *p. 391*

osteoporosis   *p. 389*

pathological fractures   *p. 389*

perception   *p. 394*

presbycusis   *p. 390*

presbyopia   *p. 390*

recent memory   *p. 394*

sarcopenia   *p. 389*

sensory memory   *p. 394*

short-term memory   *p. 394*

xerostomia   *p. 391*

zoomers   *p. 383*

CHAPTER HIGHLIGHTS

- The Canadian older adult population is steadily growing and is projected to outnumber young people by 2036.
- Older adults are categorized into young-old, old, old-old, and centenarians.
- It is important for nurses to be aware of their own values and attitudes toward aging to avoid ageism, and to examine whether myths or stereotypes influence their personal attitudes and beliefs.
- Older adults are primary users of health care services in different types of care settings, including acute care, rehabilitation, long-term care, and the community. Regardless of the setting, the older adult requires health assessment, health promotion, and injury protection.
- Several theories have been proposed to account for the biological aging process: wear-and-tear, genetic, immunity, cross-linking, free radicals, genetics cross-linking, and neuroendocrine theories.
- Older adults experience many physical changes associated with aging. All body systems undergo change.

- Psychosocial theories about aging include the disengagement, activity, and continuity theories.
- The older adult has to adjust to psychosocial changes, including retirement, grandparenting, relocation, increasing dependence on others, and coping with losses and death.
- The cognitive abilities of the healthy older adult undergo changes in perception, cognitive agility, memory, and learning.
- In the realm of moral reasoning, most older adults begin to blend concepts of justice and caring relationships into their moral decision making.
- Health problems of older adults include injuries, chronic disabling disease, drug abuse and misuse, addictions, mental health disorders, and mistreatment.
- Health-promotion information for all adults needs to include positive health practices that can promote health and wellness.

ASSESS YOUR LEARNING

1. In view of the increased incidence of prostate cancer among older Canadian men, which of the following topics would be important to include in a health-promotion presentation to a group of men?

   a. Signs and symptoms of prostate cancer

   b. Screening practices for prostate cancer

   c. Treatment for prostate cancer

   d. Rising mortality rates of prostate cancer

2. Mrs. Weathers, an 83-year-old long-term care resident, has multiple chronic health problems and disability. For which of the following health problems should she regularly be assessed?

   a. Dementia

   b. Delirium

   c. Depression

   d. Diabetes

3. Mrs. Chino has recently been admitted to a long-term care facility. She refuses to interact with other residents, appears sad, and has not been eating. How should the nurse intervene?

   a. Ask other residents to visit Mrs. Chino

   b. Speak with Mrs. Chino about her feelings

   c. Suggest that the physician prescribe an antidepressant

   d. Take Mrs. Chino to social events in the facility

4. Activity theory suggests that activity is which of the following?

   a. Constrained by economic circumstances

   b. Used by the individual to stay healthy

   c. Maintained throughout the lifespan

   d. Reduced according to age

5. Which of the following statements about abuse of older adults is true?

   a. Trusteeship reduces the occurrence of older adult abuse.

   b. Most abuse is committed by daughters and daughters-in-law.

   c. Nurses must be familiar with national laws regarding the reporting of abuse of older adults.

   d. Older adults should be assessed for the presence of abuse.

6. Six months ago, Mr. Harry experienced a right-sided cerebrovascular accident (stroke). When the home care nurse visits, she observes that Mr. Harry is reluctant to perform the exercises suggested by the physiotherapist when Mr. Harry was in hospital. How should the nurse intervene?

   a. Encourage the client to perform the exercises on a regular basis

   b. Help the client verbalize his feelings

   c. Refer the client to mental health services

   d. Talk to his wife about the reason why her husband is reluctant

7. Usual physical changes associated with aging include which of the following?

   a. Decreased muscle mass and tone

   b. Orthostatic hypertension

   c. Increased cardiac output

   d. Urinary incontinence and frequency

8. Mrs. Wu, 76 years old, has been a widow for about 7 months. She recently sold her house and moved into a seniors' complex, following the advice of her daughter, who lives about 600 km away. Influencing her decision was the fact that she has never driven a car. The nurse should be aware of what?

   a. Mrs. Wu may be vulnerable to social isolation.

   b. Mrs. Wu may be subject to abuse by her daughter.

   c. Mrs. Wu may be experiencing dementia.

   d. Retirement may be stressful to Mrs. Wu.

9. Mr. Ken, an 82-year-old retired engineer, likes to ride his bicycle to the library twice a week. What might this indicate to the nurse?

   a. Chronological age is a more accurate indicator of abilities than is functional age.

   b. Functional age is the same as chronological age.

   c. Functional age is a more accurate indicator of abilities than is chronological age.

   d. This is an example of continuity theory.

10. Mrs. Treathing, who is on a number of medications, was admitted to a long-term care facility with Alzheimer's disease (senile dementia of Alzeimer's type) about 6 months ago. Over the past several days, she has demonstrated bizarre behaviour, hallucinations, and increased verbal rambling. How should the nurse intervene?

    a. Ask other residents to visit Mrs. Treathing as she is experiencing sensory deprivation because of lack of social interaction.

    b. Assess Mrs. Treathing for signs of adverse effects from the medications she is taking.

    c. Inform the other staff of the changes in Mrs. Treathing's behaviour.

    d. Request that a sedative be given to reduce Mrs. Treathing's aggressive behaviour.

> *Check the eText in MyNursingLab for answers and explanations.*

WEBLINKS

Hartford Institute for Geriatric Nursing

http://hartfordign.org

This website provides a portal to a number of valuable geriatric initiatives and tools. One example is ConsultGeriRN.org, a website that provides nurses with immediate access to the most current and comprehensive geriatric care information available.

National Initiative for the Care of the Elderly (NICE)

http://www.nicenet.ca

NICE is an international network of researchers, practitioners, and students dedicated to improving the care of older adults in Canada and across the globe. This website is a rich information source for current projects, resources, and tools to support gerontological nursing practice.

MyNursingLab

REFERENCES

Alzheimer's Society of Canada. (2010). *Rising tide: The impact of dementia on Canadian society.* Retrieved from http://www.alzheimer.ca/english/rising_tide/rising_tide_report.htm

Bayer-Carter, J., Green, P., Montine, T., VanFossen, B, Baker, L., Watson, G., & Craft, S. (2011). Diet intervention and cerebrospinal fluid biomarkers in amnestic mild cognitive impairment. *Archives of Neurology, 68*(6), 743–752. doi: 10.1001/archneurol.2011.125

Butler, R. (1963). The life review: An interpretation of reminiscence in the aged. *Psychiatry, 26,* 65–76.

Campbell, T., Grover, S., Hill, M., & Padwal, R. (2011). *2011 Canadian hypertension education program recommendations: The short clinical summary—an annual update.* Retrieved from http://hypertension.ca/chep/recommendations-2011

Canadian Cancer Society. (2011). *Getting checked.* Retrieved from http://www.cancer.ca/Ontario/Prevention/Get%20 screened.aspx?sc_lang=en

Canadian Cancer Society's Steering Committee on Cancer Statistics. (2012). *Canadian cancer statistics 2012.* Toronto, ON: Canadian Cancer Society.

Canadian Cardiovascular Society. (2006). *2006 guidelines for the management and treatment of dyslipidemia and prevention of cardiovascular disease.* Ottawa, ON: Author.

Canadian Coalition for Seniors' Mental Health. (2009). *Mental health issues in long-term care homes: A guide for seniors and their families.* Retrieved from http://www.ccsmh.ca/en/resources/ resources.cfm

Canadian Diabetes Association. (2008). *2008 clinical practice guidelines.* Toronto, ON: Author.

Canadian Institute for Health Information. (2010). *Seniors' use of emergency departments in Ontario, 2004–2005 to 2008–2009.* Ottawa, ON: Author.

Canadian Mental Health Association. (2011). *Seniors and mental health.* Retrieved from http://www.ontario.cmha.ca/seniors.asp

Canadian Task Force on Preventive Health Care. (2011). *Screening for breast cancer: Summary of recommendations for clinicians and policy-makers.* Retrieved from http://www.canadiantaskforce.ca/recommendations/2011_01_eng.html

Demko, D. (1998). *Gerontologist coins new term, "zoomer."* Retrieved from http://www.zoomerboomermagazine.com/zoomers.htm

Ellsworth, P., & Kirshenbaum, E. M. (2008). Current concepts in the evaluation and management of erectile dysfunction. *Urologic Nursing, 28,* 357–369.

Erikson, E. H. (1982). *The life cycle completed: A review.* New York, NY: Norton.

Gilligan, C. (1982). *In a different voice: Psychological theory and women's development.* Cambridge, MA: Harvard University Press.

Government of Canada. (2008). *Investing in seniors.* Retrieved from http://www.seniors.gc.ca/content.jsp?lang=en&auxPag eId=143&geo=144http://www.seniors.gc.ca/content.jsp?lang =en&auxPageId=143&geo=144

Government of Canada. (2009). *Elder abuse: It's time to face the reality.* Retrieved from http://www.seniors.gc.ca/c.4nt.2nt@. jsp?lang=eng&geo=106&cid=154#d

Government of Canada. (2010). *National seniors council. Working for seniors.* Retrieved from http://www.seniorscouncil.gc.ca/ eng/research_publications/working_for_seniors/index.shtml

Hartford Institute for Geriatric Nursing. (2011). *About us.* Retrieved from http://hartfordign.org/About

Havighurst, R. J. (1972). *Developmental tasks and education* (3rd ed.). New York, NY: Longman.

Health Canada. (2004). *Health care system. Long-term facilities-based care.* Retrieved from http://www.hc-sc.gc.ca/hcs-sss/ home-domicile/longdur/index-eng.php

Kohlberg, L. (1984). *The psychology of moral development: The nature and validity of moral stages.* San Francisco, CA: Harper & Row.

Lawlor-Row, K. A., & Elliott, J. (2009). The role of religious activity and spirituality in the health and well-being of older adults. *Journal of Health Psychology, 14,* 43–52. doi: 10.1177/1359105308097944

Madden, M. (2010). *Older adults and social media.* Retrieved from http://www.pewinternet.org/Reports/2010/Older-Adults-and-Social-Media/Report.aspx

Mauk, K. L. (2010). *Gerontological nursing. Competencies for care* (2nd ed.). Sudbury, MA: Jones and Bartlett.

Mosby's medical dictionary (8th ed.). (2009). Maryland Height, MO: Elsevier Health Sciences.

National Guideline Clearinghouse. (2005, revised February, 2011). *Guideline synthesis: Screening for cervical cancer.* Retrieved from http://www.guideline.gov.

National Initiative for the Care of the Elderly. (2011). *About NICE.* Retrieved from http://www.nicenet.ca/detail.aspx?me nu=31&app=187&cat1=510&tp=2&lk=n

Organization for Economic Co-operation and Development. (2011, May 18). *Canada: Long term care.* Retrieved from http://www.oecd.org/canada/47877490.pdf

Peck, R. (1968). Psychological development in the second half of life. In B. L. Neugarten (Ed.), *Middle age and aging* (pp. 137–147). Chicago, IL: University of Chicago Press.

Phelan, A. (2008). Elder abuse, ageism, human rights and citizenship: Implications for nursing discourse. *Nursing Inquiry, 15,* 320–329. doi: 10.1111/j.1440-1800.2008.00423.x

Piaget, J. (1981). *Intelligence and affectivity. Their relationship during child development.* Palo Alto, CA: Annual Reviews.

Pinch, W. J. E., & Parsons, M. E. (1997). Moral orientation of elderly persons: Considering ethical dilemmas in health care. *Nursing Ethics, 4,* 380–393.

Public Health Agency of Canada. (2009). *Healthy aging and age-friendly communities.* Retrieved from http://www.phac-aspc. gc.ca/seniors-aines/ha-vs-eng.php

Registered Nurses' Association of Ontario. (2004, Revised 2010). *Caregiving strategies for older adults with delirium, dementia and depression: Nursing best practice guidelines.* Retrieved from http://www.rnao.org/Storage/69/6404_FINAL_-_ Caregiving_-_BPG_+_Supplement.pdf

Scott, V., Wagar, B., Sum, A., Metcalfe, S., & Wagar, L. (2010). A public health approach to fall prevention among older persons in Canada. *Clinical Geriatric Medicine, 26,* 705–718, doi: 10.1016/j.cger.2010.06.003

Special Senate Committee on Aging. (2009). *Canada's aging population: Seizing the opportunity.* Ottawa, ON: Author.

Statistics Canada. (2010a). *Population projections: Canada, the provinces and territories.* Retrieved from http://www.statcan. gc.ca/daily-quotidien/100526/dq100526b-eng.htm

Statistics Canada. (2010b). *Aboriginal statistics at a glance.* Retrieved from http://www.statcan.gc.ca/pub/89-645-x/89-645-x2010001-eng.htm

Tabloski, P. A. (2010). *Gerontological nursing* (2nd ed.). Upper Saddle River, NJ: Pearson Prentice Hall.

Thomas, R. E., Jefferson, T., & Lasserson, T. (2010). Influenza vaccination for healthcare workers who work with the elderly. *Cochrane Database of Systematic Reviews, Issue 2,* Art. No.: CD005187. doi: 10.1002/14651858.CD005187.pub3

Touhy, T., Jett, K., Boscart, V., & McCleary, L. (2011). *Gerontological nursing and healthy aging* (1st Canadian ed.). Toronto, ON: Elsevier Canada.

Wallace, M. A. (2008). How to try this: Sexuality assessment. *American Journal of Nursing, 108*(7), 40–48.

Woods, N., LaCroix, A., Gray, S., Aragaki, A., Cochrane, B., Brunner, R., . . . & Newman, A. (2005). Frailty: Emergence and consequences in women aged 65 and older in the Women's Health Initiative Observational Study. *Journal of the American Geriatrics Society, 53*(8), 1321–1330.

World Health Organization. (2012). *Ageing.* Retrieved from http://www.who.int/topics/ageing/en

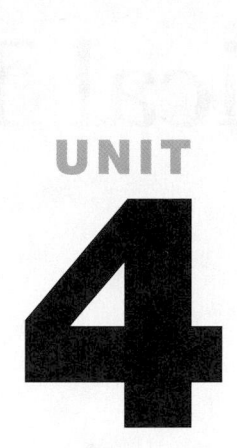

UNIT
4

Integral Aspects of Nursing

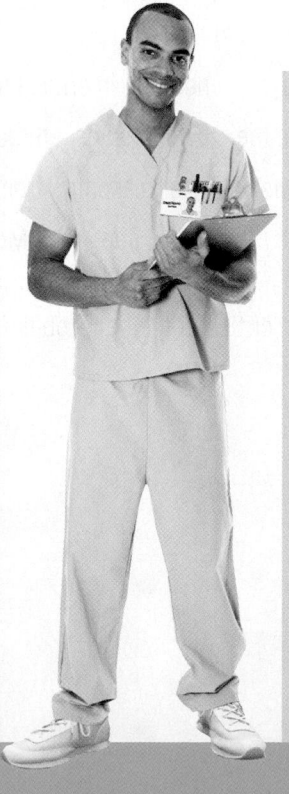

Chapter 21

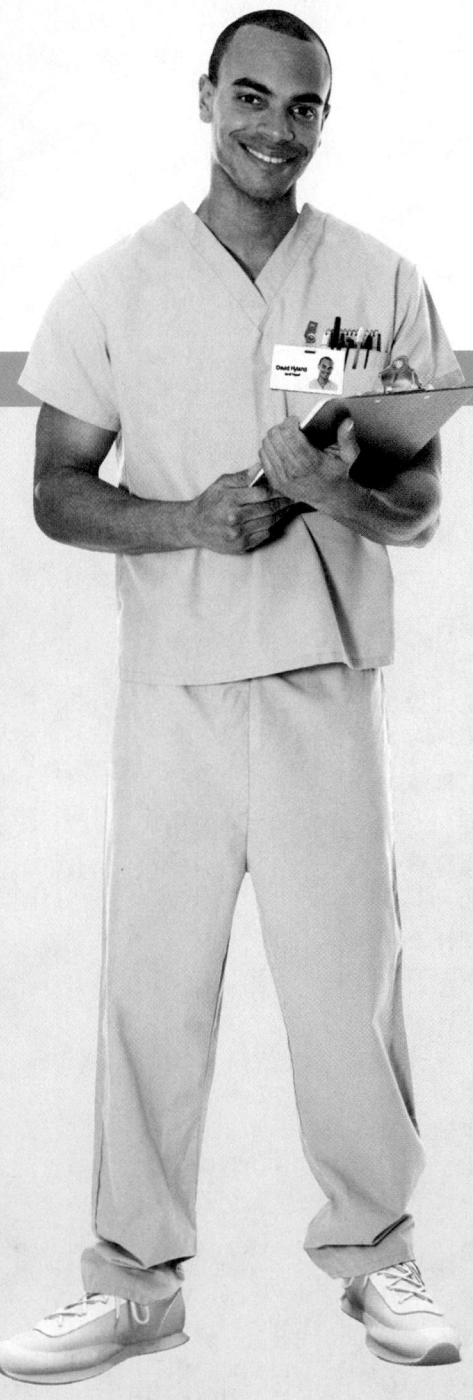

Critical Thinking

LEARNING OUTCOMES

After studying this chapter, you will be able to:

1. Describe the significance of developing critical thinking abilities to practise safe and competent nursing care.

2. State ways of engaging in critical thinking in nursing practice.

3. Describe the characteristics, attitudes, and skills of critical thinking.

4. Distinguish clinical reasoning from clinical judgment and critical thinking.

5. Describe the Clinical Judgment Model.

6. Discuss the relationship among the related concepts throughout the nursing process: critical thinking, problem solving, decision making, and reflective thinking.

The nature of nursing and the complexity of nurses' work mandate that nurses be *critical thinkers*. Nurses help clients solve problems or issues by critically analyzing contributing factors. *Critical thinking* allows the nurse and client to make better decisions. Critical thinking, problem solving, decision making, reflective thinking, and clinical reasoning are interrelated processes. Creativity in problem solving and decision making can enhance the effectiveness of proposed solutions or decisions.

Nurses use critical thinking to make meaningful observations, draw sound conclusions, create new information and ideas, evaluate lines of reasoning, question prevailing assumptions, and improve self-knowledge. The Canadian Association of Schools of Nursing (CASN, 2006) promotes and supports the use of critical thinking. It acknowledges the importance and relevance of critical thinking to the discipline and practice of nursing. This is reflected in the Canadian Registered Nurses Examination, where the emphasis is on assessing nurses' competency in decision making, problem solving, and critical thinking skills in varied clinical or client situations (Canadian Nurses Association [CNA], 2003, 2010).

Critical Thinking Definitions and Purposes

The thinking process that guides nursing practice must be organized, purposeful, and disciplined, rather than random or undirected. Simpson and Courtney (2002) explained **critical thinking** as "a process, an orientation of the mind, . . . including both the cognitive and affective domains of reasoning" (p. 91). Parse (1996) described critical thinking as "carefully choosing a direction in light of personal tacit and explicit knowing" (p. 139). Critical thinking involves calling into question the assumptions that underlie usual ways of thinking about people and acting in situations and then being prepared to think and act differently on the basis of this critical questioning (Brookfield, 1987). Critical thinking is "the art of thinking about thinking" (Paul, 1988, pp. 2–3). It is purposeful thinking wherein the thinker systematically and habitually imposes criteria and intellectual standards on thinking. The thinker is aware of and takes charge of the thinking process, guiding it according to these standards (Paul, 1993).

Critical thinking is a complex process, and it moves beyond thinking to purposeful action. A landmark study involving internationally diverse expert nurses from nine countries defined 10 habits of the mind (affective components) and 7 skills (cognitive components) of critical thinking in nursing (Scheffer & Rubenfeld, 2000) (see Box 21.1 on the next page).

Critical thinking is essential for safe and competent nursing practice. Oermann and Gaberson (2009) stated that critical thinking is "a process used to determine a course of action after collecting appropriate data, analyzing the validity and utility of the information, evaluating multiple lines of reasoning, and coming to valid conclusions" (p. 31). Nurses are expected to help clients make decisions and address problems by critically analyzing contributing factors. This critical analysis, or critical thinking, allows the nurse and client to make better decisions, particularly when neither clear answers nor standardized procedures are available and when conflicting forces make decisions complex. Alfaro-LeFevre's Four-Circle Critical Thinking Model (2008) provides a visual representation of critical thinking abilities and promotes making meaningful connections between nursing research and positions on critical thinking and practice (Figure 21.1 on the next page). The processes of higher level critical thinking skills and problem-solving skills are essential for the transition from student to practitioner and provider of safe and effective care (Kostovoch, Poradzisz, Wood, & O'Brian, 2007).

Nurses use critical thinking skills in a variety of ways:

- *Nurses use knowledge from other disciplines.* Nurses use critical thinking skills when they reflect on knowledge derived from other interdisciplinary subject areas, such as the biophysical and behavioural sciences, and the humanities to provide holistic nursing care. For example, registered nurses might use information from nutrition, physiology, and physics to promote wound healing and prevent further injury to a client with a pressure ulcer.

- *Nurses deal with change in stressful environments.* A client's condition may rapidly change and

---

BOX 21.1 SCHEFFER AND RUBENFELD'S HABITS OF THE MIND AND CRITICAL THINKING SKILLS

HABITS OF THE MIND (AFFECTIVE COMPONENTS)

1. *Confidence*—assurance of one's reasoning abilities
2. *Contextual perspective*—consideration of the whole situation including relationships, background and environment, and relevant to some happening
3. *Creativity*—intellectual inventiveness used to generate, discover, or restructure ideas; imagining alternatives
4. *Flexibility*—capacity to adapt, accommodate, modify, or change thoughts, ideas, and behaviours
5. *Inquisitiveness*—an eagerness to know by seeking knowledge and understanding through observation and thoughtful questioning to explore possibilities and alternatives
6. *Intellectual integrity*—seeking the truth through sincere, honest processes, even if the results are contrary to one's assumptions and beliefs
7. *Intuition*—insightful sense of knowing without conscious use of reason
8. *Open-mindedness*—a viewpoint characterized by being receptive to divergent views and sensitive to one's biases
9. *Perseverance*—pursuit of a course with determination to overcome obstacles
10. *Reflection*—contemplation upon a subject, especially one's assumptions and thinking for the purposes of deeper understanding and self-evaluation

**CRITICAL THINKING SKILLS
(COGNITIVE COMPONENTS)**

1. *Analyzing*—separating or breaking a whole into parts to discover their nature, function, and relationships
2. *Applying standards*—judging according to established personal, professional, or social rules or criteria
3. *Discriminating*—recognizing differences and similarities among things or situations and distinguishing carefully as to category or rank
4. *Information seeking*—searching for evidence, facts, or knowledge by identifying relevant sources and gathering objective, subjective, historical, and current data from those subjects
5. *Logical reasoning*—drawing inferences or conclusions that are supported in or justified by evidence
6. *Predicting*—envisioning a plan and its consequences
7. *Transforming knowledge*—changing or converting the condition, nature, form, or function of concepts among contexts

Source: From Scheffer, B., & Rubenfeld, M. (2000). A consensus statement on critical thinking in nursing. *Journal of Nursing Education, 39,* 358. Used by permission of SLACK Incorporated.

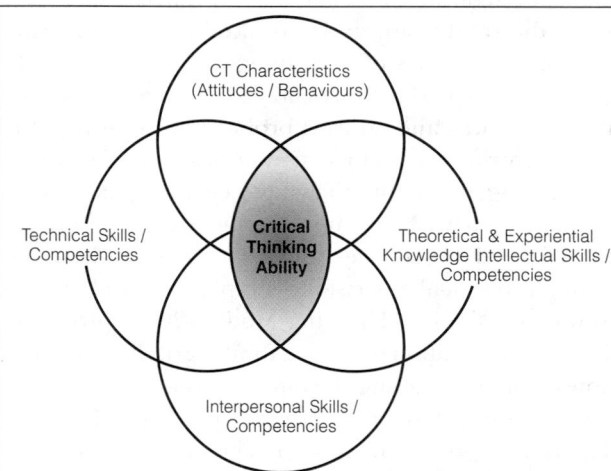

Starting at the top and going clockwise around the circles above, here's what you need to do to develop your ability to think critically:

1. Develop a critical thinking character. Hold yourself to high standards. Make a commitment to developing critical thinking characteristics such as honesty, fair-mindedness, creativity, patience, and confidence.
2. Take responsibility and seek out learning experiences to help you get the theoretical and experiential knowledge to think critically. Practise intellectual skills such as assessing systematically and comprehensively. Just as practising physical skills improves your ability to perform physically, practising thinking skills improves your ability to perform intellectually.
3. Gain interpersonal skills such as teamwork, resolving conflict, and being an advocate. Keep in mind that "being too nice" problems (e.g., not giving constructive criticism because of concerns of not offending someone) can be as bad as "not being very nice" problems (e.g., demonstrating arrogance, sarcasm, or intolerance of other ways of doing things). Learn how to give and take feedback. To improve you must get through the negative aspects of criticism.
4. Practise related technical skills (e.g., using computers, managing IV's,). Until these skills become like second natures, they create a "brain drain" making it difficult to focus on other important things such as monitoring patient responses to care.

FIGURE 21.1 Alfaro-LeFevre's Four-Circle Critical Thinking Model.

Source: Reprinted with permission from Alfaro-LeFevre, R. (2008). *Critical thinking indicators.* Florida, MI: Stuart. Retrieved from http://www.alfaroteachsmart.com/cti.htm

routine protocols may not be adequate to cover every unexpected situation. When unanticipated situations arise, critical thinking enables the nurse to recognize important cues, respond quickly by drawing on relevant knowledge, and adapt best practice interventions at the right time to meet specific client needs. Box 21.2 lists some personal critical thinking indicators.

- *Nurses make important decisions.* During the course of a workday, nurses use critical thinking skills to collect, compile, and interpret the information needed to make clinical decisions and judgments. For example, nurses must use prudent judgment to decide which observations to report to the appropriate member of the health care team immediately and which can be noted in the patient record for the appropriate member of the health care team to address later, during the routine client visit.

Critical thinking cognitively fuels the intellectual artistic activity of creativity. **Creativity**—original thinking—is a major component of critical thinking. When nurses incorporate creativity into their thinking, they are able to find unique solutions to unique problems. Creative thinking is thinking that results in the development of new ideas and products. It is a vital part of providing competent client care. Critical thinking skills and abilities are developed over time through practice and with constructive feedback. Creativity in problem solving and decision making is the ability to develop and implement new and better solutions or ideas.

BOX 21.2 PERSONAL CRITICAL THINKING INDICATORS: BEHAVIOURS DEMONSTRATING CRITICAL THINKING CHARACTERISTICS AND ATTITUDES

- *Self-aware:* Clarifies biases, inclinations, strengths, and limitations; acknowledges when thinking may be influenced by emotions or self-interest
- *Genuine:* Shows authentic self; demonstrates behaviours that indicate stated values
- *Self-disciplined:* Stays on task as needed; manages time to focus on priorities
- *Healthy:* Promotes a healthy lifestyle; uses healthy behaviours to manage stress
- *Careful and prudent:* Knows own limits—seeks help, as needed; suspends or revises judgment as indicated by new or incomplete data
- *Confident and resilient:* Expresses faith in ability to reason and learn; overcomes disappointments
- *Honest and upright:* Seeks the truth, even if it sheds unwanted light; upholds standards; admits flaws in thinking
- *Curious and inquisitive:* Looks for reasons, explanations, and meaning; seeks new information to broaden understanding
- *Alert to context:* Looks for changes in circumstances that warrant a need to modify thinking or approaches
- *Analytical and insightful:* Identifies relationships; expresses deep understanding
- *Logical and intuitive:* Draws reasonable conclusions (if this is so, then it follows that . . . because . . .); uses intuition as a guide to search for evidence; acts on intuition only with knowledge of risks involved
- *Open and fair-minded:* Shows tolerance for different viewpoints; questions how own viewpoints are influencing thinking

- *Sensitive to diversity:* Expresses appreciation of human differences related to values, culture, personality, or learning style preferences; adapts to preferences, when feasible
- *Creative:* Offers alternative solutions and approaches; comes up with useful ideas
- *Realistic and practical:* Admits when things are not feasible; looks for user-friendly solutions
- *Reflective and self-corrective:* Carefully considers meaning of data and interpersonal interactions, asks for feedback; corrects own thinking, alert to potential errors by self and others, finds ways to avoid future mistakes
- *Proactive:* Anticipates consequences, plans ahead, acts on opportunities
- *Courageous:* Stands up for beliefs, advocates for others, does not hide from challenges
- *Patient and persistent:* Waits for right moment; perseveres to achieve best results
- *Flexible:* Changes approaches, as needed, to get the best results
- *Empathetic:* Listens well; shows ability to imagine others' feelings and difficulties
- *Improvement-oriented (self, patients, systems):* Self—identifies learning needs; finds ways to overcome limitations, seeks out new knowledge. Patients—promotes health; maximizes function, comfort, and convenience. Systems—identifies risks and problems with health care systems; promotes safety, quality, satisfaction, and cost containment.

Source: Reprinted with permission from *Critical Thinking Indicators*, by R. Alfaro-LeFevre, 2009, p. 7. Retrieved from http://www.AlfaroTeachSmart.com.

Techniques in Critical Thinking

In addition to the affective and cognitive components of critical thinking skills noted in Box 21.1, the nurse uses other techniques to ensure effective problem solving and decision making. These techniques include cognitive abilities such as critical analysis, inductive and deductive reasoning, making valid inferences, differentiating facts from opinions, evaluating the credibility of information sources, clarifying concepts, and recognizing assumptions.

Critical analysis is the application of questions to a particular situation or idea to determine essential elements, and discard superfluous information and ideas. The questions are *not* sequential steps; rather, they form a set of criteria for judging an idea. Not all questions will need to be applied to every situation, but one should be aware of all the questions and choose those appropriate to a given situation.

Socrates was a Greek philosopher who developed the Socratic method of question and answer. **Socratic questioning** is a technique one can use to look beneath the surface, recognize and examine assumptions, search for inconsistencies, examine multiple points of view, and differentiate what is known from what one merely believes. Box 21.3 on the next page lists Socratic questions to use in critical analysis. Nurses can employ Socratic questioning when listening to an end-of-shift report, reviewing a client health history or progress notes, planning care, or discussing a client's care with the client, colleagues, and other health care professionals.

Two skills used in complex thinking are inductive and deductive reasoning. In **inductive reasoning**, generalizations are formed from a set of facts or observations. When viewed together, certain bits of information suggest a particular interpretation proceeding from the specific to the general. For example, the nurse who observes that a patient has dry skin, poor tissue turgor, sunken eyes, and dark amber urine may make the generalization that the patient is dehydrated.

BOX 21.3 SOCRATIC QUESTIONS

Nurses can use Socratic questions to help them think critically:

QUESTIONS ABOUT THE QUESTION (OR PROBLEM)
- Is this question clear, understandable, and correctly identified?
- Is this question important?
- Could this question be broken down into smaller parts?
- How might _____ state this question?

QUESTIONS ABOUT ASSUMPTIONS
- You seem to be assuming _____; is that so?
- What could you assume instead? Why?
- Does this assumption always hold true?

QUESTIONS ABOUT POINT OF VIEW
- You seem to be using the perspective of _____. Why?
- What would someone who disagrees with your perspective say?
- Can you see this any other way?

QUESTIONS ABOUT EVIDENCE AND REASONS
- What evidence do you have for that?
- Is there any reason to doubt that evidence?
- How do you know?
- What would change your mind?

QUESTIONS ABOUT IMPLICATIONS AND CONSEQUENCES
- What effect would that have?
- What is the probability that will actually happen?
- What are the alternatives?
- What are the implications of that?

Source: Paul, R. (1993). Socratic questioning in Critical thinking: How to prepare students for a rapidly changing world (pp. 335–365). Santa Rosa, CA: Foundation for Critical Thinking.

Deductive reasoning, by contrast, is reasoning from a general to a specific conclusion. If you begin with the premise that the sum of the angles in any triangle is always 180 degrees, you can then conclude that the sum of the angles in the triangle you happen to have is also 180 degrees. A nurse might start with a premise that all children love apple juice. If the client is a child, then the child will love apple juice. This is an example in which the premise is not always valid and, thus, the conclusion also may not be valid.

In critical thinking, the nurse also differentiates statements of fact, inference, judgment, and opinion. Table 21.1 shows how these statements may be applied to nursing care. Evaluating the credibility of information sources is an important step in critical thinking. Unfortunately, we cannot always believe what we read or are told. The nurse may need to ascertain the accuracy of information by checking other documents or with other informants. Hence, the expanding need for evidence-based nursing practice.

REASONING PROCESS A clear *reasoning* process is particularly important when problems are complex and have multiple potential solutions. Oermann and Gaberson (2009) summarized the following elements of reasoning comprising the critical thinking process:

1. Purpose of the critical thinking
2. Question, issue, or problem that requires resolution
3. Assumptions about the problem
4. Analysis of own and others' points of view
5. Data and evidence to support
6. Concepts and theories used in thinking
7. Inferences and conclusions based on given data
8. Implications and consequences of reasoning

Clinical Reasoning

Clinical reasoning and critical thinking are similar but different concepts. In nursing practice, **clinical reasoning** is a thought process used to assess a client's evolving situation and health care concerns, gather data, and make decisions to solve problems within a particular clinical context to achieve better client outcomes (Benner, Hughes, & Sutphen, 2008; Benner, Sutphen, Leonard, & Day, 2010; Tanner, 2006). Clinical reasoning focuses on the thinking

---

TABLE 21.1 Differentiating Types of Statements

Statement	Description	Example
Facts	Can be corroborated through investigation	Blood pressure is affected by blood volume.
Inferences	Conclusions drawn from the facts; going beyond facts to make a statement about something not currently known	If blood volume is decreased (e.g., in hemorrhagic shock), blood pressure will drop.
Judgments	Evaluation of facts or information that reflect values or other criteria; a type of opinion	It is harmful to the client's health if his or her blood pressure drops too low.
Opinions	Beliefs formed over time; include judgments that may fit facts or be in error	Nursing intervention can assist in maintaining the client's blood pressure within normal limits.

strategies nurses use to make judgments or decisions and/or solve problems with clients. In contrast, critical thinking is a broader process, involving both cognitive and affective components of which reasoning is a part (Simmons, 2010).

Context is an important aspect of clinical reasoning. The nurse is not only aware of how he or she performs a task with the patient but also aware of the patient's reaction to the task. For example, if the patient requires assistance with ambulating, was the proper technique employed in moving the patient from the bed to a chair? How did the patient experience this move, is the patient resting comfortably, and did the nurse follow-up to ensure the patient is still comfortable after an appropriate period? The nurse must be aware of the patient's perception of their health experience and the effect on the patient's relationship with their family. How does the patient feel about the need for assistance to move from bed to chair? How will the need for assistance impact the roles and relationships with family members and the discharge home? Clinical reasoning involves awareness, assessment, and reaction to all aspects of the patient's care on an ongoing basis (Benner et al., 2010).

Another component of clinical reasoning is *priority setting*. Nurses recognize the importance of assessing and prioritizing patient care needs. In this process, nurses think about what patient care to provide first, what patient care goals are less urgent, and how to evaluate, reassess, and adapt if need be. Time management is critical in complex practice settings. Confidence and autonomy in practice grows and develops (Benner et al., 2010). For example, one patient is due to be repositioned in bed; however, after making a respiratory assessment on another patient, the nurse notes that the patient is having difficulty breathing and complains of tightness in the chest. While recognizing the importance of repositioning the patient every 2 hours, the respiratory complaint is the more urgent situation, requiring immediate attention and change in the plan of care.

Various types of knowledge are drawn upon when using clinical reasoning (Simmons, 2010). Tanner proposes a Clinical Judgment Model based on a review and synthesis of the literature about clinical judgment. **Clinical judgment** is defined as "... the interpretation or conclusion about a patient's needs, concerns or health problems, and/or the decision to take action (or not), use or modify standard approaches, or improvise new ones as deemed appropriate by the patient's response" (Tanner, 2006, p. 204). *Clinical reasoning* is described as the thought process by which these decisions are made.

The **Clinical Judgment Model** includes four aspects that can be used within continuously evolving practice environments. *Noticing* is the nurses' initial grasp of the patient's situation and can include preconceived expectations from the nurses' previous experience with patients experiencing similar situations. A pattern of reasoning (analytic, intuitive, or narrative) is triggered after

noticing, and in the *interpreting* aspect the meaning of the data gathered from the patient is examined. This leads to taking an appropriate course of action, the *responding* aspect. There are two components in the *reflection* aspect. *Reflection-in-action* refers to the nurses' ability to determine how the patient is responding to the nursing care or intervention delivered and to make adjustments as appropriate. *Reflection-on-action* takes into account what nurses learn from the practice situation and how this experience contributes to their overall knowledge development and builds their expertise for future practice situations. Reflection involves both a sense of responsibility, where the nurse links actions and outcomes, and knowledge development, where the nurse recognizes what occurred for the patient as a result of the nurses' actions.

Nurses use clinical reasoning to think about a patient's health care situation and use their knowledge and experience to gather and assess patient data, weigh alternative interventions, and plan appropriate care. This process evolves and is ongoing as the patient's situation changes (Simmons, 2010; Tanner, 2006).

Attitudes That Foster Critical Thinking

Certain attitudes are crucial to critical thinking. These attitudes are based on the assumption that a rational person is motivated to develop, learn, and grow. A critical thinker works to develop the following attitudes or traits: independence of thought, fair-mindedness, insight, intellectual humility, intellectual courage, integrity, perseverance, confidence, and curiosity.

Independence

Critical thinking requires that individuals think for themselves. People acquire many beliefs in their childhood that are not necessarily based on reason or evidence. These provide an explanation they can comprehend or offer rational reasons for believing. Rewards may have been associated with believing. Alternatively, these beliefs may be an outcome of not questioning the authorities promoting them. As critical thinkers mature and acquire knowledge and experience, they examine their beliefs and assumptions in light of new evidence. Critical thinkers consider a wide range of ideas, learn from them, and then make their own judgments about them.

Fair-Mindedness

Critical thinkers are fair-minded, assessing all viewpoints against the same standards and not basing judgments on personal or group bias or prejudice (Catalano, 2009).

Fair-mindedness helps people consider opposing points of view and try to understand new ideas fully before rejecting or accepting them. Critical thinkers strive to be open to the possibility that new evidence or information could change their minds.

Insight

Critical thinkers are open to the possibility that their personal biases, social pressures, customs, and cultural background could unduly affect their thinking. They actively try to examine their own biases and bring them to awareness each time they think or make a decision. For example, consider a nurse who spent extensive time trying to teach a client how to prevent a recurrence of some problem but was mystified when the client appeared uninterested and did not follow the nurse's advice. The nurse's egocentric tendency to assume that all clients would be motivated and interested in preventive care (just because the nurse was) resulted in an inaccurate assessment of the client's desire and readiness to learn; both the nurse's and the client's time was wasted. Had the nurse assessed the client's understanding about what caused the disease and considered the client's cultural background, beliefs and, perhaps, even the client's support systems (i.e., had the nurse collected sufficient evidence), the nurse might have developed more meaningful insights about the issues of immediate concern to the client, identified more relevant priorities, and, thus, developed a better care plan.

Intellectual Humility

Intellectual humility means having an awareness of the limits of your own knowledge. Critical thinkers are willing to admit what they do not know; they are willing to seek new information and rethink their conclusions in light of new knowledge. They never assume that what everybody knows to be right will always be right, because new evidence may emerge. A hospital nurse might be unable to imagine how the 80-year-old wife will care for her husband, who has recently had a stroke. However, the nurse also recognizes that it is not really possible to know what the couple can achieve.

Intellectual Courage

With an attitude of courage, people are willing to consider and examine their own ideas or views, especially those to which they have a strong negative reaction. This type of courage comes from recognizing that beliefs or assumptions are sometimes false or misleading. Values, assumptions, and beliefs are not always acquired rationally.

Rational beliefs are those that have been examined and found to be supported by solid reasons and data.

After such examination, it is inevitable that some ideas, previously held to be true, are found to contain questionable elements and that some truth may emerge from ideas considered dangerous or false. Courage is needed to be true to new thinking in such cases, especially if social penalties for nonconformity are severe. As an example, some nurses may believe that allowing family members to observe an emergency (such as cardiopulmonary resuscitation) would be psychologically harmful to the family and that members would get in the health care team's way. Others may feel that blanket exclusion of family members was unnecessary and extremely stressful for some. As a result, nurses can initiate research to demonstrate that the family can be present without detrimental effects to the nurse, the client, or the family.

Integrity

Intellectual integrity requires that individuals apply the same rigorous standards of proof to their own knowledge and beliefs as they apply to the knowledge and beliefs of others. Critical thinkers question their own knowledge and beliefs or assumptions as quickly and thoroughly as they challenge those of another. They are readily able to admit and evaluate inconsistencies within their own beliefs and between their own beliefs and those of another. For example, a nurse might believe that wound care always requires sterile technique. Reading an evidence-based article on the use and outcomes of clean technique for some wounds leads the critically thinking nurse to reconsider.

Perseverance

Nurses who are critical thinkers show perseverance in seeking effective solutions to client and nursing problems. This determination enables them to clarify concepts and sort out related issues in spite of difficulties and frustrations. Confusion and frustration are uncomfortable, but critical thinkers resist the temptation to find a quick and easy answer. Important questions tend to be complex and confusing and, therefore, often require a great deal of thought and research to arrive at an answer. The nurse needs to continue to address the issue until it is resolved and to resist the temptation to come to a hasty conclusion on a complex issue.

Confidence

Critical thinkers believe that well-reasoned thinking will lead to trustworthy conclusions. Therefore, they cultivate an attitude of confidence in the reasoning process and examine emotion-laden arguments by using the standards for evaluating thought, by asking questions such as the following: Is that argument fair? Is it based on sufficient evidence?

The critical thinker develops skill in both inductive reasoning and deductive reasoning. As a critical thinker gains greater awareness of the thinking process and more experience in improving such thinking, confidence in the thinking process will grow. This confident thinker will not be afraid of disagreement and, indeed, will be concerned when all agree too quickly. Such an individual can serve as a role model to colleagues, inspiring and encouraging them to think critically as well.

Curiosity

The mind of a critical thinker is filled with questions: Why do we believe this? What causes that? Does it have to be this way? Could something else work? What would happen if we did it another way? Who says that is so? The curious individual may value tradition but is not afraid to examine traditions to be sure they are still valid. The nurse may, for example, apply these questions and strategies to the issue of moving responsibility for a procedure, such as drawing arterial blood samples, among the nursing, respiratory therapy, or laboratory department staff.

Standards of Critical Thinking

How can one know whether one's thinking is critical thinking? Elder and Paul (2007) proposed that thinkers can use universal standards as a guide in thinking to achieve excellence and to provide competent care based on evidence-based practice. The nurse considers questions, such as those in Table 21.2, to be certain that critical thinking is conscious and systematic.

Applying Critical Thinking to Nursing Practice

There are multiple ways of thinking during nursing practice. Critical thinking, problem solving, decision making, and reflective thinking are interrelated processes. In comparison, critical thinking is a broader process that relies on examination of knowledge and assumptions as well as on exploration of alternatives that can include both problem solving and decision making. Problem solving and decision making are often used interchangeably; however, they are different. **Reflective thinking** focuses on the critique and evaluation of actions taken and lessons learned.

TABLE 21.2   Universal Intellectual Standards

Standard	Sample Question
Clarity	What is an example of this?
Accuracy	How can I find out if that is true?
Precision	Can I be more specific?
Relevance	How does that help me with the issue?
Depth	What makes this a difficult problem?
Breadth	Do I need to consider another point of view?
Logic	Does that follow from the evidence?
Significance	Which of these facts is most important?
Fairness	Am I considering the thinking of others?

Source: From Paul, R. & Elder, L. (2005). *A guide for educators to critical thinking competency standards* (p. 57). Dillon Beach, CA: Foundation for Critical Thinking. Adapted with permission.

Problem Solving

Problem solving involves working through a process of recognizing, defining, and then solving a problem. Many alternative solutions may be considered and implemented in resolving the problem. In *decision making*, alternatives are examined and the one most appropriate to the situation is selected. Decision making may or may not involve a problem.

In problem solving, the nurse obtains information that clarifies the nature of the problem and suggests possible solutions. The nurse then carefully evaluates the possible solutions, chooses the best one to implement, and continues to monitor outcomes and the effectiveness of the solution. The nurse does not discard the other possible solutions but holds them in reserve in the event that the first solution is ineffective. In the same way, depending on the client context, an alternative solution may be more appropriate. Therefore, problem solving for one situation contributes to the nurse's body of knowledge for problem solving in other similar situations.

TRIAL AND ERROR   One way to solve problems is through **trial and error**; that is, a number of approaches are tried until a solution is found. However, knowing why a solution was effective may be difficult to determine if alternatives are not considered systematically. Trial and error methods in nursing care can be dangerous because the client might suffer harm if a particular solution or approach is inappropriate.

INTUITION   **Intuition** is the understanding or learning of things without the conscious use of reasoning. It is also known as sixth sense, hunch, instinct, feeling, or suspicion. Some people view intuition as a form of guessing, and, as such, an inappropriate basis for nursing decisions. However, others view intuition as an essential and legitimate aspect of clinical judgment acquired through knowledge and experience. The nurse must first have the knowledge base necessary to practise in the clinical area and then use that knowledge in clinical practice. Clinical experience allows the nurse to recognize cues and patterns and begin to reach correct conclusions.

Experience is important in improving intuition because the rapidity of the judgment depends on the nurse having seen similar client situations many times before. Sometimes, nurses use the words "I had a feeling" to describe a leap (or a condensing) in the critical thinking element of considering evidence. These nurses are able to judge quickly and decisively which evidence is most important and to act on that limited evidence. Nurses in critical care often pay closer attention than usual to a client when they sense that the client's condition could change suddenly.

Although the intuitive method of problem solving is gaining recognition as part of nursing practice, it is not recommended for novices or students, because they usually lack the knowledge base and clinical experience on which to make a valid judgment.

RESEARCH PROCESS   The **research process** is a formalized, logical, systematic approach to problem solving. It is becoming increasingly important that nurses apply the research process to identify evidence that supports effective nursing care. One critical source of this evidence is research (see Chapter 3).

Decision Making

Nurses use critical thinking skills in **decision making** to help them choose the best action to meet a desired goal. Decisions must be made whenever several mutually exclusive choices exist. For example, the individual who wants to become a nurse in Canada can choose from many different university programs throughout the country. To make an appropriate decision, a prospective student must evaluate the programs and consider personal circumstances, as well as any other relevant data (e.g., geography, entry-to-program requirements) that may influence their choice.

Nurses make decisions in their personal and professional lives. For example, when faced with meeting several clients' needs at the same time, the nurse must prioritize and decide which client to assist first. When a client is trying to make a decision about what course of treatment to follow, the nurse may need to provide the client with information or resources (see the Lifespan Considerations box). Decision making is an important process and takes place at many levels (see http://www.cno.org/Global/docs/reg/41037_EntryToPracitic_final.pdf for Decision Tree: A Guide to Practice Decision Making for the Entry-Level Registered Nurse).

In practice, nurses use evidence to guide their decision making about patient care. **Evidence-based practice** (EBP) is "the integration of best research evidence with clinical expertise and patient values to facilitate clinical decision making" (DiCenso, Ciliska, & Guyatt, 2005, p. 4). EBP involves consciously questioning practice and using evidence to guide the care provided to patients. Evidence consists of information acquired through research (quantitative and qualitative studies), and meta-analysis, EBP guidelines, or case studies. Several models exist to assist health care agencies to implement EBP in their organizations. The Iowa Model for EBP and the Ottawa Model of Research Use are two examples (Titler & Cameron, 2009). The Registered Nurses' Association of Ontario offers best practice guidelines (BPGs) for nurses to use in hospital and community agencies. These BPGs are one example of how research is summarized and synthesized into guidelines to provide nurses with an evidence-based standard of care to guide problem solving and decision making in practice.

Evidence-informed nursing practice is "the ongoing process that incorporates evidence from research, clinical expertise, client preferences, and other available resources to make nursing decisions about clients" (CNA, 2010, p. 3). Evidence-informed decision making in practice is different from EBP in that it is broader, not only including the use of evidence but also incorporating patients' values, beliefs, choices, and cultural and/or religious practices, as well as ethics, legislation, policy, health care resources, and the resources and context of the practice setting, all of which influence decision making (CNA, 2010). Evidence for evidence-informed practice may also include documents from commissioned reports, expert panels, policy/practice standards or regulations, and historical or experiential information (CNA, 2010). It is the responsibility of every nurse to use evidence (research or other) and incorporate patient values to guide their decision making in practice and thus practise from an evidence-informed perspective (CNA, 2010; Titler & Cameron, 2009).

A clinical example of the phases of the nursing process and the decision-making process, demonstrating the use of critical thinking with an individual client, is given in Table 21.3.

Developing Critical Thinking Attitudes and Skills

After gaining an appreciation of what it means to think critically, solve problems, and make decisions, nurses need to become aware of their own thinking style and abilities. Acquiring critical thinking skills and a critical

LIFESPAN CONSIDERATIONS

Health Care Decisions for Children and Older Adults

CHILDREN

Parents most often make decisions about the health care of children. Growing children can participate in those decisions in age-appropriate ways. As described by Piaget (1966), children's ability to reason and critically think about themselves and their situation develops gradually (see Chapter 17).

At each stage, nurses should be aware of the ways children think and be sensitive to how children can be involved in health care decisions:

* Infants progress from reflexive behaviour to simple, repetitive behaviour and then to imitative behaviours, learning the concepts of cause and effect and object permanence. Though not involved in making decisions, they need to be comforted and secure as care is given.

* Toddlers and preschoolers are very egocentric and engage in magical thinking. They cannot reason out the implications of care but need explanations in language they can understand. Play therapy and the use of dolls and toys can help them adjust to care, and they can sometimes be given options (e.g., Do you want your dressing changed before breakfast or after?).

* School-age children tend to be concrete thinkers. They benefit from simple, direct explanations; hands-on exploration of equipment and materials; and the chance to help the care

provider as appropriate during procedures. Involving these children in care can increase cooperation and decrease anxiety.

* Adolescents are increasingly able to think abstractly and may make many of their own health care decisions. They should be actively consulted as a part of the family system.

OLDER ADULTS

It is important to include all adult clients in decision making and planning nursing care, but it is especially difficult to do this when working with older adults who have impaired cognitive abilities, such as Alzheimer's disease. The nurse should allow them as much control and input as possible, keeping things simple and direct so that they understand everything. Older adults with impairments are usually unable to perform multiple tasks or to think of more than one step at a time. The nurse must have patience and be willing to calmly repeat instructions, if necessary. Presenting and discussing issues in basic terms helps to maintain respect and dignity and allows older adults to participate in their own care for as long as possible. If the older adult is unable to perform self-care activities, such as bathing, or health-related activities, such as a dressing change, the nurse seeks appropriate alternative methods for assisting the older adult with these.

TABLE 21.3 Phases of the Nursing Process, the Decision-Making Process, and a Clinical Example of Critical Thinking

Nursing Process	Decision-Making Process	Clinical Application
Assessing	*Identify the purpose.* The nurse identifies why a decision is needed and what needs to be determined.	*Data:* A 45-year-old Aboriginal male complains of severe headache; 10 kg overweight; blood pressure 180/95 mm Hg; states he has been taking high blood pressure pills only when he has a headache; is self-employed as a gardener; lives with wife, mother-in-law, and four children
		Given these data, a critical thinker is aware that more data must be obtained about the client's cultural health values and reasons for stated behaviour. Failure to think critically and to obtain additional data leads to inaccurate goals, diagnosis, and interventions.
Diagnosing		A critical thinker will defer identifying the client's diagnosis until more data are obtained and the client's priorities are known. This prevents a premature diagnosis based on insufficient data.
		As a critical thinker, the nurse is aware that the client's point of view may differ from the nurse's.
		Although the nurse may support the Western medical belief system that puts high priority on preventing disease, the critical thinker is also aware that the client may hold diverse views of health and illness, therapy, and preventive measures.
		The critical thinker recognizes that the client's erratic use of the prescribed medication may have multiple causes (e.g., troublesome side effects, or belief that illness is due to God's will and is not preventable) and will not infer a diagnosis with etiology until more data are obtained. Failure to think critically can lead to interpretations that are irrelevant, inadequate, and superficial (e.g., an erroneous interpretation that the client's problem is lack of sufficient knowledge).

(continued)

TABLE 21.3 (continued)

Nursing Process	Decision-Making Process	Clinical Application
		The critical thinker makes assumptions in accordance with a broad, unbiased database and mutually set client goals. The critical thinker avoids making unverified assumptions, for example, that an increase in knowledge will increase this client's compliance or that this client is motivated to prevent a cerebrovascular accident (CVA).
Planning		The critical thinker uses concepts about motivation, change theory, and multicultural nursing to understand the client's behaviour and motivation to change. Failure to think critically can lead to exclusive reliance on a simplistic concept, such as "knowledge creates change."
	Set the criteria. When the nurse sets the criteria for decision making, three questions must be answered: What is the desired outcome? What needs to be preserved? What needs to be avoided?	*Goal:* To increase compliance with medication regimen to relieve headaches and prevent a CVA. Thinking critically, a nurse will try to determine the client's goals and agree to mutual goals.
	Weight the criteria. In this step, the decision maker sets priorities or ranks activities or services from least important to most important as they relate to the specific situation. Because the weighting is specific to the situation, an activity may be ranked as most important in one situation and of less importance in another situation.	
	Seek alternatives. The decision maker identifies possible ways to meet the criteria. In clinical situations, the alternatives may be selected from a range of nursing interventions or client care strategies.	
	Examine alternatives. The nurse analyzes the alternatives to ensure that there is an objective rationale in relation to the established criteria for choosing one strategy over another.	
Implementing	*Implement.* The decision plan is placed into action.	The critical thinker considers the implications and consequences of selected nursing strategies before implementing plans of care. Plans of care, including goals and outcomes, are based on ongoing assessment of the client's cultural values, beliefs, and needs. Failure to think critically may lead to ineffective interventions, such as client teaching that focuses only on resolving a knowledge deficit about the prescribed medication. The critical thinker recognizes that a knowledge deficit may or may not be one of several problems.
Evaluating	*Evaluate the outcome.* As with all nursing care, in evaluating, the nurse determines the effectiveness of the plan and whether the initial purpose was achieved.	The critical thinker bases evaluation of client outcomes and the effectiveness of nursing interventions on well-developed, measurable criteria and considers rationally whether the outcomes have been validated. Failure to think critically may lead to client noncompliance and an inference that the client did not learn effectively and needs further instruction.

attitude becomes a matter of practice. Critical thinking is not an either/or phenomenon; people develop and use it more or less effectively along a continuum. Some people make better evaluations than others do; some people believe information from nearly any source; still others seldom believe anything without carefully evaluating the credibility of the information. Critical thinking is not easy. Solving problems and making decisions is risky. Sometimes, the outcome is not what was desired. With effort and practice, however, almost everyone can develop some level of critical thinking skills and become an effective problem solver and decision maker.

Reflection on Practice

Reflection is thinking from a critical point of view, analyzing why one acted in a certain way, and assessing the results of one's actions. To become a caring practitioner, reflection on practice must be personal and meaningful. *Reflective practice* is a form of self-evaluation and is a requirement of ongoing competence in nursing and a practice required by provincial and territorial regulation. Reflective journaling, as a tool for learning, is usually shared with a mentor or teacher, who works in partnership with the student. Reflection could be done with a partner or as a group. The nurse *can* reflect on situations in which he or she made decisions that were later regretted and to analyze thinking processes and attitudes or ask a trusted colleague to assess them. Identifying weak or vulnerable skills and attitudes is also important. Figure 21.2 shows a mind map that visually depicts the interactive concepts used in critical thinking. The action of reflection appears as part of three of the steps: the starting points, processes, and outcomes.

A framework, such as the one in Box 21.4 on the next page, provides structure for the journaling process. Writing reflections in a journal provides a space for the student to look at and acknowledge the deeper self. Guidance from a mentor or teacher can help the student view a nursing situation from many different perspectives. It helps the student find meaning in the event,

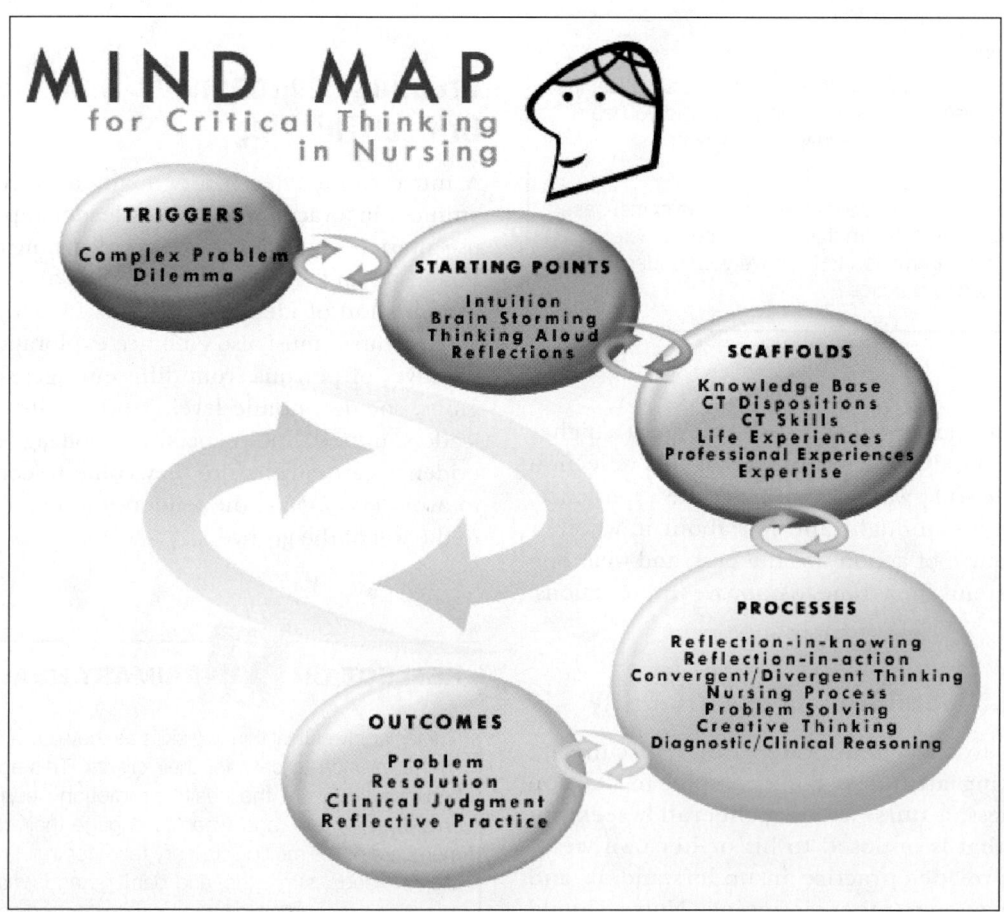

FIGURE 21.2 Mind map for critical thinking in nursing.

Source: Duphome, P. & Giddens, J. (2004). *Critical thinking in nursing resource.* Funded by an intramural grant of the College of Nursing, University of New Mexico.

BOX 21.4   A FRAMEWORK FOR REFLECTIVE JOURNALING

To engage in meaningful reflection, students must bring special skills to the process: self-awareness, description, critical analysis, synthesis, and evaluation (Bulman & Schutz, 2008). Using a framework is especially helpful to the beginner who is establishing the process of reflection. The framework listed below includes suggestions from several different models on reflection and can be further developed by the individual practitioner.

1. *What happened?*

   Describe the situation or event, including who was involved and the associated events. Avoid making judgments; simply describe.

2. *What did you do and think?*

   Describe your role in the situation, what you did, and your thoughts at the time. Again, focus on description only.

3. *What did it mean?*

   Analyze the meaning of the event to those involved. How did the environment or context of the event influence the participants? Bring in ideas from outside of the experience to enlighten and compare.

4. *How do you evaluate the situation?*

   What was good or bad about the experience, in light of your own values and feelings?

5. *What did you learn?*

   What conclusions did you reach about the situation, in a general sense? More specifically, what did you learn about yourself and your own way of working?

6. *Now what?*

   What are you going to do differently (or the same) based on what you learned from this experience? Where can you get more information to improve your understanding and approach to practice?

understand and learn through it, and emerge at a higher level of understanding. The purpose of this reflection is to determine what was learned from the experience, examine what was thought and felt about it, whether the current course of action was the best, and what one would do differently next time to improve future actions.

Tolerating Dissonance and Ambiguity

Nurses need to take deliberate efforts to cultivate critical thinking attitudes. For example, to develop fair-mindedness, a nurse could deliberately seek out information that is opposed to his or her own views. This action provides practice in understanding and learning to be open to other viewpoints. Nurses should increase their tolerance for ideas that contradict previously held beliefs, and they should practise suspending judgment.

Suspending judgment means tolerating ambiguity for a time. If an issue is complex, it may not be resolved quickly or neatly, and judgment should be postponed. For a while, the nurse will need to say, "I don't know" and be comfortable with that answer until more is known. Although postponing judgment may not be feasible in emergency situations, where fast action is required, it is often feasible in other situations.

Seeking Situations in Which Good Thinking Is Practised

Nurses will find it valuable to attend conferences in clinical or educational settings that support open examination of all sides of issues and respect opposing viewpoints. Cultivating a questioning attitude, by using either Socratic questioning or another technique, is vital (see the Reflect on Primary Health Care box). Nurses need to review the standards for evaluating thinking and apply them to their own thinking. If nurses are aware of their own thinking and assumptions—while they are doing the thinking—they can detect thinking errors.

Creating Environments That Support Critical Thinking

A nurse cannot develop or maintain critical thinking attitudes in a vacuum. Nurses in leadership positions can use a variety of strategies to create learning environments that foster and encourage differences of opinion and fair examination of ideas and options (Mundy & Denham, 2008). Nurses must also embrace exploration of the perspectives of persons from different ages, cultures, religions, socioeconomic levels, and family structures. As leaders, nurses should encourage colleagues to examine evidence carefully before they come to conclusions and to avoid *group think,* the tendency to defer unthinkingly to the will of the group.

REFLECT ON **PRIMARY HEALTH CARE**

Nurses apply critical thinking skills as they use a *primary health care approach* to care for their clients. This activity involves knowing *what* are the health-promotion needs of their clients; *how, where,* and *when* to engage their clients and the members of the multidisciplinary team for input regarding their clients' needs, strengths, and barriers; and *what* and *how* to adapt the resources or appropriate technology in order to design services and care that will meet the clients' socioeconomic and cultural needs.

Concept Mapping

Concept mapping is a technique that uses a graphic depiction of nonlinear and linear relationships to represent critical thinking. Also known as mind mapping, concept maps are context dependent and can be used to develop analytical skills. Concept maps allow one to organize (and reorganize) and connect information, making meaning of the concept that they represent. Concept maps provide an opportunity to "see" thinking; mapping is an effective method to facilitate creative, reflective, and critical thinking (Billings & Kowalski, 2008; Chabeli, 2010).

Concept Mapping and Critical Thinking

Concept mapping can be used to bridge nursing theory and practice by enhancing critical thinking processes when trying to understand complex phenomena (Billings & Halstead, 2012). Visual mapping of relationships enables students to develop and clarify links among key pieces of information. As a conceptual approach with active involvement, concept mapping promotes higher level thinking and decision-making skills. Because nurses are faced with copious amounts of information and are expected to consider more than one possibility, recognize emerging client problems, and intervene appropriately in life-threatening situations, concept mapping may be a valuable tool to improve nurses' critical thinking, clinical decision making, and performance (Rogal & Young, 2008; Wilgis & McConnell, 2008). Four basic types of maps are shown in Figure 21.3. See the Evidence-Informed Practice box on how to mobilize nursing students to employ the critical thinking process in practice situations.

EVIDENCE-INFORMED PRACTICE

How to Mobilize Nursing Students to Employ the Critical Thinking Process in Practice Situations

This qualitative study, carried out in an Eastern Canadian university, explored how students mobilize the critical thinking process in practice situations. Sixteen undergraduate baccalaureate female nursing students, ages 21 to 27 years, were interviewed. The findings revealed that eight types of knowledge were used to guide nursing students' practice: (a) intrapersonal, (b) interpersonal, (c) perceptual, (d) moral/ethical, (e) experiential, (f) practical, (g) scientific, and (h) contextual. To attain new knowledge, which was termed *combinational constructive knowledge,* a higher level of critical thinking is required for practical and moral reasoning and creativity. Students provide care by drawing on and assimilating various types of knowledge specific to the situation. Some types of knowledge may be relied on more than others; however, the process of using multiple types of knowledge through critical thinking results in this new knowledge.

NURSING IMPLICATIONS: **For students to provide competent and holistic care, nurse educators need to have a better understanding of the types of knowledge needed by their students and assist them to develop and practise critical thinking skills and abilities in both classroom and clinical settings.**

Source: Based on Lechasseur, K., Lazure, G., & Guilbert, L. (2011). Knowledge mobilized by a critical thinking process deployed by nursing students in practical care situations: A qualitative study. *Journal of Advanced Nursing, 67,* 1930–1940. doi: 10.1111/j.1365-2648.2011.05637.x

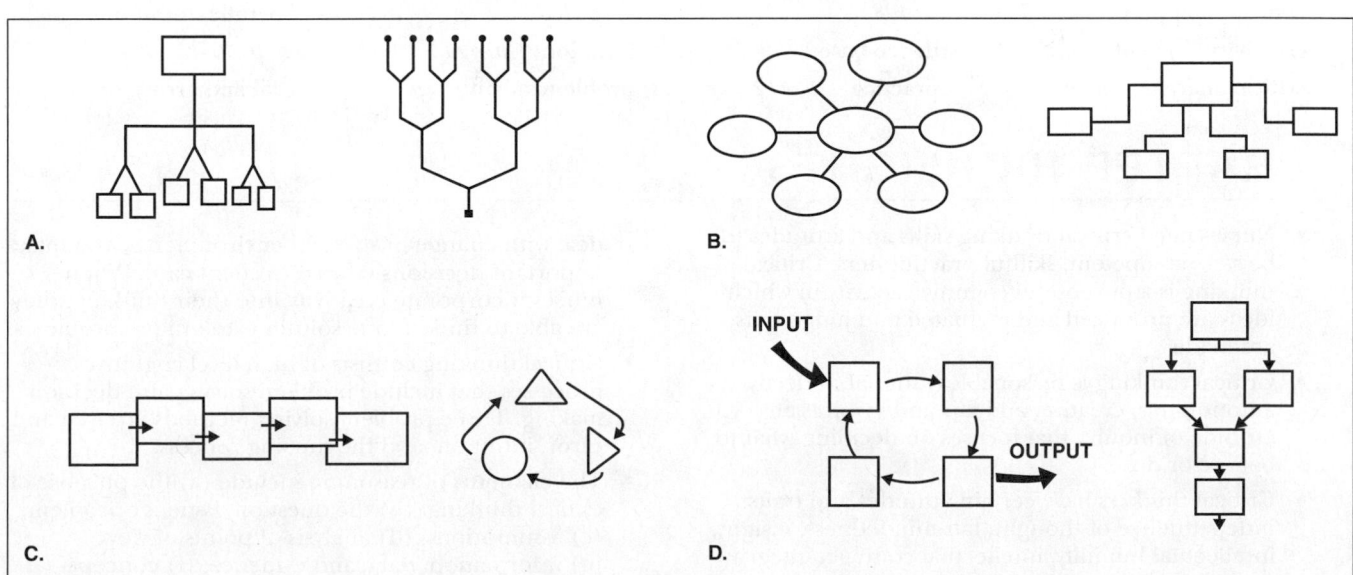

FIGURE 21.3 Types of concept maps: A, Hierarchical; B, Spider; C, Flowchart; D, Systems.

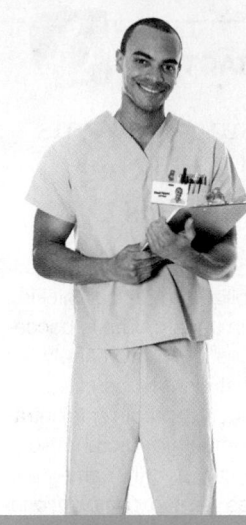

Case Study 21

You are taking the bus to downtown Vineland, an area that is unfamiliar to you. As a nursing student involved in a community health practice experience, you assess the neighbourhood along the bus route. There is graffiti on both residential and commercial buildings, trash is blowing along the road outside a number of premises, and some shops are closed, with boarded-up windows. You see a home with the front porch falling away, another home with a few broken windows, and a home with a roof that is missing many shingles. In your assessment, you notice that children reside in each of these residences, as older bikes and a few toys are scattered around each property. As the bus passes a gas station and convenience store, you notice a group of youth painting a mural depicting community development on the side of the gas station wall. When you pass by a city park in this neighbourhood, you see a child under 10 years old playing on a rusty swing set, while his young mother is close by, rocking her newborn. In the distance, a woman is pushing a grocery cart that is filled with items in garbage bags. The woman looks to be in her 50s and has a slow gait as she struggles with the cart. On your return to your nursing school, you meet with the community health faculty adviser to discuss the neighbourhood assessment experience.

CRITICAL THINKING QUESTIONS*

1. What conclusions can you draw about this neighbourhood on the basis of your assessment?

2. What further information would be relevant to support your conclusions?

3. How can a nursing student begin to address some of the actual and potential issues assessed within the neighbourhood?

4. What assumptions do you hold about this neighbourhood and the people you saw who reside in the area?

5. Do any of your assumptions reflect biases or prejudices?

6. What critical thinking skills were used to respond to this case study?

Check the eText in MyNursingLab for answers and explanations.

*Source: Questions adapted from Green, C. (2000). *Critical thinking in nursing: Case studies across the curriculum.* Upper Saddle River, NJ: Prentice Hall Health.

KEY TERMS

clinical judgment *p. 409*	critical thinking *p. 405*	evidence-informed nursing practice *p. 412*	reflection *p. 415*
Clinical Judgment Model *p. 409*	decision making *p. 412*		reflective thinking *p. 411*
clinical reasoning *p. 408*	deductive reasoning *p. 408*	inductive reasoning *p. 407*	research process *p. 412*
concept mapping *p. 417*			Socratic questioning *p. 407*
creativity *p. 406*	evidence-based practice *p. 412*	intuition *p. 411*	
critical analysis *p. 407*		problem solving *p. 411*	trial and error *p. 411*

CHAPTER HIGHLIGHTS

- Nurses need critical thinking skills and attitudes to be safe, competent, skillful practitioners. Critical thinking is a purposeful cognitive activity in which ideas are produced and evaluated and judgments are made.

- Critical thinking is reasonable, rational, reflective, autonomous, creative, and fair and inspires an attitude of inquiry that focuses on deciding what to believe or do.

- Critical thinkers have certain attitudes and traits: independence of thought, fair-mindedness, insight, intellectual humility, intellectual courage, integrity, perseverance, confidence, curiosity, and contextual awareness.

- Nurses use critical thinking as they apply knowledge from other subjects and fields to nursing practice,

deal with change in stressful environments, and make important decisions related to client care. When nurses incorporate creativity into their thinking, they are able to find unique solutions to unique problems.

- Critical thinking consists of high-level cognitive processes that include problem solving and decision making. Three problem-solving methods are trial and error, intuition, and the nursing process.

- The elements of reasoning include (a) the purpose of critical thinking, (b) the question, issue, or problem, (c) assumptions, (d) analysis of points of view, (e) information, data, and evidence, (f) concepts and theories, (g) inferences and conclusions, and (h) implications and consequences. Critical thinkers consider these elements when solving problems and making decisions.

- The nursing process and critical thinking are interrelated and interdependent, but they are not identical. Both involve problem solving, decision making, and creativity.

- Decisions must be made whenever several mutually exclusive choices exist. Nurses must make decisions in both their personal and professional lives. The steps of the decision-making process are identifying the purpose of the decision, setting the criteria, weighting the criteria, seeking alternatives, testing alternatives, troubleshooting, and evaluating the action.

- Almost everyone has at least some level of critical thinking skill, and that skill can be developed with practice. Some guidelines to enhance critical thinking skills and attitudes include making a self-assessment, tolerating dissonance and ambiguity, seeking situations in which good thinking is practised, and creating environments that support critical thinking.

- Clinical reasoning is described as a thought process used for a specific purpose in a practice setting. Context and priority setting are important components of clinical reasoning and various types of knowledge are drawn upon during this process.

ASSESS YOUR LEARNING

1. Mr. Richard runs into the emergency department. He screams, "My wife is bleeding! She is going to die! Quick, do something! She is losing our baby in the car!" What should the nurse do as a priority?

   a. Ask Mr. Richard to say where the car is and then conduct a summary assessment of the situation

   b. Tell a colleague to perform a vaginal examination as quickly as possible

   c. Inform the physician of the urgency of the situation and suggest that the operating room be prepared

   d. Tell Mr. Richard that he must calm down because his screaming is only making the situation worse and his cooperation is required

2. A patient with diarrhea has a physician's order for a bulk laxative daily. The nurse, not realizing that bulk laxatives can help solidify certain types of diarrhea, concludes that the physician does not know the patient has diarrhea. This statement is an example of which of the following?

   a. A fact

   b. An inference

   c. A judgment

   d. An opinion

3. A patient reports feeling hungry but does not eat when food is served. Using critical thinking skills, the nurse should do which of the following?

   a. Assess why the patient is not eating the food provided

   b. Continue to leave the food at the bedside until the patient is hungry enough to eat

   c. Notify the health care provider that tube feeding may be needed soon

   d. Believe the patient is not really hungry

4. The patient who is short of breath benefits from the head of the bed being elevated. Because this position can result in skin breakdown in the sacral area, the nurse decides to study the amount of sacral pressure occurring in other positions. This decision is an example of which of the following?

   a. The scientific method

   b. The trial and error method

   c. Intuition

   d. The nursing process

5. In the decision-making process, the nurse sets and weights the criteria, examines alternatives, and performs which of the following before implementing the plan?

   a. Re-examines the purpose for making the decision

   b. Consults the client and family members to determine their view of the criteria

   c. Identifies and considers various means for reaching the outcomes

   d. Determines the logical course of action should intervening problems arise

6. Mr. Scott is an 87-year-old man who had hip replacement surgery 2 weeks ago. Today is Mr. Scott's fourth day at the rehabilitation centre. His long-term plan is to return home after 6 weeks of therapy. Today is your first day caring for this patient. You have returned Mr. Scott to his room and helped him into bed for the night. Mr. Scott had a difficult time at physiotherapy this afternoon, and you have just spent an hour with him, listening to his concerns about getting up and around on his own in the future. Before leaving the room, what should you do?

   a. Inform Mr. Scott you will also be caring for him tomorrow and wish him goodnight

   b. Tell Mr. Scott you will turn out the lights and leave the door ajar as you leave

   c. Ensure Mr. Scott's call bell is within reach and the bedside rails are in the upright position

   d. Knowing Mr. Scott has an as-needed (prn) order for a sleeping pill, ask if he feels he will need a pill tonight

7. Mr. Avery is a 72-year-old man who had a myocardial infarction 3 weeks ago. He has been started on one Aspirin a day, a new anticoagulant, and a different

blood pressure (BP) medication. He continues to receive oxygen via nasal prongs. Next week he will be going home. The nurse enters his room to do his morning assessment, including his vital signs (BP, pulse, temperature, respirations, oxygen saturation). Mr. Avery tells the nurse he is having trouble catching his breath. The nurse notes his pulse is above the normal range, and his respirations seem laboured. The nurse interprets the situation, draws a conclusion about the patient's needs and decides to take action. What is the BEST description of this process?

    a. Clinical reasoning

    b. Clinical judgment

    c. Priority setting

    d. Critical thinking

8. You are the nurse asked to interview Mrs. Crocker, a 92-year-old woman who has just today come to the long-term care facility to live. You need to take a complete history from her. Which of the following should you do?

    a. Ensure you have the proper health history forms, enter the room, pull up a chair and sit down, introduce yourself, and begin the history

    b. Ensure you have the proper health history forms, knock, enter the room, introduce yourself, and explain what you would like to do

    c. Enter the room, find Mrs. Crocker sleeping, and decide to wait until tomorrow or the next day to complete the history

    d. Ensure you have the proper health history forms, enter the room, introduce yourself, stand at Mrs. Crocker's bedside, and complete the forms

9. Nancy Crane is the manager of the transplantation unit. She is concerned about having adequate staffing on the unit for the summer as several nurses have requested the same weekends off. How might the problem BEST be resolved?

    a. Call a unit meeting to consider what solutions the nursing staff might propose

    b. Propose that no holidays be permitted during the peak summer months

    c. Ask each nurse for his or her preferences and have a lottery

    d. Let everyone take the holidays they want and see what happens

10. Your classmate, Lydia, shares with you that she recently found a small lump in her breast and that she does not want to get a mammogram or see her nurse practitioner. She tells you her grandmother had breast cancer. She asks for your advice on what she should do. What is your BEST course of action?

    a. Ask if she would like to go for a walk and talk about her discovery

    b. Tell her not to worry about it, that it is probably nothing, but to keep an eye on it

    c. Offer to find some reading materials for her about mammograms and breast cancer

    d. Ask how you can support her in making a decision to deal with the issue

Check the eText in MyNursingLab for answers and explanations.

WEBLINKS

The Critical Thinking Community
http://www.criticalthinking.org
This is the Critical Thinking Community website, based on Dr. Richard Paul and Dr. Linda Elder's work on their critical concepts and tools.

The Critical Thinking Consortium
http://www.tc2.ca
This is a Canadian consortium of educational associations that promote critical thinking through research, professional development, and publications.

"A Practical Guide to Critical Thinking"
http://www.skepdic.com/essays/haskins.pdf
This paper is written as a guide to critical thinking and how to develop reasoning skills and arguments.

Rosalinda Alfaro-LeFevre, *Promoting Critical Thinking in Frontline Nurses*
http://www.alfaroteachsmart.com/index.html
This website provides resources for developing and enhancing critical thinking, specifically for registered nurses.

Registered Nurses' Association of Ontario: Nursing Best Practice Guidelines
http://rnao.ca/bpg
This site has a number of published guidelines, as well as a Toolkit and Educator's Resource to support implementation of best practices.

MyNursingLab
MyNursingLab's guided learning path makes reviewing and test preparation straightforward.

- Content summaries, animations, and videos reinforce key concepts and skills
- Practice questions help with test prep by showing gaps in knowledge
- An eText, available online and via the iPad, makes searching, highlighting, and note-taking easy

This QR code appears at the end of every chapter and provides learning resources that you can access with your smartphone to study on the go. Access self-review quizzes, flashcards, and more!

REFERENCES

Alfaro-LeFevre, R. (2008). *Critical thinking indicators.* Retrieved from http://www.alfaroteachsmart.com/cti.htm

Benner, P., Hughes, R. G., & Sutphen, M. (2008). Clinical reasoning, decision making and action: Thinking critically and clinically. In R. G. Hughes (Ed.). *Patient safety and quality: An evidenced-based handbook for nurses.* (Vol. 1, pp. 87–109). Rockville, MD: Agency for Health Care Research and Quality.

Benner, P. Sutphen, M., Leonard, V., & Day, L. (2010). Teaching and learning in clinical situations. In *Educating nurses: A call for radical transformation* (pp. 41–62). San Francisco, CA: Jossey-Bass.

Billings, D. M., & Halstead, J. A. (2012). *Teaching in nursing: A guide for faculty* (4th ed.). St. Louis, MO: Elsevier.

Billings, D. M., & Kowalski, K. (2008). Argument mapping. *Journal of Continuing Education in Nursing, 39,* 246–247. doi: 10.3928/00220124-20080601-09

Brookfield, S. D. (1987). Developing critical thinking. Challenging adults to explore alternative ways of thinking and acting (4th ed.). San Francisco, CA: Jossey-Bass.

Bulman, C., & Schutz, S. (2008). *Reflective practice in nursing* (4th ed.). Ames, IA: Blackwell Publishing.

Canadian Association of Schools of Nursing. (2006). *Position paper on baccalaureate education.* Ottawa, ON: Author.

Canadian Nurses Association. (2003). *The Canadian registered nurse examination. CRNE Bulletin.* Retrieved from http://www.cna-aiic.ca/CNA/documents/pdf/publications/CRNE_Bulletin_December_2003_e.pdf

Canadian Nurses Association. (2010). *Evidence-informed decision-making and nursing practice.* Retrieved from http://www.cna-aiic.ca/CNA/documents/pdf/publications/PS113_Evidence_informed_2010_e.pdf

Canadian Nurses Association. (2011). *Canadian registered nurse examination.* Retrieved from http://cna-aiic.ca/CNA/nursing/rnexam/default_e.aspx

Catalano, J. T. (2009). *Nursing now! Today's issues, tomorrow's trends* (5th ed.). Philadelphia, PA: Davis.

Chabeli, M. M. (2010). Concept-mapping as a teaching method to facilitate critical thinking in nursing education: A review of the literature. *Health SA Gesonheid, 15*(1). doi: 10.4102/hsag.v15il.432

DiCenso, A., Ciliska, D. K., & Guyatt, G. (2005). Introduction to evidence-based nursing. In A. DiCenso, G. Guyatt, & D. K. Ciliska (Eds.), *Evidence-based nursing: A guide to clinical practice* (pp. 3–19). St. Louis, MO: Elsevier Mosby.

Elder, L., & Paul, R. (2007). *The thinker's guide to analytic thinking.* Dillon Beach, CA: Foundation for Critical Thinking.

Kostovoch, C. T., Poradzisz, M., Wood, K., & O'Brian, K. L. (2007). Learning style preference and student aptitude for concept maps. *Journal of Nursing Education, 46,* 225–231.

Lechasseur, K., Lazure, G., & Guilbert, L. (2011). Knowledge mobilized by a critical thinking process deployed by nursing students in practical care situations: A qualitative study. *Journal of Advanced Nursing, 67,* 1930–1940. doi: 10.1111/j.1365-2648.2011.05637.x

Mundy, K., & Denham, S. A. (2008). Nurse educators—still challenged by critical thinking. *Teaching and Learning in Nursing, 3,* 94–99. doi: 10.1016/j.teln.2008.02.007

Oermann, M. H., & Gaberson, K. B. (2009). *Evaluation and testing in nursing education* (3rd ed.). New York, NY: Springer Publishing Company.

Parse, R. R. (1996). Critical thinking: What is it? *Nursing Science Quarterly, 9*(4), 139.

Paul, R. W. (1988). *What, then, is critical thinking?* From the Eighth Annual and Sixth International Conference on Critical Thinking and Educational Reform. Rohnert Park, CA: Center for Critical Thinking and Moral Critique, Sonoma State University.

Paul, R. W. (1993). *Critical thinking: How to prepare students for a rapidly changing world.* Santa Rosa, CA: Foundation for Critical Thinking.

Paul, R., & Elder, L. (2006). *A guide for educators to critical thinking competency standards.* Dillon Beach, CA: Foundation for Critical Thinking.

Piaget, J. (1966). *Origins of intelligence in children.* New York, NY: Norton.

Rogal, S. M., & Young, J. (2008). Exploring critical thinking in critical care nursing education: A pilot study. *Journal of Continuing Education in Nursing, 39,* 28–33. doi: 10.3928/00220124-20080101-08

Scheffer, B. K., & Rubenfeld, M. G. (2000). A consensus statement on critical thinking in nursing. *Journal of Nursing Education, 39,* 352–362.

Simmons, B. (2010). Clinical reasoning: Concept analysis. *Journal of Advanced Nursing, 66,* 1151–1158. doi: 10.1111/j.1365-2648.2010.05262.x

Simpson, E., & Courtney, M. (2002). Critical thinking in nursing education: Literature review. *International Journal of Nursing Practice, 8*(2), 89–98.

Tanner, C. A. (2006). Thinking like a nurse: A research-based model of clinical judgment in nursing. *Journal of Nursing Education, 45*(6), 204–211.

Titler, M. G., & Cameron, C. (2009). Use of research in practice. In G. Lobiondo-Wood, J. Haber, C. Cameron, & M. D. Singh (Eds.). *Nursing research in Canada: Methods and critical appraisal for evidence-based practice* (2nd Canadian ed, pp. 458-491). Toronto, ON: Elsevier Canada.

Wilgis, M., & McConnell, J. (2008). Concept mapping: An education strategy to improve graduate nurses' critical thinking skills during a hospital orientation program. *Journal of Continuing Education in Nursing, 39,* 119–126. doi: 10.3928/00220124-20080301-12

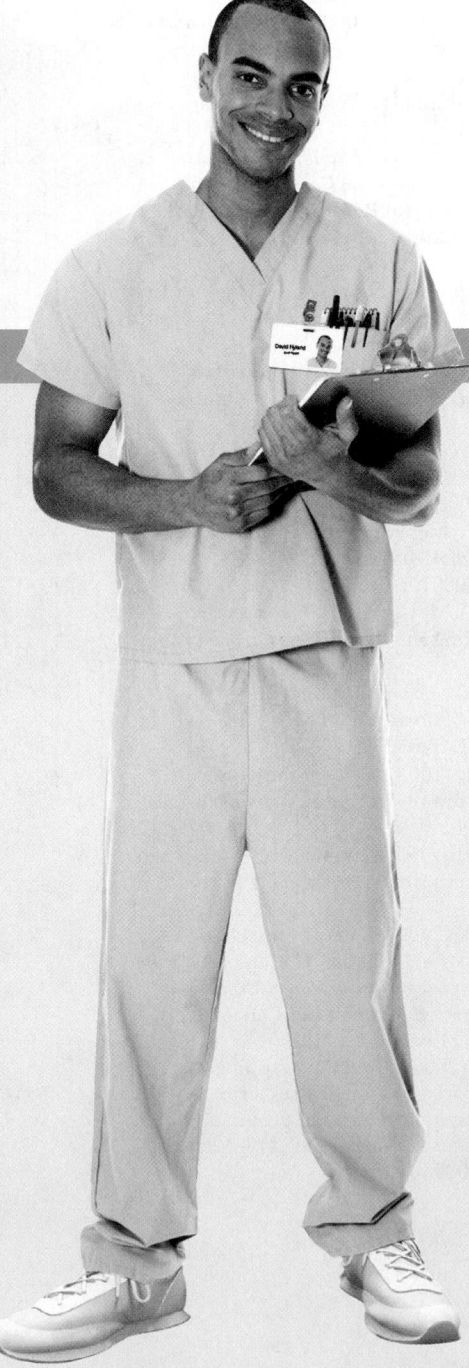

Chapter 22

Caring and Communicating

Many students enter the nursing profession because they want to care for people. In this caring profession, communication is both a critical and vital skill and is an integral part of the nurse–client relationship; it is the process by which people build relationships and experience joy. Nurses use communication to gather information, to teach and persuade, and to express caring and comfort. **Caring** is central to all helping professions, and enables people to create meaning in their lives. In caring for clients, nurses need strong communication skills to effectively convey client needs and wishes to the interdisciplinary team.

Professionalization of Caring

Caring is an essential aspect of nursing. **Caring practice** involves connection, mutual recognition, and involvement between the nurse and the client. Consider these examples of caring:

- A nurse talks quietly and holds the hand of a client who is in pain. The nurse's presence provides comfort for the client.
- A student nurse helps an elderly woman, who is immobilized, apply her makeup before greeting her daughter and grandchildren. The woman's sense of dignity is enhanced by this personal care.

The nurses involved in these situations experience caring through knowing that they have made a difference in their clients' lives. The caring process has benefits for the one giving care. By caring and being cared for, each person finds his or her place in the world. By serving others through caring, persons live the meaning of their own lives. The essence of caring is often found in the process itself—that of engagement and connection between the nurse and the client and between the nurse and the community (Hills & Watson, 2011; Watson, 2008). Caring includes assistive, supportive, and facilitative acts for individuals or groups.

Nursing Theories on Caring

The focus of any professional discipline is derived from its belief and value system, the nature of its service, and its area of knowledge development. The focus of nursing as a discipline has been defined as the study of *caring in the human health experience* (Newman, Sime, & Corcoran-Perry, 2009). Nurse scholars have reviewed the literature,

conducted research, and analyzed nurses' experiences, resulting in the development of theories and models of caring. These theories and models are grounded in humanism and the idea that caring is the basis for human science. Each theory develops different aspects of caring, describing how caring is unique in nursing. Several nursing theorists focus on caring: Leininger, Swanson, Watson, Benner and Wrubel, and Roach.

Culture Care Diversity and Universality (Leininger)

Madeleine Leininger's (Leininger & McFarland, 2006) theory of culture care diversity and universality is based on the assumption that nurses must understand various cultures to function effectively. Transcultural nursing focuses on both the differences and similarities among persons in diverse cultures. Although cultures have different ways of caring for others, certain universal behaviours are seen among all cultures of the world. To provide care that is congruent with cultural values, beliefs, and practices, the nurse must understand these differences and similarities. To understand the care desired by clients, the nurse requires knowledge of the culture and local language. When nursing care fails to be reasonably congruent with the client's beliefs, lifeways, and values, signs of conflict, noncompliance, and stress may arise.

Leininger believed that **culturally competent care** is provided in three ways: (a) by preserving the client's familiar lifeways, (b) by making accommodations in care that are satisfying to clients, and (c) by repatterning nursing care to help the client move toward wellness. Creative nursing approaches incorporating the above activities are needed to make care both meaningful and helpful to clients. She further defined caring as "those assistive, supportive, and enabling experiences or ideas towards others with evident or anticipated needs, to ameliorate or improve a human condition or lifeway" (Leininger & McFarland, 2006, p. 12).

Theory of Caring (Swanson)

Swanson (1991) defined caring as "a nurturing way of relating to a valued 'other,' toward whom one feels a personal sense of commitment and responsibility" (cited in Wojnar, 2010, p. 743). An assumption of her theory is that a client's well-being should be enhanced through the caring of a nurse who understands the common human responses to a specific health problem. The theory focuses on caring processes as nursing interventions. Swanson's theory was developed through interactions with parents at the time of pregnancy, miscarriage, and birth.

Swanson's Theory of Caring (Jansson & Adolfsson, 2011; Swanson, 1991) described the following five caring processes to guide nursing interventions:

1. *"Knowing"* involves the need for the nurse to understand the life event/situation experienced by the client and family. To do this, nurses engage themselves and centre their care on the client. As they conduct their thorough assessment, nurses must avoid making assumptions and look for cues as part of their data collection.

2. *"Being with"* encompasses how nurses convey caring and centre their presence on their clients. To do this, nurses must be empathic, and they must listen and attend to their clients' needs. Nurses must also convey their ability in providing care and share feelings or perspectives without burdening their clients.

3. *"Doing for"* refers to the need for nurses to do what needs to be done for their clients as the clients cope with their life situations. To do this, nurses carry out therapeutic caring actions such as comforting, anticipating, and performing care skillfully while protecting and preserving the dignity of their clients.

4. *"Enabling"* refers to how nurses facilitate their clients to move through life transitions and unfamiliar events. To do this, nurses empower their clients by providing information and explanation; and by supporting and allowing their clients to focus, to think through the situation and thereby to generate alternatives, and to seek validation and feedback for their actions.

5. *"Maintaining belief"* is the foundation of caring. Nurses maintain faith and a belief that people have the capacity to get through an event and find meaning and fulfillment as they move through their various life stages. To do this, nurses regard their clients in high esteem, maintain a hope-filled attitude, offer realistic optimism, help them to find meaning of the event or crisis, and offer the needed support during that particular time.

Theory of Human Care (Watson)

Watson's theory of human care views caring as the essence and the moral ideal of nursing. Human care is the basis for nursing's role in society; and nursing's contribution to society lies in its moral commitment to human care. Jean Watson (1999a, 1999b, 2008) described caring as being grounded in a set of universal human values: kindness, concern, and love of the self and others. It is the moral ideal of nursing and it involves the will to care, the intent to care, and the caring actions. Caring actions include communication, positive regard, support, or physical interventions by the nurse. Caring goes beyond the notions of curing at all costs. Within the caring situation, the nurse enters into the experience of the client, and the client can enter into the nurse's experience. The nurse maintains professional objectivity; both the nurse and the client seek a sense of harmony within the mind, body, and soul, thereby actualizing the real self. Such interpersonal contact, which touches the soul, has the power to generate the self-healing process.

The Primacy of Caring (Benner and Wrubel)

Benner and Wrubel (1989) viewed caring as the essence of excellence in nursing. Nursing is described as a relationship in which caring is primary because it sets up the possibility of giving and receiving help. Caring practice requires attending to the particular client over time, determining what matters to the person, and using this knowledge in clinical judgments.

A caring relationship requires a certain amount of openness and capacity to respond to care on the part of the client. In caring practice, being with someone can be just as important as doing something for that person, if not more so. As the nurse gains expertise, he or she learns how to be with people, to respect who they are and where they are at, and to stop doing for them. Thus, caring practice involves client advocacy and provides the necessary conditions to help the client grow and develop (Gordon, Benner, & Noddings, 1996).

Caring: The Human Mode of Being (Roach)

M. Simone Roach focused on caring as a philosophical concept and proposed that caring is the human mode of being, or the "most common, authentic criterion of humanness" (Roach, 2004, p. 28). Most persons are caring, and develop their caring abilities by being true to self, being real, and being who they truly are. Roach defined the following attributes as the "six Cs of caring": (a) compassion, (b) competence, (c) confidence, (d) conscience, (e) commitment, and (f) comportment (see Box 22.1 for definitions of each characteristic). The six Cs are used as a broad framework, suggesting categories of behaviour that describe professional caring.

Types of Knowledge in Nursing

Nursing involves different types of knowledge that are integrated to guide nursing practice. Nurses require scientific competence (empirical knowing), therapeutic use of self (personal knowing), moral/ethical awareness (ethical knowing), and creative action (aesthetic knowing). These four types of knowledge were identified by Carper (2009) from her observations of nurses' activities. An understanding of each type of knowledge is important for the student of nursing because only by integrating all ways of knowing can the nurse develop a professional practice. Figure 22.1 illustrates the interconnection of these different types of knowledge.

Empirical Knowing: The Science of Nursing

Knowledge about the empirical world is systematically organized into laws and theories for the purpose of describing, explaining, and predicting phenomena of special concern to the discipline of nursing. **Empirical knowing** ranges from factual, observable phenomena (e.g., anatomy, physiology, chemistry) to theoretical analysis (e.g., developmental theory, adaptation theory).

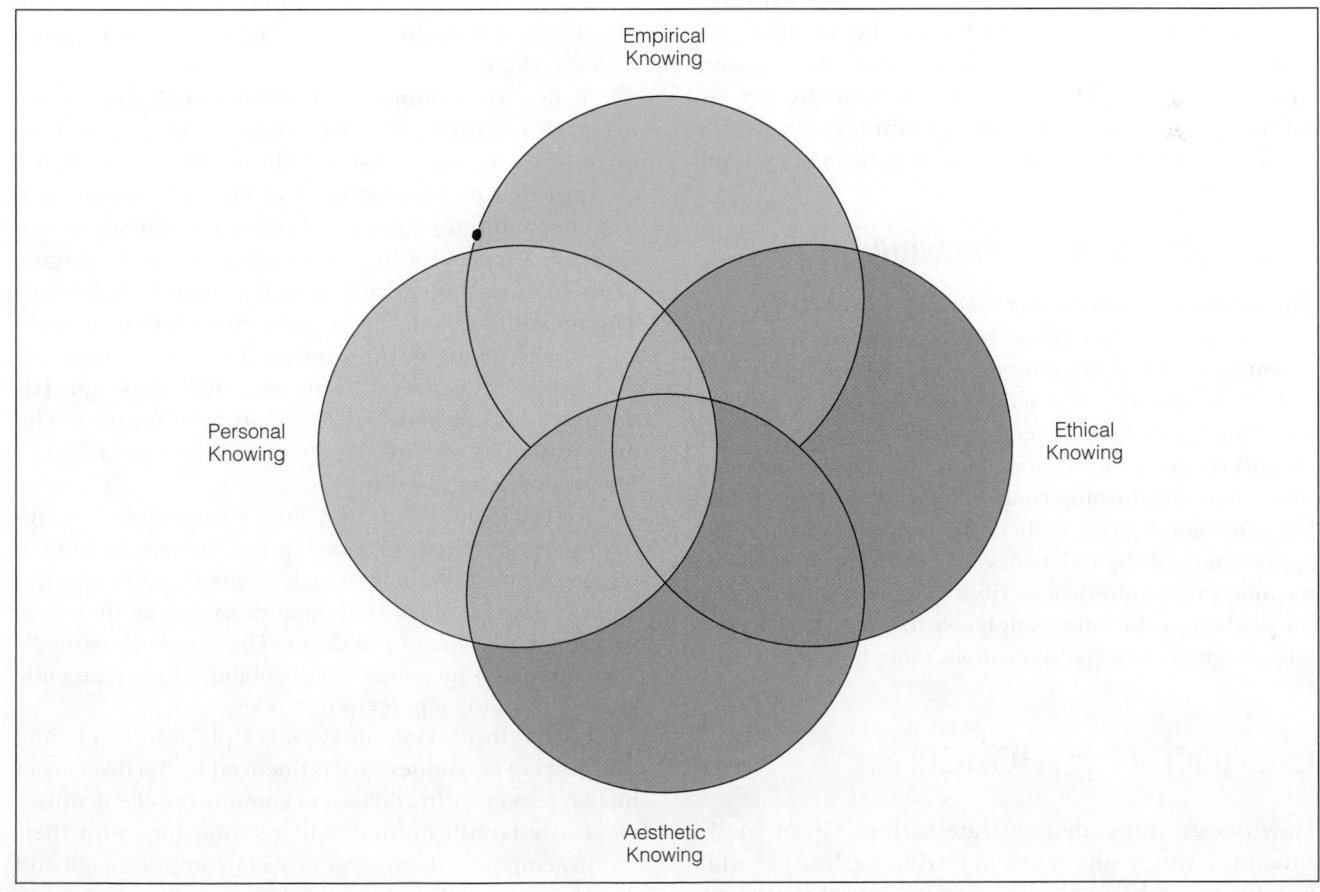

FIGURE 22.1 The four ways of knowing.

Personal Knowing: The Therapeutic Use of Self

Personal knowledge is concerned with the knowing, encountering, and actualizing of the concrete, individual self. Because nursing is an interpersonal process, the way in which nurses view their own selves and the client is of primary concern in any therapeutic relationship. **Personal knowing** promotes wholeness and integrity in the personal encounter, achieves engagement rather than detachment, and denies the manipulative or impersonal approach.

Ethical Knowing: The Moral Component

The goals of nursing include the conservation of life, alleviation of suffering, and promotion of health. **Ethical knowing** focuses on matters of obligation or what ought to be done and goes beyond following the ethical codes of the discipline. Nursing care involves a series of deliberate actions or choices that are subject to the judgment of right or wrong. Occasionally, the principles and norms that guide choices may be in conflict. The more sensitive and knowledgeable the nurse is to these issues, the more "ethical" the nurse will be.

Aesthetic Knowing: The Art of Nursing

Aesthetic knowing is the art of nursing and is expressed by the individual nurse through his or her creativity and style in meeting the needs of clients. The nurse uses aesthetic knowing to provide care that is both effective and satisfying. Empathy, compassion, holism, and sensitivity are important modes in the aesthetic pattern of knowing.

Developing Ways of Knowing

The methods for developing each type of knowledge mentioned above are unique (Chinn & Kramer, 2008). For example, personal knowing is developed through critical reflection on one's own actions and feelings in practice. Empirical knowing is gained from studying scientific models and theories and from making objective observations. Ethical knowing involves confronting and resolving conflicting values and beliefs. Aesthetic knowing arises from a deep appreciation of the uniqueness of each individual and the meanings that individual ascribes to a given situation. The nurse who practises effectively is able to integrate all types of knowledge to understand situations more holistically.

Caring in Practice

How does a nurse demonstrate caring? Given similar situations, why is one nurse judged to be "caring" while another is said to be "uncaring"? Nurse theorists and researchers have studied this question and identified caring attributes and behaviours. Consider, for example, Roach's six Cs, Watson's carative factors (see Chapter 4), and Swanson's structure of caring. Because caring is contextual, a nursing approach used with a client in one situation may be ineffective in another. Caring responses are as varied as clients' needs, environmental resources, and nurses' imaginations. When clients perceive the encounter to be caring, their sense of dignity and self-worth is increased, and feelings of connectedness are expressed. Common caring patterns include knowing the client, nursing presence, empowering the client, compassion, and competence.

Knowing the Client

Caring attends to the universality of the client's experience. The nurse asks: Who is this person? What is the client's history? needs? desires? dreams? spiritual beliefs? Who loves and cares for this person at home? Where is home, and what resources are there? What does this person need today, from me, right now? Can this person tell me what is needed? Personal knowledge of the client is a key in the caring relationship between nurse and client. The nurse aims to know who the client is, in his or her *uniqueness*. This knowledge is gained by observing and talking with the client and family while using effective listening and communication skills. The nurse cannot remain detached but is actively engaged with the client.

Take, for example, an older client experiencing postoperative pain after removal of a cancerous prostate. The nurse assesses the client's pain, using an appropriate pain scale. The client's positioning, hygiene, amount of rest, and other physiological variables are assessed for their effect on pain. Is this surgery likely to cure the cancer, or is it primarily palliative? The meaning of the diagnosis and surgery to this client affects his pain experience. The nurse discovers that this man lost his wife to cancer 2 years ago. His daughter, at the bedside, is his primary support. The nurse discusses with his daughter how she can make her father more comfortable.

Knowing the client and family ultimately involves the nurse and client in a caring transaction. By attending broadly to personal, ethical, aesthetic, and empirical knowledge, the nurse understands events as they have meaning in the life of the client. The nurse's *knowing the client* ultimately increases the possibilities for therapeutic interventions to be perceived as relevant.

Caring in nursing always takes place in a relationship. Caring encounters are influenced by the diversity of human responses. In addition to knowing the client, nurses need to establish mutuality in relationships with their clients, empower them, and provide compassionate and competent care. Caring for self is central to caring for others. Self-care includes a healthy lifestyle (e.g., nutrition, activity and exercise, recreation) and mind–body therapies (e.g., guided imagery, meditation, yoga).

Relational ethics (RE) is an action ethic. One acts in ways that lead to goodness without being absolutely sure if one is right (Storch, Rodney, & Starzomski, 2012). Nurses act using relational ethics as a guide for practice. Nurses often do not know the whole picture and therefore act knowing that something must be done.

Communicating

Communication is a critical skill for nursing. It is the process by which humans meet their survival needs, build relationships, and experience emotions. In nursing, communication is a dynamic process used to gather assessment data, to teach and persuade, and to express caring and comfort. It is an integral part of the helping relationship.

The term *communication* has various meanings, depending on the context in which it is used. To some, **communication** is the interchange of information between two or more people; in other words, it is the exchange of ideas or thoughts, a transmission of feelings, or a more personal and social interaction between two or more people. This kind of communication uses such methods as talking and listening or writing and reading; however, painting, dancing, storytelling, and body gestures are also means of communication.

Communication is often synonymous with *relating*. Frequently, one member of a couple comments that the other is not communicating (e.g., some teenagers complain about a generation gap—being unable to communicate with understanding or feeling to a parent or authority figure).

The *intent* of any communication is to elicit a response. When individuals communicate, they have a purpose. Thus, communication is a process. It has two main purposes: (a) to influence others and (b) to obtain information. Helpful communication encourages a sharing of information, thoughts, or feelings between two or more people. Unhelpful communication hinders or blocks the transfer of information and feelings.

Nurses who communicate effectively are better able to collect assessment data, initiate interventions, evaluate outcomes of interventions, initiate change that promotes health, and prevent the safety and legal problems associated with nursing practice. The communication process is built on a trusting relationship with a client and support persons. Effective communication is essential for the establishment of a nurse–client relationship.

Communication can occur on an intrapersonal level within a single individual, as well as on interpersonal and group levels. Intrapersonal communication is the communication that you have with yourself (i.e., *self-talk*). Both the sender and the receiver of a message usually engage in this type of communication. It involves thinking about the message before it is sent, while it is being sent, and after it is sent, and it occurs constantly. Consequently, intrapersonal communication can interfere with a person's ability to hear a message as the sender intended.

The Communication Process

Communication involves a sender, a message, a receiver, and a response or feedback (Figure 22.2). It is a two-way process that involves the sending and receiving of messages between at least two individuals (Burkhardt, Nathaniel, & Walton, 2010). Because the intent of communication is to elicit a response, the process is ongoing; the receiver of the message then becomes the sender of a response, and the original sender then becomes the receiver.

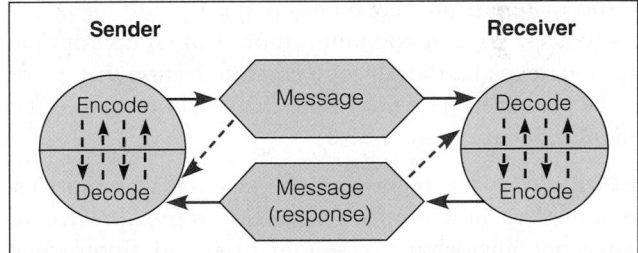

FIGURE 22.2 The communication process. The dashed arrows indicate intrapersonal communication (self-talk). The solid lines indicate interpersonal communication.

SENDER   The **sender**, a person or group who wants to convey a message to another, can be considered the *source encoder*. This term suggests that the person or group sending the message must have an idea or reason for communicating (source) and must put the idea or feeling into a form that can be transmitted. **Encoding** involves the selection of specific signs or symbols (codes) to transmit the message, such as which language and words to use, how to arrange the words, and what tone of voice and gestures to use. For example, if the receiver speaks English, the sender usually selects English words. If the message is "Mr. Johnson, smoking is not permitted in patient rooms in this hospital," the tone of voice selected will be one of firmness, and a shake of the head or a pointing index finger can reinforce it. The nurse must not only deal with dialects and foreign languages but also must cope with two language approaches—the layperson's and the health care professional's.

MESSAGE   The **message** refers to what is actually said or written, the body language that accompanies the words, and how the message is transmitted. The medium used to convey the message is the channel. It is important for the channel to be appropriate for the message, and it should help make the intent of the message clearer.

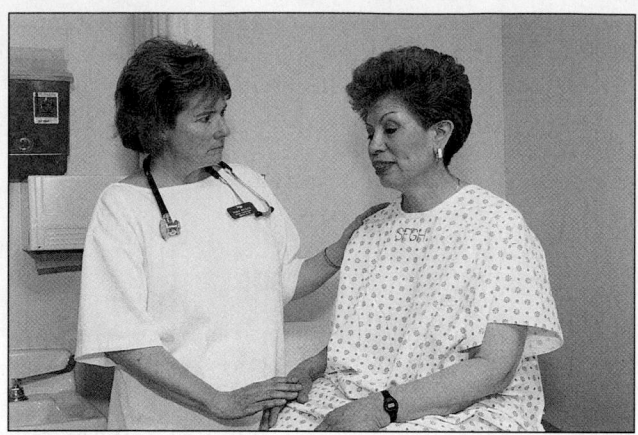

FIGURE 22.3 Appropriate forms of touch can communicate caring.

Talking face to face with a person can be more effective in some instances than telephoning or writing a message. Recording messages on tape or communicating by radio or television may be more appropriate for larger audiences. Written communication is often appropriate for long explanations or for a communication that needs to be preserved. The nonverbal channel of touch is often highly effective (Figure 22.3).

RECEIVER   The **receiver** is the listener, who must listen, observe, and attend. This person is the *decoder*, who must perceive what the sender intended (interpretation). Perception uses all the senses to receive verbal and nonverbal messages. To **decode** means to relate the message perceived to the receiver's storehouse of knowledge and experience and to sort out the meaning of the message. Whether the message is decoded accurately by the receiver, according to the sender's intent, depends largely on their similarities in knowledge and experience and sociocultural background. If the meaning of the decoded message matches the intent of the sender, then the communication has been effective. Ineffective communication occurs when the message sent is misinterpreted by the receiver. For example, Mr. Johnson may perceive the message accurately—"No smoking is allowed in my room." However, if experience has taught him that he can smoke in his room if a certain nurse is on duty, he will interpret the intent of the message differently.

RESPONSE   *Response* is the message that the receiver returns to the sender. It is also called **feedback**. Feedback can be verbal, nonverbal, or both. Nonverbal examples are a nod of the head or a yawn. Either way, feedback allows the sender to correct or reword a message. In the case of Mr. Johnson, the receiver may appear irritated or say, "Well, the nurse on evening shift lets me smoke." The sender then knows the message was interpreted accurately. However, now the original sender becomes the receiver, who is required to decode and respond.

Modes of Communication

Communication is generally carried out in two different modes: (a) verbal and (b) nonverbal. **Verbal communication** uses the spoken or written word; **nonverbal communication** uses other forms, such as gestures or facial expressions and touch. Although both kinds of communication occur concurrently, the majority of communication is nonverbal. Learning about nonverbal communication is thus important for nurses in developing effective communication patterns and relationships with clients.

Another form of communication has evolved with technology—**electronic communication**. The most common form of electronic communication is e-mail, in which an individual can send a message, by computer, to another person or group of people. Nurses must decide when it is appropriate and not appropriate to use e-mail when communicating with clients and follow agency policies regarding privacy and confidentiality as well as therapeutic nurse–client relationships and boundaries.

VERBAL COMMUNICATION   Verbal communication is largely conscious because people choose the words they use. The words used vary among individuals according to culture, socioeconomic background, age, and education. As a result, countless possibilities exist for the ways ideas are exchanged. An abundance of words can be used to form messages. In addition, a wide variety of feelings can be conveyed when people talk.

When choosing words to say or write, nurses need to consider (a) pace and intonation, (b) simplicity, (c) clarity and brevity, (d) timing and relevance, (e) adaptability, (f) credibility, and (g) humour.

Pace and Intonation   The manner of speech, as in the pace or rhythm and intonation, will modify the feeling and impact of the message. The intonation can express enthusiasm, sadness, anger, or amusement. The pace of speech can indicate interest, anxiety, boredom, or fear.

Simplicity   Many complex technical terms become natural to nurses; however, laypersons often misunderstand these terms. Words such as *vasoconstriction* or *cholecystectomy* are common terms and easy for the nurse to use but are incomprehensible when communicating with clients. Nurses need to select simple, appropriate, and understandable terms based on the age, knowledge, culture, and education of the client. For example, instead of saying to a client, "The nurses will be catheterizing you tomorrow for a urinalysis," it may be more appropriate and understandable to say, "Tomorrow we need to get a sample of your urine, so we will collect it by putting a small tube into your bladder." The latter statement is more likely to elicit a response from the client asking why it is needed and whether it will be uncomfortable because the client understands the message being conveyed by the nurse.

Clarity and Brevity   Clarity is saying precisely what is meant and brevity is using the fewest words necessary.

The result is a message that is simple and clear. An aspect of this is congruence or consistency, in which the nurse's behaviour or nonverbal communication matches the words spoken. When the nurse tells the client, "I am interested in hearing what you have to say," the nonverbal behaviour would include the nurse facing the client, making eye contact, and leaning forward. The goal is to communicate clearly so that all aspects of a situation or circumstance are understood. To ensure clarity in communication, nurses also need to speak slowly and enunciate carefully.

Timing and Relevance   No matter how clearly or simply words are stated or written, the timing needs to be appropriate to ensure that words are heard, and the messages are related to the person or to the person's interests and concerns. This involves sensitivity to the client's needs and concerns. For example, a client who is enmeshed in fear of cancer may not hear the nurse's explanations about the expected procedures before and after gallbladder surgery. In this situation, the nurse first has to encourage the client to express concerns and then to deal with those concerns. The necessary explanations can be provided at another time when the client is able to listen.

Another problem in timing is asking several questions at once. For example, a nurse enters a client's room and says in one breath, "Good morning, Mrs. Brody. How are you this morning? Did you sleep well last night? Is your partner coming to see you before your surgery?" The client no doubt wonders which question to answer first, if any. Avoid asking a question and then not waiting for an answer before making another comment.

Adaptability   Spoken messages need to be altered in accordance with behavioural cues from the client. This adjustment is referred to as *adaptability*. What the nurse says and how it is said must be individualized and carefully considered. This requires astute assessment and sensitivity on the part of the nurse. For example, a nurse who usually smiles, appears cheerful, and greets the client every afternoon with an enthusiastic "Hi, Mrs. Brown!" notices that the client is not smiling and appears distressed. It is important for the nurse to modify tone of speech and express concern in facial expression while moving toward the client.

Credibility   *Credibility* means "worthiness of belief, trustworthiness, and reliability." Nurses foster credibility by being consistent, dependable, and honest. The nurse needs to be knowledgeable about what is being discussed and to have accurate information. Nurses should convey confidence and certainty in what they are saying while being able to acknowledge their limitations: "I don't know the answer to that, but I will find someone who does."

Humour   The use of humour can be a positive and powerful tool in the nurse–client relationship, but it must be used with care. Humour can be used to help clients adjust to difficult and painful situations. The physical act of laughter can be both an emotional and physical release, reducing tension by providing a different perspective and promoting a sense of well-being. When using humour, it is important to consider the client's perception of what is considered humorous. Timing is also important to consider. Though humour and laughter can help reduce stress and anxiety, the feelings of the client need to be considered (Moore, 2008).

NONVERBAL COMMUNICATION   Nonverbal communication is sometimes called *body language*. It includes gestures, body movements, use of touch, and physical appearance, including adornment. Nonverbal communication often tells others more about what a person is *feeling* than what is actually said (Figure 22.4). Nonverbal communication either reinforces or contradicts what is said verbally. For example, if a nurse says to a client, "I'd be happy to sit here and talk to you for a while" and yet glances nervously at a watch every few seconds, the

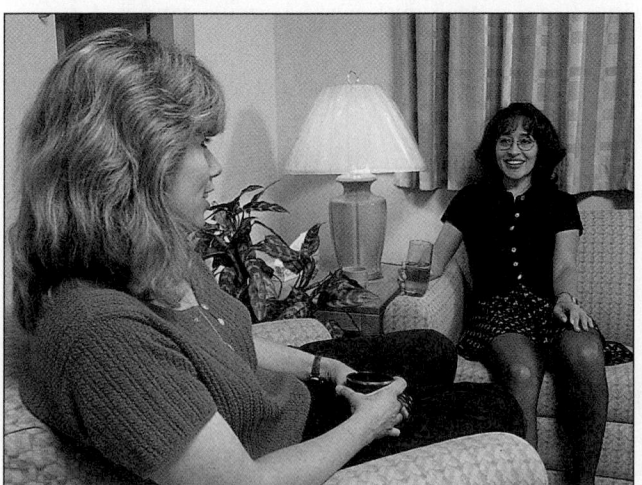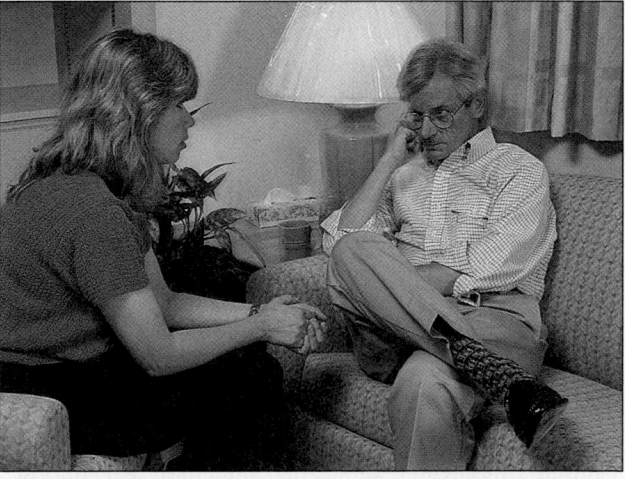

FIGURE 22.4 Nonverbal communication sometimes conveys meaning more effectively than words. A: The postures of these women indicate openness to communication. B: The listener's posture suggests resistance to communication.

actions contradict the verbal message. The client is more likely to believe the nonverbal behaviour, which conveys "I am very busy and need to leave."

Observing and interpreting the client's nonverbal behaviour is an essential skill for nurses to develop. To observe nonverbal behaviour efficiently requires a systematic assessment of the person's overall physical appearance, posture, gait, facial expressions, and gestures. Whatever is observed, the nurse needs to exercise caution in interpretation, always clarifying any observation with the client.

Transculturally, nonverbal communication varies widely (Hearnden, 2008). Even in such behaviours as smiling and hand shaking, cultures differ. For example, to many Hispanics, smiling and hand shaking are an integral part of an interaction and essential to establishing trust. The same behaviour might be perceived by a Russian as insolent and frivolous.

The nurse cannot always be sure of the correct interpretation of the feelings expressed nonverbally. The same feeling can be expressed nonverbally in more than one way, even within the same cultural group. For example, anger may be communicated by aggressive or excessive body motion, or it may be communicated by frozen stillness. Therefore, the interpretation of such observations requires validation with the client. For example, the nurse might say, "You look as if you have been crying. Do you want to talk about it?"

Clients who have altered thought processes, such as in schizophrenia or dementia, may experience times when expressing themselves verbally is difficult or impossible. During these times, the nurse needs to be able to interpret the feeling or emotion that the client is expressing nonverbally. An attentive nurse who clarifies observations very often portrays caring and acceptance to the client. This can be a beginning for establishing a trusting relationship between the nurse and the client, even in clients who have difficulty communicating appropriately.

Personal Appearance Clothing and adornments can be rich sources of information about a client. Although choice of apparel is highly personal, it can convey social and financial status, culture, religion, group association, and self-concept. Charms and amulets may be worn for decorative or for health-protection purposes. When the symbolic meaning of an object is unfamiliar, the nurse can inquire about its significance, which may foster rapport with the client.

How a person dresses is often an indicator of how the person feels. Someone who is tired or ill may not have the energy or the desire to maintain normal grooming. When a person known for immaculate grooming becomes lax about appearance, the nurse may suspect a loss of self-esteem or a physical illness. The nurse must validate these observed nonverbal data by asking the client. A change in grooming habits may signal that the client is feeling better; for example, a man may request a shave, or a woman may request a shampoo and some makeup.

Posture and Gait The ways people walk and carry themselves are often reliable indicators of self-concept, current mood, and health. Erect posture and an active, purposeful stride suggest a feeling of well-being. Slouched posture and a slow, shuffling gait suggest depression or physical discomfort. Tense posture and a rapid, determined gait suggest anxiety or anger. The posture of people when they are sitting or lying can also indicate feelings or mood. Again, the nurse clarifies the meaning of the observed behaviour by describing to the client what the nurse sees and then asking what it means or whether the nurse's interpretation is correct. For example, "You look as if it really hurts to move. Are you in pain? What would help make you feel more comfortable?"

Facial Expression No part of the body is as expressive as the face (see Figure 22.5). Feelings of surprise, fear, anger, disgust, happiness, and sadness can be conveyed by facial expressions. Although the face can express the person's genuine emotions, it is also possible to control these muscles so the emotion expressed does not reflect what the person is feeling. Many facial expressions convey a universal meaning. The smile expresses happiness. Contempt is conveyed by the mouth turned down, the head tilted back, and the eyes directed down the nose. No single expression can be interpreted accurately, however, without considering other reinforcing physical cues, the setting in which it occurs, the expression of others in the same setting, and the cultural background of the client.

Nurses need to be aware of their own expressions and what they are communicating with clients. Clients are quick to notice the nurse's facial expression, particularly when a client feels unsure or uncomfortable. The client who questions the nurse about a feared diagnostic result will watch whether the nurse maintains eye contact or looks away when answering. The client who has had disfiguring surgery will examine the nurse's face for signs of disgust. It is impossible to control all facial expression, but the nurse must learn to control expressions of feelings like fear or disgust in some circumstances.

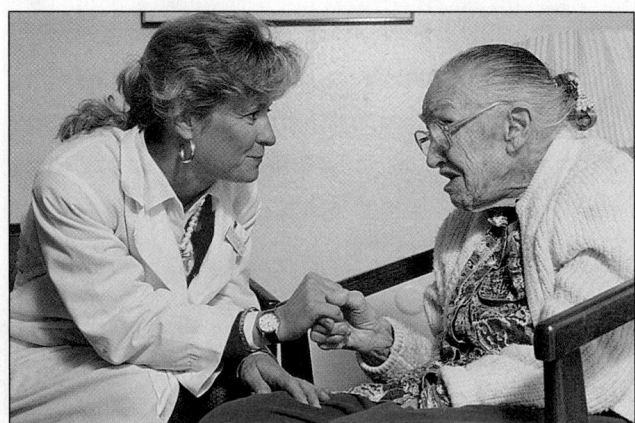

FIGURE 22.5 The nurse's facial expression communicates warmth and caring.

Eye contact is another essential element of facial communication. In many cultures, mutual eye contact acknowledges recognition of the other person and a willingness to maintain communication. Often, a person initiates contact with another person with a glance, capturing the person's attention before communicating. A person who feels weak or defenceless often averts the eyes or avoids eye contact; in some Eastern cultures, avoiding eye contact is a sign of respect to others.

Gestures Hand and body gestures can emphasize and clarify the spoken word, or they can occur without words to indicate a particular feeling or to give a sign. A parent awaiting information about his child in surgery may wring his hands or pick his nails. A gesture may more clearly indicate the size or shape of an object. A wave goodbye and the motioning of a visitor toward a chair are gestures that have relatively universal meanings. Some gestures, however, are culture specific. The North American gesture meaning "shoo" or "go away" means "come here" or "come back" in some Asian cultures. In the Hmong culture, it is considered rude to point at something with your toe.

For people with special communication problems, such as those with hearing impairment, the hands are invaluable in communication, and many learn sign language. Persons with illnesses who are unable to reply verbally can similarly devise a communication system that uses hands. The client may be able to raise an index finger once for "yes" and twice for "no." Other signals can often be devised by the client and the nurse to denote other meanings.

ELECTRONIC COMMUNICATION: E-MAIL Computers are increasingly playing a big role in nursing practice. Many health care agencies are moving toward electronic medical records in which nurses document their assessments and nursing care. Electronic mail (e-mail) can be used in health care facilities for many purposes: to schedule and confirm appointments, to report lab results, to conduct client education, and to follow up with discharged clients (Macon & Mendiola, 2008)

E-mail (including texting) is the most common form of electronic communication. It is important for the nurse to know the advantages and disadvantages of e-mail and also other guidelines to ensure client confidentiality.

Advantages of E-Mail E-mail is a fast, efficient way to communicate, and it is legible. It provides a record of the date and time of the message that was sent or received. Some health care facilities provide information to their clients on how they can reach, via e-mail, specified staff members. This improves communication and continuity of client care. E-mail promises better access, and one research study indicated that half of Internet users would like to communicate with doctors online (Reid & Wagner, 2008).

Disadvantages of E-Mail E-mail can be a risk to client confidentiality. Organizations must apply reasonable and appropriate safeguards when e-mailing protected health information. The health care agency needs to have an e-mail encryption system to ensure security.

Austin (2006) suggested that the use of e-mail be avoided in the following situations:

- When the information is urgent and the client's health could be in jeopardy if he or she does not read it immediately
- When the information is highly confidential (e.g., human immunodeficiency virus (HIV) status, mental health, chemical dependency)
- In the case of lab results showing abnormality: If the information is confusing and could prompt many questions by the client, it is better to either telephone the client or see him or her in person.

Other Guidelines Concerning E-Mail Agencies usually develop standards and guidelines for the use of e-mail in health care. It is important to know, per the agency's guidelines, what can be e-mailed to clients. Usually, clients need to sign an e-mail consent form first. This form provides information about the risks of e-mail and authorizes the health care agency to communicate with the client at a specified e-mail address.

The nurse can identify in the subject line that the e-mail is important or needs immediate attention. Instead of identifying the e-mail as "confidential" in the subject line, the nurse can include a disclaimer that the message is to be read only by the person to whom it is addressed and that no one else is authorized to read the message. Additionally, the disclaimer should state that if the e-mail is sent to anyone else by mistake, he or she should contact the sender.

Information sent to a client via e-mail is considered part of the client's medical record. Therefore, a copy of the e-mail needs to be included in the client's file. E-mails, like other documentation in the client's record, may be used as evidence during litigation.

E-mail is another form of communication that can enhance effective relationships with clients. It is not, however, a substitute for effective verbal and nonverbal communication. Nurses need to use their professional judgment about what forms of communication will best meet their client's health care needs.

Factors Influencing the Communication Process

Many factors influence the communication process. Some of these are development, gender, values and perceptions, personal space, territoriality, roles and relationships, environment, congruence, attitudes, and boundaries.

DEVELOPMENT Language, psychosocial, and intellectual development move through stages across the lifespan. Knowledge of a client's developmental stage will allow the nurse to modify the message accordingly. The use of dolls and games with simple language can help explain a procedure to an 8-year-old. With adolescents who have developed more abstract thinking skills, a more detailed explanation can be given, whereas a well-educated, middle-aged business executive may want to have detailed technical information provided. Older clients are apt to have had a wider range of experiences with the health care system, which can influence their response or understanding. With aging also come changes in vision and hearing acuity that can affect nurse–client interactions.

GENDER From an early age, females and males communicate differently. Girls tend to use language to seek confirmation, minimize differences, and establish intimacy. Boys use language to establish independence and negotiate status within a group. These differences can continue into adulthood so that the same communication may be interpreted differently by a man and a woman.

VALUES AND PERCEPTIONS Values are the standards that influence behaviour, and perceptions are the personal view of an event. Because each person has unique personality traits, values, and life experiences, each will perceive and interpret messages and experiences differently. For example, if the nurse draws the curtains around a crying woman and leaves her alone, the woman may interpret this as "The nurse thinks that I will upset others and that I shouldn't cry" or "The nurse respects my need to be alone." It is important for the nurse to be aware of a client's values and to validate or correct perceptions to avoid creating barriers in the nurse–client relationship.

PERSONAL SPACE **Personal space** is the distance people prefer in interactions with others. Middle-class North Americans use definite distances in various interpersonal relationships, along with specific voice tones and body language. Communication, thus, alters in accordance with four distances, each with a close and a far phase. Tamparo and Lindh (2008) listed the following example:

1. Intimate: Touching to 0.5 m
2. Personal: 0.5 m to 1.3 m
3. Social: 1.3 m to 4 m
4. Public: 4 m and beyond

Intimate distance communication is characterized by body contact, heightened sensations of body heat and smell, and vocalizations that are low. Intimate distance is frequently used by nurses. Examples include cuddling a baby, touching the sightless client, positioning clients, observing an incision, and restraining a toddler for an injection.

It is a natural protective instinct for people to maintain a certain amount of space immediately around them, and the amount varies with individuals and cultures. When someone who wants to communicate steps too close, the receiver automatically steps back a pace or two.

In their therapeutic roles, nurses often are required to violate this personal space. However, it is important for them to be aware when this will occur and to forewarn the client. In many instances, the nurse can respect (not come as close as) a person's intimate distance. In other instances, the nurse can come within intimate distance to communicate warmth and caring.

Personal distance is less overwhelming than intimate distance. Physical contact, such as hand shaking or touching a shoulder, is possible. More of the person is perceived at a personal distance so that nonverbal behaviours, such as body stance or full facial expressions, are seen with less distortion. Much communication between nurses and clients happens at this distance. Examples occur when nurses are sitting with clients, giving medications, or establishing an intravenous infusion. Communication at a close personal distance can convey involvement by facilitating the sharing of thoughts and feelings. At the outer extreme of 1.3 m, however, less involvement is conveyed.

Social distance is characterized by a clear visual perception of the whole person. This communication is formal and is limited to seeing and hearing. It is expedient in communicating with several people at the same time or within a short time. Examples occur when nurses make rounds or wave a greeting to someone. Social distance is important in accomplishing the business of the day. However, it is frequently misused. For example, the nurse who stands in the doorway and asks a client, "How are you today?" will receive a more noncommittal reply than the nurse who moves to a personal distance to inquire.

Public distance requires loud, clear vocalizations with careful enunciation. Although the faces and forms of people are seen at public distance, individuality is lost. Instead, the perception is of the group of people or the community.

TERRITORIALITY **Territoriality** is a concept of the space and things that an individual considers as belonging to the self. Territories marked off by people can be visible to others. For example, patients in a hospital often consider their territory as bounded by the curtains around the bed unit or by the walls of a private room. This human tendency to claim territory must be recognized by all health care workers. Patients often feel the need to defend their territory when it is invaded by others; for example, when a visitor or nurse removes a chair to use at another bed, the visitor has inadvertently violated the territoriality of the client whose chair was removed. Nurses need to obtain permission from patients to remove, rearrange, or borrow objects in their hospital area.

ROLES AND RELATIONSHIPS The roles and the relationship between sender and receiver affect the communication process. Such roles as nursing student and instructor, client and physician, or parent and child affect the content and responses in the communication process. Choice of words, sentence structure, and tone of voice vary considerably from role to role. In addition, the specific relationship between the communicators is significant. The nurse who meets with a client for the first time communicates differently from the nurse who has previously developed a longer relationship with the client.

ENVIRONMENT   People usually communicate most effectively in a comfortable environment. Temperature extremes, excessive noise, and a poorly ventilated environment can all interfere with communication. Also, lack of privacy may interfere with a client's communication about matters the client considers private. For example, a client who is worried about the ability of his wife to care for him after discharge from the hospital may not wish to discuss this concern with a nurse within hearing of other clients in the room. Environmental distraction can impair and distort communication.

CONGRUENCE   In **congruent communication**, the verbal and nonverbal aspects of the message match. Clients more readily trust the nurse when they perceive the nurse's communication as congruent. Both nurse and client can easily determine if there is congruence between verbal expression and nonverbal expression. Nurses are taught to assess clients, but clients are often just as adept at reading a nurse's expression or body language. If there is an incongruence between verbal and nonverbal expression, the body language or nonverbal communication is usually the one with the true meaning. For example, when teaching a client how to care for a colostomy, the nurse might say, "You won't have any problem with this." However, if the nurse looks worried or disgusted while saying this, the client is less likely to trust the nurse's words.

INTERPERSONAL ATTITUDES   Attitudes convey beliefs, thoughts, and feelings about people and events. Attitudes are communicated convincingly and rapidly to others. Such attitudes as caring, warmth, respect, and acceptance facilitate communication, whereas condescension, lack of interest, and coldness inhibit communication.

Caring and *warmth* convey a feeling of emotional closeness and deep and genuine concern for the person. Warmth conveys friendliness and consideration, shown by acts of smiling and attention to physical comforts (Boyd, 2008). Caring is more enduring and intense than warmth. Caring involves giving feelings, thoughts, skill, and knowledge. It requires psychological energy and poses the risk of gaining little in return.

Respect is an attitude that emphasizes the other person's worth and individuality. It conveys that the person's hopes and feelings are special and unique, even though similar to others in many ways. A nurse conveys respect by listening with an open mind to what the other person is saying, even if the nurse disagrees. Nurses can learn new ways of approaching situations when they conscientiously listen to another person's perspective.

Acceptance emphasizes neither approval nor disapproval. The nurse willingly receives the client's honest feelings and actions without judgment. An accepting attitude encourages clients to express personal feelings freely and to be themselves. The nurse may need to restrict acceptance in situations in which clients' actions are harmful to themselves or to others.

BOUNDARIES   **Boundaries** are "limits in which a person may act or refrain from acting within a designated time or place" (Boyd, 2008, p. 900). To keep clear boundaries, the nurse keeps the focus on the client and avoids sharing personal information or meeting his or her own needs through the nurse–client relationship. If the client seeks friendship with the nurse or a relationship outside the work environment, the nurse affirms his or her professional role and declines the invitation. Some boundary issues include gift-giving by the nurse or client, spending more time than necessary with a client, or the nurse believing only he or she understands the client (Boyd, 2008).

Therapeutic Communication

Therapeutic communication promotes understanding and can help establish a constructive relationship between the nurse and the client. Unlike the social relationship, which may not have a specific purpose or direction, therapeutic communication is goal-directed and can promote understanding.

Nurses need to respond not only to the content of a client's verbal message but also to the feelings and thoughts expressed. It is important to understand how the client views the situation and feels about it before responding. Sometimes, people may convey their thoughts in words, but their emotions may contradict their words. For example, a client says, "I am glad my spouse has left me; my spouse was very cruel." However, the nurse observes that the client is in tears as this is said. To respond to the client's *words*, the nurse might simply rephrase, saying, "You are pleased that your spouse has left you." To respond to the client's *feelings*, the nurse would need to acknowledge the tears in the client's eyes, saying, for example, "You seem saddened by all this." Such a response helps the client to focus on feelings. In some instances, the nurse may need to know more about the client and resources for coping with these feelings.

Strong emotions are often draining. People usually need time to deal with their feelings before they can cope with other matters, such as learning new skills or planning for the future. This is most evident in hospitals when patients learn that they have a terminal illness. Some require hours, days, or even weeks before they are ready to start other tasks. Some need time to themselves, and others need someone to listen to them; some need assistance identifying and verbalizing feelings, and others need assistance making decisions about future action.

ATTENTIVE LISTENING   **Attentive listening** is listening actively by using all the senses, as opposed to listening passively with just the ears. Attentive listening involves paying attention to the total message, both verbal and nonverbal and absorbing both the message content and the feeling the person is conveying, without selectivity. The listener does not select or listen solely to what the

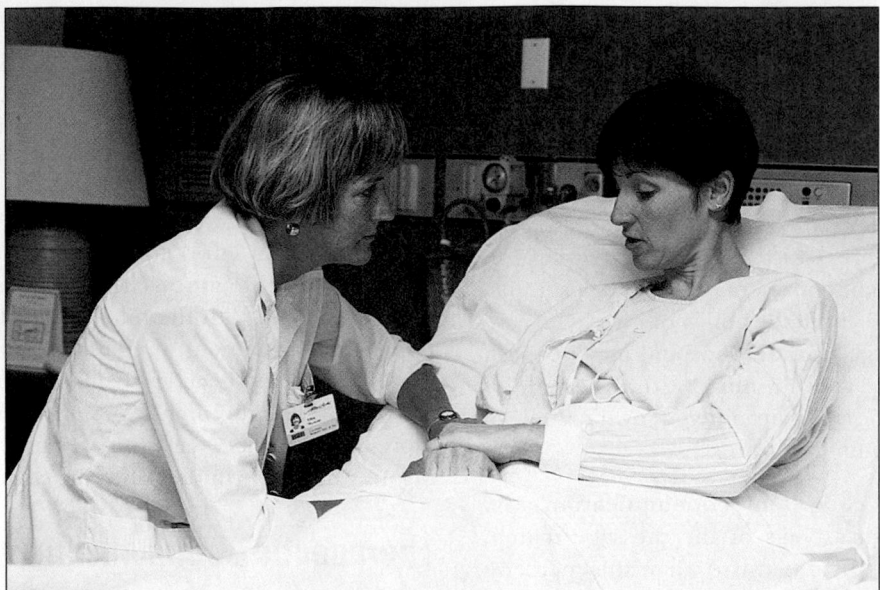

FIGURE 22.6 The nurse conveys attentive listening through a posture of involvement.

listener wants to hear; the nurse focuses not on his or her own needs but rather on the client's needs. Attentive listening conveys an attitude of caring and interest, thereby encouraging the client to talk (Figure 22.6).

Nurses must be aware of their own biases and careful not to react quickly to the message. The speaker should not be interrupted, and the nurse (the responder) should take time to think about the message before responding. As a listener, the nurse also should ask questions either to obtain additional information or to clarify. The message sender (i.e., the client) should decide when to close a conversation. When the nurse ends the conversation, the client may assume that the nurse considers the message unimportant. It is also important that nurses be aware of their own biases. A message from a client that reflects different values or beliefs should not be discredited for that reason (Dearing & Steadman, 2008).

Attentive listening is a highly developed skill, and it can be learned with practice. A nurse can communicate attentive listening to clients in various ways. Common responses are nodding the head, uttering "Uh-huh" or "Mmm," repeating the words that the client has used, or saying "I see what you mean."

PHYSICAL ATTENDING Egan (2009) has outlined five specific ways to convey physical attending, which he defines as the manner of being present to another or being with another. Listening is what a person does while attending. The five actions of physical attending, which convey a "posture of involvement" and specifically focus on comforting a client are shown in Box 22.2. Therapeutic communication techniques facilitate communication and focus on the client's concerns (as described in Table 22.1).

BOX 22.2   ACTIONS OF PHYSICAL ATTENDING

Use of the following actions of physical attending helps nurses comfort clients:

1. *Face the other person squarely*. This position says, "I am available to you." Moving to the side lessens the degree of involvement.

2. *Adopt an open posture*. The nondefensive position is one in which neither arms nor legs are crossed. It conveys that the person wants to encourage the passage of communication, as the open door of a home or an office does.

3. *Lean toward the person*. People move naturally toward each other when they want to say or hear something—by moving to the front of a class, by moving a chair nearer a friend, or by leaning across a table with arms propped in front. The nurse conveys involvement by leaning forward, closer to the client.

4. *Maintain good eye contact*. Mutual eye contact, preferably at the same level, recognizes the other person and denotes

willingness to maintain communication. Eye contact neither glares at nor stares down another person but is natural.

5. *Try to be relatively relaxed*. Total relaxation is not feasible when the nurse is listening with intensity, but the nurse can show relaxation by taking time in responding, allowing pauses as needed, balancing periods of tension with relaxation, and using gestures that are natural.

These five attending postures need to be adapted to the specific needs (and culture) of clients in a given situation. For example, leaning forward may not be appropriate at the beginning of an interview. It may be reserved until a closer relationship develops between the nurse and the client. The same applies to eye contact, which is generally uninterrupted when the communicators are very involved in the interaction.

Source: From Egan, G. (1998). *The skilled helper: A problem-management approach to helping* (6th ed., pp. 63–64). Wadsworth, a part of Cengage Learning, Inc. Reproduced by permission. www.cengage.com/permissions

TABLE 22.1 Therapeutic Communication Techniques

Technique	Description	Examples
Using silence	Accepting pauses or silences that extend for several seconds or minutes without interjecting any verbal response	Sitting quietly (or walking with the client) and waiting attentively until the client is able to put thoughts and feelings into words
Providing general leads	Using statements or questions that do the following: (1) Encourage the client to verbalize (2) Choose a topic of conversation (3) Facilitate continued verbalization	"Perhaps you would like to talk about . . ." "Would it help to discuss your feelings?" "Where would you like to begin?" "And then what?" "Tell me more. . . ."
Being specific and tentative	Making statements that are specific, rather than general, tentative, or absolute	"You scratched my arm." (specific statement) "Are you in pain?" (general statement) "You seem unconcerned about Mary's diabetes." (tentative statement)
Using open-ended questions	Asking broad questions that lead or invite the client to explore (elaborate, clarify, describe, compare, or illustrate) thoughts or feelings. Open-ended questions specify only the topic to be discussed and invite answers that are longer than one or two words.	"I'd like to hear more about that." "Tell me about . . ." "How have you been feeling lately?" "What brought you to the hospital?" "What is your opinion?" "You said you were frightened yesterday. How do you feel now?"
Using touch	Providing appropriate forms of touch to reinforce caring feelings. Because tactile contacts vary considerably among individuals, families, and cultures, the nurse must be sensitive to the differences in attitudes and practices of clients and self.	Putting an arm over the client's shoulder, or placing your hand over the client's hand, with permission
Restating or paraphrasing	Actively listening for the client's basic message and then repeating those thoughts and/or feelings in similar words. This conveys that the nurse has listened and understood the client's basic message and also offers the client a clearer idea of what was said by the client.	*Client*: "I couldn't manage to eat any dinner last night—not even the dessert." *Nurse*: "You had difficulty eating yesterday." *Client*: "Yes, I was very upset after my family left." *Client*: "I have trouble talking to strangers." *Nurse*: "You find it difficult talking to people you do not know?"
Seeking clarification	A method of making the client's broad overall meaning of the message more understandable. It is used when paraphrasing is difficult or when the communication is rambling or garbled. To clarify the message, the nurse can restate the basic message or confess confusion and ask the client to repeat or restate the message.	"I'm puzzled." "I'm not sure I understand that." "Would you please say that again?" "Would you tell me more?"
	Nurses can also clarify their own messages with statements	"I meant this rather than that." "I guess I didn't make that clear—I'll go over it again."
Checking perception or seeking consensual validation	A method similar to clarifying that verifies the meaning of specific words, rather than the overall meaning of a message	*Client*: "My husband never gives me any presents." *Nurse*: "You mean he has never given you a present for your birthday or Christmas?" *Client*: "Well—not never. He does get me something for my birthday and Christmas, but he never thinks of giving me anything at any other time."

(continued)

TABLE 22.1 *(continued)*

Technique	Description	Examples
Offering the self	Suggesting a presence, interest, or wish to understand the client without making any demands or attaching conditions that the client must comply with to receive the nurse's attention	"I'll stay with you until your daughter arrives." "We can sit here quietly for a while; we don't need to talk unless you would like to." "I'll help you dress to go home."
Giving information	Providing, in a simple and direct manner, specific factual information the client may or may not request. When information is not known, the nurse states this and indicates who has it or when the nurse will obtain it.	"Your surgery is scheduled for 11 a.m. tomorrow." "You will feel a pulling sensation when the tube is removed from your abdomen." "I do not know the answer to that, but I will find out from Mrs. King, the nurse in charge."
Acknowledging	Giving recognition, in a nonjudgmental way, of a change in behaviour, an effort the client has made, or a contribution to a communication. Acknowledgment may be with or without understanding and verbal or nonverbal.	"You trimmed your beard and moustache and washed your hair." "I notice you keep squinting your eyes. Are you having difficulty seeing?" "You walked twice as far today with your walker."
Clarifying time or sequence	Helping the client clarify an event, situation, or happening in relationship to time	*Client*: "I vomited this morning." *Nurse*: "Was that after breakfast?" *Client*: "I feel that I have been asleep for weeks." *Nurse*: "You had your operation Monday, and today is Tuesday."
Presenting reality	Helping the client to differentiate the real from the unreal	"That telephone ring came from the program on television." "That's not a dead mouse in the corner; it is a discarded washcloth." "Your magazine is here in the drawer. It has not been stolen."
Focusing	Helping the client expand on and develop a topic of importance. It is important for the nurse to wait until the client finishes stating the main concerns before attempting to focus. The focus may be an idea or a feeling; however, the nurse often emphasizes a feeling to help the client recognize an emotion disguised behind words.	*Client*: "My wife says she will look after me, but I don't think she can, what with the children to take care of, and they're always after her about something—clothes, homework, what's for dinner that night." *Nurse*: "You are worried about how well she can manage."
Reflecting	Directing ideas, feelings, questions, or content back to clients to enable them to explore their own ideas and feelings about a situation	*Client*: "What can I do?" *Nurse*: "What do you think would be helpful?" *Client*: "Do you think I should tell my husband?"
Summarizing and planning	Stating the main points of a discussion to clarify the relevant points discussed. This technique is useful at the end of an interview or to review a health teaching session. It often acts as an introduction to future care planning.	"You seem unsure about telling your husband." "During the past half hour we have talked about . . ." "Tomorrow afternoon we may explore this further." "In a few days I'll review what you have learned about the actions and effects of your insulin."

Barriers to Communication

Nurses need to recognize barriers or nontherapeutic responses to effective communication. See Table 22.2.

Failure to listen, improperly decoding the client's intended message, and placing the nurse's needs above the client's needs are major barriers to communication.

TABLE 22.2   Barriers to Communication

Barrier	Description	Examples
Stereotyping	Offering generalized and oversimplified beliefs about groups of people that are based on experiences too limited to be valid. These responses categorize clients and negate their uniqueness as individuals.	"Two-year-olds are brats." "Women are complainers." "Men don't cry." "Most people don't have any pain after this type of surgery."
Agreeing and disagreeing	Implying that the client is either right or wrong and that the nurse is in a position to judge this. Akin to judgmental responses, these responses deter clients from thinking through their position and may cause a client to become defensive.	*Client*: "I don't think Dr. Broad is a very good doctor. He doesn't seem interested in his patients." *Nurse*: "Dr. Broad is head of the Department of Surgery and is an excellent surgeon."
Being defensive	Attempting to protect a person or health care services from negative comments. These responses prevent the client from expressing true concerns. The nurse is saying, "You have no right to complain." Defensive responses protect the nurse from admitting weaknesses in the health care services, including personal weaknesses.	*Client*: "Those night nurses must just sit around and talk all night. They didn't answer my light for over an hour." *Nurse*: "I'll have you know we literally run around on nights. You're not the only client, you know."
Challenging	Giving a response that makes clients prove their statement or point of view. These responses indicate that the nurse is failing to consider the client's feelings, making the client feel it necessary to defend a position.	*Client*: "I felt nauseated after that red pill." *Nurse*: "Surely you don't think I gave you the wrong pill?" *Client*: "I feel as if I am dying." *Nurse*: "How can you feel that way when your pulse is 60?" *Client*: "I believe my husband doesn't love me." *Nurse*: "You can't say that; why, he visits you every day."
Probing	Asking for information chiefly out of curiosity, rather than with the intent to assist the client. These responses are considered prying and violate the client's privacy. Asking "why" is often probing and places the client in a defensive position.	*Client*: "I was speeding along the street and didn't see the stop sign." *Nurse*: "Why were you speeding?" *Client*: "I didn't ask the doctor when he was here." *Nurse*: "Why didn't you?"
Testing	Asking questions that make the client admit to something. These responses permit the client only limited answers and often meet the nurse's need, rather than the client's.	"Who do you think you are?" (forces people to admit their status is only that of client) "Do you think I am not busy?" (forces the client to admit that the nurse really is busy)
Rejecting	Refusing to discuss certain topics with the client. These responses often make clients feel that the nurse is rejecting not only their communication but also the clients themselves.	"I don't want to discuss that. Let's talk about . . ." "Let's discuss other areas of interest to you rather than the two problems you keep mentioning." "I can't talk now. I'm on my way for coffee break."
Changing topics and subjects	Directing the communication into areas of self-interest, rather than considering the client's concerns, is often a self-protective response to a topic that causes anxiety. These responses imply that what the nurse considers important will be discussed and that clients should not discuss certain topics.	*Client*: "I'm separated from my wife. Do you think I should have sexual relations with another woman?" *Nurse*: "You like gardening. This sunshine is good for my roses. I have a beautiful rose garden."
Unwarranted reassurance	Using clichés or comforting statements of advice as a means to reassure the client. These responses block the fears, feelings, and other thoughts of the client.	"You'll feel better soon." "I'm sure everything will turn out all right." "Don't worry."
Passing judgment	Giving opinions and approving or disapproving responses, moralizing, or implying one's own values. These responses imply that the client must think as the nurse thinks, fostering client dependence.	"That's good (bad)." "You shouldn't do that." "That's not good enough." "What you did was wrong (right)."
Giving common advice	Telling the client what to do. These responses deny the client's right to be an equal partner. Note that giving expert, rather than common, advice is therapeutic.	*Client*: "Should I move from my home to a nursing home?" *Nurse*: "If I were you, I'd go to a nursing home where you'll get your meals cooked for you."

The Helping Relationship

Nurse–client relationships are referred to by some as *interpersonal relationships,* by others as *therapeutic relationships,* and by still others as *helping relationships.* Helping is a growth-facilitating process that strives to achieve two basic goals (Egan, 2009):

1. Helping clients manage their problems in living more effectively and develop unused or underused opportunities more fully
2. Helping clients become better at helping themselves in their everyday lives

A helping relationship can develop over weeks of working with a client, or over minutes. The keys to the helping relationship are (a) the development of trust and acceptance between the nurse and the client, and (b) an underlying belief that the nurse cares about and wants to help the client.

The helping relationship is influenced by the personal and professional characteristics of the nurse and the client. Age, gender, appearance, diagnosis, education, values, ethnic and cultural background, personality, expectations, and setting can all affect the development of the nurse–client relationship. Consideration of all these factors, combined with good communication skills and sincere interest in the client's welfare, will enable the nurse to create a helping relationship. Characteristics of helping relationships are described in Box 22.3.

Phases of the Helping Relationship

The helping relationship process can be described in terms of four sequential phases, each characterized by identifiable tasks and skills. The relationship must progress through the stages in succession because each builds on the one before. Nurses can identify the progress of a relationship by understanding these phases: (a) pre-interaction phase, (b) introductory phase, (c) working (maintaining) phase, and (d) termination phase. Table 22.3 summarizes the tasks and skills required.

BOX 22.3 CHARACTERISTICS OF A HELPING RELATIONSHIP

A helping relationship has the following characteristics:

- It is an intellectual and emotional bond between the nurse and the client and is focused on the client.
- It respects the client as an individual, including the following:
  a. Maximizing the client's abilities to participate in decision making and treatments
  b. Considering ethnic and cultural aspects
  c. Considering family relationships and values
- It respects client confidentiality.
- It focuses on the client's well-being.
- It is based on mutual trust, respect, and acceptance.

PRE-INTERACTION PHASE Before an interview and in most situations, the nurse has information about the client before the first face-to-face meeting. Such information can include the client's name, address, age, medical history, and social history. Planning for the initial visit may generate some anxious feelings in the nurse. If the nurse recognizes these feelings and identifies specific information to be discussed, positive outcomes can evolve.

INTRODUCTORY PHASE This phase, also referred to as the *orientation phase* or the *prehelping phase,* is important because it sets the tone for the rest of the relationship. During this initial encounter, the client and the nurse closely observe each other and form judgments about the other's behaviour. The goal of the nurse in this phase is to get to know the client and develop trust and security within the nurse–client relationship (Boyd, 2008).

After introductions, the nurse may initially engage in some social interaction to put the client at ease. For example, the nurse and client may talk about what a nice day it is and what they would like to do if at home.

During the initial parts of the introductory phase, the client may display some resistive behaviours. *Resistive behaviours* are those that inhibit involvement, cooperation, or change. They may be due to difficulty in acknowledging the need for help and, thus, a dependent role, fear of exposing and facing feelings, anxiety about the discomfort involved in changing problem-causing behaviour patterns, and fear or anxiety in response to the nurse's approach, which may, in the client's opinion, be inappropriate.

Resistive behaviours can be overcome by conveying a caring attitude, genuine interest in the client, and competence. These behaviours of the nurse also foster the development of trust in the relationship. *Trust* can be described as a reliance on someone without doubt or question, or the belief that the other person is capable of assisting in times of distress and, in all likelihood, will do so. To trust another person involves risk; clients become vulnerable when they share thoughts, feelings, and attitudes with the nurse. Trust, however, enables the client to express thoughts and feelings openly.

By the end of the introductory phase, clients should begin to do the following:

- Develop trust in the nurse
- View the nurse as a competent professional capable of helping
- View the nurse as honest, open, and concerned about their welfare
- Believe the nurse will try to understand and respect their cultural values and beliefs
- Believe the nurse will respect client confidentiality
- Feel comfortable talking with the nurse about feelings and other sensitive issues
- Understand the purpose of the relationship and the roles
- Feel that they are active participants in developing a mutually agreeable plan of care

TABLE 22.3 Tasks and Skills for Each Phase of the Helping Relationship

Phase	Tasks	Skills
Pre-interaction phase	The nurse reviews pertinent knowledge, considers potential areas of concern, and develops plans for interaction.	Recognizing limitations and seeking assistance, as required
Introductory phase 1. Opening the relationship	Both client and nurse identify each other by name. When the nurse initiates the relationship, it is important to explain the nurse's role to give the client an idea of what to expect. When the client initiates the relationship, the nurse needs to help the client express concerns and reasons for seeking help. Vague, open-ended questions, such as "What's on your mind today?" are helpful at this stage.	A relaxed, attending attitude to put the client at ease (It is not easy for all clients to receive help.)
2. Clarifying the problem	Because the client initially may not see the problem clearly, the nurse's major task is to help clarify the problem.	Attentive listening, paraphrasing, clarifying, and other effective communication techniques discussed in this chapter (A common error at this stage is to ask too many questions of the client.)
3. Structuring and formulating the contract (obligations to be met by both the nurse and client)	Nurse and client develop a degree of trust and verbally agree about the following: (1) Location, frequency, and length of meetings (2) Overall purpose of the relationship (3) How confidential material will be handled (4) Tasks to be accomplished (5) Duration and indications for termination of the relationship	Communication skills listed above and ability to overcome resistive behaviours if they occur
Working phase	Nurse and client accomplish the tasks outlined in the introductory phase, enhance trust and rapport, and develop caring.	Listening and attending skills, empathy, respect, genuineness, concreteness, self-disclosure, and confrontation (Skills acquired by the client are nondefensive listening and self-understanding.)
1. Exploring and understanding thoughts and feelings	The nurse assists the client to explore thoughts and feelings and acquires an understanding of the client. The client explores thoughts and feelings associated with problems, develops the skill of listening, and gains insight into personal behaviour.	Decision-making and goal-setting skills; also, for the nurse, reinforcement skills; for the client, risk taking
2. Facilitating and taking action	The nurse plans programs within the client's capabilities and considers long-term and short-term goals. The client needs to learn to take risks (i.e., accept that either failure or success may be the outcome). The nurse needs to reinforce successes and help the client recognize failures realistically.	Decision-making and goal-setting skills; also, for the nurse, reinforcement skills; for the client, risk taking
Termination phase	Nurse and client accept feelings of loss. The client accepts the end of the relationship without feelings of anxiety or dependence.	For the nurse, summarizing skills; for the client, abilities to handle problems independently

WORKING PHASE During the working phase of a helping relationship, the nurse and the client begin to view each other as unique individuals. They begin to appreciate this uniqueness and care about each other. Caring is sharing deep and genuine concern about the welfare of another person. Once caring develops, the potential for empathy increases.

The working phase has two major stages: *exploring and understanding thoughts and feelings,* and *facilitating and taking action.* The nurse helps the client to explore thoughts, feelings, and actions and helps the client plan a program of action to meet established goals.

Exploring and Understanding Thoughts and Feelings The nurse requires the following skills for this phase of the helping relationship:

- *Empathetic listening and responding.* Nurses must listen attentively and communicate (respond) in ways that indicate they have listened to what was said and understand how the client feels. The nurse responds to content or feelings, or both, as appropriate. The nurse's nonverbal behaviours are also important. Nonverbal behaviours indicating empathy include moderate head nodding, a steady gaze, moderate gesturing, and little activity or body movement. **Empathy** is "the ability to experience, in the present, a situation as another did at some time in the past" (Boyd, 2008, p. 143). Empathetic listening focuses on a kind of "being with" clients to develop an understanding of them and their world. This understanding, however, must also be communicated effectively to the client in the form of an empathetic response. The end result of empathy is comforting and caring for the client and a helping, healing relationship.
- *Respect.* The nurse must show respect for the client's willingness to be available, as well as a desire to work with the client, and a manner that conveys the idea of taking the client's point of view seriously.
- *Genuineness.* The genuine person is spontaneous, is nondefensive, displays few discrepancies, and uses self-disclosure appropriately (Egan, 2009). Personal statements can be helpful in solidifying the rapport between the nurse and the client. Nurses need to exercise caution when making references about themselves. These statements must be used with discretion.
- *Concreteness.* The nurse must assist the client to be concrete and specific, rather than to speak in generalities. When the client says, "I'm stupid and clumsy," the nurse narrows the topic to the specific by pointing out, "You tripped on the scatter rug."
- *Confrontation.* The nurse points out discrepancies among thoughts, feelings, and actions that inhibit the client's self-understanding or exploration of specific areas. This is done empathetically, not judgmentally.

During this first stage of the working phase, the intensity of interaction increases, and such feelings as anger, shame, or self-consciousness may be expressed. If the nurse is skilled in this stage, and if the client is willing to pursue self-exploration, the outcome is a beginning of understanding on the part of the client about behaviour and feelings.

Facilitating and Taking Action Ultimately, the client must make decisions and take action to become more effective. The responsibility for action belongs to the client. The nurse, however, collaborates in these decisions, provides support, and may offer options or information.

TERMINATION PHASE The termination phase of the relationship is often expected to be difficult and filled with ambivalence. However, if the previous phases have evolved effectively, the client generally has a positive outlook and feels able to handle problems independently. On the other hand, because caring attitudes have developed, it is natural to expect some feelings of loss, and each person needs to develop a way of saying goodbye.

Many methods can be used to terminate relationships. Summarizing or reviewing the process can produce a sense of accomplishment. This can include sharing reminiscences of how things were at the beginning of the relationship and comparing them with how they are now. It is also helpful for both the nurse and the client to express their feelings about termination openly and honestly. Thus, termination discussions need to start in advance of the termination interview. This allows time for the client to adjust to independence. In some situations, referrals are necessary, or it may be appropriate to offer an occasional standby meeting to give support, as needed. Follow-up phone calls are another intervention that eases the client's transition to independence. (See the Evidence-Informed Practice box on the relationship between patient-centred care and patient outcomes.)

EVIDENCE-INFORMED PRACTICE

What Is the Relationship between Patient-Centred Care and Patient Outcomes?

The investigators examined the extent of relationship between patient-centred care (PCC) and patient outcomes (i.e., patient needs, patient health-related problems, patients' preferences, levels of self-care, and satisfaction with care). Data were collected through a self-completed questionnaire from 63 staff nurses and 44 patients in acute care settings. The patients completed the questionnaire on admission and 1 week following hospital discharge. Both nurses and patients reported a moderate association of PCC and patient outcomes.

NURSING IMPLICATIONS: PCC is linked to improved satisfaction with care and quality of life outcomes. When attending to patient needs and their health problems, providing care according to patient preferences, and encouraging self-care, it is important for nurses to consider patients' perception of their care received through communication, caring, and decision making.

Source: Based on Poochikian-Sarkissian, S., Sidani, S., Ferguson-Pare, M., & Doran, D. (2010). Examining the relationship between patient-centred care and outcomes. *Canadian Journal of Neuroscience Nursing, 32*(4), 14–21.

Developing Helping Relationships

Whatever the practice setting, the nurse establishes some type of helping relationship in which mutual goals (outcomes) are set with the client or, if the client is unable to participate, with support persons. Although special training in counselling techniques is advantageous, there are many ways of helping clients that do not require special training. The following are key elements for developing a helping relationship:

- Listen actively.
- Help to identify what the person is feeling. Often clients who are troubled are unable to label their feelings and consequently have difficulty working them out or talking about them. Responses such as "You seem angry about taking orders from your boss" or "You sound as if you've been lonely since your wife died" can help clients recognize what they are feeling and talk about it.
- Put yourself in the other person's shoes (i.e., empathize).
- Be honest and genuine.
- Use your ingenuity. There are always many courses of action to consider in handling problems. Whatever course is chosen needs to further the achievement of the client's goals (outcomes), be compatible with the client's value system, and offer the probability of success.
- Be aware of cultural differences.
- Maintain client confidentiality.
- Know your role and limitations and refer the client to the appropriate health care professional, as needed.

Group Communication

People interact with others at all stages of life in various groups: family, peer groups, work groups, recreational groups, religious groups, and so on. A **group** is two or more people who have shared needs and goals, who take each other into account in their actions and who, thus, are held together and set apart from others by virtue of their interactions. Groups exist to help people achieve goals (outcomes) that would be unattainable by individual effort alone. For example, groups can often solve problems more effectively than one person by pooling the ideas and expertise of several individuals; in addition, information can be disseminated to groups more quickly than to individuals.

Group Dynamics

The communication that takes place between members of any group is known as **group dynamics**. Members of the group can affect the group dynamics on the basis of their motivation for participating and their similarity to other group members and the goal of that group. The unique dynamics of each group will influence its maturation or group process, as well as the effectiveness of the group. Three main functions are required for any group to be effective: (a) It must maintain a degree of group unity or cohesion; (b) it needs to develop and modify its structure to improve its effectiveness; and (c) it must accomplish its goals. The characteristics of an effectively functioning group are shown in Table 22.4 on the next page.

Types of Health Care Groups

Much of a nurse's professional life is spent in a wide variety of groups. Common types of health care groups include task groups, teaching and learning groups, self-help groups, self-awareness or growth groups, therapy groups, work-related social support groups, and professional organizations. There are similarities and differences among the characteristics of these various types of groups and the nurse's role.

TASK GROUPS The **task group** is one of the most common types of work-related groups to which nurses belong. The focus of such groups is the completion of a specific task, and the leader and/or members define the format at the beginning. The methods vary according to the task to be completed. Examples are health care planning committees, nursing service committees, nursing team meetings, nursing care conference groups, and hospital staff meetings.

The leader of a task group, usually called the *chairperson,* must be accepted by the members as an appropriate leader and, therefore, should be an expert in the area of task emphasis. The chairperson's role is to identify the specific task, clarify communication, and assist in expressing opinions and offering solutions. *Committee members* are generally selected in terms of their individual functional role and employment status rather than in terms of their personal characteristics. Member participation is determined by the task. A target date for termination of the group is usually set in advance.

TEACHING GROUPS The major purpose of teaching groups is to impart information to the participants. Examples of teaching groups include continuing education and client health care groups. Numerous subjects are often handled via the group teaching format: childbirth techniques; birth control methods; effective parenting; nutrition; management of chronic illness, such as diabetes; exercise for middle-aged and older adults; and instructions to family members about follow-up care for discharged clients. A nurse who leads a group in which the primary purpose is to teach or learn must be skilled in the teaching–learning process (see Chapter 26).

TABLE 22.4 Comparative Features of Effective and Ineffective Groups

Factor	Effective Groups	Ineffective Groups
Atmosphere	Comfortable and relaxed: It is a working atmosphere in which people demonstrate their interest and involvement).	Tense: This atmosphere lacks privacy or voluntary commitment to the group.
Purpose	Goals, tasks, and outcomes are clarified, understood, and modified so that members of the group can commit themselves to purposes through cooperation.	The purposes are unclear, misunderstood, or imposed.
Leadership and member participation	Leadership is democratic with a shift in leadership from time to time depending on knowledge or experience.	Authoritarian: The leader may dominate the group, or the members may defer unduly. Member participation is unequal, with some members dominating.
Communication	Open: Ideas and feelings are encouraged.	Closed: Only idea production is encouraged. Feelings are ignored. Members may have "hidden agendas" (personal goals at cross-purposes with group goals).
Decision making	Although done by the group, various decision-making procedures appropriate to the situation may be instituted.	This is done by the highest authority in the group, or one or two strong members of the group, with minimal involvement by members. Disagreements are ignored.
Cohesion	Facilitated through valuing other group members, open expression of feelings, trust, and support.	The leader claims full credit for achievements. Comments are critical and focus on personal characteristics.
Conflict tolerance	The reasons for disagreements or conflicts are carefully examined, and the group seeks to resolve them.	Fear of conflict prevents decisions and growth.
Power	Determined by the members' abilities and the information they possess. Power is shared.	Determined by position in the group. Obedience to authority is strong. The issue is who is in control based on individual emotional needs of members.
Problem solving	High: Constructive criticism is frequent, frank, relatively comfortable, and oriented toward problem solving.	Low: Criticism may be destructive, taking the form of either overt or covert personal attacks.
Creativity	Encouraged.	Discouraged.

SELF-HELP GROUPS A self-help group is a small, voluntary organization composed of individuals who share a similar health, social, or daily living problem. One of the central beliefs of the self-help movement is that people who experience a particular social or health problem have an understanding of that condition which those without it do not. Self-help groups are available for a range of problems (e.g., stillbirth, parenting, pregnant adolescents, divorce, problematic drug use, cancer, menopause, mental illness, diabetes, acquired immunodeficiency syndrome [AIDS], women's health, caregivers of people, and grief). Alcoholics Anonymous was the first self-help group. Positive aspects of self-help groups are outlined in Box 22.4.

The major functions of the nurse's role in self-help groups include the following:

- Helping clients form such groups by identifying key people who can act as facilitators
- Sharing expertise with clients and helping them gain appropriate knowledge and skills
- Informing clients and support persons about existing self-help groups available to them
- Participating as a member of a self-help group when this is appropriate; the nurse's role is that of a resource person, that is, being "on tap but not on top"
- Helping out in times of crisis

BOX 22.4 POSITIVE ASPECTS OF SELF-HELP GROUPS

Self-help groups have many positive aspects:

- Members can experience almost instant kinship because the essence of the group is the idea that "you are not alone."

- Members can talk about their feelings and listen to the concerns of others, knowing they all share this experience.

- The group atmosphere is generally one of acceptance, support, encouragement, and caring.

- Many members act as role models for newer members and can inspire them to attempt tasks they might consider impossible.

- The group provides the opportunity for people to help as well as to *be* helped—a critical component in restoring self-esteem.

SELF-AWARENESS OR GROWTH GROUPS The purpose of self-awareness or growth groups is to develop or use interpersonal strengths. The overall aim is to improve the person's functioning in the group to which they return, whether job, family, or community. From the beginning, broad goals are usually apparent, for example, to study communication patterns, group process, or problem solving. Because the focus of these groups is interpersonal concerns around current situations, the work of the group is oriented to reality testing with a here-and-now emphasis. Members are responsible for correcting inefficient patterns of relating and communicating with each other. They learn group process through participation and involvement and guided exercises.

THERAPY GROUPS Therapy groups work toward self-understanding, more satisfactory ways of relating or handling stress, and changing patterns of behaviour toward health. Members of the therapy group are referred to as clients or, in some settings, as patients. They are selected by health care professionals after extensive selection interviews that consider the pattern of personalities, behaviours, needs, and identification of group therapy as the treatment of choice. Duration of therapy groups is not usually set. A termination date is usually mutually determined by the therapist and members.

WORK-RELATED SOCIAL SUPPORT GROUPS Many nurses, for example, hospice, emergency, and acute care nurses, experience high levels of vocational stress. Various types of group support can buffer such stress. For example, a nurse may help another team member consider alternative strategies for intervention. Members also can share the joys of success and the frustration of failure through active listening without giving advice or making judgments. This type of social support is best given outside of the work environment.

Communication and the Nursing Process

Communication is an integral part of the nursing process. Nurses use communication skills in each phase of the nursing process. Communication is also important when caring for clients who have communication problems, such as those with sensory, language, or cognitive deficits.

Assessing

To assess the client's communication, the nurse determines communication impairments or barriers and communication style. Remember that culture can influence when and how a client speaks. Obviously, language varies according to age and development. With children, the nurse observes sounds, gestures, and vocabulary.

IMPAIRMENTS TO COMMUNICATION Various barriers can alter a client's ability to send, receive, or comprehend messages. These include language deficits, sensory deficits, cognitive impairments, structural deficits, and paralysis. The nurse must assess each client to determine their presence.

Language Deficits Determine the client's primary language for communicating and whether a fluent interpreter is required. Some clients for whom English is a second language may have limited language skills to express their needs.

Sensory Deficits The ability to hear, see, feel, and smell are important adjuncts to communication. Deafness can significantly alter the message the client receives; impaired vision alters the ability to observe nonverbal behaviour, such as a smile or a gesture; the inability to feel and smell can impair the client's capabilities to report injuries or detect the smoke from a fire. For clients with severe hearing impairments, follow these steps:

- Look for a MedicAlert bracelet (or necklace or tag) indicating hearing loss.
- Determine whether the client wears a hearing aid and whether it is functioning.
- Observe whether the client is attempting to see your face to read your lips.
- Observe whether the client is using his or her hands to communicate with sign language.

Cognitive Impairments Any disorder that impairs cognitive functioning (e.g., cerebrovascular disease, Alzheimer's disease, and brain tumours or injuries) can affect a client's ability to use and understand language (see the Lifespan Considerations box on the next page). These clients lose the ability to speak, have impaired articulation, or may not be able to find the correct words.

LIFESPAN CONSIDERATIONS: COMMUNICATION WITH OLDER ADULTS

Older adults may have physical or cognitive problems that necessitate nursing interventions for improvement of communication skills. Some of the common problems are as follows:

- Sensory deficits, such as vision and hearing deficits
- Cognitive impairment, as in dementia
- Neurological deficits from strokes or other neurological conditions, such as aphasia (expressive or receptive) and lack of movement
- Psychosocial problems, such as depression

Recognizing specific needs and obtaining appropriate resources for clients can greatly increase their socialization and quality of life. Interventions directed toward improving communication in clients with these special needs are as follows:

- Make sure that assistive devices, glasses, and hearing aids are being used and are in good working order.

- Make referrals to appropriate resources, such as for speech therapy.
- Make use of communications aids, such as communication boards, computers, or pictures, when possible.
- Keep environmental distractions to a minimum.
- Speak in short, simple sentences, one subject at a time. Reinforce or repeat what is said, when necessary.
- Always face the person when speaking. Coming up behind someone can startle him or her.
- Include family and friends in conversation.
- Use reminiscing, either in individual conversations or in groups, to

maintain memory connections and to enhance self-identity and self-esteem in the older adult.

- When verbal expression and nonverbal expression are incongruent, believe the nonverbal expression. Clarification of this and attentiveness to their feelings will help promote a feeling of caring and acceptance.
- Find out what has been important and has meaning to the person and try to maintain these things as much as possible. Even simple things, such as bedtime rituals, become important if they are lost in a hospital or extended care setting.

Certain medications, such as sedatives, antidepressants, and neuroleptics, can also impair speech, causing the client to use incomplete sentences or to slur words.

The nurse assesses whether the client responds when asked a question and, if so, the nurse then assesses the following: Is the client's speech fluent or hesitant? Can the client comprehend and follow directions? In addition, the nurse assesses the client's ability to understand written words: Can the client follow written directions? Can the client read aloud? Can the client recognize words or letters if unable to read whole sentences? The nurse uses large, clearly written words when trying to establish abilities in this area.

When the client is unconscious, the nurse looks for any indication that suggests comprehension of what is communicated (e.g., tries to arouse the client verbally and through touch). The nurse can ask a closed question, such as "Can you hear me?" and watch for a nonverbal response, such as a nod of the head for yes or a shake for no, or the nurse can ask for a hand squeeze or blink of the eyes once for yes or twice for no.

Structural Deficits Structural deficits of the oral and nasal cavities and respiratory system can alter a person's ability to speak clearly and spontaneously. Examples include cleft palate; artificial airways, such as an endotracheal tube or tracheostomy; and laryngectomy (removal of the larynx). Extreme dyspnea (shortness of breath) can also impair speech patterns.

Paralysis If verbal impairment is combined with paralysis of the upper extremities that impairs the client's ability to write, the nurse should determine whether the client can point, nod, shrug, blink, or squeeze a hand. Any of these could be used to devise a communication system.

STYLE OF COMMUNICATION In assessing communication style, the nurse considers both verbal and nonverbal communication. In addition to physical barriers, some psychological illnesses (e.g., depression or psychosis) influence the ability to communicate. The client may demonstrate constant verbalization of the same words or phrases, a loose association of ideas, or flight of ideas.

Verbal Communication When assessing verbal communication, the nurse focuses on three areas: (a) the content of the message, (b) the themes, and (c) verbalized emotions. In addition, the nurse considers the following:

- Whether the communication pattern is slow, rapid, quiet, spontaneous, hesitant, evasive, and so on
- The vocabulary of the individual, particularly any changes from the vocabulary normally used; for example, a person who normally never swears may indicate increased stress or illness by an uncharacteristic use of profanity
- The presence of hostility, aggression, assertiveness, reticence, hesitance, anxiety, or loquaciousness (incessant verbalization) in communication
- Difficulties with verbal communication, such as slurring, stuttering, an inability to pronounce a particular sound, a lack of clarity in enunciation, an inability to speak in sentences, loose association of ideas, flight of ideas, or an inability to find or name words or identify objects
- Refusal or inability to speak

Nonverbal Communication Consider nonverbal communication in relation to the client's culture. Pay particular attention to facial expression, gestures, body movements, affect, tone of voice, posture, and eye contact.

Diagnosing

Impaired Verbal Communication may be used as a nursing diagnosis when "an individual experiences a decreased, delayed, or absent ability to receive, process, transmit, and use a system of symbols—anything that has meaning (i.e., transmits meaning)" (Wilkinson & Ahern, 2009, p. 110). Communication problems may be receptive (e.g., difficulty hearing) or expressive (e.g., difficulty speaking).

The nursing diagnosis *Impaired Verbal Communication* may not be useful when an individual's communication problems are caused by a psychiatric illness. For example, a client with depression may have difficulty expressing feelings or have slowed thinking or responses; clients who have anxiety have decreased ability to focus; and clients with schizophrenia may have auditory hallucinations (hearing voices) and have difficulty hearing the nurse's voice at the same time (Boyd, 2008).

If the communication issue is caused by the client having a problem coping, the diagnoses of *Fear or Anxiety* may be more appropriate. Other nursing diagnoses (NANDA International, 2012) used for clients experiencing communication problems that involve impaired verbal communication as the etiology could include the following:

- *Anxiety* related to impaired verbal communication
- *Powerlessness* related to impaired verbal communication
- *Situational low self-esteem* related to impaired verbal communication
- *Social isolation* related to impaired verbal communication
- *Impaired social interaction* related to impaired verbal communication.

Planning

When a nursing diagnosis related to impaired communication has been made, the nurse and client determine goals or outcomes and begin planning ways to promote effective communication. The overall client goal for persons with *Impaired Verbal Communication* is to reduce or resolve the factors impairing the communication. Specific nursing interventions will be planned from the stated etiology. Examples of outcome criteria to evaluate the effectiveness of nursing interventions and achievement of client goals includes the client doing the following:

- Communicates that needs are being met.
- Begins to establish a method of communication:
  a. Signals yes or no to direct questions by using vocalization or an agreed-on physical cue (e.g., eye blink, hand squeeze).
  b. Uses verbal or nonverbal techniques to indicate needs.
- Perceives the message accurately, as evidenced by appropriate verbal or nonverbal responses.
- Communicates effectively in any of the following ways:
  a. Uses the predominant language.
  b. Uses a translator or an interpreter.
  c. Uses sign language.
  d. Uses a word board or a picture board.
  e. Uses a computer.
- Regains maximum communication abilities.
- Expresses minimum fear, anxiety, frustration, and depression.
- Uses resources appropriately.

Implementing

Nursing interventions to facilitate communication with clients who have problems with speech or language include manipulating the environment, providing support, employing measures to enhance communication, and educating the client and support person.

MANIPULATE THE ENVIRONMENT A quiet environment with limited distractions will make the most of the communication efforts of both the client and the nurse and increase the possibility of effective communication. Sufficient light will help in conveying nonverbal messages, which is especially important if visual or auditory acuity is impaired. Initially, the nurse needs to provide a calm, relaxed environment that will help reduce any anxiety the client may have.

PROVIDE SUPPORT The nurse should convey encouragement to the client and provide nonverbal reassurance, perhaps by touch, if appropriate. If the nurse does not understand, it is critical to let the client know so that the nurse can provide clarification with other words or through some other means of communication. When speaking with a client who has difficulty understanding, the nurse should check frequently to determine what the client has heard and understood. The use of open-ended questions will help the nurse obtain accurate information about the effectiveness of communication. For example, Maria Perez, who has limited English skills, is being taught about a diet related to her Crohn's disease. If the nurse asks, "Do you understand what to eat?" Maria may nod her head yes. However, this does not give her nurse confirmation that the message given has been received. Rather, the nurse needs to say, "What do you think will be good for you to eat when you go home?" The nurse's body language (e.g., gestures, posture, facial expression, and eye contact) should convey acceptance and approval.

EMPLOY MEASURES TO ENHANCE COMMUNICATION Determine how the client can best receive messages: by listening, by looking, through touch, or through an interpreter. Ways to enhance communication include keeping words simple and concrete and discussing topics of interest to the client. It is often helpful to use alternative communication strategies, such as word boards, pictures, or paper and pencil (see the Reflect on Primary Health Care box on the next page).

Often, interpreters can help a client and nurse to communicate when the client lacks fluency in the predominant language. Some hospitals have a list of interpreters for various languages who can assist at the bedside. If the client's support person offers to interpret, it is important to ask the client's permission, for the sake of confidentiality. Then, instruct the person to translate as precisely as possible, without interpretation.

EDUCATE THE CLIENT AND SUPPORT PERSONS
Sometimes, clients and support people can be prepared in advance for communication problems, for example, before an intubation or throat surgery. By explaining anticipated problems, the client is often less anxious when problems do arise.

Evaluating

Evaluation is useful for both client and nurse communication.

CLIENT COMMUNICATION To establish whether client goals have been met in relation to communication, the nurse must listen actively, observe nonverbal cues, and use therapeutic communication skills to determine that communication was effective. Examples of evaluative statements indicating goal achievement could be "using picture board effectively to indicate needs" or "the client stated, 'I listened more closely to my daughter yesterday and found out how she feels about our divorce.'"

NURSE COMMUNICATION For nurses to evaluate the effectiveness of their own communication with clients, process recordings are frequently used. A **process recording** is a verbatim (word-for-word) account of a conversation. It can be taped or written and includes all verbal and nonverbal interactions of both the client and the nurse. One method of writing a process recording is to make two columns on a page. The first column lists what the nurse and the client said along with the associated nonverbal behaviour. The second column contains interpretive comments about the nurse's responses. An example of a process recording is shown in Table 22.5.

TABLE 22.5 Sample Process Recording

Mary Jane Adams, a nursing aide, reports to Irene Olsen, the staff nurse, that Sandra Barrett, the client in room 815, had finished only her orange juice when Ms. Adams collected the breakfast trays. Mrs. Barrett had been admitted 2 days earlier for diagnostic studies. Concerned about her client, Ms. Olsen walks down the corridor to room 815, knocks, and enters. Mrs. Barrett turns away from the window, tears in her eyes, as Ms. Olsen enters.

Nurse/Client Dialogue	Analysis
Nurse: Good morning, Mrs. Barrett. *Client*: Hello.	Acknowledging
Nurse: I understand you didn't eat your breakfast. *Client*: I wasn't hungry.	Making a specific statement but ignoring the nonverbal expression
Nurse: Is something wrong? *Client*: No. (Eyes fill with tears.)	Asking a closed question that fails to facilitate exploration
Nurse: You look sad, as if you're about to cry. *Client*: (Cries)	Giving feedback
Nurse: I'll sit here awhile with you. (Sits down.) *Client*: (Continues to cry.)	Offering self
Nurse: (After a 30-second pause) Sometimes it's hard to share the things you're concerned about with someone you don't know well. I'd like to be able to help. *Client*: (Angrily) You can help me by telling me the truth.	Empathizing Supporting Offering self
Nurse: (Leans forward and maintains eye contact.) *Client*: Everyone beats around the bush when I ask them what's wrong with me. The nurse manager said, "What do you think is wrong?" That kind of put-off drives me up the wall!	Actively listening and demonstrating interest

TABLE 22.5 (*continued*)

Nurse/Client Dialogue	Analysis
Nurse: You're angry because you're not getting any answers. It seems as if the staff knows something about your condition and they're keeping it from you. *Client*: They all seem to be in cahoots. Nobody tells me anything. (Pause.) (Softly) If the news was good, they wouldn't beat around the bush.	Paraphrasing
Nurse: I'm wondering if you're worried that because people haven't answered your question it means that you have a serious illness? *Client*: Good news is always easy to give.	Paraphrasing
Nurse: Yes, people do seem to be able to deliver good news easier and faster. I also know that we don't have any news—good or bad—to give you because none of the laboratory or x-ray results are back yet. I know that doesn't help answer your questions, but I hope it relieves you a bit from worrying that there is some bad news that's being withheld. *Client*: Well, when my father-in-law had surgery for a bleeding ulcer, the x-ray and laboratory results were available immediately.	Giving information Supporting
Nurse: When there's a question of emergency surgery being needed, then test results are asked for immediately. Usually, though, it's preferable to wait for an accurate reading and a thorough written report. *Client*: Are you absolutely sure?	Giving information
Nurse: You don't sound convinced. *Client*: Listen, I don't mean to give you a hard time. It's just that . . . it may not seem like an emergency to my doctor or the lab people, but it sure is to me. I can't stand not knowing. I don't know the results of the tests I had yesterday. I don't know how many more tests I have to have. Will I have to have surgery? When can I go home?	Acknowledging the implied
Nurse: The problem you need help with now is finding out the answers to four questions: What are the results of yesterday's tests? Is your doctor considering any other tests for you and, if so, what are they? Is surgery being planned? And when can you go home? Let's try to figure out how you can get the answers to these questions. *Client*: Well, I can't call my doctor on the phone. All his receptionist will do is take the message. And, anyway, I'm afraid that he'll be offended if he thinks I'm complaining about him. You won't tell him, will you?	Summarizing Encouraging problem solving
Nurse: No, not unless you and I decide together that it would be the best solution. *Client*: I suppose I could try to forget about it and be patient, just like everyone tells me to.	Encouraging collaboration
Nurse: You've tried that, but you're still worried, fearful, and angry. Let's think of some other possibilities. *Client*: Maybe you could call his office for me! Since you're a nurse, they'll probably put your call right through.	Encouraging further exploration
Nurse: So far there are three possible solutions—calling his office yourself, waiting until he comes to visit you later this afternoon, or having me call his office. Are there any other possible solutions that we haven't considered? *Client*: I can't think of any other.	Focusing on solutions
Nurse: Okay, then, which do you think would be best? *Client*: I guess I'd feel better if you called his office. I just don't want him to think that I'm criticizing him.	Demonstrating respect for the client
Nurse: You're concerned about what he might think of you because of this phone call. Let's discuss how I should handle the call and what I should say.	Paraphrasing Encouraging collaboration and problem solving

Source: Based on material by Carol Ren Kneisl, president and educational director, nursing transitions, Williamsville, NY.

Once a process recording has been completed, it should be analyzed in terms of the content and meaning of the interaction based on communication theory. Each of the nurse's statements is interpreted in terms of the communication skill used, with the rationale for and effectiveness of its use. Any barriers to effective communication can be identified, with a possible alternative response noted. The outcome for nurses should be increased awareness and insight regarding their communication strengths, as well as identification of areas for future skills development.

Communication among Health Care Professionals

Effective communication among the health care professions is as important as the promotion of therapeutic communication between the nurse and the client. For example, communication problems among health care personnel have been implicated as a cause of most client errors (Dillon, Noble, & Kaplan, 2009). Sirota (2007) reported that poor communication between nurses and physicians was the most important factor causing dissatisfaction with nurse–physician working relationships. Many nurses report verbal abuse, lateral violence, incivility, and bullying from physicians and other nurses (Johnson, Martin, & Markle-Elder, 2007; Olender-Russo, 2009a; Woelfle & McCaffrey, 2007). These disruptive behaviours have a negative impact on the work environment and are one of the reasons nurses leave the profession, which subsequently contributes to nursing shortages. Workplace violence destroys the ideal organizational climate of mutual respect and has negative health consequences and impairs productivity. Examples include absenteeism, emotional exhaustion, decreased commitment to the organization, decreased effort at work, incivility toward others, decreased communication, decreased reporting of problems, and leaving the organization (Hutton & Gates, 2008).

The Canadian Nurses Association (CNA) and Canadian Federation of Nurses Unions (CFNU) (2010) support zero workplace violence and promote a healthy workplace for all nurses. Workplace intimidation is a threat to client safety and subsequently requires health care facilities to design and implement a system-wide approach for ensuring employee awareness of disruptive behaviours. One example is the implementation of Ontario's Bill 168, Occupational Health and Safety Act, by all workplaces to halt and prevent such behaviours (Legislative Assembly of Ontario, 2009).

Disruptive Behaviours

Three common disruptive behaviours reported among nurses are (a) incivility, (b) lateral violence, and (c) bullying.

Incivility

Incivility is described as rude, discourteous, or disrespectful behaviour that reflects a lack of regard for others (Hutton & Gates, 2008; Olender-Russo, 2009b). Common actions that characterize incivility include personal insults, invading personal territory, uninvited physical contact, threats and intimidation, sarcastic jokes and teasing, abusive e-mails, humiliation, public shaming, rude interruptions, twofaced attacks, dirty looks, and treating people as if they are invisible (Sutton, 2010).

Lateral Violence

Lateral violence, also known as horizontal violence and horizontal hostility, are terms that describe physical, verbal, or emotional abuse or aggression directed at coworkers at the same organizational level. Examples of these behaviours include undermining activities, withholding information, sabotage, scapegoating, infighting, back-stabbing, and broken confidences (CNA & CFNU, 2010). Newly registered nurses are at risk for lateral violence (Sheridan-Leos, 2008).

Bullying

Bullying is an abusive, intimidating treatment of someone who is in a vulnerable position or a position with less power. The person being bullied feels threatened and humiliated and suffers stress. The perpetrator usually is at a higher level of authority (e.g., nursing supervisor to staff nurse). To be considered bullying behaviour, it must occur repeatedly (e.g., twice a week or more) and for at least 6 months, and be targeted at an individual who is unable to defend herself or himself (Olender-Russo, 2009b).

Nurse and Physician Communication

There are few guidelines for the frequent verbal communication that occurs between nurses and doctors. This lack of guidelines or format may contribute to medical errors as a result of communication problems.

Communication Styles

The differences between nurse and physician communication can make collaboration difficult. In general, nurses have been taught to be descriptive in verbal and written communication. Physicians, however, are trained to be brief, to the point, and focused on a problem. Therefore, they may become impatient waiting for the nurse to come to the point (Johnson et al., 2007; Pope, Rodzen, & Spross, 2008). One model, called SBAR (situation, background, assessment, recommendations) provides a standardized framework for effective and accurate communication of important information. (See Chapter 24, "Documenting and Reporting.")

Emotional Intelligence

Emotional intelligence is the ability to form work relationships with colleagues, display maturity in a variety of situations, manage emotions, consider the emotions of others, and resolve conflicts by interacting with colleagues constructively to achieve a positive outcome (Momeni, 2009). A nurse or primary care provider with emotional intelligence may be viewed as mature, approachable, or easygoing.

Assertive Communication

Assertive communication promotes client safety by minimizing miscommunication with colleagues. People who use assertive communication are honest, direct, and appropriate while being open to ideas and respecting the rights of others. An important characteristic of assertive communication includes the use of "I" statements versus "you" statements. The "you" statement places blame and puts the listener in a defensive position. In contrast, the "I" statement encourages discussion. For example, a nurse who states "I am concerned about . . ." will be gaining the attention of the primary care provider while also giving a message about the importance of working together for the benefit of the client. It is then important for the nurse to be clear, concise, organized, and fully informed when verbally presenting the client concern.

Nonassertive Communication

Two types of interpersonal behaviours are considered nonassertive: (a) submissive and (b) aggressive.

SUBMISSIVE When people use a submissive communication style, they meet the demands and requests of others without regard to their own feelings and needs because they believe their own feelings are not important. People who use submissive communication style usually are insecure with low self-esteem and want to avoid conflict (e.g., negative criticism and disagreement from others).

AGGRESSIVE There is a fine line between assertive and aggressive communication. Assertive communication is an open expression of ideas and opinions while respecting the rights, opinions, and ideas of others. Aggressive communication can be blaming and delivered in a rushed manner, thus becoming ineffective and leading to frustration for the nurse and the primary care provider (Cleary, Walter, & Horsfall, 2009; Mascioli, Laskowski-Jones, Urban, & Moran, 2009).

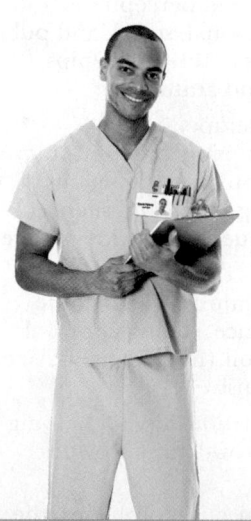

Case Study 22

You are the nursing student assigned to care for Mr. Manasovitz, a 45-year-old man, who will be returning from the recovery room after undergoing the removal of a mass from his abdomen. While you are preparing his room for his return, the nurse and physician arrive to talk with Mrs. Manasovitz about her husband's surgery. The physician explains that the mass was malignant and invasive. Mr. Manasovitz is a candidate for chemotherapy, but his prognosis is guarded because of the extent of the tumour growth. Mrs. Manasovitz looks away, closes her eyes, and only nods her head "yes." As the physician leaves, the nurse approaches Mrs. Manasovitz, sits next to her, and puts her arm around Mrs. Manasovitz, who begins to cry. The nurse uses a soothing voice to tell Mrs. Manasovitz that it is okay to cry and provides assurance by remaining with her. The two of them sit in silence until Mrs. Manasovitz is able to express her feelings. The nurse listens attentively. Later, the nurse offers to get a cup of coffee for Mrs. Manasovitz and offers to assist her at this difficult time.

CRITICAL THINKING QUESTIONS

1. Interpret Mrs. Manasovitz's nonverbal behaviour in response to the news about her husband's surgery.

2. Evaluate the nurse's response to Mrs. Manasovitz on the basis of the concepts of caring and comforting.

3. Why is it important for the nurse to effectively communicate with Mrs. Manasovitz at this time?

4. The nurse was described as listening attentively to Mrs. Manasovitz. Cite actions that portray attentive listening.

5. Think about your past experiences when you or a family member has been ill. What relationship characteristics did you most value on the part of the nurse caring for you?

Check the eText in MyNursingLab for answers and explanations.

KEY TERMS

aesthetic knowing   *p. 426*
attentive listening   *p. 433*
boundaries   *p. 433*
bullying   *p. 448*
caring   *p. 423*
caring practice   *p. 423*
communication   *p. 427*
congruent communication
   p. 433
culturally competent care
   p. 423

decode   *p. 428*
electronic communication
   p. 428
e-mail   *p. 431*
emotional intelligence
   p. 449
empathy   *p. 440*
empirical knowing   *p. 425*
encoding   *p. 427*
ethical knowing   *p. 426*
feedback   *p. 428*

group   *p. 441*
group dynamics   *p. 441*
incivility   *p. 448*
lateral violence   *p. 448*
message   *p. 427*
nonverbal communication
   p. 428
personal knowing   *p. 426*
personal space   *p. 432*
process recording   *p. 446*
receiver   *p. 428*

sender   *p. 427*
task group   *p. 441*
territoriality   *p. 432*
therapeutic
   communication
   p. 433
verbal communication
   p. 428

CHAPTER HIGHLIGHTS

- Communication is a critical nursing skill used to gather information, to teach and persuade, and to express caring and comfort.

- Caring is said to be the essence of nursing. It includes assistive, supportive, and facilitative acts for individuals or groups.

- Caring acts promote individual growth, preserve human dignity and worth, augment self-healing and comfort, and relieve distress.

- Comfort needs can be viewed in a framework of physical, psychospiritual, social, and environmental needs. Nurses need to be knowledgeable, skilled, and innovative to individualize comforting strategies.

- Caring is a key concept in the nurse–client process. When clients feel cared for, they report higher levels of health satisfaction and quality of life. Client-centred care is focused on effective nurse–client interaction.

- Communication is a two-way interpersonal process involving the sender of the message and the receiver of the message. It also involves intrapersonal messages, or self-talk, which can affect the message, the interpretation of the message, and the response.

- Because the sender must encode the message and determine the appropriate channels for conveying it, and because the receiver must perceive the message, decode it, and then respond, the communication process includes four elements: sender, message, receiver, and feedback.

- Verbal communication is effective when the criteria of pace and intonation, simplicity, clarity and brevity, timing, relevance, adaptability, and credibility are met.

- Nonverbal communication often reveals more about a person's thoughts and feelings than verbal communication; it includes personal appearance, posture and gait, facial expressions, and gestures.

- When assessing verbal and nonverbal behaviours, the nurse needs to consider cultural influences and be

aware that a single nonverbal expression can indicate any of a variety of feelings and that words can have various meanings.

- When communication is effective, verbal and nonverbal expressions are congruent.

- Electronic communication, particularly e-mail, is evolving in nursing practice. E-mail has advantages and disadvantages and nurses must be aware of the risk to client confidentiality.

- Many factors influence the communication process: development, gender, values and perceptions, personal space (intimate, personal, social, and public distances), territoriality, roles and relationships, environment, congruence, and attitudes.

- Many techniques facilitate therapeutic communication: attentive listening; paraphrasing; clarifying; using open questions and statements; focusing; being specific; using touch and silence; clarifying reality, time, or sequence; providing general leads; and summarizing.

- Techniques that inhibit communication include offering invalidated reassurance, stating approval or disapproval, giving common (not expert) advice, stereotyping, and being defensive.

- The effective nurse–client relationship is a helping relationship that facilitates growth and provides support, comfort, and hope.

- To help clients with communication problems, the nurse manipulates the environment, provides support, employs measures to enhance communication, and educates the client and support persons.

- Nurses interact with groups of clients and colleagues in a wide variety of settings. To use groups rationally and effectively, nurses must understand the features of effective groups.

- Effective groups produce outstanding results, succeed in spite of difficulties, and have members who feel responsible for the output of the group. They accomplish their goals (outcomes), maintain cohesion, and develop and modify their structure in ways that improve effectiveness.

• Process recordings are frequently made by nurses to evaluate their own communication. With them, nurses can analyze both the process and the content of the communication.

• Effective communication among health care professionals is vital and communication styles can differ between nurses and physicians.

• Assertive communication can promote client safety.

ASSESS YOUR LEARNING

1. The interpersonal communication process is situated in the context that includes which of the following components?

   a. Social, historical, physical, psychological, and cultural

   b. Physical, psychological, environmental, and cultural

   c. Cultural, historical, physical, psychological, and environmental

   d. Environmental, contextual, social, and physical

2. A young woman is crying on a chair beside her bed. As her nurse, which of the following is your most caring response?

   a. "You look sad. Why are you crying?"

   b. "Are you in pain?"

   c. "Tell me more about how you are feeling."

   d. "Do you want to go home?"

3. You are a nurse in a fast-paced medical unit. A patient approaches you and asks where his nurse is. Knowing that she is on break, which of the following is your most caring response?

   a. "I am not sure, but she will be back soon to assist you."

   b. "She is having coffee. She has had a very busy morning."

   c. "She is having coffee. Is there anything that I may assist you with?"

   d. "She is having coffee and I am very busy. Can you wait until she comes back"?

4. Which of the following describes the comforting process?

   a. A simple process of giving and receiving

   b. Unique to nursing

   c. A complex process

   d. Does not last longer than the intervention

5. A health care team on an acute geriatric unit meets on a weekly basis to review clients' progress. The nurse observes that one team member consistently dominates the discussion. Which of the following actions is MOST appropriate for the nurse to take?

   a. Continue observing and note any changes in behaviour

   b. Discuss these observations with the group

   c. Speak to group members individually to validate these observations

   d. Speak with the individual privately regarding these observations

6. A colleague says, "You do not know what you are doing!" How should you respond to build effective communication?

   a. "Of course I do! You don't know what you are saying."

   b. "Let's talk about this later when we've both had time to think."

   c. "You have hurt my feelings. I am going to speak with the manager."

   d. "Let's go to a quieter area and you can tell me what you mean."

7. What method of communicating is a barrier to communication?

   a. Judging

   b. Caring

   c. Summarizing

   d. Clarifying

8. A supervisor states to you that you are spending too much time talking with patients and not enough time training the new staff on the unit. Which of the following is your BEST response?

   a. "Don't worry about it, I will work overtime tonight to make sure they are all trained."

   b. "My priority is to the patients. How can you expect me to have enough time to do both?"

   c. "It is important for me to discuss patients' issues and concerns with them. I will arrange new staff training times."

   d. "It is my role as a nurse to speak with my patients and address their concerns as much as possible. You know that."

9. After breakfast, a client states that he wants to rest in bed for the morning and not go to physiotherapy. Which of the following is your BEST response?

   a. "It is best if you go. The physiotherapist will help you walk better."

   b. "Please tell me more about this."

   c. "Are you in pain?"

   d. "What would you like me to tell her?"

10. Which of the following qualities BEST fosters each nurse–client relationship?
    a. Nurse-centred
    b. Power based
    c. Client-focused
    d. Not based on boundaries

Check the eText in MyNursingLab for answers and explanations.

WEBLINKS

College and Association of Registered Nurses of Alberta

https://www.nurses.ab.ca/Carna-Admin/Uploads/Professional%20Boundaries%20Guidelines.pdf

This website (similar to various provincial and territorial associations of registered nurses) includes documents that provide interpretations of the expectations of registered nurses in establishing therapeutic relationships and maintaining appropriate boundaries with clients and their significant others.

College of Nurses of Ontario

http://www.cno.org/pubs/publist.html

This website includes documents concerning the nurse–client relationship, such as Therapeutic Nurse–Client Relationship, and Ethics.

Registered Nurses' Association of Ontario, Best Practice Guidelines

http://www.rnao.org/bestpractices

The following documents are related to the nurse–client relationship: Client Centred Care, Establishing Therapeutic Relationships, and Supporting and Strengthening Families Through Expected and Unexpected Life Events. They are available on this site by clicking Nursing Best Practice Guidelines, then Clinical Practice Guidelines Program, and Guidelines and Fact Sheets.

Watson Caring Science Institute: International Caritas Consortium

http://www.watsoncaringscience.org/j_watson/index.html

This website provides an overview of Jean Watson's lifetime work and her international Watson Caring Science Institute, including many resources related to Watson's Theory of Human Caring.

Registered Nurses' Association of Ontario: Video

http://rnao.ca/bpg/guidelines/resources/establishing-therapeutic-relationship-video

Establishing a therapeutic relationship.

MyNursingLab

REFERENCES

Austin, S. (2006). E-mail: So fast, so convenient, so . . . risky? *Nursing, 36*(2), 76–77.

Benner, P., & Wrubel, J. (1989). *The primacy of caring: Stress and coping in health and illness.* Menlo Park, CA: Addison-Wesley.

Boyd, M. A. (2008). *Psychiatric nursing: Contemporary practice.* Philadelphia, PA: Lippincott Williams & Wilkins.

Burkhardt, M. A., Nathaniel, A. K., & Walton, N. A. (2010). *Ethics and issues in contemporary nursing.* Toronto, ON: Nelson.

Canadian Nurses Association and Canadian Federation of Nurses Unions. (2010). *Joint position statement: Workplace violence.* Ottawa, ON: Authors. Retrieved from http://www.cna-aiic.ca/CNA/documents/pdf/publications/JPS95_Workplace_Violence_e.pdf

Carper, B. (2009). Fundamental patterns of knowing in nursing. In P. Reed & N. Shearer (Eds.), *Perspectives on nursing theory* (5th ed.) (pp. 377–384). Philadelphia, PA: Wolters Kluwer-Lippincott Williams & Wilkins.

Chinn, P., & Kramer, M. (2008). *Integrated knowledge development in nursing* (7th ed.). St. Louis, MO: Mosby.

Cleary, M., Walter, G., & Horsfall, J. (2009). Handover in psychiatric settings. *Journal of Psychosocial Nursing, 47*(3), 28–33.

Dearing, K. S., & Steadman, S. (2008). Challenging stereotyping and bias: A voice simulation study. *Journal of Nursing Education, 47,* 59–65.

Dillon, P. M., Noble, K. A., & Kaplan, L. (2009). Simulation as a means to foster collaborative interdisciplinary education. *Nursing Education Perspectives, 30*(2), 87–90.

Egan, G. (2009). *The skilled helper: A problem-management approach to helping* (9th ed.). Pacific Grove, CA: Brooks/Cole.

Gordon, S., Benner, P., & Noddings, N. (1996). *Caregiving.* Philadelphia, PA: University of Pennsylvania Press.

Hearnden, M. (2008). Coping with differences in culture and communication in health care. *Nursing Standard, 23*(11), 49–58.

Hills, M., & Watson, J. (2011). *Creating a caring science curriculum: An emancipatory pedagogy for nursing.* New York, NY: Springer Publishing.

Hutton, S., & Gates, D. (2008). Workplace incivility and productivity losses among direct care staff. *AAOHN Journal, 56*(4), 168–175. doi: 10.3928/08910162- 20080401-01

Jansson, C., & Adolfsson, A. (2011). Application of "Swanson's middle range caring theory" in Sweden after miscarriage— Swanson's middle range caring theory, miscarriage, missed miscarriage, qualitative method. *International Journal of Clinical Medicine, 2*, pp. 102-109. doi:10.4236/ijcm.2011.22021

Johnson, C. L., Martin, S. L., & Markle-Elder, S. (2007). Stopping verbal abuse in the workplace. *American Journal of Nursing, 107*(4), 32–34.

Legislative Assembly of Ontario. (2009). *Bottom of Form Bill 168, Occupational Health and Safety Amendment Act (Violence and Harassment in the Workplace) 2009.* Retrieved from http://www.ontla.on.ca/web/bills/bills_detail.do?locale=en&Intranet=&BillID=2181

Leininger, M., & McFarland, M. (2006). *Culture care diversity and universality: A worldwide nursing theory.* Sudbury, MA: Jones & Bartlett.

Macon, A., & Mendiola, R. (2008). One-stop shopping, *Health Management Technology, 29*(11), 22–24.

Mascioli, S., Laskowski-Jones, L., Urban, S., & Moran, S. (2009). Improving handoff communication. *Nursing 2009, 39*(2), 52–55.

Momeni, N. (2009). The relation between managers' emotional intelligence and the organizational climate they create. *Public Personnel Management, 38*(2), 35–48

Moore, K. (2008). Is laughter the best medicine? Research into the therapeutic use of humor and laughter in nursing practice. *Whitireia Nursing Journal, 15*, 33–38.

NANDA International. (2012). *NANDA nursing diagnosis: Definitions and classification 2012–2014.* Oxford, UK: Wiley-Blackwell.

Newman, M. A., Sime, A. M., & Corcoran-Perry, S. A. (2009). The focus of the discipline of nursing. In P. Reed & N. Shearer (Eds.), *Perspectives on nursing theory* (5th ed., pp. 601–606). Philadelphia, PA: Wolters Kluwer-Lippincott Williams & Wilkins.

Olender-Russo, L. (2009a). Creating a culture of regard: An antidote for workplace bullying. *Creative Nursing, 15*(2), 75–81. doi: 10.1891/1078-4535.15.2.75

Olender-Russo, L. (2009b). Reversing a bullying culture. *RN, 72*(8), 26–29.

Poochikian-Sarkissian, S., Sidani, S., Ferguson-Pare, M., Doran, D. (2010). Examining the relationship between patient-centred care and outcomes. *Canadian Journal of Neuroscience Nursing, 32*(4), 14–21.

Pope, B. B., Rodzen, L., & Spross, G. (2008). Raising the SBAR. How better communication improves patient outcomes. *Nursing, 38*(3), 41–43.

Reid, R. J., & Wagner, E. H. (2008). Strengthening primary care with better transfer of information. *Canadian Medical Association Journal, 179,* 987–988.

Roach, M. S. (2004). *Caring, the human mode of being* (2nd ed.). Ottawa, ON: CHA Press.

Sheridan-Leos, N. (2008). Understanding lateral violence in nursing. *Clinical Journal of Oncology Nursing, 12,* 399–403. doi: 10.1188/08.CJON.399-403

Sirota, T. (2007). Nurse/physician relationships: Improving or not? *Nursing, 37*(1), 52–55.

Storch, J., Rodney, P., & Starzomski, R. (2012). *Toward a moral horizon: Nursing ethics for leadership and practice* (2nd ed.). Toronto, ON: Pearson Education Canada.

Sutton, R. I. (2010). *The no asshole rule: Building a civilized workplace and surviving one that isn't.* New York, NY: Business Plus.

Swanson, K. M. (1991). Empirical development of a middle range theory of caring. *Nurse Researcher, 40*(3), 161–166.

Tamparo, C. T., & Lindh, W. Q. (2008). *Therapeutic communications for health professionals* (3rd ed.). Albany, NY: Delmar: Thomson Learning.

Watson, J. (1999a). Postmodern nursing and beyond. In N. Chaska (Ed.), *The nursing profession: Nursing theories and nursing practice* (pp. 343–354). Philadelphia, PA: Davis.

Watson, J. (1999b). *Nursing: Human science and human care: A theory of nursing.* Boston, MA: National League for Nursing.

Watson, J. (2008). *Nursing: The philosophy and science of caring.* Boulder, CO: University Press of Colorado.

Wilkinson, J. M., & Ahern, N. R. (2009). *Nursing diagnosis handbook with NIC interventions and NOC outcomes* (9th ed.). Upper Saddle River, NJ: Pearson Prentice Hall.

Woelfle, C. Y., & McCaffrey, R. (2007). Nurse on nurse. *Nursing Forum, 42,* 123–131.

Wojnar, D. (2010). Kristen M. Swanson: The theory of caring. In M. Alligood & A. Tomey (Eds.), *Nursing theorists and their work* (7th ed., pp. 741–752). St. Louis, MO: Mosby.

The editorial team would like to acknowledge and to thank Lucia Yiu for preparing and writing sections of Chapter 22.

Chapter 23

The Nursing Process

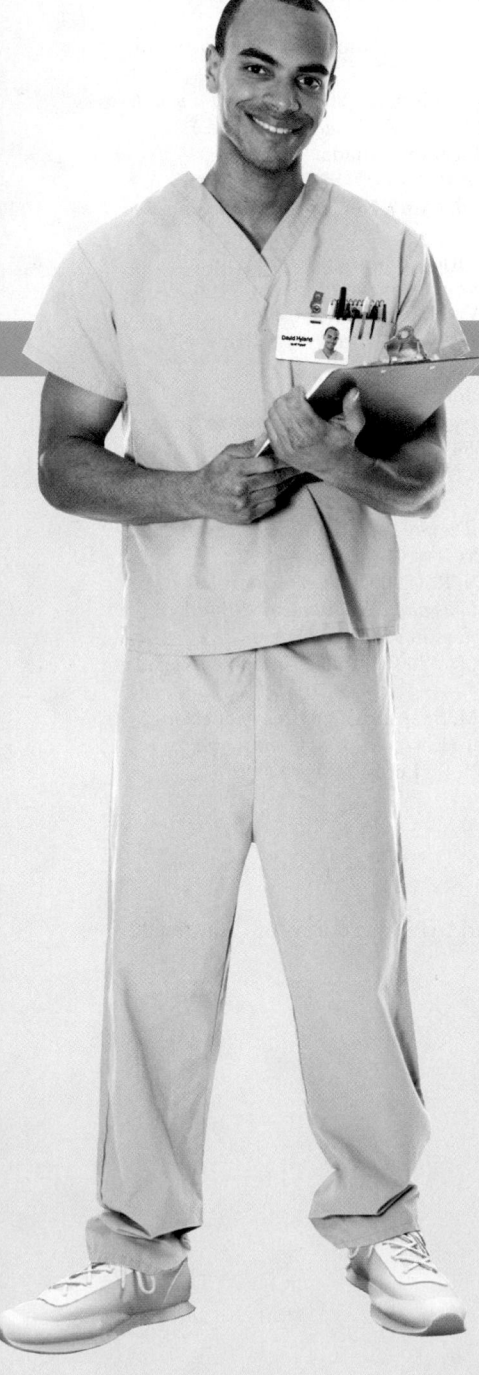

After studying this chapter, you will be able to:

1. Describe the five phases of the nursing process.

2. Identify the relevance of each phase of the nursing process in guiding nursing practice.

3. Identify methods of data collection.

4. Differentiate objective and subjective data and primary and secondary data.

5. Describe the characteristics and formulations of writing nursing diagnoses.

6. Identify factors that the nurse must consider in planning for, implementing, and evaluating patient care.

7. Outline how critical pathways and concept maps are used to create a comprehensive nursing care plan.

8. Formulate client health outcome evaluation criteria while planning nursing care.

9. Explain how evaluating relates to various phases of the nursing process.

10. Identify the importance of quality improvement processes to guide ongoing improvement in client care.

The **nursing process** is a systematic, client-centred, rational method of planning and providing individualized nursing care. Its purpose is to identify client strengths and potential or actual health problems or needs, and to develop specific nursing interventions to achieve mutually agreed-upon outcomes. At every stage of the process, the nurse works closely with the client to tailor care and build a relationship of mutual regard and trust. The client may be an individual, a family, a community, or a group.

Overview of the Nursing Process

Hall (1955) coined the term *nursing process* in 1955, whereas others (Johnson, 1959; Orlando,1961; Wiedenbach,1963) referred to phases of the process to describe the practice of nursing. There are five phases of the nursing process: (a) assessment, (b) diagnosis, (c) planning, (d) implementation, and (e) evaluation of its competencies for professional nursing practice (see Figure 23.1 on the next page). The use of the nursing process in clinical practice gained additional legitimacy in 1973 when the phases were included in the American Nurses Association's [ANA] (2010) standards of nursing practice. These phases of nursing process are also expected competencies for professional nursing practice in Canada (Canadian Nurses' Association [CNA], 2011).

Since the 1970s, the Canadian Nurses Association has endorsed the nursing process in guiding nursing practice (CNA, 1980, revised 1987). The nursing process remains a fundamental process that facilitates a thoughtful, informed, evidence-based, and ethical nursing practice. This process guides nursing care with individual, family, group, and community clients from simple to complex practice environments. It is a process that fosters critical thinking and decision making. Regulatory nursing bodies in each province have standards of nursing practice to support the centrality of the nursing process in guiding nursing practice to meet client health outcomes.

Phases of the Nursing Process

As mentioned above, the nursing process has five phases. These phases of the nursing process are not separate entities but overlapping, continuing subprocesses. For example, while administering medications (implementing), the nurse continuously notes the client's skin colour, level of consciousness (assessment), and response to medication (evaluation). Each phase of the nursing process affects the others; they are closely interrelated. If inadequate data are obtained during assessing, the nursing diagnoses will be incomplete or incorrect because of this omission, and inaccuracy could thus be reflected in the planning, implementing, and evaluating phases.

An overview of the five-phase nursing process is shown in Figure 23.2 on page 458.

Characteristics of the Nursing Process

The nursing process has distinctive characteristics that enable the nurse to respond to the changing health status of the client. These characteristics include the following:

- *Cyclical and dynamic nature.* Data from each phase provide input into the next phase. Findings from evaluation feed back into assessment. Hence, the nursing process is a regularly repeated event or sequence of events (cyclical) that is continuously changing (dynamic) rather than staying the same (static).

- *Client-centredness.* The nurse organizes the plan of care according to identified client problems. In the assessment phase, the nurse collects data to determine the client's habits or routines, preferences, and needs, enabling the nurse to incorporate client routines into the care plan as much as possible.

- *Focus on problem solving.* The nursing process uses both problem-solving technique (see Chapter 21) and systems theory (see Chapter 12) to organize care. Both processes (a) begin with data gathering and analysis, (b) base action (intervention or treatment) on a problem statement (nursing diagnosis or medical diagnosis), and (c) include an evaluative component. The nursing process is directed toward a client's responses to disease and illness and adaptations to altered health status, whereas the medical model of care tends to focus on physiological systems and the disease process.

- *Focus on decision making.* Decision making is involved in every phase of the nursing process. Nurses can be highly creative in determining when and how to use data to make decisions. Nurses are not bound by standard responses and can apply their repertoire of skills and knowledge to assist clients.

- *Interpersonal and collaborative style.* Nurses communicate directly and consistently with clients to meet

THE NURSING PROCESS IN ACTION

The nursing process is a systematic, rational method of planning and providing nursing care. Its purpose is to identify a client's healthcare status and actual or potential health problems, to establish plans to meet the identified needs, and to deliver specific nursing interventions to address those needs. The nursing process is cyclical; that is, its components follow a logical sequence, but more than one component can be involved at one time. At the end of the first cycle, care may be terminated if goals are achieved, or the cycle may continue with reassessment, or the plan of care may be modified.

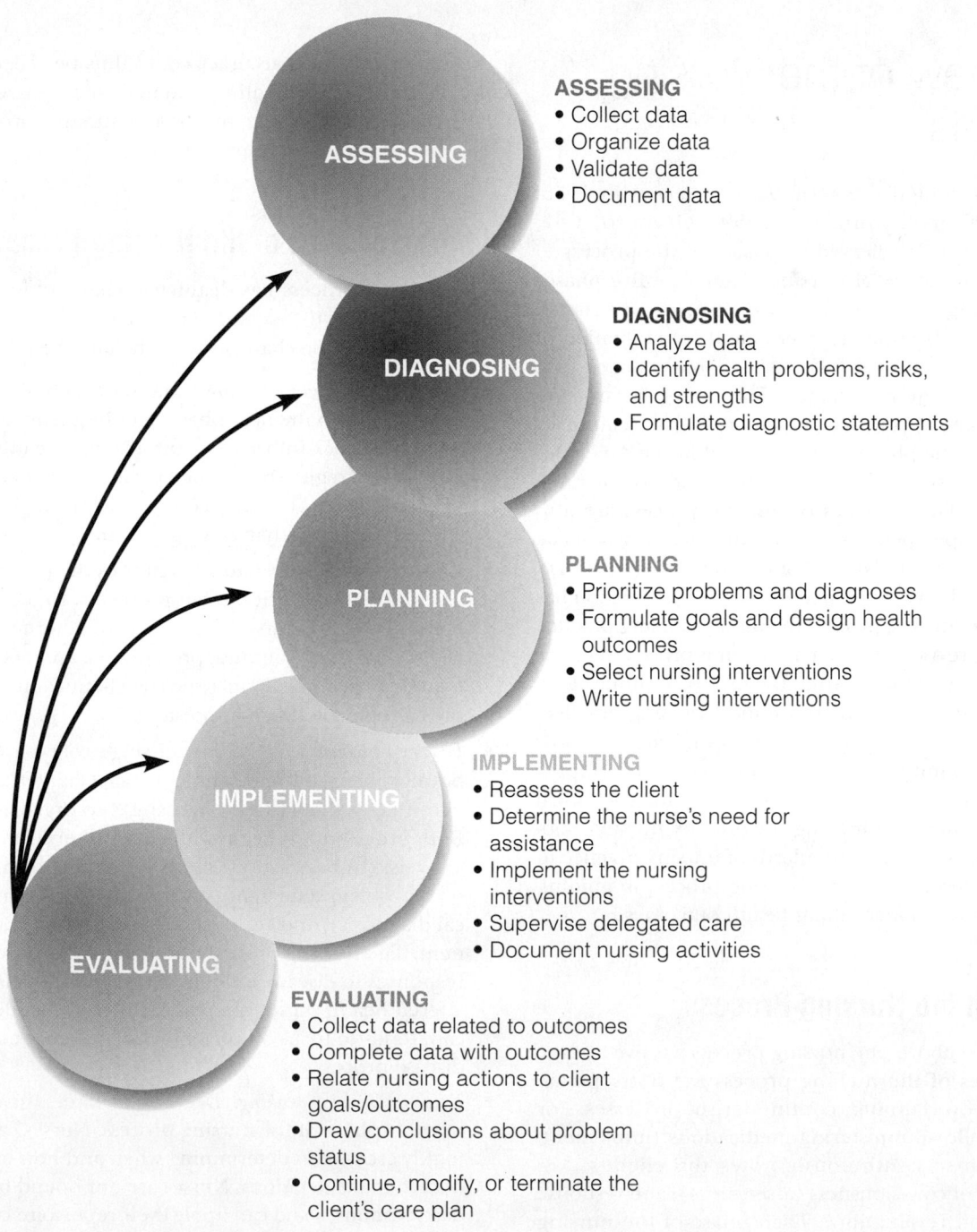

ASSESSING
- Collect data
- Organize data
- Validate data
- Document data

DIAGNOSING
- Analyze data
- Identify health problems, risks, and strengths
- Formulate diagnostic statements

PLANNING
- Prioritize problems and diagnoses
- Formulate goals and design health outcomes
- Select nursing interventions
- Write nursing interventions

IMPLEMENTING
- Reassess the client
- Determine the nurse's need for assistance
- Implement the nursing interventions
- Supervise delegated care
- Document nursing activities

EVALUATING
- Collect data related to outcomes
- Complete data with outcomes
- Relate nursing actions to client goals/outcomes
- Draw conclusions about problem status
- Continue, modify, or terminate the client's care plan

FIGURE 23.1 The nursing process in action.
*The medical abbreviation "q3h" indicates "deep breathing and coughing every three hours."

Amanda Aquilini, a 28-year-old married lawyer, was admitted to the hospital with an elevated temperature, a productive cough, and rapid, laboured respirations. In taking a nursing history, Nurse Mary Medina, RN, finds that Amanda has had a "chest cold" for two weeks, and has been experiencing shortness of breath on exertion. Yesterday she developed an elevated temperature and began to experience "pain" in her "lungs."

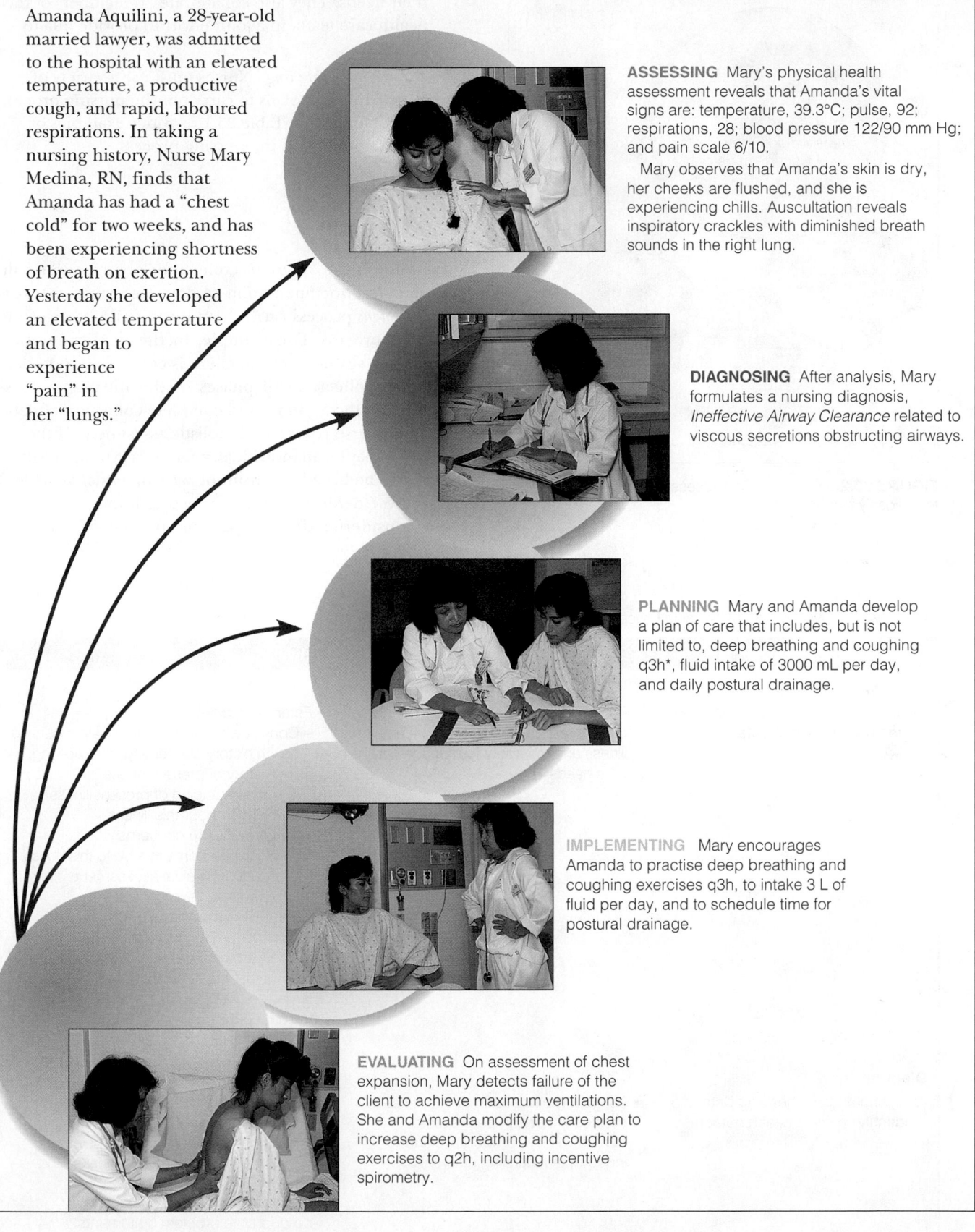

ASSESSING Mary's physical health assessment reveals that Amanda's vital signs are: temperature, 39.3°C; pulse, 92; respirations, 28; blood pressure 122/90 mm Hg; and pain scale 6/10.

Mary observes that Amanda's skin is dry, her cheeks are flushed, and she is experiencing chills. Auscultation reveals inspiratory crackles with diminished breath sounds in the right lung.

DIAGNOSING After analysis, Mary formulates a nursing diagnosis, *Ineffective Airway Clearance* related to viscous secretions obstructing airways.

PLANNING Mary and Amanda develop a plan of care that includes, but is not limited to, deep breathing and coughing q3h*, fluid intake of 3000 mL per day, and daily postural drainage.

IMPLEMENTING Mary encourages Amanda to practise deep breathing and coughing exercises q3h, to intake 3 L of fluid per day, and to schedule time for postural drainage.

EVALUATING On assessment of chest expansion, Mary detects failure of the client to achieve maximum ventilations. She and Amanda modify the care plan to increase deep breathing and coughing exercises to q2h, including incentive spirometry.

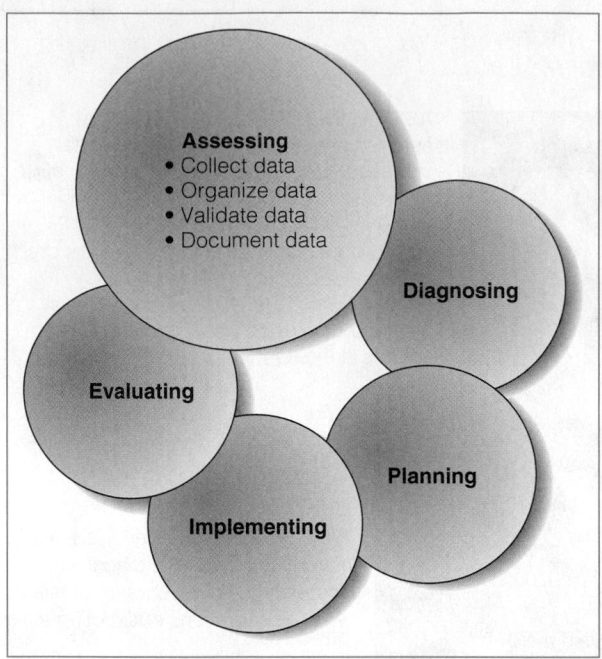

FIGURE 23.2 Assessing: The assessment process involves four closely related activities.

their needs. They also collaborate, as members of the health care team, in a joint effort to provide quality client care.

- *Use of critical thinking.* Nurses must use a variety of critical thinking skills to carry out the nursing process (see Chapter 21). Table 23.1 provides examples of critical thinking in the nursing process.

Assessing

Assessing is the *systematic* collection, organization, validation, and documentation of data (information). It is a *continuous* process carried out during all phases of the nursing process. For example, in the implementation phase, reassessment of the client is completed to update the data collected. All phases of the nursing process depend on the accurate and complete collection of data.

The nurse completes a holistic assessment of the client, who may be an individual, a family, a group, or a community. The broad spectrum of *determinants of health* and how these determinants are affecting human responses are considered during assessment (see Chapter 7).

TABLE 23.1 Overview of the Nursing Process Component and Description

Components and Description	Purpose	Activities

Assessing
Collecting, organizing, validating, and documenting client data
	• To establish a database about the client's response to health concerns or illness and the ability to manage health care needs	• Establish a database:
		  – Consult with the client to obtain a nursing health history concerning the following:
		    – History of present illness
		    – Understanding of present illness
		    – Beliefs about this illness
		    – Other health concerns
		    – Social concerns relative to this illness
		  – Conduct a physical assessment.
		  – Review client records.
		  – Review relevant literature.
		  – Consult support persons.
		  – Consult other health care professionals.
		• Update data, as needed.
		• Organize data.
		• Validate data.
		• Communicate and document data.

Diagnosing
Analyzing and synthesizing data and identifying client health outcomes
	• To identify client strengths and health problems that can be prevented or resolved by collaborative and independent nursing interventions
	
	• To develop a list of nursing diagnoses and collaborative problems that will focus care
		• Interpret and analyze data:
		  – Cluster or group data.
		  – Identify gaps and inconsistencies.
		• Determine client's strengths, risks, and problems.
		• Formulate nursing diagnoses and collaborative problem statements.
		• Document nursing diagnoses on the care plan.

TABLE 23.1 (*continued*)

Components and Description	Purpose	Activities
Planning Determining how to prevent, reduce, or resolve the identified priority client problems; how to support client strengths; and how to implement nursing interventions in an organized, individualized, and goal-directed manner to achieve client health outcomes	• To develop an individualized care plan that specifies client goals and desired health outcomes and related nursing interventions	• Set priorities and goals or health outcomes in collaboration with client. • Write goals, or desired outcomes. • Select nursing strategies or interventions. • Consult other health care professionals. • Write nursing orders and the nursing care plan. • Communicate the care plan to relevant health care providers.

Implementing
 	
Carrying out (or delegating) and documenting the planned nursing interventions
	• To assist the client to meet desired goals and desired health outcomes; promote wellness; prevent illness and disease; restore health; and facilitate coping with altered functioning	• Reassess the client to update the database.
		• Determine the nurse's need for nursing assistance.
		• Perform (or delegate) the planned nursing interventions.
		• Communicate what nursing actions were implemented:
		  – Document care and client responses to care.
		  – Give verbal reports, as necessary.

Evaluating Measuring the degree to which goals/outcomes have been achieved and identifying factors that positively or negatively influence this achievement	• To determine whether to continue, modify, or terminate the plan of care	• Collaborate with the client, and collect data related to desired health outcomes. • Document the achievement of health outcomes and modifications of the care plan. • Judge whether goals or outcomes have been achieved. • Relate nursing actions to client health outcomes. • Make decisions about the status of the problem. • Review and modify the care plan, as indicated, refer or terminate nursing care.

Assessment comes in four different types: (a) initial assessment, (b) problem-focused assessment, (c) emergency assessment, and (d) time-lapsed reassessment (see Table 23.2 on page 460). Assessments vary according to their purpose, timing, time available, and client status.

Nursing assessments focus on a client's responses to a health problem. A nursing assessment should include the client's strengths, perceived needs, health problems, related experience, health practices, values, culture, social network, and lifestyle preferences. The nursing assessment includes collaborating with the client to prioritize the client's concerns.

Collecting Data

Data collection is the process of gathering information about a client's health status. It must be both systematic and continuous to prevent the omission of significant data and reflect a client's changing health status.

A **database** contains all the information about a client; it includes the nursing health history (see Box 23.1 on page 461), physical assessment, health care provider's history and physical examination, results of laboratory and diagnostic tests, and material contributed by other health care personnel.

Client data should include past history as well as current problems. For example, a history of an allergic reaction to penicillin is a vital piece of historical data. Past surgical procedures, folk healing practices, and chronic diseases are also examples of historical data. Current data relate to present circumstances, such as pain, nausea, sleep patterns, and religious practices. Data can be subjective or objective and constant or variable, and come from a primary or secondary source (see Chapter 24).

TABLE 23.2 Types of Assessment

Type	Time Performed	Purpose	Example
Initial assessment	Performed within specified time after admission to a health care agency	To establish a complete database for problem identification, reference, and future comparison	Nursing admission assessment
Problem-focused assessment	Ongoing process integrated with nursing care	To determine the status of a specific problem identified in earlier assessment of a new problem	Hourly assessment of client's fluid intake and urinary output in an intensive care unit (ICU)
	Initial assessment when client presents for brief, episodic care	To identify new or evolving problems	Assessment of client's ability to perform self-care while assisting a client to bathe
Emergency assessment	During any physiological or psychological crisis	To identify life-threatening, new, or overlooked problems	Rapid assessment of a person's airway, breathing status, and circulation during a cardiac arrest
			Assessment of suicidal tendencies or potential for violence
Time-lapsed reassessment	Follow-up several months after initial assessment	To compare the client's current status to baseline data previously obtained	Reassessment of a client's functional health patterns in a home care or outpatient setting or in a home or hospital shift change

Types of Data

Subjective data, also referred to as *symptoms* or covert data, are based on client's perceptions, sensations, feelings, values, beliefs, attitudes, and understanding of personal health status and life situations and can be described or verified by that person. Itching, pain, and feelings of worry are examples of subjective data.

Objective data, also referred to as *signs*, are detectable by an observer or can be tested against an accepted standard. They can be seen, heard, felt, or smelled, and they are obtained by observation or physical examination. For example, discoloration of skin and blood pressure readings are objective data. Nurses should obtain the objective data needed to validate subjective data and to complete the assessment phase of the nursing process at all times.

Constant data is information that does not change over time such as race or blood type. **Variable data** can change quickly, frequently, or rarely and include such data as blood pressure, level of pain, and age.

Both subjective and objective data provide a baseline for determining client's responses to nursing and medical interventions. To identify the key symptoms that should be the primary focus of care, clients are asked to indicate what symptoms are of the most concern (see Box 23.2 on page 462).

SOURCES OF DATA Sources of data are *primary* or *secondary*. The client is the primary source of data. Family members or other support persons, other health care professionals, records and reports, laboratory and diagnostic analyses, and relevant literature are secondary or indirect sources. All sources other than the client are considered secondary sources.

Client The best source of data is usually the client, unless the client is too ill, young, or confused to communicate clearly. Some clients are reluctant to provide accurate data because they are afraid, embarrassed, or distrustful, or do not speak the nurse's language (D'Amico & Barbarito, 2012), In addition, depending on the client's cultures, he or she may be reluctant to discuss certain personal topics or share specific information. If the client is hesitant to provide data, the nurse can remind the client that the privacy of all data collected is protected and can be shared only with persons who have a legitimate health care–related need to know it.

Support People Family members, friends, and caregivers who know the client well often can supplement or verify information provided by the client. They might convey information about the client's response to illness, cultural beliefs and practices, stresses the client was experiencing before the illness, important information about

BOX 23.1 COMPONENTS OF A NURSING HEALTH HISTORY

BIOGRAPHICAL DATA

Client's name, address, age, gender, marital status, occupation, religious preference, next of kin, and usual sources of health care

CHIEF CONCERN OR REASON FOR VISIT

The answer given to the question, "What is troubling you?" or, "What brought you to the hospital or clinic?" The chief concern should be recorded in the client's own words.

HISTORY OF PRESENT ILLNESS OR HEALTH CONCERN

- *Symptoms:* description of each; steady, episodic, or worsening pattern
- *Onset of symptoms:* sudden or gradual, how long ago, circumstances at time of onset
- How often the problem occurs
- Exact location of the distress
- Character of the complaint (e.g., intensity of pain or quality of sputum, emesis, or discharge)
- Other phenomena or symptoms associated with the chief concern
- Factors that aggravate or alleviate the problem

PAST HISTORY

- *Medications:* all currently used prescription and over-the-counter medications, such as Aspirin, nasal spray, vitamins, laxatives, birth control pills, or herbal remedies
- *Hospitalization for serious illnesses:* reasons for the hospitalization, dates, surgery performed, course of recovery, and any complications
- *Immunizations:* date of the last tetanus shot, influenza immunization
- *Accidents and injuries:* how, when, and where the incident occurred, type of injury, treatment received, and complications
- *Childhood illnesses:* for example, chickenpox, mumps, measles, rubella (German measles), rubeola (red measles), streptococcal infections, scarlet fever, rheumatic fever, and other significant illnesses
- *Allergies:* drugs, animals, insects, or other environmental agents and the type of reaction that occurs
- *Infectious disease exposure*

FAMILY HISTORY OF ILLNESS

To ascertain risk factors for certain diseases, the ages of siblings, parents, and grandparents and their current state of health or (if they are deceased) the cause of death are obtained. Particular attention should be given to such disorders as heart disease, cancer, diabetes, hypertension, obesity, allergies, arthritis, tuberculosis, bleeding, alcoholism, and mental illnesses.

LIFESTYLE

- *Personal habits:* the amount, frequency, and duration of substance use (tobacco, alcohol, coffee, cola, tea, and illicit or recreational drugs)
- *Diet:* description of a typical diet on a normal day or any special diet, number of meals and snacks per day, who cooks and shops for food, ethnically distinct food patterns, and allergies
- *Sleep and rest patterns:* usual daily sleep and wake times, difficulties sleeping, remedies used for difficulties, napping
- *Activities of daily living (ADLs):* any difficulties experienced in the basic activities of eating, grooming, dressing, elimination, and mobility
- *Recreation and hobbies:* exercise activity and tolerance, hobbies and other interests

SOCIAL DATA

- *Family relationships, social networks, and friendships:* the client's support system in times of stress (who helps in time of need?); what effect the client's illness has on the family; and whether any family problems are affecting the client (See also the discussion of family assessment in Chapter 13.)
- *Ethnic and religious affiliation:* health customs and beliefs; cultural and religious practices that may affect health care and recovery (See also detailed ethnic and cultural assessment guide in Chapter 11.)
- *Educational history:* data about the client's highest level of education attained and any past difficulties with learning
- *Occupational history:* current employment status, the number of days missed from work because of illness, history of accidents on the job, occupational hazards with a potential for future disease or accident, the client's need to change jobs because of past illness, the employment status of both spouses or partners and the way childcare is handled, and the client's overall satisfaction with the work
- *Economic status:* financial concerns for medical care and coverage
- *Home and neighbourhood conditions:* home safety measures and adjustments in physical facilities that may be required to help the client manage a physical disability, activity intolerance, and ADLs; the availability of neighbourhood and community services to meet the client's needs

PSYCHOLOGICAL DATA

- *Major stressors:* those experienced in the past year and the client's perception of them
- *Usual coping pattern:* used to cope with a serious problem or a high level of stress
- *Communication style:* ability to verbalize appropriate emotion; nonverbal communication, such as eye contact, gestures, use of touch, and posture; interactions with support persons; and the congruence of nonverbal behaviour and verbal expression

PATTERNS OF HEALTH CARE

All the health care resources the client is currently using and has used in the past. These include the family health care providers, specialists (e.g., ophthalmologist or gynecologist), dentist, alternative practitioners (e.g., herbalist or faith healers), health clinic, or health centre; whether the client considers the care being provided adequate; and whether access to health care is a problem.

BOX 23.2 EXAMPLES OF SUBJECTIVE AND OBJECTIVE DATA	
SUBJECTIVE	**OBJECTIVE**
"I feel weak all over when I exert myself."	Blood pressure 90/50 mm Hg
	Apical pulse 104/min
	Skin pale and diaphoretic
Client states he has a cramping pain in his abdomen. States, "I feel sick to my stomach."	Vomited 100 mL green-tinged fluid
	Abdomen firm and slightly distended
	Active bowel sounds auscultated in all four quadrants
"I'm short of breath."	Lung sounds clear bilaterally; diminished in right lower lobe
Wife states: "He doesn't seem so sad today." (This is subjective and secondary source data.)	Client cried during interview
"I would like to see the chaplain before surgery."	Holding open Bible
	Has small silver cross on bedside table

the client's home and/or work environment, behaviour patterns, family attitudes toward health, wellness, illness, or any prior health directive. The nurse should also indicate on the nursing history what data were obtained from a support person.

Client Records Client records include information documented by various health care professionals and data regarding the client's occupation, religion, and marital status. By reviewing such records before interviewing the client, the nurse can avoid asking questions for which answers have already been supplied. Repeated questioning can be stressful and annoying to clients and cause concern about the lack of communication among health care professionals.

Medical records (e.g., medical history, physical examination, progress notes, and consultations) can provide nurses with information about the client's coping behaviours, health practices, previous illnesses, and allergies.

Records of therapies by other health care professionals, such as social workers, dietitians, or physiotherapists, help the nurse obtain relevant data not expressed by the client.

Laboratory records also provide pertinent health information for the nurse to compare with established norms for that particular test and for the client's age, gender, geographical location, or present situation, and so on. For example, the determination of blood glucose level allows health care professionals to monitor the effects of oral hypoglycemic medications on a 60-year-old newly diagnosed person with diabetes who just immigrated to Canada. Similarly, if the most recent health record is 5 years old, it is likely that the client's health practices, family situations, and coping behaviours have changed.

Health Care Professionals Nurses, social workers, physicians, and physiotherapists, for example, may have information from either previous or current contact with the client. Sharing of information among professionals is especially important to ensure continuity of care when clients are transferred to and from home and health care agencies.

Literature The review of nursing and related literature, such as professional journals and reference texts, can provide additional information for the database. A literature review includes but is not limited to the following information:

- Standards or norms against which to compare findings (e.g., height and weight tables, normal developmental tasks for an age group)
- Cultural and social health practices
- Clinical practice guidelines
- Research evidence for nursing interventions and evaluation criteria relevant to a client's health problems
- Information about medical diagnoses, treatments, and prognoses

DATA COLLECTION METHODS The primary methods used to collect data are observing, interviewing, and examining. Observation occurs whenever the nurse is in contact with the client or support persons. Interviewing is used mainly while taking the nursing health history. Examining is the major method used in the physical health assessment. The nurse uses all three methods simultaneously when assessing clients. For example, during the client interview, the nurse observes, listens, asks questions, and mentally retains information to explore in the physical examination.

Observing To observe is to gather data by using the five senses. Observation is a conscious, deliberate skill that is developed through effort and with an organized approach. Examples of client data observed through four of the five senses are shown in Table 23.3.

Observation has two aspects: (a) attending to the stimuli and (b) selecting, organizing, and interpreting the data. A nurse who observes that a client's face is flushed must relate that observation to, for example, body temperature, activity, environmental temperature, and blood pressure. Nurses often need to focus on specific stimuli to avoid being overwhelmed by a multitude

TABLE 23.3 Observational Skills

Sense	Example of Client Data
Sight	Overall appearance (body size, general weight, posture, grooming); signs of distress or discomfort; facial and body gestures; skin colour and lesions; abnormalities of movement; nonverbal demeanour (e.g., signs of anger or anxiety); religious or cultural artifacts (e.g., books, icons, beads)
Smell	Body or breath odours
Hearing	Lung and heart sounds; bowel sounds; ability to communicate; language spoken; ability to initiate conversation; ability to respond when spoken to; orientation to time, person, and place; thoughts and feelings about self, others, and health status; noise level
Touch	Skin temperature and moisture; muscle strength (e.g., hand grip); pulse rate, rhythm, and volume; palpatory lesions (e.g., lumps, masses, nodules)

of stimuli. Observing, therefore, involves distinguishing stimuli in a meaningful manner. For example, nurses caring for newborns learn to ignore the usual sounds of machines in the nursery but respond quickly to an infant's cry or movement.

The experienced nurse is often able to attend to an intervention (e.g., giving a bed bath or monitoring an intravenous infusion) and, at the same time, make important observations (e.g., noting a change in respiratory status or skin colour). The beginning student must learn to make observations and complete tasks simultaneously.

Nursing observations must be organized so that nothing significant is missed. Most nurses develop a particular sequence for observing events, usually focusing on the client first. For example, a nurse walks into a client's room and observes, in the following order:

- The client (e.g., response to greeting, verbalizations)
- Clinical signs of client distress (e.g., pallor or flushing, laboured breathing, and behaviour indicating pain or emotional distress)
- Threats to the client's safety, real or potential (e.g., a lowered side rail, a fire threat)
- The presence and functioning of associated equipment (e.g., intravenous equipment and oxygen)
- The immediate environment (e.g., appropriateness of lighting level, accessibility to personal items), including the people in it and assistive equipment

Interviewing An **interview** is a planned communication or a conversation with a purpose, to gather data, for

example, during the nursing admission assessment, to identify problems of mutual concern, evaluate change, teach, provide support, or provide counselling or therapy. Interviewing is a process that the nurse applies in most phases of the nursing process. Clients are considered to be the expert in knowing themselves. The goal of the nurse is to listen actively, demonstrate caring in the development of a caring relationship, and encourage client participation in their own care. Interviews should be characterized by mutuality between nurse and client.

Two approaches to interviewing are used: *directive* and *nondirective*. The **directive interview** is highly structured and elicits specific information. The nurse establishes the purpose of the interview and guides the interview by asking closed questions (see the next section) that call for specific data. The client responds to questions but may have limited opportunity to ask questions or discuss concerns. Nurses frequently use directive interviews to gather and to give information when time is limited (e.g., in an emergency situation).

During a **nondirective interview**, or rapport-building interview, by contrast, the nurse facilitates the client's control of purpose, subject matter, and pacing. **Rapport** is a relationship between two or more people that facilitates effective communication.

A combination of directive and nondirective approaches is usually used during the interview to collect data and to begin to establish rapport. The nurse begins by asking open-ended questions to determine areas of concern for the client. If, for example, a client expresses worry about surgery, the nurse pauses to explore the client's worry and to provide support. Simply noting the worry without dealing with it can leave the client feeling the nurse does not care about the client's concerns or dismisses them as unimportant.

Types of Interview Questions Questions are often classified as closed or open-ended and as neutral or leading.

Closed questions, used in the directive interview, are restrictive and generally require only "yes" or "no" or short factual answers giving specific information. Examples of closed questions are "Did you take this medication?" "Are you having pain now? Show me where it is." "How old are you?" "When did you fall?"

Open-ended questions, associated with the nondirective interview, lead or invite clients to discover, elaborate, clarify, or explore their thoughts or feelings. An open-ended question specifies only the broad topic to be discussed and gives clients the freedom to divulge only the information that they are ready to disclose. Responses may also convey clients' attitudes and beliefs. The open-ended question is useful at the beginning of an interview or to change topics and to elicit attitudes.

Open-ended questions usually begin with *what* or *how*. Examples of open-ended questions are "How have you been feeling lately?" "What brought you to the hospital?" "How did you feel in that situation?"

Open-ended and closed questions each have advantages and disadvantages. See Box 23.3 for a summary.

The type of question a nurse chooses depends on the needs of the client at the time. For example, the nurse asks closed questions in an emergency or other acute situation when information must be obtained quickly. Nurses may use a combination of closed and open-ended questions throughout an interview to accomplish the goals of the interview and obtain needed information.

A **neutral question** is a question the client can answer without direction or pressure from the nurse. Examples are "How do you feel about that?" and "Why do you think you had the operation?" A **leading question**, by contrast, directs the client's answer. The phrasing of the question suggests what answer is expected. Examples are "You're stressed about surgery tomorrow, aren't you?" or "You will take your medicine, won't you?" Leading questions create problems if the client, in an effort to please the nurse, gives inaccurate responses. This can result in inaccurate data.

Use the "why" questions carefully. Clients may not be able to explain the rationale behind their behaviour and can view such questions as threatening (Williams, 2008). Because the goal of questioning is to elicit as much purposeful information as possible, anything that puts the client on the defensive will interfere with reaching that goal.

Planning the Interview and Setting   Before beginning an interview, the nurse reviews available information, such as the medical history, information about the current illness, or literature about the client's health problem. Nurses may also prepare an interview guide to determine what important questions to ask.

Effective interviews are influenced by time, place, seating arrangement, distance, and language:

- *Time:* Nurses need to plan interviews with clients when the client is physically comfortable and free of pain, and when interruptions by friends, family, and other health care professionals are minimal. Nurses should schedule interviews with clients in their homes at a time mutually agreed upon with the client and family.

- *Place:* A well-lit, well-ventilated, moderate-sized room that is relatively free of noise, movements, and interruptions encourages communication. In addition, a place where others cannot overhear or see the client is desirable. Although many interviews are conducted at the client bedside, privacy is often compromised in multiclient rooms.

- *Seating Arrangement:* A seating arrangement in which the parties sit on two chairs placed at right angles

---

BOX 23.3   SELECTED ADVANTAGES AND DISADVANTAGES OF OPEN-ENDED AND CLOSED QUESTIONS

OPEN-ENDED QUESTIONS

Advantages

1. They let the interviewee do the talking.
2. The interviewer is able to listen and observe.
3. They are easy to answer and nonthreatening.
4. They reveal what the interviewee thinks is important.
5. They may reveal the interviewee's lack of information, misunderstanding of words, frame of reference, prejudices, or stereotypes.
6. They can provide information the interviewer may not ask for.
7. They can reveal the interviewee's degree of feeling about an issue.
8. They can convey interest and trust because of the freedom they provide.

Disadvantages

1. They take more time.
2. Only brief answers may be given.
3. Valuable information may be withheld.
4. They often elicit more information than necessary.
5. Responses are difficult to document and require skill in recording.
6. The interviewer requires skill in controlling an open-ended interview.
7. Responses require psychological insight and sensitivity from the interviewer.

CLOSED QUESTIONS

Advantages

1. Questions and answers can be controlled more effectively.
2. They require less effort from the interviewee.
3. They may be less threatening, since they do not require explanations or justifications.
4. They take less time.
5. Information can be asked for sooner than it would be volunteered.
6. Responses are easily documented.
7. Questions are easy to use and can be handled by unskilled interviewers.

Disadvantages

1. They may provide too little information and require follow-up questions.
2. They may not reveal how the interviewee feels.
3. They do not allow the interviewee to volunteer possibly valuable information.
4. They may inhibit communication and convey lack of interest by the interviewer.
5. The interviewer may dominate the interview with questions.

Source: From Stewart, C. J. & Cash, W. B., Jr. (2011). *Interviewing: Principles and practices* (13th ed.). Boston, MA: McGraw-Hill. Reprinted with permission from The McGraw-Hill Companies.

to a desk or table or a few feet apart, with no table between, creates a less formal atmosphere, and the nurse and client tend to feel comfortable. In groups, a horseshoe or circular chair arrangement can facilitate comfortable group discussion. When a client is in bed, the nurse can sit at a 45-degree angle to the bed. This position is less formal and intimidating than standing at the foot of the bed or positioned standing near the client's head.

- *Distance:* People feel uncomfortable when talking to someone who is too close or too far away. Most people feel comfortable maintaining a distance of about 1 m (metre) during an interview. Communication at a distance greater than this tends to be more impersonal and may suggest a lack of involvement on the part of the nurse. Some clients require more or less personal space depending on their cultural and personal needs.

- *Language:* The nurse must avoid using complicated medical terminology and instead use common English, and interpreters or translators are needed if the client and the nurse do not speak the same language or dialect. Interpreters may make judgments about precise wording to make the meaning clearer or more culturally appropriate. If giving written documents to clients, the nurse must determine that the client can read in his or her native language. Live translation is preferred since the client can then ask questions for clarification. Nurses must be cautious when asking family members, client visitors, or agency nonprofessional staff to assist with translation. Issues of confidentiality or gender mismatch can interfere with effective communication. The nurse must always confirm accurate understandings.

Stages of an Interview An interview has three major stages: (a) the opening or introduction, (b) the body or development, and (c) the closing.

The Opening The opening is the most important part of the interview because what is said and done at that time sets the tone for the remainder of the interview. The purposes of the opening are to establish rapport and orient the interviewee. Depending on the situation, the relationship between the two parties, and the interviewer's choice, the rapport and orientation stages may occur at the same time.

Establishing rapport is a process of creating relationship and trust. It can begin with a greeting ("Good morning, Mr. Johnson") or a self-introduction ("Good morning. I'm Jennifer Thomas, a nursing student.") accompanied by nonverbal gestures, such as a smile, a handshake, and a friendly manner. The nurse continues to develop rapport by asking questions about the person and may proceed with some small talk about the weather, sports, families, and the like. The nurse

must be careful not to overdo this; too much superficial talk can arouse anxiety about what is to follow and may appear insincere.

In the introduction stage, the nurse explains the purpose and nature of the interview, for example, what information is needed, how long it will take, and what is expected of the client. The nurse usually states that the client has the right to refuse to answer a question and tells the client how the information will be used.

The following is an example of an interview introduction:

Step 1—Establish Rapport

Nurse: Hello, Ms. Goodwin, I'm Jim Fellows. I'm a nursing student, and I'll be assisting with your care here.

Client: Hi. Are you a student from the university?

Nurse: Yes, I'm in my final year. Are you familiar with the campus?

Client: Oh, yes! I'm an avid hockey fan. My nephew graduated in 2012 and I often attend hockey games with him.

Nurse: That's great! Sounds like fun.

Client: Yes, I enjoy it very much.

Step 2—Orientation

Nurse: May I sit with you here for about 10 minutes to talk about how I can help you while you're here?

Client: All right. What do you want to know?

Nurse: Well, to plan your care after your operation, I'd like to get some information about your normal daily activities and what you expect here in the hospital. I'd like to make notes while we talk to get the important points and have them available to other staff members who will also look after you.

Client: OK. That's all right with me.

Nurse: If there is anything you don't want to talk about, please feel free to say so, and if there is anything you would rather I didn't write down, just tell me. Is this a good time for you?

Client: Sure, that will be fine.

The Body In the body of the interview, the client communicates what he or she thinks, feels, knows, and perceives in response to questions from the nurse. The nurse can ask an open-ended question that is related to the stated purpose, is easy to answer, and does not embarrass or place stress on the person. For example, "What brought you to the hospital today?"

Effective development of the interview demands that the nurse use communication skills that make both parties feel comfortable and serve the purpose of the

ADMISSION DATA

Date 11-04-16 Time 1515h Primary Language English

Arrived Via: ☐ Wheelchair ☐ Stretcher ☑ Ambulatory

From: ☐ Admitting ☐ ER ☑ Home ☐ Nursing Home ☐ Other

Admitting M.D. R. Katz Time Notified 1700h

ORIENTATION TO UNIT

	YES	NO		YES	NO
Arm Band Correct	☒	☐	Visiting Hours	☒	☐
Allergy Band	☒	☐	Smoking Policy	☒	☐
Telephone	☒	☐	TV, Lights, Bed Controls,		
Electrical Policy	☒	☐	Call Lights, Side Rails	☒	☐
Educational Mat'l (TV Brochure)	☒	☐	Nurses Station	☒	☐
	☒	☐			

Family M.D. R. Katz

Weight 57 kg Height 158 cm BP:R — L 122/80

Temp. 39.4°C Pulse 92, weak Resp. 28, shallow

Source Providing Information ☑ Patient ☐ Other

Unable to Obtain History ☐

Reason for Admission (Onset, Duration, Pt.'s Perception) "Chest cold" X2 weeks S.O.B on exertion. "Lung pain, fever," "Dr. says I have pneumonia."

ALLERGIES & REACTIONS

Drugs Penicillin

Food/Other

Signs & Symptoms rash, nausea

Blood Reaction ☐ Yes ☑ No Dyes/Shellfish ☐ Yes ☑ No

MEDICATIONS

Current Meds	Dose/Freq.	Last Dose
Synthroid	0.1 mg. daily	12-24, 0800h

Disposition of Meds: ☒ Home ☐ Pharmacy ☐ Safe *At Bedside

MEDICAL HISTORY

☑ No Major Problems ☐ Gastro

☐ Cardiac ☐ Arthritis

☐ Hyper/Hypotension ☐ Stroke

☐ Diabetes ☐ Seizures

☐ Cancer ☐ Glaucoma

☐ Respiratory ☑ Other Childbirth-2004

Surgery/Procedures	Date
Appendectomy	2000
Partial thyroidectomy	2004

SPECIAL ASSISTIVE DEVICES

☐ Wheelchair ☐ Contacts ☐ Venous Access Device ☐ Dentures ☐ Partial ☐ Upper ☐ Lower

☐ Braces ☐ Hearing Aid

☐ Cane/Crutches ☐ Prosthesis

☐ Walker ☐ Glasses ☐ Epidural Catheter

☐ Other None

VALUABLES

Patient informed Hospital not responsible for personal belongings.

Valuables Disposition: ☐ Patient ☐ Safe ☐ Given to

Patient/SO Signature None

PSYCHOSOCIAL HISTORY

Recent Stress None

Coping Mechanism Not assessed because of fatigue

Support System Husband, coworkers, friends

Calm: ☑ Yes ☐ No

Anxious: ☐ Yes ☐ No Facial muscles tense; trembling

Religion Catholic, Would want Last Rites

Tobacco Use: ☐ Yes ☑ No

Alcohol Use: ☐ Yes ☑ No

Drug Use: ☐ Yes ☑ No

NEUROLOGICAL

Oriented: ☑ Person ☑ Place ☑ Time ☐ Confused ☐ Sedated ☐ Alert ☐ Restless ☑ Lethargic ☐ Comatose

Pupils: ☑ Equal ☐ Unequal ☑ Reactive ☐ Sluggish ☐ Other 3mm.

Extremity Strength: ☑ Equal ☐ Unequal

Speech: ☑ Clear ☐ Slurred ☐ Other

MUSCULO-SKELETAL

Normal ROM of Extremities ☑ Yes ☐ No

☑ Weakness ☐ Paralysis ☐ Contractures ☐ Joint Swelling ☑ Pain (when coughing)

☐ Other ↓ related to fatigue

RESPIRATORY

Pattern: ☐ Even ☐ Uneven ☑ Shallow ☑ Dyspnea ☑ Other diminished breath sounds

Breathing Sounds: ☐ Clear ☑ Other inspiratory crackles

Secretions: ☐ None ☑ Other pink, thick sputum

Cough: ☐ None ☑ Productive ☐ Nonproductive

CARDIOVASCULAR

Pulses: Apical Rate 92-W ☑ Reg. ☐ Irregular ☐ Pacemaker

S = Strong W = Weak A = Absent D = Doppler

Radial R 92 L — Pedal R — L —

Edema: ☑ Absent ☐ Present Site

Perfusion: ☐ Warm ☐ Dry ☑ Diaphoretic ☐ Cool (Hot)

GASTROINTESTINAL

Oral Mucosa ☐ Normal ☑ Other pale and dry

Bowel Sounds: ☑ Normal ☐ Other Abd. soft

Wt. Change: ☐ ☑ N/V Stool Frequency/Character 1/day; soft

Last B/M 11-04-16 ☐ Ostomy (type)

Equip.

GENITOURINARY

Urine: Last Voided This morning

☐ Normal ☐ Anuria ☐ Hematuria ☐ Dysuri ☐ Incontinent

☒ Other ↓ amount & frequency since ill

☐ Catheter (type) Other

LMP 11-04-16 ☐ Vaginal/Penile Discharge

Other

SELF CARE

Need Assist with: ☐ Ambulating ☐ Elimination ☐ Meals ☒ Hygiene ☐ Dressing

While fatigued

Amanda Aquilini [F. age 28]
#4637651

BROWARD HEALTH®

FIGURE 23.3 Assessment for Amanda Aquilini. Nursing assessment tool.

Source: Courtesy of Broward Health, Broward County. Reprinted with permission.

Note: The patient and information on this form are fictitious.

NUTRITION

General Appearance: ☑ Well Nourished ☐ Emaciated
☐ Other _____
Appetite: ☐ Good ☐ Fair ☑ Poor -x2 days
Diet _Liquid_ Meal Pattern _3/day_
☐ Feeds Self ☐ Assist ☐ Total Feed

SKIN ASSESSMENT

Color: ☐ Normal ☐ Flushed ☑ Pale ☐ Dusky ☐ Cyanotic
☐ Jaundiced ☑ Other _Cheeks flushed, hot_
General Description _Surgical scars:_
RLQ abdomen; anterior neck
_____
_____
_____
Note Cultures Obtained _____
_____
_____
_____

PRESSURE SORE ™ AT RISK SCREENING CRITERIA

OVERALL SKIN CONDITION
Grade
☐ 0 Turgor (elasticity adequate, skin warm and moist)
☑ 1 Poor turgor, skin cold & dry
☐ 2 Areas mottled, red or denuded
☐ 3 Existing skin ulcer/lesions

BOWEL AND BLADDER CONTROL
Grade
☑ 0 Always able to ask for bedpan
☐ 1 Incontinence of urine
☐ 2 Incontinence of feces
☐ 3 Totally incontinent Confined to bed

REHABILITATIVE STATE
Grade
☐ 0 Fully ambulatory
☑ 1 Ambulated with assistance
☐ 2 Chair to bed ambulation only
☐ 3 Confined to bed
☐ 4 Immobile in bed

NUTRITIONAL STATE
Grade
☐ 0 Eats all
☑ 1 Eats very little
☐ 2 Refuses food often
☐ 3 Tube feeding
☐ 4 Intravenous feeding

MENTAL STATE
Grade
☑ 0 Alert and clear
☐ 1 Confused
☐ 2 Disoriented/senile
☐ 3 Stuporous
☐ 4 Unconscious

CHRONIC DISEASE STATUS
(i.e. COPD, ASCVD, Peripheral Vascular Disease, Diabetes, or Renal Disease, Cancer, Motor or Sensory Deficits, Elderly, Other)
Grade
☑ 0 Absent
☐ 1 One Present
☐ 2 Two Present
☐ 3 Three or more Present

TOTAL ___3___ Refer to Skin Care Protocol

FALLS SCREENING

If one or more of the following are checked institute fall precautions/plan of care
☐ History of Falls ☐ Unsteady Gait ☐ Confusion/Disorientation ☐ Dizziness

If two or more of the following are checked institute fall precautions/plan of care
☐ Age over 80 ☐ Utilizes cane, walker, w/c ☐ Sleeplessness
☐ Impaired vision ☐ Urgency/frequency in elimination
☐ Multiple Diagnoses ☐ Impaired hearing
☐ Inability to understand or follow directions ☐ Medication/Sedative /Diuretic etc.

EDUCATION/DISCHARGE PLANNING

1. What do you know about your present illness? _"Dr. says I have pneumonia." "I will have an I.V."_
2. What information do you want or need about your illness? _____
3. Would you like family/SO involved in your care? _Husband, Michael_
4. How long do you expect to be in the hospital? _"1-2 days"_
5. What concerns do you have about leaving the hospital? ____

CHECK APPROPRIATE BOX

Will patient need post discharge assistance with ADLs/physical functioning? ☐ Yes ☑ No ☐ Unknown
Does patient have family capable of and willing to provide assistance post discharge?
☑ Yes ☐ No ☐ Unknown ☐ No family
Is assistance needed beyond that which family can provide?
☐ Yes ☑ No ☐ Unknown
Previous admission in the last six months?
☐ Yes ☑ No ☐ Unknown
Patient lives with _Husband and 1 child_
Planned discharge to _Home_
Comments: _Fatigue and anxiety may have interfered with learning. Re-teach anything covered at admission, later._

Social Services Notified ☐ Yes ☑ No

NARRATIVE NOTES

S--c/o sharp chest pain when coughing and dyspnea on exertion. States unable to carry out regular daily exercise for past week. Coughing relieved "if I sit up and sit still." Nausea associated with coughing. Having occasional "chills." Occasionally becomes frightened, stating, "I can't breathe." Well groomed but "too tired to put on make-up."

O--Chest expansion < 3 cm, no nasal flaring or use of accessory muscles. Breath sounds and insp. crackles in Ⓡ upper and lower chest.
   Assesses own supports as "good" (eg, relationship c̄ husband). Is "worried" about daughter. States husband will be out of town until tomorrow. Left 5-year-old daughter with neighbour. Concerned too about her work (is lawyer). "I'll never get caught up." Had water at noon—no food today. Informed of need to save urine for 24 h specimen. IV D₅W LR 1000 mL started in Ⓡarm, 100 mL/h Slow capillary refill. Keeping head of bed↑ to facilitate breathing.

NURSE SIGNATURE/TITLE	DATE	TIME
Mary Medina, RN	11-04-16	1530h
NURSE SIGNATURE/TITLE	DATE	TIME

✿ **BROWARD HEALTH**

interview. See the discussion of communication skills in Chapter 22.

The Closing   The nurse terminates the interview when the needed information has been obtained. In some cases, however, a client terminates it, for example, when deciding not to give any more information or when unable to offer more information for some other reason—fatigue, for example. The closing is important in maintaining the rapport and trust and in facilitating future interactions. the following techniques are commonly used to close an interview:

1. Offering to answer questions: "Do you have any further questions?" "I would be glad to answer any questions you have." Be sure to allow time for the person to answer, or the offer will be regarded as insincere.

2. Conclude by saying, "That's about all I need to know for now" or "Those are all the questions I have for now."

3. Thank the client. "Thank you for your time." "The questions you have answered will be helpful in planning your nursing care."

4. Express concern for the person's welfare and future: "I'll see you on Thursday." "I hope all goes well for you. If you run into additional problems, be sure to contact me."

5. Plan for the next meeting or next steps in client care, if there is to be one. Include the day, time, place, topic, and purpose: "Let's get together again tomorrow, here, at 9 a.m. to see how you are managing then."

6. Reveal what will happen next. For example: "Ms. Goodwin, I will be responsible for giving you care three mornings per week while you are here. I will be in to see you Monday, Tuesday, and Wednesday between 8 o'clock and noon. At those times, we can adjust your care, if we need to, and prepare for discharge."

7. Signal that the time is up if a time limit was agreed on or explain why the interview must close at that time: "I see our time is up; it went so quickly today," or "I'm sorry, but we're going to have to end our discussion; I have another appointment in 10 minutes."

8. Provide a summary to verify accuracy and agreement. Summarizing serves several purposes: It helps terminate the interview, it reassures the client that the nurse has listened, it checks the accuracy of the nurse's perceptions, it clears the way for new ideas, and it helps the client to note progress and forward direction. "Let's review what we have covered in this interview." Summaries are particularly helpful for clients who are anxious or who have difficulty staying with the topic: "It seems to me that you are especially worried about your hospitalization and chest pain because your father died of a heart attack 5 years ago. Is that correct? I'll discuss this with you again

tomorrow, and we'll decide what plans need to be made to help you."

Examining   The *physical examination* or physical health assessment is a *systematic* data collection method that uses observational skills (i.e., the senses of sight, hearing, smell, and touch) to detect health problems. To conduct the examination, the nurse uses techniques of inspection, auscultation, palpation, and percussion. These techniques are discussed in Chapter 28.

The nurse may also focus on a specific problem area noted from the nursing assessment, for example, the client's inability to urinate. On occasion, the nurse may find it necessary to resolve a client complaint or problem (e.g., shortness of breath) before completing the examination. This type of assessment is called a **focused assessment**. Alternatively, the nurse may perform a **screening examination**, which is a brief review of essential functioning of various body parts or systems. An example of a screening examination is the nursing admission assessment form shown in Figure 23.3.

Figure 23.3 on pages 466–467 is a concise data collection tool that is organized according to body systems and specific nursing concerns (e.g., screening for falls and allergies); it does not use one particular nursing model. In Box 23.7 on page 470, the data from Amanda Aquilini are shown after being organized according to Gordon's 11 functional health patterns. Note how the categories in Box 23.7 differ from those in Figure 23.3. As a rule, the nurse organizes the data by using the same model on which the data collection tool is based.

Organizing Data

The nurse uses a written or computerized format that organizes the assessment data systematically. This format is often referred to as a *nursing health history, nursing assessment,* or *nursing data base form.* The format can be modified according to the client's physical status, such as one focused on musculoskeletal data for orthopedic clients.

NURSING CONCEPTUAL MODELS/FRAMEWORKS   Most schools of nursing and health care agencies have developed their own structured assessment tools. Many of these are based on selected nursing theories (see Chapter 4). Three examples are Gordon's functional health pattern framework (Gordon, 2010), Orem's self-care model (Orem, 2001), and Roy's adaptation model (Roy, 2008).

Gordon (2010) provided a framework of 11 functional health patterns (see Box 23.4). Gordon used the word *pattern* to signify a sequence of recurring behaviour. The nurse collects data about dysfunctional as well as functional behaviour. Thus, by using Gordon's

BOX 23.4   GORDON'S TYPOLOGY OF 11 FUNCTIONAL HEALTH PATTERNS

The following 11 functional health patterns can be used to organize data:

1. *Health-perception/health-management pattern.* Describes the client's perceived pattern of health and well-being and how health is managed

2. *Nutritional–metabolic pattern.* Describes the client's pattern of food and fluid consumption relative to metabolic need and pattern indicators of local nutrient supply

3. *Elimination pattern.* Describes the patterns of excretory function (bowel, bladder, and skin)

4. *Activity–exercise pattern.* Describes the pattern of exercise, activity, leisure, and recreation

5. *Sleep–rest pattern.* Describes patterns of sleep, rest, and relaxation

6. *Cognitive–perceptual pattern.* Describes sensory–perceptual and cognitive patterns

7. *Self-perception/self-concept pattern.* Describes the client's self-concept pattern and perceptions of self (e.g., self-conception/worth, comfort, body image, feeling state)

8. *Role–relationship pattern.* Describes the client's pattern of role participation and relationships

9. *Sexuality–reproductive pattern.* Describes the client's patterns of satisfaction and dissatisfaction with sexuality pattern; describes reproductive patterns

10. *Coping/stress-tolerance pattern.* Describes the client's general coping pattern and the effectiveness of the pattern in terms of stress tolerance

11. *Value–belief pattern.* Describes the patterns of values, beliefs (including spiritual), and goals that guide the client's choices or decisions

Source: From Gordon, M. (2010). *Manual of nursing diagnosis* (12th Ed.) (pp. 2–5). Boston, MA: Jones & Bartlett. Reprinted with Permission.

BOX 23.5   OREM'S SELF-CARE MODEL

UNIVERSAL SELF-CARE REQUISITES

1. The maintenance of a sufficient intake of air.
2. The maintenance of a sufficient intake of water.
3. The maintenance of a sufficient intake of food.
4. The provision of care associated with elimination processes and excrement.
5. The maintenance of a balance between activity and rest.
6. The maintenance of a balance between solitude and social interaction.
7. The prevention of hazards to human life, human functioning, and human well-being.
8. The promotion of human functioning within social groups in accord with human potential, known human limitations, and human desire to be normal. (*Normalcy* is used in the sense of that which is essentially human and that which is in accord with the genetic and constitutional characteristics and the talents of individuals.)

Source: Adapted from Orem, D. E. (2001). *Nursing: Concepts of practice.* (6th ed.) (p. 225). St. Louis, MO: Mosby. Permission granted by the estate of Dorothea Orem.

BOX 23.6   ROY'S ADAPTATION MODEL

The Roy adaptation model classifies observable behaviour into the following categories:

ADAPTIVE MODES

1. **Physiological/Physical**
   - Activity and rest
   - Nutrition
   - Elimination
   - Fluid and electrolytes
   - Oxygenation
   - Protection
   - Regulation: temperature
   - Regulation: the senses
   - Regulation: endocrine system
2. **Self-Concept**
   - Physical self
   - Personal self
3. **Role Function**
4. **Interdependence**

Source: Roy, Sister Callista; Andrew, Heather A., *The Roy adaptation model, 3rd ed.,* © 2009. Reprinted and Electronically reproduced by permission of Pearson Education, Inc., Upper Saddle River, New Jersey.

framework to organize data, nurses are able to discern emerging patterns.

Orem (2001) delineated eight universal self-care requisites of humans (see Box 23.5). Roy (2008) outlined the data to be collected according to the Roy adaptation model and classified observable behaviour into four categories: (a) physiological, (b) self-concept, (c) role function, and (d) interdependence (see Box 23.6).

WELLNESS MODELS   Nurses use wellness models to assist clients to identify health risks and to explore lifestyle habits and health behaviours, beliefs, values, and attitudes that influence levels of wellness. See Chapter 7 for details. Such models generally include the following:

- Health history
- Physical fitness evaluation
- Nutritional assessment
- Life-stress analysis
- Lifestyle and health habits
- Health beliefs
- Sexual health
- Spiritual health
- Relationships
- Health risk appraisal

BOX 23.7 DATA FOR AMANDA AQUILINI, ORGANIZED ACCORDING TO FUNCTIONAL HEALTH PATTERNS

HEALTH PERCEPTION AND HEALTH MANAGEMENT

- Aware and understands medical diagnosis
- Gives thorough history of illnesses and surgeries
- Complies with Synthroid regimen
- Relates progression of illness in detail
- Expects to have antibiotic therapy and "go home in a day or two"
- States usual eating pattern "3 meals a day"

NUTRITIONAL AND METABOLIC

- 158 cm tall; weighs 57 kg
- Usual eating pattern "3 meals a day"
- "No appetite" since having "cold"
- Has not eaten today; last fluids at noon
- Nauseated
- Oral temperature 39.4°C
- Decreased skin turgor

ELIMINATION

- Usually no problem
- Decreased urinary frequency and amount 2–3 days
- Last bowel movement yesterday, formed, "normal"

ACTIVITY AND EXERCISE

- No musculoskeletal impairment
- Difficulty sleeping because of cough
- "Can't breathe lying down"
- States, "I feel weak"
- Short of breath on exertion
- Exercises daily

COGNITIVE AND PERCEPTUAL

- No sensory deficits
- Pupils 3 mm, equal, brisk reaction
- Oriented to time, place, and person
- Responsive but fatigued
- Responds appropriately to verbal and physical stimuli
- Recent and remote memory intact
- States "short of breath" on exertion
- Reports "pain in lungs," especially when coughing
- Experiencing chills
- Reports nausea

SELF-PERCEPTION AND SELF-CONCEPT

- Expresses "concern" and "worry" over leaving daughter with neighbours until husband returns
- Well-groomed, says, "Too tired to put on makeup"

ROLES AND RELATIONSHIPS

- Lives with husband and 7-year-old daughter
- Husband out of town; will be back tomorrow afternoon
- Child with neighbour until husband returns
- States "good" relationships with friends and coworkers
- Working mother, lawyer

COPING AND STRESS

- Anxious: "I can't breathe"
- Facial muscles tense; trembling
- Expresses concerns about work: "I'll never get caught up"

VALUES AND BELIEFS

- Catholic
- Anointing of the sick requested
- Middle-class, professional orientation
- No wish to see chaplain or priest at present

MEDICATION AND HISTORY

- Synthroid 0.1 mg per day
- Client has history of appendectomy, partial thyroidectomy

NURSING PHYSICAL ASSESSMENT

- 28 years old
- Height 158 cm; weight 57 kg
- Temperature, Pulse, and Respiration (TPR): 39.4°C, 92, 28
- Radial pulses weak, regular
- Blood pressure: 122/80 mm Hg sitting
- Skin hot and pale, cheeks flushed
- Mucous membranes dry and pale
- Respirations shallow; chest expansion <3 cm
- Cough productive of small amounts of pale pink sputum
- Inspiratory crackles auscultated throughout right upper and lower chest
- Diminished breath sounds on right side
- Abdomen soft, not distended
- Old surgical scars: anterior neck, right left quadrant (RLQ) abdomen
- Diaphoretic

NON-NURSING MODELS Frameworks and models from other disciplines may also be helpful for organizing data. The nurse usually combines these with other approaches to obtain a complete history.

BODY SYSTEMS MODEL The body systems model focuses on abnormalities of the following systems:

- Integumentary
- Respiratory
- Cardiovascular
- Nervous
- Musculoskeletal
- Gastrointestinal
- Genitourinary
- Reproductive

MASLOW'S HIERARCHY OF NEEDS Maslow's hierarchy of needs clusters data pertaining to the following:

- Physiological needs
- Safety and security needs
- Love and belonging needs
- Self-esteem needs
- Self-actualization needs

See Chapter 12 for detailed information.

DEVELOPMENTAL THEORIES Several physical, psychosocial, cognitive, and moral developmental theories can be used by the nurse in specific situations. Examples include the following:

- Havighurst's age periods and developmental tasks
- Freud's five stages of development
- Erikson's eight stages of development
- Piaget's phases of cognitive development
- Kohlberg's stages of moral development

See Chapters 17, 18, 19, and 20 for further information.

Validating Data

The information gathered during the assessment phase must be complete and accurate for the nurse to analyze the data and determine appropriate interventions. **Validation** is the act of "double-checking" or verifying data (cues) to confirm that they are accurate and factual. Validating data helps the nurse:

- Ensure that assessment information is complete.
- Ensure that objective and related subjective data agree.
- Obtain additional information that may have been missed initially.
- Differentiate between cues and inferences. **Cues** are subjective or objective data that can be directly heard or observed by the nurse, that is, what the client says or what the nurse can see, hear, feel, smell, or measure. **Inferences** are the nurse's conclusions or interpretation of the cues (e.g., a nurse observes the cues that an incision is red, hot, and swollen; the nurse makes the inference that the incision is infected).
- Avoid jumping to conclusions and focusing too quickly on what seem like obvious problems.

The nurse validates data when discrepancies exist between data obtained in the nursing interview (subjective data) and the physical examination (objective data), or when the client's statements differ at different times in the assessment. Guidelines for validating data are shown in Table 23.4.

To collect data accurately, nurses need to be aware of their own biases, values, and beliefs and to separate fact from inference, interpretation, and assumption. They must validate assumptions regarding the client's physical or emotional behaviour. For example, a nurse

TABLE 23.4 Validating Assessment Data

Guideline	Example
Compare subjective and objective data to verify the client's statements with your observations.	Client's perceptions of "feeling hot" need to be compared with measurement of the body temperature.
Clarify any ambiguous or vague statements.	*Client:* "I've felt sick on and off for 6 weeks." *Nurse:* "Describe what your sickness is like. Tell me what you mean by 'on and off.'"
Be sure your data consist of cues and not inferences.	*Observation:* Dry skin and reduced tissue turgor *Inference:* Dehydration *Action:* Collect additional data that are needed to make the inference in the diagnosing phase. For example, determine the client's fluid intake, amount and appearance of urine, and blood pressure.
Double-check data that are extremely abnormal.	*Observation:* A resting pulse of 50 beats per minute or a blood pressure of 180/96 mm Hg *Action:* Use another piece of equipment as needed to confirm abnormalities, or ask someone else to collect the same data.
Determine the presence of factors that may interfere with accurate measurement.	A crying infant will have an abnormal respiratory rate and will need quieting before accurate assessment can be made.
Use references (textbooks, journals, research reports) to explain phenomena.	A nurse considers tiny purple or bluish-black swollen areas under the tongue of an older client to be abnormal until reading about physical changes of aging. Such varicosities are not uncommon.

seeing a man holding his arm to his chest might assume that he is experiencing chest pain, when, in fact, he has a painful hand. The nurse should ask the client why he is holding his arm to his chest. The client's response may validate the nurse's assumptions or prompt further questioning. Figure 23.3 (pages 464 and 465) shows that the nurse auscultated Amanda Aquilini's heart and lungs to validate her statement that she had "pain" in her "lungs" and "shortness of breath" on exertion. Failure to validate assumptions can lead to an inaccurate or incomplete nursing assessment and could compromise client safety.

Documenting Data

To complete the assessment phase, the nurse records client data. Accurate documentation is essential and should include all data collected about the client's health status. Data are recorded in a factual manner and not interpreted by the nurse. For example, the nurse records the client's breakfast intake (objective data) as "coffee 240 mL, juice 120 mL, 1 egg, and 1 slice of toast," rather than as "appetite good" (a judgment). A judgment or conclusion, such as "appetite good" or "normal appetite," may have different meanings for different people. To increase accuracy, the nurse records subjective data in the client's own words. Restating in other words what someone says increases the chance of changing the original meaning. Details of recording are discussed in Chapter 24.

Diagnosing

In this phase, nurses use critical thinking skills to interpret assessment data and identify client strengths, problems, and desired health outcomes. Diagnosing is a pivotal step in the nursing process. All activities preceding this phase are directed toward formulating the nursing analyses, hypotheses, or diagnoses, which are followed by all the care-planning activities (see Figure 23.4).

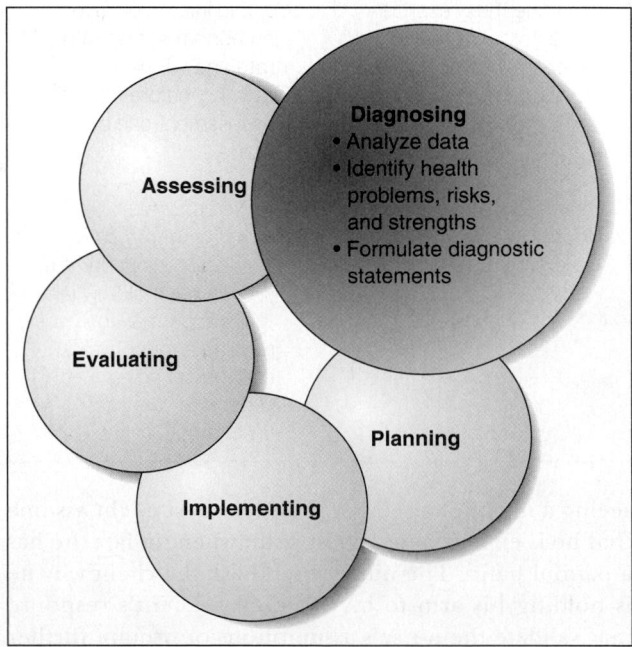

FIGURE 23.4 Diagnosing: The pivotal second phase of the nursing process.

There are various approaches to analyzing client issues, concerns, or problems in nursing. Nonetheless, the role of the nurse is to thoroughly assess and analyze the health status of each client, and to carry out holistic interventions that are specifically tailored to meet the unique needs of the individual. In some educational programs and practice areas, nursing care is organized around *nursing diagnoses, nursing analyses,* or *nursing conclusions,* including approaches using *best practice statements.* Throughout this book, we use the term *nursing diagnosis,* including the North American Nursing Diagnosis Association's (NANDA) predefined diagnoses as well as alternative ways of summarizing nursing assessments and analyses.

The First National Conference to identify nursing diagnoses was sponsored by the Saint Louis University School of Nursing and Allied Health Professions in 1973. International recognition came with the First Canadian Conference in Toronto in 1977 and the International Nursing Conference in May 1987 in Calgary, Alberta (Hannah, Reimer, Mills, & Letourneau, 1987). In 1982, the conference group accepted the name *North American Nursing Diagnosis Association (NANDA),* recognizing the participation and contributions of nurses in the United States and Canada. NANDA, transformed to NANDA International, is the premier international nursing diagnosis association (NANDA International, 2012).

The purpose of NANDA International is to define, refine, and promote a *taxonomy* (a classification system) of nursing diagnostic terminology of general use to professional nurses. Currently, there are more than 217 nursing diagnosis labels for clinical use and testing (NANDA International, 2012).

Nursing Diagnoses

The nursing diagnosis phase of the nursing process includes identifying one or more nursing diagnoses and collaborating with the client to establish priority health outcomes. **Client health outcomes** are the anticipated, predetermined outcomes that the client selects in collaboration with the nurse to guide and inform nursing practice.

NANDA International Nursing Diagnosis

To use the concept of nursing diagnoses effectively in generating and completing a nursing care plan, the nurse must be familiar with the definitions of terms used, the types, and the components of nursing diagnoses.

DEFINITIONS The term *diagnosing* refers to the reasoning process, whereas the term *diagnosis* is a statement or conclusion regarding the nature of a phenomenon. The standardized NANDA International names for the diagnoses are called **diagnostic labels**; and the client's problem statement, consisting of the diagnostic label plus **etiology** (causal relationship between a problem and its related risk factors), is called a *nursing diagnosis.*

In 1990, NANDA International adopted an official working definition of **nursing diagnosis**, which is "a clinical judgment about individual, family, or community responses to actual and potential health problems/life processes. A nursing diagnosis provides the basis for selection of nursing interventions to achieve outcomes for which the nurse is accountable" (NANDA International, 2012, p. 499). This definition implies the following:

- The domain of nursing diagnosis includes only those health states that nurses are educated and licensed to treat. For example, generalist nurses are not educated to diagnose or treat such diseases as diabetes mellitus; this task is defined legally as within the practice of medicine. Yet nurses can diagnose and treat *Deficient Knowledge, Ineffective Coping,* or *Imbalanced Nutrition,* all of which are human responses to the medical diagnosis of diabetes mellitus.

- A nursing diagnosis is a judgment made only after thorough, systematic data collection.

- Nursing diagnoses describe a continuum of health states: deviations from health, presence of risk factors, and areas of enhanced personal growth.

TYPES OF NURSING DIAGNOSES Four types of nursing diagnoses are actual, potential, risk, and wellness.

1. An **actual nursing diagnosis** is a client problem that is present at the time of the nursing assessment. Examples are *Ineffective Breathing Pattern* and *Anxiety.* An actual nursing diagnosis is based on the presence of associated signs and symptoms.

2. A **possible nursing diagnosis** is one in which evidence about a health problem is incomplete or unclear. A *potential diagnosis* requires more data either to support or to refute it. For example, an older widow who lives alone is admitted to the hospital. The nurse notices that she has no visitors and that she is pleased with attention and conversation from the nursing staff. Until more data are collected, the nurse may write a nursing diagnosis of *Possible Social Isolation* related to unknown etiology.

3. A **risk nursing diagnosis** is a clinical judgment that a problem does not yet exist, but the presence of **risk factors** indicates that a problem is likely to develop unless the nurse intervenes. For example, all people admitted to a hospital have some possibility of acquiring an infection; however, a client with diabetes or a compromised immune system is at higher risk than others. Therefore, the nurse would appropriately use the label *Risk for Infection* to describe the client's health status.

4. A **wellness nursing diagnosis** "describes human responses to levels of wellness in an individual, family or community that have a readiness for enhancement" (NANDA International, 2012, p. 501). Wellness diagnosis sometimes is referred to as *health promotion diagnosis,* which relates to clients' preparedness to implement behaviours to improve their health condition. Examples of wellness diagnoses would be *Readiness for Enhanced Spiritual Well-Being* or *Readiness for Enhanced Family Coping.*

COMPONENTS OF A NANDA INTERNATIONAL NURSING DIAGNOSIS A nursing diagnosis usually has three components: (a) the diagnostic label or the problem and its definition, (b) the etiology, and (c) the defining characteristics.

Problem (Diagnostic) The problem statement, or diagnostic label, describes the client's health problem or response for which nursing therapy is given. It describes the client's health status clearly and concisely in a few words. The purpose of the diagnostic label is to direct the formation of client goals and desired health outcomes. It may also suggest some nursing interventions. Diagnostic labels need to be specific; when the word *Specify* follows a NANDA International label, the nurse states the area in which the problem occurs, for example, *Deficient Knowledge (Medications)* or *Deficient Knowledge (Dietary Adjustments).*

Qualifiers are words that have been added to some NANDA International labels to give additional meaning to the diagnostic statement:

- Deficient (inadequate in amount, quality, or degree; not sufficient; incomplete)

- Impaired (made worse, weakened, damaged, reduced, deteriorated)

- Decreased (lesser in size, amount, or degree)

- Ineffective (not producing the desired effect)

- Compromised (to make vulnerable to threat)

Each diagnostic label approved by NANDA International carries a definition that clarifies its meaning.

Etiology (Related Factors) The **related factors** component of a nursing diagnosis identifies one or more probable causes of the health problem, gives direction to the required nursing therapy, and enables the nurse to individualize the client's care. As shown in the example in Table 23.5 on the next page, the probable causes of *anxiety* include lack of knowledge, fear, and so on. Differentiating among possible causes in the nursing diagnosis is essential because each may require different nursing interventions.

Defining Characteristics **Defining characteristics** are the cluster of signs and symptoms that indicate the presence of a particular diagnostic label. For actual nursing diagnoses, the defining characteristics are in the client's signs and symptoms. For risk nursing diagnoses, no subjective and objective signs are present. Thus, risk factors that cause the client to be more than "normally" vulnerable to the problem are identified instead.

DIFFERENTIATING NURSING DIAGNOSES FROM MEDICAL DIAGNOSES A *nursing diagnosis* is a statement of nursing judgment and refers to a condition that

TABLE 23.5 Example for Components of a Nursing Diagnosis

Client Data: 65-year-old female, newly diagnosed with diabetes

Diagnosis	Related Factors	Defining Characteristics
Anxiety	Lack of knowledge of diabetes and its treatment	– Asking the same questions repeatedly. – Stated was shocked to have been diagnosed with diabetes.
	Fear of impending lifestyle changes	– Tearful, loss of appetite, insomnia – Stated it is difficult to get old and she has no control of her life from now on

nurses are licensed to treat. A *medical diagnosis* is made by a physician and refers to a condition that only a physician or nurse practitioner can treat. **Medical diagnoses** refer to disease processes—specific pathophysiological responses that are fairly uniform from one client to another. In contrast, nursing diagnoses describe a client's physical, sociocultural, psychological, and spiritual responses to an illness or a health problem (see Table 23.6). These responses vary among individuals. A client's medical diagnosis remains the same for as long as the disease process is present, but nursing diagnoses change as the client's responses change, as in the following example:

> *Seventy-year-old Mary Cain and 20-year-old Kristi Vidan both have rheumatoid arthritis. Their disease processes are much the same. X-ray studies show that in both clients, the extent of inflammation and the number of joints involved are similar, and both clients experience almost constant pain. Ms. Cain views her condition as part of the aging process and is responding with acceptance. Ms. Vidan, however, is responding with anger and hostility because she views her disease as a threat to her personal identity, role performance, and self-esteem.*

Nurses have responsibilities related to both medical and nursing diagnoses and work collaboratively in carrying out physician-prescribed therapies and treatments. Nursing diagnoses relate to the nurse's **independent functions**, that is, the areas of health care that are unique to nursing and separate and distinct from medical management. Nurses may not prescribe *all* the care for a nursing diagnosis, but if the problem is a nursing diagnosis, the nurse can prescribe *most* of the interventions needed for prevention or resolution. For example, most clients with a nursing diagnosis of *Pain* have medical orders for analgesics, but many independent nursing interventions can also alleviate pain (e.g., guided imagery or teaching

a client to splint an incision). With regard to medical diagnoses, nurses are obligated to carry out physician-prescribed therapies and treatments, that is, **dependent functions**.

DIFFERENTIATING NURSING DIAGNOSES FROM COLLABORATIVE PROBLEMS Carpenito-Moyet (2009) has suggested that all *collaborative problems* begin with the label *Potential Complication* to indicate both the possible complications they are monitoring and the disease or treatment that is present to produce it (see Table 23.6).

For example, if the client has a head injury and could develop increased intracranial pressure, the nurse should write the following:

> *Potential complication of head injury: Increased intracranial pressure*

When monitoring for a group of complications associated with a disease or pathology, the nurse states the disease and follows it with a list of the complications:

> *Potential complications of pregnancy-induced hypertension: Seizures, fetal distress, pulmonary edema, hepatic/renal failure, premature labour, CNS hemorrhage*

The Diagnostic Process

The diagnostic process uses the critical thinking and clinical reasoning skills of analysis and synthesis. These skills are a cognitive process during which a person reviews data and considers explanations before forming an opinion (see Chapter 21). *Analysis* is the separation into components, that is, breaking down the whole into its parts (deductive reasoning). *Synthesis* is the opposite, that is, putting together the parts into the whole (inductive reasoning).

The diagnostic process has three steps:

1. Analyzing data
2. Identifying health problems, risks, and strengths
3. Formulating diagnostic statements

ANALYZING DATA In the diagnostic process, analyzing involves the following steps:

1. Compare data against standards (identify significant cues).
2. Cluster the cues (generate tentative hypotheses).
3. Identify gaps and inconsistencies.

For experienced nurses, these activities occur continuously rather than sequentially. Novice nurses, however, need guidelines to understand and formulate nursing diagnoses.

Comparing Data with Standards Nurses draw on knowledge and experience to compare client data with standards and norms and identify significant and relevant cues. A **standard** or **norm** is a generally accepted measure, rule, model, or pattern. The nurse uses a wide range of

TABLE 23.6   Comparison of Nursing Diagnoses, Medical Diagnoses, and Collaborative Problems

Category	Nursing Diagnoses	Medical Diagnoses	Collaborative Problems
Example	*Activity Intolerance* related to decreased cardiac output	Myocardial infarction	Potential complication of myocardial infarction: congestive heart failure
Description	Describe human responses to disease process or health problem; consist of a one-, two-, or three-part statement, usually including problem and etiology	Describe disease and pathology; do not consider other human responses; usually consist of not more than three words	Involve human responses—mainly physiological complications of disease, tests, or treatments; consist of a two-part statement of situation/pathophysiology and the potential complication
Orientation and responsibility for diagnosing	Oriented to the individual; nurses responsible for diagnosing	Oriented to pathology; physician responsible for diagnosing; diagnosis not within the scope of nursing practice	Oriented to pathophysiology; nurses responsible for diagnosing
Nursing focus	Treat and prevent	Implement medical orders for treatment and monitor status of condition	Prevent and monitor for onset or status of condition
Duration	Can change frequently	Remains the same while disease is present	Present when disease or situation is present
Classification system	Classification system is developed and being used but is not universally accepted	Well-developed classification system accepted by the medical profession	No universally accepted classification system

standards, such as growth and development patterns, normal vital signs, and laboratory values. A cue is any piece of information or data that influences decisions. A cue is considered significant if it does any of the following:

- *Points to negative or positive change in a client's health status or pattern.* For example, the client states "I have recently experienced shortness of breath while climbing stairs," or "I have not smoked for 3 months."

- *Varies from norms of the client population.* The client's pattern may fit within cultural norms but vary from norms of the general society. The client may consider a pattern—for example, eating very small meals and having little appetite—to be normal. This pattern, however, may not be productive and may require further exploration.

- *Indicates a developmental delay.* To identify significant cues, the nurse must be aware of the normal patterns and changes that occur as the person grows and develops. For example, by age 9 months, an infant is usually able to sit without support. The infant who has not accomplished this task needs further assessment for possible developmental delays.

Refer to Table 23.7 on the next page for specific examples of client cues and norms to which they may be compared. Significant cues and data clusters for

Amanda Aquilini that were extracted from Figure 23.3 (pages 466–467) and Box 23.4 (page 469) are shown in Table 23.8 on the next page.

Clustering Cues   Clustering or grouping cues is a process of determining the relatedness of facts and determining whether any patterns are present, whether the data represent isolated incidents, and whether the data are significant. This is the beginning of synthesis.

The nurse may cluster data *inductively* (as in Table 23.8) by combining data from different assessment areas to form a pattern, or the nurse may begin with a framework, such as Gordon's functional health patterns, and cluster the subjective and objective data into the appropriate categories (see Box 23.4 on page 469). The latter is a *deductive* approach to data clustering, or pattern formation.

Experienced nurses may cluster data as they collect and interpret it, as evidenced in such remarks or thoughts as, "I'm getting a picture of. . . ," or "This cue doesn't fit the picture." The novice nurse does not have the knowledge base or the clinical experience that aids in recognizing cues. Thus, the novice must take careful assessment notes, search data for abnormal cues, and use textbook resources for comparing the client's cues with the defining characteristics and etiological factors of the accepted nursing diagnoses.

TABLE 23.7 Comparing Cues to Standards and Norms

Type of Cue	Client Cues	Standard/Norm
Deviation from population norms	Client height is 158 cm. The woman has a small frame. She weighs 109 kg.	The body mass index (BMI) indicates that the BMI for a woman 158 cm tall who weighs 109 kg is 43.7. Normal BMI ranges from 18.5 to 24.9.
Developmental delay	The child is 18 months old. Parents state child has not yet attempted to speak. The child laughs aloud and makes cooing sounds.	Children usually speak their first word by 10 to 12 months of age.
Changes in client's usual health status	The client states, "I'm just not hungry these days." She ate only 15% of food on breakfast tray. She has lost 13 kg in the past 3 months.	The client usually eats three balanced meals per day. Adults typically maintain stable weight.
Dysfunctional behaviour	Tanya's mother reports that Tanya has not left her room for 2 days. Tanya is 16 years old. Tanya has stopped attending school and has withdrawn from social contact.	Adolescents usually like to be with their peers; social groups are very important. Functional behaviour includes school attendance.
Changes in client's usual behaviour	Mrs. Stuart reports that lately her husband gets angry easily. "Yesterday he even yelled at the dog." "He just seems so tense."	Mr. Stuart is usually relaxed and easygoing. He is friendly and kind to animals.

TABLE 23.8 Formulating Nursing Diagnoses for Amanda Aquilini

Functional Health Pattern	Client Cue Clusters	Inferences (Tentative Identification of Problems)	Formulating Diagnostic Statements
Health perception/ health management	No significant cues	No problem	No problem *Strength:* Has healthy lifestyle, understanding of and compliance with treatment regimens
Nutritional/metabolic (includes hydration)	"No appetite" since having "cold" Has not eaten today; last fluids at noon today Nauseated × 2 days	***Imbalanced Nutrition: Less than Body Requirements***	***Altered Nutrition: Less than Body Requirements*** related to decreased appetite and nausea and increased metabolism (secondary to disease process) *Strength:* Normal weight for height
	Last fluids at noon today Oral temperature 39.4°C Skin hot and pale; cheeks flushed Mucous membranes dry Poor skin turgor *Cues from elimination pattern:* Decreased urinary frequency and amount × 2 days	***Deficient fluid volume***	***Deficient fluid volume*** related to intake insufficient to replace fluid loss secondary to fever, diaphoresis, anorexia

TABLE 23.8   *(continued)*

Functional Health Pattern	Client Cue Clusters	Inferences (Tentative Identification of Problems)	Formulating Diagnostic Statements
Elimination	Decreased urinary frequency and amount × 2 days	Cues consist of elimination data but are actually symptoms of a fluid volume problem in the nutritional/metabolic functional health pattern	No elimination problem
Activity/exercise	States, "I feel weak standing at the sink and in the shower" Short of breath on exertion *Cues from cognitive/ perceptual pattern:* Responsive but fatigued "I can think OK, just weak" *Cues from cardiovascular pattern:* Radial pulses weak, regular Pulse rate 92	***Activity Intolerance***	***Activity Intolerance*** related to general weakness *Strength:* No musculoskeletal impairment
Sleep/rest	Difficulty sleeping because of cough "Can't breathe lying down"	***Disturbed Sleep Pattern***	***Disturbed Sleep Pattern*** related to cough, pain, orthopnea, fever, and diaphoresis
Cognitive/perceptual	Reports pain in chest, especially when coughing Responsive but fatigued "I can think OK, just weak"	***Acute pain***	***Acute pain (Chest)*** related to cough secondary to pneumonia *Strength:* No cognitive or sensory deficits
Roles/relationships	Husband out of town; will be back tomorrow afternoon Child with neighbour until husband returns	***Interrupted Family Processes*** related to mother's illness and temporary unavailability of father to provide childcare Cues also related to a problem in the coping/stress pattern	***Risk for Interrupted Family Processes*** related to mother's illness and temporary unavailability of father to provide childcare *Strength:* Neighbours available and willing to help
Self-perception/ self-concept	Expresses "concern" and "worry" over leaving daughter with neighbours until husband returns	Cue is a symptom of a problem in the coping/stress pattern	No self-perception/self-concept problem
Coping/stress	Anxious: "I can't breathe" Facial muscles tense; trembling Expresses concerns about work: "I'll never get caught up" *Cues from role/relationship pattern:* *Cues from self-perception/ self-concept patterns:* Expresses "concern" and "worry" over leaving daughter with neighbours	***Anxiety*** related to difficulty breathing, inability to work, and provide childcare	***Anxiety*** related to difficulty breathing and concerns over work and parenting roles

(continued)

TABLE 23.8 *(continued)*

Functional Health Pattern	Client Cue Clusters	Inferences (Tentative Identification of Problems)	Formulating Diagnostic Statements
Medication/history	No significant cues	No problem	No problem
Physical assessment			
Cardiovascular	Radial pulses weak, regular Pulse rate 92	Cues are symptoms only; symptoms of exercise/rest and oxygenation problems	No cardiovascular problem
Oxygenation	Skin hot, pale, and moist Respirations shallow; chest expansion, 3 cm Cough productive of small amounts of pale pink sputum Inspiratory crackles auscultated throughout right upper and lower chest Diminished breath sounds on right side Mucous membranes pale	***Ineffective Airway Clearance*** related to disease process	***Ineffective Airway Clearance*** related to viscous secretions and shallow chest expansion secondary to pain, deficient fluid volume, and fatigue
Skin	Old surgical scars, anterior neck, right left quadrant (RLQ) abdomen	No problem now	Old problems; resolved

Data clustering involves making inferences about the data. An inference is the nurse's judgment or interpretation of cues. The nurse interprets the possible meaning of the cues and labels the cue clusters with tentative diagnostic hypotheses. Data clustering or grouping for Amanda Aquilini is illustrated in Table 23.8, in which data are clustered according to standardized diagnostic labels.

Another technique used to cluster data is by using *concept mapping*. Data is clustered in the same manner described above, but it is developed into a visual format (see Concept Map: Ineffective Airway Clearance [Gas Exchange] on page 487).

Identifying Gaps and Inconsistencies in Data Skillful assessment minimizes gaps and inconsistencies in data. However, data analysis should include a final check to ensure that data are complete and correct.

Inconsistencies are conflicting data. Possible sources of conflicting data include measurement error, expectations, and conflicting or unreliable reports. For example, a nurse may learn from the nursing history that the client reports not having seen a doctor in 15 years, yet during the physical health examination, he states, "My doctor takes my blood pressure every week." All inconsistencies must be clarified before a valid pattern can be established.

IDENTIFYING HEALTH PROBLEMS, RISKS, AND STRENGTHS After data are analyzed, the nurse and client can together identify strengths and problems. This is primarily a decision-making process. See Chapter 21.

Determining Problems and Risks After grouping and clustering data, the nurse and client together identify tentative diagnoses. In addition, the nurse must determine whether the client's problem is a nursing diagnosis, medical diagnosis, or collaborative problem (see Table 23.6). See Figure 23.5 for a decision tree to aid in this decision.

For examples, refer to the cue clusters and tentative identification of problems for Amanda Aquilini in Table 23.8. In this example, the nurse and client identified nine tentative problems: *Imbalanced Nutrition: Less than Body Requirements; Deficient Fluid Volume; Disturbed Sleep Pattern; Self-Care Deficit; Acute Pain (Chest); Interrupted Family Processes; Anxiety; Activity Intolerance;* and *Ineffective Airway Clearance.*

Determining Strengths At this stage, the nurse and client also establish the client's strengths, resources, and abilities to cope. Most people focus more on their problems or weaknesses than on their strengths and assets, which they often take for granted. By taking an inventory of strengths, the client can develop a more well-rounded self-concept and self-image. Strengths can be an aid to mobilizing health and regenerative processes.

A client's strengths can be found in the nursing assessment record (health, home life, education, recreation, exercise, work, family and friends, religious beliefs, and sense of humour, for example), the health examination, and the client's records. See Table 23.8 for strengths identified for Amanda Aquilini.

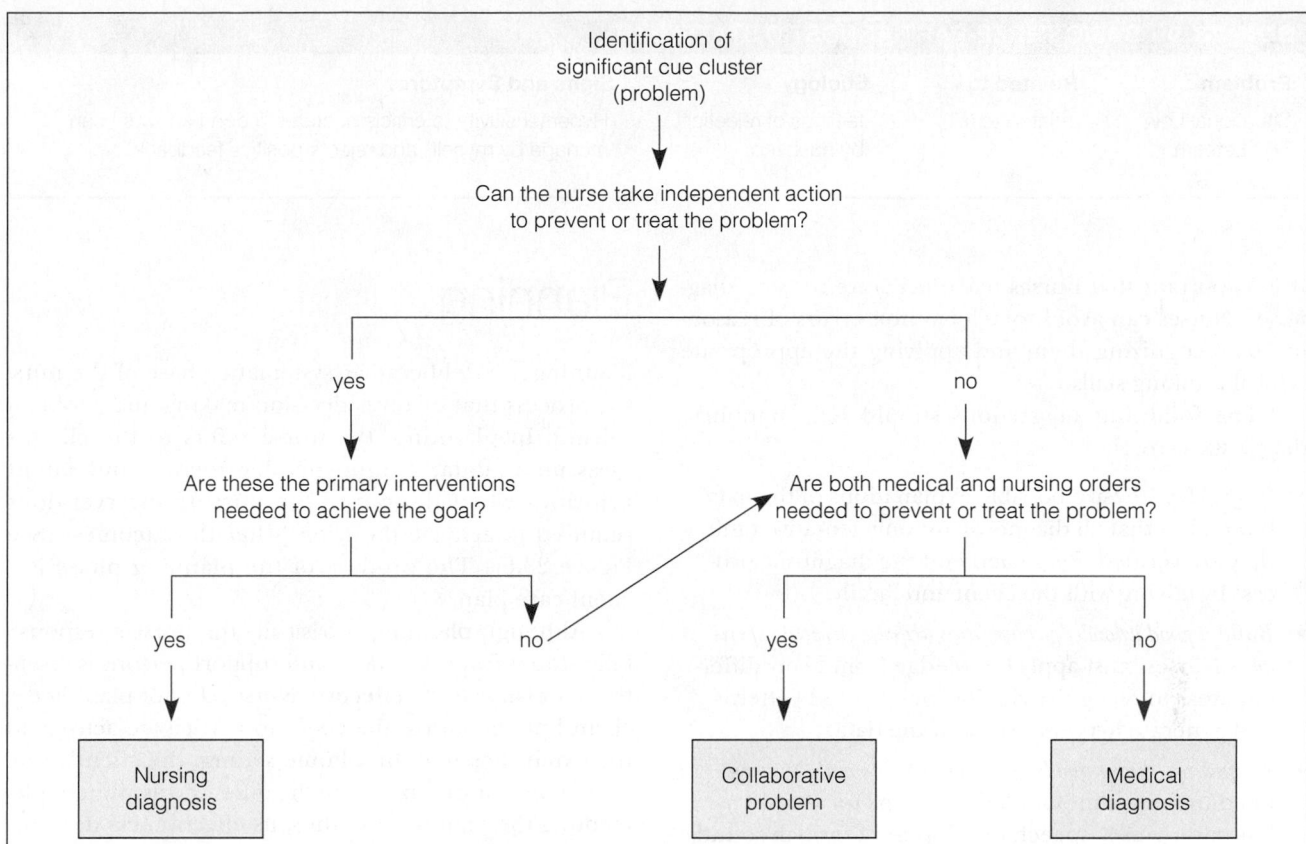

FIGURE 23.5 Decision tree for differentiating among nursing diagnoses, collaborative problems, and medical diagnoses.

FORMULATING DIAGNOSTIC STATEMENTS Most nursing diagnoses are written as two-part or three-part statements.

Basic Two-Part Statements The basic two-part statement includes the following:

1. Problem (P): statement of the client's response
2. Etiology (E): factors contributing to or probable causes of the responses

The two parts are joined by the words *related to* rather than *because of*. The phrase *because of* implies that one part causes or is responsible for the other part. By contrast, the phrase *related to* merely implies a relationship. Some examples of two-part nursing diagnoses are shown in the Box 23.8.

Basic Three-Part Statements The basic three-part nursing diagnosis statement includes the following:

1. Problem (P): statement of the client's response
2. Etiology (E): factors contributing to or probable causes of the response
3. Signs and symptoms (S): defining characteristics manifested by the client

Actual nursing diagnoses can be documented by using the three-part statement (see Box 23.9 on the next page) because the signs and symptoms have been identified. This format cannot be used for risk diagnosis because the client does not have signs and symptoms of the diagnosis. The PES format is especially recommended for beginning diagnosticians because the signs and symptoms validate why the diagnosis was chosen and make the problem statement more descriptive.

Using Diagnostic Statements Effectively Beginning nurses often prepare long lists, but checking initial statements (hypotheses) with the client helps both nurse and client narrow down the list to those that are most important in the current clinical context. Next, through negotiating with the client, the nurse clusters nursing diagnoses and identifies priority client health outcomes to guide nursing care.

AVOIDING ERRORS IN DIAGNOSTIC REASONING Error can occur at any point in the diagnostic process: data collection, data interpretation, and data clustering.

BOX 23.8	BASIC TWO-PART DIAGNOSTIC STATEMENT	
Problem	**Related to**	**Etiology**
Constipation	related to	prolonged laxative use
Ineffective breast-feeding	related to	breast engorgement

BOX 23.9	BASIC THREE-PART AGNOSTIC STATEMENT		
Problem	**Related to**	**Etiology**	**Signs and Symptoms**
Situational Low Self-Esteem	related to (r/t)	feelings of rejection by husband	Hypersensitivity to criticism; states "I don't know if I can manage by myself" and rejects positive feedback

It is important that nurses make accurate nursing diagnoses. Nurses can avoid some common errors of reasoning by recognizing them and applying the appropriate critical thinking skills.

The following suggestions should help minimize diagnostic error:

- *Verify.* Hypothesize possible explanations of the data, but realize that all diagnoses are only tentative until they are verified. Begin and end the diagnostic process by talking with the client and family.

- *Build a good knowledge base, and acquire clinical experience.* Nurses must apply knowledge from many different areas to recognize significant cues and patterns and generate hypotheses about the data.

- *Have a working knowledge of what is normal.* Nurses need to know the population norms for vital signs, laboratory tests, speech development, breath sounds, and so on. In addition, nurses must determine what is normal for a particular person, taking into account age, physical makeup, lifestyle, culture, and the person's own perception of what is normal. For example, high normal blood pressure for adults is in the range of 130–139/85–89 mm Hg (Canadian Hypertension Education Program, 2012). However, a nurse might obtain a reading of 90/50 mm Hg that is normal for a particular client. The nurse should compare findings with the client's baseline, when possible.

- *Consult resources.* Both novices and experienced nurses should consult appropriate resources whenever in doubt about a diagnosis. Professional literature, nursing colleagues, and other health care professionals are all appropriate resources.

- *Base diagnoses on patterns—that is, on behaviour over time—rather than on an isolated incident.* For example, even though Amanda Aquilini is concerned today about needing to leave her child with a neighbour, it is likely that this concern will be resolved without intervention by the next day. Therefore, the admitting nurse should not diagnose *Interrupted Family Processes*, and this tentative nursing diagnosis should be reconsidered.

- *Improve critical thinking skills.* These skills help the nurse to be aware of and avoid errors in thinking, such as overgeneralizing, stereotyping, making unwarranted assumptions, and so on. See Chapter 21.

Planning

Planning is a deliberative, systematic phase of the nursing process that involves decision making and problem solving. In planning, the nurse refers to the client's assessment data, diagnostic statements, and client priorities when designing the nursing interventions required to achieve the client's health outcomes. (See Figure 23.6.) The product of the planning phase is a client care plan.

Although planning is basically the nurse's responsibility, input from the client and support persons is essential if a plan is to be effective. Nurses do not plan *for* the client but encourage the client to participate actively to the extent possible. In a home setting, the client's support people or caregivers are the ones who assist in implementing the plan of care; thus, its effectiveness depends largely on them.

Types of Planning

Planning begins with the first client contact and continues until the nurse–client relationship ends, usually when the client is discharged from the health care agency.

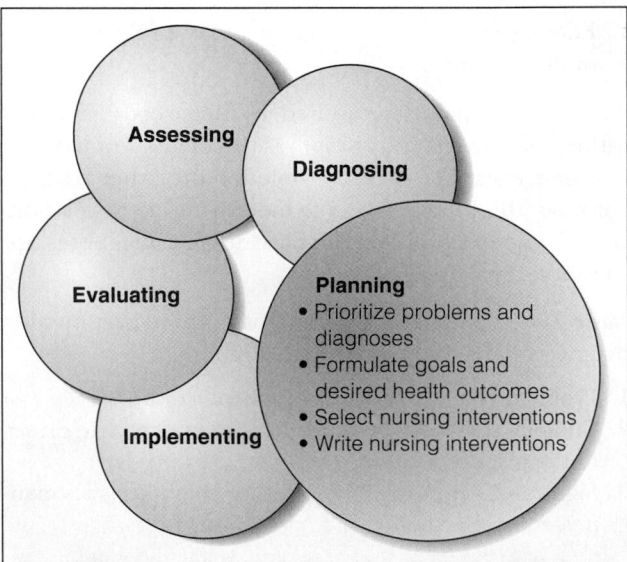

FIGURE 23.6 Planning: The third phase of the nursing process, in which the nurse and client develop a mutually agreed-upon plan of care.

Planning involves interacting with the client and family to the fullest extent possible.

INITIAL PLANNING   The nurse who performs the admission assessment usually develops the initial comprehensive plan of care. Planning should be initiated as soon as possible after the initial assessment, especially because of the trend toward shorter hospital stays.

ONGOING PLANNING   As nurses obtain new information and evaluate the client's responses to care, they can individualize the initial care plan further. Ongoing planning also occurs at the beginning of a shift, home visit, or clinic appointment. Ongoing assessment and planning serve the following purposes (Wilkinson, 2012):

1. To determine whether the client's health status has changed

2. To set the priorities for the client's care during the contact period (e.g., shift, home visit)

3. To decide which problems to focus on during the contact period

4. To coordinate the nurse's activities so that more than one problem can be addressed at each client contact

DISCHARGE PLANNING   **Discharge planning**, the process of anticipating and planning for needs after discharge, is a crucial part of comprehensive health care and should be addressed in each client's care plan. Because the average stay of clients in acute care hospitals has become shorter, people are often discharged still needing care. Although many clients are discharged to other agencies (e.g., nursing homes), such care is increasingly being delivered in the home. (See Chapters 12 to 14.)

Developing Nursing Care Plans

Nursing care planning involves formal or informal plan of care. An **informal care plan** is a plan of action that exists in the nurse's mind. For example, the nurse may think, "Mrs. Phan is very tired. I will need to reinforce her teaching after she is rested." A **formal care plan** is a written guide that organizes information about the client's care. The most obvious benefit of a formal written care plan is that it provides continuity of care.

Standardized care plans specify the nursing care for groups of clients with common needs (e.g., all clients with myocardial infarction). **Individualized care plans** are tailored to meet the unique needs of a specific client—needs that are not addressed by the standardized plans. It is important that all nursing caregivers use a consistent approach with a client. Nurses also use the written care plan for direction about what needs to be documented in client progress notes and as a guide for delegating and assigning staff to care for clients.

Care plans include the actions nurses must take to address the nursing diagnoses and produce the desired health outcomes. The nurse begins the plan when the client is admitted to the agency and constantly updates it throughout the client's stay in response to changes in the client's condition and evaluations of goal achievement. The plan of care should be mutually established with the client and with input from the client's family if appropriate. During the planning phase, the nurse must do the following:

1. Decide which of the client's problems need individualized plans and which problems can be addressed by standardized plans and routine care

2. Choose and adapt standardized, preprinted interventions and care plans, where appropriate

3. Write individualized desired health outcomes and nursing interventions for client problems that require nursing attention beyond preplanned, routine care

4. Decide when referrals to other health care professionals are needed

The complete plan of care for a client is made up of several different documents that (a) describe the routine care needed to meet basic needs (e.g., bathing, nutrition), (b) address the client's nursing diagnoses and identified health outcomes, and (c) specify nursing responsibilities in carrying out the client's plan of care (e.g., keeping the client from eating or drinking before surgery; scheduling a laboratory test). A complete plan of care integrates all nursing functions into a meaningful whole and provides a central source of client information. Figure 23.7 on the next page illustrates the various documents that may be included in a nursing care plan.

STANDARDIZED APPROACHES TO CARE PLANNING Most health care agencies have a variety of preprinted, standardized guides for providing essential nursing care to specified groups of clients who have certain needs in common (e.g., all clients with pneumonia). Standards of care, standardized care plans, protocols, policies, and procedures are developed to (a) ensure that minimally acceptable standards of care are provided and (b) promote efficient use of nurses' time by removing the need to handwrite common activities that are done over and over for many of the clients with common needs.

Standards of care describe nursing care for groups of clients rather than for individuals, and they describe achievable, rather than ideal nursing care. They define the interventions for which nurses are held accountable; they do not contain medical orders. Standards of care are usually agency records and not part of the client's care plan, but they may be referred to in the plan (e.g., a nurse might write, "See standards of care for cardiac catheterization"). Standards of care may or may not be organized according to problems or nursing diagnoses.

Standardized care plans are also preplanned, preprinted guides for the nursing care of groups of clients with common needs (e.g., a specific nursing diagnosis or all the nursing diagnoses associated with a particular medical condition). However, they should not be

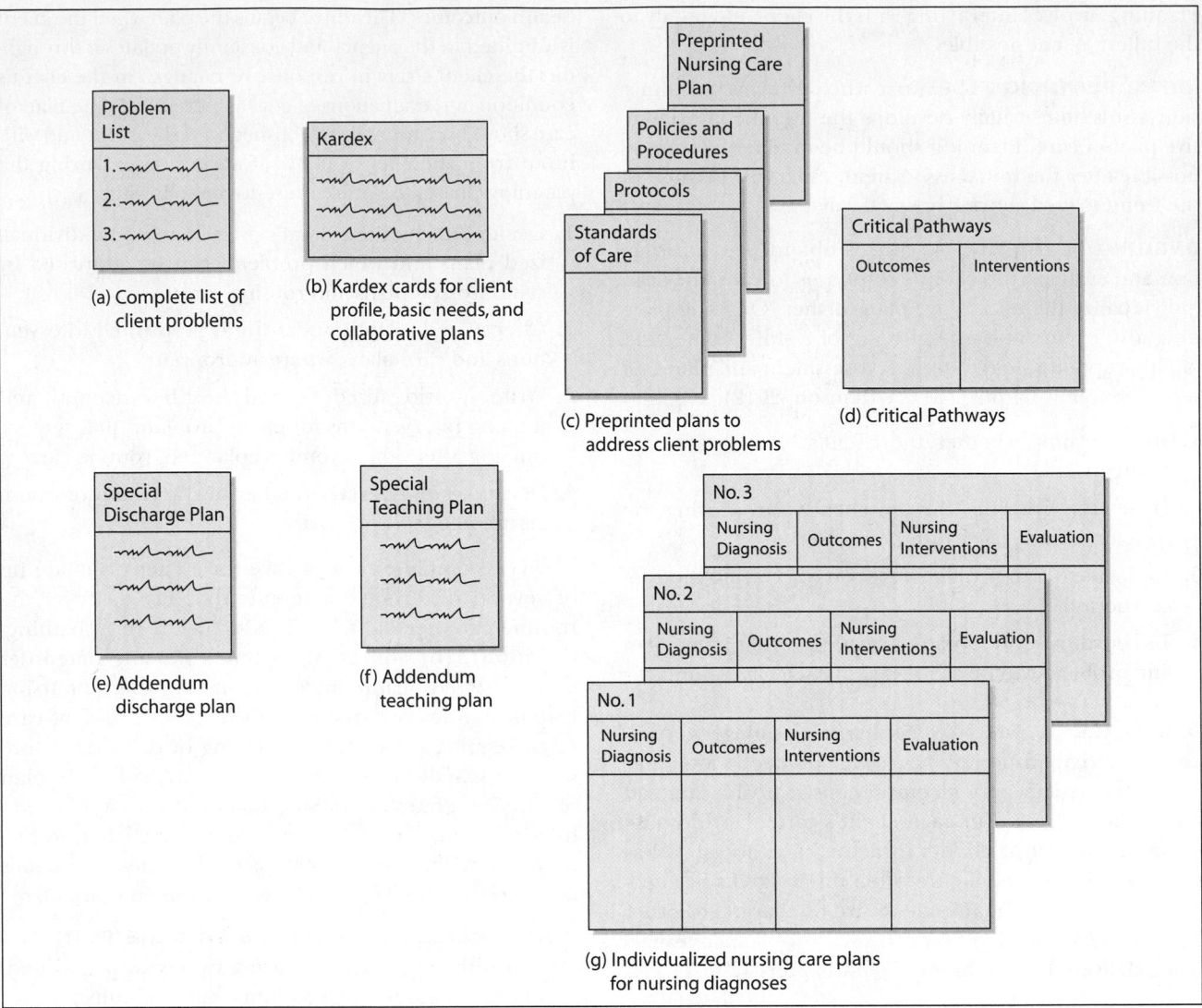

(a) Complete list of client problems

(b) Kardex cards for client profile, basic needs, and collaborative plans

(c) Preprinted plans to address client problems

(d) Critical Pathways

(e) Addendum discharge plan

(f) Addendum teaching plan

(g) Individualized nursing care plans for nursing diagnoses

FIGURE 23.7 Documents that may be included in a complete client care plan.

Source: From Wilkinson, J. M. (2012). *Nursing process & critical thinking.* (5th ed.) (p. 452). Upper Saddle River, NJ: Prentice Hall. Adapted with permission.

confused with *standards of care.* These care plans are generally included in a client's chart.

Protocols are preprinted and preplanned to indicate the actions commonly required for a particular group of clients. For example, an agency may have a protocol for admitting a client to the intensive care unit (ICU). Protocols may include both medical orders and nursing interventions.

Policies and **procedures** are developed to govern the handling of frequently occurring situations. For example, a hospital may have a policy specifying the number of visitors a client may have. Some policies and procedures are similar to protocols and specify what is to be done, for example, in the case of cardiac arrest. If a policy covers a situation pertinent to client care, it is usually noted on the care plan (e.g., "Make social work referral according to Unit Policy Manual").

A **standing order** is a written document about policies, rules, regulations, or orders regarding client care. Standing orders give nurses the authority to carry out specific actions under certain circumstances, often when a physician is not immediately available. In a hospital critical care unit, a common example is the administration of emergency antiarrhythmic medications when a client's cardiac monitoring pattern changes. In a home care setting, a physician may write a standing order for the administration of epinephrine for a client who becomes excessively dyspneic (short of breath).

Nursing care must be individualized to fit the unique needs of each client. In practice, a care plan usually consists of both preprinted and handwritten sections. The nurse uses standardized care plans for predictable, commonly occurring problems and handwrites an individual plan for unusual problems or problems needing special attention. For example, a standardized care plan for all "clients with a medical diagnosis of pneumonia" would probably include a nursing diagnosis of *Deficient Fluid Volume* and direct the nurse to assess the client's hydration status. On a respiratory or medical unit, this would be a common nursing diagnosis; therefore, Amanda Aquilini's nurse was able to obtain a standardized plan directing care commonly needed by clients with *Deficient Fluid Volume*. (See Figure 23.3 on pages 466–467 and Figure 23.8 on the next page.) However, the nursing diagnosis *Risk for Interrupted Family Processes* would not be common to all clients with pneumonia; it is specific to Amanda. Therefore, the goals and nursing interventions for that diagnosis would need to be handwritten by the nurse.

Types of Nursing Care Plans

Although formats differ from agency to agency, the care plan is often organized into four sections: (a) problem/ nursing diagnoses, (b) goals/desired outcomes, (c) nursing interventions, and (d) evaluation. Some agencies use a three-section plan in which evaluation is done with the goals or in the nurses' notes; others have five sections that add assessment data preceding the problem/nursing diagnosis.

STUDENT CARE PLANS Because student care plans are a learning activity as well as a plan of care, they may be more lengthy and detailed than care plans used by nurses. To help students learn to write care plans, educators may suggest a five-column format: (a) nursing diagnosis or hypotheses, (b) goals or desired health outcomes, (c) interventions, (d) rationale, and (e) evaluation. A **rationale** is the scientific principle given as the reason for selecting a particular nursing intervention. Students may also be required to cite supporting literature for their stated rationale.

CONCEPT MAPS A **concept map** is a visual tool in which ideas or data are graphically depicted in circles or boxes and relationships between these are indicated by connecting lines. Concept maps can encompass various forms and categories of data, according to the creator's interpretation of the client or health condition. The concept map for Amanda Aquilini (see page 487) is another way of depicting her nursing care plan and includes unique boxes that enclose assessment, nursing diagnosis, desired outcomes, and interventions.

Concept maps are often used to depict complex relationships among ideas, processes, actions, and so on. There are numerous benefits to using concept maps. For example, students can complete pathophysiology flow sheets or concept maps to see the linkages among disease processes, laboratory data, medications, signs and symptoms, risk factors, and other relevant data. They can critically analyze the "whole picture" of their clients, their conditions, and the connections between concerns,

which promotes a holistic approach to planning and evaluating care (Hicks-Moore, 2005; Hill, 2006).

COMPUTERIZED CARE PLANS Computers are increasingly being used to create and store nursing care plans. For an individualized plan, the nurse chooses the appropriate diagnoses from a menu suggested by the computer. The computer then lists possible goals and nursing interventions for those diagnoses; the nurse chooses those appropriate for the client and types in any additional goals and interventions or nursing actions not listed on the menu. The nurse can read the plan on the computer screen or print out an updated working copy each day.

A **multidisciplinary care plan** is a standardized plan that outlines the care required for clients with common, predictable—usually medical—conditions. Such plans, also referred to as **collaborative care plans** and **critical pathways**, sequence the care that must be given on each day during the projected length of stay for the specific type of condition. Like the traditional nursing care plan, a multidisciplinary care plan can specify outcomes and nursing interventions to address client problems (including nursing diagnoses). However, it includes medical treatments to be performed by other health care providers as well.

Critical pathways are used to plan and direct client care. This multidisciplinary client-centred tool helps the health care team to deliver care according to the client health outcomes. The document includes the expected outcomes predicted by the client and health care team (nursing, physiotherapy, medicine, pharmacy, and social work, for instance) to develop and integrate a plan of care as the client progresses through an illness. The plan is usually organized with a column for each day, listing the interventions that should be carried out and the client outcomes that should be achieved on that day. There are as many columns on the multidisciplinary care plan as the preset number of days allowed for the client's diagnosis-related group. For further information, see Chapter 6. Multidisciplinary care plans do not include detailed nursing activities. They should be drawn from, but do not replace, standards of care and standardized care plans.

The Planning Process

In the process of developing client care plans, the nurse engages in the following activities:

- Setting priorities
- Establishing client goals or desired health outcomes
- Selecting nursing interventions and activities
- Writing an individualized plan of care

SETTING PRIORITIES **Priority setting** is the process of establishing a preferential order for nursing diagnoses, client health outcomes, and interventions. The nurse and client begin planning by deciding which nursing

Standardized Care Plan for Nursing Diagnosis of DEFICIENT FLUID VOLUME

Related Factors	Desired Outcomes	Nursing Order (Identify Frequency)
✓Decreased oral intake	✓Urinary output > 30 mL/hr	✓Monitor intake and output q _1_ h
✓Nausea	✓Urine specific gravity 1.005 ±1.025	✓Weigh daily
__Depression		✓Monitor serum electrolyte levels X 1 or *until normal*
✓Fatigue, weakness	✓Serum Na⁺ normal	✓Check skin turgor and mucous membranes q _8_ h
__Difficulty swallowing	✓Mucous membranes moist	✓Monitor temperature q_4 h_
__Other:_____	✓Skin turgor good	✓Administer prescribed IV therapy (Monitor according to protocol for Intravenous Therapy)
✓Excess fluid loss	✓No weight loss	
✓Fever or increased metabolic rate	✓8-hour intake = _400 mL oral_	*1000 mL D₅ LR* ✓Offer oral liquids q _1_ h *at 100 mL/hr*
✓Diaphoresis	Other:	Type _clear, cold_____
✓Vomiting		✓Instruct client regarding amount, type, and schedule of fluid intake
__Diarrhea		✓Assess understanding of type of fluid loss; teach accordingly
__Burns		✓Mouth care (prn) with _water_____
__Other_____		✓Institute measures to reduce fever (e.g., lower room temperature, remove bed covers, offer cold liquids)

Defining Characteristics

Other Nursing Orders:_____

✓Insufficient intake

Monitor urine specific gravity

✓Negative balance of intake and output

q shift

✓Dry mucous membranes

_____

✓Poor skin turgor

_____

__Concentrated urine

_____

__Hypernatremia

_____

✓Rapid, weak pulse

_____

__Falling blood pressure

_____

__Weight loss

Plan Initiated by: _M. Medina RN_____ Date _11-04-16_____

Plan/outcomes evaluated_____ Date_____

Plan/outcomes evaluated_____ Date_____

Client:_Amanda Aquilini_____

FIGURE 23.8 A standardized care plan for nursing diagnosis of *Deficient Fluid Volume*.

diagnosis requires attention first, which second, and so on. Instead of rank-ordering diagnoses, nurses can group them as having high, medium, or low priority. Life-threatening problems, such as loss of respiratory or cardiac function, are designated as *high priority*. Health-threatening problems, such as acute illness and decreased coping ability, are assigned *medium priority* because they may result in delayed development or cause destructive physical or emotional changes. A *low-priority* problem is one that arises from normal developmental needs or that requires only minimal nursing support.

Nurses frequently use Maslow's hierarchy of needs when setting priorities. In Maslow's hierarchy, physiological needs, such as air, food, and water, are basic to life and receive higher priority than the need for security or activity. Growth needs, such as self-esteem, are not perceived as "basic" in this framework. Thus, such nursing diagnoses as *Ineffective Airway Clearance* and *Impaired Gas Exchange* would take priority over such nursing diagnoses as *Anxiety* or *Ineffective Coping*.

It is not necessary to resolve all high-priority diagnoses before addressing others. The nurse may partially address a high-priority diagnosis and then deal with a diagnosis of lesser priority. Furthermore, because clients usually have several problems, the nurse often deals with more than one diagnosis at a time. See Table 23.9 on the next page for priorities assigned to Amanda Aquilini's nursing diagnoses.

Priorities change as the client's responses, problems, and therapies change. The nurse must consider a variety of factors when assigning priorities:

1. *The client's health values and beliefs:* Values concerning health may be more important to the nurse than to the client. For example, a client may believe being home for the children to be more urgent than a health problem. When such a difference of opinion exists, the client and nurse should discuss it openly to resolve any conflict. However, in a life-threatening situation, the nurse usually must take the initiative.

2. *The client's priorities:* Involving the client in prioritizing and care planning enhances collaboration. Sometimes, however, the client's perception of what is important conflicts with the nurse's knowledge of potential problems or complications. For example, the client may not regard turning and repositioning in bed as important, preferring to be undisturbed. However, the nurse, who is aware of the potential complications of prolonged bed rest (e.g., muscle weakness and decubitus ulcers), needs to inform the client and gain the client's agreement to carry out the necessary interventions.

3. *The resources available to the nurse and client:* If money, equipment, or personnel resources are scarce in a health care agency, then the nurse must use critical thinking, clinical reasoning, and creative measures to address the nursing diagnoses. If the necessary resources are not available, the solution to that problem might need to be altered, or the client may need referral. Client resources, such as finances or coping ability, can also influence the setting of priorities.

4. *The urgency of the health problem:* Regardless of the framework used, life-threatening situations require that the nurse assign them high priority. For example, in Table 23.10 on page 488, although Amanda Aquilini is anxious about childcare, her *Ineffective Airway Clearance* has higher priority (see the Concept Map Box Ineffective Airway Clearance on page 487). Situations that affect the integrity of the client, that is, those that could have a negative or destructive effect on the client, also have high priority.

5. *The medical treatment plan:* The priorities for treating health problems must be congruent with treatment by other health care professionals. For example, a high priority for the client might be to become ambulatory; however, if the physician's therapeutic regimen calls for extended bed rest, then ambulation must assume a lower priority in the nursing care plan. The nurse can provide or teach exercises to facilitate ambulation later, provided the client's health permits. The nursing diagnosis related to ambulation is not ignored; it is merely deferred.

ESTABLISHING CLIENT GOALS OR DESIRED HEALTH OUTCOMES   After establishing priorities, the nurse and client set goals for each nursing diagnosis (see the Reflect on Primary Health Care box). On a care plan, the **goals** or **desired health outcomes** describe, in terms of observable client responses, what the nurse, through implementation of nursing interventions, hopes the client will achieve. The terms *goal* and *desired health outcome* are used interchangeably in this text. Some references also use the terms *expected outcome, predicted outcome, outcome criterion,* and *objective.*

Some nursing literature differentiates the terms by defining *goals* as broad statements about the client's status and *desired health outcomes* as the more specific, observable criteria used to evaluate whether the goals have been met. For example:

Goal (broad): Improve nutritional status

Desired health outcome (specific): Gain 2.5 kg by April 25

When goals are stated broadly, as in this example, the care plan must include *both* goals and desired health outcomes. They are sometimes combined into one statement linked by the words "as evidenced by," as follows: Improve nutritional status as evidenced by weight gain of 2.5 kg by April 25.

Writing the broad, general goal first can help students think of the specific outcomes that are needed, but the broad goal is just a starting point for planning.

TABLE 23.9   Assigning Priorities to Nursing Diagnoses for Amanda Aquilini

Nursing Diagnosis	Priority	Rationale
Ineffective Airway Clearance related to (a) viscous secretions secondary to deficient fluid volume, and (b) shallow chest expansion secondary to pain and fatigue	High priority	Loss of respiratory functioning is a life-threatening problem. The nurse's primary concern must be to promote Amanda's oxygenation by addressing the related factors.
Deficient Fluid Volume related to intake insufficient to replace fluid loss secondary to fever and diaphoresis	High priority	**Severe Deficient Fluid Volume** is life threatening. Although not that severe for Amanda, it is a high-priority problem because it is also a contributing factor for **Ineffective Airway Clearance**. Collaborative efforts to improve her hydration have already begun (intravenous fluids). The nurse must immediately and continuously assess and promote Amanda's hydration.
Anxiety related to (a) difficulty breathing, and (b) concerns over work and parenting roles	Medium priority	Although Amanda is concerned about work and parenting roles, these are not a threat to life. Also, treatment of her high-priority problem, **Ineffective Airway Clearance**, will relieve one of the related factors (dyspnea). Meanwhile, the nurse should provide symptomatic relief of Amanda's anxiety during periods of dyspnea because extreme anxiety could further compromise her oxygenation by causing her to breathe ineffectively and increasing the rate at which she uses oxygen.
Risk for Interrupted Family Processes related to illness and temporary unavailability of father to provide childcare	Low priority	Amanda's child is currently being cared for. If Amanda's husband returns as planned, this risk diagnosis will not develop into an actual diagnosis. No interventions are needed at present except for continued assessment and support.
Imbalanced Nutrition: Less than Body Requirements related to decreased appetite, nausea, and increased metabolism secondary to disease process	Low priority	This problem is not currently health threatening, but it could be if it were to persist. It will almost certainly resolve in a day or two as the medical problem is treated. If the medical problem does not resolve quickly, this will change to a medium priority.
Self-Care Deficit, Bathing/Hygiene related to activity intolerance secondary to ineffective airway clearance and sleep pattern disturbance	Low priority	This problem is caused by other, higher-priority problems; therefore, it will resolve as they resolve. Meanwhile, the nurse needs to assist Amanda with bathing and so on, to support and conserve her energy until she is strong enough to resume her own care.
Disturbed Sleep Pattern related to cough, pain, orthopnea, fever, and diaphoresis	Low priority	Lack of sleep is health threatening. But for the moment, the nurse does not need to address this problem. **Disturbed Sleep Pattern** does contribute to Amanda's **Ineffective Airway Clearance**, but it is not the main cause. Therefore, measures to promote sleep will be low priority at least until evening. After the nurse has attended to Amanda's oxygenation and hydration needs, this problem priority will change.
Pain (Chest) related to cough secondary to pneumonia	Not on care plan	The nurse did not write **Pain** as a problem on the care plan because **Pain** is to be addressed as the etiology of **Disturbed Sleep Pattern** and **Ineffective Airway Clearance**. The related factors to pain (cough and pneumonia) will be treated by medications (collaborative interventions). Independent nursing actions would address the problem rather than the related factors and would be the same as the nursing actions for **Ineffective Airway Clearance**.

It is the specific, observable outcomes that *must* be written on the care plan and used to evaluate client progress. Table 23.10 on page 488 shows both broad goals and desired health outcomes.

Purpose of Goals or Desired Health Outcomes   Goals or desired health outcomes serve the following purposes:

1. *They provide direction for planning nursing interventions.* Ideas for interventions come more easily if the desired

CONCEPT MAP Ineffective Airway Clearance (Gas Exchange)

AA
28-year-old female
Possible
pneumonia

→ Assess →

- Cold × 2 weeks
- Dyspnea on exertion
- Fever
- Orthopnea
- Occasional chills
- Decreased oral intake × 2 days

- T: 39.4°C P: 92 R: 28, shallow BP: 122/80
- Dry mucous membranes; skin hot, pale
- Cheeks flushed
- Decreased breath sounds
- Inspiratory crackles RUL and RLL
- Ineffective cough—small amount thick, pale pink sputum
- Lethargic, c/o being weak, fatigued

Generate nursing diagnosis

Ineffective Airway Clearance r/t viscous secretions,
& shallow chest expansion, secondary to deficient fluid volume, pain, and fatigue

Outcome

Respiratory status: Gas Exchange aeb
- Absent of pallor & cyanosis
- Use of correct breathing and coughing technique after instruction
- Productive cough
- Symmetric chest excursion

Within 48–72h

- Lungs clear to auscultation
- Respirations 12–22/min; pulse <100 bpm
- Inhales normal volume air on incentive spirometer

Nursing intervention

Respiratory Monitoring

Activity / Activity / Activity / Activity / Activity

Monitor results of blood gases, X-rays, and incentive spirometry

Auscultate breath sounds q4h

Monitor level of consciousness

Monitor rate, depth, effort of respirations, skin colour, mucous membranes, amount and colour of sputum q4h

Nursing intervention

Respiratory Monitoring

Activity / Activity / Activity / Activity / Activity / Activity

Instruct in breathing & coughing techniques. Remind and assist q3h

Administer antibiotics

Administer analgesics

Assist with postural drainage @ 0930 h

Administer expectorants

Administer O_2 per NC

---

health outcomes state clearly and specifically what the nurse plans for the client to achieve.

2. *They serve as criteria for evaluating client progress.* Although developed in the planning step of the nursing process, desired health outcomes serve as the criteria for judging nursing interventions and client progress in the evaluation step.

3. *They enable the client and nurse to determine when the problem has been resolved.*

4. *They help motivate the client and nurse by providing a sense of achievement.* As goals are met, both client and nurse can see that their efforts have been worthwhile. This provides motivation to continue following the plan.

Long-Term and Short-Term Goals   Goals may be for the short term or the long term. A short-term goal might be "Client will raise right arm to shoulder height by Friday." In the same context, a long-term goal might be "Client

REFLECT ON **PRIMARY HEALTH CARE**

While engaging in the processes of assessing, diagnosing, planning, implementing, and evaluating, the nurse includes the client or patient as a full partner in decision making. During assessment, the nurse talks with the client, observes the client and family or significant others, and analyzes the client's environment, particularly when caring for clients in their homes, workplaces, and education and leisure settings. Next, the nurse engages the client in setting health goals and identifying priority health outcomes. During the planning process, the nurse collaborates with the client in determining mutually agreeable interventions and then continues to work with the client to implement the plan of care collaboratively. Evaluation involves both the expertise of the nurse in assessing how well the client has achieved desired health outcomes and the client's self-assessment. The process will not be effective without the full *participation* of the client. The nurse must use effective communication skills in determining how to involve clients in planning for their nursing care (see Chapter 22).

will regain full use of right arm in 6 weeks." Short-term goals are useful (a) for clients who require health care for a short time and (b) for those who are frustrated by long-term goals that seem difficult to attain and who need the satisfaction of achieving a short-term goal.

In an acute care setting, much of the nurse's time is spent on the client's immediate needs, so most goals are short-term goals. However, clients in acute care settings also need long-term goals to guide planning for their discharge to long-term agencies or home care, especially in a managed care environment. Long-term goals are often used for clients who live at home and have chronic health problems and for clients in nursing homes, extended care facilities, and rehabilitation centres.

The Nursing Outcomes Classification Standardized nursing language is required if nursing data are to be included in computerized databases that are analyzed and used in nursing decisions. Researchers have developed a taxonomy, the **Nursing Outcomes Classification (NOC)**, for describing client outcomes that respond to nursing interventions.

An NOC is similar to a broadly stated *goal*. To be measured, an outcome includes a definition or label for client outcomes, a measuring scale, and indicators that apply to a client. Indicators are similar to desired health outcomes, and each outcome includes a five-point scale (a *measure*) that is used to rate the client's status on each indicator. When using the NOC taxonomy to write a desired health outcome on a care plan, the nurse writes the label for client outcome, the indicators that apply to the particular client, and the location on the measuring scale that is desired for each indicator (Moorhead, Johnson, Maas, & Swanson, 2008). For example:

> Nursing diagnosis: client diagnosed with impaired physical mobility: inability to bear weight on left leg, related to inflammation of knee joint.

Desired health outcomes would read as follows:

> Mobility Level: Transfer performance (5, completely independent)
>
> Ambulation: walking (4, independent with assistive device)

Stated in *traditional* language, that goal would be read: "Client will have improved mobility as evidenced by ability to transfer independently and walk with assistive device (walker)."

Relationship of Goals or Desired Health Outcomes to Nursing Diagnoses Goals are derived from and relate to the client's nursing diagnoses—primarily from the diagnostic label. The diagnostic label clause contains the unhealthy response; it states what should change. Therefore, the *essential* client goals are derived from the diagnostic label clause. For example, if the nursing diagnosis is *Risk for Deficient Fluid Volume* related to diarrhea and inadequate intake secondary to nausea, the *essential* goal statement might be "Maintain fluid balance as evidenced by urinary and stool output in balance with fluid intake, normal skin turgor, and moist mucous membranes."

TABLE 23.10 Deriving Desired Client Health Outcomes from Nursing Diagnoses

Nursing Diagnosis	Goals	Desired Client Outcomes
Impaired Physical Mobility: Inability to bear weight on left leg, related to inflammation of knee joint	Improved mobility Able to bear weight on left leg	Ambulate with crutches by end of the week Be able to stand without assistance by end of the month
Ineffective Airway Clearance related to poor cough effort, secondary to incision pain and fear of damaging sutures	Effective airway clearance	Lungs will be clear to auscultation during entire postoperative period No skin pallor or cyanosis by 12 hours following operation Will demonstrate good cough effort within 24 hours after surgery

For every nursing diagnosis, the nurse must write at least one desired health outcome that, when achieved, directly demonstrates resolution of the problem. When developing goals/desired outcomes, ask the following questions:

1. What is the client's problem?
2. What is the opposite, healthy response?
3. How will the client look or behave if the healthy response is achieved? (What will I be able to see, hear, measure, palpate, smell, or otherwise observe with my senses?)
4. What must the client do and how well must the client do it to demonstrate problem resolution or to demonstrate the capability of resolving the problem?

Components of Goal or Desired Health Outcome Statements
Goal or desired health outcome statements usually have the following four components:

1. *Subject.* The subject, a noun, is the client, any part of the client, or some attribute of the client, such as the client's pulse or urinary output. The subject is often omitted in goals; it is assumed that the subject is the client unless indicated otherwise.
2. *Verb.* The verb specifies an action the client is to perform, for example, what the client is to do, learn, or experience. Verbs that denote directly observable behaviours, such as *administer, demonstrate, show, walk,* must be used. See Box 23.10 for some examples.
3. *Conditions or Modifiers.* Conditions or modifiers may be added to the verb to explain the circumstances under which the behaviour is to be performed. They explain what, where, when, or how. For example:

- *Walks with the help of a walker* (how)
- Lists signs and symptoms of diabetes *after attending two group diabetes classes* (when)
- Weight will remain at existing level when *at home* (where)

BOX 23.10	EXAMPLES OF ACTION VERBS	
Apply	Explain	Share
Assemble	Help	Sit
Breathe	Identify	Sleep
Choose	Inject	State
Compare	List	Talk
Define	Move	Transfer
Demonstrate	Name	Turn
Describe	Prepare	Verbalize
Differentiate	Report	
Discuss	Select	
Drink		

- Discusses *Canada's Food Guide and recommended daily servings* (what)

Conditions need not be included if the criterion of performance clearly indicates what is expected.

4. *Criterion of desired performance.* The criterion indicates the standard by which a performance is evaluated or the level at which the client will perform the specified behaviour. These criteria may specify time or speed, accuracy, distance, and quality. To establish a time-achievement criterion, the nurse needs to ask, "How long?" To establish an accuracy criterion, the nurse asks, "How well?" Similarly, the nurse asks, "How far?" and "What is the expected standard?" to establish distance and quality criteria, respectively. Examples are as follows:

- Weighs 75 kg *by April* (time)
- Lists *five out of six* signs of diabetes (accuracy)
- Walks *one block per day* (time and distance)
- Administers insulin *using aseptic technique* (quality)

Table 23.11 on the next page lists desired outcomes that were developed for Amanda Aquilini.

Guidelines for Writing Goals or Desired Health Outcomes The following guidelines can help nurses write useful goals and desired health outcomes:

1. *Write goals and outcomes in terms of client responses, not nurse activities.* Beginning each goal statement with "the client will" can help focus it on client behaviours and responses. Avoid statements that start with *enable, facilitate, allow, let, permit,* or similar verbs followed by the word *client.* These verbs indicate what the nurse hopes to accomplish, not what the client will do.
   Correct: Client will drink 100 mL of water per hour (client behaviour).
   Incorrect: Maintain client hydration (nursing action).

2. *Be sure that desired health outcomes are realistic for the client's capabilities, limitations, and designated time span,* if it is indicated. *Limitations* refer to finances, equipment, family support, social services, physical and mental condition, and time. For example, the outcome "Measures insulin accurately" may be unrealistic for a client who has poor vision caused by cataract.

3. *Ensure that the goals and desired health outcomes are compatible with the therapies of other professionals.* For example, the outcome "Will increase the time spent out of bed by 15 minutes each day" is not compatible with a physician's prescribed therapy of bed rest.

4. *Make sure that each goal is derived from only one nursing diagnosis.* For example, the goal "The client will increase the amount of nutrients ingested and show progress in the ability to feed self" is derived from

TABLE 23.11 Desired Outcomes for Amanda Aquilini

Nursing Diagnosis*	Goal Statements/Desired Outcomes
Ineffective Airway Clearance related to viscous secretions and shallow chest expansion secondary to fluid volume deficit, pain, and fatigue	Respiratory Status: Gas exchange, as evidenced by • Absence of pallor and cyanosis (skin and mucous membranes) • Use of correct breathing/coughing technique after instruction • Productive cough • Symmetric chest excursion of at least 4 cm Within 48–72 hours: • Lungs clear to auscultation • Respirations 12–22/min, pulse less than 100 beats/min • Inhales normal volume of air on incentive spirometer
Deficient Fluid Volume: intake insufficient to replace fluid loss related to vomiting, fever, and diaphoresis	Fluid balance, as evidenced by the following: • Urine output greater than 30 mL/h • Urine specific gravity 1.005–1.025 • Good skin turgor • Moist mucous membranes • Stating the need for oral fluid intake
Anxiety related to difficulty breathing and concerns about work and parenting roles	Anxiety control, as evidenced by the following: • Listening to and following instructions for correct breathing and coughing technique, even during periods of dyspnea • Verbalizing understanding of condition, diagnostic tests, and treatments (by end of day) • Decrease in reports of fear and anxiety; none within 12 hours • Voice steady, not shaky • Respiratory rate of 12–22/min • Freely expressing concerns and possible solutions about work and parenting roles
Risk for Interrupted Family Processes related to mother's illness and temporary unavailability of father to provide childcare	Family coping, as evidenced by the following: • Report of satisfactory childcare arrangements having been made • Client and husband communicating effectively and working together to solve problems • Family members expressing feelings and providing mutual support
Imbalanced Nutrition: Less than Body Requirements related to decreased appetite, nausea, and increased metabolism secondary to disease process	Nutritional status: Nutrient intake, as evidenced by the following: • Eating at least 85% of each meal • Maintaining present weight • Verbalizing importance of adequate nutrition • Verbalizing improved appetite
Bathing/Hygiene Self-Care Deficit related to activity intolerance secondary to airway clearance and sleep pattern disturbance	Self-care: Activities of daily living, as evidenced by the following: • Ambulates to bathroom without dyspnea, fatigue, ineffective or shortness of breath • Within 24 hours, bathes with assistance in bed; within 48 hours, bathes with assistance at sink; within 72 hours, bathes in shower without dyspnea • Reports satisfaction and comfort with hygiene needs
Disturbed Sleep Pattern related to cough, pain, orthopnea, and diaphoresis	Sleep, as evidenced by the following: • Observed sleeping at night rounds • Reports feeling rested • Does not experience orthopnea

The nursing diagnoses are listed in priority order.

two nursing diagnoses: *Self-Care Deficit: Feeding* and *Imbalanced Nutrition: Less than Body Requirements.* Keeping the goal statement related to only one diagnosis facilitates evaluation of care by ensuring that planned nursing interventions are clearly related to the diagnosis.

5. *Use observable, measurable terms for outcomes.* Avoid words that are vague and require interpretation or judgment by the observer. For example, phrases such as "increase daily exercise" and "improve knowledge of nutrition" can mean different things to different people. If used in outcomes, these phrases can lead to disagreements about whether the outcome was met. These phrases may be suitable for a broad client goal but are not sufficiently clear and specific to guide the nurse when evaluating client responses.

6. *Make sure the client considers the goals or desired health outcomes important and values them.* Some outcomes, such as those for problems related to self-esteem, parenting, and communication, involve choices that are best made by the client or in collaboration with the client. Some clients may know what they want to accomplish with regard to their health problems; others may not know all the outcome possibilities. The nurse must actively listen to the client to determine personal values, goals, and desired health outcomes in relation to current health concerns. Clients are usually motivated and expend the necessary energy to reach goals they consider important.

SELECTING NURSING INTERVENTIONS AND ACTIVITIES Nursing interventions and activities are the actions that a nurse performs to achieve client goals. The specific strategies chosen should focus on eliminating or reducing the etiology, that is, the related factors of the diagnostic statement.

When it is not possible to change the related factors, the nurse chooses interventions to treat the signs and symptoms. Examples of this situation would be *Pain* related to surgical incision and *Anxiety* related to unknown etiology.

Interventions for risk nursing diagnoses should focus on measures to reduce the client's risk factors.

Correct identification of the main related factors during the diagnosing phase provides the framework for choosing successful nursing interventions. For example, the diagnostic label *Activity Intolerance* may have several related factors: pain, weakness, sedentary lifestyle, anxiety, or cardiac arrhythmias. Interventions will vary according to the cause of the problem.

Types of Nursing Interventions Nursing interventions are identified during the planning phase of the nursing process; however, they are actually performed during the implementation phase. Nursing interventions include both direct and indirect care, as well as nurse-initiated, physician-initiated, and other provider-initiated treatments. *Direct care* is an intervention performed through interaction with the client. *Indirect care* is an intervention performed away from, but on behalf of, the client, such as interdisciplinary collaboration or management of the care environment.

Independent interventions are those activities that nurses are licensed to initiate on the basis of their knowledge and skills. They include physical care, ongoing assessment, emotional support and comfort, teaching, counselling, environmental management, and making referrals to other health care professionals. In performing an autonomous activity, the nurse determines that the client requires certain nursing interventions, either carries these out or delegates them to other nursing personnel, and is accountable or answerable for the decision and the actions. An example of an independent action is planning and providing special mouth care for a client after diagnosing *Impaired Oral Mucous Membranes*.

Dependent interventions are activities carried out under the physician's orders or supervision, or according to specified routines. Physicians' orders commonly include orders for medications, intravenous therapy, diagnostic tests, treatments, diet, and activity. The nurse is responsible for explaining, assessing the need for, and administering the medical orders. Nursing interventions may be written to individualize the medical order based on the client's status. For example, for a medical order of "Progressive ambulation, as tolerated," a nurse might write the following nursing interventions:

1. Dangle for 5 min, 12 h postop.
2. Stand at bedside 24 h postop; observe for pallor, dizziness, and weakness.
3. Check pulse before and after ambulating. Do not progress if pulse >110.

Collaborative interventions are actions the nurse carries out in collaboration with other health care team members, such as physical therapists, social workers, dietitians, and physicians. Collaborative nursing activities reflect the overlapping responsibilities of, and collegial relationships among, health care personnel. For example, the physician might order physical therapy to teach the client crutch walking. The nurse would be responsible for informing the physical therapy department and for coordinating the client's care to include the physical therapy sessions. When the client returns to the nursing unit, the nurse would assist with crutch walking and collaborate with the physical therapist to evaluate the client's progress.

Considering the Consequences of Each Strategy Usually, several possible interventions can be identified for each nursing diagnosis. The nurse's task is to choose those that are most likely to achieve the desired client outcomes. The nurse begins by considering the risks and benefits of each activity. An intervention may have more than one consequence. For example, the strategy "Provide accurate information" could result in the following client behaviours:

- Increased anxiety
- Decreased anxiety
- Desire to talk with the physician
- Desire to leave the hospital
- Relaxation

Determining the consequences of each strategy requires nursing knowledge and experience. For example, the nurse's experience may suggest that providing information the night before the client's surgery may increase the client's worry and tension, whereas maintaining the usual rituals before sleep is more effective. The nurse might then consider providing information several days before surgery.

Criteria for Choosing Nursing Strategies After considering the consequences of the alternative nursing strategies, the nurse chooses one or more that are likely to be most effective. Although the nurse bases this decision on knowledge and experience, the client's input is important. (See the Evidence-Informed Practice box on what enhances the self-efficacy of first-time mothers who are breast-feeding.)

The following criteria can help the nurse choose the best nursing strategy:

- The planned action must be safe and appropriate for the individual's age, health, and condition.

- The planned action must be achievable with the resources available. For example, a home care nurse might want to include a nursing intervention for an older adult client to "Check blood glucose daily"; but, for that to occur, either the client must have intact sight, cognition, and memory to carry this out independently, or daily visits from a home care nurse must be available.

EVIDENCE-INFORMED PRACTICE

What Enhances the Self-Efficacy of First-Time Mothers Who Are Breast-Feeding?

The Canadian Paediatric Society and Health Canada advocate that mothers exclusively breast-feed their infants for the first 6 months of life. Current evidence demonstrates that about 50% of Canadian mothers are still breast-feeding at 6 months, with fewer than 20% breast-feeding exclusively. An intervention consisting of exploration of past experience, observation of others, encouragement, and physiological cues was presented. Based on initial assessments of the women, and through a randomized controlled trial (RCT) with 150 primiparous (first-time) mothers, one group received the intervention and the other group received the standardized postpartum teaching over the course of three interactions: two in hospital and one by telephone after discharge. More of the intervention group continued to breast-feed exclusively at 4 and 8 weeks, and reported higher breast-feeding self-efficacy.

NURSING IMPLICATIONS: Enhancing the first-time mother's sense of self-efficacy through patient teaching and supportive interactions postpartum, both in person and via telephone, is effective in maintaining breast-feeding in primiparous mothers. This preliminary evidence supports those interventions that focus on counselling new mothers, enhancing their sense of self-efficacy, and providing information on physiological cues that enhance breast-feeding. The importance of initially assessing the participants and providing an intervention that addressed their areas of lack of confidence or knowledge in breast-feeding was demonstrated.

Source: Based on McQueen, K.A., Dennis, C.L., Stremler, R., & Norman, C.D. (2011). A pilot randomized controlled trial of a breastfeeding self-efficacy intervention with primiparous mothers. *Journal of Obstretical, Gynecological, and Neonatal Nursing, 40*(1), 35–46.

- The planned action must be congruent with the client's values, beliefs, and culture.

- The planned action must be congruent with other therapies (e.g., if the client is not permitted food, the strategy of an evening snack must be deferred until health permits).

- It must be based on evidence from research, expert opinion, and experience.

- It must be within established standards of care as determined by government regulations and professional associations (CNA, provincial or territorial professional associations, specialty organizations, such as the Canadian Association of Neuroscience Nurses) and the policies of the agency.

WRITING AN INDIVIDUALIZED PLAN OF CARE The nurse uses the following guidelines when writing a nursing plan of care:

1. *Date and sign the plan.* The date the plan is written is essential for evaluation, review, and future planning. The nurse's signature demonstrates accountability to the client and to the nursing profession since the effectiveness of nursing actions can be evaluated.

2. *Use category headings,* such as Assessment Data, Nursing Assessment, Nursing Diagnoses, Client Goals, Desired Health Outcomes, Nursing Interventions, Selected Activities, and Evaluation. *Include a date for the evaluation of each goal.*

3. *Use accepted medical abbreviations and symbols and key words,* rather than complete sentences, to communicate your ideas. For example, write "Turn and reposition q2h," rather than "Turn and reposition the client every two hours." See Table 24.4 on page 523 for a list of commonly used medical abbreviations and Table 24.5 on page 524 for commonly used symbols.

4. *Refer to procedure books or other sources of information* rather than including all the steps on a written plan. For example, write: "See unit procedure book for tracheostomy care," or attach a standard nursing plan about such procedures as radiation-implantation care and preoperative or postoperative care.

5. *Tailor the plan to the unique characteristics of the client* by ensuring that the client's choices, such as preferences about the times of care and the methods used, are included. This reinforces the client's individuality and sense of control. For example, the written nursing intervention "Provide prune juice at breakfast, rather than orange juice" indicates that the client was given a choice of beverages.

6. *Ensure that the nursing plan incorporates preventive and health maintenance aspects as well as restorative ones.* For example, carrying out the order "provide active-assistance rom [range-of-motion] exercises to affected

limbs q2h" prevents joint contractures and maintains muscle strength and joint mobility.

7. *Ensure that the plan contains orders for ongoing assessment* of the client (e.g., "Inspect incision q8h").

8. *Include collaborative and coordination activities in the plan.* For example, the nurse may write orders to ask a nutritionist or physical therapist about specific aspects of the client's care.

9. *Include plans for the client's discharge and home care needs.* It is often necessary to consult and make arrangements with the community health nurse, social worker, and specific agencies that supply client information and needed equipment. Add teaching and discharge plans as addenda if they are lengthy and complex.

See the Sample Care Plan for Amanda Aquilini.

Sample Care Plan for Amanda Aquilini

Nursing Diagnosis: *Ineffective Airway Clearance* related to viscous secretions and shallow chest expansion secondary to deficient fluid volume, pain, and fatigue

Goals/Desired Outcomes	Nursing Interventions	Rationale
Demonstrate adequate air exchange (goal), as evidenced by the following: • Absence of pallor and cyanosis (skin and mucous membranes) • Using correct breathing/coughing technique after instruction • Productive cough • Symmetric chest expansion of at least 4 cm	Monitor respiratory status q4h: rate, depth, effort, skin colour, mucous membranes, amount and colour of sputum. Monitor results of blood gases, chest x-ray studies, and incentive spirometer volume, as available. Monitor level of consciousness. Auscultate lungs q4h. Take vital signs q4h (temperature, pulse, respiration [TPR], blood pressure [BP], pulse oximetry, pain).	*This helps identify progress toward or deviations from goal. Ineffective Airway Clearance leads to poor oxygenation, evidenced by pallor, cyanosis, lethargy, and drowsiness.* *Inadequate oxygenation causes increased pulse rate. Respiratory rate may be decreased by narcotic analgesics.*
Within 48–72 hours • Lungs clear to auscultation • Respirations 12–22/min, pulse <100 beats/min • Inhaling normal volume of air on incentive spirometer	Instruct in breathing and coughing techniques. Remind to perform, and assist q3h. Administer prescribed expectorant; schedule for maximum effectiveness. Maintain Fowler's or semi-Fowler's position. Administer prescribed analgesics. Notify physician if the pain is not relieved. Administer oxygen by nasal cannula, as prescribed. Provide portable oxygen if client goes off unit (e.g., for x-ray examination). Assist with postural drainage daily at 0930. Administer the prescribed antibiotic to maintain constant blood level. Observe for rash and gastrointestinal or other side effects.	*This enables the client to cough up secretions. The client may need encouragement and support because of fatigue and pain.* *This helps loosen secretions so they can be coughed up and expelled.* *Gravity allows for fuller lung expansion by decreasing pressure of abdomen on diaphragm.* *This controls pleuritic pain by blocking pain pathways and altering perception of pain, enabling client to increase thoracic expansion. Unrelieved pain may signal impending complication.* *Supplemental oxygen makes more oxygen available to the cells, even though less air is being moved by the client, thereby reducing the work of breathing.* *Gravity facilitates movement of secretions upward through the respiratory passage.* *This resolves infection by bacteriostatic or bactericidal effect, depending on the type of antibiotic used. A constant level is required to prevent pathogens from multiplying. Allergies to antibiotics are common.*

(continued)

Sample Care Plan for Amanda Aquilini (continued)

Nursing Diagnosis: *Deficient Fluid Volume Related to Intake Insufficient to Replace Fluid Loss*

(See standardized care plan for Deficient Fluid Volume, Figure 23.8, p. 482.)

Nursing Diagnosis: Anxiety Related to Difficulty Breathing and Concerns over Work and Parenting Roles

Goals/Desired Outcomes	Nursing Interventions	Rationale
Demonstrate decreased anxiety, as evidenced by the following:	When the client is dyspneic, stay with her; reassure her you will stay and remain calm and confident.	*Presence of a competent caregiver reduces fear of being unable to breathe.*
• Listening to and following instructions for correct breathing and coughing technique, even during periods of dyspnea	Encourage client to do slow, deep breathing.	*Focusing on breathing may help client feel in control and decrease anxiety. Control of anxiety will help the client maintain an effective breathing pattern.*
• Verbalizing understanding of condition, diagnostic tests, and treatments (by end of day)	When client is dyspneic, give brief explanations of treatments and procedures.	*Information increases client's understanding and reassurance of what to expect.*
• Decrease in reports of fear and anxiety; none within 12 hours	When the acute episode is over, give detailed information about nature of condition, treatments, and tests.	*Anxiety and pain interfere with learning. Knowing what to expect reduces anxiety.*
• Voice steady, not shaky		
• Respiratory rate of 12–22/min		
• Freely expressing concerns about work and parenting roles, but placing them in perspective in view of her illness	Encourage to express and expand on her concerns about her child and her work. Explore alternatives as needed.	*Awareness of source of anxiety enables the client to gain control over it.*
	Note whether the husband returns as scheduled. If not, institute care plan for actual *Interrupted Family Processes*.	*Husband's continued absence would constitute a defining characteristic for this nursing diagnosis.*

The Nursing Interventions Classification

The Iowa Intervention Project has developed a taxonomy of nursing interventions, referred to as the **Nursing Interventions Classification (NIC)**. The NIC provide nurses with a standardized language to describe and communicate their interventions to other nurses and providers and to compare outcomes. More than 514 interventions are grouped into 7 domains and 30 classes of interventions within the taxonomy. The 7 domains for NIC interventions include care related to the physiological (e.g. acid–base management), psychosocial (e.g., anxiety reduction), behavioural (e.g., patient education), safety (e.g., fall prevention), family (e.g., childbearing care), health system (e.g., health system management), and community (e.g., community health promotion) (Bulechek & Dochterman, 2008).

All NIC interventions are linked to NANDA nursing diagnostic labels. Based on their judgment and knowledge of the client, nurses look up a client's nursing diagnosis, choose from the list activities most appropriate for the client, and individualize them to fit the resources available in the organization.

Implementing

The nursing process is action oriented, client centred, and goal directed. Implementing is the phase in which the nurse puts the nursing care plan into action. Implementing consists of doing, delegating, and recording. After developing a plan of care based on the assessing and diagnosing phases, the nurse puts the plan into effect and evaluates the results. On the basis of this evaluation, the plan of care is either continued, modified, or terminated. The nurse concludes the implementing step by recording nursing activities and the resulting client responses. As in all phases of the nursing process, clients and support persons are encouraged to participate as much as possible.

Ongoing assessment occurs simultaneously with implementation. While implementing the nursing interventions, the nurse continues to reassess the client at every contact, gathering data about the client's responses to the nursing actions and about any new problems that may develop. For example, while bathing an older adult client, the nurse observes a reddened area on the client's sacrum or when emptying a catheter bag, the nurse measures 200 mL of strong-smelling, brown urine.

Implementing Skills

To implement the care plan successfully, nurses need good cognitive, interpersonal, and technical skills. The skills are distinct from one another; in practice, however, nurses use them in various combinations and with different emphasis depending on the activity. For instance, when inserting a urinary catheter, the nurse needs cognitive knowledge of the principles and steps of the procedure, technical skill in draping the client and manipulating the equipment, and interpersonal skills to inform and reassure the client.

The **cognitive skills** (intellectual skills) include problem solving, decision making, critical thinking, and creative thinking (see Chapter 21). They are crucial to safe, intelligent nursing care.

Interpersonal skills are necessary for all nursing activities: caring, comforting, referring, counselling, and supporting are just a few. The skills include conveying knowledge, attitudes, feelings, interest, and appreciation of the client's cultural values and lifestyle. Before nurses can be highly skilled in interpersonal relations, they must have self-awareness and sensitivity to others. (See Chapters 22 and 45.)

Technical skills are hands-on skills, such as manipulating equipment, giving injections, and bandaging, moving, lifting, and repositioning clients. These activities are also called *procedures* or *psychomotor skills*. The term *psychomotor* includes the interpersonal component, for example, the need to communicate with the client.

Technical skills require knowledge and, frequently, manual dexterity. The number of technical skills expected of a nurse has greatly increased in recent years because of the increased use of technology, especially in acute care hospitals.

Process of Implementing

The process of implementing (Figure 23.9) normally includes the following:

- Reassessing the client
- Determining the nurse's need for assistance
- Implementing the nursing interventions
- Delegating and supervising
- Communicating the nursing actions

REASSESSING THE CLIENT Just before implementing an order, the nurse must reassess the client to make sure the intervention is still needed. Even though an order is written on the care plan, the client's condition may have changed. For example, Amanda Aquilini had a nursing diagnosis of *Disturbed Sleep Pattern* related to cough, pain, orthopnea (trouble breathing when lying down), fever, and diaphoresis (sweating). During rounds, the nurse discovers that Amanda is sleeping and, therefore, defers the cooling back rub that had been planned as an intervention.

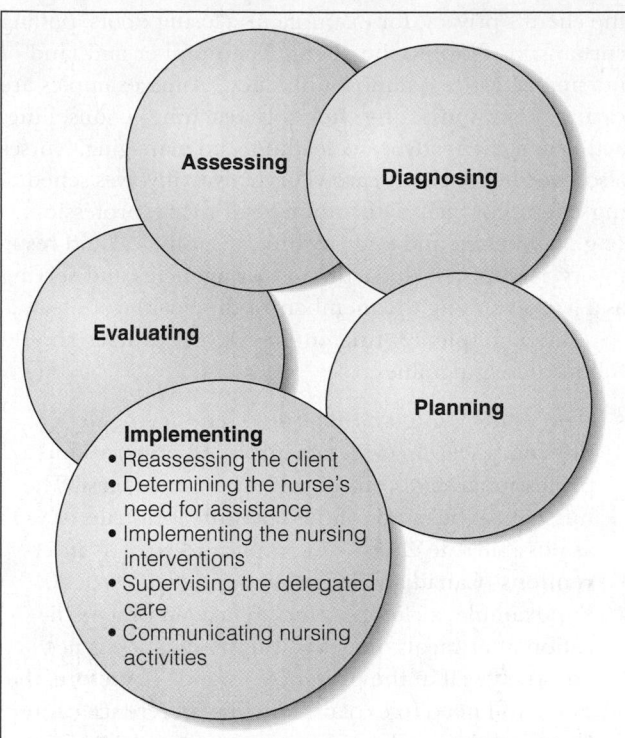

FIGURE 23.9 Implementing: The fourth phase of the nursing process, in which the nurse implements the nursing interventions and documents the care provided.

New data may indicate a need to change the priorities of care or the nursing strategies. For example, a nurse begins to teach Ms. Eves, who has diabetes, how to give herself insulin injections. Shortly after beginning the teaching, the nurse realizes that Ms. Eves is not concentrating on the lesson. Subsequent discussion reveals that she is worried about her eyesight and fears she is going blind. Realizing that the client's level of stress is interfering with her learning, the nurse ends the lesson and makes arrangements for the nurse practitioner from the diabetes clinic to meet with her. The nurse also provides supportive communication to help alleviate the client's stress.

DETERMINING THE NURSE'S NEED FOR ASSISTANCE When implementing some nursing strategies, the nurse may require assistance for one of the following reasons:

- The nurse is unable to safely implement the nursing strategies alone (e.g., turning a heavy client in bed).
- Assistance would reduce stress on the client (e.g., turning a person who experiences acute pain when moved).
- The nurse lacks the knowledge or skills to implement a particular nursing activity (e.g., a nurse who is not familiar with a particular model of oxygen mask).

IMPLEMENTING NURSING INTERVENTIONS It is important to explain to the client what will be done, what sensations to expect, and what the client is expected to do. For many nursing actions, it is also important to ensure the client's privacy, for example, by closing doors, pulling curtains, or draping the client. The number and kind of nursing activities is almost unlimited. Some examples are caring, communicating, helping, teaching, counselling, acting as a client advocate, leading, and managing. Nurses also coordinate client care. This activity involves scheduling client contacts with other health care professionals (e.g., laboratory and x-ray technicians, physical and respiratory therapists), departments, or agencies and serving as a liaison among the members of the health care team.

When implementing interventions, nurses should follow these guidelines:

- Base nursing interventions on scientific knowledge, nursing research, evidence-informed practice, and professional standards of care when these exist. The nurse must be aware of the scientific rationale, as well as possible side effects or complications, of all interventions (Canadian Nurses Association [CNA], 2010). For example, a client prefers to take an oral medication after meals; however, this medication is not absorbed well in the presence of food. Therefore, the nurse will need to explain why this preference cannot be accommodated.

- Clearly understand the interventions to be implemented and question any that are not understood. The nurse is responsible for intelligent implementation of medical and nursing plans of care. This requires knowledge of each intervention, its purpose in the client's plan of care, any contraindications (e.g., allergies), and changes in the client's condition that may affect the order.

- Adapt activities to the individual client. A client's beliefs, values, age, health status, and environment are factors that can affect the success of a nursing action. For example, the nurse determines that a client chokes when swallowing pills and so consults with the physician to change the order to a liquid form of the medication; or the nurse recognizes that many Asian persons prefer to drink hot water rather than ice water and, after confirming it with a specific client, supplies this at the bedside.

- Implement safe care. For example, when changing a sterile dressing, the nurse practises sterile technique to prevent infection; when giving a medication, the nurse administers the correct dosage by the ordered route.

- Provide teaching, support, and comfort. See Chapter 26. The nurse should always explain the purpose of interventions, what the client will experience, and how the client can participate. The client must have sufficient knowledge to agree to the plan of care and to be able to assume responsibility for as much self-care as possible. These independent nursing activities enhance the effectiveness of nursing care plans (see Figure 23.10).

- Use a holistic approach. The nurse must always view the client as a whole and consider the client's responses in

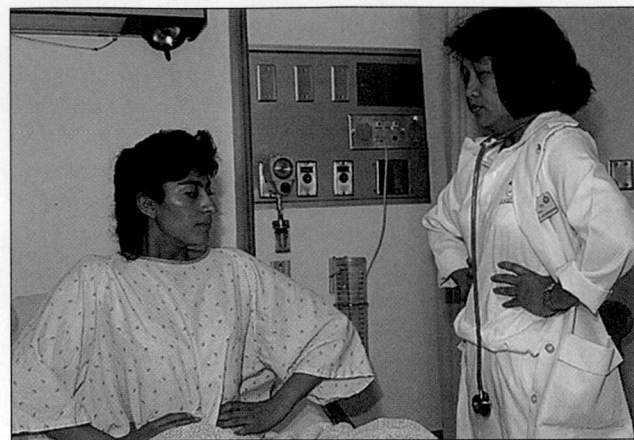

FIGURE 23.10 Amanda agrees to practise deep-breathing exercises q3h during the day. In addition, she verbalizes awareness of the need to increase her fluid intake.

that context. For example, whenever possible, the nurse honours the client's expressed preference that interventions be planned for times that fit with the client's usual schedule of visitors, work, sleep, or eating.

- Respect the dignity of the client and enhance the client's self-esteem. Providing privacy and encouraging clients to make their own decisions are ways of respecting dignity and enhancing self-esteem.

- Encourage clients to participate actively in implementing the nursing interventions. Active participation enhances the client's sense of independence and control. However, clients vary in the degree of participation they desire. Some want total involvement in their care, whereas others prefer little involvement. The amount of desired involvement may be related to the severity of the illness; the client's culture; or the client's fear, understanding of the illness, and understanding of the intervention.

SUPERVISING DELEGATED CARE While developing and writing nursing interventions on the client's care plan, the nurse must also determine who should actually perform the activity. The ability to delegate client care and assign tasks is a vital skill for registered nurses (RNs) and registered nursing assistants (RPNs) because many health care agencies have assistive personnel to perform tasks previously done only by these nurses. To delegate appropriately, the nurse must match the needs of the client and family with the skills, knowledge, and scope of practice of the available caregivers. This requires knowing the background, experience, knowledge, skills, and strengths of each person and understanding which tasks are within their legal scope of practice.

Canadian RNs provide leadership while caring for clients requiring complex care, they collaborate with other professionals to set standards of client care while ensuring quality client care. Unregulated health care providers are increasingly evident in Canadian health care settings. RNs are involved in making key decisions that determine the initial and ongoing use of unregulated health care providers. Unregulated health care provider standards vary, as they are identified by individual health care agencies across the provinces and territories (CNA, 2003).

COMMUNICATING THE NURSING ACTIONS After carrying out the nursing interventions, the nurse completes the implementing phase by reporting and recording the nursing activities and client responses in the client record in a timely fashion. When a client's health is changing rapidly, the charge nurse and/or the primary care provider may want to be kept up to date with verbal reports. Nurses also report client status at a change of shift and on a client's discharge to another unit or health care agency in person, via a voice recording, or in writing. For information on documenting and reporting, see Chapter 24.

Evaluating

To evaluate is to judge or to appraise. Evaluating is the last phase of the nursing process. In this context, **evaluation** is a planned, ongoing, purposeful activity in which clients and health care professionals determine (a) the client's progress toward goal achievement and (b) the effectiveness of the nursing care plan. Evaluation is an important aspect of the nursing process because conclusions drawn from the evaluation determine whether the nursing interventions should be terminated, continued, or changed.

Evaluation completed immediately after implementing a nursing action enables the nurse to make on-the-spot modifications in an intervention. Evaluation performed at specified intervals (e.g., once a week for the home care client) shows the extent of progress toward goal achievement and enables the nurse to correct any deficiencies and modify the care plan as needed. Evaluation performed at discharge allows the nurse to measure the degree of goal achievement and the client's self-care abilities with regard to follow-up care. Most agencies have a special discharge record for the terminal evaluation. Through evaluating, nurses accept responsibility for their actions, indicate interest in the results of the nursing actions, and demonstrate a desire not to perpetuate ineffective actions but to adopt more effective ones.

Relationship of Evaluating to Other Nursing Process Phases

Successful evaluation depends on the effectiveness of the steps that precede it. Assessment data must be accurate and complete so that the nurse can formulate appropriate nursing diagnoses and desired health outcomes. The desired health outcomes must be stated concretely in behavioural terms if they are to be useful for evaluating client responses. Without the implementing phase in which the plan is put into action, there would be nothing to evaluate.

The evaluating and assessing phases overlap. As previously stated, assessment (data collection) is ongoing and continuous at every client contact. However, data are collected for different purposes at different points in the nursing process. During the assessing phase, the nurse collects data for the purpose of making diagnoses. During the evaluating step, the nurse collects data for the purpose of comparing them with preselected goals and judging the effectiveness of the nursing care. The *act* of assessing (data collection) is the same; the differences lie in (a) when the data are collected and (b) how the data are used.

Process of Evaluating Client Responses

In the planning step, the nurse identifies the desired outcomes (indicators) that will be used to measure (evaluate) client goal achievement. Desired outcomes serve two purposes: (a) They establish the kind of evaluative data that need to be collected; and (b) they provide a standard against which the data are evaluated.

The evaluation process (see Figure 23.11) has five components:

1. Collecting data related to the desired client health outcomes
2. Comparing the data with the desired health outcomes
3. Relating nursing actions to client goals and desired health outcomes
4. Drawing conclusions about problem status
5. Continuing, modifying, or terminating the client's care plan

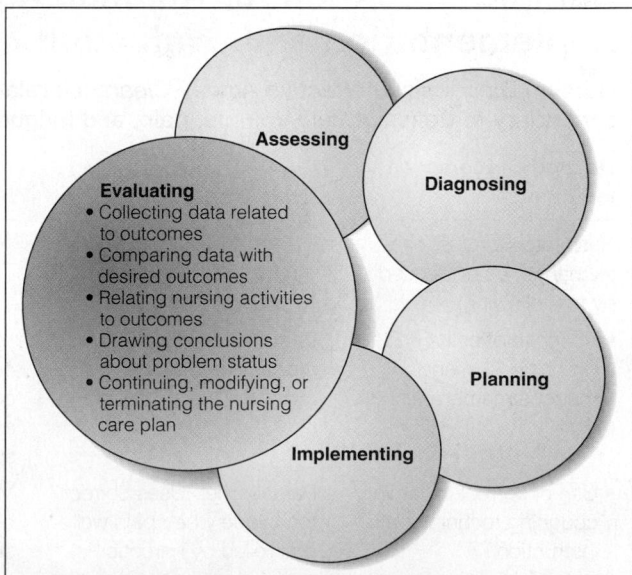

FIGURE 23.11 Evaluating: The final phase of the nursing process, in which the nurse and the client determine the client's progress toward goal achievement and the effectiveness of the plan of care. The plan may be continued, modified, or terminated.

COLLECTING DATA Using the clearly stated, precise, and measurable desired health outcomes as a guide, the nurse collects data so that conclusions can be drawn about whether goals have been met. It is usually necessary to collect both objective and subjective data.

Some data may require interpretation. Examples of objective data requiring interpretation are the degree of tissue turgor of a dehydrated client or the degree of restlessness of a client with pain. When objective data need interpretation and the nurse has not worked with the client recently, the nurse may obtain the views of other nurses to substantiate whether change has occurred. Examples of subjective data needing interpretation include complaints of nausea or pain by the client. When interpreting subjective data, the nurse must rely on either (a) the client's statements (e.g., "My pain is worse now than it was after breakfast") or (b) objective indicators of the subjective data, even though these indicators may require further interpretation (e.g., decreased restlessness, decreased pulse and respiratory rates, and relaxed facial muscles as indicators of pain relief). Data must be recorded concisely and accurately to facilitate the next part of the evaluation process.

COMPARING DATA WITH OUTCOMES If the first two parts of the evaluation process have been carried out effectively, it is relatively simple to determine whether a desired health outcome has been met. Both the nurse and the client play an active role in comparing the client's actual responses with the desired health outcomes. Did the client drink 3000 mL of fluid in 24 hours? Did the client walk unassisted the specified distance per day? When determining whether a goal has been achieved, the nurse can draw one of three possible conclusions:

1. The goal was met; that is, the client response is the same as the desired health outcome.

2. The goal was partially met; that is, either a short-term goal was achieved but the long-term goal was not, or the desired health outcome was only partially attained.

3. The goal was not met.

After determining whether a goal has been met, the nurse writes an evaluative statement (either on the care plan or in the nurse's notes). An **evaluative statement** consists of two parts: (a) a conclusion and (b) supporting data. The conclusion is a statement that the goal or desired health outcome was met, partially met, or not met. The supporting data are the list of client responses that support the conclusion, for example:

> Goal Met: Oral intake 300 mL more than output; skin turgor good; mucous membranes moist.

If the goal has not been met, alterations in interventions are necessary and more time is needed for achievement of the goal. See the Sample Care Plan: Modified Following Implementation and Evaluation for evaluative statements for Amanda Aquilini. Data in this table represent Ms. Aquilini's responses to care as observed by the night nurse on the morning after her admission to the unit. In practice, care plans usually do not have a column for evaluative statements; rather, evaluative statements are recorded in the nurses' notes.

Sample Care Plan for Amanda Aquilini: Modified Following Implementation and Evaluation

Nursing Diagnosis: *Ineffective Airway Clearance* related to viscous secretions and shallow chest expansion; secondary to deficient fluid volume, pain, and fatigue

Desired Outcomes/ Indicators	Evaluation Statements	Nursing Interventions*	Explanation for Continuing or Modifying Nursing Interventions
Respiratory status: gas exchange, as evidenced by the following:			
• Absence of pallor and cyanosis (skin and mucous membranes)	Partially met. Skin and mucous membranes not cyanotic, but still pale	Monitor respiratory status q4h; rate, depth, effort, skin color, mucous membranes, and amount and colour of sputum.	*Retain nursing interventions to continue to identify progress. Goal status indicates problem has not been resolved.*
• Use of correct breathing/ coughing technique after instruction	Partially met. Uses correct technique when pain well controlled by narcotic analgesics	Monitor the results of blood gases, chest x-ray studies, pulse oximetry, and incentive spirometer volume, as available.	
• Productive cough	Met. Cough productive of moderate amounts of thick, yellow, pink-tinged sputum	Monitor level of consciousness.	

(continued)

Sample Care Plan for Amanda Aquilini (continued)

Nursing Diagnosis: *Ineffective Airway Clearance* related to viscous secretions and shallow chest expansion; secondary to deficient fluid volume, pain, and fatigue

Desired Outcomes/ Indicators	Evaluation Statements	Nursing Interventions*	Explanation for Continuing or Modifying Nursing Interventions
• Symmetric chest excursion of at least 4 cm	Not met. Chest excursion = 3 cm	Auscultate lungs q4h.	
• Lungs clear to auscultation within 48–72 h	Not met. Scattered inspiratory crackles auscultated throughout right anterior and posterior chest	Monitor vital signs q4h (TPR, BP, pulse oximetry, pain).	*Client does not need to be reinstructed as she demonstrates correct techniques; she may still need support and encouragement because of fatigue and pain of breathing.*
• Respirations 12–22/ min, pulse, less than 100 beats/min	Partially met. Respirations 26/min, pulse 96	Instruct the client in breathing and coughing techniques. Remind her to perform the task, and assist q3h. *Support and encourage. (11/04/17, JW)*	
• Inhaling normal volume of air on incentive spirometer	Not met. Tidal volume only 350 mL *(Evaluated 11/04/17, JW)*	Administer prescribed expectorant; schedule for maximum effectiveness. Have the client maintain Fowler's or semi-Fowler's position. Administer prescribed analgesics. Notify the primary care provider if the pain not relieved. Administer oxygen via nasal cannula, as prescribed. Provide portable oxygen if the client goes off the unit (e.g., for x-ray examination). Assist with postural drainage daily at 0930 h. *On 4/17, teach to continue prn at home. (11/04/17, JW)* Administer prescribed antibiotic to maintain con- stant blood level. Observe for rash and gastrointestinal or other side effects.	*As soon as client is hydrated and fever is controlled, she will probably be discharged to self-care at home.*
Anxiety control, as evidenced by the following:			
• Listening to and following instructions for correct breathing and coughing technique, even during periods of dyspnea	Met. Performed coughing techniques as instructed during periods of dyspnea	When the client is dyspneic, stay with her; reassure her that you will remain with her. Remain calm, and appear confident.	
• Verbalizing understanding of condition, diagnostic tests, and treatments (by end of day)	Met. See nurse's notes for 3–11 shift. Client stated, "I know I need to try to breathe deeply even when it hurts." Demonstrated correct use of incentive spirometer and stated understanding of the need to use it. Understands IV is for hydration and antibiotics *(Evaluated 11/04/17, JW)*	Encourage slow, deep breathing. When the client is dyspneic, give brief explanations of treatments and procedures.	

(continued)

Sample Care Plan for Amanda Aquilini (continued)

Nursing Diagnosis: *Ineffective Airway Clearance* related to viscous secretions and shallow chest expansion; secondary to deficient fluid volume, pain, and fatigue

Desired Outcomes/ Indicators	Evaluation Statements	Nursing Interventions*	Explanation for Continuing or Modifying Nursing Interventions
• Decrease in reports of fear and anxiety	Met. Stated, "I know I can get enough air, but it still hurts to breathe."		
• Voice steady, not shaky	Met. Speaks in steady voice		
• Respiratory rate of 12–22 min	Not met. Rate 26–36/min	~~When acute episode is over, give detailed information about nature of condition, treatments, and tests.~~ *Reassess whether client needs any information on condition, treatments, or tests. (11/04/17, JW)*	*Detailed information has been given. Because client shows understanding, there is no need to repeat the information.*
• Freely expresses concerns and possible solutions about work and parenting roles	Partially met. Discussed only briefly on 3–11 shift. Not done on 11–7 shift because of client's need to rest. *(Evaluated 11/04/17, JW)*	Depending on the client's tolerance level, encourage her to express and expand on her concerns about her child and her work. Explore alternatives, as needed. Note whether the husband returns as scheduled. If he does not, institute care plan for actual *Interrupted Family Process. (Do on 4/17, day shift) (11/04/17, JW)*	*It is important that this assessment be made right away, so childcare can be arranged, if needed.*

*In this care plan, a line has been drawn through portions the nurse wished to delete; additions to the care plan are shown in italics.

RELATING NURSING ACTIONS TO CLIENT GOALS OR OUTCOMES The third aspect of the evaluating process is determining the relationship of the nursing actions to the outcomes. One should never assume that a nursing action was the only factor in meeting or not meeting a goal; clients' response must be considered.

For example, Mrs. Sophi Ringdale was obese and needed to lose 14 kg. When the nurse and client drew up a care plan, one goal was "Lose 1.4 kg in 4 weeks." A nursing strategy in the care plan was "Explain how to plan and prepare a 1000-calorie diet." Four weeks later, the client weighed herself and had lost 1.8 kg. The goal had been met—in fact, exceeded. It is easy to assume that the nursing strategy was highly effective. However, it is important to collect more data before drawing that conclusion. On questioning the client, the nurse might find any of the following: (a) the client planned a 1000-calorie diet and prepared and ate the food; (b) the client planned a 1000-calorie diet but did not prepare the correct food; (c) the client did not understand how to plan a 1000-calorie diet, so she did not bother with it.

If the first possibility is found to be true, the nurse can safely conclude that the nursing strategy "Explain how to plan and prepare a 1000-calorie diet" was effective in helping the client gain knowledge and lose weight.

However, if the nurse learns that either the second or third possibility actually happened, then it must be assumed that the nursing strategy did not affect the outcome. The next step for the nurse is to collect data about what the client actually did to lose weight. It is important to establish the relationship (or lack thereof) of the nursing actions to the client responses.

DRAWING CONCLUSIONS ABOUT THE PROBLEM'S STATUS The nurse judges if goals are achieved by determining whether the care plan was effective in resolving, reducing, or preventing client problems. When goals have been met, the nurse can draw one of the following conclusions about the status of the client's problem:

• The actual problem stated in the nursing diagnosis has been resolved; or the potential nursing problem is being prevented and the risk factors no longer exist. In these instances, the nurse documents that the goals have been met and discontinues the care for the problem.

• The potential problem stated in the nursing diagnosis is being prevented, but the risk factors are still present. In this case, the nurse keeps the problem on the care plan.

• The actual problem still exists even though some goals are being met. For example, a desired health outcome on a client's care plan is "Will ingest 3000 mL of fluid daily." Even though the data may show this outcome has been achieved, other data (dry oral mucous membranes) may indicate that the client still has a *Deficient Fluid Volume*. Therefore, the nursing interventions must be continued, even though this one goal was met.

When goals have been partially met, or when goals have not been met, one of two conclusions can be drawn:

1. The care plan may need to be revised since the problem is only partially resolved. The revisions may need to occur during assessing, diagnosing, or planning phases, as well as implementing.

2. The care plan does not need revision because the client merely needs more time to achieve the previously established goals. To make this decision, the nurse must assess why the goals are being only partially achieved, including whether the evaluation was conducted too soon. (See Figure 23.12.)

CONTINUING, MODIFYING, OR TERMINATING THE NURSING CARE PLAN After drawing conclusions about the status of the client's problems, the nurse modifies the care plan by indicating "discontinued," "goal met," or "problem resolved" and the date, per agency policy. Whether or not goals were met, a number of decisions must be made about continuing, modifying, or terminating nursing care for each problem. Before making individual modifications, the nurse must first determine why the plan as a whole was not completely effective. This requires a review of the entire care plan and a critique of the nursing process steps involved in its development. See Table 23.12 on the next page for a checklist to use when reviewing a care plan.

Assessing An incomplete or incorrect database influences all subsequent steps of the nursing process and care plan. If data are incomplete, the nurse needs to reassess the client and record the new data. In some instances, new data may indicate the need for new nursing diagnoses, new goals, and new nursing interventions.

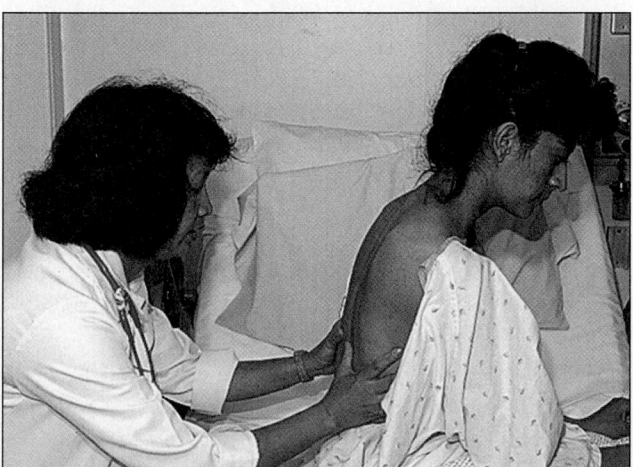

FIGURE 23.12 Upon assessment of respiratory excursion, Mary detects failure of the client to achieve maximum ventilation. Mary and Amanda re-evaluate the care plan and modify it to increase coughing and deep-breathing exercises to q2h.

Diagnosing If the database is incomplete, new diagnostic statements may be required. If the database is complete, the nurse needs to analyze whether the problems were identified correctly and whether the nursing diagnoses are relevant to that database. After making judgments about the problem's status, the nurse revises or adds new diagnoses as needed to reflect the most recent client data.

Planning: Desired Health Outcomes If a nursing diagnosis is inaccurate, the goal statement will need revision. If the nursing diagnosis is appropriate, the nurse then checks that the goals are realistic and attainable. Unrealistic goals require correction. The nurse should also determine whether priorities have changed and whether the client still agrees with the priorities. Goals must also be written for any new nursing diagnoses.

Planning: Nursing Interventions The nurse investigates whether the nursing strategies were related to goal achievement and whether the best nursing strategies were selected. Even when diagnoses and goals are appropriate, the nursing strategies selected may not have been the best ones to achieve the goal. New nursing interventions may reflect changes in the amount of nursing care the client needs, scheduling changes, or rearrangement of nursing activities to group similar activities or to permit longer rest or activity periods for the client. If new nursing diagnoses have been written, then new nursing interventions will also be necessary.

Implementing Even if all sections of the care plan appear to be satisfactory, the manner in which the plan was implemented may have interfered with goal achievement. Before selecting new interventions, the nurse should check whether they were carried out. Other personnel may not have carried them out, either because the orders were unclear or because they were unreasonable in terms of external constraints, such as money, staff, time, and equipment.

After making the necessary modifications to the care plan, the nurse implements the modified plan and begins the nursing process cycle again. Refer to Nursing Care Plan for Amanda Aquilini: Modified Following Implementation and Evaluation on page 498 to see how the plan for Amanda Aquilini was modified after evaluation of goal achievement and review of the nursing process. Additions to the care plan are shown in italics.

Evaluating the Quality of Nursing Care In addition to evaluating goal achievement for individual clients, nurses are also involved in evaluating and modifying the overall quality of care given to groups of clients. This is an essential part of professional accountability.

Quality Assurance A quality assurance (QA) program is an ongoing, systematic process designed to evaluate and promote excellence in the health care provided to clients. **Quality assurance** frequently refers to evaluation of the level of care provided in a health care agency, it may

TABLE 23.12 Evaluation Checklist

Assessing	Diagnosing	Planning	Implementing
_____ Are the data complete, accurate, and validated? _____ Do the new data require changes in the care plan?	_____ Are the nursing diagnoses relevant and accurate? _____ Are the nursing diagnoses supported by the data? _____ Has the problem status changed (i.e., potential, actual, risk)? _____ Are the diagnoses stated clearly and in the correct format? _____Have any nursing diagnoses been resolved?	*Desired Health Outcomes* _____ Do the new nursing diagnoses require new goals? _____ Are the goals realistic? _____ Was enough time allowed for goal achievement? _____ Do the goals address all aspects of the problem? _____ Does the client still concur with the goals? _____ Have client priorities changed? *Nursing Interventions* _____Do the nursing interventions need to be written for new nursing diagnoses or new goals? _____ Are the nursing interventions related to the stated goals? _____ Is there a rationale to justify each nursing intervention? _____ Are the nursing interventions clear, specific, and detailed? _____ Are the new resources available? _____ Do the nursing interventions address all aspects of the client's goals? _____ Were all nursing interventions clearly effective?	_____ Was client input obtained at each step of the nursing process? _____ Were the goals and nursing interventions acceptable to the client? _____ Did the caregivers have the knowledge and skill to perform the interventions correctly? _____ Were explanations given to the client prior to implementing?

also include the evaluation of care provided on one nursing unit in an agency, within a health region, or even in a province or territory.

Quality assurance requires evaluation of three components of care: (a) structure, (b) process, and (c) outcome. Each type of evaluation requires different criteria and methods, and each has a different focus.

Structure evaluation focuses on the setting in which care is given. It answers the question, what effect does the setting have on the quality of care? Structural standards describe desirable environmental and organizational characteristics that influence care, such as equipment and staffing.

Process evaluation focuses on how the care was given. It answers such questions as these: Is the care relevant to the client's needs? Is the care appropriate, complete, and timely? Process standards focus on the manner in which the nurse uses the nursing process and meets care standards. Some examples of process criteria are "Checks

client's identification band before giving medication" and "Performs and records chest assessment, including auscultation, once per shift."

Outcome evaluation focuses on demonstrable changes in the client's health status as a result of nursing care. Outcome criteria are written in terms of client responses or health states, just as they are for evaluation within the nursing process. For example, "How many clients develop pneumonia after undergoing hip repair?" or "How many clients who have a colostomy experience an infection that delays discharge?"

Quality Improvement In Canada, the Canadian Council on Health Services Accreditation (CCHSA), Canadian Patient Safety Institute, and nurse educators, practitioners, and researchers promote quality health care, identifying and measuring nursing-sensitive desired health outcomes and exploring various factors that affect client safety and best practices (Armstrong, Laschinger, &

Wong, 2009; Kingston-Riechers, Ospina, Jonsson, Childs, McLeod, & Maxted, 2010). Governments also play a role by requiring health care organizations to provide excellent care and to increase public awareness of their rights to safe and quality care. An example can be seen in the passing of the Excellence Care for All Act, 2010 in Ontario (Ontario Ministry of Health and Long-Term Care, 2011).

Unlike quality assurance, **quality improvement (QI)** follows client care rather than organizational structure, focuses on process rather than individuals, and uses a systematic approach with the intention of improving the quality of care rather than *ensuring* the quality of care. QI studies focus on identifying and correcting a system's problems, such as duplication of services in a hospital. QI is also known as continuous quality improvement (CQI), total quality management (TQM), performance improvement (PI), or persistent quality improvement (PQI).

Nursing Audit   An **audit** involves the examination or review of records. A **retrospective audit** is the evaluation of a client's record after discharge from an agency. *Retrospective* means "relating to past events." A **concurrent audit** is the evaluation of a client"s health care while the client is still receiving care from the agency. These evaluations use interviewing, direct observation of nursing care, and review of clinical records to determine whether specific evaluative criteria have been met.

Another type of evaluation of care is the *peer review*. In nurse **peer review**, nurses functioning in the same capacity (that is, peers) appraise the quality of care or practice performed by other equally qualified nurses. The peer review is based on established standards or criteria and come in two

types: (a) individual peer review and (b) nursing audits. The *individual peer review* focuses on the performance of an individual nurse and is intended to support professional growth. The nursing regulatory bodies promote and require peer evaluation as a means of supporting continuing professional competence. The *nursing audit* focuses on evaluating nursing care through the review of records. The success of these audits depends on accurate documentation.

Nursing Process Summarized

The nursing process is foundational to nursing practice. Its basic structure can be modified for the split-second decision making sometimes necessary in critical care environments or the complex, long-range planning and evaluation necessary for community health-promotion programs. It is characterized as being the following:

- Open and flexible to meet the unique needs of clients, families, communities, and whole populations
- Cyclical and dynamic, with a built-in plan for evaluation, reassessment, and modification
- Client centred and individualized
- Interpersonal and collaborative as a process and as a means of communication
- Planned and goal directed
- Creative
- Universally applicable

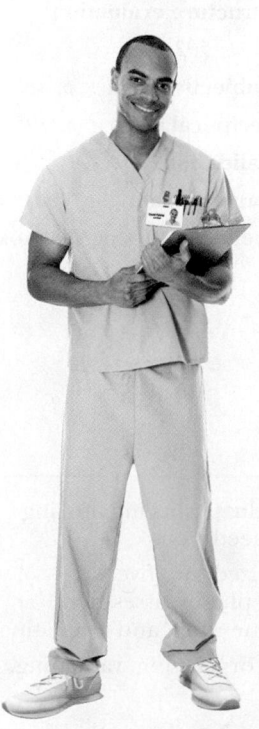

Case Study 23

Ms. Sharon Noble is a 55-year-old woman who lives with her partner, Marielle, in a condominium they own in Barrie, Ontario. They have no children but they do have a close network of friends. Sharon has a business degree and is a self-employed proprietor of Novel-Novels Book Shoppe. She is an agnostic. Her medical care in hospital is covered by the Ontario Health Insurance Plan (OHIP). She arrives at the hospital alone.

1. Presenting symptoms: Chest pain and shortness of breath × 3 hours.
2. Vital signs: Temperature: 36.4°C; pulse: 140/min; respiration: 28/min at rest. BP: 150/97 mm Hg, Cloxacillin allergy.
3. Assessment: Visibly short of breath (SOB) at rest, skin cold and clammy, capillary oxygen level is low in blood (saturation 90%) on room air. *Chest Auscultation:* Air entry throughout with medium coarse wet crackles mid- to lower lobes. Apical heart rate very rapid. O_2 via 5 L nasal prongs commenced. IV of normal saline at 20 mL/h initiated by RN. She reports a Cloxacillin allergy.
4. Client statement: "I have a heaviness that won't let up in the middle of my chest. I feel as if I could be sick to my stomach." Chest pain started after Sharon unloaded five heavy boxes of books sent from a publisher. She thought that once she stopped working, it would go away but the intensity of the pressure kept mounting and has lasted 3 hours. She rates her pain (heaviness) as 8/10 using the numeric rating scale.
5. Client concerns: Sharon is very worried about her own health. In addition, she is worried about Marielle. Marielle just had cataract surgery, and Sharon has been looking after her, instilling the eye drops, shopping, and preparing foods.

(continued)

CRITICAL THINKING QUESTIONS

1. What questions run through your mind when analyzing Sharon's subjective data?
2. What questions run through your mind when analyzing Sharon's objective data?
3. Considering the above symptoms, explain why Sharon's current condition is a medical emergency.
4. What are your nursing priorities when assessing and caring for Sharon?

Check the eText in MyNursingLab for answers and explanations.

KEY TERMS

actual nursing diagnosis *p. 473*

assessing *p. 458*

audit *p. 503*

client health outcomes *p. 472*

closed questions *p. 463*

cognitive skills *p. 495*

collaborative care plans *p. 483*

collaborative interventions *p. 491*

concept map *p. 483*

concurrent audit *p. 503*

constant data *p. 460*

critical pathways *p. 483*

cues *p. 471*

database *p. 459*

data collection *p. 459*

defining characteristics *p. 473*

dependent functions *p. 474*

dependent interventions *p. 491*

desired health outcomes *p. 485*

diagnostic labels *p. 472*

directive interview *p. 463*

discharge planning *p. 481*

etiology *p. 472*

evaluation *p. 497*

evaluative statement *p. 498*

focused assessment *p. 468*

formal care plan *p. 481*

goals *p. 485*

independent functions *p. 474*

independent interventions *p. 491*

individualized care plans *p. 481*

inferences *p. 471*

informal care plan *p. 481*

interpersonal skills *p. 495*

interview *p. 463*

leading question *p. 464*

medical diagnoses *p. 474*

multidisciplinary care plan *p. 483*

neutral question *p. 464*

nondirective interview *p. 463*

norm *p. 474*

nursing diagnosis *p. 473*

Nursing Interventions Classification (NIC) *p. 494*

Nursing Outcomes Classification (NOC) *p. 488*

nursing process *p. 455*

objective data *p. 460*

open-ended questions *p. 463*

outcome evaluation *p. 502*

peer review *p. 503*

policies *p. 482*

possible nursing diagnosis *p. 473*

priority setting *p. 483*

procedures *p. 482*

process evaluation *p. 502*

protocols *p. 482*

qualifiers *p. 473*

quality assurance *p. 501*

quality improvement (QI) *p. 503*

rapport *p. 463*

rationale *p. 483*

related factors *p. 473*

retrospective audit *p. 503*

risk factors *p. 473*

risk nursing diagnosis *p. 473*

screening examination *p. 468*

standard *p. 474*

standardized care plans *p. 481*

standing order *p. 482*

structure evaluation *p. 502*

subjective data *p. 460*

technical skills *p. 495*

validation *p. 471*

variable data *p. 460*

wellness nursing diagnosis *p. 473*

CHAPTER HIGHLIGHTS

- The nursing process is a systematic, client-centred method for structuring the delivery of nursing care. At every stage of the process, the nurse works closely with the client to tailor care and build a relationship of mutual regard and trust.

- The goals of the nursing process are to identify a client's actual or potential health care needs and strengths, to establish plans to meet the identified

needs, and to deliver and evaluate specific nursing interventions to meet those needs.

- The nursing process is organized into five interrelated, interdependent phases: assessing, diagnosing, planning, implementing, and evaluating.

- Assessing involves collecting, organizing, validating, and documenting data.

- Assessment involves mutual participation by client and nurse in obtaining subjective and objective data about the client's health status and assessing the socioenvironmental determinants of health affecting individual, family, group, and community clients.

- The client is the primary source of data. Secondary sources are family, friends, significant other, health care team members, the health record, and pertinent literature.

- Subjective data are the client's personal perceptions, often gathered during the nursing health history.

- Objective data (e.g., data observed and collected during the physical examination) are detectable by the observer.

- Some data must be validated. Objective data can be used to validate subjective data, and vice versa. Primary and secondary data can also be used to validate each other.

- Both nursing and non-nursing models provide frameworks for collecting and organizing client data.

- In the assessment phase, nurses need to listen carefully to client stories to gain an understanding of the health concerns of each individual. In the diagnosis phase, nurses use their clinical reasoning to develop a plan of care that acknowledges the uniqueness and diversity of each individual client.

- Diagnosing, or making a nursing diagnosis, is the process of making a clinical judgment (nursing diagnosis or hypothesis) about a client's potential or actual health problems and strengths, and identifying desired health outcomes.

- Nursing diagnoses can be categorized into four types: actual, possible, risk, and wellness diagnoses.

- Critical thinking skills used in diagnosing include analysis, synthesis, inductive reasoning, and decision making.

- Three phases of the diagnostic process are data analysis; identification of client's health problems, health risks, and strengths; and formulation of diagnostic statements including desired health outcomes.

- It is important to identify client strengths as well as problems.

- Planning involves the nurse, the client, support persons, and other caregivers.

- Planning involves setting priorities, establishing client goals or desired health outcomes, selecting nursing interventions, and writing a plan of care.

- The Nursing Outcomes Classification (NOC) describes measurable states, behaviours, or perceptions that respond to nursing interventions. Each NOC has a definition of client outcome, a measuring scale, and an indicator.

- Desired health outcomes describe specific and measureable client responses and help the nurse evaluate the effectiveness of the nursing interventions.

- Nurses initiate and tailor nursing care plans that operationalize critical pathways and concept maps.

- Standardized care plans should be tailored to meet individual, family, group, and community needs.

- Implementation is carrying out or delegating the nursing interventions in collaboration with clients. It incorporates all the activities performed to promote health, prevent complications, treat symptom problems, and facilitate the client's coping with chronic alterations in health status.

- Evaluating is the process of comparing client responses to preselected outcomes to determine whether goals have been met. It includes renegotiating and modifying of unmet goals and reidentifying client health outcomes of the plan of care.

- The Nursing Interventions Classification (NIC) is linked to NANDA nursing diagnostic labels. Each NIC includes a label, a definition, and a list of activities that outlines key nursing interventions.

- Nursing interventions and actions promote desired health outcomes.

ASSESS YOUR LEARNING

1. Mrs. Chekov, 25 years old, has undergone a cesarean section. She and her baby have just entered the recovery room. What is the nurse's initial action?

   a. Perform a newborn assessment

   b. Inspect Mrs. Chekov's dressing and lochia

   c. Assess Mrs. Chekov's level of pain

   d. Ask Mrs. Chekov if she would like to feed her baby

2. The nurse records the client's breakfast intake as "tea 240 mL, milk 125 mL, 1 egg, 2 slices of toast." The nurse knows that the documentation is part of which phase of the nursing process?

   a. Assessment

   b. Diagnosis

   c. Planning

   d. Evaluation

3. A nursing care plan includes the desired health outcome of "quality of life" for a client with a chronic degenerative illness who is likely to live for many more years. Which of the following is one example that would indicate the outcome has been met?

   a. The client demonstrates financial resources to pay for health care for many years.

   b. The client spends the majority of his or her time in spiritual reflection.

   c. The client has no signs or symptoms of preventative complications of the illness.

   d. The client verbalizes satisfaction with current relationships with other persons.

4. Which of the following behaviours is most representative of the *nursing diagnosis* phase of the nursing process?

   a. Identifying major problems or needs

   b. Organizing data in the client's family history

   c. Establishing short-term and long-term goals

   d. Administering an antibiotic

5. Which of the following behaviours would indicate that the nurse was using the assessment phase of the nursing process to provide nursing care?

   a. Proposing hypotheses

   b. Generating desired health outcomes

   c. Reviewing results of laboratory tests

   d. Documenting care

6. The use of a conceptual or theoretical framework for collecting and organizing assessment data ensures which of the following?

   a. Correlation of the data with other members of the health care team

   b. Demonstration of cost-effective care

   c. Use of creativity and intuition in creating a plan of care

   d. Collection of all necessary information for a thorough appraisal

7. The client with a fractured pelvis requests that family members be allowed to stay overnight in the hospital room. Before determining whether or not this request can be honoured, the nurse should consult which of the following?

   a. Hospital policies

   b. Standardized care plans

   c. Orthopedic protocols

   d. Standards of care

8. The nurse selects the nursing diagnosis of *Risk for Impaired Skin Integrity* related to immobility, dry skin, and surgical incision. Which of the following represents a properly stated outcome or goal?

   a. The client will turn in bed q2h.

   b. The client will report the importance of applying lotion to skin daily.

   c. The client will have intact skin during hospitalization.

   d. The client will use a pressure-reducing mattress.

9. When initiating the implementation phase of the nursing process, the nurse performs which of the following steps first?

   a. Carrying out nursing interventions

   b. Determining the need for assistance

   c. Reassessing the client

   d. Documenting interventions

10. Mr. Jones comes into the doctor's office to evaluate his blood sugar and update his treatment for diabetes. The nurse collects Mr. Jones's recent blood sugar values that the client has been recording daily at home. The nurse is performing which type of assessment?

    a. Initial assessment

    b. Problem-focused assessment

    c. Emergency assessment

    d. Time-lapsed assessment

Check the eText in MyNursingLab for answers and explanations.

WEBLINKS

Canadian Nurses Association and Canadian Federation of Nurses Unions

http://www2.cna-aiic.ca/CNA/documents/pdf/ publications/PS88-Practice-Environments-e.pdf

This document presents the Canadian Nurses Association's and the Canadian Federation of Nurses Unions' joint position statement on practice environments and their role in maximizing client, nurse, and systems outcomes.

College of Nurses of Ontario

http://www.cno.org/Global/docs/reg/41037_ EntryToPracitic_final.pdf

The College of Nurses of Ontario offers this comprehensive guide to its entry-to-practice competencies.

Saskatchewan Registered Nurses Association

http://www.srna.org/images/stories/pdfs/nurse_resources/ standards_competencies.pdf

The Saskatchewan Registered Nurses Association has its professional practice standards and competencies online for registered nurses in Saskatchewan.

NANDA International

http://www.nanda.org

Formerly the North American Nursing Diagnosis Association International and now known as NANDA International, this is the premier international nursing diagnosis association. Its website states that it "is committed to increasing the visibility of nursing's contribution to patient care by continuing to develop, refine and classify phenomena of concern to nurses."

MyNursingLab

REFERENCES

American Nurses Association. (2010). *Nursing: Scope and standards of nursing practice* (2nd ed.). Silver Spring, MD: Author.

Armstrong, K., Laschinger, H., & Wong, C. (2009). Workplace empowerment and magnet hospital characteristics as predictors of patient safety climate. *Journal of Nursing Care Quality, 24*(1), 55–62.

Bulechek, G. M., & Dochterman, J. C. (2008). *Nursing intervention classification (NIC)* (5th ed.). St. Louis, MO: Mosby Elsevier.

Canadian Hypertension Education Program. (2012). *CHEP 2012 recommendations.* Retrieved from http://www.hypertension.ca/chep-recommendations

Canadian Nurses Association. (1980, Revised 1987). *A definition of nursing practice, standards for nursing practice* (2nd ed.). Ottawa, ON: Author. Retrieved from http://www.cna-aiic.ca/cna/search/default_e.aspx?cx=017995081769602664776%3Amo7p1eqo4vc&cof=FORID%3A11&ie=UTF-8&q=%22Nursing+Process%22+%2B+1987

Canadian Nurses Association. (2003). *Position statement: Staffing decisions for the delivery of safe nursing care.* Retrieved from http://www.cna-aiic.ca http:// cna-aiic.ca/CNA/documents/pdf/ publications/PS67_Staffing_Decisions_Delivery_Safe_Nursing_Care_June_2003_e.pdf

Canadian Nurses Association. (2010). *Position statement: Evidence-informed decision-making and nursing practice.* Retrieved from www.cna-aiic.ca

Canadian Nurses Association. (2011). *RN Exam Competencies, June 2010 – May 2015: Professional practice.* Retrieved from http://www.cna-aiic.ca/en/becoming-an-rn/rn-exam/competencies/

Carpenito-Moyet, L. J. (2009). *Nursing diagnosis: Application to clinical practice* (12th ed.). Philadelphia, PA: Lippincott, Williams & Wilkins.

D'Amico, D., & Barbarito, C. (2012). *Health & physical assessment in nursing* (2nd ed.). Upper Saddle River, NJ: Pearson Prentice Hall.

Gordon, M. (2010). *Manual of nursing diagnosis* (12th ed.). Boston, MA: Jones & Bartlett.

Hall, L. (1955, June). Quality of nursing care. *Public Health News.* Newark, NJ: State Department of Health.

Hannah, K. J., Reimer, M., Mills, W. C., & Letourneau, S. (1987). *Clinical judgement and decision making: The future with nursing diagnosis.* Toronto, ON: John Wiley & Sons.

Hill, C. M. (2006). Integrating clinical experiences into the concept mapping process. *Nurse Educator, 31*(1), 36–39.

Hicks-Moore, S. L. (2005). Clinical concept maps in nursing education: An effective way to link theory and practice. *Nurse Education in Practice, 5,* 348–352.

Johnson, D. E. (1959). A philosophy of nursing. *Nursing Outlook, 7,* 198–200.

Kingston-Riechers, J. Ospina, M., Jonsson, E., Childs, P., McLeod, L., & Maxted, J. (2010). *Patient safety in primary care.* Edmonton, AB: Canadian Patient Safety Institute and BC Patient Safety & Quality Council.

Moorhead, S., Johnson, M., Maas, M. L., & Swanson, E. (2008). *Nursing outcome classification (NOC)* (4th ed.). St. Louis: Mosby.

NANDA International. (2012). *Nursing diagnoses: Definitions and classification 2012–2014.* Oxford, UK: Wiley-Blackwell.

Ontario Ministry of Health and Long-Term Care. (2011). *Excellence Care For All Act, 2010.* Retrieved from http://www.health.gov.on.ca/en/legislation/excellent_care

Orem, D. E. (2001). *Nursing: Concepts of practice* (6th ed.). St. Louis, MO: Mosby.

Orlando, I. (1961). *The dynamic nurse–patient relationship.* New York, NY: Putnam.

Roy, C. (2008). *The Roy adaptation model* (3rd ed.). Upper Saddle River, NJ: Prentice Hall.

Wiedenbach, E. (1963). The helping art of nursing. *American Journal of Nursing, 63*(11), 54–57.

Wilkinson, J. M. (2012). *Nursing process and critical thinking* (5th ed.). Upper Saddle River, NJ: Prentice Hall.

Williams, C. L. (2008). *Therapeutic interaction in nursing* (2nd ed.). Boston, MA: Jones & Bartlett.

Chapter 24

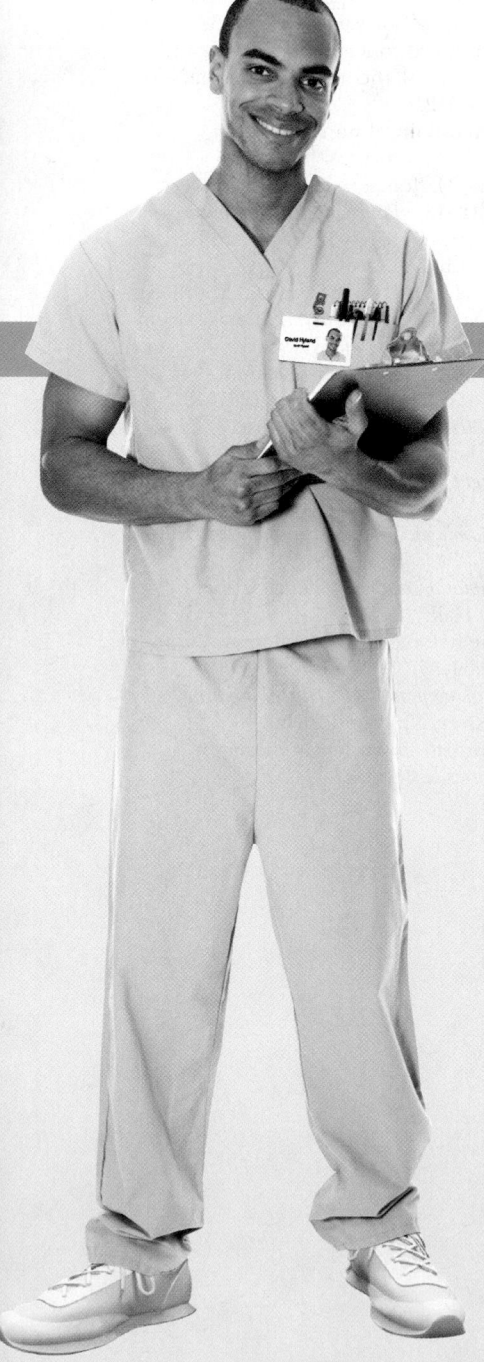

Documenting and Reporting

After studying this chapter, you will be able to:

1. Discuss the purpose and legal and ethical considerations of documentation in client records.

2. List the measures used to maintain confidentiality and security of computerized client records.

3. Compare and contrast different documentation methods: source-oriented and problem-oriented medical records; the assessments, problems, interventions, evaluation (APIE) model; focus charting; charting by exception; computerized records; and the case management model.

4. Explain how common documentation tools are used to document the steps of the nursing process.

5. Compare and contrast the documentation needed for clients in acute care, long-term care, and home care settings.

6. Discuss guidelines for effective documentation that meet legal and ethical standards.

7. Describe the nurse's role in documenting, reporting, conferring, and making referrals.

8. List the terminology and appropriate abbreviations commonly used for documentation and reporting.

9. Identify essential guidelines for reporting client data.

Effective communication among health care providers is a vital component to providing quality client care. Generally, health care providers communicate through discussion, reports, and records. A **discussion** is an informal oral conversation of a subject by two or more persons to identify a problem or establish strategies to resolve a problem. A **report** is oral, written, or computer-based communication, intended to convey information to others. For instance, nurses report on a client's progress at the end of a shift.

A **record**, also called a **chart** or **client record**, is a formal, legal document that provides evidence of a client's care and can be written or computer based. Although health care organizations use different systems and forms for documentation, all client records contain similar information. The process of making an entry on a client record is called **documenting**, **recording**, or **charting**. Documentation can be paper, electronic, audio, or visual.

Ethical and Legal Considerations

The Canadian Nurses Association's (CNA) (2008) *Code of Ethics* outlines values for practice, including safe, competent, ethical, accountable, and confidential care. Documenting and reporting are critical nursing activities guided by the *Code of Ethics*. The client's record is the cornerstone of communication among several disciplines involved in the care of the client. Nurses are responsible and accountable for documenting and reporting client care, and for implementing competent care that meets the standards for professional nursing practice (Canadian Nurses Protective Society, 2007).

The client's record is a *legal* document. Nurses need to be aware of and follow the legal and ethical standards of documentation. Documentation must be clear, concise, accurate, relevant, and completed in a timely manner. Subjective opinions must be avoided and objective language should be used when documenting or reporting client care. Statements made by clients or family members must be quoted to ensure accuracy. Diverse cultural perspectives need to be taken into consideration and clarified when documenting subjective data. Detailed descriptions of what was observed and changes to client's health status need to be documented. If care is not documented, then it is considered not completed (Cartwright-Vanzant, 2010).

Nurses can be called to court to testify several years after a case has started (see the Nursing and Canadian Society box). A nurse's memory may fade; therefore, accurate, objective documentation will allow recollection of what occurred and give credible evidence of the care provided. A well-constructed record will allow nurses to impart their testimony as documented in the client's chart. All aspects of the record, including flowsheets, graphic records, progress notes, nurses' notes, late entries, and incident reports, will provide a complete picture of events for the court.

As a legal record, most client records are retained by the health care institution or held for a minimum of

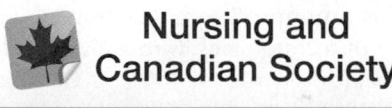

Nursing and Canadian Society

Fact	Implications for Nursing Practice
A client heath record can be entered into evidence in a court of law.	Nurses are accountable and have a responsibility to know the legislation, standards, and principles that govern documentation and reporting.
The Canada Health Infoway (2011) aims to have electronic health records for 100% of Canadians available by 2016. As of December 2010, 49% of Canadians' electronic health records are available to authorized providers.	Regardless of the documenting and recording system present in any health facility, nurses must apply the same legal principles and regulations to all client health records.
Juries' decisions in the Canadian court system are influenced by the overall quality of a client's health records.	Nurses should avoid spelling and grammar mistakes, along with unofficial and confusing abbreviations. A careless entry, poor spelling, and poor grammar tend to prejudice the entire client record, leaving everything suspect of being of poor quality or incompetent and, therefore, possibly inaccurate (Cartwright-Vanzant, 2010).

10 years by a health care professional responsible for the client's care. If the individual is under 18 years, then the record is held for 10 years after the client turns 18 years old (College of Nurses of Ontario, 2009). The public has the legal right to request access to their personal health records.

In Canada, federal privacy legislation, the Personal Information Protection and Electronic Documents Act (S.C. 2000, c. 5) (Department of Justice, 2011), applies to provincial and territorial organizations collecting and holding personal information. In addition, provinces and territories apply an additional act to protect the public's privacy. For example, Manitobans are protected by the Freedom of Information and Protection of Privacy Act, 1997, amended 2011 (Manitoba Government, 2011), and Ontarians are protected by the Personal Health Information Protection Act, 2004, amended 2010 (Service Ontario, 2010).

Ensuring Confidentiality of Electronic Health Records

Because of the increased use of electronic client information, health care agencies have implemented policies and procedures to ensure the privacy and confidentiality of client information is maintained. The Canada Health Infoway (2011) is a nonprofit organization supporting the development of technologies, with a mandate to provide electronic health records for 100% of Canadians by 2016. Health facilities in many provinces have begun the transition to electronic health records. Electronic health records are fast becoming a reality for Canadian nurses (CNA, 2009). The same documenting and recording principles apply regardless of the system of record-keeping used. Health care agencies are ultimately responsible for the computer information system selected and the overall security of the network. See the Clinical Alert box on faxing confidential information.

Nurses are accountable for the integrity and security of client records during use and must adhere to set policies and procedures. The following are some suggestions for ensuring confidentiality of computerized records:

1. A personal password is required to enter and sign out from computer files. The password should not be shared with anyone, including other health care team members.
2. After logging on, never leave a computer terminal unattended.
3. Do not leave client information displayed on the monitor screen visible for others to read.
4. Follow agency policies and procedures for documenting sensitive material, such as medical diagnoses.
5. Exit the client record, and log off the system when work is completed.

> **⚠ CLINICAL ALERT**
>
> Take safety measures before faxing confidential information. Consent is needed from the client to fax information. Make sure that personally identifiable information (e.g., client name, social insurance number) has been removed. If needed, confirm that the material is being sent to a confidential fax number or call ahead to ensure the person is present to receive the fax. Check that the fax number is correct before pressing the send button.

6. Information technology (IT) personnel must install a firewall to protect the server from unauthorized access.
7. Inform the appropriate health facility managers when a security breach has occurred.

Purpose of Client Records and Documentation

Documentation is an important nursing practice standard used to *communicate* with the interprofessional team, that demonstrates the nurse's *accountability* related to client care, and is a *legal requirement* of the nursing profession (College of Nurses of Ontario, 2009). Client records are kept for a number of purposes, including communication, planning client care, auditing health care agencies, research, education, reimbursement, legal documentation, and health care service analysis.

Communication

The client record is the primary communication vehicle for members of the health care team (see the Reflect on Primary Health Care box). Each health care provider contributes to the care of the client in various ways and uses the client record to access, communicate, and document information. Clear, concise, relevant, and accurate documentation provides continuity of care and increases the probability of quality health care.

> **REFLECT ON** **PRIMARY HEALTH CARE**
>
> As nurses work within interprofessional teams, documentation is used as a key vehicle to communicate and facilitate the type of care needed for clients. Collaborative efforts should be used to develop documentation of client care with common assessment criteria (e.g., pain assessment scale in palliative clients). The use of electronic health records could also bring experts from a distance, if needed, to engage in interprofessional team care planning. Reflect on how both *interprofessional collaboration* and *appropriate technology* can enhance the nurse's ability to assist clients to *access* the needed care for optimal health.

Planning Client Care

Each health care provider uses data from the client's record to plan care for that client. Nurses apply the nursing process by using baseline and ongoing assessment data to plan care, implement the appropriate interventions, evaluate the effectiveness, and revise nursing care according to the client's progress. For example, nursing documentation can communicate to a physician to order a specific antibiotic after establishing that the client's temperature is steadily rising or for a physiotherapist to change the client's exercise routine related to the client's pain or limitation in his or her range of movement.

Accountability

Nurses are accountable to follow the institution's policies and procedures as well as the standards set out by the regulatory body in each province or territory related to documentation legal liability (Austin, 2011; Canadian Council of Health Services Accreditation, 2007). Their documentation must be accurate, relevant, timely, and complete (College of Nurses of Ontario, 2009).

Auditing for Quality Assurance

An audit is a review of records. Client records are regularly audited for quality assurance to evaluate the health care facility and the care provided by all health care providers. Accrediting agencies, such as the Canadian Council of Health Standards Association (CCHSA), may audit client records to determine if a particular health agency is meeting the stated agency standards (see the section "Evaluating the Quality of Nursing Care" in Chapter 23).

Education and Research

Most agencies allow nursing students and health care providers to have access to client records. Nursing students or health care providers are bound by a strict ethical code and legal responsibility to hold all information in confidence and to protect clients' privacy and anonymity by not using identifiable data.

Client records contain valuable information for research and education. Client records provide a comprehensive view of the client, including nursing and medical diagnoses, signs and symptoms of the condition, diagnostic findings, behaviours, effective treatment strategies, and factors that affect outcomes. Information from client records can assist health care planners to identify service needs and client outcomes. Using data from client records, research can be conducted to determine themes and patterns, which can be further analyzed to determine effective health care interventions.

Documentation Systems

A number of documentation systems are currently used: (a) source-oriented record; (b) problem-oriented medical record; (c) the assessment, problems, interventions, evaluation (APIE) model; (d) focus charting; (e) charting by exception (CBE); (f) computerized documentation; and (g) case management. These documentation systems can be implemented using the traditional paper forms or with electronic medical records (EMRs).

Source-Oriented Record

The traditional client record is a **source-oriented record**. Each person or department makes notations in a separate section or sections of the client's chart. For example, the admission department has an admission sheet; nurses document on the initial nursing assessment and interdisciplinary notes; the physician has a physician's order sheet and a physician's history sheet; all disciplines record on interdisciplinary notes; and other departments or personnel may have their own documentation forms. In this type of record, information about a particular problem is distributed throughout the record. For example, if a client had right hemiplegia (paralysis of the left side of the body), data about this problem might be found in the initial nursing assessment, physician's history sheet, on the physician's order sheet, and in the interdisciplinary notes. See Table 24.1 on the next page for the components of a source-oriented record.

Narrative charting is a traditional part of the source-oriented record (see Figure 24.1 on page 513). It consists of written notes that include routine care, normal findings, and client problems. The information has no right or wrong order, although a chronological order is recommended and frequently used. Narrative documentation is being replaced by other systems, such as charting by exception and focus charting. Narrative documentation is expedient in emergency situations. For instance, during emergency situations, a delegated note taker records events in the order they occur.

Many agencies combine narrative charting with another system. For example, an agency using a *charting-by-exception* system (discussed later) may use *narrative charting* when describing findings of abnormalities. When using narrative charting, it is important to organize the information in a clear, coherent manner. Using the nursing process as a framework is one way to organize the information. (See Box 24.1 on page 513).

Source-oriented records are convenient because health care providers from each discipline can easily locate the forms on which to record data, and it is easy to trace the information to a specific discipline. The disadvantage is that information about a particular client problem is scattered throughout the chart, so it is difficult to find chronological information on a client's problem and progress.

TABLE 24.1 Components of the Source-Oriented Record

Form	Information
Admission (face) sheet	Legal name, birth date, age
	Social insurance number, Health Card number, other health insurance information
	Address
	Marital status; closest relatives or person to notify in case of emergency
	Date, time, and admitting diagnosis
	Food or drug allergies
	Name of admitting (attending) primary care provider
Initial nursing assessment	Findings from the initial nursing history and physical health assessment
Graphic record	Body temperature, pulse rate, respiratory rate, blood pressure, daily weight, and special measurements, such as fluid intake and output and oxygen saturation
Daily care record	Activity, diet, bathing, and elimination records
Special flowsheets	Examples: fluid balance record, skin assessment
Medication record	Name, dosage, route, time, date of regularly administered medications
	Name or initials of person administering the medication
Nurses' notes	Pertinent assessment of client
	Specific nursing care, including teaching, and client's responses
	Client's complaints and how client is coping
Medical history and physical examination	Past and family medical history, present medical problems, differential or current diagnoses, findings of physical examination by the primary care provider
Physician's order form	Medical orders for medications, treatments, and so on
Physician's progress notes	Medical observations, treatments, client progress, and so on
Consultation records	Reports by medical and clinical specialists
Diagnostic reports	Examples: laboratory reports, x-ray reports, computed tomography (CT) scan reports
Consultation reports	Reports by medical and clinical specialists
Client discharge plan and referral summary	Started on admission and completed on discharge; includes nursing problems, general information, and referral data

Problem-Oriented Medical Record

In the **problem-oriented medical record (POMR)**, or **problem-oriented record (POR)**, data are arranged according to the problem the client has rather than according to the source of the information. Members of the health care team contribute to the problem list, plan of care, and progress notes. Plans for each active or potential problem are drawn up and progress notes are recorded for each problem.

The advantages of POR are (a) it encourages collaboration; and (b) the problem list is in the front of the chart, which alerts health care providers to the client's needs and makes it easier to track the status of each problem. The disadvantages are (a) health care providers

differ in their ability to use the required charting format; (b) it takes constant vigilance to maintain an up-to-date problem list; and (c) repetitive because assessments and interventions that apply to more than one problem must be repeated.

The POR has four basic components:

1. Database
2. Problem list
3. Plan of care
4. Progress notes

DATABASE The database consists of all information known about the client when the client first enters the

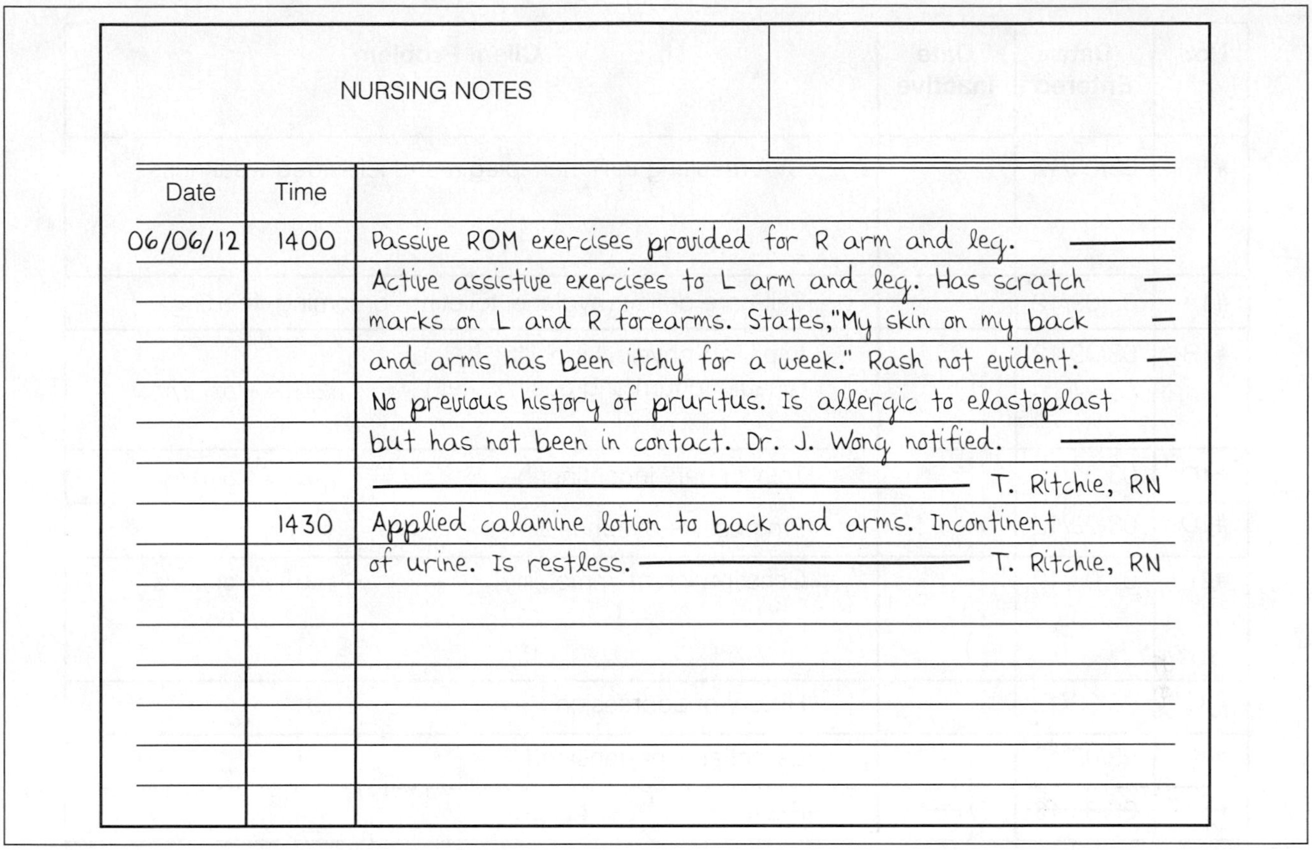

NURSING NOTES

Date	Time	
06/06/12	1400	Passive ROM exercises provided for R arm and leg.
		Active assistive exercises to L arm and leg. Has scratch
		marks on L and R forearms. States,"My skin on my back
		and arms has been itchy for a week." Rash not evident.
		No previous history of pruritus. Is allergic to elastoplast
		but has not been in contact. Dr. J. Wong notified.
		————————————————————————— T. Ritchie, RN
	1430	Applied calamine lotion to back and arms. Incontinent
		of urine. Is restless. ——————————————— T. Ritchie, RN

FIGURE 24.1 An example of narrative notes.

BOX 24.1 EXAMPLE OF ORGANIZING NARRATIVE CHARTING

Situation: Client is on day 2 after abdominal surgery. Questions to ask yourself:

- What assessment data are relevant?
- What nursing interventions have I completed?
- What is my evaluation of the result of the interventions, and/or what is the client's response to the interventions?

Example

1000h: Diminished breath sounds in all lung fields with crackles in the lower left lobe (LLL). Not using incentive spirometer (IS). Stated he is "not sure how to use it." Temperature 39°C. Instructed how to use IS. Discussed the importance of deep breathing and coughing after surgery. Administered analgesic for c/o abdominal pain rating of 5/10. After pain relief (1/10), able to demonstrate correct use of IS.

_____ S. Martin, RN

1400h: Using IS each hour. Lungs less diminished with fewer LLL crackles. Temperature 38°C.

_____ S. Martin, RN

health care agency. It includes the nursing assessment, the physician's history, social and family data, the results of the physical examination, and baseline diagnostic tests. Data are constantly updated as the client's health status changes.

PROBLEM LIST The problem list (Figure 24.2 on the next page) is derived from the database. It is usually kept at the front of the chart and serves as an index to the numbered entries in the progress notes. Problems are listed in the order in which they are identified, and the list is continually updated as new problems are identified and others resolved. All health care providers can contribute to the problem list, which includes the client's physiological, psychological, social, cultural, spiritual, developmental, and environmental needs. Nurses write problems as nursing diagnoses and physicians write problems as medical diagnoses, surgical procedures, or symptoms.

As the client's condition changes or more data are obtained, it may be necessary to redefine problems. Figure 24.2 illustrates how this has been done for problems 1B, 1C, and 2. When a problem is resolved, a line is drawn through it, and the number is not used again for that client.

PLAN OF CARE The initial list of orders or plan of care is made with reference to the current or active problems. Care plans are generated by the health care provider who lists the problems. Nurses write nursing care plans and physicians write physician's orders or medical care plans. The written plan in the record is listed under each problem in the progress notes and is not isolated as a separate list of orders.

No.	Date Entered	Date Inactive	Client Problem
#1	03/09/12		CVA resulting in Rt hemiplegia and left-sided weakness
#1A	03/09/12		Self-care deficit (hygiene, toileting, grooming, feeding)
#1B	03/09/12		Impaired physical mobility (unable to turn and position self) Redefined 02/07/13
#1C	03/09/12		Total urinary incontinence Redefined 01/17/13
#1D	03/09/12		Progressive dysphasia
#2	03/09/12		Constipation r/t immobility Redefined 06/10/13
#3	03/09/12		History of depression
#4	03/09/12		Essential hypertension
~~#5~~	~~06/06/12~~	~~7/11/12~~	~~Pruritus~~
#2	06/10/12		Risk for constipation r/t insufficient fibre intake
#1C	01/17/13		Urge urinary incontinence at night
#1B	02/07/13		Impaired physical mobility (needs 2-person assistance to transfer and walk)

FIGURE 24.2 A client's problem list in the problem-oriented medical record (POMR) system. Note that problems 1B, 1C, and 2 were redefined on the dates indicated and listed subsequently.

PROGRESS NOTES **Progress notes** in the POR are made by all health care providers involved in a client's care and everyone uses the same type of sheet for their notes. Progress notes are numbered to correspond to the problems on the problem list and may be lettered for the type of data. For example, **SOAPIER** is an acronym for subjective data, objective data, assessment, planning, interventions, evaluation, and revision. Some progress notes use SOAP only.

S: Subjective data are obtained from what the client says. They describe the client's perceptions and experience of the problem. When possible, the nurse quotes the client's words; otherwise, they are summarized. Subjective data are included only when it is important and relevant to the problem. It is important for nurses to acknowledge cultural considerations when recording subjective data to ensure accuracy and relevancy in their documentation.

O: Objective data consist of information that is measured or observed by use of the senses (e.g., vital signs, laboratory and x-ray results). See Chapter 23 for examples of subjective and objective data.

A: Assessment is the interpretation or conclusions drawn about the subjective and objective data. The problem list is created from the database; the "A" entry should be a statement of the problem. In all subsequent SOAP notes for that problem, the "A" should describe the client's condition and level of progress rather than merely restating the diagnosis or problem.

P: Planning is the plan of care designed to resolve the stated problem. The initial plan is written by the health care provider who enters the problem into the record. All subsequent plans, including revisions, are entered into the progress notes.

Over the years, the SOAP format has been modified. The acronyms SOAPIE and SOAPIER refer to formats that add interventions, evaluation, and revision.

I: Interventions refer to the specific interventions that have actually been performed by the health care provider.

E: Evaluation includes client responses to nursing interventions and medical treatments. This is primarily reassessment of client data.

R: Revision reflects care plan modifications that arose from the evaluation. Changes may be made in desired outcomes, interventions, or target dates.

See Figure 24.3 for an example of progress notes that use the SOAP, SOAPIER, and APIE formats.

APIE

The **APIE** documentation model is similar to SOAPIER charting. APIE is an acronym for *assessments, problems, interventions,* and *evaluation* of nursing care. This system consists of a client care assessment flowsheet and progress notes. The flowsheet uses specific assessment criteria in a particular format, such as human needs or functional health patterns. The time parameters for a flowsheet can vary from minutes to months. In a hospital intensive care unit, for example, a client's blood pressure may be monitored by the minute, whereas in an ambulatory clinic a client's blood glucose level may be recorded once a month.

After the assessment, the nurse establishes and documents specific problems on the progress notes. The *problem statement* is labelled "P" and referred to by number

SOAP Format	**SOAPIER Format**	**APIE Format**
6/6/12 #5 Generalized pruritus	6/6/12 #5 Generalized pruritus	6/6/12 A— Generalized pruritus r/t unknown cause
1400 S— "My skin is itchy on my back and arms, and it's been like this for a week." ___	1400 S— "My skin is itchy on my back and arms, and it's been like this for a week." ___	1400 States, "My skin is itchy on my back and arms, and it's been like this for a week." Skin appears clear. No rash or irritations noted. Marks where client has scratched noted on left and right forearms. Allergic to elastoplast but has not been in contact. No previous history of pruritus. ___
O— Skin appears clear—no rash or irritation noted. Marks where client has scratched noted on left and right forearms. Allergic to elastoplast but has not been in contact. No previous history of pruritus. ___	O— Skin appears clear—no rash or irritation noted. Marks where client has scratched noted on left and right forearms. Allergic to elastoplast but has not been in contact. No previous history of pruritus. ___	P— Instruct to not scratch skin. — Apply calamine lotion, as necessary. ___ — Cut nails to avoid scratches. — Assess further to determine whether recurrence associated with specific drugs or foods. — Refer to physician and pharmacist for assessment.
A— Altered comfort (pruritus): cause unknown. ___	A— Altered comfort (pruritus): cause unknown. ___	I— Instructed not to scratch skin. Applied calamine lotion to back and arms at 1430 h. ___ Assisted to cut fingernails. Notified physician and pharmacist of problem. ___
P— Instructed not to scratch skin. — Applied calamine lotion to back and arms at 1430 h. ___ — Cut fingernails. ___ — Assess further to determine whether recurrence associated with specific drugs or foods. — Refer to physician and pharmacist for assessment. ___ T. Ritchie, RN	P— Instruct to not scratch skin. — Apply calamine lotion, as necessary. ___ — Cut nails to avoid scratches. — Assess further to determine whether recurrence associated with specific drugs or foods. — Refer to physician and pharmacist for assessment.	E— States, "I'm still itchy. That lotion didn't help." ___ ___ T. Ritchie, RN
	I — Instructed not to scratch skin. Applied calamine lotion to back and arms at 1430 h. ___ Assisted to cut fingernails. Notified physician and pharmacist of problem.	
	1600 E— States, "I'm still itchy. That lotion didn't help." ___	
	R— Remove calamine lotion, and apply hydrocortisone cream, as ordered. T. Ritchie, RN	

FIGURE 24.3 Examples of nursing progress notes that use the SOAP, SOAPIER, and APIE formats. *SOAP*, subjective data, objective data, assessment, planning; *SOAPIER*, subjective data, objective data, assessment, planning, interventions, evaluation, and revision; *APIE*, assessments, problems, interventions, and evaluation.

(e.g., P #5). The *interventions* employed to manage the problem are labelled "I" and numbered according to the problem (e.g., I #5). The *evaluation* of the effectiveness of the interventions is also labelled and numbered according to the problem (e.g., E #5).

Focus Charting

Focus charting is intended to make the client's concerns and strengths the focus of care. Three columns for documenting are usually used: (a) date and time, (b) focus, and (c) progress notes (see the example at the end of this section). The *focus* can be a condition, a nursing diagnosis, a behaviour, a sign or symptom, an acute change in the client's condition, or a client strength. The progress notes are organized into data (D), action (A), and response (R), referred to as DAR or DARP, where (P) stands for plans for future actions or future interventions.

The *data category* consists of observations of client status and behaviours, including data from flowsheets (e.g., vital signs, pupil reactivity). The nurse records both subjective and objective data in this section. The *action category* includes immediate and future nursing actions. It can also include any changes to the plan of care. The *response category* describes the client's response to any nursing and medical care.

Focus charting systems provide a holistic perspective of the client and the client's needs. This documentation system also provides a framework for the progress notes (DAR). The three components do not need to be documented in order, and each note does not need to have all three categories. Flowsheets and checklists are frequently used in the client's chart to document routine nursing tasks and assessment data.

Date/Hour	Focus	Progress Notes
13/12/25	Pain	**D:** Guarding abdominal incision. Facial grimacing. Rates pain at "8" on scale of 0–10.
0900		**A:** Administered morphine sulphate 4 mg IV.
0930		**R:** Rates pain at "1." States willing to ambulate.

Charting by Exception

Charting by exception (CBE) is a documentation system in which only significant findings or exceptions to norms are recorded by using flowsheets as much as possible. CBE incorporates three key components: clinical observations, nursing interventions, and client response to nursing care (Guido, 2010).

1. *Flowsheets that highlight significant findings and define assessment parameters and findings.* Examples of

flowsheets include a graphic record (see Figure 24.4), fluid balance record, daily nursing assessments record (see Figure 24.5), client teaching record, client discharge record, and skin assessment record.

2. *Standards of nursing care.* Printed standardized documentation of nursing care eliminates much of the repetitive charting of routine care. An agency using CBE must develop its own specific standards of nursing practice that identify the minimum criteria unique to the type of client and care. For example, "The nurse must ensure that the unconscious client has oral care at least q2h." Documentation of care according to these specified standards involves only a check mark in the routine standard box on the graphic record. All exceptions to the standards are fully described in narrative form on the nurses' notes.

3. *Bedside access to chart forms.* All flowsheets are kept at the client's bedside to allow for immediate documentation and to eliminate the need to transcribe data from the nurse's worksheet to the permanent record.

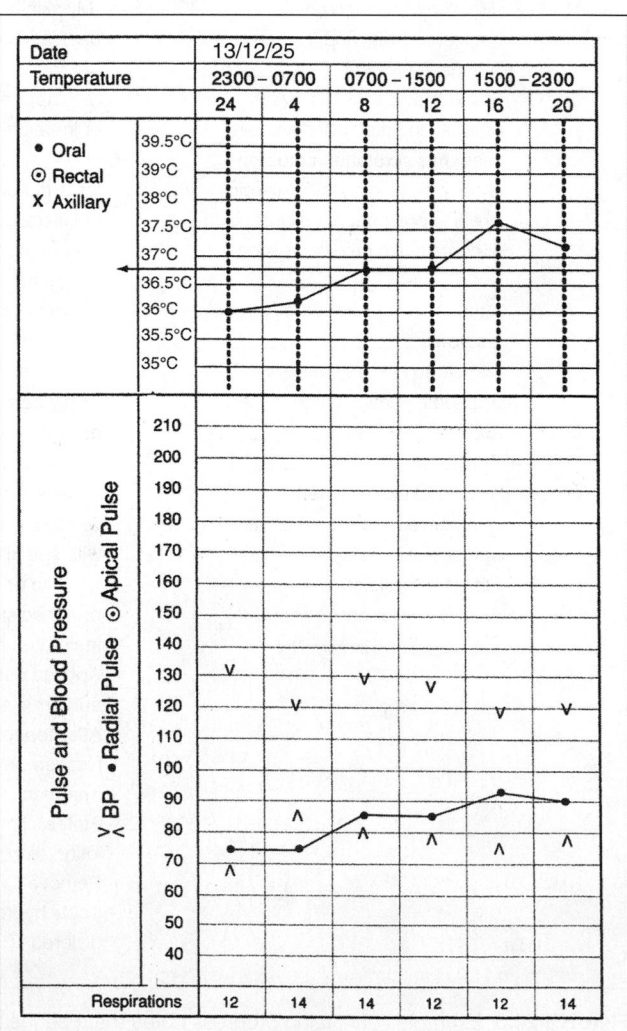

FIGURE 24.4 Sample vital signs graphics record.

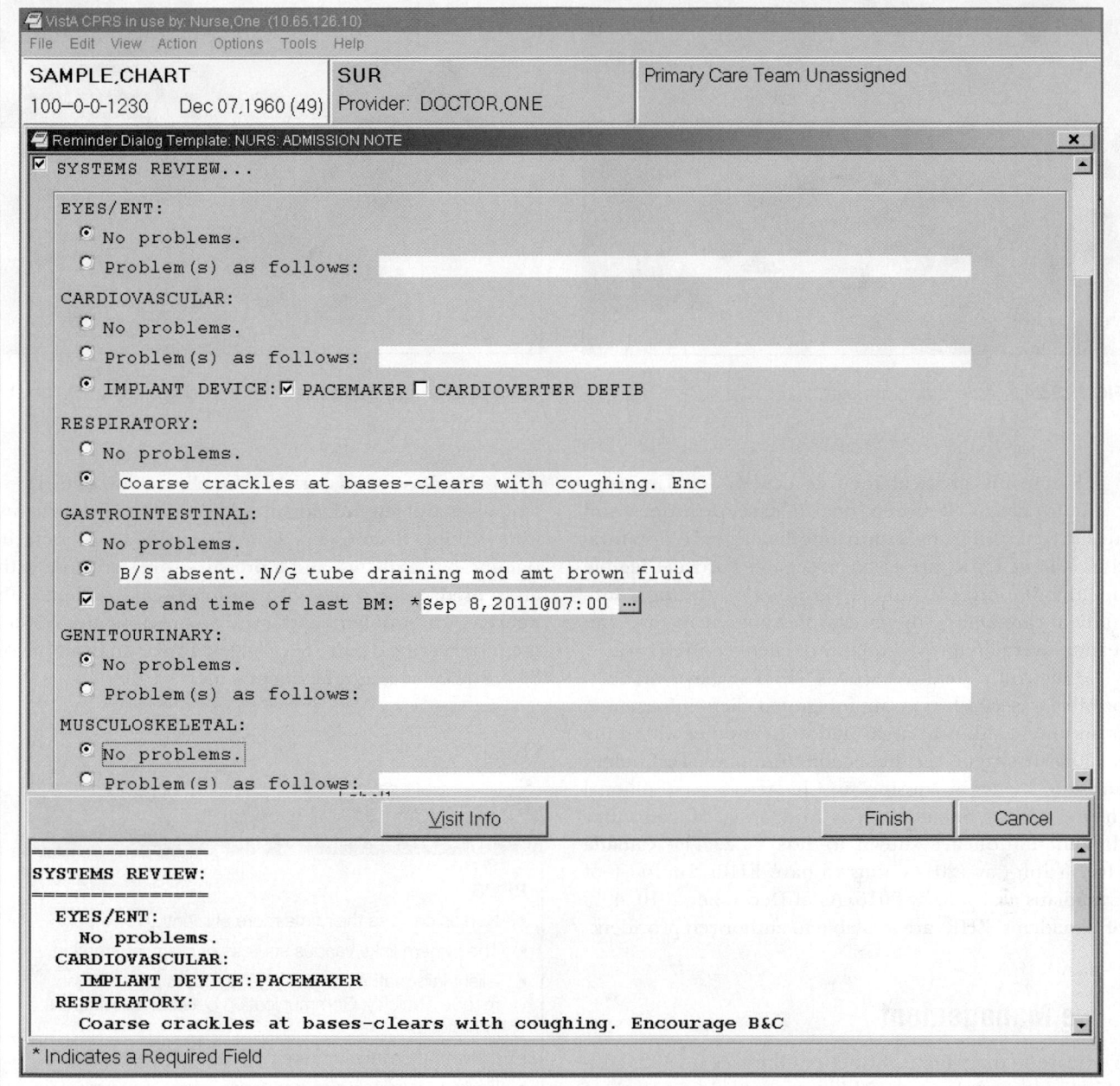

FIGURE 24.5 Sample of a portion of a daily nursing charting by exception (CBE) assessment form used in an electronic medical record (EMR).

Computerized Documentation

Computerized clinical record systems can manage the huge volume of information required in contemporary health care. Some institutions have a computer terminal at each client's bedside (see Figure 24.6 on the next page), or nurses carry a small handheld terminal or personal digital assistant (PDA), enabling the nurse to document immediately after care is given (see Figure 24.7 on the next page).

Computerized record systems can generate a work list for the shift with a list of all the treatments, procedures, and medications needed by the client. For example, the nurse can obtain results of a client's blood test, a schedule of all clients on the unit who are to have surgery during the day, a suggested list of interventions for a nursing diagnosis, a graphic chart of a client's vital signs, or a printout of all the progress notes for a client.

Computers can make planning care and documentation easier when recording nursing actions and client responses, by choosing client-specific standardized forms and recording additional narrative information as needed. Automated speech-recognition technology allows nurses to enter data by voice for conversion to written documentation. If the spoken word is used to create personal health information, the nurse must be alert and aware of others who might hear the dictation to ensure client confidentiality.

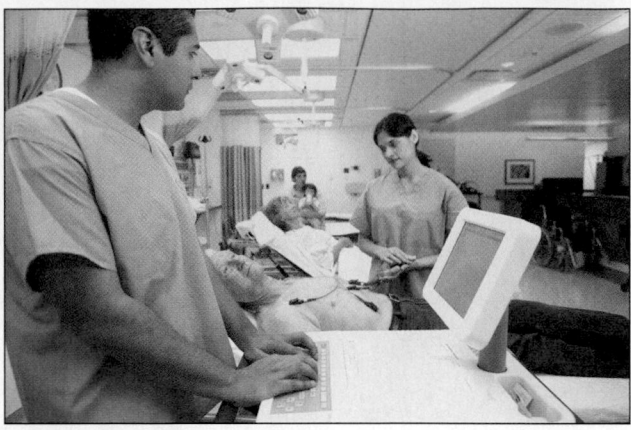

FIGURE 24.6 A bedside computer.

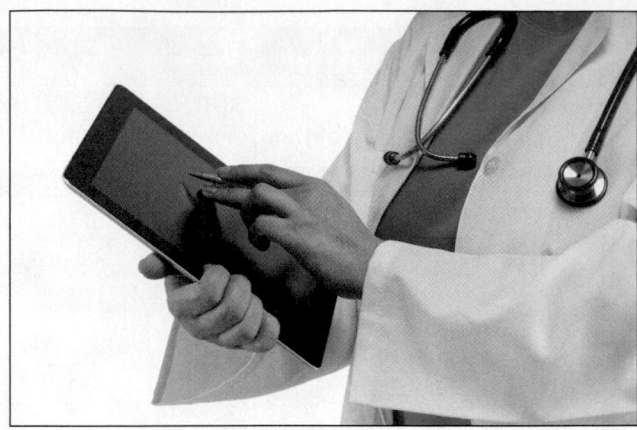

FIGURE 24.7 Electronic health record using a computer tablet.

Electronic medical records (EMRs) can improve communication between health care providers and authorized clinicians within one health care organization. Client EMRs are easily accessible, provide legible documentation, coordinate care demonstrating continuity of care among the interprofessional team, and can lead to overall improved quality of client-centred care.

Electronic health records (EHRs) have made it possible to securely transmit integrated client information from one health care organization to another within the health care system (see the section "Computer Technology and Informatics in Nursing" in Chapter 25 for additional information). Selected pros and cons of computer documentation are shown in Box 24.2. The Canada Health Infoway (2011) aims to have EHRs for 100% of Canadians available by 2016. As of December 2010, 49% of Canadians' EHRs are available to authorized providers.

Case Management

The case management model emphasizes quality, cost-effective care delivered within an established length of stay. This model uses a multidisciplinary approach to planning and documenting client care by using *critical pathways*. These forms identify the outcomes that certain groups of clients are expected to achieve on each day of care, along with the interventions necessary for each day.

The case management model also incorporates graphics and flowsheets. Progress notes typically use some type of CBE. For example, if goals are met, no further charting is required. Goals that are not met are called **variances**. They are deviations from what is planned on the critical pathway—unexpected occurrences that affect the planned care or the client's responses to care. When a variance occurs, the nurse writes a note documenting the unexpected event, the cause, and the actions taken to correct the situation or justify the actions taken.

Critical pathways work best for clients with one or two diagnoses and few individualized needs. Data from clients with multiple diagnoses (e.g., a client with a hip fracture, pneumonia, diabetes, and a pressure sore) or those with an unpredictable course of symptoms (e.g., a client with neurological problems and seizures) are difficult to document on a critical path. See Table 24.2 for an example of how a variance might be documented.

BOX 24.2 SELECTED PROS AND CONS OF COMPUTER DOCUMENTATION

PROS

- Nurses can use their time more efficiently.
- The system links various sources of client information.
- Client information, requests, and results are sent and received quickly. Communication between providers is enhanced.
- Links to monitors improve accuracy of documentation.
- Bedside terminals can synthesize information from monitoring equipment.
- Bedside terminals eliminate the need to take notes on a worksheet before recording.
- Bedside terminals permit the nurse to check an order immediately before administering a treatment or medication.
- Information is legible.
- The system incorporates and reinforces standards of care.
- Standard terminology improves communication.

CONS

- Client's privacy may be infringed on if security measures are not used.
- Breakdowns make information temporarily unavailable.
- The system is expensive.
- Extended training periods may be required when a new or updated system is installed.

TABLE 24.2 Example of Variance Documentation (Critical Pathway)

A client has had a below-the-knee amputation. On the third postoperative day, he has a temperature of 38.8°C. Lung sounds are clear, and he is not coughing. The nurse notices redness and skin breakdown over the client's sacrum. The critical pathway outcomes specified for day 3 are "Oral temperature 37.7°C" and "Skin intact over bony prominences." The nurse should chart the following variances:

Date/Time	Variation	Cause	Action Taken/Plans
12/4/16 0900	Elevated temperature (38.8°C)	Possible sepsis	4/16—Blood cultures × 3 per order • Monitor temperature q1h. • Monitor I&O, hydration, and mental status.
12/4/16 1130	Impaired skin integrity: stage 1 redness, 5 cm circular area on sacrum	Client does not move about in bed unless reminded	4/16—Positioned on L side • Turn side-to-side q2h while awake. • On every client contact, remind client to move about in bed. • Apply Duoderm after bath.

Documenting Nursing Activities

Client records should describe the client's perceptions, ongoing health status, and reflect the nursing process. Regardless of the records system used in the organization, nurses should document evidence of the nursing process using a variety of forms throughout the client's record (see Table 24.3).

Admission Nursing Assessment

A comprehensive admission assessment, also referred to as an initial database, nursing history, or nursing assessment, is completed when the client is admitted to the nursing unit. As discussed in Chapter 23, these forms may be organized according to health patterns, body systems, functional abilities, health problems and risks, nursing model, or type of health care setting.

Nursing Care Plans

There are two types of nursing care plans: (a) traditional and (b) standardized. The *traditional care plan* is written for each client. The form varies from agency to agency, according to the needs of the client and the department. Most forms have three columns: (a) nursing diagnoses, (b) expected outcomes, and (c) nursing interventions. (See the section "Developing Nursing Care Plans" in Chapter 23 for additional information.)

Standardized care plans have been developed to save documentation time. These plans can be based on an institution's standards of practice, thereby helping to provide high-quality nursing care. Standardized care plans must be individualized by the nurse, critically analyzing the client using the nursing process to competently address individual client needs.

TABLE 24.3 Documentation for the Nursing Process

Step	Documentation Forms
Assessment	Initial assessment form, various flowsheets
Nursing diagnosis	Nursing care plan, Kardex, critical path, interdisciplinary notes, problem list
Planning	Nursing care plan, critical path
Intervention	Interdisciplinary notes, flowsheets
Evaluation	Interdisciplinary notes

Kardexes

The **Kardex** is a concise method of organizing and recording data about a client. It consists of a series of cards kept in a portable index file or in a computer-generated form. The Kardex may or may not become a part of the client's permanent record. In some organizations, it is a temporary worksheet written in pencil for ease in recording frequent changes in details of a client's care. Nurses need to ensure the pencil written information is accurately transcribed from the original medical order. The information on Kardexes may be organized into various sections. For example:

• Pertinent information about the client, such as name, room number, age, religion, marital status, admission date, physician's name, diagnosis, type of surgery and date, occupation, and next of kin

• Allergies and list of medications, including date of order and times of administration

• List of intravenous fluids, with dates of infusions

• List of daily treatments and procedures, such as irrigations, dressing changes, postural drainage, or measurement of vital signs

• List of diagnostic procedures ordered, such as x-ray or laboratory tests

- Specific data on how the client's physical needs are to be met, such as type of diet, assistance needed with feeding, elimination devices, activity, hygienic needs, and safety precautions (e.g., one-person assist)
- A problem list, stated goals, and nursing interventions to meet the goals

Information on the Kardex may be updated by the nurse in charge or a delegate (e.g., the nursing unit clerk) to keep the data current. Whether the Kardex is a written paper or computerized, it is important to have a place on it to record dates and the initials of the person reviewing or revising it.

Flowsheets

Flowsheets enable nurses to document nursing data quickly and concisely and provide an easy-to-read record of the client's condition over time.

GRAPHIC RECORD This record typically indicates body temperature, pulse, respiratory rate, blood pressure, weight, and, in some agencies, other significant clinical data, such as admission or postoperative day, treatments, protective measures, diagnostic studies, bowel movements, diet, appetite, hygiene, and activity.

INTAKE AND OUTPUT RECORD All routes of fluid intake and all routes of fluid loss or output are measured and documented on this form. Information about ways to measure and record specific amounts of fluid intake and output are described in Chapter 44.

MEDICATION ADMINISTRATION RECORD (MAR) Medication administration records usually include designated areas for the date the medication was ordered, the expiration date, the medication name, dose, frequency, route, time of administration, and the nurse's signature. Some records also include a place to document the client's allergies. (A sample medication record is shown in Figure 33.6: Medication administration record, on page 885.)

Progress Notes

Progress notes made by nurses provide information about the progress a client is making toward achieving desired outcomes. In addition to assessment and reassessment data, progress notes include information about client problems and nursing interventions.

Nursing Discharge and Referral Summaries

A discharge note and referral summary are completed when the client is being discharged and transferred to another institution or to a home setting in which a visit by a community health nurse is required (see the section "Discharge Planning" in Chapter 14). Some records combine the discharge plan, including instructions for care, follow-up appointments, and the final progress note.

Regardless of format, discharge and referral summaries usually include some or all of the following:

- Description of the client's physical, mental, and emotional status at discharge or transfer
- Resolved health problems
- Unresolved continuing health problems and continuing care needs, which may include a review-of-systems checklist that considers integumentary, respiratory, cardiovascular, neurological, musculoskeletal, gastrointestinal, elimination, and reproductive problems
- Treatments that are to be continued (e.g., wound care, oxygen therapy)
- Current medications
- Restrictions that relate to (a) activity, such as lifting, stair climbing, walking, driving, work; (b) diet; and (c) bathing, such as sponge bath, tub, or shower
- Functional and self-care abilities in terms of vision, hearing, speech, mobility with or without aids, meal preparation and eating, preparation and administration of medications
- Comfort level
- Support networks, including family, significant others, spiritual adviser, community self-help groups, home care, and other community agencies available
- Client education provided in relation to the disease process, activities and exercise, special diet, medications, specialized care or treatments, and follow-up appointments
- Discharge destination (e.g., home, nursing home) and mode of discharge (e.g., walking, wheelchair, ambulance)
- Referral services (e.g., home health nurse, social worker)

Long-Term Care Documentation

Requirements for documentation in long-term care settings are based on professional standards, federal and provincial regulations, and policies of the health care agency.

Nurses need to familiarize themselves with regulations influencing the type and frequency of documentation required in long-term care facilities. The nurse usually completes a nursing care summary at least once a week for clients requiring skilled care and every 2 to 4 weeks for those requiring intermediate care. Summaries should address the following:

- Specific problems expressed by clients and/or families
- Mental health status
- Activities of daily living (ADLs)
- Hydration and nutrition status
- Elimination status
- Safety measures needed
- Medications
- Treatments
- Preventive measures

BOX 24.3 GUIDELINES FOR LONG-TERM CARE DOCUMENTATION

Long-term care facilities require nurses to follow specific guidelines:

- Complete the assessment and screening forms and plan of care within the period specified by agency policy.

- Document and report any change in the client's condition to the physician and the client's family within 24 hours.

- Document all measures implemented in response to a change in the client's condition.

- Document nursing summaries and progress notes that comply with the frequency and standards required by agency policy, using the nursing process as a guideline.

- Ensure that progress notes address the client's progress in relation to the goals or outcomes defined in the plan of care.

- Review and revise the plan of care according to agency policies or whenever the client's health status changes.

- Keep a record of any visits and phone calls from family, friends, and others regarding the client.

See Box 24.3 for guidelines for long-term care documentation.

Home Care Documentation

Home care is one of the fastest growing areas in health care in Canada because of an increasing older population and shorter hospitalizations. Health care providers often document in client-held records that remain at the residence (see Box 24.4 for guidelines for home health care documentation). Health care providers may access critical information through the use of voicemail,

BOX 24.4 GUIDELINES FOR HOME HEALTH CARE DOCUMENTATION

Home care nurses must follow these documentation guidelines:

- Complete a comprehensive nursing assessment and develop a plan of care.

- Write a progress note during each client visit, noting any changes in the client's condition, nursing interventions performed (including education and instructional brochures and materials provided to the client and home caregiver), client responses to nursing care, and vital signs as indicated.

- Keep a copy of the care plan in the client's home and update it as the client's condition changes.

- Report changes in the plan of care to the appropriate member of the health care team, and document that these were reported.

- Encourage the client or home caregiver to record data, when appropriate.

- Write a discharge summary, including the client's health status at discharge, outcomes achieved, and recommendations for further care.

wireless devices, and laptops, which enhances their ability to care for their clients and maintain accurate and current records. In addition, telehealth technologies allow the sharing of professional expertise in urban areas with health care providers practising in homes and communities in rural and remote locations.

Incidents Reports

An *incident report* is a form completed by the nurse, if the nurse was directly or indirectly involved or witnessed an error that adversely affected the client. **Incident reports**, also known as event or occurrence reports, are completed when the care provided is not consistent with standard practice, causing injury, harm, or loss to the client, and negatively affecting the quality of client care (Dunn, 2010). Near-misses, no-harm events, adverse events, medication or human errors, and miscommunication causing errors are instances when an incident report would be completed. (See the Evidence-Informed Practice box on incident reports.)

Nurses are accountable to provide safe and competent care to clients. When errors occur in nursing care, nurses are responsible to report the incident. Effective communication and documentation regarding the care provided to the client, the client's progress, and continuity of care will decrease the risk for errors and may help identify problems that could have prevented similar occurrences in the future. It is important to promote a culture of safety and to remember that incident reports are not to blame an individual; instead, the purpose is to improve future quality in client care (Casey & Wallis, 2011).

EVIDENCE-INFORMED PRACTICE

Can Incident Reports Enhance Client Health Outcomes?

One hundred and six semistructured interviews were conducted with 92 front-line nursing managers in 94 of 98 emergency departments across British Columbia to explore their perception of reporting safety events (PSE). Barriers to reporting PSE were related to time constraints, sense of futility, fear of reprisal, lack of education on PSE reporting, reports being viewed as indicators of incompetence, and inaccessibility of reporting forms.

NURSING IMPLICATIONS: Underreporting of PSEs impedes research on the events, decreases educational opportunities to learn from the incident, and, therefore, hinders the ability to implement change and prevent reoccurrence. Nurses need to be educated on the value of PSE reporting and advocate for a culture of safety and create system changes that will help overcome the barriers of reporting PSE and enhance client health outcomes.

Source: Based on Brubacher, J., Hunte, G., Hamilton, L., & Taylor, A. (2011). Barriers to and incentives for safety event reporting in emergency departments. *Health Care Quarterly, 14*(3), 57–65.

General Guidelines for Documentation

A client's record is a legal document and can be used to provide evidence in court. Health care providers must maintain the confidentiality of the client's record and meet the legal standards of documentation. Follow agency policies regarding handwritten recording, including the type of pen ink used for documentation.

Date and Time

The date and time of each documentation entry is required for legal reasons and for client safety. Record the time according to the 24-hour clock to avoid confusion about whether the time was a.m. or p.m. (see Figure 24.8).

Timing

Follow the health care institution's policy about the frequency of documentation and adjust the frequency as a client's condition indicates. For example, a client whose blood pressure is changing requires more frequent documentation than a client whose blood pressure is constant. Documenting should be done as soon as possible after an assessment or intervention. No documentation should be completed *before* providing nursing care. Blanket charting (i.e., charting all events occurring within an extended period of time) should be avoided.

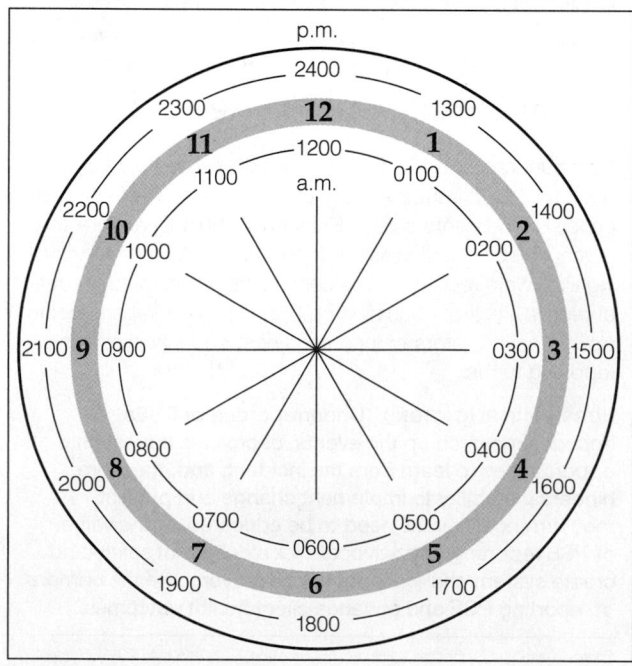

FIGURE 24.8 The 24-hour clock.

Legibility

All entries must be legible and easy to read to prevent interpretation errors. Printing or easily understood handwriting is usually permissible.

Permanence

All entries on the client's record are made in dark ink, according to agency policies, so that the record is permanent and changes can be identified. Dark ink reproduces well on microfilm and in duplication processes.

Accepted Terminology and Abbreviations

Use only commonly accepted *abbreviations, symbols,* and *terms* that are specified by the agency. Many abbreviations are standard and used universally. When in doubt about whether to use an abbreviation, write the term out in full until certain about the abbreviation. Abbreviations that are not official can lead to misunderstandings. For example, *D/C* may mean "discharge" or "discontinue"; *od* could mean "once a day" or "right eye." Refer to Table 24.4 and Table 24.5 on page 524 for the common abbreviations and symbols. Use the metric system to document measurements (e.g., height, weight, volume).

Correct Spelling

Correct spelling is essential for accuracy in documentation. Two decidedly different medications may have almost similar spellings, for example, digitoxin and digoxin. Errors in spelling can negatively affect your credibility as a nurse (Cartwright-Vanzant, 2010).

Signature

Each recording should be signed by the nurse who performed the care provided. The signature includes the *name* and *title,* for example, "Susan J. Green, RN." The following title abbreviations are often used, however, nurses need to follow the institution's policy about how to sign their name:

RN = registered nurse
RNA = registered nurse assistant
LPN = licensed practical nurse (outside Ontario)
RPN = registered practical nurse (Ontario only)
RPN = registered psychiatric nurse (Western provinces)
NA = nursing assistant
NS = nursing student
RA = resident attendant
SN = student nurse

TABLE 24.4 Commonly Used Abbreviations

Abbreviation	Term	Abbreviation	Term
abd	abdomen	m	metre
ABO	the main blood group system	meds	medications
ac	before meals (*ante cibum*)	mg	milligram
ADL	activities of daily living	mL	millilitre
ad lib	as desired (*ad libitum*)	mod	moderate
adm	admitted or admission	neg	negative
a.m.	morning (*ante meridiem*)	NPO	nothing by mouth (*nil per os*)
amb	ambulatory	NS	normal saline
amt	amount	O₂	oxygen
approx	approximately (about)	OOB	out of bed
BM (bm)	bowel movement	pc	after meals (*post cibum*)
BP	blood pressure	PE (PX)	physical examination
BR	bed rest	per	by or through
BRP	bathroom privileges	p.m.	afternoon (*post meridiem*)
c̄	with	PO	by mouth (*per ora*)
C	Celsius (centigrade)	postop	postoperative(ly)
CBC	complete blood count	preop	preoperative(ly)
CBR	complete bed rest	prep	preparation
CDA	Canadian Diabetic Association	prn	when necessary (*pro re nata*)
Cl	client	pt	patient
cm	centimetre	q	every (*quaque*)
c/o	complains of	qh (q1h)	every hour (*quaque hora*)
DAT	diet as tolerated	q2h, q3h, and so on	every 2 hours, 3 hours, and so on
drsg	dressing	qid	four times a day (*quarter in die*)
Dx	diagnosis	req	requisition
ECG (EKG)	electrocardiogram	Rt (rt, R)	right
fld	fluid	S (s̄)	without (*sine*)
g	gram	SI	Systeme International d'unites (metric system)
GI	gastrointestinal		
GP	general practitioner	spec	specimen
gtt	drops (*guttae*)	STAT	at once, immediately (*statim*)
h	hour (*hora*)	tid	three times a day (*ter in die*)
H₂O	water	TL	team leader
I&O	intake and output	TLC	tender loving care
j	joule	TO	telephone order
IV	intravenous	TPR	temperature, pulse, respirations
kg	kilogram	VO	verbal order
kJ	kilojoule	VS	vital signs
L	litre	WNL	within normal limits
Lab	laboratory	wt	weight
liq	liquid		
LMP	last menstrual period		
lt (L)	left		

Note: The Institute for Safe Medication Practice Canada (ISMP) and the Joint Commission recommend the elimination of specific abbreviations, symbols, and dose designations because they are prone to errors that may cause harm. These "do not use" symbols include >, <, @, **ss, D/C, hs, OD, OS, os, qd, q.d., Q.D., QD, U, u, IU, q.o.d, qod, QOD, per os, qhs, MS, MSO4, MgSO4, ø,** Δ, and **no**. For possible future inclusion: all abbreviations for drug names, apothecary units, the abbreviation "cc" and "ug." See Table 33.6 (page 882) for selected examples and visit the ISMP and Joint Commission websites for a complete listing: http://www.jointcommission.org/assets/1/18/do_not_use_list.pdfand http://www.ismp.org/tools/errorproneabbreviations.pdf

TABLE 24.5 Commonly Used Symbols

Symbol	Term	Symbol	Number
=	equal to	ī	1
↑	increased	īī	2
↓	decreased	īīī	3
♀	female	īv̄	4
♂	male	v̄	5
°	degree	v̄ī	6
#	number; fracture	v̄īī	7
×	times	viii	8
		ix	9
		x̄	10

Accuracy

Check that the correct client's name and identifying information are stamped or written on each page of the client's record before making any entry. Special care is needed when caring for clients with the same last name. Health care facilities may use a brightly coloured warning sticker on the health care record and information shared by clients with similar names.

Documentation must be accurate, clear, relevant, and concise. Accurate documentation consists of facts or observations rather than opinions or interpretations. It is more accurate, for example, to write that the client "refused medication" (fact) than to write that the client "was unco-operative" (opinion) or to write that a client "was crying" (observation) than to write that the client "was depressed" (interpretation). Similarly, when a client expresses worry about the diagnosis or problem, this should be quoted directly on the record: "Stated: 'I'm worried about my leg.'" When describing a situation, avoid general words, such as *large, good,* or *normal,* which can be interpreted differently. For example, chart specific data, such as "2 cm × 3 cm bruise," rather than "large bruise."

When a *recording mistake* is made, draw one line through it (leave the mistake readable), and correct the error, according to agency policy. For example, write the words *entry mistake* above it with your initials or name (depending on agency policy) and the date and time of correction. Do not erase, blot out, or use correction fluid. Do not recopy a chart page or remove chart pages because an error occurred. The original entry must remain visible. Correcting or modifying another health care provider's documentation is illegal and is considered a professional misconduct.

Sample Recording

Date: 2013/12/10   Time: 0100h

entry mistake AJR

Pulse ~~180 beats per min~~   108 beats per min

Abby J. Roberts, NS

Write *on* every line but never *between* lines. If a *blank* appears in a notation, draw a line through the blank space so that no additional information can be recorded at any other time or by any other person, and sign the notation.

Sample Recording

Date: 2013/11/07   Time: 0730h

Urine cloudy, light brown with dark flecks.

No odour. States "Burning pain in pubic region prior to voiding." _____ Lin I. Ma, NS

Sequence

Document events in the chronological order in which they occur. For example, record assessments, then the nursing interventions, and then the client's responses. Update or delete problems, as needed. Events documented out of sequence must be clearly identified as a late entry, according to agency policy. If alterations are made to the sequence of events, explain that you are making a *late note entry* and include the actual time you are making the note in the client record (Cartwright-Vanzant, 2010).

Appropriateness

Document only information that is significant to the client's health problems and care. Any other personal information that the client conveys is inappropriate for the record. Documenting irrelevant information can be considered an invasion of the client's privacy or subject to legal action from the client. A client's disclosure that she was addicted to heroin 20 years ago, for example, *would not* be recorded on the client's medical record unless it had a direct bearing on the client's health.

Completeness

Document only information that is helpful to the client and health care providers. Nurses' notes need to reflect the nursing process. Document all assessments, nursing diagnoses, plans, nursing interventions, and client comments and responses to interventions and tests, progress toward goals, and communication with other health care providers.

Care that is *omitted* because of the client's condition or refusal of treatment must also be documented. It is vitally important to clearly document the events of what happened and why a component of care was omitted. Ensure that the details are specific and state who was notified and outcomes of these actions.

Conciseness

Documentation needs to be brief, as well as complete, to save time in communication. For example, write "Perspiring profusely. Respirations shallow, wet, 28 per min." End each thought or sentence with a period.

Legal Prudence

Accurate, complete documentation should enhance legal protection for the nurse. The client's chart is admissible in court as a legal document. The nurse's documentation should present an accurate, complete representation of the quality of care given. Incompleteness or omission seriously undermines the strength of the evidence, competency of the nurse, and questions if care was actually provided. Failing to maintain a client's record or falsifying information within the client's record is considered a professional misconduct under the Nursing Act, 1991. The nurse must adhere to professional standards of nursing care and follow the institution's policies and procedures for intervention and documentation in all situations—especially in high-risk situations. For example:

> 2013/12/9 1100h—Client stated "feeling dizzy."
> Raised side rails. Instructed to stay in bed and ring call bell if requiring assistance. _____
> RS Chartrand, RN
>
> 2013/12/9 1130h—Found beside table on the floor. Client said, "I climbed over these rails all by myself." When asked about pain, replied, "I feel fine but a little dizzy." Helped client into bed. BP 100/60, P90, R24, Dr. RJ Naden notified. _____ RS Chartrand, RN

Reporting

Reports can be either verbal or written. The purpose of reporting is to communicate specific information to a person or group of people, for example at change-of-shift or when transferring a client. A report should be concise, including only pertinent information and no extraneous details.

Change-of-Shift Reports

A **change-of-shift report** is a report usually given to nurses starting the next shift. The purpose is to provide continuity of care for clients by providing the subsequent health care provider with a quick summary of the client needs and details of care to be given.

Change-of-shift reports can be written or given verbally, either in person or by audiotape recording. The face-to-face report permits the listener to ask questions during the report; written and tape-recorded reports are often brief and less time consuming. Reports are sometimes given at the bedside, and clients as well as nurses can participate in the exchange of information. See Box 24.5 for key elements of a change-of-shift report and Box 24.6 on the next page for a sample change-of-shift report. See the Clinical Alert box on shift reports.

SITUATION-BACKGROUND-ASSESSMENT-RECOMMENDATION (SBAR) The **SBAR** is a communication tool commonly used during change-of-shift reports to promote and maintain effective communication between

---

BOX 24.5 KEY ELEMENTS OF A CHANGE-OF-SHIFT REPORT

The following guidelines are important to follow in shift-change reports:

- Follow a particular order (e.g., room numbers in a hospital).
- Provide basic identifying information for each client (e.g., name, room number, bed designation).
- For newly admitted clients, provide the reason for admission or medical diagnosis (or diagnoses), age, general condition, surgery (date), diagnostic tests, plan of therapy, and significant information about the client's support people.
- Include significant changes in the client's condition and present information in order (i.e., assessment, nursing diagnoses, interventions, outcomes, and evaluation). For example, "Mr. Ronald Oakes said he had an aching pain in his left calf at 1400 hours. Inspection revealed no other signs. Calf pain is related to altered blood circulation. Rest and elevation of his legs on a footstool for 30 minutes provided relief."
- Provide exact information, such as "Ms. Jessie Jones received Demerol 100 mg intramuscularly at 2000 hours," *not* "Ms. Jessie Jones received some Demerol during the evening."

- Report the client's need for special emotional support. For example, a client who has just learned that his biopsy results revealed malignancy and who is now scheduled for a laryngectomy needs time to discuss his feelings before preoperative teaching starts.
- Include current nurse interventions/plans/care and physician-prescribed orders.
- Report clients that have been transferred or discharged from the unit.
- Clearly state priorities of care and care that is due after the shift begins. For example, in a 0700h report, the nurse might say, "Mr. Li's vital signs are due at 0730, and his IV bag will need to be replaced by 0800." Give this information at the end of that client's report, as people remember best the first and last information given.
- Be concise. Do not elaborate on background data or routine care. For example, do not report "Vital signs at 0800 and 1200" when that is the unit standard. Do not report coming and going of visitors unless there is a problem or concern or if the visitors are involved in teaching and care. Social support and visits are considered normal within the hospital.

BOX 24.6 SAMPLE CHANGE-OF-SHIFT REPORT

The following sample of a shift-change report uses the key elements listed in Box 24.5:

ROOM 201—C.W.

Admitted last night for pneumonia

Allergic to penicillin

DNR

IV of D5/0.45 NS infusing at 100 mL/h in (L) forearm

Need sputum specimen for C&S

Temperature 39.1. Tylenol 325 mg, 2 tablets given at 0600h

Lung sounds diminished in lower lobes

ROOM 202—G. H.

Admitted for left total knee arthroplasty on 2013/09/14.

Has discharge orders to go to rehab today

Dressing clean, dry, and intact

Regular diet. Taking fluids well.

Had BM yesterday

Pain rating of 4/10—last medicated with oxycodone 2.5 mg with acetaminophen 325 mg, 1 tablet, given at 0400h

---

! CLINICAL ALERT

The shift report should take place in an area that is private and free from interruption to maintain client confidentiality.

BOX 24.7 SAMPLE SBAR COMMUNICATION TOOL

S = Situation

- State your name, unit, and client name.
- Briefly state the problem.

B = Background

- State client admission diagnosis and date of admission.
- State pertinent medical history.
- Provide brief summary of treatment to date.
- Code client status (if appropriate).

A = Assessment

- Vital signs
- Pain scale
- Is there a change from prior assessments?

R = Recommendation

- State what you would like to see done or specify that the appropriate health care provider needs to come and assess the client.
- Ask if the health care provider wants to order any tests or medications.
- Ask the health care provider if she or he wants to be notified for any reason.
- In case of no improvement, ask the health care provider when you should call again.

---

the health care team when discussing a client's condition and progress. Implementation of the SBAR tool can increase quality care and client safety by decreasing miscommunication, which will help to prevent errors, such as near-misses (Boaro, Fancott, Baker, Velji, & Andreoli, 2010). The SBAR tool can be also be used during transition of care, for debriefing and conflict resolution (Andreoli, et al., 2010). (See Box 24.7 and the Weblinks at the end of the chapter for SBAR tools.)

Telephone Reports

Health care providers frequently report about a client by telephone. Nurses inform physicians about a change in a client's condition; a radiologist reports the results of an x-ray study; a nurse may confer with a nurse on another unit about a transferred client.

The nurse receiving a telephone report should document the date and time, the name of the person giving the information, and the information received and should sign the documentation. For example:

> 2013/06/06 1035h. GL Messina, laboratory technician, reported by telephone that Mrs. Sara Ames's hematocrit was 39%. _____ Barbara Ireland, RN

If any doubt exists about the information given over the telephone, the person receiving the information should repeat it back to the sender to ensure accuracy.

The nurse needs to provide concise, accurate and relevant information when giving a telephone report to another health care provider. Begin with your name and relationship to the client. For example, "This is Jana Gomez; I'm calling from xxx Hospital, Unit xxx, about your client, Dorothy Mendes. I'm her registered nurse on the 0700h to 1900h shift."

Telephone reports usually include the client's name and medical diagnosis, changes in nursing assessment, vital signs related to baseline vital signs, significant laboratory data, and related nursing interventions. The nurse should have the client's chart ready to provide any further information. Implementing the SBAR tool can assist the nurse to communicate important information regarding the client.

After reporting, the nurse should document the date, time, and content of the call. For example:

> 2013/09/14, 1200h. Dorothy Mendes admitted to Unit A. Client states she has "burning abdominal pain in upper right side of abdomen." BP 120/80, P100, R20 on admission. Demerol 100 mg IM given at 1200. _____ RS Chartrand, RN

> 2013/09/14, 1400h. BP 100/40, P120, R30. Pain unchanged. Colour pale and perspiring. _____ RS Chartrand, RN

> 2013/09/14, 1535h. Dr. Burns called regarding client's pain, pallor, diaphoresis, and vital signs. Dr. Burns stated will be in to assess in one-half hour. _____ RS Chartrand, RN

Telephone Orders

Physicians often order a therapy or medication for a client by telephone. Most agencies have specific policies about telephone orders. While the physician gives the order, *write* the complete order down and read it back to the physician to ensure accuracy. Question the physician about any order that is ambiguous, unusual (e.g., an abnormally high dosage of a medication), or contraindicated by the client's condition. Then, transcribe the order onto the physician's order sheet, indicating it as a verbal order (VO), telephone order (TO), or read back order (RBO). See Box 24.8 for selected guidelines.

Once the order is transcribed on the physician's order sheet, the order must be countersigned by the physician within a period described by agency policy. Many acute care facilities require that this be done within 24 hours.

BOX 24.8 GUIDELINES FOR TELEPHONE ORDERS

With telephone orders, it is especially important to carefully follow these guidelines:

1. Do not accept an order from a prescriber you do not know.
2. Ask the prescriber to speak slowly and clearly.
3. Ask the prescriber to spell out the medication if you are not familiar with it.
4. Question the drug, dosage, or changes if they seem inappropriate for this client.
5. Write down the order, or enter it into a computer.
6. Read the order back to the prescriber at the end. Use words for abbreviations (e.g., three times a day for tid).
7. When writing a dosage, always put a number before a decimal (e.g., 0.3 mL) but never put a zero after a decimal (e.g., 6 mg).
8. Write out units (e.g., 20 units of insulin, *not* 20 u of insulin).
9. Follow agency policy on the prescriber protocol for signing telephone orders (e.g., within 24 hours).
10. Never follow a voicemail order. Call the prescriber back for a verbal order. Write it down, and read it back for confirmation.

Conferring

Nurses often confer with colleagues and other health care providers for advice, information, ideas, or instructions about the client situation in a mentoring relationship or to elicit or validate data needed to plan nursing care. Two ways nurses share information are through (a) a nursing care conference and (b) nursing rounds.

Nursing Care Conference

A **nursing care conference** is a meeting of a group of nurses to discuss possible solutions to certain problems of a client. The nursing care conference allows each nurse an opportunity to offer possible solutions to the problem (e.g., lack of progress toward goal attainment). Other health care providers may be invited to attend the conference to offer their expertise. For example, a social worker may discuss the family problems of a severely burned child, or a dietitian may discuss the dietary problems of a client who has diabetes. Nursing care conferences are most effective when members on the team will accept and respect each person's contributions and listen with an open mind to what others are saying.

Nursing Rounds

Nursing rounds are procedures in which a group of nurses visit selected clients' bedsides to do the following:

- Obtain information that will help plan nursing care
- Provide clients the opportunity to discuss their care
- Evaluate the nursing care the client has received
- Identify alternative nursing possibilities from evidence-based practice and experienced nurses

During nursing rounds, the nurse assigned to the client provides a brief summary of the client's needs and the interventions being implemented. Nursing rounds offer advantages to both clients and nurses. Clients can participate in the discussions and nurses can meet the client and assess client's environment (e.g., view the equipment being used). To facilitate client participation in nursing rounds, nurses need to use terms that the client can understand. Medical terminology can exclude the client from the discussion.

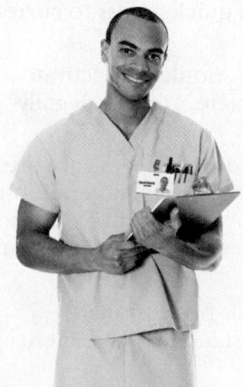

Case Study 24

Mr. Anderson, an 80-year-old male, was admitted for back pain. He has a past medical history of hypertension. He told the admitting nurse that he has lost interest in many of his normal activities because of the constant pain. You read the following documentation entry by a previous nurse:

8—Client is a complainer. I listened to him for 15 minutes with no success.
BP 210/90 and 180/70, P 72, R 18
12—Refused lunch
2—Client fell out of bed

(continued)

CRITICAL THINKING QUESTIONS

1. What guidelines were *not* used in this documentation?

2. The nursing diagnosis for Mr. Anderson is *Acute Pain*. What would you expect to document?

3. Using the following pieces of data for Mr. Anderson, sort them into a SOAPIER note:

   a. "I didn't sleep last night."

   b. Positioned on side with pillows behind back

   c. Continues to need analgesic medication to progress toward goal of pain relief

   d. States pain is 8 out of 10

   e. "I feel better." (after interventions)

   f. Last medicated 5 hours previously

   g. Heating pad applied to lower back

   h. BP 210/90, P 72, R 18

   i. Add to plan of care to offer analgesic around the clock q4h versus prn

   j. 2013/6/6 #1 pain

   k. "Sharp, stabbing pain in lower back that radiates to left leg."

   l. Medicated with ordered analgesic

4. Use the same pieces of data and sort them into a DAR note.

Check the eText in MyNursingLab for answers and explanations.

KEY TERMS

APIE *p. 515*

change-of-shift report *p. 525*

chart *p. 509*

charting *p. 509*

charting by exception *p. 516*

client record *p. 509*

discussion *p. 509*

documenting *p. 509*

flowsheets *p. 520*

focus charting *p. 516*

incident reports *p. 521*

Kardex *p. 519*

narrative charting *p. 511*

nursing care conference *p. 527*

nursing rounds *p. 527*

problem-oriented medical record (POMR) *p. 512*

problem-oriented record (POR) *p. 512*

progress notes *p. 514*

record *p. 509*

recording *p. 509*

report *p. 509*

SBAR *p. 525*

SOAPIER *p. 514*

source-oriented record *p. 511*

variances *p. 518*

CHAPTER HIGHLIGHTS

- Client records are legal documents that provide evidence of a client's care.

- The nurse has a legal and ethical duty to maintain confidentiality of the client's record; this includes special measures to protect client information stored in computers.

- Client records are kept for a number of purposes, including communication, planning client care, auditing health care agencies, research, education, reimbursement, legal documentation, and health care analysis.

- In source-oriented records, recording is organized around the source of the information.

- In problem-oriented records, recording is organized around client problems.

- Other examples of documentation systems include APIE (assessment, planning, interventions, evaluation), focus charting, charting by exception, computer documentation, and case management.

- Computer records have simplified nursing documentation. The use of computer terminals at the bedside allows for immediate documentation of nursing actions.

- The case management model focuses on standardized interventions given within a defined time frame.

- The case management record for a client incorporates graphics and flowsheets along with critical pathways that serve as both an abbreviated care plan and a documentation form.

- The Kardex record is used for quick access to current data about clients.

- The content of progress notes should be accurate, sequential, appropriate, complete, concise, legally prudent, relevant, and ethical.

- Principles of documentation for long-term care are the same as for acute care; however, documentation in long-term care is (a) less frequent and (b) focuses more on daily functioning, preventive measures, and restorative care.

- Documentation needs to follow professional, regulatory, and accreditation standards and agency policies.

- The case management model emphasizes quality, cost-effective care delivered within an established length of stay.
- Document data as soon as possible *after* nursing assessments, interventions, and evaluations.
- The purpose of reporting is to communicate specific information for the goal of improving or maintaining quality of care.
- A change-of-shift report and a telephone report are considered handoff communications.

ASSESS YOUR LEARNING

1. The Cameron family is caring for their father at home in the final stage of his life. The family has decided that they will all participate in providing care to minimize the caregiver burden for Mrs. Cameron. How should the home care nurse document this?
   a. "The agency's standardized palliative care plan will be implemented."
   b. "Each family member has agreed to spend one day per week caring for Mr. Cameron."
   c. "Mrs. Cameron is unable to cope with the care of her husband without assistance."
   d. "A care plan has been developed and presented to the Cameron family."

2. A client frequently refuses his daily medication. The nurse is finishing the narrative charting in the client record and writes the subjective client statement, "Don't come near me with that pill. I hate it. . . . Go away and stop bothering me." Which of the following is the BEST comment that the nurse could include in the narrative recording?
   a. "Client uncooperative again."
   b. "Client remains negative about treatment."
   c. "Client still very angry with nurse."
   d. "Client refuses scheduled medication."

3. Nursing documentation and reporting are guided by which of the following?
   a. Canadian Nurses Association, International Council of Nurses, health facility policies
   b. Canadian Council of Health Standards Association, health facility policies, International Council of Nursing
   c. Canadian Nurses Association, health care policies, provincial or territorial nurses' unions
   d. Canadian Nurses Association, Canadian Council of Health Standards Association, health care policies

4. The charting-by-exception (CBE) method of documenting and reporting is most appropriate and useful for which of the following health care settings?
   a. Acute care facility
   b. Outpost nursing station
   c. Primary health care clinic
   d. Long-term care facility

5. Which of the following is the primary purpose of the client health record?
   a. Communication document
   b. Nursing process tool
   c. Research database
   d. Accreditation process

6. When documenting in a client chart (health record), nurses must be sure to include a nursing note related to which of the following?
   a. Routine care
   b. Usual events
   c. Doctor's orders
   d. Treatment refusal

7. Gisele Beulieu, RN, is working evenings on a psychiatric unit in a large urban facility when she receives a telephone call. The caller identifies himself as the husband of one of her clients and would like to know how his wife is doing. Nurse Beulieu is unable to verify the caller's identification. What is the nurse's BEST response?
   a. "Policy prevents me from providing confidential client information."
   b. "Confidential information can't be provided without client permission."
   c. "If you want client information, call back in the morning."
   d. "I don't know who you are, so I can't give you any information."

8. The requirements of documenting and reporting suggest nurses resolve a problem with a chart entry by using which of the following guidelines?
   a. Erase all errors as thoroughly as possible, and write the correction in the same spot.
   b. Draw a pencil line through the wrong entry and write *entry mistake* above it.
   c. Write *mistaken entry* above the entry with your initial or name.
   d. Write *error* above the entry with your position or title.

9. Which of the following is a legal comment frequently used to describe nursing care?

   a. Nurses are too busy to chart effectively.

   b. Nurses are often sued for malpractice.

   c. Nurses' routine care that is not documented is assumed to be done.

   d. Nurses' routine care that is not documented is assumed to not be done.

10. Maria Dubois, RN, works on a surgical unit and recently she has been visiting her son (age 18 years) who is receiving treatment on a medical unit in the same facility. During your care for her son, you return from lunch and find Nurse Dubois reading her son's chart. Select the BEST response in this situation.

   a. "Maria, what you are doing is illegal."

   b. "Maria, please read the chart in a private place."

   c. "Maria, as a nurse you know the chart is confidential."

   d. "Maria put that chart back; it's not your business."

Check the eText in MyNursingLab for answers and explanations.

WEBLINKS

Accreditation Canada

http://www.accreditation.ca

This organization helps health care service organizations achieve greater degrees of excellence by concentrating on improvements in quality health care services that focuses on clients' specific needs in Canada and internationally. It offers organizations ideas about improving documentation systems and ways to become more consistent in standardizing charting across regions.

College of Nurses of Ontario—Documentation Practice Standard and Modules

http://www.cno.org/learn-about-standards-guidelines/ educational-tools/learning-modules/documentation-2010

This website provides a learning module on documentation for nurses to review and test their knowledge about their roles and responsibilities related to documentation.

Registered Nurses Association of Ontario: *The Nursing and eHealth Project*

http://rnao.ca/bpg/initiatives/nursing-and-ehealth-project

This website provides a nursing focus related to eHealth. There is a video explaining the importance of eHealth to nursing, it showcases past eHealth webinars and tutorials and highlights the nurse's role in the future of our health care.

Registered Nurses Association of Ontario (RNAO) survey—*Best Practice Guidelines and Use of Electronic Documentation Systems*

https://survey.rnao.ca/BPGELECTRONIC

The RNAO created a survey to evaluate the nurse's perspective related to eHealth and to determine the nurse's role and use of electronic medical records within the health care system.

Videos on SBAR

http://youtu.be/NBNrYOBFwDs & http://youtu.be/ 1r31pL1aZDQ

The Toronto Rehabilitation Institute created these videos to illustrate health care providers communicating with and without the SBAR tool.

MyNursingLab

REFERENCES

Andreoli, A., Fancott, C., Velji, K., Baker, G., Solway, S., Aimone, E., & Tardif, G. (2010). Using SBAR to communicate fall risk and management in inter-professional rehabilitation teams. Situation-background-assessment-recommendation. *Healthcare Quarterly*, 1394–1401.

Austin, S. (2011). Stay out of court with proper documentation. *Nursing*, 41(4), 24–30.

Boaro, N., Fancott, C., Baker, R., Velji, K., & Andreoli, A. (2010). Using SBAR to improve communication in interprofessional rehabilitation teams. Situation-background-assessment-recommendation. *Journal of Interprofessional Care*, 24(1), 111–114. doi: 10.3109/13561820902881601

Canada Health Infoway. (2011). *Summary corporate plan.* Retrieved from https://www2.infoway-inforoute.ca/Documents/Infoway_Sum.Corp.Plan.2011-2012_EN.pdf

Canadian Council of Health Services Accreditation. (2007). *Canadian health accreditation report.* Retrieved from http://www.accreditation.ca/uploadedFiles/2008_Health_Accreditation_Report_EN.pdf

Canadian Nurses Association. (2008). *Code of ethics for registered nurses* (Centennial ed.). Ottawa, ON: Author.

Canadian Nurses Association. (2009). *Enhancing workforce productivity and increasing capacity in the health system through information and communications technology. Policy Brief #6.* Retrieved from http://www.cna-aiic.ca/CNA/documents/pdf/publications/HHR_Policy_Brief6_2009_e.pdf

Canadian Nurses Protective Society. (2007). Quality documentation: Your best defence. *Infolaw*, 1(1), Ottawa, ON: Author.

Cartwright-Vanzant, R. (2010). Medical record documentation: Legal aspects in neonatal nursing. *Newborn & Infant Nursing Reviews*, 10(3), 134–137. Retrieved from EBSCO*host*. doi: 10.1053/j.nainr.2010.06.008

Casey, A., & Wallis, A. (2011). Effective communication: Principle of nursing practice. *Nursing Standard*, 25(32), 35–37.

College of Nurses of Ontario. (2009) *Documentation, Revised 2008.* Pub No. 41001. Retrieved from http://www.cno.org/Global/docs/prac/41001_documentation.pdf

Department of Justice. (2011). *Personal information protection and electronic documents act (S.C. 2000, c. 5).* Ottawa, ON: Government of Canada. Retrieved from http://laws-lois.justice.gc.ca/eng/acts/P-8.6/index.html

Dunn, D. (2010). Do no harm: Our duty to report. *Nursing Management*, 41(6), 38–43. doi: 10.1097/01.NUMA.0000381741.79787.1b

Guido, G. W. (2010). *Legal and ethical issues in nursing* (5th ed.). Upper Saddle River, NJ: Prentice Hall.

Manitoba Government. (1997, amended 2011). *Freedom of information and protection of privacy act.* Winnipeg, MB: Manitoba Government.

Service Ontario. (2004, amended 2010). *Personal health information protection act.* Toronto, ON: Government of Ontario. Retrieved from http://www.e-laws.gov.on.ca/html/statutes/english/elaws_statutes_04p03_e.htm

Chapter 25

Nursing Informatics and Technology

LEARNING OUTCOMES

After studying this chapter, you will be able to:

1. Define the concepts consistent across various definitions of nursing informatics.

2. Outline the current conceptualizations of technology by nurses.

3. Discuss some of the modern information and computer technology (ICT) used within clinical practice.

4. Explain how nurses are using core technology in different areas of practice (e.g., research, administration, practice, education).

5. Outline evidence-informed nursing practice in the presence of ICT.

6. Explain sociotechnical perspectives as related to the use of ICT in practice (e.g., workflow, human-technology relationships).

7. Describe the process of clinical informatics implementation.

8. Describe consumers' participation in health informatics.

9. Identify different nursing specific informatics organizations in Canada.

10. Discuss issues of professional practice within a technologically mediated health care environment.

A dvances in technology, the growth of scientific knowledge, the increase in chronic disease burden, and a substantial proportion of aging Canadians underscores the need for health information that is reliable, accurate, and accessible to consumers and health care providers (Forkner-Dunn, 2003; Haux, 2002; Nutbeam, 2000). Nurses are the largest provider group with the greatest interaction with information technology and client health care (Deese & Stein, 2004). It is imperative that nurses understand the opportunities information and computer technologies (ICTs) can provide to enhance their practice. This chapter will emphasize the various definitions, conceptualizations, technologies, roles, and evolution of the informatics discipline within nursing. Other topics related to informatics (i.e., social media, mobile health, evidence-informed practice, professionalism) will be discussed in relation to ICT and nursing practice.

Advances in technology, an aging population, increases in chronic disease, and an exponential rise in scientific knowledge have contributed to the advancement of the "information age" model of health care (Eysenbach, 2008; Forkner-Dunn, 2003). In fact, there is widespread consensus and evolving evidence that the Internet and information technology is revolutionizing health care practices (D'Alessandro & Dosa, 2001; Ferguson, 2000; Kassirer, 2003). Not surprisingly, the nursing profession and Canadians in general are increasingly relying on the Internet and information technology as tools for improved access to health information and health care (Canadian Home Care Association, 2008; Underhill & McKeown, 2008). The Health Council of Canada, mandated by the Canadian government to report on the progress of health care renewal, health status of Canadians, and health outcomes, has made the development of information and computer technology to all Canadians a priority (Health Council of Canada [HCC], 2005).

Definition of Nursing Informatics

The term *nursing informatics* was coined roughly 30 years ago by Scholes and Barber (1980) to describe "the application of computer technology to all fields of nursing— nursing services, nurse education, and nurse research" (p. 73). In fact, nursing has had a long lineage of using technology within the profession to support client care and knowledge generation.

Nurses first began experimenting with computer technology during the 1960s. As Saba and Westra (2011) state, the use of computers by nurses was stimulated by questions regarding the applicability of computer technology within health care settings. Increased patient complexity, for example, required nurses to become comfortable reading and interpreting various cardiac monitors and other computerized devices. During the 1970s, computer technology in health care was leveraged to automate various research and reporting elements of the profession. The 1980s brought significant growth in the informatics discipline.

The medical informatics and nursing informatics specialities began to grow and the topic of "informatics" became recognized as a unique discipline within health care.

Stemming from Scholes and Barber's (1980) original definition, there has been significant evolution of the term over the last three decades. Regardless, all definitions of nursing informatics continue to encompass the ideals of information, science, knowledge, and practice (see Figure 25.1 on the next page).

By the early 2000s, the term **eHealth** (electronic health) was commonly used as a catch-all term within the informatics disciplines. The term *eHealth* was subsequently adopted by a number of health care agencies and organizations and is a popular term within the Canadian health care system. Currently, *eHealth* is used synonymously with such terms as *informatics* and *health informatics* within the Canadian context. For the purposes of this chapter, the term *informatics* will be utilized in the context of nursing to describe the evolving science of information, technology, and nursing practice.

Within the nursing informatics discipline, multiple conceptualizations of "technology" exist. For the purposes

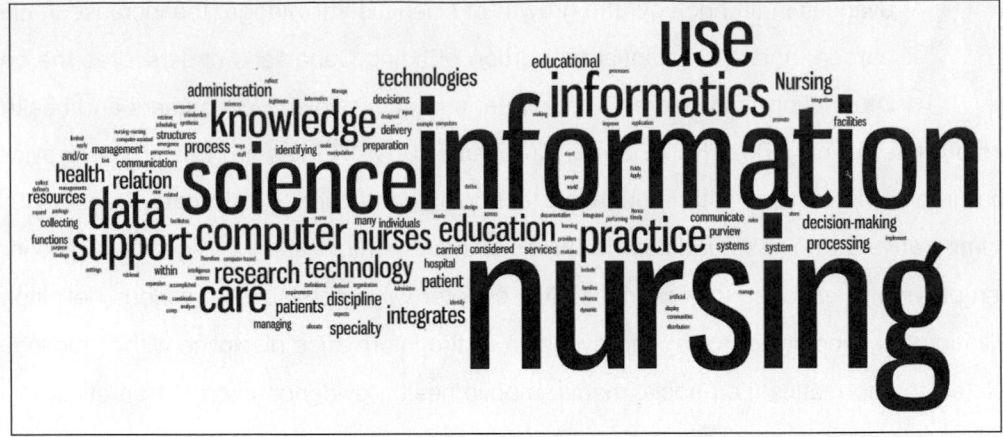

FIGURE 25.1 A word-cloud of aggregated published definitions of "nursing informatics" as listed by Thede (2010) on her website. The size of the text denotes the frequency in which the specific word was used in the definitions. Connecting such words such as "and" and "the" have been removed from the cloud. Thede's listing of nursing informatics definitions encompasses a period from 1980 to 2008. Words such as "information," "science," "practice," and "knowledge" appear to be common threads between different nursing informatics definitions.

Source: Data for the word cloud based on Thede, L. (2010). *Nursing informatics definitions.* Retrieved from http://dlthede.net/Informatics/Chap01Overview/NIDefinitions.html

of this chapter, *technology* will be used in reference to computerized (or microprocessor) systems that are used in the practice, delivery, or management of patient care. Another common term within the health literature is **information and computer technology (ICT)**. Historically, this term has been used to describe various informatics devices, software, hardware, or systems. For instance, a handheld blood pressure machine may be referred to as an ICT device. Similarly, an electronic medical record (EMR) may also be referred to as an ICT device. Given the common use of such terms as *technology* and *ICT* within the nursing informatics discipline, within this chapter *ICT* will be used to refer to computerized technology that is used by nurses in their practice.

Currently, there exists a wide continuum of reactions from nurses and patients when presented with technology in health care. These reactions range from fear and refusal to engagement and optimism. Similarly, the wide-scale penetration of the Internet and mobile technologies into Canadian consumer populations has positively influenced consumer interest and receptivity of informatics within nursing. A study completed by Canada Health Infoway (2007) found that roughly 88% of Canadians supported the use of electronic health records within health care.

Informatics Fundamentals: Data, Information, and Knowledge

To better understand nursing informatics, an explanation of the interrelationships among data, information, and knowledge is required. **Data** are raw observations that have not been interpreted, such as age, weight, blood pressure, number of admissions, and number of workload units. **Information** results when data are interpreted, organized, or structured in a meaningful way. For example, data regarding sex, age, weight, height, lab values, and blood pressure (BP = 120/80 mm Hg) can be interpreted to provide information about risk of cardiovascular disease. **Knowledge** requires synthesis of information to identify relationships that provide fuller understanding of an issue or subject (see Figure 25.2). For example, once raw data are integrated to provide information about fall risk, the nurse's knowledge about care maps or fall-reduction programs, derived from both practice and the nursing literature, allows for evidence-based decisions that advance effective patient care.

These concepts—data, information, and knowledge—can be influenced by nursing informatics applications (e.g., electronic health record [EHR]). Raw data can be collected and stored by using computer systems. Electronic monitoring of vital signs and electrocardiography (ECG) in intensive care units can be recorded directly in the electronic medical record (EMR). Integration of data to provide useful information is demonstrated by the use of aggregated or combined patient data. For example, information on the prevalence of immunizations for a specific disease across communities or the frequency of falls across a given organization can be calculated from incident records embedded into electronic documentation. Knowledge can be enhanced through integration of care maps or **decision-support systems** (e.g., medication administration decision support), which analyze raw data and nursing assessments to suggest nursing diagnoses and recommended interventions. Beyond clinical nursing practice, nursing informatics applications also support data, information, and knowledge integration for education, administration, and research.

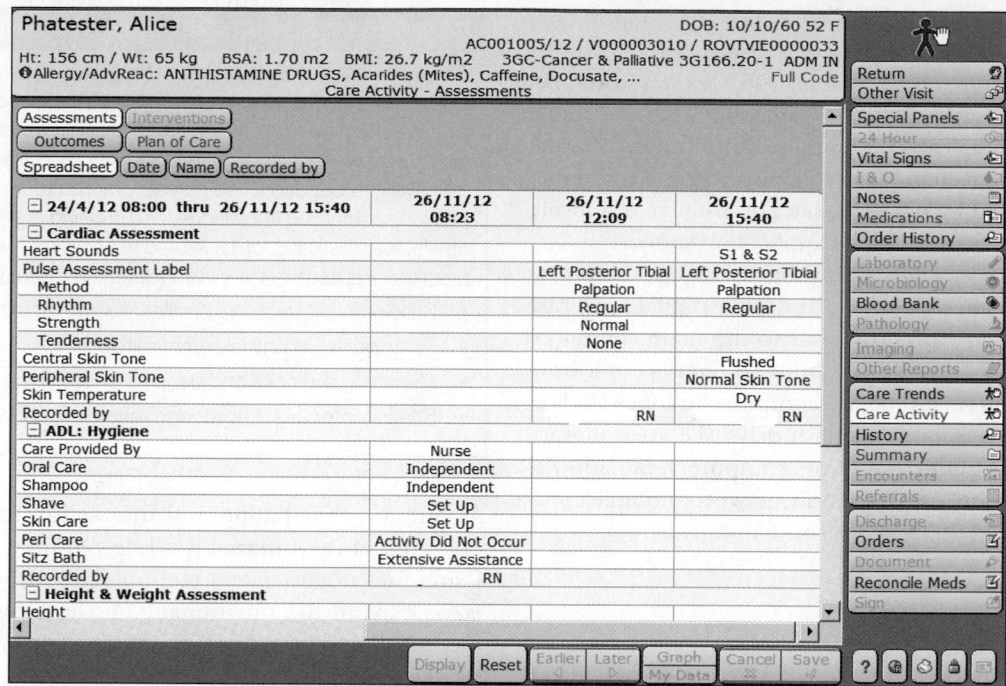

FIGURE 25.2 Both *data* and *information* are presented in this screenshot of the assessments section of a patient's electronic medical record (EMR). *Knowledge* is required on behalf of the nurse to interpret the various data and information contained in this record in order to determine appropriate nursing interventions and actions.

Source: Courtesy of Royal Victoria Regional Health Centre, Barrie, Ontario.

Standardized Languages

To utilize information and knowledge, a common language (e.g., for use in documenting patient care) is required to communicate effectively. Within nursing informatics, the term **standardized language** refers to the use of a body of terms that has been agreed upon by an overarching authority or by general consent (McGonigle & Mastrian, 2012). The International Classification for Nursing Practice (ICNP) is a set of nursing diagnoses, interventions, and outcomes that has been endorsed by the Canadian Nurses Association (CNA) since 2006. In early 2010, a new agreement was struck between the International Council of Nurses (ICNP's authoring body) and the International Healthcare Terminology Standards Development Organisation (IHTSDO) to harmonize standardized languages for use in health information systems. The agreement between the IHTSDO and the International Council of Nurses will help ensure that informatics systems will contain nursing terms and facilitate nursing's involvement in the future development of standardized languages used in health care.

For example, consider the use of standardized languages to describe a pressure ulcer. A "pressure ulcer" might be referred to as a "bed sore" or "decubitus ulcer." If a standardized language is not developed and used to ensure all pressure ulcers are named "pressure ulcers," various ICT systems will be limited in tracking all instances of the condition. Therefore, standardized nursing languages, such as ICNP, are extremely important to ensure the consistency of classification of nursing interventions, outcomes, and phenomena.

Computer Technology and Informatics in Nursing

Nursing informatics is the science and art of using various information and computer technology systems in the caring of patients and their families (IMIA-NI, 2009). Therefore, a basic understanding of some of the various technological components is required to appreciate how informatics can assist patient or client care delivery. All informatics systems use some sort of computerized technology. A computer is a collection of hardware and software that operate together to perform calculations. **Hardware** is a term that is used to describe the physical elements of a computer. For instance, microprocessors, hard drives, random access memory (RAM), and other physical elements of a computer are referred to as *hardware*. **Software** is applications or programs that control computer hardware and, in essence, are instructions that direct a computer's hardware to function. Programs are generally divided into two categories: **system software** and **application software**. System software includes instructions for the initiation (e.g., boot-up), input, output, and storage mechanisms of a computer (McHugh, 2011). Apple's Operating System (OS) X Lion would be an example of system software controlling the operating functions of Apple-based computers. Application software includes programs that allow someone using a computer to perform functions or work tasks. For instance, Microsoft Word would be an example of application software.

Other devices, such as keyboards, mouse, printers, universal serial bus (USB) flash drives, digital cameras, and iPods, can act as peripherals to the main computer device. A peripheral has the ability to connect to a host computer and is reliant on the computer to function. For instance, connecting a USB flash drive (i.e., peripheral) to a laptop computer (i.e., host computer) can allow a user to transfer information easily between multiple computer hosts (e.g., to/from a second laptop).

Internet

As a global network of interconnected computers, the Internet allows people to send and receive information almost instantaneously across geographical distances. According to the Internet World Statistics (2011), over 2 billion people use the Internet globally (1.1 billion Internet users in 2007).

Previously, accessing the Internet was only possible through hardwired connections (e.g., telephone line, broadband cable connection). Over the last decade, access to the Internet via mobile devices has become prevalent worldwide. It is now possible in many locations to access the Internet via handheld mobile devices via cellular or satellite reception. The increased access and immediacy of the Internet has stimulated new areas of opportunity for nursing informatics. Yet, access concerns remain (provincially, and within the northern Canadian territories) in situations where Internet access is limited or nonexistent resulting from a lack of information technology infrastructure or the topography of the area. For more information, see a video listed in the Weblinks section at the end of the chapter.

Web 2.0/Social Media

The first iterations of the **World Wide Web (WWW)** consisted of mostly static webpages that did not offer any real interactive capability. By the early 2000s, web functionality advanced to the point where websites were more user centred and interactive. The rise of *Web 2.0* in the early 2000s provided users the ability to create and generate content, share ideas, and collaborate with others. The emergence of collaborative web platforms, such as blogs, wikis, video sharing sites, and other social networking sites, has ushered in a new phase in the Internet's history; with these platforms, users not only access information from Internet sources but also share their content with others.

BOX 25.1 SOCIAL MEDIA IN NURSING

To explore how social media technologies can be used safely and effectively by nurses, Fraser (2011) developed a comprehensive book to explore the topic. Fraser's work explores how these sorts of technologies can be safely and effectively embedded into a nurses' practice to assist in building networks, obtaining knowledge, and creating quality content for others. Key thematic topics related to social media and nursing practice discussed in this work include the following:

- Building a professional profile, reputation, and network
- Participating in online communities
- Managing the risks and benefits of social media
- Sharing interests, knowledge, and expertise with others

As online participation and interaction increased, this novel use of the Internet was referred to as **social media**. Using the processes and technologies of Web 2.0, *social media* expand the functionality of the Internet through the use of mobile and web-based communication technologies to generate an interactive and user-centric platform for information sharing and social networking. All elements of nursing practice (and particularly educational practice settings) are influenced by connectivity offered by the Internet and related social media technologies. It is important to discuss the significance (and potential impact) of this new communication modality within the context of nursing informatics. (See Box 25.1.)

Electronic Health Records

Electronic health record (EHR) systems permit electronic data retrieval by caregivers, administrators, and other persons who require the data and have authorized access. In November 2002, the Romanow Commission issued the report titled *Building on Values: The Future of Health Care in Canada,* which emphasized the importance of EHR systems as "one of the keys to modernizing Canada's health care system and improving access and outcomes for Canadians" (p. 77). The EHR has been defined as an individual's health record that is accessible online from many separate, interoperable, automated systems within an electronic network. Simply put, the health information collected within the EHR would be accessible (with proper authorization) by many and diverse health care providers, using different EHR systems within Canada. Although the use of the term *EHR* tends to vary between countries, in Canada the EHR, defined by Canada Health Infoway, is:

> a complete health record under the *custodianship* of a health care provider(s) that holds all relevant health information about a person over their lifetime. This is often described as a person-centric health record, which can be used by many approved health care providers or health care organizations. (Hodge, 2011) (See Figure 25.3.).

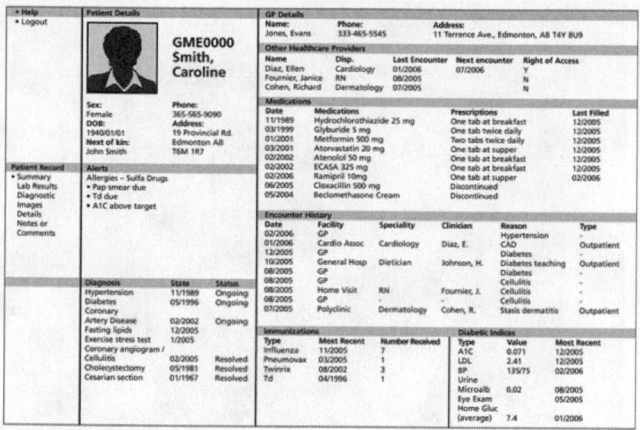

FIGURE 25.3 A screenshot of the proposed EHR interface as outlined by Canada Health Infoway.

Source: 2010 April Report of the Auditor General of Canada, http://www.oag-bvg. gc.ca/internet/English/parl_oag_201004_07_e_33720.html. Office of the Auditor General of Canada. Reproduced with the permission of the Minister of Public Works and Government Services, 2012.

BOX 25.2 COMMON EMR OR EPR FUNCTIONALITY

EMR or EPR systems usually consist of (but are not limited to) the following (Registered Nurses Association of Ontario [RNAO], 2011):

- Client demographics
- Medical history
- Allergy and immunization status
- Laboratory results and trending
- Pharmacy and medication records (including side effects and contraindications)
- Advanced directives
- Diagnostic tests and reports
- Images
- Clinical records, both historic and current

Other commonly used terms for electronic records include **electronic medical record (EMR)** and **electronic patient record (EPR)**. Both the EMR and EPR are essentially the same within the Canadian context, and are often used interchangeably within Canadian literature and policy documents. Unlike the complete health record of the EHR, an EMR or an EPR is a "partial health record under the custodianship of a health care provider(s) that holds a portion of the relevant health information about a person over their lifetime" (Hodge, 2011). In essence, the pan-Canadian EHR is considered a comprehensive record of information of an individual, drawn from various EMR or EPR systems.

Generally, EMRs or EPRs can be found within various clinical and organizational settings. For instance, a nurse practitioner–led clinic may use an EPR to help record and document patient interactions. Similarly, a large hospital organization might also operate an EPR to document all medical and nursing care delivered to a patient. Until the EMR or the EPR replaces paper-based charting and documentation of care delivery, a "hybrid" solution (i.e., the simultaneous use of both paper charts and electronic records) may be used. See Box 25.2 for a list of common functions associated with EMRs and EPRs.

Canada Health Infoway (*Infoway*) is a national, non-profit corporation that was initiated in 2001 to "foster and accelerate the development and adoption of electronic health record (EHR) systems with compatible standards and communications technologies" (Canada Health Infoway, 2011a). *Infoway* is funded by the Government of Canada to strategically invest in EHR-related initiatives across the provinces and territories. In 2006, *Infoway* released a "blueprint" document outlining the components necessary for the interoperable EHR and describing how the components will work together. According to *Infoway*, the creation of a pan-Canadian EHR will attempt to ensure that the various components of the electronic health record system are developed using consistent standards, to allow information and knowledge to flow across jurisdictions (e.g., health information captured in a rural hospital will be easily accessible in an urban health care setting with the proper security and privacy permissions).

Infoway has an invested interest in the effective use of EHRs or ICT adoption by health care professionals that aligns with their mandate to accelerate the development of the EHR within Canada (Canada Health Infoway, 2011a). *Infoway* and the Canadian Association of Schools of Nursing (CASN) have partnered to develop tools and resources for faculty and students related to the development of skill in nursing informatics for students and practising nurses (Canada Health Infoway, 2011b). In addition, health professional practice associations and health care system advisory groups have recognized the need for health care providers who are competent in the use of informatics within nursing (CNA, 2006; Health Council of Canada, 2006). The goal of the *Infoway*/CASN initiative is to develop educational resources and strategies for nursing faculty and students to ensure graduates develop competencies in informatics within nursing. As well, the RNAO (2011) has created a number of resources related to nursing and eHealth for practising nurses.

Other health technologies also work in conjunction with the EMR/EPR and are used to collect, organize, or manage different types of health information. For instance, a **computer provider order entry (CPOE)** system allows a clinician or provider to enter treatment and medication orders electronically. Orders that are entered electronically are received at their respective destinations (e.g., pharmacy for medication orders) within the health care organization (e.g., hospital) for processing and delivery. CPOE systems have the potential to reduce medication errors caused by handwriting illegibility and have been found to assist in decreasing certain prescribing and medication errors. However, Koppel Metlay, Cohen, Abaluck, Localio, Kimmel, and Strom (2005) demonstrated that such a system also brought to light new types of medication error potential. Another example of an application software system that integrates with an EMR/EPR is a **picture and archiving communication system (PACS)**. PACS allows digital images to be securely transferred and accessed by multiple health care providers. Previously, all medical imaging were physically transferred and interpreted on film. Interpretation of medical imagery can now occur remotely from the origin of the image, thus reducing time required between assessment and diagnosis.

Care documentation is also supported using EMRs or EPRs. Documentation electronically is commonly referred to as **electronic documentation** or *electronic charting.* This catch-all term is used to describe how nurses and other health care providers capture, transcribe, and add information to a patient's electronic record. As stated by the RNAO (2011), the term *electronic documentation* is a misnomer—documentation principles completed electronically are the same as documentation on paper (see Chapter 24). In advanced EMR/EPR systems, documentation can take on a number of different activities from narrative charting, vital signs trending (e.g., graphical representation of vital sign fluctuation over a period), and other standardized outcome assessments of client functioning (e.g., Resident Assessment Index, or C-HOBIC [page 538]).

Finally, patients can undergo diagnostic procedures in which ICT can play a significant role. Computed tomography (CT) scans, magnetic resonance imaging (MRI), and positron emission tomography (PET) scans use computers to perform tests and analyze findings. Blood gas analyzers, pulmonary function test machines, and intracranial pressure monitors can sometimes be linked to store data in the EMR or the EPR.

Telehealth

Telehealth refers to the use of ICT to support health care, services, and expertise over any geographical distance. For instance, in Ontario, the Ontario Telemedicine Network (OTN) operates a province-wide two-way videoconferencing telehealth network that connects over 1175 sites across the province (OTN, 2011). To date, as one of the largest telehealth networks in the world, OTN delivers over 135 000 patient "visits" per year. Patient assessments, educational workshops, and other consultations can be conducted via the OTN, thus saving patients and their families the financial and logistical burden of travel over large geographical distances to obtain health care consultation. For example,

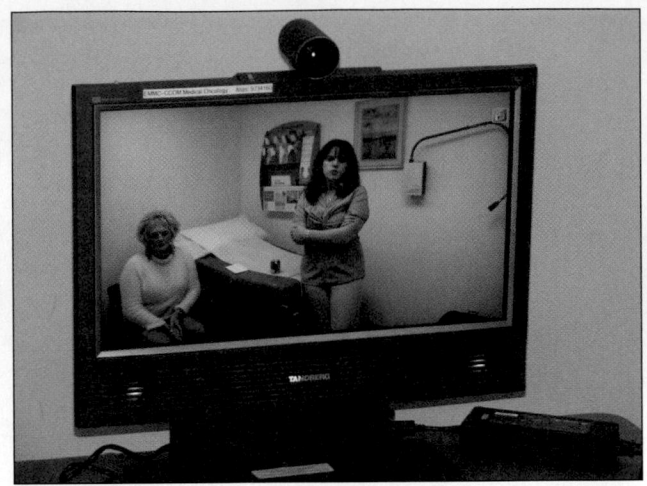

FIGURE 25.4 Consumers and clinicians are able to consult using telehealth technology in the form of a video conference.
Source: Courtesy of the U.S. Department of Agriculture.

using videoconferencing, an interprofessional team can examine and consult from kilometres away, especially in rural or remote areas where resources and expertise are scarce (see Figure 25.4). Telehealth can be used in (a) teleconsultation, teleimaging, and telepsychiatry, (b) education and training in health disciplines, such as telelearning and telementoring, (c) health information transfer for health care providers, and (d) health care information for clients. (See Box 25.3 for more benefits.)

REMOTE MONITORING Telehealth technologies can also support various types of remote monitoring of patients in their households. Various stand-alone devices (e.g., blood pressure monitor, glucometer, weight scale, etc.) can be connected to either a telephone line, mobile connection, or the Internet to automatically transmit data to authorized specialists or clinicians managing the patient's care. In the study by Logan et al. (2007), remote monitoring of patients' blood pressure was accomplished by synchronizing a Bluetooth-enabled home blood pressure monitor with a cellular phone. Blood pressure readings from the monitor were automatically sent to a data centre for processing by a case manager caring for the specific client.

BOX 25.3 BENEFITS OF TELEHEALTH

Telehealth can offer new ways to assist in improving health care of remote patients. For instance, telehealth can do the following:

- Help ensure continuity of client care
- Reduce geographical barriers to care
- Allow for collaboration among health care team members
- Potentially increase client involvement in care
- Act as a distance education tool

Point of Care Technology

Point of care (POC) technology and devices can assist nurses in collecting and documenting data at or near the location of care. For instance, computer tablets and mobile technologies are commonly used in home care to assist nurses in documenting or recording patient information at patients' homes. Similarly, within hospital settings, POC technologies can include various devices like digital or tympanic thermometers; digital scales; pulse oximetry; ECG; telemetry; hemodynamic monitoring; apnea monitors; fetal heart monitors; blood glucose analyzers; ventilators; and intravenous (IV) pumps. Some of these devices can transmit data to more sophisticated systems (e.g., EMR or EPR) or interact with the user via digital displays. Most POC technologies include error detection, warnings that the instrument is malfunctioning or that the assessed value is outside predetermined parameters. These devices can act to extend the nurse's observations and supply reliable health status related data.

Portals

Portals are websites that allow a user to view information that is personalized and/or relevant to their role. For instance, the social networking site Facebook is a type of Internet portal—upon authenticating, Facebook users are able to personalize their online presence with various feeds, friends, and images. Health care portals are similar in many respects. Patient portals include a type of technology that allows an individual patient (or sometimes their family) to log into a hospital information system to view certain elements of their treatment or care (i.e., lab values, rebook appointments) (McGonigle & Mastrian, 2012). Similarly, portals can also act as a technology link, connecting two or more various ICT systems together. Portal technology can enable a user to securely access information from two or more discrete sources (i.e., two different EMR systems) (see Box 25.4).

The **NurseONE portal**, released in 2006, was developed by the CNA to provide nurses with "timely, easily

accessible information on all aspects of health care—from public health alerts, to consultations with experts and health specialists, to best practices" (Canadian Healthcare Technology, 2006). As a bilingual, web-based health information service designed for Canadian nurses, a goal of NurseONE is to be a gateway for information and resources to assist health care professionals in all domains of practice—direct care, education, administration, research, and policy. Currently, users of the portal have access to professional practice resources, a comprehensive electronic library and *NurseConnect*, a forum for nurses to connect and discuss areas of interest and expertise (CNA, 2011).

mHealth and Mobile Technology

Recently, there has been a rise in the use of mobile technology and mobile health (**mHealth**) within health care. According to investigations by Juniper Research (as cited in Royston, 2011) it is expected that downloading of mobile health care applications for both tablets and smartphones will reach 44 million by 2012. Similarly, the research organization estimates that by 2016, the desire for mobile health care applications will meet or exceed 142 million downloads.

As an example of an mHealth application, researchers from the Abramson Center for the Future Health (2011) created an interactive smartphone called *Azmo the Dragon*. As part of the game, the child plays "Azmo," a fire-breathing dragon. By regularly testing their lung capacity using the digital spirometer connected to the phone, children are able to "power Azmo the Dragon in the game" and also "record their lung capacity regularly over time so it can be monitored by parents and doctors." The game is customizable for each child and also will have the ability to interlink with current weather and atmospheric data (e.g., pollen, pollution) to assist the child in making appropriate health-related choices to minimize asthma triggers.

Similarly, more nurses are using **mobile technologies** to support health care delivery. Doran et al. (2010) found that nurses ($n = 488$), by using **personal digital assistant (PDA)** and tablet technologies at the point-of-care, accessed drug and medical reference information most frequently during practice. Other information sources included mobile versions of best practice guidelines and the search engine Google.

How Nurses Are Currently Using Technology

Education

As outlined in this chapter, nursing informatics is a core competency within nursing practice. Nagle (2007), a champion of nursing informatics within Canada,

---

> **BOX 25.4   PATIENT PORTAL AT SUNNYBROOK HEALTH SCIENCES CENTRE**
>
> Sunnybrook Health Sciences Centre in Toronto uses a patient portal to provide patients access to elements of their health and medical records. Currently, the portal provides patients the ability to grant specific access to family caregivers or other related health care organizations and agencies (e.g., family physician, pharmacists). Patients using the portal are able to access various elements surrounding their health records, including lab results, clinic notes, and other personalized health information. Similarly, patients are also able to electronically submit appointment requests, medication refill requests, and send electronic messages to clinicians involved in their ongoing care.

advocates for informatics-embedded undergraduate nursing curricula, as opposed to a stand-alone course. A functional understanding of informatics across the educational spectrum is important in order to remain competent within the profession.

Within nursing education, there are a number of integration points for nursing informatics that have been explored over the years. The increased use of high fidelity simulation mannequins, handheld devices within clinical practicum, virtual nursing environments, and the use of Internet-enabled technologies are just a few examples of commonly used informatics technologies within education.

Over the last decade the use of computer-conferencing systems (e.g., WebCT, Blackboard, Moodle) has become commonplace within the education sector. Similarly, e-mail and the use of electronic scholarly resources (e.g., electronic journal articles, e-books) has become standard in schools around Canada. Many schools offer distance education courses mediated through computer-conferencing and other videoconferencing platforms. For instance, the Ontario Primary Health Care Nurse Practitioner consortium (consisting of nine universities in Ontario) delivers online classes to over 150 nurse practitioner students on various topics using the web-conferencing system Elluminate. The professor leading the class is able to present a slideshow, complete with voice narration, and has the ability to send and receive text messages from students. Dr. Sandra Bassendowski, a professor at the University of Saskatchewan, used the social networking tool Ning© in a fourth year nursing course to generate a dynamic and interactive environment for students to share ideas and experiences. Along with using Ning, she has also created a paperless classroom underpinned by the Canadian Nurses Association NurseONE Portal (http://www.usask.ca/nursing/research/profiles/bassendowski.php).

Research

Nursing research has been heavily influenced by informatics over the last few decades. From data analysis software packages to assist researchers in analyzing quantitative and qualitative data (e.g., SPSS, NVivo), to new methods of data collection via electronically aggregated data, informatics within the research realm has significant potential to improve patient care and practice. Research databases like the Cumulative Index for Nursing and Allied Health Literature (CINAHL) provide nurses ease of access to research information to inform practice. Similarly, the Cochrane Collaboration and other evidence-informed databases have reduced access and geographical barriers for nurses seeking research evidence.

With the increased use of Internet and related technologies, new areas of research have begun to arise within health care. The use of socially generated or aggregated knowledge has generated an interesting approach to

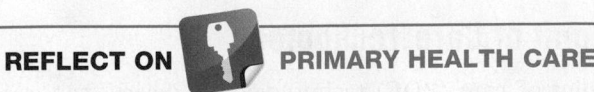

REFLECT ON **PRIMARY HEALTH CARE**

Primary health care has also seen an increase in the use of various technologies to support the health of individuals and communities. Currently, Ottawa Public Health uses Twitter to broadcast information related to health to its 6600+ (as of January 2012) followers.

Source: Twitter feed found at http://twitter.com/ottawahealth

examining public health issues. For instance, Chew and Eysenbach (2010) discovered that the microblogging system Twitter supported health information delivery during the 2009 H1N1 flu pandemic outbreak (see the Reflect on Primary Health Care box). In their study, they found that messages posted via Twitter could be used to disseminate health-related information from credible sources. Similarly, the authors indicated that Twitter may be useful in assisting public health personnel in tracking real-time developments associated with such situations as pandemics or natural disasters.

The Health Outcomes for Better Information and Care (HOBIC) is an initiative originally developed by the Ontario Ministry of Health and Long-Term Care to collect nursing sensitive outcomes related to patient care. As of 2007, HOBIC became a national initiative, called HOBIC (C-HOBIC). C-HOBIC allows nurses to collect information related to the impact nurses make on patients suffering from pain, fatigue, dyspnea, and nausea. Other outcomes measured in the HOBIC initiative include pressure ulcers, falls, continence, activities of daily living, and readiness for discharge. For more information, visit http://www2.cna-aiic.ca/c-hobic/about/default_e.aspx.

Administration

Informatics applied to an administration setting can streamline processes that were once difficult and time consuming. For instance, streamlining patient referral processes is a significant issue in parts of Canada (e.g., Resource Matching and Referrals Project, eHealth Ontario). Interoperable informatics systems can assist clinicians and administration in terms of matching patients to appropriate resources in the community. Similarly, wait times for various procedures can be captured in real time allowing administration and leadership to make decisions regarding resource allocation (e.g., staff, finances, human resources, etc.). (See Box 25.5.)

Practice

The clinical application of informatics in the direct provision of care include the use of EMRs or EPRs, order entry, decision support, reporting systems, e-mail, Internet, phones, and fax machines that act in support of

BOX 25.5 INFORMATICS ADMINISTRATION: WAIT TIMES NOW AVAILABLE ONLINE IN SOME PROVINCES

Many provinces now publish wait time listings for various common medical procedures online. From these websites, consumers and patients can view up to date wait times for various services at specific hospitals and organizations.

See, for example, the following sites:

- http://www.health.gov.on.ca/en/public/programs/waittimes
- http://waittimes.alberta.ca

BOX 25.6 HOW ONE HOME CARE AGENCY USES HANDHELD DEVICES

Saint Elizabeth Health Care, a home care agency in Canada, recently issued BlackBerry smartphones to its clinicians in an effort to equip "them with valuable tools to enable real time communication and enhance the client experience through automated data collection and increased flexibility" (Saint Elizabeth, 2010). Using software built in to the phone, nurses and clinicians are able to send and receive messages, manipulate care schedules, track mileage expenditures through global positioning (GPS) functionality, and securely access client records.

clinical decision making. Handheld, point-of-care devices and other devices like laptops, computer terminals, and monitoring systems will collect raw data that is eventually fed into a clinical informatics system. Nurses play a key role and are vital to ensuring the collection, input, and validation of data entered into clinical informatics systems. Some informatics systems will capture individual patients' data and aggregate or combine it to form unit or organizational level information on health trends among patients, or to assess if there has been an increase in preventable situations, such as falls or medication errors. See Box 25.6 for one example of how a health care agency uses handheld devices to improve client care.

Using Evidence-Informed Nursing Practice in ICT

Clinical Knowledge Translation

Chapter 3 outlines the significance of research evidence in support of *evidence-informed* nursing practice. In evidence-informed nursing practice, the nurse considers the available research literature in determining best care practices within the life context of the client. In addition to the research literature, consideration is given to the availability of fiscal, material, or human resources and to personal clinical expertise. Clinical decision making regarding

client care constitutes an intersection of multiple information sources (e.g., clinical expertise, patient preference for alternative forms of care, clinical research evidence, and available resources). DiCenso, Cullum, and Cilisko (1998) illustrated the intersection of these information sources in considering, for example, clinical expertise in determining clients' status to tolerate an intervention supported by research evidence, and the patient's preference to accept or decline treatment, mitigated by the resources available.

Nurses working today are expected to deal with overwhelming sources and amounts of information in order to provide "evidence-informed" health care. Foundational to the evidence-informed clinical decision-making processes are information literacy skills. **Information (digital) literacy** is a term that captures the proficiencies of knowing, identifying, finding and organizing, evaluating, and using information (e.g., critical evaluation of and production of new knowledge) that advance research skills and critical thinking (Mackey & Ho, 2005). Information literacy has become an important topic for nurses in providing evidence-informed care. For nurses, this involves critical thinking, an awareness of personal and professional ethics, information evaluation, conceptualizing information needs that address the existing context of health care (e.g., clinical expertise, access to resources, research evidence, client preference), organizing information, and interacting with other information professionals (Bruce, 1999).

Digital transition is a phrase that refers to the movement of significant professional and scholarly information from paper to digital form (Bawden & Robinson, 2009). Increasingly, greater availability of online information has highlighted the need for media, computer, and digital literacies (information literacy components) that allow nurses to access and evaluate web-based materials (Mackey & Ho, 2005). Nurses currently practise in complex information environments characterized by greater amounts of available information, in a variety of formats, and accessible through diverse media and communication channels.

Media literacy is defined as the application of critical thinking in assessing information gained from the mass media: television, radio, newspapers and magazines, and (increasingly) the Internet. A media-literate person can evaluate, analyze, and produce both print and electronic media (Aufderheide & Firestone 1993). Within contemporary health care, information (digital) literacy involves the development of a critical approach to *accessing* (e.g., distinguishing between information and knowledge; not being content with the first six "hits" on a search; managing the "multimedia flow"; an awareness of other people and our ability to contact them [online networks] to get information and help), *assessing* (e.g., asking key questions about the information source and the assumptions contained within; assessing the usefulness, timeliness, accuracy and integrity of information; questioning/checking answers provided by technology tools; judging validity and completeness of material referenced by hypertext links), and *using* information (Bawden, 2001; Eysenbach, 2008).

Youth and Adults

Computer and Internet-based programs are increasingly available for children and adults to learn everything from a foreign language to algebra. There are many issues of concern related to frequent and extended use of computers by all ages. In particular, repetitive motion injuries (especially of the hand) can occur with extensive typing and use of the computer mouse, eye strain can occur from computer monitor viewing, and musculoskeletal damage is related to inadequate ergonomic arrangement of desk chairs, surface height, and monitor placement. Students and adults who use computers daily should be thoroughly evaluated and instructed in the prevention of these conditions. Parents need to be reminded of potential risks to children from Internet contact with strangers and adult-only websites. They also need to monitor schoolchildren's use of computers to ensure they are not being sidetracked from homework into computer games and messaging. All persons should be wary about protecting their financial and personal information when conducting business via the computer. Similarly, there has been an increase in the prevalence of online bullying or "cyber bullying" among youth (i.e., using electronic media like the Internet, e-mail, and social networking sites to harass, threaten, or embarrass others) (Mishna, Saini, & Solomon, 2009). It has been found by Mitchell, Ybarra, and Finkelhor (2007) that a large majority of youth who are victimized by cyber bullying do not disclose the experiences to their parents.

OLDER ADULTS

Computer skills and competency classes are being taught to increasing numbers of older adults. Use of the computer can provide older adults with an avenue of communication and exposure to a vast amount of health care information. Although nurses have little control over which Internet sites will be accessed, it is important to teach clients and the general public to evaluate information from the site and to be aware that misinformation can also be presented. Important guidelines that increase the validity of a site are as follows:

- The article or information lists the author and credentials and/or the institution from which the information came.
- A date is listed that states when information was updated.
- If health care information is presented, a disclaimer should be included. The disclaimer presents limitations of the information and should say that it is not medical advice.

Computer and Internet resources can be very effective teaching aids for older adults. They may provide audiovisual instruction and may even be interactive. They are useful for teaching about medical conditions and medications and for providing information about procedures and surgeries to be performed.

Experts have expressed concern that Internet use and access to information is *inequitable*, that is, Internet use and information access are not fairly balanced in relation to gender, age, income, and education (see the Lifespan Considerations box on youth and adults). There is a tendency for individuals who are seniors and have lower education and limited income to have less skill in accessing

and assessing online information. This becomes particularly troubling given that government, business or corporation, and public information is increasingly accessible via the Internet (Balka, Rodje, & Bush, 2007). Beyond the skill limitations described above, many Canadians remain limited in their ability to access online information if living in rural and remote areas or for Canadians who have limited bandwidth.

Bandwidth refers to the amount of information that can be transmitted and is an important variable in determining access to online information. Within some of Canada's most remote communities (e.g., Aboriginal communities) 36% have high-speed Internet access, 55% rely on dial-in access, and 7% of communities have no Internet access (Aboriginal Canada Portal, 2005). Nurses practising in rural and remote Canadian communities tend to have fewer clinical resources and geographically distant relationships with colleagues (MacLeod, Kulig, Stewart, Pitblado, & Knock, 2004).

Roles in Nursing Informatics

All nurses function in an informatics role. Nurses are in instrumental positions within the health care system to develop and improve ICT used in clinical delivery. Specialized roles within the nursing and health care professions have evolved over the last two decades in order to ensure the advancement of the informatics discipline within health care. **Nurse informaticians** (also known as *informatics nurses*) are nurses who have specialized knowledge and skills within the informatics discipline (McGonigle & Mastrian, 2012). Many nurse informaticians undertake graduate preparation in management, leadership, informatics, and practice elements to prepare for the complexity of their roles. Within many health care and hospital organizations, a clinical informatics department will typically include a number of nurse informaticians working to develop and maintain ICT components housed within their health care setting. Current educational avenues within Canada to obtain specialized knowledge in health informatics include self-directed courses, college diplomas, undergraduate specialization, and graduate preparation.

How Technology Influences Humans and How Humans Influence Technology

Discussions of nursing informatics tend to focus heavily on the technology. Technology is sometimes described as a panacea or a "cure-all" within health care. It is not uncommon to hear statements such as "The technology will solve our issues" or "The computers will improve how nurses perform their roles." This is an example of **technological determinism**—a perspective that identifies *technology* as the primary actor in social changes (Croteau & Hoynes, 2003). In many respects, a balanced approach is required when examining how the social elements of nursing mix with the technological elements of informatics. A sociotechnical perspective entertains a dynamic relationship between how humans and technology interact within an environment (Berg, Aarts, & Vander Lei, 2003). Rather than viewing and evaluating an informatics or ICT system as an isolated entity, a sociotechnical perspective would evaluate the ICT performance within the context in which it operates. ICT can only be understood within the larger environment that includes nurses, consumers, health care professionals, and support staff, leading to a more holistic (and accurate) understanding of how informatics functions.

Development, Implementation, and Evaluation of Clinical Informatics

The development, implementation, and evaluation of informatics are a complex and multifaceted process. Regardless of the size, breadth, or scope of an informatics implementation, there are many individuals involved in the process.

To begin, an organization requires a readiness assessment of nurses and their practice setting (e.g., unit/organization) to determine whether key factors are in place to support the use of ICT. Perhaps the most important question within a readiness assessment is to address the "rationale" for the proposed ICT. Similarly, it is important to also explore how the proposed ICT would influence or impact client care, clinicians, staff, and other organizational processes. Cost, licensing, maintenance fees, regulatory policies, and other system integration attributes must be thoroughly explored. Staff and clinician readiness must be purposefully and carefully addressed. Although the Internet and other related technologies are commonplace in practice, some informatics technologies may present as difficult or intimidating to some staff. Therefore, ascertaining the staff and clinicians, readiness in terms of both knowledge and technical competency is a prerequisite to implementing any kind of ICT system.

Implementation of clinical informatics (e.g., EMR or EPR) can be a daunting task. Combined with significant preplanning, a project team of clinicians and informaticians are generally brought together to develop an implementation plan for the practice environment. Since the use of ICT in nursing produces a substantial change

in work patterns and relationships, attending to the elements of social change is extremely important. Bridges (2003) stated, "Before you can begin something new, you have to end what used to be . . . the problem is, people don't like endings" (p. 23). Therefore, possessing a firm understanding of change management and leadership skills is important in all informatics implementations.

Workflow or Nursing Practice Process

Nowhere is the understanding of process and change management as vitally important as in the issue of workflow. **Workflow** is a term used to describe a process of interconnected steps that depict an action or behaviour. For instance, an example of workflow within nursing might include a nurse distributing medications to his or her patients. The workflow process of this action would include the following:

1. Having access to the medication from a centralized medication cart
2. Performing the "Ten Rights of Medication Administration" while cross-comparing with the written orders on the medication Kardex
3. Walking to the client's room with the medications in a small plastic basket
4. Obtaining a cup of water prior to entering client's room
5. Checking the identity of the client on their attached ID band around their wrist and reiterating the "Ten Rights of Medication Administration"
6. Asking the client if he or she has any questions regarding the prescribed medications
7. Observing the client taking the medications
8. Mobilizing to the nursing station and documenting the medication administration in the client's chart

As seen in the example above, much of what the nurse "does" to complete the action of administering medications to the client is often accomplished without conscious thought. This type of knowledge, also known as **tacit knowledge**, is extremely difficult to evaluate or make explicit. When informatics and ICT systems are implemented into a practice area that has not previously used these innovations, issues can arise due to the "changes" that occur in the pre-established nursing workflow processes.

Let us review a situation in which a computerized provider order entry (CPOE) system was implemented in a clinical environment to automate the ordering and delivering of medications (Cheung, Goldstein, Geller, & Levitt, 2003) (see Figure 25.5 on the next page). The developers of the CPOE system conceptualized the workflow of medication administration as a linear process (i.e., physician → pharmacist → unit clerk → nurse). Not surprisingly, the

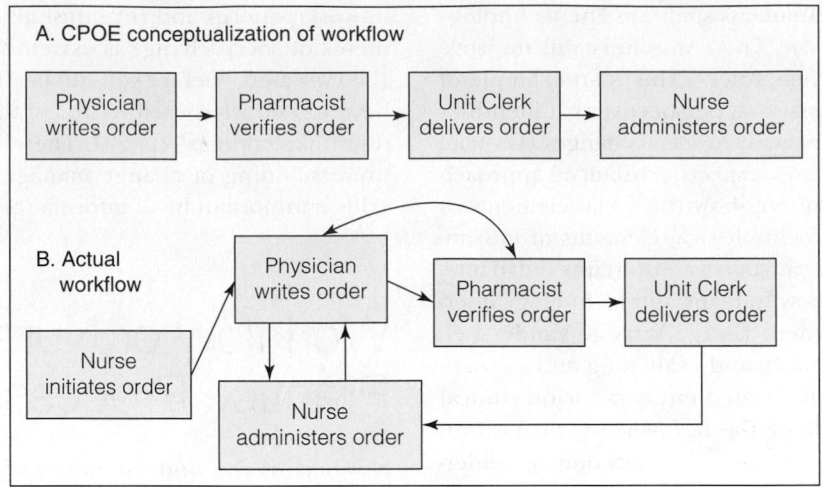

FIGURE 25.5 A demonstration of how workflow can be altered by the implementation of ICT can be observed in this example, from Cheung et al. (2003).

Source: From "The effects of CPOE on ICU workflow: an observational study," by C.H. Cheng, M.K. Goldstein, E. Geller, and R.E. Levitt. *AMIA Annu Symp Proc. 2003*; 2003: 150–154.

actual workflow of medication administration did not subscribe to a linear pathway; rather, the actual workflow was much more nurse-dependent than originally thought (see "Actual Workflow" Figure 25.5). Subsequently, the conceptualized CPOE workflow processes needed to be altered as it quickly became apparent that physicians were rarely the primary initiator of medication orders on this particular unit.

Therefore, it is important that nurses be involved in the planning, development, and implementation of ICT used in practice. As clearly outlined in the example above, the practice realities of nursing were not considered in the original conceptualization of the medication administration process. Operationalizing nurses' clinical knowledge and possessing an understanding of informatics may assist in developing better and more functional ICT to support client care.

Consumers' Health Informatics and Online Information Access

According to Statistics Canada (2011), in 2010, nearly 80% of Canadian households had access to the Internet and many used multiple devices to go online. North Americans increasingly use the Internet as a tool for improved access to health information and health care. In fact, the widespread availability of the Internet has dramatically opened public access to health and medical information that was previously the domain of expert knowledge (Anderson, Rainey, & Eysenbach, 2003; Cline & Haynes, 2001; Welch-Cline, 2003). This rise in online information seeking is not unexpected given the increased diffusion and popularity of tablets, smartphones, laptops, and other Internet-capable devices, which are becoming commonplace in

Canada. Regardless, as outlined by Valaitis and Ferguson (2008), despite the availability of the Internet, nurses should not assume that *everyone* has access to or is willing to use the Internet to access information and/or services. The Canadian Radio-television and Telecommunications Commission (CRTC) has forecasted that by the end of 2015 all Canadians will have broadband Internet access (including those living in rural and remote areas). Despite promised access based on technology infrastructure, the 2010 Canadian Internet Use Survey reported that of the one-fifth (21%) of households without home Internet access, over one-half (56%) reported they had no need for or interest in it. Other reasons for lack of Internet access included the cost of Internet service or computer equipment (20%) or the lack of a device, such as a computer (15%). About 12% of households reported they lacked the confidence, knowledge, or skills to support technology use. Limited household income persists in restricting access to technology or the Internet. A survey of health information and the Internet reported that more than one-third of Canadian adults used the Internet to search for health information in 2005 (Underhill & McKeown, 2008). Almost 6 of every 10 (58%) home Internet users went online at some point within 2005 to search for health information. A relatively high proportion of these "health users" were women, with higher levels of education and income.

The use of the Internet to search for health information appears to be unevenly distributed among Canadians. Searching for health information online is an example of what has been described as a *second-level digital divide* among Internet users. Canadians with the lowest health-literacy skills were found to be more than 2.5 times as likely to describe their health as fair or poor relative to Canadians with excellent literacy skills (Canadian Council on Learning [CCL], 2008). Similarly, these individuals were also more than 2.5 times as likely to be receiving income support (CCL, 2008). Hirji (2004) has noted that barriers to accessing health information and services are associated with low literacy levels and limited technological skills, particularly among older adults. These systemic barriers mean that certain Canadians cannot access online health or other resources related to important determinants of health (e.g., education, and employment) (Middleton & Sorensen, 2006).

Currently, contemporary models of health care advocate for a client-centred model that places increased responsibility for self–health care with the individual. Health education, a component of client-centred care, requires a skill set that enables access to and comprehension of health educational material. However, many Canadians do not have the necessary literacy skills to understand and use reading, writing, speaking, and other forms of communication to meaningfully participate in these important health care discussions (Statistics Canada, 2003). General literacy skills include prose, document, and numeric literacy. According to the most recent International Adult Literacy and Life Skills Survey (Statistics Canada), almost half of Canadian adults do not have the prose or numeric literacy skills needed for daily functioning, and nearly 20% cannot perform simple mathematical tasks. Older adults have even poorer skills: 27% of individuals aged 56 to 65 years and 52% of those aged 66 years and older have difficulty with basic reading.

Fundamental to effective use of health information is literacy and health literacy skill (Nutbeam, 2000; Calgary Charter on Health Literacy, 2008). **Health literacy** is defined as the degree to which a person has the capacity to obtain, interpret, and understand basic health-related information and to make appropriate health care decisions (Nutbeam, 2000; Calgary Charter on Health Literacy, 2008). Low levels of literacy constitute a major barrier to accessing and using health information to make informed health decisions. Canada has a significant percentage of adults (60%) who lack the skills to manage their health literacy needs with the most vulnerable being seniors (ages 66 years and older); immigrants, especially those who do not speak either French or English; and people who are not employed (CCL, 2008). Without adequate health literacy skills, ill-informed decisions may be made, health conditions may go undetected or worsen, and people may get lost in the health care system (CCL, 2008). Given the increasing role of the Internet as a primary source of information about health and medical topics, health literacy constitutes a significant health care issue for nurses and clients.

Nursing Informatics in Canada

In the CNA (2006) *e-Nursing Strategy for Canada* position paper, it is purported that "ICT is no longer an add-on to traditional methods of health care, but rather an integrated, integral part of practice" (p. 10). This report has highlighted the significance of information technology within contemporary health care and advocates for system changes to support quality nursing practice (CNA, 2006). As part of the CNA's strategic direction for the future, they propose three directions (i.e., Access, Competency, Participation) nurses need to undertake to ensure informatics is embedded into the culture and practice of nursing in Canada.

The authors of the report encourage organizations to provide "access" to broadband Internet and other necessary ICT to nurses to support practice (see the Evidence-Informed Practice box on online communities of practice). Similarly, the CNA advocates that informatics-related "competency" be improved for continuing education and also embedded into nursing undergraduate and graduate curricula. Finally, the CNA suggests that

---

EVIDENCE-INFORMED PRACTICE

Do Online Communities of Practice Facilitate Knowledge Exchange?

In this study it was found that community health nurses (CHN) working with vulnerable homeless populations were able to use an online community for knowledge exchange. The researchers in the study developed an online community of practice (CoP) that would provide CHNs a secure online space to create discussion threads, collaborate on best practices, and connect geographically dispersed members. The CoP also provided CHNs enrolled in the study the ability to participate in asynchronous discussions of current trends and issues. Interestingly, the researchers found that the type and intensity of CoP use varied between participants. Using Q-methodology, the authors were able to identify two different thematically related user groups—(a) *tacit knowledge warriors* and (b) *tacit knowledge communicators*. *Warriors* believed the CoP could be used for political awareness purposes and the validation of nursing practice considerations. The *communicators* were neutral regarding the emancipatory elements espoused by the *warriors*, stating that they wished the CoP was more interactive in regards to having their questions promptly answered, enabled by a discussion facilitator. All participants agreed that the CoP would be valuable tool to share information, knowledge, and experiences with other CHNs.

NURSING IMPLICATIONS: The authors of this study highlight the potential value of online CoP within the CHN role. Similarly, this study examined not only the functionality of the technology but also other various sociotechnical responses by CHNs (i.e., *warriors, communicators*) emerging through their participation and use of the online CoP. This deeper level examination of a health ICT system reinforces the importance to consider the ongoing and evolving relationship between humans and technology—not all users of technology will react or "use" the ICT in the same fashion, as evidenced in this study.

Source: Based on Valaitis, R. K., Akhtar-Danesh, N., Brooks, F., Binks, S., & Semogas, D. (2011). Online communities of practice as a communication resource for community health nurses working with homeless persons. *Journal of Advanced Nursing, 67*(6), 1273–1284. doi: 10.1111/j.1365-2648.2010.05582.x

BOX 25.7 LIST OF CANADIAN NURSING INFORMATICS ORGANIZATIONS

Below is a list of Canadian nursing informatics organizations:

Canadian Nursing Informatics Association (CNIA)	http://cnia.ca
Saskatchewan Nursing Informatics Group (SNIA)	http://cnia.ca/SNIA.html
Manitoba Nursing Informatics Association (MNIA)	http://www.mnia.ca
Ontario Nursing Informatics Group (ONIG)	http://www.onig.on.ca
Quebec—Association québécoise des infirmières et infirmiers en systèmes et technologies de l'information (AQIISTI)	http://cnia.ca/AQIISTI.html
New Brunswick Nursing Informatics Group (NBNIG)	http://www.nbnig-giinb.ca
Nova Scotia Nursing Informatics Group (NSNIG)	http://www.nsnig.ca

"participation" is a key determinant to improving nursing practice in the presence of ICT solutions. The report positions nursing education and nurse educators as pivotal players in advancing nursing knowledge and skill through the planned incorporation of ICT competencies within undergraduate and graduate education programs (CNA, 2006). As a knowledge-dependent profession, nurses are in key positions to influence the development and implementation of ICT into clinical practice to improve both care management and delivery. Box 25.7 lists nursing informatics organizations in Canada.

Professional Issues

As society becomes connected through various ICT and Internet-related technologies, nurses must be aware of the evolving professional practice responsibilities. Although informatics provides immense opportunities for collaboration, sharing, and exchange, care must be taken to ensure the anonymity of patients and their information.

Professionalism within a digitally connected world is essentially no different from that in a noncomputerized world. That said, the *context* in which professionalism operates within nursing and health care has changed. Unlike a decade ago, mobile devices, high-speed wireless Internet, and digital cameras were not prevalent within nursing populations. Currently, many of these mobile and Internet-connected devices are readily available within clinical environments or personally owned by the nurse. Similarly, with the increased use of social media technologies, the blurring of personal and professional roles has become a salient topic within nursing practice.

In 2010, the Canadian Nurses Protection Society (CNPS) released a legal information notice for nurses regarding social media use within the profession. The CNPS stated that "[p]rofessional practice standards may be applicable when nurses use social media in connection with their professional activities and require nurses to display professional conduct towards both patients and colleagues" and that "breach of professional standards . . . could also be a breach of privacy legislation" (p. 1). Therefore, it is important that nurses uphold the same professional standards of practice in the online world as in the physical realm. In some respects, the blurring between nurses' online presence (e.g., on Facebook, Twitter, LinkedIn) and their physical representation is quickly becoming "one and the same." Therefore, any online activity by nurses may be held and scrutinized if deemed to violate professional standards of the province or territory.

Although there are many horror stories revolving around inappropriate use of social media technologies within the profession (see Box 25.8), there are significant benefits that can come from having a functional and robust online presence. The use of professional networking sites can assist nurses in terms of finding employment, connecting with others, sharing information or resources, and expanding a nurse's professional network (Fraser, 2011). The use of social networking sites such as LinkedIn, Twitter, and NurseONE can provide a competitive advantage for nurses who are seeking to demonstrate their knowledge or expertise in a specific nursing area, or build a network of colleagues to collaborate on various projects or research studies.

BOX 25.8 VIOLATION OF PROFESSIONALISM ONLINE

Doyle Barnes, a nursing student at Johnson County Community College in Kansas, was expelled from school after posing for a picture beside a human placenta and posting this image as her Facebook profile image. Ms. Barnes's instructor had given permission for students to take the photos beside the placenta—regardless, after the school administration found that she had posted the image on Facebook, she was promptly dismissed from the nursing program. Ms. Barnes was able to regain admission to the program after a short legal battle with the school. The judge in the trial sided with Ms. Barnes, stating that it "was reasonable to anticipate that the photos would be shown to others." Ms. Barnes apologized for her lapse in judgment.

Sources: CBS News. (2011, January 3). *Nursing students kicked out for placenta photos.* Retrieved from http://www.cbsnews.com/stories/2011/01/03/ap/strange/main7208544.shtml; Forbes. (2011, January 7). *Update: Taking a photo with a placenta won't get you kicked out of nursing school.* Retrieved from http://www.forbes.com/sites/kashmirhill/2011/01/07/update-taking-a-photo-with-a-placenta-wont-get-you-kicked-out-of-nursing-school/; Wall Street Journal Online. (2011, January 5). *Odd Facebook post leads to student's ouster, suit.* Retrieved from http://online.wsj.com/article/SB10001424052748704835504576060272240924628.html

Conclusion

Nursing informatics will continue to evolve as the importance, accessibility, and understanding of informatics is realized within the profession. Since health care is an information-rich environment, possessing the skills to use ICT to support patient care will be essential in the coming decades. Informatics can provide significant benefits to the profession; regardless, sound clinical judgment of nurses must prevail when using technology to support clinical practice. Therefore, it is important that nurses remain abreast of developments in nursing informatics through involvement in professional organizations and reflective practice requirements.

The informatics role within nursing will continue to evolve and broaden over time. As outlined previously,

although there will be differing levels of engagement by nurses in the informatics discipline, the skills, knowledge, and understanding of informatics in care delivery are important for all clinicians. For instance, nurses must not only understand the underpinnings of nursing informatics, but be ready to leverage and generate the future opportunities for informatics within practice. The coming decades promise many new innovations in health care technology—including nanotechnology, the ubiquitous Internet, and an increased prevalence of mobile and wearable technologies. Therefore, without a critical mass of nurses engaged in the topic of informatics and technology, the nursing profession will not be able to provide the quality service that is expected by all Canadians into the future.

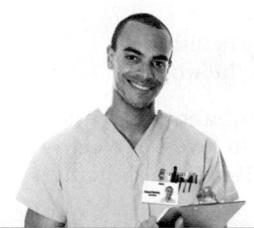

Case Study 25

As a nurse working for a home care agency in a rural town, you want your clients to receive current and accurate health information. High-speed Internet access is available in your office and many of the residents have computers in their homes with dial-up connections.

CRITICAL THINKING QUESTIONS

1. You have a difficult clinical case and want to investigate possible interventions. How can handheld or computer technology assist in this endeavour?

2. One of your clients has a complex leg wound, and you wish to obtain a consult from the covering wound care nurse. The wound care nurse is unable to physically see the client because of scheduling issues. What types of secured and approved ICTs could a home care nurse use to assist in completing this consult?

3. A client shares with you a website promising a cure for the client's illness. How would you respond?

Check the eText in MyNursingLab for answers and explanations.

KEY TERMS

application software *p. 535*
bandwidth *p. 542*
computer provider order entry (CPOE) *p. 537*
data *p. 534*
decision-support systems *p. 534*
digital transition *p. 541*
eHealth *p. 533*
electronic documentation *p. 538*

electronic health record (EHR) *p. 536*
electronic medical record (EMR) *p. 537*
electronic patient record (EPR) *p. 537*
hardware *p. 535*
health literacy *p. 545*
information *p. 534*
information and computer technology (ICT) *p. 534*

information (digital) literacy *p. 541*
knowledge *p. 534*
media literacy *p. 541*
mHealth *p. 539*
mobile technology *p. 539*
nurse informaticians *p. 542*
NurseONE portal *p. 539*
nursing informatics *p. 535*

personal digital assistant (PDA) *p. 539*
picture and archiving communication systems (PACS) *p. 538*
point of care (POC) *p. 539*
portals *p. 539*
social media *p. 536*
software *p. 535*
standardized language *p. 535*

ASSESS YOUR LEARNING

1. Which of the following BEST defines *nursing informatics*?

   a. The compilation of information about nursing

   b. The use of computer information systems in the practice of nursing

   c. The results of research in nursing available online

   d. The ability to take nursing courses in an online format

2. Which of the following is the challenge MOST associated with the use of an electronic client record system?

   a. Cost

   b. Accuracy

   c. Privacy

   d. Accessibility

3. Which of the following is associated with non-synchronous electronic (e.g., Internet-based) courses?

   a. They take longer to complete.

   b. Everyone must log on at the same time.

   c. Interpersonal communication is not possible.

   d. It is more difficult to establish a sense of community.

4. Which of the following is the primary advantage of using computers while conducting nursing research?

   a. Locating potential participants

   b. Analyzing the quantitative data

   c. Disseminating the research findings

   d. Designing the steps of the research plan

5. Which of the following is the MOST appropriate nursing response when a client insists that the practitioner use a treatment method discovered on an Internet site?

   a. "The treatment must be examined to see if it is appropriate."

   b. "Most website treatments have not been studied or researched."

   c. "Websites are like advertising; they are biased and may not be legitimate."

   d. "The person who established the website is the only one who can use it on clients."

6. Which of the following is a primary role of the nurse in telehealth practice?

   a. To inform the client's health care provider of the call

   b. To offer advice about the care being received by a client

   c. To evaluate a previous response received by a client via telehealth

   d. To deliver health information, services, and expertise over any distance

7. The electronic health record can improve patient care for which of the following reasons?

   a. It can be easily transported by the patient and others.

   b. It provides constant availability of patient health information.

   c. It is understood and accepted by everyone in health care.

   d. It is easily accessed by any health care professional anywhere in the world.

8. Which of the following organizations is funded by the Government of Canada to invest in electronic health records–related (EHR-related) initiatives across Canada?

   a. The Romanow Commission

   b. Telehealth Canada

   c. Canada Health Infoway

   d. Canadian Nurses Association

9. Synthesis of information is known as which of the following?

   a. Data

   b. Instructions

   c. Statistics

   d. Knowledge

10. When a person's *health literacy* is mentioned, what is being referred to?

    a. The ability for someone to obtain a health research article online and to be able to understand 80% of the article

    b. The ability for someone to obtain a health research article online and to be able to give an accurate summary of the article

    c. The degree to which a person has the capacity to obtain, interpret, and understand advanced health-related information

    d. The degree to which a person has the capacity to obtain, interpret, and understand basic health-related information

Check the eText in MyNursingLab for answers and explanations.

WEBLINKS

Warriors of The .Net

http://www.youtube.com/watch?v=Ve7_4ot-Dzs

This is an engaging video illustrating how the Internet works.

MyNursingLab

REFERENCES

Aboriginal Canada Portal. (2005). *2004 Report on Aboriginal connectivity*. Retrieved from http://www.aboriginalcanada.gc.ca/acp/site.nsf/eng/ao34157.html

Abramson Center for the Future Health. (2011). *Introducing Azmo*. Retrieved from http://www.theabramsoncenter.org/en/azmo/introducingazmo

Anderson, J. G., Rainey, M. R., & Eysenbach, G. (2003). The impact of cyber healthcare on the physician-patient relationship. *Journal of Medical Systems, 27*(1), 67–84.

Aufderheide, P. & Firestone, C. M. (1993). *Media literacy: A report of the National Leadership Conference on Media Literacy, the Aspen Institute Wye Center, Queenstown Maryland*. Washington, DC: Communications and Society Program, the Aspen Institute.

Balka, E., Rodje, K. & Bush, C. G. (2007). Rose-coloured glasses: The discourse on information technology in the Romanow Report. *Canadian Journal of Communication, 32*, 475–494.

Bawden, D. (2001). Information and digital literacies: A review of concepts. *Journal of Documentation, 57*(2), 218–259.

Bawden, D. & Robinson, L. (2009). The dark side of information: Overload, anxiety and other paradoxes and pathologies. *Journal of Information Science, 35*(2), 180–191.

Berg, M., Aarts, J., & Vander Lei, J. (2003). ICT in health care: Sociotechnical approaches. *Methods of Information in Medicine, 42*(4), 297–301.

Bridges, W. (2003). *Managing transitions: Making the most of change*. Cambridge, MA: Da Capo Press.

Bruce, C. S. (1999). Workplace experiences of information literacy. *International Journal of Information Management, 19*, 33–47.

Calgary Charter on Health Literacy. (2008). Retrieved from http://www.centreforliteracy.qc.ca/health_literacy/calgary_charter

Canada Health Infoway. (2007). *Canadians' support for electronic health records increases to 88 per cent, poll finds*. Retrieved from https://www.infoway-inforoute.ca/lang-en/about-infoway/news/news-releases/168-canadians-support-for-electronic-health-records-increases-to-88-per-cent-poll-finds

Canada Health Infoway. (2011a). *About Canada Health Infoway*. Retrieved from https://www.infoway-inforoute.ca/about-infoway

Canada Health Infoway. (2011b). *Education of next generation of nurses to include effective clinical use of information and communications technologies*. Retrieved from https://www.infoway-inforoute.ca/about-infoway/news/news-releases/732

Canadian Council on Learning. (2008). *Health literacy in Canada: A healthy understanding*. Retrieved from http://www.ccl-cca.ca/CCL/Reports/HealthLiteracy.html

Canadian Healthcare Technology. (2006). *Nursing IT: Ottawa announces $8.1 million for NurseOne portal*. Retrieved from http://www.canhealth.com/News446.html

Canadian Home Care Association. (2008). *Integration through information communication technology for home care in Canada*. Mississauga, ON: Author.

Canadian Nurses Association. (2006). *e-Nursing strategy for Canada*. Retrieved from http://cna-aiic.ca

Canadian Nurses Association. (2011). *NurseONE overview*. Retrieved from http://www.nurseone.ca/documents/NurseONE-Overview_en/

Canadian Nurses Protection Society. (2010). *INFO legal information sheet for nurses: Social media*. Retrieved from http://www.cnps.ca/upload-files/pdf_english/social_media.pdf

Cheung, C., Goldstein, M., Geller, E., & Levitt, R. (2003). The effects of CPOE on ICU workflow: An observational study. *AMIA Annual Symposium Proceedings* (pp. 150–154). Retrieved from http://www.ncbi.nlm.nih.gov/pmc/articles/PMC1480350/

Chew, C., & Eysenbach, G. (2010). Pandemics in the age of Twitter: Content analysis of Tweets during the 2009 H1N1 outbreak. *PloS One, 5*(11), e14118. doi: 10.1371/journal.pone.0014118

Cline, R., & Haynes, K. (2001). Consumer health information seeking on the internet: The state of the art. *Health Education Research, 16*(6), 671–692.

Croteau, D., & Hoynes, W. (2003). *Media society: Industries, images and audiences* (3rd ed.). Thousand Oaks, CA: Pine Forge Press.

D'Alessandro, D. M., & Dosa, N. P. (2001). Empowering children and families with information technology. *Archives of Pediatric & Adolescent Medicine, 155*, 1131–1136.

Deese, D., & Stein, M. (2004). The ultimate health care IT consumers: How nurses transform patient data into a powerful narrative of improved care. *Nursing Economics, 22*(6), 336–341.

DiCenso, A., Cullum, N., & Cilisko, D. (1998). Implementing evidence-based nursing: Some misconceptions. *Evidence-Based Nursing, 1*(2), 38–40.

Doran, D. M., Haynes, R. B., Kushniruk, A., Straus, S., Grimshaw, J., Hall, L. M., Dubrowski, A., . . . Jedras, D. (2010). Supporting evidence-based practice for nurses through information technologies. *Worldviews on evidence-based nursing /*

Sigma Theta Tau International, Honor Society of Nursing, 7(1), 4–15. doi: 10.1111/j.1741-6787.2009.00179.x

Eysenbach, G. (2008). Medicine 2.0: Social networking, collaboration, participation, apomediation, and openness. *Journal of Medical Internet Research, 10*(3), e22. Retrieved from http://www.jmir.org/2008/3/e22

Ferguson, T. (2000). Online patient-helpers and physicians working together: A new partnership for high quality health care. *British Medical Journal, 321*, 1129–1132.

Forkner-Dunn, J. (2003). Internet based patient self-care: The next generation of health care delivery. *Journal of Medical Informatics Research, 5*, e8.

Fraser, R. (2011). *The nurse's social media advantage: How making connections and sharing ideas can enhance your nursing practice.* Indianapolis, IN: Sigma Theta Tau International.

Haux, R. (2002). Health care in the information society: What should be the role of medical informatics? *Methods of Information in Medicine, 41*, 31–35.

Health Council of Canada. (2005). *Health care renewal in Canada: Accelerating change.* Retrieved from www.healthcouncilcanada.ca

Health Council of Canada. (2006). *Healthcare renewal in Canada: Clearing the road to quality.* Retrieved from http://healthcouncilcanada.ca/docs/rpts/2006/ExecSumEnglish2006.pdf

Hirji, F. (2004). Freedom or folly? Canadians and the consumption of online health information. *Information, Communication & Society, 7*(4), 445–465. doi: 10.1080/1369118042000305593

Hodge, T. (2011). *EMR, EHR, and PHR—why all the confusion? Infoway connects.* Retrieved from http://infowayconnects. infoway-inforoute.ca/blog/electronic-health-records/374-emr-ehr-and-phr-%E2%80%93-why-all-the-confusion/

IMIA-NI. (2009). *Nursing informatics.* Retrieved from http://www.amia.org/programs/working-groups/nursing-informatics

Internet World Statistics. (2011). *Internet world stats: Usage and population statistics.* Retrieved from http://www.internetworldstats.com/stats.htm

Kassirer, J. P. (2003). The next transformation in the delivery of health care. *New England Journal of Medicine, 332*(1), 52–54.

Koppel, R., Metlay, J. P., Cohen, A., Abaluck, B., Localio, R., Kimmel, S. E., & Strom, B. L. (2005). Role of computerized physician order entry systems in facilitating medication errors. *JAMA: The Journal of the American Medical Association, 293*(10), 1197–1203. doi: 10.1001/jama.293.10.1197

Logan, A. G., McIsaac, W. J., Tisler, A., Irvine, M. J., Saunders, A., Dunai, A., Rizo, C. . . . Cafazzo, J. A. (2007). Mobile phone-based remote patient monitoring system for management of hypertension in diabetic patients. *American Journal of Hypertension, 20*(9), 942–948. doi: 10.1016/j.amjhyper.2007.03.020

Mackey, T. & Ho, J. (2005). Implementing a convergent model for information literacy: Combining research and web literacy. *Journal of Information Science, 31*, 6, 541–555.

MacLeod, M. L. P., Kulig, J. C., Stewart, N. J., Pitblado, J. R., & Knock, M. (2004). The nature of nursing practice in rural and remote Canada. *Canadian Nurse, 100*(6), 27–31.

McGonigle, D., & Mastrian, K. (2012). *Nursing informatics and the foundation of knowledge* (2nd ed.). Burlington, VA: Jones & Bartlett Learning.

McHugh, M. (2011). Computer systems. In V. Saba & K. McCormick (Eds.), *Essentials of nursing informatics* (5th ed.) (pp. 47–76). New York, NY: McGraw Hill Medical.

Middleton, C., & Sorensen, C. (2006). How connected are Canadians? Inequities in Canadian households' Internet access. *Canadian Journal of Communication, 30*(4). Retrieved from http://www.cjc-online.ca/index.php/journal/article/view/1656/1794

Mishna, F., Saini, M., & Solomon, S. (2009). Ongoing and online: Children and youth's perceptions of cyber bullying. *Children and Youth Services Review, 31*(12), 1222–1228. doi: V10.1016/j.childyouth.2009.05.004

Mitchell, K. J., Ybarra, M., & Finkelhor, D. (2007). The relative importance of online victimization in understanding depression, delinquency, and substance use. *Child Maltreatment, 12*(4), 314–324. doi: 10.1177/1077559507305996

Nagle, L. M. (2007). Everything I know about informatics, I didn't learn in nursing school. *Journal of Nursing Leadership, 20*(3), 22–25.

Nutbeam, D. (2000). Health literacy as a public health goal: A challenge for contemporary health education and communication strategies into the 21st century. *Health Promotion International, 15*, 259–267.

Ontario Telemedicine Network. (2011). *About OTN.* Retrieved from http://otn.ca/en/otn/about-otn

Registered Nurses' Association of Ontario. (2011). *eHealth for every nurse—Nursing and eHealth education course. Module four: The electronic health record (EHR) and information and communication—The nurse and electronic documentation.* Retrieved from http://elearning.rnao.ca

Romanow, R. (2002). *Building on values: The future of health care in Canada.* Retrieved from http://publications.gc.ca/collections/Collection/CP32-85-2002E.pdf

Royston, J. (2011). *mHealth apps "expected to rise to 142 million downloads."* Retrieved from http://www.spirehealthcare.com/Patient-Information/Health-News/Healthcare/801224521-mHealth-apps-expected-to-rise-to-142-million-downloads

Saba, V., & Westra, B. (2011). Historical perspectives of nursing informatics. In V. Saba & K. McCormick (Eds.), *Essentials of nursing informatics* (5th ed.) (pp. 11–30). New York, NY: McGraw Hill Medical.

Saint Elizabeth. (2010). *Saint Elizabeth Health Care launches mobile technology to enhance client experience.* Retrieved from http://www.saintelizabeth.com/news/saint-elizabeth-health-care-launches-mobile-technology-enhance-client-experience

Scholes, M., & Barber, B. (1980). Towards nursing informatics. *MEDINFO: 1980* (pp. 7–73). Amsterdam, Netherlands: MedInfo.

Statistics Canada. (2003). *Learning a living: First results of the adult literacy and life skills survey.* Retrieved from http://www.statcan.gc.ca/bsolc/olc-cel/olc-cel?catno=89-603-XWE&lang=eng

Statistics Canada. (2011). *Canadian Internet use survey.* Retrieved from http://www.statcan.gc.ca/daily-quotidien/110525/dq110525b-eng.htm

Thede, L. (2010). *Nursing informatics definitions.* Retrieved from http://dlthede.net/Informatics/Chap01Overview/NIDefinitions.html

Underhill, C. & McKeown, L. (2008). Getting a second opinion: Health information and the Internet Statistics Canada, *Health Reports, 19*(1). Retrieved from http://www.statcan.gc.ca/pub/82-003-x/82-003-x2008001-eng.pdf

Valaitis, R., & Ferguson, L. (2008). Information and communication technology. In L. L. Stamler & L. Yiu (Eds.), *Community health nursing: A Canadian perspective* (2nd ed.) (pp. 245–262). Toronto, ON: Pearson Prentice Hall.

Welch-Cline, R. J. (2003). At the intersection of micro and macro: Opportunities and challenges for physician-patient communication research. *Patient Education and Counseling, 50*(1), 13–16.

Chapter 26

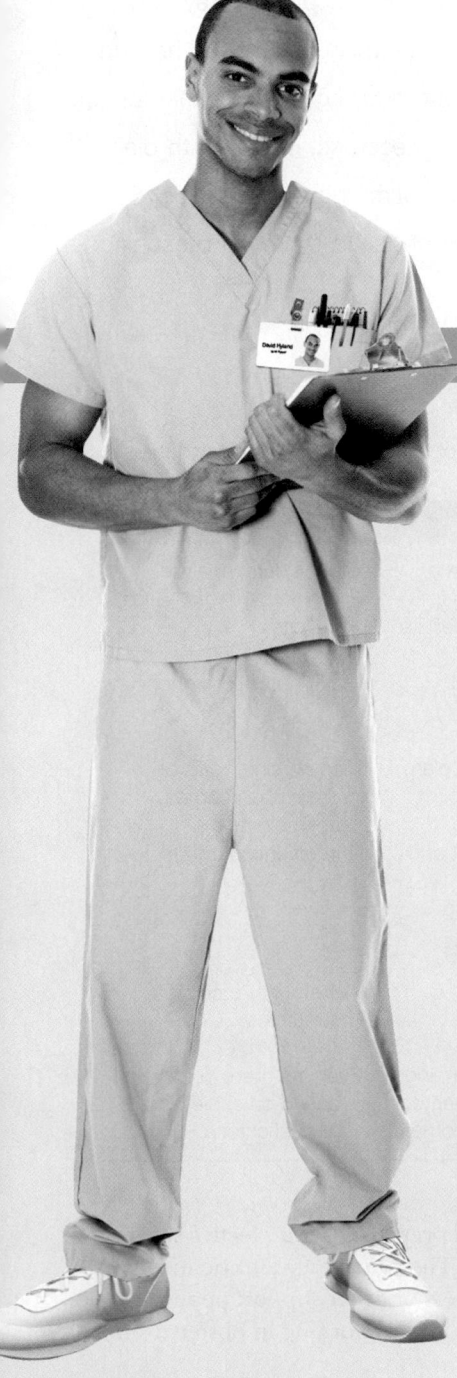

Teaching and Learning

After studying this chapter, you will be able to:

1. Discuss the importance of the teaching role of the nurse.

2. Compare and contrast andragogy, pedagogy, and geragogy.

3. Describe the three main categories of learning theories.

4. Discuss factors that facilitate or inhibit learning throughout the lifespan.

5. Discuss the nurse's role in assisting clients to use health information from the Internet.

6. Identify nursing diagnoses, outcomes, and interventions that reflect the learning needs of clients.

7. Describe essential aspects of effective teaching.

8. Discuss advantages and disadvantages of selected teaching strategies.

9. Identify methods used to evaluate learning outcomes.

Client education is a major aspect of nursing practice and an important independent nursing function. Each provincial and territorial nursing association or college in Canada specifies in its standards that teaching is a required competent skill for nursing practice. Best practice guidelines for client-centred care also stress the importance of including teaching in client care; teaching needs to focus on providing information and teaching on issues for which clients have expressed needs and in a manner that is meaningful and relevant to them (Registered Nurses Association of Ontario, 2006). Legislation related to nursing also includes client teaching as a function of nursing, thereby making teaching both a legal and professional responsibility.

Porter-O'Grady (2001), a nursing futurist, sees nursing in the twenty-first century focusing on "activities of accessing, informing, guiding, teaching, counseling, and linking" (p. 183) clients with service, with a focus on early engagement and preventative interventions. Client education, a key part of this role, is multifaceted, involving promoting, protecting, maintaining, and restoring health and helping clients cope with illness or altered health status. It involves teaching about reducing health risk factors, increasing a person's level of wellness, taking specific protective health measures, coping with diagnostic procedures and treatments, managing symptoms of illness, and optimizing health status. See the Lifespan Considerations box in Chapter 8 (page 146) for examples of health-promotion teaching topics for various age groups.

Teaching

Teaching is a system of activities intended to produce learning. The teaching process is intentionally designed to produce specific learning. The teaching–learning process involves dynamic interaction between teacher and learner. Each participant in the process communicates information, emotions, perceptions, and attitudes to the other. The teaching process and the nursing process are much alike. See Table 26.1.

Nurses teach a variety of clients and their families in a range of settings, They include hospital, primary health care clinics, community health centres, urgent care facilities, the home, and assisted-living and long-term care facilities. Nurses also teach professional colleagues and auxiliary health care personnel in academic institutions, health care facilities, and groups and the community at large.

Teaching Clients and Their Families

Nurses may teach individual clients in one-to-one teaching sessions or in groups. For example, the nurse may teach about wound care while changing a client's dressing or may teach about diet, exercise, and other lifestyle behaviours that minimize the risk of a heart attack for a client who has a cardiac problem. Clients are often

TABLE 26.1   Comparison of the Teaching Process and the Nursing Process

Step	Teaching Process	Nursing Process
1	Collect data; analyze client's learning strengths and deficits.	Collect data; analyze client's strengths and deficits.
2	Make educational diagnoses.	Make nursing diagnoses.
3	Prepare teaching plan: • Write learning outcomes. • Select content and time frame. • Select teaching strategies.	Plan nursing goals or desired outcomes, and select interventions.
4	Implement teaching plan.	Implement nursing strategies.
5	Evaluate client learning based on achievement of learning outcomes.	Evaluate client outcomes based on achievement of goal criteria.

taught in small groups in preparation for elective surgery in pre-admission clinics. The nurse may also be involved in teaching family members or other support people who are caring for the client. Nurses working in obstetric and pediatric areas teach parents and sometimes grandparents how to care for children.

Because of the decreased length of hospital stays, time constraints on client education can occur. Nurses need to provide education that will ensure the client's safe transition from one level of care to another and make appropriate plans for follow-up education in the home. Discharge plans must include both information about what the client has been taught before transfer or discharge and information about what remains for the client to learn to perform self-care in the home or other residence (see the "Discharge Planning" section in Chapter 14).

Teaching in the Community

Nurses are often involved in community health education programs. Such teaching activities may be part of the nurse's involvement in an organization, such as seniors' centres or Planned Parenthood, or with other sectors in the community concerned with the well-being of citizens. Community teaching activities may be aimed at large groups of people who have an interest in some aspect of health, such as nutrition classes, cardiopulmonary resuscitation (CPR), cardiac risk factor reduction, or bicycle or swimming safety programs. Community education programs, such as childbirth preparation classes or family planning classes, can also be for small groups or individual learners.

Teaching Health Care Personnel

Nurses are also involved in the instruction of professional colleagues through continuing education, in-service programs, and staff development. For example, experienced nurses can act as preceptors for students and new graduate nurses. Nurses with specialized knowledge and experience can share that knowledge with nurses who are new to that practice setting. Experienced nurses are often involved in the clinical teaching of nursing students. They may also teach specialized courses, such as critical care nursing, perioperative nursing, and quality improvement or quality assurance processes.

Nurses can also be involved in teaching other health care professionals. They may participate in the education of medical students or allied health students. In this capacity, the nurse educator clarifies the role of the nurse for other health care professionals or how nurses can work with them in caring for clients.

Learning

Clients have a variety of learning needs. A **learning need** is a desire or a requirement to know something that is presently unknown by the learner. Learning needs include new knowledge but can also include a new or different skill or physical ability, a new understanding about an issue,

---

> **BOX 26.1 ATTRIBUTES OF LEARNING**
>
> Learning can take many forms, and they all share the following attributes:
> - An experience that occurs inside the learner
> - The discovery of the personal meaning and relevance of ideas
> - A consequence of experience
> - A collaborative and interactive process
> - An evolutionary process that builds on past learning and experiences
> - A process that is both intellectual and emotional

new beliefs, or a way to change an ineffective behaviour. **Learning** is a change in human disposition or capability that persists and that cannot be accounted for solely by growth.

Learning is a cognitive activity that is represented by a change in behaviour. **Cognitive** refers to the act of knowing or the development of knowledge. See Box 26.1 for attributes of learning.

An important aspect of learning is the individual's desire to learn and to act on the learning, referred to as **compliance**. In the health care context, compliance is the extent to which a person's behaviour coincides with medical or health advice. Since the term *compliance* may imply that learners are not decision makers about their own health, the term **adherence** is often used to reflect the client's engagement in the learning process and willingness to follow a recommended treatment regimen. Adherence is best illustrated when the person recognizes and accepts the need to learn and then follows through with the appropriate behaviours that reflect the learning. For example, a person diagnosed as having diabetes willingly learns about the special diet needed and then plans and follows the learned diet. Bastable (2008) explained both compliance and adherence as the client's ability to maintain "health-promoting regimens, which are determined largely by a health care provider" (p. 201). Nurses should be cautious about labelling clients as *noncompliant*. Clients may intend to follow the treatment regimen but may be unable to do so for a number of reasons (e.g., no access to care or cannot afford the medicine).

Andragogy is the art and science of teaching with a special focus on adults. **Pedagogy** is concerned with all teaching and learning strategies regardless of age, though this Greek term refers to teaching children. **Geragogy** is focused on the learning of older adults. Nurses can use the following principles of adult learning as a guide for client teaching (Bastable, 2008; Knowles, Holton, & Swanson, 2011):

- As people mature, they move from dependence to independence.
- An adult's previous experiences can be used as a resource for learning.
- Learning is related to an immediate need, problem, or deficit.

- An adult is more oriented to learning when the material is useful immediately, not sometime in the future.
- Learning is reinforced by application and prompt feedback.

Learning Domains

Bloom (1956) identified three learning domains: (a) cognitive, (b) affective, and (c) psychomotor. The **cognitive domain** includes six intellectual skills, from simple to complex, beginning with knowing, comprehending, and applying. The **affective domain** involves five major learning categories: (a) feelings, (b) emotions, (c) interests, (d) attitudes, and (e) appreciations. The **psychomotor domain** includes motor skills, such as giving an injection, and also reflects a development hierarchy of skills.

Nurses should include cognitive and affective domains in every teaching plan, and when teaching a skill, all three domains. For example, teaching a client how to irrigate a colostomy is in the psychomotor domain. But an important part of a teaching plan for a client with a colostomy is to teach why a specific amount of fluid is used and when the irrigation should be carried out; this part is in the cognitive domain. Helping the client accept the colostomy and maintain self-esteem is in the affective domain.

Learning Theories

Three main theoretical constructs of learning theory are (a) behaviourism, (b) cognitivism, and (c) humanism (Bastable, 2008). Nurses use behaviourist theory to identify what is to be taught and the reward for correct responses. Cognitive theory will enable nurses to recognize the developmental level of the learner and acknowledge the learner's motivation and environment. When using humanism, nurses focus on the feelings and attitudes of learners and help motivate them to take responsibility for their own health and learning.

BEHAVIOURISM Edward Thorndike originally advanced behaviourism, a theory based on learning as reflected in changes in behaviour. Other major behaviourist theorists include Pavlov (1927), Skinner (1953), and Bandura (1971). In the behaviourist school of thought, an act is called a *response* when it can be traced to the effects of a stimulus. Behaviourists closely observe responses and then manipulate the environment to bring about the intended behaviour change. Thus, to modify a person's attitude and response, a behaviourist "would either alter the stimulus condition in the environment or change what happens after a response occurs" (Bastable, 2008, p. 54).

Skinner also introduced the importance of **positive reinforcement** in fostering repetition of an action. Bandura claimed that most learning comes from observational learning and instruction rather than from trial-and-error behaviour. Bandura's research focused on **imitation**, the process by which individuals copy or reproduce what they have observed, and **modelling**, the process by which a person learns by observing the behaviour of others.

Nurses applying behaviouristic theory will do the following:

- Provide sufficient practice time and both immediate testing and redemonstration
- Provide opportunities for learners to solve problems by trial and error
- Select teaching strategies to avoid distracting information and that evoke the desired behaviours
- Praise the learner for correct behaviour and provide positive feedback at intervals throughout the learning experience
- Provide role models of the desired behaviour

COGNITIVISM Cognitivism, or **cognitive theory**, depicts learning as a complex cognitive activity which is largely a mental, an intellectual, or a thinking process. Based on their personal characteristics and experience and how the learners perceive their environments, cognitivists emphasize the importance of the social, emotional, and physical contexts in which learning occurs, such as the teacher–learner relationship and environment. Developmental readiness and individual readiness (expressed as motivation) are other key factors with cognitive approaches.

Major cognitive theorists include Piaget, Lewin, and Bloom (Bastable, 2008). As discussed in Chapter 17, Piaget's (1966) five major phases of cognitive development include the following phases: (a) sensorimotor, (b) preconceptual, (c) intuitive, (d) concrete operations, and (e) formal intuitive. Lewin (1951) viewed learning as involving four different types of change: changes in (a) cognitive structure, (b) motivation, (c) sense of belonging to the group, and (d) voluntary muscle control. His widely known theory of change has three basic stages: (a) unfreezing, (b) moving, and (c) refreezing (see the "Models of Change" section in Chapter 27).

Nurses applying cognitive theory will do the following:

- Provide a social, emotional, and physical environment conducive to learning
- Encourage a positive teacher–learner relationship
- Select multisensory teaching strategies, since perception is influenced by the senses
- Recognize that personal characteristics have an impact on how cues are perceived and develop appropriate teaching approaches to target different learning styles
- Adapt teaching strategies to the learner's developmental level and readiness to learn
- Select learning outcomes and teaching strategies that encompass the cognitive, affective, and psychomotor domains of learning

HUMANISM **Humanism**, or humanistic learning theory, focuses on both the cognitive and the affective qualities of the learner. Prominent members of this school of thought include Abraham Maslow and Carl Rogers. According to humanistic theory, learning is self-motivated, self-initiated, and self-evaluated. Each individual is viewed as a unique composite of biological, psychological, social, cultural, and spiritual factors. Learning focuses on self-development and achieving full potential; it is best achieved when it is relevant to the learner. Autonomy and self-determination are important; the learner identifies the learning needs and takes the initiative to meet these needs. The learner is, thus, an active participant and takes responsibility for meeting his or her learning needs.

Nurses applying humanistic theory will do the following:

- Recognize the importance of the nurse–client relationship on learning, such as the feelings and attitudes of learners
- Encourage learners to identify their own learning needs and establish goals
- Encourage active learning by serving as a facilitator, mentor, or resource for the learner
- Expose learners to new, relevant information and assist the client's adoption of new behaviour

Factors Affecting Learning

The nurse should be aware of the following factors that can facilitate or hinder optimal learning by a client.

AGE AND DEVELOPMENTAL STAGE Three major developmental stage factors associated with clients' readiness to learn include physical, cognitive, and psychosocial maturation. Nurses need to consider these factors at each developmental period throughout the lifespan of their clients (Bastable, 2008). (See Chapter 17.)

MOTIVATION **Motivation** to learn is the *desire* to learn. Motivation is generally greatest when a person experiences a need and believes the need will be met through learning. Often, the nurse's task is to help the client personally work through the problem and identify the need. For instance, clients with heart disease may need to know the effects of smoking before they recognize the need to stop smoking; or adolescents may need to know the consequences of an untreated sexually transmitted infection before they see the need for treatment.

READINESS **Readiness to learn** is the demonstrated behaviours that reflect not only the client's desire or willingness to learn but also his or her ability to learn at a specific time. For example, a client may want to learn self-care during a dressing change, but, when experiencing pain, he may not be able to learn. The nurse can provide pain medication to make the client more comfortable so that he is more able to learn. Often, the nurse's role is to encourage the client to develop readiness for learning.

ACTIVE INVOLVEMENT When the learner is actively involved in the process of learning, learning becomes more

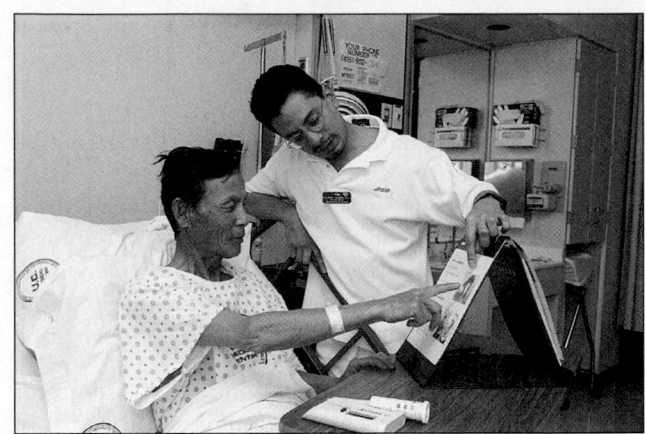

FIGURE 26.1 Learning is facilitated when the client is interested and actively involved.

meaningful, the learning is faster, and retention is better (Figure 26.1). Active learning promotes critical thinking, enabling learners to problem solve more effectively and to apply the learning to their own situation. For example, clients who are actively involved in learning about their therapeutic diets may be more able to apply the principles being taught to their cultural food preferences and their usual eating habits. Passive learning, such as listening to a lecture or watching a film, does not foster optimal learning.

RELEVANCE The client can learn more easily if he or she can connect or relate the new knowledge or skills to what he or she already knows or has experienced. For example, if a client is diagnosed with hypertension and is overweight and has symptoms of headaches and fatigue, she is more likely to understand the need to lose weight if she remembers having more energy when she weighed less. The nurse needs to validate the relevance of learning with the client throughout the learning process.

FEEDBACK Feedback is information regarding a person's performance in meeting a desired goal, and it needs to be meaningful and given in a timely manner. Feedback that accompanies the practice of psychomotor skills helps the person learn those skills. Support of desired behaviour through praise, positively worded corrections, and suggestions of alternative methods are ways of providing positive feedback. Negative feedback, such as ridicule, anger, or sarcasm, can lead people to withdraw from learning.

NONJUDGMENTAL SUPPORT People learn best when they believe they are accepted and not being judged. Once learners have succeeded in accomplishing a task or understanding a concept, they gain self-confidence in their ability to learn. This reduces their anxiety about failure and can motivate greater learning. Nonjudgmental support contributes to a positive and safe climate for learning.

SIMPLE TO COMPLEX Learning is facilitated by material that is logically organized and proceeds from *the simple to the complex*. Such organization enables the learner to comprehend new information, assimilate it with previous learning, and form new understandings. *Simple* and *complex* are relative terms depending on the level at which the person is learning. What is simple for one person may be complex for another.

REPETITION Repetition of key concepts and facts facilitates retention of newly learned material. When the same information is provided in several formats, including visual and verbal, and in examples, such repetition can reinforce learning. Practice of psychomotor skills, particularly with feedback from the nurse, improves performance of those skills and facilitates their transfer to another setting.

TIMING People retain information and psychomotor skills best when the time between learning and active use of the learning is short; the longer the time interval, the more the learning is forgotten. Immediate application facilitates learning. For example, a person who is only shown literature and videotapes about administering insulin and is not permitted to administer the insulin until discharge from the hospital is unlikely to remember what was learned. Learning will be enhanced, however, if the person can give injections while in hospital.

ENVIRONMENT An optimal learning environment facilitates learning by reducing distraction and providing physical and psychological comfort. It has a comfortable room temperature, good ventilation, and adequate lighting that is free from glare. Noise can distract the learner and interfere with listening and thinking. To facilitate optimal learning, nurses choose a time or location in which distractions in the environment are limited and interruptions are unlikely.

Privacy is essential for some learning. For example, when a client is learning to irrigate a colostomy, the presence of others can be embarrassing and, thus, interfere with learning. However, when a client is particularly anxious, having a support person present can give the client confidence. Some of the most common barriers to learning are described in Table 26.2.

TABLE 26.2 Common Barriers to Learning

Barrier	Explanation	Nursing Implications
Acute illness	The client requires all resources and energy to cope with illness.	Defer teaching until the client is less ill. Focus teaching on coping with symptoms.
Pain	Pain decreases a client's ability to concentrate.	Assess and control pain before teaching.
Prognosis	The client can be preoccupied with illness and unable to concentrate on new information.	Defer teaching to a better time. Focus the teaching on coping strategies.
Biorhythms	Mental and physical performances have a circadian rhythm.	Adapt the time of teaching to suit the client.
Emotions (e.g., anxiety, denial, depression, grief)	Emotions require energy and distract from learning.	Deal with emotional responses to learning and possible misinformation first. Provide repetition of content.
Language	The client may not be fluent in the nurse's language.	Obtain the services of an interpreter or a nurse with appropriate language skills. Increase teaching time.
Age		
• Older adults	Vision, hearing, and motor control can be impaired in older adults.	Consider sensory and motor deficits in the teaching plan.
• Children	Children have a shorter attention span and vocabulary limitations.	Plan shorter and more active learning episodes.
Culture or religion	There may be cultural or religious restrictions on certain types of knowledge, for example, birth control information.	Assess the client's cultural or religious needs when planning learning activities.
Physical disability	Visual, hearing, sensory, or motor impairments may interfere with a client's ability to learn.	Plan teaching activities appropriate to learner's physical abilities. For example, provide audio learning tools for the client who is blind, or large-print materials for the client whose vision is impaired.
Mental disability	Impaired cognitive ability may affect the client's capacity for learning.	Assess client's capacity for learning and plan teaching activities to complement the client's ability. Plan more complex learning for the client's caregivers.

EMOTIONS   Emotions, such as fear, anger, and depression, can impede learning, as can a high level of anxiety. Clients or families who are experiencing extreme emotional states may not hear spoken words or may retain only part of the communication. Emotional responses, such as fear and anxiety, may be relieved by information that relieves uncertainty.

PHYSIOLOGICAL EVENTS   Physiological events, such as a critical illness, pain, or sensory deficits, inhibit learning. Certain drugs and treatments can interfere with the client's ability to concentrate and apply energy to learning, and the learning itself is impaired. The nurse should try to reduce the physiological barriers to learning as much as possible before teaching. Some clients, however, may find it helpful to have analgesics and rest before learning.

CULTURAL BARRIERS   Cultural barriers to learning include language, beliefs, and values. The client who does not understand the nurse's language will learn little. Western medicine may conflict with cultural healing beliefs and practices. Nurses need to be competent in providing culturally safe and sensitive care; otherwise, the client may be partially or totally noncompliant with recommended treatments. Another impediment to learning is differing values held by the client and the health care providers. For example, clients who come from a culture that does not value slimness may have difficulty learning about a reducing diet. The nurse and the client therefore should together determine an acceptable weight and develop a plan for achieving that weight (Chang & Kelly, 2007; Purnell & Paulanka, 2008).

PSYCHOMOTOR ABILITY   Nurses must be aware of a client's psychomotor skills when planning teaching. Motor abilities can be affected by health. For example, an older adult who has severe osteoarthritis of the hands may not be able to put on a bandage. The following physical abilities are important for learning psychomotor skills:

1. *Muscle strength.* For example, an older client who cannot rise from a chair because of insufficient leg and muscle strength cannot be expected to learn to lift herself out of a bathtub without assistance.
2. *Motor coordination.* Gross and fine motor coordination are required for many skills. For example, a client who lacks coordination of the hand will probably find it difficult to self-administer an injection.
3. *Energy.* Energy is required for most psychomotor skills. and learning these skills uses more energy. People who have limited energy may be taught skills during the times when their energy levels are highest.
4. *Sensory acuity.* Sight is used for most learning. Clients who are visually impaired often need the assistance of a support person to carry out some tasks.

Nurse as Educator

Being an educator is an important and primary role for the nurse. Clients and families have the right to health information to make informed decisions about their health. The nurse's role is to promote healthy lifestyles through the application of health knowledge, the change process, learning theories, and the nursing and teaching processes when teaching clients and their families.

Assessing

A comprehensive assessment of learning needs incorporates data from the nursing history and physical assessment and addresses the client's support system. It also considers client characteristics that can influence the learning process: for example, readiness to learn, motivation to learn, and reading and comprehension level. Assessing a person's stage of change and any barriers to change is also important and often overlooked (see the section "The Transtheoretical Model: Stages of Health Behaviour Change" in Chapter 8). Learning needs change as the client's health status changes, so nurses must constantly reassess them.

NURSING HISTORY   Several elements in the nursing history provide clues to learning needs as well as client strengths and limitations. These elements include the client's (a) age, (b) understanding and perceptions of the health problem, (c) health beliefs and cultural practices, (d) economic factors, (e) learning style, and (f) support systems. Examples of open-ended interview questions to elicit this information are shown in the Assessment: Interview box on the next page.

Age   Age provides information on the person's developmental status that may indicate the need for distinctive health teaching content or teaching approaches. Simple questions to school-age children and adolescents will elicit information on what they know. Observing children at play provides information about their motor and intellectual development as well as their relationships with other children. For older people, questioning may reveal slow recall or limited motor abilities, sensory deficits, or learning difficulties (see the Lifespan Considerations box on page 559).

Client's Understanding of Health Problem   A client's perception of a current health problem and concern may indicate knowledge deficits or misinformation. In addition, the effects of the problem on the client's usual activities can alert the nurse to other areas requiring instruction. For example, people who cannot manage self-care at home often need information about community resources and services.

ASSESSMENT   INTERVIEW

Learning Needs and Characteristics

The use of opened-ended questions can help nurses find evidence of clients' learning needs.

PRIMARY HEALTH PROBLEM

- Tell me what you know about your current health problem. What do you think caused it?
- What concerns do you have about it?
- How has the problem affected what you can or cannot do during your usual activities (e.g., work, recreation, shopping, housework)?
- What do you or did you do at home to relieve the problem? How helpful was it?
- How have the treatments you have started helped your problem?
- What, if any, difficulties have the treatments caused you (e.g., inconvenience, cost, discomfort)?
- Tell me about the tests (surgery, treatments) you are going to have.

HEALTH BELIEFS

- How would you describe your health generally?
- What things do you usually do to keep healthy?
- What health problems do you think you may be at risk for because of family history, age, diet, occupation, inadequate exercise, or habits, such as smoking?
- What changes would you be willing to make to decrease your risk for these problems or to improve your health?

CULTURAL FACTORS

- What language do you use most often when speaking and writing?
- Do you seek the advice of another health care practitioner?

- Do you use herbs or other medications or treatments commonly used in your cultural group?
- Does your current doctor know about these?
- What advice or treatments given previously by your doctor conflicted with values or beliefs you consider important?
- When a conflict arose, what did you do?

LEARNING STYLE

- Note the client's age and developmental level.
- What is your highest level of formal education?
- Do you like to read?
- Where do you obtain health information (e.g., physician, nurse, magazines, books, pharmacist, and so on)?
- How do you best learn new things?
  a. By reading about them
  b. By asking questions and discussing them
  c. By watching a demonstration
  d. By using Internet-based or computer resources
  e. By listening to the teacher
  f. By first being shown how something works and then doing it
  g. By working on your own or in a group
  h. By reflecting on what was learned

CLIENT SUPPORT SYSTEM

- Would you like a family member or friend to help you learn about things that you need to do to take care of yourself?
- Who do you think would be interested in learning with you?

Health Beliefs and Cultural Practices The client's health beliefs and practices must be considered in any teaching plan. The health belief model described in Chapter 7 provides a predictor of preventive health behaviour. Many cultural groups have their own beliefs and practices, a number of them related to diet, health, illness, and lifestyle. Nurses need to know how the practices and values held by clients affect their learning needs. Folk beliefs of certain groups can also affect learning. Although the client may readily understand the health care information being taught, this learning may not be implemented in the home where folk health practices prevail (see the "Health Beliefs and Practices" section in Chapter 11 and the "Transcultural Teaching" section later in this chapter).

Economic Factors Economic factors can also affect a client's learning. For example, a client who cannot afford to obtain a new sterile syringe for each injection of insulin may find it difficult to follow through on learning if cost is an issue.

Learning Style The best way to learn varies with the individual. Some people are visual learners and learn best by watching; others learn by manipulating equipment and discovering how it works. Other people can learn well from reading things presented in an orderly fashion, while others learn best in groups where they can discuss the content. For many, stressing the emotional aspects promotes learning.

A client's learning style may be based in his or her cultural background. For example, clients from cultures that have a strong oral tradition may prefer educational videos presented in their own language.

The nurse may not have the time to assess each learner's particular learning style and then adapt teaching accordingly; what the nurse can do, however, is to ask clients how they like to learn. Many people know what helps them learn, and the nurse can use this information in planning teaching. In teaching a group, the nurse can use a variety of teaching techniques and vary activities to

LIFESPAN CONSIDERATIONS

Special Teaching Considerations

OLDER ADULTS

Older adults often have chronic illnesses that require multiple treatments or medications. Health teaching will focus on health and wellness promotion and prevention of illness and accidents, as with other ages. Older adults' greatest need is in learning to manage their own lives and to maintain optimal health and functioning as they live with their chronic health conditions. For older adults to be motivated to learn, the material must be practical and have meaning for them individually, especially if the information is new to them. Special considerations in teaching older adults include the following:

- Health promotion is a priority need and should include these areas:
  - Exercise
  - Nutrition
  - Safety habits
  - Regular health checkups
  - Understanding of medications
- Set achievable goals—involve the client and family in doing this.
- If developing written materials:
  - Use large print (e.g., at least 14-point font) in bulleted format.
  - Use buff-coloured paper (which avoids the glare from white paper).
- Present information at the Grade 6 reading level.
- Increase time for teaching and allow for rest periods as processing of information is slower.
- Ensure that verbal presentation of material is well organized and that there is minimal distraction.
- Repeat information if necessary.
- Use return demonstrations with psychomotor skills, such as teaching someone to learn to do insulin injections.
- Determine where clients obtain most of their health information (e.g., newspapers, magazines, television).
- Use examples that they can relate to in their daily lives.
- Be aware of sensory deficits, such as hearing and vision.
- Use the setting with which the individual is most comfortable—either a group setting or a one-on-one setting.

- If noncompliance is a problem, investigate the cause. It could be due to lack of finances, transportation problems, poor access to medical care, and so on.

Older adults come with a lifetime of experiences and learned knowledge of their own. Respect this and always have them use their strengths to work through any problems. Positive reinforcement and ongoing evaluation of what has been taught are important factors in effective health teaching with older adults.

CHILDREN

Often, the parent is a child's first and most important teacher. Every interaction between a child and a parent (or others) is a moment in which teaching and learning occurs, often unconsciously.

Children learn by observation and interaction and pick up information, values, and skills from the world around them. Nurses can assist parents to teach their children about health promotion, disease prevention, and care and procedures, using knowledge of the child's developmental level. Considerations in teaching children include the following:

Preschool Children (3–5 Years of Age)

- Are concerned about fear of pain and bodily harm. Reassure them and allow them to tell you about these fears. Use words carefully. For example, use "fix" instead of "cut"; "bandage" instead of "dressing."
- Allow the child to play with replicas or dolls to learn about body parts.
- Give praise and approval to motivate learning.

Middle and Late Childhood (6–11 Years of Age)

- Are able to think logically but abstract thought is limited.
- Like to be actively involved in the learning process.
- Teaching for health promotion often occurs through the school nurse.

Adolescent (12–19 Years of Age)

- Have a strong need to belong to a group, develop friendships, and maintain peer support.
- Need to develop a mutually respectful and trusting relationship with them.

---

meet clients' preferred ways of learning, thus addressing different learning styles. One learning situation will be effective for some clients whereas other approaches may be preferable for other clients.

Client Support System The nurse explores the client's support system to determine the extent to which others can enhance learning and offer support. Family members or a close friend may help the client perform required skills at home and maintain required lifestyle changes.

PHYSICAL EXAMINATION The visual inspection part of the physical examination provides useful clues to clients' learning needs, such as mental status, energy level, and nutritional status, as well as their physical capacity to learn and to perform self-care activities. For example, visual ability, hearing ability, and muscle coordination affect the selection of content and approaches to teaching.

READINESS TO LEARN A client who is ready may search out information by asking questions, reading books or articles, talking to others, and generally showing interest. The person who is not ready to learn is more likely to avoid the subject or situation. In addition, the unready client may change the subject when it is brought up by the nurse. For example, the nurse might say, "I was wondering about a good time to show you how to change your dressing," and the client responds, "Oh, my wife will take care of everything."

The nurse assesses for these readiness characteristics:

- *Physical readiness.* Is the client able to focus on things other than physical status? Is the client experiencing pain, fatigue, or nausea?
- *Emotional readiness.* Is the client emotionally ready to learn self-care activities? Clients who are extremely anxious, depressed, or grieving over their health status are not ready.
- *Cognitive readiness.* Can the client think clearly at this point? Is the client taking any medications that may affect his or her level of consciousness?

Nurses can promote readiness to learn by providing physical and emotional support during the critical stage of recovery. As the client stabilizes physically and emotionally, the nurse can provide opportunities to learn.

MOTIVATION As discussed earlier, motivation relates to whether the client wants to learn and is usually greatest when the client is ready, the learning need is recognized, and the information being offered is meaningful to the client. Nurses can increase a client's motivation in several ways:

- By relating the learning to something the client values and helping the client see the benefits of learning
- By helping the client make the learning situation pleasant and nonthreatening
- By encouraging self-direction and independence
- By demonstrating a positive attitude about the client's ability to learn
- By offering continuing support and encouragement as the client attempts to learn (i.e., positive reinforcement)
- By creating a learning situation in which the client is likely to succeed, as motivation for continued learning

HEALTH LITERACY **Health literacy** is the ability to read, understand, and act on health information, including such tasks as comprehending prescription labels and nutrition labels, interpreting appointment slips, completing health insurance forms, and following instructions for diagnostic tests (Redman, 2004; Weiss et al., 2005).

Limited health literacy skills are often more prevalent among certain groups: older adults, people of limited education, people from low-income groups, and immigrant population with limited English proficiency.

The Canadian Council on Learning (2007) reported that low health literacy skills are associated with poor health outcomes and higher health care costs and that low literacy has direct and indirect effects on almost all aspects of health. Clients with low literacy skills have less information about health promotion and management of a disease process for themselves and their families. They may be unable to read the educational materials or miss the opportunity for employment where literacy is involved.

It is a challenge for the nurse to teach clients with low or no reading and writing skills. However, such teaching is vitally important because clients with low literacy skills need learning opportunities to improve their health practices (see the Teaching: Clinical boxes on developing written teaching aids and teaching clients with low literacy levels).

READING LEVEL The nurse should not assume that a client's reading level is equal to the highest grade or level of formal education the client has completed. Most word-processing programs have a readability feature, e.g., for the Microsoft Word Program, under Tools, Options, and the Spelling and Grammar tab, one can look up the readability of the written material. Written health education materials should be written for lower reading levels, such as the Grade 5 or Grade 6 level (Bastable, 2008; Mayer & Villaire, 2007). People with good reading skills are not offended by simple reading material and prefer

---

TEACHING | CLINICAL

Developing Written Teaching Aids

When developing any written teaching aids, nurses should consider the following guidelines:

- Keep reading level at or below the Grade 6 level.
- Write abbreviations out in full, and define technical terms.
- Use active voice, not passive voice.
- Use easy, common words of one or two syllables (e.g., *use* instead of *utilize*, or *give* instead of *administer*).
- Use the second person (*you*) rather than the third person (*the client*).
- Use a large type size (14 to 16 point), especially for older adults.
- Write short sentences.
- Avoid using all capital letters.
- Place priority information first and repeat more than once.
- Use bold face for emphasis.
- Use simple pictures, drawings, or cartoons, if appropriate.
- Leave plenty of white space to create an easy-to-read and uncluttered appearance.

TEACHING   CLINICAL

Teaching Clients with Low Literacy Levels

Nurses can use several methods to improve their success in teaching clients with low or no reading and writing skills:

- Use multiple teaching methods: Show pictures. Read important information. Lead a small group discussion. Role play. Demonstrate a skill. Provide hands-on practice.
- Emphasize key points in simple terms and provide examples.
- Limit the amount of information in a single teaching session by providing short and frequent sessions.
- Associate new information with something the client already knows or associates with his or her job or lifestyle.
- Reinforce information through repetition.
- Involve the client actively in the learning.
- Obtain feedback: Ask the client specific questions about the information presented or ask the client to repeat it in his or her own words.
- Avoid handouts with many pages or a classroom lecture format with a large group.
- Explain acronyms (i.e., HDL [high-density lipoprotein], COPD [chronic obstructive pulmonary disease]).

easy-to-read information (see the Teaching: Clinical box on developing written teaching aids).

Box 26.2 on the next page describes assessment data clusters and teaching plans for two clients, Mr. Steinberg and Mr. Evans.

Diagnosing

Nursing diagnoses for clients with learning needs can be designated in two ways: (a) as the client's primary concern or problem, or (b) as the etiology of a nursing diagnosis associated with the client's response to health alterations or dysfunction.

LEARNING NEED AS THE DIAGNOSTIC LABEL   NANDA International (2012) (formerly the North American Nursing Diagnosis Association) includes the following diagnostic labels appropriate to a client's learning needs when the learning need is the primary concern:

- *Deficient Knowledge:* "absence or deficiency of cognitive information related to a specific topic" (NANDA International, 2012, p. 153). Whenever the diagnostic label *Deficient Knowledge* is used, either the client is seeking health information or the nurse has identified a learning need. The area of deficiency should always be included in the diagnosis.The following are examples that use the NANDA International label *Deficient Knowledge* as the primary concern:

- *Deficient Knowledge: Low-Cholesterol Diet* related to inexperience with newly ordered therapy
- *Deficient Knowledge: Home Safety Hazards* related to declining physical mobility

Wilkinson and Ahern (2008) stressed that if *Deficient Knowledge* is used as the primary concern, one client goal must be "client will acquire knowledge about." The nurse needs to provide information that has the potential to change the client's behaviour, rather than focus on the behaviours caused by the client's lack of knowledge.

A second nursing diagnostic label in which a learning need may be the primary concern or problem is as follows:

- *Readiness for Enhanced Knowledge:* "active seeking (by a person in stable health) of ways to alter personal health habits and/or the environment in order to move toward a higher level of health" (NANDA International, 2012, p. 158).

When this diagnostic label is used, the client does not necessarily have a dysfunction at the time but is seeking information to improve health or prevent illness. This diagnosis is especially appropriate for clients attending community health education programs. The following are examples that use the NANDA International label *Readiness for Enhanced Knowledge* as the primary concern:

- *Readiness for Enhanced Knowledge: Exercise and Activity* related to desire to improve health behaviours and decrease the risk of osteoporosis. This diagnosis is appropriate for the client who has identified a personal health risk for osteoporosis and wants to minimize that risk through exercise.
- *Readiness for Enhanced Knowledge: Home Safety Hazards* related to desire to minimize risk of injury. This diagnosis is appropriate for parents of a toddler who are seeking information to ensure that their home is safe for their child.

Clinical applications of these kinds of diagnoses using the assessment data are shown in Box 26.2 on the next page.

Planning

INFORMAL TEACHING   Clients frequently ask questions during the course of their care. Informal teaching is often initiated in response to these questions or other indicators of readiness to learn. These "teaching moments" may be brief but are usually highly effective due to client motivation to learn. Nurses usually have the knowledge to provide the requested information without formal planning and may use pen and paper illustrations or graphics on their personal digital assistants (PDAs) to enhance their explanations. If the nurse does not have sufficient content knowledge or if the client's need to learn requires a more formalized process, a plan for teaching will be developed.

BOX 26.2 IDENTIFYING NURSING DIAGNOSES, OUTCOMES, AND INTERVENTIONS: CLIENTS REQUIRING TEACHING

Data cluster: The nurse brings Mr. Steinberg the first dose of a new medication ordered by his physician. The nurse asks whether he understands what this medication is and why he is taking it. He says no.

Nursing Diagnosis	Long-Term Goal	Desired Outcomes	Content	Selected Teaching Interventions
Deficient Knowledge (medication information): Related to lack of exposure to newly prescribed medication and absence or deficiency of cognitive information related to specific topic	Client safely takes prescribed medications and monitors self for their effects.	Client conveys understanding about the safe use of medication.	• Identification of correct medication name • Description of medication • Description of side effects of medication • Description of medication precautions	• Inform the client of both the generic and brand names of the medication. • Instruct the client on the purpose and action of the medication. • Instruct the client on the dosage, route, and duration of the medication. • Instruct the client on specific precautions to observe when taking the medication (e.g., no driving), as appropriate.

Data cluster: George Evans is a 45-year-old man who has come to the clinic for his annual physical examination. He expresses concern about his family history of heart disease and requests information about activities to decrease his risk of heart disease.

Readiness for Enhanced Health (nutrition, activity, and exercise information): To reduce risk of heart disease; active seeking (by a person in stable health) of ways to alter personal health habits or the environment to move toward a higher level of health	The client initiates change to achieve personally important goals.	Client initiates action to promote wellness, recovery, and rehabilitation.	• Asks health-related questions, when indicated • Seeks health-related information from a variety of sources • Uses strategies to eliminate unhealthy behaviours	• Assist the client in identifying target behaviours that need to change to achieve the desired goal. • Assist the client in identifying a specific goal for change. • Appraise the client's present knowledge and skill level in relationship to the desired change. • Explore with the client potential barriers to changing behaviour.

FORMAL PLANNING Developing a teaching plan is accomplished in a series of steps. Involving the client at this time promotes the formation of a meaningful plan and stimulates client motivation. The client who helps formulate the teaching plan is more likely to achieve the desired outcomes. See the Teaching: Clinical box for a sample teaching plan for wound care.

Determining Teaching Priorities The client's learning needs must be ranked according to priority. The client and the nurse should do this together, with the client's priorities always being considered. Once a client's priorities have been addressed, the client is generally more motivated to concentrate on other identified learning needs. For example, a man who wants to know all about coronary artery

disease may not be ready to learn how to change his lifestyle until he meets his own need to learn more about the disease. Nurses can also use theoretical frameworks, such as Maslow's (1970) hierarchy of needs, to establish priorities (see the section "Needs Theories" in Chapter 12).

Setting Learning Outcomes Learning outcomes can be considered the same as desired outcomes for other nursing diagnoses. They are written in the same way. Like client outcomes, learning outcomes should do the following:

• State the client (learner) behaviour or performance, not the nurse behaviour. For example, "Identify personal risk factors for heart disease" (client behaviour), not "Teach the client about cardiac risk factors" (nurse behaviour).

| TEACHING | CLINICAL |

Sample Teaching Plan: Wound Care

Assessment of Learner: A 24-year-old male university student suffered a 7-cm laceration on the lower anterior part of the left leg during a hockey game. The laceration was cleaned, sutured, and bandaged. The client was given an appointment to return to the health clinic in 10 days for suture removal. Client states that he lives in the university dormitory and is able to care for the wound if given instructions. Client is able to understand and read English. Assessed to be in the *preparation* and *action* stages of change.

- *Nursing diagnosis:* Deficient knowledge (care of sutured wound) related to no prior experience.
- *Long-term goals:* Client's wound will heal completely without infection or other complications.
- *Intermediate goal:* At clinic appointment, client's wound will be healing without signs of infection, loss of function, or other complication.
- *Short-term goals:* Client will (a) correctly list three signs and symptoms of wound infection and (b) correctly perform a return demonstration of wound cleansing and bandaging.

Behavioural Outcomes

On completion of the instructional session, the client will do the following:

1. Describe normal wound healing
2. Describe signs and symptoms of wound infection
3. Identify equipment needed for wound care
4. Demonstrate wound cleansing and bandaging
5. Describe appropriate action if questions or complications arise
6. Identify date, time, and location of follow-up appointment for suture removal

Content Outline

i. Normal wound healing
ii. Infection
   a. Signs and symptoms include the wound being warm to the touch, malalignment of the wound edges, and purulent wound drainage.
   b. Signs of systemic infection include fever and malaise.

iii. Wound care equipment
   a. Cleansing solution, as prescribed by physician (e.g., clear water, mild soap and water, or antimicrobial solution)
   b. Bandaging material: Telfa, gauze wrap, adhesive tape
iv. Demonstration of wound cleansing and bandaging on the client's wound or a mannequin
v. Resources available for client's questions include health clinic and emergency department
vi. Follow-up treatment plan: where and when

Teaching Methods

1. Describe normal wound healing with the use of audiovisuals.
2. Discuss the mechanism of wound infection. Use audiovisuals to demonstrate infected wound appearance. Provide a handout describing signs and symptoms of wound infection.
3. Demonstrate the equipment needed for cleansing and bandaging wound. Provide a handout listing equipment needed.
4. Demonstrate wound cleansing and bandaging on the client's wound or a mannequin. Provide a handout describing the procedure for cleansing and bandaging the wound.
5. Discuss available resources. Provide a handout listing available resources and a follow-up treatment plan.
6. Provide written instructions.

Evaluation

The client will do the following:

1. Correctly describe normal wound healing and signs and symptoms of wound infection
2. Return demonstration of wound cleansing and bandaging
3. State contact person and telephone number to obtain assistance
4. State date, time, and location of follow-up appointment

- Reflect an observable, measurable activity. The performance may be visible (e.g., walking) or invisible (e.g., adding a column of figures). However, it is necessary to be able to deduce whether an unobservable activity has been mastered from some performance that represents the activity. Therefore, the performance of an outcome might be written as "selects low-fat foods from a menu" (observable), not "understands low-fat diet" (unobservable). Selected measurable verbs used for learning outcomes are shown in Box 26.3 on the next page. Avoid using such words as *knows, understands, believes,* and *appreciates;* they are neither observable nor measurable.
- Use modifiers as required to clarify what, where, when, or how the behaviour will be performed.

Examples are "demonstrates four-point crutch gait *correctly*" (modifier), "irrigates his colostomy *independently* (modifier) as taught," or "states *three* (modifier) factors that affect blood glucose level."

- Include criteria specifying the time by which learning should have occurred. For example, "the client will state three things that affect blood glucose level *by end of second class on diabetes.*"

Learning outcomes can reflect mastery of concepts, moving from the simple to the complex. For example, the learning outcome "the client will list cardiac risk factors" is a low-level knowledge outcome that simply requires the learner to identify cardiac risk factors; it does not suggest

BOX 26.3 EXAMPLES OF MEASURABLE VERBS FOR WRITING LEARNING OUTCOMES

Cognitive Domain	Affective Domain	Psychomotor Domain
Compares	Accepts	Assembles
Describes	Attends	Calculates
Evaluates	Chooses	Changes
Explains	Discusses	Demonstrates
Identifies	Displays	Measures
Labels	Initiates	Moves
Lists	Joins	Organizes
Names	Participates	Shows
Plans	Shares	
Selects	Uses	
States		
Writes		

application of the knowledge to the learner's own behaviours. The learning outcome "the client will describe *personal* cardiac risk factors" requires that the learner not only know cardiac risk factors but also know his personal behaviours that increase his risk for cardiac disease. See the Evidence-Informed Practice box on assessing postcardiac surgery patient learning needs.

In writing learning outcomes, the nurse must be specific about what behaviours and knowledge (cognitive, psychomotor, and affective) the learner must have to be able to positively influence his or her health state. In most cases, the learning needs are more complex than simple acquisition of knowledge and include the application of that knowledge to the learner (refer back to Box 26.2 on page 562).

Choosing Content What is to be taught is determined by learning outcomes. For instance, "identify appropriate sites for insulin injection" means the nurse must include content about the body sites suitable for insulin injections. Nurses can select among many sources of information, including books, nursing journals, and other nurses and health care professionals. Whatever sources the nurse chooses, content should be as follows:

- Accurate and current
- Based on learning outcomes
- Adjusted for the learner's age, developmental stage, culture, and ability
- Selected with consideration of how much time and what resources are available for teaching

Selecting Teaching Strategies The method of teaching that the nurse chooses should be suited to the individual and to the material to be learned (Figure 26.2). For example, the person who cannot read needs material presented in other ways; a one-to-one presentation session with question and answer is usually the best strategy for teaching a client how to give an injection; and group discussion is a useful way of discussing effective coping strategies. See Table 26.3 for selected teaching strategies.

Teaching Tools Having the right tools facilitates teaching. Tools can include handouts, equipment and supplies, photo albums, overhead transparencies, flip charts, bulletin boards, models of the human body, audio and videotapes, closed-circuit television, and computer programs. Tools need to be carefully selected for the individual client on the basis of the nurse's assessment.

EVIDENCE-INFORMED PRACTICE

Assessing Postcardiac Surgery Patient Learning Needs

Clinical nurses developed and tested a discharge questionnaire to elicit the specific learning needs of clients and their families following cardiac surgery in a large urban hospital in Quebec. The researchers developed the questionnaire by integrating learning issues identified by clients and families, caregivers, and nurses with those issues identified in the literature. The design of the questionnaire took into consideration client literacy levels, culture, language, and past experience of respondents.

NURSING IMPLICATIONS: When the questionnaire is properly developed to assess clients' learning needs, data collected will be valid and reliable and allow nurses to tailor their client teaching to the unique needs of patients and families.

Source: Based on Spyropoulos, V., Ampleman, S., Miousse, C., & Purden, M. (2011). Cardiac surgery discharge questionnaires: Meeting information needs of patients and families. *Canadian Journal of Cardiovascular Nursing, 21*(1), 13–19.

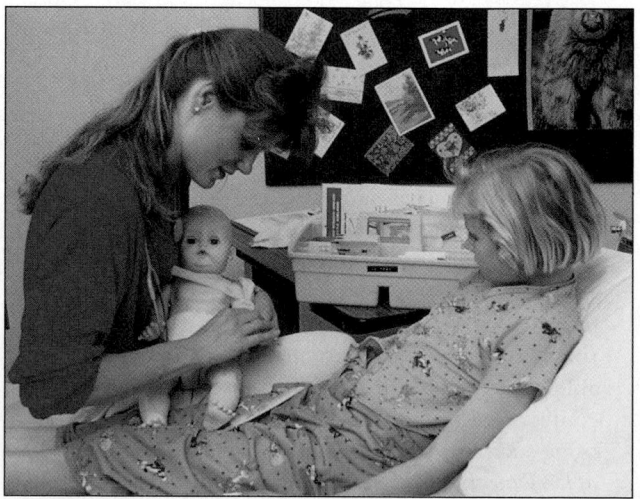

FIGURE 26.2 Teaching materials and strategies should be suited to the client's age and learning abilities.

TABLE 26.3   Selected Teaching Strategies

Strategy	Major Type of Learning	Characteristics
Explanation or description (e.g., lecture)	Cognitive	• Teacher controls content and pace. • Learner is passive and, therefore, retains less information than when actively participating. • Feedback is determined by teacher. • Can be given to individual or group.
One-to-one discussion	Affective, cognitive	• Encourages participation by learner. • Permits reinforcement and repetition at learner's level. • Permits introduction of sensitive subjects.
Answering questions	Cognitive	• Learner guides content taught. • Learner may need to overcome cultural perception that asking questions is impolite. • Can be used with individuals and groups.
Demonstration	Psychomotor	• Can be used with individuals, small or large groups. • Does not permit use of equipment by learners; learner is passive.
Discovery	Cognitive, affective	• Teacher guides problem-solving situation. • Learner is active participant. • Retention of information is high.
Group discussions	Affective, cognitive	• Learner can obtain assistance from supportive group. • Group members learn from one another. • Teacher needs to keep the discussion focused.
Practice	Psychomotor	• Allows repetition and immediate feedback. • Permits hands-on experience.
Printed and audiovisual materials	Cognitive	• Forms include books, pamphlets, films, programmed instruction, and computer learning. • Learners can proceed at their own speed. • Nurse can act as resource person. • Learner can learn independently.
Role playing	Affective, cognitive	• Permits expression of attitudes, values, and emotions. • Can assist in development of communication skills. • Teacher must create supportive, safe environment for learners.
Modelling	Affective, psychomotor	• Nurse sets example by attitude and psychomotor skill.
Computer-assisted learning programs	All types of learning	• Learner is active. • Learner controls pace. • Provides immediate reinforcement and review. • Use with individuals or groups.

Organizing Learning Experiences   To save nurses time in constructing their own teaching guides, some health agencies have developed teaching guides for teaching sessions that nurses commonly give. These guides standardize content and teaching methods and make it easier for the nurse to plan and implement client teaching. Standardized teaching plans also ensure consistency of content for the learner, thereby decreasing the risk of confusion if different practices are taught. For example, when teaching infant bathing, the nurses on the unit should be consistent about which soaps are appropriate for the infant's bath. Whether the nurse is implementing

a plan devised by another or developing an individualized teaching plan, some guidelines can help the nurse organize the learning experience:

• Start with something the learner is concerned about; for example, before learning how to self-administer insulin, an adolescent wants to know how to adjust his or her lifestyle and continue to play sports.

• Review what the learner knows, and then proceed to the unknown. This approach gives the learner confidence. Sometimes, you will not know the client's knowledge or skill base and will need to elicit this information, either by asking questions or by having the client fill out a form, such as a pretest.

- Address early in the teaching session any area that is causing the client anxiety. A high level of anxiety can impair concentration in other areas. For example, a woman highly anxious about turning her husband in bed might not be able to learn about bathing him until she has successfully learned to turn him in bed.

- Teach the basics before proceeding to the variations or adjustments. It is confusing to learners to have to consider possible adjustments and variations before they master the basic concepts. For example, when teaching a female client how to insert a retention catheter, it is best to teach the basic procedure before teaching any adjustments that might be needed if the catheter stops draining after insertion.

- Schedule time for review of content and to answer questions learners may have.

Implementing

The nurse must be flexible in implementing any teaching plan and revise the plan, as needed. The client's needs may change, or external factors may intervene. For instance, the nurse and the client, Mr. Brown, have planned to irrigate his colostomy at 1000h, but when the time comes, Mr. Brown wants additional information before actually doing it himself. In this case, the nurse alters the teaching plan and discusses the desired information, provides written information, and defers teaching the psychomotor skill until the next day. It is also important for nurses to use teaching techniques that enhance learning and reduce or eliminate any barrier to learning, such as pain or fatigue. Refer back to Table 26.2 on page 556 for barriers to learning.

GUIDELINES FOR TEACHING Knowledge alone is not enough to motivate a person to change a behaviour. Do not assume that providing information will automatically result in clients changing their behaviour. Learning what needs to be done to change behaviour and acting on that knowledge are two different processes. The stages of change, the person's willingness and perceived need to change, and barriers to change are important elements to reflect on when implementing a teaching plan (see the section "The Transtheoretical Model: Stages of Health Behaviour Change" in Chapter 8).

When implementing a teaching plan, the nurse may find the following guidelines helpful:

1. Assess the characteristics of the learners and, before the teaching session, identify factors that will affect their learning.

2. Determine the outcomes jointly with the client (learner). Reassess learning activities and replace them if they are ineffective. Active learner involvement can enhance learning.

3. The optimal time for each session depends largely on the learner. Whenever possible, ask the client for help in choosing the best time—for example, when he or she feels most rested.

4. The nurse should take time to establish rapport before teaching. A relationship between client and nurse that is respectful, constructive, and focused on client needs will facilitate learning.

5. Be sensitive to any signs that the pace is too fast or too slow. A client who appears confused or does not comprehend material when questioned may be finding the pace too fast. When the client appears bored and loses interest, the pace may be too slow, the learning period may be too long, or the client may be tired.

6. Build on the client's previous learning and encourage the client to learn and develop new skills. For example, the spouse of a person with diabetes may already have some knowledge of diabetes on which the nurse can build.

7. Communicate clearly and concisely. The words used need to have the same meaning to the learner as to the teacher. Using a layperson's vocabulary enhances communication. Even such words as *urine* or *feces* may be unfamiliar to some clients, and abbreviations, such as RR (recovery room) or PAR (postanesthesia room), are often misunderstood.

8. Use teaching aids that can help focus a learner's attention. To ensure the transfer of learning, the nurse should use the type of supplies or equipment the client will eventually use. Before the teaching session, the nurse needs to assemble all equipment and visual aids and ensure that all audiovisual equipment is functioning effectively (see the Teaching: Clinical box on teaching tools for children).

9. Create an environment conducive to learning. If in the hospital, and if possible, the client should be out of bed for learning activities. Being seated facilitates alertness but the nurse needs to be attentive to signs of fatigue in the client.

10. Use multiple senses in teaching to enhance learning. For example, when teaching about changing a surgical dressing, the nurse can tell the client about the procedure (hearing), show how to change the dressing (sight), and let the client manipulate the equipment (touch).

11. Provide a context for learning. For example, learning to select low-sodium foods can be done very effectively in a tour of a grocery store or through food selection from a restaurant menu.

12. Provide opportunities for clients to explore the content themselves. Ways to increase learning include stimulating motivation and self-direction, for example, (a) by providing specific, realistic,

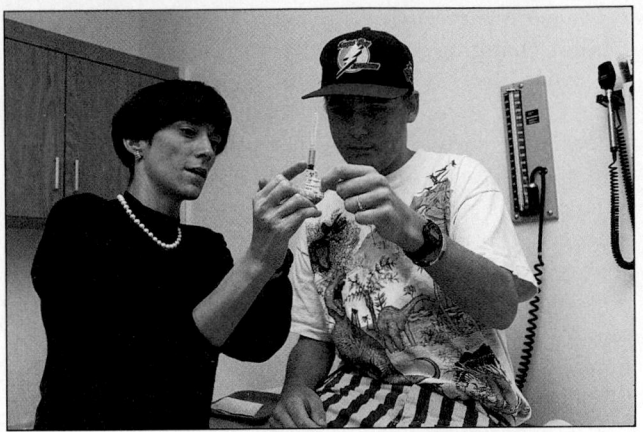

FIGURE 26.3 Teaching activities may need to include hands-on client participation.

achievable outcomes; (b) by giving feedback; and (c) by helping the learner derive satisfaction from learning. The nurse can also encourage self-directed independent learning by encouraging the client to explore different sources for the information required. Teaching activities may need to be replaced or supplemented to attain learning outcomes. Figure 26.3 illustrates that actual handling of the syringe may be more effective than explanation alone.

13. Use repetition to reinforce learning. Summarizing content, rephrasing (using other words), and teaching the material in another way are means of repeating and clarifying content. For instance, after discussing the kinds of foods that can be included in a diet, the nurse describes the foods again but in the context of the three meals eaten during one day.

14. The use of advance organizers to structure the content facilitates retention of information. Use such statements as "There are three signs of inflammation that I am going to discuss with you."

15. Assessment of learner outcomes must always be based on reasonable behavioural changes for the client to enact.

SPECIAL TEACHING STRATEGIES Nurses can choose from a number of special teaching strategies that are appropriate for the learner and the learning outcomes.

Client Contracting Client contracting involves establishing a learning contract with a client that specifies certain outcomes and when they are to be met. Here is an example of a self-contract:

> *I, Amy Martin, will exercise strenuously for 20 minutes three times per week for a period of 2 weeks and will then buy myself six yellow roses.*
>
> *Amy Martin*
>
> *July 30, 2013*

TEACHING   **CLINICAL**

Teaching Tools for Children

The use of the following teaching aids can help focus children's attention:

- *Visits.* Visiting the hospital and treatment rooms; seeing people dressed in uniforms, scrub suits, protective gear
- *Dress-up.* Touching and dressing up in the clothing they will see and wear
- *Colouring books.* Using colouring books to prepare for treatments, surgery, or hospitalization; shows what rooms, people, and equipment will look like
- *Storybooks.* Storybooks describe how the child will feel, what will be done, and what the place will look like. Parents can read these stories to children several times before the experience. Younger children like this repetition.
- *Dolls.* Practising procedures that children will later experience on dolls or teddy bears gives a sense of mastery of the situation. Custom dolls are often available for inserting tubes and giving injections, for example.
- *Puppet play.* Puppets can be used in role-play situations to provide information and show the child what the experience will be like; they help the child express emotions.
- *Health fairs.* Health fairs can educate children about their bodies and ways to stay healthy. Fairs can focus on high-risk problems that children face, such as accidents and poisoning.

The contract, drawn up and signed by the client and the nurse, can specify the learning outcomes, the responsibilities of the client and the nurse, and the methods of follow-up and evaluation. The contract can be changed in two ways: (a) if the client meets the contract outcomes and wants to negotiate new learning outcomes, and (b) if the client decides that it is not possible to meet the existing learning outcomes and wants to revise them (Bastable, 2008). A learning contract allows for freedom, mutual respect, and mutual responsibility and encourages clients to accept responsibility for learning.

Group Teaching Group instruction is economical and provides members with an opportunity to share with and learn from others. A small group allows for discussion in which everyone can participate. A large group often necessitates a lecture technique or use of films, videos, slides, or role playing by teachers. It is important that all members involved in group instruction have a need in common (e.g., prenatal health or preoperative instruction).

Internet Learning Resources The Internet has become a part of the lives of many Canadians, allowing them to communicate and obtain information quickly. The Internet has also become an important source of health information, screening tools, health services, and support groups;

REFLECT ON   **PRIMARY HEALTH CARE**

Client education is a central activity of nursing. Nurses use various teaching strategies to equip their clients with the needed knowledge and thus develop skills to improve and maintain their health. *Health promotion,* therefore, involves health education. Health education, in turn, calls for nurses to be innovative and to adapt delivery of care to meet client's social, economic, and cultural needs. Consider this example: In low-resource countries, where high-tech teaching supplies and visual models are often not affordable, nurses incorporate the principle of *appropriate technology* by teaching school-age children to draw in the sand in the schoolyard in the absence of papers or pencils. Nurses can also use available materials, such as twigs, stones, and vegetables, to create homemade teaching models if commercial models or charts are unavailable.

and many individuals are now accessing the Internet before consulting health care professionals about their health issues. Statistics Canada (2010) reported that 69.9% of Canadians searched the Internet for medical or health information in 2009. These searches focused on specific diseases, healthy lifestyles, symptoms, drugs or medications, and alternative therapies. The fastest growing group of people learning to use the Internet is those age 55 years and older (Mauk, 2010). More than 48% used the Internet first, prior to consulting with a physician. Nurses, therefore, need to be aware of such technology and be competent in integrating it into their teaching (see the Reflect on Primary Health Care box).

ONLINE HEALTH INFORMATION Computer-assisted instruction (CAI) can be used to teach new information, provide opportunities for the application of information, or support the development of complex problem-solving skills, often for continuing education of health care professionals. The learners are able to set the pace that meets their learning needs.

Computer simulations are becoming a common teaching strategy in student learning situations, such as nursing labs. Simulations provide not only a safe environment but also a realistic scenario for student learning, without jeopardizing the safety of a real client. Simulations can also standardize teaching and evaluation.

Discovery or Problem Solving In using the discovery or problem-solving technique, the nurse presents some initial information and then a situation related to the information. The learner applies the new information to the situation and decides what to do. Learners can work alone or in groups. The nurse guides the learners through the thinking process necessary to reach the best action to take in the situation. This method may also be referred to as anticipatory problem solving. For example, the nurse might ask parents with a newborn and a 2-year-old at home to identify ways of addressing issues of sibling rivalry with the toddler.

Behaviour Modification The behaviour modification system for changing behaviour has as its basic assumptions the following: (a) that human behaviours are learned and can be selectively strengthened, weakened, eliminated, or replaced; and (b) that a person's behaviour is under conscious control. Under this system, desirable behaviour is rewarded, and undesirable behaviour is ignored. The client's response is the key to behaviour change. For example, clients trying to quit smoking are not criticized when they smoke, but they are praised or rewarded when they go without a cigarette for a certain time. A learning contract may also be used to support this learning.

Transcultural Teaching The nurse and clients of different cultural and ethnic backgrounds have additional barriers to overcome in the teaching–learning process. These barriers can include language and communication problems, differing concepts of time, conflicting cultural healing practices, beliefs that may positively or negatively affect learning, or unique high-risk or high-frequency health problems that can be addressed with health-promotion instruction. Nurses should consider the following guidelines when teaching clients from various ethnic backgrounds:

- *Obtain teaching materials, pamphlets, and instructions in languages used by clients.* Nurses who are unable to read the foreign language material for themselves can have the interpreter read the material to clients.

- *Use visual aids, such as pictures, charts, or diagrams, to communicate meaning.* Audiovisual material can be helpful if English is spoken clearly and slowly. Even if understanding the verbal message is a problem for the client, seeing a skill or procedure may be helpful. In some instances, an interpreter can be asked to clarify the visual aid.

- *Use concrete rather than abstract words.* Use simple language (short sentences, short words), and present only one idea at a time.

- *Allow sufficient time for learners to ask questions and clarify any misconceptions* due to language or culture.

- *Avoid the use of medical terminology or health care language,* such as "taking your vital signs" or "apical pulse." Rather, nurses should say they are going to take a blood pressure reading or listen to the client's heart.

- *If understanding another's pronunciation is a problem, validate brief information in writing.*

- *Use humour very cautiously.* Meaning can change in the translation process.

- *Do not use slang words or colloquialisms.* These may be interpreted literally.

- *Do not assume that a client who nods, uses eye contact, or smiles is indicating an understanding of what is being taught.* These responses may simply be the client's way of indicating respect.

- *Invite and encourage questions during teaching.* Urge clients to ask questions to clarify information.

- When explaining procedures or functioning related to personal areas of the body, *it may be appropriate to have the teaching done by a nurse (and interpreter, if needed) of the same sex.*

- *Include the family in planning and teaching.* This promotes trust and mutual respect. Ask the client to identify the appropriate family member and incorporate that person into the planning and teaching to promote adherence and support of health teaching.

- *Consider the client's time orientation.* The client may be more oriented to the present than the future, so teaching preventative health behaviours may be difficult.

- *Identify cultural health practices and beliefs.* Noncompliance with health teaching may be related to conflict with folk medicine beliefs, lack of understanding, or conflict with cultural beliefs. To encourage compliance, the nurse needs to learn to the client's explanation of why the illness developed and how it might be treated.

Evaluating

Evaluating is both an ongoing and a final process in which the client, the nurse, and often the support people determine what has been learned.

EVALUATING LEARNING   The process of evaluation is the same as evaluating client achievement of desired outcomes for other nursing diagnoses. Learning is measured against the predetermined learning outcomes selected in the planning phase of the teaching process. Thus, the outcomes serve not only to direct the teaching plan but also to provide outcome criteria for evaluation. For example, the outcome "selects foods that are low in carbohydrates" can be evaluated by asking the client to name such foods or to select low-carbohydrate foods from a list.

The best method of evaluation depends on the type of learning. In *cognitive learning,* the client demonstrates acquisition of knowledge. Examples of the evaluation tools for cognitive learning include the following:

- Direct observation of behaviour (e.g., observing the client selecting the solution to a problem by using the new knowledge)

- Oral questioning (e.g., asking the client to restate information or provide correct verbal responses to questions)

- Self-reports and self-monitoring, which can be useful during follow-up phone calls and home visits

- Online self-assessment or self-screening tools, and learning post-tests

The acquisition of *psychomotor skills* is best evaluated by observing how well the client carries out a procedure, such as changing a dressing or carrying out a urinary self-catheterization.

Affective learning is more difficult to evaluate. Whether attitudes or values have been learned can be inferred by listening to the client's responses to questions, noting how the client speaks about relevant subjects, and observing the client's behaviour that expresses feelings and values. For example, do clients who state that they value health actually report use of condoms every time they have sex with a new partner?

Following evaluation, the nurse may find it necessary to modify or repeat the teaching plan if the outcomes have not been met or have been met only partially. For the hospitalized client, follow-up teaching in the home or by phone may be needed.

Behaviour change does not always take place immediately after learning. Often, individuals accept change intellectually first and then change their behaviour inconsistently (e.g., Mrs. Green, who knows that she must lose weight but diets and exercises only periodically). The nurse can assist clients with behaviour change by allowing for client vacillation and by providing encouragement.

EVALUATING TEACHING   It is important for nurses to evaluate their own teaching and the content of the teaching program. Evaluation should include a consideration of all factors: the timing, the teaching strategies, the amount of information, whether the teaching was helpful, and so on. The nurse may find, for example, that the client was overwhelmed with too much information, was bored, or was motivated to learn more. Both the client and the nurse should evaluate the learning experience. The client can tell the nurse what was helpful, interesting, and so on. Feedback questionnaires and videotapes of the learning sessions can also be useful.

The nurse should not feel ineffective as a teacher if the client forgets some of what is taught. Forgetting is normal and should be anticipated. Having the client write down information, repeating it during teaching, giving handouts on the information, and having the client be active in the learning process all promote retention.

Documenting

Documentation of the teaching process is essential because it provides a legal record that the teaching took place and communicates the teaching to other health care professionals. If teaching is not documented, then, legally, it did not occur.

It is also important to document the responses of the client and support people to teaching activities. What did the client or support person say or do to indicate that learning had occurred? Has the client demonstrated mastery of a skill or the acquisition of knowledge? The nurse records this evidence of learning in the client's chart. (See Chapter 24.)

Many agencies have multiple-copy client teaching forms that include the medical and nursing diagnoses, the treatment plan, and the client education. After the teaching session is completed, the client and the nurse sign the form and a copy of the form is given to the client as a record of teaching and as reinforcement of the content taught. A second copy of the completed and signed form is placed in the client's chart. The parts of the teaching process that should be documented in the client's chart include the following:

- Diagnosed learning needs
- Learning outcomes
- Topics taught
- Client outcomes
- Need for additional teaching
- Resources provided

The written teaching plan that the nurse uses as a resource to guide future teaching sessions might also include these elements:

- Actual information and skills taught
- Teaching strategies used
- Time framework and content for each class
- Teaching outcomes and methods of evaluation

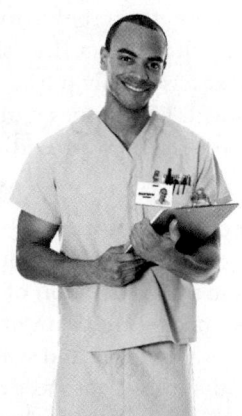

Case Study 26

Mrs. Marcos is a 59-year-old bank vice-president who is heavily relied on by her employer and coworkers. She moved to Canada from the Philippines 5 years ago. Three days ago, she was admitted to the hospital with complaints of shortness of breath and mild chest pain. A diagnostic evaluation indicated that she has significant coronary artery disease but has not yet suffered a heart attack. Her physician has indicated that Mrs. Marcos will need to make significant lifestyle changes to reduce her risk of heart attack. As her nurse, you recognize Mrs. Marcos's need to learn about her disease process, diet, exercise, and stress reduction. As you begin teaching Mrs. Marcos, you note that she is very pleasant and frequently nods her head, but she also seems preoccupied and is readily distracted.

CRITICAL THINKING QUESTIONS

1. How would you evaluate Mrs. Marcos's readiness to learn?

2. Mrs. Marcos is a well-educated client. Of what benefit would a learning needs assessment be?

3. You recognize that you have a great deal of information to teach Mrs. Marcos, and you are concerned that you will not be able to teach it all. What can you do to help Mrs. Marcos and still accomplish your teaching goals?

4. How will you know if your teaching is effective?

5. How might your teaching differ if you were teaching Mrs. Marcos at home, rather than in a hospital or acute care setting?

Check the eText in MyNursingLab for answers and explanations.

KEY TERMS

adherence *p. 553*

affective domain *p. 554*

andragogy *p. 553*

client education *p. 552*

cognitive *p. 553*

cognitive domain *p. 554*

cognitive theory *p. 554*

compliance *p. 553*

geragogy *p. 553*

health literacy *p. 560*

humanism *p. 554*

imitation *p. 554*

learning *p. 553*

learning need *p. 553*

modelling *p. 554*

motivation *p. 555*

pedagogy *p. 553*

positive reinforcement *p. 554*

psychomotor domain *p. 554*

readiness to learn *p. 555*

teaching *p. 552*

CHAPTER HIGHLIGHTS

- Teaching clients and families about their health needs is a major role of the nurse. Nurses also teach colleagues, other health care professionals, auxiliary personnel, nursing and other health care students, and groups in community education programs.
- Learning is represented by a change in behaviour or a different way of thinking.
- Three main theories of learning are behaviourism, cognitivism, and humanism.
- Bloom has identified three learning domains: cognitive, affective, and psychomotor.
- A number of factors facilitate learning: motivation, readiness, active involvement, relevance, feedback, nonjudgmental support, the progression from simple to complex concepts, repetition, timing, and environment.
- Such factors as emotions, certain physiological events, cultural barriers, and psychomotor deficits can impede learning.
- The teaching process, like the nursing process, consists of six activities: assessing the learner, diagnosing learning needs, developing a teaching plan, implementing the plan, evaluating learning

outcomes and teaching effectiveness, and documenting instructional activities.

- Learning outcomes guide the content of the teaching plan and are written in terms of client or learner behaviour.
- Teaching strategies should be suited to the client, the material to be learned, and the teacher. They should be adjusted to the client's developmental level and health status.
- A teaching plan is a written plan consisting of learning outcomes, content to teach, a time frame for teaching, and strategies to use in teaching the content. The plan must be revised when the client's needs change or the teaching strategies prove ineffective.
- Adaptations in teaching will facilitate learning for clients who have low or no reading skills, or are older or from different cultural backgrounds.
- Evaluation of the teaching–learning process is both an ongoing and a final process.
- Documentation of client teaching is essential to communicate the teaching to other health care professionals and to provide a record for legal and accreditation purposes.

ASSESS YOUR LEARNING

1. A community health nurse is giving a presentation to a group of parents. Which of the following actions would provide the nurse with the BEST initial feedback on the nurse's teaching skills?

   a. Eliciting the group's feelings about the presentation

   b. Observing the group's nonverbal behaviour

   c. Asking the group to complete a feedback questionnaire

   d. Administering a quiz on the content of the presentation

2. Which of the following activities would be classified as learning in the affective domain of Bloom's taxonomy?

   a. Learning how to calculate an appropriate drug dosage

   b. Learning to accept the loss of a limb

   c. Learning how to insert a catheter

   d. Reading handout material on the symptoms of congestive heart failure

3. Which of the following is the BEST way to help a client newly diagnosed with diabetes to learn the dietary requirements associated with the disease?

   a. Providing a videotape that addresses the dietary requirements associated with the disease

   b. Asking a nutritionist to visit the client to present information and handouts about the diabetic diet

   c. Assisting the client to determine how to work favourite foods into the diabetic diet

   d. Having the client attend a group meeting for diabetic clients to discuss adapting to this chronic health condition

4. A nurse is scheduling a teaching situation. Which of the following clients is MOST ready to learn?

   a. A 45-year-old man whose doctor just informed him that he has cancer

   b. A 3-year-old child whose parents have read her a storybook about going to the hospital

   c. A 60-year-old woman who received medication 5 minutes ago for relief of abdominal pain

   d. A 70-year-old man who is recovering from a stroke and has returned from physical therapy

5. How can the nurse BEST assess a client's style of learning?

   a. Ask the client how he or she learns best

   b. Use a variety of teaching strategies

   c. Observe the client's interactions with others

   d. Ask family members how the client learns

6. A 74-year-old client who takes multiple medications tells the nurse, "I have no idea what that little yellow pill is for." What is the BEST nursing diagnosis for this client?

   a. *Deficient Knowledge: Medication Information*

   b. *Readiness for Enhanced Knowledge: Disease Information*

   c. *Deficient Knowledge: Self-Care Measures*

   d. *Noncompliance: Medication Self-Administration*

7. A nurse is talking with a client who is scheduled to have a diagnostic procedure. Which comment by the client indicates a teachable moment?

   a. "I've had this procedure done before."

   b. "Will this procedure hurt?"

   c. "I'm trying not to think about it."

   d. "I have an appointment with another person right now."

8. A client needs to learn to self-administer insulin injections. Which statement may reflect low literacy skills?

   a. "I will read the information later. I'm too tired right now."

   b. "I've watched my brother give his own shots. I know how to do it."

   c. "I'm afraid of injections. Do I have to give my own shots?"

   d. "Do you have a video showing how I should give myself the shot?"

9. A client has a learning outcome of "select foods that are low in fat." Which of the following statements reflects that the client has met this learning outcome?

   a. "I understand the importance of maintaining a low-fat diet."

   b. "I feel better about myself now, since I have learned this."

   c. "I was able to choose a low-fat lunch off the restaurant menu."

   d. "Since I changed my diet, my husband is also losing weight."

10. A client's learning outcome is "client will state medication name, purpose, and appropriate precautions." Which of the following documented statements reflects evidence of learning?

    a. Taught name, purpose, and precautions for the new cardiac medication; client seemed to understand.

    b. Written information about the medication provided and reviewed; correct responses were given to follow-up questions.

    c. Written information read to client; stated he would read it when he got home.

    d. Information about the medication taught to client; client stated he understood it.

Check the eText in MyNursingLab for answers and explanations.

WEBLINKS

ABC Life Literacy Canada
http://abclifeliteracy.ca

This foundation is a Canada-wide educational organization that focuses on literacy skills. This site identifies literacy statistics, an overview of related workplace issues, and publications.

Canadian Nurses Association
http://www.cna-aiic.ca

Through this site, the user has access to resources of the Canadian Nurses Association in which the role of the nurse as client teacher is identified. The NurseOne portal is an excellent resource for students and nurses who are engaged in teaching.

Canadian Public Health Association (CPHA)
http://www.cpha.ca/en/pls.aspx

As part of its National Literacy and Health Program, the CPHA established the Plain Language Service (PLS) to support health care professionals in the preparation of clear and easily understood written print and Internet materials.

The Public Health Agency of Canada (PHAC)
http://www.phac-aspc.gc.ca

This agency provides educational resources for both clients and professionals around various issues of lifestyle and health. The public resources are specifically tailored to the needs of Canadians.

HLWIKI Canada
http://hlwiki.slais.ubc.ca/index.php/Patient_education

An open health information and services Wikipedia source with entries about social media for information professionals and information technology topics.

MyNursingLab

REFERENCES

Bandura, A. (1971). Analysis of modelling processes. In A. Bandura (Ed.)., *Psychological modelling: Conflicting theories* (pp. 1–62). New York: NY: Aldione-Atherton.

Bastable, S. (2008). *Nurse as educator: Principles of teaching and learning for nursing practice* (3rd ed.). Boston, MA: Jones & Bartlett.

Bloom, B. S. (Ed.). (1956). *Taxonomy of educational objectives. Book 1, Cognitive domain.* New York, NY: Longman.

Canadian Council on Learning. (2007). *Health literacy in Canada: Initial results from the international adult and skills survey.* Retrieved from http://www.ccl-cca.ca/ccl/Reports/HealthLiteracy.html

Chang, M., & Kelly, A. E. (2007). Patient education: Addressing cultural diversity and health literacy issues. *Urologic Nursing, 27*(5), 411–417.

Knowles, M., Holton, E. F., & Swanson, R. A. (2011). *The adult learner: The definitive classic in adult education and human resource development* (7th ed.). Burlington, MA: Elsevier.

Lewin, K. (1951). *Field theory in social science.* New York, NY: Harper and Row.

Mauk, K. L. (2010). *Gerontological nursing: Competencies for care* (2nd ed.). Boston, MA: Jones and Bartlett.

Maslow, A. H. (1970). *Motivation and personality* (2nd ed.). New York, NY: Harper & Row.

Mayer, G. G., & Villaire, M. (2007). *Health literacy in primary care: A clinician's guide.* New York, NY: Springer.

NANDA International. (2012). *Nursing diagnoses: Definitions and classification, 2012–2014.* Oxford, U.K.: Wiley-Blackwell.

Pavlov, I. P. (1927). *Conditioned reflexes* (G. V. Anrep, Trans.). London, UK: Oxford University Press.

Piaget, J. (1966). *Origins of intelligence in children.* New York, NY: Norton.

Porter-O'Grady, T. (2001). Profound change: 21st century nursing. *Nursing Outlook, 49,* 182–186.

Purnell, L. D., & Paulanka, B. J. (2008). *Transcultural health care: A culturally competent approach* (3rd ed.). Philadelphia, PA: F. A. Davis.

Redman, B. K. (2004). *Advances in patient education.* New York, NY: Springer.

Registered Nurses' Association of Ontario. (2006). *Client centred care. Nursing best practice guidelines: Shaping the future of nursing.* Toronto, ON: Author.

Skinner, B. F. (1953). *Science and human behavioral change.* New York, NY: Macmillan.

Statistics Canada. (2010). *Internet use by individuals, by type of activity.* CANSIM Table 358-0130. Retrieved from http://www40.statcan.gc.ca/l01/cst01/comm29a-eng.htm?sdi=internet

Weiss, B. D., Mays, M. Z., Martz, W., Castro, K. M., DeWalt, D. A., Pignone, M. P., . . . Hale, F. (2005). Quick assessment of literacy in primary care: The newest vital sign. *Annals of Family Medicine, 3*(6), 514–522.

Wilkinson, J. M., & Ahern, N. R. (2008). *Nursing diagnosis handbook with NIC interventions and NOC outcomes* (9th ed.). Upper Saddle River, NJ: Prentice Hall Health.

Chapter 27

Leading, Managing, and Delegating

LEARNING OUTCOMES

After studying this chapter, you will be able to:

1. Compare and contrast leadership and management.

2. Differentiate formal from informal leaders.

3. Compare and contrast different leadership styles.

4. Identify the characteristics of an effective leader.

5. Compare and contrast the levels of management.

6. Describe the skills and competencies needed by a nurse manager.

7. Describe the functions of management.

8. Describe change management theories and the impact of change on leadership decisions.

9. Discuss the roles and functions of nurse leaders in planning for and implementing change.

ccording to the Canadian Nurses Association (CNA, 2009), in the next decade, we will see a Canadian health system that is different from one we have ever seen. Many of these changes will have been driven by new knowledge and technology, and changes in global and regional dynamics. In the *Toward 2020: Visions for Nursing* document (Villeneuve & MacDonald, 2006), the CNA envisions nurses as working with an ever-increasing multidisciplinary team of health care providers. The CNA stressed that nurse leaders "must focus on health and the health system, not [just] on nurses and nursing. . . . Nurses will be expected to be strong advocates for patients, facilities, communities, and social issues" (p. 84). The next generation of nurses must work efficiently and effectively to meet public expectations and to become effective leaders and change agents.

Nurse as Leader

Leadership, management, and delegation are consistent aspects of the nursing role. As a part of multidisciplinary teams, the nurse may function as a manager and as a change agent in some situations, or as a leader and delegate aspects of care to others, as needed. The professional nurse frequently assumes the roles of leader and manager. These roles are linked but differ in their focus.

A **leader** influences others to work together to accomplish a specific goal. Leaders are often visionaries; they are informed, articulate, confident, and self-aware. Leaders must have excellent interpersonal skills and be astute communicators. Most importantly, they have the ability to innovate, change, motivate, facilitate, mentor, and inspire others. Within their organizations, nurse leaders engage and lead teams that assess the effectiveness of care, implement evidence-based practice, and construct process improvement strategies. (See the Reflect on Primary Health Care box.)

A **manager** is an employee of an organization who is given authority, power, and responsibility for planning, organizing, coordinating, and directing the work of others, and for establishing and evaluating standards. Managers understand organizational structure and culture. They control human, financial, and material resources. Managers set goals, make decisions, and solve problems. They initiate and implement change.

Nurse managers are also responsible for (a) efficiently accomplishing the goals of the organization, (b) efficiently using the organization's resources, (c) ensuring effective client care, and (d) ensuring compliance with institutional, professional, regulatory, and governmental standards. Managers focus on the task and concentrate on activities to increase productivity, while leaders focus on motivation, developing a vision, and building trusting relationships (Meilinger, 2001). Table 27.1 on the next page compares the roles of the leader and the manager. Figure 27.1 on the next page provides some examples of leader and manager roles.

Leadership

Leadership may be formal or informal. The **formal leader** is selected by an organization and given official authority to make decisions and act. An **informal leader** is not officially appointed to direct activities of others but is selected by a group as its leader because of seniority, age, special abilities, experience, or a charismatic personality and plays an important role in influencing colleagues to achieve goals.

Leadership Theory

Early leadership theories focused on what leaders are (trait theories), what leaders do (behavioural theories), and how leaders adapt their leadership style according to the situation (contingency theories). Theories about **leadership style** describe traits, behaviours, motivations, and choices used by individuals to effectively influence others.

REFLECT ON 🔑 **PRIMARY HEALTH CARE**

Nurses work in multiple roles with various health care providers in multidisciplinary teams to provide care for well and ill clients (*intersectoral collaboration*). Within their organizations, nurse leaders play a formal role to guide their teams in assessing the effectiveness of care, implementing evidence-based practice, and constructing process improvement strategies. These nurse leaders may be team leaders or institutional leaders. As well, they may also be informal leaders associated with professional health and social service organizations or community boards. They assist in strategic planning to create positive change. Can you identify who the nurse leaders are in your community and the role they play in creating change in their practice locations?

TABLE 27.1 Comparison of Leader and Manager Roles

Leaders	Managers
May or may not be officially appointed to the position	Are appointed officially to the position
Have power and authority to enforce decisions only as long as followers are willing to be led	Have power and authority to enforce decisions
Influence others toward goal setting, either formally or informally	Carry out predetermined policies, rules, and regulations
Are interested in risk-taking and exploring new ideas	Maintain an orderly, controlled, rational, and equitable structure
Relate to people personally in an intuitive and empathetic manner	Relate to people according to their roles
Feel rewarded by personal achievements	Feel rewarded when fulfilling organizational mission or goals
May or may not be successful as managers	Are managers as long as the appointment holds
Manage relationships	Manage resources
Focus on people	Focus on systems

CLASSICAL LEADERSHIP THEORIES The *trait theorists* found that leaders often possess specific traits and abilities, including good judgment, decisiveness, knowledge, adaptability, integrity, tact, popularity, nonconformity, and cooperativeness. The *behaviourists* believed that through education, training, and life experiences, effective leaders develop a particular style of leadership. These styles have been characterized as autocratic, democratic, laissez-faire, and bureaucratic.

Autocratic (authoritarian, directive) leaders make decisions for the group. The leader believes individuals are externally motivated and incapable of independent

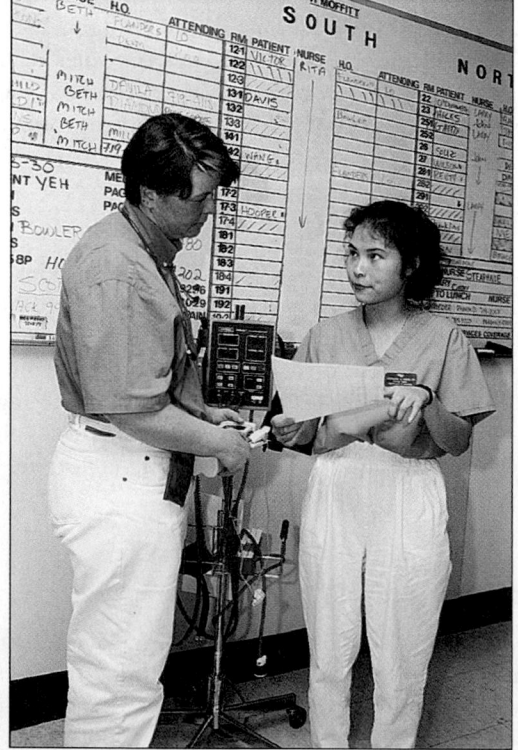

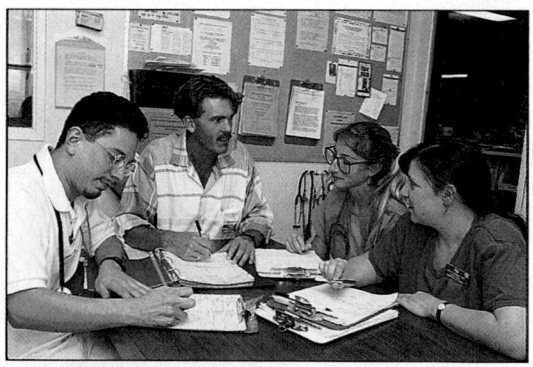

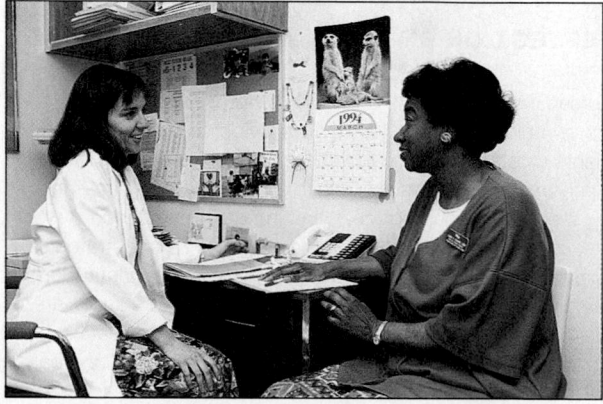

FIGURE 27.1 Nurses as leaders and managers. **A:** The nurse manager discusses work assignments during the change-of-shift report. **B:** The nurse delegates basic client care activities to other care providers. **C:** The nurse consults the social worker during discharge planning.

decision making. The autocratic leader determines policies and gives orders to the group. The group may feel secure because procedures are well defined. Productivity may also be high. However, the group's needs for creativity, autonomy, and self-motivation are not met, and openness and trust between the leader and the group members is minimal. Members are often dissatisfied with this type of leadership; however, sometimes an autocratic style is effective. When urgent decisions are necessary (e.g., during a cardiac arrest, a unit fire, or a mass casualty event), one person must assume the responsibility to make decisions without being challenged. When group members are unable or do not wish to participate in making a decision, the authoritarian style solves the problem and enables everyone to move on. This style can also be effective when a project must be completed quickly and efficiently.

Democratic (participative, consultative) leaders encourage group discussion and decision making. This type of leader assumes individuals are internally motivated, capable of making decisions, and value independence. Group productivity and satisfaction are high as members contribute to the effort. The democratic leader acts as a facilitator, actively guiding the group toward achieving goals, providing constructive criticism, offering information, making suggestions, and asking questions. This type of leadership demands that the leader have faith in the group members to accomplish the tasks. Although democratic leadership has been shown to be less efficient than authoritarian leadership, it allows for more self-motivation and more creativity and cooperation among group members. This style of leadership can be extremely effective in the health care setting.

The **laissez-faire (nondirective, permissive, ultraliberal) leader** presupposes the group is internally motivated, autonomous, and self-regulating. This leader assumes a hands-off approach while group members act independently. This may result in a lack of coordination. A laissez-faire style is most effective for groups whose members have both personal and professional maturity. When the group has made a decision, the members become committed to it.

The **bureaucratic leader** presumes the group is externally motivated. However, the bureaucrat does not trust self or others to make decisions. Instead, the bureaucrat relies on the organization's rules, policies, and procedures to direct the group's efforts. Group members may be dissatisfied with the leader's inflexibility and impersonal relations with them. Table 27.2 compares the authoritarian, democratic, laissez-faire, and bureaucratic leadership styles.

Situational leaders consider the situation and determine an appropriate leadership style for the individual or group to perform the task in that particular situation. When employees are insecure or unable or unwilling to perform the task, the leader uses a directive style, providing specific instructions and supervision. If the group is motivated and willing but unable to perform the task, the leader explains decisions and provides the opportunity for clarification. When the group is able but unwilling or lacking in confidence, the leader shares ideas and facilitates decision making. For a group that is willing, able, and confident to perform the task, the leader delegates, turning responsibility for decision making and implementation over to the group.

CONTEMPORARY LEADERSHIP THEORIES Contemporary theorists have described charismatic leaders, transactional leaders, transformational leaders, and shared leadership.

A **charismatic leader** is characterized by an emotional relationship between the leader and the group members. The charming personality of the leader evokes strong feelings of commitment to the leader and the leader's cause and beliefs. The followers of a charismatic leader often overcome extreme hardship to achieve the group's goals because of their faith in the leader.

The **transactional leader** focuses on the process and not what changes to make for the future. The main activities are supervision, organization, and monitoring of staff performance. The leader promotes compliance by using rewards and punishments. Rewards may be in the form of job promotion, preferred shifts, and special privileges or more benefits. Punishments may be in the form of suspension, demotion, or job loss.

TABLE 27.2 Comparison of Autocratic, Democratic, Laissez-Faire, and Bureaucratic Leadership Styles

	Autocratic	Democratic	Laissez-Faire	Bureaucratic
Degree of control	Makes decisions alone	Collaborative	No control	Strict reliance on policy
Leader activity level	High	High	Minimal	High
Assumption of responsibility	Primarily the leader	Shared	Relinquished	Leader
Output of the group	High quantity, good quality	Creative, high quality	Variable, may be of poor quality	Good quality through following standard procedures
Efficiency	Very efficient	Less efficient than autocratic	Inefficient	Efficient

The **transformational leader** fosters creativity, risk-taking, commitment, and collaboration by empowering the group to share in the organization's vision. The leader inspires others with a clear, attractive, and attainable goal and enlists them to participate in attaining the goal. The Registered Nurses' Association of Ontario (RNAO, 2006) stresses the need for nurse leaders to be aware of the personal attributes they bring to their role. The best practice guidelines include the following attributes for transformational leadership:

1. Nurse leaders exhibit a strong professional nursing identity.
2. Nurse leaders reflect on and work to develop their individual leadership attributes.
3. Nurse leaders take responsibility for the growth and development of their own leadership expertise and mentor others to develop leadership expertise.
4. Nurse leaders cultivate professional and personal supports.

In addition, transformational nurse leaders work to create an environment of empowerment, support others to develop and integrate knowledge, and understand the impact of change.

One subtype of the transformational leader is a **servant leader**, which is based on the concept that leaders serve their followers. Members of an organization act as both servants and leaders within a work environment of mutual respect, trust, and collaboration (Sturm, 2009). The distinctive quality of a servant leader is that the leader is focused on serving the best interests of the followers (Irving & Longbotham, 2007). In nursing, this concept is internally consistent with a focus on caring where the leader aspires to assist those they are leading to become more autonomous, empathetic, and healing.

Shared leadership recognizes that a professional workforce is made up of many leaders. No one person is considered to have knowledge or ability beyond that of other members. Appropriate leadership is thought to emerge in relationship to whatever challenges confront the group. **Shared governance** refers to the process where people participate in the planning and decision-making processes while holding one another accountable to the outcomes of the actions.

Effective Leadership

Leadership is a learned process. An effective leader needs to apply the principles of effective leadership, which include vision, influence, and power to effect positive change. This encompasses an understanding of motivation factors, such as needs, goals, and rewards; knowledge of leadership skills and of group dynamics; and possession of effective communication and interpersonal skills to influence others. Statements about effective leaders are listed in Box 27.1.

Vision is a mental image of a possible and desirable future state. Leaders transform visions that reflect their

> **BOX 27.1 CHARACTERISTICS OF EFFECTIVE LEADERS**
>
> Effective leaders:
> - Are able to function autonomously
> - Use a leadership style that is natural to them
> - Use a leadership style appropriate to the task and the members
> - Assess the effects of their behaviour on others and the effects of others' behaviour on themselves
> - Are sensitive to forces acting for and against change
> - Express an optimistic view about human nature
> - Are energetic
> - Are open and encourage openness so that real issues are confronted and trust is developed
> - Facilitate personal relationships
> - Plan and organize activities of the group
> - Are consistent in behaviour toward group members
> - Delegate tasks and responsibilities to develop members' abilities, not merely to get tasks done
> - Involve members in all decisions
> - Value and use group members' contributions
> - Encourage creativity
> - Encourage feedback about their leadership style
> - Assess for and promote the use of current technology

values and beliefs into realistic goals and communicate their visions to others, who accept them as their own.

Influence is an informal strategy used to gain the cooperation of others without exercising formal authority. Influence is exercised through persuasion and excellent communication skills; it is based on a trusting relationship with the followers.

Power is the capacity to act or to influence others to act to achieve something. There are five sources of power: (a) position power, (b) personal power, (c) task power, (d) relationship power, and (e) expert power. **Position power** is related to the authority associated with a role or title and includes the power to manage people or command resources. **Personal power** is associated with admiration by others, which comes from having such attributes as strength of character, passion, inspiration, or wisdom. **Task power** is the ability to influence who is able to help with a process or task. **Relationship power** pertains to the respect others have for an individual's personal abilities, knowledge, or skills. **Expert power** is based on the person's expertise or knowledge (Sullivan & Decker, 2009).

Nurse as Manager

The manager's job is to accomplish the work of the organization. To this end, managers perform a number of roles and functions that vary with the type of organization and the level of management.

Levels of Management

Traditional management is divided into three levels of responsibility. **First-level managers** (e.g., program or unit managers, supervisors, charge nurse, head nurse, or nurse manager) are responsible for managing the work of non-managerial personnel and the day-to-day activities of a specific work group or groups. Their primary responsibility is to implement the organization's goals. This level of manager represents staff and reports to a middle-level manager.

Middle-level managers (e.g., program directors; department, division, or regional managers) supervise a number of first-level managers and are responsible for the activities in the departments they supervise. Middle-level managers serve as liaisons between first-level managers and upper-level managers.

Upper-level managers (e.g., senior administrators such as executive directors (ED), vice presidents (VP), chief executive officer (CEO), chief operating office (COO), and chair of the board) are primarily responsible for instilling organizational changes by establishing goals and developing strategic plans. Nurse managers at this level are responsible for leading the management team to work collaboratively to achieve the organization's vision and goals with a view to achieving an excellent standard of client services.

Management Functions

Four management functions that help achieve the goal of quality client care are (a) planning, (b) organizing, (c) directing, and (d) coordinating.

PLANNING   Planning is an ongoing process that involves (a) assessing a situation, (b) establishing goals and objectives based on assessment of a situation or future trends, and (c) developing a plan of action that identifies priorities, delineates who is responsible, determines deadlines, and describes how the intended outcome is to be achieved and evaluated. In short, it involves deciding what to do; when, where, and how to do it; who will do it; and what resources will be used.

For example, when planning for the introduction of a falls prevention program, the upper-level manager develops the goals, approves the financial commitment, and directs the middle manager to implement the program. The middle manager communicates and directs the implementation of the falls prevention program to the first-level manager. The first-level manager is responsible for directing the actual implementation of the program with educators and staff.

ORGANIZING   Organizing involves determining responsibilities, communicating expectations, and establishing the chain of command for authority and communication.

DIRECTING   Directing is the process of getting the organization's work accomplished. Directing involves assigning and communicating expectations. It could also include providing instruction and guidance, and ongoing decision

making. For example, charge nurses direct shift work by assigning clients and scheduling meal and break times. Staff nurses direct the care of clients by ordering nursing care, communicating care in written care plans and shift reports, and supervising care that is given by others.

COORDINATING   Coordinating is the process of ensuring that plans are carried out and evaluating outcomes. The manager measures results or actions against standards or desired outcomes and then reinforces effective actions.

Principles of Management

A manager exercises authority, accountability, and responsibility, as described below.

Authority is the official power to act; it is the legitimate right to direct the work of others and an integral component of managing. Authority is conveyed through leadership actions; it is determined largely by the situation, and it is always associated with responsibility and accountability. The manager must exercise the authority that comes with the role.

Accountability is a person's ability and willingness to assume responsibility for his or her own actions and to accept the consequences of his or her behaviour. Accountability starts at the individual level, moves to the institutional or professional level, and ends at the societal level. At the individual level, accountability is reflected in the nurse's ethical integrity. At the institutional level, it is reflected in the statement of philosophy and objectives of the nursing department and nursing policies. At the professional level, it is reflected in standards of practice developed by national or provincial or territorial nursing associations. At the societal level, it is reflected in legislated nurse practice acts.

Responsibility is an obligation to complete a task. Managers are responsible for all operations under their authority. For example, the utilization of resources, communication to subordinates, and implementation of organizational goals.

Skills and Competencies of Nurse Managers

To be effective managers, nurses need to be able to think critically, communicate well, manage resources effectively, enhance employee performance, build and manage teams, manage conflict, manage time effectively, delegate effectively, and initiate and manage change. (Refer to the section "The Transtheoretical Model: Stages of Health Behaviour Change" in Chapter 8.)

CRITICAL THINKING   Critical thinking is a cognitive process that includes creativity, problem solving, and decision making. The nurse manager reasons with logic, exploring the assumptions, the alternatives, and the consequences of actions. See Chapter 21 for a discussion of critical thinking and decision making.

COMMUNICATING Good communication is essential to other critical interpersonal skills and often determines the manager's success as a leader. Managers use both verbal and written communication. Effective managers communicate assertively, clearly, accurately, and honestly. Managers use **networking**, a process whereby professional links are established through which people share ideas, knowledge, and information; offer support and direction to one another; and facilitate accomplishment of professional goals. Nurses can develop professional networks throughout their careers in settings such as school, work, professional organizations, and social groups.

MANAGING RESOURCES One of the greatest responsibilities of managers is their accountability for human, fiscal, and material resources. Budgeting and determining variances between the actual and the budgeted expenses are crucial skills for any manager.

Staff Mix Determining the correct staff mix of registered nurses (RNs), licensed practical nurses (LPNs), and registered practical nurses (RPNs) in a practice setting can directly influence client outcomes. Delegation between nurses must be accomplished on the basis of the knowledge of the scope of practice of other nurses, client factors such as the complexity of care, the predictability of care outcomes, and the risk of negative consequences to care, as well as practice environmental factors, such as access to resources and supports for nurses and policies and procedures needed for client decision making (CNA, 2005b; College of Nurses of Ontario [CNO], 2009; College of Registered Nurses of British Columbia [CRNBC], 2005).

Intergenerational Workers For the first time in nursing history, four generations of nurses are working in the health care system. Today's nurses can be categorized into the *Silent Generation, Baby Boomers, Generation X,* and the *Millennial Generation* (Sudheimer, 2009). Nurses from different generations must learn to appreciate each other's strengths and respectfully work through differences. Managers need to be aware that the different work ethics, values, and strengths of intergenerational nurses can create stress in the workplace. The characteristics of each generation are described below:

- **Silent Generation** (1933–1944): Nurses of this generation have a traditional work ethic and excellent critical thinking skills. They are disciplined and loyal team players. They share their knowledge and expertise readily with their colleagues.
- **Baby Boomers** (1945–1964): Nurses of this generation make up most of the nursing profession. They are extremely hard working and have been the driving force of much of the progress in nursing in the past 20 years.
- **Generation X** (1965–1978): Nurses of this generation are independent, resilient, and confident, and they are committed to their colleagues and clients before their employers. They like to share their expertise with their colleagues and clients. Their care tends to be guided more by their clients' desire than by rules and policies in the organization.
- **Millennial Generation, or Generation Y** (1979–2000): Nurses of this generation grew up with technologies and are at ease with computers, video games, and cell phones. They can multitask and strive for self-fulfillment; they can also establish rapport easily with team members, patients, and families. The next generation of nurses will be the *Generation Z,* who place more importance on loyalty, are more conservative, and hold a more traditional value system compared with those of Generation Y.

ENHANCING EMPLOYEE PERFORMANCE Managers are responsible for developing their staff by providing appropriate learning opportunities such as in-service education or professional workshops or encouraging achievement of advanced education. Nurse managers who provide support to enhance their staff performance will find that their employees have greater commitment to the institution, are more effective in their role, have increased self-esteem, and are better able to meet their goals.

The manager may also provide day-to-day coaching or serve as a mentor or preceptor. **Mentors** "give their time, energy, and material support to teach, guide, assist, counsel, and inspire younger nurses. It is a nurturing relationship . . ." (Marriner Tomey, 2009, p. 373). Having a mentor is recognized as important for career development. In the clinical area, the term **preceptor** is used to describe relationships in which the experienced nurse assists the "new" nurse in improving clinical nursing skills and judgment. The preceptor also instills understanding of the routines, policies, and procedures of the unit.

BUILDING AND MANAGING TEAMS The manager is responsible for building and managing the work team. Familiarity with group processes and the roles that group members play facilitates the manager's ability to lead the group and enhances development of the group into a work team. Groups develop in stages, during which roles and relationships are established (see the Evidence-Informed Practice box on what motivates nurses to improve their performance). (Detailed information about group stages and roles is provided in the section "Group Communication" in Chapter 22.)

Evaluating the group's work is another responsibility of the manager. Effectiveness, efficiency, and productivity are three outcome measures that are frequently used. In nursing, **effectiveness** is a measure of the quality or quantity of services provided. **Efficiency** is a measure of the resources used in the provision of nursing services. **Productivity** is a performance measure of both the effectiveness and the efficiency of nursing care. Productivity is frequently measured in the amount of nursing resources used per client or in terms of required versus actual hours of care provided.

EVIDENCE-INFORMED PRACTICE

What Motivates Nurses to Improve Their Performance?

Two University of Alberta nursing professors conducted a systematic review of studies that focused on nurse's perceptions of factors that influence nursing performance. They reviewed 6289 articles and selected eight studies that met the criteria on what motivates nurses to perform, leadership practices in health care settings, and relationships between nurse performance and leadership behaviours. The analysis revealed that autonomy, work relationships, accessibility of resources, nurse factors, and leadership practices all affect nurses' ability to meet organizational goals and deliver quality patient care.

NURSING IMPLICATIONS: Nurse performance can be improved by addressing their autonomy, available resources, relationships among peers, and leaders in the workplace. Effective leadership can directly and indirectly affect nurses' ability to perform optimally on the job. Organizations should evaluate what motivational factors for nurses help them to perform optimally.

Source: Based on Brady Germain, P., & Cummings, G. G. (2010). The influence of nursing leadership on nurse performance: A systematic review of the literature, *Journal of Nursing Management, 18,* 425–439.

MANAGING CONFLICT Nurse managers are frequently in a position to manage conflict. Conflict can arise from differing values, philosophies, or personalities. It can also arise through competition for resources. When conflict among nurses is left unresolved, it can lead to workplace incivility (bullying, inappropriate conduct and behaviours) and can have serious consequences. Collegial relationships based on trust and respect are important to ensuring safe client care. Unresolved conflict—and a lack of communication, support, and trust—can leave clients and nurses vulnerable to unnecessary risk (CNO, 2006a). It is an expectation that nurses demonstrate effective conflict-resolution skills. Communication strategies, such as active listening, attending to nonverbal behaviours, and addressing behaviours in a nonjudgmental manner, all contribute to promoting respect and collegiality among team members. However, these strategies are only the first step in resolving the conflict. Nurses need to explore and understand the root cause of conflict and abusive behaviour. The CNO's (2006b) special training on conflict management and crisis prevention would be added resources for nurses in management position.

There are many methods to manage conflict, and each has its advantages and disadvantages. Among the most common are compromise, negotiation, and collaboration. The new nurse manager may require training to become proficient in the use of these methods. Basic principles for all types of conflict management include demonstrating respect for all parties, avoiding blaming others, allowing full discussion, using ground rules during meetings to promote fairness, encouraging active listening, identifying the themes in the discussion, and exploring alternative solutions (Sullivan & Decker, 2009).

MANAGING TIME Effective nurse managers use time effectively and assists others to do the same. Many factors inhibit good use of time, such as personal preferences, emergencies or crises that divert the nurse's attention, and unrealistic demands from others. Strategies that can be employed to use time well involve setting goals and priorities, delegating appropriately, examining how time is used, minimizing paperwork (automating, whenever possible), and using regular schedules that avoid interruptions and set time limits on activities (Sullivan & Decker, 2009).

Nurse as Delegator

Delegation is the transference of responsibility and authority for the performance of an activity to a competent individual. The delegator retains accountability for the outcome. Managers use delegation so that they can devote more time to tasks that cannot be delegated. Delegation builds self-esteem, promotes morale, and enhances teamwork and organizational goal attainment. In nursing, delegation refers to care that is provided by someone else and supervised by the nurse. The delegating nurse defines the task, determines who can perform the task, describes the expectation, seeks agreement, meets timelines, monitors performance, and provides feedback to the delegatee regarding performance and outcomes of the assigned task (Sullivan & Decker, 2009).

With the complexity of the work environment, increasingly RNs delegate components of nursing care to **unregulated care providers (UCP)**, such as community health workers, health care aides, home support workers, personal support workers (PSW), visiting homemakers, palliative care workers, and unit or ward aides. An RN who delegates a task is accountable for selecting an appropriately skilled caregiver and for continued evaluation of the client's care. The actual performance of the task is the responsibility of the UCP. Guidelines for delegating nursing tasks and procedures appear in Box 27.2.

Tasks that can be delegated to UCPs vary nationally and must be considered by the delegating RN. Principles guiding the nurse's decision to delegate that ensure the safety and quality of outcomes are listed in Box 27.3. The UCP cannot delegate tasks to another person.

When an RN or RPN decides to delegate, he or she must communicate clearly to the UCP and verify that the UCP understands the following:

- The specific tasks to be done for each client
- When each task is to be done
- The expected outcomes for each task, including parameters outside of which the UCP must immediately report to the nurse (and any action that must urgently be taken)
- Who is available to serve as a resource, if needed

BOX 27.2 EXAMPLES OF TASKS THAT CAN AND CANNOT BE DELEGATED TO UNREGULATED CARE PROVIDERS

As the following lists show, not all tasks can be delegated.

TASKS THAT CAN BE DELEGATED TO UNREGULATED CARE PROVIDERS:

- Taking vital signs
- Measuring and recording intake and output
- Client transfers and ambulation
- Conducting postmortem care
- Bathing
- Feeding
- Giving gastrostomy feedings in established systems
- Attending to safety
- Weighing
- Performing simple dressing changes
- Suctioning chronic tracheostomies
- Performing basic life support (cardiopulmonary resuscitation [CPR])

TASKS THAT CANNOT BE DELEGATED TO UNREGULATED CARE PROVIDERS:

- Assessment
- Interpretating data
- Making a nursing diagnosis
- Creating a nursing care plan
- Evaluating care effectiveness
- Care of invasive lines
- Administering parenteral medications
- Inserting nasogastric tubes
- Client education
- Performing triage
- Giving telephone advice

BOX 27.3 PRINCIPLES USED BY THE NURSE TO DETERMINE DELEGATION TO UNREGULATED CARE PROVIDERS

The following principles should inform every decision to delegate:

1. The nurse must assess the individual client before delegating tasks.
2. The client must be medically stable or in a chronic condition and not fragile.

The task must have the following characteristics:

3. Be considered routine for this client
4. Not require a substantial amount of scientific knowledge or technical skill
5. Be considered safe for this client
6. Have a predictable outcome

The nurse must ensure the following:

7. Know the agency's procedures and policies about delegation

8. Know the scope of practice and the customary knowledge, skills, and job description for each health care discipline represented on his or her team
9. Be aware of individual variations in work abilities; each individual has different experiences and may not be capable of performing every task cited in the job description
10. Observe while the UCP performs a task when unsure about the person's abilities to perform it, or demonstrate it to the person and get a return demonstration before allowing the person to perform it independently
11. Clarify reporting expectations to ensure the task is accomplished
12. Create an atmosphere that fosters communication, teaching, and learning; for example, encouraging staff to ask questions and be listened to carefully regarding their concerns, and making use of every opportunity to teach

- When and in what format (written or verbal) a report on the task is expected

The CNA (2008) noted that a specific task that can be delegated to one UCP may not be appropriate for a different UCP as it depends on each UCP's experience and individual skill sets. Also, a task that is appropriate for the UCP to perform with one client (who is in a stable condition) may not be appropriate with a different client or the same client under altered circumstances.

It is important to note that the nurse is not held legally responsible for the acts of the unregulated person but is accountable for the quality of the act of delegation and has the ultimate responsibility for ensuring that proper care is provided. The nurse must know their

specific scopes of practice to delegate effectively and to ensure that proper care is provided.

Delegation can be an extremely useful strategy in providing thorough and effective nursing care. Skill in delegation, however, must be learned and developed over time. The nurse should not hesitate to consult with others regarding the appropriateness of delegation. See the Clinical Alert box regarding the role of the nurse with regard to delegation.

CLINICAL ALERT

Each nurse is responsible for his or her own actions. Anyone who feels unqualified to perform a delegated task must decline to perform it.

Change

Change is the process of making something different from what it was (Sullivan & Decker, 2009). Change can involve gaining new knowledge or skills, or adapting what is currently known in light of new information. Change can involve individual clients, families, communities, organizations, nursing as a profession, and the entire health care delivery system. Change is an integral aspect of nursing, and nurses are often **change agents**, that is, individuals who initiate, motivate, and implement change. It is essential for managers to understand the impact of change on employees and to develop strategies of support. Change often produces feelings of grief among those affected and requires a manager to have additional understanding of the impact change may have on employees' lives. Change agents have the following characteristics:

- Excellent communication and interpersonal skills with individuals, groups, administration, and all levels of the organization involved in change
- Knowledge of available resources and how to use them: people, time, money, facilities, and information
- Skill in problem solving
- Skill in teaching
- Respect of those involved in the change
- Ability to encourage and nurture those going through change
- Self-confidence, ability to take risks and inspire trust in self and others
- Ability to make decisions
- A broad base of knowledge
- A good sense of timing

See the Clinical Alert box regarding the role of the nurse with regard to change.

 CLINICAL ALERT

Change that is viewed as a threat by one nurse may be viewed as an opportunity by another nurse.

Types of Change

Unplanned change is an alteration imposed by external events or persons. It occurs when unexpected events force a reaction. Drift is a type of unplanned change in which change occurs without effort on anyone's part. Situational, or natural, change can also be considered unplanned and occurs without any control by the person or group affected. An example is the change that occurs because of a war or a natural disaster. Not all situational changes are negative.

Planned change is an intended attempt to achieve desired change. These changes may be specific to the organization (e.g., strategic planning, visiting schedules), cross-institutional (e.g., merging of linen services), or system-wide (e.g., restructuring of health care services). Problem-solving skills, decision-making skills, and interpersonal skills are important factors for effective planned change. To instill organizational changes, nurse leaders must do the following:

- Understand that change does not always occur in a linear fashion
- Invest in organizational relationships with employees, clients, and key partners
- Reinforce the organization vision, mission, and values through regular review of strategic plans
- Encourage and support behaviours that align with strategic planning
- Remove barriers that hinder strategic actions (L. Yiu, personal communication, January 20, 2012)

Change can also be considered covert or overt. A *covert change* is hidden or occurs without the individual's awareness. For example, a person can become increasingly deaf without being aware of this fact. Overt change is change a person is aware of. Examples are the development of abdominal pain and of shortness of breath while walking up stairs. People who experience overt change may also experience anxiety. Overt change often necessitates behavioural changes that are at variance with the person's needs or goals.

Models of Change

The following section describes the contemporary change models commonly used in practice. Please also refer to the Prochaska's model of change described in Chapter 8 of this book.

LEWIN'S THEORY OF CHANGE In his classic work, Lewin (1951) described that change involves three stages: (a) unfreezing, (b) moving, and (c) refreezing. He also stated that it requires a change agent to implement any planned change. During the unfreezing stage, the change agent will identify the desired change and the related driving and restraining forces, generate alternative solutions, and motivate the participants to change. In the second stage, the moving stage, the change agent helps the participants to see that the status quo is undesirable, and together they carry out actions to resolve the identified problem. In the final stage, refreezing, the change agent will integrate and stabilize the change and withdraw when change is completed. See an example in Figure 27.2.

APPRECIATIVE INQUIRY Appreciative inquiry (**AI**) is an approach to organization change where one would focus on what is positive (appreciative) by asking participants to share their experiences and successes, examine the challenges, and explore what is working well (inquiry) (Cooperrider, Whitney, Stavros, & Fry, 2008). AI adopts a *positive* approach to individual and organizational

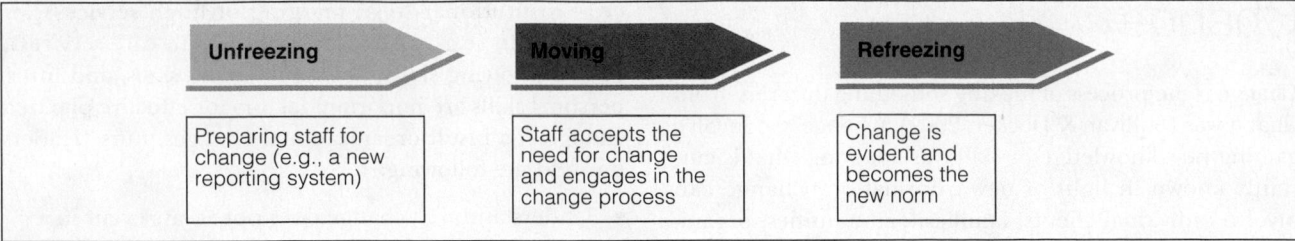

FIGURE 27.2 An Example Using Lewin's Theory of Change Model.

Source: Based on work from Lewin, K. (1951). *Field theory in social science: Selected theoretical papers.* New York, NY: Harper & Row.

change. It encourages the participants to visualize where they want to be in the future, set goals, and act toward their *destiny*. AI focuses on building strengths rather than on problems. AI is an effective approach to changing organizational culture, to planning for organizational strategic directions, and to mentoring programs. AI has a cycle of four phases:

1. *Discover:* People are to exchange stories and ideas about when the organization is at its best and to discover what is working well.

2. *Dream:* People are to envision what would work well in the future or what could be the peak moments for the organization.

3. *Design:* People are empowered to plan and set priorities to realize what would work well in the future or to realize the dream.

4. *Destiny:* People are to implement the actions for change. (Seel, 2008)

KOTTER'S EIGHT-STEP CHANGE PROCESS To combat common organization behaviours and resistance to change, Kotter and Rathgeber (2006) provided the following eight steps to guide leaders and managers in leading change successfully:

Set the Stage

1. *Create a sense of urgency:* Help others see the need for change and the importance of acting immediately.

2. *Pull together the guiding team:* Form a powerful group to guide the change. Members of this group need to possess leadership skills, credibility, communications ability, authority, and analytical skills.

Decide What to Do

3. *Develop the change vision and strategy:* Allow everyone to share his or her vision regarding how to transform the past into a reality for the future.

Make It Happen

4. *Communicate for understanding and buy-in:* Ensure as many people as possible will understand and accept the proposed vision and the strategy.

5. *Empower others to act:* Facilitate the process to achieve the vision by removing barriers and providing the needed resources and support.

6. *Produce short-term wins:* Create some visible successes as quickly as possible.

7. *Don't let up:* Institute the change tirelessly until the vision is achieved.

Make It Stick

8. *Create a new culture:* Foster the new ways of behaving and help the group to develop it into a part of their culture.

An important aspect of planning change is establishing the likelihood of the acceptance of the change and then determining the criteria by which that acceptance can be identified. Accepting change often takes time, particularly when it does not fit into a person's attitudinal framework. The course of acceptance is easier for people if they are involved in the process. If possible, change should be instituted on a small scale before full implementation. To facilitate acceptance of the change, the change agent also needs to identify common driving and restraining forces (see Box 27.4). Guidelines for dealing with resistance are found in Box 27.5.

BOX 27.4 COMMON DRIVING AND RESTRAINING FORCES FOR CHANGE

Identifying driving and restraining forces can help the change agent make acceptance of the change possible.

DRIVING FORCES

- Perception that the change is challenging
- Economic gain
- Perception that the change will improve the situation
- Visualization of the future impact of change
- Potential for self-growth, recognition, achievement, and improved relationships

RESTRAINING FORCES

- Fear that something of personal value will be lost (e.g., threat to job security or self-esteem)
- Misunderstanding of the change and its implications
- Low tolerance for change related to intellectual or emotional insecurity
- Perception that the change will not achieve goals; failure to see the big picture
- Lack of time or energy
- Perceived loss of freedom to engage in particular behaviours

---

BOX 27.5 GUIDELINES FOR DEALING WITH RESISTANCE TO CHANGE

The following guidelines are useful for dealing with resistance to change:

1. Communicate with those who oppose the change. Get to the root of their reasons for opposition.

2. Clarify information and provide accurate information.

3. Be open to revisions, but be clear about what must remain.

4. Present the negative consequences of resistance (threats to organizational survival, compromised client care, and so on).

5. Emphasize the positive consequences of the change and how the individual or group will benefit. However, do not spend too much energy on rational analysis of why the change is good and why the arguments against it do not hold up. People's resistance frequently flows from feelings that are not rational.

6. Keep resisters involved in face-to-face contact with supporters. Encourage proponents to empathize with opponents, recognize valid objections, and relieve unnecessary fears.

7. Maintain a climate of trust, support, and confidence.

8. To access optimal power, use the following strategies:

- Analyze the organizational chart; know the formal lines of authority. Identify informal lines as well.

- Identify key persons who will be affected by the change. Pay attention to those immediately above and below the point of change.

- Find out as much as possible about these key people. What interests them, gets them excited, or turns them off? What is on their personal and organizational agendas? Who typically aligns with whom on important decisions?

- Begin to build a coalition of support before you start the change process. Identify the key people who will most likely support your idea and those who are most likely to be persuaded easily. Talk informally with them to flush out possible objections to your idea and potential opponents. What will the costs and benefits be to them—especially in political terms?

- Follow the organizational chain of command in communicating with administrators. Don't bypass anyone to avoid having an excellent proposal undermined.

Source: Sullivan, Eleanor J., *Effective Leadership and Management in Nursing, 7th Ed.,* © 2009. Reprinted and Electronically reproduced by permission of Pearson Education, Inc., Upper Saddle River, New Jersey.

A Vision for Change

As nurses work at the forefront of the health care system, they are constantly affected by change. Knowledgeable nurses make rational plans to deal with opportunities both to initiate and guide needed change as they embrace and respond to change.

It is time for a shift of focus to have a new generation of nurse leaders and managers (Villeneuve & MacDonald, 2006). One of the visions for the year 2020 is to have at least 20% of nursing leaders from the Aboriginal and visible minority populations, and at least 10% of nursing leaders be male. The nursing curriculum must foster opportunity to develop skills required for nursing leadership (Villeneuve & MacDonald, 2006). Nurses can learn and grow to be leaders by doing the following:

- Seize opportunities created by change

- Enable others to influence change

- Support each other, especially younger nurses

- Practise personal accountability

- Put the *Code of Ethics for Registered Nurses* to work every day

- Apply research; participate in research

- Embrace lifelong learning

- Build strategic relationships

- Cultivate flexibility and innovation

- Advocate for improved client care (CNA, 2005a, p. 4)

Now, more than ever, we need the knowledge, expertise, and capacity of nurses to bring solutions to our health care challenges. Nurses are, and will continue to be, at the heart of the system's transformation, driving and managing change (CNA, 2009).

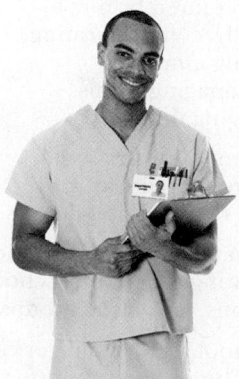

Case Study 27

You recently interviewed for two nursing positions and are trying to decide which job to pursue. During your first interview, the nurse manager, Mr. Caruso, was cheerful, spoke highly of his current staff, complimented them on their abilities, listened to your ideas, and explored ways that you could contribute to this team's effectiveness. The second nurse manager, Mrs. Turner, was also cheerful and talkative. She provided you with a job description as a primary nurse caregiver, explained expectations of new employees, and spoke of new programs she was attempting to implement. Both nurse managers talked about changes taking place in their facilities and the need for employees to remain flexible.

(continued)

1. Based on the brief data provided, speculate about the leadership style of each of these nurse managers.

2. Think about managers (or leaders) you have known and admired. What characteristics did they have that you would like to integrate into your own management style?

3. Both nurse managers spoke of changes that were taking place in their facility. As a nurse, how can you assist your peers who are unhappy and seem to resist change even when it is positive?

4. What factors should you consider before making a decision about accepting a position in a team nursing environment as opposed to a primary nursing environment?

Check the eText in MyNursingLab for answers and explanations.

KEY TERMS

accountability   *p. 579*

appreciative inquiry (AI)
   p. 583

authority   *p. 579*

autocratic (authoritarian,
   directive) leaders
   p. 576

Baby Boomers   *p. 580*

bureaucratic leader
   p. 577

change   *p. 583*

change agent   *p. 583*

charismatic leader
   p. 577

coordinating   *p. 579*

critical thinking
   p. 579

delegation   *p. 581*

democratic (participative,
   consultative) leaders
   p. 577

directing   *p. 579*

effectiveness   *p. 580*

efficiency   *p. 580*

expert power   *p. 578*

first-level managers
   p. 579

formal leader   *p. 575*

Generation X   *p. 580*

influence   *p. 578*

informal leader   *p. 575*

laissez-faire (nondirective,
   permissive, ultraliberal)
   leader   *p. 577*

leader   *p. 575*

leadership style   *p. 575*

manager   *p. 575*

mentors   *p. 580*

middle-level managers
   p. 579

Millennial Generation, or
   Generation Y   *p. 580*

networking   *p. 580*

organizing   *p. 579*

personal power   *p. 578*

planned change   *p. 583*

planning   *p. 579*

position power   *p. 578*

power   *p. 578*

preceptor   *p. 580*

productivity   *p. 580*

relationship power   *p. 578*

responsibility   *p. 579*

servant leaders   *p. 578*

shared governance   *p. 578*

shared leadership   *p. 578*

Silent Generation
   p. 580

situational leaders   *p. 577*

task power   *p. 578*

transactional leader
   p. 577

transformational leader
   p. 578

unplanned change   *p. 583*

unregulated care providers
   (UCP)   *p. 581*

upper-level managers
   p. 579

vision   *p. 578*

CHAPTER HIGHLIGHTS

• The professional nurse frequently assumes the roles of leader and manager. Leaders influence others to accomplish a specific goal, whereas managers are employees of an organization with responsibility and accountability for accomplishing the tasks of the organization.

• Several leadership styles have been described: autocratic, democratic, laissez-faire, and bureaucratic. Leadership styles vary and are often blended to fit the situation. Nurses need to know which style is most consistent with their behaviour and learn to incorporate aspects of other styles into their practice.

• Descriptions of leadership, including charismatic, transactional, transformational, connective, and shared, address the traits, behaviours, and relationships between leaders and followers.

• Four major management functions are discussed: planning, organizing, directing, and coordinating.

• Nurse managers work in the organizational framework of the employing agency. Principles of management include authority, accountability, and responsibility.

• The skills and competencies required by nurse managers are thinking critically, communicating, managing resources, enhancing employee performance, building and managing teams, managing conflict, and managing time.

• Networking is the establishment of professional linkages to obtain information, share ideas, and facilitate the accomplishment of professional goals.

• Nurses can develop professional networks throughout their careers in a variety of settings, including school, work, professional organizations, and social groups.

• Delegation is a management tool that a manager can use to improve productivity. The manager transfers responsibility and authority to another but retains accountability for the task.

- Organizational changes include unplanned change and planned change.

- Planned change requires problem-solving skills, decision-making skills, and interpersonal competence. Nurse leaders and managers must be able to understand the driving and restraining forces and engage their staff in the change process.

- Lewin's change theory addressed the unfreezing, moving, and freezing stages. Kotter described eight steps of change from setting the stage to making it happen and making it stick.

- Appreciative inquiry (AI) uses a positive approach to organization change. It encourages people to discover what works well, visualize their dreams, design action plans, and act to reach the destiny.

- Nurses function as change agents to initiate, motivate, and implement change

ASSESS YOUR LEARNING

1. As *leaders,* nurses influence which of the following?
   a. Clients and their family members
   b. Physicians and other health care professionals
   c. Politicians and health care institution administrators
   d. A wide range of people seeking health care or with concerns about health and/or health care

2. Which of the following are three characteristics of successful leaders?
   a. Knowing when to talk, knowing when to listen, and having excellent interpersonal skills
   b. Having a goal, having power over people, and having the resources to succeed
   c. Having a leadership position, creating a vision, and supporting the people
   d. Having the ability to motivate, trusting in destiny, and enjoying the process

3. Which of the following is a leadership style that has been described as autocratic?
   a. Deprived
   b. Exploitive
   c. Directive
   d. Enlightened

4. A nurse is assigned a new role as a manager of an outpatient department where many issues have been identified. Which of the following would be important as the first goal to achieve?
   a. Working all of the unit shifts
   b. Setting up a meeting with staff
   c. Requesting feedback from the team
   d. Reviewing the unit budget

5. Both responsibility and which of the following come with the leadership position?
   a. Power
   b. Dependence
   c. Wealth
   d. Anxiety

6. A client hospitalized after a cerebrovascular accident is being admitted to home care. Who will be the MOST likely person to coordinate home care services for the client?
   a. Registered nurse
   b. Physician
   c. Physiotherapist
   d. Dietitian

7. What should a staff nurse know before delegating tasks to an unregulated care provider?
   a. The worker should have practised each procedure beforehand.
   b. The worker's level of knowledge must be verified before delegation.
   c. Workers must be directly supervised in all aspects of nursing care.
   d. Workers can perform procedures if they are guided by a registered nurse.

8. Which of the following approaches BEST illustrates transformational leadership?
   a. The leader stimulates group interest in establishing unit goals that contribute to the agency's mission.
   b. The leader forms subgroups or task forces that make decisions about unit problems.
   c. The leader provides funding for continuing education conferences to staff members who have not used any sick leave.
   d. The leader adjusts his or her strategies to fit the current situation.

9. After taking the client's history, the nurse recognizes that the client is at risk of developing an infection. Which of the following should the nurse know about the problem?
   a. It is the responsibility of the client's physician.
   b. It is a nursing diagnosis.
   c. It is a collaborative problem.
   d. It is a concern that should be left for the next day shift.

10. The nurse who is the stroke coordinator at a community care access centre explains that there will be a move toward best practice guidelines in the management of stroke care and takes the time to facilitate information sessions regarding this change. Several physicians are resistant to the changes. Which strategy would help the nurse encourage change?

   a. Requesting feedback from stakeholders, holding information sessions to share the feedback, and determining which change theory to apply

   b. Using information sessions to inform the audience, gathering input, and recording questions from the attendees

   c. Introducing the changes, completing research, and using the information sessions to inform the audience about the change

   d. Applying a change theory to the process, completing a current literature search, and using the information sessions as a beginning step

Check the eText in MyNursingLab for answers and explanations.

WEBLINKS

Canadian Health Leadership Network

http://www.chlnet.ca/front_page

This website provides information for health sector leaders to enhance leadership networking and development. It provides rapid access to leading leadership practices in Canada.

Canadian Nurses Association

http://www.cna-aiic.ca

This website provides information regarding the Canadian Nurses Association, its policies and guidelines, current news, and links to provincial and territorial sites.

Registered Nurses' Association of Ontario

http://rnao.ca

This website provides information on health and nursing policy, nursing best practice guidelines, educational material, and information on the Centre for Nursing Excellency.

MyNursingLab

REFERENCES

Canadian Nurses Association. (2005a). Nursing leadership in a changing world. *Nursing Now: Issues and Trends in Canadian Nursing, 18.* Retrieved http://www2.cna-aiic.ca/CNA/documents/pdf/publications/NN_Nursing_Leadership_05_e.pdf

Canadian Nurses Association. (2005b). Nursing staff mix: A key link to patient safety. *Nursing Now: Issues and Trends in Canadian Nursing, 19,* 1–6. Retrieved from http://www2.cna-aiic.ca/CNA/documents/pdf/publications/NN_Nursing_Staff_Mix_05_e.pdf

Canadian Nurses Association. (2008). *Valuing health-care team members: Working with unregulated health workers.* Ottawa, ON: Author. Retrieved from http://www.cna-aiic.ca/CNA/documents/pdf/publications/UHW_Valuing_2008_e.pdf

Canadian Nurses Association. (2009). *The next decade: CNA's vision for nursing and health.* Retrieved from http://www.cna-aiic.ca/CNA/documents/pdf/publications/Next_Decade_2009_e.pdf

College of Nurses of Ontario. (2006a). *Therapeutic nurse-client relationship.* Toronto, ON: Author.

College of Nurses of Ontario. (2006b). *Practice guideline: Conflict prevention and management guideline.* Toronto, ON: Author.

College of Nurses of Ontario. (2009). *Practice guideline: Utilization of RNs and RPNs.* Toronto, ON: Author.

College of Registered Nurses of British Columbia. (2005). *Practice standard for registered nurses and nurse practitioners: Assignment between nurses.* Retrieved from https://www.crnbc.ca/downloads/414.pdf

Cooperrider, D. L., Whitney, D., Stavros, J. M., & Fry, D. (2008). *Appreciative inquiry handbook: For leaders of change* (2nd ed.). Brunswick, OH: Crown Custom Publishing Inc.

Irving, J. A., & Longbotham, G. J. (2007). Team effectiveness and six essential servant leadership themes: A regression model based on items in the organizational leadership assessment. *International Journal of Leadership Studies, 2*(2), 98–113.

Kotter, J., & Rathgeber, H. (2006). *Our icebergs are melting.* New York, NY: St. Martin's Press.

Lewin, K. (1951). *Field theory in social science.* New York, NY: Harper & Row.

Marriner Tomey, A. M. (2009). *Guide to nursing management and leadership* (8th ed.). St. Louis, MO: Mosby.

Meilinger, P. S. (2001). The ten rules of good followership. In R. I. Lester, & A. Glenn Morton (Eds.), *AU-24 concepts for air force leadership* (pp. 99–101). Maxwell AFB, AL: Air University Press.

Registered Nurses' Association of Ontario. (2006). *Developing and sustaining nursing leadership*. Toronto, ON: Author. Retrieved from http://www.rnao.org/Storage/16/1067_BPG_Sustain_Leadership.pdf

Seel, R. (2008). *Introduction to appreciative inquiry. New paradigm consulting*. Norfolk, UK. Retrieved from http://www.new-paradigm.co.uk/introduction_to_ai.htm

Sturm, B. (2009). Principles of servant-leadership in community health nursing: Management issues and behaviors discovered in ethnographic research. *Home Health Care Management and Practice, 21*, 82–89. doi: 10.1177/1084822308318187

Sudheimer, E. E. (2009). Appreciating both sides of the generation gap: Baby boomer and Generation X nurses working together. *Nursing Forum, 44*, 57–63. doi: 10.1111/j.1744-6198.2009.00127.x

Sullivan, E. J., & Decker, P. J. (2009). *Effective leadership and management in nursing* (7th ed.). Upper Saddle River, NJ: Prentice-Hall.

Villeneuve, M., & MacDonald, J. (2006). *Toward 2020: Visions for nursing*. Ottawa, ON: Canadian Nurses Association. Retrieved from http://www.cna-nurses.ca/CNA/documents/pdf/publications/Toward-2020-e.pdf

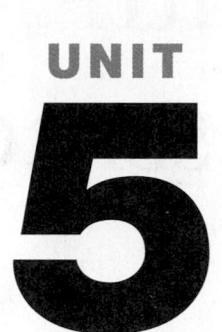

UNIT 5

Nursing Assessment and Clinical Studies

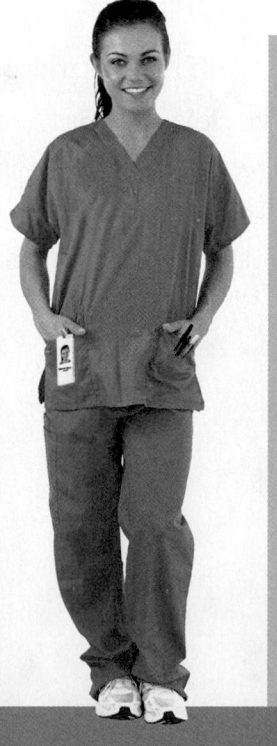

Chapter 28

Health Assessment

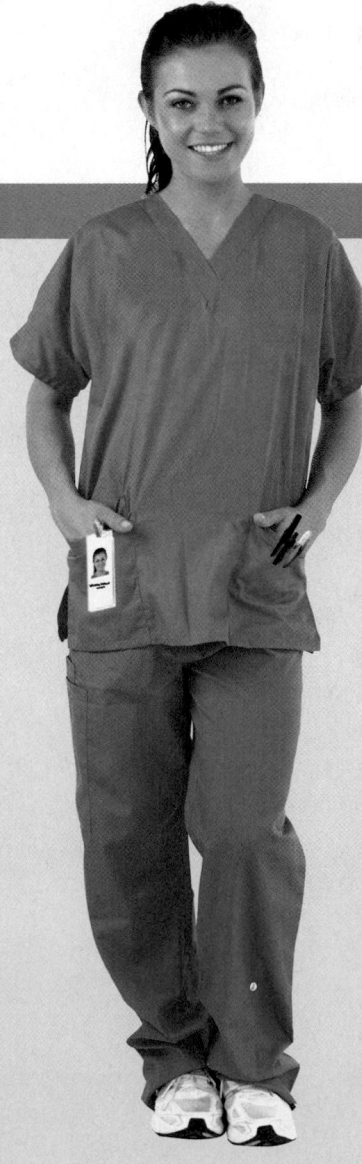

Assessing a client's health status, which is a major component of nursing care, has two aspects: (a) the nursing health history, discussed in Chapter 23, and (b) the physical health assessment discussed in this chapter. A physical assessment can be any of three types: (a) a complete assessment (e.g., when a client is admitted to a health care agency); (b) examination of a body system (e.g., the cardiovascular system); (c) examination of a body area (e.g., the lungs, when difficulty with breathing is observed).

Note: Some nurses consider *assessment* to be the broad term used in applying the nursing process to health data and *examination* to be the physical process used to gather the data. In this text, the terms *assessment* and *examination* are sometimes used interchangeably, referring to both a critical investigation and an evaluation of client status.

Physical Health Assessment

A physical health assessment can be done for many different reasons:

- To obtain baseline data about the client's functional abilities
- To supplement, confirm, or refute data obtained in the nursing history
- To obtain data that will help the nurse establish nursing and client goals and a plan of care
- To evaluate the physiological outcomes of health care interventions and, thus, the progress of a client's health situation
- To make clinical judgments about a client's health status
- To identify areas for health promotion and disease prevention

A complete health assessment can be conducted starting at the head and proceeding in a systematic manner downward in what is referred to as a head-to-toe assessment. However, the procedure can vary according to the age of the individual, the severity of the illness, the preferences of the nurse, the location of the examination, and the clinical agency guidelines. The order of the standard head-to-toe assessment is given in Box 28.1. Regardless of the procedure used, the client's energy and time need to be considered. The health assessment is, therefore, conducted in a systematic and efficient manner that requires the fewest position changes for the client.

The sequence of the assessment differs with children and adults. With children, always proceed from the least invasive or uncomfortable to the more invasive. Examination of the head and neck, heart, lungs, and range of motion can be done early in the process, and the ears, mouth, abdomen, and genitals should be left for the end of the exam.

BOX 28.1 HEAD-TO-TOE FRAMEWORK

- General survey
- Vital signs
- Head
  - Hair, scalp, cranium, face
  - Eyes and vision
  - Ears and hearing
  - Nose and sinuses
  - Mouth and oropharynx
  - Cranial nerves
- Neck
  - Muscles
  - Lymph nodes
  - Trachea
  - Thyroid gland
  - Carotid arteries
  - Neck veins

- Upper extremities
  - Skin and nails
  - Muscle strength and tone
  - Joint range of motion
  - Brachial and radial pulses
  - Tendon reflexes
  - Sensation

- Thorax and back
  - Skin
  - Thorax shape and size
  - Lungs
  - Heart
  - Spinal column
  - Breasts and axillae

BOX 28.1 *(continued)*

- Abdomen
  - Skin
  - Abdominal sounds
  - Specific organs (e.g., liver, bladder)
- External genitals
- Anus and rectum
- Lower extremities
  - Skin and toenails
  - Gait and balance
  - Joint range of motion
  - Femoral, popliteal, posterior tibial, and pedal pulses
  - Tendon and plantar reflexes
  - Sensation

Frequently, nurses assess a specific body area instead of the entire body. These specific assessments are made in relation to client concerns, the nurse's own observation of problems, the client's presenting problem, nursing interventions provided, and medical therapies. Examples of these situations and assessments are provided in Table 28.1.

Nurses use evidence-based practice guidelines and standards to focus health assessment on specific conditions. For example, when screening for cancer, nurses should keep in mind the Canadian Cancer Society screening guidelines (see Box 28.2). (See also the Evidence-Informed Practice box on breast cancer screening guidelines.)

TABLE 28.1 Nursing Assessments Addressing Specific Client Situations

Situation	Physical Assessment
The client complains of abdominal pain.	Inspect, auscultate, percuss, and palpate the abdomen; assess vital signs.
The client is admitted with a head injury.	Assess level of consciousness using the Glasgow Coma Scale (see Table 28.12, p. 673); assess pupils for reaction to light and accommodation; assess vital signs.
The nurse prepares to administer a cardiotonic drug to a client.	Assess apical pulse, and compare with baseline data.
The nurse administers a bronchodilator for an acute asthmatic episode.	Auscultate lungs before and after the medication.
The client has just had a cast applied to the lower leg.	Assess peripheral perfusion of toes, blanch test (capillary refill), pedal pulse, temperature and sensation of toes, movement of toes, and vital signs.

BOX 28.2 CANADIAN CANCER SOCIETY'S SELECTED EARLY DETECTION AND SCREENING GUIDELINES FOR AVERAGE-RISK CANADIANS

Type of Cancer	Early detection and screening (screening tests can find signs of cancer before symptoms develop, but further testing will be needed to confirm the presence of cancer)	Possible Signs and Symptoms (note that the presence of any of the signs or symptoms can be indicative of a range of health problems other than cancer; Canadians should know what is normal for their bodies so that they can report changes to how their bodies look or feel)
Prostate cancer		
The most common cancer in Canadian men	Prostate cancer can be detected early using a PSA test to measure prostate-specific antigen produced by the prostate and a digital rectal exam to palpate the prostate through the rectum. However, research does not clearly show if the benefits of testing for prostate cancer outweigh the harms. Men who are 50 or older should talk to their doctor about their risk of prostate cancer and about the benefits and harms of early detection.	Need to urinate often, especially at night Intense need to urinate (urgency) Difficulty in starting or stopping the urine flow Inability to urinate Weak, decreased or interrupted urine stream A sense of incompletely emptying the bladder Burning or pain during urination Blood in the urine or semen Painful ejaculation

Breast cancer		
The most common cancer in Canadian women; less than 1% of breast cancers occur in men	Women age 40–49 years should discuss the benefits and risks of mammography as well as their risk of breast cancer. Women age 50–69 years should have a mammogram every 2 years. Women age ≥70 years should speak with their doctor about how often they should be tested. See the Evidence Informed Practice Box for further elaboration.	Painless lump in the breast or axilla Changes in breast size or shape Dimpling or puckering of the skin Redness, swelling and increased warmth in the affected breast Inverted nipple Crusting or scaling on the nipple
Colorectal cancer		
The second leading cause of death from cancer in Canadians	Stool test (fecal occult blood test [FOBT] or fecal immunochemical test [FIT]) at least every two years in men and women age 50 years and older	General discomfort in the abdomen (gas pains, bloating, fullness, or cramps); change in bowel habits, such as diarrhea or constipation, for no apparent reason; bright red or very dark blood in stools; stools that are narrower than usual; vomiting; feeling very tired; weight loss
Cervical cancer		
Rates are declining owing to screening; introduction of human papillomavirus (HPV) vaccine may reduce incidence even further	Sexually active women require a Pap test every 1 to 3 years, depending on previous test results, from the time they are 21 years old. Women who are no longer sexually active continue to require Pap testing. Women who have received the HPV vaccine continue to require Pap testing.	Abnormal bleeding from the vagina Bleeding or spotting between regular menstrual periods Bleeding after sex Menstrual periods that last longer and are heavier than before Bleeding after menopause More discharge from the vagina than normal Pain in the pelvis or lower back Pain during sexual intercourse

Source: Summarized from the Canadian Cancer Society's website at http://www.cancer.ca/Canada-wide/About%20cancer.aspx?sc_lang=en. Used with permission.

EVIDENCE-INFORMED PRACTICE

What Are the Best Screening Guidelines for Breast Cancer?

With breast cancer representing 26% of all newly diagnosed cancer cases and the second leading cause of cancer death in Canadian women (Canadian Cancer Society, 2012), it is no wonder that women and health care professionals are concerned about how this disease process is detected. For years, women were encouraged to perform breast self-examination (BSE) on a regular basis—even as frequently as every month—and have a clinical breast examination (CBE) performed by a trained health care professional, generally on an annual basis. With the advent of newer forms of technology, new guidelines came out in 2001 recommending regular mammograms (every 2 years) for women age 50 to 69 years; these recommendations discouraged BSE, and many provinces stopped funding nurses to teach this self-assessment skill. In 2011, the Canadian Task Force on Preventive Health Care conducted a systematic review of the evidence (randomized and quasi-randomized control trials) related to the use of mammograms, magnetic resonance imaging (MRI), BSE, and CBE as methods for screening for breast cancer in average-risk women (i.e., women who do not have a personal history of breast cancer, history of breast cancer in a first-degree relative [mother, sister, daughter], known *BRCA1/BRCA2* mutation, or prior chest wall radiation). In conducting the review, the researchers took into account the benefits of screening as well as the harms and cost of false-positive results, overdiagnosis, and overtreatment. The systematic

(continued)

EVIDENCE-INFORMED PRACTICE (continued)

review made the following recommendations on screening for breast cancer in women with average risk:

- No screening for women age 40 to 49 years
- No use of CBE or BSE alone or in conjunction with mammography
- No use of MRI
- Routine screening with mammography every 2 to 3 years for women age 50 to 74 years

NURSING IMPLICATIONS: Nurses play an important role in helping Canadian women stay up to date and understand the recommendations related to periodic

health assessment, such as those released by the Canadian Task Force on Preventive Health Care on breast cancer screening. With many women being concerned about their breast health and having grown up in the decades when BSE was espoused as an effective means of early detection, nurses can play a role in helping them understand the varying recommendations over the years. The most important thing that nurses could do is ensure that women can identify their risk level: "average" or "higher than average."

Source: Based on The Canadian Task Force on Preventive Health Care. (2011). Recommendations on screening for breast cancer in average-risk women aged 40–74 years. *Canadian Medical Association Journal, 183* (17), 1991–2001.

Preparing the Client

Before the assessment, the nurse should explain when and where it will take place, why it is important, and what will happen during the assessment. Often, clients are anxious about what the nurse will find. They can be reassured during the examination by explanations provided at each step. Instruct the client that all information gathered and documented during the assessment is kept confidential.

Health assessments are usually painless; however, it is important to determine in advance any positions that are contraindicated for a particular client. The nurse helps the client, as needed, to undress and put on a gown. Clients should empty their bladders before the examination. Doing so helps them feel more relaxed and makes palpation of the abdomen and the pubic area more comfortable. If a urinalysis is required, urine should be collected at the time the client empties his or her bladder. Since an empty rectum facilitates rectal examination, the client should be encouraged to defecate before a complete examination.

When assessing adults, it is important to recognize that people of the same age can differ markedly. Box 28.3 provides special considerations for assessing adults, especially older adults.

> **BOX 28.3 HEALTH ASSESSMENT OF THE ADULT**
>
> Keep these guidelines in mind when examining adults:
> - Be aware of normal physiological changes that occur with age.
> - Expose only areas of the body to be examined to avoid chilling the client.
> - Permit ample time for the client to assume the required positions.
> - Be aware of cultural differences. The client may want a family member present during disrobing.
> - Arrange for an interpreter if the client's language is different from yours.
> - Adapt assessment techniques to any sensory impairment; for example, make sure clients have their eyeglasses or hearing devices.
> - If a client is older or frail, several assessment times may be necessary to avoid overtiring him or her.

Family and friends should not be present unless the client specifically asks for someone to be present in the room. A client who is physically relaxed will usually experience little discomfort.

Preparing the Environment

It is important to prepare the environment before starting the assessment. The time for the physical assessment should be convenient to both the client and the nurse. The environment should be a warm and comfortable temperature, well lit, and the equipment should be systematically arranged for the examination.

It is important to provide the client with privacy. Most people are embarrassed if their bodies are exposed or if others can overhear or view them during the assessment.

Positioning

Several positions are frequently required during the physical assessment. It is important to consider the client's ability to assume a position. The client's physical condition, energy level, and age should also be taken into consideration. Some positions are embarrassing and uncomfortable and, therefore, should not be maintained for long. The assessment is organized so that several body areas can be assessed in one position, thus minimizing the number of position changes needed (see Table 28.2).

TABLE 28.2 Client Positions and Body Areas Assessed

Position	Description	Areas Assessed	Cautions
Dorsal recumbent	Back-lying position with knees flexed and hips externally rotated; small pillow under the head; soles of feet on the surface	Female genitals, rectum, and female reproductive tract	May be contraindicated for clients who have cardiopulmonary problems
Supine (horizontal recumbent)	Back-lying position with legs extended; with or without pillow under the head	Head, neck, axillae, anterior thorax, lungs, breasts, heart, vital signs, abdomen, extremities, peripheral pulses	Tolerated poorly by clients with cardiovascular or respiratory problems
Sitting	A seated position, back unsupported and legs hanging freely	Head, neck, posterior and anterior thorax, lungs, breasts, axillae, heart, vital signs, upper and lower extremities, reflexes	Older adults and weak clients may require support
Lithotomy	Back-lying position with feet supported in stirrups; the hips should be in line with the edge of the table	Female genitals, rectum, and female reproductive tract	May be uncomfortable and tiring for older adults and often embarrassing
Sims'	Side-lying position with lowermost arm behind the body, uppermost leg flexed at hip and knee, upper arm flexed at shoulder and elbow	Rectum, vagina	Difficult for older adults and people with limited joint movement
Prone	Lying on abdomen with head turned to the side, with or without a small pillow	Posterior thorax, hip joint movement	Often not tolerated by older adults and people with cardiovascular or respiratory problems

Draping

Drapes should be arranged so that the area to be assessed is exposed and other body areas are covered. Exposure of the body is frequently embarrassing to clients. Drapes provide not only a degree of privacy but also warmth. Drapes are made of paper, cloth, or bed linen.

Instrumentation

All equipment required for the health assessment should be clean, in good working order, and readily accessible. Equipment is frequently set up on trays, ready for use. Photographs of various instruments are shown in Table 28.3.

TABLE 28.3 Equipment and Supplies Used for a Health Examination

Instruments and Supplies		Purpose
Flashlight or penlight		To assist viewing of the pharynx or to determine the reactions of the pupils of the eye
Nasal speculum		To permit visualization of the lower and middle turbinates; usually, a penlight is used for illumination
Ophthalmoscope		A lighted instrument to visualize the interior of the eye
Otoscope		A lighted instrument to visualize the eardrum and external auditory canal (a nasal speculum can be attached to the otoscope to inspect the nasal cavities)
Percussion (reflex) hammer		An instrument with a rubber head to test reflexes
Ruler or measuring tape		To measure skin lesions, if present
Sphygmomanometer and cuff (see Figure 29.15, p. 724)		To measure blood pressure
Stethoscope (see Figure 4 in Skill 29.3, p. 715)		To auscultate body sounds (e.g., blood pressure, chest, bowel sounds)
Thermometer (see Figures 29.5 through 29.9, pp. 704–707)		To measure body temperature
Tuning fork		A two-pronged metal instrument used to test hearing acuity and vibratory sense
Vaginal speculum (various sizes) (see Figure 28.36, p. 687)		To assess the cervix and the vagina

Instruments and Supplies		Purpose
Cotton applicators		To obtain specimens; to test sensory function
Disposable pads		To absorb fluids
Drapes		To cover the client
Gloves		To protect the nurse and the client
Lubricant		To ease insertion of instruments (e.g., vaginal speculum)
Tongue blades (depressors)		To depress the tongue during assessment of the mouth and the pharynx

Methods of Examination

Four primary techniques are used in the physical examination: (a) inspection, (b) palpation, (c) percussion, and (d) auscultation. These techniques are discussed throughout this chapter as they apply to each body system.

INSPECTION **Inspection** is a visual examination, that is, an assessment made by observing with the eyes. It should be deliberate, purposeful, and systematic. The nurse inspects with the naked eye and with a lighted instrument, such as an otoscope (used to view the ear). In addition to visual observations, olfactory (smell) and auditory (hearing) cues are noted. Nurses frequently use visual inspection to assess moisture, colour, and texture of body surfaces, as well as shape, position, size, colour, and symmetry of the body. Lighting must be sufficient for the nurse to see clearly; either natural or artificial light can be used. When using the auditory senses, it is important to have a quiet environment for accurate hearing. Observation can be combined with the other assessment techniques.

PALPATION **Palpation** is the examination of the body by using the sense of touch. The pads of the fingers are used because their concentration of nerve endings makes them highly sensitive to tactile discrimination. Palpation is used to determine (a) texture (e.g., of hair); (b) temperature (e.g., of a skin area); (c) vibration (e.g., of a joint); (d) position, size, consistency, and mobility of organs or masses; (e) distension (e.g., of the urinary bladder); (f) pulsation; and (g) the presence of tenderness or pain.

There are two types of palpation: light and deep. *Light* (superficial) *palpation* should always precede *deep palpation* because heavy pressure on the fingertips can dull the sense of touch. For light palpation, the nurse extends the fingers of the dominant hand parallel to the skin surface and presses gently while moving the hand in a circle (Figure 28.1 on the next page). Skin is slightly depressed in light palpation. If it is necessary to determine the details of a mass, the nurse presses lightly several times, rather than holding the pressure constant. See Box 28.4 for the characteristics of masses.

Deep palpation is done with two hands (bimanually) or one hand. In deep bimanual palpation, the nurse extends the dominant hand as for light palpation, and

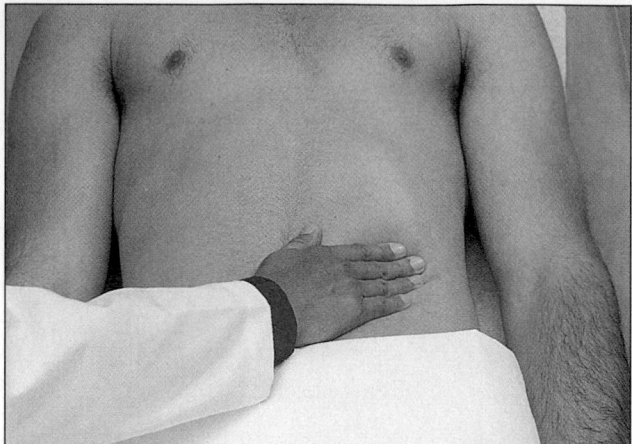

FIGURE 28.1 The position of the hand for light palpation.

BOX 28.4 CHARACTERISTICS OF MASSES

Nurses should note the following characteristics of any masses:

- *Location:* Site on the body, dorsal or ventral surface
- *Size:* Length and width in centimetres
- *Shape:* Oval, round, elongated, irregular
- *Consistency:* Soft, firm, hard
- *Surface:* Smooth, nodular
- *Mobility:* Fixed, mobile
- *Pulsatility:* Present, absent
- *Tenderness:* Degree of tenderness to palpation

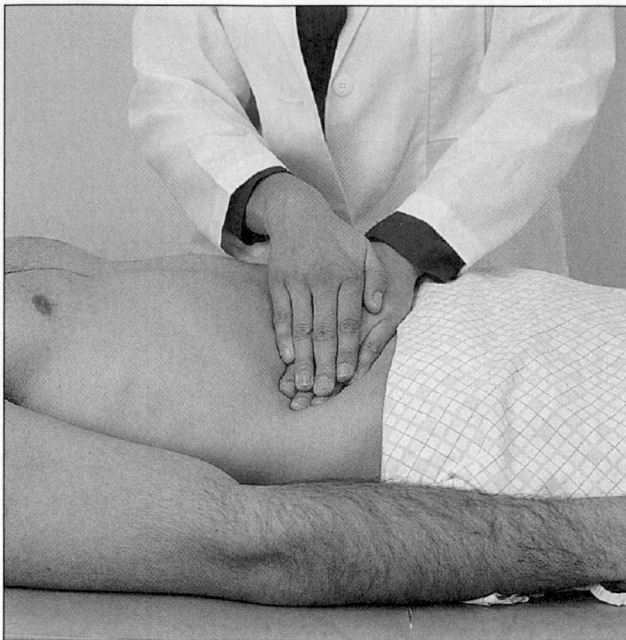

FIGURE 28.2 The position of the hands for deep bimanual palpation.

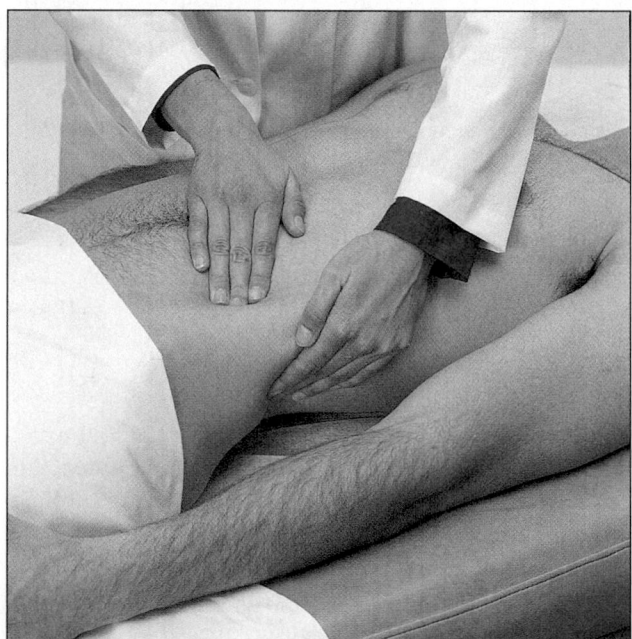

FIGURE 28.3 Deep palpation by using the lower hand to support the body while the upper hand palpates the organ.

---

then places the fingerpads of the nondominant hand on the dorsal surface of the distal interphalangeal joint of the middle three fingers of the dominant hand (Figure 28.2). The top hand applies pressure while the lower hand remains relaxed to perceive the tactile sensations. For deep palpation using one hand, the fingerpads of the dominant hand are pressed over the area to be palpated. Often, the other hand is used to support a mass or organ from below (Figure 28.3). *Deep palpation is usually not done during a routine examination and requires significant practitioner skill because pressure can damage internal organs. It is usually not indicated in clients who have acute abdominal pain or pain that is not yet diagnosed.*

To test skin temperature, it is best to use the dorsum or back of the hand and fingers where skin is thinnest. To test for vibration, the nurse should use the palmar surface of the hand. General guidelines for palpation include the following:

- The nurse's hands should be clean and warm and the fingernails short.
- Areas of tenderness should be palpated last.
- Deep palpation, if indicated, should be done after superficial palpation.

The effectiveness of palpation depends largely on the client's level of relaxation. Nurses can assist clients to relax by (a) gowning and draping the client appropriately, (b) positioning the client comfortably, (c) ensuring that their own hands are warm before beginning, and (d) communicating with the client during the exam. During palpation, the nurse should be sensitive to the client's verbal and facial expressions indicating discomfort.

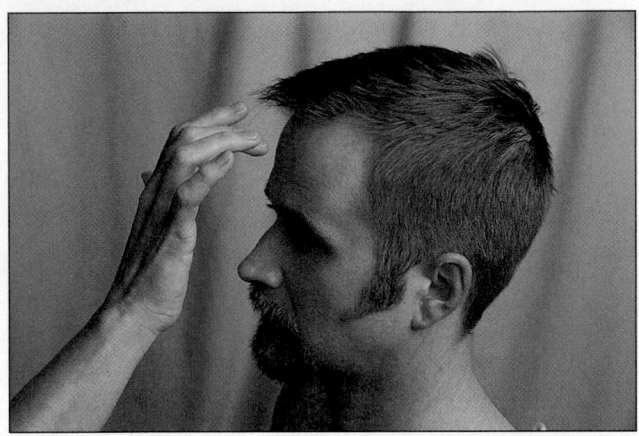

FIGURE 28.4 Direct percussion: Using one hand to strike the surface of the body.

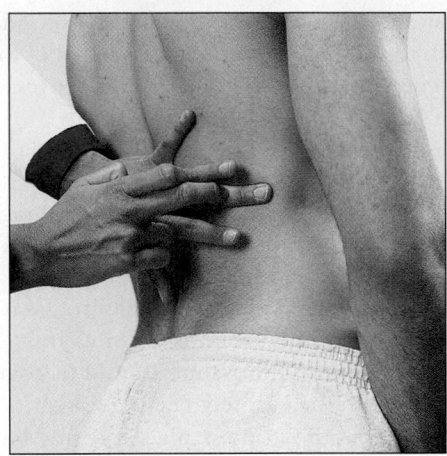

FIGURE 28.5 Indirect percussion: Using the finger of one hand to tap the finger of the other hand.

PERCUSSION **Percussion** is the act of striking the body surface to elicit sounds that can be heard or vibrations that can be felt. Percussion has two types: direct and indirect. In *direct percussion,* the nurse strikes the area to be percussed directly with the pads of two, three, or four fingers or with the pad of the middle finger. The strikes are rapid, and the movement is from the wrist. See Figure 28.4. This technique is not generally used to percuss the thorax but is useful in percussing an adult's sinuses.

The second type, *indirect percussion,* is the striking of an object (e.g., a finger) held against the body area to be examined. In this technique, the middle finger of the nondominant hand, referred to as the **pleximeter**, is placed firmly on the client's skin. Only the distal phalanx and joint of this finger should be in contact with skin. The nurse strikes the pleximeter at the distal interphalangeal joint with the tip of the flexed middle finger of the other hand. The tip of the middle finger that strikes the pleximeter is known as the **plexor** (Figure 28.5). Some nurses may find a point between the distal and proximal joints to be a more comfortable pleximeter point. The motion comes from the wrist; the forearm remains stationary. The angle between the plexor and the pleximeter should be 90 degrees, and the taps must be firm, rapid, and short to obtain a clear sound.

Percussion is used to determine the size and shape of internal organs by establishing their borders. It indicates whether tissue is fluid filled, air filled, or solid. Percussion elicits five types of sound: flatness, dullness, resonance, hyperresonance, and tympany. **Flatness** is an extremely dull sound produced by very dense tissue, such as muscle or bone. **Dullness** is a thud-like sound produced by dense tissue, such as the liver, spleen, or heart. **Resonance** is a hollow sound, such as that produced by lungs filled with air. **Hyperresonance** is not present in a healthy individual. It is described as booming and can be heard over a diseased lung (e.g., in the client with emphysema). **Tympany** is a musical or drum-like sound produced from an air-filled stomach. On a continuum, flatness reflects the most dense tissue (the least amount of air) and tympany the least dense tissue (the greatest amount of air). A percussion sound is described according to its intensity, pitch, duration, and quality. See Table 28.4.

AUSCULTATION **Auscultation** is the process of listening to sounds produced within the body. Auscultation may be direct or indirect. *Direct auscultation* is the use of the unaided ear, for example, to listen to a respiration wheeze or the grating of a moving joint. *Indirect auscultation* is the

TABLE 28.4 Percussion Sounds and Tones

Sound	Intensity	Pitch	Duration	Quality	Example of Location
Flatness	Soft	High	Short	Extremely dull	Muscle, bone
Dullness	Medium	Medium	Moderate	Thud-like	Liver, heart
Resonance	Loud	Low	Long	Hollow	Normal lung
Hyperresonance	Very loud	Very low	Very long	Booming	Emphysematous lung
Tympany	Loud	High (distinguished mainly by musical timbre)	Moderate	Musical	Stomach filled with gas (air)

use of a stethoscope to listen to sounds from within the body, such as bowel sounds or valve sounds of the heart. A stethoscope amplifies the sounds and conveys them to the nurse's ears.

The stethoscope should be 30 cm to 35 cm long with an internal diameter of about 0.3 cm. It should have both a flat-disc and a bell-shaped diaphragm. (See Figure 4 in Skill 29.3, p. 715) The flat-disc diaphragm is best for transmitting high-pitched sounds (e.g., bronchial sounds), and the bell-shaped diaphragm is best for transmitting low-pitched sounds, such as heart sounds. The earpieces of the stethoscope should fit comfortably into the ears, with the earpieces facing forward. The diaphragm of the stethoscope is placed firmly but lightly against the client's skin. If a client is very hairy, it may be necessary to dampen hairs with a moist cloth so that they will lie flat against skin and not cause scratching sounds.

Auscultated sounds are described according to their pitch, intensity, duration, and quality. The **pitch** is the frequency of the vibrations (the number of vibrations per second). Low-pitched sounds, such as some heart sounds, have fewer vibrations per second than high-pitched sounds, such as bronchial sounds. The **intensity** (amplitude) refers to the loudness or softness of a sound. Some body sounds are loud, for example, bronchial sounds heard from the trachea; others are soft, for example, normal breath sounds heard in the lungs. The **duration** of a sound is its length (long or short). The **quality** of a sound is a subjective description, for example, whistling, gurgling, or snapping.

General Survey

A physical assessment begins with a general survey, which involves observation of the client's general appearance and mental status and measurement of vital signs, height, weight (height and weight measures are used to calculate body mass index), and waist circumference. Many components of the general survey are assessed while taking the client's health history, such as the client's body build, posture, hygiene, and mental status (see the Lifespan Considerations box).

Appearance and Mental Status

The general appearance and behaviour of an individual must be assessed in relationship to culture, educational level, socioeconomic status, and current circumstances. For example, an individual who has recently experienced a personal loss may appropriately appear depressed (sad expression, slumped posture). The

---

LIFESPAN CONSIDERATIONS

General Survey

INFANTS

- Observation of children's behaviour can provide important data for the general survey, including physical development, neuromuscular function, and social and interactional skills.
- It may be helpful to have parents hold older infants and very young children for part of the assessment.
- Measure the height of children under age 2 years in the supine position with knees fully extended.
- Weigh without clothing.
- Include a measurement of head circumference until age 2 years. Standardized growth charts include head circumference up to age 3 years.

CHILDREN

- Anxiety in preschool-age children can be decreased by letting them handle and become familiar with the examination equipment.
- School-age children may be very modest and shy about exposing parts of their bodies.
- Adolescents should be examined without parents present.
- Children should be weighed without their shoes and with as little clothing as possible.

OLDER ADULTS

- Allow extra time for clients to answer questions.
- Adapt questioning techniques as appropriate for clients with hearing or visual limitations.
- Older adults with osteoporosis can lose several centimetres in height. Be sure to document height and ask if they are aware of becoming shorter.
- When asking about weight loss, be specific about amount and time frame (e.g., "Have you lost more than 10 kilograms in the last 2 months?").

---

client's age, gender, and ethnicity or race are useful factors in interpreting findings that suggest increased risk for known conditions. Skill 28.1 describes how to assess general appearance and mental status. Skill 28.17 (see p. 676) later in this chapter describes a mental status examination in detail.

Vital Signs

Vital signs are measured (a) to establish baseline data against which future measurements are compared and (b) to detect actual and potential health problems. Refer to Chapter 29 for measurements of temperature, pulse, respirations, blood pressure, and oxygen saturation. See Chapter 30 for pain assessment.

SKILL 28.1 ASSESSING APPEARANCE AND MENTAL STATUS

PLANNING

Equipment: None

IMPLEMENTATION

Performance

1. Before performing the procedure, introduce yourself and verify the client's identity using two identifiers or per agency protocol. Explain to the client what you are going to do, why it is necessary, and how he or she can participate. Discuss how the results will be used in planning further care or treatments.

2. Perform hand hygiene, and follow other appropriate infection prevention and control procedures.

3. Provide for client privacy.

Assessment	Normal Findings	Deviations from Normal
General Appearance		
4. Observe body build, height, and weight in relation to the client's age, lifestyle, and health.	Proportionate, varies with lifestyle	Excessively thin or obese
5. Observe the client's posture and gait, standing, sitting, and walking.	Relaxed, erect posture; coordinated movement	Tense, slouched, bent posture; uncoordinated movement; tremors, unbalanced gait
6. Observe the client's overall hygiene and grooming.	Clean, neat	Dirty, unkempt
7. Note body and breath odour.	No body odour or minor body odour relative to work or exercise; no breath odour	Foul body odour; ammonia odour; acetone breath odour; foul breath
8. Observe for signs of distress in posture or facial expression.	No distress noted	Bending over because of abdominal pain; wincing, frowning, or laboured breathing
9. Note obvious signs of health or illness (e.g., in skin colour or breathing).	Healthy appearance	Pallor, weakness, lesions, cough
10. Assess the client's attitude (frame of mind).	Cooperative, able to follow directions	Negative, hostile, withdrawn, anxious
11. Note the client's affect or mood; assess the appropriateness of the client's response and level of orientation to time, place, persons, and situation.	Appropriate to situation, orientated	Inappropriate to situation, sudden mood change, not orientated
12. Listen for quantity of speech (amount and pace), quality (loudness, clarity, inflection), and organization (coherence of thought, overgeneralization, vagueness).	Understandable, moderate pace; exhibits thought association	Rapid or slow pace; overly loud or soft; lacks association
13. Listen for relevance and organization of thoughts.	Logical sequence; makes sense; has sense of reality	Illogical sequence; flight of ideas; confusion; generalizations; vague

EVALUATION

- Perform a detailed follow-up examination of other individual systems based on findings that deviated from expected or normal for the client.

- Report significant deviations from normal to the appropriate members of the health care team.

Height, Weight, Body Mass Index, and Waist Circumference

In adults, the ratio of weight to height provides a general measure of health. By asking clients about their height and weight before actually measuring them, the nurse obtains some idea of the person's self-image. Excessive discrepancies between the client's responses and the measurements may provide clues to actual or potential problems in self-concept. It is also important that the nurse and client be aware of any significant unintentional weight gain or loss.

The nurse measures height with a measuring stick attached to weight scales or to a wall. The client removes

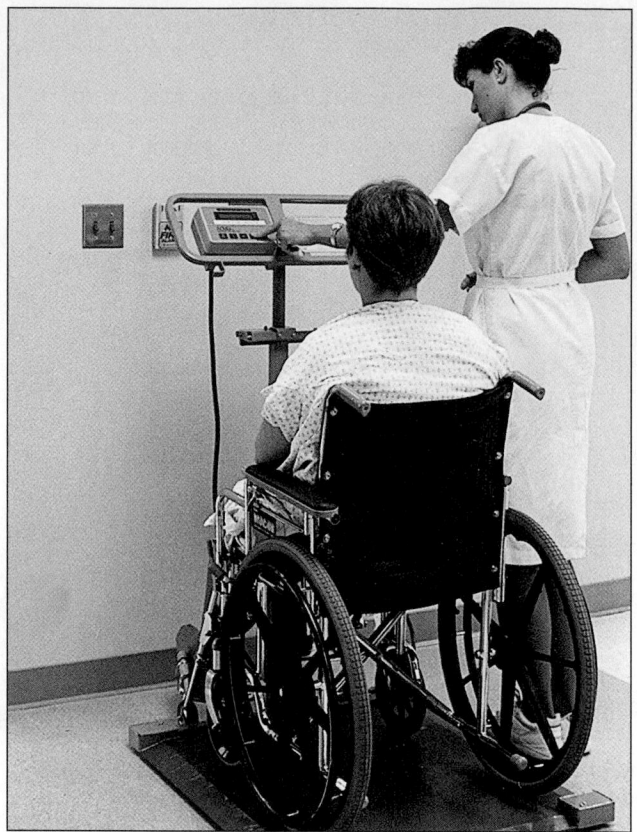

FIGURE 28.6 A chair scale.

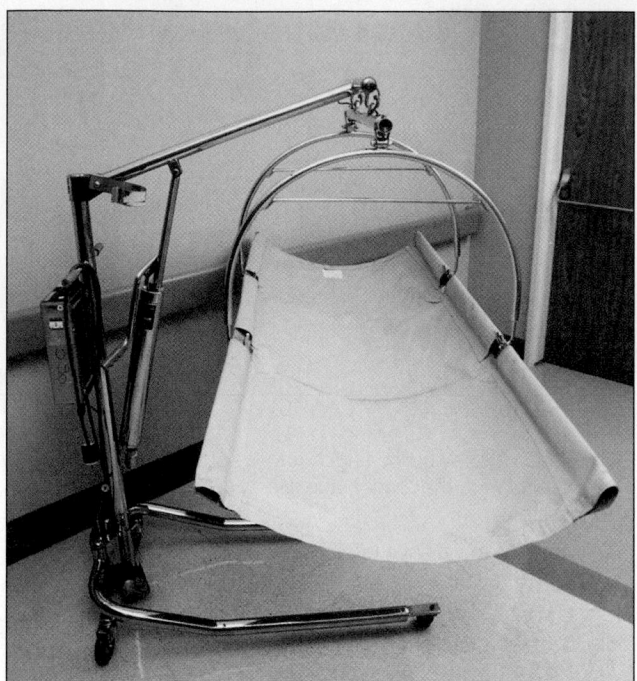

FIGURE 28.7 A bed scale.

his or her shoes and stands erect, with heels together, buttocks and the back of the head against the measuring stick, and eyes looking straight ahead. The nurse raises the L-shaped sliding arm on the measuring stick until it rests on top of the client's head, or the nurse places a small flat object, such as a ruler or book, on the client's head. The edge of the flat object should abut the measuring guide.

Weight is usually measured when a client is admitted to a health care agency and often regularly, for example, each morning before breakfast. The nurse should use the same scale each time (because there may be some variation among scales), take the measurements at the same time each day, and make sure the client wears the same kind of clothing and no shoes. The client stands on a platform, and the weight is read from a digital display panel or a balancing arm. Clients who cannot stand are weighed on chair scales (Figure 28.6) or bed scales. Bed scales (Figure 28.7) have canvas straps or a stretcher-like apparatus. A machine lifts the client above the bed, and the weight is reflected either on a digital display panel or on a balance arm like that of a standing scale. Some agencies have beds with built-in scales.

Standardized charts have the average heights and weights of children and adults. It is important to remember that these averages provide only general guidelines for assessing growth, development, and nutritional status.

Body mass index (BMI) is a useful indicator of the overall health status of adults age 20 to 65 years. BMI does not apply to infants, children, adolescents, pregnant and breastfeeding women, and adults over the age of 65 years. BMI is calculated by taking the weight of the individual in kilograms and dividing it by the height in metres squared. The formula is BMI = weight (kg)/ height (m^2).

For example, an individual weighing 75 kg and measuring 150 cm tall would have a BMI of 33.3, which, as may be seen in Table 40.6 (p. 1232), would put him or her at high risk for health problems. See Table 40.5 (p. 1231) for the BMI nomogram and more discussion of BMI. Because adipose tissue located in the visceral area of the abdomen places a person at risk, measurement of waist circumference is now becoming a part of the general health assessment. Chapter 40 "Nutrition" discusses waist circumference and its influences on health in greater detail. See Figure 40.9 (p. 1232) for the waist circumference measurement technique.

The Integument

The integument includes skin, hair, and nails. The examination begins with a generalized inspection by using a good source of lighting, preferably indirect natural sunlight.

Skin

Assessment of skin involves inspection and palpation. In some instances, the nurse may also need to use the olfactory sense to detect unusual skin odours; these are usually most evident in the skinfolds or in the axillae. Pungent body odour is frequently related to poor hygiene, **hyperhidrosis** (excessive perspiration), or **bromhidrosis** (foul-smelling perspiration). The entire skin surface can be assessed at one time or as each aspect of the body is assessed.

Pallor is the result of inadequate circulating blood or hemoglobin and subsequent reduction in tissue oxygenation. It may be difficult to determine in clients with dark skin. It is usually characterized by the absence of underlying red tones in skin and may be most readily seen in the buccal mucosa (mucous membrane of the inside of the cheek). In brown-skinned clients, pallor may appear as a yellowish-brown tinge; in black-skinned clients, skin may appear ashen grey. Pallor in all people is usually most evident in areas with the least pigmentation, such as the conjunctiva, oral mucous membranes, nail beds, palms of hands, and soles of feet.

Cyanosis (a bluish tinge) is most evident in the nail beds, lips, and buccal mucosa. In dark-skinned clients, close inspection of the palpebral conjunctiva (the lining of the eyelids), palms, and soles may also show evidence of cyanosis. **Jaundice** (a yellowish tinge) may first be evident in the sclera of the eyes and then in the mucous membranes and skin. Nurses should take care not to confuse jaundice with the normal yellow pigmentation in the sclera of a dark-skinned client. If jaundice is suspected, the posterior part of the hard palate should also be inspected for a yellowish colour tone. **Erythema** is a redness associated with a variety of skin disorders.

Dark-skinned clients have areas of lighter pigmentation, such as the palms, lips, and nail beds. Localized areas of hyperpigmentation (increased pigmentation) and hypopigmentation (decreased pigmentation) may also occur as a result of changes in the distribution of melanin (the dark pigment) or in the function of the melanocytes in the epidermis. An example of hyperpigmentation in a defined area is a birthmark; an example of hypopigmentation is vitiligo. **Vitiligo**, seen as patches of hypopigmented skin, is caused by the destruction of melanocytes in the area. **Albinism** is the complete or partial lack of melanin in skin, hair, and eyes. Other localized colour changes can indicate a problem, such as edema or a localized infection. **Edema** is the presence of excess interstitial fluid. When edema is present, the tissues appear swollen, and skin is shiny, taut, and blanched. If the edema is accompanied by inflammation, skin will appear reddened (erythematous). Generalized edema is most often an indication of impaired venous circulation and, in some cases, reflects cardiac dysfunction or vein abnormalities.

A skin lesion is an alteration in a client's normal skin appearance. **Primary skin lesions** are those that appear initially in response to some change in the external or internal environment of skin (Figure 28.8, 1–8, on the next page). **Secondary skin lesions** are those that do not appear initially but result from changes to the primary lesion, such as those caused by trauma or infection of the primary lesion. For example, a vesicle or blister (primary lesion) may rupture and cause an erosion (secondary lesion). Table 28.5 on page 607 describes secondary lesions. Nurses are responsible for describing skin lesions accurately in terms of location (e.g., face), distribution (i.e., body regions involved), and configuration (the arrangement or position of several lesions), as well as colour, shape, size, firmness, texture, and characteristics of individual lesions. See Box 28.5 on page 607.

See Chapter 35 for discussion of skin assessment relative to wounds and pressure ulcers. Skill 28.2 on page 608 describes how to assess skin (also see the Lifespan Considerations box on assessing skin on page 610).

Hair

Assessing a client's hair includes inspecting it, considering developmental changes, and determining the individual's hair care practices and the factors influencing them. Much of the information about hair can be obtained by questioning the client.

Normal hair is resilient and evenly distributed. In people with *kwashiorkor* (severe protein deficiency), hair colour is faded and appears reddish or bleached, and the texture is coarse and dry. Some therapies cause **alopecia** (hair loss), and some disease conditions affect the coarseness of hair. For example, hypothyroidism can cause very thin and brittle hair. Skill 28.3 on page 610 describes how to assess hair (also see the Lifespan Considerations box on assessing hair on page 611).

Nails

Nails are inspected for nail plate shape, angle between the nail and the nail bed, nail texture, nail bed colour, and the intactness of the tissues around the nails. The parts of the nail are shown in Figure 28.9 on page 611.

The nail plate is normally colourless and has a convex curve. The angle between the nail and the nail bed is normally 160 degrees (Figure 28.10A on page 612). One nail abnormality is the spoon shape, in which the nail curves upward from the nail bed (Figure 28.10B). This condition, called **koilonychia**, may be seen in clients with iron deficiency anemia. **Clubbing** is a condition in which the angle between the nail and the nail bed is 180 degrees or greater (Figure 28.10C and

Macule, Patch Flat, unelevated change in colour. Macules are 1 mm to 1 cm in size and circumscribed. Examples: freckles, measles, petechiae, flat moles. Patches are larger than 1 cm and may have an irregular shape. Examples: port wine birthmark, vitiligo (white patches), rubella. ❶

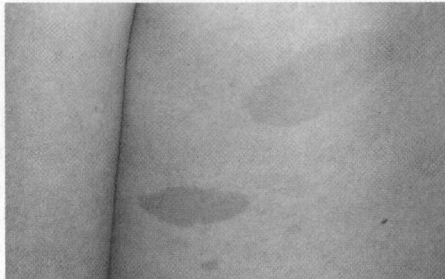

❶ Multiple café-au-lait macules

Nodule, Tumour Elevated, solid, hard mass that extends deeper into the dermis than a papule. Nodules have a circumscribed border and are 0.5 cm to 2 cm. Examples: squamous cell carcinoma, fibroma. Tumours are larger than 2 cm and may have an irregular border. Examples: malignant melanoma, hemangioma. ❹

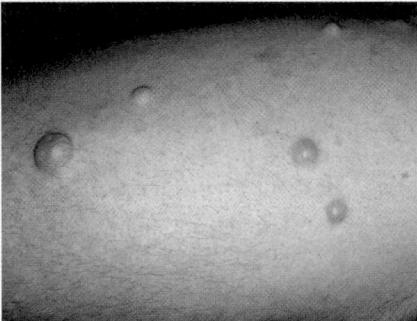

❹ Peripheral neurofibromas

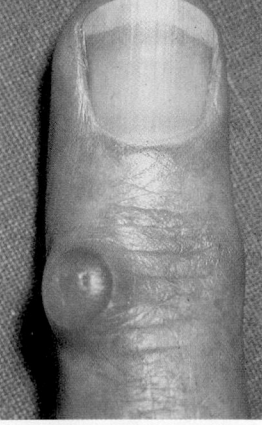

❼ Digital mucous cyst

Papule Circumscribed, solid elevation of skin. Papules are less than 1 cm. Examples: warts, acne, pimples, elevated moles. ❷

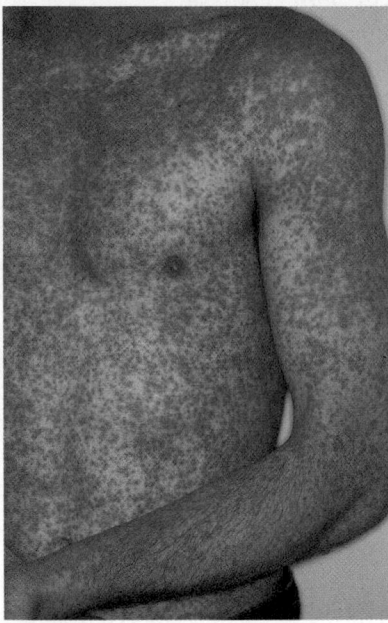

❷ Papular drug eruption

Pustule Vesicle or bulla filled with pus. Examples: acne vulgaris, impetigo. ❺

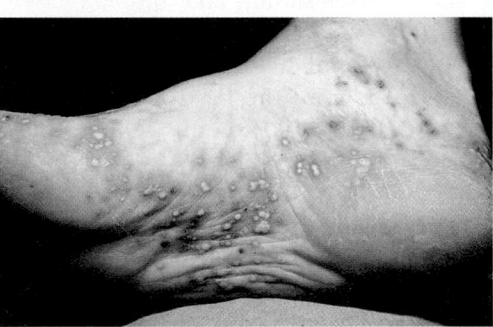

❺ Chronic pustular psoriasis

Cyst A 1 cm or larger, elevated, encapsulated, fluid-filled or semisolid mass arising from the subcutaneous tissue or dermis. Examples: sebaceous and epidermoid cysts, chalazion of the eyelid. ❼

Plaque Plaques are larger than 1 cm. Examples: psoriasis, rubeola. ❸

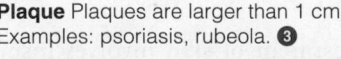

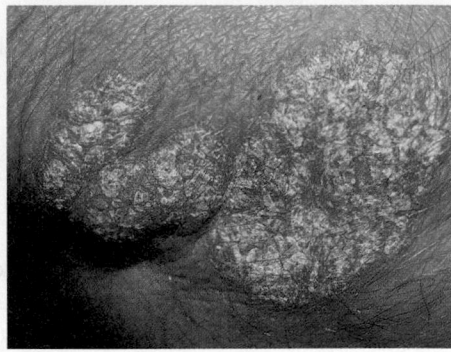

❸ Psoriasis vulgaris

Vesicle, Bulla A circumscribed, round or oval, thin, translucent mass filled with serous fluid or blood. Vesicles are less than 0.5 cm. Examples: herpes simplex, early chicken pox, small burn blister. Bullae are larger than 0.5 cm. Examples: large blister, second-degree burn, herpes simplex. ❻

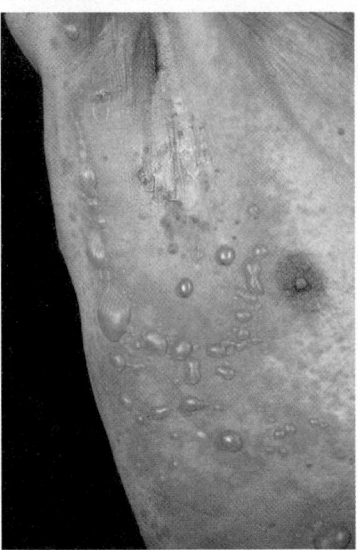

❻ Bullous pemphigoid

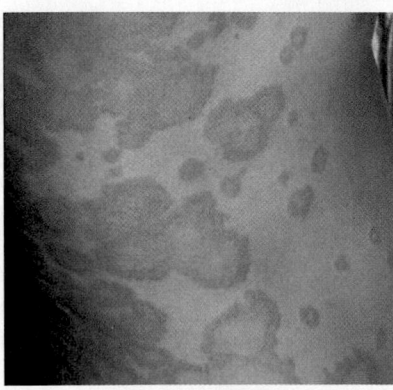

Wheal A reddened, localized collection of edema fluid; irregular in shape. Size varies. Examples: hives, mosquito bites. ❽

❽ Allergic wheals, urticaria

FIGURE 28.8 Primary skin lesions.

TABLE 28.5 Secondary Skin Lesions

Atrophy 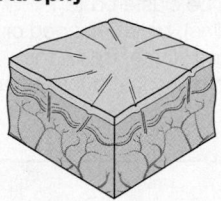	A translucent, dry, paper-like, sometimes wrinkled skin surface resulting from thinning or wasting of skin caused by loss of collagen and elastin **Examples:** striae, aged skin	**Ulcer** 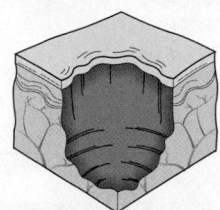	Deep, irregularly shaped area of skin loss extending into the dermis or subcutaneous tissue; may bleed; may leave scar **Examples:** pressure ulcers, stasis ulcers, chancres
Erosion 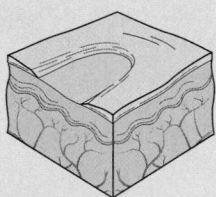	Wearing away of the superficial epidermis causing a moist, shallow depression; because erosions do not extend into the dermis, they heal without scarring **Examples:** scratch marks, ruptured vesicles	**Fissure** 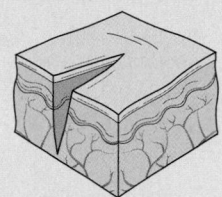	Linear crack with sharp edges extending into the dermis **Examples:** cracks at the corners of the mouth or in the hands, athlete's foot
Lichenification 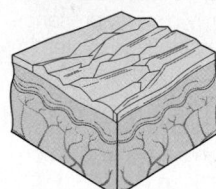	Rough, thickened, hardened area of epidermis resulting from chronic irritation, such as scratching or rubbing. **Example:** chronic dermatitis	**Scar** 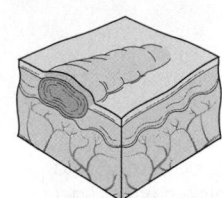	Flat, irregular area of connective tissue left after a lesion or wound has healed; new scars may be red or purple; older scars may be silvery or white **Examples:** healed surgical wound or injury, healed acne
Scales 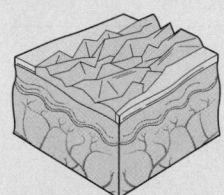	Shedding flakes of greasy, keratinized skin tissue; colour may be white, grey, or silver; texture may vary from fine to thick **Examples:** dry skin, dandruff, psoriasis, and eczema	**Keloid** 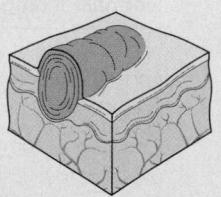	Elevated, irregular, darkened area of excess scar tissue caused by excessive collagen formation during healing; extends beyond the site of the original injury; higher incidence in black people **Examples:** keloid from ear piercing or surgery
Crust 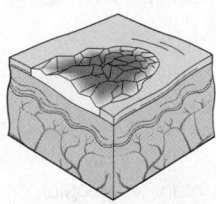	Dry blood, serum, or pus left on the skin surface when vesicles or pustules burst; can be red-brown, orange, or yellow; large crusts that adhere to the skin surface are called scabs **Examples:** eczema, impetigo, herpes, or scabs following abrasion	**Excoriation** 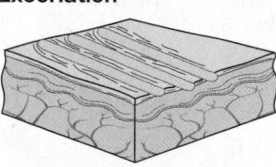	Linear erosion. **Examples:** scratches, some chemical burns

---

BOX 28.5 DESCRIBING SKIN LESIONS

Describe lesions according to the following characteristics:

- *Type or structure.* Skin lesions are classified as *primary* (those that appear initially in response to some change in the external or internal environment of skin) and *secondary* (those that result from modifications, such as chronicity, trauma, or infection, of the primary lesion). For example, a pustule (primary lesion) can burst and cause a secondary crust lesion.

- *Size, shape, and texture.* Note size in millimetres and whether the lesion is circumscribed or irregular; round or oval shaped; flat, elevated, or depressed; solid, soft, or hard; rough or thickened; fluid filled; or has flakes.

- *Colour.* Lesions can have no discoloration; one discrete colour (e.g., red, brown, or black); several colours, as with *ecchymosis* (a bruise), in which an initial dark red or blue fades to yellow. When colour changes are limited to the edges of a lesion, they are described as *circumscribed;* when spread over a large area, they are described as *diffuse.*

(continued)

BOX 28.5 *(continued)*

- *Distribution.* Distribution is described according to the location of the lesions on the body and symmetry or asymmetry of findings in comparable body areas.
- *Configuration.* Configuration refers to the arrangement of lesions in relation to one another. Configurations of lesions

can be annular (arranged in a circle), be clustered together or grouped, be linear (arranged in a line), be arc shaped or bow shaped, merge together or be indiscrete, follow the course of cutaneous nerves, or be meshed in the form of a network.

SKILL 28.2 ASSESSING SKIN

PLANNING

- Review the characteristics of primary and secondary lesions, if necessary (see Figure 28.8, p. 606 and Table 28.5, p. 607).
- Ensure that adequate lighting is available.

Equipment

- Millimetre ruler
- Clean gloves
- Magnifying glass

IMPLEMENTATION

Performance

1. Before performing the procedure, introduce yourself and verify the client's identity using two identifiers or per agency protocol. Explain to the client what you are going to do, why

it is necessary, and how he or she can participate. Discuss how the results will be used in planning further care or treatments.

2. Perform hand hygiene, and observe other appropriate infection prevention and control procedures.

3. Provide for client privacy.

4. Inquire whether the client has any history of the following: pain or itching; presence and spread of lesions, bruises, abrasions, pigmented spots; previous experience with skin problems; associated clinical signs; family history; presence of skin problems in other family members; related systemic conditions; use of medications, lotions, home remedies; excessively dry or moist feel to skin; tendency to bruise easily; association of the problem to season of year, stress, occupation, medications, recent travel, housing, and so on; recent contact with allergens.

Assessment	Normal Findings	Deviations from Normal
5. Inspect skin colour (best assessed under natural light and on areas not exposed to the sun).	Varies from light to deep brown; from ruddy pink to light pink; from yellow overtones to olive	Pallor, cyanosis, jaundice, erythema
6. Inspect uniformity of skin colour.	Generally uniform except in areas exposed to the sun; areas of lighter pigmentation (palms, lips, nail beds) in dark-skinned people	Areas of either hyperpigmentation or hypopigmentation
7. Assess edema, if present (i.e., location, colour, temperature, shape, and the degree to which skin remains indented or pitted when pressed with a finger). Measuring the circumference of the extremity with a millimetre tape may be useful for future comparison.	No edema	See the scale for grading edema in ❶.
8. Inspect, palpate, and describe skin lesions. Put on gloves if lesions are open or draining. Palpate lesions to determine shape and texture. Describe lesions according to location, distribution, colour, configuration, size, shape, type, or structure (see Box 28.5, p. 607).	Freckles, some birthmarks, some flat and raised nevi; no abrasions or other lesions	Interruptions in skin integrity; irregular, multicoloured, or raised nevi
9. Observe and palpate for skin moisture.	Moisture in skinfolds and axillae (varies with environmental temperature and humidity, body temperature, and activity)	Excessive moisture (e.g., in hyperthermia); excessive dryness (e.g., in dehydration)

Assessment	Normal Findings	Deviations from Normal
10. Palpate for skin temperature. Compare the two feet and the two hands, using the backs of your fingers.	Uniform; within normal range	Generalized hyperthermia (e.g., in fever); generalized hypothermia (e.g., in shock); localized hyperthermia (e.g., in infection); localized hypothermia (e.g., in arteriosclerosis)
11. Note skin turgor (fullness or elasticity) by lifting and pinching the skin on an extremity.	When pinched, skin springs back to previous state; may be slower in older adults	Skin stays pinched or tented or moves back slowly (e.g., in dehydration)

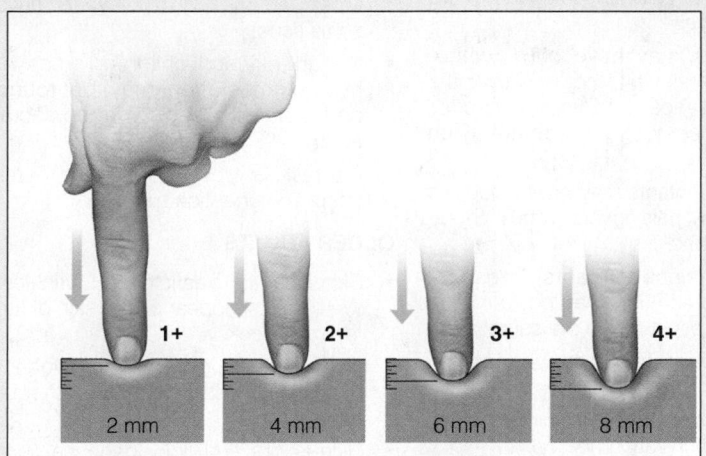

❶ Scale for grading edema.

12. Document your findings in the client record by using forms or checklists supplemented by narrative notes, when appropriate. Draw location of skin lesions on body surface diagrams, shown in ❷.

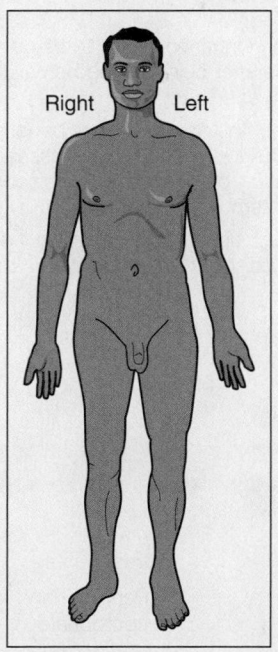 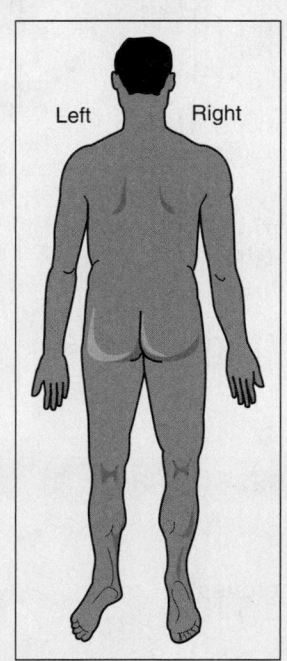

❷ Diagram for charting skin lesions.

EVALUATION

- Perform a detailed follow-up examination of other individual systems based on findings that deviated from expected or normal for the client. Relate findings to previous assessment data, if available.

- Report significant deviations from normal to the appropriate members of the health care team.

LIFESPAN CONSIDERATIONS

Assessing Skin

INFANTS

- Physiological jaundice may appear in newborns 2 to 3 days after birth and usually lasts about 1 week. Pathological jaundice, or that which indicates a disease, appears within 24 hours of birth and may last more than 8 days.
- Newborns may have *milia* (white-heads), small white nodules over the nose and face, and vernix caseosa (white cheesy, greasy material on skin).
- Premature infants may have *lanugo*, a fine downy hair covering their shoulders and back.
- In dark-skinned infants, areas of hyperpigmentation may be found on the back, especially in the sacral area.
- Diaper dermatitis may be seen in infants.
- If a rash is present, inquire in detail about immunization history.
- Assess skin turgor by pinching the skin on the abdomen.

CHILDREN

- Children may have minor skin lesions (e.g., bruising or abrasions) on arms and legs because of their high activity level. Lesions on other parts of the body may be signs of disease or abuse, and a thorough history should be taken.

- Secondary skin lesions may occur frequently as children scratch or expose a primary lesion to microbes.
- With puberty, oil glands become more productive, and acne may develop. Most persons 12 to 24 years have some acne.
- In dark-skinned children, areas of hyperpigmentation may be found on the back, especially in the sacral area.
- If a rash is present, inquire in detail about immunization history.

OLDER ADULTS

- Skin loses its elasticity and wrinkles. Wrinkles first appear on the skin of the face and neck.
- Skin appears thin and translucent because of loss of dermis and subcutaneous fat.
- Skin is dry and flaky because sebaceous and sweat glands are less active.
- Skin takes longer to return to its natural shape after being tented between the thumb and finger.
- Because of the normal loss of peripheral skin turgor in older adults, assess for hydration by checking skin turgor over the sternum or clavicle.
- Flat, tan- to brown-coloured macules, referred to as *senile lentigines* or *melanotic freckles,* are normally apparent on the back of the hands and other skin areas that are exposed to the sun. These macules may be as large as 1 cm to 2 cm.
- *Seborrheic keratosis* (warty lesions) with irregularly shaped borders and a scaly surface often occur on the face, shoulders, and trunk. These benign lesions begin as yellowish to tan and progress to a dark brown or black.
- Vitiligo tends to increase with age and is thought to result from an auto-immune response.
- *Acrochordons* (cutaneous tags) are most commonly seen in the neck and axillary regions. These skin lesions vary in size and are soft, often flesh coloured, and pedicled (on a stem or stalk of tissue).
- *Telangiectasias* (visible, bright red, fine, dilated blood vessels) commonly occur as a result of the thinning of the dermis and the loss of support for the blood vessel walls.
- *Actinic keratoses* (pink to slightly red lesions with indistinct borders) may appear at about age 50 years, often on the face, ears, backs of the hands, and arms. They can become malignant if left untreated.

SKILL 28.3 ASSESSING HAIR

PLANNING

Equipment: Clean gloves

IMPLEMENTATION

Performance

1. Before performing the procedure, introduce yourself and verify the client's identity using two identifiers or per agency protocol. Explain to the client what you are going to do, why it is necessary, and how he or she can participate. Discuss how the results will be used in planning further care or treatments.
2. Perform hand hygiene, put on gloves, and observe other appropriate infection prevention and control procedures.
3. Provide for client privacy.
4. Inquire if the client has any history of the following: use of hair dyes, rinses, or curling or straightening preparations; recent chemotherapy (if alopecia is present); presence of disease, such as hypothyroidism, which can be associated with brittle hair.

Assessment	Normal Findings	Deviations from Normal
5. Inspect the evenness of growth over the scalp.	Evenly distributed hair	Patches of hair loss (i.e., alopecia)
6. Inspect hair thickness or thinness.	Thick hair	Very thin hair (as in hypothyroidism)

Assessment	Normal Findings	Deviations from Normal
7. Inspect hair texture and oiliness.	Silky, resilient hair	Brittle hair (as in hypothyroidism); excessively oily or dry hair
8. Note the presence of infections or infestations by parting the client's hair in several areas and checking behind the ears and along the hairline at the neck.	No infection or infestation	Flaking, sores, lice, nits (louse eggs), or ringworm
9. Inspect amount of body hair.	Variable	**Hirsutism** (abnormal hairiness) in women and children; naturally absent or sparse leg hair (poor circulation)
10. Document your findings in the client record by using handwritten or electronic forms and checklists supplemented by narrative notes, when appropriate.		

EVALUATION

Report significant deviations from normal to the appropriate members of the health care team.

LIFESPAN CONSIDERATIONS

Assessing Hair

INFANTS

- It is normal for infants to have either very little or a great deal of body and scalp hair.

CHILDREN

- As puberty approaches, axillary and pubic hairs will appear.

OLDER ADULTS

- The age at which the scalp hair greys is influenced largely by genetic factors.
- There may be loss of scalp, pubic, and axillary hairs.
- Older women may present with coarse facial hair.
- Hairs of the eyebrows, ears, and nostrils become bristle-like and coarse.

28.10D). Clubbing can be caused by a long-term lack of oxygen and may be seen in clients with chronic respiratory or cardiac conditions.

Nail texture is normally smooth. Excessively thick nails can appear in older adults, in the presence of poor circulation, or in relation to a chronic fungal infection. Excessively thin nails or the presence of grooves or furrows can reflect prolonged iron deficiency anemia. *Beau's lines* are horizontal depressions in the nail that can result from injury or severe illness (Figure 28.10E on page 612).

The nail bed is highly vascular, a characteristic that accounts for its pink colour in Caucasian people. A bluish or purplish tint to the nail bed may reflect cyanosis, and pallor may reflect poor arterial circulation. Should the client report a history of onychomycosis (nail fungus), a referral to a podiatrist or dermatologist for treatment of

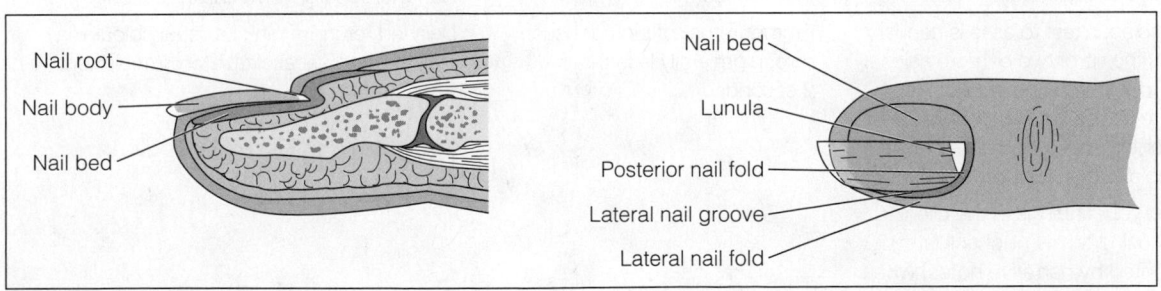

FIGURE 28.9 The parts of a nail.

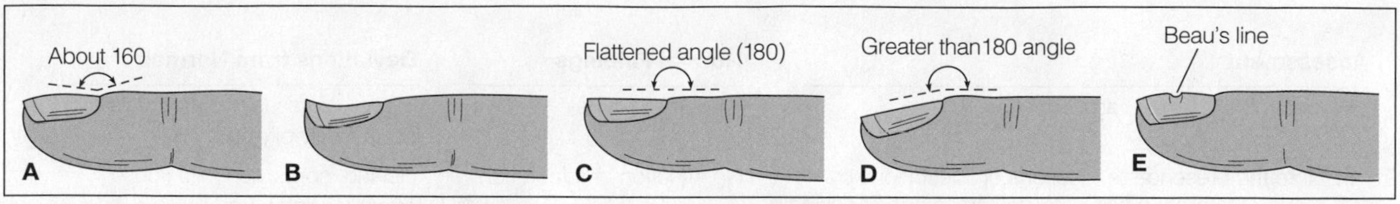

FIGURE 28.10 A: A normal nail, showing the convex shape and the nail plate angle of about 160 degrees; **B:** A spoon-shaped nail, which may be seen in clients with iron deficiency anemia; **C:** Early clubbing; **D:** Late clubbing (may be caused by long-term lack of oxygen); **E:** Beau's line on nail (may result from severe injury or illness).

nail fungus may be appropriate. Symptoms of nail fungus include brittleness, discoloration, thickening, distortion of nail shape, crumbling of the nail, and detaching (loosening) of the nail.

The tissue surrounding the nails is normally intact epidermis. **Paronychia** is an inflammation of the tissues surrounding a nail (often referred to as "ingrown nail"). The tissues appear inflamed and swollen, and tenderness is usually present. A **blanch test** assesses capillary refill, an indicator of peripheral circulation. Normal nail bed capillaries blanch when the tip of the nail is pressed but quickly (usually 2–3 seconds) turn pink or their usual colour when pressure is released. A slow rate of capillary refill may indicate peripheral circulatory problems.

Skill 28.4 describes how to assess the nails (also see the Lifespan Considerations box on assessing nails on page 613).

SKILL 28.4 ASSESSING NAILS

PLANNING
Equipment: None

IMPLEMENTATION
Performance

1. Before performing the procedure, introduce yourself and verify the client's identity using two identifiers or per agency protocol. Explain to the client what you are going to do, why it is necessary, and how he or she can participate. Discuss how the results will be used in planning further care or treatments. In most situations, clients with artificial nails or polish on fingernails or toenails are not required to remove these for assessment. If the assessment cannot be conducted because of the presence of polish or artificial nails, document this in the record.

2. Perform hand hygiene, and observe other appropriate infection prevention and control procedures.

3. Provide for client privacy.

4. Inquire whether the client has any history of the following: diabetes mellitus, peripheral circulatory disease, previous injury, or severe illness.

Assessment	Normal Findings	Deviations from Normal
5. Inspect fingernail plate shape to determine its curvature and angle.	Convex curvature; angle between nail and nail bed of about 160° (see Figure 28.10A)	Spoon nail (see Figure 28.10B); clubbing (180 degrees or greater) (see Figure 28.10C and 28.10D)
6. Inspect fingernail and toenail texture.	Smooth texture	Excessive thickness or thinness or presence of grooves or furrows; Beau's lines (see Figure 28.10E); discoloured or detached nail, often caused by fungus
7. Inspect fingernail and toenail bed colour.	Highly vascular and pink; dark-skinned clients may have brown or black pigmentation in longitudinal streaks	Bluish or purplish tint (may reflect cyanosis); pallor (may reflect poor arterial circulation)
8. Inspect tissues surrounding nails.	Intact epidermis	Hangnails; paronychia (inflammation)
9. Perform a blanch test to assess capillary refill. Press the tip of two or more nails between your thumb and index finger causing the nail bed to blanch; release and observe for the speed with which the pink or usual colour of the nail bed returns.	Prompt return of pink or usual colour, generally less than 2 seconds.	Delayed return of pink or usual colour may indicate peripheral circulatory impairment
10. Document your findings in the client record by using forms or checklists supplemented by narrative notes, when appropriate.		

EVALUATION

- Perform a detailed follow-up examination of other individual systems based on findings that deviated from expected or normal for the client. Relate findings to previous assessment data, if available.

- Report significant deviations from normal to the appropriate members of the health care team.

LIFESPAN CONSIDERATIONS

Assessing Nails

INFANTS

- Newborns' nails grow very quickly, are extremely thin, and tear easily.

CHILDREN

- Bent, bruised, or ingrown toenails can indicate shoes that are too tight.
- Nail biting should be discussed with a caregiver.

OLDER ADULTS

- The nails grow more slowly and thicken.
- Longitudinal bands commonly develop in older adults, and the nails tend to split.
- Bands across the nails may indicate protein deficiency; white spots, zinc deficiency; and spoon-shaped nails, iron deficiency.
- Toenail fungus is more common and difficult to eliminate (although not dangerous to health).

Head

Assessment of the head includes inspection, palpation, and percussion. The nurse examines the skull, face, eyes, ears, nose, sinuses, mouth, and pharynx.

Skull and Face

Normal skulls come in a range of shapes. A normal head size is referred to as **normocephalic**. The names of the areas of the head are derived from the names of the underlying bones: frontal, parietal, occipital, mastoid process, mandible, maxilla, and zygomatic (Figure 28.11).

Many disorders cause a change in facial shape or condition. Renal or cardiac disease can cause edema of eyelids. Hyperthyroidsm can cause **exophthalmos**, protrusion of eyeballs with elevation of the upper eyelids, resulting in a startled or staring expression. Hypothyroidism, or *myxedema,* can cause a puffy face with dry skin and coarse features and thinning of the scalp hair and eyebrows. Increased adrenal hormone production or administration of steroids can cause a round face with reddened cheeks, referred to as a *moon face,* and excessive hair growth on the upper lips, chin, and sideburn areas. Prolonged illness, cachexia, and dehydration can result in sunken eyes, cheeks, and temples.

Skill 28.5 on the next page describes how to assess the skull and face (also see the Lifespan Considerations box on assessing the skull and face on page 615).

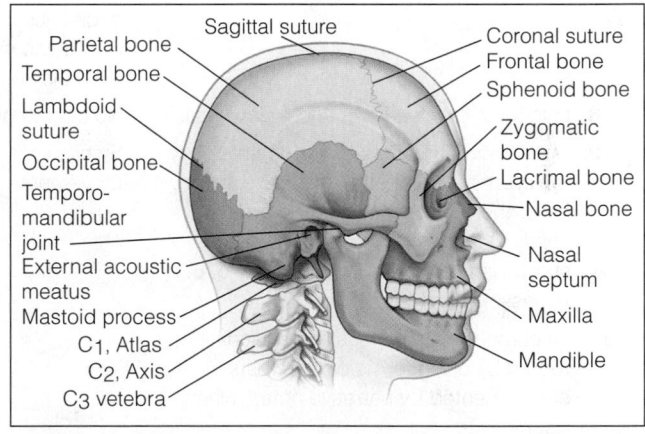

FIGURE 28.11 The bones of the head.

Eyes and Vision

To maintain optimal vision, people need to have their eyes examined regularly throughout life. It is recommended that people under age 40 years have their eyes tested every 3 to 5 years, or more frequently if there is a family history of diabetes, hypertension, blood dyscrasia, or eye disease (e.g., glaucoma). After age 40 years, an eye examination is recommended every 2 years to rule out the possibility of glaucoma.

An eye assessment should be carried out as part of the client's initial physical examination; periodic reassessments need to be made for clients in long-term care. Examination of the eyes includes assessment of **visual acuity** (the degree

SKILL 28.5 ASSESSING THE SKULL AND FACE

PLANNING

Equipment: None

IMPLEMENTATION

Performance

1. Before performing the procedure, introduce yourself and verify the client's identity using two identifiers or per agency protocol. Explain to the client what you are going to do, why it is necessary, and how he or she can participate. Discuss how the results will be used in planning further care or treatments.

2. Perform hand hygiene, and observe other appropriate infection prevention and control procedures.

3. Provide for client privacy.

4. Inquire whether the client has any past problems with lumps or bumps, itching, scaling, or dandruff; any history of loss of consciousness, dizziness, seizures, headache, facial pain, or injury; when and how any lumps occurred; the length of time any other problem existed; any known cause of the problem; and associated symptoms, treatment, and recurrences.

Assessment	Normal Findings	Deviations from Normal
5. Inspect the skull for size, shape, and symmetry. If the skull is of abnormal size, measure its circumference just above the eyebrows.	Rounded (normocephalic and symmetrical, with frontal, parietal, and occipital prominences); smooth skull contour	Lack of symmetry; increased skull size with more prominent nose and forehead; longer mandible (may indicate excessive growth hormone or increased bone thickness)
6. Palpate the skull for nodules or masses and depressions. Use a gentle rotating motion with the fingertips. Begin at the front and palpate down the midline, and then palpate each side of the head.	Smooth, uniform consistency; absence of nodules or masses	Sebaceous cysts; local deformities from trauma; masses, nodules
7. Inspect the facial features (e.g., symmetry of structures and distribution of hair).	Symmetric or slightly asymmetric facial features; palpebral fissures equal in size; symmetric nasolabial folds; even distribution of hair	Increased or uneven distribution of facial hair; thinning of eyebrows; asymmetric features; exophthalmos (bulging eyes); myxedema facies; "moon face"
8. Inspect eyes for edema and hollowness.	No edema or hollowness	Periorbital edema; sunken eyes
9. Note symmetry of facial movements. Ask the client to elevate the eyebrows, frown, lower the eyebrows, close the eyes tightly, puff the cheeks, and smile and show the teeth. See Skill 28.17 (p. 676), Assessing the Neurological System.	Symmetrical facial movements	Asymmetrical facial movements (e.g., eye on affected side cannot close completely); drooping of lower eyelid and mouth; involuntary facial movements (i.e., tics or tremors)

10. Document your findings in the client record by using forms or checklists supplemented by narrative notes, when appropriate.

EVALUATION

- Perform a detailed follow-up examination of other systems based on findings that deviated from expected or normal for the client. Relate findings to previous assessment data, if available.

- Report significant deviations from normal to the appropriate members of the health care team.

of detail the eye can discern in an image), ocular movement, **visual fields** (the area an individual can see when looking straight ahead), and external structures. If the client wears contact lenses or has an artificial eye, consideration should be given to individual hygiene practices. For the anatomical structures of the eye, see Figure 28.12 and Figure 28.13.

Many people wear eyeglasses or contact lenses to correct common refractive errors of the lens of the eye. These errors include **myopia** (nearsightedness), **hyperopia** (farsightedness), and **presbyopia** (loss of elasticity of the lens and, thus, loss of ability to see close objects). Presbyopia begins at about 45 years of age. People with presbyopia have difficulty reading newsprint. Often, two corrective

Assessing the Skull and Face

INFANTS

- Newborns delivered vaginally can have elongated, moulded heads, which take on more rounded shapes after a week or two. Infants delivered by cesarean section tend to have smooth, rounded heads.

- The posterior fontanelle (soft spot) is about 1 cm in size and usually closes by eight weeks. The anterior fontanelle is larger, about 2 cm to 3 cm in size. It closes by 18 months.

- Newborns can lift their heads slightly and turn them from side to side. Voluntary head control is well established by 4 to 6 months.

- Occipital flattening of positional origin results when an infant spends prolonged periods with the head in the same position against a flat surface. Flattening can occur before birth from wedging against a maternal pelvic bone, or it can occur postnatally.

lenses (bifocals) are required—one for near vision or reading, the other for far vision. **Astigmatism**, an uneven curvature of the cornea that prevents horizontal and vertical rays from focusing on the retina, is a common problem that can occur in conjunction with myopia and hyperopia.

Three types of eye charts are available to test visual acuity (Figure 28.14 on the next page). A child acquires normal 20/20 vision by 6 years of age. Visual acuity can be tested on a standard Snellen chart. Visual acuity is documented as two numbers (e.g., 20/20). The first number indicates the distance of the client from the chart (i.e., 20 ft, which is about 6 m), and the second number indicates the distance at which a normal eye can read the chart. For example, a test result of 20/200 means that at 20 ft, the client can read the chart that a person with normal vision could read at 200 ft. In other words, the larger the second number, or denominator, the worse the visual acuity. People with denominators of 40 or more on the Snellen chart, with or without corrective lenses, need to be referred to an ophthalmologist.

Inflammatory visual problems include conjunctivitis, dacryocystitis, hordeolum, iritis, and contusions or hematomas of the eyelids and surrounding structures. **Conjunctivitis** (inflammation of the bulbar and palpebral conjunctiva) can be caused by foreign bodies, chemicals, allergenic agents, bacteria, or viruses. Redness, itching, tearing, and discharge occur. During sleep, the eyelids may become encrusted and matted together. **Dacryocystitis** (inflammation of the lacrimal sac) is manifested by tearing and discharge from the nasolacrimal duct. **Hordeolum (sty)** is a redness, swelling, and tenderness of the hair follicle and glands that empty at the edge of the eyelids. **Iritis** (inflammation of the iris) can be caused by local or systemic infections and results in pain, tearing, and **photophobia** (sensitivity to light). Contusions or hematomas are "black eyes" resulting from injury.

Cataracts are an opacity of the lens of the eye. Most cataracts occur in individuals over age 65 years. However,

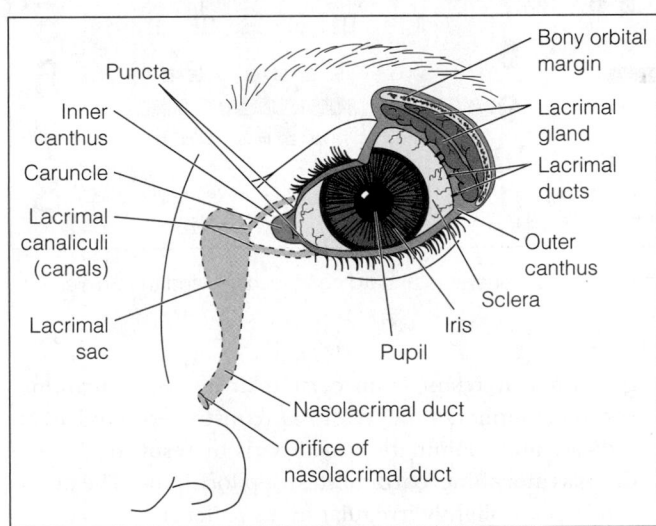

FIGURE 28.12 The external structures and lacrimal apparatus of the left eye.

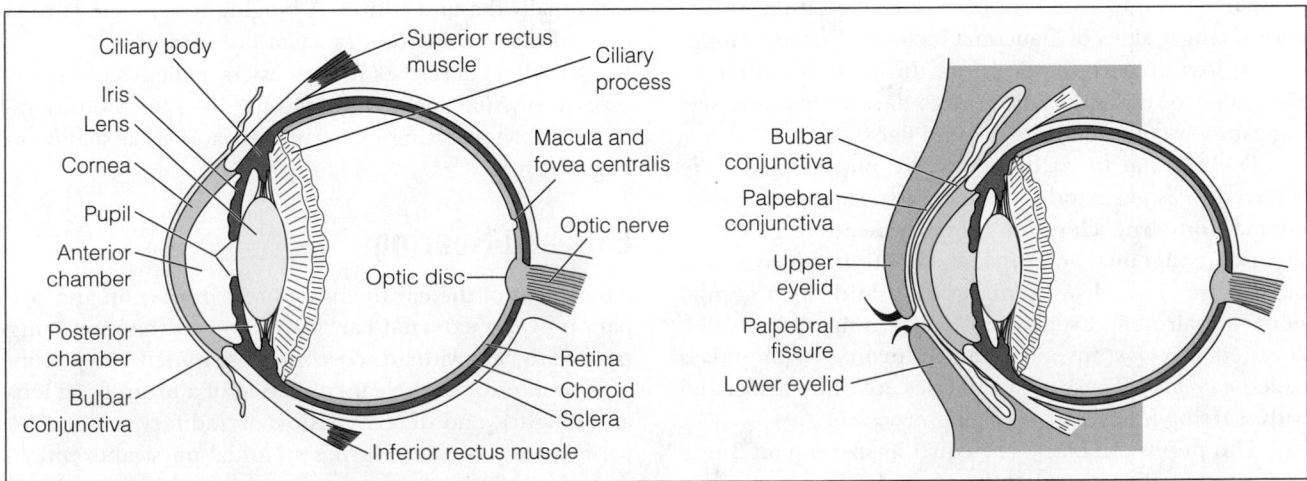

FIGURE 28.13 Anatomical structures of the right eye, lateral view.

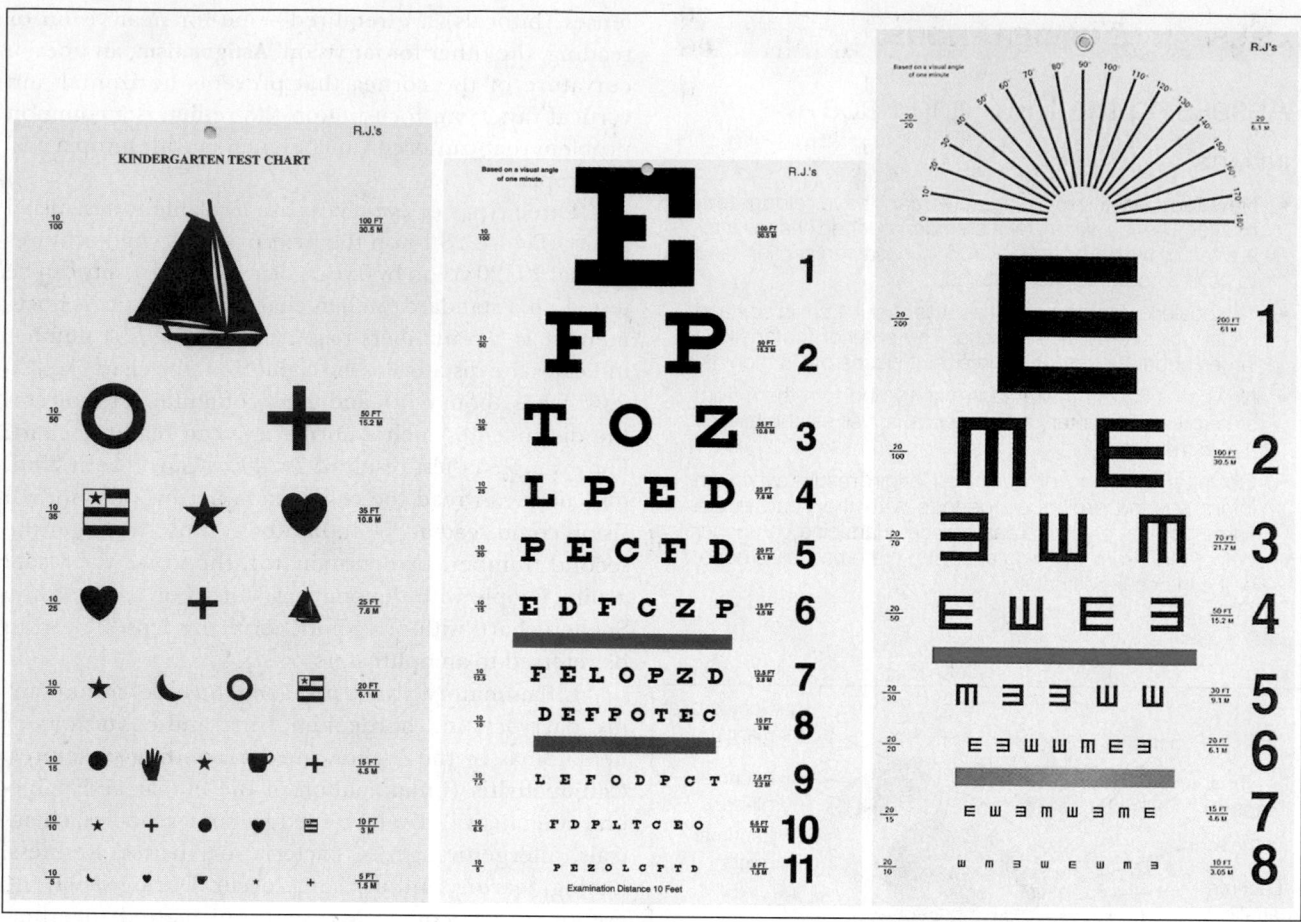

FIGURE 28.14 Three types of eye charts; the preschool children's chart (*left*), the Snellen standard chart (*centre*), and the Snellen E chart for clients unable to read (*right*).

cataracts also occur in infants because of a malformation of the lens, for example, if a mother contracts rubella in the first trimester of pregnancy. A common treatment is removal of the lens and replacement of the lens with an implant. **Glaucoma** is a disruption in the circulation of the aqueous fluid, which causes an increase in intra-ocular pressure and a reduced blood supply to the optic disc. Glaucoma is the most common cause of blindness in people over 40 years. It can be managed if diagnosed early. Danger signs of glaucoma include blurred or foggy vision, loss of peripheral vision, difficulty focusing on close objects, difficulty adjusting to dark rooms, and see-ing rainbow-coloured rings around lights.

Eyelids that lie at or below the pupil margin are referred to as *ptosis* and are usually associated with aging, edema from drug allergy or systemic disease (e.g., kidney disease), congenital lid muscle dysfunction, neuromuscu-lar disease (e.g., myasthenia gravis), and third cranial nerve impairment. Eversion, an out-turning of the eyelid, is called *ectropion*; inversion, an in-turning of the lid, is called *entropion*. These abnormalities are often associated with scarring injuries or the aging process.

The pupils are black, are equal in size (about 3 mm to 7 mm in diameter), and have round, smooth bor-ders. **Mydriasis** (enlarged pupils) can indicate injury or glaucoma or result from certain drugs (e.g., atropine, cocaine, amphetamines). **Miosis** (constricted pupils) can indicate an inflammation of the iris or result from such drugs as morphine, barbiturates, or pilocarpine. The pupils can become slightly irregular and smaller in older adults, making it more difficult to examine the eyes. **Anisocoria** (unequal pupils) can result from a central nervous system disorder; however, slight variations may be normal. The iris is normally flat and round. A bulging toward the cornea can indicate increased intraocular pressure.

Skill 28.6 describes how to assess a client's eye struc-tures and visual acuity (also see the Lifespan Considera-tions box on assessing eye structures and visual acuity on page 618).

Ears and Hearing

Assessment of the ear includes direct inspection and pal-pation of the external ear, inspection of the remaining parts of the ear with an **otoscope** (instrument for examin-ing the interior of the ear consisting of a magnifying lens and a light), and determination of auditory acuity. The ear is usually assessed during an initial physical examina-tion; periodic reassessments may be necessary for long-term clients or those with hearing problems.

SKILL 28.6 ASSESSING EYE STRUCTURES AND VISUAL ACUITY

PLANNING

Place the client in an appropriate room for assessing eyes and vision. The nurse must be able to control the natural or overhead lighting during some portions of the exam.

Equipment

- Millimetre ruler
- Penlight
- Snellen or E chart
- Opaque card

IMPLEMENTATION

Performance

1. Before performing the procedure, introduce yourself and verify the client's identity using two identifiers or per agency protocol. Explain to the client what you are going to do, why it is necessary, and how he or she can participate. Discuss how the results will be used in planning further care or treatments.

2. Perform hand hygiene, put on gloves, and observe other appropriate infection prevention and control procedures.

3. Provide for client privacy.

4. Inquire whether the client has any history of the following: family history of diabetes, hypertension, blood dyscrasia, or eye disease, injury, or surgery; client's last visit to an ophthalmologist; current use of eye medications; use of contact lenses or eyeglasses; hygienic practices for corrective lenses; current symptoms of eye problems (e.g., changes in visual acuity, blurring of vision, tearing, spots, photophobia, itching, or pain).

Assessment	Normal Findings	Deviations from Normal
External Eye Structures		
5. Inspect the eyebrows for hair distribution and alignment and for skin quality and movement. (Ask the client to raise and lower eyebrows.)	Hair evenly distributed; skin intact; eyebrows symmetrically aligned; equal movement	Loss of hair; scaling and flakiness of skin; unequal alignment and movement of eyebrows
6. Inspect eyelashes for evenness of distribution and direction of curl.	Equally distributed; curled slightly outward	Turned inward
7. Inspect eyelids for surface characteristics (e.g., skin quality and texture), position in relation to the cornea, ability to blink, and frequency of blinking. For proper visual examination of the upper eyelids, elevate the eyebrows with your thumb and index fingers, and have the client close the eyes (see ❶). Inspect the lower eyelids while the client's eyes are closed.	Skin intact; no discharge; no discoloration; lids close symmetrically; approximately 15 to 20 involuntary blinks per minute; bilateral blinking; when lids open, no visible sclera above corneas, and upper and lower borders of cornea are slightly covered	Redness, swelling, flaking, crusting, plaques, discharge, nodules, lesions; lids close asymmetrically, incompletely, or painfully; rapid, monocular, absent, or infrequent blinking; ptosis, ectropion, or entropion; rim of sclera visible between lid and iris (possible hyperthyroidism)

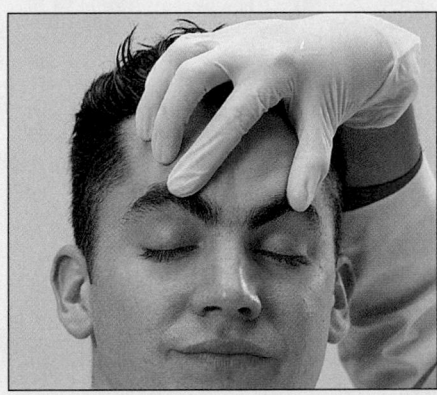

❶ Inspecting the upper eyelids.

8. Inspect the bulbar conjunctiva (lying over the sclera) for colour, texture, and the presence of lesions. Retract the eyelids with your thumb and index finger, exerting pressure over the upper and lower bony orbits, and ask the client to look up, down, and from side to side.	Transparent; capillaries sometimes evident; sclera appears white (yellowish in dark-skinned clients)	Jaundiced sclera (e.g., in liver disease); excessively pale sclera (e.g., in anemia); reddened sclera; lesions or nodules (may indicate damage by mechanical, chemical, allergenic, or bacterial agents)

(continued)

SKILL 28.6 ASSESSING EYE STRUCTURES AND VISUAL ACUITY (*continued*)

Assessment	Normal Findings	Deviations from Normal
9. Inspect the cornea for clarity and texture. Ask the client to look straight ahead. Hold a penlight at an oblique angle to the eye, and move the light slowly across the corneal surface. Tangential lighting best shows corneal regularity.	Transparent, shiny, and smooth; details of the iris are visible; in older people, a thin, greyish-white ring around the margin, called *arcus senilis,* may be evident	Opaque; surface not smooth (may be the result of trauma or abrasion); arcus senilis in clients under age 40 years
10. Inspect the pupils for colour, shape, and symmetry of size. Pupil charts are available in some agencies. See ❷ for variations in pupil diameters.	Black in colour; equal in size; normally 3 to 7 mm in diameter; round, smooth border; iris flat and round	Cloudiness, mydriasis, miosis, anisocoria; bulging of iris toward cornea

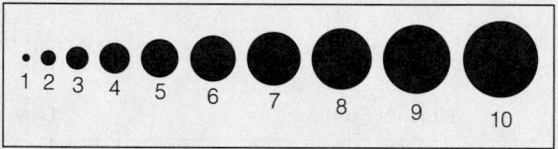

❷ Variations in pupil diameters in millimetres.

Assessment	Normal Findings	Deviations from Normal
11. Assess each pupil's direct and consensual reaction to light to determine the function of the oculomotor (third) and trochlear (fourth cranial) nerves. • Partially darken the room. • Ask the client to look straight ahead. • By using a penlight and approaching from the side, shine a light on the pupil. • Observe the response of the illuminated pupil. It should constrict (direct response). • Shine the light on the pupil again, and observe the response of the other pupil. It should also constrict (consensual response).	Illuminated pupil constricts (direct response); nonilluminated pupil constricts (consensual response)	Neither pupil constricts; unequal responses; absent responses
12. Assess each pupil's reaction to accommodation. • Hold an object (a penlight or pencil) about 10 cm from the bridge of the client's nose. • Ask the client to look first at the top of the object and then at a distant object (e.g., the far wall) behind the penlight. Have the client alternate the gaze from the near object to the far object. • Observe the pupil response. The pupils should constrict when looking at the near object and dilate when looking at the far object. • Next, move the penlight or pencil toward the client's nose. The pupils should converge. To record normal assessment of the pupils, use the acronym **PERRLA** (pupils equally round and react to light and accommodation).	Pupils constrict when looking at near object; pupils dilate when looking at far object; pupils converge when near object is moved toward nose	One or both pupils fail to constrict, dilate, or converge

Assessment	Normal Findings	Deviations from Normal

Visual Fields

13. Assess peripheral visual fields to determine the functioning of the retina and neuronal visual pathways to the brain and the optic (second cranial) nerve.

When looking straight ahead, client can see objects in the periphery

Visual field smaller than normal (possible glaucoma); one-half vision in one or both eyes (possible nerve damage)

- Have the client sit directly facing you at a distance of 60 cm to 90 cm.
- Ask the client to cover the right eye with a card and look directly at your nose.
- Cover or close your eye directly opposite the client's covered eye (i.e., your left eye), and look directly at the client's nose.
- Hold an object (e.g., a penlight or pencil) in your fingers, extend your arm, and move the object into the visual field from various points in the periphery (see ❸). The object should be at an equal distance from the client and you. Ask the client to tell you when the moving object is first spotted.
  - **a.** To test the temporal field of the left eye, extend and move your right arm in from the client's right periphery. Temporally, peripheral objects can be seen at right angles (90 degrees) to the central point of vision.
  - **b.** To test the superior (upward) field of the left eye, extend and move the right arm down from the upward periphery. The upward field of vision is normally 50 degrees because the orbital ridge is in the way.
  - **c.** To test the inferior (downward) field of the left eye, extend and move the right arm up from the lower periphery. The downward field of vision is normally 70 degrees because the cheekbone is in the way.
  - **d.** To test the nasal field of the left eye, extend and move your left arm in from the periphery. The nasal field of vision is normally 50 degrees away from the central point of vision because the nose is in the way.
- Repeat the above steps for the right eye, reversing the process.

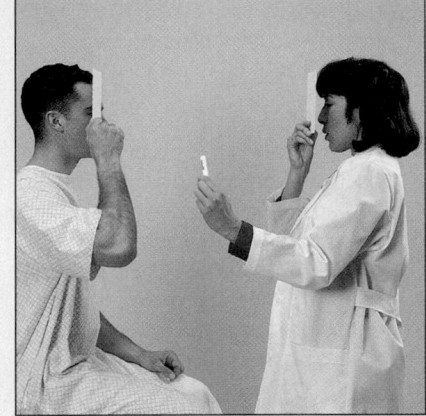

❸ Assessing the client's left peripheral visual field.

Extraocular Muscle Tests

14. Assess six ocular movements to determine eye alignment and coordination.

Both eyes are coordinated, move in unison, with parallel alignment.

Eye movements not coordinated or parallel; one or both eyes fail to follow a penlight in specific directions (e.g., strabismus or cross-eye); **nystagmus** (rapid involuntary rhythmic eye movement) other than at end point may indicate neurological impairment

- Stand directly in front of the client and hold the penlight at a comfortable distance, such as 30 cm in front of the client's eyes.
- Ask the client to hold the head in a fixed position facing you and to follow the movements of the penlight with the eyes only.
- Move the penlight in a slow, orderly manner through the six cardinal fields of gaze, that is, from the centre of the eye along the lines of the arrows in ❹ and back to the centre.
- Stop the movement of the penlight periodically so that nystagmus can be detected.

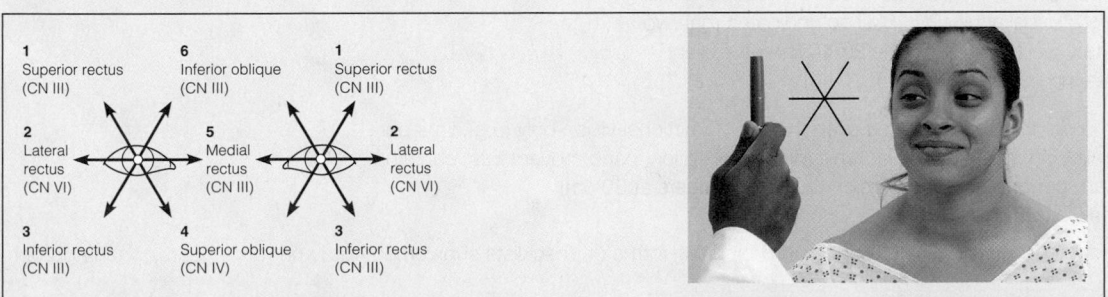

❹ The six muscles that govern eye movement.

(continued)

SKILL 28.6 ASSESSING EYE STRUCTURES AND VISUAL ACUITY (continued)

Assessment	Normal Findings	Deviations from Normal
15. Assess for location of light reflex by shining penlight on pupil on the corneal surface (Hirschberg test).	Light falls symmetrically on both pupils (e.g., at 6 o'clock on both pupils)	Light falls off centre on one eye (indicates misalignment)
16. Have the client fixate on a near or far object. Cover one eye, and observe for movement in the uncovered eye (cover test).	Uncovered eye does not move	If misalignment is present, when the dominant eye is covered, the uncovered eye will move to focus on the object

Visual Acuity

17. Assess near vision by providing adequate lighting and asking the client to read from a magazine or newspaper (if the client can read and in a language the client can read) held at a distance of 36 cm. If the client normally wears corrective lenses, the glasses or lenses should be worn during the test.	Able to read newsprint	Difficulty reading newsprint
18. Assess distance vision by asking the client to wear corrective lenses, unless they are used for reading only (i.e., for distances of only 36 cm).	20/20 vision on Snellen-type chart	Denominator of 40 or more on Snellen-type chart with corrective lenses

- Ask the client to stand or sit 6 m (20 ft) from a Snellen or character chart (see ❺), cover the eye not being tested, and identify the letters or characters on the chart.
- Take three readings: right eye, left eye, both eyes.
- Record the readings of each eye and both eyes (i.e., the smallest line from which the person is able to read one half or more of the letters).

At the end of each line of the chart are standardized numbers (fractions). The top line is 20/200. The numerator (top number) is always 20, the distance the person stands from the chart. The denominator (bottom number) is the distance from which the normal eye can read the chart. Therefore, a person who has 20/40 vision can see at 20 ft from the chart what a normal-sighted person can see at 40 ft from the chart. Visual acuity is recorded as "s̄c" (without correction), or "c̄c" (with correction). You can also indicate how many letters were misread in the line (e.g., "visual acuity 20/40, 2 c̄c" indicates that two letters were misread in the 20/40 line by a client wearing corrective lenses).

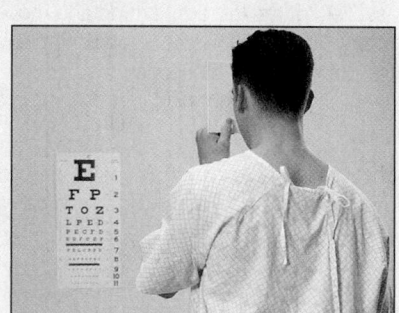

❺ Testing distance vision.

19. If the client is unable to see even the top line (20/200) of the Snellen-type chart, perform functional vision tests (see Box 28.6).	Functional vision only (e.g., light perception, hand movements, counting fingers at 30 cm)	

20. Document findings in the client record by using forms or checklists supplemented by narrative notes, when appropriate.

EVALUATION

- Perform a detailed follow-up examination of neurological and other systems based on findings that deviated from expected or normal for the client. Relate findings to previous assessment data, if available.

- Report significant deviations from normal to the appropriate members of the health care team. Persons with denominators of 40 or more on the Snellen or character chart, with or without corrective lenses, may need to be referred to an optometrist or ophthalmologist.

LIFESPAN CONSIDERATIONS

Assessing Eye Structures and Visual Acuity

INFANTS

- Infants 4 weeks of age should gaze at and follow objects.
- Ability to focus with both eyes should be present by 6 months of age.
- Infants do not have tears until about 3 months of age.
- A cover test and the corneal light reflex (Hirschberg) test should be conducted on infants to detect misalignment early and prevent amblyopia.
- Visual acuity is about 20/300 at 4 months and progressively improves.

CHILDREN

- Epicanthal folds, common in persons of Asian cultures, may cover the medial canthus and cause eyes to appear misaligned. Epicanthal folds may also be seen in young children of any race before the bridge of the nose begins to elevate.
- Preschool children's acuity can be checked with picture cards or the E chart. Acuity should approach 20/20 by 6 years of age.
- A cover test and the corneal light reflex (Hirschberg) test should be conducted on young children to detect misalignment early and prevent amblyopia.
- Always perform the acuity test with glasses on if a child has a prescription to wear lenses.

- Children should be tested for colour vision deficit. From 8% to 10% of Caucasian males and from 0.5% to 1% of Caucasian females have this deficit; it is much less common in non-Caucasian children. The Ishihara or Hardy-Rand-Rittler test can be used.

OLDER ADULTS

Visual Acuity

- Visual acuity decreases as the lens ages, becomes more opaque, and loses elasticity (presbyopia).
- The ability of the iris to accommodate to darkness and dim light diminishes.
- Peripheral vision diminishes.
- The adaptation to light (glare) and dark decreases.
- Accommodation to far objects often improves, but accommodation to near objects decreases.
- Colour vision declines; older people are less able to perceive purple colours and to discriminate pastel colours.
- Many older people wear corrective lenses; they are most likely to have hyperopia. Visual changes are caused by loss of elasticity (presbyopia) and transparency of the lens.

External Eye Structures

- The skin around the orbit of the eye may darken.
- The eyes may appear dry and lustreless because of the decrease in tear production from the lacrimal glands.
- The eyeball may appear sunken because of the decrease in orbital fat.
- Skinfolds of the upper lids may seem more prominent, and the lower lids may sag.
- **Arcus senilis** (a thin, greyish-white arc or ring) appears around part or all of the cornea. It results from an accumulation of a lipid substance on the cornea. The cornea tends to cloud with age.
- The iris may appear pale with brown discolorations as a result of pigment degeneration.
- The conjunctiva of the eye may appear paler than in younger adults and may take on a slightly yellow appearance because of the deposition of fat.
- Pupil reaction to light and accommodation is normally symmetrically equal but may be less brisk.
- The pupils can appear smaller in size, unequal, and irregular in shape because of sclerotic changes in the iris.

BOX 28.6 PERFORMING FUNCTIONAL VISION TESTS

LIGHT PERCEPTION

Shine a penlight into the client's eye from a lateral position, and then turn the light off. Ask the client to tell you when the light is on or off. If the client knows when the light is on or off, the client has light perception, and the vision is recorded as "LP."

HAND MOVEMENTS (H/M)

Hold your hand 30 cm from the client's face, and move it slowly back and forth, stopping it periodically. Ask the client to tell you when your hand stops moving. If the client knows when your hand stops moving, record the vision as "H/M 30 cm."

COUNTING FINGERS (C/F)

Hold up some of your fingers 30 cm from the client's face, and ask the client to count your fingers. If the client can do so, note on the vision record "C/F 30 cm."

The ear is divided into three parts: (a) external ear, (b) middle ear, and (c) inner ear. Most of the structures mentioned next are illustrated in Figure 28.15 on the next page. The external ear includes the **auricle** or **pinna**, the external auditory canal, and the **tympanic membrane**, or eardrum. Landmarks of the auricle include the **lobule** (earlobe), **helix** (the posterior curve of the auricle's upper aspect), **antihelix** (the anterior curve of the auricle's upper aspect), **tragus** (the cartilaginous protrusion at the entrance to the ear canal), **triangular fossa** (a depression of the antihelix), and **external auditory meatus** (the entrance to the ear canal). Although not part of the ear, the **mastoid**, a bony prominence behind the ear, is another important landmark. The external ear canal is curved, is about 2.5 cm long in the adult, and ends at the tympanic membrane. The tympanic membrane separates the external ear from the middle ear. It is covered with skin that has many fine hairs, glands, and nerve endings. The glands secrete **cerumen** (earwax), which lubricates and protects the canal.

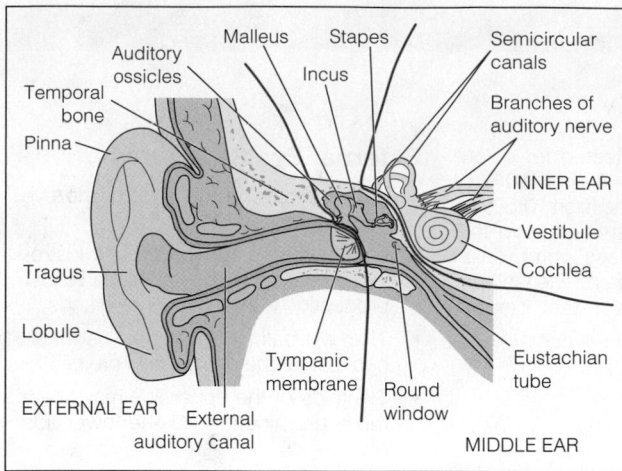

FIGURE 28.15 Anatomical structures of the external, middle, and inner ear.

The curvature of the external ear canal differs with age. In the infant and toddler, the canal has an upward curvature. By the age of 3 years, the ear canal assumes the more downward curvature of adulthood.

The middle ear is an air-filled cavity that starts at the tympanic membrane and contains three **ossicles** (bones of sound transmission): the **malleus** (hammer), which is the most easily seen, the **incus** (anvil), and the **stapes** (stirrup). The **eustachian tube**, another part of the middle ear, connects the middle ear to the nasopharynx. The tube stabilizes the air pressure between the external atmosphere and the middle ear, thus preventing rupture of the tympanic membrane and discomfort produced by marked pressure differences.

The inner ear contains the **cochlea**, a seashell-shaped structure essential for sound transmission and hearing,

and the **vestibule** and **semicircular canals**, which contain the organs of equilibrium.

Sound transmission and hearing are complex processes. In brief, sound can be transmitted by air conduction or bone conduction. The process of air-conducted transmission is as follows:

1. A sound stimulus enters the external canal and reaches the tympanic membrane.
2. The sound waves vibrate the tympanic membrane and reach the ossicles.
3. The sound waves travel from the vibrating ossicles to the opening in the inner ear (round window).
4. The cochlea receives the sound vibrations.
5. The stimulus travels to the auditory nerve (the eighth cranial nerve) and the cerebral cortex.

Bone-conducted sound transmission occurs when skull bones transport the sound directly to the auditory nerve.

Audiometric evaluations, which measure hearing at various decibels, are recommended for older adults. A common hearing deficit with age is loss of ability to hear high-frequency sounds, such as *f, s, sh,* and *ph*. This neurosensory hearing deficit does not respond well to the use of a hearing aid.

Conduction hearing loss is the result of interrupted transmission of sound waves through the outer and middle ear structures. Possible causes are a tear in the tympanic membrane or an obstruction, because of swelling or other causes, in the auditory canal. **Sensorineural hearing loss** is the result of damage to the inner ear, the auditory nerve, or the hearing centre in the brain. **Mixed hearing loss** is a combination of conduction and sensorineural loss.

Skill 28.7 describes how to assess the ears and hearing (see also the Lifespan Considerations box on assessing ears and hearing on page 626).

SKILL 28.7   ASSESSING EARS AND HEARING

PLANNING

It is important to conduct the ear and hearing examination in a quiet area. In addition, the location should allow the client to be positioned sitting or standing at the same level as the nurse.

Equipment

Otoscope with several sizes of ear specula

IMPLEMENTATION

Performance

1. Before performing the procedure, introduce yourself and verify the client's identity using two identifiers or per agency protocol. Explain to the client what you are going to do, why

it is necessary, and how he or she can participate. Discuss how the results will be used in planning further care or treatments.

2. Perform hand hygiene, and follow other appropriate infection prevention and control procedures.

3. Provide for client privacy.

4. Inquire whether the client has a family history of hearing problems or loss; presence of any ear problems; medication history, especially if there are complaints of ringing in ears; any hearing difficulty; its onset, factors contributing to it, and how it interferes with activities of daily living; use of a corrective hearing device: when and from whom it was obtained.

5. Position the client comfortably, seated if possible.

Assessment	Normal Findings	Deviations from Normal

Auricles

6. Inspect the auricles for colour, symmetry of size, and position. To inspect position, note the level at which the superior aspect of the auricle attaches to the head in relation to the eye.

Colour same as facial skin; symmetrical; auricle aligned with outer canthus of eye, about 10 degrees from vertical (see ❶).

Bluish colour of earlobes (e.g., cyanosis); pallor (e.g., frostbite); excessive redness (inflammation or fever); asymmetry; low-set ears (associated with a congenital abnormality, such as Down syndrome)

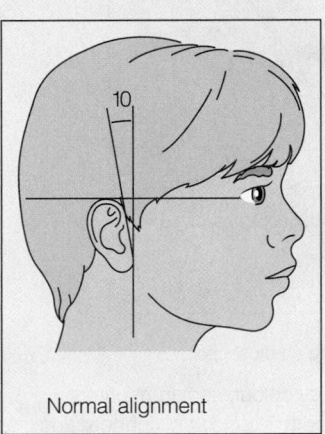

Normal alignment

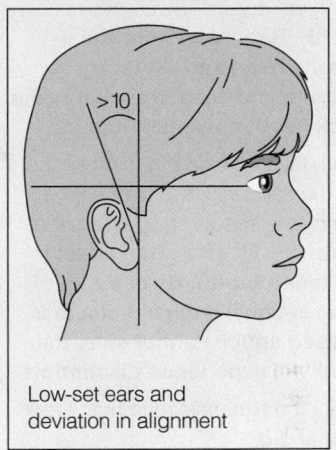

Low-set ears and deviation in alignment

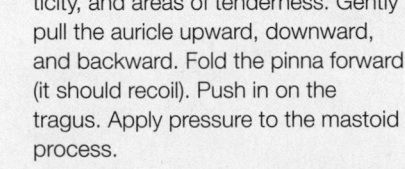

❶ Alignment of ears.

7. Palpate the auricles for texture, elasticity, and areas of tenderness. Gently pull the auricle upward, downward, and backward. Fold the pinna forward (it should recoil). Push in on the tragus. Apply pressure to the mastoid process.

Mobile, firm, and not tender; pinna recoils after it is folded

Lesions (e.g., cysts); flaky, scaly skin (e.g., seborrhea); tenderness when moved or pressed (may indicate inflammation or infection of external ear)

External Ear Canal and Tympanic Membrane

8. Use an otoscope to inspect the external ear canal for cerumen, skin lesions, pus, and blood. Visualize the tympanic membrane.

- Attach a speculum to the otoscope. Use the largest diameter that will fit the ear canal without causing discomfort. **Rationale: This achieves maximum vision of the entire ear canal and tympanic membrane.**

- Tip the client's head away from you, and straighten the ear canal. For an adult, straighten the ear canal by pulling the pinna up and back (see ❷). **Rationale: Straightening the ear canal facilitates vision of the ear canal and the tympanic membrane.**

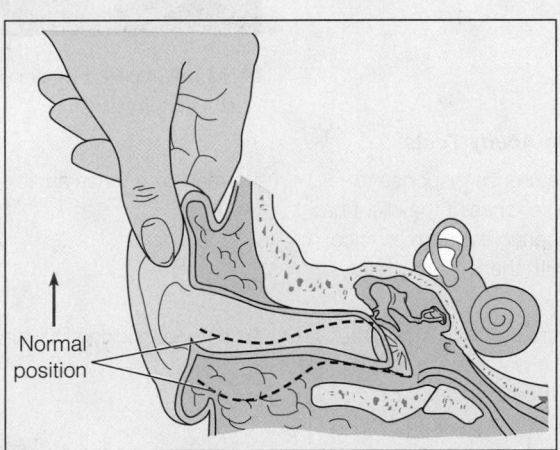

Normal position

❷ Straightening the ear canal of an adult by pulling the pinna up and back.

(continued)

SKILL 28.7   ASSESSING EARS AND HEARING (continued)

Assessment	Normal Findings	Deviations from Normal
• Hold the otoscope either (a) right side up, with your fingers between the otoscope handle and the client's head or (b) upside down, with your fingers and the ulnar surface of your hand against the client's head (see ❸). **Rationale: This stabilizes the head and protects the eardrum and canal from injury if a quick head movement occurs.** • Gently insert the tip of the otoscope into the ear canal, avoiding pressure by the speculum against either side of the ear canal. **Rationale: The inner two-thirds of the ear canal is bony; if the speculum is pressed against either side, the client will experience discomfort.**	Distal third contains hair follicles and glands; dry cerumen, greyish-tan colour; or sticky, wet cerumen in various shades of brown 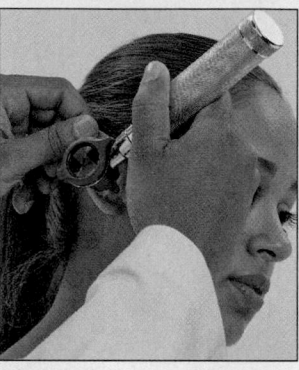 ❸ Inserting an otoscope.	Redness and discharge; scaling; excessive cerumen obstructing canal
9. Inspect the tympanic membrane for colour and gloss.	Pearly grey colour, semitransparent, light reflex at 5 o'clock in right ear and 7 o'clock in left ear (see ❹) 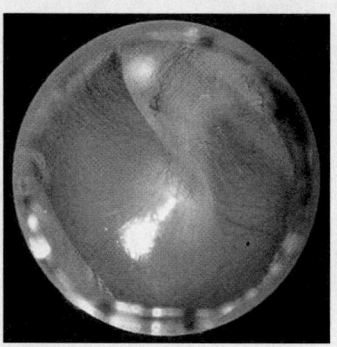 ❹ Normal tympanic membrane with light reflex at 7 o'clock (left ear).	Pink to red, some opacity; yellow-amber, white, blue, or deep red; dull surface

Gross Hearing Acuity Tests

10. Assess the client's response to normal voice tones. If the client has difficulty hearing the normal voice, proceed with the following tests.	Normal voice tones audible	Normal voice tones not audible (e.g., client requests nurse to repeat words or statements, leans toward the speaker, turns the head, cups the ears, or speaks in loud voice)
10A. Perform the watch tick test. The ticking of a watch has a higher pitch than the human voice. Have the client occlude one ear. Out of the client's sight, place a ticking watch 2 cm to 3 cm from the unoccluded ear. Ask what the client can hear. Repeat with the other ear.	Able to hear ticking in both ears	Unable to hear ticking in one or both ears

Assessment	**Normal Findings**	**Deviations from Normal**
10B. *Tuning Fork Tests* Perform **Weber's test** (a test to assess bone conduction) by examining the lateralization (sideward transmission) of sounds.	Sound is heard in both ears or is localized at the centre of the head (Weber negative)	Sound is heard better in impaired ear, indicating a bone-conductive hearing loss, or sound is heard better in ear without a problem, indicating a sensorineural disturbance (Weber positive)

• Hold the tuning fork at its base. Activate it by tapping the fork gently against the back of your hand near the knuckles or by stroking the fork between your thumb and index fingers. It should be made to ring softly.

• Place the base of the vibrating fork on top of the client's head (see ❺) and ask where the client hears the noise.

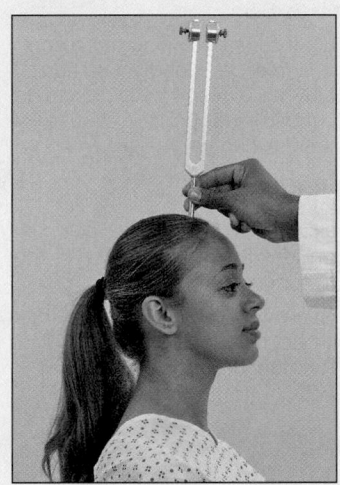

❺ Placing the base of a tuning fork on the client's skull (Weber's test).

Assessment	**Normal Findings**	**Deviations from Normal**
Conduct the **Rinne test** (a test to compare air conduction to bone conduction).	Air-conducted (AC) hearing time is greater than bone-conducted (BC) hearing time, that is, AC > BC (positive Rinne)	Bone conduction time is equal to or longer than the air conduction time, that is, BC > AC or BC = AC (negative Rinne; indicates conductive hearing loss)

• Ask the client to block the hearing in one ear intermittently by moving a fingertip in and out of the ear canal.

• Hold the handle of the activated tuning fork on the mastoid process of one ear (see ❻) until the client states that the vibration can no longer be heard.

• Immediately hold the vibrating fork prongs in front of the client's ear canal (see ❼).

• Push aside the client's hair, if necessary. Ask whether the client now hears the sound. Sound conducted by air is heard more readily than sound conducted by bone. The tuning fork vibrations conducted by air are normally heard longer.

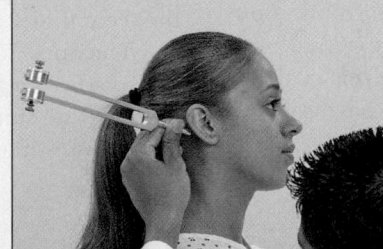

❻ Base of the tuning fork on the mastoid process (Rinne test).

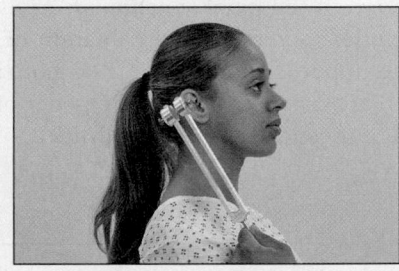

❼ Tuning fork prongs placed in front of the client's ear (Rinne test).

11. Document findings in the client record by using forms or checklists supplemented by narrative notes, when appropriate.

EVALUATION

• Perform a detailed follow-up examination of neurological and other systems based on findings that deviated from expected or normal for the client.

• Report significant deviations from normal to the appropriate members of the health care team.

Assessing Ears and Hearing

INFANTS

- To assess gross hearing, ring a bell from behind the infant, or have the parent call the child's name to check for a response. Newborns will quieten to the caregiver's voice and may open their eyes wider. By 3 to 4 months of age, the child will turn the head and eyes toward the sound.
- All newborns should be assessed for hearing with auditory brain response testing before being discharged from the hospital.

CHILDREN

- To inspect the external canal and tympanic membrane in children younger than 3 years old, pull the pinna down and back. Insert the speculum only 0.5 cm to 1 cm.
- Hearing loss is becoming more common in adolescents and young adults, probably as a result of exposure to loud music and prolonged use of headsets at loud volumes.

OLDER ADULTS

- The skin of the ear may appear dry and be less resilient because of the loss of connective tissue.
- Increased coarse and wire-like hair growth occurs along the pinna, anti-helix, and tragus.
- The tympanic membrane is more translucent and less flexible.
- Earwax is drier.
- The pinna increases in both width and length, and the earlobe elongates.
- Sensorineural hearing loss occurs.
- **Presbycusis** (generalized hearing loss) occurs in all frequencies, although the first symptom is the loss of high-frequency sounds: the *f, s, sh,* and *ph* sounds. To such persons, conversation can be distorted and result in what appears to be inappropriate or confused behaviour.

Nose and Sinuses

The nasal passages can be inspected very simply with a flashlight. However, a nasal *speculum* and a penlight or an otoscope with a nasal attachment facilitates examination of the nasal attachment. Assessment of the nose includes inspection and palpation of the external nose (the upper third of the nose is bone; the remainder is cartilage); determination of patency of the nasal cavities; and inspection of the nasal cavities.

If the client reports difficulty or abnormality in his or her sense of smell, the nurse may test the client's olfactory sense by asking the client to identify common odours, such as coffee or mint. This is done by asking the client to close the eyes and then placing vials containing the scent under the client's nose.

The nurse inspects, palpates, and percusses the facial sinuses (Figure 28.16). Skill 28.8 describes how to assess the nose and sinuses (see also the Lifespan Consideration box on assessing the nose and sinuses on page 628).

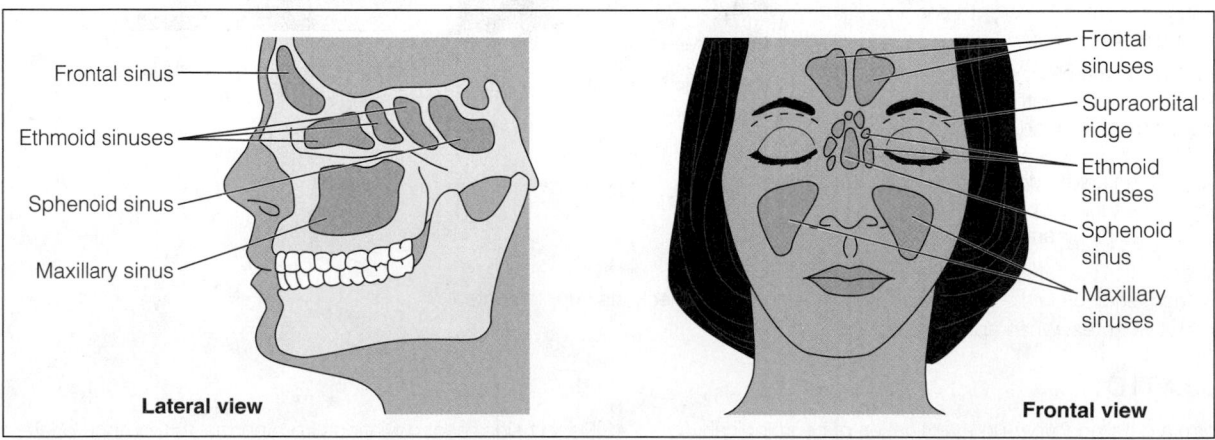

Frontal sinus
Ethmoid sinuses
Sphenoid sinus
Maxillary sinus

Lateral view

Frontal sinuses
Supraorbital ridge
Ethmoid sinuses
Sphenoid sinus
Maxillary sinuses

Frontal view

FIGURE 28.16 The facial sinuses.

SKILL 28.8   ASSESSING THE NOSE AND SINUSES

PLANNING

Equipment

- Nasal speculum
- Flashlight or penlight

IMPLEMENTATION

Performance

1. Before performing the procedure, introduce yourself and verify the client's identity using two identifiers or per agency protocol. Explain to the client what you are going to do, why it is necessary, and how he or she can participate. Discuss how the results will be used in planning further care or treatments.

2. Perform hand hygiene, and observe other appropriate infection prevention and control procedures.

3. Provide for client privacy.

4. Inquire whether the client has a history of allergies, difficulty breathing through the nose, sinus infections, injuries to nose or face, nosebleeds; any medications taken; any changes in the sense of smell; any facial or nasal surgery.

5. Position the client comfortably, seated if possible.

Assessment	Normal Findings	Deviations from Normal
Nose		
6. Inspect the external nose for any deviations in shape, size, or colour and flaring or discharge from the nares.	Symmetric and straight; no discharge or flaring; uniform colour	Asymmetric; discharge from nares; localized areas of redness or presence of skin lesions
7. Lightly palpate the external nose to determine any areas of tenderness, masses, and displacements of bone and cartilage.	Not tender; no lesions	Tenderness on palpation; presence of lesions
8. Determine patency of both nasal cavities. Ask the client to close the mouth, exert pressure on one naris, and breathe through the opposite naris. Have the client repeat this to assess patency of the opposite naris.	Air moves freely as the client breathes through the nares	Air movement is restricted in one or both nares

9. Inspect the nasal cavities by using a flashlight or a nasal speculum.

   - Hold the speculum in your right hand to inspect the client's left nostril and your left hand to inspect the client's right nostril.

   - Tip the client's head back.

   - Facing the client, insert the tip of the closed speculum (blades together) about 1 cm or up to the point at which the blade widens. Care must be taken to avoid pressure on the sensitive nasal septum (see ❶).

   - Stabilize the speculum with your index finger against the side of the nose. Use the other hand to position the head, and then to hold the light.

   - Open the speculum as much as possible and inspect the floor of the nose (vestibule), the anterior portion of the septum, the middle meatus, and the middle turbinates. The posterior turbinate is rarely visualized because of its position (see ❷).

   - Inspect the lining of the nares and the integrity and the position of the nasal septum.

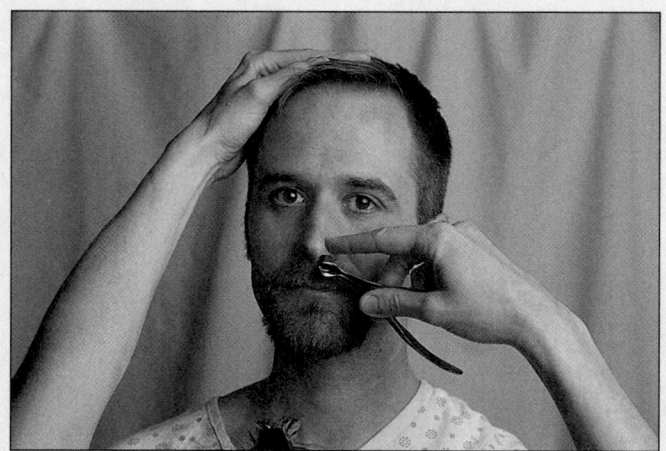

❶ Using a nasal speculum to inspect the nasal passages.

(continued)

SKILL 28.8 **ASSESSING THE NOSE AND SINUSES** (*continued*)

Assessment	Normal Findings	Deviations from Normal
10. Observe for the presence of redness, swelling, growths, and discharge.	Mucosa pink; clear, watery discharge; no lesions	Mucosa red, edematous; abnormal discharge (e.g., pus); presence of lesions (e.g., polyps)

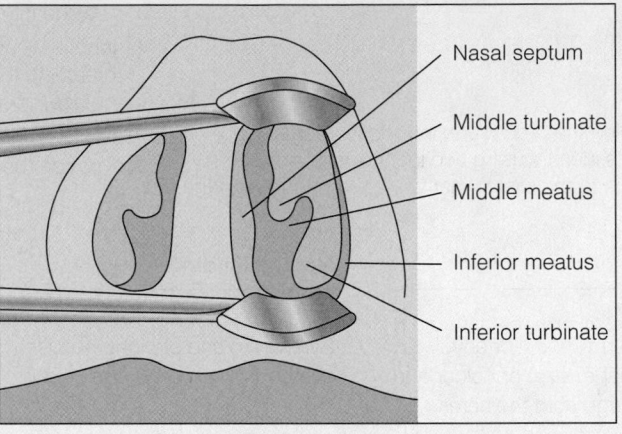

❷ The inferior and middle turbinates of the nasal passage.

- Nasal septum
- Middle turbinate
- Middle meatus
- Inferior meatus
- Inferior turbinate

Assessment	Normal Findings	Deviations from Normal
11. Inspect the nasal septum between the nasal chambers.	Nasal septum intact and in midline	Septum deviated to the right or to the left.
Facial Sinuses		
12. Palpate the maxillary and frontal sinuses for tenderness.	Not tender	Tenderness in one or more sinuses
13. Document your findings in the client record by using forms or checklists supplemented by narrative notes, when appropriate.		

EVALUATION

- Perform a detailed follow-up examination of other systems based on findings that deviated from expected or normal for the client.
- Report significant deviations from normal to the appropriate members of the health care team.

LIFESPAN CONSIDERATION

Assessing the Nose and Sinuses

INFANTS

- A speculum is usually not necessary to examine the septum, turbinates, and vestibule. Instead, push the tip of the nose upward with the thumb and shine a light into the nares.
- Ethmoid and maxillary sinuses are present at birth; frontal sinuses begin to develop by 1 to 2 years of age; and sphenoid sinuses develop later in childhood. Infants and young children have fewer sinus problems than older children and adolescents.

CHILDREN

- A speculum is usually not necessary to examine the septum, turbinates, and vestibule. It might cause the child to be apprehensive. Instead, push the tip of the nose upward with the thumb and shine a light into the nares.

- Ethmoid sinuses develop by age 6 years. Sinus problems in children younger than 6 years are rare.
- Cough and runny nose are the most common signs of sinusitis in preadolescent children.
- Adolescents may have headaches, facial tenderness, and swelling, similar to the signs seen in adults.

OLDER ADULTS

- The sense of smell diminishes markedly because of a decrease in the number of olfactory nerve fibres and atrophy of the remaining fibres. Older persons are less able to identify and distinguish odours.
- Nosebleeds can result from hypertensive disease or other arterial vessel changes in older adults.

Mouth and Oropharynx

The mouth and pharynx are composed of a number of structures: lips, inner and buccal mucosa, the tongue, floor of the mouth, teeth and gums, hard and soft palates, uvula, salivary glands, tonsillar pillars, and tonsils. The anatomical structures of the mouth are shown in Figure 28.17.

By age 25 years, most people have all their permanent teeth. For information about structures of the teeth, see Chapter 31.

Normally, three pairs of salivary glands empty into the oral cavity: the parotid, submandibular, and sublingual glands (see Figure 28.17). The *parotid gland* is the largest and empties through the Stensen's duct opposite the second molar. The *submandibular gland* empties through Wharton's duct, which is situated at the side of the frenulum on the floor of the mouth. The *sublingual salivary gland* lies in the floor of the mouth and has numerous openings.

Dental **caries** (cavities) and **pyorrhea** (periodontal disease) are the two problems that most frequently affect teeth. Both problems are commonly associated with plaque and tartar deposits. **Plaque** is an *invisible* soft film that adheres to the enamel surface of teeth; it consists of bacteria, molecules of saliva, and remnants of epithelial cells and leukocytes. When plaque accumulates on teeth, dental calculus (tartar) forms. **Tartar** is a visible, hard deposit of plaque and dead bacteria that forms at the gum line. Tartar buildup can alter the fibres that attach teeth to the gum and eventually disrupt bone tissue. Periodontal disease is characterized by **gingivitis** (inflamed gums), bleeding, receding gum lines, and

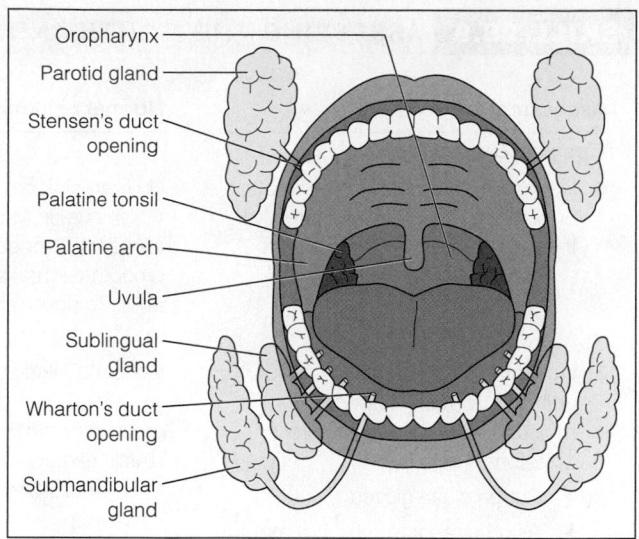

FIGURE 28.17 Anatomical structures of the mouth.

the formation of pockets between teeth and gums. In advanced periodontal disease, teeth are loose, and pus is evident when gums are pressed.

Other problems nurses may see are **glossitis** (inflammation of the tongue), **stomatitis** (inflammation of the oral mucosa), **parotitis** (inflammation of the parotid salivary gland) and **sordes** (accumulation of foul matter, such as food, microorganisms, and epithelial elements, on teeth and gums).

Skill 28.9 describes assessment of the mouth and oropharynx (see also the Lifespan Considerations box on assessing the mouth and oropharynx on page 633).

SKILL 28.9 ASSESSING THE MOUTH AND OROPHARYNX

PLANNING

If possible, arrange for the client to sit with his or her head against a firm surface, such as a headrest or an examination table. This makes it easier for the client to hold the head still during the examination.

Equipment

- Clean gloves
- Tongue depressor
- 5 cm × 5 cm gauze pads
- Penlight

IMPLEMENTATION

Performance

1. Before performing the procedure, introduce yourself and verify the client's identity using two identifiers or per agency protocol. Explain to the client what you are going to do, why it is necessary, and how he or she can participate. Discuss how the results will be used in planning further care or treatments.

2. Perform hand hygiene, and follow other appropriate infection prevention and control procedures.

3. Provide for client privacy.

4. Inquire whether the client has any history of the following: routine pattern of dental care, last visit to dentist; length of time ulcers or other lesions have been present; any denture discomfort; any medications the client is taking.

5. Position the client comfortably, seated if possible.

(continued)

SKILL 28.9 ASSESSING THE MOUTH AND OROPHARYNX *(continued)*

Assessment	Normal Findings	Deviations from Normal
Lips and Buccal Mucosa		
6. Inspect the outer lips for symmetry of contour, colour, and texture. Ask the client to purse the lips as if to whistle.	Uniform pink colour (darker, e.g., bluish hue, in Mediterranean groups and dark-skinned clients); soft, moist, smooth texture; symmetry of contour; ability to purse lips	Pallor; cyanosis; blisters; generalized or localized swelling; fissures, crusts, or scales (may result from excessive moisture, nutritional deficiency, or fluid deficit); inability to purse lips (may indicate facial nerve damage)
7. Inspect and palpate the inner lips and buccal mucosa for colour, moisture, texture, and the presence of lesions. • Put on clean gloves. • Ask the client to relax the mouth, and, for better visualization, pull the lip outward and away from teeth. • Grasp the lip on each side between the thumb and index finger (see ❶). • Palpate any lesions for size, tenderness, and consistency. • Inspect the front teeth and gums.	Uniform pink colour (freckled brown pigmentation in dark-skinned clients); moist, smooth, soft, glistening, and elastic texture (drier oral mucosa in older clients because of decreased salivation)	Pallor; **leukoplakia** (white patches or spots on mucous membranes), red, bleeding; excessive dryness; mucosal cysts; irritations from dentures; abrasions, ulcerations; nodules

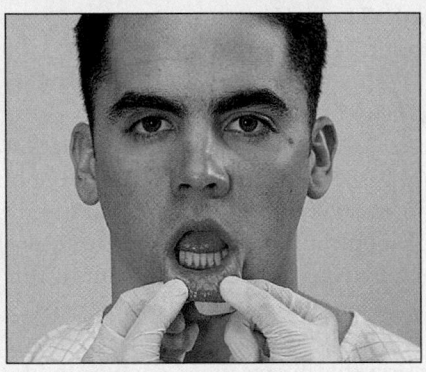

❶ Inspecting the mucosa of the lower lip.

Assessment	Normal Findings	Deviations from Normal
Teeth and Gums		
8. Inspect teeth and gums while examining the inner lips and buccal mucosa. • Ask the client to open his or her mouth. Use a tongue depressor to retract the cheek (see ❷). View the surface buccal mucosa from top to bottom and back to front. A flashlight or penlight will help illuminate the surface. Repeat the procedure for the other side. • Ask the client to open his or her mouth again. Use a penlight for better visualization, and move a finger along the inside cheek. Another finger may be moved outside the cheek. • Examine the back teeth. For proper vision of the molars, use the index fingers of both hands to retract the cheek (see ❸). Ask the client to relax his or her lips and first close then open the jaw. **Rationale: Closing the jaw assists in observation of tooth alignment and loss of teeth; opening the jaw assists in observation of dental fillings and caries.**	Thirty-two adult teeth; smooth, white, shiny tooth enamel; pink gums (bluish or brown patches in dark-skinned clients); moist, firm texture to gums; no retraction of gums (pulling away from teeth)	Missing teeth; ill-fitting dentures; brown or black discoloration of the enamel (may indicate staining or the presence of caries); excessively red gums; spongy texture; bleeding; tenderness (may indicate periodontal disease); receding, atrophied gums; swelling that partially covers teeth

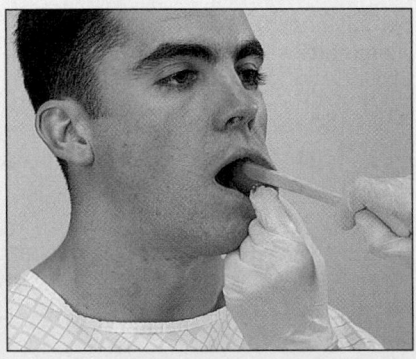

❷ Inspecting the buccal mucosa by using a tongue depressor.

Assessment	Normal Findings	Deviations from Normal

- Observe the number of teeth, tooth colour, the state of fillings, dental caries, and tartar along the base of teeth. Note the presence and fit of partial or complete dentures.
- Inspect the gums around the molars. Observe for bleeding, colour, retraction (pulling away from teeth), edema, and lesions.

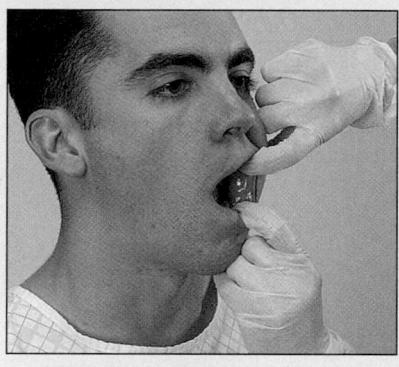

❸ Inspecting the back teeth.

9. Inspect the dentures. Ask the client to remove complete or partial dentures. Inspect their condition, noting in particular broken or worn areas.

Smooth, intact dentures

Ill-fitting dentures; irritated and excoriated area under dentures

Tongue/Floor of the Mouth

10. Inspect the surface of the tongue for position, colour, and texture. Ask the client to stick out the tongue.

Central position; pink colour (some brown pigmentation on tongue borders in dark-skinned clients); moist; slightly rough; thin whitish coating; smooth, lateral margins; no lesions; raised papillae (taste buds)

Deviated from centre, which may indicate damage to the hypoglossal (12th cranial) nerve; excessive trembling; smooth, red tongue (may indicate iron, vitamin B_{12}, or vitamin B_3 deficiency); dry, furry tongue (associated with fluid deficit); white coating (may be oral yeast infection); nodes, ulcerations, discolorations (white or red areas); areas of tenderness

11. Inspect tongue movement. Ask the client to roll the tongue upward and move it from side to side.

Moves freely; no tenderness

Restricted mobility

12. Inspect the base of the tongue, the mouth floor, and the frenulum. Ask the client to place the tip of the tongue against the roof of the mouth.

Smooth tongue base with prominent veins

Swelling, ulceration

13. Palpate the tongue and floor of the mouth for any nodules, lumps, or excoriated areas. To palpate the tongue, use a piece of gauze to grasp its tip (stabilize it), and with the index finger of your other hand, palpate the back of the tongue, its borders, and its base (see ❹).

Smooth with no palpable nodules

Swelling, nodules

To assess the functioning of the glossopharyngeal and hypoglossal nerves, see the section on neurological assessment later in this chapter.

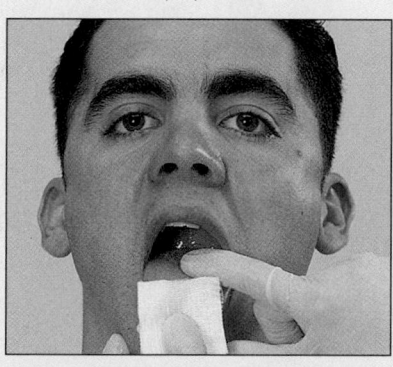

❹ Palpating the tongue.

(continued)

SKILL 28.9   ASSESSING THE MOUTH AND OROPHARYNX (*continued*)

Assessment	Normal Findings	Deviations from Normal
Palates and Uvula		
14. Inspect the hard and soft palates for colour, shape, texture, and the presence of bony prominences. Ask the client to open the mouth wide and tilt his or her head backward. Then, depress the tongue with a tongue blade, as necessary, and use a penlight for better visualization.	Light pink, smooth, soft palate; lighter pink hard palate, more irregular texture	Discoloration (e.g., jaundice or pallor); palates the same colour; irritations; exostoses (bony growths) growing from the hard palate
15. Inspect the uvula for position and mobility while examining the palates. To observe the uvula, ask the client to say "ah" so that the soft palate rises.	Positioned in midline of soft palate	Deviation to one side from tumour or trauma; immobility, which may indicate damage to trigeminal (fifth cranial) nerve or vagus (10th cranial) nerve
Oropharynx and Tonsils		
16. Inspect the oropharynx for colour and texture. Inspect one side at a time to avoid eliciting the gag reflex. To expose one side of the oropharynx, press a tongue blade against the tongue on the same side about halfway back while the client tilts the head back and opens his or her mouth wide. Use a penlight for illumination, if needed.	Pink and smooth posterior wall • *Grade 1 (normal):* The tonsils are behind the tonsillar pillars (the soft structures supporting the soft palate)	Reddened or edematous; presence of lesions, plaques, or drainage
17. Inspect the tonsils (behind the fauces) for colour, discharge, and size.	Pink and smooth; no discharge; of normal size or not visible	Inflamed; presence of discharge; swollen • *Grade 2:* The tonsils are between the pillars and the uvula • *Grade 3:* The tonsils touch the uvula • *Grade 4:* One or both tonsils extend to the midline of the oropharynx
18. Elicit the gag reflex by pressing the posterior tongue with a tongue blade.	Present	Absent, which may indicate problems with glossopharyngeal (ninth cranial) or vagus (10th cranial) nerves
19. Document your findings in the client record by using forms or checklists supplemented by narrative notes, when appropriate.		

EVALUATION

• Perform a detailed follow-up examination of neurological and other systems based on findings that deviated from expected or normal for the client. Relate findings to previous assessment data, if available.

• Report significant deviations from normal to the appropriate members of the health care team.

The Neck

Examination of the neck includes the muscles, lymph nodes, trachea, thyroid gland, carotid arteries, and jugular veins. Areas of the neck are defined by the sternocleidomastoid muscles, which divide each side of the neck into two triangles: the anterior and the posterior (Figure 28.18). The trachea, thyroid gland, anterior cervical nodes, and carotid artery lie within the anterior triangle (Figure 28.19); the carotid artery runs parallel and anterior to the sternocleidomastoid muscle. The

LIFESPAN CONSIDERATIONS

Assessing the Mouth and Oropharynx

INFANTS

- Inspect the palate and uvula for a cleft. A bifid (forked) uvula may indicate an unsuspected cleft palate (i.e., a cleft in the cartilage that is covered by skin).
- Newborns may have a pearly white nodule on their gums, which resolves without treatment.
- The first teeth erupt at about 6 to 7 months of age. Assess for dental hygiene; parents should cleanse the infant's teeth daily with a soft cloth or soft toothbrush.
- Children should see a dentist by 1 year of age.

CHILDREN

- Tooth development should be appropriate for age. See Chapter 31. Permanent teeth are darker than deciduous teeth.
- White spots on teeth may indicate excessive fluoride ingestion.
- Drooling is normal up to 2 years of age.
- The tonsils are normally larger in children than in adults and usually extend beyond the palatine arch until the age of 11 or 12 years.

OLDER ADULTS

- The oral mucosa may be drier than that of younger persons because of decreased salivary gland activity. Decreased salivation occurs in older adults who are taking prescribed medications, such as antidepressants, antihistamines, decongestants, diuretics, antihypertensives, tranquilizers, antispasmodics, and antineoplastics. Extreme dryness is associated with dehydration.
- Some receding of the gums occurs, giving an appearance of increased toothiness.
- There may be a brownish pigmentation to the gums, especially in black persons.
- Taste sensations diminish with aging due to atrophy of the taste buds and a decreased sense of smell. It indicates diminished function of the fifth and seventh cranial nerves.
- Tiny purple or bluish-black swollen areas (varicosities) under the tongue, known as *caviar spots,* are not uncommon.
- Teeth may show signs of staining, erosion, chipping, and abrasions because of loss of dentin. Tooth loss occurs as a result of gum disease but is preventable with good dental hygiene.
- Older adults who are housebound or are in long-term care facilities often have teeth or dentures in need of repair because of the difficulty of obtaining dental care in these situations. Do a thorough assessment of missing teeth and those in need of repair, whether they are natural teeth or dentures.

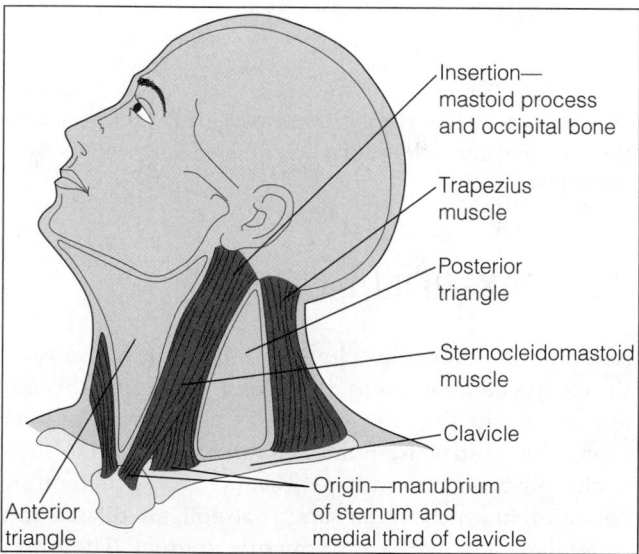

FIGURE 28.18 Major muscles of the neck.

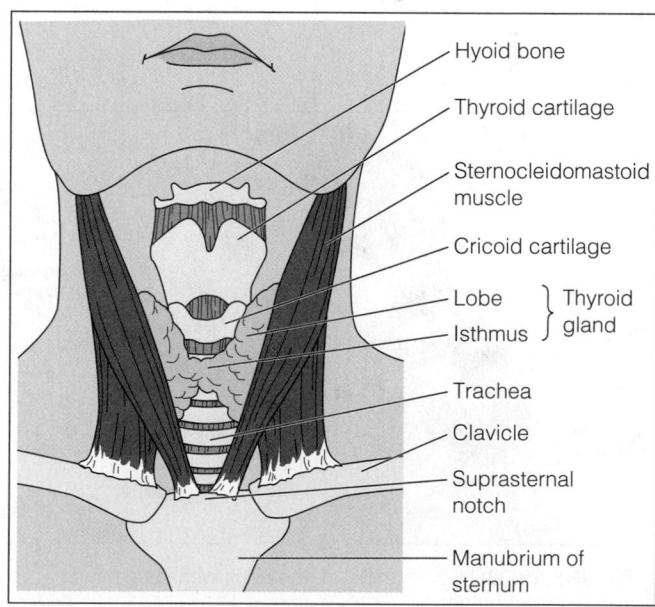

FIGURE 28.19 Structures of the neck.

posterior lymph nodes lie within the posterior triangle (Figure 28.20 on the next page).

Each sternocleidomastoid muscle extends from the upper sternum and the medial third of the clavicle to the mastoid process of the temporal bone behind the ear. These muscles turn and laterally flex the head. Each trapezius muscle extends from the occipital bone of the skull to the lateral third of the clavicle. These muscles draw the head to the side and back, elevate the chin, and elevate the shoulders for shrugging.

TABLE 28.6 Lymph Nodes of the Head and Neck

Node Centre	Location	Area Drained
Head		
The occipital region of the scalp and the deep structures of the following:	At the posterior base of the skull	The occipital region of the scalp and the deep structures of the back of the neck
Postauricular (mastoid)	Behind the auricle of the ear or in front of the mastoid process	The parietal region of the head and part of the ear
Preauricular	In front of the tragus of the ear	The forehead and upper face
Floor of Mouth		
Submandibular (submaxillary)	Along the medial border of the lower jaw, halfway between the angle of the jaw and the chin	The chin, upper lip, cheek, nose, teeth, eyelids, part of the tongue, and part of the floor of the mouth
Submental	Behind the tip of the mandible, in the midline, under the chin	The anterior third of the tongue, gums, and floor of the mouth
Neck		
Superficial (anterior) cervical chain	Along the anterior to the sternocleidomastoid muscle	Skin and neck
Posterior cervical chain	Along the anterior aspect of the trapezius muscle	The posterior and lateral regions of the neck, occiput, and mastoid
Deep cervical chain	Under the sternocleidomastoid muscle	The larynx, thyroid gland, trachea, and upper part of the esophagus
Supraclavicular	Above the clavicle, in the angle between the clavicle and the sternocleidomastoid muscle	The lateral regions of the neck and lungs

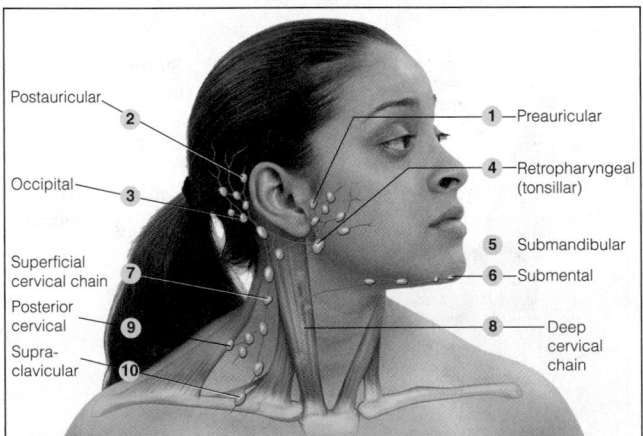

FIGURE 28.20 Lymph nodes of the neck with suggested sequence for palpation.

Lymph nodes in the neck that collect lymph from the head and neck structures are grouped serially and referred to as *chains*. See Figure 28.20 and Table 28.6. The deep cervical chain is not shown in Figure 28.20 because it lies beneath the sternocleidomastoid muscle.

Skill 28.10 describes how to assess the neck (see also the Lifespan Considerations box on assessing the neck on page 638).

Thorax and Lungs

Assessing the thorax and lungs is important in assessing the client's aeration status. Changes in the respiratory system can occur slowly or quickly. In clients with asthma or chronic obstructive pulmonary disease (COPD), such as chronic bronchitis or *emphysema* (a chronic pulmonary condition in which the air sacs, or alveoli, are dilated and distended), changes are frequently gradual. The onset of such conditions as pneumonia or *pulmonary embolus* (a blockage of an artery in the lungs by fat, air, tumour tissue, or a blood clot) is generally more acute or sudden.

Chest Landmarks

Before beginning the assessment, the nurse must be familiar with a series of imaginary lines on the chest wall and be able to locate the position of each rib and

SKILL 28.10 ASSESSING THE NECK

PLANNING
Equipment: None

IMPLEMENTATION
Performance

1. Before performing the procedure, introduce yourself and verify the client's identity using two identifiers or per agency protocol. Explain to the client what you are going to do, why it is necessary, and how he or she can participate. Discuss

how the results will be used in planning further care or treatments.
2. Perform hand hygiene, and observe other appropriate infection prevention and control procedures.
3. Provide for client privacy.
4. Inquire whether the client has any history of the following: problems with neck lumps; neck pain or stiffness; when and how any lumps occurred; previous diagnoses of thyroid problems; and other treatments provided (e.g., surgery, radiation).

Assessment	Normal Findings	Deviations from Normal
Neck Muscles		
5. Inspect the neck muscles (sternocleidomastoid and trapezius) for abnormal swellings or masses. Ask the client to hold the head erect.	Muscles equal in size; head centred	Unilateral neck swelling; head tilted to one side (indicates presence of masses, injury, muscle weakness, shortening of sternocleidomastoid muscle, scars)
6. Observe head movement. Ask the client to do the following:	Coordinated, smooth movements with no discomfort	Muscle tremor, spasm, or stiffness
• Move the chin to the chest. **Rationale: This determines the functioning of the sternocleidomastoid muscle.**	Head flexes 45 degrees	Limited range of motion; painful movements; involuntary movements (e.g., up-and-down nodding movements associated with Parkinson's disease)
• Move the head back so that the chin points upward. **Rationale: This determines the functioning of the trapezius muscle.**	Head hyperextends 60 degrees	Head hyperextends less than 60 degrees
• Move the head so that the ear is moved toward the shoulder on each side. **Rationale: This determines the functioning of the sternocleidomastoid muscle.**	Head laterally flexes 40 degrees	Head laterally flexes less than 40 degrees
• Turn the head to the right and to the left. **Rationale: This determines the functioning of the sternocleidomastoid muscle.**	Head laterally rotates 70 degrees	Head laterally rotates less than 70 degrees
7. Assess muscle strength. Ask the client to turn the head to one side against the resistance of your hand. Repeat with the other side. **Rationale: This determines the strength of the sternocleidomastoid muscle.**	Equal strength	Unequal strength
• Ask the client to shrug the shoulders against the resistance of your hands. **Rationale: This determines the strength of the trapezius muscles.**	Equal strength	Unequal strength
Lymph Nodes		
8. Palpate the entire neck for enlarged lymph nodes (see Figure 28.20).	Not palpable	Enlarged, palpable, possibly tender (associated with infection and tumours)
• Face the client, and bend the client's head forward slightly or toward the side being examined. **Rationale: This relaxes soft tissue and muscles.**		

(continued)

SKILL 28.10 | **ASSESSING THE NECK** (*continued*)

Assessment	Normal Findings	Deviations from Normal
• Palpate the nodes by using the pads of your fingers. Move the fingertips in a gentle rotating motion.		
• When examining the submental and submandibular nodes, place the fingertips under the mandible on the side nearest the palpating hand, and pull the skin and subcutaneous tissue laterally over the mandibular surface so that the tissue rolls over the nodes.		
• When palpating the supraclavicular nodes, have the client bend the head forward to relax the tissues of the anterior neck and to relax the shoulders so that the clavicles drop. Use your hand nearest the side to be examined when facing the client (i.e., your left hand for the client's right nodes). Use your free hand to flex the client's head forward, if necessary. Hook your index and third fingers over the clavicle lateral to the sternocleidomastoid muscle (see ❶). 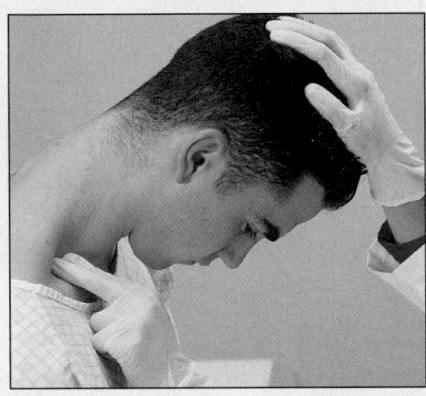 ❶ Palpating the supraclavicular lymph nodes.		
• When palpating the anterior cervical nodes and posterior cervical nodes, move your fingertips slowly in a forward circular motion against the sternocleidomastoid and trapezius muscles, respectively.		
• To palpate the deep cervical nodes, bend or hook your fingers around the sternocleidomastoid muscle.		
Trachea		
9. Palpate the trachea for lateral deviation. Place your fingertip or thumb on the trachea in the suprasternal notch (see Figure 28.19, p. 633), and then move your finger laterally to the left and the right in spaces bordered by the clavicle, the anterior aspect of the sternocleidomastoid muscle, and the trachea.	Central placement in midline of neck; spaces equal on both sides	Deviation to one side, indicating possible neck tumour; thyroid enlargement; enlarged lymph nodes
Thyroid Gland		
10. Inspect the thyroid gland. Stand in front of the client. Observe the lower half of the neck overlying the thyroid gland for symmetry and visible masses.	Not visible on inspection	Visible diffuseness or local enlargement
• Ask the client to hyperextend the head and swallow. If necessary, offer a glass of water to make it easier for the client to swallow. **Rationale: This action determines how the thyroid and cricoid cartilages move and whether swallowing causes a bulging of the gland.**	Gland ascends during swallowing but is not visible	Gland is not fully moveable with swallowing

Assessment	Normal Findings	Deviations from Normal
11. Palpate the thyroid gland for smoothness. Note any areas of enlargement, masses, or nodules. Stand in front of or behind the client, and ask the client to lower the chin slightly. **Rationale: Lowering the chin relaxes the neck muscles, facilitating palpation.**	Lobes may not be palpated; if palpated, lobes are small, smooth, centrally located, painless, and rise freely with swallowing	Solitary nodules

Posterior Approach

- Place your hands around the client's neck, with your fingertips on the lower half of the neck over the trachea (see ❷).

- Ask the client to swallow (taking a sip of water, if necessary). Feel for any enlargement of the thyroid isthmus as it rises. The isthmus lies across the trachea, below the cricoid cartilage. See Figure 28.19 (p. 633).

- To examine the right thyroid lobe, have the client lower the chin slightly and turn the head slightly to the right (the side being examined). With your left fingers, displace the trachea slightly to the right. With your right fingers, palpate the right thyroid lobe. Have the client swallow while you are palpating.

- Repeat the last step, in reverse, to examine the left thyroid lobe.

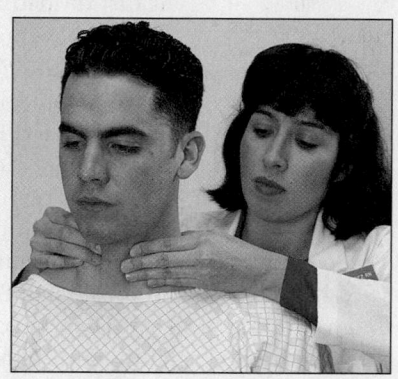

❷ Placement of the fingertips over the trachea to begin palpation of the thyroid gland (posterior approach).

Anterior Approach

- Place the tips of your index and middle fingers over the trachea, and palpate the thyroid isthmus as the client swallows.

- To examine the right thyroid lobe, have the client lower the chin slightly and turn the head slightly to the right. With your right fingers, displace the trachea slightly to the client's right (your left). With your left fingers, palpate the right thyroid lobe (see ❸).

- To examine the left thyroid lobe, repeat the above step in reverse.

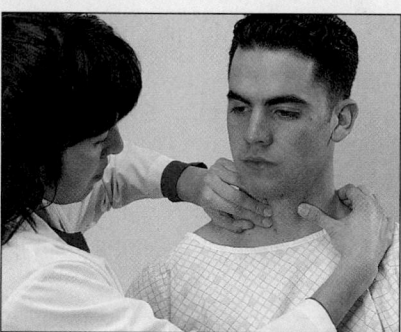

❸ Palpating the thyroid (anterior approach).

	Normal Findings	Deviations from Normal
12. If enlargement of the gland is suspected, auscultate over the thyroid area for a *bruit* (a soft rushing sound created by turbulent blood flow). Use the bell of the stethoscope because it transmits this low-frequency sound better than the diaphragm does.	Absence of bruit	Presence of bruit
13. Document your findings in the client record by using forms or checklists supplemented by narrative notes, when appropriate.		

(continued)

SKILL 28.10   ASSESSING THE NECK (*continued*)

EVALUATION

- Perform a detailed follow-up examination of other systems based on findings that deviated from expected or normal for the client.

- Report significant deviations from normal to the appropriate members of the health care team.

LIFESPAN CONSIDERATION

Assessing the Neck

INFANTS AND CHILDREN

- Examine the neck while the infant or child is lying supine. Lift the client's head, and turn it from side to side to determine neck mobility.

- An infant's neck is normally short, lengthening by about age 3 years. This lack of length makes palpation of the trachea difficult.

some spinous processes. These landmarks help the nurse identify the position of underlying organs (e.g., lobes of the lung) and to record abnormal assessment findings. Figure 28.21 shows the anterior, lateral, and posterior series of lines. The *midsternal line* is a vertical line running through the centre of the sternum. The *midclavicular lines* (right and left) are vertical lines from the midpoints of the clavicles. The *anterior axillary lines* (right and left) are vertical lines from the anterior axillary folds (Figure 28.21A). Figure 28.21B shows the three imaginary lines of the lateral chest. The *posterior axillary line* is a vertical line from the posterior axillary fold. The *midaxillary line* is a vertical line from the apex of the axilla. The anterior axillary line is as described for part A. Figure 28.21C shows the posterior thorax landmarks. The *vertebral line* is a vertical line along the spinous processes. The *scapular lines* (right and left) are vertical lines from the inferior angles of the scapulae.

Locating the position of each rib and certain spinous processes is essential for identifying the underlying lobes of lungs. Figure 28.22A shows an anterior view of the chest and underlying lungs; Figure 28.22B, a posterior view; and Figure 28.22C, right and left lateral views. Each lung is first divided into upper and lower lobes by an oblique fissure that runs from the level of the spinous process of the third thoracic vertebra (T-3) to the level of the sixth rib at the midclavicular line (MCL). The right upper lobe is abbreviated RUL; the right lower lobe, RLL. Similarly, the left upper lobe is abbreviated LUL; the left lower lobe, LLL. The right lung is further divided by a minor fissure into the right upper lobe and right middle lobe (RML). This fissure runs anteriorly from the right midaxillary line at the level of the fifth rib to the level of the fourth rib.

These specific landmarks, that is, T-3 and the fourth, fifth, and sixth ribs, are located as follows: The starting point for locating the ribs anteriorly is the **angle of Louis**, the junction between the body of the **sternum** (breastbone) and the **manubrium** (the handle-like superior part of the sternum that joins with the clavicles). The superior border of the second rib attaches to the sternum at this manubriosternal junction (Figure 28.23). The nurse can identify the manubrium by first palpating the clavicle and following its course to its attachment at the manubrium. The nurse then palpates and counts distal ribs and intercostal spaces from the second rib. It is important to note that an intercostal space is numbered according to the number of the rib immediately *above* the space. When palpating for rib identification, the nurse should palpate along the midclavicular line rather than the sternal border

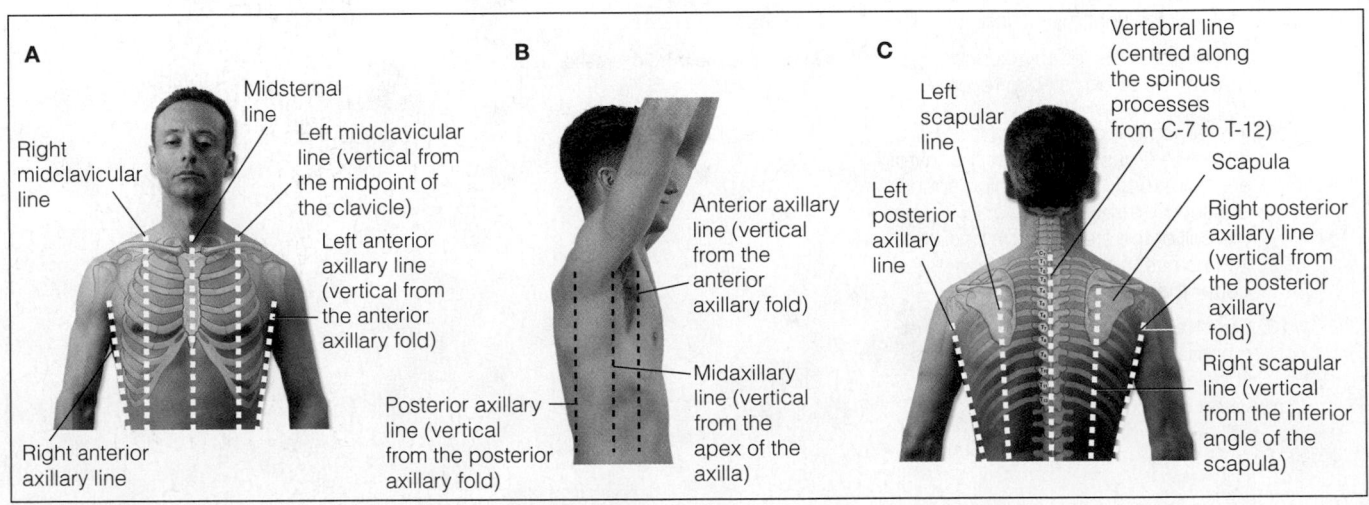

FIGURE 28.21 Chest wall landmarks: **A:** Anterior chest; **B:** Lateral chest; **C:** Posterior chest.

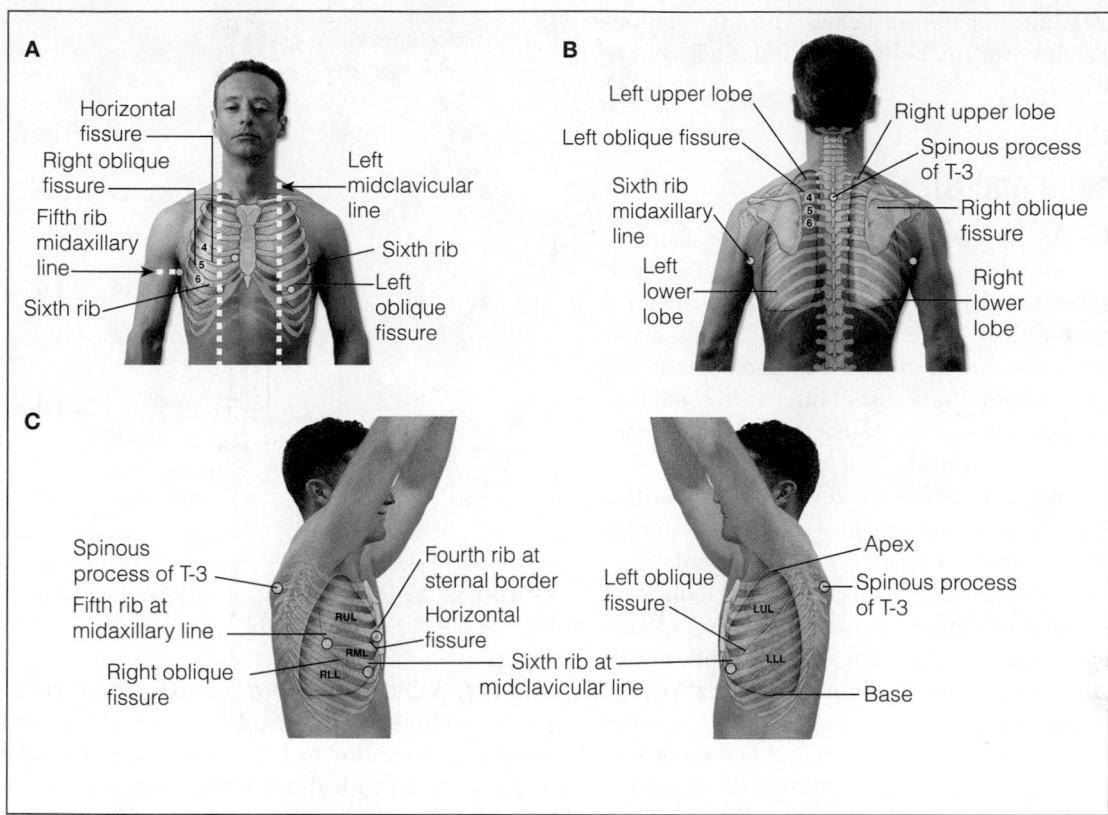

FIGURE 28.22 Chest landmarks: **A:** Anterior chest landmarks and underlying lungs; **B:** Posterior chest landmarks and underlying lungs; **C:** Lateral chest landmarks and underlying lungs.

because the rib cartilages are very close at the sternum. Only the first seven ribs attach directly to the sternum.

The counting of ribs is more difficult on the posterior thorax than on the anterior thorax. For identifying underlying lung lobes, the pertinent landmark is T-3. The starting point for locating T-3 is the spinous process of the seventh cervical vertebra (C-7) (Figure 28.24). When the client flexes the neck anteriorly, a prominent process can be observed and palpated. This is the spinous process

of the seventh cervical vertebra. If two spinous processes are observed, the superior one is C-7, and the inferior one is the spinous process of the first thoracic vertebra (T-1). The nurse then palpates and counts the spinous processes from C-7 to T-3. Each spinous process up to T-4 is adjacent to the corresponding rib number; e.g., T-3 is adjacent to the third rib. After T-4, however, the spinous processes project obliquely, causing the spinous process of the vertebra to lie not over its correspondingly

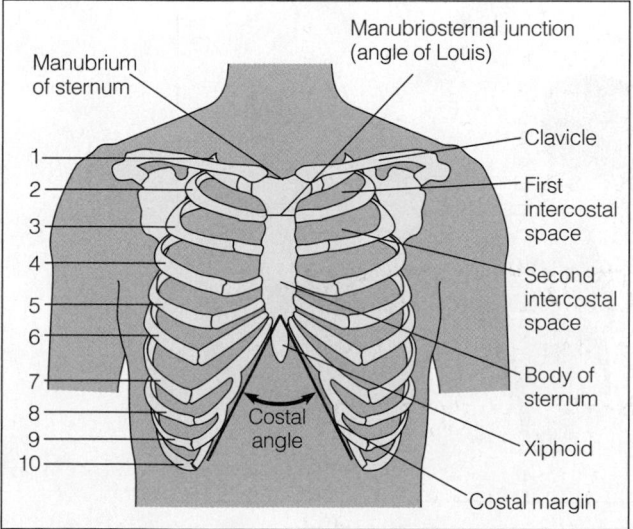

FIGURE 28.23 Location of the anterior ribs in relation to the angle of Louis and the sternum.

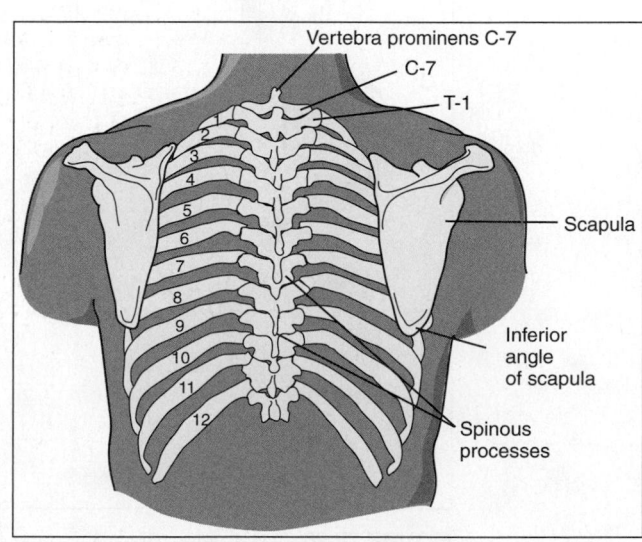

FIGURE 28.24 Location of the posterior ribs in relation to the spinous processes.

numbered rib, but over the rib below. Thus, the spinous process of T-5 lies over the body of T-6 and is adjacent to the sixth rib.

Chest Shape and Size

In adults, the thorax is oval. Its anteroposterior diameter is half its transverse diameter (Figure 28.25). The overall shape of the thorax is elliptical; that is, its diameter is smaller at the top than at the base. In older adults, *kyphosis* (excessive convex curvature of the thoracic spine) and *osteoporosis* (a condition that causes bones to become thin and porous) alter the size of the chest cavity as the ribs move downward and forward.

The chest can acquire several deformities (Figure 28.26). *Pectus carinatum* (pigeon chest), a permanent deformity, can be caused by *rickets* (a softening of bones due to deficiency or impaired metabolism of vitamin D, magnesium, phosphorus, or calcium). A narrow transverse diameter, an increased anteroposterior diameter, and a protruding sternum characterize pigeon chest. *Pectus excavatum* (a funnel chest), a congenital defect, is the opposite of pigeon chest in that the sternum is depressed, narrowing the anteroposterior diameter. Because the sternum points posteriorly in clients with a

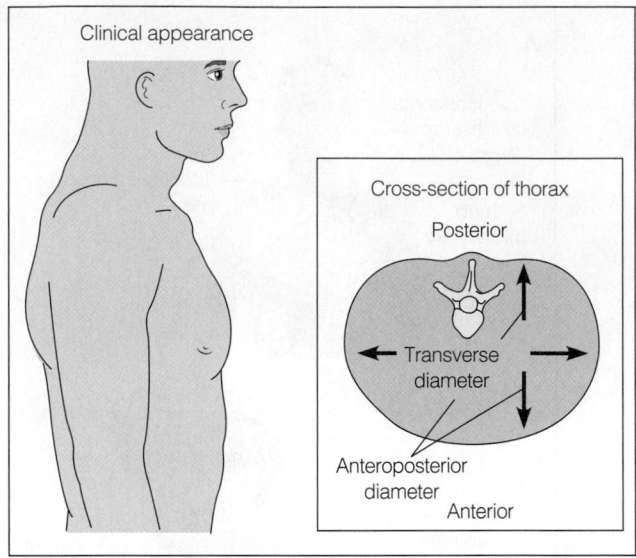

FIGURE 28.25 Configurations of the thorax showing anteroposterior diameter and transverse diameter.

funnel chest, abnormal pressure on the heart can result in altered function. A barrel chest, in which the ratio of the anteroposterior to transverse diameter is 1 to 1, is seen in clients with thoracic kyphosis and emphysema. Scoliosis is a lateral deviation of the spine.

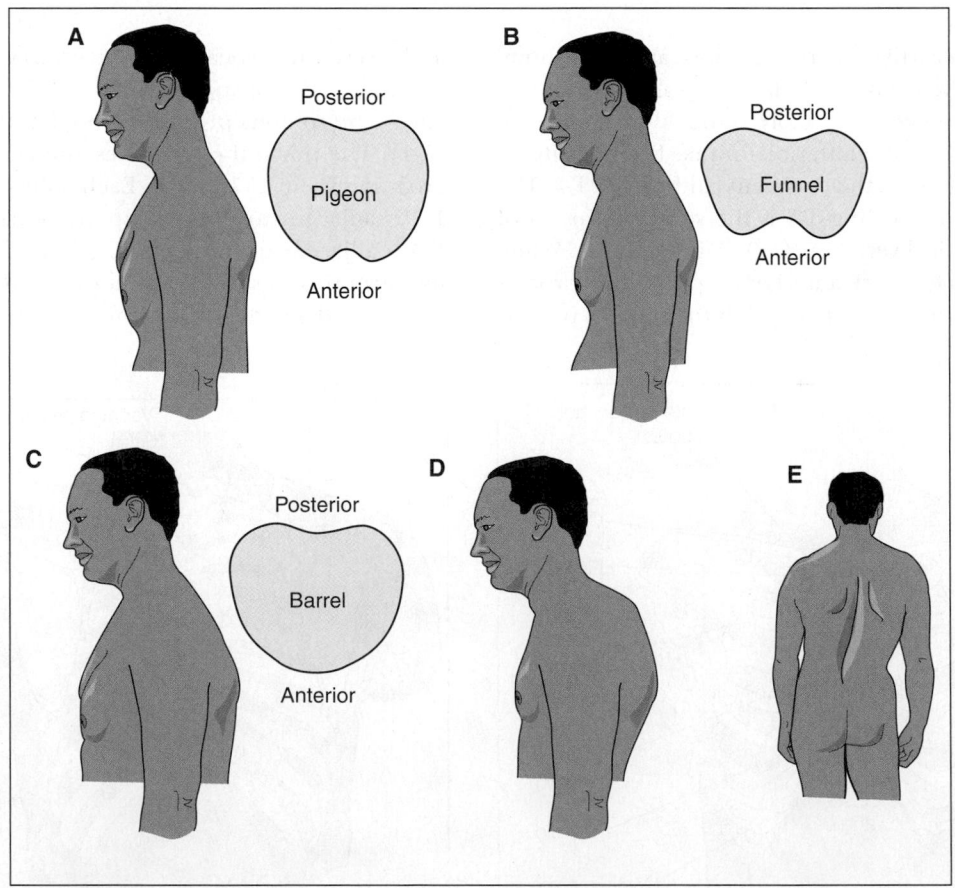

FIGURE 28.26 Chest deformities: **A:** Pigeon chest; **B:** Funnel chest; **C:** Barrel chest; **D:** Kyphosis; **E:** Scoliosis.

Breath Sounds

Abnormal breath sounds, called **adventitious breath sounds**, occur when air passes through narrowed airways or airways filled with fluid or mucus, or when pleural linings are inflamed. Table 28.7 describes normal breath sounds. Adventitious sounds are often superimposed over normal sounds. The main types of adventitious sounds—crackles (fine, coarse), friction rub, wheezes (sonorous, sibilant), and stridor—are described in Table 28.8. The absence of breath sounds over some lung areas is also a significant finding that is associated with collapsed or surgically removed lobes.

Assessment of the lungs and thorax includes all methods of examination: inspection, palpation, percussion, and auscultation. Skill 28.11 on the next page describes how to assess the thorax and lungs (see also the Lifespan Considerations box on assessing the thorax and lungs on page 648).

TABLE 28.7 Normal Breath Sounds

Type	Description	Location	Characteristics
Vesicular	Soft-intensity, low-pitched, "gentle sighing" sounds created by air moving through smaller airways (bronchioles and alveoli)	Over peripheral lung; best heard at base of lungs	Best heard on inspiration, which is about 2.5 times longer than the expiratory phase (5:2 ratio)
Bronchovesicular	Moderate-intensity and moderate-pitched "blowing" sounds created by air moving through larger airways (bronchi)	Between the scapulae and lateral to the sternum at the first and second intercostal spaces	Equal inspiratory and expiratory phases (1:1 ratio)
Bronchial (tubular)	High-pitched, loud, "harsh" sounds created by air moving through the trachea	Anteriorly over the trachea; not normally heard over lung tissue	Louder than vesicular sounds; have a short inspiratory phase and long expiratory phase (1:2 ratio)

TABLE 28.8 Adventitious Breath Sounds

Name	Description	Cause	Location
Fine crackles (formerly referred to as *rales*)	Dry, high-pitched, discontinuous crackling, popping; sound can be simulated by rolling a lock of hair near the ear; predominantly heard on inspiration but can be heard on both inspiration and expiration; may not be cleared by coughing	Air passing through moisture (fluid or mucus) in small airways that suddenly reinflate	Most commonly heard in the bases of the lower lung lobes
Coarse crackles	Discontinuous, moist, low-pitched crackling, gurgling; predominantly heard on inspiration but can be heard on both inspiration and expiration; may be altered by coughing	Air passing through moisture (fluid or mucus) in large airways that suddenly reinflate	Loud sounds can be heard over most lung areas but predominate over the trachea and bronchi
Friction rub	Superficial grating or creaking sounds heard during inspiration and expiration; not relieved by coughing	Rubbing together of inflamed pleural surfaces	Heard most often in areas of greatest thoracic expansion (e.g., lower anterior and lateral thorax)
Sonorous wheeze (formerly referred to as *rhonchi*)	Continuous, low-pitched snoring sound; best heard on expiration; may be cleared by coughing	Air passing through narrowing of large airways or obstruction of the bronchus	Heard over all lung fields
Sibilant wheeze	Continuous, high-pitched, musical sounds; best heard on expiration; not usually altered by coughing	Air passing through narrowing of large airways or obstruction of the bronchus	Heard over all lung fields
Stridor	Continuous crowing sound, high pitched; predominantly heard on inspiration.	Partial obstruction of larynx or trachea	Louder in neck than over chest wall

SKILL 28.11 ASSESSING THE THORAX AND LUNGS

PLANNING

For efficiency, the nurse usually examines the posterior thorax first, then the anterior thorax. For posterior and lateral thorax examinations, the client is uncovered to the waist and in a sitting position. A sitting or lying position can be used for anterior thorax examination. The sitting position is preferred because it maximizes chest expansion. Good lighting is essential, especially for inspection.

Equipment

- Stethoscope
- Skin marker or pencil
- Centimetre ruler

IMPLEMENTATION

Performance

1. Before performing the procedure, introduce yourself and verify the client's identity using two identifiers or per agency protocol. Explain to the client what you are going to do, why it is necessary, and how he or she can participate. Discuss how the results will be used in planning further care or treatments.

2. Perform hand hygiene, and follow other appropriate infection prevention and control procedures.

3. Provide for client privacy. For women, drape the anterior chest when it is not being examined.

4. Inquire whether the client has any history of the following: family history of illness, including cancer, allergies, tuberculosis; lifestyle habits, such as smoking and occupational hazards (e.g., inhaling fumes); medications being taken; current problems (e.g., swellings, coughs, wheezing, pain).

Assessment	Normal Findings	Deviations from Normal
Posterior Thorax		
5. Inspect the shape and symmetry of the thorax from the posterior and lateral views. Compare the anteroposterior diameter to the transverse diameter.	Anteroposterior to transverse diameter in ratio of 1:2; chest symmetrical	Barrel chest; increased anteroposterior to transverse diameter; thorax asymmetric
6. Inspect the spinal alignment for deformities. Have the client stand. From a lateral position, observe the three normal curvatures: cervical, thoracic, and lumbar.	Spine vertically aligned	Exaggerated spinal curvatures (kyphosis, *lordosis* [an inward curvature of a portion of the lumbar and cervical vertebral column])
• To assess for scoliosis, stand behind the client and have him or her stand. Observe the spinal alignment. Have the client bend forward at the waist, and then observe the alignment again.	Spinal column is straight; right and left shoulders and hips are at same height	Spinal column deviates to one side, often accentuated when bending over; shoulders or hips are not even
7. Palpate the posterior thorax.		
• For clients who have no respiratory complaints, rapidly assess the temperature and integrity of all chest skin.	Skin intact; uniform temperature	Skin lesions; areas of hyperthermia
• For clients who do have respiratory complaints, palpate all chest areas for bulges, tenderness, or abnormal movements. Avoid deep palpation in painful areas, especially if a fractured rib is suspected. In such a case, deep palpation could lead to displacement of the bone fragment against the lungs.	Chest wall intact; no tenderness; no masses	Lumps, bulges; depressions; areas of tenderness; moveable structures (e.g., rib)
8. Palpate the posterior thorax for *respiratory excursion* (thoracic expansion). Place the palms of both your hands over the lower thorax with your thumbs adjacent to the spine and your fingers stretched laterally	Full and symmetric chest expansion (i.e., when the client takes a deep breath, your thumbs should move apart an equal distance and	Asymmetric or decreased chest expansion

Assessment	Normal Findings	Deviations from Normal
(see ❶). Ask the client to take a deep breath while you observe the movement of your hands and any lag in movement.	at the same time; normally the thumbs separate 3 cm to 5 cm during deep inspiration)	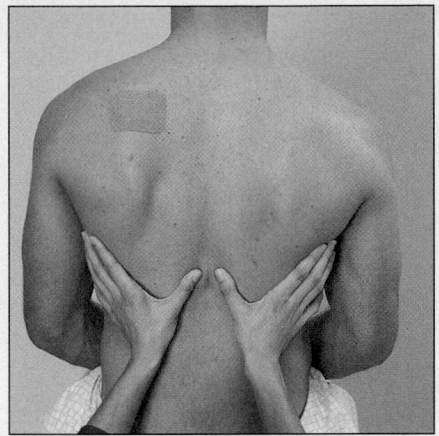

❶ Position of the nurse's hands when assessing respiratory excursion on the posterior thorax.

Assessment	Normal Findings	Deviations from Normal
9. Palpate the thorax for vocal (tactile) **fremitus**, the faintly perceptible vibration felt through the chest wall when the client speaks.	Bilateral symmetry of vocal fremitus; fremitus is heard most clearly at the apex of the lungs	Decreased or absent fremitus (associated with pneumothorax); increased fremitus (associated with consolidated lung tissue, as in pneumonia)
• Place the ulnar surface of the hand or the palmar surface of the hand at the base of the metacarpophalangeal joints (see ❷) on the posterior chest, starting near the apex of the lungs (see ❸, position A).	Low-pitched voices of males more readily palpated than higher-pitched voices of females	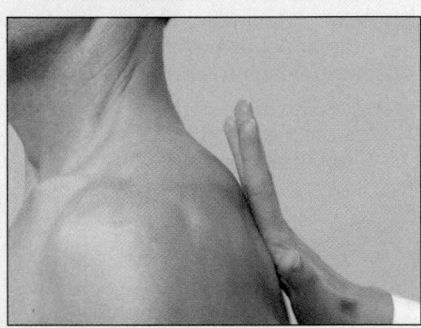
• Ask the client to repeat such words as "blue moon" or "one, two, three."		
• Repeat the two steps, moving your hands sequentially to the base of the lungs, through positions B to E in ❸.		

❷ Palpation for tactile fremitus by using metacarpophalangeal joint area.

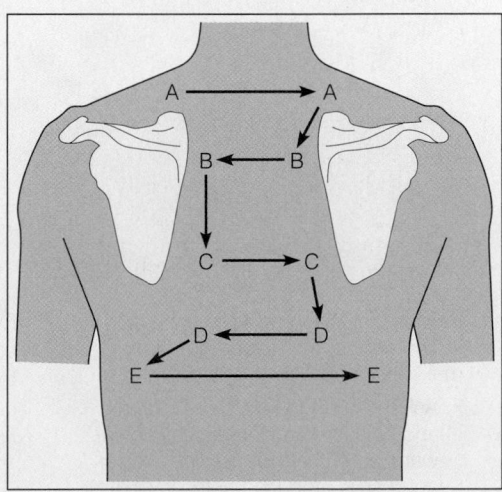

❸ Areas and sequence for palpating tactile fremitus on the posterior thorax.

(continued)

SKILL 28.11   ASSESSING THE THORAX AND LUNGS (continued)

Assessment	Normal Findings	Deviations from Normal
• Compare the fremitus on both lungs and between the apex and the base of each lung, using either one hand and moving it from one side of the client to the corresponding area on the other side *or* using two hands that are placed simultaneously on the corresponding areas of each side of the chest.		

10. Percuss the thorax. Percussion of the thorax is performed to determine whether underlying lung tissue is filled with air, liquid, or solid material and to determine the positions and boundaries of certain organs. Because percussion penetrates to a depth of 5 cm to 7 cm, it detects superficial rather than deep lesions. Percussion sounds and tones are described in Table 28.4 (p. 601). Normal percussion sounds in the posterior chest are shown in ❹.

- Ask the client to bend the head and fold the arms forward across the chest. **Rationale: This separates the scapula and exposes more lung tissue to percussion.**
- Percuss in the intercostal spaces at about 5 cm intervals in a systematic sequence (see ❺).
- Compare one side of the lung with the other.
- Percuss the lateral thorax every few centimetres, starting at the axilla and working down to the eighth rib.

Normal Findings: Percussion notes resonate, except over scapula; lowest point of resonance is at the diaphragm (i.e., at the level of the 8th to 10th ribs posteriorly); *note:* percussion on a rib normally elicits dullness

Deviations from Normal: Asymmetry in percussion; areas of dullness or flatness over lung tissue (associated with consolidation of lung tissue or a mass)

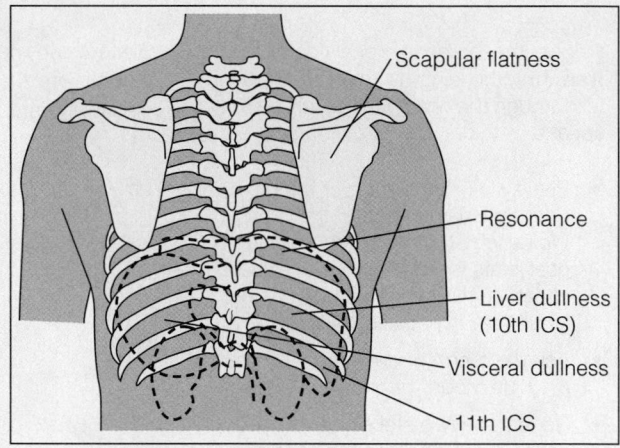

❹ Normal percussion sounds in the posterior thorax.

Labels: Scapular flatness; Resonance; Liver dullness (10th ICS); Visceral dullness; 11th ICS

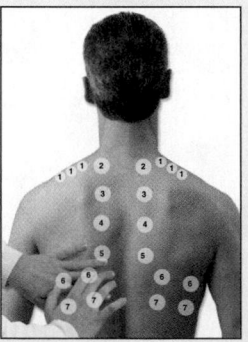

❺ Pattern for percussion: Posterior thorax.

11. Percuss for diaphragmatic excursion (movement of the diaphragm during maximal inspiration and expiration).

- Ask the client to take a deep breath and hold it while you percuss downward along the scapular line until dullness is produced at the level of the diaphragm. Mark this point with a marking pencil, and repeat the procedure on the other side of the thorax.

Normal Findings: Excursion is 3 cm to 5 cm bilaterally in women and 5 cm to 6 cm in men; diaphragm is usually slightly higher on the right side

Deviations from Normal: Restricted excursion (associated with lung disorder)

Assessment	Normal Findings	Deviations from Normal

- Ask the client to take a few normal breaths and then expel the last breath completely and hold it while you percuss upward from the marked point to assess and mark the diaphragmatic excursion during deep expiration on each side.

- Measure the distance between the two marks.

12. Auscultate the thorax by using the flat-disc diaphragm of the stethoscope (best for transmitting high-pitched breath sounds). See ❻.

Vesicular and bronchovesicular breath sounds (see ❼, and Table 28.7, p. 641)

Adventitious breath sounds (e.g., crackles, wheezes, friction rub; see Table 28.8, p. 641)

Absence of breath sounds

- Ask the client to take slow, deep breaths through the mouth. Listen at each point to the breath sounds during a complete inspiration and expiration cycle.

- Compare findings at each point with the corresponding point on the opposite side of the chest.

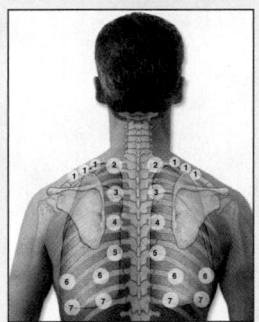

❻ Pattern for auscultation: Posterior thorax.

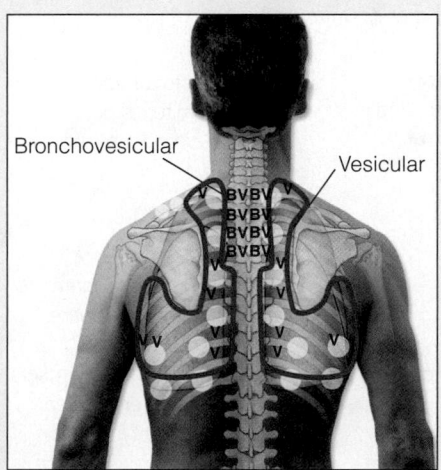

Bronchovesicular

Vesicular

❼ Auscultatory sounds: Posterior thorax.

Anterior Thorax

13. Inspect breathing patterns (e.g., respiratory rate and rhythm).

Quiet, rhythmic, and effortless respirations (see Chapter 29)

See Chapter 29, Box 29.5 (p. 719), for altered breathing patterns and sounds

14. Inspect the costal angle (angle formed by the intersection of the costal margins) and the angle at which the ribs enter the spine.

Costal angle is less than 90 degrees, and the ribs insert into the spine at approximately a 45-degree angle (see Figure 28.23, p. 639)

Costal angle is widened (associated with COPD)

15. Palpate the anterior thorax (see the Posterior Thorax section).

16. Palpate the anterior thorax for respiratory excursion.

Full symmetric excursion; thumbs normally separate 3 cm to 5 cm

Asymmetric or decreased respiratory excursion

- Place the palms of both your hands on the lower thorax, with your fingers laterally along the lower rib cage and your thumbs along the costal margins (see ❽).

(continued)

SKILL 28.11 ASSESSING THE THORAX AND LUNGS (*continued*)

Assessment	Normal Findings	Deviations from Normal

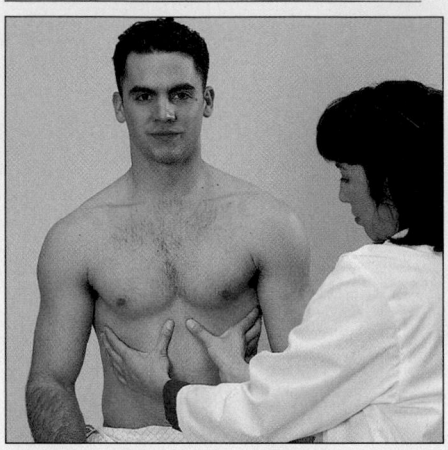

❽ Position of nurse's hands when assessing respiratory excursion on the anterior thorax.

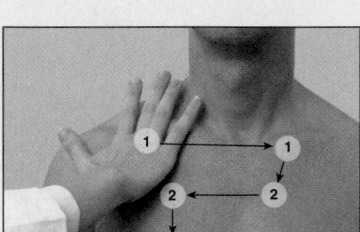

❾ Palpation for tactile fremitus: Anterior thorax.

- Ask the client to take a deep breath while you observe the movement of your hands.

17. Palpate tactile fremitus in the same manner as for the posterior thorax and by using the sequence shown in ❾. If the breasts are large and cannot be retracted adequately for palpation, this part of the examination is usually omitted.

Same as posterior vocal fremitus; fremitus is normally decreased over heart and breast tissue

Same as posterior fremitus

18. Percuss the anterior thorax systematically.

- Begin above the clavicles in the supraclavicular space, and proceed downward to the diaphragm (see ❿).

Percussion notes resonate down to the sixth rib at the level of the diaphragm but are flat over areas of heavy muscle and bone, dull over the heart and the liver, and tympanic over the underlying stomach (see ⓫).

Asymmetry in percussion notes; areas of dullness or flatness over lung tissue

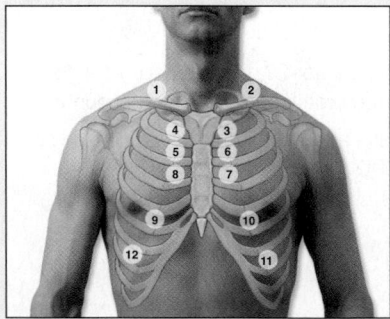

❿ Pattern for percussion: Anterior thorax.

Assessment	Normal Findings	Deviations from Normal
• Compare one side of the lung to the other. In women, displace breasts for proper examination.		

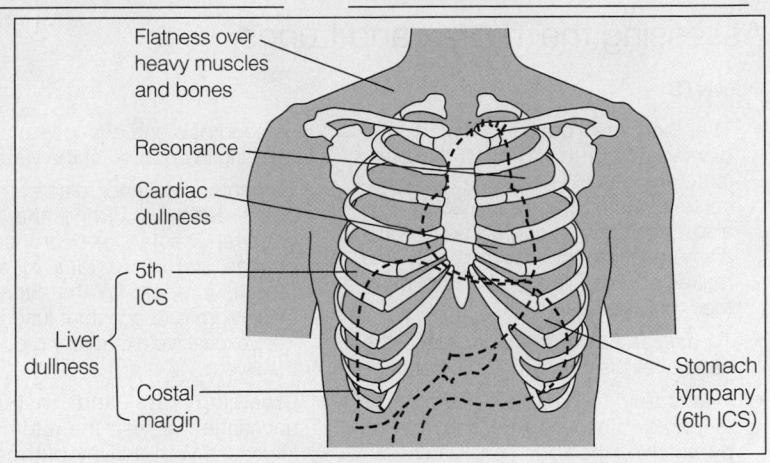

❶❶ Normal percussion sounds on the anterior thorax.

Assessment	Normal Findings	Deviations from Normal
19. Auscultate the trachea.	Bronchial and tubular breath sounds (see ❶❷ and Table 28.7, p. 641)	Adventitious breath sounds (see Table 28.8, p. 641)
20. Auscultate the anterior thorax. Use the sequence used in percussion (see ❶⓪), beginning over the bronchi between the sternum and the clavicles.	Bronchovesicular and vesicular breath sounds (see ❶❷ and Table 28.7, p. 641)	Adventitious breath sounds (see Table 28.8, p. 641)
21. Document your findings in the client record by using forms or checklists supplemented by narrative notes, when appropriate.		

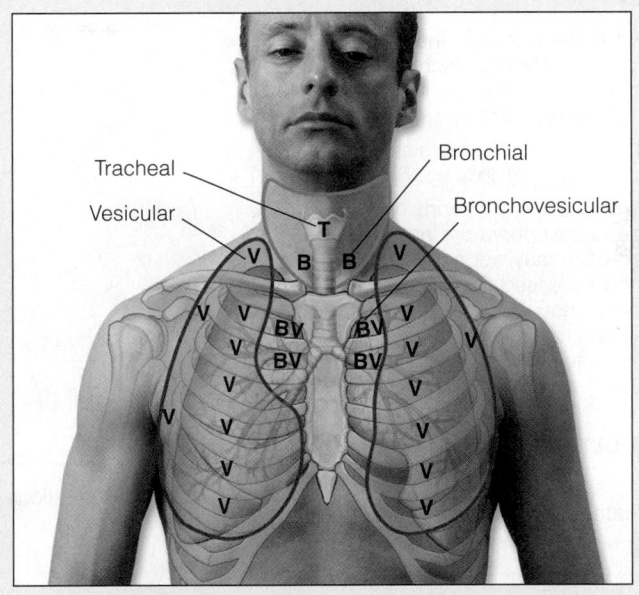

❶❷ Auscultatory sounds: Anterior thorax.

EVALUATION

Relate findings to previous assessment data, if available. Report significant deviations from normal to the appropriate members of the health care team.

LIFESPAN CONSIDERATIONS

Assessing the Thorax and Lungs

INFANTS

- The thorax is rounded; that is, the diameter from the front to the back (anteroposterior) is equal to the transverse diameter. See Figure 28.27. It is also cylindrical, having a nearly equal diameter at the top and the base. This makes it harder for infants to expand their thoracic space.

- To assess tactile fremitus, place the hand over the crying infant's thorax.

- Infants tend to breathe by using their diaphragm; assess rate and rhythm by watching the abdomen, rather than the thorax, rise and fall.

- The right bronchial branch is short and angles down as it leaves the trachea, making it easy for small objects to be inhaled. Sudden onset of cough or other signs of respiratory distress may indicate the infant has inhaled a foreign object.

CHILDREN

- By about 6 years of age, the anteroposterior diameter has decreased in proportion to the transverse diameter, with a 1:2 ratio present.

- Children tend to breathe more abdominally than thoracically up to age 6 years.

- During the rapid growth spurts of adolescence, spinal curvature and rotation (scoliosis) may appear. Children should be assessed for scoliosis by age 12 and annually until their growth slows. Curvature greater than 10% should be referred for further medical evaluation.

OLDER ADULTS

- The thoracic curvature may be accentuated (kyphosis) because of

osteoporosis and changes in cartilage resulting in collapse of the vertebrae.

- The anteroposterior diameter of the chest deepens, giving the person a barrel-chested appearance. This change is due to loss of skeletal muscle strength in the thorax and diaphragm and constant lung inflation from excessive expiratory pressure on the alveoli.

- Breathing rate and rhythm are unchanged at rest; the rate normally increases with activity but may take longer to return to the resting rate.

- Inspiratory muscles become less powerful, and the inspiration reserve volume decreases. A decrease in depth of respiration is therefore apparent.

- Expiration may require the use of accessory muscles. The expiratory reserve volume significantly increases

because of the increased amount of air remaining in the lungs at the end of a normal breath.

- Small airways lose their cartilaginous support and elastic recoil; as a result, they tend to close, particularly in the basal, or dependent, portions of the lung.

- Alveolar tissue loses its elasticity and changes to fibrous tissue. This thicker alveolar membrane decreases the pulmonary diffusion capacity. As a result, arterial *oxyhemoglobin* (a compound of oxygen and hemoglobin that transports oxygen) saturation and *PaO₂* (partial pressure of oxygen) are slightly lower than those of young adults.

- Cilia in the airways decrease in number and are less effective in removing mucus; older clients are, therefore, at greater risk for pulmonary infections.

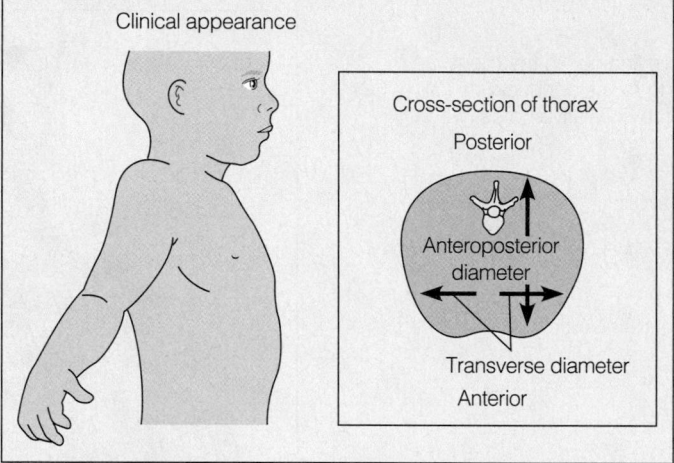

FIGURE 28.27 Configurations of the child's thorax showing anteroposterior diameter and transverse diameter.

Cardiovascular and Peripheral Vascular Systems

Nurses assess the cardiovascular system through observations (inspection), palpation, and auscultation. The examination includes palpation of upper and lower extremity pulses; inspection of jugular venous distension; measurement of blood pressure bilaterally and with the client standing versus lying flat or sitting; and inspection, palpation, and auscultation of the heart. Although heart examinations are initially performed while the client is in a semi-reclined position, other positions, such as left lateral recumbent position, leaning forward, and standing, can also be used.

Heart

To assess the client's heart, the nurse must first determine its exact location. In the average adult, most of the heart lies behind and to the left of the sternum. A small portion (the right atrium) extends to the right of the sternum. The upper portion of the heart (both atria), referred to as its **base**, lies toward the back. The lower portion (the ventricles), referred to as its **apex**, points forward. The apex of the left ventricle actually touches the anterior chest wall at or medial to the left midclavicular line (MCL) and at or near the fifth left intercostal space, which is slightly below the left nipple. See Figure 29.11 (p. 710). This point where the apex touches the anterior chest wall is known as the **point of maximal impulse (PMI)**. The point of maximal impulse refers to the point at which the apical impulse is most readily seen or felt.

The **precordium**, the area of the chest overlying the heart, is inspected and palpated simultaneously for the presence of abnormal pulsations or lifts or heaves. The terms **lift** and **heave**, often used interchangeably, refer to a rising along the sternal border with each heartbeat. A lift occurs when cardiac action is very forceful. It should be confirmed by palpation with the palm of the hand. Enlargement or overactivity of the left ventricle produces a heave lateral to the apex, whereas enlargement of the right ventricle produces a heave at or near the sternum.

Heart sounds can be heard by auscultation. The normal first two heart sounds are produced by closure of the valves of the heart. The first heart sound, S_1, occurs when the atrioventricular (A-V) valves close and is best heard at the apex. These valves close when the ventricles have been sufficiently filled. Although the right and left A-V valves do not close simultaneously, the closures occur closely enough to be heard as one sound (S_1), a dull, low-pitched sound described as "lub." After the ventricles empty their blood into the aorta and pulmonary arteries, the semilunar valves close, producing the second heart sound, S_2, described as "dub." S_2 has a higher pitch than S_1 and is also shorter. The S_2 is best heard in the aortic and pulmonic areas. These two sounds, S_1 and S_2 ("lub-dub"), occur within one second or less, depending on the heart rate.

Heart sounds are audible anywhere on the precordial area, but they are best heard over the aortic, pulmonic, tricuspid, and apical areas (Figure 28.28). Each area is associated with the closure of heart valves: the aortic area with the aortic valve (inside the aorta as it arises from the left ventricle); the pulmonic area with the pulmonic valve (inside the pulmonary artery as it arises from the right ventricle); the tricuspid area with the tricuspid valve (between the right atrium and the right ventricle); and the apical (mitral) area with the mitral valve (between the left atrium and the left ventricle).

Associated with these sounds are *systole* and *diastole*. **Systole** is the period in which the ventricles contract. It begins with the first heart sound and ends at the second heart sound. Systole is normally shorter than diastole. **Diastole** is the period in which the ventricles relax. It starts with the second sound and ends at the subsequent first sound. Normally, no sounds are audible during these periods (Figure 28.29). The experienced nurse,

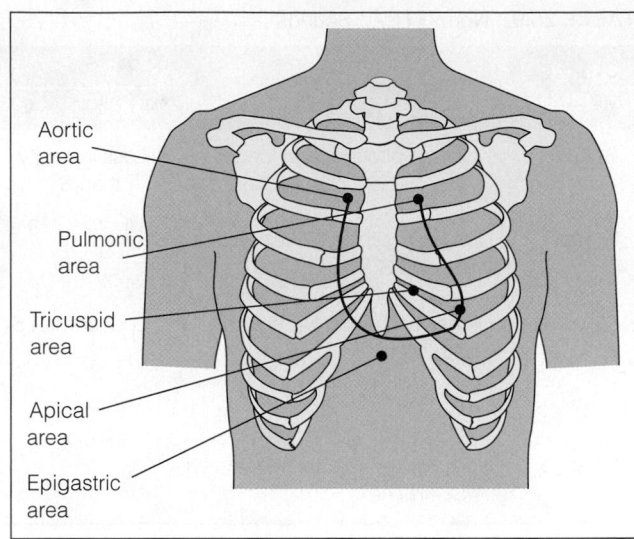

FIGURE 28.28 Anatomical sites of the precordium.

however, may auscultate extra heart sounds (S_3 and S_4) during diastole. Both sounds are low in pitch and heard best at the apex, with the bell of the stethoscope, and with the client either supine or lying on the left side. S_3 (often referred to as a *gallop rhythm*) occurs early in diastole right after S_2 and sounds like "lub-dub-*ee*" (S_1, S_2, S_3) or "Kentuc-*ky*." It often disappears when the client sits up. S_3 is normal in children and young adults. In older adults, it may indicate heart failure. S_4 is rarely heard in healthy young adults. It occurs near the very end of diastole just before S_1 and creates the sound of "*dee*-lub-dub" (S_4, S_1, S_2) or "*Ten*-nessee." S_4 may be heard in many older adult clients and can be a sign of hypertension. An S_4 may be heard following acute myocardial infarction (MI) or in older adults with cardiovascular disease. The presence of an S_4 indicates an increased resistance to ventricular filling, which occurs because of a loss of compliance in the ventricular walls (e.g., hypertensive disease, coronary heart disease).

Normal heart sounds are summarized in Table 28.9 on the next page. The nurse may also hear abnormal

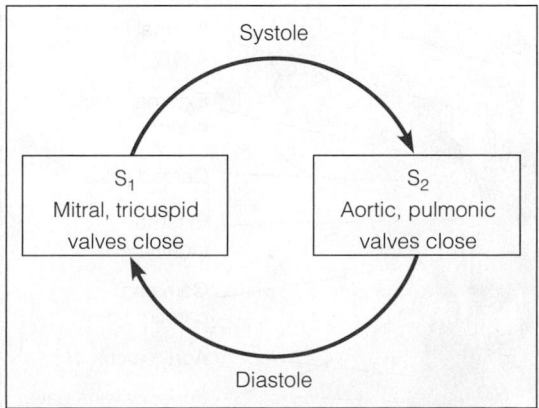

FIGURE 28.29 Relationship of heart sounds to systole and diastole.

TABLE 28.9 Normal Heart Sounds

Sound or Phase	Description	Area			
		Aortic	Pulmonic	Tricuspid	Apical
S_1	Dull, low-pitched, and longer than S_2; sounds like "lub"	Less intensity than S_2	Less intensity than S_2	Louder than or equal to S_2	Louder than or equal to S_2
Systole	Normally silent interval between S_1 and S_2				
S_2	Higher pitch than S_1; sounds like "dub"	Louder than S_1	Louder than S_1; abnormal if louder than the aortic S_2 in adults more than 40 years of age	Less intensity than or equal to S_1	Less intensity than or equal to S_1
Diastole	Normally silent interval between S_2 and next S_1				

heart sounds, such as clicks, rubs, and murmurs. These are caused by valve disorders or impaired blood flow within the heart and require advanced training to diagnose.

Central Vessels

The *carotid arteries* supply oxygenated blood to the head and neck (Figure 28.30). Because they are the only source of blood to the brain, prolonged occlusion of one of these arteries can result in serious brain damage. The carotid pulses correlate with central aortic pressure, thus reflecting cardiac function better than peripheral pulses can. When cardiac output is diminished, the peripheral pulses may be difficult or impossible to feel, but the carotid pulse should be felt easily.

The carotid is also auscultated for a bruit, and if a bruit is found, the carotid artery is then palpated for a *thrill*. A **bruit** (a blowing or swishing sound), best heard with the diaphragm of the stethoscope, is created by turbulence of blood flow created by either a narrowed arterial lumen (a common development in older people) or to a condition, such as anemia or hyperthyroidism, that elevates cardiac output. A **thrill**, which frequently accompanies a bruit, is a vibrating sensation, similar to the purring of a cat or water running through a hose. It, too, indicates turbulent blood flow because of arterial obstruction.

The *jugular veins* drain blood from the head and neck directly into the superior vena cava (SVC) and right side of the heart. The external jugular veins are superficial and may be visible above the clavicle. The internal jugular veins lie deeper along the carotid artery and may transmit pulsations onto the skin of the neck. Normally, external neck veins are distended and visible when a person lies down; they are flat and not as visible when a person stands up because gravity encourages venous drainage. By inspecting the jugular veins for pulsations and distension, the nurse can assess the adequacy of function of the right side of the heart and venous pressure. Bilateral jugular vein distension (JVD) may indicate right-sided heart failure.

Skill 28.12 describes how to assess the heart and central vessels (see also the Lifespan Considerations box on assessing the heart and central vessels on page 654).

Peripheral Vascular System

Assessing the peripheral vascular system includes measuring blood pressure; palpating peripheral pulses; inspecting, palpating, and auscultating the carotid pulse; inspecting the jugular and peripheral veins; and inspecting skin and tissues to determine **perfusion** (blood supply to an area) to the extremities. Certain aspects of peripheral vascular assessment are often incorporated into other parts of the assessment procedure. For example, blood pressure is usually measured

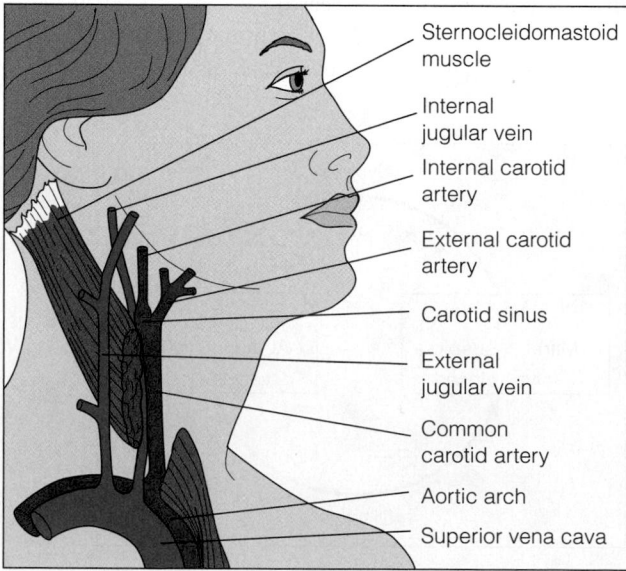

Sternocleidomastoid muscle

Internal jugular vein

Internal carotid artery

External carotid artery

Carotid sinus

External jugular vein

Common carotid artery

Aortic arch

Superior vena cava

FIGURE 28.30 Arteries and veins of the right side of the neck.

SKILL 28.12   ASSESSING THE HEART AND CENTRAL VESSELS

PLANNING

Heart examinations are usually performed while the client is in a semi-reclined position. The practitioner stands at the client's right side, where palpation of the cardiac area is facilitated and optimal inspection allowed.

Equipment

- Stethoscope
- Centimetre ruler

IMPLEMENTATION

Performance

1. Before performing the procedure, introduce yourself, and verify the client's identity using a minimum of two identifiers or per agency protocol. Explain to the client what you are going to do, why it is necessary, and how he or she can participate. Discuss how the results will be used in planning further care or treatments.

2. Perform hand hygiene, and follow other appropriate infection prevention and control procedures.

3. Provide for client privacy.

4. Inquire whether the client has any history of the following: family history of incidence and age of heart disease, high cholesterol levels, hypertension, cerebrovascular accident (CVA, or stroke), obesity, congenital heart disease, arterial disease, and rheumatic fever; client's past history of rheumatic fever, heart murmur, heart attack, varicosities, or heart failure; present signs or symptoms indicative of heart disease (e.g., fatigue, dyspnea, orthopnea, edema, cough, chest pain, palpitations, syncope, elevated blood pressure, wheezing, hemoptysis); presence of problems that affect the heart (e.g., obesity, diabetes, lung disease, endocrine disorders); lifestyle habits that are risk factors for cardiac disease (e.g., smoking, excessive alcohol intake, eating and exercise patterns, areas and degree of stress perceived).

Assessment	Normal Findings	Deviations from Normal
5. Simultaneously inspect and palpate the precordium for the presence of abnormal pulsations, lifts, or heaves. Locate the valve areas of the heart: • Locate the angle of Louis. It is felt as a prominence on the sternum. • Move your fingertips down each side of the angle until you can feel the second intercostal spaces. The client's right second intercostal space is the aortic area, and the left second intercostal space is the pulmonic area (see ❶).		
• Inspect and palpate the aortic and pulmonic areas, observing them at an angle and to the side, to note the presence or absence of pulsations. **Rationale: Observing these areas at an angle increases the likelihood of seeing pulsations.** • From the pulmonic area, move your fingertips down three left intercostal spaces along the side of the sternum. The left fifth intercostal space close to the sternum is the tricuspid or right ventricular area.	No pulsations	Pulsations
• Inspect and palpate the tricuspid area for pulsations and heaves or lifts.	No pulsations; no lift or heave	Pulsations; diffuse lift or heave, indicating enlarged or overactive right ventricle

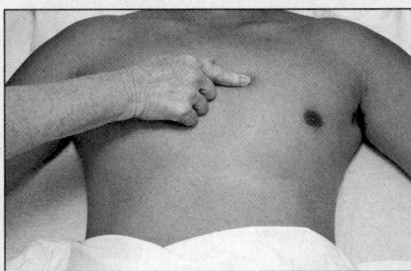

❶ Second intercostal space.

(continued)

SKILL 28.12 ASSESSING THE HEART AND CENTRAL VESSELS (*continued*)

Assessment	Normal Findings	Deviations from Normal
• From the tricuspid area, move your fingertips laterally 5 cm to 7 cm to the left MCL. This is the apical or mitral area or PMI (see ❷). If you have difficulty locating the PMI, have the client roll onto the left side to move the apex closer to the chest wall.	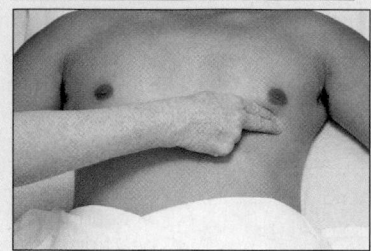 ❷ Fifth intercostal space, MCL.	
• Inspect and palpate the apical area for pulsation, noting its specific location (it may be displaced laterally or lower) and diameter. If displaced laterally, record the distance between the apex and the MCL in centimetres.	Pulsations visible in 50% of adults and palpable in most PMI in fifth left intercostal space at or medial to the MCL; diameter of 1 cm to 2 cm; no lift or heave	PMI displaced laterally or lower (indicates enlarged heart or aneurysm); diameter of more than 2 cm; diffuse lift or heave lateral to apex (indicates enlargement or overactivity of left ventricle)
• Inspect and palpate the epigastric area at the base of the sternum for abdominal aortic pulsations.	Aortic pulsations	Bounding abdominal pulsations (e.g., aortic aneurysm)
6. Auscultate the heart in all four anatomical sites: aortic, pulmonic, tricuspid, and apical (mitral). Auscultation need not be limited to these areas; however, you may need to move the stethoscope to find the most audible sounds for each client.	S_1: usually heard at all sites, usually louder at apical area; S_2: usually heard at all sites, usually louder at base of heart; Systole: silent interval, slightly shorter duration than diastole at normal heart rate (60–100 beats/min); Diastole: silent interval, slightly longer duration than systole at normal heart rates; S_3 in children and young adults; S_4 in many older adults	Increased or decreased intensity; varying intensity with different beats; increased intensity at aortic area; increased intensity at pulmonic area; sharp-sounding ejection clicks; S_3 in older adults; S_4 may be a sign of hypertension
• Eliminate all sources of room noise. **Rationale: Heart sounds are of low intensity, and other noise hinders the nurse's ability to hear them.**		
• Keep the client in a supine position with head elevated 30 degrees to 45 degrees.		
• Use both the diaphragm and the bell of the stethoscope to listen to all areas.		
• In every area of auscultation, distinguish both S_1 and S_2 sounds.		
• When auscultating, concentrate on one particular sound at a time in each area: the first heart sound, followed by systole, then the second heart sound, then diastole. Systole and diastole are normally silent intervals.		

Assessment	Normal Findings	Deviations from Normal
• Later, re-examine the heart while the client is in the upright sitting position. **Rationale: Certain sounds are more audible in certain positions.**		

Carotid Arteries

Assessment	Normal Findings	Deviations from Normal
7. Palpate the carotid artery, using extreme caution (see Figure 28.30, p. 650).	Symmetrical pulse volumes; full pulsations, thrusting quality; quality remains same when client breathes, turns head, and changes from sitting to supine position; elastic arterial wall	Asymmetric volumes (possible stenosis or thrombosis); decreased pulsations (may indicate impaired left cardiac output); increased pulsations; thickening, hard, rigid, beaded, inelastic walls (indicate arteriosclerosis)
• Palpate only one carotid artery at a time. **Rationale: This ensures adequate blood flow through the other artery to the brain.**		
• Avoid exerting too much pressure and massaging the area. **Rationale: Pressure can occlude the artery and carotid sinus massage can precipitate bradycardia.**		
• The carotid sinus is a small dilation at the beginning of the internal carotid artery just above the bifurcation of the common carotid artery, in the upper third of the neck.		
• Ask the client to turn the head slightly toward the side being examined. This makes the carotid artery more accessible.		
8. Auscultate the carotid artery.	No sound heard on auscultation	Presence of bruit in one or both arteries (suggests occlusive artery disease)
• Turn the client's head slightly away from the side being examined. **Rationale: This facilitates the placement of the stethoscope.**		
• Auscultate the carotid artery on one side and then the other.		
• Listen for the presence of a bruit. If you hear a bruit, gently palpate the artery to determine the presence of a thrill.		

Jugular Veins

Assessment	Normal Findings	Deviations from Normal
9. Inspect the jugular veins for distension while the client is placed in the semi-Fowler's position (30-degree to 45-degree angle), with the head supported on a small pillow.	Veins not visible (indicating right side of heart is functioning normally)	Veins visibly distended (indicating advanced cardiopulmonary disease)

(continued)

SKILL 28.12 **ASSESSING THE HEART AND CENTRAL VESSELS** (*continued*)

Assessment	Normal Findings	Deviations from Normal
10. If jugular vein distension is present, assess the jugular venous pressure (JVP).		Bilateral measurements of more than 3 cm to 4 cm are considered elevated (may indicate right-sided heart failure); unilateral distension (may be caused by local obstruction)

- Locate the highest visible point of distension of the internal jugular vein. Although either the internal or the external jugular vein can be used, the internal jugular vein is more reliable. **Rationale: The external jugular vein is more easily affected by obstruction or kinking at the base of the neck.**

- Measure the vertical height of this point in centimetres from the sternal angle, the point at which the clavicles meet (see ❸).

- Repeat the preceding steps on the other side.

11. Document your findings in the client record by using forms or checklists supplemented by narrative notes, when appropriate.

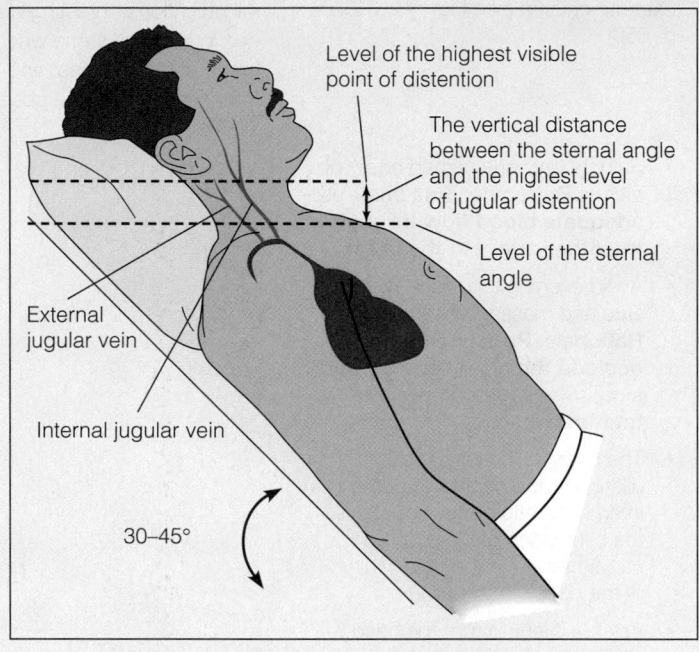

❸ Assessing the highest point of distension of the jugular vein.

EVALUATION

- Perform a detailed follow-up examination based on findings that deviated from expected or normal for the client. Relate findings to previous assessment data, if available.

- Report significant deviations from normal to the appropriate members of the health care team.

LIFESPAN CONSIDERATIONS

Assessing the Heart and Central Vessels

INFANTS

- Physiological splitting of the second heart sound (S_2) may be heard when the child takes a deep breath, and the aortic valve closes a split second before the pulmonic valve. If splitting of S_2 is heard during normal respirations, it is abnormal and may indicate an atrial-septal defect, pulmonary stenosis, or another heart problem.

- Infants may normally have sinus arrhythmia that is related to respiration. The heart rate slows during expiration and increases when the child breathes in.

- Murmurs may be heard in newborns as the structures of fetal circulation, especially the ductus arteriosus, close.

CHILDREN

- Heart sounds are louder because of the thinner chest wall.

- A third heart sound (S_3), caused as the ventricles fill, is best heard at the apex and is present in about one-third of all children.
- The PMI is higher and more medial in children younger than 8 years old.

OLDER ADULTS

- If no disease is present, heart size remains the same throughout life.

- Cardiac output and strength of contraction decrease, thus lessening the older person's activity tolerance.
- The heart rate returns to its resting rate more slowly after exertion than it did when the individual was younger.
- S_4 heart sound may be audible in older adults as a result of a more rigid ventricle.

- Extra systoles commonly occur. Ten or more extra systoles per minute are considered abnormal.
- Sudden emotional and physical stresses can result in cardiac arrhythmias and heart failure.

at the beginning of the physical examination (see the section on assessing blood pressure in Chapter 29). Pulse sites and pulse assessments are also described in Chapter 29.

Skill 28.13 describes how to assess the peripheral vascular system (see also the Lifespan Considerations box on assessing the peripheral vascular system on page 657).

SKILL 28.13 ASSESSING THE PERIPHERAL VASCULAR SYSTEM

PLANNING

Equipment: None

IMPLEMENTATION

Performance

1. Before performing the procedure, introduce yourself and verify the client's identity using two identifiers or per agency protocol. Explain to the client what you are going to do, why it is necessary, and how he or she can participate. Discuss

how the results will be used in planning further care or treatments.

2. Perform hand hygiene, and follow other appropriate infection prevention and control procedures.
3. Provide for client privacy.
4. Inquire whether the client has any history of the following: past history of heart disorders, varicosities, arterial disease, and hypertension; lifestyle habits, such as exercise patterns, activity patterns and tolerance, smoking, and use of alcohol.

Assessment	Normal Findings	Deviations from Normal
5. Palpate the peripheral pulses individually and systematically on both sides of the client's body simultaneously (except the carotid pulse) to determine the symmetry of pulse volume. If you have difficulty palpating some of the peripheral pulses, use a Doppler ultrasound probe.	Symmetric pulse volumes; full pulsations	Asymmetric volumes (indicate impaired circulation); absence of pulsation (indicates arterial spasm or occlusion); decreased, weak, thready pulsations (indicate impaired cardiac output); increased pulse volume (may indicate hypertension, high cardiac output, or circulatory overload)
Peripheral Veins		
6. Inspect the peripheral veins in the arms and legs for the presence or appearance of superficial veins when limbs are dependent and when limbs are elevated.	In dependent position, presence of distension and nodular bulges at calves; when limbs elevated, veins collapse (veins may appear tortuous or distended in older people)	Distended veins in the thigh or lower leg or on posterolateral part of calf from knee to ankle
7. Assess the peripheral leg veins for signs of *phlebitis* (vein inflammation). • Inspect the calves for redness and swelling over vein sites.	Limbs not tender; symmetric in size	Tenderness on palpation; warmth and redness over vein; swelling of one calf or leg

(continued)

SKILL 28.13 ASSESSING THE PERIPHERAL VASCULAR SYSTEM (*continued*)

Assessment	Normal Findings	Deviations from Normal
• Palpate the calves for firmness or tension of the muscles, the presence of edema over the dorsum of the foot, and areas of localized warmth. **Rationale: Palpation augments inspection findings, particularly in darker-skinned people in whom redness may not be visible.**		
• Push the calves from side to side to test for tenderness.		

Peripheral Perfusion

| 8. Inspect the skin of the hands and feet for colour, temperature, edema, and skin changes. | Skin colour pink; skin temperature not excessively warm or cold; no edema; skin texture resilient and moist | Cyanotic (venous insufficiency); pallor that increases with limb elevation; dependent *rubor,* a dusky red colour when limb is lowered (arterial insufficiency); brown pigmentation around ankles (arterial or chronic venous insufficiency); skin cool (arterial insufficiency); marked edema (venous insufficiency); mild edema (arterial insufficiency); skin thin and shiny or thick, waxy, shiny, and fragile, with reduced hair and ulceration (venous or arterial insufficiency) |
| 9. Assess the adequacy of arterial flow if arterial insufficiency is suspected. | | |

Capillary Refill Test (Blanch Test)

| • Press at least one nail on each hand and foot between your thumb and index finger sufficiently to cause blanching (about 5 seconds). | Immediate return of colour (less than 2 to 3 seconds) | Delayed return of colour (arterial insufficiency) |
| • Release the pressure, and observe how quickly normal colour returns. | | |

Other Assessments

• Inspect fingernails for changes indicative of circulatory impairment. See the section on assessment of nails earlier in this chapter (Skill 28.4, p. 612).

• See also peripheral pulse assessment in Chapter 29 (Skill 29.2, p. 712).

10. Document findings in the client record by using forms or checklists supplemented by narrative notes, when appropriate.

EVALUATION

• Perform a detailed follow-up examination of the heart or central vessels, integument, or other systems based on findings that deviated from expected or normal for the client. Relate findings to previous assessment data, if available.

• Report significant deviations from normal to the appropriate members of the health care team.

LIFESPAN CONSIDERATIONS

Assessing the Peripheral Vascular System

INFANTS

- Screen for *coarctation* (narrowing) of the aorta by palpating the peripheral pulses and comparing the strength of femoral pulses with radial and apical pulses. If coarctation is present, femoral pulses will be diminished and radial pulses will be stronger.

CHILDREN

- Palpation of pulses in the lower extremities (particularly femoral pulses) is essential to screen for coarctation of the aorta.
- Changes in the peripheral vasculature, such as bruising, *petechiae* (small purple or red spots caused by a broken blood vessel), and *purpura* (larger red or purple spots caused by bleeding under the skin), can indicate serious

systemic diseases in children (e.g., leukemia, meningococcemia).

OLDER ADULTS

- The overall effectiveness of blood vessels decreases as smooth muscle cells are replaced by connective tissue. The lower extremities are more likely to show signs of arterial and venous impairment because of the more distal and dependent position.
- Proximal arteries become thinner and dilate.
- Peripheral arteries become thicker and dilate less effectively because of arteriosclerotic changes in the vessel walls.
- Blood vessels lengthen and become more tortuous and prominent. Varicosities occur more frequently.

- In some instances, arteries may be palpated more easily because of loss of the supportive surrounding tissues. Often, however, the most distal pulses of the lower extremities are more difficult to palpate because of decreased arterial perfusion.
- Systolic and diastolic blood pressures may increase. See Chapter 29 for Canadian guidelines for measurement of blood pressure, follow-up, and lifestyle counselling.
- Peripheral edema is frequently observed and is most commonly the result of chronic venous insufficiency or low protein levels in the blood (hypoproteinemia).
- Carotid artery assessment is an essential aspect of peripheral vascular examination in the older adult.

Breasts and Axillae

The breasts of both men and women need to be inspected and palpated. Men have some glandular tissue beneath each nipple, a potential site for malignancy, whereas mature women have glandular tissue throughout the breast. In females, the largest portion of glandular breast tissue is located in the upper outer quadrant of each breast. From this quadrant, there is a projection of breast tissue into the axilla, called the **axillary tail of Spence** (Figure 28.31). The majority of breast tumours are located in this upper outer breast quadrant and in the tail of Spence. During assessment, the nurse can localize specific findings by using this division of the breast into quadrants and the axillary tail.

Skill 28.14 describes a nursing assessment of breasts and axillae (see also the Lifespan Considerations box on assessing breasts and axillae on page 661).

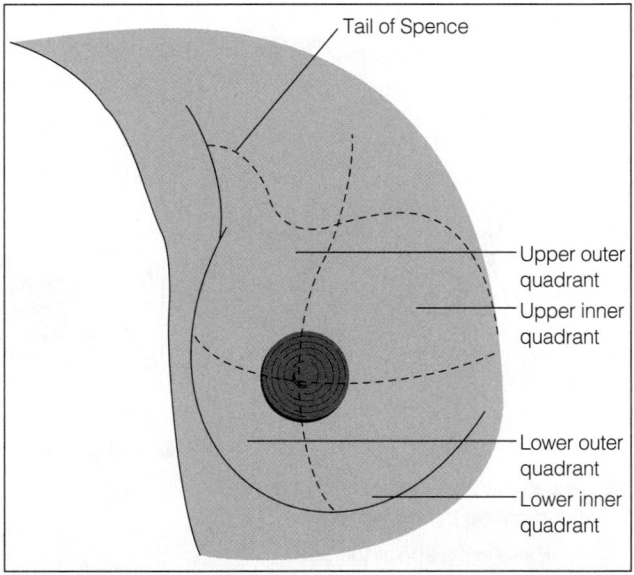

FIGURE 28.31 Four breast quadrants and the axillary tail of Spence.

SKILL 28.14 ASSESSING BREASTS AND AXILLAE

PLANNING

Equipment: Centimetre ruler

IMPLEMENTATION

Performance

1. Before performing the procedure, introduce yourself and verify the client's identity using two identifiers or per agency protocol. Explain to the client what you are going to do, why it is necessary, and how he or she can participate. Inquire

whether the client has ever had a clinical breast exam. Discuss how the results will be used in planning further care or treatments.

2. Perform hand hygiene, and follow other appropriate infection prevention and control procedures.

3. Provide for client privacy.

4. Inquire whether the client has a history of breast masses and what was done about them; pain or tenderness in the breasts and relation to the woman's menstrual cycle; discharge from the nipple; medication history (some

(continued)

medications, e.g., oral contraceptives, steroids, digitalis, and diuretics, can cause nipple discharge; estrogen replacement therapy may be associated with the development of cysts or cancer); risk factors that may be associated with development of breast cancer (e.g., mother, sister, aunt with breast cancer; alcohol consumption, high-fat diet, obesity, use of oral contraceptives, menarche before age 12 years, menopause after age 55 years, age 30 years or older at first pregnancy, or never having been pregnant). Inquire whether the client monitors the look and feel of her breasts and notes the normal changes in relation to her menstrual cycle.

Assessment	Normal Findings	Deviations from Normal
5. Inspect breasts for size, symmetry, and contour or shape while the client is in the sitting position.	*Females:* Rounded shape; slightly un-equal in size; generally symmetrical *Males:* Breasts even with the chest wall; if obese, may be similar in shape to female breasts	Recent change in breast size; swell-ings; marked asymmetry
6. Inspect the skin of the breast for localized discolorations or hyperpig-mentation, retraction or dimpling, localized hypervascular areas, swell-ing, or edema (see ❶).	Skin uniform in colour (same in appear-ance as skin of abdomen or back); skin smooth and intact; diffuse symmetric horizontal or vertical vascular pattern in light-skinned people; *striae* (stretch marks); moles and nevi	Localized discolorations or hyperpig-mentation; retraction or dimpling (result of scar tissue or an invasive tumour); unilateral, localized hypervascular areas (associated with increased blood flow); swelling or edema appearing as "pig skin" or "orange peel" because of exaggeration of the pores

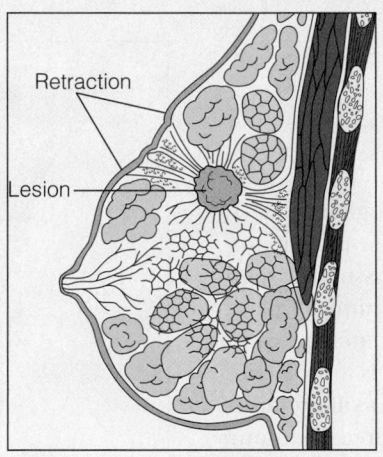

❶ A lesion causing retraction of the skin.

7. Accentuate any retraction by having the client do the following:
- Raise arms above the head.
- Push hands together, with elbows flexed (see ❷).
- Press hands down on hips (see ❸).

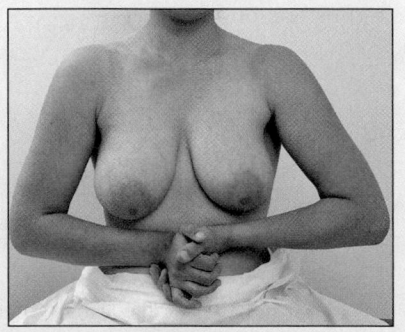

❷ Pushing hands together to accentuate retraction of breast tissues.

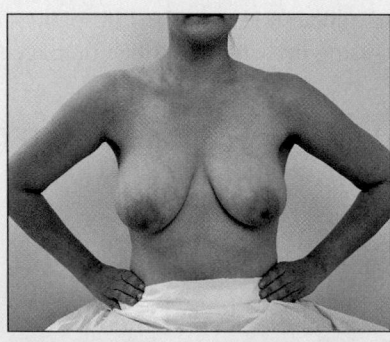

❸ Pressing hands down on hips to accentuate retraction of breast tissue.

Assessment	Normal Findings	Deviations from Normal
8. Inspect the areola area for size, shape, symmetry, colour, surface characteristics, and any masses or lesions.	Round or oval and bilaterally the same; colour varies widely, from light pink to dark brown; irregular placement of sebaceous glands on the surface of the areola (Montgomery's tubercles)	Any asymmetry, mass, or lesion
9. Inspect nipples for size, shape, position, colour, discharge, and lesions.	Round, everted, and equal in size; similar in colour; soft and smooth; both nipples point in same direction (out in young women and men, downward in older women); no discharge, except from pregnant or breast-feeding females; inversion of one or both nipples that is present from puberty	Asymmetrical size and colour; presence of discharge, crusts, or cracks; recent inversion of one or both nipples
10. Palpate the axillary, subclavicular, and supraclavicular lymph nodes (see ❹) while the client sits with arms abducted and supported on the nurse's forearm. For palpation of clavicular lymph nodes, see Skill 28.10 (p. 635). Use the flat surfaces of all fingertips to palpate the four areas of the axilla:	No tenderness, masses, or nodules	Tenderness, masses, or nodules

- The edge of the musculus pectoralis major (greater pectoral muscle) along the anterior axillary line
- The thoracic wall in the midaxillary area
- The upper part of the humerus
- The anterior edge of the latissimus dorsi muscle along the posterior axillary line

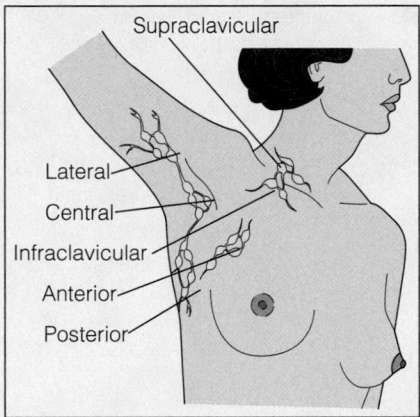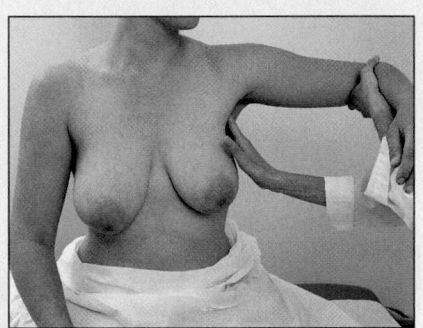

❹ Location and palpation of lymph nodes that drain the lateral breast: **A:** Lymph nodes; **B:** palpating the axilla.

Assessment	Normal Findings	Deviations from Normal
11. Palpate the breast for masses, tenderness, and any discharge from the nipples. Palpation of the breast is generally performed while the client is supine. **Rationale: In the supine position, the breasts flatten evenly against the chest wall, facilitating palpation.**	No tenderness, masses, nodules, or nipple discharge	Tenderness, masses, nodules, or nipple discharge

- For clients who have a past history of breast masses, who are at high risk for breast cancer, or who have pendulous breasts, examination in both supine and sitting positions is recommended.
- If the client reports a breast lump, start with the rest of the breast to obtain baseline data that will serve as a comparison to the reportedly involved breast.
- To enhance flattening of the breast, instruct the client to abduct the arm and place her hand behind her head. Then place a small pillow or rolled towel under the client's shoulder.

(continued)

SKILL 28.14 ASSESSING BREASTS AND AXILLAE *(continued)*

Assessment	Normal Findings	Deviations from Normal

Assessment

- For palpation, use the palmar surface of the middle three fingertips (held together) and make a gentle rotary motion on the breast.
- Choose one of three patterns for palpation:
  a. Hands of the clock or spokes on wheel (see ❺)
  b. Concentric circles (see ❻)

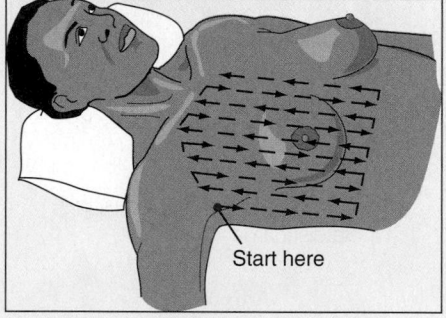

  c. Vertical strips pattern (see ❼)
- Start at one point for palpation, and move systematically to the end point to ensure that all breast surfaces are assessed.
- Pay particular attention to the upper outer quadrant area and the tail of Spence.

Start here

❼ Vertical strips pattern of breast palpation.

12. Palpate the areola and nipples for masses. Compress each nipple to determine the presence of any discharge. If discharge is present, milk the breast along its radius to identify the discharge-producing lobe. Assess any discharge for amount, colour, consistency, and odour. Note also any tenderness on palpation.

13. Document your findings in the client record by using forms or checklists supplemented by narrative notes, when appropriate.

Normal Findings

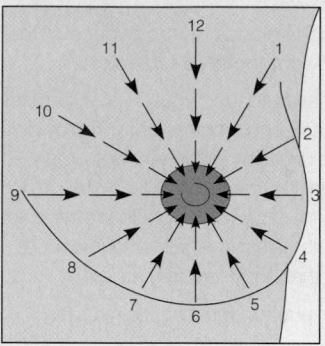

❺ Hands-of-the-clock or spokes-on-a-wheel pattern of breast palpation.

No tenderness, masses, nodules, or nipple discharge

Deviations from Normal

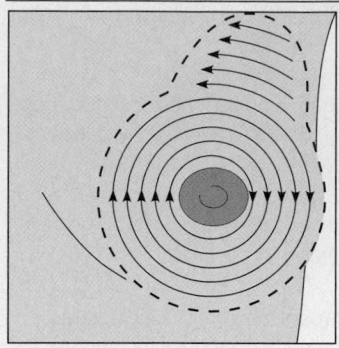

❻ Concentric circles pattern for breast palpation.

If you detect a mass, record the following data:

a. *Location:* The exact location relative to the quadrants and axillary tail, or the clock (as in ❺), and the distance from the nipple in centimetres

b. *Size:* The length, width, and thickness of the mass in centimetres. If you are able to determine the discrete edges, record this fact

c. *Shape:* Whether the mass is round, oval, lobulated, indistinct, or irregular

d. *Consistency:* Whether the mass is hard or soft

e. *Mobility:* Whether the mass is movable or fixed

f. *Skin over the lump:* Whether it is reddened, dimpled, or retracted

g. *Nipple:* Whether it is displaced or retracted

h. *Tenderness:* Whether palpation is painful to the client

Tenderness, masses, nodules, or nipple discharge

EVALUATION

- Perform a detailed follow-up examination based on findings that deviated from expected or normal for the client. Relate findings to previous assessment data, if available.

- Report significant deviations from normal to the appropriate members of the health care team.

LIFESPAN CONSIDERATIONS

Assessing the Breasts and Axillae

INFANTS

- Newborns, both boys and girls, up to 2 weeks of age may have breast enlargement and *galactorrhea* (white discharge from the nipples or neonatal milk).

- *Supernumerary* (extra) nipples are present infrequently as small dimples along the mammary chain; these may be associated with renal anomalies.

PREADOLESCENTS AND ADOLESCENTS

- Female breast development begins between ages 8 and 13 years and occurs in five stages. Development may be asymmetrical.

  Stage 1 Prepubertal with no noticeable change

  Stage 2 Breast bud with elevation of nipple and enlargement of the areola

  Stage 3 Enlargement of the breast and areola; nipple flush with the breast surface

Stage 4 Projection of the areola and nipple forming a secondary mound over the breast

Stage 5 Recession of areola in most women by about age 14 or 15 years, leaving only the nipple projecting

- Boys can develop breast buds and have slight enlargement of the areola in early adolescence. Gynecomastia (further enlargement of breast tissue) can occur. This growth is transient, usually lasting about 2 years, resolving completely by late puberty.

- Axillary hair usually appears by age 13 years and is related to adrenal rather than gonadal changes.

PREGNANT FEMALES

- Breast, areola, and nipple sizes increase.

- The areolae and nipples darken; nipples may become more erect; areolae contain small, scattered, elevated Montgomery's glands.

- Superficial veins become more prominent and jagged linear stretch marks may develop.

- *Colostrum* (a thick yellow fluid) may be expressed from the nipples after the first trimester.

OLDER ADULTS

- In the postmenopausal female, breasts change in shape and often appear pendulous or flaccid; breasts lack the firmness they had in younger years.

- The presence of breast lesions may be detected more readily because of the decrease in connective tissue.

- General breast size remains the same. Although glandular tissue atrophies, the amount of fat in breasts (predominantly in the lower quadrants) increases in most women.

Abdomen

The nurse locates and describes abdominal findings in a client by using two common methods of subdividing the abdomen: *quadrants* and *regions*. To divide the abdomen into quadrants, the nurse imagines two lines: (a) a vertical line from the xiphoid process to the pubic symphysis, and (b) a horizontal line across the umbilicus (Figure 28.32). These quadrants are labelled right upper quadrant (1), left upper quadrant (2), right lower quadrant (3), and left lower quadrant (4). Using the second method, division into nine regions, the nurse imagines two vertical lines that extend superiorly from the midpoints of the inguinal ligaments, and two horizontal lines, one at the level of the edge of the lower ribs and the other at the level of the iliac crests (Figure 28.33). Specific organs or parts of organs lie in each abdominal region. See Table 28.10 and Table 28.11 on the next two pages.

In addition, practitioners often use certain landmarks to locate abdominal signs and symptoms. These are the xiphoid process of the sternum, the costal margins, the midline (a line drawn from the tip of the sternum through the umbilicus to the pubic symphysis), the anterosuperior iliac spine, the inguinal ligaments (Poupart's

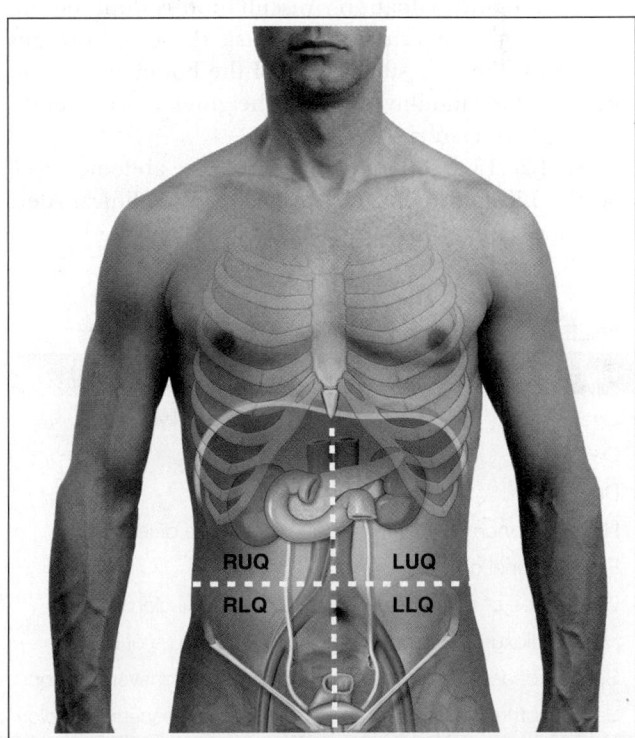

FIGURE 28.32 The four abdominal quadrants and the underlying organs: **1,** Right upper quadrant (RUQ); **2,** Left upper quadrant (LUQ); **3,** Right lower quadrant (RLQ); **4,** Left lower quadrant (LLQ).

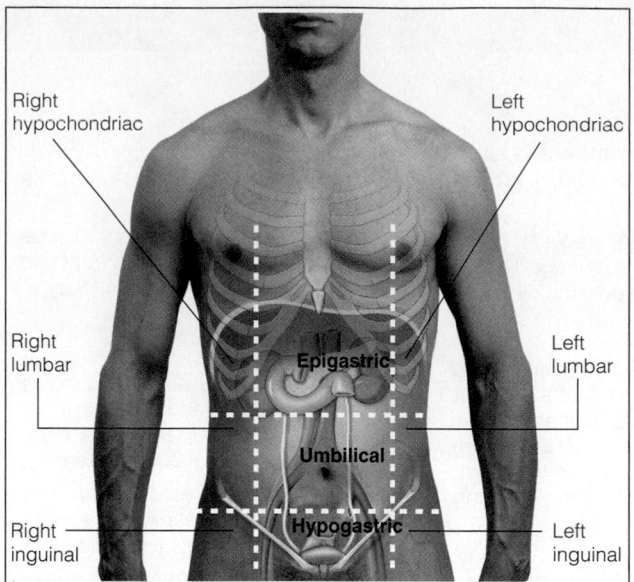

FIGURE 28.33 The nine abdominal regions: epigastric; left and right hypochondriac; umbilical; left and right lumbar; hypogastric (pubic); left and right inguinal or iliac.

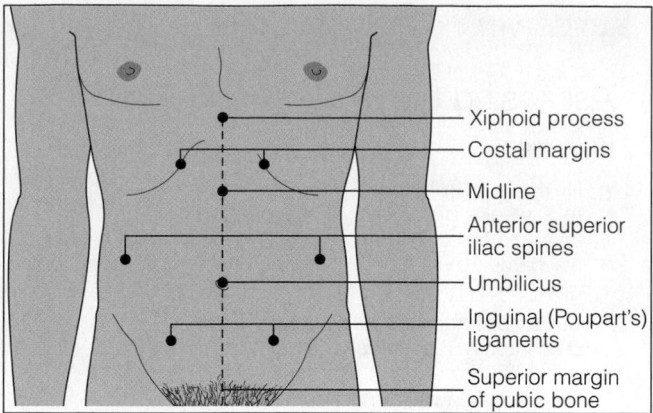

FIGURE 28.34 Landmarks commonly used to identify abdominal areas.

> **! CLINICAL ALERT**
>
> If abdominal distension is observed on inspection, evaluation of the abdominal girth is necessary. Place a measuring tape around the abdomen at the level of the umbilicus. Mark the location of the measuring tape so that additional measurements can be taken in the same location.

ligaments), and the superior margin of the pubic symphysis (Figure 28.34).

Assessment of the abdomen involves all four methods of examination (inspection, auscultation, palpation, and percussion). When assessing the abdomen, the nurse performs inspection first, followed by auscultation, percussion, and palpation. Auscultation is done before palpation and percussion because these techniques cause movement or stimulation of the bowel, which can increase bowel motility and, thus, heighten bowel sounds, creating false results.

Skill 28.15 describes how to assess the abdomen (see also the Lifespan Considerations box and Clinical Alert box on assessing the abdomen that follows).

Musculoskeletal System

The musculoskeletal system encompasses the muscles, bones, and joints. The completeness of an assessment of this system depends largely on the needs and problems of the individual client. The nurse usually assesses the musculoskeletal system for muscle strength, tone, size, and symmetry of muscle development, fasciculations, and tremors. A **fasciculation** is an abnormal *contraction* (shortening) of a bundle of muscle fibres. A **tremor** is an involuntary

TABLE 28.10 Organs in the Four Abdominal Quadrants

Right Upper Quadrant	Left Upper Quadrant	Left Lower Quadrant	Right Lower Quadrant
Liver	Left lobe of liver	Lower lobe of left kidney	Lower lobe of right kidney
Gallbladder	Stomach	Sigmoid colon	Cecum
Duodenum	Spleen	Section of descending colon	Appendix
Head of pancreas	Upper lobe of left kidney	Left ovary	Section of ascending colon
Right adrenal gland	Pancreas	Left fallopian tube	Right ovary
Upper lobe of right kidney	Left adrenal gland	Left ureter	Right fallopian tube
Hepatic flexure of colon	Splenic flexure of colon	Left spermatic cord	Right ureter
Section of ascending colon	Section of transverse colon	Part of uterus	Right spermatic cord
Section of transverse colon	Section of descending colon		Part of uterus

TABLE 28.11   Organs in the Nine Abdominal Regions

Right Hypochondriac	Right Inguinal	Umbilical	Splenic flexure of colon
Right lobe of liver	Cecum	Omentum	Upper half of left kidney
Gallbladder	Appendix	Mesentery	Suprarenal gland
Part of duodenum	Lower end of ileum	Lower part of duodenum	
Hepatic flexure of colon	Right ureter	Part of jejunum and ileum	
Upper half of right kidney	Right spermatic cord		
Suprarenal gland	Right ovary		

Right Lumbar	Epigastric	Hypogastric (Pubic)	Left Lumbar
Ascending colon	Aorta	Ileum	Descending colon
Lower half of right kidney	Pyloric end of stomach	Bladder	Lower half of left kidney
Part of duodenum and jejunum	Part of duodenum	Uterus	Part of jejunum and ileum
	Pancreas		
	Part of liver		

		Left Hypochondriac	Left Inguinal
		Stomach	Sigmoid colon
		Spleen	Left ureter
		Tail of pancreas	Left spermatic cord
			Left ovary

SKILL 28.15   ASSESSING THE ABDOMEN

PLANNING

- Ask the client to urinate, since an empty bladder makes the assessment more comfortable.
- Ensure that the room is warm, as the client will be exposed.

Equipment

- Examining light
- Tape measure (metal, paper, or unstretchable cloth)
- Water-soluble skin-marking pencil
- Stethoscope

IMPLEMENTATION

Performance

1. Before performing the procedure, introduce yourself and verify the client's identity using two identifiers or per agency protocol. Explain to the client what you are going to do, why it is necessary, and how he or she can participate. Discuss how the results will be used in planning further care or treatments.

2. Perform hand hygiene, and follow other appropriate infection prevention control procedures.

3. Provide for client privacy.

4. Inquire whether the client has any history of the following: incidence of abdominal pain; its location, onset, sequence, and chronology; its quality (description); its frequency; associated symptoms (e.g., nausea, vomiting, diarrhea); bowel habits; incidence of constipation or diarrhea (have client describe what client means by these terms); change in appetite, food intolerances, and foods ingested in last 24 hours; specific signs and symptoms (e.g., heartburn, flatulence or belching, difficulty swallowing, *hematemesis*—vomiting blood—blood or mucus in stools, and aggravating and alleviating factors); previous problems and treatment (e.g., stomach ulcer, gallbladder surgery, history of jaundice).

5. Assist the client to the supine position, with the arms placed comfortably at the sides. Place small pillows beneath the knees and the head to reduce tension in the abdominal muscles. Expose only the client's abdomen from the chest line to the pubic area to avoid chilling and shivering, which can tense the abdominal muscles.

Assessment	Normal Findings	Deviations from Normal
Inspection of the Abdomen		
6. Inspect the abdomen for skin integrity (refer to the discussion on skin assessment, earlier in this chapter).	Unblemished skin; uniform colour; silver-white striae (stretch marks) or surgical scars	Presence of rash or other lesions; tense, glistening skin (may indicate *ascites*—an accumulation of fluid in the peritoneal cavity—and edema); purple striae (associated with Cushing's disease or rapid weight gain and loss)

(continued)

SKILL 28.15 ASSESSING THE ABDOMEN (*continued*)

Assessment	Normal Findings	Deviations from Normal
7. Inspect the abdomen for contour and symmetry:		
• Observe the abdominal contour (profile line from the rib margin to the pubic bone) while standing at the client's side, with the client in the supine position.	Flat, rounded (convex), or scaphoid (concave)	Distended
• Ask the client to take a deep breath and to hold it. **Rationale: This makes an enlarged liver or spleen more obvious.**	No evidence of enlargement of liver or spleen	Evidence of enlargement of liver or spleen
• Assess the symmetry of contour while standing at the foot of the examination table.	Symmetrical contour	Asymmetrical contour (e.g., localized protrusions around umbilicus, inguinal ligaments, or scars, which can be caused by a hernia or tumour)
• If distension is present, measure the abdominal girth by placing a tape around the abdomen at the level of the umbilicus (see ❶).		

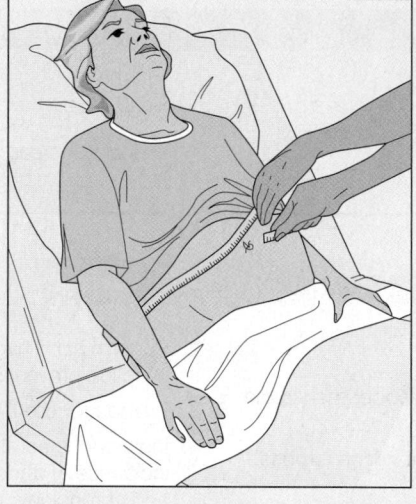

❶ Measuring abdominal girth.

Assessment	Normal Findings	Deviations from Normal
8. Observe abdominal movements associated with respiration, peristalsis, or aortic pulsations.	Symmetrical movements caused by respiration; visible peristalsis in very lean people; aortic pulsations in thin persons at epigastric area	Limited movement because of pain or disease process; visible peristalsis in heavier clients (possible bowel obstruction); marked aortic pulsations
9. Observe the vascular pattern.	No visible vascular pattern	Visible venous pattern (dilated veins) is associated with liver disease, ascites, and venocaval obstruction

Auscultation of the Abdomen

Assessment	Normal Findings	Deviations from Normal
10. Auscultate the abdomen for bowel sounds, vascular sounds, and peritoneal friction rubs. Warm your hands and the stethoscope diaphragms. **Rationale: Cold hands and a cold stethoscope may cause the client's abdominal muscles to contract, and these contractions may be heard during auscultation.**	Audible bowel sounds; absence of arterial bruits; absence of friction rub	Hypoactive (i.e., extremely soft and infrequent—one per minute), which can indicate decreased motility and are usually associated with manipulation of the bowel during surgery, inflammation, paralytic ileus, or late bowel obstruction; hyperactive or increased (i.e., high-pitched, loud, rushing sounds that occur frequently—every 3 seconds), also known as **borborygmi**; hyperactive bowel sounds indicate increased intestinal motility and are usually associated with diarrhea, early bowel obstruction, or the use of laxatives; true absence of sounds (none heard in 3 to 5 minutes) indicates cessation of intestinal motility; loud bruit over aortic area (possible aneurysm); bruit over renal or iliac arteries

For Bowel Sounds

• Use the flat-disc diaphragm. **Rationale: Intestinal sounds are relatively high pitched and best accentuated by the diaphragm. Light pressure with the stethoscope is adequate.**

Assessment	Normal Findings	Deviations from Normal

- Ask when the client last ate. **Rationale: Shortly after or long after eating, bowel sounds can normally increase.**

  They are loudest when a meal is long overdue. Four to seven hours after a meal, bowel sounds may be heard continuously over the ileo-cecal valve area while the digestive contents from the small intestine empty through the valve into the large intestine.

- Place diaphragm of the stethoscope in each of the four quadrants of the abdomen over all of the auscultatory sites shown in ❷. Listen for active bowel sounds.

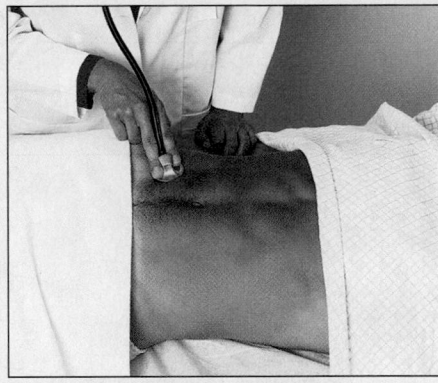

❷ Auscultating the abdomen for bowel sounds.

Irregular gurgling noises occurring about every 5 to 20 seconds. The duration of a single sound may range from less than a second to more than several seconds.

For Vascular Sounds
- Use the bell of the stethoscope over the aorta, renal arteries, iliac arteries, and femoral arteries (see ❸).
- Listen for bruits.

Peritoneal Friction Rubs
- Peritoneal friction rubs are rough, grating sounds like those produced by rubbing two pieces of leather together. Friction rubs may be caused by inflammation, infections, or abnormal growths.

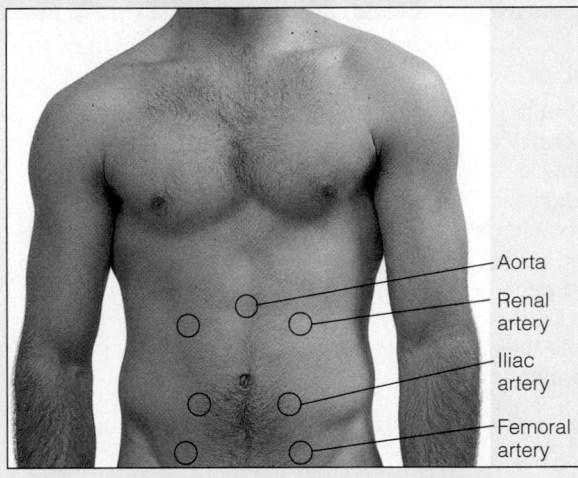

Aorta
Renal artery
Iliac artery
Femoral artery

❸ Sites for auscultating for vascular sounds.

Percussion of the Abdomen
11. Percuss several areas in each of the four quadrants to determine presence of tympany (gas in stomach and intestines) and dullness (decrease, absence, or flatness of resonance over solid masses or fluid). Use a systematic pattern: begin in the lower left quadrant, proceed to the lower right quadrant, the upper right quadrant, and the upper left quadrant (see ❹).

Tympany over the stomach and gas-filled bowels; dullness, especially over the liver and spleen, or a full bladder

Large dull areas (associated with presence of fluid or a tumour)

Percussion of the Liver
12. Percuss the liver to determine its size. Begin in the right MCL below the level of the umbilicus and proceed as follows:

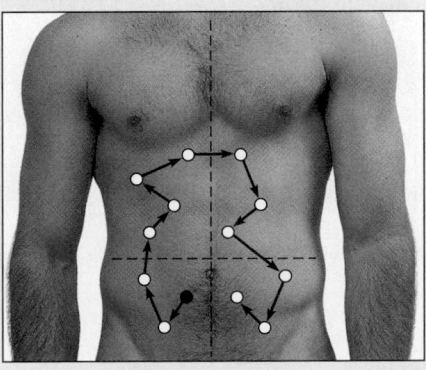

❹ Systematic percussion sites for all four quadrants.

(continued)

SKILL 28.15   ASSESSING THE ABDOMEN (continued)

Assessment	Normal Findings	Deviations from Normal
• Percuss upward over tympanic areas until a dull percussion sound indicates the lower liver border. Mark the site with a skin-marking pencil (see ❺).	6 cm to 12 cm in the MCL 4 cm to 8 cm at the midsternal line	Enlarged size (associated with liver disease)

• Then, percuss downward at the right MCL, beginning from an area of lung resonance and progressing downward until a dull percussion sound indicates the upper liver border (usually at the fifth to seventh interspace). Mark this site.

• Measure the distance between the two marks (upper and lower liver border) in centimetres to establish the liver span or size.

• Repeat these steps at the midsternal line.

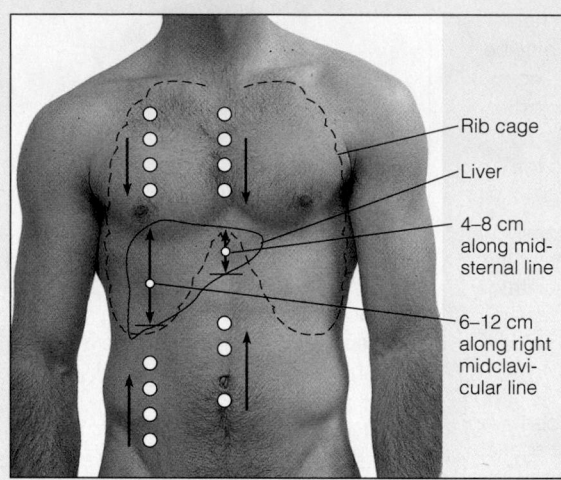

❺ Percussion pattern to determine liver size.

Labels on image: Rib cage; Liver; 4–8 cm along mid-sternal line; 6–12 cm along right midclavicular line

Palpation of the Abdomen

13. Perform light palpation first to detect areas of tenderness or muscle guarding. Systematically explore all four quadrants. Ensure that the client's position is appropriate for relaxation of the abdominal muscles, and warm your hands. **Rationale: Cold hands can elicit muscle tension and thus impede palpatory evaluation.**

No tenderness; relaxed abdomen with smooth, consistent tension

Tenderness and hypersensitivity; superficial masses; localized areas of increased tension

Light Palpation

• Hold the palm of your hand slightly above the client's abdomen, with your fingers parallel to the abdomen.

• Depress the abdominal wall lightly, about 1 cm or to the depth of the subcutaneous tissue, with the pads of your fingers (see ❻).

• Move the finger pads in a slight circular motion.

• Note areas of tenderness or superficial pain, masses, and muscle guarding. To determine areas of tenderness, ask the client to tell you about them, and watch for changes in the client's facial expressions.

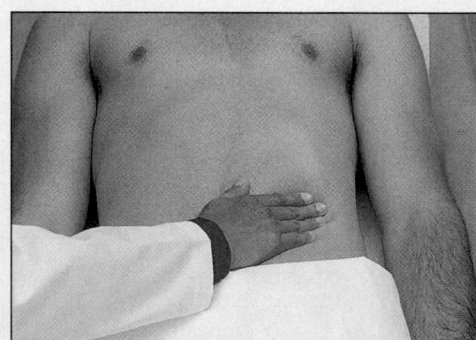

❻ Light palpation of the abdomen.

• If the client is excessively ticklish, begin by pressing your hand on top of the client's hand while pressing lightly. Then, slide your hand off the client's and onto the abdomen to continue the examination.

Assessment	Normal Findings	Deviations from Normal
14. If deep palpation is required, then follow this step: *Note:* Deep palpation is not usually part of a general health assessment unless there are abnormalities found on light palpation; some agencies only allow experienced nurses or physicians to perform deep palpation as it can be risky to organs if not performed correctly.	Tenderness may be present near xiphoid process, over cecum, and over sigmoid colon	Generalized or localized areas of tenderness; mobile or fixed masses

- Palpate sensitive areas last.

- Press the distal half of the palmar surface of the fingers of one hand into the abdominal wall, *or* use the bimanual method of palpation discussed earlier in this chapter.

- Depress the abdominal wall about 4 cm to 5 cm (see ❼).

- Note masses and the structure of underlying contents. If a mass is present, determine its size, location, mobility, contour, consistency, and tenderness. Normal abdominal structures that can be mistaken for masses include the lateral borders of the rectus abdominis muscles, the feces-filled colon, the aorta, and the uterus.

- Check for rebound tenderness in areas where the client complains of pain. With one hand, press slowly and deeply over the area indicated and then lift the hand quickly. If the client does not complain of pain during the deep pressure but indicates pain at the release of the pressure, rebound tenderness is present. This can indicate peritoneal inflammation and should be reported to the primary health care provider immediately.

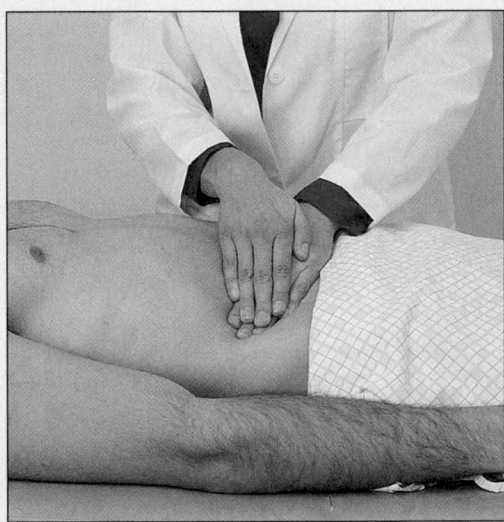

❼ Deep palpation of the abdomen.

Palpation of the Liver

15. Palpate the liver to detect enlargement and tenderness. Two bimanual approaches are used in palpation of the liver. In using the first method, place one hand along the anterior rib cage and the other hand on the posterior rib cage.	May not be palpable; border feels smooth	Enlarged (abnormal finding, even if liver is smooth and not tender); smooth but tender; nodular or hard

- Stand on the client's right side.

- Place your left hand on the posterior thorax at about the 11th or 12th rib. This hand is used to push upward and provide support of underlying structures for the subsequent anterior palpation.

(continued)

SKILL 28.15   ASSESSING THE ABDOMEN (continued)

Assessment	Normal Findings	Deviations from Normal
• Place your right hand along the rib cage at about a 45-degree angle to the right of the rectus abdominis muscle or parallel to the rectus muscle with the fingers pointing toward the rib cage (see ❽). • While the client exhales, exert a gradual and gentle downward and forward pressure beneath the costal margin until you reach a depth of 4 cm to 5 cm. **Rationale: During expiration, the abdominal wall relaxes, facilitating deep palpation.** • Maintain your hand position, and ask the client to inhale deeply. **Rationale: This makes the liver border descend and moves the liver into a palpable position.** • While the client inhales, feel the liver border move against your hand. It should feel firm and have a regular contour. If you do not palpate the liver initially, ask the client to take two or three more deep breaths while you maintain or apply slightly more palpation pressure. The liver is harder to palpate in obese, tense, or very physically fit people. • If the liver is enlarged (i.e., palpable below the costal margin), measure the number of centimetres it extends below the costal region. A second method is the bimanual palpation method discussed previously, in which one hand is superimposed on the other (see Figure 28.2, p. 600). The techniques and principles used for palpating the liver with one hand apply to the two-hand method as well.	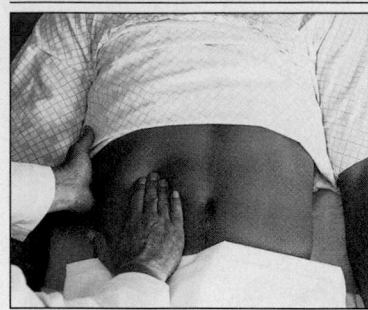 ❽ Palpating the liver. 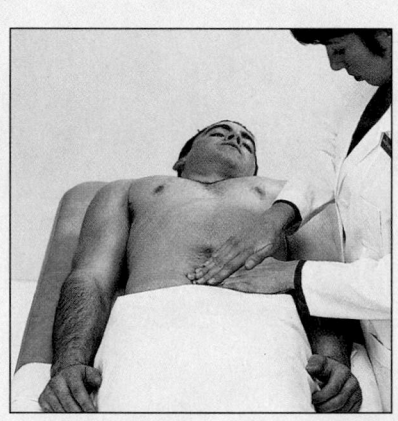 ❾ Palpating the bladder.	

Palpation of the Bladder

16. Palpate the area above the pubic symphysis if the client's history indicates possible urinary retention (see ❾).	Not palpable	Distended and palpable as smooth, round, tense mass (indicates urinary retention)

17. Document your findings in the client record by using forms or checklists supplemented by narrative notes, when appropriate.

EVALUATION

• Perform a detailed follow-up examination of other systems based on findings that deviated from expected or normal for the client. Relate findings to previous assessment data, if available.

• Report significant deviations from normal to the appropriate members of the health care team.

LIFESPAN CONSIDERATIONS

Assessing the Abdomen

INFANTS

- Internal organs of newborns and infants are proportionately larger than those of older children and adults, so their abdomens are rounded and tend to protrude.
- The infant's liver may be palpable 1 cm to 2 cm below the right costal margin.
- Umbilical hernias may be present at birth.

CHILDREN

- Toddlers have a characteristic "pot belly" appearance, which can persist until age 3 to 4 years.
- Late-preschool-age and school-age children are leaner and have a flat abdomen.
- Peristaltic waves may be more visible than in adults.
- Children may not be able to pinpoint areas of tenderness; by observing facial expressions the examiner can determine areas of maximum tenderness.
- The liver is relatively larger than in adults. It can be palpated 1 cm to 2 cm below the right costal margin.

- If the child is ticklish, guarding, or fearful, use a task that requires concentration (such as squeezing the hands together) to distract the child, or have the child place his or her hands on yours as you palpate the abdomen, "helping" you to do the exam.

OLDER ADULTS

- The rounded abdomens of older adults are caused by an increase in adipose tissue and a decrease in muscle tone.
- The abdominal wall is slacker and thinner, making palpation easier and more accurate than in younger clients. Muscle wasting and loss of fibroconnective tissue occur with aging.
- The pain threshold in older adults is often higher; major abdominal problems, such as appendicitis or other acute emergencies, may therefore go undetected.
- Gastrointestinal pain needs to be differentiated from cardiac pain. Gastrointestinal pain may be located in the chest or abdomen, whereas cardiac pain is usually located in the chest. Factors aggravating gastrointestinal pain are usually related to

either ingestion or lack of food intake; gastrointestinal pain is usually relieved by antacids, food, or assuming an upright position. Common factors that can aggravate cardiac pain are activity or anxiety; rest or nitroglycerine relieves cardiac pain.
- Stool passes through the intestines at a slower rate in older adults, and the perception of stimuli that produce the urge to defecate often diminishes.
- Fecal incontinence can occur in confused or neurologically impaired older adults.
- Many older adults erroneously believe that the absence of a daily bowel movement signifies constipation. When assessing for constipation, the nurse must consider the client's diet, activity, medications, and characteristics and ease of passage of feces as well as the frequency of bowel movements.
- The incidence of colon cancer is higher among older adults than younger adults. Symptoms include a change in bowel function, rectal bleeding, and weight loss. Changes in bowel function, however, are associated with many factors, such as diet, exercise, and medications.

trembling of a limb or body part. Tremors may involve large groups of muscle fibres or small bundles of muscle fibres. An **intention tremor** becomes more apparent when an individual attempts a voluntary movement, such as holding a cup of coffee. A **resting tremor** is more apparent when the client is at rest and it diminishes with activity.

Bones are assessed for normal form. Joints are assessed for tenderness, swelling, thickening, *crepitation*

(the sound of bone grating on bone), presence of nodules, and range of motion. Body posture is assessed for normal standing and sitting positions. For information about body posture, see Chapter 39.

Skill 28.16 describes how to assess the musculoskeletal system (see also the Lifespan Considerations box on assessing the musculoskeletal system on page 672).

SKILL 28.16 ASSESSING THE MUSCULOSKELETAL SYSTEM

PLANNING

Equipment:

- Goniometer
- Tape measure

IMPLEMENTATION

Performance

1. Before performing the procedure, introduce yourself and verify the client's identity using two identifiers or per agency protocol. Explain to the client what you are

going to do, why it is necessary, and how he or she can participate. Discuss how the results will be used in planning further care or treatments.

2. Perform hand hygiene, and follow other appropriate infection prevention and control procedures.

3. Provide for client privacy.

4. Inquire whether the client has any history of the following: presence of muscle pain: onset, location, character, associated phenomena (e.g., redness and swelling of joints), and aggravating and alleviating factors; limitations to movement or inability to perform activities of daily living; previous sports injuries; loss of function without pain.

(continued)

SKILL 28.16 **ASSESSING THE MUSCULOSKELETAL SYSTEM** (*continued*)

Assessment	Normal Findings	Deviations from Normal
Muscles		
5. Inspect muscles for size. Compare the muscles on one side of the body (e.g., of the arm, thigh, and calf) to the same muscles on the other side. To identify any discrepancies, measure muscles with a tape.	Equal size on both sides of body	*Atrophy* (a decrease in size) or *hypertrophy* (an increase in size), asymmetry
6. Inspect muscles and tendons for *contractures* (shortening).	No contractures	Malposition of body part, such as *foot drop* (foot flexed downward)
7. Inspect muscles for tremors, for example, by having the client hold the arms out in front of the body.	No tremors	Presence of tremor
8. Palpate muscles at rest to determine muscle tonicity (the normal condition of tension, or tone, of a muscle at rest).	Normally firm	Atonic (lacking tone)
9. Palpate muscles while the client is active and when passive for flaccidity, spasticity, and smoothness of movement.	Smooth coordinated movements	*Flaccidity* (weakness or laxness) or *spasticity* (sudden involuntary muscle contraction)
10. Test muscle strength. Compare the right side with the left side.	Equal strength on each body side	25% or less of normal strength
Sternocleidomastoid: The client turns the head to one side against the resistance of your hand. Repeat with the other side.		**Grading Muscle Strength**
Trapezius: The client shrugs the shoulders against the resistance of your hands.		0: 0% of normal strength; complete paralysis
		1: 10% of normal strength; no movement, contraction of muscle is palpable or visible
Deltoid: The client holds arm up and resists while you try to push it down.		2: 25% of normal strength; full muscle movement against gravity, with support
Biceps: The client fully extends each arm and tries to flex it while you attempt to hold arm in extension.		3: 50% of normal strength; normal movement against gravity
Triceps: The client flexes each arm and then tries to extend it against your attempt to keep arm in flexion.		4: 75% of normal strength; normal full movement against gravity and against minimal resistance
Wrist and finger muscles: The client spreads the fingers and resists as you attempt to push the fingers together.		5: 100% of normal strength; normal full movement against gravity and against full resistance
Grip strength: The client grasps your index and middle fingers while you try to pull your fingers from the client's grasp.		
Hip muscles: The client is supine, both legs extended; client raises one leg at a time while you attempt to hold it down.		
Hip abduction: The client is supine, both legs extended. Place your hands on the lateral surface of each knee; the client spreads the legs apart against your resistance.		

Assessment	Normal Findings	Deviations from Normal

Hip adduction: The client is in same position as for hip abduction. Place your hands between the knees; the client brings the legs together against your resistance.

Hamstrings: The client is supine, with both knees bent. The client resists while you attempt to straighten the legs.

Quadriceps: The client is supine, knee partially extended; the client resists while you attempt to flex the knee.

Muscles of the ankles and feet: The client resists while you attempt to dorsiflex the foot and again resists while you attempt to flex the foot.

Bones

11. Inspect the skeleton for structure.	No deformities	Bones misaligned
12. Palpate bones to locate any areas of edema or tenderness.	No tenderness or swelling	Presence of tenderness or swelling (may indicate fracture, neoplasms, or osteoporosis)

Joints

13. Inspect joints for swelling. Palpate each joint for tenderness, smoothness of movement, swelling, crepitation, and presence of nodules.	No tenderness, swelling, crepitation, or nodules; joints move smoothly	One or more swollen joints; presence of tenderness, swelling, crepitation, or nodules
14. Assess joint range of motion. See Chapter 39 for the types of joint movements.	Varies to some degree in accordance with person's genetic makeup and degree of physical activity	Limited range of motion in one or more joints

- Ask the client to move selected body parts. The amount of joint movement can be measured by a goniometer, a device that measures the angle of the joint in degrees (see ❶).

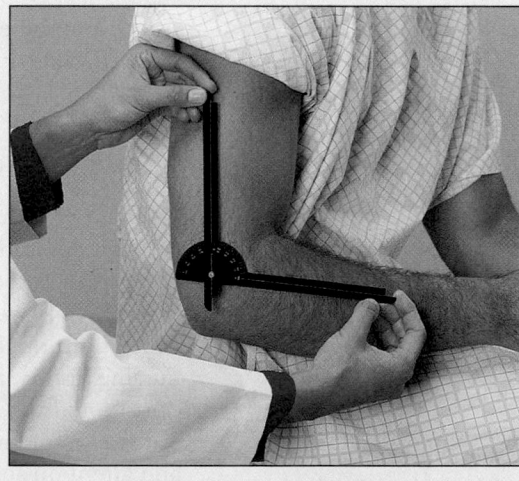

❶ A goniometer is used to measure range of motion.

15. Document your findings in the client record by using forms or checklists supplemented by narrative notes, when appropriate.

EVALUATION

- Perform a detailed follow-up examination of other systems based on findings that deviated from expected or normal for the client. Relate findings to previous assessment data if available.

- Report significant deviations from normal to the appropriate members of the health care team.

Assessing the Musculoskeletal System

INFANTS

- Palpate the clavicles of newborns. A mass and crepitus may indicate a fracture experienced during vaginal delivery. The newborn may also have limited movement of the arm and shoulder on the affected side.

- When the arms and legs of newborns are pulled to extension and released, the newborns naturally return to the flexed fetal position.

- Check muscle strength by holding the infant lightly under the arms with feet placed lightly on a table. Infants should not fall through the hands and should be able to bear body weight on their legs if normal muscle strength is present.

- Check infants for developmental dysplasia of the hip (congenital dislocation) by examining for asymmetrical gluteal folds, asymmetrical abduction of the legs (Ortolani and Barlow tests), or apparent shortening of the femur.

- Infants should be able to sit without support by 8 months of age, crawl by 7 to 10 months, and walk by 12 to 15 months.

- Observe for symmetry of muscle mass, strength, and function.

CHILDREN

- Pronation with "toeing in" of the feet is common in children between 12 and 30 months of age.

- Genu varum (bowleg) is normal in children for about 1 year after they begin to walk.

- Genu valgus (knock-knee) is normal in preschool and young school-age children.

- Lordosis (swayback) is common in children before age 5 years.

- Observe the child in normal activities to determine motor function.

- During the rapid growth spurts of adolescence, spinal curvature and rotation (scoliosis) may appear. Children should be assessed for scoliosis by age 12 years and annually until their growth slows. Curvature greater than 10% should be referred for further medical evaluation.

- Muscle mass increases in adolescence, especially as children engage in strenuous physical activity, and requires increased nutritional intake.

- Children are at risk for injury related to physical activity and should be

assessed for nutritional status, physical conditioning, and safety precautions to prevent injury.

- Adolescent girls who participate in strenuous athletic activities are at risk for delayed onset of menses, osteoporosis, and eating disorders; assessment should include a history of these factors.

OLDER ADULTS

- Muscle mass decreases progressively with age, but wide variations exist among different individuals.

- The decrease in speed, strength, resistance to fatigue, reaction time, and coordination in the older person is due to a decrease in nerve conduction and muscle tone.

- The bones can become more fragile, and osteoporosis (if present) leads to a loss of total bone mass. As a result, some older adults are predisposed to fractures and compressed vertebrae.

- In most older adults, osteoarthritic changes in the joints can be observed.

- Note any surgical scars from joint replacement surgeries.

Neurological System

A thorough neurological examination can take one to two hours; however, routine screening tests are usually done first. If the results of these tests raise questions, more extensive evaluations are made. Three major considerations determine the extent of a neurological exam: (a) the client's chief complaints, (b) the client's physical condition (i.e., level of consciousness and ability to ambulate), because many parts of the examination require movement and coordination of the extremities, and (c) the client's willingness to participate and cooperate.

Examination of the neurological system includes assessment of (a) mental status, including level of consciousness, (b) cranial nerves, (c) reflexes, (d) motor function, and (e) sensory function. Parts of the neurological assessment are performed throughout the health examination. For example, the nurse performs a large part of the mental status assessment during history taking and when observing the client's general appearance. Also, the nurse assesses the function of many cranial nerves. The second, third, fourth, fifth, and sixth cranial nerves (ophthalmic branch) are assessed with eyes and

vision, and the eighth cranial nerve (cochlear branch) is assessed with ears and hearing.

Mental Status

Assessment of mental status reveals the client's general cerebral function. These functions include intellectual (cognitive) and emotional (affective) functions.

If problems with the use of language, memory, concentration, or thought processes are noted during the nursing history, a more extensive examination is required during neurological assessment. Major areas of mental status assessment include language, orientation, memory, and attention span and calculation.

LANGUAGE Any defects in or loss of the power to express self through speech, writing, or sign language or to comprehend spoken or written language because of disease or injury of the cerebral cortex is called **aphasia**. Aphasia can be categorized as sensory or receptive aphasia and motor or expressive aphasia.

Sensory or *receptive aphasia* is the loss of the ability to comprehend written or spoken words. Two types of sensory aphasia are auditory (or acoustic) aphasia and visual aphasia. Clients with *auditory aphasia* have lost the ability to understand the symbolic content associated with sounds. Clients with *visual aphasia* have lost the ability to understand printed or written letters and numbers.

Motor or *expressive aphasia* involves loss of the power to express self through writing, making signs, or speaking. Clients may find that even though they can recall words, they have lost the ability to combine speech sounds into words.

ORIENTATION This aspect of the assessment determines the client's ability to recognize other persons (*person*) (see the Clinical Alert box below), awareness of when and where they presently are (*time* and *place*), and who they are (*self*).

> ### ! CLINICAL ALERT
>
> Nurses often chart that the client is "awake, alert, and oriented ×3 [or times three]." This refers to accurate awareness of persons, time, and place. Remember, "person" indicates that the client recognizes others, not that the client can state what his or her own name is.

MEMORY The nurse assesses the client's recall of information presented seconds previously (immediate recall), events or information from earlier in the day or examination (recent memory), and knowledge recalled from months or years back (remote or long-term memory).

ATTENTION SPAN AND CALCULATION This component determines the client's ability to focus on a mental task that is expected to be able to be performed by persons of normal intelligence.

Level of Consciousness

Level of consciousness (LOC) can lie anywhere along a continuum from a state of alertness to coma. A fully alert client responds to questions spontaneously; a comatose client may not respond to verbal stimuli. The Glasgow Coma Scale was originally developed to predict recovery from a head injury; however, it is used by many professionals to assess LOC. It tests three major areas: (a) eye response, (b) motor response, and (c) verbal response. An assessment totalling 15 points indicates the client is alert and completely oriented. A comatose client scores 7 or fewer points. See Table 28.12.

Cranial Nerves

The nurse needs to be aware of nerve functions to detect abnormalities (see Table 28.13 on the next page). In some cases, each cranial nerve (CN) is assessed; in other cases only selected nerve functions are evaluated.

TABLE 28.12 Levels of Consciousness: Glasgow Coma Scale

Faculty Measured	Response	Score
Eye opening	Spontaneous	4
	To verbal command	3
	To pain	2
	No response	1
Motor response	To verbal command	6
	To localized pain	5
	Flexes and withdraws	4
	Flexes abnormally	3
	Extends abnormally	2
	No response	1
Verbal response	Oriented, converses	5
	Disoriented, converses	4
	Uses inappropriate words	3
	Makes incomprehensible sounds	2
	No response	1
Glasgow Coma Scale Score		/15

Reflexes

A **reflex** is an automatic response of the body to a stimulus. It is not voluntarily learned or conscious. The deep tendon reflex is activated when a tendon is stimulated (tapped) and its associated muscle contracts. The quality of a reflex response varies among individuals and by age. As a person ages, reflex responses may become less intense.

> ### ! CLINICAL ALERT
>
> All questions and tests used in a neurological examination must be appropriate for age, language, education level, and culture. Individualize questions and tests before using them.

Reflexes are tested by using a percussion hammer. The response is described on a scale of 0 to 4. Experience is necessary to determine the appropriate scoring for an individual. When assessing reflexes, it is important for the nurse to compare one side of the body with the other to evaluate the symmetry of response. Several reflexes are normally tested during the physical examination: (a) the biceps reflex, (b) the triceps reflex, (c) the brachioradialis reflex, (d) the patellar reflex, (e) the Achilles reflex, and (f) the plantar (Babinski) reflex.

Motor Function

Neurological assessment of the motor system evaluates proprioception and cerebellar function. Structures involved in proprioception are the proprioceptors, the

TABLE 28.13 Cranial Nerve Functions and Assessment Methods

Cranial Nerve	Name (Mnemonic)*	Type	Function	Assessment Method
I	Olfactory (On)	Sensory	Smell	Ask the client to close the eyes and identify different mild aromas, such as coffee, vanilla, orange, lemon, lime, chocolate.
II	Optic (Old)	Sensory	Vision and visual fields	Ask the client to read the Snellen chart; check visual fields by confrontation; and conduct an ophthalmoscopic examination.
III	Oculomotor (Olympus's)	Motor	Extraocular eye movement (EOM); movement of sphincter of pupil; movement of ciliary muscles of lens; opening of upper eyelid	Assess the six ocular movements and pupil reaction.
IV	Trochlear (Towering)	Motor	EOM; specifically moves eyeball downward and laterally	Assess the six ocular movements.
V	Trigeminal (Tops)			
	Ophthalmic branch	Sensory	Sensation of cornea, skin of face, and nasal mucosa	While the client looks upward, lightly touch the lateral sclera of the eye to elicit the blink reflex. To test light-touch sensation, have the client close the eyes, pass a wisp of cotton (formed by twirling together a few fibres of cotton from a cotton ball or Q-Tip) over client's forehead and paranasal sinuses. To test deep sensation, use the blunt and sharp ends of a safety pin alternatingly over same areas.
	Maxillary branch	Sensory	Sensation of skin of face and anterior oral cavity (tongue and teeth)	Assess skin sensation as for ophthalmic branch above.
	Mandibular branch	Sensory	Muscles of mastication; sensation of skin of face	Ask the client to clench his or her teeth.
VI	Abducens (A)	Motor	EOM; moves eyeball laterally	Assess the directions of gaze.
VII	Facial (Finn)	Motor and sensory	Facial expression; taste (anterior two-thirds of tongue); closing of eyelid	Ask the client to smile, raise the eyebrows, frown, puff out the cheeks, and close the eyes tightly. Ask the client to identify various tastes placed on the tip and sides of the tongue: sugar (sweet), salt, lemon juice (sour), and quinine (bitter); identify areas of taste.
VIII	Auditory (And)			
	Vestibular branch	Sensory	Equilibrium	Assessment methods are discussed with cerebellar functions (see next section).
	Cochlear branch	Sensory	Hearing	Assess the client's ability to hear the spoken word and the vibrations of a tuning fork.

TABLE 28.13 *(continued)*

Cranial Nerve	Name (Mnemonic)*	Type	Function	Assessment Method
IX	Glossopharyngeal (German)	Motor and sensory	Swallowing ability; tongue movement; taste (posterior tongue)	Apply different things on the posterior tongue for taste identification. Ask the client to move the tongue from side to side and up and down.
X	Vagus (Viewed)	Motor and sensory	Sensation of pharynx and larynx; swallowing; vocal cord movement	Assessed with CN IX; assess the client's speech for hoarseness.
XI	Spinal accessory (Some)	Motor	Head movement; shrugging of shoulders	Ask the client to shrug the shoulders against resistance from your hands and to turn the head to the side against resistance from your hand (repeat for the other side).
XII	Hypoglossal (Hops)	Motor	Protrusion of tongue; moves tongue up and down and side to side	Ask the client to protrude the tongue at the midline and then move it from side to side.

Mnemonic: On Old Olympus's Towering Tops A Finn And German Viewed Some Hops.

posterior columns of the spinal cord, the cerebellum, and the vestibular apparatus (which is innervated by the eighth CN) in the labyrinth of the internal ear.

Proprioceptors are sensory nerve terminals that occur chiefly in the muscles, tendons, joints, and internal ear and give information about the movements and position of the body. Stimuli from the proprioceptors travel through the posterior columns of the spinal cord. Deficits of function of the posterior columns of the spinal cord result in impairment of muscle and position sense. Clients with such an impairment often must watch their own arm and leg movements to ascertain the position of the limbs.

The cerebellum (a) helps control posture; (b) acts with the cerebral cortex to make body movements smooth and coordinated; and (c) controls skeletal muscles to maintain equilibrium.

Sensory Function

Sensory functions include touch, pain, temperature, position, and tactile discrimination. The first three are routinely tested. The spinothalamic tract conducts sensations of superficial pain and temperature to the sensory cortex. The posterior column conducts the sensation of position. Generally, the face, arms, legs, hands, and feet are tested for touch and pain, although all parts of the body can be tested. If the client complains of numbness, peculiar sensations, or paralysis, the nurse should check sensation more carefully over flexor and extensor surfaces of limbs, mapping out clearly any abnormality of touch or pain by examining responses in the area about every 2.5 cm. This is a lengthy procedure. Abnormal responses to touch stimuli include **anesthesia** (loss of

sensation); **hyperesthesia** (more than normal sensation); **hypoesthesia** (less than normal sensation); or **paresthesia** (an abnormal sensation, such as numbness and prickling as in "pins and needles").

A more detailed neurological examination includes position sense, temperature sense, and tactile discrimination. Three types of tactile discrimination are generally tested: (a) **one-** and **two-point discrimination**, the ability to sense whether one or two areas of the skin are being stimulated by pressure; (b) **stereognosis**, the act of recognizing objects by touching and manipulating them; and (c) **extinction**, the failure to perceive touch on one side of the body when two symmetrical areas of the body are touched simultaneously.

Skill 28.17 describes how to assess the neurological system (see also Lifespan Considerations box on assessing the neurological system on page 684).

Female Genitals and Inguinal Lymph Nodes

The examination of the genitals and reproductive tract of women includes assessment of the inguinal lymph nodes and inspection and palpation of the external genitals. Completeness of the assessment of the genitals and reproductive tract depends on the health care needs of the individual client. In most practice settings, generalist nurses perform only inspection of the external genitals and palpation of the inguinal lymph nodes.

Assessment of adolescent girls is limited to an inspection of the external genitals. For sexually active adolescents and adult women, a Papanicolaou test (Pap test) is advised

SKILL 28.17 | **ASSESSING THE NEUROLOGICAL SYSTEM**

PLANNING

If possible, determine whether a screening or full neurological examination is indicated. This will determine the preparation of the client, the equipment required, and timing.

Equipment (depending on components of examination):

- Sugar, salt, lemon juice (sour), tonic water (bitter)
- Percussion hammer
- Tongue depressors (one broken diagonally for testing pain sensation)
- Wisps of cotton wool to assess light-touch sensation
- Test tubes of hot and cold water for skin temperature assessment (optional)
- Sterile safety pin for tactile discrimination

IMPLEMENTATION

Performance

1. Before performing the procedure, introduce yourself and verify the client's identity using two identifiers or per agency protocol. Explain to the client what you are going to do, why it is necessary, and how he or she can participate. Discuss how the results will be used in planning further care or treatments.

2. Perform hand hygiene, and follow other appropriate infection prevention and control procedures.

3. Provide for client privacy.

4. Inquire whether the client has any history of the following: presence of pain in the head, back, or extremities, as well as onset and aggravating and alleviating factors; disorientation to time, place, or person; speech disorder; history of loss of consciousness, fainting, convulsions, trauma, tingling or numbness, tremors or tics, limping, paralysis, uncontrolled muscle movements, loss of memory, mood swings, or problems with smell, vision, taste, touch, or hearing.

Language

5. If the client displays difficulty speaking, do the following:

   - Point to common objects, and ask the client to name them.
   - Ask the client to read some words and to match the printed or written words with pictures.
   - Ask the client to respond to simple verbal and written commands (e.g., "Point to your toes" or "Raise your left arm").

Orientation

6. Determine the client's orientation to *person, time,* and *place* by tactful questioning. Ask the client the city and province or territory of residence, time of day, date, day of the week, duration of illness, and names of family members. To evaluate the response, you must know the correct answer. More direct questioning may be necessary for some people (e.g., "Where are you now?" "What day is it today?"). Most people readily accept these questions if initially the nurse asks, "Do you get confused at times?" If the client cannot answer these questions accurately, also include assessment of *self* by asking the client to state his or her full name.

Memory

7. Identify lapses in memory. Ask the client about difficulty with memory. If problems are apparent, three categories of memory are tested: (a) immediate recall, (b) recent memory, and (c) remote memory.

To assess immediate recall:

- Ask the client to repeat a series of three digits (e.g., 7, 4, 3), spoken slowly.
- Gradually increase the number of digits (e.g., 7, 4, 3, 5; then 7, 4, 3, 5, 6; and 7, 4, 3, 5, 6, 7, 2), until the client fails to repeat the series correctly.
- Start again with a series of three digits, but this time ask the client to repeat them backward. The average person can repeat a series of five to eight digits in sequence and four to six digits in reverse order.

To assess recent memory:

- Ask the client to recall recent events of the day, such as how the client got to the clinic. This information must be validated.
- Ask the client to recall information given early in the interview (e.g., the name of a doctor or nurse).
- Provide the client with three facts to recall (e.g., a colour, an object, and an address), or a three-digit number, and ask the client to repeat all three. Later in the interview, ask the client to recall all three items.

To assess remote memory, ask the client to describe a previous illness or surgery (e.g., 5 years ago), or a birthday or anniversary.

Attention Span and Calculation

8. Test the ability to concentrate or maintain *attention span* by asking the client to recite the alphabet or to count backward from 100. Test the ability to calculate by asking the client to subtract 7 or 3 progressively from 100 (i.e., 100, 93, 86, 79, or 100, 97, 94, 91), referred to as *serial sevens* or *serial threes*. Normally, an adult can complete serial sevens test in about 90 seconds with three or fewer errors. Because educational level, language, or cultural differences affect calculating ability, this test may be inappropriate for some people.

Level of Consciousness

9. Apply the Glasgow Coma Scale: eye response, motor response, and verbal response. An assessment totalling 15 points indicates the client is alert and completely oriented. A comatose client scores 7 or fewer points (see Table 28.12, p. 673).

Cranial Nerves

10. For the specific functions and assessment methods of each CN, see Table 28.13 (p. 674). Test each nerve not already evaluated in another component of the health assessment. A quick way to remember which CNs are assessed in the face is shown in ❶.

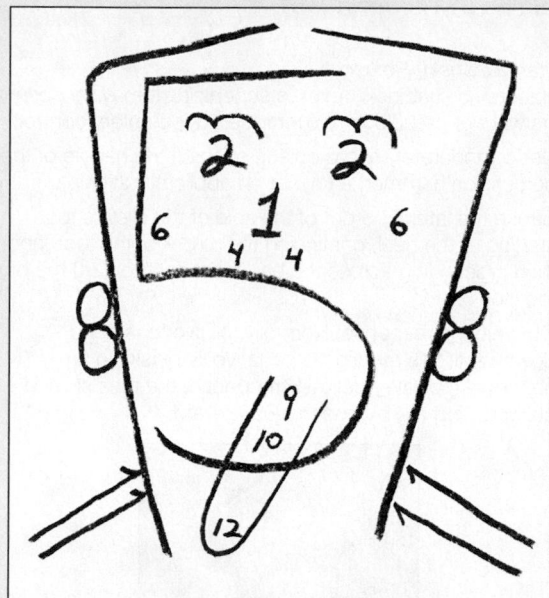

❶ Cranial nerves by the numbers. The next time you are trying to remember the locations and functions of the CNs, picture this drawing. All the CNs are represented (e.g., shoulders formed by the number "11" for CN 11, which controls neck and shoulder movement; the sides of the face and the top of the head are formed by the number "7", as controlled by CN 7).

Source: From Bolek, B. (2006). Strictly clinical: Facing cranial nerve assessment. *American Nurse Today, 1(2)*, 21–22. *Used by permission.*

Reflexes

11. Test reflexes by using a percussion hammer, comparing one side of the body with the other to evaluate the symmetry of response:

0	No reflex response
1	Hypoactive (minimal activity)
2	Normal response
3	More active than normal
4	Hyperactive (maximal activity)

Biceps Reflex:

The biceps reflex tests the spinal cord level C-5 and C-6.

- Partially flex the client's arm at the elbow, and rest the forearm over the thighs, placing the palm of the hand down.
- Place the thumb of your nondominant hand horizontally over the biceps tendon.
- Deliver a blow (slight downward thrust) with the percussion hammer to your thumb (see ❷).
- Observe the normal slight flexion of the elbow, and feel the bicep's contraction through your thumb.

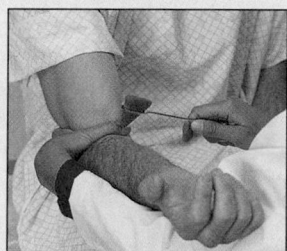

❷ The biceps reflex.

Triceps Reflex:

The triceps reflex tests the spinal cord level C-7 and C-8.

- Flex the client's arm at the elbow, and support it in the palm of your nondominant hand (see ❸).
- Palpate the triceps tendon about 2 cm to 5 cm above the elbow.
- Deliver a blow with the percussion hammer directly to the tendon.
- Observe the normal slight extension of the elbow.

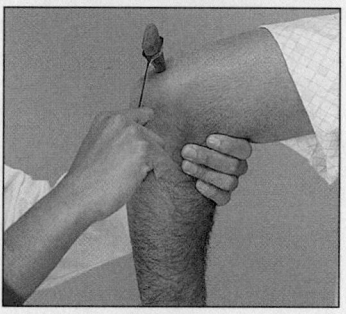

❸ The triceps reflex.

Brachioradialis Reflex:

The brachioradialis reflex tests the spinal cord level C-3 and C-6.

- Rest the client's forearm in a relaxed position externally rotated on a firm surface.
- Deliver a blow with the percussion hammer directly on the radius 2 cm to 5 cm above the wrist or the styloid process, the bony prominence on the thumb side of the wrist (see ❹).
- Observe the normal flexion and supination of the forearm. The fingers of the hand may also extend slightly.

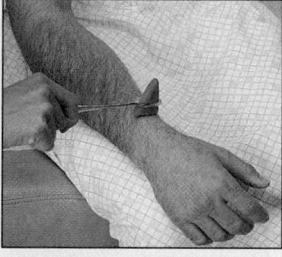

❹ The brachioradialis reflex.

Patellar Reflex:

The patellar reflex tests the spinal cord level L-2, L-3, and L-4.

- Ask the client to sit on the edge of the examining table so that the legs hang freely.
- Locate the patellar tendon directly below the patella (kneecap).
- Deliver a blow with the percussion hammer directly to the tendon (see ❺).
- Observe the normal extension or kicking out of the leg as the quadriceps muscle contracts.
- If no response occurs and you suspect the client is not relaxed, ask the client to interlock the fingers and pull. **Rationale: This action often enhances relaxation so that a more accurate response is obtained.**

(continued)

SKILL 28.17 ASSESSING THE NEUROLOGICAL SYSTEM (*continued*)

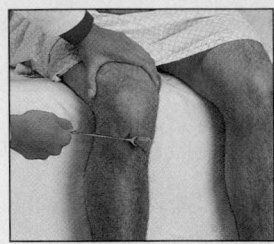

5 The patellar reflex.

Achilles Reflex:

The Achilles reflex tests the spinal cord level S-1 and S-2.

- With the client in the same position as for the patellar reflex, slightly dorsiflex the client's ankle by supporting the ball of the foot lightly in the hand.
- Deliver a blow with the percussion hammer directly to the Achilles tendon just above the heel (see **6**).
- Observe and feel the normal plantar flexion (downward jerk) of the foot.

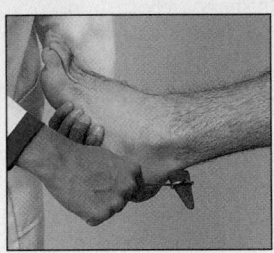

6 The Achilles reflex.

Plantar (Babinski) Reflex:

The planter, or Babinski, reflex is superficial. It may be absent in adults without pathology or overridden by voluntary control.

- Use a moderately sharp object, such as the handle of the percussion hammer, a key, or an applicator stick.
- Stroke the lateral border of the sole of the client's foot, starting at the heel, continuing to the ball of the foot, and then proceeding across the ball of the foot toward the big toe (see **7**).
- Observe the response. Normally, all five toes bend downward; this reaction is negative Babinski. In an abnormal (positive) Babinski response, the toes spread outward and the big toe moves upward.

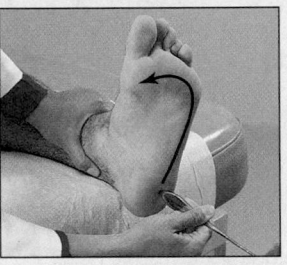

7 The plantar (Babinski) reflex.

Assessment	Normal Findings	Deviations from Normal
Motor Function		
12. *Gross Motor and Balance Tests* Generally, the Romberg test and one other gross motor function and balance tests are used.		
Walking Gait		
Ask the client to walk across the room and back, and assess the client's gait.	Has upright posture and steady gait with opposing arm swing; walks unaided, maintaining balance	Has poor posture and unsteady, irregular, staggering gait with wide stance; bends legs only from hips; has rigid or no arm movements
Romberg Test		
Ask the client to stand with feet together and arms resting at the sides, first with eyes open, then closed. Stand close during this test. **Rationale: You may need to prevent the client from falling.**	Negative Romberg: may sway slightly but is able to maintain upright posture and foot stance	Positive Romberg: cannot maintain foot stance; moves the feet apart to maintain stance; if client cannot maintain balance with the eyes shut, client may have sensory ataxia (lack of coordination of the voluntary muscles); if balance cannot be maintained whether the eyes are open or shut, client may have cerebellar ataxia
Standing on One Foot with Eyes Closed		
Ask the client to close the eyes and stand on one foot. Repeat on the other foot. Stand close to the client during this test.	Maintains stance for at least 5 seconds	Cannot maintain stance for 5 seconds

Assessment	Normal Findings	Deviations from Normal

Heel-to-Toe Walking

Ask the client to walk a straight line, placing the heel of one foot directly in front of the toes of the other foot (see ❽).

Maintains heel-toe walking along a straight line

Assumes a wider foot gait to stay upright

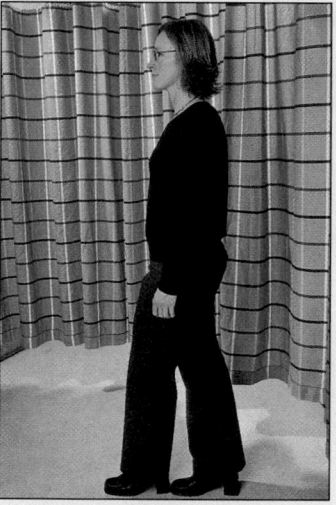

❽ Heel-to-toe walking.

Toe or Heel Walking

Ask the client to walk several steps on toes and then on heels.

Able to walk several steps on toes or heels

Cannot maintain balance on toes and heels

13. *Fine Motor Tests for the Upper Extremities*

Finger-to-Nose Test

Ask the client to abduct and extend the arms at shoulder height and then rapidly touch the nose alternately with one index finger and then the other. The client repeats the test with the eyes closed if the test is performed easily (see ❾).

Repeatedly and rhythmically touches the nose

Misses the nose or gives slow response

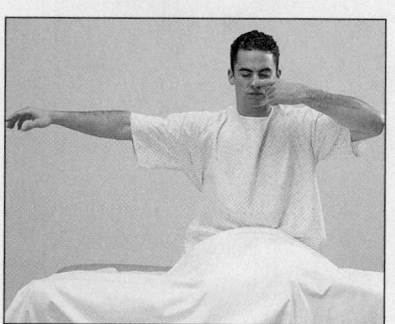

❾ Finger-to-nose test.

Alternating Supination and Pronation of Hands on Knees

Ask the client to pat both knees with the palms of both hands and then with the backs of the hands alternately at an ever-increasing rate (see ❿).

Can alternately supinate and pronate hands at rapid pace

Performs with slow, clumsy movements and irregular timing; has difficulty alternating from supination to pronation

(continued)

SKILL 28.17 ASSESSING THE NEUROLOGICAL SYSTEM (*continued*)

Assessment	Normal Findings	Deviations from Normal
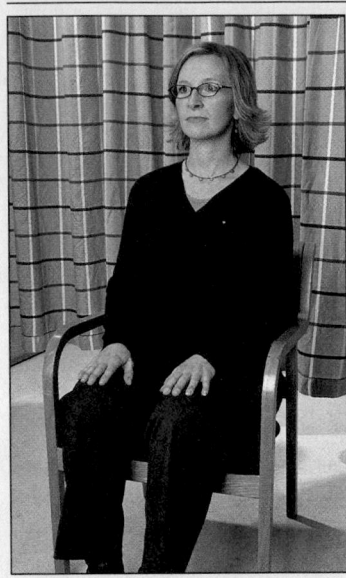 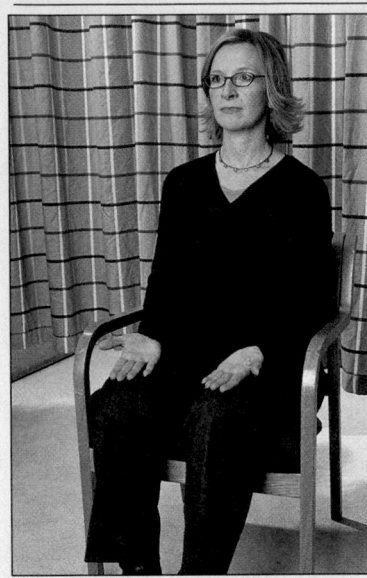		

⑩ Alternating supination and pronation of hands on knees test.

Finger to Nose and to the Nurse's Finger

Ask the client to touch the nose and then your index finger, held at a distance of about 45 cm, at a rapid and increasing rate (see ⑪).	Performs with coordination and rapidity	Misses the finger and moves slowly

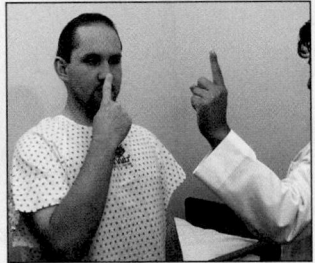 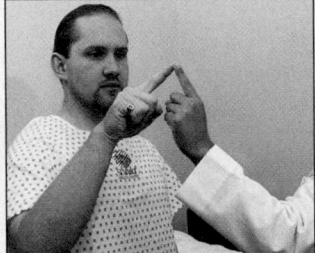

⑪ Finger-to-nose and to the nurse's finger test.

Fingers to Fingers

Ask the client to spread the arms broadly at shoulder height and then bring the fingers together at the midline, first with the eyes open and then closed, first slowly and then rapidly (see ⑫).	Performs with accuracy and rapidity	Moves slowly and is unable to touch fingers consistently

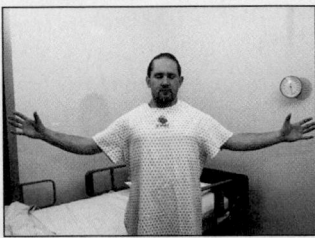 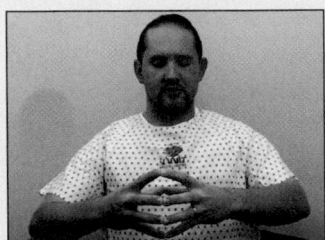

⑫ Fingers-to-fingers test.

Fingers to Thumb (Same Hand)

Ask the client to touch each finger of one hand to the thumb of the same hand as rapidly as possible (see ⑬).	Rapidly touches each finger to thumb with each hand.	Cannot coordinate this fine discrete movement with either one or both hands

Assessment	Normal Findings	Deviations from Normal

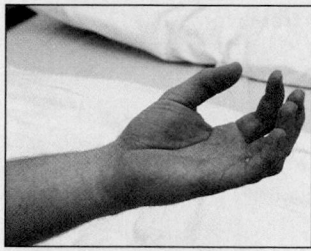 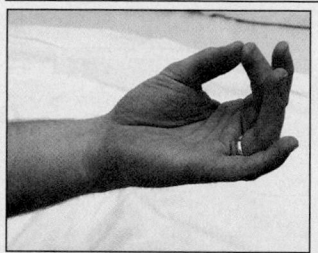

⑬ Fingers-to-thumb (same hand) test.

14. *Fine Motor Tests for the Lower Extremities*

Ask the client to lie supine and to perform these tests.

Heel Down Opposite Shin

Ask the client to place the heel of one foot just below the opposite knee and run the heel down the shin to the foot. Have the client repeat with the other foot. The client may also use a sitting position for this test (see ⑭).

Demonstrates bilateral equal coordination

Has tremors or is awkward; heel moves off shin

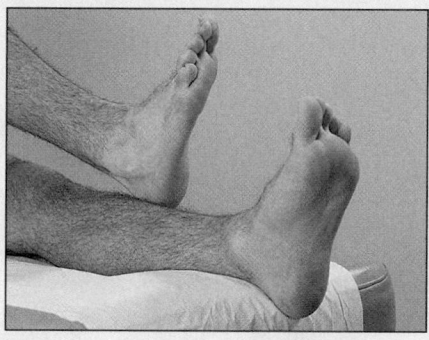

⑭ Heel down opposite shin.

Toe or Ball of Foot to the Nurse's Finger

Ask the client to touch your finger with the large toe of each foot (see ⑮).

Moves smoothly, with coordination

Misses your finger; cannot coordinate movement

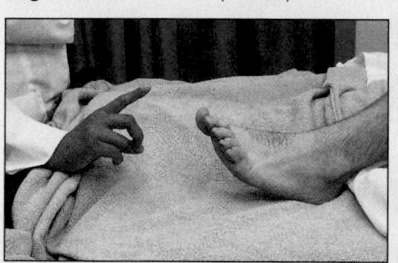 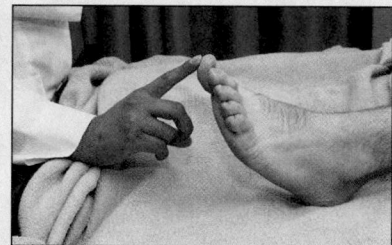

⑮ Toe or ball of foot to the nurse's finger test.

15. *Light-Touch Sensation*

Compare the light-touch sensation of symmetrical areas of the body. **Rationale: Sensitivity to touch varies among different skin areas.**

(continued)

SKILL 28.17 ASSESSING THE NEUROLOGICAL SYSTEM (*continued*)

Assessment	Normal Findings	Deviations from Normal

- Ask the client to close the eyes and to respond by saying "yes" or "no" whenever the client feels the wisp of cotton wool touching the skin. With a cotton wool wisp, lightly touch one specific spot and then the same spot on the other side of the body (see ⓰). Test areas on the forehead, cheek, hand, lower arm, abdomen, foot, and lower leg. Check a distal area of the limb first (i.e., the hand before the arm and the foot before the leg). **Rationale: The sensory nerve may be assumed to be intact if sensation is felt at its most distal part.**

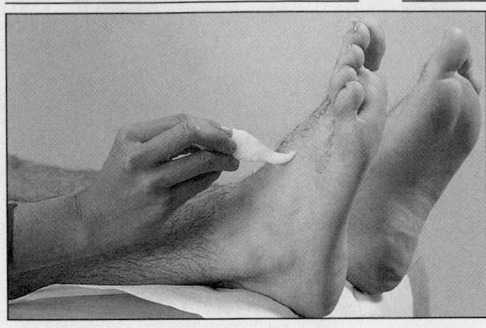

⓰ Assessing light-touch sensation.

- Ask the client to point to the spot where the touch was felt. **Rationale: This demonstrates whether the client is able to determine tactile location (point localization); that is, the client can accurately perceive where he or she was touched. If areas of sensory dysfunction are found, determine the boundaries of sensation by testing responses about every 2.5 cm in the area. Make a sketch of the sensory loss area for recording purposes.**

Light tickling or touch sensation

Anesthesia, hyperesthesia, hypoesthesia, or paresthesia

16. *Pain Sensation*

Assess pain sensation as follows:
- Ask the client to close the eyes and to say "sharp," "dull," or "don't know" when the sharp or dull end of the broken tongue depressor is felt.

- Alternatingly, use the sharp and dull end to lightly prick designated anatomic areas at random (e.g., hand, forearm, foot, lower leg, abdomen) (see ⓱). The face is not tested in this manner.

- Allow at least 2 seconds between each test to prevent summation effects of stimuli (i.e., several successive stimuli perceived as one stimulus).

Able to discriminate "sharp" and "dull" sensations

Areas of reduced, heightened, or absent sensation (map them out for recording purposes)

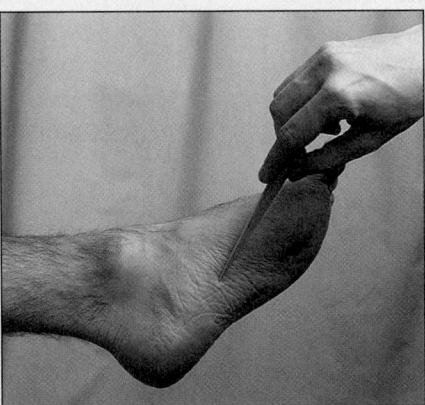

⓱ Assessing pain sensation by using a broken tongue depressor.

17. *Temperature Sensation*

Temperature sensation is not routinely tested if pain sensation is found to be within normal limits. If pain sensation is not normal or is absent, testing sensitivity to temperature may prove more reliable.

- Touch skin areas with test tubes, one filled with warm water (40°C to 45°C) and one with cold water (5°C to 10°C).

- Have the client respond by saying "warm," "cold," or "don't know."

Able to distinguish "warm" and "cold" sensations

Areas of dulled or lost sensation (when sensations of pain are dulled, temperature sense is usually also impaired because distribution of these nerves over the body is similar)

Assessment	Normal Findings	Deviations from Normal
18. *Position or Kinesthetic Sensation* Commonly, the middle fingers and the large toes are tested for the kinesthetic sensation (sense of position). • To test the fingers, support the client's arm and hand with one hand. To test the toes, place the client's heels on the examining table. • Ask the client to close his or her eyes. • Grasp a middle finger or a big toe firmly between your thumb and index finger, and exert the same pressure on both sides of the finger or toe while moving it (see ⑱). • Move the finger or toe until it is up, down, or straight out, and ask the client to identify the position. • Use a series of brisk up-and-down movements before bringing the finger or toe suddenly to rest in one of the three positions.	Can readily determine the position of fingers and toes 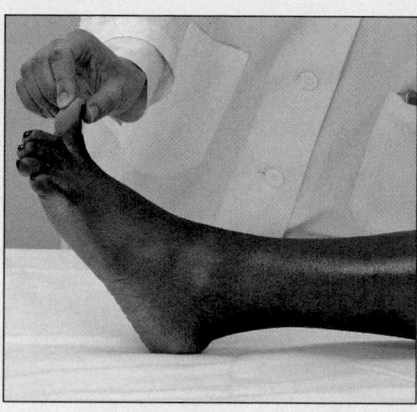 ⑱ Position or kinesthetic sensation test.	Unable to determine the position of one or more fingers or toes
19. *Tactile Discrimination* For all tests, the client needs to keep the eyes closed.	Perception varies widely in adults over different parts of the body; normally, a person can distinguish between a one-point stimulus and a two-point stimulus within the following minimum distances: Fingertips, 2.8 mm; palms of hands, 8–12 mm; chest, forearm, 40 mm; back, 50–70 mm; upper arm, thigh, 75 mm; toes, 3–8 mm	Unable to sense whether one or two areas of the skin are being stimulated by pressure
One- and Two-Point Discrimination Alternatingly stimulate skin with two pins simultaneously and then with only one pin. Ask whether the client feels one or two pinpricks.		
Stereognosis Place a series of familiar objects, such as a key, paper clip, or coin, in the client's hand, and ask the client to identify each one.	Recognizes common objects	Unable to recognize common objects
If the client has a motor impairment of the hand and is unable to manipulate an object, write a number or letter on the client's palm, using a blunt instrument, and ask the client to identify it.	Able to identify numbers or letters written on palm (graphesthesia)	Unable to identify numbers or letters written on palm
Extinction Phenomenon Simultaneously stimulate two symmetrical areas of the body, such as thighs, cheeks, or hands.	Both points of stimulus are felt	Failure to perceive touch on one side of the body when two symmetrical areas of the body are touched simultaneously (frequently noted in clients with lesions of the sensory cortex)

(continued)

SKILL 28.17	ASSESSING THE NEUROLOGICAL SYSTEM (*continued*)

Assessment	Normal Findings	Deviations from Normal

20. Document your findings in the client record by using forms or checklists supplemented by narrative notes, when appropriate. Describe any abnormal findings in objective terms (e.g., "When asked to count backwards by threes, client made 7 errors and completed the task in 4 minutes").

EVALUATION

- Perform a detailed follow-up examination of other systems based on findings that deviated from expected or normal for the client. Relate findings to previous assessment data, if available.

- Report significant deviations from normal to the appropriate members of the health care team.

LIFESPAN CONSIDERATIONS

Assessing the Neurological System

INFANTS

Reflexes commonly tested in newborns include the following:

- *Rooting:* Stroke the side of the face near mouth; the infant opens mouth and turns to the side that is stroked.
- *Sucking:* Place finger 3 cm to 4 cm into the infant's mouth, or have the mother place her nipple in the infant's mouth; infant sucks vigorously.
- *Tonic neck:* Place the infant in the supine position, and turn the head to one side; the arm on the side to which head is turned extends; on the opposite side, the arm curls up (fencer's pose).
- *Palmar grasp:* Place your finger on the infant's palm, and press; the infant curls his or her fingers around your finger.
- *Stepping:* Hold the infant above a surface as if weight bearing; the infant steps along, one foot at a time.
- *Moro:* Present loud noise or unexpected movement; the infant spreads his or her arms and legs, extends fingers, and then flexes and brings the hands together; the infant may cry.

  Most of these reflexes disappear between 4 and 6 months of age.

CHILDREN

- Present the procedures as games, whenever possible.
- A positive Babinski reflex is abnormal after the child ambulates or at age 2 years.
- For children younger than age 5 years, the Denver Developmental Screening Test II provides a comprehensive neurological evaluation, particularly for motor function.
- Note the child's ability to understand and follow directions.

- Assess immediate recall or recent memory by using names of cartoon characters. Normal recall in children is one item fewer than their age in years (e.g., a 4-year-old should be able to recall three items).
- Assess for signs of hyperactivity or abnormally short attention span.
- Children should be able to walk backward by age 2 years, balance on one foot for 5 seconds by age 4 years, heel-to-toe walk by age 5 years, and heel-to-toe walk backward by age 6 years.
- The Romberg test is appropriate for children over age 3 years.

OLDER ADULTS

- A full neurological assessment can be lengthy. Conduct it in several sessions, if indicated; stop the tests if the client is noticeably fatigued.
- A decline in mental status is not a normal result of aging. Changes are more likely the result of physical or psychological disorders (e.g., fever, fluid and electrolyte imbalances, medications). Acute, abrupt-onset mental status changes are usually caused by delirium. These changes are often reversible with treatment. Chronic, subtle, insidious mental health changes are usually caused by dementia and are usually irreversible.
- Intelligence and learning ability remain unaltered with aging. Many factors, however, inhibit learning (e.g., anxiety, illness, pain, cultural barrier).
- Short-term memory is often less efficient. Long-term memory is usually unaltered.
- Because aging is often associated with loss of support persons, depression is

a common disorder. Mood changes, weight loss, anorexia, constipation, and early morning awakening may be symptoms of depression.
- The stress of being in unfamiliar situations can cause confusion in older adults.
- As a person ages, reflex responses may become less intense.
- Because older adults tire more easily than younger clients, a total neurological assessment is often done at a different time from the other parts of the physical assessment.
- Although there is a progressive decrease in the number of functioning neurons in the central nervous system and in the sense organs, older adults usually function well because of the abundant reserves in the number of brain cells.
- Impulse transmission and reaction to stimuli are slower.
- Many older adults have some impairment of hearing, vision, smell, temperature and pain sensation, memory, and mental endurance.
- Coordination changes, including a reduced speed of fine finger movements. Standing balance remains intact, and Romberg's test remains negative.
- Reflex responses may slightly increase or decrease. Many show loss of Achilles reflex, and the plantar reflex may be difficult to elicit.
- When testing sensory function, the nurse needs to give older adults time to respond. Normally, older adults have unaltered perception of light touch and superficial pain, decreased perception of deep pain, and decreased perception of temperature stimuli. Many also reveal a decrease or absence of position sense in the large toes.

every one to three years (depending on results) for early detection of cancer of the cervix. If an increased or abnormal vaginal discharge is present, specimens should be taken to check for sexually transmitted infections (STIs).

Examination of genitals usually creates uncertainty and apprehension in females, and the lithotomy position required for the examination can cause embarrassment. The nurse must explain each part of the examination in advance and perform the examination in an objective and efficient manner. Appropriate draping is essential to prevent undue exposure of the client, and good lighting is required for the nurse to ensure accuracy of inspection.

Skill 28.18 describes how to assess the female genitals and inguinal lymph nodes (see also the Lifespan Considerations box on assessing female genitals and inguinal lymph nodes on the next page).

SKILL 28.18 ASSESSING FEMALE GENITALS AND INGUINAL LYMPH NODES

PLANNING

Equipment

- Clean gloves
- Drape
- Supplemental lighting, if needed

IMPLEMENTATION

Performance

1. Before performing the procedure, introduce yourself and verify the client's identity using two identifiers or per agency protocol. Explain to the client what you are going to do, why it is necessary, and how she can participate. Discuss how the results will be used in planning further care or treatments.

2. Perform hand hygiene, put on gloves, and follow other appropriate infection prevention and control procedures.

3. Provide for client privacy. Request the presence of another woman, if you so desire, if required by agency policy, or if requested by the client.

4. Inquire about the following: age of onset of menstruation, last menstrual period (LMP), regularity of cycle, duration, amount of daily flow, and whether menstruation is painful; incidence of pain during intercourse; vaginal discharge; number of pregnancies, number of live births, labour or delivery complications; urgency and frequency of urination at night; blood in urine, painful urination, incontinence; history of STIs, past and present.

5. Cover the pelvic area with a sheet or drape at all times when it is not actually being examined. Position the client in the supine position, with feet elevated on the stirrups of the examination table. Alternatively, assist the client into the dorsal recumbent position, with the client's knees flexed and thighs externally rotated.

Assessment	Normal Findings	Deviations from Normal
6. Inspect the distribution, amount, and characteristics of pubic hair.	Wide variations exist; generally kinky in the menstruating adult, thinner and straighter after menopause; distributed in the shape of an inverse triangle	Scant pubic hair (may indicate hormonal problem); hair growth should not extend over the abdomen
7. Inspect the skin of the pubic area for parasites, inflammation, swelling, and lesions. To assess pubic skin adequately, separate the labia majora and labia minora.	Pubic skin intact, no lesions; skin of vulva area slightly darker than the rest of the body; labia round, full, and relatively symmetrical in adult females	Lice, lesions, scars, fissures, swelling, erythema, *excoriations* (abrasions from scratching), *varicosities* (swollen and twisted veins), or leukoplakia
8. Inspect the clitoris, urethral orifice, and vaginal orifice when separating the labia minora.	Clitoris does not exceed 1 cm in width and 2 cm in length; urethral orifice appears as a small slit and is the same colour as surrounding tissues; no inflammation, swelling, or discharge	Presence of lesions; presence of inflammation, swelling, or discharge
9. Palpate the inguinal lymph nodes (see ❶). Use the pads of the fingers in a rotary motion, noting any enlargement or tenderness.	No enlargement or tenderness	Enlargement and tenderness

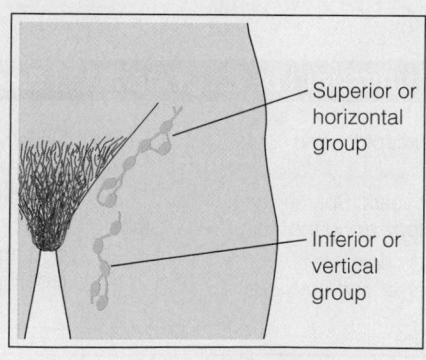

Superior or horizontal group

Inferior or vertical group

❶ Inguinal lymph nodes.

(continued)

SKILL 28.18 **ASSESSING FEMALE GENITALS AND INGUINAL LYMPH NODES** (*continued*)

Assessment	Normal Findings	Deviations from Normal
10. Remove and discard gloves. Perform hand hygiene.		
11. Document your findings in the client record by using forms or checklists supplemented by narrative notes, when appropriate.		

EVALUATION

* Perform a detailed follow-up examination based on findings that deviated from expected or normal for the client. Relate findings to previous assessment data, if available.

* Significant deviations from normal indicate the need for an internal vaginal examination.

LIFESPAN CONSIDERATIONS

Assessing Female Genitals and Inguinal Lymph Nodes

INFANTS

* Infants can be held in a supine position on the parent's lap with the knees supported in a flexed position and separated.

* Because of maternal estrogen, the labia and clitoris in newborns may be edematous and enlarged, and newborns may have a small amount of white or bloody vaginal discharge.

* Assess the mons and inguinal area for swelling or tenderness that may indicate the presence of an inguinal hernia.

CHILDREN

* Ensure that you have the approval of a parent or guardian to perform the examination, and then tell the child what you are going to do. Preschool children are taught not to allow others to touch their "private parts."

* Assessment of adolescent girls is limited to inspection of the external genitals, unless the girl is sexually active.

The presence of the parent during the exam will depend on the nature of the clinical situation and the provincial or territorial age of consent for medical investigation (e.g., some provinces require that the adolescent be at least 14 years old before being examined without parental presence or permission).

* Girls should be assessed for Tanner staging of pubic hair development (see Box 28.7).

* Girls should have a Papanicolaou (Pap) test done if sexually active, or by age 18 years.

OLDER ADULTS

* Loss of pubic hair and a flattening of the labia occur with aging.

* The clitoris is a potential site for cancerous lesions in older females.

* The vulva atrophies as a result of a reduction in vascularity, elasticity, adipose tissue, and estrogen levels.

Because the vulva is more fragile, it is more easily irritated.

* The vaginal environment becomes drier and more alkaline, resulting in an alteration of the type of flora present and a predisposition to vaginitis. Dyspareunia (difficult or painful coitus) is also a common occurrence.

* The cervix and uterus decrease in size.

* The fallopian tubes and ovaries atrophy.

* Ovulation and estrogen production cease.

* Vaginal bleeding unrelated to estrogen therapy is abnormal in older women.

* Prolapse of the uterus can occur in older females, especially those who have had multiple pregnancies.

* Older females may be arthritic and find the lithotomy position uncomfortable. A semi-lithotomy position may be necessary.

BOX 28.7 **TANNER STAGES OF PUBIC HAIR DEVELOPMENT IN FEMALES**

Stage 1   Preadolescence. No pubic hair except for fine body hair.

Stage 2   Usually occurs at ages 11 and 12 years. Sparse, long, slightly pigmented curly hair develops along the labia.

Stage 3   Usually occurs at ages 12 and 13 years. Hair becomes darker in colour and curlier and develops over the pubic symphysis.

Stage 4   Usually occurs between ages 13 and 14 years. Hair assumes the texture and curl of the adult but is not as thick and does not appear on the thighs.

Stage 5   Sexual maturity. Hair assumes adult appearance and appears on the inner aspect of the upper thigh (see Figure 28.35)

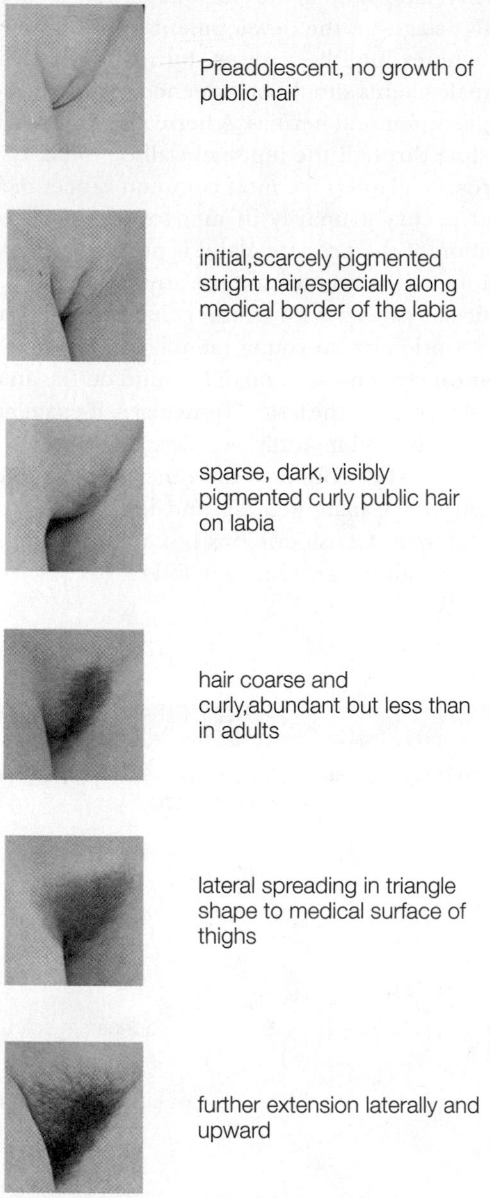

Preadolescent, no growth of public hair

initial,scarcely pigmented stright hair,especially along medical border of the labia

sparse, dark, visibly pigmented curly public hair on labia

hair coarse and curly,abundant but less than in adults

lateral spreading in triangle shape to medical surface of thighs

further extension laterally and upward

FIGURE 28.35 Maturation stages in the female.

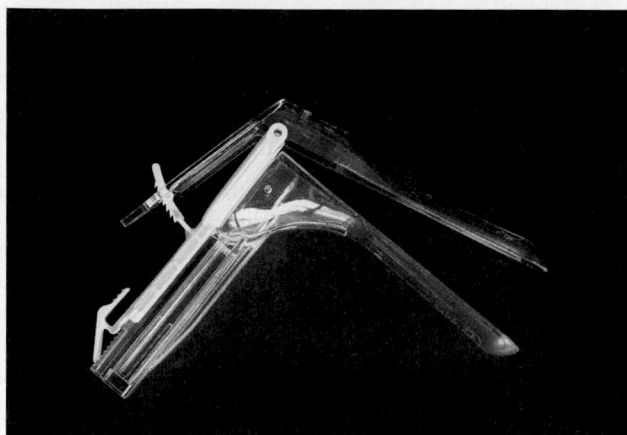

FIGURE 28.36 A vaginal speculum.

two blades and an adjustable thumb screw (Figure 28.36). Various sizes are available (small, medium, and large); the appropriate size needs to be selected for each client. The speculum can be lubricated with water-soluble lubricant if specimens are *not* being collected. Most examiners lubricate the speculum with warm water.

The nurse's responsibilities when assisting with an examination of the internal female genitals include the following:

1. *Assembling equipment.* These include drapes, gloves, vaginal speculum of correct size, warm water or lubricant, and supplies for cytology studies.
2. *Preparing the client.* Advise the client not to douche before the procedure. Explain the procedure. It should take only 5 minutes and is normally not painful. Assist the client to a lithotomy position as needed, and drape her appropriately.
3. *Supporting the client during the procedure.* This involves explaining the procedure as needed, and encouraging the client to take deep breaths that will help the pelvic muscles relax.
4. *Monitoring and assisting the client after the procedure.* Assist the client from the lithotomy position and with perineal care as needed. Observe any discharge from the vagina.
5. *Documenting the procedure.* Include the date and time it was performed, the name of the physician, and any nursing assessments and interventions.

Male Genitals and Inguinal Area

In adult men, complete examination should include assessment of the external genitals, the presence of any hernias, and the prostate gland. The male reproductive and urinary systems (Figure 28.37) share the urethra,

In many agencies, only midwives, labour and delivery nurses, and nurse practitioners examine the internal genitals. However, generalist nurses often assist with this examination and need to be familiar with the procedure. Examination of the internal genitals involves (a) palpating Skene's and Bartholin's glands; (b) assessing the pelvic musculature; (c) inserting a vaginal speculum to inspect the cervix and vagina; and (d) obtaining a Pap smear.

The *speculum examination* of the vagina involves the insertion of a plastic or metal speculum that consists of

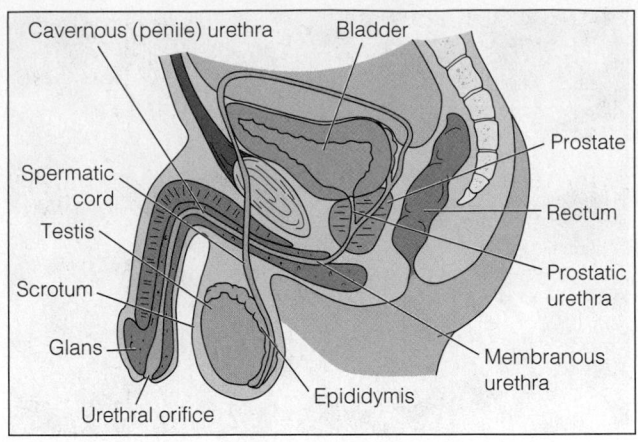

Labels on figure: Cavernous (penile) urethra, Bladder, Spermatic cord, Prostate, Testis, Rectum, Scrotum, Prostatic urethra, Glans, Membranous urethra, Urethral orifice, Epididymis

FIGURE 28.37 The male urogenital tract.

which is the passageway for both urine and semen. Therefore, in physical assessment of the male, these two systems are frequently assessed together.

Development of secondary sex characteristics is assessed in relationship to the client's age. See Table 28.14 for the five stages of the development of pubic hair, the penis, the testes, and the scrotum during puberty.

All male clients should be screened for the presence of inguinal or femoral hernias. A **hernia** is a protrusion of the intestine through the inguinal wall or canal. Cancer of the prostate gland is the most common cancer in adult men and occurs primarily in men over age 50 years. Examination of the prostate gland is performed with the examination of the rectum and the anus.

Testicular cancer is much rarer than prostate cancer and occurs primarily in young men aged 15 to 35 years. Testicular cancer is most commonly found on the anterior and lateral surfaces of the testes. **Testicular self-examination** should be conducted monthly. See Chapter 46.

Skill 28.19 describes how the nurse can conduct an assessment of the male genitals and inguinal area (see also the Lifespan Considerations box on assessing male genitals and inguinal area on page 691).

TABLE 28.14 Tanner Stages of Development of Pubic Hair, Penis, and Testes or Scrotum (12 to 16 Years)

Stage	Pubic Hair	Penis	Testes/Scrotum
1	None, except for body hair, such as that on the abdomen	Size is relative to body size, as in childhood	Size is relative to body size, as in childhood
2	Scant, long, slightly pigmented at base of penis	Slight enlargement occurs	Becomes reddened in colour and enlarged
3	Darker, begins to curl and becomes more coarse; extends over pubic symphysis	Elongation occurs	Continuing enlargement
4	Continues to darken and thicken; extends on the sides, above, and below	Increase in both breadth and length; glans develops	Continuing enlargement; colour darkens

TABLE 28.14 *(continued)*

Stage	Pubic Hair	Penis	Testes/Scrotum
5	Adult distribution that extends to inner thighs, umbilicus, and anus	Adult appearance	Adult appearance

SKILL 28.19 ASSESSING MALE GENITALS AND INGUINAL AREA

PLANNING
Equipment: Clean gloves

IMPLEMENTATION
Performance

1. Before performing the procedure, introduce yourself and verify the client's identity using two identifiers or per agency protocol. Explain to the client what you are going to do, why it is necessary, and how he can participate. Discuss how the results will be used in planning further care or treatments.

2. Perform hand hygiene, put on gloves, and follow other appropriate infection prevention and control procedures.

3. Provide for client privacy. Request the presence of another person if you so desire, if required by agency policy, or if requested by the client.

4. Inquire whether the client has any history of the following: urinary incontinence, frequency, urgency, abdominal pain; symptoms of STIs; swellings that could indicate presence of hernia; family history of nephritis, malignancy of the prostate, or malignancy of the kidney. Inquire about usual voiding patterns and changes, and bladder control.

5. Cover the pelvic area with a sheet or drape at all times when it is not actually being examined.

Assessment	Normal Findings	Deviations from Normal
Pubic Hair		
6. Inspect the distribution, amount, and characteristics of pubic hair.	Triangular distribution, often spreading up the abdomen	Scant amount or absence of hair
Penis		
7. Inspect the penile shaft and glans penis for lesions, nodules, swellings, and inflammation.	Penile skin intact; appears slightly wrinkled and varies in colour as widely as other body skin; foreskin easily retractable from the glans penis; small amount of thick white smegma between the glans and foreskin	Presence of lesions, nodules, swellings, or inflammation
8. Inspect the urethral meatus for swelling, inflammation, and discharge. • Compress, or ask the client to compress, the glans slightly to open the urethral meatus to inspect it for discharge.	Pink and slit-like appearance; positioned at the tip of the penis	Inflammation; discharge; variation in meatal locations (e.g., hypospadias, on the underside of the penile shaft, and epispadias, on the upper side of the penile shaft)
Scrotum		
9. Inspect the scrotum for appearance, general size, and symmetry. • Inspect all skin surfaces by spreading the *rugated* (ridged) surface skin and lifting the scrotum, as needed, to observe posterior surfaces.	Scrotal skin is darker in colour than that the skin of the rest of the body and is loose Size varies with temperature changes (the dartos muscles contract when the area is cold and relax when the area is warm) Scrotum appears asymmetric (left testis is usually lower than right testis)	Discolorations; any tightening of skin (may indicate edema or mass)

(continued)

SKILL 28.19 ASSESSING MALE GENITALS AND INGUINAL AREA (*continued*)

Assessment	Normal Findings	Deviations from Normal
10. Palpate the scrotum to assess status of underlying testes, epididymis (the narrow tube connecting the back of each testicle to its vas deferens), and spermatic cord. Palpate both testes simultaneously for comparative purposes.	Testicles are rubbery, smooth, and free of nodules and masses; testis is about 2 cm × 4 cm; epididymis is resilient, normally tender, and softer than the spermatic cord; spermatic cord is firm	Testicles are enlarged, with uneven surface (possible tumour); epididymis is nonresilient and painful

- Using your first two fingers and thumb, palpate each testis for size, consistency, shape, smoothness, and presence of masses. During assessment of male adolescents, establish the descent of the testicles into the scrotum; note undescended testes.

- Palpate the epididymis between your thumb and index finger. It is located at the top of the testis and extends behind it.

- Palpate the spermatic cord between your thumb and index finger. It is usually found at the top lateral portion of the scrotum and feels firm.

- If swelling, irregularities, or nodules are detected during the scrotal examination, attempt to transilluminate the lesion. This is done by darkening the room and shining a flashlight behind the scrotum through the mass. **Rationale: Serous fluid causes the light to show with a red glow; tissue or blood does not transilluminate.**

- Describe all scrotal masses in terms of their size, shape, placement, consistency, tenderness, and presence of transillumination.

Inguinal Area

11. Inspect both inguinal areas for bulges while the client is standing, if possible.	No swelling or bulges	Swelling or bulge (possible inguinal or femoral hernia)

- First, have the client remain at rest.

- Next, have the client hold his breath and strain or bear down as though having a bowel movement. Bearing down may make the hernia more visible.

12. Remove and discard gloves. Perform hand hygiene.

13. Document your findings in the client record by using forms or checklists supplemented by narrative notes, when appropriate.

EVALUATION

- Perform a detailed follow-up examination based on findings that deviated from expected or normal for the client. Relate findings to previous assessment data, if available.

- Report significant deviations from normal to the appropriate members of the health care team.

Assessing Male Genitals and Inguinal Area

INFANTS

- The foreskin of the uncircumcised infant is normally tight at birth and should not be retracted. It will gradually loosen as the baby grows and is usually fully retractable by age 2 to 3 years. Assess for cleanliness, redness, or irritation.
- Assess for placement of the urethral meatus.
- Palpate the scrotum to determine if the testes are descended; in the newborn and infant, the testes may retract into the inguinal canal, especially with stimulation of the *cremasteric reflex* (lightly stroking the superior and medial part of the thigh causes the cremaster muscle to pull up the scrotum and testis on that side).
- Assess the inguinal area for swelling or tenderness that may indicate the presence of an inguinal hernia.

CHILDREN

- Ensure that you have the parent or guardian's approval to perform the examination, and then tell the child what you are going to do. Preschool children are taught to not allow others to touch their "private parts."

- In young boys, the cremasteric reflex can cause the testes to ascend into the inguinal canal. If possible, have the boy sit cross-legged, which stretches the muscle and decreases the reflex.

OLDER ADULTS

- The penis decreases in size with aging; the size and firmness of the testes decrease.
- Testosterone is produced in smaller amounts.
- More time and direct physical stimulation are required for an older man to achieve an erection, but the client can maintain the erection for a longer period before ejaculation than he could at a younger age.
- Seminal fluid is reduced in amount and viscosity.
- Urinary frequency, nocturia, dribbling, and problems with beginning and ending the stream are usually the result of prostatic enlargement.

The Anus

For the generalist nurse, anal examination, an essential part of every *comprehensive* physical examination, generally involves only inspection.

Skill 28.20 describes how to assess the anus (see also the Lifespan Considerations box on assessing the anus on the next page).

SKILL 28.20 ASSESSING THE ANUS

PLANNING

Equipment

- Clean gloves
- Water-soluble lubricant

IMPLEMENTATION

Performance

1. Before performing the procedure, introduce yourself and verify the client's identity using two identifiers or per agency protocol. Explain to the client what you are going to do, why it is necessary, and how he or she can participate. Discuss

how the results will be used in planning further care or treatments.
2. Perform hand hygiene, put on gloves, and follow other appropriate infection prevention and control procedures for all anal and rectal examinations.
3. Provide for client privacy. Drape the client appropriately to prevent undue exposure of body parts.
4. Inquire whether the client has any history of the following: bright red blood in stools, tarry black stools, diarrhea, constipation, abdominal pain, excessive gas, hemorrhoids, or rectal pain; family history of colorectal cancer; when last stool specimen for occult blood was performed and the results; and for males, if not obtained during the genitourinary examination, signs or symptoms of

(continued)

SKILL 28.20   ASSESSING THE ANUS (*continued*)

prostate enlargement (e.g., slow urinary stream, hesitance, frequency, dribbling, and nocturia).

5. Position the client. In adults, a left lateral or Sims' position with the upper leg acutely flexed is required for the examination. For females, a dorsal recumbent position with hips externally rotated and knees flexed or a lithotomy position may be used (see Table 28.2 on page 597). For males, a standing position while the client bends over the examining table may also be used. This position is commonly used to examine the prostate gland.

Assessment	Normal Findings	Deviations from Normal
6. Inspect the anus and surrounding tissue for colour, integrity, and skin lesions. Then, ask the client to bear down as though defecating. Bearing down creates slight pressure on the skin that may accentuate rectal fissures, rectal prolapse, polyps, or internal hemorrhoids. Describe the location of all abnormal findings in terms of a clock, with the 12 o'clock position toward the pubic symphysis.	Intact perianal skin; usually slightly more pigmented than the skin of the buttocks; anal skin is normally more pigmented, coarser, and more moist than perianal skin and is usually hairless	Presence of fissures (cracks), ulcers, excoriations, inflammations, abscesses, protruding hemorrhoids (dilated veins seen as reddened protrusions of the skin), lumps or tumours, fistula openings, or rectal prolapse (varying degrees of protrusion of the rectal mucous membrane through the anus)

7. Remove and discard gloves. Perform hand hygiene.

8. Document findings in the client record by using forms or checklists supplemented by narrative notes, when appropriate

EVALUATION

• Perform a detailed follow-up examination based on findings that deviated from expected or normal for the client. Relate findings to previous assessment data, if available.

• Report significant deviations from normal to the appropriate members of the health care team.

LIFESPAN CONSIDERATIONS

Assessing the Anus

INFANTS

• Lightly touching the anus should result in a brief anal contraction ("wink" reflex).

CHILDREN

• Erythema and scratch marks around the anus may indicate a pinworm parasite. Children with this condition may be disturbed by itching during sleep.

OLDER ADULTS

• Chronic constipation and straining at stool cause an increase in the frequency of hemorrhoids and rectal prolapse.

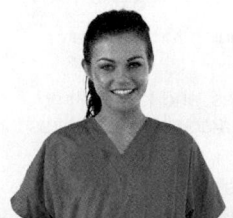

Case Study 28

Mrs. J., a 32-year-old Inuit woman, has come to the clinic because she has felt a lump in her breast. When you begin the breast examination, the client shrieks and asks, "What do you think you are doing?"

CRITICAL THINKING QUESTIONS

1. How would you respond to this client?

2. How would you develop nursing interventions to help put clients at ease for an invasive procedure that has a vital role in physical assessment?

3. How will you address clients in a manner that is likely to gain their trust and cooperation?

Check the eText in MyNursingLab for answers and explanations.

KEY TERMS

adventitious breath
  sounds *p. 641*
albinism *p. 605*
alopecia *p. 605*
anesthesia *p. 675*
angle of Louis *p. 638*
anisocoria *p. 616*
antihelix *p. 621*
apex *p. 649*
aphasia *p. 672*
arcus senilis *p. 621*
astigmatism *p. 615*
auricle *p. 621*
auscultation *p. 601*
axillary tail of Spence
  p. 657
base *p. 649*
blanch test *p. 612*
borborygmi *p. 664*
bromhidrosis *p. 605*
bruit *p. 650*
caries *p. 629*
cataracts *p. 615*
cerumen *p. 621*
clubbing *p. 605*
cochlea *p. 622*
conduction hearing loss
  p. 622
conjunctivitis *p. 615*
cyanosis *p. 605*
dacryocystitis *p. 615*
diastole *p. 649*
dullness *p. 601*
duration *p. 602*
edema *p. 605*

erythema *p. 605*
eustachian tube *p. 622*
exophthalmos *p. 613*
external auditory meatus
  p. 621
extinction *p. 675*
fasciculation *p. 662*
flatness *p. 601*
fremitus *p. 643*
gingivitis *p. 629*
glaucoma *p. 616*
glossitis *p. 629*
heave *p. 649*
helix *p. 621*
hernia *p. 688*
hirsutism *p. 611*
hordeolum *p. 615*
hyperesthesia *p. 675*
hyperhidrosis *p. 605*
hyperopia *p. 614*
hyperresonance *p. 601*
hypoesthesia *p. 675*
incus *p. 622*
inspection *p. 599*
intensity *p. 602*
intention tremor *p. 669*
iritis *p. 615*
jaundice *p. 605*
koilonychia *p. 605*
leukoplakia *p. 630*
lift *p. 649*
lobule *p. 621*
malleus *p. 622*
manubrium *p. 638*
mastoid *p. 621*

miosis *p. 616*
mixed hearing loss *p. 622*
mydriasis *p. 616*
myopia *p. 614*
normocephalic *p. 613*
nystagmus *p. 619*
one-point discrimination
  p. 675
ossicles *p. 622*
otoscope *p. 616*
pallor *p. 605*
palpation *p. 599*
paresthesia *p. 675*
paronychia *p. 612*
parotitis *p. 629*
PERRLA *p. 618*
percussion *p. 601*
perfusion *p. 650*
photophobia *p. 615*
pinna *p. 621*
pitch *p. 602*
plaque *p. 629*
pleximeter *p. 601*
plexor *p. 601*
point of maximal impulse
  (PMI) *p. 649*
precordium *p. 649*
presbycusis *p. 626*
presbyopia *p. 614*
primary skin lesions
  p. 605
proprioceptors *p. 675*
pyorrhea *p. 629*
quality *p. 602*
reflex *p. 673*

resonance *p. 601*
resting tremor *p. 669*
Rinne test *p. 625*
S_1 *p. 649*
S_2 *p. 649*
secondary skin lesions
  p. 605
semicircular canals *p. 622*
sensorineural hearing loss
  p. 622
sordes *p. 629*
stapes *p. 622*
stereognosis *p. 675*
sternum *p. 638*
stomatitis *p. 629*
sty *p. 615*
systole *p. 649*
tartar *p. 629*
testicular self-examination
  p. 688
thrill *p. 650*
tragus *p. 621*
tremor *p. 662*
triangular fossa *p. 621*
two-point discrimination
  p. 675
tympanic membrane
  p. 621
tympany *p. 601*
vestibule *p. 622*
visual acuity *p. 613*
visual fields *p. 614*
vitiligo *p. 605*
Weber's test *p. 625*

CHAPTER HIGHLIGHTS

- The health examination is conducted to assess the function and integrity of the client's body parts.
- The health examination may entail a complete head-to-toe assessment or individual assessment of a body system or body part.
- The health assessment is conducted in a systematic manner that requires the fewest position changes for the client.

- Data obtained in the physical health examination supplement, confirm, or refute data obtained during the nursing history.
- Nursing history data help the nurse focus on specific aspects of the physical health examination.
- Data obtained in the physical health examination help the nurse establish nursing diagnoses, plan the client's care, and evaluate the outcomes of nursing care.

- Initial assessment findings provide baseline data about the client's functional abilities against which subsequent assessment findings are compared.
- Skills in inspection, palpation, percussion, and auscultation are required for the physical health examination; these skills are used in that order throughout the examination except during abdominal assessment, when the order is inspection, auscultation, percussion, and palpation.
- Knowledge of the normal structure and function of body parts and systems is a prerequisite to conducting a physical assessment.

ASSESS YOUR LEARNING

1. The nurse documents the client's complaints of numbness and tingling in the right arm and right leg as which of the following?
   a. Hyperesthesia
   b. Hypoesthesia
   c. Paresthesia
   d. Extinction

2. The nurse has the client in the upright sitting position during palpation of which of the following areas?
   a. Abdomen
   b. Genitals
   c. Breast
   d. Head

3. Which of the following is the correct order to conduct an assessment of the abdomen?
   a. Inspection, palpation, percussion, auscultation
   b. Inspection, percussion, palpation, auscultation
   c. Auscultation, inspection, palpation, percussion
   d. Inspection, auscultation, palpation, percussion

4. In older adults, the nurse must remember which of the following while conducting the health assessment?
   a. The vital organs are in different locations because of aging.
   b. This population fatigues easily, and the exam must be tailored to best support the client.
   c. Members of this population usually have memory lapses.
   d. The nurse should always help the client off the examination table.

5. When the nurse is broaching sensitive topics, it is BEST to do which of the following?
   a. Clearly state any personal feelings on the topic of discussion.
   b. Be vague with the questions to make sure the client is not embarrassed.
   c. Be nonjudgmental and provide privacy for the interview.
   d. Omit this kind of assessment so that neither the nurse nor the client will feel uncomfortable.

6. After auscultating the abdomen, the nurse should report which of the following for further follow-up?
   a. Bruit over the aorta
   b. Absence of bowel sounds for 60 seconds
   c. Continuous bowel sounds over the ileocecal valve
   d. An irregular pattern of bowel sounds

7. If unable to locate the client's popliteal pulse during a routine examination, the nurse should perform which of the following next?
   a. Check for a pedal pulse.
   b. Check for a femoral pulse.
   c. Take the client's blood pressure on that thigh.
   d. Ask another nurse to try to locate the pulse.

8. Which of the following techniques should the nurse use to palpate the lymph nodes?
   a. Use the flat part of all four fingers in a vertical and then side-to-side motion.
   b. Use the back of the hand and feel for temperature variation between the right and left sides.
   c. Use the pads and tips of the index and middle fingers in a circular motion.
   d. Compress the nodes between the index fingers of both hands.

9. If the client complains of having difficulty remembering recent events, the nurse would assess this by doing which of the following?
   a. Have the client repeat a series of three numbers, if possible.
   b. Have the client describe his or her childhood illnesses.
   c. Ask the client to describe how he or she arrived at your location.
   d. Ask the client to count backward from 100 subtracting 7 each time.

10. Which of the following indicates a normal finding on general percussion of the lungs?

    a. Tympany over the right upper lobe

    b. Resonance over the left upper lobe

    c. Hyperresonance over the left lower lobe

    d. Dullness above the left 10th intercostal space

> *Check the eText in MyNursingLab for answers and explanations.*

WEBLINKS

Canadian Cancer Society

http://www.cancer.ca

This site provides educational resources related to cancer, including risk reduction.

Canadian Task Force on Preventive Health Care

http://www.canadiantaskforce.ca/recommendations_current_eng.html

This site is supported by the Public Health Agency of Canada and provides clinical practice guidelines for screening of health issues (e.g., breast cancer, obesity).

McGill University Virtual Stethoscope

http://sprojects.mmi.mcgill.ca/dir/mvs.html

This site allows listeners to hear normal and adventitious lung sounds. Links are made with pathophysiology.

MyNursingLab MyNursingLab's guided learning path makes reviewing and test preparation straightforward.

- Content summaries, animations, and videos reinforce key concepts and skills

- Practice questions help with test prep by showing gaps in knowledge

- An eText, available online and via the iPad, makes searching, highlighting, and note-taking easy

 This QR code appears at the end of every chapter and provides learning resources that you can access with your smartphone to study on the go. Access self-review quizzes, flashcards, and more!

REFERENCES

Canadian Cancer Society. (2012). *Canadian cancer statistics 2012*. Toronto, ON: Author.

D'Amico, D., Barbarito, C., Twomey, C., & Harder, N. (2012). *Health and physical assessment in nursing*. Toronto, ON: Pearson Education.

Chapter 29

Vital Signs

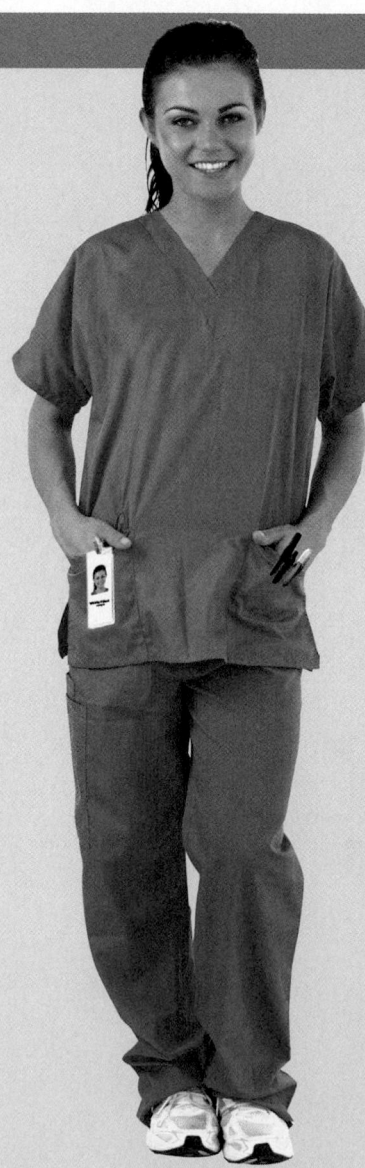

LEARNING OUTCOMES

After studying this chapter, you will be able to:

1. Describe factors that affect the vital signs and accurate measurement of them.

2. Identify the normal range variations in body temperature, pulse, respirations, and blood pressure that occur across the lifespan.

3. Describe the body's system of thermoregulation and identify factors influencing the body's heat production.

4. Explain and distinguish oral, rectal, axillary, tympanic membrane, and temporal artery methods of measuring body temperature and their relative merits.

5. Outline appropriate nursing care for alterations in body temperature.

6. Perform accurate body temperature assessment using the correct method for the client.

7. Identify nine sites commonly used to assess the pulse and state the reasons for use of each.

8. Describe the characteristics that should be included when assessing pulses.

9. Perform accurate apical pulse and apical–radial pulse measurement.

10. Describe the mechanics of breathing and the mechanisms that control respirations.

11. Identify the components of a respiratory assessment.

12. Perform accurate respiration rate and quality assessment.

13. Summarize the physiology of blood pressure and what it indicates about client health.

14. Identify noninvasive methods for measuring blood pressure, and differentiate between systolic and diastolic blood pressure, including the five phases of Korotkoff sounds.

15. Perform accurate blood pressure measurement.

16. Discuss measurement of blood oxygenation by using pulse oximetry and the correct interpretation of oximetry measurements.

The traditional **vital signs** are body temperature, pulse, respirations, and blood pressure. Pulse oximetry or oxygen saturation is also commonly measured at the same time as the traditional vital signs and is sometimes called the *fifth vital sign*. Recently, some health care agencies have designated pain as the fifth vital sign (see Box 29.1), to be assessed at the same time as each of the other four. Pain assessment is covered in Chapter 30. Vital signs are assessed to monitor the functions of the body; they are interrelated with each other and are an important part of a comprehensive patient assessment. Vital signs reflect changes in function that otherwise might not be observed. Monitoring a client's vital signs should be a thoughtful, scientific assessment, not merely an automatic or routine procedure. When assessed, vital signs must be evaluated with reference to the client's present and prior health status and also compared with accepted normal standards. Vital signs cannot be interpreted in isolation of each other but must be interpreted together.

When and how often to assess a specific client's vital signs are primarily nursing judgments, depending on the client's health status. Some agencies have policies about taking clients' vital signs and about when this must occur. Physicians may specify frequency (e.g., "blood pressure q2h"), but this should be considered the minimum; a nurse should measure vital signs more often if the client's health status requires it. Examples of times to assess vital signs are listed in Box 29.2.

BOX 29.1   THE FIFTH VITAL SIGN

The debate about what constitutes the "real" fifth vital sign has been ongoing for several years. Those who advocate for pain as the fifth vital sign point to the longstanding underassessment of pain and its significant negative impact on physiological and psychological processes as meriting this rank. Those who advocate that oxygen saturation has this status point to it as a true "sign of life" in that one cannot survive without oxygen. Interestingly, some argue that only pulse and respirations are vital signs, as blood pressure and temperature require instruments for measuring and, as such, are results of diagnostic testing. Depending on the nature of the clinical agency, specialty, or both, other contenders for the "fifth" spot include level of emotional distress, blood glucose level, urine output, body mass index, pupil size and reaction, and the list goes on! One thing for sure is that since pain and oxygenation have been emphasized as meriting consideration as "vital signs," clinicians have given these important areas greater attention—all in an effort to improve the client's health status and ability to rally when ill.

BOX 29.2   WHEN TO ASSESS VITAL SIGNS

- On admission to a health care agency or nursing unit, to obtain baseline data
- When a client's health status changes or he or she reports symptoms
- Before and after invasive diagnostic procedures or demanding treatments
- Before or after the administration of a medication that has a direct effect or side effects, such as altering respirations, heart rate, or blood pressure (medications such as digoxin and morphine and other opioids are examples)
- Before and after any nursing intervention that could affect the vital signs (e.g., ambulating a client who has been on bed rest)
- According to policy and standard procedure on the unit

Body Temperature

Body temperature reflects the balance between the heat produced and the heat lost from the body, and it is measured in units called *degrees*. The body has two kinds of temperatures: (a) core temperature and (b) surface temperature. **Core temperature** is the temperature of the deep tissues of the body, such as the cranium, thorax, abdominal cavity, and pelvic cavity. It remains relatively constant. The **surface temperature** is the temperature of skin, subcutaneous tissue, and fat. It, in contrast to core body temperature, fluctuates in response to the environment.

The normal core body temperature of an adult is approximately between 36.7°C and 37°C (Braine, 2009). Small fluctuations of 0.2°C to 0.4°C can occur without

TABLE 29.1 Range of Normal Body Temperatures by Route of Measurement

Route of Measurement	Temperature Range
Core	36.5°C–37.5°C
Oral	35.5°C–37.5°C
Rectal	36.6°C–38.0°C
Tympanic	35.5°C–38.0°C
Temporal artery	35.0°C
Axillary	34.7°C–37.3°C

Sources: Adapted from Canadian Paediatric Society. (2010). Temperature measurement in paediatrics. *Position Statement: Canadian Pediatric Society.* Retrieved from http://www.cps.ca/english/statements/CP/cp00-01.htm; Health Canada. (2001). *Pediatric clinical practice guidelines for nurses in primary care.* First Nations Inuit Health Branch; Sessler, D. I. (2008). Temperature monitoring and perioperative thermoregulation. *Anesthesiology, 109* (2), 318–338.

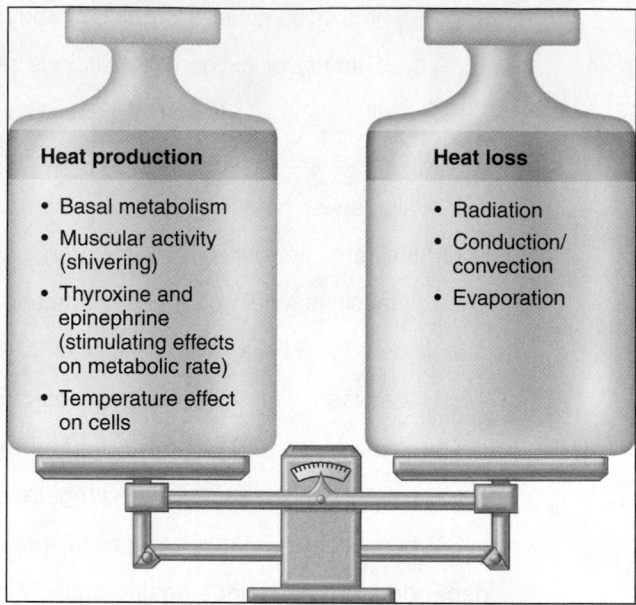

FIGURE 29.1 As long as heat production and heat loss are properly balanced, body temperature remains constant. Factors contributing to heat production (and temperature rise) are shown on the left side of the scale; those contributing to heat loss (and temperature drop) are shown on the right side.

Source: Marieb, Elaine N.; Hoehn, Katja N., *Human Anatomy and Physiology*, 8th Ed. © 2010. Reprinted and Electronically reproduced by permission of Pearson Education, Inc., Upper Saddle River, New Jersey.

the body mounting a response to bring it back to normal (Braine, 2009; Sessler, 2008). Measured orally, the normal range in adults is between 36.5°C and 37.5°C, although in practice, the acceptable norms can range from 34.8°C to 37.8°C (Frommelt, Ott, & Hays, 2008). Given the variations in the literature for what constitutes a 'normal' oral temperature, many practice settings accept a range of 36°C to 38°C as 'normal' in adults (Figure 29.3). More importantly, temperature measurements must be interpreted in light of the client's other vital signs and in consideration of the client's usual and previous temperatures. For example, older people often have a body temperature below 37°C and, as such, a temperature of 37°C may, in fact, represent a febrile state. As such, when working with older people, it is beneficial to also observe for signs such as increased heart and respiration rates, change in blood pressure, signs of confusion, and a decline in functional status. Table 29.1 identifies accepted norms for body temperature in children by route of measurement.

The body continually produces heat as a byproduct of metabolism. When the amount of heat produced by the body exactly equals the amount of heat lost, the person is said to be in **heat balance** (Figure 29.1).

A number of factors affect the body's heat production. The five most important are as follows:

1. *Basal metabolic rate.* The **basal metabolic rate (BMR)** is the rate of energy utilization in the body required to maintain essential activities, such as breathing. Metabolic rates decrease with age. In general, the younger the person, the higher is the BMR.

2. *Muscle activity.* Muscle activity, including shivering, increases the BMR.

3. *Thyroxine output.* Increased thyroxine output increases the rate of cellular metabolism throughout the body. This effect is called **chemical thermogenesis**, the stimulation of heat production in the body through increased cellular metabolism.

4. *Sympathetic stimulation, including release of epinephrine and norepinephrine.* Sympathetic stimulation of the autonomic nervous system (e.g., during stress) causes the release of epinephrine and norepinephrine. These hormones directly affect liver and muscle cells, thereby increasing cellular metabolism and heat production.

5. *Fever.* Fever increases the cellular metabolic rate and thus further increases the body's temperature.

Heat is lost from the body through *radiation, conduction, convection,* and *vaporization.*

- **Radiation** is the transfer of heat from the surface of one object to the surface of another without contact between the two objects, mostly in the form of infrared rays.

- **Conduction** is the transfer of heat from one molecule to a molecule of lower temperature. Conductive transfer cannot take place without contact between the molecules and normally accounts for minimal heat loss, except, for example, when the body is immersed in cold water. The amount of heat transferred depends on the temperature difference and the amount and duration of the contact.

- **Convection** is the dispersion of heat by air currents. The body usually has a small amount of warm air adjacent to it. This warm air rises and is replaced by cooler air, and so people always lose a small amount of heat through convection. This can be useful in clinical practice, as in the use of fans to help cool a client who has a high temperature.

- **Evaporation** is continuous vaporization of moisture from the respiratory tract, from the mucosa of the mouth, and from skin. This continuous and unnoticed water loss is called **insensible water loss**, and the accompanying heat loss is called **insensible heat loss**. Insensible heat loss accounts for about 10% of basal heat loss. When the body temperature increases, vaporization accounts for greater heat loss.

Regulation of Body Temperature

The system that regulates body temperature has three main parts: (a) sensors on the skin and in the body's core, (b) an integrator in the hypothalamus, and (c) an effector system that adjusts the production and loss of heat. Most *sensors* or *sensory receptors* are in skin. Skin has more receptors for cold than for warmth. Therefore, skin sensors detect cold more efficiently than warmth.

When skin becomes chilled over the entire body, three physiological processes take place to increase the body temperature:

1. Shivering increases heat production.
2. Sweating is inhibited to decrease heat loss.
3. Vasoconstriction decreases heat loss.

The **hypothalamic integrator**, the centre that controls the core temperature, is located in the anterior region of the hypothalamus (Braine, 2009). When the sensors in the hypothalamus detect heat, they send out signals intended to reduce the temperature, that is, to decrease heat production and increase heat loss. When the cold sensors are stimulated, signals are sent out to increase heat production and decrease heat loss.

The signals from the cold-sensitive receptors of the hypothalamus initiate *effectors*, such as vasoconstriction, shivering, and the release of epinephrine, which increases cellular metabolism and, hence, heat production. When the warmth-sensitive receptors in the hypothalamus are stimulated, the effector system sends out signals that initiate sweating and peripheral vasodilation. Also, when this system is stimulated, the person consciously makes appropriate adjustments, such as putting on additional clothing in response to cold or turning on a fan in response to heat.

Factors Affecting Body Temperature

Nurses should be aware of the factors that can affect a client's body temperature to recognize normal temperature variations and understand the significance of body temperature measurements that deviate from normal.

Among the factors that affect body temperature are the following:

1. *Age.* The infant is greatly affected by the temperature of the environment and must be protected from extreme changes. Until puberty, children's temperatures continue to be more *labile* (changeable) than those of adults. Many older people, particularly those older than 75 years, are at risk of hypothermia (temperatures below 36°C) for a variety of reasons, such as inadequate diet, loss of subcutaneous fat, lack of activity, and reduced thermoregulatory efficiency. Older people are also particularly sensitive to extremes in the environmental temperature because of decreased thermoregulatory controls.

2. *Diurnal variations (circadian rhythms).* Body temperatures normally change throughout the day, varying by as much as 1°C between the early morning and the late afternoon. The point of highest body temperature is usually reached between 1600 and 1800 hours (4 p.m. and 6 p.m.), and the lowest point is reached during sleep between 0400 and 0600 hours (4 a.m. and 6 a.m.) (see Figure 29.2).

3. *Exercise.* Hard work or strenuous exercise can increase body temperature to as high as 38.3°C to 40°C, when measured rectally.

4. *Hormones.* Women usually experience more hormone fluctuations than men do. In women, progesterone secretion at the time of ovulation raises body temperature by about 0.3°C to 0.6°C above basal temperature.

5. *Stress.* Stimulation of the sympathetic nervous system can increase the production of epinephrine and norepinephrine, thereby increasing metabolic activity and heat production. Nurses can anticipate that a highly stressed or anxious client could have an elevated body temperature for that reason.

6. *Environment.* Extremes in environmental temperatures can affect a person's temperature regulatory systems. If the temperature is assessed in a very warm room and the body temperature cannot be modified by convection, conduction, or radiation, the temperature will be elevated. Similarly, if the client has been outside in extremely cold weather without suitable clothing, the body temperature may be low.

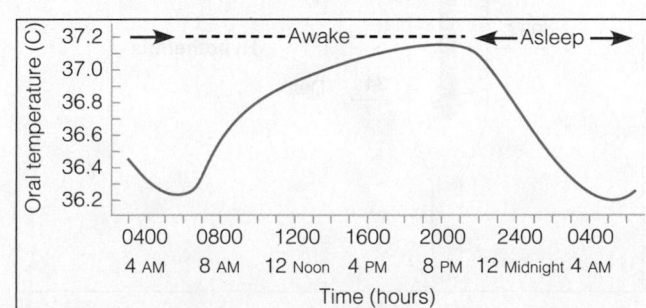

FIGURE 29.2 Range of oral temperatures during 24 hours for a healthy young adult.

Alterations in Body Temperature

Two primary alterations in body temperature occur: *pyrexia* (hyperthermia, fever) and *hypothermia*

PYREXIA A body temperature above the normal range is called **pyrexia**, or hyperthermia. In many cases, hyperthermia, or pyrexia, indicates fever, but not always. **Fever** is a regulated rise in core body temperature or change in temperature set point, which is regulated by the hypothalamus, the body's thermostat. **Hyperthermia**, in contrast, is an unregulated rise in body temperature caused by the body's inability to eliminate heat adequately, such as in the case of heat stroke (Henker & Carlson, 2007). The client who has a fever is referred to as febrile; many agencies consider a client to be **febrile** if he or she has an oral temperature of 38.3°C once or ≥38.0°C sustained for more than one hour. A very high fever, above 41°C, is called hyperpyrexia (Figure 29.3). Clients who do not have a fever are referred to as **afebrile**.

Fever is a physiological response to a stimulus, such as infection, and can be a beneficial mechanism to a certain point (Henker & Carlson, 2007). Four common types of fevers are *intermittent, remittent, relapsing,* and *constant.* During **intermittent fever**, the body temperature alternates at regular intervals between periods of fever and periods of normal or subnormal temperatures. This occurs, for example, with malaria. During a **remittent** fever, such as with a cold or influenza, a wide range of temperature fluctuations (more than 2°C) occurs in 24 hours, all of which are above normal. In a **relapsing fever**, short febrile periods of a few days are interspersed with periods of one or two days of normal temperature. During a **constant fever**, the body temperature fluctuates minimally but always remains above normal. This can occur with typhoid fever. A temperature that rises to fever level rapidly following a normal temperature and then returns to normal within a few hours is called a **fever spike**. Bacterial blood infections often cause fever spikes.

An elevated temperature is not always a true fever. Three examples of this are heat exhaustion, heat stroke, and malignant hyperthermia. **Heat exhaustion** is a result of excessive heat and dehydration. Signs of heat exhaustion include pallor, dizziness, nausea, vomiting, fainting, and a moderately increased temperature (38.5°C to 39°C). Persons experiencing **heat stroke** generally have been exercising in hot weather, have warm, flushed skin, and often do not sweat. They usually have a temperature of 41°C or higher and may be delirious, unconscious, or having seizures. A very rare form of hyperthermia is **malignant hyperthermia**, a pharmacogenetic disorder, which can be triggered by exposure to certain anesthetic agents. Individuals who develop this condition display elevated carbon dioxide production, profuse sweating, tachycardia, and skeletal muscle rigidity, prior to developing a life-threatening rapid increase in core body temperature (Glahn et al., 2010).

The clinical signs of fever vary with the onset, course, and abatement stages of the fever (see the Clinical Manifestations box).

These signs occur as a result of changes in the *set point* of the temperature control mechanism regulated by the hypothalamus. Under normal conditions, whenever the core temperature rises above 37°C, the rate of heat loss becomes greater than heat production, resulting in a fall in temperature toward the set point level. Conversely, when the core temperature falls below 37°C, the rate of heat production becomes greater than heat loss, resulting in a rise in temperature toward the set point.

In a fever, however, the set point of the hypothalamic thermostat changes suddenly from the normal level to a higher-than-normal value (e.g., 39.5°C) as a result of the effects of tissue destruction, pyrogenic substances, or dehydration on the hypothalamus. Although the set point changes rapidly, the core body temperature reaches this new set point only after several hours. During this interval, the usual heat production responses that cause elevation of the body temperature occur.

When the core temperature reaches the new set point, the person feels neither cold nor hot and no longer experiences chills (the *plateau phase*). Depending on the degree of temperature elevation, various other signs may occur at this stage. Very high temperatures, such as 41°C to 42°C, damage the parenchyma of cells throughout the body, particularly in the brain, where destruction

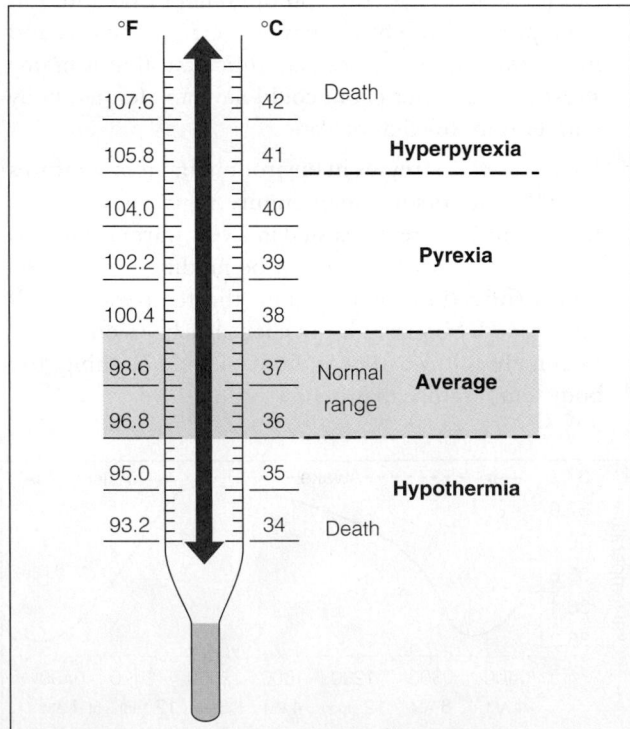

FIGURE 29.3 Terms used to describe alterations in body temperature (oral measurements) and ranges in Celsius and Fahrenheit scales.

CLINICAL MANIFESTATIONS

Fever

Fever can manifest in several different ways:

ONSET (COLD OR CHILL STAGE)

- Increased heart rate
- Increased respiratory rate and depth
- Shivering
- Pallid, cold skin
- Complaints of feeling cold
- Cyanotic nail beds
- Gooseflesh appearance of the skin
- Cessation of sweating

COURSE (PLATEAU PHASE)

- Absence of chills
- Skin that feels warm
- Photosensitivity
- Glassy-eyed appearance
- Increased pulse and respiratory rates
- Increased thirst
- Mild to severe dehydration
- Drowsiness, restlessness, delirium, or convulsions
- Herpetic lesions of the mouth
- Loss of appetite (if the fever is prolonged)
- Malaise, weakness, and aching muscles

DEFERVESCENCE (FEVER ABATEMENT OR FLUSH PHASE)

- Skin that appears flushed and feels warm
- Sweating
- Decreased shivering
- Possible dehydration

BOX 29.3   NURSING INTERVENTIONS FOR CLIENTS WITH FEVER

Nurses can do several things to help a client through each stage of a fever:

- Monitor vital signs, every 2 hours if the client is critically ill.
- Assess skin colour, temperature, and other physiological signs associated with fever.
- Monitor white blood cell count, hematocrit value, and other pertinent laboratory reports for indications of infection or dehydration.
- Remove any excess blankets when the client feels warm, but provide extra warmth when the client feels chilled.
- Provide adequate nutrition and fluids (e.g., 2500 mL to 3000 mL per day, if not contraindicated) to meet the increased metabolic demands and prevent dehydration.
- Measure intake and output.
- Reduce physical activity to limit heat production, especially during the flush stage.
- Administer antipyretics (drugs that reduce the level of fever), if this is part of the client's treatment plan.
- Provide oral hygiene to keep the mucous membranes moist.
- Provide dry clothing and bed linens.

---

of neuronal cells is irreversible. Damage to the liver, kidneys, and other body organs can also be great enough to disrupt functioning and eventually cause death. When the cause of the high temperature is suddenly removed, the set point of the hypothalamic thermostat is suddenly reduced to a lower value, perhaps even back to the original normal level. In this instance, the hypothalamus now attempts to lower the temperature to 37°C, and the usual heat loss responses causing a reduction of the body temperature occur. This sudden change of events is known as the *flush* or *defervescent stage* of a pyrexic condition. The clinical signs and symptoms associated with each phase of fever are listed in the Clinical Manifestations box.

Nursing interventions for a client who has a fever are designed to support the body's normal physiological processes, provide comfort, and prevent complications. During the course of the fever, the nurse must monitor the client's vital signs closely. Nursing measures during the chill phase are designed to help the client decrease heat loss. At this time, the body's physiological processes are attempting to raise the core temperature to the new set-point temperature. During the flush or crisis phase, the body processes are attempting to lower the core temperature to the reduced or normal set-point temperature. At this time, the nurse takes measures to increase heat loss and decrease heat production. Nursing interventions for a client with fever are shown in Box 29.3.

HYPOTHERMIA   **Hypothermia** is a core body temperature below the lower limit of normal. The three physiological mechanisms of hypothermia are (a) excessive heat loss, (b) inadequate heat production to counteract the heat loss, and (c) impaired hypothalamic thermoregulation. The clinical signs of hypothermia are given in the Clinical Manifestations Box.

CLINICAL MANIFESTATIONS

Hypothermia

Hypothermia typically manifests in the following ways:
- Decreased body temperature
- Severe shivering (initially)
- Feelings of cold and chills
- Pale, cool, waxy skin
- Hypotension
- Decreased urinary output
- Lack of muscle coordination
- Disorientation
- Drowsiness progressing to coma

Hypothermia can be induced or accidental. *Induced hypothermia* is the deliberate lowering of the body temperature to decrease the need for oxygen by the body tissues. Induced hypothermia can involve the whole body or a body part. It may be indicated for certain surgical cases (e.g., neurosurgery) but remains controversial. *Accidental hypothermia* can occur as a result of (a) exposure to a cold environment, (b) immersion in cold water, and (c) lack of adequate clothing, shelter, or heat. In older people, the problem can be compounded by a decreased metabolic rate. Additionally, chronic hypothermia progresses over days or weeks in older adults (Guly, 2011). If skin and underlying tissues are damaged by freezing cold, it results in frostbite. Frostbite most commonly occurs in the hands, feet, nose, and ears of an exposed person. A diagnosis of hypothermia requires the measurement of core or near-core body temperature.

Managing hypothermia involves removing the client from the cold and warming the client's body. For the client with mild hypothermia, the body is warmed by applying blankets and covering the head; for the client with severe hypothermia, an electric hyperthermia blanket is applied, and warm intravenous fluids are given. Rapid rewarming may be dangerous and even life threatening (Kemp, 2008). Do not immerse a hypothermic patient in warm or hot water, apply heating pads to extremities, or rub or massage the patient (Kemp, 2008). Wet clothing should be replaced with dry clothing. The focus of care should be on heat retention, restoring normal core body temperature, and the preservation of tissue.

Assessing Body Temperature

The most common sites for measuring body temperature are oral, rectal, axillary, tympanic membrane, and skin or temporal artery sites. Each of the sites has advantages and disadvantages (see Table 29.2). A wide range of preferred practices and norms exist in the measurement of temperature. Nurses need to consider numerous factors when deciding which route to use to obtain a temperature measurement and when interpreting the obtained readings. See the Clinical Alert box (page 703) on deciding which route to use when measuring temperature; in addition, see the Clinical Alert box (page 705) on ensuring reliability of temperature measurement over time.

The body temperature is frequently measured *orally*. If a client has ingested hot food or fluids or has been smoking, the nurse should wait 30 minutes before taking the temperature orally to ensure that the temperature

TABLE 29.2 Advantages and Disadvantages of the Five Sites for Body Temperature Measurement

Site	Advantages	Disadvantages
Oral	Accessible and convenient; consistent measurement; close to core temperature	Thermometers can break, if bitten; inaccurate if client has ingested hot or cold food or fluid or smoked within the last 30 minutes; could injure the mouth following oral surgery; not appropriate for some clients who are confused, unconscious, or unable to follow directions
Rectal	Reliable measurement; closest to core temperature	Inconvenient and more unpleasant for clients; difficult for client who cannot turn to the side; could injure the rectum; presence of stool may interfere with thermometer placement; if the stool is soft, the thermometer may be embedded in stool rather than against the mucosal wall of the rectum. If the stool is impacted, the depth of thermometer insertion may be insufficient; may stimulate a vagal reaction leading to bradycardia and syncope; in newborns and infants, insertion of rectal thermometer has caused ulcerations and rectal perforations
Axillary	Safe and noninvasive	The thermometer must be left in place a long time to obtain an accurate measurement; readings are accurate but must be adjusted as they are consistently lower than oral (by 0.5C°) and rectal (by 1.0°C); may be inaccurate if client has bathed within the last 30 minutes or if client is experiencing vasoconstriction, vasodilation, or sweating (El-Radhi & Barry, 2006)
Tympanic membrane	Readily accessible; reflects core temperature; very fast	Can be uncomfortable and involves risk of injuring the membrane if the probe is inserted too far; repeated measurements may vary between and within clients; right and left measurements can differ; more variable results than oral or rectal thermometry; presence of cerumen can affect the reading; subject to considerable error if tympanic thermometer is used incorrectly (see Box 29.4 on page 705).
Temporal artery	Safe and noninvasive; very fast; does not require client cooperation	Requires electronic equipment that may be expensive or unavailable; variation in technique needed if the client has perspiration on the forehead

of the mouth has not been affected by the temperature of the food, fluid, or warm smoke.

Rectal temperature readings are considered to be very accurate. Because inserting a rectal thermometer can produce vagal stimulation, which can cause bradycardia and syncope, taking rectal temperatures is generally contraindicated in clients with cardiac arrhythmias or recovering from a myocardial infarction. Rectal temperatures are usually contraindicated in clients who are undergoing rectal surgery, have diarrhea or diseases of the rectum, are immunosuppressed, have a clotting disorder, or have significant hemorrhoids.

The *axilla* is often the preferred site for measuring temperature in newborns because it is accessible and offers no possibility of rectal perforation. However, research indicates that the axillary method is inaccurate when assessing a fever (Ball & Bindler, 2008). Nurses should check agency protocol when taking the temperature of newborns, infants, toddlers, and children. The axillary temperature assessment method is appropriate for adult clients for whom other temperature sites are contraindicated (e.g., following oral surgery, agitation).

The *tympanic membrane,* in the ear canal, is a frequent site for estimating core body temperature. Like the sublingual oral site, the tympanic membrane has an abundant arterial blood supply, primarily from branches of the external carotid artery. Because temperature sensors applied directly to the tympanic membrane can be uncomfortable and involve risk of membrane injury or perforation, noninvasive *infrared thermometers* are used to detect the temperature of the thermal radiation emitted from the tympanic membrane (eardrum) and surrounding ear canal.

The temperature can also be measured on the forehead by using a chemical thermometer or a temporal artery thermometer. Forehead temperature measurements are most useful for infants and children on occasions when a more invasive measurement is not necessary.

TYPES OF THERMOMETERS   Traditionally, body temperatures have been measured by using mercury-in-glass thermometers. These are rarely seen anymore, as mercury thermometers can be hazardous if the thermometer cracks or breaks, leaking out toxic mercury. Another drawback of mercury-in-glass thermometers is the length

of time to obtain an accurate oral temperature, which can be as long as 8 minutes (Khorshid, Eşer, Zaybak, & Yapucu, 2005). These thermometers can also be difficult to read and use properly. You may still see mercury-in-glass thermometers used in client's homes or in some international settings. Whenever these thermometers are encountered, the nurse should recommend their immediate replacement with less hazardous thermometers and their safe disposal.

Electronic thermometers can provide a reading in as little as two seconds, depending on the model. The equipment consists of a battery-operated portable electronic unit (Figure 29.4), a probe, and a disposable probe cover.

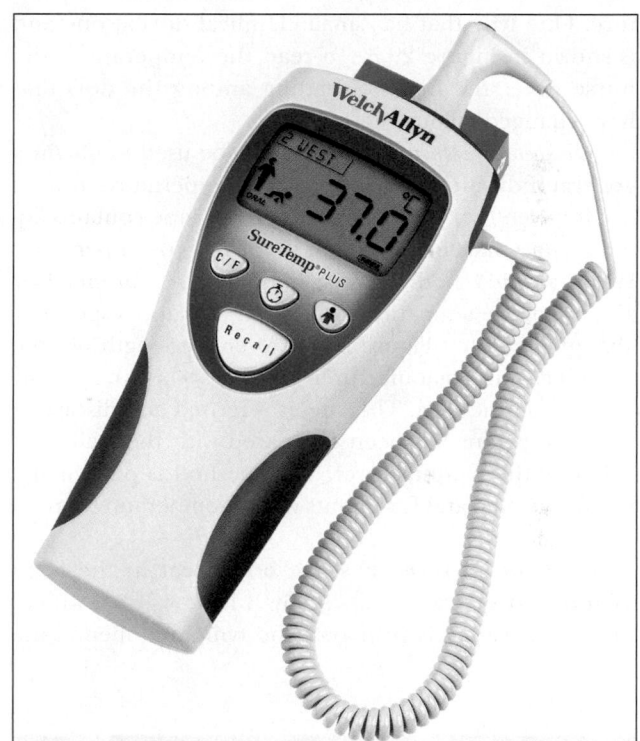

A

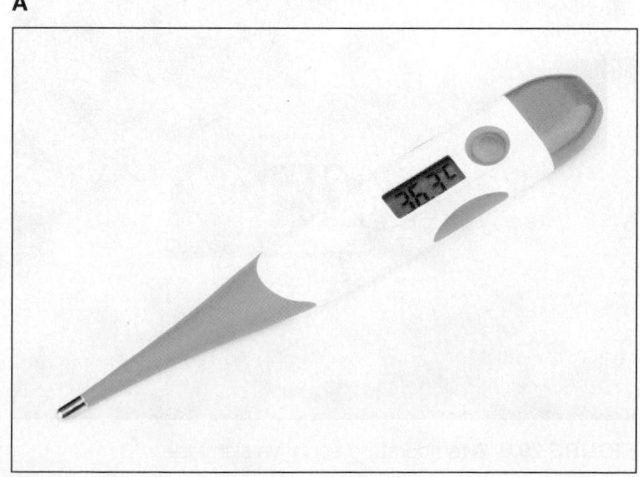

B

FIGURE 29.4 Electronic thermometers. **A**, Institutional model; **B**, One-piece home digital thermometer.

> ### ! CLINICAL ALERT
>
> When deciding which route to use to measure a client's body temperature, the nurse should use the least invasive route for clients who are not critically ill or merely being screened for fever, and the route that will yield the most accurate measurement for clients who are critically ill, unstable, or requiring a definitive diagnosis of fever. If trying to determine the presence or absence of fever in a client, use the same route of measurement as used previously with the client to make the most accurate assessment, and compare previous measurements to the most recent measurement.

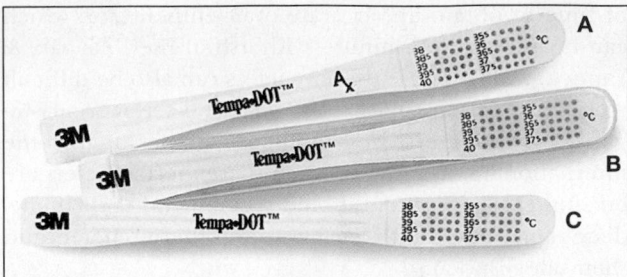

FIGURE 29.5 Chemical dot thermometers: **A**, Axillary (note the "Ax"); **B**, Rectal (note the plastic cover); **C**, oral.

Chemical disposable thermometers have liquid crystal dots or bars that change colour to indicate temperature. One type that has small chemical dots at one end is shown in Figure 29.5. To read the temperature, the nurse notes the highest reading among the dots that have changed colour.

Temperature-sensitive tape can also be used to obtain a general indication of body surface temperature. It does not indicate the core temperature. The tape contains liquid crystals that change colour according to temperature. When applied to dry skin, usually on the forehead or abdomen, the temperature digits on the tape respond by changing colour (Figure 29.6). After the length of time specified by the manufacturer (e.g., 15 seconds), a colour appears on the tape. The tape is removed and discarded after the colour has been compared with the scale provided by the manufacturer. This method is particularly useful at home and for infants whose temperatures are to be monitored.

Infrared thermometers sense body heat in the form of infrared energy given off by a heat source, which, in the ear canal, is primarily the tympanic membrane

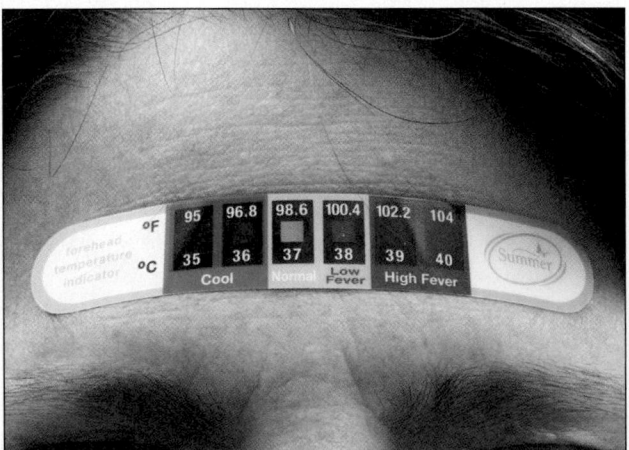

FIGURE 29.6 A temperature-sensitive skin tape.

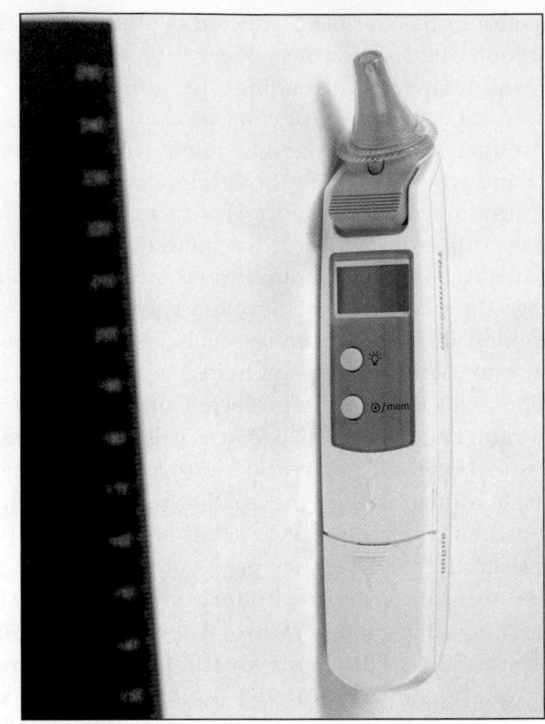

FIGURE 29.7 An infrared (tympanic) thermometer used to measure the tympanic membrane temperature.

(Figure 29.7). The infrared thermometer makes no contact with the tympanic membrane but detects the temperature of the thermal radiation emitting from it. Infrared tympanic membrane thermometry is a common method of assessing body temperature in care settings because of its relative convenience. However, there are numerous sources of error that can lead to false readings. These errors must be minimized for good patient care. See Box 29.4.

Temporal artery (TA) thermometers use scanning infrared rays to compare arterial temperature in the temporal artery of the forehead with the temperature in the room and calculate the heat balance to approximate the core temperature of blood in the pulmonary artery. The probe of the thermometer is placed in the middle of the forehead and then drawn laterally to the hairline. If the client has perspiration on the forehead, the probe is also touched behind the earlobe so the thermometer can compensate for evaporative cooling (Figure 29.8).

Clients may need to be taught how to use and read a thermometer properly when they are sent home. See the Teaching: Home Care box.

Skill 29.1 on page 706 explains how to measure body temperature (see also the Lifespan Considerations box on assessing body temperature on page 707).

BOX 29.4 SOURCES OF ERROR IN INFRARED TYMPANIC MEMBRANE THERMOMETRY

IMPROPER TECHNIQUE:

- Ineffective positioning inside the ear and improper seal against the outer ear
- Using the opposite ear instead of that which is closest
- The client talking or yawning during the procedure
- Incorrect "ear tug"

ANATOMICAL FEATURES:

- The auditory canal being highly variable among clients
- Neonates, children, and adults requiring different techniques because of their different anatomical structures

- The probe having to be the right size for the ear canal
- The presence of cerumen, which can undermine accuracy

EQUIPMENT:

- Dirty lens
- Instrument temperature being different from ambient environment temperature
- Improper instrument calibration
- Variations among different brands in terms of design, technology, offsets, and operating instructions

Sources: Canadian Paediatric Society. (2010). Temperature measurement in paediatrics. *Position Statement: Canadian Pediatric Society.* Retrieved, from http://www.cps.ca/english/statements/CP/cp00-01.htm; Casa, D. J., Becker, S. M., Ganio, M. S., Brown, C. M., Yeargin, S. W., Roti, M. W., Siegler, J., Blowers, J. A., Glaviano, N. R., ... Maresh, C. M. (2007). Validity of devices that assess body temperature during outdoor exercise in the heat. *Journal of Athletic Training, 42*(3), 333–342; Heusch, A. I., & McCarthy, P. W. (2005). The patient: A novel source of error in clinical temperature measurement using infrared aural thermometry. *The Journal of Alternative and Complementary Medicine, 11*(3), 473–476; Hooper, V. D., & Andrews, J. O. (2006). Accuracy of noninvasive core temperature measurement in acutely ill adults: The state of the science. *Biological Research for Nursing, 8*(1), 24–34; Latman, N. S. (2003). Clinical thermometry: Possible causes and potential solutions to electronic, digital thermometer inaccuracies. *Biomedical Instrumentation and Technology, 37*(3), 190–196; Lawson, L., Bridges, E. J., Ballou, I., Eraker, R., Greco, S., Shively, J., & Sochulak, V. (2007). Accuracy and precision of noninvasive temperature measurement in adult intensive care patients. *American Journal of Critical Care, 16*(5), 485–496; Lockwood, C., Conroy-Hiller, T., & Page, T. (2004). Vital signs. *JBI Reports, 2,* 207–230; Mackechnie, C., & Simpson, R. (2006). Traceable calibration of blood pressure and temperature monitoring. *Nursing Standard, 21*(11), 42–47; and Sessler, D. I. (2008). Temperature monitoring and perioperative thermoregulation. *Anesthesiology, 109*(2), 318–338.

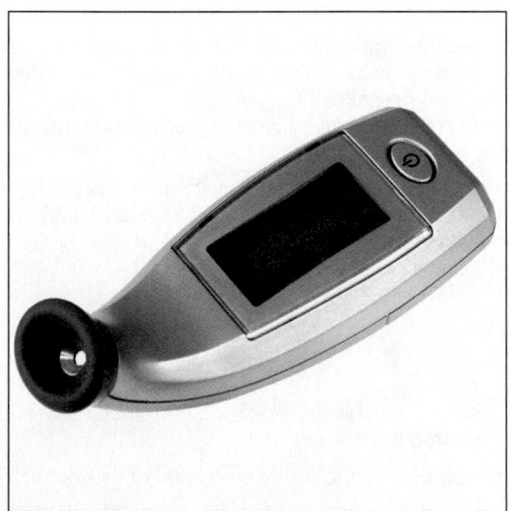

FIGURE 29.8 A temporal artery thermometer.

CLINICAL ALERT

To increase the reliability of temperature measurements in a client over time the nurse should use the same method and route of measurement as much as possible. Otherwise, measurements cannot be compared with one another and used to establish a consistent trend within the client.

TEACHING | HOME CARE

Temperature

Being able to take their temperature at home is an important skill for clients to have:

- Teach the client to accurately use and read the type of thermometer to be used. Many clients have tympanic thermometers but are not aware that these instruments require a level of skill to ensure accurate readings. Examine the thermometer used by the client in the home for safety and proper functioning. Facilitate the replacement of mercury thermometers with nonmercury ones.
- Observe the client or caregiver taking and reading a temperature. Reinforce the importance of reporting the site and type of thermometer used and the value of using one consistently.
- Discuss means of keeping the thermometer clean, such as warm water and soap, and avoiding cross-contamination.
- Ensure that the client has water-soluble lubricant if using a rectal thermometer.
- Instruct the client or family member to notify the health care provider if the temperature is 38°C or higher.
- Check that the client knows how to record the temperature, if required.
- Discuss relevant and appropriate measures to take during illness.

SKILL 29.1 ASSESSING BODY TEMPERATURE

PURPOSE

- To establish baseline data for subsequent evaluation
- To identify whether the core temperature is within normal range
- To determine changes in the core temperature in response to specific therapies (e.g., antipyretic medication, immunosuppressive therapy, invasive procedure)
- To monitor clients at risk for alterations in temperature (e.g., clients at risk for infection or diagnosis of infection)

ASSESSMENT

Assess

- Clinical signs of fever (pyrexia)
- Clinical signs of hypothermia
- Site most appropriate for measurement
- Factors that can alter core body temperature

Equipment

- Thermometer
- Thermometer sheath or cover
- Water-soluble lubricant and tissue, if the rectal site is used
- Disposable gloves
- Tissues or wipes

IMPLEMENTATION

Preparation

Check that all equipment is functioning normally.

Performance

1. Before performing the procedure, introduce yourself and verify the client's identity using two identifiers or per agency protocol. Explain to the client what you are going to do, why it is necessary, and how he or she can participate.

2. Perform hand hygiene, and follow other appropriate infection prevention and control procedures. Put on gloves, if performing a rectal temperature.

Thermometer Placement

Oral

Place the bulb under the tongue in the sublingual pocket beside the frenulum (see ❶).

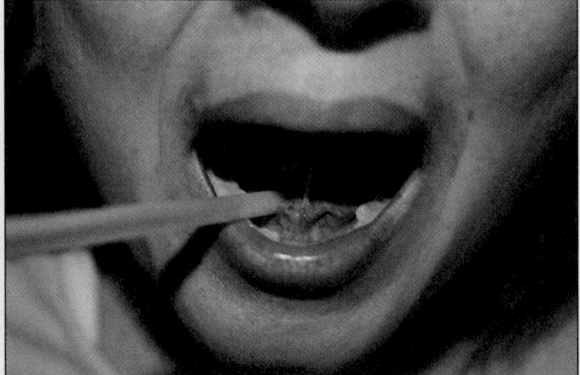

❶ Oral thermometer placement

3. Provide for client privacy.

4. Place the client in the appropriate position (e.g., lateral or Sims' position for inserting a rectal thermometer).

5. Place the thermometer (see ❶ through ❺).
   - Apply a protective sheath or probe cover, if appropriate.
   - Lubricate the rectal thermometer.

6. Wait the appropriate amount of time. Electronic and tympanic thermometers will indicate that the reading is complete through a light or tone. Check package instructions for length of time to wait before reading chemical dot or tape thermometers.

7. Remove the thermometer, and discard the cover or wipe with a tissue, if necessary.

8. Read the temperature (prior to recapping if electronic) and record it. If the temperature is obviously too high, too low, or inconsistent with the client's condition, recheck it with a thermometer known to be functioning properly.

9. Wash the thermometer, if necessary, and return it to the storage location.

10. Document the temperature in the client record. A rectal temperature may be recorded with an "R" next to the value or with the mark on a graphic sheet circled. An axillary temperature may be recorded with "AX" or marked on a graphic sheet with an "X."

EVALUATION

- Compare the temperature measurement to baseline data, the normal range for the age of the client, and the client's previous temperatures. Analyze by considering the time of day and any additional influencing factors and other vital signs.

- Conduct appropriate follow-up, such as notifying the appropriate members of the health care team, giving a medication, removing heavy coverings, or altering the client's environment.

Rectal Put on clean gloves. Apply a thermometer cover, if required by device.

Apply lubricant to the insertion end of the thermometer.

Instruct the client to take a slow deep breath during insertion (see ❷).

Never force the thermometer if resistance is felt.

Insert 3.5 cm in adults.

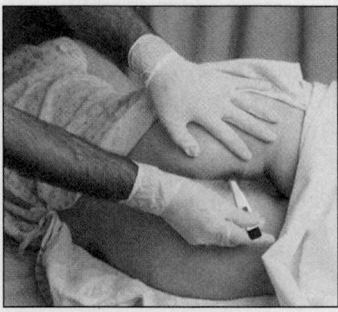

❷ Inserting a rectal thermometer

Thermometer Placement

Axillary   Pat the axilla dry if very moist.

Place the bulb in the centre of the axilla (see ❸), then adduct the arm over the thermometer.

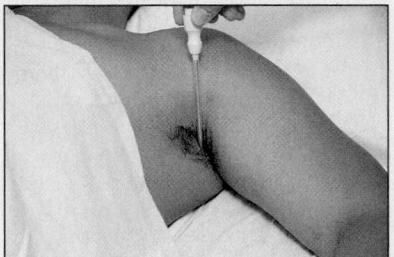

❸ Placing the bulb of the thermometer in the centre of the axilla

Tympanic   Pull the pinna slightly upward and backward (see ❹).

Point the probe slightly anteriorly, toward the eardrum.

Insert the probe slowly by using a circular motion until snug.

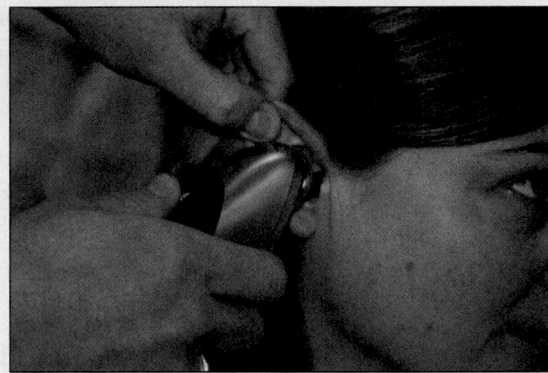

❹ Inserting and pointing the tympanic thermometer

Temporal Artery   Brush hair aside if it is covering the temporal artery area. With the probe flush on the centre of the forehead, depress the red button, and keep it depressed. Slowly slide the probe midline across the forehead to the hairline, not down the side of the face (see ❺A). Lift the probe from the forehead and touch it on the neck, just behind the earlobe (see ❺B). Release the button.

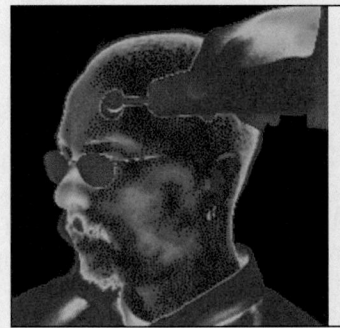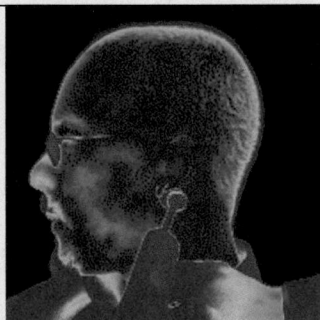

❺A and ❺B Positioning the temporal artery thermometer

LIFESPAN CONSIDERATIONS

Assessing Body Temperature

INFANTS

- The body temperature of newborns is labile, and newborns must be kept warm and dry to prevent hypothermia.

- When using the axillary site, hold the infant's arm against the chest (see Figure 29.9).

- The axillary route may not be as accurate as other routes for detecting fevers in children.

- The tympanic route is fast and convenient but needs to be avoided if

the child has an active ear infection or drainage tubes. Place the infant in the supine position, and stabilize the head. Pull the pinna straight back and slightly downward. Direct the probe tip anteriorly and insert far enough to seal the canal. The tip will not touch the tympanic membrane.

- The tympanic membrane route may be more accurate in determining temperature in febrile infants.

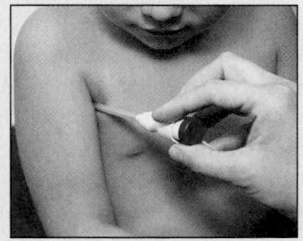

FIGURE 29.9 Axillary thermometer placement for a child.

- Infants tolerate temporal artery thermometry well.
- The rectal route is least desirable in infants. However, sometimes it is used to obtain definitive temperature measurements.

CHILDREN

- Tympanic or temporal artery sites are preferred.
- For the tympanic route, have the child held on an adult's lap with the child's head held gently against the adult for support. Pull the pinna straight back and upward for children over age 3 years.
- Avoid the tympanic route in a child with active ear infections or tympanic membrane drainage tubes.
- The oral route can be used for children over age 3 years, but unbreakable

electronic thermometers are recommended.

- For a rectal temperature, place the child prone across your lap or in the side-lying position with the knees flexed. Insert the thermometer 2.5 cm into the rectum.

OLDER ADULTS

- Older adults' temperatures tend to be lower than those of middle-aged adults; they also tend to have a diminished fever response due to physiological changes associated with aging.
- Their temperatures are strongly influenced by environmental temperature changes as thermoregulation control processes are not as efficient as when they were younger, and they are at higher risk for both hypothermia and hyperthermia.

- Older adults can develop significant buildup of ear cerumen that may interfere with tympanic thermometer readings.
- Older adults are more likely to have hemorrhoids. Inspect the anus before taking a rectal temperature.
- Older adults' temperatures may not be a valid indication of the seriousness of the pathology of a disease. In the presence of fever, there is a strong possibility of infection, the source of which should be determined and treated promptly.
- Other symptoms, such as confusion and restlessness, may be displayed and need follow-up.

Pulse

The **pulse** is a wave of blood created by contraction of the left ventricle of the heart. Generally, the pulse wave represents the stroke volume output (the amount of blood entering the arteries with each ventricular contraction). **Compliance** of the arteries is their ability to contract and expand. When a person's arteries lose their distensibility, as can happen in old age, greater pressure is required to pump the blood into the arteries.

Cardiac output is the volume of blood pumped into the arteries by the heart and equals the result of the stroke volume (SV) multiplied by the heart rate (HR) per minute. For example, 65 mL × 70 beats per minute = 4.55 L per minute. When an adult is resting, the heart pumps about 5 L of blood each minute.

In a healthy person, the pulse reflects the heartbeat; that is, the pulse rate is the same as the rate of the ventricular contractions of the heart. However, in some types of cardiovascular disease, the heartbeat and pulse rates can differ. For example, a client's heart may produce very weak or small pulse waves that are not detectable in a peripheral pulse distal to the heart. In these instances, the nurse should assess the heartbeat *and* the peripheral pulse. See the section on assessing the apical pulse later in this chapter. A **peripheral pulse** is located in the periphery of the body, such as in the foot, hand, or neck. The **apical pulse**, in contrast, is a central pulse; that is, it is located at the apex of the heart. It is also referred to as the **point of maximal impulse (PMI)**.

Factors Affecting Pulse Rate

The rate of the pulse is expressed in beats per minute (beats/min). A pulse rate varies according to a number of factors. The nurse should consider each of the following factors when assessing a client's pulse:

- *Age.* As age increases, the pulse rate gradually decreases. See Table 29.3 for specific variations in pulse rates from birth to adulthood.
- *Sex.* After puberty, the average male's pulse rate is slightly lower than the average female's.
- *Exercise.* The pulse rate normally increases with activity. The rate of increase in the professional athlete is often less than in the average person because of greater cardiac size, strength, and efficiency.
- *Fever.* The pulse rate increases (a) in response to the lowered blood pressure that results from peripheral vasodilation associated with elevated body temperature and (b) with an increased metabolic rate.
- *Medications and other ingestants.* Many substances affect the heart rate and pulse. For example, cardiotonics (e.g., digitalis) and beta-blockers decrease the heart rate, whereas caffeine, nicotine, and epinephrine increase the heart rate.
- *Hypovolemia.* Low blood volume or loss of blood from the vascular system (*hemorrhage*) normally increases pulse rate. An adult has about 5 L of blood in the system and can usually lose up to 10% without adverse effects. Fluid volume deficits caused by extensive diarrhea and vomiting or prolonged lack of fluid intake can also cause increased pulse rate.

TABLE 29.3 Variations in Pulse and Respirations by Age

Age	Pulse Average (and Ranges)	Respirations Average (and Ranges)
Newborn (0–4 weeks)	130 (80–180)	35 (30–80)
<1 year	120 (80–140)	30 (20–40)
1–4 years	110 (80–120)	25 (20–30)
5–8 years	100 (75–120)	20 (15–25)
9–10 years	70 (50–90)	19 (15–25)
11–19 years	75 (50–90)	18 (15–20)
20–64 years	80 (60–100)	16 (12–20)
>65 years	70 (60–100)	16 (15–20)

- *Stress.* In response to stress, sympathetic nervous stimulation increases the overall activity of the heart. Stress increases the rate as well as the force of the heartbeat. Fear and anxiety, as well as the perception of severe pain, stimulate the sympathetic system.

- *Position.* When a person assumes a sitting or standing position, blood usually pools in dependent vessels of the venous system. Pooling results in a transient decrease in the venous blood return to the heart and a subsequent reduction in blood pressure and increase in heart rate.

- *Pathology.* Certain diseases, such as some heart conditions or those that impair oxygenation, can alter the resting pulse rate.

Pulse Sites

A pulse can be measured in nine sites—eight peripheral sites (Figure 29.10) and one at the apex of the heart (Figure 29.11 on the next page):

1. *Temporal,* where the temporal artery passes over the temporal bone of the head. The site is superior (above) and lateral (away from the midline of) to the eye.

2. *Carotid,* at the side of the neck where the carotid artery runs between the trachea and the sternocleidomastoid muscle. See the Clinical Alert Box below.

3. *Apical,* at the apex of the heart. In an adult, this is located on the left side of the chest, no more than 8 cm to the

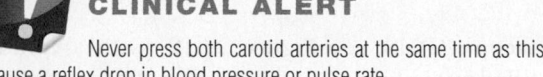

CLINICAL ALERT

Never press both carotid arteries at the same time as this can cause a reflex drop in blood pressure or pulse rate.

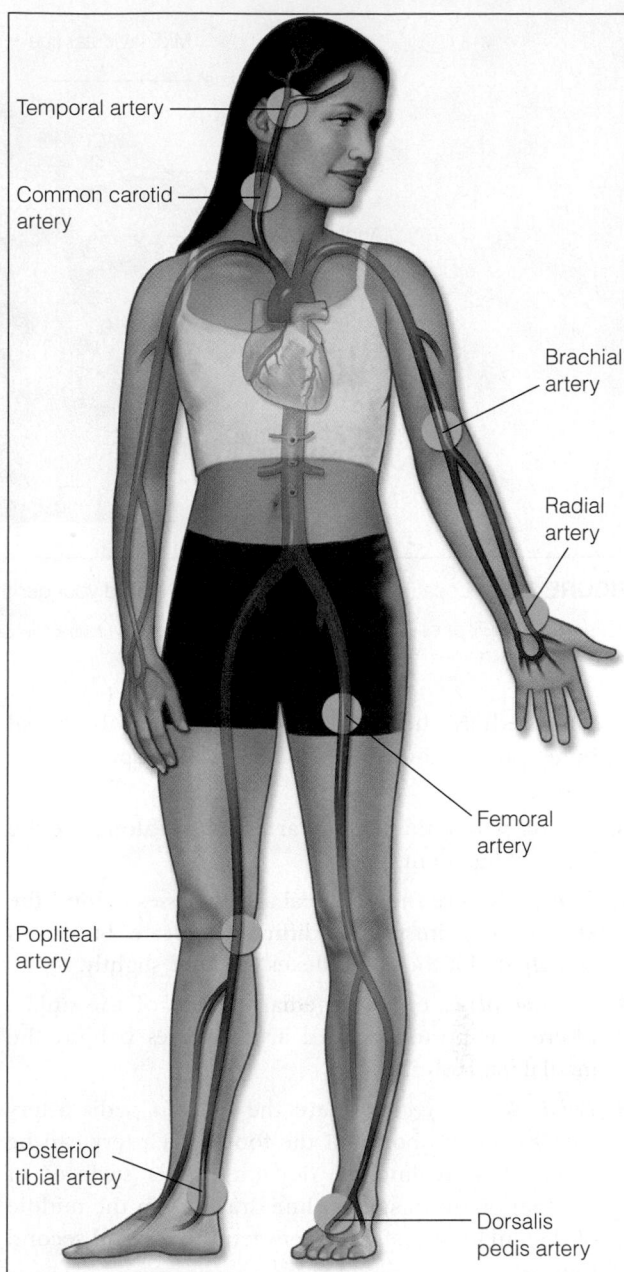

FIGURE 29.10 Body sites where the peripheral pulse is most easily palpated.

Source: From D'Amico, D., Barbarito, C., Twomey, C., & Harder, N. (2012). *Health & Physical Assessment in Nursing, Canadian Edition,* Pearson Education Canada. Reprinted with permission by Pearson Canada Inc.

left of the sternum (breastbone) and at the fourth, fifth, or sixth intercostal space (area between the ribs). In older adults, the apex may be further left if there are conditions that have led to an enlarged heart. Before 4 years of age, the apex is left of the midclavicular line (MCL); between 4 and 6 years, it is at the MCL (see Figure 29.11). For a child 7 to 9 years of age, the apical pulse is located at the fourth or fifth intercostal space.

4. *Brachial,* at the inner aspect of the biceps muscle of the arm (especially in infants) or medially in the antecubital space.

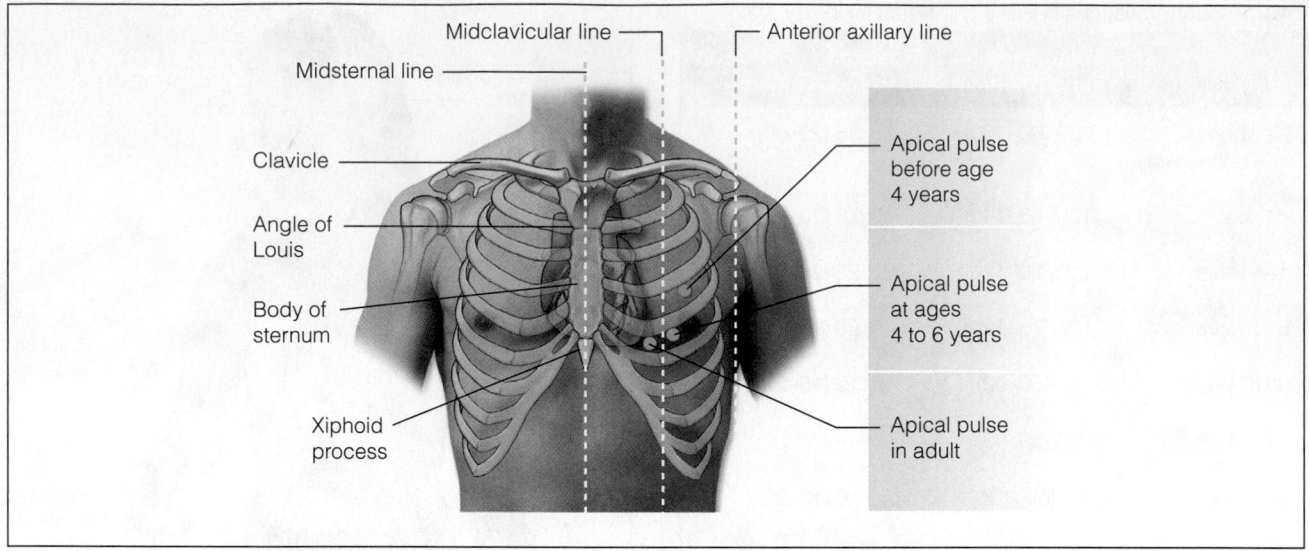

FIGURE 29.11 Locations of the apical pulse in a child younger than 4 years, a child 4 to 6 years, and an adult.

Source: From D'Amico, D., Barbarito, C., Twomey, C., & Harder, N. (2012). *Health & Physical Assessment in Nursing, Canadian Edition*, Pearson Education Canada. Reprinted with permission by Pearson Canada Inc.

5. *Radial,* where the radial artery runs along the radial bone, on the thumb side of the inner aspect of the wrist.

6. *Femoral,* where the femoral artery passes alongside the inguinal ligament.

7. *Popliteal,* where the popliteal artery passes behind the knee. This point may be difficult to locate, but it can be palpated if the client flexes the knee slightly.

8. *Posterior tibial,* on the medial surface of the ankle, where the posterior tibial artery passes behind the medial malleolus.

9. *Pedal (dorsalis pedis),* where the dorsalis pedis artery passes over the bones of the foot. This artery can be palpated by feeling the dorsum (upper surface) of the foot on an imaginary line drawn from the middle of the ankle to the space between the big and second toes.

The radial site is most commonly used. It is easily detected in most people and readily accessible. The reasons for use of each site are given in Table 29.4.

Assessing the Pulse

A pulse is commonly assessed by palpation or auscultation. A peripheral pulse is normally palpated by applying moderate pressure with the three middle fingers of the hand. The pads on the most distal aspects of the finger are the most sensitive areas for detecting a pulse. The thumb is not used to palpate as it has its own pulse, which can be confused with the client's pulse. Excessive pressure can obliterate a pulse, whereas too little pressure may make it undetectable. A stethoscope is used for assessing apical pulses. A Doppler ultrasound

TABLE 29.4 Reasons for Using Specific Pulse Site

Pulse Site	Reasons for Use
Radial	Readily accessible
Temporal	Used when radial pulse is not accessible
Carotid	Used during cardiac arrest or shock in adults
	To determine circulation to the brain
Apical	Routinely used in infants and children up to 3 years of age
	To determine discrepancies with radial pulse
	To monitor some medication effects
Brachial	To measure blood pressure
	During cardiac arrest in infants
Femoral	Used in cases of cardiac arrest or shock
	To determine circulation to the leg
Popliteal	To determine circulation to the lower leg
Posterior tibial	To determine circulation to the foot
Pedal	To determine circulation to the foot

stethoscope (DUS; see Figure 29.12) with a volume-controlled audio unit is used for pulses that are difficult to assess.

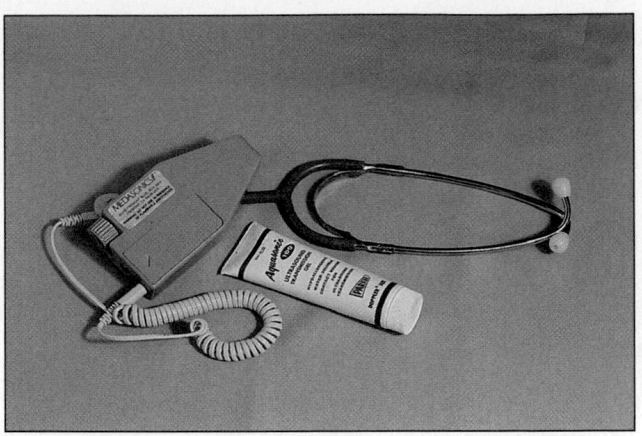

FIGURE 29.12 A Doppler ultrasound stethoscope (DUS).

TABLE 29.5 Scales for Measuring Pulse Volume

Three-Point Scale	Description of Pulse
0	Absent, not discernible
+1	Thready or weak, difficult to feel
+2	Normal, detected readily, obliterated by strong pressure
+3	Bounding, difficult to obliterate

Four-Point Scale	Description of Pulse
0	Absent, not discernible
+1	Thready or weak, difficult to feel
+2	Normal, detected readily, obliterated by strong pressure
+3	Increased
+4	Bounding

Before the nurse assesses the *resting* pulse, the client should assume a comfortable position. The nurse should also be aware of the following:

- Any drugs (prescribed, over-the-counter [OTC], caffeine, etc.) that could affect the heart rate
- Whether the client has been physically active; if so, wait 10 to 15 minutes until the client has rested and the pulse has returned to its usual rate
- Any baseline data about the usual heart rate for the client; for example, a physically fit athlete may have a heart rate below 60 beats/min
- Whether the client should assume a particular position (e.g., sitting); in some clients, the rate changes with the position because of changes in blood flow volume and autonomic nervous system activity

When assessing the pulse, the following data are collected: rate, rhythm, volume, arterial wall elasticity, and presence or absence of bilateral equality. **Tachycardia** is an excessively fast heart rate (e.g., more than 100 beats/min in an adult); **bradycardia** is a heart rate that is lower than normal (e.g., less than 60 beats/min in an adult). If a person has tachycardia or bradycardia, the apical pulse should be assessed.

The **pulse rhythm** is the pattern of the beats and the intervals between the beats. Equal time elapses between beats of a normal pulse. A pulse with an irregular rhythm is referred to as a **dysrhythmia** or **arrhythmia**. It may consist of random, irregular beats or a predictable pattern of irregular beats referred to as *regular-irregular arrhythmia*. When a dysrhythmia is detected, the apical pulse should be assessed. An electrocardiogram (ECG) is necessary to further define the dysrhythmia.

Pulse volume, also called *pulse strength* or *amplitude*, refers to the force of blood with each beat. Usually, pulse volume is the same with each beat. It can range from absent to bounding. A normal pulse can be felt with moderate pressure of the fingers and can be obliterated with greater pressure. A forceful or full blood volume that is obliterated only with difficulty is called a *full* or *bounding* pulse. A pulse that is readily obliterated with pressure from the fingers is referred to as *weak, feeble,* or *thready*. A pulse volume can be measured on a scale of 0 to 3 (indicated by x/3) or 0 to 4 (indicated by x/4), depending on the agency (see Table 29.5).

The **elasticity of the arterial wall** reflects its expansibility or its deformities. A healthy, normal artery feels straight, smooth, soft, and pliable. Older people often have inelastic arteries that feel *tortuous* (twisted) and irregular on palpation.

When assessing a peripheral pulse to determine the adequacy of blood flow to a particular area of the body, the corresponding pulse on the other side of the body should be assessed to compare the pulses. For example, when assessing the blood flow to the right foot, the nurse assesses the right dorsalis pedis pulse and then the left dorsalis pedis pulse. If the client's right and left pulses are the same, the client's dorsalis pedis pulses are *bilaterally equal*.

When a peripheral pulse is located, it indicates that pulses more proximal to that location will also be present. For example, if the dorsalis pedis, the most distal pulse of the lower extremity, cannot be felt, the nurse next palpates for the posterior tibial pulse. If it is not felt, the popliteal pulse must be assessed. If the popliteal pulse is found, it is not necessary to assess the femoral pulse, since it must also be present for the more distal pulse to exist.

Skill 29.2 on the next page provides guidelines for assessing a peripheral pulse.

SKILL 29.2 ASSESSING A PERIPHERAL PULSE

PURPOSES

- To establish baseline data for subsequent evaluation
- To identify whether the pulse rate is within normal range
- To determine whether the pulse rhythm is regular and the pulse volume is appropriate
- To compare the equality of corresponding peripheral pulses bilaterally
- To monitor and assess changes in the client's health status
- To monitor clients at risk for pulse alterations (e.g., those with a history of heart disease or experiencing cardiac arrhythmias, hemorrhage, acute pain, infusion of large volumes of fluids, fever)
- To evaluate blood perfusion to the extremities

ASSESSMENT

Assess

- Clinical signs of cardiovascular alterations, such as dyspnea, fatigue, pallor, cyanosis, palpitations, syncope, or impaired peripheral tissue perfusion, as evidenced by skin discoloration and cool temperature
- Factors that may alter pulse rate (e.g., emotional state and activity level)
- Which site is most appropriate for assessment based on the purpose

Equipment

- Watch with a second hand or indicator
- If using a DUS: transducer probe, stethoscope headset, transmission gel, and tissues or wipes

IMPLEMENTATION

Preparation

If using a DUS, ensure that the equipment is functioning normally.

Performance

1. Before performing the procedure, introduce yourself and verify the client's identity using two identifiers or per agency protocol. Explain to the client what you are going to do, why it is necessary, and how he or she can participate.
2. Perform hand hygiene, and follow other appropriate infection prevention and control procedures.
3. Provide for client privacy.
4. Select the pulse point. Normally, the radial pulse is taken, unless it cannot be exposed or circulation to another body area is to be assessed.
5. Assist the client to a comfortable resting position. When the radial pulse is assessed, with the palm facing downward, the client's arm can rest alongside the body or the forearm can rest at a 90-degree angle across the chest. For the client who can sit, the forearm can rest across the thigh, with the palm of the hand facing downward or inward.
6. Palpate and count the pulse. Place two or three middle fingertips lightly and squarely over the pulse point (see ❶). **Rationale: Using the thumb is contraindicated because the nurse's thumb has a pulse that could be mistaken for the client's pulse.**
   - Count for 30 seconds and multiply by 2 to obtain beats per minute. If taking a client's pulse for the first time, when obtaining baseline data, or if the pulse is irregular or difficult to assess, count for a full minute. If an irregular pulse is found, take the apical pulse also.

❶ Assessing the pulses

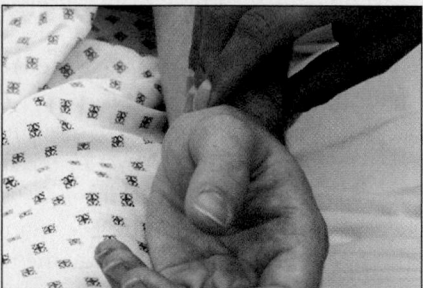

A Radial

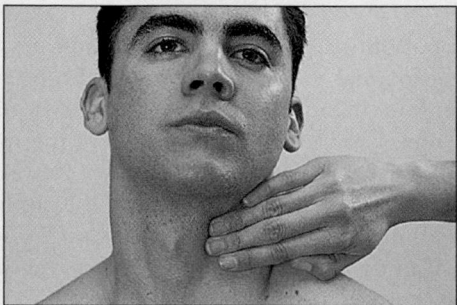

C Carotid

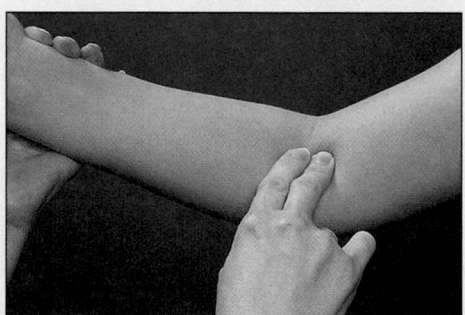

B Brachial

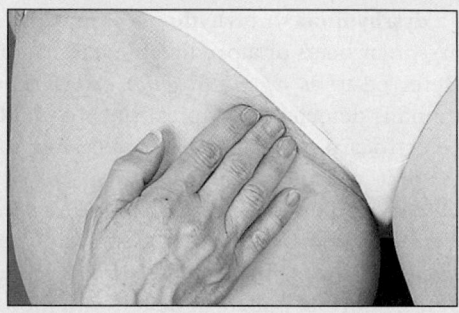

D Femoral

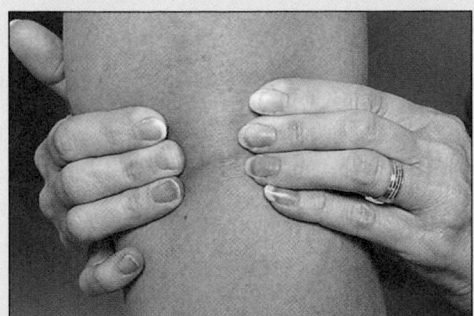

E Popliteal

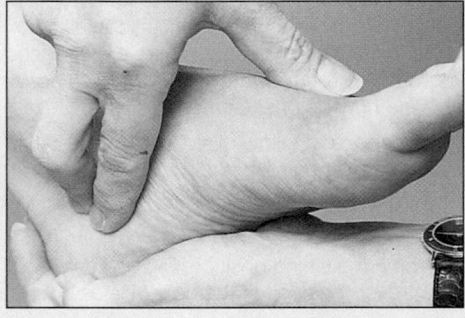

F Posterior tibial

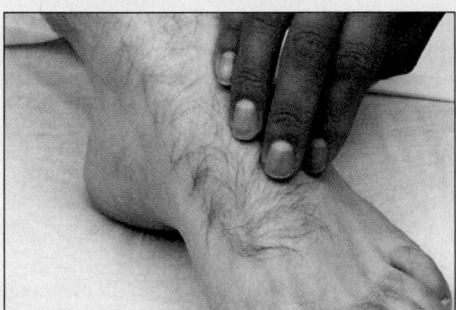

G Pedal (dorsalis pedis)

7. Assess pulse rhythm and volume.
   - Assess pulse rhythm by noting the pattern of the intervals between the beats. A normal pulse has equal periods between beats. If this is an initial assessment, assess for 1 minute.
   - Assess pulse volume. A normal pulse can be felt with moderate pressure, and the pressure is equal with each beat. See Table 29.5 for scales for measuring pulse volume.

8. Document pulse rate, rhythm, and volume (see Table 29.5) and your actions in the client record. Also record pertinent related data, such as any variation in pulse rate compared with normal for the client and abnormal skin colour and skin temperature.

Variation: Using a DUS

- Apply transmission gel either to the probe at the narrow end of the plastic case housing the transducer or to the client's skin. **Rationale: The gel makes an airtight seal, which then promotes optimal ultrasound wave transmission.**
- Press the "On" button.
- Hold the probe against the client's skin over the pulse site. Use light pressure, and keep the probe in contact with the skin (see ❷). **Rationale: Too much pressure can stop the blood flow and obliterate the signal.**
- Adjust the volume, if necessary. Distinguish artery sounds from vein sounds. The artery sound (signal) is distinctively pulsating and has a pumping quality. The venous sound is intermittent and varies with respirations. Both artery and vein sounds are heard simultaneously through the DUS because major arteries and veins are situated close together throughout the body. If arterial sounds cannot be easily heard, reposition the probe.
- After assessing the pulse, remove all of the gel from the probe and clean the transducer with a water-based solution. **Rationale: Alcohol or other disinfectants may damage the face of the transducer. Remove all of the gel from the client's skin.**

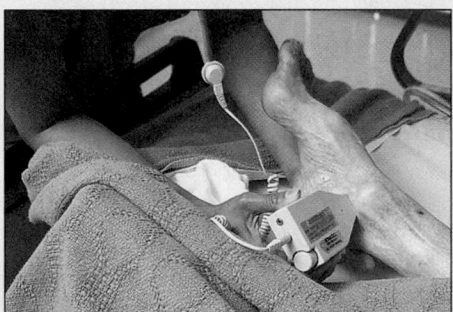

❷ Using a (Doppler) ultrasound stethoscope to assess the posterior tibial pulse

EVALUATION

- Compare the pulse rate to baseline data or the usual range for the age of the client.
- Relate pulse rate and volume to other vital signs, and relate pulse rhythm and volume to baseline data and health status.
- If assessing peripheral pulses, evaluate equality, rate, and volume in corresponding extremities.
- Conduct appropriate follow-up, such as notifying the appropriate members of the health care team or giving medication.

APICAL PULSE ASSESSMENT Assessment of the apical pulse is indicated for clients whose peripheral pulse is irregular as well as for clients with known cardiovascular, pulmonary, and renal diseases. It is commonly assessed before administering medications that affect heart rate. The apical site is also used to assess the pulse for newborns, infants, and children up to age 2 to 3 years. Skill 29.3 presents guidelines for assessing the apical pulse.

APICAL–RADIAL PULSE ASSESSMENT An **apical–radial pulse** may need to be assessed for clients with certain cardiovascular disorders. Normally, the apical and radial rates are identical. An apical pulse rate greater

---

SKILL 29.3   ASSESSING AN APICAL PULSE

PURPOSES

- To obtain the heart rate of newborns, infants, and children age 2 to 3 years or of an adult with an irregular peripheral pulse
- To establish baseline data for subsequent evaluation
- To determine whether the cardiac rate is within normal range and the rhythm is regular
- To monitor clients with cardiac disease and those receiving medications to improve heart action

ASSESSMENT

Assess

- Clinical signs of cardiovascular alterations (e.g., dyspnea, fatigue or weakness, pallor, cyanosis, syncope)
- Factors that may alter pulse rate (e.g., emotional state, activity level, and medications that affect heart rate, such as beta-blockers or calcium channel blockers)

Equipment

- Watch with a second hand or indicator
- Stethoscope
- Antiseptic wipes
- If using a DUS: the transducer probe, the stethoscope headset, transmission gel, and tissues or wipes

IMPLEMENTATION

Preparation

If using a DUS, ensure that the equipment is functioning normally.

Performance

1. Before performing the procedure, introduce yourself and verify the client's identity using two identifiers or per agency protocol. Explain to the client what you are going to do, why it is necessary, and how he or she can participate.
2. Perform hand hygiene, and follow other appropriate infection prevention and control procedures.
3. Provide for client privacy.
4. Position the client appropriately and comfortably in the supine position or in the sitting position. Expose only the area of the chest over the apex of the heart. Be as discrete as possible.
5. Locate the apical impulse. This is the point over the apex of the heart where the apical pulse can be most clearly heard.
   - Palpate the angle of Louis (the angle between the manubrium, the top of the sternum, and the body of the sternum). It is palpated just below the suprasternal notch and is felt as a prominence (see Figure 29.11).
   - Slide your index finger just to the left of the sternum, and palpate the second intercostal space (see ❶).
   - Place your middle or next finger in the third intercostal space, and continue palpating downward until you locate the fifth intercostal space (see ❷).
   - Move your index finger laterally along the fifth intercostal space toward the MCL (see ❸). Normally, the apical impulse is palpable at or just medial to the MCL.
6. Auscultate and count heartbeats.
   - Use antiseptic wipes to clean the earpieces and diaphragm of the stethoscope. **Rationale: This promotes infection control.**

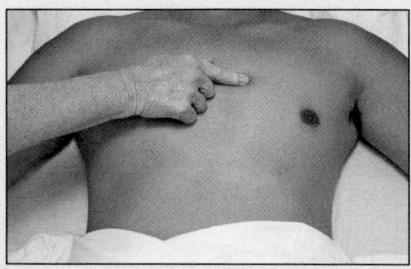
❶ Second intercostal space

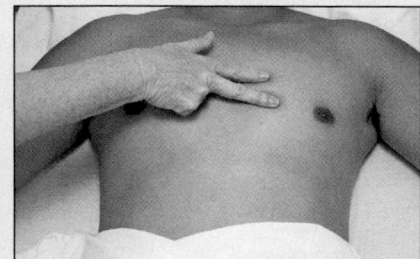
❷ Third intercostal space

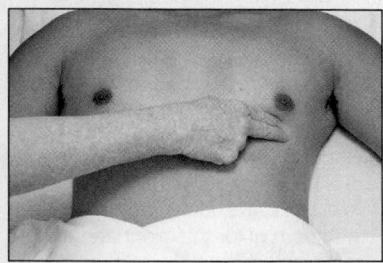
❸ Fifth intercostal space, MCL

- Warm the diaphragm of the stethoscope by holding it in the palm of the hand for a moment. **Rationale: This promotes comfort, as the metal of the diaphragm is usually cold.**
- Insert the earpieces of the stethoscope into your ears in the direction of the ear canals, or slightly forward. **Rationale: This facilitates hearing.**
- Tap your finger lightly on the diaphragm *to be sure it is the active side of the head*. If necessary, rotate the head to select the diaphragm side (see ❹).
- Place the diaphragm of the stethoscope over the apical impulse and listen for S_1 and S_2 heart sounds (see Chapter 28); each pairing of S_1 and S_2 represents one heartbeat (see ❺). **Rationale: The heartbeat is normally loudest over the apex of the heart. S_1 represents closure of the atrioventricular valves; S_2 occurs when the semilunar valves close after the ventricles empty.**
- If you have difficulty hearing the apical pulse, ask the supine client to roll onto his or her left side or the sitting client to lean slightly forward. **Rationale: This positioning moves the apex of the heart closer to the chest wall.**
- If the rhythm is regular, count the heartbeats for 30 seconds and multiply by 2. If the rhythm is irregular or for giving certain medications, such as digoxin, count the beats for 60 seconds. **Rationale: A 60-second count provides a more accurate assessment of an irregular pulse compared with a 30-second count.**

7. Assess the rhythm of the heartbeat by noting the pattern of intervals between the beats. A normal pulse has equal periods between beats.

8. Document the pulse site, rate, and rhythm and nursing actions in the client record. Also record pertinent related data, such as variation in pulse rate compared with the usual for the client and any abnormal skin colour and skin temperature.

EVALUATION

- Relate pulse rate to other vital signs. Relate pulse rhythm to baseline data and health status.
- Report to the appropriate members of the health care team any abnormal findings, such as irregular rhythm, reduced ability to hear the heartbeat, pallor, cyanosis, dyspnea, tachycardia, or bradycardia.
- Conduct appropriate follow-up, such as administering medication ordered on the basis of the apical heart rate.

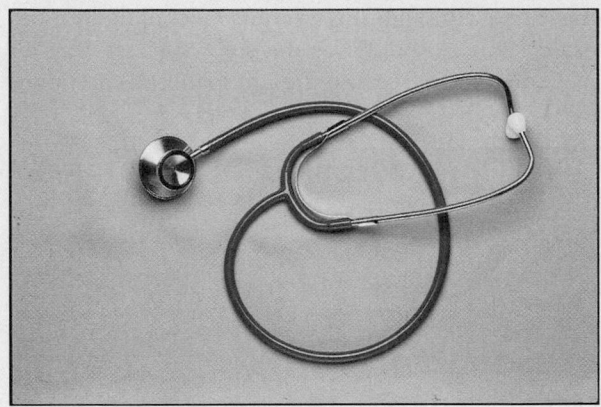

❹ **A** Stethoscope with both a bell-shaped and flat-disc amplifiers

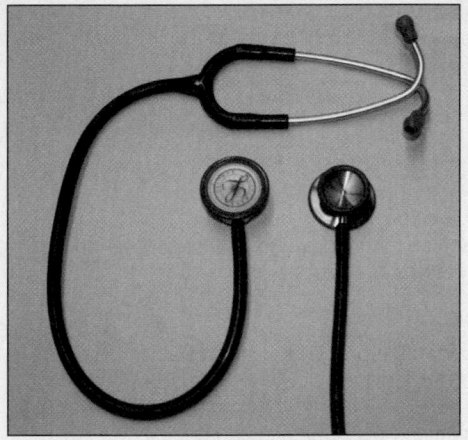

❹ **B** Close up of a diaphragm (L) and a bell (R).

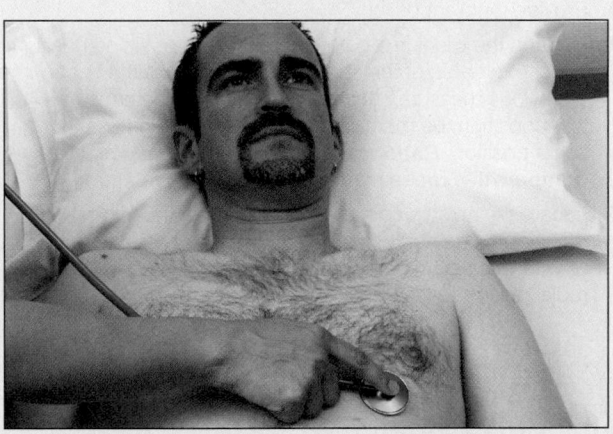

❺ Taking an apical pulse using the diaphragm of the stethoscope

than a radial pulse rate can indicate that the thrust of the blood from the heart is too weak for the wave to be felt at the peripheral pulse site, or it can indicate that vascular disease is preventing impulses from being transmitted. A **pulse deficit** is a discrepancy between the two pulse rates and needs to be reported promptly. In no instance is the radial pulse greater than the apical pulse.

An apical–radial pulse can be taken by two nurses or one nurse, although the two-nurse technique is more accurate. Skill 29.4 outlines the steps for assessing an apical–radial pulse (see also the Lifespan Considerations box on assessing an apical–radial pulse that follows). Guidelines for teaching clients about measuring their pulse in the home are found in the Teaching: Home Care box on page 717.

SKILL 29.4	**ASSESSING AN APICAL–RADIAL PULSE**

PURPOSE

- To determine adequacy of peripheral circulation or presence of pulse deficit

ASSESSMENT

Assess

- Clinical signs of hypovolemic shock (hypotension, pallor, cyanosis, and cold, clammy skin)

Equipment

- Watch with a second hand or indicator
- Stethoscope
- Antiseptic wipes

IMPLEMENTATION

Preparation

If using the two-nurse technique, ensure that another nurse is available at this time.

Performance

1. Before performing the procedure, introduce yourself and verify the client's identity using two identifiers or per agency protocol. Explain to the client what you are going to do, why it is necessary, and how he or she can participate.

2. Perform hand hygiene, and follow other appropriate infection prevention and control procedures.

3. Provide for client privacy.

4. Position the client in a comfortable supine or sitting position. Expose the area of the chest over the apex of the heart. If previous measurements had been taken, determine what position the client had assumed then, and use the same position. **Rationale: This ensures an accurate comparative measurement.**

5. Locate the apical and radial pulse sites. In the two-nurse technique, one nurse locates the apical impulse by palpation or with the stethoscope while the other nurse palpates the radial pulse site (see Skills 29.2 and 29.3).

6. Count the apical and radial pulse rates.

Two-Nurse Technique

- Place the watch where both nurses can see it, and decide on a time to begin counting (e.g., when the second hand is on 12 or an even number on a digital clock). One nurse says "Start." **Rationale: This ensures that simultaneous counts are taken.**

- Each nurse counts the pulse rate for 60 seconds ending with one nurse saying "Stop." **Rationale: A full 60-second count ensures accurate assessment of any discrepancies between the two pulse sites.**

- The nurse who assesses the apical rate also assesses the apical pulse rhythm. If the pulse is irregular, note whether the irregular beats come at random (called *irregular-irregular*) or at predictable times (called *regular-irregular*).

- The nurse assessing the radial pulse rate assesses the radial pulse rhythm and volume.

One-Nurse Technique

- Assess the apical pulse for 60 seconds then assess the radial pulse for 60 seconds.

7. Document the apical–radial (AR) pulse data and any pulse deficit in the client record. Also record related data, such as variation in pulse rate compared with the normal for the client and other pertinent observations, such as pallor, cyanosis, or dyspnea.

EVALUATION

- Relate pulse rate and rhythm to other vital signs, to baseline data, and to general health status.

- Report to the appropriate members of the health care team any changes from previous measurements or any discrepancy between the two pulses.

- Conduct appropriate follow-up, such as administering medication or other actions to be taken for a discrepancy in the apical and radial pulse rates.

Respirations

Respiration is the act of breathing. **External respiration** refers to the interchange of oxygen and carbon dioxide between the alveoli of the lungs and the pulmonary blood. **Internal respiration**, by contrast, takes place throughout the body; it is the interchange of these same gases between the circulating blood and the cells of body tissues.

Inhalation or **inspiration** refers to the intake of air into the lungs. **Exhalation** or **expiration** refers to breathing out, or the movement of gases from the lungs to the atmosphere. **Ventilation** is also used to refer to the movement of air in and out of the lungs.

Breathing is of basically two types: **costal (thoracic) breathing** and **diaphragmatic (abdominal) breathing**. Costal breathing involves the external intercostal muscles and other accessory muscles, such as the sternocleidomastoid muscles. It can be observed by the movement of the chest upward and outward. By contrast, diaphragmatic breathing involves the contraction and relaxation of the diaphragm, and it is observed by the movement of the abdomen, which occurs as a result of the diaphragm's contraction and downward movement.

LIFESPAN CONSIDERATIONS

Assessing an Apical–Radial Pulse

INFANTS

- Use the apical pulse for the heart rate of newborns, infants, and children age 2 to 3 years to establish baseline data for subsequent evaluation, to determine whether the cardiac rate is within normal range, and to determine whether the rhythm is regular.

- Place the baby in the supine position, and offer a pacifier if the baby is crying or restless to avoid any increase in the pulse rate.

- Locate the apical pulse in the fourth intercostal space, lateral to the midclavicular line during infancy.

- Brachial, popliteal, and femoral pulses may be palpated. Because of a normally low blood pressure and rapid heart rate, infants' other distal pulses may be hard to feel.

- Newborn infants may have heart murmurs that are not pathological but reflect functional incomplete closure of the ductus arteriosus or foramen ovale.

CHILDREN

- To take a peripheral pulse, position the child comfortably in the adult's arms, or have the adult remain close by. This may decrease anxiety in the child and yield more accurate results.

- To assess the apical pulse, assist a young child to the comfortable supine or sitting position.

- Demonstrate the procedure to the child by using a stuffed animal or doll, and allow the child to handle the stethoscope before beginning the procedure. This will decrease anxiety and promote positive engagement with the procedure.

- The apex of the heart is normally located in the fourth intercostal space in young children and in the fifth intercostal space in children age 7 years and older.

- Locate the apical impulse along the fourth intercostal space, between the MCL and the anterior axillary line (see Figure 29.11).

- Count the pulse *before* performing other uncomfortable procedures so that the rate is not artificially elevated by the discomfort.

OLDER ADULTS

- Cardiac changes in older adults, such as a decrease in cardiac output, sclerotic changes to heart valves, and dysrhythmias, often indicate that obtaining an apical pulse will be more accurate.

- Older adults often have decreased peripheral circulation, so pedal pulses should also be checked for regularity, volume, and symmetry.

- The pulse returns to baseline after exercise more slowly than with other age groups.

TEACHING	HOME CARE

- If appropriate, teach the client or family member how to take a pulse measurement. Ensure correct technique by having him or her demonstrate the procedure to you.

- Teach the client to monitor pulse rate before taking medications that affect the heart rate. Tell the client to report any notable changes in heart rate or rhythm (regularity) to the appropriate member of the health care team.

Mechanics and Regulation of Breathing

During *inhalation*, the following processes normally occur (Figure 29.13 on the next page): the diaphragm *contracts* (flattens), the ribs move upward and outward, and the sternum moves outward, thus enlarging the thorax and permitting the lungs to expand. During *exhalation* (Figure 29.14 on the next page), the diaphragm relaxes, the ribs move downward and inward, and the sternum moves inward, thus decreasing the size of the thorax as the lungs are compressed. Normally, breathing is carried out automatically and effortlessly. An inspiration lasts 1 to 1.5 seconds, and an expiration lasts 2 to 3 seconds.

Respiration is controlled by (a) the respiratory centres in the medulla oblongata and the pons of the brain, and (b) the chemoreceptors located centrally in the medulla and peripherally in the carotid and aortic bodies. These centres and receptors respond to changes in the concentrations of oxygen (O_2), carbon dioxide (CO_2), and hydrogen (H^+) in the arterial blood. See Chapter 43 for details.

Assessing Respirations

Respirations should be assessed when the client is relaxed because exercise affects respirations, increasing their rate and depth. Anxiety is likely to affect respiratory rate and depth as well. Respirations may also need to be assessed after exercise to identify the client's tolerance to activity. Before assessing a client's respirations, a nurse should be aware of the following:

- The client's normal breathing pattern
- The influence of the client's health problems on respirations
- Any medications or therapies that might affect respirations
- The relationship of the client's respirations to cardiovascular function

The rate, depth, rhythm, and special characteristics of respirations should be assessed. The *respiratory rate* is normally described in breaths per minute. Breathing that is normal in rate and depth is called **eupnea**. Abnormally slow respirations are referred to as **bradypnea**, and abnormally rapid respirations are called **tachypnea**. **Apnea** is the absence of breathing. **Hyperventilation** refers to very deep, rapid respirations; **hypoventilation** refers to very shallow, slow respirations. For the respiratory rates for different age groups, see Table 29.3 on page 709.

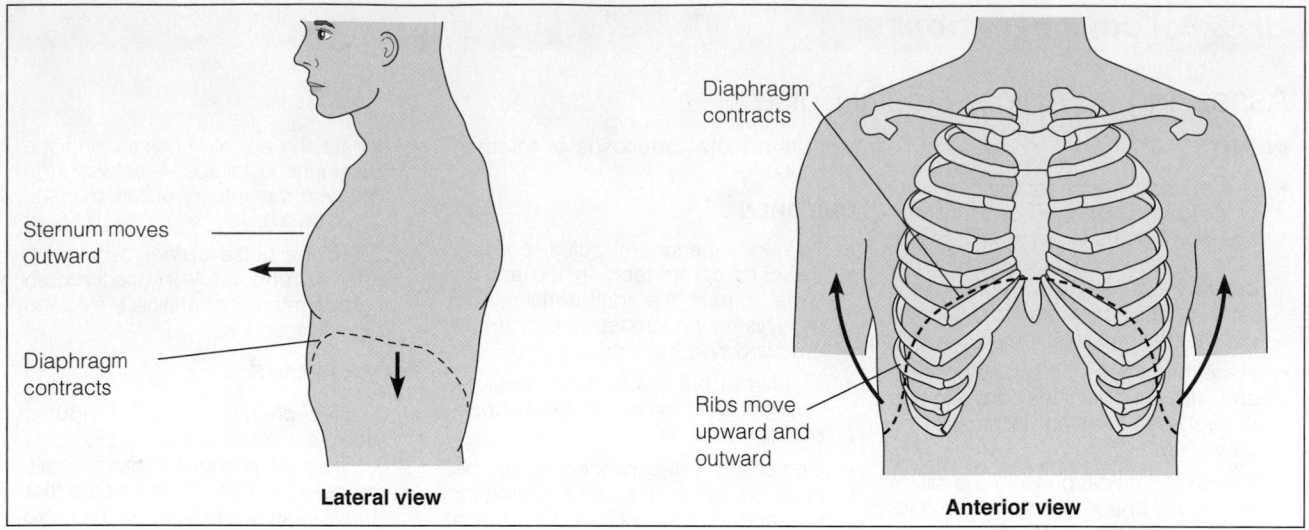

FIGURE 29.13 Respiratory inhalation: *Left*, Lateral view; *Right*, Anterior view.

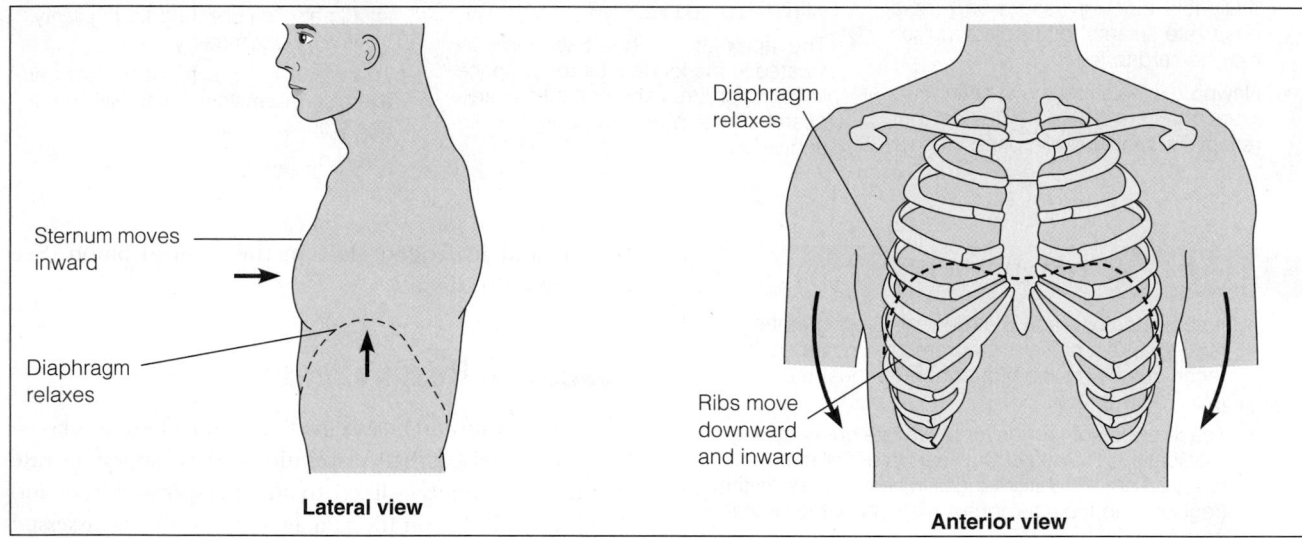

FIGURE 29.14 Respiratory exhalation: *Left*, Lateral view; *Right*, Anterior view.

Factors Affecting Respirations

Several factors influence respiratory rate. Those that increase the rate include increased metabolism (as caused by exercise, fever), stress (as a result of epinephrine release), increased environmental temperature, and lowered arterial oxygen concentration. Factors that may decrease the respiratory rate include certain medications (e.g., opioids, barbiturates), sleep, and increased intracranial pressure.

The *depth* of a person's respirations can be established by watching the movement of the chest. Respiratory depth is generally described as normal, deep, or shallow. *Deep respirations* are those in which a large volume of air is inhaled and exhaled, inflating most of the lungs. *Shallow respirations* involve the exchange of a small volume of air and often the minimal use of lung tissue. During a normal inspiration and expiration, an adult takes in about 500 mL of air. This volume is called the **tidal volume**. For

further information about pulmonary volumes and pulmonary capacities, see Chapter 43.

Body position also affects the amount of air that can be inhaled. People in the supine position experience two physiological processes that suppress respiration: an increase in the volume of blood inside the thoracic cavity and compression of the chest. Consequently, clients lying on their back have poorer lung aeration, which predisposes them to the stasis of fluids and subsequent infection, such as pneumonia.

Respiratory rhythm or pattern refers to the regularity of the expirations and the inspirations. Normally, respirations are evenly spaced. Respiratory rhythm can be described as *regular* or *irregular*. An infant's respiratory rhythm may be less regular than an adult's. See Chapter 43 for details about abnormal respiratory rhythms.

Respiratory quality or character refers to those aspects of breathing that are different from normal, effortless breathing. Two of these are the amount of effort a client must exert to breathe and the sound of breathing. Usually, breathing does not require noticeable effort; some clients, however, exhibit visible effort in breathing (e.g., using accessory muscles), called *laboured breathing*.

The *sound* of breathing is also significant. Normal breathing is silent, but a number of abnormal sounds, such as a wheeze, are obvious to the nurse's ear. Many sounds occur as a result of the presence of fluid in the lungs and are most clearly heard using a stethoscope. See Chapter 28 for methods (e.g., auscultation, percussion, etc.) used to assess lung sounds. For details about altered breathing patterns and terms used to describe various patterns and sounds, see Box 29.5.

The effectiveness of respirations is measured, in part, by the uptake of oxygen from the air into blood and the release of carbon dioxide from blood into the expired air. The amount of hemoglobin in arterial blood that is saturated with oxygen can be measured indirectly through pulse oximetry. A pulse oximeter provides a digital readout of both the client's pulse rate and the oxygen saturation (see Skill 29.7 on page 731).

Skill 29.5 provides guidelines for assessing respirations (see also the Lifespan Considerations box on assessing respirations on page 720 and the Assessment: Home Care box on the special accommodations that should be made in home care settings, on page 721).

BOX 29.5 ALTERED BREATHING PATTERNS AND SOUNDS

The following lists describe altered breathing patterns and sounds:

BREATHING PATTERNS

Rate

- *Tachypnea:* rapid respiration marked by quick, shallow breaths
- *Bradypnea:* abnormally slow breathing
- *Apnea:* cessation of breathing

Volume

- *Hyperventilation:* an increase in the amount of air in the lungs, characterized by increased rate and depth of breaths
- *Hypoventilation:* a reduction in the amount of air in the lungs, characterized by shallow respirations
- *Kussmaul's respiration:* abnormally deep, very rapid sighing respirations characteristic of diabetic ketoacidosis

Rhythm

- *Cheyne-Stokes respiration:* rhythmic waxing and waning of respirations, from very deep to very shallow breathing and temporary apnea; associated with increased intracranial pressure or brain damage and can indicate impending death

Ease or Effort

- *Dyspnea:* the subjective sensation of difficult or uncomfortable breathing or breathlessness (shortness of breath)
- *Orthopnea:* ability to breathe only in upright sitting or standing positions

BREATH SOUNDS

Audible without Amplification

- *Stridor:* a shrill, harsh sound heard during inspiration with laryngeal obstruction
- *Stertor:* snoring or sonorous respiration, usually caused by a partial obstruction of the upper airway
- *Wheeze:* continuous, high-pitched musical squeak or whistling sound occurring on expiration and sometimes on inspiration when air moves through a narrowed or partially obstructed airway
- *Bubbling sounds:* gurgling sounds heard as air passes through moist secretions in the respiratory tract

Chest Movements

- *Intercostal retraction:* indrawing between the ribs
- *Substernal retraction:* indrawing beneath the breastbone
- *Suprasternal retraction:* indrawing above the clavicles
- *Flail chest:* the ballooning out of the chest wall through injured rib spaces; results in *paradoxical breathing*, during which the chest wall balloons on expiration but is depressed or sucked inward on inspiration

Secretions and Coughing

- *Hemoptysis:* the presence of blood in sputum
- *Productive cough:* a cough accompanied by expectorated secretions
- *Nonproductive cough:* a dry, harsh cough without secretions

---

SKILL 29.5 ASSESSING RESPIRATIONS

PURPOSES

- To acquire baseline data against which future measurements can be compared
- To monitor abnormal respirations and respiratory patterns and identify changes
- To assess respirations before or after the administration of a medication that influences breathing, such as morphine or general anesthetics
- To monitor clients at risk for respiratory alterations (e.g., those with fever, pain, acute anxiety, chronic obstructive pulmonary disease, respiratory infection, pulmonary edema or emboli, chest trauma or constriction, brain stem injury)

ASSESSMENT

Assess

- Skin and mucous membrane colour (e.g., cyanosis or pallor)

(continued)

SKILL 29.5 **ASSESSING RESPIRATIONS** (*continued*)

- Position assumed for breathing (e.g., use of orthopneic [upright] position)
- Signs of cerebral hypoxia (e.g., irritability, restlessness, drowsiness)
- Chest movements (e.g., intercostal retractions)
- Activity tolerance
- Chest pain
- Subjective respiratory complaints (e.g., dyspnea)
- Medications affecting respiratory rate

Equipment

- Watch with a second hand or indicator

IMPLEMENTATION

Preparation

For a routine assessment of respirations, determine the client's activity schedule, and choose a suitable time to monitor the respirations. A client who has been exercising will need to rest for a few minutes to permit the accelerated respiratory rate to return to normal.

Performance

1. Before performing the procedure, introduce yourself and verify the client's identity using two identifiers or per agency protocol. Explain to the client what you are going to do, why it is necessary, and how he or she can participate. (For the conscious and alert client, it is best if the nurse counts respirations as an extension of taking the client's pulse.)

2. Perform hand hygiene, and follow other appropriate infection prevention and control procedures.

3. Provide for client privacy.

4. Observe or palpate and count the respiratory rate.
   - The client's awareness that the nurse is counting the respiratory rate could cause the client to purposefully alter the respiratory pattern. If you anticipate this, place the client's arm across the chest and observe the chest movements while supposedly taking the radial pulse.
   - Count the respiratory rate for 30 seconds if the respirations are regular. Count for 60 seconds if they are irregular. An inhalation and an exhalation count as one respiration.

5. Observe the depth, rhythm, and character of respirations.
   - Observe the respirations for depth by watching the movement of the chest. **Rationale: This helps assess if respirations are deep, shallow, or normal.**
   - Observe the respirations for regular or irregular rhythm. **Rationale: Normally, respirations are evenly spaced.**
   - Observe the character of respirations—the sound they produce and the effort they require. **Rationale: Normally, respirations are silent and effortless.**

6. Document respiratory rate, depth, rhythm, and character on the appropriate record.

EVALUATION

- Relate respiratory rate to other vital signs, in particular, pulse rate; relate respiratory rhythm and depth to the client's baseline data and health status.
- Report to the appropriate members of the health care team any respiratory rate significantly above or below the normal range and any notable change in respirations from previous assessments; irregular respiratory rhythm; inadequate respiratory depth; abnormal character of breathing (orthopnea, wheezing, stridor, or bubbling); and any complaints of dyspnea.
- Conduct appropriate follow-up, such as administering oxygen or other appropriate medications, treatments, or positioning the client to ease breathing, and requesting involvement of other members of the health care team, such as the respiratory therapist.

LIFESPAN CONSIDERATIONS

Assessing Respirations

INFANTS

- An infant or a child who is crying will have an abnormal respiratory rate and rhythm and needs to be quieted before respirations can be accurately assessed.
- Infants and young children use their diaphragms for inhalation and exhalation. If necessary, place your hand gently on the infant's abdomen to feel the rapid rise and fall during respirations.
- Most newborns are obligate nose breathers, and nasal obstruction can be life threatening.
- Some newborns display periodic breathing, in which they pause for a few seconds between respirations. This condition can be normal, but parents should be alert to prolonged or frequent pauses between 15 and 20 seconds (apnea) or pauses with a decrease in heart rate below 100 beats/min, as this requires immediate medical attention.
- Compared with adults, infants have fewer alveoli, and their airways have a smaller diameter. As a result, infants' respiratory rate and effort of breathing will increase with respiratory infections.

CHILDREN

- Because young children are diaphragmatic breathers, observe the rise and fall of the abdomen. If necessary, place your hand gently on the abdomen to feel the rapid rise and fall during respirations.
- Count respirations before performing other uncomfortable procedures so that the respiratory rate is not artificially elevated by the discomfort.
- Have an adult hold the child gently to reduce movement while counting respirations.

OLDER ADULTS

- Ask the client to remain quiet, or surreptitiously count respirations after taking the pulse.
- Older adults experience anatomical and physiological changes that cause the respiratory system to be less efficient. Any changes in rate or type of breathing should be reported immediately.

Blood Pressure

Blood pressure is a measurement of the pressure exerted by the blood on the vessel walls as it flows through the arteries. Because the blood moves in waves, two blood pressure measures exist. **Systolic pressure** is the pressure of the blood exerted on the artery wall as a result of contraction of the maximum left ventricle, that is, the pressure of the height of the blood wave. **Diastolic pressure** is the pressure when the ventricles are at rest. Diastolic pressure is the lower pressure present at all times within the arteries. The difference between systolic and diastolic pressures is called **pulse pressure**. Normal pulse pressure is about 40 mm Hg but can be as high as 100 mm Hg during exercise. A consistently elevated pulse pressure occurs in arteriosclerosis. A low pulse pressure (e.g., less than 25 mm Hg) occurs in such conditions as severe heart failure.

Blood pressure is measured in millimetres of mercury (mm Hg) and recorded as a fraction: the systolic pressure over the diastolic pressure. Traditionally, novice health care professionals assumed that the average blood pressure of a healthy adult is 120/80 mm Hg (pulse pressure of 40). However, it is more complex than that. The Canadian Hypertension Education Program (CHEP, 2012) considers adult blood pressure measurements between 130 mm Hg and 139 mm Hg systolic or 85 mm Hg and 89 mm Hg diastolic as high–normal. Blood pressure should be medically treated (usually involving at least one antihypertensive agent, until it is below 140/90 mm Hg in most clients and below 130/80 mm Hg in clients with diabetes (CHEP, 2012). Table 29.6 contains an approximate guide to the classification of blood pressure. A single blood pressure reading is not enough to make a diagnosis of hypertension.

A number of health conditions can be indicated by changes observed in blood pressure recordings in individuals. It is important for the nurse to know a specific client's baseline blood pressure as blood pressure can vary considerably. For example, if a client's usual blood pressure is 120/80 mm Hg and it is assessed following surgery to be 80/40 mm Hg, this significant drop in measure may indicate complications and the primary health care provider needs to be informed. The trend or pattern of blood pressure readings is usually of greater significance than a single result.

TABLE 29.6 Classification of Blood Pressure

Category	Systolic (mm Hg)	Diastolic (mm Hg)
Normal	<130	and/or <85
High Normal	130–139	and/or 85–89
Grade 1 HTN	140–159	and/or 90–99
Grade 2 HTN	160–179	and/or 100–109
Grade 3 HTN	≥180	and/or ≥110
Isolated Systolic HTN (ISH)	>140	and/or >90

Sources: Adapted from Canadian Hypertension Education Program. *(2012). 2012 CHEP recommendations for the management of hypertension.* Ottawa: Author. Retrieved from http://www.hypertension.ca/chep-recommendations; Drouin, D., & Milot (2007) and Kaplan et al. (2003).

Determinants of Blood Pressure

Arterial blood pressure is determined by blood flow and the resistance to blood flow as indicated in the following formula: MAP = CO × SVR, where MAP refers to *mean arterial pressure* (the pressure in the arteries throughout the cardiac cycle), CO refers to *cardiac output*, and SVR refers to *systemic vascular resistance.*

CARDIAC OUTPUT *Cardiac output* is the volume of blood pumped into the arteries by the heart. It is seen as an indicator of the pumping action of the heart. When the pumping action of the heart is weak, less blood is pumped into arteries, and the blood pressure decreases. When the heart's pumping action is strong and the volume of blood pumped into the circulation increases, blood pressure increases.

SYSTEMIC VASCULAR RESISTANCE **Systemic vascular resistance (SVR)**, which is the resistance against which the heart must pump to eject the blood into the systemic circulation (excluding the pulmonary vasculature), is influenced by the size of the arterioles and capillaries, the compliance of the arteries, the blood volume, and the blood viscosity. Increased SVR leads to an increased blood pressure; decreased SVR leads to a decreased blood pressure. Diastolic pressure is especially affected by the resistance in the peripheral vasculature.

The internal diameter or capacity of the arterioles and the capillaries influences SVR in that the smaller the lumen of a vessel, the greater is the resistance. Normally, the arterioles are in a state of partial constriction. Increased vasoconstriction, as occurs with smoking, raises the SVR and, hence, blood pressure; vasodilation, as occurs during a long and hot shower, lowers the SVR (leading to lower blood pressure).

If the normal elastic and muscular tissues of the arteries are replaced with fibrous tissue, as occurs in arteriosclerosis, their compliance (distensibility, elasticity) is decreased. The arteries account for most of the systemic resistance.

When the blood volume decreases (e.g., as a result of a hemorrhage or dehydration), blood pressure decreases because of decreased fluid exerting pressure on the arteries. Conversely, when the volume increases (e.g., as a result of a rapid intravenous infusion), blood pressure increases because of the greater fluid volume within the circulatory system, until homeostasis is restored.

Viscosity is a physical property that results from friction of molecules in a fluid. A viscous (or thick) fluid has a great deal of friction among the molecules as they slide by one another. The viscosity of blood is mostly determined by **hematocrit** (the proportion of red blood cells to blood plasma). Blood pressure is higher when blood is highly viscous (i.e., when the hematocrit is more than 0.6 to 0.65).

Factors Affecting Blood Pressure

Age, exercise, stress, race, obesity, sex, medications, sodium intake, diurnal variations, and medical conditions are factors influencing blood pressure.

- *Age.* Newborns have a mean systolic pressure of about 75 mm Hg. The pressure rises with age, reaching a peak at the onset of puberty, and then tends to decline somewhat. It rises again in older adults, with half of Canadians over age 65 years having hypertension and an estimated 90% of those with normal blood pressure at 55 years who will go on to develop hypertension at some later point (CHEP, 2012). In older adults, elasticity of the arteries is decreased—the arteries are more rigid and less yielding to the pressure of the blood. This produces elevated systolic pressure. Because the walls no longer retract as flexibly with decreased pressure, diastolic pressure may also be high.

- *Exercise.* Physical activity increases the cardiac output and hence blood pressure; thus, 20 to 30 minutes of rest following exercise is indicated before the resting blood pressure can be reliably assessed.

- *Stress.* Stimulation of the sympathetic nervous system increases cardiac output and vasoconstriction of the arterioles, thus increasing blood pressure. The *white coat effect* describes the elevation in blood pressure that occurs by virtue of the stress generated by going to a hospital or clinic for assessment. Severe pain, however, can decrease blood pressure greatly and cause shock by inhibiting the vasomotor centre and producing vasodilation.

- *Race.* Black men over 35 years of age usually exhibit higher blood pressures compared with other men of the same age.

- *Obesity.* Generally, overweight and obese people have higher blood pressure than people of normal weight. Both childhood and adult obesity predispose people to hypertension.

- *Sex.* After puberty, females usually have lower blood pressures compared with males of the same age; this difference is thought to be caused by hormonal variations. Women generally have higher blood pressure following menopause.

- *Medications.* Many medications can increase or decrease blood pressure (e.g., sympathomimetic decongestants and caffeine increase blood pressure; opioids and beta-blockers lower blood pressure); nurses should be aware of over-the-counter and "natural" products that a client is taking and review their possible impact on blood pressure.

- *Sodium intake.* A high sodium intake can increase the release of natriuretic hormone, which indirectly contributes to hypertension. Additionally, sodium stimulates vasopressor mechanisms, which cause vasoconstriction. A sodium intake of no more than 2300 mg is recommended for the prevention of hypertension (CHEP, 2012).

- *Diurnal variations.* Blood pressure is usually lowest early in the morning, when the metabolic rate is lowest, then rises throughout the day, and peaks in the late afternoon or early evening.

- *Medical conditions.* Any condition affecting the cardiac output, blood volume, blood viscosity, or compliance of the arteries has a direct effect on blood pressure.

The Teaching: Wellness box identifies several strategies to maintain a healthy blood pressure.

Hypertension

Blood pressure that is persistently above normal is called **hypertension**. A single elevated blood pressure reading indicates the need for reassessment. Blood pressure that is consistently more than 140/90 mm Hg is considered high and diagnostic of hypertension. Hypertension is a widespread health problem that affects more than 5 million Canadians, with many people not even knowing they have it (CHEP, 2012). Usually asymptomatic, hypertension—sometimes called "the silent killer"—is the number-one risk factor for cerebrovascular accidents and a major risk factor for myocardial infarction, heart failure, peripheral vascular disease, and blindness.

The CHEP makes annual recommendations related to the diagnosis, treatment, and follow-up of hypertension in the most efficient and effective way. The CHEP supports the use of ambulatory and home assessment of blood pressure, if these are available, to monitor people with diabetes, chronic renal disease, and "white coat

Maintaining Healthy Blood Pressure

The following are some ways to maintain healthy blood pressure and reduce the risk for hypertension:

1. Maintain a healthy diet that is high in fresh fruits, vegetables, low-fat dairy products, dietary fibre, whole grains, nonanimal protein (e.g., soy), and low in saturated fat and cholesterol, in keeping with Health Canada's *Eating Well with Canada's Food Guide.*

2. Reduce sodium intake to no more than 2300 mg/day and be aware that adequate sodium intake is: 1500 mg/day if aged 19 to 50 years; 1300 mg if aged 51 to 70 years; and to 1200 mg per day if older than 71 years (CHEP, 2012).

3. Take part in regular physical activity according to Canadian Physical Activity Guidelines (see Chapter 39).

4. Reduce alcohol consumption to ≤2 standard drinks per day and ≤14/week for men and ≤9/week for women.

5. Attain and maintain a healthy BMI (18.5–24.9 kg/m^2) and waist circumference (<94 cm for men and <80 cm for women) in all normotensive and hypertensive individuals for prevention and management of hypertension. For people of South Asian and Chinese descent, waist circumference should be <90 cm for men and <80 cm for women (CHEP, 2012). (See Chapter 40.)

6. Abstain from smoking, and maintain a smoke-free environment.

7. Practise stress management (see Chapter 48).

Source: Summarized with permission from Canadian Hypertension Education Program. (2012). *2012 CHEP recommendations for the management of hypertension.* Ottawa: Author. Retrieved from http://www.hypertension.ca/chep-recommendations

effect" or masked hypertension (blood pressure controlled at clinic visits but not at home). Nurses play an important role in ensuring the appropriate assessment and follow-up of people with hypertension.

Elevated blood pressure of unknown cause is called *primary hypertension*. Elevated blood pressure of known cause is called *secondary hypertension*. The majority (90%) of hypertension diagnoses are of the primary type. Factors associated with primary hypertension include thickening of the arterial walls, which reduces the size of the arterial lumen, loss of elasticity of the arteries, as well as lifestyle factors, such as cigarette smoking, obesity, heavy alcohol consumption, caffeine consumption, lack of physical exercise, high blood cholesterol levels, and continued exposure to stress. Follow-up care should include counselling for lifestyle changes as well as monitoring blood pressure itself. Secondary hypertension causes include renal failure and tumours of the adrenal medulla.

Hypotension

Hypotension is blood pressure that is below normal, that is, a systolic reading consistently between 85 mm Hg and 110 mm Hg in an adult. **Orthostatic hypotension** is blood pressure that falls when the client sits or stands. It is usually the result of peripheral vasodilation in which the blood leaves the central body organs, especially the brain, and moves to the periphery, often causing the person to feel faint. Hypotension can also be caused by opioids, bleeding, severe burns, and prolonged diarrhea and vomiting. It is important to monitor hypotensive clients carefully to prevent falls. When assessing for orthostatic hypotension, follows these steps:

- Place the client in a supine position for at least 5 minutes to allow blood pressure and pulse to stabilize in this position.

- Record the client's pulse and blood pressure.

- Assist the client to slowly sit or stand. Support the client in case of faintness.

- After 1 to 3 minutes in the upright position, recheck the pulse and blood pressure in the same sites as previously.

- Record the results. A rise in pulse of 20 beats/min or a decrease in systolic or diastolic blood pressure of 10 mm Hg indicates orthostatic hypotension. However, interpret these changes with caution, since wide discrepancies exist in the literature about the magnitude of the orthostatic response and its correlation with intravascular volume status (e.g., a healthy individual can have a drop in blood pressure despite normal vascular volume; a person with significantly low vascular volume may not have a postural drop) (Estes & Buck, 2008).

Assessing Blood Pressure

EQUIPMENT   Blood pressure is measured with a *blood pressure cuff*, a *sphygmomanometer*, and a stethoscope. The traditional blood pressure cuff consists of a rubber bladder that can be inflated with air (Figure 29.15 on the next page). The bladder is covered with cloth and has two tubes attached to it. One tube connects to a bulb that inflates the bladder. A small valve on the side of this bulb releases the air from the bladder. When the valve is closed, air pumped into the bladder remains there.

The other tube is attached to a sphygmomanometer. The sphygmomanometer indicates the pressure of

> **! CLINICAL ALERT**
>
> The registered nurse (RN) is responsible for the overall assessment, determination of client status, care planning, interventions, and care evaluation when tasks are delegated to an unregulated care provider (such as a health care aide). Under certain conditions, an RN may delegate selected tasks (if permitted by the agency), such as some aspects of vital signs assessment, if it is in the best interests of the client, if the client is stable, if his or her condition is straightforward, and if the unregulated care provider has sufficient training, supervision, and support to perform the delegated task safely. However, the nurse remains responsible for client care and assessment.

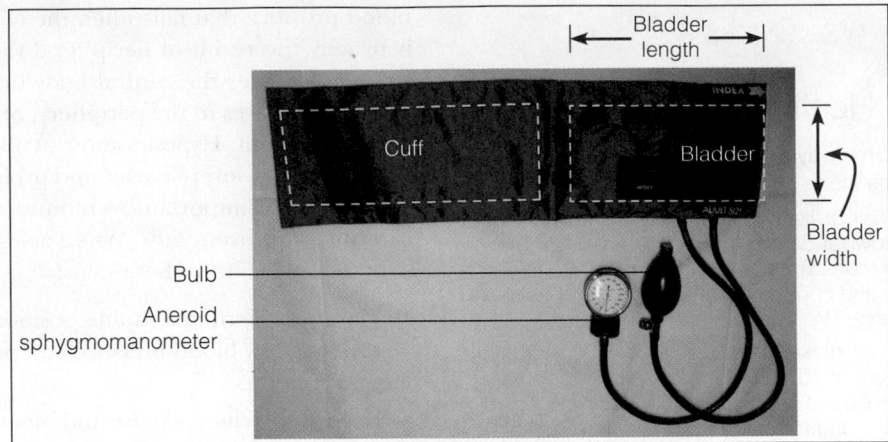

FIGURE 29.15 An aneroid sphygmomanometer, bulb, and cuff. Note the location, length, and width of the bladder.

the air within the bladder. Sphygmomanometers come in two types: *aneroid* and *digital*. The aneroid sphygmomanometer is a calibrated dial with a needle that points to markings that correlate with blood pressure values (see Figure 29.15). Most agencies use digital (electronic) sphygmomanometers (Figure 29.16), which eliminate the need to listen to the sounds of the client's systolic and diastolic blood pressures through a stethoscope.

See the Evidence-Informed Practice box for an indication of how the Canadian Hypertension Education Program disseminates its recommendations to Canadian physicians and other health care professionals.

Doppler ultrasound stethoscopes (DUSs) are also used to assess blood pressure (see Figure 29.12 on page 711). These are of particular value when blood pressure sounds are difficult to hear, such as in infants, obese clients, and clients in shock. A systolic blood pressure assessed with a DUS is recorded with a capital "D," (e.g., 85D). Systolic pressure may be the only blood pressure obtainable with some ultrasound models.

Blood pressure cuffs come in various sizes; the bladder must be the correct width and length for the client's

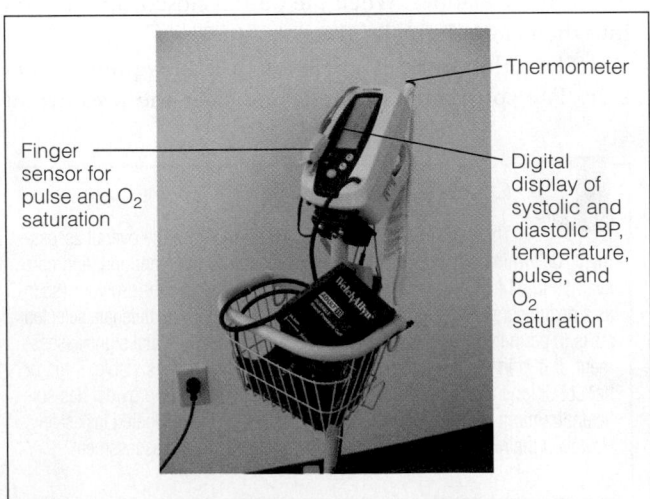

FIGURE 29.16 Electronic blood pressure monitors register systolic and diastolic pressures and often other vital signs.

EVIDENCE-INFORMED PRACTICE

How the Canadian Hypertension Education Program (CHEP) Provides Current Information to Canadian Health Care Professionals

The Canadian Hypertension Education Program (CHEP) provides annual recommendations to ensure that Canadian health care professionals have up-to-date resources for the prevention, diagnosis, and treatment of hypertension. Health care professionals often have difficulty keeping abreast of hypertension prevention and management recommendations and resources. The CHEP focuses on developing and enhancing mechanisms to assist health care professionals and clients to stay up to date with the latest evidence and resources to prevent, diagnose, and manage hypertension. Based on new evidence, changes are made to the CHEP recommendations on an annual basis.

- The full CHEP recommendations are available at www.hypertension.ca
- Health care professionals can receive important updates by signing up at www.htnupdate.ca
- Clients with hypertension can sign up at www.myBPsite.ca to receive regular hypertension updates and help them manage their health.

Nursing Implications: Nurses must remain up-to-date on the latest recommendations for preventing, screening for, and controlling hypertension. The Canadian Hypertension Education Program is an excellent evidence-based resource for all nurses and other health professionals.

arm (Figure 29.17). If the bladder is too narrow, the blood pressure reading will be erroneously elevated; if it is too wide, the reading will be underestimated. The circumference of the limb determines the cuff size. The bladder width should be 40% of the limb circumference or 20% wider than the diameter of the midpoint of the limb, and the bladder length should cover 80% to 100% of the limb circumference (Figure 29.18). When using an electronic

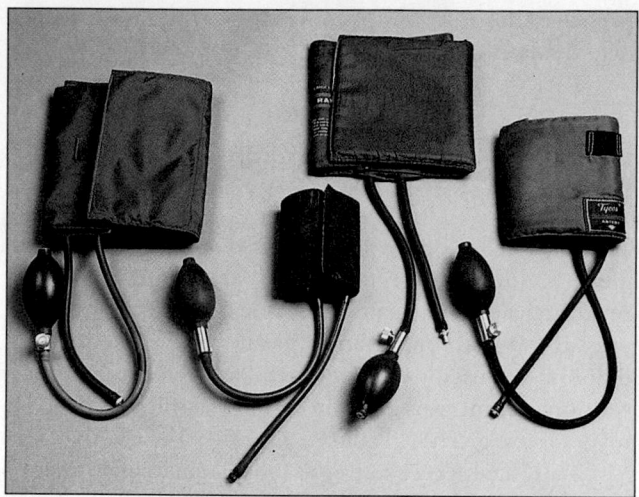

FIGURE 29.17 A variety of cuff sizes: a small cuff for a small child, or frail adult; a normal adult-size cuff; and a large cuff for measuring blood pressure on the leg or on the arm of an obese adult.

device, the cuff size should be determined on the basis of the manufacturer's recommendations (CHEP, 2012).

Blood pressure cuffs are made of nondistensible material so that an even pressure is exerted around the limb. Most cuffs are held in place by Velcro.

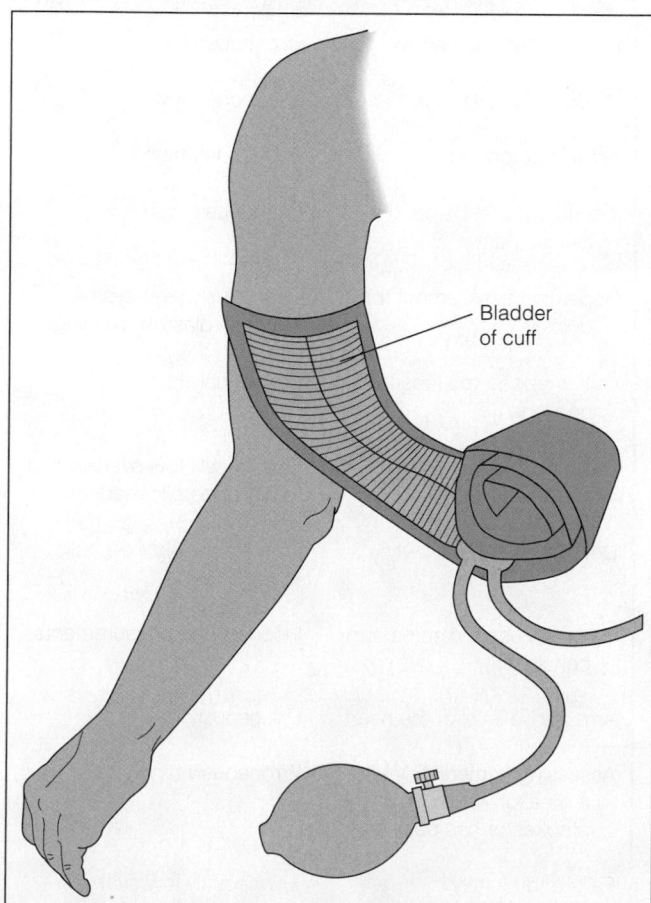

Bladder of cuff

FIGURE 29.18 Determining that the bladder of a blood pressure cuff is 40% of the arm circumference or 20% wider than the diameter of the midpoint of the limb.

BLOOD PRESSURE SITES   Blood pressure is usually assessed in the client's arm at the brachial artery site and by using a standard stethoscope. If the arm is very large or grossly misshapen and the conventional cuff cannot be properly applied, leg or forearm measurements can be taken. To obtain a *thigh blood pressure*, apply an appropriate-sized cuff to the thigh and auscultate the pulsations of blood over the popliteal artery.

Assessing blood pressure on a client's thigh is usually indicated when blood pressure cannot be measured on either arm (e.g., because of burns or other trauma) or if blood pressure in one thigh is to be compared with blood pressure in the other thigh.

Blood pressure is *not* measured on a particular limb (arm or leg) in the following situations:

- The shoulder, arm, or hand (or the hip, knee, or ankle) is injured or diseased.
- A cast or bulky bandage is on any part of the limb.
- Axilla or inguinal lymph nodes have been removed on the side of the limb (such as after radical mastectomy).
- Intravenous infusion is being given in that limb.
- The client has an arteriovenous fistula (e.g., for renal dialysis) in that limb.

METHODS   Blood pressure can be assessed directly or indirectly. *Direct (invasive monitoring) measurement* involves the insertion of a catheter into the brachial, radial, or femoral artery. Arterial pressure is represented as wavelike forms displayed on an oscilloscope. With correct placement, this pressure reading is highly accurate.

Two *noninvasive indirect methods* of measuring blood pressure are auscultatory and palpatory methods. The *auscultatory method* is most commonly used in hospitals, clinics, and homes. Required equipment is a sphygmomanometer, a cuff, and a stethoscope. When carried out correctly, the auscultatory method is relatively accurate.

When taking a blood pressure by using a stethoscope, the nurse identifies the five phases in the series of sounds called **Korotkoff sounds** (Figure 29.19 on the next page). First, the nurse pumps the cuff up to about 30 mm Hg above the palpatory systolic pressure (when the pulse is no longer felt—this is the point when the blood flow in the artery is stopped). Pressure is released slowly (2 mm Hg/beat), while the nurse observes the readings on the manometer and relates them to the sounds heard through the stethoscope. Five phases occur but may not always be audible. *Phase I* is the pressure at which the first sounds are heard. Initially, a tapping or thumping sound, this gradually becomes louder. Thus, phase I Korotkoff sounds signify systolic blood pressure. *Phase II* occurs during deflation of the cuff, and the sounds have a muffled or swishing quality. During *phase III*, blood flows freely through the increasingly open artery, and the sounds increase in crispness and develop a thumping quality. In *phase IV*, the sounds become muffled again and have a much softer quality. Finally, *phase V* represents diastolic blood pressure, and

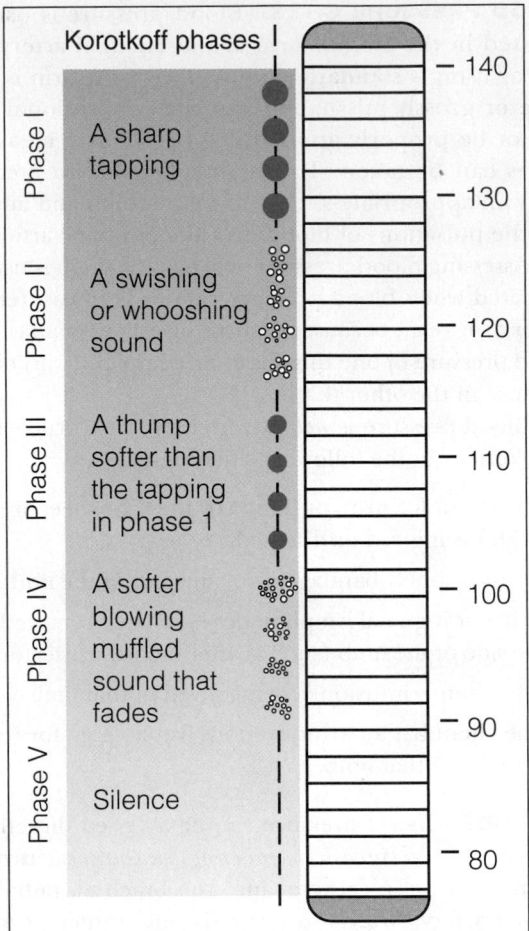

FIGURE 29.19 Korotkoff sounds can be differentiated into five phases. In the illustration, blood pressure is 138/90 mm Hg or 138/102/90 mm Hg.

it is the point at which the sounds disappear. If Korotkoff sounds continue until the level approaches 0 mm Hg, then phase IV is used to indicate diastolic pressure. Some agencies require the recording of phase I, phase IV, and phase V measurements.

The *palpatory method* is sometimes used when Korotkoff sounds cannot be heard and electronic equipment to amplify the sounds is not available, or when an auscultatory gap occurs. An **auscultatory gap**, which occurs particularly in hypertensive clients, is the temporary disappearance of sounds normally heard over the brachial artery when the cuff pressure is high, followed by the reappearance of the sounds at a lower level. This temporary disappearance of sounds occurs in the latter part of phase I and phase II and may cover a range of 40 mm Hg. Instead of listening for blood flow sounds, the nurse palpates the pulsations of the artery as the pressure in the cuff is released. Systolic pressure is read from the sphygmomanometer when the first pulsation is felt. A single whiplike vibration, felt in addition to the pulsations, identifies the point at which the pressure in the cuff nears diastolic pressure. This vibration is no longer felt when the cuff pressure is below diastolic pressure. To palpate diastolic

pressure, the nurse applies light to moderate pressure over the pulse point.

Common Errors in Assessing Blood Pressure

The importance of the accuracy of blood pressure assessments cannot be overemphasized. Many determinations regarding a client's health are made on the basis of blood pressure. It is an important indicator of the client's condition and is used extensively as a basis for nursing interventions. Some reasons for erroneous blood pressure readings are given in Table 29.7.

Many health care settings use automated manometers in place of aneroid manometers. The mercury column manometer, rarely seen in modern health care settings, has long been considered the gold standard in accuracy for blood pressure measurements, and these devices tend to maintain their accuracy over time. Aneroid units consist of mechanical parts, require frequent calibration, and

TABLE 29.7 Selected Sources of Error in Blood Pressure Assessment

Error	Effect
Bladder cuff too narrow	Erroneously high
Bladder cuff too wide	Erroneously low
Arm unsupported	Erroneously high
Insufficient rest before the assessment	Erroneously high
Repeating assessment too quickly	Erroneously high systolic or low diastolic readings
Cuff wrapped too loosely or unevenly	Erroneously high
Deflating cuff too quickly	Erroneously low systolic and high diastolic readings
Deflating cuff too slowly	Erroneously high diastolic readings
Failure to use the same arm consistently	Inconsistent measurements
Arm above level of the heart	Erroneously low
Assessing immediately after a meal or while client smokes or has pain	Erroneously high
Failure to identify auscultatory gap	Erroneously low systolic pressure and erroneously low diastolic pressure

can break when mishandled. Using an aneroid manometer requires the nurse to listen for sounds to interpret blood pressure. Automated and digital devices are oscillometric and measure blood pressure based on pulse pattern, not sound. Each device has its own method for calculating blood pressure; they are difficult to calibrate and are not suitable for some clients (Mackechnie & Simpson, 2006; Nelson et al., 2008). Automated blood pressure machines can be convenient, but their use does not replace knowledge of the correct method to obtain manual blood pressure measurements. Nurses should do the following:

1. Retain the important skill of manual blood pressure measurement to ensure clients are accurately diagnosed and treated.

2. Make sure that the blood pressure equipment is validated, in good working order, and calibrated.

3. Maintain proper technique in blood pressure assessment, regardless of the device used.

4. Confirm findings that are critical or that do not align with the client's history or health status.

Regardless of the device used in the assessment of a client's blood pressure, the nurse is responsible for the findings of the assessment. When verification of blood pressure is required, the nurse may find it useful to do so with a recently calibrated manual sphygmomanometer.

Skill 29.6 provides guidelines for assessing blood pressure using auscultatory and palpatory methods and using aneroid and digital blood pressure equipment (see also the Lifespan Considerations box on assessing blood pressure on page 729 and the Teaching: Home Care box on page 730 for how to instruct clients to take their own blood pressure at home).

SKILL 29.6 | ASSESSING BLOOD PRESSURE

PURPOSES

- To obtain a baseline measure of arterial blood pressure for subsequent evaluation
- To determine the client's hemodynamic status (e.g., blood vessel resistance)
- To identify and monitor changes in blood pressure resulting from a disease process and medical therapy (e.g., presence or history of cardiovascular disease, renal disease, shock, or acute pain; rapid infusion of fluids or blood products)

ASSESSMENT

Assess

- Signs and symptoms of hypertension (e.g., occipital headache, ringing in the ears, flushing of face, nosebleeds, keeping in mind that hypertension may have NO symptoms)
- Signs and symptoms of hypotension (e.g., tachycardia, dizziness, mental confusion, restlessness, cool and clammy skin, pale skin, syncope)
- Factors affecting blood pressure (e.g., activity, emotional stress, pain, and time the client last smoked or ingested caffeine)

Equipment

- Stethoscope or DUS
- Blood pressure cuff of the appropriate size
- Sphygmomanometer

IMPLEMENTATION

Preparation

1. Ensure that the equipment is intact and functioning properly. Check for leaks in the tubing of the sphygmomanometer.

2. Make sure that the client has not smoked or ingested caffeine within 30 minutes before measurement. **Rationale: Smoking constricts blood vessels, and caffeine**

increases the pulse rate. Both cause a temporary increase in blood pressure.

3. The patient should be seated comfortably with back support for at least 5 minutes before commencing the blood pressure assessment (CHEP, 2012).

Performance

1. Before performing the procedure, introduce yourself and verify the client's identity using two identifiers or per agency protocol. Explain to the client what you are going to do, why it is necessary, and how he or she can participate. Discuss how the results will be used in planning further care or treatments.

2. Perform hand hygiene, and follow other appropriate infection prevention and control procedures.

3. Provide for client privacy.

4. Position the client appropriately.
   - The adult client should be sitting with back support, unless otherwise specified. Both feet should be flat on the floor (CHEP, 2012). **Rationale: Legs crossed at the knee result in elevated systolic and diastolic blood pressures).**
   - The elbow should be slightly flexed with the palm of the hand facing up and the forearm supported at heart level (see ❶). Readings in any other position should be specified. Blood pressure is normally similar in sitting, standing, and lying positions, but it can vary significantly by position in certain persons. **Rationale: Blood pressure increases when the arm is below the heart level and decreases when the arm is above the heart level.**
   - Expose the upper arm.

5. Wrap the deflated cuff evenly around the bare upper arm. Locate the brachial artery (see Figure 29.10 on page 709). Apply the centre of the bladder directly over the artery. **Rationale: The bladder inside the cuff must be**

(continued)

SKILL 29.6   ASSESSING BLOOD PRESSURE (*continued*)

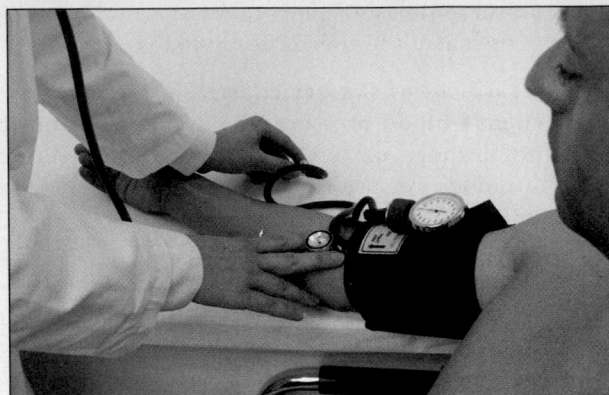

① Location of the brachial artery and application of the cuff

directly over the artery to be compressed to obtain an accurate reading.

- For an adult, place the lower border of the cuff 3 cm above the antecubital space (CHEP, 2012).

6. If this is the client's initial examination, perform a preliminary palpatory determination of systolic pressure. **Rationale: The initial estimate indicates the maximal pressure to which the manometer needs to be elevated in subsequent determinations. It also prevents underestimation of systolic pressure or overestimation of diastolic pressure should an auscultatory gap occur.**
    - Palpate the brachial artery with your fingertips.
    - Close the valve on the bulb.
    - Pump up the cuff until the brachial pulse is no longer felt. At that pressure the blood cannot flow through the artery. Note the pressure on the sphygmomanometer at which the pulse is no longer felt. **Rationale: This gives an estimate of systolic pressure.**
    - Release the pressure completely in the cuff, and wait 1 to 2 minutes before making further measurements. **Rationale: A waiting period gives the blood trapped in the veins time to be released. Otherwise, false high systolic readings will occur.**

7. Position the stethoscope appropriately.
    - Clean the earpieces with antiseptic wipe.
    - Insert the ear attachments of the stethoscope in your ears so that they tilt slightly forward. **Rationale: Sounds are heard more clearly when the ear attachments follow the direction of the ear canal.**
    - Ensure that the stethoscope hangs freely from the ears to the diaphragm. **Rationale: If the stethoscope tubing rubs against an object, the noise can block the sounds of the blood within the artery.**
    - Place the bell side of the amplifier of the stethoscope over the brachial pulse site. **Rationale: Because blood pressure is a low-frequency sound, it is best heard with the bell-shaped diaphragm. Place the stethoscope directly on skin, not on clothing over the site to avoid noise made from rubbing the**

amplifier against cloth. Hold the diaphragm with the thumb and index finger.

8. Auscultate the client's blood pressure.
    - Pump up the cuff rapidly until the sphygmomanometer reads 30 mm Hg above the point where the brachial pulse disappeared (CHEP, 2012). **Rationale: This reduces the chance of a systolic auscultatory gap.**
    - Release the valve on the cuff carefully so that the pressure decreases at the rate of 2 mm Hg per heart beat (CHEP, 2012). **Rationale: If the rate is faster or slower, an error in measurement may occur.**
    - As the pressure falls, identify the manometer reading at Korotkoff phases I, IV, and V. **Rationale: There is no clinical significance to phases II and III.**
    - Auscultate at least 10 mm Hg below phase V. **Rationale: This excludes a diastolic auscultatory gap.**
    - Deflate the cuff rapidly and completely.
    - Wait at least 1 to 2 minutes before making further determinations. **Rationale: This permits the blood trapped in the veins to be released.**
    - Repeat the above steps two more times to confirm the accuracy of the reading. Reject the first reading and average the next two (CHEP, 2012). These additional steps are especially important if the blood pressure reading falls outside of the normal range (although this may not be routine procedure for hospitalized or well clients). If there is >5 mm Hg difference between the two readings, additional measurements may be taken and the results averaged.

9. If this is the client's initial examination, repeat the procedure on the client's other arm and with the client in the standing position (arm must be supported). The difference between the arms should be no more than 10 mm Hg. The arm found to have the higher pressure should be used for subsequent examinations.

Variation: Obtaining Blood Pressure by the Palpation Method

If it is not possible to use a stethoscope to obtain blood pressure or if Korotkoff sounds cannot be heard, palpate the radial or brachial pulse site as the cuff pressure is released. The manometer reading at the point where the pulse reappears is an estimate of systolic value.

Variation: Taking Thigh Blood Pressure

- Help the client to assume the prone position. If the client cannot assume this position, measure blood pressure while the client is in the supine position with his or her knee slightly flexed. Slight flexing of the knee will facilitate placing the stethoscope on the popliteal space (see **②**).
- Expose the thigh, taking care not to expose the client unduly.
- Locate the popliteal artery (see Figure 29.10 on page 709).
- Wrap the cuff evenly around the mid-thigh with the compression bladder over the posterior aspect of the thigh and the bottom edge above the knee. **Rationale: The bladder must be directly over the posterior popliteal artery for the reading to be accurate.**

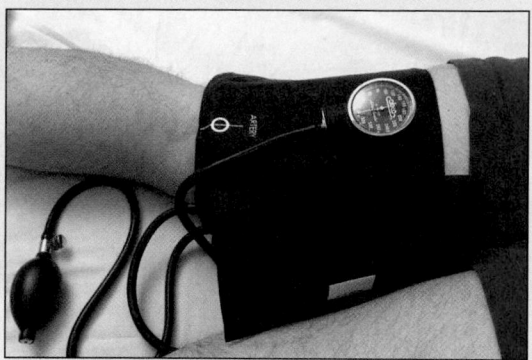

❷ Measuring blood pressure in the client's thigh

- If this is the client's initial examination, perform a preliminary palpatory determination of systolic pressure by palpating the popliteal artery.

- In adults, systolic pressure in the popliteal artery is usually 20 mm Hg to 30 mm Hg higher than that in the brachial artery because of use of a larger bladder; diastolic pressure is usually the same.

Variation: Using an Electronic Indirect Blood Pressure Monitoring Device

- Place the blood pressure cuff on the extremity, according to the manufacturer's guidelines.

- Turn on the blood pressure measuring device.

- If appropriate, set the device for the desired number of minutes between blood pressure determinations.

- When the device has determined the blood pressure reading, note the digital results.

10. Remove the cuff.

11. Wipe the cuff with an approved disinfectant. **Rationale: This helps prevent transmission of microorganisms.**

12. Document and report all pertinent assessment data, according to agency policy. Record blood pressure to the nearest 2 mm Hg (or 1 mm Hg on electronic devices). Record two pressures in the form "130/80" where "130" is systolic pressure (phase 1) and "80" is diastolic (phase V) pressure. Record three pressures in the form "130/90/0," where "130" is systolic pressure, "90" is the first diastolic pressure (phase IV), and "0" denotes that sounds are audible even after the cuff is completely deflated. Use the abbreviations RA or RL for right arm or right leg and LA or LL for left arm or left leg. Record a difference of greater than 10 mm Hg between the two arms or legs.

> **! CLINICAL ALERT**
>
> An electronic or automatic blood pressure cuff can be left in place for many hours. Remove the cuff and check skin condition periodically.

EVALUATION

- Relate blood pressure to the client's other vital signs, to baseline data, and to health status.

- Report any significant change in the client's blood pressure. Also report these findings:
  - Systolic blood pressure (of an adult) above 130 mm Hg
  - Diastolic blood pressure (of an adult) above 85 mm Hg
  - Systolic blood pressure (of an adult) below 100 mm Hg
  - Conduct appropriate follow-up, such as administration of medication.

LIFESPAN CONSIDERATIONS

Assessing Blood Pressure

INFANTS

- Use a pediatric stethoscope with small diaphragm.

- The lower edge of the blood pressure cuff can be closer to the antecubital space of an infant.

- Use the palpation method if auscultation with a stethoscope or DUS is unsuccessful.

- Arm and thigh pressures are equivalent in children less than 1 year of age.

- One quick way to determine the normal systolic blood pressure of a child is to use the following formula: Normal systolic blood pressure = 80 + (2 × child's age in years).

CHILDREN

- Blood pressure should be measured in all children age more than 3 years and in children age less than 3 years with certain medical conditions (e.g., heart disease, renal malformation, medications that affect blood pressure).

- Explain each step of the process and what it will feel like. Demonstrate on a doll.

- Use the palpation technique for children age less than 3 years.

- Take the blood pressure before performing other uncomfortable procedures so that the blood pressure is not artificially elevated by the discomfort.

- In children, diastolic pressure is considered to be the onset of phase IV, where the sounds become muffled.

- In children, thigh pressure is about 10 mm Hg higher than arm pressure.

OLDER ADULTS

- Skin may be very fragile. Do not allow cuff pressure to remain high any longer than necessary.

- Determine whether the client is taking antihypertensives and, if so, when the last dose was taken.

- Medications that cause vasodilation (e.g., certain antihypertensive agents) along with the loss of baroreceptor efficiency in older adults place them at increased risk for having orthostatic hypotension. Measuring blood pressure while the client is in the lying, sitting, and standing positions and noting any changes can determine this.

- If the client has arm contractures, assess the blood pressure by palpation, with the arm in a relaxed position. If this is not possible, take thigh blood pressure.

Blood Pressure

If taught properly, clients can take blood pressure readings at home:

- Home blood pressure measurement done by the client or family can detect elevated pressures not identified when the client is seen in a medical setting. Home blood pressure measurements can also be used when a client is suspected of having white coat hypertension—an elevated blood pressure when measured in a medical setting but an otherwise normal blood pressure at home.

- Observe the client or family member taking the blood pressure, and provide feedback if further instruction is needed.

- Clients should purchase home blood pressure monitoring devices, preferably with data-recording capabilities, that have "Recommended by the Canadian Hypertension Society" noted on the packaging. (Visit the CHEP website for photos of approved equipment.)

- If the client is in a chair or low bed, position yourself so that you maintain the client's arm at heart level and you can read the sphygmomanometer at eye level.

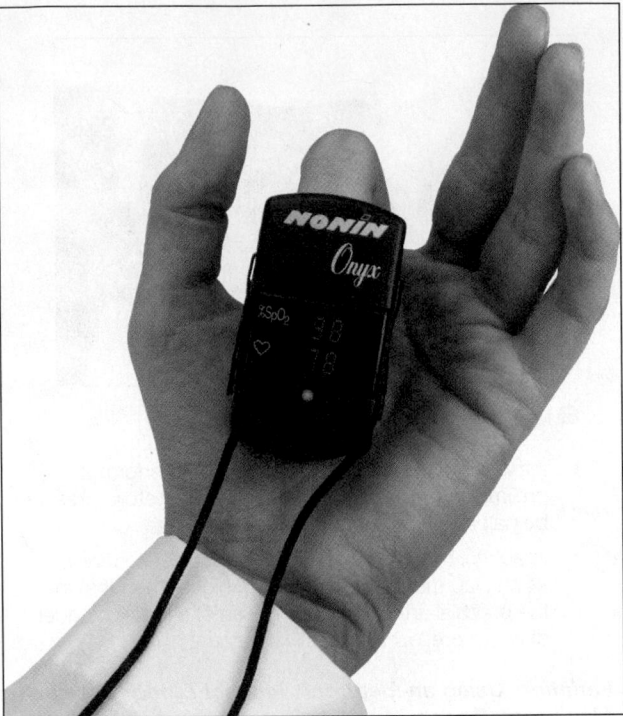

FIGURE 29.20 Fingertip oximeter sensor (adult).

CLINICAL ALERT

Automated and digital assessment of vital signs is replacing conventional and manual assessments in most clinical sites. Make sure you verify any unexpected vital signs using conventional measurement and confirm any vital signs that are inconsistent with the client's presentation. Maintain your skills in the assessment of vital signs, as human touch and clinical wisdom cannot be replaced by technology.

BOX 29.6 OXIMETRY: UNDERSTANDING THE NUMBERS

SpO_2, %	Oxygenation
95–100	Normal
91–94	Mild hypoxia
86–90	Moderate hypoxia
<85	Severe hypoxia

Note: Oximetry measurements should always be interpreted in conjunction with other client factors, including signs and symptoms of hypoxia.

Source: Adapted from DeMeulenaere, S. (2007). Pulse oximetry: Uses and limitations. *The Journal for Nurse Practitioners, 3*(5), 312–317.

Oxygen Saturation

A **pulse oximeter** is a noninvasive device that estimates a client's arterial blood oxygen saturation by means of a sensor attached to the client's finger (Figure 29.20), toe, nose, earlobe, or forehead (or around the hand or foot of a neonate). Pulse oximetry is often used instead of the riskier, more painful, and invasive arterial blood gas measurement of blood oxygen saturation. The pulse oximeter can detect hypoxemia before clinical signs and symptoms, such as *dusky* (darker) skin colour and dusky nail bed colour, develop. Box 29.6 contains guidelines for understanding the values obtained from oximetry. Oxygen saturation assessed using the invasive approach is documented as SaO_2 (arterial oxygen saturation); oxygen saturation assessed by pulse oximetry is documented as SpO_2 (peripheral oxygen saturation).

The pulse oximeter's sensor has two parts: (a) two light-emitting diodes (LEDs)—one red, the other infrared—that transmit light through nails, tissue, venous blood, and arterial blood; and (b) a photodetector placed directly opposite the LEDs (e.g., the other side of the finger, toe, or nose). The photodetector measures the amount of red and infrared light absorbed by oxygenated and deoxygenated hemoglobin in peripheral arterial blood and reports it as SpO_2. Normal SpO_2 as measured by pulse oximetry is 95% to 100%, and SpO_2 values below 70% are unreliable (DeMeulenaere, 2007). It is important to note that oximeters do not measure the actual tissue oxygenation or how well a client is ventilated. Therefore, it is essential that oximetry measurements be interpreted in conjunction with other client factors, including signs and symptoms of hypoxia.

Pulse oximeters with various types of sensors are available from several manufacturers. The oximeter unit consists of an inlet connection for the sensor cable and a faceplate that indicates (a) the oxygen saturation measurement (expressed as a percentage) and (b) the pulse rate. Cordless units are also available (Figure 29.21). A preset alarm system signals high and low SpO_2 measurements and a high and low pulse rate. High and low SpO_2

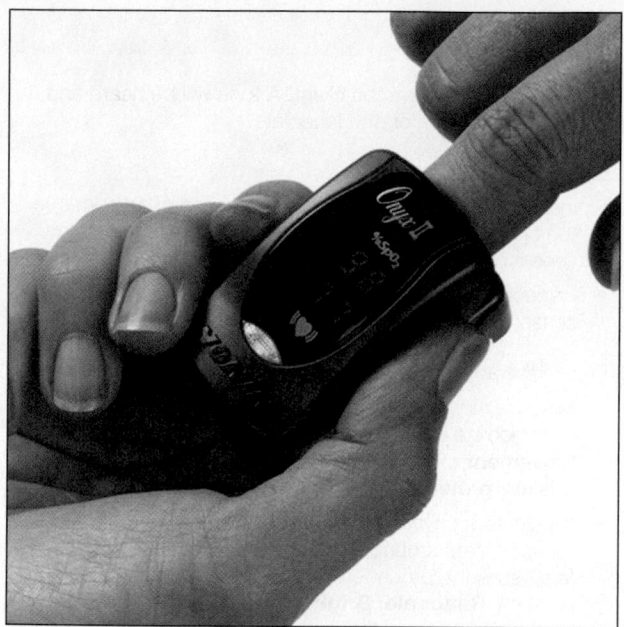

FIGURE 29.21 Fingertip oximeter sensor (cordless).

Factors Affecting Oxygen Saturation Readings

Several factors can affect oxygen saturation readings:

- *Hemoglobin.* If the hemoglobin is fully saturated with oxygen, the SpO_2 will appear normal, even if the total hemoglobin level is low. Thus, the client could be severely anemic and have inadequate oxygen to supply tissues, but the pulse oximeter would return a normal value.

- *Circulation.* The oximeter will not provide an accurate reading if the area under the sensor has impaired circulation.

- *Activity.* Shivering or excessive movement of the sensor site can interfere with accurate readings.

- *Carbon monoxide poisoning.* Pulse oximeters cannot discriminate between hemoglobin saturated with carbon monoxide (CO) versus oxygen. In this case, other measures of oxygenation are needed.

Skill 29.7 outlines the steps in measuring oxygen saturation (see also the Lifespan Considerations box on pulse oxymetry on the next page and the Home Care Considerations box for how pulse oximetry can be used in a home setting). See Chapter 43 for a more extensive discussion of oxygenation.

levels are generally preset at 100% and 85%, respectively, for adults. High and low pulse rate alarms are usually preset at 140 and 50 beats/min for adults. These alarm limits can, however, be changed according to the manufacturer's directions.

SKILL 29.7 MEASURING OXYGEN SATURATION

PURPOSES

- To estimate the arterial blood oxygen saturation
- To detect the presence of hypoxemia before visible signs develop

ASSESSMENT

Assess

- The best location for a pulse oximeter sensor, based on the client's age and physical condition; unless contraindicated, the finger is usually selected for adults
- The client's overall condition, including risk factors for development of hypoxemia (e.g., respiratory or cardiac disease) and hemoglobin level
- Vital signs, skin colour and temperature, nail bed colour, and tissue perfusion of extremities as baseline data
- Adhesive allergy

PLANNING

Many hospitals and clinics have pulse oximeters readily available for use with other vital signs equipment (or even as an integrated part of the electronic blood pressure device). Other facilities may have a limited supply of oximeters, and the nurse may need to request it from the central supply department.

Equipment

- Nail polish remover
- Sheet or towel, as needed
- Alcohol wipe
- Pulse oximeter

IMPLEMENTATION

Preparation

Check that the oximeter equipment is functioning normally.

Performance

1. Before performing the procedure, introduce yourself and verify the client's identity using two identifiers or per agency protocol. Explain to the client what you are going to do, why it is necessary, and how he or she can participate.

2. Perform hand hygiene, and follow other appropriate infection prevention and control procedures.

3. Provide for client privacy.

4. Choose a sensor appropriate for the client's weight and size, and the desired location. Because weight limits of sensors overlap, a pediatric sensor could be used for a small adult.

   - If the client is allergic to adhesive, use a clip or sensor without adhesive. If using an extremity, assess the proximal pulse and capillary refill at the point closest to the site.

   - If the client has low tissue perfusion because of peripheral vascular disease or therapy that uses vasoconstrictive medications, use a nasal sensor or a

(continued)

SKILL 29.7 MEASURING OXYGEN SATURATION (*continued*)

reflectance sensor on the forehead. Avoid using lower extremities that have compromised circulation and extremities that are used for infusions or other invasive monitoring.

5. Prepare the site.
   - Clean the site with an alcohol wipe before applying the sensor.
   - It may be necessary to remove a client's dark nail polish and artificial acrylic fingernails. **Rationale: These can interfere with accurate measurements.** Alternatively, position the sensor on the side of the finger rather than perpendicular to the nail bed (Booker, 2008; Hinkelbein, Koehler, Genzwuerker, & Fiedler, 2007).

6. Apply the sensor, and connect it to the pulse oximeter.
   - Make sure the LED and photodetector are accurately aligned, that is, opposite each other on either side of the finger, toe, nose, or earlobe. Many sensors have markings to facilitate correct alignment of the LEDs and photodetector.
   - Attach the sensor cable to the connection outlet on the oximeter. Turn on the machine, according to the manufacturer's directions. Appropriate connection will be confirmed by an audible beep indicating each arterial pulsation. Some devices have a wheel that can be turned clockwise to increase the pulse volume and counterclockwise to decrease it.
   - Ensure that the bar of light or waveform on the face of the oximeter fluctuates with each pulsation.

7. Set and turn on the alarm when using continuous monitoring.
   - Check the preset alarm limits for high and low oxygen saturation and high and low pulse rates. Change these alarm limits, according to the manufacturer's directions, as indicated. Ensure that the audio and visual alarms are

on before you leave the client. A tone will be heard and a number will blink on the faceplate.

8. Ensure client safety.
   - Inspect and move or change the location of an adhesive toe or finger sensor every 4 hours and a spring-tension sensor every 2 hours.
   - Inspect the sensor site tissues for irritation from adhesive sensors.

9. Ensure the accuracy of measurement.
   - Minimize motion artifacts by using an adhesive sensor, or immobilize the client's monitoring site. **Rationale: Movement of the client's finger or toe may be misinterpreted by the oximeter as arterial pulsations.**
   - If indicated, cover the sensor with a sheet or towel to block large amounts of light from external sources (e.g., sunlight, procedure lamps, or bilirubin lights in the nursery). **Rationale: Bright room light may be sensed by the photodetector and alter the SpO$_2$ value (Booker, 2008).**
   - Compare the pulse rate indicated by the oximeter to the radial pulse periodically. **Rationale: A large discrepancy between the two values may indicate oximeter malfunction.**

10. Document the SpO$_2$ as measured by pulse oximetry on the appropriate record at designated intervals.

EVALUATION

- Compare the SpO$_2$ with the client's previous oxygen saturation level, including any invasive SaO$_2$ measurements. Relate findings to the pulse rate and other vital signs.
- Conduct appropriate follow-up, such as notifying the appropriate members of the health care team or adjusting oxygen therapy.

LIFESPAN CONSIDERATIONS

Pulse Oximetry

INFANTS

- If an appropriate-sized finger or toe sensor is not available, consider using an earlobe or forehead sensor.
- High and low SpO$_2$ levels are generally preset at 95% and 80% for neonates.
- High and low pulse rate alarms are usually preset at 200 and 100 beats/min for neonates.
- The oximeter may need to be taped, wrapped with an elastic bandage, or covered by a stocking to keep it in place.

CHILDREN

- Instruct the child that the sensor does not hurt. Disconnect the probe, whenever possible, to allow for movement.

OLDER ADULTS

- Use of vasoconstrictive medications, poor circulation, or thickened nails in older adults may make finger or toe sensors inaccurate.

HOME CARE CONSIDERATIONS

Pulse Oximetry

Pulse oximetry can be used in a home setting:

- Pulse oximetry is a quick, inexpensive, noninvasive method of assessing oxygenation. Like an automatic blood pressure cuff, it also provides a pulse rate reading. Use in the ambulatory or home setting, whenever indicated.
- Encourage caregivers to assess not only the measurement obtained through pulse oximetry but to evaluate the client for signs and symptoms of hypoxia.
- If the client requires frequent or continuous home monitoring, teach the client and family how to apply and maintain the equipment. Remind them to rotate the site periodically and assess for skin trauma.

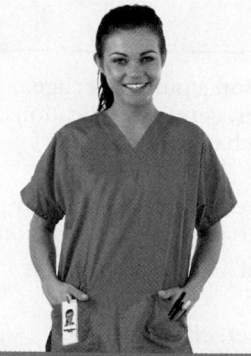

Case Study 29

Mrs. Awosoga, 75 years old, has just been transferred to her own bed from the postanesthetic care unit stretcher, following total hip replacement for osteoarthritis. After a verbal report from the registered nurse, you assess her vital signs. On taking her blood pressure, you are unable to hear any Korotkoff sounds during release of the valve. You repeat the procedure after 3 minutes and obtain a reading of 180/110 mm Hg LA supine. Her temperature (tympanic) is 35.8°C and pulse (radial) is 90 beats/min, regular, 2+/4 amplitude. Her respirations are 28 and shallow. The pulse oximeter indicates an SpO$_2$ of 95%. She is awake and oriented, and her skin is warm; but it is difficult to discern skin colour as it relates to oxygenation because of the dark pigmentation of her skin.

CRITICAL THINKING QUESTIONS

1. What would you say to her when you were unable to hear the Korotkoff sounds?

2. What is your analysis of the blood pressure reading of 180/110 mm Hg? What further data do you need to collect?

3. How would you interpret her temperature, pulse, and respiratory rate?

Check the eText in MyNursingLab for answers and explanations.

KEY TERMS

afebrile *p. 700*
apical pulse *p. 708*
apical–radial pulse *p. 714*
apnea *p. 717*
arrhythmia *p. 711*
auscultatory gap *p. 726*
basal metabolic rate (BMR) *p. 698*
blood pressure *p. 721*
body temperature *p. 697*
bradycardia *p. 711*
bradypnea *p. 717*
cardiac output *p. 708*
chemical thermogenesis *p. 698*
compliance *p. 708*
conduction *p. 698*
constant fever *p. 700*
convection *p. 698*
core temperature *p. 697*
costal (thoracic) breathing *p. 716*

diaphragmatic (abdominal) breathing *p. 716*
diastolic pressure *p. 721*
dysrhythmia *p. 711*
elasticity of the arterial wall *p. 711*
eupnea *p. 717*
evaporation *p. 699*
exhalation *p. 716*
expiration *p. 716*
external respiration *p. 716*
febrile *p. 700*
fever *p. 700*
fever spike *p. 700*
heat balance *p. 698*
heat exhaustion *p. 700*
heat stroke *p. 700*
hematocrit *p. 722*
hyperpyrexia *p. 700*
hypertension *p. 722*
hyperthermia *p. 700*
hyperventilation *p. 717*
hypotension *p. 723*

hypothalamic integrator *p. 699*
hypothermia *p. 701*
hypoventilation *p. 717*
inhalation *p. 716*
insensible heat loss *p. 699*
insensible water loss *p. 699*
inspiration *p. 716*
intermittent fever *p. 700*
internal respiration *p. 716*
Korotkoff sounds *p. 725*
malignant hyperthermia *p. 700*
orthostatic hypotension *p. 723*
peripheral pulse *p. 708*
point of maximal impulse (PMI) *p. 708*
pulse *p. 708*
pulse deficit *p. 715*

pulse oximeter *p. 730*
pulse pressure *p. 721*
pulse rhythm *p. 711*
pulse volume *p. 711*
pyrexia *p. 700*
radiation *p. 698*
relapsing fever *p. 700*
remittent fever *p. 700*
respiration *p. 716*
respiratory quality or character *p. 718*
respiratory rhythm or pattern *p. 718*
surface temperature *p. 697*
systematic vascular resistance (SVR) *p. 721*
systolic pressure *p. 721*
tachycardia *p. 711*
tachypnea *p. 717*
tidal volume *p. 718*
ventilation *p. 716*
vital signs *p. 697*

CHAPTER HIGHLIGHTS

- Vital signs reflect changes in body function that otherwise might not be observed.
- Body temperature is the balance between heat produced by the body and heat lost from the body.
- Factors affecting body temperature include age, diurnal variations, exercise, hormones, stress, and environmental temperatures.
- Four common types of fever are intermittent, remittent, relapsing, and constant.
- During a fever, the set point of the hypothalamic thermostat changes suddenly from the normal level to a higher-than-normal level, but several hours elapse before the core temperature reaches the new set point.
- Hypothermia involves three mechanisms: excessive heat loss, inadequate heat production by body cells, and increasing impairment of hypothalamic thermoregulation.
- The nurse selects the most appropriate site to measure temperature, according to the client's age and condition.
- Pulse rate and volume reflect the stroke volume output, the compliance of the client's arteries, and the adequacy of blood flow.
- Normally, the peripheral pulse reflects the client's heartbeat, but it may differ from the heartbeat in clients with certain cardiovascular diseases; in these instances, the nurse takes an apical pulse reading and compares it with the peripheral pulse.

- Many factors may affect a person's pulse rate: age, sex, exercise, presence of fever, certain medications, hypovolemia, stress, position changes (in some situations), and pathology.
- Although the radial pulse is the site most commonly used, eight other sites can be used in certain situations.
- The difference between apical and radial pulses is called *pulse deficit.*
- Respirations are normally quiet, effortless, and automatic and are assessed by observing respiratory rate, depth, rhythm, quality, and effectiveness.
- Blood pressure reflects cardiac output and peripheral vascular resistance.
- Among the factors influencing blood pressure are age, exercise, stress, race, sex, medications, obesity, diurnal variations, and disease processes.
- Orthostatic hypotension occurs when blood pressure falls as the client assumes an upright position.
- A blood pressure cuff too large or too small will give false readings.
- During blood pressure measurement, the artery must be held at heart level.
- Pulse oximetry is a noninvasive means of measuring the percentage of hemoglobin saturated with oxygen. A normal SpO_2 result is 95% to 100%.
- Pulse oximeter sensors can be placed on the finger, hand, foot, or nose.

ASSESS YOUR LEARNING

1. The client's temperature at 0800 hours taken by using an oral electronic thermometer is 36.1°C. All other vital signs are within normal range. What would the nurse do next?

   a. Wait 15 minutes and retake it.

   b. Check what the client's temperature was the last time.

   c. Retake it by using a different thermometer.

   d. Chart the temperature, as it is normal.

2. For which of the following clients would the nurse take an apical pulse rather than a radial pulse?

   a. A client in shock

   b. To establish baseline data on a client

   c. A client with a dysrhythmia

   d. A client less than 24 hours after surgery

3. For a client with a previous blood pressure of 138/74 mm Hg and pulse of 64, approximately how long should the nurse take to release the blood pressure cuff in order to obtain an accurate reading?

   a. 20 seconds

   b. 45 seconds

   c. 60 seconds

   d. 120 seconds

4. An 85-year-old client has had a cerebrovascular accident (stroke) resulting in right-sided facial drooping and difficulty swallowing. The client is unable to move or maintain a position unaided. Which of the following would be an appropriate site(s) for taking the temperature?

   a. Oral

   b. Rectal

   c. Axillary, oral, or temporal artery

   d. Axillary, tympanic, or temporal artery

5. A client with ineffective peripheral tissue perfusion would be expected to have which of the following findings?

   a. Bounding radial pulse

   b. Irregular apical pulse

   c. Radial pulse that is obliterated by strong pressure

   d. Absent posterior tibial and pedal pulses

6. The proper assessment of the respiratory rate should include which of the following?

   a. Measurement of oxygen saturation by using pulse oximetry

   b. Asking the client to take five deep breaths before starting the measurement

   c. Counting the respiration for 15 seconds and multiplying by 4

   d. Counting the respirations for a full minute if they are irregular

7. A client states, "I feel so breathless all the time." The nurse documents that the client is experiencing which of the following?

   a. Hypoventilation

   b. Laboured breathing

   c. Dyspnea

   d. Orthopnea

8. When auscultating a blood pressure on an older man, on two separate visits, the nurse records the blood pressure as 166/102 mm Hg on visit one and 164/98 mm Hg on visit two. The nurse knows that this means which of the following?

   a. Grade 1 hypertension

   b. Grade 2 hypertension

   c. Grade 3 hypertension

   d. High normal

9. The nurse who is providing wellness teaching to a 72-year-old client with newly diagnosed hypertension would recommend which of the following?

   a. The client should go from a lying to a standing position gradually.

   b. The client should aim to reduce sodium intake to 1200 mg per day.

   c. The client should avoid all stressful situations.

   d. The client should aim to participate in moderate to vigorous intensity aerobic physical activity at least one hour a week.

10. The nurse obtains an oxygen saturation value (SpO_2) of 70% by pulse oximeter in a client who is alert and oriented and who has come to an ambulatory clinic because of feeling short of breath. The client's respiratory rate is 16 per minute; her heart rate is 74 beats per minute, regular and +2/4 amplitude. What is the first thing the nurse should do in this situation?

    a. Seek help

    b. Administer oxygen therapy

    c. Auscultate the lungs

    d. Retake the oxygen saturation

Check the eText in MyNursingLab for answers and explanations.

WEBLINKS

Hypertension Canada / Canadian Hypertension Education Program

http://www.hypertension.ca

This site provides the general population and health care professionals with up-to-date information on blood pressure assessment, management, and the effects of uncontrolled blood pressure.

Canadian Heart and Stroke Foundation

http://www.heartandstroke.ca

The website of the Heart and Stroke Foundation of Canada is a reliable source of information on heart disease and stroke. The Foundation's mission is to improve the health of Canadians by preventing and reducing disability and death from heart disease and stroke through research, health promotion, and advocacy.

Canadian Council of Cardiovascular Nurses

http://www.cccn.ca

The Canadian Council of Cardiovascular Nurses maintains this site for its members and others interested in the specialty. Their mission is to advance the profession and the cardiovascular health of Canadians through education, standards, research, and health promotion. Information includes future conferences, news, journals, standards, national and provincial and territorial committee links, and employment opportunities.

MyNursingLab

REFERENCES

Ball, J. W., & Bindler, R. C. (2008). *Pediatric nursing: Caring for children* (4th ed.). Upper Saddle River, NJ: Prentice Hall Health.

Booker, R. (2008). Pulse oximetry. *Nursing Standard, 22*(30), 39–41.

Braine, M. E. (2009). The role of the hypothalamus, part 1: The regulation of temperature and hunger. *British Journal of Neuroscience Nursing, 5*(2), 66–72.

Canadian Hypertension Education Program. (2012). *2012 CHEP recommendations for the management of hypertension.* Ottawa: Author. Retrieved from http://www.hypertension.ca/chep-recommendations

Canadian Paediatric Society. (2010). Temperature measurement in paediatrics. Position Statement: Canadian Pediatric Society. Retrieved from http://www.cps.ca/english/statements/CP/cp00-01.htm

Casa, D. J., Becker, S. M., Ganio, M. S., Brown, C. M., Yeargin, S. W., Roti, M. W., Siegler, J., . . . Maresh, C. M. (2007). Validity of devices that assess body temperature during outdoor exercise in the heat. *Journal of Athletic Training, 42*(3), 333–342.

DeMeulenaere, S. (2007). Pulse oximetry: Uses and limitations. *The Journal for Nurse Practitioners, 3*(5), 312–317.

Drouin, D., & Milot, A. (Eds.). (2007). *Hypertension therapeutic guide* (3rd ed.). Montreal, PQ: The Quebec Hypertension Society.

El-Radhi, A. S., & Barry, W. (2006). Thermometry in paediatric practice. *Archives of Disease in Childhood, 91*(4), 351–356.

Estes, M. E., & Buck, M. (2008). *Health assessment and physical examination.* Toronto, ON: Nelson.

Frommelt, T., Ott, C., & Hays, V. (2008). Accuracy of different devices to measure temperature. *MEDSURG Nursing, 17*(3), 171–182.

Glahn, K. P., Ellis, F. R., Halsall, P. J., Müller, C. R., Snoeck, M. M., Urwyler, A., & Wappler, F. (2010). Recognizing and managing a malignant hyperthermia crisis: Guidelines from the European Malignant Hyperthermia Group. *The British Journal of Anaesthesia, 105*(4), 417–420.

Guly, H. (2011). History of accidental hypothermia. *Resuscitation, 82,* 122–125.

Health Canada. (2001). Pediatric clinical practice guidelines for nurses in primary care. First Nations Inuit Health Branch.

Henker, R., & Carlson, K. K. (2007). Fever: Applying research to bedside practice. *AACN Advanced Critical Care, 18*(1), 76–87.

Heusch, A. I., & McCarthy, P. W. (2005). The patient: A novel source of error in clinical tempterature measurement using infrared aural thermometry. *The Journal of Alternative and Complementary Medicine, 11*(3), 473–476.

Hinkelbein, J., Koehler, H., Genzwuerker, H. V., & Fiedler, F. (2007). Artificial acrylic finger nails may alter pulse oximetry measurement. *Resuscitation, 74,* 75–82.

Hooper, V. D., & Andrews, J. O. (2006). Accuracy of noninvasive core temperature measurement in acutely ill adults: The state of the science. *Biological Research for Nursing, 8*(1), 24-34.

Kaplan, N., Mendis, S., Poulter, N., Whiteworth, J. (2003). 2003 World Health Organization (WHO)/ International Society of Hypertension (ISH) statement on management of hypertension. *Journal of Hypertension, 21*(11), 1983–1992.

Kemp, P. (2008). Hypothermia: Causes and management. *British Journal of Healthcare Assistants, 2*(12), 586–588.

Khorshid, L., Eşer, ï., Zaybak, A., & Yapucu, Û. (2005). Comparing mercury-in-glass, tympanic and disposable thermometers in measuring body temperature in healthy young people. *Journal of Clinical Nursing, 14*(4), 496–500.

Latman, N. S. (2003). Clinical thermometry: Possible causes and potential solutions to electronic, digital thermometer inaccuracies. *Biomedical Instrumentation and Technology, 37*(3), 190–196.

Lawson, L., Bridges, E. J., Ballou, I., Eraker, R., Greco, S., Shively, J., & Sochulak, V. (2007). Accuracy and precision of noninvasive temperature measurement in adult intensive care patients. *American Journal of Critical Care, 16*(5), 485–496.

Lockwood, C., Conroy-Hiller, T., & Page, T. (2004). Vital signs. *JBI Reports, 2,* 207–230.

Mackechnie, C., & Simpson, R. (2006). Traceable calibration of blood pressure and temperature monitoring. *Nursing Standard, 21*(11), 42–47.

Nelson, D., Kennedy, B., Regnerus, C., & Schweinle, A. (2008). Accuracy of automated blood pressure monitors. *Journal of Dental Hygiene, 82*(4), 35.

Sessler, D. I. (2008). Temperature monitoring and perioperative thermoregulation. *Anesthesiology, 109*(2), 318–338.

Chapter 30

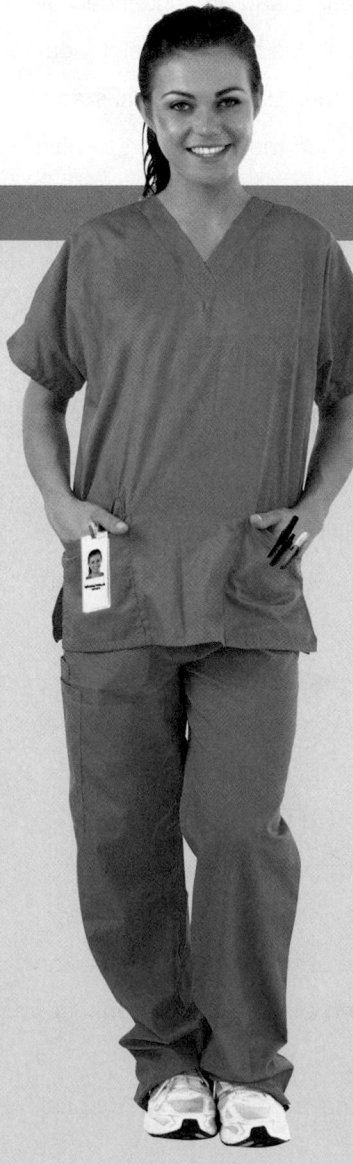

Pain Assessment and Management

A ccording to the principles of beneficence and nonmaleficence, nurses, as health care professionals, must provide comfort and pain relief for all clients, regardless of status, heritage, and type of health problem. In support of this, the International Association for the Study of Pain (IASP) issued a statement that pain relief is a fundamental human right (IASP, 2011). Being the first-line advocate for humane and quality care of their clients (Canadian Nurses Association [CNA], 2008), it is an essential responsibility of the nurse to ensure that their clients have the best pain relief possible.

Canada has a rich history in the interprofessional study and treatment of pain. Seminal work by Melzack and Wall (1965), in addition to their strong humanitarian commitment to caring for clients suffering from pain, paved the way for other exceptional Canadian researchers to understand pain mechanisms and their implications for effective pain management. **Pain** is known as an unpleasant, multidimensional, and subjective experience, and only the person experiencing pain can describe it (if he or she is able to communicate by verbal or other means). No two people experience pain the same way; the experience of pain and its related responses are unique to each client and are influenced by the person's context and past pain experiences. While the person's self-report is the most valid measure of pain, some people may be unable to communicate, depending on their developmental stage, the presence of a degenerative disease or temporary clinical conditions. When the self-report of pain cannot be obtained, the nurse should rely on other indicators to detect the presence of pain, including the use of valid behavioural pain scales developed for specific populations and in a given context (Herr, Coyne, Manworren, McCaffery, Merkel, Pelosi-Kelly, & Wild, 2006). Therefore, effective pain management requires skillful communication and assessment on the part of the nurse.

Although great advancements in pain research have been made over the past 5 decades, unrelieved acute pain remains a ubiquitous problem with numerous physiological, psychological, and economic consequences (Dahl, Gordon, Ward, Skemp, Wochos, & Schurr, 2003; McGillion, Watt-Watson, LeFort, & Stevens, 2007). Significant numbers of hospitalized clients unnecessarily experience moderate to severe pain after surgery or interventional procedures, which can delay recovery and discharge from hospital (Morrison et al., 2003). One of the main consequences of undetected and unrelieved acute pain is the development of chronic pain, which often leads to the impairment of cognitive functioning, emotional distress, fatigue, and depression (Dunwoody, Krenzischek, Pasero, Rathmell, & Polomano, 2008). Major contributors to unrelieved pain are knowledge gaps and pain-related misbeliefs among health care professionals, clients, and families.

Despite advancements in the understanding of pain and its consequences among scientists, health care professional groups, and client advocacy organizations in Canada, pain management practices generally need improvement. Historically, many health care professionals have not asked clients about their pain, and major discrepancies have been noted between clients' pain experiences and health care professionals' pain assessments (McGillion, Watt-Watson, Kim, & Graham, 2004). The problem has been compounded by the fact that many clients expect to have pain while in hospital, do not admit to having pain, and are reluctant to ask for help. Recent efforts in client care improvement, such as the *Best Practice Guidelines* launched by the Registered Nurses' Association of Ontario (RNAO) in 2004, paved the way for many improvements in pain detection and pain control for the clients inside and outside of the hospital (RNAO, 2007). In addition to these Canadian guidelines, a position statement from the American Society of Pain Management Nursing (ASPMN) was published (Herr et al., 2006) to provide nurses with clinical recommendations for the assessment of pain in nonverbal client populations.

A major priority for nurses is the development of in-depth knowledge about pain mechanisms, assessment, and pharmacological and nonpharmacological management strategies. The Canadian Pain Society (CPS) emphasizes that clients have a right to the best pain relief possible (Watt-Watson, Clark, Finley, & Watson, 1999) and that nurses should be familiar with the following principles:

1. Unrelieved acute pain complicates recovery.
2. Routine assessment that includes clients' self-reports and the use of behavioural pain scales for nonverbal clients is essential for effective pain management.
3. The best pain management strategies involve clients, families, and health care professionals, with the clients and families being encouraged to communicate the presence of pain and health care professionals are knowledgeable about pain relief options.

The Nature of Pain

Pain has been defined as "an unpleasant sensory and emotional experience associated with actual or potential tissue damage" (IASP, 1979). In accordance with this definition, Pasero and McCaffery (2010) highlighted that pain is "whatever the experiencing person says it is, existing whenever he (or she) says it does." On the basis of this, the person's self-report of pain represents the most valid measure or "gold standard" for the presence of pain and it should be obtained, whenever possible. The latter definition helped to change practice by emphasizing that health care professionals must believe clients with respect to their report and must pay particular attention to the client's subjective experience of pain.

A major limitation of the original definition of pain by the IASP (1979) is that it denies the presence of pain in clients unable to self-report, such as infants and pre-verbal children, older adults with cognitive deficits, and clients with altered levels of consciousness. To overcome this limitation, experts have proposed an alternative definition of pain stating that behavioural changes caused by pain are valuable forms of self-report and should be considered as alternative indicators of the presence of pain (Anand & Craig, 1996). A recent report by the IASP (2011) has put forth a statement that "the inability to communicate verbally does not negate the possibility that an individual is experiencing pain and is in need of

appropriate pain-relieving treatment." Therefore, pain assessment must be designed to conform to the communication capabilities of the client. When the person is not able to self-report, the nurse should select and use behavioural pain scales that have been shown to be valid for their client population.

The experience of pain is complex and multidimensional, with sensory–discriminative, motivational–affective, and cognitive–evaluative components (Melzack & Casey, 1966). The traditional nineteenth-century definition describes pain as an unpleasant feeling that is the opposite of enjoyment. This highlights that pain is a sensory experience, yet pain is different from other senses because it is inseparable from its *affective* and *cognitive* properties. The sensory component of pain is supported by the nerve pathways dedicated to delivering the pain signal to the brain and to determining its quality, magnitude, and location. Once the brain perceives the pain signal, other cortical structures detect the unpleasant effect of pain and determine whether it is a trigger for action, such as withdrawal, avoidance or aggression. This motivational–affective component of pain is directed by the limbic system and the reticular formation in the brain stem (Melzack & Casey, 1966). By activating these structures, pain can disrupt everyday tasks, demand attention, and can become overwhelming. The central control exerted by the cortex provides the cognitive–evaluative component of pain, which refers to the significance or meaning of the pain experience. The cultural background, personal beliefs, anxiety, attention, and anticipation of pain can all modify its multidimensional properties. Structures in the frontal cortex are thought to be implicated in mediating between the cognitive and affective features of pain.

When treating a client with pain, the nurse must understand that pain is defined in terms of its sensory, affective, and cognitive determinants and that it cannot be ascribed to only one of them. The therapeutic implications of this definition of pain is choosing a pain management plan that treats pain as not only a sensory but a cognitive and affective experience; this means providing the client with holistic care that includes analgesia as well as nonpharmacological interventions, such as relaxation or anxiety management.

Origin of Pain

Pain can be classified by its inferred origin into two major types: (a) nociceptive pain and (b) neuropathic pain. Common pain syndromes of both types are briefly described in the Clinical Manifestations box. See also the Evidence-Informed Practice box about administering analgesia to people with pain and whether that interferes with the diagnosis of pain.

NOCICEPTIVE PAIN **Nociceptive pain** is the result of the normal physiological processing of harmful or potentially harmful noxious stimuli that are perceived as being painful (Pasero & McCaffery, 2010). This type of pain is a result of the stimulation of **nociceptors** (nerves that transmit noxious stimuli) that is often the case with tissue damage due to trauma or inflammation (Pasero, 2004). Further, nociceptive pain can be categorized according to its origin as somatic or visceral. **Somatic pain** originates in the skin, muscles, bone, or connective tissue. The sharp sensation of a paper cut or aching and throbbing of a sprained ankle are examples of somatic pain. **Visceral pain** results from the stimulation of pain receptors in the organs. Visceral pain tends to be diffuse and often feels like deep somatic pain, that is, burning, aching, or a feeling of pressure. Visceral pain is frequently caused by stretching of the tissues, ischemia, or muscle spasms. For example, an obstructed bowel or blocked coronary artery will result in visceral pain (Pasero & McCaffery, 2010).

NEUROPATHIC PAIN **Neuropathic pain** is the result of injury to the nerves or an abnormal processing of stimuli by the nervous system (Adler, Nico, VandeVord, & Skoff, 2009). The nerves may be abnormal because of illness (e.g., postherpetic neuralgia, diabetic peripheral neuropathy), injury (e.g., phantom limb pain, spinal cord injury pain), or undetermined reasons. Neuropathic pain that arises after surgery or another invasive procedure that resulted in nerve damage is called *iatrogenic*. Neuropathic pain is chronic in nature; it is characterized by ongoing pain with the sensation of burning, prickling, and often a concomitant sensory discrimination deficit

---

CLINICAL MANIFESTATIONS OF COMMON PAIN SYNDROMES

The following are some common pain syndromes:

* *Postherpetic neuralgia.* An episode of herpes zoster (shingles) has two phases: (a) a vesicular eruption and (b) neurological pain that often encircles the body. The pain ranges from mild to severe. In postherpetic syndrome, severe pain persists for months or years with burning or electric-shock pain in the area of the original eruption. The main risk factors for the development of postherpetic neuralgia in individuals with herpes zoster are old age, the acuity of the initial pain, and the severity of the rash at the onset of shingles (Dworkin et al., 2008).

* *Phantom pain.* Phantom sensation, the feeling that a lost body part is present, occurs in most people after amputation. For many, this sensation is painful; it may occur spontaneously or be evoked (e.g., by using a poorly fitting prosthesis). When the amputation involves a limb, it is termed *phantom limb pain,* whereas following breast removal, it is called *postmastectomy pain*. Phantom pain varies and may be burning, severe, crushing, or a cramping sensation. This pain is neuropathic in nature and its etiology is complex because of the loss of sensory input into the central nervous system (CNS) from the amputated region (Melzack Katz, & Vaccarino, 2001; Saarto & Wiffen, 2010; Wolff et al., 2011).

* *Trigeminal neuralgia.* Trigeminal neuralgia is episodic; it is an intense stabbing pain that is transmitted by one or more branches of the trigeminal (fifth cranial) nerve. The pain is usually experienced in small parts of the face and head, for example, gums, cheek, and surface of the head. The attacks of pain are often precipitated by sensory stimulation of the areas innervated by the trigeminal nerve, called "trigger zones" (Love & Coakham, 2001).

* *Headaches and migraines.* Headache is a common somatic pain that can be caused by either intracranial or extracranial problems. Although often similar to a regular headache, migraines are thought to be a neurovascular disorder characterized by severe throbbing headaches that are normally (but not always) unilateral. Attacks of migraines may be accompanied by nausea, vomiting, and photophobia (Schurks, Rist, Bigal, Buring, Lipton, & Kurth, 2009). Up to 20% of clients also present with an aura that is associated with the presence of neurological manifestations (Russell & Olesen, 1996). In addition to appropriate medication (e.g. administration of nonspecific treatments, such as Aspirin and acetaminophen, or migraine-specific drugs, such as ergotamine), both headaches and migraines can be treated by nonpharmacological approaches (e.g., avoidance of the triggers, education, and proper diet) (Goadsby, Lipton, & Ferrari, 2002).

* *Fibromyalgia.* Fibromyalgia is a chronic disorder that is characterized by widespread musculoskeletal pain, fatigue, and multiple tender points. A *tender point* is tenderness that occurs in a precise, localized area, particularly in the neck, spine, shoulders, and hips. People with this syndrome can also experience sleep disturbances, morning stiffness, irritable bowel syndrome, anxiety, and other symptoms. Although the symptoms present as muscle pain, stiffness, and weakness, it is considered by many to be a problem of abnormal CNS functioning, particularly as it relates to the way nerves process pain (Mease, 2005).

EVIDENCE-INFORMED PRACTICE

Does Administering Analgesia to People with Acute Pain Interfere with the Diagnosis of the Pain?

Although some clinicians think that administering analgesia to people with acute pain, such as acute abdominal pain (AAP), might "mask" the pain and interfere with diagnosis, others think that it is unethical to leave a person in acute pain and that giving analgesia might actually help in making a diagnosis, especially if a physical examination can be performed with increased ease. To establish any conclusion on this matter, Manterola et al. (2011) conducted a systematic review of all published randomized control trials (RCTs) that compared the outcomes of opioid treatment versus no treatment of adults with AAP. The review concluded that "in addition to improving their comfort while the diagnostic process is concluded, (the use of opioids) does not increase the risk of diagnosis error or the risk of error in decisions for treatment."

NURSING IMPLICATIONS: Acute abdominal pain is a relatively common clinical situation. While the pain itself can be distressing to the client, not knowing the reason for the pain can be equally distressing. Nurses who work in clinical settings where analgesia is viewed as "masking" symptoms and interfering with diagnosis can be placed in a challenging situation as they try to help their clients deal with both the untreated pain and uncertainty about diagnosis. Using the knowledge derived from this meta-analysis will mean greater comfort for our clients with the assurance that having the pain managed will not interfere with diagnostic accuracy—a win-win situation for both nurses and their clients.

Source: Based on Manterola, C., Vial, M., Moraga, J., & Astudillo, P. (2011). Analgesia in patients with acute abdominal pain. *Cochrane Database of Systematic Reviews*, Issue 1. Art. No.: CD005660. DOI: 10.1002/14651858.CD005660.pub3

BOX 30.1   CONCEPTS ASSOCIATED WITH PAIN

The following are terms used in the study of pain and pain management:

- *Acute pain:* Pain that is directly related to tissue injury and resolves when tissue heals; it should not last for more than 6 months
- *Chronic pain:* Pain that persists beyond 6 months secondary to chronic disorders or nerve malfunctions that produce ongoing pain after healing is complete
- *Cancer pain:* Pain associated with the disease, treatment, or some other factor in individuals with cancer
- *Nociceptive pain:* Pain that is directly related to tissue damage and nociception; may be somatic (e.g., damage to skin, muscle, bone) or visceral (e.g., damage to organs)
- *Neuropathic pain:* Pain that is related to damaged or malfunctioning nervous tissue in the peripheral nervous system (PNS) or the CNS
- *Pain threshold:* The lowest intensity of noxious stimulation that reliably invokes pain
- *Pain tolerance:* The most pain an individual is willing or able to endure before taking evasive actions
- *Phantom pain:* Painful sensations felt from a part of the body that has been amputated; can arise from the residual limb (e.g., stump pain) or nerves that lost communication with the missing part

   The following states indicate abnormal nerve functioning, and the associated cause needs to be identified or treated (as possible) before irreversible damage occurs:

- *Allodynia:* Sensation of pain from a stimulus that normally does not produce pain (e.g., light touch)
- *Dysesthesia:* An unpleasant, abnormal sensation that can be either spontaneous or evoked
- *Hyperalgesia:* Increased sensation of pain in response to a normally painful stimulus

---

in the affected area. The most common presentations of this condition are **hyperalgesia** and **allodynia** (Box 30.1) (Campbell & Meyer, 2006). It is thought that the phenomenon of neuroplasticity is a contributing factor to some of the abnormal changes that take place in many types of neuropathic pain (Pasero & McCaffery, 2010). **Neuroplasticity** is the ability of the brain to reorganize its signalling and the processing of stimuli in accordance with the input from the environment. These changes take place on a cellular level, but they have the ability to rearrange the functionality of larger CNS regions (Coderre, Katz, Vaccarino, & Melzack, 1993). Peripheral painful stimuli may sensitize neural structures involved in pain perception. For example, a prolonged noxious stimulus can result in changes to the sensitivity of the dorsal horn neurons that can be maintained even after the stimulus is removed (Melzack, Coderre, Katz, & Vaccarino, 2001). Smaller noxious stimuli to the same area may result in a higher amount of pain as well as a further increase in dorsal horn neuron sensitivity

(**hyperexcitability**), thus initiating a vicious cycle of maintained pain. Continued noxious stimulation can also increase the receptive field of dorsal horn neurons. If not eliminated, it may produce prolonged excitability that is maintained without further stimulation (Coderre et al., 1993; Melzack et al., 2001). Neuropathic pain conditions tend to be difficult to treat. Unfortunately, evidence suggests that in some instances, neuropathic pain results from a failure to effectively treat acute pain episodes, such as that during the perioperative period (Manias, Bucknall, & Botti, 2005).

Neuropathic pain can be classified into two subcategories based on the assumed mechanism that is responsible for the pain: (a) peripheral neuropathic pain and (b) central neuropathic pain.

Peripheral neuropathic pain (e.g., phantom limb pain, postherpetic neuralgia, carpal tunnel syndrome) follows damage, sensitization, or abnormal changes of peripheral nerve fibres (Pasero & McCaffery, 2010). Peripheral neuropathic pain is typically chronic; it is described as burning, an electric shock, or tingling, dull, and aching; episodes of sharp, shooting pain can also be experienced (Adler et al., 2009; Herr, 2002)

Central neuropathic pain (e.g., spinal cord injury pain, poststroke pain, multiple sclerosis pain) results from malfunctioning nerves in the CNS (brain and spinal cord). The neurons in the CNS may exhibit abnormal hyperexcitability as a result of complex changes induced by the ongoing firing of afferent nociceptors. These changes can occur anywhere in the CNS. One of the well-characterized central neuropathic pain mechanisms is the increased release and binding of the excitatory neurotransmitters in the milieu of the central neurons that are responsible for pain processing. Another mechanism, termed **central disinhibition,** causes hyperexcitability of the central pain neurons because of the loss of control mechanisms that usually inhibit the conduction of a pain signal (Pasero & McCaffery, 2010).

Complex regional pain syndrome (CRPS) is a term used for a number of pain conditions whose etiology is poorly understood (Dunwoody et al., 2008; Harden, Bruehl, Stanton-Hicks, & Wilson, 2007). The causative mechanisms of this group of pain conditions may include both PNS and CNS abnormalities. To be diagnosed with this condition, clients must have continuous moderate to severe pain along with edema and vasomotor, motor, or sensory changes in the affected area. In addition, all other diagnoses that explain the symptoms must be excluded (Harden et al., 2007). Pain in clients suffering from CRPS proves a difficult target to treat completely, and it usually requires multimodal pharmacological and holistic approaches (Gibbs, Drummond, Finch, & Phillips, 2008).

Duration of Pain

When pain lasts only through the expected recovery period (usually 30 days), it is described as **acute pain**. Acute pain is purposeful, informing the person that something is wrong. Typically, the onset of acute pain is sudden because of a noxious stimulus, such as trauma, and the location of the pain can usually be easily identified. This type of pain should not exceed 6 months, and if not adequately treated can become chronic (Joshi & Ogunnaike, 2005; Kehlet, Jensen, & Woolf, 2006).

Chronic pain lasts beyond 6 months (Bonica, 1990; Merskey & Bogduk, 1994) and has no purpose. Chronic pain can be further classified as chronic cancer pain or noncancer pain. Because its onset can be subtle, it may be difficult for the client to determine when the chronic pain started. It can also often be difficult to pinpoint the

TABLE 30.1 Differences between Acute and Chronic Pain

Acute Pain	Chronic Pain
Usually sudden onset	Onset may be sudden or gradual
Duration usually transient (never more than six months)	Duration prolonged (months to years)
Mild to severe	Mild to severe
Sympathetic nervous system responses: • Increased pulse rate • Increased respiratory rate • Elevated blood pressure • Diaphoresis • Dilated pupils • Purposeful warning or related to tissue injury; resolves with healing • Client commonly exhibits behaviour indicative of pain: crying, rubbing area, holding area • Client may appear restless and anxious	Parasympathetic nervous system responses: • Vital signs normal (because of adaptation) • Dry, warm skin • Pupils normal or dilated • No purpose; continues beyond healing • Client may appear depressed and withdrawn • Behaviour indicative of obvious pain often absent

location of chronic pain, as it is typically more diffuse compared with acute pain. Chronic pain is complex and can become all-consuming, causing irritability, insomnia, and withdrawal from family, friends, and interests (Watt-Watson, Evans, & Watson, 1988).

Table 30.1 outlines some common differences between acute and chronic pain.

See the Reflect on Primary Health Care box on intersectoral collaborations in the assessment, treatment, and follow-up of a person with pain.

REFLECT ON PRIMARY HEALTH CARE

Intersectoral collaboration is essential in the assessment, treatment, and follow-up of a person experiencing pain. Find out whether any pain clinics or networks are available in your region. In pain clinics, professionals, such as physicians, nurses, social workers, physiotherapists, psychologists, pharmacologists, and chaplains, work together to treat the client dealing with chronic pain.

Concepts Associated with Pain

Two additional terms used in the context of pain are *pain threshold* and *pain tolerance*. **Pain threshold** is the minimum level of noxious stimulation that reliably evokes pain (Cleeland, Serlin, Nakamura, & Mendoza, 1997). A person's pain threshold is generally fairly uniform, relative to the location of the pain and the kind of noxious stimulus experienced. The pain thresholds of two different individuals may be markedly different (Mader, Blank, Smithline, & Wolfe, 2003). Therefore, the same stimulus can cause various levels of pain in different individuals. The understanding of the pain threshold variability should remind a nurse to always elicit a client's report of his or her pain level to detect pain and provide adequate analgesia (Pasero & McCaffery, 2010). **Pain tolerance** is the maximum amount of painful stimuli that a person is willing or able to endure without seeking avoidance of the pain or relief. Pain tolerance can vary widely within individuals and cultures, as it relates to the cognitive–affective and subjective experience of each individual. For example, a woman may withstand severe pain for a prolonged period during childbirth to make the experience more natural or drug-free; however, she may want pain relief for a regular headache.

See Box 30.1 for a summary of concepts associated with pain. Some of these terms will be expanded on later in the chapter. See the Clinical Alert box about major contributors to unrelieved pain.

CLINICAL ALERT

Unrelieved acute pain should not be tolerated; it has numerous physiological, psychological, and economic consequences. Major contributors to unrelieved pain are client, health care professional, and societal knowledge gaps and misbeliefs about pain.

Physiology of Pain: Nociception

Nociception represents the neural and cortical activity that is necessary, but not sufficient, for pain. Pain is the conscious experience that emerges from nociception (Charlton, 2005). Four processes are involved in nociception: (a) transduction, (b) transmission, (c) perception, and (d) modulation (Pasero & McCaffery, 2010). The process of pain transduction and transmission involves three types of neurons: (a) the afferent or sensory neurons, (b) the efferent or motor neurons, and (c) the interneurons or connector neurons.

Transduction

The peripheral nervous system includes primary afferent sensory neurons specialized to detect noxious, or injurious, stimuli, which can be thermal, chemical, or mechanical in nature (see Table 30.2). The nerve fibres that transmit noxious information are called primary afferent nociceptors. Nociceptors are located throughout skin and mucosa and less frequently in deep structures, such as joints, arteries, and viscera; their terminals possess a broad array of very selective molecular receptors. When a sufficiently noxious stimulus is in the peripheral microenvironment (e.g., injury to cells or tissue), the nociceptors can be activated by the direct stimulus (e.g., heat,

TABLE 30.2 Types of Noxious Stimuli

Stimulus Type	Physiological Causes of Pain
Mechanical	
1. Trauma to body tissues (e.g., surgery)	Tissue damage; direct irritation of the pain receptors; inflammation
2. Alterations in body tissues (e.g., edema)	Pressure on pain receptors
3. Blockage of a body duct	Distension of the lumen of the duct
4. Tumour growth	Pressure on pain receptors; irritation of nerve endings
5. Muscle spasm	Stimulation of pain receptors (also see chemical stimuli)
Thermal	
Extreme heat or cold (e.g., burns, frostbite)	Tissue destruction; stimulation of thermosensitive pain receptors
Chemical	
1. Tissue ischemia (e.g., blocked coronary artery)	Stimulation of pain receptors because of accumulated lactic acid (and other chemicals, such as bradykinin and enzymes) in tissues
2. Muscle spasm	
3. Toxins	Tissue ischemia secondary to mechanical stimulation (see above)

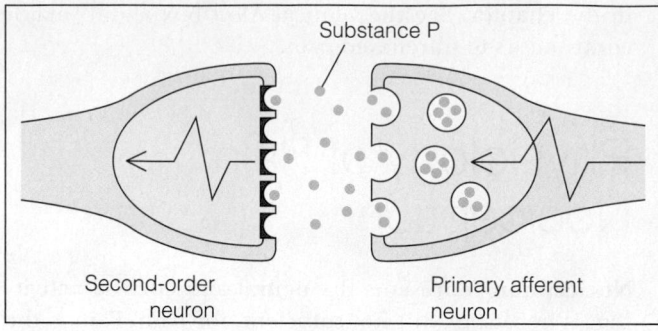

FIGURE 30.1 Substance P assists the transmission of impulses across the synapse from the primary afferent neuron to a second-order neuron.

cold, or pressure) or by the biochemical mediators released from the milieu (local tissues, immune cells, and nerve endings) via their receptors (Caterina, Gold, & Meyer, 2005). The mediators that activate and further sensitize the nociceptors include serotonin, histamine, potassium, bradykinin, prostaglandins, and substance P (Marchand, 2008) (Figure 30.1). **Transduction** occurs when the excited nociceptor converts the surrounding noxious stimuli into an action potential (i.e., electrochemical impulse) that is then transmitted to the spinal cord to ultimately reach the CNS.

Transmission

Transmission occurs when information about a noxious stimulus is conducted through the spinal cord to the brain via two types of peripheral afferent nociceptive fibres: (a) A-delta fibres and (b) C fibres. A-delta fibres have a relatively large diameter, are myelinated, and rapidly conduct the impulse. These fibres are associated with the sensation of sharp, pricking pain. The other set of nociceptive fibres is the small-diameter, unmyelinated C fibres. C fibres transmit the impulse more slowly and mediate long-lasting, burning pain.

The terminals of afferent nociceptors enter the dorsal horn of the spinal cord through the dorsal root and synapse onto second-order neurons in substantia gelatinosa (Figure 30.2). Impulse transmission from the sensory (afferent) nerve fibres to the second-order neurons in the dorsal horn happens via the release of neurotransmitters, acetylcholine, norepinephrine, epinephrine, serotonin, and dopamine. The fast A-delta fibres primarily conduct impulses from mechanical and thermal pain. They synapse with second-order neurons (long fibres) in the dorsal horn that cross immediately to the opposite side of the spinal cord. They later enter the lateral spinothalamic tract and ascend to the brain, where the information about the pain stimulus is perceived

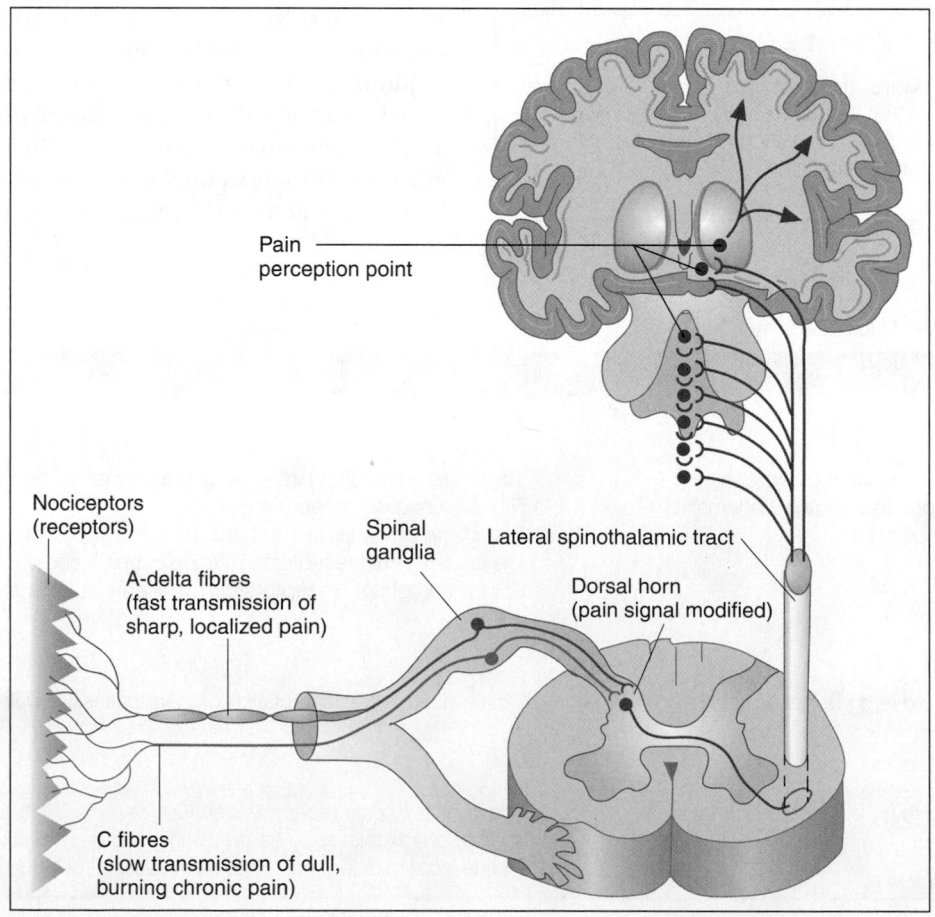

FIGURE 30.2 Nociception mechanisms.

and processed. A few fibres terminate in the reticular areas of the brain stem, but most nerve fibres of the spinothalamic tract terminate in the thalamus. From there, signals are sent to the basal areas of the brain and to the somatic sensory cortex. A-delta fibres allow for the detection of "first pain"—this is a mechanism of quick detection and localization of pain that would allow for a fast protective response, such as a withdrawal reflex (Dahl & Moiniche, 2004; Manias et al., 2005; Marchand, 2008).

The slow C fibres conduct impulses from mechanical, thermal, and chemical stimuli. C-fibre pain, or the "second" pain, is an aching pain that is poorly localized (Dahl & Moiniche, 2004; Marchand, 2008). The impulses from C fibres often pass through one or more additional short neurons in the dorsal horn before travelling up to the brain via the spinothalamic tract.

Perception

Perception occurs when a client becomes conscious of the pain. Four key regions of the cerebral cortex are thought to be activated by noxious stimuli via the ascending pathways: (a) the insular cortex, (b) the anterior cingulate cortex, (c) the primary somatosensory cortex, and (d) the secondary somatosensory cortex (Craig & Sorkin, 2011). These regions, together with other areas of the forebrain, produce the sensory–discriminative, motivational–affective, and cognitive–evaluative aspects of the pain experience, as well as motoric integration of noxious stimuli and pain memory (Basbaum & Bushnell, 2002; Basbaum & Jessell, 2000; Craig & Sorkin, 2011).

Modulation

Modulation is a process by which painful messages that travel from the nociceptors to the CNS may be enhanced or inhibited. Modulation happens at every level of the pain pathway and includes the structures of the spinal cord, the brain stem, and the cortex. Pain can be modulated by ascending and descending mechanisms. A typical example of ascending pain modulation is rubbing an injury site, thus activating large non-nociceptive nerve fibres in the periphery. Stimulation of these large A-beta fibres activates inhibitory interneurons in the dorsal horn of the spinal cord, effectively preventing noxious signal transmission from the periphery to the higher brain regions. The physiological basis of this mechanism of pain modulation was elucidated by Melzack and Wall (1965) in their work on gate control theory (GCT), which is described later in the chapter.

Inhibition may also be produced at the level of the spinal cord and the brain stem (spinothalamic pathway) via the release of endogenous opioids and neurotransmitters. Endogenous opioids are naturally occurring morphine-like pentapeptides found throughout the nervous system. They exist in three general classes: (a) enkephalins, (b) dynorphins, and (c) beta-endorphins. These substances block neuronal activity related to noxious impulses by binding to opiate receptor sites in the central and peripheral nervous systems (Melzack & Wall, 1996). The opiate-binding receptor sites are identified as mu (μ), kappa (κ), and delta (δ) and are the same sites to which exogenous opioid analgesics (e.g., oxycodone) bind to provide pain relief. In the ascending pain modulation mechanism, endogenous opioids may be produced in the brain stem and the dorsal horn or exogenous opioids may be introduced by an administration of an opioid analgesic. The released or introduced opioids bind to the μ-opioid receptors on nociceptive nerve fibres, blocking the release of substance P. In the descending mechanism, the efferent spinothalamic nerve fibres that descend from the brain can inhibit the propagation of the pain signal by triggering the release of endogenous opioids in the brain stem and in the spinal cord. Serotonin and norepinephrine are two other important nonopioid pain-inhibitory neurotransmitters that are involved in endogenous analgesic mechanisms. These substances are released by the descending fibres of the descending spinothalamic pathway (Jung, Staiger, & Sullivan, 1997; Marks et al., 2009; Saarto & Wiffen, 2010).

Endogenous pain control by higher cortical structures accounts for many differences in pain perception and interpretation. For example, many clients report lesser pain intensity when they are distracted or when they use imagery techniques to control their pain (Lorenz, Minoshima, & Casey, 2003). We have incomplete understanding of the mechanisms of cortical pain modulation, but it is thought to involve multiple levels of the CNS. One such pathway is the opioid-sensitive descending pathway from the prefrontal cortex to the amygdala, the rostral ventral medulla and the periaqueductal grey matter (Villemure & Bushnell, 2002). Other affective–motivation structures involved in the modulation of pain perception are located in the thalamus.

Gate Control Theory

In 1965, Melzack and Wall's gate control theory (GCT) (Melzack, 1990; Melzack & Wall, 1965, 1973, 1982) proposed that interneurons of the substantia gelatinosa act as a gate, regulating the input of large and small nerve fibres to lamina V cells (Figure 30.3 on the next page).

According to GCT, pain is not a simple sensory experience but one that involves central perception and cognitive–appraisal mechanisms. This theory suggests that if small nociceptive fibre activity in the dorsal horn reaches a critical threshold without being blocked, nociceptive impulses are transmitted to the thalamus and cerebral cortex (Melzack & Wall, 1965, 1973, 1982). Pain perception can be modulated centrally through descending mechanisms that can be influenced by peoples' past

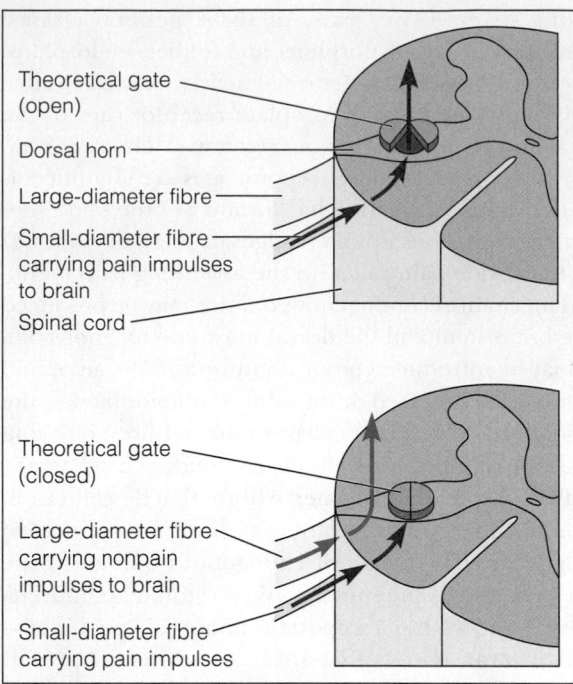

FIGURE 30.3 A schematic illustration of gate control theory.

experience, attention, and emotion. The modulation of the nociceptive signal happens via a "gating mechanism" in the substantia gelatinosa within the dorsal horn (Melzack & Wall, 1965, 1973, 1982).

This gating mechanism can be open, partially open, or closed. The position of the gate is influenced by the relative amounts of activity in large non-nociceptive (A-beta) and small nociceptive (A-delta and C) fibres. Increased activity in the large fibres closes the gate and inhibits the transmission of noxious messages carried by the small fibres to transmission cells (T cells) in the substantia gelatinosa (Melzack & Wall, 1965, 1973, 1982). However, if noxious impulses are not blocked by large fibre activity (i.e., the gate is open or partially open) and reach a critical level, they will be transmitted to second-order neurons in the substantia gelatinosa. The noxious impulse is then transmitted to the thalamus and the cerebral cortex, via ascending nociceptive second-order neurons.

Since GCT was developed, pain knowledge has greatly evolved. Cumulative research has led to more advanced understanding of the nature of pain and its mechanisms, including sensitization, cortical processing, as well as spinal and supraspinal mechanisms of pain control, beyond Melzack and Wall's original theory. Although GCT greatly enhanced the understanding of the complexity of the pain experience and the potential consequences of unrelieved pain, it is largely a theory of acute pain. GCT cannot, for example, explain why a person develops chronic pain long after the original injury has healed.

Nervous System Plasticity: Peripheral and Central Sensitization

The role of plasticity of the nervous system in *peripheral and central sensitization* is now being recognized, along with the individuality of pain perception and response (Basbaum & Jessell, 2000). In the context of pain, **nervous system plasticity** refers to the fact that pain mechanisms in the PNS and CNS can change in response to continued noxious stimulation, a process known as **sensitization**. For example, **peripheral sensitization** of peripheral nociceptors can occur after injury, surgery, or inflammation because of inflammatory mediators released from damaged cells, such as bradykinin, histamine, and prostaglandins. Peripheral sensitization can change the properties of nociceptors so that they transmit spontaneous discharges and respond at a lowered threshold to both noxious and non-noxious stimuli (Basbaum & Jessell, 2000). Moreover, prolonged firing of nociceptors with severe or persistent injury, such as surgery, causes dorsal horn spinal cord neurons to become more responsive to all inputs, resulting in a phenomenon known as **central sensitization**. Central sensitization can result in abnormal interpretation of normal stimuli (allodynia), the amplification or prolongation of the pain signal (hyperalgesia), and chronic pain that lasts long after the original trauma (Basbaum & Jessell, 2000). The two major neurotransmitters that play a role in this mechanism are (a) substance P and (b) glutamate. These neurotransmitters cause an increase in intracellular calcium levels and lower the threshold for the firing of an action potential (Argoff, Albrecht, Irving, & Rice, 2009; Khasabov et al., 2002; Latremoliere & Woolf, 2009). One of the possible consequences of central sensitization is **wind-up**, a condition where, because of the repeated firing of C fibres, the spinal cord neurons become hyperresponsive, and their receptive fields in the corresponding organs expand. As a result, the client may present with secondary hyperalgesia (Herrero, Laird, & Lopez-Garcia, 2000).

Factors Affecting the Pain Experience

Numerous factors can affect a person's perception of and reaction to pain as well as his or her preferences for treatment. These include the person's ethnic and cultural values, developmental stage, environment and support people, previous pain experiences, and the meaning of the current pain.

Ethnic and Cultural Values

Ethnic background and cultural heritage have long been recognized as factors that influence both a person's reaction to pain and the expression of that pain. Behaviour related to pain is a part of the socialization process.

CLINICAL ALERT

It is imperative that nurses are aware of their "hidden" biases in pain assessment, that is, biases that he or she may not be conscious of and that may cause the nurse to either under- or overestimate their clients' pain or to omit pain assessment altogether. These biases may include the client's physical appearance, gender, age, race, or culture, as well as the nurse's personal experiences with pain.

In addition to some variations in pain threshold, cultural background can affect the level of pain that an individual is willing to tolerate. In some Middle Eastern and African cultures, self-infliction of pain is a sign of mourning or grief. In other groups, pain is anticipated as part of the ritualistic practices, and therefore, tolerance of pain signifies strength and endurance. Moreover, the expression of pain varies widely. Studies have shown that individuals of northern European descent tend to be more stoic and less expressive of their pain than individuals from southern European backgrounds. Persons of Asian descent, especially those of Chinese origin, may believe that pain is an essential part of life and tend to underreport their levels of pain (Gordon, 1997; IASP, 2001; Kumasaka, 1996; Munoz & Luckmann, 2005).

Nurses must realize that they have their own attitudes and expectations about pain (see the Clinical Alert box). For example, nurses may place a higher value on silent suffering or self-control in response to pain. Nurses expect people to be objective about pain and to be able to provide a detailed description of the pain. Since many clients have individual and cultural differences in pain reporting and in treatment preferences, the nurse must be competent to elicit a report and to accurately assess pain in each of their clients. To become culturally competent, nurses must become knowledgeable about differences in the meaning of and appropriate responses to pain in their client's culture while being sympathetic to their concerns and developing the skills needed to address pain in a culturally sensitive way.

Developmental Stage

The ages and developmental levels of clients are important factors that will influence their reactions to and expressions of pain. Some age variations and related nonpharmacological nursing interventions are presented in Table 30.3 on the next page.

The field of pain management for infants and children has grown significantly over the past years. It is now accepted that anatomical, physiological, and biochemical elements necessary for pain transmission are present in newborns, regardless of gestational age (Bartocci, Bergqvist, Lagercrantz, & Anand, 2006;

Grunau et al., 2005; Hall & Anand, 2005; Slater et al., 2006). However, children's pain is often undertreated because they may be less able to articulate their pain experience and needs compared with adults (Ellis et al., 2002; Stevens, 1999).

The likelihood of experiencing pain increases with age as older adults are more likely to suffer from chronic conditions that can cause pain, such as arthritis, diabetes, and joint disorders (Kane, Ouslander, & Itamar, 2004; Ramage-Morin, 2008). In addition, as the body system ages, older adults may require more medical interventions, such as surgery, that may result in acute pain. Older adults may also experience age-related changes in nociception. Although current knowledge of how aging affects pain transmission and perception is incomplete, recent investigations showed that aging affects central pain processing and pain pathway plasticity (Gibson & Farrell, 2004; Zheng, Gibson, Helme, & McMeeken, 2009). Certain changes in nociception may result in a higher pain threshold. For example, the transduction and transmission of the pain signal in the older adult may be delayed by a reduction in substance P and the density of myelinated and nonmyelinated fibres. The nurse should not conclude that an older adult has lower pain intensities. In fact, if such a client chooses to report pain, the nurse should be alerted by the possibility of a greater underlying pathology. In addition, older adults often have more than one source of pain and they may have trouble localizing and explaining it (American Geriatric Society, 2002; Ramage-Morin, 2008).

For clients of all ages, the nurse may attempt to assess pain by using self-report and observational or behavioural and physiological measures (Herr et al., 2006; von Baeyer & Spagrud, 2007). Ideally, the nurse should use a composite measure that includes self-report and one or more of the other indicators (Champion, Goodenough, von Baeyer, & Thomas, 1998). When self-report cannot be obtained (e.g., infants, preverbal children, and children or older adults with cognitive impairment, and older adults), behavioural observation should be the primary source for pain assessment (Herr et al., 2006; von Baeyer & Spagrud, 2007).

Environment and Support People

The psychological state of a person can affect their attention to, and the interpretation and perception of pain. The surrounding environment has been shown to greatly affect the psychological state of an individual; it can cause many reactions from relaxation to excitation and anxiety (Oberle et al., 1990). Notably, a strange environment, such as a hospital with its noises, lights, and activity, can compound the state of stress or anxiety (Topf, 2000). Although there is no proven causal relationship between anxiety and pain, being in an unfamiliar environment may

TABLE 30.3 Age Variations in the Pain Experience

Age Group	Pain Perception and Behaviour	Selected Nursing Interventions
Infant	Perceives pain Responds to pain with increased sensitivity Older infant tries to avoid pain; for example, turns away and physically resists	Promote breastfeeding during painful procedures. Use tactile stimulation (e.g., gently rub the other side of the affected area). Play music or tapes of a heartbeat.
Toddler and preschooler	Develops the ability to describe pain and its intensity and location Often responds with crying and anger because a child perceives pain as a threat to security Reasoning at this stage is not always successful May consider pain a punishment Feels sad May learn there are gender differences in pain expression Tends to hold someone accountable for the pain	Distract the child with toys, books, pictures. Involve the child in blowing bubbles as a way of "blowing away the pain." Appeal to the child's belief in magic by using a "magic" blanket or glove to take away the pain. Hold the child to provide comfort. Explore misconceptions about pain.
School-age child	Tries to be brave when facing pain Rationalizes in an attempt to explain the pain Responsive to explanations Can usually identify the location and describe the pain With persistent pain, may regress to an earlier stage of development	Use imagery to turn off "pain switches." Provide a behavioural rehearsal of what to expect and how it will look and feel. Provide support.
Adolescent	May be slow to acknowledge pain Recognizing pain or "giving in" may be considered weakness Wants to appear brave in front of peers and not report pain	Provide opportunities to discuss pain. Provide privacy. Present choices for dealing with pain. Encourage music or TV viewing as a distraction.
Adult	Behaviours exhibited when experiencing pain may be gender-based behaviours learned as a child May ignore pain because to admit it is perceived as a sign of weakness or failure May use pain for secondary gain, for example, to get attention Fear of what pain means may prevent some adults from taking action	Deal with any misbeliefs about pain. Focus on the client's control in dealing with the pain. Allay fears and anxiety, when possible. Spend time with the client, and listen carefully.
Older adult	May perceive pain as part of the aging process May have decreased sensations or perceptions of the pain Lethargy, anorexia, and fatigue may be indicators of pain May withhold complaints of pain because of fear of the treatment, of any lifestyle changes that may be involved, or of becoming dependent May describe pain differently, that is, as "ache," "hurt," or "discomfort" May consider it unacceptable to admit to or show pain	Explore and clarify misbeliefs. Encourage independence, whenever possible.

cause a psychological discomfort that can have an indirect effect on the affective component of pain and increase the psychological suffering of the person who is experiencing it (Oberle et al., 1990). In addition, it was shown that lonely persons who are without a support network may perceive pain as severe, whereas persons who have supportive people around perceive less pain. People who consider their family and friends supportive also show less pain behaviours and higher levels of activity and report lower levels of emotional distress (Jamison & Virts, 1990). Finally, satisfaction with perceived social support was shown to be associated with lower pain intensity and lower depression levels (Lopez-Martinez, Esteve-Zarazaga, & Ramirez-Maestre, 2008).

Expectations of society or significant others can affect a person's perceptions of and responses to pain. In some situations, for example, girls may be permitted to express pain more openly compared with boys. Family roles can also affect how a person perceives or responds to pain. For instance, a single mother supporting three children may ignore pain because of her need to stay on the job. The presence of support people often changes a client's reaction to pain. For example, toddlers often tolerate pain more readily when supportive parents or nurses are nearby (Lopez-Martinez et al., 2008; Schiff, Holtz, Peterson, & Rakusan, 2001).

Past Pain Experiences

The adaptation model of pain proposed by Rollman (1979) suggests that an individual's judgment of a pain signal is based on the stimulus, its contextual meaning, the motivational state of the subject, and a number of experiential factors. This model implies that previous pain experiences can influence a client's response to pain. People who have personally experienced pain or who have been exposed to the suffering of someone close are often more threatened by anticipated pain than are people without a pain experience (Rollman, Abdel-Shaheed, Gillespie, & Jones, 2004).

Meaning of Pain

The meaning of pain can contribute to the overall pain experience (Arntz & Claassens, 2004; McGillion et al., 2007). Some clients may accept pain more readily than others, depending on the circumstances and the client's interpretation of its significance. A client who associates pain with a positive outcome may withstand it amazingly well. For example, a woman giving birth to a child or an athlete undergoing knee surgery to prolong his career may tolerate pain better because of the benefit associated with it. These clients may view pain as a temporary inconvenience rather than a potential threat or disruption to daily life.

In contrast, clients with unrelenting chronic pain may suffer more intensely. Chronic pain affects the body, mind, spirit, and social relationships in an undesirable way. Physically, the pain limits functioning and contributes to disuse or deconditioning. For many, changes in activities of daily living (e.g., eating, sleeping, toileting) also take a toll. The side effects of the various medications used to try to control pain also place a heavy burden on the sufferer's body. Socially, pain often strains valued relationships, in part because of the impaired ability to fulfill role expectations. Together, these changes caused by pain may create a sense of loss (e.g., loss of work, friends, identity, or pleasure) to the client.

Mentally, individuals with chronic pain change their outlook, becoming more pessimistic, often to the point of helplessness and hopelessness. Mood often becomes impaired when pain persists: the sadness of being unable to do important or enjoyable activities combined with self-doubts and learned helplessness, can contribute to depression. The anxiety surrounding the timing of pain flares, the worry about the physical ability to do what is needed, and the uncertainty about coping with multiple competing demands (including pain control) can escalate emotionally, to the point of panic.

Spiritually, pain can be viewed in a variety of ways. It may be perceived as a punishment for wrongdoing, a betrayal by a higher power, a test of fortitude, or a threat to the essence of who the person is. As such, pain can be a source of spiritual distress or be a source of strength and enlightenment (Gatchel, Peng, Peters, Fuchs, & Turk, 2007).

Pain Assessment

Accurate pain assessment is the foundation of effective pain management. In fact, many health facilities are making pain assessment the fifth* vital sign (American Pain Society, 1999; Dahl, 2000). Because pain is a complex, subjective, and multidimensional experience, no simple method can objectively determine how much pain an individual experiences. Nurses should tailor pain assessments to the unique developmental levels, communication capabilities, and cultural needs of their clients.

In general, pain should be assessed on hospital admission and routinely thereafter, as well as before, during, and after therapeutic interventions (Canadian Pain Society [CPS], 2005). However, the extent and frequency of the pain assessment will vary according to the situation. For clients experiencing acute or severe pain, the nurse may focus only on location, quality, severity, and early intervention. Clients with less severe or chronic pain can usually provide a more detailed description of the experience. The frequency of pain assessment usually depends on the pain management intervention being used and the clinical circumstances. For example, in the initial postoperative period, pain is often assessed whenever vital signs are taken, which may be as often as every 15 minutes and then extended to every 2 to 4 hours. Following pain management interventions, pain intensity should be reassessed at an interval appropriate for the intervention. For example, following the intravenous administration of 2.5 mg of intravenous morphine, the severity of pain should be reassessed at the peak effect, which is within 10 to 15 minutes.

Because it has been found that many people will not voice their pain unless asked about it, pain assessments *must* be initiated by the nurse. Some of the many reasons why clients may be reluctant to report pain are listed in Box 30.2 on the next page. Knowledge deficits and personal beliefs may underlie some of these reasons, especially those regarding pharmacological pain management interventions. When conducting pain assessments, it is essential that nurses listen to and rely on the client's perceptions of pain because it is a subjective experience. Believing the person who is conveying their perceptions of pain is also crucial in establishing a sense of trust.

---

*The editors draw the readers' attention to the debate about the *fifth vital sign*—some argue that pain is the fifth vital sign, but others indicate that oxygen saturation is the fifth vital sign (see Chapter 29).

BOX 30.2 WHY CLIENTS MAY BE RELUCTANT TO REPORT PAIN

Some clients are hesitant to report pain for a number of reasons:

- Unwillingness to trouble staff who are perceived as busy
- Concern about being labelled as a complainer or "bad patient"
- Fear of the injectable route of analgesic administration—children, in particular
- Belief that pain is to be expected as part of the recovery process
- Belief that pain is a normal part of aging or a necessary part of life—older adults, in particular
- Belief that expressing pain reveals weakness
- Difficulty expressing personal discomfort
- Concern about potential risks associated with opioid drugs (e.g., addiction)
- Fear about the cause of pain or that reporting pain will lead to further tests
- Concern about the possibility of unwanted side effects, especially of opioid drugs
- Concern that use of drugs now will render the drug inefficient if or when the pain becomes worse

Whenever possible, the nurse should question the client about his or her pain experience. In the nonverbal client (i.e. infants, older adults with cognitive deficits, unconscious clients), the nurse will look for observational indicators to detect the presence of pain. The goal of pain assessment is to get a comprehensive description of this subjective experience.

Pain Assessment in Clients Able to Self-Report

The gold standard of pain assessment is the client's self-report (IASP, 1979). The nurse must provide an opportunity for clients to express, in their own words, how they perceive their pain. The commonly used symptom assessment mnemonic PQRSTU symptom assessment can help the nurse elicit questions during a pain assessment.

P: PRECIPITATING/PALLIATING FACTORS *Precipitating factors* are events that normally cause the pain or that aggravate it. For example, physical exertion may precede chest pain and cause muscle spasms in the neck, shoulders, or back; abdominal pain may occur after eating. These observations can help prevent pain and determine its cause. Environmental factors, such as extreme cold or heat, can affect some types of pain. For example, sudden exercise on a hot day can cause muscle spasm. Physical and emotional stressors can also precipitate pain. Strong emotions can trigger a migraine headache or an episode of angina. Some clients, especially those with chronic pain, may not be able to tell what brings on their pain. By working together with the client and going over their daily routines and events that precede the pain, a nurse may be able to help them determine whether their pain is related to any precipitating factors.

Assessing *palliating factors* consists of taking note of all the strategies that the client has tried to decrease the pain and whether or not they were helpful. These may include medical procedures, home remedies, such as herbal teas, medications, rest, applications of heat or cold, prayer, or distractions like watching television. It is important to explore the effect that both pharmacological and non-pharmacological strategies have had on the pain. This information may provide the nurse with valuable clues on how to tailor the client's pain management plan to his or her unique situation. Any side effects of pain-relieving strategies should also be documented.

Q: QUALITY/QUANTITY *Quality* refers to the client's description of the pain sensation. Descriptive adjectives help people communicate the quality of their pain and can provide information on the nature of the pain (i.e., nociceptive, neuropathic, or a combination of both). A headache may be described as "hammer-like" or an abdominal pain as "piercing, like a knife." Sometimes, clients have difficulty describing their pain because they have never experienced any sensation like it. This is particularly true for children, older adults, and adults who have neuropathic pain.

Nurses need to record the exact words clients use to describe pain. Exact information can be significant in both the diagnosis of the pain etiology and the treatment choices. For example, key descriptors, such as "burning" and "electrical," may help the nurse to identify neuropathic pain. To help gather information, a nurse can use a validated pain questionnaire (e.g., McGill Pain Questionnaire or MPQ; see Table 30.4 on page 753) (Melzack, 1975).

Quantity refers to pain intensity. Valid and reliable self-report measures of pain intensity include the 0–10 Numerical Rating Scale (NRS), the Visual Analogue Scale (VAS), the Verbal Rating Scale (VRS), and Faces Pain Scales (FPSs). Such scales provide consistency for nurses to communicate with the client and other health care providers (Jensen & Karoly, 1986). Nurses can affect the quality of the pain report by selecting pain scales that are appropriate for their target populations. Some clients may require the nurse to teach them how to use the scale or to fill in the pain assessment with them. Some of the commonly used pain scales are described below.

The NRS is widely used in clinical practice and consists of an 11-point scale from 0 (no pain) to 10 (worst possible pain) (Figure 30.4B). The VAS (Huskisson, 1983) consists of a 10-cm line with one end indicating "no pain" and the other end indicating "pain as bad as it could possibly be." The distance on the line is calculated in millimetres (from 0 to 100) (Figure 30.4A). The advantages of both scales include the ease of use, their applicability to many communicative client populations, and their sensitivity and validity. The VRS gives the client a list of adjectives that describe pain in a ranked order. Each adjective can also be assigned a score. For example, a VRS may consist of "no pain," "mild," "moderate," and "severe" pain that are assigned the scores of 0, 1, 2, and 3, respectively (Ohnhaus & Adler, 1975).

Various FPSs that are based on facial expressions associated with different pain levels have been developed. Each face can refer to a number to help document the pain intensity. Among them, the Faces Pain Scale—Revised (FPS-R) (Hicks, von Baeyer, Spafford, van Korlaar, & Goodenough, 2001), shown in Figure 30.4B, can be used with school-age children (Stinson, Kavanagh, Yamada, Gill, & Stevens, 2006). The Faces Pain Thermometer (FPT) depicted in Figure 30.4C was developed for use with adults (Gelinas, 2007).

Not all clients can understand or relate to numbers (i.e., NRS). These include children who are unable to verbally communicate their pain and clients with impairments in cognition or communication. FPSs may be easier to use for these clients (Hadjistavropoulos & Craig, 2002; Jensen & Karoly, 2001). For example, when measuring pain intensity in children, it is critical that the nurse use a self-report measure recommended for the child's age and developmental level.

Many scales, including the NRS, FPT, and FPS-R, have been shown to be valid and reliable when used with clients who have cognitive deficits (Taylor & Herr, 2003; Zhou, Petpichetchian, & Kitrungrote, 2011).

Interestingly, it was found that older adults find it easier to use the vertical pain intensity scale, rather than its horizontal version, because it reminds them of a thermometer (Herr & Mobily, 1993).

R: REGION/RADIATION Pain can be described according to where it is experienced in the body. *Radiating pain* is perceived at the source of the pain and extends to nearby tissues. For example, cardiac pain may be felt not only in the chest but also along the left shoulder and down the left arm. **Referred pain** is pain felt in a part of the body that is considerably removed from the tissues causing the pain. For example, pain from one part of the abdominal viscera may be perceived in an area of the skin remote from the organ causing the pain (Figure 30.5 on the next page). Referred pain is complex and occurs most often with damage to visceral organs. The mechanisms of referred pain relate to the spatial organization of the grey matter of the spinal cord into five distinct laminae (I to V) or layers. It is thought that noxious stimuli from both somatic and visceral structures may converge via lamina V neurons, making it difficult for higher brain centres to discriminate the original sources of these noxious inputs (Basbaum & Jessell, 2000).

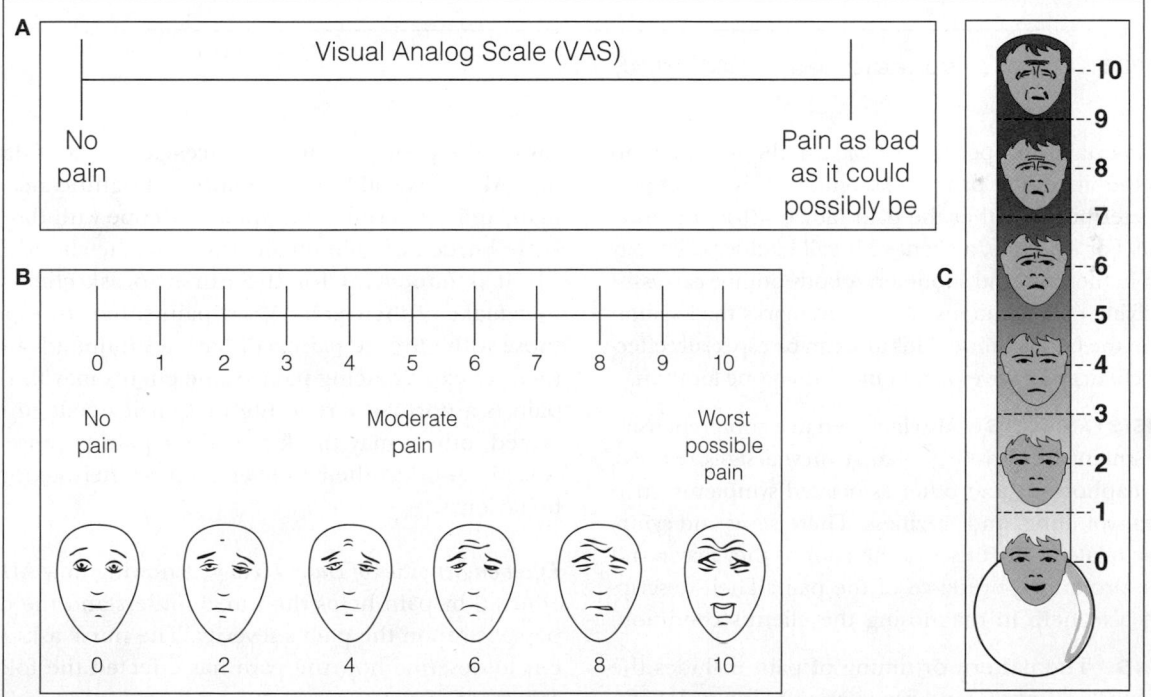

FIGURE 30.4 Commonly used self-report pain scales. **A:** The Visual Analogue Scale. **B:** The 0–10 Numeric Rating Scale (NRS) and the Faces Pain Scales-Revised (FPS-R) combined. **C:** The Faces Pain Thermometer.

Sources: A and B: From Pasero, C. & McCaffery, M. (2010). *Pain assessment and pharmacological management* (pp. 56–57). Mosby: St. Louis. A is in the public domain. *B* has been reproduced with the permission of the International Association for the Study of Pain. Permission to use the FPS-R for purposes other than clinical practice or research can be obtained by emailing IASPdesk@iasp-pain.org. The NRS is in the public domain. C The Faces Pain Thermometer from Gelinas, C. (2007). Le thermomètre d'intensité de douleur: Un nouvel outil pour les patients adultes en soins critiques. *Perspective infirmière, 4*(4), 12–20. Permission by C. Gelinas.
A: The Visual Analogue Scale (VAS). The client is asked to rate their pain on a 10-cm long line from "no pain" to "pain as bad as it could possibly be." The pain rating is calculated on the basis of how many millimetres the client's pain is removed from the "no pain" end of the line (e.g., 40 mm means the client's pain rating is 40 out of a possible 100).
B: The 0–10 Numeric Rating Scale (NRS) and the Faces Pain Scales-Revised (FPS-R) combined in a horizontal format. Clients may have a choice of the pain rating scale, when the scale is presented in this format. The left-most face shows "no pain," and the right-most face shows "worst possible pain." Clients are asked to point to the face that shows how much they hurt right now.
C: The Faces Pain Thermometer (Gelinas, 2007) has a vertical orientation that may be easier for older adults to use.

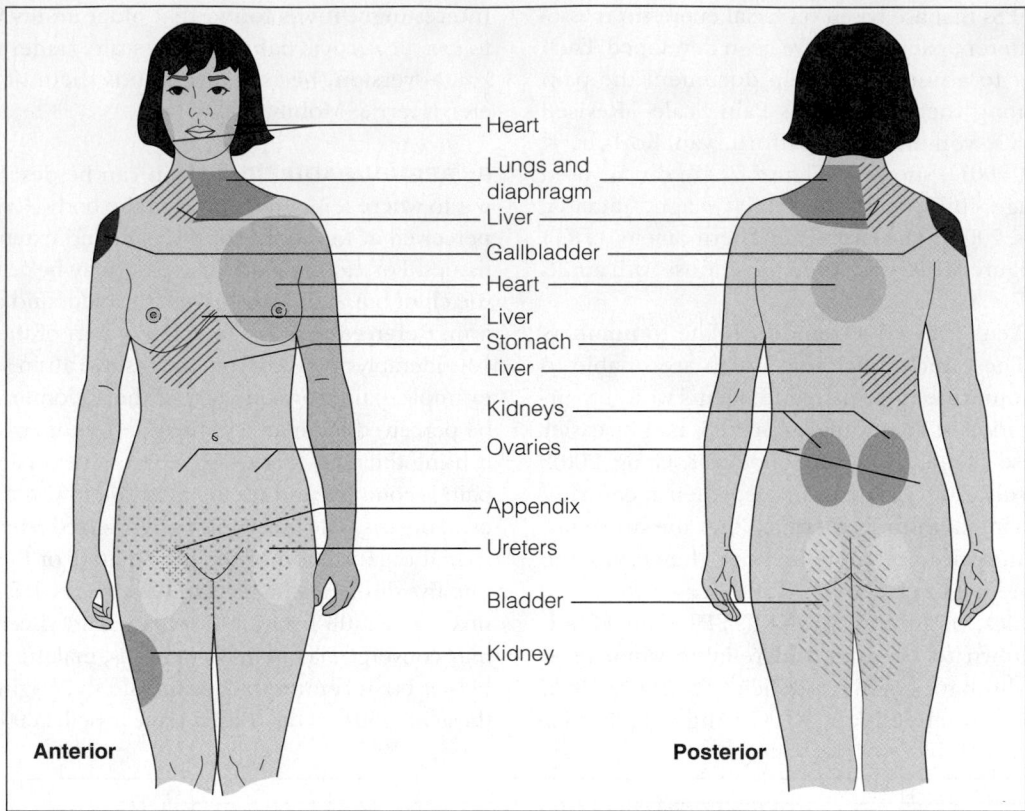

FIGURE 30.5 Common sites of referred pain from various body organs.

To ascertain the specific *location,* ask the individual to point to the site of the pain or discomfort. It is also important to determine whether the pain radiates from the indicated site. For example, a client with gall bladder colic may feel pain in the back and shoulder. A body outline can assist in identifying pain locations. The client marks the location of pain on the body outline. This tool can be especially effective with clients who have pain in more than one location.

S: SIGNS/SYMPTOMS Also included in a comprehensive pain assessment are signs (e.g., changes in vital signs, redness, edema, diaphoresis) and other associated symptoms, such as nausea, vomiting, and dizziness. These signs and symptoms may relate to the onset of the pain or they may result from the prolonged presence of the pain. Their description can also help in diagnosing the client's condition.

T: TIMING The pattern or timing of pain includes the time of onset, duration, and recurrence or intervals without pain. The nurse therefore determines when the pain began; how long the pain lasts; whether it recurs and, if so, the length of the interval without pain; and when the pain last occurred. With this information, the nurse can tailor pain interventions, such as analgesics administration, to precede the onset of pain. For example, a nurse might suggest taking an analgesic before exercise or physiotherapy to some clients.

U: UNDERSTANDING The assessment of understanding includes eliciting the client's opinion on what causes the pain, how it influences activities of daily living (ADLs), social life, the emotional significance of the pain, and the resources available to cope with the cumulative burden of pain on all aspects of the client's life.

It is important for the nurse to ask clients what they make of their pain. Many pain sufferers, especially those with chronic pain, will have a unique idea of why they are experiencing pain. Some clients may think that pain is a normal part of life or that it needs to be tolerated; others may think that their pain is caused by a specific event in their lives or even by their actions and behaviours.

Effect on Activities of Daily Living Knowing how ADLs are affected by pain helps the nurse understand the client's perspective on the pain's severity. The nurse asks the client to describe how the pain has affected the following aspects of life:

- Sleep
- Appetite
- Concentration
- Work or school
- Interpersonal relationships
- Marital relations and sex
- Home activities
- Driving or walking
- Leisure activities
- Emotional status (mood, irritability, depression, anxiety)

A rating scale of none, a little, or a great deal, or another range, can be used to determine the degree of alteration.

Client's History

In addition to the description of the pain experience using PQRSTU, the nurse needs to gather other information related to the client's history. AMPLE is an abbreviated client health history assessment that may help the nurse establish a picture of the client's health, present and past problems, and the events that may affect the client's condition. The letters in the AMPLE mnemonic correspond to the following:

- **A**llergies/reactions
- **M**edications/substances
- **P**ast medical history
- **L**ast meal
- **E**nvironment or events leading to the incident or illness

If this is a first encounter, a nurse must establish whether the client has allergies to medications, animals, fruits, vegetables, or environmental allergens, and the client's reactions to those allergies. Medication use (past and present) may affect a client's current status and also provide the nurse with clues about the client's current pain management regime (if any) and other medical problems. These may include prescription and over-the-counter medications, vitamins, and herbal remedies. It is also important to inquire whether the client consumes alcohol, nonprescription drugs, and tobacco; these substances may cause or affect many physical symptoms and can interfere with action of the medications that the client is prescribed. Past medical history includes questions about the past and present diagnoses, surgeries, injuries, and, if pertinent, family history of certain diseases. Last meal may be important as a precipitating factor in certain cases. For example, a client with epigastric pain may be suffering from gastroesophageal reflux or an ulcer that is aggravated by a large cup of coffee in the morning. Environment may refer to the client's social status, their living situation, or their work place. The pertinence of these questions should be determined by the nurse. For a client who has chronic back pain, it would be important to know about his or her work and whether the person has to lift heavy weights or to spend a long time sitting or standing. For acute pain, a nurse can also inquire about events leading to the incident, such as falling or having surgery. Examples of these questions are shown in the Assessment: Interview box on the next page.

Pain Questionnaires for Nursing Practice

Pain questionnaires are useful tools for a nurse to elicit a more descriptive picture of the client's pain, to organize it, and to make conclusions about possible nursing diagnoses related to pain. Some questionnaires have the ability to distinguish between different types of

pain (e.g., neuropathic or somatic), whereas others can help the nurse understand the nature of the pain as it is experienced by the client. For example, the McGill Pain Questionnaire (MPQ) (Melzack, 1975) and the Present Pain Intensity (PPI) scale (Melzack, 1987; see Table 30.4) were shown to be reliable and valid multidimensional questionnaires of pain for different types of pain in adults. The Brief Pain Inventory (BPI) collects information about pain severity, treatment relief, and the effect of pain on key areas of function (general activity, mood, walking ability, normal work, relations with people, sleep, enjoyment of life). This tool is especially useful for initial pain assessment and tracking the progress of pain (Cleeland & Ryan, 1994; Wu, Beaton, Smith, & Hagen, 2010). Another commonly used pain questionnaire is the Leeds Assessment of Neuropathic

TABLE 30.4 PPI (Present Pain Intensity)

Client's Name:			Date:	
	None	Mild	Moderate	Severe
Throbbing	0)	1)	2)	3)
Shooting	0)	1)	2)	3)
Stabbing	0)	1)	2)	3)
Sharp	0)	1)	2)	3)
Cramping	0)	1)	2)	3)
Gnawing	0)	1)	2)	3)
Hot-Burning	0)	1)	2)	3)
Aching	0)	1)	2)	3)
Heavy	0)	1)	2)	3)
Tender	0)	1)	2)	3)
Splitting	0)	1)	2)	3)
Tiring-Exhausting	0)	1)	2)	3)
Sickening	0)	1)	2)	3)
Fearful	0)	1)	2)	3)
Punishing-Cruel	0)	1)	2)	3)
	No pain		Worst Possible Pain	

PPI (Present Pain Intensity)

0 No Pain	4 Horrible
1 Mild	5 Excruciating
2 Discomforting	
3 Distressing	

Source: From the "Short Form McGill Pain Questionnaire". Copyright R. Melzack, 1984; 1987, reprinted with permission from Dr. Melzack and www.mapigroup.com.

ASSESSMENT	INTERVIEW

It is important for the nurse to obtain accurate data on a client's pain. Examples of PQRSTU pain assessment questions:

- **P**recipitating/**P**alliating (aggravating/alleviating) factors: How did your pain start? What were you doing when the pain appeared? What makes the pain worse? What makes the pain better? What have you tried to alleviate your pain, and has it helped?

- **Q**uality/**Q**uantity: In your own words, describe what the pain feels like. Some of the descriptors the client may use are *burning, aching, dull, sharp, gnawing, shooting,* or *stabbing.* On a scale from 0 to 10 (with 0 meaning "No pain" and 10 meaning "Worst possible pain"), how would you rate the level of pain you are having?

- **R**egion/**R**adiation: Where do you feel the pain? (point/describe). Does the pain radiate to any other regions of your body?

- **S**igns, **S**ymptoms: Do you have any swelling, redness, fever? Do you have any other symptoms or sensations (e.g., nausea, dizziness, blurred vision, shortness of breath, anxiety, fatigue) in addition to your pain?

- **T**iming: When did or does the pain start? How long have you had it, or how long does it usually last? How long are the pain-free periods, if there are any? What is the frequency of the pain attacks?

- **U**nderstanding: How do you interpret your pain? Have you felt a similar kind of pain before, and if so, can you describe the situation? What outcomes (implications) do you anticipate from this pain? What do you fear most about your pain? How does the pain make you feel (e.g., anxious, depressed, frightened, tired)?

The nurse must inform himself or herself about the client's health history to be able to perform a comprehensive assessment. Examples of AMPLE health history assessment questions are as follows:

- **A**llergies/reactions: Do you have any known allergies? Are you sensitive to any foods/products/environments? What is your reaction to the food/product/environment that you are allergic to?

- **M**edications/substances:
  - Do you take any prescription medications? If so, what is the name/dosage/reason for the prescription? When did you take the last dose?
  - Do you take any nonprescription medications, vitamins, or herbal supplements? (name/dose/reason/time of last dose)
  - Do you consume alcohol, smoke cigarettes, or use drugs? (quantity/frequency/since when?)
  - Are your vaccinations up to date? Type (tetanus, flu, hepatitis, etc.)
  - Do you drink caffeinated beverages (coffee, tea, energy drinks)? How much, and how many a day? At what time of the day?

- **P**ast medical history: Do you have a diagnosed medical problem? To your knowledge, do you have any diseases? If yes, what type? When were you diagnosed? Did you receive treatment? Is the problem still present? Are there medical problems in your family? Have you ever been hospitalized, and if so, for what reason/when? Have you ever had surgery? If yes, for what reason/when?

- **L**ast meal: When did you eat last? What did you eat before the incident? Did you tolerate the meal well? Do you follow a diet? If yes, what kind, and for what reason?

- **E**nvironment/**E**vents leading to injury or illness: Where do you live? Do you live alone? If not, who do you live with? What were you doing before the incident? Where do you work? Do you find work stressful? Do you have friends or family who can provide support? Do you feel well supported? What were you doing right before the pain started?

Symptoms and Signs (LANSS) used to differentiate between nociceptive and neuropathic pain when the pain pathology is unclear (Bennett, 2001; Kaki, El-Yaski, & Youseif, 2005).

Daily Pain Diary

For clients who experience chronic pain, a daily diary may help the client and the nurse identify pain patterns and factors that exacerbate or moderate the pain experience. In home care, the family or the caregiver can be taught to complete the diary. The record can include time or onset of pain, activity before pain, pain-related positions or behaviours, pain intensity level, duration of pain, and the use of pharmacological and nonpharmacological pain management strategies. Recorded data can provide the basis for developing or modifying the plan for care. For this tool to be effective, it is important for the client to use it routinely. Therefore, the nurse should educate the client and the family about the value and use of the diary in achieving effective pain control. Determining the client's abilities to use the diary is essential.

Pain Assessment in Clients Who Cannot Self-Report

Clients who are unable to self-report their pain are a particularly vulnerable group of clients that present multiple challenges in pain detection and control. Clients who may experience pain but are unable to communicate it, among others, include older adults with cognitive deficits, infants and preverbal toddlers, intubated or unconscious clients, and clients at the end of life (Hadjistavropoulos et al., 2007; Herr et al., 2006; Mularski et al., 2009).

Recommendations for pain assessment in the non-verbal client are described in the position statement of the American Society for Pain Management Nursing (ASPMN; Herr et al., 2006). The approach to pain assessment is hierarchical (see Box 30.3), with no single pain scale being sufficient by itself. Rather, pain assessment

1. Attempt to elicit the client's self-report of pain.

2. Search for potential causes of pain (e.g., pathological conditions or procedures that can cause pain, such as surgery, physiotherapy activities, turning and positioning, blood draws, pressure ulcers). Assume that pain is present if any pain-causing condition is identified.

3. Observe the client's pain behaviours. Use valid evidence-based behavioural pain scales developed for specific client groups and contexts.

4. Use surrogate reporting from family, parents, or caregivers.

5. Attempt an analgesic trial if the presence of pain is suspected. Administer appropriate analgesics and re-evaluate behaviours. If there is an improvement in a potentially pain-related behaviour, then pain was present.

Source: Herr, K., P. J. Coyne, et al. (2006). Pain assessment in the nonverbal patient: Position statement with clinical practice recommendations. *Pain Management Nursing* 7(2): 44–52.

should be based on a combination of pain evaluation techniques. Attempting to elicit the client's self-report is encouraged in all clients.

BEHAVIOURAL RESPONSES TO PAIN People show wide variations in *behavioural responses* to pain. In the case of clients who are very young, aphasic, confused, or have an altered level of consciousness, nonverbal expressions may be the only means of communicating pain. Facial expression is often the first indicator of pain, and it may be the only one. Frowning, brow lowering, eyes tightly shut, clenched teeth or open mouth, and grimacing may be indicative of pain (Prkachin, 1992). Vocalizations, such as moaning, groaning, crying, or screaming, are also associated with pain (Mateo & Krenzischek, 1992). A client who remains immobile with the purpose of avoiding movement may also be in pain and should be assessed (Puntillo et al., 1997). The client with chest pain often holds the left arm across the chest. A person with abdominal pain may assume the position of greatest comfort, often flexing the knees and hips and moving reluctantly.

Purposeless or rhythmic body movements are other cues of pain. For example, clients may toss and turn in bed or fling their arms about. Involuntary movements, such as a reflexive jerking away from a needle inserted through the skin, may also indicate pain (Feldt, 2000; Odhner, Wegman, Freeland, Steinmetz, & Ingersoll, 2003). An adult may be able to control this reflex; however, a child may be unable or unwilling to do so. An adult or child may assume the fetal position and rock back and forth when experiencing abdominal pain (Cohen et al., 2008). Rubbing an affected area is also a known pain indicator (Feldt, 2000). During labour, a woman may massage her abdomen rhythmically with her hands.

Behavioural changes, such as confusion and restlessness, may be indicative of pain in both cognitively intact and cognitively impaired older adults. A change in

behaviours with others including becoming hostile or aggressive may also be observed in older adults with chronic pain (Gibson & Helme, 2001; Odhner et al., 2003).

It is important to note that some behavioural responses can be controlled, and the nurse must develop competent interpersonal observation skills to detect reflexive pain behaviours (Hadjistavropoulos & Craig, 2002; Hadjistavropoulos et al., 2007). For example, vocalization or body movements in response to pain can be controlled, but facial expressions, especially the reflexive movements of the upper face, were shown to be under less conscious control (Rinn, 1984). Also, many behavioural responses (e.g., crying) are not unique to pain. When pain is chronic, overt behavioural responses are rare, as pain behaviours habituate over time, and the individual develops personal coping styles for dealing with the pain. When looking for indicators of chronic pain, the nurse can focus on changes in the patterns of daily living, such as sleep, appetite, activity levels, social interactions, and avoidance behaviours (Shankland, 2011).

Valid and reliable assessment tools can be used to measure a client's behavioural responses to pain. Currently, no behavioural observation tool is acceptable for all client populations. Indeed, a pain assessment tool can only be shown to be valid when used for a specific purpose in a specified group of respondents and in a given context (American Educational Research Association, American Psychological Association, & National Council on Measurment in Education, 1999). The scope of this chapter cannot provide an exhaustive list of the available behavioural pain assessment tools. The Pain Resource Center at the City of Hope (http://prc.coh.org/PAIN-NOA.htm) provides a summary and critiques of the existing pain tools for nonverbal adult clients. A few examples of pain assessment tools developed for nonverbal client groups are described in Table 30.5 on the next page.

PHYSIOLOGICAL RESPONSES TO PAIN Elevated or lowered vital signs as well as changes from the client's baseline may indicate but are not specific to pain. Early in the onset of acute pain, the sympathetic nervous system is stimulated, resulting in increased blood pressure, heart rate, respiratory rate, pallor, diaphoresis, and pupil dilation. Although the nociceptors do not adapt to painful stimuli, the sympathetic nervous system does, making the physiological responses less evident or even absent. With visceral pain, signs of parasympathetic stimulation may be observed, such as decreased blood pressure and heart rate, pupil constriction, and warm dry skin (McCance & Huether, 2006). Physiological responses are likely to be absent in people with chronic pain because of CNS adaptation (McEwen, 2001).

The evidence supporting the use of vital signs as valid indicators of pain is varied. Vital signs can be affected by many physiological and psychological changes other than pain (e.g., distress, medication, biochemical changes in the body, medical conditions). Therefore, vital signs alone should not be used as pain indicators, but, rather, they should be used as cues to prompt for further pain

TABLE 30.5 List of Behavioural Pain Assessment Scales

FLACC (Face, Legs, Activity, Cry, and Consolability)	A five-item scale; each item is scored from 0 to 2 with final scale score from 0 to 10. Developed for infants and children from 2 months to 7 years old and used to quantify pain behaviours in children who cannot verbalize the presence of pain or its severity during or after a variety of surgical and medical procedures (Merkel, Voepel-Lewis, & Malviya, 2002; Merkel, Voepel-Lewis, Shayevitz, & Malviya, 1997).
PIPP (Premature Infant Pain Profile)	A seven-item scale scored from 0 to 21, developed for premature and term neonates and used for the detection of acute pain in neonates and the assessment of procedural pain in the neonatal intensive care unit (NICU; Ballantyne, Stevens, McAllister, Dionne, & Jack, 1999; Stevens, Johnston, Petryshen, & Taddio, 1996; Stevens, Johnston, Taddio, Gibbins, & Yamada, 2010).
CPOT (Critical-Care Pain Observation Tool)	A four-item scale scored from 0 to 8 developed for critically ill adults who are mechanically ventilated or not and used for the detection of pain in medical, surgical, and trauma ICUs (Gelinas, Fillion, Puntillo, Viens, & Fortier, 2006; Gelinas & Arbour, 2009; Gelinas & Johnston, 2007). The scale is easy to use while it describes four different behavioural domains.
BPS (Behavioral Pain Scale)	A three-item scale scored from 3 to 12 developed for critically ill and mechanically ventilated adults and used for the detection of pain in medical, surgical, and trauma ICUs (Payen, Bru, Bosson, et al., 2001).
Doloplus	A 10-item scale with each item scored from 0 to 3 with a maximum score of 30. Developed for older adults with cognitive impairment, including nonverbal older adults and mainly used in the chronic care settings (Torvik et al., 2010; Wary, Serbouti, & Doloplus, 2001).
PACSLAC (Pain Assessment Checklist for Seniors with Limited Ability to Communicate)	A checklist of 60 items developed for older adults whose communication capacity is limited because of dementia. The scale is intended for the use by caregivers, and it was developed based on the observations of behavioural (facial and body movements or aggression) as well as ADL changes (eating/sleeping) and includes physiological indicators (Fuchs-Lacelle & Hadjistavropoulos, 2004).

assessment and in conjunction with other pain assessment tools (Herr et al., 2011).

Diagnosing

When writing a diagnostic statement related to pain, the nurse should specify the location (e.g., right ankle pain, or left frontal headache), etiological factors and precipitating factors, when known, and may include both physiological and psychological factors. For example, in addition to the injurious agent, related factors may include knowledge deficit of pain management techniques or fear of drug tolerance or addiction. Examples of a few possible nursing diagnoses related to pain include acute somatic pain related to surgical repair of right hip fracture and movement; chronic neuropathic pain interfering with quality of life and mental status; ineffective acute visceral pain management related to fear of analgesics and personal beliefs about the need to endure pain regardless of its intensity; insomnia, impaired physical mobility, and social isolation related to allodynia; high pain tolerance when experiencing visceral anginal pain negatively impacting on client's use of nitroglycerine potentiating the risk of myocardial infarction; risk of unintentional injury (e.g., scald, cut) related to reduced nociception from peripheral nerve block.

Planning

The established goals will vary according to the diagnosis, but possible examples include the following:

- Modify or minimize pain to enable partial or complete resumption of daily activities.
- Enhance abilities to control pain or to cope with pain.
- Demonstrate actions to control pain and associated symptoms.

Examples of desired outcomes for each of these goals, although established in the planning phase, are provided in Table 30.10 in the "Evaluating" section of this chapter.

Examples of nursing interventions to assist clients experiencing pain include specific nursing activities associated with each of these interventions, which can be selected to meet the individual needs of the client. See the "Implementing" section of this chapter for details. A Sample Nursing Care Plan is provided on the next page.

When planning, nurses need to choose pain relief measures appropriate for the client on the basis of the assessment data and input from the client or support persons. Nursing interventions can include a variety of pharmacological and nonpharmacological pain management strategies. Developing a plan that incorporates a wide range

Sample Care Plan for Acute Pain

Assessment Data

Nursing Assessment

Mr. Chin is a 57-year-old Chinese-Canadian businessman who was admitted to the surgical unit of an urban hospital for the treatment of a strangulated inguinal hernia. Two days ago, he had a partial bowel resection. Postoperative orders include NPO (no food orally), intravenous infusion of 5% dextrose in 0.45% sodium chloride (D5 1/2NS) at 125 mL/h left arm, nasogastric tube to low intermittent suction with continuous drainage of 20–30 mL/h. Mr. Chin is in the dorsal recumbent (supine) position and is attempting to draw up his legs. He appears restless and is complaining of pain (7 on a scale of 0 to 10) along his abdominal incision line; he describes the pain as "throbbing" and aggravated by movement and coughing—as a result, he is not using his incentive inspirometer and avoiding getting out of bed; alleviated somewhat (5/10) with splinting (he "hugs" a pillow); no radiation; accompanied by nausea and poor quality of sleep; his understanding of the pain is: "It is expected after a big operation—I will try not to move too much, and it will likely go away on its own in a couple of days. I don't want to be a bother to anyone."

Physical Examination

Height: 188 cm
Weight: 90 kg
Body mass index (BMI): 25.5
Temperature: 37°C Oral
Heart rate: 90 beats/min, 2+ amplitude, regular
Respirations: 24/min, shallow
Blood pressure: 158/82 mm Hg
Oxygen Saturation (SpO$_2$): 96%
Skin pale, pupils dilated; intact midline abdominal incision, sutures dry, no exudate, no erythema along wound edges

Diagnostic Data

Chest x-ray and urinalysis negative, white blood count (WBC) 6.2×10^9/L

Nursing Diagnosis

Acute severe somatic pain related to surgical incision stimulation of mechanosensitive receptors; accompanied by behavioural (grimacing, restlessness), and physiological cues (e.g., elevated pulse, respirations, systolic blood pressure; and dilated pupils); Mr. C.'s coping strategy of limiting physical activity to deal with the uncontrolled acute pain places him at risk for postoperative complications (e.g., atelectasis, urinary retention, venous thromboembolism); nausea could lead to vomit increasing intra-abdominal pressure placing client at risk for wound dehiscence; his fear of being a burden may limit his disclosure of pain or request for help in managing it. *Strengths*: No apparent signs/symptoms of wound infection (a possible reason for incisional pain); nasogastric tube is patent (a blocked nasogastric [NG] tube can cause abdominal distension and visceral pain)

Client Goal

Client goal

The client will experience minimal incisional pain and discomfort.

Desired Health Outcomes

1. Pain control as evidenced by demonstrating willingness and ability to report pain to the health care team and use pharmacological and nonpharmacological pain relief measures appropriately.

2. Pain level controlled as evidenced by no or mild reported pain; increased movement and use of inspirometer, decreased nausea, protective body positioning; return to baseline of blood pressure (BP), heart rate (HR), respirations (R).

Nursing Interventions	Rationale
Pain Assessment and Management	
• Perform ongoing comprehensive pain assessment using PQRSTU.	*Pain is a subjective experience and, whenever possible, must be described by the client to plan and monitor treatment; ongoing assessment will ensure that the nurse monitors the pain in the event that Mr. Chin continues to underreport it.*

(continued)

Sample Care Plan for Acute Pain (continued)

Nursing Interventions	Rationale
Pain Assessment and Management	
• Consider cultural influences on Mr. Chin's pain response (e.g., cultural beliefs about pain can result in a stoic attitude).	*Each person experiences and expresses pain in an individual manner by using a variety of sociocultural adaptation techniques.*
• Reduce or eliminate factors that may precipitate or worsen Mr. Chin's pain experience (e.g., fear, fatigue, blocked NG tube, abrupt movements).	*Personal factors can influence pain and pain tolerance. Those factors that may be precipitating or increasing pain should be reduced or eliminated to enhance the overall pain management program.*
• Teach the use of nonpharmacological techniques (e.g., relaxation, guided imagery, music therapy, distraction) before, after, and, if possible, during potentially painful activities (e.g., deep breathing and coughing exercises, wound care, ambulation); before pain occurs or increases; and along with other pain relief measures.	*The use of nonpharmacological pain relief measures can increase the release of endorphins and enhance the therapeutic effects of analgesics.* *Each client has a right to expect maximum pain relief. Optimal pain relief is achieved by using analgesics includes determining the preferred route, drug, dosage, and frequency for each individual.*
• Medicate before an activity to increase participation, but evaluate the hazard of sedation.	*Turning and ambulation activities will be enhanced if pain is controlled.*
• Evaluate the effectiveness of the pain control measures used through ongoing assessment of Mr. Chin's pain experience.	*He is at risk of silently tolerating the pain if not specifically asked about it. It is therefore important that the nurse routinely assesses pain.*
Analgesic Administration	
• Check the prescription for drug (e.g., opioid, nonsteroidal anti-inflammatory drug [NSAID], other), dose, route, and frequency of analgesic prescribed.	*The choice of analgesia varies with the type of pain (e.g., acute, chronic, neuropathic) and the quantity (e.g., mild, moderate, severe), and client variables, such as renal and liver function. Around-the-clock (rather than "as-needed") analgesia provides better control for acute somatic pain.* *Mr. Chin will not be able to receive oral analgesia as long as he has a draining NG tube—topical, rectal, and parenteral (e.g., subcutaneous) routes must be used.*
• Institute regular dosing (around-the-clock) and monitoring, as appropriate, relative to the analgesic pharmacodynamics and pharmacokinetics.	
• Evaluate the effectiveness of the analgesic at regular, frequent intervals after each administration at the peak effect and especially after the initial doses, also observing for any signs and symptoms of untoward effects (e.g., sedation, respiratory depression, nausea and vomiting, dry mouth, and constipation).	*The analgesic dose may not be adequate to achieve pain control or may be causing intolerable or dangerous side effects or both. Ongoing evaluation will assist in making necessary adjustments for effective pain management.*
• Encourage Mr. Chin to communicate before his pain is at a 4/10 or greater and request prn (as needed) analgesia for breakthrough pain.	*Severe pain is more difficult to control and requires around-the-clock administration of analgesia as well as additional "as-needed" analgesia until pain is better controlled. Mr. Chin is already reluctant to report his pain, so ongoing encouragement may help him reduce his concerns of being a burden.*
• Document Mr. Chin's response to analgesics and any untoward effects. Implement actions to decrease untoward effects of analgesics (e.g., constipation, urinary retention).	*Side effects of opioid narcotics, among others, include drowsiness, sedation, respiratory depression, constipation, and urinary retention. A treatment plan to prevent occurrence of side effects and their monitoring should be instituted at the beginning of analgesic therapy.*
Nonpharmacological pain relief measures	
• Inquire if Mr. Chin has a preference for the type of strategy to be used. Investigate if he is receptive to nonpharmacological pain management strategies other than splinting, such as relaxation therapy.	*Mr. Chin may have preferences for nonpharmacological pain management strategies. He has already learned that splinting is helpful and may have other preferred pain management strategies that he practises at home.*

Nursing Interventions	Rationale
Pain Assessment and Management	
• Consider Mr. Chin's willingness and ability to participate, preference, past experiences, and contraindications before selecting a specific relaxation strategy.	*The client must feel comfortable trying a different approach to pain management. To avoid ineffective strategies, the client should be involved in the planning process.*
• Elicit conditioned behaviours that produce relaxation, such as deep breathing, peaceful imaging, or meditation.	*Relaxation techniques help reduce skeletal muscle tension and anxiety, which will reduce the intensity of the pain.*
• Create a quiet, nondisruptive environment with dim lights and comfortable temperature, when possible.	*Each person may find different images or approaches to relaxation more helpful than others.*
• Demonstrate and practise the relaxation technique with Mr. Chin, if he is agreeable.	*Return demonstrations by the participant provide an opportunity for the nurse to evaluate the effectiveness of teaching sessions.*
• Discuss the possible use of distraction (e.g., reading, Sudoku, television).	*Distraction reduces the perception of nociception.*
• Evaluate and document his response to relaxation therapy.	*Conveys to the health care team effective strategies in reducing or eliminating pain.*

Evaluation

Outcomes partially met. Mr. Chin accepted "around-the-clock" parenteral analgesia with his pain dropping to 2–3/10 about 30 minutes after analgesia; although he originally requested breakthrough analgesic in the daytime, he did not ring his call bell in the night to obtain additional analgesia and awoke with pain 6/10; in addition, when asked if he had pain, he continued to underreport its effects. His use of the incentive inspirometer increased, but he continued to limit his coughing and activity in bed. He attempted to use distraction and found that watching TV was most helpful; he did not like the rhythmic breathing activities but was able to start using meditation techniques that he had learned in the past. Ongoing use of his splinting technique continued.

of interventions is usually most effective. Whether in acute care or in home care, it is important for everyone involved in pain management to understand the plan of care. The plan should be documented in the client's record; in home care, a copy needs to be made available to the client, support persons, and caregivers. Involvement of the client and support persons is essential in pain management.

When the client's pattern and level of pain can be anticipated or is already known, regular or scheduled administration of analgesics can provide a therapeutic plasma level. The importance and meaning of a stable drug level in pain management should be explained to the client. With acute pain, this may be possible in the first 24 to 48 hours following surgery, when the client is likely to have pain requiring opioid analgesics. Frequency of medication administration can be adjusted to prevent pain from recurring. When persistent cancer-related pain exists,

analgesics should be given around the clock (ATC) with additional breakthrough (as needed: prn) doses available. Nonpharmacological interventions should also be regularly scheduled. The additional advantage of scheduling measures is that the client spends less time in pain and does not experience the anxiety or fear of the pain recurring.

Planning for Home Care

In preparation for discharge, the nurse needs to determine the client's and family's needs, strengths, and resources. The Assessment: Home Care box describes the specific assessment data required when establishing a discharge plan. By using the assessment data, the nurse tailors a teaching plan for the client and family (see the Teaching: Home Care box on monitoring pain on the next page).

ASSESSMENT | HOME CARE

PAIN

The nurse needs to determine the client's and family's ability to effectively cope with pain once the client is discharged:

CLIENT

• *Level of knowledge:* Mastery of pharmacological and nonpharmacological pain relief measures prescribed and

selected; adverse effects and measures to counteract these effects; warning signs to report to health care provider

• *Self-care abilities for analgesic administration:* Ability and mental capacity to use analgesics appropriately (e.g., to prepare correct dosages of analgesics and adhere to scheduled administration); physical dexterity to take pills or to administer intravenous medications and to store

(continued)

| ASSESSMENT | HOME CARE *(continued)* |

medications safely; ability to obtain prescriptions or over-the-counter medications at the pharmacy; and need for assistance in any one of the described tasks

FAMILY

- *Caregiver availability, skills, and willingness:* Primary and secondary persons able and willing to assist with pain management; shopping if the client has restricted activity; ability to comprehend selected therapies (e.g., infusion pumps, imagery, massage, positioning, and relaxation

techniques) and perform them or assist the client with them, as needed

- *Family role changes and coping:* Effect on financial status, parenting and spousal roles, sexuality, social roles

COMMUNITY

- *Resources:* Availability of and familiarity with resources, such as supplies, home care aid, or financial assistance

| TEACHING | HOME CARE |

Monitoring Pain

Understanding pain and monitoring it for changes are important tasks when a client returns home:

- Teach the client to keep a pain diary to monitor pain onset, activity before pain, pain intensity, aggravating and alleviating factors, use of analgesics or other pain relief measures.
- Instruct the client to contact a health care professional if planned pain control measures are ineffective or adverse effects arise and are problematic.

Pain Control

- Teach the use of selected nonpharmacological techniques, such as relaxation, guided imagery, distraction, music therapy, massage, and so on.
- Discuss the actions, potential adverse effects, dosages, frequency, and route of administration of prescribed analgesics.
- Suggest ways to handle adverse effects of medications and describe warning signs of medication overdose.

- Provide accurate information about tolerance, physical dependence, and addiction if opioid analgesics are prescribed and these topics are of concern.
- Instruct the client to use pain control measures *before* the pain becomes moderate to severe.
- Inform the client of the consequences of untreated pain.
- Demonstrate and have the client or caregiver redemonstrate appropriate skills to administer analgesics (e.g., skin patches, injections, infusion pumps, or patient-controlled analgesia [PCA]), when appropriate.

Resources

Nurses should provide appropriate information about how to access community resources, home care agencies, and associations that offer self-help strategies and educational materials. See the Weblinks section of this chapter for useful websites.

Generally speaking, a combination of strategies is best for the client in pain. Sometimes, strategies need to be tried and changed until the client obtains effective pain relief.

Implementing

Pain management is the alleviation of pain or a reduction in pain to a level of comfort that is acceptable to the client. It includes two basic types of nursing interventions: *pharmacological* and *nonpharmacological*. Nursing management of pain consists of both independent and collaborative nursing actions. In general, nonpharmacological pain relief measures can be executed as an independent nursing function, whereas administration of analgesic medications requires a physician's prescription. However, the decision to administer the prescribed medication is frequently the nurse's, often requiring judgment as to the dose to be given and the time of administration.

Barriers to Pain Management

Misbeliefs and knowledge deficits of nurses, other health care professionals, and clients can interfere with effective pain management. Some of these involve attitudes of the nurse or the client as well as knowledge deficits. Clients respond to pain on the basis of their culture, personal

experiences, and the meaning the pain has for them. For many people, pain is expected and accepted as a normal aspect of illness and treatments, such as surgery. Clients and families may lack knowledge of the adverse effects of pain and may have misinformation and fears regarding the use of analgesics. Clients may not report pain because they expect that nothing can be done, they think it is not severe enough, they do not want to take medication, or they feel it would distract or prejudice the health care provided. Other common misbeliefs are shown in Table 30.6.

Key Strategies in Pain Management

ACKNOWLEDGING AND ACCEPTING Basic to effective pain management is comprehensive pain assessment (see the Pain Assessment section in this chapter), which begins with believing the client. Four ways of communicating this belief follow:

1. Verbally acknowledge the presence of the pain, and use standardized measures to clarify pain intensity, quality, and impact.

TABLE 30.6   Common Misbeliefs about Pain

Misbelief	Correction
Clients experience severe pain only when they have had major surgery.	Even after minor surgery, clients can experience intense pain.
The nurse or other health care professionals are the authorities on a client's pain.	The person who experiences the pain is the only authority on its existence and nature.
Administering analgesics regularly for pain will lead to addiction.	Clients are unlikely to become addicted to an analgesic provided to treat pain.
The amount of tissue damage is directly related to the amount of pain.	Pain is a subjective experience, and the intensity and duration of pain vary considerably among individuals.
Unconscious or sedated clients cannot experience pain.	Unconscious or sedated individuals may still experience pain; recent evidence has shown that clients with altered levels of consciousness may have the ability for conscious pain perception (Boly et al., 2008; Laureys et al., 2002). The absence of pain-related behaviours in unconscious or sedated clients does not necessarily indicate absence of pain.
Visible physiological or behavioural signs accompany pain and can be used to verify its existence.	Even with severe pain, periods of physiological and behavioural adaptation can occur.

2. Listen attentively to what the client says about the pain, restating your understanding of the reported pain. Use empathetic statements, such as "I'm sorry you are hurting. It must be upsetting. I want to help you feel better."
3. Convey that you need to understand the client's pain experience and whether pain treatments are effective or not. Ask, for example, "Has the pain treatment reduced the intensity of your pain?"
4. Attend to the client's needs for pain relief promptly. It is unconscionable to believe the client's report of pain and then do nothing!

ASSISTING CAREGIVERS   Caregiver persons often need assistance to respond to the client experiencing pain. Nurses can help by giving them accurate information about the pain and providing opportunities for them to discuss their emotional reactions, which may include anger, fear, frustration, and feelings of inadequacy. Enlisting the aid of support persons in the provision of pain relief to the client may diminish their feelings of helplessness and foster a more positive attitude toward the client's pain experience. Support persons also may need the nurse's understanding and reassurance, and perhaps access to resources that will help them cope as they add the caregiver role to an already stressful life circumstance.

REDUCING MISBELIEFS ABOUT PAIN   Misbeliefs refer to incorrect beliefs that are thought to be true despite evidence to the contrary. It is important to recognize that people's beliefs about pain and their related responses to pain and treatments can be deeply entrenched in a complex array of contextual and societal factors. Reducing a client's misbeliefs about the pain and its treatment will help to prevent inadequate pain management. The nurse should explain to clients that the perception of pain is

highly individualized and that they need to help clinicians understand their pain experience. Misbeliefs are also dealt with when nurses and clients have comprehensive discussions about the client's pain experience, including the intensity and quality of the pain, the impact of the pain, its aggravating and alleviating factors, and any fears and concerns the client may be struggling with, such as fears of opioid addiction, or common opioid adverse effects, such as constipation (Watt-Watson, 1992; Watt-Watson et al., 2001). Nurses must be aware of any personal misbeliefs that they may have about the client's pain. This includes becoming aware of any prejudices they may have and discarding them when caring for a client, educating themselves about different manifestations of pain, and getting to know the client and his or her background.

REDUCING FEAR AND ANXIETY   It is important to address the meaning of pain, along with emotional components, such as anxiety or fear, associated with the pain experience. When clients have no opportunity to talk about the pain and associated fears, their perceptions and reactions to the pain can intensify; in particular, the meaning of pain can affect pain intensity (Arntz & Claassens, 2004). If the nurse establishes an effective pattern of assessment and communication and promptly attends to the client's pain-related needs, effective pain relief is more likely. By providing accurate explanations, the nurse can also reduce many of the client's fears, such as a fear of addiction or a fear that the pain will always be present.

PREVENTING PAIN   A preventive approach to pain relief involves the provision of measures to treat the pain before it occurs or before it becomes moderate to severe. **Preemptive analgesia** is the administration of analgesics before an activity or an invasive or operative procedure to treat pain before it occurs. For example, evidence suggests that treating clients perioperatively with local infiltration of an anesthetic or parenteral administration of an opioid can reduce postoperative pain and decrease the potential for the development of chronic pain (Katz, 2003). Intraoperative and postoperative administration of analgesics is also important for optimal pain relief. Nurses can use a preventative approach by providing analgesic as prescribed around the clock, rather than as needed.

Pharmacological Pain Management

Pharmacological pain management involves the use of opioids, NSAIDs, and coanalgesics (see Box 30.4).

Opioid Analgesics

Opioid analgesics include naturally occurring and synthetic opium derivatives, such as morphine and codeine. In clinical settings, opioids were commonly referred to as *narcotics*; this language is not appropriate, as narcotics include drugs not used for pain treatment. Opioids relieve pain by binding to opiate receptors in the spinal cord and by blocking its transmission to the brain where decreased pain level is perceived. Opioids also activate endogenous pain modulation in the CNS. Opiate receptors are of several different types, including mu (μ), delta (δ), and kappa (κ) receptors. The μ–opioid receptor is most commonly associated with pain relief. These drugs are prescribed by a physician or nurse practitioner practising under medical directive. The nurse requires knowledge of appropriate dose, duration of effect, time to onset, and strategies to manage adverse effects of opioid medications.

Opioids come in three primary types:

1. Full agonists. **Full agonists** bind to opioid receptors, mimicking the effects of endogenous opioids, or endorphins. Examples of full agonists include morphine, codeine, methadone, and hydromorphone. Meperidine (Demerol) is also a full agonist, but its use is *not recommended* (see the Clinical Alert box). Full agonists have no **ceiling dose**, the level at which increasing the dose results in no further increase in analgesia. Hence, their dose can be steadily increased to relieve pain.

2. *Mixed agonists–antagonists.* **Agonist–antagonist analgesic** drugs can act similar to opioids and relieve pain (agonist effect) when given to a client who has not taken any pure opioids. However, they can block or inactivate other opioid analgesics when given to a client who has been taking pure opioids (antagonist effect). These drugs include dezocine (Dalgan), pentazocine hydrochloride (Talwin), butorphanol tartrate (Stadol), and nalbuphine hydrochloride (Nubain). They block the μ–receptor site and activate a κ–receptor site. If a client has been receiving a μ-agonist (e.g., morphine) daily for more than a couple of weeks, the administration of a mixed agonist–antagonist may result in the inactivation of the morphine effect and in increased pain. These drugs have a **ceiling effect** (larger doses of a medication have progressively smaller incremental effects) that limits the dose. They are not recommended for use in terminally ill clients.

3. *Partial agonists.* **Partial agonists** have a ceiling effect. These drugs, such as buprenorphrine (Buprenex), block the μ–receptors or are neutral at that receptor but bind at a κ–receptor site. Buprenorphrine has good analgesic potency and is emerging as an alternative to methadone for opioid maintenance treatment programs.

Opioids are the most effective analgesic for the relief of moderate to severe pain and must be given on a regular basis to prevent pain from recurring. Acetaminophen is a nonopioid analgesic that is often used in a combination with a number of opioids, such as oxycodone and codeine.

BOX 30.4 CATEGORIES AND EXAMPLES OF ANALGESICS

The following are just some of the analgesics available (trade names are given in parentheses):

OPIOID ANALGESICS
- Fentanyl citrate (Duragesic)
- Oxycodone (OxyContin)
- Hydromorphone hydrochloride (Dilaudid)
- Morphine sulphate (morphine)
- Codeine (Tylenol No. 3)
- Methadone (Dolophine, Methadose)

NONOPIOID ANALGESICS
- Acetaminophen (Tylenol)
- Acetylsalicylic acid (Aspirin)
- Diclofenac sodium (Voltaren)
- Ibuprofen (Motrin, Advil)
- Indomethacin sodium trihydrate (Indocid)
- Naprosyn (Naproxen)
- Piroxicam (Feldene)
- Tolmetin sodium (Tolectin)
- Celecoxib (Celebrex)
- Ketorolac (Toradol)

COANALGESICS
- Antidepressants (amitriptyline [Elavil] nortriptyline [Aventyl])
- Anticonvulsants (carbamazepine [Tegretol], gabapentin [Neurontin], pregabaline [Lyrica])

> ## ⚠ CLINICAL ALERT
>
> Nurses must challenge the general use of meperidine in the clinical setting. This drug has a short duration (2 to 3 hours), and its toxic metabolite, normeperidine, accumulates with repetitive dosing, causing CNS excitability and the lower seizure threshold. Several organizations issued cautions against the use of meperidine, including IASP and the Institute for Safe Medication Practices (ISMP) Canada. Meperidine use is still recommended for very few clinical cases, such as in the prevention and treatment of postoperative shivering and rigors caused by certain drugs and blood product administration; or for the management of acute pain episodes for clients with significant adverse reactions to other opioid analgesics (Ashley & Given, 2008; Dobbins, 2010). In these cases, meperidine should only be given if the frontline medications (e.g., clonidine or tramadol) are ineffective or cause an adverse reaction. Meperidine should never be given to clients with poor kidney function or those taking MAOI (monoamine oxidase inhibitor) medications (Daniel & Schmelzer, 2009; Pasero & McCaffery, 2010).

Adverse effects of opioids vary with the physiological state of the client. Box 30.5 provides suggested measures to prevent side effects of opioid analgesics. Respiratory depression is one of the most dangerous side effects of opioid administration, and if the client is not monitored and treated promptly, negative outcomes may occur (Box 30.6 on the next page). As sedation is another common side effect, nurses should assess and document the client's level of awareness. If sedation is a problem, respiratory status must also be frequently monitored. Early recognition of

an increasing level of sedation or respiratory depression will enable the nurse to implement appropriate measures promptly.

When administering opioids, it is important to distinguish among the effects of *tolerance, physical dependence,* and *addiction.*

TOLERANCE With **tolerance**, progressively larger doses are needed to produce the same analgesic effects. The consensus paper written by the American Academy of Pain Medicine (AAPM), the American Pain Society (APS), and the American Society for Addiction Medicine (ASAM) defines tolerance as a "state of adaptation in which exposure to a drug induces changes that result in a diminution of one or more of the drug's effects over time" (AAPM, APS, & ASAM, 2001). The full mechanism of tolerance is not well known. A possible theory suggests that it is caused by the progressive desensitization of opioid receptors (DuPen, Shen, Ersek, 2007). In humans, tolerance to certain opioid drug effects can start taking place on the first administration, but usually it is not clinically significant. Clinicians are more concerned about tolerance that happens over time with prolonged opioid administration and that requires increasingly high doses of the drug. The need for dose escalation is often misdiagnosed as tolerance; however, it can often be caused by disease or pain progression and not the body's adaptation to

---

BOX 30.5 COMMON OPIOID ADVERSE EFFECTS: PREVENTIVE AND TREATMENT MEASURES

Opioids can have a number of side effects that nurses can help to alleviate:

CONSTIPATION

- If the client's condition allows it, increase fluid intake (e.g., 6 to 8 glasses daily).
- Add more fibre and bulk-forming agents to the diet (e.g., fresh fruits and vegetables). Increased exercise is often ineffective in controlling this type of constipation.
- Administer prophylactic daily stool softeners combined with a mild laxative (e.g., senna [Senokot], docusate sodium [Colace]) as a first line of prevention against constipation for clients on opioid maintenance therapy.
- Stimulants (e.g., bisacodyl), osmotic laxatives (e.g., lactulose, sorbitol, and polyethylene glycol), enemas (e.g., tap water and sodium phosphate), and even prokinetic agents (e.g., metoclopramide) may be needed for treating refractory constipation.

NAUSEA AND VOMITING

- Inform the client that tolerance to this emetic effect generally develops after several days of opioid therapy.
- Antiemetics (e.g., dimenHYDRINATE [Gravol], ondansetron [Zofran]) or gastrointestinal stimulants (e.g., metoclopramide) are sometimes prescribed to treat opioid-induced nausea. Because they are CNS depressants and may precipitate or increase respiratory depression, their concomitant use with opioids is not recommended. Evidence suggests that the least dangerous strategy to

reduce opioid-induced nausea and emesis is to change the dose and the route of administration or to change the opioid (Laugsand, Kaasa, & Klepstad, 2011).

SEDATION

- Inform the client that tolerance usually develops over several days.
- Observe the client's frequency of respiration and oxygen saturation as their decreased values may indicate respiratory depression, a life-threatening side effect of opioid administration. See Box 30.6 for details.

PRURITUS

- Apply cool packs and lotion, and provide a diversional activity.
- Administer an antihistamine (e.g., diphenhydrAMINE hydrochloride [Benadryl]), as ordered. As with antiemetic medications, caution must be exercised if the client is prescribed an antihistamine because of its depressant effect on the CNS.
- Inform the client that tolerance to pruritus also develops.

URINARY RETENTION

- The nurse may need to catheterize the client or change or lower the opioid dose (Fernandes, da Costa, & Saraiva, 2007). The first steps in diagnosing urinary retention are abdominal examination (palpation and percussion), the observation of a client's intake and output (I&O), and performing a bladder scan (ultrasound).

BOX 30.6 OPIOID-INDUCED RESPIRATORY DEPRESSION

Definition

Opioid-induced respiratory depression is a decrease in the effectiveness of an individual's ventilatory function after opioid administration that is usually (but not always) preceded by sedation. It is characterized by poor respiratory effort (shallow breathing) and a respiratory rate below 10 breaths per minute.

Risk Factors

Physical and Lifestyle Characteristics

- Age >65 years (>55 years if client has sleep apnea)
- Hypertension
- Obesity (BMI >30 kg/m^2)
- Smoking (>20 pack/year)
- Untreated obstructive or central sleep apnea and their predisposing factors

Primary and Comorbid Medical Conditions

- Dependent functional status (unable to walk four blocks or two flights of stairs without assistance)
- Preexisting pulmonary or cardiac disease or dysfunction (e.g., history of chronic obstructive pulmonary disease [COPD] or heart failure)
- Major organ failure (e.g., decreased hepatic or renal function)
- Poor nutritional status

Medical Factors

- Prolonged surgery >2 hours
- Thoracic and other large incisions that may interfere with circulation
- Concomitant administration of other agents with a depressant effect on the central nervous system (antihistamines, benzodiazepines, some antiemetics)
- Large single-bolus techniques (e.g., 10 mg IV morphine)
- Continuous opioid infusion in opioid-naïve clients (those who have not recently received any opioid doses).
- Prior naloxone administration (naloxone is a short-acting medication, which puts clients at risk of repeated respiratory depression once the action wears off)
- Opioid-naïve clients who require large opioid administration
- Opioid-tolerant clients who are given large administrations of opioids in addition to their own opioid regimen
- General anesthesia (as opposed to other types of anesthesia)
- Timing of opioid administration (clients are at a greater risk in the first 24 hours)

Required Monitoring

Purposeful and systematic serial assessments of pain intensity, level of sedation, and respiratory status (quality, character, rate, and effectiveness).

- Pain intensity using a valid scale (refer the "Pain Questionnaires for Nursing Practice" section)
- Oxygenation (pulse oximetry)
- Capnography monitoring (end-tidal carbon dioxide [CO_2] measures)
- Respiratory rate (rhythm, rate, depth of chest excursion)
- Ventilation efficacy (depth and rhythm of respirations, snoring, loud breathing)
- Sedation status (e.g., Sedation-Agitation Scale [SAS], Ramsay Scale, Richmond Agitation and Sedation Scale [RASS], or Pasero Opioid-Induced Sedation Scale)

Treatment

- Immediately arouse all clients with signs of advancing sedation, poor respiratory effort, or noisy respiration (e.g., snoring)
- Instruct the client to take deep breaths (inspirometer may be used to motivate the client)
- Alert other members of the care team
- Monitor the client closely until the respiratory status is recovered
- Administer Naloxone as per hospital protocol, if needed

Source: From Jarzyna, D., Jungquist, C.R., Pasero, C., Willens, J., Nisbet, A., Oakes, L., Dempsey, S.J., Santangelo, D., & Polomano, R.. (2011). American Society for Pain Management nursing guidelines on monitoring for opioid-induced sedation and respiratory depression. *Pain Management Nursing, 12*(3), 118–145.

opioids (Pasero & McCafferey, 2010). Because full agonist opioids do not have a ceiling or maximum amount, drug tolerance should not preclude achievement of adequate analgesia, with incremental dosage increases as ordered. Many clients with nonprogressive pain are able to find a stable dose of opioids that provide adequate analgesia.

PHYSICAL DEPENDENCE With **physical dependence**, people experience a need to continue to use the drug to prevent symptoms of withdrawal. The AAPM, the APS, and the ASAM (2001, p. 2) define it as "a state of adaptation that is manifested by a drug class–specific withdrawal syndrome that can be produced by abrupt cessation, rapid dose reduction, decreasing blood level of the drug and/or administration of an antagonist." Withdrawal symptoms can include vomiting, diarrhea, abdominal cramping, tremors, chills, diaphoresis, myalgia, arthralgia (joint pain not caused by inflammation), and coryza (inflammation of the mucous membranes of the nose). The term "dependence" is often used to describe a person who is addicted or has psychological dependence on the drug. Therefore, although it is appropriate to say that a person who has or could have withdrawal symptoms after the discontinuation of a drug is "physically dependent," the nurse must be careful to strictly avoid using the term "dependent" on its own.

Physical dependence and drug tolerance are involuntary behaviours and are the physiological result of frequent, ongoing opioid administration. Although physical dependence and tolerance develop, symptoms of withdrawal rarely occur because as pain decreases, the dosage is gradually tapered and no symptoms are experienced. *Physical dependence and drug tolerance do not represent addiction.*

ADDICTION No universally accepted definition of addiction to opioids exists. According to the AAPM, the APS, and the ASAM (2001, p. 2) **addiction** is characterized by the presence of adverse behaviours that feature a compulsion for the drug, craving, and a preoccupation with drug use predominantly for psychological effect, despite actual or potential harm. Determination of opioid addiction requires expert assessment of the client's history, risk factors for addiction, and potential biopsychological factors. Clinicians should not presume that clients' persistence or expression of the urgent need for pain relief is drug seeking or addictive behaviour. True opioid addiction is rare if opioids are prescribed and monitored appropriately. For most clients, opioid-seeking behaviours usually stop when the pain is adequately controlled. It is important to note that opioids can be effective for those with a history of chemical dependency on opioids; this requires prescription, supervision, and support by clinicians with expertise in pain management and chemical dependency. Guidelines for safe administration of opioids are available from a number of pain societies, such as the Canadian Pain Society and the International Association for the Study of Pain.

EQUIANALGESIC DOSING As nurses are responsible for evaluating the effectiveness of analgesics, monitoring for adverse effects, and advocating for change when an analgesic is not effective, it is important to understand the concept of **equianalgesia**, which refers to the relative potency of various opioid analgesics compared with a standard dose of morphine. An **equianalgesic dose** is the dose of one analgesic that has the same pain-relieving effect as another drug. This concept makes it possible to change one analgesic for another or to change the route of administration, for example, from parenteral to oral opioid doses. Equianalgesic dosing also allows comparisons to be made between weak analgesics, such as codeine, for mild pain, and stronger analgesics, such as morphine, for moderate to severe pain. See Table 30.7 for equianalgesic doses of common opioid medications.

The two basic techniques for calculating doses based on equianalgesic equivalents are (a) the ratio method and (b) the cross-multiplication method. For example, with the ratio technique, it is known that the oral–IV morphine ratio is 3:1, meaning IV morphine is three times as potent as oral morphine. Thus, a client who has required 100 mg of IV morphine per day will require 300 mg of oral morphine per day to control the same level of pain. If a different client who had an opioid requirement of 40 mg IV morphine per day were to be switched to oral

TABLE 30.7 Equianalgesic Chart for Some Common Opioids

Equianalgesic Dosages		
Opioid	Oral	Parenteral
Morphine	30 mg	10 mg
Codeine	200 mg NR	130 mg
Fentanyl*	—	100 μg/h (0.1 mg) is equal to 2–4 mg/h morphine IV
Hydromorphone	7.5 mg	1.5–2 mg
Meperidine	300 mg NR	75–100 mg
Methadone	20 mg	10 mg
Hydrocodone	30 mg	—
Oxycodone	15–20 mg	—

Note: For comparison, a dosage of 10 mg of parenteral morphine is established.

NR = not recommended.

*Fentanyl is also available in the transdermal route (Duragesic).

Source: Critical Care Nursing of Older Adults: Best Practice, 3rd Edition. Marquis D. Foreman, Koen Milisen, Terry T. Fulmer. Copyright © 2010, Reproduced with the permission of Springer Publishing Company, LLC.

hydromorphone, the equianalgesia chart informs the nurse that 10 mg IV morphine is equivalent to 7.5 mg hydromorphone. By using the cross-multiplication technique (x represents the unknown dose), the following steps are calculated:

10 mg IV morphine = 7.5 mg oral hydromorphone
40 mg IV morphine = x mg hydromorphone
Cross-multiply:
$10x = 7.5 \times 40$
$10x = 300$
$x = 30$ mg hydromorphone

Thus, 30 mg of oral hydromorphone per day would provide equivalent analgesia to 40 mg of IV morphine per day. The hydromorphone dose is then divided on the basis of the duration of action of the available preparations (e.g., every 4 hours).

ROUTES FOR OPIOID DELIVERY Opioids have traditionally been administered by oral routes; subcutaneous routes, including continuous subcutaneous infusions; intramuscular routes; and intravenous routes. In addition, newer methods of delivering opioids, for example, transnasal, transdermal, and rectal drug therapy, as well as intraspinal infusion, have been developed.

Oral Oral administration of opioids remains the preferred route of delivery because of ease of administration. Because the duration of action of most immediate-release (IR) opioids is approximately 4 hours, people with chronic pain have had to awaken several times during the night to medicate themselves for pain. To circumvent this problem, *long-acting*, or slow-release, forms of opioids with a duration of 8 to 12 hours have been developed. Examples of long-acting preparations are MS Contin, OxyContin, and Hydromorph Contin. Clients receiving long-acting preparations also require as-needed (prn) doses of IR analgesics (e.g., short-acting morphine, Percocet) for acute breakthrough pain.

Subcutaneous The subcutaneous (SC) route has been used extensively to deliver opioids, and another technique uses SC catheters and infusion pumps to provide *continuous subcutaneous infusion* (CSCI). The SC route is helpful for people who need long-term use of parenteral opioids and are unable to take opioids orally over the long-term, such as those experiencing dysphagia or gastrointestinal obstruction. CSCI involves the use of a small, light, battery-operated pump that administers the drug through a 23- or 25-gauge butterfly needle. The needle should be rotated between sites on the abdomen and thigh areas every 3 to 7 days. Client mobility can be maintained by attaching the pump to a belt, or using a shoulder bag or holster to hold the pump.

Because the client or the caregivers must operate the pump and change and care for the injection site, the nurse needs to provide appropriate instruction on assessment of pump functioning and care. Clients or their caregivers need to be able to do the following:

- Describe the basic parts and symbols of the system
- Identify ways to determine whether the pump is working
- Change the battery
- Change the medication
- Demonstrate stopping and starting the pump
- Demonstrate tubing care, site care, and changing of the injection site
- Identify signs indicating the need to change an injection site
- Describe general care of the pump when the client is ambulatory, bathing, sleeping, or travelling
- Identify actions to take when the alarm signals

Intramuscular The intramuscular (IM) route should not be used; it is the least desirable route for opioid administration because of variable absorption, pain involved with administration, and the need to repeat administration every 3 to 4 hours.

Intravenous The intravenous (IV) route provides rapid and effective relief of acute pain. The analgesic can be administered by continuous IV infusion, or by patient-controlled analgesia (PCA) (see the discussion on PCA later in this chapter).

Transnasal Transnasal administration has the advantage of rapid action of the medication because of direct absorption through the vascular nasal mucosa. A commonly used agent is the mixed agonist–antagonist butorphanol (Stadol) for acute headaches.

Transdermal Transdermal drug therapy is advantageous in that it delivers a relatively stable plasma drug level and is noninvasive. Fentanyl (Duragesic) is an opioid currently available as a skin patch with various dosages. It provides drug delivery for up to 72 hours. The time before the medication given via this route begins to take effect is between 12 to 16 hours; in the meanwhile, the client should be provided with short-acting opioids to relieve pain. The transdermal route is distinguished from the topical route in that the effects of the medications are systemic after the medication is absorbed; topical medications placed on the skin work locally at the point they are placed on the body.

Rectal Several opioids are now available in suppository form. The rectal route is particularly useful for clients who have dysphagia (difficulty swallowing), nausea, or vomiting.

Intraspinal An increasingly popular method of delivery is the infusion of opioids into the epidural or intrathecal (subarachnoid) space. Analgesics administered via the intraspinal route are delivered adjacent to the opioid receptors in the dorsal horn of the spinal cord. Two commonly used medications are morphine sulphate and fentanyl. All medicines administered by the intraspinal route need to be sterile and preservative free (preservatives are neurotoxic). The major benefit of intraspinal drug therapy is superior analgesia with less medication used. The epidural space is most commonly used because the dura mater acts as a protective barrier against infection, including meningitis, and there is less risk of developing a spinal headache. Intraspinal catheters are not in constant contact with blood, and thus an infusion can be stopped and restarted later without the concern that the catheter is no longer patent.

Intrathecal administration delivers medication directly into the cerebrospinal fluid (CSF) that bathes and nourishes the spinal cord. Medicines quickly and efficiently bind to the opioid receptor sites in the dorsal horn when administered in this way, speeding the onset and peak effect, while prolonging the duration of action of the analgesic. An example of how the route of administration affects the relative potency of opioids is as follows: A client who needs 300 mg of oral morphine per day to control pain will need 100 mg of parenteral morphine, 10 mg of epidural morphine, and only 1 mg of intrathecal morphine in a 24-hour period. Very little drug is absorbed by blood vessels into the systemic circulation. In fact, the drug must circulate through the CSF to be excreted. As a result, onset of respiratory depression can be delayed (24 hours after the administration) as medication that has left the spinal opioid sites travels through the brain to be eliminated. Therefore, it is essential that the nurse continues diligent monitoring of respiratory depression in clients receiving intrathecal opioids.

In contrast, the epidural space is separated from the spinal cord by the dura mater, which acts as a barrier to drug diffusion. In addition, it is filled with fatty tissue and an extensive venous system. With this diffusion delay, some medications (especially fat-soluble medications, such as fentanyl) from the epidural space enter the systemic circulation via the venous plexus. Thus, a higher dose of opiate is required to create the desired effect, which can produce side effects, such as itching, urinary retention, and respiratory depression. Often, a mixture of an opioid (e.g., fentanyl) and a local anesthetic (e.g., bupivacaine) are combined to lower the dose of opioid needed. As a result, there may be an increase in fall risk for some clients who develop muscular weakness in their legs or orthostatic hypotension in response to the local anesthetic.

Intraspinal analgesia can be administered by three modes of operation:

1. *Bolus*. A single dose, or repeated bolus doses, can be provided. When clients have spinal anesthesia (e.g., during a cesarean section), a bolus of 1 mg intrathecal morphine can provide significant pain control for up to 24 hours. For shorter-acting medications,

an epidural catheter may be intact and accessed by a qualified health care professional (e.g., anesthesiologist) to administer bolus doses on an as-needed basis. Check agency policy regarding who can provide these bolus doses, how they are documented, and the post-bolus monitoring procedures.

2. *Continuous infusion administered by pump*. The pump can be external (for acute or chronic pain) or surgically implanted (for chronic pain) to provide a continuous infusion of pain relievers into the epidural or intrathecal space.

3. *Continuous plus intermittent bolus*. With this mode of operation, the client receives a continuous infusion, with bolus rescue doses administered for breakthrough pain. Often, a pump with *patient-controlled epidural analgesia (PCEA)* capabilities is used for this mode of operation. This is similar to PCA (detailed later) in which a basal rate may or may not be used to meet the client's anticipated analgesic need, with the client's ability to request an incremental dose by pressing a button at set intervals. PCEA is often used to manage acute postoperative pain, chronic pain, and intractable cancer pain. The so-called *walking epidurals* used for women in labour are typically PCEA devices that are programmed in the bolus mode without a continuous infusion (basal rate) set.

The needle is inserted into the intrathecal or epidural space (typically in the lumbar region), and a catheter is threaded through the needle to the desired level. The catheter is connected to tubing that is then positioned along the spine and over the client's shoulder for the nurse to access. The entire catheter and tubing are taped securely to prevent dislodgement. Often, an occlusive transparent dressing is placed over the insertion site for easy identification of catheter displacement or local inflammation. Temporary catheters, used for short-term acute pain management, are usually placed at the lumbar or thoracic vertebral level and often removed after 2 to 4 days. Permanent catheters, for clients with chronic pain, may be tunnelled subcutaneously through the skin and exit at the client's side, or be connected to a pump implanted in the abdomen. Tunnelling of the catheter reduces the risk of infection and displacement of the catheter. After the catheter is inserted, the nurse is responsible for monitoring the infusion and assessing the client per institutional policy. Nursing care of clients with intraspinal infusions is summarized in Table 30.8.

There are misconceptions that either overstate or ignore the risks of spinal analgesia. This is, in part, due to the importance of the technique of the professional inserting the catheter, which varies considerably. In general, clients receiving epidural analgesia do not need to be monitored in an intensive care setting, but they do need vigilant assessment of their pain, neurological and

TABLE 30.8 Nursing Interventions for Clients Receiving Analgesics through an Epidural Catheter

Nursing Goal	Interventions
Maintain client safety	Label the tubing, the infusion bag, and the front of the pump with tape marked EPIDURAL to prevent confusion with similar-looking IV lines. Post a sign above the client's bed indicating that the epidural is in place. Secure all connections with tape. If there is no continuous infusion, apply tape over all injection ports on the epidural line to avoid the injection of substances intended for IV administration into the epidural catheter. Do not use alcohol in any care of catheter or insertion site, as it can be neurotoxic.
Maintain catheter placement	Secure temporary catheters with tape. When bolus doses are used, gently aspirate before medication administration to determine that the catheter has not migrated into the subarachnoid space. (Expect <1 mL of fluid return in the syringe.) Assist client in repositioning or moving out of bed. Assess insertion site for leakage with each bolus dose or at least every 8–12 hours.
Prevent infection	Use strict aseptic techniques with all epidural-related procedures. Maintain a sterile occlusive dressing over the insertion site. Assess the insertion site for signs of infection (e.g., redness, discoloration, secretions at the site, swelling, pain or fever [sign of a systemic infection]).
Maintain client's urinary and bowel functions	Monitor intake and output. Assess for bowel and bladder distension.
Prevent respiratory depression	Assess sedation level and respiratory status q1h for the first 24 hours and q4h thereafter. Do not administer other opioids or central nervous system depressants, unless ordered. Keep a 0.4-mg ampule of naloxone hydrochloride (Narcan) at the client's bedside. Notify the clinician in charge if the respiratory rate falls below 10 per minute or if the client is difficult to rouse.

respiratory status, and the insertion site frequently during the course of therapy.

PATIENT-CONTROLLED ANALGESIA Patient-controlled analgesia (PCA) is a method that allows clients to self-administer their own opioids whenever they feel it is necessary. PCA involves an infusion system with a pump. With a PCA pump, the client pushes a button to release a set amount of opioid by bolus via the intravenous, subcutaneous, or epidural route. PCA pumps usually have a chamber or cartridge that contains the analgesic, a mechanism for setting the ordered dose, and a control for client activation. When clients want a dose of analgesic, they can push a button attached to the infusion pump and the preset dose is delivered. A programmable lockout interval (usually 10 to 15 minutes) follows the dose, when an additional dose cannot be given even if the client activates the button. It is also possible to program the maximum dose that can be delivered over a period of hours (usually 4 hours). Many pumps are capable of delivering a low continuous infusion, or basal rate, to provide sustained analgesia during times of rest and sleep. Older children can be taught to use PCAs.

People using PCA tend to take less total analgesia than those receiving intermittent injections (Pasero & McCaffery, 2010). PCA is used for the management of postoperative pain and for other types of acute pain, such as sickle-cell crisis, and for cancer pain. A major advantage to PCA is that it can meet pain relief needs of clients in a more flexible manner compared with conventional analgesic methods (McIntyre, 2001). Whether in an acute care hospital setting, an ambulatory clinic, or home care, the nurse is responsible for the initial instruction regarding the use of the PCA and for the ongoing monitoring of the therapy (see the Teaching: Clinical box). The client's pain must be assessed at regular intervals and analgesic use documented in the client's record. Client concerns about addiction and adverse effects also need to be assessed and addressed. If the PCA pump is used with a child, the nurse must engage in interactive teaching with the child and parents. Additionally, the child's ability to use the PCA client control button must be assessed. Older adults may have more comorbidities and need to be monitored for medication side effects as well as impaired renal and pulmonary functions. Older adults must also be assessed for cognitive and physical ability to push the client control button.

TEACHING **CLINICAL**

Client Self-Management of Pain by Using a Patient-Controlled Analgesia Pump

Choose a time to teach the client about pain management when the pain is controlled so that the client is able to focus on the teaching.

Teaching the client about self-management of pain can include the following:

- Demonstrate the operation of the patient-controlled analgesia (PCA) pump and explain that the client can safely push the button without fear of overmedicating. Sometimes, it helps clients who are reluctant to repeatedly push the button to know that they must dose themselves (i.e., push the button) 5 to 10 times

to receive the same amount of medication (10 mg morphine equivalent) they would receive in a standard injection.

- Describe the use of the pain scale and encourage the client to respond to demonstrate understanding.
- Explore a variety of nondrug pain relief techniques that the client is willing to learn and use to promote pain relief and optimize functioning.
- Explain to the client the need to notify staff when ambulation is desired (e.g., for bathroom use), if applicable.

Nonopioid Analgesics

NONSTEROIDAL ANTI-INFLAMMATORY DRUGS
Nonsteroidal anti-inflammatory drugs (NSAIDs), sometimes referred to as nonopioids, include drugs from the following categories: (a) first-generation (COX-1 and COX-2 inhibitors; e.g., Aspirin, ibuprofen, naproxen, ketorolac), and (b) second-generation (COX-2 inhibitors, e.g., celecoxib). These medications have anti-inflammatory, analgesic, and antipyretic effects. They relieve pain mainly by blocking the action of cyclooxygenase (COX, which has two forms: COX-1 and COX-2), the enzyme necessary for the synthesis of prostaglandins that sensitize nerve endings and trigger pain at the periphery (i.e., transduction). The inhibition of COX-1 is responsible for many of the side effects, such as gastric ulceration, bleeding due to platelet inhibition, and acute renal failure. In contrast, the inhibition of COX-2 is responsible for the suppression of pain and inflammation (Lehne, 2009). The use of medication that is a combination of an NSAID and an opioid is indicated for clients with acute musculoskeletal and soft tissue inflammation. Individual drugs in this category vary widely in their analgesic properties, metabolism, excretion, and adverse effects. In addition, the analgesic activity of these drugs has a ceiling effect. Not all clients are candidates for NSAIDs because of side effects. Caution is advised with older adults or clients with renal impairment because of slower clearance rates in these individuals.

The most common adverse effect of NSAIDs is dyspepsia, which can be minimized by taking the medication with food. Stomach ulcers and gastric bleeding have also been reported; those on longer-term NSAID therapy may be prescribed proton-pump inhibitors to preserve the gastric mucosa. NSAIDs may be contraindicated for those with impaired blood clotting, gastrointestinal bleeding or ulcer risk, renal disease, thrombocytopenia (low platelet levels), Aspirin triad (i.e., bronchial asthma, Aspirin intolerance, and rhinitis), and possible infection. Many

NSAIDs require a prescription and all have a maximum daily dose limit. Clients and nurses should be aware that dark tarry stools may indicate gastrointestinal bleeding, one of the more dangerous effects of NSAIDs. Depending on the nature of the pain problem, NSAIDs may be prescribed in combination with opioids or coanalgesics. It is also common for an NSAID, such as ibuprofen, to be prescribed together with acetaminophen (Tylenol) to achieve more efficient analgesia.

ACETAMINOPHEN
Acetaminophen (Tylenol) has a different mechanism of action and side effect, or toxicity profile, from that of NSAIDs. It does not affect platelet function and rarely causes gastrointestinal distress, ulcers, skin, or cardiovascular problems. Hepatotoxicity, and possibly renal toxicity, does occur with higher doses or with long-term use. Generally, 10 g of acetaminophen is considered a lethal dose, with 6 g per day causing measurable liver damage. It is recommended that otherwise young and healthy people limit acetaminophen consumption to less than 4 g/day, with susceptible individuals (e.g., older adults, those with a history of alcoholism, those with liver disease) limiting their consumption to 2.4 g/day or less (Pasero & McCaffery, 2010).

Coanalgesics

A **coanalgesic** agent (formerly known as an *adjuvant*) is a medication that is not classified as a pain medication but that has properties that can reduce pain, alone or in combination with other analgesics; relieve other discomforts; potentiate the effect of pain medications; or reduce the pain medication's side effects. Examples of coanalgesics are antidepressants, anticonvulsants, and others.

Tricyclic antidepressants, such as amitriptyline (Elavil) or nortriptyline (Aventyl), interfere with the reuptake of epinephrine and serotonin in the CNS, leading to reduced pain perception when given in low doses.

Anticonvulsants, such as carbamazepine (Tegretol), stabilize nerve membranes, reducing excitability and spontaneous firing. Gabapentin (Neurontin) and pregabaline (Lyrica) are thought to modulate the electrical activity of the brain by modulating the release of excitatory neurotransmitters (Pasero & McCaffery, 2010). These agents appear to be particularly beneficial in the management of neuropathic pain. Anxiolytics, sedatives, and antispasmodics are examples of medicines that relieve other discomforts but do not alleviate pain and thus should be used in addition to, rather than instead of analgesics. Examples of medications used to reduce the side effects of analgesics include stimulants, laxatives, and antiemetics.

Placebo Response

The **placebo response** occurs when people experience pain relief from an intervention that may not be directly related to the actual pain relief method employed. Health care professionals can cause a positive placebo response by the ways they interact with clients. The nurse's empathic approach toward the client, such as listening without judgment, giving opportunities to express pain and permission to do so, and recognizing the person's unique responses, help to facilitate pain relief. Medication placebos, such as giving a saline injection instead of an opioid, are unethical and must not be used in practice.

Nonpharmacological Pain Management

Nonpharmacological pain management consists of a variety of physical, cognitive–behavioural, and lifestyle pain management strategies that target the body, mind, spirit, and social interactions (Table 30.9). Physical

TABLE 30.9 Nonpharmacological Interventions for Pain Control

Target Domain of Pain Control	Intervention	Pain Pathway Implicated
Body	Reducing pain triggers, promoting comfort Massage Applying heat or ice Electric stimulation (TENS) Positioning, bracing (selective immobilization) Acupressure Invasive interventions (e.g., blocks) Sleep hygiene Diet, nutritional supplements, exercise	May involve various pain pathways Perception (see GCT) Transmission, transduction, perception Perception, ascending modulation Transduction, transmission Ascending modulation, perception Transmissions and other processes Perception and modulation May involve multiple pain pathways
Mind	Relaxation, imagery Self-hypnosis Distracting attention Pain diary, journal writing Repatterning thinking Attitude adjustment Reducing fear, anxiety, stress Reducing sadness, helplessness Information about pain	*Mind* activities primarily involve perception and modulation
Spirit	Prayer, meditation Self-reflection about life and pain Meaningful rituals Energy work (e.g., therapeutic touch, reiki) Spiritual healing Functional restoration	*Spirit* pain intervention domains involve perception and modulation but may evolve to implicate other pain pathways
Social Interactions	Improved communication Family therapy Problem solving Vocational training Volunteering Support groups	May implicate various pain pathways

modalities include cutaneous stimulation, immobilization or therapeutic exercises, transcutaneous electrical nerve stimulation (TENS), and acupuncture. Mind–body (cognitive–behavioural) interventions include distracting activities, relaxation techniques, imagery, meditation, biofeedback, hypnosis, cognitive reframing, emotional counselling, and spiritually directed approaches, such as therapeutic touch or reiki. Lifestyle management approaches include symptom monitoring, stress management, exercise, nutrition, pacing activities, disability management, and other approaches used by many clients with persistent pain that has caused a drastic change in their lives. Detailed information on selected mind–body interventions is provided in Chapter 16. The discussion here is limited to selected physical and cognitive–behavioural interventions.

Physical Interventions

The goals of physical intervention include providing comfort, altering physiological responses to reduce pain perception, and optimizing functioning.

CUTANEOUS STIMULATION Cutaneous stimulation can provide effective temporary pain relief. It distracts the client and focuses attention on the tactile stimuli, away from the painful sensations, thus reducing pain perception. Cutaneous stimulation is also believed to create the release of endorphins that block pain stimuli transmission and stimulate large-diameter A-beta sensory nerve fibres, thus decreasing the transmission of pain impulses through the smaller A-delta and C fibres. Cutaneous stimulation techniques include the following:

- Massage
- Application of heat or cold
- Acupressure
- Contralateral stimulation

Cutaneous stimulation can be applied directly to the painful area, proximal to the pain, distal to the pain (along the nerve path or dermatome), and contralateral (exact location, opposite side of the body) to the pain. Cutaneous stimulation is contraindicated in areas of skin breakdown and for those clients with impaired neurological functioning.

Massage Massage is a comfort measure that can aid relaxation and decrease muscle tension as well as ease anxiety as the physical contact communicates caring. Massage can also decrease pain intensity by increasing superficial circulation to the area. Massage can involve the back and neck, hands and arms, or feet (see Chapter 38 for a discussion on back massage).

Heat and Cold Applications A warm bath, warm pads, ice bags, ice massage, warm or cold compresses, and warm or cold sitz baths, in general, relieve pain and promote healing of injured tissues (see Chapter 35). These are modalities of pain management that are not time consuming and are easily obtained in any setting; they should not be overlooked by clinicians as a complementary strategy for the standard pain management techniques. Application of heat should, however, be used with caution, especially in the emergency department setting.

Acupressure Acupressure developed from the ancient Chinese healing system of acupuncture. The therapist applies finger pressure to points that correspond to many of the points used in acupuncture (see Chapter 16).

Contralateral Stimulation Contralateral stimulation can be accomplished by stimulating the skin in an area opposite to the painful area (e.g., stimulating the left knee if the pain is in the right knee). The contralateral area may be scratched for itching, massaged for cramps, if appropriate, or treated with cold packs or analgesic ointments. This method is particularly useful when the painful area cannot be touched because it is hypersensitive, when it is inaccessible by a cast or bandages, or when the pain is felt in a missing part (phantom pain).

IMMOBILIZATION AND BRACING Immobilizing or restricting the movement of a painful body part (e.g., arthritic joint, traumatized limb) may help to manage episodes of acute pain. Splints or supportive devices should hold joints in the position of optimal function and should be removed regularly in accordance with agency protocol to provide range-of-motion (ROM) exercises, if not contraindicated. Prolonged immobilization can result in joint contracture, muscle atrophy, and cardiovascular problems. Therefore, clients should be encouraged to participate in self-care activities and remain as active as possible, with frequent ROM exercises.

TRANSCUTANEOUS ELECTRICAL NERVE STIMULATION Transcutaneous electrical nerve stimulation (TENS) is a method of applying low-voltage electrical stimulation directly over identified pain areas, at an acupressure point, along peripheral nerve areas that innervate the pain area, or along the spinal column. The TENS unit consists of a portable, battery-operated device with lead wire and electrode pads that are applied to the chosen area of skin. Cutaneous stimulation from the TENS unit is thought to activate large-diameter fibres that modulate the transmission of the nociceptive impulse in the peripheral nervous system and CNS (closing the pain gate), resulting in pain relief. This stimulation may also cause a release of endorphins from the CNS centres.

ACUPUNCTURE Acupuncture, a form of traditional Chinese medicine, involves the insertion of thin sterile needles into specific points of the skin with the goal of relieving pain (see Chapter 16).

Cognitive–Behavioural Interventions

The goals of cognitive–behavioural interventions include providing comfort, altering psychological responses to reduce pain perception, and optimizing functioning. Selected cognitive–behavioural interventions include distraction, elicitation of the relaxation response, and psychoeducation.

DISTRACTION Distraction draws the person's attention away from the pain and lessens the perception of pain. In some instances, distraction can make a client completely unaware of pain. For example, a client recovering from surgery may feel no pain while watching a football game on television, yet feel pain again when the game is over. Different types of distraction include visual distraction (reading or watching TV, guided imagery), auditory distraction (listening to music, humour), tactile distraction (slow rhythmic breathing, massage, holding and stroking a pet or a toy), and intellectual distraction (playing table or card games, doing a puzzle, hobbies).

ELICITATION OF THE RELAXATION RESPONSE Stress increases pain, in part by increasing muscle tension, activating the sympathetic nervous system, and putting the client at risk for stress-related types of pain (e.g., tension headaches). The relaxation response decreases and counteracts the harmful effects of stress, including the effect it has on physical, cognitive, and emotional functioning. Eliciting this response requires more than simply helping a person to relax; rather, it involves a structured technique designed to focus the mind and relax muscle groups. Basic techniques with helpful scripts are detailed by Pasero and McCaffery (2010), with common techniques including progressive relaxation, breath-focus relaxation, and meditation. The nurse can coach the client, urge self-directed meditation, or provide an audiotaped guide to help elicit the relaxation response. Many clients can achieve the desired state after a few attempts, but mastery of this skill requires daily practice over a few weeks. In general, relaxation techniques by themselves do not have distinct pain-relieving properties; however, they can reduce pain that may have been exacerbated by stress. Some clients may become more consciously aware of their pain while practising relaxation techniques before they have mastered controlling mind chatter and remaining mentally focused.

PSYCHOEDUCATION Once the client has mastered the basic skills for eliciting the relaxation response, techniques of imagery or self-hypnosis can be considered. Both imagery and hypnosis begin with attaining a deep state of relaxation and are capable of altering the experience of pain, for example, by having the client replace their pain with a feeling of pleasant

---

LIFESPAN CONSIDERATIONS

Pain Management

INFANTS

- Giving an infant, particularly a very low-birth-weight infant, a water and sucrose solution administered through a pacifier provides some evidence of pain reduction during procedures that may be painful, but it should not be a substitute for anesthetic or analgesic medications.

CHILDREN

- Distract the child with toys, books, or pictures.
- Hold the child to console him or her and provide comfort.
- Explore misbeliefs about pain and correct them in understandable concrete terms. Be aware of how your explanations may be misunderstood. For example, telling a child that surgery will not hurt because he or she will be "put to sleep" will be very upsetting to a child who knows of an animal that was "put to sleep."
- Children can use their imagination during guided imagery. To use the pain switch, ask the child to imagine a pain switch (even give it a colour) and tell him or her to visualize turning the switch off in the area where he or she has pain. A "magic glove" or "magic blanket" is an imaginary object that the child applies on areas of the body (e.g., hand, thigh, back, hip) to lessen discomfort.

OLDER ADULTS

- Promote the client's use of pain-control measures that have worked in the past.
- Spend time with the client, and listen carefully.
- Clarify misbeliefs. Encourage independence, whenever possible.
- Carefully review the treatment plan to avoid drug–drug, food–drug, or disease–drug interactions.

If desired health outcomes are *not* achieved, the nurse and the client need to explore the reasons before modifying the care plan. The following are some questions the nurse might consider:

- Is adequate analgesic being given? Would the client benefit from a change in dose or in the time interval between doses?
- Were the client's beliefs and values about pain therapy considered?
- Did the client understate the pain experience for some reason?
- Were appropriate instructions provided to allay misbeliefs about pain management?
- Did the client and support people understand the instructions about pain management techniques?
- Is the client receiving adequate support from his or her significant others?
- Has the client's physical condition changed, necessitating modifications in interventions?
- Should selected intervention strategies be re-evaluated?

numbness (Arnstein, 2004). Additional posthypnotic suggestions can then be made, linking these pleasant numb sensations to coping efforts used during the day (e.g., "Every time you stop to take a slow, deep, diaphragmatic breath, you will feel this pleasant numbness instead of pain").

Psychoeducation is increasingly being used as an adjunctive means of managing the impact of chronic pain on health-related quality of life and disability (McGillion, Watt-Watson, Kim, & Yamada, 2004; McGillion et al., 2007). Psychoeducational interventions are group self-management education programs delivered by a trained facilitator; clients can be accompanied by family members or friends if they want. The focus is to provide participants with an opportunity to enhance their skills for self-care. Through rehearsal and application of various cognitive and behavioural self-management techniques, participants learn to set realistic self-management goals in relation to their chronic pain. The goal-setting process allows for the self-attribution of success thereby improving perceived self-efficacy in managing symptoms. Nurses facilitating psychoeducation programs require expertise in psychoeducational techniques, group process, and assessment of participants' readiness to engage in self-management.

See the Lifespan Considerations box for age-specific ways to manage pain.

Evaluating

By using the desired outcomes established during the planning stage as a guide, the nurse and the client determine whether client goals and outcomes have been achieved. Examples of client goals and related outcomes are shown in Table 30.10.

To assist in the evaluation process, a flowsheet or a client diary may be helpful. Columns for day, time, onset of pain, activity before pain, pain-relief measure, and duration of pain can be devised to help the client and nurse determine the effectiveness of pain-relief strategies.

TABLE 30.10 Evaluation Goals and Outcomes: Pain

Goal	Examples of Desired Health Outcomes
Modify or minimize pain to enable partial or complete resumption of daily activities	Reports pain relief at level of (specify) or less, on a scale of 0 to 10; or expresses feelings of reasonable comfort Reports decreased frequency and length of pain episodes or decreased fear and anxiety Absence of nonverbal pain responses, such as restlessness, muscle tension, protective body position, facial grimacing (specify) Reports increase in mobility and physical activity, in hours of uninterrupted sleep at night, and in quality of life
Enhance abilities to control pain	Identifies factors that precipitate or intensify the pain experience Identifies both pharmacological and nonpharmacological pain management techniques Identifies ways to prevent side effects of drugs
Demonstrate actions to control pain and associated symptoms	Reduces or eliminates factors that precipitate or intensify the pain experience Uses a pain diary to monitor pain pattern and effectiveness of pain measures Uses planned nonpharmacological pain relief measures (specify) Uses analgesics appropriately

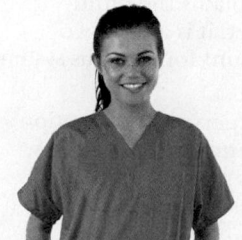

Case Study 30

Mrs. Lundahl, 45 years old, underwent an emergency anterior bowel resection approximately 6 hours ago. She has a 15-cm midline incision that is covered with a dry and intact surgical dressing. On assessing Mrs. Lundahl, you note that she is perspiring, lying in a rigid position, holding her abdomen, and grimacing. Her blood pressure is 150/90; heart rate, 100; and respiratory rate, 32. She rates her pain as 8 on a scale of 0 to 10.

(continued)

CRITICAL THINKING QUESTIONS

1. What conclusions, if any, can be drawn about Mrs. Lundahl's pain status?

2. What type of pain is Mrs. Lundahl experiencing?

3. What interventions, in addition to pain medication, may be useful in reducing Mrs. Lundahl's pain?

4. How will you know if your interventions have been effective in reducing Mrs. Lundahl's pain?

Check the eText in MyNursingLab for answers and explanations.

KEY TERMS

acute pain   *p. 742*

addiction   *p. 765*

agonist–antagonist
   analgesic   *p. 762*

allodynia   *p. 741*

ceiling dose   *p. 762*

ceiling effect   *p. 762*

central disinhibition
   p. 742

central neuropathic
   pain   *p. 742*

central sensitization
   p. 746

chronic pain   *p. 742*

coanalgesic   *p. 769*

complex regional pain
   syndrome   *p. 742*

equianalgesia   *p. 765*

equianalgesic dose
   p. 765

full agonist   *p. 762*

hyperalgesia   *p. 741*

hyperexcitability   *p. 741*

modulation   *p. 745*

nervous system
   plasticity   *p. 746*

neuropathic pain   *p. 740*

neuroplasticity   *p. 741*

nociception   *p. 743*

nociceptive pain   *p. 740*

nociceptors   *p. 740*

nonsteroidal anti-
   inflammatory drug
   (NSAID)   *p. 769*

pain   *p. 738*

pain management   *p. 760*

pain threshold   *p. 743*

pain tolerance   *p. 743*

partial agonist   *p. 762*

patient-controlled
   analgesia (PCA)   *p. 768*

perception   *p. 745*

peripheral neuropathic
   pain   *p. 741*

peripheral sensitization
   p. 746

physical dependence
   p. 765

placebo response   *p. 770*

preemptive analgesia
   p. 761

referred pain   *p. 751*

sensitization   *p. 746*

somatic pain   *p. 740*

tolerance   *p. 763*

transcutaneous
   electrical nerve
   stimulation (TENS)
   p. 771

transduction   *p. 744*

transmission   *p. 744*

visceral pain   *p. 740*

wind-up   *p. 746*

CHAPTER HIGHLIGHTS

- Pain is a subjective, multidimensional experience with sensory–discriminative, cognitive–evaluative, and motivational–affective components; many clients need encouragement or help to communicate their pain experience, particularly with respect to its intensity, duration, qualities, and related individual responses.

- Unrelieved pain has multiple serious consequences and can prolong recovery from surgery, disease, and trauma.

- Pain can be categorized according to its origin (e.g., somatic, visceral, neuropathic) or according to its duration (e.g., acute pain, chronic pain).

- Pain threshold is relatively similar in all people and changes little in the same individual over time; conversely, pain tolerance and response vary considerably from person to person *and* in the same person at different times and in different circumstances.

- For pain to be experienced, primary afferent nociceptors must be stimulated. Three types of pain stimuli are mechanical, thermal, and chemical.

- The pain process is complex and involves transduction, transmission, perception, and modulation.

- Endogenous opioids, critical to pain modulation, include enkephalins, endorphins, and dynorphins.

- Gate control theory is the basis of many pain-intervention strategies and explains the multi-dimensional nature of pain; yet, it is a theory of acute pain, and it cannot account for nervous system plasticity.

- Numerous factors influence a person's perception and reaction to pain: ethnic and cultural values, developmental stage, environment and support people, past pain experiences, and meaning of pain.

- Pain is subjective, and the most reliable indicator of the presence or intensity of pain is the client's self-report. Assessment of a client who is experiencing pain should include a comprehensive pain history. Clients who cannot self-report (e.g., comatose clients) require specialized assessment techniques.

- Multiple nursing diagnoses related to pain can be formulated; many also relate to the consequences of the pain experience (e.g., social isolation).

- Overall client goals include preventing, modifying, or eliminating pain so that the client is able to partially or completely resume usual daily activities and to cope more effectively with the pain experience.

- When planning, nurses need to choose pain-relief measures appropriate for the client. Nursing interventions should include a variety of pharmacological and nonpharmacological interventions. Selecting several strategies from both broad categories is usually most effective.

- Scheduling the measures to *prevent* pain is far more supportive of the client than trying to deal with pain once it is established.

- Pain management includes two basic types of nursing interventions: pharmacological and nonpharmacological.

- Major nursing functions for all clients are to acknowledge and convey belief in the client's pain, assist support people, reduce misbeliefs about pain, and reduce fear and anxiety associated with the pain.

- Pharmacological interventions include the use of opioids, nonopioids or NSAIDs, and coanalgesics.

- The nurse assesses the client's pain needs, administers the prescribed analgesics, and evaluates the client's response to analgesics provided.

- Analgesic medication can be delivered through a variety of routes and methods to meet the specific needs of the client. These routes include oral, subcutaneous with a continuous infusion, intravenous, transnasal, transdermal or topical, rectal, and intraspinal.

- Patient-controlled analgesia (PCA) enables the client to exercise control and minimize feelings of helplessness.

- Nonpharmacological pain interventions include cutaneous stimulation, such as warm and cold applications, massage, acupressure, and contralateral stimulation; transcutaneous electrical nerve stimulation (TENS); and immobilization or bracing.

- Examples of cognitive–behavioural interventions include distraction techniques and psychoeducation.

- Evaluation of the client's pain therapy includes the response of the client, the changes in the pain, and the client's perceptions of the effectiveness of the therapy. Ongoing verbal or written feedback from the client and family is integral to this process.

ASSESS YOUR LEARNING

1. When an excited nociceptor converts a noxious stimulus into an action potential, this is referred to as which of the following?

   a. Modulation

   b. Perception

   c. Transduction

   d. Transmission

2. Which of the following indicates a placebo response?

   a. The person's pain is not real.

   b. Inflammation has subsided.

   c. The person experiences pain relief after the nurse verbally states the pain will subside.

   d. The client has failed to respond to opioids.

3. Which of the following will the nurse perform to check for the presence of the most dangerous adverse effect of opioids?

   a. A respiratory assessment

   b. A bladder scan or palpation

   c. An assessment of the level of pruritus

   d. An assessment of the client's bowel function

4. A client who is receiving treatment for unmanaged chronic pain is prescribed morphine and nortriptyline, an antidepressant. The client states, "I'm here for pain, not depression! Give me the morphine but I refuse the other pill!" The nurse responds with which of the following statements about the antidepressant?

   a. "This pill is meant to prevent you from getting depressed because of the pain you have been experiencing."

   b. "This pill will help reduce any inflammation that you might have."

   c. "This pill will help your nervous system by increasing your body's own pain-reducing substances."

   d. "This pill helps to block the pain signals from going up your spinal cord."

5. A patient recovering from a surgical intervention requires increasing doses of analgesia in the postoperative period to control pain. Of the following possibilities, which is the most likely hypothesis to explain this pattern?

   a. Tolerance to the analgesia has occurred.

   b. Physical dependence on the analgesia has occurred.

c. Addiction to the analgesia has occurred.

d. Compulsive drug abuse has been established.

6. The patient is prescribed morphine 2.5 mg to 5 mg IV every 4 hours. He received 2.5 mg IV 4 hours ago for pain rated at 3 on a scale of 0 to 10. He is now watching TV and visiting with family members. When asked about his pain, he rates it as a 5. His vital signs (VS) are stable. What nursing intervention is the MOST appropriate?

a. Give morphine 3.5 mg IV and inform him to continue watching TV because it is a distraction from the pain

b. Give 2.5 mg of morphine IV to avoid the client becoming addicted

c. Give nothing at this time because he is not exhibiting any signs of pain

d. Give morphine 5 mg IV and reassess in 20 minutes

7. During an admission nursing assessment, a client with diabetes describes his leg pain as a "dull, burning sensation." The nurse recognizes this description as characteristic of which type of pain?

a. Referred

b. Somatic

c. Visceral

d. Neuropathic

8. Which of the following is the need to continue the use of an opioid to prevent the symptoms of withdrawal?

a. A psychological response

b. A physiological response

c. A threshold response

d. An addictive response

9. Ms. Aitken, 45 years old, has acute pain following a fractured ankle. The physician's order is acetaminophen (Tylenol #3) with 30 mg of codeine one to two tablets, q3–4h prn. Although the last dose was given 1 hour ago, she reports severe pain. What nursing action is most appropriate?

a. Consult the nurse-in-charge

b. Reassess Ms. Aitken's pain in 15 minutes

c. Notify the physician of Ms. Aitken's pain level

d. Administer an additional dose while awaiting a new order

10. A client who has been receiving 100 mg IV morphine per day is now being prescribed oral hydromorphone (Dilaudid). The equianalgesia chart indicates that 10 mg IV morphine is equivalent to 7.5 mg oral hydromorphone. How many milligrams of hydromorphone will this client receive daily that is equivalent to the IV dosage of morphine?

a. 0.75 mg oral hydromorphone (Dilaudid) per day

b. 7.5 mg oral hydromorphone (Dilaudid) per day

c. 75 mg oral hydromorphone (Dilaudid) per day

d. 750 mg oral hydromorphone (Dilaudid) per day

Check the eText in MyNursingLab for answers and explanations.

WEBLINKS

The Canadian Pain Society

http://www.canadianpainsociety.ca

The Canadian Pain Society is a chapter of the International Association for the Study of Pain. The site provides information on research opportunities, conferences, interest groups, and news about pain practices.

International Association for the Study of Pain

http://www.iasp-pain.org

This association is the largest multidisciplinary nonprofit international association in the field of pain. Its goal is to advance research on pain and improve the care of clients with pain. The site provides an overview of the association and its activities, as well as links to publications and continuing education initiatives.

Institute for the Study and Treatment of Pain

http://www.istop.org

This is a Canadian nonprofit society dedicated to research, treatment, training, and education in chronic pain. Information about the society and treatment options for people with chronic pain is available at this site.

Canadian Pain Coalition

http://www.canadianpaincoalition.ca

The Canadian Pain Coalition is "a partnership of patient pain groups, health professionals who care for people in pain, and scientists studying better ways of treating pain."

Chronic Pain Association of Canada

http://www.chronicpaincanada.com

The Chronic Pain Association of Canada is a nonprofit group that focuses on treatments and the management of chronic intractable pain.

MyNursingLab

REFERENCES

Adler, J. E., Nico, L., VandeVord, P., & Skoff, A. M. (2009). Modulation of neuropathic pain by a glial-derived factor. *Pain Medicine, 10*(7), 1229–1236. doi: 10.1111/j.1526-4637.2009.00708.x

American Academy of Pain Medicine, American Pain Society, & American Society of Addiction Medicine. (2001). Definitions related to the use of opioids for the treatment of pain: A consensus document from the American Academy of Pain Medicine, the American Pain Society, and the American Society of Addiction Medicine. Retrieved from http://www.painmed.org/Workarea/DownloadAsset.aspx?id=3204

American Educational Research Association, American Psychological Association, & National Council on Measurment in Education. (1999). *Standards for educational and psychological testing.* Washington, DC: American Educational Research Association.

American Geriatric Society. (2002). The management of persistent pain in older persons. *Journal of the American Geriatric Society, 50,* S205–S224.

Anand, K. J. S., & Craig, K. D. (1996). New perspectives on the definition of pain. *Pain, 67,* 3–6.

American Pain Society. (1999). *Principles of analgesic use in treatment of acute pain and cancer pain* (4th ed.). Glenview, IL: American Pain Society.

Argoff, C. E., Albrecht, P., Irving, G., & Rice, F. (2009). Multimodal analgesia for chronic pain: Rationale and future directions. *Pain Medicine, 10*(S2), S53–S66. doi: 10.1111/j.1526-4637.2009.00669.x

Arnstein, P. M. (2004). Chronic neuropathic pain: Issues in patient education. *Pain Management Nursing, 5*(4), 34–41.

Arntz, A., & Claassens, L. (2004). The meaning of pain influences its experienced intensity. *Pain, 109*(1–2), 20–25. doi: 10.1016/j.pain.2003.12.030

Ashley, E., & Given, J. (2008). Pain management in the critically ill. *Critical Illness, 18*(11), 504–509. ISSN 1467-1026.

Ballantyne, M., Stevens, B., McAllister, M., Dionne, K., & Jack, A. (1999). Validation of the premature infant pain profile in the clinical setting. *Clinical Journal of Pain, 15*(4), 297–303.

Bartocci, M., Bergqvist, L. L., Lagercrantz, H., & Anand, K. J. S. (2006). Pain activates cortical areas in the preterm newborn brain. *Pain, 122*(1-2), 109–117. doi: 10.1016/j.pain.2006.01.015

Basbaum, A., & Bushnell, M. C. (2002). Pain: Basic mechanisms. In Giamberardino, M. A. (Ed.), *Pain 2002, An updated review: Refresher course and syllabus* (pp. 3–9). Seattle, WA: IASP Press.

Basbaum, A., & Jessell, T. (2000). The perception of pain. In Kandel, E. R., Schwartz, J. H., & Jessell, T. (Eds.). *Principles of neural science* (4th ed.). NewYork, NY: McGraw-Hill, Health Professions Division.

Bennett, M. (2001). The LANSS Pain Scale: the Leeds assessment of neuropathic symptoms and signs. [Clinical Trial Validation Studies]. *Pain, 92*(1-2), 147–157.

Boly, M., Faymonville, M. E., Schnakers, C., Peigneux, P., Lambermont, B., Phillips, C., . . . Laureys, S. (2008). Perception of pain in the minimally conscious state with PET activation: An observational study. *Lancet Neurology, 7*(11), 1013–1020.

Bonica, J. J. (1990). *The management of pain.* Philadelphia, PA: Lea & Febiger.

Campbell, J. N., & Meyer, R. A. (2006). Mechanisms of neuropathic pain. *Neuron, 52*(1), 77–92.

Canadian Nurses Association. (2008). Code of Ethics for Registered Nurses, Centennial Edition. *Nursing values and ethical responsibilities.* Ottawa, ON: Canadian Nurses Association.

Canadian Pain Society. (2005). *Accreditation pain standard: Making it happen!* Retrieved from http://www.canadianpainsociety.ca/accreditation_manual.pdf

Caterina, M. J., Gold, M. S., & Meyer, R. A. (2005). Molecular biology of nociceptors. In Hunt, S. & Koltzenburg, M. (Eds.). *The neurobiology of pain* (pp. 1–5). Oxford, NY: Oxford University Press.

Champion, G. D., Goodenough, B., von Baeyer, C. L., & Thomas, W. (1998). Measurement of pain by self-report. In Finley, G. A. & McGrath, P. J. (Eds.). *Measurement of pain in infants and children. Progress in pain research and management* (Vol. 10) (pp. 123–160). Seattle, WA: IASP Press.

Charlton, J. E. (2005). *Core curriculum for professional education in pain.* Seattle, WA: IASP Press.

Cleeland, C. S., & Ryan, K. M. (1994). Pain assessment: Global use of the Brief Pain Inventory. [Review]. *Annals of the Academy of Medicine Singapore, 23*(2), 129–138.

Cleeland, C. S., Serlin, R., Nakamura, Y., & Mendoza, T. (1997). Effects of culture and language on ratings of cancer pain and patterns of functional interference. In Jensen, T. S., Turner, J. A. & Wiesenfeld-Hallin, Z. (Eds.). *Progress in Pain Research and Management* (Vol. 8). Seattle, WA: IASP Press.

Coderre, T. J., Katz, J., Vaccarino, A. L., & Melzack, R. (1993). Contribution of central neuroplasticity to pathological pain: Review of clinical and experimental evidence. *Pain, 52*(3), 259–285. doi: 10.1016/0304-3959(93)90161-h

Cohen, L. L., Lemanek, K., Blount, R. L., Dahlquist, L. M., Lim, C. S., Palermo, T. M., . . . Weiss, K. E. (2008). Evidence-based assessment of pediatric pain. *Journal of Pediatric Psychology, 33*(9), 939–955. doi: 10.1093/jpepsy/jsm103

Craig, A. D., & Sorkin, L. S. (2011, March). Pain and analgesia. In *Encyclopedia of Life Sciences (ELS).* Chichester, UK: John Wiley & Sons, Ltd. doi: 10.1002/9780470015902.a0000275.pub3

Dahl, J. B. (2000, November 2–5). *Implementing the JCAHO pain management standards.* Paper presented at the American Pain Society 19th Annual Meeting, Atlanta, GA.

Dahl, J. B., & Moiniche, S. (2004). Pre-emptive analgesia. *British Medical Bulletin, 71*(1), 13–27. doi: 10.1093/bmb/ldh030

Dahl, J. L., Gordon, D., Ward, S., Skemp, M., Wochos, S., & Schurr, M. (2003). Institutionalizing pain management: The post-operative pain management quality improvement project. *Journal of Pain, 4,* 361–371.

Daniel, K. & Schmelzer, M. (2009). Research in practice: Why are we still using meperidine (Demerol) for conscious sedation? *Gastroenterology Nursing, 32*(4), 298–301.

Dobbins, E. H. (2010). Where has all the meperidine gone? *Nursing, 40*(1), 65–66.

Dunwoody, C. J., Krenzischek, D. A., Pasero, C., Rathmell, J. P., & Polomano, R. C. (2008). Assessment, physiological monitoring, and consequences of inadequately treated acute pain. *Journal of Perianesthesia Nursing: Official journal of the American Society of PeriAnesthesia Nurses / American Society of PeriAnesthesia Nurses, 23*(1), S15–S27.

DuPen, A., Shen, D., & Ersek, M. (2007). Mechanisms of opioid-induced tolerance and hyperalgesia. *Pain Management Nursing, 8*(3), 113–121.

Dworkin, R. H., Gnann, J. W., Oaklander, A. L., Raja, S. N., Schmader, K. E., & Whitley, R. J. (2008). Diagnosis and assessment of pain associated with herpes zoster and postherpetic neuralgia. *The Journal of Pain: Official Journal of the American Pain Society, 9*(1), 37–44.

Ellis, J. A., O'Connor, B. V., Cappelli, M., Goodman, J. T., Blouin, R., & Reid, C. W. (2002). Pain in hospitalized pediatric patients: How are we doing? *The Clinical Journal of Pain, 18*(4), 262–269.

Feldt, K. S. (2000). The checklist of nonverbal pain indicators (CNPI). *Pain Management Nursing, 1*(1), 13–21. doi: 10.1053/jpmn.2000.5831

Fernandes, M., da Costa, V., & Saraiva, R. A. (2007). Postoperative urinary retention: Evaluation of patients using opioid analgesics. *Revista Latino-Americana Enfermagem, 15*(2), 318–322.

Fuchs-Lacelle, S., & Hadjistavropoulos, T. (2004). Development and preliminary validation of the pain assessment checklist for seniors with limited ability to communicate (PACSLAC). *Pain Management Nursing, 5*(1), 37–49. doi: 10.1016/j.pmn.2003.10.001

Gatchel, R. J., Peng, Y. B., Peters, M. L., Fuchs, P. N., & Turk, D. C. (2007). The biopsychosocial approach to chronic pain: Scientific advances and future directions. *Psychology Bulletin, 133*(4), 581–624. doi: 10.1037/0033-2909.133.4.581

Gelinas, C. (2007). Le thermomètre d'intensité de douleur: Un nouvel outil pour les patients adultes en soins critiques. *Perspective infirmière, 4*(4), 12–20.

Gelinas, C. & Arbour, C. (2009). Behavioral and physiologic indicators during a nociceptive procedure in conscious and unconscious mechanically ventilated adults: Similar or different? *Journal of Critical Care, 24*(4), 628.e7–e17. Epub 2009 Mar 27.

Gélinas, C., Fillion, L., Puntillo, K., Viens, C., & Fortier, M. (2006). Validation of a Critical-Care Pain Observation Tool in adult patients. *American Journal of Critical Care, 15*(4), 420–427.

Gelinas, C. & Johnston, C., (2007). Pain assessment in the critically ill ventilated adult: Validation of the Critical-Care Pain Observation Tool and physiologic indicators. *Clinical Journal of Pain, 23*(6), 497–505.

Gibbs, G. F., Drummond, P. D., Finch, P. M., & Phillips, J. K. (2008). Unravelling the pathophysiology of complex regional pain syndrome: Focus on sympathetically maintained pain. *Clinical and Experimental Pharmacology and Physiology, 35*(7), 717–724. doi: 10.1111/j.1440-1681.2007.04862.x

Gibson, S. J., & Farrell, M. (2004). A review of age differences in the neurophysiology of nociception and the perceptual experience of pain. *The Clinical Journal of Pain, 20*(4), 227–239.

Gibson, S. J., & Helme, R. D. (2001). Age-related differences in pain perception and report. *Clinics in Geriatric Medicine, 17,* 433–456.

Goadsby, P. J., Lipton, R. B., & Ferrari, M. D. (2002). Migraine—current understanding and treatment. *New England Journal of Medicine, 346*(4), 257–270.

Gordon, C. (1997). The effect of cancer pain on quality of life in different ethnic groups: A literature review. [Review]. *Nurse Practice Forum, 8*(1), 5–13.

Grunau, R. E., Holsti, L., Haley, D. W., Oberlander, T., Weinberg, J., Solimano, A., Whitfield, M. F., Fitzgerald, C., Yu, W. (2005). Neonatal procedural pain exposure predicts lower cortisol and behavioral reactivity in preterm infants in the NICU. *Pain, 113*(3), 293–300.

Hadjistavropoulos, T., & Craig, K. D. (2002). A theoretical framework for understanding self-report and observational measures of pain: A communications model. *Behaviour Research and Therapy, 40*(5), 551–570. doi: 10.1016/s0005-7967(01)00072-9

Hadjistavropoulos, T., Herr, K., Turk, D. C., Fine, P. G., Dworkin, R. H., Helme, R., . . . Williams, J. (2007). An interdisciplinary expert consensus statement on assessment of pain in older persons. *The Clinical Journal of Pain, 23,* S1–S43. doi: 10.1097/AJP.1090b1013e31802be31869

Hall, R. W., & Anand, K. J. S. (2005). Physiology of pain and stress in the newborn. *Neoreviews, 6*(2), e61–e68. doi: 10.1542/neo.6-2-e61

Harden, R. N., Bruehl, S., Stanton-Hicks, M., & Wilson, P. R. (2007). Proposed new diagnostic criteria for complex regional pain syndrome. *Pain Medicine, 8*(4), 326–331. doi: 10.1111/j.1526-4637.2006.00169.x

Herr, K. (2002). Chronic pain: Challenges and assessment strategies. *Journal of Gerontologocal Nursing, 28*(1), 54–55.

Herr, K., & Mobily, P. R. (1993). Comparison of selected pain assessment tools to be used with the elderly. *Applied Nursing Research, 6*(1), 39–46.

Herr, K., Coyne, P. J., Manworren, R., McCaffery, M., Merkel, S., Pelosi-Kelly, J., & Wild, L. (2006). Pain assessment in the nonverbal patient: Position statement with clinical practice recommendations. *Pain Management Nursing, 7*(2), 44–52.

Herr, K., Coyne, P. J., McCaffery, M., Manworren, R., & Merkel, S. (2011). Pain assessment in the patient unable to self-report: Position statement with clinical practice recommendations. *Pain Management Nursing, 12*(4), 230–250.

Herrero, J. F., Laird, J. M. A., & Lopez-Garcia, J. A. (2000). Wind-up of spinal cord neurons and pain sensation: Much ado about something? *Progress in Neurobiology, 61*(2), 169–203. doi: 10.1016/s0301-0082(99)00051-9

Hicks, C. L., von Baeyer, C. L., Spafford, P. A., van Korlaar, I., & Goodenough, B. (2001). The Faces Pain Scale—Revised: Toward a common metric in pediatric pain measurement. *Pain, 93*(2), 173–183. doi: 10.1016/s0304-3959(01)00314-1

Huskisson, E. C. (1983). Visual analogue scales. In Melzack, R. (Ed.). *Pain measurement and assessment* (pp. 33–37). New York, NY: Raven Press.

International Association for the Study of Pain. (1979). Pain terms: A list with definitions and notes on usage. *Pain, 6,* 249–252.

International Association for the Study of Pain. (2001). Ethnicity and pain. *Pain Clinical Updates, 9*(4).

International Association for the Study of Pain. (2011). IASP Taxonomy. Retrieved from http://www.iasp-pain.org/Content/NavigationMenu/GeneralResourceLinks/PainDefinitions/default.htm

Jamison, R. N., & Virts, K. L. (1990). The influence of family support on chronic pain. *Behaviour Research and Therapy, 28*(4), 283–287. doi: 10.1016/0005-7967(90)90079-x

Jensen, M. P., & Karoly, P. (1986). The measurement of clinical pain intensity: A comparison of six methods. *Pain, 27*(1), 117–126.

Jensen, M. P., & Karoly, P. (2001). Self-report scales and procedures for assessing pain in adults. In Turk, D. C. &

Melzack, R. (Eds.). *Handbook of pain assessment.* New York, NY: Gilfrod Press.

Joshi, G. P., & Ogunnaike, B. O. (2005). Consequences of inadequate postoperative pain relief and chronic persistent postoperative pain. *Anesthesiology Clinics of North America, 23*(1), 21–36.

Jung, A. C., Staiger, T., & Sullivan, M. (1997). The efficacy of selective serotonin reuptake inhibitors for the management of chronic pain. *Journal of General Internal Medicine, 12*(6), 384–389. doi: 10.1007/s11606-006-5088-3

Kaki, A. M., El-Yaski, A. Z., & Youseif, E. (2005). Identifying neuropathic pain among patients with chronic low-back pain: Use of the Leeds Assessment of Neuropathic Symptoms and Signs pain scale. *Regional Anesthesia and Pain Medicine, 30*(5), 422–428. doi: 10.1016/j.rapm.2005.05.013

Kane, R. L., Ouslander, J. G., & Itamar, B. A. (2004). Clinical implications of the ageing process. *Essentials of Clinical Geriatrics* (5th ed.) (pp. 3–15). Highstown, NJ: McGraw Hill.

Katz, J. (2003). Timing of treatment and preemptive analgesia. In Rowbotham, D. J. & Macintyre, P. E. (Eds.). *Clinical pain management: Acute pain* (pp. 113–163). London, UK: Arnold.

Kehlet, H., Jensen, T. S., & Woolf, C. J. (2006). Persistent postsurgical pain: Risk factors and prevention. *The Lancet, 367*(9522), 1618–1625. doi: 10.1016/s0140-6736(06)68700-x

Khasabov, S. G., Rogers, S. D., Ghilardi, J. R., Peters, C. M., Mantyh, P. W., & Simone, D. A. (2002). Spinal neurons that possess the substance P receptor are required for the development of central sensitization. *The Journal of Neuroscience, 22*(20), 9086–9098.

Kumasaka, L. (1996). My pain is God's will. *American Journal of Nursing, 96*(6), 45–47.

Latremoliere, A., & Woolf, C. J. (2009). Central densitization: A generator of pain hypersensitivity by central neural plasticity. *The Journal of Pain, 10*(9), 895–926. doi: 10.1016/j.jpain.2009.06.012

Laugsand, E. A., Kaasa, S., & Klepstad, P. (2011). Management of opioid-induced nausea and vomiting in cancer patients: Systematic review and evidence-based recommendations. *Palliative Medicine, 25,* 442–453.

Laureys, S., Faymonville, M. E., Peigneux, P., Damas, P., Lambermont, B., Del, F. G., . . . Maquet, P. (2002). Cortical processing of noxious somatosensory stimuli in the persistent vegetative state. *Neuroimange, 17*(2), 732–741.

Lehne, R. (2009). *Pharmacology for nursing care.* St. Louis, MO: Elsevier Mosby.

Lopez-Martinez, A. E., Esteve-Zarazaga, R., & Ramirez-Maestre, C. (2008). Perceived social support and coping responses are independent variables explaining pain adjustment among chronic pain patients. *The Journal of Pain: Official Journal of the American Pain Society, 9*(4), 373–379.

Lorenz, J., Minoshima, S., & Casey, K. L. (2003). Keeping pain out of mind: The role of the dorsolateral prefrontal cortex in pain modulation. *Brain, 126*(5), 1079–1091. doi: 10.1093/brain/awg102

Love, S., & Coakham, H. B. (2001). Trigeminal neuralgia. *Brain, 124*(12), 2347–2360. doi: 10.1093/brain/124.12.2347

Mader, T. J., Blank, F. S. J., Smithline, H. A., & Wolfe, J. M. (2003). How reliable are pain scores? A pilot study of 20 healthy volunteers. *Journal of Emergency Nursing, 29*(4), 322–325. doi: 10.1067/men.2003.107

Manias, E., Bucknall, T., & Botti, M. (2005). Nurses' strategies for managing pain in postoperative setting. *Pain Management Nursing, 6,* 18–29.

Marchand, S. (2008). The physiology of pain mechanisms: From the periphery to the brain. *Rheumatic Disease Clinics of North America, 34*(2), 285–309. doi: 10.1016/j.rdc.2008.04.003

Marks, D. M., Shah, M. J., Patkar, A. A., Masand, P. S., Park, G.-Y., & Pae, C.-U. (2009). Serotonin-norepinephrine reuptake inhibitors for pain control: Premise and promise. *Current Neuropharmacology, 7,* 331–336. doi: 10.2174/157015909790031201

Mateo, O., & Krenzischek, D. A. (1992). A pilot study to assess the relationship between behavioral manifestations and self-report of pain in postanesthesia care unit patients. *Journal of Post Anasthesia Nursing, 7*(1), 15–21.

McCance, K. L., & Huether, S. E. (2006). *Pathophysiology: The biological basis of disease in adults and children.* St. Louis, MO: Mosby.

McEwen, B. S. (2001). Plasticity of the hippocampus: Adaptation to chronic stress and allostatic load. *Annals of the New York Academy of Science, 933,* 265–277.

McGillion, M. H., Watt-Watson, J. H., Kim, J., & Graham, A. (2004). Learning by heart: A focused group study to determine the self-management learning needs of chronic stable angina patients. *Canadian Journal of Cardiovascular Nursing, 14,* 12–22.

McGillion, M. H., Watt-Watson, J. H., Kim, J., & Yamada, J. (2004). A systematic review of psychoeducational interventions for the management of chronic stable angina. *Journal of Nursing Management, 12,* 1–9.

McGillion, M., Watt-Watson, J., LeFort, S., & Stevens, B. (2007). Positive shifts in the perceived meaning of cardiac pain following a psychoeducation program for chronic stable angina. *CJNR (Canadian Journal of Nursing Research), 39*(2), 48–65.

McIntyre, P. E. (2001). Safety and efficacy of patient controlled analgesia. *British Journal of Anaesthesia, 87,* 36–46.

Mease, P. (2005). Fibromyalgia syndrome: Review of clinical presentation, pathogenesis, outcome measures, and treatment. *The Journal of Rheumatology, 75,* 6–21.

Melzack, R. (1975). The McGill pain questionnaire: Major properties and scoring methods. *Pain, 1,* 277–299.

Melzack, R. (1987). The short-form McGill pain questionnaire. *Pain, 30,* 191–197.

Melzack, R. (1990). The tragedy of needless pain. *Scientific American, 262,* 27–33.

Melzack, R., & Casey, K. L. (1966). Sensory, motivational, and central control determinants of pain. In Kenshalo, D. R. (Ed.), *The skin sense.* Springfield, IL: Charles C. Thomas.

Melzack, R., & Wall, P. D. (1965). Pain mechanisms: A new theory. *Science, 150,* 171–179.

Melzack, R., & Wall, P. D. (1973). *The puzzle of pain.* London, UK: Basic Books.

Melzack, R., & Wall, P. D. (1982). *The challenge of pain.* New York, NY: Penguin Books.

Melzack, R., & Wall, P. D. (1996). *The challenge of pain.* (Updated 2nd ed.). New York, NY: Penguin Books.

Melzack, R., Coderre, T. J., Katz, J., & Vaccarino, A. L. (2001). Central neuroplasticity and pathological pain. *Annals of the New York Academy of Sciences, 933*(1), 157–174. doi: 10.1111/j.1749-6632.2001.tb05822.x

Merkel, S., Voepel-Lewis, T., & Malviya, S. (2002). Pain control: Pain assessment in infants and young children: The FLACC Scale. *The American Journal of Nursing, 102*(10), 55–58.

Merkel, S. I., Voepel-Lewis, T., Shayevitz, J. R., & Malviya, S. (1997). The FLACC: A behavioral scale for scoring postoperative pain in young children. *Pediatric nursing, 23*(3), 293–297.

Merskey, H., & Bogduk, N. (Eds.). (1994). *Classification of chronic pain: Description of chronic pain syndromes and definitions of pain terms* (2nd ed.). Seattle, WA: IASP Press.

Morrison, R. S., Magazinger, J., McLaughlin, M. A., Orosz, G., Silberzweig, S. B., Koval, K. J., & Siu, A. L. (2003). The impact of post-operative pain on outcomes following hip fracture. *Pain, 103,* 303–311.

Mularski, R. A., Puntillo, K., Varkey, B., Erstad, B. L., Grap, M. J., Gilbert, H. C., . . . Sessler, C. N. (2009). Pain management within the palliative and end-of-life care experience in the ICU. *Chest, 135*(5), 1360–1369. doi: 10.1378/chest.08-2328

Munoz, C., & Luckmann, J. (2005). *Transcultural communication in nursing* (2nd ed.). Clifton Park, NY: Thomson Learning.

Oberle, K., Wry, J., Paul, P., Grace, M., Smith, R. A. P., & Shaver, J. F. (1990). Environment, anxiety, and postoperative pain. *Western Journal of Nursing Research, 12*(6), 745–757. doi: 10.1177/019394599001200604

Odhner, M., Wegman, D., Freeland, N., Steinmetz, A., & Ingersoll, G. (2003). Assessing pain control in nonverbal critically ill adults. *Dimensions of Critical Care Nursing, 22*(6), 260–267.

Ohnhaus, E. E., & Adler, R. (1975). Methodological problems in the measurement of pain: A comparison between the verbal rating scale and the visual analogue scale. *Pain, 1*(4), 379–384. doi: 10.1016/0304-3959(75)90075-5

Pasero, C. (2004). Pathophysiology of neuropathic pain. *Pain Management Nursing, 5*(47), 3–8.

Pasero, C., & McCaffery, M. (2010). *Pain assessment and pharmacologic management.* St. Louis, MO: Elsevier Mosby.

Payen, J. F., Bru, O., Bosson, J. L., Lagrasta, A., Novel, E., Deschaux, I., Lavagne, P., & Jacquot, C. (2001). Assessing pain in critically ill sedated patients by using a behavioral pain scale. *Critical Care Medicine, 29*(12), 2258–2263.

Prkachin, K. M. (1992). The consistency of facial expressions of pain: A comparison across modalities. *Pain, 51*, 297–306.

Puntillo, K. A., Miaskowski, C., Kehrle, K., Stannard, D., Gleeson, S., & Nye, P. (1997). Relationship between behavioral and physiological indicators of pain, critical care patients' self-reports of pain, and opioid administration. *Critical Care Medicine, 25*(7), 1159–1166.

Ramage-Morin, P. (2008). Chronic pain in Canadian seniors. *Health Reports, 19*(1), 1–16.

Registered Nurses' Association of Ontario. (2007). *Assessment and management of pain.* Toronto, ON: Registered Nurses' Association of Ontario.

Rinn, W. E. (1984). The neuropsychology of facial expression: A review of the neurological and psychological mechanisms for producing facial expressions. *Psychological Bulletin, 95*(1), 52–77. doi: 10.1037/0033-2909.95.1.52

Rollman, G. B. (1979). Signal detection theory pain measures: Empirical validation studies and adaptation-level effects. *Pain, 6*(1), 9–21. doi: 10.1016/0304-3959(79)90136-2

Rollman, G. B., Abdel-Shaheed, J., Gillespie, J. M., & Jones, K. S. (2004). Does past pain influence current pain? Biological and psychosocial models of sex differences. *European Journal of Pain, 8*(5), 427–433. doi: 10.1016/j.ejpain.2004.03.002

Russell, M. B. R., & Olesen, J. (1996). A nosographic analysis of the migraine aura in a general population. *Brain, 119*(2), 355–361. doi: 10.1093/brain/119.2.355

Saarto, T., & Wiffen, P. J. (2010). Antidepressants for neuropathic pain: A Cochrane review. *Journal of Neurology, Neurosurgery & Psychiatry, 81*(12), 1372–1373. doi: 10.1136/jnnp.2008.144964

Schiff, W. B., Holtz, K. D., Peterson, N., & Rakusan, T. (2001). Effect of an intervention to reduce procedural pain and distress for children with HIV infection. *Journal of Pediatric Psychology, 26*(7), 417–427. doi: 10.1093/jpepsy/26.7.417

Schurks, M., Rist, P. M., Bigal, M. E., Buring, J. E., & Lipton, R. B., & Kurth, T. (2009). Migraine and cardiovascular disease: Systematic review and meta-analysis. *British Medical Journal, 339*(b3914).

Shankland, W. E., 2nd. (2011). Factors that affect pain behavior. *CRANIO: The Journal of Craniomandibular Practice, 29*(2), 144–154.

Slater, R., Cantarella, A., Gallella, S., Worley, A., Boyd, S., Meek, J., & Fitzgerald, M. (2006). Cortical pain responses in human infants. *The Journal of Neuroscience, 26*(14), 3662–3666. doi: 10.1523/jneurosci.0348-06.2006

Statistics Canada. (2003). A profile of disability in Canada. Retrieved from http://www.statcan.gc.ca/pub/89-577-x/4151364-eng.htm - limitations_related_to_pain

Stevens, B. (1999). Pain in infants. In McCaffery, M. & Pasero, C. (Eds.). *Pain: Clinical manual* (pp. 626–673). St. Louis, MO: Mosby.

Stevens, B., Johnston, C., Petryshen, P., & Taddio, A. (1996). Premature Infant Pain Profile: Development and initial validation. *The Clinical Journal of Pain, 12*(1), 13–22.

Stevens, B., Johnston, C. L., Taddio, A., Gibbins, S., & Yamada, J. (2010). The Premature Infant Pain Profile: Evaluation 13 years after development. *The Clinical Journal of Pain, 26*(9), 813–830 doi: 810.1097/AJP.1090b1013e3181ed1070

Stinson, J. N., Kavanagh, T., Yamada, J., Gill, N., & Stevens, B. (2006). Systematic review of the psychometric properties, interpretability and feasibility of self-report pain intensity measures for use in clinical trials in children and adolescents. *Pain, 125*(1-2), 143–157. doi: 10.1016/j.pain.2006.05.006

Taylor, L. J., & Herr, K. (2003). Pain intensity assessment: A comparison of selected pain intensity scales for use in cognitively intact and cognitively impaired African American older adults. *Pain Management Nursing, 4*(2), 87–95. doi: 10.1016/s1524-9042(02)54210-7

Topf, M. (2000). Hospital noise pollution: An environmental stress model to guide research and clinical interventions. *Journal of Advanced Nursing, 31*(3), 520–528. doi: 10.1046/j.1365-2648.2000.01307.x

Torvik, K., Kaasa, S., Kirkevold, O., Saltvedt, I., Holen, J. C., Fayers, P., & Rustoen, T. (2010). Validation of Doloplus-2 among nonverbal nursing home patients—an evaluation of Doloplus-2 in a clinical setting. [Comparative Study/Multicenter Study/Validation Studies]. *BMC Geriatrics, 10*, 9. doi: 10.1186/1471-2318-10-9

Villemure, C., & Bushnell, M. C. (2002). Cognitive modulation of pain: How do attention and emotion influence pain processing? *Pain, 95*, 195–199.

von Baeyer, C. L., & Spagrud, L. J. (2007). Systematic review of observational (behavioural) measures of pain for children and adolescents aged 3 to 18 years old. *Pain, 127*(1–2), 140–150.

Wary, B., Serbouti, S., & Doloplus, C. (2001). Validation d'une échelle d'évaluation comportementale de la douleur chez la personne âgée. *Douleurs, 1*, 35–38.

Watt-Watson, J. (1992). Misbeliefs about pain. In Watt-Watson, J. & Donovan, M. (Eds.). *Pain management: Nursing perspective* (pp. 36–58), St. Louis, MO: Mosby Yearbook.

Watt-Watson, J. H., Clark, A. J., Finley, G. A., & Watson, C. P. N. (1999). Canadian Pain Society position statement on pain relief. *Pain Research and Management, 4*(2), 75–78.

Watt-Watson, J., Evans, R., & Watson, C. P. (1988). Relationships among coping responses and perceptions of pain intensity, depression and family functioning. *Clinical Journal of Pain, 4*, 101.

Watt-Watson, J., Stevens, B., Streiner, D., Garfinkel, P., & Gallop, R. (2001). Relationship between pain knowledge and pain management outcomes for their postoperative cardiac patients. *Journal of Advanced Nursing, 36*, 535–545.

Wolff, A., Vanduynhoven, E., van Kleef, M., Huygen, F., Pope, J. E., & Mekhail, N. (2011). Phantom pain. *Pain Practice, 11*(4), 403–413. doi: 10.1111/j.1533-2500.2011.00454.x

Wu, J. S., Beaton, D., Smith, P. M., & Hagen, N. A. (2010). Patterns of pain and interference in patients with painful bone metastases: A brief pain inventory validation study. *Journal of Pain Symptom Management, 39*(2), 230–240. doi: 10.1016/j.jpainsymman.2009.07.006

Zheng, Z., Gibson, S. J., Helme, R. D., & McMeeken, J. M. (2009). The effect of local anaesthetic on age-related capsaicin-induced mechanical hyperalgesia—a randomised, controlled study. *Pain, 144*(1–2), 101–109. doi: 10.1016/j.pain.2009.03.021

Zhou, Y., Petpichetchian, W., & Kitrungrote, L. (2011). Psychometric properties of pain intensity scales comparing among postoperative adult patients, elderly patients without and with mild cognitive impairment in China. *International Journal of Nursing Studies, 48*(4), 449–457. doi: 10.1016/j.ijnurstu.2010.08.002

Chapter 31

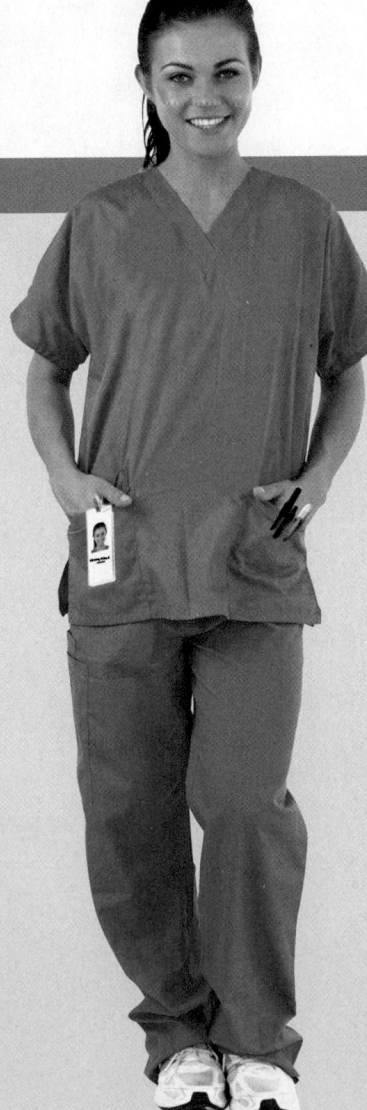

▉▉ Hygiene*

After studying this chapter, you will be able to:

1. Explain the main purpose of hygiene.

2. Relate determinants of health to the practice of personal hygiene.

3. Discuss comprehensive assessment related to hygiene.

4. Discuss common conditions affecting clients' hygiene needs.

5. Apply the nursing process to care for common hygiene problems related to skin, feet, nails, the mouth, hair, eyes, ears, and the nose.

6. Describe hygiene care for various types of baths.

7. Verbalize the steps used in providing perineal–genital, foot, oral, and hair hygiene care, as well as care related to contact lenses and hearing aids.

8. Identify safety and comfort measures underlying bed-making procedures.

*Hand hygiene is an essential component of "hygiene." This practice is discussed in great detail in Chapter 34.

Hygiene is the science of health and its maintenance. It is a highly personal matter determined by individual values and practices. It involves the care of skin, hair, nails, teeth, oral and nasal cavities, eyes, and ears, as well as perineal and genital care. **Personal hygiene** is self-care that includes bathing, toileting, general body cleaning, and grooming. Individuals engage in personal hygiene activities to fulfill the need for physical, social, and emotional comfort, as well as for safety.

Nurses frequently encounter people who require varying degrees of assistance, from minimal intervention to complete care, to attain their optimal hygiene needs. Responsibility for assisting clients to meet their hygiene needs encompasses not only the *activities* related to hygiene but also comprehensive assessment, mutual goal setting and planning, interventions, and evaluation of the extent to which the hygiene needs are met. This approach is based on thorough knowledge of relevant anatomy and physiology, developmental considerations, factors affecting hygiene practices, and knowledge of current research regarding these practices and the determinants of health (Table 31.1; see the Lifespan Considerations box on bathing on page 784).

TABLE 31.1   Determinants of Health Influencing Individual Hygiene Practices

Determinant of Health	Influence on Hygiene Practices
Culture	Body odour is considered offensive in some cultures and not in others. Culture affects health-related choices and strongly influences choices regarding frequency and type of bathing, privacy during personal hygiene, and acceptability of body odour. Certain foods, such as garlic and spicy foods, typically consumed in some cultures also contribute to noticeable body odour.
Religion	Ceremonial washing is practised in some religions.
Income and Social Status	Finances can affect the availability of resources for maintaining hygiene practices, such as not being able to purchase cleansing products (e.g., soap, shampoo). Some individuals may also lack privacy for bathing, if privacy for such practices is a cultural norm.
Physical Environment	The availability of facilities may be limited (e.g., to homeless clients) and access to assistive devices (e.g., tub, chairs, and lifts) to ensure safety may be limited.
Developmental Level	Hygiene needs depend on the age and stage of development. Particular considerations need to be given to infants and older adults (see the Lifespan Considerations box on bathing).
Personal Health Practices	Individual preferences regarding when and how to perform personal hygiene give the nurse an opportunity to individualize care. However, particular considerations should be given to individuals who are unable to completely meet their own needs for hygiene because of illness. Compromised physical or emotional health (e.g., in neuromuscular diseases) may lead to lack of motivation or energy to engage in personal hygiene practices. Individual preferences regarding evening or morning tub bath, showers, or other must be considered. Choice of products, preferred activities (e.g., washing hair, trimming nails, dental and oral hygiene) are individual.

LIFESPAN CONSIDERATIONS

Bathing

NEWBORNS

Newborns do not need to be bathed daily, and they do not need tub baths. Sponge baths are recommended. The diaper area is cleansed with each diaper change, and any milk that remains on the face or in neck creases can be wiped away by using water and a mild soap.

After the bath, the infant should be immediately dried and wrapped. Parents need to be advised that the infant's ability to regulate body temperature is not fully developed and that newborns' bodies lose heat quickly. The use of lotions, baby oil, and powders is not recommended because these can cause skin irritation and rashes.

Never leave a newborn unsupervised in the bath.

CHILDREN

Encourage a child's participation, as appropriate for developmental level. Closely supervise children in the bathtub. Do not leave them unattended.

ADOLESCENTS

Assist adolescents, as needed, to choose deodorants and antiperspirants. Secretions from newly active sweat glands react with bacteria on the skin, causing a pungent odour; the teen may need to be informed of the odour as he or she may not be aware of it.

OLDER ADULTS

Older adults are at risk for scalds from hot water and falls in the bath, and factors such as arthritis, fatigue, weakness, effects of a cerebrovascular accident (stroke), dyspnea, and other form of compromise may also influence the older adult's ability for hygiene self-care.

Safety devices can include the use of nonskid mats and abrasive bathtub strips, tub or shower chairs (Figure 31.1), and hand bars (Figure 31.2). Nurses in home care settings must thoroughly assess the environment and the capability of older adult clients and implement strategies to further promote their safety while meeting their personal hygiene needs.

Changes associated with aging can decrease the protective function of skin as it becomes fragile, loses elasticity, and contains less moisture. Important considerations related to skin changes in older adults are summarized in Table 31.2.

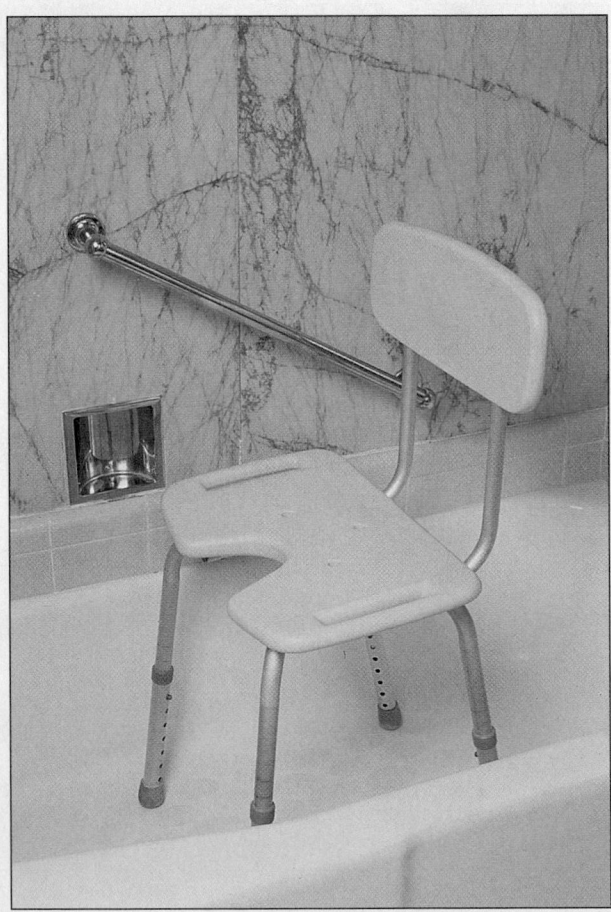

FIGURE 31.1 A shower chair.

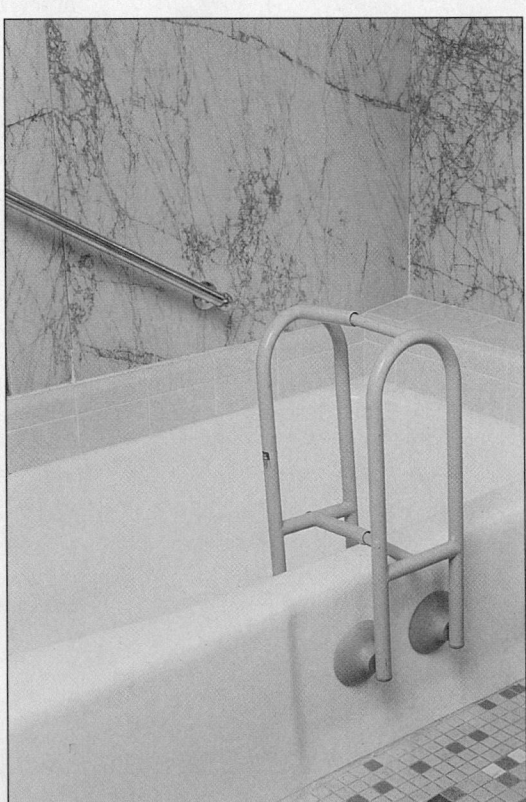

FIGURE 31.2 Hand bars on the side of a bathtub.

TABLE 31.2 Developmental Consideration: Assessment of Skin in Older Adults

Skin Alterations Related to Aging	Implications for the Older Adult
Subcutaneous and dermal tissue become thin	Skin tends to wrinkle and sag; increased risk of skin tears, less capacity to insulate
Decreased activity of sebaceous and sweat glands	Decreased perspiration, dryer skin, and increased incidence of pruritus
Decreased vascularity to skin	Skin temperature is cooler; skin appears pale in light-skinned older adults and dull, grey, or darker in dark-skinned older adults
Decreased production of melanin	Heightened susceptibility to sunlight, and skin cancer rates increase with age
Decreased circulation in extremities	Nails may become thicker, harder, yellowed, oddly shaped, or opaque; they may be brittle and prone to breaking or splitting
Melanocytes (cells that make the pigment that colours hair and skin) decrease in number	Hair thins and turns grey; facial hair may become thicker

Source: Adapted from D'Amico, C. B., Twomey, C., & Harder, N. (2012). *Health and physical assessment in nursing,* Canadian Edition (p. 174). Toronto, ON: Pearson Canada.

Skin

Skin is the largest organ of the body. It serves five major functions:

1. It protects underlying tissues from injury by preventing the passage of microorganisms. Skin and mucous membranes are considered the body's first line of defence.

2. It regulates the body temperature. Cooling the body occurs through the heat loss processes of evaporation of perspiration, and by radiation and conduction of heat from the body when the blood vessels of skin are vasodilated. Body heat is conserved through lack of perspiration and by vasoconstriction. See Chapter 29.

3. It secretes **sebum**, an oily substance that softens and lubricates hair and skin, prevents hair from becoming brittle, and decreases water loss from skin when the external humidity is low. Because fat is a poor conductor of heat, sebum lessens the amount of heat lost from skin. Sebum also has a **bactericidal** (bacteria-killing) action.

4. It transmits sensations through nerve receptors, which are sensitive to pain, temperature, touch, and pressure.

5. It produces and absorbs vitamin D in conjunction with ultraviolet rays from the sun, which activate a vitamin D precursor present in skin.

Normal skin of a healthy person has transient and resident microorganisms that are not usually harmful. See Table 34.1 (page 954) for some common resident organisms.

Sudoriferous (sweat) glands are on all body surfaces, except lips and parts of the genitals. The body has 2 to 5 million of these glands, which are all present at birth. They are most numerous on the palms of hands and the soles of feet. Sweat glands are classified as *apocrine* and *eccrine.* **Apocrine glands**, located largely in the axillae and anogenital areas, begin to function at puberty under the influence of androgens. Although their secretion is produced almost constantly, apocrine glands are of little use in thermoregulation. The secretion of these glands is odourless, but when decomposed or acted on by bacteria on skin, it takes on a musky, unpleasant odour. **Eccrine glands** are more numerous than apocrine glands and are found chiefly on the palms of hands, the soles of feet, and the forehead. The sweat they produce cools the body through evaporation. Sweat is made up of water, sodium, potassium, chloride, glucose, urea, and lactate.

Assessing

Assessment of the client's ability to engage in self-care activities includes taking a nursing history to determine the client's usual hygiene practices and self-care abilities, and the existence of any problems or potential problems associated with skin, the oral cavity, hair, nails, and other structures requiring hygiene. Important considerations include the client's balance, ability to sit unsupported, activity tolerance, coordination, strength, range of motion, and vision and hearing. Difficulties the client may encounter in performing activities related to hygiene include the inability to wash any or all of the body, to obtain or get to a source of water, to regulate the temperature or flow of the water, to unfasten or remove clothing, and to get dressed again following bathing. Clients who have difficulty with elimination may also have difficulties associated with removing or unfastening clothing to access the toilet or commode.

Assessment data about the client's skin care practices enable the nurse to incorporate the client's preferences into an overall plan of care designed to meet the need for hygiene. Clients whose cognitive function is

---

ASSESSMENT | **INTERVIEW**

Hygiene Practices

The following questions can help the nurse learn about the client's hygiene practices:

SKIN CARE PRACTICES

- What is your usual time to shower or bathe?
- What products, such as soap, shampoo, deodorant, do you prefer to use?
- What products, if any, do you use on your face?
- How frequently do you clean or discard applicators or puffs that you use on your face?
- Are there any products or practices that you avoid because of how they affect your skin?

SELF-CARE ABILITIES

- Do you have any problems managing your own hygiene?
- What assistance can the nurse give you to help you meet your need for hygiene?

SKIN PROBLEMS

- Do you have any tendency toward dry skin, acne, itchiness, rashes, bruising, excessive perspiration, or lack of perspiration?
- Do you have any allergies? If so, to what?

---

impaired or whose illness alters energy levels and motivation will require assistance. It is important for the nurse to determine the client's functional level to maintain and promote as much client independence as possible and as safely as possible. When working with clients who have skin conditions, the nurse must attend to the client's self-concept (see Chapter 45). Some skin conditions cause physical challenges and concerns for clients, who may experience psychological and social ramifications as well.

Questions to elicit data about hygiene practices are shown in the Assessment: Interview box.

The *presence of past, current, or potential skin problems* alerts the nurse to specific nursing interventions or referrals the client may require. The client may provide descriptions of these problems during the nursing history, or the nurse may observe deviations from normal during the physical examination. Common skin problems and implications for nursing interventions are summarized in Table 31.3.

TABLE 31.3 Common Problems Affecting Skin

Problem and Appearance	Nursing Implications
Abrasion Superficial layers of skin scraped or rubbed away; area is reddened and may have localized bleeding or serous weeping	1. Wounds should be kept clean and dry, as they are prone to infection. 2. Do not wear rings or jewellery when providing care to avoid causing abrasions to clients. 3. Lift, and not pull, a client across a bed. See Chapter 39.
Excessive Dryness Flaky and rough appearance of skin	1. If skin cracks, it becomes prone to infection; therefore, provide alcohol-free lotions to moisturize skin and prevent cracking. 2. Bathe the client less frequently; do not use soap, or use nonirritating soap to a limited extent. Rinse skin thoroughly because soap can be irritating and drying. 3. Encourage increased fluid intake, if the client's health permits, to prevent dehydration.
Ammonia Dermatitis (Diaper Rash) Caused by skin bacteria reacting with the urea in urine; skin becomes reddened and sore	1. Keep skin dry, and clean by applying protective ointments containing zinc oxide to areas at risk (e.g., buttocks and perineum). 2. Change diapers as soon as they become soiled. Ensure that cloth diapers are washed with an antibacterial detergent.
Acne Inflammatory condition with papules and pustules	1. Keep skin clean to prevent secondary infection. 2. Treatment varies widely, so integrate prescribed or recommended approaches into care.
Erythema Redness associated with a variety of conditions, such as rashes, exposure to sun, elevated body temperature	1. Wash the affected area carefully to remove excess microorganisms. 2. Apply antiseptic spray or lotion to prevent itching, promote healing, and prevent skin breakdown.
Hirsutism Excessive hair on a person's body and face, particularly in women	1. Remove unwanted hair by using depilatories, shaving, electrolysis, or tweezing. 2. Enhance client's self-concept. See Chapter 45.

ASSESSMENT HOME CARE

Hygiene

Nurses need to consider all of the following elements in meeting the hygiene needs of clients living in the community:

CLIENT AND ENVIRONMENT

- *Self-care abilities for hygiene:* Assess the client's ability to bathe, to manipulate water taps, to dress and undress, to groom, and to use the toilet.

- *Self-care aids required:* Determine whether the client needs a shower chair (Figure 31.3), a hand shower, a nonskid surface or mat in the tub or shower, hand bars on the sides of the tub, or a raised toilet seat.

- *Facilities:* Check for the presence of laundry facilities and running water.

- *Mechanical barriers:* Note furniture that obstructs access to the bathroom and toilet, or a doorway that is too narrow for a wheelchair.

FAMILY

- *Caregiver availability, skills, and responses:* Determine whether individuals are available and able to assist with bathing, dressing, toileting, nail care, shampooing, shopping for hygienic or grooming aids, and so on.

- *Education needs:* Assess whether the caregiver needs instructions in how to assist the client in and out of the tub, on and off the toilet, and so on.

- *Family role changes and coping:* Assess the effects of client's illness on financial status, parenting, spousal roles, sexuality, and social roles.

COMMUNITY

- Explore resources that will provide assistance with bathing, laundry, and foot care (e.g., home health aid, podiatrist).

- Consult a social worker or a home care nurse as needed to coordinate placement of a client unable to remain in the home or to identify community resources that will help the client stay in the home.

- Consider consulting with (a) a physical therapist to assess, develop, and improve the client's motor function; (b) a home care nurse to provide follow-up for care, teaching, and support; and (c) an occupational therapist to assess and develop the client's abilities to perform activities of daily living (ADLs).

ASSESSMENT IN THE COMMUNITY OR HOME CARE SETTING To meet the hygiene needs of clients living in the community, the nurse must consider the client's environment, the family or caregiver, and the community. See the Assessment: Home Care box on hygiene.

Diagnosing

Nursing diagnoses that are related to hygiene include deficit in self-care related to hygiene or inability to perform personal hygiene related to any number of factors, for example, weakness, fatigue, neuromuscular and/or musculoskeletal problems, environmental barriers, perceptual or cognitive impairment, pain, inability to perceive body parts, inability to transfer or mobilize effectively and safely, and emotional states (e.g., severe anxiety or depression). Diagnoses related to skin integrity are discussed in Chapter 35.

Planning

Planning activities can include assisting dependent clients with bathing, skin care, and perineal care, providing back massages to promote circulation, and instructing clients on appropriate hygiene practices and therapies to prevent skin lesions. Consider the client's personal preferences, health, and limitations in determining the best time to give the care and the

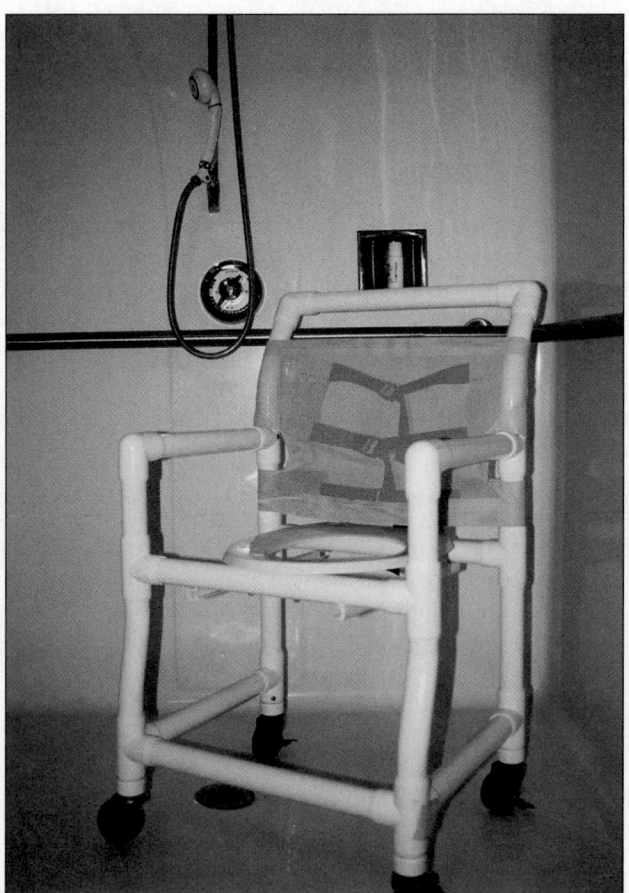

FIGURE 31.3 A shower chair.

equipment, facilities, and personnel available. A client's personal preferences—for example, about when and how to bathe—should be followed as long as they are compatible with the client's health and the equipment available. Nurses need to provide whatever assistance the client requires, either directly or by delegating this task to other nursing personnel. See the Reflect on Primary Health Care box below.

REFLECT ON **PRIMARY HEALTH CARE**

Nurses engage in health-promotion activities to fulfill clients' basic needs for cleanliness and comfort and to prevent infections. They seek opportunities to assess, diagnose, plan, implement, and evaluate clients' hygiene needs, such as bathing and care of nails, hair, and skin. They also work with interdisciplinary teams to coordinate the type and level of hygiene care to be provided to clients in both home and hospital settings. Consider how you can engage in health-promotion and intersectional collaboration activities in your nursing care planning process.

PLANNING FOR HOME CARE To provide for continuity of care, the nurse must assess the client's and family's abilities for care (see the Assessment: Home Care box) and the need for referrals and home health services. In addition, the nurse needs to determine the client's learning needs.

Implementing

Nursing interventions discussed in this chapter focus on hygiene measures; the etiology of the nursing diagnoses established may point to other interventions that promote circulation, promote self-esteem, restore nutritional status, correct fluid deficits or excesses, or prevent problems associated with immobility. Nursing strategies that deal with these etiologies are provided in other chapters.

GENERAL PRINCIPLES OF SKIN CARE

1. *Intact, healthy skin is the body's first line of defence.* Nurses need to ensure that all skin care measures prevent injury and irritation. Scratching of skin with jewellery or long or sharp fingernails must be avoided. Harsh rubbing or use of rough towels and washcloths can cause tissue damage, particularly when skin is irritated or when circulation or sensation is diminished. Bottom bedsheets are kept taut and free from wrinkles to reduce friction and abrasion to skin. Top bed linens are arranged to prevent undue pressure on toes. When necessary, bed cradles or footboards are used to keep bedclothes off the client's feet.

2. *The degree to which skin protects underlying tissues from injury depends on the general health of cells, the amount of subcutaneous tissue, and the dryness of skin.* Skin that is poorly nourished and dry is less easily protected and more vulnerable to injury. When skin is dry, lotions or creams with lanolin can be applied, and bathing is limited to once or twice a week because frequent bathing removes the natural oils of skin and causes dryness.

3. *Moisture in contact with skin for a long period can result in increased bacterial growth and irritation.* After a bath, the client's skin is dried carefully. Particular attention is paid to such areas as the axillae, the groin, and the areas beneath the breasts and between the toes, where the potential for irritation is greatest. Clients who have fecal or urinary incontinence or who perspire excessively are provided with immediate skin care to prevent skin irritation.

4. *Body odours are caused by skin bacteria acting on body secretions.* Cleanliness is the best deodorant. Commercial deodorants and antiperspirants should be applied only after skin is cleaned. Deodorants diminish odours, whereas antiperspirants reduce the amount of perspiration. Neither is applied immediately after shaving because of the possibility of skin irritation, and they are not used on skin that is already irritated.

5. *Skin sensitivity to irritation and injury varies among individuals and in accordance with their health.* Skin sensitivity is generally greater in infants, very young children, and older people. A person's nutritional status also affects sensitivity. Emaciated or obese persons tend to experience more skin irritation and injury. The same tendency is seen in individuals with poor dietary habits and insufficient fluid intake. Even in healthy persons, skin sensitivity is highly variable. Some people's skin is sensitive to the chemicals in skin care agents and cosmetics. Hypoallergenic cosmetics and soaps or soap substitutes are available. The nurse needs to ascertain whether the client has any sensitivities and what agents are appropriate to use.

6. *Agents used for skin care have selective actions and purposes.* Commonly used agents are described in Table 31.4.

BATHING Bathing removes accumulated oil, perspiration, sweat, dirt, dead skin cells, and microorganisms from skin. When skin is cleaned, body odours are decreased. Bathing also stimulates circulation by dilating superficial arterioles, bringing more blood and nourishment to skin. A bath can be refreshing and relaxing and frequently improves morale, sense of well-being, appearance, and self-respect. Some people take a morning shower for its refreshing, stimulating effect. Others prefer an evening bath because it is relaxing.

While bathing is generally seen as a positive experience, clients with acute confusion or dementia can find bathing anxiety provoking and exhibit

TABLE 31.4 Agents Used on Skin

Type	Description
No-rinse cleansers	Preferred over soaps (except possibly emollient soaps) in the care of the skin of older adults; reduce the risk of skin deterioration (skin dryness, skin tears) (Hodgkinson, Nay, & Wilson, 2007)
Soap	Lowers surface tension and, thus, helps in cleaning; some soaps contain antibacterial agents that can change the natural flora of the skin; soaps, if used for bathing, should not be perfumed and should be rich in emollients (Penzer, 2001)
Detergent	Used instead of soap for cleaning; some people who are allergic to soaps may not be allergic to detergents, and vice versa; should not be used on older clients
Bath oil	Used in bathwater; provides an oily film on the skin that softens and prevents chapping; oils can make the tub surface slippery, and clients should be instructed about safety measures (e.g., using a nonskid tub surface or mat)
Skin cream or lotion	Provides a film on the skin that prevents evaporation and, therefore, chapping
Powder	Although not generally recommended because of a risk of clumping of the product, powder can be used to absorb water and prevent friction, for example, powder under the breasts can prevent skin irritation; some powders are antibacterial
Deodorant	Masks or diminishes body odours
Antiperspirant	Reduces the amount of perspiration

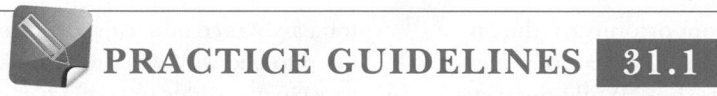

PRACTICE GUIDELINES 31.1

Bathing People with Dementia

Guideline	Rationale
Provide the bath at a calm and agreeable time of the day, and be consistent in the ritual.	Being situation responsive to the client's preferences may cause less stress. Predictability can be reassuring.
Ensure that all materials needed for the bath are at hand before the client enters the bath.	Organization will ensure that no fuss is generated in having to call for missing items and having others come and go during the bath.
Fill the bathtub with water prior to the client entering the bathroom.	Many people with dementia are fearful of the noise of running water.
Ensure that the temperature of the bathroom and bath water is comfortable.	Shivering is stressful for people with dementia. Increased comfort generally limits distress.
Shower using a handheld showerhead rather than an overhead mounted showerhead.	Water in the face can cause distress.
Allow the person as much independence as possible in an unrushed environment.	This approach acknowledges the client's dignity and avoids learned helplessness.
Give one direction at a time, and use modelling or cueing, if necessary, to help the client understand what needs to be done.	Clients with poor concentration or short-term memory changes will benefit from clear and timely instructions.
Never leave the client alone in the bath, and ensure that all security devices (e.g., bath seat, grab bars) are in place.	Safety must be ensured.
Consider sponge bathing on alternative days.	This practice maintains the client's personal hygiene without the stress of a daily shower or bath.
Focus on the client and the relationship rather than on the task.	Focusing on the bath at the expense of the individual being bathed may give rise to rushing for the sake of completing the task and neglecting the importance of the experience for the client who may feel frustrated, humiliated, or fearful.

Sources: Guidelines summarized from Alzheimer Society of Canada. (2011). Guidelines for care: Person-centered care of people with dementia living in care homes. Retrieved from http://www.alzheimer.ca/english/care/framework.pdf; Hodgkinson, B., Nay, R., & Wilson, J. (2007). A systematic review of topical skin care in aged care facilities. *Journal of Clinical Nursing, 16,* 129–136; and Radner, J., Barrick, A. L., Hoeffer, B., Sloane, P., McKenzie, D., Talerico, K. A., & Glover, J. U. (2006). The bathing of older adults with dementia: Easing the unnecessary unpleasant aspects of assisted bathing. *American Journal of Nursing, 106*(4), 40–48.

resistance, aggression, or agitation as a result. Washing of hair, the perineum, the axillae, and feet are particularly likely to provoke negative behavioural responses (Sloane, Hoeffer, & Somboontanont, 2006). Practice Guidelines 31.1 summarizes practice guidelines related to bathing of clients with dementia. See also the Clinical Alert box that follows.

! CLINICAL ALERT

When Joanne Rader, a prominent researcher, was doing a study on the bathing experience of older adults with dementia, she accepted to receive a shower herself in a nursing home and found the experience cold and depressing. She cautions health care professionals to reflect on how the older adult with dementia perceives the bathing experience and hypothesizes that what health care professionals view as "aggressive"' or "resistive" may well be defensive actions related to feeling threatened and anxious.

Excessive bathing, however, can interfere with the intended lubricating effect of the sebum, causing dryness of skin. This is an important consideration, especially for older adults, who produce less sebum.

Bathing offers an excellent opportunity for the nurse to assess clients with illnesses. The nurse can observe for such conditions as edema or rashes. While assisting a client with a bath, the nurse may also assess the client's psychosocial needs, such as orientation to time and ability to cope with the illness. The nurse can also assess learning needs, such as the need of a client with diabetes to learn foot care.

Caution is needed when bathing clients who are receiving intravenous therapy. Easy-to-remove gowns that have Velcro or snap fasteners along the sleeves may be used. If a special gown is not available, the nurse needs to pay particular attention when changing the client's gown after the bath or whenever the gown becomes soiled. Guidelines for clients with an intravenous (IV) pump are provided in Box 31.1.

Categories of Baths   Two categories of baths are given to clients: cleansing and therapeutic. **Cleansing baths** are given chiefly for hygiene purposes and include the following:

- *Complete bed bath.* The nurse washes the entire body of an individual who needs total assistance.
- *Self-help bed bath.* Clients confined to bed are able to bathe themselves, with assistance for washing the back and, perhaps, feet.
- *Partial bath.* Only the parts of the client's body that might cause discomfort or odour are washed: the face, hands, axillae, perineal area, and back. The arms, chest, abdomen, legs, and feet are omitted. The nurse provides this bath for clients who need

---

BOX 31.1   CHANGING A HOSPITAL GOWN FOR A CLIENT WITH AN INTRAVENOUS INFUSION WITHOUT A PUMP

Changing a gown for a client receiving intravenous therapy requires special attention:

- Slip the gown completely off the arm without the infusion and onto the tubing connected to the arm with the infusion.
- Holding the container above the client's arm, slide the sleeve up over the container to remove the used gown.
- Place the clean gown sleeve for the arm with the infusion over the container as if it were an extension of the client's arm, from the inside of the gown to the sleeve cuff.
- Rehang the container. Slide the gown carefully over the tubing toward the client's hand.
- Guide the client's arm and tubing into the sleeve, taking care not to pull on the tubing or IV site.
- Assist the client to put the other arm into the second sleeve of the gown, and fasten as usual.
- Count the rate of flow of the infusion to make sure it is correct before leaving the bedside.

---

total assistance and assists self-sufficient clients confined to bed with washing their backs. Some ambulatory clients prefer to take a partial bath at the sink with the nurse assisting as needed, particularly with cleaning their backs.

- *Bag bath.* The bag bath is a packaged disposable bathing system that contains 8 to 12 no-rinse cleansing washcloths with emollients and moisturizers to protect skin. The solution and washcloths are warmed in a microwave. The warming time is about 1 minute, but to ensure the safety of the client, the nurse needs to determine how long it takes to attain a desirable temperature. Each area of the body is cleaned with a different cloth and then air dried. Bag baths save time and are easy to perform.
- *Tub bath.* Tub baths are often preferred to bed baths because it is easier to wash and rinse the entire body in a tub. Tubs are also used for therapeutic baths. The amount of assistance the nurse offers depends on the abilities of the client. Specially designed tubs are available for those needing total assistance. These tubs greatly reduce the work of the nurse in lifting clients in and out of the tub and offer greater benefits than a sponge bath in bed. See Figures 31.4 and 31.5 for using a bath lift to assist the client into a raised tub.
- *Shower.* Many ambulatory clients are able to use shower facilities and require only minimal assistance from the nurse. Shower chairs are available for clients who are not able to stand in the shower (see Figure 31.1, page 784).

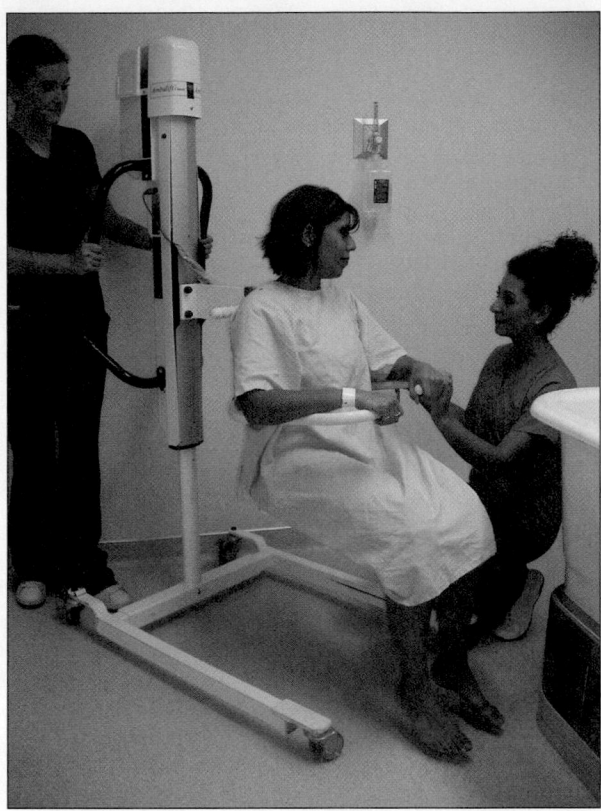

FIGURE 31.4 Using a bath lift.

The water for a bath should feel comfortably warm to the client. People vary in their sensitivity to heat; generally, the temperature should be 43°C to 46°C. Most clients are able to verify a suitable temperature. Clients with reduced sensation, such as people with peripheral neuropathy, can use a thermometer to measure bath water temperature to avoid scalds. (See Chapter 32 for recommendations on hot water tank temperature settings and faucet devices that help avoid scalds.) The water for a bed bath should be changed when cleansing from a dirtier to a cleaner area or when bath water becomes dirty or cool.

Therapeutic baths are given for physical effects, such as to soothe irritated skin or to treat a specific area, such as the perineum. Medications can be placed in the water. A therapeutic bath is generally taken in a tub one-third or one-half full. The client remains in the bath for a designated time, often 20 to 30 minutes. If the client's back, chest, and arms are to be treated, these areas need to be immersed in the solution. The bath temperature is generally included in the order; 37.7°C to 46°C may be ordered for adults and 40.5°C is usually ordered for infants.

Skill 31.1 provides guidelines for bathing an adult or pediatric client.

See the Teaching: Home Care box on hygiene on page 796.

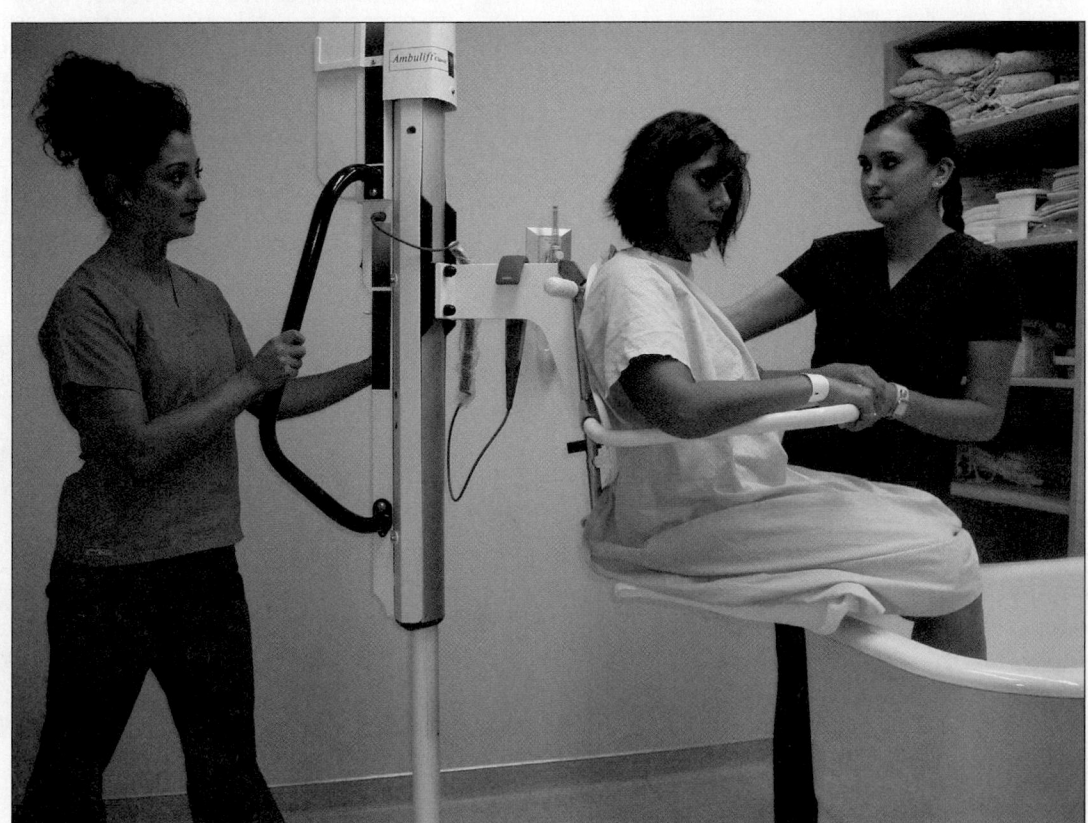

FIGURE 31.5 Using a bath lift to assist the client into a raised tub.

SKILL 31.1 BATHING AN ADULT OR PEDIATRIC CLIENT

PURPOSES

- To remove transient microorganisms, body secretions and excretions, and dead skin cells
- To stimulate circulation to the skin
- To promote a sense of well-being
- To produce relaxation and comfort
- To prevent and eliminate unpleasant body odours

ASSESSMENT

Assess

- Condition of the skin (colour, texture, and turgor; presence of pigmented spots; temperature; lesions; excoriations, abrasions, and bruises)
- Physical or emotional factors (e.g., fatigue, sensitivity to cold, need for control, anxiety or fear)
- Presence of pain and need for adjunctive measures (e.g., an analgesic) before the bath
- Range of motion of the joints
- Any other aspect of health that may affect the client's bathing process (e.g., mobility, strength, cognition)
- Need for use of clean gloves during the bath

Equipment

- Basin or sink with warm water (between 43°C and 46°C)
- Soap and soap dish
- Linens: bath blanket, two bath towels, washcloth, clean gown or pyjamas or clothes, as needed, and additional bed linen and towels, if required
- Gloves, if appropriate (e.g., presence of bodily fluids or open lesions)
- Personal hygiene articles (e.g., deodorant, powder, lotions)
- Shaving equipment
- Table for bathing equipment
- Laundry hamper

IMPLEMENTATION

Preparation

Before bathing a client, determine (a) the purpose and type of bath the client needs; (b) the self-care ability of the client; (c) any movement or positioning precautions specific to the client; (d) other care the client may be receiving, such as physical therapy or radiation therapy, to coordinate all aspects of health care and prevent unnecessary fatigue; (e) the client's comfort level with regard to being bathed by someone else; and (f) the necessary bath equipment and linens.

Performance

1. Before performing the procedure, introduce yourself and verify the client's identity using two identifiers or per agency protocol. Explain to the client what you are going to do, why it is necessary, and how he or she can participate. Discuss with the client the plan for bathing, and explain any unfamiliar procedures to the client. Ensure the client that privacy and dignity will be maintained.

2. Perform hand hygiene, and follow other appropriate infection prevention and control procedures.

3. Provide for client privacy by drawing the curtains around the bed or closing the door to the room. Some agencies provide signs indicating the need for privacy. **Rationale: Hygiene is a personal matter, and clients can experience anxiety and possibly shame at being naked in front of caregivers.**

4. Prepare the client and the environment.
   - Invite a family member or significant other to participate if the client prefers it.
   - Close windows and doors to ensure the room is a comfortable temperature. **Rationale: Air currents increase loss of heat from the body by convection and can lead to discomfort and shivering.**
   - Offer the client a bedpan or urinal, or ask whether the client wants to use the toilet or commode. **Rationale: Warm water and activity can stimulate the need to void. The client will be more comfortable after voiding; voiding before cleaning the perineum is advisable.**
   - Encourage the client to perform as much personal self-care as possible. **Rationale: This promotes independence, exercise, and self-esteem.**
   - During the bath, assess each area of skin carefully.

For a Bed Bath

5. Prepare the bed and position the client appropriately.
   - Position the bed at a comfortable working height. Lower the side rail on the side closest to you. Keep the other side rail *up*. Help the client move near you. **Rationale: This avoids undue reaching and straining and promotes good body mechanics.**
   - Place a bath blanket over the top sheet. Remove the top sheet from under the bath blanket by starting at the client's shoulders and moving the linen down toward the client's feet (see ❶). Ask the client to grasp and hold the top of the bath blanket while you pull the linen to the foot of the bed.

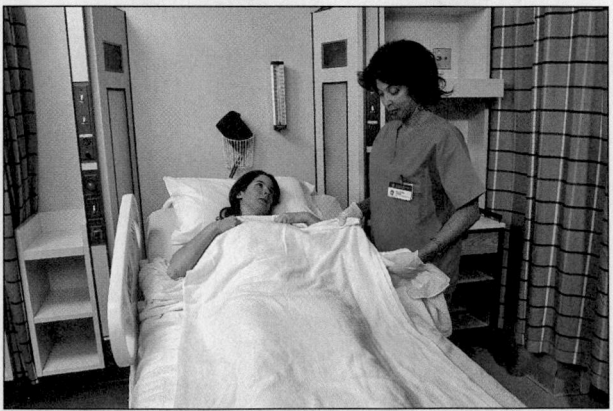

❶ Remove the top sheet from under the bath blanket.

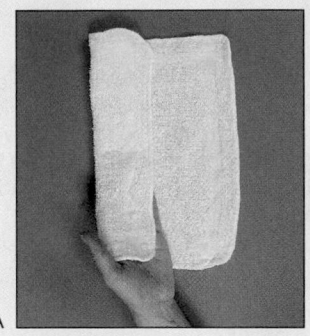 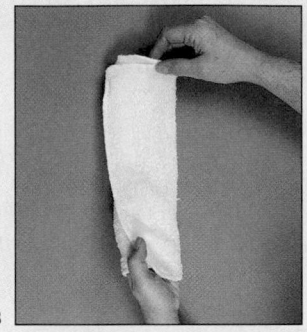 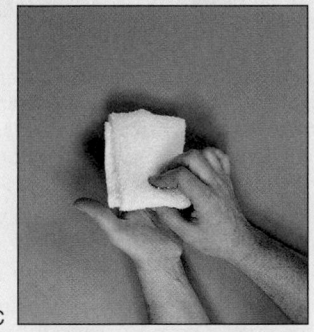

② Making a bath mitt. **A:** Lay the back of your hand on the washcloth, and fold one side over your hand. **B:** Fold the second side over your hand. **C:** Fold the top of the cloth down, and tuck it under the folded side against your palm to secure the mitt.

Rationale: The bath blanket provides comfort, warmth, and privacy. *Note:* If the bed linen is to be reused, place it over the bedside chair. If it is to be changed, place it in the linen hamper, not on the floor.

- Remove client's gown while keeping the client covered with the bath blanket. Place the gown in the linen hamper. If a client has an intravenous infusion, follow the procedures in Box 31.1 (page 790) regarding changing the hospital gown.

6. Make a bath mitt with the washcloth (see **②**). **Rationale: A bath mitt retains water and heat better than a cloth loosely held and prevents the ends of the washcloth from dragging across the client's skin.**

7. Wash the face. **Rationale: Begin the bath at the cleanest area, and work downward toward the feet.**

- Place the towel under the client's head.
- Wash the client's eyes with water only and dry them well. Use a separate corner of the washcloth for each eye. **Rationale: The use of separate corners prevents the transmission of microorganisms**

from one eye to the other. Wipe from the inner to the outer canthus (see **③**). **Rationale: To prevent secretions from entering the nasolacrimal ducts.**

- Ask whether the client wants soap used on the face. **Rationale: Soap has a drying effect, and the face, which is exposed to the air more than other body parts, tends to be drier.**
- Wash, rinse, and dry the client's face, ears, and neck.
- Remove the towel from under the client's head.

8. Wash the arms and hands. Omit the arms for a partial bath.

- Place a towel lengthwise under the client's arm away from you. **Rationale: It protects the bed from becoming wet.**
- Wash, rinse, and dry the client's arm by elevating it and supporting the client's wrist and elbow. Use long, firm strokes from wrist to shoulder, including the axillary area (see **④**). **Rationale: Firm strokes from distal to proximal areas promote circulation by increasing venous blood return.**
- Apply deodorant or powder, if desired.
- (Optional) Place a towel on the bed, and put a washbasin on it. Place the client's hands in the basin.

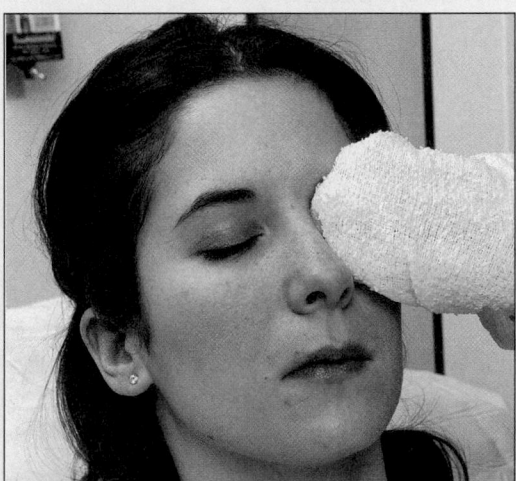

③ Use a separate corner of the washcloth for each eye, and wipe from the inner canthus to the outer canthus

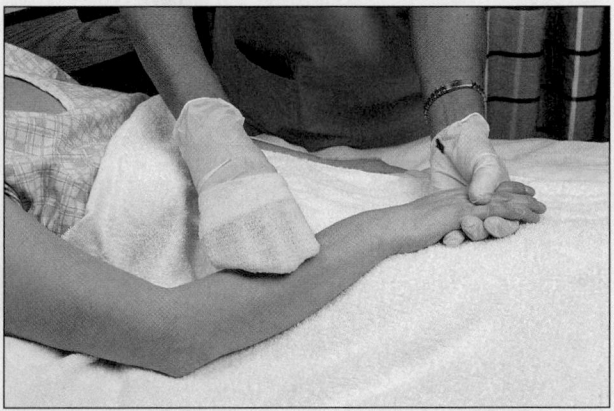

④ Washing the far arm by using long, firm strokes from wrist to shoulder area

SKILL 31.1 BATHING AN ADULT OR PEDIATRIC CLIENT (continued)

Rationale: Many clients enjoy immersing their hands in the basin and washing themselves. Soaking loosens dirt under the nails. Assist the client as needed to wash, rinse, and dry his or her hands, paying particular attention to the spaces between fingers.

- Repeat for the hand and arm nearest you. Exercise caution if an intravenous infusion is present, and check its flow after moving the arm.

9. Wash the chest and abdomen. Omit the chest and abdomen for a partial bath. However, the areas under a woman's breasts may require cleaning if this area is irritated or if the client has significant perspiration under the breasts.

- Place the bath towel lengthwise over the chest. Fold the bath blanket down to the client's pubic area. **Rationale: This keeps the client warm while preventing unnecessary exposure of the chest**.

- Lift the bath towel off the chest, and bathe the chest and the abdomen with your mitted hand by using long, firm strokes (see ❺). Give special attention to the skin under the breasts and any other skinfolds, particularly if the client is overweight. Rinse and dry well.

- Replace the bath blanket when the areas have been dried.

10. Wash legs and feet. Omit for a partial bath.

- Expose the leg farthest from you by folding the bath blanket toward the other leg, being careful to keep the perineum covered. **Rationale: Covering the perineum promotes privacy and maintains the client's dignity**.

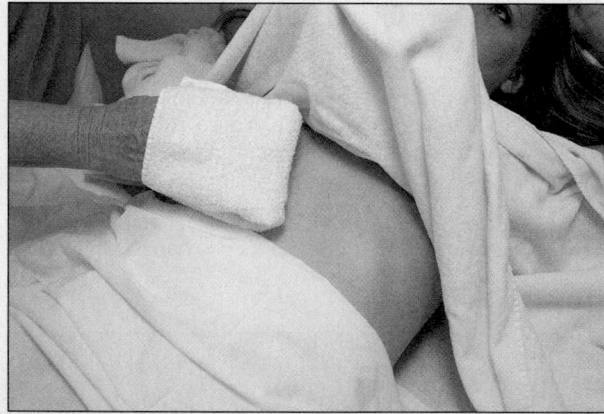

❺ Washing the chest and the abdomen

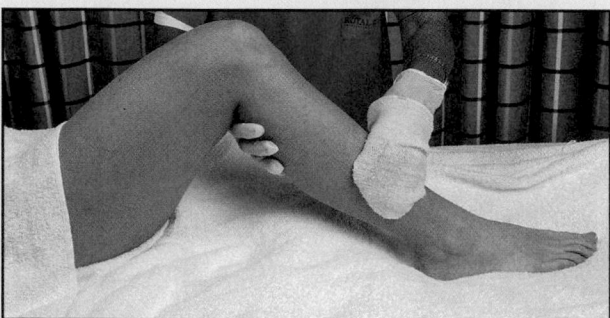

❻ Washing the leg on the far side

- Lift the leg and place the bath towel lengthwise under the leg. Wash, rinse, and dry the leg by using long, smooth, firm strokes from the ankle to the knee to the thigh (see ❻). **Rationale: Washing from the distal to proximal areas promotes circulation by stimulating venous blood flow**.

- Reverse the coverings and repeat for the other leg.

- Wash the feet by placing them in the basin of water (see ❼).

- Dry each foot. Pay particular attention to the spaces between the toes. If preferred, wash one foot after that leg before washing the other leg.

- Obtain fresh, warm water, whenever necessary. **Rationale: Water may become dirty or cold.** Because surface skin cells are removed with washing, the bathwater from dark-skinned clients may become dark, however, this does not mean the client is dirty. Lower the bed when refilling the basin. **Rationale: This practice ensures the safety of the client**.

11. Wash the back and then the perineum.

- Assist the client into the prone or side-lying position facing away from you. Place the bath towel lengthwise alongside the back and buttocks while keeping the client covered with the bath blanket as much as possible. **Rationale: To provide warmth and prevent undue exposure**.

- Wash and dry the client's back, moving from the shoulders to the buttocks and upper thighs, paying attention to the gluteal folds (see ❽).

- Perform a back massage now or after completion of the bath. (See Skill 38.1).

- Assist the client to the supine position, and determine whether the client can wash the perineal area independently. If the client cannot do so, drape the client, and wash the area.

12. Assist the client with grooming aids, such as powder, lotion, or deodorant.

- Use powder sparingly. Release as little as possible into the air. **Rationale: To avoid irritation of**

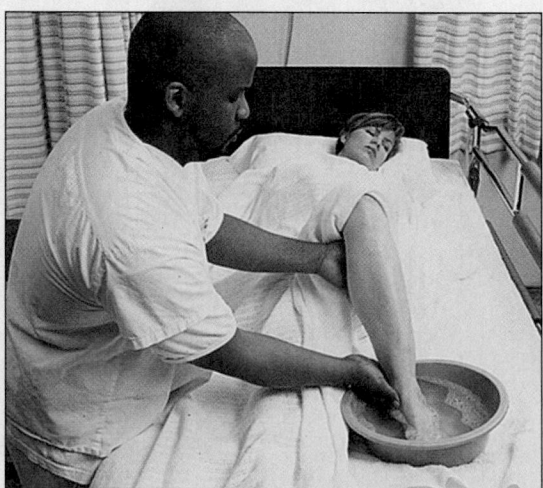

❼ Soaking the foot in a basin

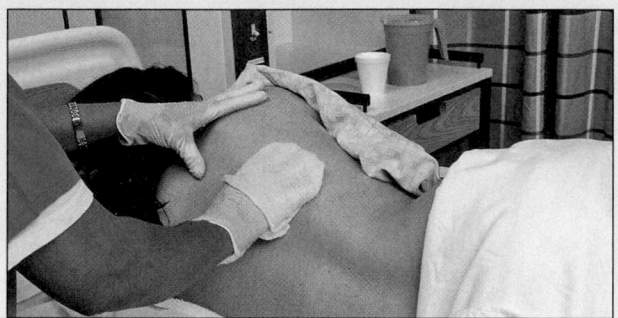

8 Washing the back

the respiratory tract by powder inhalation. Excessive powder can cause caking on skin, which leads to skin irritation.

- Help the client put on a clean gown or pyjamas.
- If required, assist the client to care for hair, mouth, and nails.

For a Tub Bath or Shower

13. Prepare the client and the tub.
    - Fill the tub about one-third to one-half full with water at 43°C to 46°C. **Rationale: The water level should be sufficient to cover the perineal area**.
    - Cover all intravenous catheters or wound dressings with plastic coverings, and instruct the client to prevent wetting these areas, if possible.
    - Put a rubber bath mat or towel on the floor of the tub if safety strips are not on the tub floor. **Rationale: These prevent slipping during the bath or shower**.

14. Assist the client into the shower or tub.
    - Assist the client taking a standing shower with the initial adjustment of the water temperature and water flow pressure, as needed. Some clients need a chair in the shower because of weakness. Hot water can cause older adults to feel faint.
    - If the client requires considerable assistance with a tub bath, a hydraulic bathtub chair may be required (see "Variation").
    - Explain how the client can signal for help, leave the client for 2 to 5 minutes, and place an "occupied" sign on the door. For safety reasons, do not leave a client with decreased cognition or clients who may be at risk (e.g., history of seizures, syncope).

15. Assist the client with washing and then getting out of the tub.
    - Wash the client's back, lower legs, and feet, if necessary.
    - Assist the client out of the tub. If the client is unsteady, place a bath towel over the client's shoulders and drain the tub of water before the client attempts to get out of it. **Rationale: Draining the water first lessens the likelihood of a fall. The towel prevents chilling**.

16. Dry the client, and assist with follow-up care.
    - Follow step 12.
    - Assist the client back to his or her bed.
    - Clean the tub or shower in accordance with agency practice, discard the used linen in the laundry hamper, and place the "unoccupied" sign on the door.

17. Document the following:
    - The type of bath given (i.e., complete, partial, or self-help); this is usually recorded on a flowsheet
    - Skin assessment, such as excoriation, erythema, exudates, rashes, drainage, or skin breakdown
    - Nursing interventions related to skin integrity
    - The ability of the client to assist or participate with bathing
    - The client's response to bathing
    - Educational needs regarding hygiene
    - Information or teaching shared with the client or the family

Variation: Bathing by Using a Hydraulic Bathtub Chair

A hydraulic lift, often used in long-term care or rehabilitation settings, can facilitate the safe transfer of a client who is unable to ambulate to a tub. The lift also helps eliminate strain on the nurse's back.

- Ensure that the client is covered with a towel or blanket before and after the bath *to maintain privacy and body temperature*
- Bring the client to the tub room in a wheelchair or shower chair.
- Fill the tub, and check the water temperature *to avoid thermal injury to the client.*
- Lower the hydraulic chair lift to its lowest point, outside the tub.
- Transfer the client to the chair lift, and secure the seat belt (see **9**).
- Raise the chair lift above the tub.
- Support the client's legs as the chair is moved over the tub *to avoid injury to the legs.*
- Position the client's legs down into the water, and slowly lower the chair lift into the tub.
- Assist in bathing the client, if appropriate.
- Reverse the procedure when taking the client out of the tub.
- Dry the client, and transport him or her to the room.

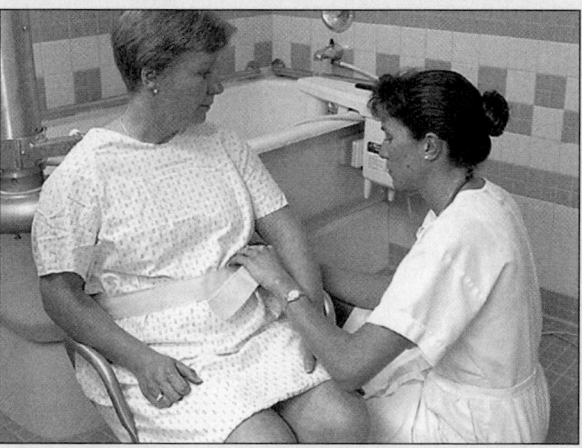

9 Secure the seat belt before moving the client in a hydraulic bathtub chair.

(continued)

SKILL 31.1 **BATHING AN ADULT OR PEDIATRIC CLIENT** (*continued*)

EVALUATION

- Note the client's tolerance of the procedure (e.g., respiratory rate and effort, pulse rate, behaviours of acceptance or resistance, statements regarding comfort).

- Conduct appropriate follow-up:
  - Condition and integrity of skin (dryness, turgor, redness, lesions, and so on)
  - Client's strength
  - Percentage of bath done without assistance
- Relate to prior assessment data, if appropriate.

TEACHING **HOME CARE**

Hygiene

Suggest the client or family do the following:

- Consider purchasing a bath seat that fits in the tub or shower.
- Install a hand shower for use with a bath seat and shampooing.
- Use a nonskid surface on the tub or shower floor.
- Install hand bars on both sides of the tub or shower to facilitate transfers in and out of the tub or shower.
- Carefully monitor the temperature of the bathwater. See Chapter 32 for hot water tank setting recommendations.
- Apply lotion *after* the client is out of the tub or shower since lotions may make the tub surface or shower floor slippery.

PERINEAL–GENITAL CARE Perineal–genital care is also called *perineal care,* or *pericare.* Perineal care as part of the bed bath can be embarrassing for many clients. Nurses also may find it embarrassing initially, particularly with clients of the opposite sex (Grant, Giddings, & Beale, 2005). However, most clients who require a bed bath from the nurse are able to clean their own genital areas with minimal assistance. The nurse may need to hand a moistened washcloth to the client, rinse the washcloth, and provide a towel.

Because some clients are unfamiliar with terminology for the genitals and perineum, it may be difficult for nurses to explain what is expected. Most clients, however, understand what is meant if the nurse simply says, "I'll give you a washcloth to finish your bath." Older clients may use the term *private parts.* Whatever expression the nurse uses, it needs to be one that the client understands and one that is comfortable for the nurse to use.

The nurse needs to provide perineal care efficiently and in a matter-of-fact manner. Nurses should wear gloves while providing this care for the comfort of the client and to protect themselves. Skill 31.2 explains how to provide perineal–genital care.

Evaluating

By using data collected during care, the nurse judges whether desired outcomes have been achieved. If the outcomes are not achieved, the nurse explores reasons why:

- Did the nurse overestimate the client's functional abilities (physical, mental, emotional) for self-care?

SKILL 31.2 **PROVIDING PERINEAL–GENITAL CARE**

PURPOSES

- To remove normal perineal secretions and odours
- To promote client comfort

ASSESSMENT

Assess for the presence of the following:

- Irritation, excoriation, inflammation, swelling
- Excessive discharge
- Odour, pain, or discomfort
- Urinary or fecal incontinence
- Recent rectal or perineal surgery
- Indwelling catheter

Determine the following:

- Perineal–genital hygiene practices
- Self-care abilities

Equipment

For perineal–genital care provided in conjunction with the bed bath:

- Bath towel
- Bath blanket
- Clean gloves
- Bath basin with water at 43°C to 46°C
- Soap
- Washcloth

For special perineal–genital care:

- Bath towel
- Bath blanket
- Clean gloves
- Cotton balls or swabs
- Solution bottle, pitcher, or container filled with warm water or a prescribed solution
- Bedpan to receive rinse water
- Moisture-resistant bag or receptacle for used cotton swabs
- Perineal pad

IMPLEMENTATION

Preparation

- Determine whether the client is experiencing any discomfort in the perineal–genital area.
- Obtain and prepare the necessary equipment and supplies.

Performance

1. Before performing the procedure, introduce yourself and verify the client's identity using two identifiers or per agency protocol. Explain to the client what you are going to do, why it is necessary, and how he or she can participate, being particularly sensitive to any embarrassment felt by the client.
2. Perform hand hygiene, and follow other appropriate infection prevention and control procedures (e.g., clean gloves).
3. Provide for client privacy by drawing the curtains around the bed or closing the door to the room. Some agencies provide signs indicating the need for privacy. **Rationale: Hygiene is a personal matter**.
4. Prepare the client.
   - Fold the top bed linen to the foot of the bed, and fold the client's gown up to expose the genital area.
   - Place a bath towel under the client's hips. **Rationale: The bath towel prevents the bed from becoming soiled**.
5. Position and drape the client, and clean the upper inner thighs.

For Females

- Position the client in the back-lying position, with her knees flexed and spread well apart.
- Cover her body and legs with the bath blanket positioned such that a corner is at her chin, the opposite corner at her feet, and the other two on the sides. Drape the legs by tucking the bottom corners of the bath blanket under the inner sides of the legs (see ❶). **Rationale: Minimum exposure lessens embarrassment and helps provide warmth**. Bring the middle portion of the base of the blanket up over the pubic area.
- Put on gloves; wash and dry the upper inner thighs.

For Males

- Position the client in the supine position, with knees slightly flexed and hips slightly externally rotated.
- Put on gloves; wash and dry the upper inner thighs.

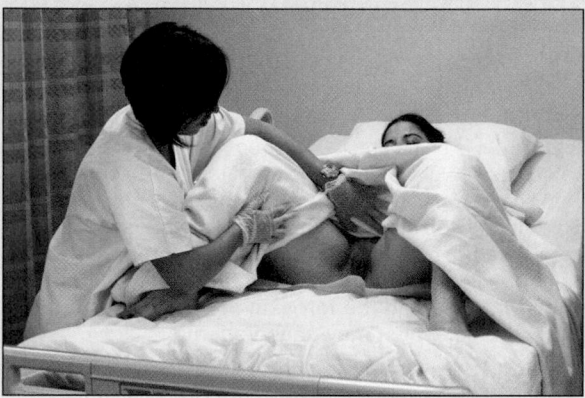

❶ Draping the female client for perineal–genital care

6. Inspect the perineal area.
   - Note areas of inflammation, excoriation, or swelling, especially between the labia in females and the scrotal folds in males.
   - Also, note any excessive discharge or secretions from orifices and the presence of odours.
7. **Wash and dry the perineal–genital area.**

For Females

- Clean the labia majora. Then, spread the labia to wash the folds between the labia majora and the labia minora (see ❷). **Rationale: Secretions that tend to collect around the labia minora facilitate bacterial growth**.
- Use separate quarters of the washcloth for each stroke, and wipe from the pubis to the rectum. For menstruating women and clients with indwelling catheters, use a fresh wipe for each stroke. **Rationale: Using separate quarters of the washcloth or new wipes prevents the transmission of microorganisms from one area to another. Wipe from the area of least contamination (the pubis) to that of greatest (the rectum)**.
- Rinse the area well. You may place the client on a bedpan and use a periwash or solution bottle to pour warm water over the area. Dry the perineum thoroughly, paying particular attention to the folds between the labia. **Rationale: Moisture promotes the growth of many microorganisms**.

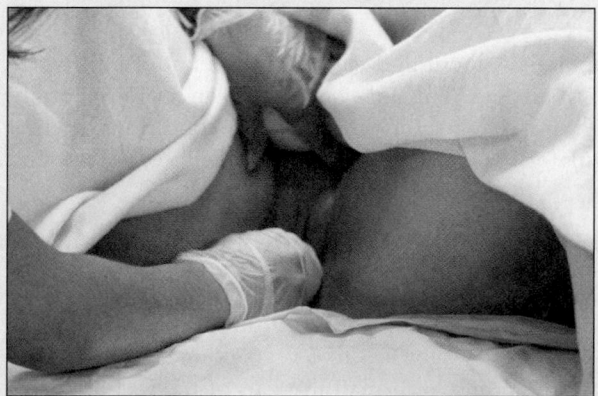

❷ Cleaning the labia

(continued)

SKILL 31.2 PROVIDING PERINEAL–GENITAL CARE (*continued*)

For Males

- Wash and dry the penis, using firm strokes.
- If the client is uncircumcised, retract the prepuce (foreskin) to expose the glans penis (the tip of the penis) for cleaning. Replace the foreskin after cleaning the glans penis (see ❸). **Rationale: Retracting the foreskin is necessary to remove the smegma (thick, cheesy secretion) that collects under the foreskin and facilitates bacterial growth. Replacing the foreskin prevents constriction of the penis, which may cause edema**.
- Wash and dry the scrotum. The posterior folds of the scrotum may need to be cleaned when the buttocks are cleaned (see step 9). **Rationale: The scrotum tends to be more soiled than the penis because of its proximity to the rectum; thus, it is usually cleaned after the penis**.

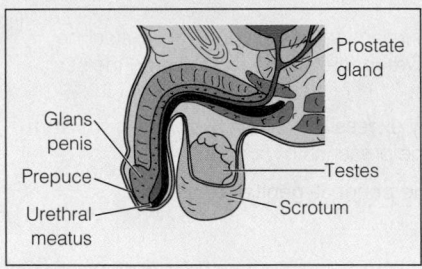

❸ Male genitals

8. Inspect perineal orifices for intactness.
   - Inspect particularly around the urethra in clients with indwelling catheters. **Rationale: A catheter can cause excoriation around the urethra**.
9. Clean between the buttocks.
   - Assist the client to turn onto the side facing away from you.
   - Pay particular attention to the anal area and posterior folds of the scrotum in males. Before washing the anus, clean it with toilet tissue, if necessary.
   - Dry the area well.
   - In female clients, after childbirth or during menstruation, apply a perineal pad, as needed, from front to back. **Rationale: This prevents contamination of the vagina and urethra from the anal area**.
10. Document any unusual findings, such as redness, excoriation, skin breakdown, discharge or drainage, and any localized areas of tenderness.

EVALUATION

- Relate current assessments to previous assessments.
- Conduct appropriate follow-up, such as applying prescribed ointment for excoriation.
- Report any deviation from normal to the appropriate members of the health care team.

- Were provided instructions clear to the client?
- Were appropriate assistive devices or supplies available to the client?
- Did the client's condition change?
- Were required analgesics provided before hygiene care?
- What currently prescribed medications and therapies could affect the client's abilities or tissue integrity?

Feet

Proper assessment and care of feet is important for clients of all ages. This care becomes even more important with aging clients and when certain conditions, such as circulatory disturbances or diabetes mellitus, are present.

Developmental Variations

At birth, a baby's foot is relatively unformed. The arches are supported by fatty pads and do not attain their full shape until the baby is 5 to 6 years of age. During childhood, the bones and small muscles of the feet are easily damaged by tight, binding stockings and ill-fitting shoes. For normal development, it is important that the arches be supported and that the bony structures and the feet

grow with no external restrictions. Feet are not fully grown until about age 20 years. Normal changes in the feet associated with aging include wider and longer feet, mild settling of the arches, and loss of natural padding on the bottom of the heels. The cartilage around the joints also deteriorates, producing loss of normal range of motion of the foot and ankle. Older clients often require special attention for their feet. For example, reduced blood supply and accompanying arteriosclerosis can make a foot prone to infection following trauma. Decreased flexibility or poor vision can make self-care of the feet impossible or dangerous for the older client.

Assessing

NURSING HISTORY The nurse determines the client's history of (a) normal nail and foot care practices, (b) type of footwear worn, (c) self-care abilities, (d) presence of factors that place the client at risk for foot problems, (e) any foot discomfort, and (f) any perceived problems with foot mobility (see the Assessment: Interview box on foot hygiene).

PHYSICAL ASSESSMENT Each foot and toe is inspected for shape, size, and presence of lesions and is palpated to assess areas of tenderness, edema, and circulatory status. Normally, the toes are straight and flat. See Table 31.5

ASSESSMENT INTERVIEW

Foot Hygiene

FOOT CARE PRACTICES

- How often do you wash your feet and cut your toenails?
- What hygiene products do you usually use on your feet (cleanser, foot powder or deodorant, lotion, or cream)?
- What type of shoes and socks do you wear?
- How often do you change your socks or put on clean socks?
- Do you ever go barefoot? If so, when, where, and how often?

SELF-CARE ABILITIES

- Do you have any problems managing your foot care? If so, what are these?
- How can the nurses best help you?

FOOT PROBLEMS AND RISK FACTORS

- Do you have any problems with foot odour?
- Do you have any foot discomfort? If so, where? When does this occur? What do you do to relieve the discomfort? Does this discomfort affect how you walk?
- Have you noticed any problems with foot mobility (e.g., joint stiffness)?
- Do you have diabetes, any circulatory problems affecting your feet (e.g., swelling, changes in skin colour, arthritis), or any instances of prolonged exposure to chemicals or water?

for physical assessment methods for the feet. Common foot problems include calluses, corns, unpleasant odours, plantar warts, fissures between the toes, and fungal infections, such as athlete's foot.

A **callus** is a thickened portion of the epidermis, a mass of keratotic material. Most calluses are painless and flat and are found on the bottom or side of the foot over a bony prominence. Calluses are usually caused by pressure from shoes. They can be softened by soaking the foot in warm water with Epsom salts. Creams with lanolin help keep skin soft and prevent the formation of calluses.

A **corn** is a keratosis caused by friction and pressure from a shoe. It commonly occurs on the fourth or fifth toe, usually over a bony prominence, such as a joint.

Corns are usually conical (circular and raised). The base is the surface of the corn and the apex is in deeper tissues, sometimes even attached to bone. Corns are generally removed surgically. They are prevented from reforming by relieving the pressure on the area (generally by wearing properly fitting shoes) and massaging the tissue to promote circulation. The use of oval corn pads should be avoided because they increase pressure and decrease circulation.

Unpleasant odours occur as a result of perspiration and its interaction with microorganisms. Regular and frequent washing of the feet and wearing clean hosiery help minimize odour. Medicated foot powders and deodorants also help prevent this problem.

TABLE 31.5 Assessment of Feet

Method	Normal Findings	Deviations from Normal
Inspect all skin surfaces, particularly between toes, for cleanliness, odour, dryness, inflammation, swelling, abrasions, or other lesions.	Intact skin Absence of swelling or inflammation	Excessive dryness Areas of inflammation or swelling (e.g., corns, calluses) Fissures Scaling and cracking of skin (e.g., athlete's foot) Plantar warts
Palpate anterior and posterior surfaces of ankles and feet for edema.	No swelling	Swelling or pitting edema
Palpate dorsalis pedis pulse on dorsal surface of foot and posterior tibial pulse behind the medial malleolus.	Strong, regular pulses in both feet	Weak or absent pulses in one foot or both feet
Compare skin temperatures of both feet.	Warm skin	Cool skin temperature in one or both feet
Assess the sensation of touch.	Sensation of touch	Absence of sensation
Assess movement.	Movement of feet or toes	Decreased movement of feet or toes

Plantar warts appear on the sole of the foot. These warts are caused by human papilloma virus (HPV). They are moderately contagious; they are frequently painful and often make walking difficult. A physician may curettage the warts (scrape them out), use a carbon dioxide laser to excise them, use cryotherapy, which involves freezing the lesion with liquid nitrogen several times, or apply salicylic acid.

Fissures, or deep grooves, frequently occur between toes as a result of dryness and cracking of skin. The treatment of choice is practising foot hygiene and application of an antiseptic to prevent infection. Often, a small piece of gauze is inserted between toes while applying the antiseptic and is left in place to assist healing by allowing air to reach the area.

Tinea pedis (athlete's foot, or ringworm of the foot) is caused by a fungus. The symptoms are scaling and cracking of skin, particularly between toes. Sometimes small blisters form, containing a thin fluid. In severe cases, lesions can also appear on other parts of the body, particularly hands. Treatments usually involve the application of commercial antifungal ointments or powders. Prevention is important. Common preventive measures are keeping feet well ventilated, drying feet well after bathing, wearing clean socks or stockings, and not going barefoot in public showers.

Onychocryptosis, the inward growing of the nail into the soft tissue around it, most often results from improper nail trimming. Pressure applied to the area causes localized pain. Treatment involves frequent, hot antiseptic soaks and, possibly, surgical removal of the portion of nail embedded in skin. Preventing recurrence involves appropriate instruction and adherence to proper nail-trimming techniques.

Diagnosing

A number of nursing diagnoses can apply to clients with foot or foot care problems. Selected diagnoses include foot self-care deficit related to such factors as visual impairment, poor hand coordination, or reduced flexibility; risk for impaired skin integrity related to such factors as poor-fitting footwear, pedal edema, or lack of sensory perception.

Planning

Planning involves (a) identifying nursing interventions that will help the client maintain or restore healthy foot care practices, and (b) establishing desired outcomes for each client. Interventions may include teaching the client about correct nail and foot care, proper footwear, and ways to prevent potential foot problems (e.g., infection, injury, and decreased circulation). For clients with self-care difficulties, the nurse plans a schedule for soaking the client's feet and assisting with regular cleaning and trimming of nails, if not contraindicated. Foot care and nail care are often provided during the client's bath but can be provided at any time in the day to accommodate the client's preference or schedule. The frequency of foot care is determined by the nurse and client and is based on objective assessment data and the client's specific problems. For some clients, their feet need to be bathed daily; for those whose feet perspire excessively, bathing more than once a day may be necessary.

Examples of desired health outcomes to evaluate the achievement of goals and the effectiveness of the nursing interventions include the client doing the following:

- Participating in self-care (foot hygiene) at optimal level of capacity

- Describing hygiene and other interventions (e.g., proper footwear) to maintain skin integrity, prevent infection, and maintain peripheral tissue perfusion

- Demonstrating optimal hygiene, as evidenced by the following:

  - Intact, smooth, pink, soft, hydrated, and warm skin

  - Intact cuticles and skin surrounding nails

  - Correct foot care and nail care practices

Implementing

Skill 31.3 describes how to provide foot care.

See the Teaching: Wellness box on foot care on page 802.

SKILL 31.3 PROVIDING FOOT CARE

PURPOSES

- To maintain the skin integrity of feet
- To prevent foot infections
- To prevent foot odours
- To assess or monitor foot problems

ASSESSMENT

Assess

- History of any problems with foot discomfort, foot odour, foot mobility, circulatory problems (e.g., swelling, changes in skin colour or temperature, and pain), structural problems (e.g., bunion, hammer toe, or overlapping digits)

- Usual foot care practices (e.g., frequency of washing feet and cutting nails, foot hygiene products used, how often socks are changed, whether the client ever goes barefoot, whether the client sees a podiatrist)
- Skin surfaces for cleanliness, odour, dryness, and intactness

Determine

- Shape, size, presence of lesions (e.g., corn, callus, wart, or rash), areas of tenderness, ankle edema for each foot and toe
- Skin temperatures of both feet to assess circulatory status
- Pedal pulses: dorsalis pedis and posterior tibial (see Chapter 29)
- Self-care abilities (e.g., any problems managing foot care)

Equipment

- Washbasin containing warm water
- Pillow
- Moisture-resistant disposable pad
- Towels
- Soap
- Washcloth
- Toenail cleaning and trimming equipment, if agency policy permits
- Lotion or foot powder

IMPLEMENTATION

Performance

1. Before performing the procedure, introduce yourself and verify the client's identity using two identifiers or per agency protocol. Explain to the client what you are going to do, why it is necessary, and how he or she can participate.

2. Perform hand hygiene, and follow other appropriate infection prevention and control procedures.

3. Provide for client privacy by drawing the curtains around the bed or closing the door to the room. Some agencies provide signs indicating the need for privacy. **Rationale: Hygiene is a personal matter**.

4. Prepare the equipment and the client.
   - Fill the washbasin with warm water at about 40°C to 43°C. **Rationale: Warm water promotes circulation, comforts, and refreshes**.
   - Assist the ambulatory client to the sitting position in a chair, or the client in bed to the supine or semi-Fowler's position.
   - Place a pillow under the bed client's knees. **Rationale: To provide support and prevent muscle fatigue**.
   - Place the washbasin on the moisture-resistant pad at the foot of the bed (see **7,** page 794) for a client in bed or on the floor in front of the chair for an ambulatory client.
   - For a client in bed, pad the rim of the washbasin with a towel. **Rationale: The towel prevents undue pressure on skin**.

5. Wash the foot, and then soak it.
   - Place one of the client's feet in the basin, and wash it with soap, paying particular attention to the interdigital areas. Prolonged soaking is generally not recommended for clients with diabetes or those with peripheral vascular disease. **Rationale: Prolonged soaking may remove natural skin oils, thus drying the skin and making it more susceptible to cracking and injury**.
   - Rinse the foot well to remove all of the soap. **Rationale: Soap irritates skin if not completely removed**.
   - Rub callused areas of the foot with the washcloth. **Rationale: This helps remove dead skin layers**.
   - If nails are brittle or thick and require trimming, replace the water, and allow the foot to soak for 10 to 20 minutes. **Rationale: Soaking softens nails and loosens the debris under them**.
   - Clean nails, as required, with an orange stick. **Rationale: This removes excess debris that harbours microorganisms**.
   - Remove the foot from the basin, and place it on the towel.

6. Dry the foot thoroughly, and apply lotion or foot powder.
   - Blot the foot gently with the towel to dry it thoroughly, particularly between toes. **Rationale: Harsh rubbing can damage skin. Thorough drying reduces the risk of infection**.
   - Apply lotion or lanolin cream to the foot but not between toes. **Rationale: This lubricates dry skin and keeps the area between toes dry**.
   - *Or* apply a foot powder containing a nonirritating deodorant if the client's feet tend to perspire excessively. **Rationale: Foot powders have greater absorbent properties compared with regular bath powders; some also contain menthol, which makes feet feel cool**.

7. If agency policy permits, trim the nails of the first foot while the second foot is soaking.
   - See the discussion on nails for the appropriate method to trim nails. Note that in many agencies, toenail trimming requires a physician's order or is contraindicated for clients with diabetes mellitus, toe infections, and peripheral vascular disease, unless performed by a podiatrist, physician, or advanced practice nurse.

8. Document any foot problems observed.
   - Foot care is not generally recorded unless problems are noted.
   - Record any signs of inflammation, infection, breaks in the skin, corns, troublesome calluses, bunions, and pressure areas. This is of particular importance for clients with peripheral vascular disease and diabetes.

EVALUATION

- Inspect nails and skin after the soak.
- Compare current data with prior assessment data.
- Report any abnormalities to the appropriate members of the health care team.

TEACHING | WELLNESS

Foot Care

- Wash your feet daily, in warm water (not hot) and dry them well, especially between toes.
- When washing, inspect the skin of your feet, including between toes, for breaks or red or swollen areas. Use a mirror, if needed, to visualize all areas.
- To prevent burns, check the water temperature before immersing your feet or stepping into the bathwater.
- Use creams or lotions to moisten the skin of your feet, except between toes. Lotions will also soften calluses. A lotion that is a mixture of lanolin and mineral oil reduces dryness effectively.
- To prevent or control an unpleasant odour caused by excessive foot perspiration, wash your feet frequently and change socks and shoes at least daily. Special deodorant sprays or absorbent foot powders are also helpful. It is generally advisable not to use perfumed products.
- File your toenails, rather than cutting them, to avoid skin injury. File nails straight across the ends of toes. If nails are too thick or too misshapen to file, consult a podiatrist.
- Wear clean stockings or socks daily. Avoid socks with holes or darns that can cause pressure areas. The Canadian Diabetes Association (2008) recommends that, when possible, people with diabetes wear white socks so that they can easily note drainage in the event of a cut or sore.
- Wear correctly fitting shoes that neither restrict your feet nor rub on any area; rubbing can cause corns

and calluses. Check worn shoes for rough spots in the lining. Break in new shoes gradually by increasing the wearing time by 30 to 60 minutes each day.
- Avoid walking barefoot (people with diabetes should NEVER go barefoot) because injury and infection may result. Wear footwear (e.g., shower sandals) in public showers and in change areas to avoid contracting athlete's foot or other infections.
- Several times each day, exercise your feet to promote circulation. Point your feet upward, then point them downward, and move them in circles.
- Avoid wearing constricting garments, such as knee-high stockings, and avoid sitting with the legs crossed at the knees or ankles, which may decrease circulation.
- When your feet are cold, use extra blankets or wear warm socks rather than using heating pads or hot water bottles, which may cause burns.
- Wash any cut on the foot thoroughly, apply a mild antiseptic, and notify the health care provider, if indicated.
- Avoid self-treatment for corns or calluses, especially if reduced peripheral vascular circulation is present. Pumice stones and some callus and corn applications are injurious to skin. Consult a podiatrist or the health care provider first.
- Notify the health care provider if you notice abnormal sores or drainage, pain, or changes in temperature, colour, and sensation of the foot.

Evaluating

See examples of desired health outcomes earlier in the "Planning" section.

Nails

Nails are normally present at birth. They continue to grow throughout life and change very little until people are much older. At that time, nails tend to be tougher, more brittle, and, in some cases, thicker. The nails of an older person normally grow less quickly than those of a younger person and may be ridged and grooved.

Assessing

During the nursing history, the nurse explores the client's usual nail care practices, self-care abilities, and any problems associated with them. See the Assessment: Interview box on nail hygiene. Physical assessment involves inspection of nails (see Chapter 28).

Diagnosing

Nursing diagnoses related to nail care and nail problems include difficulties or inability to perform self-care related to nail care related to such issues as impaired vision, lack of hand–eye coordination; impaired nail integrity related to presence of fungal infection.

ASSESSMENT | INTERVIEW

Nail Hygiene

Ask about your client's nail care practices:
- What are your usual nail care practices?
- Do you have any problems managing your nail care? If so, what are these?
- Have you had any problems associated with your nails (e.g., inflammation of the tissue surrounding the nail, injury, prolonged exposure to water or chemicals, circulatory problems)?

Planning

The nurse identifies measures that will help the client to develop or maintain healthy nail care practices. A schedule of nail care needs to be established. The following are examples of desired client outcomes used to evaluate the effectiveness of nursing interventions:

- Demonstrates healthy nail care practices as shown by the following:
  a. Clean, short nails with smooth edges
  b. Intact cuticles and hydrated surrounding skin
- Describes factors contributing to the nail problem
- Describes preventive interventions for the specific nail problem
- Demonstrates nail care as instructed
- Has pink nail beds and quick return of nail bed colour after blanch test

Implementing

To provide nail care, the nurse needs a nail cutter or sharp scissors, a nail file, an orange stick to push back the cuticle, hand lotion or mineral oil to lubricate any dry tissue around the nails, and a basin of water to soak the nails if they are particularly thick or hard.

Hands or feet are soaked, if needed, and dried; then the nail is cut or filed straight across beyond the end of the finger or toe. See Figure 31.6. Avoid trimming or digging into nails at the lateral corners, as this practice predisposes the client to ingrown toenails. Clients who have diabetes or circulatory problems should have their nails filed, rather than cut; inadvertent injury to tissues can occur if scissors are used. After the initial cut or filing, the nail is filed to round the corners, and the nurse cleans under the nail. The nurse then gently pushes back the cuticle, taking care not to injure it. The next finger or toe is cared for in the same manner. Any abnormalities, such as an infected cuticle or inflammation of the tissue around the nail, are recorded and reported.

Evaluating

See examples of desired health outcomes earlier in the "Planning" section.

Mouth

Developmental Variations

Teeth usually appear 5 to 8 months after birth. Each tooth has three parts: (a) the crown, (b) the root, and (c) the pulp cavity (Figure 31.7). The **crown** is the exposed part of the tooth that is outside the gum. It is covered with a hard substance called **enamel**. The ivory-coloured internal part of the crown below the enamel is **dentin**. The root of a tooth is embedded in the jaw and covered by a bony tissue called **cementum**. The **pulp cavity** in the centre of the tooth contains the blood vessels and nerves.

By the time children are 2 years old, they usually have all 20 of their temporary teeth. At about age 6 or 7 years, children start losing their deciduous teeth, and these are gradually replaced by the 32 permanent teeth. By age 25 years, most people have all their permanent teeth (see Figure 31.8 on the next page).

The incidence of periodontal disease increases during pregnancy because the rise in female hormones affects gingival tissue and increases its reaction to bacterial plaque. Many pregnant women experience more bleeding from the gingival sulcus (the space between a tooth and the gum) during brushing and increased redness and swelling of the **gingiva** (the gum).

Some older adults may have few permanent teeth left, and some wear dentures. Older individuals may lose teeth mainly because of **periodontal disease** (gum disease), rather than **dental caries** (cavities); however, caries can also be the cause of lost teeth in middle-aged adults.

Some recession of gums and a brownish pigmentation of gums occur with age. Because saliva production

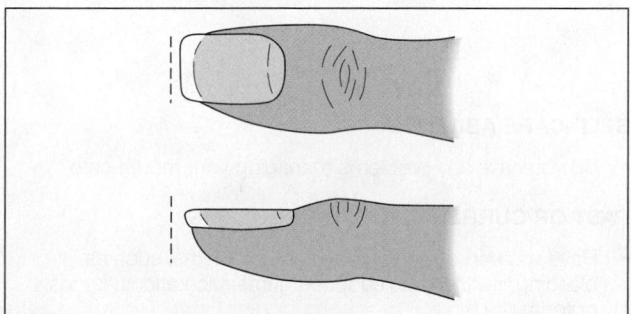

FIGURE 31.6 Fingernails are trimmed straight across.

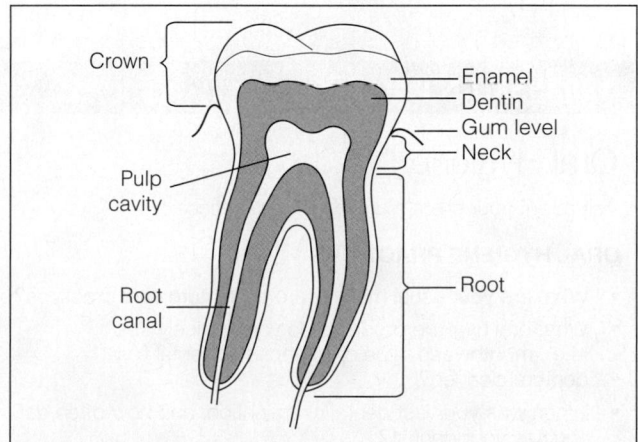

FIGURE 31.7 The anatomy of a tooth.

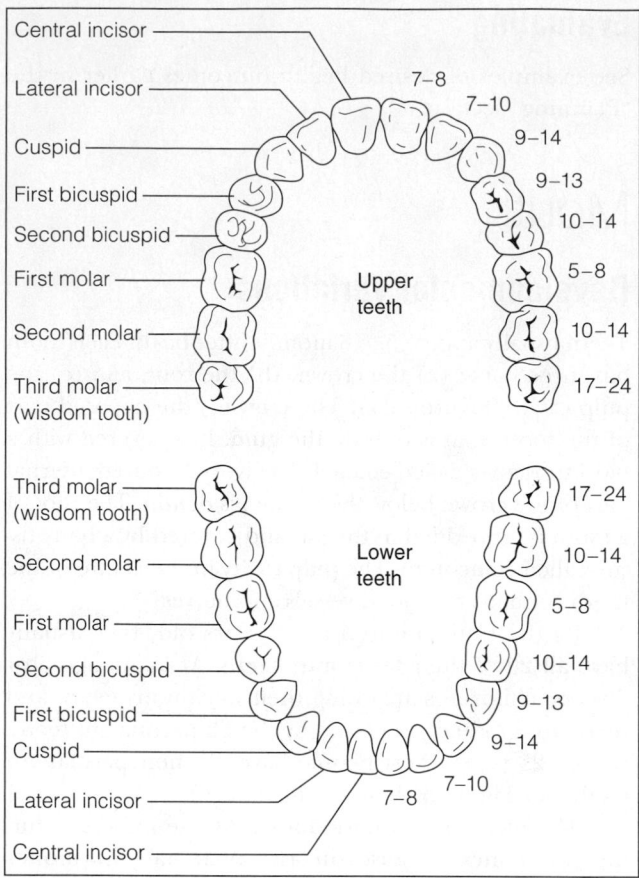

Central incisor
Lateral incisor
Cuspid
First bicuspid
Second bicuspid
First molar
Second molar
Third molar
(wisdom tooth)

7–8
7–10
9–14
9–13
10–14
5–8
10–14
17–24

Upper teeth

Third molar
(wisdom tooth)
Second molar
First molar
Second bicuspid
First bicuspid
Cuspid
Lateral incisor
Central incisor

17–24
10–14
5–8
10–14
9–13
9–14
7–10
7–8

Lower teeth

FIGURE 31.8 Permanent teeth and their times of eruption (stated in years).

decreases with age, dryness of the oral mucosa is a common finding in older people.

Assessing

Assessment of the client's mouth and hygiene practices includes (a) a nursing history, (b) physical assessment of the mouth, and (c) identification of clients at risk for developing oral problems.

NURSING HISTORY The nurse collects data about the client's oral hygiene practices, including dental visits, self-care abilities, and past or current mouth problems. Data about the client's oral hygiene help the nurse determine learning needs and incorporate the client's needs and preferences in the plan of care. Assessment of the client's *self-care abilities* determines the amount and type of nursing assistance to provide. Clients whose hand coordination is impaired, whose cognitive function is impaired, whose illness alters energy levels and motivation, or whose therapy imposes restrictions on activities will need assistance from the nurse. Information about *past or current problems* alerts the nurse to specific interventions or referrals that may be necessary. Questions to elicit oral hygiene information are shown in the Assessment: Interview box.

PHYSICAL ASSESSMENT For information about mouth assessment, see Chapter 28. Dental caries and periodontal disease are the two problems that most frequently affect teeth. Both problems are commonly associated with plaque and tartar deposits. **Plaque** is an *invisible* soft film that adheres to the enamel surface of teeth; it consists of bacteria, molecules of saliva, and remnants of epithelial cells and leukocytes. **Tartar** is a visible, hard deposit of plaque and dead bacteria that forms at the gum lines. Tartar buildup can alter the fibres that attach teeth to gums and eventually disrupt bone tissue. Periodontal disease is characterized by **gingivitis** (red, swollen gingiva), bleeding, receding gum lines, and the formation of pockets between teeth and gums. In advanced periodontal disease (**pyorrhea**), teeth are loose and pus is evident when gums are pressed. See Table 31.6 for additional problems of the mouth.

IDENTIFYING CLIENTS AT RISK Certain clients are prone to oral problems because of lack of knowledge or the inability to maintain oral hygiene. Among these are clients who are seriously ill, confused, comatose, or depressed. In addition, clients with nasogastric tubes, those who are dehydrated, or those receiving oxygen are likely to develop dry oral mucous membranes, especially

---

ASSESSMENT | **INTERVIEW**

Oral Hygiene

Ask about your client's oral hygiene practices:

ORAL HYGIENE PRACTICES

- What are your usual mouth care or denture care practices?
- What oral hygiene products do you routinely use (e.g., mouthwash, type of toothpaste, dental floss, denture cleaner)?
- When was your last dental examination, and how often do you see your dentist?

SELF-CARE ABILITIES

- Do you have any problems managing your mouth care?

PAST OR CURRENT MOUTH PROBLEMS

- Have you had or do you have any problems, such as bleeding, swollen, or reddened gums, ulcerations, lumps, or tooth pain?

TABLE 31.6 Problems of the Mouth

Problem	Description	Nursing Implications
Halitosis	Bad breath	Teach or provide regular oral hygiene.
Glossitis	Inflammation of the tongue	As above
Gingivitis	Inflammation of gums	As above
Periodontal disease	Gums that appear spongy and bleeding	As above
Reddened or excoriated mucosa		Check for ill-fitting dentures.
Xerostomia	Mouth dryness	Have the client sip water or sugarless drinks, as general health permits; avoid caffeine, nicotine, and alcohol, as these can lead to further dryness; and chew on sugarless gum or suck on sugarless hard candies.
Cheilosis	Cracking of lips	Advise the client to lubricate lips and use antimicrobial ointment to prevent infection.
Dental caries	Teeth have darkened areas; may be painful	Advise the client to see a dentist.
Sordes	Accumulation of foul matter (food, microorganisms, and epithelial elements) in the mouth	Teach or provide regular flossing and brushing.
Stomatitis	Inflammation of the oral mucosa	Teach or provide regular oral hygiene.
Parotitis	Inflammation of the parotid salivary glands	Teach or provide regular oral hygiene.

if they breathe through their mouths. Clients who have had oral surgery must receive meticulous oral hygiene care to prevent the development of infections. Intubated clients who cannot swallow their saliva and may experience lesions in the oropharynx are at particular risk, as the mouth can become colonized with bacteria that are then aspirated into the trachea, and this can lead to the development of pneumonia. People who have neurological problems, such as after a cerebrovascular accident (stroke), can have difficulty with oral self-care and may need to rely on others for assistance (Brady et al., 2009).

Individuals with inadequate nutrition, excessive intake of refined sugars, and family history of periodontal disease may also be at risk for dental health problems. Some older people may be at risk, for example, those who choose salty or enamel-eroding sugary foods because of a decline in their number of taste buds. The decreased saliva production in older adults, which produces a dry mouth and thinning of the oral mucosa, is another factor.

A dry mouth can be aggravated by poor fluid intake, heavy smoking, alcohol use, high salt intake, anxiety, and many medications. Medications that can cause dryness of the mouth include diuretics; laxatives, if used excessively; and tranquilizers, such as chlorpromazine (Thorazine) and diazepam (Valium). Some chemotherapeutic agents used to treat cancer also cause oral dryness and mucositis (lesions of the mucous membranes).

Diagnosing

Nursing diagnoses related to problems with oral hygiene and the oral cavity can include self-care deficit related to such factors as poor motor coordination or altered level of consciousness; lack of knowledge about dental hygiene; inadequate dental hygiene practices related to poor toothbrushing techniques or fatigue (as when the client falls asleep without brushing teeth before bedtime). Impaired oral mucous membranes may also be a diagnosis and can be related to a range of issues, such as adverse effects of chemotherapy, lack of salivation, and physical injury (e.g., from oral intubation) or inflammatory processes.

Implementing

Good oral hygiene includes daily stimulation of gums, mechanical brushing and flossing of teeth, and flushing of the mouth. The nurse has various opportunities to teach good oral hygiene by inspecting whether clients (especially children) have brushed their teeth or by actually providing mouth care to clients who are ill or incapacitated. The nurse can also be instrumental in identifying problems that require the intervention of a dentist or an oral surgeon and arranging a referral.

PROMOTING ORAL HEALTH THROUGH THE LIFESPAN
A major role of the nurse in promoting oral health is to teach clients about specific oral hygienic measures.

Infants and Toddlers Dental hygiene is very important in this age group, and children are dependent on their family members or caregivers to ensure the health of their primary teeth.

Dental caries can occur during the toddler period, often as a result of the excessive intake of sweets or a prolonged use of a bottle filled with milk or juice during naps and at bedtime. The nurse should provide parents the following instructions to promote and maintain dental health:

- From birth to 3 years, children should have their gums and teeth brushed twice a day by an adult. The use of fluoridated toothpaste in this age group is determined by the level of risk, which should be discussed with the dentist (Canadian Dental Association, 2010).

- Fluoridated toothpaste should be introduced after age 3 years and only a small amount (the size of a pea) should be used; young children should be supervised by an adult to ensure that they do not ingest the toothpaste, as excess fluoride intake can cause *fluorisis* (a defect in tooth enamel) (Canadian Dental Association, 2010).

- A fluoride supplement should be given daily or as recommended by the physician or dentist, unless the drinking water is fluoridated.

- The Canadian Dental Association recommends that the child's first visit to the dentist be within 6 months of the eruption of the first tooth or by 1 year of age.

- Professional dental attention should be sought for any problems, such as discoloration of teeth; chipping; or signs of infection, such as redness and swelling.

Preschoolers and School-Age Children Because deciduous teeth guide the entrance of permanent teeth, dental care is essential to keep these teeth in good repair. Abnormally placed or lost deciduous teeth can cause misalignment of permanent teeth. Fluoride is essential to prevent dental caries. Preschoolers need to be taught to brush their teeth at least twice a day and to limit their intake of refined sugars. Parental supervision may be needed to ensure the completion of these self-care activities. Regular dental checkups are required during these years when permanent teeth appear.

Adolescents and Adults Proper diet and tooth and mouth care should be taught to adolescents and adults. Brushing and flossing after every meal or at least before going to bed is generally recommended. See specific measures to prevent tooth decay in the Teaching: Wellness box.

CARE OF TEETH

Brushing and Flossing Teeth Thorough brushing of teeth is important in preventing tooth decay. The mechanical action of brushing removes food particles that can harbour and incubate bacteria. It also stimulates circulation in gums,

---

TEACHING | **WELLNESS**

Measures to Prevent Tooth Decay

Several oral hygiene practices can help prevent tooth decay:

- Brush teeth and tongue after each meal and at bedtime; at a minimum, once a day and always before going to bed.
- Use a soft brush with rounded bristles with a size and shape that allow you to reach all the way to the back teeth.
- Floss teeth at least daily because "if you don't floss, you are missing more than a third of your tooth surface." Brush teeth after flossing (Canadian Dental Association, 2012).
- Ensure an adequate intake of nutrients, particularly calcium, phosphorus, and vitamins A, C, and D.
- Avoid sweet foods and drinks between meals. Take them in moderation at meals.
- Eat coarse, fibrous foods (cleansing foods), such as fresh fruits and raw vegetables.
- Have topical fluoride applications, as prescribed by the dentist, in locales where fluoridated water is not available.
- Have a checkup by a dentist every 6 to 9 months.

---

thus maintaining their healthy firmness. One of the techniques recommended for brushing teeth is called the **sulcular technique**, which removes plaque and cleans under the gingival margins. Fluoride toothpaste is recommended because of its antibacterial protection. An effective dentifrice (toothpaste) can also be made by using baking soda.

Caring for Dentures Some people have artificial teeth, or *dentures*. A *plate*, or denture, is a complete set of teeth. Some clients may have a *bridge*, which is a partial set of artificial teeth. Artificial teeth either are fixed and cannot be removed or are removable. People who wear dentures or other types of oral prostheses should be encouraged to use them. Those who do not wear their prostheses are prone to shrinkage of gums, which results in further tooth loss.

Like natural teeth, artificial dentures collect microorganisms and food debris. Dentures, therefore, need to be cleaned regularly, at least once a day. They can be removed from the mouth, scrubbed with a toothbrush, rinsed, and reinserted. Some people use a dentifrice for cleaning teeth, and others use commercial cleaning compounds for plates.

ASSISTING CLIENTS WITH ORAL CARE When providing mouth care for partially or completely dependent clients, the nurse should wear gloves to guard against infections. Other required equipment includes a curved basin that fits snugly under the client's chin (e.g., a kidney basin or emesis basin) to receive the rinse water and a towel to protect the client and the bedclothes. See Skill 31.4. When providing care of dentures, it is important to assess the client's need for privacy when dentures are removed and cleaned.

SKILL 31.4 BRUSHING AND FLOSSING TEETH

PURPOSES

- To remove food particles from around and between teeth
- To remove dental plaque
- To promote the client's feelings of well-being
- To prevent sores and infection of oral tissues

ASSESSMENT

- Determine the extent of the client's self-care abilities.
- Assess the client's usual mouth care practices.
- Inspect the client's lips, gums, oral mucosa, and tongue for deviations from normal.
- Identify the presence of any oral problems, such as tooth caries, halitosis, gingivitis, and loose or broken teeth.
- Check whether the client has any bridgework or wears dentures. If the client has dentures, ask if any tenderness or soreness is present and, if so, the location of the areas for ongoing assessment.

Equipment

For Brushing and Flossing

- Towel
- Disposable gloves
- Curved basin
- Toothbrush (soft brush with rounded bristles; the shape and size should allow easy reach all the way to the back teeth)
- Cup of tepid water
- Dentifrice
- Mouthwash
- Dental floss, at least two pieces 20 cm long
- Floss holder (optional)

For Cleaning Dentures

- Disposable gloves
- Tissue or piece of gauze
- Denture container
- Clean washcloth
- Toothbrush or stiff-bristled brush
- Dentifrice or denture cleaner
- Tepid water
- Container of mouthwash
- Curved basin
- Towel

IMPLEMENTATION

Preparation

Assemble all the necessary equipment.

Performance

1. Before performing the procedure, introduce yourself and verify the client's identity using two identifiers or per agency protocol. Explain to the client what you are going to do, why it is necessary, and how he or she can participate.

2. Perform hand hygiene, and follow other appropriate infection prevention and control procedures (e.g., disposable gloves). **Rationale: Wearing gloves while providing mouth care prevents the nurse from acquiring infections. Gloves also prevent transmission of microorganisms to the client**.

3. Provide for client privacy by drawing the curtains around the bed or closing the door to the room. Some agencies provide signs indicating the need for privacy. **Rationale: Hygiene is a personal matter**.

4. Prepare the client.
   - Assist the client to the sitting position in bed, if the client's health permits. If not, assist the client to the side-lying position with the head turned *so that liquid is prevented from draining down the client's throat.*

5. Prepare the equipment.
   - Place a towel under the client's chin.
   - Put on disposable gloves.
   - Moisten the bristles of the toothbrush with tepid water, and apply the dentifrice to the toothbrush.
   - Use a soft toothbrush (a small one for a child) and the client's choice of dentifrice.
   - For the client who must remain in bed, place or hold the curved basin under the client's chin, fitting the small curve around the chin or neck.
   - Inspect the mouth and teeth.

6. Floss the client's teeth.
   - Assist the client to floss independently, or floss the teeth of an alert and cooperative client as described below. Waxed floss is less likely to fray than unwaxed floss; particles between the teeth attach more readily to unwaxed floss than to waxed floss.
     a. Wrap one end of the floss around the third finger of each hand (see ❶).
     b. To floss the upper teeth, use your thumb and index finger to stretch the floss. Slide the floss between teeth and wrap it into a "C" shape around the base of the tooth and gently under the gumline. Wipe the tooth with the floss from the base to tip two or three times (Canadian Dental Association, 2012). Start at the back on the right side and work around to the

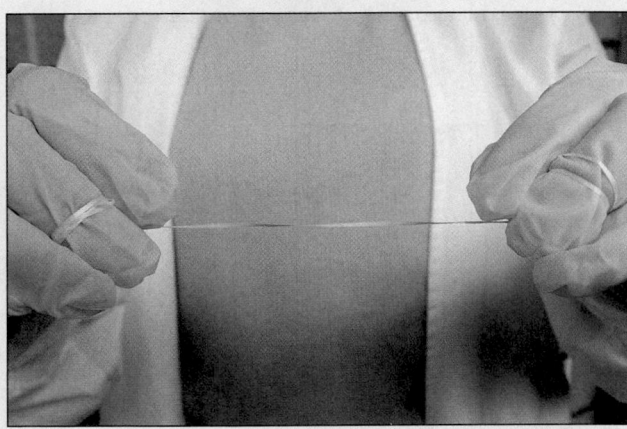

❶ Stretching the floss between the third finger of each hand

(continued)

SKILL 31.4 **BRUSHING AND FLOSSING TEETH** (*continued*)

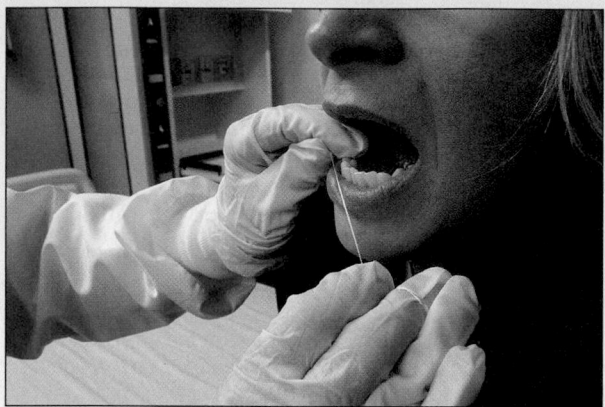

❷ Flossing the lower teeth by using the index fingers to stretch the floss

> back of the left side, or work from the centre teeth to the back of the jaw on either side.
>
> c. To floss the lower teeth, use your index fingers to stretch the floss (see ❷).

- Give the client tepid water or mouthwash to rinse the mouth and a curved basin in which to spit the water.
- Assist the client in wiping the mouth.

7. Brush the client's teeth.

- Hand the toothbrush to the client, or brush the client's teeth as follows:
  a. Hold the brush against teeth, with the bristles at a 45-degree angle. The tips of the outer bristles should rest against and penetrate under the gingival sulcus (see ❸). The brush will clean under the sulcus of two or three teeth at one time. **Rationale: This sulcular technique removes plaque and cleans under the gingival margins**.
  b. Use a gentle, circular, massaging motion up and down. Do not scrub (see ❹).
  c. Repeat until all outer and inner surfaces of the teeth and sulci of the gums are cleaned.
  d. Clean the biting surfaces by moving the brush back and forth over them in short strokes (see ❺).
  e. Brush the tongue gently with the toothbrush. **Rationale: Brushing removes bacteria and freshens breath. A coated tongue may be**

caused by poor oral hygiene and low fluid intake. Brushing gently and carefully helps prevent gagging or vomiting.

- Hand the client the water cup or mouthwash to rinse the mouth vigorously. Then, ask the client to spit the water and excess dentifrice into the basin. Some agencies supply a standard mouthwash. Alternatively, a mouth rinse of normal saline can be an effective cleaner and moisturizer. **Rationale: Vigorous rinsing loosens food particles and washes out already loosened particles**.
- Repeat the preceding steps until the mouth is free of dentifrice and food particles.
- Remove the curved basin, and help the client wipe the mouth.

8. Remove and dispose of equipment appropriately.

- Remove and clean the curved basin.
- Remove and discard the gloves.

EVALUATION

Document your assessment of the client's teeth, tongue, gums, and oral mucosa. Record any problems, such as sores or inflammation, bleeding, and swelling of the gums. Brushing and flossing of teeth are not usually recorded.

Variation: Artificial Dentures

1. Remove the client's dentures.

- Put on gloves. **Rationale: Wearing gloves decreases the likelihood of spreading infection**.
- If the client cannot remove the dentures, take tissue or gauze, grasp the upper plate at the front teeth with your thumb and second finger, and move the denture up and down slightly (see ❻). **Rationale: The slight movement breaks the suction that holds the plate on the roof of the mouth**.
- Lower the upper plate, move it out of the mouth, and place it in the denture container.
- Lift the lower plate, turning it so that the left side, for example, is slightly lower than the right, to remove the plate from the mouth without stretching the client's lips. Place the lower plate in the denture container.
- Remove a partial denture by exerting equal pressure on the border of each side of the denture, not on the clasps, which can bend or break.

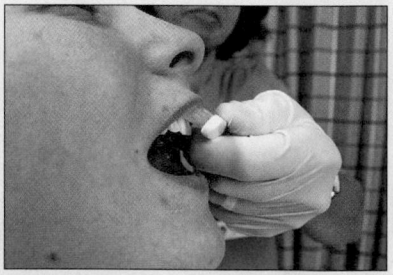

❸ The sulcular technique: Place the bristles at a 45-degree angle with the tips of the outer bristles under the gumline, where the gums and teeth meet.

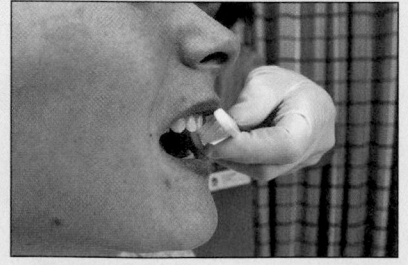

❹ Brushing from the sulcus to the crown of teeth

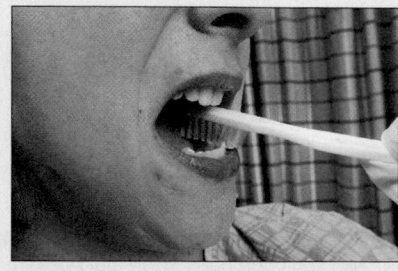

❺ Brushing the biting surfaces

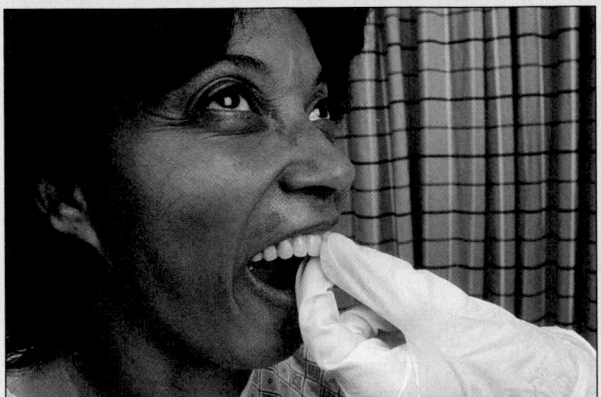

❻ Removing the top dentures by first breaking the suction

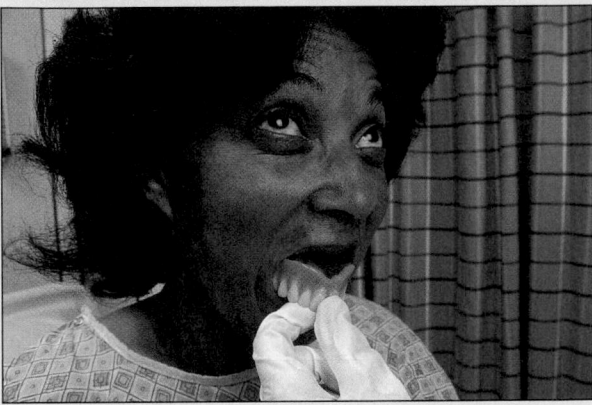

❼ Inserting the dentures at a slight angle

2. Clean the dentures.

- Take the denture container to a sink. Take care not to drop the dentures. Place a washcloth in the bowl of the sink *to prevent damage if the dentures are dropped.*
- Use a toothbrush or special stiff-bristled brush to scrub the dentures with the cleaning agent and tepid water.
- Rinse the dentures with tepid running water. **Rationale: Rinsing removes the cleaning agent and food particles**.
- If the dentures are stained, soak them in a commercial cleaner. Be sure to follow the manufacturer's directions. To prevent corrosion, dentures with metal parts should not be soaked overnight.

3. Inspect the dentures and the client's mouth.

- Observe the dentures for any rough, sharp, or worn areas that could irritate the tongue or the mucous membranes of the mouth, lips, and gums.
- Inspect the mouth for any redness, irritated areas, or indications of infection.
- Assess the fit of the dentures. People who have dentures should see a dentist at least once a year to

check the fit and the presence of any irritation to the soft tissues of the mouth. Clients who need repairs to their dentures or new dentures may need a referral for financial assistance.

4. Return the dentures to the client's mouth.

- Offer some mouthwash and a curved basin to rinse the mouth. If the client cannot insert the dentures independently, insert the plates one at a time. Hold each plate at a slight angle while inserting it, to avoid injuring the lips (see **❼**).

5. Assist the client, as needed.

- Wipe the client's hands and mouth with the towel.
- If the client does not want to or cannot wear the dentures, store them in a denture container with water. Label the container with the client's name and identification number.

6. Remove and discard gloves.

EVALUATION

Document and report all assessments, including any problems, such as an irritated area on the mucous membrane.

Foam swabs are often used in health care agencies to clean the mouths of dependent clients. While these swabs are convenient, they are ineffective in removing dental plaque and, ideally, a soft bristle toothbrush should be used (Pear, 2007). Lemon-glycerine swabs are not recommended, as they irritate and dry the oral mucosa and can decalcify teeth.

Special Oral Hygiene For the client who is debilitated or unconscious or who has excessive dryness, sores, or irritations of the mouth, it may be necessary to clean the oral mucosa and the tongue in addition to teeth. Agency practices differ concerning special mouth care and the frequency with which it is provided. Depending on the health of the client's mouth, special care may be needed every 2 to 8 hours.

Mouth care for unconscious or debilitated clients is important because their mouths tend to become dry and consequently predisposed to infections. Dryness occurs because the client cannot take fluids by mouth, is often breathing through the mouth, or may be receiving oxygen, which tends to dry the mucous membranes. For clients with special oral hygiene needs, the nurse needs to focus on removal of plaque and microorganisms and promote client comfort. If possible, a soft-bristled toothbrush should be used as it provides the best means of plaque removal. A sodium bicarbonate toothpaste will help breakdown mucus and reduce the acidity of saliva, which helps decrease bacteria (Pear, 2007). If the client cannot tolerate the use of a toothbrush, the nurse can use a foam swab or gauze soaked with saline to swab teeth and the tongue.

The nurse can use commercially prepared mouth-washes, tepid water, or normal saline (according to agency policy) for oral hygiene. Long-term use of commercially prepared mouthwashes can lead to further dryness of the mucosa and changes in tooth enamel. Mineral oil is contraindicated because aspiration of it can initiate an infection (lipid pneumonia). Regular strength hydrogen peroxide is *not* recommended for use in oral care because it irritates healthy oral mucosa and may alter the micro-flora of the mouth. Skill 31.5 focuses on oral care for the unconscious person, but it can be adapted for conscious persons who are seriously ill or have mouth problems.

SKILL 31.5 PROVIDING ORAL CARE FOR AN UNCONSCIOUS CLIENT

PURPOSES

- To maintain the intactness and health of the lips, tongue, and mucous membranes of the mouth
- To prevent oral infections
- To clean and moisten the membranes of the mouth and lips

ASSESSMENT

- Inspect lips, gums, oral mucosa, and tongue for deviations from normal.
- Identify the presence of oral problems, such as tooth caries, halitosis, gingivitis, and loose or broken teeth.
- Assess for a gag reflex, when appropriate.

Equipment

- Towel
- Curved basin
- Disposable clean gloves
- Bite-block to hold the mouth open and teeth apart (optional)
- Toothbrush
- Cup of tepid water
- Dentifrice or denture cleaner
- Tissue or piece of gauze to remove dentures (optional)
- Denture container as needed
- Mouthwash
- Rubber-tipped bulb syringe
- Suction catheter with suction apparatus when aspiration is a concern
- Foam swabs and cleaning solution for cleaning the mucous membranes
- Water-soluble lip moisturizer

IMPLEMENTATION

Performance

1. Before performing the procedure, introduce yourself and verify the client's identity using two identifiers or per agency protocol. Explain to the client and the family what you are going to do and why it is necessary.

2. Perform hand hygiene, and follow other appropriate infection prevention and control procedures (e.g., disposable gloves).

3. Provide for client privacy by drawing the curtains around the bed or closing the door to the room. Some agencies provide signs indicating the need for privacy. **Rationale: Hygiene is a personal matter**.

4. Prepare the client.
   - Position the unconscious client in the side-lying position, with the head of the bed lowered. **Rationale: In this position, the saliva automatically runs out by gravity rather than being aspirated into the lungs.** This position is chosen for the unconscious client receiving mouth care. If the client's head cannot be lowered, turn it to one side. **Rationale: The fluid will readily run out of the mouth or pool in the side of the mouth, where it can be suctioned**.
   - Place the towel under the client's chin.
   - Place the curved basin against the client's chin, and lower the client's cheek to receive the fluid from the mouth (see ❶).
   - Put on gloves.

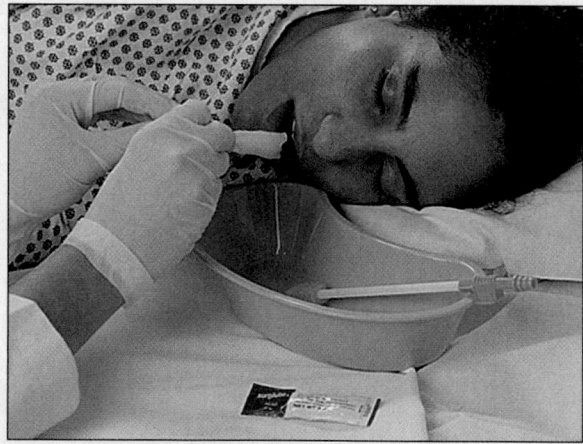

❶ Position of client and placement of curved basin when providing special mouth care

5. Clean the client's teeth, and rinse the mouth.
   - If the person has natural teeth, brush them as described in Skill 31.4 (p. 807). Brush gently and carefully to avoid injuring the gums. If the client has artificial teeth, clean them as described in the "Variation" component of Skill 31.4 (p. 808).
   - Rinse the client's mouth by drawing about 10 mL of water or alcohol-free mouthwash into the syringe and injecting it gently into each side of the mouth. **Rationale: If the solution is injected with force, some of it may flow down the client's throat and be aspirated into the lungs**.

- Watch carefully to make sure that all the rinsing solution has run out of the mouth into the basin. If not, suction the fluid from the mouth. **Rationale: Fluid remaining in the mouth can be aspirated into the lungs**.
- Repeat rinsing until the mouth is free of dentifrice, if used.

6. Inspect and clean the oral tissues.

- If the tissues appear dry or unclean, clean them with foam swabs or gauze and cleaning solution, following agency policy.
- Picking up a moistened foam swab, wipe the mucous membrane of one cheek. Discard the swab in a waste container; use a fresh one to clean the next area. **Rationale: Using separate applicators for each area of the mouth prevents the transfer of microorganisms from one area to another**.
- Clean all of the mouth tissues in an orderly progression, using separate applicators: cheeks, roof of the mouth, base of the mouth, and tongue.
- Observe the tissues closely for inflammation and dryness.
- Rinse the client's mouth as described in step 5.
- Remove and discard gloves.

7. Ensure client comfort.

- Remove the basin, and dry around the client's mouth with the towel. Replace artificial dentures, if indicated.
- Lubricate the client's lips with water-soluble moisturizer. **Rationale: Lubrication prevents cracking and subsequent infection.**

8. Document your assessment of the client's teeth, tongue, gums, and oral mucosa. Include any problems, such as sores or inflammation and swelling of the gums.

EVALUATION

- Consider the client's medical diagnosis and treatment (e.g., chemotherapy, oxygen) and the necessary nursing interventions related to oral hygiene.
- Conduct an ongoing assessment, if appropriate, of the oral mucosa, gums, tongue, and lips.
- Report deviations from normal to the appropriate members of the health care team.
- Conduct appropriate follow-up, such as a referral to a dentist for dental caries.

TABLE 31.7 Evaluation Goals and Outcomes: Oral Hygiene and Health

Goal	Desired Outcomes
Improves oral hygiene practices	The oral mucosa, tongue, and lips are pink, moist, and intact.
	Dental surfaces are free of debris and plaque.
	Breath is free of halitosis.
	The client brushes teeth after meals and at bedtime.
	The client flosses teeth daily.
	The client obtains regular dental care.
	The client uses fluoridation or fluoride supplements, as recommended.
Maintains integrity of oral tissues	The oral mucosa is intact, smooth, well hydrated, and uniform in colour.
	Gums are firm, well hydrated, not bleeding, and of uniform colour.
	The tongue is well hydrated.
	Lips are smooth and well hydrated.
	Oral tissues are free of inflammation and pain.

Evaluating

By using data collected during care—status of the oral mucosa, lips, tongue, teeth, and so on—the nurse judges whether desired outcomes have been achieved. Examples of client goals and related outcomes are shown in Table 31.7.

See the Evidence-Informed Practice box on preventing ventilator acquired pneumonia through mouth care on the next page.

Hair Care

The appearance of a person's hair often reflects his or her feelings of self-concept and well-being. Many people take pride in their hair and go to great lengths to keep it looking healthy and groomed. People who feel ill may not groom their hair as they used to because they lack energy, are in pain and find it difficult to perform hair care, or do not have access to usual hair washing or grooming resources. Some people who are depressed may not be motivated to care for their hair, and it may appear unkempt. A dirty scalp and hair can be itchy, uncomfortable, and malodorous. Hair may also reflect state of health, for example, excessive coarseness and dryness may indicate hypothyroidism.

EVIDENCE-INFORMED PRACTICE

Preventing Ventilator Acquired Pneumonia through Mouth Care

Clients who are intubated are critically ill and reliant on others for their hygiene, including mouth care. Oral hygiene is important in intubated clients as they are generally not able to swallow normally and saliva accumulates in the mouth; as well, the endotracheal tube can cause local trauma to the oropharyngeal mucosa and tongue leading to an increased risk of discomfort and infection. Ventilator associated pneumonia (VAP) is a complication in clients receiving mechanical ventilation, and there is strong evidence that oropharyngeal colonization and colonization of dental plaque with such bacteria as *Staphylococcus aureus* and *Pseudomonas aeruginosa* can lead to VAP. According to Shi et al. (2010), "fundamental nursing practices such as hand hygiene, semi-recumbent positioning of patients, subglottal suctioning and reducing dental plaque colonized with respiratory pathogens are thought to play a critical role in minimizing the incidence of VAP." Oral hygiene using chlorhexidine, povidone–iodine, Listerine, saline, and oral antibiotics has been studied. A meta-analysis conducted by Pineda, Saliba, and El Solh (2006) concluded that oral decontamination does reduce the incidence of VAP and recommended that oral decontamination be integrated into the care of intubated clients. However, there were no conclusions related to the best product. The systematic review by Shi et al. is important, as it will help assess all quality studies related to oral hygiene care and products used in minimizing VAP in intubated clients.

NURSING IMPLICATIONS: Nurses in critical care settings can become focused on so many aspects of care that they may overlook basic hygiene needs, such as mouth care. This systematic review will be helpful in delineating the requirements and methods for providing the best oral hygiene to intubated clients so as to minimize complications and improve quality of life.

Source: Based on Shi, Z., Xie, H., Wang, P., Wu, Y., Chen, E., Ng, L., ... Needleman, I. (2010). Oral hygiene care for critically ill patients to prevent ventilator associated pneumonia (Protocol). *Cochrane Database of Systematic Reviews 2010, Issue 2.* Art. No.: CD008367. doi: 10.1002/14651858.CD008367

Developmental Variations

Newborns may have **lanugo** (the fine hair on the body of the fetus over the shoulders, back, and sacrum). Lanugo disappears, and the hair distribution on the eyebrows, head, and eyelashes of young children subsequently becomes noticeable. Some newborns have hair on their scalps; others are free of hair at birth, but hair grows over the scalp during the first year of life.

Pubic hair usually appears in early puberty, followed, in about 6 months, by the growth of axillary hair. Boys develop facial hair in later puberty.

In adolescence, sebaceous glands increase in activity because of increased hormone levels. As a result, hair follicle openings enlarge to accommodate the increased amount of sebum, which can make the adolescent's hair oilier.

In older adults, hair is generally thinner, grows more slowly, and loses its colour as a result of aging tissues and diminishing circulation. Men often lose their scalp hair and may become completely bald. This phenomenon may also occur when a man is relatively young. The older person's hair tends to be drier than normal. With age, axillary and pubic hairs become finer and more scant, in contrast to the hair of the eyebrows, which becomes bristly and coarse. Many women develop hair on their faces, which may be a concern to them.

Assessing

NURSING HISTORY When taking the nursing history, the nurse elicits data about usual hair care, self-care abilities, history of hair or scalp problems, and conditions known to affect hair. Chemotherapeutic agents and radiation of the head may cause alopecia (hair loss). Hypothyroidism may cause hair to become thin, dry, and brittle. Use of some hair dyes and curling or straightening preparations can cause hair to become dry and brittle. Questions to elicit these data are shown in the Assessment: Interview box for hair care.

PHYSICAL ASSESSMENT Physical assessment of the hair is discussed in Chapter 28. Some problems related to hair include dandruff, hair loss, ticks, pediculosis, scabies, and hirsutism.

Dandruff Often accompanied by itching, dandruff appears as a diffuse scaling of the scalp. In severe cases, it involves the auditory canals and the eyebrows. Dandruff can usually be treated effectively with a commercial shampoo. In severe or persistent cases, the client may need the advice of a physician.

Hair Loss Hair loss and growth are continual processes. Some permanent thinning of hair normally occurs with aging. Baldness, common in men, is thought to be a hereditary condition for which there is no known remedy other than wearing a hairpiece or undergoing costly surgical hair transplantation, in which hair is taken from the back or the sides of the scalp and surgically affixed to the hairless area. Hair loss may also occur as a result of certain cancer chemotherapy agents.

Ticks Ticks are small grey-brown parasites that bite into tissue and suck blood. Ticks can transmit several diseases to people, in particular, Rocky Mountain spotted fever, Lyme disease, and tularemia. Ticks should

Hair Care

Ask the client about hair care:

HAIR CARE PRACTICES

- How do you usually take care of your hair?
- What hair care products do you routinely use (e.g., hair spray, lubricant, shampoo, conditioners, hair dye, curling or straightening preparations)?

SELF-CARE ABILITIES

- Do you have any problems managing your hair?

PAST OR CURRENT HAIR PROBLEMS

- Have you had any of the following conditions or therapies: recent chemotherapy, hypothyroidism, radiation of the head, unexplained loss of hair, growth of excessive body hair?
- How do you manage these hair problems?

---

never be forcibly pulled from the skin because the sucking apparatus may remain and become infected. To remove the tick, use blunt tweezers or gloved fingers to grasp the tick as close to the skin as possible. Gently pull the tick away by using a perpendicular traction to remove the tick. Be careful not to twist or squeeze the tick's body. Wash the area with antibacterial soap. Save the tick in a bottle of rubbing alcohol in case there is a need to analyze the tick for disease. Applying heat with a match or petroleum jelly are ineffective and can be dangerous.

Pediculosis (Lice) **Lice** are parasitic insects that infest mammals. Infestation with lice is called **pediculosis**. Hundreds of varieties of lice can infest humans. Three common kinds are *Pediculus capitis* (the head louse), *Pediculus corporis* (the body louse), and *Pediculus pubis* (the crab louse).

Head and pubic lice lay their eggs on hair; the eggs look like oval particles, similar to dandruff, clinging to hair. Bites and pustular eruptions may also be noticed at the hairlines and behind the ears. Lice are very small, greyish white, and difficult to see. The crab louse in the pubic area has red legs. Lice can be contracted from infested clothes and direct head-to-head (hair-to-hair) contact with a person who has the infestation; lice do not leap or fly, nor do animals act as vectors for human lice (Canadian Paediatric Society, 2008).

Pediculus capitis is found on the scalp and tends to stay hidden in hair; similarly, *Pediculus pubis* stays in pubic hair. *Pediculus corporis* tends to cling to clothing so that when a client undresses, the lice may not be evident on the body; these lice suck blood from the person and lay their eggs on the clothing. The nurse can suspect their presence in the clothing if (a) the person habitually scratches, (b) he or she has scratches on skin, and (c) he or she has hemorrhagic spots on skin areas where the lice have sucked blood.

Treatment consists of the application of pediculocides and manual removal of nits. Permethrin 1% cream rinse (e.g., Kwellada, Nix) is an insecticide commonly used in Canada; permethrin is neurotoxic to lice but not to humans. While generally effective, some lice have become resistant to permethrin in some countries—the resistance rates in Canada are unknown because formal studies have not been performed (Canadian Paediatric Society, 2008). A new noninsecticide containing isopropyl myristate 50% and ST-cyclomethicone 50% (Resultz rinse) has become available in Canada; this agent (not recommended for children under age 4 years) works by dissolving the exoskeleton of the louse. See Box 31.2 on the next page for prevention of pediculosis.

Scabies **Scabies** is a contagious skin infestation by the eight-legged *Sarcoptes scabiei*, or the "itch mite." The characteristic lesion is the burrow produced by the female mite as it penetrates into the upper layers of skin. The burrows are short, wavy, brown or black, thread-like lesions most commonly observed between the webs of fingers and the folds of wrists and elbows. The mites cause intense itching that is more pronounced at night because the increased warmth of skin has a stimulating effect on the parasites. Secondary lesions caused by scratching include vesicles, papules, pustules, excoriations, and crusts. Treatment involves thorough cleansing of the body with soap and water to remove scales and debris from crusts, followed by an application of a scabicide lotion. All bed linens and clothing should be washed in very hot or boiling water.

Hirsutism The growth of excessive body hair is called **hirsutism**. The acceptance of body hair in the axillae and on the legs is largely dictated by culture. The cause of excessive body hair is not always known. Older women may have some on their faces, and women in menopause may also experience some growth of facial hair. Excessive body hair may be caused by the action of the endocrine system. Heredity is also thought to influence the pattern of distribution.

BOX 31.2 PREVENTING PEDICULOSIS

Clients can take steps to prevent pediculosis:

- "Excessive cleaning of personal items in the environment is not warranted. The cleaning of items in prolonged or intimate contact with the head (e.g., hats, pillowcases, brushes and combs) may be warranted" (Canadian Paediatric Society, 2008). Washing items in hot water (66°C), drying them in a hot dryer for 15 minutes, or storing them in an occlusive plastic bag for 2 weeks will kill lice and nits.
- Discourage head-to-head (hair-to-hair) contact and sharing of headgear (e.g., hats, headbands, barrettes), scarves, towels, brushes, and combs among all children.
- Teach children to put their hats and scarves in their coat sleeves or back pack.
- Conduct regular pediculosis screening in daycare centres and schools; parents should check their child's hair weekly as a routine practice and daily in the event of an outbreak at daycare or school.
- Keep long hair tied back or braided. (Short hair does not prevent infestation.)
- There are no published trials on the safety or efficacy of home remedies, such as mayonnaise, oil, petrolatum jelly (Canadian Paediatric Society, 2008).
- "Exclusion from school and daycare due to the detection of the presence of 'nits' does not have sound medical rationale. Even the detection of active head lice should not lead to the exclusion of the affected child. Treatment should be recommended, and close head-to-head contact should be discouraged pending treatment" (Canadian Paediatric Society, 2008).

Diagnosing

Nursing diagnoses related to hair hygiene and hair and scalp problems can include self-care deficit in hair grooming and hygiene related to such factors as poor range of motion, lack of motivation, lack of access to hygiene products and/or facilities, or altered level of consciousness; impaired skin integrity related to such factors as presence of scabies or persistent itchiness; and poor body image related to hirsutism or hair loss.

Planning

In planning care, the nurse identifies nursing activities that will assist the client to achieve these goals:

- Maintaining or improving hair care
- Maintaining or improving a sense of well-being
- Preventing specific hair and scalp problems

Examples of desired health outcomes to evaluate the effectiveness of nursing interventions have the client doing the following:

- Performing hair grooming with assistance (specify)
- Having clean, well-groomed, resilient hair with a healthy sheen
- Having reduced or absent scalp lesions or infestations
- Describing the contributing factors, interventions, and preventive measures for a specific hair problem (e.g., dandruff)

Plans for assisting the client should take into account the client's personal preferences, health, and energy resources, as well as the time, equipment, and personnel available. Often, clients like to receive hair care after a bath, before receiving visitors, and before retiring. At some agencies, shampoos can be given for clients only after a physician's order.

Implementing

Hair needs to be brushed or combed daily and washed, as needed, to be kept clean. Nurses may need to provide hair care for clients who cannot meet their own hygiene needs.

BRUSHING AND COMBING HAIR Brushing hair a minimum of once a day is necessary to stimulate the circulation of blood in the scalp, distribute oil produced by the scalp along the hair shaft, and arrange hair strands to avoid tangles or matting. Long hair can present a problem for clients confined to bed, as it may become matted. It should be combed and brushed at least once a day to prevent this. One method is to comb the back of the head while the client is positioned on the side. A brush with stiff bristles provides the best stimulation to blood circulation in the scalp. The bristles should not be so sharp that they injure the client's scalp, however. A comb with dull, even teeth is advisable. A comb with sharp teeth might injure the scalp; combs that are too fine can pull and break the client's hair. Some clients prefer to have their hair tied neatly in the back or braided until other assistance is available or until they feel better and can look after it themselves.

Dark-skinned people often have thicker, drier, curlier, or kinkier hair compared with light-skinned people and may use combs with a wide tooth. Spiralled or very curly hair may stand out from the scalp. Although the shafts of spiralled hair look strong and wiry, they have less strength than straight hair shafts and can break easily. Oil-based products may be used in such cases. This type of hair tends to be dry, so shampooing is generally needed less often than for straight hair. Skill 31.6 describes how to provide hair care for clients.

SHAMPOOING HAIR Hair should be washed as often as needed to be kept clean. There are several ways to shampoo clients' hair, depending on health, strength, and age. The client who is well enough to take a shower can shampoo while in the shower. The client who is

SKILL 31.6 PROVIDING HAIR CARE FOR CLIENTS

PURPOSES

- To increase the client's comfort
- To stimulate the blood circulation to the scalp
- To assess or monitor hair or scalp problems (e.g., matted hair or dandruff)
- To distribute hair oils and provide a healthy sheen

ASSESSMENT

Determine

- History of the following conditions or therapies: recent chemotherapy, hypothyroidism, radiation of the head, unexplained hair loss, and growth of excessive body hair
- Usual hair care practices and routinely used hair care products (e.g., hair spray, shampoo, conditioners, hair oil preparation, hair dye, curling or straightening preparations)

Assess

- Condition of the hair and scalp. Is the hair straight, curly, kinky? Is the hair matted or tangled? Is the scalp dry?
- Evenness of hair growth over the scalp, in particular, any patchy loss of hair; hair texture, oiliness, thickness, or thinness; presence of lesions, infections, or infestations on the scalp; presence of hirsutism.
- Self-care abilities (e.g., any problems managing hair care).

PLANNING

Brushing and combing hair, shampooing hair, and shaving facial hair can be delegated to another member of the health care team unless the client has a condition in which the procedure would be contraindicated (e.g., cervical spinal injury or trauma). The nurse needs to assess the health care team member's knowledge and experience of hair care for clients of other cultures, if appropriate.

Equipment

- Clean brush and comb
- A wide-toothed comb is usually used for people with very curly or kinky hair to avoid breaking the hair strands
- Towel
- Hair oil preparation, if appropriate

IMPLEMENTATION

1. Before performing the procedure, introduce yourself and verify the client's identity using two identifiers or per agency protocol. Explain to the client what you are going to do, why it is necessary, and how he or she can participate.
2. Perform hand hygiene, and follow other appropriate infection prevention and control procedures.
3. Provide for client privacy by drawing the curtains around the bed or closing the door to the room. Some agencies provide signs indicating the need for privacy. **Rationale: Hygiene is a personal matter**.
4. Position and prepare the client appropriately.
   - Assist the client who can sit to move to a chair. **Rationale: Hair is more easily brushed and combed when the client is sitting.** If health permits, assist a client confined to a bed to a sitting position by raising the head of the bed. Otherwise, assist the client to alternate side-lying positions, and do one side of the head at a time.
   - If the client remains in bed, place a clean towel over the pillow and the client's shoulders. Place a towel over the shoulders of the sitting client. **Rationale: The towel collects any removed hair, dirt, and scaly material**.
   - Remove any pins or ribbons in the hair.
5. Remove any mats or tangles gradually.
   - Mats can usually be pulled apart with fingers or worked out with repeated brushings.
   - If the hair is very tangled, rub an oil, such as mineral oil, or commercial detangling product on the strands to help loosen the tangles.
   - Comb out tangles in a small section of hair toward the ends. Stabilize the hair with one hand and comb toward the ends of the hair with the other hand. **Rationale: This avoids discomfort and scalp trauma**.
6. Brush and comb the hair.
   - For short hair, brush and comb one side at a time. Divide long hair into two sections by parting it down the middle from the front to the back. If the hair is very thick, divide each section into front and back subsections or into several layers.
7. Arrange the client's hair as neatly and attractively as possible, according to the individual's preferences.
   - Braiding long hair helps prevent tangles.
8. Document assessments and special nursing interventions. Daily combing and brushing of the hair are not normally recorded.

Variation: Hair Care for Clients with Very Curly and Kinky Hair

- Position and prepare the client.
- Separate the hair into four sections, proceeding from one section to the next.
- Untangle the hair first, if appropriate.
- Use fingers to reduce hair breakage and discomfort. Move fingers in a circular motion starting at the roots and gently moving up to the tip of the hair.
- Comb hair.
- Dampen hair with water or a leave-in conditioner. **Rationale: This will help loosen any tangles**.
- Apply hair oil preparation as the client indicates.
- Using a large and wide-toothed comb, grasp a small section of hair and, holding the hair at the tip, start untangling at the tip and work down toward the scalp.
- Ask the client if he or she would like the hair braided. **Rationale: Braiding will decrease tangling; however, the choice is the client's**.

EVALUATION

- Conduct ongoing assessments for problems, such as dandruff, alopecia, pediculosis, scalp lesions, or excessive dryness or matting.
- Evaluate effectiveness of medication (e.g., for treating pediculosis), if appropriate.

unable to shower may be given a shampoo while sitting on a chair in front of a sink. The back-lying client who can move to a stretcher can be given a shampoo on a stretcher wheeled to a sink. The client who must remain in bed can be given a shampoo with water brought to the bedside.

Shampoo basins to catch the water and direct it to the washbasin or other receptacle are usually made of plastic or metal. A pail or large washbasin can be used as a receptacle for the shampoo water. If possible, the receptacle should be large enough to hold all the shampoo water so that it does not have to be emptied during the procedure.

Water used for the shampoo should be 40.5°C for an adult or child to be comfortable and not injure the scalp. A medicated shampoo may be used as prescribed by the physician to treat lice or other conditions of the scalp. Dry shampoos are also available. They will remove some of the dirt, odour, and oil. Their main disadvantage is that they dry the hair and scalp, if used frequently. How often a person needs a shampoo is highly individual, depending largely on the person's activities and the amount of sebum secreted by the scalp. Oily hair tends to look stringy and dirty, and it feels unclean to the person.

Skill 31.7 explains how to give a shampoo for a client confined to bed.

SKILL 31.7 SHAMPOOING THE HAIR OF A CLIENT CONFINED TO BED

PURPOSES

- To stimulate the blood circulation to the scalp through massage
- To clean the hair and increase the client's sense of well-being

ASSESSMENT

- Determine routinely used shampoo products
- Assess any scalp problems
- Assess the activity tolerance of the client

Equipment

- Comb and brush
- Plastic sheet or pad
- Two bath towels
- Shampoo basin
- Washcloth or pad
- Bath blanket
- Receptacle for the shampoo water
- Pitcher of water
- Bath thermometer
- Liquid or cream shampoo
- Hair dryer

IMPLEMENTATION

Preparation

- Determine whether a physician's order is needed before a shampoo can be given. **Rationale: Some agencies require an order, depending on the client's condition.**
- Determine the type of shampoo to be used (e.g., medicated shampoo).
- Determine the best time of day for the shampoo. Discuss this with the client. A person who must remain in bed may find the shampoo tiring. Choose a time when the client is rested and can rest after the procedure.

Performance

1. Before performing the procedure, introduce yourself and verify the client's identity using two identifiers or per agency protocol. Explain to the client what you are going to do, why it is necessary if appropriate, and how he or she can participate.

2. Perform hand hygiene, and follow other appropriate infection prevention and control procedures, as needed.

3. Provide for client privacy by drawing the curtains around the bed or closing the door to the room. Some agencies provide signs indicating the need for privacy. **Rationale: Hygiene is a personal matter.**

4. Position and prepare the client appropriately.

   - Assist the client to the side of the bed where you will work.
   - Remove pins and ribbons from the hair, and brush and comb it to remove any tangles.

5. Arrange the equipment.

   - Put a plastic sheet or pad on the bed under the client's head. **Rationale: The plastic keeps the bedding dry.**
   - Remove the pillow from under the client's head, and place it under the shoulders unless there is some underlying condition (e.g., neck surgery, arthritis of the neck). **Rationale: This hyperextends the neck.**
   - Tuck a bath towel around the client's shoulders. **Rationale: This keeps the shoulders dry.**
   - Place the shampoo basin under the head (see ❶), putting a folded washcloth or pad where the client's neck rests on the edge of the basin. If the client is on a stretcher, the neck can rest on the edge of the sink with the washcloth as padding. **Rationale: Padding supports the muscles of the neck and prevents undue strain and discomfort.**
   - Fanfold the top bedding down to the waist, and cover the upper part of the client with the bath blanket. **Rationale: The folded bedding will stay dry, and the bath blanket, which can be discarded after the shampoo, will keep the client warm.**

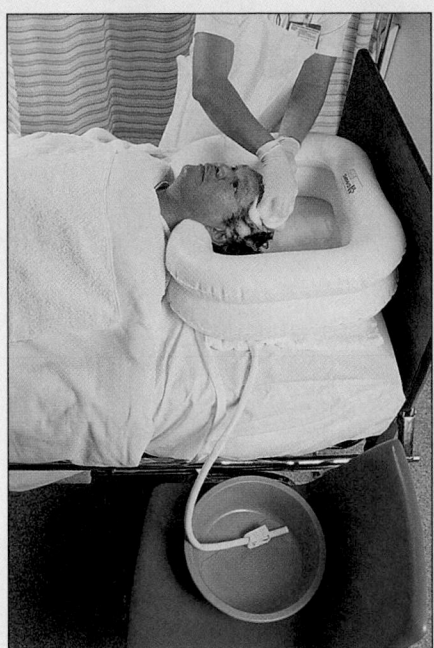

❶ Shampooing the hair of a client confined to bed (note the shampoo basin and the receptacle below)

- Place the receiving receptacle on a table or chair at the bedside. Put the spout of the shampoo basin over the receptacle.

6. Protect the client's eyes.
   - Place a damp washcloth over the client's eyes. **Rationale: The washcloth protects the eyes from soapy water. A damp washcloth will not slip**.

7. Shampoo the client's hair.
   - Wet the hair thoroughly with the water.

- Apply shampoo to the scalp. Make a good lather with the shampoo while massaging the scalp with the pads of your fingertips. Massage all areas of the scalp systematically, for example, starting at the front and working toward the back of the head. **Rationale: Massaging stimulates the blood circulation in the scalp. The pads of the fingers are used so that the fingernails will not scratch the scalp**.
- Rinse the hair briefly, and apply shampoo again.
- Make a good lather and massage the scalp as before.
- Rinse the hair thoroughly this time to remove all shampoo. **Rationale: Shampoo remaining in the hair may dry and irritate the scalp**.
- Squeeze as much water as possible out of the hair with your hands.

8. Dry the client's hair thoroughly.
   - Rub the hair with a heavy towel.
   - Dry the hair with the dryer. Set the temperature at "warm."
   - Continually move the dryer to prevent burning the client's scalp.

9. Ensure client comfort.
   - Assist the person confined to bed to a comfortable position.
   - Arrange the client's hair using a clean brush and comb.

10. Document the shampoo procedure and any assessments.

EVALUATION

Conduct ongoing assessments, such as any scalp problems or intolerance to the procedure. Report any problems noted to the nurse in charge.

BEARD AND MOUSTACHE CARE The beard and the moustache also require daily care. The most important aspect of the care is to keep them clean. Food particles tend to collect in the beard and moustache, so they need to be washed and combed regularly. Clients may also want their beards or moustaches trimmed to maintain a well-groomed appearance. The client's beard or moustache should not be shaved off without his consent.

Clients often shave or are shaved after a bath. Frequently, clients supply their own electric or safety razors. See Box 31.3 on the next page for the steps involved in shaving facial hair with a safety razor.

Evaluating

See examples of desired health outcomes earlier in the "Planning" section.

Eyes

Normally, eyes require no special hygiene because lacrimal fluid continually washes them, and eyelids and eyelashes prevent the entrance of foreign particles. Special interventions are needed, however, for unconscious clients, for clients recovering from eye surgery, and for those with eye injuries, irritations, infections, or systemic diseases affecting eyes. In unconscious clients, the blink reflex may be absent, and excessive drainage may accumulate along eyelid margins. In clients with eye trauma or eye infections, excessive discharge or drainage is common. Excessive secretions on eyelashes need to be removed before they form crusts. Clients who wear eyeglasses or contact lenses may require instruction from and care by the nurse.

BOX 31.3 USING A SAFETY RAZOR TO SHAVE FACIAL HAIR

Follow these steps when shaving a client with a safety razor:

- When possible, it is preferable to shave a client with an electric razor.

- Wear gloves in case there are facial nicks and contact with blood.

- Apply shaving cream or soap and water to soften the bristles and make the skin more pliable.

- Hold the skin taut, particularly around creases, to prevent cutting the skin.

- Hold the razor such that the blade is at a 45-degree angle to the skin, and shave in short, firm strokes in the direction of hair growth, being careful not to cut or nick the skin (Figure 31.9).

- After shaving the entire area, wipe the client's face with a wet washcloth to remove any remaining shaving cream and hair.

- Dry the face well, then apply aftershave lotion or powder as the client prefers.

- To prevent irritating the skin, pat on the lotion with the fingers and avoid rubbing the face.

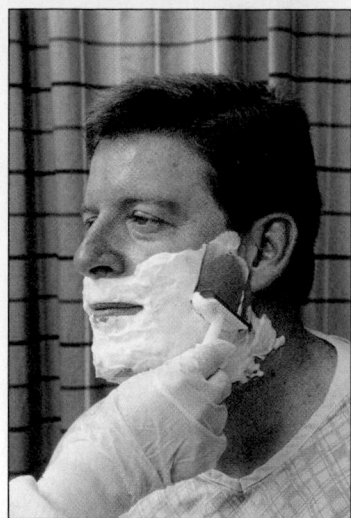

FIGURE 31.9 Shaving in the direction of hair growth.

Assessing

NURSING HISTORY During the nursing history, the nurse obtains data about the client's eyeglasses or contact lenses, recent examination by an ophthalmologist, and any history of eye problems and related treatments. Questions to elicit these data are shown in the Assessment: Interview box.

PHYSICAL ASSESSMENT In physical assessment, all external eye structures are inspected for signs of inflammation, excessive drainage, encrustations, or other obvious abnormalities. Inspection of the external eye structures is discussed in Chapter 28.

Diagnosing

Nursing diagnoses related to eye problems may include self-care deficit in caring for contact lenses related to such factors as reduced fine motor abilities or altered level of consciousness; risk for eye trauma related to lack of blink reflex; and risk for eye infection related to improper contact lens hygiene or accumulation of secretions on eyelids.

ASSESSMENT INTERVIEW

Eyes

Ask the client about eye care:

FOR CLIENTS WHO WEAR EYEGLASSES

- When do you use your glasses?
- What is your vision like with and without the glasses?

FOR CLIENTS WHO WEAR CONTACT LENSES

- How often do you wear lenses? daily? on special occasions?
- How long do you wear your lenses in a given day, including sleep time?
- Do you have any problems with the lenses (e.g., cleaning, insertion, removal, damage)?
- Do you carry an emergency identification label to alert others to remove the lenses and ensure appropriate care in an emergency? (If not, advise the client to acquire one.)
- What are your insertion and removal procedures?
- What are your cleaning and storage procedures?

- Have you had any problems with one or both eyes or eyelids, such as excessive tearing, burning, redness, discomfort, sensitivity to light, swelling, or feelings of dryness? Describe them.
- Are you using any eye drops or ointments? (These medications can combine chemically with *soft* lenses and cause lens damage and eye irritation.)

FOR ALL CLIENTS

- When did you last have your eyesight tested?
- Are you currently taking any eye medication? If so, provide name, dosage, and frequency.
- Do you have any of the following eye problems: difficulty reading or seeing objects, blurring of vision, tearing, spots or floaters, photophobia (sensitivity to light), burning, itching, dryness, pain, double vision, flashing lights, or halos around lights?

Planning

In planning care, the nurse identifies nursing activities that will assist the client to maintain the integrity of the eye structures or a prosthesis and to prevent eye injury and infection. Nursing activities may include teaching clients about how to insert, clean, and remove contact lenses or a prosthesis and ways to protect the eyes from injury and strain. Examples of desired outcomes to evaluate the effectiveness of nursing interventions include:

- Conjunctiva and sclera free of inflammation
- Eyelids free of secretions
- No tearing
- No eye discomfort
- Demonstration of appropriate methods of caring for contact lenses
- Description of interventions to prevent eye injury and infection

Implementing

EYE CARE Dried secretions that have accumulated on eyelashes need to be softened and wiped away. Soften dried secretions by placing a sterile cotton ball moistened with sterile water or normal saline over the lid margins. Wipe the loosened secretions from the inner canthus of the eye to the outer canthus to prevent the particles and fluid from draining into the lacrimal sac and nasolacrimal duct.

If the client is unconscious and lacks the blink reflex or cannot close the eyelids completely, drying and irritation of the cornea must be prevented. Lubricating eyedrops may be ordered. See Box 31.4 for providing eye care for the comatose client.

BOX 31.4 EYE CARE FOR THE COMATOSE CLIENT

When a comatose client's corneal reflex is impaired, eye care is essential to keep moist the areas of the cornea that are exposed to air:

- Administer moist compresses to cover the client's eyes every 2 to 4 hours.
- Clean the eyes with saline solution and cotton balls. Wipe from the inner to outer canthus. This method prevents debris from being washed into the nasolacrimal duct.
- Use a new cotton ball for each wipe to prevent extending infection in one eye or to the other eye.
- Instill prescribed ophthalmic ointment or artificial tears into the lower lids. This keeps eyes moist.
- If the client's corneal reflex is absent, keep the eye moist with artificial tears and protect the eye with a protective shield. These interventions should be ordered by a physician.
- Monitor the eyes for redness, exudate, or ulceration.

EYE SAFETY Eye safety is also an important consideration of eye care. The body's natural eye defences can be augmented by instructing the client to wear safety lenses, goggles, or shields for high-risk activities.

EYEGLASS CARE It is essential that the nurse exercise caution when cleaning eyeglasses to prevent breaking or scratching the lenses. Glass lenses can be cleaned with warm water and dried with a soft cloth that will not scratch the lenses. Plastic lenses are easily scratched and may require special cleaning solutions and drying cloths. When not being worn, all glasses should be placed in a case, labelled appropriately, and stored in the client's bedside table drawer.

CONTACT LENS CARE Most contact lenses, hard or soft, are used to replace eyeglasses for full-time wear. The most commonly used kind is soft lenses, which can be clear or coloured, conventional or disposable, daily wear or extended wear, and with or without correction for astigmatism. Disposable contact lenses are worn one time only and then disposed. Some disposable lenses are designed to be changed every 2 weeks. Extended wear brands are generally removed at least once a week for cleaning, which must be scrupulous to avoid infection.

Gas-permeable lenses are rigid enough to provide clear vision but are more flexible than the traditional hard lens. They permit oxygen to reach the cornea, thus providing greater comfort, and will not cause serious damage to the eye if left in place for several days.

Most clients normally care for their own contact lenses. In general, lens manufacturers provide detailed cleaning instructions. Depending on the type of lens and cleaning method used, warm tap water, normal saline, or special rinsing or soaking solutions may be used.

All contact lens users should have a special container for their lenses. Some contain a solution so that the lenses are stored wet; in others, the lenses are dry. Each lens container has a label indicating whether it is for the right or left lens. It is essential that the correct lens be stored in the appropriate cup so that it can be worn in the correct eye. Clean gloves should be worn when removing or inserting contact lenses.

Removing Contact Lenses Hard contact lenses must be positioned directly over the cornea for proper removal. If the lens is displaced, the nurse asks the client to look straight ahead and gently exerts pressure on the upper and lower lids to move the lens back onto the cornea. Figure 31.10 on the next page shows the steps needed to remove a hard lens. To avoid lens mixups, the nurse places the first lens in its designated cup in the storage base before removing the second lens (Figure 31.11).

Removal of soft lenses differs in two ways. First, have the client look forward. Retract the lower lid with one hand. Using the pad of your index finger of the other hand, move the lens down to the inferior part of the sclera so as to reduce the risk of damage to the

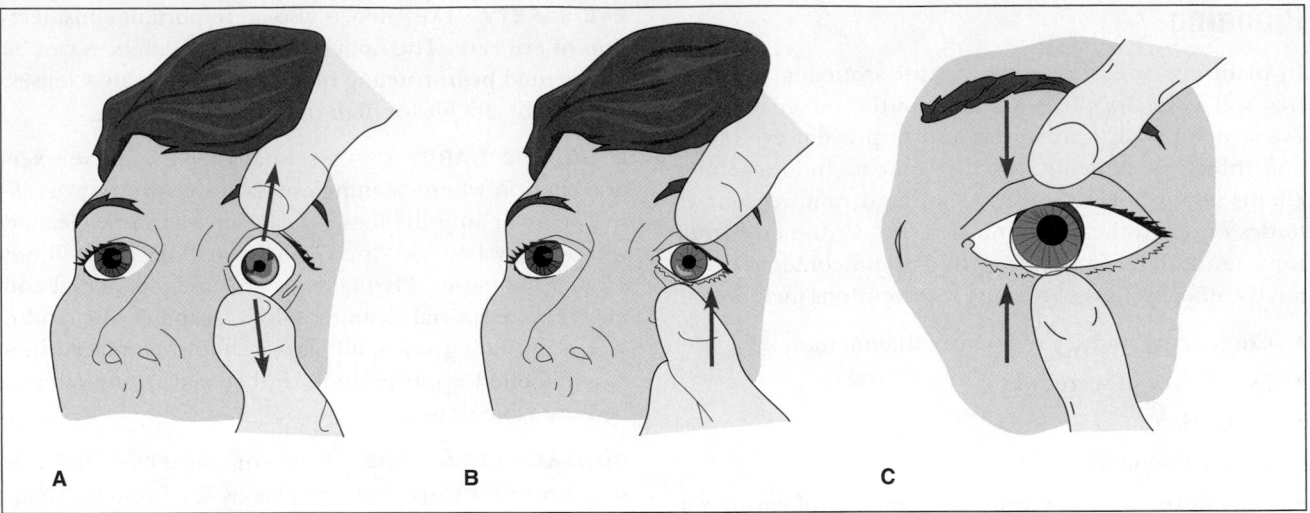

FIGURE 31.10 Removing hard contact lenses.

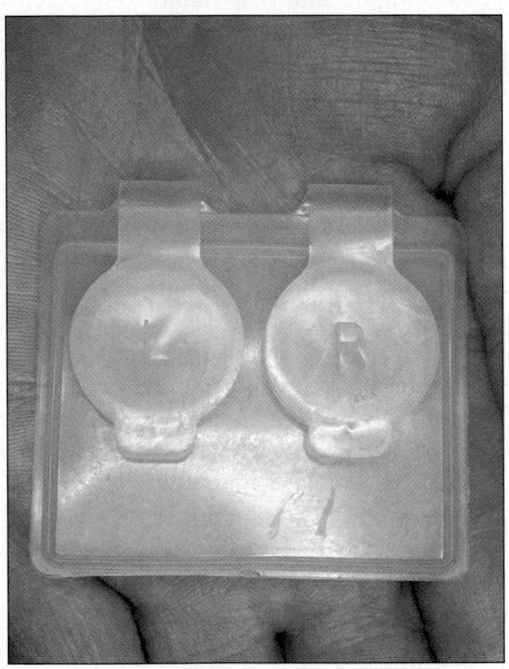

FIGURE 31.11 Storing lenses.

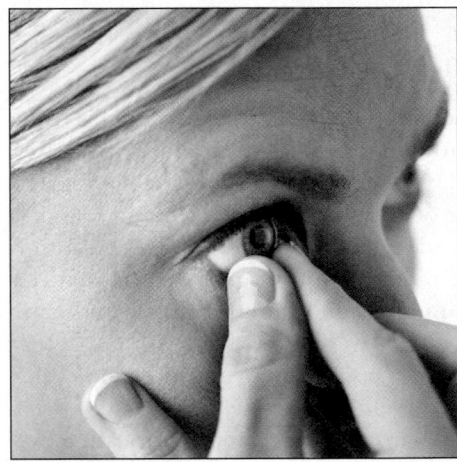

FIGURE 31.12 Removing a soft lens by pinching between the pads of the thumb and index finger.

cornea. Second, remove the lens by gently pinching the lens between the pads of the thumb and index finger. Pinching causes the lens to double up, so that air enters underneath the lens, overcoming the suction and allowing removal. Use the pads of the fingers to prevent scratching the eye or the lens with the fingernails. Figure 31.12 shows a client removing her own contact lens by using the method described. Note that a nurse would need to wear gloves.

Inserting Contact Lenses Seriously ill clients whose contact lenses have been removed will not need them reinserted until they become more active in their care and require the lenses to see properly. Contact lenses need to be lubricated in a sterile, nonirritating wetting solution (usually a saline solution) before they are inserted. The wetting solution helps the lens glide over the cornea, thus reducing the risk of injury. Most clients, when well, will reinsert the lenses independently.

GENERAL EYE CARE Many clients may need to learn specific information about care of the eyes. They need to be instructed as follows:

- Avoid home remedies for eye problems. Eye irritations or injuries at any age should be treated medically and immediately.

- If dirt or dust gets into your eyes, clean them copiously with clean, tepid water as an emergency treatment.

- Take measures to guard against eyestrain and to protect vision, such as maintaining adequate lighting for reading and wearing protective goggles or safety glasses.

- Schedule regular eye examinations, particularly after age 40 years, to detect such problems as cataracts and glaucoma.

Evaluating

By using data collected during care, the nurse judges whether desired outcomes have been achieved. The following are examples of desired outcomes to evaluate the effectiveness of nursing interventions:

- Conjunctiva and sclera are free of inflammation
- Eyelids are free of secretions
- No tearing
- No eye discomfort
- Demonstration of appropriate methods of caring for contact lenses
- Description of interventions to prevent eye injury and infection

Ears

Normally, ears require minimal hygiene. Clients who have excessive cerumen (earwax) and dependent clients who have hearing aids may require assistance from the nurse. Hearing aids are usually removed before surgery.

Cleaning Ears

The auricles of ears are cleaned during the bed bath. The nurse or client must remove excessive cerumen that is visible or that causes discomfort or hearing difficulty. Visible cerumen can be loosened and removed by retracting the auricle downward. If this measure is ineffective, irrigation may be necessary. Clients need to be advised never to use hair pins, toothpicks, or cotton-tipped applicators to remove cerumen. Hair pins and toothpicks can injure the ear canal and rupture the tympanic membrane; cotton-tipped applicators can cause wax to become impacted within the canal.

Caring for Hearing Aids

For people with hearing loss, properly selected hearing aids improve the ability to hear and to communicate. Hearing aids are battery-powered, sound-amplifying devices consisting of a microphone that picks up sound and converts it to electric energy; an amplifier that magnifies the electric energy electronically; a receiver that converts the amplified energy back to sound energy; and an earmould that directs the sound in the ear. There are several types of hearing aids:

- *Behind-the-ear (BTE) open fit.* BTEs are the newest in hearing aid technology. A BTE has no earmould,

and it is barely visible with a clear tube that runs down into the ear canal. It does not occlude the ear canal (Figure 31.13)

- *Behind-the-ear (BTE) with earmould.* This type is widely used because it fits snugly behind the ear. The hearing aid case, which holds the microphone, amplifier, and receiver, is attached to the earmould by a plastic tube (Figure 31.14 on the next page).
- *In-the-ear (ITE) aid.* This one-piece aid has all its components housed in the earmould (Figure 31.15). It is more visible than other types but has more room for such features as volume control.
- *In-the-canal (ITC) aid.* This aid is the most compact and least visible aid, fitting completely inside the ear canal. In addition to having cosmetic appeal, the ITC does not interfere with telephone use or the wearing of eyeglasses. However, it is not suitable for clients with progressive hearing loss; it requires adequate ear canal diameter and length for a good fit; and it tends to plug with cerumen compared with other aids.
- *Completely-in-the-canal (CIC) aid.* Almost invisible to an observer, the CIC aid has to be custom designed to fit the individual's ear (Figure 31.16).
- *Body hearing aid.* This pocket-sized aid, used for more severe hearing losses, clips onto an undergarment, shirt, pocket, or harness carrier supplied by the manufacturer. The case, containing the microphone and amplifier, is connected by a cord to the receiver, which snaps onto the earpiece.

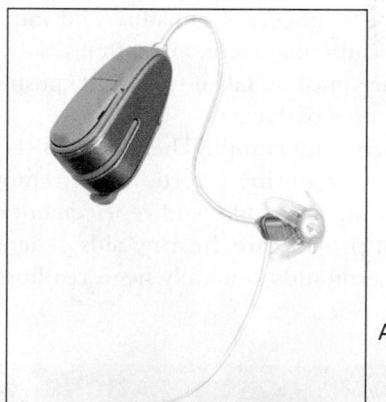

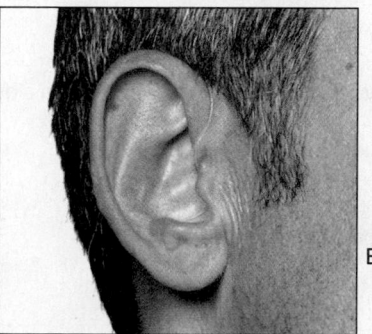

FIGURE 31.13 A: A behind-the-ear (BTE) open fit hearing aid; **B:** A BTE open fit hearing aid in place.

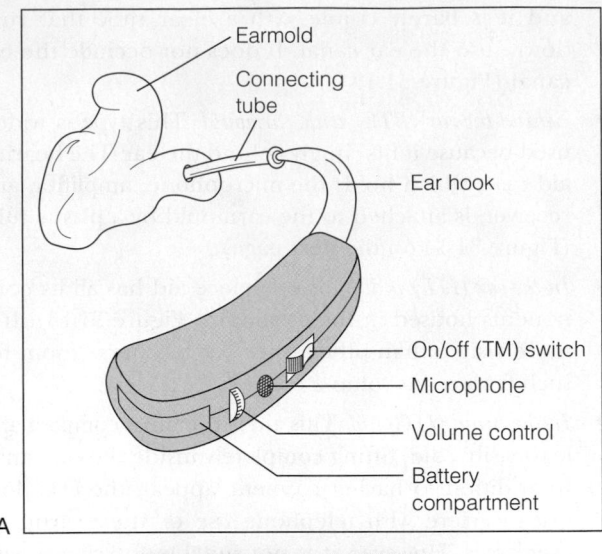

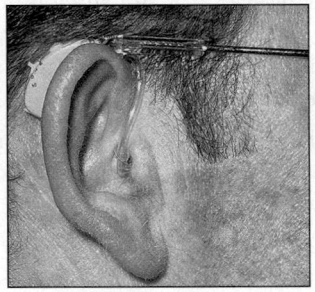

FIGURE 31.14 A: A behind-the-ear (BTE) hearing aid with earmould; **B:** A BTE hearing aid attached to glasses.

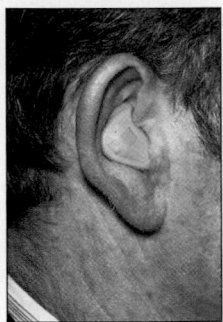

FIGURE 31.15 An in-the-ear (ITE) hearing aid.

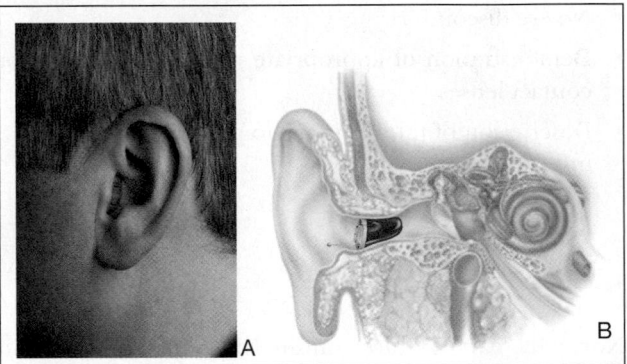

FIGURE 31.16 A: A completely in-the-canal (ITC) hearing aid; **B:** CIC in place.

Hearing aids containing microcomputers are very sensitive to the effects of moisture and impact, both of which can cause extensive, and often costly, damage to the aid. Care must be taken to avoid exposing these aids to either source of damage.

For correct functioning, hearing aids require appropriate handling during insertion and removal, regular cleaning of the earmould, and replacement of dead batteries. With proper care, hearing aids generally last 5 to 10 years. Earmoulds generally need readjustment every 2 to 3 years. See the Home Care Considerations box and Skill 31.8 for hearing aid care.

Nose

Nurses usually need not provide special care for the nose because clients can ordinarily clear nasal secretions by blowing gently into a soft tissue. When the external

---

HOME CARE CONSIDERATIONS

Hearing Aids

Clients may need to learn about their hearing aids:

- People who need a hearing aid may not wear one because they view the hearing aid as a stigma of growing older.

- It is important for the client who just purchased a hearing aid to know that it often takes weeks or even months to adjust to the hearing aid. At first, sounds will seem shrill as they start hearing high-frequency sounds they had forgotten. Remind them that it is a hearing aid, not a hearing cure. Encourage them to not give up.

- The client needs to adjust to the hearing aid gradually by increasing the amount of time each day until the aid can be worn for a full day.

- Encourage clients to purchase their hearing aids from a company that has a minimum warranty of a 30-day return policy.

- Emphasize the importance of maintaining the hearing aid by having it cleaned and checked regularly.

SKILL 31.8 REMOVING, CLEANING, AND INSERTING A HEARING AID

PURPOSE

- To maintain proper hearing aid function

ASSESSMENT

Determine whether the client has experienced any problems with the hearing aid and hearing aid practices. Assess for the presence of inflammation, excessive wax, drainage, or discomfort in the external ear.

Equipment

- Client's hearing aid
- Soap, water, and towels or a damp cloth
- Pipe cleaner or toothpick (optional)
- New battery (if needed)

IMPLEMENTATION

Performance

1. Before performing the procedure, introduce yourself and verify the client's identity using two identifiers or per agency protocol. Explain to the client what you are going to do, why it is necessary, and how he or she can participate.

2. Perform hand hygiene, and follow other appropriate infection prevention and control procedures.

3. Provide for client privacy by drawing the curtains around the bed or closing the door to the room. Some agencies provide signs indicating the need for privacy. **Rationale: Hygiene is a personal matter**.

4. Remove the hearing aid.
   - Turn the hearing aid off and lower the volume. The on/off switch may be labelled O (off), M (microphone), T (telephone), or TM (telephone/microphone). **Rationale: The batteries continue to run if the hearing aid is not turned off**.
   - Remove the earmould by rotating it slightly forward and pulling it outward.
   - If the hearing aid will not to be used for several days, remove the battery. **Rationale: Removal prevents corrosion of the hearing aid from battery leakage**.
   - Label the hearing aid with the client's name, and store it in a safe place. Avoid exposure to heat and moisture. **Rationale: Proper storage prevents loss or damage**.

5. Clean the earmould.
   - Detach the earmould, if possible. Disconnect the earmould from the receiver of a body hearing aid or from the hearing aid case of behind-the-ear and eyeglass hearing aids, where the tubing meets the hook of the case. Do not remove the earmould if it is glued or secured by a small metal ring. **Rationale: Removal facilitates cleaning and prevents inadvertent damage to the other parts**.
   - If the earmould is detachable, soak it in a mild soapy solution. Rinse and dry it well. Do not use isopropyl alcohol. **Rationale: Alcohol can damage the hearing aid**.
   - If the earmould is not detachable or is for an in-the-ear aid, wipe the earmould with a damp cloth.
   - Check that the earmould opening is patent. Remove any excess moisture through the opening or remove debris (e.g., earwax) with a pipe cleaner or toothpick.

   - Reattach the earmould if it was detached from the rest of the hearing aid.

6. Insert the hearing aid.
   - Determine from the client whether the earmould is for the left ear or the right ear.
   - Check that the battery is inserted in the hearing aid. Turn off the hearing aid, and make sure the volume is turned all the way down. **Rationale: A volume that is too loud is distressing**.
   - Inspect the earmould to identify the ear canal portion. Some earmoulds are fitted for only the ear canal and concha; others are fitted for all the contours of the ear. The canal portion, common to all, can be used as a guide for correct insertion.
   - Line up the parts of the earmould with the corresponding parts of the client's ear.
   - Rotate the earmould slightly forward, and insert the ear canal portion.
   - Gently press the earmould into the ear while rotating it backward.
   - Check that the earmould fits snugly by asking the client if it feels secure and comfortable.
   - Adjust the other components of a behind-the-ear or body hearing aid.
   - Turn the hearing aid on, and adjust the volume according to the client's preferences.

7. Correct problems associated with improper functioning.
   - If the sound is weak or there is no sound:
     a. Ensure that the volume is turned high enough.
     b. Ensure that the earmould opening is not clogged.
     c. Check the battery by turning the hearing aid on, turning up the volume, cupping your hand over the earmould, and listening. A constant whistling sound indicates the battery is functioning. If necessary, replace the battery. Be sure that the negative (–) and positive (+) signs on the battery match those where indicated on the hearing aid.
     d. Ensure that the ear canal is not blocked with wax, which can obstruct sound waves.
   - If the client reports a whistling sound or squeal after insertion, do the following:
     a. Turn the volume down.
     b. Ensure that the earmould is properly attached to the receiver.
     c. Reinsert the earmould.

8. Document pertinent data.
   - Removal and insertion of a hearing aid are not normally recorded.
   - Report and record any problems the client has with the hearing aid.

EVALUATION

- Speak to the client in a normal conversational tone, and observe client behaviours.
- Compare the client's hearing ability to previous assessments.
- Report any deviations from normal for the client to the appropriate members of the health care team.

nares are encrusted with dried secretions, they should be cleaned with a cotton-tipped applicator or moistened with saline or water. The applicator should not be inserted beyond the length of the cotton tip; inserting it farther can cause injury to the mucosa.

Supporting a Hygienic Environment

Because people are usually confined to bed when ill, often for long periods, the bed becomes an important element in the client's life. A place that is clean, safe, and comfortable contributes to the client's ability to rest and sleep and to a sense of well-being. Basic furniture in a health care facility includes the bed, bedside table, overbed table, one or more chairs, and a storage space for the client's clothing and other personal items. Most bed units also have a nurse call system, light fixtures, electric outlets, and hygienic equipment in the bedside table. Four types of equipment often installed in an acute care facility are a *suction outlet* for several kinds of suction, an *oxygen outlet* for most oxygen equipment, an air outlet for nebulizers and humidifiers, and a *sphygmomanometer* to measure the client's blood pressure. Some long-term care agencies also permit clients to have *personal furniture*, such as a television, a chair, and lamps, at the bedside. In the home, a client often has both personal and medical equipment.

Environment

When providing a comfortable environment, it is important to consider the client's age, severity of illness, and level of activity.

TEMPERATURE The very young, the very old, and the acutely ill frequently need a room temperature higher than normal. A room temperature between 20°C and 23°C is comfortable for most clients.

VENTILATION Good ventilation is important to remove unpleasant odours and stale air. Odours caused by urine, draining wounds, or vomitus, for example, can be offensive. Room deodorizers can help eliminate odours. However, good hygienic practices are the best way to prevent offensive body and breath odours. Hospitals are required to monitor smoking. Hospitals frequently no longer have smoking areas and prohibit smoking in any client (patient) areas.

NOISE Ill persons are usually sensitive to noise, such as clanging of metal equipment, loud talking, and laughter. Nurses should try to control noise in health care settings (see Chapter 37).

Hospital Beds

The frame of a hospital bed is divided into three sections to permit the head and the foot to be elevated separately. Most hospital beds have electric motors to operate the movable joints. The motor is activated by pressing a button or moving a small lever, located either at the side of the bed or on a small panel separate from the bed but attached to it by a cable, which the client can readily use. See Table 31.8 for common bed positions.

Hospital beds are usually 65 cm high and 1 m wide, narrower than the usual bed so that the nurse can reach the client from either side of the bed without undue stretching. The length is usually 2 m. Some beds can be extended in length to accommodate very tall clients. Long-term care facilities for ambulatory residents usually have low beds to facilitate safe movement in and out of bed. Most hospital beds have high and low positions that can be adjusted either mechanically or electrically by a button or lever. The high position permits the nurse to reach the client without undue stretching or stooping. The low position allows the client to step easily to the floor.

MATTRESSES Mattresses are usually covered with a water-repellent material that resists soiling and can be cleaned easily. Most mattresses have handles on the sides called lugs by which the mattress can be moved.

Many special mattresses are also used in hospitals to relieve pressure on the body's bony prominences, such as the sacrum and heels. They are particularly helpful for clients confined to bed for long periods. For additional information about mattresses, see Table 35.3 in Chapter 35.

SIDE RAILS Side rails are used on both hospital beds and stretchers. They are of various shapes and sizes and are usually made of metal or high-density plastic and can be the full length of the bed or split length. Devices to raise and lower them differ. Often, one or two knobs are pulled to release the side and permit it to be moved. While side rails are often raised to help prevent a patient from falling out of bed, such as after receiving a preoperative sedative, there is a risk that an unattended disoriented or confused client may become entrapped in the openings or gaps around the bed resulting in asphyxiation or climb over the rails leading to a higher fall than had the rails not been elevated. Chapter 32 has a complete discussion on the recommendations for side rail positions and alternative strategies (e.g., motion sensors, bed alarms) to prevent falls. If all the bedside rails are raised and restrict the client's freedom to leave the bed and the client did not voluntarily request all rails to be up, they are considered a form of physical restraint. If, however, the side rail is up to assist the client to get in and out of bed or move within the bed, then the side rails are not considered a restraint. The routine use of side rails in acute and long-term care settings is decreasing as a result of the evidence indicting physical and psychological risks associated with their use.

TABLE 31.8 Common Bed Positions

Position	Description	Purpose
Flat Head of bed Foot of bed	Mattress is completely horizontal.	Client sleeping in a variety of bed positions, such as back-lying, side-lying, and prone (face down) To maintain spinal alignment for clients with spinal injuries To assist clients to move and turn in bed For bed making
Fowler's position	Semi-sitting position in which head of bed is raised to an angle of at least 45 degrees; client's knees may be flexed or horizontal	Convenient for eating, reading, visiting, watching TV Relief from lying positions To promote lung expansion for clients with respiratory problems To assist a client to a sitting position on the edge of the bed
Semi-Fowler's position	Head of bed is raised only to 30-degree angle.	Relief from lying position To promote lung expansion
Trendelenburg's position	Head of bed is lowered; foot is raised in a straight incline	To promote venous circulation in certain clients To provide postural drainage of basal lung lobes
Reverse Trendelenburg's position	Head of bed is raised and the foot is lowered; straight tilt in direction opposite to Trendelenburg's position	To promote stomach emptying and prevent esophageal reflux in clients with hiatal hernias

FOOTBOARD OR FOOT BOOT The footboard, or foot boot, is used to support the immobilized client's foot in a normal right angle to the legs to prevent plantar flexion contractures. See the section "Positioning Clients" in Chapter 39.

BED CRADLES A bed cradle is a device designed to keep the top bedclothes off the feet, legs, and even the abdomen of a client. The bedclothes are arranged over the device and may be pinned or tucked in place. Bed cradles come in several types. One of the most common is a curved metal rod that fits over the bed (Figure 31.17). Part of the cradle fits under the mattress, and small metal brackets press down on each side of the mattress to keep the cradle in place. The frame of some cradles extends over half of the width of the bed, above one leg.

INTRAVENOUS POLES Intravenous poles, usually made of metal, support intravenous (IV) infusion containers while fluid is being administered to a client. These rods

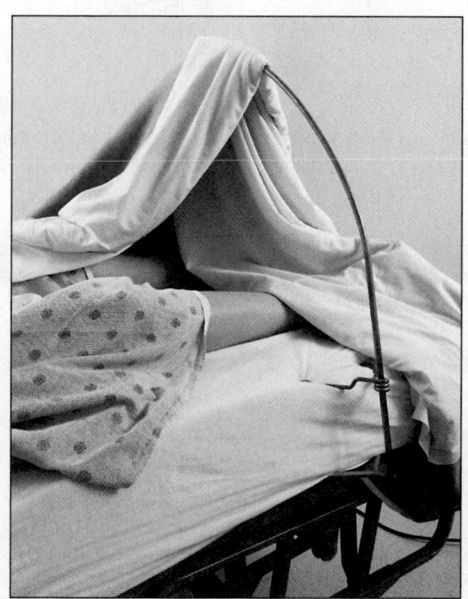

FIGURE 31.17 Bed cradle.

were traditionally freestanding on the floor beside the bed. Intravenous rods may also be attached to the hospital beds. Some hospital units have overhead hanging rods on a track for IVs.

MAKING BEDS Nurses need to be able to prepare hospital beds in different ways for specific purposes. In most instances, beds are made after the client receives certain care and when beds are unoccupied. At times, however, nurses need to make an occupied bed or prepare a bed for a client who is having surgery (postoperative or surgical bed).

Regardless of what type of bed equipment is available, whether the bed is occupied or unoccupied, or the purpose for which the bed is being prepared, certain practice guidelines pertain to all bed making and disposal of linen. See Practice Guidelines 31.2 on bed making and disposal of linens.

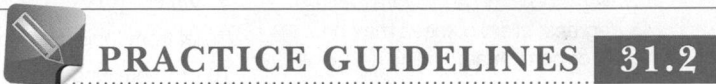

PRACTICE GUIDELINES 31.2

Bed Making and Disposal of Linens

The following guidelines apply to any bed making and disposal of bed linens:

Guideline	Rationale
Wash hands thoroughly after handling a client's bed linen (Public Health Agency of Canada, 2007; Ontario Agency for Health Protection and Promotion, Provincial Infectious Diseases Advisory Committee, 2011). Hold used linen away from uniform. Linen for one client is *never* (even momentarily) placed on another client's bed or furniture	Used linen from health care settings can harbour large numbers of microorganisms that can be transmitted to others directly or by the health care professional's hands or uniform.
Never place used linens on the floor (Public Health Agency of Canada, 2007).	For aesthetic purposes as well as to reduce transfer of microorganisms, placing used linens on the floor is to be avoided.
Do not shake linen in the air (Public Health Agency of Canada, 2007).	Shaking can disseminate secretions and excretions and the microorganisms they contain.
Except for linen from persons with a diagnosis of rare, viral, hemorrhagic fevers (Public Health Agency of Canada, 2007), all linen that is soiled with blood, bodily fluids, secretions, or excretions should be handled in the same way regardless of source or setting by bagging the laundry at the point of care in a leak proof container (Public Health Agency of Canada, 2007; Ontario Agency for Health Protection and Promotion, Provincial Infectious Diseases Advisory Committee, 2011).	Sealed and leak proof bags or receptacles avoid leakage and prevent contamination. Highly infective material on linens need special washing procedures.
Heavily soiled linen should be rolled or folded to contain the heaviest soil in the centre of the bundle (Public Health Agency of Canada, 2007). Large amounts of solid soil, feces, or blood clots should be removed from linen with a gloved hand and toilet tissue and placed into a bedpan or toilet for flushing (Public Health Agency of Canada, 2007; Ontario Agency for Health Protection and Promotion, Provincial Infectious Diseases Advisory Committee, 2011).	All attempts must be made to avoid contaminating the health care worker or other items in the environment.
Ensure that no sharps are folded into the linen in error (Ontario Agency for Health Protection and Promotion, Provincial Infectious Diseases Advisory Committee, 2011).	Sharps in soiled linen can easily cause injury to any health care worker, especially those working in the laundry.

Sources: Based on Public Health Agency of Canada. (2007). *Infection prevention and control best practices for long term care, home and community care including health care offices and ambulatory clinics June, 2007*. Retrieved from *http://www.phac-aspc.gc.ca/amr-ram/ipcbp-pepci/appendix_ii-annexe_ii-eng.php#laundry*; and Ontario Agency for Health Protection and Promotion, Provincial Infectious Diseases Advisory Committee. (2011). *Routine practices and additional precautions in all health care settings*. Toronto: ON: Queens Printer for Ontario. Retrieved from *http://www.oahpp.ca/resources/pidac-knowledge/best-practice-manuals/routine-practices-and-additional-precautions.html*

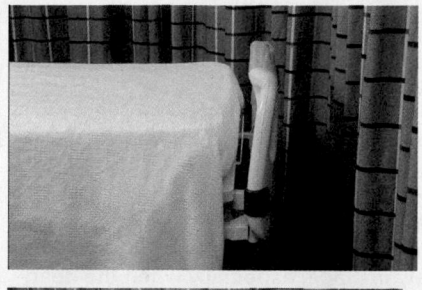
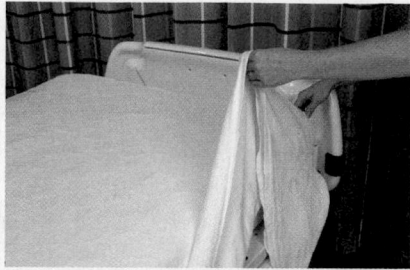
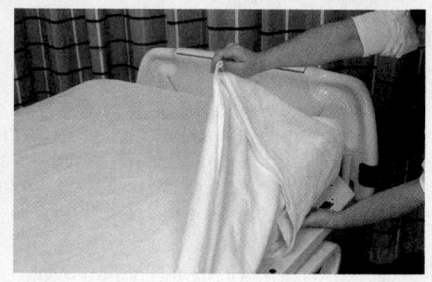
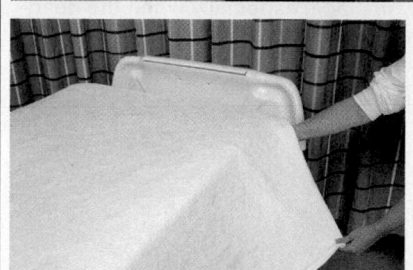
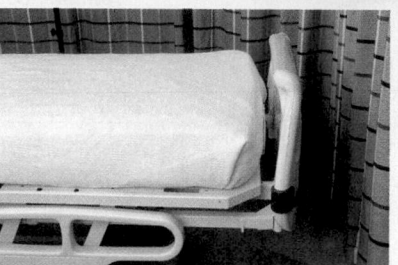

FIGURE 31.18 Mitring the corner of a bed.

An *unoccupied bed* can be either a closed bed or an open bed. Generally, the top covers of an open bed are folded back (thus the term *open bed*) to make it easier for a client to get in. Open and closed beds are made the same way, except that the top sheet, blanket, and bedspread of a *closed bed* are drawn up to the top of the bed and under the pillows.

Bedsheets are often changed after bed baths. The linen can be collected before the bath. The linen is not usually changed unless it is soiled. Check the policy at each health agency. Unfitted sheets, blankets, and bedspreads are mitred at the corners of the bed. The purpose of mitring is to secure the bedclothes while the bed is occupied. Figure 31.18 shows how to mitre the corner of a bed. Skill 31.9 explains how to change an unoccupied bed.

CHANGING AN OCCUPIED BED Some clients may be too weak to get out of bed. Either the nature of their illness may contraindicate their sitting out of bed, or they may be restricted in bed by the presence of traction or other therapies. When changing an *occupied bed,* the nurse works quickly, disturbs the client as little as possible to conserve the client's energy, and uses the following guidelines:

- Maintain the client in good body alignment. Never move or position a client in a manner that is contraindicated by the client's health. Obtain help, if necessary, to ensure the client's safety.

SKILL 31.9 CHANGING AN UNOCCUPIED BED

PURPOSES

- To promote the client's comfort
- To provide a clean, neat environment for the client
- To provide a smooth, wrinkle-free bed foundation, thus minimizing sources of skin irritation

ASSESSMENT

- Assess the client's health status to determine whether the person can safely get out of bed. In some hospitals or other health care facilities, it is necessary to have a written order if the client has been in bed continuously.
- Assess the client's pulse and respirations, if indicated.
- Note all the tubes and equipment connected to the client. **Rationale: These may influence the need for additional linens or waterproof pads, or assistance**.

Equipment

- Clean gloves, if needed
- Two flat sheets; or one fitted sheet and one flat sheet
- Cloth drawsheet (optional)
- One blanket
- One bedspread (optional)
- Waterproof pads (optional)
- Pillowcase(s) for the head pillow(s)
- Plastic laundry bag or portable linen hamper, if available

IMPLEMENTATION

Preparation

Determine what linens the client already has in the room *to avoid stockpiling of unnecessary extra linens.*

(continued)

SKILL 31.9 CHANGING AN UNOCCUPIED BED (*continued*)

Performance

1. If the client is in bed prior to performing the procedure, introduce yourself and verify the client's identity using two identifiers or per agency protocol. Explain to the client that you will be changing the bed linens.

2. Perform hand hygiene, and follow other appropriate infection prevention and control procedures.

3. Provide for client privacy.

4. Place the fresh linen on the client's chair or overbed table; do not use another client's bed. **Rationale: This prevents *cross-contamination* (the movement of microorganisms from one client to another) via soiled linen.**

5. Assess and assist the client out of bed.

   - Make sure that this is an appropriate and convenient time for the client to be out of bed.

   - Assist the client to a comfortable chair—if the client cannot get out of bed, proceed to Skill 31.10: Changing an Occupied Bed.

6. Raise the bed to a comfortable working height.

7. Apply clean gloves if linens and equipment have been soiled with secretions and/or excretions.

8. Strip the bed.

   - Check bed linens for any items belonging to the client, and detach the call bell or any drainage tubes from the bed linen.

   - Loosen all bedding systematically, starting at the head of the bed on the far side and moving around the bed up to the head of the bed on the near side. **Rationale: Moving around the bed systematically prevents stretching, reaching, and possible muscle strain.**

   - Remove the pillowcases, if soiled, and place the pillows on the bedside chair near the foot of the bed.

   - Fold reusable linens, such as the bedspread and top sheet on the bed. **Rationale: Folding linens saves time and energy when reapplying the linens on the bed and keeps them clean.**

   - Remove the waterproof pad and discard it, if soiled.

   - Roll all soiled linen inside the bottom sheet, hold it away from your uniform, and place it directly in the linen hamper, not on the floor (see ❶). **Rationale: These actions are essential to prevent the transmission of microorganisms to the nurse, client, and others.**

   - Grasp the mattress securely, using the lugs if present, and move the mattress up to the head of the bed.

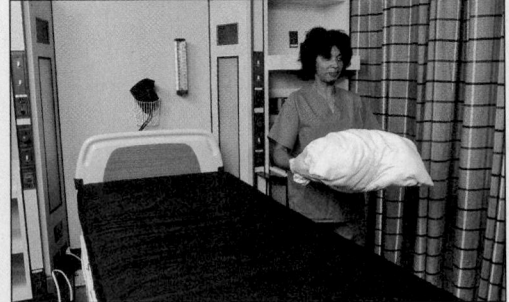

❶ Roll soiled linen inside the bottom sheet and hold away from the body.

9. Apply the bottom sheet and drawsheet.

   - Place the folded bottom sheet with its centre fold on the centre of the bed. Make sure the sheet is hem-side down for a smooth foundation. Spread the sheet out over the mattress, and allow a sufficient amount of sheet at the top to tuck under the mattress (see ❷). **Rationale: The top of the sheet needs to be well tucked under to remain securely in place, especially when the head of the bed is elevated.** Place the sheet along the edge of the mattress at the foot of the bed and do not tuck it in (unless it is a contour or fitted sheet).

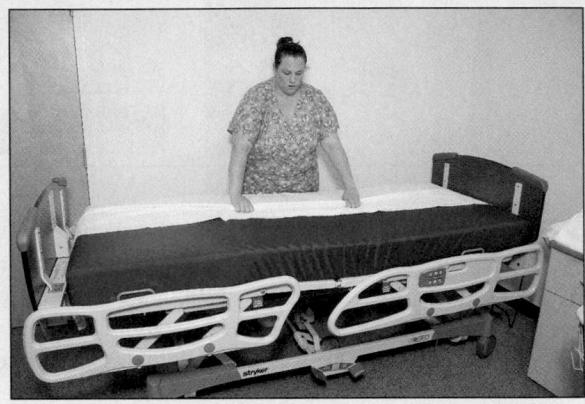

❷ Placing a bottom sheet on the bed

   - Mitre the sheet at the top corner on the near side (see Figure 31.18, p. 827) and tuck the sheet under the mattress, working from the head of the bed to the foot.

   - If a waterproof drawsheet is used, place it over the bottom sheet so that the centrefold is at the centreline of the bed and the top and bottom edges extend from the middle of the client's back to the area of the mid-thigh or knee. Fanfold the uppermost half of the folded drawsheet at the centre or far edge of the bed and tuck in the near edge (see ❸).

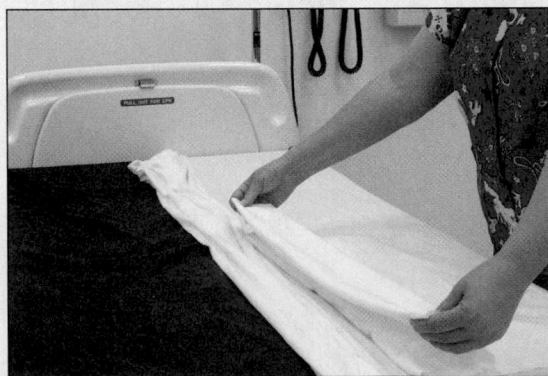

❸ Placing a clean drawsheet on the bed

   - Lay the cloth drawsheet over the waterproof sheet in the same manner.

   - *Optional:* Before moving to the other side of the bed, place the top linens on the bed hem-side up, unfold them, tuck them in, and mitre the bottom corners. **Rationale: Completing one entire side of the bed at a time saves time and energy.**

10. Move to the other side and secure the bottom linens.

- Tuck the bottom sheet under the head of the mattress, pull the sheet firmly, and, if not using a fitted sheet, mitre the corner of the sheet.
- Pull the remainder of the sheet firmly so that there are no wrinkles. **Rationale: Wrinkles can cause discomfort for the client and breakdown of skin.** Tuck in the sheet at the side.
- Complete this same process for the drawsheet.

11. Apply or complete the top sheet, blanket, and spread.

- Place the top sheet, hem-side up, on the bed so that its centrefold is at the centre of the bed and the top edge is even with the top edge of the mattress.
- Unfold the sheet over the bed.
- *Optional:* Make a vertical or a horizontal toe pleat in the sheet to provide additional room for the client's feet.

  a. *Vertical toe pleat:* Make a fold in the sheet 5 cm to 10 cm perpendicular to the foot of the bed (see ❹).
  b. *Horizontal toe pleat:* Make a fold in the sheet 5 cm to 10 cm across the bed near the foot (see ❺).

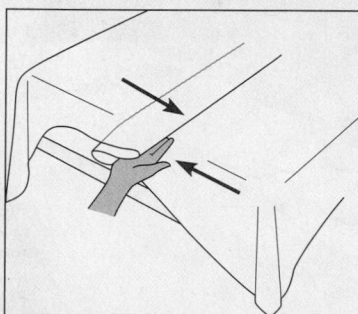

❹ A vertical toe pleat

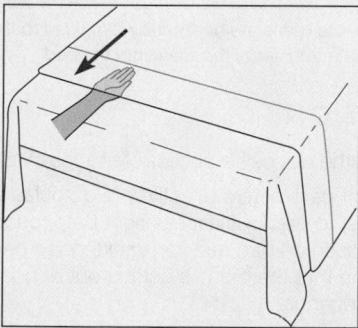

❺ A horizontal toe pleat

Loosening the top covers around the feet after the client is in bed is another way to provide additional space.

- Follow the same procedure for the blanket and the spread, but place the top edges about 15 cm from the head of the bed to allow a cuff of sheet to be folded over them.
- Tuck in the sheet, blanket, and spread at the foot of the bed, and mitre the corner, using all three layers of linen. Leave the sides of the top sheet, blanket, and spread hanging freely unless toe pleats were provided.
- Fold the top of the top sheet down over the spread, providing a cuff (see ❻). **Rationale: The cuff of the**

sheet makes it easier for the client to pull the covers up.

- Move to the other side of the bed and secure the top bedding in the same manner.

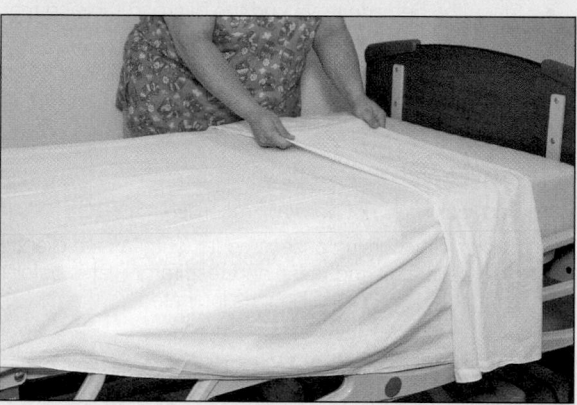

❻ Making a cuff of the top linens

12. Put clean pillowcases on the pillows as required.

- Grasp the closed end of the pillowcase at the centre with one hand.
- Gather up the sides of the pillowcase and place them over the hand grasping the case. Then, grasp the centre of one short side of the pillow through the pillowcase (see ❼).
- With the free hand, pull the pillowcase over the pillow.
- Adjust the pillowcase so that the pillow fits into the corners of the case and the seams are straight. **Rationale: A smoothly fitting pillowcase is more comfortable than a wrinkled one**.
- Place the pillows appropriately at the head of the bed.

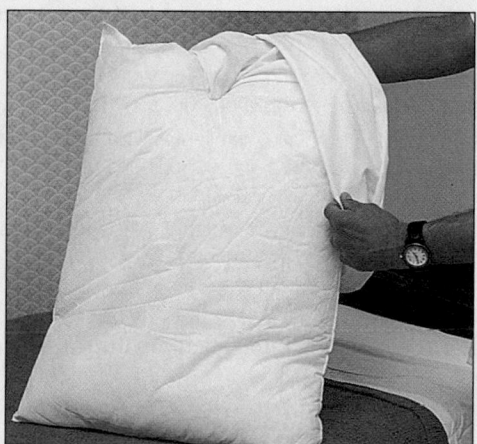

❼ Method for putting a clean pillowcase on a pillow

13. Provide for client comfort and safety.

- Attach the signal cord so that the client can conveniently reach it. Some cords have clamps that attach to the sheet or pillowcase. Others are attached by a safety pin.
- If the bed is currently being used by a client, either fold back the top covers at one side or fanfold them down to

(continued)

SKILL 31.9 CHANGING AN UNOCCUPIED BED (continued)

the centre of the bed. **Rationale: This makes it easier for the client to get into the bed.**

- Place the bedside table and the overbed table so that they are available to the client.
- Leave the bed in the high position if the client is returning by stretcher, or place in the low position if the client is returning to bed after being up.

14. Document and report pertinent data.

- Bed making is not normally recorded.
- Record any nursing assessments, such as the client's physical status and pulse and respiratory rates before and after being out of bed, as indicated.

Variation: Surgical Bed

While the client is in the operating room, the client's bed is prepared for the postoperative phase. In some agencies, the client is brought back to the unit on a stretcher and transferred to the bed in the room. In other agencies, the client's bed is brought to the surgery suite, and the client is transferred there. In the latter situation, the bed needs to be made with clean linens as soon as the client goes to surgery so that it can be taken to the operating room when needed.

1. Strip the bed.

2. Place and leave the pillows on the bedside chair. **Rationale: Pillows are left on a chair to facilitate transferring the client into the bed.**

3. Apply the bottom linens as for an unoccupied bed. Place a bath blanket on the foundation of the bed if this is agency practice. **Rationale: A flannel bath blanket provides additional warmth.**

4. Place the top covers (sheet, blanket, and bedspread) on the bed as you would for an unoccupied bed. Do not tuck them in, mitre the corners, or make a toe pleat.

5. Make a cuff at the top of the bed as you would for an unoccupied bed. Fold the top linens up from the bottom.

6. On the side of the bed where the client will be transferred, fold up the two outer corners of the top linens so they meet in the middle of the bed, forming a triangle (see ❽).

7. Pick up the apex of the triangle and fanfold the top linens lengthwise to the other side of the bed *to facilitate the client's transfer into the bed* (see ❾).

8. Leave the bed in high position with the side rails down. **Rationale: The high position facilitates the transfer of the client.**

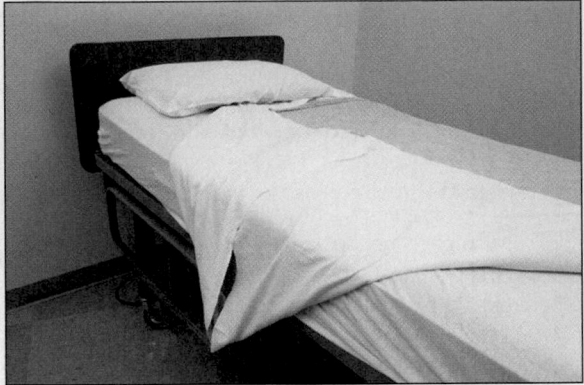

❽ Fold up the two outer corners of the top linens, forming a triangle.

9. Lock the wheels of the bed if the bed is not to be moved. **Rationale: Locking the wheels keeps the bed from rolling when the client is transferred from the stretcher to the bed.**

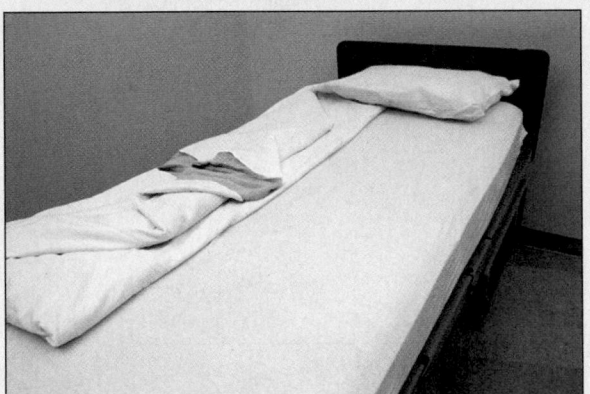

❾ Surgical bed: the linens are horizontally fanfolded to the other side of the bed to facilitate transfer of the client into the bed.

EVALUATION

- Make sure the call bell is accessible to the client.
- Relate client parameters of activity (e.g., pulse and respirations) to previous assessment data, particularly if the client has been on bed rest for an extended period or if it is the first time that the client is getting out of bed after surgery or other procedure.

- Move the client gently and smoothly. Rough handling can cause the client discomfort and abrade the skin.
- Explain to the client what you plan to do during the procedure *before* you do it. Use terms that the client can understand.

- Use the bed making time to assess and meet the client's needs.

   Skill 31.10 describes how to change an occupied bed.

SKILL 31.10   CHANGING AN OCCUPIED BED

PURPOSES

- To conserve the client's energy
- To promote client comfort
- To provide a clean, neat environment for the client
- To provide a smooth, wrinkle-free bed foundation, thus minimizing sources of skin irritation

ASSESSMENT

- Note specific orders or precautions for moving and positioning the client.
- Determine client's ability to reposition self so as to determine if additional assistance is needed.
- Determine the presence of incontinence or excessive drainage from other sources, indicating the need for protective waterproof pads.
- Assess skin condition and the need for a special mattress (e.g., egg crate), footboard, bed cradle, or heel protectors.

Equipment

- Clean gloves, if needed
- Two flat sheets; or one fitted sheet and one flat sheet
- Cloth drawsheet (optional)
- One blanket
- One bedspread (optional)
- Waterproof drawsheet or waterproof pads (optional)
- Pillowcase(s) for the head pillow(s)
- Plastic laundry bag or portable linen hamper, if available

IMPLEMENTATION

Performance

1. Before changing the bed, introduce yourself and verify the client's identity using two identifiers or per agency protocol. Explain to the client what you are going to do, why it is necessary, and how he or she can participate.
2. Perform hand hygiene, and follow other appropriate infection prevention and control procedures. Put on disposable gloves if the linen is soiled with bodily fluids.
3. Provide for client privacy.
4. Remove the top bedding.
   - Remove any equipment attached to the bed linen, such as a call light.
   - Loosen all the top linen at the foot of the bed, and remove the spread and the blanket.
   - Leave the top sheet over the client (the top sheet can remain over the client if it is being changed and if it will provide sufficient warmth), or replace it with a bath blanket as follows:

      a. Spread the bath blanket over the top sheet.
      b. Ask the client to hold the top edge of the blanket.

   c. Reaching under the blanket from the side, grasp the top edge of the sheet and draw it down to the foot of the bed, leaving the blanket in place (see ❶).
   d. Remove the sheet from the bed and place it in the soiled linen hamper.

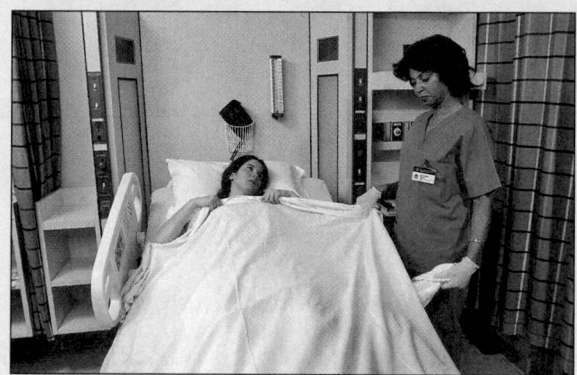

❶ Removing top linens under a bath blanket

5. Change the bottom sheet and drawsheet.
   - Raise the side rail nearest the client. **Rationale: This protects the client from falling.** If the bed does not have a side rail, have another nurse support the client at the edge of the bed.
   - Assist the client to turn on the side facing away from the side where the clean linen is.
   - Loosen the foundation of the linen on the side of the bed near the linen supply.
   - Fanfold the drawsheet and the bottom sheet at the centre of the bed (see ❷), as close to and under the client as possible. **Rationale: Doing this leaves the near half of the bed free to be changed**.

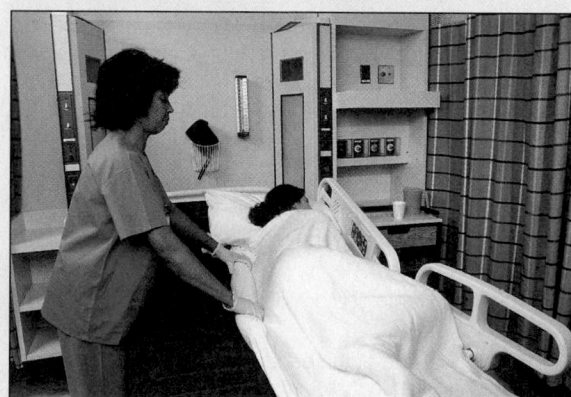

❷ Moving soiled linen as close to the client as possible

   - Place the clean bottom sheet on the bed, and vertically fanfold the half to be used on the far side of the bed as close to the client as possible (see ❸). Tuck the sheet under the near half of the bed and mitre the corner if a contour sheet is not being used.

(continued)

SKILL 31.10 **CHANGING AN OCCUPIED BED** (*continued*)

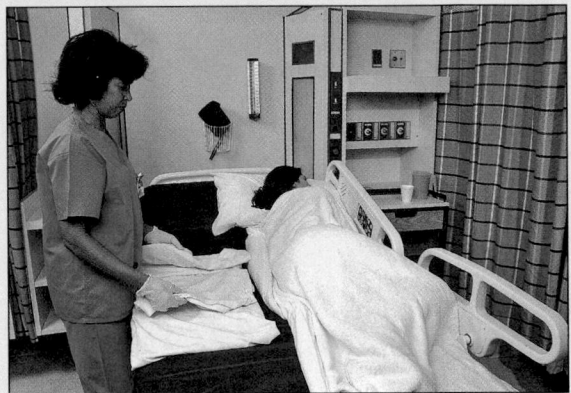

❸ Placing a clean bottom sheet on half of the bed

- Place the clean drawsheet on the bed with the centrefold at the centre of the bed. Fanfold the uppermost half vertically at the centre of the bed and tuck the near side edge under the side of the mattress (see ❹).

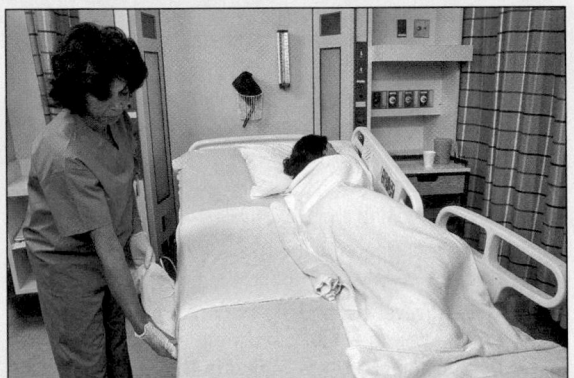

❹ Placing a clean drawsheet on the bed

- Assist the client to roll over toward you onto the clean side of the bed. The client rolls over the fanfolded linen at the centre of the bed.
- Move the pillows to the clean side for the client's use. Raise the side rail before leaving the side of the bed.
- Move to the other side of the bed, and lower the side rail.
- Remove the used linen, and place it in the portable hamper.
- Unfold the fanfolded bottom sheet from the centre of the bed.
- Facing the side of the bed, use both hands to pull the bottom sheet so that it is smooth and tuck the excess under the side of the mattress.

- Unfold the drawsheet fanfolded at the centre of the bed, and pull it tightly with both hands. Pull the sheet in three sections: (a) Face the side of the bed to pull the middle section, (b) face the far top corner to pull the bottom section, and (c) face the far bottom corner to pull the top section.
- Tuck the excess drawsheet under the side of the mattress.

6. Reposition the client in the centre of the bed.
   - Reposition the pillows at the centre of the bed.
   - Assist the client to the centre of the bed. Determine what position the client requires or prefers and assist the client to that position.

7. Apply or complete the top bedding.
   - Spread the top sheet over the client and either ask the client to hold the top edge of the sheet or tuck it under the shoulders. The sheet should remain over the client when the bath blanket or used sheet is removed (see ❺).
   - Complete the top of the bed.

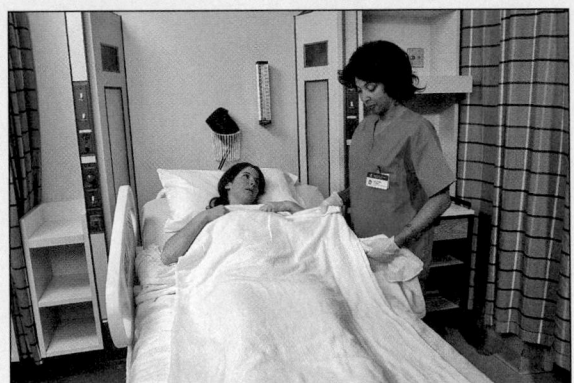

❺ Client holds top edge of sheet while nurse removes bath blanket

8. Ensure the continued safety of the client.
   - Raise the side rails. Place the bed in the low position before leaving the bedside.
   - Attach the call bell to the bed linen within the client's reach.
   - Put the items used by the client within easy reach.

9. Bed making is not normally recorded.

EVALUATION

Conduct appropriate follow-up, such as determining the client's comfort and safety, the patency of all drainage tubes, and the client's access to the call bell to summon help when needed.

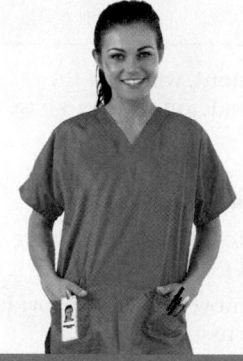

Case Study 31

It is the fourth day following Mrs. Perinic's abdominal surgery. She is progressing well, is ambulating several times each day, has been providing for her own hygienic needs, and is planning to go home tomorrow. During your early morning assessment, you note that Mrs. Perinic's hair is oily and she has an unpleasant body odour. Her dentures in a container at the bedside are in need of cleaning. You check her abdominal incision and verify that there is no drainage, redness, or signs of infection. You inquire about her ability to take care of her own bath and personal needs, and offer to assist her with her bath. She replies that she had a bath yesterday, does not feel that she needs another one today, and requests to omit her personal care for the day.

CRITICAL THINKING QUESTIONS

1. Support or contradict the use of the nursing diagnosis hygiene self-care deficit as an appropriate nursing diagnosis for Mrs. Perinic.

2. Explain why it would be in Mrs. Perinic's best interests for you to assist her with hygienic care, even though she does not feel she needs a bath.

3. What factors should you consider before you attempt to encourage Mrs. Perinic to attend to her personal care?

4. What approaches might you use if you feel that Mrs. Perinic does need her hair shampooed and needs to have her personal care attended to?

5. What advantages does performing baths and personal hygiene for clients offer the nurse?

Check the eText in MyNursingLab for answers and explanations.

KEY TERMS

apocrine glands *p. 785*

bactericidal *p. 785*

callus *p. 799*

cementum *p. 803*

cleansing baths *p. 790*

corn *p. 799*

crown *p. 803*

dental caries *p. 803*

dentin *p. 803*

eccrine glands *p. 785*

enamel *p. 803*

fissures *p. 800*

foam swabs *p. 809*

gingiva *p. 803*

gingivitis *p. 804*

hirsutism *p. 813*

hygiene *p. 783*

lanugo *p. 812*

lice *p. 813*

onychocryptosis *p. 800*

pediculosis *p. 813*

periodontal disease *p. 803*

personal hygiene *p. 783*

plantar warts *p. 800*

plaque *p. 804*

pulp cavity *p. 803*

pyorrhea *p. 804*

scabies *p. 813*

sebum *p. 785*

sudoriferous (sweat) glands *p. 785*

sulcular technique *p. 806*

tartar *p. 804*

therapeutic baths *p. 791*

ticks *p. 812*

tinea pedis *p. 800*

CHAPTER HIGHLIGHTS

- Clients' hygiene practices are influenced by relevant health determinants.

- The major functions of the skin are to help regulate body temperature, to protect underlying tissues, to secrete sebum, to transmit sensations through nerve receptors for sensory perception, and to produce and absorb vitamin D in conjunction with ultraviolet rays of the sun.

- The nurse considers clients' preferences when planning for their hygiene care.

- Nurses provide perineal–genital care for clients who are unable to care for themselves.

- Oral hygiene includes daily dental flossing and mechanical brushing of teeth.

- Nurses provide special oral care to clients who are unable to manage their own care (e.g., they are unconscious) and who have oral problems.

- Regular dental checkups are recommended to maintain healthy teeth.

- Hair care includes daily combing and brushing and regular shampooing.

- Nurses can often teach clients how to prevent foot problems.

- Nurses may need to assist dependent clients with their eyeglasses and contact lenses.

- Clients with hearing aids may require nursing assistance with the devices.

- Changing bed linens is a part of maintaining hygiene.

- It is important to keep beds clean and comfortable for clients.

ASSESS YOUR LEARNING

1. A nurse who is conducting a wellness teaching session promoting dental health recommends all of the following *except:*

   a. Brush teeth and tongue at a minimum once a day and always before going to bed

   b. Floss teeth at least daily and brush teeth after flossing

   c. Avoid sweet foods and drinks between meals

   d. Use a hard bristled toothbrush with a size and shape that allows for easy access to the molars

2. The client is unresponsive and requires complete care. Before proceeding with mouth care on an unconscious client, the nurse will assess for which of the following?

   a. Presence of any pain

   b. Condition of skin

   c. Condition of the mouth

   d. Presence of a gag reflex

3. A client with diabetes has very dry skin on her feet. To promote skin integrity of this client's feet, the nurse will suggest that the client do which of the following?

   a. Soak her feet frequently

   b. Rub skin on the feet briskly several times a day

   c. Use nonperfumed alcohol-free lotion

   d. Avoid knee-high stockings

4. Appropriate treatment for a client with acne includes which of the following?

   a. Frequent washing with hot water and a mild commercial soap

   b. Soaking with warm water, followed by gentle squeezing of pustules

   c. Washing with medicated soap daily, with active abrading once a week

   d. Washing with medicated soap, followed by application of medicated cream

5. Which of the following is a treatment for pediculosis (lice infestation) in a 3-year-old child?

   a. Isopropyl myristate 50% and ST-cyclomethicone 50% solution applied to the scalp as directed

   b. Permethrin 1% cream rinse and use of a fine-toothed comb

   c. Paraffin 2% solution left on scalp for 6 hours and then washed out

   d. Peroxide 1% and baking soda in a paste that is brushed out when dried

6. In planning foot care for a client, which of the following is the correct rationale on which to base decisions about the care?

   a. Use of lotion is avoided as this creates a moist environment for growth of bacteria.

   b. It is sometimes necessary to extend the cutting of a nail into the sulcus (nail groove).

   c. Calluses should not be removed, as they provide protection for underlying tissue.

   d. Unpleasant foot odours in older adults are usually the result of poor hygiene practices.

The next four questions are related to this scenario:

Tal Chakar-Aimaq is a 77-year-old man who had a cerebrovascular accident (stroke) 2 weeks ago. Although he has made a remarkable recovery, he has residual right-sided weakness and requires assistance to meet his hygiene needs.

7. The most relevant nursing diagnosis for this client is which of the following?

   a. Deficient knowledge related to not understanding how to manage his own care

   b. Potential for altered self-esteem related to inability to complete his own care

   c. Self-care deficit related to inability to complete care independently

   d. Altered skin integrity related to inadequate hygiene

8. In considering hygiene care for Mr. Chakar-Aimaq, the nurse will adhere to which of the following principles?

   a. The level of independence before illness is generally quite different from the present level.

   b. If the nurse is doing the care, it is not necessary to assess the environment for safety.

   c. To prevent frustration for the client, the nurse should recognize the client's limits.

   d. The client should be allowed to do what he can or wants to do to, regardless of the time it takes.

9. Mr. Chakar-Aimaq tends to remain positioned on either his left side or on his back, and he moves very little without assistance. Which of the following is the priority nursing action intended to reduce the risk of skin breakdown?

   a. Keeping his skin dry and clean and the bed linens free of wrinkles

   b. Ensuring adequate hydration and mobilizing him frequently

   c. Using powder on his back and changing the bed linens twice a day

   d. Using pillows to prop him in his preferred position and rubbing his back

10. In planning hair care for Mr. Chakar-Aimaq, which of the following principles is a priority for the nurse to consider at this point in his recovery?

  a. Shampooing should be done daily to maintain hygiene.

  b. Brushing the hair improves circulation to the scalp.

  c. Neglecting hair care is culturally unacceptable to him.

  d. Asking Mr. Chakar-Aimaq what he prefers is inappropriate.

Check the eText in MyNursingLab for answers and explanations.

WEBLINKS

Canadian Diabetes Association

http://www.diabetes.ca

This site provides best practice guidelines for foot care in people with diabetes mellitus (DM). Resources are available for both health care professionals and people with DM.

Canadian Dental Association (CDA)

http://www.cda-adc.ca/

The CDA provides a variety of teaching resources and position statements on various topics related to oral health.

Canadian Hearing Society (CHS)

http://www.chs.ca

The CHS provides valuable information and links to resources, including information on hearing aids.

MyNursingLab

REFERENCES

Alzheimer Society of Canada. (2011). *Guidelines for care: Person-centered care of people with dementia living in care homes.* Retrieved from http://www.alzheimer.ca/english/care/framework.pdf

Brady, M. C., Furlanetto, D., Hunter, R., Lewis, S. C., Milne, V. (2006). Staff-led interventions for improving oral hygiene in patients following stroke. *Cochrane Database of Systematic Reviews 2006, Issue 4.* Art. No.: CD003864. doi: 10.1002/14651858. CD003864.pub2

Canadian Dental Association. (2010). *Position paper on use of fluorides in caries prevention.* Retrieved from http://www.cda-adc. ca/en/oral_health/cfyt/dental_care_children/fluoride.asp

Canadian Dental Association. (2012). Flossing and brushing. Retrieved from http://www.cda-adc.ca/en/oral_health/cfyt/ dental_care/flossing_brushing.asp

Canadian Diabetes Association. (2008). *Foot care: A step toward good health Canadian practice guideline.* Retrieved from http://www.diabetes.ca/images/about-diabetes/CDA_ FootcareFINAL_flexitol.pdf

Canadian Paediatric Society – Infectious Diseases and Immunization Committee. (2008). Head lice infestations: A clinical update. *Paediatric Child Health 2008, 13*(8), 692–696.

Grant, B. M., Giddings, L. S., & Beale, J. E. (2005). Vulnerable bodies: Competing discourses of intimate bodily care. *Journal of Nursing Education, 44* (11), 498–504.

Hodgkinson, B., Nay, R., & Wilson, J. (2007). A systematic review of topical skin care in aged care facilities. *Journal of Clinical Nursing, 16,* 129–136.

Ontario Agency for Health Protection and Promotion, Provincial Infectious Diseases Advisory Committee. (2011).

Routine practices and additional precautions in all health care settings. Toronto, ON: Queens Printer for Ontario. Retrieved from http://www.oahpp.ca/resources/pidac-knowledge/ best-practice-manuals/routine-practices-and-additional-precautions.html

Pear, S. (2007). Oral care is critical care: The role of oral care in the prevention of hospital-acquired pneumonia. *Infection Control Today, 11,* 10.

Penzer, R. F. M. (2001). Promoting healthy skin in older people. *Nursing Standard, 15*(34), 46–52.

Pineda, L. A., Saliba, R. G., & El Solh, A. A. (2006). Effect of oral decontamination with chlorhexidine on the incidence of nosocomial pneumonia: A meta analysis. *Critical Care, 10*(1), R35.

Public Health Agency of Canada. (2007). *Infection prevention and control best practices for long-term care, home and community care including health care offices and ambulatory clinics, June, 2007.* Retrieved from http://www.phac-aspc.gc.ca/amr-ram/ipcbp-pepci/appendix_ii-annexe_ii-eng.php#laundry

Radner, J., Barrick, A. L., Hoeffer, B., Sloane, P., McKenzie, D., Talerico, K. A., & Glover, J. U. (2006). The bathing of older adults with dementia: Easing the unnecessary unpleasant aspects of assisted bathing. *American Journal of Nursing, 106* (4), 40–48.

Sloane, P. D., Hoeffer, B. & Somboontanont, B. (2006). Bathing without a battle: Providing more person-centered experiences for long-term care residents with dementia. *Research and Practice in Alzheimer's Disease, 11,* 294–299.

Chapter 32

Safety

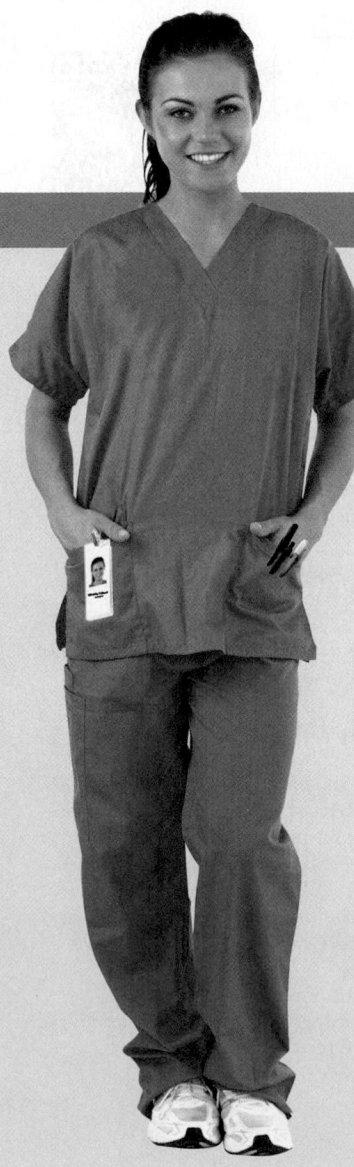

After studying this chapter, you will be able to:

1. Discuss nine factors that affect people's ability to protect themselves from unintentional injury.

2. Describe the five parts to assessing clients at risk for unintentional injury.

3. List Accreditation Canada's six required organizational practices related to patient safety.

4. Identify common potential hazards throughout the lifespan.

5. Give examples of nursing diagnoses, outcomes, and interventions for clients at risk for unintentional injury.

6. Plan strategies to maintain safety in the home, community, and health care setting, including prevention strategies across the lifespan for unintentional injuries related to motor vehicles, thermal injury, falls, poisoning, suffocation or choking, excessive noise, electric hazards, and firearms.

7. Explain measures to prevent falls.

8. Discuss implementation of seizure precautions.

9. Describe 11 alternatives to restraints.

10. Describe the procedural steps in applying physical restraints and discuss the use and legal implications of restraints.

11. List desired health outcomes to use in evaluating the selected strategies for injury prevention.

Patient safety is fundamental to nursing care and health care across all settings. It is not merely a mandate; it is a moral and ethical imperative in caring for others (Canadian Nurses Association [CNA], 2009). Defined as the reduction and mitigation of unsafe acts within the health care system, and the use of best practices shown to lead to optimal patient outcomes, **patient safety** is a critical aspect of quality health care (Canadian Patient Safety Institute, 2011). Because nurses work with individuals, families, groups, communities, and populations in a range of settings (e.g., the home, schools, acute care and long-term care facilities, and community clinics) and with people across all points in the lifespan in both health and illness situations, they can play a major role in promoting the safety of the Canadian population. Through their vigilance, nurses act to keep patients safe, identify areas of risk, and recognize situations in need of improvement (CNA, 2009).

Promoting safety includes preventing injury across all stages of the lifespan. An **injury** is defined as the physical damage to the body from a sudden exposure to energy (e.g., mechanical, chemical, thermal, or environmental) at levels that exceed the normal human tolerance or as a result of the lack of one or more vital elements, such as oxygen (World Health Organization [WHO], 2008). Although the terms *injury* and *accident* are sometimes used interchangeably, safety experts indicate that most injuries are predictable and therefore preventable, unlike **accidents**, which are random or chance events that are not preventable (Pless & Hagel, 2005). Injury can be differentiated by intent: **unintentional injuries** result from unplanned events, such as motor vehicle collisions, falls, drowning, fire, or the ingestion of foreign objects; **intentional injuries** are the result of purposeful harm, such as in the case of child abuse, assault, or suicide. Although Canada is considered one of the best places to live in the world, we continue to have high rates of injury, particularly among the youth, with unintentional injury being the leading cause of mortality in Canadian children and youth ages 0 to 19 years (Public Health Agency of Canada, 2009a). Safe Kids Canada goes as far as saying that Canada has a daunting injury epidemic and that preventing child injury is a priority (Fuselli & Wanounou, 2011).

As a result of an increased awareness of the frequency and significance of adverse events, patient safety has become a key priority for all stakeholders. **Adverse events** are unintended injuries or complications that result in death, disability, or prolonged hospital stays and that are the result of health care management (Royal College of Physicians and Surgeons—*Canadian Patient Safety Dictionary,* 2003). Specific to the health care system, efforts are aimed at the reduction and mitigation of unsafe acts and at the use of evidence-informed practices that lead to optimal patient outcomes. Nurses themselves have their own safety concerns, owing to the nature of risks in the workplace setting. Providing a safe work environment for nurses so that they, in turn, can ensure the safety of the people they work with has emerged as another priority in the health care setting. See the Nursing and Canadian Society box on the next page for some facts on safety research and improvements and their implications for nursing practice.

Nursing and Canadian Society

Canadian Safety Initiatives: Implications for Nursing Practice

Fact	Implications for Nursing Practice
Safer Healthcare Now! offers Canadian health care organizations the opportunity to participate in and support a campaign dedicated to improving patient safety through the implementation of targeted interventions in patient care.	Nurses must be prepared to be challenged by all stakeholders when safety is an issue. Many Canadians are concerned and nurses must be aware that they are taking action. The interventions (e.g., preventing ventilator associated pneumonia, surgical site infections, and venous thromboembolism) are of interest to nurses.
The Institute for Safe Medication Practices (ISMP) Canada is a national nonprofit organization committed to the advancement of medication safety in all health care settings. The ISMP collaborates with Health Canada and other stakeholders in the Canadian Medication Incident Reporting and Prevention System (CMIRPS), where people can voluntarily report medication incidents.	Nurses can take advantage of the many resources and recommendations offered by the ISMP as they seek to ensure medication safety. Nurses can report medication incidents so that others can learn from them.
Safe Kids Canada is working toward a 25% reduction in preventable injuries by 2016 and offers a range of resources, including fact sheets, about multiple issues related to child safety.	Nurses can take advantage of the many safety initiatives of Safe Kids Canada, especially during the Safe Kids Week. This organization advocates for the three E's in preventing childhood injuries: Educate, Engineer, Enforce.
The Registered Nurses' Association of Ontario released its *Prevention of Falls and Fall Injuries in the Older Adult—Guideline Supplement* outlining best practices in falls prevention in 2011.	Nurses can draw on much evidence to inform their practice, particularly in such nurse-sensitive areas as fall prevention.
The *Canadian Patient Safety Dictionary* (Royal College of Physicians and Surgeons, 2003) provides definitions of terms used in the area of patient safety.	This dictionary helps to ensure that members of the health care team use a common language when assessing, monitoring, and evaluating patient safety issues.
The Canadian Patient Safety Institute (CPSI) aims at raising awareness and facilitating the implementation of ideas and best practices to achieve a transformation in patient safety.	Nurses need the most up-to-date knowledge to guide their practice. The CPSI provides a forum in which key stakeholders can identify issues and evolve research programs to enhance patient safety.
The Canadian Framework for Managing Patient Incidents (the Framework) is a tool to help identify and address the contributing factors relating to critical incidents in health care. The Framework was developed by the Canadian Patient Safety Institute in partnership with the Institute for Safe Medication Practices Canada, Saskatchewan Health, and Groupe Vigilance pour la sécurité des soins.	Identifying the multiple contributing factors that give rise to a critical incident, including near misses, enhances the learning from that incident, which can then be translated into changed practices to avoid further incidents.
The Canadian Hospitals Injury Reporting and Prevention Program (CHIRPP) collects and analyzes data on injuries to people (mainly children) who are seen at the emergency rooms of 14 hospitals across Canada.	Nurses can use the data collected by the CHIRPP to develop health-promotion programs and keep current on major issues related to injury in the general population.

Factors Affecting Safety

People's ability to protect themselves from injury is affected by such factors as age and development, lifestyle, mobility and health status, sensory–perceptual alterations, cognitive awareness, emotional state, ability to communicate, safety awareness, and environmental factors. Nurses need to assess each of these factors when they plan care or help clients learn to protect themselves.

Age and Development

The age-dependent cognitive, psychological, language, and physical changes that occur across the lifespan influence an individual's ability to identify, anticipate, prevent, and recover from a range of health risks. Unfortunately, injury is the leading cause of death for Canadians ages 1 to 44 years, with suicide, an intentional injury, as the leading cause of all injury deaths followed by unintentional injuries resulting from transport incidents and falls (Smartrisk, 2011).

Consider the following examples: Toddlers and preschool-age children are attracted to the water but generally lack a sense of danger. This is compounded by the fact that a top-heavy physique makes them more vulnerable to falling into the water, and their relatively small lungs fill quickly with water. This age group has the highest incidence of drowning (Safe Kids Canada, 2011a). Very young children can easily sustain burns if exposed to very hot water (greater than 49°C) as their dermis is thin and they cannot move away from hot water. The adolescent, whose thoughts usually include the *personal fable,* may believe he or she is immune to adverse outcomes when engaging in risky behaviour. In older adults, the combination of reduced reflex activity and diminished sensory acuity can lead to increased risk of falling. Box 32.1 summarizes selected safety hazards throughout the lifespan.

Lifestyle

Lifestyle factors that place people at risk include unsafe work environments, residence in neighbourhoods with high crime rates, access to guns and ammunition, abuse of alcohol and street drugs, and lack of income to buy safety equipment or make necessary repairs. Risk-taking behaviour is a factor in some accidents.

BOX 32.1 SELECTED SAFETY HAZARDS THROUGHOUT THE LIFESPAN

The following, organized by age groups most affected, are some important safety hazards. Preventive measures are discussed later in this chapter.

- *Developing fetus:* Exposure to teratogens (maternal smoking, alcohol, certain medications, radiation)
- *0–14 years:* The three leading causes of injury-related death are drowning (15%), motor vehicle collisions (14%), and suffocation (13%); falls (in the home, at school, in playgrounds) account for 44% of injury-related hospitalizations (Safe Kids Canada, 2011a)
- *Newborns and infants:* Drowning; motor vehicle collisions (passenger); burns (e.g., spilled hot liquids, bath water), threats to breathing (choking, suffocation, strangulation), falls, electric shock, poisoning
- *Toddlers and preschoolers:* Motor vehicle collisions (passenger and pedestrian or cyclist), drowning, falling, threats to breathing (choking, suffocation, strangulation), farm-related injuries and fatalities, lacerations, burns, poisoning, electric shock, harm from other people or animals
- *School-age children:* Motor vehicle collisions (passenger and pedestrian or cyclist), drowning, off-highway vehicle (including snowmobile) accidents, burns
- *Adolescents:* Motor vehicle collisions (passenger and pedestrian or cyclist), off-highway vehicle (including snowmobile) accidents, falls, drowning, cycling accidents, problematic substance use
- *Older adults:* Falls, burns, and motor vehicle collisions (passenger and pedestrian)

Mobility and Health Status

People with impaired mobility because of paralysis, muscle weakness, or poor balance or coordination are at increased risk of injury. People with paraplegia may be unable to move even when they perceive discomfort. People with hemiplegia or with leg casts often have poor balance and fall easily. Clients weakened by illness or surgery may not be fully aware of their limitations.

Sensory–Perceptual Alterations

Accurate sensory perception of environmental stimuli is vital to safety. People with impaired touch perception, hearing, taste, smell, and vision are highly susceptible to injury. A person who does not see well may trip over an object; a person with hearing impairment will not hear a siren in traffic; and people with anosmia (impaired olfactory sense) may not smell burning food or the sulphur aroma of a natural gas leak.

Cognitive Awareness

Awareness is the ability to perceive environmental stimuli and body reactions and to respond appropriately through thought and action. Clients with impaired awareness include people lacking sleep, unconscious or semiconscious persons, disoriented people who may not understand where they are or what to do to protect themselves, people who perceive stimuli that do not exist, and people whose judgment is altered by disease or medications (e.g., opioids, tranquilizers, hypnotics, and sedatives).

Emotional State

Extreme emotional states can alter the ability to perceive environmental hazards. Stressful situations can reduce a person's level of concentration, cause errors of judgment, and decrease awareness of external stimuli. People with depression may think and react to environmental stimuli more slowly than usual.

Ability to Communicate

Individuals with diminished ability to receive and convey information are at risk for injury. They include people with *aphasia* (loss or impairment of the power to use or understand words, usually resulting from brain damage), people with language barriers, and those unable to read. For example, the person unable to interpret the sign "No smoking: oxygen in use" could cause a fire or an explosion.

Safety Awareness

Information about water safety, car safety, fire prevention, and the many age-specific hazards and their preventive measures is crucial to safety. Clients in unfamiliar environments (e.g., hospital) or dealing with new treatments (e.g., oxygen

REFLECT ON PRIMARY HEALTH CARE

Mothers Against Drunk Driving (MADD) is an example of how *public participation* can raise awareness about the role of alcohol and risk-taking behaviours in many unintentional injuries caused by motor vehicle collisions. Reflect on the benefits of *intersectoral cooperation,* such as a nurse and a parent who has lost a child to drunk driving both speaking at a high school preparing for its graduation dance or a rally to raise the minimum age for obtaining a driver's licence, in reducing the incidence of drunk driving.

therapy, hot packs) frequently need specific safety information. The Reflect on Primary Health Care box describes how public participation can also raise safety awareness.

Environmental Factors

Depending on the client's situation, the nurse may need to assess the environment of the home, workplace, or community. Client safety is affected by the health care setting. Bioterrorism has become a safety concern related to the environment.

HOME A safe home requires, among many things, well-maintained flooring and carpets, a nonskid bathtub or shower surface, strategically placed and functioning smoke alarms and carbon monoxide detectors, and knowledge of fire escape routes. Outdoor areas, such as swimming pools, need to be safely secured and maintained. Adequate lighting, both inside and out, will minimize the potential for unintentional injury. Families that live on farms are exposed to particular risks as their home is also a workplace where there is often heavy equipment, large vehicles, open water, and animals. Unfortunately, there is a disproportionately high number of fatal injuries (e.g., from tractor run-over, drowning, falls from barn loft) in children living on farms compared with children not living on a farm (Canadian Agricultural Injury Surveillance Program, 2007).

WORKPLACE A range of chemical, biological, physical, ergonomic, and psychosocial hazards exist in the workplace. Workers exposed to temperature extremes, those who lack adequate training on the use of mechanical equipment, or those who are the victims of sexual harassment or discrimination in the workplace are all at risk for ill health. Farming, governed almost entirely by voluntary workplace standards, is considered one of Canada's most dangerous occupations. The work environment of the nurse includes such risks to safety as exposure to microbial agents and potentially aggressive clients.

COMMUNITY Adequate street lighting; safe water and sewage treatment; restrictions on pollution, including smoke-free environments; and regulation of consumer products and sanitation in food buying and handling all contribute to a healthy, hazard-free community. A safe and secure community strives to be free of excess noise, crime, traffic congestion, dilapidated housing, or unprotected creeks and landfills.

HEALTH CARE SETTING, INCLUDING HOME CARE

Safety issues within the Canadian health care setting have come to the forefront since the release of the *Canadian Adverse Events Study* (Baker, Norton, Flintoft, Blais, Brown, Cox, et al., 2004) indicating that as many as 1 in 13 hospitalized patients can experience adverse events, including death, with many of these events deemed preventable.

Safety problems arise from *acts of omission* (failure to institute the appropriate therapeutic intervention), such as lack of assessment to predict risk of falls, lack of discharge teaching; or *acts of commission* (incorrect diagnosis or treatment, or poor performance), such as errors in medication dosage, wrong-site surgery, restraint-related injuries or death, burns, mistaken identity, and health-care associated infection. There are multiple factors that can contribute to errors, such as a gap between the increased complexity of care in health care settings and outdated communication systems, poor product design, a shortage of qualified health care personnel, the quality of communication patterns among health care professionals, the quality of the nursing practice environment, nursing staffing and skill mix, among others. Client safety is viewed as going beyond the blaming of individual professionals to looking at the multiple system factors whose complex interplay ultimately influences whether safety is assured.

Interprofessional collaboration also promotes client safety and quality assurance in health care, especially when health care professionals demonstrate the competencies needed for such collaboration: interprofessional communication; patient-, client-, family-, and community-centred care; role clarification; team functioning; collaborative leadership; and interprofessional conflict resolution (Canadian Interprofessional Health Collaborative, 2010). Many professional schools have tried to develop opportunities where nursing students and other students in the health care professions learn with, from, and about each other—all in an effort to improve collaboration and quality of client care.

Client safety concerns also occur in home care situations. Family members, friends, and informal caregivers under the indirect supervision of medical personnel are taking on complex care, from administering intravenous antibiotics, through caring for a partner who is paralyzed, to caring for a child who is ventilator dependent. Family members' safety may also be at risk as they take on such activities as lifting heavy equipment or moving their family member in and out of bed or a bath. Research is needed on the impact of home care on the physical, emotional, and functional safety of the client, family, and other caregivers (Macdonald, Lang, & MacDonald, 2011).

BIOTERRORISM When bioterrorism with anthrax paralyzed the United States postal system after the September 11, 2001, terrorist attacks in the country, awareness of bioterrorism as a threat to safety emerged. Terrorism includes chemical, biological, or nuclear weapons, but **bioterrorism** is "the use of a microorganism with the deliberate intent of causing infection in order to achieve certain goals" (Public Health Agency of Canada, 2005).

Bioterrorism is of concern because it has potentially far-reaching effects because of easy transmission, high mortality rates, and public panic.

Assessing

Assessing clients at risk for unintentional injury involves (a) noting pertinent indicators in the nursing history and physical examination, (b) using specifically developed risk-assessment tools, (c) evaluating the client's home environment, (d) assessing standards related to client safety goals in hospitals, and (e) addressing bioterrorism.

Nursing History and Physical Examination

The nursing history and physical examination can reveal considerable data about the client's safety practices and risks for injury. Data include age and developmental level; general health status; mobility status; presence of physiological or perceptual deficits, such as olfactory, visual, tactile, taste, or other sensory impairments; altered thought processes or impaired cognitive or emotional capabilities; problematic substance use; indications of abuse or neglect; and a history of unintentional injury. A safety history also includes the client's awareness of hazards, knowledge of safety precautions at home and at work, and any perceived threats to safety (Figure 32.1).

Risk-Assessment Tools

Risk-assessment tools are available to determine which clients are at risk for specific kinds of injury, such as falls, or for the general assessment necessary to keep clients safe in their homes and in health care settings. In general, these tools direct the nurse to appraise multiple factors affecting safety. The tools summarize specific data contained in the client's nursing history and physical examination. Client risk factors and environmental hazards for falls are discussed later in this chapter.

Home Hazard Appraisal

Hazards in the home are major causes of falls, fire, poisoning, suffocation, and other incidents, such as those caused by improper use of household equipment, tools, and cooking utensils. See Box 14.4 (page 280), for a summary of specific data necessary for a home hazard appraisal.

National Patient Safety Goals

Accreditation Canada (formerly the Canadian Council on Health Services Accreditation) plays a major role in improving patient safety through the accreditation of Canadian health services organizations. The accreditation program evaluates how organizations meet standards of excellence in ensuring patient safety and providing quality services relative to meeting six *Required Organizational Practices* (Accreditation Canada, 2011):

1. *Creating a culture of safety within the organization,* as evidenced by such indicators as a formal policy and process of disclosure of adverse events to clients and families; support mechanisms for clients, family, staff, service providers involved in adverse events.

2. *Improving the effectiveness of coordination of communication among care and service providers and with the recipients of care or services across the continuum,* as evidenced by such indicators as the following:

   • Clients and families being informed about their role in promoting safety, with staff taking client or family questions or comments about potential error seriously (e.g., a client who is surprised that he is being sent for a test may be an indication that the wrong client is being solicited!)
   • Not using dangerous abbreviations so as to avoid medication errors (see Chapter 33)
   • Effective mechanisms for transfer of information at transition points, such as change of shift, transfer between units or institutions, and discharge home

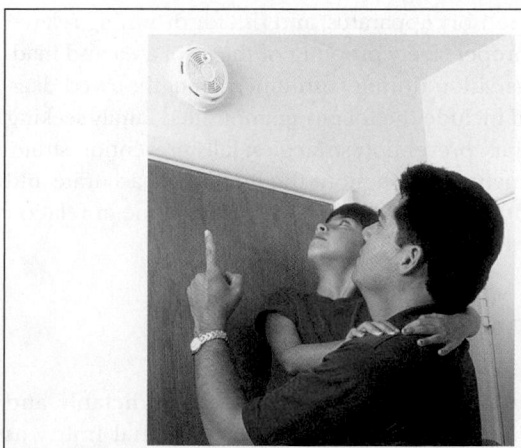
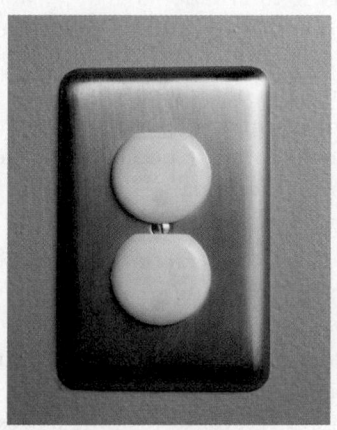

FIGURE 32.1 Nurses need to teach clients about safety and how to prevent unintentional injury, such as by using smoke detectors and safety covers for electrical outlets.

- Reconciliation of clients' medications at admission and transfer or discharge (discussed in detail in Chapter 33)
- A safe-surgery checklist used to confirm safety steps in the case of surgical procedures (see Chapter 36)
- Clients properly identified using two client indicators
- Verification processes for high-risk activities (e.g., two-person verification for blood transfusions or automated alert systems for communication of critical test results)

3. *Ensuring the safe use of high-risk medications,* as evidenced by the following indicators:
   - Absence of concentrated electrolytes (e.g., potassium chloride, sodium chloride >0.9%) from client service areas
   - A limited number of heparin concentrations being available on the care unit, with high-dose formats (e.g., unfractionated heparin 10 000 U/mL) being removed
   - Adequate training for staff on all infusion pumps
   - High-dose, high-potency opioids removed from patient care units (Chapter 33 discusses safety with respect to medications in great detail)

4. *Creating a work life and physical environment that supports the safe delivery of care and service,* as evidenced by the following:
   - Training on client safety for all staff
   - Staff having a clear understanding of the roles, responsibilities, and accountabilities of the health team members in relation to the care and safety of patients or clients
   - Preventive maintenance programs for medical devices, equipment, and technology
   - Comprehensive strategy to prevent workplace violence

5. *Reducing the risk of health-care associated infections and their impact across the continuum of care or service,* as evidenced by the following:
   - Ongoing evaluation of compliance with hand hygiene practices for staff, service providers, and volunteers
   - Adherence to international, federal, and provincial or territorial infection control guidelines
   - Tracking and analysis of infection rates
   - Implementation of protocols to ensure the administration of vaccines for pneumococcal infection and influenza in at-risk populations (including health care professionals)
   - Monitoring of processes for reprocessing equipment

6. *Identifying safety risks inherent in the client population,* as evidenced by the following:
   - Falls prevention strategy
   - Safety risk assessment for clients receiving services in the home
   - Assessment of risk for developing a pressure ulcer, with implementation of interventions to prevent pressure ulcers

- Assessment and monitoring of clients for risk of suicide
- Identification of clients at risk for venous thromboembolism with provision of appropriate prevention strategies

Accreditation Canada focuses on system-wide indicators of safety, marking a shift from the method of finding out who made any particular error (i.e., creating an environment of fear and scapegoating) to analyzing the system to find out why any particular error occurred (i.e., creating an environment of learning and improvement).

Bioterrorism

Health care workers, especially emergency medical responders and front-line workers, many of whom are nurses, need to be alert to circumstances or patterns that can indicate bioterrorism, such as an unusual geographical clustering of illness (e.g., persons who attended the same public event), the hospital or community clinic receiving an increase in the number of clients with similar symptoms, or an unusual age distribution for common diseases (e.g., an increase in a childhood illness, such as varicella, among adults). The health problems seen in one facility may be part of a bigger picture; calling public health authorities to report observations and suspicions may reveal a larger pattern.

Diagnosing

Given the broad range of safety issues facing individuals, families, and communities, a large number of potential risk nursing diagnoses can be made in relation to safety!

Any of the following, and many more, are possible analyses: risk for poisoning related to lack of childproofing the home environment; risk for suffocation related to use of stuffed animals and improperly fitted mattress in crib; risk for fall related to polypharmacy, muscle weakness, and unsafe home environment; risk for unintentional injury related to incorrect car seat choice and improper installation; risk for scalding related to high hot water temperature and reduced peripheral sensory apparatus; and risk for drowning related to lack of proper safety proofing of the pool area and inadequate supervision during bath time. Strengths-based diagnoses could include the following: motivated family seeking to learn injury prevention strategies; falls prevention strategies implemented throughout the home; and accurate and effective anticipatory childproofing of the home in relation to increased mobility of the toddler.

Planning

Nurses must use knowledge about the predictable and contributing factors related to unintentional injury as they plan their care. Nurses can help individuals and families anticipate risks for injury in relation to changing developmental skills and demands and help them minimize or eliminate the risks. The major goal for clients with safety risks is to prevent unintentional injury.

Nursing interventions to meet desired outcomes are largely directed toward helping the individual and family do the following:

- Identify and remove or reduce environmental hazards in the home, workplace, community, and health care agency

- Demonstrate safety practices appropriate to the home, health care agency, community, and workplace

- Experience the absence of injury or, at least, a decrease in the frequency or severity of injury

- Demonstrate safe childrearing practices or lifestyle practices

Implementing

Promoting Safety across the Lifespan

Hazards to safety occur at all ages and vary according to the age and development level of the individual. Measures to ensure the safety of people of all ages focus on (a) observation or prediction of potentially harmful situations so that harm can be avoided and (b) health teaching that promotes wellness by empowering clients and families to protect themselves from injury. Safety measures covering the lifespan from infancy to older adults are listed in the Teaching: Wellness box.

NEWBORNS AND INFANTS   Unintentional injuries are a leading cause of death and reason for hospitalization

---

TEACHING   **WELLNESS**

Safety Measures throughout the Lifespan

Across the lifespan, several measures can help promote safety:

NEWBORNS AND INFANTS

- Infant car seats must meet strict Canadian Motor Vehicle Safety Standards and be used correctly at all times. A rear-facing infant seat, properly secured at a 45-degree angle in the back seat of the vehicle, is recommended from birth and until the child grows out of the rear-facing seat (Transport Canada, 2011a). Before 2011, rear-facing seats were recommended until the child was 1 year old; however, more stringent guidelines are now in place as newer rear-facing seats are safer, even for children who weigh as much as 20 kg and are walking! Parents must ensure that the child is properly secured in the car seat (Figure 32.2), check seat labels for specific weight and height limits and detailed installation instructions for particular models.

- Bath safety includes constant supervision and checking the water temperature (ideally between 37°C and 40°C) before placing the child in the bath; turn cold water off last to avoid a burn if tap is inadvertently turned on. Do not use bath seats as they can mistakenly be seen as a substitute for supervision and lead to drowning (Safe Kids Canada, 2011b).

- Hold the infant upright during feeding and do not prop the bottle if the infant is bottle fed. Bottle nipples displaying signs of wear and tear should be discarded. Cut food into small pieces, and do not feed the infant foods that could be choked on, such as peanuts, raisins, or popcorn. Hotdogs and gluey foods, such as white bread with peanut butter, can occlude an airway; cutting a wiener down the middle and then into small bits, and toasting the bread and spreading only a thin layer of peanut butter are safer alternatives.

- Health Canada (2010a) indicates that cribs, cradles, and bassinettes must meet stringent Canadian safety standards. Bumper pads are not recommended. To prevent strangulation, babies should never be harnessed or tied in a crib or placed near window blind or electric cords. Any crib or cradle should not be used if there are

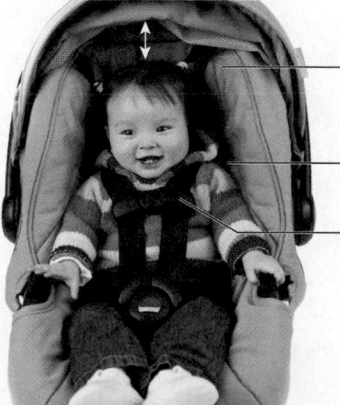

HEAD
At least 2.5 cm of space between the top of the child's head and the top of the car seat

SHOULDERS
Make sure the harness straps are snug on the child's shoulders. Only one finger should be able to fit between the harness and the child at the collarbone

CHEST
Make sure the chest clip is at the child's armpit level and closed properly

FIGURE 32.2 Proper restraint in a rear-facing seat.

Source: Transport Canada. (2011a). Car seats, seatbelts, and your child: Keep kids safe. Stage 1: Rear-facing seats. Retrieved from http://www.tc.gc.ca/eng/roadsafety/safedrivers-childsafety-car-time-stage1-1084.htm

(continued)

any loose or missing parts. The crib mattress should be no thicker than 15 cm and be of such a size that when it is pushed firmly against any side of the crib, it does not leave a gap of more than 3 cm between the mattress and any part of the sides of the crib. Parents should avoid using pillows, comforters, or soft mattresses in the crib to avoid suffocation. Unless otherwise contraindicated, the baby should be placed on his or her back to reduce the risk of sudden infant death syndrome.

- Use a sturdy playpen with sides made of mosquito type netting; the playpen should not have any sharp edges or hinges; the playpen mattress pad should be firm; do not put large toys or stuffed animals in the play pen as these can be used to climb out of the playpen (Health Canada, 2010b).

- Provide large soft toys with no small detachable or sharp-edged parts.

- To avoid strangulation, never tie or hang pacifiers or any other objects around the neck of a baby or a young child; Health Canada (2010c) recommends that pacifiers be replaced at least every 2 months and that a teething ring is a safer alternative for a baby who is chewing on a pacifier.

- Use guard gates on stairs and screens on windows. Gates that have large diamond-shaped or large V-shaped openings at the top are not allowed to be sold in Canada. Supervise the infant in swings and highchairs.

- Cover electrical outlets and keep cords out of reach.

- Place plants, household cleaners, and other potentially poisonous substances out of reach.

- The sale of baby walkers has been banned in Canada since 2004. Anyone with a hand-me-down baby walker is advised to destroy it.

TODDLERS AND PRESCHOOLERS

- A properly installed, forward-facing car seat that meets Canadian Motor Vehicle Safety Standards is used for children who have outgrown the height and weight limits for rear-facing seats. The seat is installed in the back seat of the car and must be tethered following the manufacturer's instructions. The child must be properly restrained in the seat (Figure 32.3) (Transport Canada, 2011b). While provincial or territorial car seat legislation may allow for booster seats when a child reaches 18 kg, Transport Canada indicates that the child is safer in the forward-facing seat as long as he or she is still below the child seat's weight and height limits. Forward-facing car seats for children as heavy as 30 kg are also available.

- Provide constant supervision when in or near water, including pools, baths, beaches, ditches, and wells. Safe Kids Canada (2011c) recommends the following to prevent drowning: adults remain within sight and arms' reach of any child under 5 years of age or any older child who does not swim well; installation of fencing that is least 1.2 m high, enclosing all four sides of the pool, devoid of objects that a child might use to climb, and with a self-closing self-latching gate that is as high as the pool fencing; use of properly secured life jackets when boating. While it is strongly recommended that children receive swimming training, adults should not assume that this will prevent drowning.

- Avoid choking by not allowing children to run with anything in the mouth; teach children not to put small objects in their mouth or nose; ensure food is chewed properly: nuts, carrots, hard fruits, popcorn, and large pieces of hotdog are leading causes of choking in this age group; supervise balloon use: latex balloons are not recommended for play.

- To avoid strangulation, keep blind and curtain cords out of reach, remove drawstrings or cords on the child's clothing, avoid long scarves in winter (they can become snagged on play equipment). To avoid asphyxiation, remove doors from unused equipment, such as refrigerators.

- Children under 6 years of age should not be allowed to use a trampoline, even when supervised (Health Canada, 2006).

- Keep sharp objects (such as knives and scissors) out of children's reach.

- On the stove, place hot pots on back burners with the handles turned inward. Cover electrical outlets with plugs.

- Teach children about the dangers of playing with matches, fire, and heating appliances.

- Keep cleaning solutions, insecticides, medications, and other poisons in locked cupboards.

- Keep windows and balconies screened.

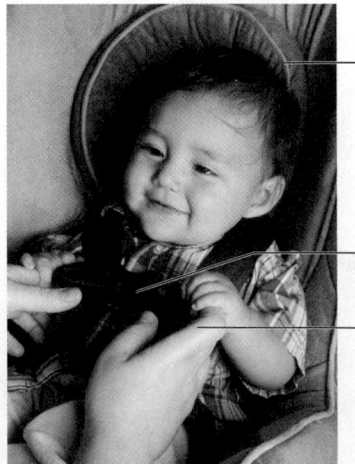

HEAD
Make sure the middle of the child's ear is not above the back (top) of the child's seat

CHEST CLIP HEIGHT
Make sure the chest clip is at the child's armpit level and closed properly

CHEST CLIP TIGHTNESS
Only one finger should be able to fit between the harness and the child's chest

FIGURE 32.3 Proper restraint in a forward-facing seat.

Source: Transport Canada. (2011b). Car seats, seatbelts, and your child: Keep kids safe. Stage 2: Forward-facing seats. Retrieved from http://www.tc.gc.ca/eng/roadsafety/safedrivers-childsafety-stage2-forward-facing-1085.htm

(continued)

- Teach children not to run or ride into the street and supervise street crossing, including teaching about traffic lights and the importance of looking both ways.
- Obtain a low bed when the child begins to climb.
- Teach children to play in safe areas, not on streets and railroad tracks, and to avoid strangers.

SCHOOL-AGE CHILDREN

- A booster seat properly secured in the rear seat of a car is used when a child weighs at least 18 kg; if the child weighs over 18 kg but still falls within the height and weight limits of the forward-facing car seat, then the child should remain in that seat until the limits are exceeded. Booster seat installation must follow the manufacturer's instructions so that the lap and shoulder belts are properly in place across the child's hips, chest, and shoulders (Figure 32.4; see also the Clinical Alert box on car seats on page 846). Front-seat airbags can be dangerous for children 12 years old or younger so they must sit in the back seat (Transport Canada, 2011c).
- Teach children safety rules for recreational and sports activities: never swim alone, always wear a life jacket when in a boat, and wear protective gear (e.g., helmet, knee and elbow pads) when engaging in risky activities (e.g., hockey, skateboarding, inline skating, using a scooter).
- Supervise contact sports and activities in which children aim at a target.
- Teach children to obey all traffic and safety rules for bicycling, skateboarding, inline skating, and so on.
- Help children learn safe ways to use the stove, garden tools, and other equipment.
- Supervise children when they use saws, electric appliances, tools, and other potentially dangerous equipment.
- Teach children not to play with fireworks, gunpowder, or firearms. Keep firearms unloaded, locked up, and out of reach.
- Teach children to avoid excavation sites, quarries, vacant buildings, and playing around heavy machinery.
- Teach children the health hazards of smoking. If you smoke, stop.
- Teach children the effects of drugs and alcohol on judgment and coordination.

ADOLESCENTS

- Have adolescents complete a drivers' education course, and take practice drives with them in various kinds of weather.
- Set firm limits on automobile use (including off-highway vehicles): never drive after drinking or using drugs, always use seatbelts properly (Figure 32.5), and never ride with a driver who is under the influence of alcohol or drugs. Encourage adolescents to call home for a ride if they have been drinking, assuring them they can do so without a reprimand.
- Allow only adolescents over age 16 to drive an off-highway vehicle (OHV) (e.g., snowmobile, dirt bike) (Safe Kids Canada, 2011d). Given that current legislation allows those under 16 to drive an OHV, Safe Kids Canada recommends educating younger riders in rural and farming communities who use OHVs for the purpose of work and travel.
- Teach adolescents to wear proper safety equipment (e.g., helmet, padding) when participating in sports (e.g., inline skating, hockey, football) or when riding scooters and other sports vehicles.
- Encourage adolescents to swim, jog, and go boating (always wearing a life jacket) in groups so they can get help in an emergency.
- Inform the adolescent of the dangers of alcohol, other drugs, and unprotected sex. Include teaching about date rape prevention and defence.
- Teach about the dangers of sunbathing and tanning beds. Encourage them to use sun block and wear protective clothing when doing outdoor activities.
- Be alert to changes in the adolescent's mood and behaviour. Listen to and maintain open communication with the adolescent. Open communication is a powerful preventive measure.
- Set a good example of behaviour that the adolescent can follow.

YOUNG ADULTS

- Reinforce motor vehicle safety: Use designated drivers or public transport if alcohol is consumed, routinely check brakes and tires, and use seat and shoulder belts or car seats for all passengers.

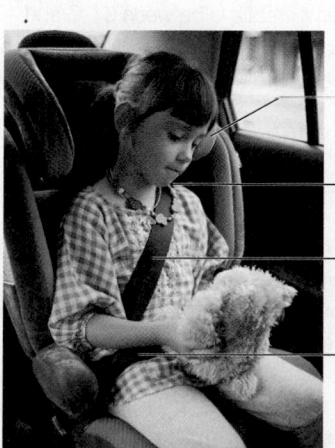

BOOSTER BACK
If the booster seat has a back, make sure the middle of the child's ears are lower than the top of the back of the booster seat

SEAT BELT GUIDE
If there is a seat belt guide, it should be at or above the child's shoulder

SHOULDER BELT
Make sure the shoulder belt rests on the child's shoulder, and never on the neck or arm, or under the arm

LAP BELT
The lap belt should be snug against the child's hips, and not on his or her stomach

FIGURE 32.4 Proper restraint in a booster seat.

Source: Transport Canada. (2011c). Car seats, seatbelts, and your child: Keep kids safe. Stage 3: Booster seats. Retrieved from http://www.tc.gc.ca/eng/roadsafety/ safedrivers-childsafety-stage3-booster-seats-1086.htm

(continued)

TEACHING WELLNESS *(continued)*

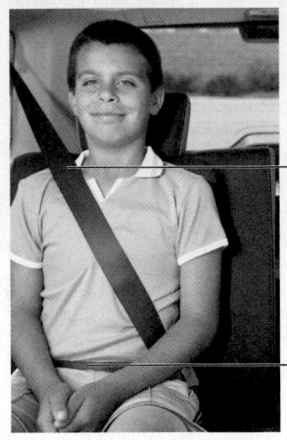

SHOULDER BELT
The shoulder belt should rest on the child's shoulder, never on the neck or arm; it should never be behind the back or tucked in under the arm

LAP BELT
The lap belt should be snug against the child's hips, and not on the stomach

FIGURE 32.5 Proper restraint when using a seatbelt.

Source: Transport Canada. (2011). Car seats, seatbelts, and your child: Keep kids safe. Stage 4: Seat belts. Retrieved from http://www.tc.gc.ca/eng/roadsafety/safedrivers-childsafety-stage4-seat-belts-1087.htm

- Remind the young adult to repair potential fire hazards, such as electric wiring.
- Reinforce water safety: Know the depth of a pool or lake before diving; supervise backyard pools and other water activities; wear a life jacket when in a boat.
- Discuss evaluating the potential for workplace injuries or death when making decisions about a career or an occupation. Encourage the young adult to participate actively in programs that reduce occupational hazards.
- Reinforce the importance of limiting sun exposure, using sunblocking agents, and wearing protective clothing.
- Encourage young adults who are having trouble coping with the pressures, responsibilities, and expectations of adulthood to seek counselling.

MIDDLE-AGED ADULTS

- Reinforce motor vehicle safety: Use seatbelts and drive within the speed limit, especially at night. Test visual acuity periodically.
- Make certain stairways are well lit and uncluttered.
- Equip bathrooms with hand grasps and nonskid bath mats.
- Test smoke detectors, fire alarms, and carbon monoxide detectors regularly.
- Keep all machines and tools in good working condition at work and at home. Follow safety precautions when using machinery.
- Reinforce safety measures taught earlier in life, such as the hazards of excessive sun exposure.

OLDER ADULTS

- Encourage the client to have regular vision and hearing tests.
- Assist the client to have a home hazard appraisal.
- Encourage the client to keep as active as possible.
- Ensure appropriate lighting and mark doorways and edges of steps, as needed.
- Keep the environment tidy and uncluttered, and securely fasten rugs.
- Encourage clients to wear shoes or well-fitting slippers with nonskid soles.
- Have clients use ambulatory devices as necessary (cane, crutches, walker, braces, wheelchair).
- Monitor gait and balance.
- Have clients adapt to living arrangements on one floor, if necessary.
- Encourage exercise and activity as tolerated to maintain muscle strength, joint flexibility, and balance.
- Encourage clients to request assistance rather than take a risk.
- Keep the client's bed in the low position.
- Ensure that grab bars have been installed in bathrooms, and set the hot water tank at no more than 49°C—the comfortable bath temperature is between 37°C and 40°C.
- Instruct the client to rise slowly from the lying position, to the sitting position, and finally to the standing position, and to stand in place for several seconds before walking.
- Encourage annual or more frequent review of all medications prescribed.

during the first year of life. Infants are completely dependent on others for care and are oblivious to such dangers as falling or ingesting harmful substances. Parents need

! CLINICAL ALERT

Many families are not aware that car seats have expiry or useful-life dates, generally between 6 and 8 years. Car seats should not be used past these dates, and it is preferable that the car seat be permanently discarded rather than donated or given to friends or relatives.

to learn the amount of observation necessary to maintain infant safety. They must continually anticipate risks and identify and remove common hazards in and around the home. Parents must learn first aid, including interventions for airway obstruction and cardiopulmonary resuscitation (CPR). The leading causes of hospitalization related to unintentional injury in children less than 1 year are falls, followed by poisoning in males and injury related to fire or hot objects for females; the leading causes of unintentional injury deaths in this age group are suffocation followed by motor vehicle traffic collisions

(Public Health Agency of Canada, 2009a). Education and support of parents can help them become knowledgeable and better prepared to protect their children.

TODDLERS Toddlers are curious and like to feel and taste everything. Their rapidly changing mobility skills, from crawling to walking to running, mean they can gain access to physical locations they were not able to reach as infants. They are fascinated by potential dangers, such as pools and busy streets, so they need constant supervision and protection. For this age group, falls and poisoning account for the majority of unintentional injuries requiring hospitalization; drowning followed by motor vehicle traffic collisions are the leading cause of unintentional injury deaths (Public Health Agency of Canada, 2009a). Parents can prevent many injuries by toddler-proofing the child's environment. This practice extends to using proper car restraints, promoting a safe environment to avoid falls, ensuring water safety, and removing or securing all items that can pose a safety hazard to the child.

PRESCHOOLERS Preschool-age children are active and sometimes clumsy, making them susceptible to injury. Environmental control continues, keeping hazards, such as matches, medicines, and other potential poisons, out of sight and reach. Safety education includes learning such things as how to cross streets or how to ride bicycles safely. Children must be cautioned to avoid known hazards, such as swimming without adult supervision. Parents must maintain careful surveillance as the developmental level of the preschooler does not allow for self-reliance in matters of safety. For example, telling a preschooler to stay away from the pool when no one is around *cannot replace* a latched enclosure in promoting the child's safety. The preschool-age child's cognitive and motor skills increase quickly; hence, safety measures must keep up with the acquisition of new skills.

SCHOOL-AGE CHILDREN By the time children attend school, they are learning to think before they act and must make safety decisions on their own as they are away from the constant supervision of parents and caregivers. They want to play with other children in such activities as bicycling, swimming, and skating. Although sensitive to peer pressure, the school-age child generally responds to rules. Falls and being struck by or against an object are the leading cause of unintentional injury hospitalizations in this age group, with motor vehicle traffic collisions being the leading cause of unintentional death followed by drowning in boys and fire or flame in girls. School-age children often sustain unintentional injury during outdoor activities, such as bicycling, skateboarding, and inline skating, as well playing in playgrounds.

ADOLESCENTS Obtaining a driver's licence can be an important event in the life of an adolescent, but the privilege comes with many risks. Motor vehicle collisions remain the leading cause of death and disability in Canadian teenagers. Because teens lack driving experience and may use driving as an outlet for stress, as a way to assert independence, or as a way to impress peers, parents need to assess the teenager's level of responsibility, problem solving, and ability to resist peer pressure as they determine driving privileges. The age of the teenager alone does not determine readiness to handle this responsibility.

Adolescents are at risk for sports injuries because their coordination skills are not fully developed. However, sports activities are important to the adolescent's self-esteem and overall development so all efforts must be made to provide protective equipment and foster safe play. Young workers have been identified as a particularly high-risk group for traumatic occupational injuries in Canada. Part-time employment status, lack of preparation and education in workplace risks, eagerness to please, and viewing aches or pain simply as part of the job can all contribute to occupational injuries (Breslin, Polzer, MacEachen, Morrongiello, & Shannon, 2006). Parents can coach their adolescents to ensure that they get the necessary safety training specific for their jobs.

The adolescent's mental health may give rise to safety concerns related to suicide risk. Suicide, a form of intentional injury, is the second leading cause of death among teenagers, especially boys, and families need to be aware of the signs of suicidal ideation. Economic deprivation, family breakup, depression, being a victim of bullying, and access to firearms are factors that can influence the suicide rate in this age group. Concerns about potential suicidal risk should be referred to a mental health professional or a crisis centre.

YOUNG ADULTS Motor vehicle collisions are the leading cause of mortality for this group followed by suicide (Statistics Canada, 2008); other causes of death from unintentional injury include drowning (especially men), burns, poisonings, and firearms. Exposure to natural radiation from sunbathing or outdoor activities is a safety hazard for many young adults. Suicide is another leading cause of death in this age group, and it is thought that many suicides are mistaken for accidental death (e.g., automobile accidents, drug overdoses). As during adolescence, the prevention of suicide includes identifying behaviours that indicate potential problems: depression, decreased interest in previously pleasurable activities, and an increase in isolation. A young adult identified as being at risk for suicide should be referred to a mental health professional or a crisis centre.

MIDDLE-AGED ADULTS Changing physiological factors, as well as preoccupations with personal, family, and work-related responsibilities, may contribute to the accident rate of middle-aged persons. Motor vehicle collisions are the most common cause of death from unintentional injury in this age group. Decreased reaction times and decreased visual acuity can make the middle-aged adult prone to accidents. Other causes of death related to injury in this age group include falls, burns, poisonings, and drowning. Occupational accidents continue to be a significant safety hazard during the middle years.

OLDER ADULTS Injury prevention is a major concern for older adults. For some, because vision is limited, reflexes are slowed, or bones are brittle, climbing stairs, driving a car, and even walking require caution. Driving, particularly at night, requires caution because the accommodation of the eye to light is impaired and the peripheral vision is diminished. Older adults need to learn to turn their head before changing lanes and should not rely on side vision, for example, when crossing a street or changing lanes.

Fires are a hazard if memory problems are present; appliances may be left on or cigarettes may not be extinguished. Because of reduced sensitivity to pain and heat, care must be taken to prevent burns when the person bathes or uses heating devices. People at risk for wandering because of organic brain syndromes need to wear identification devices. They can also be registered with the local Alzheimer Society of Canada's Safely Home program.

Decrease in temperature regulation in the older adult can increase the risk of hypothermia and hyperthermia. Reduced renal function increases the risk of toxicity from medications (e.g., the older adult who takes analgesics or sedatives may become lethargic or confused). The nurse teaches the importance of taking only prescribed medications and that over-the-counter medications must be reported because they can influence the pharmacokinetics and/or pharmacodynamics of prescribed medications.

A home environment that was previously safe may need modifications for older adults to decrease the risk of injury. A plan and telephone numbers of those to call should be available for emergency situations.

Unfortunately, the incidence of suicide in older adults, especially men, is increasing (Statistics Canada, 2008). It often goes unnoticed when the causes are such behaviours as starvation, overdosing with medications, and noncompliance with the medical treatment plan. Factors that have been linked to suicide risk in older adults are uncontrollable pain, loss of a loved one, major life changes, major depression, and social isolation. Unlike other age groups, older adults rarely threaten suicide; they just do it.

Safety Problems across the Lifespan

Domestic violence is a safety concern involving individuals of all ages. It includes child abuse, intimate partner abuse, and abuse of older adults, and it affects the health and safety of families and the community. Statistics are likely inaccurate because of the underreporting of incidents. Nurses should be involved in working with all phases of domestic violence: prevention, screening, referrals for treatment, and follow-up care. Situations of domestic violence usually necessitate interprofessional collaboration among the health care team, law enforcement agencies, and other community agencies.

Safety in the Health Care Setting

Since the release of the *Canadian Adverse Events Study* (Baker et al., 2004), health care agencies have rallied to address client safety. The basis for the provision of safe nursing care is addressed throughout a range of chapters in this book, for example, Chapter 33 addresses safe medication administration practices, and Chapter 34 focuses on nursing care to minimize health care–associated infection. Leonard, Hoffman, and the National Steering Committee on Patient Safety (2002) and Kohn, Corrigan, and Donaldson (2000) suggest that beyond learning specific details of direct nursing care and knowing the Accreditation Canada safety goals, nurses need to work toward building new systems to improve patient safety by doing the following:

- Creating a culture of safety in which human error is viewed as inevitable and, subject to limited qualifications, no blame is assigned when adverse events are reported. Disclosures of errors and near-miss situations are encouraged so that in-depth analysis can take place to minimize risks of subsequent similar events.

- Conducting a comprehensive assessment of known and potential safety issues and providing education, anticipatory guidance, and learning opportunities, such as the use of simulated high-risk scenarios to rehearse or learn skills that are essential to patient safety.

- Promoting effective teamwork and communication. Patient safety may be at risk if critical, relevant information is not communicated appropriately among members of the health care team.

- Involving health care workers in the design of work processes and workspaces to promote efficiency and safety.

Preventing Specific Hazards

Implementing measures to prevent specific hazards or unintentional injuries, such as scalds and burns, fires, falls, poisoning, suffocation, electrocution, and so on are critical aspects of nursing care. Nurses have many opportunities and responsibilities to implement health teaching about a range of known safety hazards.

SCALDS AND BURNS A **scald** is a second or third-degree burn from a hot liquid or vapour, such as steam. A **burn** results from excessive exposure to thermal (scald, flame, contact), chemical, electric, or radioactive agents.

Examples of home hazards that can cause scalds include pot handles that stick out over the edge of a stove, electric appliances (used to heat liquids or oils) with dangling cords, and excessively hot bath water. Use of stove guards and cord attachment devices along with diligent efforts at turning pot handles in can help in promoting safety in the kitchen. Hot water tanks (except electric water heaters) should be set at *no more than 49°C** (or set at Warm or Medium if there is no

---

*The Asthma Society of Canada recommends that clothing and bedding be washed in water at least 55°C to kill dust mites and their allergens. Instead of using very hot water, several other options should be considered. A dust mite control additive can be used in a low-temperature wash. Dust mites will also be killed by drying fabrics at a high setting for 1 hour.

temperature reading) to avoid scalds from tap water (Safe Kids Canada, 2011e). Unfortunately, the majority of water tanks in Canadian homes are set at 60°C, the temperature at which a person can sustain a third-degree burn within 1 to 5 seconds! A meat or candy thermometer can be used to measure tap water temperature and Safe Kids Canada offers special testing cards. In homes where the hot water tank cannot be adjusted—generally, large apartment buildings with a central hot water tank—*antiscald* devices can be added to the faucet or tap. Tap guards are available to child-proof a hot water faucet. Lowering the risk of scalds from tap water must be balanced with the risk of bacterial growth in water tanks (i.e., lowering gas and oil-fired water heaters below 49°C or electric water heaters below 60°C), which can lead to the growth of the bacterium *Legionella* that causes legionnaires' disease.

Touching a stovetop element can cause a contact burn; ingestion of a caustic cleaning product can cause a chemical burn. The risk of scalds and burns is greater for clients whose skin sensitivity to temperature is impaired, such as a person with peripheral neuropathy who cannot sense that a heat pack is too hot. The nurse must assess how well clients can protect themselves and what special precautions, if any, need to be taken.

FIRES Fires continue to be a constant risk in both health care settings and homes. Agency fires usually result from malfunctioning electrical equipment or combustion of anesthetic gas. Home fires most frequently result from careless disposal of burning cigarettes or matches, from grease, or from faulty electrical wiring.

Agency Fires In health care agencies, fire is particularly hazardous when people are incapacitated and unable to leave the building without assistance. It is extremely important for nurses to be aware of the fire safety regulations and fire-prevention practices of the agency in which they work. When a fire occurs, the nurse follows four sequential priorities that can easily be remembered by using the RACE mnemonic:

R **R**escue and **R**emove persons who are in immediate danger.
A **A**ctivate the fire alarm, and call for help.
C **C**ontain or **C**onfine the fire and smoke (e.g., close doors).
E **E**xtinguish the fire, if possible; otherwise **E**vacuate.

Extinguishing the fire requires knowledge of four categories of fire, classified according to the type of material that is burning:

- *Class A:* Ordinary combustibles (e.g., paper, wood, upholstery, rags, rubbish)
- *Class B:* Flammable and combustible liquids (e.g., oils, grease, gasoline)
- *Class C:* Electrical material (e.g., electrical wiring, equipment, fuse box)
- *Class D:* Combustible metals (e.g., magnesium)

The right type of extinguisher must be used to fight the fire. Extinguishers have picture symbols showing the type of fire for which they are to be used. Directions for use are also attached. Fire Prevention Canada (2011a) recommends that people *learn how to PASS*:

P **P**ull the pin
A **A**im the extinguisher nozzle at the base of the fire
S **S**queeze or press the handle
S **S**weep from side-to-side at the base of the fire and discharge the contents of the extinguisher

Home Fires Nursing interventions for home fires focus on teaching fire safety, including the following:

- Keep lighters and matches out of sight and reach of children, have regular inspections of electrical systems, and adopt a no smoking policy (especially in bed or on the couch).
- Keep emergency numbers near the telephone or stored for speed dialling.
- Ensure that smoke alarms, fire extinguishers, and carbon monoxide detectors are operable and appropriately located.
- Test smoke alarms and carbon monoxide detectors monthly and change batteries twice a year (if not hard-wired). Choosing special days, such as birthdays or the days the clocks change for daylight savings time, can help people remember this important safety detail.
- Have a family fire drill plan aimed at evacuating the home within 3 minutes (Fire Prevention Canada, 2011b). Every member needs to know the nearest exit from different locations of the home.
- In the event of a fire, close the windows and doors if possible; cover your mouth and nose with a damp cloth when exiting through a smoke-filled area; and avoid heavy smoke by assuming a bent position with the head as close to the floor as possible.

FALLS A **fall** is an unexpected event in which the person comes to rest on the ground, floor, or lower level (Lamb, Hauer, & Becker, 2005). People of any age can fall, but infants, toddlers, and older adults are particularly at risk for falls causing serious injury. Falls are the leading cause of unintentional injuries among older adults and they account for more than 85% of major injury hospitalizations among Canadian older adults (Scott, Wager, & Elliot, 2010). With falls as the leading cause of death due to injury in Canadians older than 65 years, those who recover from a fall may have long-term sequelae to cope with, such as reduced mobility and chronic pain (Smartrisk, 2011). Falls in older adults are linked to multiple modifiable and nonmodifiable biological or medical, behavioural, environmental, and socioeconomic factors (Public Health Agency of Canada, 2009b; Registered Nurses' Association of Ontario [RNAO], 2011).

Biological or medical factors include gait instability and lower-limb weakness; reduced general physical fitness; impaired balance and/or gait; vision problems, such as reduced acuity, difficulty accommodating to light and darkness; cognitive impairment; chronic illness, in particular arthritis, cerebrovascular accident (stroke) and Parkinson's disease; and acute illness events.

Behavioural factors include a positive fall history; a fear of falling, which can lead to tension and stiffness, making the person more susceptible; risk-taking behaviour, such as not heeding warnings of risk; taking culprit medications, such as antihypertensive agents or diuretics, that can lead to orthostatic hypotension or cardiac syncope, and benzodiazepines, such as alprazolam or diazepam; polypharmacy (taking five or more medications); excessive alcohol intake; and footwear (poor fitting, slippery footing), clothing (can cause tripping or can get caught on objects or in doorways), and handbags (can cause imbalance or get caught in doorways).

Environmental factors include uneven or excessively high or narrow stairs, stairs with unmarked edges, lack of hand railings or poorly fitted hand rails, in-home features like lack of grab bars, inadequate lighting (too dark or too bright), clutter, and scatter rugs.

Socioeconomic factors include low income, poor housing, and reduced sense of connectedness (which links to going out unassisted). The role that social and economic factors play in falls is poorly understood but could relate to such factors as poor nutrition resulting in weakened muscles or lack of funds to install protective equipment such as grab bars. (See the Evidence-Informed Practice box on effective interventions in preventing falls among older people.)

Although hip and femur fractures are the most frequent complication of falls in older adults (followed by wrist fracture) (Public Health Agency of Canada, 2011), a hip fracture may actually *precede* a fall, thus *causing* it. In fact, it is estimated that 40% of falls leading to hospitalization are the *result* of hip fractures and that the number of hip fractures will increase dramatically from 23 375 in 1993 to more than 88 000 cases by the year 2041, as the Canadian population ages (Smartrisk, 2011).

Most falls occur in the home and usually involve falling down stairs and in the bedroom or bathroom. Fear of falling is common in older adults, especially those who live alone. For these individuals the nurse should encourage daily or more frequent contact with a friend or family member, installation of a personal emergency response system, and measures to maintain a physical environment that prevents falls. Selected risk factors and associated preventive measures for falls are shown in Table 32.1. Regardless of efforts to prevent falls, they may still occur—in the event of such, clients should try to land on their buttocks, wait to get up to make sure there is no injury, and, most important, not cope with the fall by becoming less active as this will only serve to weaken muscles needed to prevent falls (Public Health Agency

of Canada, 2011). (See the Clinical Alert box about fractures in older adults related to falls.)

The nurse can use an assessment tool, called the *Get Up and Go Test (GUGT)*, in a hospital, a subacute care setting, or the home setting. The GUGT consists of the following steps:

1. Observe the client's posture while he or she sits in a straight-backed chair.

2. Ask the client to stand. Observe whether the client stands by using only the leg muscles or if the client needs to push himself or herself up with the hands.

EVIDENCE-INFORMED PRACTICE

What Interventions Are Most Effective in Preventing Falls Among Older People?

There have been several studies on factors influencing falls risk as well as fall-prevention strategies. A few systematic reviews have sought to determine the effectiveness of specific interventions (e.g., Tai Chi, vitamin D supplements), but no systematic review has been completed to determine the effectiveness of the range of fall-prevention interventions that have been studied. This proposal for a systematic review will evaluate several fall-prevention interventions, including supervised or unsupervised exercises; medications; surgery; management of urinary incontinence; fluid or nutrition therapy; psychological factors; environment and assistive technologies; social environment; knowledge or education interventions; and others. The authors will review whether any single intervention is more effective than no intervention or if a combination of interventions is more effective.

NURSING IMPLICATIONS: Falls, especially in older adults, are far too frequent and unintentional injuries that often result from falls have major implications on quality of life and even mortality. As Canada's population ages, nurses must be aware of the strategies that are most effective in reducing falls. This review will help to develop fall-prevention programs, likely in many settings. Nurses working in primary health care can use the results to develop intersectoral collaborations, such as by promoting public transit safety.

Source: Based on Udell, J. E., Drahota, A., Dean, T. P., Sander, R., & Mackenzie, H. (2011). Interventions for preventing falls in older people: An overview of Cochrane Reviews (Protocol). *Cochrane Database of Systematic Reviews*, Issue 4. Art. No.: CD009074. doi: 10.1002/14651858.CD009074

! CLINICAL ALERT

Falls can cause broken bones, but sometimes, broken bones can cause falls. When a client is brought to hospital for treatment of a bone fracture, it is important to determine if a fracture caused the fall or if the fall caused the fracture. The health history of the former scenario generally reveals pain or a "cracking noise" before the fall. Falls in older adults may be due to arrhythmias, problems with the vestibular apparatus, hypoglycemic episodes, hypotensive episodes, or being pushed (in the case of abuse).

TABLE 32.1 Risk Factors and Preventive Measures for Falls

Risk Factors	Preventive Measures
History of falling	Conduct a detailed analysis of the reasons underlying any previous falls to determine modifiable factors or circumstances that can become preventive measures.
	Protective measures (such as hip pads and knee pads) should be considered if previous preventive measures have not been successful.
Poor vision	Ensure that the client's eyeglasses are functional. Encourage the client to allow time for visual adjustment if he or she is wearing bifocals.
	Ensure that lighting is appropriate, including having a light switch at the top and bottom of stairs. Night lighting of stairs and hallways that does not need to be switched on is also recommended.
	Mark doorways and stair edgings, as needed.
	Encourage the client to keep the environment tidy.
Presence of stairs, in particular, stair geometry that is nonuniform, steep, winding, or curved	Look for securely attached handrails on each side of the stairway; handrails should extend, without a break, the full length of the stairs as well as beyond the bottom and top of the stairs with a tactile indicator (i.e., slight bend) to indicate the stair is coming to an end.
	If the stairs are problematic, ask the client to consider renovating them to Canada Mortgage and Housing Corporation (2011) recommendations (riser no higher than 180 mm and run no shorter than 280 mm); clients with severe limitations should consider installing a stair lift.
Cognitive dysfunction (confusion, disorientation, impaired memory, or judgment)	Clients should set safe limits to activities.
	Remove unsafe objects.
	Consider the need for constant surveillance.
Gait instability (impaired gait or balance) or lower-limb weakness or dysfunction	Ask the client to wear shoes or well-fitting slippers with nonskid soles.
	Antislip shoe devices in icy conditions can reduce the rate of falls (Gillespie, Gillespie, & Parker, 2010)
	Have the client use ambulatory devices, as necessary (cane, crutches, walker, braces, wheelchair).
	Ensure the environment is uncluttered and rugs are securely fastened.
	Suggest that the client adapt living arrangements to one floor, if feasible. It may require installing an additional phone or bathroom, and having frequently used items nearby.
	Encourage exercise and activity as tolerated to maintain muscle strength and joint flexibility. Tai Chi exercises can enhance balance (Li, Harmer, Fisher, McAuley, Chaumeton, Eckstrom, et al., 2005; Public Health Agency of Canada, 2011).
	Hip protectors (underwear types exist) or elbow and knee protectors may be used as protective measures. However, the effectiveness of hip protectors in reducing the incidence of hip fracture in older people is not clearly established; they may work best in frail older people in nursing care (Gillespie, et al., 2010).
Difficulty getting in and out of a chair or bed	Encourage the client to request assistance.
	Keep the bed in the low position.
	Install a side rail on the bed to provide grip.
	Install grab bars in bathrooms and raised toilet seats.
Orthostatic hypotension	Instruct the client to rise slowly from the lying position, to the sitting position, and finally to the standing position and to stand in place for several seconds before walking.
Urinary frequency, nocturia (having to get up in the night to urinate), receiving diuretics	Provide a bedside commode (without wheels).
	Assist the client with voiding on a frequent and scheduled basis.
Weakness from disease process or therapy	Encourage the client to summon help.
	Monitor activity tolerance.

(continued)

TABLE 32.1 *(continued)*

Risk Factors	Preventive Measures
Polypharmacy (clients taking more than five medications) or those prescribed benzodiazepines, tricyclic antidepressants, selective serotonin reuptake inhibitors, trazodone	Monitor orientation and alertness status.
	Discuss how alcohol contributes to fall-related injuries, and encourage the client not to mix alcohol and medications or avoid alcohol, if necessary.
	Encourage annual or more frequent review of all medications prescribed.
	Discuss alternative solutions (other than benzodiazepines) for such symptoms as anxiety and insomnia.

3. Once the client is comfortably standing, ask him or her to close the eyes. Does the client sway?

4. Ask the client to open his or her eyes, walk 3 metres, turn around, and return to the chair. Observe gait, balance, speed, and stability. How smoothly does the client turn?

5. When the client gets to the chair, ask him or her to turn and sit down. Observe how smoothly the client performs this motion.

The GUGT score ranges from 0 to 4. The client who is able to perform all five steps with ease receives a score of 0; the score is 1 if the client must use his or her hands to get out of the chair; the client who is able to stand but requires multiple pushes to get up scores a 3; and the client who is unable to get up without assistance receives a 4. This quick assessment, along with an assessment of the client's environment, can help the nurse recommend safety measures to the client and family.

Prevention of falls in health care agencies is an ongoing concern. Other than the illness process that necessitates hospitalization, being in a hospital poses additional fall risks (e.g., an unfamiliar environment, reluctance to ask for help for fear of being a burden, and a lack of usual safety reminders). Health care environments are designed with many safety features to reduce the risk of falls, such as railings along corridors; call bells at each bedside; safety bars in toilet areas; locks on bed, wheelchair, and stretcher wheels; side rails on beds; and night lights. In addition, nurses can implement measures to decrease the incidence of falls (see Practice Guidelines 32.1).

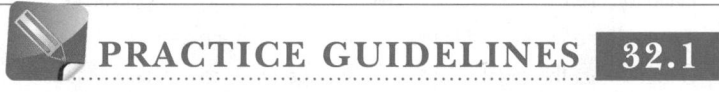

PRACTICE GUIDELINES 32.1

Preventing Falls in Health Care Agencies

Guidelines	Rationales
Ensure that multiple prevention strategies are implemented rather than rely on only one or two strategies.	Multifactorial interventions reduce falls and risk of falling in hospitals and may do so in nursing care facilities (Cameron, Murray, Gillespie, Robertson, Hill, Cumming, & Kerse, 2010)
On admission, orient clients to their surroundings and explain the call system. Encourage the client to use the call bell to request assistance. Ensure that the bell is within easy reach.	Familiarity with surroundings increases awareness of risks and resources; access to help when required is important to ensure safety. Informing clients that help is readily available will help reduce clients' reluctance to ask for assistance.
All individuals should be screened for risk of falls by a nurse at admission to identify factors known to contribute to falls risk. Perform a fall-risk assessment by using a standardized tool—a variety of tools are available (e.g., Morse Fall Scale, or STRATIFY [St. Thomas Risk Assessment Tool in Falling Elderly Inpatients]); however, few of the standardized tools have been thoroughly assessed for reliability across different settings with varying populations (Cameron, et al., 2010).	Previous history of falls is predictive of future falls; risk assessment can identify modifiable factors that will determine relevant, client-specific fall-prevention strategies.
Assess the client's ability to ambulate and transfer. Provide walking aids and assistance, as required. Consult with other members of the health care team, such as physical and occupational therapists, to help address mobility issues.	Mobility risks increase the risk of falls. Environmental resources can buffer client deficits, such as a walker providing stability. Interprofessional collaboration results in a sharing of expertise to augment the quality of patient care.
Closely supervise clients at risk for falls, especially at night.	Clients are at increased risk of falling at night because of possible disorientation, poor lighting, and effects of sleeping aids.

(continued)

PRACTICE GUIDELINES 32.1

Preventing Falls in Health Care Agencies (continued)

Guidelines	Rationales
Place bedside tables and overbed tables near the bed or chair (but avoid obstructing movement). Keep the environment tidy; in particular, keep light cords from underfoot and furniture out of the way.	Easy access to personal supplies will prevent the client from overreaching, which can cause loss of balance with a resultant fall. Any clutter can cause imbalance and a possible fall.
Always keep hospital beds in the low position and the wheels locked when not providing care.	Clients can move in or out of bed easily. If a fall occurs, it will be from the lowest height.
Use beds designed to promote patient safety (Figure 32.6).	Equipment that is designed with patient safety in mind (e.g., low height, easy-grip rails, smaller openings in side rails, automatic night light) can augment the safety repertoire.

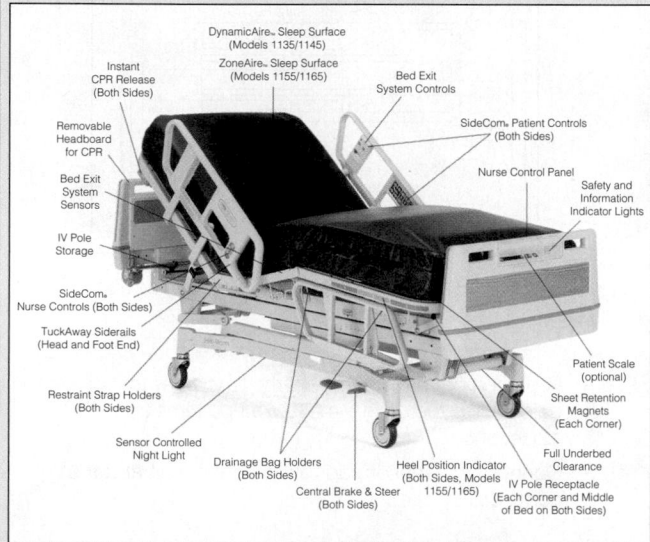

FIGURE 32.6 The Advanta Bed is designed for improved patient safety.

Bed rails should not be raised routinely for the purpose of reducing falls. Use individualized interventions (e.g., an alarm sensitive to client position, a bed exit alarm) rather than side rails for confused clients. If side rails are used to help with movement, consider half or three-quarter side rails in the event the client will attempt to crawl around or over full-length side rails.	People with memory impairment, altered mobility, nocturia, and other sleep disorders can become entrapped in side rails and many, in fact, are more likely to fall trying to get out around or over the raised rails. Alternative technology is available to alert the team when the client attempts to crawl out of bed. The half or three-quarter rail provides a movement aid while giving the patient who is trying to get up a safer way out than over or between full-length rails.

Electronic devices are available to detect when clients are attempting to get out of bed. A bed or chair safety monitoring device has a position-sensitive switch that triggers an audio alarm when the client attempts to get out of the bed or chair. Skill 32.1 describes how to use these devices. See the Home Care Considerations box on page 855.

SKILL 32.1 USING A BED OR CHAIR EXIT SAFETY MONITORING DEVICE

PURPOSES

- To alert the nurse that the client is attempting to get out of bed
- To help decrease the risk of client falls

ASSESSMENT

Assess

- Mobility status
- Judgment about ability to get out of bed safely

- Clients usual pattern of exiting the bed or chair
- Proximity of client's room to nurses' station
- Position of side rails
- Functioning status of call light

Clinical Reasoning

What possible meaning will the client and/or family place on the use of the monitoring device (e.g., will they see it negatively, such as a form of restraint or invasion of privacy, or positively

(continued)

SKILL 32.1 **USING A BED OR CHAIR EXIT SAFETY MONITORING DEVICE** (*continued*)

as a safety resource)? Are there any modifiable factors (e.g., presence of infection; medications altering judgment) that have been overlooked as a possible reason for why the client needs the extra monitoring?

PLANNING

Determine the best type of device and appropriate location for the device. No matter where the device will be applied, choose a location where skin is intact.

Equipment

- Alarm and control device
- Sensor device
- Connection to nurse call system

IMPLEMENTATION

Performance

1. Before performing the procedure, introduce yourself and verify the client's identity using two identifiers or per agency protocol. Explain to the client and family the purpose and procedure of using a safety monitoring device.

   - Explain that the device does not limit mobility in any manner; rather, it alerts the staff when the client is about to get out of bed.

   - Explain that the nurse must be called when the client needs to get out of bed.

2. Perform hand hygiene, and follow other appropriate infection prevention and control procedures.

3. Provide for client privacy.

4. Test the battery device and alarm sound. **Rationale: Testing ensures that the device is functioning properly before use**.

5. Apply the sensor pad or leg band.

   - Place the leg band according to the manufacturer's recommendation (see ❶). Place the client's leg in a straight horizontal position. **Rationale: The alarm device is position sensitive; that is, when it approaches a near-vertical position (such as in walking, crawling, or kneeling as the client attempts to get out of bed), the audio alarm will be triggered**.

   - For the bed or chair device, the sensor is usually placed under the buttocks area (see ❷).

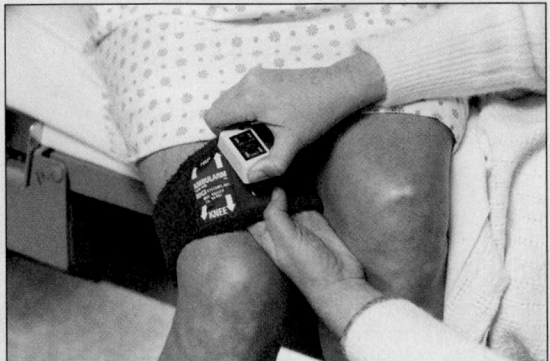
❶ Placing the leg band alarm

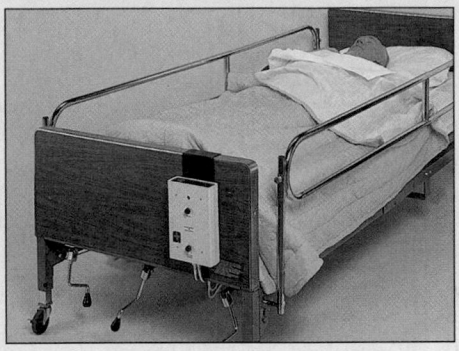

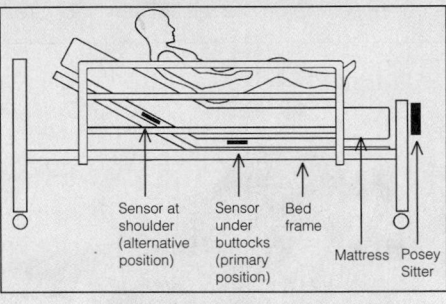

Sensor at shoulder (alternative position) — Sensor under buttocks (primary position) — Bed frame — Mattress — Posey Sitter

❷ Placement of a bed exit monitoring device

   - For a bed or chair device, set the time delay for determining the client's movement patterns from 1 to 12 seconds.

   - Connect the sensor pad to the control unit and the nurse call system.

6. Instruct the client to call the nurse when the client wants or needs to get up, and assist, as required.

   - When assisting the client up, deactivate the alarm.

   - Assist the client back to bed, and reattach the alarm device.

7. Ensure client safety with additional safety precautions.

   - Place the call light within client reach, lift the side rails per agency policy, and lower the bed to its lowest position. **Rationale: The alarm device is not a substitute for other precautionary measures**.

   - Place ambulation monitoring stickers on the client's door, chart, and Kardex.

8. Document the type of alarm used, where it was placed, and its effectiveness in the client record by using forms or checklists supplemented by narrative notes when appropriate. Record all additional safety precautions and interventions discussed and employed.

EVALUATION

- If the alarm is too sensitive to client movements that are not an attempt to move from the bed or chair, reassess and modify alarm controls accordingly.

- Conduct appropriate follow-up relating to effectiveness of the safety precautions.

- Report any difficulties in using the device or any falls to the appropriate members of the health care team.

HOME CARE CONSIDERATIONS

Using a Bed or Chair Exit Safety Monitoring Device

If the device is used in the home, instruct caregivers to do the following:

- Test the monitoring device every 12 to 24 hours to ensure that it is working.

- Check the volume of the alarm to be certain they can hear it.

    Use of the device does not take the place of proper supervision of clients at

risk for falling. Assessment of the reasons for falling, especially among older adults, can lead to effective prevention.

SEIZURES A **seizure** is a sudden onset of excessive electrical discharges in one or more areas of the brain. Seizures can develop at any time during a person's life. Clients may be prone to seizures because of permanent or temporary medical conditions, such as drug reactions or epilepsy; seizures can occur with no known cause.

Seizures are classified into two categories: *partial* and *generalized*. Partial seizures (also called *focal seizures*) involve electrical discharges from one area of the brain. In contrast, generalized seizures affect the whole brain. Each of these seizure categories includes different types of seizure depending on the characteristics of the seizure activity (e.g., loss of consciousness or no impairment to consciousness). Thus, it is important for the nurse to thoroughly describe the observations before, during, and after a seizure episode. Clients are at risk for injury if they experience seizures that involve the entire body, such as *grand mal* (tonic–clonic) seizures or any seizure that includes loss of consciousness. **Seizure precautions** are safety measures taken by the nurse to protect clients from injury should they have a seizure. Skill 32.2 describes how to implement seizure precautions. (See also the Home Care Considerations box on page 856.)

POISONING With an estimated annual incidence of five Canadian children under 14 dying and another 1280 ending up in hospital with serious consequences from poisoning, poison prevention takes on special meaning in families (Safe Kids Canada, 2011f). Inadequate supervision and improper storage of medications (including vitamin and iron supplements) and household products (e.g., cleaning products, alcohol, pesticides) are the major reasons for poisoning in children. Implementing poison prevention for children is focused on childproofing the environment, including disposing of unused medications by returning them to a pharmacy and properly storing risky products.

Adolescent and adult poisonings are usually caused by excess intake of drugs used for recreation or in suicide attempts. Implementing poison prevention in these age groups focuses on providing information and counselling. Poisoning in the older adult usually results from unintended ingestion of a toxic substance (e.g., because of failing eyesight) or an overdose of prescription or over-the-counter medications. People with altered mental status, such as dementia, are at risk for poisoning as they may lack judgment or memory about risky substances. Poison prevention focuses on safeguarding the environment, monitoring the underlying problems, and regularly

---

SKILL 32.2   IMPLEMENTING SEIZURE PRECAUTIONS

PURPOSE
Protect the client from injury

ASSESSMENT
Assess the history of seizures during the admission assessment. If the client has experienced a seizure previously, ask for detailed information, including characteristics of an aura or warning symptoms that indicate the seizure is beginning, duration and frequency of the seizures, consequences of the seizures (e.g., incontinence or difficulty breathing), and actions that should be taken to prevent or reduce seizure activity.

Clinical Reasoning
How do the client and his or her family interpret the need for seizure precautions? Are they frightened by what the cause of the seizures might be? Are they familiar with seizure activity and what to do if one occurs, or are they dealing with uncertainty about how to know if a seizure is happening and what to do in that

event? While the precautions are aimed at promoting safety, is it possible that the client will become isolated or fearful as a result?

Planning
Review emergency procedures: a respiratory arrest or other injury can result from a seizure.

Equipment
- Blankets or other linens to pad side rails
- Oral suction equipment
- Oxygen equipment

IMPLEMENTATION
Performance

1. Before performing the procedure, introduce yourself and verify the client's identity using two identifiers or per agency protocol. Explain to the client what you are

(continued)

SKILL 32.2 IMPLEMENTING SEIZURE PRECAUTIONS (*continued*)

going to do, why it is necessary, and how he or she can participate.

2. Perform hand hygiene, and follow other appropriate infection prevention and control procedures. If the client is actively seizing, apply clean gloves in preparation for performing respiratory care measures.

3. Provide for client privacy.

4. Pad the bed of any client who might have a seizure. Secure blankets or other linens around the head, foot, and side rails of the bed (see ❶).

5. Put oral suction equipment in place and test to ensure that it is functional. **Rationale: Suctioning may be needed to prevent aspiration of oral secretions**.

6. If a seizure occurs,

   • Remain with the client and call for assistance. Do not restrain the client.

   • If the client is not in bed, assist him or her to the floor, and protect the client's head in your lap or on a pillow.

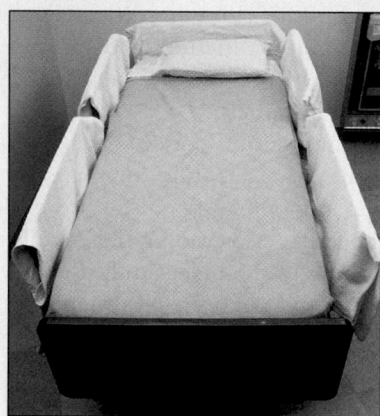

❶ Padding a bed for seizure precautions

Loosen any clothing around the client's neck and chest.

• Turn the client to the lateral position, if possible. **Rationale: Turning to the side allows secretions to drain out of the mouth, decreasing the risk of aspiration, and helps keep the tongue from occluding the airway**.

• Move items in the environment to ensure the client does not experience an injury.

• Do not insert anything into the client's mouth.

• Time the seizure duration.

• Observe the progression of the seizure, noting the sequence and type of limb involvement. Observe skin colour. When it is possible during the seizure, check pulse and respirations.

• Apply oxygen, according to agency policy.

• Use equipment to suction the oral airway if the client vomits or has excessive oral secretions.

• Administer anticonvulsant medications, as prescribed.

• When the seizure has subsided, assist the client to a comfortable position. Reorient the client. Explain what happened, and reassure the client. Provide hygiene, as necessary. Allow the client to verbalize his or her feelings about the seizure.

7. Document the event in the client record by using forms or checklists, supplemented by narrative notes, when appropriate.

EVALUATION

• Perform a detailed follow-up examination of the client. Administer medications, if indicated and prescribed.

• Report any significant deviations from normal to the appropriate members of the health care team.

HOME CARE CONSIDERATIONS

Implementing Seizure Precautions

• If clients have frequent or recurrent seizures or take anticonvulsant medications, they should wear a medical identification tag (bracelet or necklace) and carry a card listing any medications they take.

• When making home visits, inspect anticonvulsant medications and confirm that clients are taking them

correctly. Blood level measurements may be required periodically.

• Assist clients in determining which persons in the community should or must be informed of their seizure disorder (e.g., employers, motor vehicle department if driving, friends).

• Discuss safety precautions for inside and out of the home. If seizures are

not well controlled, activities that may require restriction or direct supervision by others include tub bathing, swimming, cooking, using electric equipment or machinery, and driving.

• Discuss the factors that may precipitate a seizure with clients and their families.

---

reviewing prescription and over-the-counter medications. A telephone number for the nearest poison control centre should be readily available so that accurate, up-to-date information about potential hazards and recommended treatment can be obtained, as needed.

Nurses intervene in community settings by educating the public about what to do in the event of poisoning.

Identify the specific poison by searching for an opened container, empty bottle, or other evidence. Contact the poison control centre, indicate the exact quantity of poison the person ingested, and state the person's age and apparent symptoms. Keep the person as quiet as possible and lying on his or her side or sitting with his or her head placed between the legs to prevent aspiration of vomitus.

TEACHING WELLNESS

Preventing Poisoning

Clients can take steps to help prevent poisonings:

- Lock potentially toxic products, including prescription and over-the-counter drugs and cleaning agents, in a cupboard, or attach childproof latches or devices to cabinet doors to keep them securely closed. Do not let children watch you open the latches. Kids learn fast!

- Keep medications and potential poisons in their original containers so that warning labels and child-resistant packaging remain intact. Do not reuse empty containers to store different substances. The labels of poisons usually specify first aid and precautionary measures.

- Do not rely on cooking to destroy toxic chemicals in plants. Never use anything prepared from nature as a medicine or tea.

- Teach children never to eat any part of an unknown plant or mushroom and not to put leaves, stems, bark, seeds, nuts, or berries from any plant into their mouths.

- Teach children to do the following: Stop *when you see a container, and don't touch*; Look for a hazard symbol; stay safe, *go get a grown up* (Health Canada, 2010d). Hazard symbol stickers geared to children are available through Health Canada's Stay Safe program for children.

- Do not refer to medicine as candy or pretend false enjoyment when taking medications in front of children; allow them to see the necessity of the medicine without glamorizing it.

- Read and follow label directions on all products before using them.

- Remove poisonous plants from the home, and avoid planting poisonous plants in the yard.

- Be aware of the local Poison Control emergency phone number, and display it near or on all telephones in the home so that it is available to babysitters, family, and friends.

The Teaching: Wellness box provides additional guidelines for helping clients to prevent poisoning.

CARBON MONOXIDE POISONING **Carbon monoxide** (CO) is a colourless, odourless, toxic gas that is a product of incomplete combustion. Exposure to CO can cause symptoms of headaches, dizziness, weakness, nausea, vomiting, and loss of muscle control. Prolonged exposure can lead to unconsciousness, brain damage, and death. Learning how to prevent CO exposure is important because all gasoline-powered vehicles or generators; lawn mowers; kerosene lanterns, heaters, and stoves; propane stoves; charcoal barbecues; and burning wood emit CO.

People are at risk for CO poisoning any time they use an appliance in which incomplete combustion of its fuel can occur. Sources of CO include malfunctioning furnaces, exhaust vents for gas appliances, wood-burning fireplaces that are not properly vented, exhaust fumes from idling cars, and charcoal briquettes (Health Canada, 2010e). Health Canada recommends that homes have CO detectors installed; they are mandatory in some Canadian cities.

CHOKING OR SUFFOCATION **Choking** occurs when a person's trachea is obstructed by either a foreign body (e.g., a chunk of food) or a liquid (e.g., vomitus), and it leads to suffocation. The universal sign of distress for a choking victim is the grasping of the anterior neck and being unable to speak or cough.

Suffocation, also referred to as **asphyxiation**, is lack of oxygen intake that can ultimately lead to unconsciousness and death. Suffocation occurs in situations of crush injuries to the chest, drowning, CO poisoning, or smothering (such as when a child covers his or her face with a plastic bag).

Other causes of suffocation are drowning, gas or smoke inhalation, strangulation by the shoulder harness of a seatbelt, and being trapped in a confined space (e.g., a discarded refrigerator). If a person does not receive immediate relief from suffocation, the interrupted breathing leads to respiratory and cardiac arrest and death. Any obstruction to the air passages must be immediately removed and life support measures instituted when an arrest occurs.

EXCESSIVE NOISE Excessive noise is a health hazard that can cause hearing loss, depending on the overall level of noise, the frequency range of the noise, and the duration of exposure and individual susceptibility. Sound levels above 120 decibels (dB) are painful and may cause hearing damage even if a person is exposed for only a short period. Exposure to 85 dB to 95 dB for several hours a day can lead to progressive or permanent hearing loss. No known risk of hearing loss is associated with sound levels below 70 dB.

Noise in hospital can be one of several factors contributing to sensory overload. Physiological effects of noise include increased heart and respiratory rates, increased muscular activity, nausea, and hearing loss (if the noise is sufficiently loud).

Noise can be minimized by acoustic tile on ceilings, walls, and floors; drapes and carpeting to absorb sound; background music to mask noise and have a calming effect (on some people); keeping your voice down while giving care or talking in the background; and appropriate alarm settings to reduce false alarms.

ELECTRICAL HAZARDS All electric equipment must be properly grounded. The electric plug of grounded equipment has three prongs. The two short prongs transmit the power to the equipment. The third, longer prong is the grounding device, which carries short circuits or stray electric current to the ground. Grounding

TEACHING	WELLNESS

Reducing Electrical Hazards

Take the following steps to reduce electrical hazards:

- Check cords for fraying or other signs of damage before using an appliance. Do not use it if the cord is damaged.
- Avoid overloading outlets and fuse boxes with too many appliances; use grounded outlets and plugs.
- Always pull a plug from the wall outlet by firmly grasping the plug and pulling it straight out. Pulling a plug by its cord can damage the cord and plug unit.
- Ensure that ground fault circuit interrupters (GFCIs) have been installed wherever electrical appliances or equipment can inadvertently come in contact with water, such as near sinks, bathtubs, or showers, or outdoors.

- Keep electric cords and appliances out of the reach of children, and place protective covers over wall outlets to protect young children.
- Carefully read instructions before operating electric equipment.
- Always disconnect appliances before cleaning or repairing them.
- Unplug any appliance that has given a tingling sensation or shock and have an electrician evaluate it.
- Keep electric cords coiled or taped to the ground away from areas of traffic to prevent people from damaging the cords or tripping over them.

prongs offer a path of least resistance to stray electric currents.

Faulty equipment, such as equipment with a frayed cord, presents a danger of electric shock or may start a fire. For example, an electric spark near certain anesthetic gases or a high concentration of oxygen can cause a fire or explosion. Actions to reduce electrical hazards are described in the Teaching: Wellness box.

When major electrical injury does occur, such as *macro-shock* (when the current finds a pathway through the body), the victim may sustain both superficial and deep burns, muscle contractions, and cardiac and respiratory arrest, necessitating CPR and life support. Small currents can cause *microshock* (when the current flows through a direct pathway to the heart), such as during intracardiac catheterization. Using machines in good repair, wearing shoes with rubber soles, standing on a nonconductive floor, and using nonconductive gloves can prevent shock. Rescuers must not touch the victim until the electricity is shut off or the victim has been removed from contact with the electric current; otherwise, the rescuer can also receive electrical injury.

FIREARMS Canadian regulations about firearm ownership are very strict, and gun registration is required. Any gun owner is required to follow a range of safety precautions to ensure that no harm or injury results from improper gun use or storage. Access to firearms is a serious concern in homes with children and in situations of suicidal ideation or domestic violence. Members of any household in which guns are present must take full responsibility for following basic firearm safety rules: Store all guns in sturdy locked cabinets, and make sure the keys are inaccessible to children; store bullets in a different location from the gun; and do not use firearms while under the influence of alcohol or other drugs of any kind, including over-the-counter medications that can change sensorium.

RADIATION Radiation injury can occur from overexposure to radioactive materials used in diagnostic and therapeutic procedures. Clients being examined by using radiography or fluoroscopy generally receive minimal exposure and few precautions are necessary. Nurses need to protect themselves, however, from radiation when some clients are receiving radiation therapy. Exposure to radiation can be minimized by (a) limiting the time near the source, (b) providing as much distance as possible from the source, and (c) using shielding devices, such as lead aprons, when near the source. Nurses need to become familiar with agency protocols related to radiation therapy.

Procedure-Related and Equipment-Related Risks

Risk assessment in the health care setting must include risks related to procedures and equipment. Whether giving a medication or assisting a person out of bed, nurses need to follow safeguards to prevent errors or unintentional injury. Nurses must be aware of and adhere to provincial or territorial regulations of occupational health and safety. The Workplace Hazardous Materials Information System (WHMIS) is an example of a legislated hazard communication system to ensure safety when using a range of dangerous products. Canada has recently adopted the Globally Harmonized System of Classification and Labelling of Chemicals (GHS) to communicate the related information about chemical hazards. Figure 32.7 is an example of a pictogram used by the GHS.

When an error or unintentional injury does occur, most agencies require that the incident be reported. Indeed, in some agencies where client safety is a priority, near misses are encouraged to be reported so that an analysis can be conducted and preventive measures put

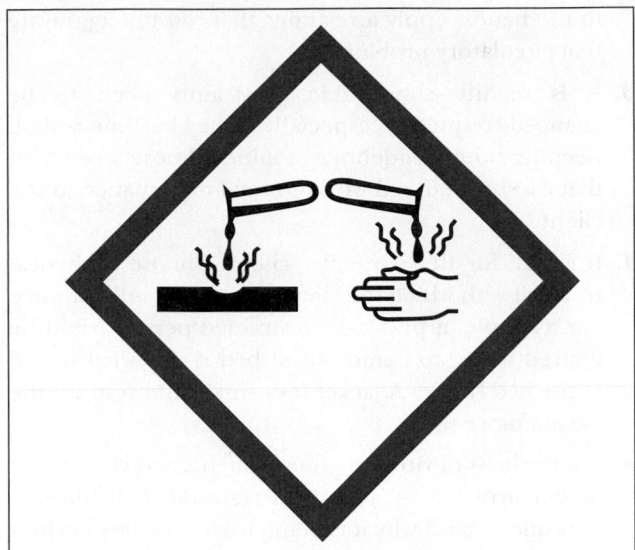

FIGURE 32.7 Globally Harmonized System of Classification and Labelling of Chemicals (GHS): Sample pictogram indicating corrosive material.

Source: Label Source (Online). *Globally Harmonised System: New classification and labelling of chemicals. Pictogram indicating corrosive material.* Retrieved from http://www.labelsourceonline.co.uk/ProdImages/hgs5001_gs.gif. Copyright 2008 Label Source Ltd.

in place to ensure client safety. For additional information about incident reports, see Chapter 6.

Restraining Clients

Restraints are physical, chemical, or environmental measures used to control the physical or behavioural activity of a person or a portion of his or her body. **Physical restraints** are any manual method or physical or mechanical device, material, or equipment attached to the client's body (e.g., vest or wrist restraint); they cannot be removed easily, and they restrict the client's movement. **Environmental restraints** control a person's mobility, such as when two full bedside rails or four split bedside rails are raised or the client is on a secured unit. **Chemical restraints** are medications, such as neuroleptics, anxiolytics, sedatives, and psychotropic agents, used to control disruptive behaviour. Generally, the only justifiable reasons for applying restraints are to avoid or prevent purposeful or accidental harm to a client when *all other methods have been tried* or to do what is required to provide medically necessary treatment that could not be provided *through any other means*. To reiterate, *restraints should be used only after every other possible means of ensuring safety have been unsuccessful and documented*. If restraints are deemed necessary, then a policy of **least restraint**—the use of the minimum amount of restraint needed to ensure safety (e.g., by securing one hand rather than both)—should be applied. Most agencies have strict policies and procedures related to use of restraints. See the alternatives to the use of restraints in Box 32.2.

Restraints can contribute to muscle atrophy, skin deterioration, urinary incontinence, constipation, and

respiratory infection because the client is more likely to remain recumbent or confined to bed when restrained. Coroners' reports have linked restraints to deaths, such as suffocation from becoming trapped between bedrails when trying to climb out of bed, strangulation when the ties of a restraint vest encircle the neck, or aspiration from vomitus when protective movements are limited by restraints. In addition to the physical safety concerns, many consider restraints to be demeaning and to limit a client's autonomy. They can be harmful psychologically, such as by making clients feel ashamed or guilty. For clients with a history of sexual abuse or other forms of violence, being placed in restraints has been linked to flashbacks and potential exacerbation of post-traumatic stress disorder (PTSD) symptoms. The focus in health care is to explore ways to prevent, reduce, and eliminate the use of restraints while protecting a client's safety, rights, and dignity.

LEGAL IMPLICATIONS OF RESTRAINTS Because restraints restrict the individual's freedom, their use has legal implications. Nurses need to know agency policies and provincial or territorial laws about restraining clients.

BOX 32.2 ALTERNATIVES TO RESTRAINTS

Some alternatives to restraints are as follows:

- Assign the care of a client to a team who can share in providing continuous or periodic surveillance and monitoring.
- Place the client in an area that is constantly or closely supervised; prepare the client if relocation is required to limit possible confusion or anxiety.
- Stay with a client who is using a bedside commode or the bathroom if the client is confused or sedated or has a gait disturbance or a high-risk score for falling.
- Monitor all medications and, if possible, lower or eliminate dosages of sedatives or psychotropics.
- Position the bed at the lowest level to facilitate getting in and out of bed.
- Replace full-length side rails with half- or three-quarter–length rails to prevent confused clients from climbing over rails or falling from the end of the bed.
- Wedge pillows or pads against the sides of a wheelchair to keep a client well positioned.
- To quiet agitated clients, try a warm beverage, soft lights, a back rub, or a walk.
- Use objects in the environment, such as pieces of furniture or large plants, as barriers to keep clients from wandering beyond appropriate areas.
- Try to determine the causes of a client's *sundowner syndrome* (nocturnal wandering and disorientation as darkness falls, associated with dementia). Possible causes include poor hearing, poor eyesight, or pain.
- Regularly monitor clients for changes in physical and cognitive functional abilities and risk factors.
- Engage family members or other supports such as friends or sitters who can help to calm or support the client, such as holding his or her hand to avoid pulling out an IV or nasogastric tube.

A clear understanding of what constitutes a restraint is important. For example, if a client has the side rails up to help with side-to-side movement in the bed, then this situation is not one of restraint; if, however, the side rails are up to confine the client, then the use of side rails is considered an environmental restraint. Most agencies and provincial or territorial legislation require informed consent of the client or legal representative before implementing restraints in nonemergency situations. A collective prescription or policy will generally identify the steps to be followed before using restraints. Some institutions allow for individual decision making in emergency situations, but the trend is toward documented interdisciplinary and client or family dialogue *before* their use. Continued use of restraints must also be addressed, often within specific time frames (e.g., involuntary restraint may require reassessment every 2 to 4 hours, voluntary restraint is generally reviewed every 8 or 24 hours). Most agencies require visual or auditory supervision of any client in restraint so that any safety issues can be quickly addressed. (See the Clinical Alert box regarding restrained clients.)

Clients have the right to be free from restraints that are not necessary. As a result, there must be justification that the use of restraints will protect the client and that less restrictive measures were attempted and found ineffective. Restraints *cannot* be used for staff convenience or client punishment. To reiterate, generally, the only justifiable reasons for applying restraints are to avoid or prevent purposeful or accidental harm to a client when all other methods have been tried and to do what is required to provide medically necessary treatment that could not be provided through any other means. Given that the above conditions are met and physical restraints are needed, it is important for the nurse to be able to correctly apply the restraints without endangering client safety.

SELECTING A PHYSICAL RESTRAINT Before selecting a physical restraint, nurses need to understand its purpose clearly and measure it against the following five criteria:

1. It restricts the client's movement as little as possible. If a client needs to have one arm restrained, do not restrain the entire body.

2. It does not interfere with the client's treatment or health problem. If a client has poor blood circulation to the hands, apply a restraint that will not aggravate that circulatory problem.

3. It is readily changeable. Restraints need to be changed frequently, especially if they become soiled. Keeping other guidelines in mind, choose a restraint that can be changed with minimal disturbance to the client.

4. It is safe for the particular client. Choose a physical restraint with which the client cannot self-inflict injury. For example, a physically restrained person could be injured trying to climb out of bed if one wrist is tied to the bed frame. A jacket restraint would restrain the person more safely.

5. It is the least obvious to others. Clients and visitors can be embarrassed by a physical restraint, even though they understand why it is being used. The less obvious the restraint, the more comfortable people feel.

KINDS OF PHYSICAL RESTRAINTS The most common types of physical restraints for adults are jacket or vest restraints, belt restraints, mitt or hand restraints, and limb restraints. Although bed rails can be used to aid in turning or repositioning and reduce the risk of clients falling out of bed during transport, they are also seen as restraints in that they can limit purposeful movement. Geri-chairs and wheelchairs with lap trays are also classified as forms of restraints. Physical restraints for infants and children include mummy restraints, elbow restraints, and crib nets. When using restraints, the nurse will find Practice Guidelines 32.2 helpful.

Several types of vest restraints are used, but all are essentially sleeveless jackets or vests with straps (tails) that can be tied to the bed frame under the mattress. These body restraints are used to ensure the safety of confused or sedated clients in beds or wheelchairs. "Front" and "back" labels on vest restraints ensure that they are applied correctly and safely.

Psychological trauma must be avoided; some clients can feel isolated, become panicky if left alone, and become fearful, especially if they have claustrophobic tendencies. Clients can have negative emotions even when restraints are no longer being used.

Belt or safety strap body restraints (Figure 32.8 on page 862) are used to ensure the safety of clients who are being moved on stretchers or in wheelchairs. Some wheelchairs have a soft, padded safety bar that attaches to side brackets that are installed under the armrests. To prevent the person from slumping forward, the nurse then attaches a shoulder Y strap to the bar and over the client's shoulders to the rear handles. Other safety belt models have a three-loop design. One loop surrounds the person's waist and the other two attach to the rear handles. If such restraints are unavailable, the nurse can place a folded towel or small sheet around the client's waist and fasten it at the back of the wheelchair. Belt restraints can also be used for certain clients confined to bed or to chairs.

! CLINICAL ALERT

Restrained clients may become more restless and anxious as a result of the loss of self-control. The nurse must keep in mind that such behaviours may be the result of pain or hypoxia from improper restraint application. A client who was agitated and suddenly becomes quiet must be assessed to ensure that the change in behaviour is the result of calmness rather than a hypoxic or other physiological event.

PRACTICE GUIDELINES 32.2

Applying Restraints

Guidelines	Rationales
Ensure that all alternative measures other than restraints have been exhausted and that the least restraint option is being used. Assure the client and the family that the restraint is temporary and protective.	Underlying reasons for restraints must be addressed and corrected, if possible, as their use is associated with psychological (guilt, anger, shame, feeling punished) and physiological (strangulation, skin breakdown, constipation) risks.
Obtain consent from the client or guardian and ensure that necessary collective or physician prescriptions are in order.	Legal and ethical considerations require informed consent, unless in an emergency situation. Health agencies generally have specific protocols and lines of authority to ensure practices are consistent and safe.
If restraints are applied, ensure the following:	
• Apply the restraint so that the client can move as freely as possible without defeating the purpose of the restraint.	Inability to move can cause anxiety and agitation, and enhance the risk of physiological complications, such as aspiration if vomiting.
• Apply a restraint using quick-release buckles or a half-bow (quick-release) knot that does not tighten when pulled and supports the normal anatomy of the body part.	Time is of the essence in emergency situations and tight physical restraints can impede blood circulation and are uncomfortable; contractures and discomfort can arise from poor body alignment.
• Pad bony prominences (e.g., wrists, ankles) before applying a restraint over them. Immediately report and document any persistent reddened or broken skin areas under the restraint.	The movement of a physical restraint without padding over bony prominences can abrade the skin. Any sign of skin breakdown or poor circulation may mean restraints are improperly attached or contraindicated.
At the first indication of cyanosis or pallor, coldness of a skin area, or a client's complaint of tingling, pain, or numbness, loosen the physical restraint, and exercise the limb.	Poor circulation must be corrected immediately to avoid tissue or neurological damage.
Tie the ends of a body restraint to the part of the bed that moves to elevate the head.	Tying the ends to a side rail or to the fixed frame of the bed will cause injury if the bed position is changed.
Assess the response to restraints per agency protocol and time frame, generally at least once an hour. Assessment must include determining a continued need for the restraints.	Regular assessment is necessary to ensure safety and that the underlying cause of the behaviour necessitating the original use of the restraints persists or no longer exists.
Provide range-of-motion (ROM) exercises and skin care, and assist with basic needs: hygiene, positioning, nutrition, hydration, elimination.	Maintenance of general health needs must be met to prevent further deterioration.
Provide emotional support throughout and after restraints are removed.	Maintenance of psychological health is imperative.

A mitt or hand restraint (Figure 32.9 on the next page) is used to prevent confused clients from using their hands or fingers to scratch and injure themselves. For example, a confused client may need to be prevented from pulling at intravenous tubing or at a head bandage following neurosurgery. Hand or mitt restraints allow the client to be ambulatory and to move the arm freely rather than be confined to a bed or a chair. Mittens need to be removed on a regular basis to permit the client to wash and exercise the hands. The nurse also needs to take off the mitten to check the circulation to the hand.

Limb restraints (Figure 32.10 on the next page) can be used to immobilize a limb, primarily for therapeutic reasons (e.g., to maintain an intravenous infusion). See Skill 32.3 for applying restraints. See also the Lifespan Considerations box on the use of restraints and the Home Care Considerations box on applying restraints that follow.

Evaluating

To prevent client injury, the nurse's role is largely educative, and desired outcomes reflect the client's acquisition of knowledge of hazards, behaviours that incorporate safety practices, and skills to perform in the event of

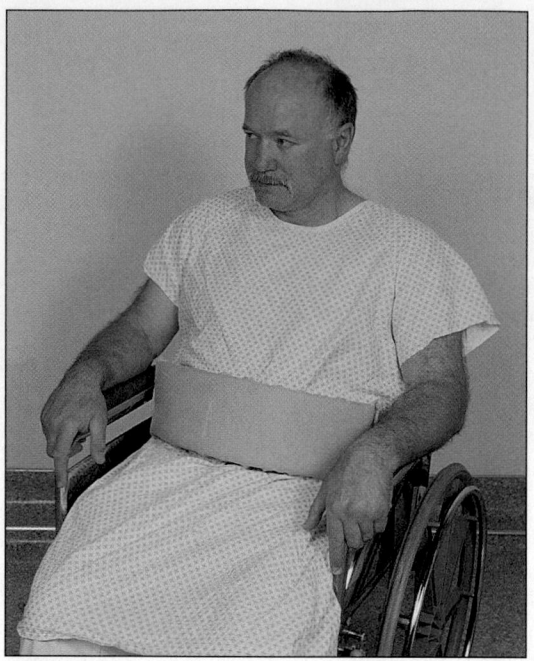

FIGURE 32.8 A belt restraint.

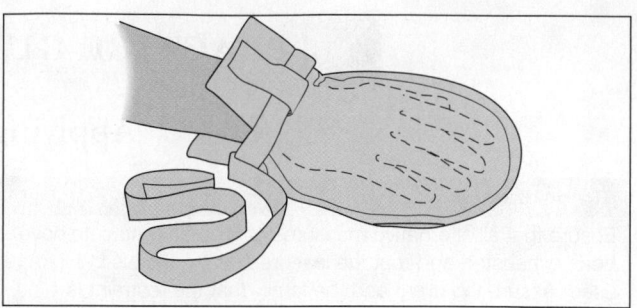

FIGURE 32.9 A mitt restraint.

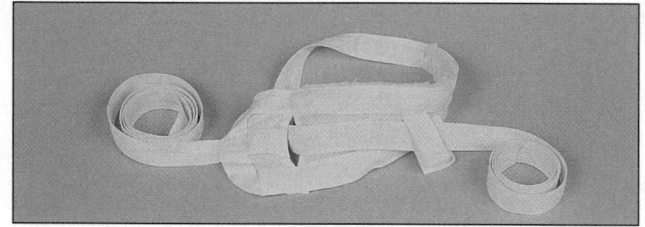

FIGURE 32.10 A limb restraint.

SKILL 32.3 APPLYING PHYSICAL RESTRAINTS

PURPOSES

- To promote safety and prevent injury *only when all other less restrictive measures have been exhausted*
- To allow a medical or surgical treatment to proceed without client interference (e.g., to prevent movements that would disrupt therapy to a limb connected to tubes or an appliance)

ASSESSMENT

Assess

- The behaviour indicating the possible need for a restraint
- Underlying causes for the assessed behaviour
- What other protective measures can be implemented before applying a restraint
- The status of skin to which a restraint is to be applied
- The circulatory status distal to restraints and of extremities
- The effectiveness of other available safety precautions

Clinical Reasoning

Is there something that has been missed (e.g., hypoxemia, psychological distress) during the assessment phase that might explain why this client seems to need restraints but if assessed or addressed could mean that restraints are not needed? If the client is agitated or angry, has he or she been given the opportunity to share feelings and frustrations? How will the client and his family interpret the use of the physical restraint, and how can the nurse buffer the potentially negative feelings? Is it possible that the family and the client see the restraints as helpful and are relieved that the restraints will be used, for example, when it is feared that the client might extubate himself or herself unless the hand is gently restrained?

PLANNING

Review institutional policy for restraints and seek consultation as appropriate before independently deciding to apply a restraint. Many Canadian institutions require interdisciplinary discussions and informed client or legal guardian consent before instituting restraints.

Equipment

- Appropriate type and size of restraint

IMPLEMENTATION

Performance

1. Before performing the procedure, introduce yourself and verify the client's identity using two identifiers or per agency protocol. Explain to the client and family what you are going to do, why it is necessary, and how they can participate. Allow time for the client to express feelings about being restrained. Provide needed emotional reassurance that the physical restraints will be used only when absolutely necessary and that there will be close contact with the client in case assistance is required.

2. Perform hand hygiene, and follow other appropriate infection prevention and control procedures.

3. Provide for client privacy, if indicated.

4. Apply the selected restraint.

Belt Restraint (Safety Belt)

- Determine that the safety belt is in good order. If a Velcro safety belt is to be used, make sure that both pieces of Velcro are intact.

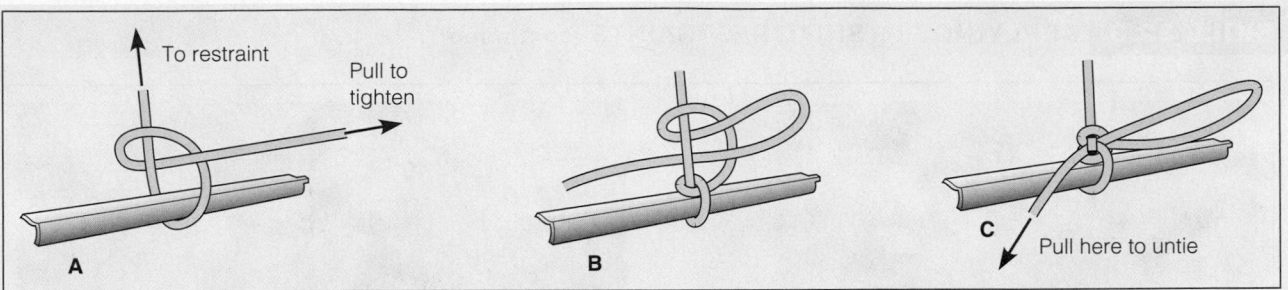

1 To make a half-bow (quick-release) knot, first place the restraint tie under the side frame of the bed (or around a chair leg). **A:** Bring the free end up, around, under, and over the attached end of the tie and pull it tight. **B:** Again take the free end over and under the attached end of the tie, but this time make a half-bow loop. **C:** Tighten the free end of the tie and the bow until the knot is secure. To untie the knot, pull the end of the tie and then loosen the first cross over the tie.

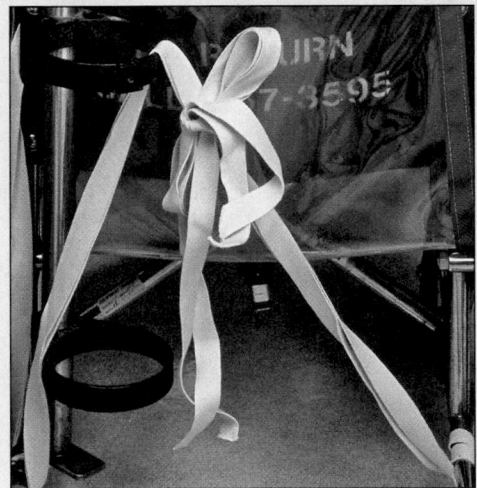

2 Half-bow (quick-release) knot

- If the belt has a long portion and a shorter portion, place the long portion of the belt behind (under) the client confined to bed and secure it to the movable part of the bed frame. **Rationale: The long attached portion will then move up when the head of the bed is elevated and will not tighten around the client.**

- Place the shorter portion of the belt around the client's waist, over the gown. There should be a finger's width between the belt and the client.

- *Or* attach the belt around the client's waist, and fasten it at the back of the chair.

- *Or* if the belt is attached to a stretcher, secure the belt firmly over the client's hips or abdomen. **Rationale: Belt restraints must be applied to all clients on stretchers, even when the side rails are up.**

Jacket Restraint

- Place the vest on the client, with opening at the front or the back, depending on the vest type.

- Pull the tie on the end of the vest flap across the chest, and place it through the slit in the opposite side of the chest.

- Repeat for the other tie.

- Use a half-bow (quick-release) knot to secure each tie around the movable bed frame or behind the chair to a chair leg (see **1** and **2**). **Rationale: A half-bow (quick-release) knot does not tighten or slip when the attached end is pulled but unties easily when the loose end is pulled.**

- *Or* fasten the ties together behind the chair by using a slip or quick-release knot.

- Ensure that the client is positioned appropriately to enable maximum chest expansion for breathing.

Mitt Restraint

- Apply the commercial thumbless mitt (see Figure 32.9) to the hand to be restrained. Make sure the fingers can be slightly flexed and are not caught under the hand.

- Follow the manufacturer's directions for securing the mitt.

- If a mitt is to be worn for several days, remove it at regular intervals per agency protocol. Wash and exercise the client's hand, then reapply the mitt. Check agency practices about recommended intervals for removal.

- Assess the client's circulation to the hands shortly after the mitt is applied and at regular intervals. **Rationale: Client complaints of numbness, discomfort, or inability to move the fingers could indicate impaired circulation to the hand.**

Wrist or Ankle Restraint

- Pad bony prominences on the wrist or ankle, if needed, to prevent skin breakdown.

- Apply the padded portion of the restraint around the ankle or wrist.

- Pull the tie of the restraint through the slit in the wrist portion or through the buckle and ensure that the restraint is not too tight (see **3**).

- By using a half-bow knot (quick-release knot), attach the other end of the restraint to the movable portion of the bed frame. **Rationale: If the ties are attached to the movable portion, the wrist or ankle will not be pulled when the bed position is changed.**

5. Adjust the plan of care, as required, for example, to include releasing the restraint, providing skin care, helping with range-of-motion exercises, and attending to the

(continued)

| SKILL 32.3 | APPLYING PHYSICAL RESTRAINTS (*continued*) |

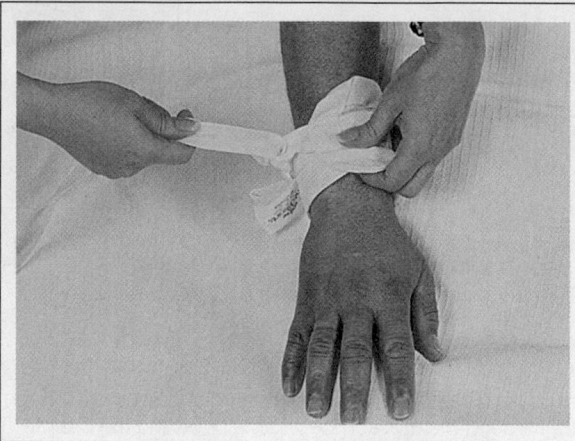 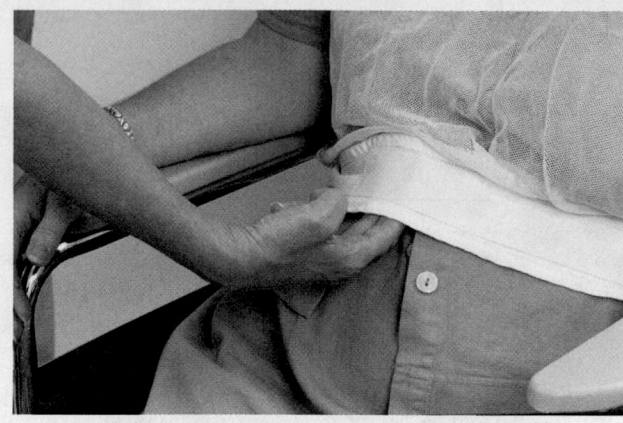

❸ Ensure that two fingers can be inserted between the restraint and *A* (wrist) and *B* (chest).

client's physical needs by providing fluids, nutrition, and toileting.

6. Record on the client's chart the behaviour(s) indicating the need for the restraint, all other interventions implemented in an attempt to avoid the use of restraints and their outcomes, and the time the physician was notified of the need for restraint. Also, record the following:

- The type of restraint applied, the time it was applied, and the goal for its application
- The client's response to the restraint, as well as the rationale for its continued use
- The times that the restraints were removed and skin care given
- Any other assessments and interventions
- Explanations given to the client and significant others

EVALUATION

- Perform a detailed follow-up of the need for the restraints and the client's physical and emotional responses. Relate these findings to previous data, if available.
- Evaluate circulatory status of restrained limbs at least on an hourly basis.
- Evaluate skin status beneath restraints at least on an hourly basis.
- Remove the restraints as soon as they are no longer needed, and document the removal.
- When restraints are released, ensure that the client is not experiencing any emotional or physical consequences. Reaffirm that the physical restraints were a last resort to protect the client and that they were not a form of punishment.
- Report significant deviations from normal to the appropriate members of the health care team.

LIFESPAN CONSIDERATIONS

Restraints

INFANTS

Elbow restraints (Figure 32.11) are used to prevent infants or small children from flexing their elbows to touch or reach their face or head, especially after surgery. Ready-made elbow restraints are available commercially.

A mummy restraint (Figure 32.12) is a folding of a blanket or sheet around the infant to prevent movement during a procedure, such as eye irrigation or collection of a blood specimen.

- Obtain a blanket or sheet large enough so that the distance between opposite corners is about twice the length of the infant's body. Lay the blanket or sheet on a flat, dry surface.
- Fold down one corner, and place the baby on it in the supine position.
- Fold the right side of the blanket over the infant's body, leaving the left arm free (see Figure 32.12A). The right arm is in a natural position at the side.

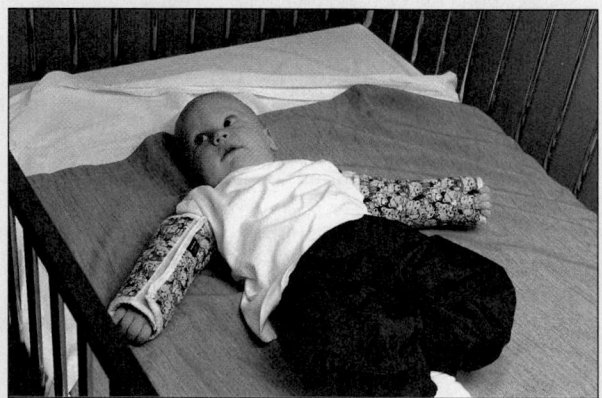

FIGURE 32.11 Infant with elbow restraints.

- Fold the excess blanket at the bottom up under the infant (see Figure 32.12B, 2).
- With the left arm in a natural position at the baby's side, fold the left side of the blanket over the infant, including the arm, and tuck the blanket under the body (see Figure 32.12B, 3).
- Remain with the infant who is in a mummy restraint until the specific procedure is completed.

CHILDREN

A crib net is simply a device placed over the top of a crib to prevent active young children from climbing out of the crib. At the same time, it allows them freedom to move about in the crib. The crib net or dome is not attached to the movable parts of the crib so that the caregiver can have access to the child without removing the dome or net.

- Place the net over the sides and ends of the crib.
- Secure the ties to the springs or frame of the crib. The crib sides can then be freely lowered without removing the net.
- Test with your hand that the net will stretch if the child stands against it in the crib.

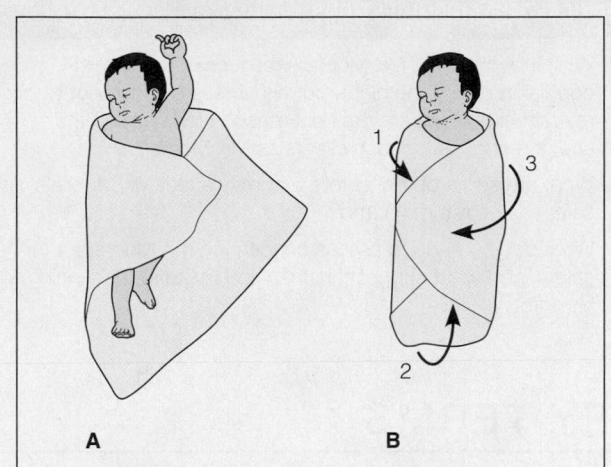

FIGURE 32.12 Making a mummy restraint

HOME CARE CONSIDERATIONS

Applying Restraints

Physical restraints may be necessary for clients in wheelchairs or in the home. Safety guidelines apply in all cases. Assess the knowledge and skill of all caregivers in the use of restraints, and educate them, as indicated.

- Use means other than restraints as much as possible, and stay with the client.
- Pad bony prominences, such as wrists and ankles, if needed before applying a restraint over them.
- Tie restraints with knots that will not tighten when pulled, and tie them to parts of the wheelchair that do not move. Release the knots quickly in case of emergency.
- Assess restrained limbs for signs of impaired blood circulation.
- Always stay with a client whose restraint is temporarily removed.

certain emergencies. The nurse needs to individualize these for clients. Examples of desired outcomes include the client being able to do the following:

- Describe methods to prevent specific hazards (e.g., falls, suffocation, scalds, fires, drowning, electric shock)
- Report use of home safety measures (e.g., fire safety measures, smoke detector and CO detector maintenance, fall-prevention strategies, burn-prevention measures, poison-prevention measures, firearm safety precautions, water safety precautions, motor vehicle safety)
- Alter home physical environment to reduce the risk of unintentional injury
- Describe emergency procedures such as for poisoning or fire
- Describe age-specific risks, work safety risks, or community safety risks
- Demonstrate correct use of child safety seats

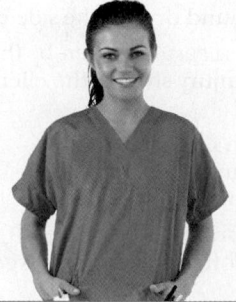

Case Study 32

Mr. Moore is a 72-year-old widower who is recovering from a fall in which he fractured his hip and underwent surgical repair 1 week ago. He will be staying with his son for 2 weeks after he is discharged from the hospital, but he is eager to return to his own home. Once he is home, his son will visit nightly after work, he will receive Meals on Wheels once a day, and a home care attendant will visit weekly to assist with hygienic care until he is more independent. Mr. Moore's wife died 3 years ago; he has remained independent and continued his social functions. He lives in a small single-level house with his dog, and he enjoys gardening. Before fracturing his hip, he walked his dog daily. You will be his home care nurse.

(continued)

CRITICAL THINKING QUESTIONS

1. While hospitalized, Mr. Moore experienced some mild confusion during the night, but his nurses decided not to restrain him. What are the best reasons for avoiding the use of restraints for such clients as Mr. Moore?

2. What are some of the factors that may affect Mr. Moore's safety as he returns home?

3. What do you need to assess concerning Mr. Moore's safety, and what suggestions can you make for enhancing his safety?

4. What strengths do you note about Mr. Moore that may protect him from injury when he returns home?

Check the eText in MyNursingLab for answers and explanations.

KEY TERMS

accidents *p. 837*

adverse event *p. 837*

asphyxiation *p. 857*

bioterrorism *p. 840*

burn *p. 848*

carbon monoxide *p. 857*

chemical restraints *p. 859*

choking *p. 857*

environmental restraints *p. 859*

fall *p. 849*

injury *p. 837*

intentional injuries *p. 837*

least restraint *p. 859*

patient safety *p. 837*

physical restraints *p. 859*

restraints *p. 859*

scald *p. 848*

seizure *p. 855*

seizure precautions *p. 855*

suffocation *p. 857*

unintentional injuries *p. 837*

CHAPTER HIGHLIGHTS

- Unintentional injuries are a major cause of death among Canadians.

- Nurses need to be aware of what constitutes a safe environment for specific individuals and for groups of people in the home, community, health care agency, and workplace.

- Hazards to safety occur at all ages and vary according to the age and development of the individual.

- Nursing assessment of safety includes assessing factors that can affect safety: age and development, lifestyle, mobility and health status, sensory–perceptual alterations, cognitive awareness, emotional state, ability to communicate, safety awareness, and environmental factors.

- Nurses assess clients at risk for injury through such methods as taking a nursing history and conducting a physical examination, using risk assessment tools, evaluating the home environment, assessing standards of safety in the health care setting, and addressing bioterrorism.

- Many medical errors in hospitals are preventable, and agencies that adopt a culture of safety focus on achieving patient safety goals by addressing system-wide issues.

- Multiple nursing diagnoses related to client safety focus on specific risks for unintentional injury, such as risk for poisoning, suffocation, drowning, and falls.

- When planning for safety needs of clients, nurses need to consider physical factors in the environment and the psychological and physiological state of the individual. Clients often need to change their health behaviour and may need to modify the environment.

- Measures to ensure the safety of people of all ages focus on (a) observation or prediction of situations that are potentially harmful and (b) client education that empowers clients to safeguard themselves and their families from injury. Education is a major health-protection strategy in preventing unintentional injury.

- Nurses must be familiar with fire procedures in their health care agency. In the event of a fire, the nurse must RACE: **R**escue or **R**emove persons who are in immediate danger; **A**ctivate the alarm and call for help; **C**ontain or **C**onfine the fire and smoke; **E**xtinguish the fire if possible; otherwise **E**vacuate.

- Falls are a common cause of unintentional injury among older adults. Prevention of falls in the home and health care setting is a continuous concern. Strategies for fall risk assessment, fall prevention, and fall protection are numerous. Side rails do not protect hospitalized patients from falls; it is more likely the patient will fall trying to get around or over the side rail.

- Seizure precautions are safety measures taken by the nurse to protect clients from injury should the client have a seizure.

- Major reasons for poisoning in children are inadequate supervision and improper storage of medications and household toxic substances.

- Suffocation can occur when foreign objects are swallowed or inhaled, cutting off the person's oxygen supply.

- Prolonged exposure to excessive noise can produce hearing loss.
- Faulty electric equipment and improper grounding pose health hazards in the hospital and at home. Accidents can be prevented by using grounded outlets and plugs, putting protective covers over outlets, keeping appliances in good repair, and making sure that electric wiring and circuits meet safety standards.
- Firearms pose a risk to individuals of all ages. Adults must take full responsibility for following safety procedures when keeping firearms in the home, including storage of ammunition in a separate location.
- Various alternatives to restraints must be considered before a restraint is applied.
- Because physical restraints restrict a client's basic freedom to move, careful assessment and accurate, complete documentation are important when restraints are used with all efforts aimed at resolving the need for restraints.

ASSESS YOUR LEARNING

1. What is the correct sequence of the following nursing priorities if a fire occurs in a health care setting?

   a. Remove clients from the site of danger, pull the fire alarm, contain the fire, and extinguish the fire.

   b. Pull the fire alarm, contain the fire, remove clients from the site of danger, and extinguish the fire.

   c. Remove clients from the site of danger, pull the fire alarm, extinguish the fire, and contain the fire.

   d. Pull the fire alarm, contain the fire, extinguish the fire, and remove clients from the site of danger.

2. A hospitalized 90-year-old woman who uses a walker is receiving diuretic medication and must use the bathroom several times each night. To promote safety, which of the following should the nurse do?

   a. Leave the bathroom light on

   b. Withhold her diuretic medication

   c. Provide a bedside commode

   d. Keep the side rails up

3. A 75-year-old man is hospitalized following a cerebrovascular accident (stroke). He is unable to ambulate without help but becomes disoriented at times and tries to get out of bed. What is the MOST appropriate safety measure the nurse must perform for this patient?

   a. Restraining him in bed

   b. Asking a family member to stay with him

   c. Checking the patient every 15 minutes

   d. Using a bed exit safety monitoring device

4. Which of the following nursing interventions is the highest in priority for a client at risk for falls in a hospital setting?

   a. Keeping all the side rails up

   b. Reviewing prescribed medications

   c. Completing the Get Up and Go test

   d. Placing the bed in the lowest position

5. Accreditation Canada's client safety goals address the need to decrease the number of errors in hospitals. Which of the following practices will help increase client safety?

   a. Improving the nurse's ability to multitask

   b. Identifying the health care practitioners who are incompetent

   c. Establishing strict policies and procedures

   d. Creating a culture of safety

6. The nurse, at the change-of-shift report, learns that one of the clients in his care has bilateral soft wrist restraints. The client is confused, has been trying to get out of bed, and had pulled out the intravenous (IV) line, which was subsequently reinserted. Which of the following actions by the nurse is appropriate?

   a. Keeping the wrist restraint on at all times and removing it only if it becomes soiled

   b. Ensuring that no fingers can be inserted between the restraint and the wrist

   c. Using a square knot to ensure the client cannot get the restraint undone

   d. Ensuring that the restraints are tied to the part of the bed that moves to elevate the head

7. A client is being admitted to the hospital because of a seizure that occurred at home. The client has no previous history of seizures. In planning the client's nursing care, which of the following measures is the MOST essential at this time of admission?

   a. Placing a padded tongue depressor at the head of the bed

   b. Padding the bed with blankets

   c. Informing the client about the importance of wearing a medical identification tag

   d. Teaching the client about epilepsy

8. Marcel, 8 years old, is admitted to the pediatric unit following a convulsive (i.e., seizure) episode at home. When entering Marcel's room, the nurse notes that he is having a convulsion.

What should the nurse do as a priority in this situation?

a. Draw the curtains to provide Marcel with privacy

b. Place a pillow under Marcel's head to prevent trauma

c. Reassure Marcel by talking to him gently

d. Ensure airway patency for Marcel

9. Mr. Taylor, 85 years old, has a history of dementia. He is known to strike out during personal care. What is the BEST way to minimize risk to the nurse when giving Mr. Taylor a tub bath?

a. Encouraging the client to remain calm

b. Asking a colleague for assistance

c. Giving him a shower instead

d. Administering a sedative prior to his bath

10. Mr. Sanders has had Alzheimer's disease for 3 years. He is 75 years old and lives with his 72-year-old wife. He takes little part in his care and is confused at times. The nurse suggests prevention strategies to Mrs. Sanders, who is worried about her husband roaming at night. Which of the following suggestions by the nurse would reduce the risk of unintentional injury?

a. Install an alarm bell on the bedroom door.

b. Ensure adequate lighting in the house.

c. Administer sleeping medication to Mr. Sanders before he retires.

d. Ensure that someone stays with him.

Check the eText in MyNursingLab for answers and explanations.

WEBLINKS

Canadian Nurses Association's Patient Safety Resource Guide

http://www.cna-aiic.ca/en/improve-your-workplace

This site offers a searchable database containing references related to all aspects of client safety.

Canadian Centre for Occupational Health and Safety—Young Workers Zone

http://www.ccohs.ca/youngworkers

Youth and their families can consult this website for information about keeping safe during seasonal work (e.g., summer jobs), including who is responsible for on-the-job training.

Canadian Patient Safety Institute

http://www.patientsafetyinstitute.ca

This resource provides a range of information about a variety of safety issues in Canada. It offers an electronic newsletter, research updates, safety resources, and relevant links to other websites.

Canada Safety Council

http://www.safety-council.org

This site offers a range of tips on safety for all age groups. It addresses topical safety issues, such as bullying and Internet safety.

Child Car Seat Clinics Across Canada

http://www.tc.gc.ca/eng/roadsafety/safedrivers-childsafety-seat-clinics-1058.htm

Transport Canada has compiled a list of car seat clinics across Canada as a resource to ensure that seats have been installed correctly.

Hazardcheck, Health Canada

http://www.hc-sc.gc.ca/ewh-semt/hazards-risques/index-eng.php

This is a public awareness site related to home safety; a virtual house tour is available allowing for an interactive exploration of the risks in every room of the home!

Public Health Agency of Canada: Injury Surveillance On-Line

http://dsol-smed.phac-aspc.gc.ca/dsol-smed/is-sb/index_e.html

Injuries treated in the emergency departments of the Canadian Hospitals Injury Reporting and Prevention Program (CHIRPP) are summarized at this site. Nurses can monitor trends so that relevant health-promotion and injury-prevention programs can be developed.

Safe Kids Canada

http://www.safekidscanada.ca

Parents, children, and health care professionals can all benefit from this site, which offers practical, fun, and up-to-date material on injury prevention for all childhood age groups.

Smartrisk

http://www.smartrisk.ca

Smartrisk is a Canadian nonprofit organization dedicated to preventing injuries and saving lives. This site provides a range of creative and educational safety learning opportunities.

MyNursingLab

REFERENCES

Accreditation Canada. (2011). *Required organizational practices, 2011.* Ottawa, ON: Author.

Baker, G. R., Norton, P. G., Flintoft, V., Blais, R., Brown, A., Cox, J., . . . Etchells, E. (2004). The Canadian adverse event study: The incidence of adverse events among hospital patients in Canada. *Canadian Medical Association Journal, 170*(11), 1678–1686.

Breslin, F. C., Polzer, J., MacEachen, E., Morrongiello, B., & Shannon, H. (2006). Workplace injury or "part of the job"? Towards a gendered understanding of injuries and complaints among young workers. *Social Science & Medicine, 64,* 782–793.

Cameron, I. D., Murray, G. R., Gillespie, L. D., Robertson, M. C., Hill, K. D., Cumming, R. G., & Kerse, N. (2010). Interventions for preventing falls in older people in nursing care facilities and hospitals. *Cochrane Database of Systematic Reviews,* Issue 1. Art. No.: CD005465. doi: 10.1002/14651858.CD005465.pub2

Canada Mortgage and Housing Corporation. (2011). *Preventing falls on stairs.* Ottawa, ON: Author.

Canadian Agricultural Injury Surveillance Program. (2007). Fatal and hospitalized agricultural injuries among children and youth in Canada. Kingston, ON: Author.

Canadian Interprofessional Health Collaborative. (2010). A national interprofessional competency framework. Vancouver, BC: Author.

Canadian Nurses Association. (2009). *Position statement: Patient safety.* Ottawa, ON: Author.

Canadian Patient Safety Institute. (2011). *The patient safety competencies framework.* Retrieved from http://www.patientsafetyinstitute.ca/English/toolsResources/safetyCompetencies/Pages/default.aspx

Fire Prevention Canada. (2011a). *Fire extinguishers.* Retrieved from http://www.fiprecan.ca/index.php?section=2&show=fireExtinguishers

Fire Prevention Canada. (2011b). *Modern homes burn faster—the 3 minute drill.* Retrieved from http://www.fiprecan.ca/index.php?section=2&show=threeminutedrill

Fuselli, P., & Wanounou, A. (2011). Canada and the world: A comparative approach to injury prevention. *Health Care Quarterly, 14* (Special Issue 3), 84–89.

Gillespie, W. J., Gillespie, L. D., & Parker, M. J. (2010). Hip protectors for preventing hip fractures in older people. *Cochrane Database of Systematic Reviews,* Issue 10. Art. No.: CD001255. doi: 10.1002/14651858.CD001255.pub4

Health Canada. (2006). *Trampolines.* Retrieved from http://www.hc-sc.gc.ca/cps-spc/pubs/cons/trampolines-eng.php

Health Canada. (2010a). *Cribs, cradles, bassinettes regulations.* Ottawa, ON: Health Canada. Retrieved from http://www.hc-sc.gc.ca/cps-spc/legislation/acts-lois/_cribs-berceaux/index-eng.php

Health Canada. (2010b). *Playpens—Consumer product safety.* Ottawa, ON: Health Canada. Retrieved from http://www.hc-sc.gc.ca/cps-spc/child-enfant/equip/playpens-parcs-eng.php

Health Canada. (2010c). *Pacifiers—Consumer product safety.* Ottawa, ON: Health Canada. Retrieved from http://www.hc-sc.gc.ca/cps-spc/child-enfant/equip/pacif-suce-eng.php

Health Canada. (2010d). *Stay Safe: An educational program about hazard symbols.* Retrieved from http://www.hc-sc.gc.ca/cps-spc/house-domes/chem-chim/hazard-danger-eng.php

Health Canada. (2010e). *Carbon monoxide.* Retrieved from http://www.hc-sc.gc.ca/ewh-semt/air/in/poll/combustion/carbon-eng.php

Kohn, L. T., Corrigan, J. M., & Donaldson, M. S. (Eds.). (2000). To err is human. Building a safer health system. Washington, DC: National Academy Press.

Lamb, S. E., Hauer. K,, & Becker, C. (2005). *Manual for the fall prevention classification system.* Retrieved from www.profane.eu.org/profane_documents/Falls_Taxonomy.pdf

Leonard, P., Hoffman, C., & the National Steering Committee on Patient Safety. (2002). *Building a safer system: A national integrated strategy for improving patient safety in Canadian health care.* Retrieved from http://rcpsc.medical.org/publications/building_a_safer_system_e.pdf

Li, F., Harmer, P, Fisher, J., McAuley, E., Chaumeton, N., Eckstrom, E., & Wilson, N. (2005). Tai Chi and fall reductions in older adults: A randomized controlled trial. *Journal of Gerontology, 60*(2), 187–194.

Macdonald, M., Lang, A., & MacDonald, J. (2011). Mapping a research agenda for home care safety: Perspectives from researchers, providers, and decision makers. *Canadian Journal on Aging, 30*(2), 233–245.

Pless, I. B., & Hagel, B. E. (2005). Injury prevention: A glossary of terms. *Journal of Epidemiology and Community Health, 59,* 182–185.

Public Health Agency of Canada. (2005). Bioterrorism and emergency preparedness. Retrieved from http://www.phac-aspc.gc.ca/ep-mu/bioem-eng.php

Public Health Agency of Canada. (2009a). *Child and youth injury in review.* Ottawa, ON: Author. Retrieved from http://www.phac-aspc.gc.ca/publicat/cyi-bej/2009/pdf/injreprapbles2009_eng.pdf

Public Health Agency of Canada. (2009b). *Report on seniors' falls in Canada: Chapter 3 Risk factors for falls and fall-related injuries in seniors. Technical Report.* Ottawa, ON: Minister of Public Works and Government Services. Retrieved from http://www.phac-aspc.gc.ca/seniors-aines/publications/pro/injury-blessure/falls-chutes/chap3-eng.php

Public Health Agency of Canada. (2011). *You CAN prevent falls!* Retrieved from http://www.phac-aspc.gc.ca/seniors-aines/publications/public/injury-blessure/prevent-eviter/index-eng.php

Registered Nurses' Association of Ontario. (2011). *Prevention of falls and fall injuries in the older adult—Guideline supplement.* Toronto, ON: Author.

Royal College of Physicians and Surgeons. (2003). *Canadian patient safety dictionary.* Retrieved from http://rcpsc.medical.org/publications/PatientSafetyDictionary_e.pdf

Safe Kids Canada. (2011a). Most common injuries to children in Canada. Retrieved from http://www.safekidscanada.ca/Professionals/Safety-Information/About-Injuries/Index.aspx

Safe Kids Canada. (2011b). *Drowning prevention.* Retrieved from http://www.safekidscanada.ca/Professionals/Safety-Information/Drowning-Prevention/Index.aspx

Safe Kids Canada. (2011c). *Pool safety.* Retrieved from http://www.safekidscanada.ca/Professionals/Safety-Information/Drowning-Prevention/Pool-Safety/Pool-Safety.aspx

Safe Kids Canada. (2011d). *Off-highway vehicles.* Retrieved from http://www.safekidscanada.ca/Professionals/Safety-Information/Off–Highway-Vehicles/Index.aspx

Safe Kids Canada. (2011e). *Scalds and burns—hot tap water.* Retrieved from http://www.safekidscanada.ca/Professionals/Safety-Information/Scalds-and-Burns/Tap-Water/Hot-Tap-Water.aspx

Safe Kids Canada. (2011f). *Preventing a parents' nightmare—unintentional poisoning.* Retrieved from http://www.safekidscanada.ca/Parents/Newsroom/Media-Releases/2011/Poison-Prevention-Week.aspx

Scott, V., Wager, L.., & Elliot, S. (2010). *Falls and related injuries among older Canadians: Fall-related hospitalizations and intervention initiatives*. Prepared on behalf of the Public Health Agency of Canada, Division of Aging and Seniors. Victoria, BC: Victoria Scott Consulting.

Smartrisk. (2011). *Facts on injury*. Retrieved from http://www.smartrisk.ca/index.php/aboutSR/C11

Statistics Canada. (2008). *Leading causes of death in Canada, 2008*. Ottawa, ON: Author.

Transport Canada. (2011a). *Car seats, seatbelts, and your child—Keep kids safe, Stage 1:* Rear-facing seats. Retrieved from http://www.tc.gc.ca/eng/roadsafety/safedrivers-childsafety-car-time-stage1-1084.htm

Transport Canada. (2011b). *Car seats, seatbelts, and your child—Keep kids safe, Stage 2: Forward-facing seats*. Retrieved from http://www.tc.gc.ca/eng/roadsafety/safedrivers-childsafety-stage2-forward-facing-1085.htm

Transport Canada. (2011c). *Car seats, seatbelts, and your child—Keep kids safe, Stage 3: Booster seats*. Retrieved from http://www.tc.gc.ca/eng/roadsafety/safedrivers-childsafety-stage3-booster-seats-1086.htm

World Health Organization. (2008). *World report on child injury prevention*. Geneva, Switzerland: Author.

Chapter 33

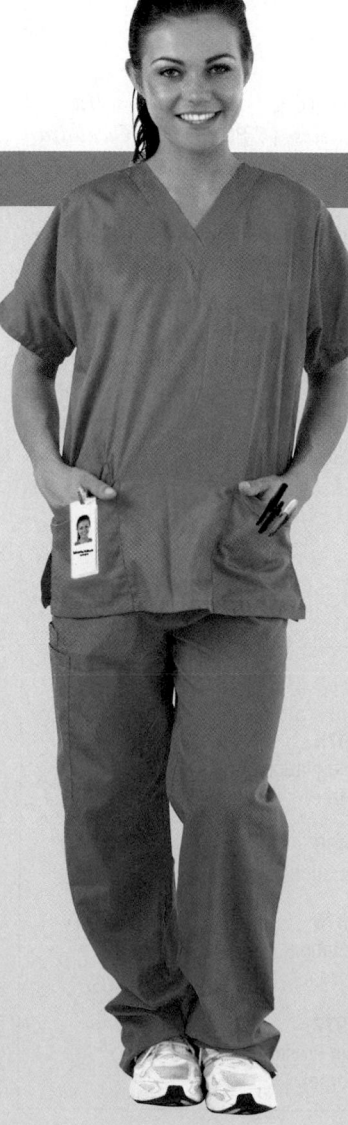

Medications

LEARNING OUTCOMES

After studying this chapter, you will be able to:

1. Define selected terms related to the administration of medications.

2. Identify physiological factors and individual variables affecting medication action.

3. Describe the various routes of medication administration.

4. Identify the essential parts of a medication order.

5. Describe three methods for calculating drug dosages.

6. List six essential steps to follow when administering medications.

7. State the 10 "rights" to accurate medication administration.

8. Describe the physiological changes in older adults that alter medication administration and effectiveness.

9. Outline the steps required for nasogastric or gastrostomy tube medication administration.

10. Describe the essential steps in safely administering parenteral medications by subcutaneous, intramuscular, intradermal, and intravenous routes.

11. Describe the essential steps in safely administering topical medications: dermatological, ophthalmic, otic, nasal, rectal, vaginal, and respiratory inhalation preparations.

Pharmacology is the study of the effect of drugs on living organisms. **Pharmacy** is the art of preparing, compounding, and dispensing drugs. The word also refers to the place where drugs are prepared and dispensed. The licensed **pharmacist** prepares, makes, and dispenses drugs as ordered by the physician, dentist, nurse practitioner, and other health care professionals, on the basis of provincial or territorial legislation. A clinical pharmacist is a specialist who often guides the physician in prescribing drugs.

A **drug** is any chemical that affects physiological processes. A **medication** is a substance administered for the prevention, diagnosis, cure, treatment, or relief of a symptom or disease. In the health care context, the words *medication* and *drug* are generally used interchangeably. Given that many people associate "drugs" with illicitly obtained substances such as marijuana or cocaine, clients will often state that they take "medications" rather than "drugs." Medications have been known and used since antiquity. Crude drugs, such as opium, castor oil, and vinegar, were used in ancient times to treat disease. Over the centuries, the number of medications available has increased greatly, and knowledge about these drugs has become correspondingly more accurate and detailed.

Key Concepts in Pharmacology

In Canada, medications are usually dispensed on the order of physicians and dentists or other health care professionals who have prescribing authority, such as nurse practitioners. The written direction for the preparation and administration of a drug is called a **prescription**. One drug can have as many as four kinds of names: its generic name, official name, chemical name, and trademark or brand name. The **generic name** is assigned before a drug becomes official. The generic name is approved by Health Canada under the Food and Drug Regulations. The **trade name** (sometimes called the **brand name**) is the name given by the drug manufacturer, which means that the drug has a registered trademark and patent and is the property of that company. The name selected is usually short and easy to remember. A patent gives the manufacturing company the exclusive right to sell the drug for 20 years in Canada. The trade name is identified by manufacturers with the symbol ™ or ® in the upper right corner of the name (for example, Aspirin®). When the drug is no longer protected by patent, the company may market its product under either the generic or trade name. Other companies that wish to market the off-patent drug must use the same generic name but can produce their own trade name. Consequently, one drug may be manufactured by several companies and have several trade names. For example, the drug hydrochlorothiazide (generic name) is known by the trade names Aldactazide and Apo-Hydro. The **official name** is the name under which a drug is listed in one of the official publications (e.g., the *Compendium of Pharmaceuticals and Specialties* [CPS], the *Canadian Formulary*). The **chemical name** is the name by which a chemist knows it; this name describes the chemical constituents and molecular structure of the drug precisely. The chemical name of Aspirin, for example, is acetylsalicylic acid. Each drug evaluated by Health Canada Therapeutic Products Directorate and approved for sale in Canada receives an eight-digit Drug Identification Number (DIN). This number is found on the label of all prescription and over-the-counter drugs (OTCs) as well as natural health products. See Figure 33.1.

Medications are often available in a variety of forms (Table 33.1).

Hepatitis B Vaccine

DIN: 02243576
Pediatric Presentation
(thimerosal-free)

DIN: 00749486
Adult Presentation

DIN: 02243676
Adult Presentation
(thimerosal-free)

DIN: 02245977
Adult Dialysis Presentation
(thimerosal-free)

FIGURE 33.1 Drug Identification Number.

TABLE 33.1 Types of Medication Preparations

Type	Description	Type	Description
Aerosol spray or foam	A liquid, powder, or foam deposited in a thin layer on skin by air pressure	Lozenge (troche)	A flat, round, or oval preparation that dissolves and releases a drug when held in the mouth
Aqueous solution	One or more drugs dissolved in water	Ointment (salve, unction)	A semisolid preparation of one or more drugs used for application to skin and mucous membranes
Aqueous suspension	One or more drugs dispersed in a liquid, such as water	Paste	A preparation like an ointment, but thicker and stiff, that penetrates skin less than an ointment
Caplet	A solid form, shaped like a capsule, coated and easily swallowed	Pill	One or more drugs mixed with a cohesive material, in oval, round, or flattened shapes
Capsule	A gelatinous container to hold a drug in powder, liquid, or oil form	Powder	A finely ground drug or drugs; some are used internally, others externally
Cream	A nongreasy, semisolid preparation used on skin	Suppository	One or several drugs mixed with a firm base, such as gelatin, and shaped for insertion into the body (e.g., the rectum); the base dissolves gradually at body temperature, releasing the drug
Elixir	A sweetened and aromatic solution of alcohol used as a vehicle for medicinal agents	Syrup	An aqueous solution of sugar often used to disguise unpleasant-tasting drugs
Extract	A concentrated form of a drug made from vegetables or animals	Tablet	A powdered drug compressed into a hard small disc; some are readily broken along a scored line; others are enteric coated to prevent them from dissolving in the stomach
Gel or jelly	A clear or translucent semisolid that liquefies when applied to skin	Tincture	An alcoholic or water-and-alcohol solution prepared from drugs derived from plants
Liniment	A medication mixed with alcohol, oil, or soapy emollient and applied to skin	Transdermal disc or patch	A semipermeable membrane shaped in the form of a disc or patch that contains a drug to be absorbed through skin over a long period
Lotion	A medication in a liquid suspension applied to skin		

Drug Standards

Drugs vary in strength and activity. Drugs derived from plants, for example, vary in strength according to the age of the plant, the variety, the place in which it is grown, and the method by which it is preserved. Drugs must be pure and of uniform strength if drug dosages are to be predictable in their effect. Drug standards have therefore been developed to ensure uniform quality. In Canada, official drugs are those so designated by the Canadian Federal Food, Drug, and Cosmetic Act. There is a trend for people to purchase natural health products from health food stores or over the counter (OTC) at pharmacies. An example of this is a thyroid supplement. The natural form varies in strength and is difficult to regulate, whereas the synthetic thyroid is much more predictable in strength and management of symptoms for clients who need to take a thyroid supplement.

Legal Aspects of Drug Administration

Within Canada, laws have been enacted to control the development and administration of drugs. Table 33.2 on the next page provides a summary of Canadian drug

TABLE 33.2 Canadian Medication Legislation

Legislation	Content
Proprietary or Patent Medicine Act (1908)	Protects the public against unsafe and ineffective over-the-counter drugs
Canada Food and Drugs Act (1953)	Responsible for the regulation of drugs in Canada; prohibits advertising any food, drug, cosmetic, or device as a cure for certain specified diseases; sets standards for manufacture, distribution, and sale of all drugs, with the exception of opioids
Canadian Narcotic Control Act (1961)	Allows only authorized people to possess opioids; specifies records about opioids that must be kept
Controlled Drugs and Substances Act (1996)	The Controlled Drugs and Substances Act replaced the former Canadian Narcotic Control Act. Regulations regarding possession, sale, manufacture, production, and distribution of opioids are all covered in the Controlled Drugs and Substances Act. Health Canada is responsible for the administration of policies, and the Royal Canadian Mounted Police enforce the act.
Marijuana Medical Access Regulations (2001)	Canada is the first country to allow legal access to cannabis for medicinal purposes. In 2005, Canada was the first country to approve Sativex for the use of neuropathic pain in multiple sclerosis. Since 2005, selected Canadian pharmacies have been allowed to distribute medicinal marijuana for use by MMAR authorized clients. This initiative makes Canada the second country (after the Netherlands) to allow access to medical marijuana in pharmacies.
Natural Health Products Regulations (2004)	Ensures that natural health products are safe, effective, and of high quality

legislation. Nurses need to (a) know how nursing practice acts in their jurisdictions define and limit their functions and (b) be able to recognize the limits of their own knowledge and skill. To function beyond the limits of nursing practice acts or one's ability is to endanger clients' lives and leave oneself open to malpractice lawsuits. Under the law, nurses are responsible for their own actions, regardless of whether there is a written order. If the prescribing health care professional writes an incorrect order (e.g., digoxin 25 mg, instead of digoxin 0.25 mg), *a nurse who administers the written incorrect dosage is responsible for the error as well as the prescribing health care professional.* Therefore, nurses should question any order that appears unreasonable and refuse to give the medication until the order is clarified.

Another aspect of nursing practice governed by law is the use of controlled substances. In hospitals, controlled substances are kept in a locked drawer, cupboard, medication cart, or computer-controlled dispensing system. Agencies may have special inventory forms for recording the use of controlled substances. The information required usually includes the name of the client, the date and time of administration, the name of the drug, the dosage, and the signature of the person who prepared and gave the drug. The name of the prescribing health care professional who ordered the drug may also be part of the record. Some agencies may require a verifying signature of another registered nurse for administration of a controlled substance. Most agencies maintain a list of **high-alert medications** (medications that carry a high risk of harming the patient when they are used in error), including controlled substances, which require the verification of two registered nurses. Before removing a controlled substance, the nurse verifies the number actually available with the number indicated on the narcotic or controlled substance inventory record (Figure 33.2). If the number is not the same, the nurse must investigate and correct the discrepancy before proceeding. Any portion or all of a controlled substance dose that

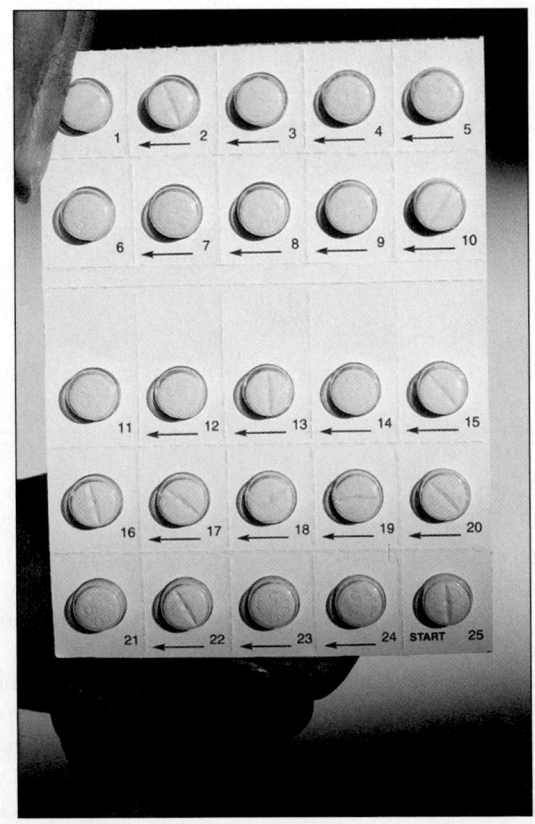

FIGURE 33.2 Some narcotics are kept in specially designed packages or plastic containers that are sectioned and numbered.

is discarded must be witnessed and documented by both nurses. In most agencies, counts of controlled substances are also taken at the end of each shift. If the count is not accurate and the discrepancy cannot be resolved, it must be reported immediately to the appropriate person, according to agency policy. Computerized dispensing systems generally run a continuous count; however, discrepancies must be accounted for.

Effects of Drugs

The **therapeutic effect** of a drug, also referred to as the **desired effect**, is the primary effect intended, that is, the reason the drug is prescribed. For example, the therapeutic effect of morphine sulphate is analgesia, and the therapeutic effect of diazepam is relief of anxiety. See Table 33.3 for kinds of therapeutic actions.

An **adverse effect**, or **secondary (side) effect**, of a drug is one that is unintended and undesired. Adverse effects are usually predictable and are either harmless or potentially harmful. For example, digitalis has a positive *inotropic effect* (increases the strength of myocardial contractions), which is a desired effect; however, it can have the adverse effect of causing *bradycardia* (decreasing the heart rate too much). Some adverse effects are tolerated for the drug's therapeutic effect. Sometimes, a medication is given because of its adverse effect; for example, minoxidil (Rogaine), an antihypertensive agent, is used for its *side* effect of stimulating hair growth. Intolerable or severe adverse effects may justify the discontinuation of a drug. The nurse should monitor for dose-related adverse effects and report these to the prescriber who may discontinue the medication or change the dosage.

Drug toxicity, deleterious effects of a drug on an organism or a tissue, results from overdosage, ingestion of a drug intended for external use, or buildup of the drug in the blood because of impaired metabolism or excretion (cumulative effect). Some toxic effects are apparent immediately; some are not apparent for weeks or months. Fortunately, most drug toxicity is avoidable if careful attention is paid to dosage and client monitoring for toxicity. An example of a toxic effect is respiratory depression caused by the cumulative effect of morphine sulphate in the body.

A **drug allergy** is an immunological reaction to a drug. When a person is first exposed to an antigen (foreign substance), the body may react by producing antibodies. A drug can be antigenic and induce an allergic reaction. A person can react to a drug in the same manner as to an antigen and thus develop symptoms of an allergic reaction.

Allergic reactions can be either mild or severe. A mild reaction has a variety of symptoms, from skin rashes to diarrhea (Table 33.4 on the next page). An allergic reaction can occur from a few minutes to 2 weeks after the administration of the drug. A severe allergic reaction usually occurs immediately after the administration of the drug and is called an **anaphylactic reaction**. This response can be fatal if the symptoms are not noticed immediately and treatment is not obtained promptly. The earliest symptoms are a subjective feeling of swelling in the mouth and tongue, acute shortness of breath, acute hypotension, and tachycardia.

Drug tolerance exists in a person who has unusually low physiological response to a drug and who requires increases in the dosage to maintain a given therapeutic effect. Drugs that commonly produce tolerance are opiates, barbiturates, and ethyl alcohol. A **cumulative effect** is the increasing response to repeated doses of a drug that occurs when the rate of administration exceeds the rate of metabolism or excretion. As a result, the amount of the drug builds up in the client's body unless the dosage is adjusted. Toxic symptoms can occur. An **idiosyncratic effect** is one that is unexpected and may be individual to a client. Underresponse and overresponse to a drug may be idiosyncratic. Also, the drug may have a completely different effect from the normal one or cause unpredictable and unexplainable symptoms in a particular client.

A **drug interaction** occurs when the administration of one drug before, at the same time as, or after another drug alters the effect of one or both drugs. Drug interactions may be beneficial or harmful. The effect of one or both drugs may be either increased (**potentiating effect**)

TABLE 33.3 Therapeutic Actions of Drugs

Drug Type	Description	Examples
Curative	Cures a disease or condition	Penicillin (for infection)
Chemotherapeutic	Destroys malignant cells	Methotrexate for leukemia
Palliative	Relieves the symptoms of a disease but does not affect the disease itself	Morphine sulphate, acetaminophen (for pain)
Restorative	Returns the body to health	Vitamin, mineral supplements
Supportive	Supports body function until other treatments or the body's response can take over	Norepinephrine bitartrate (for low blood pressure), acetaminophen (for high body temperature)
Substitutive	Replaces bodily fluids or substances	Thyroxine (for hypothyroidism), insulin (for diabetes mellitus)

TABLE 33.4 Mild Allergic Responses

Symptom	Description/Rationale
Skin rash	Either an intraepidermal vesicle rash or a rash typified by an urticarial wheal or macular eruption; rash is usually generalized over the body
Pruritus	Itching of the skin with or without a rash
Angioedema	Edema caused by increased permeability of the blood capillaries
Rhinitis	Excessive watery discharge from the nose
Lacrimal tearing	Excessive tearing
Nausea, vomiting	Stimulation of these centres in the brain
Wheezing and dyspnea	Shortness of breath and wheezing on inhalation and exhalation caused by accumulated fluids and swelling of the respiratory tissues
Diarrhea	Irritation of the mucosa of the large intestine

or decreased (**inhibiting effect**). Potentiating effects may be additive or synergistic. When two of the same types of drug increase the action of each other, it is known as an **additive effect**. A **synergistic effect** occurs when two different drugs given together increase the action of one of the drugs. For example, probenecid, which blocks the excretion of penicillin, can be given with penicillin to increase blood levels of the penicillin for longer periods (synergistic effect). Two analgesics, such as acetaminophen and codeine, are often given together because together they provide greater pain relief (additive effect). In addition, certain foods may interact adversely with a medication (see Table 40.2 in Chapter 40).

Iatrogenic disease, disease caused unintentionally by medical therapy, can be due to drug therapy. Hepatic toxicity resulting in biliary obstruction, renal damage, and malformations of the fetus as a result of specific drugs taken during pregnancy are examples.

Drug Misuse

Drug misuse is the improper use of common medications in ways that lead to acute and chronic toxicity. Both OTC drugs and prescription drugs may be misused. Laxatives, antacids, vitamins, headache remedies, and cough and cold medications are often self-prescribed and overused. Most people suffer no harmful effects from these drugs, but some people do. For example, a client might use an OTC cough medicine to treat a cough that might be caused by a serious underlying problem, such as throat cancer.

Drug abuse (sometimes referred to as **problematic substance use**) is an inappropriate intake of a substance, either continually or periodically. By definition, drug use is abusive when society considers it abusive. For example, the intake of alcohol at work may be considered alcohol abuse, but intake at a social gathering may not. Drug abuse has two main facets: (a) drug dependence and (b) drug habituation. **Drug dependence** is a person's reliance on or need to take a drug or substance. Drug dependence comes in two types: *psychological* and *physical*. **Physiological dependence** is caused by biochemical changes in body tissues, especially in the nervous system. These tissues come to require the substance for normal functioning. A dependent person who stops using the drug experiences withdrawal symptoms. **Psychological dependence** is emotional reliance on a drug to maintain a sense of well-being, accompanied by feelings of need or cravings for that drug. There are varying degrees of psychological dependence, ranging from mild desire to craving and compulsive use of the drug.

Drug habituation denotes a mild form of psychological dependence. The individual develops the habit of taking the substance and feels better after taking it. The habituated individual tends to continue the habit even though it may be injurious to health.

Illicit drugs, or *street drugs*, are those sold illegally. Illicit drugs are of two types: (a) drugs unavailable for purchase under any circumstances, such as heroin (in Canada); and (b) drugs normally available with a prescription that are being obtained through illegal channels. Illicit drugs often are taken because of their mood-altering effect; that is, they make the person feel happy or relaxed.

Actions of Drugs in the Body

The action of a drug in the body relates to its pharmacodynamics and pharmacokinetics.

Pharmacodynamics

Pharmacodynamics is the mechanism of drug action and relationships between drug concentration and the body's responses. Such responses require that the drug interact with specific molecules and chemicals normally found in the body (Adams & Koch, 2010). A **receptor** is the drug's specific target, usually a protein located on the surface of a cell membrane or within the cell. As the drug binds to the receptor, it enhances or inhibits the normal cellular function. The binding is usually reversible and the action of the drug terminated once the drug leaves the receptor.

Most drugs exert their effects by chemically binding with receptors at the cellular level. When a drug binds to its receptor, the pharmacological effects are either *agonism* or *antagonism*. When a drug produces the same type of response as the physiological or endogenous substance, it is referred to as an **agonist**. For example, epinephrine-like drugs act on the heart to increase heart rate. Conversely, a drug that inhibits cell function by occupying receptor sites is called an **antagonist**. The antagonist prevents natural body substances or other drugs from activating the functions of the cell by occupying the receptor sites. For example, naloxone (Narcan) is an opioid antagonist used as an antidote for respiratory depression caused by an opioid drug (e.g., morphine). This drug competes with opioid receptor sites in the brain and thereby prevents the opioid from binding to its receptors. By blocking the effect of the opioid, respiratory depression is reversed.

Pharmacokinetics

Pharmacokinetics is the study of the absorption, distribution, biotransformation, and excretion of drugs.

ABSORPTION

Absorption is the process by which a drug passes into the bloodstream. Unless the drug is administered directly into the bloodstream, absorption is the first step in the movement of the drug through the body. For absorption of a drug to occur, the correct form of the drug must be given by the correct route. The rate of absorption of a drug in the stomach is variable. Food, for example, can delay the dissolution and absorption of some drugs as well as their passage into the small intestine, where most drug absorption occurs. Food can also combine with molecules of certain drugs, thereby changing their molecular structure and subsequently inhibiting or preventing their absorption. The acidity of the stomach can also affect the absorption of some drugs. The absorption of some drugs can occur in the tissues of the mouth prior to reaching the stomach. For example, nitroglycerin is administered under the tongue or as a buccal spray, where it is absorbed into the blood vessels that carry it directly to the heart, the intended site of action. If swallowed, this drug will be absorbed into the bloodstream and carried to the liver, where it will be destroyed. The **first-pass effect** occurs when oral drugs first pass through the liver and are partially metabolized prior to reaching the target organ. This requires higher oral doses to achieve the appropriate effect.

A drug administered directly into the bloodstream, that is, intravenously, is immediately in the vascular system without having to be absorbed. This, then, is the route of choice for rapid action. The intramuscular route is the next most rapid route because of the highly vascular nature of muscle tissue. Because subcutaneous tissue has a poorer blood supply compared with muscle tissue, absorption from subcutaneous tissue is slower. The rate of absorption of a drug can be accelerated by the application of heat, which increases blood flow to the area; conversely, absorption can be slowed by the application of cold. In addition, the injection of a vasoconstrictor drug, such as epinephrine, into the tissue can slow absorption of other drugs. Some drugs intended to be absorbed slowly are suspended in a low-solubility medium, such as oil. The absorption of drugs from the rectum into the bloodstream tends to be unpredictable. Therefore, this route is normally used when other routes are unavailable or when the intended action is localized to the rectum or sigmoid colon.

DISTRIBUTION

Distribution is the transportation of a drug from its site of absorption to its site of action. When a drug enters the bloodstream, it is carried to the most vascular organs—that is, liver, kidneys, and brain. Body areas with lower blood supply—that is, skin and muscles—receive the drug later. The chemical and physical properties of a drug largely determine the area of the body to which the drug will be attracted. For example, fat-soluble drugs accumulate in fatty tissue, whereas other drugs bind with plasma proteins.

BIOTRANSFORMATION

Biotransformation, also called **detoxification** or **metabolism**, is a process by which a drug is converted to a less active form. Most biotransformation takes place in the liver, where many drug-metabolizing enzymes in the cells detoxify the drugs. The products of this process are called **metabolites**. There are two types of metabolites: *active* and *inactive*. An *active metabolite* has a pharmacological action, whereas an *inactive metabolite* does not.

Biotransformation may be altered if a person is a child, is an older adult, or has an unhealthy liver. Nurses must be alert to the accumulation of the active drug in these clients and to subsequent toxicity.

EXCRETION

Excretion is the process by which metabolites and drugs are eliminated from the body. Most drug metabolites are eliminated by the kidneys in the urine; however, some are excreted in feces, breath, perspiration, saliva, and breast milk. Certain drugs, such as general anesthetic agents, are excreted in an unchanged form via the respiratory tract. The efficiency with which the kidneys excrete drugs and metabolites diminishes with age. Older adults may require smaller doses of a drug because the drug and its metabolites may accumulate in the body.

Key terms related to pharmacokinetics include:

- **Onset of action**: The time after administration when the body initially responds to the drug
- **Peak plasma level**: The highest plasma level achieved by a single dose when the elimination rate of a drug equals the absorption rate
- **Half-life**: The time required for the elimination process to reduce the concentration of the drug to one half what it was at initial administration—for example, if a drug's half-life is 8 hours, then the amount of drug in the body is as follows:

  - Initially: 100%
  - After 8 hours: 50%
  - After 16 hours: 25%
  - After 24 hours: 12.5%
  - After 32 hours: 6.25%

- **Plateau (steady state)**: A maintained concentration of a drug in the plasma whereby the amount of drug removed by processes of elimination equals the amount of drug absorbed with each dose administered

When an orally administered drug is absorbed from the gastrointestinal tract into the blood plasma, its concentration in the plasma increases until the elimination rate equals the rate of absorption. This point is known as the *peak plasma level* (Figure 33.3). When a drug is given intravenously (IV), its level is high immediately after administration and decreases through time. Another dose is given in order to maintain therapeutic levels. If the client does not receive another dose of the drug (either orally or IV), the concentration steadily decreases. Because the purpose of most drug therapy is to maintain a constant drug level in the body (i.e., plateau or steady state), repeated doses are required to maintain that level. The frequency of the doses will vary with the half-life of the drug.

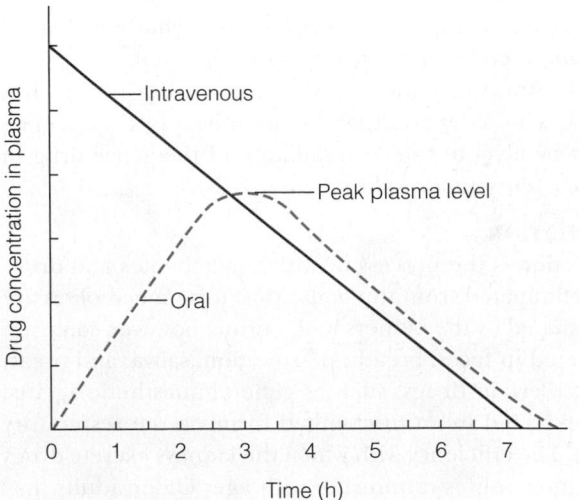

FIGURE 33.3 A graphic plot of drug concentration in the blood plasma following a single dose.

Factors Affecting Medication Action

A number of factors other than the drug can affect its action. A person may not respond in the same manner to successive doses of a drug. In addition, the identical drug and dosage may affect different clients differently. A number of factors other than the drug itself can affect its action.

Developmental Factors

Drugs taken during pregnancy pose a risk throughout the pregnancy, but they pose the highest risk during the first trimester because of the formation of vital organs and functions of the fetus during this time. Most drugs are contraindicated because of the possible adverse effects on the fetus.

Infants usually require smaller drug dosages because of their body size and the immaturity of their organs, especially the liver and kidneys. Differences in gastric acidity and liver enzymes required for drug metabolism may require different medication choices and dosages than adults. In adolescence or adulthood, allergic reactions may occur to drugs formerly tolerated.

Older adults have different responses to medications due to physiological changes that accompany aging. These changes include decreased liver and kidney function, which can result in the accumulation of the drug in the body. In addition, the older person may be on multiple drugs, and drug incompatibilities may occur. Older adults often experience decreased gastric mobility and decreased gastric acid production and blood flow, which can impair drug absorption. Increased adipose tissue and decreased total bodily fluid proportionate to the body mass can increase the possibility of drug toxicity. Older adults may also have a decreased number of protein-binding sites and changes in the blood–brain barrier. The latter permits fat-soluble drugs to move readily to the brain, often resulting in dizziness and confusion. This is particularly evident with beta (β)–blockers.

Sex

Differences in the way men and women respond to drugs are chiefly related to the distribution of body fat and fluid and hormonal differences. Historically, because most drug research was done on men, more research on women is required to reflect the effects of hormonal changes on drug actions in women.

Genetic and Ethnic Factors

A client's response to a drug can be influenced by genetic and ethnic factors. **Pharmacogenetics**, the study of how the actions of and reactions to drugs vary with the individual's genes, has determined that drug metabolism and variations in enzymes are genetically determined. For example, the genes that control metabolic cytochromes in the liver vary from one individual to another based on their genetic makeup. The individual genetic variation in liver enzymes, in particular P450-2C9, explains why some people who are prescribed the anticoagulant warfarin metabolize the drug very slowly thus requiring a low dose. Genetic differences in cytochromes have also been linked to how individuals metabolize codeine (an analgesic) and isoniazid (a drug used in the treatment of tuberculosis). Researchers continue to learn about cytochromes, especially the genetic variation that seems to account for differences in how medications are metabolized (Greener, 2009, p. 110). For example, some clients may have slow liver metabolism and not achieve an adequate response to a medication, whereas others are rapid metabolizers and may require lower doses of a medication to avoid adverse reactions. A genetic blood test can analyze genes in a client's blood to determine if they could cause variations in the metabolism of certain drugs. This information can help health care providers to individualize medication treatment and avoid adverse reactions.

Ethnopharmacology is the study of the effect of racial and ethnic differences or responses to prescribed medication. For example, certain medications may work well at usual therapeutic dosages for certain ethnic groups but may be toxic for others. Ethnopharmacology also incorporates pharmacogenetics, which is the study of the genetic ability to produce enzymes that affect drug metabolism. Pharmacogenetics can also vary by race or ethnic group. Examples of how the effects of certain medications vary with ethnicity include isoniazid (INH), hydralazine hydrochloride (Apresoline), procainamide (Pronestyl), and caffeine, which metabolize slowly in Scandinavians, Jews, Northern Africans, and Caucasians and rapidly in Japanese; amitriptyline (Elavil), imipramine (Tofranil), perphenazine, haloperidol (Haldol), propranolol (Inderal), metoprolol (Lopressor), codeine, morphine, diazepam (Valium), barbiturates, and warfarin (Coumadin), which are metabolized slowly in Asians and blacks. Cultural factors and practices (e.g., values and beliefs) can also affect a drug's action. For example, a natural health product used in certain cultures (e.g., the Chinese herb ginseng) may speed up or slow down the metabolism of prescribed medications.

Diet

Nutrients can affect the action of a medication. For example, vitamin K, found in green leafy vegetables, can counteract the effect of an anticoagulant, such as warfarin. See Table 40.2 in Chapter 40.

Environment

The client's environment can affect the action of drugs, particularly those used to alter behaviour and mood.

Therefore, nurses assessing the effects of a drug need to consider the drug in the context of the client's personality and surroundings.

Environmental temperature may also affect drug activity. When environmental temperature is high, the peripheral blood vessels dilate, thus intensifying the action of vasodilators. In contrast, a cold environment and the subsequent vasoconstriction inhibit the action of vasodilators but enhance the action of vasoconstrictors. A person who takes a sedative or analgesic in a busy, noisy environment may not benefit as fully as when the environment is quiet and peaceful.

Psychological Factors

A person's expectations about what a drug can do can affect the response to the medication. For example, a client who believes that codeine is ineffective as an analgesic may experience no relief from pain after it is given.

Illness and Disease

Illness and disease can also affect the action of drugs. For example, acetaminophen can reduce the body temperature of a person with fever but has no effect on the body temperature of a person without fever. Drug action is altered in people with circulatory, liver, or kidney dysfunction.

Time of Administration

The time of administration of oral medications affects the relative speed with which they act. Some orally administered medications are absorbed more quickly if the stomach is empty, whereas, other medications have a more rapid absorption when administered with food. For example, the anti-infective drug ampicillin is absorbed more rapidly on an empty stomach, whereas the antidepressant trazodone hydrochloride is absorbed more rapidly with food. Iron supplements are known to cause gastrointestinal irritation. Gastrointestinal irritation can be reduced by administering the iron supplement after a meal.

Routes of Administration

Pharmaceutical preparations are generally designed for one or two specific routes of administration (Table 33.5 on the next page). The route of administration should be indicated when the drug is ordered. When administering a drug, the nurse should ensure that the pharmaceutical preparation is appropriate for the route specified.

TABLE 33.5 Routes of Administration and Selected Advantages and Disadvantages

Route	Advantages	Disadvantages
Oral	Most convenient Usually least expensive Safe, does not break the skin barrier Administration usually does not cause stress	Inappropriate for clients with nausea or vomiting Drug may have unpleasant taste or odour Inappropriate when gastrointestinal tract has reduced motility Inappropriate if client cannot swallow or is unconscious Cannot be used before certain diagnostic tests or surgical procedures Drug may discolour teeth, harm tooth enamel Drug may irritate gastric mucosa Drug can be aspirated by clients with serious illnesses
Sublingual	Same as for oral, *plus* Drug can be administered for local effect Drug is rapidly absorbed into the bloodstream More potent than oral route because drug directly enters the blood and bypasses the liver	If swallowed, drug may be inactivated by gastric secretions Drug must remain under the tongue until dissolved and absorbed
Buccal	Same as for sublingual	Drug must remain against the cheek until dissolved and absorbed
Subcutaneous	Onset of drug action is faster than oral	Must involve sterile technique because it breaks the skin barrier More expensive than oral Only small volume can be administered Slower absorption than intramuscular administration Some drugs can irritate tissues and cause pain Can be anxiety producing
Intramuscular	Pain from irritating drugs is minimized Can administer larger volume than subcutaneous Drug is rapidly absorbed	Breaks the skin barrier Can be anxiety producing Can cause discomfort Obese clients may receive subcutaneous injection if needle is not long enough
Intradermal	Absorption is slow (this is an advantage in testing for allergies)	Amount of drug administered must be small Breaks the skin barrier
Intravenous	Rapid effect	Limited to highly soluble drugs Drug distribution inhibited by poor circulation Irretrievable if there is an administration error
Rectal	Can be used when drug has objectionable taste or odour Drug released at slow, steady rate	Dose absorbed is unpredictable May be perceived as unpleasant by client
Vaginal	Provides local therapeutic effect	Limited use
Topical	Provides a local effect Few adverse effects	May be messy and may soil clothes Drug can enter body through abrasions and cause systemic effects
Transdermal	Prolonged systemic effect Few adverse effects Avoids gastrointestinal absorption problems	Leaves residue on skin, thus soiling clothes
Inhalation	Introduces drug throughout respiratory tract Rapid localized relief Drug can be administered to unconscious client	Drug intended for localized effect can have systemic effect Of use only for the respiratory system

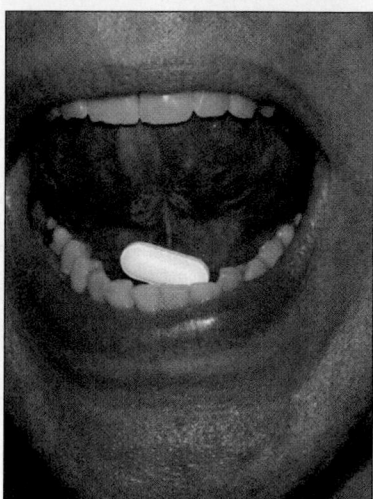

FIGURE 33.4 Sublingual administration of a tablet.

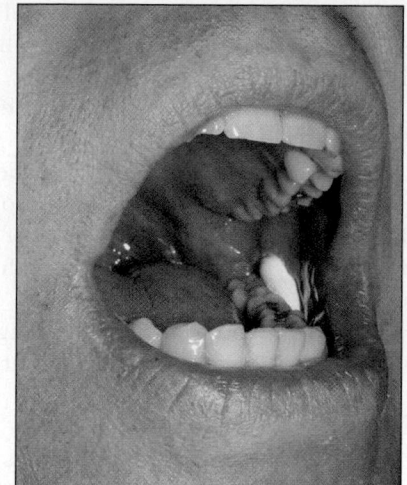

FIGURE 33.5 Buccal administration of a tablet.

Oral

Oral administration is the most common, least expensive, and most convenient **enteral** (by way of the gastrointestinal tract) route for most clients. In oral administration, the drug is swallowed. Because skin is not broken as it is for an injection, oral administration is also a safe method. The major disadvantages can include an unpleasant taste of the drugs, irritation of the gastric mucosa, irregular absorption from the gastrointestinal tract, slow absorption, and, in some cases, harm to the client's teeth. For example, the liquid preparation of ferrous sulphate (iron) can stain teeth. In **sublingual** administration, a drug is placed under the tongue where it dissolves (Figure 33.4). In a relatively short time, the drug is largely absorbed into the blood vessels on the underside of the tongue. The medication should not be swallowed. Nitroglycerin is one example of a drug commonly given in this manner.

Buccal

Buccal means "pertaining to the cheek." In buccal administration, a medication (e.g., a tablet) is held in the mouth against the mucous membranes of the cheek until the drug dissolves (Figure 33.5). The drug may act locally on the mucous membranes of the mouth or systemically, such as buccal fentanyl, when it is swallowed with saliva.

Parenteral

The **parenteral** route is defined as other than through the alimentary or respiratory tract; that is, by injection. The following are some of the more common routes for parenteral administration:

- **Subcutaneous**: into the subcutaneous tissue, just below skin

- **Intramuscular** (IM): into a muscle
- **Intradermal** (ID): under the epidermis (into the dermis)
- **Intravenous** (IV): into a vein

Some of the less commonly used routes for parenteral administration are **intra-arterial** (into an artery), **intracardiac** (into the heart muscle), **intraosseous** (into a bone), **intrathecal** or **intraspinal** (into the spinal canal), **intrapleural** (into the pleural space), **epidural** (into the epidural space), and **intra-articular** (into a joint). Sterile equipment and sterile drug solution are essential for all parenteral therapy. The main advantage of parenteral administration is fast absorption.

Topical

Topical applications are those applied to a circumscribed surface area of the body. They affect only the area to which they are applied. Topical applications include the following:

- *Dermatological preparations:* applied to skin
- *Instillations and irrigations:* applied into body cavities or orifices, such as the urinary bladder, eyes, ears, nose, rectum, or vagina
- *Inhalations:* administered into the respiratory tract by a nebulizer or positive pressure breathing apparatus.

Air, oxygen, and vapour are generally used to carry the drug into the lungs

Medication Order

A physician usually determines the client's medication needs and orders medications, although in some settings nurse practitioners now order some drugs as determined by their provincial or territorial scope of practice. Also, each health care agency will have its own policies. Usually, the order is written, although telephone and verbal orders are acceptable in some agencies (see the Clinical Alert box about verbal or telephone medication orders). Nursing students need to know the agency policies about medication orders. Students should recognize the importance of checking doctor's orders prior to administering any drug. Solid guidelines must be in place to reduce or eliminate errors stemming from verbal orders. Nursing practice standards set out the requirements for registered nurses

CLINICAL ALERT

Given the client safety risks associated with verbal or telephone medication orders, most health care agencies have strict policies and procedures related to their use. General procedures related to ensuring safety when verbal or telephone orders are used include the following: The nurse ascertains the full name of the client; writes down the details of the order on the order sheet in the correct client's chart or file, including the date, time, details of the order (i.e., generic name of drug, dose, route); reads the order back to the prescriber to ensure accuracy; records the prescriber's name; and signs the entry. Many agencies require that TWO nurses listen to the order and that the telephone or verbal order be signed by the prescriber within a specified time frame.

TABLE 33.6 Do Not Use: Dangerous Abbreviations, Symbols, and Dose Designations

Abbreviation	Intended Meaning	Potential Problem	Correction
U	Unit	Mistaken for "0" (zero), "4" (four), or cc	Use "unit."
IU	International unit	Mistaken for "IV" (intravenous) or "10" (ten)	Use "unit."
Abbreviations for drug names		Misinterpreted because of similar abbreviations of multiple drugs: e.g., MS, MSO_4 (morphine sulphate), $MgSO_4$ (magnesium sulphate) may be confused for one another	Do not abbreviate drug names.
QD	Every day	QD and QOD (every other day) have been mistaken for each other, or as "QID" (four times a day); the Q has also been misinterpreted as "2" (two)	Use "daily" and "every other day."
QOD	Every other day		
OD	Every day	Mistaken for "right eye" (OD = oculus dexter).	Use "daily."
OS, OD, OU	Left eye, right eye, both eyes	May be confused with one another.	Use "left eye," "right eye," or "both eyes."
D/C	Discharge	Interpreted as "discontinue whatever medications follow" (typically discharge medications)	Use "discharge."
cc	Cubic centimetre	Mistaken for "u" (units).	Use "mL" or "millilitre."
μg	Microgram	Mistaken for "mg" (milligram) resulting in 1000-fold overdose.	Use "mcg."
Symbol	Intended Meaning	Potential Problem	Correction
@	At	Mistaken for "2" (two) or "5" (five).	Use "at."
>	Greater than	Mistaken for "7" (seven) or the letter "L."	Use "greater than" / "more than."
<	Less than	Confused with "greater than."	Use "less than" / "lower than."
Dose Designation	Intended Meaning	Potential Problem	Correction
Trailing zero	x.0 mg	Decimal point is overlooked resulting in a 10-fold dose error (e.g., 3.0 mg is interpreted as 30 mg).	Never use a zero by itself after a decimal point. Use "x mg."
Lack of leading zero	.x mg	Decimal point is overlooked resulting in a 10-fold dose error (e.g., .3 mg is interpreted as 3 mg).	Always use a zero before a decimal point. Use "0.x mg."

Source: Reprinted with permission from ISMP Canada.

to accept telephone and verbal orders. For example, for all verbal or telephone orders the nurse must first write down the order and then read it back, verbatim, to the prescriber.

Policies about the ordering of medications vary considerably from agency to agency. For example, a client's medications may be automatically cancelled after surgery, after which new orders must be written. Most agencies also have a list of abbreviations that are acceptable to use within that agency. To prevent medication errors, the Institute for Safe Medication Practices Canada (ISMP Canada) has generated a list of potentially dangerous abbreviations, symbols, and dose designations that are frequently associated with harmful medication errors. Many institutions in Canada are implementing ISMP Canada's recommendations. Table 33.6 summarizes ISMP Canada's recommendations.

Types of Medication Orders

Five types of medication orders are the stat order, the single order, the standing order, the prn order, and the protocol order (sometimes referred to as a *collective prescription*). (See Table 33.7 for common abbreviations used in medication orders.)

1. A **stat order** indicates that the medication is to be given immediately and only once (e.g., morphine sulphate 4 milligrams IV stat).
2. The **single order** or *one-time order* is for medication to be given once at a specified time (e.g., lorazepam 1 mg at bedtime before surgery).
3. The **standing order** may or may not have a termination date. A standing order may be carried out indefinitely (e.g., multiple vitamins daily) until an order is written to cancel it, or it may be carried out for a specified number of days (e.g., furosemide 40 mg orally twice daily for 2 days). In some agencies, standing orders are automatically cancelled after a specified number of days and must be reordered.
4. A **prn order**, or *as-needed order*, permits the nurse to give a medication when, in the nurse's judgment, the client requires it (e.g., acetaminophen 650 mg orally every 4–6 hours prn). The nurse must use judgment about when the medication is needed and when it can be safely administered.
5. A **protocol order** or **collective prescription** is a set of criteria and orders under which a medication is to be administered. For example, heparin protocols and insulin protocols are often used in hospital settings for a variety of patients.

TABLE 33.7 Common Abbreviations Used in Medication Orders

Abbreviation	Explanation
ac (*ante cibum*)	before meals
ad lib	freely, as desired
bid	twice a day
cap	capsules
hs	at bedtime
IM	intramuscular
IV	intravenous
pc (*post cibum*)	after meals
PO (*per os*)	by mouth
prn	when needed
q2h	every 2 hours
q4h	every 4 hours
q6h	every 6 hours
q8h	every 8 hours
stat	immediately

Essential Parts of a Drug Order

The drug order has seven essential parts, as listed in Box 33.1. In addition, unless it is a standing order, it should state the number of doses or the number of days the drug is to be administered.

The *client's full name*, that is, the first and last names and middle initials or names, should always be used to avoid confusion between two clients who have the same last name. In some agencies, the client's identification number and prescriber's name are placed on the order as further identification. Some hospitals imprint the

---

BOX 33.1 ESSENTIAL PARTS OF A DRUG ORDER

A drug order has the following essential parts:

1. Full name of the client
2. Date and time the order is written
3. Generic name of the drug to be administered (some agencies accept the trade name)
4. Dosage of the drug
5. Route of administration
6. Frequency of administration
7. Signature of the person writing the order

client's name, identification number, and room number on all forms; some agencies use stickers with similar information.

In addition to *the day, the month,* and *the year* the order was written, some agencies also require that the *time of day* be written. Writing the time of day on the order can eliminate errors when the nursing shifts change and makes clear when certain orders automatically terminate. For example, in some settings, narcotics can be ordered only for 48 hours after surgery. Therefore, a drug that is ordered at 1600 hours November 1, 2012, is automatically cancelled at 1600 November 3, 2012. Many health agencies use the 24-hour clock, which eliminates confusion between morning and afternoon times. The 24-hour clock begins at midnight, which is 0000 hours. Adding 12 to any "p.m." time will yield the equivalent time on the 24-hour clock (e.g., 5:00 p.m. is 1700 and 11 p.m. is 2300 on the 24-hour clock).

The *name of the drug to be administered* must be clearly written. In some settings, only generic names are permitted; however, trade names are widely used in hospitals and other health care settings.

The *dosage of the drug* includes the amount, the times or *frequency of administration,* and, in many instances, the strength; for example, tetracycline *250 mg* (amount) *four times a day* (frequency); potassium chloride *10%* (strength) *5 mL* (amount) *three times a day with meals* (time and frequency). Also included in the order is the *route of administration* of the drug. This part of the order, like other parts, is frequently abbreviated. It is not unusual for a drug to have several possible routes of administration; therefore, it is essential that the route be included in the order.

The *signature* of the ordering health care professional makes the drug order a legal request. *An unsigned order has no validity,* and the ordering health care professional needs to be notified if the order is unsigned.

When the prescribing health care professional writes a prescription for a client, the prescription also includes information for the pharmacist such as "Dispense 30 capsules."

Communicating a Medication Order

A drug order is written on the client's chart by a health care professional with prescriptive rights or by a registered nurse receiving a telephone or verbal order from an authorized prescriber. Most acute care agencies have a specified time frame (e.g., 12 to 24 hours) in which the prescriber issuing the telephone or verbal order must co-sign the order written by the nurse. The medication order is then transcribed onto the *medication administration record (MAR).* Increasingly, prescribers are using computer resources to prescribe medication orders; the nurse then prepares the medications using the

electronic record. This method avoids errors and saves nursing time.

MARs vary in form, but all include the client's name, room, and bed number; drug name and dose; and times and method of administration (Figure 33.6). In some agencies, the date the order was prescribed and the date the order expires are also included. The nurse should always question the prescribing health care professional about any order that is ambiguous, unusual (e.g., an abnormally high dosage of a medication), or contraindicated by the client's condition. When the nurse judges that a prescribed medication is inappropriate, the nurse must do the following:

- Contact the prescribing health care professional and discuss the rationale for determining the medication or dosage to be inappropriate
- Document in the notes the following: when the prescribing health care professional was notified, what was conveyed, and how the prescriber responded
- If the prescribing health care professional cannot be reached, document all attempts to contact the individual and the reason for withholding the medication
- If someone else gives the medication, document data about the client's condition before and after the medication.
- If an incident report (see Chapter 6) is indicated, clearly document factual information

Systems of Measurement

Two systems of measurement are used in Canada: (a) the metric system and (b) the household system.

Metric System

The metric system is the official system of measurement in Canada. The metric system is logically organized into units of 10; it is a decimal system. Basic units can be multiplied or divided by 10 to form secondary units. Multiples are calculated by moving the decimal point to the right, and division is accomplished by moving the decimal point to the left. Basic units of measurement are the *metre,* the *litre,* and the *gram.* Prefixes derived from Latin designate subdivisions of the basic unit: *deci* (1/10 or 0.1), *centi* (1/100 or 0.01), and *milli* (1/1000 or 0.001). Multiples of the basic units are designated by prefixes derived from Greek: *deca* (10), *hecto* (100), and *kilo* (1000). Only the measurements of volume (the litre) and of weight (the gram) are discussed in this chapter. These are the measures used in medication administration (Figure 33.7 on page 886). The *kilogram* (kg) is a multiple of the *gram* (g), and the *milligram* (mg)

Name: Waters, Juni Location: 236 B	**MEDICATION ADMINISTRATION RECORD**		PAGE 1 OF 1

VERIFIED BY: _____ **DATE:** _____

PRN#:
MRN#:   **AGE:**
ADM: 08/15/2012   **SEX:**
DOB: **HT:**
DR.   **WT:**

DIAGNOSIS: ALOC
                          PNEUMONIA
ALLERGIES: NO KNOWN DRUG ALLERGIES

GENERATED: 08/15/2012   07:32
FOR PERIOD: 08/15/2012   08:00
THROUGH: 08/17/2012   07:59

START	STOP	MEDICATION/IV/IVPB/IRRIGATION		0800–1559	1600–2359	0000–0759
08/15	08/17	FERROUS SULPHATE 300 MG = 5 ML TWICE A DAY PO (FESO4)	(973539)	09	17	
08/15	08/17	DOCUSATE SODIUM 100 MG = 1 UDCUP TWICE A DAY PO (COLACE) 100 MG/30 ML UD HOLD FOR LOOSE STOOL	(973532)	09	17	
08/15	08/17	ASCORBIC ACID 500 MG = 1 TAB TWICE A DAY PO (VITAMIN C) 500 MG TAB	(972096)	09	17	
08/15	08/17	LEVOTHYROXINE 0.05 MG = 1 TAB DAILY PO (SYNTHROID) 0.05 MG TAB	(972095)	09		
08/15	08/17	ASPIRIN 325 MG = 1 TAB DAILY PO (ASPIRIN) 325 MG TAB *W/FOOD TO AVOID GI UPSET	(972094)	09		
08/15	08/17	CEFUROXIME ADDV. 1.500 G =1 VIAL EVERY 8 HOURS IV (KEFUROX) 1.5 G ADDV *ATTACH TO D$_5$W 50 ML ADDV BAG *ACTIVATE BEFORE INFUSION* * INFUSE OVER 30 MIN*	(971776)	14	22	06
		—— PRN ORDERS ——				
08/15	08/17	ACETAMINOPHEN 650 MG = 1SUPP EVERY 4 HOURS AS NEEDED PR (TYLENOL) 650 MG SUPP	(971779)			

INITIALS	SIGNATURE	SHIFT	INITIALS	SIGNATURE	SHIFT	INITIALS	SIGNATURE	SHIFT

FIGURE 33.6 Medication administration record (MAR).

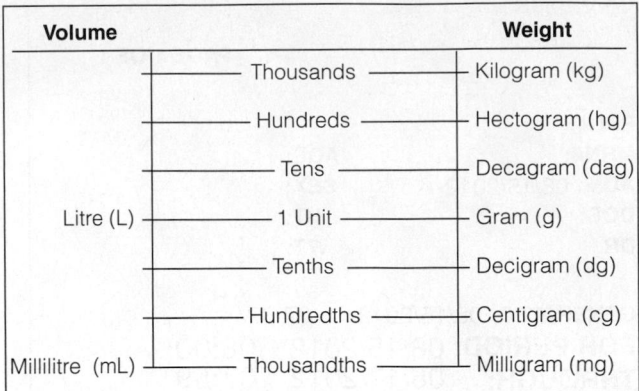

Volume	Weight
Thousands	Kilogram (kg)
Hundreds	Hectogram (hg)
Tens	Decagram (dag)
Litre (L) — 1 Unit	Gram (g)
Tenths	Decigram (dg)
Hundredths	Centigram (cg)
Millilitre (mL) — Thousandths	Milligram (mg)

FIGURE 33.7 Basic metric measurements of volume and weight and their symbols.

and *microgram* (mcg) are subdivisions. Fractional parts of the litre are usually expressed in *millilitres* (mL), for example, 2.5 litres or 2500 mL. In nursing practice, it is important to understand the difference between *weight* and *volume*. A drug dosage may be ordered by weight (i.e., grams, milligrams), but administered by volume (mL). For example, a health care provider prescribes 250 mg (weight) of amoxicillin in an oral suspension form. The suspension is available as 250 mg per 5 mL. The nurse administers 5 mL (volume) of amoxicillin.

CONVERTING UNITS OF WEIGHT WITHIN THE METRIC SYSTEM It is relatively simple to arrive at equivalent units of weight within the metric system because the system is based on units of 10. Three metric units of weight are used for drug dosages: (a) the gram (g), (b) milligram (mg), and (c) microgram (mcg); 1000 mg or 1 000 000 mcg equals 1 gram (g). Equivalents are computed by dividing or multiplying; for example, to change milligrams to grams, the number of milligrams is divided by 1000. The simplest way to divide by 1000 is to move the decimal point three places to the left (e.g., 4500 mg = 4.5 g; 500 mg = 0.5 g). In the last example, it is important to put a leading 0 in front of the decimal point (i.e., 0.5 g); otherwise, the reader may miss the decimal point if the value is written as ".5" and administer an incorrect dose of medication (i.e., 5 g).

Conversely, to convert grams to milligrams, multiply the number of grams by 1000, or move the decimal point three places to the right: 0.006 g = 6 mg (note that a trailing zero should NOT be used, as 6.0 mg could be misinterpreted as 60 mg).

Household System

Household measures may be used when more accurate systems of measure are not required. Included in household measures are teaspoons (tsp) and tablespoons (tbsp). Nurses must be aware of the relative metric conversion for household measures: 1 tsp = approximately

5 mL (4.92892159 mL); 1 tbsp = approximately 15 mL 14.7867648 mL).

Methods of Calculating Dosages

Several methods can be used to calculate drug dosages—three are presented below. Nurses are encouraged to review all methods and to choose the method that works best for them. Using one method consistently generally avoids confusion in calculations and, thus, promotes client safety. When calculating drug dosages, there are times when the nurse may need to round the numbers (see Box 33.2 for guidelines). Many institutions, in particular pediatric settings, require an independent double-check of calculations to ensure patient safety.

Basic Formula

The basic formula for calculating drug dosages is commonly used and easy to remember:

D = desired dose (i.e., dose ordered)
H = dose on hand (i.e., dose on label of bottle, vial, ampule)
V = vehicle (i.e., form in which the drug comes, such as tablet or liquid).

$$\text{Basic formula} = \frac{D \times V}{H} = \text{amount to administer}$$

Example:
Order: clarithromycin 500 mg
On hand: clarithromycin 250 mg in 5 mL

D = 500 mg; H = 250 mg; V = 5 mL

$$\text{Amount to administer} = \frac{500\,\text{mg} \times 5\,\text{mL}}{250\,\text{mg}} = 10\,\text{mL}$$

Another Example:
Order: Coumadin 7.5 mg
On hand: Coumadin 5 mg in 1 tablet

D = 7.5 mg; H = 5 mg; V = 1 tablet

$$\text{Amount to administer} = \frac{7.5\,\text{mg} \times 1\,\text{tablet}}{5\,\text{mg}} = 1.5\,\text{tablet}$$

Ratio and Proportion Method

The ratio and proportion method is considered the oldest method used for calculating dosages. The equation is set up with the known quantities on the left side

BOX 33.2   GUIDELINES FOR ROUNDING NUMBERS IN DRUG CALCULATIONS

Note: Rounding of numbers is only performed AFTER all calculations have been completed.

- Intravenous medications:
  - Gravity infusion
    - Round to the nearest whole number (e.g., 37.5 drops/minute is rounded up to 38 drops/minute; 53.4 drops/minute is rounded down to 53 drops/minute).
  - Infusion by intravenous pump
    - If the pump uses only whole numbers then round to the nearest whole number (e.g., 87.6 mL/hour is rounded up to 88 mL/hour).
    - Some pumps in critical care settings can be set to a tenth of the rate (e.g., 11.14 mL/hour is rounded down to 11.1 mL/hour). Round to the nearest tenth decimal point.
- Oral medications:
  - A capsule cannot be divided.
  - Tablets that are scored (a line marked on the table) can be divided, generally into halves. A tablet must be scored by the manufacturer to be divided properly.
  - For tablets that are not scored and for capsules, it may not be realistic to administer the exact amount as calculated. For example, if the calculation for *x* is 1.9 tablets, the nurse cannot reasonably divide the tablet accurately and would therefore give two tablets. Before doing this, the nurse should consult with the pharmacy to see if there is another preparation (e.g., alternative tablet concentrations of the same drug) that can provide the exact dosage. If the medication is considered high-alert then consultation with the health care team is advisable.

- For liquid medications, check to see if it is possible to administer the accurate dosage. Syringes, such as a 1-mL syringe, include markings for hundredths of a millilitre. These syringes are often used in pediatric settings to give the most accurate dosage that is possible.
- Injectable medications:
  - Medications that are administered by injection (either into the client or into an intravenous solution) are generally rounded to the nearest tenth (e.g., 0.83 mL is rounded down to 0.8 mL; 0.86 mL is rounded up to 0.9 mL; 1.65 mL is rounded up to 1.7 mL).
  - High-alert medications (e.g., insulin) are rounded to the hundredth and specially calibrated syringes are used (e.g., 44 units 100 u/mL insulin is administered as 0.44 mL using an insulin syringe—do not give 0.4 mL in this case as the insulin syringe is calibrated to give tenths of a mL).
- Rounding down:
  - Rounding down may be used in pediatric clients or when administering high-alert medications to adults so as to avoid the danger of overdose.
  - To round down to hundredths, drop all of the numbers after the hundredth place. For tenths, drop all of the numbers after the tenth place, and for whole numbers, all of the numbers after the decimal are dropped. For example, 6.6477 rounded down to the nearest is as follows:
    - Hundredth = 6.64
    - Tenth = 6.6
    - Whole number = 6

(i.e., H and V). The right side of the equation consists of the desired dose (i.e., D) and the unknown amount to administer (i.e., *x*). The equation looks like this:

$$H:V::D:x$$

Once the equation is set up, multiply the extremes (i.e., H and *x*) and the means (i.e., V and D). Then solve for *x*.

Example:

Order: cephalexin 750 mg
On hand: cephalexin 250 mg in one tablet

$$H = 250 \text{ mg} : V = 1 \text{ tablet} :: D = 750 \text{ mg} : x$$
$$250 \text{ mg} : 1 \text{ tablet} :: 750 \text{ mg} : x \text{ tablet}$$

Multiply the extremes (i.e., H and *x*) and the means (V and D) and solve for *x*:

$$250 x = 750$$
$$x \text{ tablet} = \frac{750 \text{ mg}}{250 \text{ mg}} = 3 \text{ tablets}$$

Another Example:

Order: Gentamycin 60 mg
On hand: Gentamycin 80 mg/mL

$$H = 80 \text{ mg} : V = 1 \text{ mL} :: D = 60 \text{ mg} : x$$
$$80 \text{ mg} : 1 \text{ mL} :: 60 \text{ mg} : x \text{ mL}$$

Multiply the extremes (i.e., H and *x*) and the means (V and D) and solve for *x*:

$$80 x = 60$$
$$x \text{ mL} = \frac{60 \text{ mg}}{80 \text{ mg}} = 0.75 \text{ mL}$$

Fractional Equation Method

The fractional equation method is similar to ratio and proportion except it is written as a fraction:

$$\frac{H}{V} = \frac{D}{x}$$

The formula consists of cross multiplying and solving for *x*:

$$Hx = DV$$
$$x = \frac{DV}{H}$$

Example:

Order: furosemide 20 mg
On hand: furosemide 40 mg in one tablet

$$D = 20 \text{ mg}; H = 40 \text{ mg}; V = 1 \text{ tablet}$$
$$\frac{40 \text{ mg}}{1 \text{ tablet}} = \frac{20 \text{ mg}}{x \text{ tablet}}$$

Cross multiply: 40 $x = 20$
Solve for x

$$x \text{ tablet} = \frac{20 \text{ mg}}{40 \text{ mg}}$$

$$x = 0.5 \text{ (or } \frac{1}{2}\text{) tablet}$$

Another Example:

Order: Lanoxin 0.25 mg
On hand: Lanoxin 0.125 mg in one tablet

$$D = 0.25 \text{ mg}; H = 0.125 \text{ mg}; V = 1 \text{ tablet}$$

$$\frac{0.125 \text{ mg}}{1 \text{ tablet}} = \frac{0.25}{x}$$

Cross multiply:

$$0.125 \; x = 0.25$$

Solve for x

$$x \text{ tablet} = \frac{0.25 \text{ mg}}{0.125 \text{ mg}}$$

$$x = 2 \text{ tablets}$$

Another Example:

Order: Heparin 800 units per hour by intravenous infusion
On hand: Heparin 25,000 units in 500 mL dextrose 5% in water

$$D = 800 \text{ units}; H = 25,000 \text{ units}; V = 500 \text{ mL}$$

$$\frac{25,000 \text{ units}}{500 \text{ mL}} = \frac{800 \text{ units}}{x \text{ mL}}$$

Cross multiply:

$$25,000 \; x = 500 \times 800$$

Solve for x:

$$x \text{ mL} = \frac{800 \text{ units} \times 500 \text{ mL}}{25,000 \text{ units}}$$

$x = 16$ mL (remember that this is 16 mL per hour).

Calculations Involving Conversion

Sometimes a medication is prescribed using one type of unit but the medication is available in another type of unit. In these situations, the units need to be converted with a conversion factor so that like units are used for calculations. The units that are converted to are usually the units of the vehicle available for administration.

Example:

Order: Ampicillin 0.5 gram
On hand: Ampicillin 250 mg in 5 mL

Because the "on hand" preparation (vehicle) is in *mg* the prescribed dosage needs to be converted from *grams* to *mg*. Because 1 gram = 1000 mg, the decimal is moved to the right: 0.5 grams = 500 mg.

Now, use your preferred formula. If using the fractional equation method, proceed as follows:

$$D = 500 \text{ mg}; H = 250 \text{ mg}; V = 5 \text{ mL}$$

$$\frac{250 \text{ mg}}{5 \text{ mL}} = \frac{500 \text{ mg}}{x \text{ mL}}$$

Cross multiply:

$$250 \; x = 500 \times 5$$

Solve for x

$$x \text{ mL} = \frac{500 \text{ mg} \times 5 \text{ mL}}{250 \text{ mg}} = 10 \text{ mL}$$

Calculation for Individualized Drug Dosages

Nurses may need to individualize the dosage of a medication, particularly for children. Other clients who may require an individualized dosage include those receiving chemotherapy for cancer and clients who are critically ill. The two methods for individualizing drug dosages are (a) body weight and (b) body surface area.

BODY WEIGHT Unlike adult dosages, children's dosages are not always standard. Body weight significantly affects dosage; therefore, dosages are calculated on an individual basis. Dosages based on weight use kilograms of body weight and per kilogram medication recommendations to arrive at appropriate and safe doses.

The steps involved in calculating an individualized dose are as follows:

1. Determine the drug dose per body weight by multiplying drug dose × body weight × frequency.
2. Choose a method of drug calculation to determine the amount of medication to administer.

Example:

Order: cephalexin, 25 mg/kg/day in four divided doses. The client weighs 9.6 kg.
On hand: cephalexin oral suspension 125 mg per 5 mL

Multiply drug dose × body weight × frequency:
25 mg × 9.6 kg × 1 day = 240 mg/day
240 ÷ 4 divided doses = 60 mg/dose

3. The nurse chooses the preferred method of calculation (e.g., basic formula, ratio and proportion, fractional equation) to determine how many millilitres per dose of medication (e.g., if using the fractional equation method: 125 mg/5 mL = 60 mg/x mL = 2.4 mL of cephalexin oral suspension per dose).

Another Example:

A child weighing 20 kg is prescribed cloxacillin 0.75 grams IV q6h. The therapeutic dose range of cloxacillin is 50–200 mg/kg/day.

To find out if the prescribed dosage falls within the therapeutic dosage range, proceed as follows:

As the therapeutic dosage is presented as mg/kg/day, first start by finding the safe range relative to the child's weight: (50 mg/kg/day × 20 kg) to (200 mg/kg/day × 20 kg) = 1000 mg to 4000 mg/day.

Now, given that the therapeutic dosage range is in *mg* and the prescribed dose is in *grams*, one could convert grams to mg: 0.75 grams = 750 mg per dose OR convert mg to grams: 1000 mg to 4000 mg = 1 to 4 grams per day.

Now, calculate if the prescribed dose is in the therapeutic range. There are two ways to do this given that the therapeutic range is expressed as a daily range whereas the prescribed dose is every 6 hours.

a. One method is to divide the therapeutic range by 4 (i.e., a medication given every 6 hours in a 24-hour period will be given in 4 doses): therapeutic range for each of 4 doses would be 1000/4 to 4000/4 = 250 mg to 1000 mg per dose. Given that 0.75 mg is equal to 750 mg and 750 falls between 250 and 1000, the prescribed dosage falls within the safe therapeutic dose range.

b. An alternative method is to multiply the unit dose by 4: 750 mg × 4 = 3000 mg per day. As 3000 mg falls between the therapeutic daily range of 1000 mg to 4000 mg per day, the dosage is safe to give.

BODY SURFACE AREA Sometimes, the body surface calculation may be used instead of body weight to individualize the medication dosage. It is considered to be the most accurate method of calculating a pediatric dose. Body surface area is determined by using a nomogram and the child's height and weight. A standard nomogram will give a child's body surface area based on the weight and height of the child (Figure 33.8). The formula is the ratio of the child's body surface area to the surface area of an average adult (1.7 m²), multiplied by the normal adult dose of the drug:

$$\text{Child's dose} = \frac{\text{surface area of child (m}^2)}{1.7\text{ m}^2} \times \text{Normal adult dose}$$

For example, a child who weighs 10 kg and is 50 cm tall has a body surface area of 0.4 m² (see the nomogram in Figure 33.8). Therefore, the child's dose of tetracycline, corresponding to an adult dose of 250 mg, would be as follows:

$$= \frac{0.4\text{ (m}^2)}{1.7\text{ m}^2} \times 250\text{ mg} = 0.23 \times 250 = 58.82\text{ mg}$$

Administering Medications Safely

The nurse should always assess a client's health status and obtain a medication history before administering any medication. The extent of the assessment depends on the

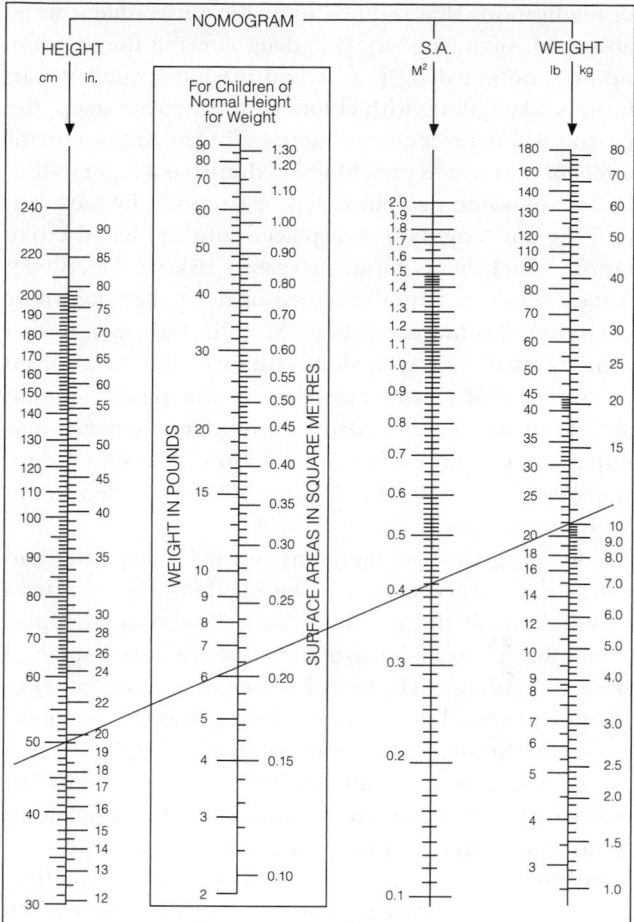

FIGURE 33.8 A nomogram with estimated body surface area. A straight line is drawn between the child's height (*on the left*) and the child's weight (*on the right*). The point at which the line intersects the surface area column is the estimated body surface area.

client's illness or current condition, the intended drug, and the route of administration. For example, if a client is experiencing dyspnea, the nurse assesses respirations carefully before administering any medication that might affect breathing. It is important to determine whether the route of administration is suitable. For example, a client who is nauseated may not be able to tolerate a drug taken orally. In general, the nurse assesses the client *prior* to administering any medication to obtain baseline data by which to evaluate the effectiveness of the medication. The **medication history** includes information about the drugs the client is taking currently or has taken recently. This includes prescription drugs; OTC drugs, such as antacids, alcohol, and tobacco; vitamins and natural health products; and illicit drugs, such as marijuana. Some people may not list vitamins, herbs, food supplements, or folk remedies because they do not believe they are "drugs"; however, these substances still exert an effect on the body and can have adverse effects, including drug–drug interactions when taken in conjunction with other drugs. **Drug–drug interactions** (Lehne, 2010) can involve the following: one drug altering the absorption of another drug (e.g., antacids raise stomach pH and reduce absorption of medications that require an acidic environment to be absorbed, such as iron); one drug altering the distribution of another drug (e.g., when the anticoagulant warfarin is taken along with chloral hydrate to aid sleep, the person will experience an increase in the anticoagulant effect of warfarin as the chloral hydrate has a higher affinity for the same protein receptor site used by warfarin; and the anticoagulant is displaced into the blood circulation, which leads to an increased risk for bleeding); some drugs can either enhance or delay metabolism or excretion of other drugs (e.g., St. John's wort, an herbal remedy used for depression, enhances the metabolism of certain oral contraceptives thus placing the woman at risk for pregnancy). **Drug–food interactions** can also enhance or diminish the absorption of certain medications (see Table 40.2 in Chapter 40, for selected drug–food interactions).

Keeping track of the many possible drug–drug and drug–food interactions can be challenging, so nurses should consult the pharmacy as well as computer programs that are available to analyze a client's list of medications (including OTC, herbal remedies, and vitamins) to identify potential drug–drug and drug–food interactions.

The clients' knowledge of drug allergies is also important. The nurse should clarify with the client any adverse effects or allergic responses to any medications. Some clients may not be sure about their allergic reactions and may interpret an illness or secondary effect (e.g., nausea) occurring after a drug was taken as an allergy when it is not.

It is essential for the nurse to identify any problems the client may have in self-administering a medication. Someone with poor eyesight may require special labels for the medication container; older adults with unsteady hands may not be able to hold a syringe or to inject themselves. Obtaining information as to how and where medications are stored in clients' homes is also important. If clients have difficulty opening certain containers, they may change the containers but leave old labels on, which increases the risk of medication errors; some medications must not be exposed to direct sunlight (e.g., nitroglycerine).

Socioeconomic factors should be assessed, such as whether the client has adequate finances to purchase medications or equipment (e.g., syringes). When aware of these problems, the nurse can refer the client to relevant proper resources.

System Factors Related to Medication Safety

The landmark *Canadian Adverse Events Study* (Baker, Norton, Flintoft, Blais, Brown, Cox, & Tamblin, 2004) found that one out of nine drugs administered to adults in Canadian hospitals and skilled nursing facilities is in error, with upwards of 24% of these errors being preventable. In the past, the investigation of a medication error emphasized finding out who made the error—often implicating the person administering the medication—and "shaming and blaming" that person in an attempt to prevent further incidents. This approach often resulted in people hiding their errors to avoid the shame. More recently, evidence indicates that many medication errors and adverse events are related to system factors rather than to any one individual. The Canadian Patient Safety Institute and the Institute for Safe Medication Practices Canada (both founded after the release of the *Canadian Adverse Events Study*) emphasize a culture of safety, in which one is encouraged to report medication errors and near-misses so that the multiple factors influencing the situation can be analyzed.

Errors in medication administration can happen at multiple stages including at the time of prescription and administration as well as during the monitoring phase. Some examples (drawn from *real life*) of how medication errors can occur as a result of multiple systems issues are given below:

- *Wrong-drug error:* The prescriber, who is exhausted after working a double shift because two of her colleagues called in sick with the flu, overlooks important clinical data related to poor renal function and prescribes a high-alert medication that is contraindicated for the client. The nurse administering the medication suspects that the drug is contraindicated but remembers being yelled at by the prescriber the last time she questioned a prescription, so she does not question the prescriber this time. Would such errors be avoided if more health care professionals received the flu vaccine? if the hospital had additional relief staff? an improved communication system existed between the renal lab and the clinical unit? there was a computerized medication system that relates relevant lab findings and high-alert medications, providing "red flags" in the event of a wrong-drug error? the environment was more conducive to respectful interprofessional communication?

- *Wrong-dose error:* Poor prescriber handwriting results in "5.0 mg" being transcribed as "50 mg" giving rise to a 10-fold increase in medication dosage prescribed; the medication is supplied in bulk on the unit and the nurse prepares five tablets for administration; the patient thinks, "Five pills seems like a lot!" He says nothing and tells himself, "They must know what they are doing." Could this error have been avoided if the following system factors were in place: a computerized prescription system? individual medication packages rather than bulk containers? an environment in which patients feel they are part of the team and should be contributing to—and questioning—their care?

- *Wrong-dose error:* The nurse mixes two types of insulin in a syringe in a medication room that is poorly lit and has multiple distractions. The insulin is for a patient whose glucometer indicated a blood glucose of 15.6. The unit is very busy and the nurse races to the patient's room stopping on the way to get a double-check from another nurse who is equally busy and acknowledges that the insulin dose is correct. Within 30 minutes of the insulin administration, the patient becomes severely hypoglycemic and needs a STAT infusion of dextrose. Although there was no way to confirm if the amount of insulin drawn into the syringe was in error, the fact that six patients had had similar episodes of hypoglycemia after receiving insulin doses based on glucometer readings, pointed to a malfunctioning glucometer! Could this error have been avoided if there was a better way of ensuring proper functioning of equipment? What if no one had seen the pattern of hypoglycemia?

Other errors in medication administration result from a lack of coordination and continuity of care related to medications as the client moves across various settings in the health care system resulting in the possible omission of important drugs OR the addition of medications that are contraindicated. **Medication reconciliation** is a process that aims to prevent potential medication errors and adverse drug events through "a formal process in which health care professionals partner with clients to ensure accurate and complete medication information transfer at interfaces of care. It involves a systematic process for obtaining a medication history, and using that information to compare to medication orders to identify and resolve discrepancies" (ISMP Canada, 2012). Accreditation Canada (see Chapter 32) now includes medication reconciliation as part of its required organizational practices. Protocols and processes for medication reconciliation must be in place, particularly in the following transition areas: on admission; during transfer between units, in shift reports, and in new MARs; and at discharge. A complete list of the client's medications (including prescriptions, natural health products, and OTC agents) is documented on admission. This list is then compared with any new medications ordered on admission and during the client's hospital stay. Medications that are to be administered around the change-of-shift report need to be discussed at the report. For example, insulin is a common medication scheduled between night and day shifts. It is important that the oncoming nurse know if the medication was given or not. If a client is transferred to another setting, within or outside of the facility, a complete list of the client's medications must be communicated to the next provider of care. This list is also provided to clients on discharge from the facility. In addition, the client should receive, at discharge, written and oral information on each medication to be taken at home. It is important for the nurse to emphasize to clients the importance of keeping the list of their medications handy and taking it with them to their follow-up visits and to future hospitalizations, if any.

A range of client safety initiatives have emerged across Canada (and the world!)—see Chapter 32 for a discussion of various initiatives. The Practice Guidelines 33.1 summarize important Canadian medication safety guidelines from national initiatives.

PRACTICE GUIDELINES 33.1

Medication Safety

Guideline	Rationale
Accurately identify client using a minimum of two identifiers (not the person's physical location) (Accreditation Canada, 2011)	Using at least two identifiers (e.g., client's full name [first and last], date of birth, hospital identification number, and/or photo) ensures that the correct person for whom the medication is intended actually receives the medication.
Use computerized order entry (ISMP, 2000)	Reduced errors related to illegible handwriting and during transcription; many programs have built in warnings for drug–drug interactions; some order entry systems synchronize with patient data (e.g., lab results, weight) to issue safety warnings, as necessary.
Avoid dangerous abbreviations, symbols, and dose designations when computerized order entry not used (ISMP Canada, 2012). (See Table 33.6 for full list of "do not use" abbreviations, symbols, and dose designation.)	Medication errors occur due to misinterpretation of abbreviations (e.g., DC medications can mean 'discontinue' OR 'discharge' medications), symbols (e.g., > mistaken for 7), and dose designations (e.g., 5.0 mg interpreted as 50 mg giving rise to a 10-fold error).

(continued)

PRACTICE GUIDELINES 33.1

Medication Safety (continued)

Guideline	Rationale
Use Tall Man lettering for look-alike sound-alike medications (ISMP Canada, 2012)	Uppercase lettering of the *dissimilar* part of medications that have a look-alike sound-alike name draws attention to the difference and leads to less chance of error (e.g., dimenhyDRINATE and diphenhydrAMINE; vinBLAStine and vinCRIStine).
Medication reconciliation at all transfer points of care (within an institution, across institutions) (ISMP Canada, 2012)	Comparing the client's medications on admission and as he or she moves through the system, including transfers at shift change, from one unit to another, from one institution to another, and home, ensures that medications being added, changed, or discontinued are carefully evaluated.
Use extreme caution when using high-alert medications: • Independent double-check by two registered nurses prior to administering high-alert medication • Removal of high-dose concentrations of high-alert medications from units • Training on infusion pumps used for administration of high-alert medications (Accreditation Canada, 2011).	When used in error, high-alert medications such as hypoglycemics (e.g., insulin), inotropes (e.g., digoxin), opioids (e.g., morphine), heparin, and potassium chloride for injection (among many others) bear a heightened risk of causing harm to the patient.
Listen to the client (Accreditation Canada, 2011)	People are often very knowledgeable about their situations and how their bodies function—a person or family member who expresses concern or makes a comment about a medication (e.g., "my blood pressure pill is usually blue") is likely providing a clue that "something is not right"!
Be aware of the 10 rights of medication administration (see Box 33.3 on page 895)	Ensuring that the right patient receives the right drug in the right dosage at the right time and by the right route is important, but so are additional rights: right assessment, right patient education, right evaluation, right documentation, and right to refuse.
Report all near-misses and medication errors and support a culture of safety. (See Chapter 32 for a complete discussion on the culture of safety.)	Analyzing actual errors AND near-misses—an "almost error"—can help ensure that measures are taken to avoid the same thing from happening in the future. The Canadian Framework for Managing Patient Incidents (previously referred to as *Root Cause Analysis*) is a tool to help identify contributing factors. A "no shame no blame" culture of safety supports the disclosure of errors, all in an effort to promote patient safety.

Sources: Table compiled by M. Buck based on documentation from Institute for Safe Medication Practices. (2011). *Oral dosage forms that should not be crushed.* Retrieved from http:// www.ismp.org/tools/donotcrush.pdf; Institute for Safe Medication Practices. (2000). *A call to action: Eliminating hand written prescriptions within 3 years.* Retrieved from http://www.ismp.org/newsletters/acutecare/articles/whitepaper.asp; and Accreditation Canada. (2011). *Required organizational practices.* Retrieved from http://www.accreditation. ca/accreditation-programs/international/required-organizational-practices

Medication Dispensing Systems

Medical facilities vary in their medication dispensing systems. The systems can include the following:

• *Medication cart.* The medication cart (Figure 33.9) is on wheels, allowing the nurse to move the cart to the client's room. The cart contains small numbered drawers that correlate to the room numbers on the nursing unit, and each drawer holds individual client's medications for the shift or for 24 hours. Medications are usually in unit-dose packaging with the drug name, dose, and expiration date indicated (Figure 33.10). There is generally a larger locked drawer in the cart containing controlled substances and additional supply drawers that contain bulk containers or equipment (e.g., syringes). The MAR is usually located in a binder or a computer located on top of the medication cart. The nurse either carries a

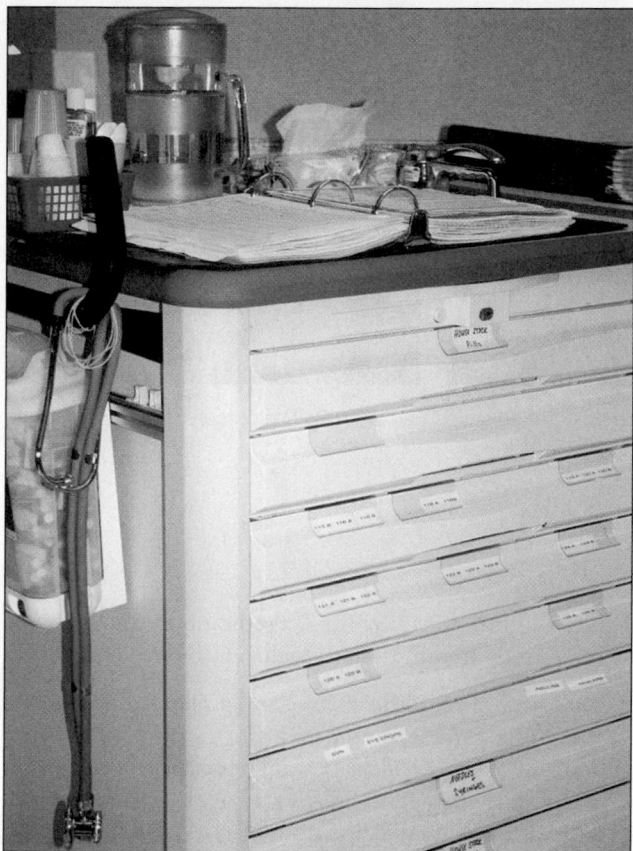

FIGURE 33.9 Medication cart, including lock to ensure safety when not in use.

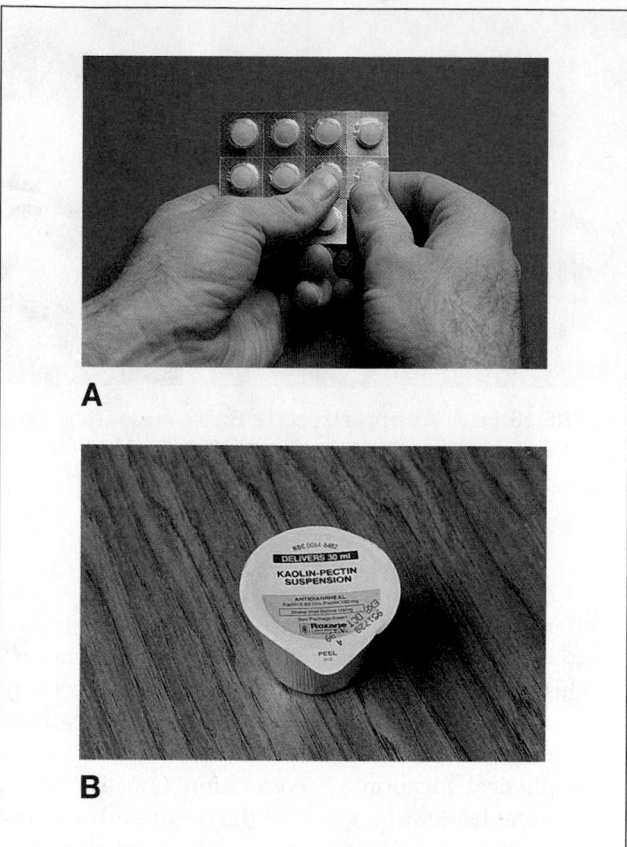

A

B

FIGURE 33.10 Unit-dose packages: **A:** Tablets; **B:** Liquid medications.

key or enters a special code to open the cart because it must be kept locked when not in use.

- *Medication cabinet.* Some facilities have a locked cabinet in the client's room that holds the person's medications and the MAR. Generally, controlled substances are not kept in this cabinet but at another location on the nursing unit. The medication cabinet must be locked when not in use.

- *Medication room.* Depending on the facility, a medication room may be used for a variety of purposes. For example, the medication carts, when not in use, may be placed in this room. This room may also be the central location for stock medications, controlled medications, or drugs used for emergencies. The medication room may have a refrigerator for medications requiring a cold storage environment. The room may also contain other medication administration supplies (e.g., syringes, needles). Nurses access the medication room by either a key or a code, as the room is often kept locked.

- *Automated dispensing cabinet (ADC).* A computerized access system that automates the distribution, management, and control of medications.

Similar to automated teller machines, the nurse uses a password to access the system, selects the client's name from an on-screen list, and selects the medication(s).

Process of Administering Medications

When administering any drug, regardless of the route of administration, the nurse must do the following:

1. *Check the prescriber orders.* Preventable hospital medication errors occur in the administration and order entry or transcription stages of medication use. The nurse must check and verify the drug with the prescriber's order prior to proceeding with administration. It is becoming more common for health care facilities to use computerized systems that lower the risk of error by validating the drug information automatically.

2. *Accurately identify the client.* Errors can and do occur, usually because one client gets a drug intended for another. One of Accreditation Canada's Required Organizational Practices (2011) is "to implement a client verification protocol for all services and procedures. The organization has a documented method of

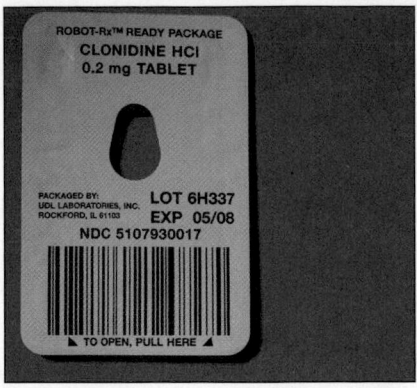
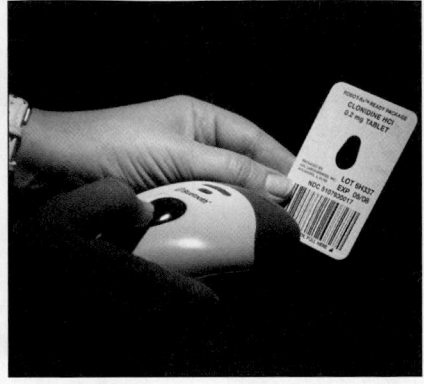
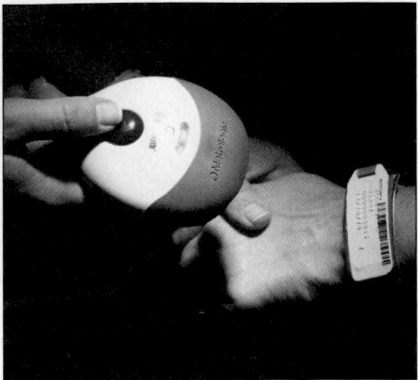

FIGURE 33.11 A: A sample barcode; **B:** The nurse scans the barcode on the medication package; **C:** The nurse scans the barcode on the client's wristband before administering the medication.

Source: Courtesy of Shirlee Snyder.

client identification (e.g., wrist bands, photo identification) that is standardized across the organization." This goal requires a nurse to use at least two client identifiers whenever administering medications. Neither identifier can be the client's room number or physical location (Accreditation Canada, 2011). Acceptable identifiers may be the client's first and last name, date of birth, and assigned hospital identification number. In long-term care facilities and home care settings where continuing care is provided, the requirement is generally that two identifiers be used to identify the client at the first encounter with the health care professional; check agency policy.

Some hospitals use barcode technology for medication administration. A nurse preparing to administer a medication using barcode technology scans or enters the nurse's own ID, the client's wristband, and each package of medication to be administered. Barcoding often includes two or more person-specific identifiers that meet the identifier requirement (Figure 33.11). See

CLINICAL ALERT

Accreditation Canada's 2011 Required Organizational Practice: Communication

Use at least two patient identifiers when providing care, treatment, and services.

Rationale: Wrong-patient errors occur in virtually all stages of diagnosis and treatment. The intent for this goal is twofold: first, to reliably identify the individual as the person for whom the service or treatment is intended; second, to match the service or treatment to that individual. Acceptable identifiers may be the individual's name, an assigned identification number, telephone number, or other person-specific identifier. When verifying the client's name, do not ask, "Are you Derek James?" because the person may answer "yes" to the wrong name. It is recommended that the client be asked to state his or her name.

the Clinical Alert box for Accreditation Canada's 2011 Required Organizational Practice: Communication.

3. *Inform the client.* If the client is unfamiliar with the medication, the nurse should explain the intended action and any adverse effects that might occur. It is important to listen to the client. It is easy to get so focused on the task of timely medication administration that the nurse may miss relevant information provided by the client. For example, if the client says that he does not take a pill for high blood pressure, this should be an alert for the nurse to stop and check if this is the correct medication for that client.

4. *Perform right assessments.* Prior to the administration of some drugs, a specific assessment may be indicated. It is the nurse's responsibility to ensure that the assessment has been done prior to the administration of the drug. For example, **PRIOR TO** the administration of digoxin, the apical pulse is taken for 1 minute noting rate, rhythm, and quality; **PRIOR TO** administering medications with a narrow therapeutic index (e.g., aminoglycoside antibiotics, digoxin, phenobarbitol), the nurse should verify if the blood levels have been assessed; **PRIOR TO** administering insulin, the client's blood glucose level should be checked.

5. *Administer the drug.* The MAR should be read carefully and three checks performed against the labelled medication: (a) when it is taken from the medication cart, (b) before withdrawing the medication (such as from a vial), and (c) after withdrawing the medication. Then, the medication should be administered in the prescribed dosage, by the route ordered, at the correct time. Certain aspects of medication administration are important for the nurse to check each time a medication is administered. These are referred to as

the "rights." Traditionally, there were five "rights" to medication administration. With the aim of improving client safety, more "rights" have been added over the past few years, with a total of "10 rights" being the current standard (Box 33.3).

6. *Provide adjunctive interventions, as indicated.* Clients may need assistance when receiving medications. They may require physical assistance, for instance, in assuming positions for intramuscular injections, or they may need guidance about measures to enhance drug effectiveness and prevent complications, such as increasing intake of potassium when taking certain diuretics. Some clients convey fear about their medications. The nurse can allay fears by listening carefully to concerns and giving correct information.

7. *Record the drug administered.* The facts recorded in the chart, in ink or by computer printout, are the name of the drug, the dosage, the method of administration,

specific relevant data, such as pulse rate (taken in most settings before the administration of cardiac glycosides), and any other pertinent information. The record should also include the exact time of administration and the signature of the nurse providing the medication. Many medication records are designed such that the nurse signs once on the page and initials each medication administered. Often, medications that are given regularly are recorded on a special flow record. PRN (as needed) or stat (at once) medications are recorded separately.

8. *Evaluate the client's response to the drug.* The kinds of client behaviours that reflect the action or lack of action of a drug and its untoward effects (both minor and major) are as variable as the purposes of the drugs. The anxious client may show the desired effects of an anxiolytic by behaviour that reflects a lowered stress level (e.g., slower speech, less agitation); the

---

BOX 33.3   TEN "RIGHTS" OF MEDICATION ADMINISTRATION

These 10 rights must be checked every time:

1. **Right medication**
   - Ensure that the medication given is the medication ordered.

2. **Right dose**
   - Ensure the dose ordered is appropriate for the client.
   - Give special attention if the calculation indicates multiple pills or tablets or a large quantity of a liquid medication. This can be a "cue" that the math calculation may be incorrect.
   - Double-check calculations that appear questionable.
   - Know the usual dosage range of the medication.
   - Question a dosage outside of the usual dosage range.

3. **Right time**
   - Give the medication at the right frequency and at the time ordered, according to agency policy.
   - Know that medications given within 30 minutes before or after the scheduled time are considered to meet the right time standard.

4. **Right route**
   - Give the medication by the ordered route.
   - Make certain that the route is safe and appropriate for the client.

5. **Right client**
   - Ensure that the medication is given to the intended client.
   - Accurately identify the client using a minimum of two identifiers with each administration of a medication.
   - Know the agency's name alert procedure when clients with the same or similar last names are on the nursing unit.

6. **Right client education**
   - Provide information about the medication to the client (e.g., why receiving, what to expect, any precautions).

7. **Right documentation**
   - Document medication administration after giving it, not before.
   - If the time of administration differs from the prescribed time, note the time on the MAR and explain the reason and follow-through activities (e.g., pharmacy states medication will be available in 2 hours) in progress notes.
   - If a medication is not given, follow the agency's policy for documenting the reason.

8. **Right to refuse**
   - Adults have the right to refuse any medication.
   - The nurse's role is to ensure that the client is fully informed of the potential consequences of refusal and to communicate the client's refusal to the appropriate member of the health care team.

9. **Right assessment**
   - Some medications require specific assessments before administration (e.g., apical pulse, blood pressure, laboratory results).
   - Medication orders may include specific parameters for administration (e.g., do not give if pulse rate is less than 60 or systolic blood pressure is less than 100 mm Hg).

10. **Right evaluation**
    - Conduct appropriate follow-up (e.g., Was the desired effect achieved or not? Did the client experience any adverse effects?).

effectiveness of an analgesic can be measured by how much self-rated pain changes while monitoring for dry mouth, sedation, and constipation; the action of a diuretic can be measured by the change in urine output while potassium levels are monitored for hypokalemia. In all nursing activities, nurses need to be aware of the medications that a client is taking and record their effectiveness on the client's chart, as assessed by the client and the nurse. The responses must be communicated with the appropriate members of the health care team to ensure that the treatment plans are effective.

Developmental Considerations

It is important for the nurse to be aware of how growth and development affect administration of medications for all age groups, particularly infants and the older population.

INFANTS AND CHILDREN Knowledge of growth and development is essential for the nurse administering medications to children. Oral medications for children are usually prepared in sweetened liquid form to make them more palatable. Parents may provide suggestions about what method is best for their child. Do not use necessary foods such as milk or orange juice to mask the taste of medications because the child may develop unpleasant associations and refuse that food in the future.

Children tend to fear any procedure in which a needle is used because they anticipate pain or because the procedure is unfamiliar and threatening. The nurse needs to acknowledge that the child will feel some pain; denying this fact only deepens the child's distrust. After the injection, the nurse (or the parent) can cuddle and speak softly to the infant or give the child a toy to dispel the association of the nurse only with pain.

OLDER ADULTS Older adults may have special problems, most of which are related to physiological changes, presence of comorbidities, and reduced functional abilities. Some physiological changes in older adults that may influence response to medications include reduced renal and liver functions that can result in a slower speed of metabolism and excretion of certain medications, necessitating a lower dosage of medication and more frequent monitoring; slower absorption from the gastrointestinal tract; increased proportion of fat to lean body mass, which facilitates retention of lipophilic drugs and increases potential for toxicity; reduced circulation may delay the absorption and action of medications given intramuscularly or subcutaneously. Older adults may have multiple forms of illness, each requiring a particular medication regimen. It is not uncommon for older adults to be taking several medications

(sometimes referred to as *polypharmacy*) at once, and close monitoring of drug–drug interactions must take place to ensure safety. Changes in functional abilities include reduction in manual dexterity or reduced visual acuity, which could affect the ability of an older adult to self-administer injections (e.g., insulin) and measure medications accurately.

Polypharmacy combined with changes in memory can also pose a challenge to older adults with respect to medication safety. Helping them to organize their medication scheduling (such as using a Dosette box) and finding memory cues (e.g., alarms, associating medications with mealtimes) can be helpful; the nurse must also assess if other resources (e.g., home care, family members) may need to be used to ensure safety.

Reactions of older adults to medications, particularly sedatives, are unpredictable and often bizarre and increase the risk for falls. The attitudes of older adults toward medical care and medications can vary. Some may strongly believe in the wisdom of the physician more readily than others and passively accept their medications without questioning in spite of having concerns. As a safety measure, ISMP Canada recommends that people ask questions when a new medication is prescribed, for example, whether the medication replaces a previously prescribed medication or interacts with others (including OTC and natural products) currently taken.

See the Evidence-Informed Practice box on how work interruptions for the nurse during medication administration can impact client safety.

Enteral Medications

Oral Medications

The oral route is the most common route by which medications are given. As long as a client can swallow and retain the drug in the stomach, this is the route of choice (Skill 33.1). Oral medications are contraindicated when a client is vomiting, has gastric or intestinal suction, or is unconscious and unable to swallow. Such patients in hospital are usually on orders for "nothing by mouth" (the Latin term is *nil per os:* NPO). Medications that are inactivated in the stomach or toxic to it are prescribed using an alternative route.

See the Lifespan Considerations box and the Home Care Considerations box on administering oral medications on page 901.

Nasogastric or Gastrostomy Tube Medications

For clients who cannot take anything by mouth (NPO) and have a **nasogastric tube** or a **gastrostomy tube** in place, an alternative route for administering medications is through

EVIDENCE-INFORMED PRACTICE

Work Interruptions During Medication Administration

Work interruptions (WIs) while nurses are involved in medication administration (which includes medication preparation) are a client safety issue. WIs can lead to nurses omitting an important step in the administration process, making a calculation error, and feeling anxious or frustrated at not being able to complete the task in an efficient and effective manner. Biron, Lavoie-Tremblay, and Loiselle used a descriptive observational design to document the characteristics of nurses' work interruptions during medication administration while working on a medical unit of a tertiary care university teaching hospital in Quebec. The findings indicated that, on average, nurses experienced 5.2 WIs per hour during the medication preparation phase and 6.8 WIs per hour during the actual administration phase. Of the 109 "medication administrative rounds" that were observed, WIs were noted in over half (53.9%)! The leading causes of WIs were other nurses (29.3% in the preparation phase), such as getting a report on a patient or talking about personal matters; system failures (22.8% in the preparation phase), such as missing medications or searching for narcotics cupboard keys; and direct patient care (44.4% in the administration phase), such as being asked questions by the family or the patient unrelated to the medication administration.

NURSING IMPLICATIONS: **Nurses spend a great deal of time preparing and administering medications and do not want to make errors. This study is one of very few to formally document work interruption rates of nurses administering medications, so it is significant as a start to "benchmarking" standards. Awareness of the quantity and quality of the WIs can help raise nurses' self-awareness and provide the "system" information about areas of improvement. Possible solutions could include inculcating a "do not disturb" culture surrounding medication administration, automated medication carts to reduce "key searching," improved pharmacy resources to avoid the search for medications, and possibly moving preparation of medications from open common areas (e.g., medication room, hallway) to more isolated areas, such as the patient's room.**

Source: Based on Biron, A. D., Lavoie-Tremblay, M., & Loiselle, C. G. (2009). Characteristics of work interruptions during medication administration. *Journal of Nursing Scholarship, 41,* 330–336. doi: 10.1111/j.1547-5069.2009.01300.x

SKILL 33.1 ADMINISTERING ORAL MEDICATIONS

PURPOSE

To provide a medication that has systemic effects or local effects on the gastrointestinal tract or both (see specific drug action)

ASSESSMENT

Assess

- Allergies to medications
- Client's ability to swallow the medication
- Presence of vomiting or diarrhea that would interfere with the ability to absorb the medication
- Specific drug action, adverse effects, and interactions
- Client's knowledge of and learning needs about the medication
- Any relevant data that is specific to the medication (e.g., heart rate prior to administering digoxin; blood pressure prior to antihypertensive agent)
- Determine if the assessment data influence administration of the medication (i.e., whether it is appropriate to administer the medication or if the medication needs to be held and the prescriber notified).

Clinical Reasoning

Are there any issues you might anticipate regarding how the client will respond to taking this medication orally? How will your nursing care of the client be influenced by his or her understanding of the health situation and the reasons why the medication is prescribed? If the client understands why the medication is necessary, is there anything in his or her situation that may make it difficult to tolerate the oral medication?

Equipment

- Dispensing system
- Disposable medication cups: small paper or plastic cups for tablets and capsules, waxed or plastic calibrated medication cups for liquids
- Medication administration record (MAR) or computer printout
- Pill crusher or cutter
- Straws to administer medications that may discolour teeth or to facilitate the ingestion of liquid medication for certain clients
- Drinking glass and water or juice
- Soft foods, such as applesauce or pudding, to use as a vehicle for crushed medications (if there are no contraindications such as drug–food interaction) for clients who may choke on liquids

IMPLEMENTATION

Preparation

1. Know the reason the client is receiving the medication, the drug classification, contraindications, usual dosage

(continued)

SKILL 33.1 ADMINISTERING ORAL MEDICATIONS (*continued*)

range, adverse effects, and nursing considerations for administering and evaluating the intended outcomes for the medication. **Rationale: A thorough knowledge of the medication to be administered assists in evaluating its therapeutic effect. The nurse can also use this knowledge to educate the client.**

2. Check the MAR.
   - Check for the drug name, dosage, frequency, route of administration, and expiration date for administering the medication, if appropriate. **Rationale: Orders for certain medications (e.g., narcotics, antibiotics) expire after a specified time frame, and they need to be reordered.**
   - If the MAR is unclear or pertinent information is missing, compare the MAR with the prescriber's most recent written order.
   - Report any discrepancies to the charge nurse or the prescriber, as agency policy dictates.

3. Verify the client's ability to take medication orally. Determine whether the client can swallow, is NPO, is nauseated or vomiting, has gastric suction, or has diminished or absent bowel sounds.

4. Organize the supplies. Gather the MAR(s) for each client together so that medications can be prepared for one client at a time. **Rationale: Organization of supplies saves time and reduces the chance of error.**

Performance

1. Perform hand hygiene, and follow other appropriate infection prevention and control procedures.

2. Unlock the dispensing system (if applicable).

3. Obtain the appropriate medication.
   - Read the MAR, and take the appropriate medication from the shelf, drawer, or refrigerator. The medication may be dispensed in a bottle, box, or unit-dose package.
   - Compare the label of the medication container or unit-dose package against the order on the MAR or computer printout. See ①. **Rationale: A safety check ensures that the right medication is given.** If these are not identical, recheck the prescriber's written order

in the client's chart. If there is still a discrepancy, check with the nurse in charge or the pharmacist.
   - Check the expiration date of the medication. Return expired medications to the pharmacy. **Rationale: Outdated medications are not safe to administer.**
   - Use only medications that have clear, legible labels. **Rationale: The labels help ensure accuracy.**

4. Prepare the medication.
   - Calculate the medication dosage accurately.
   - Prepare the correct amount of medication for the required dose, without contaminating the medication. **Rationale: Aseptic technique maintains drug cleanliness.**
   - While preparing the medication, recheck each prepared drug and container against the MAR again. **Rationale: This second safety check reduces the chance of error.**

Tablets or Capsules

- Place packaged unit-dose capsules or tablets directly into the medicine container. Do not remove the medication from the package until at the bedside. **Rationale: The wrapper keeps the medication clean. Not removing the medication facilitates identification of the medication in the event the client refuses the drug or assessment data indicate to hold the medication. Unopened unit-dose packages can usually be returned to the medication cart.**

- If using a stock container, pour the required number into the bottle cap, and then transfer the medication to the disposable cup without touching the tablets.

- Keep narcotics and medications that require specific assessments, such as pulse measurements, respiratory rate or depth, or blood pressure, separate from the others. **Rationale: This reminds the nurse to complete the needed assessments in order to decide whether to give the medication or to withhold the medication if indicated.**

- Break only scored tablets, if necessary, to obtain the correct dosage. Use a cutting or splitting device, if needed (see ②). Check the agency policy as to whether unused portions of a medication are to be discarded and, if so, how they are to be discarded.

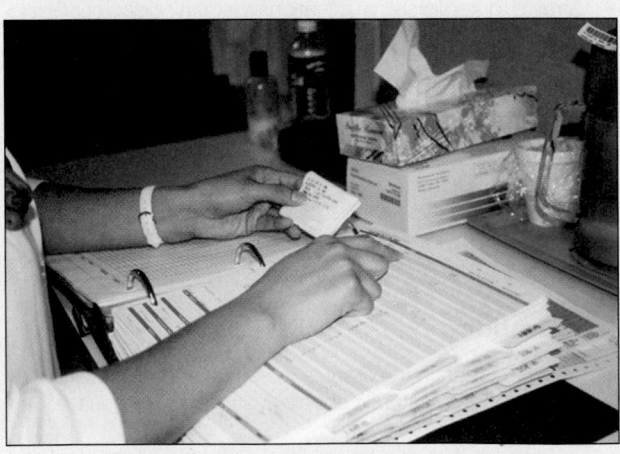

❶ Compare the medication label to the MAR.

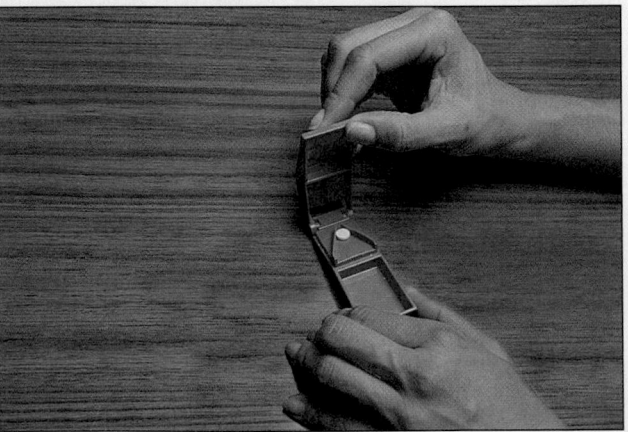

❷ A cutting device can be used to divide tablets.

- If the client has difficulty swallowing, check if the medication can be crushed. Some drug handbooks have an appendix that lists the "Do Not Crush" medications; alternatively, consult with the pharmacy before crushing tablets. See Box 33.4.
- If it is acceptable, crush the tablets to a fine powder with a pill crusher (mortar and pestle or between two medication cups). Then, mix the powder with a small amount of soft food (e.g., custard, applesauce).

Liquid Medication

- Thoroughly mix the medication before pouring. Discard any medication that has changed colour or turned cloudy.
- Remove the cap and place it upside down on the countertop. **Rationale: This action helps avoid contaminating the inside of the cap.**
- Hold the bottle so the label is next to your palm and pour the medication away from the label (see ❸). **Rationale: This step prevents the label from becoming soiled and illegible as a result of spilled liquid**.
- Place the medication cup on a flat surface at eye level, and fill it to the desired level, using the *bottom* of the meniscus (crescent-shaped upper surface of a column of liquid) to align with the container scale (see ❹). **Rationale: This method ensures accuracy of measurement**.
- Before capping the bottle, wipe its lip with a paper towel. **Rationale: This prevents the cap from sticking**.

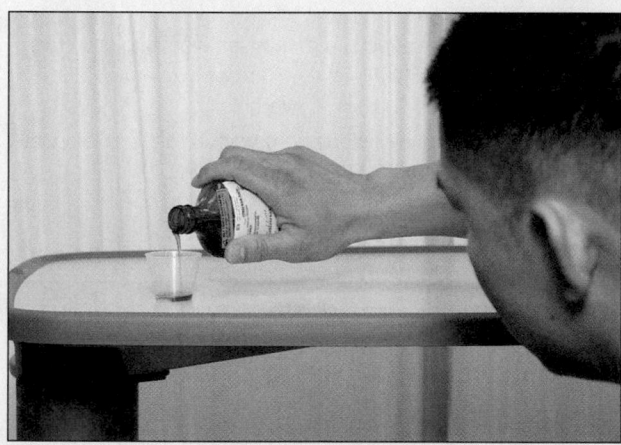

❸ Pouring a liquid medication from a bottle

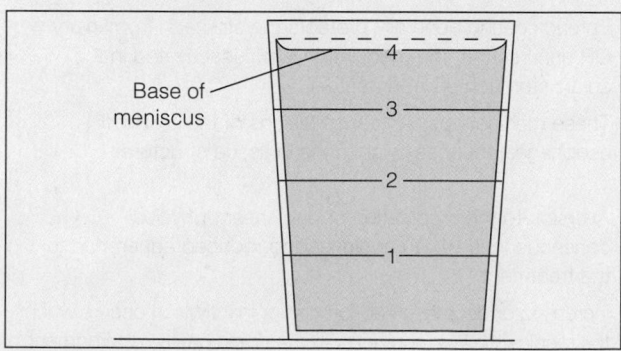

Base of meniscus

❹ The base of the meniscus is the measuring guide.

- When giving small amounts of liquids (e.g., less than 5 mL), prepare the medication in a sterile syringe without the needle or in a specially designed oral syringe. Label the syringe with the name of the medication and the route (PO). **Rationale: Any oral solution removed from the original container and placed into a syringe should be labelled to avoid medications being given by the wrong route (e.g., IV). This practice facilitates client safety and avoids tragic errors**.
- Keep unit-dose liquids in their package, and open them at the bedside.

Controlled Substances

- If an agency uses a manual recording system for controlled substances, check the control substance record for the previous drug count and compare it with the supply available.
- Remove the oral preparation (e.g., tablet, capsule), and drop it in the medicine cup.
- After removing a medication, record the necessary information on the appropriate control record and sign it.
- *Note:* Computer-controlled dispensing systems allow access only to the selected drug and automatically record its use.

All Medications

- Place the prepared medication and MAR together on the medication cart.
- Recheck the label on the container before returning the bottle, box, or envelope to its storage place. **Rationale: This third check further reduces the risk of error.**
- Avoid leaving prepared medications unattended. **Rationale: This precaution prevents potential mishandling errors.**
- Lock the medication cart before entering the client's room. **Rationale: This is a safety measure because medication carts are not to be left open when unattended.**
- Check the room number against the MAR if agency policy does not allow the MAR to be removed from the medication cart. **Rationale: This is another safety measure to ensure that the nurse is entering the correct client's room.**

5. Provide for client privacy.

6. Prepare the client.
- Introduce yourself and verify the client's identity using two identifiers or per agency policy. **Rationale: This step ensures that the right client receives the medication**.
- Assist the client to a sitting position or, if not possible, to the side-lying position. **Rationale: These positions facilitate swallowing and prevent aspiration**.
- If not previously assessed, take the required assessment measures (e.g., apical pulse rate before administering digitalis; blood pressure before giving antihypertensive drugs; respiratory rate before administering opioids). If any of the findings are above or below the predetermined parameters, consult the appropriate member of the health care team before administering the medication.

7. Explain the purpose of the medication and how it will help, using language that the client can understand. Include relevant information about effects; for example, tell the client

(continued)

SKILL 33.1 ADMINISTERING ORAL MEDICATIONS (*continued*)

receiving a diuretic to expect an increase in urine output. **Rationale: Information can facilitate acceptance of, and adherence to, the therapy**.

8. Administer the medication at the correct time.

- Take the medication to the client within the period of 30 minutes before or after the scheduled time.

- Give the client sufficient water or preferred juice to help swallow the medication. Before using juice, check for any food and medication incompatibilities. **Rationale: Fluids ease swallowing and facilitate absorption from the gastrointestinal tract but drug–food interactions must be avoided**. Liquid medications other than antacids or cough preparations may be diluted with 15 mL of water to facilitate absorption.

- If the client is unable to hold the pill cup, use the pill cup to introduce the medication into the client's mouth, and give only one tablet or capsule at a time. **Rationale: Putting the cup to the client's mouth maintains the cleanliness of the nurse's hands. Giving one medication at a time eases swallowing**.

- If an older child or adult has difficulty swallowing, ask the client to place the medication on the back of the tongue before taking the water. **Rationale: Stimulation of the back of the tongue elicits the swallowing reflex**.

- If the medication has an unpleasant taste, ask the client to suck a few ice chips beforehand, or give the medication with juice, applesauce, or bread if there are no contraindications. **Rationale: The cold of the ice chips will desensitize the taste buds, and juices or bread can mask the taste of the medication**.

- If the client says that the medication you are about to give is different from what the client has been receiving, do not give the medication without first checking the original order. **Rationale: Most clients are familiar with the appearance of medications taken previously. Unfamiliar medications may signal a possible error**.

- Stay with the client until all medications have been swallowed. **Rationale: The nurse must see the client swallow the medication before the drug administration can be recorded**. Some agencies may have a policy that allows medications to be left at the bedside, such as when a client is learning self-medication prior to discharge.

9. Document each medication given.

- Record the medication given, dosage, time, any complaints or assessments of the client, and your signature.

- If medication was refused or omitted, record this fact on the appropriate record; document the reason, when possible, and your actions, according to agency policy.

10. Dispose of all supplies appropriately.

- Replenish stock (e.g., medication cups), and return the cart to the appropriate place.

- Discard used disposable supplies.

EVALUATION

- Return to the client when the medication is expected to take effect (determined by the onset of action of the medication—usually 30 minutes) to evaluate the effects of the medication on the client.

- Observe for desired effect (e.g., relief of pain or decrease in body temperature).

- Note any adverse effects (e.g., nausea, vomiting, skin rash, or change in vital signs).

- Relate to previous findings, if available.

- Report significant deviations from normal to the appropriate members of the health care team.

BOX 33.4 MEDICATIONS THAT SHOULD NOT BE CRUSHED*

TYPE OF MEDICATION	CONSEQUENCE OF CRUSHING
Sustain-released (SR)—also referred to as extended-release (XR), long-acting (LA), delayed-action (DA), delayed-release (DR), enteric-release (ER) medications, and granules with capsules (GC)	The medication is absorbed quickly and a surge of effect occurs rather than one spread out over time as intended.
Enteric-coated medications (e.g., enteric-coated Aspirin [ECASA])	Enteric coating generally protects the stomach from injury OR ensures that the medication is not inactivated in the acidic stomach environment.
Medications that are irritants (e.g., risedronate [Actonel]) or cytotoxic (e.g., mycophenolate mofetil [CellCept]) to oral mucosa	These medications can cause lesions of the oral and esophageal mucosa or changes in tissue structure.
Medications that are foul tasting (e.g., docusate [Colace]) or stain teeth (e.g., ferrous sulphate)	Aversion to the medication or unpleasant physical consequences—both could lead to reduced adherence to the treatment.
Buccal or sublingual medications (e.g. nitroglycerine)	Increased or decreased absorption or inactivation occurs when the medication is in contact with the acidic gastric environment.

Note that a complete list of Do Not Crush Medications can be found at the ISMP Canada website: http://www.ismp.org/tools/donotcrush.pdf

Sources: Table created by M. Buck based on Institute for Safe Medication Practices. (2011). *Oral dosage forms that should not be crushed*. Retrieved from http://www.ismp.org/tools/donotcrush.pdf; and Lehne, R. (2010). *Pharmacology for nursing care*. St. Louis, MO: Elsevier.

Administering Oral Medications

INFANTS

- Knowledge of growth and development is essential for the nurse administering medications to infants and children.

- Nurses must know the range of safe medication dosages for infants and children.

- Oral medications can be effectively administered in several ways:
  - An oral syringe or dropper
  - A medication nipple, which allows the infant to suck the medication
  - Mixed in small amounts of food
  - A spoon or medication cup, for older children

- Never mix medications into foods that are essential, since the infant may associate the food with an unpleasant taste and refuse that food in the future. Never mix medications with formula.

- Place a small amount of liquid medication along the inside of the baby's cheek and wait for the infant to swallow before giving more to prevent aspiration or spitting out.

- When using a spoon, retrieve and refeed medication that is thrust outward by the infant's tongue.

CHILDREN

- Whenever possible, give children a choice with the use of a spoon, dropper, or oral syringe.

- Dilute the oral medication, if indicated, with a small amount of water. Many oral medications are readily swallowed if they are diluted with a small amount of water. If large quantities of water are used, the child may refuse to drink the entire amount and receive only a portion of the medication.

- Oral medications for children are usually prepared in sweetened liquid form to make them more palatable. Crush medications that are not supplied in liquid form and mix them with substances available on most pediatric units, such as honey, flavoured syrup, jam, or a fruit puree.

- Necessary foods, such as milk or orange juice, should not be used to mask the taste of medications because the child may develop unpleasant associations and refuse that food in the future.

- Disguise disagreeable-tasting medications with sweet-tasting substances mentioned previously. However, present any altered medication to the child honestly and not as a food or treat.

- Place the young child or toddler on your lap or a parent's lap in a sitting position.

- Administer the medication slowly with a measuring spoon, plastic syringe, or medicine cup.

- To prevent nausea, pour a carbonated beverage over finely crushed ice, and give it before or immediately after the medication is administered.

- Follow medication with a drink of water, juice, a soft drink, or a Popsicle or frozen juice bar to remove any unpleasant aftertaste.

- For children who take sweetened medications on a long-term basis, follow the medication administration with oral hygiene. These children are at high risk for dental caries.

OLDER ADULTS

- The physiological changes associated with aging influence medication administration and effectiveness. Examples include altered memory, less acute vision, decrease in renal function, less complete and slower absorption from the gastrointestinal tract, and decreased liver function. Many of these changes enhance the possibility of cumulative effects and toxicity.

- Older adults usually require smaller dosages of drugs, especially sedatives and other central nervous system depressants.

- Older adults are mature adults capable of reasoning. The nurse, therefore, needs to explain the reasons for and the effects of the client's medications.

- Socioeconomic factors, such as lack of transportation and decreased finances, may influence obtaining medications when needed.

- An increase in marketing and availability of natural health products alerts the nurse to include this information in a medication history.

Administering Medication

The nurse should instruct the client to do the following:

- Learn the names of the medications as well as their actions and possible adverse effects. Carry a complete list of all prescriptions, OTC medications, and natural health products at all times.

- Keep all medications out of reach of children and pets.

- If using a syringe to administer the medication to an infant or child, use an oral syringe rather than an injection syringe as infants and small children

have been known to choke on the cap of an injection syringe.

- Take the medications only as prescribed. Know which medications need to be taken on an empty stomach and which can be taken with food or meals. Immediately consult the appropriate member of the health care team about any problems with the medication.

- Always check the medication label to make sure the correct medication is being taken.

- Request labels printed with larger type on medication containers if experiencing difficulty reading the label.

- Check the expiration date, and discard outdated medications in a responsible way. Previously, most people discarded old medicines by flushing them down the toilet. Health Canada (2011) recommends that unused and expired medications be disposed of in an environmentally safe manner. Check with the municipality or pharmacy about a drug take-back program that collects and disposes

(continued)

HOME CARE CONSIDERATIONS (*continued*)

of unused and expired drugs in a safe manner.

- Ask the pharmacist to substitute childproof caps with ones that are more easily opened, if necessary.

- If one dose or more of the medication has been missed, do not take two or more doses; ask the pharmacist or other appropriate member of the health care team for instructions.

- Do not crush or cut a medication without first checking with the prescriber or pharmacist. Doing so may affect the medication's absorption.

- Never stop taking the medication without first discussing it with the prescriber or appropriate member of the health care team.

- Always check with the pharmacist or appropriate member of the health

care team before taking any non-prescription medications. Some OTC medications can interact with the prescribed medication.

- Additionally, the nurse can set up a medication plan to assist clients and family members to remember a schedule. Weekly pill containers (available at pharmacies) or a written plan may be helpful.

---

the nasogastric or gastrostomy tube. A nasogastric (NG) tube is inserted by way of the nasopharynx and is placed into the client's stomach for the purpose of feeding the client or to remove gastric secretions. A gastrostomy tube is surgically placed directly into the client's stomach and provides another route for administering medications and nutrition (see Chapter 40 for further discussion of nasogastric and gastrostomy tubes). Practice guidelines for administering medications by nasogastric tubes and gastrostomy tubes are shown in Practice Guidelines 33.2.

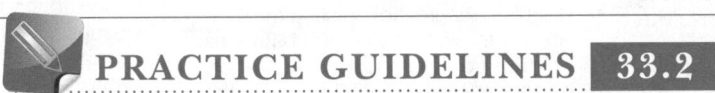

PRACTICE GUIDELINES 33.2

Administering Medications by Nasogastric or Gastrostomy Tube

Guidelines	Rationales
Always check with the pharmacist to see if the client's medications come in liquid form.	This form is less likely to cause tube obstruction.
If medications do not come in liquid form, check to see whether they may be crushed.	Crushing enteric-coated, sustained-action, enzyme-specific, buccal, and sublingual tablets affects pharmacokinetics or causes gastric irritation (see Box 33.4).
Read medication labels carefully before opening a capsule. Open capsules and mix the contents with water *only* with the pharmacist's advice.	The pellets inside some capsules (e.g., Effexor XR) can be poured down the tube, provided they are not crushed. Manufacturer's instructions may indicate drug-specific information that is relevant.
Crush a tablet into a fine powder, and dissolve in at least 30 mL of warm water. Generally, use water for mixing and flushing.	Cold liquids can cause patient discomfort and may not dissolve medication. Some medications are mixed with other fluids, such as normal saline, to maximize dissolution. Whole or undissolved medications will clog the tube.
If bulk-forming laxatives (e.g., Metamucil) are prescribed, consult the appropriate member of the health care team for an alternative prescription.	These medication preparations form a semisolid mass and can occlude the tube.
If the nasogastric or gastrostomy tube is also being used for enteral feeding, then ensure that the medication is compatible with the feeding solution.	A physical incompatibility may exist, leading to precipitation that can occlude the tube (e.g., ferrous sulphate and potassium chloride liquids are incompatible with most enteral formulae).
Assess the tube placement (see Chapter 40 for methods to assess tube placement).	Misplacement of the tube can lead to inadvertently administering medications outside the gastrointestinal tract (e.g., into the lungs).
Before giving the medication, aspirate all the stomach contents, and measure the residual volume. Check agency policy if the residual volume is greater than 200 mL.	Excess residual volume may mean that peristalsis is not effective in moving stomach contents forward. Adding medication to a high residual volume can lead to poor absorption.

PRACTICE GUIDELINES 33.2

Administering Medications by Nasogastric or Gastrostomy Tube (continued)

Guidelines	Rationales
When administering the medication(s), remove the plunger from the syringe, and connect the syringe to a pinched or kinked tube.	Pinching or kinking the tube prevents excess air from entering the stomach and causing distension.
Put 15 mL to 30 mL (5 mL to 10 mL for children) of water into the syringe barrel to flush the tube before administering the first medication. Raise or lower the barrel of the syringe to adjust the flow, as needed. Pinch or clamp the tubing before all the water is instilled.	Flushing ensures that the medication does not come in contact with any other substance; clamping will prevent excess air from entering the stomach.
Pour liquid or dissolved medication into the syringe barrel and allow to flow by gravity into the enteral tube.	This helps avoid trauma to the gastrointestinal mucosa.
If giving several medications, administer each one separately and flush with at least 15 mL to 30 mL (5 mL for children) of tap water between each medication. Consult the appropriate health care professional if the patient is on fluid restriction.	This will avoid any possible drug–drug interactions.
When all medications have been administered, flush with another 15 mL to 30 mL (5 mL to 10 mL for children) of warm water.	Clearing the tube ensures that the entire medication dose has been given and that no blockage occurs.
If the tube is connected to suction, disconnect the suction, and keep the tube clamped for a minimum of 20 to 30 minutes after giving the medication; some agencies recommend 1 to 2 hours.	This ensures that the medication is absorbed rather than be suctioned out of the stomach when suction is reconnected.

Parenteral Medications

Parenteral administration of medications is a common nursing procedure. Nurses give parenteral medications intradermally (ID), subcutaneously (SC), intramuscularly (IM), or intravenously (IV). Because these medications are absorbed more quickly than oral medications and are irretrievable once injected, the nurse must prepare and administer them carefully and accurately. Administering parenteral drugs requires the same nursing knowledge as for oral and topical drugs; however, because injections are invasive procedures, aseptic technique must be used to minimize the risk of infection.

Equipment

To administer parenteral medications, nurses use syringes and needles to withdraw medication from ampules and vials.

SYRINGES Syringes have three parts: (a) the tip, which connects with the needle; (b) the barrel, or outside part, on which the scales are printed; and (c) the plunger, which fits inside the barrel (Figure 33.12). When handling a syringe, the nurse may touch the outside of the barrel and the handle of the plunger; however, the nurse must *avoid letting any unsterile object contact the tip or inside of the barrel, the shaft of the plunger, or the shaft or tip of the needle.*

There are several kinds of syringes, differing in size, shape, and material. Syringes range in sizes from 1 to 60 mL. A nurse typically uses a syringe ranging from 1 to 3 mL in size for injections (e.g., SC or IM). The choice of syringe depends on many factors, such as medication, location of injection, and type of tissue. A scale on the syringe marks off gradations (e.g., 0.1 mL) to allow for fractions of a millilitre to be administered. The larger-sized syringes (e.g., 10, 20, and 50 mL) are not used to administer drugs directly but can be useful for adding medications to IV solutions or for irrigating wounds.

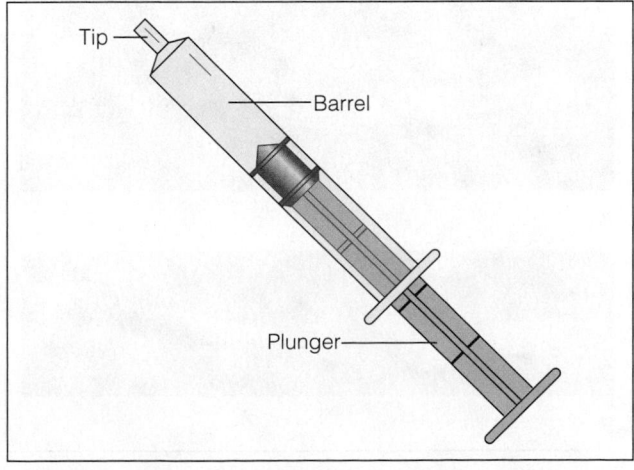

FIGURE 33.12 The three parts of a syringe.

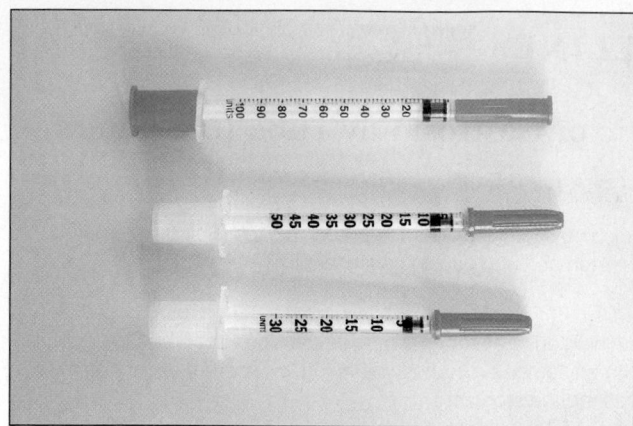

FIGURE 33.13 Different insulin syringes based on the amount of insulin required.

An **insulin syringe** has a "unit" scale specially designed for insulin and is the only syringe that should be used to administer insulin. All insulin syringes are calibrated on the 100-unit scale; low-dose insulin syringes are available (e.g., 30-unit, 50-unit). These smaller syringes often have a nonremovable needle. The correct choice of syringe is based on the amount of insulin required (Figure 33.13).

The **tuberculin syringe** was originally designed to administer tuberculin as in PPD (purified protein derivative) testing for tuberculosis. It is a narrow syringe calibrated in tenths and hundredths of a millilitre (up to 1 mL). This type of syringe can also be useful in administering other drugs, particularly when small or precise measurement is indicated (e.g., pediatric dosages).

Syringes are made in other sizes as well (e.g., 5 mL, 10 mL, 20 mL, and 50 mL). These are not generally used to administer drugs directly but can be useful for adding medications to intravenous solutions or for irrigating wounds. The tip of a syringe varies and is classified as either a Luer-Lok or non–Luer-Lok. A Luer-Lok syringe has a tip that requires the needle to be twisted onto it to avoid accidental removal of the needle (Figure 33.14).

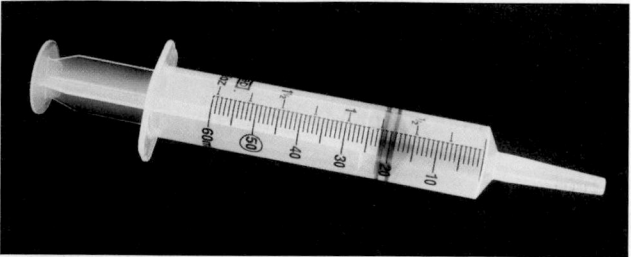

FIGURE 33.15 A 50-mL non–Luer-Lok syringe, which can be used for irrigation of tubes or wounds.

The non–Luer-Lok syringe has a smooth graduated tip, and needles are slipped onto it. The larger 50-mL non–Luer-Lok syringe is often used for **irrigation** (**lavage**) purposes (e.g., wounds, tubes) (Figure 33.15).

Most syringes used today are made of plastic, are individually packaged for sterility in a paper wrapper, and are disposable. The syringe and needle may be packaged together or separately. Safety-engineered systems include a shielded needle device (Figure 33.16), a retractable needle system (see Figure 33.21 on page 906), and a needleless system (see Figure 33.23 on page 906) in which the needle is replaced by a plastic cannula.

Injectable medications may be supplied in disposable **prefilled unit-dose systems**. These are available as ready for use or as prefilled cartridges requiring assembly, per the manufacturer's specific instructions. Because most prefilled cartridges are overfilled, excess medication must be ejected before the injection to ensure the right dosage. As the needle is generally fused to the prefilled unit-dose syringe, the nurse is unable to change the **gauge**, or diameter of the needle, or the length of the needle. The nurse, however, can transfer the medication into a regular syringe if the assessment of the client necessitates a different needle gauge or length.

NEEDLES Needles are made of stainless steel, and most are disposable. A needle has three discernible parts: (a) the **hub**, which fits onto the syringe; (b) the **cannula**, or **shaft**, which is attached to the hub; and (c) the **bevel**, which is the slanted part at the tip of the needle (Figure 33.17).

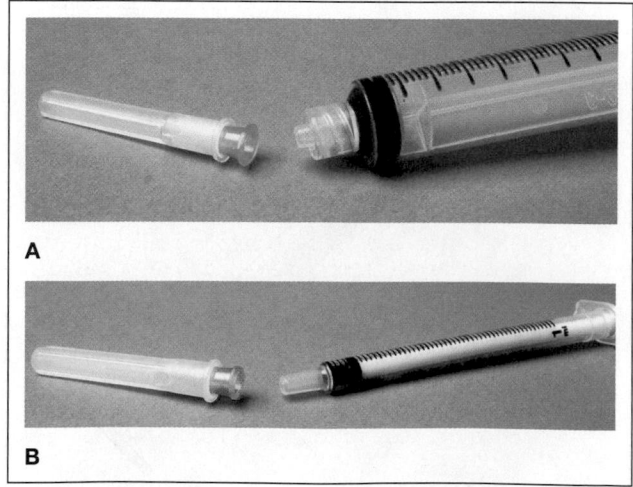

FIGURE 33.14 Tips of syringes: **A:** Luer-Lok (note threaded tip); **B:** Non–Luer-Lok syringe (note the smooth graduated tip).

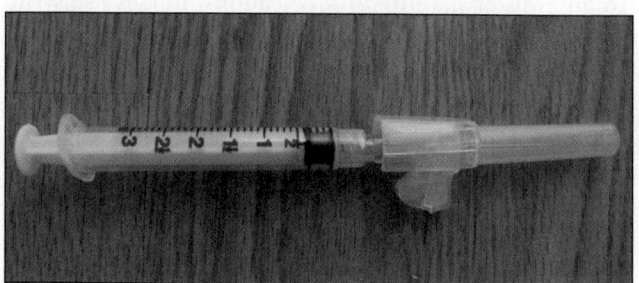

FIGURE 33.16 A shielded needle device.

Source: Reprinted with permission from Julie Wood.

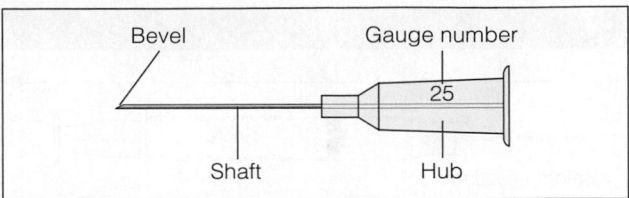

Bevel   Gauge number

25

Shaft   Hub

FIGURE 33.17 The parts of a needle.

A disposable needle has a plastic hub. Needles used for injections have three variable characteristics:

1. *Slant or length of the bevel.* The bevel of the needle may be short or long. Longer bevels provide the sharpest needles, cause less discomfort, and are commonly used for subcutaneous and intramuscular injections. Short bevels are used for intradermal and intravenous injections because a long bevel can become occluded if it rests against the side of a blood vessel.

2. *Length of the shaft.* The shaft length of commonly used needles varies from 10 mm to 5 cm. The appropriate needle length is chosen according to the client's muscle development, the client's weight, and the type of injection.

3. *Gauge (or diameter) of the shaft.* The gauge of needles used for humans varies from #16 (1.651 mm in diameter) to #28 (0.356 mm in diameter). The larger the gauge number, the smaller is the diameter of the shaft. Smaller gauges cause less tissue trauma and are ideal for daily subcutaneous injections, such as insulin; larger gauges are necessary for viscous medications, such as penicillin.

For intramuscular injections, the needle should be long enough to reach the muscle but not so long that it penetrates to underlying blood vessels or bone. For the majority of infants, a 2.5 cm needle length is sufficient to penetrate the thigh muscle; most young children require a 2.2 cm to 2.5 cm long needle for injections in the deltoid while older children and adolescents generally require a 2.5 cm needle; men and women weighing 60 kg to 70 kg generally require a 2.5 cm long needle to reach the deltoid muscle. A 22-gauge to a 25-gauge needle is generally adequate for injecting medications that are not highly viscous.

For an adult requiring a subcutaneous injection, it is generally appropriate to use a needle that is 16 mm long with a #25 to #27 gauge. Intradermal injections generally require a 26-gauge or 27-gauge micro-needle.

Preventing Needlestick Injuries

One of the most potentially hazardous procedures that health care personnel face involves using and disposing of needles and sharps. Needlestick injuries present a major risk for infection with hepatitis B and C viruses, human immunodeficiency virus (HIV), and many other pathogens. Standards have been set by the Canadian Centre for Occupational Health and Safety to prevent such injuries, and any medical procedure involving the use of hollow-bore needles requires the use of safety-engineered needles or needleless systems. Some of these standards are summarized in Box 33.5. If an accidental needlestick injury occurs, the nurse needs to follow specific steps outlined by the agency.

BOX 33.5   AVOIDING PUNCTURE INJURIES

Use appropriate puncture-proof disposal containers to dispose of uncapped needles and sharps. These are provided in all client areas (Figure 33.18). Never throw sharps in wastebaskets. Sharps include any items that can cut or puncture skin, such as the following: needles, surgical blades, lancets, razors, broken glass, reusable items (e.g., large-bore needles, hooks, rasps, drill points), and ANY SHARP INSTRUMENT!

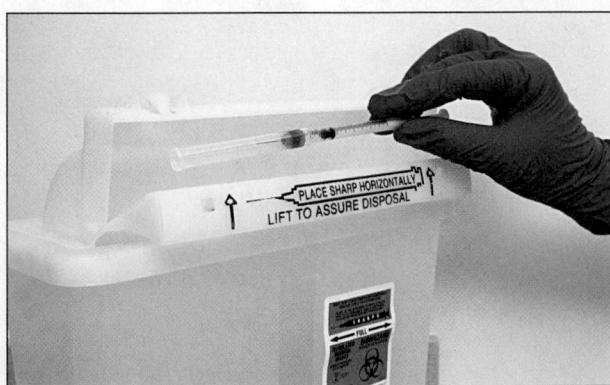

FIGURE 33.18 Dispose of used syringe and needle in sharps container.

- Never bend or break needles before disposal.
- Never recap needles that have been inserted into clients except under specified circumstances (e.g., when transporting a syringe to the laboratory for an arterial blood gas or blood culture).
- When recapping a needle (e.g., after drawing up a medication into a syringe *prior* to administration):
  - Use a safety mechanical device that firmly grips the needle cap and holds it in place until it is ready to be recapped (Figure 33.19).
  - Use a one-handed "scoop" method. This is performed by (a) placing the needle cap and syringe with needle horizontally on a flat surface, (b) inserting the needle into the cap using one hand (Figure 33.20), and then (c) using the other hand to pick up the cap and tighten it to the needle hub. Be careful not to contaminate the needle. If the needle becomes contaminated, replace the needle with a new one.
  - Use safety syringes that require NO contact with the needle. Passive devices have needles that retract immediately into the barrel after injection (Figure 33.21); active safety devices require the nurse to manually activate the safety feature (see Figure 33.22).

(continued)

BOX 33.5 AVOIDING PUNCTURE INJURIES (continued)

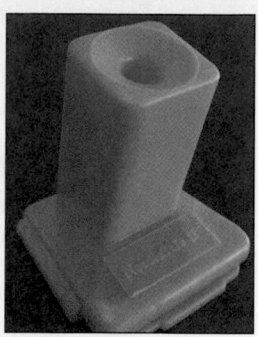 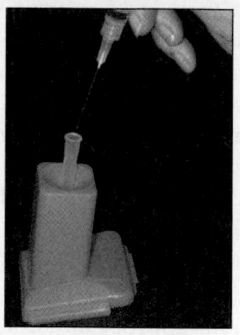

FIGURE 33.19 A safety mechanical device that holds the needle cap in place until the nurse is ready to recap.

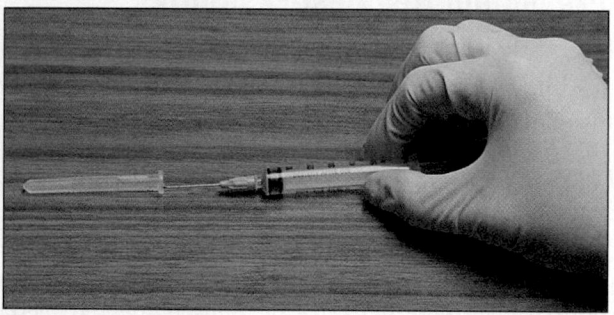

FIGURE 33.20 Recapping a used needle by using the scoop method.

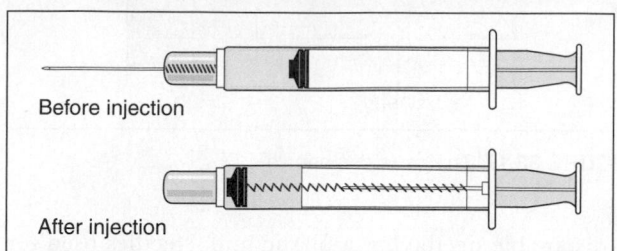

FIGURE 33.21 Passive safety device: the needle retracts immediately into the barrel after injection.

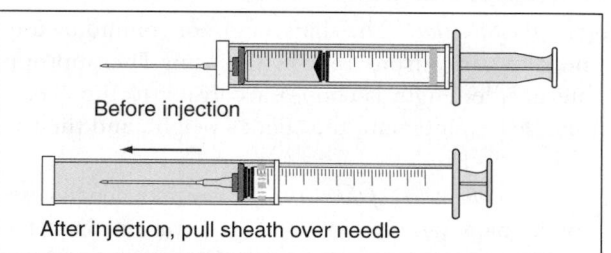

FIGURE 33.22 Active safety device: the nurse manually pulls the sheath or guard over the needle after injection.

Preparing Injectable Medications

Injectable medications can be prepared by withdrawing the medication from an ampule or a vial into a sterile syringe, using prefilled syringes, or using needleless injection systems. Figure 33.23 shows an example of a needleless system used to access medication from a vial.

AMPULES AND VIALS Ampules and vials (Figure 33.24) are frequently used to package sterile parenteral medications. An **ampule** is a glass container usually designed to hold a single dose of a drug. It is made of clear glass and has a distinctive shape with a constricted neck. Ampules vary in size, ranging from 1 mL to 10 mL or more. Most ampule necks have coloured marks around them where they are scored for easy opening.

While more and more pharmacies are preparing medications that are supplied in ampules and vials, the nurse may be drawing up these medications in certain settings. To access the medication in an ampule, the ampule must be broken at its constricted neck. Traditionally, files were used to score the ampule. Today, plastic ampule openers are available that prevent injury from broken glass. The device consists of a plastic cap that fits over the top of an ampule. The head of the ampule, when broken, remains inside the cap (Figure 33.25) and is placed into a

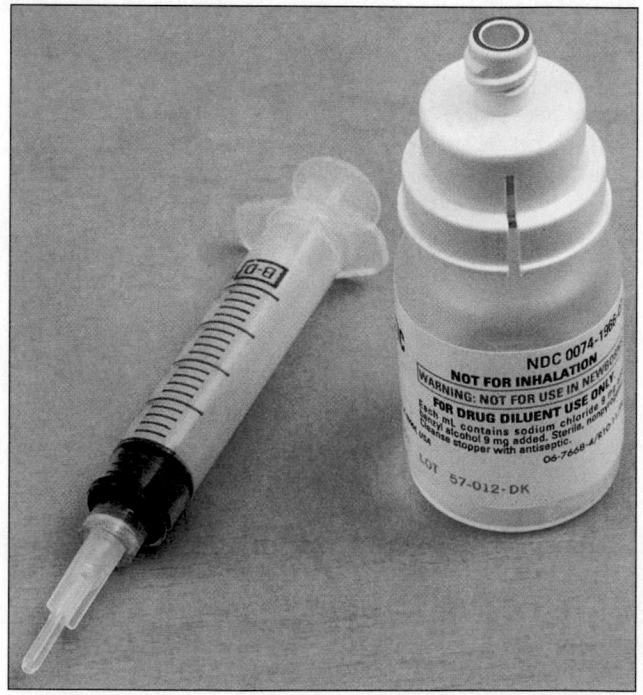

FIGURE 33.23 A needleless system can extract medication from a vial.

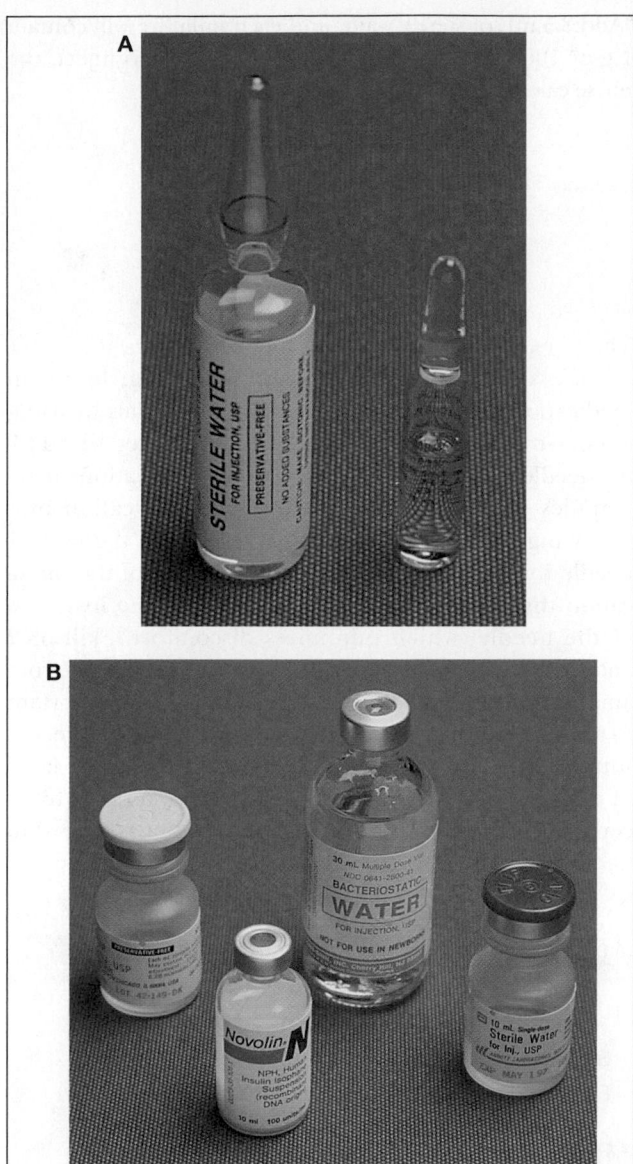

FIGURE 33.24 A: Ampules; **B:** Vials.

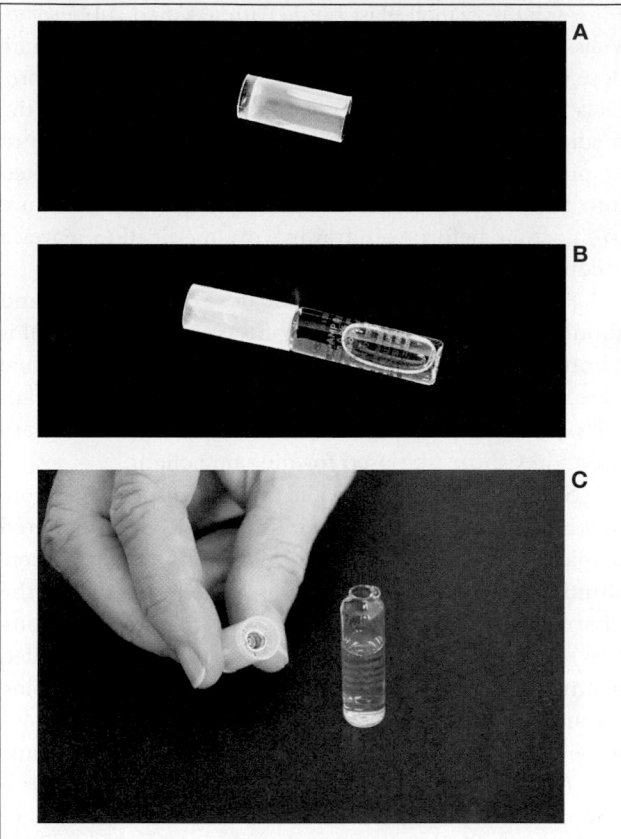

FIGURE 33.25 A: Ampule opener; **B:** Plastic opener is placed over top of ampule; **C:** Top of ampule remains in opener after ampule is broken.

sharps container (see Figure 33.18). If an ampule opener is not available, the nurse can clean the ampule neck with an antiseptic swab and, using dry sterile gauze, snap off the top of the ampule. Once the ampule is broken, the fluid is aspirated into a syringe by using a filter needle or filter straw (Figure 33.26). Both prevent aspiration of any glass particles.

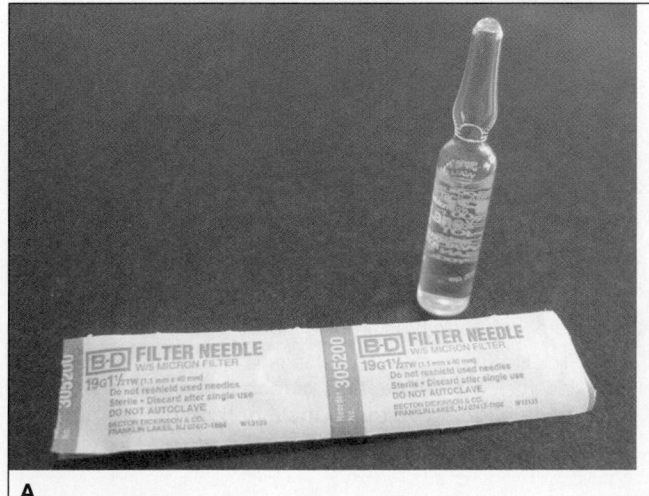
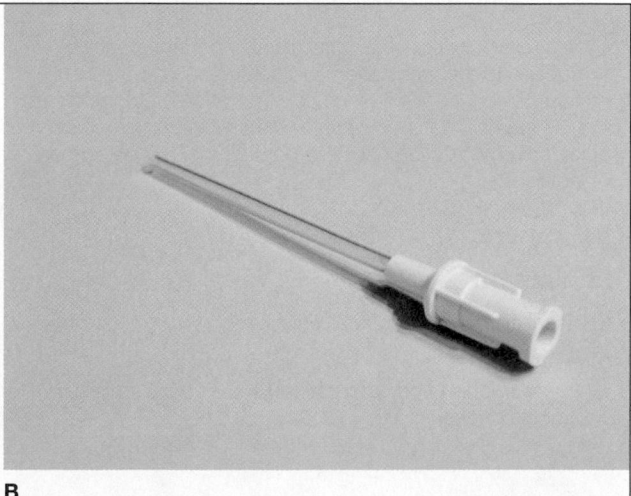

FIGURE 33.26 A filter needle, *A*, or a filter straw, *B*, prevents glass from being withdrawn with the medication.

A **vial** is a small glass bottle with a sealed rubber cap. Vials come in different sizes, from single-use vials to multi-dose vials. They usually have a metal or plastic cap that protects the rubber seal and must be removed to access the medication. To access the medication in a vial, the vial must be pierced with a needle. In addition, air must be injected into a vial before the medication can be withdrawn. Failure to inject air before withdrawing the medication leaves a vacuum within the vial that makes withdrawal difficult.

A single-use vial contains one dose of medication and should only be used once. In contrast, a multidose vial is a bottle of liquid medication that contains more than one dose, such as insulin. Whenever possible, single-dose vials are preferred over multidose vials; if multidose vials are used, they should be used for the same client.

Some drugs (e.g., penicillin) may be dispensed as powders in vials. A diluent (liquid) must be added to a powdered medication before it can be injected, a process called **reconstitution**. Reconstitution is frequently completed in the pharmacy, however, nurses are responsible for reconstitution in some agencies. Powdered drugs usually have printed instructions (enclosed with each packaged vial) describing the amount and kind of diluent (e.g., sterile water or saline) to be added. The following is an example of the preparation of a powdered drug: A dose of 750 mg of a drug is ordered for a client. On hand is a 10-g multidose vial of powdered medication. The directions for preparation are: "Add 8.5 mL of sterile water and each millilitre will contain 1 g or 1000 mg." To determine the amount to inject, the nurse calculates as follows:

$$1 \text{ mL} = 1000 \text{ mg}$$
$$x \text{ mL} = 750 \text{ mg}$$
(cross multiply and solve for x)
$$x = \frac{750 \text{ mg} \times 1 \text{ mL}}{1000 \text{ mg}}$$
$$x = 0.75 \text{ mL}$$

The nurse will give 0.75 mL of the medication.

Glass and rubber particulate have been found in medications withdrawn from ampules and vials by using a regular needle, so it is strongly recommended that a filter needle be used when withdrawing medications from ampules and vials. After drawing the medication into the syringe, the filter needle is replaced with the regular needle for injection. This prevents tracking of the medication through the client's tissues during the insertion of the needle, which minimizes discomfort. Skill 33.2 and Skill 33.3 describe how to prepare medications from ampules and vials, respectively. In addition, it is important to remember that when powdered drugs have been reconstituted, the date and time should be written on the label of the vial. Many of these drugs have to be used within a certain period following reconstitution, so nurses need to know the expiration time after it has been reconstituted.

SKILL 33.2 PREPARING MEDICATIONS FROM AMPULES

ASSESSMENT

Assess

- Client allergies to medication
- Specific drug action, adverse effects, and interactions
- Client's knowledge of and learning needs about the medication
- Intended route of parenteral medication to determine appropriate size of syringe and needle for the client
- Ordered medication for clarity and expiration date
- Any relevant data (e.g., vital signs, laboratory results) specific to the medication and determine how the assessment data influence administration of the medication (i.e., whether it is appropriate to administer the medication or if the medication needs to be held and the prescriber notified).

PLANNING

Equipment

- Client's MAR or computer printout
- Ampule of sterile medication
- File (if ampule is not scored) and small gauze square, or ampule opener

- Antiseptic swabs
- Syringe
- Filter needle for withdrawing medication from the ampule

IMPLEMENTATION

Preparation

1. Check the MAR.
   - Check the label on the ampule carefully against the MAR to make sure that the correct medication is being prepared.
   - Follow the three checks for administering medications. Read the label on the medication (a) when it is taken from the medication cart, (b) before withdrawing the medication, and (c) after withdrawing the medication.

2. Organize the equipment.

Performance

1. Perform hand hygiene, and follow other appropriate infection prevention and control procedures.

2. Prepare the medication ampule for drug withdrawal.
   - Flick the upper stem of the ampule several times with a fingernail. **Rationale: This manoeuvre will bring all medication down to the main portion of the ampule.**

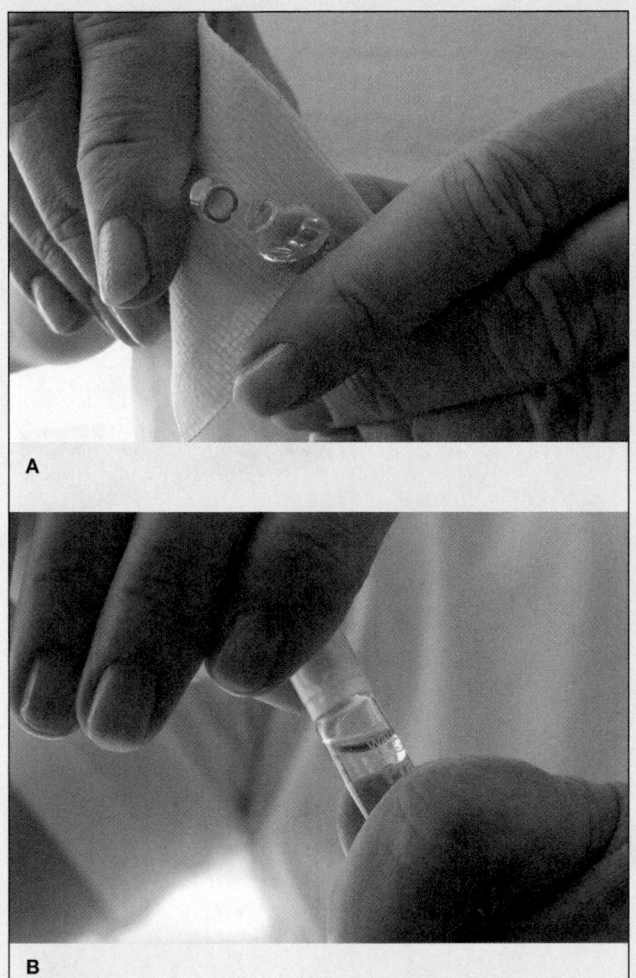

A

B

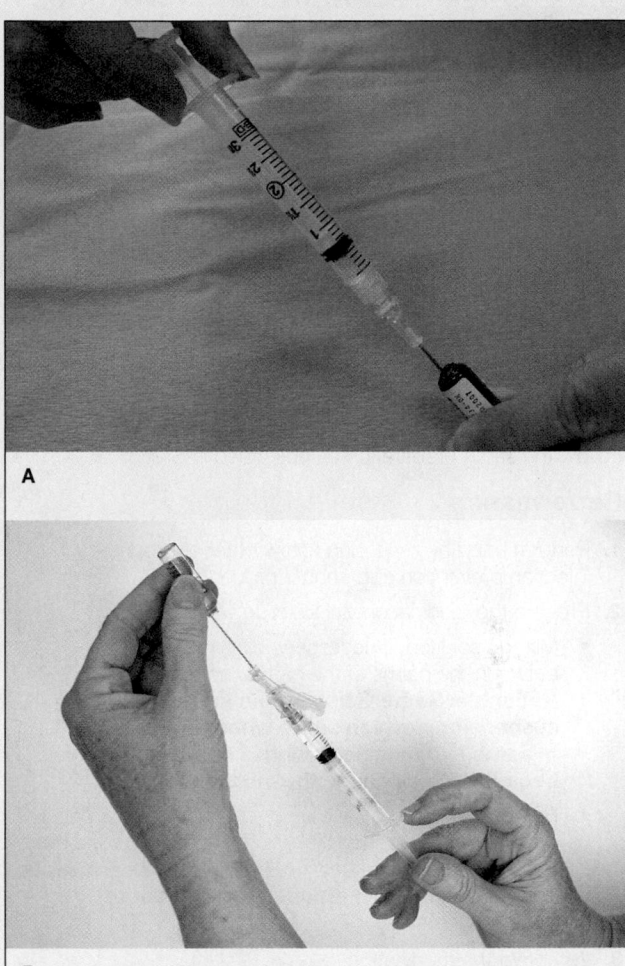

A

B

❶ **A:** Breaking the neck of an ampule using a gauze pad; **B:** Breaking the neck of an ampule using an ampule opener.

- Use an ampule opener or place a piece of sterile gauze or antiseptic wipe between your thumb and the ampule neck or around the ampule neck, and break off the top by bending it toward you to ensure the ampule is broken away from you and away from others (see ❶). **Rationale: The sterile gauze protects the fingers from the broken glass, and any glass fragments will spray away from the nurse**.

Or

- Place the antiseptic wipe packet over the top of the ampule before breaking off the top. **Rationale: This method ensures that all glass fragments fall into the packet and reduces the risk of cuts**.
- Dispose of the top of the ampule in the sharps container.

3. Withdraw the medication.
  - Place the ampule on a flat surface.
  - Attach the filter needle or straw to the syringe. **Rationale: The filter needle or straw prevents**

❷ **A:** Withdrawing a medication from an ampule on a flat surface; **B:** From an inverted ampule.

glass particles from being withdrawn with the medication.

- Remove the cap from the filter needle and insert the needle into the centre of the ampule. Do not touch the rim of the ampule with the needle tip or shaft. **Rationale: The needle must remain sterile**.
- Withdraw the amount of drug required for the dosage.
- With a single-dose ampule, hold the ampule slightly on its side, if necessary, to obtain more than the ordered amount of medication (see ❷).
- Dispose of the filter needle by placing it in a sharps container.
- If giving an injection, replace the filter needle with a regular needle, tighten the cap at the hub of the needle, and push the solution into the needle, to the prescribed amount.

SKILL 33.3 PREPARING MEDICATIONS FROM VIALS

PLANNING

Equipment

- Client's MAR or computer printout
- Vial of sterile medication
- Antiseptic swabs
- Safety needle and syringe
- Filter needle (check agency policy)
- Sterile water or normal saline, if drug is in powdered form

IMPLEMENTATION

Preparation

Follow the same preparation as described in Skill 33.2.

Performance

1. Perform hand hygiene, and follow other appropriate infection prevention and control procedures.

2. Prepare the medication vial for drug withdrawal.

   - Mix the solution, if necessary, by rotating the vial between the palms of the hands, not by shaking. **Rationale: Some vials contain aqueous suspensions, which settle when they stand. In some instances, shaking is contraindicated because it may cause the mixture to foam.**

   - Remove the protective cap, or clean the rubber cap of a previously opened vial with an antiseptic wipe by rubbing in a circular motion. **Rationale: The antiseptic cleans the cap and reduces the number of microorganisms.**

3. Withdraw the medication.

   - Attach a filter needle, as agency practice dictates, to draw up premixed liquid medications from multidose vials. **Rationale: The filter prevents any solid particles from being drawn up through the needle.**

   - Ensure that the needle is firmly attached to the syringe.

   - Remove the cap from the needle; then draw up into the syringe the amount of air equal to the volume of the medication to be withdrawn.

   - Carefully insert the needle into the upright vial through the centre of the rubber cap, maintaining the sterility of the needle.

   - Inject the air into the vial, keeping the bevel of the needle above the surface of the medication (see ❶). **Rationale: The air will allow the medication to be drawn out easily because negative pressure will not be created inside the vial. The bevel is kept above the medication to avoid creating bubbles in the medication.**

   - Withdraw the prescribed amount of medication by using either of the following methods:

     a. Hold the vial down (i.e., with the base lower than the top), move the needle tip so that it is below the fluid level, and withdraw the medication. Avoid drawing up the last drops of the vial (see ❷). **Rationale: Proponents of this method suggest that keeping the vial in the upright position while withdrawing the medication allows particulate matter to precipitate out of the solution. Leaving the last few drops reduces the chance of withdrawing foreign particles.**

   Or

     b. Invert the vial and ensure the needle tip is below the fluid level; gradually withdraw the medication (see ❸). **Rationale: Keeping the tip of the needle below the liquid level prevents air from being drawn into the syringe.**

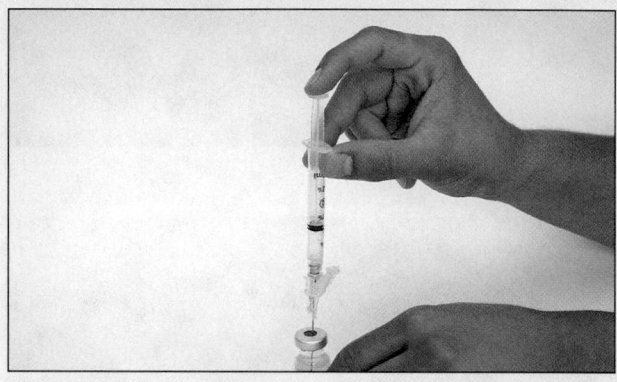

❶ Injecting air into a vial.

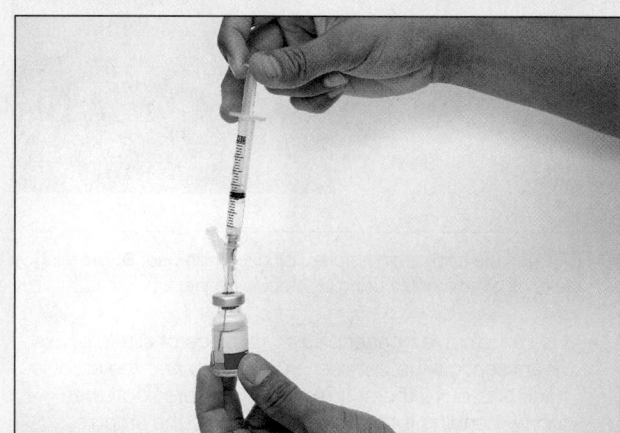

❷ Withdrawing a medication from a vial that is held with the base down.

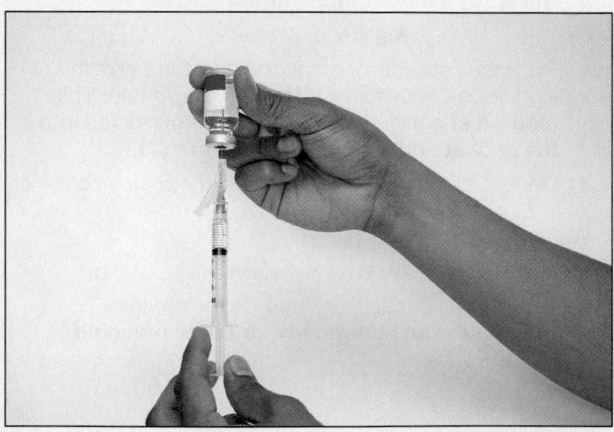

❸ Withdrawing a medication from an inverted vial.

- Hold the syringe and vial at eye level to determine that the correct dosage of drug is drawn into the syringe. Eject the air remaining at the top of the syringe into the vial.

- When the correct volume of medication plus a little more (e.g., 0.25 mL) is obtained, withdraw the needle from the vial, and replace the cap over the needle by using the scoop method, thus maintaining its sterility.

- If necessary, tap the syringe barrel to dislodge any air bubbles present in the syringe. **Rationale: The tapping action will cause the air bubbles to rise to the top of the syringe where they can be ejected out of the syringe**.

- If giving an injection, replace the filter needle, if used, with a regular or safety needle of the correct gauge and length. Eject air from the new needle and verify the correct medication volume before injecting the client.

Variation: Preparing and Using Multidose Vials

- Read the manufacturer's directions.

- Withdraw an equivalent amount of air from the vial before adding the diluent, unless otherwise indicated by the directions.

- Add the amount of sterile water or saline indicated in the directions.

- If a multidose vial is reconstituted, label the vial with the date and time it was prepared, the amount of drug contained in each millilitre of solution, and your initials. **Rationale: Time is an important factor to consider in the expiration of medications**.

- Once the medication is reconstituted, store it in a refrigerator or as recommended by the manufacturer.

- Discard vial if sterility is compromised or questionable.

- Remember to use a sterile syringe and needle/cannula for each access to the multidose vial.

Mixing Medications in One Syringe

Clients may need more than one drug injected at the same time. To spare the client the experience of being injected twice, two drugs (if compatible) are often mixed together in one syringe and given as one injection. It is common, for instance, to combine two types of insulin in this manner or to combine injectable preoperative medications, such as morphine with atropine or scopolamine. Drugs can also be mixed in intravenous solutions. When uncertain about drug incompatibilities, the nurse should consult a pharmacist or check a compatibility chart before mixing the drugs.

The nurse must also exercise caution when mixing rapid-acting or short-acting and intermediate-acting insulins because they vary in content. Chemically, insulin is a protein, which yields a number of amino acids when hydrolyzed in the body. Intermediate-acting insulin preparations contain an additional modifying protein, such as globulin or protamine, which slows absorption. This fact is particularly relevant to mixing two insulin preparations for injection because many insulin syringes have needles that cannot be changed. A vial of insulin that does not have the added protein (e.g., Humulin R) should never be contaminated with insulin that does have the added protein (e.g., Humulin N or Novolin ge or NPH). Fortunately, insulin is available in premixed cartridges for people living with diabetes mellitus and who have to self-inject on a daily basis; these premixed cartridges are placed in "insulin pens" and are available through community pharmacists—they are usually not available in hospitals. Skill 33.4 describes how to mix medications in one syringe.

SKILL 33.4   MIXING MEDICATIONS USING ONE SYRINGE

PURPOSE

To mix medications using one syringe

ASSESSMENT

Assess

- Client allergies to medications
- Specific drug action, side effects, interactions, and adverse reactions
- Client's knowledge of and learning needs about the medications
- Intended route of parenteral medication to determine appropriate size of syringe and needle for the client
- Ordered medications for clarity and expiration date
- Determine that the two medications are compatible

PLANNING

Equipment

- Client's MAR or computer printout
- One vial and one ampule of medication or two ampules of medication (depending on the presentation)
- Antiseptic swabs
- Sterile syringe and safety needle or insulin syringe (ONLY use insulin syringes for administering insulin)
- Additional sterile subcutaneous or intramuscular needle (optional)

(continued)

SKILL 33.4 MIXING MEDICATIONS USING ONE SYRINGE (*continued*)

IMPLEMENTATION

Preparation

1. Check the MAR.

- Check the label on the medications carefully against the MAR to make sure that the correct medication is being prepared.

- Follow the three checks for administering medications. Read the label on the medication (a) when it is taken from the medication cart, (b) before withdrawing the medication, and (c) after withdrawing the medication.

- Before preparing and combining the medications, ensure that the total volume of the injection is appropriate for the injection site.

2. Organize the equipment.

Performance

1. Perform hand hygiene, and follow other appropriate infection prevention and control procedures.

2. Prepare the medication ampule or vial for drug withdrawal.

- See Skill 33.2, Performance section, step 2, for an ampule.

- Inspect the appearance of the medication for clarity. Note, however, that some medications are always cloudy. **Rationale: Preparations that have changed in appearance should be discarded.**

- If using insulin, thoroughly mix the solution in each vial before administration. Rotate the vials between the palms of the hands. **Rationale: Mixing ensures an adequate concentration and thus an accurate dose. Shaking insulin vials can make the medication frothy, making precise measurement difficult.**

- Clean the tops of the vials with antiseptic swabs.

3. Withdraw the medications.

Mixing Medications from Two Vials

- Take the syringe and draw up a volume of air equal to the volume of medications to be withdrawn from both vials A and B.

- Inject a volume of air equal to the volume of medication to be withdrawn into vial A. Make sure the needle does not touch the solution. **Rationale: Cross-contamination of the medications must be avoided.**

- Withdraw the needle from vial A, and inject the remaining air into vial B.

- Withdraw the required amount of medication from vial B. **Rationale: The same needle is used to inject air into and withdraw medication from the second vial. It must not be contaminated with the medication in vial A.**

- Using a newly attached sterile needle, withdraw the required amount of medication from vial A. Avoid pushing the plunger as that will introduce medication B into vial A. If using a syringe with a fused needle, withdraw the medication from vial A. The syringe now contains a mixture of medications from vials A and B. **Rationale: With this method, neither vial is contaminated by microorganisms or by medication from the other vial.** Be careful to withdraw only the ordered amount and to not create air bubbles. **Rationale: The syringe now contains two medications and an excess amount cannot be returned to the vial.**

See also the Variation later in this Skill box.

Mixing Medications from One Vial and One Ampule

- First prepare and withdraw the medication from the vial. **Rationale: Ampules do not require the addition of air before withdrawal of the drug.**

- Then withdraw the required amount of medication from the ampule.

Variation: Mixing Insulins

The following is an example of mixing 10 units of Humulin R insulin and 30 units of Humulin N insulin which contains protamine:

- Inject 30 units of air into the Humulin N vial and withdraw the needle. (There should be no insulin in the needle.) The needle should not touch the insulin (see ❶).

- Inject 10 units of air into the Humulin R, and immediately withdraw 10 units of Humulin R insulin (see ❷ and ❸). **Rationale: This step minimizes the possibility of the Humulin R insulin becoming contaminated with the additional protein in the Humulin N insulin.**

- Reinsert the needle into the Humulin N vial, and withdraw 30 units of Humulin N insulin (see ❹). (The air was previously injected into the vial.) Be careful to withdraw

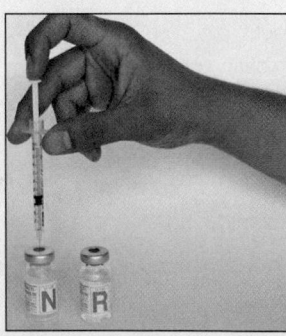

❶ Mixing intermediate-acting and short-acting insulin together: step 1.

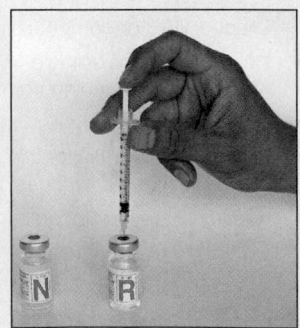

❷ Step 2.

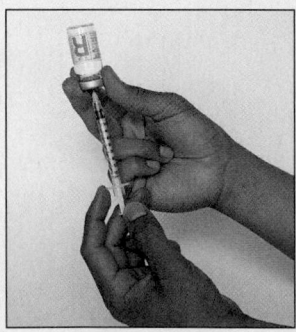

❸ Step 3.

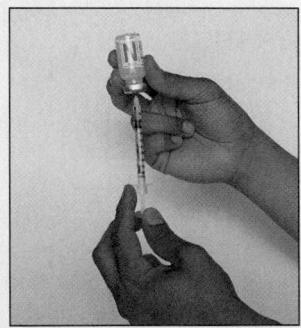

❹ Step 4.

only the ordered amount and to not create air bubbles. If excess medication has been drawn up, discard the syringe and begin the procedure over again. **Rationale: The syringe now contains two medications, and an excess amount cannot be returned to the vial because the syringe contains regular insulin, which, if returned to the Humulin N vial, would dilute the Humulin N with Humulin R insulin. The Humulin N vial would not provide accurate future dosages of Humulin N insulin**.

By using this method, you avoid adding NPH insulin to the regular insulin.

> ### ! CLINICAL ALERT
>
> One way to determine which insulin to withdraw first is to remember the saying "Clear before cloudy." Short-acting and rapid-acting analogue insulins are clear and intermediate-acting insulin is cloudy because of the proteins in the insulin. New extended long-acting insulins, insulin glargine, and insulin detemir are also clear and colourless and should not be confused with rapid-acting or short-acting insulins. These insulins are NOT to be mixed with ANY other insulin or mixed in a solution, such as an intravenous solution.

Intradermal Injections

An *intradermal (ID) injection* is the administration of a drug into the dermal layer of skin, just beneath the epidermis. Usually, only a small amount of drug is injected, for example 0.1 mL. This method of administration is frequently indicated for allergy testing and tuberculosis (TB) screening. The most common site for intradermal injections are the flexor aspect of the forearm (inner lower forearm). The left arm is commonly used for TB screening and the right arm is used for all other tests. The steps for administering an intradermal injection are described in Skill 33.5.

SKILL 33.5   ADMINISTERING AN INTRADERMAL INJECTION FOR SKIN TESTS

PURPOSE

To provide a medication that the client requires for allergy testing and tuberculosis screening.

ASSESSMENT

Assess

- Appearance of injection site
- Specific drug action and expected response
- Client's knowledge of drug action and response

Check agency protocol about sites to use for skin tests.

PLANNING

Equipment

- Client's MAR or computer printout
- Vial or ampule of the correct medication
- Sterile 1-mL syringe calibrated into hundredths of a millilitre (i.e., tuberculin syringe) and a #25- to #27-gauge safety needle that is 12 mm to 16 mm long
- Antiseptic swabs
- 10-cm sterile gauze square (optional)
- Clean gloves (according to agency protocol)
- Bandage (optional)
- Epinephrine on hand in case of allergic anaphylactic reaction per agency policy

IMPLEMENTATION

Preparation

1. Check the MAR.
   - Check the label on the medication carefully against the MAR to make sure that the correct medication is being prepared.

- Follow the three checks for administering medications. Read the label on the medication (a) when it is taken from the medication cart, (b) before withdrawing the medication, and (c) after withdrawing the medication.

2. Organize the equipment.

Performance

1. Perform hand hygiene, and follow other appropriate infection prevention and control procedures (e.g., clean gloves).
2. Prepare the medication from the vial or ampule for drug withdrawal.
   - See Skills 33.2 and 33.3.
3. Prepare the client.
   - Prior to performing the procedure, introduce yourself and verify the client's identity using two identifiers or per agency protocol.
4. Explain to the client that the medication will produce a small wheal, sometimes called a *bleb. A wheal* is a small raised area, like a blister. The client will feel a slight prick as the needle enters the skin. Some medications are absorbed slowly through the capillaries into the general circulation, and the bleb gradually disappears. Other drugs remain in the area and interact with the body tissues to produce redness and induration (hardening), which will need to be interpreted at a particular time (e.g., in 24 or 48 hours). This reaction will also gradually disappear. **Rationale: Information can facilitate acceptance of, and adherence to, the therapy**.
5. Provide for client privacy.
6. Select and clean the site (e.g., the forearm about a hand's width above the wrist and three or four finger widths below the antecubital space).
   - Avoid using sites that are tender, inflamed, or swollen and those that have lesions.

(continued)

SKILL 33.5 ADMINISTERING AN INTRADERMAL INJECTION FOR SKIN TESTS (*continued*)

- Put on gloves, as indicated by agency policy.
- Cleanse the skin at the site by using a firm circular motion, starting at the centre and widening the circle outward. Allow the area to dry thoroughly.

7. Prepare the syringe for the injection.
   - Remove the needle cap while waiting for the antiseptic to dry.
   - Expel any air bubbles from the syringe. Small bubbles that adhere to the plunger are of no consequence. **Rationale: A small amount of air will not harm the tissue**.
   - Grasp the syringe in your dominant hand, close to the hub, holding it between thumb and forefinger. Hold the needle almost parallel to the skin surface, with the bevel of the needle up. **Rationale: The possibility of the medication entering the subcutaneous tissue increases when using an angle greater than 15 degrees**.

8. Inject the fluid.
   - With the nondominant hand, pull the skin at the site until it is taut. For example, if using the ventral forearm, grasp the client's dorsal forearm and gently pull it to tighten the ventral skin (see ❶A). **Rationale: Taut skin allows for easier entry of the needle and less discomfort for the client**.
   - Insert the tip of the needle far enough to place the bevel through the epidermis into the dermis. The outline of the bevel should be visible under the skin surface (see ❶B).
   - Stabilize the syringe and needle. Inject the medication carefully and slowly so that it produces a small wheal on the skin (see ❶C). **Rationale: This wheal indicates that the medication entered the dermis**.
   - Withdraw the needle quickly at the same angle at which it was inserted. Activate the needle safety device. Apply a bandage, if indicated.
   - Do not massage the area. **Rationale: Massage can dispense the medication into the tissue or out through the needle insertion site**.
   - Dispose of the syringe and needle into the sharps container. **Rationale: This helps prevent needlestick injuries. Do not recap the needle**.
   - Remove and discard gloves. Perform hand hygiene.
   - Circle the injection site with ink to observe for redness or induration (hardening), per agency policy.

9. Document all relevant information.
   - Record the testing material given, time, dosage, route, site, and nursing assessments.

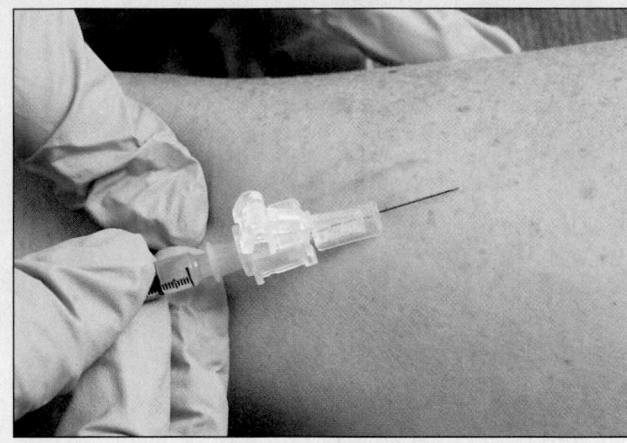

❶ A

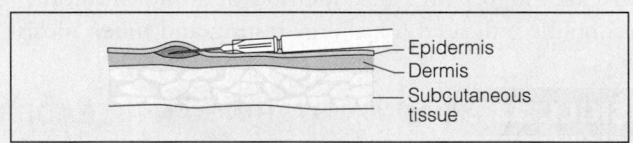

Epidermis
Dermis
Subcutaneous tissue

❶ B

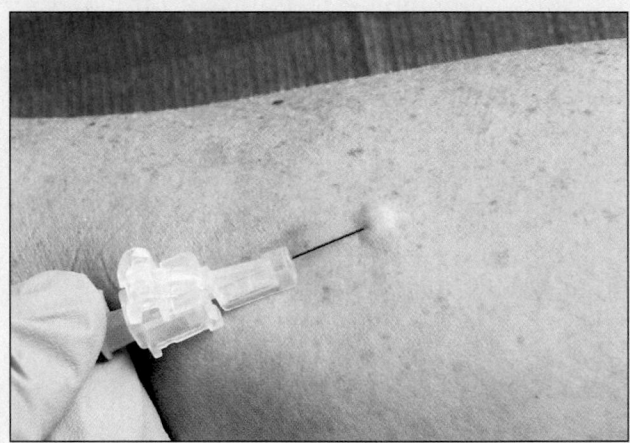

❶ C

❶ For an intradermal injection: **A:** The needle enters the skin at a 5- to 15-degree angle; **B and C:** The medication forms a bleb, or wheal, under the epidermis.

EVALUATION

- Evaluate the client's response to the testing substance. **Rationale: Some medications used in testing can cause allergic reactions**. Epinephrine may need to be used.
- Evaluate the condition of the site in 24 or 48 hours, depending on the test. Measure the area of redness and induration in millimetres at the largest diameter and document findings.

Subcutaneous Injections

Among the many kinds of drugs administered subcutaneously (just beneath skin) are certain vaccines, insulin, and heparin. Common sites for subcutaneous injections are the abdomen, outer aspect of the upper arms, and the anterior aspect of the thighs. These areas are convenient and normally have good blood circulation. Other areas that can be used are the scapular areas of the upper back, and the upper ventrogluteal and dorsogluteal areas (see Figure 33.27). Only small doses (less than 1 mL) of medication are usually injected via the subcutaneous route.

The type of syringe used for subcutaneous injections depends on the medication being given. Generally, a 1- or 2-mL syringe is used for most subcutaneous injections. However, if insulin is being administered, an insulin syringe is used; if heparin is being administered, a prefilled cartridge may be used.

Needle sizes and lengths are selected based on the client's body mass, the intended angle of insertion, and the planned site. For an adult of normal weight requiring a subcutaneous injection, it is generally appropriate to use a needle that is 16 mm long with a #23 to #25 gauge.

One method nurses use to determine length of needle is to pinch the tissue at the site and select a needle length that is half the width of the skinfold. To determine the angle of insertion, a general rule to follow relates to the amount of tissue that can be bunched or grasped at the site. A 45-degree angle is used when 2.5 cm of tissue can be grasped at the site; a 90-degree angle is used when 5 cm of tissue can be grasped.

For administering insulin to adults, a small-gauge needle is used (e.g., #28 gauge or #30 gauge) to minimize tissue injury and leakage. Unless otherwise indicated, the insulin should be injected at a 90-degree angle. Insulin syringes are smaller, have fine needles, and also have special coatings on the needles to allow for an injection that is as pain free as possible. Insulin pens (similar in appearance to a writing pen) are also available to clients. An insulin cartridge (supplied in 1.5 mL or 3.0 mL) is inserted into the pen and remains there until all the insulin is used. A short needle is attached to the end of the pen and changed for each injection. The cartridges may contain different types of insulin, such as Humulin N or Humulin R, and premixed formulations with a fixed ratio of insulin, such as Humulin 30/70 (30% R and 70% N insulin).

Subcutaneous injection sites need to be rotated in an orderly fashion to minimize tissue damage, aid absorption, and avoid discomfort. This is especially important for clients who must receive repeated injections. Insulin is absorbed most quickly when injected into the abdomen and then into the arms, and the slowest when injected into the thighs or buttocks.

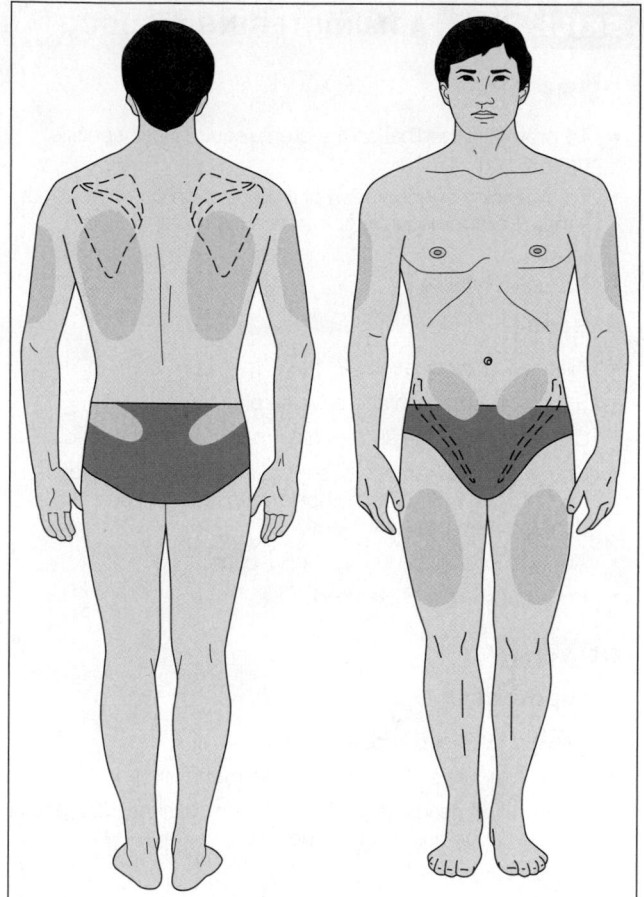

FIGURE 33.27 Body sites commonly used for subcutaneous injections.

Varying injection sites within the same anatomical site (approximately 2.5 cm apart) rather than between anatomical sites is recommended to limit variations in blood glucose levels (e.g., rotate sites for 1 to 2 weeks within one anatomical area, such as the right abdomen, then move to another anatomical area such as the left abdomen) (Registered Nurses' Association of Ontario [RNAO], 2009). Aspiration is not performed with insulin administration.

Swabs soaked with 70% alcohol or a mixture of alcohol and chlorhexidine are generally used to cleanse the injection site before injecting the medication. Although swabbing the area for 5 seconds may result in reduction of bacteria, no prevention of infection occurs. Infection from injections is more likely related to contaminated syringes or needles rather than lack of cleansing of the skin site. *Cleansing of the injection site is now considered an optional step for home injection of insulin* (RNAO, 2009).

The steps for administering a subcutaneous injection are described in Skill 33.6.

See the Home Care Considerations box on subcutaneous injections on page 918.

SKILL 33.6 ADMINISTERING A SUBCUTANEOUS INJECTION

PURPOSE

- To provide a medication the client requires (see specific drug action)
- To allow slower absorption of a medication compared with either the intramuscular or intravenous route

ASSESSMENT

Assess

- Allergies to medication
- Specific drug action and adverse effects
- Client's knowledge and learning needs about the medication
- Status and appearance of subcutaneous site for lesions, erythema, swelling, ecchymosis, inflammation, and tissue damage from previous injections
- Ability to cooperate during the injection
- Previous injection sites used

PLANNING

Equipment

- Client's MAR or computer printout
- Vial or ampule of the correct sterile medication
- Syringe and needle (e.g., 1-mL to 2-mL syringe, #25-gauge to #27-gauge needle or smaller, 16 mm long)
- Antiseptic swabs
- Dry sterile gauze for opening an ampule (optional)
- Clean gloves

IMPLEMENTATION

Preparation

1. Check the MAR.
   - Check the label on the medication carefully against the MAR to make sure that the correct medication is being prepared.
   - Follow the three checks for administering medications. Read the label on the medication (a) when it is taken from the medication cart, (b) before withdrawing the medication, and (c) after withdrawing the medication.

2. Organize the equipment.

Performance

1. Perform hand hygiene, and follow other appropriate infection prevention and control procedures (e.g., clean gloves).

2. Prepare the medication from the ampule or vial for drug withdrawal.
   - See Skill 33.2 (ampule) or Skill 33.3 (vial).
   - If the medication is insulin or heparin, the dosage needs to be verified by another nurse. **Rationale: An independent double-checking of the dosage avoids medication errors**.

3. Provide for client privacy.

4. Prepare the client.
   - Prior to performing the procedure, introduce yourself and verify the client's identity using two identifiers or per

---

> **! CLINICAL ALERT**
>
> When asking another nurse to verify the dosage of insulin or heparin, leave the needle and syringe in the vial and ask "What dosage do I have in the syringe?" The nurse needs to independently check the vial medication name and concentration as well as calculate the dosage. This is a safer and more accurate method of double-checking than saying to another nurse, "I have 10 units of insulin," which "presets" the other nurse's checking of the medication dosage and can lead to an error.

agency protocol. **Rationale: This ensures that the right client receives the right medication**.
   - Assist the client to a position in which the arm, leg, or abdomen can be relaxed, depending on the site to be used. **Rationale: A relaxed position of the site minimizes discomfort**.
   - Obtain assistance for holding an uncooperative client. **Rationale: This prevents injury caused by sudden movement after needle insertion**.

5. Explain the purpose of the medication and how it will help, using language that the client can understand. Include relevant information about effects of the medication. **Rationale: Information can facilitate acceptance of, and adherence to, therapy**.

6. Select and clean the site.
   - Select a site free of tenderness, hardness, swelling, scarring, itching, burning, or localized inflammation. Select a site that has not been used frequently. **Rationale: These conditions could hinder the absorption of the medication and may also increase the likelihood of injury and discomfort at the injection site**.
   - Put on clean gloves.
   - As agency protocol indicates, clean the site with an antiseptic swab. Start at the centre of the site, and clean in a widening circle to about 5 cm. Allow the area to dry thoroughly. **Rationale: The mechanical action of swabbing removes skin secretions, which contain microorganisms**.
   - Place and hold the swab between the third and fourth fingers of the nondominant hand, or position the swab on the client's skin above the intended site. **Rationale: Using this technique keeps the swab readily accessible when the needle is withdrawn**.

7. Prepare the syringe for injection.
   - Remove the needle cap while waiting for the antiseptic to dry. Pull the cap straight off to avoid contaminating the needle by the outside edge of the cap. **Rationale: The needle will become contaminated if it touches anything but the inside of the cap, which is sterile**.
   - Dispose of the needle cap.

8. Inject the medication.
   - Grasp the syringe in your dominant hand by holding it between your thumb and fingers. With palm facing to the side or upward for a 45-degree angle insertion, or with palm downward for a 90-degree angle insertion, prepare to inject (see ❶).
   - Using the nondominant hand, pinch or spread the skin at the site, and insert the needle by using the dominant

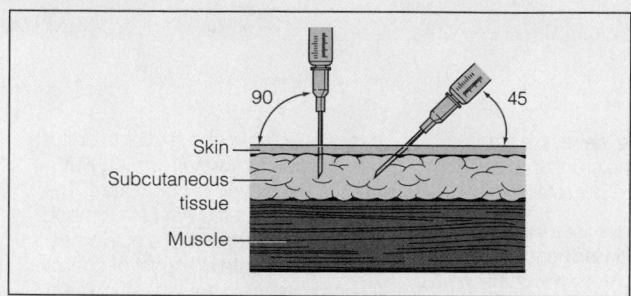

❶ Inserting a needle into the subcutaneous tissue using 90- and 45-degree angles.

hand and a firm steady push. Recommendations vary about whether to pinch or spread the skin and at what angle to administer subcutaneous injections. The most important consideration is the depth of the subcutaneous tissue in the area to be injected. If the client has more than 5 cm of adipose tissue in the injection site, it would be safe to administer the injection at a 90-degree angle with the skin spread. If the client is thin or lean and lacks adipose tissue, the subcutaneous injection should be given with the skin pinched and at a 45- to 60-degree angle. One way to check whether the pinch of skin is subcutaneous tissue is to ask the client to flex and extend the elbow. If any muscle is being held in the pinch, you will feel it contract and relax. If so, release the pinch and try again (see ❷).

- When the needle is inserted, move the nondominant hand to the end of the plunger. Some nurses find it easier to move the nondominant hand to the barrel of the syringe and the dominant hand to the end of the plunger.

- Inject the medication by holding the syringe steady, with a slow, even pressure. **Rationale: Holding the syringe steady and injecting the medication at an even pressure minimizes discomfort for the client**.

- It is recommended that with many subcutaneous injections, especially insulin, the needle should be embedded in the skin for 5 seconds after complete depression of the plunger to ensure complete delivery of the dose. **Rationale: This ensures that the medication dissipates into the tissue**.

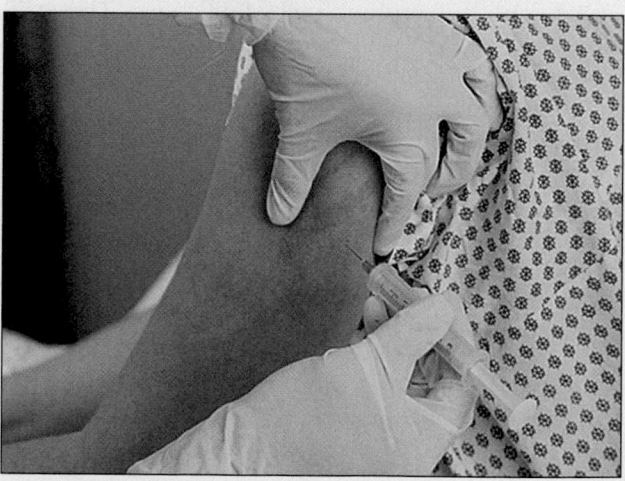

❷ Administering a subcutaneous injection into pinched tissue.

9. Remove the needle.
   - Remove the needle smoothly, pulling along the line of insertion while depressing the skin with your nondominant hand. **Rationale: Depressing the skin places countertraction on it and minimizes the client's discomfort when the needle is withdrawn**.
   - If bleeding occurs, apply pressure to the site with dry sterile gauze until it stops. **Rationale: Bleeding rarely occurs after subcutaneous injection**.

10. Dispose of supplies appropriately.
    - Activate the needle safety device or discard the uncapped needle and attached syringe into the sharps container. **Rationale: Proper disposal protects the nurse and others from needlestick injury**.
    - Remove and discard gloves. Perform hand hygiene.

11. Document all relevant information.
    - Document the medication given, dosage, time, route, and any assessments.
    - Many agencies prefer that medication administration be recorded on the medication record. The progress notes are used when prn medications are given or when there is a special problem.

12. Assess the effectiveness of the medication at the time it is expected to act and document it.

Variation: Administering a Heparin Injection

The subcutaneous administration of heparin and low-molecular-weight heparin (e.g., enoxaparin) requires special precautions because of the drug's anticoagulant properties.

- Select a site on the abdomen at least 10 cm *away* from the umbilicus and above the level of the iliac crests. Some agencies support the practice of subcutaneous injection of heparin in the thighs or arms as alternative sites to the abdomen. Avoid injecting into bruises, scars, masses, or areas of tenderness.

- Use a 10-mm #25-gauge or #26-gauge needle or smaller, and insert it at a 90-degree angle. If a client is lean or has a wasted appearance, use a needle longer than 10 mm and insert it at a 45-degree angle. The arms or thighs may be used as alternative sites.

- Do *not* aspirate when giving heparin by subcutaneous injection. **Rationale: Aspiration can possibly damage the surrounding tissue and cause bleeding as well as ecchymoses (bruises)**.

- Inject the anticoagulant over 30 seconds. **Rationale: This helps reduce the risk of bruising.**
  - Do not massage the site after the injection. **Rationale: Massaging could cause bleeding and ecchymoses (bruises) and hasten drug absorption**.

- Alternate the sites of subsequent injections.

EVALUATION

- Conduct appropriate follow-up, such as checking for desired effect (e.g., relief of pain, sedation, lowered blood glucose, a prothrombin time within established limits), any adverse effects (e.g., nausea, vomiting, skin rash).

- Relate to previous findings, if available.

- Report deviations from normal to the appropriate member of the health care team.

Subcutaneous Injections

- If the client has impaired vision, consider prefilling syringes and storing them in an appropriate environment or obtaining prefilled medication syringes from the pharmacy. Prefilled insulin syringes can be stored in the refrigerator for up to 1 month with the needle tips up (to avoid the medication precipitating in the needle)—the insulin must be resuspended (by gently rolling the syringe) prior to use (RNAO, 2009, p. 72)

- For frequent injections, develop a plan for site rotation with the client and explain the reason for injection site rotation.

- For clients who require insulin, ensure that at least one knowledgeable support person can correctly inject insulin in an emergency situation and recognize and treat hypoglycemia.

- Teach the client and family how to safely dispose of needles. Do not throw needles in the garbage or flush used needles down the toilet. Put needles in recycling containers. The Canadian Diabetes Association and local health boards have guidelines outlining the safe disposal of sharps. Recommend to clients to find out what services are offered in the client's community. For example, most large chain pharmacies offer a sharp disposal service to their customers.

Intramuscular Injections

Injections into muscle tissue, or *intramuscular (IM) injections,* are absorbed more quickly than subcutaneous injections because of greater blood supply to the body tissues. Muscles can also hold a larger volume of fluid without discomfort than subcutaneous tissues can, although the amount varies among individuals, chiefly based on muscle size and condition and the site used. An adult with well-developed muscles can usually safely tolerate up to 3 mL of medication in the gluteus medius and gluteus maximus muscles (Figure 33.28). A volume of 1 mL to 2 mL is usually recommended for adults with less developed muscles. In the deltoid muscle, volumes of 0.5 mL to 1 mL are recommended. Usually, a 3-mL to 5-mL syringe is needed. The size of syringe used depends on the amount of medication being administered. The standard prepackaged intramuscular needle is 2.5 cm or 3.8 cm and #21 or #22 gauge. Several factors dictate the size and length of the needle to be used:

- The muscle
- The type of solution
- The amount of adipose tissue covering the muscle
- The age of the client

For example, a #22-gauge to #25-gauge needle 2.5 cm long, is commonly used for the deltoid muscle in adults. More viscous solutions require a larger gauge (e.g., #22 gauge). Clients who are obese may require a needle longer than 3.8 cm (e.g., 5 cm), and clients who are emaciated may require a shorter needle (e.g., 2.5 cm). The essential issue is that the needle is long enough to reach muscle—if the needle is too short, it will only penetrate the subcutaneous tissue; if it is too long, it will possibly penetrate underlying blood vessels or bone.

A major consideration in the administration of IM injections is the selection of a safe site located away from large blood vessels, nerves, and bone. Several body sites can be used for intramuscular injections. These sites are discussed in detail next. Contraindications for using a specific site include tissue injury and the presence of nodules, lumps, abscesses, tenderness, or other pathology. Generally, the muscles of the buttock are not recommended for active immunization because the presence of adipose tissue in this area can make absorption of vaccines variable (i.e., fat tissue makes it difficult to ensure that the needle length choice is accurate so the risk is that a subcutaneous rather than an intramuscular injection is given).

VENTROGLUTEAL SITE The ventrogluteal site is in the gluteus medius muscle, which lies over the gluteus minimus (see Figure 33.28). The ventrogluteal site is the

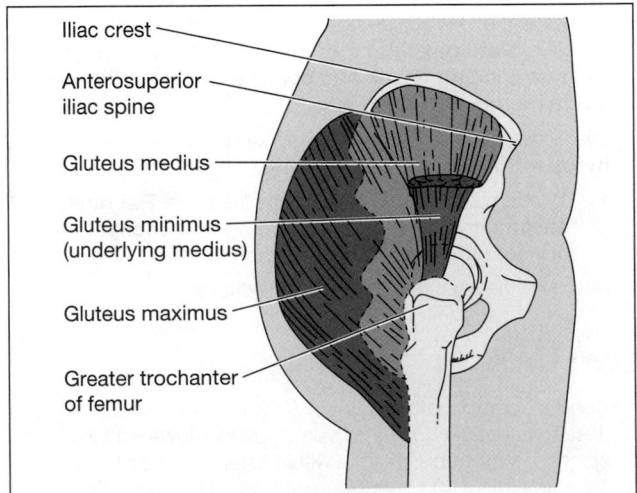

Iliac crest

Anterosuperior iliac spine

Gluteus medius

Gluteus minimus (underlying medius)

Gluteus maximus

Greater trochanter of femur

FIGURE 33.28 Lateral view of the right buttock showing the three gluteal muscles used for intramuscular injections.

preferred site for intramuscular injections in the buttock area because of the following reasons:

- This area contains no large nerves or blood vessels.
- It provides the greatest thickness of gluteal muscle, consisting of both the gluteus medius and the gluteus minimus.
- It is sealed off by bone.
- It contains consistently less fat than the buttock area, thus eliminating the need to determine the depth of subcutaneous fat.

The client position for an injection into the ventrogluteal site can be the supine, prone, or side-lying position. The side-lying position, however, helps locate the ventrogluteal site more easily. Position the client on the appropriate side, with his or her knee bent and raised slightly toward the chest. The trochanter will protrude, which facilitates locating the ventrogluteal site. To establish the exact site, place the heel of the hand on the client's greater trochanter, with the fingers pointing toward the client's head. The right hand is used for the left hip, and the left hand for the right hip. With the index finger on the client's anterior superior iliac spine, stretch the middle finger dorsally (toward the buttocks), palpating the iliac crest and then pressing below it. The triangle formed by the index finger, the third finger, and the iliac crest is the injection site (see Figures 33.29 and 33.30).

VASTUS LATERALIS SITE The vastus lateralis muscle is usually thick and well developed in both adults and children. It is recommended as the site of choice for intramuscular injections for infants 1 year and younger. Because

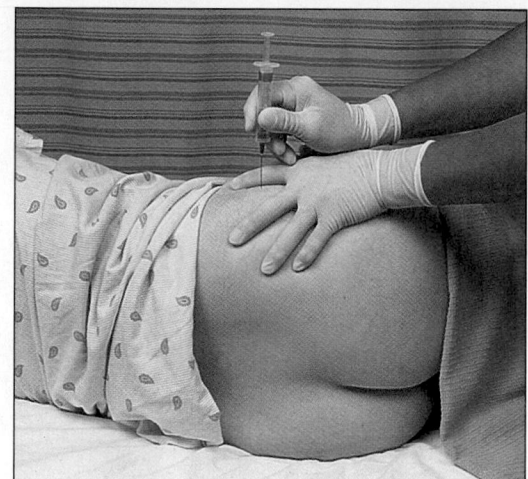

FIGURE 33.30 Administering an intramuscular injection into the ventrogluteal muscle.

there are no major blood vessels or nerves in the area, it is desirable for infants whose gluteal muscles are poorly developed. It is situated on the anterior lateral aspect of the infant's thigh (Figure 33.31). The middle third of the muscle is suggested as the site. In the adult, the landmark is established by dividing the area between the greater trochanter of the femur and the lateral femoral condyle into thirds and selecting the middle third (Figures 33.32 and 33.33). The client can assume the back-lying or sitting position for an injection into this site.

DORSOGLUTEAL SITE Historically, the dorsogluteal site was primarily used for intramuscular injections. However, this site is close to the sciatic nerve and the superior gluteal nerve and artery. As a result,

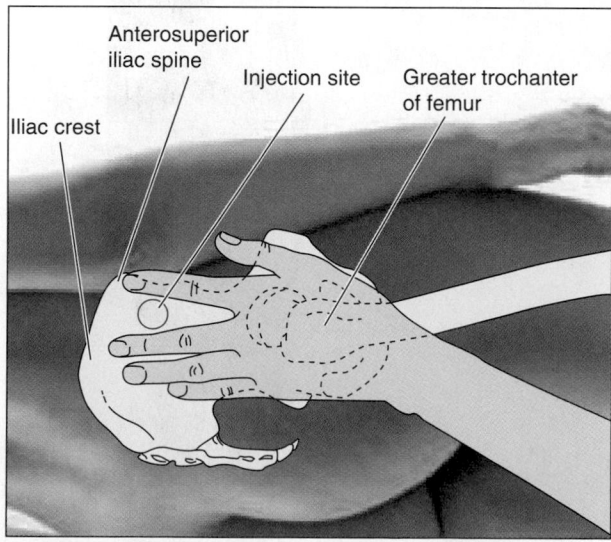

FIGURE 33.29 Landmarks for the ventrogluteal site of an intramuscular injection.

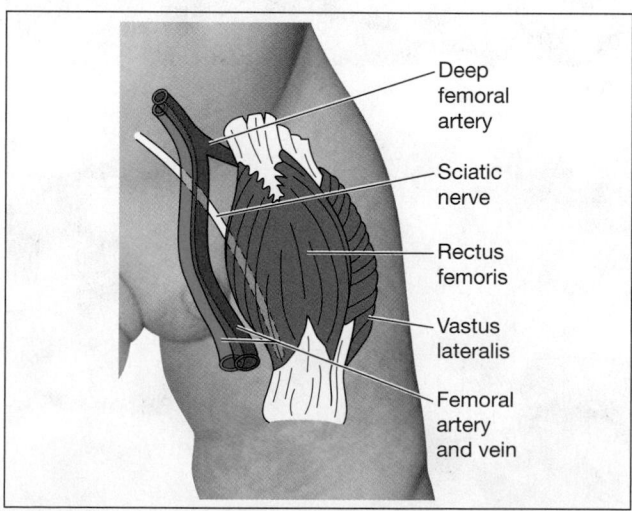

FIGURE 33.31 The vastus lateralis muscle of the infant's upper thigh, used for intramuscular injections.

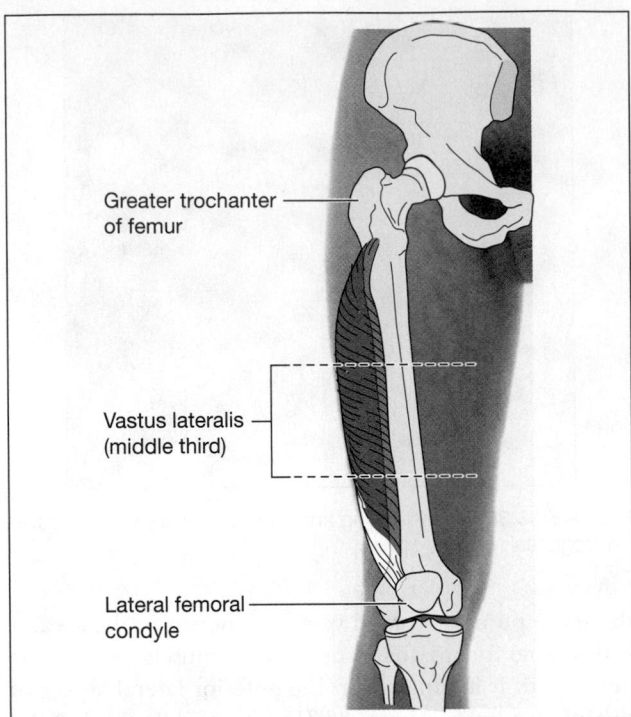

FIGURE 33.32 Landmarks of the vastus lateralis site of an adult's right thigh, used for an intramuscular injection.

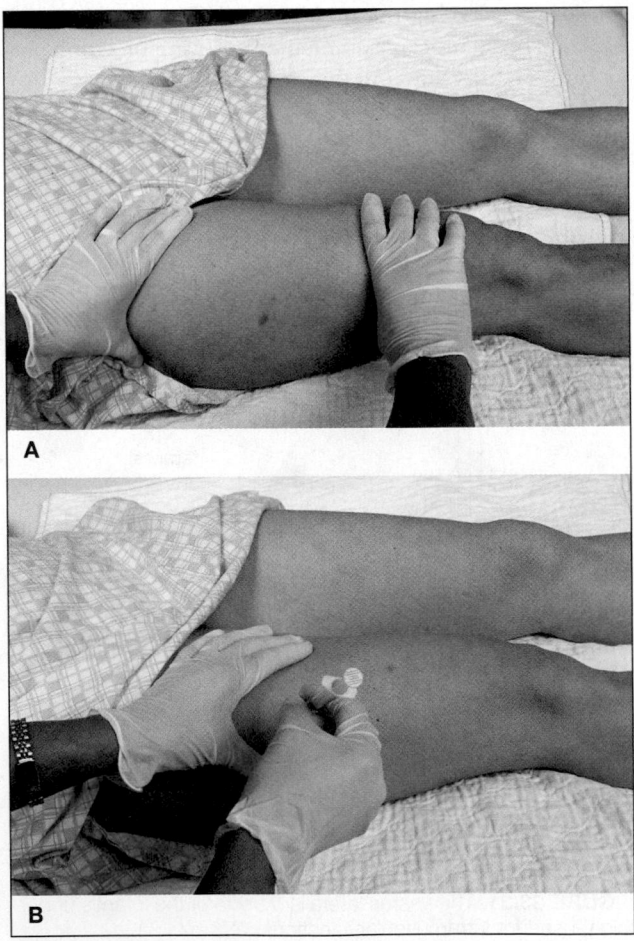

FIGURE 33.33 **A:** Determining landmarks; **B:** Administering an intramuscular injection into the vastus lateralis site.

complications (e.g., numbness, pain, paralysis) occurred if the nurse injected a medication near or into the sciatic nerve. In addition, there tends to be more subcutaneous tissue at the dorsogluteal site. The medication may be injected into the subcutaneous tissue instead of the muscle, which can then affect the intended therapeutic effect. Developmentally, infants and children have larger ventrogluteal than dorsogluteal muscle mass (Malkin, 2008). For all of these reasons, the dorsogluteal site is NOT recommended for intramuscular injection. It is interesting to note, however, that many nurses still use the dorsogluteal site. Several reasons for this practice include ease of site identification, more experience with using the dorsogluteal site, less confidence using the ventrogluteal site, and failure to emphasize the use of the ventrogluteal site rather than the dorsogluteal site during teaching about intramuscular injections.

RECTUS FEMORIS SITE The rectus femoris muscle, which belongs to the quadriceps muscle group, is used occasionally for intramuscular injections. It is situated on the anterior aspect of the thigh (Figure 33.34). Its chief advantage is that clients who administer their own injections can reach this site easily. Its main disadvantage is that an injection here can cause considerable discomfort for some people.

DELTOID SITE The deltoid muscle is found on the lateral aspect of the upper arm. It is most frequently used for the administration of several vaccines in children over 1 year of age and in adults. As it is a relatively small muscle, generally, no more than 1 mL of solution should be administered so as to minimize discomfort.

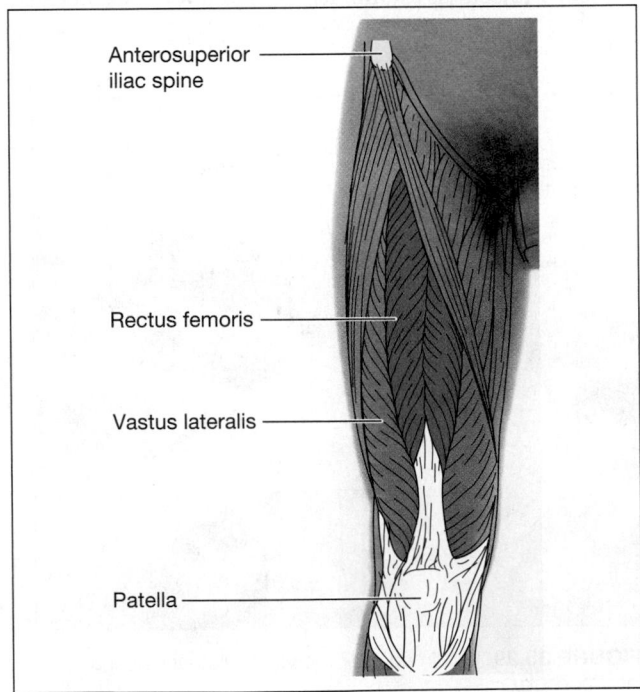

FIGURE 33.34 Landmarks for the rectus femoris muscle of the upper right thigh, used for intramuscular injections.

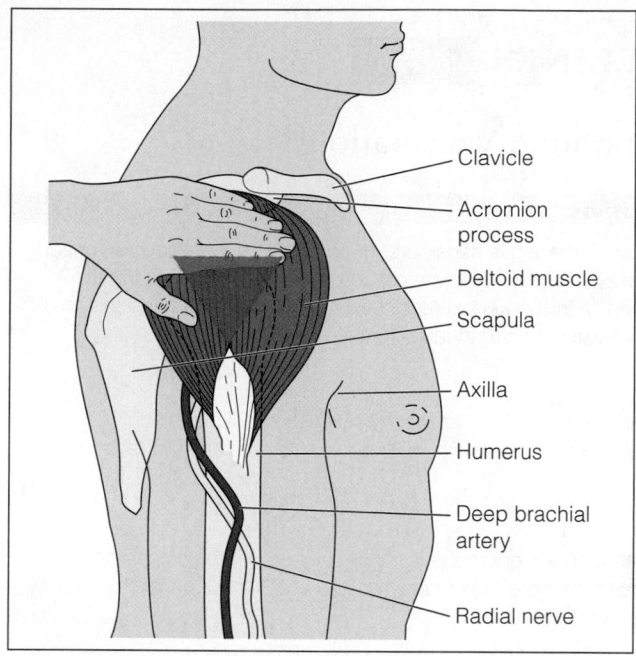

FIGURE 33.35 A method of establishing the deltoid muscle site for an intramuscular injection.

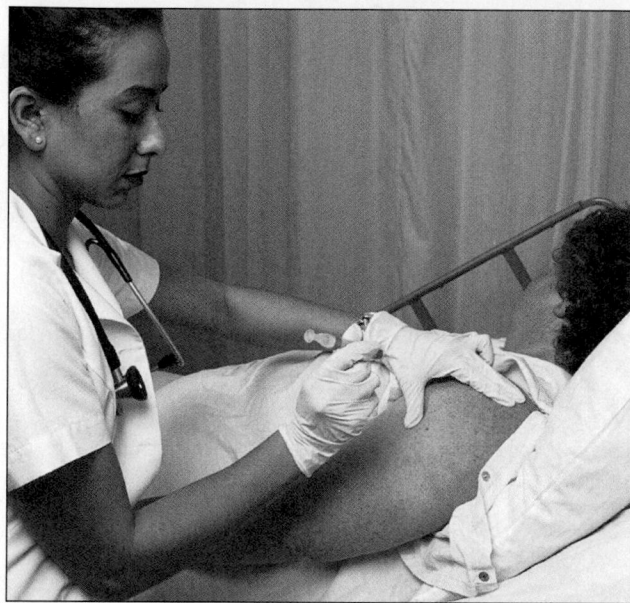

FIGURE 33.36 Administering an intramuscular injection into the deltoid site.

The upper landmark for the deltoid site is located by the nurse placing three or four fingers (approximately 3 to 5 cm) across the deltoid muscle with the first finger on the acromion process (Figure 33.35). The top of the axilla is the line that marks the lower border landmark. A triangle within these boundaries indicates the deltoid muscle, about 3 to 5 cm below the acromion process. The deltoid is easier to access compared with the ventrogluteal site (Figure 33.36).

INTRAMUSCULAR INJECTION TECHNIQUE Skill 33.7 on page 923 describes how to administer an intramuscular injection by using the Z-track technique, which is recommended for intramuscular injections. The Z-track method has been found to be less painful than the traditional straight injection technique and decreases leakage of irritating and discolouring medications into the subcutaneous tissue (Barron & Cocoman, 2008; Nicoll & Hesby, 2002; Zimmerman, 2010).

RAPID INJECTION TECHNIQUE The longstanding recommendations for administering immunizations by the intramuscular route have been (a) aspiration to ensure that no blood vessel was penetrated and (b) slow injection time to promote dissipation of medication and comfort. New evidence for the pragmatic technique of "no aspiration, rapid injection, and rapid withdrawal" is shedding some controversy on the age old "slow" technique. Ipp, Taddio, Sam, Goldback, and Parkin (2007) conducted a randomized controlled trial comparing the acute pain response during IM diphtheria, tetanus, pertussis, and *Haemophilus influenzae* type b (DPTaP-Hib) immunization in infants using the standard "slow" injection procedure versus the rapid technique. The result of this study is that the rapid injection technique of administering IM injections to the infants was less painful compared with the slow technique. Recently, the pan-Canadian Help ELiminate Pain in KIDS (HELPinKIDS) Team issued the following practice guideline: "to reduce pain at the time of injection, administer intramuscular vaccines to children using a rapid injection technique without aspiration" (Taddio, Ilersich, Ipp, Kikuta, Shah, & HELPinKIDS, 2009). For a summary of the work of the HELPinKIDS recommendations for reducing pain of childhood immunizations see Practice Guidelines 33.3.

ASPIRATING FOR BLOOD Until recently, most nursing textbooks and practice guidelines recommended that after inserting the needle into a muscle and prior to injecting the medication, the practitioner would aspirate by pulling back on the plunger of the syringe to check for the presence of blood in the event that a low-flow blood vessel or artery had been punctured. If there was bloody return, the practitioner would have to withdraw the needle and restart the procedure. More recently, several authors have argued against this practice, as it prolongs the injection time and there is no evidence to support aspiration (Diggle & Richards, 2007; World Health Organization [WHO], 2006). In addition, the recommended anatomical sites for injection are devoid of large blood vessels; most health care professionals administer immunizations without aspiration, and no complications have arisen (Taddio et al., 2009). To date, several international organizations (World Health Organization, 2006; U.S. Centers for Disease Control and Prevention, 2010) have adopted a "no aspiration" technique for immunization and vaccines. According to the *Canadian Immunization Guide,* "there are no studies that have assessed the need for aspiration prior to IM injection

PRACTICE GUIDELINES 33.3

Reducing the Pain of Childhood Vaccination*

Guidelines	Rationales
Encourage breast-feeding mothers to breast-feed their infants during vaccination (breast-feeding should be started before and should continue during and after the vaccine injections, for up to several minutes after the last injection is completed).	Breast-feeding is considered a combined analgesic intervention because several aspects of breast-feeding (e.g., holding the child, skin-to-skin contact, the sweet-tasting milk, and the act of sucking) may individually attenuate pain responses.
Among infants up to 12 months of age who cannot be breastfed during vaccination, administer a sweet-tasting solution (e.g., one packet or cube of sugar with 10 mL (two tsp) of water) during vaccination.	It is hypothesized that oral sweet-tasting solutions stimulate release of endogenous opioids and also provide distraction.
Do not place children in the supine position during vaccination.	Although the optimal position is not known, the supine position results in more pain than when the child sits upright or is held by a parent.
Administer intramuscular vaccines to children using a rapid injection technique without aspiration.	Less pain is experienced during rapid injection than with the slow injection technique.
When administering multiple vaccine injections to children sequentially, inject the most painful vaccine last (e.g., MMR, Prevnar) to reduce pain at the time of injection.	This may enhance the cooperation of the child and reduce distress.
Among children 4 years of age and older, offer to rub or stroke the skin near the injection site with moderate intensity before and during vaccination	Tactile stimulation before and during injection results in less pain; no studies have been performed on younger children.
Encourage parents to use topical anesthetics (applied correctly, according to instructions provided by the agent) during vaccination.	Topical anesthetics (e.g., lidocaine–prilocaine 5% cream or patch) are effective in reducing vaccination pain.
Use clinician-led or child-led distraction during vaccination.	Distraction reduces pain.
Have children 3 years of age and older engage in slow, deep breathing or blowing during vaccination.	This promotes relaxation and can act as a distraction.
Do not tell children that "it won't hurt."	This is not effective in reducing pain at the time of injection; deceiving the child is unethical and can lead to lack of trust in the health care professional.

*Insufficient evidence exists for the following practices: skin cooling techniques, simultaneous injection if multiple injections are required, use of intramuscular or subcutaneous route when various route options are available, and administering oral analgesia prior to the injection.

Source: Guidelines are summarized by M. Buck from Taddio, A., Appleton, M., Bortolussi, R., Chambers, C., Dubey, V., Halperin, S., Hanrahan, A., Ipp, M., Lockett, D., Macdonald, N., Midmer, D., Mousmanis, P., Palda, V., Pielak, K., Riddell, R. P., Rieder, M., Scott, J., & Shah, V. (2010). Reducing the pain of childhood vaccination: An evidence-based clinical practice guideline (summary). *Canadian Medical Association Journal 182,*1989–1995. doi:10.1503/cmaj.092048

of vaccines in relation to vaccine safety. As well, the syringes provided for immunization may not allow aspiration." Although most immunization guides currently do not include aspiration in their recommendations, some argue that research findings related to immunization guidelines may not apply to injection of other types of medications (Malkin, 2008). Skill 33.7 provides "with aspiration" and "without aspiration" instructions.

See also the Lifespan Considerations box on intramuscular injections on page 927.

Intravenous Medications

Medications administered intravenously (IV) enter the client's bloodstream directly by way of a vein and are appropriate when a rapid effect is required or when

SKILL 33.7 ADMINISTERING AN INTRAMUSCULAR INJECTION

PURPOSE

To provide a medication the client requires (see specific drug action)

ASSESSMENT

Assess

- Client allergies to medications
- Specific drug action and adverse effects
- Client's knowledge of and learning needs about the medication
- Tissue integrity of the selected site
- Client's age and weight to determine site and needle size
- Client's ability or willingness to participate

Determine whether the size of the muscle is appropriate to the amount of medication to be injected. An average adult's deltoid muscle can usually absorb 0.5 mL of medication, although some authorities believe 1 mL can be absorbed by a well-developed deltoid muscle. The gluteus medius muscle can often absorb 1 mL to 4 mL, although 4 mL may be painful and may be contraindicated by agency protocol.

Clinical Reasoning

Although intramuscular injections are an effective way of administering parenteral medications, they can be painful and frightening to some clients. Ask yourself if there is an alternative and equally effective route by which this medication could be administered so as to avoid the IM injection; for example, instead of administering the antiemetic dimenhyDRINATE by IM injection, could the client receive the medication as a suppository?

PLANNING

Equipment

- Client's MAR or computer printout
- Sterile medication (usually provided in an ampule, a vial, or a prefilled syringe)
- Syringe and needle of a size appropriate for the amount and type of solution to be administered
- Antiseptic swabs
- Clean gloves

IMPLEMENTATION

Preparation

1. Check the MAR.
   - Check the label on the medication carefully against the MAR to make sure that the correct medication is being prepared.
   - Follow the three checks for administering the medication and dose. Read the label on the medication (a) when it is taken from the medication cart, (b) before withdrawing the medication, and (c) after withdrawing the medication.
   - Confirm that the dose is correct.
2. Organize the equipment.

Performance

1. Perform hand hygiene, and follow other appropriate infection prevention and control procedures (e.g., clean gloves).
2. Prepare the medication from the ampule or vial for drug withdrawal.
   - See Skill 33.2 (ampule) or Skill 33.3 (vial).
   - Whenever feasible, change the needle on the syringe before the injection. **Rationale: Because the outside of a new needle is free of medication, it does not irritate subcutaneous tissues as it passes into the muscle.**
   - Invert the syringe, needle uppermost, and expel all excess air.
3. Provide for client privacy.
4. Prepare the client.
   - Prior to performing the procedure, introduce yourself and verify the client's identity using two identifiers or per agency protocol. **Rationale: This ensures that the right client receives the medication.**
   - Assist the client to the supine, lateral, prone, or sitting position, depending on the chosen site. If the target muscle is the gluteus medius (ventrogluteal site), have the client assume the supine position and flex the knee(s); in the lateral position, have the client flex the upper leg; and in the prone position, have the client hold the toes in. **Rationale: Appropriate positioning promotes relaxation of the target muscle.**
   - Obtain assistance for holding an uncooperative client. **Rationale: This prevents injury caused by sudden movement after needle insertion.**
5. Explain the purpose of the medication and how it will help, using language that the client can understand. Include relevant information about effects of the medication. **Rationale: Information can facilitate acceptance of, and adherence to, the therapy.**
6. Select, locate, and clean the site.
   - Select a site free of skin lesions, tenderness, swelling, hardness, or localized inflammation and one that has not been used frequently.
   - If injections are to be frequent, alternate the sites. Avoid using the same site twice in a row. **Rationale: This helps reduce the discomfort of intramuscular injections.**
   - Locate the exact site for the injection. See the discussion of sites earlier in this chapter.
   - Put on clean gloves.
   - Clean the site with an antiseptic swab. Use a circular motion, start at the centre, and move outward about 5 cm.
   - Transfer and hold the swab between the third and fourth fingers of the nondominant hand in readiness for needle withdrawal, or position the swab on the client's skin above the intended site. Allow skin to dry before injecting medication. **Rationale: This will help reduce the discomfort of the injection.**

(continued)

SKILL 33.7 ADMINISTERING AN INTRAMUSCULAR INJECTION (*continued*)

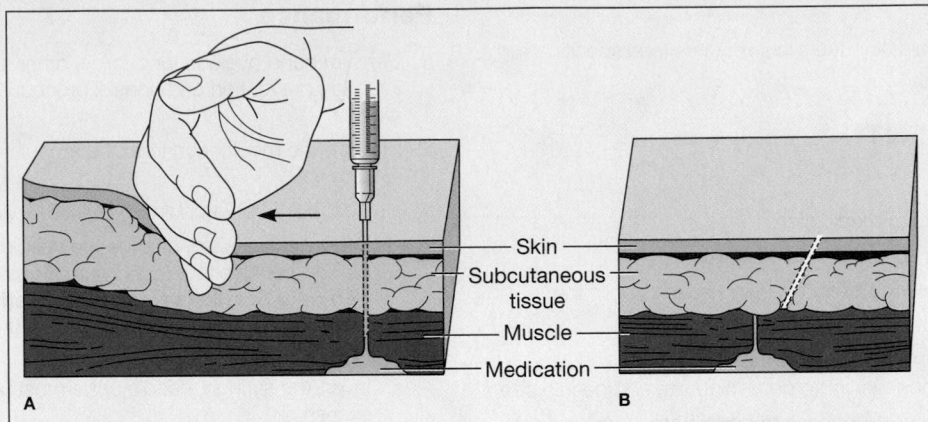

❶ Inserting an intramuscular needle at a 90-degree angle by using the Z-track method; **A:** Skin pulled to the side; **B:** Skin released. *Note:* When the skin returns to its normal position after the needle is withdrawn, a seal is formed over the intramuscular site. This prevents seepage of the medication into the subcutaneous tissues and subsequent discomfort.

7. Prepare the syringe for injection.
   - Remove the needle cover, and discard without contaminating the needle.
   - If using a prefilled unit-dose medication, take caution to avoid dripping medication on the needle before injection. If this does occur, wipe the medication off the needle with sterile gauze. Some sources recommend changing the needle, if possible. **Rationale: Medication left on the needle can cause pain when it is tracked through the subcutaneous tissue**.

8. Inject the medication by using a Z-track technique.
   - Use the ulnar side of the nondominant hand to pull the skin approximately 2.5 cm to the side. Under some circumstances, such as with a client who is emaciated or with an infant, the muscle may be pinched (see **❶**). **Rationale: Pulling the skin and subcutaneous tissue or pinching the muscle makes it firmer and facilitates needle insertion**.
   - Holding the syringe between the thumb and forefinger (as if holding a pen), pierce the skin quickly and smoothly at a 90-degree angle (see **❷**), and insert the needle into the muscle. **Rationale: Using a quick motion lessens the client's discomfort**.
   - *If the practice agency does not require aspiration as part of its IM injection protocol, then proceed to the next point below; if the agency does require aspiration,* hold the barrel of the syringe steady with the nondominant hand, and aspirate by pulling back on the plunger with your dominant hand). Aspirate for 5 to 10 seconds. If blood appears in the syringe, withdraw the needle, discard the syringe, and prepare a new injection. **Rationale: See discussion on aspiration** (page 921).
   - Inject the medication steadily and slowly (approximately 10 seconds per millilitre) OR rapidly if using the *rapid injection technique*. **Rationale: See discussion on rapid injection technique** (page 921).
   - After injection, wait 10 seconds and withdraw the needle OR withdraw the needle rapidly if using the *rapid injection technique*. **Rationale: Some hypothesize that waiting allows the medication to disperse into the muscle**

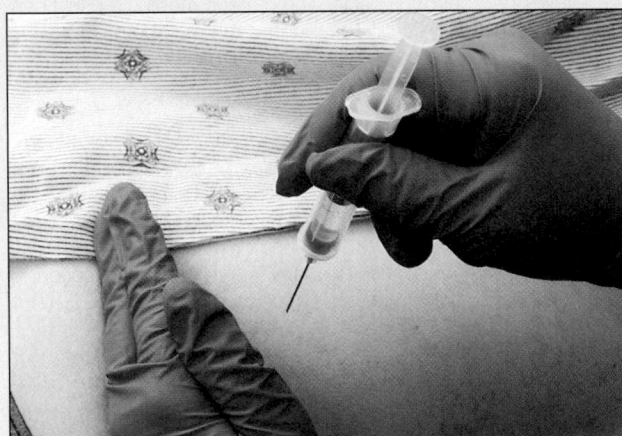

❷ Holding the syringe between the thumb and forefinger. Note that the nurse is using the Z-track technique.

tissue, thus decreasing the client's discomfort; others view rapid injection as less painful.
   - Apply gentle pressure at the site with a dry gauze. **Rationale: Use of an antiseptic swab may cause pain or a burning sensation**.
     - It is not necessary to massage the area at the site of injection. **Rationale: Massaging the site may cause the leakage of medication from the site and result in irritation** (Hunter, 2008).
   - If bleeding occurs, apply pressure with a dry gauze until the bleeding stops.

9. Activate the needle safety device, or discard the uncapped needle and attached syringe into the sharps container.
   - Remove and discard gloves. Perform hand hygiene.

10. Document all relevant information.
    - Include the time of administration, drug name, dose, route, and the client's reactions.

11. Assess the effectiveness of the medication at the time it is expected to act.

EVALUATION

- Conduct appropriate follow-up, such as the following:
  - Desired effect (e.g., relief of pain or vomiting)
  - Any adverse effects
  - Local skin or tissue reactions at injection site (e.g., redness, swelling, pain, or other evidence of tissue damage)

- Relate to previous findings, if available.
- Report significant deviations from normal to the appropriate members of the health care team.

LIFESPAN CONSIDERATIONS

Intramuscular Injections

INFANTS

- The vastus lateralis site is recommended as the site of choice for intramuscular injections for infants. There are no major blood vessels or nerves in this area, and it is the infant's largest muscle mass. It is situated on the anterior lateral aspect of the thigh.
- Obtain assistance to immobilize an infant or a young child. The parent may hold the child. This prevents accidental injury during the procedure.

CHILDREN

- Use needles that will place the medication in the main muscle mass; children usually require needles with #22 gauge to #25 gauge and 16 mm long for injections into the deltoid muscle and 2.5 cm long for injections into the vastus lateralis.
- The deltoid is recommended as the site of choice for IM injection of immunizations in toddlers and children.
- For the older child and for the adolescent, the recommended sites are the same as that for the adult: ventrogluteal or deltoid. Ask clients which arm they would like the injection in.

OLDER ADULTS

- Older clients may have a decreased muscle mass or muscle atrophy. A shorter needle may be needed. Assessment of the appropriate injection site is critical. Absorption of medication may occur more quickly than expected.

medications are too irritating to tissues to be given by other routes. When an IV line is already established, this route is desirable because it avoids the discomfort of other parenteral routes. Following are methods to administer medications intravenously:

- Large-volume infusion of intravenous fluid
- Intermittent intravenous infusion (piggyback or tandem setups)
- Volume-controlled infusion (often used for children)
- Intravenous push (IVP) or bolus
- Intermittent injection ports (device)

In all of these methods, the client has an existing IV line or an IV access site, such as a saline lock. Most agencies have procedures and policies about who may administer an IV medication. Skill 44.1 (page 1450) describes the technique for performing a venipuncture and establishing an IV line.

With all IV medication administration, it is important to observe clients closely for signs of adverse effects. Because the drug enters the bloodstream directly and acts immediately, there is no way it can be withdrawn or its action terminated. Therefore, the nurse must take special care to avoid any errors in the preparation of the drug and the calculation of the dosage. When the administered drug is particularly potent, an antidote to the drug should be available. In addition, assess the vital signs before, during, and after infusion of the drug. Before adding any medications to an existing intravenous infusion, the nurse must check for the "10 rights" and check compatibility of the drug and the existing intravenous fluid. Be aware of any incompatibilities of the drug and the existing IV fluid. For example, the drug phenytoin is incompatible with glucose and will form a precipitate if injected through a port in an intravenous line with glucose or dextrose infusing.

LARGE-VOLUME INFUSIONS At times, medications are diluted in a large-volume IV container of 250 mL, 500 mL, or 1000 mL of compatible fluids because the medication requires a large volume for dilution (e.g., certain antibiotics, such as vancomycin, potassium chloride [KCl]) or it is to be administered as a continuous drip (e.g., insulin, xylocaine). Ideally, such medications are premixed by the manufacturer or in the pharmacy (as with xylocaine, dopamine, KCL*); however, the nurse may have to add the medication to the infusing fluid container (ideally before it is hung rather than while it is infusing to ensure that the volume the medication is being diluted into is accurate). It may be necessary to consult a pharmacist to confirm compatibility of the medication with IV fluids and possibly with the type of IV container and tubing (i.e., some medications may not be compatible with the plastic bag and tubing and require a glass container and special tubing). Common IV fluids into which medications are infused include normal saline (NS) and dextrose 5% in water (D_5W). See Skill 33.8 for adding medications to IV fluid containers. Other than

---

*Accreditation Canada and the Institute for Safe Medication Practices recommend that vials of concentrated KCl, a high-alert medication, NOT be kept on units and that agencies use IV solutions premixed with KCl by the manufacturer.

SKILL 33.8 ADDING MEDICATIONS TO INTRAVENOUS FLUID CONTAINERS

PURPOSE

- To provide and maintain a constant level of a medication in the blood
- To administer well-diluted medications at a continuous and slow rate

ASSESSMENT

- Inspect and palpate the intravenous insertion site for signs of infection, infiltration, or a dislocated catheter.
- Inspect the surrounding skin for redness, pallor, or swelling.
- Palpate the surrounding tissues for coldness and the presence of edema, which could indicate leakage of the IV fluid into the tissues.
- Take vital signs for baseline data for medication that is particularly potent.
- Determine whether the client has allergies to the medication.
- Check the compatibility of the medication and IV fluid.

> **! CLINICAL ALERT**
>
> When checking the compatibility of the medication with the IV fluid, remember that any additives already in the IV fluid must be considered. For example, if vitamins are to be added to a maintenance infusion of dextrose 5% in 0.45% normal saline premixed with 20 mmol KCl/L (D5 1/2NS with 20 KCl), you must verify if the vitamin is compatible with the dextrose, the saline, AND the KCl.

PLANNING

Equipment

- Client's MAR or computer printout
- Correct sterile medication
- Diluent for medication in powdered form (see manufacturer's instructions)
- Correct solution container, if a new one is to be attached
- Antiseptic swabs
- Sterile syringe of appropriate size (e.g., 5 mL or 10 mL) and a 2.5-cm or 3.8-cm, #20- or #21-gauge sterile needle or equivalent needleless system
- IV additive label

IMPLEMENTATION

Preparation

1. Check the MAR.
   - Check the label on the medication carefully against the MAR to make sure the correct medication is being prepared.
   - Follow the three checks for administering medications. Read the label on the medication (a) when it is taken from the medication cart, (b) before withdrawing the medication, and (c) after withdrawing the medication.
   - Confirm that the dosage and route are correct.
   - Verify which infusion solution is to be used with the medication.

- Consult a pharmacist, if required, to confirm compatibility of the drugs and solutions being mixed.

2. Organize the equipment.

Performance

1. Perform hand hygiene, and follow other appropriate infection prevention and control procedures.

2. Prepare the medication ampule or vial for drug withdrawal.
   - See Skill 33.2 (ampule) or Skill 33.3 (vial).
   - Check the agency's practice for using a filter needle to withdraw premixed liquid medications from multidose vials or from ampules.

3. Add the medication.
   - Locate the injection port. Clean the port with the antiseptic swab (see ❶). **Rationale: This reduces the risk of introducing microorganisms into the container when the needle is inserted**.
   - Remove the needle cap from the syringe, insert the needle through the centre of the injection port, and inject the medication into the bag. Activate the needle safety device (see ❷).

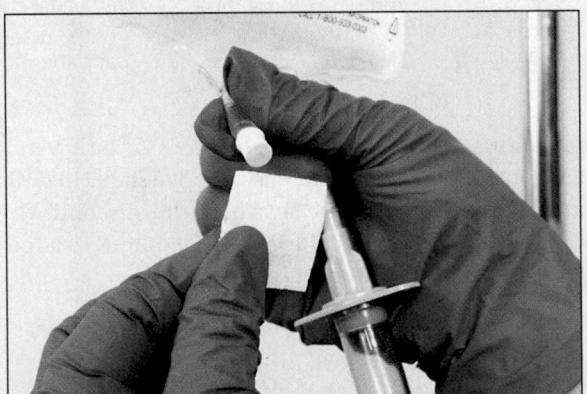

❶ Cleanse the injection port with an antiseptic swab.

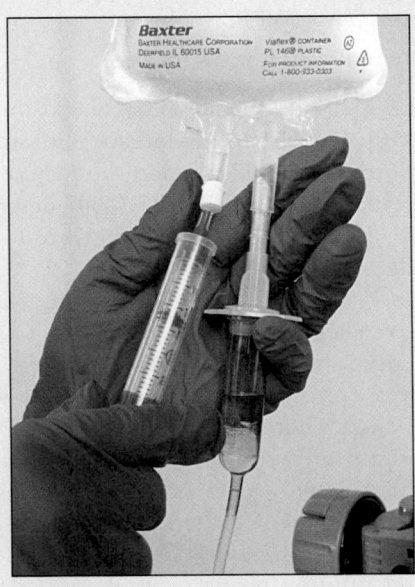

❷ Inserting a medication through the injection port of a fluid container.

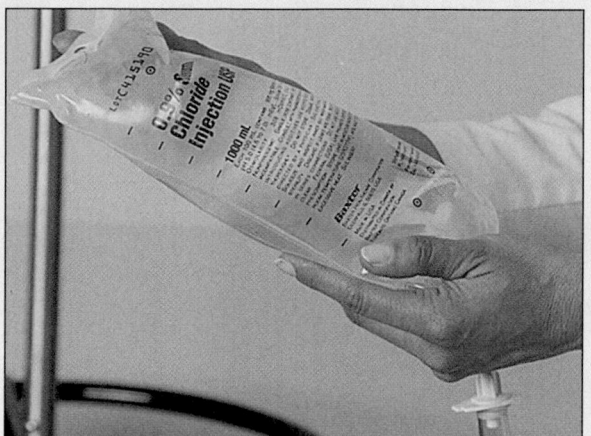

❸ Rotating an intravenous bag to distribute a medication.

- Mix the medication and solution by gently rotating the bag or bottle (see ❸). **Rationale: This should disperse the medication throughout the solution**.

- Complete the IV additive label with the name and dose of medication, date, time, and nurse's initials (see ❹). **Rationale: This documents that the medication has been added to the solution**.

- Clamp the IV tubing. Spike the bag or bottle with IV tubing and hang the IV. **Rationale: Clamping prevents rapid infusion of the solution**.

- Regulate infusion rate, as ordered. Often, a controller device, such as an IV pump, is used to ensure an accurate rate of infusion.

4. Dispose of the equipment and supplies, according to agency practice. **Rationale: This prevents inadvertent injury to others and the spread of microorganisms**.

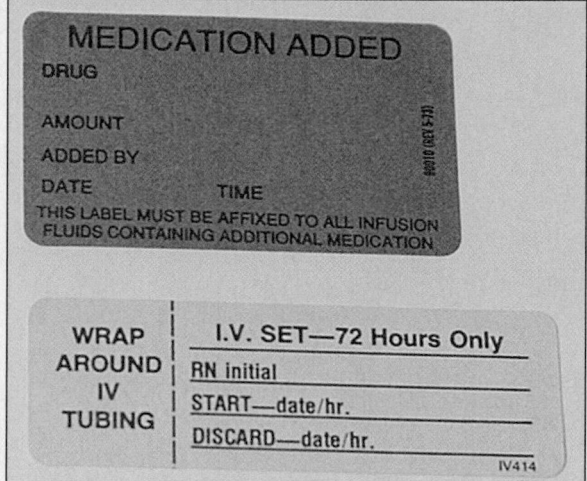

❹ **Top:** Label indicating a medication added to an IV infusion; **Bottom:** Label indicating time for IV tubing change.

5. Document the medication on the appropriate form in the client's record.

EVALUATION

- Conduct appropriate follow-up, such as desired effect of medication, any adverse effects, or change in vital signs.

- Reassess the status of IV site and patency of IV infusion.

- Relate to previous findings, if available.

- Report significant deviations from normal to the appropriate member of the health care team.

---

monitoring the effects of the medication, the main danger of infusing a large volume of fluid is circulatory overload (hypervolemia). See Chapter 44.

INTERMITTENT INTRAVENOUS INFUSIONS An intermittent infusion is a method of administering a medication mixed in a small amount of IV solution, such as 50 mL or 100 mL (Figure 33.37). The drug is administered at regular intervals, such as every 4 hours, with the drug being infused for a short period, such as 30 to 60 minutes. Two commonly used additive setups are the *tandem* and the *piggyback*. In a **tandem** setup or alignment, a second container is attached to the line of the first container at the lower, secondary port (see Figure 33.38A). It permits medications to be administered intermittently or simultaneously with the primary solution. In the **piggyback** alignment, a second set connects the second container to the tubing of the primary container at the upper port (see Figure 33.38B). This setup is used solely for intermittent drug administration. Various manufacturers describe these sets differently, so the nurse must check the manufacturer's labelling and directions

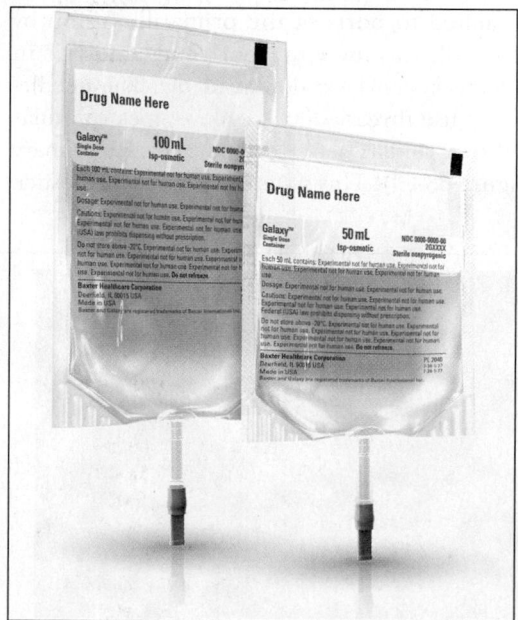

FIGURE 33.37 Infusion bags for medications.

Source: Copyright 2011 Baxter Healthcare Corporation. Reprinted with permission.

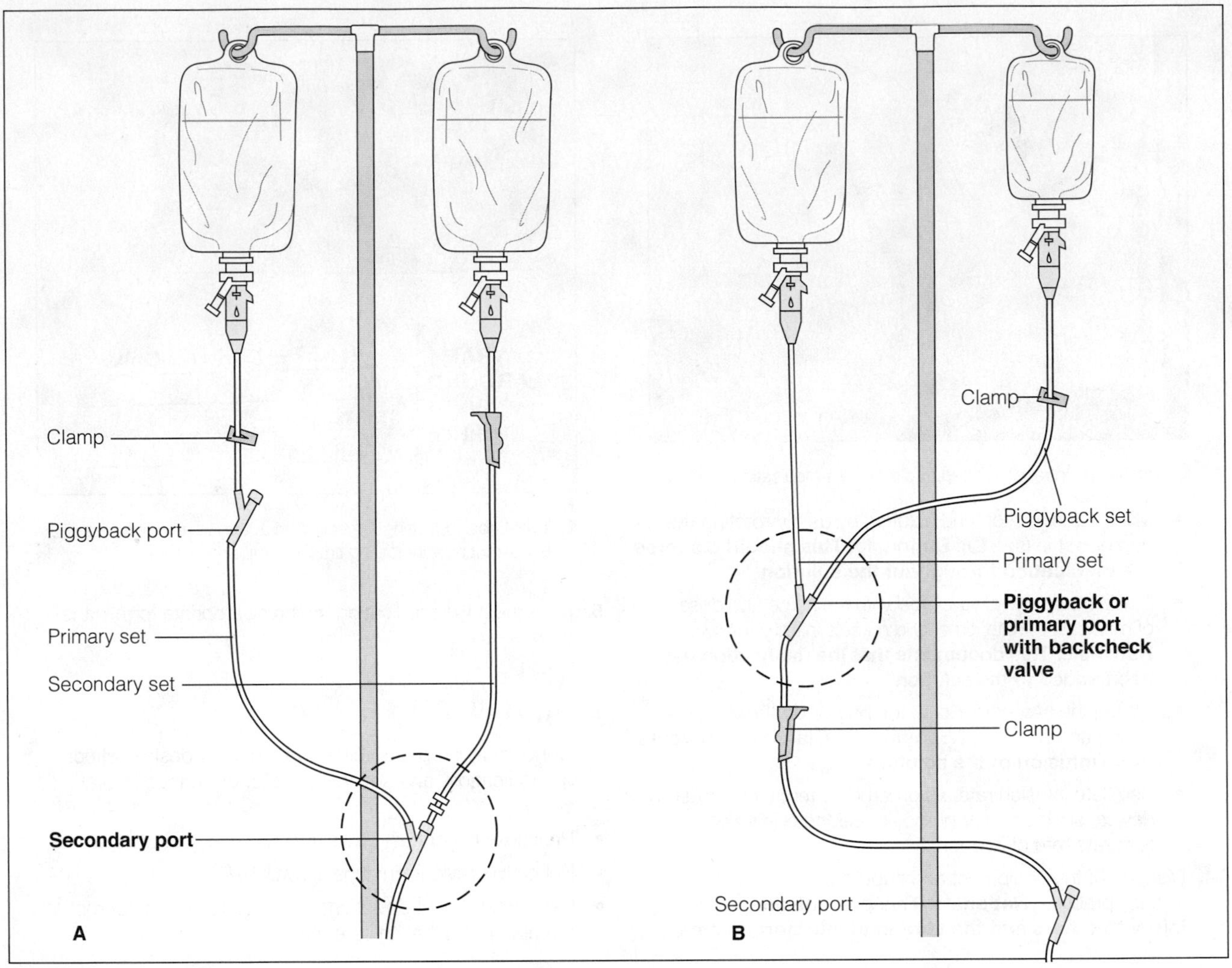

Clamp

Piggyback port

Primary set

Secondary set

Secondary port

A

Clamp

Piggyback set

Primary set

**Piggyback or
primary port
with backcheck
valve**

Clamp

Secondary port

B

FIGURE 33.38 Secondary intravenous lines: **A:** A tandem intravenous alignment; **B:** An intravenous piggyback (IVPB) alignment.

carefully. Traditionally the tubing of the secondary set has been attached to ports of the primary infusion by inserting a needle through the port and taping it in place. Needleless systems are now available. The needleless systems can use threaded-lock or lever-lock cannulas to connect the secondary set to the ports of the primary infusion (Figure 33.39). This system prevents needlestick

injuries as well as touch contamination at the IV connection site. Skill 33.9 explains how to administer an intermittent intravenous infusion using a secondary set.

Another method of intermittently administering an IV medication is by a syringe pump or mini-infuser. The medication is mixed in a syringe that is connected to the primary IV line via a mini-infuser (Figure 33.40 on page 931).

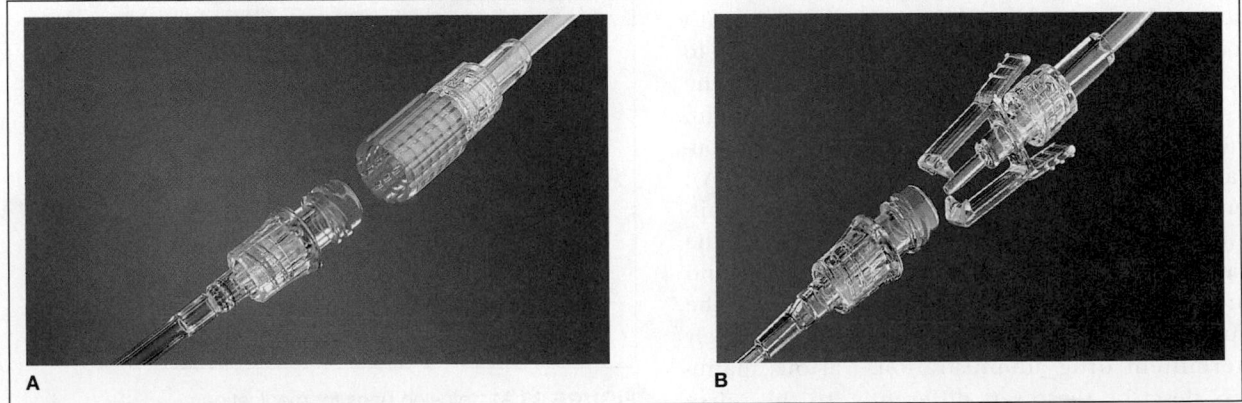

A

B

FIGURE 33.39 Needleless cannulas used to connect the tubing of secondary sets to primary infusions: **A:** Threaded-lock cannula; **B:** Lever-lock cannula.

SKILL 33.9 ADMINISTERING INTERMITTENT INTRAVENOUS MEDICATIONS USING A SECONDARY SET

PURPOSE

To administer an intravenous medication at variable intervals

ASSESSMENT

- Inspect and palpate the IV insertion site for signs of infection, infiltration, or a dislocated catheter.
- Inspect the surrounding skin for redness, pallor, or swelling.
- Palpate the surrounding tissues for tenderness, coldness, and the presence of edema, which could indicate leakage of the IV fluid into the tissues.
- Take vital signs for baseline data if the medication being administered is particularly potent.
- Determine if the client has allergies to the medication(s).
- Check the compatibility of the medication, primary IV fluid, and any medication(s) in the primary IV bag.
- Determine specific drug action, side effects, normal dosage, recommended administration time, and peak action time.
- Check patency of the IV line by assessing flow rate.

PLANNING

Equipment

- Client's MAR or computer printout
- 50-mL to 250-mL infusion bag with medication (most medication infusion bags are prepared by the pharmacist)
- Secondary administration set
- Antiseptic swabs
- Sterile needle, if system is not needleless
- Tape
- Sterile needle or needleless adapter, syringe, and saline, if medication is incompatible with the primary infusion

IMPLEMENTATION

Preparation

- Check the MAR.
- Check the label on the medication carefully against the MAR to make sure that the correct medication is being prepared.
- Confirm that the dosage is correct.
- Ensure medication compatibility with the primary infusion solution (including any additives such as KCl).
- Consult a pharmacist, if required, to confirm compatibility of the drugs and solutions being mixed.
- Organize the equipment.
- Remove the medication bag from the refrigerator 30 minutes before administration, if appropriate.

Performance

1. Perform hand hygiene, and follow other appropriate infection control procedures.
2. Provide for client privacy.
3. Prepare the client.
   - Prior to performing the procedure, introduce yourself and verify the client's identity using two identifiers or per agency protocol. **Rationale: This ensures that the right client receives the right medication.**
   - If not previously assessed, take the appropriate assessment measures necessary for the medication.
4. Explain the purpose of the medication and how it will help, using language that the client can understand. Include relevant information about the effects of the medication. **Rationale: Information can facilitate acceptance of, and compliance with, the therapy.**
5. Assemble the secondary infusion:
   - Close the clamp on the secondary infusion tubing.
   - Spike the secondary medication infusion bag and fully flush the tubing, making sure no air is trapped in the tubing. Do not allow more than one or two drops of the solution to exit the tubing to ensure that the client receives the full dose of medication.
   - Hang the secondary container at or above the level of the primary infusion. Use the extension hook to lower the primary infusion if a piggyback setup is required. Some infusion pumps do not require this.
   - Attach the needleless cannula to the tubing.
   - Attach the appropriate label to the secondary tubing. Secondary tubing is generally changed every 24 hours. Check agency policy.
6. Attach the secondary infusion to the primary infusion.
   - Clean the Y-port on the primary IV line with an antiseptic swab. Clean the **primary port** (the port farthest from the client) for a piggyback alignment and the **secondary port** (the port closest to the client) for a tandem setup.
   - If the medication is not compatible with the primary infusion, temporarily discontinue the primary infusion. Flush the primary line with a sterile saline solution before attaching the secondary set. To flush the line, wipe the port with an antiseptic swab, clamp the primary line, and, using a sterile syringe and needleless adapter, instill sufficient sterile saline solution through the port to flush any primary fluid out of the infusion tubing.
   - Insert the needleless cannula of the secondary line into the primary tubing port. See ❶.

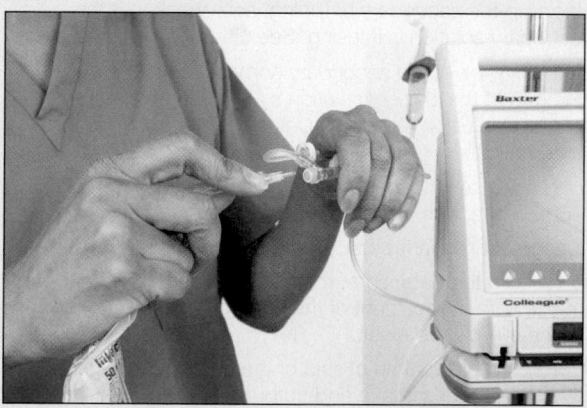

❶ Insert the needleless cannula of the secondary line into the primary tubing port.

(continued)

| **SKILL 33.9** | **ADMINISTERING INTERMITTENT INTRAVENOUS MEDICATIONS USING A SECONDARY SET** (*continued*) |

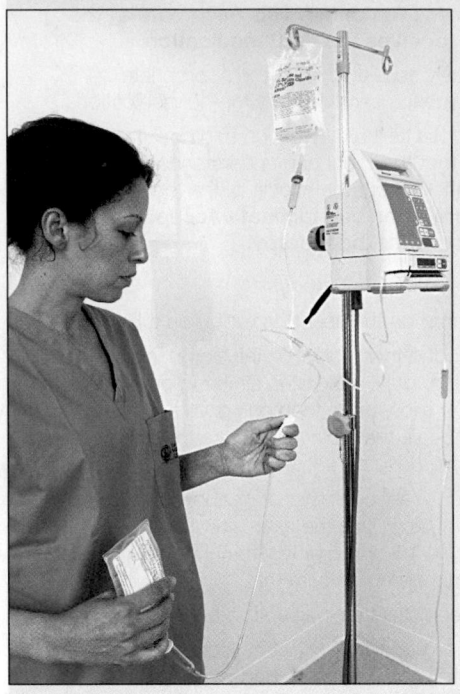

❷ Lower the IV medication bag to back prime the secondary tubing.

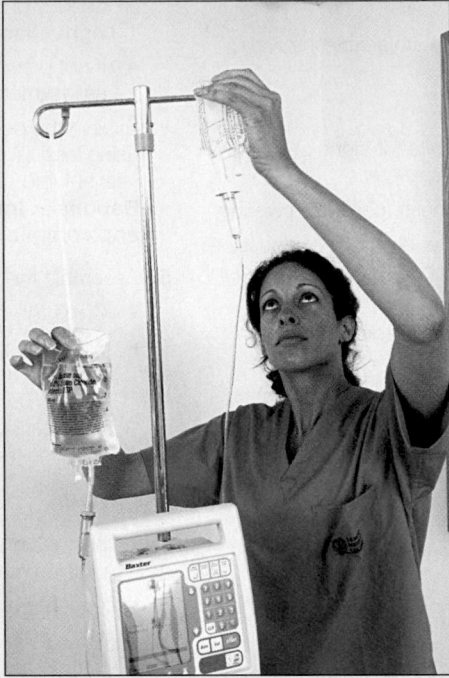

❸ Hang the IV medication bag on the IV pole.

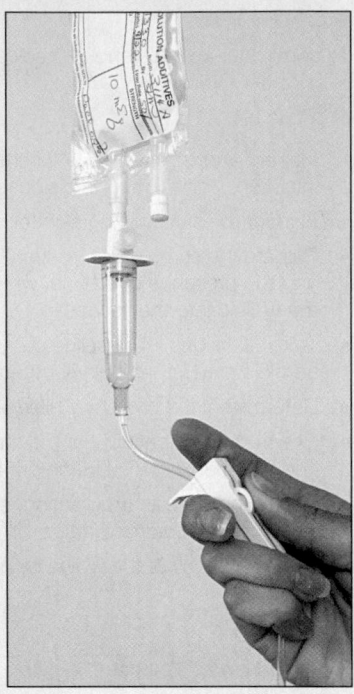

❹ Open the clamp on the secondary tubing.

7. Back prime the secondary tubing if the primary and secondary fluids are compatible.

- Lower the medication infusion bag below the primary IV bag.
- Open the clamp of the medication bag.
- Allow the solution from the primary IV bag to backfill the secondary IV tubing and one-third to one-half of the secondary tubing chamber. See ❷. **Rationale: This method of priming the secondary tubing prevents any loss of medication.**
- Clamp the secondary IV tubing.
- Hang the secondary IV bag on the IV pole. See ❸.

8. Program the IV pump for the infusion rate of the IV medication bag.

9. Unclamp the secondary IV tubing, and check that the secondary solution is infusing. See ❹.

10. After infusion of the secondary IV medication bag, regulate the rate of the primary solution by adjusting the clamp or IV pump infusion rate. Some infusion pumps will do this automatically.

11. Leave the secondary bag and tubing in place for future administration or discard, as appropriate.

12. Document relevant data.

- Record the date, time, medication, dose, route, and solution; assessment of the IV site, if appropriate; and the client's response.
- Record the volume of fluid of the medication infusion bag on the client's intake and output record.

Variation: Using a Saline Lock

Intermittent infusion devices (see ❺) may be attached to an intravenous catheter to allow medications to be administered intravenously without requiring a continuous IV infusion. The device may also have a port at one end of the lock and a needleless injection cap at the other end with the extension tubing between the two ends. See ❻.

- Prepare two normal saline prefilled syringes (1 mL each).
- Spike the medication bag with microdrip (60 drops/mL) IV tubing.
- Attach the needleless adapter to the tubing, prime the tubing, and close the clamp.
- Clean the needleless injection port of the saline lock with an antiseptic swab. Open the saline lock clamp, if appropriate.
- Insert the first saline syringe into the port, and gently aspirate to check for patency. Flush slowly noting any resistance, swelling, pain, or burning. **Rationale: This ensures placement of the IV in the vein**.
- After connecting the IV tubing to the injection port of the lock, administer the medication, regulating the drip rate to allow medication to infuse for the appropriate period. Macrodrip (10–20 drops/mL) tubing may also be used if using an IV pump to regulate the flow.
- When the medication has been infused, disconnect the IV tubing, maintaining sterility of the end of the IV tubing.

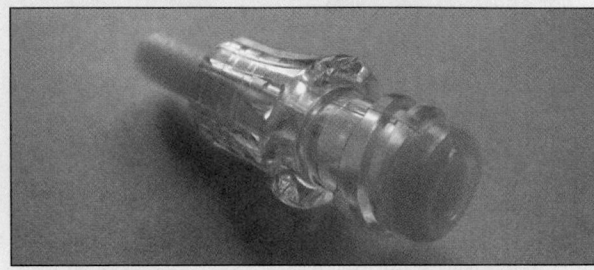

❺ Intermittent infusion device with an injection port.

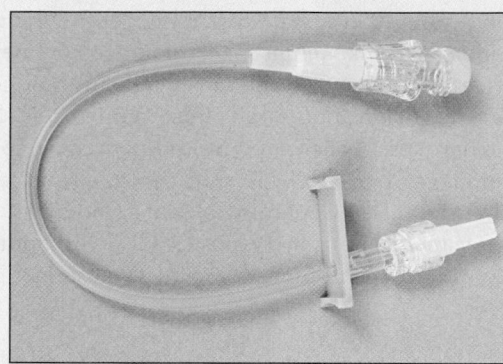

❻ Intermittent infusion device with an injection port and extension tubing.

- Insert the second saline syringe into the port and gently flush the saline lock. **Rationale: Flushing clears the tubing and maintains patency.**
- Clamp the saline lock after flushing, if appropriate.
- Dispose of syringes in the appropriate container.

Variation: Adding a Medication to a Volume-Control Infusion

- Withdraw the required dose of the medication into a syringe.
- Ensure that there is sufficient fluid in the volume-control fluid chamber to dilute the medication. Generally, at least 50 mL of fluid is used. Check the directions from the drug manufacturer, or consult the pharmacist.
- Close the inflow to the fluid chamber by adjusting the upper roller or slide clamp above the fluid chamber; also, ensure that the clamp on the air vent of the chamber is open.
- Clean the medication port on the volume-control fluid chamber with an antiseptic swab.
- Inject the medication into the port of the appropriately filled volume-control set (i.e., the ordered amount of solution).
- Gently rotate the fluid chamber until the fluid is well mixed.
- Regulate the flow by adjusting the lower roller clamp below the fluid chamber.
- Attach a medication label to the volume-control fluid chamber.
- Document relevant data, and monitor the client and the infusion.

EVALUATION

- Conduct appropriate follow-up, such as desired effect of medication, any adverse reactions or side effects, and change in vital signs.
- Reassess status of the IV lock site and patency of the IV infusion.
- Relate to previous findings, if available.
- Report significant deviations from normal to the appropriate member of the heath care team.

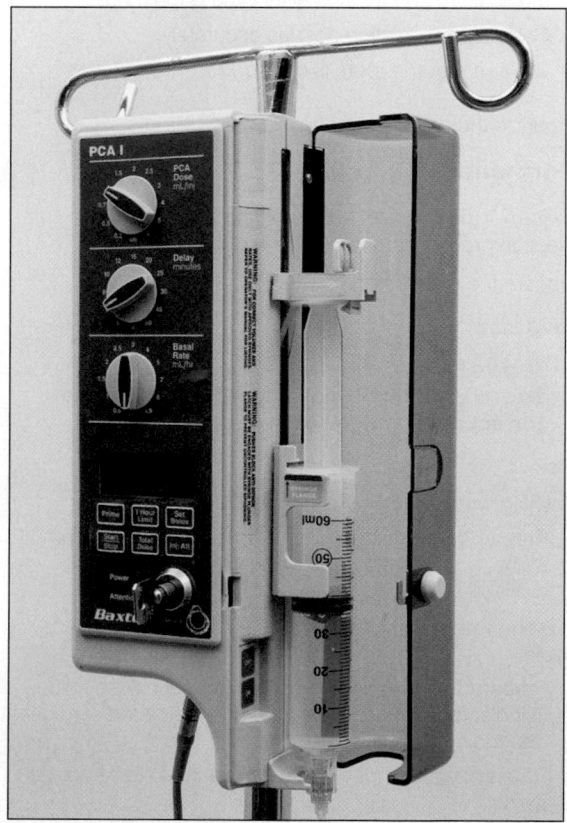

FIGURE 33.40 Syringe pump or mini-infuser for administration of IV medications

VOLUME-CONTROL INFUSIONS Intermittent medications can also be administered by a **volume-control infusion set**, such as Buretrol and Soluset (Figure 33.41). They are small fluid containers (100 mL to 150 mL in size) attached below the primary infusion container so that the medication is administered through the client's IV line. Volume-control sets are frequently used to infuse solutions into children and older clients when the volume administered is critical and must be carefully monitored. See Skill 33.9.

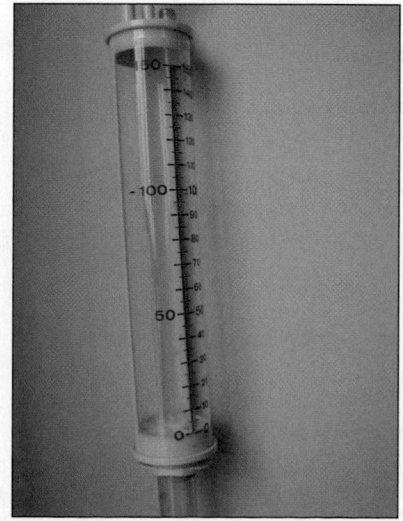

FIGURE 33.41 A volume-control infusion set.

INTRAVENOUS PUSH Intravenous push (IVP) or bolus is the intravenous administration of an undiluted drug directly into the systemic circulation. It is used when a medication cannot be diluted or in an emergency. An IV bolus can be introduced directly into a vein by venipuncture or into an existing IV line through an injection port or through an IV lock.

There are two major disadvantages to this method of drug administration: (a) Any error in administration cannot be corrected after the drug has entered the client; and (b) the drug may be irritating to the endothelial lining of the blood vessels. Before administering a bolus, the nurse should look up the maximum concentration recommended for the particular drug and the rate of administration. The administered medication takes effect immediately. Many agencies have strict policies and procedures related to what medications can be given by IV push, by whom, and under what circumstances. Generally, nursing students do not administer medications by IV push. Skill 33.10 addresses administering IV medications using the IV push method.

SKILL 33.10   ADMINISTERING INTRAVENOUS MEDICATIONS USING IV PUSH

PURPOSE
To achieve immediate and maximum effects of a medication

ASSESSMENT

- Inspect and palpate the IV insertion site for signs of infection, infiltration, or a dislocated catheter.
- Inspect the surrounding skin for redness, pallor, or swelling.
- Palpate the surrounding tissues for coldness and the presence of edema, which could indicate leakage of the IV fluid into the tissues.
- Take vital signs for baseline data if the medication being administered is particularly potent.
- Determine if the client has allergies to the medication(s).
- Check the compatibility of the medication(s) and IV fluid.
- Determine specific drug action, adverse effects, normal dosage, recommended administration time, and peak action time.
- Check patency of IV.

PLANNING

Clinical Reasoning

Given that the IV push medication's effects will be instantaneous, reflect on what the desired effects and potential adverse effects are so that you can anticipate how you will monitor the client for safety.

Equipment

IV Push for an Existing Line

- Client's MAR
- Medication in a vial or an ampule
- Sterile syringe (3 to 5 mL) (to prepare the medication)
- Sterile needles #21 to #25 gauge, 2.5 cm (needle not needed if using a needleless system)
- Antiseptic swabs
- Watch with a digital readout or second hand
- Clean gloves

IV Push for an IV Lock

- Same equipment as IV push for an existing line, but add two sterile syringes (usually 3 mL) and a vial of flush liquid or preloaded syringes of flush solution (generally normal saline)

to flush the IV catheter before and after administering the medication, depending on agency practice. **Rationale: The flush ensures that no medication remains in the tubing and then maintains the patency of the lock**.

IMPLEMENTATION

Preparation

1. Check the MAR.
   - Check the label on the medication carefully against the MAR to make sure that the correct medication is being prepared.
   - Follow the three checks for correct medication and dose. Read the label on the medication (a) when it is taken from the medication cart, (b) before withdrawing the medication, and (c) after withdrawing the medication.
   - Calculate medication dosage accurately.
   - Confirm that the route is correct.

2. Organize the equipment.

Performance

1. Perform hand hygiene, and follow other appropriate infection prevention and control procedures.
2. Prepare the medication.

Existing Line

- Prepare the medication according to the manufacturer's direction. **Rationale: It is important to have the correct dose and the correct dilution**.

IV Lock

a. Flushing with saline
   - Prepare two syringes, each with 1 mL of sterile normal saline, or use preloaded syringes, depending on availability.
b. Flushing with heparin (if indicated by agency policy) and saline
   - Prepare one syringe with 1 mL of heparin flush solution (if indicated by agency policy). Use preloaded syringes depending on availability.
   - Prepare two syringes with 1 mL each of sterile normal saline.
   - Draw up the medication into a syringe.

3. Put a small-gauge needle on the syringe, if using a needle system.

4. Perform hand hygiene, and put on clean gloves. **Rationale: This reduces the transmission of microorganisms and reduces the likelihood of the nurse's hands contacting the client's blood**.

5. Provide for client privacy.

6. Prepare the client.
   - Prior to performing the procedure, introduce yourself and verify the client's identity using two identifiers or per agency protocol.
   - If not previously assessed, take the appropriate assessment measures necessary for the medication. If any of the findings are above or below the predetermined parameters, consult the appropriate member of the health care team before administering the medication.

7. Explain the purpose of the medication and how it will help, using language that the client can understand. Include relevant information about the effects of the medication. **Rationale: Information can facilitate acceptance of, and adherence to, the therapy**.

8. Administer the medication by IV push.

IV Lock with Needle

- Clean the injection port with an antiseptic swab. **Rationale: This prevents microorganisms from entering the circulatory system during needle insertion**.

- Insert the needle of the syringe containing normal saline through the centre of the diaphragm (see ❶) and aspirate for blood. **Rationale: The presence of blood confirms that the catheter or needle is in the vein. In some situations, blood will not return, even though the lock is patent**.

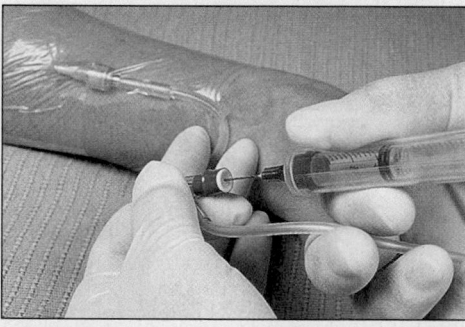

❶ Inserting a needle through the diaphragm of an IV lock

- Flush the lock by injecting 1 mL of saline slowly. **Rationale: This removes blood and heparin (if present) from the needle and the lock**.

- Remove the needle and syringe. Activate the needle safety device.

- Clean the lock's diaphragm with an antiseptic swab. **Rationale: This prevents the transfer of microorganisms**.

- Insert the needle of the syringe containing the prepared medication through the centre of the injection port.

- Inject the medication slowly at the recommended rate of infusion (see ❷). Use a watch or digital readout to time the

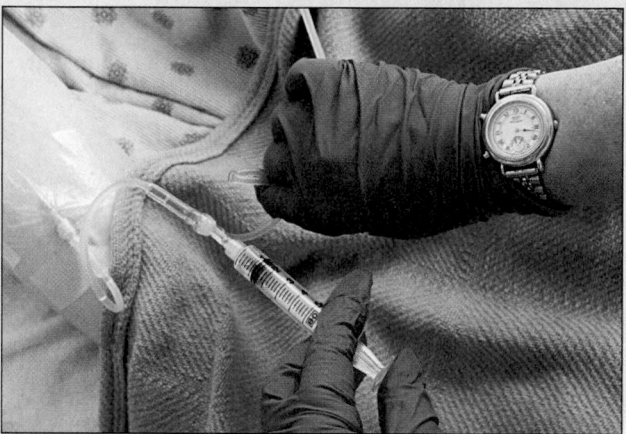

❷ Using a watch to time the rate of a medication injection

injection. Observe the client closely for adverse reactions. Remove the needle and syringe when all of the medication has been administered. **Rationale: Injecting the drug too rapidly can cause a serious untoward reaction**.

- Activate the needle safety device.

- Clean the diaphragm of the lock.

- Attach the second saline syringe, and inject 1 mL of saline. **Rationale: The saline injection flushes the medication through the catheter and prepares the lock for heparin if this medication is used. Heparin is incompatible with many medications**.

- If heparin is to be used, insert the heparin syringe, and inject the heparin slowly into the lock.

IV Lock with Needleless System

- Clean the injection port with an antiseptic swab.

- Remove the protective cap from the needleless port.

- Insert syringe containing normal saline into the lock.

- Flush the lock with 1 mL sterile saline. **Rationale: This clears the lock of blood**.

- Remove the syringe.

- Insert the syringe containing the medication into the valve (see ❸).

- Inject the medication, following the precautions described previously.

- Withdraw the syringe.

- Repeat injection of 1 mL of saline.

Existing Line

- Identify the injection port closest to the client. Some ports have a circle indicating the site for the needle insertion.

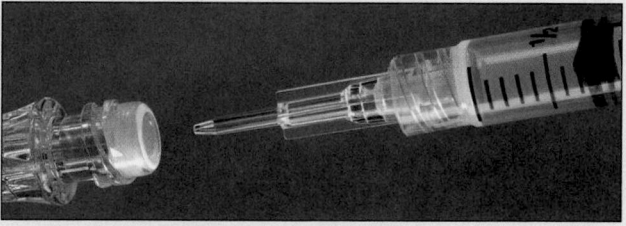

❸ A needleless tip syringe—a blunt plastic cannula replaces the sharp steel needle

(continued)

SKILL 33.10 ADMINISTERING INTRAVENOUS MEDICATIONS USING IV PUSH (*continued*)

Rationale: An injection port must be used because it is self-sealing. Any puncture to the plastic tubing will leak.

- Clean the port with an antiseptic swab.
- Stop the IV flow by closing the clamp or pinching the tubing above the injection port.
- Connect the needless syringe or insert the needle to the IV port (see ❹).

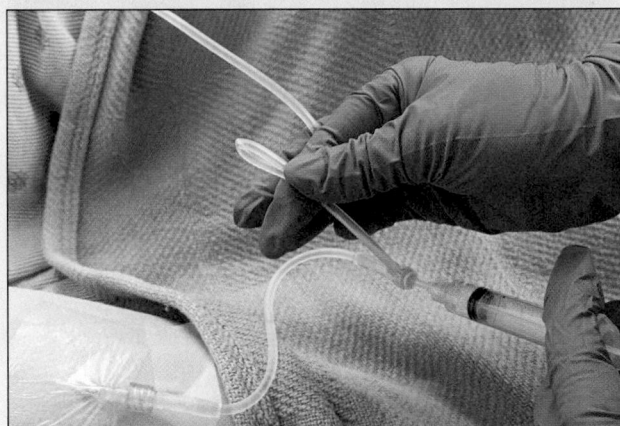

❹ Stopping the IV flow by pinching the tubing above the injection port and injecting a medication by IV push

- Inject the medication at the ordered rate. Use the watch second hand or digital readout to time the medication administration. **Rationale: This ensures safe drug administration because a too rapid injection could be dangerous.**

- After injecting the medication, flush the tubing with 3 mL to 5 mL of flush solution with the first 1 mL of flush administered at the same rate as the medication was given. **Rationale: To ensure that all of the medication is administered safely.** Release the clamp or tubing and re-establish the flow of the existing line at the prescribed rate.

9. Dispose of syringes according to agency practice—needles are placed uncapped into the sharps container. **Rationale: This reduces needlestick injuries and the spread of microorganisms.**

10. Remove and discard gloves. Perform hand hygiene.

11. Observe the client closely for adverse reactions.

12. Determine agency practice about recommended times for changing the IV lock. Some agencies advocate a change every 48 to 72 hours for peripheral IV devices.

13. Document all relevant information.
    - Record the date, time, drug, dose, and route; client response; and assessments of infusion or heparin lock site, if appropriate.

EVALUATION

- Conduct appropriate follow-up, such as desired effect of medication, any adverse reactions or side effects, or change in vital signs.
- Reassess the status of IV lock site and patency of the IV infusion, if running.
- Relate to previous findings, if available.
- Report significant deviations from normal to the appropriate members of the health care team.

HOME CARE CONSIDERATIONS

Administering IV Antibiotics

Shortened hospital stays and improved ambulatory services have led to the need for clients or their caregivers to learn how to administer IV antibiotics at home, such as by continuous ambulatory drug delivery (CADD) pump mechanisms or by positive pressure elastomeric technologies (e.g., Intermate infusion pump). These clients generally have an indwelling peripheral venous catheter or a central venous access device, such as a peripherally inserted central catheter (PICC) (see Chapter 44). The venous access device must be flushed before and after administration to maintain patency to ensure that no drug–drug interaction occurs within the tubing and to administer the complete prescribed dosage.

The nurse must do the following:

- Assess the caregiver or client's eyesight, manual dexterity, and general ability to use the technology, and ability to monitor the response to the medication delivery. All are needed for safe administration of the antibiotic.

- Provide thorough teaching about the following: care of the venous access device, administration rate (minutes/dose), schedule for medication administration, flushing technique, adverse reactions, signs that indicate an emergency and how to proceed, and proper storage of medications

---

See the Home Care Considerations box on administering IV antibiotics.

INTERMITTENT INFUSION DEVICES Intermittent infusion devices (see **5**, Skill 33.9) may be attached to an intravenous catheter or needle to allow medications to be administered intravenously without requiring a continuous intravenous infusion. The device may also have a port at one end of the lock and a needleless injection cap at the other end with the extension tubing between the two ends (see **6**, Skill 33.9). Intermittent injection ports have either a resealable latex injection site for needle access or a port that allows a syringe or a needleless adapter to be connected for administering medications. Needleless systems are preferred because they significantly reduce the risk of needlestick injuries among health care workers. Skill 44.5 (see Chapter 44, page 1461) describes how to convert an intravenous infusion to an intermittent injection port. With the needleless system, the injection adapter may be attached at the time of intravenous catheter placement, allowing a closed system to be maintained.

Intermittent injection ports may be flushed with sterile saline before and after medication administration. Most agencies use saline flushes with medication administration through peripheral IV lines. When administering a medication through a central venous access device (CVAD), some agencies use the SASH (saline, administer drug, saline, heparin) flushing procedure. Flushing the port maintains patency of the intravenous catheter and port, and reduces the risks of mixing incompatible medications within the system (see Skill 33.10).

Clients who require long-term venous access for administering medications, such as cancer chemotherapy, may have a specialized catheter or port to allow central venous access (see the Reflect on Primary Health Care box). The catheter may be tunnelled subcutaneously and accessed through an intermittent injection port attached to the distal end of the venous catheter. Other devices have an *implantable port* or *vascular access port* surgically inserted under the skin so that no portion of the device exits the body. To administer medications,

the port is accessed by using a specialized needle through the skin. Nurses administering medications through central lines must consult the detailed policies and procedures provided by the clinical agency, as these can vary significantly. See Chapter 44 for more information on central venous lines.

Topical Medications

A topical medication is applied locally to the skin or to mucous membranes in such areas as the eye, external ear canal, nose, vagina, and rectum. Most topical applications used therapeutically are not absorbed well, completely, or predictably when applied to intact skin because the skin's thick outer layer serves as a natural barrier to drug diffusion. This **percutaneous** (through the skin) route of absorption can be increased if the skin is altered by a laceration, burn, or some other problem. However, if high concentrations or large amounts of a topical medication are applied to skin, especially if it is done repeatedly, sufficient amounts of the drug can enter the bloodstream to cause systemic effects, often undesirable ones.

One type of topical medication delivery system is the **transdermal patch**. This system administers sustained-action medications (e.g., nitroglycerin, nicotine) via multilayered films containing the drug and an adhesive layer. The rate of delivery of the drug is controlled and varies with each product (e.g., from 12 hours to 1 week). Generally, the patch is applied to a hairless, clean area of skin that is not subject to excessive movement or wrinkling (e.g., the trunk or lower abdomen) (Figure 33.42). It may also be applied on the side, lower back, or buttocks. Patches should not be applied to areas with cuts, burns, or abrasions, or on distal parts of extremities (e.g., the forearms). Women who use a patch containing estrogen or nicotine should not apply the patch to the breasts. If hair is likely to interfere with patch adhesion or removal, clipping (not shaving) may be necessary before application. See the Clinical Alert box on wearing gloves when applying a transdermal patch (on the next page).

REFLECT ON 🔑 **PRIMARY HEALTH CARE**

Medication delivery systems, such as the continuous ambulatory drug delivery (CADD) pump and Intermate positive pressure system, allow clients who would otherwise require hospitalization to remain in their homes as they receive intravenous therapy. Find out if this form of *technology* is accessible in your institution or community. If it is, find out how accessible care is for the home care client who has problems with his or her medication delivery system.

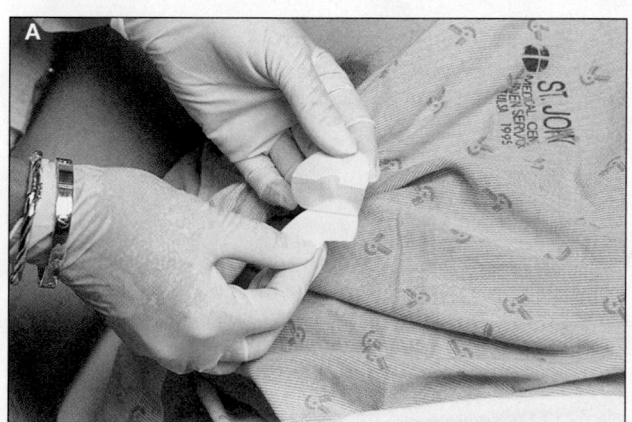
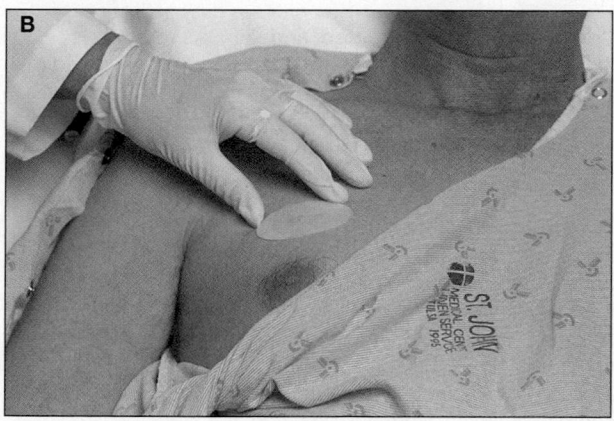

FIGURE 33.42 Transdermal patch administration: **A:** Protective coating removed from patch; **B:** Patch immediately applied to clean, dry, hairless skin and labelled with date, time, and initials

Reddening of skin with or without mild local itching or burning, as well as allergic contact dermatitis, may occasionally occur. Upon removal of the patch, any slight reddening of skin usually disappears within a few hours. All applications should be changed regularly to prevent local irritation, and each successive application should be placed on a different site.

The transdermal patch should be dated, timed, and initialled by the nurse before it is applied to the client. All clients need to be assessed for allergies to the drug and to materials in the patch before the patch is applied. If a client has a transdermal patch on and develops a fever, the medication may be absorbed and metabolize at a faster rate than normal. The client will need to be monitored for changes in effects of the medication.

When transdermal patches are removed, care needs to be taken as to how and where they are discarded. In the home environment, if they are simply discarded into a trash can, pets or children can be exposed to them, causing effects from any drug remaining on the patch. When removed, they should be folded with the medication side to the inside, put into a closed container, and kept out of reach of children and pets.

Skin Applications

Topical skin or dermatological preparations include ointments, pastes, creams, lotions, powders, sprays, and patches. See Table 33.1 (page 873) earlier in this chapter. See the Practice Guidelines 33.4 for applying topical medications. Before applying a dermatological preparation, thoroughly clean the area with soap and water, and dry the area by using a patting motion. Skin encrustations harbour microorganisms, and these as well as previously applied applications can prevent the medication from coming in contact with the area to be treated. Nurses should wear gloves when administering skin applications and always use surgical asepsis when an open wound is present.

Ophthalmic Instillations

Medications may be administered to the eyes by using irrigations or instillations. An eye irrigation is administered to wash out the conjunctival sac to remove

PRACTICE GUIDELINES 33.4

Applying Skin Preparations

Guidelines	Rationales
Powder Make sure the skin surface is dry. Spread apart any skinfolds, and sprinkle the site until the area is covered with a fine, thin layer of powder. Cover the site with a dressing, if ordered.	Applying powder to a damp or moist area gives rise to clumping; powder can be easily brushed off if not protected.
Suspension-Based Lotion Shake the container before use. Put a small amount of lotion on a small gauze dressing or pad, and apply the lotion to skin by stroking it evenly in the direction of the hair growth.	Shaking distributes suspended particles; using a gauze or pad will avoid hand absorption.
Creams, Ointments, Pastes, and Oil-Based Lotions Warm and soften the preparation in gloved hands. Spread it evenly over skin by using long strokes that follow the direction of the hair growth. Explain that skin may feel somewhat greasy after application. Apply a sterile dressing, if ordered by the prescribing health care professional.	Warming the preparation makes it easier to apply and to prevent chilling (if a large area is to be treated).
Transdermal Patches Ensure that all previous patches have been removed. Select a clean, dry area that is free of hair and matches the manufacturer's recommendations. Remove the patch from its protective covering, holding it without touching the adhesive edges, and apply it by pressing firmly with the palm of the hand for about 10 seconds. Advise the client to avoid using a heating pad over the area. Remove the patch at the appropriate time, folding the medicated side to the inside so that it is covered.	The presence of multiple patches leads to increased dosage of medication than that prescribed. The hand provides heat that can cause an increase in circulation and the rate of absorption. The effects of the medication are time limited; folding the patch will ensure that no one is exposed to the topical medication.

secretions or foreign bodies or to remove chemicals that may injure the eye. **Ophthalmic** medications, that is, medications for the eyes, are instilled in the form of liquids or ointments. Eye drops are packaged in monodrip plastic containers that are used to administer the preparation. Ointments are usually supplied in small tubes. All containers must indicate that the medication is for ophthalmic use. Sterile preparations and sterile technique are indicated. Prescribed liquids are usually diluted, for example, less than 1% strength. Skill 33.11 illustrates the method to administer ophthalmic instillations.

SKILL 33.11 ADMINISTERING OPHTHALMIC INSTILLATIONS

PURPOSE

To provide an eye medication the client requires (e.g., an antibiotic) to treat an infection or for other reasons (see specific drug action)

ASSESSMENT

In addition to the assessment performed by the nurse related to the administration of any medication, before applying ophthalmic medications, assess the following:

- Appearance of eye and surrounding structures for lesions, exudate, erythema, or swelling
- The location and nature of any discharge, lacrimation, and swelling of the eyelids or of the lacrimal gland
- Client complaints (e.g., itching, burning pain, blurred vision, or photophobia)
- Client behaviour (e.g., squinting, blinking excessively, frowning, or rubbing the eyes)

Determine if assessment data influence administration of the medication (i.e., whether it is appropriate to administer the medication or if the medication needs to be held and the appropriate member of the health care team notified).

PLANNING

Equipment

- Client's MAR or computer printout
- Clean gloves
- Sterile absorbent sponges soaked in sterile normal saline
- Prescribed medication
- Dry sterile absorbent sponges
- Sterile eye dressing (pad) as needed and paper eye tape to secure it

For an irrigation, add the following:

- Irrigating solution (e.g., normal saline) and irrigating syringe or tubing
- Dry sterile absorbent sponges
- Moisture-resistant towel
- Basin (e.g., emesis basin)

IMPLEMENTATION

Preparation

1. Check the MAR.
   - Check the MAR for the drug name, dose, and strength. Also confirm the prescribed frequency of the instillation and which eye is to be treated.
   - Check the client's allergy status.
   - If the MAR is unclear or pertinent information is missing, compare it with the most recent written order by the primary care provider.
   - Report any discrepancies to the appropriate member of the health care team, as agency policy dictates.
2. Know the reason the client is receiving the medication, the drug classification, contraindications, usual dose range, adverse effects, and nursing considerations for administering and evaluating the intended outcomes of the medication.

Performance

1. Compare the label on the medication tube or bottle with the medication record and check the expiration date.
2. If necessary, calculate the medication dosage.
3. Introduce yourself, and explain to the client what you are going to do, why it is necessary, and how the client can participate. The administration of an ophthalmic medication is not usually painful. Ointments are often soothing to the eye, but some liquid preparations may sting initially. Discuss how the results will be used in planning further care or treatments.
4. Perform hand hygiene, and follow other appropriate infection prevention and control procedures.
5. Provide for client privacy.
6. Prepare the client.
   - Prior to performing the procedure, verify the client's identity using two identifiers or per agency protocol. **Rationale: This ensures that the right client receives the right medication.**
   - Assist the client to a comfortable position, either to the sitting or the lying position.
7. Clean the eyelid and the eyelashes.
   - Put on clean gloves.
   - Use sterile cotton balls moistened with sterile irrigating solution or sterile normal saline, and wipe from the inner canthus to the outer canthus. **Rationale: If not removed, material on the eyelid and lashes can be washed into the eye. Cleaning toward the outer canthus prevents contamination of the other eye and the lacrimal duct.**
8. Administer the eye medication.
   - Check the ophthalmic preparation for the name, strength, and number of drops if a liquid is used. **Rationale: Checking medication data is essential to prevent a medication error.**
   - Draw the correct number of drops into the shaft of the dropper if a dropper is used. If ointment is used, discard the first bead. **Rationale: The first bead of ointment from a tube is considered contaminated.**

(continued)

SKILL 33.11   ADMINISTERING OPHTHALMIC INSTILLATIONS (*continued*)

- Instruct the client to look up to the ceiling. Give the client a dry sterile absorbent sponge. **Rationale: The person is less likely to blink if looking up. While the client looks up, the cornea is partially protected by the upper eyelid. A sponge is needed to press on the nasolacrimal duct after a liquid instillation to prevent systemic absorption or to wipe excess ointment from the eyelashes after an ointment is instilled.**

- Expose the lower conjunctival sac by placing the thumb or fingers of your nondominant hand on the client's cheekbone just below the eye and gently drawing down the skin on the cheek. If the tissues are edematous, handle the tissues carefully to avoid damaging them. **Rationale: Placing the fingers on the client's cheekbone minimizes the possibility of touching the cornea, avoids putting any pressure on the eyeball, and prevents the person from blinking or squinting.**

- Holding the medication in the dominant hand, place your hand on the client's forehead to stabilize the client's head and your hand. Approach the eye from the side, and instill the correct number of drops onto the outer third of the lower conjunctival sac. Hold the dropper 1 cm to 2 cm above the sac (see ❶). **Rationale: The client is less likely to blink if a side approach is used. When instilled into the conjunctival sac, drops will not harm the cornea, as they might if dropped directly on it. The dropper must not touch the sac or the cornea.**

Or

- Holding the tube above the lower conjunctival sac, squeeze 2 cm of ointment from the tube into the lower conjunctival sac from the inner canthus outward (see ❷).

- Instruct the client to close the eyelids but not to squeeze them shut. **Rationale: Closing the eye spreads the medication over the eyeball. Squeezing can injure the eye and push out the medication.**

- For liquid medications, press firmly, or have the client press firmly on the nasolacrimal duct for at least 30 seconds (see ❸). **Rationale: Pressing on the nasolacrimal duct prevents the medication from running out of the eye and down the duct, preventing systemic absorption.**

Variation: Irrigation

- Place absorbent pads under the head, neck, and shoulders. Place an emesis basin next to the eye to catch any drainage. Some eye medications cause systemic reactions, such as confusion or a decrease in heart rate and blood pressure, if the eye drops go down the nasolacrimal duct and get into the systemic circulation.

- Expose the lower conjunctival sac. To irrigate in stages, first hold the lower lid down, and then hold the upper lid up. Exert pressure on the bony prominences of the cheekbone and beneath the eyebrow when holding the eyelids. **Rationale: Separating the lids prevents reflex blinking. Exerting pressure on the bony prominences minimizes the possibility of pressing the eyeball and causing discomfort.**

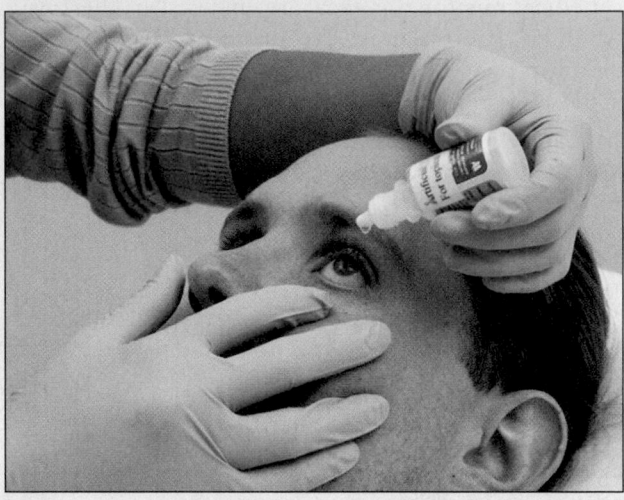

❶ Instilling an eye drop into the lower conjunctival sac

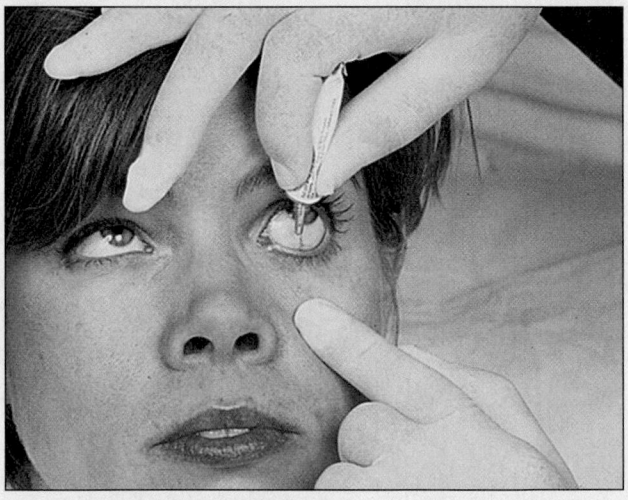

❷ Instilling an eye ointment into the lower conjunctival sac

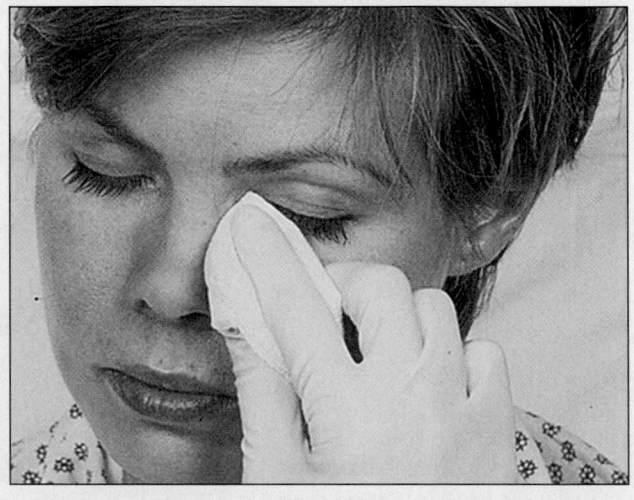

❸ Pressing on the nasolacrimal duct

- Fill and hold the eye irrigator about 2.5 cm above the eye. **Rationale: At this height, the pressure of the solution will not damage the eye tissue, and the irrigator will not touch the eye**.
- Irrigate the eye, directing the solution onto the lower conjunctival sac and from the inner canthus to the outer canthus (see Figure 33.43). **Rationale: Directing the solution this way prevents possible injury to the cornea and prevents fluid and contaminants from flowing down the nasolacrimal duct**.
- Irrigate until the solution leaving the eye is clear (no discharge is present) or until all the solution has been used.
- Instruct the client to close and move the eye periodically. **Rationale: Eye closure and movement help move secretions from the upper conjunctival sac to the lower conjunctival sac**.

9. Clean and dry the eyelids, as needed. Wipe the eyelids gently from the inner canthus to the outer canthus to collect excess medication.

10. Remove and discard gloves. Perform hand hygiene.

11. Apply an eye pad, if needed, and secure it with paper eye tape.

12. Assess the client's response immediately after the instillation or irrigation and again after the medication should have acted.

13. Document all relevant assessments and interventions. Include the name of the drug or irrigating solution, the strength, the number of drops if a liquid medication, the time, and the response of the client.

EVALUATION

- Perform follow-up based on findings of the effectiveness of the administration or outcomes that deviated from expected or normal for the client. Relate findings to previous data, if available.
- Report significant deviations from normal to the appropriate members of the health care team.

LIFESPAN CONSIDERATIONS

Administering Ophthalmic Medications

INFANTS AND CHILDREN

- Explain the technique to the parents of an infant or a child.
- For a young child or an infant, obtain assistance to immobilize the arms and head. The parent may hold the infant or young child. **Rationale: This prevents accidental injury during medication administration**.
- For a young child, use a doll to demonstrate the procedure. **Rationale: This facilitates cooperation and decreases anxiety**.

- Drops may be tolerated better by children than ointment, since drops are less likely to cause blurred vision.
- An IV bag and tubing may be used to deliver irrigating fluid to the eye (Figure 33.43).

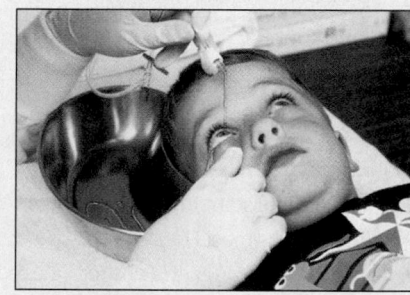

FIGURE 33.43 Eye irrigation by using IV tubing.

See the Lifespan Considerations box on administering ophthalmic medications.

Otic Instillations

Instillations or irrigations of the external auditory canal are referred to as **otic instillations** and are generally carried out for cleaning purposes. Sometimes, applications of heat and antiseptic solutions are prescribed. Irrigations performed in a hospital require aseptic technique so that microorganisms are not introduced into the ear. Sterile technique is used if the eardrum is perforated. The position of the external auditory canal varies with age. In the child younger than 3 years, it is directed upward. In the

adult, the external auditory canal is an S-shaped structure about 2.5 cm long. Skill 33.12 on the next page explains the technique used to administer otic instillations.

See the Lifespan Considerations box on administering otic medications on page 942.

Nasal Instillations

Nasal instillations (nose drops and sprays) usually are instilled for their astringent effect (to shrink swollen mucous membranes), to loosen secretions and facilitate drainage, or to treat infections of the nasal cavity or sinuses. Nasal decongestants are the most common nasal instillations. Many of these products are available without a

SKILL 33.12 ADMINISTERING OTIC INSTILLATIONS

PURPOSE

- To soften cerumen (earwax) so that it can be readily removed at a later time
- To provide local therapy to reduce inflammation, destroy infective organisms in the external ear canal, or both
- To relieve pain

ASSESSMENT

In addition to the assessment performed by the nurse related to the administration of any medications, before applying otic medications, assess the following:

- Appearance of the pinna of the ear and meatus for signs of redness and abrasions
- Type and amount of any discharge

Determine whether assessment data influence administration of the medication (i.e., whether it is appropriate to administer the medication or if the medication needs to be held and the appropriate member of the health care team notified).

PLANNING

Equipment

- Client's MAR or computer printout
- Clean gloves
- Cotton-tipped applicator
- Correct medication bottle with a dropper
- Flexible rubber tip (optional) for the end of the dropper, which prevents injury from sudden motion, for example, by disoriented client
- Cotton fluff

For irrigation, add the following:

- Moisture-resistant towel
- Basin (e.g., emesis basin)
- Irrigating solution at the appropriate temperature, about 500 mL or as ordered
- Container for the irrigating solution
- Syringe (rubber bulb or Asepto syringe is frequently used)

IMPLEMENTATION

Preparation

1. Check the MAR.
   - Check the MAR for the drug name, strength, number of drops, and prescribed frequency.
   - Check the client's allergy status
   - If the MAR is unclear or pertinent information is missing, compare it with the most recent written order.
   - Report any discrepancies to the appropriate member of the health care team, as agency policy dictates.
2. Know the reason the client is receiving the medication, the drug classification, contraindications, usual dose range, adverse effects, and nursing considerations for administering and evaluating the intended outcomes of the medication.

Performance

1. Compare the label on the medication container with the medication record, and check the expiration date.
2. If necessary, calculate the medication dosage.
3. Explain to the client what you are going to do, why it is necessary, and how the client can participate. The administration of an otic medication is not usually painful. Discuss how the results will be used in planning further care or treatments.
4. Perform hand hygiene, and follow other appropriate infection prevention and control procedures.
5. Provide for client privacy.
6. Prepare the client.
   - Prior to performing the procedure, introduce yourself and verify the client's identity using two identifiers or per agency protocol.
   - Assist the client to a comfortable position for eardrops, in the lying position, with the ear being treated uppermost.
7. Clean the pinna of the ear and the meatus of the ear canal.
   - Put on gloves if infection is suspected.
   - Use cotton-tipped applicators and solution to wipe the pinna and auditory meatus. **Rationale: This removes any discharge present before the instillation so that it will not be washed into the ear canal**.
   - Ensure that the applicator does not go into the ear canal. **Rationale: This avoids damage to the tympanic membrane or wax becoming impacted within the canal**.
8. Administer the ear medication.
   - Warm the medication container in your hand, or place it in warm water for a short time. **Rationale: This promotes client comfort and prevents nerve stimulation and pain**.
   - Partially fill the ear dropper with medication.
   - Straighten the ear canal by pulling the pinna upward and backward for clients older than 3 years of age, and instill the correct number of drops along the side of the ear canal (see ❶). **Rationale: The auditory canal is straightened so that the solution can flow the entire length of the canal**.

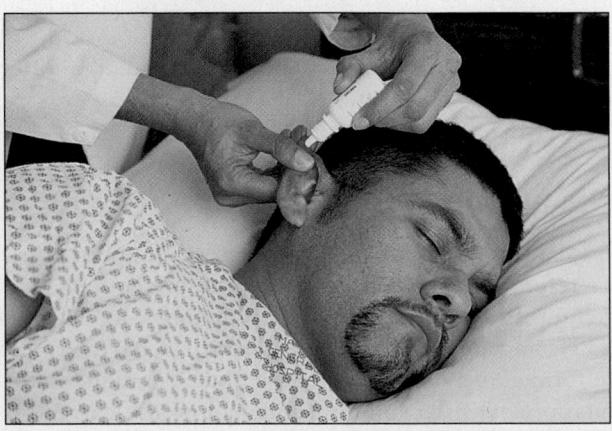

❶ Instilling ear drops while straightening the adult's ear canal by pulling the pinna upward and backward

- Press gently but firmly a few times on the tragus of the ear (the cartilaginous projection in front of the exterior meatus of the ear). **Rationale: Pressing on the tragus assists the flow of medication into the ear canal**.
- Ask the client to remain in the side-lying position for about 5 minutes. **Rationale: This prevents the drops from escaping and allows the medication to reach all sides of the canal cavity**.
- Insert a small piece of cotton fluff loosely at the meatus of the auditory canal for 15 to 20 minutes. Do not press it into the canal. **Rationale: The cotton helps retain the medication when the client is up. If pressed tightly into the canal, the cotton would interfere with the action of the drug and the outward movement of normal secretions**.

Variation: Ear Irrigation

- Explain that the client may experience a feeling of fullness, warmth, and, occasionally, discomfort when the fluid comes in contact with the tympanic membrane.
- Assist the client to the sitting or lying position, with head tilted toward the affected ear (see ❷). **Rationale: The solution can then flow from the ear canal to a basin**.
- Place the moisture-resistant towel around the client's shoulder under the ear to be irrigated, and place the basin under the ear to be irrigated.
- Fill the syringe with solution.

Or

- Hang up the irrigating container, and run solution through the tubing and the nozzle. **Rationale: Solution is run through to remove air from the tubing and nozzle**.
- Straighten the ear canal.
- Insert the tip of the syringe into the auditory meatus, and direct the solution gently upward against the top of the canal. **Rationale: The solution will flow around the entire canal and out at the bottom. The solution is instilled gently because strong pressure from the fluid can cause discomfort and damage the tympanic membranes**.
- Continue instilling the fluid until all the solution is used or until the canal is cleaned, depending on the purpose of the irrigation. Take care not to block the outward flow of the solution with the syringe.

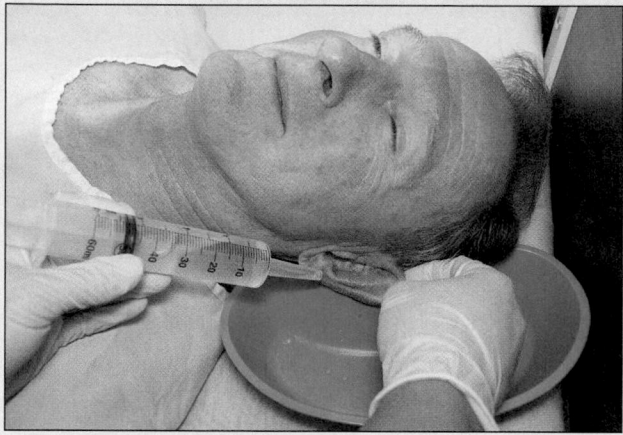

❷ Ear irrigation

- Assist the client to the side-lying position on the affected side. **Rationale: Lying with the affected side down helps drain the excess fluid by gravity**.
- Place a cotton fluff in the auditory meatus to absorb the excess fluid.

10. Remove and discard gloves. Perform hand hygiene.
11. Assess the client's response and the character and amount of discharge, appearance of the canal, and discomfort, immediately after the instillation and again when the medication is expected to act. Inspect the cotton fluff for any drainage.
12. Document all nursing assessments and interventions relative to the procedure. Include the name of the drug or irrigating solution, the strength, the number of drops if a liquid medication, the time, and the response of the client.

EVALUATION

- Perform follow-up based on findings of the effectiveness of the administration or outcomes that deviated from expected or normal for the client. Relate findings to previous data, if available.
- Report significant deviations from normal to the appropriate members of the health care team.

prescription. Clients need to be taught to use these agents with caution. Chronic use of nasal decongestants can lead to a rebound effect, that is, an increase in nasal congestion. If excessive decongestant solution is swallowed, systemic effects may also develop, especially in children. Saline drops are safer as a decongestant for children.

Often, clients self-administer nasal sprays. People should blow their noses prior to administration of nasal sprays, unless contraindicated. In the seated position with the head tilted back, the client holds the tip of the container just inside the nares and inhales as the spray enters the nasal passages. For clients who use nasal sprays repeatedly, the nares need to be assessed for irritation.

In children, nasal sprays are given with the head in an upright position to prevent excess spray from being swallowed.

Nasal drops may be used to treat sinus infections. Clients need to learn ways to position themselves to effectively treat the affected sinus:

- To treat the ethmoid and sphenoid sinuses, instruct the client to assume the back-lying position, with the head turned toward the side to be treated lie back with the head over the edge of the bed or a pillow under the shoulders so that the head is tipped backward (Figure 33.45 on the next page).

LIFESPAN CONSIDERATIONS

Administering Otic Medications

INFANTS AND CHILDREN

- Obtain assistance to immobilize an infant or a young child to prevent accidental injury caused by sudden movement during the procedure.

- Because in infants and children younger than 3 years the ear canal is directed upward, to administer medication, gently pull the pinna down and back (Figure 33.44). For a child *older* than 3 years, pull the pinna upward and backward.

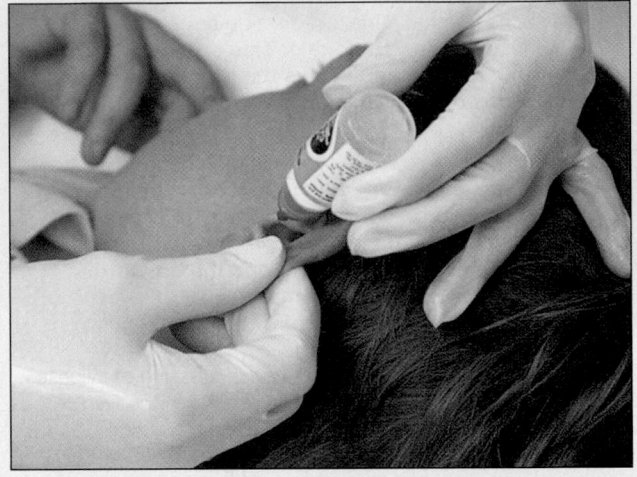

FIGURE 33.44 Straightening the ear canal of a child by pulling the pinna down and back.

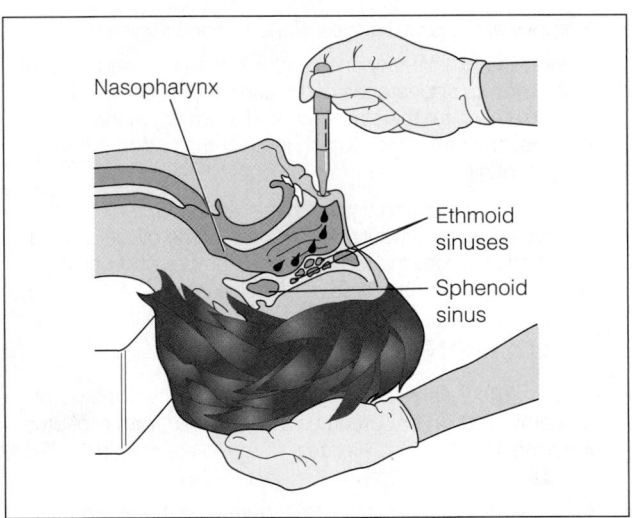

FIGURE 33.45 Position of the head to instill drops into the ethmoid and sphenoid sinuses.

- To treat the maxillary and frontal sinuses, instruct the client to assume the back-lying position, with the head turned toward the side to be treated (Figure 33.46). The client should also be instructed to (a) breathe through the mouth to prevent aspiration of medication into the trachea and bronchi, (b) remain in the back-lying position for at least 1 minute so that the solution will come into contact with the entire nasal surface, and (c) avoid blowing the nose for several minutes.

Vaginal Instillations

Vaginal medications, or instillations, are inserted as creams, jellies, foams, or suppositories to treat infection or to relieve vaginal discomfort (e.g., itching or pain).

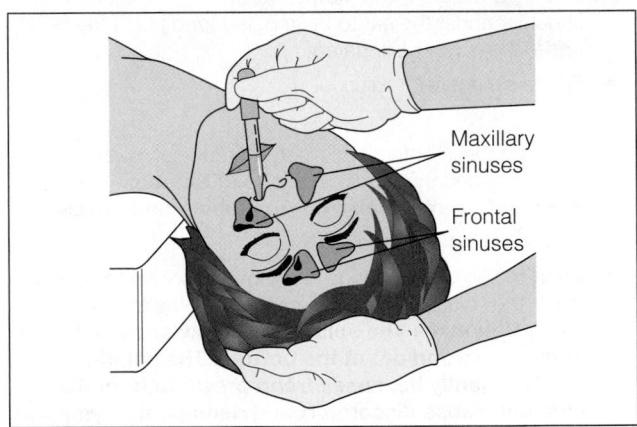

FIGURE 33.46 Position of the head to instill drops into the maxillary and frontal sinuses.

Medical aseptic technique is usually used. Vaginal creams, jellies, and foams are applied by using a tubular applicator with a plunger. Suppositories are inserted with the index finger of a gloved hand. Suppositories are designed to melt at body temperature, so they are generally stored in the refrigerator to keep them firm for insertion. See Skill 33.13 for administering vaginal instillations.

A vaginal irrigation (douche) is the washing of the vagina with a liquid at a low pressure. Vaginal irrigations are not necessary for ordinary female hygiene but are used to prevent infection by applying an antimicrobial solution that discourages the growth of microorganisms, to remove an offensive or irritating discharge, and to reduce inflammation or prevent hemorrhage by the application of heat or cold. In hospitals, sterile supplies and equipment are used; in a home, sterility is not usually necessary because people are accustomed to the microorganisms in their environments. Sterile technique, however, is indicated if there is an open wound.

SKILL 33.13 ADMINISTERING VAGINAL INSTILLATIONS

PURPOSE

- To treat or prevent infection
- To reduce inflammation
- To relieve vaginal discomfort

ASSESSMENT

In addition to the assessment performed by the nurse related to the administration of any medications, before applying vaginal medications, assess the following:

- The vaginal orifice for inflammation and the amount, character, and odour of vaginal discharge
- Complaints of vaginal discomfort (e.g., burning or itching)

Determine if assessment data influence administration of the medication (i.e., whether it is appropriate to administer the medication or if the medication needs to be held and the appropriate member of the health care team notified).

PLANNING

Equipment

- Client's MAR or computer printout
- Drape
- Correct vaginal suppository or cream
- Applicator for vaginal cream
- Clean gloves
- Lubricant for a suppository
- Disposable towel
- Clean perineal pad

For an irrigation, add the following:

- Moisture-proof pad
- Vaginal irrigation set (these are often disposable) containing a nozzle, tubing and a clamp, and a container for the solution
- Irrigating solution

IMPLEMENTATION

Preparation

1. Check the MAR.
   - Check the MAR for the drug name, strength, and prescribed frequency.
   - Check the client's allergy status.
   - If the MAR is unclear or pertinent information is missing, compare it with the most recent written order.
   - Report any discrepancies to the appropriate member of the health care team, as agency policy dictates.
2. Know the reason the client is receiving the medication, the drug classification, contraindications, usual dose range, adverse effects, and nursing considerations for administering and evaluating the intended outcomes of the medication.

Performance

1. Compare the label on the medication container with the medication record, and check the expiration date.
2. If necessary, calculate the medication dosage.

3. Explain to the client what you are going to do, why it is necessary, and how she can participate. Explain to the client that a vaginal instillation is normally a painless procedure and, in fact, may bring relief from itching and burning if an infection is present. Many people feel embarrassed about this procedure, and some may prefer to perform the procedure themselves if instruction is provided. Discuss how the results will be used in planning further care or treatments.
4. Perform hand hygiene, and follow other appropriate infection prevention and control procedures.
5. Provide for client privacy.
6. Prepare the client.
   - Prior to performing the procedure, introduce yourself and verify the client's identity using two identifiers or per agency protocol.
   - Ask the client to void. **Rationale: If the bladder is empty, the client will experience less discomfort during the treatment, and the possibility of injuring the vaginal lining is decreased**.
   - Assist the client to the back-lying position with her knees flexed and the hips rotated laterally.
   - Drape the client appropriately so that only the perineal area is exposed.
7. Prepare the equipment.

   Unwrap the suppository, and put it on the opened wrapper.

   Or

   Fill the applicator with the prescribed cream, jelly, or foam. Directions are provided with the manufacturer's applicator.
8. Assess and clean the perineal area.
   - Put on gloves. **Rationale: Gloves prevent contamination of the nurse's hands from vaginal and perineal microorganisms**.
   - Inspect the vaginal orifice, note any odour of discharge from the vagina, and ask about any vaginal discomfort.
   - Provide perineal care to remove microorganisms. **Rationale: This decreases the chances of microorganisms moving into the vagina**.
9. Administer the vaginal suppository, cream, foam, jelly, or irrigation.

Suppository

- Lubricate the rounded (smooth) end of the suppository, which is inserted first. **Rationale: Lubrication facilitates insertion**.
- Lubricate your gloved index finger.
- Expose the vaginal orifice by separating the labia with your nondominant hand.
- Insert the suppository about 8 cm to 10 cm along the posterior wall of the vagina, or as far as it will go (see ❶). **Rationale: The posterior wall of the vagina is about 2.5 cm longer than the anterior wall because the cervix protrudes into the uppermost portion of the anterior wall**.
- Ask the client to remain lying in the supine position for 5 to 10 minutes following insertion. The hips may also be elevated on a pillow. **Rationale: This position allows the medication to flow into the posterior fornix after the suppository has dissolved**.

(continued)

SKILL 33.13 **ADMINISTERING VAGINAL INSTILLATIONS** (*continued*)

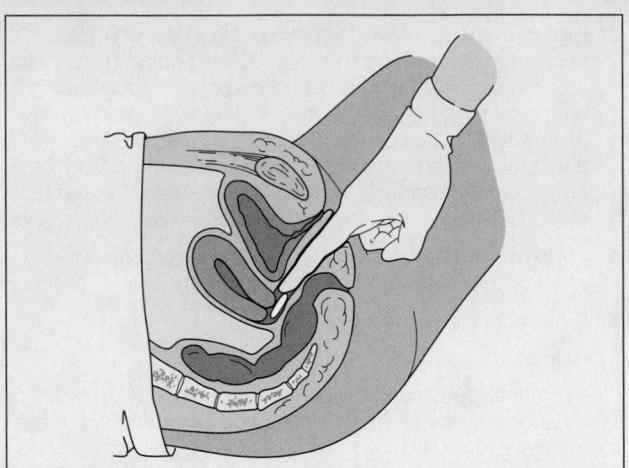

❶ Instilling a vaginal suppository

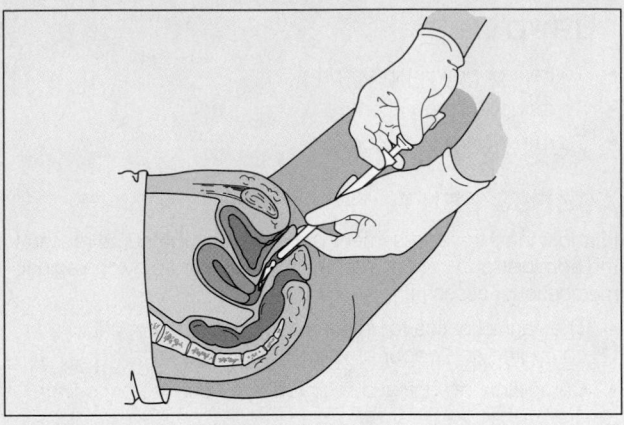

❷ Using an applicator to instill a vaginal cream

Vaginal Cream, Jelly, or Foam

- Gently insert the applicator about 5 cm.
- Slowly push the plunger until the applicator is empty (see ❷).
- Remove the applicator and place it on the towel. **Rationale: The applicator is put on the towel to prevent the spread of microorganisms**.
- Discard the applicator, if disposable, or clean it according to the manufacturer's directions.
- Ask the client to remain lying in the supine position for 5 to 10 minutes following the insertion.

Irrigation

- Place the client on a bedpan.
- Clamp the tubing. Hold the irrigating container about 30 cm above the vagina. **Rationale: At this height, the pressure of the solution should not be great enough to injure the vaginal lining**.
- Run fluid through the tubing and nozzle into the bedpan. **Rationale: Fluid is run through the tubing to remove air and to moisten the nozzle**.
- Insert the nozzle carefully into the vagina. Direct the nozzle toward the sacrum, following the direction of the vagina.
- Insert the nozzle about 7 cm to 10 cm, start the flow, and rotate the nozzle several times. **Rationale: Rotating the nozzle irrigates all parts of the vagina**.

- Use all of the irrigating solution, permitting it to flow out freely into the bedpan.
- Remove the nozzle from the vagina.
- Assist the client to the sitting position on the bedpan. **Rationale: Sitting on the bedpan will help drain the remaining fluid by gravity**.

10. Ensure client comfort.

   - Dry the perineum with tissues, as required.
   - Apply a clean perineal pad if there is excessive drainage.

11. Remove and discard gloves. Perform hand hygiene.

12. Document all nursing assessments and interventions relative to the procedure. Include the name of the drug or irrigating solution, the strength, the time, and the response of the client.

EVALUATION

- Perform follow-up based on findings of the effectiveness of the administration or outcomes that deviated from expected or normal for the client. Relate findings to previous data, if available.
- Report significant deviations from normal to the appropriate members of the health care team.

Rectal Medications

The insertion of medications into the rectum in the form of suppositories is a frequent practice. Rectal administration is a convenient and safe method of giving certain medications. Advantages include the following:

- It avoids irritation of the upper gastrointestinal tract in clients who encounter this problem (e.g., in clients who are nauseated or vomiting).
- It is advantageous when the medication has an objectionable taste or odour.

- The drug is released at a slow but steady rate.
- Rectal suppositories are thought to provide higher levels of medication in the bloodstream (titres) because the venous blood from the lower rectum is not transported through the liver.

   To insert a rectal suppository, do the following:

- Assist the client to a left lateral or left Sims' position, with the upper leg flexed.
- Fold back the top bedclothes to expose the buttocks.

- Put a glove on the hand that will be used to insert the suppository.

- Unwrap the suppository and lubricate the smooth rounded end, or check the manufacturer's instructions. The rounded end is usually inserted first and the lubricant reduces irritation of the mucosa.

- Lubricate the gloved index finger.

- Encourage the client to relax by breathing through the mouth. This usually relaxes the external anal sphincter.

- Insert the suppository gently into the anal canal, rounded end first (or according to manufacturer's instructions), along the rectal wall using the gloved index finger. For an adult, insert the suppository beyond the internal sphincter (approximately 10 cm) (Figure 33.47).

- Avoid embedding the suppository in feces, as this would prevent the suppository from being absorbed effectively.

- Press the client's buttocks together for a few minutes.

- Ask the client to remain in the left lateral or supine position for at least 5 minutes to help retain the suppository. The suppository should be retained for varying lengths of time, according to manufacturer's instructions.

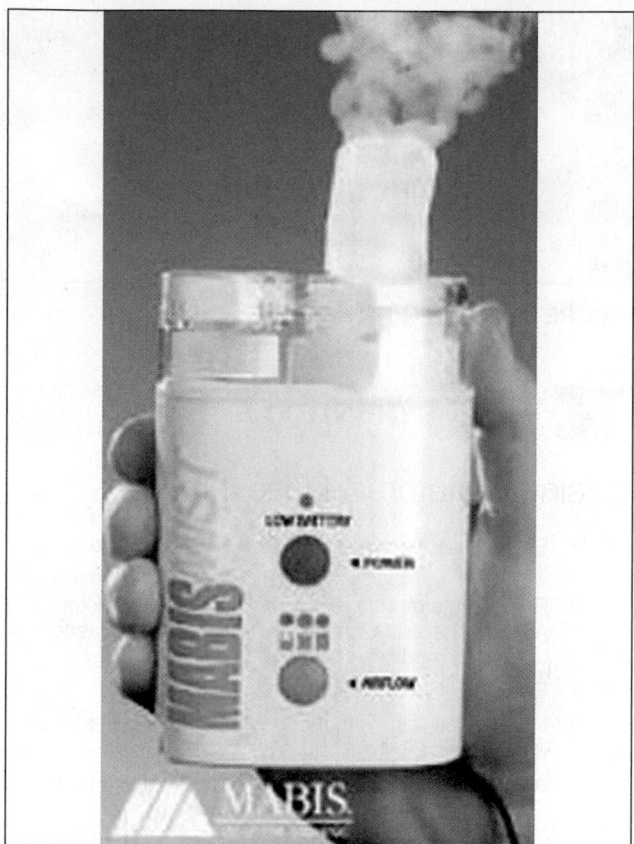

FIGURE 33.48 Ultrasonic nebulizer.

Inhaled Medications

Nebulizers deliver most medications administered through the inhaled route. A nebulizer is used to deliver a fine spray (fog or mist) of medication or moisture to a client. There are two kinds of nebulization: *atomization* and *aerosolization*. In atomization, a device called an *atomizer* produces rather large droplets for inhalation. In aerosolization, the droplets are suspended in a gas, such as

oxygen or compressed air. The smaller the droplets, the further they can be inhaled into the respiratory tract. When a medication is intended for the nasal mucosa, it is inhaled through the nose; when it is intended for the trachea, bronchi, or lungs, it is inhaled through the mouth. A large-volume nebulizer can provide a heated or cool mist. It is used for long-term therapy, such as that following a tracheostomy. The ultrasonic nebulizer (Figure 33.48) provides 100% humidity and can provide particles small enough to be inhaled deeply into the respiratory tract.

The **metered-dose inhaler (MDI)**, a handheld nebulizer (Figure 33.49), is a pressurized container of medication that can be used by the client to release the medication through a mouthpiece. The force with which the air moves through the nebulizer causes the large particles of medicated solution to break up into finer particles, forming a mist or fine spray. MDIs can deliver accurate doses, provide for target action at the needed sites, and result in fewer systemic effects than medication delivered by other routes.

To ensure correct delivery of the prescribed medication by MDIs, nurses need to instruct clients to use them properly. The client compresses the medication canister by hand to release medication through a mouthpiece. An extender or spacer can be attached to the mouthpiece (see the Aerochamber in Figure 33.49 on the next page)

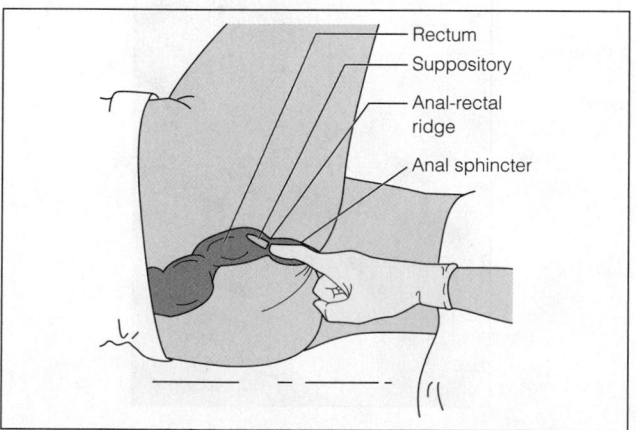

FIGURE 33.47 Inserting a rectal suppository beyond the internal sphincter along the rectal wall.

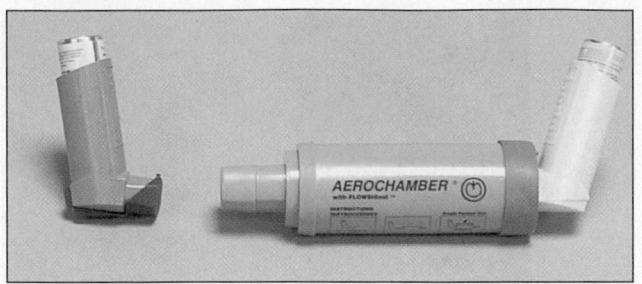

FIGURE 33.49 Metered-dose inhaler.

to facilitate medication absorption. Spacers are holding chambers into which the medication is fired and from which the client inhales so that the dose is not lost by exhalation. The Teaching: Clinical box provides instructions for clients about using an MDI (see also the Home Care Considerations box). Newer breath-activated MDIs are being produced in which inhalation triggers the release of a premeasured dose of medication.

See the Lifespan Considerations box on administering metered-dose inhalers and nebulizers.

TEACHING | **CLINICAL**

Using a Metered-Dose Inhaler

- Ensure that the canister is firmly and fully inserted into the inhaler.
- Remove the mouthpiece cap. Holding the canister upright, shake the inhaler vigorously for 3 to 5 seconds to mix the medication evenly.
- Exhale comfortably (as in a normal full breath).
- Hold the canister with the mouthpiece down, as illustrated in Figure 33.50.
  - **a.** Hold the MDI 2 cm to 4 cm from the open mouth (see Figure 33.50).

Or
  - **b.** Place the mouthpiece far enough into the mouth with its opening toward the throat such that the lips can tightly close around the mouthpiece (Figure 33.51). An MDI with a spacer or extender is always placed in the mouth (Figure 33.52).

ADMINISTERING THE MEDICATION

- Press down *once* on the MDI canister (which releases the dose), and inhale slowly (for 3 to 5 seconds) and deeply through the mouth.
- Hold your breath for 10 seconds or as long as possible. **Rationale: This allows the aerosol to reach deeper airways**.
- Remove the inhaler from or away from the mouth.
- Exhale slowly through *pursed* lips. **Rationale: Controlled exhalation keeps the small airways open during exhalation**.
- Repeat the inhalation if ordered. Wait 20 to 30 seconds between inhalations of bronchodilator medications. **Rationale: The first inhalation has a chance to work and the subsequent dose reaches deeper into the lungs**.

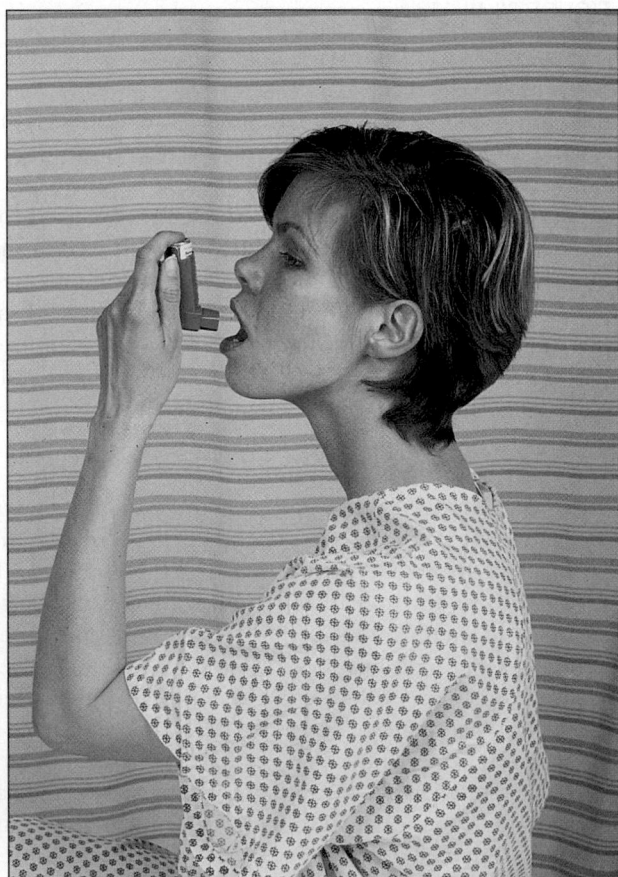

FIGURE 33.50 Inhaler positioned away from the open mouth.

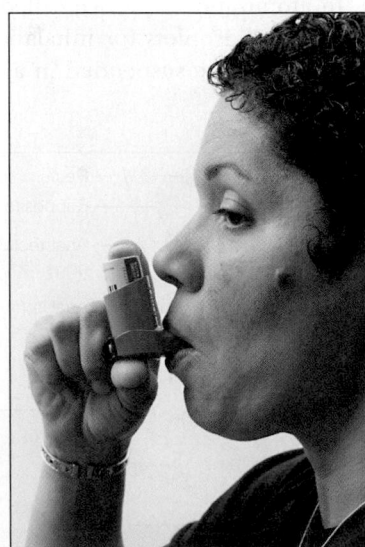

FIGURE 33.51 Placing MDI in mouth with lips sealed around mouthpiece.

- Following use of the inhaler, rinse mouth with tap water to remove any remaining medication and reduce irritation and risk of infection.
- Clean the MDI mouthpiece after each use. Use mild soap and water, rinse it, and let it air dry before replacing it on the device.
- Store the canister at room temperature. Avoid extremes of temperature.
- Report adverse reactions, such as restlessness, palpitations, nervousness, or rash to the appropriate member of the health care team.
- Many MDIs contain steroids for an anti-inflammatory effect. Prolonged use increases the risk of fungal infections in the mouth, indicating a need for attentive mouth care.

If two inhalers are to be used, the bronchodilator medication (which opens the airways) should be given before other medications. A mnemonic to help remember this is *B before C* (i.e., bronchodilator before corticosteroid).

Inhaled steroids may not be correctly used by clients because they do not associate these medications with immediate symptom relief. Bronchodilators act to open the airways in the short term. However, it is the inhaled steroids that act to keep airway inflammation under control.

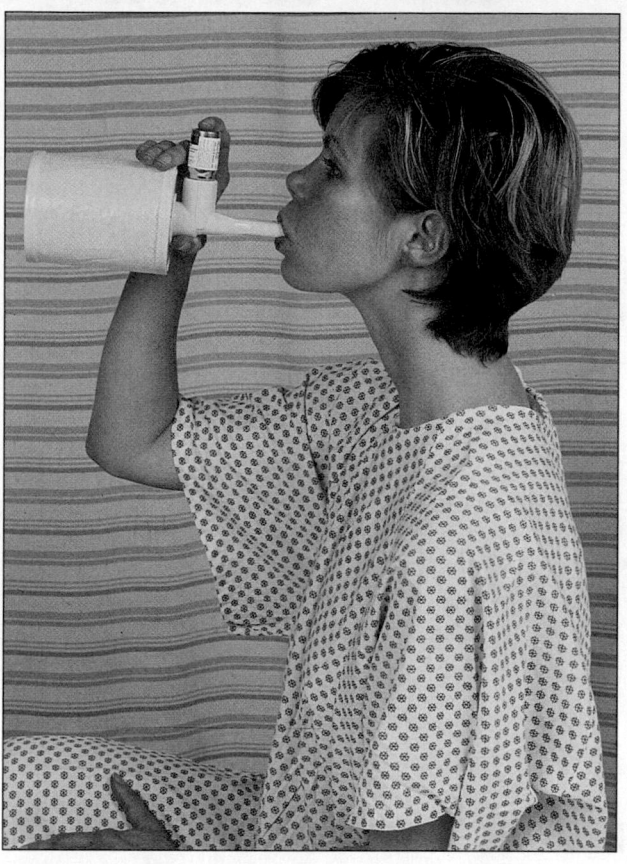

FIGURE 33.52 An extender spacer attached to a mouthpiece placed in the mouth.

HOME CARE CONSIDERATIONS

Metered-Dose Inhalers

- Disinfect the metered-dose inhaler mouthpieces weekly by soaking for 20 minutes in 500 mL of water with 60 mL of vinegar added.
- Teach clients how to determine the amount of medication remaining in a metered-dose inhaler canister:
  - Calculate the number of days' doses in a canister. Divide the number of doses (puffs) in the canister (on the label) by the number of puffs taken per day. Newer inhalers (e.g., Advair) have a dose-counting mechanism. The previous method of floating the canister in water is not considered accurate because some of the propellant may remain (even after the medication is gone), which leads the client to incorrectly believe medication is being received.
- Review instructions and periodically assess the client's techniques for using an inhaler spacer or chamber correctly. These devices assist in delivering the medication deeply into the lungs rather than only to the oropharynx.

LIFESPAN CONSIDERATIONS

Administering Metered-Dose Inhalers and Nebulizers

CHILDREN

- Spacers hold a medication in suspension and provide the child an opportunity to take several deep breaths to inhale all the medication. Children over age 2 years can be taught how to use an MDI effectively.
- A mask is used for nebulizer treatments, allowing the child to breathe normally. Some infants and children may be frightened or uncomfortable with the mask and become resistant. Use a doll or stuffed animal to demonstrate the use of the mask, and allow the child to play with the equipment before putting it in place. Having the child sit in the parent's lap during the procedure can help the child relax and be more cooperative.

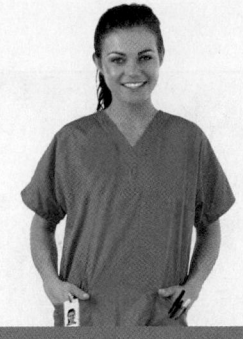

Case Study 33

Mr. Ketron, a 20-year-old client, just returned to the nursing unit from surgery after undergoing an emergency appendectomy. He is awake and complaining of mild incisional pain for which he is prescribed analgesics. His dressing is dry and intact, and he has an intravenous infusion of Ringer's solution infusing at 125 mL/h. He is to receive cefazolin (a cephalosporin antibiotic) 1 g intravenously every 4 h until he is able to tolerate fluids, at which time he will be placed on oral cefixime 200 mg twice daily until discharged and for 1 week after returning home. Because of a history of alcoholism, he also has an order for vitamin K intramuscular.

CRITICAL THINKING QUESTIONS

1. It is always possible that a person receiving antibiotic drugs may experience adverse effects or an allergic reaction. How does an allergic reaction differ from a drug adverse effect?

2. Predict the possible consequences of not obtaining a medication history from Mr. Ketron, despite the fact that he will be receiving antibiotics and analgesics.

3. How will you select the best site to give the vitamin K injection?

4. What precautions should you take, if any, before administering Mr. Ketron's intravenous antibiotic medication?

5. Mr. Ketron will be placed on the oral antibiotic when he can tolerate food and oral fluids. What difference, if any, does it make if this drug is given before or after meals?

Check the eText in MyNursingLab for answers and explanations.

KEY TERMS

absorption   *p. 877*
additive effect   *p. 876*
adverse effect   *p. 875*
agonist   *p. 877*
ampule   *p. 906*
anaphylactic reaction
   p. 875
antagonist   *p. 877*
bevel   *p. 904*
biotransformation
   p. 877
brand name   *p. 872*
buccal   *p. 881*
cannula   *p. 904*
chemical name   *p. 872*
collective prescription
   p. 883
cumulative effect   *p. 875*
desired effect   *p. 875*
detoxification   *p. 877*
distribution   *p. 877*
drug   *p. 872*
drug abuse   *p. 876*

drug allergy   *p. 875*
drug dependence   *p. 876*
drug habituation   *p. 876*
drug interaction   *p. 875*
drug misuse   *p. 876*
drug tolerance   *p. 875*
drug toxicity   *p. 875*
drug–drug interaction
   p. 889
drug–food interaction
   p. 890
enteral   *p. 881*
epidural   *p. 881*
ethnopharmacology
   p. 879
excretion   *p. 877*
first-pass effect   *p. 877*
gastrostomy tube   *p. 896*
gauge   *p. 904*
generic name   *p. 872*
half-life   *p. 878*
high-alert medications
   p. 874

hub   *p. 904*
iatrogenic disease   *p. 876*
idiosyncratic effect   *p. 875*
illicit drugs   *p. 876*
inhibiting effect   *p. 876*
insulin syringe   *p. 904*
intra-arterial   *p. 881*
intra-articular   *p. 881*
intracardiac   *p. 881*
intradermal   *p. 881*
intramuscular   *p. 881*
intraosseous   *p. 881*
intrapleural   *p. 881*
intraspinal   *p. 881*
intrathecal   *p. 881*
intravenous   *p. 881*
irrigation   *p. 904*
lavage   *p. 904*
medication   *p. 872*
medication history
   p. 889
medication reconciliation
   p. 891

metabolism   *p. 877*
metabolites   *p. 877*
metered-dose inhaler
   (MDI)   *p. 945*
nasogastric tube   *p. 896*
official name   *p. 872*
onset of action   *p. 878*
ophthalmic   *p. 937*
oral   *p. 881*
otic instillations   *p. 939*
parenteral   *p. 881*
peak plasma level   *p. 878*
percutaneous   *p. 935*
pharmacist   *p. 872*
pharmacodynamics
   p. 877
pharmacogenetics
   p. 878
pharmacokinetics   *p. 877*
pharmacology   *p. 872*
pharmacy   *p. 872*
physiological dependence
   p. 876

CHAPTER HIGHLIGHTS

- Medications have several names. Nurses need to know the generic and trade names of a medication and be aware of its therapeutic and adverse effects.

- Federal drug legislation in Canada regulates the production, prescription, distribution, and administration of drugs.

- Nursing practice acts define limits on the nurse's responsibilities regarding medications.

- Adverse effects of medications include drug toxicity, drug allergy, drug tolerance, idiosyncratic effect, and drug interactions.

- Several factors other than the drug itself can affect its action. These include pregnancy; age; sex; genetic and ethnic factors; diet; client environment; psychological factors; illness and disease; and time of administration.

- Various routes are used to administer medications: oral, sublingual, buccal, parenteral, topical, or via a nasogastric or gastrostomy tube. When administering a medication, the nurse must ensure that it is appropriate for the route specified.

- Medication orders must include the client name, date and time the order is written, name of the medication, dosage, route, frequency of administration, and signature of the person writing the order. Nurses must question any unclear orders before implementing the order.

- Telephone or verbal orders must be co-signed by the prescriber within a time frame specified by agency policy.

- The metric system is the measurement system used in Canada; nurses may encounter situations where the household system is used.

- Mathematical methods to calculate medication dosages include the basic formula, ratio and proportion method, and fractional equation. Pediatric dosages are often calculated by incorporating the child's weight or body surface area.

- Nurses must always assess a client's physical status before giving any medication and obtain a medication history.

- Health care system factors contribute to medication safety and a culture of safety within the health care setting encourages disclosure of errors and near misses so that factors contributing to the error can be identified and corrected. This approach is different from the "shame-and-blame," *individual finger pointing* approach that increases the tendency to cover up or hide errors.

- Clinical practice guidelines to promote patient safety with respect to medications include avoiding the use of certain abbreviations, using Tall Man lettering for look-alike or sound-alike medications, using caution when administering high alert medications, and listening to patients!

- Medication reconciliation is another method that the nurse uses to ensure that clients receive the appropriate medications and dosages. Three important areas for medication reconciliation to occur are (a) on admission, (b) during shift reports and transfers, and with new medication orders, and (c) on discharge.

- When administering medications, the nurse observes specified *"10 rights"* to ensure accurate administration. When preparing medications, the nurse checks the medication container label against the medication administration record (MAR) or printout three times.

- The nurse always identifies the client appropriately using a minimum of two identifiers before administering a medication and stays with the client until the medication is taken.

- Medications, once given, are documented as soon as possible after administration.

- Medications given parenterally act more quickly than those given orally or topically and must be prepared using aseptic technique.

- When preparing two insulins to be mixed in the same syringe, a vial of unmodified insulin should never be contaminated with modified insulin.

- Proper site selection is essential for an intramuscular injection to prevent tissue, blood vessel, bone, and nerve damage. The nurse should always palpate anatomical landmarks when selecting a site.

  - The ventrogluteal site is the safest site of choice because it provides the greatest thickness of gluteal muscle and is free of penetrating nerves.

  - The dorsogluteal site should **not** be used for injection because it poses unnecessary and unacceptable risk for clients.

- The Z-track method for intramuscular injection is recommended because it is less painful than the traditional injection technique and decreases leakage of irritating or staining medication into subcutaneous tissues.
- Clients receiving a series of injections should have the injection sites alternated.
- After use, needles should not be recapped and must be placed in puncture-resistant sharps containers.
- Intravenous medications can be administered by various methods: in a large-volume infusion of intravenous fluid; by intermittent intravenous infusion; by volume-controlled infusion; by intravenous push (IVP) or bolus; or by intermittent venous access. In all of these methods, the client has an existing intravenous line or an IV access site, such as a saline lock.
- Topical medications are applied to the skin and mucous membranes in areas such as the eye, external ear canal, nose, vagina, and rectum.
- A metered-dose inhaler (MDI) is a handheld nebulizer that can be used by clients to self-administer measured doses of an aerosol medication. To ensure correct delivery of the prescribed medication by MDIs, nurses need to instruct clients to use aerosol inhalers correctly.
- Irrigations of body cavities may be performed (a) to remove a foreign object or excessive secretions or discharge, (b) to apply heat or cold, (c) to apply a medication, such as an antiseptic, (d) to reduce inflammation, or (e) to relieve discomfort.

ASSESS YOUR LEARNING

1. A patient tells the nurse, "This pill is a different colour from the one that I usually take at home." Which of the following is the BEST response by the nurse?

   a. "Go ahead and take your medicine."

   b. "I will recheck your medication orders."

   c. "Maybe the doctor ordered a different medication."

   d. "I'll leave the pill here while I check with the doctor."

2. Which of the following medications listed on a patient's medication administration record (MAR) should the nurse question?

   a. Furosemide 40 mg, PO, stat

   b. Ampicillin 500 mg, q6h, IVPB

   c. Humulin R insulin 36 units, SC, ac breakfast

   d. Codeine q4h, PO, prn for pain

3. The physician prescribed 5 mL of immunoglobulin (a slightly viscous solution) to be given as a deep ventrogluteal intramuscular injection to a 40-year-old female who is 170 cm tall and weighs 61 kg. Which of the following is the most appropriate method of administration?

   a. A tuberculin syringe, #25 gauge to #27 gauge, 16-mm needle

   b. Two 3-mL syringes, #22 gauge to #23 gauge, 2.54-cm to 3.8-cm needle

   c. Two 2-mL syringes, #25 gauge to #27 gauge, 16-mm needle

   d. Two 3-mL syringes, #25 gauge to #27 gauge, 2.5-cm needle

4. The nurse is to administer 0.75 mL of medication subcutaneously in the upper arm to a 50-year-old patient who weighs 180 kg. The nurse can grasp approximately 10 cm of the patient's tissue at the upper arm. Which is the most appropriate syringe for the nurse to use?

   a. A tuberculin syringe, #25 gauge to #27 gauge, 16-mm needle

   b. 3-mL syringes, #20 gauge to #23 gauge, 3.8-cm needle

   c. 2-mL syringe, #25 gauge to #27 gauge, 16-mm needle

   d. 2-mL syringe, #20 gauge to #23 gauge, 2.5-cm needle

5. The nurse is to administer a tuberculin test to a 22-year-old male who is 182 cm tall and weighs 82 kg. Which of the following is the most appropriate for the nurse to use?

   a. A tuberculin syringe, #25 to #27 gauge, 6-mm to 16-mm needle

   b. Two 3-mL syringes, #20 to #23 gauge, 3.8-cm needle

   c. 2-mL syringe, #25 to #27 gauge, 16-mm needle

   d. 2-mL syringe, #20 to #23 gauge, 2.5-cm needle

6. The nurse calculates that 93.75% of a medication with a half-life of 12 hours will be eliminated from a patient's body in how many hours following administration?

   a. 24 hours

   b. 36 hours

   c. 48 hours

   d. 60 hours

7. Which of the following dosages is MOST appropriate for the nurse to administer to an older adult patient with renal insufficiency about to receive a cardiac medication?

   a. A decreased dosage

   b. The standard dosage

   c. An increased dosage

   d. A divided dosage

8. Which of the following is the correct method when administering an otic medication to a 2-year-old client?

   a. Pulling the ear straight back

   b. Pulling the ear down and back

   c. Pulling the ear up and back

   d. Pulling the ear straight upward

9. A physician writes a prescription for 0.15 mg of digoxin to be administered intravenously every day. The medication is available in a concentration of 400 mcg/mL. How many millilitres will the nurse administer?

   a. 0.4 mL

   b. 0.04 mL

   c. 0.16 mL

   d. 4 mL

10. Christian, 4 years old and weighing 15 kg, has been admitted for bacterial respiratory infection. The pediatrician orders IV cefotaxime sodium (Claforan) 60 mg/kg/day. What amount of medication should the nurse administer every 6 hours?

   a. 175 mg

   b. 200 mg

   c. 225 mg

   d. 250 mg

Check the eText in MyNursingLab for answers and explanations.

WEBLINKS

Canadian Pharmacists Association

http://www.pharmacists.ca

The association is the national organization for pharmacists. Its website provides a source for drug information, pharmacy practices, and patient information.

Health Canada Drug Product Database

http://www.hc-sc.gc.ca/dhp-mps/prodpharma/ databasdon/index_eng.php

The Drug Product Database (DPD) contains product-specific information on drugs approved for use in Canada.

SickKids Hospital

http://www.sickkids.ca/Nursing/Education-and-learning/ Nursing-Student-Orientation/module-two-clinical-care/ medadmin/index.html

The SickKids Hospital has created a nursing student orientation module with medication calculations and a self-test.

MyNursingLab

REFERENCES

Accreditation Canada. (2011). *Required organizational practices*. Retrieved from http://www.accreditation .ca/accreditation-programs/international/ required-organizational-practices/

Adams, M. P., & Koch, R. (2010). *Pharmacology: Connections to nursing practice*. Upper Saddle River, NJ: Pearson Prentice Hall.

Baker, G. R., Norton, P. G., Flintoft, V., Blais, R., Brown, A., Cox, J., & Tamblin, R. (2004). The Canadian adverse events study: The incidence of adverse events among hospital patients in Canada. *Canadian Medical Association Journal, 170*(11), 1678–1686.

Barron, C., & Cocoman, A. (2008). Administering intramuscular injections to children: What does the evidence say? *Journal of Children's and Young People's Nursing, 2*, 138–143.

Diggle, L., & Richards, S. (2007). Best practice when immunising children. *Primary Health Care, 17*(7), 41–46.

Greener, M. (2009). Understanding the principles of drug metabolism. *Nurse Prescribing, 7*, 109–114.

Health Canada. (2011). *Proper use and disposal of medication*. Retrieved from http://www.hc-sc.gc.ca/hl-vs/iyh-vsv/med/ disposal-defaire-eng.php#pr

Hunter, J. (2008). Intramuscular injection techniques. *Nursing Standard, 22*(24), 35–40.

Institute for Safe Medication Practices. (2000). *A call to action: Eliminating hand written prescriptions within 3 years*. Horsham, PA: Author. Retrieved from http://www.ismp.org/ newsletters/acutecare/articles/whitepaper.asp

Institute for Safe Medication Practices. (2011). *Oral dosage forms that should not be crushed.* Retrieved from http://www.ismp .org/tools/donotcrush.pdf

Institute for Safe Medication Practices Canada. (2012). *Medication reconciliation.* Retrieved from http://www.ismp-canada.org/medrec/

Ipp, M., Taddio, A., Sam, J., Goldbach, M., & Parkin, P. (2007). Vaccine-related pain: Randomised controlled trial of two injection techniques. *Archives of Diseases of Children, 92,* 1105–1108. doi:10.1136/adc.2007.118695

Lehne, R. (2010). *Pharmacology for nursing care.* St. Louis, MO: Saunders Elsevier.

Malkin, B. (2008). Are techniques used for intramuscular injection based on evidence? *Nursing Times, 104* (50/51), 48–51.

Nicoll, L. H., & Hesby, A. (2002). Intramuscular injection: An integrative research review and guideline for evidence-based practice. *Applied Nursing Research, 16*(2), 149–162.

Registered Nurses' Association of Ontario. (2009). *Nursing best practice guideline: Subcutaneous administration of insulin in adults with Type 2 Diabetes—Guideline Supplement.* Toronto, ON: Author.

Taddio, A., Appleton, M., Bortolussi, R., Chambers, C., Dubey, V., Halperin, S., Hanrahan, A., Ipp, M., Lockett, D., Macdonald, N., Midmer, D., Mousmanis, P., Palda, V., Pielak, K., Riddell, R. P., Rieder, M., Scott, J., & Shah, V. (2010). Reducing the pain of childhood vaccination: An evidence-based clinical practice guideline (summary). *Canadian Medical Association Journal 182,* 1989–1995. doi:10.1503/cmaj.092048

Taddio, A., Ilersich, A.L., Ipp, M., Kikuta, A., Shah, V., & HELPinKIDS Team. (2009). Physical interventions and injection techniques for reducing injection pain during routine childhood immunizations: Systematic review of randomized controlled trials and quasi-randomized controlled trials. *Clinical Therapeutics, 31*(Suppl 2), S48–S76.

U.S. Centers for Disease Control and Prevention. (2010). *Injection safety: Information for providers.* Retrieved from http://www.cdc.gov/injectionsafety/providers.html

World Health Organization. (2006). *Immunization in practice. Module 4: Ensuring safe injections.* Retrieved from http://www.who.int/vaccines-documents/DoxTrng/IIP.../www9556-05.pdf

Zimmerman, P. G. (2010). Revisiting IM injections. *American Journal of Nursing, 110* (2), 60–61.

Chapter 34

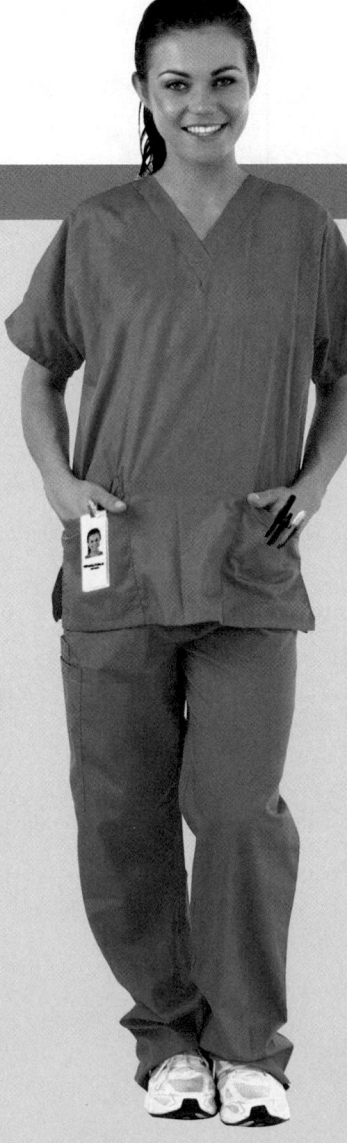

Infection Prevention and Control

LEARNING OUTCOMES

After studying this chapter, you will be able to:

1. Identify risks for health care–associated infections.

2. Describe the specific and nonspecific body defences against microorganisms.

3. Outline the pathophysiology of infection and describe the characteristics of the five major types of microorganisms that can cause an infection.

4. Describe the six links in the chain of infection and identify measures that break each link.

5. Describe the six routes of transmission of microorganisms.

6. Describe factors that place people at risk for developing an infection.

7. List indications for hand hygiene and describe respiratory hygiene.

8. Correctly perform hand hygiene, donning and removing personal protective equipment including facial protection, gowns and gloves (clean and sterile), establishing and maintaining a sterile field, and managing equipment used for patients.

9. Describe the system of routine practices and additional precautions and compare these with other systems.

10. Identify nursing responsibilities in infection prevention and control.

11. Outline relevant nursing diagnoses and contributing factors for people at risk for infection and those who have an infection.

12. Explain the measures to take to prevent or manage a potential exposure to a blood-borne pathogen.

Nurses are directly involved in providing a biologically safe environment. Microorganisms exist everywhere in the environment: in air, in water, in soil, and on body surfaces. Skin, the intestinal tract, and mucous membranes lining other areas open to the outside (e.g., mouth, upper respiratory tract, vagina, and lower urinary tract) have different types of **normal** or **resident flora** (the collective microorganisms in a given area). See Table 34.1 for common resident organisms. Most microorganisms are harmless, and some are even beneficial. An important role of resident flora, for example, is to prevent a potential **pathogen**, a microorganism with the potential to cause disease, from taking up residence. Bacteria on skin or mucous membranes produce toxic metabolites or alter local pH, thus repressing the growth of other species. Some microorganisms found in the intestines (e.g., *Enterobacteriaceae*) produce substances that are lethal to related strains of bacteria. Other gut flora produce B vitamins and vitamin K.

TABLE 34.1 Examples of Common Resident Organisms

Body Area	Organisms
Skin	Coagulase-negative staphylococci *Propionibacterium acnes* *Staphylococcus aureus* *Corynebacterium xerosis* *Pityrosporum ovale* (yeast)
Nasal passages	*Staphylococcus aureus* Coagulase-negative staphylococci
Oropharynx	*Streptococcus pneumoniae*
Bronchi, lungs	None
Mouth	*Streptococcus mutans* *Lactobacillus* *Bacteroides* *Actinomyces*
Stomach	None
Esophagus	*Bacteroides*
Intestine	*Fusobacterium* *Eubacterium* *Lactobacillus* *Streptococcus* *Enterobacteriaceae* *Shigella* *Escherichia coli*
Urethral orifice	Coagulase-negative staphylococci
Urethra (lower)	*Proteus*
Bladder, ureters, kidneys	None
Vagina	*Lactobacillus* *Bacteroides* *Clostridium* *Candida albicans*
Blood, lymph system	None

An **infection** is an invasion of body tissue by a micro-organism and its subsequent proliferation there, causing damage to host tissue. Such a microorganism is called an **infectious agent**. Some infections are caused by normal resident flora when they move to a different part of the body. For example, *Escherichia coli* is a normal inhabitant of the large intestine but a common cause of infection of the urinary tract. Other infections are caused by microorganisms that are acquired from the environment or from another person.

Infectious diseases are a major cause of death world-wide and a leading cause of illness in Canada. The control of the spread of microorganisms and the protection of people from communicable diseases and infections are carried out on international, national, provincial or territorial, community, and individual levels. The World Health Organization (WHO) is the major regulatory agency at the international level. In Canada, the Public Health Agency of Canada (PHAC) is the principal public health agency at the national level, with its Health Care–Associated Infections and Infection Prevention and Control division concerned with infection prevention and control. At the provincial and territorial level, health departments track epidemics and illnesses as reports are made throughout a particular area. At the local level, hospitals and continuing care facilities have infection control practitioners who are responsible for monitoring infection rates and implementing appropriate education, prevention and control strategies, or other programs.

The Community and Hospital Infection Control Association–Canada (CHICA–Canada) has articulated core competencies in infection prevention and control for health care workers, which include knowledge and skills related to the transmission of microorganisms, hand hygiene (see the Evidence-Informed Practice box on this page about hand washing by health care workers), routine practices and additional precautions, personal protective equipment, personal safety, sterilization and disinfection, and critical assessment of risk. Key strategies for the prevention and control of infections involve eliminating microorganisms, reducing transmission of microorganisms to an individual, and reducing the susceptibility of that individual. **Asepsis** is freedom from disease-causing microorganisms. To decrease the possibility of transferring microorganisms from one place to another, aseptic technique is used in such procedures as dressing changes and insertion of intravenous lines. Hand hygiene is another method used to reduce transmission of organisms.

Health Care–Associated Infections

Infections that are associated with the delivery of health care services in a health care facility were traditionally called **nosocomial infections**. Nosocomial infections

EVIDENCE-INFORMED PRACTICE

How Well Do Health Care Workers Wash Their Hands?

In this study, Mertz and colleagues assessed hand hygiene practices in 13 acute care hospital sites and 123 hospital units in Ontario, Canada. Using a standardized instrument, nine trained research assistants observed a total of 3697 health care worker–client contacts and 9511 opportunities for hand hygiene. Overall adherence to the recommended indications for hand hygiene was 31%, ranging from 18.9% to 39.2% on different units. Adherence was higher in intensive care units (ICUs) and in single rooms, and when the client was on Contact Precautions. Adherence by nurses was higher than among other categories of health care workers.

Other studies have shown considerable variation in hand hygiene adherence before and after contact with clients or by indication for hand hygiene, both before and after a variety of strategies to improve adherence. Sustained adherence appears to require repeated and varied measures to promote hand hygiene (Gould, Moralejo, Drey, & Chudleigh, 2010). Knowledge alone is insufficient to ensure optimal behaviour.

NURSING IMPLICATIONS: Hand hygiene needs to be continuously reinforced. Besides education about when and how to perform hand hygiene, work environments need to be structured so as to facilitate hand hygiene (e.g., easy access to sinks or alcohol-based hand rub).

Sources: Based on Mertz D., Johnstone J., Krueger P., Brazil K., Walter S.D., Loeb M. (2011). Adherence to hand hygiene and risk factors for poor adherence in 13 Ontario acute care hospitals. *American Journal of Infection Control, 39*(8): 693–696; and Gould D. J., Moralejo D., Drey N., Chudleigh J. H. (2010). Interventions to improve hand hygiene compliance in patient care. *Cochrane Database of Systematic Reviews,* Sept 8 (9): CD005186.

can either develop during a patient's stay in a facility or manifest after discharge. Standard definitions are available for different sites of infection (e.g., pneumonia, surgical site infection). The broader term of **health care–associated infections** (HAIs) is now preferred, as it includes infections in all settings, including hospitals, long-term care or continuing care facilities, community, home care, health care professionals' offices, or test centres. HAIs are not limited to patients; microorganisms may also be acquired by personnel working in the facility and can cause significant illness (e.g., hepatitis B infection and human immunodeficiency virus [HIV] infection).

HAIs are receiving increasing attention. The most common settings in which such infections develop are surgical or medical intensive care units in hospitals, but they also occur in clients in all settings of the health care system. Infections of the urinary tract, surgical site, and lower respiratory tract are the most common types of HAIs. Although less common, line-associated bacteremias, infections with antibiotic-resistant organisms, and *Clostridium difficile*–associated diarrhea are associated with higher mortality and health care costs.

The microorganisms that cause HAIs can originate from an endogenous (internal) source or from an exogenous (external) source. Most of these infections appear to have endogenous sources, and many factors contribute to HAIs. A number of infections are the direct result of diagnostic or therapeutic procedures. One example of such an infection is **bacteremia** (bacteria in the bloodstream) that results from contamination of an intravascular line. Not all HAIs are procedure related, and not all infections are preventable. A key factor contributing to the development of these infections is the *presence of compromised hosts,* that is, people whose normal defences have been lowered by surgery or illness. The hands of personnel serve as a common vehicle for the spread of microorganisms. *Insufficient hand hygiene* is, thus, an important factor contributing to the spread of microorganisms in health care settings.

A point prevalence study conducted by the Canadian Nosocomial Infection Surveillance Program found that 10.5% of hospitalized adults (Gravel, Taylor et al, 2007) and 9.1% of children (Gravel, Matlow et al, 2007) had an HAI. Few comprehensive prevalence studies have been conducted in Canada or elsewhere. More common are reports of specific types of infections or infections by specific microorganisms, such as *C. difficile* (Zoutman & Ford, 2009). The cost of HAIs to the patient, the facility, and the health care system is significant. These infections extend hospitalization time, increase patients' time away from work, cause disability and discomfort, and can even result in loss of life. See Table 34.2 for common HAIs.

TABLE 34.2 Health Care–Associated Infections

Most Common Microorganisms	Contributing Factors
Urinary Tract	
Escherichia coli	Catheterization technique
Enterococcus species	Contamination of closed drainage system
Pseudomonas aeruginosa	Inadequate hand hygiene
Surgical Sites	
Staphylococcus aureus (including methicillin-resistant strains [MRSA])	Inadequate hand hygiene
Enterococcus species (including vancomycin-resistant strains [VRE])	Inadequate preoperative skin preparation or antibiotic prophylaxis
Pseudomonas aeruginosa	Contaminated water
Bloodstream	
Coagulase-negative staphylococci	Inadequate hand hygiene
Staphylococcus aureus	Improper intravenous fluid, tubing, and site care technique
Enterococcus species	Inadequate hand hygiene, contamination from feces
Hepatitis B	Needle puncture
Respiratory Tract	
Staphylococcus aureus	Inadequate hand hygiene
Pseudomonas aeruginosa	Improper suctioning technique
Enterobacter species	
Gastrointestinal Tract	
Norovirus	Inadequate hand hygiene

Types of Microorganisms Causing Infections

Five major categories of microorganisms cause infection in humans: (a) bacteria, (b) viruses, (c) fungi, (d) protozoa, and (e) helminths. **Bacteria**, by far the most common infection-causing microorganisms, are large enough to be seen with a light microscope, can replicate outside of host cells, and are fairly easily grown in a laboratory. Several hundred species can cause disease in humans and can live and be transported through air, water, food, soil, body tissues and fluids, and inanimate objects. Most of the microorganisms in Table 34.2 are bacteria.

Viruses consist primarily of nucleic acid and lipoproteins and, therefore, must enter living cells to reproduce. They can be seen only with an electron microscope, require tissue culture for growth, and cannot easily be grown in most hospital laboratories. Common viruses include rhinoviruses (which cause the common cold), influenza, hepatitis, herpes, and HIV. **Fungi** include yeasts

and moulds. *Candida albicans* is a yeast considered to be normal flora in the human vagina.

Protozoa are single-celled organisms, and **helminths** (worms) are multicelled organisms. Both are classified as **parasites** as they live on other living organisms with benefit only to themselves. Few cause HAIs, although some, such as the protozoa that cause malaria, present enormous public health challenges.

Bacteria, some fungi, and some protozoa are susceptible to antibiotics, whereas viruses are not. A limited number of available antiviral drugs are effective for certain viral infections. Other classes of drugs are used to treat infections caused by protozoa and helminths.

Some microorganisms affect only specific tissues, resulting in a predictable clinical picture. For example, rhinoviruses infect the nasopharynx, causing signs and symptoms of the common cold, whereas the hepatitis B virus infects only the liver, resulting in hepatitis. Other microorganisms can infect a variety of tissues. For example, *Staphylococcus* species can cause skin infections, pneumonia, and gastroenteritis. Many different microorganisms can, therefore, cause a similar disease, such as pneumonia or diarrhea. Health assessment and laboratory testing are necessary to determine the exact infectious agent in any particular case of infection.

Microorganisms also vary in the severity of the diseases they produce and their degree of **communicability**, that is, their ability to be spread from one person to another. For example, the common cold virus is more readily transmitted than the bacillus that causes Hansen's disease (leprosy) (*Mycobacterium leprae*). If the infectious agent can be transmitted to an individual by direct or indirect contact, through a vector or vehicle, or as an airborne infection, as described later in the chapter, and transmission results in the same disease, the resulting condition is called a **communicable disease**.

Pathogenicity is the ability to produce disease. Many microorganisms that are normally harmless can cause disease under certain circumstances. A *true pathogen* causes disease or infection in a healthy individual. An **opportunistic pathogen** causes disease only in a susceptible individual. Pathogens vary in their **virulence**, that is, their power to overcome the host's defences. Different species have different **virulence factors** or evasion mechanisms, such as proteins that strengthen adherence to target cells, affect motility, or promote resistance to acid, enzymes, or antibiotics. Bacteria that acquire resistance to certain antibiotics frequently become resistant to many classes of antibiotics, reducing treatment options and effectiveness. Some microorganisms, such as the measles virus, have the ability to infect almost all susceptible people after exposure. By contrast, microorganisms, such as the tuberculosis bacillus, infect a relatively small number of the population who are susceptible and exposed, usually people who are poorly nourished or immunocompromised.

Body Defences against Infection

Individuals normally have defences that protect the body from infection when exposed to an infectious agent. These defences can be categorized as *nonspecific* and *specific*. **Nonspecific defences** protect the person against all microorganisms regardless of prior exposure. The **specific defences** of the immune system, by contrast, are directed against identifiable bacteria, viruses, fungi, or other infectious agents recognized by the host from prior exposure.

Nonspecific Defences

Nonspecific body defences include anatomical and physiological barriers and the inflammatory response.

ANATOMICAL AND PHYSIOLOGICAL BARRIERS Intact skin and mucous membranes are the body's first line of defence against microorganisms. Unless skin and mucosa become cracked and broken, they are effective barriers against bacteria. Fungi can live on skin, but they cannot penetrate it. The dryness of skin also acts as a deterrent to bacteria, which are most plentiful in moist areas of the body, such as the perineum and axillae. Resident bacteria of skin also prevent other bacteria from multiplying. They use up the available nourishment, and the end products of their metabolism inhibit other bacteria. Normal secretions make skin slightly acidic; acidity also inhibits bacterial growth.

The nasal passages have a defensive function. As entering air follows the tortuous route of the passage, it comes in contact with moist mucous membranes and *cilia* (tiny hairs). These trap microorganisms, dust, and foreign materials. The *lungs* have alveolar **macrophages** (large phagocytes). **Phagocytes** are cells that ingest microorganisms, other cells, and foreign particles.

Each body orifice also has protective mechanisms. The oral cavity regularly sheds mucosal epithelium to rid the mouth of colonizers. The flow of saliva and its partial buffering action help prevent infections. Saliva contains microbial inhibitors, such as lactoferrin, lysozyme, and secretory immunoglobulin A (IgA).

The *eye* is protected from infection by tears, which continually wash microorganisms away and contain inhibiting lysozymes (enzymes). The gastrointestinal tract also has defences against infection. The high acidity (low pH) of the stomach normally prevents microbial growth. The resident flora of the large intestine helps prevent the establishment of disease-producing microorganisms. Peristalsis also tends to move microbes out of the body.

The *vagina* also has natural defences against infection. When a girl reaches puberty, lactobacilli ferment sugars in the vaginal secretions, creating a vaginal pH of 3.5 to 4.5. This acidic environment inhibits the growth of many disease-producing microorganisms. The entrance to the urethra normally harbours many microorganisms. These include coagulase-negative staphylococci (from skin) and *Escherichia coli* (from feces). It is believed that the urine flow has a flushing and bacteriostatic action that keeps the bacteria from ascending the urethra. An intact mucosal surface also acts as a barrier.

INTERFERONS **Interferons** are a class of molecules produced by virus-infected cells. These proteins, of which there are 20 types, move to and enter neighbouring cells, where they prevent binding of the virus to the uninfected cell or interfere with viral replication in the cell. Interferons have no effect on the cells that produce them but do protect neighbouring cells from becoming infected by the virus.

INFLAMMATORY RESPONSE **Inflammation** is a local and nonspecific defensive response of the tissues to injury or infection. It is an adaptive mechanism that destroys or dilutes the injurious agent, prevents further spread of the

BOX 34.1 CARDINAL SIGNS OF INFLAMMATION

Sign	Rationale
Pain or tenderness	Secondary to stimulation of local nociceptors by the chemical mediators associated with the injurious stimulus, most frequently by the prostaglandins synthesized from damaged cell membranes
Edema	Secondary to increased vascular permeability caused by the chemical mediators associated with the injurious stimulus, which allows fluid and cells to move from the intravascular space to the interstitial space
Erythema (redness) and heat	Results from hyperemia (increase in blood supply) to the area caused by the chemical mediators associated with the injurious stimulus, which brings warm blood close to the skin or tissue surface
Altered tissue function	Related to either or both of the following: (a) the damage that led to inflammation (e.g., damaged liver cells cannot conjugate bilirubin, so the unconjugated bilirubin cannot be excreted and accumulates, leading to jaundice); or (b) the inflammation itself (e.g., air exchange is diminished with inflammation in the lung because of bronchospasm, increased mucus and/or local edema)

injury, and promotes the repair of damaged tissue. Five cardinal signs characterize inflammation: (a) pain or tenderness, (b) edema (swelling), (c) erythema (redness), (d) heat, and (e) altered tissue function of the body part, if the injury is severe. Box 34.1 summarizes the cardinal signs and provides the rationale for why they occur. Exudate may also be produced though it is generally not listed in the "cardinal signs." Mucus may also be produced secondary to stimulation of local goblet cells if there are any in the area (e.g., in the respiratory or gastrointestinal tracts).

Commonly, words with the suffix -*itis* describe an inflammatory process. For example, *appendicitis* means inflammation of the appendix; *gastritis* means inflammation of the stomach lining.

Injurious stressors to body tissues can be categorized as physical agents, chemical agents, and microorganisms. *Physical agents* include mechanical objects causing trauma to tissues, excessive heat or cold, and radiation. *Chemical agents* include external irritants (e.g., acids, alkalis, poisons, and irritating gases) and internal irritants (substances produced within the body, such as excessive hydrochloric acid in the stomach). *Microorganisms* include the broad groups of bacteria, viruses, fungi, protozoa, and helminths.

The inflammatory response involves a series of dynamic events commonly referred to as the three stages of the inflammatory response:

1. *First stage:* vascular and cellular responses
2. *Second stage:* exudate production
3. *Third stage:* reparative phase

Vascular and Cellular Responses At the start of the first stage of inflammation, the damage to tissue cells caused by the infectious agent leads to synthesis of prostaglandins and leukotrienes from the damaged cell membranes, release of serotonin and histamine from platelets and mast cells or basophils, respectively, and/or activation of bradykinin. These chemical mediators cause constriction of the blood vessels at the site of injury, lasting only a few moments. This initial vasoconstriction is rapidly followed by dilation of small blood vessels, caused by the same chemical mediators. Thus, more blood flows to the injured area. This marked increase in blood supply is referred to as **hyperemia** and is responsible for the characteristic signs of redness and heat as warm blood flows to the area. Not all chemical mediators are involved in any given reaction; which ones are involved depends on the site and nature of the damage.

Prostaglandins and histamine also cause increased vascular permeability at the injured site. The result of this altered permeability is an outpouring of fluid, proteins, and leukocytes into the interstitial spaces, clinically manifested by the characteristic inflammatory signs of edema (swelling) and pain. The pain is caused by the pressure of accumulating fluid on local nerve endings and by stimulation of pain receptors by the chemical mediators. Too much fluid pouring into such areas as the pleural or pericardial cavity can seriously affect organ function. In other areas, such as joints, mobility is impaired. These chemical mediators will also stimulate mucus production if the site of infection involves a mucous membrane (e.g., infection of the bronchi) or stimulate smooth muscle contraction if the site of infection has smooth muscle. For example, in the lung, smooth muscle contraction leads to bronchospasm, and in the gastrointestinal tract, smooth muscle contraction leads to increased peristalsis and, thus, diarrhea.

Blood flow slows in the dilated vessels, allowing more **leukocytes** (white blood cells) to arrive at the injured tissues. When the blood flow slows, leukocytes aggregate or line up along the inner surface of the blood vessels. This process is known as **margination**. Leukocytes then move between the cells of the now permeable blood vessel wall into the affected tissue spaces, a process called **emigration**.

The actual passage of blood cells through the blood vessel wall is referred to as **diapedesis**. Leukocytes are attracted to injured cells by **chemotaxis**. In response to the exit of leukocytes from the blood vessels, the bone marrow produces large numbers of leukocytes and releases them into the bloodstream (**leukocytosis**). A number of **cytokines** (chemical mediators) produced by the leukocytes are responsible for stimulating this increase. An increase in white blood cell count is a sign associated with inflammation. A normal leukocyte count of 4.5×10^9/L to 11×10^9/L of blood can rise to 20×10^9/L or more when extensive inflammation occurs. Cytokines released from the leukocytes or molecules associated with bacterial cell walls also act as **pyrogens**, stimulating the production of fever.

Exudate Production In the second stage of inflammation, the inflammatory **exudate** is produced, consisting of fluid that escaped from the blood vessels, dead phagocytic cells, dead bacteria and dead tissue cells, and the products that they release. Exudate that contains leukocytes is called **pus**; it is frequently yellow because of the colour of the cells as they age. The nature and amount of exudate vary according to the tissue involved and the intensity and duration of the inflammation. The major types of exudate are *serous* (clear, containing serum but no cells), *sanguinous* (containing red blood cells), and *purulent* (containing pus).

Thromboplastin (a product released by injured tissue cells) initiates the coagulation pathway, resulting in a plasma protein called **fibrinogen** being converted to fibrin. Threads of fibrin and platelets together form an interlacing network to make a barrier, wall off the area, and prevent spread of the injurious agent. During the second stage, the injurious agent is destroyed by leukocytes, and the exudate is cleared away by lymphatic drainage.

Reparative Phase The third stage of the inflammatory response involves the repair of injured tissues by regeneration or replacement with fibrous tissue (scar) formation. **Regeneration** is the replacement of destroyed tissue cells by cells that are identical or similar in structure and function. It involves not only replacement of damaged cells one by one but also organization of these cells so that the architectural pattern and function of the tissue are restored. The ability to reproduce cells varies considerably from one type of tissue to another. For example, epithelial tissues of the skin and of the digestive and respiratory tracts have a good regenerative capacity, provided that their underlying support structures are intact. The same holds true for osseous, lymphoid, and bone marrow tissues. Tissues that have little regenerative capacity include nervous, muscular, and elastic tissues.

When regeneration is not possible, repair occurs by *fibrous tissue formation*. **Fibrous (scar) tissue** has the capacity to proliferate under the unusual conditions of ischemia and altered pH. The inflammatory exudate with its interlacing network of fibrin provides the framework for this tissue to develop. Damaged tissues are replaced with the connective tissue elements of collagen, blood capillaries, lymphatics, and other tissue-bound substances. In the early stages of this process, the tissue is called **granulation tissue**. It is a fragile, gelatinous tissue, appearing pink or red because of the many newly formed capillaries. Later in the process, the tissue shrinks (the capillaries are constricted, even obliterated) and the collagen fibres contract so that a firmer fibrous tissue remains. This is called **cicatrix** or scar.

Specific Defences

Specific defences of the body involve the immune system, which responds to foreign proteins in the body (e.g., bacteria or transplanted tissues). In some cases, the immune system even responds to the body's own proteins. Foreign proteins in the body are called **antigens** and are considered invaders. If the proteins originate in a person's own body, the antigen is called an **autoantigen**. Immunity is the specific resistance of the body to infection (pathogens or their toxins). Acquired immunity is of two major types: *active* and *passive*. See Table 34.3. In **active immunity**, the

TABLE 34.3 Types of Acquired Immunity

Type	Antigen or Antibody Source	Duration
1. Active	Antibodies are produced by the body in response to an antigen.	Long (months to decades)
a. Natural	Antibodies are formed in the presence of active infection in the body.	Long
b. Artificial	Antigens (vaccines or toxoids) are administered to stimulate antibody production.	Long: the immunity must be reinforced by booster inoculations
2. Passive	Antibodies are produced by another source, animal or human.	Short
a. Natural	Antibodies are transferred naturally from an immune mother to her baby through the placenta or in colostrum.	6 months to 1 year
b. Artificial	Immune serum (antibody) from an animal or another human is injected.	2 to 3 weeks

host produces its own antibodies in response to natural antigens (e.g., infection) or artificial antigens (e.g., vaccines). With **passive immunity**, the host receives antibodies produced by another source, either natural (e.g., from a nursing mother) or artificial (e.g., from an injection of immune serum).

ANTIBODY-MEDIATED DEFENCES Another name for the *antibody-mediated defences* is **humoral (circulating) immunity**. **Antibodies**, also called **immunoglobulins**, are part of the body's plasma proteins. B lymphocytes are activated when they recognize an antigen. They then differentiate into plasma cells, which secrete antibodies that bind specifically to the foreign antigen. This results in *neutralization* of a virus or toxin so it cannot enter or injure the target host cell, or *opsonization* (coating) of a bacterial cell to make it more attractive to leukocytes. The antigen-antibody complex also activates the complement system, which initiates inflammation and further helps eliminate the foreign invader. The antibody-mediated responses defend primarily against bacterial infection by opsonizing bacteria that are replicating in tissue and against viral infection by neutralizing viruses in the bloodstream before they enter host cells (i.e., in the extracellular phase).

Immunoglobulins (Ig) include IgM, IgG, IgA, IgD, and IgE. IgM, IgG, and IgA act in the protective function just described. They differ in that IgM and IgG are found in the bloodstream, while IgA is generally found in mucous membrane secretions. IgM is produced early and lasts only a short time; IgM to measles virus infection, for example, lasts about 1 month after the infection. The presence of IgM in a laboratory analysis, therefore, shows current or very recent infection. IgG or IgA are produced later and can last a very long time (years or decades for some infectious agents). On second or subsequent exposure to the same antigen, only IgG or IgA are produced, at a much faster rate than occurs after the initial infection.

IgD has no direct protective function and appears to regulate some aspects of B lymphocyte activity. IgE is also not involved in the protective response to infectious agents. It is the key mediator in allergic reactions.

CELL-MEDIATED DEFENCES The **cell-mediated defences**, or **cellular immunity**, occur through the T-cell system. On exposure to an antigen, the lymphoid tissues release large numbers of activated T cells into the lymph system. These T cells pass into the general circulation. T cells come in three main groups: (a) *helper T cells*, which help in the activation of both B cells and cytotoxic T cells; (b) *cytotoxic T cells*, which attack and kill microorganisms and sometimes the body's own cells; and (c) *suppressor T cells*, which can suppress the functions of the helper T cells and the cytotoxic T cells. The cytotoxic T cells act against their specific antigen, which may be a part of a bacterial cell wall or an altered host cell (e.g., virus-infected host cell). Prostaglandins are synthesized from the cell membrane damaged by the cytotoxic T cells, initiating inflammation. The cytotoxic T cell–mediated response defends against bacterial infections and against the intracellular phases of viral infections. When cell-mediated immunity is lost, as occurs with HIV infection, an individual is defenceless against most viral, bacterial, and fungal infections.

Pathophysiology of Infection

When an infection occurs, the infectious agent enters the host body, moves to its preferred target site, and overcomes the host defences. It will encounter defences at the site of entry as well as when moving to its target site (e.g., moving in the bloodstream to the liver in the case of hepatitis B virus). At the site of infection, the infectious agent multiplies, causing physical damage to the host cells. Bacteria replicate outside host cells within the tissue, taking up space and putting physical pressure on host cells, thereby damaging them. Some bacteria also produce a toxin that gets absorbed into the bloodstream and moves to other cells, damaging them. Viruses enter host cells and take over their protein-synthesizing machinery (ribosomes) so that the host cell then produces **virions** (new virus particles). The virions exit the host cell through *exocytosis* (budding from the cell membrane) or by causing *lysis* (destruction) of the host cell. The virions move into neighbouring cells to infect them, repeating the cycle.

Damage to the host cell initiates the inflammatory response, while recognition of the infectious agent by the immune system leads to antibody-mediated or cytotoxic T cell–mediated immune responses, both of which ultimately also promote inflammation. The white blood cells called in by the inflammatory and immune responses destroy the infectious agents and initiate phagocytosis and repair of the damaged tissue.

Clinical manifestations of infection result from both altered function of the damaged tissue and from the inflammatory response that is initiated in defence. Classic signs and symptoms of infection related to inflammation are redness and swelling at the site of infection, local pain, presence of purulent exudate, fever, and elevated leukocyte count. The clinical manifestations associated with altered tissue function depend on the tissue involved. For example, mucus production and edema of the airways with pneumonia lead to altered gas exchange and, thus, hypoxia, whereas with hepatitis, the damage that occurs to the ability of liver cells to conjugate bilirubin, a process required for its excretion, leads to the accumulation of bilirubin and results in jaundice.

The Clinical Spectrum of Infection

Colonization is the process by which strains of microorganisms become resident flora. In this state, the microorganisms may grow and multiply but do not cause physiological changes in host tissue. The presence of colonizing bacteria does not mean the person has an infection. Infection occurs when newly introduced or resident microorganisms succeed in invading a part of the body in which the host's defence mechanisms are ineffective and the pathogen causes tissue damage. If tissue damage is localized to a few cells or a small part of the tissue, then changes may not be noticeable unless they are looked for specifically with relevant types of testing. When this occurs and there is no clinical evidence of disease, the infection is called *asymptomatic* or *subclinical*. Some subclinical infections can cause significant damage, however. For example, cytomegalovirus infection in a pregnant woman can lead to significant disease in the fetus. When a detectable alteration in normal tissue function occurs, the infection is called *overt* and presents as disease.

Infections can be local or systemic. A **local infection** is limited to the specific part of the body in which the microorganisms remain. If the microorganisms spread and damage different parts of the body, it is a **systemic infection**. When a culture of the person's blood reveals microorganisms, the condition is called *bacteremia*. When bacteremia results in systemic symptoms, it is referred to as **septicemia**.

Infections are also acute or chronic. Acute infections generally appear suddenly or last a short time. A chronic infection may occur slowly, over a very long period, and can last months or years.

A **carrier** is a person or an animal that harbours a specific infectious agent and serves as a potential source of infection yet does not manifest any clinical signs of disease. The carrier state can also exist in the incubation period, convalescence, and postconvalescence of an individual with a clinically recognizable disease. This type of carrier is referred to as an *incubatory* or *convalescent carrier*. Under either circumstance, the carrier state can be of short duration (*temporary* or *transient carrier*) or long duration (*chronic carrier*).

Infection: An Imbalance between Microorganisms and Defences

Given the defence mechanisms available, it should be clear that the very presence of a microorganism entering the body is not enough to determine that an infection will occur. For an infection to occur, the microorganisms have to overcome the defences. This defeat can occur in the following cases:

- The microorganisms are highly virulent (even if present in small numbers) and so are able to overcome normal defence mechanisms.
- The **microbial load** (number of infectious agents present) is greater than the number that the available defence mechanisms can handle quickly, so the microorganisms are able to proliferate.
- Defence mechanisms are reduced or compromised, and thus, host resistance is low; so the host cannot overcome a microbial load that he or she would be expected to normally be able to handle.

Reducing the risk of infection therefore involves ensuring that defences are greater than the microorganisms' ability to overcome them. This goal can be accomplished by either reducing microbial load or strengthening host resistance. Both can be accomplished in clinical practice, while it is not possible to directly affect virulence.

The chain of infection is an important framework for understanding how microorganisms enter a host or move from one to another. Breaking any link in the chain is the key to infection prevention and control.

The Chain of Infection

Six links make up the chain of infection (Figure 34.1 on the next page): (a) the etiological agent or microorganism, (b) the reservoir (place) in which the organism naturally resides, (c) a portal of exit from the reservoir, (d) a mode (route) of transmission, (e) a portal of entry into a host, and (f) the susceptibility of the host.

Etiological Agent

The extent to which any microorganism is capable of producing an infectious process depends on the number of microorganisms present, the virulence and pathogenicity of the microorganisms, the ability of the microorganisms to enter the body, the susceptibility of the host, and the ability of the microorganisms to live in the host's body. The presence of an infectious agent is a necessary condition for an infection to occur, but the mere presence of an infectious agent alone is insufficient to ensure that an infection will develop.

Reservoir

Many **reservoirs**, or sources of microorganisms, exist. Common sources are other humans, the client's own microorganisms, plants, animals, or the general environment.

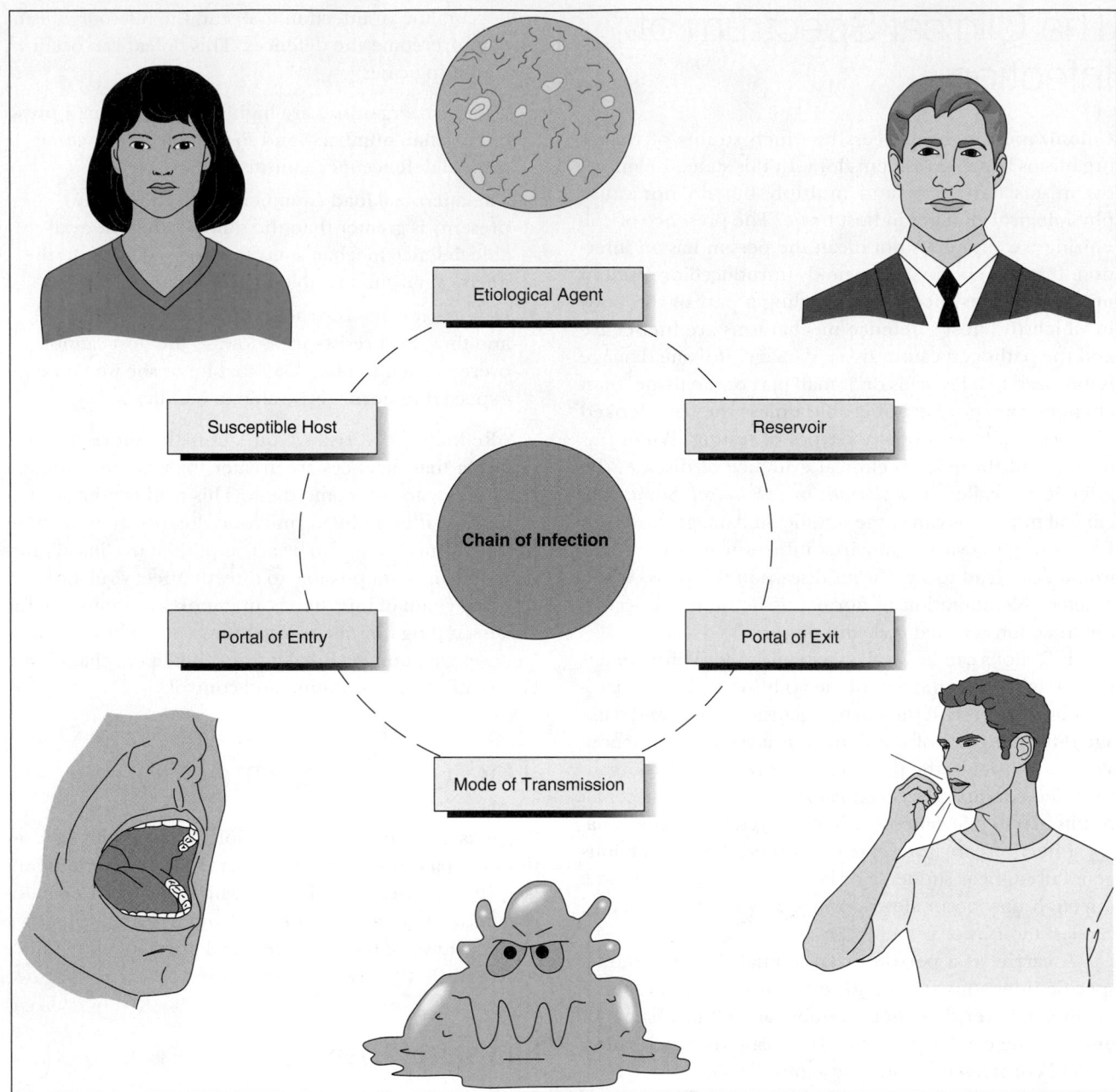

FIGURE 34.1 The chain of infection.

People are the most common source of infection for others and for themselves. For example, the person with an influenza virus frequently spreads it to others. When their resistance is lowered by fatigue and other factors, an infection may develop.

Insects, birds, and other animals are common reservoirs of infection. For example, the *Anopheles* mosquito carries the malaria parasite. Food, water, milk, and feces also can be reservoirs. In hospitals, urinary catheters, wound dressings contaminated with purulent exudates, oxygen humidity canisters, and contaminated bedside surfaces are all examples of reservoirs.

Portal of Exit

Before an infection can establish itself in a host, the microorganisms must leave the reservoir. Common human reservoirs and their associated **portals of exit** are summarized in Table 34.4.

Mode of Transmission

After a microorganism leaves its source or reservoir, it requires a route of transmission to reach another person or host through a *receptive* **portal of entry**. There are

TABLE 34.4 Human Reservoirs, Common Infectious Microorganisms, and Portals of Exit

Body Area Reservoir	Common Infectious Microorganisms	Portals of Exit
Respiratory tract	Parainfluenza virus *Mycobacterium tuberculosis* *Staphylococcus aureus*	Nose or mouth through sneezing, coughing, breathing, or talking; endotracheal tubes or tracheostomies
Gastrointestinal tract	Hepatitis A virus *Salmonella* species	Mouth—saliva, vomitus; anus—feces; ostomies; drainage tubes (e.g., nasogastric or T-tubes)
Urinary tract	*Escherichia coli* Enterococci *Pseudomonas aeruginosa*	Urethral meatus and urinary diversion ostomies
Reproductive tract (including genitals)	*Neisseria gonorrhoeae* *Treponema pallidum* Herpes simplex virus type 2 Hepatitis B virus	Vagina—vaginal discharge; urinary meatus—semen, urine; urethral discharge; contaminated urine
Blood	Hepatitis B virus Human immunodeficiency virus (HIV) *Staphylococcus aureus* Coagulase-negative staphylococci	Open wound, needle puncture site, any disruption of intact skin or mucous membrane surfaces
Tissue	*Staphylococcus aureus* *Escherichia coli* *Proteus* species Beta-hemolytic *streptococcus* group A or B	Drainage from cut or wound

six possible routes: (a) direct contact, (b) indirect contact, (c) droplet transmission, (d) airborne transmission, (e) vehicle-borne transmission, and (f) vector-borne transmission.

DIRECT CONTACT TRANSMISSION **Direct contact transmission** involves immediate and direct transfer of microorganisms from person to person through touching, biting, kissing, or sexual intercourse, that is, body surface to body surface or direct exchange of bodily fluids.

INDIRECT CONTACT TRANSMISSION **Indirect contact transmission** involves passive transfer from the reservoir to an intermediate inanimate object in the recipient's immediate environment and then to the recipient (e.g., hands touch a contaminated doorknob, pick up microorganisms, and transfer them to the recipient's mucous membrane). The length of time that the microorganism remains infectious on inanimate surfaces depends on the microorganism, the relative humidity and temperature of the environment, and the nature of the surface.

DROPLET TRANSMISSION **Droplet transmission** is also a form of direct contact but is usually considered separately as it requires different interventions. Droplets are large drops of respiratory secretions, larger than 5 microns in diameter. They are generated from sneezing (see Figure 34.2), coughing, spitting, singing, talking,

or procedures such as suctioning. Droplets can be projected a short distance but do not remain suspended in air for long. The larger the particle, the faster it falls. About 85% of the droplets generated by an average sneeze or closed-mouth cough, and almost all of those generated by an open-mouth cough, are larger than 20 microns and will take less than 4 minutes to fall 3 metres. If the source and the recipient are within this distance of each other, the droplet spray can be deposited into the conjunctiva or onto the mucous membranes of the eye, nose, or mouth of the recipient. This route transmits the majority of agents causing respiratory infections. Droplets also

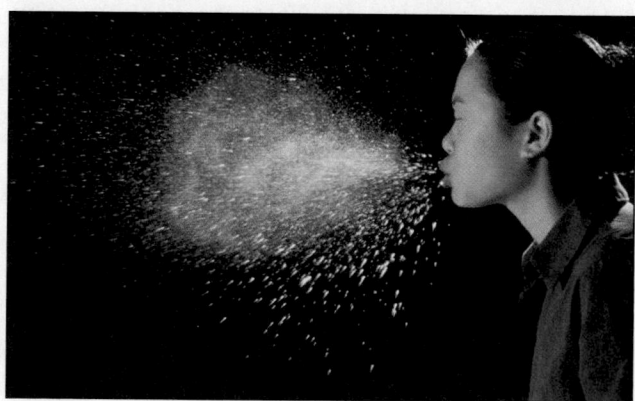

FIGURE 34.2 Droplet dispersion from a sneeze.

contaminate the local environment, contributing to indirect contact transmission.

AIRBORNE TRANSMISSION **Airborne transmission** can involve droplet nuclei, which have an average size of less than 5 microns, or dust. **Droplet nuclei**, the residue of evaporated droplets emitted from an infected host, such as someone with tuberculosis, can remain in the air for long periods. Dust particles containing an infectious agent (e.g., varicella virus) can also become airborne. The material is transmitted by air currents to a suitable portal of entry, usually the respiratory tract, of another person. The droplet nuclei are inhaled into the lower respiratory tract and are also deposited on the person's mucous membranes. Very few infectious agents are spread by airborne transmission: tuberculosis, varicella, measles, and, prior to its eradication, smallpox.

It should be noted that splashes and sprays of blood or bodily fluids represent neither droplet transmission, which is usually reserved for droplets of respiratory secretions, nor airborne transmission, which is very specific, as described above. This is often a source of confusion and misuse of terms, since the splashes or sprays are often in the form of droplets and "fly through the air." Depending on the conditions under which the splash or spray occurs, the mode of transmission would be considered either direct or indirect contact.

VEHICLE-BORNE TRANSMISSION In **vehicle-borne transmission**, a *vehicle* is any substance that serves as an intermediate means to transport and introduce an infectious agent into a susceptible host through a suitable portal of entry. *Fomites* (inanimate materials or objects), such as handkerchiefs, toys, soiled clothes, cooking or eating utensils, and surgical instruments or dressings, can act as vehicles. Water, food, milk, blood, serum, and plasma are other vehicles. For example, a food handler who carries the hepatitis A virus may contaminate food or water with fecal particles. A susceptible host then ingests the food. This is called the **fecal–oral route** of transmission, with the contaminated food acting as the vehicle.

VECTOR-BORNE TRANSMISSION A *vector* is an animal or insect that serves as an intermediate means of transporting the infectious agent. **Vector-borne transmission** can occur when salivary fluid is injected during biting or when feces or other materials are deposited on skin through the bite wound or a traumatized skin area.

Portal of Entry

Before a person can become infected, microorganisms must enter the body. The skin is a barrier to infectious agents; however, any break in skin can readily serve as a portal of entry. Other examples of portals of entry are the mucous membranes of the eyes, the respiratory tract, the gastrointestinal tract, or the bloodstream (e.g., with intravenous administration). Often, microorganisms enter the body of the host by the same route they used to leave the source.

Susceptibility of the Host

A **susceptible host** is any person who is at risk for infection. **Compromised hosts** are persons at increased risk, individuals who, for one or more reasons, are more likely than others to develop an infection. Impairment of the body's natural defences and a number of other factors can affect susceptibility to infection.

FACTORS INCREASING SUSCEPTIBILITY TO INFECTION Whether a microorganism causes an infection depends on a number of factors previously mentioned. One of the most important factors is host susceptibility, which is affected by age, immune status, heredity, level of stress, nutritional status, current medical therapy, obesity, smoking, existing disease processes, and previous surgery.

Age influences the risk of infection (see the Lifespan Considerations box). Newborns and older adults have reduced defences against infection. Infections are a major cause of death among newborns, who have immature immune systems and are protected only for the first 2 or 3 months by immunoglobulins passively received from the mother. Between 1 and 3 months of age, infants begin to synthesize their own immunoglobulins, and immunizations begin at 2 months. Immunizations are discussed later in the chapter.

With advancing age, the immune responses again weaken. Although much is still to be learned about aging, it is known that immunity to infection decreases with age. Because of the prevalence of influenza and pneumococcal pneumonia and their potential for causing death, the National Advisory Committee on Immunization (2011) recommends annual immunization against influenza for adults older than age 65 years; children aged 6 to 23 months; persons with chronic conditions, such as cardiac, respiratory, metabolic, and renal diseases; healthy pregnant women; Aboriginal peoples; and those capable of transmitting influenza to these individuals, such as health care providers and close family members. Adults 65 years and older and adults younger than 65 years with chronic conditions should receive one dose of pneumococcal vaccine.

Immune status is an important factor for host susceptibility or resistance to a specific infectious agent. The presence of antibodies from prior exposure, either by natural infection or **vaccination** (administration of an antigen—in the form of a vaccine—for the purpose of achieving immunization), will act to destroy the infectious agent when encountered again before it can lead to infection. **Immunization**, the process of developing antibodies to a particular disease through exposure to an antigen, is, therefore, an important strategy for decreasing host susceptibility, although not all infections are vaccine preventable.

Heredity influences the development of infection in that some people have a genetic susceptibility to certain infections. For example, some may be deficient in serum immunoglobulins, which play a significant role in the internal defence mechanisms of the body.

LIFESPAN CONSIDERATIONS

Infections

CHILDREN

Most children experience some kind of infection from time to time. The majority of these infections are caused by viruses and, for the most part, are transient, relatively benign, and overcome by the body's natural defences and supportive care. In some cases, severe, even life-threatening, infections occur. Considerations related to children include the following:

- Newborns may not be able to respond to infections because of an underdeveloped immune system. As a result, in the first few months of life, infections may not be associated with typical signs and symptoms (e.g., an infant with an infection may not have a fever).
- Newborns have some naturally acquired immunity transferred from the mother across the placenta.
- Breast-fed infants have higher levels of immunity against infections than formula-fed infants do.
- Children who are immunocompromised (e.g., leukemia, HIV) or have a chronic health condition (e.g., cystic fibrosis, sickle-cell anemia, congenital heart disease) need extra precautions to prevent exposure to infectious agents.
- Hand hygiene, comprehensive immunizations, good nutrition, adequate hydration, and appropriate rest are essential to preventing and treating infections in children.

- Handwashing and good hygiene in daycare and schools are important to prevent the spread of infections.
- Adolescents are at high risk for sexually transmitted infections; they should be well educated about how to prevent infections.

OLDER ADULTS

Normal aging may predispose older adults to increased risk of infection and delayed healing. Anatomical and physiological mechanisms that are protective when a person is younger often change in structure and function with increasing age, and the protective ability of those mechanisms decreases. Changes take place in skin, the respiratory tract, the gastrointestinal system, kidneys, and the immune system. If unchallenged, these systems work well to maintain homeostasis for the individual, but if compromised by stress, illness, infections, treatments, or surgeries, they often cannot keep up and, therefore, are not able to provide adequate protection. Special considerations for older adults are as follows:

- Nutrition can be poor in older adults and certain components, especially adequate protein, are necessary to maintain the immune system.
- Diabetes mellitus, which occurs more frequently in older adults, increases the risk of infection and delayed healing by causing an alteration in white blood cell function, and by impairing

peripheral circulation, which decreases the oxygen transport to the tissues.
- The immune system reacts slowly to the introduction of antigens, allowing the antigen to reproduce itself several times before it is recognized by the immune system. T cell effectiveness is often decreased because of immaturity.
- The normal inflammatory response is delayed. This delay often causes atypical responses to infections with unusual presentations. Instead of displaying redness, swelling, and fever usually associated with infections, atypical symptoms, such as confusion and disorientation, agitation, incontinence, falls, lethargy, and general fatigue, are often seen first.

Recognizing these changes in older adults is important in early detection and treatment of infections and to avoid delayed healing. The following nursing interventions promote prevention:

- Provide and teach ways to improve nutritional and hydration status and to avoid damaging skin.
- Use strict aseptic technique to decrease the chance of infections (especially HAIs in health care facilities).
- Encourage older adults to have immunizations for influenza annually and against pneumococcal pneumonia once.
- Be alert to subtle atypical signs of infection and act quickly to diagnose and treat.

The nature, number, and duration of physical and emotional *stressors* can influence susceptibility to infection. Stressors elevate blood cortisol. Prolonged elevation of blood cortisol decreases inflammatory and immune responses and, thus, decreases resistance to infection. For example, a person recovering from a major operation or injury is more likely to develop an infection than is a healthy person.

Resistance to infection depends on adequate *nutritional status*. Because antibodies are proteins, the ability to synthesize antibodies can be impaired by inadequate nutrition, especially when protein reserves are depleted (e.g., as a result of injury, surgery, or debilitating diseases, such as cancer).

Some *medical therapies* predispose a person to infection. Radiation treatments for cancer destroy not only cancerous cells but also some normal cells, including leukocytes, thereby damaging normal defences or barriers. Some *diagnostic procedures* can also predispose the client to an infection, especially when the skin is broken

or sterile body cavities are penetrated during the procedure. Certain *medications* also increase susceptibility to infection. Antineoplastic (anticancer) medications can depress bone marrow function, resulting in inadequate production of white blood cells necessary to combat infections. Anti-inflammatory medications, such as corticosteroids, inhibit the inflammatory response that is an essential defence against infection. Even some antibiotics that are used to treat infections can have adverse effects as they may destroy resident flora, allowing the proliferation of strains that would not grow and multiply in the body under normal conditions. *Clostridium difficile* infection, for example, is associated with antibiotic use. Certain antibiotics can also induce antibiotic resistance in some strains of microorganisms, making such infections difficult to treat (e.g., methicillin-resistant *Staphylococcus aureus* [MRSA], vancomycin-resistant *Staphylococcus aureus* [VRSA], vancomycin-resistant enterococci [VRE], and carbapenem-resistant *Enterobacteriaceae* [CRE]).

Obesity contributes to infection because it is associated with decreased blood flow to skin and underlying tissue. Delivery of oxygen, nutrients, and leukocytes is therefore compromised, interfering with both rapid elimination of infectious agents and tissue repair.

Smoking increases susceptibility to infection by damaging respiratory defences and by impairing tissue oxygenation. Oxygen is important to tissue maintenance and repair, and to the energy production required for the inflammatory and immune responses. Any situation that leads to tissue hypoxia, such as smoking, compromised blood flow, or *anemia*, will increase susceptibility to infection.

Any *disease* that lessens the body's defences against infection places the client at risk. Examples are chronic pulmonary disease, which impairs ciliary action and weakens the mucous barrier; peripheral vascular disease, which restricts blood flow; burns, which impair skin integrity; chronic or debilitating diseases, which deplete protein reserves; and such immune system diseases as leukemia and aplastic anemia, which alter the production of white blood cells. *Diabetes mellitus* is a major underlying disease predisposing clients to infection for a number of reasons. For example, glycosylation of hemoglobin and other proteins impairs oxygenation of tissues and disrupts leukocyte function (critical to phagocytosis). Increased serum glucose levels also provide a source of energy that will support bacterial growth.

Previous surgery at the same site can increase risk of infection because scar tissue has reduced blood supply, interfering with delivery of leukocytes, oxygen, and nutrients.

Breaking the Chain: Prevention and Control of Health Care–Associated Infections

The key to the prevention and control of infection is breaking one of the links in the chain of infection. Doing so can either prevent a new infection from occurring or realign an imbalance between the numbers of microorganisms and the host defence mechanisms to promote more rapid recovery from an existing infection. Many HAIs can be disrupted by (a) eliminating microorganisms and their reservoirs; (b) reducing transmission through the use of proper hand hygiene, the use of personal protective equipment to protect portals of entry, and the use of aseptic and sterile technique when warranted; and (c) supporting host defences or reducing susceptibility. Identification of clients at risk and implementation of appropriate strategies are essential aspects of infection prevention and control. Tables 34.5 and 34.6 summarize nursing interventions that break the chain of infection.

TABLE 34.5 Nursing Interventions That Break the Chain of Infection: Infectious Agent and Reservoir

Link	Interventions	Rationale
Etiological agent (microorganism)	Ensure that articles are correctly cleaned and disinfected or sterilized before use.	Correct cleaning, disinfecting, and sterilizing reduce or eliminate microorganisms.
	Educate clients and support persons about appropriate methods to clean, disinfect, and sterilize articles.	Knowledge of ways to reduce or eliminate microorganisms is a step in the direction of gaining compliance with aseptic practices.
Reservoir (source)	Change dressings and bandages when they are soiled or wet.	Moist dressings are ideal environments for microorganisms to grow and multiply.
	Assist clients to carry out appropriate hand, skin, and oral hygiene.	Hygiene measures reduce the numbers of resident and transient microorganisms and the likelihood of infection.
	Dispose of damp, soiled linens appropriately.	Damp, soiled linens provide a source of infectious agents that can be transmitted by indirect contact.
	Dispose of feces and urine in appropriate receptacles.	Urine and feces contain many microorganisms. Feces may also be the source of certain microorganisms, such as hepatitis A virus, in asymptomatic carriers.
	Empty suction and drainage containers at the end of each shift or before they become full, or according to agency policy.	Drainage harbours microorganisms that, if left for long periods, proliferate and are at risk for transmission to others.
Portal of exit	Avoid talking, coughing, or sneezing over open wounds or sterile fields, and cover the mouth and nose when coughing and sneezing.	These measures limit the number of microorganisms that escape from the respiratory tract.

TABLE 34.6 Nursing Interventions That Break the Chain of Infection: Transmission and Susceptible Host

Link	Interventions	Rationale
Mode of transmission	Perform hand hygiene between client contacts; after touching blood, any bodily fluids, or contaminated items; and before and after performing invasive procedures or touching open wounds. Instruct clients and support persons to perform hand hygiene before handling food or eating, after eliminating, and after touching infectious material.	Hand hygiene is an important means of controlling and preventing the transmission of microorganisms.
	Place discarded soiled materials in moisture-proof refuse bags.	Moisture-proof bags prevent the spread of microorganisms by capillary action.
	Cover used bedpans and hold away from clothing to prevent spillage, and dispose of urine and feces in appropriate receptacles.	Feces in particular contain many microorganisms.
	Place used bedpans on disposable bed pad, not directly on patient-use surfaces (e.g., overbed table). Avoid splashing when emptying.	Preventing contamination of the patients' environment can reduce transmission of organisms.
	Use routine practices (see page 989) for *all* clients at *all* times, regardless of their diagnosis or presumed infection status.	All clients can harbour potentially infectious microorganisms that can be transmitted to others.
	Wear masks and eye protection when in close contact with clients who have infections transmitted by droplets from the respiratory tract.	These reduce the spread of droplet-transmitted microorganisms.
	Wear masks and eye protection when splashes or sprays of body fluid are possible (e.g., during irrigation procedures).	Masks and eye protection provide protection from microorganisms in clients' blood, bodily fluids, nonintact skin, and mucous membranes.
	Wear gloves when handling secretions and excretions. Wear gowns if there is danger of soiling or contact of clothing with blood, any bodily fluids, nonintact skin, and mucous membranes.	Gloves and gowns prevent soiling of the hands and clothing.
	Place used disposable needles and syringes in puncture-resistant containers for disposal.	Injuries from needles contaminated by blood or bodily fluids from an infected client or carrier are a primary cause of hepatitis B virus (HBV) and HIV transmission to health care workers.
	Use sterile technique for invasive procedures (e.g., injections, catheterizations).	Invasive procedures penetrate the body's natural protective barriers to microorganisms.
Portal of entry	Use sterile technique when exposing open wounds or handling dressings	Open wounds are vulnerable to microbial infection.
	Provide all clients with their own personal care items.	People have less resistance to another person's microorganisms than to their own.
Susceptible host	Maintain the integrity of the client's skin and mucous membranes.	Intact skin and mucous membranes protect against invasion by microorganisms.
	Ensure that the client receives a balanced diet.	A balanced diet supplies proteins and vitamins necessary to build or maintain body tissues.
	Educate the public about the importance of immunizations.	Immunizations protect people against some infectious diseases.

It should be noted that there are multiple layers of prevention and control measures, often referred to as the *hierarchy of controls*. Some, such as engineering controls, relate to construction of a physically safe environment, such as having adequate ventilation and appropriate placement of sharps containers. Others, such as administrative controls, promote safe practice, for example, via adequate resources, education, and policies and procedures. The use of personal protective equipment is the third layer of control. While under the control of the individual nurse, its effectiveness is reduced if engineering and administrative controls are ineffective.

Elimination of Microorganisms and Reservoirs

The first links in the chain, the etiological agent (i.e., microorganism) and the reservoir, are disrupted by a variety of strategies. Some reservoirs can be physically eliminated or reduced, for example, through removal and proper disposal of contaminated dressings, frequent emptying of catheter bags, or replacement of contaminated oxygen equipment. Other reservoirs can be affected through decontamination or antimicrobial agents.

DECONTAMINATION Decontamination has three levels: (a) cleaning, (b) disinfecting, and (c) sterilizing. These are important for reducing infections caused by exogenous flora from the environment or transmitted through equipment or other materials. Items should be cleaned before being disinfected or sterilized. Items intended for single-use should be discarded and not processed for reuse.

Cleaning Cleaning physically removes contaminants (e.g., fluids and microorganisms) with detergent and mechanical removal. Cleaning is the lowest level of decontamination and is appropriate for items used on intact skin. When cleaning visibly soiled objects, nurses must always wear appropriate personal protective equipment, such as gloves, impervious gowns, and facial protection, to avoid direct contact with infectious microorganisms. Most objects used in the care of patients, whether forceps or draw sheets, can be cleaned by rinsing them in cold water to remove any organic material, washing them with hot soapy water, then rinsing them again to remove the soap; equipment should be cleaned following manufacturers' recommendations and using appropriate cleaning agents. The following general steps should be followed when cleaning objects in a hospital or in a home:

1. Rinse the article with cold water to remove organic material. Hot water coagulates the protein of organic material and tends to make it adhere. Examples of organic material are blood, pus, and respiratory secretions.

2. Wash the article in hot water and soap. The emulsifying action of soap reduces surface tension and facilitates the removal of dirt. Washing dislodges the emulsified dirt.

3. Use an abrasive, such as a stiff-bristled brush, to clean equipment with grooves and corners. Friction helps dislodge foreign material.

4. Rinse the article well with warm to hot water.

5. Dry the article. It is now considered clean.

6. Clean the brush and sink. These are considered soiled until they are cleaned appropriately, usually with a disinfectant.

Disinfecting Disinfection reduces the number of microorganisms but will not eliminate them all, and it does not kill most spores. It provides a medium level of decontamination and is appropriate for items that have contact with mucous membranes or nonintact skin, or are contaminated by microorganisms that are easily transmitted. A **disinfectant** is a chemical preparation, such as phenol or iodine compounds, used on inanimate objects. In comparison, an **antiseptic** is a chemical preparation used on skin or tissue. Disinfectants are frequently caustic and toxic to tissues. Disinfectants and antiseptics often have similar chemical components, but the disinfectant is a more concentrated solution. Disinfectants are able to destroy a variety of pathogens but are ineffective against spores. Table 34.7 lists commonly used antiseptics and disinfectants.

Both antiseptics and disinfectants are said to have bactericidal or bacteriostatic properties. A *bactericidal* preparation destroys bacteria, whereas a *bacteriostatic* preparation prevents the growth and reproduction of some bacteria.

TABLE 34.7 Commonly Used Antiseptics and Disinfectants: Effectiveness and Effective against

Agent	Effective against					Use on
	Bacteria	Tuberculosis	Spores	Fungi	Viruses	
Isopropyl and ethyl alcohol	×	×		×	×	Hands, vial stoppers
Chlorine (bleach)	×	×	×	×	×	Blood spills
Hydrogen peroxide	×	×	×	×	×	Surfaces
Iodophors	×	×	×	×	×	Equipment; intact skin and tissues if diluted
Phenol	×	×		×	×	Surfaces
Chlorhexidine gluconate	×				×	Hands
Triclosan	×					Hands, intact skin

When disinfecting articles, nurses need to follow agency protocols and manufacturer recommendations and consider the following:

1. The type and number of infectious organisms (Some microorganisms are readily destroyed, whereas others require longer contact with the disinfectant.)

2. The recommended concentration of the disinfectant and the duration of contact

3. The temperature of the environment (Most disinfectants are intended for use at room temperature.)

4. The presence of soap (Some disinfectants are ineffective in the presence of soap or detergent.)

5. The presence of organic materials (The presence of saliva, blood, pus, or excretions can prevent contact between the disinfectant and the actual surface to be decontaminated.)

6. The surface areas to be treated (The disinfecting agent must come into contact with all surfaces and areas; the presence of lumens, hinges and crevices must be accommodated.)

Sterilizing **Sterilization** is a process that destroys *all* microorganisms, including spores and viruses. It provides the highest level of decontamination and is indicated for items that penetrate skin or mucous membranes, or enter sterile body areas. Three commonly used methods of sterilization are (a) moist heat, (b) gas, and (c) boiling water.

Moist Heat For sterilizing, moist heat (steam) can be employed in two ways: (a) as steam under pressure or (b) as free steam. Steam under pressure (autoclave) attains temperatures higher than the boiling point. The time required to sterilize an item relates to how long it takes to destroy spores at the temperature of the autoclave, which varies from 15 minutes at 121°C to 3 minutes at 134°C.

Free steam, 100°C, is used to sterilize objects that would be destroyed at the higher temperature and pressure of the autoclave. Usually, it is necessary to steam the article for 30 minutes on 3 consecutive days. The intervals are required so that unkilled spores will return to their vegetative state and again become vulnerable to the heat.

Gas Ethylene oxide gas destroys microorganisms by interfering with their metabolic processes. It is also effective against spores. Its advantages are good penetration and effectiveness for heat-sensitive items. Its major disadvantage is its toxicity to humans.

Boiling Water Boiling water is the most practical and inexpensive method for sterilizing in the home but is not recommended for use in health care facilities. The main disadvantage is that spores and some viruses are not killed by this method. The water temperature rises no higher than 100°C. Boiling a minimum of 15 minutes is advised for disinfection of articles in the home.

Nurses should be familiar with the cleaning, disinfecting, and sterilizing protocols of the agency where they practise.

ANTIMICROBIAL AGENTS **Antimicrobial agents** kill or slow the growth of infectious agents. Antibiotics or antiviral drugs can reduce the number of infectious agents present in the host, allowing the body's defences to eliminate them. Antibiotics, for example, are given at the start of surgery to reduce the number of bacteria at the surgical site at the time of the incision, thereby reducing surgical site infection. Antiseptics, antimicrobial agents that remove both transient and resident flora on living tissue (e.g., skin), are also used to reduce the number of infectious agents present near the site of a surgical incision or insertion point (e.g., for an intravenous line or chest tube). Their use reduces the number of infections caused by the client's endogenous flora.

Reduction of Transmission

The transmission of microorganisms can be reduced through the use of proper hand hygiene, the use of personal protective equipment to protect portals of entry, and the use of aseptic technique when warranted. Nurses must do a **point of care risk assessment**, that is, a risk assessment prior to each individual encounter with a client, to identify the most appropriate strategies to implement to reduce transmission.

HAND HYGIENE The importance of hand hygiene in every setting, including homes and hospitals, cannot be overemphasized. It is considered to be the single most effective infection prevention and control measure one can implement. Any person can harbour microorganisms that are currently harmless yet potentially harmful to that person or to others *if they find a portal of entry*. As a health care worker's hands are in continuous contact with clients and their environments, those hands are most at risk for contamination with organisms. Subsequent transfer of the microorganisms to other clients and health care personnel, to the environment, or to the health care worker involved might then occur. It is critical that hands be cleaned frequently and correctly. The term **hand hygiene** refers to both handwashing and the use of alcohol-based hand rub.

Handwashing with soap and water physically removes transient microorganisms carried on the hands but not resident flora. **Alcohol-based hand rub (ABHR)**, available in liquid, gel, and foam formulations, kills microorganisms on the hands and is more effective than soap and water in reducing hand contamination. ABHR facilitates hand hygiene compliance because of ease of accessibility, reduced time required to perform, and reduced skin irritation. Use of ABHR, at the point of care, is therefore the preferred method of hand hygiene. ABHR does, however, have reduced effectiveness when there is physical material on the hands, such as secretions. When there is visible

BOX 34.2 RECOMMENDATIONS FOR HAND HYGIENE

Indications for the frequency of hand hygiene depend on the following:

- The type, intensity, duration, and sequence of activity
- The degree of contamination associated with the contact
- The susceptibility to infection of the health care recipient

According to the Four Moments of Hand Hygiene (Figure 34.3), hand hygiene must be performed at these times:

1. Before initial contact with the client/client's environment

- Before contact with a client or the client's environment, even if gloves are worn. This includes between direct contact with individual clients

2. Before aseptic procedures or contact with a portal of entry

- Before performing invasive procedures
- Before preparing, handling, serving, or eating food, and before feeding a patient or preparing food or oral medications

3. After exposure or potential exposure to contamination

- After contact with blood or bodily fluids, or items known or considered likely to be contaminated with blood, bodily fluids, secretions, or excretions
- Between certain procedures on the same patient where soiling of hands is likely, to avoid cross-contamination of body sites
- After situations or procedures in which microbial or blood contamination of hands is likely
- Immediately after removing gloves

4. After contact with the client/client's environment. Perform hand hygiene with soap and water rather than ABHR:

- When hands are visibly soiled or contaminated with organic material
- After caring for a patient with *C. difficile* or norovirus infection
- Immediately after using toilet facilities

Source: Canadian Hospital Infection Control Association (CHICA) - Canada: Information about hand hygiene. Available at http://www.chica.org/links_handhygiene.php.

soiling, or the client has a *C. difficile* or norovirus infection, hands should be washed before or instead of using ABHR. The World Health Organization has identified five indications for hand hygiene, called the "Five Moments for Hand Hygiene": (1) before patient contact, (2) before aseptic technique, (3) after body fluid exposure risk, (4) after patient contact, and (5) after contact with patient surroundings. The Canadian Patient Safety Institute has collapsed the last two moments into one, so most Canadian jurisdictions promote the "Four Moments of Hand Hygiene," shown in Figure 34.3 (Provincial Infectious Diseases Advisory Committee [PIDAC], 2009). Box 34.2 summarizes the indications for hand hygiene and provides examples of activities relevant to each "moment". Practice guidelines related to nail and hand care are summarized in Practice Guidelines 34.1.

Skill 34.1 describes correct hand hygiene techniques. Removal of jewellery, using an adequate amount of product (ABHR or soap), covering all surfaces of the hand (particularly between fingers, fingertips, and back

of hands), and allowing adequate contact time are elements common to both methods for hand hygiene. Manufacturers' instructions should be followed for the amount of ABHR to use and hands should be rubbed until the hands feel dry, usually 15 to 30 seconds. Paper towels should not be used with ABHR and the product should be applied to dry hands so as not to dilute the alcohol. With handwashing, additional elements of correct technique are rubbing the hands together to create friction, ensuring that rinsing occurs under running water, and turning off the tap with a paper towel. Plain soap will successfully remove most transient microbial flora; antimicrobial (antiseptic) soap is not indicated for most hand hygiene but may be used prior to prolonged invasive procedures, when residual antimicrobial activity may be desirable. Soap and sink manufacturers' recommendations should be adhered to for proper use.

The decisions as to what product to use, the amount of ABHR or soap to use, the frequency of performing hand hygiene, as well as the actual technique implemented

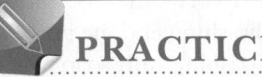

PRACTICE GUIDELINES 34.1

Nail and Hand Care for Nurses

Guideline	Rationale
Nails should be kept short.	Short, natural nails are less likely to harbour microorganisms, scratch a client, or puncture gloves.
Fingernail polish or artificial nails should not be used.	Both can harbour microorganisms.
Hands should be regularly assessed for breaks in skin, such as hangnails or cuts. Lotions should be used frequently to prevent hangnails and cracked, dry skin.	A nurse who has broken skin areas may have to change work assignments with decreased risk for transmission of infectious organisms or wear gloves for protection.

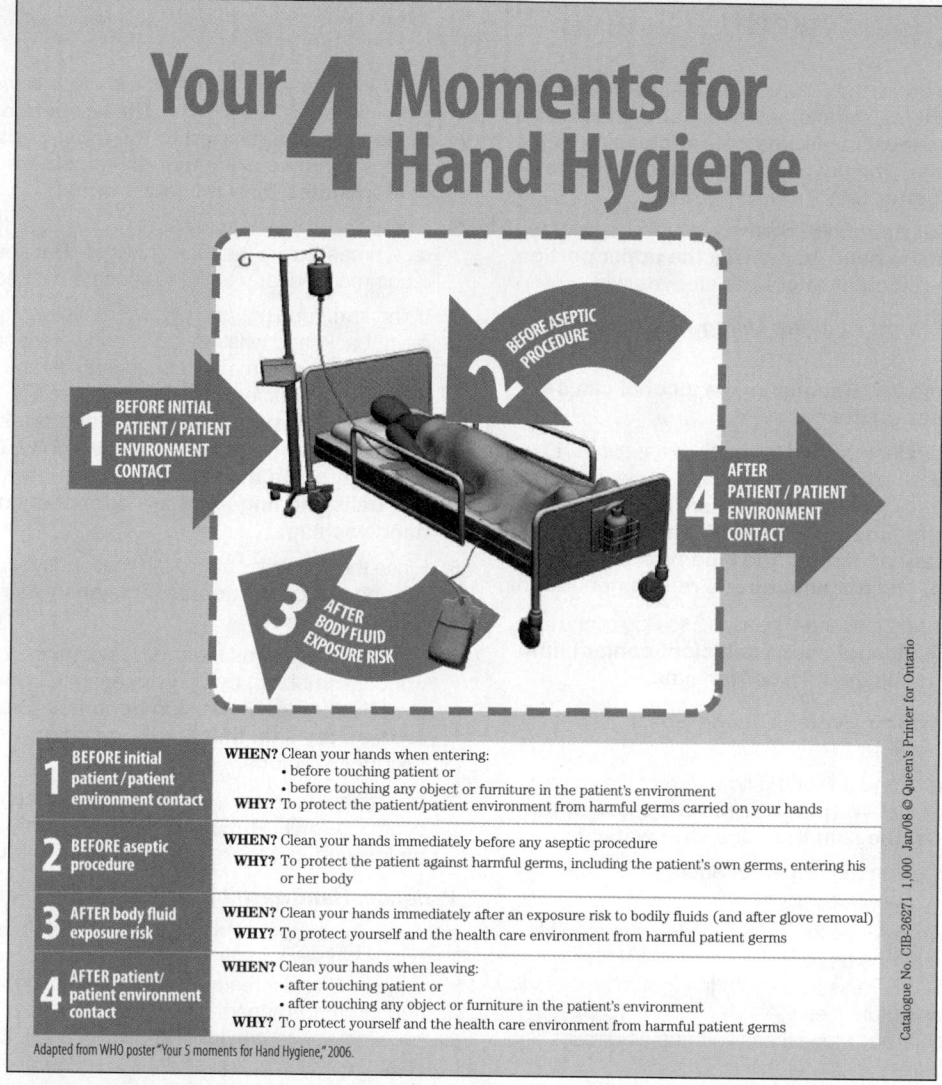

FIGURE 34.3 Four Moments of Hand Hygiene.

Source: Reproduced with permission from "Just Clean Your Hands." Ontario's hand hygiene program for hospitals. Retrieved from http://www.justcleanyourhands.ca/pdf/10_1_4_moment_poster_Eng.pdf

SKILL 34.1   HAND HYGIENE

PURPOSES

- To reduce the number of microorganisms on the hands
- To reduce the risk of transmission of microorganisms to clients and between clients
- To reduce the risk of transmission of infectious organisms to oneself

ASSESSMENT

Assess the nature of the interaction with the client, the degree of likely contamination associated with the contact, and whether the interaction is one of the indications for hand hygiene.

PLANNING

Determine the location of alcohol-based hand rub (ABHR) or running water and soap.

Equipment

- Alcohol-based hand rub

or

- Soap, warm running water, and disposable towels if washing hands

IMPLEMENTATION

Preparation

- If performing hand hygiene where the client can observe you, introduce yourself and explain to the client what you are going to do and why it is necessary.
- Remove all jewellery. Some nurses prefer to slide their watches up above their elbows. Others pin the watch to the uniform. Rings should be removed or moved so that the

(continued)

SKILL 34.1 HAND HYGIENE (continued)

skin below can be washed. **Rationale: Microorganisms can lodge in the settings of jewellery and under rings on fingers. Removal facilitates proper cleaning of the hands and arms. The jewellery itself also needs to be washed. It is better to not wear it at all.**

- Push up sleeves. **Rationale: Sleeves inhibit contact with all surfaces of the hand, especially the upper portion, as nurses are reluctant to get the sleeves wet.**

Performance of Hand Hygiene Using Alcohol-Based Hand Rub

1. Ensure hands are dry. **Rationale: The alcohol can be diluted by water on the hands.**

2. Use sufficient product to cover all parts of the hands (including between fingers, fingertips, and back of hands) and rub thoroughly (see ❶). **Rationale: This ensures use of adequate amounts of ABHR. The amount to be used will vary according the type of product (e.g., liquid or foam) and manufacturer's recommendations.**

3. Rub until the hands feel dry—usually 15 to 30 seconds. **Rationale: The alcohol needs sufficient contact time with the skin to kill the microorganisms.**

Performance of Hand Hygiene Using Soap and Water

1. Turn on the water and adjust the flow so that the water is warm. **Rationale: Warm water removes less of the protective oil of the skin than does hot water.**

   - There are five common types of faucet controls:
     a. Hand-operated handles
     b. Knee levers: Move these with the knee to regulate flow and temperature
     c. Foot pedals: Press these with the foot to regulate flow and temperature (see ❷).
     d. Elbow controls: Move these with the elbows instead of the hands.
     e. Infrared controls (ideal): The water runs when motion is detected at a preset distance.

2. Wet the hands thoroughly by holding them under the running water, and apply soap to the hands. Hold the hands lower than the elbows so that the water flows from the arms to the fingertips. **Rationale: The water should flow from the least contaminated to the most contaminated area; the hands are generally considered more contaminated than the lower arms.**

3. If the soap is liquid, apply 2 mL to 5 mL, or the amount recommended by the manufacturer. (Bar soap is not recommended for use by health care workers.)

4. Using firm, rubbing, and circular movements, wash the palm, back, and wrist of each hand. Interlace the fingers and thumbs, and move the hands back and forth continuing this motion for *at least* 15 seconds (see ❸). Ensure all areas are covered. **Rationale: Friction and brisk action help remove microorganisms mechanically. Interlacing the fingers and thumbs cleans the interdigital spaces. The nails and fingertips are commonly missed during handwashing.**

5. Rinse the hands for at least 10 seconds by using a rubbing motion. **Rationale: This ensures removal of microorganisms.**

6. Dry hands and arms thoroughly from fingertips to wrist, without scrubbing, by using a separate paper towel for each arm. **Rationale: Moist skin becomes chapped readily, as does dry skin that is rubbed vigorously; chapping produces lesions.**

7. Use a dry, clean paper towel to grasp a hand-operated control (see ❹). **Rationale: This prevents the nurse from picking up microorganisms from the faucet handles.**

Variation: Handwashing before Sterile Techniques

- Apply the soap and wash as described above, but hold the hands higher than the elbows during this handwash. Wet the hands and forearms under the running water, letting it run from the fingertips to the elbows so that the hands become cleaner than the elbows (see ❺). Ensure that at least 2 minutes of friction is used for surgical handwashing. **Rationale: In this way, the water runs from the area with the fewest microorganisms to areas with a relatively greater number.**

- After washing and rinsing, use a towel to dry one hand thoroughly in an encircling motion from the fingers to the elbow. Use a clean towel to dry the other hand and arm. **Rationale: A clean towel prevents the transfer of microorganisms from one elbow (least clean area) to the other hand (cleanest area).**

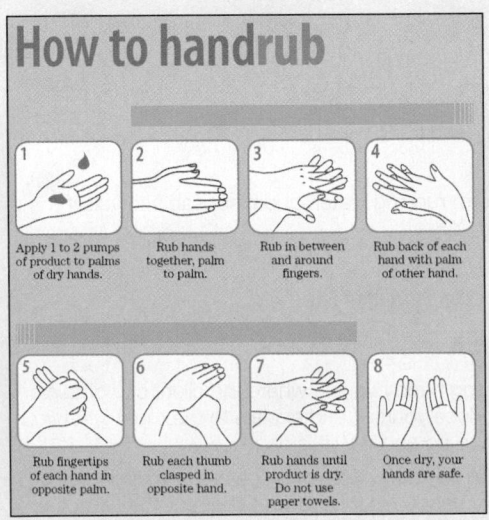

How to handrub

1. Apply 1 to 2 pumps of product to palms of dry hands.
2. Rub hands together, palm to palm.
3. Rub in between and around fingers.
4. Rub back of each hand with palm of other hand.
5. Rub fingertips of each hand in opposite palm.
6. Rub each thumb clasped in opposite hand.
7. Rub hands until product is dry. Do not use paper towels.
8. Once dry, your hands are safe.

❶ How to handrub.

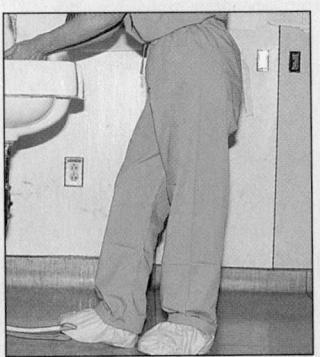

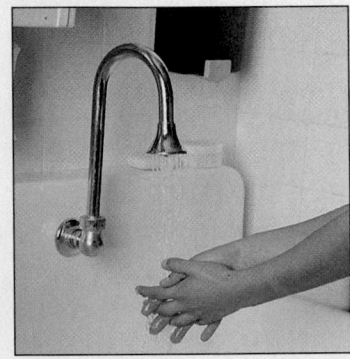

❷ A foot-pedal faucet control.

❸ Interlacing the fingers during handwashing.

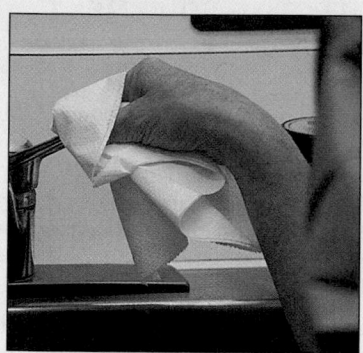

4 Using a paper towel to grasp the handle of a hand-operated faucet.

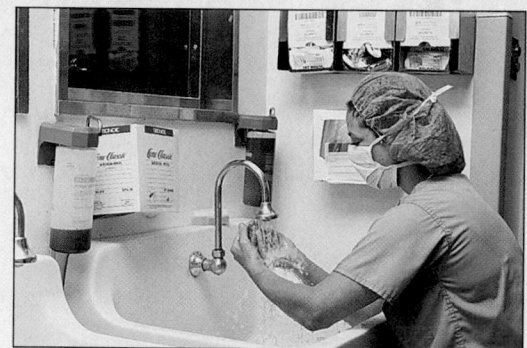

5 Hands are held higher than elbows during a handwash before sterile technique.

EVALUATION

No traditional evaluation exists for the effectiveness of the individual nurse's hand hygiene in preventing infection in a particular client. Some studies, however, have shown reductions in HAIs when hand hygiene rates increase. Health care facilities increasingly perform regular audits of hand hygiene by health care workers, assessing whether hand hygiene was performed when indicated as well as adequacy of technique.

remain with the health care worker, based on their point of care risk assessment. They are decisions that must be made with an unrelentingly conscientious attitude.

PERSONAL PROTECTIVE EQUIPMENT **Personal protective equipment (PPE)** acts as a barrier to reduce a health care worker's exposure to microorganisms and reduce carriage of microorganisms by the health care worker on hands and clothes. PPE includes gloves, gowns, facial protection (face masks and eyewear) and respirators. The point of care risk assessment also helps the health care worker determine what PPE are appropriate for the encounter.

Gloves Gloves are worn for three reasons. First, they protect the hands when the nurse is likely to handle or have contact with any of the body substances, for example, blood, urine, feces, sputum, mucus, and nonintact skin. Second, gloves reduce the likelihood of nurses transmitting their own endogenous microorganisms to individuals receiving care. Nurses who have open sores or cuts on the hands must wear gloves to both prevent exposure of others to their own microorganisms and to reduce exposure to others' microorganisms. Third, gloves reduce the chance

that the nurse's hands will transmit microorganisms from one client or a fomite to another client. In all situations, gloves are changed between client contacts. Hand hygiene must be performed each time gloves are removed for two primary reasons: (a) The gloves may have imperfections or be damaged during wearing so that they could allow microorganisms to pass through to the skin; and (b) the hands may become contaminated during glove removal.

For most activities, disposable *clean* gloves are used. The type of glove chosen should be based on the task to be performed; the correct size should be worn. Sterile gloves, discussed later in the chapter, are used when the hands will come in contact with an open wound or when the hands might introduce microorganisms into a body orifice that is normally considered sterile.

No special technique is required to don clean disposable gloves. If a gown is worn, the nurse pulls up the gloves to cover the cuffs of the gown. If a gown is not worn, the nurse pulls up the cuffs to cover the wrists. Skill 34.2 describes application and removal of nonsterile gloves.

Many of the gloves used are made of latex rubber. As a result of the frequent use of gloves, health care workers and clients with chronic illnesses have increasingly

SKILL 34.2 DONNING AND REMOVING PERSONAL PROTECTIVE EQUIPMENT (GLOVES, GOWN, MASK, EYEWEAR)

PURPOSE

- To protect health care workers and clients from transmission of potentially infective materials

ASSESSMENT

Consider which activities will be required while the nurse is in the client's room and what the potential exposure might be to blood, body fluids, nonintact skin, mucous membranes, and contaminated objectives or surfaces. Identify the personal protective equipment (PPE) needed, if any, given the potential exposure.

PLANNING

- Application and removal of PPE can be time consuming. Prioritize care and arrange for personnel to care for your other clients' if indicated.

(continued)

SKILL 34.2 **DONNING AND REMOVING PERSONAL PROTECTIVE EQUIPMENT (GLOVES, GOWN, MASK, EYEWEAR)** (*continued*)

- Determine which supplies are present within the client's room and which must be brought to the room.
- Consider whether special handling is indicated for removal of any specimens or other materials from the room.

Equipment

As indicated, according to which activities will be performed. Ensure that extra supplies are easily available.

- Gown
- Facial protection (mask and eye protection)
- Clean gloves

IMPLEMENTATION

Preparation

Remove and secure all loose items, such as name tags or jewellery.

Performance

1. Before performing the procedure, introduce yourself and verify the patient's identity using two identifiers or per agency protocol. Explain to the client what you are going to do, why it is necessary, and how he or she can participate.

2. Perform proper hand hygiene.

3. Don a clean gown.
   - Pick up a clean gown, and allow it to unfold in front of you without allowing it to touch any area soiled with body substances.
   - Slide the arms and the hands through the sleeves.
   - Fasten the ties at the neck to keep the gown in place.
   - Overlap the gown at the back as much as possible, and fasten the waist ties or belt (see ❶). **Rationale: Overlapping securely covers the uniform at the back. Waist ties keep the gown from falling away from the body, which can cause inadvertent soiling of the uniform.**

4. Don the face mask.
   - Locate the top edge of the mask. The mask usually has a narrow metal strip along the edge.
   - Hold the mask by the top two strings or loops.
   - Place the upper edge of the mask over the bridge of the nose, and tie the upper ties at the back of the head or secure the loops around the ears. If glasses are worn, fit the upper edge of the mask under the glasses. **Rationale: With the edge of the mask under the glasses, clouding of the glasses is less likely to occur.**
   - Secure the lower edge of the mask under the chin, and tie the lower ties at the nape of the neck (see ❷). **Rationale: To be effective, a mask must cover both the nose and the mouth because air moves in and out of both.**
   - If the mask has a metal strip, adjust this firmly over the bridge of the nose. **Rationale: A secure fit prevents both the escape and the inhalation of**

microorganisms around the edges of the mask and the fogging of eyeglasses.

   - Wear the mask only once, and do not wear any mask longer than the manufacturer recommends or once it becomes wet. **Rationale: A mask should be used only once because it becomes ineffective when moist.**
   - Do not leave a used face mask hanging around the neck.

5. Don protective eyewear if it is not combined with the face mask.

6. Don clean disposable gloves.
   - No special technique is required.
   - If wearing a gown, pull up the gloves to cover the cuffs of the gown. If not wearing a gown, pull up the gloves to cover the wrists.

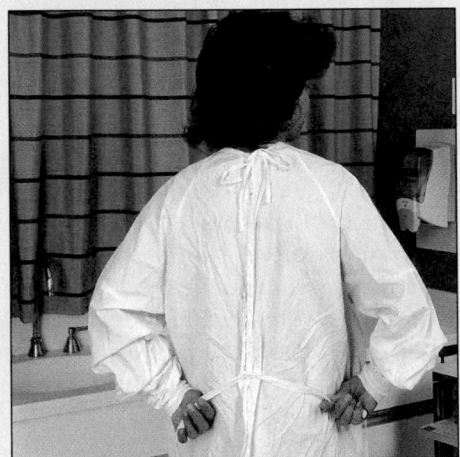

❶ Overlapping the gown at the back to cover the nurse's uniform.

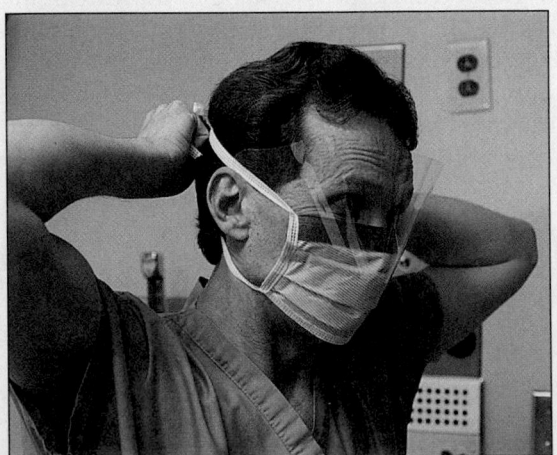

❷ A face mask and eye protection covering the nose, mouth, and eyes.

7. To remove soiled PPE, remove the gloves first since they are the most soiled.

   - If wearing a gown that is tied at the waist in front, undo the ties before removing gloves. If wearing a gown that is tied at the back, remove the gloves first.

   - Remove the first glove by grasping it on its palmar surface, taking care to touch only glove to glove (see ❸). **Rationale: This keeps the soiled parts of the used gloves from touching the skin of the wrist or hand.**

   - Pull off the first glove completely by inverting or rolling the glove inside out.

   - Continue to hold the inverted removed glove by the fingers of the remaining gloved hand. Place the first two fingers of the bare hand inside the cuff of the second glove (see ❹). **Rationale: Touching the outside of the second soiled glove with the bare hand is avoided.**

   - Pull off the second glove to the fingers by turning it inside out. This pulls the first glove inside the second glove. **Rationale: The soiled part of the glove is folded to the inside to reduce the chance of transferring any microorganisms by direct contact.**

   - By using the bare hand, continue to remove the gloves, which are now inside out, and dispose of them in the refuse container (see ❺).

8. Remove the gown when preparing to leave the room or following completion of the task for which use of the gown was indicated, whichever is appropriate. Even if a gown is not grossly soiled, it should be removed as though the outside of the gown had been contaminated during use. Do the following:

   - Avoid touching the outside of the gown, if possible. **Rationale: The outside of the gown may be soiled or contaminated, for example, if you have been holding an infant who has a respiratory infection.**

   - Grasp the gown along the inside of the neck and pull down over the shoulders.

   - Roll up the gown with the soiled or potentially contaminated part inside, and discard it in the appropriate container.

9. Perform proper hand hygiene. **Rationale: Hands may have become contaminated during the removal of the gown and gloves. Hand hygiene performed at this point will prevent transmission of microorganisms to the face, eyes, nose, or mouth during removal of facial protection.**

10. Remove facial protection at the doorway of the client's room or following completion of the task for which facial protection was indicated. Note: If using an N95 respirator, remove it AFTER leaving the room and CLOSING the door.

    - If the facial protection used is a single piece of equipment, remove it and dispose of it properly or place in an appropriate receptacle for cleaning.

    - If mask and protective eyewear are used as separate pieces of equipment, remove the protective eyewear first then remove the mask. Dispose of items properly or place in the appropriate receptacle for cleaning.

    - If using a mask with strings, first untie the *lower* strings of the mask. **Rationale: This prevents the top part of the mask from falling onto the chest.**

    - Untie the top strings and, while holding the ties securely, remove the mask from the face. If side loops

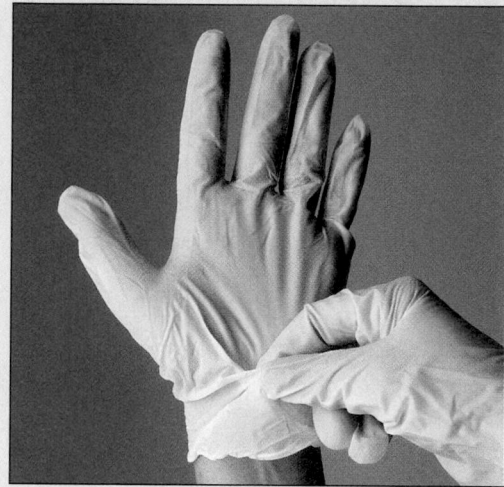

❸ Plucking the palmar surface below the cuff of a contaminated glove.

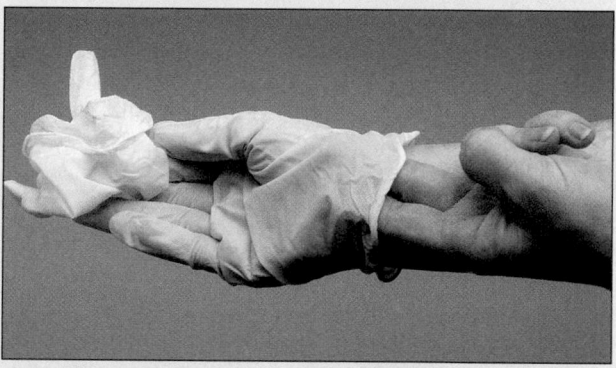

❹ Inserting fingers to remove the second contaminated glove.

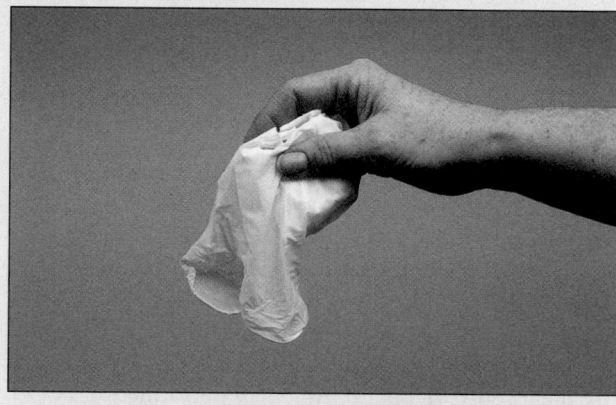

❺ Holding contaminated gloves, which are inside out.

are present, lift the side loops up and away from the ears and face. Do not touch the front of the mask. **Rationale: The front of the mask through which the nurse has been breathing is contaminated.**

- Remove an N95 respirator in a fashion similar to removal of a mask, handling the N95 respirator by its straps and not touching the front part of the N95 respirator.

(continued)

SKILL 34.2	**DONNING AND REMOVING PERSONAL PROTECTIVE EQUIPMENT (GLOVES, GOWN, MASK, EYEWEAR)** (*continued*)

- Discard a disposable mask or N95 respirator in the waste container.
- Perform proper hand hygiene again. **Rationale: Hands may have become contaminated during the removal** of the facial protection. Hand hygiene is done at this point to prevent transmission of microorganisms to the environment or other clients.

EVALUATION

- Conduct any follow-up indicated during your care of the client. If any failure of the equipment has occurred and exposure to potentially infective materials is suspected, follow the steps in Box 34.5 later in this chapter (p. 997).

- Ensure that an adequate supply of equipment is available for the next health care provider.

---

reported allergic reactions to latex. In addition, latex gloves lubricated by powder or cornstarch are particularly allergenic because the latex allergen adheres to the powder, which is aerosolized during glove use and inhaled by the user. Though labelled *hypoallergenic*, latex gloves still contain measurable latex and should not be used by or on persons with known latex sensitivity. The people at greatest risk for developing latex allergies are those with other allergic conditions and those who have had frequent or long-term exposure to latex.

Latex allergies can be either local or systemic and may take the form of dermatitis, urticaria (hives), bronchospasm, or anaphylaxis. Clients and health care workers should be assessed for possible allergies by taking a thorough history. Clients should be asked if they have had any adverse reactions to such items as balloons, condoms, and dishwashing or utility gloves. Strategies to avoid sensitization or exposure to latex include use of latex-free products, latex-free barriers between latex products and skin, and unpowdered gloves. People with significant allergies should have no contact with latex products. Health care agencies are increasingly providing alternatives to latex equipment and supplies, including vinyl or nitrile gloves.

Gowns   Clean or disposable water-resistant gowns or plastic aprons are worn during procedures when the nurse's uniform is likely to become soiled. *Single use of a gown* (using a gown only once before it is discarded or laundered) is the usual practice in health care agencies. After the gown is worn, the nurse discards paper gowns or places linen gowns in a laundry hamper. Before leaving the patient's room, the nurse makes sure that hand hygiene is performed.

Sterile gowns may be indicated when the nurse changes the dressings of a patient with extensive wounds (e.g., burns).

A gown worn for protection is always assumed to have become contaminated during use. Skill 34.2 provides guidelines for donning and removing a gown.

Facial Protection: Face Masks and Eyewear   During certain techniques requiring sterile technique, masks are worn to prevent droplet contact transmission of exhaled microorganisms to the sterile field or to a patient's open wound. Masks are also worn as part of routine practices to protect the nurse from splashes of body substances from the patient. Surgical and procedure masks protect the wearer's mouth and nose and, thus, are worn to reduce the risk for transmission of organisms by droplet contact and by splashes or sprays of body substances. In addition to health care personnel, family members and others who are close to the client should wear masks if the infection (e.g., mumps or acute respiratory diseases in children) is transmitted by droplet transmission.

Protective eyewear (goggles, glasses, or face shields) are indicated along with masks in situations in which respiratory secretions or other bodily fluids, including blood, may have contact with the face, thereby allowing entry of microorganisms through the eyes as well as the nose, mouth, or respiratory tract. If the nurse wears prescription eyeglasses, goggles must still be worn over the glasses because the protection must extend around the sides of the glasses. Guidelines for donning and removing face masks and eyewear are found in Skill 34.2. Special care must be taken to avoid self-contamination when removing the mask or eyewear.

Various types of masks differ in their filtration effectiveness and fit. Single-use disposable surgical masks are effective for use when the nurse provides care to most clients but should be changed if they become wet or soiled. These masks are discarded in the waste container after use.

Respirators   Surgical masks do not create a tight seal around the mouth and nose so that not all of the air breathed by the wearer is filtered through the mask itself. The loose weave of the material is also such that they are not effective against smaller droplets and droplet nuclei. Disposable particulate **respirators** are masks made of a high-filtration material and are designed to create a tight seal around the mouth and nose. An N95-level respirator filters out at least 95% of airborne particles under standard conditions, excluding oil particles (the *N* of N95 stands for *not resistant to oil*).

Respirators need to be fitted—health care providers need to choose a size and style of respirator mask that allows a good seal. Since faces vary in shape and size and facial hair, not every individual can use the same size and style of respirator and obtain a good seal. Most institutions provide a selection of respirators; assessing an individual for an appropriate respirator is called **fit testing**. Fit testing is done by an appropriately trained individual. Although done in some places on an annual basis, regulations vary by jurisdiction as to the frequency with which fit testing must occur. **Fit checking** means assessing the adequacy of the seal (see photo and caption in item 6 of Figure 34.4). It is done by the wearer on donning the respirator and should be done each time a respirator is worn.

Respirators should be worn by all persons entering the room when the infection (e.g., pulmonary tuberculosis) is transmitted by the airborne route and the individual

is not immune (e.g., to measles or varicella). Respirators should also be worn during certain aerosol-generating medical procedures (e.g., bronchoscopy or suctioning).

Guidelines for donning and removing a respirator are similar to those for donning and removing a facemask; however, the respirator is removed after leaving the patient's room and special care must be taken to avoid self-contamination when removing the respirator (see Figure 34.4).

Sterile and Aseptic Technique *Asepsis* means "without infection" and implies the absence of disease-causing microorganisms. To decrease the possibility of transferring

Application

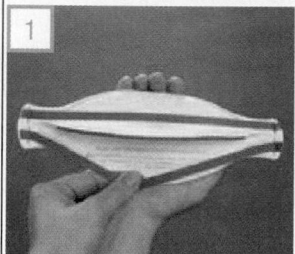

1. Remove the respirator from its packaging and hold with straps facing upward. Place the bottom strap under the centre flaps next to the "WARNING" statement.

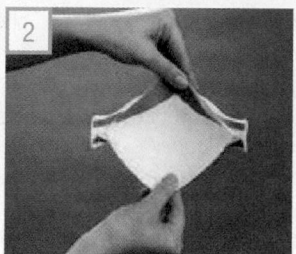

2. Fully open the top and bottom panels, bending the nosepiece around your thumb at centre of the foam. Straps should separate when panels are opened. Make certain the bottom panel is unfolded and completely opened.

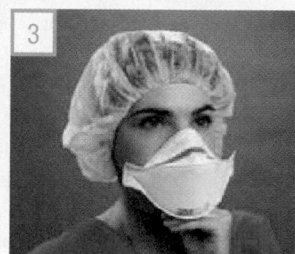

3. Place the respirator on your face so that the foam rests on your nose and the bottom panel is securely under your chin.

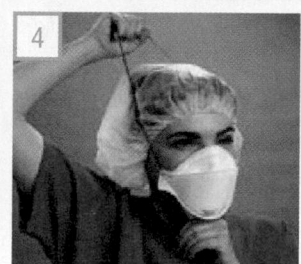

4. Pull the top strap over your head and position it high on the back of the head. Then, pull the bottom strap over your head and position it around your neck and below your ears.

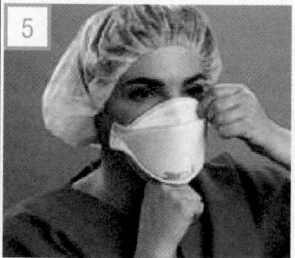

5. Adjust for a comfortable fit by pulling the top panel toward the bridge of your nose and positioning the bottom panel under your chin.

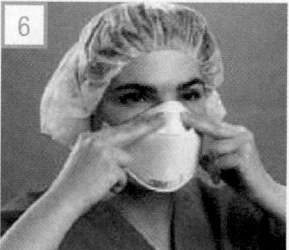

6. Place fingertips from both hands at the top of your nose and mould the nosepiece around your nose to achieve a secure seal.

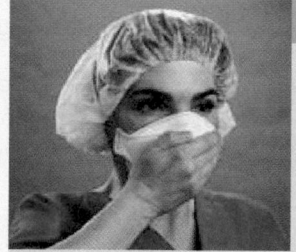

Place one or both hands completely over the middle panel. Inhale and exhale sharply. If air leaks around your nose, readjust the nosepiece. If air leaks between the face and faceseal of the respirator, reposition it by adjusting the panels and straps. If you cannot achieve a proper seal, do not enter the contaminated area. See your supervisor.

Please Note:

Check the seal of your three-panel facepiece respirator each time you don the respirator.

Removal

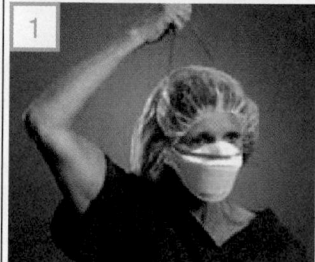

1. Without touching the respirator, slowly lift the bottom strap from around your neck up over your head.

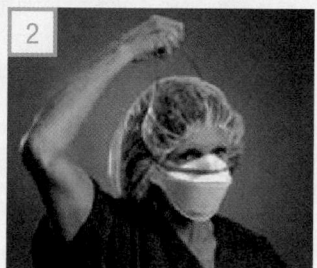

2. Lift off the top strap. Do not touch the respirator.

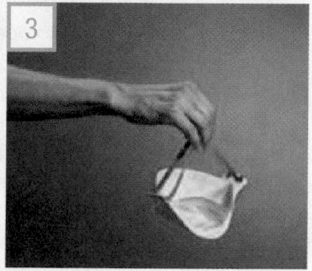

3. Store or discard according to your facility's infection control policy.

FIGURE 34.4 Application and removal of an N95 respirator.

microorganisms from one place to another, aseptic technique or sterile technique is used. The two terms are not the same. **Sterile technique** employs the strictest possible measures to maintain sterility throughout the procedure. It refers to using sterile items within a sterile field, such as an operative site in an operating room, or in an intensive care unit when a sterile drape is applied for insertion of a central venous access device. **Aseptic technique** is sometimes referred to as **clean technique**, where clean denotes the absence of almost all, but not all, microorganisms. While efforts are made to reduce transfer of microorganisms, items in use may not be sterile (e.g., use of clean forceps) and activity occurs outside of a sterile field (e.g., a wound during a dressing change).

Approaches to asepsis will vary, depending on the procedure and setting. For example, before an operating room procedure, the scrub nurse generally puts on a mask and cap, performs a surgical hand scrub, and then dons a sterile gown and gloves. In a general care area, the nurse may only perform hand hygiene and don sterile gloves. In both areas, the nurse works with sterile equipment and a sterile field. The basic principles of sterile technique appear in Table 34.8, with examples from nursing practice that relate to each principle.

TABLE 34.8 Principles and Practices of Establishing and Maintaining a Sterile Field

Principle	Practices
All objects used in a sterile field must be sterile.	All articles are sterilized appropriately by dry or moist heat, chemicals, or radiation before use.
	Sterile articles can be stored for only a prescribed time; after that, they are considered unsterile.
	Always check a package containing a sterile object for intactness, dryness, and expiration date. Any package that appears open, torn, punctured, or wet is considered unsterile. Never assume an item is sterile; if in doubt, consider the item unsterile.
	Storage areas should be clean, dry, off the floor, and away from sinks.
	Always check chemical indicators of sterilization before using a package. The indicator is often a tape used to fasten the package or contained inside the package. The indicator changes colour during sterilization, indicating that the contents have undergone a sterilization procedure. If the colour change is not evident, the package is considered unsterile. Commercially prepared sterile packages may not have indicators but are marked with the word *sterile*.
Sterile objects become unsterile when touched by unsterile objects.	Handle sterile objects that will touch open wounds or enter body cavities only with sterile forceps or sterile gloved hands.
	Discard or resterilize objects that come into contact with unsterile objects.
	Whenever the sterility of an object is questionable, assume the article is unsterile.
Sterile items that are out of vision or below the waist level of the nurse are considered unsterile.	Once left unattended, a sterile field is considered unsterile.
	Sterile objects are always kept in view. Nurses should not turn their backs on a sterile field.
	Only the front part of a sterile gown (from the waist to the shoulder) and 5 cm above the elbows to the cuff of the sleeves are considered sterile.
	Always keep sterile gloved hands in sight and above waist level; touch only objects that are sterile.
	Sterile draped tables are considered sterile only at surface level.
	Once a sterile field becomes unsterile, it must be set up again before proceeding.
Sterile objects can become unsterile by prolonged exposure to airborne dust containing microorganisms.	Keep doors closed and traffic to a minimum in areas where a sterile procedure is being performed; moving air can carry dust and microorganisms.
	Keep areas in which sterile procedures are carried out as clean as possible by frequent damp cleaning with detergent germicides to minimize contaminants in the area.
	Keep hair clean and short, tied back, or enclosed in a net to prevent hair from falling on sterile objects. Microorganisms on the hair can make a sterile field unsterile.
	Wear surgical caps in operating rooms, delivery rooms, and burn units.
	Refrain from sneezing or coughing over a sterile field. This can render the field unsterile because of the spray of droplets containing microorganisms from the respiratory tract. Some nurses recommend that masks covering the mouth and the nose be worn when working over a sterile field or an open wound.
	Nurses with mild upper respiratory tract infections should refrain from carrying out sterile procedures, or should wear masks.
	When working over a sterile field, talking should be kept to a minimum. Turn the head from the field if talking is necessary.
	To prevent microorganisms from falling over a sterile field, refrain from reaching over a sterile field, unless sterile gloves are worn, and refrain from moving unsterile objects over a sterile field.

Principle	Practices
Fluids flow in the direction of gravity.	Hold instruments with the tips below the handles. When the tips are held higher than the handles, fluid can flow onto the handle and become contaminated by the hands. When the forceps are again pointed downward, the fluid flows back down and contaminates the tips. During a surgical handwash, hold your hands higher than your elbows to prevent contaminants from the forearms from reaching the hands.
Moisture that passes through a sterile object draws microorganisms from unsterile surfaces above or below to the sterile surface by capillary action.	Sterile moisture-proof barriers are used beneath sterile objects. Liquids (sterile saline or antiseptics) are frequently poured into containers on a sterile field. If they are spilled onto the sterile field, the barrier keeps the liquid from seeping beneath it. Keep the sterile covers on sterile equipment dry. Damp surfaces can attract microorganisms in the dust in the air. Replace sterile drapes that do not have a sterile barrier underneath when they become moist.
The edges of a sterile field are considered unsterile.	A 2.5-cm margin at each edge of an opened drape is considered unsterile because the edges are in contact with unsterile surfaces. Place all sterile objects more than 2.5 cm inside the edges of a sterile field. Any article that falls outside the edges of a sterile field is considered unsterile.
Skin is unsterile and cannot be sterilized.	Use sterile gloves or sterile forceps to handle sterile items. Prior to a surgical aseptic procedure, perform appropriate hand hygiene to reduce the number of microorganisms on them.
Conscientiousness, alertness, and honesty are essential qualities in maintaining surgical asepsis.	When a sterile object becomes unsterile, it does not necessarily change in appearance. The person who sees a sterile object become contaminated must correct or report the situation. Do not set up a sterile field ahead of time for future use.

HOME CARE CONSIDERATIONS

Sterile Field

Creating a sterile field is essential in many procedures conducted in the home:

- Clean and wipe dry a flat surface for the sterile field.
- Keep pets and uninvolved small children out of the area when setting up for and performing sterile procedures.
- Dispose of all soiled materials in a waterproof bag. Check with the agency as to how to dispose of medical refuse.
- Remove all instruments from the home or other setting in which others might accidentally find them. *New or used instruments can be sharp or capable of causing injury. Used instruments may transmit infection.* Check with the agency for instructions on the cleansing of reusable supplies and disposal of single-use instruments.
- If appropriate, teach the client and family members the principles and rationale underlying the use of a sterile field.

Sterile Field A **sterile field** is a microorganism-free area. Nurses often establish a sterile field by using the innermost side of a sterile wrapper or by using a sterile drape. When the field is established, sterile supplies and sterile solutions can be placed on it. Sterile forceps are used in many instances to handle and transfer the sterile supplies.

To maintain their sterility, supplies are wrapped in a variety of materials. Commercially prepared items are frequently wrapped in plastic, paper, or glass. In the past, it was not unusual for sterile liquids (e.g., sterile water for irrigations) to be supplied in large containers. This practice is considered undesirable today because once a container has been opened, there can be no guarantee that it is sterile. Liquids are preferably packaged in amounts adequate for single use only; leftover liquid is discarded.

The Home Care Considerations box contains information that the nurse should teach the client to maintain a sterile field at home.

Skill 34.3 on the next page describes how to establish and maintain a sterile field.

Sterile Gloves Sterile gloves are worn during many procedures to maintain the sterility of equipment and protect the client. Sterile gloves are packaged with a cuff of about 5 cm and with the palms facing upward when the package is opened. The package usually indicates the size of the glove (e.g., size 6 or 7 1/2).

Sterile gloves can be donned by the open method or the closed method. The open method is most frequently used outside the operating room because the closed method requires that the nurse wear a sterile gown. Skill 34.4 on page 984 describes how to don and remove sterile gloves by using the open method.

SKILL 34.3 ESTABLISHING AND MAINTAINING A STERILE FIELD

PURPOSE

To maintain the sterility of supplies and equipment

ASSESSMENT

Review the client's record or discuss with the client or other health care team members exactly what procedure will be performed that requires a sterile field. Determine the client's presence of or risk for infection and ability to cope with the procedure.

Determine, if possible, what supplies and techniques have been used in the past to perform the procedures for this client. Attempt to determine if the procedure will be performed again in the future, so appropriate client teaching can be done and adequate supplies will be available.

Schedule the procedure at a time consistent with the order, the need for the procedure, and the client's other activities.

Equipment

- Package containing a sterile drape
- Sterile equipment as needed (e.g., packaged gauze, wrapped sterile bowl, antiseptic solution, sterile forceps)

IMPLEMENTATION

Preparation

- Ensure that the package is clean and dry; if moisture is noted on the inside of a plastic-wrapped package or the outside of a cloth-wrapped package, it is considered contaminated and must be discarded.
- Check the sterilization expiration dates on the package, and look for any indications that it has been previously opened. Spots or stains on cloth-wrapped or paper-wrapped objects may indicate contamination and should not be used.
- Follow agency practice for disposal of possibly contaminated packages.

Performance

1. Before performing the procedure, introduce yourself and verify the patient's identity using two identifiers or per agency protocol. Explain to the client what you are going to do, why it is necessary, and how he or she can participate.
2. Observe other appropriate infection prevention and control procedures (see Skills 34.1 and 34.2).
3. Provide for client privacy.
4. Open the package. If the package is inside a plastic cover, remove the cover.

To Open a Wrapped Package on a Clean Surface

- Place the package in the centre of the work area so that the top flap of the wrapper opens away from you. **Rationale: This position prevents the nurse from reaching directly over the exposed sterile contents, which could contaminate them.**
- Reaching from the side of the package (not over it), pinch the first flap on the outside of the wrapper between the thumb and index finger (see ❶). **Rationale: Touching only the outside of the wrapper maintains the sterility of**

the inside of the wrapper. Pull the flap open, laying it flat on the far surface.

- Repeat for the side flaps, opening the top one first. Use the right hand for the right flap, and the left hand for the left flap (see ❷). **Rationale: By using both hands, the nurse avoids reaching over the sterile contents.**
- Pull the fourth flap toward you by grasping the corner that is turned down (see ❸). Make sure that the flap does not touch any object. **Rationale: If the inner surface touches any unsterile article, it is contaminated.**

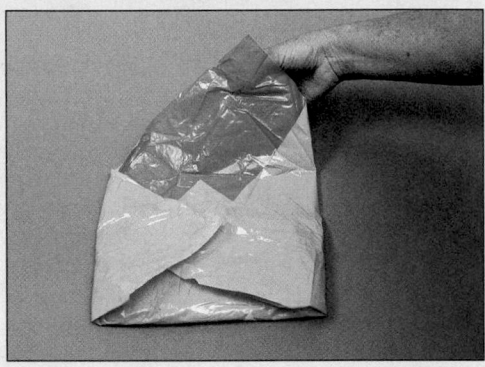

❶ Opening the first flap of a sterile wrapped package.

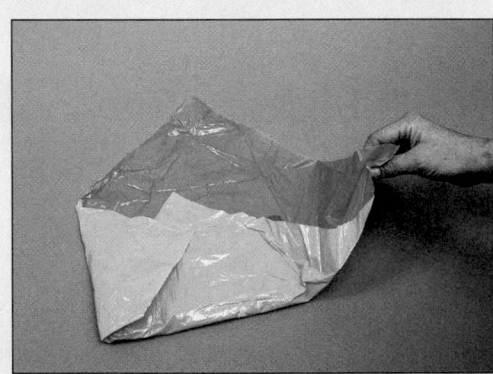

❷ Opening the second flap to the side.

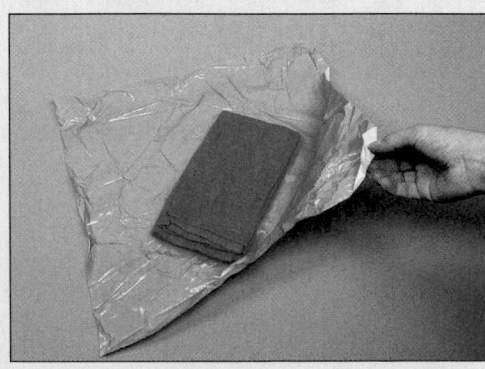

❸ Pulling the last flap toward you by grasping the corner.

Variation: Opening a Wrapped Package while Holding It

- Hold the package in one hand with the top flap opening away from you.
- By using the other hand, open the package as described above, pulling the corners of the flaps well back and not reaching across the contents of the package (see ❹). **Rationale: The hands are considered contaminated, and at no time should they touch the contents of the package**.

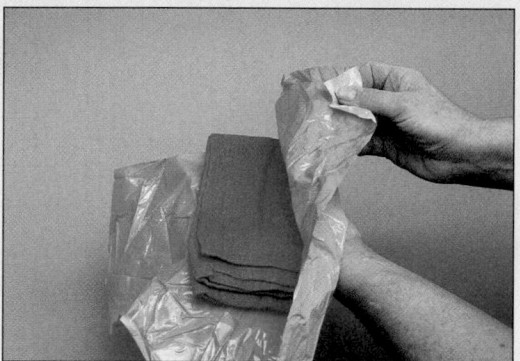

❹ Opening a wrapped package while holding it.

- If the package has a peel back edge, grasp both sides of the edge, one with each hand, and pull apart gently (see ❻).
5. Establish a sterile field by using a sterile drape.
   - Open the package containing the drape, as described above.
   - With one hand, pluck the corner of the drape that is folded back on the top touching only one side of the drape.

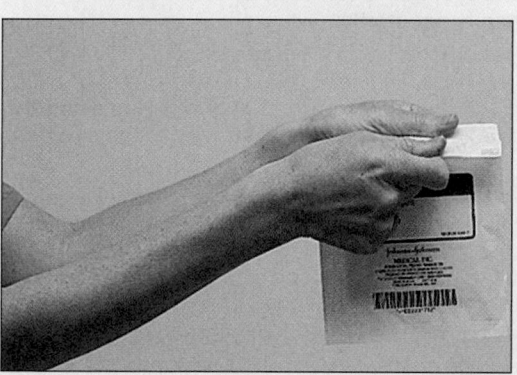

❻ Opening a sterile package that has a partially sealed edge.

- Lay the drape on a clean and dry surface, placing the bottom (i.e., the freely hanging side) farthest from you (see ❽). **Rationale: By placing the lowermost side farthest away, the nurse avoids leaning over the sterile field and contaminating it.**
6. Add necessary sterile supplies, being careful not to touch the drape with the hands.

Variation: Opening Commercially Prepared Packages

Commercially prepared sterile packages and containers usually have manufacturer's directions for opening.

- If the flap of the package has a peel back corner, hold the container in one hand and pull back on the flap with the other hand (see ❺).

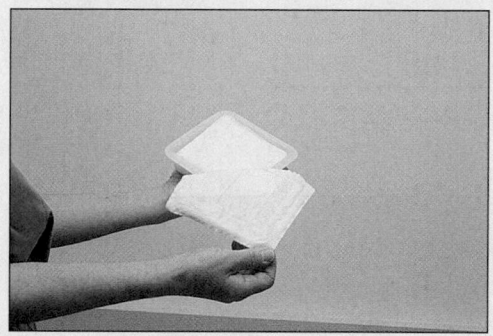

❺ Opening a sterile package that has a peel back corner.

- Lift the drape out of the cover and allow it to open freely without touching any objects (see ❼). **Rationale: If the drape touches the outside of the package or any unsterile surface or object, it is considered contaminated**.
- Discard the cover.
- With the other hand, carefully pick up another corner of the drape, holding it well away from you, and again, touching only the same side of the drape as the first hand.

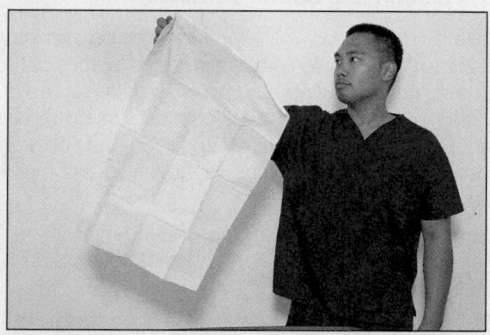

❼ Allowing a drape to open freely without touching any objects.

Adding Commercially Packaged Supplies to a Sterile Field

- Open each package as previously described.
- Hold the package 15 cm above the field, and allow the contents to drop on the field (see ❾). Keep in mind that 2.5 cm around the edge of the field is considered contaminated. **Rationale: At a height of 15 cm, the outside of the package is not likely to touch and contaminate the sterile fields.**

(continued)

SKILL 34.3 ESTABLISHING AND MAINTAINING A STERILE FIELD (*continued*)

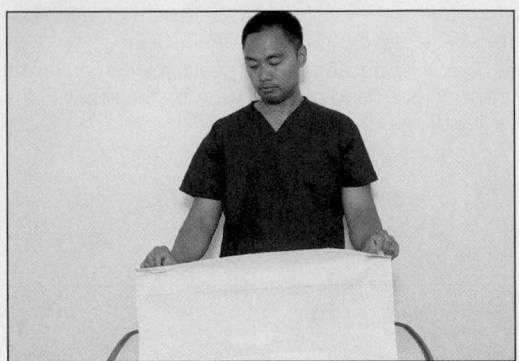

⑧ Placing a drape on a surface.

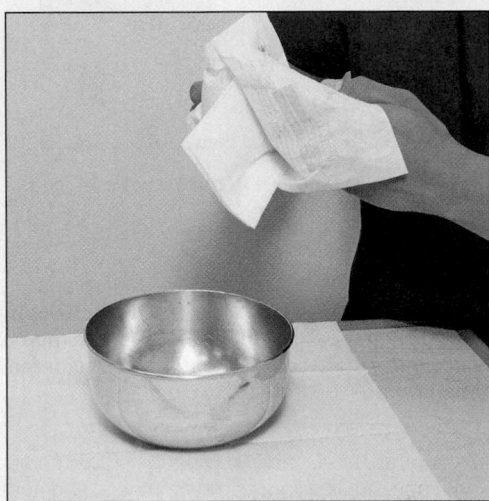

⑨ Adding commercially packaged gauze to a sterile filed.

Adding Solution to a Sterile Container

Liquids (e.g., normal saline) may need to be poured into containers within a sterile field. Unwrapped bottles or flasks that contain sterile solution are considered sterile on the inside and contaminated on the outside because the bottle has been handled. Bottles used in an operating room may be sterilized on the outside as well as the inside, however, and these are handled with sterile gloves.

- Before pouring any liquid, read the label three times to ensure you have the correct solution and concentration.

- Obtain the exact amount of solution, if possible. **Rationale: Once a sterile container has been opened, its sterility cannot be ensured for future use unless it is used again immediately.**

- Remove the lid or cap from the bottle and invert the lid before placing it on a surface that is not sterile. **Rationale: Inverting the lid maintains the sterility of the inside surface because it is not allowed to touch an unsterile surface.**

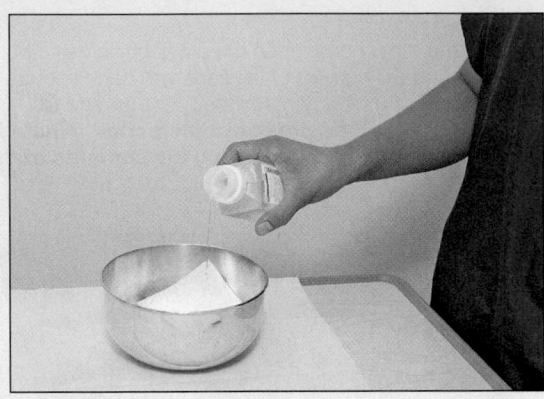

⑩ Adding liquid to a sterile bowl.

- Hold the bottle at a slight angle so that the label is uppermost (see ⑩). **Rationale: Any solution that flows down the outside of the bottle during pouring will not damage or obliterate the label.**

- Hold the bottle of fluid at a height of 10 cm to 15 cm over the container and to the side of the sterile field so that as little of the bottle as possible is over the field. **Rationale: At this height, there is less likelihood of contaminating the sterile field by touching the field or by reaching an arm over it.**

- Pour the solution gently to avoid splashing the liquid. **Rationale: If the sterile drape is on an unsterile surface, any moisture will contaminate the field by facilitating the movement of microorganisms through the drape.**

- Tilt the neck of the bottle back to vertical quickly when done pouring so that none of the liquid flows down the outside of the bottle. **Rationale: Such drips would contaminate the sterile field if the outside of the bottle is not sterile.**

- If the bottle will be used again, replace the lid securely on the bottle, and record the date and time of opening, according to agency policy. **Rationale: Replacing the lid immediately maintains the sterility of the inner aspect of the lid and the solution.**

- Depending on agency policy, a sterile container of solution that is opened may be used only once and then discarded (such as in the operating room). In other settings, policy may permit recapped bottles to be reused within 24 hours.

- If the bottle of solution is used again, the lip of the container should be cleansed by pouring a small amount of solution (and then discarding) before pouring solution into the sterile container.

7. Use sterile forceps to handle certain sterile supplies.

- Forceps are commonly used for such techniques as changing a sterile dressing and shortening a drain. Transfer forceps are used to move a sterile article from one place to another, for example, transferring sterile gauze from its package to a sterile dressing tray. Forceps may be discarded or resterilized after use. Commonly used forceps include hemostats or artery forceps (see ⑪) and tissue forceps (see ⑫).

- Keep the tips of wet forceps lower than the wrist at all times unless you are wearing sterile gloves (see ⑬). **Rationale: Gravity prevents liquids on the tips of the forceps from flowing to the handles and later back to the tips, thus making the forceps unsterile. The handles are unsterile once they are held by the bare hand.**

- Hold sterile forceps above waist level. **Rationale: Items held below waist level are considered contaminated.**

- Hold sterile forceps within your visual field. **Rationale: While out of sight, forceps may, unknown to the user, become contaminated. Any forceps that go out of sight should be considered unsterile.**

- When using forceps to lift sterile supplies out of a commercially prepared package, be sure that the forceps do not touch the edges or outside of the wrapper. **Rationale: The edges and outside of the package are exposed to the air and are handled and are, thus, unsterile.**

- Deposit a sterile item on a sterile field without permitting moist forceps to touch the sterile field when the surface under the sterile field is unsterile and a barrier drape is not used. A *barrier drape* is resistant to moisture and should be used whenever a procedure involves moisture. **Rationale: Made of chemically treated cotton or synthetic materials, barrier drapes prevent a sterile field from becoming contaminated when the drape becomes wet. Sterile cloth becomes unsterile when dampened (even with sterile water) if it is on an unsterile surface or has contact with any unsterile object. Microorganisms can move through a damp sterile cloth from an unsterile surface by capillary action.**

- When placing forceps whose handles were in contact with the bare hand, position the handles outside the sterile area. **Rationale: The handles of these forceps harbour microorganisms from the bare hand.**

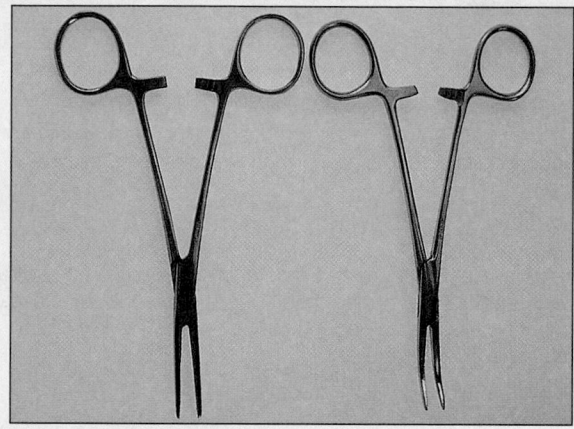

⑪ Hemostats: **A:** Straight; **B:** Curved.

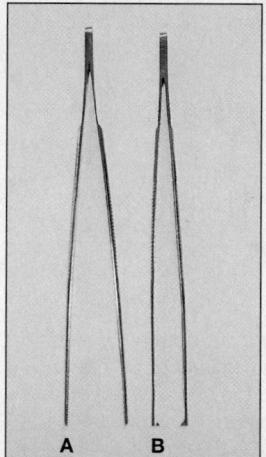

⑫ Tissue forceps: **A:** Plain; **B:** Toothed.

A   B

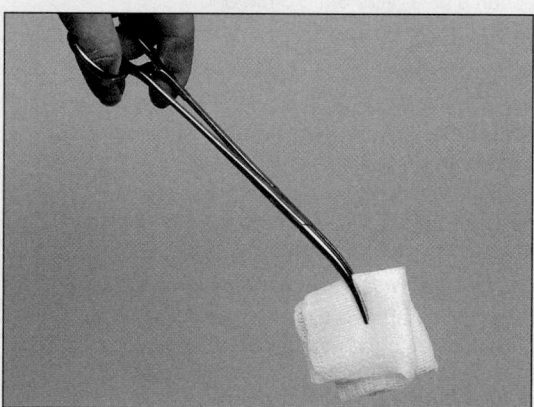

⑬ Holding forceps with an ungloved hand, keeping the tips pointing downward.

EVALUATION

Conduct any follow-up indicated during your care of the client. Ensure that adequate numbers and types of sterile supplies are available for the next health care provider.

SKILL 34.4 DONNING AND REMOVING STERILE GLOVES (OPEN METHOD)

PURPOSES

- To enable the nurse to handle sterile objects freely
- To prevent clients at risk (e.g., those with open wounds) from becoming infected by microorganisms on the nurse's hands

ASSESSMENT

Review the client's record and orders to determine exactly what procedure will be performed that requires sterile gloves. Check the client record and ask about latex allergies. Use latex-free gloves, whenever possible.

PLANNING

Think through the procedure, planning which steps need to be completed before the gloves can be applied. Determine what additional supplies are needed to perform the procedure for this client. Always have an extra pair of sterile gloves available.

Equipment

- Packages of sterile gloves

IMPLEMENTATION

Preparation

Ensure the sterility of the package of gloves.

Performance

1. Before performing the procedure, introduce yourself and verify the client's identity using two identifiers or per agency protocol. Explain to the client what you are going to do, why it is necessary, and how he or she can participate.

2. Observe other appropriate infection prevention and control procedures (see Skills 34.1, 34.2, and 34.3).

3. Provide for client privacy.

4. Open the package of sterile gloves.
   - Place the package of gloves on a clean, dry surface. **Rationale: Any moisture on the surface could contaminate the gloves.**
   - Some gloves are packed in an inner as well as an outer package. Open the outer package without contaminating the gloves or the inner package. See Skill 34.3.
   - Remove the inner package from the outer package.
   - Open the inner package as in step 4 of Skill 34.3, or according to the manufacturer's directions. Some manufacturers provide a numbered sequence for opening the flaps and folded tabs to grasp for opening the flaps. If no tabs are provided, pluck the flap so that the fingers do not touch the inner surfaces. **Rationale: The inner surfaces, which are next to the sterile gloves, will remain sterile.**

5. Put the first glove on the dominant hand.
   - If the gloves are packaged so that they lie side by side, grasp the glove for the dominant hand by its cuff (on the palmar side) with the thumb and first finger of the nondominant hand. Touch only the inside of the cuff (see ❶). **Rationale: The hands are not sterile. By touching only the inside of the glove, the nurse avoids contaminating the outside.**

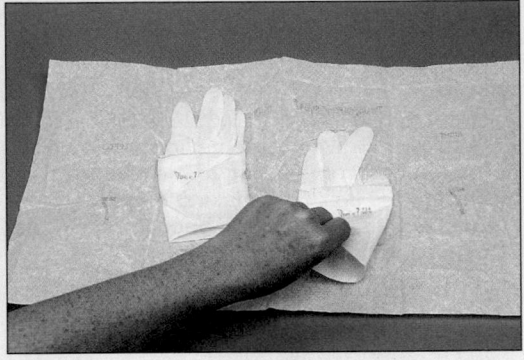

❶ Picking up the first sterile glove.

Or

- If the gloves are packaged one on top of the other, grasp the cuff of the top glove as above, using the opposite hand.
- Insert the dominant hand into the glove and pull the glove on. Keep the thumb of the inserted hand against the palm of the hand during insertion (see ❷). **Rationale: If the thumb is kept against the palm, it is less likely to contaminate the outside of the glove.**
- Leave the cuff turned down. **Rationale: Attempting to further unfold the cuff is likely to contaminate the gloves.**

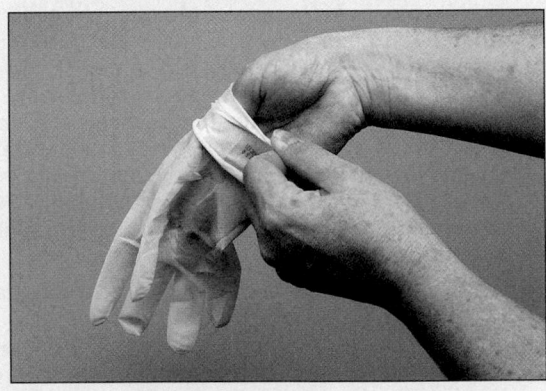

❷ Putting on the first sterile glove.

6. Put the second glove on the nondominant hand.
   - Pick up the other glove with the sterile gloved hand, inserting the gloved fingers under the cuff and holding the gloved thumb close to the gloved palm (see ❸). **Rationale: This helps prevent accidental contamination of the glove by the bare hand.**
   - Pull on the second glove carefully. Hold the thumb of the gloved first hand as far as possible from the palm (see ❹). **Rationale: In this position, the thumb is less likely to touch the arm and become contaminated.**
   - Adjust each glove so that it fits smoothly, and carefully pull up the cuffs by sliding the fingers under the cuffs.

7. Remove and dispose of used gloves.
   - Remove them by turning them inside out. See Skill 34.2.

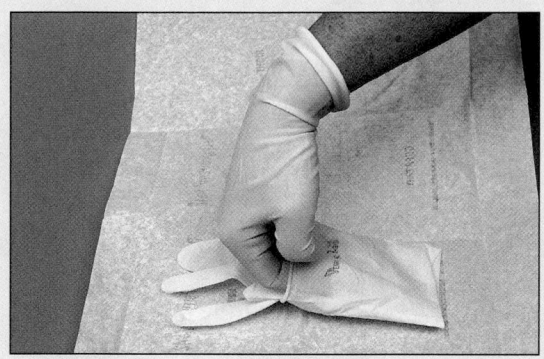

❸ Picking up the second sterile glove.

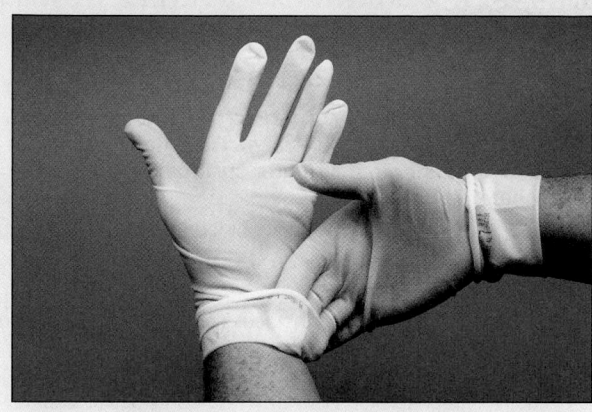

❹ Putting on the second sterile glove.

EVALUATION

Conduct any follow-up indicated during your care of the client. Ensure that adequate numbers and types of sterile supplies are available for the next health care provider.

Latex and latex-free (e.g., nitrile and vinyl) sterile gloves are available to protect the nurse from contact with blood and bodily fluids. Latex and nitrile are more flexible than vinyl, mould to the wearer's hands, allow freedom of movement, and have the added feature of resealing tiny punctures automatically. Therefore, wear latex or nitrile gloves when performing tasks that (a) demand flexibility, (b) place stress on the material (e.g., turning stopcocks, handling sharp instruments or tape), and (c) involve a high risk of exposure to pathogens. Vinyl gloves should be chosen for tasks unlikely to stress the glove material, requiring minimal precision, or with minimal risk of exposure to pathogens.

Sterile Gowns Sterile gowning and closed gloving are chiefly carried out in operating or delivery rooms. The closed method of gloving can be used only when a sterile gown is worn because the gloves are handled through the sleeves of the gown. Before these procedures, the nurse dons a hair cover and a mask, and performs a surgical handwash.

Skill 34.5 describes the steps in donning a sterile gown and sterile gloves by the closed method.

SKILL 34.5 DONNING A STERILE GOWN AND STERILE GLOVES (CLOSED METHOD)

PURPOSES
- To enable the nurse to work close to a sterile field and handle sterile objects freely
- To protect clients from becoming contaminated with microorganisms on the nurse's hands, arms, and clothing

ASSESSMENT
Review the client's record and orders to determine exactly what procedure will be performed that requires sterile gloves. Check the client record and ask about latex allergies. Use latex-free gloves, whenever possible.

PLANNING
Think through the procedure, planning which steps need to be completed before the gown and gloves can be applied. Determine what additional supplies are needed to perform the procedure for this client. Always have an extra pair of sterile gloves and an extra sterile gown available.

Equipment
- Sterile pack containing a sterile gown
- Sterile gloves

IMPLEMENTATION
Ensure the sterility of the gown and gloves.

Performance
1. Before performing the procedure, introduce yourself and verify the client's identity using two identifiers or per agency protocol. Explain to the client what you are going to do, why it is necessary, and how he or she can participate.
2. Observe other appropriate infection prevention and control procedures (see Skills 34.1, 34.2, and 34.3).
3. Provide for client privacy.

Donning a Sterile Gown
4. Open the package of sterile gloves.
   - Remove the outer wrap from the sterile gloves and leave the gloves in their inner sterile wrap on the sterile field. **Rationale: If the inner wrapper is not touched, it will remain sterile.** See Skill 34.3, step 4 (p. 980).
5. Unwrap the sterile gown pack.
6. Perform proper hand hygiene. (See "Variation" at the end of Skill 34.1.)
7. Put on the sterile gown.

(continued)

SKILL 34.5 **DONNING A STERILE GOWN AND STERILE GLOVES (CLOSED METHOD)** *(continued)*

- Grasp the sterile gown at the neck, hold it away from you, and permit it to unfold freely without touching anything, including the uniform. **Rationale: The gown will be unsterile if its outer surface touches any unsterile objects.**
- Put your hands inside the shoulders of the gown (see ❶)
- Work your hands down the sleeves only to the beginning of the cuffs (see ❷).
- Have a coworker grasp the neck ties without touching the outside of the gown and pull the gown upward to cover the neckline of your uniform in front and back. The coworker ties the neck ties (see ❸). Gowning continues at step 11.

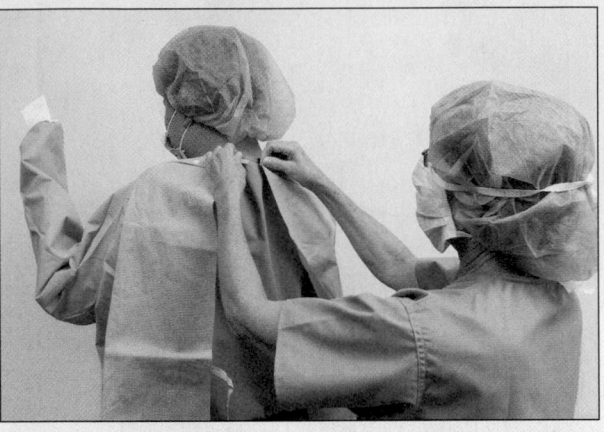

❸ A coworker ties the neck ties of a sterile gown.

Donning Sterile Gloves (Closed Method)

8. Open the sterile glove wrapper while the hands are still covered by the sleeves (see ❹).
9. Put the glove on the nondominant hand. Figures ❺ through ❼ show a right-handed person.

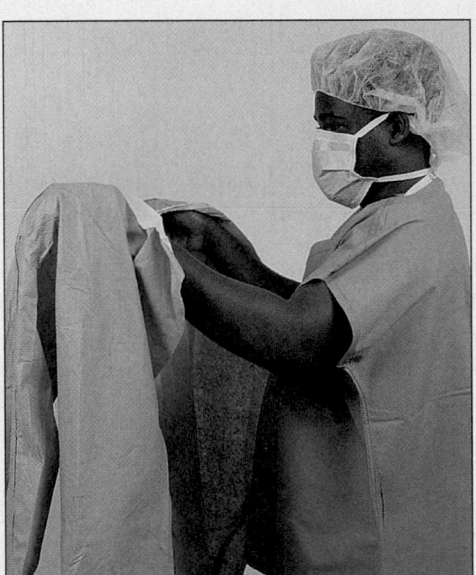

❶ Putting on a sterile gown.

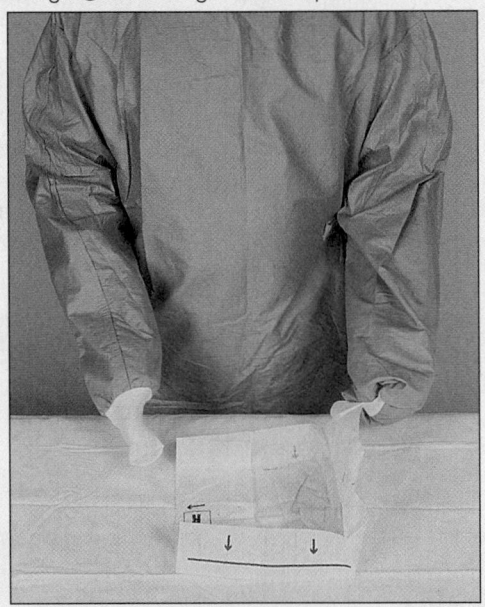

❹ Opening the sterile glove wrapper.

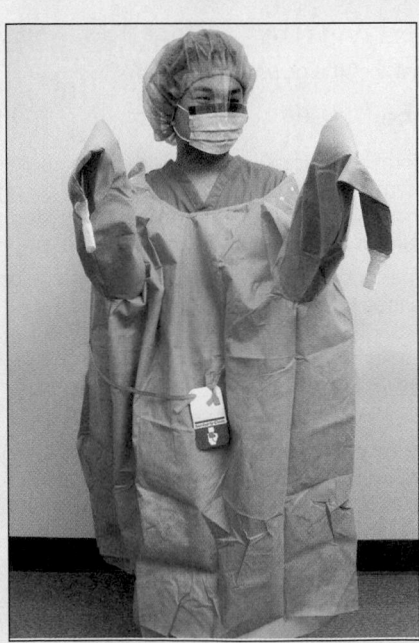

❷ Working the hands down the sleeves of a sterile gown.

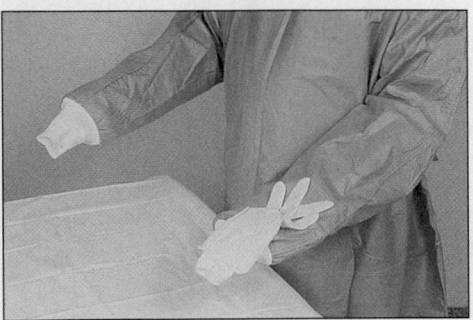

❺ Positioning the first sterile glove for the nondominant hand.

- With the *dominant* hand, pick up the *opposite* glove with the thumb and index finger, handling it through the sleeve of the gown.
- Lay the glove on the opposite gown cuff, thumb side down, with the glove opening pointed toward the fingers (see ❺).
- Use the nondominant hand to grasp the cuff of the glove through the gown cuff, and firmly anchor it.
- With the dominant hand working through its gown sleeve, grasp the upper side of the glove's cuff, and stretch it over the cuff of the gown.
- Pull the sleeve up to draw the cuff over the wrist as you extend the fingers of the nondominant hand into the glove's fingers (see ❻).

10. Put the glove on the dominant hand.
- Place the fingers of the gloved hand under the cuff of the remaining glove.
- Place the glove over the cuff of the second sleeve.
- Extend the fingers into the glove as you pull the glove up over the gown cuff (see ❼).

Completion of Gowning

11. Complete gowning as follows:
- Have a coworker hold the long end of the waist tie of your gown by using sterile gloves or a sterile forceps or drape. **Rationale: This approach keeps the ties sterile.**
- Make a three-quarter turn, then take the tie from the coworker, and secure it in front of the gown.

Or

- Have a coworker wearing sterile gloves take the two ties at each side of the gown and tie them at the back of the gown, making sure that your uniform is completely covered. **Rationale: Both methods ensure that the back of the gown remains sterile.**
- When worn, sterile gowns should be considered *sterile* only in front from the waist to the shoulder. The sleeves should be considered sterile from the cuff to 5 cm above the elbow, since the arms of a scrubbed person must move across a sterile field. Moisture collection and friction areas, such as the neckline, shoulders, underarms and back, should be considered unsterile.

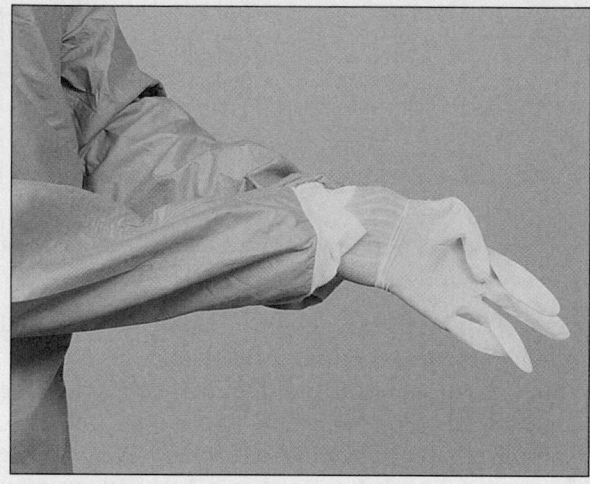

❻ Pulling on the first sterile glove.

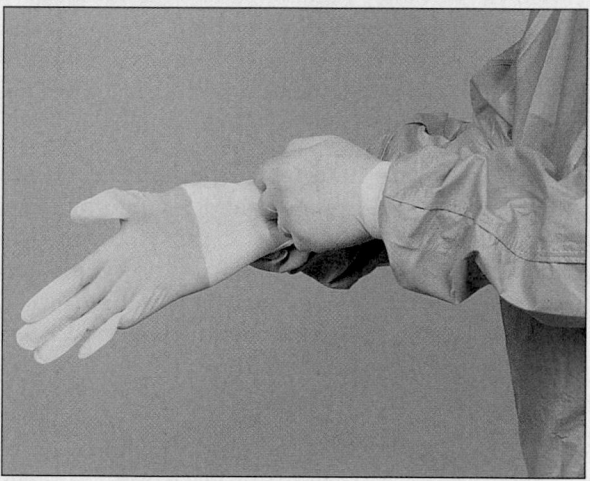

❼ Extending the fingers into the second glove of the dominant hand.

12. Remove and dispose of used gown and gloves (see Skill 34.2).

EVALUATION

Conduct any follow-up indicated during your care of the client. Ensure that adequate numbers and types of sterile supplies are available for the next health care provider.

Support of the Defences of a Susceptible Host

People are constantly in contact with microorganisms in the environment (see the Clinical Alert box on the next page). Normally, a person's natural defences ward off the development of an infection. *Susceptibility* is the degree to which an individual can be affected, that is, the likelihood of an organism causing an infection in that person. Factors affecting a person's susceptibility have previously been identified. Although it is not possible to specifically

> ### ! CLINICAL ALERT
>
> A person does not need to have an identified infection in order to pass potentially infective microorganisms to another person. Even microorganisms that are normal flora for one person can infect another person.

manipulate age or heredity as risk factors, a number of strategies can support host defences.

HYGIENE Maintaining the intactness of skin and mucous membranes retains a barrier against microorganisms entering the body. In addition, oral care, including flossing teeth, reduces the likelihood of an oral infection. Regular and thorough bathing and shampooing remove microorganisms, and the dirt that contains them, that can cause an infection.

NUTRITION A balanced diet enhances the health of all body tissues, helps keep skin intact, and promotes skin's ability to repel microorganisms. Adequate nutrition enables tissues to maintain and rebuild themselves and helps keep the immune system functioning well.

FLUID An adequate fluid intake permits a fluid output that flushes out the bladder and urethra, removing microorganisms that could cause an infection. Adequate hydration also helps maintain the natural barriers since dehydrated skin or mucous membranes have breaks through which microorganisms can enter. Adequate sleep is essential to health and to renewing energy. See Chapter 38.

STRESS Excessive stress predisposes people to infections. Nurses can assist clients to learn stress-reducing techniques. See Chapter 48.

OPTIMIZING TISSUE OXYGENATION AND BLOOD FLOW Optimizing blood flow allows sufficient numbers of leukocytes to reach a given tissue; these are key cells for reducing the number of microorganisms locally. Adequate tissue oxygenation will promote production of adenosine triphosphate (ATP) for use by the leukocytes and either replacement or strengthening of the tissue. Stopping smoking, ensuring adequate hydration, managing pain, reducing stress, avoiding obesity, and correcting anemia are all strategies that promote blood flow and tissue oxygenation.

GLYCEMIC CONTROL Uncontrolled glucose levels is a risk factor for a variety of infections. Maintaining glycemic control can reduce the physiological changes that increase risk. Studies have shown that hemoglobin A_{1C} levels of less than 7% are significantly associated with lower rates of infection in surgical patients (Dronge, Perkal, Kancir, Concato, Asian, & Rosenthal, 2006). Diabetic clients need to be taught to monitor their blood glucose levels and appropriate diet, exercise, and medication strategies for controlling them.

IMMUNIZATIONS Immunizations have dramatically decreased the incidence of infectious diseases. It is recommended that immunizations begin shortly after birth and be completed in early childhood, except for boosters (see Table 34.9 for recommended immunizations for Canadian infants and children). Immunizations are frequently given in combination to minimize multiple injections. National guidelines for immunization schedules are established by the Public Health Agency of Canada National Advisory Committee on Immunization. However, nurses must be aware of the immunization guidelines in the jurisdiction in which they are working as provinces and territories determine their specific immunization guidelines.

All adults, especially older adults and adults with health problems, should ensure they are adequately immunized for specific risk situations such as influenza and hepatitis (see Table 34.10). Immunization programs are also available for high-risk groups, such as health care personnel, people who have had

TABLE 34.9 Routine immunization schedules for infants and children

Age at vaccination	DTaP-IPV	Hib	MMR	Var	HB	Pneu-C-7	Men-C	Tdap	HPV	Inf
Birth										
2 months	yes	yes				yes	yes*			
4 months	yes	yes			yes Infancy 3 doses	yes	yes*			
6 months	yes	yes				yes	yes* and			yes 6–23 months 1–2 doses
12 months			yes	yes		yes 12–15 months	yes			
18 months	yes	yes	yes or yes		or					
4–6 years	yes						and			
12 years					Pre-teen/teen 2-3 doses		yes		yes (Females, 9–13 years, 3 doses)	
14–16 years								yes		
*Asterisks imply that these doses may not be required, depending upon the age of the child or adult.										

DTaP-IPV – Diphtheria, tetanus, acellular pertussis vaccine and inactivated polio virus vaccine

Hib – *Haemophilus influenzae* type b conjugate vaccine

MMR – Measles, mumps, and rubella vaccine

Var – Varicella vaccine

HB – Hepatitis B vaccine

Pneu-C-7 – Pneumococcal conjugate vaccine: 7-valent

Men-C – Meningococcal C conjugate vaccine

Tdap – Diphtheria, tetanus, acellular pertussis vaccine: adult/adolescent formulation

HPV – Human papilloma virus vaccine

Inf – Influenza vaccine

Note: Provincial and territorial variations to this immunization schedule may exist.

Source: Canadian Immunization Guide, 7th Edition. Public Health Agency of Canada, 2006. Reproduced with the permission of the Minister of Health, 2012.

TABLE 34.10 Adult Immunization Schedule—Specific Risk Situations

Vaccine or Toxoid	Indication	Schedule
Influenza	Adults ≥ 65 years; Adults < 65 years at high risk of Influenza-related complications, their household contacts, health care workers, and all those wishing to be protected against influenza.	Every autumn using current recommended vaccine formulation
Pneumococcal polysaccharide	Adults 65 ≥ years; Adults < 65 who have conditions putting them at increased risk of pneumococcal disease.	1 dose
Hepatitis A	Occupational risk, lifestyle, travel and living in areas lacking adequate sanitation. Outbreak control, post-exposure immunoprophylaxis. Patients with chronic liver disease.	2 doses 6–12 months apart
Hepatitis B	Occupational risk, lifestyle, post-exposure immunoprophylaxis. Patients with chronic liver disease.	3 doses at 0, 1 and 6 months

Note: *Provincial and territorial variations to this immunization schedule may exist.*

Source: *Canadian Immunization Guide,* 7th Edition. Public Health Agency of Canada, 2006. Reproduced with the permission of the Minister of Health, 2012.

a splenectomy, and people travelling, each of which require individual assessment. In view of the increased risk of exposure to communicable diseases, the following vaccines are generally recommended for all health care workers and others providing personal care: hepatitis A and B, influenza, and varicella if seronegative.

New vaccines are reviewed as they appear and may be recommended for specific populations. For example, the vaccine against human papilloma virus (HPV) infection, one of the most common sexually transmitted infections (STIs) in Canada, is, as of 2010, now available for men (Public Health Agency of Canada, 2010).

Routine Practices and Additional Precautions

Since the late 1990s, Canada has adopted the use of *routine practices* and *additional precautions* (replacing the previous *standard precautions* and *transmission-based precautions*) as measures to limit the spread of microorganisms. First published in 1999 by Health Canada, guidelines

for routine practices and additional precautions provide comprehensive practice recommendations regardless of setting. The Public Health Agency of Canada is currently revising these guidelines but they have not yet been published. Many provinces have developed their own guidelines for *routine practices and additional precautions,* which are based are current evidence and thus very similar from one set to another, even though the jurisdictions themselves vary. Manitoba, Ontario and Newfoundland, for example, have readily accessible guidelines for *routine practices and additional precautions.*

Routine Practices

Routine practices are infection prevention and control activities used in the care of *all* clients regardless of their diagnosis or possible infection status. They apply to blood, all bodily fluids, secretions, and excretions (*except sweat*), nonintact skin, and mucous membranes whether or not blood is present or visible. Recommended practices for routine practices are shown in Box 34.3. The point of care risk assessment helps the nurse identify which are appropriate to implement for any particular client or situation.

BOX 34.3 **RECOMMENDED ROUTINE PRACTICES**

The recommendations below are designed for *all* clients (i.e., in hospitals, long-term care facilities, community, and any other care setting). The precautions apply to blood; all bodily fluids, excretions, and secretions except sweat; nonintact (broken) skin; and mucous membranes. They are designed to reduce risk of transmission of microorganisms from recognized and unrecognized sources.

1. Perform hand hygiene:

   a. Perform hand hygiene after contact with blood, bodily fluids, secretions, excretions, nonintact skin, mucous

membranes, and contaminated objects whether or not gloves are worn, and before contact with the client, the client's environment, or a portal of entry (see the indications for hand hygiene in Box 34.2). Hand hygiene is performed between client contacts.

   b. Perform hand hygiene at the point of care.

   c. Use of alcohol-based hand rub is the preferred method for hand hygiene unless hands are visibly soiled or the client has a *C. difficile* or norovirus infection.

(continued)

BOX 34.3 RECOMMENDED ROUTINE PRACTICES (*continued*)

2. Use appropriate personal protective equipment:

 a. Wear clean gloves when touching blood, bodily fluids, secretions, excretions, nonintact skin and mucous membranes, and contaminated items (e.g., soiled gowns).

 b. Clean gloves can be unsterile unless their use is intended to prevent the entrance of microorganisms into the body. See the discussion on sterile gloves in this chapter.

 c. Remove gloves before touching uncontaminated items and surfaces.

 d. Perform hand hygiene immediately after removing gloves.

 e. Wear a mask with eye protection, or a face shield, if splashes or sprays of blood, bodily fluids, secretions, or excretions can be expected.

 f. Wear a clean, nonsterile gown if client care is likely to result in splashes or sprays of blood, bodily fluids, secretions, or excretions, or contact of the health care provider's body (clothing and arms) with any of these materials. The gown is intended to protect clothing and arms.

 g. Remove a soiled gown carefully to avoid the transfer of microorganisms to others (i.e., clients, other health care workers, or yourself).

 h. Perform hand hygiene after removing gown.

3. Use clean equipment:

 a. Handle client care equipment that is soiled with blood, bodily fluids, secretions, or excretions carefully to prevent the transfer of microorganisms to others and to the environment.

 b. Make sure reusable equipment is cleaned and reprocessed correctly.

 c. Dispose of single-use equipment correctly.

4. Promote a clean and safe environment:

 a. Handle, transport, and process linen that is soiled with blood, bodily fluids, secretions, or excretions in a manner to prevent contamination of clothing and the transfer of microorganisms to others and to the environment.

 b. Ensure regular cleaning of the environment.

 c. Prevent injuries from used scalpels, needles, or other equipment, and place in puncture-resistant containers.

 d. Ensure proper handling and disposal of waste.

5. Control sources of infection:

 a. Consider client accommodation and flow, in terms of who they will be in contact with and their susceptibility to infection.

 b. Promote respiratory hygiene (cough etiquette) and provide resources such as tissues and alcohol-based hand rub so that clients can contain their respiratory secretions.

6. Provide education:

 a. Educate the client, visitors, and other health care workers, as appropriate.

Source: Summarized from Provincial Infectious Diseases Advisory Committee (PIDAC). Routine Practices and Additional Precautions in All Healthcare Settings, Ministry of Health and Longterm Care, Ontario, May 2010. Available at: http://www.oahpp.ca/resources/documents/pidac/Routine%20Practices%20and%20Additional%20Precautions.pdf
Manitoba Health. Routine Practices and Additional Precautions: Preventing the Transmission of Infection in Health Care. April 2012. Available at: http://www.gov.mb.ca/health/publichealth/cdc/docs/ipc/rpap.pdf
Newfoundland Labrador. Guidelines for Routine Practices and Additional Precautions. Department of Health and Community Services. February 2009. Available at http://www.health.gov.nl.ca/health/publichealth/cdc/routine_practices_additional_precautions.pdf

Additional Precautions

Additional precautions are infection prevention and control activities used in addition to routine practices for clients with *known* or *suspected* infections that are spread in one of three ways: (a) by airborne transmission, (b) by droplet transmission, or (c) by contact (direct or indirect). These three types of additional precautions can be used alone or in combination with each other, depending on the mode of transmission of the microorganism, but they are always used *in addition* to routine practices. Recommended practices for additional precautions are shown in Box 34.4. Signs indicating appropriate actions to be taken, such as PPE to be worn, should be placed where they are visible.

Airborne precautions are used for clients known or suspected to have illnesses transmitted by airborne droplet nuclei smaller than 5 microns, for example, measles, varicella (including disseminated zoster), and tuberculosis.

Droplet precautions are used for clients known or suspected to have illnesses transmitted by particle droplets larger than 5 microns. Examples of such illnesses are diphtheria (pharyngeal); pertussis (whooping cough); mumps; rubella; influenza, viral pneumonia, scarlet fever in infants and young children; and pneumonic plague.

Contact precautions are used for clients known or suspected to have illnesses easily transmitted by direct client contact or by contact with items in the client's environment. Such illnesses include gastrointestinal, respiratory, skin, or wound infections; colonization with multidrug-resistant bacteria; specific enteric infections, such as with *C. difficile* or norovirus; enteric infections, such as with enterohemorrhagic *E. coli* O157:H7, *Shigella*, and hepatitis A virus in clients who are diapered or incontinent; respiratory syncytial virus, parainfluenza virus, or enteroviral infections in infants and young children; and highly contagious skin infections, such as herpes simplex virus, impetigo, pediculosis, and scabies.

SPECIAL CONSIDERATIONS: RESPIRATORY HYGIENE
To further reduce transmission by droplets, respiratory secretions should be contained as much as possible. **Respiratory hygiene** involves coughing or sneezing into tissues or cloth (e.g., sleeves) rather than hands, which become contaminated. Used tissues should be immediately discarded and not saved for reuse, and hands washed or decontaminated with an alcohol-based hand rub. Further containment of infection can be achieved by recognizing when you pose a risk

BOX 34.4 RECOMMENDED ADDITIONAL PRECAUTIONS

The following are additional precautions:

AIRBORNE PRECAUTIONS

Use routine practices as well as the following:

1. Place the client in a private room that has negative air pressure, six to nine air changes per hour, and either discharge of air to the outside or a filtration system for the room air. Keep doors closed.

2. If a private room is not available, place the client with another client who is infected with the same microorganism.

3. Wear an N95 respirator when entering the room of a client who is known or suspected of having primary tuberculosis.

4. Susceptible (i.e., nonimmune) people should not enter the room of a client who has rubella (measles) or varicella (chickenpox). If they must enter, they should wear an N95 respirator.

5. Limit movement of client outside the room to essential purposes. Place a surgical mask on the client during transport.

6. Perform hand hygiene after removing a respirator.

DROPLET PRECAUTIONS

Use routine practices as well as the following:

1. Place the client in a private room.

2. If a private room is not available, place the client with another client who is infected with the same microorganism.

3. Wear a mask as well as eye protection if working within 1 to 2 metres of the client

4. Limit movement of the client outside the room to essential purposes. Place a surgical mask on the client during transport.

5. Perform hand hygiene after removing mask and eye protection.

CONTACT PRECAUTIONS

Use routine practices as well as the following:

1. Place the client in a private room.

2. If a private room is not available, place the client with another client who is infected with the same microorganism.

3. Wear gloves on entering the client's room.

   a. Change gloves after contact with infectious material.

   b. Remove gloves before leaving the client's room.

   c. Perform hand hygiene immediately after removing gloves.

   d. After hand hygiene, do not touch possibly contaminated surfaces or items in the room.

4. Wear a gown when entering a room if there is a possibility of contact with infected surfaces or items, or if the client is incontinent or has diarrhea, a colostomy, or wound drainage not contained by a dressing.

   a. Remove the gown in the client's room, and perform hand hygiene immediately after removal.

   b. Make sure uniform does not contact possible contaminated surfaces.

5. Limit movement of the client outside the room.

6. Dedicate the use of noncritical client care equipment to a single client or to clients with the same infecting microorganisms. In the latter situation, clean the equipment between use on different clients.

Source: Summarized from Provincial Infectious Diseases Advisory Committee (PIDAC). Routine Practices and Additional Precautions in All Healthcare Settings, Ministry of Health and Longterm Care, Ontario, May 2010. Available at: http://www.oahpp.ca/resources/documents/pidac/Routine%20Practices%20and%20Additional%20Precautions.pdf
Manitoba Health. Routine Practices and Additional Precautions: Preventing the Transmission of Infection in Health Care. April 2012. Available at: http://www.gov.mb.ca/health/publichealth/cdc/docs/ipc/rpap.pdf
Newfoundland Labrador. Guidelines for Routine Practices and Additional Precautions. Department of Health and Community Services. February 2009. Available at http://www.health.gov.nl.ca/health/publichealth/cdc/routine_practices_additional_precautions.pdf

to others and staying home from work and not socializing. Respiratory hygiene may be referred to as *cough etiquette* in lay terms.

SPECIAL CONSIDERATIONS: MULTIDRUG-RESISTANT ORGANISMS AND EMERGING PATHOGENS In addition to the preceding precautions, additional measures can be used for specific communicable diseases caused by multidrug-resistant or antibiotic-resistant organisms, such as vancomycin-resistant enterococci (VRE) or methicillin-resistant *S. aureus* (MRSA). Nurses should follow their agency's guidelines with respect to these pathogens, as protocols vary by jurisdiction. Additional precautions may also be warranted for infectious agents, such as severe acute respiratory syndrome (SARS), or microorganisms that are difficult to eliminate from the environment, such as *C. difficile* or norovirus.

SPECIAL CONSIDERATIONS: IMMUNOCOMPROMISED CLIENTS Compromised clients are those who are highly susceptible to infection, such as the following:

• Those who have diseases (e.g., leukemia) or have received treatments (e.g., cancer chemotherapy) that depress the resistance to infectious organisms

• Those who have extensive skin impairments, such as severe dermatitis or major burns that cannot be effectively covered with dressings

Such clients are often infected by their own microorganisms (endogenous source), but they can also be infected by microorganisms carried on the inadequately decontaminated hands of health care personnel and through nonsterile items (food, water, air, and client care equipment). Guidelines for severely compromised (immunocompromised) clients include the use of routine practices and additional precautions appropriate to their condition. Additional cleaning and use of protective clothing are not necessary beyond routine practices. The need for a single room depends on the extent to which the individual is compromised. Hand hygiene by health care workers and visitors, as well as protection from those with infection, are essential to reducing transmission of microorganisms.

Practical Issues for Implementation of Precautions

Disposal of Soiled Equipment and Supplies

Many pieces of equipment are supplied for single use only and are disposed of after use. Some items, however, are reusable. Agencies have specific policies and procedures for handling soiled equipment (e.g., disposal, cleaning, disinfecting, and sterilizing); the nurse needs to be familiar with these practices and with what items can be reused. Appropriate handling of soiled equipment and supplies is essential for these reasons:

- To prevent inadvertent exposure of health care workers to articles contaminated with body substances
- To prevent contamination of the environment

See Skill 34.2 for removing soiled PPE. Information about cleaning, disinfecting, and sterilizing is presented earlier in this chapter.

BAGGING Most articles do not need to be placed in bags unless they are contaminated or likely to have been contaminated with infective material, such as pus, blood, bodily fluids, feces, or respiratory secretions. Contaminated articles need to be enclosed in a sturdy bag impervious to microorganisms before removal from the client's room. Some agencies use labels or bags of a particular colour that designate them as infective wastes.

Follow agency protocol, or use the following guidelines to handle and bag soiled items:

- Use a single bag if it is sturdy and impervious to microorganisms, and if the contaminated articles can be placed in the bag without soiling or contaminating its outside.
- Double-bag if the above conditions are not met.
- Place garbage and soiled *disposable* equipment, including dressings and tissues, in the plastic bag that lines the waste container. Some agencies separate dry and wet waste material and incinerate dry items, such as paper towels and disposable items. No special precautions are required for disposable equipment that is not contaminated.
- Place *nondisposable* or *reusable* equipment that is visibly soiled in a labelled bag before removing it from the client's room or cubicle, and send it to a central processing area for decontamination. Some agencies may require that glass and metal items be placed in separate bags from rubber and plastic items. Glass and metal can be sterilized in an autoclave, but rubber and plastic are damaged by this process and must be cleaned by other methods, such as gas sterilization.

- Disassemble *special procedure trays* into component parts. Some components are disposable; others need to be sent to the laundry or central services for cleaning and decontaminating.
- Bag soiled *clothing* before sending it home or to the agency laundry.

LINENS Handle soiled linen as little as possible and with minimal manipulation before placing it in the laundry hamper. This prevents gross microbial contamination of the environment and persons handling the linen. Close the bag before sending it to the laundry, in accordance with agency protocol.

LABORATORY SPECIMENS Laboratory specimens, if placed in a leakproof container with a secure lid, need no special precautions. Use care when collecting specimens to avoid contaminating the outside of the container. Containers that are visibly contaminated on the outside should be placed inside a sealable plastic bag before sending them to the laboratory. This prevents personnel from having hand contact with potentially infective material.

DISHES Dishes require no special precautions. Soiling of dishes can largely be prevented by encouraging clients to wash their hands before eating. Some agencies use paper dishes for convenience, which are disposed of in the refuse container.

BLOOD PRESSURE EQUIPMENT AND GLUCOMETERS Other than routine cleaning between use on different clients, blood pressure equipment and glucometers need no special precautions unless the unit becomes contaminated with infective material. If it does become contaminated, follow agency practice.

DISPOSABLE NEEDLES, SYRINGES, AND SHARPS Place needles, syringes, and sharps (e.g., lancets, scalpels, and broken glass) into a puncture-resistant container. To avoid puncture wounds, do not detach needles from the syringe or recap the needle before disposal. See Chapter 33 for preventing needlestick injuries.

TOYS Personal toys that are visibly contaminated are bagged and sent home. Agency toys, if visibly soiled, may require cleaning. Check agency practice. Depending on the type of microorganism, its transmission, and the child's hygiene behaviours, special precautions may be required. For example, a child who has an enteric infection that can be spread by contact transmission or by fomites should not be allowed to share toys with others.

HAZARDOUS MATERIAL In addition to precautions discussed in this chapter, significant emphasis is placed on avoiding injury caused by sharp instruments, measures to be taken in case of exposure to **blood-borne pathogens** (disease causing microorganisms that are transmitted in the blood such as HIV), and communication of biohazards to employees. Health Canada (2010) requires that Workplace Hazardous Materials Information System (WHMIS) labels be affixed to containers of regulated waste and to refrigerators and freezers containing blood or other potentially infectious materials.

Transporting Clients with Infections

Transporting clients with infections outside their own rooms is avoided unless absolutely necessary. If a client must be moved, the nurse implements appropriate measures to prevent soiling of the environment. For example, the nurse ensures that any draining wound is securely covered or places a surgical mask on the client who has an airborne infection. In addition, the nurse notifies personnel at the receiving area of any infection risk so that they can maintain necessary precautions. Follow agency protocol.

Psychosocial Needs of Clients Requiring Isolation Precautions

Clients requiring **isolation precautions** (practices that prevent the spread of infection and communicable disease such as requiring that the client remain in a single room) can develop several problems as a result of the separation from others and of the special precautions taken in their care. Two of the most common are sensory deprivation and feelings of inferiority. *Sensory deprivation* occurs when the environment lacks normal stimuli for the client, for example, communication with others. Nurses should, therefore, be alert to common clinical signs of sensory deprivation: boredom, inactivity, slowness of thought, daydreaming, increased sleeping, thought disorganization, anxiety, hallucinations, and panic. Furthermore, nurses should be aware that staff members might contribute to sensory deprivation by spending less time with the client than might otherwise occur, especially if the client is in a single room, or if gowns and facial protection are required. Since the latter require additional time for client care, nurses may not be able to frequently or quickly check on a client.

A client's *feeling of inferiority* can be caused by the perception of the infection itself or to the required precautions. In North America, many people place a high value on cleanliness, and the idea of being "soiled," "contaminated," or "dirty" can give clients the feeling that they are at fault and are substandard. Although this is inaccurate, the infected persons may feel they are not as good as others and blame themselves.

Nurses need to provide care that prevents these two problems or that deals with them positively. Nursing interventions include the following:

- Assess the individual's need for stimulation.
- Initiate measures to help meet the need, including regular communication with the client and diversionary activities, such as toys for a child and books, television, or radio for an adult; providing a variety of foods to stimulate the client's sense of taste; stimulating the client's visual sense by providing a view or an activity to watch.

- Explain the infection and the associated procedures to help clients and their significant others understand the situation.
- Demonstrate warm, accepting behaviour. Avoid conveying to the client any sense of annoyance about the precautions or any feelings of revulsion about the infection.
- Do not use stricter precautions than are indicated by the diagnosis or the client's condition.

Nursing Responsibility for Infection Prevention and Control

Initiation of practices to prevent the transmission of microorganisms is generally a nursing responsibility and is based on a comprehensive assessment of the client. This assessment takes into account the status of the client's normal defence mechanisms, the client's ability to implement necessary precautions, and the source and mode of transmission of the infectious agent. The nurse then decides whether to wear gloves, gowns, masks, or protective eyewear. In all client situations, nurses must *perform appropriate hand hygiene*. Nurses should be aware of resources in their practice setting, such as an infection prevention and control policy and procedure manual or infection control practitioners, and refer to these resources for guidance, when necessary.

Besides initiating and maintaining routine practices and additional precautions, nurses have a responsibility for evaluating changes in the client's condition that could indicate a need for further precautions or indicate that additional precautions are no longer warranted. In some agencies or practice settings, especially community health, nurses are responsible for notifying the local public health officials about notifiable diseases so that accurate incidence rates can be calculated and contacts managed, as appropriate. Nurses might also be responsible for alerting infection control practitioners about incidences or clusters of infections or situations that might increase risk of infection. Nurses share responsibility for ensuring visitors wash their hands and follow posted instructions, and for

---

REFLECT ON 🔑 **PRIMARY HEALTH CARE**

Canadians have become increasingly aware of the importance of hand hygiene in the prevention and control of infection. Consider the role of *intersectoral collaboration* the next time you see a sign in a washroom reminding you to wash your hands. Automated wall mounted alcohol-based hand rub dispensers at entrance ways to public facilities and automatic sensor water faucets are examples of *appropriate technology* to limit the spread of infection. The next time a client or patient asks, "Have you washed your hands?" consider that this person is a true *participant* in his or her health care.

assisting clients to clean their hands after using the toilet and before eating (see the Reflect on Primary Health Care box on the previous page). Furthermore, nurses can demonstrate prevention behaviours by updating their immunizations and not reporting to work when ill.

In addition to the precautions cited within this chapter, the nurse implements specific actions relevant to infection prevention and control when performing many specific therapies discussed throughout this book. The following are some examples:

- Use strict aseptic technique when performing any invasive procedure (e.g., inserting an intravenous needle or catheter, suctioning an airway, and inserting a urinary catheter) and when changing surgical dressings.

- Handle needles and syringes carefully to avoid needlestick injuries. See Chapter 33.

- Change intravenous cannulae, tubing, and solution containers according to agency policy. See Chapter 44.

- Check all sterile supplies for expiry date and intact packaging before use.

- Prevent urinary infections by maintaining a closed urinary drainage system with a downward flow of urine. Do not irrigate a catheter unless ordered to do so. Provide regular catheter and perineal care. Keep the drainage bag and spout off the floor. See Chapter 42.

- Implement measures to prevent impairment of skin integrity and to prevent accumulation of secretions in the lungs (e.g., encourage the client to move, breathe deeply, and cough at least every 2 hours).

Assessing

NURSING HISTORY During the nursing history, the nurse assesses (a) the degree to which a client is at risk for developing an infection, and (b) any client complaints suggesting the presence of an infection. To identify clients at risk, the nurse reviews the client's chart and structures the nursing interview to collect data regarding the factors influencing the development of infection, especially existing disease process, history of recurrent infections, current medications and therapeutic measures, current emotional stressors, nutritional status, and history of immunizations. To obtain subjective data that may indicate the presence of an infection, the nurse asks whether the client has experienced loss of energy, loss of appetite, nausea, headache, or other signs associated with specific body systems (e.g., difficulty urinating, urinary frequency, or a sore throat). Specific questions to be asked depend on the clinical situation and should be directly related to what the suspected infection might be or the type of infection for which the client is likely at risk. See the Assessment: Interview box for sample assessment questions.

PHYSICAL ASSESSMENT Signs and symptoms of an infection vary according to the body area involved. For example, sneezing, watery or mucoid discharge from the nose, and nasal stuffiness commonly occur with an infection of the nose and sinuses; urinary frequency and sometimes cloudy or discoloured urine often occur with a urinary infection. Signs and symptoms of *localized inflammation* include the following:

- Localized swelling
- Localized redness
- Pain or tenderness with palpation or movement
- Palpable heat at the infected area
- Loss of function of the body part affected, depending on the site and extent of involvement
- Drainage from open wounds; exudate may be of various colours

Signs and symptoms of *systemic infection* are as follows:

- Fever
- Increased pulse and respiratory rate, if the fever is high
- Lassitude, malaise, and loss of energy
- Anorexia and, in some situations, nausea and vomiting

ASSESSMENT	**INTERVIEW**

Clients at Risk for Infections

The questions a nurse needs to ask will depend on the client, but the following provide examples of questions that might be asked to assess susceptibility to infection or possible exposure to an infectious agent:

- When were you last immunized for (e.g., diphtheria, tetanus, poliomyelitis, rubella, measles, influenza, hepatitis, and pneumococcal pneumonia)?*

- Have you travelled recently outside North America?

- What infections have you had in the past, and how were these treated?

- Have any of these infections recurred?

- Are you taking any antineoplastic, anti-inflammatory, or antibiotic medications?

- Do you smoke?

- Are you overweight?

- Do you have diabetes? If yes, how well controlled is it?

- Have you recently been exposed to someone with an infection?

- Have you had any recent diagnostic procedure or therapy that penetrated your skin or a body cavity?*

- What surgeries have you had? How recent were they?

- How would you describe your nutritional status in terms of a well-balanced diet?

- On a scale of 0 to 10, how would you rate the stress you have experienced in the last 6 months?

---

*These questions would be tailored according to the nature of the infection the person is at risk for or suspected of having.

- Enlargement and tenderness of lymph nodes that drain the area of infection

LABORATORY DATA Laboratory data that indicate the presence of an infection include the following:

- Elevated leukocyte (white blood cell, or WBC) count, if it is higher than $11 \times 10^9/L$.
- Increases in specific types of leukocytes as revealed in the differential white blood cell count. Specific types of white blood cells are increased or decreased in certain infections.
- Urine, blood, sputum, or other drainage *cultures* that indicate the presence of pathogenic microorganisms.

Culture and sensitivity testing involves laboratory cultivation of bacteria or yeast in a special growth medium. Laboratories report the specific species as well as its sensitivity or resistance to specific antibiotics. A Gram stain smear is also done to identify the presence of bacteria, white blood cells, and epithelial cells in the original specimen. The presence of numerous white blood cells is indicative of infection, whereas the presence of numerous epithelial cells is indicative of a poor-quality specimen (e.g., sputum may be contaminated with saliva). Collecting a good specimen is important if results are to be credible and useful. See also Skill 35.1 (page 1021), "Obtaining a Wound Drainage Specimen for Culture."

Diagnosing

Several nursing diagnoses can be associated with the transmission of microorganisms, such as risk for infection, risk for transmission of infection to others, risk for septicemia, learning required related to gaps in knowledge related to routine practices, hand hygiene, and/or respiratory hygiene, among others. Clients who have, or are at risk for, an infection are prime candidates for other physical and psychological problems. Examples of nursing diagnoses include social isolation related to additional precautions; fluid and nutritional imbalance related to anorexia associated with having an acute infection; at risk for anxiety related to uncertainty of infection trajectory.

Planning

The major goals for clients susceptible to infection are to do the following:

- Maintain or restore defences
- Avoid the spread of infectious organisms
- Reduce or alleviate problems associated with the infection

Desired health outcomes depend on the individual client's condition. Examples of desired health outcomes, although established in the planning phase, are provided in Table 34.11 on the next page

Nursing strategies to meet the three broad goals stated above generally include the measures previously described for breaking the chain of infection, such as using meticulous hand hygiene and aseptic techniques to prevent the spread of potentially infectious microorganisms, implementing measures to support the defences of a susceptible host, and teaching clients about protective measures to prevent infections and the spread of infectious agents when an infection is present.

Examples of interventions related to clients at risk for infection include the following:

- Environmental management
- Infection prevention and control (e.g., minimizing the acquisition and transmission of infectious agents)
- Risk identification
- Teaching of individuals
- Wound care

Specific nursing activities associated with each of these interventions can be selected to meet the individual needs of the client.

PLANNING FOR HOME CARE Clients being discharged following hospital care for an infection often require continued care to completely eliminate the infection or to adapt to a chronic state. In addition, such clients may be at increased risk for reinfection or development of an opportunistic infection following therapy for existing pathogens.

In preparation for discharge, the nurse needs to know the client's and family's risks, needs, strengths, and resources. The nurse tailors the teaching plan for the client and family (see the Teaching: Home Care box on the next page).

Implementing

Whenever possible, the nurse invokes strategies to prevent infection. If infection cannot be prevented, the nurse works to prevent the spread of the infection within and between persons and to treat the existing infection. In the previous sections, specific nursing activities were described that interfere with the chain of infection to prevent and control transmission of infectious organisms and that promote care of the infected client. These activities were summarized earlier in Tables 34.5 and 34.6.

Evaluating

By using data collected during care—vital signs, breath sounds, skin status, characteristics of urine or other drainage, laboratory blood values, and so on—the nurse judges whether client health outcomes have been achieved. Examples of client goals and related health outcomes are shown in Table 34.11 on the next page.

If the health outcomes are not achieved, the nurse may need to consider such questions as the following:

TEACHING | **HOME CARE**

Environmental Management

The way the client takes care of an infection after going home is important. The nurse can help by teaching the client how to do it correctly:

- Discuss injury-proofing the home to prevent the possibility of further tissue injury (e.g., use of padding, handrails, removal of hazards).
- Explore ways to control the environmental temperature and airflow (especially if the client has an airborne infection).
- Determine the advisability of visitors and family members in proximity to the client.
- Describe ways to manipulate the bed, the room, and other household facilities.

Infection Prevention and Control

- On the basis of the assessment of the client and family knowledge, teach proper hand hygiene (e.g., before handling foods, before eating, after toileting, before and after any required home care treatment, and after touching any of the body substances, such as wound drainage) and related hygiene measures to all family members.
- Promote nail care: Teach about keeping fingernails short, clean, and well manicured to eliminate rough edges or hangnails, which can harbour microorganisms.
- Instruct not to share personal care items, such as toothbrushes, washcloths, and towels, and describe the rationale of how infections can be transmitted from shared personal items.
- Discuss alcohol-based hand rub, different types of soaps, and effective disinfectants.
- Ensure access to and proper use of gloves and other barriers as indicated by the type of infection or risk.
- Discuss the relationship among hygiene, rest, activity, and nutrition in the chain of infection.
- Instruct about proper administration of medication.

- Instruct about cleaning reusable equipment and supplies, using soap and water, and disinfecting with a chlorine bleach solution.
- Teach the client and family members how to avoid infections.
- Suggest techniques for safe food preservation and preparation (e.g., wash raw fruits and vegetables before eating them; refrigerate all opened and unpackaged foods).
- Encourage respiratory hygiene by covering the mouth and nose with a tissue or the sleeve to prevent the transmission of microorganisms by the airborne or droplet route when coughing or sneezing.
- Teach about the importance of maintaining sufficient fluid intake to promote urine production and output. This helps flush the bladder and urethra of microorganisms and maintains tissue hydration.
- Advise the client and family members to put used needles in a puncture-resistant container with a screw-top lid and label it to avoid discarding it in the garbage.
- Emphasize the need for proper immunizations of all family members.

Wound Care

- Teach the client and family about the signs of wound healing and of wound infection and why monitoring the wound is important.
- Delineate the factors that promote wound healing.
- Explain the proper technique for changing the dressing and disposing of the soiled dressing. Reinforce the need to place contaminated dressings and other disposable items containing bodily fluids in moisture-proof plastic bags.

Referrals

- Provide appropriate information regarding how to access community resources, home care agencies, sources of supplies, and community or public health departments for immunizations.

TABLE 34.11 Evaluation of Goals and Health Outcomes: Risk for Infection

Goal	Examples of Desired Health Outcomes
Maintain body defences	Skin integrity intact
	Mucous membranes intact
	WBC values within normal range
	T cell levels within normal range
	Respiratory assessment findings within normal range (e.g., respiratory rate, rhythm, depth, and breath sounds)
Avoid spread of microorganisms	Gastrointestinal tract assessment findings within normal range (e.g., stool colour, odour, and consistency, and absence of emesis)
	Immunizations recommended for age are current
	Describes mode of transmission of microorganism
	Demonstrates infection prevention and control practices that reduce transmission
	Follows prescribed treatment for diagnosed infection

BOX 34.5 STEPS TO FOLLOW AFTER EXPOSURE TO BLOOD-BORNE PATHOGENS

The following are important steps to follow after potential exposure to blood-borne pathogens (e.g., HIV, hepatitis B, hepatitis C):

- Report the incident immediately to appropriate personnel within the agency.
- Complete an injury report.
- Seek appropriate evaluation and follow-up. This includes the following:
  - Identification and documentation of the source individual when feasible and legal
  - Testing of the source individual's blood when feasible and consent is given
  - Making results of the test available to the source individual's health care provider

- Testing of blood of exposed health care personnel (with consent)
- Postexposure prophylaxis (PEP) if medically indicated (e.g., hepatitis B vaccine for hepatitis B virus, or recommended agents for HIV)
- Medical counselling regarding personal risk of infection or risk of infecting others
- For a puncture or laceration,
  - Encourage bleeding.
  - Clean the area with soap and water.
  - Initiate first aid and seek treatment, if indicated.
- For a mucous membrane exposure (eyes, nose, mouth), flush with saline solution or water for 5 to 10 minutes.

- Were appropriate measures implemented to prevent skin breakdown and lung infection?
- Was strict aseptic technique implemented for invasive procedures?
- Are prescribed medications affecting the immune system?
- Is client placement appropriate to reduce the risk of transmission of microorganisms?
- Did the client and family misunderstand or fail to follow necessary instructions?

Occupational Health Issues Related to Infection

The Public Health Agency of Canada provides guidelines to protect health care workers from occupational exposure to blood-borne pathogens in the workplace. **Occupational exposure** is defined as reasonably anticipated skin, eye, mucous membrane, or parenteral contact with blood or other potentially infectious materials that may result from the performance of an employee's duties. Nurses should be immunized against hepatitis B, varicella, and other vaccine-preventable diseases prior to beginning work in nursing.

The transmission of infectious fluids in the clinical setting has three major modes:

1. *Puncture wounds* from contaminated needles or other sharps, commonly referred to as needlestick injuries
2. *Skin contact*, which allows infectious fluids to enter through wounds and broken or damaged skin
3. *Mucous membrane* contact, which allows infectious fluids to enter through mucous membranes of the eyes, mouth, and nose

Conscientious use of routine practices, appropriately using PPE (gloves, masks, gowns, goggles, face shields, special

resuscitative equipment), and avoiding carelessness in the clinical area will reduce the risk of injury to the caregiver. Used needles and sharp items should be disposed of immediately after use, without recapping of needles. Puncture resistant containers need to be placed for easy access in areas where the items are used. Measures to be taken in case of possible exposure to blood-borne pathogens are outlined in Box 34.5. Nurses should follow their agency's specific protocols for managing exposure and for handling blood or body fluid spills. Management and **postexposure prophylaxis (PEP)** (treatment given after exposure to an infectious agent aimed at reducing the probability of infection) vary according to the potential or known infectious agent.

Nurses who themselves are infected with a blood-borne pathogen must ensure that they practise in a manner that does not put their clients at risk. Most health care agencies and some nursing regulatory bodies have expert panels to advise nurses and other health care professionals in these situations.

Roles of the Infection Control Practitioner

Infection control practitioners (ICPs) are important in both acute care and continuing care facilities. Many organizations, however, do not meet the recommendation of one ICP per 100 to 150 beds for acute care, and one per 100 to 250 beds for long-term care (Zoutman & Ford 2009). The role of the ICP is less developed in community health settings, outside of control of communicable diseases. The majority of ICPs come from a nursing background, though some may have a background in microbiology or epidemiology.

Key roles and activities of ICPs relate to the following:

- Surveillance of infections to monitor rates and trends in order to identify problems or affirm success of interventions

- Outbreak identification and management
- Staff education related to infection prevention and control, for example, with respect to using routine practices and additional precautions, promoting hand hygiene, or addressing and preventing specific problems
- Consultation with staff on individual client management
- Development, implementation, and evaluation of policies and procedures with specific implications for infection prevention and control (e.g., IV insertion or maintenance, operating room procedures, infection prevention and control manual)
- Acting as consultants to a variety of committees on issues related to, or that may have an impact on, infection prevention and control (e.g., policy and procedure committee, selection of products for purchase)

ICPs also collaborate with occupational health and safety staff on specific issues, such as prevention and management of needlestick injuries, or annual influenza immunization campaigns. Finally, ICPs are an integral part of infection prevention and control committees, which all health care organizations must have. Such committees are multidisciplinary, including representatives from the clinical laboratory, housekeeping, maintenance, nutritional services, pharmacy, nursing, medicine, and client care areas. Their mandate is to monitor the infection prevention and control programs, advise ICPs on direction, and facilitate consultation between key groups.

Infection Prevention and Control Is a Shared Responsibility

Nurses are key players in preventing and controlling infections, given the nature and extent of their contact with clients. Their focus is most commonly on individuals and small groups (e.g., by identifying risks, performing hand hygiene, minimizing exposure of portals of entry to microorganisms, and using routine practices and additional precautions). They also contribute to promoting a safe work environment. Administrators share responsibility in promoting a safe work environment by ensuring appropriate staffing (in numbers and skills), implementing evidence-informed guidelines, and advocating for adequate supplies and structures (e.g., ventilation or environmental controls). Use of PPE alone is insufficient for preventing and controlling infections in the absence of administrative supports and engineering controls. Infection control practitioners focus on larger groups and institutions, both helping to identify problems and intervening to resolve them. Together, health care providers, clients and families, administrators, and infection control practitioners can reduce the incidence of infections and their impact.

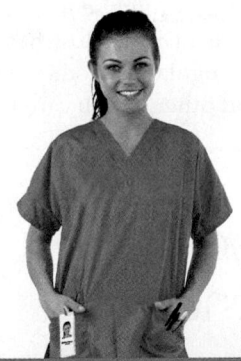

Case Study 34

Mrs. Cortez is a 76-year-old woman who is independent, lives alone, and prefers not to rely on others unless absolutely necessary. She was active and healthy until about 6 months ago, at which time she developed a persistent upper respiratory tract infection. Because she was unable to obtain or prepare food, she lost weight and became very weak. She finally sought medical attention, but she has not yet fully recovered. Mrs. Cortez was admitted to the acute care facility for fever, shortness of breath, productive cough, dehydration, and nutritional deficiency. An initial Gram stain of a sputum specimen suggests that she does not have tuberculosis but may have pneumococcal pneumonia.

CRITICAL THINKING QUESTIONS

1. Mrs. Cortez's physician suspects that she has pneumonia, a serious lower respiratory tract infection. Identify factors that increase Mrs. Cortez's risk for such an infection, and explain how each factor contributes to the risk.

2. What assessment data would be helpful to the nurse when planning care for Mrs. Cortez?

3. What routine practices and additional precautions should be instituted for Mrs. Cortez? Explain your reasoning in terms of the chain of infection.

4. What should the nurse teach Mrs. Cortez and her visitors with respect to preventing infection?

5. The nurse notes that the housekeeping aide is leaving Mrs. Cortez's room. The aide stops to wash her hands, soaping them and rubbing them together under running water for about 5 seconds. She then turns off the water before reaching for the paper towels to dry her hands. Should the nurse intervene, and if so, in what way?

Check the eText in MyNursingLab for answers and explanations.

KEY TERMS

active immunity *p. 959*

additional
  precautions *p. 990*

airborne
  precautions *p. 990*

airborne
  transmission *p. 964*

alcohol-based hand rub
  (ABHR) *p. 969*

antibodies
  (immunoglobulins)
  p. 960

antigens *p. 959*

antimicrobial
  agents *p. 969*

antiseptic *p. 968*

asepsis *p. 955*

aseptic technique *p. 978*

autoantigen *p. 959*

bacteremia *p. 956*

bacteria *p. 956*

blood-borne
  pathogens *p. 992*

carrier *p. 961*

cell-mediated
  defences *p. 960*

cellular immunity *p. 960*

chemotaxis *p. 958*

cicatrix *p. 959*

clean technique *p. 978*

colonization *p. 961*

communicability *p. 957*

communicable
  disease *p. 957*

compromised
  hosts *p. 964*

contact
  precautions *p. 990*

cytokines *p. 959*

diapedesis *p. 958*

direct contact
  transmission *p. 963*

disinfectant *p. 968*

disinfection *p. 968*

droplet nuclei *p. 964*

droplet
  precautions *p. 990*

droplet
  transmission *p. 963*

emigration *p. 958*

exudate *p. 959*

fecal–oral route *p. 964*

fibrinogen *p. 959*

fibrous (scar)
  tissue *p. 959*

fit checking *p. 977*

fit testing *p. 977*

fungi *p. 956*

granulation
  tissue *p. 959*

hand hygiene *p. 969*

health care–associated
  infections *p. 955*

helminths *p. 956*

humoral (circulating)
  immunity *p. 960*

hyperemia *p. 958*

immunization *p. 964*

immunoglobulins *p. 960*

indirect contact
  transmission *p. 963*

infection *p. 955*

infection control
  practitioners *p. 997*

infectious agent *p. 955*

inflammation *p. 957*

interferons *p. 957*

isolation
  precautions *p. 993*

leukocytes *p. 958*

leukocytosis *p. 959*

local infection *p. 961*

macrophages *p. 957*

margination *p. 958*

microbial load *p. 961*

nonspecific
  defences *p. 957*

normal flora *p. 954*

nosocomial
  infections *p. 955*

occupational
  exposure *p. 997*

opportunistic
  pathogen *p. 957*

parasites *p. 956*

passive immunity *p. 960*

pathogen *p. 954*

pathogenicity *p. 957*

personal protective
  equipment
  (PPE) *p. 973*

phagocytes *p. 957*

point of care risk
  assessment *p. 969*

portal of entry *p. 962*

portals of exit *p. 962*

postexposure
  prophylaxis *p. 997*

protozoa *p. 956*

pus *p. 959*

pyrogens *p. 959*

regeneration *p. 959*

reservoirs *p. 961*

resident flora *p. 954*

respirators *p. 976*

respiratory
  hygiene *p. 990*

routine practices *p. 989*

septicemia *p. 961*

specific defences *p. 957*

sterile field *p. 979*

sterile technique *p. 978*

sterilization *p. 969*

susceptible host *p. 964*

systemic infection *p. 961*

vaccination *p. 964*

vector-borne
  transmission *p. 964*

vehicle-borne
  transmission *p. 964*

virions *p. 960*

virulence *p. 957*

virulence factors *p. 957*

viruses *p. 956*

CHAPTER HIGHLIGHTS

- Microorganisms exist everywhere. Most are harmless and some are beneficial; however, many can cause infection in susceptible persons.

- Some normal body flora produce toxic metabolites, alter local pH, or physically compete for space, thereby inhibiting growth of foreign bacteria.

- Effective control of infectious disease is an international, national, community, and individual responsibility.

- Health care–associated infections (HAIs) have significant impact on morbidity, mortality, quality of life, and health care costs. Major sites for these infections are the respiratory and urinary tracts, the bloodstream, and surgical or open wounds.

- Bacteria and viruses are responsible for most HAIs. They differ in their ability to be spread from individual to individual and in their ability to produce disease.

- Humans have both specific and nonspecific defences that combat infectious agents.

- Intact skin and mucous membranes are the body's first line of defence against microorganisms.

- Some body secretions (e.g., saliva and tears) contain enzymes that act as antibacterial agents.

- The inflammatory response limits physical, chemical, and microbial injury and promotes repair of injured tissue.

- Immunity is the specific resistance of the body to infectious agents. Antibodies neutralize viruses or toxins so that they cannot enter or damage cells, while cytotoxic T cells target and kill specific bacteria or virus-infected cells.

- Acquired immunity is active or passive and, in either case, can be naturally or artificially induced.

- Clinical manifestations of infection result from both altered function of the damaged tissue and from the inflammatory response that is initiated in defence.

- In colonization, microorganisms grow and multiply but do not cause physiological changes in host tissue. In infection, microorganisms cause tissue damage.

- Infection occurs when there is an imbalance between microorganisms and host defences (e.g., high microbial load or low resistance).

- An infection can develop if the six links in the chain of infection—infectious agent, reservoir, portal of exit, mode of transmission, portal of entry, and susceptible host—are not interrupted.

- The six routes of transmission are direct contact, indirect contact, droplet, airborne, vehicle-borne, and vector-borne.

- Factors that contribute to HAI risks are invasive procedures, medical therapies, the existence of susceptible persons, inappropriate use of antibiotics, and insufficient hand hygiene before and after client contact and after contact with body substances.

- Especially at risk of acquiring an infection are the very young or old; those with poor nutritional status, a deficiency of serum immunoglobulins, multiple stressors, insufficient immunizations, obesity, anemia, poorly controlled diabetes, or an existing disease process; those who smoke; and those receiving certain medical therapies.

- Infectious agents can be eliminated by physically removing reservoirs, by using antimicrobial drugs to kill microorganisms or slow their growth, by physically cleaning materials, by disinfecting, or by sterilizing.

- Hand hygiene, considered to be the single most effective infection control measure, includes both handwashing (to physically remove transient microorganisms) and use of an alcohol-based hand rub (to kill microorganisms), done correctly and at indicated times to reduce hand carriage of microorganisms.

- Personal protective equipment (gloves, gowns, face masks, respirators, and eyewear) disrupts transmission of microorganisms from patient to caregiver and from patient to patient via the caregiver.

- Facial protection (surgical masks and eye protection) protect against infections transmitted via the droplet route, while respirators, if properly fitted and used, protect against infections transmitted by both the airborne and the droplet routes.

- Asepsis is the freedom from infection or infectious material.

- Aseptic (clean) technique keeps the area free from most microorganisms, whereas sterile technique refers to working within a sterile field, using sterile items, and keeping an area or objects free of all microorganisms.

- Supporting host defences by addressing individual risk factors for infection is important in breaking the chain of infection.

- Routine practices rely on hand hygiene and use of appropriate personal protective equipment, and they are used to protect against exposure to all blood and bodily fluids from all clients, regardless of infection status.

- Other routine practices relate to source control, cleaning equipment, ensuring a clean and safe environment, and education.

- Additional precautions are used in addition to routine practices when clients have infections that are transmitted through the airborne, droplet, and/or contact routes.

- Respiratory hygiene (cough etiquette) involves containing respiratory secretions by coughing or sneezing into a tissue (which is then discarded) or cloth (e.g., sleeve), accompanied by hand hygiene.

- Additional protocols may be in effect, depending on the practice setting, for clients who are immunocompromised or who have infections caused by multidrug-resistant organisms.

- Clients requiring isolation precautions are susceptible to sensory deprivation and decreased self-esteem.

- Nursing responsibilities for infection prevention and control include assessing clients' risks for infection or status of an infection and problems or complications associated with the infection; implementing routine practices and additional precautions and other interventions appropriate to the client's needs and situation; evaluating outcomes; and preventing the transmission of microorganisms from infected clients to others.

- The nurse must be knowledgeable about sources and modes of transmission of microorganisms.

- Nurses must also take measures to protect themselves and others from needlestick injuries.

- Infection control practitioners are key personnel for infection prevention and control, helping to identify problems and intervene to resolve them. They are an excellent resource for nurses.

- Infection prevention and control is a shared responsibility.

ASSESS YOUR LEARNING

1. A patient is a chronic carrier of an infection. To prevent the spread of the infection to other patients or health care providers, the nurse emphasizes interventions that do which of the following?

   a. Eliminate the reservoir.

   b. Block the portal of exit from the reservoir.

   c. Block the portal of entry into the host.

   d. Decrease the susceptibility of the host.

2. The most effective nursing action for controlling the spread of infection includes which of the following?

   a. Performing hand hygiene before and after client contact

   b. Wearing gloves and masks for all client care

   c. Implementing isolation precautions

   d. Administering broad-spectrum prophylactic antibiotics

3. In caring for a patient on contact precautions for a draining infected foot ulcer, the nurse should perform which of the following?

   a. Wear a mask during dressing changes.

   b. Provide disposable meal trays and silverware.

   c. Follow routine practices in all interactions with the patient.

   d. Use aseptic technique for all direct contact with the patient.

4. When caring for a single patient during one shift, it is appropriate for the nurse to reuse which of the following personal protective equipment?

   a. Goggles

   b. Gown

   c. Surgical mask

   d. Clean gloves

5. While donning sterile gloves (open method), the cuff of the first glove rolls under itself about 0.5 cm. Which is the BEST action for the nurse?

   a. Remove the glove and start over with a new pair.

   b. Wait until the second glove is in place and then unroll the cuff with the other sterile hand.

   c. Ask a colleague to assist by unrolling the cuff.

   d. Leave the cuff rolled under.

6. Which of the following statements by a 69-year-old client with no major health problems requires further teaching?

   a. "I need to make sure that I get my flu shot at least every two years."

   b. "I don't think I need to get vaccinated against Hepatitis A unless I plan on doing some travelling to risky areas."

   c. "I had one dose of vaccine against pneumonia when I turned 65 so I think I am fine with that."

   d. "I had chickenpox when I was a child so I don't think I need that new vaccine."

7. The nurse has taught a client and family general infection prevention strategies. Which of the following statements by the client indicates effective learning has occurred?

   a. "We will use antimicrobial soap and hot water to wash our hands at least three times per day."

   b. "We must wash or peel all raw fruits and vegetables before eating."

   c. "A wound or sore is not infected unless we see it draining pus."

   d. "We should not share toothbrushes but it is OK to share towels and washcloths."

8. Which of the following areas are considered sterile on a person in the operating room? Assume that all articles were sterile when applied.

   a. The chest area of the surgeon's sterile gown

   b. The back area of the surgeon's sterile gown

   c. The sterile face mask on the surgeon's face

   d. The full arm of the surgeon's gown

9. The nurse determines that a field remains sterile if which of the following conditions exist?

   a. The tips of wet forceps are held upward when held in ungloved hands.

   b. The field was set up 1 hour before the procedure.

   c. Sterile items are kept at least 5 cm from the edge of the field.

   d. The nurse reaches over the field rather than around the edges.

10. Sue and Mary are coworkers who have desks beside each other and share a telephone. Sue comes to work with a cold. She is tired, has a low-grade fever, and is sneezing frequently. What can Sue do to minimize the risk that Mary will develop the same respiratory infection?

    a. She should stay a minimum of 0.5 metres from Mary.

    b. She should take an antipyretic agent to lower her fever.

    c. She should sneeze into a tissue or her sleeve.

    d. She should not come to work if the symptoms do not subside within 2 days.

Check the eText in MyNursingLab for answers and explanations.

WEBLINKS

Canada's Hand Hygiene Challenge

http://www.handhygiene.ca/English/Pages/default.aspx

This site is a joint venture of the Canadian Patient Safety Institute, Safer Healthcare Now! and other stakeholders with interest in patient safety. The site offers a wide range of tools, links to evidence, and educational materials for the public as well as health care professionals.

Public Health Agency of Canada: Provincial Immunization Guides

http://www.phac-aspc.gc.ca/im/iyc-vve/is-cv-eng.php

This site provides access to provincial and territorial immunizations guides and schedules—the date of birth of a child can be entered along with the province or territory he or she resides in, and an individualized immunization schedule is produced.

Community and Hospital Infection Control Association–Canada (CHICA–Canada)

http://www.chica.org

This website, although targeted primarily to infection control practitioners, also has links to information useful for education about infection control issues.

MyNursingLab

REFERENCES

Dronge, A. S., Perkal, M. F., Kancir, S., Concato, J., Asian, M., & Rosenthal, R. A. (2006). Long-term glycemic control and postoperative infectious complications. *Archives of Surgery, 141*(4), 365–380.

Gravel, D., Taylor, G., Ofner, M., Johnston, L., Loeb, M., Roth, V. R., ... Matlow. A. (2007). Point prevalence survey for healthcare-associated infections within Canadian adult acute-care hospitals. *Journal of Hospital Infection, 66*(3), 343–248. Epub 2007 Jun 18.

Gravel, D., Matlow, A., Ofner-Agostini, M., Loeb, M., Johnston, L., Bryce, E., ... Canadian Nosocomial Infection Surveillance Program. (2007). A point prevalence survey for health care-associated infections in pediatric populations in major Canadian acute care hospitals. *American Journal of Infection Control, 35*(3), 157–162.

Health Canada. (2010). The Workplace Hazardous Materials Information System. Retrieved from http://www.hc-sc.gc.ca/ewh-semt/occup-travail/whmis-simdut/index-eng.php

National Advisory Committee on Immunization. (2011). Statement on influenza vaccination for the 2011–2012 season. *Canada Communicable Disease Report, 37 ACS-5*(September). Retrieved from http://www.phac-aspc.gc.ca/publicat/ccdr-rmtc/11vol37/acs-dcc-5/index-eng.php

Provincial Infectious Diseases Advisory Committee. (2009). "Just Clean Your Hands" Ontario's hand hygiene program for hospitals. Retrieved from http://www.justcleanyourhands.ca/pdf/10_1_4_moment_poster_Eng.pdf

Public Health Agency of Canada. (2010). The facts on the safety and effectiveness of HPV vaccine. Retrieved from http://www.phac-aspc.gc.ca/std-mts/hpv-vph/fact-faits-vacc-eng.php

Zoutman, D. E., & Ford, B. D. (2009). A comparison of infection control program resources, activities, and antibiotic resistant organism rates in Canadian acute care hospitals in 1999 and 2005. *The Canadian Journal of Infection Control, 24*(2), 109–115.

Chapter 35

Skin Integrity and Wound Care

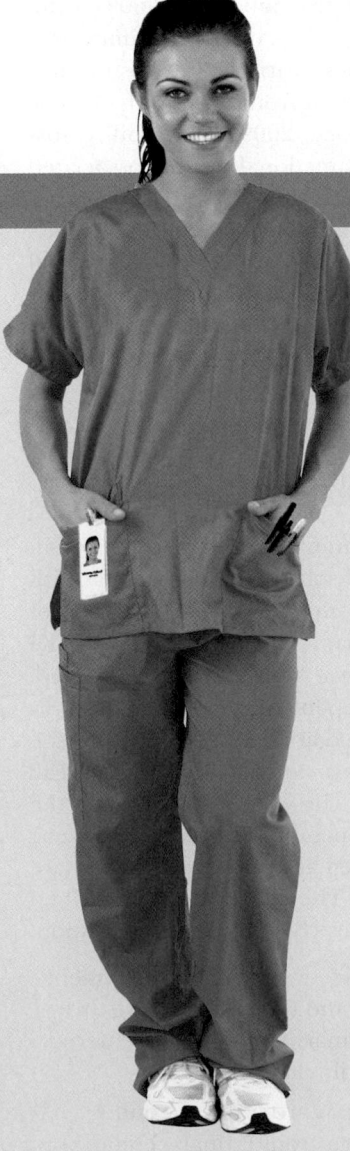

After studying this chapter, you will be able to:

1. Discuss factors affecting skin integrity.

2. Classify wounds according to depth, chronicity, and level of contamination.

3. Identify 10 risk factors for pressure ulcer development.

4. Compare and contrast the six categories of pressure ulcer classification.

5. Describe the process of wound healing and five factors that can affect healing.

6. Differentiate among wound colonization, contamination, and infection.

7. Identify assessment data pertinent to the integument.

8. Describe special considerations associated with lower limb ulcers.

9. List the essential steps of obtaining wound specimens, selecting and applying dressings, and irrigating a wound.

10. Contrast the indications and contraindications of commonly used dressing materials and supportive or immobilizing devices.

11. List adjunctive therapies that are used to promote wound healing.

12. Explain physiological responses to heat and cold and describe the methods of applying dry and moist heat and cold.

Skin, or the integument, is the largest organ in the body and serves a variety of important functions in maintaining health and protecting the individual from harm. Although impaired skin integrity is uncommon in most healthy individuals, it poses a particular threat to vulnerable populations (e.g., older adults) as well as those experiencing a health crisis or an invasive procedure.

Healthy skin integrity is an essential nursing goal of any skin care program and nurses must routinely encourage health-promotion practices to maintain their clients' skin integrity. When disruptions occur, however, effective wound management requires a comprehensive knowledge of the wound healing process, sensitivity to the experience of the client, and excellent care informed by the most recent and valid evidence.

Skin Function and Integrity

Intact skin refers to surface skin and skin layers that are free of disruption or alteration. See Chapter 28 for details regarding physical examination of the integumentary system. Skin provides a protective interface between the environment and the internal organs of the body. It also plays a major role in thermoregulation, vitamin D synthesis, immune function, and the transmission of the sensory impulses of touch, pain, pressure, vibration, and temperature. As an organ of communication, the appearance of skin is closely linked with self-perception. When the integrity of skin is damaged or scarred, changes may occur in self-esteem, body image, and social interactions.

Skin integrity is influenced by factors *intrinsic* to the individual, such as age, genetics, and general health, as well as *extrinsic* factors, such as hygiene, living conditions, and mechanical forces, such as shear. Genetics and heredity determine many aspects of a person's skin, including skin colour, sensitivity to sunlight, and allergies. Age influences skin integrity in that the skin of both the very young and the very old is more fragile and susceptible to injury than that of most adults. Sensory or cognitive impairments, poor nutrition, obesity, infection, medications (e.g., corticosteroids), and many chronic illnesses and their treatment can also interfere with the appearance and function of the integument. People with impaired peripheral circulation may have skin on the legs that appears shiny, has lost its hair distribution, and damages easily. Some medications, corticosteroids for example, cause thinning of skin and allow it to be much more readily harmed. Many medications increase sensitivity to sunlight and can predispose the person to severe sunburns. Some of the most common ones that cause this damage are certain antibiotics, chemotherapy drugs for cancer, and some psychotherapeutic drugs. Poor nutrition alone can interfere with the appearance and function of normal skin.

Skin integrity must be viewed in the context of the whole person. A history and focused physical assessment provide invaluable data about skin integrity problems. Psychosocial assessments are equally important to determine the client's ability and motivation to understand and adhere to any treatment program (Price, 2009). Pain, immobility, sleep disturbance, lack of energy, limitations in work and leisure activities, worries and frustrations, and poor self-esteem may result from living with chronic impaired skin integrity (Price, 2009). Immobility, loss of independence, and the functional decline associated with limitations resulting from chronic wounds can have significant impacts on overall health, including altered eating habits, depression, social isolation and a gradual reduction in activity (Price, 2009). These, in turn, further compromise the person's intrinsic ability to heal the wound.

Types of Wounds

Body wounds are either intentional or unintentional. *Intentional* wounds are the result of therapy, such as with surgery or venipunctures—in which the wounding of skin, though causing trauma, is done to implement the therapeutic plan. *Unintentional* wounds are not planned, nor are they part of a therapeutic intervention, such as the traumatic wound incurred as a result of a motor vehicle collision. If the tissues are traumatized without a break in skin, the wound is *closed*. The wound is *open* when the skin surface or the mucous membrane surface is broken.

Wounds can be described according to how they are acquired (see Table 35.1). They also can be described according to the likelihood and degree of contamination:

- **Clean wounds** are uninfected wounds in which there is minimal inflammation and the respiratory, gastrointestinal, genital, and urinary tracts are not entered. Clean wounds are primarily closed wounds.
- **Clean-contaminated wounds** are surgical wounds in which the respiratory, gastrointestinal, genital, or urinary tract has been entered under controlled

TABLE 35.1 Types of Wounds Based on How Acquired

Type	Cause	Description and Characteristics
Incision	Sharp instrument (e.g., knife or scalpel), usually intentional	Open wound; painful; deep or shallow
Contusion	Blow from a blunt instrument	Closed wound, skin appears ecchymotic (bruised) because of damaged blood vessels
Abrasion	Surface scrape, either unintentional (e.g., scraped knee from a fall) or intentional (e.g., dermal abrasion to remove pockmarks)	Open wound involving skin; painful
Puncture	Penetration of skin and often the underlying tissues by a sharp instrument, either intentional or unintentional	Open wound
Laceration	Tissues torn apart, often from accidents (e.g., with machinery)	Open wound; edges are often jagged
Penetrating	Penetration of skin and the underlying tissues, usually unintentional (e.g., from a bullet or metal fragments)	Open wound

conditions. Such wounds show no evidence of infection.

- **Contaminated wounds** include open, fresh, accidental wounds and surgical wounds that involve a major break in sterile technique or gross spillage from the gastrointestinal tract, and incisions in which acute, nonpurulent inflammation is visible.
- **Dirty or infected wounds** include old traumatic wounds with retained dead tissue and wounds that involve existing clinical infection or perforated viscera.

Wounds, excluding pressure ulcers and burns, can also be classified by depth, that is, the tissue layers involved in the wound (see Box 35.1).

Wounds are considered to be *acute* or *chronic*, depending on the healing process and the inflammatory response to trauma. An **acute wound** is one that heals within an expected time frame, whereas the term **chronic wound** describes any break or alteration in skin that is of long duration (often 3 months or more) or recurs frequently.

BOX 35.1 CLASSIFYING WOUNDS BY DEPTH

Wounds can be classified by depth:

- **Partial-thickness wound:** Confined to skin, that is, the dermis and epidermis; heals by regeneration
- **Full-thickness wound:** Involving the dermis, epidermis, subcutaneous tissue, and possibly muscle and bone; requires connective tissue repair

Pressure Ulcers

Pressure ulcers are a serious, costly, and, unfortunately, common problem in many health care settings. Pressure ulcers are also called *decubitus ulcers, pressure sores,* and *distortion sores,* although the preferred term is *pressure ulcers.* Note that use of the term *bedsores* has fallen out of favour, as pressure ulcers can develop even in the patient who is not bedridden. According the National Pressure Ulcer Advisory Panel (NPUAP, 2007), a **pressure ulcer** is "a clinical sign indicating tissue damage which results from prolonged and excessive tissue deformation (compression, shear, and tension), including possible ischemic distortion of the vasculature" (Sibbald, on behalf of the Shifting the Original Paradigm Expert [SOPE] Panel, 2011). People who are predisposed to pressure ulcers are at high risk for increased morbidity and mortality. Unrelenting pain from a nonhealing wound affects quality of life and also contributes to further delays in the wound-healing processes (Woo & Sibbald, 2008). People who develop pressure ulcers have a 4.5 times higher risk of death than those with similar risk factors but no pressure ulcers (Salcido, 2011).

The incidence and prevalence of pressure ulcers in health care settings can vary widely. In hospitals, incidence rates of between 1% and 30% have been reported, with higher rates reported in intensive care units, where patients are less mobile and are critically ill. Older adult patients admitted to acute care hospitals for hip replacements and long bone fractures are at even greater risk, with a 66% incidence of pressure ulcers (Salcido, 2011). In Canada, estimates of pressure ulcer prevalence across various settings are 25.1% for acute care settings, 29.9% for non–acute care settings, 22.1% in mixed health care settings, and 15.1% in community care settings. The overall estimate of prevalence in all health care institutions in Canada is 26% (Woodbury & Houghton, 2004).

In this chapter, we use pressure ulcers as an example to identify healing strategies for chronic wounds, recognizing, however, that chronic ulcers have many causes. Venous leg ulcers and diabetic foot ulcers are other common types of chronic ulcers that will be discussed briefly. The Canadian Association of Wound Care (2006) has published a *Quick Reference Guide* summarizing best practice recommendations for wound bed preparation, as well as for the prevention and treatment of pressure ulcers, venous leg ulcers, and diabetic foot ulcers (see Box 35.2).

BOX 35.2 CANADIAN ASSOCIATION OF WOUND CARE QUICK REFERENCE GUIDE RECOMMENDATIONS FOR PRACTICE

QRG
Quick Reference Guide
RECOMMENDATIONS FOR PRACTICE

CAWC·ACSP

1 PREPARING THE WOUND BED
R. Gary Sibbald, BSc MD FRCPC (Med) FRCPC (Derm);
Heather L. Orsted, RN BN ET MSc; Patricia M. Coutts, RN;
David H. Keast, MSc MD FCFP

No. Recommendations

Identify and Treat the Cause

No.	Recommendation
1.	Assess the patient's ability to heal. Adequate blood supply must be present as well as the correction of other important host factors to support healing.
2.	Diagnose and correct or modify treatable causes of tissue damage.

Address Patient-centred Concerns

No.	Recommendation
3.	Assess and support the management of patient-centred concerns (pain and quality of life) to enable healing.
4.	Provide patient education and support to increase adherence to treatment plan.

Provide Local Wound Care

No.	Recommendation
5.	Assess and monitor the wound history and physical characteristics (location + MEASURE*).
6.	Debride healable wounds by removing non-viable, contaminated or infected tissue (through surgical, autolytic, enzymatic, mechanical or larval [biologic] methods). Non-healable wounds should have only non-viable tissue removed; active debridement to bleeding tissue is contraindicated.
7.	Cleanse wounds with low toxicity solutions (such as normal saline or water). Topical antiseptic solutions should be reserved for wounds that are non-healable or those in which the local bacterial burden is of greater concern than the stimulation of healing.
8.	Assess and treat the wound for increased bacterial burden or infection (distinguish from persistent inflammation of non-bacterial origin).
9.	Select a dressing that is appropriate for the needs of the wound, the patient and the caregiver or clinical setting.
10.	Evaluate expected rate of wound healing. If suboptimal, reassess recommendations 1 to 9.
11.	Use active wound therapies (biological agents, skin grafts, adjunctive therapies) when other factors have been corrected and healing still does not progress.

Provide Organizational Support

No.	Recommendation
12.	For improved outcomes, education and evidence base must be tied to interprofessional teams with the co-operation of health-care systems.

* MEASURE is an acronym for Measure, Exudate, Appearance, Suffering, Undermining, Re-evaluate and Edge.

2 PREVENTION & TREATMENT OF PRESSURE ULCERS
David H. Keast, MSc MD FCFP; Nancy Parslow, RN ET;
Pamela E. Houghton, BScPT PhD; Linda Norton, OT Reg (Ont);
Chris Fraser, BSc RD

No. Recommendation

Identify and Treat the Cause

No.	Recommendation
1.	Complete a patient history and a targeted physical examination to determine general health and risk factors that may lead to pressure ulcer formation or that may affect healing of existing ulcers.
2.	Assess and modify situations where pressure may be increased.
3.	Maximize nutritional status.
4.	Manage moisture and incontinence.
5.	Maximize activity and mobility, reducing or eliminating friction and shear.

Address Patient-centred Concerns

No.	Recommendation
6.	Assess and control pain.
7.	Assess and assist with psychosocial needs.

Provide Local Wound Care

No.	Recommendation
8.	Stage, assess and treat the wound. Provide an optimal wound environment consistent with the principles of *Preparing the Wound Bed*.
9.	Introduce adjunctive modalities or biologically active dressings where appropriate.
10.	Consider surgical intervention for deep non-healing ulcers (Stage III and Stage IV).

Provide Organizational Support

No.	Recommendation
11.	Develop an interdisciplinary team specific to the needs of the patient.
12.	Educate patients, caregivers, and healthcare providers on the prevention and treatment of pressure ulcers.

Etiology of Pressure Ulcers

Pressure ulcers are the result of localized **ischemia**, a deficiency in the blood supply to the tissue. External pressure (such as compression between the surface of the bed and the bony skeleton) that exceeds capillary closing pressure causes occlusion of blood vessels, decreased tissue perfusion, and, possibly, tissue necrosis. Blood cannot reach the tissue, the cells are deprived of oxygen and nutrients, the waste products of metabolism accumulate in the cells, and the tissue consequently dies.

After skin has been compressed, blood flow is interrupted, and skin becomes pale. When pressure is relieved, skin takes on a bright-red flush called **reactive hyperemia**, which is the body's way of quickly restoring blood flow to an area. The flush is caused by *vasodilation*, a process in which extra blood floods the area to compensate for the preceding period of impeded blood flow. Reactive hyperemia usually lasts one-half to three-quarters as long as the duration of impeded blood flow to the area. If the redness disappears in that time, no tissue damage is likely. If, however, the redness does not disappear, then tissue damage (abnormal reactive hyperemia) has already occurred.

Risk Factors

Key contributors to the development of pressure ulcers include mechanical loads (e.g., pressure, friction, and shear), immobility, inadequate nutrition, fecal and urinary incontinence, decreased mental status, diminished sensation, excessive body heat, advanced age, and the presence of certain chronic medical conditions.

MECHANICAL LOADS **Mechanical loads** are extrinsic forces, such as pressure, friction, and shear, that cause soft tissue damage and potentially lead to blood flow impedance, tissue necrosis, and pressure ulcer development

CAWC Quick Reference Guide

PROVIDES RECOMMENDATIONS FOR BEST PRACTICES

The directors and members of the Canadian Association of Wound Care have updated the four articles covering the recommendations for best practice in the areas of (1) Preparing the Wound Bed, (2) Pressure Ulcers, (3) Venous Leg Ulcers, and (4) Diabetic Foot Ulcers.

These quick reference guides (QRGs) are excerpts from the articles published in *Wound Care Canada* and reprinted here with the permission. The complete articles can be accessed through the CAWC Web site at **www.cawc.net**.

The QRGs are not intended to be complete protocols in themselves but aids in the diagnosis, prevention and treatment of specific wounds.

3 PREVENTION & TREATMENT OF VENOUS LEG ULCERS

Cathy Burrows, RN BScN; Rob Miller, MD FRCP (c); Debbie Townsend, RN; Ritchie Bellefontaine, BSc RVT; Gerald MacKean, MD FRCS (c); Heather L. Orsted, RN BN ET MSc; David H. Keast, MSc MD FCFP

No.	Recommendations
Identify and Treat the Cause	
1.	Obtain a careful history to determine the venous characteristics and to rule out other diagnoses: assess pain and identify the systemic and local factors that may impair wound healing.
2.	Perform a physical assessment. This will include a bilateral lower limb assessment as well as an ankle-brachial pressure index (ABPI) test on all patients with venous ulcers to help rule out the presence of arterial disease.
3.	Determine the cause(s) of chronic venous insufficiency based on etiology: abnormal valves (reflux), obstruction, or calf-muscle-pump failure.
4.	Implement appropriate compression therapy.
5.	Implement medical therapy if indicated for chronic venous insufficiency (superficial and deep thrombosis, woody fibrosis).
6.	Consider surgical management if significant superficial or perforator vein disease exists in the absence of extensive deep disease.
Address Patient-centred Concerns	
7.	Communicate with the patients, the family and the caregivers to establish realistic expectations for healing and provide information for care and management of venous disease. The presence or absence of a social support system is important for treatment and prevention of venous leg ulcers.
Provide Local Wound Care	
8.	Assess the wound.
9.	Provide local wound care. Optimize the local wound healing environment through debridement, bacterial balance, and moisture balance. Consider appropriate adjunctive therapies.
Provide Organizational Support	
10.	Consult appropriate disciplines to maximize and individualize the treatment plan to address factors and co-factors that may affect healing (e.g., mobility and nutrition).

4 PREVENTION, DIAGNOSIS & TREATMENT OF DIABETIC FOOT ULCERS

Heather L. Orsted, RN BN ET MSc; Gordon E. Searles, OD MD MSc FRCPC FACP CCI; Heather Trowell, BSc OT (c); Leah Shapera, RN MSN; Pat Miller, RN ET; John Rahman, CO

No.	Recommendations
Identify and Treat the Cause	
1.	Take a careful history to determine general health, diabetic control, complications and co-factors that may cause skin breakdown or affect the healing of an ulcer.
2.	Complete a physical assessment that includes vascular status, bony/structural deformities (and footwear), and sensation.
3.	Classify persons with diabetes into a risk category to support co-ordination of care.
4.	Modify factors that cause skin breakdown and/or influence healing and make referral(s) to the team to ensure comprehensive care.
5.	Provide pressure downloading if there is loss of protective sensation.
Address Patient-centred Concerns	
6.	Provide individualized education as indicated by patient need and by risk category.
Provide Local Wound Care	
7.	Assess diabetic foot ulceration(s).
8.	Provide an optimum wound environment: debridement, moisture balance, infection control.
9.	Determine effectiveness of interventions, reassess if healing is not occurring at expected rate.
10.	Consider the use of biological agents and adjunctive therapies.
Provide Organizational Support	
11.	Establish, train and empower a team to work with patients with diabetes.

www.cawc.net

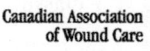

Canadian Association of Wound Care   Association canadienne du soin des plaies

Source: Canadian Association of Wound Care. (2006). *Quick reference guide: Recommendations for practice.*, Toronto, ON: Author. Available online at http://cawc.net/index.php/resources/store/cawc-quick-reference-guides-qrg

---

(Registered Nurses' Association of Ontario [RNAO], 2011). **Friction** is a mechanical force that occurs when two surfaces move across each other and often results in damage to the superficial layers of skin (RNAO, 2011). Poor lifting techniques and voluntary or involuntary movements by the client are common causes of friction injuries. **Shearing** is a combination of friction and pressure that typically results when skin and superficial tissues remain stationary while the deeper tissues attached to bone move downward. Shearing between two tissue layers leads to stretching, kinking, and tearing of the vessels at a subcutaneous level, resulting in ischemia, endothelial damage, and, possibly, cell death (RNAO, 2011). Dragging patients up in bed or allowing them to slide down in the bed are common sources of shearing injury.

IMMOBILITY Although pressure is the major cause of pressure ulcers, immobility and inactivity are also important risk factors. *Immobility* refers to a reduction in the amount and control of movement a person has. Normally, people move when they experience discomfort caused by pressure on an area of the body. Healthy people rarely exceed their tolerance for pressure. However, paralysis, extreme weakness, immobility, or any cause of decreased activity can hinder a person's ability to change positions independently and relieve the pressure, even if the person can perceive the pressure.

INADEQUATE NUTRITION Nutritional factors are crucial in the development of pressure ulcers. Generally, prolonged inadequate nutrition causes weight loss, muscle atrophy, and the loss of subcutaneous tissue. These three changes reduce the amount of padding between skin and bone and increase the risk of pressure ulcer development. Nutritional risk factors for pressure ulcer development include low prealbumin levels, low serum transferrin levels, low hemoglobin, low lymphocyte counts, dehydration, poor food (including low zinc and vitamin C intake) or fluid intake, and unintentional weight loss. Among older adult patients, malnutrition is a particularly significant problem, with poor nutritional status being found to increase the risk of death in residents of long-term care facilities in Canada (Allard et al., 2004).

Hypoproteinemia (abnormally low protein content in the blood), caused by either inadequate intake or abnormal loss, predisposes the client to dependent edema. Edema (the presence of excess fluid in the tissues) makes skin more prone to injury by decreasing its elasticity, resilience, and vitality. Edema increases the distance between the capillaries and the cells, thereby slowing the diffusion of oxygen to the tissue cells and of metabolites away from the cells.

FECAL AND URINARY INCONTINENCE Moisture, particularly from incontinence, promotes skin **maceration** (tissue softened by prolonged wetting or soaking) and causes the epidermis to be more easily eroded and susceptible to injury. Digestive enzymes in feces also contribute to skin excoriation. Any accumulation of secretions or excretions is irritating to skin, harbours microorganisms, and makes an individual prone to skin breakdown and infection.

DECREASED MENTAL STATUS Individuals with a reduced level of awareness, for example, those who are unconscious or heavily sedated, are at risk for pressure ulcers because they are less able to recognize and respond to the pain associated with prolonged pressure.

DIMINISHED SENSATION Paralysis, cerebrovascular accident, or other neurological disease may cause loss of sensation in a body area. Loss of sensation reduces a person's ability to respond to injurious heat and cold and to feel the tingling ("pins and needles") that signals loss of circulation.

EXCESSIVE BODY HEAT Body heat is another factor in the development of pressure ulcers. An elevated body temperature increases the body's metabolic rate, thus increasing the need of the cells for oxygen. This increased need is particularly severe in the cells of an area under pressure, which are already oxygen deficient. Therefore, severe infections with accompanying elevated body temperatures can affect the body's ability to deal with the effects of tissue compression.

ADVANCED AGE The aging process brings about several changes in skin and its supporting structures, making the older person more prone to impaired skin integrity and altered wound healing. These changes include the following:

- Loss of lean body mass
- Generalized thinning of the epidermis
- Decreased strength and elasticity of skin because of changes in the collagen fibres of the dermis
- Increased dryness because of a decrease in the amount of oil produced by the sebaceous glands

- Diminished pain perception because of a reduction in the number of cutaneous end organs responsible for the sensation of pressure and light touch
- Diminished venous and arterial flow because of aging vascular walls

CHRONIC MEDICAL CONDITIONS The presence of certain chronic conditions, such as diabetes mellitus and cardiovascular disease, places individuals at particular risk for developing pressure ulcers. These conditions result in poor perfusion, compromising oxygen and nutrient delivery to tissues.

OTHER FACTORS Other factors contributing to the formation of pressure ulcers are poor lifting techniques, incorrect positioning, repeated injections in the same area, hard support surfaces, and incorrect application of pressure-relieving devices. See the Clinical Alert box below.

> **! CLINICAL ALERT**
>
> Although much effort goes into treating a pressure, arterial, or venous ulcer, keep in mind that, unless the cause is identified and treated, the ulcer might never be cured.

Classification of Pressure Ulcers

The most widely accepted system for classifying the degree of observed tissue damage is NPUAP's classification system (Figure 35.1):

- *Suspected deep tissue injury:* Purple or maroon localized area of discoloured intact skin or blood-filled blister caused by damage of underlying soft tissue from pressure or shear (Figure 35.2 on the next page). The discoloration may be preceded by tissue that is painful, firm, mushy, boggy, warmer, or cooler as compared with adjacent tissue.

- *Category/Stage I:* Intact skin with nonblanchable redness of a localized area, usually over a bony prominence. Darkly pigmented skin may not have visible blanching; its colour may differ from the surrounding area.

- *Category/Stage II:* Partial-thickness skin loss presenting as a shallow open ulcer with a red-pink wound bed, without slough. It may also present as an intact or open or ruptured serum-filled blister.

- *Category/Stage III:* Full-thickness tissue loss. Subcutaneous fat may be visible but bone, tendon, or muscle is not exposed. Slough may be present but does not obscure the depth of tissue loss. It may include undermining and tunnelling.

- *Category/Stage IV:* Full-thickness tissue loss with exposed bone, tendon, or muscle. Slough or **eschar** (a covering of dried plasma proteins and dead cells) may be present on some parts of the wound bed. It often includes undermining and tunnelling.

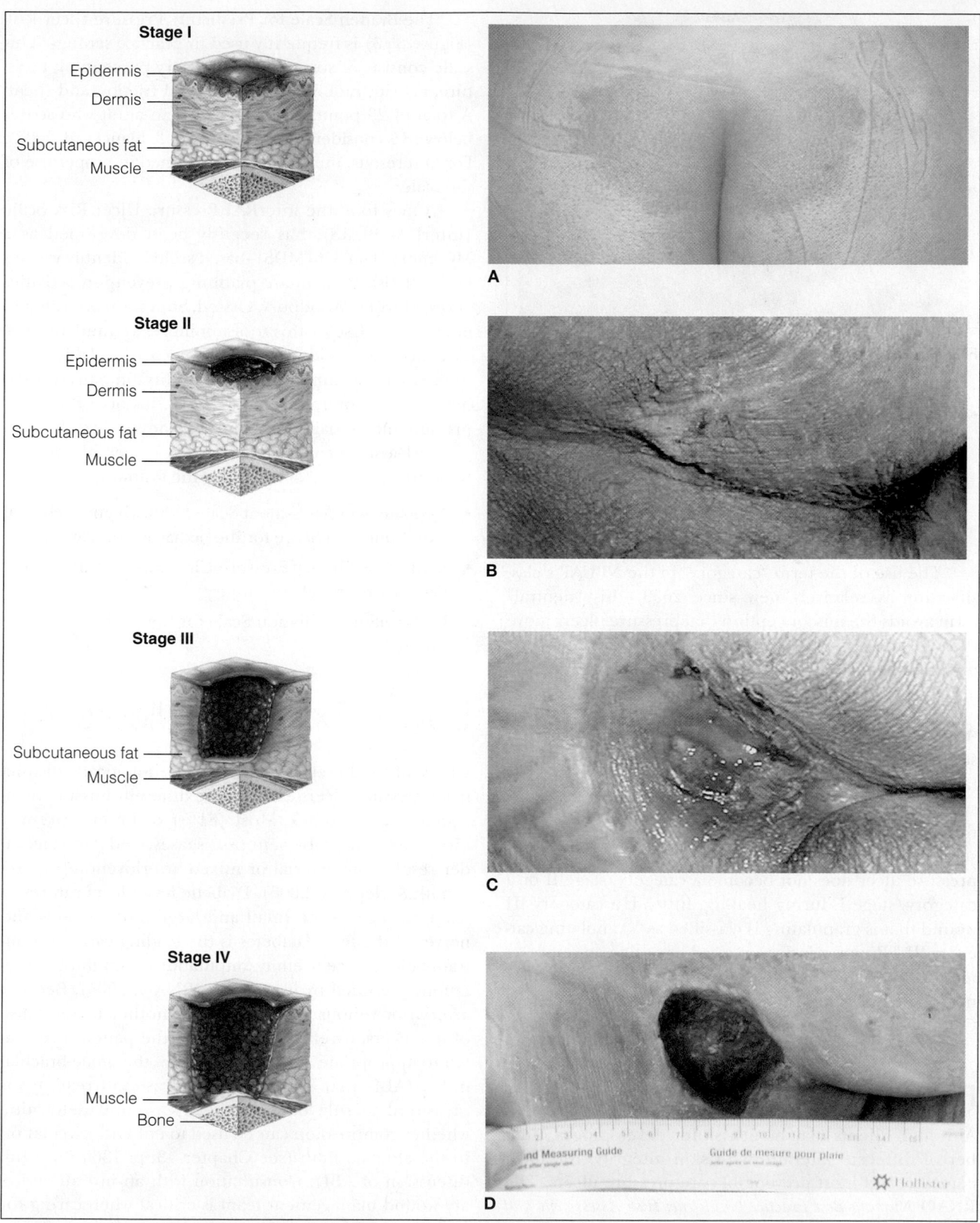

FIGURE 35.1 Categories/stages I to IV of pressure ulcers. **A:** Category/stage I: A defined area of persistent redness signalling potential ulceration; **B:** Category/stage II: Partial-thickness skin loss (abrasion, blister, or shallow crater) involving the epidermis and possibly the dermis; **C**: Category/stage III: Full-thickness skin loss involving damage or necrosis of subcutaneous tissue that may extend down to, but not through, underlying fascia; **D:** Category/stage IV: Full-thickness skin loss with extensive destruction, tissue necrosis, or damage to muscle, bone, or supporting structures, such as a tendon or joint capsule. Undermining and sinus tract may also be present.

Source: Pressure Ulcer Category/ Staging Illustrations." Used with permission of the National Pressure Ulcer Advisory Panel, 2012.

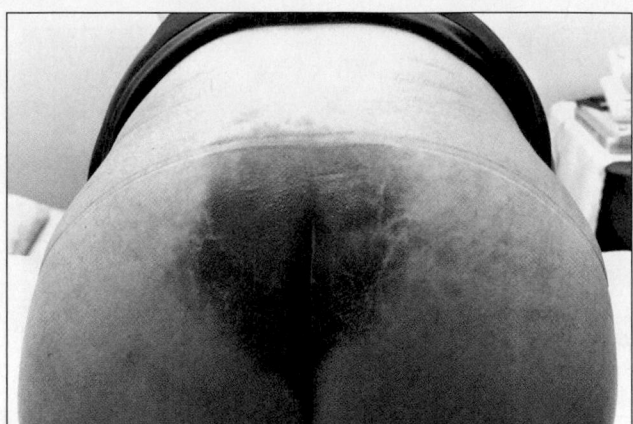

FIGURE 35.2 Suspected deep tissue injury

- *Unstageable:* Full-thickness tissue loss in which the base of the ulcer is covered by slough (yellow, tan, grey, green, or brown) or eschar (tan, brown, or black) in the wound bed. Until enough slough and/or eschar has been removed to expose the base of the wound, the true depth cannot be determined.

The use of the term "category" in the NPUAP's classification is relatively new since 2009—this "neutral" term avoids the misconception that pressure ulcers move through progressive stages in their development. While many clinicians will continue to use the term "stage," the aim is to replace this terminology with "category."

REVERSE (DOWN) CATEGORIZATION/STAGING Clinical studies indicate that as deep ulcers heal, the lost muscle, fat, and dermis is *not* replaced. Instead, granulation tissue fills the defect before epithelialization occurs. Given this information, it is not appropriate to reverse or *down* stage a healing ulcer. For example, a category/stage III pressure ulcer does not become a category/stage II or a category/stage I during healing. Instead, a category III wound that is granulating is classified as "granulating category III." Progress is documented by noting an improvement in the actual characteristics: size, depth, amount of necrotic tissue, amount of exudate, and so on (Wound, Ostomy, and Continence Nurses Society [WOCN], 2007).

Risk-Assessment Tools

Although clients may be at risk for developing a number of different alterations in skin integrity, the most common and most preventable are pressure ulcers. The RNAO *Nursing Best Practice Guideline: Risk Assessment and Prevention of Pressure Ulcers* (2011) recommends that a comprehensive head-to-toe skin assessment be conducted on admission of clients at risk for skin breakdown. The client's risk is determined by a combination of clinical judgment and the use of a structured, valid, and reliable risk-assessment tool, such as the Braden Scale for Predicting Pressure Ulcer Risk.

The Braden Scale for Predicting Pressure Ulcer Risk (Figure 35.3) is frequently used in practice settings. This scale consists of six subscales: sensory perception, moisture, activity, mobility, nutrition, and friction and shear. A total of 23 points is possible and an adult who scores below 18 is considered at risk (Braden & Blanchard, 2007). For best results, nurses should be trained in proper use of the scale.

A new tool, the interRAI Pressure Ulcer Risk Scale (interRAI PURS), has recently been developed as a Minimum Data Set (MDS)–based scale to identify various levels of risk to facilitate planning prevention activities (Poss, Murphy, Woodbury, Orsted, Stevenson, & Williams, et al. 2010). Use of this tool minimizes redundant pressure ulcer risk scales when MDS data are available. Scale items include impaired bed mobility, impaired walking, bowel incontinence, weight loss, history of resolved pressure ulcers, daily pain, and shortness of breath.

Risk-assessment tools specific to vulnerable populations are also available including the following:

- Neonate Skin Assessment Scale (NSRAS) and Neonatal Skin Condition Score for the pediatric population
- Spinal Cord Injury Pressure Ulcer Scale (SCIPUS) for clients with spinal cord injury
- Performance Palliation Scale for the palliative care population

Lower Extremity Ulcers

Ulcers of the lower extremities are etiologically distinct from pressure ulcers and require different nursing management approaches. Most (81%) of lower extremity ulcers are caused by venous diseases, and the remainder result from arterial or mixed arteriovenous disease (Smith & Nephew, 2006). Diabetic foot ulcers can result from damage to the small and large blood vessels and nerves of the foot. Diabetes is the leading cause of nontraumatic lower extremity amputations, with most amputations preceded by foot ulcers (RNAO, 2005). Because arterial or venous insufficiency is another major cause of leg ulcers, careful assessment of the patient is essential to appropriate care. For example, the ankle-brachial index (ABI) that uses Doppler ultrasound readings is measured to rule out arterial disease and determine whether compression can be used to enhance circulation to the affected limb (see Chapter 43, p. 1365 for a full discussion of ABI). Consultation with an interdisciplinary wound management team is critical when caring for patients with any type of lower extremity ulcer.

Table 35.2 on page 1012 describes the differences in limb appearance between patients with arterial ulcers and those with venous ulcers. Some common ulcers include those on the **gaiter area**, which extends from 2.5 cm below the malleolus to the lower third of the calf; **ankle flares**, which appear near or on the ankle and are associated with

BRADEN SCALE FOR PREDICTING PRESSURE SORE RISK

Patient's Name _____   Evaluator's Name _____   Date of Assessment

SENSORY PERCEPTION
Ability to respond meaningfully to pressure-related discomfort

1. Completely Limited: Unresponsive (does not moan, flinch, or grasp) to painful stimuli, due to diminished level of consciousness or sedation,
OR
limited ability to feel pain over most of body surface.

2. Very Limited: Responds only to painful stimuli. Cannot communicate discomfort except by moaning or restlessness,
OR
has a sensory impairment which limits the ability to feel pain or discomfort over 1/2 of body.

3. Slightly Limited: Responds to verbal commands but cannot always communicate discomfort or need to be turned,
OR
has some sensory impairment which limits ability to feel pain or discomfort in 1 or 2 extremities.

4. No Impairment: Responds to verbal commands. Has no sensory deficit which would limit ability to feel or voice pain or discomfort.

MOISTURE
Degree to which skin is exposed to moisture

1. Constantly Moist: Skin is kept moist almost constantly by perspiration, urine, etc. Dampness is detected every time patient is moved or turned.

2. Moist: Skin is often but not always moist. Linen must be changed at least once a shift.

3. Occasionally Moist: Skin is occasionally moist, requiring an extra linen change approximately once a day.

4. Rarely Moist: Skin is usually dry; linen requires changing only at routine intervals.

ACTIVITY
Degree of physical activity

1. Bedfast: Confined to bed.

2. Chairfast: Ability to walk severely limited or nonexistent. Cannot bear own weight and/or must be assisted into chair or wheelchair.

3. Walks Occasionally: Walks occasionally during day but for very short distances, with or without assistance. Spends majority of each shift in bed or chair.

4. Walks Frequently: Walks outside the room at least twice a day and inside room at least once every 2 hours during waking hours.

MOBILITY
Ability to change and control body position

1. Completely Immobile: Does not make even slight changes in body or extremity position without assistance.

2. Very Limited: Makes occasional slight changes in body or extremity position but unable to make frequent or significant changes independently.

3. Slightly Limited: Makes frequent though slight changes in body or extremity position independently.

4. No Limitations: Makes major and frequent changes in position without assistance.

NUTRITION
Usual food intake pattern

1. Very Poor: Never eats a complete meal. Rarely eats more than 1/3 of any food offered. Eats 2 servings or less of protein (meat or dairy products) per day. Takes fluids poorly. Does not take a liquid dietary supplement,
OR
is NPO and/or maintained on clear liquids or IVs for more than 5 days.

2. Probably Inadequate: Rarely eats a complete meal and generally eats only about 1/2 of any food offered. Protein intake includes only 3 servings of meat or dairy products per day. Occasionally will take a dietary supplement,
OR
receives less than optimal amount of liquid diet or tube feeding.

3. Adequate: Eats over half of most meals. Eats a total of 4 servings of protein (meat, dairy products) each day. Occasionally will refuse a meal, but will usually take a supplement if offered,
OR
is on a tube feeding or TPN regimen, which probably meets most of nutritional needs.

4. Excellent: Eats most of every meal. Never refuses a meal. Usually eats a total of 4 or more servings of meat and dairy products. Occasionally eats between meals. Does not require supplementation.

FRICTION AND SHEAR

1. Problem: Requires moderate to maximum assistance in moving. Complete lifting without sliding against sheets is impossible. Frequently slides down in bed or chair, requiring frequent repositioning with maximum assistance. Spasticity, contractures, or agitation leads to almost constant friction.

2. Potential Problem: Moves feebly or requires minimum assistance. During a move, skin probably slides to some extent against sheets, chair, restraints, or other devices. Maintains relatively good position in chair or bed most of the time but occasionally slides down.

3. No Apparent Problem: Moves in bed and in chair independently and has sufficient muscle strength to lift up completely during move. Maintains good position in bed or chair at all times.

Total Score _____

FIGURE 35.3 Braden Scale for Predicting Pressure Ulcer Risk.

Source: Braden Scale for Predicting Pressure Sore Risk. Copyright © Barbara Braden and Nancy Bergstrom, 1988. Reprinted with permission.

TABLE 35.2   Comparison of the Manifestations of Arterial and Venous Disease in the Lower Limbs

Arterial Disease	Venous Disease
Ulcers with a "punched out" appearance	Usually shallow, moist ulcers
Base of wound poorly perfused, pale, dry	Situated on the gaiter area of the leg (the gaiter area is 2.5 cm below the malleolus to the lower one-third of the calf)
Cold legs/feet in a warm environment	Edema
Shiny, taut skin	Eczema
Dependent rubour	Ankle flare (the characteristic clinical sign evident in the region of the ankle associated with venous hypertension or varicose veins as a result of a number of engorged veins in the area)
Pale or blue feet	Lipodermatosclerosis (deposit of fibrin in the deep dermis and fat, resulting in a woody induration of the gaiter area of the calf)
Gangrenous toes	Hyperpigmentation
	Atrophie blanche (white atrophic lesions often associated with venous disease); tiny visible blood vessels, called *teleangiectasia,* often seen in the centre

Source: From Registered Nurses' Association of Ontario. (2007). *Nursing best practice guideline: Assessment and management of venous leg ulcers* (rev. suppl.). Toronto, Canada: Author.

venous hypertension or varicose veins; **lipodermatosclerosis**, which occurs in the gaiter area, is caused by areas of connective tissue in the deep dermis and fat, and produces a woody hardening of tissue; and **atrophie blanche**, which appears as white atrophic lesions and is often associated with venous disease. Box 35.2 Sections 3 and 4 provide guidelines for prevention and treatment of venous leg ulcers as well as the prevention, diagnosis, and treatment of diabetic foot ulcers.

Skin Tears

Skin tears are the result of blunt trauma, shearing, or friction and can easily develop in at-risk clients with such activities as removing tape, removing stockings, banging into a coffee table, or sliding an ankle against the footrest of a wheelchair. While traditionally skin tears have been seen as less significant when compared with pressure ulcers or arterial and venous ulcers, skin tears can be equally difficult to manage and can lead to such complications as pain and wound infection (Leblanc, Christensen, Orsted, & Keast, 2008). Risk factors for developing skin tears include poor nutritional status, being older than 85 years, being female, being immobilized, polypharmacy, requiring transfer assistance, and having vascular problems, to name a few. Prevention of skin tears through skin hygiene and hydration, the use of appropriate clothing (e.g., long sleeves, long pants), ensuring proper transfer, avoiding adhesive products on fragile skin (use paper tape or silicone dressings, if necessary), and removal of environmental risk factors (e.g., by padding sharp corners on furniture) have been proposed as strategies to minimize skin tears (Leblanc et al., 2008).

Wound Healing

Healing is a quality of living tissue; it is also referred to as **regeneration** (renewal) of tissues. Healing can be considered in terms of *types of healing*, which refer to the decision to allow the wound to heal itself or to purposefully close the wound, and *phases of healing*, which refer to the steps in the body's natural processes of tissue repair. The phases are the same for all wounds, but the rate of healing depends on such factors as the type of healing, the location and size of the wound, and the health of the client.

Types of Wound Healing

The two types of healing are distinguished by the amount of tissue loss. **Primary intention healing** occurs when the tissue surfaces have been approximated (closed) and minimal or no tissue loss has occurred; it is characterized by the formation of minimal granulation tissue and scarring. It is also called *primary union* or *first intention healing*. An example of wound healing by primary intention is a closed surgical incision. Another example would be the use of tissue adhesive, a glue that can be used to seal clean lacerations or incisions, which may result in less noticeable scars.

A wound that is extensive and involves considerable tissue loss, and in which the edges cannot or should not be approximated, heals by **secondary intention healing**. An example of wound healing by secondary intention is a pressure ulcer. Secondary intention healing differs from primary intention healing in three ways: (a) the repair time is longer; (b) the scarring is greater; and (c) the susceptibility to infection is greater.

Those wounds that are left open for 3 to 5 days to allow edema or infection to resolve or exudate to drain and are then closed with sutures, staples, or adhesive skin closures heal by **tertiary intention healing**. This method is also called **delayed primary intention healing**.

Phases of Wound Healing

Wound healing involves three overlapping but distinct phases: (a) inflammatory, (b) proliferative, and (c) maturation.

INFLAMMATORY PHASE The *inflammatory phase* is initiated immediately after injury and lasts 3 to 6 days. Two major processes occur during this phase: (a) hemostasis and (b) phagocytosis.

Hemostasis (the cessation of bleeding) results from vasoconstriction of the larger blood vessels in the affected area, retraction (drawing back) of injured blood vessels, the deposition of **fibrin** (connective tissue), and the formation of blood clots in the area. The blood clots, formed from blood platelets, provide a matrix of fibrin that becomes the framework for cell repair. A scab also forms on the surface of the wound. Consisting of clots and dead and dying tissue, this scab serves to aid hemostasis and inhibit contamination of the wound by microorganisms. Below the scab, epithelial cells migrate into the wound from the edges. The epithelial cells serve as a barrier between the body and the environment, preventing the entry of microorganisms.

The inflammatory phase also involves vascular and cellular responses intended to remove any foreign substances and dead and dying tissues. The blood supply to the wound increases, bringing with it substances and nutrients needed in the healing process. The area appears reddened and edematous as a result. Exudate of fluid and cell debris is a normal accumulation and helps cleanse the wound.

During cell migration, leukocytes (specifically, neutrophils) move into the interstitial space. These are replaced about 24 hours after injury by macrophages, which arise from the blood monocytes. These macrophages engulf microorganisms and cellular debris by a process known as *phagocytosis*. The macrophages also secrete an angiogenesis factor (AGF), which stimulates the formation of epithelial buds at the end of injured blood vessels. The microcirculatory network that results sustains the healing process and the wound during its life. This inflammatory response is essential to healing, and measures that impair inflammation, such as steroid medications, can place the healing process at risk.

PROLIFERATIVE PHASE The *proliferative phase,* the second phase in healing, extends from day 3 or 4 to about day 21 after injury. Fibroblasts (connective tissue cells),

which migrate into the wound starting about 24 hours after injury, begin to synthesize collagen and a substance called *proteoglycan* about day 5 after injury. **Collagen** is a whitish protein substance that adds tensile strength to the wound. As the amount of collagen increases, so does the strength of the wound; thus, the chance that the wound will open decreases progressively. If the wound is sutured, a raised healing ridge appears under the intact suture line. In a wound that is not sutured, the new collagen is often visible.

Capillaries grow across the wound, increasing the blood supply, which brings with it oxygen and nutrients needed for healing. Fibroblasts move from the bloodstream into the wound, depositing fibrin. As the capillary network develops, the tissue becomes a translucent red colour. This tissue, called **granulation tissue**, is fragile and bleeds easily.

When the skin edges of a wound are not sutured, the area fills in with granulation tissue. When the granulation tissue matures, marginal epithelial cells migrate to it, proliferating over this connective tissue base to fill the wound. If the wound does not close by epithelialization, the area becomes covered with dried plasma proteins and dead cells, called *eschar.* Initially, wounds healing by secondary intention ooze blood-tinged drainage. Later, if they are not covered by epithelial cells, they become covered with thick, grey, fibrinous tissue that is eventually converted into dense scar tissue.

MATURATION PHASE The *maturation phase* begins about day 21 and healing can extend 1 or 2 years after the injury. Fibroblasts continue to synthesize collagen. The collagen fibres themselves, which were initially laid in a haphazard fashion, reorganize into a more orderly structure. During maturation, the wound is remodelled and contracted. The scar becomes stronger but the repaired area is never as strong as the original tissue. Scar tissue is at increased risk of reulceration because it will not achieve more than 80% of the tissue's preinjury tensile strength (Health Quality Council, 2006). In some individuals, particularly dark-skinned persons, an abnormal amount of collagen is laid down, resulting in a hypertrophic scar, or **keloid**.

One method of documenting the progress of healing in pressure ulcers is to use the Pressure Ulcer Scale for Healing (PUSH) tool. This well-validated tool (Figure 35.4) assigns scores to the ulcer length, width, amount of exudate, and tissue type. The change in the total score over time can be used as an indication of healing.

Types of Wound Drainage

Exudate is material, such as fluid and cells, that has escaped from blood vessels during the inflammatory process and is deposited in tissue or on tissue surfaces. The nature and amount of exudate vary according to the

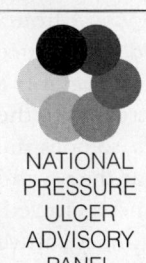

NATIONAL
PRESSURE
ULCER
ADVISORY
PANEL

Pressure Ulcer Scale for Healing (PUSH)
PUSH Tool 3.0

Patient Name_____ Patient ID#_____

Ulcer Location _____ Date _____

Directions:

Observe and measure the pressure ulcer. Categorize the ulcer with respect to surface area, exudate, and type of wound tissue. Record a sub-score for each of these ulcer characteristics. Add the sub-scores to obtain the total score. A comparison of total scores measured over time provides an indication of the improvement or deterioration in pressure ulcer healing.

	0	**1**	**2**	**3**	**4**	**5**	**Sub-score**
LENGTH X WIDTH	0	< 0.3	0.3 – 0.6	0.7 – 1.0	1.1 – 2.0	2.1 – 3.0	
	6	**7**	**8**	**9**	**10**		
(in cm²)	3.1 – 4.0	4.1 – 8.0	8.1 – 12.0	12.1 – 24.0	> 24.0		
EXUDATE AMOUNT	**0** None	**1** Light	**2** Moderate	**3** Heavy			**Sub-score**
TISSUE TYPE	**0** Closed	**1** Epithelial Tissue	**2** Granulation Tissue	**3** Slough	**4** Necrotic Tissue		**Sub-score**
							TOTAL SCORE

Length x Width: Measure the greatest length (head to toe) and the greatest width (side to side) using a centimeter ruler. Multiply these two measurements (length x width) to obtain an estimate of surface area in square centimeters (cm²). Caveat: Do not guess! Always use a centimeter ruler and always use the same method each time the ulcer is measured.

Exudate Amount: Estimate the amount of exudate (drainage) present after removal of the dressing and before applying any topical agent to the ulcer. Estimate the exudate (drainage) as none, light, moderate, or heavy.

Tissue Type: This refers to the types of tissue that are present in the wound (ulcer) bed. Score as a "4" if there is any necrotic tissue present. Score as a "3" if there is any amount of slough present and necrotic tissue is absent. Score as a "2" if the wound is clean and contains granulation tissue. A superficial wound that is reepithelializing is scored as a "1." When the wound is closed, score as a "0."

- **4 – Necrotic Tissue (Eschar):** black, brown, or tan tissue that adheres firmly to the wound bed or ulcer edges and may be either firmer or softer than surrounding skin
- **3 – Slough:** yellow or white tissue that adheres to the ulcer bed in strings or thick clumps, or is mucinous
- **2 – Granulation Tissue:** pink or beefy red tissue with a shiny, moist, granular appearance
- **1 – Epithelial Tissue:** for superficial ulcers, new pink or shiny tissue (skin) that grows in from the edges or as islands on the ulcer surface
- **0 – Closed/Resurfaced:** the wound is completely covered with epithelium (new skin)

www.npuap.org
11F

PUSH Tool Version 3.0:9/15/98
@National Pressure Ulcer Advisory Panel

FIGURE 35.4 Pressure Ulcer Scale for Healing (PUSH) tool.

Source: Pressure Ulcer Scale for Healing (PUSH) Tool. From the National Pressure Ulcer Advisory Panel. © NPUAP, 2003. Used with permission

tissue involved, the intensity and duration of the inflammation, and the presence of microorganisms.

There are three major types of exudate: (a) serous, (b) purulent, and (c) sanguineous. A **serous exudate** consists chiefly of serum (the clear portion of the blood) derived from blood and the serous membranes of the body, such as the peritoneum. It looks watery and has few cells. An example is the fluid in a blister from a burn.

A **purulent exudate** is thicker than serous exudate because of the presence of pus, which consists of leukocytes, liquefied dead tissue debris, and dead and living bacteria. The process of pus formation is referred to as **suppuration**, and the bacteria that produce pus are called **pyogenic bacteria**. Not all microorganisms are pyogenic. Purulent exudates vary in colour, some acquiring tinges of blue, green, or yellow. The colour may depend on the causative organism.

A **sanguineous exudate** consists of large amounts of red blood cells, indicating damage to capillaries that is severe enough to allow the escape of red blood cells from plasma. This type of exudate is frequently seen in open wounds. Nurses often need to distinguish whether the sanguineous exudate is dark or bright. A bright sanguineous exudate indicates fresh bleeding, whereas dark sanguineous exudate denotes older bleeding.

Mixed types of exudates are often observed. A **serosanguineous exudate** (consisting of clear and blood-tinged drainage) is commonly seen in surgical incisions. A *purosanguineous* discharge (consisting of pus and blood) is often seen in a new wound that is infected. See the Clinical Alert box.

> ### ! CLINICAL ALERT
>
> Sanguinous (bloody) discharge from a wound must be assessed carefully. A bright sanguineous exudate indicates fresh bleeding and must be attended to immediately, whereas dark sanguineous exudate denotes older bleeding.

Complications Relating to Wound Healing

HEMORRHAGE Some escape of blood from a wound is normal. **Hemorrhage** (extensive bleeding), however, is abnormal. It may be caused by a dislodged clot, a slipped ligature, or erosion of a blood vessel, for example.

Internal hemorrhage can often be detected by swelling or distension in the area of the wound and, possibly, sanguineous drainage from a surgical drain. Some clients will have a **hematoma**, a localized collection of blood underneath skin, which may appear as a reddish-blue swelling. A large hematoma can be dangerous in that it places pressure on blood vessels and can, thus, obstruct blood flow.

External hemorrhage is often easily identified from the blood that either appears under a dressing or escapes from the dressing and pools under the client. The risk

of hemorrhage is greatest during the first 48 hours after surgery. Hemorrhage is an emergency; the nurse should apply extra sterile pressure dressings to the area and monitor the client's vital signs. In many instances, the client must be taken to the operating room for surgical intervention.

INFECTION A wound can be infected with microorganisms at the time of injury, during surgery, or postoperatively, that is, during open wound healing. An **infection** is the disease process produced by those microorganisms.

A number of systemic and local factors predispose clients to wound infections. Systemic factors include vascular disease, edema, malnutrition, diabetes mellitus, alcoholism, prior surgery or radiation, drugs (e.g., corticosteroids), and inherited immune defects. Local factors include a large wound area, increased wound depth, degree of chronicity, anatomical location (distal extremity, perineal), presence of foreign bodies, necrotic tissue, reduced perfusion, and degree of postwound contamination. In addition to the classic signs of infection (erythema, induration, and increased pain), friable (jelly-like) granulation tissue, unstable epithelial bridges, or a failure to respond to therapy are subtle signs of infection (Dolynchuk et al., 2000). Clients who are immunosuppressed, such as those with human immunodeficiency virus (HIV) infection or receiving myelosuppressive treatment for cancer, are especially susceptible to wound infections.

Wounds that occur as a result of injury (e.g., bullet and knife wounds) are most likely to be contaminated at the time of injury. Surgical site infections (SSIs) are health care-associated infections that can occur in surgical patients. Most SSIs are caused when the patient's own flora enters the body through the incision, but outside sources of contamination also pose significant risk. Hyperglycemia, smoking, prolonged preoperative hospital stay, using shaving for hair removal, and intra and postoperative hypothermia (i.e., <36° C) all increase a patient's risk of developing an SSI (Safer HealthCare Now!, 2011). Surgical infection is most likely to become apparent 2 to 11 days postoperatively. Box 35.3 on the next page summarizes Safer HealthCare Now! (2011) recommendations for preventing surgical site infections.

Systemic antibiotics should not be routinely used for pressure ulcers with only clinical signs of local infection, but they may be required when patients are diagnosed with bacteremia, sepsis, advancing cellulitis, or osteomyelitis. Topical antibiotics (effective for Gram-negative, Gram-positive, and anaerobic organisms) may be given a 2-week trial in the case of clean pressure ulcers that do not show evidence of healing or are continuing to produce exudate after 2 to 4 weeks of optimal treatment (RNAO, 2007).

DEHISCENCE WITH POSSIBLE EVISCERATION Dehiscence is the partial or total rupturing of a sutured wound. Dehiscence usually involves an abdominal wound in which the layers below the skin also separate. **Evisceration** is the protrusion of the internal viscera through an incision. A

BOX 35.3 PREVENTING SURGICAL SITE INFECTION (SSI): RECOMMENDATIONS FROM SAFER HEALTHCARE NOW!

Appropriate hair removal	No hair removal is ideal; if hair must be removed then use clippers (NOT razors) only within 2 hours of the surgery (not in the operating room); no shaving in the vicinity of the incision 7 days before surgery
Perioperative normothermia	Core body temperature should remain 36° to 38°C preoperatively, intraoperatively, and in the postanesthetic care unit (PACU)
Perioperative antimicrobial coverage	Through use of appropriate prophylactic antibiotics within 1 hour of surgery and antiseptic prophylaxis of the skin by cleansing with a chlorhexidine-based solution, preferably with no-rinse disposable chlorhexidine gluconate impregnated wash cloths; surgical skin preparation with alcohol-based chlorhexidine that is not washed off until at least 6 hours after surgery
Maintenance of perioperative glucose control	Blood glucose levels should be checked on all postoperative patients who are diabetic or at risk for diabetes; glucose control is recommended for hyperglycemia

Source: Safer HealthCare Now! (2010). Preventing surgical site infections: Getting started kit. Available online at http://www.saferhealthcarenow.ca/EN/Interventions/SSI/Documents/SSI%20Getting%20Started%20Kit.pdf

BOX 35.4 FACTORS INHIBITING WOUND HEALING IN OLDER ADULTS

Wounds in older adults can heal more slowly for several reasons:

- Vascular changes associated with aging, such as atherosclerosis and atrophy of capillaries in skin, can impair blood flow to the wound.
- Collagen tissue is less flexible, which increases the risk of damage from pressure, friction, and shear.
- Scar tissue is less elastic.
- Changes in the immune system may reduce the formation of the antibodies and monocytes necessary for wound healing.
- Nutritional deficiencies may reduce the numbers of red blood cells and leukocytes, thus impeding the delivery of oxygen and the inflammatory response essential for wound healing. Oxygen is needed for the synthesis of collagen and the formation of new epithelial cells.
- Having diabetes or cardiovascular disease increases the risk of delayed healing because of impaired oxygen delivery to these tissues.
- Cell renewal is slower, leading to delayed healing.

LIFESPAN CONSIDERATIONS Healthy children and adults often heal more quickly than older adults, who are at higher risk of having chronic diseases that hinder healing. For example, impaired liver function can impair the synthesis of blood clotting factors. Box 35.4 lists factors inhibiting wound healing in older adults.

NUTRITION Wound healing increases the body's energy and protein needs. Clients require a diet rich in protein, carbohydrates, lipids, vitamins A and C, and minerals, such as iron, zinc, and copper. NPUAP (2007) recommends that each individual with nutritional risk and pressure ulcer risk be offered a minimum of 30 to 35 kcal per kg body weight per day, with 1.25 to 1.5 g/kg/day protein and 1 mL/kcal/day of fluid intake. Malnourished clients may require time to improve their nutritional status before surgery, if this is possible. Obese clients are at increased risk of wound infection and slower healing because adipose tissue usually has a minimal blood supply.

LIFESTYLE People who exercise regularly tend to have good circulation, and because blood brings oxygen and nourishment to the wound, they are more likely to heal quickly. Smoking constricts arterioles, and it reduces the amount of functional hemoglobin in the blood, thus limiting the oxygen-carrying capacity of the blood.

MEDICATIONS Anti-inflammatory drugs (e.g., steroids and Aspirin), heparin, and antineoplastic agents interfere with healing. Prolonged use of antibiotics can make a person susceptible to wound infection by resistant organisms.

CONTAMINATION, COLONIZATION, AND INFECTION Considerable debate has occurred about the influences of bacterial contamination, colonization, and infection on wound healing. All chronic wounds are presumed

number of factors, including obesity, smoking, poor nutrition, multiple traumas, failure of suturing, excessive coughing, vomiting, and dehydration, heighten a client's risk of wound dehiscence. Wound dehiscence is more likely to occur 4 to 5 days postoperatively, before extensive collagen is deposited in the wound. Clients at risk for dehiscence may be prescribed an abdominal binder for support.

An increase in the flow of serosanguineous drainage into the wound dressing can indicate an impending dehiscence. Dehiscence may also be preceded by sudden straining (e.g., sneezing), and it is not unusual for a client to feel that "something has given way." When dehiscence or evisceration occurs, the wound should be quickly supported by large sterile dressings soaked in sterile normal saline. The client is placed in bed with knees bent to decrease pull on the incision and emotional support is provided. The surgeon should be notified, as immediate surgical repair of the area may be necessary.

Factors Affecting Wound Healing

Characteristics of the individual, such as age, nutritional status, lifestyle, and medications, influence the speed of wound healing.

to be in a state of bacterial **contamination**, in which bacteria are present but are neither attached to the wound surface nor replicating (Dolynchuk et al., 2000), but not all chronic wounds become infected. This contrasts with **colonization**, in which bacteria are attached to the wound surface and are replicating. In neither contamination nor colonization, however, do bacteria interfere with wound healing. When bacteria become invasive and cause an inflammatory response, the wound may proceed to shows signs of local infection, which can progress to systemic infection. The most common microcolonies of bacteria in wounds are *Staphylococcus* and *Pseudomonas*.

Assessing

Assessment of Skin Integrity

In addition to the history and psychosocial assessment, the nurse conducts an examination of the integument as part of a routine assessment and during regular care. Removing barriers to assessment is very important. Antiembolism stockings, braces, or devices must be removed to assess the underlying skin condition.

NURSING HISTORY AND PHYSICAL EXAMINATION
Completion of a client history and targeted physical examination to determine general health and risk factors that may lead to impaired skin integrity is a key component of the nursing history. During the review of systems as part of the nursing history, information is collected regarding skin diseases, previous bruising, general skin condition, skin lesions, and usual healing of ulcers. Inspection and palpation of skin focus on determination of skin colour, temperature, texture, turgor, presence of edema, vascularity, and characteristics of any lesions that are present. Particular attention is paid to skin condition in areas most likely to break down: in skin folds, such as under the breasts; in areas that are frequently moist, such as the perineum; and in areas that are subject to pressure: areas over bony prominences (e.g., occiput of the skull, scapulae, spinous processes, shoulders, elbows, sacrum, ischial tuberosities, trochanters, knees, malleoli, heels); and skin adjacent to external devices (RNAO, 2011).

Practice Guidelines 35.1 on the next page describes the principles of assessing common pressure sites.

Pain

Pain is a patient-centred concern that is all too often neglected in the provision of wound care. Patients with impaired skin integrity frequently experience pain occurring with dressing change. Best practice guidelines from the RNAO (2007) recommend that all patients receiving wound care should be routinely assessed for pain by using a validated assessment tool that is easy to use and appropriate for the cognitive ability of the client.

Assessment of Wounds

Nurses commonly assess both untreated and treated wounds. Untreated wounds usually are seen shortly after an injury (e.g., at the scene of an accident). Assessment for these wounds is shown in Box 35.5. Guidelines for care of untreated wounds includes the following:

- Control severe bleeding by (a) applying direct pressure over the wound, and (b) elevating the involved extremity.
- Prevent infection by (a) cleaning or flushing abrasions or lacerations with water and (b) covering the wound with a clean dressing, if possible (a sterile dressing is preferred). When applying a dressing, wrap the wound tightly enough to apply pressure and approximate the wound edges, if possible. If the first layer of dressing becomes saturated with blood, apply a second layer. Do so without removing the first layer of dressing because blood clots might be disturbed, resulting in more bleeding.
- Control swelling and pain by applying cold over the wound and surrounding tissues (see the section "Heat and Cold Applications" later in the chapter).
- If bleeding is severe, if internal bleeding is suspected, and if emergency equipment is available, assess the client for signs of shock (rapid, thready pulse; cold clammy skin; pallor; lowered blood pressure).

TREATED WOUNDS
Treated wounds, or *wounds healing by primary intention,* are regularly assessed to determine the progress of healing. Assessment of a treated wound involves observation of its size and location; the approximation of wound edges; presence of healing ridge; the condition of the wound closure devices (e.g., sutures,

---

BOX 35.5 ASSESSING UNTREATED WOUNDS

INITIAL ASSESSMENT

Untreated wounds need to be assessed carefully:

- Assess the location and extent of tissue damage (e.g., partial thickness or full thickness). Measure the wound length, width, and depth.
- Inspect the wound for bleeding. The amount of bleeding varies according to the type of wound and location. Penetrating wounds may cause internal bleeding.
- Inspect the wound for foreign bodies (soil, broken glass, shreds of cloth, or other foreign substances).
- Assess associated injuries, such as fractures, internal bleeding, spinal cord injuries, or head trauma.
- If the wound is contaminated with foreign material, determine when the client last had a tetanus toxoid injection. A tetanus immunization or booster may be necessary.

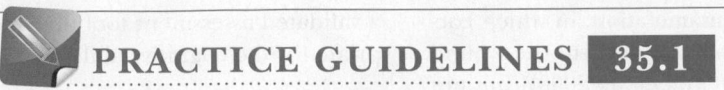

PRACTICE GUIDELINES 35.1

Assessing Common Pressure Sites

Guidelines	Rationales
Ensure the lighting is good, preferably natural or fluorescent.	Incandescent lights can create a transilluminating effect.
Regulate the environment before beginning the assessment so that the room is neither too hot nor too cold.	Heat can cause skin to flush; cold can cause skin to blanch or become cyanotic.
Inspect pressure areas (see Figure 35.5) for any abrasions, excoriations, or discoloration (which can be caused by impaired blood circulation to the area). The pressure areas should a have brisk capillary refill or blanch response when gently palpated by using the end of a finger or thumb.	A thorough and purposeful inspection of pressure areas ensures that any changes in skin are noted.
Inspect areas adjacent to any external device for any evidence of changes in skin integrity.	Pressure can be caused by external devices, such as face masks, nasogastric tubes, and the like.
Palpate for surface skin temperature over the pressure areas (warm your hands first). Normally, the temperature is the same as that of surrounding skin.	Increased temperature is abnormal and may be caused by inflammation or blood trapped in the area.
Palpate over bony prominences and dependent body areas for the presence of edema, which feels spongy or boggy.	Edema slows the diffusion of oxygen to the tissue cells and of metabolites away from the cells.

A Heels (calcaneus) Sacrum Elbows (olecranon process) Scapulae Back of head (occipital bone)

C Toes (phalanges) Knees (patellas) Genitalia (men) Breasts (women) Shoulder (acromial process) Cheek and ear (zygomatic bone)

B Malleolus (medial and lateral) Knee (medial and lateral condyles) Greater trochanter Ilium Shoulder (acromial process) Side of head (parietal and temporal bones)

D Heels (calcaneus) Vertebrae (spinal processes) 30 Pelvis (ischial tuberosity) Sacrum

FIGURE 35.5 Body pressure areas in **A:** Supine position; **B:** Lateral position; **C:** Prone position; **D:** Fowler's position.

staples), as well as the presence of any odour, swelling, redness, bruising, or pain. The status of any drains and the type and amount of drainage are also important to note. In some long-term care facilities, home care situations, and outpatient clinics, photographs are taken weekly for a visual record of the progress of pressure ulcers and wounds. Other assessments are documented and dated along with the photograph.

If the wound itself cannot be directly inspected, the dressing is inspected and other data regarding the wound (e.g., the presence of pain) are assessed. Many treated wounds are covered with a transparent occlusive dressing that permits observation of the wound without exposure to air.

Estimating the amount of wound drainage can be difficult. One recommendation is to describe the degree to which the dressing is saturated. Minimal drainage only stains the dressing, moderate drainage saturates the dressing without leakage before scheduled dressing changes, and heavy drainage overflows the dressing before scheduled changes. These terms, plus the description of the drainage and the amount and type of dressing material used, should be well understood by all care providers.

Further details about surgical wound assessment are discussed in Chapter 36.

PRESSURE ULCERS When a pressure ulcer (or any chronic ulcer) is present, the nurse needs to use a tool that will accurately and consistently assess the wound and surrounding skin. The quantifiable tool should compare two or more measurements over time, be able to detect small changes in the wound, and be reproducible in a clinical setting. This assessment will provide baseline data to evaluate the repair process and be used to drive treatment decisions. An example is the PUSH tool, which was shown in Figure 35.4.

When a pressure ulcer or wound healing by secondary intention is present, the nurse notes the following:

- The location of the wound
- The size of the wound: measure length, width, and depth, beginning with length (head to toe) and then width (side to side); to measure depth, gently insert a sterile probe at the deepest part of the wound, and then measure against a measuring guide
- The presence of undermining or sinus tracts, assessed using a sterile probe (see Figure 35.6). Note the location using the face on a clock, with 12 o'clock at the client's head
- The category/stage of the ulcer (if applicable) (see Figure 35.1)
- The colour of the wound bed assessing for presence of healthy granulation tissue (bright red or pink, moist and bumpy in appearance) or for unhealthy tissue, such as eschar (necrotic tissue that is dry, dark, tan, or

black) or slough (stringy clumps of debris scattered in the wound, can be yellow, green, tan, or brown)

- The condition of the wound margins (e.g., colour, temperature, edema, level of moisture)
- The integrity of surrounding skin
- Clinical signs of infection, such as redness, warmth, swelling, pain, odour, exudate (note colour of exudate), and blanching

Document the status of the client's skin and wounds on the standard agency form. A sample form for use with pressure ulcers is seen in Figure 35.7 on the next page.

LABORATORY DATA Laboratory data can often support the nurse's clinical assessment of the wound's progress in healing. A *decreased leukocyte (white blood cell) count* can delay healing and increase the possibility of infection. A *hemoglobin* level below normal range indicates poor oxygen delivery to the tissues. *Blood coagulation studies* are also significant. Prolonged coagulation times can result in excessive blood loss and prolonged clot absorption. Hypercoagulability can lead to intravascular clotting. Intra-arterial clotting can result in a deficient blood supply to the wound area. *Serum protein analysis,* including *albumin* and *prealbumin,* provides an indication of the body's nutritional reserves for rebuilding cells. *Wound cultures* can either confirm or rule out the presence of infection. Sensitivity studies are helpful in the selection of appropriate antibiotic therapy. The nurse obtains a wound culture whenever an infection is suspected. *Glycemic control* is measured by fasting serum glucose levels and hemoglobin A_{1C}; elevated levels of glucose (e.g., Hgb $A_{1C} > 7.0$) are associated with increased risk for microvascular and macrovascular complications, which lead to reduced circulation to skin.

Skill 35.1 on page 1021 provides guidelines on obtaining a specimen of wound drainage for culture.

Diagnosing

Multiple nursing diagnoses that relate to clients who are at risk for or have problems related to the integument can arise. Examples, among many, include at risk for pressure ulcer; wound healing by primary intention; at risk for impaired wound healing related to contaminated wound status; and at risk for wound dehiscence. Additional nursing diagnoses may be appropriate for clients with existing impaired skin or tissue integrity. Examples of these diagnoses include the following: at risk for infection, such as in the client with immunosuppression or when the wound is caused by trauma; at risk for pain related to inflammatory process; at risk for impaired body image related to negative feelings about appearance; and anxiety related to apprehension in caring for the wound or uncertainty about the eventual outcome of the healing process.

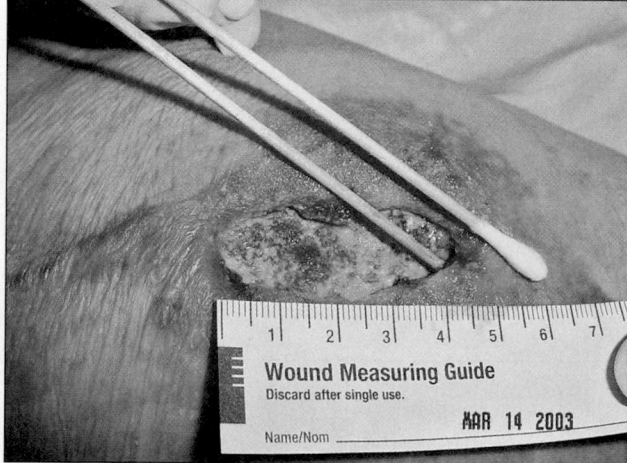

FIGURE 35.6 Presence of undermining in a wound.

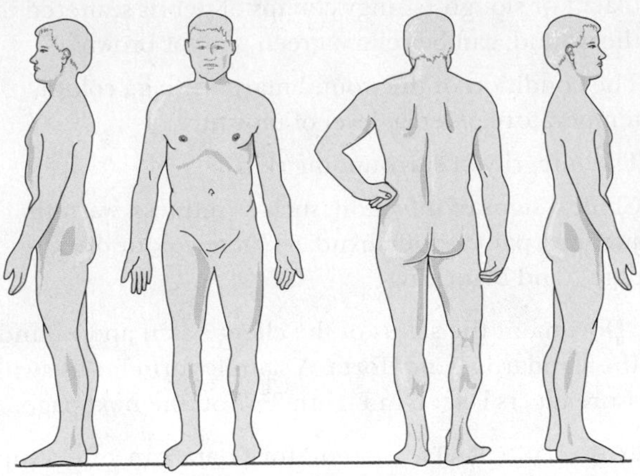

Description of Pressure Ulcers & Classification

Category/Stage I: A defined area of persistent redness; skin remains intact.

Category/Stage II: Partial-thickness skin loss involving the epidermis and possibly the dermis.

Category/Stage III: Full-thickness skin loss involving damage or necrosis of subcutaneous tissue but does not extend through the underlying fascia.

Category/Stage IV: Full-thickness skin loss with extensive destruction, tissue necrosis, or damage to muscle, bone, or supporting structures, such as a tendon or joint capsule. Undermining and sinus tract may also be present.

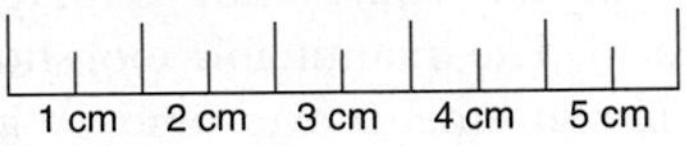

1 cm 2 cm 3 cm 4 cm 5 cm

- IDENTIFY LOCATION OF ALL PRESSURE ULCERS ABOVE BY NUMBERING (1, 2, 3): IF MORE THAN 3, USE ADDITIONAL SHEET.

- COMPLETE CHART BELOW FOR SITE #1, USE REVERSE SIDE FOR SITES 2 & 3.

Patient Admitted On: _____

Date Sheet Initiated: _____

Pressure relief methods in use:

❑ Low Airloss Bed

❑ Low Airloss Mattress Overlay

❑ Turning q2h when pt. supine and q1h if HOB↑

❑ Pressure Reducing Mattress Overlay

❑ Other _____

Date MD notified of ulcer:

_____

DOCUMENT WEEKLY AND PRN SIGNIFICANT CHANGE IN ULCER'S APPEARANCE

SITE #1: LOCATION	DESCRIBE TREATMENT:			FREQUENCY:
DATE / TIME				
DIMENSIONS: LENGTH (cm)				
WIDTH				
DEPTH				
ODOUR (none or foul)				
DESCRIBE DRAINAGE (purulent, serous, serosanguineous) and AMOUNT (scant, moderate, copious)				
STAGE (see above)				
COMMENTARY: (i.e., describe tissue surrounding ulcer: is there undermining? % necrotic vs % granular, etc.)				
NURSE				

WOUND/SKIN DOCUMENTATION SHEET

FIGURE 35.7 Wound and skin documentation sheet.

SKILL 35.1 OBTAINING A WOUND DRAINAGE SPECIMEN FOR CULTURE

PURPOSES

- To identify the microorganisms potentially causing an infection and the antibiotics to which they are sensitive
- To evaluate the effectiveness of antibiotic therapy

ASSESSMENT

Assess

- Appearance of the wound and surrounding tissue; check the character and amount of wound drainage
- Client complaints of pain or discomfort at the wound site
- Signs of infection, such as fever or elevated leukocytes (white blood cell count, [WBC])

PLANNING

Equipment

- Personal protective equipment, goggles, and gown
- Clean gloves
- Sterile gloves
- Moisture-resistant bag
- Sterile dressing set
- Normal saline and irrigating syringe
- Culture tube with swab and culture medium (aerobic and anaerobic tubes are available) or sterile syringe with needle for anaerobic culture
- Completed labels for each container
- Completed requisition to accompany the specimens to the laboratory

IMPLEMENTATION

Preparation

Check the medical orders to determine whether the specimen is to be collected for an *aerobic* (growing only in the presence of oxygen) or *anaerobic* (growing only in the absence of oxygen) culture. Aerobic organisms are generally found on the surface of the wound, whereas anaerobic organisms would be found in deep wounds, tunnels, and cavities. Administer an analgesic 30 minutes before the procedure if the client is complaining of pain at the wound site.

Performance

1. Before performing the procedure, introduce yourself and verify the client's identity using two identifiers or per agency protocol. Explain to the client what you are going to do, why it is necessary, and how he or she can participate. Discuss how the results will be used in planning further care or treatments.
2. Perform hand hygiene, and follow other appropriate infection prevention and control procedures (e.g., gloves).
3. Provide for client privacy.
4. Remove any moist outer dressings that cover the wound.
   - Put on clean gloves.
   - Remove the outer dressing, and observe any drainage on the dressing. Hold the dressing so that the client does not see the drainage. **Rationale: The appearance of the drainage could upset the client.**
   - Determine the amount of the drainage, for example, "one 5 cm × 2 cm gauze saturated with pale yellow malodorous drainage."
   - Discard the dressing in the moisture-proof bag. Handle it carefully so that the dressing does not touch the outside of the bag. **Rationale: Touching the outside of the bag will contaminate it.**
   - Remove and discard gloves. Perform hand hygiene.
5. Open the sterile dressing set by using sterile technique (see Skill 34.3, page 980).
6. Assess the wound.
   - Put on sterile gloves (see Skill 34.4, page 984).
   - Assess the appearance of the tissues in and around the wound and the drainage. Infection can cause reddened tissues with a thick discharge, which may be foul smelling, whitish, or coloured.
7. Cleanse the wound (see the Clinical Alert box on the next page).
   - By using gauze swabs or irrigation (see Skill 35.4, page 1037), cleanse the wound with normal saline until all exudate has been removed. **Rationale: Doing this removes any debris so that any microorganisms that are actually a part of the wound are accurately determined, rather than any contamination.**
   - After cleansing, apply a sterile gauze pad to the wound. **Rationale: Doing this helps absorb excess cleansing solution.**
   - If a topical antimicrobial ointment or cream is being used to treat the wound, use a swab to remove it. **Rationale: Residual antiseptic must be removed before culture.**
   - Remove and discard sterile gloves. Perform hand hygiene.
8. Obtain the aerobic culture.
   - Apply clean gloves.
   - Open a specimen tube and place the cap upside down on a firm, dry surface so that the inside will not become contaminated or if the swab is attached to the lid, twist the cap to loosen the swab. Hold the tube in one hand, and take out the swab in the other.
   - Rotate the swab over a healthy area of tissue 1 cm². Apply sufficient pressure to express fluid from within the wound tissue (see ❶ and ❷). **Rationale: Microorganisms that are most likely to be responsible for a wound infection reside in viable tissue.**
   - Do not use pus or pooled exudates to culture. **Rationale: These secretions contain a mixture of contaminants that are not the same as those causing the infection.**
   - Avoid touching the swab to intact skin at the wound edges. **Rationale: Doing this prevents the introduction of superficial skin organisms into the culture.**
   - Return the swab to the culture tube, taking care not to touch the top or the outside of the tube (see ❸). **Rationale: The outside of the container must remain free of pathogenic microorganisms to prevent their spread to others.**

(continued)

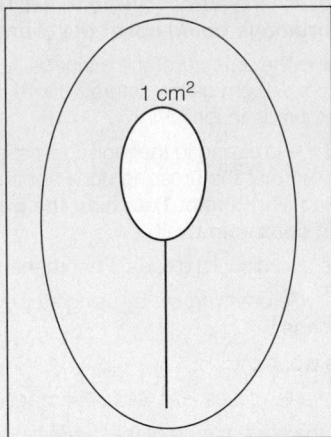

1 Rotate the swab over an area of granulation tissue 1 cm².

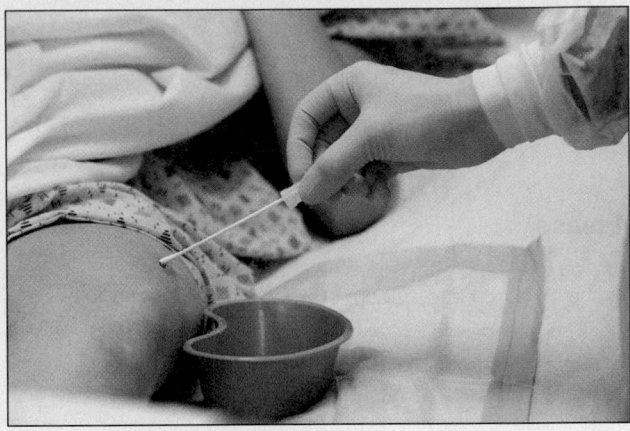

2 Obtaining a culture specimen from the base of the wound.

- Include the date and time, the appearance of the wound, the colour, consistency, amount, and odour of any drainage, the type of culture collected, and any discomfort experienced by the client.

Variation: Obtaining a Specimen for Anaerobic Culture

- Insert a sterile 10-mL syringe (without needle) into the wound, and aspirate 1 mL to 5 mL of drainage into the syringe.
- Attach the needle to the syringe, and expel all air from the syringe and needle.
- Immediately inject the drainage into the anaerobic culture tube and cap the tube tightly.

  Or

- Use an anaerobic culture swab system in which the swab is immediately placed into a tube filled with an oxygen-free gas or a gel environment.
- Label the tube or syringe appropriately.
- Send the tube or syringe of drainage to the laboratory immediately. Do not refrigerate the specimen.

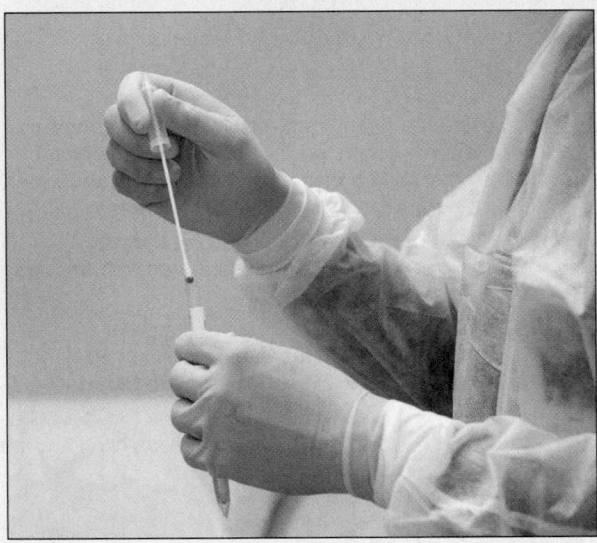

3 Return the swab to the culture tube.

- Crush the inner ampule containing the medium for organism growth at the bottom of the tube. **Rationale: Doing this ensures that the swab with the specimen is surrounded by culture medium**.
- Twist the cap to secure.
- If a specimen is required from another site, repeat the steps. Specify the exact site (e.g., inferior drain site or lower aspect of incision) on the label of each container. Be sure to put each swab in the appropriately labelled tube.

9. Dress the wound.
   - Apply any prescribed medication to the wound.
   - Cover the wound with a sterile wound dressing. See Table 35.4 on page 1029 for selected types of wound dressings.

10. Arrange for the specimen to be transported to the laboratory immediately. Be sure to include the completed requisition.

11. Document all relevant information.
    - Record on the client's chart the taking of the specimen and source.

EVALUATION

- Compare the findings of wound assessment and drainage to previous assessments to determine any changes.
- Report the culture results to the appropriate health care team members.
- Conduct appropriate follow-up, such as administering antibiotics or modifying wound treatment, as prescribed.

> **! CLINICAL ALERT**
>
> Wound cleansing must be done before obtaining a specimen for culture. The goal of a culture is to evaluate the microorganisms present in the wound tissue. Failure to cleanse means that the results are indicative of contaminants, such as wound exudate, topical therapies, or nonviable tissue, which could lead to inappropriate or unnecessary treatment.

Planning

The major goals for clients at risk for impaired skin integrity (e.g., pressure ulcer development) are to maintain skin integrity and to avoid potential associated risks. Clients with actual impaired skin integrity need to demonstrate progressive wound healing and regain intact skin. In the event that the client is unable to heal, the goal may be to palliate the wound.

Examples of specific desired health outcomes related to these goals, although established in the planning phase, are provided in the "Evaluating" section of this chapter.

Planning for Home Care

Increasingly, wound care is provided in the home rather than in health care facilities. The client and family assume much of the responsibility for assessing and treating existing wounds and for helping to prevent pressure ulcers. The Assessment: Home Care box outlines appropriate assessment for clients who have wounds or pressure ulcers or who are at risk for developing alterations in skin integrity. In planning for client discharge, nurses are accountable for teaching the client and family wound preventive and skin integrity care measures (see the Teaching: Clinical box).

ASSESSMENT   HOME CARE

Wound Care and Prevention of Pressure Ulcers

Assess the client's and the family's understanding of wounds and wound care:

CLIENT AND ENVIRONMENT

- *Current level of knowledge:* Understanding of the cause of the wound or risk for developing a pressure ulcer; prevention or treatment strategies
- *Self-care abilities for mobility:* Physical ability to change position, ambulate, and transfer, including the use of assistive devices
- *Self-care abilities for wound care:* Manual dexterity and visual acuity necessary to perform skin assessments and wound treatments
- *Facilities:* Presence of running water, garbage, and bathroom needed to perform wound care and contain potentially infectious materials
- *Current level of nutrition:* Eating habits and preferences, laboratory values indicating need for teaching or other intervention

FAMILY

- *Caregiver availability, skills, and responses:* Willingness to assist with wound care and actions to prevent pressure ulcers
- *Family role changes and coping:* Effect on financial status, parenting and spousal roles, sexuality, social roles
- *Alternative potential primary or respite caregivers:* For example, other family members, volunteers, church members, paid caregivers or housekeeping services, available community respite care (adult daycare, senior centres, and so on)

COMMUNITY

- *Resources:* Availability and familiarity with possible sources of assistance, such as equipment and supply companies, organizations that offer medical supplies or financial assistance, home care agencies

---

TEACHING   CLINICAL

Skin Integrity

Nurses must teach the client and family wound preventive and skin integrity care measures before discharge:

Maintaining Intact Skin

- Discuss the relationship between adequate nutrition (especially fluids, protein, vitamins B and C, iron, zinc, and calories) and healthy skin.
- Demonstrate appropriate positions for pressure redistribution.
- Establish a turning or repositioning schedule.
- Demonstrate the application of appropriate skin protection agents and devices.
- Instruct to report persistent reddened areas.
- Identify potential sources of skin trauma and means of avoidance.

Promoting Wound Healing

- Discuss the importance of adequate nutrition (especially fluids, protein, vitamins B and C, iron, zinc, and calories).
- Instruct in wound assessment and provide mechanism for documenting.
- Emphasize the principles of infection prevention and control, especially hand hygiene and the proper methods of handling used dressings.
- Provide information about signs of wound infection and other complications to report.
- Reinforce the appropriate aspects of pressure ulcer prevention.
- Demonstrate wound care techniques, such as wound cleansing and dressing change.
- Discuss pain control measures, if needed.

Implementing

Many interventions exist to help preserve a client's skin and underlying tissues. An initial step involves identifying clients at risk for breakdown since risk factors provide the basis for prophylaxis (RNAO, 2011). Refer to the Braden Scale in Figure 35.3 (page 1011).

Nursing interventions for maintaining skin integrity and wound care involve supporting wound healing, preventing pressure ulcers, treating pressure ulcers, dressing and cleaning wounds, applying heat and cold, and supporting and immobilizing wounds. Wounds must be reassessed on a regular basis to determine the adequacy of the treatment plan.

Supporting Wound Healing

The four major areas in which nurses can help clients develop optimal conditions for wound healing are (a) maintaining moist wound healing, (b) providing sufficient nutrition and hydration, (c) preventing wound infections, and (d) using proper positioning.

MAINTAINING MOIST WOUND HEALING The frequency of dressing change should support moist wound bed conditions. Wound beds that are too dry, too wet, or disturbed too often fail to heal.

PROVIDING NUTRITION AND FLUIDS Clients should be assisted to take in at least 2500 mL of fluids a day unless conditions contraindicate this amount. Although no evidence shows that excessive doses of vitamins or minerals enhance wound healing, adequate amounts are extremely important. The nurse should ensure that clients receive sufficient protein, vitamins C, A, B_1, and B_5, and zinc. Consultations with a registered dietitian or speech language pathologist (in the case of swallowing difficulties) may be very helpful.

PREVENTING INFECTION Controlling wound infection has two main aspects: (a) preventing microorganisms from entering the wound, and (b) preventing the transmission of blood-borne pathogens to or from the client to others. See Box 35.6 and Chapter 34 for more information about infection prevention and control.

POSITIONING To promote wound healing, clients must be positioned to keep pressure off the wound (sometimes referred to as *offloading*). Changes of position and transfers can be accomplished without shear or friction damage. In addition to proper positioning, the client should be assisted to be as mobile as possible because activity enhances circulation. If the client cannot move independently, range-of-motion exercises and a turning schedule are implemented.

BOX 35.6 GUIDELINES FOR PREVENTING INFECTION AND THE TRANSMISSION OF BLOOD-BORNE PATHOGENS

Preventing infection is an extremely important part of wound care:

- Perform hand hygiene before and after caring for wounds.

- Masks and protective eyewear (e.g., goggles, safety glasses) or face shields should be worn to protect mucous membranes, nonintact skin, and conjunctiva during procedures that are likely to generate splashes of blood or fluids capable of transmitting blood-borne pathogens. Wherever a possibility exists for exposure to blood or fluid capable of transmitting blood-borne pathogens, masks and protective eyewear should be worn.

- Touch an open or fresh surgical wound only when wearing sterile gloves or using sterile forceps.

- Remove, change, or reinforce dressings over closed wounds when they become wet.

Source: These recommendations are based on the principles outlined in Public Health Agency of Canada. (2002). Prevention and control of occupational infections in health care. *Canada Communicable Disease Report, 28S1.* Retrieved from http://www.phac-aspc.gc.ca/publicat/ccdr-rmtc/02vol28/28s1/index.html

---

Preventing Pressure Ulcers

To reduce the likelihood of pressure ulcer development in all clients, the nurse employs a variety of preventive measures (i.e., skin hygiene and pressure redistribution devices) to maintain the skin integrity and instructs the client, support people, and caregivers in how to prevent pressure ulcers.

PROVIDING NUTRITION Optimal nutrition promotes wound healing, maintains immune competence, and decreases the risk of infection (RNAO, 2007). Because an inadequate intake of calories, protein, vitamins, and iron is believed to be a risk factor for pressure ulcer development, nutritional supplements should be considered for nutritionally compromised clients. The diet should be similar to one that supports wound healing, as discussed earlier. Monitor weight regularly to help assess nutritional status. Pertinent lab work should also be monitored, including lymphocyte count, protein (especially albumin), and hemoglobin.

MAINTAINING SKIN HYGIENE Obtain baseline data by using an established tool and then reassess the skin at least daily in the hospital and weekly at home. When bathing the client, the nurse should minimize the force and friction applied to skin and use mild cleansing agents that minimize irritation and dryness and that do not disrupt skin's natural barriers. Also, the nurse should avoid using hot water, which increases skin dryness and irritation. Nurses can minimize skin dryness by avoiding exposure to cold and low humidity. Dry skin is best treated with moisturizing lotions applied while skin is moist after bathing. The client's skin should be kept clean and dry and free of irritation and maceration by urine, feces, sweat, and incomplete drying after a bath. Apply skin protection, if indicated. Dimethicone-based creams or alcohol-free barrier films are available in liquid, spray, and moist wipe format and are very effective in preventing moisture or drainage from collecting on the skin. In most cases, the nurse can apply these without a physician's prescription. Petroleum-based creams and ointments are no longer advised because of poor overall skin protection and interference with diaper or incontinence product absorption. Chapter 31 discusses hygiene care in detail.

AVOIDING SKIN TRAUMA Massage over bony prominences or reddened (indicative of inflammation) areas should be avoided (RNAO, 2011). Traditionally, nurses have used massage to stimulate blood circulation, with the intention of preventing pressure ulcers. Scientific evidence does not support this belief and, in fact, suggests that massage may lead to deep tissue trauma.

Appropriate positioning is critical in addressing issues related to pressure. Providing the client with a smooth, firm, and wrinkle-free foundation on which to sit or lie helps prevent skin trauma. To prevent injury caused by friction and shear, clients must be moved, positioned, transferred, and turned correctly. For clients confined to bed, shear force can be reduced by elevating the head of the bed to no more than 30 degrees, if this position is not contraindicated by the client's condition. (For example, clients with respiratory disorders may find it easier to breathe in Fowler's position.) When the head of the bed is raised, skin and the superficial fascia stick to the bed linen, whereas the deep fascia and skeleton slide down toward the bottom of the bed. As a result, blood vessels in the sacral area become twisted, and tissues in the area can become ischemic and necrotic. Baby powder and cornstarch are never used as friction or moisture prevention. These powders create harmful abrasive grit that is damaging to tissues and are considered a respiratory hazard when airborne.

Frequent shifts in position, even if only slight, effectively change pressure points. The client should shift weight 10 to 15 degrees every 15 to 30 minutes and, whenever possible, exercise or ambulate to stimulate blood circulation.

When moving a client to change position, nurses should use a lifting device, such as a trapeze, rather than dragging the client across or up in bed. The friction that results from dragging the skin against a sheet can cause blisters and abrasions, which may contribute to more extensive tissue damage. Therefore, the use of devices that lift the client's weight off the bed surface is the method of choice.

A client who has a pressure ulcer on a seating surface should be discouraged from sitting, when possible. It is important to obtain a seating assessment if a client has a pressure ulcer on a sitting surface that requires relief from pressure (RNAO, 2011). A repositioning schedule of at least every 2 hours should be implemented when a client is on a standard mattress, emergency stretcher, or operating table; if a pressure management surface is used (e.g., redistribution mattress), a repositioning schedule of at least every four hours or as necessary depending on the client's individual situation is recommended (RNAO, 2011). Despite years of using repositioning as an intervention in the treatment of pressure ulcers, "no randomised trials exist that assess the effects of repositioning patients on the healing rates of pressure ulcers" (Moore & Cowman, 2009). The six body positions that can usually be used are the prone, supine, right and left lateral (side lying), and right and left Sims' positions. When the lateral position is used, the nurse should avoid positioning the client directly on the trochanter and instead position the client on a 30-degree angle (RNAO, 2011). A written schedule should be established for turning and repositioning. Chapter 39 discusses moving clients in detail.

PROVIDING SUPPORTIVE DEVICES For circulation to remain uncompromised, pressure on the bony prominences should remain below capillary pressure for as much time as possible through a combination of turning, positioning, and using pressure-relieving surfaces. Mean capillary pressure can be estimated at 20 mm Hg. The nurse should review the manufacturer's product descriptions that report the amount of time that the pressure between the surface and the bony prominence is above or below specified levels and determine whether this is adequate to protect a particular client.

There are two major types of support surfaces used to redistribute pressure when the client is in bed. Reactive support surfaces are powered or nonpowered support surfaces that are capable of changing load distribution only in response to applied load (e.g., a client lying on the surface); active support devices use power to change the load distribution properties with or without applied load (pressure changes regardless of whether the patient moves or not) (NPUAP, 2007). Reactive support surfaces include overlay pads or mattresses (generally made of high density foam, air, or gel) and low-air-loss devices.

Active support surfaces include mattress replacements and overlay devices, such as an alternating pressure air mattress and specialty rotational mattresses (Norton, Coutts, & Sibbald, 2011). An alternating pressure mattress is composed of a number of cells in which the pressure alternately increases and decreases (Figure 35.8). Rotational mattresses turn the patient based on a programmed angle of movement, frequency,

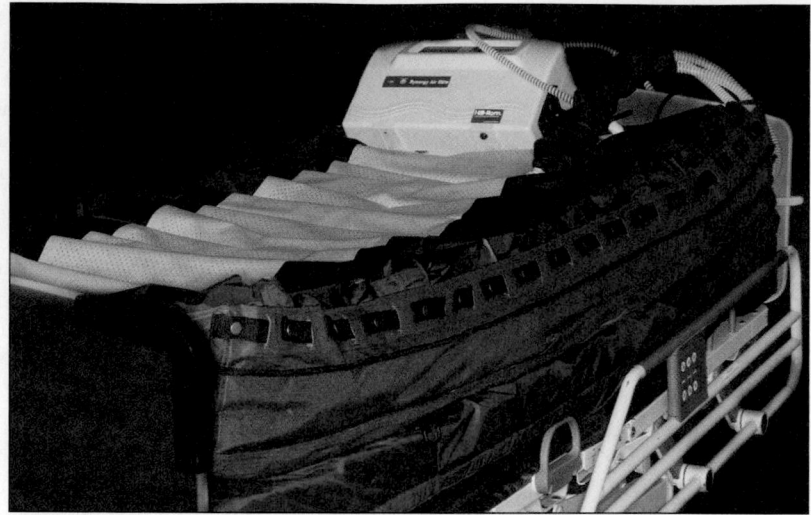

FIGURE 35.8 Alternating pressure mattress.

Note: electronic device pictured on the mattress is not attached to the bed when mattress is in use.

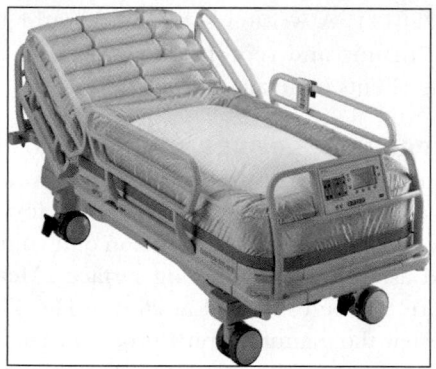

FIGURE 35.9 Low-air-loss and air-fluidized combo bed.

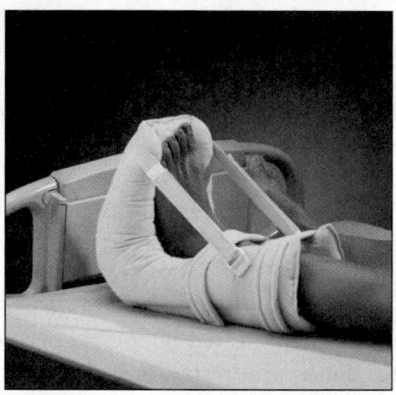

FIGURE 35.10 Heel protector.

and duration. The redistribution devices can be further classified into zoned and multizoned. Zoned mattresses redistribute pressure within one body area, whereas multizoned surfaces have different sections (zones) that can vary the distribution of pressure across different body segments. Specialized beds are available that offer "combinations" of pressure redistribution mechanisms, including the use of silicone-coated beads that absorb moisture from the client, thus reducing the risk of maceration (Figure 35.9). Norton, Coutts, and Sibbald (2011) have created a tool to help clinicians select the appropriate pressure redistribution device based on the client's risk assessment or actual presence of pressure ulcer (see Table 35.3). Ongoing research is needed, as there is no conclusive evidence about the superiority of any support surface for the treatment of existing pressure ulcers (McInnes, Dumville, Jammali-Blasi, & Bell-Syer, 2009).

Regardless of the supportive device used in redistributing pressure while the client is in bed, the heels should be managed independent of the surface in use (Norton et al., 2011). Heel protectors (Figure 35.10) include

sheepskin boots, padded splints, off-loading inflatable boots, and foam blocks and can raise or "float" the heel off the surface.

Pillows and wedges (made of foam, gel, air, fluid) are available to support positioning and offload bone on bone (e.g., avoids knee against knee when a client is in the side-lying position).

When a client is confined to bed or to a chair, pressure-reducing devices, such as pillows made of high-density foam, gel, air, or a combination of these, can be used. When the client is sitting, weight should be distributed over the entire seating surface so that pressure does not centre on just one area. To protect a client's heels, pressure must be offloaded in all positions (e.g., sitting, lying) by completely elevating the heel off the pressure surface (RNAO, 2011). Air or foam mattress overlays, heel protection devices, foam wedges, and pillows can be used to raise the heels. Ongoing research is needed to determine what offloading devices are the most effective (Junkin & Gray, 2009). Doughnut-type devices should not be used, since they limit blood flow and could cause tissue damage to the areas in direct contact with the device.

TABLE 35.3 Therapeutic Support Surface Selection Tool

		Validated Risk Assessment Score or Pressure Ulcer Description			
		At risk *Or* Redness present that fades quickly when pressure removed	Moderate risk *Or* One pressure ulcer (excluding the heels) where the client can be positioned off the ulcer	High risk *Or* One pressure ulcer (excluding the heels) and redness over another area	Very high risk *Or* Multiple pressure ulcers (excluding the heels) or the client cannot be positioned off of an ulcerated area
Ability to Change Position in Bed (i.e., bed mobility)	Total assistance to change position in bed	Reactive Support Surface (nonpowered) (e.g., air/gel/foam overlay)	Reactive Support Surface (e.g., air/gel/foam overlay)	Active Support Surface Multizoned surface (e.g., alternating pressure mattress, rotational surface) or a powered reactive support surface (e.g., low air loss)	Active Support Surface Multizoned surface (e.g., alternating pressure mattress, rotational surface)
	Moderate assistance with bed mobility required	Reactive Support Surface (nonpowered) (e.g., air/gel/foam overlay or high density foam mattress)	Reactive Support Surface (e.g., foam overlay with air section insert in the area of the wound)	Reactive Support Surface (nonpowered) (e.g., foam overlay with air section insert in the area of the wound)	Active Support Surface Multizoned surface (e.g., alternating pressure mattress, rotational surface)
	Client independent with or without a device with bed positioning (light assistance may be required)	Reactive Support Surface (e.g., high density foam mattress)	Reactive Support Surface (e.g., foam overlay with air section insert)	Reactive Support Surface (nonpowered) (e.g., air/gel/foam overlay)	Active Support Surface (if the controls can be placed within the client's reach)

User's guide:

1. With a validated risk assessment tool, determine the client's level of risk, or grade the clients with ulcers based on the clinical descriptors.
2. Assess the level of mobility in bed and follow the column-and-row intersection to determine the appropriate reactive or active support system.

Source: Norton, L., Coutts, P., & Sibbald, G. (2011). Beds: Practical pressure management for surfaces/mattresses. *Advances in Skin and Wound Care Management, 24*(7), 324–332. Copyright © Norton, Coutts, & Sibbald. Reprinted with permission.

Treating Pressure Ulcers

Pressure ulcers are a challenge for nurses because of the number of variables involved (e.g., risk factors, types of ulcers, and degrees of impairment) and the numerous treatment measures advocated. Existing and potential infections are the most serious complications of pressure ulcers. For clients with compromised skin integrity of the lower limbs, a vascular assessment is essential to rule out arterial disease and to determine appropriate therapy.

In treating pressure ulcers, nurses should follow the agency skin and wound management protocols. Prompt treatment can prevent further tissue damage and pain and facilitate wound healing. See Box 35.2 (pages 1006–1007) for the Canadian Association of Wound Care recommendations for practice regarding the prevention and treatment of pressure ulcers.

THE RYB COLOUR CODE The universal classification of wounds by colour uses red, yellow, black (RYB) (Figure 35.11 on the next page) and offers a user-friendly, practical method of assessing wounds and determining treatment options. The colour classification describes the wound in terms of its surface appearance. The red denotes granulation tissue; the yellow indicates slough; and the black indicates necrotic tissue. The goals of wound care by using this system are to *protect* (cover) red, *cleanse* yellow, and *debride* black.

Wounds that are red are usually in the late regeneration phase of tissue repair (i.e., developing granulation tissue). They need to be protected to avoid disturbance to regenerating tissue. The nurse protects red wounds by (a) gentle cleansing (i.e., use of a noncytotoxic wound cleanser applied without pressure), (b) protecting peri-wound skin with an alcohol-free barrier film, (c) filling

R | **Red wounds** may vary from pale pink to a beefy red with the colour indicating the presence and depth of granulation tissue. Red wounds can be in the inflammatory or proliferative phase of wound healing. There is a need to cover a red wound for protection and to keep it moist. Both protection from trauma and a moist wound bed enhance wound healing.

Y | **Yellow wounds** vary in colour from pale ivory to various shades of yellow, green, and brown. The yellow/green/brown colour indicates the presence of slough (dead but moist tissue). Yellow wounds actively generate wound fluid and need to be debrided to remove the slough and reduce the bacterial load.

B | **Black wounds** are covered with tissue that is a black/brown or tan. The colour indicates the presence of dead tissue that is dehydrated to various degrees. Often, black wounds are referred to as being covered with eschar, a thick, hard, leathery material. When eschar is covering a wound, the depth cannot be accurately assessed until the eschar is removed. In most cases, eschar provides an excellent medium for bacterial proliferation and needs to be removed to prevent infection and promote wound healing. In patients with diabetes with inadequate blood supply, dry eschar is kept intact until a thorough vascular exam has been completed.

FIGURE 35.11 RYB colour wound classification system.

dead space with hydrogel or alginate, (d) covering with an appropriate dressing, such as transparent film, hydrocolloid dressing, or a clear absorbent acrylic dressing, and (e) changing the dressing as infrequently as possible.

Yellow wounds are characterized primarily by liquid to semiliquid slough that is often accompanied by purulent drainage. Generally, yellow wounds are cleansed to remove exudate and nonviable tissue. Methods used include applying wet-to-damp dressings; irrigating the wound; using absorbent dressing materials, such as impregnated nonadherent hydrogel dressings or other exudate absorbers; and consulting with the physician about the need for a topical antimicrobial to minimize bacterial growth. Slough that is not removed by cleansing will need to be removed by debridement.

Black wounds are covered with thick necrotic tissue or eschar. Black wounds require **debridement** (removal of necrotic or devitalized tissue that interferes with wound healing), except in cases of foot ulcers with dry eschar (RNAO, 2007). Removal of nonviable tissue from a wound must occur before the wound can heal.

Debridement can be achieved in four different ways: (a) sharp, (b) mechanical, (c) chemical, and (d) autolytic. The method of debridement will depend on (a) the client's condition and goals of treatment; (b) the type, quantity,

and location of necrotic tissue; and (c) the depth and amount of fluid (RNAO, 2007). Refer to Box 35.2 (p. 1006–1007) for the Canadian Association of Wound Care's recommendations for preparing the wound bed.

In *sharp debridement,* a sharp instrument (scalpel or scissors) is used to separate and remove dead tissue. Generally, this high-risk procedure is performed only by specially trained health care professionals (e.g., wound, ostomy, and continence nurses [WOCNs]; qualified physical therapists). Sharp debridement should be used if there is urgent need for debridement, such as advancing cellulitis or sepsis; sharp debridement entails a serious risk of bleeding, may require anesthesia, and has the potential to cause injury to nervous or other viable tissue (RNAO, 2007).

Mechanical debridement refers to the removal of foreign material and devitalized or contaminated tissue from a wound by physical forces. Whirlpool baths, dextranomers, and wound irrigations are examples of mechanical debridement. This treatment may be used as a preparation for sharp debridement. Mechanical debridement has a number of important disadvantages. It is a slow and often painful process that must be discontinued once the necrotic tissue has been removed. Pain management should be an integral part of nursing care for the client undergoing mechanical debridement.

Chemical or *enzymatic debridement* is the topical application of proteolytic substances (enzymes) to break down devitalized tissues. Collagenase enzyme agents, such as papain-urea, are currently most recommended for this use. This method is relatively slow, but it can be helpful for clients who are not candidates for sharp debridement, clients in long-term care or home care, and clients in whom ulcer infection is not present (RNAO, 2007).

In *autolytic debridement,* synthetic dressings are used to cover a wound and allow eschar to self-digest by the action of enzymes present in wound fluids. Although this method takes longer than the other three, it is the most selective and, therefore, causes the least damage to healthy surrounding and healing tissues. Because occlusive synthetic dressings create an anaerobic environment, they should never be used if an infection in the wound is suspected. Recently, the use of sterile fly larvae (maggots, *Phaenicia sericata*) has received increased attention. Larval therapy can be extremely effective in cleansing chronic wounds because the maggots secrete enzymes that break down necrotic tissue (while leaving healthy tissue untouched), ingest bacteria, and decrease bacterial growth through the rise in surface pH that results from their presence (Hunter, Langemo, Thompson, Hanson, & Anderson, 2009).

Most wounds display a combination of colours and are called mixed-colour wounds. In these wounds, care is planned to address the most serious problem first. Thus, the highest priority is to address the black, then the yellow, and finally the red. Black and yellow wounds need to be debrided and both types kept moist. The appearance of the wound is documented by percentage (e.g., 50% red, 25% yellow, and 25% black).

The RYB system is an excellent conceptual framework for guiding the local treatment of the wound, although its use has limitations in that this system does not address the underlying pathology and treatment needed for specific pathologies, such as the compression that would be needed to treat a venous ulcer or revascularization to treat an arterial ulcer. Consultation with a wound care specialist is important in determining appropriate therapies, particularly when the ulcer is a manifestation of a systemic disease.

Dressing Wounds

Dressings are applied for the following purposes:

- To protect the wound from mechanical injury
- To protect the wound from microbial contamination
- To provide or maintain moist wound healing

- To provide thermal insulation
- To absorb drainage or debride a wound, or both
- To prevent hemorrhage (when applied as a pressure dressing or with elastic bandages)
- To splint or immobilize the wound site and thereby facilitate healing and prevent injury
- To provide psychological (aesthetic) comfort

The development of interactive wound dressings has produced dressings that work with the environment of the wound to promote wound healing. Moisture-retentive dressings promote wound healing by optimizing the local wound environment (RNAO, 2007).

TYPES OF DRESSING A wide, and sometimes confusing, array of dressings are available for wound management. Table 35.4 provides a summary of selected types of wound dressings. A number of factors influence the type of dressing that is appropriate for any given wound.

TABLE 35.4 Selected Types of Wound Care Products

Product Type	Description	Purpose	Examples
Wound cleansers	These are noncytotoxic liquids. *They must not be confused with skin cleansers, which are meant for intact skin only.*	Normal saline in the preferred cleanser, although commercial products containing surfactants may be helpful with removal of debris	Normal saline, Shur-Clens, Safe-Clens, Restore
Moisture retentive dressings: Transparent films	Adhesive moisture vapour permeable polyurethane or other synthetic films are *nonabsorbent* dressings that allow exchange of oxygen and moisture vapour between the atmosphere and wound bed. They are impermeable to bacteria and water.	To provide protection against contamination and friction; to maintain a clean moist surface that facilitates cellular migration; to provide insulation by preventing fluid evaporation; and to facilitate wound assessment	Op-Site, Tegaderm, Bioclusive, Flexifix
Moisture retentive: Nonadherents (impregnated or nonimpregnated)	Woven or nonwoven cotton or synthetic materials may be impregnated with medicated or unmedicated ointments. These require secondary dressings to secure them in place.	Designed to provide a contact dressing of low adherence and support the delivery of topical antibacterials and antibiotics	Nonimpregnated: Mepore, ETE, Mepitel, Primapore, Alldress Impregnated: Xeroform, Adaptic, Jelonet, Bactigras, Sofratulle, Viscopaste
Wound hydration: Hydrocolloids	Dressings—made up of a dispersion of gelatin, pectin, and carboxymethylcellulose together with other polymers and adhesives forming a flexible wafer—are designed to be worn for up to 7 days and consist of two layers. The inner adhesive layer has particles that absorb exudate and form a hydrated gel over the wound; the outer film provides a waterproof seal; wear time is 3 to 7 days. These may also be available in pastes and powders.	To absorb light to moderate exudate; to produce a moist environment that facilitates debridement and healing but does not cause maceration of surrounding skin; to protect the wound from bacterial contamination, foreign debris, and urine or feces	DuoDERM, Comfeel, Tegasorb, Restore, SignaDress

(continued)

TABLE 35.4 Selected Types of Wound Care Products (*continued*)

Product Type	Description	Purpose	Examples
Wound hydration: Hydrogels	Hydrophilic moisture-donating polymers—prepared in sheets or gels for use in granulating wounds, minimally exudating wounds, or wounds requiring debridement—can be used in combination with transparent films, foams, hydrocolloids, or other nonadherent cover dressings; wear time varies from 1 to 3 days.	To assist with the liquefaction of necrotic tissue or slough; rehydrate the wound bed; and fill in dead space	IntraSite, Vigilon, Normlgel, Hypergel, DuoDERM Hydroactive Gel, Tegagel
Absorbent dressings: Foams	Sheet or cavity dressings of nonadherent polyurethane foams used for wounds with moderate to copious amounts of drainage to maintain autolytic debridement during wound cleansing phase; they reduce dressing bulk; wear time can be extended as volume of drainage decreases to a maximum of 4 to 7 days.	To absorb moderate amounts of exudate	Lyofoam, Allevyn, Biatain, Mepilex, Hydrasorb
Absorbent dressings: Alginates	Nonadherent sheets, ropes, granules, or powders absorb moderate to large amounts of exudate—up to 20 times their weight; many products have hemostatic properties; require a secondary dressing; remove residue by flushing wound with saline; maximum wear time is 4 days.	To absorb exudate and facilitate hemostasis	Algisite, Kaltostat, Tegagen, Fibracol
Absorbent dressings: Hydrofibre, hypertonic gauze	Nonadherent sheets or ribbon gauze used for copiously draining wounds; promote comfort by decreasing dressing bulk; requires a moisture retentive cover dressing; layering dressing increases absorption capacity; wear time of 1 to 4 day.	To provide a moist wound surface by interacting with exudate; to form a gelatinous mass; to absorb exudate; to eliminate dead space or pack wounds; and to support debridement	Aquacel, Mesalt
Antimicrobials	Topical antimicrobial agents reduce bacterial burden in wounds.	To decrease surface bacteria without excessive toxicity to the cells in the wound base	Iodosorb, Acticoat, Aquacel Ag. silver sulfadiazine, metronidazole gel, polymyxin B sulphate—Bacitracin zinc
Collagen	Gels, pastes, powders, granules, sheets, and sponges are derived from animal sources, often cow or pig.	Assists with stopping bleeding; helps recruit cells into the wound; and stimulates their proliferation to facilitate healing	Biostep, Cellerate, RX, NU-GEL, Promogran
Skin barriers	Liquids, creams, pastes, ointments or solids; products containing alcohol can cause burning if skin is not intact; liquid product must be dry before dressing is applied	To protect periwound skin from exudate and stripping by adhesives	Skin Prep, Skin Gel, Sween, Calmoseptine, Triple Care, Critic-Aid, Coloplast

Box 35.7 lists RNAO guidelines (2007) regarding factors to consider when selecting a dressing for local wound care.

In many settings, dressing cost is also a concern, particularly if extended treatment is required. A wound management consultant can help to select the dressing that best meets both the needs of the client and the need for cost containment.

Transparent Films Transparent films are often applied to superficial wounds and skin breaks with minimal damage to maintain a moist healing environment (Figure 35.12).

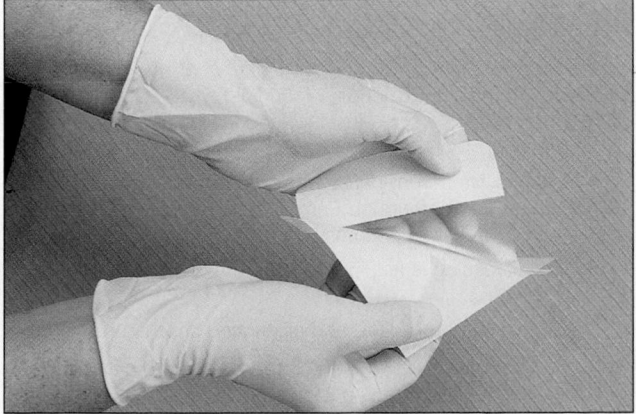

FIGURE 35.12 A transparent wound dressing.

The following considerations are important when using transparent films:

- Transparent films are nonporous, self-adhesive dressings that are often left in place for up to 7 days.
- Because they are transparent, the wound can be assessed through them.
- Because they are semiocclusive, the wound remains moist and retains the serous exudate, which promotes epithelial growth, supports autolytic debridement, and reduces the risk of infection. They should not be used if there is evidence of a yeast infection as this condition may be exacerbated.
- Because they are elastic, they can be placed over a joint without disrupting the client's mobility.
- They adhere only to the skin area around the wound and not to the wound itself because they keep the wound moist. The use of a liquid skin barrier on the periwound skin can increase adhesion and wear time.
- They allow the client to shower or bathe without removing the dressing.
- They can be removed without damaging wound tissues, although caution must be used if the client has fragile periwound skin.

Skill 35.2 on the next page describes how to apply a transparent wound dressing.

Hydrocolloid Dressings Hydrocolloid dressings (Figure 35.13 on page 1033) provide wound hydration (refer back to Table 35.4) and are frequently used in wounds with minimal drainage and those requiring debridement (see the Reflect on Primary Health Care box on page 1033). These dressings have several advantages:

- Dressing sheets can be cut to fit difficult areas. (*Note:* The dressing must always extend at least 2.5 cm to 5 cm beyond the wound margins to promote adherence and extend wear time.) Taping the edges with a paper tape may improve wear time.
- They do not need a cover dressing and are water resistant, so the client can shower or bathe.
- They can remain in place for 3 to 7 days, with the frequency of dressing changes dependent on the amount of drainage. The dressing should be changed before leakage occurs.
- They can be moulded to uneven body surfaces.
- They absorb moderate drainage so can be used on slowly draining wounds.
- They act as temporary skin and provide an effective bacterial barrier.
- Hydrocolloids decrease pain and, thus, reduce the need for analgesics.
- They can contain wound odour.

SKILL 35.2 APPLYING AND REMOVING A TRANSPARENT WOUND BARRIER DRESSING

PURPOSES

- To maintain a moist wound environment and promote wound healing
- To protect the wound from trauma and infectious agents
- To facilitate assessment of wound healing

ASSESSMENT

Assess

- Appearance and size of the wound
- Amount and character of exudate
- Complaints of discomfort
- Signs of systemic infection (e.g., elevated body temperature, malaise, leukocytosis)

PLANNING

- Before applying or changing a moist transparent wound barrier, determine agency protocol about solutions used to clean the wound and whether clean or sterile technique is to be used. Many agencies recommend clean rather than sterile technique for chronic wounds, such as a pressure ulcer.
- Obtain assistance as needed. If the size of the wound necessitates it, acquire the assistance of a coworker to help apply the dressing.

Equipment

- Disposable gloves
- Hair scissors or clippers
- Alcohol or acetone
- Moisture-proof bag
- Sterile gloves (optional)
- Sterile gauze and the wound-cleaning agents specified by the physician or agency (e.g., sterile saline)
- Wound barrier dressing
- Scissors
- Paper tape

IMPLEMENTATION

Performance

1. Before performing the procedure, introduce yourself and verify the client's identity using two identifiers or per agency protocol. Explain to the client what you are going to do, why it is necessary, and how he or she can participate. Discuss how the results will be used in planning further care or treatments.

2. Perform hand hygiene, and follow other appropriate infection prevention and control procedures.

3. Thoroughly clean the skin area around the wound. Put on disposable gloves.
   - Clean the skin around the wound well with normal saline or a nonirritating wound cleansing agent. Always rinse and dry the adjacent skin completely before applying a dressing.

- Clip the hair about 5 cm around the wound area, if indicated. Do NOT use razors. **Rationale: Razor blades can cause small nicks in the skin and create or spread infection** (Woo, Sibbald, Ayello, Coutts, & Garde, 2009).
- If adherence of the dressing is a concern, clean the area adjacent to the wound with alcohol or acetone, and allow it to dry. **Rationale: Alcohol or acetone defats the skin. Defatted, clean, dry skin ensures better adhesion of the dressing.**
- Remove gloves, and dispose of them in the moisture-proof bag.

4. Clean the wound, if indicated.
   - Put on clean disposable or sterile gloves in accordance with agency practice.
   - Clean the wound with the prescribed solution. Either (a) pour the sterile solution directly on the wound and collect drainage with an emesis basin, or (b) with forceps, use a moist sterile gauze to clean the wound.
   - Dry the surrounding skin with a dry gauze.

5. Assess the wound.
   - See "Assessment" earlier in the procedure.

6. Apply the wound barrier.
   - Some agencies require transparent dressings be dated to ensure timeliness of dressing changes. If this is required, write the date and time of application on the dressing with a ballpoint pen.
   - Remove part of the paper backing on the dressing. If you have an assistant, remove all of the paper backing; the two of you should hold the coloured tabs attached to the dressing.
   - Apply the dressing at one edge of the wound site, allowing at least 2.5 cm coverage of the skin surrounding the wound.
   - Gently lay or press the barrier over the wound. Keep it free of wrinkles, but avoid stretching it too tightly. **Rationale: A stretched dressing restricts mobility.**
   - Cut off the coloured tabs after the wound is completely covered.
   - Remove and dispose of gloves appropriately.

7. Reinforce the dressing only if absolutely needed.
   - Apply paper or other porous tape to the edges of the dressing.

8. Assess the wound area at least daily.
   - Determine the extent of serous fluid accumulation under the dressing, wound healing, and the need to repair the dressing.
   - If excessive serum has accumulated, consider replacing the transparent wound barrier with a more absorbent type of dressing, such as hydrocolloid.
   - If the dressing is leaking, remove it and apply another dressing.

9. Document the procedure and all nursing assessments.

10. To remove the dressing, stretch the product to break the adhesive bond and prevent skin stripping.

EVALUATION

Perform follow-up based on findings in relation to the amount of granulation tissue or degree of healing; amount of serous fluid under dressing; and discomfort associated with wound care.

These dressings should not be used for wounds with copious drainage but are suitable for wounds with small amounts of drainage.

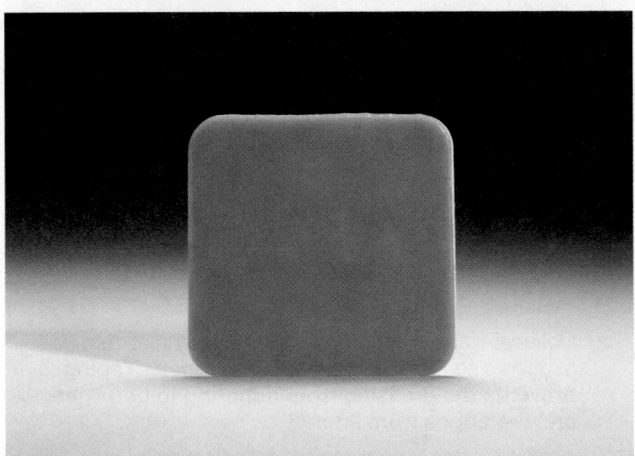

FIGURE 35.13 A hydrocolloid dressing.

REFLECT ON **PRIMARY HEALTH CARE**

Appropriate use of technology in wound care, particularly in the case of chronic wounds, has meant an increase in quality of life for many clients. For example, helping a home care client learn how to use hydrocolloid or hydrogel products can mean a reduction in dressing changes from two or three times a day to once every 1, 2, or even 7 days. This type of intervention also reduces the costs to the health care system. Because the nurse is not spending as much time performing wound care, he or she can address other aspects of the client's health.

These dressings have certain limitations, however:

- Hydrocolloids are occlusive and opaque, and obscure wound visibility.
- They have a limited absorption capacity.
- Hydrocolloids have a characteristic odour that is often mistaken for a sign of wound infection. Clinical judgment must be used in assessing for the presence of an infection.
- They can facilitate anaerobic bacterial growth and they should *not* be used when any type of infection is suspected.
- They can soften and wrinkle at the edges with wear and movement.
- They can be difficult to remove and may leave a residue on the skin.

Skill 35.3 describes how to apply hydrocolloid dressings.

SKILL 35.3 APPLYING A HYDROCOLLOID DRESSING

PURPOSES

- To maintain a moist wound surface and promote healing
- To prevent the entrance of microorganisms into the wound
- To minimize discomfort caused by the wound
- To promote autolysis of necrotic material by white blood cells
- To decrease the frequency of dressing changes

ASSESSMENT

Assess

- Appearance and size of the wound
- Amount and character of exudate
- Complaints of discomfort
- Signs of systemic infection (e.g., elevated body temperature, malaise, leukocytosis)

PLANNING

A hydrocolloid dressing should be changed whenever it becomes dislodged, leaks, or develops an odour. If the wound has substantial drainage or yellow slough, the dressing may need to be changed every 24 to 72 hours. When drainage subsides, the dressing can be left in place for 3 to 7 days. The procedure may be clean or sterile depending on agency policy.

Equipment

- Clean disposable gloves
- Moisture-proof bag

(continued)

SKILL 35.3 **APPLYING A HYDROCOLLOID DRESSING (*continued*)**

- Dressing set
- Sterile normal saline or other cleaning agent used by the agency
- Sterile gloves (optional)
- Hydrocolloid dressing at least 2.5 cm to 5 cm larger than wound on all four sides
- Paper tape

IMPLEMENTATION

Performance

1. Before performing the procedure, introduce yourself and verify the client's identity using two identifiers or per agency protocol. Explain to the client what you are going to do, why it is necessary, and how he or she can participate. Discuss how the results will be used in planning further care or treatments.

2. Perform hand hygiene, and follow other appropriate infection prevention and control procedures.

3. Remove the old dressing.
   - Put on disposable gloves.
   - Pull the dressing off gradually in the direction of hair growth. **Rationale: Doing this minimizes skin irritation**.
   - Dispose of the soiled dressing in the moisture-proof bag.

4. Clean the skin area around the wound.
   - Gently wash the skin surrounding the wound with a mild cleansing agent or with normal saline, and dry it thoroughly with gauze squares.
   - Leave the residue that is difficult to remove on the skin. It will wear off in time. **Rationale: Attempts to remove residue can irritate the surrounding skin**.

- Remove gloves and dispose of them in the moisture-proof bag.

5. Clean the wound, if indicated.
   - Open the sterile dressing supplies.
   - Pour saline or other cleaning agent into the sterile container.
   - Put on disposable or sterile gloves in accordance with agency protocol.
   - With forceps, clean the wound with the prescribed solution.

6. Assess the wound.
   - Observe the appearance and the size of the wound and the amount and character of exudate.
   - Determine presence of pain.

7. Apply the dressing.
   - Follow the manufacturer's instructions.
   - Remove and dispose of the gloves.
   - *Optional*: Tape all four sides of the dressing as required or according to agency protocol. **Rationale: Taping prevents the dressing from adhering to bed linens and the edges from lifting**.

8. Assess and change the dressing, as indicated.
   - Inspect the dressing at least daily for leakage, dislodgement, odour, and wrinkling.
   - Change the dressing if any of these signs are present.

9. Document the technique and all nursing assessments.

EVALUATION

Perform follow-up based on findings in relation to the amount of granulation tissue or degree of healing; amount of serous fluid under dressing; and discomfort associated with wound care.

SECURING DRESSINGS The nurse tapes the dressing over the wound, ensuring that it covers the entire wound and does not become dislodged. The correct type of tape should be selected and, ideally, the ends of the tape should be folded over slightly in advance of securing to aid ease of removal. Elastic tape can provide pressure; hypoallergenic tape is used when a client is allergic to other tape. The nurse follows these steps:

1. Place the tape so that the dressing cannot be folded back to expose the wound. Place strips at the ends of the dressing, and space tapes evenly in the middle.

2. Ensure that the tape is long and wide enough to adhere to several centimetres of skin on each side of the dressing, but not so long or wide that the tape loosens with activity (Figure 35.14).

3. Place the tape in the opposite direction from the body action, for example, across a body joint or crease, not lengthwise (Figure 35.15).

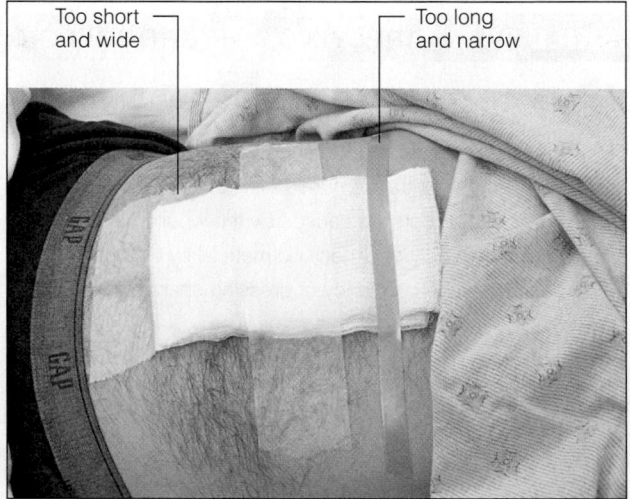

Too short and wide — Too long and narrow

FIGURE 35.14 The strips of tape should be placed at the ends of the dressing and must be sufficiently long and wide to secure the dressing. The tape should adhere to intact skin.

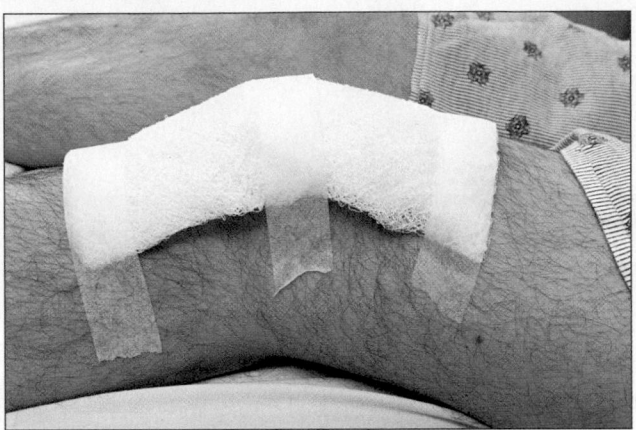

FIGURE 35.15 Dressings over moving parts must remain secure in spite of the movement. Place the tape over a joint at a right angle to the direction the joint moves.

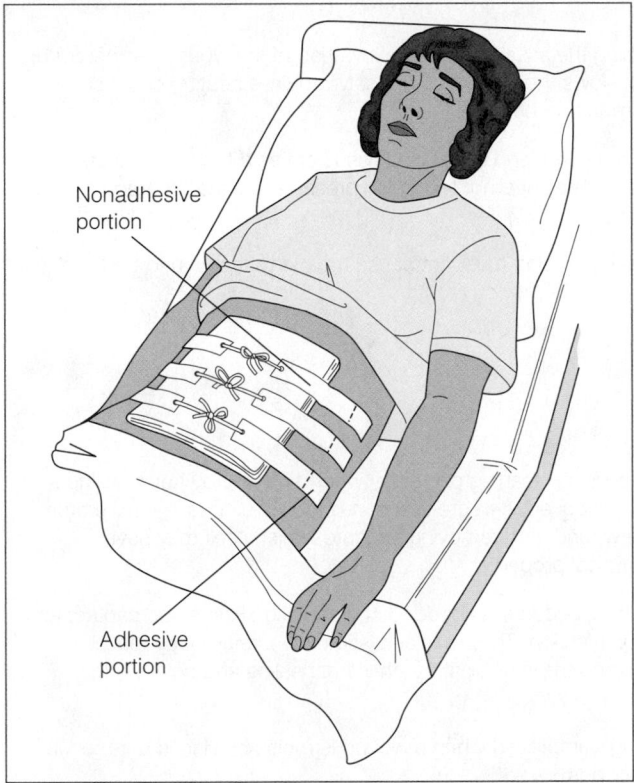

Nonadhesive portion

Adhesive portion

FIGURE 35.16 Montgomery straps, or tie tapes, are used to secure large dressings that require frequent changing.

Montgomery straps (*tie tapes*) are commonly used for wounds requiring frequent dressing changes (Figure 35.16). These straps prevent skin irritation and the discomfort caused by removing the adhesive each time the dressing is changed.

Medical tapes can cause injuries if used incorrectly. Blisters will form when too much tension is applied while placing the tape, when edema has collected after the tape was placed, and when alcohol or benzoic-based prep solutions are used under the tape. Medical tape manufacturers issue safety guidelines for specific tape products.

Before using medical tapes read the safety guidelines for indications of use and safe application and removal.

Cleansing Wounds

Wound cleansing is a critical aspect of wound management and forms the basis for good healing. Wound cleansing involves removing debris, such as foreign materials, excess slough, necrotic tissue, bacteria, and other microorganisms. A goal of routine wound cleansing is to minimize chemical and mechanical trauma while providing a clean wound bed. In the past, antimicrobial agents, such as povidone-iodine (Betadine), hydrogen peroxide, alcohol, and Dakin's solution were commonly used to cleanse wounds; however, they are now recognized to be cytotoxic. The choices of cleansing solution and method depend largely on the nature of the wound and agency protocol. See Practice Guidelines 35.2 on the next page for cleansing wounds.

The major principle of wound cleansing is moving from an area of least contamination to an area of most contamination (clean to dirty). Depending on the wound, these areas are sometimes difficult to distinguish.

Commonly used methods to clean a surgical wound and drain site are outlined in Chapter 36.

WOUND IRRIGATION AND PACKING Preparing the wound bed for healing is an essential component of any wound management strategy. The goal of preparation is to optimize the wound bed to ensure unimpeded tissue repair and regeneration (Sibbald, Mahoney, & the V.A.C. Therapy Canadian Consensus Group, 2003). The wound bed preparation paradigm advocated by the Canadian Association of Wound Care (2006) urges clinicians to first address patient-centred concerns and the etiology of the wound before tackling local wound healing strategies.

Irrigation (lavage) is the washing or flushing out of an area. It is a means of cleansing the wound. Sterile technique is required for wound irrigation because there is a break in the skin integrity.

The use of piston syringes instead of bulb syringes to irrigate a wound reduces the risk of aspirating drainage and provides safe, effective pressure. For deep wounds with small openings, a sterile straight catheter may also be necessary. Irrigation pressures should range from 4 psi to 8 psi (pounds per square inch). Below 4 psi, the irrigation may not be effective, and above 8 psi it may damage tissues. A 30- to 60-mL syringe with a #18-gauge or #19-gauge needle or catheter provides approximately 8 psi (Moreira & Markovchick, 2007). Some providers advocate the use of a commercial oral water jet for wound cleansing. This device can be effective if kept at the lowest setting that provides the desired pressure. There is no good trial evidence to support use of any particular wound cleansing solution (Moore & Cowman, 2005). Frequently used irrigation solutions are sterile normal saline, lactated Ringer's solution, and antibiotic solutions.

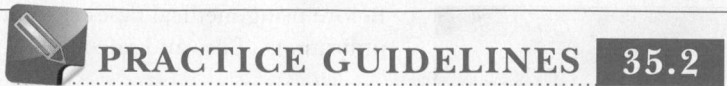

PRACTICE GUIDELINES 35.2

Cleansing Wounds

Guidelines	Rationale
Follow routine practices and additional precautions for personal protection, wear gloves, gown, goggles, and mask, as indicated.	The patient and the health care practitioner both require protection from pathogens.
Use solutions, such as isotonic saline or lactated Ringer's solution, to clean or irrigate wounds. Commercial wound cleansers often contain surfactants that help remove debris and may be useful in some circumstances.	Use of physiological solutions will ensure that there are no fluid shifts caused by osmotic gradients.
Do not use skin cleansers or antiseptic agents (e.g., povidone-iodine, iodophor, sodium hypochlorite [Dakin's] solution, hydrogen peroxide, acetic acid) to clean wounds (RNAO, 2007).	These agents are cytotoxic.
When possible, warm the solution to body temperature just before use. Microwave heating is not recommended.	Warming the solution prevents lowering of the wound temperature, which slows the healing process. Microwave heating could cause the solution to become too hot.
Cleanse wounds at each dressing change. To reduce surface bacteria and tissue trauma, the wound should be gently irrigated with 100 mL of solution (RNAO, 2007).	Foreign bodies and devitalized tissue act as a focus for infection and can delay healing; too much pressure can lead to trauma.
Use sufficient irrigation pressure to enhance wound cleansing. Effective and safe ulcer irrigation pressure ranges from 4 psi to 8 psi (pounds per square inch). Pressures in this range can be generated by using either (a) a 30- to 60-mL syringe with a #18- or #19-gauge angiocath or (b) a single-use 100-mL squeeze bottle (Moreira & Markovchick, 2007).	Wound cleansing must not cause trauma to the wound bed.
If a wound is clean, has little exudate, and reveals healthy granulation tissue, avoid repeated cleaning.	Unnecessary cleaning can delay wound healing by traumatizing newly produced, delicate tissue, reducing the surface temperature of the wound, and removing exudate, which itself may have bactericidal properties.
Use gauze squares. Avoid using cotton balls and other products that shed fibres onto the wound surface.	The fibres become embedded in granulation tissue and can act as foci for infection. They may also stimulate foreign body reactions, prolonging the inflammatory phase of healing and delaying the healing process.
Avoid drying a wound after cleansing it. Dry the skin around the wound only.	Healing is improved when a wound is moist; healing is deterred in dry wounds.
Clean the wound in an outward direction.	Cleaning in this direction avoids transferring organisms from the surrounding skin into the wound.

Skill 35.4 details the steps involved in irrigating a wound. See also the Evidence-Informed box, the Lifespan Considerations box, and the Home Care Considerations box on dressings and wound on pages 1038–1039.

Gauze packing by using the wet-to-damp technique has been used to pack wounds that require debridement, however, newer advanced dressing materials have significant advantages over the use of gauze. Box 35.8 on page 1039 summarizes issues related to using damp gauze versus advanced dressings.

Adjunctive Therapies

Many of the techniques described here for dressing and cleansing wounds can be combined, depending on the specific type of wound. In addition, a number of

SKILL 35.4 IRRIGATING A WOUND

PURPOSES

- To clean the area
- To apply heat and hasten the healing process
- To apply an antimicrobial solution

ASSESSMENT

Assess

- Previous appearance and size of the wound
- Character of the exudate
- Presence of pain and the time of the last analgesia
- Clinical signs of systemic infection
- Allergies to the wound irrigation agent or tape

PLANNING

- Before irrigating a wound, determine (a) the type of irrigating solution to be used, (b) the frequency of irrigations, and (c) the temperature of the solution.
- If possible, schedule the irrigation at a time convenient for the client. Some irrigations require only a few minutes and others can take much longer.

Equipment

- Sterile dressing equipment and dressing materials
- Sterile irrigating syringe (e.g., a 30-mL to 60-mL syringe) with a catheter of an appropriate size (#18 or #19 gauge) or an irrigating (catheter) tip or a 100-mL squeezable bottle with irrigating tip
- Sterile graduated container for the irrigating solution
- Moisture-proof bag
- Irrigating solution, usually 100 mL to 150 mL of solution, warmed to body temperature, according to agency policy
- Goggles, gown, and mask
- Clean gloves
- Sterile gloves
- Waterproof pad(s)

Although a wound may already be contaminated, sterile equipment is usually used during irrigation to prevent the possibility of adding new nonresident microorganisms to the site. In settings outside of hospitals, some reusable supplies, such as irrigating syringes or basins, may be cleaned and used again for a specific wound.

IMPLEMENTATION

Performance

1. Before performing the procedure, introduce yourself and verify the client's identity using two identifiers or per agency protocol. Explain to the client what you are going to do, why it is necessary, and how he or she can participate. Discuss how the results will be used in planning further care or treatments.

2. Perform hand hygiene, and follow other appropriate infection prevention and control procedures (e.g., goggles).

3. Provide for client privacy.

4. Prepare the client.

- Assist the client to a position in which the irrigating solution will flow by gravity from the upper end of the wound to the lower end and then into the basin.
- Place the waterproof pad(s) under the client below the area where you will be irrigating (see ❶).
- Put on clean gloves, and remove and discard the old dressing.
- If indicated, clean the wound from the cleanest area to the least clean. If the wound is circular, this would be from the centre of the wound outward. For a linear wound, cleanse from top to bottom, beginning in the middle and moving progressively laterally (see ❷).

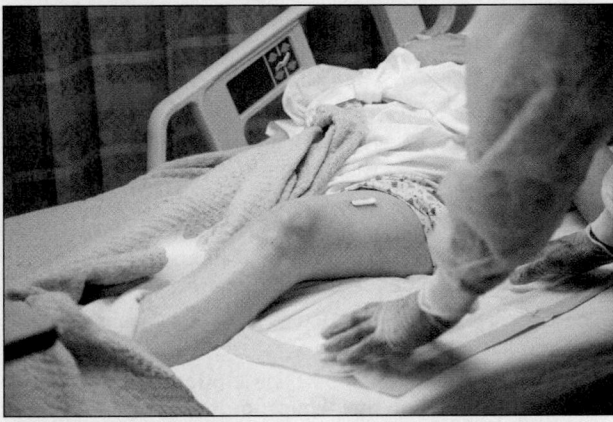

❶ Placing the waterproof pad under the client prior to wound care.

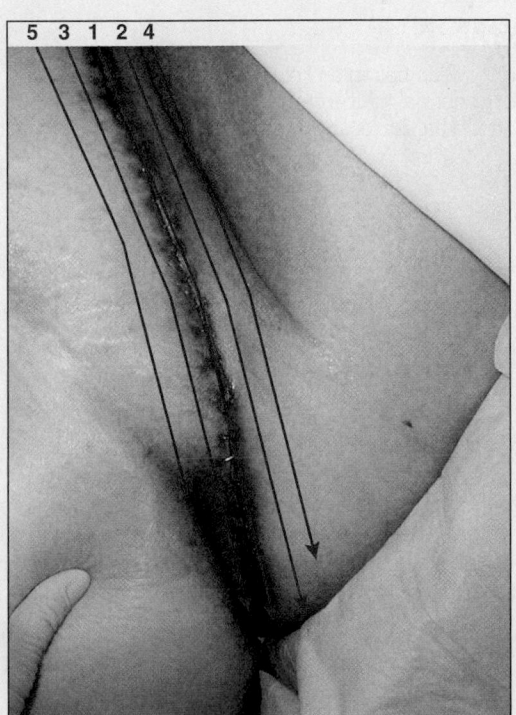

❷ Cleaning a wound from the midpoint outward and from top to bottom.

Source: Courtesy of Cory Patrick Hartley, San Ramon Regional Medical Center, San Ramon, CA.

(continued)

SKILL 35.4 IRRIGATING A WOUND (continued)

- Use a separate swab for each stroke, and discard each swab after use. **Rationale: Doing this prevents the introduction of microorganisms to other wound areas.**
- Assess the wound and drainage.
- Remove and discard gloves.

5. Prepare the equipment.
   - Open the sterile dressing set and supplies.
   - Pour the ordered solution into the solution container.
   - Position the basin below the wound to receive the irrigating fluid.
   - Put on sterile gloves

6. Irrigate the wound.
   - Instill a steady stream of irrigating solution into the wound. Make sure all areas of the wound are irrigated.
   - Use either a syringe with a catheter attached or with an irrigating tip to flush the wound (see), or a 100-mL squeezable bottle with irrigating tip.
   - If you are using a catheter to reach tracks or crevices, insert the catheter into the wound until resistance is met. Do not force the catheter. **Rationale: Forcing the catheter can cause tissue damage.**
   - Continue irrigating until the solution becomes clear (no exudate is present).
   - Dry the area around the wound. **Rationale: Moisture left on the skin promotes the growth of microorganisms and can cause skin irritation and breakdown.**

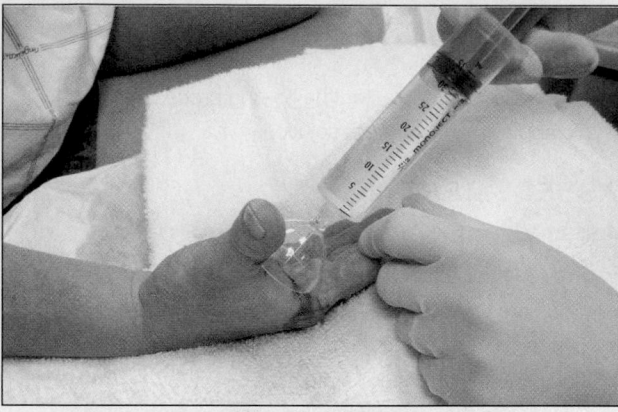

3 Irrigating an open wound

7. Assess and dress the wound.
   - Assess the appearance of the wound again, noting in particular the type and amount of exudate still present and the presence and extent of granulation tissue.
   - Using sterile technique, apply a dressing to the wound based on the amount of drainage expected (see Table 35.4 on page 1027).

8. Document the irrigation and the client's response in the client record by using forms or checklists supplemented by narrative notes when appropriate. Many agencies use a designated wound and skin documentation sheet (see Figure 35.7 on page 1020).

EVALUATION

- Perform follow-up based on findings that deviate from expected or normal for the client. Relate findings to previous assessment data, if available.

- Report significant deviations from normal to the appropriate health care team members.

EVIDENCE-INFORMED PRACTICE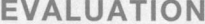

What Types of Dressings Protect against the Development of Pressure Ulcers?

The authors of this protocol will conduct a systematic review to "evaluate the effects of dressings and topical agents on the prevention of pressure ulcers, in people of any age without existing pressure ulcers, but considered to be at risk of developing a pressure ulcer, in any care setting." While several types of dressings such as semipermeable film dressings, hydrocolloid dressings, and foam dressings have been used for years with the goal of preventing pressure ulcers, there has not been a rigorous analysis of the effectiveness of these dressings nor the populations of "at-risk" clients for whom they are best suited.

NURSING IMPLICATIONS: Preventing pressure ulcers is of utmost importance so as to ensure quality of life for the client and avoid immense costs associated with a pressure ulcer. Age-old interventions must be assessed to ensure that they remain relevant.

Source: Based on Moore Z. E. H., & Webster J. (2011). Dressings and topical agents for preventing pressure ulcers (Protocol). *Cochrane Database of Systematic Reviews,* Issue 10. Art. No.: CD009362. doi: 10.1002/14651858.CD009362

LIFESPAN CONSIDERATIONS

Pressure Ulcer and Wound Care

INFANTS

- The skin of infants is more fragile than that of older children and adults, and it is more susceptible to infection, shear, and burns.

CHILDREN

- *Staphylococcus* and fungus are two major infectious agents affecting the skin of children. Abrasions or small lacerations, commonly experienced by children, provide an entry in the skin for these organisms. Minor wounds should be cleansed with warm, soapy water, and covered with a sterile bandage. Children should be instructed not to touch the wound.

- With more serious skin lesions, remind the child not to touch the wound, drains, or dressing. Cover with an appropriate bandage that will remain intact during the child's usual activities. Cover a transparent dressing with opaque material if viewing the site is distressing to the child. Restrain only when all alternatives have been tried and when absolutely necessary.

- For younger children, demonstrate wound care on a doll. Reassure that the wound will not be permanent and that nothing will fall out of the body.

OLDER ADULTS

- Hold wrinkled skin taut during application of a transparent dressing. Obtain assistance, if needed.

- Skin is more fragile and can easily tear with removal of tape (especially adhesive tape). Use paper tape and tape remover as indicated, keeping tape use to the minimum required. Use extreme caution during tape removal.

- Older adults who are in long-term care facilities often have immobility, malnutrition, and incontinence, all of which increase the risk for development of skin breakdown.

- Skin breakdown can occur as quickly as within 2 hours, so assessments should be done with each repositioning of the client.

- A thorough assessment of a client's heels should be done every shift. The skin can break down quickly from friction of movement in bed.

HOME CARE CONSIDERATIONS

Wound Care

- Perform appropriate client teaching for promoting wound healing and maintenance of healthy skin.

- Instruct family about hygiene and asepsis; hand hygiene before and after dressing changes; and the use of a clean area for storage of dressing supplies.

- Instruct the client and family on where to obtain needed supplies.

- Be sensitive to the cost of dressings (e.g., transparent barriers are costly), and suggest less expensive alternatives, if necessary. Be creative in the use of household items for padding pressure areas.

- Instruct the client and family in proper disposal of contaminated dressings. All contaminated items should be double bagged in moisture-proof bags.

- Verify how the client can bathe with the wound (i.e., does the wound need to be covered with a waterproof barrier, or should it be cleansed in the shower?).

- Potable tap water can be used to cleanse wounds instead; in the absence of potable tap water, boiled and cooled water as well as distilled water can be used as wound cleansing agents (Fernandez & Griffiths, 2008).

BOX 35.8 ISSUES RELATED TO THE USE OF DAMP GAUZE VERSUS ADVANCED DRESSINGS

The nurse should be aware of the following issues in choosing a wound dressing:

- To keep the gauze damp, change or remoisten with saline frequently. *If the gauze is allowed to dry out, removal results in pain and disruption of wound healing through drying of the surface and tissue adherence to the gauze.*

- A wound requires moisture and warmth for optimal healing. Evaporation of the saline causes wound cooling, vasoconstriction, and dehydration.

- Moistened gauze cannot prevent introduction of bacteria into the wound.

- Although gauze is less expensive than advanced dressings (e.g., polymers, alginates, collagens), the cost per week can be higher because of the number of dressing changes required. Including the price of the dressing, gloves, saline, and tape, the materials cost for a gauze dressing change twice per day versus an advanced dressing three times per week is very similar. However, when taking into account the cost per nurse home visit, the gauze dressing is almost five times as expensive.

- Wounds have been shown to heal twice as quickly with advanced dressings compared with gauze.

- *Conclusions:* Nurses should become familiar with the range and uses of advanced dressing materials. The selection of material must consider time, material cost, client comfort, and speed of wound healing.

adjunctive therapies can be used to facilitate wound healing. Electrical stimulation, therapeutic ultrasound, ultraviolet light, pulsed electromagnetic fields, and surgery may be helpful for some clients.

Vacuum-assisted closure (**VAC**) is a commonly used adjunctive therapy that employs negative pressure (vacuum) to remove fluid from difficult-to-heal wounds (World Union of Wound Healing Societies [WUWHS], 2008). The fluid passes through a sealed dressing and tubing connected to a collection container (see Figure 35.17). According to WUWHS (2008), the objectives of VAC are to achieve the following:

- Remove exudate and reduce periwound edema
- Increase local microvascular blood flow or test vascularity
- Promote formation of granulation tissue
- Reduce complexity or size of the wound
- Optimize the wound bed prior to and following surgery
- Reduce complexity of surgical wound closure procedures

To implement VAC therapy, it is important for the wound to have been thoroughly debrided, to be free of active untreated infection (e.g., cellulitis), and to not involve fistulae to internal organs or cavities.

A number of factors increase the likelihood of success. These are described in Table 35.5.

VAC dressings are changed three times per week or when the seal has broken. VAC removes exudate to help optimize fluid balance. VAC is not usually initiated until the more conventional treatments, such as dressings,

have proven ineffective because of the significant financial costs and the mobility limitations imposed on the client by the VAC equipment. Contraindications to the use of VAC include intracutaneous fistulae, necrotic tissue, untreated ostemyelitis, and malignancy (WUWHS, 2008).

Supporting and Immobilizing Wounds

Bandages and binders serve various purposes:

- Supporting a wound (e.g., a fractured bone)
- Immobilizing a wound (e.g., a strained shoulder)
- Applying pressure (e.g., elastic bandages on the lower extremities to improve venous blood flow)
- Securing a dressing (e.g., for an extensive abdominal surgical wound)
- Retaining warmth (e.g., a flannel bandage on a rheumatoid joint)

Practitioners should become familiar with the range and uses of advanced dressing materials. The selection of dressing materials must consider time, material cost, client comfort, and speed of wound healing.

Bandages and binders come in several different types and have several ways in which they are applied. When correctly applied, they promote healing, provide comfort, and prevent injury.

BANDAGES A **bandage** is a strip of cloth used to wrap some part of the body. Bandages are available in various widths, most commonly 1.5 cm to 7.5 cm, and are usually supplied in rolls for easy application to a body part.

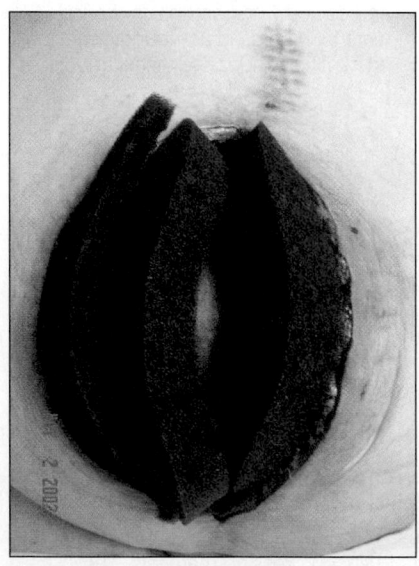
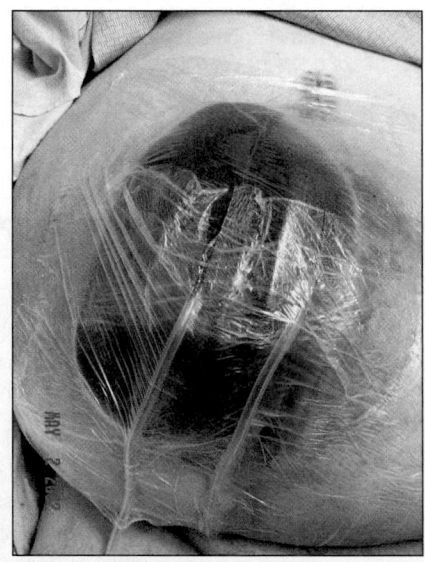
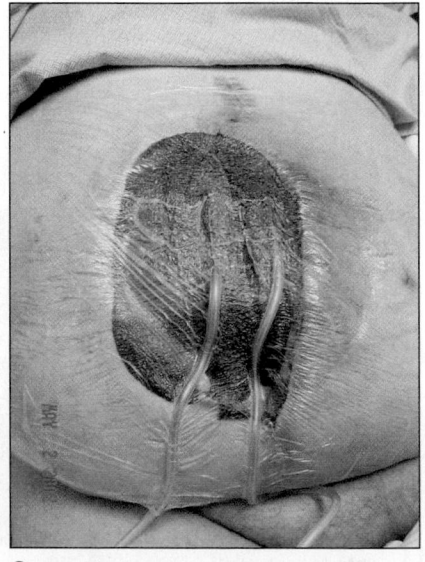

A   B   C

FIGURE 35.17 Vacuum-assisted closure system for wounds. **A:** Foam strips laid into the wound; **B:** Occlusive draping applied and suction tubing in place; **C:** Finished dressing with negative pressure (suction) applied.
Note: the suction tubing is attached to a suction unit (not shown).

TABLE 35.5 Factors That May Increase Success of Therapy

Wound Factors	Client Factors
Wound has good blood supply.	Client has been maximally medically stabilized (e.g., nutrition, blood pressure, blood glucose, fluid balance, infection).
Wound has healthy, granular bed.	Client has few or well-controlled comorbidities.
Wound has been freshly debrided (as recommended*).	Client is comfortable (e.g., not in pain).
Wound produces high levels of exudate.	Client is adherent to therapy.
Wound is wider than 2 cm.	

*Note: Occasionally, in some chronic wounds, surgical debridement may not be appropriate. Prior to starting VAC therapy, it is important to ensure that the wound has a clean wound bed and that it does not contain necrotic tissue or excessive debris.

Source: Based on World Union of Wound Healing Societies (WUWHS). *Principles of best practice: Vacuum assisted closure: recommendations for use. A consensus document.* London: MEP Ltd, 2008. Page 1.

Many types of materials are used for bandages. Gauze is one of the most commonly used; it is light and porous and readily moulds to the body. It is also relatively inexpensive, so it is generally discarded when soiled. Gauze is frequently used to retain dressings on wounds and to bandage the fingers, hands, toes, and feet. It supports dressings and, at the same time, permits air to circulate; it can also be impregnated with gels or other medications for application to wounds.

Many kinds of elasticized bandages are applied to provide pressure to an area. They are commonly used as tensor bandages or as partial stockings to provide support and improve the venous circulation in the legs.

The width of the bandage used depends on the size of the body part to be bandaged. For example, a 2.5-cm bandage is used for a finger, a 5-cm bandage for an arm, and a 7.5-cm or 10-cm bandage for a leg. The larger the circumference of a part, the wider the bandage. Padding (e.g., abdominal pads and gauze squares) is frequently used to cover bony prominences (e.g., the elbow) or to separate skin surfaces (e.g., the fingers).

Compression bandaging is widely used for management of venous leg ulcers. Compression bandaging speeds up the healing process by (a) reducing hypertension in the superficial veins; (b) improving venous return by increasing flow velocity in the deep veins; (c) reducing leg edema; and (d) accelerating blood flow in the microcirculation, reducing tissue fibrosis and subsequent lipodermatosclerosis (Smith & Nephew, 2006). There are several types of compression bandaging, but most used is the knee graduate multilayer compression bandage (Figure 35.18), which delivers the highest pressure at the

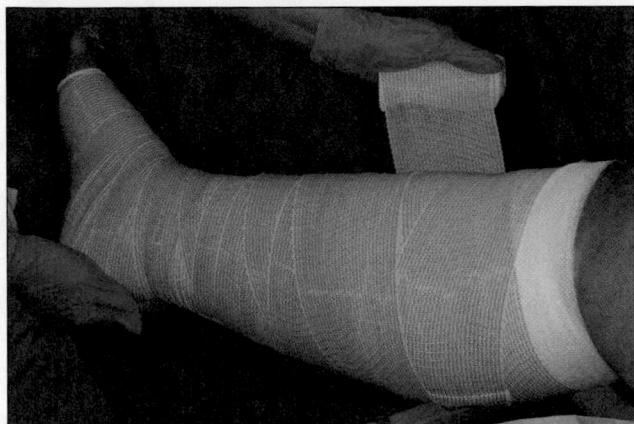

FIGURE 35.18 A compression bandage.

ankle and gaiter area, which is gradually reduced towards the knee (Smith & Nephew, 2006).

When applying a bandage, the nurse needs to know its purpose and assess the area requiring support (see Practice Guidelines 35.3 on the next page).

Basic Turns for Roller Bandages Applying bandages to various parts of the body involves one or more of five basic bandaging turns: circular, spiral, spiral reverse, recurrent, and figure of eight. *Circular turns* are used to anchor bandages and to terminate them. Circular turns usually are not applied directly over a wound because of the discomfort the bandage would cause.

Spiral turns are used to bandage parts of the body that are fairly uniform in circumference, for example, the upper arm or upper leg. *Spiral reverse turns* are used to bandage cylindrical parts of the body that are not uniform in circumference, for example, the lower leg or forearm. *Recurrent turns* are used to cover distal parts of the body, for example, the end of a finger, the skull, or the stump of an amputation. *Figure-of-eight turns* are used to bandage an elbow, knee, or ankle, because they permit some movement after application.

Circular Turns

- Hold the bandage in your dominant hand, keeping the roll uppermost, and unroll the bandage about 8 cm. This length of unrolled bandage allows good control for placement and tension.

- Apply the end of the bandage to the part of the body to be bandaged. Hold the end down with the thumb of the other hand (Figure 35.19).

- Encircle the body part a few times, or as often as needed, making sure that each layer overlaps one-half to two-thirds of the previous layer. This provides even support to the area.

- The bandage should be firm, but not too tight. Ask the client if the bandage feels comfortable. A tight bandage can interfere with blood circulation,

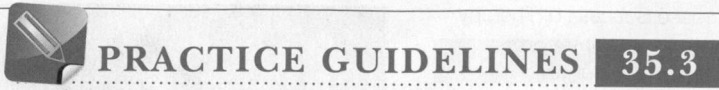

PRACTICE GUIDELINES 35.3

Bandaging

Guidelines	Rationales
Wear gloves when bandages are used to secure dressings.	Gloves help prevent contact with body fluids.
Assess the area to be bandaged thoroughly for colour, presence of drainage, nature of the wound (if present); document observations.	Baseline data will guide subsequent assessments and provide a basis for selection of appropriate bandaging material.
Whenever possible, bandage the part in its normal position, with the joint slightly flexed.	The use of this position avoids putting strain on the ligaments and the muscles of the joint.
Pad between skin surfaces and over bony prominences.	Pads prevent friction from the bandage and consequent abrasion of the skin.
Always bandage body parts by working from the distal end to the proximal end.	This method aids the return flow of venous blood.
Bandage with even pressure.	Even pressure prevents interference with blood circulation.
Whenever possible, leave the end of the body part (e.g., the toes) exposed.	This exposure allows for the adequacy of the blood circulation to the extremity to be determined.
Cover dressings with bandages at least 5 cm beyond the edges of the dressing.	This covering prevents the dressing and wound from becoming contaminated.
Face the client when applying a bandage.	This position maintains uniform tension and the appropriate direction of the bandage.
Inspect and palpate for adequacy of circulation distal to the bandage, that is, assess skin temperature, blanching (capillary refill), peripheral pulses, colour, and sensation. Ask the client about any numbness, tingling, or pain.	Pale or cyanotic skin, cool temperature, pain, tingling, and numbness could indicate impaired circulation from either a bandage that is too restrictive (tight) or edema under the bandage.

whereas a loose bandage does not provide adequate protection.

- Secure the end of the bandage with tape or clips if there is no Velcro fastener.

Spiral Turns

- Make two circular turns. Two circular turns anchor the bandage.

- Continue spiral turns at about a 30-degree angle, each turn overlapping the preceding one by two-thirds the width of the bandage (Figure 35.20).

- Terminate the bandage with two circular turns, and secure the end of the bandage with tape or a safety pin over an uninjured area.

Spiral Reverse Turns

- Anchor the bandage with two circular turns, and bring the bandage upward at about a 30-degree angle.

- Place the thumb of your free hand on the upper edge of the bandage (Figure 35.21A). The thumb will hold the bandage while it is folded on itself.

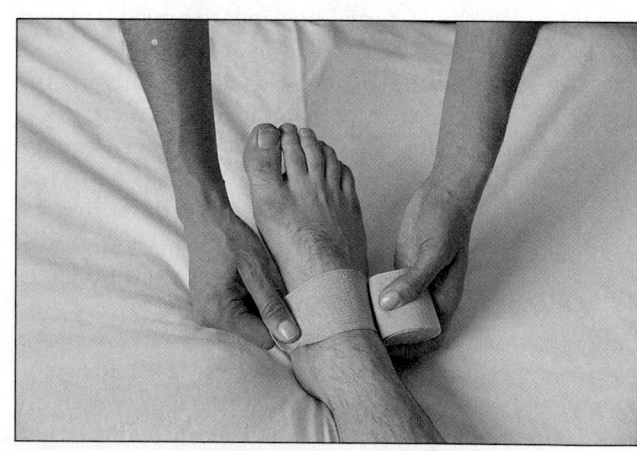

FIGURE 35.19 Starting a bandage with two circular turns.

- Unroll the bandage about 15 cm, and then turn your hand so that the bandage falls over itself (see Figure 35.21B).

- Continue the bandage around the limb, overlapping each previous turn by two-thirds the width of the bandage. Make each bandage turn at the same position

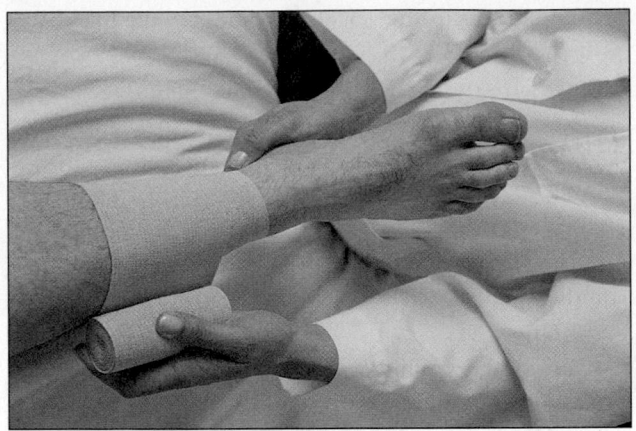

FIGURE 35.20 Applying spiral turns.

on the limb so that the turns of the bandage will be aligned (see Figure 35.21C).

- Terminate the bandage with two circular turns, and secure the end of the bandage with tape or a safety pin over an uninjured area.

Recurrent Turns

- Anchor the bandage with two circular turns.
- Fold the bandage back on itself, and bring it centrally over the distal end to be bandaged (Figure 35.22).
- Holding it with the other hand, bring the bandage back over the end to the right of the centre bandage but overlapping it by two-thirds the width of the bandage.
- Bring the bandage back on the left side, also overlapping the first turn by two-thirds the width of the bandage.
- Continue this pattern of alternating right and left until the area is covered. Overlap the preceding turn by two-thirds the bandage width each time.
- Terminate the bandage with two circular turns (Figure 35.23). Secure the end appropriately.

Figure-of-Eight Turns

- Anchor the bandage with two circular turns.

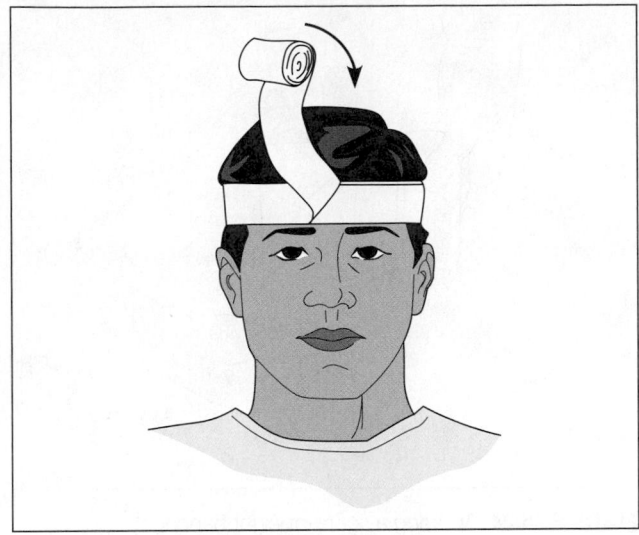

FIGURE 35.22 Starting a recurrent bandage.

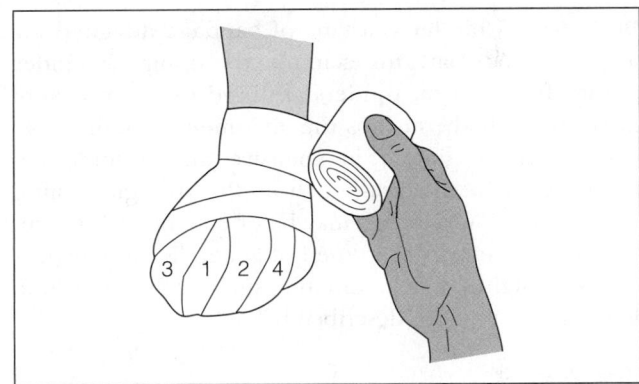

FIGURE 35.23 Completing a recurrent bandage.

- Carry the bandage above the joint, around it, and then below it, making a figure of eight (Figure 35.24 on the next page).
- Continue above and below the joint, overlapping the previous turn by two-thirds the width of the bandage.
- Terminate the bandage above the joint with two circular turns, and then secure the end with tape or a safety pin over an uninjured area.

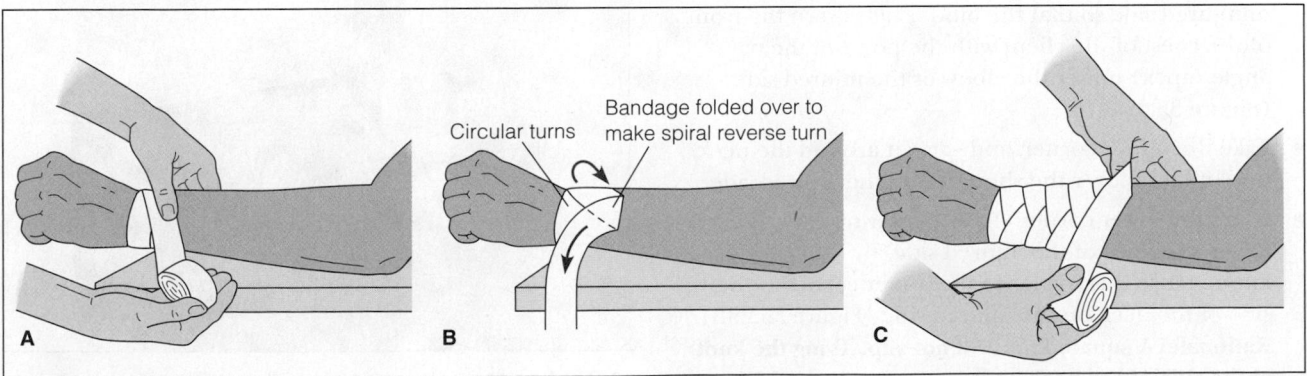

Circular turns

Bandage folded over to make spiral reverse turn

A   B   C

FIGURE 35.21 Applying spiral reverse turns.

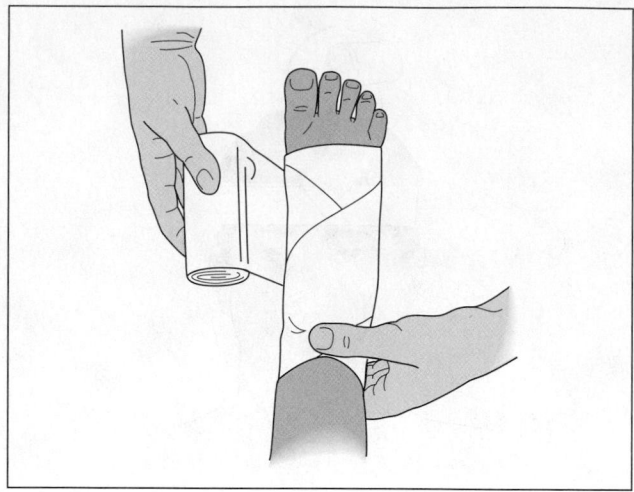

FIGURE 35.24 Applying a figure-of-eight bandage.

BINDERS A binder is a type of bandage designed for a specific body part, for example, the triangular binder (sling) fits the arm. Binders are used to support large areas of the body, such as the abdomen, arm, or chest. Binders can be simple, inexpensive, and customizable by using plain material, such as the triangular sling described below. Or they may be of commercial design, which are often easier to use but generally more expensive and slightly less modifiable, such as the hook-and-loop (Velcro) binder described below.

Arm Sling

- Ask the client to flex the elbow to an 80-degree angle or less, depending on the purpose. The thumb should be facing upward or inward toward the body. **Rationale: An 80-degree angle is sufficient to support the forearm, to prevent swelling of the hand, and to relieve pressure on the shoulder joint (e.g., to support the paralyzed arm of a stroke client whose shoulder might otherwise become dislocated).** A more acute angle is preferred if there is swelling of the hand.

- If a triangle sling is used, place one end of the unfolded triangular binder over the shoulder of the uninjured side so that the binder falls down the front of the chest of the client with the point of the triangle (apex) under the elbow of the injured side (Figure 35.25A).

- Take the upper corner, and carry it around the neck until it hangs over the shoulder on the injured side.

- Bring the lower corner of the binder up over the arm to the shoulder of the injured side. By using a square knot, secure this corner to the upper corner at the side of the neck on the injured side (Figure 35.25B). **Rationale: A square knot will not slip. Tying the knot at the side of the neck prevents pressure on the bony**

prominences of the vertebral column at the back of the neck.

- Make sure the wrist is supported, to maintain alignment.

- Fold the sling neatly at the elbow, and secure it with safety pins or tape. It may be folded and fastened at the front (see Figure 35.25B).

- Remove the sling periodically to inspect the skin for indications of irritation, especially around the site of the knot.

- If a commercial sling is used, it may also include a second strap that goes around the back of the client's chest from the finger end of the sling to the elbow (Figure 35.26). Make sure the wrist is supported, to maintain alignment, and remove the sling periodically to inspect for indications of irritation, especially around the site of the knot.

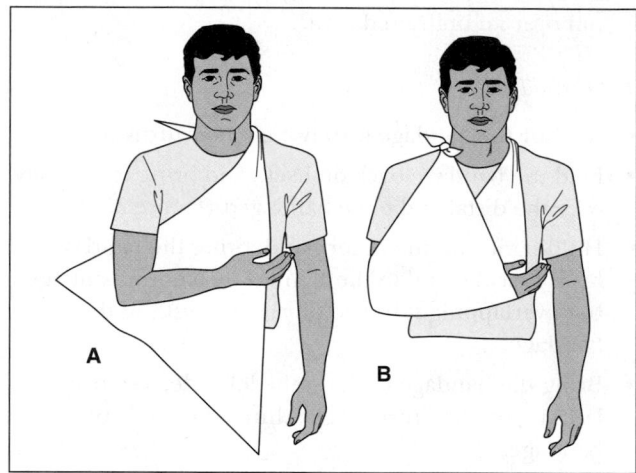

FIGURE 35.25 Large arm sling.

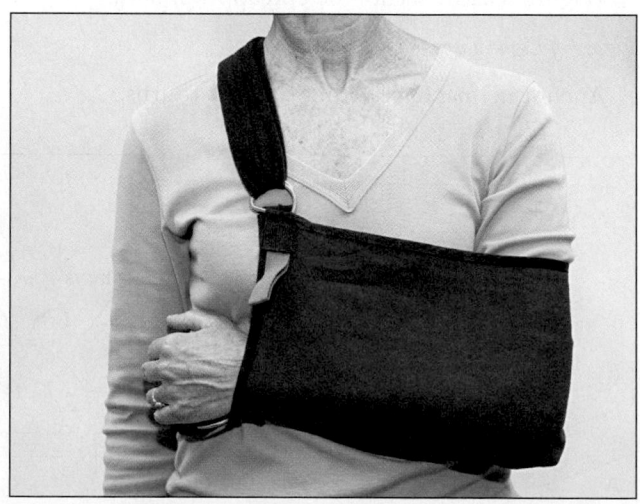

FIGURE 35.26 A commercial arm sling.

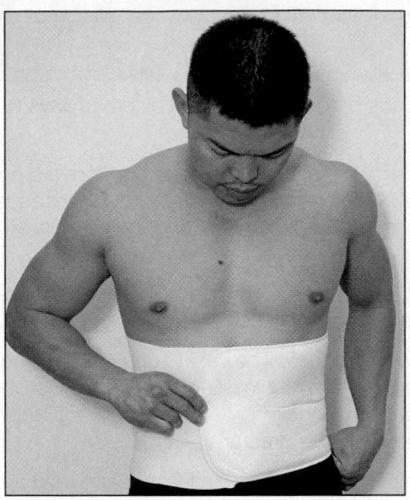

FIGURE 35.27 A straight abdominal binder.

Straight Abdominal Binder

- With the client in a supine position, place the binder smoothly under the body, with the upper border of the binder at the waist and the lower border at the level of the gluteal fold. **Rationale: A binder placed over the waist interferes with respiration; one placed too low interferes with elimination and walking.**
- Apply padding over the iliac crests if the client is thin.
- Bring the ends around the client, overlap them, and secure them with pins or Velcro (Figure 35.27). Place the top pin horizontally at the waist to allow for comfort when moving.

See the Lifespan Considerations box for guidelines on applying bandages and binders to children and older adults, and the Home Care Considerations box for information that clients will need when discharged with a bandage or binder.

Applying Bandages and Binders

Children and older adults need special considerations when the nurse is applying a bandage or binder:

CHILDREN

- Allow the child to help with the procedure by holding supplies, opening boxes, counting turns, and so on.
- If a young client is apprehensive, demonstrate the procedure on a doll or stuffed animal toy.
- Encourage the child to decorate the bandage.
- Teach the caregivers to apply bandages and binders safely.

OLDER ADULTS

- Older clients may need extra support during the procedure, especially if arthritis, contractures, or tremors are present.
- Avoid constricting the client's circulation with a tight bandage or binder. Observe skin and bony prominences frequently for signs of impaired circulation. The risk for skin breakdown increases with age.

Heat and Cold Applications

Heat and cold are applied to the body for local and systemic effects. Table 35.6 on the next page lists the physiological effects of heat and cold.

Physiological Responses

LOCAL EFFECTS OF HEAT   Heat is an old remedy for aches and pains, and people often equate heat with comfort and relief. Heat causes vasodilation and increases

Applying Bandages and Binders

Before a client is discharged, he or she will need to understand the bandage or binder:

- Assess the client's or caregiver's knowledge level of the reason for bandages or binders, and ability and willingness to perform the bandaging procedure.
- Ensure that the client has the proper supplies; assess for adequate and safe storage of supplies in the home, and ensure the client knows how to obtain replacement supplies.

- The client should have two binders so that he or she has one to wear while the other is being washed. Bandages and binders should be washed inside a mesh laundry bag to keep them from becoming twisted and to prevent Velcro or hooks from catching on other laundry.
- Instruct the client's caregiver on the importance of and how to do the following:

a. Perform hand hygiene thoroughly before handling dressing supplies and applying the bandage.
b. Report skin breakdown and redness, pain, or pallor of the affected area.
c. Check for adequate peripheral circulation after applying the bandage.

TABLE 35.6 Physiological Effects of Heat and Cold

Heat	Cold
Vasodilation	Vasoconstriction
Increases capillary permeability	Decreases capillary permeability
Increases cellular metabolism	Decreases cellular metabolism
Increases inflammation	Slows bacterial growth, decreases inflammation
Sedative effect	Local anesthetic effect

BOX 35.9 VARIABLES AFFECTING PHYSIOLOGICAL TOLERANCE TO HEAT AND COLD

Different parts of the body react in different ways to heat and cold:

- *Body part.* The back of the hand and foot are not very temperature sensitive. In contrast, the inner aspect of the wrist and forearm, the neck, and the perineal area are temperature sensitive.

- *Size of the exposed body part.* The larger the area exposed to heat and cold, the lower the tolerance.

- *Individual tolerance.* The very young and the very old generally have the lowest tolerance. Persons who have neurosensory impairments may have a high tolerance, but the risk of injury is greater.

- *Length of exposure.* People feel hot and cold applications most while the temperature is changing. After a period, tolerance increases.

- *Intactness of skin.* Injured skin areas are more sensitive to temperature variations.

blood flow to the affected area, bringing oxygen, nutrients, antibodies, and leukocytes.

Application of heat promotes soft tissue healing and increases suppuration. A possible disadvantage of heat is that it increases capillary permeability, which allows extracellular fluid and substances, such as plasma proteins, to pass through the capillary walls and can result in edema or an increase in pre-existing edema. Heat is often used for clients with musculoskeletal problems, such as low back pain, contractures, and joint stiffness from arthritis.

LOCAL EFFECTS OF COLD Generally, the physiological effects of cold are opposite to the effects of heat. Cold lowers the temperature of the skin and underlying tissues and causes vasoconstriction. Vasoconstriction reduces blood flow to the affected area and thus reduces the supply of oxygen and metabolites, decreases the removal of wastes, and produces skin pallor and coolness. Prolonged exposure to cold results in impaired circulation, cell deprivation, and subsequent damage to the tissues from lack of oxygen and nourishment. The signs of tissue damage caused by cold are a bluish-purple mottled appearance of the skin, numbness, and sometimes blisters and pain. Cold is most often used for sports injuries (e.g., sprains, strains, fractures) to limit postinjury swelling and bleeding.

SYSTEMIC EFFECTS OF HEAT AND COLD Heat applied to a localized body area, particularly a large body area, may cause excessive peripheral vasodilation, which produces a drop in blood pressure. A significant drop in blood pressure may cause fainting. Clients who have heart or pulmonary disease and who have circulatory disturbances, such as arteriosclerosis, are more prone to this effect than healthy people are. With extensive cold applications and vasoconstriction, a client's blood pressure can increase because blood is shunted from the cutaneous circulation to the internal blood vessels. Shivering, a generalized effect of prolonged cold, is a normal response as the body attempts to warm itself.

THERMAL TOLERANCE Various parts of the body differ in tolerance to heat and cold. The physiological tolerance of individuals also varies (see Box 35.9).

Specific conditions necessitate precautions in the use of hot or cold applications:

- *Neurosensory impairment.* People with sensory impairments are unable to perceive that heat is damaging the tissues and are at risk for burns or are unable to perceive discomfort from cold and prevent tissue injury.

- *Impaired mental status.* People who are confused or have an altered level of consciousness need monitoring during applications to ensure safe therapy.

- *Impaired circulation.* People with peripheral vascular disease, diabetes, or congestive heart failure lack the normal ability to dissipate heat via the blood circulation, which puts them at risk for tissue damage with heat and cold applications.

- *Immediately after injury or surgery.* Heat increases bleeding and swelling.

- *Open wounds.* Cold can decrease blood flow to the wound, thereby inhibiting healing.

ADAPTATION OF THERMAL RECEPTORS Heat and cold receptors adapt to temperature changes. When they are subjected to an abrupt change in temperature, the receptors are strongly stimulated initially. This strong stimulation declines rapidly during the first few seconds and then more slowly during the next half hour or more as the receptors adapt to the new temperature.

Nurses and clients need to understand this adaptive response when applying heat and cold. Clients may be tempted to change the temperature of a thermal application because of the change in thermal sensation following adaptation. Increasing the temperature of a hot application after adaptation can result in serious burns. Decreasing the temperature of a cold application can result in pain and serious impairment of circulation to the body part. Table 35.7 lists temperatures for hot and cold applications.

TABLE 35.7 Temperatures for Hot and Cold Applications

Description	Temperature	Application
Very Cold	Less than 15°C	Ice bags
Cold	15°C–18°C	Cold pack
Cool	18°C–27°C	Cool compresses
Tepid	27°C–37°C	Sponge bath
Warm	37°C–40°C	Warm bath, aquathermia pads
Hot	40°C–46°C	Hot soak, irrigations, hot compresses
Very hot	More than 46°C	Hot water bag for adults

REBOUND PHENOMENON The rebound phenomenon occurs at the time the maximum therapeutic effect of the hot or cold application is achieved and the opposite effect begins. For example, heat produces maximum vasodilation in 20 to 30 minutes; continuation of the application beyond 30 to 45 minutes brings tissue congestion, and the blood vessels then constrict for reasons unknown. If the heat application is continued, the client is at risk for burns because the constricted blood vessels are unable to dissipate the heat adequately via the blood circulation.

With cold applications, maximum vasoconstriction occurs when the involved skin reaches a temperature of 15°C. Below 15°C, vasodilation begins. This mechanism is protective: It helps to prevent freezing of body tissues normally exposed to cold, such as the nose and ears. It also explains the ruddiness of the skin of a person who has been walking in cold weather.

An understanding of the rebound phenomenon is essential for the nurse and client. *Thermal applications must be halted before the rebound phenomenon begins.*

Applying Heat and Cold

Heat can be applied to the body in both dry and moist forms. Dry heat is applied locally by means of a hot water bottle, aquathermia pad, disposable heat pack, or electric pad. Moist heat can be provided by compress, hot pack, soak, or sitz bath. Selected indications for the use of heat and cold are found in Table 35.8.

Dry cold is generally applied locally by means of a cold pack, ice bag, ice glove, or ice collar. Moist cold can be provided by compress or a cooling sponge bath.

For all local applications of heat or cold, the nurse needs to follow these guidelines:

- Determine the client's ability to tolerate the therapy.
- Identify conditions that might contraindicate treatment (e.g., bleeding, circulatory impairment).
- Explain the application to the client.
- Assess the skin area to which the heat or cold will be applied.
- Ask the client to report any discomfort.
- Return to the client 15 minutes after starting the heat or cold, and observe the local skin area for any untoward signs (e.g., redness). Stop the application if any problems occur.
- Remove the equipment at the designated time, and dispose of it appropriately.
- Examine the area to which the heat or cold was applied, and record the client's response.

For contraindications to the use of heat or cold, see Box 35.10 on the next page.

TABLE 35.8 Selected Indications of Heat and Cold

Indication	Effect of Heat	Effect of Cold
Muscle spasm	Relaxes muscles and increases their contractility	Relaxes muscles and decreases muscle contractility
Inflammation	Increases blood flow, softens exudates	Vasoconstriction decreases capillary permeability, decreases blood flow, slows cellular metabolism
Pain	Relieves pain, possibly by promoting muscle relaxation, increasing circulation, and promoting psychological relaxation and a feeling of comfort; acts as a counterirritant	Decreases pain by slowing nerve conduction rate and blocking nerve impulses; produces numbness, acts as a counterirritant, increases pain threshold
Contracture	Reduces contracture and increases joint range of motion by allowing greater distension of muscles and connective tissue	
Joint stiffness	Reduces joint stiffness by decreasing viscosity of synovial fluid and increasing tissue distensibility	
Traumatic injury		Decreases bleeding by constricting blood vessels; decreases edema by reducing capillary permeability

---

BOX 35.10 CONTRAINDICATIONS TO THE USE OF HEAT AND COLD

Determine the presence of any conditions contraindicating the use of heat:

- *The first 24 hours after traumatic injury.* Heat increases bleeding and swelling.
- *Active hemorrhage.* Heat causes vasodilation and increases bleeding.
- *Noninflammatory edema.* Heat increases capillary permeability and edema.
- *Localized malignant tumour.* Because heat accelerates cell metabolism and cell growth and increases circulation, it may accelerate metastases (secondary tumours).
- *Skin disorder that causes redness or blisters.* Heat can burn or cause further damage to skin.

Determine the presence of any conditions contraindicating the use of cold:

- *Open wounds.* Cold can increase tissue damage by decreasing blood flow to an open wound.
- *Impaired circulation.* Cold can further impair nourishment of the tissues and cause tissue damage. In clients with Raynaud's disease, cold increases arterial spasm.
- *Allergy or hypersensitivity to cold.* Some clients have an allergy to cold that may be manifested as an inflammatory response, for example, erythema, hives, swelling, joint pain, and occasional muscle spasm. Some react with a sudden increase in blood pressure, which can be hazardous if the person is hypertensive.

Determine the presence of any conditions indicating the need for special precautions during heat and cold therapy:

- *Neurosensory impairment.* Persons with sensory impairments are unable to perceive that heat is damaging the tissues and are at risk for burns, or they are unable to perceive discomfort from cold and are unable to prevent tissue injury.
- *Impaired mental status.* Persons who are confused or have an altered level of consciousness need monitoring and supervision during applications to ensure safe therapy.
- *Impaired circulation.* Persons with peripheral vascular disease, diabetes, or congestive heart failure lack the normal ability to dissipate heat via the blood circulation, which puts them at risk for tissue damage with heat applications. Cold applications are contraindicated for these people.
- *Open wounds.* Tissues around an open wound are more sensitive to heat and cold.

HOT WATER BAG A hot water bag or bottle is a common source of dry heat used in the home. It is convenient and relatively inexpensive. However, because of the danger of burning from improper use, many agencies use other means.

The following temperatures of the water in the bag are considered safe in most situations and provide the desired effect: normal adult and child over 2 years, 46°C to 52°C, debilitated or unconscious adult, or child under 2 years, 40.5°C to 46°C.

To apply a hot water bag, the nurse should do the following:

- Measure the temperature of the water by using a bath thermometer.
- Fill the bag about two-thirds full.
- Expel the remaining air and secure the top. With the air removed, the bag can be moulded to the body part.
- Dry the bag and hold it upside down to test for leakage.
- Wrap the bag in a towel or cover and place it on the body site (Figure 35.28).
- Remove after 30 minutes or in accordance with agency protocol.

AQUATHERMIA PAD The aquathermia or aquamatic pad (also referred to as the *K-pad*) is a pad constructed with tubes containing water. The pad is attached by tubing

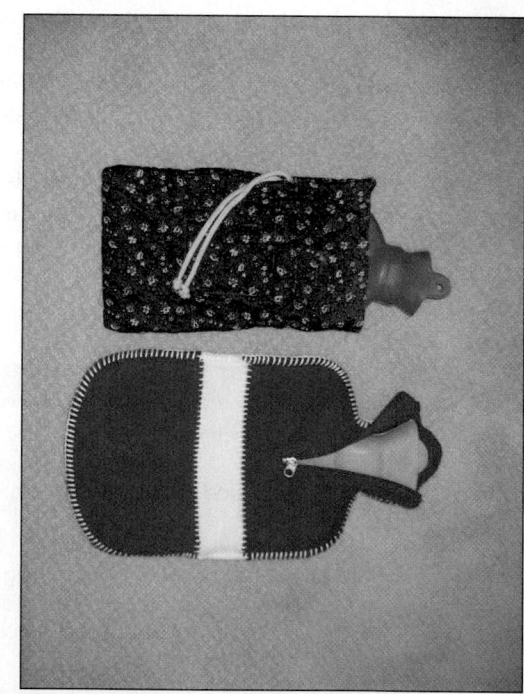

FIGURE 35.28 Hot water bottle with cloth covers.

to an electrically powered control unit that has an opening for water and a temperature gauge (Figure 35.29). Some aquathermia pads have an absorbent surface through which moist heat can be applied. The other surface of the pad is waterproof. These pads are disposable.

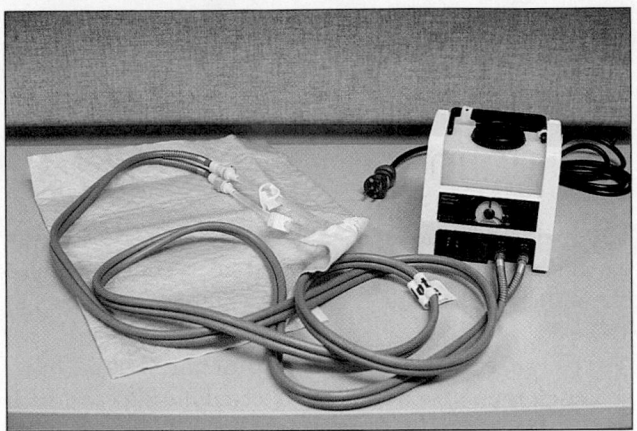

FIGURE 35.29 An aquathermia unit.

To apply an aquathermia pad, the nurse carries out the following steps:

- Fill the reservoir of the unit two-thirds full of distilled water.
- Set the desired temperature. Check the manufacturer's instructions. Most units are set at 40.5°C for adults.
- Cover the pad and plug in the unit. Some manufacturers suggest warming the pad before applying it.
- Apply the pad to the body part. The treatment is usually continued for 30 minutes. Check orders and agency protocol.

HOT AND COLD PACKS Commercially prepared hot and cold packs (Figure 35.30) provide heat or cold for a designated time. Directions on the package tell how to initiate the heating or cooling process, for example, by striking, squeezing, or kneading the pack.

ELECTRIC PADS Electric pads provide a constant, even heat, are lightweight, and can be moulded to a body part. Electric pads, however, can burn if the setting is too high. Some models have waterproof covers for use when the pad is placed over a moist dressing.

In applying electric pads, the nurse follows these guidelines:

- Do not insert sharp objects (e.g., pins) into the pad. The pin could damage a wire and cause an electric shock.
- Ensure that the body area is dry unless the pad has a waterproof cover on the pad. Electricity in the presence of water can cause a shock.
- Use pads with a preset heating switch so a client cannot increase the heat.
- Do not place the pad under the client. Heat will not dissipate, and the client may be burned.

ICE BAGS, ICE GLOVES, AND ICE COLLARS Ice bags, ice gloves, and ice collars are filled either with ice chips or with an alcohol-based solution. They are applied to

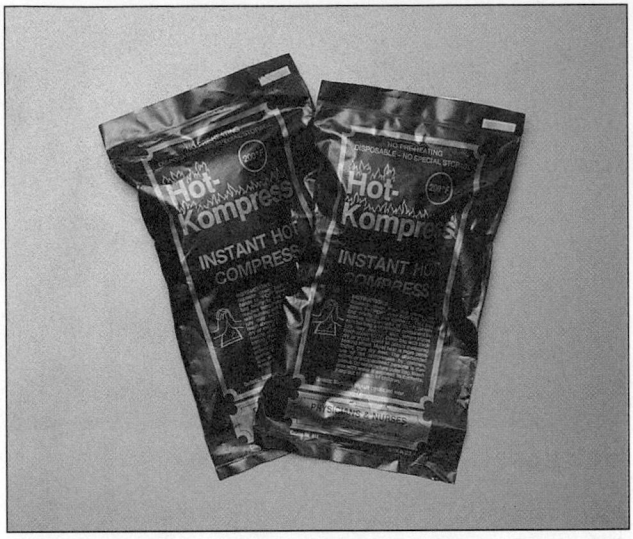

FIGURE 35.30 Commercially prepared disposable hot packs.

the body to provide cold to a localized area (e.g., a collar is often applied to the throat following a tonsillectomy). Always wrap the container in a towel or cover.

COMPRESSES Compresses can be either warm or cold. A **compress** is a moist gauze dressing applied to a wound. When hot compresses are ordered, the solution is heated to the temperature indicated by the order or according to agency protocol, for example, 40.5°C. When there is a break in the skin or when the body part (e.g., an eye) is vulnerable to microbial invasion, sterile technique is necessary; therefore, sterile gloves are needed to apply the compress and all materials must be sterile.

SOAK A **soak** refers to immersing a body part (e.g., an arm) in a solution or to wrapping a part in gauze dressings and then saturating the dressing with a solution. Sterile technique is generally indicated for open wounds, such as a burn or an unhealed surgical incision. Determine agency protocol regarding the temperature of the solution. Hot soaks are frequently done to soften and remove encrusted secretions and dead tissue.

SITZ BATH A **sitz bath**, or hip bath, is used to soak a client's perineal or rectal area. The client sits in a special tub or chair and is usually immersed from mid-thighs to the iliac crests or umbilicus. Special tubs or chairs are preferred because when the legs are also immersed, as in a regular bathtub, blood circulation to the perineum or pelvic area is decreased. Disposable sitz baths are also available (Figure 35.31 on the next page).

The temperature of the water should be from 40°C to 43°C, unless the client is unable to tolerate the heat. Determine agency protocol. Some sitz tubs have temperature indicators attached to the water taps. The duration of the bath is generally 15 to 20 minutes, depending on

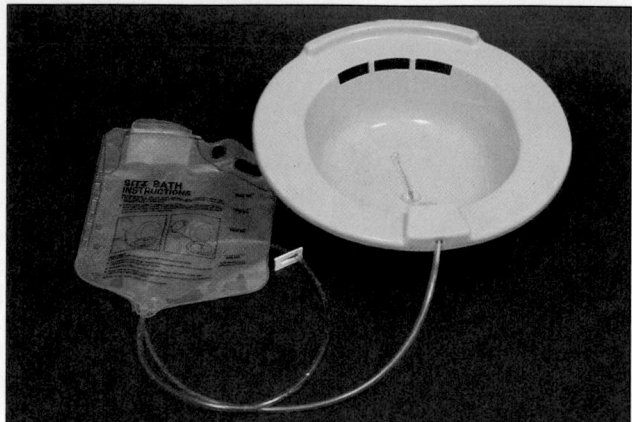

FIGURE 35.31 A plastic single-client sitz bath.

the client's health. Follow these steps to provide a sitz bath:

- Assist the client into the tub. Provide support for the client's feet; a footstool can prevent pressure on the backs of the thighs.
- Provide a bath blanket for the client's shoulders, and eliminate drafts to prevent chilling.
- Observe the client closely during the bath for signs of faintness, dizziness, weakness, accelerated pulse rate, and pallor.
- Maintain the water temperature.

- Following the sitz bath, assist the client out of the tub. Help the client dry himself or herself.

Evaluating

The goals established during the planning phase are evaluated according to specific desired health outcomes also established in that phase. Examples of these are shown in Table 35.9.

To judge whether client outcomes have been achieved, the nurse uses data collected during care, such as skin status over bony prominences and perineal area, nutritional and fluid intake, mental status, signs of healing if an ulcer is present, and so on. If outcomes are *not* achieved, the nurse should explore the reasons:

- Has the client's physical condition changed?
- Were risk factors correctly identified?
- Did the client fail to comply with instructions about moving and turning? Why?
- Were appropriate devices used to redistribute pressure?
- Was the repositioning schedule adhered to?
- Are the client's nutritional and fluid intake adequate?
- Were appropriate measures used to control incontinence and protect the client's skin?

TABLE 35.9 Evaluation Goals and Outcomes: Skin Integrity and Wound Healing

Goal	Examples of Desired Outcomes
Maintain skin integrity	Skin intact over bony prominences
	Skin supple, without signs of edema or dehydration
	Skin colour in expected range (e.g., no redness, or redness that blanches and returns to normal within a few minutes)
	Skin temperature within normal range
Promote primary intention wound healing	Wound edges approximated
	Decrease (or absence) of serosanguineous drainage
	Decrease in surrounding skin inflammation
	Absence of purulent drainage
	Absence of wound odour
Promote secondary intention wound healing	Decrease in length, width, and depth of wound
	Presence of and increase in granulation tissue
	Intact skin surrounding wound
	Decrease (or absence) of drainage
Support the nonhealing wound (palliation)	Pain control
	Infection control
	Odour control
	Absence of further breakdown

- Was the wound supported and immobilized effectively?
- Were stringent infection prevention and control practices implemented when cleaning and changing dressings to prevent infection?

- Was the client receiving anti-inflammatory medications that interfere with healing?
- Was the appropriate wound care product applied to keep the wound moist or absorb exudate, or both, as needed?

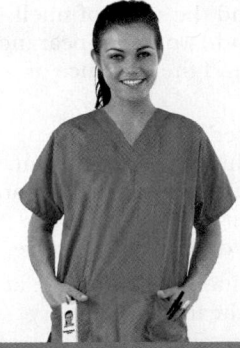

Case Study 35

You have been assigned to care for Mr. Johns, a 74-year-old client being treated for a urinary tract disorder. Mr. Johns suffered a cerebrovascular accident (stroke) 6 months ago and has had difficulty ambulating and attending to his own needs because of right-sided weakness. While assessing Mr. Johns, you note that he is thin for his height, is incontinent of foul-smelling urine, and has deeply reddened areas on his right hip, coccyx, and entire peritoneal area. Mr. Johns is alert and oriented to person, place, and time, but he has decreased sensation on his entire right side. He spends most of his time in bed or sitting at his bedside in a chair because of his difficulty with ambulation.

CRITICAL THINKING QUESTIONS

1. What data suggest that Mr. Johns is particularly vulnerable to pressure ulcer development?
2. What additional information do you need to use the Braden Scale to determine Mr. Johns's potential for pressure ulcer development?
3. What independent measures can you take to protect Mr. Johns's skin from further breakdown?

4. Considering that Mr. Johns does have impaired skin integrity, why is it important to institute treatment for pressure ulcers at this time?

Check the eText in MyNursingLab for answers and explanations.

KEY TERMS

acute wound *p. 1005*
ankle flare *p. 1010*
atrophie blanche
  p. 1012
bandage *p. 1040*
chronic wound *p. 1005*
clean wounds *p. 1004*
clean-contaminated
  wounds *p. 1004*
collagen *p. 1013*
colonization *p. 1017*
compress *p. 1049*
contaminated wounds
  p. 1005
contamination *p. 1017*
debridement *p. 1028*
dehiscence *p. 1015*

delayed primary intention
  healing *p. 1013*
dirty (infected) wounds
  p. 1005
eschar *p. 1008*
evisceration *p. 1015*
exudate *p. 1013*
fibrin *p. 1013*
friction *p. 1007*
full-thickness wound
  p. 1005
gaiter area *p. 1010*
granulation tissue
  p. 1013
hematoma *p. 1015*
hemorrhage *p. 1015*
hemostasis *p. 1013*

infection *p. 1015*
ischemia *p. 1006*
keloid *p. 1013*
lipodermatosclerosis
  p. 1012
maceration *p. 1008*
mechanical loads
  p. 1006
partial-thickness wound
  p. 1005
pressure ulcer *p. 1005*
primary intention healing
  p. 1012
purulent exudate *p. 1015*
pyogenic bacteria *p. 1015*
reactive hyperemia
  p. 1006

regeneration *p. 1012*
sanguineous exudate
  p. 1015
secondary intention
  healing *p. 1012*
serosanguineous exudate
  p. 1015
serous exudate *p. 1015*
shearing *p. 1007*
sitz bath *p. 1049*
soak *p. 1049*
suppuration *p. 1015*
tertiary intention healing
  p. 1013
vacuum-assisted closure
  p. 1040

CHAPTER HIGHLIGHTS

- Maintaining skin integrity is an important independent function of nursing.

- Wounds are described as acute or chronic; closed or open; and clean, clean-contaminated, contaminated, or dirty (infected). Wounds are also classified by depth as partial-thickness or full-thickness wounds. In addition, wounds are classified according to how they are acquired, as incisions, contusions, abrasions, punctures, lacerations, and penetrating wounds.

- Pressure ulcers are areas of localized damage to the skin and underlying tissue and are usually the result of external forces, such as pressure, friction, and shear.

- Mechanical loads are extrinsic forces, such as pressure, friction, and shear, that cause soft tissue damage and potentially lead to blood flow impedance, tissue necrosis, and pressure ulcer development.

- Factors increasing the risk for the development of pressure ulcers include immobility and inactivity, inadequate nutrition, fecal and urinary incontinence, decreased mental status, diminished sensation, excessive body heat, advanced age, and certain chronic medical conditions.

- Pressure ulcers have six recognized categories or stages, which reflect the degree of tissue damage, suspected deep tissue injury, and unstageable wounds.

- Two types of wound healing are distinguished by the amount of tissue loss: (a) primary intention healing and (b) secondary intention healing. Tertiary intention healing is delayed primary intention healing.

- The wound-healing process has three phases: (a) inflammatory, (b) proliferative, and (c) maturation.

- Major types of wound exudate are serous, purulent, and sanguineous. Exudate can be a combination of two or three (e.g., serosanguineous). The process of pus formation is referred to as *suppuration.*

- The main complications of wound healing are hemorrhage, infection, dehiscence, and evisceration, each of which is identifiable by specific clinical signs and symptoms.

- Although all chronic wounds are presumed to be bacterially contaminated (a state in which bacteria are not attached or replicating), colonization refers to the state in which bacteria are attached to the wound surface and replicating. When bacteria become invasive and cause an inflammatory response, the wound may proceed to shows signs of local infection, which can itself progress to systemic infection.

- Factors affecting wound healing include developmental stage, nutritional status, lifestyle, medications, the presence of infection, and the presence of chronic medical conditions.

- Risk-assessment tools are available to identify clients at risk for pressure ulcer development. These should be used on a regular basis.

- Meticulous skin examination of common pressure points by the nurse is an important ongoing assessment activity for clients at risk.

- When a pressure ulcer is present, the nurse describes the ulcer in terms of location, size, depth, category or stage, colour, status of wound margins and surrounding skin, and specific signs of infection, if present.

- Wound assessment is an ongoing process to evaluate healing; the nurse assesses wounds by visual inspection, palpation, and the sense of smell. Essential data for wounds include wound appearance, size, drainage, swelling, pain, and the presence of tubes and drains.

- Laboratory data that may be used to assess the progress of wound healing include leukocyte count, blood coagulation studies, serum protein analysis, and wound cultures. Nurses are usually responsible for obtaining specimens of wound drainage for culture.

- Possible nursing diagnoses include the following: at risk for pressure ulcer; wound healing by primary intention; at risk for impaired wound healing related to contaminated wound status; and at risk for wound dehiscence. Diagnoses that can be the result of alterations in skin integrity include the following: at risk for infection, such as for the client with immunosuppression, or when the wound is caused by trauma; at risk for pain; at risk for impaired body image; anxiety related to apprehension; and uncertainty.

- Major goals for clients at risk for skin impairments are to maintain skin integrity and avoid potential associated risks.

- Nursing interventions aimed at preventing skin disruptions include conducting ongoing assessment of risk factors and skin status; providing skin care to maintain skin integrity; ensuring adequate nutrition; implementing measures to avoid skin trauma; providing supportive devices; and teaching the client.

- Treatment for pressure ulcers varies according to the category or stage of the ulcer and agency protocol.

- Major nursing responsibilities related to wound care include preventing infection, preventing further tissue damage, preventing hemorrhage, promoting healing, and preventing skin excoriation around draining wounds.

- Wound care may involve cleaning wounds, changing dressings, maintaining drains, irrigating, inserting packing, and applying bandages and binders.

- The RYB colour code of wounds can assist nurses to provide appropriate nursing interventions for wounds that heal by secondary intention. In this scheme, the nurse protects *red*, cleanses *yellow*, and debrides *black*, according to agency policy and physician's orders.

- Various wound care products are available to protect wounds and to keep the wound bed moist, thus facilitating healing.

- Dressings have been developed for use with specific types of wounds. These include transparent adhesive films, impregnated nonadherent dressings, hydrocolloids, hydrogels, polyurethane foams, and exudate absorbers. The nurse must be aware of the specific indications and contraindications for use.

- The type of dressing used depends on (a) location, size, and type of the wound; (b) amount of exudate; (c) whether or not the wound requires debridement, is infected, or has sinus tracts; and (d) such considerations as frequency of dressing change, ease or difficulty of dressing applications, and cost.
- Heat and cold produce specific local physiological and systemic responses that account for their therapeutic effects.

- Various parts of the body differ in tolerance to heat and cold. The physiological tolerance of individuals also varies. Specific conditions, such as neurosensory and circulatory impairments, necessitate precautions when applying heat or cold.
- When applying heat and cold, clients and nurses need to be aware of the effects of thermal receptor adaptation and the rebound phenomenon.

ASSESS YOUR LEARNING

1. Your client has a Braden Scale score of 17. What is the appropriate nursing action?
   a. Assess the client again in 24 hours; the score is within normal limits.
   b. Implement a turning schedule; the client is at an increased risk of skin breakdown.
   c. Apply a transparent wound barrier to major pressure sites.
   d. Request a prescription for a special low-air-loss bed.

2. Proper technique for performing a wound culture includes which of the following?
   a. Cleansing the wound before obtaining the specimen
   b. Swabbing for the specimen in the area with the largest collection of drainage
   c. Removing crusts or scabs with sterile forceps and then culturing the site beneath
   d. Waiting 8 hours following a dose of antibiotic to obtain the specimen

3. A client has a pressure ulcer with a shallow partial-skin-thickness eroded area but no necrotic areas. The nurse would treat the area with which of the following dressings?
   a. Alginate
   b. Dry gauze
   c. Hydrocolloid
   d. No dressing is indicated.

4. Thirty minutes after the application of a heating pad is initiated, the client requests that the nurse leave it in place. What should the nurse explain to the client?
   a. Heat application for longer than 30 minutes can actually cause the opposite effect (constriction) of the one desired (dilation).
   b. It will be acceptable to leave the pad in place if the temperature is reduced.
   c. It will be acceptable to leave the pad in place for another 30 minutes if the site appears satisfactory when assessed.

   d. It will be acceptable to leave the pad in place as long as it is moist heat.

5. Which statement, if made by the client or family member, would indicate the need for further teaching?
   a. "If a skin area gets red and the red does not go away after turning, I should report it to the nurse."
   b. "Putting foam pads under the heels or other bony areas can help decrease pressure."
   c. "If a person cannot turn himself or herself in bed, someone should help the person change position every 4 hours."
   d. "The skin should be washed with only warm water (not hot) and lotion put on while the skin is still a little wet."

6. Your client has a pressure ulcer on his heel. It is 3 cm deep and 2 cm wide, and is covered with black eschar. According to the National Pressure Ulcer Advisory Panel staging system, how would this wound be classified?
   a. Stage III
   b. Stage IV
   c. Suspected deep tissue injury
   d. Unstageable

7. Which of the following is an appropriate nursing diagnosis for a client with large areas of skin excoriation resulting from scratching an allergic rash?
   a. Risk for impaired skin integrity
   b. Impaired skin integrity
   c. Impaired tissue integrity
   d. Social isolation

8. Mr. Boyle, 55 years old, smoked a pack of cigarettes each day. Two weeks ago, he experienced a cerebrovascular accident. Mr. Boyle has left hemiplegia and will be transferred to a rehabilitation hospital within the week. How would the nurse BEST prevent the development of a pressure ulcer for Mr. Boyle?
   a. Encourage Mr. Boyle to reposition himself, as necessary

b. Turn Mr. Boyle every 1–2 hours or as necessary, depending on his needs

c. Massage bony prominences with moisturizing cream

d. Place Mr. Boyle in a semi-Fowler's position

9. Which of the following items are used to perform wound irrigation?

a. Unsterile drape

b. Sterile gloves

c. Refrigerated irrigating solution

d. 5-mL syringe

10. Which of the following indicates proper use of a triangle arm sling?

a. The elbow is kept flexed at 90 degrees or more.

b. The knot is placed on either side of the vertebrae of the neck.

c. The sling extends to just proximal of the hand.

d. The sling is removed every 2 hours to check for circulation and skin integrity.

Check the eText in MyNursingLab for answers and explanations.

WEBLINKS

Canadian Association of Wound Care

http://www.cawc.net

The Canadian Association of Wound Care (CAWC) is Canada's only interdisciplinary organization dedicated to the advancement of wound care practice. The CAWC facilitates best practice through excellence in education, clinical practice, public policy, research, and international partnerships. CAWC offers the public an "ask the expert" option.

National Pressure Ulcer Advisory Panel

http://www.npuap.org

This U.S. organization provides multidisciplinary leadership for improved patient outcomes in pressure ulcer prevention and management through education, public policy, and research.

European Pressure Ulcer Advisory Panel

http://www.epuap.com

The mission of this European organization is to provide relief to persons suffering from or at risk of pressure ulcers, in particular through research and the education of the public.

Wound Healing Society

http://www.woundheal.org

The Wound Healing Society is a nonprofit, international organization that provides a forum for discussions among scientists, physicians, licensed practitioners, industrial representatives, and others with interest in the field of wound healing.

MyNursingLab

REFERENCES

Allard, J. P., Aghdassi E., McArthur, M., McGeer, A., Simor, A., Abdolell, M., ..., Stephens, D., & Liu, B. (2004). Nutrition risk factors for survival in the elderly living in Canadian long-term care facilities. *Journal of the American Geriatrics Society, 52,* 59–65.

Braden, B. J. & Blanchard, S. (2007). Risk assessment in pressure ulcer prevention. In D. L. Krasner, G. Rodeheaver, & R. G. Sibbald (Eds.), *Chronic wound care: A clinical source book for health care professionals* (4th ed.) (pp. 593–608). Wayne, PA: HMP Communications.

Canadian Association of Wound Care. (2006). *Quick reference guide: Recommendations for practice.* Toronto, ON: Author. Retrieved from http://www.cawc.net/open/library/clinical/QRG2006E.pdf

Dolynchuk K., Keast, D., Campbell, K., Houghton, P., Orsted, H., Sibbald, G., . . . & Atkinson, A. (2000). Best practices for the prevention and treatment of pressure ulcers. *Ostomy Wound Management, 46*(11), 38–52.

Fernandez, R., & Griffiths, R. (2008). Water for wound cleansing. *Cochrane Database of Systematic Reviews 2008,* Issue 1. Art. No.: CD003861. doi: 10.1002/14651858.CD003861.pub2

Health Quality Council. (2006). *Saskatchewan skin and wound care guidelines.* Saskatoon, SK: Health Quality Council.

Hunter, S., Langemo, D., Thompson, P., Hanson, D., & Anderson, J. (2009). Maggot therapy for wound management. *Advances in Skin & Wound Care, 22,* 25–27.

Junkin, J. & Gray, J. (2009). Are pressure redistribution surfaces or heel protection devices effective for preventing heel pressure ulcers? *Journal of Wound, Ostomy and Continence Nursing, 36*(6), 602–608.

Leblanc, K., Christensen, D., Orsted, H., & Keast, D. H. (2008). Best practice recommendations for the prevention and treatment of skin tears. *Wound Care Canada, 6*(1), 14–30.

McInnes, E., Dumville, J. C., Jammali-Blasi, A., & Bell-Syer, S. E. M. (2009). Support surfaces for treating pressure ulcers.

Cochrane Database of Systematic Reviews 2011, Issue 12. Art. No.: CD009490. doi: 10.1002/14651858.CD009490

Moore, Z. E. H., Cowman, S. (2009). Repositioning for treating pressure ulcers. *Cochrane Database of Systematic Reviews 2009*, Issue 2. Art. No.: CD006898. doi: 10.1002/14651858. CD006898.pub2

Moore, Z. E. H., Cowman, S. (2005). Wound cleansing for pressure ulcers. *Cochrane Database of Systematic Reviews 2005*, Issue 4. Art. No.: CD004983. doi: 10.1002/14651858. CD004983.pub2

Moreira, M., & Markovchick, V. (2007). Wound management. *Emergency Medicine Clinics of North America, 25,* 873–899.

National Pressure Ulcer Advisory Panel. (2007). *Updated staging system.* Retrieved from http://www.npuap.org/pr2.htm

Norton, L., Coutts, P., & Sibbald, G. (2011). Beds: Practical pressure management for surfaces/mattresses. *Advances in Skin and Wound Care Management, 24*(7), 324–332.

Poss, J., Murphy, K. M., Woodbury, G. M., Orsted, H., Stevenson, K., Williams, S., MacAlpine, S., Curtin-Telegdi, N., & Hirdes, J. P. (2010). Development of the interRAI Pressure Ulcer Risk Assessment Scale (PURS) for use in long-term care and home care settings. *BMC Geriatrics. 10,* 67. Retrieved from http://www.biomedcentral.com/1471-2318/10/67

Price, P. (2009). Psychosocial aspects of wounds. Retrieved from http://www.woundsresearch.com/content/ message-patricia-price-bahons-phd

Registered Nurses' Association of Ontario. (2004). *Nursing best practice guideline: Assessment and management of venous leg ulcers.* Toronto, ON: Author.

Registered Nurses' Association of Ontario. (2005). *Nursing best practice guideline: Assessment and management of foot ulcers for people with diabetes.* Toronto, ON: Author.

Registered Nurses' Association of Ontario. (2007). *Assessment and management of stage I to IV pressure ulcers* (Rev. ed.). Toronto, ON: Author.

Registered Nurses' Association of Ontario. (2011). *Nursing best practice guideline: Risk assessment and prevention of pressure ulcers—Guideline Supplement.* (Rev. ed.). Toronto, ON: Author. Retrieved from http://www.rnao.org/Storage/83/7749_ PRESSURE-ULCERS_Supplement_2011.pdf

Safer HealthCare Now! (2011). Prevent surgical site infections: Getting started kit. Retrieved from http:// www.saferhealthcarenow.ca/EN/Interventions/SSI/ Documents/SSI%20Getting%20Started%20Kit.pdf

Salcido, R. (2011). Pressure ulcers and wound care. *Medscape Reference.* Retrieved from http://emedicine.medscape.com/ article/319284-overview

Sibbald R. G., on behalf of the Shifting the Original Paradigm Expert Panel (SOPE Panel). (2011). Pressure ulcer staging revisited: Superficial skin changes & deep pressure ulcer framework. *Advances in Skin and Wound Care, 24*(12), 571–580.

Sibbald R. G., Mahoney, J., & the V.A.C. Therapy Canadian Consensus Group. (2003). A consensus report on the use of vacuum-assisted closure in chronic, difficult to heal wounds. *Ostomy/Wound Management, 49*(11), 52–66.

Smith & Nephew Ltd. Grace P, editor(s). (2006). *Leg ulcer guidelines: A pocket guide for practice.* Dublin, Ireland: Smith & Nephew Ltd. Retrieved from http://www.guideline.gov/ content.aspx?id=9830

Woo, K. Y., & Sibbald, R. G. (2008). Chronic wound pain: A conceptual model. *Advances in Skin and Wound Care, 21*(4), 175–188.

Woo, K. Y., Sibbald, R. G., Ayello, E., Coutts, P. M., & Garde, D. (2009). Peristomal skin complications and management. *Advances in Skin & Wound Care, 22,* 522–532.

Woodbury, M. G., & Houghton, P. E. (2004). Prevalence of pressure ulcers in Canadian health care settings. *Ostomy/ Wound Management, 50*(1), 22–38.

World Union of Wound Healing Societies (WUWHS). (2008). Principles of best practice: Vacuum assisted closure: recommendations for use. A consensus document. London, UK: MEP Ltd. Retrieved from www.wuwhs.org/datas/2_1/11/ VAC_English_WEB.pdf

Wound, Ostomy, and Continence Nurses Society. (2007). *New position statement on pressure ulcer staging.* Retrieved from http://www.wocn.org/pdfs/WOCN_Library/Position_ Statements/PressureUlcerStaging.pdf

Chapter 36

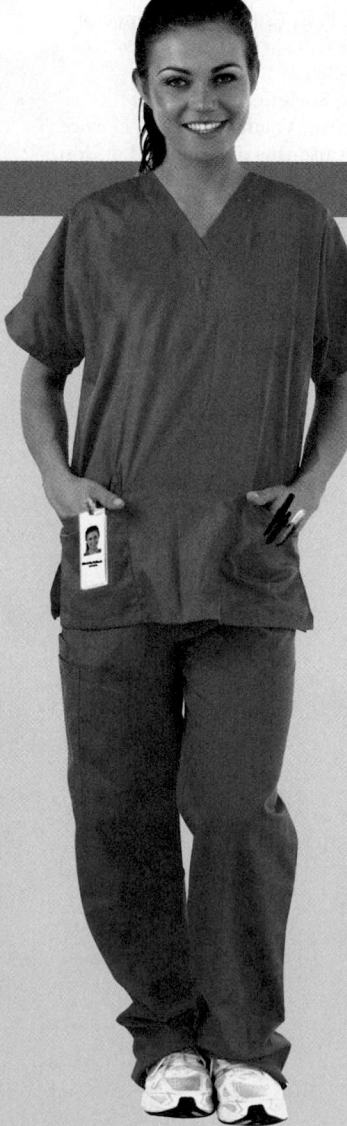

Caring for Perioperative Clients

LEARNING OUTCOMES

After studying this chapter, you will be able to:

1. Describe the three phases of the perioperative period.

2. Discuss types of surgery according to purpose, degree of urgency, invasiveness, body part, equipment used, and degree of risk.

3. Identify the nursing history, physical assessment, and screening tests essential to a thorough preoperative assessment.

4. Outline nursing responsibilities in planning perioperative nursing care.

5. Describe essential preoperative teaching, including pain control, moving, leg exercises, and deep-breathing and coughing exercises.

6. Outline the physical preparation needs for a client having surgery, including nutrition and fluids, elimination, skin preparation (hygiene, hair, nails), medications, sleep, care of valuables and prostheses, and special orders.

7. Compare three types of anesthesia.

8. Identify essential nursing assessments and interventions during the immediate postanesthetic phase.

9. Demonstrate ongoing nursing assessments and interventions for the postoperative client.

10. Discuss potential postoperative complications and describe 10 nursing interventions to prevent them.

11. Identify the essential aspects of managing gastrointestinal suction.

12. Describe appropriate surgical wound care for a postoperative client.

Surgery is a unique experience of a planned physical alteration encompassing three phases: (a) preoperative, (b) intraoperative, and (c) postoperative. These three phases are together referred to as the **perioperative period**. Perioperative nursing addresses the many patient safety and care issues related to each period of the surgical experience.

The **preoperative phase** begins when the decision to have surgery is made and ends when the client is transferred to the surgical suite. The nursing activities associated with this phase include assessing the client, identifying potential or actual health problems, planning specific care based on the individual's needs, and providing preoperative teaching for the client, the family, and significant others. Efforts are being made nationally to reduce the wait time (preoperative phase) for adult and pediatric surgery. Adult cardiac (coronary artery bypass graft), joint (hip and knee replacements and hip fixation), and sight restoration (cataract) related surgeries have been identified as priority areas with national benchmarks established for each; for example, people awaiting hip or knee replacement should have no greater than a 26 week wait time; people at high risk and awaiting cataract surgery should have no greater than a 16 week wait time (Wait Time Alliance, 2011). The Canadian Pediatric Surgical Wait Times Project addresses issues related to shortening the preoperative phase for children awaiting surgical intervention. See the Reflect on Primary Health Care box.

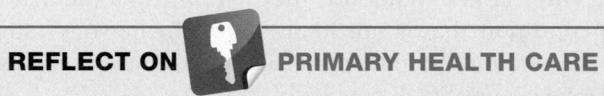

REFLECT ON   PRIMARY HEALTH CARE

Find out how *accessible* operative care is in your community. Are relatively common surgeries, such as joint replacement surgery, sight restoration (e.g., cataract surgery), or cardiac surgery, available in your region? If so, how long do people wait for such procedures? Is there a centralized registry in your province or territory for ensuring access to surgical procedures is timely? Consider the impact on the client and family if people need to travel a distance or wait several weeks or months to have one of these interventions.

The **intraoperative phase** begins when the patient is transferred to the surgical suite and ends when the patient is admitted to the postanesthesia care unit (PACU), also called the *postanesthesia room* or *recovery room* (RR). The nursing activities related to this phase include a variety of specialized procedures designed to create and maintain a safe therapeutic environment for the patient and the health care team. These activities include interventions that provide for the patient's safety, maintaining an aseptic environment, ensuring proper functioning of equipment, and providing the surgical team with instruments and supplies needed during the procedure.

The **postoperative phase** begins with the admission of the patient to the postanesthesia area and ends when healing is complete. During the postoperative phase, nursing activities include assessing the patient's response (physiological and psychological) to surgery, performing interventions to facilitate healing and prevent complications, teaching and providing support to the patient and support people, and planning for home care. The goal is to assist the person to achieve the optimal health status.

Perioperative nursing is practised in hospital-based inpatient or outpatient surgical, laser, or endoscopic suites and freestanding outpatient or ambulatory surgical centres. Outpatient procedures do not require an overnight stay. The client goes to the outpatient site the day of surgery, has the operation, and leaves the same day. In these instances, the three phases of the perioperative period are shortened, and the postoperative phase continues at home. The nurse's role in assessing, teaching, and following up is vital to successful outcomes for clients who undergo day surgery.

Types of Surgery

Surgical procedures are commonly grouped according to (a) purpose, (b) degree of urgency, (c) level of invasiveness, (d) body part, (e) equipment used, and (f) degree of risk.

Purpose

Surgical procedures can be categorized according to their purpose (see Box 36.1).

Degree of Urgency

Surgery is classified by its urgency and necessity to preserve the client's life, body part, or body function. **Emergency surgery** is performed immediately to preserve function or the life of the client. Surgeries to control internal hemorrhage, trauma, or ruptured aneurysm are examples of emergency surgeries. **Urgent surgery** occurs when the surgical problem requires attention within 24 to 48 hours, such as surgery to remove a kidney stone that is not likely to be passed naturally by the individual. **Elective surgery** is performed when surgical intervention is the preferred treatment for a condition that is not imminently life threatening (but may ultimately threaten life or well-being) or to improve the client's life. Examples of elective surgeries include laparoscopic techniques (used either as a diagnostic tool or therapeutic access method), which are among the most common procedures in surgery worldwide, such as laparoscopic cholecystectomy for chronic gallbladder disease. Further elective surgeries include hip replacement surgery and plastic surgery procedures, such as breast reduction.

Level of Invasiveness

Surgery is also classified based on how invasive the procedure is with respect to the body. **Invasive (open) surgery** involves large incisions made to visualize and provide

---

> **BOX 36.1 PURPOSES OF SURGICAL PROCEDURES**
>
> Surgery is performed for various reasons:
>
> - *Diagnostic (exploratory):* Confirms or establishes a diagnosis (e.g., biopsy of a mass in a breast)
> - *Palliative:* Relieves or reduces pain or symptoms of a disease but does not cure (e.g., resection of nerve roots)
> - *Ablative or curative:* Removes a diseased body part (e.g., removal of a gallbladder: cholecystectomy)
> - *Constructive:* Restores function or appearance that has been lost or reduced (e.g., breast implant)
> - *Transplantation:* Replaces malfunctioning structures (e.g., kidney transplantation)

---

direct access to the area requiring surgery. Cardiac and abdominal surgeries are often invasive in nature. **Minimally invasive surgery** (sometimes referred to as *laparoscopic, closed,* or *keyhole surgery*) involves multiple small incisions through which specialized telescopic equipment is inserted to provide indirect visualization and manipulation of a specific body site or organ. Cholecystectomy (gallbladder removal) and arthroscopy (examination or repair of a joint) are examples of procedures commonly performed by using minimally invasive approaches. Some agencies perform cardiac and neurosurgery by using minimally invasive techniques. Generally, the patient experiences less trauma, pain, and scarring with minimally invasive techniques compared with more invasive approaches. However, both approaches can involve complications, such as infection, bleeding, and internal organ damage. Minimally invasive procedures are not necessarily minor surgery in that general anesthesia may be required.

Body Part

Surgical procedures may also be classified by the body part involved, for example, cardiac surgery (surgery performed on the heart); neurosurgery (surgery performed on the nervous system); and orthopedic surgery (surgery performed on bones and joints).

Type of Equipment

At times, the operative procedure is classified by the specialized equipment that is used. For example, robotic surgery involves the use of a surgical robot, which is programmed to perform procedures requiring a high degree of precision, such as in laparoscopic surgery. Laser surgery involves the use of a laser, commonly used in eye surgery.

Degree of Risk

Surgery is also classified as major or minor according to the degree of risk to the client. **Major surgery** involves a high degree of risk, for a variety of reasons: It may be complicated or prolonged; large losses of blood may occur; vital organs may be involved; or postoperative complications may be likely. Examples are an organ transplantation, open heart surgery, and the removal of a kidney. In contrast, **minor surgery** normally involves little risk, produces few complications, and is often performed in a day surgery. Examples are a breast biopsy, the removal of tonsils, and knee surgery.

The degree of risk involved in a surgical procedure is affected by the individual's age, general health, nutritional status, use of medications, and mental health.

AGE Neonates or infants and older adults are greater surgical risks than are children and adults. Age and developmental status affect children's ability to cope with the physiological and psychological stresses of surgery. Neonates and infants have a higher metabolic rate and a different physiological makeup compared with adults. These differences cause a substantially different response to a surgical procedure. For example, the blood volume in an infant is small, and its fluid reserves are limited, which increase the risk of volume depletion during surgery, resulting in inadequate oxygenation of body tissues. Because of the infant's relatively large body surface area and immature temperature regulatory mechanisms, the risk of hypothermia during surgery is significant. Other organ systems, such as the kidneys, the liver, and the immune system, have not achieved maturity in infants, affecting their ability to metabolize and eliminate drugs and resist infection.

Toddlers and older children are better able to withstand surgery physiologically, but they often fear separation from their parents, painful events (e.g., insertion of an intravenous), strangers, bodily injury or mutilation, and death. The child's developmental level and age-appropriate communication are important in implementing the pediatric plan of care. The parent–child relationship, the parents' coping abilities, and the preoperative teaching and support will affect how well the child is able to deal with these surgical fears and the level of anxiety experienced.

The older adult often has fewer physiological reserves to meet the extra demands caused by surgery. The physiological deficits of aging increase the surgical risk for the older adult. For example, because of a lower percentage of body water, decreased kidney function, and a decreased thirst response, older adults are at greater risk for fluid and electrolyte imbalances. Many older adults demonstrate changes in liver and kidney functions, both of which can affect response to anesthesia and other medications that may be administered during the perioperative period. The older adult may be poorly nourished, which can impair healing. Declines in sensory function (e.g., hearing and vision) or the presence of dementia make it more difficult to understand directions and teaching. In addition, the older adult is more likely to have a chronic disease, such as cardiovascular disease, chronic lung disease, or diabetes, that affects healing and responses to medication and surgery.

GENERAL HEALTH   Surgery is least risky when the client's general health is good. Any health problem (e.g., illness or desease) can increase the risks associated with surgery. Of particular concern are respiratory tract infections, which, together with general anesthesia, can adversely affect respiratory function. Common health problems that increase surgical risk and may lead to the decision to postpone or cancel surgery are listed in Box 36.2.

NUTRITIONAL STATUS   Adequate nutrition is required for normal tissue repair. Surgery increases the body's need for nutrients for tissue healing and recovery during the postoperative period. Obesity and malnutrition increase surgical risk.

BOX 36.2   HEALTH PROBLEMS THAT INCREASE SURGICAL RISK

These health problems can place the perioperative client at increased risk:

- Malnutrition can lead to delayed wound healing, infection, and reduced energy. Protein and vitamins are needed for wound healing; vitamin K is essential for blood clotting.
- Obesity can lead to hypertension, impaired cardiac function, and impaired respiratory ventilation. Clients who are obese are also more likely to have delayed wound healing and wound infection because adipose tissue impedes blood circulation and its delivery of the nutrients, antibodies, and enzymes required for wound healing.
- Cardiac conditions, such as angina pectoris, history of myocardial infarction, hypertension, and heart failure, weaken the heart. Well-controlled cardiac problems generally pose minimal operative risk.
- Blood coagulation disorders can lead to severe bleeding, hemorrhage, and subsequent shock.
- Respiratory tract infections or chronic obstructive lung disease adversely affect pulmonary function, especially when exacerbated by the effects of general anesthesia. They also predispose the client to postoperative lung infections.
- Renal disease impairs regulation of the body's fluids and electrolytes and excretion of drugs and other toxins.
- Diabetes mellitus predisposes the client to wound infection and delayed healing.
- Liver disease (e.g., cirrhosis) impairs the liver's abilities to detoxify medications used during surgery, produce the prothrombin necessary for blood clotting, and metabolize nutrients essential for healing.
- Uncontrolled neurological disease, such as epilepsy, can result in seizures during surgery or recovery.

Obesity contributes to postoperative complications, such as pneumonia, wound infections, and wound dehiscence (separation of wound edges). Both overweight and underweight clients are vulnerable to pressure ulcer formation because of positioning required for surgery.

Protein, vitamins, and minerals are essential for healthy wound healing (see Chapter 35). A malnourished client is at risk for delayed wound healing, wound infection, and fluid and electrolyte alterations. If a client has serious malnutrition, the surgery may be postponed to improve the client's nutritional status. If the surgery cannot be delayed, parenteral or enteral nutrition may be initiated.

MEDICATION HISTORY   The regular use of certain prescribed and over-the-counter (OTC) medications can increase surgical risk. Each client situation is assessed for the risks and benefits of these medications relative to the nature of the surgery. The following medications pose challenges in the management of the perioperative client:

- *Anticoagulants* increase the risk for hemorrhage. A risk-benefit analysis must be conducted relative to the risks of anticoagulation (bleeding), the benefits (prevention of thrombus), and the nature of the surgery. For people taking *antiplatelet agents,* such as acetylsalicylic acid (Aspirin), if the risk of bleeding exceeds the risk associated with thrombosis, it will generally be recommended that they discontinue the therapy for 7 to 10 days before the surgery. Unlike acetylsalicylic acid, the effects of which are irreversible, the antiplatelet effects of nonsteroidal anti-inflammatory drugs (NSAIDS, e.g., ibuprofen) last only hours, so preoperative cessation is of shorter duration, generally 24 to 48 hours.

- *Antidepressants,* particularly monoamine oxidase inhibitors (MAOIs) and St. John's wort, a herbal product, increase the hypotensive action of certain anesthetic agents.
- *Antihypertensives* interact with anesthetic agents and can cause bradycardia, hypotension, and impaired circulation.
- *Tranquilizers* can interact with anesthetics, increasing the risk of respiratory depression.
- *Insulin* may need to be adjusted in the perioperative period to account for the fasting or altered nutritional intake of the client; the stress of surgery can cause a rise in blood glucose.
- *Diuretics,* particularly thiazides, can affect fluid and electrolyte balance (particularly potassium) after surgery.
- *Corticosteroids,* with prolonged use, decrease the anti-inflammatory effect and can interfere with wound healing and increase the risk of infection. Abrupt cessation of glucocorticoids can lead to adrenal crisis.
- *Herbal medications,* such as garlic, ginkgo, and ginseng, can affect bleeding time; ephedra can cause cardiovascular instability; ginseng can cause hypoglycemia; kava and valerian can potentiate the sedative effect of anesthetics.

Clients may be unaware of the potential adverse interactions of medications and fail to report the use of medications for conditions unrelated to the indication for surgery. The nurse who collects a preoperative history should ask the client about the use of commonly prescribed medications and OTC preparations, including natural products and recreational drugs that the client takes.

MENTAL HEALTH STATUS Alterations in cognitive function (e.g., dementia or a developmental disability) or presence of a mental health problem (e.g., panic disorder or schizophrenia) can affect the client's ability to understand and cope with the stresses of surgery. Symptoms of confusion, disorientation, and agitation can be aggravated by the change of environment in the hospital, interfering with the client's ability to cooperate with preoperative and postoperative care.

Extreme anxiety increases surgical risk and interferes with the client's ability to process information and respond appropriately to instructions. In some instances,

professional counselling is indicated before surgery. It is also important to determine whether clients have coping skills and support systems to help them.

Preoperative Phase

Preoperative Consent

Before any surgical procedure, clients must sign a consent form, which is generally supplied by the agency. This requirement protects the individual's autonomy and ensures that they have a clear understanding about the surgery, the benefits, and the risks. It also protects the hospital and the health care personnel from a claim by the client or family that permission was not granted. The consent form becomes a part of the client's record and goes to the operating room with the client.

The surgeon maintains legal responsibility for ensuring that the client is giving *informed* consent and ensuring that the client understands the procedure to be performed. If it is not clear that the client understands and consents to the surgery, the nurse has the responsibility of contacting the surgeon before surgery proceeds.

Preoperative informed consent should include the following:

- Nature of and reason for the surgery
- Name and qualifications of the surgeon performing the surgery
- Risks of the procedure and its potential outcomes (both positive and negative)
- Possible alternative measures
- The right of the client to refuse consent or later withdraw consent

Informed consent is possible only when the client understands the information being provided, that is, speaks the language and is conscious, mentally competent, and not under the influence of sedatives. The client must also be legally capable. In Canada, depending on the laws of the province or territory, a minor under a certain age cannot legally give consent or can give consent only for certain procedures (e.g., in some provinces, a 14-year-old can give consent for procedures not requiring admission, such as abortion, but not for procedures requiring admission, such as cardiac surgery). Nurses must be aware of their responsibilities regarding consents and of the particular hospital policies. See Chapter 6 for further information on informed consent.

Assessing

Preoperative assessment includes collecting and reviewing specific client data to determine the client's needs throughout the perioperative experience.

NURSING HISTORY The nursing history obtained before surgery provides client data that help the nurse plan preoperative and postoperative care. Most agencies have preoperative assessment forms to ensure comprehensive assessment. The Assessment: Interview box summarizes essential preoperative information that should be collected in the nursing history. It is also important that the nursing history include an assessment of any preoperative concerns of the client and the family or significant others.

PHYSICAL ASSESSMENT Preoperatively, a complete physical assessment is performed, paying particular attention to systems that could affect the client's response to anesthesia or surgery. A brief, or mini, mental status examination provides valuable baseline data for evaluating the client's mental status and alertness after surgery. It is also important to evaluate the client's ability to understand what is happening. For example, assessment of hearing and vision help guide perioperative teaching.

Respiratory and cardiovascular assessment not only provides baseline data for evaluating the client's perioperative status but may also alert caregivers to a problem (e.g., respiratory infection or irregular pulse rate) that could affect the client's response to surgery and anesthesia. Other systems (e.g., gastrointestinal, genitourinary, and musculoskeletal) are examined to provide baseline data (see Chapter 28).

SCREENING TESTS The surgeon or anesthesiologist orders preoperative diagnostic tests. Abnormalities may warrant treatment before surgery. The nurse's responsibility is to check the orders carefully, to see that they are carried out, and to ensure that the results are obtained and entered into the client's record before surgery. Table 36.1 on the next page lists preoperative screening tests that may be prescribed on the basis of the Canadian Anesthesiologists' Society recommendations (Merchant, Chartrand, Dain, Dobson, Kurrek, LeDez, Morgan, & Shukla, 2012).

ASSESSMENT INTERVIEW

Preoperative Assessment Data

The following information must be gathered in the nursing history before surgery:

- *Current health status.* Essential information includes general health status and the presence of any chronic diseases, such as diabetes or asthma, which may affect the client's response to surgery or anesthesia. Note any physical limitations that may affect the client's mobility or ability to communicate after surgery, as well as any prostheses, such as hearing aids or contact lenses.

- *Allergies.* Include allergies to prescription and nonprescription drugs, food allergies, and allergies to tape, latex, soaps, or antiseptic agents. Some food allergies indicate a potential reaction to drugs or substances used during surgery or diagnostic procedures; for example, an allergy to seafood alerts the nurse to a potential allergy to iodine-based dyes or soaps commonly used in hospitals; people who are allergic to such foods as kiwi, banana, avocados, and chestnuts may also have an allergy to latex in what is called latex-food syndrome.

- *Medications.* List all current medications (prescribed and OTC). It may be vital to maintain a blood level of some medications (e.g., anticonvulsants) throughout the surgical experience; others, such as anticoagulants or Aspirin, increase the risks of surgery and anesthesia and need to be discontinued several days before surgery. It is important to include in the list any herbal remedies the client currently takes.

- *Previous surgeries and anesthesia history.* Previous surgical and anesthesia (general and local) experiences can influence the client's physical and psychological responses to surgery or may reveal unexpected responses to anesthesia, such as cardiac arrest or malignant hyperthermia crisis.

- *Mental status.* The client's mental status and ability to understand and respond appropriately can affect the entire perioperative experience. Note any developmental disabilities, mental health problems, history of dementia, or excessive anxiety related to the procedure.

- *Understanding of the surgical procedure and anesthesia.* The client should have a clear understanding of the planned procedure and what to expect during and after surgery, as well as the expected outcome of the procedure.

- *Smoking.* Smokers may have more difficulty clearing respiratory secretions after surgery, increasing the risk of postoperative complications, such as pneumonia and atelectasis. Smoking also results in reduced oxygen-carrying capacity, increasing the risk of hypoxemia and delayed wound healing. Nicotine stimulates the surgical stress response, leading to increased workload for the heart.

- *Alcohol and other mind-altering substances.* Use of substances that affect the central nervous system, liver, or other body systems can affect the client's response to anesthesia, surgery, and postoperative recovery.

- *Coping.* Clients with a healthy self-concept who have successfully employed appropriate coping mechanisms in the past are better able to deal with the stressors associated with surgery.

- *Social resources.* Determine the availability of family or other caregivers as well as the client's social support network. These resources are important to the client's recovery, particularly for the client undergoing same-day or short-stay surgery.

- *Cultural and spiritual considerations.* Culture and spirituality influence the client's response to surgery; respecting cultural and spiritual beliefs and practices can reduce preoperative anxiety and improve recovery.

TABLE 36.1 Preoperative Screening Tests

Test	Rationale
Complete blood count (CBC)	Red blood cells (RBCs), hemoglobin (Hgb), and hematocrit (Hct) are important to the oxygen-carrying capacity of blood; white blood cells (WBCs) are an indicator of immune function; generally required for people with chronic cardiovascular, pulmonary, renal, or hepatic disease; malignancy; known or suspected anemia; and those undergoing major open surgery
Blood grouping and cross-matching	Determined in case blood transfusion is required during or after surgery
Serum electrolytes: sodium (Na^+), potassium (K^+), calcium (Ca^{2+}), magnesium (Mg^{2+}), chloride (Cl^-), bicarbonate (HCO_3^-)	To evaluate fluid and electrolyte status; generally required in any person at risk of imbalance (e.g., chronic illness, digoxin or diuretic therapy)
Fasting blood glucose	High levels may indicate undiagnosed diabetes mellitus
Blood urea nitrogen (BUN) and creatinine	To evaluate renal function
Alanine aminotransferase (ALT), aspartate aminotransferase (AST), and bilirubin	To evaluate liver function
Serum albumin and total protein	To evaluate nutritional status; generally only in high-risk clients
International normalized ratio (INR) and activated partial thromboplastin time (APTT)	To evaluate coagulation; generally recommended for people with liver disease or taking anticoagulant therapy
Urinalysis	To determine urine composition and possible abnormal components (e.g., protein or glucose) or infection
Chest x-ray	To evaluate pulmonary status and heart size
Electrocardiograph (ECG)	To identify pre-existing cardiac problems or disease
Pregnancy test (serum beta-human chorionic gonadotropin [β-HCG])	To determine whether the client is pregnant; generally recommended in all females of childbearing age
Screening for sickle cell disease	To determine risk of sickle cell disease in genetically predisposed clients

Diagnosing

Several nursing diagnoses that may be appropriate for the preoperative client include anxiety or uncertainty related to lack of familiarity with the surgical experience, effects of surgery on ability to function in usual roles, outcome of diagnostic/exploratory surgery, risk of death, loss of control during anesthesia or waking up during anesthesia; perceived inadequate postoperative analgesia; change in health status or body image; disturbed sleep related to hospital routines, psychological stress; and anticipatory grieving related to perceived loss of body part associated with planned surgery.

Planning

The overall goal in the preoperative period is to ensure that the client is mentally and physically prepared for surgery. Examples of nursing activities to meet this goal are discussed in the "Implementing" section that follows.

Planning should involve the client, family, and significant others. Preoperative care planning and teaching interventions are usually done on an outpatient basis, either in person or via a telephone interview by the perioperative nurse.

PLANNING FOR HOME CARE For the perioperative client, discharge planning begins before admission for the planned procedure. Early planning to meet the discharge needs of the client is particularly important for outpatient procedures, as generally these clients are discharged within hours after the procedure is performed.

Discharge planning incorporates an assessment of the client's and his or her family's or significant other's abilities and resources for care, financial resources, and the need for referrals and home health services. However, the extent of discharge planning and home care will vary significantly for clients having different types of surgery.

Implementing

The major nursing activity to ensure that the client is prepared for surgery is preoperative teaching.

PREOPERATIVE TEACHING Preoperative teaching is a vital part of nursing care. Preoperative teaching reduces clients' anxiety and postoperative complications, as well as increasing their satisfaction with the surgical experience. Effective preoperative teaching also facilitates the client's return to work and other activities of daily living (ADLs). Four dimensions of preoperative teaching have been identified as important to clients:

1. *Information, including what will happen to the client, when, and what the client will experience, such as expected sensations and discomfort.* The nurse needs to listen carefully and attentively to the client to identify specific concerns and fears. Typical questions include the following: What will happen during surgery? How will I feel after the operation? What will the surgeon find? How long will I be in the hospital? Will I have pain? The nurse and other members of the health care team (e.g., surgeon, anesthesiologist) should respond to questions accordingly. The nurse can introduce the client to the pain scale in use in the setting and discuss the nature of the pain the client can anticipate as well as provide information about pain management techniques (see Chapter 30).

2. *Psychosocial support to reduce anxiety.* The nurse provides support by actively listening and providing accurate information. It is important to rectify any misbeliefs the client may have.

3. *The roles of the client and support people in preoperative preparation, the surgical procedure, and during the postoperative phase.* Understanding his or her role during the perioperative experience increases the client's sense of control and reduces anxiety. This includes what will be expected of the client, desired behaviours, self-care activities, and what the client can do to facilitate recovery.

4. *Skills training.* These skills include moving, breathing deeply, coughing, splinting incisions with the hands or a pillow, and using an incentive spirometer.

If the client is scheduled for outpatient surgery, preoperative teaching is often provided before the day of surgery by using some combination of audiovisual and verbal and written instructions. The client may have an appointment with the outpatient surgery staff (usually scheduled to coincide with preoperative diagnostic testing) to discuss preoperative concerns and implement the teaching plan. Written instructions are always provided to reinforce verbal teaching. Teaching is further reinforced on admission the day of surgery and before discharge from the PACU. Preoperative instructions are summarized in the Teaching: Clinical box.

TEACHING | **CLINICAL**

Preoperative Instructions

Clients need to understand the preoperative instructions they are given and what to expect immediately after surgery:

PREOPERATIVE REGIMEN

- Explain the need for preoperative tests (e.g., laboratory, x-ray, ECG).
- Discuss bowel preparation, if required.
- Discuss skin preparation, including operative area and preoperative bath or shower.
- Discuss preoperative medications, if prescribed.
- Explain the need to avoid smoking and alcohol consumption preoperatively. Provide support, if necessary.
- Explain individual therapies ordered by the physician, such as intravenous therapy, the insertion of a urinary catheter or nasogastric tube, use of a spirometer, or antiembolism stockings.
- Discuss the visit by the anesthesiologist.
- Explain the need to restrict or eliminate food and oral fluid intake before surgery. Follow the institution's or the Canadian Anesthesiologists' Society's guidelines (Merchant et al., 2012), discussed later.
- Provide a general timetable for perioperative events, including the time of surgery.

- Discuss the need to remove jewellery (including body piercings), makeup, and prostheses (e.g., eyeglasses, hearing aids, dentures, wigs) immediately before surgery. In some cases, the surgeon may leave instructions for the client to leave hearing aids and eyeglasses on to enable better communication.
- Inform the client about the preoperative holding area, and give the location of the waiting room for support people (a surgical liaison nurse may visit support people intraoperatively to update them on the condition of the surgical patient).
- Teach deep-breathing and coughing exercises, leg exercises, ways to turn and move (see Skill 36.1 on the next page), and splinting techniques.
- Complete the preoperative checklist.

POSTOPERATIVE REGIMEN

- Discuss the postanesthesia care unit (PACU) routines and emergency equipment.
- Review type and frequency of assessment activities.
- Discuss pain management.
- Explain usual activity restrictions and precautions related to getting up for the first time postoperatively.
- Describe usual dietary alterations.

(continued)

TEACHING CLINICAL *(continued)*

- Discuss postoperative wound care and any drainage devices.
- Provide an explanation and tour of the intensive care unit (ICU) if the client is to be transferred there postoperatively.

OUTPATIENT SURGICAL CLIENTS

- Confirm the place and time of surgery, including when to arrive (generally 1 to 1.5 hours before scheduled surgery) and where to register (e.g., reception desk).
- Discuss what to wear (e.g., clients having hand surgery should wear a garment with large sleeve openings to fit over a bulky dressing; all clients need to leave valuables at home).

- Explain the need for a responsible adult to drive or accompany the client home, and arrange a place for them to meet. Discuss discharge criteria and how long the client should expect to stay in the health care facility postoperatively.
- Discuss medications, including specific preoperative medications and the client's current medication regimen.
- Provide anticipatory guidance about the expected recovery trajectory so that the client can make necessary plans (e.g., childcare may need to be arranged; special dietary foods may need to be purchased).
- Communicate (generally a telephone call) the day before surgery to confirm time of surgery and arrival time, and call again the evening after surgery to assess progress.

When the client is a child, addressing the fears and anxieties of both the child and the family is vital. Parents need to know what to expect and to be able to express their concerns. Parents should be considered members of the perioperative team and be allowed to participate in providing as much care as possible.

Skill 36.1 provides guidelines for teaching clients about moving, leg exercises, deep breathing, and coughing. See also the Lifespan Considerations box on preoperative teaching and the Teaching: Home Care box on postoperative teaching on page 1067.

SKILL 36.1 TEACHING MOVING, LEG EXERCISES, DEEP BREATHING, AND COUGHING

PURPOSES

Moving
- To promote venous return
- To enhance lung expansion and mobilize secretions
- To stimulate gastrointestinal mobility
- To facilitate early ambulation

Leg Exercises
- To promote venous return, thereby preventing thrombophlebitis and thrombus formation

Deep Breathing and Coughing
- To enhance lung expansion and mobilize secretions, thereby preventing **atelectasis** (collapse of the alveoli) and pneumonia

ASSESSMENT

Assess
- Vital signs
- Pain or discomfort
- Temperature and colour of feet and legs
- Breath sounds
- Presence of dyspnea or cough
- Learning needs of the client
- Client's readiness to learn (e.g., level of anxiety)
- The client's experience with previous surgeries and anesthesia

PLANNING

Before commencing to teach moving, leg exercises, deep-breathing exercises, and coughing, determine (a) the type of surgery, (b) the time of the surgery, (c) the name of the surgeon, (d) the preoperative orders, (e) the agency's policies for preoperative care, and (f) the learning needs of the client. Also, verify that the physician has completed the medical history and physical examination and that the consent form has been signed by the client or the family or substitute decision maker.

Equipment
- Pillow
- Teaching materials (e.g., DVD, online video, written materials) if available at the agency

IMPLEMENTATION

Preparation
Ensure that potential distracters (e.g., pain, TV, visitors) to teaching are not present. Family and significant others should be included in the teaching plan, if the client agrees and it is appropriate.

Performance
1. Before performing the procedure, introduce yourself and verify the client's identity using two identifiers or per agency protocol. Explain to the client what you are going to teach and the importance of the client's participation in the exercises he or she is going to be taught.

2. Perform hand hygiene, and follow other appropriate infection prevention and control procedures.

3. Provide for client privacy.

4. Show the client ways to turn in bed and to get out of bed.
   - Instruct a client who will have a right abdominal incision or a right-sided chest incision to turn to the left side of the bed and sit up as follows:
     a. Flex the knees.
     b. Splint the wound by holding the left arm and hand or a small pillow against the incision.
     c. Turn to the left while pushing with the right foot and grasping a partial side rail on the left side of the bed with the right hand.
     d. Come to a sitting position on the side of the bed by using the right arm and hand to push down against the mattress and swinging the feet over the edge of the bed.
   - Teach a client with a left abdominal or left-sided chest incision to perform the same procedure but splint with the right arm and turn to the right.
   - For clients with orthopedic surgery (e.g., hip surgery), use special aids, such as a trapeze, to assist with movement.

5. Teach the client the following three leg exercises:
   - Alternate dorsiflexion and plantar flexion of the feet. **Rationale: This exercise is sometimes referred to as *calf pumping* because it alternately contracts and relaxes the calf muscles, including the gastrocnemius muscles.** See ❶.

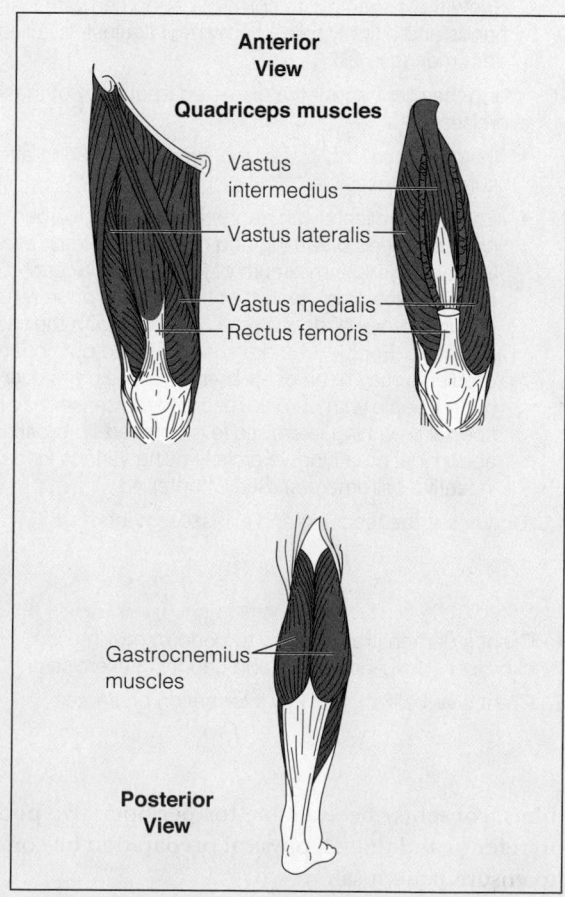

Anterior View

Quadriceps muscles

Vastus intermedius

Vastus lateralis

Vastus medialis

Rectus femoris

Gastrocnemius muscles

Posterior View

❶ Leg muscles: anterior and posterior views

   - Have the client flex and extend the knees and press the backs of the knees into the bed while dorsiflexing the feet (see ❷). Instruct clients who cannot raise their legs to do isometric exercises that contract and relax the muscles.

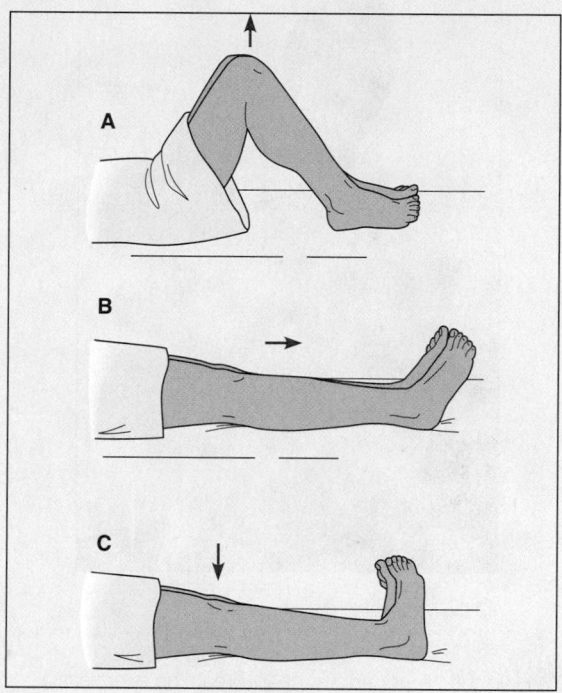

A

B

C

❷ Flexing and extending the knees

   - Have the client raise and lower the legs alternately from the surface of the bed. Have the client flex the knee of the stable leg and extend the knee of the moving leg (see ❸). **Rationale: This exercise contracts and relaxes the quadriceps muscles**.

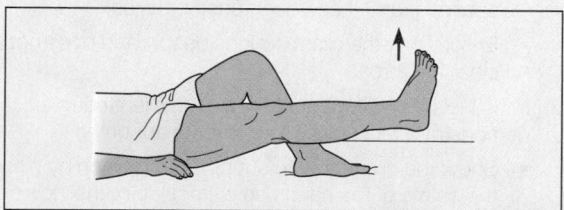

❸ Raising and lowering the legs

6. Demonstrate deep-breathing (diaphragmatic) exercises as follows:
   - Place your hands palms down on the border of your rib cage, and inhale slowly and evenly through the nose until the greatest chest expansion is achieved (see ❹).
   - Hold your breath for 2 to 3 seconds.
   - Then, exhale slowly through the mouth.
   - Continue exhalation until maximum chest contraction has been achieved.

(continued)

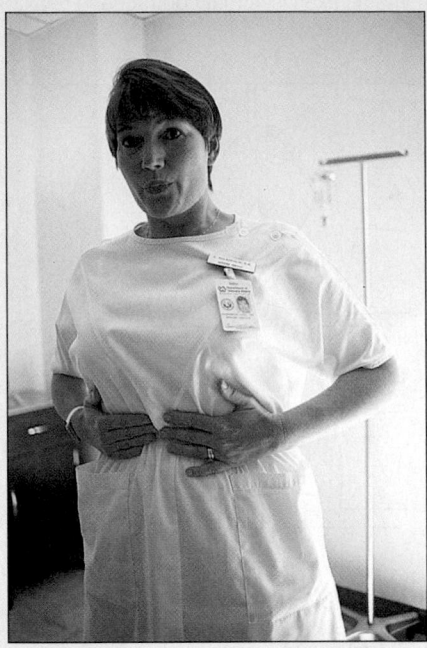

④ Demonstrating deep breathing

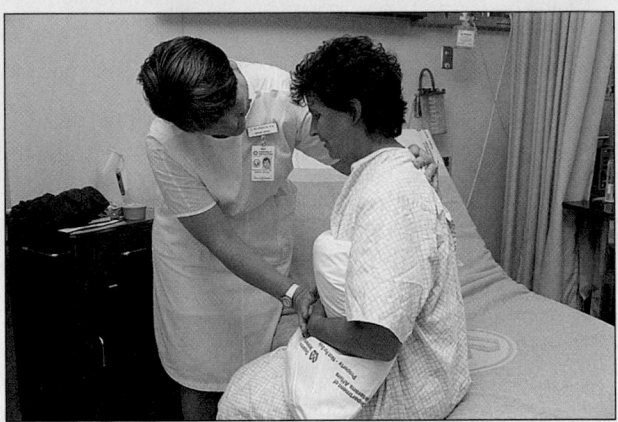

⑤ Splinting an incision with a pillow while coughing

7. Help the client perform deep-breathing exercises.
- Ask the client to assume a sitting position.
- Place the palms of your hands on the border of the client's rib cage to assess respiratory depth.
- Ask the client to perform deep breathing, as described in step 6.

8. Instruct the client to cough voluntarily after five deep inhalations.
- Ask the client to inhale deeply, hold the breath for a few seconds, and then cough once or twice.
- Ensure that the client coughs deeply and does not just clear the throat.

9. If the incision will be painful when the client coughs, demonstrate techniques to splint the abdomen.
- Show the client how to support the incision by placing the palms of the hands on either side of the incision

site or directly over the incision site, holding the palm of one hand over the other. **Rationale: Coughing uses the abdominal and other accessory respiratory muscles. Splinting the incision can reduce pain while coughing if the incision is near any of these muscles.**
- Show the client how to splint the abdomen with clasped hands and a firmly rolled pillow held against the client's abdomen (see ⑤).

10. Inform the client about the expected frequency of these exercises.
- Instruct the client to start the exercises as soon after surgery as possible.
- Encourage clients with abdominal or chest surgery to carry out deep breathing and coughing at least every 2 hours, taking a minimum of five breaths at each session. Note, however, that the number of breaths and frequency of deep breathing varies with the client's condition. People who are susceptible to pulmonary problems may need deep-breathing exercises every hour. People with chronic respiratory disease may need special breathing exercises (e.g., pursed-lip breathing, abdominal breathing, exercises using various kinds of incentive spirometers). See Chapter 43.

11. Document the teaching and all assessments.

EVALUATION

Document the outcome of the teaching plan, such as the following:

- Client's demonstrated ability to perform moving, leg exercises, deep-breathing, and coughing exercises
- Client's verbalization of key information presented

PHYSICAL PREPARATION Preoperative preparation includes the following areas: nutrition and fluids, elimination, hygiene, medications, rest, care of valuables and prostheses, special orders, and surgical skin preparation. In many agencies, a preoperative checklist is used on the day of surgery. The nurse checks the agency's forms and follows appropriate documenting procedures. It is essential that all pertinent records (laboratory records, x-ray

films, consents) be available for perioperative personnel to refer to and that all physical preparation be completed to ensure patient safety.

Nutrition and Fluids Adequate hydration and nutrition promote healing. Nurses need to identify and record any signs of malnutrition or fluid imbalance. Intake and output is recorded in patients receiving IV fluids or if the

LIFESPAN CONSIDERATIONS

Preoperative Teaching

CHILDREN

- Parents need to know what to expect and to be able to express their concerns.
- Separation from parents often is the child's greatest fear; the time of separation should be minimized and parents allowed to interact with the child both immediately preceding and following the surgery.
- Teaching and communicating with children (both timing and content) should be geared to the child's developmental level and cognitive abilities (e.g., "You will have a sore tummy.").
- Play is an effective teaching tool with children (e.g., the child can put a bandage on an incision on a doll).

OLDER ADULTS

- Assess hearing and visual abilities to ensure the older client hears and sees the necessary information.
- Assess short-term memory. Presenting one focused idea at a time and repeating or reinforcing information may be necessary.
- Older adults are at greater risk for postoperative complications, such as pneumonia. Reinforce moving and deep-breathing and coughing exercises.
- Assess potential postoperative needs at this time. Arrangements can be made preoperatively to obtain necessary items. Examples are medical equipment, such as walkers, raised

toilet seats, bed trapezes, Meals on Wheels, and help with transportation.
- If the older client will need to be in extended care for a period of time after surgery, this is the time to initiate these plans.
- Assess the client for risk of pressure ulcer development (e.g., Braden Scale) postoperatively and ensure that preventive intraoperative and postoperative measures are in place to prevent skin breakdown (see Chapter 35).

TEACHING | HOME CARE

Postoperative Instructions

Adult clients want information about activities they normally perform while they are recovering at home. This is important information for all surgical clients and particularly clients having the surgery as outpatients. Discuss the following areas:

- *Food.* Eat small portions at first because anesthesia and certain analgesics slow gastric emptying.
- *Bowel movements.* Constipation occurs frequently because of decreased gastrointestinal mobility from different causes (e.g., anesthesia, decreased activity, opioids). Discuss strategies to prevent constipation.
- *Sexual activity.* Intimacy, such as hugging and kissing, is allowed for clients when they feel like it. Full sexual intercourse cannot be resumed until wound soreness and tenderness are resolved, which generally takes approximately 2 to 4 weeks. Check with the surgeon for gynecological procedures.

- *Wound care.* Discuss relevant wound care, including the signs and symptoms of infection and when to notify the surgeon.
- *Lifting.* Be specific about weight limits, if appropriate. Relate the weight limit to everyday items (e.g., 4 L of milk weighs 4 kg).
- *Pain.* Provide information about the client's analgesia. Ask the client to describe his or her daily activities and discuss ways to avoid or reduce painful activities.
- *Bathing.* Check with the surgeon because some prefer the wound to be kept dry. If allowed, tell the client to shower, letting the warm water wash over the incision and gently pat the incision dry.
- *Activities.* Advise the client that he or she will tire easily and to plan short activities with frequent rest breaks.

person is at risk for fluid imbalance (e.g., renal failure). The order "NPO [no food by mouth] after midnight" has been a long-standing tradition because it was believed that a lengthy fasting period was needed to reduce the risk for vomiting and aspiration following the use of anesthetic agents. Reevaluation and research, however, do not support this tradition for patients at normal risk of aspiration or regurgitation. Drinking clear fluids up to a few hours before surgery does not increase the risk of regurgitation during or after surgery and leads to improved comfort and behaviour in the postoperative period (Brady, Kinn, O'Rourke, Randhawa, & Stuart, 2005). The Canadian Anesthesiologists' Society (Merchant, et al., 2012) guidelines for minimum fasting times before elective surgical procedures are summarized in Box 36.3

on the next page. Emergent or urgent procedures should be undertaken after considering the risk of delaying surgery versus the risk of aspiration of gastric contents.

Elimination Enemas before surgery are no longer routine, but cleansing enemas may be ordered if bowel surgery is planned to help prevent contamination of the surgical area by fecal matter.

Before pelvic or abdominal surgery, a retention catheter may be ordered to ensure that the urinary bladder remains empty so as to prevent inadvertent injury to the bladder during surgery. Patients undergoing high-risk or lengthy surgeries (e.g., cardiac) may have a retention catheter inserted to monitor urine production during the surgical event. If the patient does not have a catheter, it

BOX 36.3 MINIMUM FASTING GUIDELINES FOR ELECTIVE SURGICAL PROCEDURES

Before elective surgery, these fasting times should be followed:

- 8 hours after a meal that includes meat, fried food, or fatty foods
- 6 hours after a light meal (such as toast and a clear fluid)
- 6 hours after ingestion of infant formula or nonhuman milk
- 4 hours after ingestion of breast milk
- 2 hours after clear fluids

Source: Based on Merchant, R., Chartrand, D., Dain, S., Dobson, J., Kurrek, M., LeDez, K., Morgan, P., & Shukla, R. (2012). *Guidelines to the practice of anesthesia* (Rev. ed. 2012). *Canadian Journal of Anesthesia, 59*(1), 62–102.

is important to empty the bladder before receiving preoperative medications.

Skin preparation (hygiene, hair, nails) To reduce the risk for surgical site infections, preoperative *antiseptic prophylaxis of the skin* and *no hair removal OR appropriate hair removal if necessary* are recommended (Safer HealthCare Now! 2010). Preoperative antiseptic prophylaxis of the skin is achieved by a thorough cleansing with a chlorhexidine-based solution, preferably with no-rinse disposable chlorhexidine gluconate impregnated washcloths. Depending on the product, the patient either showers or bathes the entire body paying increased attention to the surgical site. This preoperative skin preparation is combined with intraoperative surgical skin preparation with alcohol-based chlorhexidine that is not washed off until at least 6 hours after surgery.

In the past, shaving hair from around the surgical site was a routine practice. It is now known that shaving causes microscopic skin abrasions that provide a portal of entry for microorganisms, a risk factor in the development of surgical site infections. Now, NO hair removal is recommended (Safer Healthcare Now! 2010). If, however, hair needs to be removed (such as for neurosurgery), Safer Healthcare Now! recommends that it be removed with clippers (NOT razors) and the hair is clipped only within 2 hours of the surgery (not in the operating room). In addition, no shaving in the vicinity of the incision is recommended for 7 days before surgery.

The patient's nails should be trimmed and free of polish, and all cosmetics should be removed so that the nail beds, skin, and lips are visible when circulation is assessed during the perioperative phases.

Intraoperatively the patient may be required to wear a surgical cap to contain the patient's hair. Before going into the operating room all hairpins or clips are removed as they may cause pressure or accidental damage to the scalp when the patient is unconscious. The patient also removes personal clothing and puts on a hospital gown.

Medications The anesthesiologist may temporarily discontinue routinely taken medications on the day of surgery. In some settings, preoperative medications are given to the patient before going to the operating room. Common preoperative medications include the following:

- *Sedatives and tranquilizers,* such as lorazepam (Ativan) and diazepam (Valium), to reduce anxiety and ease anesthesia induction
- *Opioids,* such as morphine, to provide sedation and reduce the required amount of anesthetic
- *Anticholinergics,* such as atropine, scopolamine, and glycopyrrolate, to reduce oral and pulmonary secretions and prevent laryngospasm
- *Histamine-receptor antagonists,* such as cimetidine and ranitidine, to reduce gastric fluid volume and gastric acidity
- *Neuroleptanalgesic agents,* such as droperidol and fentanyl, to induce general calmness and sleepiness
- *Antibiotics,* such as cephalosporins administered within 1 hour of the surgical incision for prophylaxis against surgical site infection (Safer Healthcare Now! 2010).

Preoperative medications must be given at a scheduled time or *on call,* that is, when the operating room notifies the nurse to give the medication.

Sleep Nurses should do everything to help the patient sleep the night before surgery. Often, a sedative is ordered. Adequate sleep helps the patient manage the stress of surgery and helps healing.

Care of Valuables Valuables, such as jewellery and money, should be labelled and placed in safekeeping if the client's support people cannot take them home. Removing jewellery also includes body-piercing jewellery; there is a risk of injury from burns if an electrosurgical unit is used. If a patient cannot or does not want to remove a wedding band, the nurse can tape it in place. Bands must be removed, however, if there is danger of the fingers swelling after surgery. Situations warranting removal include surgery on or cast application to an arm and a mastectomy that involves removal of the lymph nodes.

Care of Prostheses All prostheses (artificial body parts, such as partial or complete dentures, contact lenses, and artificial limbs), as well as eyeglasses, wigs, and false eyelashes, must be removed before surgery. Hearing aids are often left in place and the operating room personnel notified.

In some hospitals, dentures are placed in a locked storage area; in others, they are placed in labelled containers and kept at the patient's bedside. Partial dentures can become dislodged and obstruct an unconscious patient's breathing. The nurse also checks for the presence of chewing gum or loose teeth, a common problem with 5- or 6-year-olds undergoing tonsillectomy. Loose teeth can become dislodged and be aspirated during anesthesia.

Special Orders The nurse checks the surgeon's orders for special requirements (e.g., the insertion of a nasogastric tube before surgery, the administration of medications, such as insulin).

SAFETY PROTOCOLS Protocols to ensure correct patient, correct site, and correct procedure have been developed after sentinel events involving wrong person, wrong site, and wrong procedure surgical errors. The Surgical Safety Checklist and Scorecard (Canadian Patient Safety Institute, 2012) (Box 36.4) is increasingly being used across Canada to ensure patient safety throughout the operative experience. The checklist

---

BOX 36.4 SURGICAL SAFETY CHECKLIST AND SCORECARD

BRIEFING – Before induction of anesthesia
Hand-off from ER, Nursing Unit or ICU

☐ Anesthesia equipment safety check completed
☐ Patient information confirmed
- Identity (2 identifiers)
- Consent(s)
- Site and procedure
- Site, side, and level marked
- Clinical documentation
- History, physical, labs, biopsy, and x-rays

☐ Review final test results
☐ Confirm essential imaging displayed
☐ ASA Class
☐ Allergies
☐ Medications
- Antibiotic prophylaxis: double dose?
- Glycemic control
- Beta-blockers
- Anticoagulant therapy (e.g., Warfarin)?

☐ VTE Prophylaxis
- Anticoagulant
- Mechanical

☐ Difficult Airway / Aspiration Risk
- Confirm equipment and assistance available

☐ Monitoring
- Pulse oximetry, ECG, BP, arterial line, CVP, temperature and urine catheter

☐ Blood loss
- Anticipated to be more than 500 mL (adult) or more than 7 mL/kg (child)
- Blood products required and available
- Patient grouped, and screened and cross_matched

☐ Surgeon(s) review(s)
- Specific patient concerns, critical steps, and special instruments or implants

☐ Anesthesiologist(s) review(s)
- Specific patient concerns and critical resuscitation plans

☐ Nurses(s) review(s)
- Specific patient concerns, sterility indicator results and equipment / implant issues

☐ Patient positioning and support / Warming devices
☐ Special precautions
☐ Expected procedure time / Postoperative destination

TIME OUT – Before skin incision

☐ All team members introduce themselves by name and role
☐ Surgeon, Anesthesiologist, and Nurse verbally confirm
- Patient
- Site, side and level
- Procedure
- Antibiotic prophylaxis: repeat dose?
- Final optimal positioning of patient

☐ "Does anyone have any other questions or concerns before proceeding?"

DEBRIEFING – Before patient leaves OR

☐ Surgeon reviews with entire team
- Procedure
- Important intraoperative events
- Fluid balance / management

☐ Anesthesiologist reviews with entire team
- Important intraoperative events
- Recovery plans (including postoperative ventilation, pain management, glucose and temperature)

☐ Nurse(s) review(s) with entire team
- Instument / sponge / needle counts
- Specimen labelling and management
- Important intraoperative events (including equipment malfunction)

☐ Changes to postoperative destination?
☐ What are the KEY concerns for this patient's recovery and management?
☐ Could anything have been done to make this case safer or more efficient?

Hand-off to PACU / RR, Nursing Unit, or ICU

CHECKLIST SCORE

Add all checkmarks for 3 sections and enter below

Briefing _____ /17 = _____
Time Out _____ /3 = _____
Debriefing _____ /6 = _____
TOTAL _____ /26 = _____ × 100 = _____

PATIENT INFORMATION

EVIDENCE-INFORMED PRACTICE

Does the Use of a Surgical Safety Checklist Make a Difference in Patient Safety?

The authors of this relevant study compared the incidence of perioperative complications of 3760 patients before implementation of a surgical safety checklist (similar to the one in Box 36.4) with 3820 patients after implementation of the safety checklist. The number of complications dropped from 27.3 per 100 patients to 16.7 per 100 patients after the checklist was introduced! The overall proportion of patients with one or more complications decreased significantly from 15.4% to 10.6% ($p <0.001$) after implementation of the surgical safety checklist. Mortality rates also dropped from 1.5% to 0.8%.

NURSING IMPLICATIONS: Patient safety is a key nursing priority, and perioperative nurses play an important role in identifying at-risk patients as well as ensuring patient safety throughout the perioperative period. Checklists, such as the surgical safety checklist, provide memory cues and ensure that all members of the perioperative team collaborate for the sake of patient safety. This study provides the evidence to support the practice of using checklists in the perioperative care of patients so as to reduce complications and mortality rates.

Source: Based on de Vries, E. N., Prins, H. A., Crolla, R., den Outer, A. J., van Helden, S., Schlack, W., … & Boermeester, M.A., for the SURPASS Collaborative Group. (2010). Effect of a comprehensive surgical safety system on patient outcomes. *New England Journal of Medicine, 363,* 1928–1937.

CLINICAL ALERT

Multiple safety checks are recommended before and during surgery to ensure that the correct patient receives the correct procedure for the correct operative site, especially in surgeries with high risk of wrong site surgery such as orthopedic surgery (e.g., hip or knee replacement), lung lobectomy, and mastectomy. The SURgical PAtient Safety System (SURPASS) recommendations indicate that the person performing the procedure should do the site marking, making the mark at or near the incision site. DO NOT mark any nonoperative sites(s) unless necessary for some other aspect of care. The mark should be unambiguous (e.g., use initials or "YES" or a line representing the proposed incision). Note that "X" is considered ambiguous as it may mean *marks the spot* for some, whereas for others, it may mean *not here.* The mark should be positioned to be visible after the patient is prepped and draped. The mark should be made using a marker that is sufficiently permanent to remain visible after completion of the skin prep. Single use markers are available for this purpose.

recommends three key safety checks: briefing—before induction of anesthesia; timeout—before the incision is made; and debriefing—before the patient leaves the operating room. All health care professionals (i.e., anesthesiologist, surgeon, and nurse) involved in the surgical event participate in completing the briefing, timeout, and debriefing checkpoints, each addressing a number of relevant issues (e.g., properly functioning equipment, availability of blood products in the event of hemorrhage, any anticipated complications or special precautions, etc.) that must be addressed to ensure comprehensive patient safety. The use of such tools fosters interprofessional communication and team work as well as put patient safety front and centre in perioperative care. The Evidence-Informed Practice box summarizes the results of one study investigating the impact of using a patient safety protocol in clinical practice.

Accurate patient identification is key, and safety protocols recommend verification using two identifiers at the time surgery is scheduled, during admission, immediately before the incision is made, and whenever there are patient handoffs (e.g., when the patient is transferred to or from another caregiver or unit). Site identification involves marking of the operative site in an unambiguous

manner (see Clinical Alert box) to ensure proper site of the procedure. Although the type of mark may vary across institutions, the surgical site marking method *must* be consistent throughout the facility.

VITAL SIGNS Preoperatively assess and document vital signs for baseline data. Report any abnormal findings, such as elevated blood pressure or elevated temperature.

ANTIEMBOLISM STOCKINGS Antiembolism stockings are firm elastic hose that compress the veins of the legs and, when applied accurately, facilitate the return of venous blood to the heart, thus preventing edema of the legs and feet as well as reduce the risk of venous thromboembolism (see Chapter 43). These stockings are frequently applied to surgical patients.

The stockings come in several types. One type extends from the foot to the knee and another from the foot to mid-thigh. These stockings usually have a partial foot that exposes the heel or toes so that extremity circulation can be assessed. These stockings usually come in small, medium, and large sizes. Skill 36.2 details the steps required to apply antiembolism stockings. See also the Lifespan Considerations box and the Home Care Considerations box on antiembolism stockings on page 1072.

SEQUENTIAL COMPRESSION DEVICES Clients who are undergoing surgery (especially orthopedic interventions) may be prescribed a sequential compression device (SCD) to promote venous return from the legs. SCDs inflate and deflate plastic sleeves wrapped around the legs to promote venous flow. SCDs are discussed in Chapter 43. Skill 43.6 (see page 1401) outlines how to apply a sequential compression device.

Evaluating

The goals established during the planning phase are evaluated according to specific desired health outcomes, which are also established in that phase.

SKILL 36.2   APPLYING ANTIEMBOLISM STOCKINGS

PURPOSES

- To facilitate venous return from the lower extremities
- To prevent venous stasis and venous thrombosis
- To reduce peripheral edema

ASSESSMENT

Assess both lower extremities for the following:

- Rates, volumes, and rhythms of posterior tibial and dorsalis pedis pulses (note if unequal bilaterally)
- Skin colour (note pallor, cyanosis, or other pigmentation)
- Sensation (note any numbness, tingling, pain)
- Skin temperature (e.g., warm, cool)
- Presence of edema (pitting or nonpitting)
- Skin condition (e.g., thickened, shiny, taut, hairless)

PLANNING

Before applying antiembolism stockings, determine any potential or present circulatory problems and the surgeon's orders involving the lower extremities.

Equipment

- Single-use tape measure (to prevent cross-contamination)
- Clean antiembolism stockings of appropriate size and type ordered (e.g., knee or mid-thigh)

IMPLEMENTATION

Preparation

Take measurements as needed to obtain the appropriate size stockings:

- Measure the length of both legs from the heel to the gluteal fold (for thigh-length stockings) or from the heel to the popliteal space (for knee-length stockings).
- Measure the circumference of each calf and each thigh at the widest point.
- Compare the measurements to the size chart to obtain stockings of correct size. Obtain two sizes if there is a significant difference. **Rationale: Large stockings do not place adequate pressure on the legs to facilitate venous return and may bunch, increasing the risk of pressure and skin irritation. Stockings that are too small may impede blood flow to the feet and cause discomfort.**

Performance

1. Before performing the procedure, introduce yourself, and verify the client's identity using two identifiers or per agency protocol. Explain to the client what you are going to do, why it is necessary, and how he or she can participate.
2. Perform hand hygiene, and follow other appropriate infection prevention and control procedures.
3. Provide for client privacy.
4. Select an appropriate time to apply the stockings.
   - Apply stockings in the morning, if possible, before the client rises. **Rationale: In the sitting and standing positions, the veins can become distended, so edema occurs; the stockings should be applied before this happens.**
   - Assist the client who has been ambulating to lie down and elevate the legs for 15 to 30 minutes before applying the stockings. **Rationale: This facilitates venous return and reduces swelling.**
5. Prepare the client.
   - Assist the client to the lying position in bed.
   - Wash and dry the legs, as needed.
6. Apply the stockings.
   - Reach inside the stocking from the top, and grasping the heel, turn the upper portion of the stocking inside out over the foot portion. **Rationale: Firm elastic stockings are easier to fit over the foot and calf when inverted in this manner, rather than bunching the stocking up.**
   - Ask the client to point the toes, and position the stocking on the client's foot, taking care to place the toe and heel portions of the stocking appropriately (see ❶) **Rationale: Pointing of the toes makes application easier.**
   - Grasp the upper edge of the stocking, and gently pull

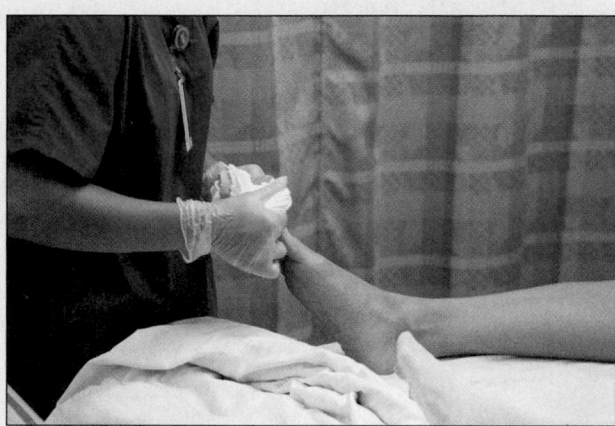

❶ Applying the stocking over the toes

   the stocking over the leg, turning it right side out in the process (see ❷, ❸).
   - Inspect the client's leg and stocking, smoothing any folds or creases. Ensure that the stocking is not rolled down or bunched at the top or ankle. **Rationale: Folds and creases can cause skin irritation under the stocking; bunching of the stocking can further impair venous return.**
   - Remove the stockings for 30 minutes every 8 hours, inspecting the legs and skin while the stockings are off.
   - Soiled stockings can be laundered by hand with warm water and mild soap. Hang to dry.
7. Document the procedure. Record the procedure, your assessment data, and when the stockings are removed and reapplied.

(continued)

SKILL 36.2   APPLYING ANTIEMBOLISM STOCKINGS *(continued)*

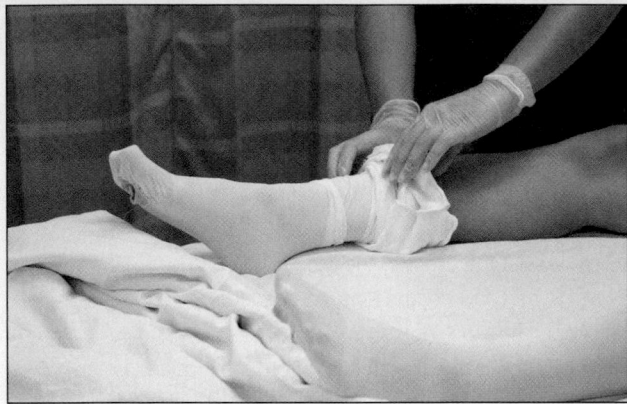

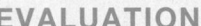 Pulling the stocking snugly over the leg

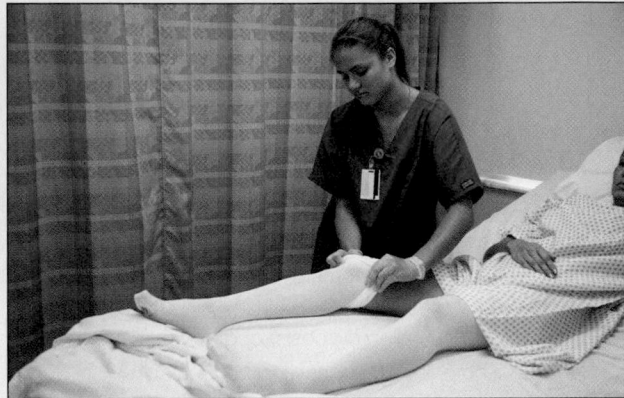 3

EVALUATION

- Remove antiembolism stockings one to three times a day for 30 minutes for skin care and inspection.

- Note the appearance of the legs and skin integrity, any edema, peripheral pulses, skin colour and temperature, and compare with previous assessment data.
- If complications occur, remove the stockings, and report your findings to the appropriate members of the health care team.

LIFESPAN CONSIDERATIONS

Antiembolism Stockings

CHILDREN

- Antiembolism stockings are rarely used on children.

OLDER ADULTS

- Because the elastic is quite strong in antiembolism stockings, older adults may need assistance with putting on

the stockings. Clients with arthritis may need to have another person put the stockings on for them.

- Many older adults have circulation problems and wear antiembolism stockings. It is important to check for wrinkles in the stockings and to see if the stocking has rolled down or twisted. If so, correct immediately

because the stockings must be evenly distributed over the limb to promote rather than hinder circulation.

- Stockings should be removed once each shift so that a thorough assessment can be made of legs and feet. Redness and skin breakdown on the heels can occur quickly and go undetected if not thoroughly assessed on a regular basis.

HOME CARE CONSIDERATIONS

Antiembolism Stockings

- Teach the client or caregiver how to apply the antiembolism stockings.
- Stress the importance of no wrinkles or rolling down of the stockings and the rationale.
- Instruct the client or caregiver to remove the stockings daily and inspect the skin on the legs.

- Provide instructions about the following:
  - Laundering the stockings
  - The need for two pairs of stockings to allow for one pair to be worn while the other is being laundered
  - Replacing the stockings when they lose their elasticity

Intraoperative Phase

The intraoperative nurse is a vital member of the surgical team, advocating for the client, maintaining safety, and continually assessing the needs of the client and the team.

Types of Anesthesia

Anesthesia is classified as *general* or *regional* or *local*. Anesthetic agents are administered by an anesthesiologist. **General anesthesia** is a state of total unconsciousness resulting from anesthetic agents. Under general anesthesia, protective reflexes, such as cough and gag reflexes, are lost. General anesthetic agents act by blocking awareness centres in the brain so that amnesia (loss of memory), analgesia (insensibility to pain), hypnosis, and relaxation occur. General anesthetics are usually administered by intravenous infusion or by inhalation of gases through a mask or through an endotracheal tube inserted into the trachea.

General anesthesia has certain advantages. Because the patient is unconscious, rather than awake and anxious, respiration and cardiac function are readily regulated. Also, the anesthesia can be adjusted to the length of the operation and the patient's age and physical status. Its chief disadvantage is that it depresses the respiratory and circulatory systems. Some patients become more anxious about general anesthesia than about the surgery itself. Often, this is because they fear losing the capacity to control their own bodies.

Local anesthesia interrupts the transmission of nerve impulses to a specific small area (e.g., index finger). Local anesthesia is used for minor surgical procedures, such as performing a biopsy, or during tooth extraction. **Regional anesthesia** is the temporary interruption of the transmission of nerve impulses to and from a specific area or region of the body (e.g., an arm). In both local and regional anesthesia, the patient loses sensation in an area of the body but remains conscious.

Local anesthesia can be given in the following ways:

- **Topical (surface) anesthesia** can be applied directly to the skin and mucous membranes, open skin surfaces, wounds, and burns. The most commonly used topical agents are lidocaine and benzocaine. A topical patch, such as a eutectic mixture of local anesthetics (or the EMLA patch), can be applied before injection or intravenous insertion. Topical anesthetics are readily absorbed and act rapidly.

- In **local infiltration**, an anesthetic agent is injected into a specific area. Lidocaine is used most commonly.

Several techniques are used in regional anesthesia:

- A **nerve block** is a technique in which the anesthetic agent is injected into and around a nerve or small nerve group that supplies sensation to a small area of the body. Major blocks involve multiple nerves or a *plexus* (e.g., the brachial plexus anesthetises the arm); minor blocks involve a single nerve (e.g., a facial nerve).

- An **intravenous block (Bier block)** is used most often for procedures involving the arm, wrist, and hand. An occlusion tourniquet is applied to the extremity to prevent infiltration and absorption of the injected intravenous agent beyond the involved extremity.

- **Spinal anesthesia** is also referred to as a **subarachnoid block** (SAB). It requires a lumbar puncture through one of the interspaces between lumbar disc 2 (L-2) and the sacrum (S-1). An anesthetic agent is injected into

the subarachnoid space surrounding the spinal cord. Spinal anesthesia is often categorized as a low, mid-, or high spinal. *Low spinals* (saddle or caudal blocks) are primarily used for surgeries involving the perineal or rectal areas. *Mid-spinals* (below the level of the umbilicus—T-10) can be used for hernia repairs or appendectomies, and *high spinals* (reaching the nipple line—T-4) can be used for surgeries such as cesarean sections.

- **Epidural (peridural) anesthesia** is injection of an anesthetic agent into the epidural space, the area inside the spinal column but outside the dura mater.

Conscious sedation may be used alone or in conjunction with regional anesthesia for some diagnostic tests (e.g., endoscopies, balloon angioplasty) and minor surgical procedures (e.g., drainage of an abscess). **Conscious sedation** is defined as minimal depression of the level of consciousness, in which the patient retains the ability to consciously maintain a patent airway and respond appropriately to commands. Intravenous opioids, such as morphine or fentanyl, and antianxiety agents, such as diazepam or midazolam, are commonly used to induce and maintain conscious sedation. Conscious sedation increases the patient's pain threshold and induces a degree of amnesia but allows for prompt reversal of its effects and a rapid return to normal ADLs. See the Clinical Alert box on the induction phase of general anesthesia.

! CLINICAL ALERT

During the induction (onset) phase of general anesthesia, reflexes can become hyperactive before becoming absent. It is during this phase that the patient is at risk for falling, vomiting, urinating, and/or defecating. Appropriate safety measures must be taken at this time.

Assessing

On the patient's admission to the surgical suite or procedure room, the perioperative nurse confirms the patient's identity and assesses the client's physical and emotional status. The nurse verifies the information on the preoperative checklist and evaluates the patient's knowledge about the surgery and events to follow. The patient's response to preoperative medications is assessed, as well as the placement and patency of tubes, such as IV lines, nasogastric tubes, and urinary catheters.

Assessment continues throughout surgery as the nurse and the anesthesiologist continuously monitor the patient's vital signs, ECG, and oxygen saturation. Fluid intake and urinary output are monitored throughout surgery, and blood loss is estimated. In addition, arterial and venous pressures, pulmonary artery pressures, and laboratory values, such as blood glucose, hemoglobin, hematocrit, serum electrolytes, and arterial blood gases, may be evaluated during surgery. Continual assessment is necessary to rapidly identify adverse responses to surgery or anesthesia and intervene promptly to prevent complications.

During the intraoperative period, the nurse is aware of potential risks, many being related to the position of the patient, the effects of the anesthesia, equipment used, disruption of tissue perfusion during surgery, and the surgical wound. The nurse also considers the complications that can occur (e.g., hemorrhage, surgical site infection, and neuromuscular injury).

Diagnosing

Several nursing diagnoses can apply to the patient experiencing surgery. As a result of general anesthesia, patients are at risk for such complications as aspiration, falling, defecation, hypotension, and bradycardia. As a result of the surgical procedure itself, the patient is at risk for impaired skin integrity, surgical site infection, hemorrhage, and complications related to the body part having the surgery (e.g., surgery on the heart places the patient at risk for inadequate circulation).

Planning

The overall goals of care in the intraoperative period are to maintain the patient's safety and to maintain homeostasis. Examples of nursing practices to achieve these goals include the following:

- Positioning the patient appropriately for surgery
- Performing preoperative skin preparation
- Assisting in preparing and maintaining the sterile field
- Opening and dispensing sterile supplies during surgery
- Providing medications and solutions for the sterile field
- Monitoring and maintaining a safe, aseptic environment
- Managing catheters, tubes, drains, and specimens
- Performing sponge, sharp, and instrument counts
- Documenting nursing care provided and the patient's response to interventions

Implementing

Intraoperative interventions are carried out by the circulating nurse and the scrub nurse. The **circulating nurse** coordinates activities and manages patient care by continually assessing patient safety, aseptic practice, and the environment (e.g., temperature, humidity, and lighting). The **scrub nurse** assists the surgeon. A scrub nurse wears a sterile gown, gloves, a cap, and eye protection. His or her responsibilities include draping the patient with sterile drapes and handling sterile instruments and supplies (see Chapter 34). The circulating nurse and scrub nurse are responsible for accounting for all sponges, needles, and instruments at the close of the surgery. This precaution avoids inadvertently leaving any surgical supplies inside the patient.

SURGICAL SKIN PREPARATION Surgical skin preparation involves cleaning the surgical site, removing hair *only* if necessary, and applying an antimicrobial agent. In most surgery centres, skin preparation is done by surgery personnel close to the time of surgery. The Safer Healthcare Now! (2010) campaign to reduce surgical site infections indicates that *no* surgical site hair removal should be performed by shaving with a razor. In cases when surgical site hair removal is required, then it is to be done with clippers. In such situations, hair is to be removed within 2 hours of the surgery and outside the surgical suite, to avoid dispersal of loose hair and potential contamination of the sterile field.

The surgical site and surrounding area is ideally prepared with alcohol-based chlorhexidine that is not washed off until at least 6 hours after surgery (Safer Healthcare Now! 2010) so as to remove transient microbes from the skin, reduce the resident microbial count to subpathogenic amounts, and inhibit rapid rebound growth of microbes.

POSITIONING Proper positioning of the patient during surgery is integral to patient safety. The ideal intraoperative patient position provides the following:

- Optimal visualization of and access to the surgical site
- Optimal access for assessing and maintaining anesthesia and vital functions
- Protection of the patient from harm (anatomical and physiological considerations)

Positioning is generally performed after general anesthesia is induced and before surgical draping of the patient. The patient is lifted into position to prevent shearing forces on the skin from sliding or rolling. The exact position for the patient depends on the surgical approach. For example, a lithotomy position is usually used for vaginal surgery.

Positions on the operating table are maintained by straps, and body prominences are frequently padded. The position should consider normal joint range of motion and good body alignment, thereby avoiding strain or injury to muscles, bones, and ligaments. For surgeries lasting more than 90 minutes, pressure management devices (e.g., pressure distributing mattress) should be used to prevent pressure ulcer development (Registered Nurses' Association of Ontario [RNAO], 2011).

Evaluating

The intraoperative nurse uses the goals developed during the planning stage (e.g., maintain patient safety) and collects data to evaluate whether the desired outcomes have been achieved.

DOCUMENTATION Throughout the intraoperative phase, the nurse documents patient care activities, such as IV fluid infusions, positioning, gastric suction, and urinary catheterization.

Postoperative Phase

Nursing during the postoperative phase is especially important for the client's recovery. Anesthesia impairs the ability of patients to respond to environmental stimuli and to help themselves, although the degree of consciousness of patients will vary. Moreover, surgery itself traumatizes the body by disrupting protective mechanisms and homeostasis.

Immediate Postanesthesia Phase

Recovery or PACU nurses have specialized skills to care for patients recovering from anesthesia and surgery (Figure 36.1). Once the health status has stabilized, the client is returned to the nursing unit or, in the case of a patient who had outpatient surgery, to the outpatient surgery area before discharge. Clinical assessment of the patient in the immediate postanesthesia period is summarized in Box 36.5.

Patients are usually discharged from the PACU when they are conscious and oriented; they are able to maintain a clear airway and deep breath and cough freely; vital signs have been stable or consistent with preoperative vital signs for at least 30 minutes; their protective reflexes (e.g., gag, swallowing) are active; they are able to move all extremities; their intake and urinary output are adequate; and their dressings are dry and intact.

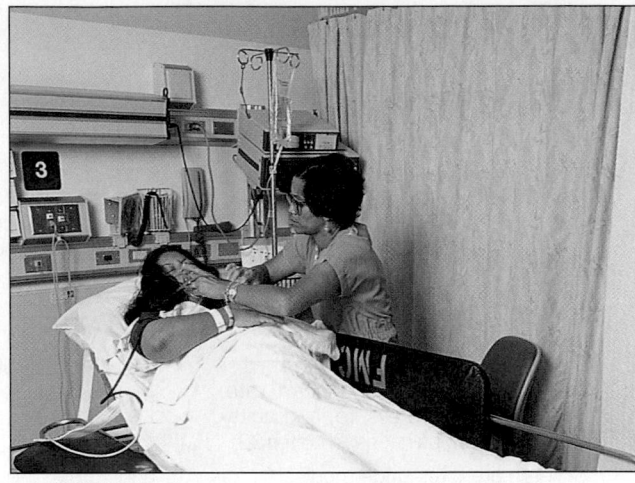

FIGURE 36.1 Postanesthesia care unit (PACU) nurse provides constant assessment and care for patients recovering from anesthesia and surgery.

ONGOING CARE OF THE POSTOPERATIVE PATIENT

While the patient is in the operating room, the patient's bed and room are prepared for the postoperative phase. Generally, the patient is brought back to the unit on a stretcher and transferred to the bed in the room which has been made with clean linens (see Chapter 31 for a description of how to prepare a bed for the postoperative patient). The nurse must ensure that equipment is available for measuring vital signs and set up any special equipment, such as suction, oxygen equipment, and IV stand. See the Lifespan Considerations box on the next page for important postoperative issues for children and older adults.

BOX 36.5 IMMEDIATE POSTANESTHETIC PHASE

Postanesthesia care unit (PACU) nurses assess the following right after surgery:

- Adequacy of airway (patency, presence of laryngeal edema or spasm); assess adequacy of artificial airway (i.e., endotracheal tube, if in place)
- Oxygen saturation
- Adequacy of ventilation
  - Respiratory rate, rhythm, and depth
  - Use of accessory muscles
  - Breath sounds
- Cardiovascular status
  - Heart rate and rhythm
  - Peripheral pulse amplitude and equality
  - Blood pressure
  - Capillary filling
- Level of consciousness
  - Not responding
  - Arousable with verbal stimuli
  - Fully awake
  - Oriented to time, person, and place

- Temperature—ideally between 36°C and 38°C (Safer Healthcare Now! 2010)
- Presence of protective reflexes (e.g., gag, cough)
- Activity, ability to move extremities
- Skin colour (pink, pale, dusky, blotchy, cyanotic, jaundiced)
- Fluid status
  - Intake and output
  - Status of IV infusions (type of fluid, rate, amount in container, patency of tubing)
  - Signs of dehydration or fluid overload (see Chapter 44)
- Condition of surgical site
  - Status of dressing
  - Drainage (amount, type, and colour)
- Patency of and character and amount of drainage from catheters, tubes, and drains
- Pain or discomfort (type, location, and severity), nausea, vomiting
- Safety (i.e., necessity for side rails, call bell within reach)

LIFESPAN CONSIDERATIONS

Postoperative Care

Postoperative care of children and older adults requires some special considerations:

CHILDREN

- Infants and young children may not be able to state their level of pain postoperatively, may be physically active, and may appear not to have much pain. Use nonverbal signs, such as crying, fussiness, refusal to eat, disturbed sleep, increased heart rate, increased blood pressure, and agitation, to assess pain (see Chapter 30).
- Children are often undermedicated for pain postoperatively. Nurses should be alert to subtle signs of pain and provide medication in a timely manner. Well-controlled pain levels facilitate the healing process in children.
- Some PACUs encourage parents to be present when their child wakes

from surgery. Having the parent at the bedside has been shown to calm the child and reduce parental anxiety.

OLDER ADULTS

- Older adults have less efficient reserves and may take longer to recover postoperatively. Be attentive to vital signs, intake and output, and mental status, and note significant changes.
- People with dementia often experience an increase in confusion and agitation from the medications and the anesthetic used during surgery. This poses a safety risk during the postoperative period and requires nursing staff to monitor these patients more

frequently. It is important to maintain a calm, reassuring attitude. These changes are often long lasting, taking days or weeks to return to the preoperative level of cognition.
- Older adults may experience more fatigue and weakness after surgery. Encouraging activity is crucial but needs to be paced to prevent exhaustion.
- When surgery is done on an outpatient basis, nurses should follow up with phone calls that evening and the next day to check on the patient's condition and make sure that postoperative instructions were understood.

Assessing

As soon as the patient returns to the nursing unit, the nurse conducts an initial assessment. The sequence of these activities varies with the situation. For example, the nurse may need to check the physician's stat orders before conducting the initial assessment; in such a case, nursing interventions to implement the orders can be carried out at the same time as the assessment.

The nurse consults the surgeon's postoperative orders to learn the following:

- Food and fluids permitted by mouth
- Intravenous solutions and intravenous medications
- Positioning
- Medications ordered (e.g., analgesics, antibiotics)
- Laboratory tests
- Intake and output, which in some agencies are monitored for all postoperative patients
- Activity permitted, including ambulation

The nurse also checks the operative and PACU record for the following data:

- Operation performed, including length of the procedure and positioning
- Presence and location of any drains
- Anesthetic agents used
- Postoperative diagnosis
- Estimated blood loss
- Medications administered in the recovery room
- Occurrence of any complications (intraoperatively and in the PACU)

Many hospitals have postoperative protocols for regular assessment of patients. In some agencies, assessments are made every 15 minutes until vital signs stabilize, every hour for the next 4 hours, then every 4 hours for the next 2 days. It is important that the assessments be made as often as the patient's condition requires. The nurse assesses the following:

- *Level of consciousness.* Assess orientation to time, place, and person. Most patients are fully conscious but drowsy when returned to their unit. Assess reaction to verbal stimuli and ability to move extremities.
- *Vital signs.* Take the patient's vital signs (including oxygen saturation) every 15 minutes until stable or in accordance with agency protocol. Vital signs may need to be taken more frequently based on the patient's condition. Compare initial findings with preoperative, intraoperative, and PACU data. In addition, assess the patient's lung sounds, and assess for signs of common circulatory problems, such as postoperative hypotension, hemorrhage, or shock. Hypovolemia from fluid losses during surgery is a common cause of postoperative hypotension. Hemorrhage can result from insecure ligation of blood vessels or disruption of sutures or staples used to close a wound. Massive hemorrhage or cardiac insufficiency can lead to shock postoperatively. Potential postoperative complications with their manifestations and preventive measures are listed in Table 36.2.
- *Skin colour and temperature, particularly that of the lips and nail beds.* The colour of the lips and nail beds is an indicator of tissue perfusion. Pale, cyanotic, cool, and moist skin may be a sign of circulatory problems.

TABLE 36.2 Potential Postoperative Problems

Problem	Description	Cause	Clinical Signs	Preventive Interventions
Respiratory				
Pneumonia	Inflammation of the alveoli	Infection, toxins, or irritants causing inflammatory process; immobility and impaired ventilation result in atelectasis and promote growth of pathogens	Elevated temperature, cough, expectoration of blood-tinged or purulent sputum, dyspnea, chest pain	Deep-breathing exercises and coughing, moving in bed, early ambulation
Atelectasis	A condition in which alveoli collapse and are not ventilated	Mucous plugs blocking bronchial passageways, inadequate lung expansion, analgesics, immobility	Dyspnea, tachypnea, tachycardia; diaphoresis, anxiety; pleural pain, decreased chest wall movement; dull or absent breath sounds; decreased oxygen saturation	Deep-breathing exercises and coughing, moving in bed, early ambulation
Pulmonary embolism	Blood clot that has moved to the lungs and blocks a pulmonary artery, thus obstructing blood flow to a portion of the lung	Stasis of venous blood from immobility, venous injury from fractures or during surgery, use of oral contraceptives high in estrogen, preexisting coagulation or circulatory disorder	Sudden chest pain, shortness of breath, cyanosis, shock (tachycardia, low blood pressure)	Turning, ambulation, antiembolism stockings, sequential compression devices
Circulatory				
Hypovolemia	Inadequate circulating blood volume	Fluid deficit, hemorrhage	Tachycardia, decreased urine output, decreased blood pressure	Early detection of signs; fluid or blood replacement
Hemorrhage	Internal or external bleeding	Disruption of sutures, insecure ligation of blood vessels	Overt bleeding (dressings saturated with bright blood; bright, free-flowing blood in drains or chest tubes), increased pain, increasing abdominal girth, swelling or bruising around incision	Early detection of signs
Hypovolemic shock	Inadequate tissue perfusion resulting from markedly reduced circulating blood volume	Severe hypovolemia from fluid deficit or hemorrhage	Rapid weak pulse, dyspnea, tachypnea; restlessness and anxiety; urine output less than 30 mL/h; decreased blood pressure; cool, clammy skin, thirst, pallor	Maintain blood volume through adequate fluid replacement, prevent hemorrhage; early detection of signs
Thrombophlebitis	Inflammation of the veins, usually of the legs and associated with a blood clot	Slowed venous blood flow caused by immobility or prolonged sitting; trauma to vein, resulting in inflammation and increased blood coagulability	Aching, cramping pain; affected area is swollen, red, and hot to touch; vein feels hard	Early ambulation, leg exercises, antiembolism stockings, SCDs, adequate fluid intake

(continued)

TABLE 36.2 Potential Postoperative Problems (*continued*)

Problem	Description	Cause	Clinical Signs	Preventive Interventions
Thrombus	Blood clot attached to wall of vein or artery (most commonly the leg veins)	As for thrombophlebitis for venous thrombi; disruption or inflammation of arterial wall for arterial thrombi	*Venous:* same as thrombophlebitis *Arterial:* pain and pallor of affected extremity; decreased or absent peripheral pulses	*Venous:* same as thrombophlebitis *Arterial:* maintain prescribed position; early detection of signs
Embolus	Foreign body or clot that has moved from its site of formation to another area of the body (e.g., the lungs, heart, or brain)	Venous or arterial thrombus; broken intravenous catheter, fat, or amniotic fluid	In venous system, usually becomes a pulmonary embolus (see pulmonary embolism); signs of arterial emboli may depend on the location	Turning, ambulation, leg exercises, sequential compression devices; careful maintenance of IV catheters
Urinary				
Urinary retention	Inability to empty the bladder, with excessive accumulation of urine in the bladder	Depressed bladder muscle tone from narcotics and anesthetics; handling of tissues during surgery on adjacent organs (rectum, vagina)	Fluid intake larger than output; inability to void or frequent voiding of small amounts, bladder distension, suprapubic discomfort, restlessness	Monitoring of fluid intake and output, interventions to facilitate voiding, urinary catheterization, as needed
Urinary tract infection	Inflammation of the bladder, ureters, or urethra	Immobilization and limited fluid intake, instrumentation of the urinary tract	Burning sensation when voiding, urgency, cloudy urine, lower abdominal pain	Adequate fluid intake, early ambulation, aseptic straight catheterization only as necessary, optimal perineal hygiene
Gastrointestinal				
Nausea and vomiting	The urge to vomit and actual emesis of stomach contents	Pain, abdominal distension, ingesting food or fluids before return of peristalsis, certain medications, anxiety	Complaints of feeling sick to the stomach, retching, or gagging	IV fluids until peristalsis returns; then clear fluids, full fluids, and regular diet; antiemetic drugs, if ordered; analgesics for pain
Constipation	Infrequent or no stool passage for abnormal length of time (e.g., later than 48 hours after solid diet started)	Lack of dietary roughage, analgesics (decreased intestinal motility), immobility	Absence of stool elimination, abdominal distension and discomfort	Adequate fluid intake, high-fibre diet, early ambulation
Tympanites	Retention of gases within the intestines	Slowed motility of the intestines caused by handling of the bowel during surgery and the effects of anesthesia	Obvious abdominal distension, abdominal discomfort (gas pains), absence of bowel sounds	Early ambulation; avoid using a straw, provide ice chips or water at room temperature
Postoperative ileus	Intestinal obstruction characterized by lack of peristaltic activity	Handling the bowel during surgery, anesthesia, electrolyte imbalance, wound infection	Abdominal pain and distension; constipation; absent bowel sounds; vomiting	Avoid general anesthesia if possible
Wound				
Wound infection	Inflammation and infection of incision or drain site	Poor aseptic technique; laboratory analysis of wound swab identifies causative microorganism	Purulent exudate, redness, tenderness, elevated body temperature, wound odour	Keep wound clean and dry, use surgical aseptic technique when changing dressings

Problem	Description	Cause	Clinical Signs	Preventive Interventions
Wound dehiscence	Separation of a suture line before the incision heals	Malnutrition (emaciation, obesity), poor circulation, excessive strain on suture line	Increased incision drainage, tissues underlying skin become visible along parts of the incision	Adequate nutrition, appropriate incisional support and avoidance of strain
Wound evisceration	Extrusion of internal organs and tissues through the incision	Same as for wound dehiscence	Opening of incision and visible protrusion of organs	Same as for wound dehiscence
Psychological				
Postoperative depression	Mental disorder characterized by altered mood	Weakness, surprise nature of emergency surgery, news of malignancy, severely altered body image, other personal matter; may be a physiological response to some surgeries	Anorexia, tearfulness, loss of ambition, withdrawal, rejection of others, feelings of dejection, sleep disturbances (insomnia or excessive sleeping)	Adequate rest, physical activity, opportunity to express anger and other negative feelings

- *Comfort.* Assess pain with the patient's vital signs and, as needed, between vital sign measurements. Assess the location, type, and intensity of the pain. Do not assume that reported pain is incisional; other causes can include muscle strains, flatus, and angina. Shoulder pain following minimally invasive abdominal surgery can result from residual carbon dioxide gas remaining in the abdominal cavity and causing referred pain. Ask the patient to rate the pain on a scale of 0 to 10, with 0 being no pain and 10 pain as bad as it could possibly be. Evaluate the patient for objective indicators of pain: pallor, perspiration, muscle tension, and reluctance to cough, move, or ambulate. Determine when and what analgesics were last administered, and assess the patient for any side effects of medication, such as nausea and vomiting.

- *Fluid balance.* Assess the type and amount of IV fluids, flow rate, and infusion site. Monitor the patient's fluid intake and output. In addition to watching for shock, assess the patient for signs of circulatory overload, and monitor serum electrolytes. Anesthetics and surgery affect the hormones regulating fluid and electrolyte balance (aldosterone and antidiuretic hormone [ADH], in particular), placing the client at risk for decreased urine output and fluid and electrolyte imbalances. Assess for the presence of nausea and vomiting.

- *Dressings and bedclothes.* Inspect the patient's dressings and the bedclothes underneath the patient. Excessive sanguineous drainage on dressings or bedclothes, often appearing underneath the patient, can indicate hemorrhage. The amount of drainage on dressings is recorded by describing the diameter of the stains or by denoting the number and type of dressings saturated with drainage.

- *Drains and tubes.* Determine colour, consistency, and amount of drainage from all tubes and drains. All tubes should be patent, and tubes and suction equipment should be functioning. Drainage bags must be hanging properly.

Document the patient's time of arrival and all assessments. Many agencies have progress flow records for this purpose. Alter the frequency, parameters, and priorities to meet the individual needs of the client.

Diagnosing

Because surgery can involve many body systems, both directly and indirectly, and is a complex experience for the patient, the nursing diagnoses focus on a wide variety of actual or potential problems.

Examples of nursing diagnoses for the postoperative patient include acute pain, risk for infection (e.g., surgical site), impaired oxygen exchange, fluid imbalance (fluid volume excess, fluid volume deficit), immobility (often related to unmanaged acute pain), disturbed body image, and reduced self-efficacy related to self-care. A range of diagnoses can relate to the particular body part or site of the surgery; for example, a patient recovering from neurosurgery may be at risk for mental status changes or increased intracranial pressure; the patient recovering from hip arthroplasty may be at risk for reduced range of motion.

Planning

Postoperative care planning and discharge planning begin in the preoperative phase when preoperative teaching is implemented. Patient goals during the postoperative period often include the following:

- Maintain comfort
- Promote surgical wound healing
- Prevent associated risks, such as respiratory or cardiovascular complications, infection, and other common problems associated with surgery
- Restore the highest possible level of wellness

PLANNING FOR HOME CARE To provide for continuity of care for the surgical patient after discharge, the nurse needs to consider the patient's needs for assistance with care in the home setting. Discharge planning both for the client after outpatient surgery and for the client who has been hospitalized for several days following surgery incorporates an assessment of the client's and family's abilities for self-care, financial resources, and the need for referrals and home health services. The Assessment: Home Care box outlines the assessment for a surgical client; however, it is important to remember that surgical clients have diverse needs and additional assessment data may be required.

Home Care Teaching Once the home care assessment is complete, nurses must meet the learning needs of clients and their support people to ensure continuity of care and restoration of the client's health. Teaching should focus on actions to maintain comfort, to promote healing and restore wellness, and to make use of appropriate community agencies and other sources of help.

Maintaining Comfort

- Instruct the client to use analgesics, as ordered, not allowing pain to become severe before taking the prescribed dose.
- If not contraindicated, discuss the use of OTC analgesics, such as acetaminophen, as postoperative pain becomes less severe or if the client is reluctant to use prescription drugs because of side effects.
- Teach the client to avoid using alcohol or other central nervous system depressants while taking opioids.
- Discuss the importance of gradually resuming activities and avoiding overexertion.
- Emphasize the importance of paying attention to increasing pain or discomfort. Instruct the client to contact the physician if pain increases after a period of decreasing discomfort.
- Teach the client to use nonpharmacological measures, such as conscious relaxation, distraction, meditation, or visualization, to help manage pain.

| **ASSESSMENT** | **HOME CARE** |

Surgical Clients

The following are guidelines for assessing home care for surgical clients before discharge:

CLIENT
- *Self-care abilities:* Ability to manage hygiene and other self-care, to perform wound care, as needed, to manage tubes and stomas, and to manage prescribed medications
- *Supplies required:* Wound care supplies, such as dressings, hypoallergenic tape, cleansing solutions, binders or slings, elastic wraps, irrigating syringe and solution
- *Assistive devices required:* Walker, cane, raised toilet seat, commode, overhead trapeze, grab bars
- *Current level of knowledge:* Postoperative pain management, wound care, dressing changes, urinary catheters or other drains, activity restrictions, dietary prescriptions, prescribed exercises (e.g., range-of-motion, postmastectomy exercises), infection prevention and control measures, such as hand hygiene

FAMILY
- *Caregiver availability, skills, and responses:* Willingness and ability to assume responsibility for care, as needed (e.g., wound care, catheter and tube management, meal preparation, assistance with ADLs, shopping, transportation to and from appointments), other available caregivers
- *Family role changes and coping:* Effect on parenting and spousal roles, sexuality, social roles, financial status
- *Financial resources:* Ability to purchase necessary supplies and equipment; other sources of funding or financial assistance (e.g., private insurance)

HOME
- Elicit information from the client, family, or significant other regarding the physical environment of the home and potential issues postoperatively, which may include the presence of stairs, access to the home, and accessibility of the kitchen, bathroom, and bedroom.

COMMUNITY
- Available community resources, such as equipment and supply companies, support and educational organizations and groups (e.g., ostomy clubs and Reach for Recovery), home health agencies or providers, access to pharmacy services, transportation services for medical care, Meals on Wheels, and other support organizations

Promoting Healing

- If indicated, teach the client how to change wound dressings and perform wound care.

- Emphasize the importance of hygiene and hand hygiene to prevent infections.

- Instruct the client to report promptly to the appropriate member of the health care team any increasing redness, swelling, pain, or discharge from the incision or drain sites.

- Discuss any prescribed activity restrictions, such as avoiding lifting.

- Discuss the importance of keeping follow-up appointments to monitor healing and recovery after surgery.

Restoring Wellness

- Discuss the relationship of increasing activities to restoring wellness and promoting a sense of well-being.

- Teach the client that surgery and stressors can depress immune function and to avoid exposure to illness (e.g., crowded areas and people with upper respiratory illnesses), whenever possible.

- Emphasize the importance of adequate rest for healing and immune function.

- If appropriate, discuss lifestyle changes to promote wellness, such as stopping smoking, increasing activity level, reducing stress, and consuming a healthy diet high in fruits, vegetables, and whole grains with adequate protein to promote healing.

Using Community Agencies and Other Sources of Help

- Provide information about where durable medical equipment can be purchased, rented, or obtained free of charge; how to access home care and other services; and where to obtain supplies, such as dressings or nutritional supplements.

- Suggest additional sources of information, such as the Canadian Association of Wound Care, Reach to Recovery, United Ostomy Association of Canada, and so on.

Making Referrals   The nurse needs to consider appropriate referrals for the client, such as the following:

- Home health agencies for wound care and assessment and for assistance with ADLs, if necessary

- Community social services for assistance in obtaining medical and assistive equipment

- Respiratory, physical, or occupational therapy services, as indicated

Implementing

Nursing interventions designed to promote client recovery and prevent complications include (a) pain management, (b) appropriate positioning, (c) incentive spirometry and deep-breathing and coughing exercises, (d) leg exercises, (e) early ambulation, (f) adequate hydration, (g) proper diet, (h) promotion of urinary and gastrointestinal elimination, (i) suction maintenance, and (j) wound care.

PAIN MANAGEMENT   Although pain is a sensory and emotional experience that serves to alert people to harm and initiate responses to avoid or minimize harm, pain in the surgical client has little protective value. It can, in fact, have detrimental effects, leading to stimulation of the sympathetic nervous system, tachycardia, shallow breathing, atelectasis, altered gas exchange, immobility, and immunosuppression. See Chapter 30 for an in-depth discussion of pain and pain management.

Pain is usually greatest 12 to 36 hours after surgery, decreasing after the second or third postoperative day. During the initial postoperative period, patient-controlled analgesia (PCA) or continuous analgesic administration through an intravenous catheter is often prescribed. The nurse monitors the infusion or amount of analgesic administered by PCA, assesses the client's pain relief, and notifies the physician if the client is experiencing unacceptable side effects or inadequate pain relief. Around-the-clock parenteral or oral analgesics should be administered on a routine basis (the timing will vary depending on the medication, route, and dose) for the first 24 to 36 hours according to the physician's prescription. Additional as-needed (prn) analgesia should be administered for breakthrough pain. When routine analgesic administration is no longer necessary, the prescribed analgesic is generally given before scheduled activities and rest periods.

An anti-inflammatory agent, such as ibuprofen, is often administered as a coanalgesic with opioids. This combination enhances pain relief. Clients need to be reminded that analgesics are most effective when taken on a regular basis or before pain becomes severe. Because muscle tension increases pain perception and responses, nurses need to use nonpharmacological measures in addition to prescribed analgesia. These include ensuring that the client is warm and providing back rubs, position changes, diversional activities, and adjunctive measures, such as imagery.

POSITIONING   The patient should be positioned, as ordered. An unconscious or semiconscious client is placed on the side with no pillow and no elevation of the head, in a position that allows fluids to drain from the mouth. Unless contraindicated, elevation of affected extremities (e.g., following foot surgery) with the distal extremity higher than the heart promotes venous drainage and reduces swelling.

DEEP-BREATHING AND COUGHING EXERCISES   Deep-breathing exercises help remove mucus, which can form and remain in the lungs because of the effects of general anesthetic agents and analgesics. These drugs depress the action of both the cilia of the mucous membranes lining the respiratory tract and the respiratory centre in the brain. By increasing lung expansion and preventing the accumulation of secretions, deep breathing helps prevent pneumonia and atelectasis.

An incentive spirometer is often ordered for the postoperative client to encourage deep breathing. This device measures the flow of air inhaled through a mouthpiece (see Chapter 43). The client is instructed to breathe in through the mouthpiece until a certain level is achieved (usually measured by a ball within an enclosed chamber). Inhalation and ventilation are enhanced by using the incentive spirometer.

Deep breathing frequently initiates the coughing reflex. Voluntary coughing in conjunction with deep breathing facilitates the movement and expectoration of respiratory tract secretions. Coughing may be contraindicated postoperatively, depending on the type of surgery (e.g., craniotomy, eye surgery).

Encourage the client to do deep-breathing and coughing exercises hourly, or at least every 2 hours, during waking hours for the first few days. Assist the client to a sitting position in bed or on the side of the bed. The client can splint the incision with a pillow when coughing, or the nurse can splint the incision for the client to reduce discomfort.

LEG EXERCISES Encourage the client to do leg exercises taught in the preoperative period every 1 to 2 hours during waking hours. Muscle contractions compress the veins, preventing the stasis of blood in the veins, a cause of **thrombus** (astationary clot adhered to the wall of a vessel) formation and subsequent **thrombophlebitis** (inflammation of a vein followed by formation of a blood clot) and **emboli** (blood clots that have moved). Contractions also promote arterial blood flow.

MOVING AND AMBULATION Encourage and assist the client to turn from side to side at least every 2 hours. Alternating positions ensures maximum ventilation and perfusion to lungs. Avoid placing pillows or rolls under the client's knees because pressure on the popliteal blood vessels can interfere with blood circulation to and from the lower extremities. Clients who practise turning before surgery usually find it easier to do after surgery. See Chapter 35 for a complete discussion on preventing pressure ulcers in at-risk clients.

The client should ambulate as soon as possible after surgery, in accordance with the surgeon's orders. Generally, clients begin ambulation the evening of the day of surgery or the first day after surgery unless contraindicated. Early ambulation prevents respiratory, circulatory, urinary, and gastrointestinal complications. It also prevents general muscle weakness. Schedule ambulation for periods after the client has taken an analgesic or when the client is comfortable. Ambulation should be gradual, starting with the client sitting on the bed and dangling the feet over the side. A client who cannot ambulate is periodically assisted to a sitting position in bed, if allowed, and turned frequently. The sitting position permits the greatest lung expansion.

HYDRATION Maintain intravenous infusions, as ordered, to replace bodily fluids lost either before or during surgery. When oral intake is permitted, initially offer only small sips of water. Large amounts of water can induce vomiting because anesthetics and opioid analgesics temporarily inhibit gut motility. The patient who cannot take fluids by mouth *may* be allowed by the surgeon's orders to suck ice chips. Provide mouth care, and place a mouthwash at the client's bedside. Postoperative clients often complain of thirst and a dry, sticky mouth. These discomforts are a result of the preoperative fasting period, preoperative medications (such as atropine), and loss of bodily fluid.

Measure the patient's fluid intake and output for at least 2 days or until fluid balance is stable without an intravenous infusion. Ensuring adequate fluid balance is important to maintain renal and cardiovascular function.

PROPER DIET The surgeon orders the client's postoperative diet. Depending on the extent of surgery and the organs involved, the client may be allowed nothing by mouth for several days or may be able to resume oral intake when nausea is no longer present. When "diet as tolerated" is ordered, offer clear liquids initially. If the client tolerates these with no nausea or vomiting, the diet can often progress to full liquids and then to a regular diet, provided that gastrointestinal functioning is normal. Assess the return of peristalsis by auscultating the abdomen (see Chapter 28). Although in the past oral fluids and food were started only after the return of peristalsis, more recent evidence indicates that fluids and food actually assist in the return of peristalsis (Anderson, Lewis, & Thomas, 2006).

Observe the client's tolerance of the food and fluids ingested and note and report the passage of flatus, abdominal distension, bowel movements, and eructation (burping).

URINARY AND GASTROINTESTINAL ELIMINATION Anesthetic agents temporarily depress urinary bladder tone, which usually returns within 6 to 8 hours after surgery. Surgery of the prostate, vagina, rectum, or lower abdomen, during which the surgeon may manipulate the urinary bladder, often causes urinary retention. Patients who have had spinal or epidural anesthetic may also develop retention. Provide measures that promote urinary elimination. For example, help male clients stand at the bedside, or assist female clients to the bedside commode, if allowed, and ensure that fluid intake is adequate. Determine whether the client has any difficulties voiding, and assess the client for bladder distension. Report to the surgeon if a client does not void within 8 hours following surgery, unless another time frame is specified.

If all measures to promote voiding fail, a urinary catheterization is often ordered (see Chapter 42). Measure the fluid intake and output (I&O) of all new postoperative clients. Generally, I&O records are kept for at least 2 days or until the client re-establishes fluid balance without an IV or a catheter in place.

Anesthetic agents, opioids, handling of the intestines during abdominal surgery, fasting, and inactivity all inhibit bowel peristalsis. Most clients regain bowel function several hours after surgery, except in abdominal procedures where the return may be delayed for several days. Assess the return of peristalsis by auscultating the abdomen. Gurgling and rumbling sounds indicate peristalsis, as does passing of flatulence. Bowel sounds should be carefully assessed every 4 to 6 hours.

SUCTION   Some patients return from surgery with a nasogastric tube in place and orders to connect the tube to suction. For more information on gastrointestinal tubes, see Chapter 40. The suction ordered can be continuous or intermittent. Intermittent suction is applied when a single-lumen gastric tube is used to reduce the risk of damaging the mucous membrane near the distal port of the tube. Continuous suction may be applied if a double-lumen tube is in place (Figure 36.2). Fluids and electrolytes, especially potassium, must be replaced intravenously when gastric suction or continuous drainage is ordered. Nasogastric tubes can be irrigated if the lumen becomes clogged. They are generally irrigated before and after tube feedings or the instillation of medications. Nasogastric irrigation may

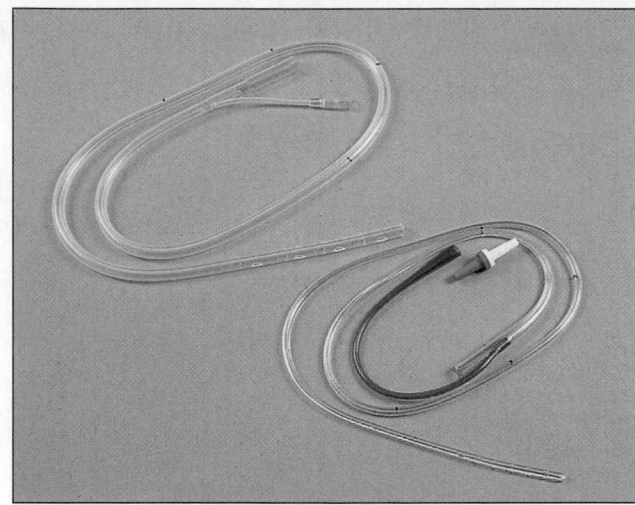

FIGURE 36.2 Nasogastric tubes used for gastric decompression: **Top left:** Levin (single-lumen) tube; **lower right:** Salem sump (double-lumen) tube with antireflux valve.

require a physician's order, particularly following gastrointestinal surgery. Agency policy for irrigations must be followed. Skill 36.3 describes the management of gastrointestinal suction. See also the Teaching: Home Care box on gastrointestinal suction on page 1086.

SKILL 36.3   MANAGING GASTROINTESTINAL SUCTION

PURPOSES

- To relieve abdominal distension
- To maintain gastric decompression after surgery
- To remove blood and secretions from the gastrointestinal tract
- To relieve discomfort (e.g., when a client has a bowel obstruction)
- To maintain the patency of the nasogastric tube

ASSESSMENT

Assess

- Presence of abdominal distension on palpation
- Bowel sounds
- Abdominal discomfort
- Vital signs for baseline data
- Amount and characteristics of drainage
- Nausea, vomiting

PLANNING

Before initiating gastric suction, determine (a) whether the suction is continuous or intermittent; (b) the ordered suction pressure (a low suction pressure is between 80 mm Hg and 100 mm Hg, and a high pressure is between 100 mm Hg and 120 mm Hg); (c) whether there is an order to irrigate the gastrointestinal tube, and if so, the type of solution to use; and (d) agency policy and physician's orders.

Equipment

Initiating Suction

- Gastrointestinal tube in place in the client
- Basin
- 50-mL syringe with an adapter
- Stethoscope
- Suction device for either continuous or intermittent suction
- Connector and connecting tubing
- Clean gloves

Maintaining Suction

- Graduated container, as required, to measure gastric drainage
- Basin of water
- Cotton-tipped applicators
- Ointment or lubricant
- Clean gloves

Irrigation

- Clean gloves
- Stethoscope
- Disposable irrigating set containing a sterile 50-mL syringe, moisture-resistant pad, basin, and graduated container
- Sterile normal saline (500 mL) or the ordered solution

(continued)

SKILL 36.3 MANAGING GASTROINTESTINAL SUCTION (*continued*)

IMPLEMENTATION

Performance

1. Before performing the procedure, introduce yourself and verify the client's identity using two identifiers or per agency protocol. Explain to the client what you are going to do, why it is necessary, and how he or she can participate. Discuss the purpose for the gastrointestinal suction.

2. Perform hand hygiene, and follow other appropriate infection prevention and control procedures (e.g., clean gloves).

3. Provide for client privacy.

Initiating Suction

4. Position the client appropriately.

   - Assist the client to the semi-Fowler's position if it is not contraindicated. **Rationale: In the semi-Fowler's position, the tube is not as likely to lie against the wall of the stomach and will, therefore, suction most efficiently. Semi-Fowler's position also prevents reflux of gastric contents, which could lead to aspiration**.

5. Confirm that the tube is in the stomach.

   - Put on clean gloves.
   - Aspirate stomach contents and check their acidity by using a pH test strip.
   - Insert air into the tube with the syringe, and listen with a stethoscope over the stomach (just below the xiphoid process) for a swish of air.
   - Use other methods in accordance with agency protocol. See Skill 40.2 in Chapter 40 (page 1245).

6. Set and check the suction equipment.

   - Connect the appropriate suction regulator to the wall suction outlet and the collection device to the regulator. *Intermittent suction regulators* generally are used with single-lumen tubes and apply suction for a set interval (15 to 60 seconds), followed by an interval of no suction. Intermittent suction is set at 80 mm Hg to 100 mm Hg (check agency policy) or as ordered by the physician. Check the suction level by occluding the drainage tube and observing the regulator dial during a suction cycle. *Continuous suction regulators* are used with double-lumen (e.g., Salem sump) nasogastric tubes. Set continuous suction as ordered by the physician, or at 80 mm Hg to 120 mm Hg (check agency policy).
   - If using a portable suction machine, turn on the machine and regulate the suction, as above. The Gomco pump has two settings: (a) low intermittent for single-lumen tubes, and (b) high for double-lumen tubes.
   - Test for proper suctioning by occluding the tube.

7. Establish gastric suction.

   - Connect the gastrointestinal tube to the suction tubing by using the connector.
   - If a Salem sump tube is in place, connect the larger lumen to the suction equipment. This double-lumen tube has a smaller tube running inside the primary suction tube. **Rationale: The smaller tube provides a continuous flow of atmospheric air through the drainage tube at its distal end and prevents excessive suction force on the gastric mucosa at the drainage outlets. Damage to the gastric mucosa is thus avoided**.

   - Always keep the air vent tube of a Salem sump tube open and above the level of the stomach when suction is applied. **Rationale: Closing the vent would stop the sump action and cause mucosal damage. Keeping the end of the air vent tube higher than the stomach prevents reflux of gastric contents into the air lumen of the tube**.
   - After suction is applied, watch the tubing for a few minutes until the gastric contents appear to be running through the tubing into the receptacle. A Salem sump tube makes a soft, hissing sound when it is functioning correctly.
   - If the suction is not working properly, check that all connections are tight and that the tubing is not kinked.
   - Anchor the tubing to the patient's gown so that it does not loop below the suction bottle. **Rationale: If the tubing falls below the suction bottle, the suction may be obstructed because of the pressure required to push the fluid against gravity**.

8. Assess the drainage.

   - Observe the amount, colour, odour, and consistency of the drainage. Normal gastric drainage has a mucoid consistency and is either colourless or yellow-green because of the presence of bile. A coffee-grounds colour and consistency may indicate bleeding.
   - Test the gastric drainage for pH and blood (by using Hematest), when indicated. A person who has had gastrointestinal surgery can be expected to have some blood in the drainage.

Maintaining Suction

9. Assess the client and the suction system regularly.

   - Assess the client every 30 minutes until the system is running effectively and then every 2 hours, or as the client's health indicates, to ensure that the suction is functioning properly. If the client complains of fullness, nausea, or epigastric pain, or if the flow of gastric secretions is absent in the tubing or in the collection bottle, ineffective suctioning or blockage of the nasogastric tube is likely.
   - Inspect the suction system for patency of the system (e.g., kinks or blockages in the tubing) and tightness of the connections. **Rationale: Loose connections can permit air to enter and thus decrease the effectiveness of the suction by decreasing the negative pressure**.

10. Relieve blockages, if present.

    - Put on clean gloves.
    - Check the suction equipment. To do this, disconnect the nasogastric tube from the suction over a collecting basin (to collect gastric drainage), and then, with the suction on, place the end of the suction tubing in a basin of water. If water is drawn into the drainage bottle, the suction equipment is functioning properly, but the nasogastric tube is either blocked or positioned incorrectly.
    - Reposition the client (e.g., to the other side), if permitted. **Rationale: This position may facilitate drainage**.
    - Rotate the nasogastric tube, and reposition it. This step is contraindicated for clients with gastric surgery. **Rationale: Moving the tube may interfere with gastric sutures**.
    - Irrigate the nasogastric tube as agency protocol states or on the order of the physician (see steps 14 to 16).

(continued)

11. Prevent reflux into the vent lumen of a Salem sump tube. **Rationale: Reflux of gastric contents into the vent lumen can occur when stomach pressure exceeds atmospheric pressure. In this situation, gastric contents follow the path of least resistance and flow out the vent lumen rather than the drainage lumen**.

    To prevent reflux, do the following:

    - Place the vent tubing higher than the client's stomach to prevent gastric fluid backup into the blue lumen air vent.
    - Keep the drainage lumen free of particulate matter that may obstruct the lumen (see steps 14 to 16 for irrigating a nasogastric tube).

12. Ensure client comfort.

    - Clean the client's nostrils, as needed, using the cotton-tipped applicators and water. Apply a water-soluble lubricant or ointment.
    - Provide mouth care every 2 hours and as needed. Some postoperative clients are permitted to suck ice chips or a moist cloth to maintain the moisture of the oral mucous membranes. A physician's order is required.

13. Empty the drainage receptacle, according to agency policy.

    - Clamp the nasogastric tube and turn off the suction.
    - Put on clean gloves.
    - If the receptacle is graduated, determine the amount of drainage.
    - Disconnect the receptacle.
    - If the receptacle is not graduated, empty the contents into a graduated container and measure.
    - Inspect the drainage carefully for colour, consistency, and presence of substances (e.g., blood clots).
    - Discard and replace receptacle, *or* rinse the receptacle with cool water and reattach it to the suction. Check agency policy.
    - Turn on the suction, and unclamp the nasogastric tube.
    - Observe the system for several minutes to make sure function is re-established.
    - Go to step 17.

Irrigating a Gastrointestinal Tube

14. Prepare the client and the equipment.

    - Verify physician's orders and agency policy.
    - Place the moisture-resistant pad under the end of the gastrointestinal tube.
    - Turn off the suction.
    - Put on clean gloves.
    - Disconnect the gastrointestinal tube from the connector.
    - Determine that the tube is in the stomach. See step 5. **Rationale: This step ensures that the irrigating solution enters the client's stomach.**

EVALUATION

- Conduct appropriate follow-up, such as relief of abdominal distension or discomfort, bowel sounds, character and amount of gastric drainage, integrity of nares, hydration of oral mucous membranes, patency of the tube, system functioning, and relief of nausea and vomiting.

15. Irrigate the tube.

    - Draw up the ordered volume of irrigating solution into the syringe; 30 mL of solution per instillation is usual, but up to 60 mL may be given per instillation, if ordered.
    - Attach the syringe to the nasogastric tube and slowly inject the solution.
    - Gently aspirate the solution, if indicated by agency policy. **Rationale: Forceful withdrawal could damage the gastric mucosa**.
    - If you encounter difficulty in withdrawing the solution, inject 20 mL of air and aspirate again, or reposition the client or the nasogastric tube. **Rationale: Air and repositioning may move the end of the tube away from the stomach wall**. If the aspirating difficulty continues, reattach the tube in intermittent low suction and notify the nurse in charge or the physician.
    - Repeat the preceding steps until the ordered amount of solution is used.
    - *Note:* A Salem sump tube can also be irrigated through the vent lumen without interrupting suction. However, only small quantities of irrigant can be injected via this lumen compared with the drainage lumen.
    - After irrigating a Salem sump tube, inject 10 mL to 20 mL of air into the vent lumen while applying suction to the drainage lumen. **Rationale: This tests the patency of the vent and ensures sump functioning**.

16. Re-establish suction.

    - Reconnect the nasogastric tube to the suction equipment.
    - Observe the system for several minutes to make sure it is functioning.

17. Document all relevant information.

    - Record the time suction was started. Also, record the pressure established, the colour and consistency of the drainage, and nursing assessments.
    - During maintenance, record assessments, supportive nursing measures, and data about the suction system.
    - When irrigating the tube, record verification of tube placement; the time of the irrigation; the amount and type of irrigating solution used; the number of times irrigated; the amount, colour, and consistency of the returns; the patency of the system following the irrigation; and nursing assessments.
    - Record client response and teaching.

- Compare with previous findings, if available.
- Report significant deviations from normal to the appropriate members of the health care team.

TEACHING	HOME CARE

Gastrointestinal Suction

Instruct the caregiver to do the following:

- Maintain suction, as ordered; do *not* increase or decrease the suction without instructions from the nurse or the physician.
- Offer mouth care every 2 hours.

- Avoid tension and pulling on the tube by securing it to the gown.
- Check the patency of the tube if nausea or vomiting occur.
- Report an increasing amount of drainage or bloody drainage.

Suction can also be applied to other drainage tubes, such as chest tubes or a wound drain. The type and amount of suction is ordered by the physician. Most agencies have *wall suction units* available (Figure 36.3). A suction regulator with a drainage receptacle connects to a wall outlet that provides negative pressure. Check the receptacle frequently to prevent excess drainage from interfering with the suction apparatus; empty or change the receptacle according to agency policy. *Portable electric suction units* or *pumps* (e.g., the Gomco pump) can be used in the home or when wall suction is not available.

WOUND CARE Most clients return from surgery with a wound that has been closed with sutures, staples, or fibrin sealant and covered by a dressing, although in some cases, such as when there is an infection, the wound is left open to heal by secondary intention. Dressings are inspected

regularly to ensure that they are clean, dry, and intact. Excessive drainage may indicate hemorrhage, infection, or an open wound.

When dressings are changed, the nurse assesses the wound for appearance, size, drainage, swelling, pain, and the status of drains or tubes (see Box 36.6). See the Clinical Alert box on incisions.

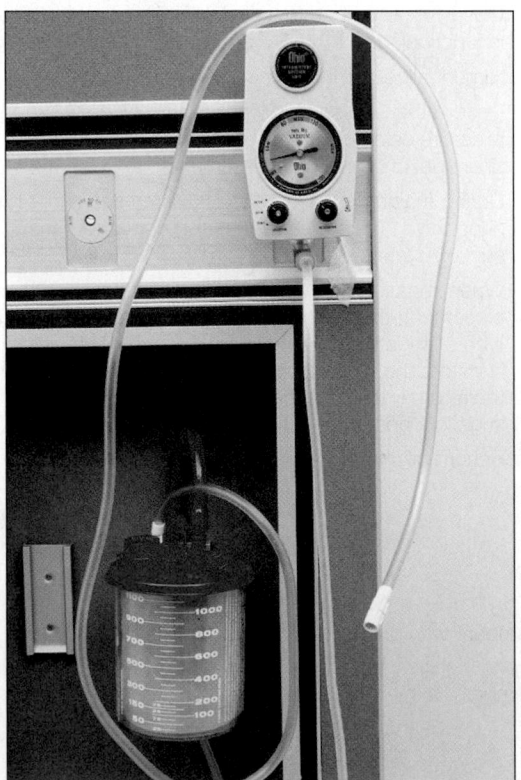

FIGURE 36.3 Wall suction unit for generating negative pressure for nasogastric suction.

BOX 36.6 ASSESSING SURGICAL WOUNDS

Assess surgical wounds for the following:

APPEARANCE

- Inspect the colour of the wound and surrounding area and the approximation of wound edges. If present, note the security of the sutures or staples.

SIZE

- Note the size and location of dehiscence, if present.

DRAINAGE

- Observe the location, colour, consistency, odour, and degree of saturation of dressings. Note the number of gauzes saturated or the diameter of drainage on the gauze.

EDEMA

- Observe the amount of swelling; minimal to moderate swelling is normal in early stages of wound healing.

PAIN

- Expect severe to moderate postoperative pain for 3 to 5 days; persistent severe pain or sudden onset of severe pain may indicate internal hemorrhaging or infection. Note specific areas of incision that cause pain when cleansed or dressed.

DRAINS OR TUBES

- Inspect drain security and placement, amount and character of drainage, and functioning of collecting apparatus, if present. Note the method of security (e.g., sutures, safety pin).

! CLINICAL ALERT

Assess the client immediately if she or he reports a giving or popping sensation in the incisional area. The client may be experiencing dehiscence or evisceration of the wound.

For surgical incisions healing by primary intention, the nurse can expect the following sequential signs of healing:

1. *Absence of bleeding and the appearance of a clot binding the wound edges.* The wound edges are well approximated and bound by fibrin in the clot within the first few hours after surgical closure.

2. *Inflammation (redness and swelling) at the wound edges for 1 to 3 days.*

3. *Reduction in inflammation when the clot diminishes,* as granulation tissue starts to bridge the area. The wound is bridged and closed within 7 to 10 days. Increased inflammation associated with fever and drainage is indicative of wound infection; the wound edges then appear brightly inflamed and swollen.

4. *Scar formation.* Collagen synthesis starts 4 days after injury and continues for 6 months or longer.

5. *Diminished scar size* over a period of months or years. An increase in scar size indicates keloid formation.

See Chapter 35 for information on wound healing, wound drainage, cleaning wounds, wound irrigation, hot and cold applications, and supporting and immobilizing wounds.

Surgical Dressings Not all surgical dressings require changing. Sometimes, surgeons in the operating room apply a dressing that remains in place until the sutures or staples are removed, and no further dressings are required. In many situations, however, surgical dressings are changed regularly to prevent the growth of microorganisms.

In some instances, a client may have a Penrose drain inserted (see page 1090). In this situation, the main surgical incision is considered cleaner than the surgical stab wound made for the drain insertion because the drainage is usually considerable. The main incision is, therefore, cleaned first, and *under no circumstances are materials that were used to clean the stab wound used subsequently* to clean the main incision. In this way, the main incision is kept free of the microorganisms around the stab wound. Box 36.5 (see page 1075) summarizes important data to be collected in assessing surgical wounds. Cleaning a surgical wound and applying a sterile dressing are detailed in Skill 36.4. See also the Teaching: Home Care box on cleaning a closed wound on page 1089.

SKILL 36.4 CLEANING A CLOSED SURGICAL WOUND AND APPLYING A STERILE DRESSING

PURPOSES

- To promote wound healing by primary intention
- To prevent infection
- To assess the healing process
- To protect the wound from mechanical trauma

ASSESSMENT

Assess

- Client allergies to wound cleaning agents
- The appearance and size of the wound
- The amount and character of exudates
- Client complaints of pain or discomfort
- The time of the last analgesia
- Signs of systemic infection (e.g., elevated body temperature, diaphoresis, malaise, leukocytosis)

PLANNING

Before changing a dressing, determine any specific orders about the wound or dressing.

Equipment

- Moisture-proof bag
- Mask (optional)
- Acetone or another solution (if necessary, to loosen adhesive)
- Clean gloves, sterile gloves

- Sterile dressing set including drape or towel, sterile gauze squares, cleaning solution (e.g., normal saline) and container, antiseptic solution for cleansing table surface, two pairs of sterile forceps (thumb or artery), sterile gauze dressings and surgipads (if necessary).
- Additional supplies required for the particular dressing (e.g., extra gauze dressings, medicated ointment, if ordered)
- Tape, tie tapes, or binder

IMPLEMENTATION

Preparation

- Confirm the physician's order, and check agency policy.
- Acquire assistance for changing a dressing on a restless or confused adult. **Rationale: The person might move and contaminate the sterile field or the wound**.
- Assist the client to a comfortable position in which the wound can be readily exposed. Expose only the wound area by using a sheet or bath blanket to cover the client, if necessary. **Rationale: Undue exposure causes unnecessary physical and psychological distress to most people**.
- Make a cuff on the moisture-proof bag for disposal of the soiled dressings, and place the bag within reach. It can be taped to the bedclothes away from the sterile field. **Rationale: Making a cuff helps keep the outside of the bag free from contamination by the soiled dressings and prevents subsequent contamination of the nurse's hands or of sterile instrument tips when discarding dressings or sponges. Placing the bag within reach prevents the nurse from reaching across the sterile**

(continued)

SKILL 36.4 CLEANING A CLOSED SURGICAL WOUND AND APPLYING A STERILE DRESSING (*continued*)

field and the wound and potentially contaminating these areas.

- Clean the table surface for the sterile field with antiseptic solution.
- Put on a mask, if required. **Rationale: Some agencies require that a mask be worn for surgical dressing changes to prevent contamination of the wound by droplet spray from the nurse's respiratory tract.**

Performance

1. Before performing the procedure, introduce yourself and verify the client's identity using two identifiers or per agency protocol. Explain to the client what you are going to do, why it is necessary, and how he or she can participate. Discuss how the results will be used in planning further care or treatments.

2. Perform hand hygiene, and follow other appropriate infection prevention and control procedures.

3. Provide for client privacy.

4. Remove binders and tape.
   - Remove binders, if used, and place them aside. Untie tie tapes, if used. Montgomery straps (tie tapes) are commonly used for wounds requiring frequent dressing changes (see ❶). **Rationale: These straps prevent skin irritation and discomfort caused by removing the adhesive each time the dressing is changed.**
   - If adhesive tape was used, remove it by holding down the skin and pulling parallel to the skin and toward the dressing. **Rationale: Pressing down on the skin provides countertraction against the pulling motion. Tape is pulled toward the incision to prevent strain on the wound.**
   - Use a solvent to loosen tape, if required. **Rationale: Moistening the tape with acetone or a similar solvent lessens the discomfort of removal, particularly from hairy surfaces.**

5. Remove and dispose of soiled dressings appropriately.
   - Put on clean disposable gloves, and remove the outer abdominal dressing or surgipad.

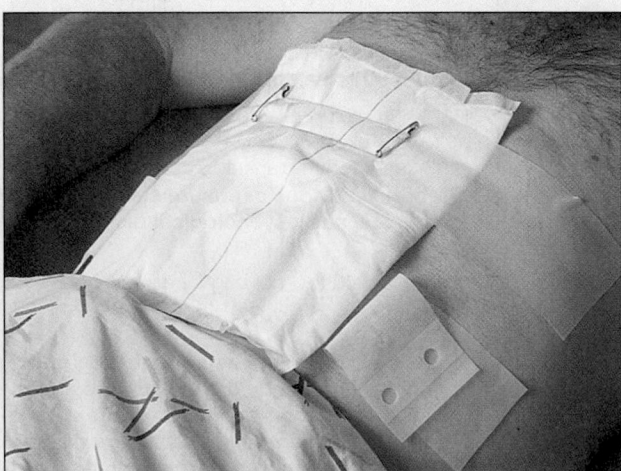

❶ Montgomery tapes holding dressing

- Lift the outer dressing so that the underside is away from the client's face. **Rationale: The appearance and odour of the drainage may be upsetting to the client. Note any drainage.**
- Place the soiled dressing in the moisture-proof bag without touching the outside of the bag. **Rationale: Contamination of the outside of the bag is avoided to prevent the spread of microorganisms to the nurse and subsequently to others.**
- Remove the *under* dressings with a sterile forceps, taking care not to dislodge any drains. If the gauze sticks to the drain, support the drain with one hand and remove the gauze with the other.
- Assess the location, type (colour, consistency), and odour of wound drainage and the number of gauzes saturated or the diameter of drainage collected on the dressings.
- Discard the soiled dressings in the bag as before.
- Remove gloves, dispose of them in the moisture-proof bag, and perform hand hygiene.

6. Set up the sterile supplies by using aseptic technique.
   - Open the sterile dressing set by using surgical aseptic technique.
   - Place the sterile drape beside the wound.
   - Open the sterile cleaning solution and pour it over the gauze sponges in the plastic container.

7. Clean the wound, if indicated.
   - Clean the wound by using your gloved hands or forceps and gauze swabs moistened with cleaning solution.
   - If using forceps, keep the forceps tips lower than the handles at all times. **Rationale: This prevents contamination by fluid travelling up to the handle and nurse's wrist and back to the tips.**
   - Use the cleaning methods illustrated and described in ❷ or one recommended by agency protocol.
   - Use a separate swab for each stroke, and discard each swab after use. **Rationale: Doing this prevents the introduction of microorganisms to other wound areas.**
   - If a drain is present, clean it next, taking care to avoid reaching across the cleaned incision. Clean the skin around the drain site by swabbing in half or full circles from around the drain site outward, using separate swabs for each wipe (see ❷C).
   - Support and hold the drain erect while cleaning around it. Clean as many times as necessary to remove the drainage. Clean the drain, cleansing at the stab wound and then up the drain away from skin.
   - Dry the drain area with dry gauze swabs, as required. Do not dry the incision or wound itself. **Rationale: Moisture facilitates wound healing.**

8. Apply dressings to the drain site and the incision.
   - Place a precut 10 cm × 10 cm gauze snugly around the drain (see ❸). **Rationale: This dressing absorbs the drainage and helps prevent it from excoriating (tearing off) skin. Using precut gauze instead of cutting the gauze prevents any threads from coming loose and getting into the wound where**

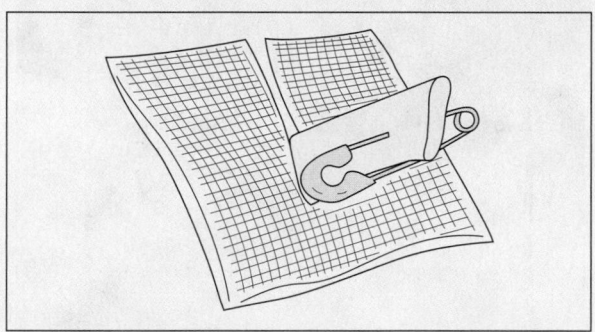

❷ Methods of cleaning surgical wounds: **A:** Cleaning the wound from top to bottom, starting at the centre; **B:** Cleaning a wound outward from the incision; **C:** Cleaning around a drain site. For all methods, a clean sterile swab is used for each stroke.

❸ Precut gauze in place around a drain

they could cause inflammation and provide a site for infection.

- Apply the sterile dressings one at a time over the drain site. Place the bulk of the dressings over the drain area and below the drain, depending on the client's usual position. **Rationale: Layers of dressings are placed for best absorption of drainage, which flows by gravity**.

- Apply the final surgipad or abdominal pad over the entire site. Secure the dressing with tape or ties.

9. Document the procedure and all nursing assessments.

EVALUATION

- Conduct appropriate follow-up, such as amount of granulation tissue or degree of healing; amount of drainage and its colour, consistency, and odour; presence of inflammation; and degree of discomfort associated with the incision or drain site.

- Compare with previous findings, if available.
- Report significant deviations from normal to the appropriate members of the health care team.

TEACHING | **HOME CARE**

Cleaning a Closed Wound

Instruct caregivers to do the following:

- Provide analgesics approximately 30 minutes before the procedure if the wound care causes pain or discomfort.
- Perform hand hygiene and dry your hands before handling wound care supplies and providing wound care.
- Clean and wipe dry a flat surface for the sterile field.
- Keep pets out of the area when setting up for and performing sterile procedures.
- Acquire all needed supplies before starting a *sterile* procedure.
- Maintain sterile or clean technique, as instructed.

- Handle all *sterile* supplies from the outside of the wrapper or the edges.
- Do not touch the parts of supplies or equipment that will touch the patient.
- Avoid skin injury by using paper tape or Montgomery tie tapes instead of adhesive tape.
- Report any increasing wound drainage, pain, redness, increasing swelling, or opening or gaping of wound edges.
- Place any soiled dressing materials in a waterproof bag and dispose of it according to public health recommendations.

Wound Drains and Suction Surgical drains are inserted to permit the drainage of excessive serosanguineous fluid and purulent material and to promote healing of underlying tissues. These drains may be inserted and sutured through the incision line, but they are most commonly inserted through stab wounds a few centimetres away from the incision line so that the incision itself can be kept dry. Without a drain, some wounds would heal on the surface and trap the discharge inside, and an abscess might form. There are two types of wound drainage systems: open-drainage and closed-drainage. An **open-drainage system** has one end of the drain in the wound or in the vicinity of the surgical procedure and the other end opening outside the body (generally covered by a dressing) with the wound drainage draining by gravity (e.g., a Penrose drain: see 2C of Skill 36.4).

A **closed-drainage system** consists of a drain connected to either an electric suction or a portable drainage suction, such as a Hemovac (Figure 36.4) or Jackson-Pratt (Figure 36.5). The closed system reduces the possible entry of microorganisms into the wound through the drain. The drainage tubes are sutured in place and connected to a reservoir. For example, the Jackson-Pratt

drainage tube is connected to a reservoir that maintains constant low suction. These portable wound suctions also provide for accurate measurement of the drainage and prevent leakage of drainage over the incision site.

The surgeon inserts the wound drainage tube during surgery. Generally, the suction is discontinued from 3 to 5 days postoperatively or when the drainage is minimal. Nurses are responsible for maintaining the wound suction, which hastens the healing process by draining excess exudate that might otherwise interfere with the formation of granulation tissue.

Closed-drainage systems have directions for use printed on the drainage container. When emptying the container, the nurse should wear gloves and avoid touching the drainage port (Figure 36.6). To re-establish suction,

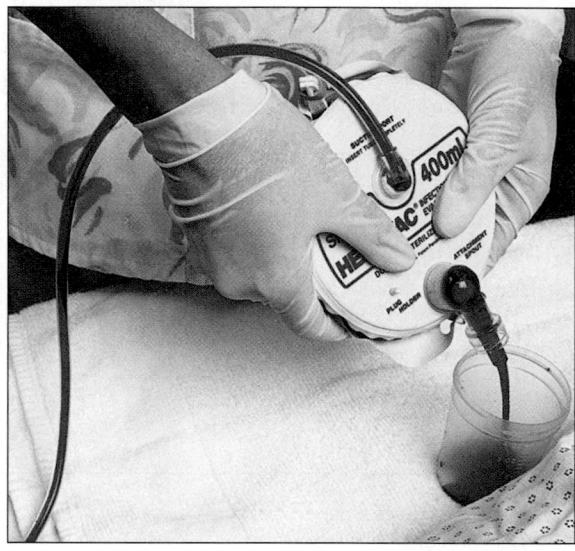

FIGURE 36.6 Emptying drainage from a Hemovac drainage system.

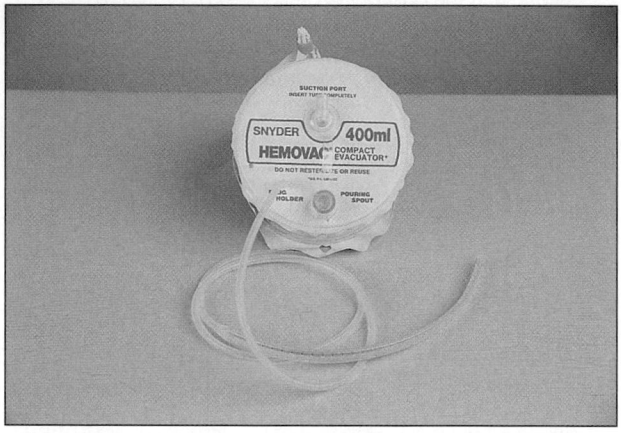

FIGURE 36.4 Hemovac closed-drainage system.

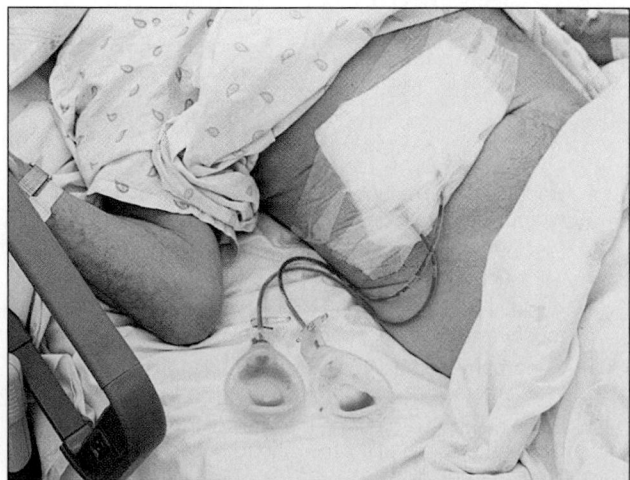

FIGURE 36.5 Two Jackson-Pratt devices compressed to facilitate collection of exudates.

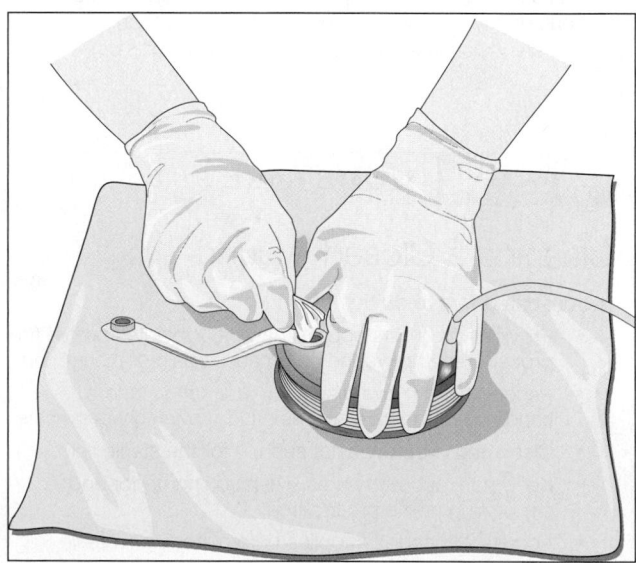

FIGURE 36.7 With one hand, press the top and bottom together. With the other hand, clean the opening and plug with an alcohol swab. Replace the plug before releasing hand.

the nurse places the container on a solid, flat surface with the port open. The palm of one hand presses the top and bottom together while the other hand cleanses the opening and plug with an alcohol swab (Figure 36.7). Replace the drainage plug before releasing hand pressure to re-establish the vacuum necessary for the closed drainage system to work.

Sutures A **suture** (referred to as a *stitch* in lay terms) is a material (e.g., thread) used to approximate body tissues together. Sutures used to attach tissues beneath the skin are often made of an absorbable material (e.g., animal gut) that disappears in several days. Skin sutures, by contrast, are made of a variety of nonabsorbable materials, such as silk, cotton, linen, wire, nylon, and Dacron (polyester fibre). Silver wire clips or staples are also available. Usually, skin sutures are removed 7 to 10 days after surgery and up to 14 days for sutures over joints.

Suturing can be done by using various methods. Skin sutures can be broadly categorized as either *interrupted* (each stitch is tied and knotted separately) or *continuous* (one thread runs in a series of stitches and is tied only at the beginning and at the end of the run).

Retention sutures are very large sutures used in addition to skin sutures for some incisions (Figure 36.8). They attach underlying tissues of fat and muscle as well as skin and are used to support incisions in individuals who are obese or when healing may be prolonged. They are frequently left in place longer than skin sutures (14 to 21 days) but, in some instances, are removed at the same time as the skin sutures. To prevent these large sutures from irritating the incision, the surgeon may place rubber tubing over them or a roll of gauze under them extending down the incision line.

The physician orders the removal of sutures. In some agencies, only physicians remove sutures; in others, registered nurses and nursing students with appropriate supervision can do so. Agency policies about removal of retention sutures vary. The nurse should verify whether they are to be removed and who can remove them.

Sterile technique and special suture scissors are used in suture removal. The scissors have a short, curved cutting tip that readily slides under the suture (Figure 36.9). Wire clips or staples are removed with a special instrument that squeezes the centre of the clip to remove it from the skin (Figure 36.10).

Guidelines for removing sutures follow:

• Before removing skin sutures, verify (a) the orders for suture removal (in some instances, only *alternate* interrupted sutures are removed one day, and the remaining sutures are removed a day or two later), and (b) whether a dressing is to be applied following the suture removal. Some physicians prefer no dressing;

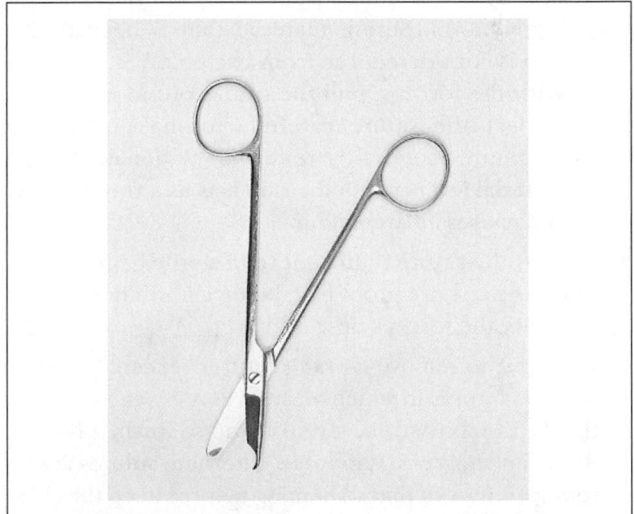

FIGURE 36.9 Suture scissors.

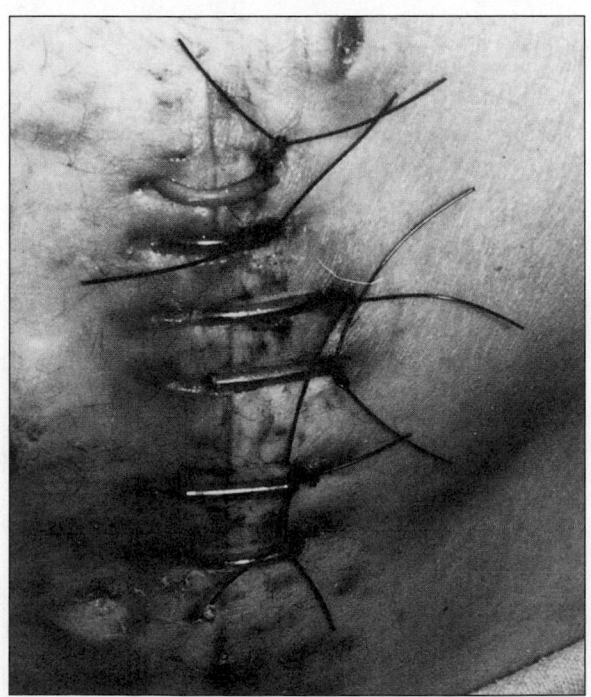

FIGURE 36.8 A surgical incision with retention sutures.

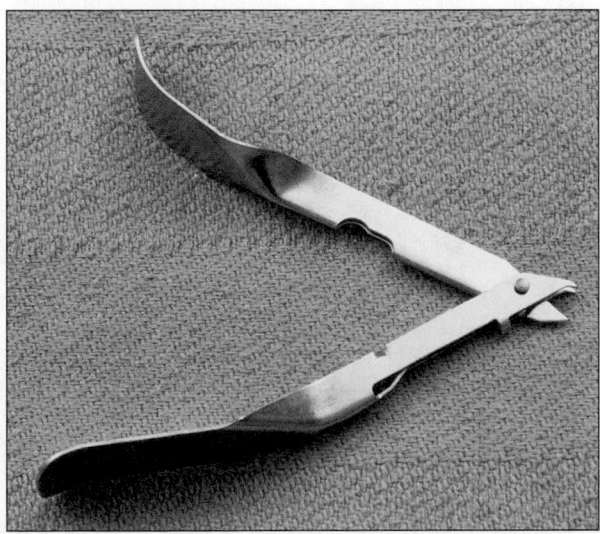

FIGURE 36.10 Staple remover.

others prefer a small, light gauze dressing to prevent friction by clothing.

- Inform the client that suture removal may produce slight discomfort, such as a pulling or stinging sensation, but it should not be painful.

- Remove the dressings and clean the incision, in accordance with agency protocol. Cleaning the suture line with normal saline before and after suture removal may help prevent infection.

- Put on sterile gloves.

- Remove the sutures as follows:
   a. Grasp the suture at the knot with a pair of forceps.
   b. Place the curved tip of the suture scissors under the suture as close to the skin as possible, either on the side opposite the knot (Figure 36.11) or directly under the knot. Cut the suture. Sutures are cut as close to the skin as possible on one side of the visible part because the suture material that is visible to the eye is in contact with resident bacteria of the skin and must not be pulled beneath the skin during removal. Suture material that is beneath the skin is considered free from bacteria.
   c. With the forceps, pull the suture out in one piece. Inspect the suture carefully to make sure that all suture material is removed. **Rationale: Suture material left beneath the skin acts as a foreign body and causes inflammation.**

- Discard the suture onto a piece of sterile gauze or into the moisture-proof bag, being careful not to contaminate the forceps tips.

- Continue to remove *alternate* sutures (except for continuous sutures in which all sutures are removed), that is, the third, fifth, seventh, and so forth, if no dehiscence occurs. **Rationale: Alternate sutures are removed first so that remaining sutures keep the skin edges in close approximation and prevent any dehiscence from becoming large.**

- If no dehiscence occurs, remove the remaining sutures. If dehiscence does occur, do not remove the remaining sutures, and report the dehiscence to the nurse in charge.

- If Steri-Strips are ordered by the physician, apply them to the wound after removing the sutures or clips. Some physicians order Steri-Strip application to provide additional support to the healing wound.

- Reapply a dressing, if indicated.

- Document the suture removal; number of sutures removed; appearance of the incision; application of a dressing, Steri-Strips, or butterfly tapes (if appropriate); client teaching; and client tolerance of the procedure.

- Remove the staples as follows:
   a. Remove the dressings, and clean the incision, in accordance with agency protocol.
   b. Place the lower tips of a sterile staple remover under the staple.
   c. Squeeze the handles together until they are completely closed (Figure 36.12). Pressing the handles together causes the staple to bend in the middle and pulls the edges of the staple out of the skin. Do not lift the staple remover when squeezing the handles.
   d. When both ends of the staple are visible, gently move the staple away from the incision site.
   e. Hold the staple remover over a disposable container, release the staple remover handles, and release the staple.

If the sutures are to be removed outside a clinical setting, sterile technique is used (see the Home Care Considerations box for client information).

Evaluating

By using the goals developed during the planning stage—maintaining comfort, promoting healing, restoring wellness, and preventing risks associated with surgery—the

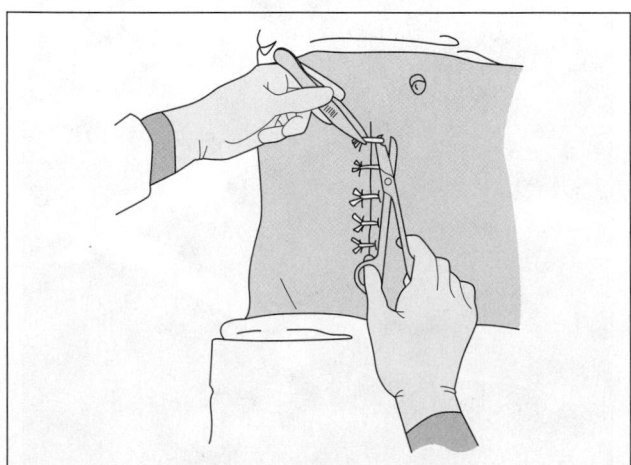

FIGURE 36.11 Removing a skin suture.

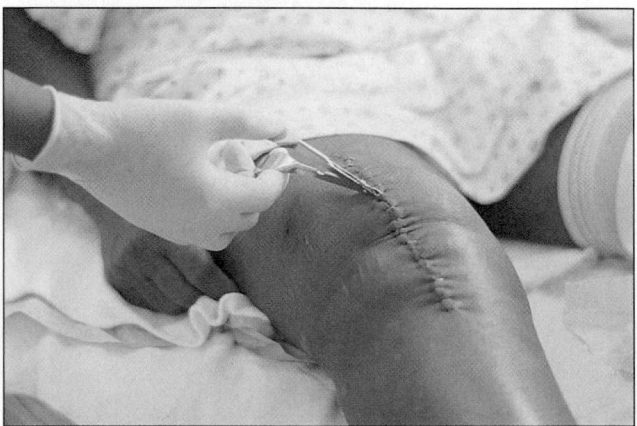

FIGURE 36.12 Removing surgical clips or staples.

HOME CARE CONSIDERATIONS

Removing Sutures or Staples

- Perform the procedure in a well-lit, private area of the home.
- Instruct the client to observe the incision daily and to call the appropriate member of the health care team if increased redness, drainage, or open areas are observed.
- Provide instructions and supplies for care of the incision, and tell the client when to shower for the first time.
- Assess the client's ability to keep the incision clean and protected at home.

nurse collects data to evaluate whether the identified goals and desired outcomes have been achieved. Examples of client goals and related outcomes are shown in Table 36.3.

If the desired outcomes are not achieved, the nurse, client, and support people need to explore the reasons why before modifying the care plan. For example, if the goal "Maintain comfort" is *not* met, questions to be considered include the following:

- What is the client's perception of the problem?
- Is the prescribed analgesic dose adequate for the client?
- Is the client allowing pain to become intense before requesting medication or using PCA?
- Where is the client's pain? Could it be due to a problem unrelated to surgery (e.g., chronic arthritis, anginal pain)?
- Is there evidence of a complication that could cause increased pain (an infection, abscess, or hematoma)?

TABLE 36.3 Evaluation Goals and Outcomes for Clients after Surgery

Goal	Examples of Desired Outcomes
Maintain comfort	Verbalizes satisfaction with pain control measures
	Absence of nonverbal indications of pain (e.g., protective body position, restlessness, facial expressions of pain)
	Absence of physiological indications of pain (e.g., muscle tension; perspiration; change in blood pressure, heart rate, respiratory rate, and pupil size; loss of appetite)
	Moves and ambulates with minimal difficulty
	Rests for extended periods
Promote healing	Incision clean, dry, and intact
	Wound edges approximated well with absence of exudate
	Balanced fluid intake and output
	Tolerating diet rich in fibre, protein, and vitamins A and C
	Active bowel sounds within 48 hours
	Normal defecation within 3 days following ingestion of food
	Hemoglobin, hematocrit, and serum electrolytes within normal limits
Prevent risks associated with surgery	Performs deep breathing, coughing, and incentive spirometry, as instructed
	Normal auscultated breath sounds heard bilaterally
	Adequate respiratory excursion (depth)
	Performs leg exercises, as instructed
	Walks increasing distances (specify) each day
	Stable vital signs
	Strong and equal peripheral pulses in all four extremities
Restore highest possible level of wellness	Increasingly participates in self-care activities (specify)
	Asks pertinent questions concerning ongoing care
	Seeks help, as appropriate
	Demonstrates ability to care for incision
	Reports ability to manage ongoing care

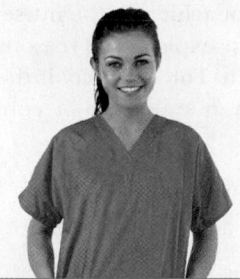

Case Study 36

Mr. Teng is a 77-year-old client with a history of chronic obstructive pulmonary disease. Currently, his respiratory condition is being controlled with medications, and he is free of infection. He has just been transferred to the PACU following an inguinal hernia repair performed under spinal anesthesia. His blood pressure is 132/88 mm Hg, pulse 84, respirations 28, and tympanic temperature is 36.8°C. He is awake and alert.

CRITICAL THINKING QUESTIONS

1. What factors place Mr. Teng at increased risk for the development of complications during and after surgery?

2. Speculate about why Mr. Teng's surgeon and anesthesiologist decided to perform Mr. Teng's surgery under regional anesthesia as opposed to general anesthesia.

3. What preparations were taken during the preoperative period to protect Mr. Teng from possible complications during and after his surgery?

4. How will Mr. Teng's postoperative assessments differ from those of a person who received general anesthesia?

5. What postoperative precautions are especially important to Mr. Teng in view of his chronic lung condition?

Check the eText in MyNursingLab for answers and explanations.

KEY TERMS

atelectasis   *p. 1064*

circulating nurse   *p. 1074*

closed-drainage system
   p. 1090

conscious sedation
   p. 1073

elective surgery   *p. 1058*

emboli   *p. 1082*

emergency surgery
   p. 1058

epidural (peridural)
   anesthesia   *p. 1073*

general anesthesia
   p. 1072

intraoperative phase
   p. 1057

intravenous block (Bier
   block)   *p. 1073*

invasive (open) surgery
   p. 1058

local anesthesia   *p. 1073*

local infiltration
   p. 1073

major surgery   *p. 1058*

minimally invasive surgery
   p. 1058

minor surgery   *p. 1058*

nerve block   *p. 1073*

open-drainage system
   p. 1090

perioperative period
   p. 1057

postoperative phase
   p. 1057

preoperative phase
   p. 1057

regional anesthesia
   p. 1073

scrub nurse   *p. 1074*

spinal anesthesia   *p. 1073*

subarachnoid block
   p. 1073

suture   *p. 1091*

thrombophlebitis
   p. 1082

thrombus   *p. 1082*

topical (surface)
   anesthesia   *p. 1073*

urgent surgery   *p. 1058*

CHAPTER HIGHLIGHTS

- Surgery is a unique experience that creates stress and necessitates physical and psychological changes.
- The perioperative period includes three phases: preoperative, intraoperative, and postoperative.
- Surgical procedures are categorized by purpose, degree of urgency, level of invasiveness, body part, equipment used, and degree of risk.
- Such factors as age, general health, nutritional status, medication history, and mental status affect a client's risk during surgery.
- Clients must agree to surgery and sign an informed consent.
- Nursing history and physical assessment data are important sources for planning preoperative and postoperative care.

- The overall goal of nursing care during the preoperative phase is to prepare the client mentally and physically for surgery.
- Preoperative teaching includes situational information and psychosocial support, the role of the client throughout the perioperative period, expected sensations and discomfort, and training for the postoperative period.
- Preoperative teaching should include moving, leg exercises, and coughing and deep-breathing exercises. Many aspects of preoperative teaching are intended to prevent postoperative complications.
- Physical preparation includes the following areas: nutrition and fluids, elimination, medications, skin preparation (hygiene, hair, nails), sleep, care of valuables and prostheses, and following special orders.

- Antiembolism stockings or sequential compression devices may be ordered for some clients to facilitate venous return and prevent venous thromboembolism.

- A preoperative checklist provides a guide to and documentation of a client's preparation before surgery.

- Maintaining the client's safety is the overall goal of nursing care during the intraoperative phase.

- Anesthesia may be general, local, or regional. General anesthesia involves the loss of consciousness. Local anesthesia techniques include topical anesthesia and local infiltration; regional anesthesia techniques include nerve block, intravenous block, spinal anesthesia (subarachnoid block), and epidural. Conscious sedation is used as an adjunctive.

- Positioning of the client during surgery is important to reduce the risk of tissue and nerve damage.

- Immediate postanesthetic care focuses on assessment and monitoring parameters to prevent complications from anesthesia or surgery.

- Initial and ongoing assessment of the postoperative client includes level of consciousness, vital signs, oxygen saturation, skin colour and temperature, comfort, fluid balance, dressings, drains, and tubes.

- The overall goals of nursing care during the postoperative period are to promote comfort and healing, restore the highest possible level of wellness, and prevent associated risks, such as infection or respiratory and cardiovascular complications.

- Ongoing postoperative nursing interventions include (a) managing pain, (b) positioning appropriately, (c) encouraging incentive spirometry and deep-breathing and coughing exercises, (d) promoting leg exercises, (e) encouraging early ambulation, (f) maintaining adequate hydration, (g) promoting a proper diet, (h) promoting urinary elimination, (i) continuing gastrointestinal suction, and (j) providing wound care.

- Sterile technique is used when changing dressings on surgical wounds to promote healing and reduce the risk of infection.

- Jackson-Pratt and Hemovac closed drainage systems are examples of drains that may be placed in or near surgical wounds to promote drainage of excess serosanguinous or purulent exudate.

- Sutures, wire clips, or staples are used to approximate skin and underlying tissues after surgery. These are generally removed 7 to 10 days after surgery.

ASSESS YOUR LEARNING

1. Which of the following tests is the best for determining the status of a client's preoperative liver function?

   a. Serum electrolytes, Complete blood count (CBC) and Thyroid stimulating hormone (TSH)

   b. Blood urea nitrogen (BUN), creatinine, and Complete blood count (CBC)

   c. Alanine aminotransferase (ALT), aspirate aminotransferase (AST), bilirubin

   d. Serum albumin, Thyroid stimulating hormone (TSH), and Fasting glucose (FBG)

2. A client who is having a mastectomy expresses sadness about losing her breast. Based on this information, the nurse would identify that the client is at risk for which nursing diagnosis?

   a. Disturbance in body image

   b. Anticipatory grieving

   c. Fear

   d. Ineffective coping

3. Which of the following statements by the client indicates that the preoperative teaching regarding elective abdominal surgery has been effective?

   a. "I cannot eat or drink anything after midnight."

   b. "I'm not going to cough after surgery because it might open my incision."

   c. "I might have a stroke if I stop taking my anticoagulant."

   d. "The nurse showed me how to contract and relax my calf muscles."

4. The nurse assesses a postoperative client who has a rapid and weak pulse, urine output of less than 30 mL/h, and decreased blood pressure. The client's skin is cool and clammy. What complication should the nurse suspect?

   a. Thrombophlebitis

   b. Hypovolemic shock

   c. Aspiration pneumonia

   d. Wound dehiscence

5. The client is most likely to require the greatest amount of analgesia for pain during which of the following times?

   a. Immediately after surgery

   b. 4 hours after surgery

   c. 12 to 36 hours after surgery

   d. 48 to 60 hours after surgery

6. Ms. Johnson, 28 years old, returns to the unit after a large bowel resection and creation of a colostomy with a Hemovac in place. Which of the following nursing assessments should be included in the initial postoperative documentation?

   a. Vital signs.

   b. Ability to perform deep breathing and coughing exercises.

   c. Position of the client postoperatively.

   d. Amount of drainage in the Hemovac.

7. A semiconscious client in the postanesthesia care unit (PACU) is experiencing dyspnea. Which of the following actions should the nurse perform first?

   a. Place a pillow under the client's head.

   b. Remove the oropharyngeal airway.

   c. Apply oxygen by mask.

   d. Reposition the client to keep the tongue forward.

8. The client's postoperative orders state "diet as tolerated." The client has been NPO. The nurse will advance the client's diet to clear liquids based on which of the following assessments?

   a. No complaints of nausea or vomiting

   b. Pain level is maintained at a rating of 2 to 3 out of 10

   c. Ambulates with minimal assistance

   d. Presence of bowel sounds

9. Which of the following is the overall goal of nursing care during the intraoperative phase?

   a. To promote the client's safety

   b. The ensure that the client has granted informed consent

   c. To enhance the client's quality of life

   d. To enhance the client's coping abilities

10. The nurse plans to remove the client's sutures. Which of the following actions demonstrates appropriate standards of care?

    a. Perform hand hygiene first, and then use clean technique.

    b. Remove sutures one after the other along the length of the incision line.

    c. Place the curved tip of the suture scissors under the suture as close to the skin as possible.

    d. Pull the suture material that is visible beneath the skin during removal.

> *Check the eText in MyNursingLab for answers and explanations.*

WEBLINKS

The Canadian Anesthesiologists' Society
http://www.cas.ca

This not-for-profit voluntary organization's website provides current information and guidelines for the practice of anesthesia and patient information about anesthesia.

Operating Room Nurses Association of Canada
http://www.ornac.ca

This website provides information related to the history, mission, values, and standards of practice of operating room nurses.

MyNursingLab

REFERENCES

Anderson, H. K., Lewis, S. J., & Thomas, S. (2006). Early enteral nutrition within 24h of colorectal surgery versus later commencement of feeding for postoperative complications. *Cochrane Database of Systematic Reviews, 4,* Art. No.: CD004080.

Brady, M., Kinn, S., O'Rourke, K., Randhawa, N., & Stuart, P. (2005). Preoperative fasting for preventing perioperative complications in children. *Cochrane Database of Systematic Review, 2,* Art. No.: CD005285.

Canadian Patient Safety Institute. (2012). *Surgical safety checklist & scorecard: Canada.* Retrieved from http://signup.patientsafetyinstitute.ca/English/toolsResources/sssl/Pages/SurgicalSafetyChecklist.aspx

Merchant, R., Chartrand, D., Dain, S., Dobson, J., Kurrek, M., LeDez, K., Morgan, P., & Shukla, R. (2012). *Guidelines to the practice of anesthesia* (Rev. ed. 2012). *Canadian Journal of Anesthesia, 59*(1), 62–102.

Registered Nurses' Association of Ontario. (2011). *Nursing best practice guideline: Risk assessment and prevention of pressure ulcers—guideline supplement.* (Rev. ed.). Toronto, ON: Author. Retrieved from http://www.rnao.org/Storage/83/7749_PRESSURE-ULCERS_Supplement_2011.pdf

Safer Healthcare Now! (2010). Preventing surgical site infections: Getting started kit. Retrieved from http://www.saferhealthcarenow.ca/EN/Interventions/SSI/Pages/default.aspx

Wait Time Alliance. (2011). Wait Time Alliance: Report card on wait times in Canada, 2011. Author. Retrieved from http://www.waittimealliance.ca/publications.htm

UNIT
6

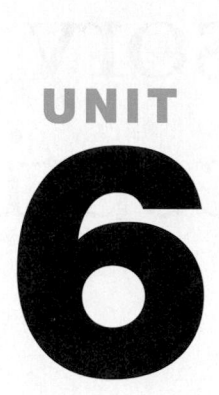

Promoting Physiological Health

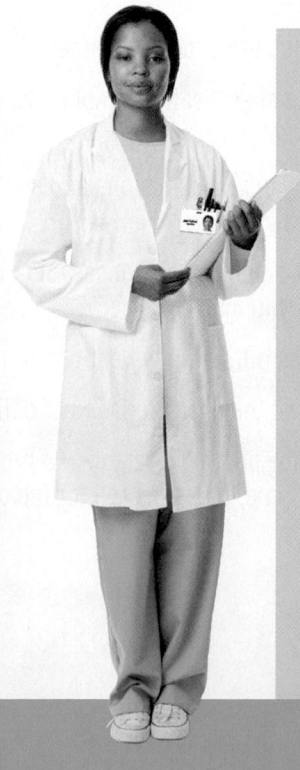

Chapter 37

Sensory Perception

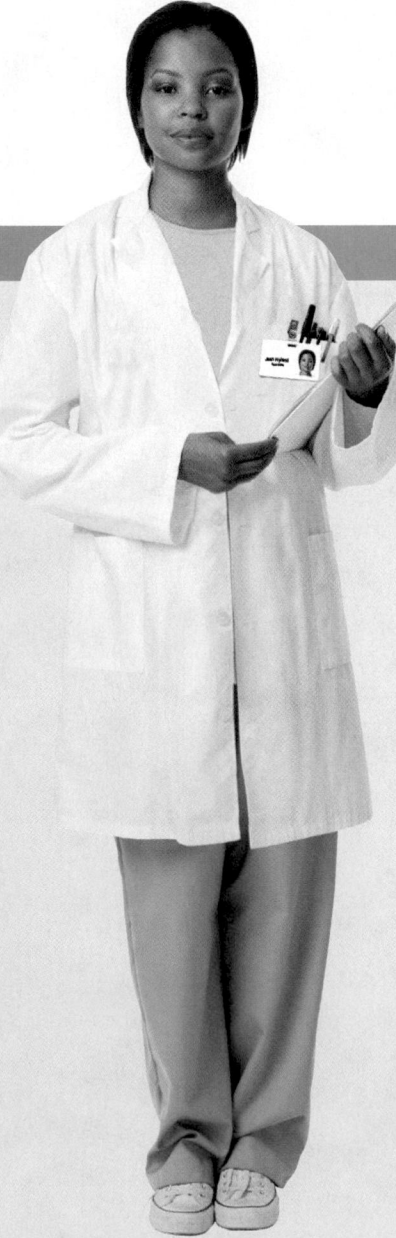

LEARNING OUTCOMES

After studying this chapter, you will be able to:

1. Discuss anatomical and physiological components of the sensory-perceptual process.

2. Describe three factors that affect a client's sensory functioning.

3. Outline six essential components in assessing a client's sensory-perceptual function.

4. Identify the clinical signs and symptoms of sensory overload and sensory deprivation.

5. Develop nursing diagnoses and outcome criteria for clients with impaired sensory function.

6. Discuss nursing interventions to promote and maintain sensory function.

7. Contrast the characteristics of delirium with the characteristics of dementia.

8. Describe nursing strategies to promote and maintain orientation to person, place, time, and situation for the client who is disoriented.

A n individual's senses are essential for growth, development, and survival. Sensory stimuli give meaning to events in the environment. Any alteration in people's sensory functions can affect their ability to function within the environment. Nurses can help them find ways to function safely in this often confusing environment.

Components of the Sensory-Perceptual Process

Reception and Perception

The sensory process involves two components: (a) reception and (b) perception. **Sensory reception** is the process of receiving stimuli or data. These stimuli are either external or internal to the body. **External stimuli** are *visual* (sight), *auditory* (hearing), *olfactory* (smell), *tactile* (touch), and *gustatory* (taste). **Internal stimuli** are kinesthetic or visceral. **Kinesthetic** refers to awareness of the position and movement of body parts. For example, a person walking is aware of which leg is forward. A related sense is **stereognosis**, the awareness of an object's size, shape, and texture by touch. For example, a person holding a tennis ball is aware of its size, round shape, and soft surface without seeing it. **Visceral** refers to any large organ within the body. Visceral organs can produce stimuli that make a person aware of them (e.g., a full stomach). **Sensory perception** involves the conscious organization and translation of the data or stimuli into meaningful information.

For an individual to be aware of the surroundings, four aspects of the sensory process must be present: (a) a stimulus, (b) a receptor, (c) impulse conduction, and (d) perception.

- **Stimulus**. A stimulus is an agent or act that stimulates a nerve receptor (e.g., a sound wave that produces vibrations on your tympanic membrane).
- **Receptor**. A nerve cell acts as a receptor by converting the stimulus to a nerve impulse. Most receptors are specific, that is, sensitive to only one type of stimulus, such as visual, auditory, or touch. Sound waves create vibrations that are carried through the ear to the receptor hairs of the organ of Corti.
- **Impulse conduction**. The impulse travels along nerve pathways to the spinal cord or directly to the brain (Figure 37.1). The vibrations received in the organ of Corti in the inner ear are translated into electric impulses, which travel along the acoustic nerve to the brain.
- **Perception**. Perception, or awareness and interpretation of stimuli, takes place in the brain where specialized brain cells interpret the nature and the quality

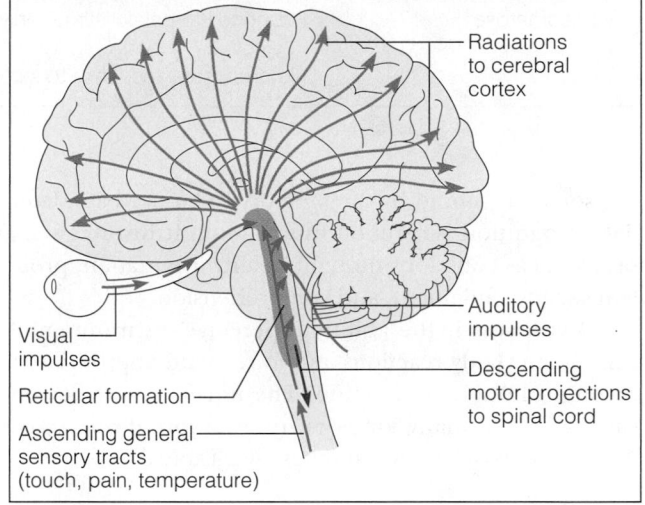

FIGURE 37.1 Nerve impulses run along the ascending sensory tracts to reach the reticular activating system (RAS); when certain impulses reach the cerebral cortex, they are perceived.

Source: From Marieb, E. N., & Hoehn, K. (2010). *Human anatomy & physiology* (8th ed.) (p. 45). Copyright © 2010 by Pearson Education. Reprinted with permission.

of the sensory stimuli. The level of consciousness affects the perception of the stimuli. The cerebral cortex of the brain then interprets the meaning of sound and initiates the appropriate response.

Arousal Mechanism

For a person to receive and interpret stimuli, the brain must be alert. The **reticular activating system (RAS)** in the brain stem acts to mediate the arousal mechanism. The RAS has two components: (a) the *reticular excitatory area* (REA) and (b) the *reticular inhibitory area* (RIA). The REA is responsible for stimulus arousal and wakefulness, and the RIA has the opposite function.

People have their own zone of optimum arousal, the level at which the person feels comfortable. **Sensoristasis** is the term used to describe optimum arousal for an individual. Beyond this comfort zone, people must adapt to increased or decreased sensory stimuli. An absence of stimuli from the RAS to the cerebrum results in the brain becoming inactive or useless.

The brain has the capacity to adapt to most sensory stimuli. For example, a person living in a city may not notice traffic noises that someone from a rural area finds loud and disturbing. Not all sensory stimuli are acted

TABLE 37.1 States of Awareness

State	Description
Full consciousness	Alert; oriented to time, place, person; understands verbal and written words
Disoriented	Not oriented to time, place, or person
Confused	Reduced awareness, easily bewildered; poor memory, misinterprets stimuli; impaired judgment
Somnolent	Extreme drowsiness but will respond to stimuli
Semicomatose	Responds to painful stimuli only
Coma*	No purposeful response to stimuli; may still react to deep pain but only with atypical posturing

*See Chapter 28, Glasgow Coma Scale (page 673).

on; some are stored by the memory to be used at a later date. Cognition is cerebral functioning. It involves such processes as conscious thought, reality orientation, problem solving, judgment, and comprehension.

Awareness is the ability to perceive environmental stimuli and body reactions and to respond appropriately through thought and action. The normal, alert person can assimilate many kinds of information at one time. Awareness exists in several states (see Table 37.1).

Sensory Alterations

People become accustomed to certain sensory stimuli, and when these change markedly, the individual may experience discomfort. When clients enter a hospital, for example, they usually experience stimuli that differ in quantity and quality from those to which they are accustomed. These changes can cause clients to become confused and disoriented.

Nurses should be aware of the behaviours that often result from different stimuli. Colour, sound, privacy, and social interaction for clients can be modified to more closely resemble those in their home environment. Factors that contribute to alterations in behaviour include sensory deprivation, sensory overload, and sensory deficits.

Sensory Deprivation

Sensory deprivation is generally thought of as a decrease in or lack of meaningful stimuli. When a person experiences sensory deprivation, the balance in the RAS is disturbed. The RAS is unable to maintain normal stimulation to the cerebral cortex. This reduced stimulation causes the person to become more acutely aware of the remaining stimuli and often perceive these in a distorted manner. Thus, the person often experiences alterations in perception, cognition, and emotion. See the Clinical Manifestations box on sensory deprivation.

CLINICAL MANIFESTATIONS

Sensory Deprivation

Sensory deprivation can manifest in several ways:

- Excessive yawning, drowsiness, sleeping
- Decreased attention span, difficulty concentrating, decreased problem solving
- Impaired memory
- Periodic disorientation, general confusion, or nocturnal confusion
- Preoccupation with somatic complaints, such as palpitations
- Hallucinations or delusions
- Crying, annoyance over small matters, depression
- Apathy, emotional lability

Sensory Overload

Sensory overload generally occurs when a person is unable to process or manage the amount or intensity of sensory stimuli. Three factors contribute to sensory overload:

1. Increased quantity or quality of internal stimuli, such as pain, dyspnea, anxiety
2. Increased quantity or quality of external stimuli, such as a noisy health care setting, intrusive diagnostic studies, contact with many strangers
3. Inability to disregard stimuli selectively, perhaps as a result of nervous system disturbances or medications that stimulate the arousal mechanism

Sensory overload can limit the brain's capability to filter or respond to specific stimuli. The individual may experience difficulty perceiving the environment in a way that makes sense; their thoughts race in many directions, and restlessness occurs. The person may feel overwhelmed and out of control. The nurse must recognize that the sights and sounds that are familiar to them often represent overload to clients. Such factors as pain, lack of

Sensory Overload

Sensory overload can manifest in several ways:
- Complaints of fatigue, sleeplessness
- Irritability, anxiety, restlessness
- Periodic or general disorientation
- Reduced problem-solving ability and task performance
- Increased muscle tension
- Scattered attention and racing thoughts

sleep, and worry can also contribute to sensory overload. People who have sensory overload may appear fatigued and may not be able to internalize new information. See the Clinical Manifestations box on sensory overload.

Sensory Deficits

A **sensory deficit** involves impaired reception, perception, or both of one or more of the senses. Two forms of sensory deficit are blindness and deafness. **Blindness** is legally defined as visual acuity of 20/200 with the best correction possible. **Deafness** is medically diagnosed when that person has little or no functional hearing and depends on visual (e.g., sign language, lip reading, and reading and writing) rather than auditory communication (e.g., voice, hearing, and hearing aids and devices) (Canadian Association of the Deaf, 2012a). Note that, whereas some people may see deafness as a deficit, within the Deaf culture, "deafness itself is a non-issue in that a person's status within the culture depends not upon his/her amount of hearing loss but upon his/her attitude towards the elements of the Deaf culture, involvement in the local Deaf community, and skill in Sign language" (Canadian Association of the Deaf, 2012a).

With a gradual loss of sensory function, individuals often develop behaviours to compensate for the loss; sometimes, these behaviours are unconscious. For example, a person with gradual hearing loss in the right ear may unconsciously turn the left ear toward a speaker. Some neurological diseases cause changes in the kinesthetic sense and tactile perception. Diseases of the inner ear, for example Meniere's disease, can cause loss of kinesthetic sense so that standing or walking is impossible.

Clients with sensory deficits are at risk of both sensory deprivation and sensory overload. Persons with vision problems may be unable to read, watch television, or recognize persons by sight. An unfamiliar environment can add to their confusion. Blind people often have highly structured home environments; the diversity and unfamiliarity of the hospital environment can create sensory overload. Impaired vision limits the person's ability to move around readily or socialize with others.

Factors Affecting Sensory Function

A number of factors affect the amount and quality of sensory stimulation, including a person's developmental stage, culture, level of stress, medications and illness, and lifestyle and personality.

Developmental Stage

Perception of sensation is critical to the intellectual, social, and physical development of infants and children. Newborns should be screened for hearing deficits before hospital discharge. If a hearing loss is detected, treatment can begin early and complications, such as speech loss, can be prevented.

Infants learn to recognize the face of the mother or caregiver and establish bonding essential to later emotional development. Young children respond to music by singing and dancing as they begin to interact with their peers. As children grow, they learn to interpret visual and auditory signals when preparing to cross the street. Adults have many learned responses to sensory cues. The sudden loss or impairment of any sense can have profound effects on both children and adults.

Normal changes of aging often result in varying degrees of impairments in sensory perception of the senses: hearing, vision, smell, taste, and touch. These physiological changes in older adults put them at higher risk for altered sensory function. Accurate figures are difficult to obtain, but it is estimated that there are approximately 3.5 million Canadians with some degree of hearing loss and approximately 350 000 profoundly deaf and deafened (Canadian Association of the Deaf, 2012b). Hearing loss is one of the most common health complaints reported by older adults. The diminishing of sensory perception that can come with aging or chronic disease or conditions (e.g., diabetes, cerebrovascular accidents, and other neurological disorders, such as Parkinson's disease) is generally gradual. *Presbycusis,* a type of inner ear hearing loss, is common with aging. The ability to hear high-frequency sounds and distinguish from background sounds is most affected. With respect to vision, it is estimated that more than 1 in 11 Canadians over age 65 years and more than 1 in 8 over age 75 years experience severe vision loss that cannot be corrected with standard eyeglasses (The National Coalition for Visual Health, 2011).

Culture

An individual's culture often determines the amount of stimulation that a person considers usual or "normal." For example, a child raised in a cultural community with large, active families may be accustomed to more stimulation compared with one raised in a culture where families are very small and insular. In addition, the normal amount of stimulation associated with ethnic origin, religious affiliation, or income level may also affect the amount of stimulation an individual desires and believes to be meaningful. The sudden change in cultural surroundings experienced by immigrants, migrants, or visitors to a new country, in which differences in language, dress, and cultural behaviours abound, can result in sensory overload or culture shock.

Cultural deprivation or cultural care deprivation is a lack of culturally assistive, supportive, or facilitative acts. Nurses must be aware of and sensitive to what stimulation is culturally acceptable to a client. In some cultures, touching is comforting and acceptable, whereas in others it may be offensive. Some clients find the presence of cultural or religious symbols reassuring (see the section "Spiritual Symbols" in Chapter 47). Nurses should accommodate clients' needs, provided these practices do not endanger health.

Stress

During times of increased stress, people may find their senses already overloaded and seek to decrease sensory stimulation. For example, people dealing with physical illness, pain, hospitalization, and diagnostic tests may want to have only close support people visit. They may also need the nurse's help to decrease unnecessary stimuli (e.g., noise) as much as possible. Alternatively, clients may seek sensory stimulation during times of low stress.

Medications and Illness

Certain medications can alter an individual's awareness of environmental stimuli. Opiates, antidepressants, and sedatives, for example, can decrease awareness or alter perception of stimuli.

Anyone taking several medications concurrently may show alterations in sensory function; older adults are especially at risk and need to be monitored carefully. Certain medications (e.g., Aspirin, furosemide, aminoglycosides, and certain cancer chemotherapeutic agents), if taken in large doses or for a long time, can become toxic to the auditory nerve, impairing hearing and/or causing tinnitus or balance disturbances.

Certain diseases and trauma affect sensory reception or perception. Direct sensory organ damage can occur as a result of the following:

- Diabetic retinopathy is a complication of diabetes mellitus in which tiny retinal hemorrhages can lead to blindness. "Nearly half a million Canadians currently have some form of diabetic retinopathy with 100 000 having a vision-threatening form of the disease. More

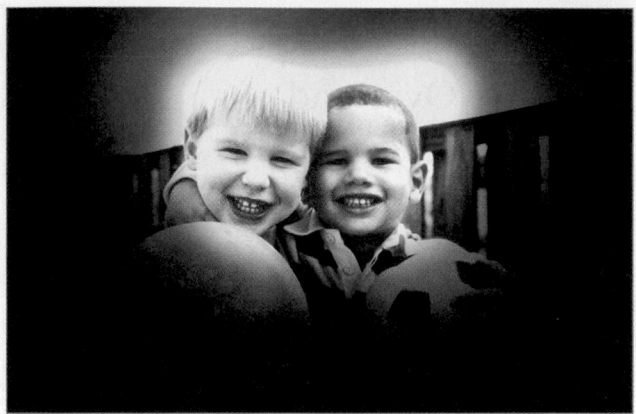

FIGURE 37.2 Narrowing of the optical field is a typical symptom of untreated glaucoma.

than 6000 are now blind due to the disease. The number of Canadians with diabetic retinopathy is expected to increase by 61% by 2031" (The National Coalition for Visual Health, 2011).

- Glaucoma, characterized by increased intraocular pressure that causes visual changes (such as narrowing of the optical field; see Figure 37.2), eventually leads to permanent damage to the optic nerve. At least 250 000 Canadians are affected with glaucoma, with 50% of these people being unaware of their disease. The number of Canadians blinded from this disease is expected to double by 2031, reaching nearly 20 000 (The National Coalition for Visual Health, 2011).

- Cataracts, an opacity of the lens of the eye, blurs vision. More than 2.5 million Canadians currently have cataracts. This number is expected to increase to 5 million by 2031 (The National Coalition for Visual Health, 2011).

- Recurrent ear infections may damage the tympanic membrane and contribute to hearing loss.

- Atherosclerosis restricts blood flow to the receptor organs and the brain, decreasing awareness and slowing responses.

- Multiple sclerosis, a central nervous system disease, is characterized by varying degrees of sensory loss and paralysis.

Lifestyle and Personality

Lifestyle influences the quality and quantity of stimulation to which an individual is accustomed. A client who is employed in a large company may be accustomed to many diverse stimuli, whereas a client who is self-employed and works in the home is exposed to fewer, less diverse stimuli. People's personalities also differ in terms of the quantity and quality of stimuli they are comfortable with. Some people delight in constantly changing stimuli and excitement, whereas others prefer a more structured life with few changes.

Assessing

Nursing assessment of sensory-perceptual functioning includes six components: (a) a nursing history, (b) a mental status examination, (c) a physical examination, (d) the identification of clients at risk, (e) an evaluation of the client's environment, and (f) an assessment of the social support network.

Nursing History

The nurse assesses present sensory perceptions, usual functioning, sensory deficits, and potential problems. In some instances, significant others can provide data the client cannot. For example, support people may reveal signs of recent changes in the client's hearing ability, such as inattention to others, recent mood swings, difficulty following clear instructions, frequent requests to have something repeated, and unusually loud radio or television volumes. To assess for risk of sensory loss, the nurse should also inquire about family history (e.g., glaucoma, diabetes), occupational or recreational exposures (e.g., noise level), and self-care practices (e.g., ear wax removal). Examples of interview questions to elicit data about the client's sensory-perceptual functioning are shown in the Assessment: Interview box.

Mental Status Examination

Mental status is critical to any evaluation of the sensory-perceptual process. Usually, data on mental status, including level of consciousness, orientation, memory, and attention span, can be obtained during the nursing history (see Chapter 28). It is important to note that sensory alterations may cause changes in cognitive functioning, and vice versa.

Physical Examination

Physical assessment determines whether the senses are impaired. During the physical examination, the nurse assesses vision and hearing, olfactory, gustatory, tactile, and kinesthetic senses. The examination should reveal the client's specific vision and hearing abilities; perception of heat, cold, light touch, and pain in the limbs; and awareness of the position of the body parts. Specific sensory tests include the following:

- *Visual acuity* and *visual fields,* by using a Snellen chart or other reading material (e.g., a newspaper)
- *Hearing acuity,* by observing the client's conversation with others and by performing the whisper test, and Weber and Rinne tuning fork tests
- *Olfactory sense,* by having the client identify specific aromas

---

ASSESSMENT **INTERVIEW**

Sensory-Perceptual Functioning

The following questions can be used to find out more information about a client's sensory-perceptual functioning:

VISUAL
- How would you rate your vision (excellent, good, fair, or poor)?
- Do you wear eyeglasses or contact lenses? If not, do you need to use a magnifying glass to read?
- Describe any recent changes in your vision.
- Do you have any difficulty seeing near or far objects?
- Have you ever experienced blurred vision, double vision, spots moving in front of your eyes, blind spots, light sensitivity, flashing lights, halos around objects, or difficulty seeing at night?
- When did you last visit an eye doctor?

AUDITORY
- How would you rate your hearing (excellent, good, fair, or poor)?
- Do you wear a hearing aid?
- Describe any recent changes in your hearing.
- Can you locate the direction of sounds and distinguish various voices?
- Do you experience any ringing, buzzing, humming, crackling noises, fullness in the ears, dizziness, or vertigo?

GUSTATORY
- Have you experienced any changes in taste (e.g., difficulty in differentiating sweet, sour, salty, and bitter tastes)?
- Do you enjoy the taste of foods as you did previously?

OLFACTORY
- Have you experienced any changes in your ability to smell?
- Do things (e.g., foods, flowers, and perfumes) smell the same as previously?
- Can you distinguish foods by their odours or tell when something is burning?
- Have you experienced any changes in appetite? (Changes in appetite may be related to an impaired sense of smell.)

TACTILE
- Are you experiencing any pain or discomfort?
- Have you experienced any decrease in your ability to perceive heat, cold, or pain in your limbs?
- Do you have any numbness or tingling in your extremities?

KINESTHETIC
- Have you noticed any difficulty in perceiving the position of parts of your body?

- *Gustatory sense,* by identifying three tastes, such as those of lemon, salt, and sugar
- *Tactile sense,* by testing light touch, sharp and dull sensation, two-point discrimination, hot and cold sensation, vibration sense, position sense, and stereognosis

These tests are described in detail in Chapter 28. The nurse should also determine whether sensory adaptive devices that the client uses, such as eyeglasses or hearing aids, function properly.

Identification of Clients at Risk for Sensory Deprivation or Overload

Clients at risk for sensory-perceptual alterations need to be identified to ensure that preventive measures can be initiated. Box 37.1 describes clients at risk for sensory alterations.

Client Environment

The nurse assesses the client's environment for quantity, quality, and type of stimuli. The client's environment may produce insufficient stimuli, placing the client at risk for sensory deprivation, or excessive stimuli, placing the client at risk for sensory overload. Nonstimulating environments include those that (a) severely restrict physical activity and (b) limit social contact with family and friends. Because appropriate or meaningful stimuli decrease the incidence of sensory deprivation, the nurse

must consider the client's health care environment for the presence of the following stimuli:

- Television, radio, or other auditory device (e.g., MP3 or CD player)
- Clock or calendar
- Reading material (age and language appropriate)
- Toys or activities for children (age appropriate)
- Number and compatibility of roommates
- Number of visitors in home or care facility

To assess a health care facility or home environment that produces excessive stimuli, the nurse considers, where appropriate, bright light, noise, therapeutic measures, frequency of assessments and procedures, the presence of a TV, pets, bright colours, adequacy of lighting, and so on. See the Clinical Alert box on sensory overload.

> **CLINICAL ALERT**
>
> Are you aware of the noise level around you or the noise level you create while providing nursing care? The standard of 45 decibels (dB) for rest and sleep is often not met. Sounds in critical care units range from 60 dB to 83 dB, contributing to sensory overload.

Social Support Network

The degree of isolation a person feels is significantly influenced by the level of support from family members and friends. The nurse assesses (a) whether the client

---

BOX 37.1 CLIENTS AT RISK FOR SENSORY DEPRIVATION AND OVERLOAD

Sensory deprivation occurs in the following:

- Clients who are confined to a nonstimulating, monotonous environment in the home or health care agency
- Clients who have impaired vision or hearing
- Clients who have mobility restrictions (e.g., those who have quadriplegia or paraplegia, are on bed rest, or are in a traction apparatus)
- Clients who are unable to process stimuli (e.g., clients who have brain damage or who are taking medications that affect the central nervous system)
- Clients who have emotional disorders (e.g., depression) and withdraw within themselves
- Clients who have limited social contact with family and friends (e.g., clients from a different culture)

Sensory overload occurs in the following:

- Clients who have pain or discomfort
- Clients who are acutely ill and have been admitted to an acute care facility
- Clients who are being closely monitored in an intensive care unit (ICU) (see Figure 37.3) and have intrusive tubes

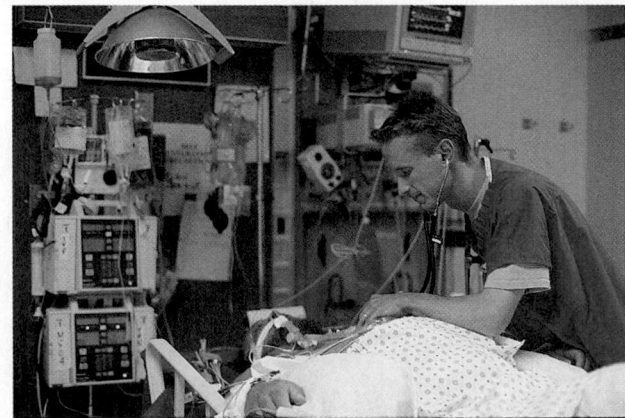

FIGURE 37.3 A patient in an intensive care unit (ICU) may experience sensory overload.

(e.g., intravenous tubes [IVs], catheters, nasogastric or endotracheal tubes)

- Clients who have decreased cognitive ability (e.g., head injury)

lives alone, (b) who visits and when, and (c) any signs indicating social deprivation, such as withdrawal from contact with others to avoid embarrassment or dependence on others, negative self-image, reports of lack of meaningful communication with others, and absence of opportunities to discuss fears or concerns.

Diagnosing

Nursing diagnoses for sensory perception alterations include those related specifically to the sensory change(s), whereas others relate to the impact of the alteration(s) on quality of life and self-care abilities. Possible diagnoses include the following:

- Altered visual sensory perception (such as when the client has impaired ability to interpret visual stimuli). Altered sensory perception can also be caused by impaired, distorted, diminished, or exaggerated responses to gustatory, olfactory, tactile, auditory, or kinesthetic stimuli.
- Any or all of anxiety, distress, fear, or social isolation related to altered sensory perception (such as when the client who is deaf or blind experiences fear for his safety when venturing from home, thus avoiding any outings, and becomes increasingly isolated)
- Acute confusion related to experiencing overwhelming sensory stimuli
- At risk for nutritional deficits related to reduced olfactory and/or gustatory sense (such as the person who has reduced appetite owing to loss of sense of smell and who no longer eats the required quality or quantity of food)
- At risk for injury related to impaired sensory perception (e.g., the person who has no olfactory sense may not smell smoke in a fire; the person who is deaf will not hear the fire alarm; the person who has reduced sensation in the limbs may experience a burn if the bath water temperature is too high)

Planning

Planning includes goals associated with the care of clients independent of setting and those specific to the home environment. The overall outcome criteria for clients with sensory-perception alterations independent of setting include the following:

- Prevention of injury
- Maintaining or improving the function of existing senses

- Maintaining or improving effective communication
- Prevention of sensory overload or deprivation
- Reducing social isolation
- Performing activities of daily living independently and safely

Nursing activities may include interventions, such as cognitive stimulation; enhancing coping with hearing, visual, olfactory, gustatory, kinesthetic, or auditory losses by promoting the use of resources (e.g., visual aids) and use of strategies to minimize losses (e.g., turn head left to right so as to scan in the case of reduced visual fields); providing emotional and/or instrumental support; implementing a fall prevention program; supporting or enhancing cognitive reframing to help the person see the strengths in the situation.

Planning for Home Care

The nurse should also consider the client's needs for assistance with care in the home (or residence) setting. Some clients with severe alterations in sensory-perceptual functioning may be discharged to an assisted-living facility that provides the specific support the client requires. Discharge planning incorporates a reassessment of the client's abilities for self-care, the availability and skills of support people, financial resources, and the need for referrals and home health services. A major aspect of discharge planning involves the instructional needs of the client and family. The Assessment: Home Care box for sensory-perception alterations outlines major needs of the clients and families.

ASSESSMENT | **HOME CARE**

Sensory-Perception Alterations

Clients with sensory-perception alterations usually have the following needs:

- *Self-care abilities:* Ability to care for self while adapting to sensory impairment
- *Safety:* Physical safety of client's environment, including lighting, noise, access, lack of clutter or obstructions, use of stairs, assistive devices with respect to sensory impairment, such as flashing fire alarms or telephones for those with hearing impairments
- *Level of knowledge:* Assistive devices that are available; ways to maximize the use of other senses; local, regional, or national organizations that provide education, training, support, or other assistance (e.g., Canadian National Institute for the Blind, the Canadian Hearing Society)
- *Resources:* Availability of family, friends, community assistance, such as senior centres, transportation, and religious or cultural organizations

Implementing

Nurses can assist clients with sensory alterations by promoting healthy sensory function, by adjusting environmental stimuli, and by helping clients to manage acute sensory deficits.

Promoting Healthy Sensory Function

The arousal mechanism for sensation is normally present at birth; however, it is undifferentiated. All senses are also present at birth, although some changes in function occur during the growth process. Early screening to detect problems in the visual and hearing functions is essential and key to prevent serious problems. For example, periodic vision screening of all newborns and children is recommended to detect congenital blindness, strabismus, and refractive errors. Children with chronic ear infections and people who live or work in an environment where there is a high noise level should undergo routine auditory testing. Women who are considering pregnancy should be advised of the importance of testing for syphilis and rubella, which may cause hearing impairments in newborns.

Healthy sensory function can be promoted with environmental stimuli that provide appropriate sensory input. This input should vary and be neither excessive nor too limited. As many senses as possible should be stimulated. Various colours, sounds, textures, smells, and body positions can provide various sensations. Nurses can teach parents and family members ways to stimulate infants and children. Social activities often help stimulate the mind and the senses in older adults.

Nurses should also teach clients at risk of sensory loss how to prevent the loss and should discuss preventive health measures, such as getting regular eye examinations and controlling chronic diseases (e.g., diabetes). See the Teaching: Wellness box on preventing sensory impairments.

Ensuring Client Safety

Nurses must implement safety precautions in health care settings for clients with sensory deficits. Examples of precautions include keeping the bed in the lowest position and placing the call light within reach.

Adjusting Environmental Stimuli

The client functions best when the environment is somewhat similar to that of the individual's ordinary daily life. Sometimes, nurses need to take steps to adjust the client's environment to prevent either sensory overload or sensory deprivation.

PREVENTING SENSORY OVERLOAD For clients who are at risk of overstimulation, nurses should reduce the number and type of environmental stimuli. The nurse can counteract sensory overload by blocking stimuli and

---

TEACHING WELLNESS

Preventing Sensory Impairments

Clients could take some steps to prevent sensory impairments:

- Have regular health examinations
- Have regular eye examinations to screen for eye problems. For clients age 40 and older, a medical eye examination is generally recommended every 3 to 5 years, or every 1 to 2 years for those with diabetes or a family history of glaucoma
- Seek early medical attention (a) if signs suggesting visual impairment arise, for example, failure to react to light or reduced eye contact from an infant; (b) if the child complains of an earache or has an ear infection; and (c) for persistent eye redness, discharge, or increased tearing; growths on or near the eye; pupil asymmetry or other irregularity; or any pain or discomfort
- Obtain regular childhood immunizations against diseases capable of causing hearing loss (e.g., rubella, mumps, and measles)
- Avoid giving infants and toddlers toys with sharp edges. Keep pointed instruments out of reach, and supervise preschoolers when they use scissors
- Supervise and teach toddlers and preschoolers not to walk or run with pointed objects in their hands
- Teach children and adolescents the proper use of sports equipment (e.g., hockey sticks)
- Wear protective eye goggles when using power tools, riding motorcycles, or spraying chemicals
- Wear ear protectors when working in an environment with high noise levels or brief loud impulse noises (e.g., blasting)
- Wear glasses with ultraviolet (UV) protection to avoid damage from ultraviolet rays; avoid looking directly at the sun

---

by helping the client organize the stimuli and alter his or her responses to the stimuli.

Dark glasses can partially block light rays, and a window shade or drape can reduce visual stimulation. Earplugs reduce auditory stimuli, as do soft background music and earphones. The odour from a draining wound can be minimized by keeping the dressing dry and clean and using a room deodorizer.

Another method of blocking stimuli is to reduce novelty and surprise and provide rest intervals free of interruptions. Sometimes, the number of visitors and the length of visits must be restricted. Also, carrying out several nursing measures together allows the client an uninterrupted period of rest before the next activity.

By explaining sounds in the environment, the nurse could help the client organize them mentally (e.g., a buzzer signals the need to change an IV). When clients understand their meaning, stimuli are frequently less confusing and more easily ignored. People can also learn to alter their responses to the stimuli. Clients could employ relaxation techniques to reduce anxiety and stress, despite continual sensory stimulation. See Box 37.2.

BOX 37.2 PREVENTING SENSORY OVERLOAD

Take the following steps to help prevent sensory overload in clients:

- Minimize unnecessary light, noise, and distraction. Provide dark glasses and earplugs, as needed.
- Control pain, as indicated.
- Introduce yourself by name and role (e.g., nurse), and address the client by name.
- Provide orienting cues, such as clocks, calendars, equipment, and furniture in the room.
- Limit the number of visitors at any given time.
- Plan care to allow for uninterrupted periods of rest, at least 2 hours at a time, if possible.
- Schedule a routine of care so the client knows when and what to expect (post a schedule for the client, wherever possible).
- Speak in a low tone of voice and in an unhurried manner.
- Provide new information gradually to enable the client to process the meaning. When providing information, ask the client to repeat it so that there is no misunderstanding.
- Describe any tests and procedures to the client beforehand.
- Reduce noxious odours. Empty a commode or bedpan immediately after use; keep wounds clean and covered; use a room deodorizer, when indicated; and provide good ventilation.
- Take time to discuss the client's problems and to correct any misinterpretation.
- Assist the client with stress-reducing techniques.

BOX 37.3 PREVENTING SENSORY DEPRIVATION

Take the following steps to help prevent sensory deprivation in clients:

- Encourage the client to use eyeglasses and hearing aids.
- Address the client by name and touch the client while speaking, if this is not culturally offensive.
- Communicate frequently with the client and maintain meaningful interactions (e.g., discuss current events).
- Provide a telephone, radio or TV, clock, and calendar.
- Provide murals, pictures, sculptures, and wall hangings. Many libraries and museums will lend artwork free of charge, or a local school may provide art projects developed by the students.
- Have family and friends bring freshly cut flowers and plants.
- Consider having a resident pet (e.g., a fish, a cat, or a bird), or make arrangements for pets to visit on a regular basis.
- Include different textured objects to feel (e.g., a sheepskin pillow, a silk scarf, or a soft blanket).
- Increase tactile stimulation through physical care measures (e.g., back massages, hair care, or foot soaks).
- Encourage social interaction through activity groups or visits by family and friends.
- Encourage doing crossword puzzles or other such games to stimulate mental function.
- Encourage environment changes, such as a walk through a mall or, for an immobilized client, sitting near a window or at a place on the nursing unit where the client can watch local traffic.
- Encourage the use of self-stimulation techniques, such as singing, humming, whistling, or reciting.

PREVENTING SENSORY DEPRIVATION For clients who are at risk for sensory deprivation, nurses can increase environmental stimuli in a number of ways. For example, newspapers, books, and television can stimulate the visual and auditory senses. Providing objects that are pleasant to touch, such as a pet to stroke, can provide tactile and interactive stimulation. Clocks that differentiate night from day by colour can help orient a client to time. The olfactory sense can be stimulated by the presence of fresh flowers or plants.

Arrangements should also be made for people to visit and talk with the client regularly. Many church and community groups provide visitors to *shut-ins,* that is, people who are confined to their homes or who reside in nursing homes. See Box 37.3 for measures to prevent sensory deprivation.

Managing Acute Sensory Deficits

When assisting clients who have a sensory deficit, the nurse needs to (a) encourage the use of sensory aids to support residual sensory function, (b) promote the use of other senses, (c) communicate effectively, and (d) ensure client safety. See the Reflect on Primary Health Care box.

ENCOURAGING THE USE OF SENSORY AIDS Many sensory aids are available for clients who have visual and

hearing deficits. See examples in Box 37.4 on the next page. Whether in the health care setting or the home setting, the assistance of support people needs to be enlisted, whenever possible, to help the client deal with the deficit.

PROMOTING THE USE OF OTHER SENSES When one sense is lost, the nurse can teach the client to use other senses to compensate the loss. This stimulation is similar to that provided to prevent sensory deprivation discussed earlier. However, the type of stimulation needs to be adapted to the client's specific deficit. For example, for the visually impaired client, stimulation of hearing, taste, smell, and touch can be encouraged. A radio, audiotapes of music or books, clocks that chime, music boxes, and

REFLECT ON PRIMARY HEALTH CARE

When working with people who have sensory alterations, the principles of accessibility and appropriate technology can be used. Significant advances in technology have been made to assist persons with sensory deficits and their families. Ensuring acceptance and accessibility of the technological advances is an important nursing contribution to health promotion, another principle of primary health care.

BOX 37.4 SENSORY AIDS FOR VISUAL AND HEARING DEFICITS

Sensory aids can help clients with vision and hearing deficits:

VISION

- Eyeglasses of the correct prescription that are clean and in good repair
- Adequate room lighting, including night lights
- Sunglasses or shades on windows to reduce glare
- Bright contrasting colours in the environment
- A magnifying glass
- A phone dialler with large numbers
- A clock and wristwatch with large numbers
- Colour code or texture code on stoves, washer, medicine containers, and so on
- Coloured or raised rims on dishes
- Reading material with large print
- A wristwatch that allows touch to determine time or gives audible time
- Braille or recorded books
- A guide dog

HEARING

- Hearing aid and battery in good order
- Lip reading
- Sign language
- Amplified telephones
- Telecommunication device for the deaf (TDD)
- Amplified telephone ringers and doorbells
- Flashing alarm clocks
- Flashing smoke detectors

BOX 37.5 COMMUNICATING WITH CLIENTS WHO HAVE IMPAIRED VISION OR HEARING

Some accommodations must be made for clients who have impaired vision or hearing:

VISION IMPAIRMENT

- Always announce your presence, and identify yourself by name and role (e.g., nurse).
- Stay in the person's field of vision.
- Speak in a warm and pleasant tone of voice; avoid speaking louder than necessary.
- Always explain what you are about to do before touching the person.
- Explain the sounds in the environment.
- Indicate when the conversation has ended and when you are leaving the room.

HEARING IMPAIRMENT

- Before initiating conversation, move to a position where the person can see you.
- Decrease background noises (e.g., radio) before speaking.
- Talk at a moderate rate and in a normal tone of voice.
- Address the person directly. Do not turn away in the middle of the conversation. Make sure the person can see your face easily and that it is in good light.
- Avoid covering up your mouth or talking when you have something in your mouth, such as chewing gum.
- Keep your voice at the same volume throughout each sentence, without dropping your voice at the end of each sentence.
- Always speak as clearly and accurately as possible. Articulate consonants with particular care. Use other words when the client has difficulty hearing phrases.
- Do not overarticulate. Mouthing or overdoing articulation is just as troublesome as mumbling. Mime, write ideas, or use sign language, if necessary.
- Use simple words and short sentences.
- Pronounce every name with care. Make a reference to the name for easier understanding, for example, "Joan, the girl from the office" or "Tim Hortons, the coffee shop."
- Change to a new subject at a slower rate, making sure that the person follows the change to the new subject.

wind chimes can be used for auditory stimulation. Diets that include a variety of flavours, temperatures, and textures can be planned to stimulate the taste buds. Taking sips of water between foods and eating foods separately can emphasize the taste sensation. Fresh flowers, room fragrances, brewing coffee, and baking can stimulate the sense of smell. Measures, such as providing a hug, massage, hair brushing, grooming, different textures in clothing and upholstery fabrics, and pets, can be used to stimulate tactile receptors.

COMMUNICATING EFFECTIVELY Communication with people who have sensory deficits should convey respect, enhance the person's self-esteem, and ensure the exchange of correct information. A person with a hearing impairment has to concentrate more than other people and, therefore, tires more readily. Fatigue compounded by an illness can further reduce the person's ability to hear. A person with a visual impairment is unable to observe most nonverbal cues during communication and relies largely on the spoken word and tone of voice. Guidelines for communicating with people who are visually or hearing impaired are shown in Box 37.5.

ENSURING CLIENT SAFETY Nurses should implement safety precautions in health care settings for clients with sensory deficits and teach them special precautions to ensure their safety at home.

Impaired Vision For clients with vision impairments who are in a health care setting, nurses should do the following:

- Orient the person to the arrangement of room furnishings and maintain an uncluttered environment.
- Keep pathways clear.
- Do not rearrange furniture without orienting the client. Ensure that housekeeping personnel are informed about this.

- Organize self-care articles within the client's reach, and orient the client to their location.
- Keep the call light within easy reach, and place the bed in the low position.
- Assist with ambulation by standing to the client's side, walking about 30 cm ahead, and allowing the client to grasp your arm. Confirm whether the client prefers grasping your arm with his or her dominant or non-dominant hand.

People with vision impairment can have difficulty in performing activities of daily living (e.g., bathing, dressing, eating) and instrumental tasks (e.g., shopping, housekeeping). Visual impairment can challenge a client's adherence to a medication regimen, as it creates difficulty in reading labels and can lead to taking the incorrect amount of a medication or the incorrect medication. Visual impairment can also increase the risk of depression among older adults living alone (Hayman, Kerse, LaGrow, Wouldes, Robertson, & Campbell, 2007). Explanations for this relationship vary. One explanation is that vision loss leads to increased disability, which leads to depression. Another explanation states that loss of vision causes fear—a fear of losing autonomy and becoming dependent on others. Vision loss also affects how a person obtains information (e.g., reading the newspaper). In addition, reading is often a leisure activity and its loss can affect a person's quality of life. It is important for the nurse to be aware of and assess for signs of depression and intervene as appropriate.

Impaired Hearing   Clients with hearing impairments who are unable to hear the alarms of IV pumps and cardiac monitors need to be assessed frequently. They can be taught to use their visual sense to identify kinks in the IV tubing or a loose ECG (electrocardiograph) lead. For home safety, clients with impaired hearing need to obtain devices that either amplify sounds or respond with flashing lights to such sounds as a doorbell or smoke detectors, a baby crying, or a burglar alarm. The sounds of doorbells and alarm clocks may be amplified or changed to a lower frequency or buzzer-like sound. These devices can be obtained from hearing aid dealers, telephone companies, and appliance stores.

An important consequence of a decline in hearing as a person ages is the person having difficulty understanding speech. Factors that influence this difficulty are the environment, rate of speech, and presence of an accent. Environments that are noisy and reverberant (echoing, hollow sounds) cause difficulty for older adult listeners. Older adults with a hearing loss have difficulty understanding fast speech. The older adult's ability to process fast verbal information is slower than that of a younger person, and rapid speech allows for less time for the older adult to recognize the acoustic or auditory cues of the speech. A person who speaks with an accent may vary their pronunciation of syllables or words, making it challenging for the older adult.

Impaired Olfactory Sense   People with an impaired sense of smell need to be taught about the dangers of cleaning with chemicals, such as ammonia. Because a gas leak can go undetected, clients need to keep gas stoves and furnaces in good working order. Strong chemicals, such as ammonia, used in confined spaces, such as a bathroom, can affect the client before the client smells them. Food poisoning is a concern with clients who have difficulty detecting spoiled meat or dairy products. These clients need to carefully inspect food for freshness and check expiration dates on food packages. Installing a smoke detector near the stove is particularly important, as is taking care to not leave the stove unattended.

Impaired Tactile Sense   People with an impaired sense of touch may not be aware of hot temperatures, which can cause burns, or pressure on bony prominences, which can produce pressure ulcers. Clients with decreased sensation to temperature should have the temperature adjusted on their hot water heater and test water temperature with a thermometer before bathing. Clients with decreased sensation to pressure must change their position frequently. Avoid using heating pads and hot water bottles, as burns may result.

Helping the Client Who Is Confused

Confusion can occur in people of all ages, but it is more commonly seen in older people. Confusion often presents with subtle symptoms, but it is important for the nurse to differentiate between *acute confusion (delirium)* and chronic confusion (dementia). **Acute confusion** (or **delirium**) is a temporary state of mental confusion and fluctuating consciousness that has an abrupt onset and a cause that, when treated, reverses the confusion. **Dementia**, often called chronic confusion, has symptoms that are gradual and irreversible, such as in Alzheimer's disease or infarcts of the brain.

The terms *acute confusion* and *delirium* are often used interchangeably by health care professionals—*delirium* is a medical diagnosis, whereas *acute confusion* is descriptive of a behavioural state. Delirium occurs in up to 42% of older hospitalized clients (Witlox, Eurelings, de Jonghe, Kalisvaart, Eikelenboom, & van Gool, 2010) and can result in poor health outcomes, including falls, pressure ulcers, extended length of stay, and placement in a long-term care facility. The components of delirium include a reduced ability to focus, sustain, or shift attention; a change in cognition that may include memory impairment, disorientation, or the development of a perceptual disturbance, such as visual, auditory, and/or tactile hallucinations.

Older adults are at risk for acute confusion when hospitalized for numerous reasons. They often have other chronic medical problems (e.g., dementia, chronic obstructive pulmonary disease, and cardiovascular disease, such as heart failure or cerebrovascular accident), and they are taking numerous medications (polypharmacy), such as anticholinergics, opiates, thiazide diuretics, antidepressants, benzodiazepines, anticonvulsants, histamine 2 antagonists, and insulin, which may increase the risk for delirium. Many older adults have vision or hearing loss; the unfamiliarity of a hospital or new living environment, possible sleep deprivation, stress, and sensory overload or deprivation increase their risk for developing delirium. An acute infection, dehydration, hypoglycemia, hypoxemia, hypercalcemia, hypo-and hypernatremia, alcohol withdrawal, head injury, and a change in environment (such as moving into a senior's residence) can also precipitate acute confusion or delirium.

Standardized tools for identifying acute confusional states include the Confusion Assessment Method (CAM), which assesses fluctuating cognition, attention difficulties, disorganized or incoherent thinking, and altered level of consciousness. Other tools are the Mini-Mental State Examination (MMSE), Delirium Index (DI), and NEECHAM Confusion Scale.

Subsyndromal delirium (SSD) and persistent delirium (PerD) have emerged as new topics of importance in the study of delirium (Registered Nurses' Association of Ontario, 2010; Cole, Ciampi, Belzile, & Zhong, 2009). With **subsyndromal delirium**, the person has one or more of the signs or symptoms of delirium, but he or she does not progress to delirium. Although SSD is a relatively new concept under study, it is estimated that upwards of one-third of patients in ICUs develop SSD (Ouimet, Riker, Bergeron, Cossette, Kavanagh, & Skrobik, 2007). With PerD, the client does not recover from the delirium. See the Evidence-Informed Practice box on persons at risk for developing SSD.

It can be a challenge to differentiate between delirium and dementia and, as the two can coexist, it is important to understand what behaviours are related to which experience (see Table 37.2). Clients who are confused often know something is wrong and face the risk that their behaviour be interpreted as "normal" or "expected" if they are elderly; this is not the case, as acute confusion/delirium is *not* part of healthy aging and because addressing predisposing and precipitating factors resolves the delirium.

Box 37.6 lists nursing interventions to help promote a therapeutic environment for the client with acute confusion or delirium. See also the Clinical Alert box on clients who experience a sudden change in mental status.

Evaluating

By using the measurable desired outcomes developed during the planning stage, the nurse collects data needed to judge whether client goals and outcomes

---

EVIDENCE-INFORMED PRACTICE

Who Is at Risk for Developing Subsyndromal Delirium?

The authors of this prospective study followed over a 6-month period two cohorts of residents older than 65 years residing in long-term care facilities in two major cities in Quebec to determine how many developed subsyndromal delirium (SSD) and what risk factors might correlate with the development of SSD. One group of residents had no to moderate cognitive impairment; the other group had severe cognitive impairment. Of the residents who participated in the study, 65% developed SSD when the authors used a definition of SSD of "one or more new symptoms in the Confusion Assessment Method (CAM) that did not meet the criteria for delirium nor progress to delirium"; 24% developed SSD when the authors used a more stringent definition of SSD requiring two or more new symptoms. The core symptoms were fluctuation, inattention, disorganized thinking, and altered level of consciousness. Statistically significant risk factors for the development of SSD were presence of depression symptoms, impaired abilities to perform activities of daily living, and dementia. Residents aged 80 to 89 years were at higher risk for developing SSD compared with those over 90 years; the authors hypothesize that this finding may be the result of the "healthy survivor" effect. Men and those with severe cognitive impairment were more likely to develop SSD, and risk factors for SSD were similar to those for delirium.

NURSING IMPLICATIONS: Although more research on detecting, preventing, and treating SSD is needed, nurses must be attuned to the client who is at risk for developing changes in mental status that might not meet "diagnostic" criteria for delirium but place the client at risk and can cause reduced quality of life. Addressing the needs of clients with dementia who develop acute changes in mental status poses a particular challenge that nurses must constantly be aware of. This study points to the need to remain vigilant in the assessment of clients, especially males 80 to 89 years, and that future studies are needed to determine ways to prevent SSD (possibly through improved treatment of depression).

Source: Based on Cole, M., McCusker, J., Voyer, P., Monette, J., Champoux, N., Ciampi, A., Vu, M., & Belzile, E. (2011). Subsyndromal delirium in older long-term care residents: Incidence, risk factors, and outcomes. *Journal of the American Geriatrics Society, 59* (10), 1829–1836. doi: 10.1111/j.1532-5415.2011.03595.x

---

! CLINICAL ALERT

A client who experiences a sudden change in mental status or a worsening of baseline cognitive state must be assessed for acute delirium. Families and caregivers must know that an acute change is not part of normal aging and can be the result of an acute infection, drug toxicity, change in environment, head injury, dehydration, electrolyte imbalance, and more. Acute delirium can be frightening for the client and can often be reversed relatively quickly if addressed properly, such as receiving treatment for an infection or correction of electrolyte imbalance.

TABLE 37.2 Differentiating between Delirium and Dementia

Feature	Delirium/Acute Confusion	Dementia
Onset	Acute/subacute	Chronic, insidious
Course	Short, fluctuating, and often worse at night	Long, progressive, yet stable loss, over time
Progression	Abrupt	Slow but even decline
Duration	Hours to <1 month (short); may be longer in older adults May be persistent	Months to years
Awareness	Reduced	Clear
Alertness	Fluctuates; lethargic or hypervigilant	Generally normal
Attention	Impaired: unfocused, fluctuating, distracted	Generally normal, varies with extent of disease
Orientation	Impaired, fluctuates in severity	Impaired over time
Memory	Recent and immediate impaired	Recent and remote impaired
Thinking	Disorganized, distorted, fragmented, rambling, incoherent	Difficulty with abstraction; thoughts impoverished; poor judgments
Delusions	Common	Sometimes
Perception-hallucination	Distorted-visual, tactile, olfactory	Uncommon

Sources: Created by Dianne Rossy, RN, MScn, GNC(C). *APN Geriatrics.* Ottawa, ON: The Ottawa Hospital; Registered Nurses' Association of Ontario. (2010). (Supplement). *Screening for delirium and depression in older adults* (Rev. Ed.) (p. 8). Toronto, ON: Author.

BOX 37.6 PROMOTING A THERAPEUTIC ENVIRONMENT FOR PERSONS WITH ACUTE CONFUSION

Take the following nursing interventions to help a client who has acute confusion or delirium:

- Ensure that the client has been assessed for all of the possible precipitating factors of acute confusion (e.g., infection, hypoglycemia, alcohol withdrawal, drug adverse effects, head injury, etc. (see "Helping the Client Who is Confused").
- Wear a readable nametag.
- Assign consistent caregivers, if possible
- Address the client by name, and introduce yourself frequently.
- Identify time and place: "Today is December 5, and it is 8 o'clock in the morning. You are on 6 Medical at the Royal Victoria Hospital in Montreal."
- Place a calendar and a clock in the client's room. Provide a means of marking the current date or holidays.
- Speak clearly and calmly to the client, allowing time for your words to be processed and for the client to respond.
- Provide frequent face-to-face contact.
- Keep glasses and hearing aids within reach.

- Provide clear, concise explanations of each treatment procedure or task.
- Eliminate unnecessary noise.
- Reinforce reality by interpreting unfamiliar sounds, sights, and smells; correct any misconceptions of events or situations.
- Schedule activities (e.g., meals, bath, activity, treatments, and rest periods) at the same time each day to provide a sense of security. If possible, assign the same caregivers.
- Provide adequate rest.
- Keep familiar items in the client's environment (e.g., photographs), and keep the environment uncluttered. A disorganized, cluttered environment increases confusion.
- Encourage the client to wear familiar or personal clothing and to arrange personal hygiene articles in order of use.
- Encourage participation in familiar activities or hobbies to emphasize the client's strengths.
- Tell the client when you are leaving and when you will return.

TABLE 37.3 Evaluation Goals and Outcomes: Sensory-Perceptual Alterations

Goal	Examples of Desired Outcomes
Maintain or promote sensory functioning	Uses protective devices (e.g., protective eyewear and ear protectors) appropriately
	Identifies hazards to sensory organs
	Demonstrates effective use of assistive devices (specify)
Prevent sensory deprivation or overload	Experiences a 3- to 4-hour uninterrupted sleep period in 24 hours (sensory overload)
	Is oriented to time, place, and person
	Reports increased energy and reduced feelings of anxiety (sensory overload)
	Reports decreased boredom and depression (sensory deprivation)
	Demonstrates increased attention span (sensory deprivation)
Maintain or improve communication	Demonstrates appropriate emotional responses
	Uses assistive devices for communication (e.g., hearing aid, writing implements, large print)
	Expresses thoughts and feelings about sensory deficits or unusual sensory experiences
Prevent injury	Identifies factors that increase risk for injury
	Makes appropriate use of sensory aids
	Alters home environment and practices to prevent injury
Reduce social isolation	Identifies factors or behaviours that produce social isolation
	Formulates a plan to become more involved with others
	Identifies community resources that will assist in decreasing social isolation

have been achieved. Examples of client goals and related outcomes are shown in Table 37.3. If outcomes are not achieved, the nurse, client, and support people, if appropriate, need to explore the reasons why before modifying the care plan. See the Sample Care Plan for nursing management of clients with sensory perceptual impairments.

Sample Care Plan for Sensory-Perceptual Alteration

ASSESSMENT DATA

Nursing Assessment

Sophia Demetrios is an 82-year-old widow who has recently become a resident of an extended care facility. Just before her admission, she underwent hip replacement surgery and also experienced more difficulty with hearing as her hearing aid was damaged. Her children were concerned about her physical safety and lack of socialization and urged her to enter a nursing residence. Mrs. Demetrios had cared for herself independently for 15 years in her own home. Three days after admission, the nurse finds the client confused and disoriented to person, place, and time; her remote memory is intact. She appears restless, withdrawn, and her syntax is sometimes inappropriate. She states, "I'm afraid of all of these strange creatures in this orphanage. I hate it here." There is no report that she has fallen; she does not drink alcohol. Receives only synthroid daily; no new medications.

Physical Examination

Height: 160 cm
Weight: 55.3 kg
Temperature: 37°C

Pulse: 72 beats/min, regular, 2+ amplitude

Respirations: 18/min

Blood Pressure: 128/74 mm Hg

Focused Assessment: No evidence of any physical injury or deformity; remote memory intact; responds to commands appropriately. Ear canals patent and tympanic membranes pale grey and translucent. Hip replacement incision line intact with a healing ridge; good range of motion of the hip joint; gait steady. Good air entry bilaterally; no fremitus

Diagnostic Data

Complete blood count (CBC), sequential multiple analysis of chemistry (SMAC), and urinalysis all within normal ranges
S_pO_2: 97% on room air

Nursing Diagnosis

Acute disorientation likely related to sensory overload from a change in environment and compounded by hearing loss and multiple recent stressors (e.g., surgery, move to a new residence). No apparent acute illness or infection (e.g., urinary tract infection [UTI]), no electrolyte imbalance (e.g., hyponatremia/hypernatremia; hypercalcemia), no apparent head injury that could account for acute change in mental status.

Client Goals

The client will demonstrate (a) decreased symptoms and increased level of orientation; (b) improved ability to hear and communicate; and (c) improved adjustment to her new living arrangement.

Desired Health Outcomes

1. Is oriented to place, significant others, month, and year
2. Is able to demonstrate effective strategies to cope with hearing loss, such as effectively using her hearing aid, positioning herself to advantage hearing, eliminating background noises.
3. Begins to make positive comments about her new living environment, including socializing with other residents.

Reality Orientation

- Provide a consistent physical environment and a daily routine.
  Rationale: Routine eliminates the element of surprise, overstimulation, and further confusion.
- Provide caregivers who are familiar to Mrs. Demetrios.
  Rationale: Familiarity with caregivers helps reduce confusion and facilitates the establishment of rapport.
- Provide a low-stimulation environment for Mrs. Demetrios because disorientation may be increased by overstimulation.
  Rationale: A disruption in the quality or quantity of incoming stimuli can affect a person's cognitive status. Sensory overload blocks out meaningful stimuli.
- Provide for adequate rest, sleep, and daytime naps.
  Rationale: Rest reduces overstimulation and fatigue, which may be contributing factors to confusion.
- Use a calm approach when interacting with Mrs. Demetrios.
  Rationale: This method promotes communication that enhances the person's sense of dignity.
- Speak to the client in a slow, distinct manner with appropriate volume.
  Rationale: The client who has difficulty hearing will be better able to lipread and comprehend speech.

- Engage her in concrete and reality-oriented activities, such as ADLs, that focus on something outside the self.
  Rationale: These activities assist the individual to differentiate between own thoughts and reality.

Enhancing Coping with Hearing Loss

- Consult with audiologist for repair of her hearing device and ensure its proper use and care once repaired.
  Rationale: Hearing will be enhanced with properly functioning equipment.
- Listen attentively.
  Rationale: Effective listening is essential in a nurse–client relationship. Poor listening skills can undermine trust and block therapeutic communication.
- Use simple words and short sentences.
  Rationale: The use of simple terms and short sentences facilitates understanding and minimizes anxiety.
- Obtain Mrs. Demetrios's attention through touch.
  Rationale: Gaining the attention of a client with a hearing impairment is an essential first step toward effective communication. However, the client's personal space should be respected and permission to touch should be obtained.
- Help Mrs. Demetrios learn/use strategies to improve hearing when with other residents (e.g., position herself facing the speaker; reduce background noise if possible).
  Rationale: These relatively simple strategies may be helpful in ensuring that she can understand the speech of other residents; although she may have used these strategies in the past, she may need gentle reminding given her changes in mental status.

Adjusting to New Living Arrangement

- Provide Mrs. Demetrios with a tour of the facility and introduce her to the residents.
  Rationale: Familiarity with the physical and social surroundings will help her remain oriented and promote her sense of security.
- Encourage her to participate in activities that are of interest to her and fit with her hearing challenges (e.g., one-on-one or small group activities rather than large groups).
  Rationale: Meaningful participation in activities and socializing may help her continually orient herself to her setting as well as increase her favourable adaptation to her new living arrangement.

EVALUATION

Goal met. Mrs. Demetrios identified her location and was aware of the season and time of year. Her hearing aid was repaired, and with her improved mental status, she was able to share that she had already developed multiple coping strategies to deal with her hearing loss and was starting to use them again (e.g., avoid the TV room but spend more time in the quiet reading room). Though she stated, "I would give anything to be back in my own home," she also said, "I knew it was going to be difficult for me to adapt to this new place but I now realize that it is better than I thought! I am gradually coming to terms with the fact that I need more help." She began to socialize with two women with similar interests.

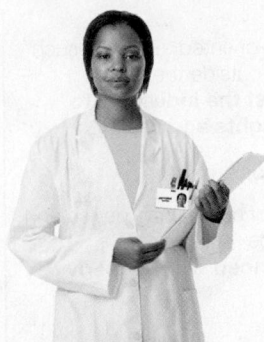

Case Study 37

Mrs. Donais is a 61-year-old client who is being cared for in the critical care unit following an automobile accident in which she suffered extensive traumatic injuries. Mrs. Donais is connected to several monitoring devices, has an intubation tube and ventilator to assist her with respirations, and is receiving various medications, including analgesics for pain.

CRITICAL THINKING QUESTIONS

1. Identify factors that place Mrs. Donais at risk for the development of sensory deprivation or overload.

2. What assessment findings would suggest that Mrs. Donais is experiencing sensory overload as opposed to sensory deprivation?

3. How can you intervene to reduce Mrs. Donais's risk for disturbed sensory perception during this stressful event?

4. How might the care of a client in the home setting differ from the care of a client, such as Mrs. Donais, who is receiving care in a critical care unit?

Check the eText in MyNursingLab for answers and explanations.

KEY TERMS

acute confusion *p. 1109*

awareness *p. 1100*

blindness *p. 1101*

deafness *p. 1101*

delirium *p. 1109*

dementia *p. 1109*

external stimuli
    p. 1099

impulse conduction
    p. 1099

internal stimuli *p. 1099*

kinesthetic *p. 1099*

perception *p. 1099*

receptor *p. 1099*

reticular activating system
    (RAS) *p. 1099*

sensoristasis *p. 1099*

sensory deficit *p. 1101*

sensory deprivation
    p. 1100

sensory overload
    p. 1100

sensory perception
    p. 1099

sensory reception
    p. 1099

stereognosis *p. 1099*

stimulus *p. 1099*

subsyndromal delirium
    p. 1110

visceral *p. 1099*

CHAPTER HIGHLIGHTS

- The sensory experience consists of two components: sensory reception and sensory perception.

- Sensory stimuli can be either external or internal. Visual, auditory, olfactory, tactile, and gustatory stimuli orient a person to the *external* environment. Kinesthetic and visceral stimuli orient the person to the *internal* environment. Kinesthetic stimuli make the person aware of the position and movement of body parts.

- Sensory perception involves the awareness and interpretation of stimuli into meaningful information. This process occurs in the cerebral cortex.

- The reticular activating system (RAS), with its many ascending and descending connections to other areas of the brain, monitors and regulates incoming stimuli. The RAS maintains, enhances, or inhibits cortical arousal.

- The normal, alert person can assimilate many kinds of information at one time and respond appropriately through thought and action.

- Sensory deprivation occurs when a person receives decreased sensory input or monotonous or meaningless sensory input.

- Sensory overload occurs when a person experiences excessive sensory input and is unable to process or manage the stimuli. The person feels overwhelmed and not in control.

- Responses to both sensory deprivation and sensory overload include perceptual changes (e.g., mild distortions or hallucinations), cognitive changes (e.g., decreased concentration and problem-solving ability), and affective changes (e.g., apathy, anxiety, anger, depression, and rapid mood swings).

- Clients at risk for sensory deprivation include (a) those who are housebound or institutionalized, (b) those on bed rest or isolation precautions, (c) those with sensory deficits, (d) those who come from a different culture, (e) those with certain affective disorders or disturbances of the nervous system, and (f) those on certain medications that affect the central nervous system.

- Clients at risk for sensory overload include (a) those in pain, (b) those in intensive care units, (c) those with intrusive and uncomfortable monitoring or treatment equipment, and (d) those with disturbances of the nervous system.

- Factors affecting sensory stimulation include developmental stage, culture, level of stress, medications and illness, and lifestyle and personality.

- Assessment for sensory-perceptual alterations includes (a) a nursing history to identify sensory deficits, (b) a physical examination, (c) a mental status examination, (d) the identification of clients at risk, (e) an evaluation of immediate environment, and (f) an assessment of the social support network.

- Nursing diagnoses related to a client's sensory-perceptual impairments include those related specifically to the sensory change(s) (e.g., altered visual sensory perception) or those related to the impact of the impairment on quality of life and self-care abilities (e.g., anxiety, distress, social isolation).

- Goals for persons with sensory-perceptual alterations include (a) maintaining or promoting the function of existing senses, (b) maintaining or improving communication, (c) preventing injury, (d) avoiding sensory deprivation or overload, (e) reducing social isolation, and (f) maintaining or restoring ability to function safely in the environment and to perform self-care.

- Interventions to prevent or modify sensory deprivation, sensory overload, and sensory deficits include promoting healthy sensory function, adjusting environmental stimuli, and managing sensory deficits.

- Clients with sensory deficits need instruction about sensory aids available to support residual sensory function, ways to promote the use of other senses, and methods to ensure safety from bodily harm.

- Nurses and support persons need to devise and implement effective communication mechanisms for clients who have visual and hearing impairments.

- Clients who are confused must be assessed for precipitating factors and need care that is directed to promoting their orientation to time, place, person, and situation.

ASSESS YOUR LEARNING

1. Mr. Jackson, 69 years old, had a recent right cerebrovascular accident with sensory-perceptual deficits. Which of the following nursing interventions is an appropriate strategy to address Mr. Jackman's deficits?

    a. Identifying Mr. Jackman's previous strengths

    b. Referring Mr. Jackman to a speech pathologist

    c. Approaching Mr. Jackman from the unaffected side

    d. Minimizing auditory sensory stimulation

2. Which client is at greatest risk for experiencing sensory overload?

    a. A 40-year-old client in a private room with no family

    b. A 28-year-old client with quadriplegia in a private room

    c. A 16-year-old listening to loud music

    d. An 80-year-old client admitted for emergency surgery

3. An alert 80-year-old client is transferred to a long-term care facility. On the second night, he becomes confused and agitated. What is the most appropriate nursing diagnosis?

    a. Chronic confusion

    b. Impaired memory

    c. Disturbed sensory perception

    d. Sensory deprivation

4. The nursing diagnosis risk for impaired skin integrity related to sensory-perception disturbance would BEST fit which of the following clients?

    a. One who cut his foot by stepping on broken glass

    b. One who uses a wheelchair because of paraplegia

    c. One who wears glasses because of poor vision

    d. One who is blind

5. Which of the following statements indicates that the client needs a sensory aid in the home?

    a. "I tripped over that rug again."

    b. "I can't hear the doorbell."

    c. "My eyesight is good if I wear my glasses."

    d. "I can hear the TV if I turn it up high."

6. A hospitalized client is disoriented and believes she is in a train station. Which of the following is the MOST appropriate response by the nurse?

    a. "You wouldn't be getting a bath at the train station."

    b. "Let's finish your bath before the train arrives."

    c. "Don't you know where you are?"

    d. "It may seem like a train station sometimes, but this is Valley Hospital."

7. A client with impaired vision is admitted to the hospital. Which intervention is MOST appropriate to meet the client's needs?

 a. Identifying yourself by name

 b. Decreasing background noise

 c. Explaining the sounds in the environment

 d. Keeping your voice at the same level

8. A client is exhibiting signs and symptoms of acute confusion (or delirium). The nurse implements which of the following strategies to promote a therapeutic environment?

 a. Keeping the lights in the room dimmed

 b. Keeping the environmental noise level high

 c. Keeping the room organized and clean

 d. Using restraints for client safety

9. Which of the following clinical signs are most likely to be present in a client at risk for sensory deprivation?

 a. Sleeplessness

 b. Increased muscle tension

 c. Irritability

 d. Crying

10. An 85-year-old client has impaired hearing. When creating his care plan, which of the following should have the highest priority?

 a. Obtaining an amplified telephone

 b. Teaching the importance of changing his position

 c. Providing reading material with large print

 d. Checking expiration dates on food packages

Check the eText in MyNursingLab for answers and explanations.

WEBLINKS

Canadian Hearing Society (CHS)

http://www.chs.ca

CHS is a nonprofit agency and the leading provider of services, products, and information that remove barriers to communication, advance hearing health, and promote equity for people who are culturally Deaf, orally deaf, deafened, or hard of hearing.

Canadian National Institute for the Blind

http://www.cnib.ca

This site provides information related to vision impairments.

Canadian Association of the Deaf

http://www.cad.ca

This site provides links and information on Deaf needs and interests.

Canadian Hard of Hearing Association

http://www.chha.ca

A nonprofit association that is operated by those with hearing deficits; its role is to inform and to promote the interests of its members.

Alzheimer Society of Canada

http://www.alzheimer.ca

The Alzheimer Society of Canada identifies, develops, and facilitates national priorities that enable its members to effectively alleviate the personal and social consequences of Alzheimer's disease and related disorders. It also promotes research and leads the search for a cure.

MyNursingLab

MyNursingLab's guided learning path makes reviewing and test preparation straightforward.

 - Content summaries, animations, and videos reinforce key concepts and skills
 - Practice questions help with test prep by showing gaps in knowledge
 - An eText, available online and via the iPad, makes searching, highlighting, and note-taking easy

This QR code appears at the end of every chapter and provides learning resources that you can access with your smartphone to study on the go. Access self-review quizzes, flashcards, and more!

REFERENCES

Canadian Association of the Deaf. (2012a). Statistics on deaf Canadians. Retrieved from http://www.cad.ca/statistics_on_deaf_canadians.php

Canadian Association of the Deaf. (2012b). Definition of "deaf." Retrieved from http://www.cad.ca/definition_of_deaf.php

Cole, M. Ciampi, A., Belzile, E., & Zhong, L. (2009). Persistent delirium in older hospital patients: A systematic review of frequency and prognosis. *Age and Ageing, 38*(1), 19–26. doi: 10.1093/ageing/afn253

Hayman, K. J., Kerse, N. M., LaGrow, S. J., Wouldes, T., Robertson, M. C., & Campbell, A. J. (2007). Depression in older people: Visual impairment and subjective ratings of health. *Optometry and Vision Science, 84,* 1024–1030.

The National Coalition for Visual Health. (2011). The vision loss epidemic in Canada. Retrieved from http://www.visionhealth.ca/faq.htm

Ouimet, S., Riker, R., Bergeron, N., Cossette, M., Kavanagh, B., & Skrobik, Y. (2007). Subsyndromal delirium in the ICU: Evidence for a disease spectrum. *Intensive Care Medicine 33*(6), 1007–1013.

Registered Nurses' Association of Ontario. (2010). Screening for delirium, dementia and depression in older adults (revised). Toronto, ON: Author.

Witlox, J., Eurelings, L., de Jonghe, J., Kalisvaart, K. J., Eikelenbroom, P., & van Gool, W. A. (2010). Delirium in elderly patients and the risk of postdischarge mortality, institutionalization, and dementia: A meta-analysis. *Journal of the American Medical Association, 304,* 443–451.

Chapter 38

Sleep

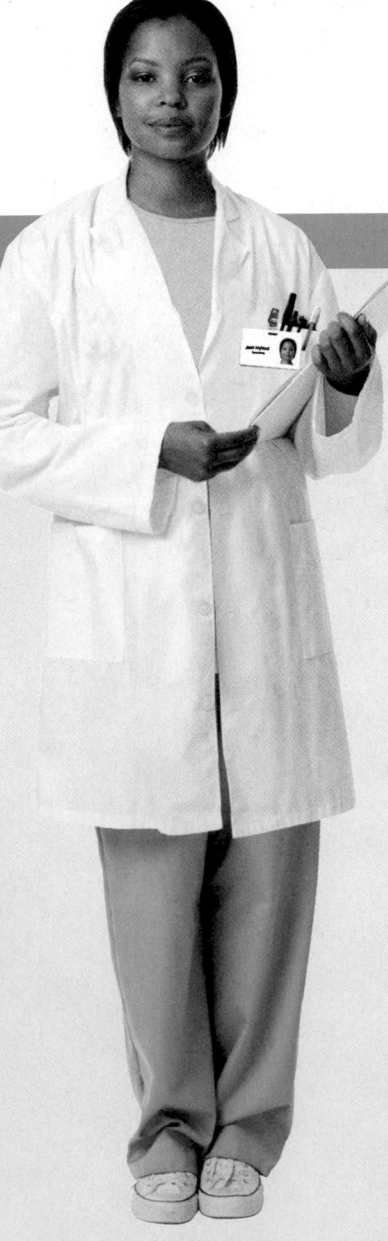

LEARNING OUTCOMES

After studying this chapter, you will be able to:

1. Explain the physiology and the functions of sleep.

2. Identify the characteristics of non–rapid eye movement (NREM) and rapid eye movement (REM) sleep.

3. Describe variations in sleep patterns throughout the lifespan.

4. Explain nine factors that affect normal sleep.

5. Describe six common sleep disorders.

6. Outline the four components of a sleep pattern assessment.

7. Develop nursing diagnoses, outcomes, and nursing interventions related to sleep problems.

8. Describe five interventions that promote normal sleep.

leep is a basic human need. Historically, sleep was viewed as a state of unconsciousness. More recently, **sleep** has come to be considered an altered state of consciousness in which the individual's perception of and reaction to the environment are decreased. Sleep is characterized by minimal physical activity, variable levels of consciousness, changes in the body's physiological processes, and decreased responsiveness to external stimuli. Some environmental stimuli, such as a smoke detector alarm, will usually awaken a sleeper, whereas other noises that have no significance will be selectively disregarded.

Sleep is critical for normal development, health, function, and healing. Despite sleep's pivotal role in health, many Canadians receive less sleep than they need. The consequences of sleep disorders and sleep insufficiency are significant, such as a serious car crash that results when someone "falls asleep at the wheel" (driver sleepiness) or the decrease in work quality and productivity when someone experiences sleepiness at work. Despite the efforts of a growing number of sleep clinicians, researchers, and national organizations, such as the Canadian Sleep Society, many members of the general public and health care professions are unaware of the consequences of chronic sleep loss (e.g., increased risk of hypertension, diabetes, obesity, depression, heart attack, and cerebrovascular accident).

Physiology of Sleep

The cyclic nature of sleep is thought to be controlled by centres located in the lower part of the brain. Neurons within the reticular formation, located in the brain stem, integrate sensory information from the peripheral nervous system and relay the information to the cerebral cortex. The upper part of the reticular formation consists of a network of ascending nerve fibres called the reticular activating system (RAS), which is involved with the sleep–wake cycle. An intact cerebral cortex and reticular formation are necessary for the regulation of sleep and waking states.

Neurotransmitters, located within neurons in the brain, affect the sleep–wake cycles. For example, serotonin is thought to lessen the response to sensory stimulation and gamma-aminobutyric acid (GABA) to shut off the activity in the neurons of the reticular activating system (RAS). Another key factor to sleep is exposure to darkness. Darkness and the reduced mental and physical activity associated with sleep preparation (e.g., lying down, decreasing noise) cause a decrease in stimulation of the RAS. During this time, the pineal gland in the brain begins to actively secrete the natural hormone melatonin, and the person feels less alert. During sleep, growth hormone is secreted, and cortisol, a stimulating hormone, is inhibited.

With the beginning of daylight, melatonin is at its lowest level in the body, and cortisol is at its peak. Wakefulness is also associated with high levels of acetylcholine, dopamine, and noradrenaline. Acetylcholine is released in the reticular formation, dopamine in the midbrain, and noradrenaline in the pons. These neurotransmitters are localized within the reticular formation and influence cerebral cortical arousal.

Functions of Sleep

The effects of sleep on the body are not completely understood. Sleep exerts physiological effects on both the nervous system and other body structures. Sleep in some way restores normal levels of activity and normal balance among parts of the nervous system. Sleep is also necessary for protein synthesis, which allows repair processes to occur. The role of sleep in psychological well-being is best manifested as the deterioration in mental functioning related to sleep loss.

Homeostatic Drive of Sleep

Patterns of sleep and wake are dependent on complex homeostatic factors. Although the effects of sleep on the body are not completely understood, we do know that sleep exerts physiological effects on the nervous system and other body structures. Sleep seems to have a homeostatic role, restoring normal levels of activity and normal balance among parts of the nervous system, including the autonomic nervous system. This **homeostatic drive** of sleep is linked to a powerful mechanism that increases the likelihood of falling asleep as the length of time a person is awake increases, and, conversely, that stimulates wakefulness following a period of restful sleep.

The underlying basis for the homeostatic drive is not completely understood, although it is known that wakefulness is associated with energy loss, fatigue, and a buildup of metabolites, including adenosine. The temporary effectiveness of caffeine, an adenosine antagonist, as a stimulant to combat sleepiness has grown dramatically in popularity, although paradoxically often itself contributing to sleep problems. The homeostatic drive is extremely powerful and is the reason that individuals will fall asleep while driving, despite certain injury or death. Conversely, a nap that lasts too long or is taken late in the day can reduce this drive, making it difficult to fall asleep at the normal bedtime.

Circadian Rhythms

Biological rhythms exist in plants, animals, and humans. In humans, these are controlled from within the body and are synchronized with environmental factors, such as light and dark. The most familiar biological rhythm, the **circadian rhythm**, or sleep–wake cycle, is regulated in all mammals by the suprachiasmatic nuclei of the hypothalamus. The term *circadian* is from the Latin *circa dies*, meaning "about a day."

Sleep is a complex biological rhythm. When a person's biological clock coincides with sleep–wake patterns and light–dark cycles, the person is said to be in circadian synchronization; that is, the person is awake when the physiological and psychological rhythms are most active and is asleep when the physiological and psychological rhythms are most inactive. Circadian regularity begins to develop by the sixth week of life, and by 3 to 6 months, most infants have a regular sleep–wake cycle. See the Clinical Alert box about sleep disturbances related to Canada's northern latitudes.

Types of Sleep

Sleep architecture refers to the basic organization of normal sleep. People have two sleep states: (a) **NREM (non–rapid eye movement) sleep** and (b) **REM (rapid eye movement) sleep**. During sleep, NREM sleep and REM

sleep alternate in cycles. Irregular cycling or absent sleep stages are associated with sleep disorders.

NREM SLEEP NREM sleep occurs when activity in the RAS is inhibited. About 75% to 80% of sleep during a night is NREM sleep. NREM sleep is divided into four stages, each associated with distinct brain activity and physiology.

Stage I is the stage of very light sleep and lasts only a few minutes. During this stage, the person feels drowsy and relaxed, the eyes roll from side to side, and heart and respiratory rates drop slightly. The sleeper can be readily awakened and may deny that he or she was sleeping.

Stage II is the stage of light sleep during which body processes continue to slow down. The eyes are generally still, heart and respiratory rates decrease slightly, and body temperature falls. Stage II lasts only about 10 to 15 minutes but constitutes 44% to 55% of total sleep. Stage II requires more intense stimuli than stage I for the person to be awakened.

Stages III and IV are the deepest stages of sleep, differing only in the percentage of delta waves recorded during a 30-second period. During *deep sleep* or **slow-wave sleep (SWS)**, the sleeper's heart and respiratory rates drop 20% to 30% below those exhibited during waking hours. The sleeper is difficult to arouse. The person is not disturbed by sensory stimuli, the skeletal muscles are very relaxed, reflexes are diminished, and snoring is most likely to occur. These stages are essential for restoring energy and releasing important growth hormones. See Box 38.1.

REM SLEEP REM sleep usually recurs about every 90 minutes and lasts 5 to 30 minutes. Most dreams take place during REM sleep but usually will not be remembered unless the person arouses briefly at the end of the REM period.

During REM sleep, the brain is highly active, and brain metabolism can increase as much as 20%. For example, during REM sleep, levels of acetylcholine and dopamine increase, with the highest levels of acetylcholine release occurring during REM sleep (see Box 38.2). Since both these neurotransmitters are associated with cortical activation, it makes sense that their levels would be high during

---

CLINICAL ALERT

Given Canada's northern latitudes, daylight length varies markedly across the year. The farther north, the more variation there is. The prolonged darkness of northern winters and the frequently cloudy fall and winter days of coastal regions contribute to sleep disturbances associated with seasonal affective disorder (SAD). Conversely, the long daylight in the summer evenings promotes late-night activity, making it especially challenging to obtain sufficient amounts of sleep and to keep to regular sleep and wake schedules.

BOX 38.1 PHYSIOLOGICAL CHANGES DURING NREM SLEEP

In the four stages of NREM sleep, some essential changes occur:

- Arterial blood pressure falls.
- Pulse rate decreases.
- Peripheral blood vessels dilate.
- Cardiac output decreases.
- Skeletal muscles relax.
- Basal metabolic rate decreases 10% to 30%.
- Growth hormone levels peak.
- Intracranial pressure decreases.

dreaming sleep. This type of sleep is also called *paradoxical sleep* because electroencephalogram (EEG) activity resembles that of wakefulness. Distinctive eye movements occur, voluntary muscle tone is dramatically decreased, and deep tendon reflexes are absent. In this phase, the sleeper may be difficult to arouse or may wake spontaneously, gastric secretions increase, and heart and respiratory rates often are irregular. It is thought that the regions of the brain that are used in learning, thinking, and organizing information are stimulated during REM sleep.

Sleep Cycles

During a sleep cycle, a sleeper passes from stage I NREM sleep through stages II and III to stage IV in about 20 to 30 minutes. Stage IV may last about 30 minutes. These stages are then followed by stages III and II, in that order. Thereafter, the first REM stage occurs, lasting about 10 minutes, completing the first sleep cycle. The healthy adult sleeper usually experiences four to six cycles of sleep during 7 to 8 hours (see Figure 38.1). Each cycle lasts about 90 minutes. The sleeper who is awakened during any stage begins anew at stage I NREM sleep and proceeds through all the stages to REM sleep.

The duration of NREM stages and REM sleep varies throughout the sleep period. As the night progresses, the sleeper spends less time in stages III and IV of NREM sleep. REM sleep increases, and dreams tend to lengthen. Before sleep ends, periods of near-wakefulness occur, and stages I and II NREM sleep and REM sleep predominate.

Recent research has shown that sleep deprivation is associated with significant cognitive and health problems.

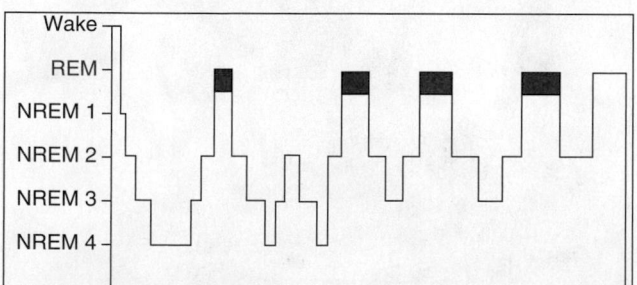

FIGURE 38.1 Time spent in REM and NREM stages of sleep by an adult.

Therefore, although re-establishing the sleep–wake rhythm (e.g., after the disruption of surgery) is important for healthy sleep, it is not appropriate to restrict daytime napping in hospitalized clients as their sleep needs are often increased.

Normal Sleep Patterns and Requirements

Newborns

Newborns sleep 16 to 18 hours a day, on an irregular schedule with periods of 1 to 3 hours of wake. Unlike older children and adults, newborns enter REM sleep (called *active sleep* in the newborn) immediately. Rapid eye movements are observable through closed lids, and body movements and irregular respirations may be seen. Quiet sleep (NREM with not yet fully differentiated sleep stages) is characterized by regular respirations, closed eyes, and the absence of body and eye movements. Premature babies spend nearly 80% of the time in REM sleep, and this amount decreases to 50% at term. Cycles of active and quiet sleep last about 50 minutes. See the Clinical Alert box on sudden infant death syndrome.

The birth of a baby is often an exciting but exhausting time for parents. Nurses should encourage parents to set realistic goals, seek and accept help with other duties, and nap when possible. Performing nighttime feeds and changes quietly and with lowered lights can also help establish day and night rhythms in babies and foster a more rapid return to sleep for the parent.

Infants

At first, infants awaken every 3 or 4 hours, eat, and then go back to sleep. Periods of wakefulness gradually increase during the first months. By 6 months, most infants sleep through the night (from midnight to 5 a.m.) and begin

CLINICAL ALERT

Sudden infant death syndrome (SIDS) continues to be the leading cause of death in babies 1 month to 1 year of age. The Back to Sleep campaign has been successful in reducing deaths attributed to SIDS (Hunt & Hauck, 2006). Bed sharing remains controversial and may be a contributing factor to infant deaths during sleep. Parents who want to share the bed with the baby need to be made aware of the risks, and the Canadian Paediatric Society recommends that the safest approach is for infants to sleep on their back in their own crib, and in the parent's room for the first 6 months of life. Parents should also be made aware that the risk of SIDS is increased when infants share the bed with mothers who smoke cigarettes or with an adult who is extremely fatigued or impaired by alcohol or drugs. The use of soft bedding, pillows, and covers that can cover the head increase the risk of death in all sleeping environments (Canadian Paediatric Society, 2011).

to establish a pattern of daytime naps. At the end of the first year, an infant usually takes two naps per day and should get about 14 to 15 hours of sleep in 24 hours.

Much of the infant's sleep time is spent in light sleep. During light sleep, the infant may exhibit movement, gurgles, and coughing. Parents should check that infants are truly awake before picking them up for feeding and changing. For both newborns and infants, being put to bed when they are drowsy but not asleep helps them to become self-soothers; this means that they fall asleep independently and if they do awaken at night, they can more easily put themselves back to sleep. Infants who become used to parental assistance at bedtime may become dependent on their parents to help them return to sleep at night (National Sleep Foundation, n.d.a).

Toddlers

Between 12 and 14 hours of sleep per 24 hours are recommended for children 1 to 3 years of age. About 30% is REM sleep. Most still need an afternoon nap, but the need for midmorning naps gradually decreases. The toddler may exhibit a great deal of resistance to going to bed and may awaken during the night. Nighttime fears and nightmares are common. A security object, such as a blanket or stuffed animal, may help. Parents need assurance that maintaining a daily sleep or rest schedule and a consistent, relaxing, and positive bedtime routine will promote good sleep habits for the entire family.

Preschoolers

The preschool child (3 to 5 years of age) requires 11 to 13 hours of sleep per night, particularly if the child is in preschool. Sleep needs fluctuate in relation to activity and growth spurts. Many children of this age dislike bedtime and resist by requesting another story or television program. The 4- to 5-year-old may become restless and irritable if sleep requirements are not met. A nap or quiet time during the day may be needed to restore energy levels.

Children in this age group benefit from bedtime rituals. Parents can help children by cueing them that bedtime is approaching and by continuing to use the same positive, clear, and consistent approach suggested for the toddler. Preschool children wake up frequently at night and they may be afraid of the dark or experience night terrors or nightmares. A relaxing bedtime story and discussion and problem solving of fears can help reduce the number of nightmares.

School-Age Children

The school-age child (5 to 12 years of age) needs between 10 to 12 hours of sleep, but most receive less because of increasing demands (e.g., homework, sports, social activities). They may also be spending more time at the computer and watching television. Some may be drinking caffeinated

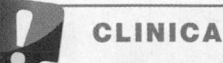

CLINICAL ALERT

Children who have a television, computer, or other electronic device (e.g., cellular phone) in their bedrooms are more likely to get less sleep than needed.

beverages or eating foods containing chocolate. All these activities can lead to difficulty falling asleep and insufficient sleep. Nurses can teach parents and school-age children about healthy sleep habits. A healthy diet, a consistent sleep schedule, and a bedtime routine need to be continued. See the Clinical Alert box on sleep disturbance in children.

Adolescents

Adolescents (12 to 18 years of age) require 9 to 10 hours of sleep each night, however, few actually get that much sleep. As many as 70% of Canadian high school students are sleep deprived (Gibson, Powles, Thabane, O'Brien, Molnar, Trajanovic, et al., 2006). Lack of sleep can lead to significant sleepiness at school and negatively affect grades, attendance, sports, extracurricular activities, and work. Fatigue contributes to negative moods (e.g., unhappiness, irritability) and poorer coping. Sleepy teens are also at greater risk for car accidents. Nurses can educate parents, teens, and teachers about sleep and the reasons why sleep health needs to be a priority.

As children reach adolescence, their circadian rhythms tend to shift. Research in the 1990s found that later sleep and later wake patterns among adolescents are biologically determined (National Sleep Foundation, n.d.b). This shift is often in contrast to the early hours demanded by school and work routines, making adolescents especially vulnerable to receiving insufficient amounts of sleep (Figure 38.2). High schools that have implemented later morning start times to better align with adolescent circadian rhythms have students who achieve more sleep, have improved mood, and are involved in

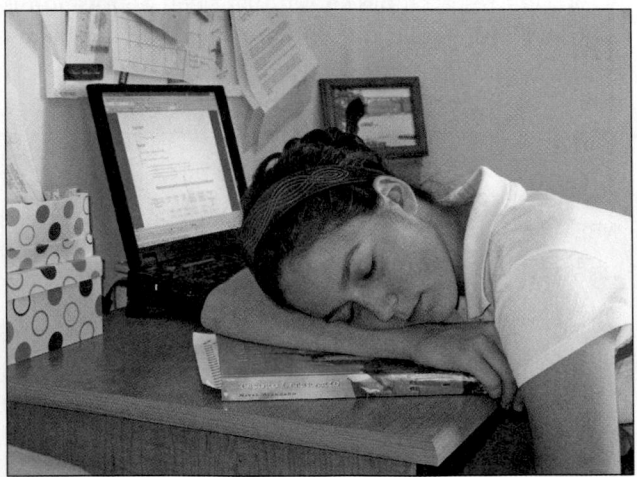

FIGURE 38.2 Many adolescents do not get enough sleep.

fewer motor vehicle accidents (Danner & Phillips, 2008; Owens, Belon, & Moss, 2010).

During adolescence, boys begin to experience **nocturnal emissions** (orgasm and emission of semen during sleep), known as *wet dreams,* several times each month. Boys need to be informed about this normal development to prevent embarrassment and fear.

Adults

The sleep–wake cycle remains very important to health throughout life. Most adults in their early to middle adult years (19 to 64 years of age) require 7 to 9 hours of sleep each night. About 20% of time is spent in REM sleep. During adulthood, most individuals experience a slight but steady increase in arousals over time and between the fourth and fifth decades, the amount of SWS begins to decrease. Shift work, school, and childcare or elder-care (or both) often lead to irregular sleep schedules. Late-night social and sports activities, alcohol, caffeine, nicotine, computer, and television are other factors contributing to the sleep deprivation and sleep disturbances experienced by many adult Canadians.

Older Adults

The older adult (ages 65 years and over) sleeps between 7 and 9 hours per night. SWS is markedly decreased with increased age and may be absent entirely. A hallmark change with age is a tendency toward earlier bedtime and wake times. Older adults usually awaken 1.3 hours earlier and go to bed approximately 1 hour earlier than younger adults. Older adults may show an increase in disturbed sleep (lighter sleep, more awakenings, difficulty falling back to sleep) that can have a negative effect on their quality of life, mood, and alertness. Although the ability to sleep becomes more difficult, the need to sleep does not decrease with age. Many older adults compensate with a daytime nap.

A strong relationship exists among sleep, health, and aging. Healthy older adults are more likely to sleep well, whereas as the number of medical conditions experienced increases, so does the likelihood of sleep problems (National Sleep Foundation, n.d.c). Nurses should assess routinely for sleep problems and be aware that sleep disorders can exacerbate other health conditions and complicate their treatment. Many older adults with dementia experience *sundown syndrome.* Although not a primary sleep disorder, the late afternoon onset of agitation, anxiety, and confusion associated with the disorder can last throughout the night, further disturbing sleep and the sleep of those nearby.

Factors Affecting Sleep

Both the quality and the quantity of sleep are affected by a number of factors. *Sleep quality* is a subjective characteristic and is often determined by whether a person wakes up feeling energetic or not. *Quantity of sleep* is the total time the individual sleeps.

Health and Illness

Normal states of health, such as rapid growth, menstruation, perimenopause, pregnancy, and parenthood, can temporarily alter sleep patterns. Nurses should reassure parents that young children and teens sleep more during periods of rapid growth and that this additional sleep is normal, needed, and temporary. For women, sleep quality is reported to be poorer 3 to 6 days before menstruation and during the first 4 days of menstruation.

Disruptions in menstrual function are linked to circadian rhythm disturbances (Baker & Driver, 2007). Hot flashes, common to perimenopause, can be especially sleep disturbing. Wearing breathable nightwear and layering bedcovers can help to support a faster return to sleep. Pregnancy is associated with sleep pattern change. Women are sleepier than usual early in pregnancy because of increased levels of circulating progesterone; they often experience nocturia (the need to urinate during the night) in the first and third trimesters because of pressure on the bladder from the growing fetus; and they experience increasing sleep disturbance in the third trimester in the form of more nighttime awakenings, lighter sleep, and less total sleep time. Postpartum recovery and the sleep-disrupting care demands of a newborn and infant make parenthood, and the early months of childcare, especially tiring for parents.

Illness that causes pain or physical distress can result in sleep problems. People who are ill require more sleep than normal, and the normal rhythm of sleep and wakefulness is often disturbed. As well, the caregivers of the ill may also experience problems with sleep as they may have to awaken several times during the night to provide care. In addition, the worry that something might happen during the night to their loved one may require the caregiver to "sleep with one eye open" (Hearson, McClement, McMillan, & Harlos, 2011). Respiratory disorders can disturb an individual's sleep. Shortness of breath makes sleep difficult, and people who have nasal congestion or sinus drainage may have trouble breathing and hence difficulty sleeping.

People who have gastric or duodenal ulcers may find their sleep disturbed because of pain, often a result of the increased gastric secretions that occur during REM sleep. Certain endocrine disturbances can also affect sleep. Hyperthyroidism lengthens presleep time, often making it difficult for a client to fall asleep. Hypothyroidism, conversely, decreases stage IV sleep. Women with low levels of estrogen often report excessive fatigue. In addition, they may experience sleep disruptions, in part, because of the discomfort associated with hot flashes or night sweats that can occur with reduced estrogen levels. Elevated body temperatures can cause some reduction in SWS and REM sleep.

Nocturia disrupts sleep and is a common problem for individuals with urinary tract infection or irritation, with bladder emptying difficulties (e.g., prostate hypertrophy), or in the early and late stages of pregnancy, as previously described. Individuals may waken several times through the night to urinate and may have difficulty getting back to sleep.

Emotional Stress

Stress is considered by most sleep experts to be the number one cause of short-term sleeping difficulties (National Sleep Foundation, n.d.d). Anxiety and depression frequently disturb sleep. A person preoccupied with personal problems may be unable to relax sufficiently to get to sleep. Anxiety increases the norepinephrine levels in the blood through stimulation of the sympathetic nervous system. This chemical change results in less stage IV NREM and REM sleep and more stage changes and awakenings.

People who are depressed typically have disturbed sleep, manifested either as insomnia or excessive sleeping. They may report difficulty getting to sleep, frequent awakenings and the inability to get back to sleep, or early morning wakening. This association may be physiological, through neurotransmitter imbalance, as well as psychological, through worry and negative thoughts.

Environment

Environment can promote or hinder sleep. The person must be able to achieve a state of relaxation prior to entering a period of sleep. The absence of usual stimuli or the presence of unfamiliar stimuli can prevent people from sleeping. Hospital and long-term care environments can be quite noisy, and special care needs to be taken to reduce noise in the hallways and nursing care units.

Discomfort from environmental temperature (e.g., too hot or cold) and poor or excessive ventilation can also affect sleep. Light levels can be another factor. A person accustomed to darkness while sleeping may find it difficult to sleep in the light. Another influence includes the comfort and size of the bed and firmness of the pillow. A person's partner who has different sleep habits, who snores, or who has other sleep difficulties, such as periodic limb movement, can cause sleep problems.

Homelessness is a growing problem in all major Canadian cities. One immediate and major health consequence of this social housing crisis is chronic, severe sleep disturbance and deprivation—if you are cold, hungry, wet, in pain, or do not feel safe, you do not sleep well, if at all.

Lifestyle

People who have irregular sleep–wake schedules are more likely to experience poor-quality sleep. Moderate exercise in the morning or early afternoon is conducive

to sleep, but vigorous exercise late in the day can delay sleep onset. The person's ability to relax before retiring is an important factor affecting the ability to fall asleep. It is best, therefore, to avoid doing homework or office work before or after getting into bed.

Shift work and travel across time zones disrupt the normal circadian rhythm. Night-shift workers frequently get less sleep compared with other workers and have difficulty falling asleep after getting off work. Wearing dark wrap-around sunglasses during the drive home and using light-blocking shades can minimize the alerting effects of exposure to daylight, thus making it easier to fall asleep when body temperature is rising.

Stimulants and Alcohol

Caffeine-containing beverages act as stimulants of the central nervous system. Drinking caffeinated beverages in the afternoon or evening can interfere with sleep. People who drink an excessive amount of alcohol often experience sleep disturbance. Excessive alcohol disrupts REM sleep, although it may initially hasten sleep onset. While making up for lost REM sleep after some of the effects of the alcohol have worn off, people often experience nightmares.

Diet

Weight gain has been associated with reduced total sleep time, fragmented sleep, and earlier awakening. During periods of sleep deprivation, ghrelin, a hormone that stimulates hunger, is oversecreted, and leptin, a satiety hormone, is suppressed, contributing to overeating when staying up late at night. Conversely, weight loss is associated with an increase in total sleep time and less fragmented sleep. L-tryptophan—found, for example, in cheese and milk—may induce sleep, a fact that might explain why warm milk helps some people get to sleep.

Smoking

Nicotine has a stimulating effect on the body, and smokers often have more difficulty falling asleep and staying asleep compared with nonsmokers. Heavy smokers often awaken early because of nicotine withdrawal. By reducing daily intake and refraining from smoking after the evening meal, the person usually sleeps better. Although the immediate withdrawal period when stopping smoking can result in disturbed sleep related to the nicotine withdrawal, sleeping patterns often improve once people get past the withdrawal period.

Motivation

Motivation can increase alertness in some situations (e.g., a moderately tired person may be able to stay alert while attending an interesting concert or surfing the Internet

BOX 38.3 DRUGS THAT AFFECT SLEEP AND WAKEFULNESS

These drugs can disrupt REM sleep, delay sleep onset, decrease sleep time, cause nightmares, or increase daytime drowsiness:

- Alcohol
- Amphetamines
- Antidepressants
- Antihistamines
- Beta-blockers
- Bronchodilators
- Caffeine
- Decongestants
- Opioids
- Steroids

late at night). Motivation alone, however, is usually not sufficient to overcome the normal circadian drive to sleep during the night. Neither is motivation sufficient to overcome sleepiness caused by insufficient sleep. Boredom alone is not sufficient to cause sleepiness, but with the combination of insufficient sleep with boredom, sleep is more likely to occur.

Medications

Some medications affect the quality of sleep. Hypnotics can interfere with SWS and suppress REM sleep. Beta-blockers and steroids have been known to cause insomnia and nightmares. Opioids, such as morphine, are known to suppress REM sleep and to cause frequent awakenings and drowsiness. Tranquilizers interfere with REM sleep. Although antidepressants suppress REM sleep, this effect is considered a therapeutic action; selectively depriving a depressed client of REM sleep will result in an immediate but transient improvement in mood. Clients accustomed to taking hypnotic medications and antidepressants may experience a REM rebound (increased REM sleep) when these medications are discontinued. Warning clients to expect a period of more intense dreams when these medications are discontinued may reduce their anxiety about this symptom. See Box 38.3 for drugs that can affect sleep.

Common Sleep Disorders

Knowledge of common sleep disorders helps nurses obtain and recognize pertinent data. Sleep disorders can be categorized as primary disorders, secondary disorders, and parasomnias. **Primary sleep disorders** are those in which the person's sleep problem is the main disorder. These disorders include insomnia and excessive daytime sleepiness such as with hypersomnia, narcolepsy, sleep apnea, or insufficient sleep. **Secondary sleep disorders** are sleep disturbances caused by another clinical disorder, such as thyroid dysfunction, depression, or alcoholism. Parasomnias, such as somnambulism, bruxism (teeth grinding), or periodic limb movement disorder, are described as unwanted physical events (e.g., movements) or experiences (e.g., sleep terrors) occurring during sleep onset, within sleep, or during arousal from sleep.

Insomnia

Insomnia, the most common sleep problem, is the inability to fall asleep or remain asleep. People suffering from insomnia do not feel refreshed on arising. The three types of insomnia are as follows:

1. Difficulty falling asleep (initial or onset insomnia)
2. Difficulty staying asleep because of frequent or prolonged waking (intermittent or maintenance insomnia)
3. Early morning or premature waking (terminal insomnia)

Acute insomnia lasts one to several nights and is often caused by personal stressors or worry. If the insomnia persists for longer than a month, it is considered chronic insomnia. More often, people experience chronic–intermittent insomnia, which means difficulty sleeping for a few nights, followed by a few nights of adequate sleep before the problem returns. The two main risk factors of insomnia are older age and female gender (National Sleep Foundation, n.d.e).

Insomnia is often characterized by predisposing, precipitating, and perpetuating factors. *Predisposing* factors include hyperarousal, predisposition to depression, and tendency to be a night owl. *Precipitating* factors can include periods of stress or grief, the loss of a loved one, a new job, a new child, or a perceived need for increased vigilance. *Perpetuating* factors include fear of not being able to sleep, irregular sleeping patterns to try to catch up, and association of the bedroom with the struggle to sleep.

Treatment for insomnia frequently requires the client to develop new behaviour patterns that induce sleep and maintain sleep. Examples of behavioural treatments include the following:

- *Stimulus control:* creating a sleep environment that promotes sleep
- *Cognitive therapy:* learning to develop positive thoughts and beliefs about sleep
- *Sleep restriction:* following a program that limits time in bed in order to get to sleep and stay asleep throughout the night (National Sleep Foundation, n.d.e).

Short-term use of hypnotics during periods of stress may be helpful in reducing the impact of a precipitating event, but the long-term efficacy of hypnotic medications is questionable as they do not deal with the cause of the problem, and their prolonged use can create drug dependencies.

Excessive Daytime Sleepiness

Clients may experience excessive daytime sleepiness as a result of hypersomnia, narcolepsy, sleep apnea, and insufficient sleep.

HYPERSOMNIA **Hypersomnia** refers to conditions where the affected individual obtains sufficient sleep at night but still cannot stay awake during the day. Hypersomnia can be caused by medical conditions, for example, central nervous system (CNS) damage and certain kidney, liver, or metabolic disorders, such as diabetic acidosis and hypothyroidism. Rarely does hypersomnia have a psychological origin.

NARCOLEPSY **Narcolepsy** is a disorder of sleep–wake instability caused by the lack of the chemical hypocretin in the area of the CNS that regulates sleep. Patients with narcolepsy have sleep attacks or excessive daytime sleepiness, and their sleep at night usually begins with a sleep-onset REM period. The majority of patients also have cataplexy, or the sudden onset of muscle weakness or paralysis in association with strong emotion; sleep paralysis (transient paralysis when falling asleep or waking up); hypnagogic hallucinations (visual, auditory, or tactile hallucinations at sleep onset or when waking up); and fragmented nighttime sleep. Their fragmented nocturnal sleep is not the cause of their excessive daytime sleepiness; many clients, particularly younger clients, have sound restorative nocturnal sleep but still cannot stay awake during the daytime. Onset of symptoms tends to occur between ages 15 and 30 years, and symptom severity usually stabilizes within the first 5 years of onset. CNS stimulants, such as methylphenidate (Ritalin), or amphetamines have been used to reduce daytime sleepiness.

SLEEP APNEA **Sleep apnea** is characterized by frequent periodic cessation of breathing during sleep. Although all individuals have occasional periods of apnea during sleep, more than five apneic episodes or five breathing pauses longer than 10 seconds per hour is considered abnormal and should be evaluated by a sleep specialist. Symptoms suggestive of sleep apnea include awakening with a sensation of choking, gasping, or smothering; snoring loud enough to be heard through closed doors; frequent nocturnal awakenings; excessive daytime sleepiness; morning headaches; memory and cognitive problems; irritability or other personality changes (Fleetham et al., for the Canadian Thoracic Society, 2011). People with sleep apnea may have a history of hypertension, cardiovascular disease, cerebrovascular disease, renal disease, type 2 diabetes mellitus, or gastroesophageal reflux disease (Lochan, 2011). An estimated 3% of adult Canadians report that they have sleep apnea with twice as many men experiencing this condition (Public Health Agency of Canada, 2009).

Three common types of sleep apnea are (a) obstructive apnea, (b) central apnea, and (c) mixed apnea. *Obstructive apnea* occurs when the structures of the pharynx or oral cavity block the flow of air. The person continues to try to breathe; that is, the chest and abdominal muscles move. Increased carbon dioxide levels lead to partial arousal, thus opening the airway. Definite risk factors for obstructive apnea include obesity, craniofacial abnormalities (e.g., short mandible), and upper airway soft tissue abnormalities (e.g., tonsillar or adenoid hypertrophy); potential risk factors include heredity, current smoking, and nasal congestion. *Central apnea* is thought to involve a defect in the respiratory centre of the brain. All actions involved in breathing, such as chest movement and airflow, cease. Clients who have brain stem injuries and muscular dystrophy, for example, often have central sleep apnea. *Mixed apnea* is a combination of central apnea and obstructive apnea.

Treatment for sleep apnea is directed at the cause of the apnea. For example, a tonsillectomy or adenoidectomy may be performed. Other surgical procedures, including laser removal of excess tissue in the pharynx, may be effective in relieving apnea. In other cases, the use of a nasal continuous positive airway pressure (CPAP) device at night is effective in maintaining an open airway. Weight loss may also decrease the severity of symptoms.

INSUFFICIENT SLEEP Healthy individuals who obtain less sleep than they need will experience sleepiness and fatigue during the daytime hours. Depending on the severity and chronicity of this voluntary, albeit unintentional sleep deprivation, individuals may develop attention and concentration deficits, reduced vigilance, distractibility, reduced motivation, fatigue, malaise, and occasionally diplopia and dry mouth. The cause of these symptoms may or may not be attributed to insufficient sleep as many people may believe that they are getting sufficient sleep.

Although the effects of obtaining less than optimal amounts of sleep are generally considered benign, there is growing evidence that insufficient sleep can have significant deleterious effects. Staying awake 19 consecutive hours produces the same impairments in reaction times and cognitive function as a blood alcohol level of 0.05%, and staying awake for 24 consecutive hours has the same effects on reaction times and cognitive function as being legally "drunk"!

When clients report obtaining more sleep on weekends or days off, it usually indicates that they are not obtaining sufficient sleep. Convincing the client to obtain more sleep may be difficult, but it can result in the resolution of their daytime symptoms.

BOX 38.4 PARASOMNIAS

- *Somnambulism:* Somnambulism (sleepwalking) occurs during stages III and IV of NREM sleep. It is episodic and usually occurs 1 to 2 hours after falling asleep. Sleepwalkers tend not to notice dangers (e.g., stairs) and often need to be protected from injury.

- *Sleeptalking:* Talking during sleep occurs during NREM sleep before REM sleep. It rarely presents a problem to the person unless it becomes troublesome to others.

- *Enuresis:* Bed wetting during sleep can occur in children over 3 years old. More males than females are affected. It often occurs 1 to 2 hours after falling asleep when rousing from NREM stages III to IV.

- *Bruxism:* Usually occurring during stage II NREM sleep, this clenching and grinding of the teeth can eventually erode dental crowns, cause teeth to come loose, and lead to deterioration of the temperomandibular joint.

- *Periodic limb movement disorder (PLMD):* In this condition, the legs jerk two or three times per minute during sleep. It is most common among older adults. This kicking motion can wake the client and result in poor sleep. PLMD differs from restless leg syndrome (RLS), which occurs whenever the person is at rest, not just at night when asleep. RLS may occur during pregnancy or be due to other medical problems that can be treated. Many clients with PLMD or RLS respond well to medications, such as levodopa and gabapentin.

Parasomnias

Parasomnia is a kind of sleep disorder in which abnormal events occur during sleep, such as sleepwalking or talking. The *International Classification of Sleep Disorders* subdivides parasomnias into arousal disorders (e.g., sleepwalking, sleep terrors), sleep–wake transition disorders (e.g., sleeptalking), parasomnias associated with REM sleep (e.g., nightmares), and others (e.g., bruxism). Box 38.4 describes examples of parasomnias.

Assessing

In addition to a comprehensive health history, the assessment of a client's sleep and rest includes a sleep and rest history, a sleep diary, a physical examination, and a review of diagnostic studies.

Sleep History

A brief general sleep history should be obtained for all clients entering a health care facility or being seen in the community. This enables the nurse to incorporate the client's needs and preferences in the plan of care. Although sleep is a health priority, many patients will not report sleep problems unless specifically asked, assuming that sleep is not that important or that little can be done

to improve it. A general sleep history should include the following:

- Usual sleeping pattern, specifically sleeping and waking times; length of time to fall asleep; hours of undisturbed sleep; number and reason for sleep interruptions; quality of or satisfaction with sleep, presence of excessive daytime sleepiness

- Usual sleeping environment, including whether single or shared sleep space, location (e.g., bed, couch, single or shared room); safety, comfort level, noise level

- Bedtime rituals performed to help the person fall asleep (e.g., a glass of hot milk, reading or other method of relaxing, and special equipment or positioning aids)

- Use of sleep medication, or other drugs (e.g., prescription, over the counter, herbal, recreational, dietary)

- Preferred sleep environment (e.g., room temperature, noise level, night light)

- Recent changes in sleep patterns or difficulties in sleeping such as presence of snoring, somnambulation, narcolepsy

If the client indicates a recent pattern change or difficulties in sleeping, a more detailed history is required. This detailed history should explore the exact nature of the problem and its cause, when it first began and its frequency, how it affects daily living, what the client is doing to cope with the problem, and whether these methods have been effective. Questions the nurse might ask the client with a sleeping disturbance are shown in the Assessment: Interview box on the next page. Information from the bed partner on snoring, breathing patterns, leg movements, sleeptalking, and sleepwalking is also important in detecting sleep disorders.

Sleep Diary

Sometimes, clients with a sleeping problem can provide more precise information if they keep a written record of their sleep pattern and the habits associated with it. Such a sleep diary or log can be kept by clients who are sleeping at home and should be maintained for at least 1 week. A sleep diary may include all of the following information or selected aspects of it that pertain to the client's specific problem:

- Total number of sleep hours per night
- Number, length, and timing of naps
- Activities performed 2 to 3 hours before bedtime (type, duration, and time)
- Bedtime rituals (e.g., ingestion of food, fluid, or medication) before going to bed
- Consumption of caffeinated beverages and alcohol and amounts of those beverages

ASSESSMENT | **INTERVIEW**

Sleep Disturbances

QUESTIONS	COMMENTS
A. Understanding the problem from the client's perspective	
• What is the biggest problem with your sleep at this time?	This helps the client focus.
• When did you first notice this problem?	Determine whether the problem is acute or chronic; you may probe as to what was happening in the client's life about the time the problem started (e.g., change in job, weight gain).
• How often does it occur?	(e.g., every night, only when overtired)
• What makes it worse?	(e.g., alcohol makes sleep apnea worse)
• What have you found that helps deal with this sleep problem?	(e.g., sleeping in front of the television or away from home suggests the bedroom has become associated with the struggle to sleep)
• What do you think might be causing or contributing to the problem?	Clients are often aware of probable etiologies.
• How is this problem affecting you? others in your family and workplace?	Sleep disorders often affect others (e.g., snoring, worry about safety).
B. Understanding the problem from the bed partner's perspective	
• What concerns do you have about your partner's sleep?	The bed partner can provide valuable information about behaviours during sleep as well as waking hours.
• What have you noticed that seems to make it better? worse?	
C. Screening questions to assist in planning care and determining need for referral	
• What do you do to prepare for sleep?	Listen for rituals, tendency to be busy right up to bedtime.
• Do you have difficulty getting to sleep?	Probe as to length of time to go to sleep (10 to 30 minutes is within normal range).
• Do you have difficulty with wakening during the night and being unable to get back to sleep?	If yes, probe as to what the client does if awake for long periods (e.g., racing thoughts).
• Do you waken earlier in the morning than you would like?	This is particularly common with depression.
• How do you feel when you wake up in the morning?	Morning headaches and feeling unrefreshed are common symptoms of sleep apnea.
• Do you sleep more than usual? less than usual?	Inquire regarding family or work pressures and fatigue.
• Do you have periods of overwhelming tiredness? If yes, when does this happen? Do you ever feel suddenly weak when laughing or upset?	A positive response may suggest narcolepsy, especially if the client also has symptoms of cataplexy.
• Has anyone ever told you that you snore? stop breathing in your sleep? sleepwalk? sleeptalk?	Snoring and apneas suggest sleep apnea; parasomnias, such as somnambulism, are uncommon in adults and can be worsened by stress.
D. Additional Information	
• Collect data on current medications (including OTC and street drugs), alcohol use, time and amount of caffeine use, and smoking.	Many medications and other substances affect sleep.
• Explore lifestyle regarding shift work or frequent travel across time zones.	Note circadian effects.

- Any prescribed medications, OTC medications, and herbal remedies taken during the day
- (a) Time of going to bed, (b) approximate time to fall asleep after lights out, (c) any instances of waking up and duration of these periods, (d) final time of waking during the night, and (e) time out of bed
- How rested the client feels on awakening (e.g., 0 "not rested at all" to 10 "completely rested")

- Any difficulties remaining awake during the day and times when difficulties occurred
- Worries that the client believes may affect sleep
- Factors that the client believes have a positive or negative effect on sleep

If the client is a child, the sleep diary may be completed by a parent.

Physical Examination

Rarely are sleep abnormalities noted during the physical exam unless the client has obstructive sleep apnea or some other health problem. Examination of the client includes observation of the client's body structure, facial appearance, behaviour, and energy level. Obesity, enlarged tongue or tonsils, obstructed nares, and such conditions as Down syndrome all increase the risk of obstructive sleep apnea.

Diagnostic Studies

Sleep is measured objectively by **polysomnography** (PSG), in which an electroencephalogram (EEG), electromyogram (EMG), and electrooculogram (EOG) are recorded simultaneously. This simultaneous recording divides sleep into REM and NREM sleep. Electrodes are placed on the scalp to record brain waves (EEG), on the outer canthus of each eye to record eye movement (EOG), and on the chin muscles to record the structural EMG. The following may also be monitored, depending on findings of the initial interview: respiratory effort and airflow, ECG, leg movements, and oxygen saturation. Oxygen saturation is determined by monitoring arterial blood or with a *pulse oximeter*, a light-sensitive electric cell that attaches to the ear or a finger. Oxygen saturation and ECG assessments are of particular importance if sleep apnea is suspected. Through PSG, the client's activity (movements, struggling, noisy respirations) during sleep can be assessed. Activity the client is unaware of may be the cause of arousal during sleep. The Canadian Thoracic Society (Fleetham, Ayas, Bradley, Fitzpatrick, Oliver, Morrison. Ryan, Series, Shomro, Tsai, & the Canadian Thoracic Society Disordered Breathing Committee, 2011) recommends that PSG testing at a sleep laboratory be used for diagnosing sleep apnea; however, there is a wide disparity in access to this resource across Canada and portable home monitoring devices may need to be used.

Diagnosing

Insomnia, a diagnosis given to clients with sleep problems, is usually made more explicit with descriptions, such as "difficulty falling asleep" or "difficulty staying asleep." Various factors or etiologies may be involved and should be specified for the individual. These include physical

discomfort or pain; anxiety about actual or anticipated loss of a loved one, loss of a job, or worry about a family member's behaviour or illness; frequent changes in sleep time because of shift work or overtime; and changes in sleep environment or bedtime rituals (e.g., noise or overstimulation of hospital environment; alcohol or other drug dependency; drug withdrawal; misuse of sedatives prescribed for insomnia; and effects of medications, such as steroids or stimulants). Examples of assessment data and exemplar nursing diagnoses for sleep pattern disturbances are shown in Table 38.1.

Sleep pattern disturbances can also be stated as the etiology of another diagnosis, in which case the nursing interventions are directed toward the sleep disturbance itself. Examples include the following:

TABLE 38.1 Clinical Application: Assessment Data and Exemplar Nursing Diagnoses for Clients with Sleep Problems

Data Cluster	Nursing Diagnosis
Francine Leduc, 51, states she has had a problem falling asleep since her mastectomy 2 months ago. She says fears of prognosis become prominent when she is not active and busy. She has tried reading or watching TV, but neither make her sleepy or relaxed. She appears agitated and restless.	Insomnia (difficulty falling asleep) related to fear of prognosis, rumination about her health situation, and difficulty relaxing
Joseph Nitchke, 83, was admitted to a four-bed room in the extended care unit 3 days ago. He states he falls asleep about 10 p.m. but is awakened by roommate's snoring. He states, "At home I used to have a hot cup of Ovaltine whenever I awakened."	Unable to maintain sleep related to change in sleep environment and sleep-time rituals
Lourdes Cabrera, a high school student whose parents recently divorced, broke up with her boyfriend 2 weeks ago. She states she does not have the energy to get up in the morning and just wants to sleep all the time. She has Grade 12 examinations next week.	Insomnia related to difficulty coping with multiple situational stresses
Tom Longboat states that recent shortage of firefighters has resulted in extensive overtime and frequent "double shifts" and rotations from his usual 2-week 7–3 and 3–7 shifts. He states, "All I want to do is go to sleep when I get home, but I can't. I guess I'm too riled up."	Altered sleep–wake pattern related to frequent changes in sleep time

- Risk for falls or injury related to somnambulism
- Risk for not being able to carry out roles effectively owing to fatigue
- Impaired gas exchange related to sleep apnea

Planning

The major goal for clients with sleep disturbances is to maintain (or develop) a sleeping pattern that provides sufficient energy for daily activities. The nurse plans specific nursing interventions based on the etiology of each nursing diagnosis. These interventions may include reducing environmental distractions; promoting bedtime rituals; providing comfort measures; scheduling nursing care to provide for uninterrupted sleep periods; and teaching stress reduction, relaxation techniques, or ways to develop good sleep habits. If the sleep disturbance is the etiology of the nursing diagnosis, the nurse plans specific strategies to relieve insomnia and deal with sleep deprivation.

Examples of interventions to assist clients with sleep disturbances include the following:

- Anxiety reduction
- Managing the environment to promote sleep
- Sleep enhancement
- Simple massage
- Simple relaxation therapy

Specific nursing activities associated with each of these interventions can be selected to meet the individual needs of the client. See the accompanying Sample Care Plan.

SAMPLE CARE PLAN FOR SLEEP

ASSESSMENT DATA

Nursing Assessment

Jack Harrison is a 36-year-old police officer assigned to a high-crime police precinct. One week ago, he received a surface bullet wound to his arm. Today, he arrives at the outpatient clinic to have the wound redressed. While speaking with the nurse, Mr. Harrison mentions that he has recently been promoted to the rank of detective and has assumed new responsibilities. He states that since his promotion he has been feeling stressed and has experienced increasing difficulty falling asleep and sometimes staying asleep. He expresses concern over the danger of his occupation and his desire to do well in his new position. He complains of waking up feeling tired and irritable.

Physical Examination

Height: 185.4 cm
Weight: 85.7 kg
Temperature: 37°C
Pulse: 80 beats/min
Respirations: 18/minute
Blood pressure: 144/80 mm Hg

Diagnostic Data

X-ray left arm: evidence of superficial soft tissue injury

Nursing Diagnosis

Disturbed sleep pattern likely related to stress from taking on a new professional role or possibly linked to the psychological trauma of having been shot. Fatigue and irritability could negatively influence his ability to assume his new role.

Client Goals

The client will (a) establish a satisfactory sleep and rest pattern and awaken feeling rested and (b) identify sources of stress and possible coping strategies.

Desired Health Outcomes

1. Describes one or two factors that contribute to insomnia
2. Identifies two or three measures that induce sleep
3. Verbalizes decreased irritability and a greater sense of well-being
4. Identifies effective new and old coping strategies

Selected Nursing Interventions and Activities with Rationales [in bold]

Enhancing Sleep

- Determine the client's sleep and activity pattern.
  Rationale: The amount of sleep an individual needs varies with lifestyle, health, and age.
- Encourage Mr. Harrison to establish a bedtime routine to facilitate transition from wakefulness to sleep.
  Rationale: Rituals and routines induce comfort, relaxation, and sleep.
- Encourage him to stop working on projects or other stressful activities at least 1 hour before bedtime.
  Rationale: Stress interferes with a person's ability to relax, rest, and sleep.
- Teach Mr. Harrison and significant others about factors (e.g., physiological, psychological, lifestyle, frequent work shift changes, excessively long work hours, and other environmental factors) that contribute to sleep pattern disturbances.
  Rationale: Knowledge of predisposing factors can enable the client to begin to control factors that inhibit sleep.
- Discuss with Mr. Harrison and his family comfort measures, sleep-promoting techniques, and lifestyle changes that can contribute to optimal sleep.

(continued)

SAMPLE CARE PLAN FOR SLEEP (continued)

Rationale: Knowledge of factors that affect sleep enables the client to implement changes in lifestyle and before bedtime activities.

- Monitor bedtime food and beverage intake for items that facilitate or interfere with sleep.
  Rationale: Milk and protein foods contain L-tryptophan, a precursor of serotonin, which is thought to induce and maintain sleep. Stimulants should be avoided because they inhibit sleep.

Stress Reduction

- Seek to understand Mr. Harrison's perspective of his situation as stressful.
  Rationale: Anxiety is a feeling aroused by a vague, nonspecific threat. Identifying his perspective on the promotion will facilitate planning for the best approach to anxiety reduction. While the "mean-

ing" of a promotion is generally seen as positive, the transition can be stressful owing to learning a new repertoire of coping strategies.

- Encourage verbalization of feelings, perceptions, and fears related to having been shot.
  Rationale: Open expression of feelings facilitates identification of specific emotions, such as anger or helplessness and realistic or unrealistic fears. Sleep disturbance may indicate post-traumatic stress and it will be important to identify the issues and refer accordingly

- Help Mr. Harrison identify possible resources to help manage his stress.
  Rationale: Police departments likely have resources to help its members cope with the stress of being in a "dangerous" profession; he may need professional support in coping with having been shot.

Evaluation

Goal met. Mr. Harrison was able to see the link between his insomnia and his anxiety regarding job promotion, a fear of failing, and feeling vulnerable after having been shot. He states that talking with the police department counsellor has been helpful. He is practising relaxation techniques each night and sleeps an average of 7 hours a night. If he starts to ruminate during the night about his stress then he gets up, reads for about 20 to 30 minutes, then returns to bed and falls asleep. Mr. Harrison expresses a greater sense of well-being.

Implementing

Nursing interventions to enhance the quantity and quality of clients' sleep involve largely nonpharmacological measures. These involve health teaching about sleep habits; support of bedtime rituals; the provision of a restful environment; specific measures to promote comfort and relaxation; and essential considerations about the use of sleep medications.

For hospitalized patients, sleep problems are often related to the hospital environment or their illness. Assisting the client to sleep in such instances can be challenging to a nurse, often involving scheduling activities, administering analgesics, and providing a supportive environment. Some interventions to reduce environmental distractions are listed in Box 38.5.

Teaching Clients about Sleep Habits

Healthy individuals need to learn the importance of rest and sleep in maintaining active and productive lifestyles. They need to learn (a) the conditions that promote sleep and those that interfere with sleep, (b) the safe use of sleep medications, (c) the effects of other prescribed medications on sleep, and (d) the effects of their disease states on sleep. See the Teaching: Wellness box on the next page for ways to promote sleep and rest.

Supporting Bedtime Rituals

Most people are accustomed to bedtime rituals or presleep routines that are conducive to comfort and relaxation. Altering or eliminating such routines can affect a client's

---

BOX 38.5   REDUCING ENVIRONMENTAL DISTRACTIONS IN HOSPITALS

Many patients have trouble sleeping in a hospital. The nurse can try the following interventions to help:

- Close the window curtains if street lights shine through
- Close the curtains between clients in semiprivate and larger rooms
- Reduce or eliminate overhead lighting; provide a night light at the bedside or in the bathroom
- Close the door of the patient's room
- Adhere to agency policy about times to turn off communal televisions or radios
- Lower the ring tone of nearby telephones

- Discontinue use of the paging system after a certain hour (e.g., 2100h), or reduce its volume
- Keep required staff conversations at low levels; conduct nursing reports or other discussions in a separate area away from patient rooms
- Wear rubber-soled shoes
- Ensure that all cart wheels and door hinges are well oiled
- Perform only essential nursing tasks during sleeping hours; avoid scheduling of tests and procedures in early morning
- Pair patients with frequent nocturnal needs in the same room to minimize disturbances for other patients

Promoting Sleep

SLEEP PATTERN

- Establish a regular bedtime and wake-up time for all days of the week to prevent disruptions in your biological rhythm. Eliminate lengthy naps or, if a daytime nap is necessary, take it at the same time each day and limit the time to 30 minutes, preferably once a day.
- Get adequate exercise during the day to reduce stress, but avoid excessive physical exertion 2 hours before bedtime.
- Avoid dealing with work or family problems before bedtime.
- Establish a regular routine before sleep, such as reading, listening to soft music, taking a warm bath, or doing some other quiet activity you enjoy.
- When you are unable to sleep, pursue some relaxing activity until you feel drowsy.
- If you have trouble falling asleep, get up and pursue nonstrenuous activity until you feel sleepy.
- Use the bed mainly for sleep (or sexual activity) so that you associate it with sleep. Take work material, computers, and TVs out of the bedroom. Lying awake, tossing and turning, will strengthen the association between wakefulness and lying in bed.
- When you are unable to sleep, get out of bed, go into another room, and pursue some relaxing activity until you feel drowsy.

ENVIRONMENT

- Create a sleep-conducive environment that is dark, quiet, comfortable, and cool.

- Keep noise to a minimum; block out extraneous noise, as necessary, with white noise from a fan, air conditioner, or other machine.
- Sleep on a comfortable mattress and pillows.

DIET

- Avoid heavy meals 2 to 3 hours before bedtime.
- Avoid alcohol and caffeine-containing foods and beverages (coffee, tea, chocolate) at least 4 hours before bedtime.
- Decrease fluid intake 2 to 4 hours before sleep, if necessary, to avoid the need to use the bathroom during sleeping hours.
- If a bedtime snack is necessary, consume only light carbohydrates or a milk drink. Heavy or spicy foods can cause gastrointestinal upsets that disturb sleep.

MEDICATIONS

- Use sleeping medications only as a last resort. Take them judiciously (e.g., three times a week at most). Use OTC medications sparingly because many contain antihistamines that cause daytime drowsiness.
- Take analgesics 30 minutes before bedtime to relieve aches and pains, if necessary.
- Consult with your health care provider about adjusting other medications that may cause insomnia.
- Take diuretics and stimulating medications early in the day.

sleep. Common prebedtime activities of adults include taking an evening stroll, listening to music, watching television, taking a soothing bath, and praying. Children, too, are socialized into presleep routines, such as hearing a bedtime story, holding onto a favourite toy or blanket, and kissing everyone goodnight. Sleep is also usually preceded by hygiene routines, such as washing the face and hands (or bathing), brushing the teeth, and voiding.

In institutional settings, nurses can provide similar bedtime rituals—assisting with a hand and face wash, providing a massage or hot drink, plumping pillows, and providing extra blankets, as needed. Conversing about accomplishments of the day or enjoyable events, such as visits from friends, can also help relax clients and bring peace of mind.

Creating a Restful Environment

To create a restful environment, the nurse needs to reduce environmental distractions, reduce sleep interruptions, ensure a safe environment, and provide a room temperature that is satisfactory to the client.

The environment must also be safe so that the client can relax. People who are unaccustomed to narrow hospital beds may feel more secure with side rails. Additional safety measures include the following:

- Placing the beds in the low position
- Using a night light
- Placing the call bell within easy reach

Promoting Comfort and Relaxation

Comfort measures are essential to help the client fall asleep and stay asleep, especially if the effects of the person's illness interfere with sleep. A concerned, caring attitude, along with the following interventions, can significantly promote client comfort and sleep:

- Provide loose-fitting nightwear.
- Assist patients with hygiene routines.
- Make sure the bed linen is smooth, clean, and dry.

- Assist or encourage the patient to void before bedtime.
- Offer to provide a back massage before sleep (see Skill 38.1).

- Position dependent patients appropriately to aid muscle relaxation, and provide supportive devices to protect pressure areas.

SKILL 38.1 PROVIDING A BACK MASSAGE

PURPOSES

- To relieve muscle tension
- To promote physical and mental relaxation
- To relieve insomnia

ASSESSMENT

Assess

- Behaviours indicating the potential need for a back massage, such as difficulty sleeping related to tenseness or anxiety
- Whether the client wants a massage; some individuals do not enjoy a massage
- Contraindications for back massage (e.g., coagulation issues, clots, impaired skin integrity, neck or spinal issues, risk of fracture)

PLANNING

Ensure that you have the full amount of time available for the massage. Although the actual technique may require only about 5 minutes, the entire process should be conducted in a calm and unhurried manner.

Equipment

- Lotion or oil
- Towel for excess lotion

IMPLEMENTATION

Preparation

Determine (a) previous assessments of the skin, (b) special lotions to be used, and (c) positions contraindicated for the client. Arrange for a quiet environment with no interruptions to promote maximum effect of the back massage.

Performance

1. Before performing the procedure, introduce yourself and verify the client's identity using two identifiers or per agency protocol. Explain to the client what you are going to do, why it is necessary, and how he or she can participate. Encourage the client to give you feedback as to the amount of pressure you are using during the back rub.

2. Perform hand hygiene, and follow other appropriate infection prevention and control procedures.

3. Provide for client privacy.

4. Prepare the client.
   - Assist the client to move to the near side of the bed within your reach and adjust the bed to a comfortable working height. **Rationale: This step prevents back strain in the nurse.**
   - Establish which position the client prefers. The prone position is recommended for a back rub. The side-lying position can be used if a client cannot assume the prone position.

- Expose the back from the shoulders to the inferior sacral area. Cover the remainder of the body. **Rationale: This measure will prevent chilling and minimize exposure.**

5. Massage the back.
   - Pour a small amount of lotion onto the palms of your hands and hold it for a minute. The lotion bottle can also be placed in a bath basin filled with warm water. **Rationale: Back rub preparations tend to feel uncomfortably cold to people. Warming the solution facilitates client comfort.**
   - Use your palm and begin in the sacral area, using smooth, circular strokes (referred to as *effleurage*).
   - Move your hands up the centre of the back and then over both scapulae.
   - Massage in a circular motion over the scapulae.
   - Move your hands down the sides of the back.
   - Massage the areas over the right and left iliac crests (see ❶).
   - Apply firm, continuous pressure without breaking contact with the client's skin.
   - Repeat above for 3 to 5 minutes obtaining more lotion, as necessary.
   - While massaging the back, assess for skin redness and areas of decreased circulation.
   - Pat dry any excess lotion with a towel.

6. Document that a massage was performed and the client's response.

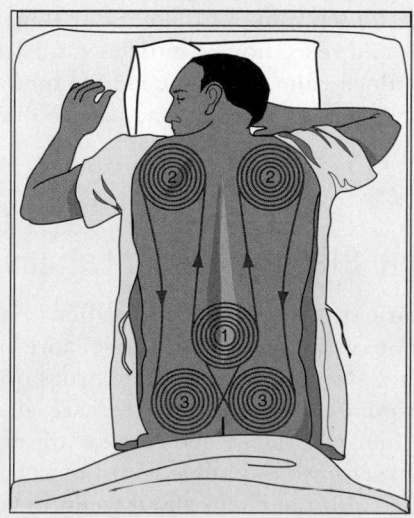

❶ One suggested pattern for a back rub

EVALUATION

Compare the client's current response to his or her previous response. Is there a positive client outcome, such as increased relaxation because of the back massage?

- Schedule medications, especially diuretics, to prevent nocturnal awakenings.

- For people who have pain, administer analgesics 30 minutes before sleep.

- For people who have breathing problems, administer prescribed medications, such as bronchodilators, before bedtime, and position clients appropriately (e.g., semi-Fowler's position) to facilitate breathing.

- Listen to the patient's concerns, and deal with problems as they arise.

People of any age, but especially older adults, are unable to sleep well if they feel cold. Changes in circulation, metabolism, and body tissue density reduce the older person's ability to generate and conserve heat. To compound this problem, hospital gowns have short sleeves and are made of thin fabric. Sheets also are often made of polyester, rather than a warm fabric, such as cotton flannel. The following interventions can be used to keep older adult clients warm during sleep:

- Provide a warmed bath blanket, if possible.

- Use 100% cotton flannel sheets or apply thermal blankets between the sheet and bedspread.

- Encourage the person to wear his or her own clothing, such as a flannel nightgown or pyjamas, nonconstricting thermal socks, leg warmers, long underwear, sleeping cap, or a sweater, or to use a favourite quilt or blanket.

Emotional stress obviously interferes with a person's ability to relax, rest, and sleep, and inability to sleep further aggravates feelings of tension. Sleep rarely occurs until a person is relaxed. Relaxation techniques can be encouraged as part of the nightly routine. Slow, deep breathing for a few minutes followed by slow, rhythmic contraction and relaxation of muscles can alleviate tension and induce calm. Imagery, meditation, and yoga can also be taught. These techniques are discussed in Chapters 16 and 48.

Enhancing Sleep with Medications

Sleep medications often prescribed on a prn (as-needed) basis for clients include sedative–hypnotics, which induce sleep, and antianxiety drugs or tranquilizers (benzodiazepines), which decrease anxiety and tension. When prn sleep medications are ordered in institutional settings, the nurse is responsible for making decisions with the client about when to administer them. These medications should be administered only with complete knowledge of their actions and effects and only when indicated. These medications are contraindicated in pregnant women because of their associated risk of congenital anomalies and in nursing mothers because the medication could be excreted in breast milk. New,

shorter-acting benzodiazepines should be considered if a medication is needed because they cause less daytime sedation. Drug hangover is particularly problematic in older adults or those with reduced clearance capacity. Whenever possible, nonpharmacological interventions to induce and maintain sleep, discussed earlier, are the preferred interventions.

Both nurses and clients need to be aware of the actions, effects, and risks of the specific medication prescribed. Although medications vary in their activity and effects, considerations include the following:

- Sedative–hypnotic medications produce a general CNS depression and an unnatural sleep; REM or NREM sleep is altered to some extent and daytime drowsiness and a "morning hangover" effect may occur. Newer hypnotics, such as zolpidem (Ambien), do not alter REM sleep or produce rebound insomnia when discontinued.

- Antianxiety medications decrease levels of arousal by facilitating the action of neurons in the CNS that suppress responsiveness to stimulation.

- Sleep medications vary in their onset and duration of action and will impair waking function as long as they are chemically active. Some medication effects can last many hours beyond the time that the client's perception of daytime drowsiness and impaired psychomotor skills have disappeared. Clients need to be cautioned about such effects and about driving or handling machinery while the drug is in their system.

- Sleep medications affect REM sleep more than NREM sleep. Clients need to be informed that 1 or 2 nights of increased dreaming (REM rebound) is usual after the drug is discontinued.

- Initial doses of medications should be low and increases added gradually, depending on the client's response. Older adults, in particular, are susceptible to side effects because of metabolic changes; they need to be closely monitored for changes in mental alertness and coordination. Clients need to be instructed to take the smallest effective dose and then only for a few nights or intermittently as required.

- Regular use of any sleep medication can lead to tolerance over time (e.g., 4 weeks) and rebound insomnia. In some instances, this may lead clients to increase the dosage or complement the drug with alcohol. Clients must be cautioned about developing a pattern of drug dependency.

- Abrupt cessation of *barbiturate* sedative–hypnotics can create withdrawal symptoms, such as restlessness, tremors, weakness, insomnia, increased heart rate, seizures, convulsions, and even death. Long-term users need to taper withdrawal under the supervision of a specialist.

EVIDENCE-INFORMED PRACTICE

What Is the Effectiveness and Safety of Chinese Herbs for Insomnia?

Sleep is valued and it is, indeed, relatively common in many Canadian households to hear on awakening, "How did you sleep?" or "Did you have a good night's sleep?" Not getting enough sleep—insomnia—is well known as a problematic issue for many Canadians who seek out prescription and over-the-counter (OTC) medications as well as other interventions to help them get that good night's sleep. While some treatments help (e.g., benzodiazepine), they also come with unwanted adverse effects (e.g., increased risk of fall, daytime somnolence, and dependence). Xu et al. (2009) acknowledged the important role that sleep plays and developed a protocol outlining how they will find evidence that supports healthy and effective ways of promoting sleep. While Chinese herbal medicines have been used for centuries to promote sleep and treat insomnia, there has been no formal review of research studies to determine effectiveness and safety of Chinese herbs for insomnia. The authors indicate that they will review randomized control trials to determine if there is evidence to support or negate the use of herbal medicines in promoting sleep, including any harmful effects.

NURSING IMPLICATIONS: Many Canadians seek nurse's opinions related to the use of complementary and alternative therapies. We need to be up-to-date on their benefits and risks so that we can help our clients make informed decisions. If Chinese herbal medicines are effective and safe, they may provide a nice alternative to those who have been using other medications that are less safe. While many Canadians view herbal remedies as "natural" and "safe," we know that they can have adverse effects. This systematic review will help to inform nurses of the effectiveness and safety of recommending Chinese herbal medicines, which will ensure high-quality care.

Source: Based on Xu, L., Li, J., Zhang, M., Wang, L., Yuan, W., Ai, C. L., ... & Zhang, L. (2009). Chinese herbs for insomnia (Protocol). *Cochrane Database of Systematic Reviews,* Issue 2. Art. No.: CD007841. doi: 10.1002/14651858.CD007841

See the Evidence-Informed Practice box on the effectiveness and safety of Chinese herbs for insomnia.

TABLE 38.2 Evaluation Goals and Outcomes: Sleep Pattern Disturbances

Goal	Example of Desired Outcomes
Develop a sleep–wake pattern that ensures sufficient energy for daily activities	Identifies possible causes of sleeping problem
	Identifies stress-relieving measures that enhance ability to fall asleep
	Uses planned relaxation techniques before bedtime
	Falls asleep within 20 to 30 minutes of going to bed
	Sleeps specified number of hours per night or for longer intervals between nursing care functions
	Reports feelings of being rested or refreshed after waking
Increase physical and psychological comfort level before and during sleep	Reports satisfaction with pain control measures and positioning techniques
	Reports satisfaction with physical surroundings
	Reports effectiveness of bedtime rituals and relaxation techniques (e.g., backrubs, soft music, warm soothing bath) in reducing anxiety

Evaluating

Using data collected during care and the desired outcomes developed during the planning stage as a guide, the nurse judges whether client goals and outcomes have been achieved. Data collection may include (a) observations of the duration of the client's sleep and the presence of signs of REM and NREM sleep, and (b) questions about how the client feels on awakening or about the effectiveness of specific interventions, such as the use of relaxation techniques, adherence to a consistent sleep–wake cycle, or the ingestion of milk products before bedtime. Examples of client goals and related outcomes are shown in Table 38.2.

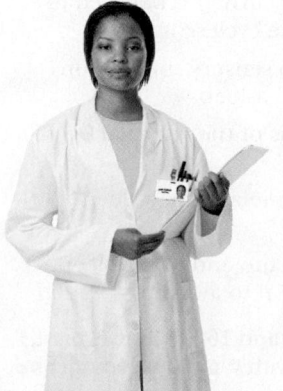

Case Study 38

While making rounds at 1 a.m., you note that Jo Su-Mi, a 23-year-old woman recovering from surgery, is awake and watching television. Concerned that she may be experiencing too much pain to sleep, you question her about how she is feeling. She states that she is not having pain; she just cannot sleep. On further questioning, you learn that she has a pattern of sleepless nights. She explains that she usually goes to bed by 11 p.m. after exercising but frequently has difficulty falling asleep. Sometimes, she listens to the radio or watches TV until she is able to sleep. She usually has a soft drink at bedtime but avoids coffee or tea because it keeps her awake. Jo states that she is frequently sleepy during the day and has considered getting a prescription for a sleeping pill from her doctor so that she can develop a better sleep routine.

(continued)

KEY TERMS

circadian rhythm *p. 1120*

homeostatic drive *p. 1119*

hypersomnia *p. 1126*

insomnia *p. 1125*

narcolepsy *p. 1126*

nocturnal emissions
  p. 1123

NREM sleep (non rapid eye movement sleep)
  p. 1120

parasomnia *p. 1127*

polysomnography *p. 1129*

primary sleep disorders
  p. 1125

REM sleep (rapid eye movement sleep)
  p. 1120

secondary sleep disorders
  p. 1125

sleep *p. 1119*

sleep apnea *p. 1126*

sleep architecture *p. 1120*

slow-wave sleep (SWS)
  p. 1120

CHAPTER HIGHLIGHTS

- Sleep is a naturally occurring altered-consciousness state in which a person's perception of and reaction to the environment are decreased.
- The sleep cycle is controlled by specialized areas in the brain stem and is affected by the individual's circadian rhythm.
- Sleep is restorative, protective, and energy conserving.
- During a normal night's sleep, an adult has four to six sleep cycles, each with NREM and REM sleep.
- NREM sleep consists of four stages, progressing from stage I, very light sleep, to stage IV, deep sleep. NREM sleep constitutes most of a sleep cycle.
- REM sleep recurs about every 90 minutes and is often associated with dreaming.
- The ratio of NREM to REM sleep varies with age.
- Many factors can affect sleep, including health and illness, environment, lifestyle, emotional stress, alcohol and stimulants, diet, smoking, motivation, and medications.
- Common sleep disorders include insomnia, hypersomnia, narcolepsy, sleep apnea, and parasomnias, such as somnambulism, nocturnal enuresis, bruxism, and periodic limb movements.
- Assessment of a client's sleep includes obtaining a sleep history, reviewing a sleep diary, conducting a physical examination to detect signs of sleep deprivation, and reviewing diagnostic studies.
- Nursing responsibilities to help clients sleep include (a) teaching clients ways to enhance sleep, (b) supporting bedtime rituals, (c) creating a restful environment, (d) promoting comfort and relaxation, and (e) using prescribed sleep medications.
- Nonpharmacological interventions to induce and maintain sleep are the preferred interventions.

ASSESS YOUR LEARNING

1. Mr. Janssen is 34 years old, married with two children, and has been diagnosed with multiple sclerosis. The reason for his hospitalization is an acute exacerbation–remitting episode. Mr. Janssen has been up in his chair visiting with his family for 3 hours and is visibly fatigued. How can the nurse promote a balance between rest and activity for Mr. Janssen?

   a. Inform the family when the unit rest periods are scheduled.

   b. Insist that Mr. Janssen abide by the scheduled rest periods.

   c. Wait until Mr. Janssen's family leaves the unit to discuss rest periods with him.

   d. Discuss the importance of rest periods with Mr. Janssen and his family.

2. Gamma-aminobutyric acid (GABA) is believed to have what role in sleep–wake cycles?

   a. It lessens the response to sensory stimulation causing the person to fall asleep.

   b. It deactivates the neurons of the reticular activating system.

   c. It triggers the release of melatonin, a sleep-inducing hormone.

   d. It stimulates the brain at the end of the sleep period, causing the person to awaken.

3. Sarah Horowitz, 35 years old and 16 weeks pregnant, was admitted to emergency with vaginal bleeding. She has been in the observation area and has been sleeping for the past hour and a half. Her vital signs have been

stable, and the bleeding has stopped. When you check in on Sarah, you notice that her eyes are closed but moving in short, sharp bursts; her respiratory rate is 14 breaths/min but irregular; the monitor shows that her heart rate is fluctuating between 64 and 82 beats/min. What should you do next?

a. Gently rouse the patient and assess vital signs.

b. Prepare the emergency cart and alert the medical team.

c. Immediately wake the patient fully and assess vital signs.

d. Do not disturb the patient and continue with observations and vital signs q1 to q2h.

4. One day after prostate surgery, at 1400h, you notice that the 74-year-old patient is having his second nap of the day. You allow the patient to continue to sleep for which of the following reasons?

a. Individuals need more total sleep as they age.

b. Older patients who nap are usually depressed.

c. Patients need more sleep than normal following surgery.

d. The patient will need to be given a sleeping medication at night.

5. Emily Bruin, age 15 years, has come to your health care centre. She is in Grade 10, has a full course load, enjoys volunteer work, and is on the school hockey team. She looks pale, has dark circles under her eyes, and states that she feels exhausted and irritable most of the time. Which factor is likely contributing most to Emily's sleep disturbance?

a. She is a straight-A student and spends 2 hours per day on homework.

b. She has hockey practice Mondays and Thursdays from 8 p.m. to 9 p.m.

c. She is a regular Saturday morning volunteer at the local Humane Society.

d. She drinks two large coffees with double sugar and double cream every morning.

6. Kaki Ashoona, a 68-year-old Inuit woman, has been flown in from Cape Dorset to undergo a hysterectomy to treat a localized uterine cancer. Following surgery, Kaki is assigned to a four-bed room. The interpreter relays that Kaki is having considerable difficulty falling asleep at night. The nurse recognizes that further teaching to enhance optimal sleep health is needed when Kaki does which of the following?

a. Takes an analgesic if the pain is "really bad"

b. Confirms her discharge plans with the interpreter

c. Asks for an extra blanket and wears a wool cap at night

d. Has a cranberry bun and a small cup of wintergreen tea at bedtime

7. Pritam Singh Sageer is attending an evening concert at the Sikh Pavilion at Winnipeg's Folklorama. The lights lower and within minutes, he is snoring loudly. He snorts, gasps, and then awakens when shaken by his wife. Mr. Sageer is 54 years old, is 173 cm tall, and weighs 95 kg. You suspect that Mr. Sageer may have obstructive sleep apnea. Which one of the following health assessments would support this condition?

a. A history of enlarged tonsils

b. Difficulty falling asleep

c. A history of sleepwalking

d. Frequent evening headaches

8. Laura DeLaat is a 40-year-old surgical nurse who has come to your sleep centre because of difficulty with her sleep–wake patterns. Laura works rotating day and night shifts, is a single parent of two teenage girls, and has an ailing mother who lives with their family. Following your assessment, you discuss several sleep health practices with Laura. Which statement suggests that Laura needs additional sleep health education?

a. "I will take the bus home rather than drive when I work nights."

b. "If I work overtime, I can make up the sleep on my days off."

c. "Regular daytime exercise will help reduce stress and make it easier for me to sleep."

d. "I need to forward my phone to the answering machine and turn down the ring tone when I sleep days."

9. Which of the following recommendations is accurate for the client dealing with maintenance insomnia?

a. Establish a night-time routine.

b. Take a prescribed sleep medication on awakening.

c. When unable to sleep, get out of bed and pursue a relaxing activity and return to bed when drowsy.

d. Make an appointment for polysomnography.

10. Rachel and Justin Peters are the exhausted parents of Grace, a 7-month-old baby girl. Grace is healthy and is gaining weight as expected. Rachel gets up four times each night to briefly breastfeed the baby, and then Justin changes the baby and walks her to sleep. Rachel is pale and teary, and Justin admits that he is irritable and that he has difficulty concentrating at work. The nurse should advise the couple to do which of the following?

a. Take turns sleeping with Grace to allow each to get more rest.

b. Put Grace back in her crib after feeding when she is drowsy but not asleep.

c. Provide Grace with a bottle of formula at night to drink if she awakens.

d. Seek psychiatric counselling immediately as Rachel is suffering from postpartum depression.

Check the eText in MyNursingLab for answers and explanations.

WEBLINKS

Canadian Sleep Society
http://www.css.to
This is an organization for health care professionals and researchers in sleep and circadian rhythms. It also contains some information for lay people, including downloadable brochures and a list of sleep specialists willing to answer questions.

Canadian Lung Association
http://www.lung.ca/diseases-maladies/apnea-apnee_e.php
This website provides an interesting section on sleep apnea.

National Sleep Foundation
http://www.sleepfoundation.org
The Sleep Foundation website offers general sleep information for the lay public, such as self-assessment guides.

MyNursingLab

REFERENCES

Baker, F. C., & Driver, H. S. (2007). Circadian rhythms, sleep, and the menstrual cycle. *Sleep Medicine, 8,* 613–622.

Canadian Paediatric Society. (2011). *Recommendations for safe sleeping environments for infants and children.* Retrieved from http://www.cps.ca/english/statements/cp/cp04-02.htm

Danner, F., & Phillips, B. (2008). Adolescent sleep, school start times, and teen motor vehicle crashes. *Journal of Clinical Sleep Medicine, 4*(6), 533–535.

Fleetham, J., Ayas, N., Bradley, D., Fitzpatrick, M., Oliver, T. K., Morrison, D., . . . & Tsai, W.; The Canadian Thoracic Society Sleep Disordered Breathing Committee. (2011). Canadian Thoracic Society 2011 guideline update: Diagnosis and treatment of sleep disordered breathing. *Canadian Respiratory Journal, 18*(1), 25–47

Gibson, E. S., Powles, A. C. P., Thabane, L., O'Brien, S., Molnar, D. S., Trajanovic, N., . . . & Chilcott-Tanser, L. (2006). "Sleepiness" is serious in adolescence: Two surveys of 3235 Canadian students. *BMC Public Health, 6,* 116.

Hearson, B., McClement, S., McMillan, D., & Harlos, M. (2011). Sleeping with one eye open: The sleep experience of family members providing palliative care at home. *Journal of Palliative Care, 27*(2), 69–78.

Hunt, C. E., & Hauck, F. R. (2006). Sudden infant death syndrome. *Canadian Medical Association Journal, 174*(13), 1861–1868.

Lochan, S. (2011). Understanding sleep-disordered breathing as a risk factor for hypertension and metabolic diseases:

Implications for clinical assessment. *Canadian Journal of Cardiovascular Nursing , 21*(2), 7–10.

National Sleep Foundation. (n.d.a). *Children and sleep.* Retrieved from http://www.sleepfoundation.org/article/sleep-topics/children-and-sleep

National Sleep Federation. (n.d.b.). *School start time and sleep.* Retrieved from http://www.sleepfoundation.org/article/sleep-topics/school-start-time-and-sleep

National Sleep Foundation. (n.d.c). *Aging and sleep.* Retrieved from http://www.sleepfoundation.org/article/sleep-topics/aging-and-sleep

National Sleep Foundation. (n.d.d). *ABCs of ZZZZ—When you can't sleep.* Retrieved from http://www.sleepfoundation.org/abcs-zzzzs-when-you-cant-sleep

National Sleep Foundation (n.d.e). *Can't sleep? What to know about insomnia.* Retrieved from http://www.sleepfoundation.org/article/sleep-related-problems/insomnia-and-sleep

Owens, J. A., Belon, K., & Moss, P. (2010). Impact of delaying school start time on adolescent sleep, mood, and behavior. *Archives of Pediatric and Adolescent Medicine, 164*(7), 608–614.

Public Health Agency of Canada. (2009). *What is the impact of sleep apnea on Canadians—fast facts from the 2009 Canadian Community Health Survey Sleep Apnea Rapid Response.* Retrieved from http://www.phac-aspc.gc.ca/cd-mc/sleepapnea-apneesommeil/pdf/sleep-apnea.pdf

Chapter 39

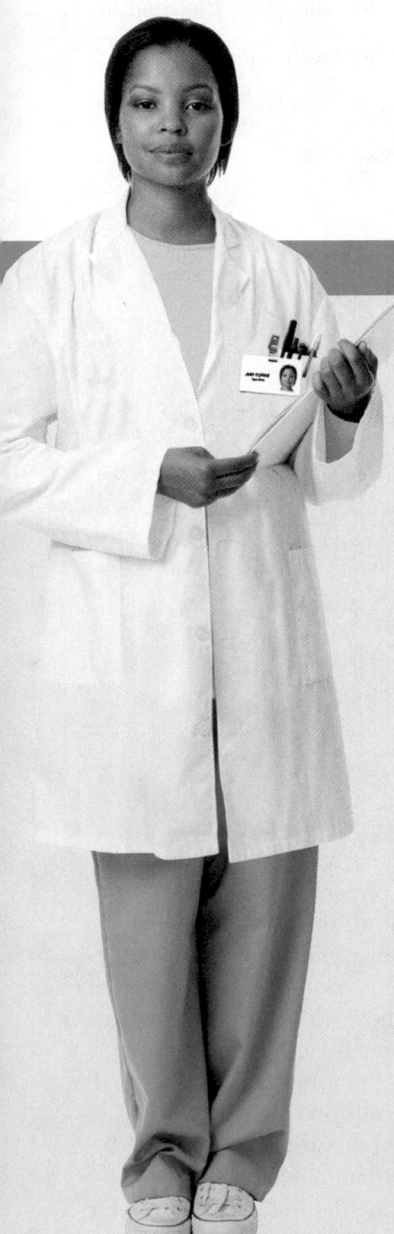

Activity and Exercise

A well-developed body of literature supports the benefits of physical activity and exercise in maintaining and improving health status. A reduced risk of cardiovascular disease, type 2 diabetes, hypertension, stroke, respiratory illness, bone and joint disease (osteoporosis and osteoarthritis), and cancer (colon and breast) is associated with regular physical activity (Warburton, Nicol, & Bredin, 2006). Canadians who are physically active report less chronic illness, improved mental health, greater life satisfaction, and less stress both at home and at work (Canadian Fitness and Lifestyle Research Institute [CFLRI], 2006). Unfortunately, the activity level and fitness of Canadians has decreased over the past several decades, with only about half of Canadians currently performing 30 minutes of moderate-vigorous physical activity on one or more days per week (Statistics Canada, 2011b). During the same period, the prevalence of obesity has risen, with approximately one-quarter of Canadian adults now considered obese (Statistics Canada, 2011a). It is estimated that inactivity costs the health care system at least $2.1 billion a year in direct health care costs and leads to an economic drain of approximately $5.3 billion a year (Katzmarzyk & Janssen, 2004). Although the majority of Canadians know about the benefits of activity, such barriers as work commitments and tight deadlines and lack of safe roads or sidewalks to perform physical activity (e.g., walking or bicycling) are cited (CFLRI, 2006). See the Reflect on Primary Health Care for a creative solution.

REFLECT ON PRIMARY HEALTH CARE

A nurse and a social worker demonstrated *intersectoral collaboration* when they worked with the management of a local shopping mall in an urban centre. They offered a walkabout program three times a week to older adults, people with physical disabilities, and new parents as a way of socializing, staying fit, and getting support during winter months, when many would otherwise be isolated or lack any physical activity because of a fear of falling on the slippery sidewalks. Find out whether any creative programs are available to people in your community. If not, what *health-promotion* activities related to physical activity and exercise are available? Do these resources address the special needs of the very young, the older adult, or the person with a physical disability?

In 2005, the Integrated Pan-Canadian Healthy Living Strategy set the goal of increasing by 20% the proportion of Canadians who participate in regular physical activity based on 30 minutes a day of moderate to vigorous activity by the year 2015. The messages *Active Transportation, Active Play, and Active Family Time* encourage Canadians to simply *Get Moving!*

The term **activity-exercise pattern** refers to a person's routine of exercise, activity, leisure, and recreation. It includes (a) activities of daily living (ADLs) that require energy expenditure, such as hygiene, cooking, shopping, eating, working, and maintaining the home; and (b) the type, quality, and quantity of exercise, including sports. **Active living** refers to adding physical activity to the time spent at home, at work, at school, and at play.

Mobility, the ability to move freely, easily, rhythmically, and purposefully in the environment, is an essential part of living. People must move to protect themselves from trauma and to meet their basic needs. Mobility is vital to independence; a fully immobilized person is vulnerable and dependent physically on others.

People often define their health and physical fitness by their activity because mental well-being and the effectiveness of body functioning depend largely on their mobility status. For example, when a person is upright, the lungs expand more easily, peristalsis (intestinal activity) is more effective, and the kidneys are able to empty completely. In addition, motion is essential for the proper functioning of bones and muscles.

The ability to move also influences self-esteem and body image, both components of self-concept. For most people, self-esteem depends on a sense of independence and a feeling of usefulness or being needed. People with mobility impairments may feel helpless and burdensome to others, and their ability to work and earn a living may be compromised. Body image can be altered by paralysis, amputations, or any motor impairment. The reaction of others to impaired mobility can also alter self-esteem and body image significantly. For individuals with impaired mobility, movement must be fostered to the full extent of their capability to facilitate a satisfying life.

Normal Movement

Normal movement and stability are the result of an intact musculoskeletal system, an intact nervous system, and intact inner ear structures responsible for equilibrium. Body movement requires coordinated muscle activity and neurological integration. It involves four basic elements: (a) body alignment (posture), (b) joint mobility, (c) balance (stability), and (d) coordinated movement.

Alignment and Posture

Proper body alignment and posture bring body parts into line in a manner that promotes optimal balance and maximal body function in whatever position the client assumes: standing, sitting, or lying down. The line of gravity and the body's centre of gravity influence standing alignment and balance. A person maintains balance as long as the **line of gravity** (an imaginary vertical line drawn through the body's centre of gravity) passes through the **centre of gravity** (the point at which all of the body's mass is centred) and the **base of support** (the foundation on which the body rests). In humans, the usual line of gravity begins at the top of the head and falls between the shoulders, through the trunk, slightly anterior to the sacrum, and between the weight-bearing joints and base of support (Figure 39.1). For a person in the upright position, the centre of gravity is located in the centre of the pelvis, approximately midway between the umbilicus and the symphysis pubis. For greatest balance and stability, a standing adult must centre body weight symmetrically along the line of gravity.

When the body is well aligned, strain on the joints, muscles, tendons, or ligaments is minimized, and the internal structures and organs are supported. People are usually unaware of the functions of the abdominal

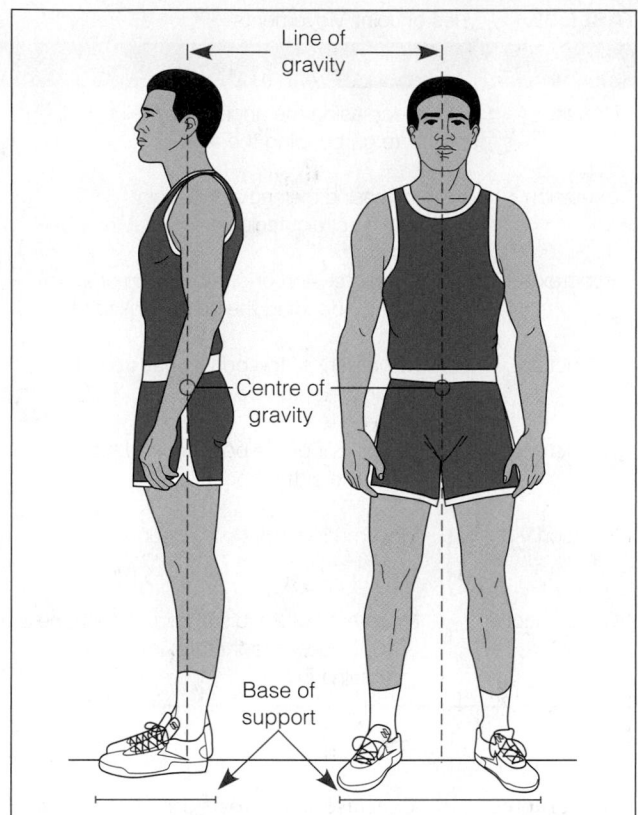

FIGURE 39.1 The centre of gravity and the line of gravity influence standing alignment.

and skeletal muscles that function almost continuously, making tiny adjustments that enable an erect or seated posture despite the endless downward pull of gravity. Sustained contraction of the muscles supporting this upright position is called **postural tonus**. The extensor muscles, often referred to as the *antigravity* muscles, carry the major load.

Proper body alignment enhances lung expansion and promotes efficient circulatory, respiratory, renal, and gastrointestinal functions. Conversely, poor body alignment detracts from a pleasing appearance and affects an individual's health adversely. A person's posture is one criterion for assessing general health, physical fitness, and attractiveness. Posture reflects the mood, self-esteem, and personality of an individual.

Joint Mobility

Joints are the functional units of the musculoskeletal system. The bones of the skeleton articulate at the joints and most of the skeletal muscles attach to the bones at the joint. Muscles are categorized according to the type of joint movement they produce on contraction. Muscles are called flexors, extensors, internal rotators, and the like. The flexor muscles are stronger than the extensor muscles. Thus, when a person is inactive, the joints are pulled into a flexed position. If this tendency is not

TABLE 39.1 Types of Joint Movements

Movement	Action	Movement	Action
Flexion	Decreasing the angle of the joint (e.g., bending the elbow)	Eversion	Turning the sole of the foot outward by moving the ankle joint
Extension	Increasing the angle of the joint (e.g., straightening the arm at the elbow)	Inversion	Turning the sole of the foot inward by moving the ankle joint
Hyperextension	Overextension or straightening of a joint (e.g., bending the head backward)	Pronation	Moving the bones of the forearm so that the palm of the hand faces downward when held in front
Abduction	Movement of the bone away from the midline of the body	Supination	Moving the bones of the forearm so that the palm of the hand faces upward when held in front
Adduction	Movement of the bone toward the midline of the body		
Rotation	Movement of the bone around its central axis	Protraction	Moving a part of the body forward in the same plane parallel to the ground
Circumduction	Movement of the distal part of the bone in a circle while the proximal end remains fixed	Retraction	Moving a part of the body backward in the same plane parallel to the ground

counteracted with exercise and position changes, the muscles permanently shorten, and the joint becomes fixed in a flexed position (contracture). The types of joint movement are shown in Table 39.1.

The **range of motion (ROM)** of a joint is the maximum movement that is possible for that joint. Joint ROM varies from individual to individual and is determined by genetic makeup, developmental patterns, the presence or absence of disease, and the amount of physical activity in which the person normally engages. Table 39.2 shows the various joint movements and the usual ranges of motion.

TABLE 39.2 Selected Joint Movements and Examples of Corresponding Activity of Daily Living (ADL)

Body Part—Type of Joint/Movement	Normal Range	Illustration
Neck—Pivot Joint		
Flexion. Move the head from the upright midline position forward so that the chin rests on the chest (Figure 39.2).	45 degrees from midline *Example:* Nodding head "yes"	**FIGURE 39.2**
Extension. Move the head from the flexed position to the upright position (see Figure 39.2).	45 degrees from midline *Example:* Nodding head "yes"	
Hyperextension. Move the head from the upright position back as far as possible (see Figure 39.2).	45 degrees from midline	
Lateral flexion. Move the head laterally to the right and left shoulders (Figure 39.3).	40 degrees from midline	**FIGURE 39.3**
Rotation. Turn the face as far as possible to the right and left (Figure 39.4).	70 degrees from midline *Example:* Shaking head "no"	**FIGURE 39.4**

Body Part—Type of Joint/Movement	Normal Range	Illustration
Shoulder—Ball and Socket Joint		
Flexion. Raise each arm from a position by the side forward and upward to a position beside the head (Figure 39.5).	180 degrees from the side *Example:* Reaching to turn on overhead light	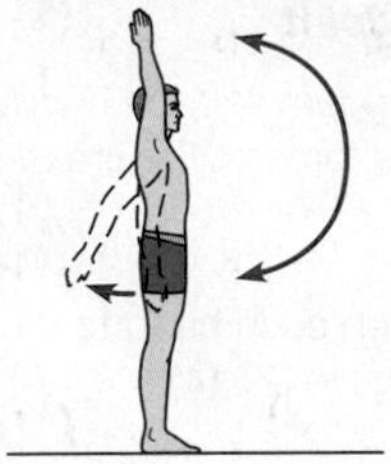
Extension. Move each arm from a vertical position beside the head forward and down to a resting position at the side of the body (see Figure 39.5).	180 degrees from vertical position beside the head	**FIGURE 39.5**
Hyperextension. Move each arm from a resting side position to behind the body (see Figure 39.5).	50 degrees from side position	
Abduction. Move each arm laterally from a resting position at the sides to a side position above the head, palm of the hand away from the head (Figure 39.6).	180 degrees *Example:* Reaching to bedside stand on same side of bed as arm	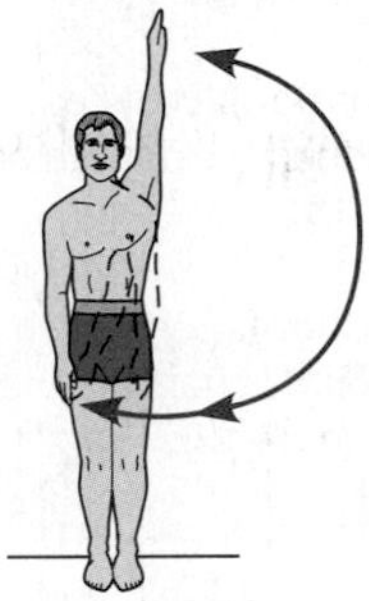
Adduction (anterior). Move each arm from a position beside the head downward laterally and across the front of the body as far as possible (see Figure 39.6).	50 degrees *Example:* Reaching across body toward opposite side of bed	**FIGURE 39.6**
Circumduction. Move each arm forward, up, back, and down in a full circle (Figure 39.7).	360 degrees	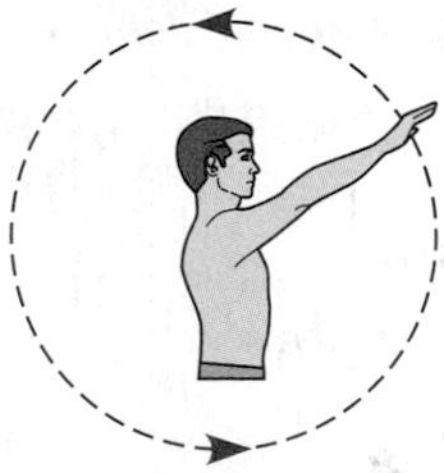 **FIGURE 39.7**
External rotation. With each arm held out to the side at shoulder level and the elbow bent to a right angle, fingers pointing down, move the arm upward so that the fingers point up (Figure 39.8).	90 degrees *Example:* Reaching over opposite shoulder to scratch upper back	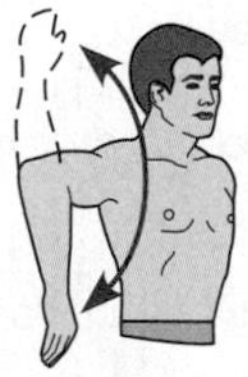 **FIGURE 39.8**
Internal rotation. With each arm held out to the side at shoulder level and the elbow bent to a right angle, fingers pointing up, bring the arm forward and down so that the fingers point down (see Figure 39.8).	90 degrees *Example:* Reaching to scratch same side lower back	
Elbow—Hinge Joint		
Flexion. Bring each lower arm forward and upward so that the hand is at the shoulder (Figure 39.9).	150 degrees *Example:* Eating, bathing, shaving	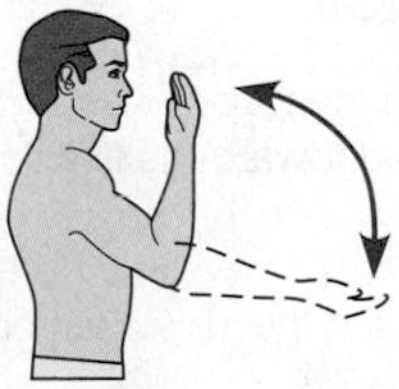 **FIGURE 39.9**
Extension. Bring each lower arm forward and downward, straightening the arm (see Figure 39.9).	150 degrees *Example:* Eating, bathing, shaving	
Rotation for supination. Turn each hand and forearm so that the palm is facing upward (Figure 39.10).	70–90 degrees	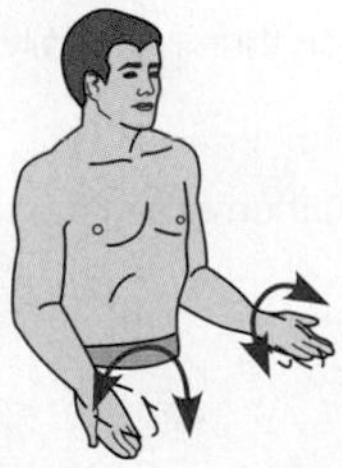
Rotation for pronation. Turn each hand and forearm so that the palm is facing downward (see Figure 39.10).	70–90 degrees	**FIGURE 39.10**

(continued)

TABLE 39.2 Selected Joint Movements and Examples of Corresponding Activity of Daily Living (ADL) (*continued*)

Body Part—Type of Joint/Movement	Normal Range	Illustration
Wrist—Condyloid Joint		
Flexion. Bring the fingers of each hand toward the inner aspect of the forearm (Figure 39.11).	80–to 90 degrees *Example:* Eating, bathing, shaving, writing	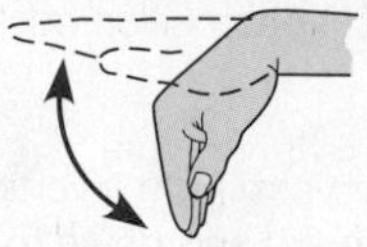 **FIGURE 39.11**
Extension. Straighten each hand to the same plane as the arm (see Figure 39.11).	80–90 degrees *Example:* Eating, bathing, shaving	
Hyperextension. Bend the fingers of each hand back as far as possible (Figure 39.12).	70–90 degrees	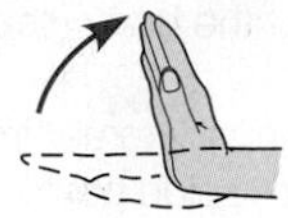 **FIGURE 39.12**
Radial flexion (abduction). Bend each wrist laterally toward the thumb side with hand supinated (Figure 39.13).	0–20 degrees	
Ulnar flexion (adduction). Bend each wrist laterally toward the fifth finger with the hand supinated (see Figure 39.13).	30–50 degrees	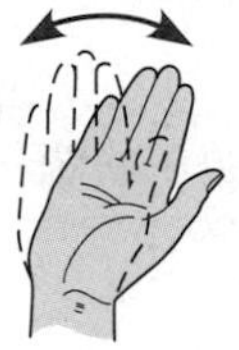 **FIGURE 39.13**
Hand and Fingers: Metacarpophalangeal Joints—Condyloid; Interphalangeal Joints—Hinge		
Flexion. Make a fist with each hand (Figure 39.14).	90 degrees *Example:* Squeezing, gripping, writing	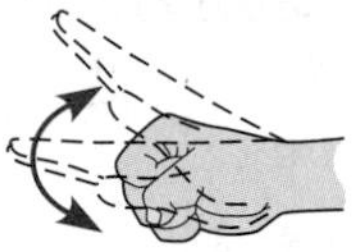 **FIGURE 39.14**
Extension. Straighten the fingers of each hand (see Figure 39.14).	30 degrees	
Hyperextension. Bend the fingers of each hand back as far as possible (see Figure 39.14).	30 degrees	
Abduction. Spread the fingers of each hand apart (Figure 39.15).	20 degrees	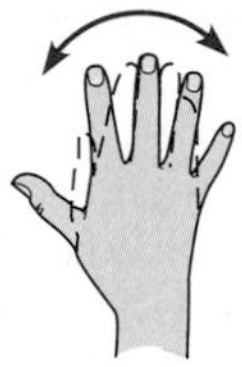
Adduction. Bring the fingers of each hand together (see Figure 39.15).	20 degrees *Example:* Writing, gripping, eating, many hobbies involving fine motor coordination (e.g., art, music)	**FIGURE 39.15**
Thumb—Saddle Joint		
Flexion. Move each thumb across the palmar surface of the hand toward the fifth finger (Figure 39.16).	90 degrees	
Extension. Move each thumb away from the hand (see Figure 39.16).	90 degrees	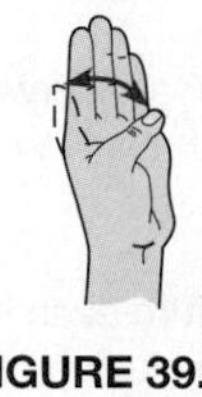
Abduction. Extend each thumb laterally (Figure 39.17).	30 degrees	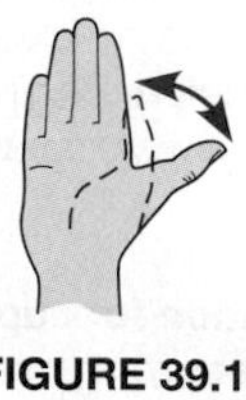 **FIGURE 39.16** **FIGURE 39.17**
Adduction. Move each thumb back to the hand (see Figure 39.17).	30 degrees	

Body Part—Type of Joint/Movement	Normal Range	Illustration
Opposition. Touch each thumb to the top of each finger of the same hand. The thumb joint movements involved are abduction, rotation, and flexion (Figure 39.18).		FIGURE 39.18

Hip—Ball-and-Socket Joint

Body Part—Type of Joint/Movement	Normal Range	Illustration
Flexion. Move each leg forward and upward. The knee may be extended or flexed (Figure 39.19).	Knee extended, 90 degrees; knee flexed, 120 degrees *Example:* Walking, leg lifts in front of body	FIGURE 39.19
Extension. Move each leg back beside the other (Figure 39.20).	90–120 degrees *Example:* Walking, lining the leg up with the body	FIGURE 39.20
Hyperextension. Move each leg back behind the body (see Figure 39.20).	30–50 degrees *Example:* Walking, lying on side and reaching leg behind body	
Abduction. Move each leg out to the side (Figure 39.21).	45–50 degrees *Example:* Moving leg away from body.	FIGURE 39.21
Adduction. Move each leg back to the other leg and beyond in front of it (see Figure 39.21).	20–30 degrees beyond other leg *Example:* Moving leg over the other leg toward the middle of the body	
Circumduction. Move each leg backward, up, to the side, and down in a circle (Figure 39.22).	360 degrees *Example:* Leg circles clockwise and counterclockwise	FIGURE 39.22
Internal rotation. Turn each foot and leg inward so that the toes point as far as possible toward the other leg (Figure 39.23).	45 degrees	FIGURE 39.23
External rotation. Turn each foot and leg outward so that the toes point as far as possible away from the other leg (see Figure 39.23).	45 degrees	

(continued)

TABLE 39.2   Selected Joint Movements and Examples of Corresponding Activity of Daily Living (ADL) (*continued*)

Body Part—Type of Joint/Movement	Normal Range	Illustration
Knee—Hinge Joint		
Flexion. Bend each leg, bringing the heel toward the back of the thigh (Figure 39.24).	120–130 degrees *Example:* Knee bends, walking	**FIGURE 39.24**
Extension. Straighten each leg, returning the foot to its position beside the other foot (see Figure 39.24).	120–130 degrees *Example:* Straightening leg from bent position, walking	
Ankle—Hinge Joint		
Extension (plantar flexion). Point the toes of each foot downward (Figure 39.25).	45–50 degrees *Example:* Pressing toes away from face, walking	**FIGURE 39.25**
Flexion (dorsiflexion). Point the toes of each foot upward (see Figure 39.25).	20 degrees *Example:* Pulling toes toward face, walking	
Foot—Gliding		
Eversion. Turn the sole of each foot laterally (Figure 39.26).	5 degrees *Example:* Foot circles clockwise and counterclockwise	**FIGURE 39.26**
Inversion. Turn the sole of each foot medially (see Figure 39.26).		
Toes: Interphalangeal Joints—Hinge ***Metatarsophalangeal Joints—Hinge*** ***Intertarsal Joints—Gliding***		**FIGURE 39.27**
Flexion. Curl the toe joints of each foot downward (Figure 39.27).	35–60 degrees	
Extension. Straighten the toes of each foot (see Figure 39.27).	35–60 degrees	
Trunk—Gliding Joint		
Flexion. Bend the trunk toward the toes (Figure 39.28).	70–90 degrees *Example:* Touching toes	
Extension. Straighten the trunk from a flexed position (see Figure 39.28).	70–90 degrees	**FIGURE 39.28**
Hyperextension. Bend the trunk backward (see Figure 39.28).	20–30 degrees *Example:* Gentle supported back bend with hands on buttocks	
Lateral flexion. Bend the trunk to the right and to the left (Figure 39.29).	35 degrees on each side *Example:* Gently allow right hand to slide down right side of thigh; repeat on left side	
Rotation. Turn the upper part of the body from side to side (Figure 39.30).	30–45 degrees *Example:* Gently swing torso right and left, maintaining forward hip alignment	**FIGURE 39.29** **FIGURE 39.30**

Balance

The mechanisms involved in maintaining balance and posture are complex and beyond the scope of this book. Mechanisms of *equilibrium* (sense of balance) respond, frequently without our awareness, to various head movements. The equilibrium sense depends on informational inputs from the inner ear labyrinth, vision (vestibulo-ocular input), and stretch receptors of muscles and tendons (proprioceptors and vestibulospinal input). The labyrinth consists of the cochlea, vestibule, and semicircular canals. The cochlea is concerned with hearing and the vestibule and semicircular canals with equilibrium. Under normal conditions, the equilibrium receptors in the semicircular canals and vestibule, collectively called the *vestibular apparatus,* send signals to the brain that initiate reflexes needed to make required changes in position. The receptors respond to displacement of the head in any direction. When the head moves, the fluid flow within the vestibule and semicircular canals stimulates the receptor cells.

Information from these balance receptors goes directly to reflex centres in the brain stem, rather than to the cerebral cortex as with other special senses. This enables fast reflexive responses to body imbalance. **Proprioception** is the term used to describe awareness of posture, movement, and changes in equilibrium and the knowledge of position, weight, and resistance of objects in relation to the body.

Coordinated Movement

Balanced, smooth, purposeful movement is the result of proper functioning of the cerebral cortex, cerebellum, and basal ganglia. The cerebral cortex initiates voluntary motor activity; the cerebellum coordinates the motor activities of movement; and the basal ganglia maintain posture. The cerebral cortex operates in terms of movements, not muscles. The cortex, for example, may direct the arm to pick up a cup of coffee. The cerebellum, which operates below the level of consciousness, blends and coordinates the muscles involved in voluntary movement. It does not direct the movement but translates the instructions from the cerebral cortex into detailed actions by the many different muscles in the hand, arm, and shoulder. When a client's cerebellum is injured, movements become clumsy, unsure, and uncoordinated.

Exercise

Physical activity is the bodily movement produced by skeletal muscles that requires energy expenditure and can produce progressive health benefits. Physical activity can include things like walking the dog, gardening,

playing tag, building a snowman, sliding, and even household chores (e.g., sweeping and raking).

Exercise is a type of physical activity defined as a planned, structured, and repetitive bodily movement done to improve or maintain one or more components of physical fitness. People participate in exercise programs to decrease risk factors for cardiovascular and other chronic diseases and to improve their health and well-being. **Functional strength** is another goal of exercise and is defined as the ability of the body to perform work. **Activity tolerance** is the type and amount of exercise or daily living activities an individual is able to perform without experiencing adverse effects.

Types of Exercise

Exercise involves the active contraction and relaxation of muscles. Exercises can be classified according to the type of muscle contraction (isotonic, isometric, or isokinetic) and according to the source of energy (aerobic or anaerobic).

Isotonic (dynamic) exercises are those in which the muscle shortens to produce muscle contraction and active movement. Most physical conditioning exercises—running, walking, swimming, cycling, and other such activities—are isotonic, as are ADLs and *active* ROM exercises (those initiated by the client). Examples of isotonic *bed* exercises are pushing or pulling against a stationary object, using a trapeze to lift the body off the bed, lifting the buttocks off the bed by pushing with the hands against the mattress, and pushing the body to a sitting position.

Isotonic exercises increase muscle tone, mass, and strength and maintain joint flexibility and circulation. During isotonic exercise, both heart rate and cardiac output quicken to increase blood flow to all parts of the body. Little or no change in blood pressure occurs.

Isometric (static or setting) exercises are those in which a change in muscle tension occurs but no change in muscle length and no muscle or joint movement takes place. These exercises are useful for strengthening abdominal, gluteal, and quadriceps muscles used in ambulation; for maintaining strength in immobilized muscles in casts or traction; and for endurance training. An example of an isometric bed exercise would be squeezing a towel or pillow between the knees and at the same time tightening the muscles in the fronts of the thighs by pressing the knees downward (Figure 39.31) and holding for 10 seconds. These are often called *quad sets.* Isometric exercises produce a moderate increase in heart rate and cardiac output but no appreciable increase in blood flow to other parts of the body.

Isokinetic (resistive) exercises involve muscle contraction or tension against resistance; thus, they can be either isotonic or isometric. During isokinetic exercises, the person moves (isotonic) or tenses (isometric)

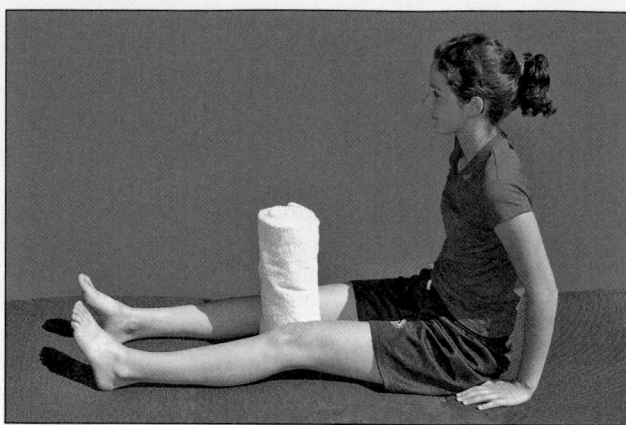

FIGURE 39.31 Example of an isometric exercise for the legs: the client sits or lies on a flat surface with the legs straight out. With a rolled towel between the knees, the client pushes the knees together and tightens the muscles in the front of the thighs by forcing the knees downward and holding for 10 seconds.

against resistance. Special machines or devices provide the resistance to the movement. These exercises are used in physical conditioning and are often done to build certain muscle groups; for example, the pectorals (chest muscles) may be increased in size and strength by lifting weights. An increase in blood pressure and blood flow to muscles occurs with resistance training.

Aerobic exercise is an activity in which the amount of oxygen taken into the body is greater than or equal to the amount the body requires. Aerobic exercises use large muscle groups, are performed continuously, and are rhythmic in nature. Examples are walking, jogging, running, bicycling, dancing, cross-country skiing, jumping rope, rowing, swimming, and skating. Aerobic exercises improve cardiovascular conditioning and physical fitness.

The *intensity* of exercise can be measured in three ways:

1. *Target heart rate.* The goal is to work up to and sustain a target heart rate during exercise, based on the person's age. To determine the target heart rate, first calculate the person's maximum heart rate by subtracting her or his current age in years from 220. Then, obtain the target heart rate by taking 60% to 85% of the maximum. Because heart rates vary among individuals, the tests that follow are replacing this measure.

2. *Talk test.* This test is easier to implement and keeps most people at 60% of maximum heart rate or more. When exercising, the person should experience laboured breathing, yet still be able to carry on a conversation.

3. *Borg scale of perceived exertion* (Borg, 1998). This scale measures how difficult the exercise feels to the person in terms of heart and lung exertion. The scale progresses from 1 to 20 with the following markers: 7 = very, very light; 9 = very light; 11 = fairly light; 13 = somewhat hard; 15 = hard; 17 = very hard; and 19 = very, very hard.

"Very, very hard" corresponds closely to 100% of maximum heart rate. "Very light" is close to 40%. Most people need to strive for the "somewhat hard" level (13/20), which corresponds to 75% of maximum heart rate.

Anaerobic exercise involves activity in which the muscles cannot draw out enough oxygen from the bloodstream, and anaerobic pathways are used to provide additional energy for a short time. This type of exercise, such as weight lifting and sprinting, is used in endurance training for athletes.

To promote healthy active living in the Canadian population, the *Canadian Physical Activity Guidelines* have been developed (Canadian Society for Exercise Physiology [CSEP], 2011a) (Figure 39.32). These guidelines recommend specific types and frequency of physical activity for individuals based on specific age groups, regardless of gender, race, ethnicity or socioeconomic status. The *Canadian Physical Activity Guidelines* provide a minimum target to gain substantial health benefits and is consistent with the message "more is better" (Tremblay, Warburten, Janssen, Paterson, Latimer, Rhodes, … & Duggan et al., 2011). Box 39.1 on page 1150 highlights the recommendations for each age group. A reduction in sedentary activities is also important and is reflected in the *Canadian Sedentary Behaviour Guidelines* (CSEP, 2011b), which provide recommendations for individuals from infancy to age 17 years, regarding the amount of time spent in sedentary activities. Specific guidelines for adults with a spinal cord injury are outlined in the *Physical Activity Guidelines for Adults with Spinal Cord Injury* (McMaster University, 2011). See www.csep.ca/guidelines for all guidelines.

Benefits of Exercise

Regular exercise is essential for healthy functioning of major body systems. The benefits of exercise on these systems follow.

MUSCULOSKELETAL SYSTEM The size, shape, tone, and strength of skeletal and cardiac muscles are maintained with mild exercise and increased with strenuous exercise. With strenuous exercise, muscles **hypertrophy** (enlarge), and the efficiency of muscular contraction increases. Hypertrophy is commonly seen in the arm muscles of a tennis player, the leg muscles of a skater, and the arm and hand muscles of a carpenter.

Exercise can increase balance and coordination, key determinants in older adults' risk of falling (Howe, Rochester, Neil, Skelton, & Ballinger, 2011), reduce pain (Busch, Barber, Overend, Peloso, & Schachter, 2007), and improve joint flexibility and ROM (Paterson & Warburton, 2010). Aquatic exercise can improve functioning of some people with osteoarthritis (Bartels, Lund, Hagen, Dagfinrud, Christensen, & Danneskiold-Samsøe, 2007). Impaired balance is a risk factor for injury related to falls and often results with client's self-imposing restrictions on their activity, particularly among older adults.

Canadian Physical Activity Guidelines

FOR ADULTS - 18 – 64 YEARS

Guidelines

 To achieve health benefits, adults aged 18-64 years should accumulate at least 150 minutes of moderate- to vigorous-intensity aerobic physical activity per week, in bouts of 10 minutes or more.

 It is also beneficial to add muscle and bone strengthening activities using major muscle groups, at least 2 days per week.

 More physical activity provides greater health benefits.

Let's Talk Intensity!

Moderate-intensity physical activities will cause adults to sweat a little and to breathe harder. Activities like:

- Brisk walking
- Bike riding

Vigorous-intensity physical activities will cause adults to sweat and be 'out of breath'. Activities like:

- Jogging
- Cross-country skiing

Being active for at least **150 minutes** per week can help reduce the risk of:

- Premature death
- Heart disease
- Stroke
- High blood pressure
- Certain types of cancer
- Type 2 diabetes
- Osteoporosis
- Overweight and obesity

And can lead to improved:

- Fitness
- Strength
- Mental health (morale and self–esteem)

Pick a time. Pick a place. Make a plan and move more!

- ☑ Join a weekday community running or walking group.
- ☑ Go for a brisk walk around the block after dinner.
- ☑ Take a dance class after work.
- ☑ Bike or walk to work every day.

- ☑ Rake the lawn, and then offer to do the same for a neighbour.
- ☑ Train for and participate in a run or walk for charity!
- ☑ Take up a favourite sport again or try a new sport.
- ☑ Be active with the family on the weekend!

Now is the time. Walk, run, or wheel, and embrace life.

 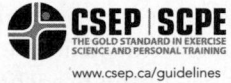

www.csep.ca/guidelines

FIGURE 39.32 Canadian physical activity guidelines for adults 18–64 years.

Source: Canadian Physical Activity Guidelines, © 2011. Used with permission from the Canadian Society for Exercise Physiology, Retrieved from http://www.csep.ca/guidelines

BOX 39.1 CANADIAN PHYSICAL ACTIVITY GUIDELINES

Infants less than 1 Year	Toddlers 1–2 Years and Preschoolers 3–4 Years	Children 5–11 And Youth 12–17	Adults 18–64 Years and * Older Adults 65 Years +
Should be physically active several times daily	At least 180 minutes of physical activity daily, at any intensity, including:	A minimum of 60 minutes of moderate to vigorous intensity physical activity daily, including:	A minimum 150 minutes of moderate to vigorous intensity aerobic physical activity per week in bouts of 10 minutes or more
	A variety of activities in different environments, and activities that develop movement skills.	Vigorous-intensity activities at least 3 days per week	Muscle and bone strengthening activities at least 2 days per week is beneficial
	Progression toward at least 60 minutes of energetic play by age 5.	Activities that strengthen muscle and bone at least 3 days per week	*Older adults with poor mobility should perform activities to enhance balance and prevent falls

More daily physical activity provides greater health benefits.

Source: Canadian Physical Activity Guidelines, © 2011. Used with permission from the Canadian Society for Exercise Physiology, Retrieved from http://www.csep.ca/guidelines

Bone density is maintained through weight bearing by maintaining a balance between *osteoblasts* (bone-building cells) and *osteoclasts* (bone-resorption and breakdown cells). Weight-bearing exercise (e.g., walking and dancing) can be effective in reducing the rate of bone loss associated with osteoporosis in women at risk, such as postmenopausal women.

CARDIOVASCULAR SYSTEM The Heart and Stroke Foundation of Canada (2011) guidelines for primary prevention of stroke and heart disease place great emphasis on physical activity as a means of promoting cardiovascular health and reducing important risk factors, such as high blood cholesterol, hypertension, and obesity.

Adequate moderate-intensity exercise (40% to 60% of maximum capacity, such as walking 1.6 km in 15 to 20 minutes) increases the heart rate, the strength of heart muscle contraction, and the blood supply to the heart and muscles through increased cardiac output. High-density lipoprotein (HDL) levels can be increased with regular endurance-type exercise. Exercise promotes heart health by mediating the harmful effects of stress. It can also improve the quality of life for people who already have heart disease, such as clients with mild to moderate heart failure (Warburton, Charlsworth, Ivey, Nettlefold, & Bredin, 2010).

RESPIRATORY SYSTEM Ventilation and oxygen intake increases during exercise, thereby improving gas exchange. Adequate exercise also prevents pooling of secretions in the bronchi and bronchioles, decreasing breathing effort and risk of infection. Attention to exercising muscles of respiration (by deep breathing) throughout activity as well as rest enhances oxygenation (improving stamina) and circulation of lymph (improving immune function). A strong body of evidence supports the use of lower extremity exercise forms (e.g., walking, treadmill, stationary bike, stair climbing) for treating individuals with chronic obstructive pulmonary disease (Freeman, 2008).

GASTROINTESTINAL SYSTEM Exercise improves the appetite and increases gastrointestinal tract tone, improving digestion and elimination. Such activities as rowing, swimming, and walking work the abdominal muscles and can help relieve constipation. Abdominal compressive exercise, such as with twisting and forward-bending yoga postures, has been shown to improve symptoms of irritable bowel syndrome (Micozzi, 2010).

METABOLIC SYSTEM Exercise elevates the metabolic rate, thus increasing the production of body heat and waste products. During strenuous exercise, the metabolic rate can increase to as much as 20 times the normal rate. This elevation lasts after exercise is completed. Exercise increases the use of triglycerides and fatty acids, resulting in a reduced level of serum triglycerides and cholesterol. Exercise also improves blood glucose control, and makes cells more responsive to insulin and decreases body fat content (Thomas, Elliott, & Naughton, 2006). The Canadian Diabetes Association (2008) recommends that individuals with diabetes accumulate a minimum of 150 minutes of moderate- to vigorous-intensity aerobic exercise each week, spread over at least 3 days of the week with no more than 2 consecutive days without exercise, for enhanced blood glucose control.

URINARY SYSTEM As adequate exercise promotes efficient blood flow, the body excretes wastes more effectively. In addition, urinary stasis (stagnation) is usually prevented, which decreases the risk for urinary tract infections and renal calculi (kidney stones).

IMMUNE SYSTEM As respiratory and musculoskeletal effort increase with exercise and as gravity is enlisted with postural changes, lymph fluid is more efficiently pumped from tissues into lymph capillaries and vessels throughout the body. Circulation through the lymph nodes, where the destruction of pathogens and the removal of foreign antigens can occur, is also improved. Research in older adults has shown the benefits of moderate exercise on natural killer cell function, circulating T cell function, and cytokine production, potentially increasing resistance to viral infections and preventing formation of malignant cells (Freeman, 2008).

Although moderate exercise seems to enhance immunity, strenuous exercise may reduce immune function, leaving a window of opportunity for infection during the recovery phase. Adequate rest is important after vigorous training to allow the body to recover (Edelman & Mandle, 2010).

PSYCHONEUROLOGICAL SYSTEM Mental or affective disorders, such as depression or chronic stress, can affect a person's desire to move. The depressed person may lack enthusiasm for taking part in any activity and may even lack energy for usual hygiene practices. Lack of visible energy is seen in a slumped posture with head bowed. Chronic stress can deplete the body's energy reserves to the point that fatigue discourages the desire to exercise, even though exercise can energize the person and facilitate coping. By contrast, individuals with eating disorders may exercise excessively in an effort to prevent weight gain.

A strong and growing body of evidence supports the role of exercise in elevating mood, reducing symptoms of depression, and relieving stress and anxiety across the lifespan through one or more of the following mechanisms: exercise increases levels of metabolites for neurotransmitters, such as norepinephrine and serotonin; exercise releases endogenous opioids, thus increasing levels of endorphins; exercise increases levels of oxygen to the brain and other body systems, inducing euphoria; and through muscular exertion (especially with movement modalities, such as yoga and Tai Chi) the body releases stored stress associated with accumulated emotional demands. Regular exercise can also improve the length and quality of sleep for individuals.

By eliciting the **relaxation response (RR)**, exercise is beneficial for counteracting some of the harmful effects of stress on the body and mind. First described by Dr. Herbert Benson, the RR is a healthful physiological state that can be elicited through deep relaxation breathing with emphasis on a prolonged exhalation phase (Edelman & Mandle, 2010). Emphasis on the exhalation recruits the parasympathetic nervous system response, the "rest and digest" reflex. Progressive muscle relaxation techniques involve contracting and then releasing groups of muscles throughout the body until all parts of the body feel relaxed. These movements are subtle and, along with relaxation breathing, can be done by almost anyone at any time, regardless of mobility or fitness status, providing potent stress relief and neurocardiovascular health benefits.

Factors Affecting Body Alignment and Activity

A number of factors affect an individual's body alignment, mobility, and daily activity level. These include growth and development, nutrition, personal values and attitudes, certain external factors, prescribed limitations, physical health, and mental health.

Growth and Development

A person's age and musculoskeletal and nervous system development affect posture, body proportions, body mass, body movements, and reflexes. Newborns' movements are reflexive and random. All extremities are generally flexed but can be passively moved through a full ROM. As the neurological system matures, control over movement progresses during the first year. Gross motor development precedes fine motor skills. Gross motor development occurs in a head-to-toe fashion, that is, it progresses from head control, to crawling, to pulling up to a standing position, to standing, and to walking, usually after the first birthday. Initially, walking involves a wide stance and unsteady gait, thus the term *toddler*. From ages 1 to 5 years, both gross and fine motor skills are refined. For example, preschoolers master riding a tricycle, dancing, running, jumping, using crayons to draw, and brushing their teeth.

From 6 to 12 years, refinement of motor skills continues, and exercise patterns for later life are generally determined. All schools provide some form of physical education to enhance physical activity. Posture in school-age children is usually excellent. In adolescence, growth spurts and such behaviours as carrying heavy book bags on one shoulder and extended computer use can result in poor postural changes that often persist into adulthood.

Adults between 20 and 40 years of age generally have few physical changes affecting mobility if they have no significant weight gain, with the exception of pregnant women. Pregnancy alters the centre of gravity and affects balance so that activities in which the body is supported (e.g., swimming and cycling) are favoured. Evidence shows that pregnant women who engage in aerobic exercise can improve their physical fitness (Kramer & McDonald, 2006). Exercise can also help pregnant women avoid excess weight gain. Leaner babies may also be at a lower risk for obesity later in life.

Advancing age is associated with a gradual loss of muscle tone, joint flexibility, and decreasing reaction time. A decrease in bone density is also common, particularly in women who have osteoporosis. **Osteoporosis** is a condition in which the bones become brittle and fragile because of calcium depletion. Osteoporosis is common in older women and primarily affects the weight-bearing joints of the lower extremities and anterior aspects of spinal bones, causing compression fractures of the vertebrae and hip fractures. All these changes affect older adults' posture, gait, and balance. Posture becomes forward leaning and stooped, which shifts the centre of gravity forward. To compensate for this shift, the knees flex slightly for support and the base of support is widened. Gait becomes wide-based, short-stepped, and shuffling. A strong body of research supports the benefits of regular activity for older adults to maintain and regain strength, flexibility, cardiovascular fitness, and bone density.

Nutrition

Both undernutrition and overnutrition can influence body alignment and mobility. Poorly nourished people may have muscle weakness and fatigue. Vitamin D deficiency causes bone deformity during growth. Inadequate calcium intake and vitamin D synthesis increase the risk of osteoporosis. Obesity can distort movement and stress joints, adversely affecting posture, balance, and joint health.

Personal Values and Attitudes

Whether people value regular exercise is often the result of family influences. In families that incorporate regular exercise in their daily routine or spend time together in physical endeavours (baseball, hiking, swimming), children learn to value physical activity. Sedentary families, conversely, participate in sports only as spectators, watching the ball game or hockey game on television, and this lifestyle is often transmitted to their children. With the increase in TV, computer, and video activities, youth are increasingly sedentary, with attendant declines in health. The *Canadian Sedentary Behaviour Guidelines* for children (5–11 years) and youth (12–17 years), recommend minimizing the time spent being sedentary each day; limiting recreational screen time to no more than 2 hours per day; and limiting sedentary (motorized) transport, extended sitting, and time spent indoors throughout the day (CSEP, 2011b). Guidelines also exist for children from infancy to age 4 years.

Values about physical appearance also influence some people's participation in regular exercise. People who value a muscular build or physical attractiveness may participate in regular exercise programs to produce the appearance they desire. The choice of physical activity or type of exercise is also influenced by values. Choices may be influenced by geographical location and cultural role expectations.

External Factors

Many external factors affect a person's mobility. Excessively high temperature and high humidity discourage activity, whereas comfortable temperature and humidity are conducive to activity, such as a brisk walk or a game of tennis. The availability of recreational facilities also influences activity; for example, lack of money may deter a person from joining an exercise group or swimming in an indoor pool. Neighbourhood safety promotes outdoor activity, whereas an unsafe environment discourages people from going outdoors.

Prescribed Limitations

Limitations to movement are medically prescribed for some health problems. To promote healing, such devices as casts, braces, splints, and traction are often used to immobilize body parts. Clients who have dyspnea may be advised not to walk up stairs. Bed rest may be the therapeutic choice for certain clients, for example, to relieve edema, to reduce metabolic and oxygen needs, or to promote tissue repair.

The term **bed rest** varies in meaning to some extent. In some agencies, bed rest means strict confinement to bed or *complete bed rest*. Others allow the client to use a bedside commode or nearby bathroom. Nurses need to familiarize themselves with the meaning of the term *bed rest* in their practice setting. In any case, the effects of limiting activity are immediate and negative. For example, muscle strength atrophies at approximately 3% per day with complete bed rest.

Physical Health

Mobility and activity tolerance are affected by any disorder that impairs the ability of the nervous system, musculoskeletal system, cardiovascular system, respiratory system, and vestibular apparatus. Congenital problems, such as spina bifida, cerebral palsy, and the muscular dystrophies, affect motor functioning. Disorders of the nervous system, such as Parkinson's disease, multiple sclerosis, cerebrovascular accidents, infectious processes (e.g., meningitis), and head and spinal cord injuries, can leave muscle groups weakened, **spastic** (with too much muscle tone), **flaccid** (without muscle tone), or with **paresis** (partial paralysis). Musculoskeletal disorders affecting mobility include strains, sprains, fractures, joint dislocations, amputations, and joint replacements. Inner ear infections and dizziness can impair balance. Many other acute and chronic illnesses that limit the supply of oxygen and nutrients needed for muscle contraction and movement can seriously affect activity tolerance. Examples include chronic obstructive lung disease, anemia, heart failure, and angina.

Mental Health

Mental or affective disorders, such as depression or chronic stress, can affect a person's desire to move. The person who is depressed may lack enthusiasm for taking part in any activity and may even lack energy for usual hygiene practices. Lack of visible energy is seen in a slumped posture with head bowed. By contrast, happy, confident people usually stand erect. Chronic stress can deplete the body's energy reserves to the point that fatigue discourages the desire to exercise even though exercise can energize the person and facilitate coping.

Effects of Immobility

Individuals who have inactive lifestyles or who are faced with inactivity because of illness or injury are at risk for many problems that can affect major body systems. Whether immobility causes problems often depends on the duration of the inactivity, the client's health status, and the client's sensory awareness. The most obvious signs of prolonged immobility are often manifested in the musculoskeletal system, and the deconditioning effects can be observed even after a few days. Clients experience a significant decrease in muscular strength and agility whenever they do not maintain a moderate amount of physical activity. In addition, immobility adversely affects the cardiovascular, respiratory, metabolic, urinary, and psychoneurological systems. Nurses need to understand these effects and encourage client movement as much as possible. Early ambulation after illness or surgery is an essential measure to prevent complications. No matter what an individual's level of mobility, nurses must encourage clients to breath fully, using their abdominal muscles, and move as much as possible to prevent the hazards of immobility. See Table 39.3 for desired outcomes and nursing interventions to prevent problems of immobility.

TABLE 39.3 Desired Outcomes and Nursing Interventions to Prevent the Problems of Immobility (Disuse Syndrome)

Desired Health Outcome	Nursing Interventions	Rationale
Maintains **normal musculoskeletal function,** as evidenced by usual range of motion in all body joints and maintenance of baseline muscle mass and strength	Implement appropriate exercise program (isometric, isotonic, or passive exercises) at least every 2 hours, as indicated.	Isotonic exercises prevent contractures and muscle atrophy. Isometric exercises maintain muscle tone. Passive exercises maintain joint mobility.
	Encourage active participation in self-care activities.	Self-care activities involve active movement of joints and muscles.
	Compare muscle size and strength to baseline data and on each side of the body daily. See Skill 28.16 (page 669) for details about testing and grading muscle strength.	Early detection of muscle atrophy or decreased strength facilitates early intervention to correct the problem.
	Position clients in good alignment.	Good alignment prevents contractures and maintains structural integrity of muscles and joints.
	Ambulate clients, as tolerated, or assist to stand at bedside.	Weight bearing prevents disuse osteoporosis.
Experiences **minimal cardiovascular alterations,** as evidenced by maintenance of baseline vital signs and signs of adequate venous blood flow (absence of edema, calf pain, inflammation, venous distension, skin changes)	Monitor vital signs according to client needs and agency protocol (e.g., bid or tid).	Regular monitoring enables the nurse to detect alterations early.
	Instruct client how and when to avoid the Valsalva manoeuvre.	The Valsalva manoeuvre increases the stress on the heart.
	Apply antiembolism stockings as indicated (see Skill 36.2, page 1071).	Use of antiembolism stockings prevents thrombus formation, venous engorgement, dependent edema, and orthostatic hypotension.
	Elevate legs several times each day for 20 minutes.	Elevation increases peripheral venous circulation.
	Implement measures to prevent postural hypotension.	
	Assess skin of lower limbs and measure calf circumferences, as indicated.	Regular inspection and measurement enable the nurse to detect changes.
	See also interventions for musculoskeletal function.	These interventions also stimulate blood circulation and prevent cardiovascular complications.
Maintains **normal respiratory function,** as evidenced by normal breath sounds during auscultation; normal chest expansion; and absence of chest pain, fever, or other respiratory signs indicative of pulmonary infarction, emboli, or atelectasis	Assess breath sounds and chest expansion at least every 4 hours.	This allows the nurse to detect onset of abnormal breath sounds and inadequate chest expansion.
	Teach clients to take five deep breaths and to cough every waking hour.	Deep breaths and coughing increase alveolar expansion, prevent stasis of secretions, promote adequate gaseous exchange, and maintain a patent airway.
	Establish a position schedule, and alter client's position at least every 2 hours. Ambulate client, if possible, or place client in chair.	Changes in position allow previously dependent lung areas to expand and promote movement and subsequent removal of secretions by coughing.

(continued)

TABLE 39.3 Desired Outcomes and Nursing Interventions to Prevent the Problems of Immobility (Disuse Syndrome) *(continued)*

Desired Health Outcome	Nursing Interventions	Rationale
Maintains **normal elimination pattern,** as evidenced by clear amber urinary output of at least 1500 mL per day; urine specific gravity of 1.010 to 1.030; an acidic urine; absence of signs of urinary retention, calculi, or infection; and excretion of formed semisolid stool at least every 2 or 3 days	Monitor colour, clarity, amount, acidity, and specific gravity of urine; colour and characteristics of feces; and frequency of defecation. Ask whether client has pain when urinating.	Decreased urinary output, cloudy urine, and painful urination are indicative of urinary retention and infection. Alkaline urine increases the risk for calculi. Constipation is associated with immobility. Increase fluid to increase urinary output to decrease incidence of renal calculi.
	Refer to Chapter 41 for interventions to prevent constipation. Teach clients to select high-fibre foods.	High-fibre foods promote intestinal peristalsis and defecation.
Maintains **intact integument,** as evidenced by clean, intact, well-hydrated skin and absence of pressure signs (pallor, redness, increased warmth, or tenderness) over pressure areas	See "Preventing Pressure Ulcers" in Chapter 35.	Preventing skin breakdown is imperative to promote recovery and optimize quality of life.
Maintains **social, emotional, and intellectual well-being,** as evidenced by actively participating in and making decisions about care, verbalizing concerns, maintaining positive relationships with others, and performing satisfying activities	Encourage the client to make as many decisions as possible, such as placement of personal items, daily plan of activities, clothes to wear.	Decision making enhances self-esteem.
	Plan time to be available to the client other than task-oriented time.	Being available for the client may encourage open expression of feelings.
	Explore diversional activities of interest to the client, and develop a daily activity plan.	A satisfying daily activity prevents boredom and gives the client something to look forward to.

Musculoskeletal System

Prolonged immobility often affects the musculoskeletal system first, sometimes within days:

- *Disuse osteoporosis.* Without the stress of weight-bearing activity, the bones demineralize. They are depleted chiefly of calcium, which gives the bones strength and density. Regardless of the amount of calcium in a person's diet, the demineralization process, known as osteoporosis, continues with immobility. The bones become spongy and may gradually deform and fracture easily.

- *Disuse atrophy.* Unused muscles **atrophy** (decrease in size), losing most of their strength and normal function.

- *Contractures.* When the muscle fibres are not moved, eventually a **contracture** (permanent shortening of the muscle) forms, limiting joint mobility. This process eventually involves the tendons, ligaments, and joint capsules; it is often irreversible except by surgical intervention. Joint deformities, such as plantar flexion contracture (foot drop) (Figure 39.33), wrist drop, and external hip rotation, occur when a stronger muscle dominates the opposite muscle.

- *Stiffness and pain in the joints.* Without movement, the collagen (connective) tissues at the joint become *ankylosed* (permanently immobile). In addition, as the

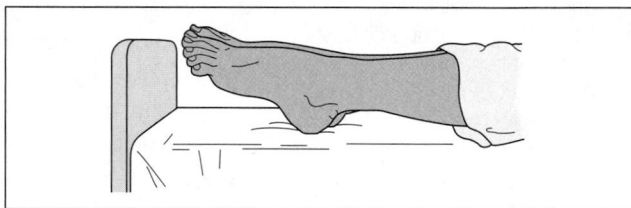

FIGURE 39.33 Plantar flexion contracture (foot drop).

bones demineralize, excess calcium may deposit in the joints, contributing to stiffness and pain.

Cardiovascular System

The cardiovascular system also shows the deconditioning effects of immobility:

- *Diminished cardiac reserve.* Decreased mobility creates an imbalance in the autonomic nervous system, resulting in a preponderance of sympathetic activity over cholinergic activity that increases heart rate. A rapid heart rate reduces diastolic pressure, coronary blood flow, and the capacity of the heart to respond to any metabolic demands above the basal levels. Because of this diminished cardiac reserve, the immobilized person may experience tachycardia with even minimal exertion.

- *Increased use of Valsalva manoeuvre.* The **Valsalva manoeuvre** refers to holding the breath and straining against a closed glottis. For example, clients tend to hold their breath when attempting to move up in a bed or sit on a bedpan. This builds up sufficient pressure on the large veins in the thorax to interfere with the return blood flow to the heart and coronary arteries. When the client exhales and the glottis again opens, pressure is suddenly released, and a surge of blood flows to the heart. The manoeuvre can also stimulate the vagus nerve leading to deceleration of heart rate and even bradycardia.

- *Orthostatic (postural) hypotension.* **Orthostatic hypotension** is a common result of immobilization. Under normal conditions, sympathetic nervous system activity causes automatic vasoconstriction in the blood vessels in the lower half of the body when a mobile person changes from a horizontal to a vertical posture. Vasoconstriction prevents pooling of the blood in the legs and effectively maintains central blood pressure to ensure adequate perfusion of the heart and brain. During any prolonged immobility, this reflex becomes dormant. When the immobile person attempts to sit or stand, this reconstricting mechanism fails to function properly in spite of increased adrenalin output. The blood pools in the lower extremities, and central blood pressure drops. Cerebral perfusion is seriously compromised, and the person feels dizzy or lightheaded and may even faint. This sequence is usually accompanied by a sudden and marked increase in heart rate, the body's effort to protect the brain from an inadequate blood supply.

- *Venous vasodilation and stasis.* The skeletal muscles of an active person contract with each movement, compressing the blood vessels in those muscles and helping to pump the blood back to the heart against gravity. The tiny valves in the leg veins aid in venous return to the heart by preventing backward flow of blood and pooling. In an immobile person, the skeletal muscles do not contract sufficiently, and the muscles atrophy. The skeletal muscles can no longer assist in pumping blood back to the heart against gravity. Blood pools in the leg veins, causing vasodilation and engorgement. The valves in the veins can no longer work effectively to prevent backward flow of blood and pooling (Figure 39.34). This phenomenon is known as *incompetent valves.* As the blood continues to pool in the veins, its greater volume increases venous blood pressure, which can become much higher than that exerted by the tissues surrounding the vessel.

- *Dependent edema.* When the venous pressure is sufficiently great, some of the serous part of the blood is forced out of the blood vessel into the interstitial spaces surrounding the blood vessel, causing edema. Edema is most common in parts of the body positioned below heart level and maintained in that position. Dependent edema is most likely to occur

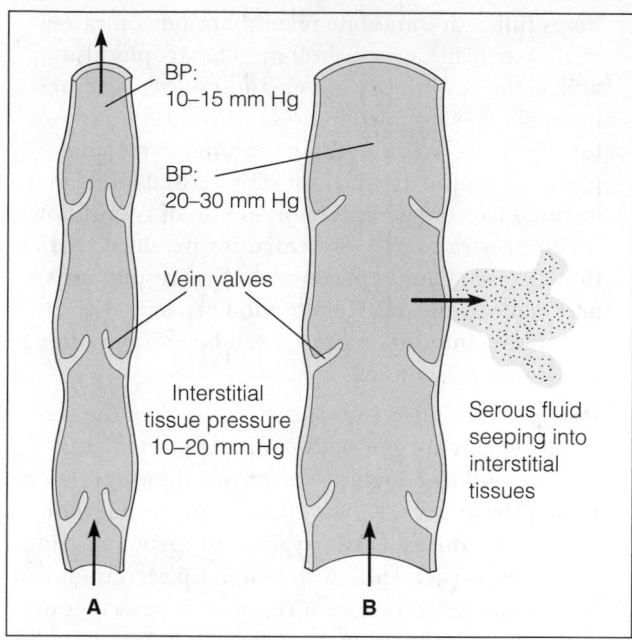

FIGURE 39.34 Leg veins: **A:** In a mobile person; **B:** In an immobile person.

around the sacrum or heels of a client who sits up in bed or in the feet and lower legs of a client who sits on the side of the bed. Edema further impedes venous return of blood to the heart, causing more pooling and more edema. Edematous tissue is uncomfortable and more susceptible to injury than normal tissue.

- *Thrombus formation.* Three factors, known as *Virchow's triad,* collectively predispose a client to the formation of a **thrombophlebitis** (a clot that is loosely attached to an inflamed vein wall): (a) impaired venous return to the heart, (b) hypercoagulability of the blood, and (c) injury to the endothelial wall of the vessel. A **thrombus** (clot) is particularly dangerous if it breaks loose from the vein wall and enters the general circulation as an **embolus** (a clot that has moved from its place of origin, causing obstruction to circulation elsewhere). Large emboli that enter the pulmonary circulation may occlude the vessels that nourish the lungs and cause an infarcted area of the lung. If the infarcted area is large, pulmonary function is seriously compromised, and death may ensue. Emboli travelling to the coronary vessels or brain can produce a similarly dangerous outcome.

Respiratory System

Prolonged immobility can harm the respiratory system:

- *Decreased respiratory movement.* In a recumbent, immobile client, ventilation of the lungs is passively altered. The body presses against the rigid bed and curtails chest movement. The abdominal organs push against the diaphragm, further restricting lung movement and making it difficult to expand the lungs fully. An immobile recumbent person rarely sighs, partly because overall muscle atrophy also affects the respiratory muscles and partly because he or she has no need to do so without the stimulus of activity. Without these periodic stretching movements, the cartilaginous intercostal joints may become fixed in an expiratory phase of respiration, further restricting the potential for maximal ventilation. These changes produce shallow respirations and may significantly reduce **vital capacity** (the maximum amount of air that can be exhaled after a maximum inhalation).

- *Pooling of respiratory secretions.* Secretions of the respiratory tract are normally expelled by changing posture and by coughing. Inactivity allows secretions to pool by gravity (Figure 39.35), interfering with the normal diffusion of oxygen and carbon dioxide in the alveoli. The ability to cough up secretions can also be hindered by loss of respiratory muscle tone, dehydration (which thickens secretions), or sedatives that depress the cough reflex. Poor oxygenation and retention of carbon dioxide in the blood can result in respiratory acidosis, a potentially lethal disorder.

- *Atelectasis.* When ventilation is decreased, pooled secretions can accumulate in a dependent area of a bronchiole and effectively block it. Because of changes in regional blood flow, bed rest decreases the

amount of surfactant produced. (Surfactant enables the alveoli to remain open.) The combination of decreased surfactant and blockage of a bronchiole with mucus can cause atelectasis (the collapse of a lobe or of an entire lung) distal to the mucus blockage. Immobile, older adult, postoperative clients are at greatest risk of atelectasis.

- *Hypostatic pneumonia.* Pooled secretions provide excellent media for bacterial growth. Under these conditions, a minor upper respiratory infection can evolve rapidly into a severe infection of the lower respiratory tract. Hypostatic pneumonia caused by static respiratory secretions can severely impair oxygen–carbon dioxide exchange in the alveoli and is a fairly common cause of death among weakened, immobile persons, especially smokers.

Metabolic System

The metabolic system suffers when a person is immobile as well:

- *Decreased metabolic rate.* **Metabolism** refers to the sum of all the physical and chemical processes by which living substance is formed and maintained and by which energy is made available for use by the body. **Basal metabolism** is the minimal energy expended for the maintenance of these processes. The metabolic rate is the rate of basal metabolism expressed in calories per hour per square metre of body surface. In immobile clients, the basal metabolic rate and gastrointestinal motility and secretions of various digestive glands decrease as the energy requirements of the body decrease.

- *Negative nitrogen balance.* An active person's body maintains a balance between anabolism and catabolism (see Chapter 40). Immobility creates a marked imbalance, and catabolic processes exceed anabolic processes. Catabolized muscle mass releases nitrogen. Over time, more nitrogen is excreted than is ingested, producing negative nitrogen balance. The negative nitrogen balance represents a depletion of protein stores that are essential for building muscle tissue and for wound healing.

- *Anorexia.* Anorexia (loss of appetite) occurs as a result of the decreased metabolic rate and the increased catabolism that accompany immobility. Reduced caloric intake is usually a response to the decreased energy requirements of the inactive person. If protein intake is reduced, the nitrogen imbalance may become more pronounced, sometimes so severely that malnutrition ensues.

- *Negative calcium balance.* A negative calcium balance occurs as a direct result of immobility. Greater amounts of calcium are extracted from bone than can be replaced. The absence of weight bearing and of

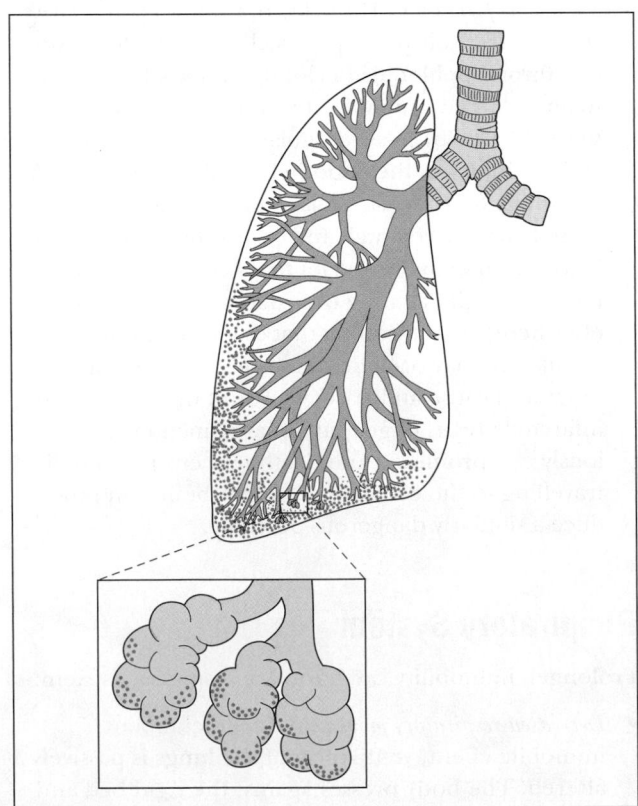

FIGURE 39.35 Pooling of secretions in the lungs of an immobile person.

stress on the musculoskeletal structures is the direct cause of the calcium loss from bones. Weight bearing and stress are also required for calcium to be replaced in bone. A similar process occurs with the body's stores of phosphate, causing a negative phosphate balance during immobility.

Urinary System

When a person is immobile, the urinary system is impaired:

- *Urinary stasis.* In a mobile person, gravity plays an important role in the emptying of the kidneys and the bladder. The shape and position of the kidneys and active kidney contractions are important in completely emptying the urine from the calyces, renal pelvis, and ureters (Figure 39.36A). The shape and position of the urinary bladder (the detrusor muscle) and active bladder contractions are also important in achieving complete emptying (Figure 39.37A). When the person remains in a horizontal position, gravity impedes the emptying of urine from the kidneys and the urinary bladder. To urinate, the person who is supine must push upward, against gravity (see Figure 39.36B and Figure 39.37B). The renal pelvis may fill with urine before it is pushed into the ureters. Emptying is not as complete, and **urinary stasis** (stoppage or slowdown of flow) occurs after a few days of bed rest. Because of the overall decrease in muscle tone during immobilization, including the tone of the detrusor muscle, bladder emptying is further compromised.

- *Renal calculi.* In a mobile person, calcium in the urine remains dissolved because calcium and citric acid are balanced in appropriately acidic urine. With immobility and the resulting excessive amounts of calcium (and phosphate) in the urine, this balance is no longer maintained. The urine becomes more alkaline, and the calcium salts precipitate out as crystals to form renal calculi. In an immobile person in a horizontal position, the renal pelvis filled with

stagnant, alkaline urine is an ideal location for calculi to form. The stones usually develop in the renal pelvis and pass through the ureters into the bladder. As the stones pass along the long, narrow ureters, they cause extreme pain and bleeding and can sometimes obstruct the urinary tract.

- *Urinary retention.* The immobile person may experience **urinary retention** (accumulation of urine in the bladder), bladder distension, and occasionally **urinary incontinence** (involuntary urination). The decreased muscle tone of the urinary bladder inhibits its ability to empty completely. In addition, the discomfort of using a bedpan or urinal, the embarrassment and lack of privacy associated with this function, and the unnatural position for urination, combine to make it difficult for the client to relax the perineal muscles sufficiently to urinate while lying in bed. When urination is not possible, the bladder gradually becomes distended with urine. The bladder may stretch excessively, eventually inhibiting the urge to void. When bladder distension is considerable, some involuntary urinary "dribbling" may occur (retention with overflow). This does not relieve the urinary distension because most of the stagnant urine remains in the bladder.

- *Urinary infection.* Static urine provides an excellent medium for bacterial growth. The flushing action

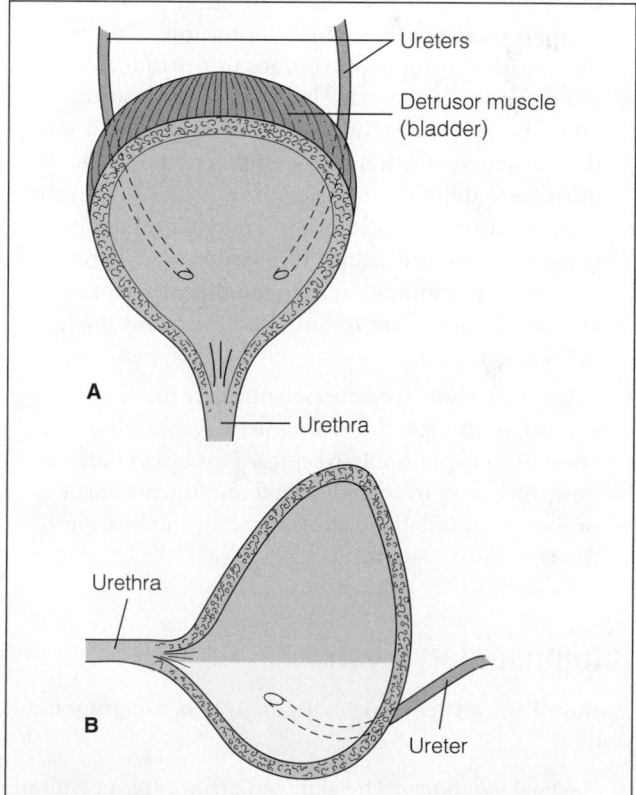

FIGURE 39.37 Pooling of urine in the urinary bladder: **A:** The client is in the upright position. **B:** The client is in the back-lying position.

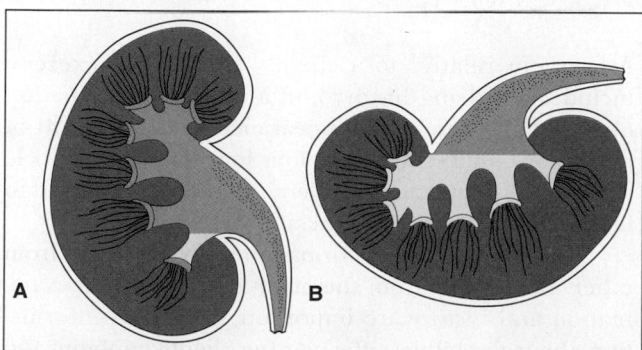

FIGURE 39.36 Pooling of urine in the kidney: **A:** The client is in the upright position. **B:** The client is in the back-lying position.

of normal, frequent urination is absent, and urinary distension often causes minute tears in the bladder mucosa, allowing infectious organisms to enter. The increased alkalinity of the urine caused by the hypercalcuria supports bacterial growth. The organism most commonly causing urinary tract infections is *Escherichia coli*, which normally resides in the colon. The normally sterile urinary tract may be contaminated by improper perineal care, the use of an indwelling urinary catheter, or occasionally, **urinary reflux** (backward flow). During reflux, contaminated urine from an overly distended bladder backs up into the renal pelvis to contaminate the kidney pelvis as well.

Gastrointestinal System

Prolonged immobility can affect the gastrointestinal system:

- *Constipation.* Constipation is a frequent problem for immobilized people because of decreased peristalsis and colon motility. The overall skeletal muscle weakness affects the abdominal and perineal muscles used in defecation. When the stool becomes very hard, more strength is required to expel it. The immobile person may lack this strength.
- *Weakened defecation reflex.* The bedridden person's unnatural and uncomfortable position on the bedpan does not facilitate elimination. The backward-leaning posture does not promote effective use of the muscles used in defecation. Some people are reluctant to use the bedpan in the presence of others. The embarrassment, lack of privacy, dependence on others to assist with the bedpan, and disruption of normal bowel habits may cause the individual to postpone or ignore the urge for elimination. Repeated postponement eventually suppresses the urge and weakens the defecation reflex.
- *Valsalva manoeuvre.* Some persons may make excessive use of the Valsalva manoeuvre by straining in an attempt to expel the hard stool. This effort dangerously increases intra-abdominal and intrathoracic pressures and places undue stress on the heart and the circulatory system.

Integumentary System

Immobility can lead to changes in the integumentary system:

- *Reduced skin turgor.* The skin can atrophy as a result of prolonged immobility. Shifts in body fluids between the fluid compartments can affect the consistency and health of the dermis and subcutaneous tissues in dependent parts of the body, eventually causing a gradual loss in skin **turgor** (elasticity).
- *Skin breakdown.* Normal blood circulation relies on muscle activity. Immobility impedes circulation and diminishes the supply of nutrients to specific areas. As a result, skin breakdown and formation of pressure (decubitus) ulcers can occur. Older adults who are immobile have an increased risk for the formation of pressure ulcers. Prevention of pressure ulcers is a primary goal of nursing care.

Psychoneurological System

Immobility can affect a person's self-esteem and neurological functioning:

- *Lowered self-esteem.* Because of a decline in the production of mood-elevating substances, such as endorphins, people experience negative effects on mood when unable to engage in physical activity. People who are unable to carry out the usual activities related to their roles (e.g., as breadwinner, father, or student) become aware of an increased dependence on others. These factors lower the person's self-esteem. Frustration and the decrease in self-esteem may, in turn, provoke exaggerated emotional reactions. Emotional reactions vary considerably. Some individuals become apathetic and withdrawn, some regress, and some become angry and aggressive.
- *Reduced cognitive abilities.* Because the immobilized person's participation in life becomes much narrower and the variety of stimuli decreases, the person's perception of time intervals deteriorates. Problem-solving and decision-making abilities often decline as a result of the lack of intellectual stimulation and the stress of the illness and immobility. In addition, the loss of control over events can cause anxiety and depression. Alterations in normal sleeping patterns may exaggerate these behavioural changes.

Assessing

Assessment relative to a client's activity and exercise includes a nursing history and a physical examination of body alignment, gait, appearance and movement of joints, capabilities and limitations for movement, muscle mass and strength, activity tolerance, problems related to immobility, and physical fitness.

The nurse collects information from the client, from other nurses, and from the client's records. The examination and history are important sources of information about disabilities affecting the client's mobility and activity status, such as contractures, edema, pain in the extremities, or generalized fatigue.

Activity and Exercise

The nurse can use these questions to gather data about the client's activity and exercise patterns:

DAILY ACTIVITY LEVEL

- What activities do you usually carry out during a routine day?
- Are you able to carry out the following tasks of daily life independently?
  a. Eating
  b. Dressing and grooming
  c. Bathing
  d. Toileting
  e. Ambulating
  f. Transferring in and out of bed, bath, and car
  g. Maintaining the home (e.g., cleaning, meal preparation, shopping)
- Where problems exist in your ability to carry out such tasks, what resources are available to you?

ACTIVITY TOLERANCE

- How much and what types of activities make you tired?
- Do you ever experience dizziness, shortness of breath, marked increase in respiratory rate, or other problems following mild or moderate activity?

EXERCISE

- What type of exercise do you carry out to enhance your physical fitness?
- What is the frequency and length of this exercise session?
- Do you believe exercise is beneficial to health? Explain.

FACTORS AFFECTING MOBILITY

- *Environmental factors.* Do stairs, lack of railings or other assistive devices, or an unsafe neighbourhood impede your mobility or exercise regimen?
- *Health problems.* Do you have any physical or mental health problems, past or current, that affect your muscle strength or endurance (e.g., heart disease, lung disease, cerebrovascular accident, cancer, neuromuscular problems, musculoskeletal problems, visual or mental impairments, depression, trauma, or pain)?
- *Financial factors.* Are your finances adequate to obtain equipment or other aids that you require to enhance your mobility?
- *Lifestyle variables.* Do cultural, leisure, or employment practices influence activity and mobility patterns?

Nursing History

An activity and exercise history is usually part of the comprehensive nursing history form. Examples of interview questions to elicit these data are shown in the Assessment: Interview box. If the client indicates a recent pattern change or difficulties with mobility, a more detailed history is required. This detailed history should include the specific nature of the problem, when it first began, its frequency, its causes, if known, how the problem affects daily living, what the client is doing to cope with the problem, and whether these methods have been effective.

Physical Examination

BODY ALIGNMENT   Assessment of body alignment includes an inspection of the client if the client is able to stand. The purpose of body alignment assessment is to identify the following:

- Normal developmental variations in posture
- Poor posture and learning needs to maintain good posture
- Factors contributing to poor posture, such as fatigue or low self-esteem
- Muscle weakness or other motor impairments

To assess alignment, the nurse inspects the client from lateral (Figure 39.38A on the next page), anterior,

and posterior perspectives. From the anterior and posterior views, the nurse should observe the presence or absence of the following:

- The head is erect and midline.
- The shoulders and hips are level.
- The feet are placed slightly apart and the toes point forward.
- The spine is straight, not curved to either side.

The slumped posture (Figure 39.38B) is the most common problem that occurs when people stand. The neck is flexed far forward, the abdomen protrudes, the pelvis is thrust forward to create **lordosis** (an exaggerated curvature of the lumbar spine), and the knees are markedly hyperextended. Lower back pain and fatigue occur quickly in people with poor posture.

GAIT   The characteristic pattern of a person's **gait** (walk) is assessed to determine the client's mobility and risk for injury from falling. Two phases of normal gait are stance and swing (Figure 39.39 on the next page). In the *stance phase,* (a) the heel of the right foot strikes the ground, and (b) body weight is spread over the ball of the right foot, while the left heel pushes off and leaves the ground. In the *swing phase,* the leg from behind moves in front of the body. When one leg is in the swing phase, the other is in the stance phase.

The nurse assesses gait as the client walks into the room or asks the client to walk a distance of 3.5 metres

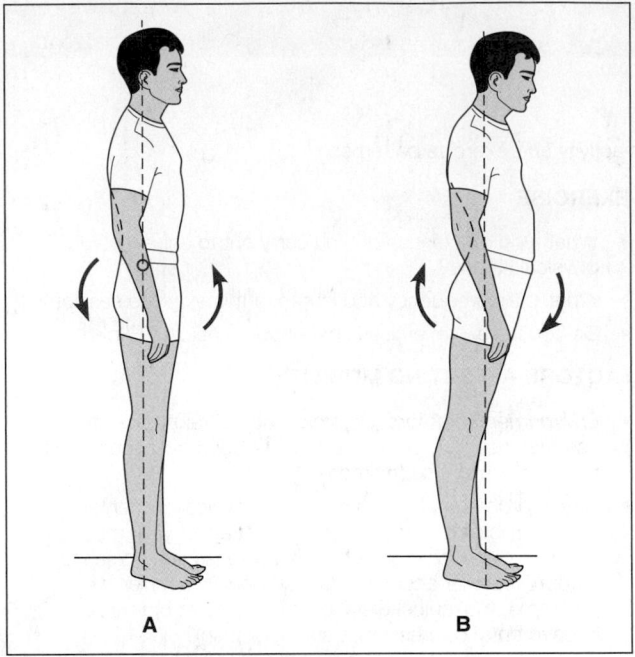

FIGURE 39.38 A standing person with **A:** good trunk alignment; **B:** poor trunk alignment. The arrows indicate the direction in which the pelvis is tilted.

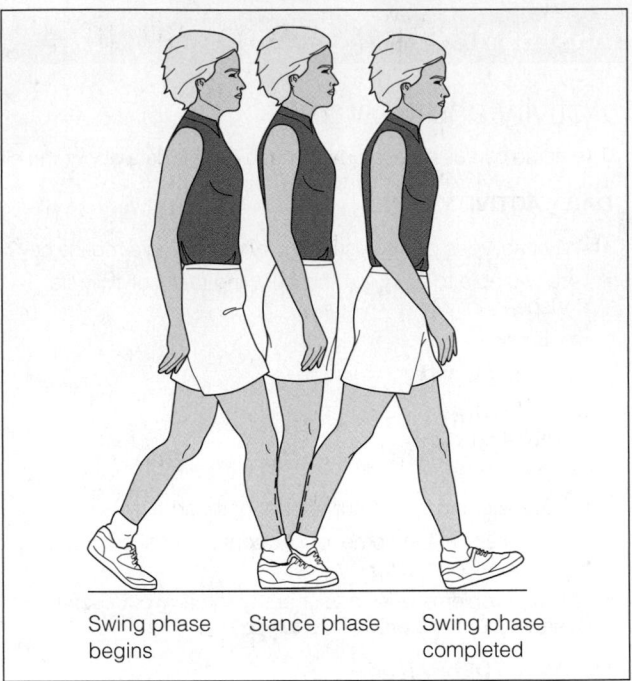

Swing phase begins   Stance phase   Swing phase completed

FIGURE 39.39 The stance and swing phases of a normal gait.

down a hallway and observes for the presence or absence of the following:

- The chin is level, the gaze is straight ahead, the sternum is lifted, and shoulders are down and back, relaxed away from the ears.
- The heel strikes the ground before the toe does.
- Feet are dorsiflexed in the swing phase.
- The arm opposite the swing-through foot moves forward at the same time.
- The gait is smooth, coordinated, and rhythmic, with even weight borne on each foot. Hips gently sway with spinal rotation; the body moves forward smoothly, stopping and starting with ease.

The nurse may also assess **pace** (the number of steps taken per minute). A normal walking pace is 70 to 100 steps per minute. The pace of an older person may slow to about 40 steps per minute.

The nurse should also note the client's need for a prosthesis or assistive device, such as a cane or walker. For a client who uses assistive aids, the nurse assesses gait without the device and compares the assisted and unassisted gaits.

APPEARANCE AND MOVEMENT OF JOINTS Physical examination of the joints involves inspection, palpation, assessment of range of active motion, and, if active motion is not possible, assessment of range of passive motion. The nurse should assess the following:

- Any joint swelling or redness, which could indicate the presence of an injury or inflammation

- Any deformity, such as a bony enlargement or contracture, and symmetry of involvement
- The muscle development associated with each joint and the relative size and symmetry of the muscles on each side of the body
- Any reported or palpable tenderness
- Presence of **crepitation** (a palpable or an audible crackling or grating sensation produced by joint motion and frequently experienced in joints that have suffered repeated trauma over time)
- Increased temperature over the joint; palpate the joint by using the backs of the fingers and compare the temperature with that of the symmetric joint
- The degree of joint movement; ask the client to move selected body parts as shown in Table 39.2. If indicated, measure the amount of movement with a goniometer in degrees (see Skill 28.16, page 671).

Assessment of ROM should not be unduly fatiguing, and the joint movements need to be performed smoothly, slowly, and rhythmically. No joint should be forced. Uneven, jerky movement and forcing can injure the joint and its surrounding muscles and ligaments.

CAPABILITIES AND LIMITATIONS FOR MOVEMENT The nurse needs to obtain data that may indicate hindrances or restrictions to the client's movement and the need for assistance, including the following:

- How the client's illness influences the ability to move and whether the client's health contraindicates any exertion, position, or movement

- Hindrances to movement, such as an intravenous line in place or a cast on one leg
- Mental alertness and ability to follow directions— check whether the client is receiving medications that hinder the ability to walk safely. (Opioids, sedatives, and some antihistamines cause drowsiness, dizziness, weakness, and orthostatic hypotension.)
- Balance and coordination
- The presence of orthostatic hypotension before transfers—specifically, to assess for any increase in pulse rate, marked fall in blood pressure, dizziness, light-headedness, and dimming of vision when the client moves from a supine to a vertical posture
- Degree of comfort—as people who have pain may not want to move and require an analgesic before they are moved
- Vision: Is it adequate to prevent falls?

The nurse also assesses the amount of assistance the client requires for the following:

- Moving in the bed. In particular, observe for the amount of assistance the client requires for turning:
  a. from the supine position to the lateral position
  b. from the lateral position on one side to the lateral position on the other
  c. from the supine position to the sitting position in bed
- Rising from the lying position to the sitting position on the edge of the bed—healthy people can normally rise without support from the arms
- Rising from a chair to a standing position—which normally can be done without pushing with the arms
- Coordination and balance—to determine the client's abilities to hold the body erect, to bear weight and keep balance in a standing position on one or both legs, to take steps, and to push off from a chair or bed

MUSCLE MASS AND STRENGTH Before the client undertakes a change in position or attempts to ambulate, it is essential that the client's strength and ability to move are assessed. Providing appropriate assistance lowers the risk of muscle strain and body injury to both the client and nurse. Assessment of upper extremity strength is especially important for clients who use ambulation aids, such as walkers and crutches. For information on how to determine muscle mass and strength in lower and upper extremities, see Chapter 28.

ACTIVITY TOLERANCE By determining an appropriate activity level for a client, the nurse can predict whether the client has the strength and endurance to participate in activities that require similar expenditures of energy. This assessment is useful in encouraging increasing independence in people who (a) have a cardiovascular or respiratory disability, (b) have

been completely immobilized for a prolonged period, (c) have decreased muscle mass or a musculoskeletal disorder, (d) have experienced inadequate sleep, (e) have experienced pain, or (f) are depressed, anxious, or unmotivated.

The most useful measures in predicting activity tolerance are heart rate, strength, and rhythm; respiratory rate, depth, and rhythm; and blood pressure. The following data are obtained at the following times:

- Before the activity starts (baseline data) while the client is at rest
- During the activity
- Immediately after the activity stops
- Three minutes after the activity has stopped and the client has rested

The activity should be stopped immediately in the event of any physiological change indicating the activity is too strenuous or prolonged for the client. These changes include the following:

- Sudden facial pallor
- Feelings of dizziness or weakness
- Change in level of consciousness
- Heart rate or respiratory rate that significantly exceeds baseline or established levels
- Change in heart or respiratory rhythm from regular to irregular
- Weakening of the pulse
- Dyspnea, shortness of breath, or chest pain
- Diastolic blood pressure change of 10 mm Hg or more

If, however, the client tolerates the activity well, and if the client's heart rate returns to baseline levels within 3 minutes after the activity ceases, the activity is considered safe. This activity, then, can serve as a standard for predicting the client's tolerance for similar activities.

PROBLEMS RELATED TO IMMOBILITY When collecting data pertaining to the problems of immobility, the nurse uses the assessment methods of inspection, palpation, and auscultation; checks results of laboratory tests; and takes measurements, including body weight, fluid intake, and fluid output. Specific techniques for assessing immobility problems and abnormal assessment findings related to the complications of immobility are listed in Table 39.4 on the next page.

It is extremely important to obtain and record baseline assessment data soon after the client first becomes immobile. These baseline data serve as the standard against which all data collected throughout the period of immobilization are compared.

Because a major nursing responsibility is to prevent the complications of immobility, the nurse needs to identify clients at risk of developing such complications before

TABLE 39.4 Assessing Problems of Immobility

Assessment	Problem	Assessment	Problem
Musculoskeletal System		**Metabolic System**	
Measure arm and leg circumferences.	Decreased circumference caused by decreased muscle mass	Measure height and weight.	Weight loss caused by muscle atrophy and loss of subcutaneous fat
Palpate and observe body joints.	Stiffness or pain in joints	Take anthropometric measurements.	Loss of body muscle and subcutaneous fat
Take goniometric measurements of joint range of motion (ROM).	Decreased joint ROM, joint contractures	Palpate skin.	Generalized edema caused by low blood protein levels
Cardiovascular System		**Urinary System**	
Auscultate the heart.	Increased heart rate	Measure intake and output.	Dehydration
Measure blood pressure.	Orthostatic hypotension	Inspect urine.	Cloudy, dark urine, high specific gravity
Palpate and observe sacrum, legs, and feet.	Peripheral dependent edema, increased peripheral vein engorgement	Palpate urinary bladder.	Distended urinary bladder caused by urinary retention
Palpate extremity pulses.	Weak peripheral pulses	**Gastrointestinal System**	
Check capillary refill.	Decreased peripheral circulation	Observe stool.	Hard, dry, lumpy stool
Measure calf muscle circumferences.	Edema; thrombus formation	Auscultate bowel sounds.	Decreased bowel sounds because of decreased intestinal motility
Observe calf muscle for redness, tenderness, and swelling.	Thrombophlebitis	**Integumentary System**	
Respiratory System		Inspect skin for intactness, redness, pallor, warmth, tenderness.	Break in skin integrity, pressure areas
Observe chest movements.	Asymmetric chest movements	**Psychoneurological System**	
Auscultate chest.	Diminished breath sounds	Observe behaviours, affect, and cognition	Anger, flat affect, confusion crying, anxiety, decline in cognitive function, or vegetative signs such as sleep and appetite disturbances that warrant further evaluation
		Monitor developmental skills in children.	

problems arise. Clients at risk include those who (a) are poorly nourished, (b) have decreased sensitivity to pain, temperature, or pressure, (c) have existing cardiovascular, pulmonary, or neuromuscular problems, or (d) have an altered level of consciousness.

Diagnosing

Mobility problems may be appropriate as the diagnostic label or as the etiology for a range of other nursing diagnoses. Sample nursing diagnoses related to activity and exercise might include:

- Activity intolerance, as evidenced by dyspnea on climbing one flight of stairs (state other indicators as relevant)

- Impaired physical mobility, as evidenced by reduced movement of the body (e.g., hemiparesis, reduced range of motion, inability to weight bear)

- Inadequate physical activity to meet minimal fitness recommendations, as evidenced by sedentary lifestyle related to such factors as chronic pain, lack of motivation, fear of falling, and many other factors

Depending on the data obtained, problems with mobility often affect other areas of functioning and indicate other diagnoses. In these instances, the mobility problem becomes the etiology. For example, a client may be at risk for falls related to poor muscle strength; at risk for pressure ulcers, urinary tract infection, constipation, bone demineralization, orthostatic hypotension, and atelectasis related to immobility; or at risk for social isolation related to confinement to bed.

Planning

Positioning, transferring, and ambulating clients are almost always independent nursing functions. The physician usually orders specific body positions only after surgery, anesthesia, or trauma involving the nervous and musculoskeletal systems. All clients should have an activity order written by their physician when they are admitted to the agency for care and following surgery and invasive diagnostic procedures (e.g., angiography, lumbar puncture).

As part of planning, the nurse is responsible for identifying those clients who need assistance with body alignment and determining the degree of assistance they need. The nurse must be sensitive to the client's need to function as independently as possible yet provide assistance when the client needs it.

Most clients require some nursing guidance and assistance to learn about, achieve, and maintain proper body mechanics. The nurse should also plan to teach clients applicable skills. For example, a client with a back injury needs to learn how to get out of bed safely and comfortably; someone with an injured leg needs to learn how to transfer from bed to wheelchair safely; and a client with a newly acquired walker needs to learn how to use it safely. Nurses often teach family members or caregivers safe moving, lifting, and transfer techniques in the home setting.

The goals established for clients vary according to the diagnosis and defining characteristics related to each individual. Examples of overall goals for clients with actual or potential problems related to mobility or activity follow:

- Increase in tolerance for physical activity
- Restoring or improving the capability to ambulate or participate in activities of daily living (ADLs)

- Avoidance of injury from falling or improper use of body mechanics
- Improvement in physical fitness
- Avoidance of any complications associated with immobility

Planning for Home Care

Clients who have been hospitalized for activity or mobility problems often need continued care in the home. In preparation for discharge, the nurse needs to determine the client's actual and potential health problems, strengths, and resources. The Assessment: Home Care box describes the specific assessment data required before establishing a discharge plan for clients with mobility or activity problems. A major aspect of discharge planning involves instructional needs of the client and family; see the Teaching: Home Care box on the next page.

Implementing

Nurses can initiate and apply a wide variety of exercise and activity interventions as needed to address a multitude of client concerns. Some nursing interventions that pertain to exercise and activity include cognitive stimulation; preventing (or managing) constipation; exercise promotion (strength and stretching); exercise therapy (ambulation, balance, joint mobility, muscle control); fall prevention; health education; prevention of pressure ulcer; and assistance with self-care (among many others).

ASSESSMENT HOME CARE

Ability and Activity Problems

To create a discharge plan, the nurse needs to collect these data:

CLIENT AND ENVIRONMENT

- *Capabilities or tolerance for required and desired activities:* Self-care (feeding, bathing, toileting, dressing, grooming, home maintenance, shopping, cooking), recreational activities
- *Mobility aids required:* Cane, walker, crutches, wheelchair, transfer boards
- *Equipment required if immobilized:* Special bed, side rails, pressure-reducing mattress
- *Current level of knowledge:* Body mechanics for use of mobility aids; specific exercises prescribed
- *Home mobility hazard appraisal:* Adequacy of lighting; presence of handrails; safety of pathways and stairs; congested areas; unanchored rugs, mats, or electrical cords; and any other obstacles to safe movement; structural adjustments needed for wheelchair access

FAMILY OR CAREGIVER

- *Caregiver availability, skills, and willingness to assist:* Assessment of learning needs and development of an appropriate teaching plan; primary people able to assist client with self-care, movement, shopping, and so on; physical and emotional status to assist with care
- *Family role changes and coping:* Effect on financial status, parenting and spousal roles, social roles
- *Availability of caregiver support:* Other support people available for occasional duties, such as shopping, transportation, housekeeping, cooking, budgeting, respite care

COMMUNITY

- *Resources:* Availability and familiarity with sources of medical equipment, financial assistance, homemaker services, hygiene care, and other services (e.g., Meals on Wheels, sources of respite for caregiver)

Activity and Exercise

Discharge planning includes teaching the client and family about the following:

Maintaining Musculoskeletal Function

- Teach the systematic performance of passive or assistive ROM exercises to maintain joint mobility.

- As appropriate, demonstrate the proper way to perform isotonic, isometric, or isokinetic exercises to maintain muscle mass and tone (collaborate with the physician and physical therapist on these). Incorporate ADLs into exercise program, if appropriate.

- Provide a written schedule for the type, frequency, and duration of exercises; encourage the use of a progress graph or chart to facilitate adherence with the therapy.

- Offer an ambulation schedule, as appropriate.

- Instruct in the availability of assistive ambulatory devices and correct use of them.

- Discuss pain-control measures required before exercise, as appropriate.

Preventing Injury

- Provide assistive devices for moving and transferring, whenever possible, and teach safe transfer and ambulation techniques.

- Discuss safety measures to avoid falls (e.g., locking wheelchairs, wearing appropriate footwear, using rubber tips on crutches, keeping the environment safe, and using mechanical aids, such as a raised toilet seat, grab bars, a urinal, a bedpan or commode, to facilitate toileting).

- Teach the use of proper body mechanics, especially for those times when assistive equipment is not used.

- Teach ways to prevent postural hypotension.

Managing Energy to Prevent Fatigue

- Discuss activity and rest patterns and develop a plan, as indicated; intersperse rest periods with activity periods.

- Discuss ways to minimize fatigue, such as performing activities more slowly and for shorter periods, resting more often, and using more assistance, as required.

- Provide information about available resources to help with ADLs and home maintenance management.

- Teach ways to increase energy (e.g., increasing intake of high-energy foods, ensuring adequate rest and sleep, controlling pain).

- Teach techniques to monitor activity tolerance as appropriate.

Referrals

Provide appropriate information about accessing community resources such as home care agencies and sources of adaptive equipment.

Nursing strategies to maintain or promote body alignment and mobility involve positioning clients appropriately, moving and turning clients in bed, transferring clients, providing range-of-motion (ROM) exercises, ambulating clients with or without mechanical aids, and creating strategies to prevent the complications of immobility. Whenever positioning, moving, lifting, and ambulating clients, nurses must use proper body mechanics to avoid musculoskeletal strain and injury.

Using Body Mechanics

Body mechanics is the term used to describe the efficient, coordinated, and safe use of the body to move objects and carry out ADLs. The major purpose of body mechanics is to facilitate the safe and efficient use of appropriate muscle groups to maintain balance, reduce the energy required, reduce fatigue, and decrease the risk of injury. Although good body mechanics is essential for clients, it is of utmost concern for nurses who, even with careful attention to body mechanics, experience one of the highest incidences of work-related back injuries (Canadian Nurses Association [CNA], 2006; O'Brien-Pallas, Shamian, Thomson, Alksnis, Koehoorn, Kerr, et al., 2004). Until recently, nurses believed that "correct" body mechanics alone would decrease the risk of injury for both clients and nurses, especially during client handling tasks (lifting, transferring, and repositioning). Training in body mechanics alone, however, does not prevent job-related injury (Verbeek, Martimo, Karppinen, Kuijer, Viikari-Juntura, & Takala, 2011).

Annually, in Canada, more than 16 million nursing hours are lost due to injury and illness (Registered Nurses' Association of Ontario, 2008). One of the leading causes of absenteeism is work-related musculoskeletal disorders. **Musculoskeletal disorders (MSDs)** are a painful group of disorders affecting muscles, joints, tendons, ligaments, and nerves and typically affect the back, neck, shoulders, upper limbs, and knees. In addition to the economic costs due to absenteeism, nurses with MSDs can experience great personal suffering. MSDs are known to play a role in the decisions of nurses to change nursing jobs and even depart from the profession. The risk of MSDs, compounded with an aging workforce and declining retention and recruitment, may worsen the current nursing shortage (Verbeek et al., 2011). It is therefore essential for reductions in MSDs to be a priority in all health care settings.

Although the complete elimination of musculoskeletal injury in health care is not realistic, the risk and incidence can be reduced by implementing safe practices in the workplace. Increasingly, health care facilities are implementing evidence-informed practices as an approach to ensuring a safe and healthy workplace for nurses. Evidence-informed practices in client handling include the use of assistive equipment or devices, client assessment protocols, "no lift" policies and the development of "lift" teams, and staff training (Nelson & Baptiste, 2004).

Until all work settings provide safe environments in which nurses have the resources they need, content pertaining to body mechanics will be included in this chapter. Readers are encouraged to support "no manual lift" and "no solo lift" policies in their workplaces and to become involved in legislation and equipment-purchase and education initiatives. Nurses must participate in this shift in ergonomic awareness and are encouraged to visit the CNA website to read about workplace initiatives to promote nurses' health.

Principles of body mechanics include maintaining (a) a stable centre of gravity, (b) the line of gravity, (c) a wide base of support, and (d) proper body alignment. When a person moves, the centre of gravity shifts continuously in the direction of the moving body parts. Balance depends on the interrelationship of the centre of gravity, the line of gravity, and the base of support. When a person moves, the closer the line of gravity is to the centre of the base of support, the greater the person's stability (Figure 39.40). Conversely, the closer the line of gravity is to the edge of the base of support, the more precarious the balance. If the line of gravity falls outside the base of support, the person falls.

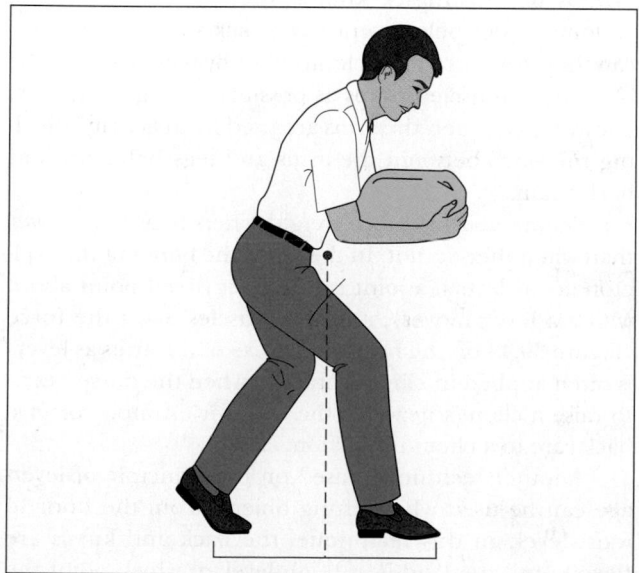

FIGURE 39.40 Balance is maintained when the line of gravity falls close to the base of support.

The broader the base of support and the lower the centre of gravity, the greater are the stability and balance. Body balance, therefore, can be greatly enhanced by (a) widening the base of support, and (b) lowering the centre of gravity, bringing it closer to the base of support. The base of support is easily widened by spreading the feet farther apart. The centre of gravity is readily lowered by flexing the hips and knees until a squatting position is achieved. The importance of these alterations cannot be overemphasized for nurses.

Two movements to avoid because of their potential for causing back injury are twisting (rotation) of the thoracolumbar spine and acute flexion of the back with hips and knees straight (stooping). Undesirable twisting of the back can be prevented by squarely facing the direction of movement, whether pushing, pulling, or sliding, and moving the object directly toward or away from the centre of gravity.

LIFTING Lifting clients is one of the leading causes of musculoskeletal injury for nurses. Client handling tasks create huge potential for injury because of client characteristics, such as their shape and physical characteristics. The Canadian Centre for Occupational Health and Safety [CCOHS] (2012) emphasizes the difference between lifting and transferring patients. A transfer is defined as "a dynamic effort in which the client aids in the transfer and is able to bear weight on at least one leg"; a lift is defined as "moving a client who cannot bear weight on at least one leg." The CCOHS recommends that lifts should *always* involve mechanical lifting devices. Proper assessment of the client is essential to avoid a transfer becoming a lift, such as could happen if the client develops syncope during the transfer. Many health care agencies have developed and implemented "no lift" policies to address work-related risk of injury associated with client handling. The term "no lift" is commonly used, however other terms such as "no manual lift" and "lift free" are also used.

Fortunately, the development of assistive client handling equipment and devices has rendered strict manual client handling unnecessary. Types of assistive equipment include mechanical lifts (Figure 39.41 on the next page), permanently mounted ceiling lifts (Figure 39.42), sit-to-stand powered lifts, and friction-reducing devices (Figure 39.43). The cost of equipment appears to be less than the cost of work-related injury (Nelson, 2007). Use of this equipment is also thought to provide greater client safety, dignity, and comfort.

Other than the weight bearing capacity of the client as a determining factor for whether a client can transfer or requires a mechanical lift, the CCOHS recommends taking into consideration such factors as: how easily the client can follow instructions and be cooperative with step-by-step transfer directions; whether the client has a history of falls; if there is the presence of tubes (e.g., intravenous, urinary drainage systems) that could complicate

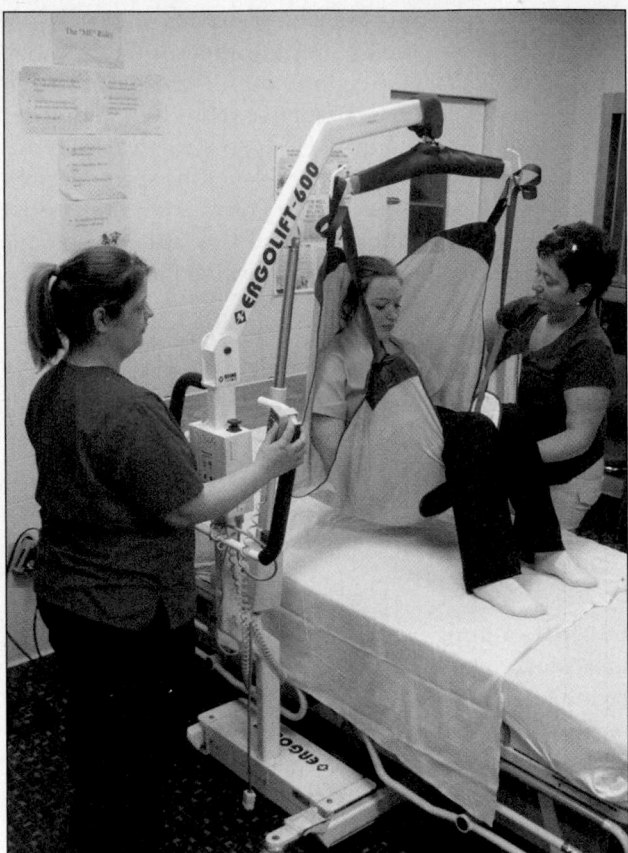

FIGURE 39.41 A mechanical lift that moves clients from a bed, a chair, a toilet, or the floor.

Source: Reprinted with permission of Glenys Moran and participants in the photo.

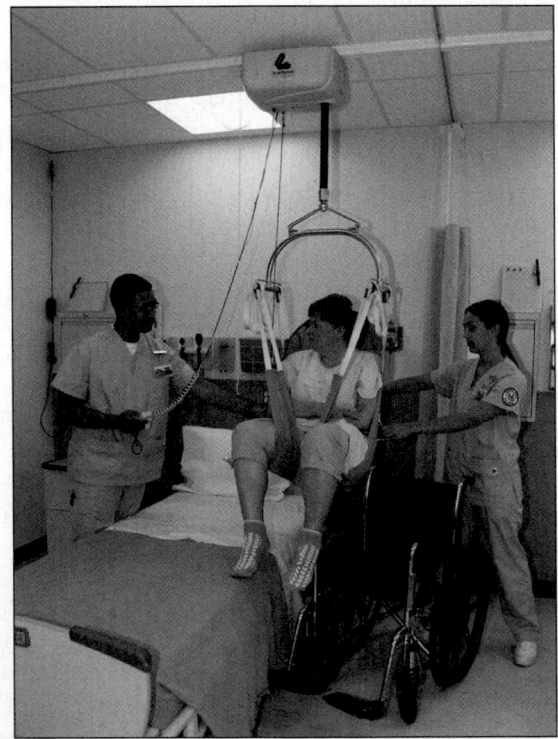

FIGURE 39.42 A ceiling-mounted lift.

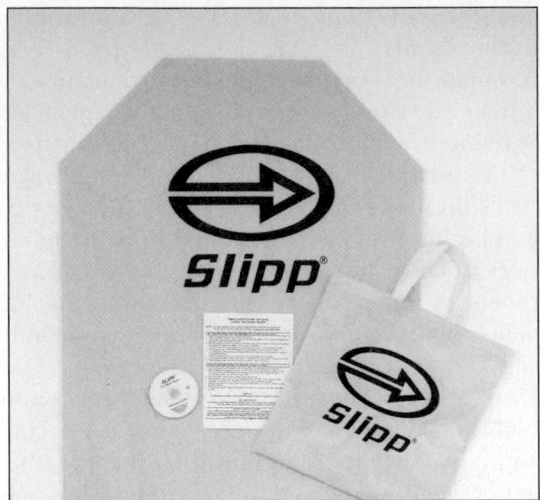

FIGURE 39.43 The Slipp Patient Mover is a transfer assistive device that reduces the nurse's exposure to back injuries and maximizes client comfort.

a transfer; the layout of the physical environment so as to allow for proper body mechanics and transfer techniques.

When a person lifts or carries an object, for example, a suitcase, the weight of the object becomes part of the person's body weight. This weight affects the location of the person's centre of gravity, which is displaced in the direction of the added weight. To counteract this potential imbalance, body parts (e.g., arm and trunk) move in a direction away from the weight. In this way, the centre of gravity is maintained over the same point in the base of support. By holding the lifted object as close as possible to the body's centre of gravity, the lifter avoids undue displacement of the centre of gravity and achieves greater stability. Because lifting involves movement against gravity, the nurse must use major muscle groups of the thighs, knees, upper and lower arms, abdomen, and pelvis to prevent back strain. The nurse can increase overall muscle strength by synchronized use of as many muscle groups as possible during an activity. For instance, when the arms are used in an activity, dividing the work between the arms and legs helps prevent back strain.

People can lift more weight when they use a lever than when they do not. In the body, the bones of the skeleton act as levers, a joint is a *fulcrum* (fixed point about which a lever moves), and the muscles exert the force (Figure 39.44 on the next page). Use of the arms as levers is often applied in clinical practice when the nurse needs to raise a client's head off the bed, for example, or give back care to a client in traction.

Another technique based on the principle of leverage can be used when lifting objects from the floor to waist level. In this technique, the back and knees are flexed until the load is at thigh level, at which point the knees remain flexed to provide thrust as the back begins

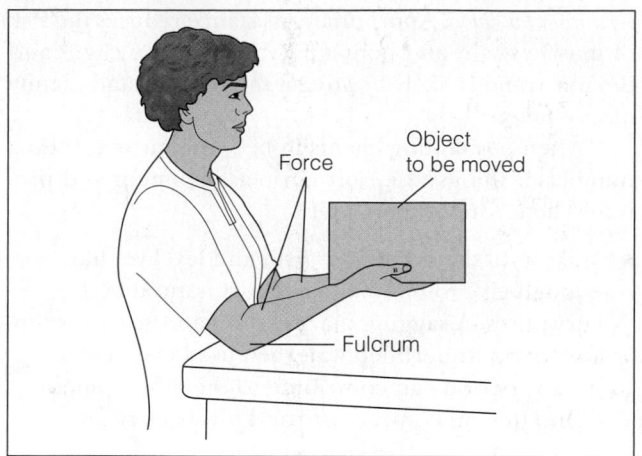

FIGURE 39.44 Using the arm as a lever.

to straighten. This technique provides for better balance, leverage, and synchronized use of muscles, which help avoid back pain and injury. When a nurse lifts an object to knee level, the shoulder and arm muscles pull, the abdominal and pelvic muscles contract for leverage and pull, and the thigh and leg muscles exert the upward thrust to bring the object off the floor. When one lifts an object from midthigh to waist level, force is provided essentially by the leg and thigh muscle groups, but the back and pelvic muscles remain contracted.

In all positions, it is important to maintain a wide base of support (feet approximately shoulder width apart) and to keep the load close to the body, especially when it is at knee level. Before attempting the lift, the nurse must ensure that the floor is free of hazards, the path for moving the object is clear, and the nurse's base of support is secure.

PULLING AND PUSHING Pushing and pulling can cause musculoskeletal injury, particularly in the shoulder and back areas, and should be performed carefully. When pulling or pushing an object, a person maintains balance with least effort when the base of support is enlarged in the direction in which the movement is to be produced or opposed. For example, when pushing an object, a person can enlarge the base of support by moving the front foot forward. When pulling an object, a person can enlarge the base of support by (a) moving the rear leg back as the person is facing the object or (b) moving the front foot forward if the person is facing away from the object. It is easier and safer to pull an object toward the person's centre of gravity than to push it away, as the person can exert more control of the object's movement when pulling it. See the Clinical Alert box on assistive equipment.

PIVOTING Pivoting is a technique in which the body is turned in a way that avoids twisting of the spine, which can cause severe injury. To pivot, place one foot ahead of the other, raise the heels very slightly, and put the body weight on the balls of the feet. When the weight is off the heels, the frictional surface is decreased and the knees are not twisted when turning. Keeping the body aligned, turn (pivot) about 90 degrees in the desired direction. The foot that was forward will now be behind.

> **! CLINICAL ALERT**
>
> Lateral-assist devices, such as horizontal air-transfer mattresses and transfer chairs, are essential equipment for most client care areas to prevent acute and chronic back pain and disability. Observing the principles of body mechanics is recommended even when using assistive equipment, as any movement is potentially injurious, especially when repeated over time.

Preventing Back Injury

Many factors increase the potential for lower back injuries. A major contributor is habitually poor standing and sitting postures, which produce lordosis. Overweight individuals who carry their extra weight over their abdomen, pregnant women, and women who consistently wear high-heeled shoes are at risk because of the exaggerated lumbar curvature these situations produce. Sedentary persons are at greater risk because of weak back and abdominal muscles.

Nurses are at a significant risk for back injury, particularly lower back injury, as a result of client handling. Client handling tasks create the potential for injury because of the awkward nature of lifting, the unpredictability of clients, and the amount of weight lifted. The changing profile of clients continues to create new challenges for safe client handling. An aging population, increasing numbers of bariatric (clinically obese) clients, and increased levels of acuity reflect the type of clients routinely seen in all care settings.

Prior to client handling, the nurse should assess a number of factors to determine the risk of musculoskeletal injury, including the physical demands of the task, the work environment and organization, and client characteristics (CCOHS, 2012). The physical demands of the task include such factors as awkward positioning and the effort required to move a client. An assessment of the work environment can include such features as the space where the client handling task will take place, the heights of the chairs and beds, and the availability of assistive equipment and additional personnel. Factors such as spreading tasks evenly over the work shift and among all staff, are included in an assessment of the work organization. Client characteristics needed to be considered before client handling include the client's physical and mental capabilities to participate. The client's weight, height, shape, and ability to bear weight and maintain balance are important. As well, their ability and willingness to follow instructions and predictability of their behaviour are essential to assess. For example, disoriented clients may initially appear cooperative with movement; however, they may suddenly become confused or aggressive, putting the nurse and themselves at risk for injury. All of these characteristics must be considered to determine whether a task can be safely performed with one or more persons assisting, and/or if an assistive device(s) is required.

Guidelines for preventing back injuries are presented in the Teaching: Clinical box.

Positioning Clients

Positioning a client in good body alignment and changing the position regularly and systematically are essential aspects of nursing practice. Clients who can move easily automatically reposition themselves for comfort. Such people generally require minimal positioning assistance from nurses other than guidance about ways to maintain body alignment and to exercise their joints. However, people who are weak, frail, in pain, paralyzed, or unconscious rely on nurses to provide or assist with position changes. For all clients, it is important to assess the skin and provide skin care before and after a position change.

Any position, correct or incorrect, can be detrimental if maintained for a prolonged period. Frequent change of position helps prevent muscle discomfort, undue pressure resulting in pressure ulcers, damage to superficial nerves and blood vessels, and contractures. Position changes also maintain muscle tone and stimulate postural reflexes.

When the client is not able to move independently or assist with moving, the *preferred method is to use appropriate assistive equipment, as well as to have two or more people reposition the client.* Appropriate assistance reduces the risk of muscle strain and body injury to both the client and the nurse and is likely to protect the comfort and dignity of the client.

When positioning clients in bed, the nurse can do a number of things to ensure proper alignment and promote client comfort and safety:

- Make sure the mattress is firm and level yet has enough give to fill in and support natural body curvatures. A sagging mattress, a mattress that is too soft, or an underfilled waterbed used over a prolonged period can contribute to the development of hip flexion contractures and low back strain and pain.

- Ensure that the bed is clean and dry. Wrinkled or damp sheets increase the risk of pressure ulcer formation. Make sure extremities can move freely (e.g., the top bed sheets need to be loose enough for the client to move the feet).

- Use appropriate support devices (see Box 39.2) to maintain alignment.

- Avoid placing one body part, particularly one with bony prominences, directly on top of another body part. Excessive pressure can damage veins and predispose the client to thrombus formation and pressure ulcers. Pressure against the popliteal space may damage nerves and blood vessels in this area. Pillows can provide needed cushioning.

- Plan a *systematic 24-hour schedule* for position changes. Frequent position changes are essential to prevent pressure ulcers in immobilized clients. Throughout the day and night, these clients should be positioned every 2 hours and more frequently as needed.

TEACHING	CLINICAL

Preventing Back Injuries

These guidelines can help prevent back injuries:
- Understand that lifting loads of more than 20 kg can lead to back or musculoskeletal injury. Keep in mind that even lifting loads of less than this amount can cause injury even when proper body mechanics are used.
- Use assistive equipment, get help from coworkers, and participate in the purchasing or ordering process of appropriate assistive equipment for your work setting.
- Become consciously aware of your posture and body mechanics.
- When standing for a long time, periodically flex one hip and knee and rest your foot on an object, if possible.
- When sitting, keep your knees slightly higher than your hips.

- Use a firm mattress and soft pillow that provide good body support at natural body curvatures.
- Exercise regularly to maintain overall physical condition; include exercises that strengthen the pelvic, abdominal, and spinal muscles.
- Avoid exercises that cause pain or require spinal flexion with straight legs (e.g., toe touching) or spinal rotation (twisting).
- When moving an object, spread your feet apart to provide a wide base of support.
- When lifting an object, distribute the weight between large muscles of the legs and arms.
- Wear clothing that allows you to use good body mechanics and comfortable low-heeled shoes that provide good foot support and will not cause you to slip, stumble, or turn your ankle.

BOX 39.2 SUPPORT DEVICES

The following are some commonly used support devices:

- *Pillows.* Different sizes are available. They are used for support or elevation of a body part (e.g., an arm) and to splint incisional areas (reducing pain and discomfort with activity and deep breathing and coughing). Specially designed dense pillows are also available, for example, an *abduction (wedge) pillow* (see ❶), a triangular-shaped foam pillow, is placed between the legs to maintain hip abduction following total hip replacement.

- *Mattresses.* There are two types of mattresses: ones that fit on the bed frame (e.g., standard bed mattress) and those that fit on the standard bed mattress (e.g.,

egg-crate mattress). Mattresses should be evenly supportive.

- *Hand roll.* These can be made by rolling a washcloth. They maintain the hand in a functional position preventing contractures.

- *Chair beds.* These beds can be placed into the position of a chair for clients who cannot move from the bed but require a sitting position.

- *Foot boot.* These are made of a variety of substances. They usually have a firm exterior and padding of foam to protect the skin. They provide support and keep the feet in dorsiflexion, preventing foot drop (see ❷). Persons who are able to sit may benefit from high-top shoes to maintain foot alignment.

- *Footboard.* This is a flat panel often made of plastic or wood. It keeps the feet in dorsiflexion to prevent plantar flexion.

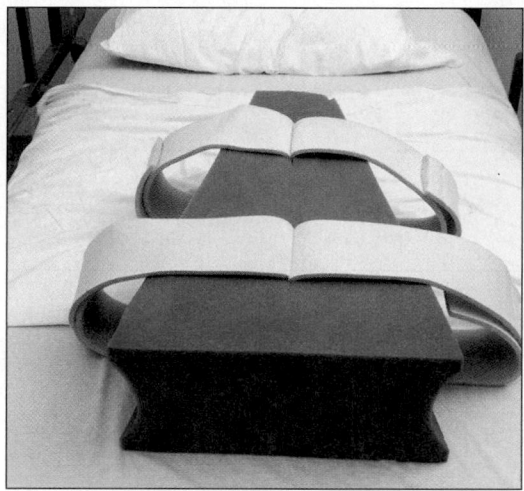

❶ An abduction pillow.

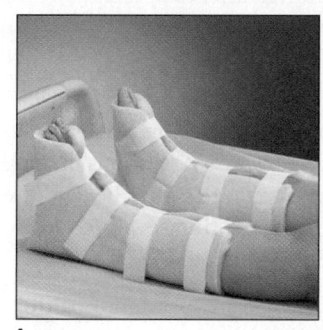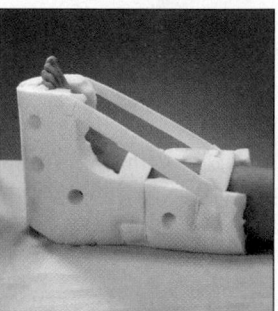

A   **B**

❷ **A:** Suspension boot; **B:** Heel guard.

Source: Images provided by Posey Company, Arcadia, California.

Both appearance (in relation to alignment criteria) and comfort are important in achieving effective alignment. Always obtain information from the client to determine which position is most comfortable and appropriate. Sometimes, a person who appears well aligned may be experiencing real discomfort.

FOWLER'S POSITION   **Fowler's position**, or a semisitting position, is a bed position in which the head and trunk are raised 45 to 60 degrees (Figure 39.45B). In **low-Fowler's**, or **semi-Fowler's position** (Figure 39.45A), the head and trunk are raised 15 to 45 degrees; in **high-Fowler's position**, the head and trunk are raised 90 degrees. In this position, the knees may or may not be flexed.

Fowler's position is the position of choice for people who have difficulty breathing and for some people with heart problems. When the client is in this position, gravity pulls the diaphragm downward, allowing greater chest expansion and lung ventilation. It is not the position of choice if the client is at risk for developing pressure ulcers

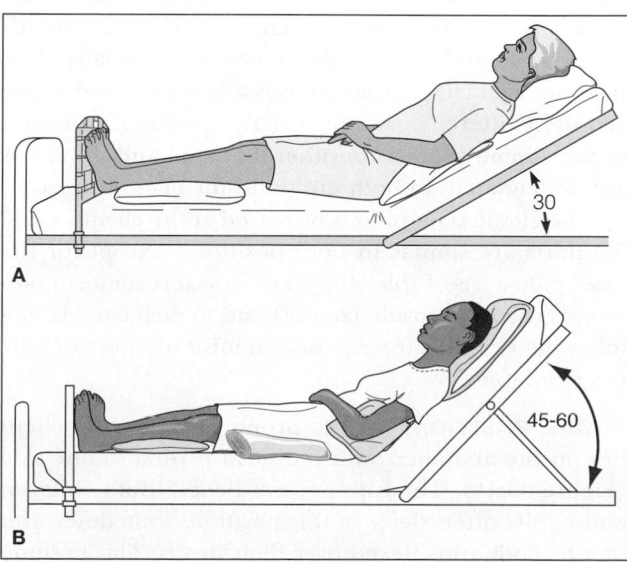

FIGURE 39.45 A: Low-Fowler's (semi-Fowler's) position; **B:** Fowler's position.

TABLE 39.5 Fowler's Position

Unsupported Position	Problem to Be Prevented	Corrective Measure*
Bed-sitting position involves upper part of body elevated 45 to 60 degrees commencing at hips.	Posterior flexion of lumbar curvature	Pillow at lower back (lumbar region) to support lumbar region
Head rests on bed surface.	Hyperextension of neck	Pillows to support head, neck, and upper back
Arms fall at sides.	Shoulder muscle strain, possible dislocation of shoulders, edema of hands and arms with flaccid paralysis, flexion contracture of the wrist	Pillow under forearms to eliminate pull on shoulder and assist venous blood flow from hands and lower arms
Legs lie flat and straight on lower bed surface.	Hyperextension of knees	Small pillow under thighs to flex knees
Heels rest on bed surface.	Pressure on heels	Pillow under lower legs
Feet are in plantar flexion.	Plantar flexion of feet (foot drop)	Footboard to provide support for dorsal flexion

The amount of support depends on the needs of the individual client.

(because of the shearing force). A common error nurses make when aligning clients in Fowler's position is placing an overly large pillow or more than one pillow behind the client's head. These errors promote the development of neck flexion contractures (See Table 39.5.).

ORTHOPNEIC POSITION   In the **orthopneic position**, the client sits in bed or on the side of the bed with an overbed table across the lap (Figure 39.46). This position facilitates respiration by allowing maximum chest expansion. It is particularly helpful to clients who have problems exhaling because they can press the lower part of the chest against the edge of the overbed table.

DORSAL RECUMBENT POSITION   In the **dorsal recumbent (back-lying) position** (Figure 39.47), the client's head and shoulders are slightly elevated on a small pillow. In some agencies, the terms *dorsal recumbent* and *supine* are used interchangeably; strictly speaking, however, in the **supine (dorsal) position** the head and shoulders are not elevated. In both positions, the client's forearms may be elevated on pillows or placed at the client's sides. Supports are similar in both positions, except for the head pillow (see Table 39.6). The dorsal recumbent position is used to provide comfort and to facilitate healing following certain surgeries or administration of anesthetics (e.g., spinal).

PRONE POSITION   In the **prone position**, the client lies on the abdomen with the head turned to one side (Figure 39.48). The hips are not flexed. Both children and adults often sleep in this position, sometimes with one or both arms flexed over their heads. This position has several advantages. It is the only bed position that allows full extension of the hip and knee joints. When

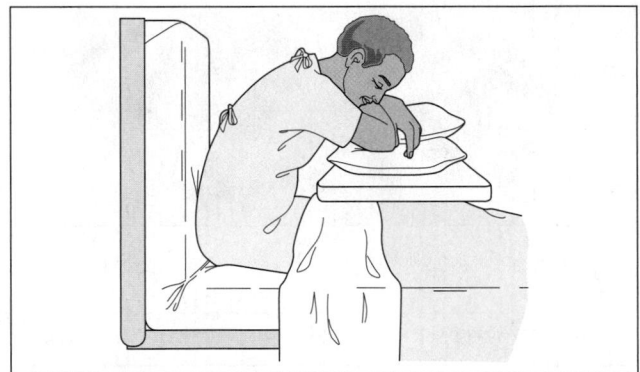

FIGURE 39.46 Orthopneic position.

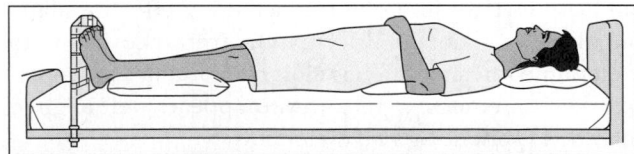

FIGURE 39.47 Dorsal recumbent position (supported).

used periodically, the prone position helps prevent flexion contractures of the hips and knees, thereby counteracting a problem caused by all other bed positions. The prone position also promotes drainage from the mouth and is especially useful for unconscious clients or those clients recovering from surgery of the mouth or throat (see Table 39.7).

The prone position poses some distinct disadvantages. The pull of gravity on the trunk produces a marked lordosis in most people, and the neck is rotated laterally

TABLE 39.6 Dorsal Recumbent Position

Unsupported Position	Problem to Be Prevented	Corrective Measure*
Head is flat on bed surface.	Hyperextension of neck in thick-chested person	Pillow of suitable thickness under head and shoulders if necessary for alignment
Lumbar curvature of spine is apparent.	Posterior flexion of lumbar curvature	Roll or small pillow under lumbar curvature
Legs may be externally rotated.	External rotation of legs	Roll or sandbag placed laterally to trochanter of femur (optional)
Legs are extended.	Hyperextension of knees	Small pillow under thigh to flex knee slightly
Feet assume plantar flexion position.	Plantar flexion (foot drop)	Footboard or rolled pillow to support feet in dorsal flexion
Heels on bed surface.	Pressure on heels	Pillow under lower legs

*The amount of support depends on the needs of the individual client.

TABLE 39.7 Prone Position

Unsupported Position	Problem to Be Prevented	Corrective Measure*
Head is turned to side and neck is slightly flexed.	Flexion or hyperextension of neck	Small pillow under head unless contraindicated because of promotion of mucus drainage from mouth
Body lies flat on abdomen, accentuating lumbar curvature.	Hyperextension of lumbar curvature; difficulty breathing; pressure on breasts (women); pressure on genitals (men)	Small pillow or roll under abdomen just below diaphragm
Toes rest on bed surface; feet are in plantar flexion.	Plantar flexion (foot drop)	Allow feet to fall naturally over end of mattress, or support lower legs on a pillow so that toes do not touch the bed

*The amount of support depends on the needs of the individual client.

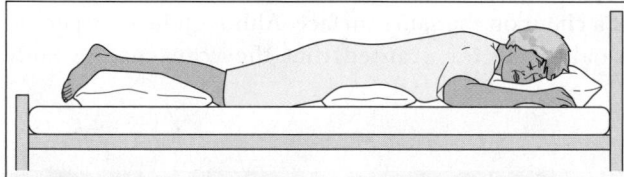

FIGURE 39.48 Prone position (supported).

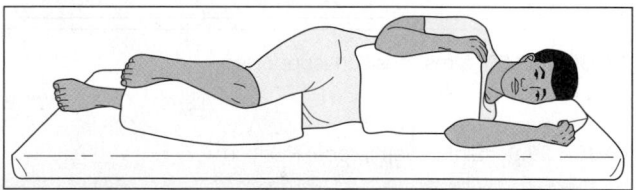

FIGURE 39.49 Lateral position (supported).

to a significant degree. For this reason, the prone position may not be recommended for people with problems of the cervical or lumbar spine. This position also causes plantar flexion. Some clients with cardiac or respiratory problems find the prone position confining and suffocating because chest expansion is inhibited during respirations. The prone position should be used only when the client's back is correctly aligned, only for short periods, and only for people with no evidence of spinal abnormalities.

LATERAL POSITION In the **lateral (side-lying) position** (Figure 39.49), the client lies on one side of the body. Flexing the top hip and knee and placing this leg in front

of the body creates a wider, triangular base of support and achieves greater stability. The greater the flexion of the top hip and knee, the greater the stability and balance in this position. This flexion reduces lordosis and promotes good back alignment. For this reason, the lateral position is good for resting and sleeping clients. The lateral position helps relieve pressure on the sacrum and heels in people who sit for much of the day or who are confined to bed and rest in Fowler's or dorsal recumbent positions much of the time. In the lateral position, most of the body's weight is borne by the lateral aspect of the lower scapula, the lateral aspect of the ilium, and the greater trochanter of the

TABLE 39.8 Lateral Position

Unsupported Position	Problem to Be Prevented	Corrective Measure*
Body is turned to side, both arms in front of body, weight resting primarily on lateral aspects of scapula and ilium.	Lateral flexion and fatigue of sternocleidomastoid muscles	Pillow under head and neck to provide good alignment
Upper arm and shoulder are rotated internally and adducted.	Internal rotation and adduction of shoulder and subsequent limited function; impaired chest expansion	Pillow under upper arm to place it in good alignment; lower arm should be flexed comfortably
Upper thigh and leg are rotated internally and adducted.	Internal rotation and adduction of femur; twisting of the spine	Pillow under leg and thigh to place them in good alignment; shoulders and hips should be aligned

The amount of support depends on the needs of the individual client.

femur. People who have sensory or motor deficits on one side of the body usually find that lying on the uninvolved side is more comfortable (see Table 39.8).

SIMS' POSITION In **Sims' (semiprone) position** (Figure 39.50), the client assumes a posture halfway between the lateral and the prone positions. The lower arm is positioned behind the client, and the upper arm is flexed at the shoulder and the elbow. Both legs are flexed in front of the client. The upper leg is more acutely flexed at both the hip and the knee than the lower one is.

Sims' position is occasionally used for unconscious clients because it facilitates drainage from the mouth and prevents aspiration of fluids. It is also used for clients who are paralyzed (paraplegic or hemiplegic) because it reduces pressure over the sacrum and greater trochanter of the hip. It can be used for clients undergoing examinations or treatments of the perineal area. Many people, especially pregnant women, find Sims' position comfortable for sleeping. People with sensory or motor deficits on one side of the body usually find that lying on the uninvolved side is more comfortable (see Table 39.9).

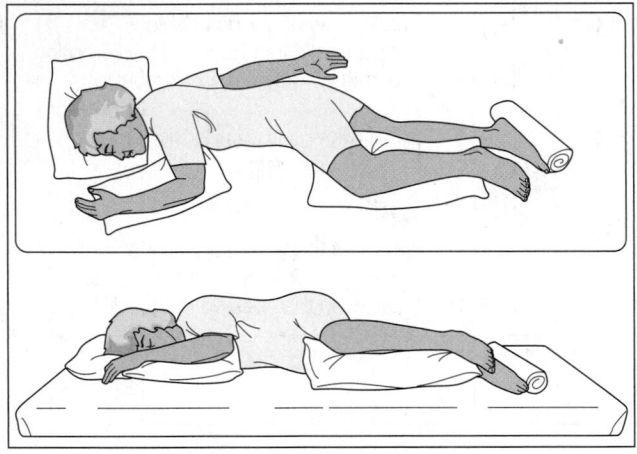

FIGURE 39.50 Sims' position (supported)

Moving and Turning Clients in Bed

Repositioning is a term used to describe the movement of a client on the same surface. Although healthy people usually take for granted that they can change body

TABLE 39.9 Sims' (Semiprone) Position

Unsupported Position	Problem to Be Prevented	Corrective Measure*
Head rests on bed surface; weight is borne by lateral aspects of cranial and facial bones.	Lateral flexion of neck	Pillow to support the head, maintaining it in good alignment unless drainage from the mouth is required
Upper shoulder and arm are internally rotated.	Internal rotation of shoulder and arm; pressure on chest, restricting expansion during breathing	Pillow under upper arm to prevent internal rotation
Upper leg and thigh are adducted and internally rotated.	Internal rotation and adduction of hip and leg	Pillow under upper leg to support it in alignment
Feet assume plantar flexion.	Foot drop	Sandbags to support feet in dorsal flexion

The amount of support depends on the needs of the individual client.

position and go from one place to another with little effort, people who are ill may have difficulty moving even in bed. How much assistance clients require depends on their own ability to move and their health status. In general, nurses should be sensitive to both people's need to function independently and their need for assistance to move.

When a nurse assists a client to move, the nurse needs to use appropriate numbers of personnel and assistive devices (such as those shown in Figures 39.41 to 39.43), as well as correct body mechanics to avoid personal and client injury. Correct body alignment for the client must also be maintained so that undue stress is not placed on the musculoskeletal system.

Mechanical lifts are examples of assistive equipment that take the place of manual lifts and transfers. A lift can be used to reposition a client and to transfer a client between the bed and a wheelchair, the bed and the bathtub, and the bed and a stretcher. Lifts usually consist of a base on casters (or mounted on the ceiling), a hydraulic mechanical pump, a mast boom, and a sling (see Figure 39.41). Most agencies recommend that two nurses operate a lift. It is important to be familiar with the model used and the practices that accompany use, as well as specific institutional policies that pertain to client handling. Before using a lift, the nurse must ensure it is in good working order.

A friction-reducing device is another type of assistive equipment used by nurses to move clients. They are used to facilitate easier movement of clients (on the same surface and from one surface to another) and can be used in combination with each other. Many varieties of friction-reducing devices exist including a turn sheet, a transfer board, and so on. These devices improve client safety and reduce the risk of injury to caregivers.

Actions and rationales applicable to repositioning clients include the following:

- Before moving a client, assess the degree of exertion permitted, the client's physical abilities (e.g., muscle strength, presence of paralysis), ability to assist with the move, ability to understand instructions, degree of comfort or discomfort when moving, weight, presence of orthostatic hypotension (particularly important when the client will be standing), and your own strength and ability to move the client.

- If indicated, provide an analgesic before moving the client.

- Prepare any needed supportive devices and supportive equipment (e.g., pillows).

- Plan around hindrances to movement, such as an IV or a heavy cast.

- Be alert to the effects of any medications the client takes that may impair alertness, balance, strength, or mobility.

- Explain the procedure to the client, and listen to any suggestions the client or support people have.

- Provide privacy, and perform hand hygiene.

- Raise the height of the bed to bring the client close to your centre of gravity (e.g., between the hips and waist). If more than one caregiver is involved, raise the bed to the height of the centre of gravity of the shortest person; additional caregivers will bend at the knee.

- When moving a client up in bed, allow gravity to assist by tilting the bed to the "head down" (Trendelenburg) position, unless contraindicated.

- Lock the wheels on the bed, and lower the rail on the side of the bed where you are standing.

- Face in the direction of the movement to prevent spinal twisting.

- Assume a broad stance to increase stability and provide balance.

- When using a draw or slider sheet, use the "palms up" grip instead of the "palms down" grip, as it is stronger and helps to keep the elbows close to the body and to maintain a neutral shoulder position (WorkSafeBC, 2006b).

- Lean your trunk slightly forward, and flex your hips, knees, and ankles to lower your centre of gravity, increase stability, and ensure use of large muscle groups during movements.

- Tighten your gluteal, abdominal, pelvic, leg, and arm muscles to prepare them for action and to prevent injury.

- Rock from the front leg to the back leg when pulling or from the back leg to the front leg when pushing to overcome inertia, counteract the client's weight, and help attain a balanced, smooth motion.

- After moving the client, determine the client's comfort, body alignment, tolerance of the activity (e.g., check pulse rate, respirations, oxygen saturation, blood pressure), and safety precautions required (e.g., side rails).

See Skill 39.1 on moving a client up in bed on the next page and Skill 39.2 on turning a client to a lateral or prone position in bed on page 1175. Skill 39.3 on page 1177 describes how to logroll a client (**logrolling** is a technique used to turn a client whose body must at all times be kept in straight alignment, like a log). The Evidence-Informed Practice Box on page 1178 summarizes a study that assessed the use of logrolling when a client has a spinal cord injury. Skill 39.4 on page 1178 explains how to help a client to sit up on the edge of the bed.

Note: The Assessment, Planning, and Equipment sections as listed in Skill 39.1 are the same for each of these four procedures and are not repeated. The Evaluation section at the end of Skill 39.4 is also the same for all four procedures and, hence, is not repeated.

SKILL 39.1 MOVING A CLIENT UP IN BED

PURPOSE

- Clients who have slid down in bed from the Fowler's position often need assistance to move up in bed.

ASSESSMENT

Before moving a client, assess the following:

- The client's physical abilities (e.g., muscle strength, presence of paralysis)
- Ability to understand and willingness to follow instructions
- Degree of comfort or discomfort when moving (if needed, administer analgesics or perform other pain-relief measures; see Chapter 30)
- Client's weight and size
- The availability of equipment and other personnel to assist you

PLANNING

Review the client record to determine whether previous nurses have recorded information about the client's ability to move. Use proper assistive equipment and additional personnel, whenever needed, to safely perform repositioning and to prevent injury to caregivers and the client.

Equipment

- Assistive devices, such as overhead trapeze, pull or turn sheet, friction-reducing device, or a mechanical lift.

IMPLEMENTATION

Preparation

Determine the following:

- Assistive devices that will be required
- Hindrances to movement, such as an IV or a heavy cast on one leg
- Medications the client is receiving, because certain medications may hamper movement or alertness of the client
- Assistance required from other health care personnel

Performance

1. Before performing the procedure, introduce yourself and verify the client's identity using two identifiers or per agency protocol. Explain the procedure to the client, why it is necessary, and how he or she can participate. Listen to any suggestions made by the client or support people.

2. Perform hand hygiene, and follow other appropriate infection prevention and control procedures.

3. Provide for client privacy.

4. Adjust the bed and the client's position.
   - Adjust the head of the bed to a flat position or as low as the client can tolerate. Moving the client upward against gravity requires more force and can cause back strain.
   - Raise the bed to the height of your centre of gravity.
   - Lock the wheels on the bed and raise the rail on the side of the bed opposite you.
   - Remove all pillows, then place one against the head of the bed. **Rationale: This pillow protects the client's head from inadvertent injury against the top of the bed during the upward move**.

5. For the client who is able to reposition without assistance:
   - Stand by and instruct the client to move independently. Encourage the use of an overhead trapeze and the use of arms and hands during the move, as appropriate. Assess if the client is able to move without causing friction to the skin.
   - Ask if a positioning device is needed (e.g., pillow)

6. For the client who is partially able to assist (a minimum of two caregivers is needed):
   - Use a friction-reducing device and determine the number of personnel required. **Rationale: Moving a client up in bed is not a one person task.** During any client handling, if the caregiver is required to lift more than recommended by the agency policy, assistive devices/equipment should be used to reduce the risk of injury to the caregiver and client.
   - Ask the client to flex the hips and knees and position the feet so that they can be used effectively for pushing. **Rationale: Flexing the hips and knees keeps the entire lower leg off the bed surface, preventing friction during movement, and ensures use of the large muscle groups in the client's legs when pushing, thus increasing the force of movement**.
   - Place the client's arms across their chest. Ask the client to flex the neck during the move and keep the head off the bed surface. **Rationale: This keeps the arms and head off the bed surface and minimizes friction during movement**.
   - Use the friction-reducing device and assistants to reposition the client. Ask the client to push on the count of three.

7. Position yourself appropriately, and then move the client.
   - Face the direction of the movement, and then assume a broad stance with your foot nearest the bed behind the forward foot and weight on the forward foot (see ❶). Lean your trunk forward from the hips. Flex your hips, knees, and ankles.
   - Tighten your gluteal, abdominal, leg, and arm muscles, and rock from the back leg to the front leg and back again. Then, on the count of three, shift your weight to the front leg as the client pushes with the heels so that the client moves toward the head of the bed (see ❷).

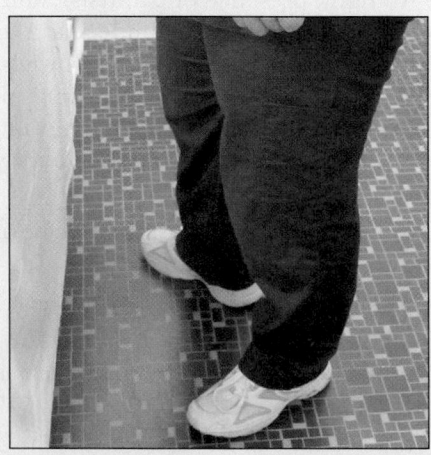

❶ Foot position.

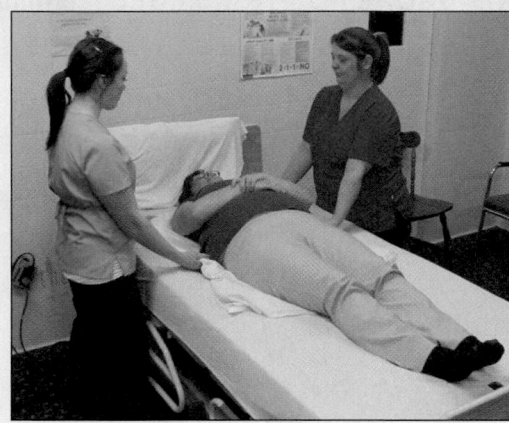

2 Moving a client up in bed

8. For the client who is unable to assist, do the following:
   - Use the ceiling lift with supine sling or mobile floor-based lift and two or more caregivers. Follow agency policy and the manufacturer's guidelines for using the lift.

9. Ensure client comfort.
   - Elevate the head of the bed and provide appropriate support devices for the client's new position.
   - See the sections on positioning clients earlier in this chapter.

Variation: Two Nurses Using a Turn Sheet

- Two nurses can use a turn sheet to move a client up in bed. **Rationale: A turn sheet distributes the client's weight more evenly, decreases friction, and exerts a more even force on the client during the move. In addition, it prevents injury of the client's skin because the friction created between two sheets when one is moved is less than that created by the client's body moving over the sheet**.
- Place a drawsheet or a full sheet folded in half under the client, extending from the shoulders to the thighs. Each

person rolls up or fanfolds the turn sheet close to the client's body on either side.

- Both individuals grasp the sheet close to the shoulders and buttocks of the client with a "palms up" grip. **Rationale: This draws the weight closer to the nurses' centre of gravity and increases the nurses' balance and stability, permitting a smoother movement. The "palms up" grip is stronger than the "palms down" grip and keeps the elbows close to the body and helps to maintain a neutral shoulder position**.
- Assist the client to flex the hips and knees as in step 6. Place the client's arms across their chest. **Rationale: This keeps them off the bed surface and minimizes friction during movement**. Ask the client to flex the neck during the move and keep the head off the bed surface.
- Position yourself appropriately, and then move the client.
- Face the direction of the movement, and then assume a broad stance with the foot nearest the bed behind the forward foot and weight on the forward foot. Lean your trunk forward from the hips. Flex hips, knees, and ankles.
- Tighten your gluteal, abdominal, leg, and arm muscles, and rock from the back leg to the front leg and back again. Then, on the count of three, shift your weight to the front leg as the client pushes with the heels so that the client moves toward the head of the bed.
- Ensure client comfort.
- Elevate the head of the bed and provide appropriate support devices for the client's new position (see the sections on positioning clients earlier in this chapter).

10. Document all relevant information, including the following:
    - Time and change of position moved from and position moved to
    - Any signs of pressure areas
    - Use of support devices
    - Ability of client to assist in moving and turning
    - Response of client to moving and turning (e.g., anxiety, discomfort, dizziness)

SKILL 39.2 **TURNING A CLIENT TO THE LATERAL OR PRONE POSITION IN BED**

PURPOSE

- Movement to the lateral (side-lying) position may be necessary when placing a bedpan beneath the client, when changing the client's bed linen, or when repositioning the client.

IMPLEMENTATION

Preparation

Determine the following:

- Assistive devices that will be required
- Hindrances to movement, such as an IV or a heavy cast on one leg
- Medications the client is receiving, because certain medications may hamper movement or alertness of the client
- Assistance required from other health care personnel

Performance

1. Before performing the procedure, introduce yourself and verify the client's identity using two identifiers or per agency protocol. Explain the procedure to the client, why it is necessary, and how he or she can participate.

2. Perform hand hygiene, and follow other appropriate infection prevention and control procedures.

3. Provide for client privacy.

4. Position yourself and the client appropriately before performing the move. Other person(s) stands on the opposite side of the bed.
   - Raise the bed to the height of your centre of gravity.
   - Adjust the head of the bed to a flat position or as low as the client can tolerate.

(continued)

SKILL 39.2 TURNING A CLIENT TO THE LATERAL OR PRONE POSITION IN BED (*continued*)

- Move the client closer to the side of the bed opposite the side the client will face when turned. **Rationale: This ensures that the client will be positioned safely in the centre of the bed after turning.** Use a drawsheet and/or friction reducing device beneath the client's trunk and thighs to reposition the client to the side of the bed. Roll up the sheet as close as possible to the client's body and grasp the sheet close to the shoulders and buttocks with a "palms up" grip. Reposition the client to the side of the bed by shifting your weight from the front foot (closest to the bed), to the rear foot. Adjust the client's head and reposition the legs appropriately. (Depending on the level of client assistance required, a mechanical lift may be needed.)

- While standing on the side of the bed nearest the client, place the client's near arm across the chest. Abduct the client's far shoulder slightly from the side of the body and externally rotate the shoulder (Figure 39.8). **Rationale: Pulling the one arm forward facilitates the turning motion. Pulling the other arm away from the body and externally rotating the shoulder prevent that arm from being caught beneath the client's body during the roll.**

- Place the client's near ankle and foot across the far ankle and foot. **Rationale: This facilitates the turning motion. Making these preparations on the side of the bed closest to the client helps prevent unnecessary reaching.**

- Raise the side rail next to the client before going to the other side of the bed. **Rationale: This action ensures that the client, who is close to the edge of the mattress, will not fall.** (If a second caregiver is present, this is not necessary).

- The person on the side of the bed toward which the client will turn should be positioned directly in line with the client's waistline and as close to the bed as possible.

- Lean your trunk forward from the hips. Flex your hips, knees, and ankles. Assume a broad stance with one foot forward and the weight placed on this forward foot.

5. Roll the client toward yourself to the lateral position. If needed, a second caregiver standing on the opposite side of the bed helps roll the client from the other side.

- Place one hand on the client's far hip and the other hand on the client's far shoulder (see ❶ A). **Rationale: This position of the hands supports the client at the two heaviest parts of the body, providing greater control in movement during the roll.**

- Tighten your gluteal, abdominal, leg, and arm muscles; rock backward, shifting your weight from the forward to the backward foot, and roll the client onto the side of the body to face you (see ❶ B). **Rationale: Turning the client toward yourself promotes the client's sense of security.**

- Position the client on his or her side with arms and legs positioned and supported properly (see Table 39.8 on page 1172).

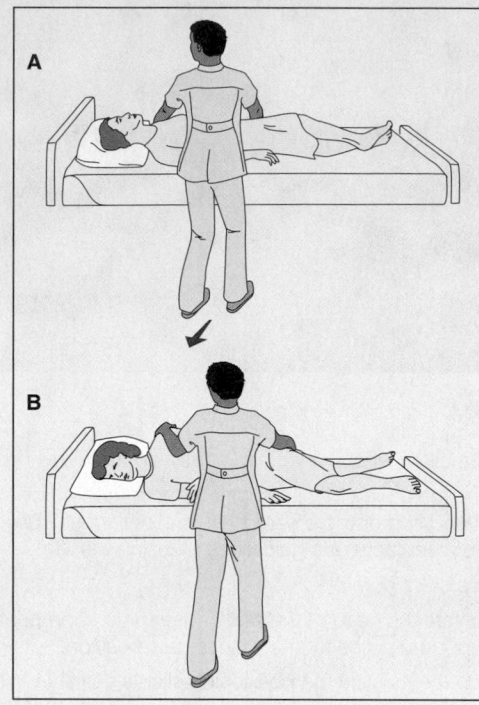

❶ Moving a client to the lateral position.

Variation: Turning the Client to the Prone Position

- To turn a client to the prone position, follow the preceding steps, with two exceptions:

- Instead of abducting the far arm, keep the client's arm alongside the body for the client to roll over. **Rationale: Keeping the arm alongside the body prevents it from being pinned under the client when the client is rolled.**

- Roll the client completely onto the abdomen. **Rationale: It is essential to move the client as close as possible to the edge of the bed before the turn so that the client will be lying on the centre of the bed after rolling.** Never pull a client across the bed while the client is in the prone position. **Rationale: Doing so can injure a woman's breasts or a man's genitals.**

- Turn the client's head to one side and support the head and body (see Table 39.7 on page 1171).

6. Document all relevant information, including the following:

- Time and change of position moved from and position moved to

- Any signs of pressure areas

- Use of support devices

- Ability of client to assist in moving and turning

- Response of client to moving and turning (e.g., anxiety, discomfort, dizziness)

SKILL 39.3 LOGROLLING A CLIENT

PURPOSE

Logrolling is used to turn a client whose body must at all times be kept in straight alignment. An example is the client with a spinal injury. Considerable care must be taken to prevent additional injury. This technique requires at least three nurses or, if the client is large, additional nurses are required. For the client who has a cervical injury, one nurse must maintain the client's head and neck alignment.

IMPLEMENTATION

Preparation

Determine the following:

- Assistive devices that will be required
- Hindrances to movement, such as an IV or a heavy cast on one leg
- Medications the client is receiving, because certain medications may hamper movement or alertness of the client
- Assistance required from other health care personnel

Performance

1. Before performing the procedure, introduce yourself and verify the client's identity using two identifiers or per agency protocol. Explain to the client what you are going to do, why it is necessary, and how he or she can participate. Discuss how the results will be used in planning further care or treatments.

2. Perform hand hygiene, and follow other appropriate infection prevention and control procedures.

3. Provide for client privacy.

4. Position yourselves and the client appropriately before the move.

   - Raise the bed to the height of your centre of gravity. Ensure that bed brakes are on.
   - Place the client's arms across the chest. **Rationale: Doing so maintains alignment during the turn and ensures that the arms will not be injured or become trapped under the body when the body is turned**.

5. Reposition the client to the side of the bed opposite the side the client will face when turned.

   - Use a draw sheet and/or a friction-reducing device to reposition the client to the side of the bed. First, stand with another nurse on the same side of the bed. Assume a broad stance with one foot forward. Roll up the sheet as close as possible to the client's body, and grasp the sheet close to the shoulders and buttocks of the client with the "palms up" grip and reposition the client to the side of the bed (see ❶).
   - Tighten your gluteal, abdominal, leg, and arm muscles.
   - One nurse counts, "One, two, three"; then, at the same time, all staff members reposition the client to the side of the bed by shifting their weight from the front foot to the back foot. **Rationale: Moving the client in unison maintains the client's body alignment**.

6. Move to the other side of the bed, and place supportive devices for the client and prepare for the turn.

   - Two nurses are positioned on the side of the bed the client will turn toward and assume a stable walking stance with one foot forward. The third nurse is positioned on the opposite side of the bed.
   - Place a pillow where it will support the client's head after the turn. **Rationale: The pillow prevents lateral

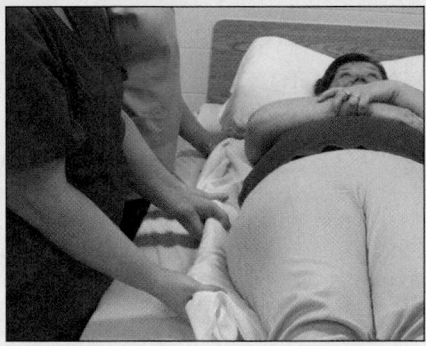

❶ By using a draw sheet, the nurses reposition the client to the edge of the bed.

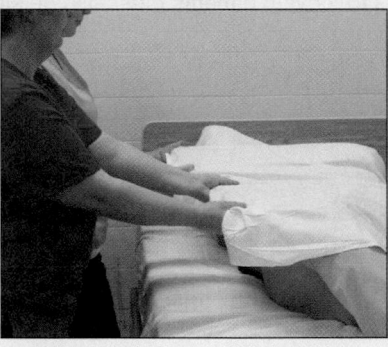

❷ The nurses use the far end of the sheet to roll the client toward them.

flexion of the neck and ensures alignment of the cervical spine.

   - Place one or two pillows between the client's legs to support the upper leg when the client is turned. **Rationale: This pillow prevents adduction of the upper leg, keeps the legs parallel and aligned, and prevents twisting of the spine**.

7. Roll and position the client in proper alignment.

   - Reaching over the client, the two nurses grasp the far edges of the draw sheet or friction-reducing device with the "palms up" grip, with one nurse grasping at the lower hip and thigh and the other grasping at the client's shoulders and lower back.
   - One nurse counts, "One, two, three"; then, at the same time, roll the client to a lateral position by shifting weight from the forward foot to the back foot (see ❷).
   - The nurse behind the client helps turn the client and supports the client's head, back, and upper and lower extremities with pillow supports to ensure good alignment in the lateral position.
   - Raise the siderails and place the call bell within the client's reach.

8. Document all relevant information, including the following:

   - Time and change of position moved from and position moved to
   - Any signs of pressure areas
   - Use of support devices
   - Ability of client to assist in moving and turning
   - Response of client to moving and turning (e.g., anxiety, discomfort, dizziness)

EVIDENCE-INFORMED PRACTICE

What Is the Safest Way to Move a Patient Off a Spine Board Following Trauma?

The authors of this randomized control trial studied the impact of using a "traditional" log roll intervention versus a lift-and-slide technique for moving patients off a spine board following trauma. "Current Advanced Trauma Life Support's recommendations are to log roll the patient 90 degrees, remove the spine board, inspect and palpate the back, and then log roll back to supine position." However, the authors note that "there are several publications showing unacceptable motion in an unstable spine when log rolling." The researchers found that the lift-and-slide technique was safer than the log roll approach and concluded that "spine boards can be removed using a lift-and-slide maneuver with less motion and potentially less risk to the patient's long-term neurologic function than expected using the log roll."

NURSING IMPLICATIONS: Nurses working in emergency departments and trauma centres must be up-to-date on the latest findings around all aspects of care, even such basic issues of moving and positioning patients. Nurses in other settings also use logrolling, such as on neuroscience units, and the effectiveness of logrolling versus alternative approaches to moving patients must also be studied.

Source: Based on Horodyski, M., Conrad, B. P., Del Rossi, G., DiPaola, C. P., & Rechtine, G. R. (2011) Removing a patient from the spine board: Is the lift and slide safer than the log roll? *The Journal of Trauma, 70*(5), 1282–1285.

SKILL 39.4   ASSISTING THE CLIENT TO SIT ON THE SIDE OF THE BED

PURPOSE

The client assumes a sitting position on the edge of the bed before walking, moving to a chair or wheelchair, eating, or performing other activities.

IMPLEMENTATION

Preparation

Determine the following:

- Assistive devices that will be required
- Hindrances to movement, such as an IV or a heavy cast on one leg
- Medications the client is receiving, because certain medications may hamper movement or alertness of the client
- Assistance required from other health care personnel

Performance

1. Before performing the procedure, introduce yourself and verify the client's identity using two identifiers or per agency protocol. Explain to the client what you are going to do, why it is necessary, and how he or she can participate. Discuss how the results will be used in planning further care or treatments.

2. Perform hand hygiene, and follow other appropriate infection prevention and control procedures.

3. Provide for client privacy.

4. Position yourself and the client appropriately before performing the move.
   - Assist the client to a lateral position facing you.
   - Raise the head of the bed slowly to the highest position the client can tolerate, if not contraindicated. **Rationale: This decreases the distance that the client needs to move to sit up on the side of the bed**. (Position the bed height to the lowest position, if the client will be ambulating)
   - Position the client's feet and lower legs at the edge of the bed. **Rationale: This enables the client's feet to move easily off the bed during the movement, and the client is aided by gravity into a sitting position**.
   - Stand beside the client's hips and face the far corner of the bottom of the bed (the angle in which movement will occur). Assume a broad stance, placing the foot nearest the client and head of the bed forward. Lean your trunk slightly forward from the hips. Flex your hips, knees, and ankles (see ❶ A).

5. Move the client to the sitting position.
   - Place the arm nearest to the head of the bed under the client's shoulders and the other arm under both of the client's thighs, near the knees. **Rationale: Supporting the client's shoulders prevents the client from falling backward during the movement. Supporting the client's thighs ensures that the legs and torso move in synchrony**.
   - Tighten your gluteal, pelvic, abdominal, leg, and arm muscles.
   - Instruct the client to push up with the hand closest to you on the count of three.
   - On the count of three, pivot on the balls of your feet in the desired direction, facing the foot of the bed while pulling the client's feet and legs off the bed At the same time, shift weight to the rear leg and elevate the client. (see ❶ B). **Rationale: Pivoting prevents twisting of the nurse's spine. The weight of the client's legs swinging downward increases downward movement of the lower body and helps make the client's upper body vertical**.
   - Keep supporting the client until the client is well balanced and comfortable. **Rationale: This movement may cause some clients to faint**.
   - Assess vital signs (e.g., pulse, respirations, and blood pressure), as indicated by the client's health status.

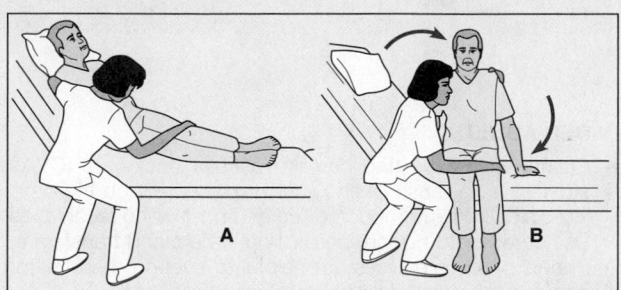

❶ Helping a client to the sitting position on the edge of the bed.

Variation: Teaching a Client How to Sit on the Side of the Bed Independently

- A client who has had recent abdominal surgery or who is weak may have too much abdominal pain or too little strength to sit straight up in bed. This person can be taught to assume a dangle position without assistance. Instruct the client to do the following:
  - Roll to the side and lift the far leg over the near leg (❷ A).
  - Grasp the mattress edge with the lower arm and push the fist of the upper arm into the mattress (❷ B).
  - Push up with the arms as the heels and legs slide over the mattress edge (❷ B).

EVALUATION

- Check the skin integrity of the pressure areas from the previous position.
- Conduct follow-up assessment for previous and new skin breakdown areas.
- Check for proper alignment after the position change. Do a visual check and ask the client for a comfort assessment.

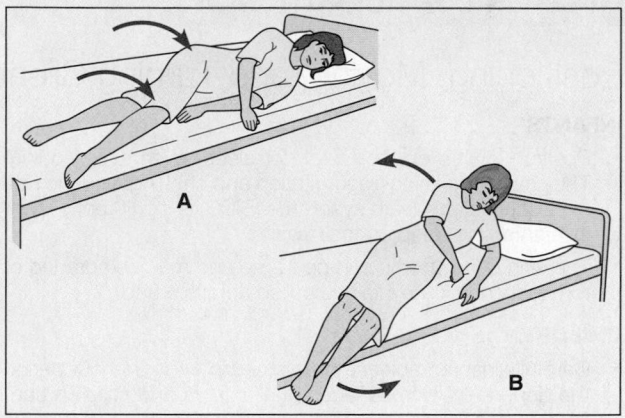

❷ Moving to a sitting position independently.

- Maintain the sitting position by pushing both fists into the mattress behind and to the sides of the buttocks.

6. Document all relevant information, including the following:
   - Ability of the client to assist in moving and turning
   - Response of client to moving and turning (e.g., anxiety, discomfort, dizziness)

- Determine that all required safety precautions (e.g., call bell) are in place.
- Determine client's tolerance of the activity (e.g., vital signs before and after dangling), particularly the first time the client changes position.
- Report significant changes to the appropriate member of the health care team.

See the Lifespan Considerations box and the Home Care Considerations box on page 1180 on positioning, moving, and turning clients.

Transferring Clients

The movement of a client from one surface to another is known as a **transfer**. Many clients require some assistance in transferring between bed and chair or wheelchair, between wheelchair and toilet, and between bed and stretcher. Before transferring any client, however, the nurse must assess and determine the client's physical and mental capabilities to participate in the transfer technique. In addition, the nurse must determine whether the transfer can be safely performed with one or more persons assisting, or if a transfer assist device or a mechanical lift is needed. An assessment of the task, the environment, and the client is essential prior to any client handling task. Refer to the section "Preventing Back Injury" (page 1167) for the assessment required. In addition, the nurse must analyze and organize the activity.

Transfer assist devices may reduce the amount of force exerted by nurses when moving partially or totally dependent clients. Assistive devices help maintain the dignity of clients and provides an increased feeling of comfort and security. A **transfer belt** is an assistive device used when moving or transferring a client. Transfer belts usually have handles, which the nurse can hold, to increase stability for both the nurse and client (Figure 39.51 on the next page). It enhances safety during transfer of a client and helps prevent back injury to the nurse. When used during ambulation, it is often referred to as a **gait belt**. The terms *transfer belt* and *gait belt* are often used interchangeably. The belt is positioned around the client's waist, over clothes, and allows the nurse to control movement of the client. When positioned properly, the nurse should only be able to place two fingers between the belt and the client. Most health care agencies require personnel to use a transfer belt to ambulate or move clients.

A sliding/transfer board is another device that can be used when transferring a client between a bed and stretcher, and bed to chair (Figure 39.52 on the next page). These devices are used to reduce friction and bridge gaps when sliding clients between surfaces such as from a bed to a stretcher.

LIFESPAN CONSIDERATIONS

Positioning, Moving, and Turning Clients

INFANTS

- Position infants on their back for sleep, even after feeding. They have little risk of regurgitation and choking, and the rate of sudden infant death syndrome (SIDS) is significantly lower in infants who sleep on their backs.
- The skin of newborns can be fragile and may be abraded or torn (sheared) if the infant is pulled across a bed.

CHILDREN

- Carefully inspect at least three times in each 24-hour period the dependent skin surfaces of all infants and children confined to bed.

OLDER ADULTS

- Clients who have had cerebrovascular accidents (CVAs, strokes) have a risk of shoulder displacement on the paralyzed side from improper moving or repositioning techniques. Use care when moving, positioning in bed, and transferring. Pillows or foam devices are helpful to support the affected arm and shoulder and prevent injury.
- Decreased subcutaneous fat and thinning of the skin place older adults at risk for skin breakdown. Repositioning approximately every 2 hours (more or less, depending on the unique needs of the individual client) helps reduce pressure on bony prominences and avoid tissue trauma.

HOME CARE CONSIDERATIONS

Positioning, Moving, and Turning Clients

- Assess the height of the bed and the person's leg length to ensure that self-movement in and out of the bed are smooth.
- Inspect the client's mattress for support.
- Assess the caregivers' knowledge and application of body mechanics to prevent injury.
- Demonstrate how to turn and position the client in bed. Observe the caregiver performing a return demonstration. Re-evaluate this technique periodically to reinforce correct application of body mechanics.
- Teach caregivers the basic principles of body alignment and how to check for proper alignment after the client has been changed to a new position.

- Warn caregivers of the dangers of lifting and repositioning and encourage the use of assistive devices and a "no solo lift" policy.
- Teach the caregiver to check the client's skin for redness and integrity after repositioning the client. Stress the importance of informing the nurse about the length of time skin redness remains over pressure areas after the person has been repositioned. Emphasize that reddened areas should not be massaged as it may lead to tissue trauma.

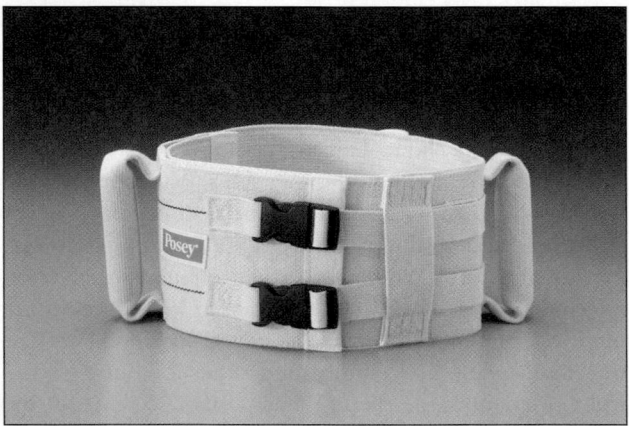

FIGURE 39.51 Transfer or gait belt with handles.

Source: Image provided by Posey Company, Arcadia, California.

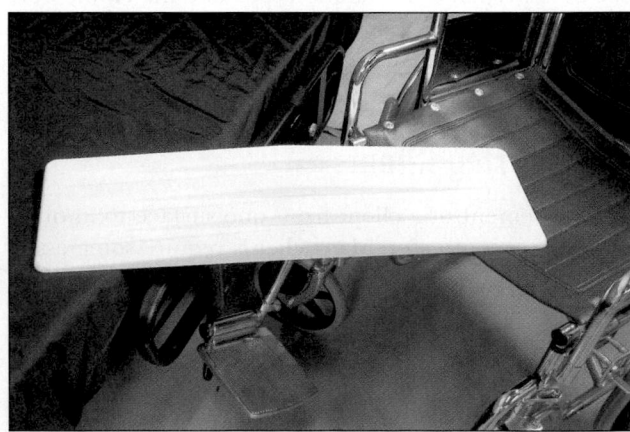

FIGURE 39.52 Plastic transfer board.

Source: Image provided by Posey Company, Arcadia, California.

Before using any assistive device, the nurse should receive training in their use and ensure the device is in working order and always be familiar with manufacturer's guidelines and agency policy before using. See Skill 39.5 on transferring a client between a bed and a chair and Skill 39.6 on on page 1183 transferring a client between a bed and a stretcher.

SKILL 39.5 **TRANSFERRING BETWEEN BED AND CHAIR**

PURPOSE

A client may need to be transferred between the bed and a wheelchair or chair, the bed and the commode, or a wheelchair and the toilet. This technique has numerous variations. Which variation the nurse selects depends on factors related to the client, the environment, and the health care provider, which are assessed before beginning the transfer.

ASSESSMENT

Before transferring a client, assess the following:

- Client's body size
- Client's ability to follow instructions
- Client's activity tolerance
- Client's muscle strength and ability to bear weight
- Client's joint mobility
- Presence of paralysis or paresis
- Client's level of comfort
- Presence of orthostatic hypotension
- Transfer technique with which the client is familiar
- Space in which the transfer will need to be manoeuvred (bathrooms, for example, are usually cramped)
- The number of assistants needed to accomplish the transfer safely
- The skill and ability of the nurses

PLANNING

Review the client record to determine whether previous nurses have recorded information about the client's ability to tolerate the transfer. Implement pain relief measures so that they are effective when the transfer begins. The decision must be made at this time regarding the client's ability to participate. If the client can participate in the transfer, a transfer belt or sliding board can be used; if not, a mechanical lift would be safer for the client and nurse.

Equipment

- Robe or appropriate clothing
- Slippers or shoes with nonskid soles
- Transfer/gait belt
- Chair, commode, or wheelchair, as appropriate to client need
- Sliding board, or mechanical lift, as appropriate

Preparation

- Plan what to do and how to do it.
- Obtain essential equipment before starting (e.g., transfer belt, wheelchair), and check that it is functioning correctly.
- Remove obstacles from the area used for the transfer.

Performance

1. Before performing the procedure, introduce yourself and verify the client's identity using two identifiers or per agency protocol. Explain the transfer process to the client. During the transfer, explain step by step what the client should do, for example, "Move your right foot forward."

2. Perform hand hygiene, and follow other appropriate infection prevention and control procedures.

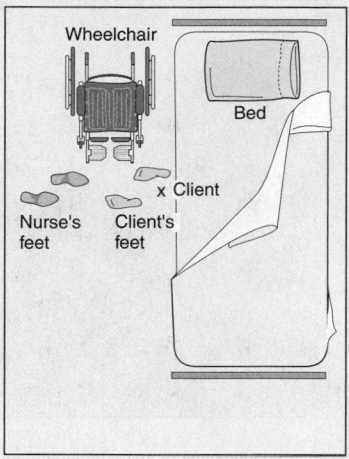

❶ The wheelchair is placed parallel to the bed as close to the bed as possible. Note that placement of the nurse's feet mirrors that of the client's feet.

3. Provide for client privacy.

4. Position the equipment appropriately.
   - Lower the bed to its lowest position so that the client's feet will rest flat on the floor. Lock the wheels of the bed.
   - Place the wheelchair parallel to the bed and as close to the bed as possible (see ❶). Put the wheelchair on the side of the bed that allows the client to move toward his or her stronger side. Lock the wheels of the wheelchair and remove or raise the footplates.

5. Prepare and assess the client.
   - Assist the client to a sitting position on the side of the bed (see Skill 39.4 on page 1178).
   - Assess the client for orthostatic hypotension before moving the client from the bed.
   - Assist the client in putting on a bathrobe and nonskid slippers or shoes.
   - Place a transfer belt snugly around the client's waist. Check to be certain that the belt is securely fastened.

6. Give explicit instructions to the client. Ask the client to do the following:
   - Move forward and sit on the edge of the bed with feet placed flat on the floor. **Rationale: This brings the client's centre of gravity closer to the nurse's.**
   - Lean forward slightly from the hips. **Rationale: This brings the client's centre of gravity more directly over the base of support and positions the head and trunk in the direction of the movement.**
   - Place the foot of the stronger leg beneath the edge of the bed, and put the other foot forward. **Rationale: In this way, the client can use the stronger leg muscles to stand and power the movement. A broader base of support makes the client more stable during the transfer.**
   - Place the client's hands on the bed surface so that the client can push while standing, unless contraindicated **Rationale: This action provides additional force for the movement and reduces the potential for strain**

(continued)

SKILL 39.5 TRANSFERRING BETWEEN BED AND CHAIR (*continued*)

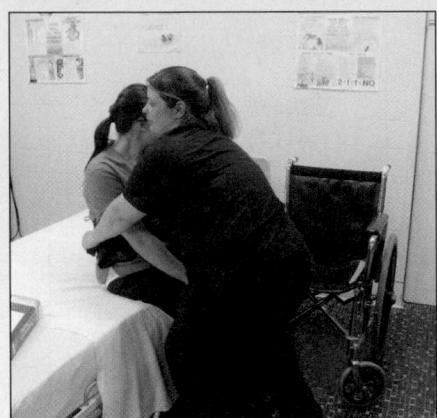

❷ Using a transfer belt

on the nurse's back. The client should not grasp your neck or shoulders for support. **Rationale: Doing so can cause injury to the nurse**.

7. Position yourself correctly.

   • Stand directly in front of the client and to the side requiring the most support. Lean the trunk slightly forward from the hips. Flex the hips, knees, and ankles. Assume a broad stance, placing one foot forward and one back. Brace the client's feet with your feet, while supporting the client's weaker knee or leg with your leg to prevent the client from sliding forward or laterally. Mirror the placement of the client's feet, if possible. **Rationale: This action helps prevent loss of balance during the transfer**.

   • Encircle the client's waist with your arms, and grasp the transfer belt at the client's back or toward his or her side (see ❷), with thumbs pointing downward. **Rationale: The belt provides a secure handle for holding onto the client and controlling the movement. Downward placement of the thumbs prevents potential wrist injury as the nurse lifts. By supporting the client in this manner, you keep the client from tilting backward during the transfer**.

   • Tighten your gluteal, pelvic, abdominal, leg, and arm muscles.

8. Assist the client to stand, and then move together toward the wheelchair.

   • On the count of three, ask the client to push with the back foot, rock to the forward foot, and extend (straighten) the joints of the lower extremities, while you transfer your weight from one foot to the other (while keeping your back straight) and stand upright moving the client forward (directly toward your centre of gravity) into the standing position. Ask the client to push up with hands, if possible. If the client requires more than a very small degree of pulling, a mechanical device should be used.

   • Support the client in an upright standing position for a few moments. **Rationale: This action allows the**

nurse and the client to extend the joints and provides the nurse with an opportunity to ensure that the client is stable before moving away from the bed.

   • Together, pivot on your foot farthest from the chair, or take a few steps toward the wheelchair.

9. Assist the client to sit.

   • Move the wheelchair forward, or have the client back up to the wheelchair and place his or her legs against the seat. **Rationale: Having the client place the legs against the wheelchair seat minimizes the risk of the client's falling when sitting down**.

   • Ensure the wheelchair brakes are on.

   • Place the foot of the stronger leg slightly behind the other. **Rationale: This supports body weight during the movement and provides a broad base of support**.

   • Have the client place both hands on the wheelchair arms (if possible). **Rationale: This increases stability and lessens the strain on the nurse**.

   • Stand directly in front of the client. Place one foot forward and one back.

   • Tighten your grasp on the transfer belt, and tighten your gluteal, pelvic, abdominal, leg, and arm muscles.

   • On the count of three, have the client sit down while you bend your knees and hips and lower the client to the wheelchair seat.

10. Ensure client safety.

   • Ask the client to push back into the wheelchair seat. **Rationale: Sitting well back on the seat provides a broader base of support and greater stability and minimizes the risk of falling from the wheelchair. A wheelchair can topple forward when the client sits on the edge of the seat and leans far forward**.

   • Lower the footplates, and place the client's feet on them, if applicable.

   • Remove the transfer belt and apply a seatbelt as required.

Variation: Angling the Wheelchair

   • For clients who have difficulty walking, place the wheelchair at a 45-degree angle to the bed. **Rationale: This enables the client to pivot into the chair and lessens the amount of body rotation required**.

Variation: Transferring Using a Belt and Two Nurses

   • When the client is ready to stand, position yourselves on both sides of the client, facing the same direction as the client. Flex your hips, knees, and ankles; grasp the client's transfer belt at the back with the hand closest to the client, and with the other hand, support the client's elbows.

   • Coordinating your efforts, all three of you stand simultaneously, pivot, and move to the wheelchair. Reverse the process to lower the client onto the wheelchair seat.

Variation: Transferring a Client with an Injured Lower Extremity or Hemiparesis

- When the client has an injured lower extremity, movement should always occur toward the client's unaffected (strong) side. For example, if the client's right leg is injured and the client is sitting on the edge of bed preparing to transfer to a wheelchair, position the wheelchair on the client's left side. **Rationale: In this way, the client can use the unaffected leg most effectively and safely.**

Variation: Using a Sliding Board

- For clients who cannot stand but are able to cooperate and have sufficient upper body strength, use a sliding board to help them move without assistance. This method not only promotes the client's sense of independence but preserves your energy (see ❸).

11. Document relevant information, including the following:
    - Client's ability to bear weight and pivot
    - Number of staff needed for transfer
    - Length of time up in chair
    - Client response to transfer and being up in chair or wheelchair

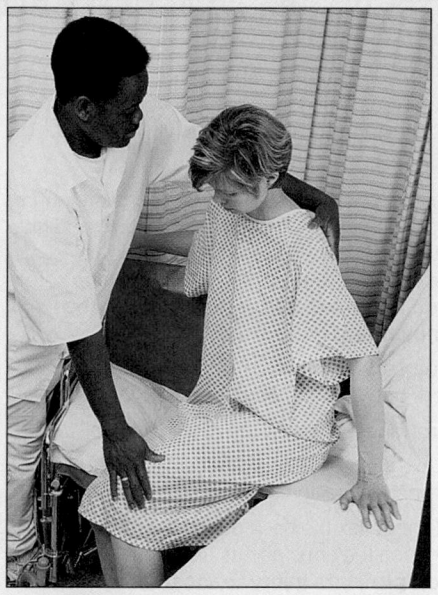

❸ Using a sliding board

SKILL 39.6   TRANSFERRING BETWEEN BED AND STRETCHER

PURPOSE

The stretcher, or *gurney,* is used to transfer supine clients from one location to another. Whenever the client is capable of accomplishing the transfer from bed to stretcher independently, either by lifting onto it or by rolling onto it, the client should be encouraged to do so. If the client cannot move onto the stretcher independently, at least three nurses are needed to assist with the transfer. Transfer assistive devices such as a friction-reducing device and/or lateral transfer (sliding) board should be used. A mechanical lift may be required.

ASSESSMENT

Before transferring a client, assess the following:
- Client's body size and weight
- Client's ability to follow instructions
- Client's activity tolerance
- Client's level of comfort
- The space in which the transfer is manoeuvred
- The number of assistants needed to accomplish the transfer safely
- The skill and ability of the nurses

PLANNING

Review the client record to determine whether previous nurses have recorded information about how the client tolerated similar transfers. If indicated, implement pain relief measures so that they are effective when the transfer begins.

Equipment

- Stretcher
- Transfer assistive devices (e.g., drawsheet, friction-reducing devices, transfer/sliding board, mechanical lift).

Preparation

Obtain the necessary equipment and nursing personnel to assist in the transfer.

Performance

1. Before performing the procedure, introduce yourself and verify the client's identity using two identifiers or per agency protocol. Explain to the client what you are going to do, why it is necessary, and how he or she can participate. Explain the transfer to the nursing personnel who are helping and specify who will give directions (one person needs to be in charge).

2. Perform hand hygiene, and follow other appropriate infection prevention and control procedures.

3. Provide for client privacy.

4. Adjust the client's bed in preparation for the transfer.
   - Lower the head of the bed until it is flat or as low as the client can tolerate.
   - Raise the bed so that it is slightly higher (2.5 cm) than the surface of the stretcher. **Rationale: It is easier for the client to move down an incline**.
   - Ensure that the wheels on the bed are locked.
   - Pull the drawsheet out from both sides of the bed.

5. Move the client to the edge of the bed, and position the stretcher.
   - Roll the drawsheet as close to the client's side as possible.
   - Reposition the client to the edge of the bed, and cover the client with a sheet or bath blanket to maintain comfort.
   - Place the stretcher parallel to the bed, next to the client, and lock its wheels.
   - Fill any gap that exists between the bed and the stretcher loosely with bath blankets (optional).

(continued)

SKILL 39.6 **TRANSFERRING BETWEEN BED AND STRETCHER** (*continued*)

6. Transfer the client securely to the stretcher.
   - If the client can transfer independently, encourage him or her to do so and stand by for safety.
   - If the client is partially able or not able to transfer:
     - Two nurses are positioned at the side of the stretcher: one positioned between the client's shoulders and hip and the other between the client's hip and lower legs, each pressing tightly against the stretcher. **Rationale: This action achieves better control over the client's movement**.
     - The third nurse is positioned on the other side of the client's bed, between the client's shoulder and hip
     - Roll the drawsheet close to the client with the "palms up" grip.
     - All nurses should position their feet in a walking stance.
     - Ask the client to flex the neck during the move, if possible, and place the arms across the chest. **Rationale: This action prevents injury to those body parts**.
     - On a planned command, the nurses at the stretcher's side pull (shifting weight from the forward foot to the rear foot), and the nurse at the bedside pushes the client toward the stretcher (shifting weight to the front foot).
   - A slider sheet may be used to decrease friction between the bed and client, facilitating easier movement.
7. Ensure client comfort and safety.
   - Make the client comfortable, unlock the stretcher wheels, and move the stretcher away from the bed.
   - Immediately raise the stretcher side rails and fasten the safety straps across the client. **Rationale: Because the stretcher is high and narrow, the client is in danger of falling unless these safety precautions are taken**.

Variation: Using a Transfer Board

- The transfer board is a lacquered or smooth polyethylene board measuring 45 cm to 55 cm by 182 cm with handholds along its edges. Transfer mattresses are also available, as are mechanical assistive devices. It is

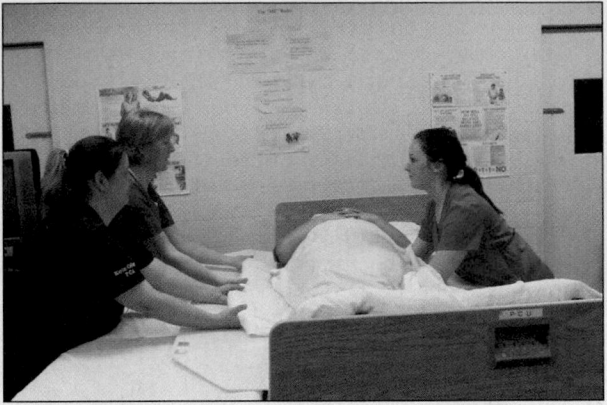

❶ Transfer from bed to stretcher using a transfer board.

imperative to have enough people assisting with the transfer to prevent injury to staff as well as clients. Ensure that two nurses are in position on the side of the bed where the stretcher is and the third nurse on the opposite side of the bed. Turn the client to a lateral position toward the one nurse using the drawsheet. Position the board under the drawsheet, close to the client's back, and between the bed and stretcher, and roll the client onto the board. The transfer board acts as a bridge, reducing the amount of friction when transferring. Transfer the client to the stretcher using the drawsheet with the "palms up" grip and shifting weight from the front foot to the rear foot (see ❶). The nurse on the opposite side of the bed holds the transfer board in position during transfer. Safety belts may be placed over the chest, abdomen, and legs when the client is positioned on the centre of the stretcher.

8. Document relevant information, including the following:
   - Equipment used
   - Number of people needed for transfer
   - Destination if reason for transfer is transport from one location to another

EVALUATION

- Compare client capabilities, such as weight-bearing ability, pivoting ability, and strength and control to previous transfers.

- Report any significant deviations from normal to the appropriate members of the health care team.

General guidelines for transfer techniques include the following:

- Plan what to do and how to do it. Determine the space in which the transfer will take place (bathrooms, for instance, are usually cramped); the number of assistants needed to accomplish the transfer safely; the skill and ability of the nurse(s); whether a mechanical lift is required; and the client's capabilities.
- Check physician's orders and agency policies.

- Obtain essential equipment before starting (e.g., wheelchair, transfer/gait belt, mechanical lift), and check its function.
- Remove obstacles from the area used for the transfer.
- Explain the transfer to the client, including what the client should do.
- Explain the transfer to the nursing personnel who are helping; specify who will give directions (one person needs to be in charge).

- Place equipment to allow client to move toward stronger side.

- Always support or hold the client rather than the equipment and ensure the client's safety and dignity.

- During the transfer, explain step by step what the client should do, for example, "Move your right foot forward."

- Make a written plan of the transfer, including the client's tolerance (e.g., pulse and respiratory rates, blood pressure, and oxygen saturation).

Because wheelchairs and stretchers are unstable, they can cause falls and injury. Guidelines for the safe use of wheelchairs and stretchers are shown in Box 39.3.

Providing Range-of-Motion Exercises

When people are unwell, they often need to perform range-of-motion (ROM) exercises until they regain their normal activity levels. **Active ROM exercises** are isotonic exercises in which the client moves each joint in the body through its complete range of movement, maximally stretching all muscle groups within each plane over the joint. These exercises maintain or increase muscle strength, length, and endurance, and they help maintain cardiorespiratory function in an immobilized client. They also prevent deterioration of joint capsules, ankylosis, and contractures.

Full ROM does not occur spontaneously in the immobilized individual who independently achieves ADLs, moves about in bed, transfers between bed and wheelchair or chair, or ambulates a short distance because only a few muscle groups are maximally stretched during these activities. Although the client may successfully achieve some active ROM movements of the upper extremities while combing the hair, bathing, and dressing, the immobilized client is very unlikely to achieve any active ROM movements of the lower extremities when these are not used in the normal functions of standing and walking about. For this reason, most wheelchair and many ambulatory clients need active ROM exercises until they regain their normal activity levels.

At first, the nurse may need to teach the client and family to perform the needed ROM exercises; eventually, the client may be able to accomplish these independently. Instructions for the client performing active ROM exercises are shown in the Teaching: Clinical box on the next page.

During **passive ROM exercises**, another person moves each of the client's joints through its complete range of movement, maximally stretching all muscle groups within each plane over each joint. Because the client does not contract the muscles, passive ROM exercises are of no value in maintaining muscle strength but are useful in maintaining joint flexibility. For this reason, passive ROM exercises should be performed only when the client is unable to accomplish the movements actively.

Passive ROM exercises should be accomplished for each movement of the arms, legs, and neck *that the client is unable to achieve actively*. As with active ROM exercises, passive ROM exercises should be accomplished to the

---

BOX 39.3 WHEELCHAIR SAFETY AND THE SAFE USE OF STRETCHERS

Wheelchairs and stretchers are unsteady, and the nurse must take care when using them with clients:

WHEELCHAIRS

- Always lock the brakes on both wheels of the wheelchair when the client transfers into or out of it. Locks should be used at all times, except when the client is being moved.

- Remove (if possible) or raise the footplates before transferring the client into the wheelchair.

- Lower the footplates after the transfer, and place the client's feet on them.

- Ensure the client is positioned well back in the seat of the wheelchair.

- Ensure body alignment is maintained. Protect extremities when transporting client (for example, through doorways).

- Use seatbelts that fasten behind the wheelchair to protect confused clients from falls. *Note:* Seatbelts are a form of restraint and must be used in accordance with policies and procedures that apply to the use of restraints (see Chapter 32).

- Back the wheelchair into or out of an elevator, rear large wheels first.

- Place your body between the wheelchair and the bottom of an incline.

STRETCHERS

- Lock the wheels of the bed and stretcher before the client is transferred into or out of them.

- Fasten safety straps across the client on a stretcher, and raise the side rails.

- Never leave a client unattended on a stretcher unless the wheels are locked and the side rails are raised on both sides or the safety straps are securely fastened across the client.

- Always push a stretcher from the end at which the client's head is positioned. This position protects the client's head in the event of a collision.

- If the stretcher has two swivel wheels and two stationary wheels, do the following:
  a. Always position the client's head at the end with the stationary wheels.
  b. Push the stretcher from the end with the stationary wheels. The stretcher is manoeuvred more easily when pushed from this end.

- Manoeuvre the stretcher when entering the elevator so that the client's head goes in first.

TEACHING CLINICAL

Active Range-of-Motion Exercises

These instructions are for clients who need to perform ROM exercises:

- Perform each ROM exercise as taught to the point of slight resistance, but not beyond, and never to the point of discomfort.
- Perform the movements systematically by using the same sequence during each session.
- Perform each exercise three to five times.
- Perform each series of exercises at least three times daily, as tolerated.
- For older clients, it is not essential to achieve full ROM in all joints, Instead, emphasize that ROM exercise is also achieved while the client carries out ADLs, such as walking, dressing, combing hair, showering, and preparing a meal.

point of slight resistance, but not beyond and never to the point of discomfort. The movements should be systematic, and the same sequence should be followed during each exercise session. Each exercise should consist of three to five repetitions, and the series of exercises should be done at least three times daily, as tolerated by the client.

Performing one series of exercises along with the bath is helpful. Passive ROM exercises are accomplished most effectively when the client lies supine in bed. General guidelines for providing passive exercises are shown in Practice Guidelines 39.1.

During **active-assistive ROM exercises**, the client uses a stronger, opposite arm or leg to move each of the joints of a limb incapable of active motion. The client learns to support and move the weak arm or leg with the strong arm or leg as far as possible. Then, the nurse continues the movement passively to its maximal degree. This activity increases active movement on the strong side of the client's body and maintains joint flexibility on the weak side. Such exercise is especially useful for clients who are hemiplegic.

Ambulating Clients

Ambulation (the act of walking) is a function that most people take for granted. However, when people are ill, they are often confined to bed and are thus nonambulatory. The longer clients are in bed, the more difficulty they have walking.

Even one or two days of bed rest can make a person feel weak and unsteady when first getting out of bed. A client who has had surgery, is older, or who has been immobilized for a longer time will feel more pronounced weakness. The potential problems of immobility are far less likely to occur when clients become ambulatory as soon as possible. The nurse can assist clients to prepare for ambulation by helping them become as independent as possible while in bed. Nurses should encourage clients to perform ADLs, maintain good body alignment, and carry out active ROM exercises to the maximum degree possible yet within the limitations imposed by their illness and recovery program.

PREAMBULATORY EXERCISES Clients who have been in bed for long periods often need a plan of isometric exercises to strengthen the muscles used for walking before attempting to walk. A physician's order may be required. One of the most important muscle groups is the quadriceps femoris, which extends the knee and flexes the thigh. This group is also important for elevating the legs, for example, for walking upstairs. These exercises are frequently called *quadriceps drills* or *sets*. To strengthen these muscles, the client consciously tenses them, drawing the kneecap upward and inward. The client pushes the popliteal space of the knee against the bed surface, relaxing the heels on the bed surface (Figure 39.53). On the count of 1, the muscles are tensed; they are held during the counts of 2, 3, 4; and they are relaxed at the count of 5. The exercise should be done within the client's tolerance, that is, without fatiguing the muscles. Carried out several times an hour during waking hours, this simple exercise significantly strengthens the muscles used for walking.

ASSISTING CLIENTS TO AMBULATE Clients who have been immobilized for even a few days may require assistance with ambulation. The amount of assistance will depend on the client's condition, including age, health status, cognition, and length of inactivity. Assistance may mean walking alongside the client while providing physical support (see Skill 39.7 on page 1188) or providing instruction to the client about the use of assistive devices, such as a cane, walker, or crutches (discussed later in this chapter). See also the Lifespan Considerations box on helping clients ambulate on page 1190.

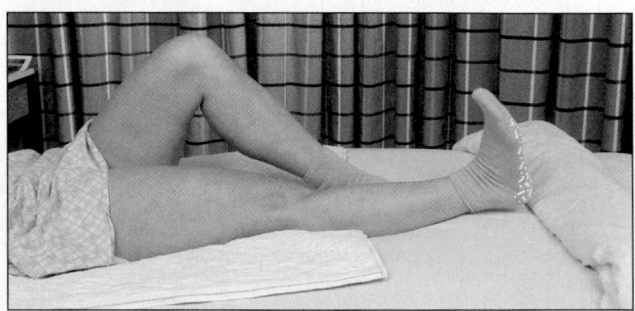

FIGURE 39.53 Tensing the quadriceps femoris muscles before ambulation.

PRACTICE GUIDELINES 39.1

Providing Passive Range-of-Motion Exercises

Guidelines	Rationales
• Ensure that the client understands the reason for doing ROM exercises.	• Understanding improves collaboration.
• If there is a possibility of hand swelling, make sure rings are removed.	• This measure prevents any discomfort for the client.
• Clothe the client in a loose gown, and cover the body with a bath blanket.	• Covering the client promotes comfort and dignity.
• Use correct body mechanics when providing ROM exercise.	• Doing this will avoid muscle strain or injury to both you and the client.
• Expose only the limb being exercised.	• Keeping the client covered avoids embarrassing the client.
• Support the client's limbs above and below the joint, as needed. (Figure 39.54). This may also be done by cupping joints in the palm of your hand or cradling limbs along your forearm (Figure 39.55). If a joint is painful, support the limb in the muscular areas above and below the joint.	• Supporting the limbs will prevent muscle strain or injury.
• Use a firm, comfortable grip when handling the limb, and move the body parts smoothly, slowly, and rhythmically.	• Jerky movements cause discomfort and, possibly, injury. Fast movements can cause spasticity (sudden, prolonged involuntary muscle contraction) or rigidity (stiffness or inflexibility).
• Avoid moving or forcing a body part beyond the existing ROM. This is particularly important for people with flaccid paralysis, whose muscles can be stretched and joints dislocated without their awareness.	• Forcing a body part can cause muscle strain, pain, and injury.
• If muscle spasticity occurs during movement, stop the movement temporarily, but continue to apply slow, gentle pressure on the part until the muscle relaxes; then proceed with the motion.	• This process avoids any trauma to the muscle.
• If a contracture is present, apply slow firm pressure, without causing pain.	• This measure prevents injury yet increases the ROM of the joint.
• If rigidity occurs, apply slight pressure against the rigidity and continue the exercise slowly, if possible.	• This action helps muscles become slightly more relaxed, thus increasing the ROM.

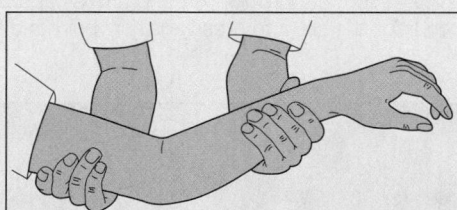

FIGURE 39.54 Supporting a limb above and below the joint for passive exercise.

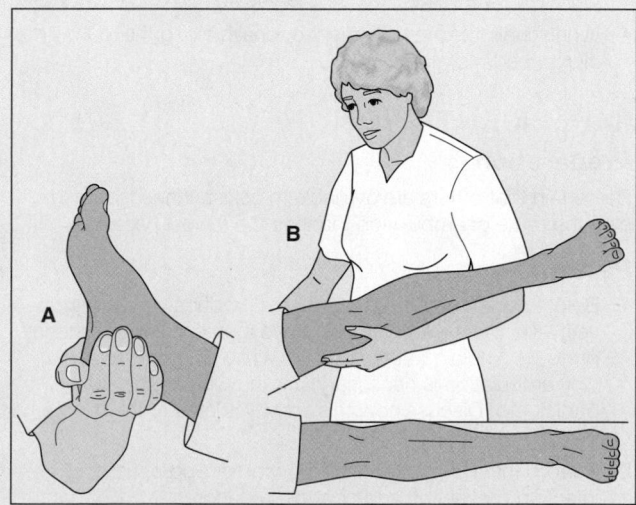

FIGURE 39.55 Holding limbs for support during passive exercise: **A:** Cupping; **B:** Cradling.

Some clients experience postural (orthostatic) hypotension on assuming a vertical position from a lying position and may need information about ways to control this problem (see the Teaching: Clinical box on controlling postural hypotension on page 1190). The client may exhibit some or all of the following symptoms: pallor,

SKILL 39.7 ASSISTING THE CLIENT TO AMBULATE

PURPOSE

- To provide a safe condition for the client to walk with whatever support is needed.

ASSESSMENT

Assess

- Length of time in bed and time up previously
- Baseline vital signs
- ROM of joints needed for ambulating (e.g., hips, knees, ankles)
- Muscle strength of lower extremities
- Need for ambulation aids (e.g., cane, walker, crutches)
- Client's intake of medications (e.g., opioids, sedatives, and antihypertensives) that may cause drowsiness, dizziness, weakness, and orthostatic hypotension and hinder the client's ability to walk safely
- Presence of joint inflammation, fractures, muscle weakness, or other conditions that impair physical mobility
- Ability to understand directions
- Level of comfort

PLANNING

Implement pain relief measures so that they are effective when the transfer begins. The amount of assistance needed while ambulating will depend on the client's condition, for example, age, health status, length of inactivity, and emotional readiness. Review any previous experiences with ambulation and the success of such efforts. Plan the length of the walk with the client, in light of the nursing or physician's orders. Be prepared to shorten the walk according to the person's activity tolerance.

Equipment

- Gait belt, whether or not the client is known to be unsteady.
- Wheelchair for following client or chairs along the route if the client needs to rest

IMPLEMENTATION

Preparation

Be certain that others are available to assist, if needed. Also, plan the route of ambulation that has the fewest hazards.

Performance

1. Before performing the procedure, introduce yourself and verify the client's identity using two identifiers or per agency protocol. Explain to the client how you are going to assist, why ambulation is necessary, and how he or she can participate. Discuss how this activity relates to the overall plan of care.
2. Perform hand hygiene, and follow other appropriate infection prevention and control procedures.
3. Ensure that the client is appropriately dressed to walk and has shoes or slippers with nonskid soles.

4. Prepare the client for ambulation.
   - Assist the client to sit up in bed for at least 1 minute, and then assist the client to sit on the edge of the bed (see Skill 39.4 on page 1178) for a least 1 minute with legs dangling, before standing.
   - Assess the client carefully for signs and symptoms of orthostatic hypotension (dizziness, light-headedness, pallor, or a sudden increase in blood pressure and heart rate) before leaving the bedside.
   - Ensure that the client is appropriately dressed to walk and wears shoes or slippers with nonskid soles. **Rationale: Proper attire and footwear prevent chilling and falling**.
   - Assist the client to stand by the side of the bed until the client feels secure.
   - Use a gait belt and ensure the belt is pulled snugly around the client's waist and fastened securely. Grasp the gait belt at the client's back. The client's hand/arm can be supported with the other hand in a palm to palm grip (see ❶) or by supporting the client's forearm with your hand.
5. Ensure client safety while assisting the client to ambulate.
   - Encourage the client to ambulate independently if the client is able, but walk beside the client's weak side and slightly behind, if appropriate.
   - Remain physically close to the client in case assistance is needed at any point.
   - If it is the client's first time out of bed following surgery, injury, or an extended period of immobility, or if the client is quite weak or unstable, have an assistant follow you and the client with a wheelchair in case it is needed quickly.
   - If the client is moderately weak and unstable, walk on the client's weaker side, holding the gait belt near the client's back and support the client's hand/arm as appropriate Encourage the client to press against your hand for

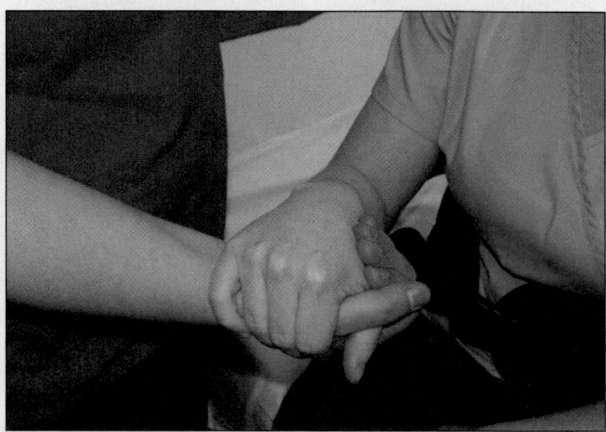

❶ Palm to palm grip.

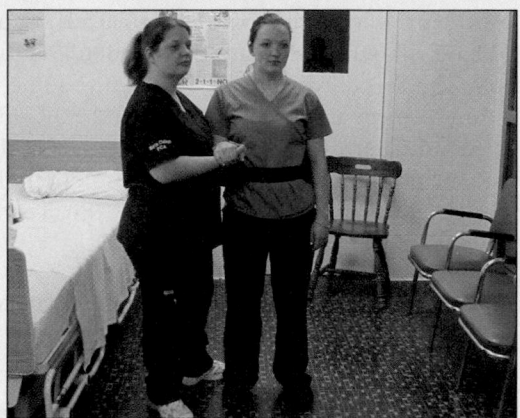

❷ Using a transfer (gait) belt to support the client.

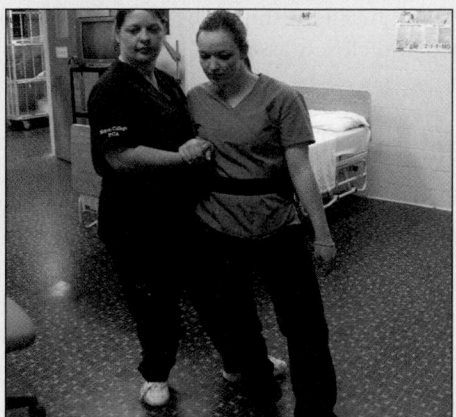

❸ Lowering a fainting client to the floor.

stability, if desired (see ❷). **Rationale: This measure provides stability and support for the client and the nurse and can prevent a fall if the client feels faint.**

- Encourage the client to assume a normal walking stance and gait as much as possible. Ask the client to straighten the back and raise the head so that the eyes are looking forward in a normal horizontal plane. **Rationale: Clients who are unsure of their ability to ambulate tend to look down at their feet, which makes them more likely to fall.**

- If the client is very weak and unstable, two people should assist with walking. **Rationale: The nurse and client are at risk of injury if the client is so compromised.**

6. Protect the client who begins to fall while ambulating.

- If a client begins to experience the signs and symptoms of orthostatic hypotension or extreme weakness, quickly assist the client into a nearby wheelchair or other chair, and help the client to lower the head between the knees if not contraindicated. **Rationale: Lowering the head facilitates blood flow to the brain.**

- Stay with the client. **Rationale: A client who faints while in this position could fall, head first, out of the chair.**

- When the weakness subsides, assist the client back to bed.

- If a chair is not close by, assist the client to a horizontal position on the floor before fainting occurs (see ❸). **Rationale: A vertical position may increase feelings of faintness.**

  a. Assume a broad stance with one foot in front of the other. **Rationale: A broad stance widens the nurse's base of support for stability. Placing one foot behind the other allows the nurse to rock backward and uses the femoral muscles when supporting the client's weight and lowering the centre of gravity thus preventing back strain.**

  b. Bring the client backward so that your body supports the person. **Rationale: Clients who do faint or start to fall and cannot regain their strength or**

balance usually drop straight downward or pitch slightly forward because of the momentum of ambulating; thus, their head, hips, and knees are most vulnerable to injury. Bringing the client's weight backward against the nurse's body allows gradual movement to the floor without injury to the client.**

  c. Extend one leg and allow the client to slide down your leg, and lower the person gently to the floor, making sure the client's head does not hit any objects. (see ❸). **Rationale: Bringing the client's weight against the nurse's body allows gradual movement to the floor without injury to the client.**

Variation: Two Nurses

- After the client stands, assume a position with one nurse at either side and each nurse grasps the side handle of the gait belt with the near hand and supports the client's hands/ arms with their other hand in a palm to palm grip or by supporting the client's forearm with their hand. **Rationale: This provides a secure grip for each nurse.**

- Walk in unison with the client, using a smooth, even gait, at the same speed and with steps the same size as the client's. **Rationale: This gives the client a greater feeling of security.**

- If the client starts to fall and cannot regain strength or balance, guide the client to the floor as previously described.

7. Document the distance and duration of ambulation in the client record. Include a description of the client's gait (including body alignment) when walking; pace; activity tolerance when walking (e.g., pulse rate, facial colour, any shortness of breath, feelings of dizziness, or weakness); degree of support required; and respiratory rate and blood pressure after initial ambulation to compare with baseline data.

EVALUATION

Establish a plan for continued ambulation based on expected or normal ability for the client.

diaphoresis, nausea, tachycardia, and dizziness. If any of these are present, the client should be assisted to a supine position in bed and closely assessed.

Using Mechanical Aids for Walking

Mechanical aids for ambulation include canes, walkers, and crutches.

CANES Three types of canes are used: (a) the standard straight-legged cane; (b) the tripod or crab cane, which has three feet; and (c) the quad cane, which has four feet and provides the most support (Figure 39.56). Cane tips should have rubber caps to improve traction and prevent slipping. The standard cane is 91 cm long; some aluminum canes can be adjusted from 56 cm to 97 cm. The length should permit the elbow to be slightly flexed. Clients may use either one or two canes depending on how much support they require. See the Teaching: Clinical box on using canes.

WALKERS Walkers are mechanical devices for ambulatory clients who need more support than a cane

---

LIFESPAN CONSIDERATIONS

Assisting the Client to Ambulate

CHILDREN

* Children and adolescents who have suffered a sports injury (e.g., sprained ankle) may want to be more active than they should be. A cast, splint, or boot may be put in place to limit activity and assist in healing. Teach the child the importance of appropriate activity, and the use of assistive devices (e.g., crutches), if necessary. Help them focus on what they *can* do rather than what they cannot do (e.g., you can stand at the free-throw line and shoot baskets).

OLDER ADULTS

* Inquire how the client has ambulated previously and modify assistance accordingly.
* Take into account a decrease in speed, strength, resistance to fatigue, reaction time, and coordination because of a decrease in nerve conduction.
* Be cautious when using a transfer belt with a client with osteoporosis. Too much pressure from the belt can increase the risk of vertebral compression fractures.

* If assistive devices, such as a walker or cane, are used, make sure clients are supervised in the beginning to learn the proper method of using them. Crutches may be much more difficult for older adults because of decreased upper body strength.
* Be alert to signs of activity intolerance, especially in older adults with cardiac and lung problems.
* Set small goals and increase slowly to build endurance, strength, and flexibility.
* Be aware of any fall risks older adults may have, such as effects of medications, neuromuscular problems, environmental hazards (see Chapter 32 for a full discussion of fall risks in older adults).
* In older adults, the body's responses return to normal more slowly. For instance, an increase in heart rate from exercise may stay elevated for hours before returning to normal.

TEACHING CLINICAL

Controlling Orthostatic Hypotension

Teach the client ways to control orthostatic (postural) hypotension:

* Rest with the head of the bed elevated 20 to 30 degrees. This position makes the position change on rising less severe.
* Avoid sudden changes in position. Arise from bed in three stages:
  a. Sit up in bed for at least 1 minute (or until symptoms subside).
  b. Sit on the side of the bed with legs dangling for at least 1 minute.
  c. Stand with care, holding onto the edge of the bed or another unmovable object for at least 1 minute.
* Never bend down all the way to the floor or stand up too quickly after stooping as baroreceptors cannot accommodate rapid change.

* Apply compression stockings before getting out of bed to inhibit venous pooling in the legs.
* Be aware that the symptoms of hypotension are most severe at the following times:
  a. 30 to 60 minutes after a heavy meal
  b. 1 to 2 hours after taking an antihypertension medication
* Get out of a warm bath very slowly because warm temperatures can lead to venous pooling. Avoid hot water for bathing.
* Use a rocking chair to improve circulation in the lower extremities. Even mild leg exercises can strengthen muscle tone and enhance circulation.
* Refrain from any strenuous activity that results in holding the breath and bearing down as the Valsalva manoeuvre slows the heart rate, leading to subsequent lowering of blood pressure.

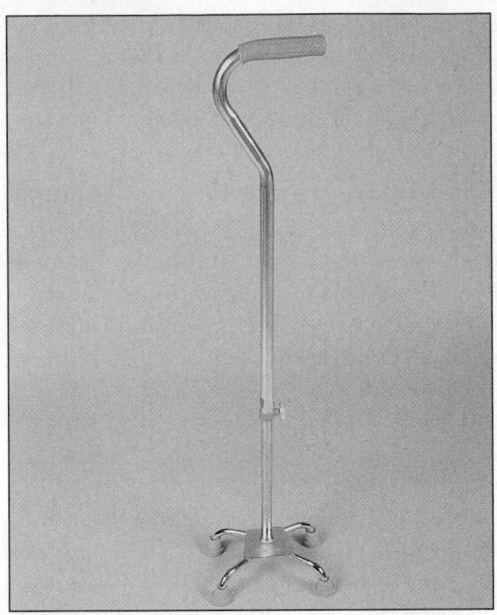

FIGURE 39.56 A quad cane.

provides. See the Teaching: Clinical box on using walkers on the next page. Many types of walkers are available in different shapes and sizes, with devices suited to individual needs. The standard type is made of polished aluminum. It has four legs with rubber tips and plastic handgrips (Figure 39.59A on the next page). Many walkers have adjustable legs.

The standard walker needs to be picked up to be used. The client, therefore, requires partial strength in both hands and wrists; strong elbow extensors, such as triceps brachii; and strong shoulder depressors, such as the pectoralis minor. The client also needs the ability to bear at least partial weight on both legs.

Four-wheeled and two-wheeled models of walkers (roller walkers) do not need to be picked up to be moved, but they are less stable than the standard walker. They are used by clients who are too weak or unstable to pick up and move the walker with each step. Some roller walkers have a seat at the back so the client can sit down to rest when desired. An adaptation of the standard and

---

TEACHING CLINICAL

Using Canes

Knowing how to use a cane properly is important for client safety:

- Hold the cane with the hand on the stronger side of the body to provide maximum support and appropriate body alignment when walking.
- Position the tip of a standard cane (and the nearest tip of other canes) about 15 cm to the side and 15 cm in front of the near foot, so that the elbow is slightly flexed.

WHEN MAXIMUM SUPPORT IS REQUIRED

- Move the cane forward about 30 cm, or a distance that is comfortable while the body weight is borne by both legs (Figure 39.57A).
- Then move the affected (weak) leg forward to the cane while the weight is borne by the cane and stronger leg (Figure 39.57B).
- Next, move the unaffected (stronger) leg forward ahead of the cane and weak leg while the weight is borne by the cane and weak leg (Figure 39.57C).
- Repeat the steps. This pattern of moving provides at least two points of support on the floor at all times.

AS YOU BECOME STRONGER AND REQUIRE LESS SUPPORT

- Move the cane and weak leg forward at the same time, while the weight is borne by the stronger leg (Figure 39.58A).
- Move the stronger leg forward, while the weight is borne by the cane and the weak leg (Figure 39.58B).

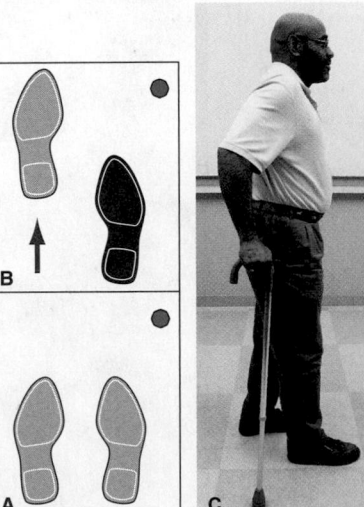

FIGURE 39.57 Steps involved in using a cane to provide maximum support.

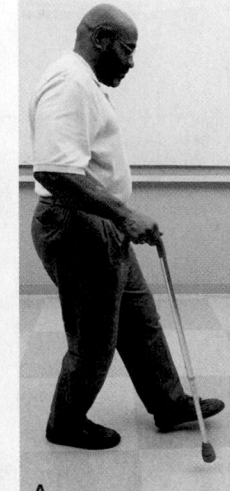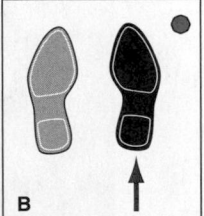

FIGURE 39.58 Steps involved in using a cane when less than maximum support is needed.

Using Walkers

Knowing how to use a walker properly is important for client safety:

WHEN MAXIMUM SUPPORT IS REQUIRED

- Move the walker ahead about 15 cm while your body weight is borne by both legs.
- Then, move the right foot up to the walker while your body weight is borne by the left leg and both arms.
- Next, move the left foot up to the right foot while your body weight is borne by the right leg and both arms.

IF ONE LEG IS WEAKER THAN THE OTHER

- Move the walker and the weak leg ahead together about 15 cm while your weight is borne by the stronger leg.
- Then, move the stronger leg ahead while your weight is borne by the affected leg and both arms.

four-wheeled walker is one that has two tips and two wheels (Figure 39.59B). This type provides more stability than the four-wheeled model yet still permits the client to keep the walker in contact with the ground at all times. The client tilts the walker forward, lifting the tips while the wheels remain on the ground, then pushes the walker forward.

The nurse may need to adjust the height of a client's walker so that the hand bar is just below the client's waist and the client's elbows are slightly flexed. This position helps the client assume a more normal stance. A walker that is too low causes the client to stoop; one that is too high makes the client stretch and reach.

CRUTCHES Crutches may be a temporary need for some people and a permanent one for others. Crutches should enable a person to ambulate independently; therefore, it is important to learn to use them properly. See the Teaching: Clinical box on using crutches. Several kinds of crutches are available. The most frequently used are the underarm crutch, or *axillary crutch,* with hand bars, and the *Lofstrand,* or *forearm crutch,* which extends only to the forearm (Figure 39.60). On the Lofstrand crutch, the metal forearm cuff and the metal bar stabilize the wrists and, thus, make walking safer and easier. The platform, or elbow extensor, crutch also has a cuff for the upper arm (Figure 39.60). This crutch is usually used by clients who require support for weak extensor muscles of the arm (e.g., weak triceps brachii). All crutches require suction tips, usually made of rubber, which help prevent the crutches from slipping on a floor surface.

In crutch walking, the client's weight is borne by the muscles of the shoulder girdle and the upper extremities. Before beginning crutch walking, exercises that strengthen the upper arms and hands are recommended.

Measuring Clients for Crutches When measuring clients for axillary crutches, it is most important to obtain the correct length for the crutches and the correct placement

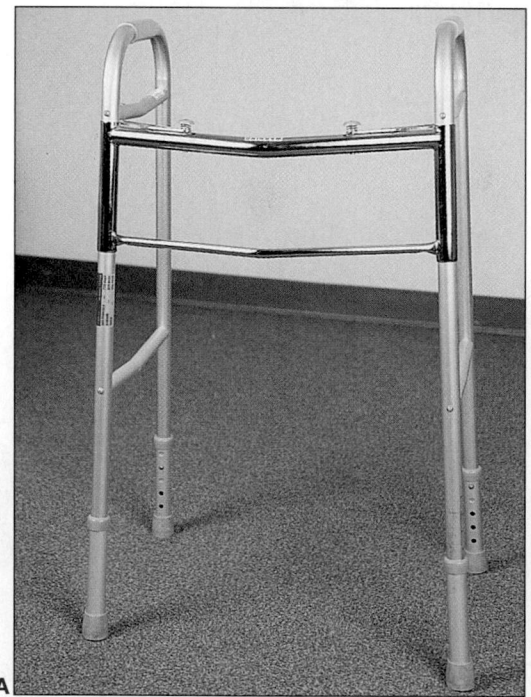

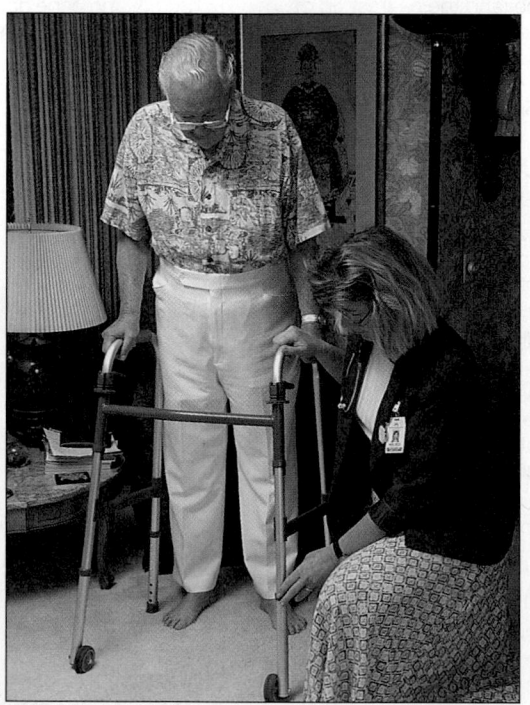

FIGURE 39.59 A: Standard walker; **B:** two-wheeled walker.

Using Crutches

Knowing how to use crutches properly is important for client safety:

- Follow the plan of exercises developed for you to strengthen your arm muscles before beginning crutch walking.
- Have a health care professional establish the correct length for your crutches and the correct placement of the hand pieces. Crutches that are too long force your shoulders upward and make it difficult for you to push your body off the ground. Crutches that are too short will make you hunch over and develop an improper body stance.
- The weight of your body should be borne by the arms rather than the axillae (armpits). Continual pressure on the axillae can injure the radial nerve and eventually cause crutch palsy, a weakness of the muscles of the forearm, wrist, and hand.
- Maintain an erect posture as much as possible to prevent strain on muscles and joints and to maintain balance.
- Each step taken with crutches should be a comfortable distance for you. It is wise to start with a small rather than large step.
- Inspect the crutch tips regularly, and replace them if worn.
- Keep the crutch tips dry and clean to maintain their surface friction. If the tips become wet, dry them well before use.
- Wear a shoe with a low heel that grips the floor. Rubber soles decrease the chances of slipping. Adjust shoelaces so they cannot come untied or reach the floor where they might catch on the crutches. Consider shoes with alternative forms of closure (e.g., Velcro), especially if you cannot easily bend to tie laces. Slip-on shoes are acceptable only if they are snug and the heel does not come loose when the foot is bent.

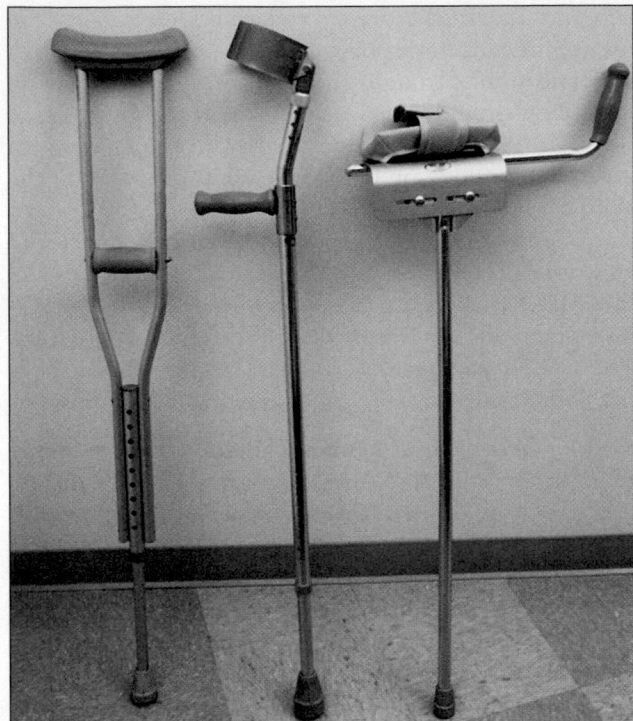

FIGURE 39.60 Types of crutches: axillary, Lofstrand, and platform.

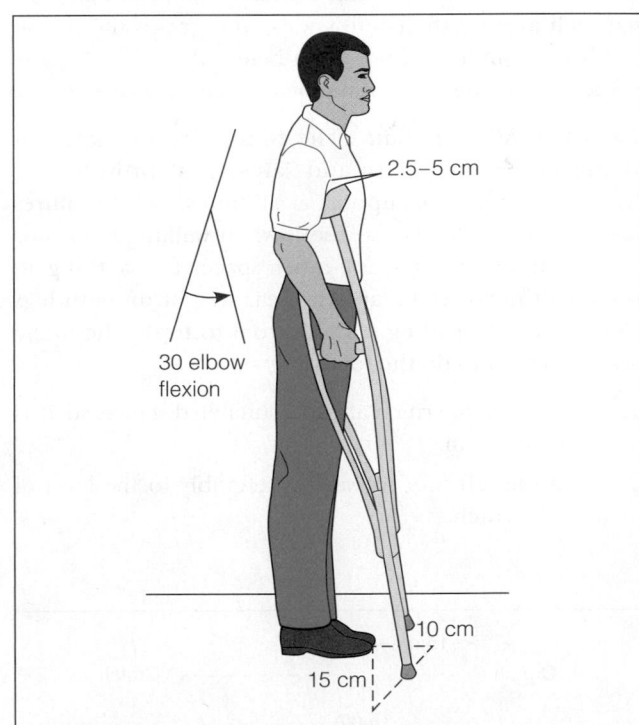

FIGURE 39.61 The standing position for measuring the correct length for crutches.

of the hand piece. Two methods of measuring crutch length are used:

1. The client lies in a supine position and the nurse measures from the anterior fold of the axilla to the heel of the foot and adds 2.5 cm.

2. The client stands erect and positions the crutch as shown in Figure 39.61. The nurse makes sure the axillary rest of the crutch is at least three finger widths, that is, 2.5 cm to 5 cm, below the axilla. This is the preferred method of measuring crutch length.

To determine the correct placement of the hand bar, the following must be done:

1. The client stands upright and supports the body weight by the handgrips of the crutches.

2. The nurse measures the angle of elbow flexion. It should be about 30 degrees. A goniometer can be used to verify

the correct angle or with the arm straight, the handgrip should be just above the wrist.

Crutch Gaits The crutch gait is the gait a person assumes on crutches by alternating body weight on one or both legs and the crutches. Five standard crutch gaits are the four-point gait, three-point gait, two-point gait, swing-to gait, and swing-through gait. The gait used depends on the following individual factors: (a) the ability to take steps, (b) the ability to bear weight and keep balance in a standing position on both legs or only one, and (c) the ability to hold the body erect.

Clients also need instruction about how to get into and out of chairs and go up and down stairs safely. All these crutch skills are best taught before the client is discharged and preferably before the client has surgery. The crutch gait may be ordered by the physician or physiotherapist.

Crutch Stance (Tripod Position)   Before crutch walking is attempted, the client needs to learn facts about posture and balance. The proper standing position with crutches is called the **tripod (triangle) position** (Figure 39.62). The crutches are placed about 15 cm in front of the feet and out laterally about 15 cm, creating a wide base of support. The feet are slightly apart. A tall person requires a wider base than a short person. Hips and knees are extended, the back is straight, and the head is held straight and high. There should be no hunch to the shoulders and thus no weight borne by the axillae. The elbows are extended sufficiently to allow weight bearing on the hands. If the client is unsteady, the nurse places a gait belt around the client's waist and grasps the belt at the back from above, not from below. A fall can be prevented more effectively if the belt is held from above.

Four-Point Gait   The **four-point alternate gait** is the most elementary and safest gait, providing at least three points of support at all times, but it requires coordination. Clients can use it when walking in crowds because it does not require much space. To use this gait, the client needs to be able to bear weight on both legs (Figure 39.63, reading from bottom to top). The nurse asks the client to do the following:

1. Move the right crutch ahead a suitable distance, such as 10 cm to 15 cm.

2. Move the left foot forward, preferably to the level of the left crutch.

3. Move the left crutch forward.

4. Move the right foot forward.

Three-Point Gait   To use the **three-point gait**, the client must be able to bear the entire body weight on the

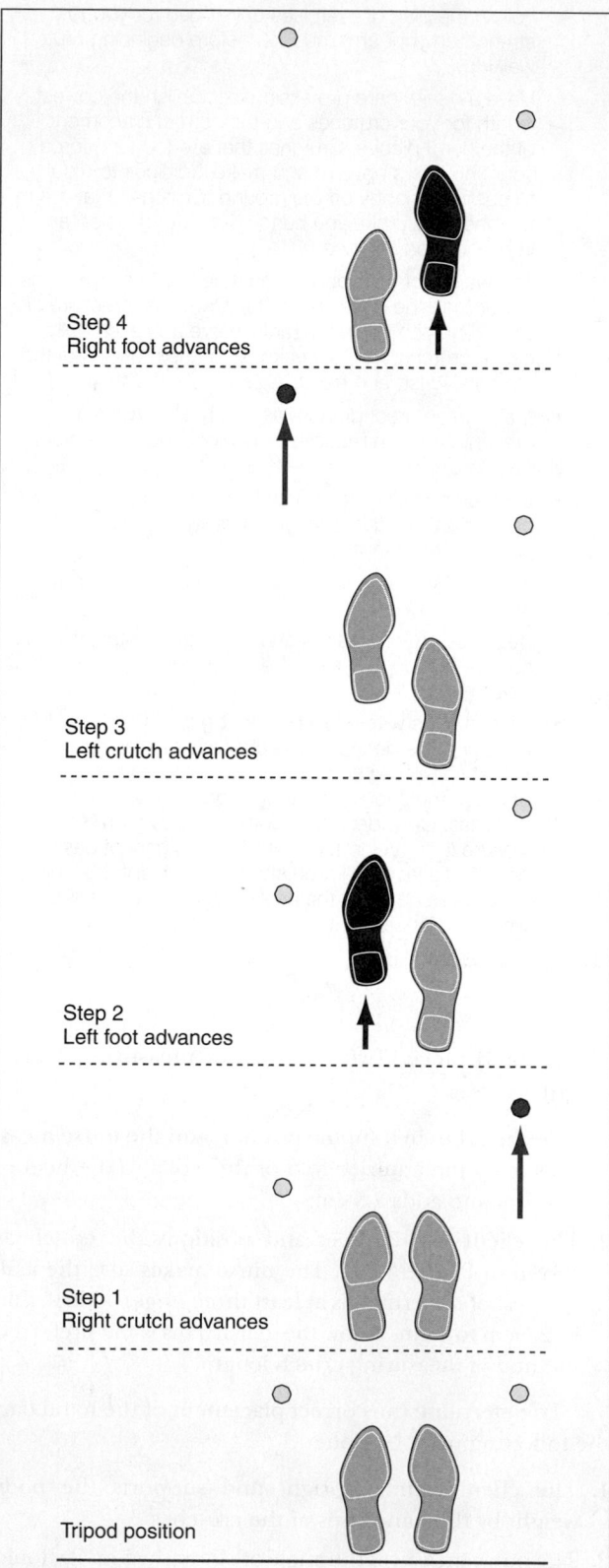

Step 4
Right foot advances

Step 3
Left crutch advances

Step 2
Left foot advances

Step 1
Right crutch advances

Tripod position

FIGURE 39.63 The four-point alternate crutch gait.

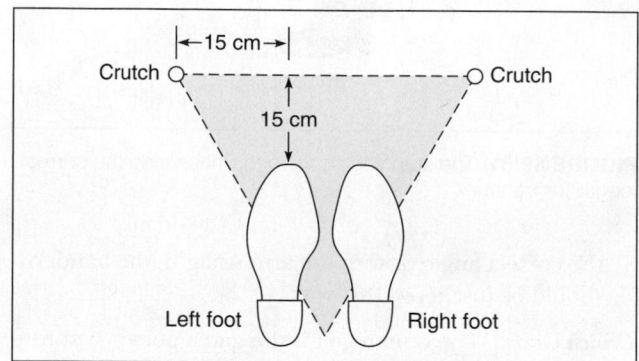

|←—15 cm—→|
Crutch   Crutch

15 cm

Left foot   Right foot

FIGURE 39.62 The tripod position.

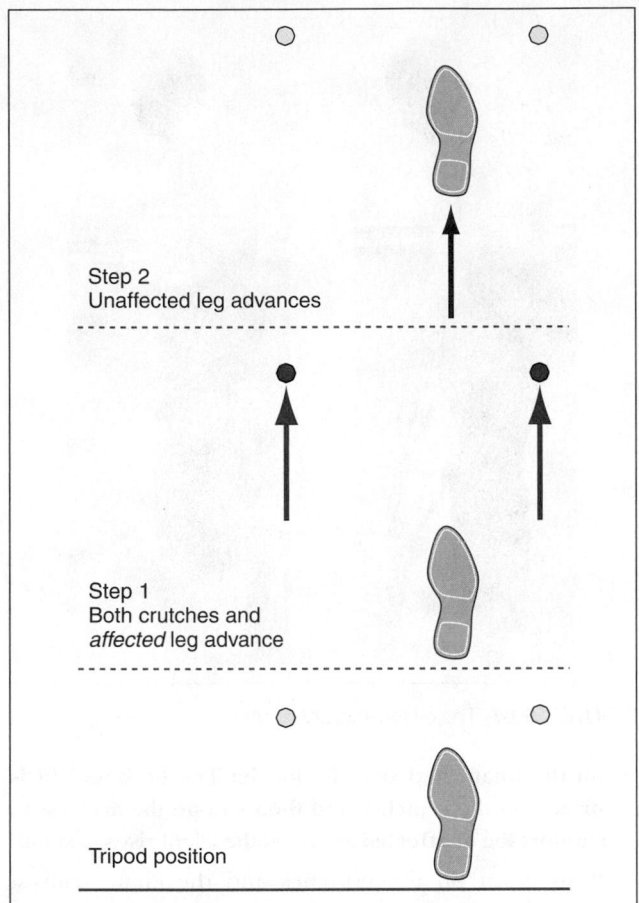

FIGURE 39.64 The three-point crutch gait.

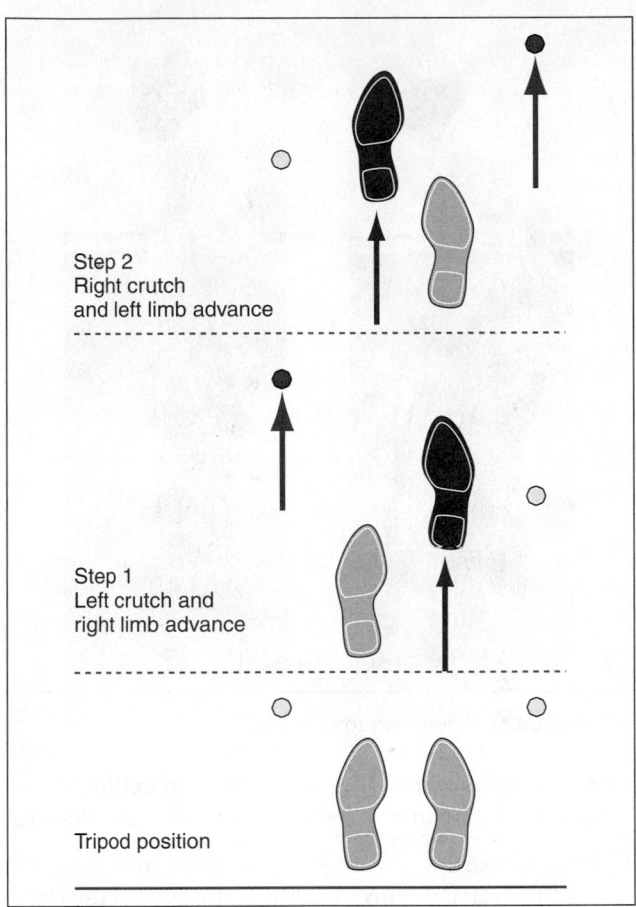

FIGURE 39.65 The two-point alternate crutch gait.

unaffected leg. The two crutches and the unaffected leg bear weight alternately (Figure 39.64, reading from bottom to top). The nurse asks the client to do the following:

1. Move both crutches and the weaker leg forward.

2. Move the stronger leg forward.

Two-Point Alternate Gait The **two-point alternate gait** is faster than the four-point gait. It requires more balance because only two points support the body at any one time; it also requires at least partial weight bearing on each foot. In this gait, arm movements with the crutches are similar to the arm movements during normal walking (Figure 39.65, reading from bottom to top). The nurse asks the client to do the following:

1. Move the left crutch and the right foot forward together.

2. Move the right crutch and the left foot ahead together.

Swing-To Gait The swing gaits are used by clients with paralysis of the legs and hips. Prolonged use of these gaits results in atrophy of the unused muscles. The **swing-to gait** is the easier of these two gaits. The nurse asks the client to do the following:

1. Move both crutches forward together (Figure 39.66A on the next page).

2. Lift body weight by the arms and swing to the crutches (Figure 39.66B).

Swing-Through Gait The **swing-through gait** requires considerable skill, strength, and coordination. The nurse asks the client to do the following:

1. Move both crutches forward together (Figure 39.67A on the next page).

2. Lift body weight by the arms and *swing through and beyond* the crutch (Figure 39.67B).

Getting into a Chair Chairs that have armrests and are secure or braced against a wall are essential for clients using crutches. For this procedure, the nurse instructs the client as follows:

1. Stand with the back of the unaffected leg centred and against the chair. The chair helps support the client during the next steps.

2. Transfer the crutches to the hand on the affected side, and hold the crutches by the hand bars. Grasp the arm of the chair with the hand on the unaffected side (Figure 39.68 on the next page). This allows the client to support the body weight on the arms and the unaffected leg.

3. Lean forward, flex the knees and hips, and lower into the chair.

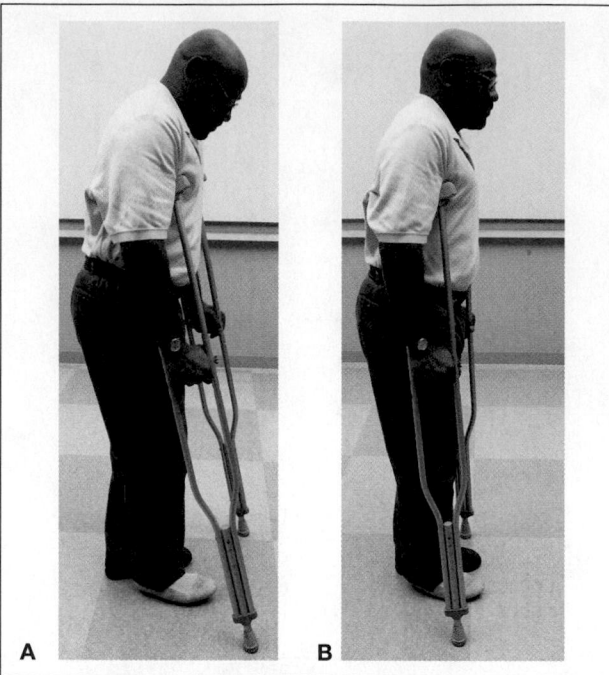

FIGURE 39.66 The swing-to crutch gait.

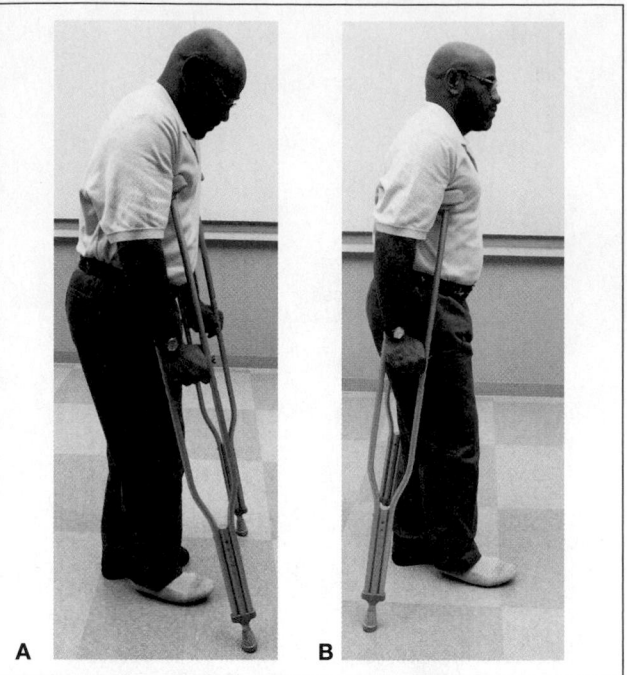

FIGURE 39.67 The swing-through crutch gait.

Getting out of a Chair To guide a client in getting out of a chair, the nurse instructs the client to do the following:

1. Move forward to the edge of the chair, and place the unaffected leg slightly under or at the edge of the chair. **Rationale: This position helps the client stand up from the chair and achieve balance since the unaffected leg is supported against the edge of the chair.**

2. Grasp the crutches by the hand bars in the hand on the affected side, and grasp the arm of the chair by the hand

on the unaffected side. **Rationale: The body weight is placed on the crutches and the hand on the armrest to support the unaffected leg when the client rises to stand.**

3. Push down on the crutches and the chair armrest while elevating the body out of the chair.

4. Assume the tripod position before moving.

Going up Stairs To help the client go up stairs, the nurse stands behind the client and slightly to the affected side, if needed. (Use a gait belt.) The nurse instructs the client as follows:

1. Assume the tripod position at the bottom of the stairs.

2. Transfer body weight to the crutches and move the unaffected leg onto the step (Figure 39.69).

3. Transfer body weight to the unaffected leg on the step, and move the crutches and affected leg up to the step. **Rationale: The affected leg is always supported by the crutches.**

4. Repeat steps 2 and 3 until you reach the top of the stairs.

Going Down Stairs To help the client go down stairs, the nurse stands one step below the client on the affected side, if needed. (Use a gait belt.) The nurse instructs the client as follows:

1. Assume the tripod position at the top of the stairs.

2. Shift the body weight to the unaffected leg, and move the crutches and affected leg down onto the next step (Figure 39.70).

3. Transfer the body weight to the crutches, and move the unaffected leg to that step. **Rationale: The affected leg is always supported by the crutches.**

4. Repeat steps 2 and 3 until you reach the bottom of the stairs.

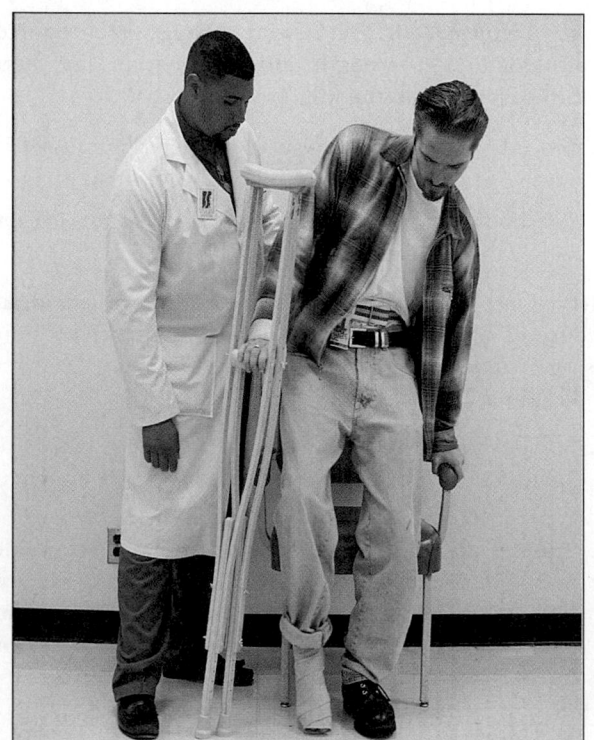

FIGURE 39.68 A client using crutches to get into a chair

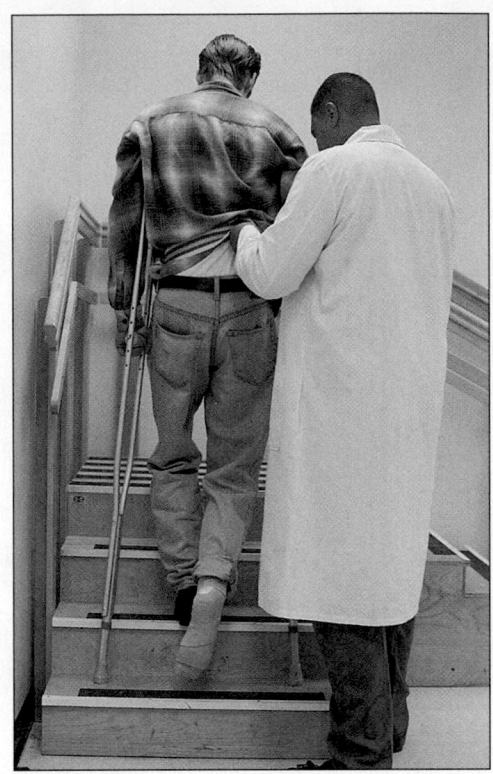

FIGURE 39.69 Climbing stairs: placing weight on the crutches while first moving the unaffected leg onto a step.

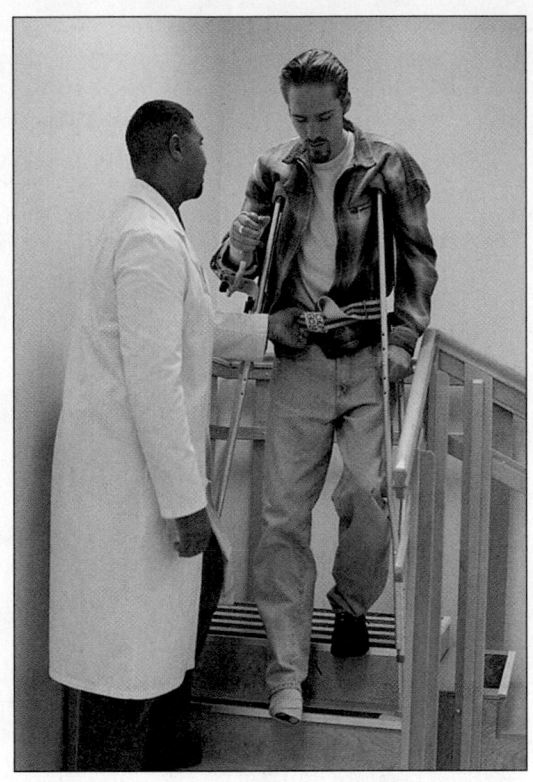

FIGURE 39.70 Descending stairs: moving the crutches and affected leg to the next step.

Evaluating

The goals established during the planning phase are evaluated according to specific desired outcomes also established in that phase. Examples of these are shown in Table 39.10.

If outcomes are *not* achieved, the nurse, client, and support person, if appropriate, need to explore the reasons why before modifying the care plan. For example, the following questions may be considered if an immobilized client fails to maintain muscle mass and tone and joint mobility:

- Has the client's physical or mental condition changed motivation to perform required exercise?
- Were appropriate ROM exercises implemented?
- Was the client encouraged to participate in self-care activities as much as possible?
- Was the client encouraged to make as many decisions as possible when developing a daily activity plan and to express concerns?
- Did the nurse provide appropriate supervision and monitoring?
- Was the client's diet adequate to provide appropriate nourishment for energy requirements?

TABLE 39.10 Evaluation Goals and Outcomes: Mobility and Activity

Goal	Examples of Desired Outcomes
Avoid any complications associated with immobility	Skin intact
	Muscle size within pre-immobility range
	Full active ROM of all joints
	Chest expansion symmetrical
	Depth of respirations within expected range
	Absence of adventitious breath sounds
	Abnormal heart rate, heart sounds, and dysrhythmia not present
	Skinfold measurements within pre-immobility range
	Urinary amount, colour, and odour within expected range
	Regular elimination

(continued)

TABLE 39.10 Evaluation Goals and Outcomes: Mobility and Activity (*continued*)

Goal	Examples of Desired Outcomes
Restore ability to ambulate	Walks with effective gait with walker
	Walks up and down stairs with assistance of support person
Avoid injury from falling or improper use of body mechanics	Transfers safely to and from bed and chair and from chair to chair or to and from wheelchair
	Demonstrates use of good body mechanics when moving and lifting objects
	Wears appropriate footwear
	Alters home environment to eliminate hazards
Increase tolerance for physical activity	Balances activity and rest periods
	Adapts lifestyle to energy level
	Recognizes energy limitations
	Maintains adequate nutrition

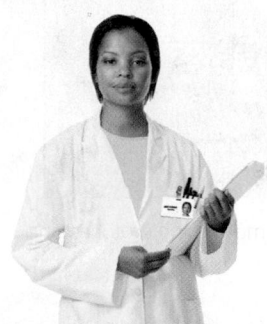

Case Study 39

Mrs. Gomez, 71, underwent surgery 2 days ago for repair of a fractured hip she suffered in a fall. She has an incision over her left hip area that is free of redness with well-approximated edges. She experiences pain on movement even though she is receiving around-the-clock analgesia. The physician has ordered daily physical therapy and that Mrs. Gomez be ambulated three times daily. Mrs. Gomez does not want to get out of bed because she does not want to experience another fall.

CRITICAL THINKING QUESTIONS

1. Why is it essential to maintain proper body alignment when turning Mrs. Gomez or helping her out of bed to ambulate?

2. What assessment findings would alert you that Mrs. Gomez is developing problems associated with her current state of decreased mobility?

3. Cite examples of exercises you can recommend for Mrs. Gomez that will reduce her risk for disuse syndrome during her recovery.

4. What are some of the factors you should consider before moving Mrs. Gomez to a sitting position on the edge of the bed in preparation for ambulation?

5. Mrs. Gomez will be using a walker to assist her with ambulation when she goes home. What teaching should be done before Mrs. Gomez's discharge from the hospital in regard to use of a walker?

Check the eText in MyNursingLab for answers and explanations.

KEY TERMS

CHAPTER HIGHLIGHTS

- The ability to move freely, easily, and purposefully in the environment is essential for people to meet their basic needs.

- Exercise and activity are essential for maintaining and regaining health and wellness.

- Purposeful, coordinated movement of the body relies on the integrated functioning of the musculoskeletal system, the nervous system, and the vestibular apparatus of the inner ear.

- Body movement involves four basic elements: body alignment, joint mobility, balance, and coordinated movement.

- People maintain alignment and balance when the line of gravity passes through the centre of gravity and the base of support.

- The broader the base of support and the lower the centre of gravity, the greater are the stability and balance achieved.

- Exercise is physical activity performed to maintain muscle tone and joint mobility, to enhance physiological functioning of body systems, and to improve physical fitness. Activity tolerance is the type and amount of exercise or daily living activities an individual is able to perform without experiencing adverse effects. Functional strength is the ability to do work.

- Exercise is classified as isotonic, isometric, isokinetic, and aerobic or anaerobic. Isotonic exercises increase muscle mass, tone, and strength, joint flexibility, and body circulation. Isometric exercises increase muscle mass, tone, and strength, and circulation to the exercised part but do not involve joint mobility.

- Many factors influence body alignment and activity. These include growth and development, physical health, mental health, personal values and attitudes, and prescribed limitations to movement.

- Immobility affects almost every body organ and system adversely; complications also include psychosocial problems. Exercise, by contrast, provides many benefits to the same body organs and systems and can be used to prevent and treat many disease processes.

- Problems of immobility include disuse osteoporosis and atrophy; contractures; diminished cardiac reserve; orthostatic hypotension; venous stasis, edema, and thrombus formation; decreased respiratory movement and pooling of secretions; decreased metabolic rate and negative nitrogen balance; urinary stasis, retention, and infection; constipation; and varying emotional reactions.

- Complete bed rest is almost never required, and it is usually dangerous because of the hazards of immobility. A risk-benefit assessment and ongoing assessment of rationale for complete bed rest is essential.

- The nurse has responsibilities (a) to determine root causes of immobility and address these whenever possible with the goal of getting the client moving as much and as soon as possible, (b) to prevent the complications of immobility and reduce the severity of any problems resulting from immobility, and (c) to partner with the client and appropriate support persons to design exercise programs that promote wellness in clients.

- Assessment relative to a client's activity and exercise includes a nursing history and physical examination of body alignment, gait, joint appearance and movement, capabilities and limitations for movement, muscle mass and strength, activity tolerance, and problems related to immobility.

- An activity and exercise history includes daily activity level, activity tolerance, type and frequency of exercise, and factors affecting mobility.

- Nursing diagnoses that relate to activity and mobility problems include activity intolerance, impaired physical mobility, and inadequate physical activity to meet minimal fitness recommendations.

- *Body mechanics* is the efficient, coordinated, and safe use of the body to move objects and carry out the activities of daily living.

- Nurses must use good body mechanics in their daily work and especially when moving and turning clients in bed and assisting clients to make transfers. Proper body mechanics does not ensure protection from injury; however, and nurses and caregivers are encouraged to avoid manual lifting and repositioning of clients. At the very least, they should avoid solo lifting, repositioning, and transferring.

- Positioning a client in good body alignment and changing the position regularly and systematically are essential aspects of nursing practice.

- Before positioning dependent clients, the nurse should plan a systematic 24-hour schedule for position changes, including positions that provide for full extension of the neck, hips, and knees. The nurse also uses appropriate supportive devices to maintain alignment and prevent strain on the client's muscles and joints.

- Before moving, turning, or transferring a client, the nurse must consider the client's health status, degree of exertion permitted, physical ability to assist, ability to comprehend instruction, degree of discomfort, and weight, and whether to use assistive devices or another caregiver to assist.

- Assistance from others or the use of mechanical lifting aids is essential for most, if not all, nonpediatric clients.

- Safety measures must always be employed when the nurse uses a wheelchair or stretcher to move and transfer clients.

- Ambulating techniques that facilitate normal walking gait yet provide needed support are most effective. The nurse can assist clients to prepare for ambulation by helping them become as independent as possible while in bed.

- Preambulatory exercises that strengthen the muscles for walking are essential for clients who have been immobilized for a prolonged period.

- Clients need specific instructions about appropriate use of canes, walkers, and crutches.

ASSESS YOUR LEARNING

1. A client is concerned that because she has had a myocardial infarction (heart attack) she will not be able to enjoy active living in the future. Which of the following is the nurse's BEST response?

    a. "People who have had a myocardial infarction should not start any physical activity program for 6 months."

    b. "Many risks and injuries can occur with exercise."

    c. "To stay physically healthy after a myocardial infarction, various activities are necessary, but consult your physician before you begin the exercise."

    d. "The older you are, the less active you need to be."

2. An 80-year-old male informs his nurse that he has "slowed down" since he had a mild cerebrovascular accident (stroke). He indicates that he has hired people to "look after everything so that all I have to do is watch TV." The nurse should explain which of the following?

    a. Obesity will likely occur if he does not do 1 hour of exercise five times per week.

    b. His strategy is a good one, as this will ensure no further cerebrovascular accidents.

    c. Adding physical activity within his tolerance level would help to decrease the risk of several serious diseases while improving a sense of well-being.

    d. At 80, he should still be able to look after his home independently and perform activities of daily living.

3. Knowing that the shoulder is a ball-and-socket joint, the nurse understands that a healthy shoulder can perform which of the following?

    a. Circumduction

    b. Supination

    c. Inversion

    d. Right-side flexion

4. The client is ambulating for the first time after surgery. She tells the nurse that she feels faint. Which of the following is the nurse's BEST action?

    a. Find another nurse for help.

    b. Return the client to her room as quickly as possible.

    c. Tell the client to take rapid, shallow breaths.

    d. Assist the client to a nearby chair.

5. A 58-year-old male is in hospital with a fractured right ankle. He was placed in a cast yesterday but is not to weight-bear. You walk into the room to find him hopping on his left foot to the bathroom and he refuses to use a bedpan. What should you do?

    a. Instruct the patient on the use of a cane in his left hand to assist with ambulation.

    b. Instruct the patient on the use of the bedpan, and insist that he use it as this would be the simplest way to ensure his safety.

    c. Instruct the patient on the use of crutches with a swing-through gait and urge him to use the call bell for assistance to use the washroom.

    d. Instruct the patient on the use of a cane in his right hand to assist with ambulation.

6. During vigorous upper body exercises, which of the following would describe the reaction of the various body systems?

   a. Musculoskeletal: increased blood flow to lower extremities

      Cardiovascular: decreased heart rate with increased cardiac muscle perfusion

      Respiratory: increased lung volume with increased fluid retention

   b. Musculoskeletal: increased blood flow to upper and lower extremities

      Cardiovascular: increased heart rate with increased cardiac muscle perfusion

      Respiratory: increased lung expansion with increased respiratory rate

   c. Musculoskeletal: increased blood flow to upper extremities

      Cardiovascular: increased heart rate with decreased cardiac muscle perfusion

      Respiratory: increased lung expansion with increased respiratory rate

   d. Musculoskeletal: increased blood flow to upper and lower extremities

      Cardiovascular: increased heart rate with decreased cardiac muscle perfusion

      Respiratory: increased lung expansion with increased respiratory rate

7. Isotonic exercises are intended to achieve which of the following?

   a. Strengthen immobilized muscles
   b. Increase blood pressure
   c. Increase muscle mass and strength
   d. Decrease heart rate and cardiac output

8. To increase stability during patient transfer, the nurse increases the base of support by doing which of the following?

   a. Leaning slightly backward
   b. Spacing the feet further apart
   c. Tensing the abdominal muscles
   d. Bending the knees

9. The client weighs 110 kg. Which of the following statements by the nurse reflects an awareness of workplace injury prevention?

   a. "The use of proper body mechanics will prevent me from injuring myself."
   b. "I am physically fit so am at lesser risk for injury when transferring the client."
   c. "I must use the mechanical lift and get another person to transfer the client from the bed to the chair."
   d. "I will use the back belt to avoid hurting my back while I am transferring a client from the bed to the chair."

10. When assessing a client's gait, the nurse should look for and encourage which of the following?

    a. The hips sway with spinal rotation.
    b. The gaze is slightly downward.
    c. The toes strike the ground before the heel.
    d. The arm on the same side as the swing-through foot moves forward at the same time.

Check the eText in MyNursingLab for answers and explanations.

WEBLINKS

Canadian Centre for Occupational Health and Safety (CCOHS)

http://www.ccohs.ca

This site offers information about general and specific occupational health and safety issues. Risks specific to registered nurses are identified.

Canadian Society for Exercise Physiology

http://www.csep.ca

This society participates in and promotes research, education, and training related to exercise and science. This site provides links to Canadian physical activity and sedentary living guidelines.

Health Canada: Healthy Living—Physical Activity

http://www.hc-sc.gc.ca/hl-vs/physactiv/index-eng.php

This site identifies the federal programs and initiatives related to fitness in Canada.

Canadian Fitness and Lifestyle Research Institute

http://www.cflri.ca

The mission of the institute is to enhance the well-being of Canadians through research and communication of information about physically active lifestyles to the public and private sectors.

Active Living Alliance for Canadians with a Disability

http://www.ala.ca

The alliance promotes inclusion and active living lifestyles for Canadians with disabilities by facilitating communication and collaboration among organizations, agencies, and individuals. The site provides provincial and territorial links to helpful local resources.

WorkSafeBC

http://www2.worksafebc.com/Portals/HealthCare/Home.asp

A site developed by the Workers' Compensation Board of British Columbia, dedicated to promoting workplace safety for employees and employers. A number of initiatives to enhance safety in health care are found on this site.

MyNursingLab

REFERENCES

Bartels, E. M., Lund, H., Hagen, K. B., Dagfinrud, H., Christensen, R., & Danneskiold-Samsøe, B. (2007). Aquatic exercise for the treatment of knee and hip osteoarthritis. *Cochrane Database of Systematic Reviews, 4*, Art. No.: CD005523.

Borg, G. (1998). *Borg's perceived exertion and pain scales.* Champaign, IL: Human Kinetics.

Busch, A. J., Barber, K. A., Overend, T. J., Peloso, P. M. J., & Schachter, C. L. (2007). Exercise for treating fibromyalgia syndrome. *Cochrane Database of Systematic Reviews, 4*, Art. No.: CD003786. doi: 10.1002/14651858.CD003786.pub2

Canadian Centre for Occupational Health and Safety. (2012). Ergonomic safe patient handling. *Occupations and workplaces: Registered nurses.* Retrieved from http://www.ccohs.ca/oshanswers/hsprograms/patient_handling.html

Canadian Diabetes Association Clinical Practice Guidelines Expert Committee. (2008). Canadian Diabetes Association clinical practice guidelines for the prevention and management of diabetes in Canada. *Canadian Journal of Diabetes, 32*(Suppl 1), S1–S201.

Canadian Fitness and Lifestyle Research Institute. (2006). *2006 Physical activity and sport monitor.* Retrieved from http://www.cflri.ca/eng/statistics/surveys/pam2006.php

Canadian Nurses Association. (2006). *Trends in illness and injury-related absenteeism and overtime among publicly employed registered nurses.* Ottawa, ON: Author.

Canadian Society for Exercise Physiology. (2011a). *Canadian physical activity guidelines.* Retrieved from http://www.csep.ca/CMFiles/Guidelines/PAGuidelines_0-65plus_en.pdf

Canadian Society for Exercise Physiology. (2011b). *Canadian sedentary behaviour guidelines.* Retrieved from http://www.csep.ca/CMFiles/Guidelines/CanadianSedentaryGuidelinesStatements_E_2012.pdf

Edelman, C., & Mandle, C. (2010). *Health promotion throughout the lifespan* (7th ed.). Philadelphia, PA: Mosby/Elsevier.

Freeman, L. (2008). *Mosby's complementary & alternative medicine: A research-based approach* (3rd ed.). St. Louis, MO: Mosby.

Heart and Stroke Foundation of Canada. (2011). *Position statement: Physical activity, heart disease and stroke.* Retrieved from http://www.heartandstroke.com/atf/cf/%7B99452D8B-E7F1-4BD6-A57D-B136CE6C95BF%7D/PhysicalActivity4pager.pdf

Howe, T. E., Rochester, L., Neil, F., Skelton, D. A., & Ballinger, C. (2011). Exercise for improving balance in older people. *Cochrane Database of Systematic Reviews 2011*, Issue 11. Art. No.: CD004963. doi: 10.1002/14651858.CD004963.pub3

Katzmarzyk, P. T., & Janssen, I. (2004). The economic costs of physical inactivity and obesity in Canada: An update. *Canadian Journal of Applied Physiology, 29*(1), 90–115.

Kramer, M. S., & McDonald, S. W. (2006). Aerobic exercise for women during pregnancy. *Cochrane Database of Systematic Reviews, 3*, Art. No.: CD000180. doi: 10.1002/14651858.CD000180.pub2

McMaster University. (2011). *Physical activity guidelines for adults with spinal cord injury.* Retrieved from http://www.csep.ca/CMFiles/Guidelines/SCIPAGuidelinesClient.pdf

Micozzi, M. (2010). *Fundamentals of complementary and alternative medicine* (4th ed.). Philadelphia, PA: Mosby.

Nelson, A. (2007). Update on evidence-based practices for safe patient handling and movement. *Orthopaedic Nursing, 25*(6), 367–368.

Nelson, A., & Baptiste, A. (2004, September 30). Evidence-based practices for safe patient handling and movement. *Online Journal of Issues in Nursing, 9*(3). Retrieved from www.nursingworld.org/MainMenuCategories/ANAMarketplace/ANAPeriodicals/OJIN/TableofContents/Volume92004/No3Sept04/EvidenceBasedPractices.aspx

O'Brien-Pallas, L., Shamian, J., Thomson, D., Alksnis, C., Koehoorn, M., Kerr, M., ... & Bruce, S. (2004). Work-related disability in Canadian nurses. *Journal of Nursing Scholarship, 36*(4), 352–357.

Paterson, D. H., & Warburton, D. E. R., (2010). Physical activity and functional limitations in older adults: A systematic review related to Canada's physical activity guidelines. *International Journal of Behavioural Nutrition and Physical Activity, 7*(38). doi: 10.1186/1479-5868-7-38

Registered Nurses' Association of Ontario. (2008). *Workplace health, safety and well-being of the nurse.* Toronto, ON: Author.

Statistics Canada. (2011a). Canadian health measures survey: Adult obesity prevalence in Canada and the United States. *The Daily*, March 2. Retrieved from http://www.statcan.gc.ca/daily-quotidien/110302/dq110302c-eng.htm

Statistics Canada. (2011b). Canadian health measures survey: Physical activity of youth and adults. *The Daily*, January 19. Retrieved from http://www.statcan.gc.ca/daily-quotidien/110119/dq110119b-eng.htm

Thomas, D., Elliott, E. J., & Naughton, G. A. (2006). Exercise for type 2 diabetes mellitus. *Cochrane Database of Systematic Reviews, 3*, Art. No.: CD002968. doi: 10.1002/14651858.CD002968.pub.2

Tremblay, M. S., Warburton, D. E. R., Janssen, I., Paterson, D. H., Latimer, A. E., Rhodes, R. E., ... & Duggan, M. (2011). New Canadian physical activity guidelines, *Applied Physiology, Nutrition, & Metabolism, 36*, 36–46. doi:10.1139/H11-009

Verbeek, J. H., Martimo, K. P., Karppinen, J., Kuijer, P. P. F. M., Viikari-Juntura, E., & Takala, E. P. (2011). Manual material handling advice and assistive devices for preventing and treating back pain in workers. *Cochrane Database of Systematic Reviews, 6*, Art. No.: CD005958, doi: 10.1002/14651858.CD005958.pub.3

Warburton, D. E. R., Charlsworth, S., Ivey, A., Nettlefold, L., & Bredin, S. S. D. (2010). A systematic review of the evidence for Canada's physical activity guidelines for adults. *International Journal of Behavioural Nutrition and Physical Activity, 7*(39), doi:10.1186/1479-5868-7-39

Warburton, D. E. R., Nichol, C. W., & Bredin, S. S. D. (2006). Health benefits of physical activity: The evidence. *Canadian Medical Association Journal, 174*(6), 801–809. doi: 10.1503/cmaj.051351

WorkSafeBC. (2006a). *Handle with care: Patient handling and the application of ergonomics (MSI) requirements.* Retrieved from http://www.worksafebc.com/publications/health_and_safety/by_topic/assets/pdf/handle_with_care.pdf

WorkSafeBC. (2006b). *Transfer assist devices for safer handling of patients. A guide for selection and safe use.* Retrieved from http://www.worksafebc.com/publications/health_and_safety/by_topic/assets/pdf/transfer_assist_devices.pdf

Chapter 40

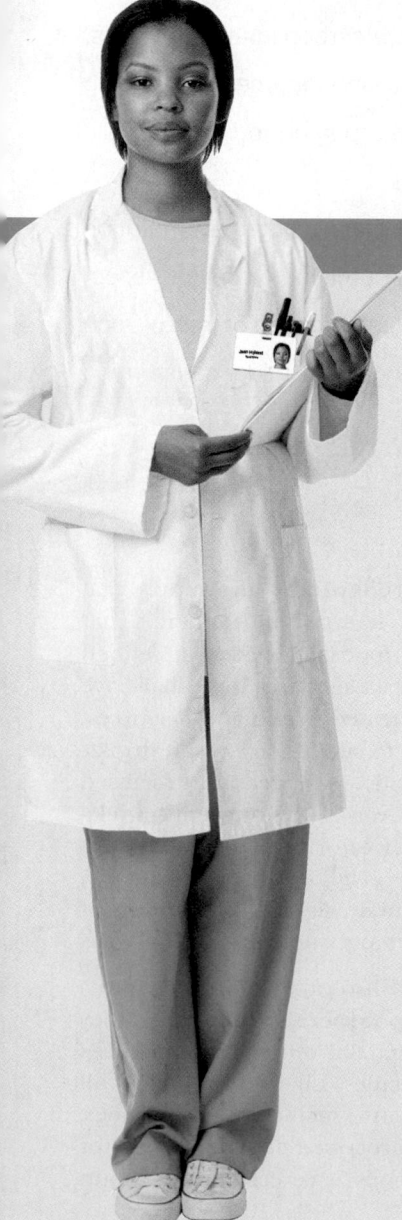

Nutrition

LEARNING OUTCOMES

After studying this chapter, you will be able to:

1. Identify six essential nutrients and dietary sources of each.

2. Describe normal digestion, absorption, and metabolism of carbohydrates, proteins, and lipids.

3. Explain the essential aspects of energy balance.

4. Discuss body weight and body mass standards.

5. List 13 factors that influence nutrition.

6. Outline developmental nutritional considerations.

7. Evaluate a diet using *Eating Well with Canada's Food Guide*.

8. Discuss the essential components and purposes of nutritional screening and nutritional assessment.

9. Outline nursing interventions to promote optimal nutrition.

10. Identify risk factors for and clinical signs of malnutrition and plan, implement, and evaluate nursing care related to nutritional problems.

11. Develop interventions to address the childhood and adult obesity problems in Canada.

12. Perform the skills of inserting enteral tubes, administering feedings and medications through enteral tubes, and removing enteral tubes.

Nutrition is the sum of all the interactions between an organism and the food it consumes. In other words, nutrition is what a person eats and how the body uses it. **Nutrients** are organic, inorganic, and energy-producing substances found in foods and required for body functioning. People require the essential nutrients in food for the growth and maintenance of all body tissues and the normal functioning of all body processes. An adequate food intake consists of a balance of essential nutrients: water, carbohydrates, proteins, lipids, vitamins, and minerals. Foods differ greatly in their **nutritive value** (the nutrient content of a specified amount of food), and no one food provides all essential nutrients. In addition, the way in which foods are processed or cooked can make a difference in their nutritional value. Nutrients have three major functions: (a) providing energy for body processes and movement, (b) providing structural material for body tissues, and (c) regulating body processes.

The body's most basic nutrient need is water (see Chapter 44 for full discussion on fluid balance). Because every cell requires a continuous supply of fuel, the most urgent nutritional need after water is for nutrients that provide fuel, or energy. The energy-providing nutrients are carbohydrates, proteins, and fats. These are called **macronutrients**. Hunger impels people to eat enough energy-providing nutrients to satisfy their energy needs, but no clear-cut body signals lead a person to ingest certain vitamins or minerals, both of which are often referred to as **micronutrients**.

Nurses can promote the health of Canadians by evaluating and facilitating adequate nutrition through the lifespan. Being well informed about the ever-changing topic of nutrition is a critical aspect of health promotion for nurses. It is essential that nurses' nutrition knowledge be based on reliable science so that they can be critical consumers of available information and engage in evidence-informed practice.

Essential Nutrients: Macronutrients

Carbohydrates

Carbohydrates are composed of the elements carbon (C), hydrogen (H), and oxygen (O) and are of two basic kinds: (a) simple carbohydrates (sugars), and (b) complex carbohydrates (starches and fibre).

TYPES OF CARBOHYDRATES

Sugars **Sugars**, the simplest of all carbohydrates, are water soluble and are produced naturally by both plants and animals. Sugars can be **monosaccharides** (single molecules) or **disaccharides** (double molecules). Of the three monosaccharides (glucose, fructose, and galactose), glucose is, by far, the most abundant.

Most sugars are produced naturally by plants, especially fruits, sugar cane, and sugar beet. However, lactose, a combination of glucose and galactose, is found in milk. Natural sources of carbohydrates also supply vital nutrients, such as protein, vitamins, and minerals that are not found in processed foods. Processed or refined sugars (e.g., table sugar, molasses) are those that have been extracted and concentrated from natural sources. Processed sugars are added to such foods as soft drinks, cookies, candy, ice cream, and some cereals. Processed carbohydrate foods are relatively low in nutrients in relation to the large number of calories they contain and thus are often referred to as *empty calories*. For example, alcoholic beverages can contain significant amounts of carbohydrate, but they are empty calories.

Starches **Starches** are the insoluble, nonsweet forms of carbohydrate. They are **polysaccharides**; that is, they are composed of branched chains of dozens, sometimes hundreds, of glucose molecules. Like sugars, nearly all starches exist naturally in plants, such as grains, legumes, and potatoes. Starches are processed in various ways, for example, in making such foods as cereals, breads, flour, and puddings.

Fibre **Fibre**, another type of polysaccharide, is a complex carbohydrate derived from plants that cannot be digested by humans. Fibre comes in two forms: insoluble and soluble. **Insoluble fibre** acts as *roughage* and draws water into the colon, preventing constipation. Sources include wheat bran and the skins of some fruits (e.g., apples) and vegetables (e.g., broccoli, peas). This bulk satisfies the appetite and also helps the digestive tract function effectively and eliminate wastes. **Soluble fibre** is found in oats, legumes (peas, kidney beans, and lentils), some seeds, brown rice, barley, fruits (such as apples), some green vegetables (such as broccoli), and potatoes. As it passes through the digestive track, soluble fibre breaks down and forms a gel that is thought to reduce the amount of cholesterol that is absorbed. Soluble fibre delays gastric emptying and slows the entry of glucose into the bloodstream. Ultimately, this delay may prevent a rapid postprandial (postmeal) increase in blood glucose, improving glucose control for individuals with diabetes mellitus (Weicker & Pfeiffer, 2008).

CARBOHYDRATE DIGESTION Through the digestive process, carbohydrates other than soluble and insoluble fibres are broken down into absorbable molecules. Most carbohydrate digestion occurs in the small intestine and occurs with the use of digestive enzyme. **Enzymes** are biological catalysts that speed up chemical reactions. Major enzymes of carbohydrate digestion include ptyalin (salivary amylase), pancreatic amylase, and the disaccharidases: maltase, sucrase, and lactase. The desired end products of carbohydrate digestion are monosaccharides. Some simple sugars are already monosaccharides and require no digestion. Essentially, all monosaccharides are absorbed by the small intestine in healthy people.

CARBOHYDRATE METABOLISM Monosaccharides, in the form of glucose, fructose, and galactose, arrive at the liver, where fructose and galactose are converted into glucose. The liver releases the glucose into the blood where the glucose levels are kept fairly constant by various hormones. After the ingestion of foods, the glucose levels are increased. Some glucose continues to circulate in the blood to maintain blood levels and to provide a readily available source of energy, while the remainder is either used as energy or stored. **Insulin**, a hormone secreted by the pancreas, enhances the transport of glucose into the cells.

STORAGE AND CONVERSION Carbohydrates are stored either as glycogen or as fat. **Glycogen** is a large polymer (compound molecule) of glucose. The process of glycogen formation is called **glycogenesis**. Almost all body cells are capable of storing glycogen; however, most of it is stored in the liver and skeletal muscles, where it is available for conversion back to glucose. Only a limited supply of glycogen can be formed, and glucose that cannot be stored as glycogen is converted to fat. When blood glucose levels fall below normal, the pancreas is stimulated to release **glucagon**, and this causes the liver to

release glycogen. This process returns the blood glucose levels to normal. This simplified overview of carbohydrate metabolism describes how it occurs in healthy individuals; this process becomes much more complicated when abnormal nutritional states exist or when an underlying pathological condition is present.

Proteins

Proteins are organic substances composed of amino acids. Like carbohydrates, proteins contain carbon, hydrogen, and oxygen, but proteins also contain nitrogen. Every cell in the body contains some protein, and about three-quarters of body solids are proteins.

Amino acids are categorized as essential or nonessential. **Essential amino acids** are those that cannot be manufactured in the body and must be supplied as part of the protein ingested in the diet. Nine essential amino acids—threonine, leucine, isoleucine, valine, lysine, methionine, phenylalanine, tryptophan, and histidine—are necessary for tissue growth and maintenance. A tenth essential amino acid, arginine, is required by the young but not by adults.

Nonessential amino acids are those that the body can manufacture. The body takes apart amino acids derived from the diet and reconstructs new ones from their basic elements (carbohydrates and nitrogen). Nonessential amino acids include glycine, alanine, aspartic acid, glutamic acid, proline, hydroxyproline, cystine, tyrosine, and serine.

Proteins can be complete or incomplete. **Complete proteins** contain all the essential amino acids plus many nonessential ones. Most animal proteins, including meats, poultry, fish, dairy products, and eggs, are complete proteins. Some animal proteins, however, contain less than the required amount of one or more essential amino acids and, therefore, cannot alone support continued growth. These proteins are sometimes referred to as **partially complete proteins**. Examples are some fish, which have small amounts of methionine, and the milk protein casein, which has little arginine.

Incomplete proteins lack one or more essential amino acids (most commonly lysine, methionine, or tryptophan) and are usually derived from vegetables. If, however, an appropriate mixture of plant proteins is provided in the diet, a balanced ration of essential amino acids can be achieved. For example, a combination of corn (low in tryptophan and lysine) and beans (low in methionine) is a complete protein. Such combinations of two or more vegetables are called *complementary proteins*. Another way to take full advantage of vegetable proteins is to eat them with a small amount of animal protein. Examples are spaghetti with cheese, rice with pork, noodles with tuna, and cereal with milk. See the discussion of vegetarian diets later in this chapter.

PROTEIN DIGESTION Digestion of protein foods begins in the stomach. However, most protein is digested in the small intestine, where enzymes break it down into successively smaller molecules and finally into amino acids, the end products of protein digestion. The pancreas secretes the proteolytic enzymes trypsin, chymotrypsin, and carboxypeptidase; glands in the intestinal wall secrete aminopeptidase and dipeptidase.

PROTEIN METABOLISM The liver coordinates the metabolism of amino acids and the creation of protein. Protein synthesis is a complicated process that assembles amino acids that are used to create proteins needed by the body. Protein metabolism includes three activities: (a) **anabolism** (energy reactions that build tissue), (b) **catabolism** (energy-producing reactions from breaking down tissue), and (c) **nitrogen balance**.

Anabolism All body cells synthesize proteins from amino acids. The types of proteins formed depend on the characteristics of the cell and are controlled by its genes.

Catabolism Because a cell can accumulate only a limited amount of protein, excess amino acids are degraded for energy or converted to fat. Protein degradation occurs primarily in the liver.

Nitrogen Balance Because nitrogen is the element that distinguishes protein from lipids and carbohydrates, nitrogen balance reflects the status of protein nutrition in the body. Nitrogen balance is a measure of the degree of protein anabolism and catabolism; it is the net result of intake and loss of nitrogen. When nitrogen intake equals nitrogen output, a state of nitrogen balance exists. If the protein synthesis exceeds the protein breakdown, as in pregnancy, growth, and recovery from injury, then a positive nitrogen state exists. However, a negative nitrogen state occurs when the protein synthesis is less than the protein breakdown. This negative state could occur during starvation or malnutrition or in the catabolic phase of recovery.

PROTEIN STORAGE Amino acids are absorbed by active transport through the small intestine into the portal blood circulation. The liver uses some amino acids to synthesize specific proteins (e.g., liver cells and the plasma proteins albumin, globulin, and fibrinogen). Plasma proteins are a storage medium that can rapidly be converted back into amino acids.

Other amino acids are transported to tissues and cells throughout the body, where they are used to make protein for cell structures. In a sense, protein is stored as body tissue. The body cannot actually store excess amino acids for future use. However, a limited amount is available in the *metabolic pool* that exists because of the constant breakdown and buildup of the protein in body tissues.

Lipids

Lipids are organic substances that are greasy and insoluble in water but soluble in alcohol or ether. Lipids include triglycerides (fats and oils), phospholipids (lecithin), and sterols (cholesterols). Lipids have the same elements (carbon, hydrogen, and oxygen) as carbohydrates. Triglycerides have proportionally less oxygen and so provide more than double the amount of calories for an equivalent amount of carbohydrate.

Fatty acids, made up of carbon chains and hydrogen, are the basic structural units of most lipids. Fatty acids are described as saturated or unsaturated, according to the relative number of hydrogen atoms they contain. **Saturated fatty acids** are those in which all carbon atoms are filled to capacity (i.e., saturated) with hydrogen; an example is butyric acid, found in butter. An **unsaturated fatty acid** is one that could accommodate more hydrogen atoms than it currently does. It has at least two carbon atoms that are not attached to a hydrogen atom; instead, a double bond exists between the two carbon atoms. Fatty acids with one double bond are called **monounsaturated fatty acids**; those with more than one double bond (or many carbons not bonded to a hydrogen atom) are **polyunsaturated fatty acids**. An example of a polyunsaturated fatty acid is linoleic acid, found in vegetable oil.

Saturated fats are generally solid at room temperature. The exceptions are coconut and palm oils. Unsaturated fats have been hydrogenated by adding hydrogen to some of the double bonds to improve the stability and increase the function of the fat or oil. A consequence of hydrogenation is the alteration of the double hydrogen bonds, which results in a shift from the *cis* position to the *trans* position. The result is **trans fats**, which are not normally found in nature. In the typical North American diet, 2% to 4% of total caloric intake comes from these fats. Trans fats are reported to raise the "bad" cholesterol levels and lower "good" cholesterol. Trans fats appear in hard margarine, fried foods, and many prepared bakery goods, such as doughnuts, cookies, muffins, croissants, and french fries. Health Canada recognized the risks of trans fats and made changes to help Canadians make healthier choices. Canada was the first country in the world to introduce mandatory labelling of trans fats. As of 2005, the trans fat content of foods was required to be listed on the Nutrition Facts Table of packaged foods.

Lipids that are required for normal growth and development but that cannot be synthesized by the body are called **essential fatty acids**. They also play a critical role in inflammation and the clotting mechanism. **Omega-3 fatty acids** and **omega-6 fatty acids** are essential fatty acids. Omega-3 fatty acids (e.g., alpha-linolenic acid (ALA) eicosapentaenoic acid (EPA), docosahexaenoic acid (DHA) are polyunsaturated fats that have been shown to lower serum triglyceride levels, reduce blood pressure, and decrease factors contributing to blood clotting and strokes. Omega-3 fatty acids are found primarily in cold water fish (e.g., albacore tuna, sardines, and lake trout), walnuts, flax, hemp, and canola oil.

Omega-6 fatty acids (e.g., linoleic acid, gamma-linolenic acid, arachidonic acid), also polyunsaturated fats, are generally consumed in adequate quantities in Western diets. Sources of linoleic acid include poultry, eggs, avocado, nuts, and most vegetable oils (sunflower, safflower, corn, cottonseed, and soybean oils). It was previously thought that excessive consumption of omega-6 fatty acids or an imbalance in the ratio of omega-3 to omega-6 FAs in the diet was linked to the development of several chronic diseases, including coronary artery disease, diabetes mellitus, osteoporosis, and some autoimmune disorders. Arachidonic acid, converted from the metabolism of linoleic acid, is a substrate in the production of proinflammatory mediators, such as prostaglandin E_2, thromboxane A_2, and leukotriene B_4. However, it is also a substrate for the production of multiple anti-inflammatory and anti-aggregatory molecules. Higher levels of anti-inflammatory markers have been noted in individuals with diets high in omega-6s in observational studies (Pischon, Hankison, Hotamisligil, Rifai, Willett, & Rimm, 2003). Furthermore, since the production of arachidonic acid from linoleic acid does not vary widely despite huge variations in dietary intake of its precursor, there are small variations in tissue concentration (Harris, Mozaffarian, Rimm, Kris-Etherton, Rudel, & Appel, 2009). It was postulated that a ratio of omega-3 to omega-6 less than 1:4 in the diet was in fact ideal for the prevention of coronary artery disease and inflammatory conditions (Simopoulos, 2008). However, new research about the benefits of omega-6 suggests that both omega-3 and omega-6 acids are important in the prevention of chronic disease and that the concept of a ratio to guide the consumption of polyunsaturated acids is mathematically problematic (Harris, 2006).

Given the benefits of omega-3 FAs in particular, Canadians should be encouraged to increase their consumption of these polyunsaturated fats. Adult male Canadians should strive to consume 1.6 g/day of all omega 3s and females should aim for 1.1 g/day (IOM, 2006). Pregnant women have increased needs for omega 3 fatty acids as they promote healthy fetal development (up to 1.4 g/day). Thus, Health Canada recommends that pregnant women consume 150 g of cooked fish per week, choosing among the fish that generally have less contaminants (e.g., methyl mercury). These fish include salmon, trout, herring, haddock, canned light tuna, pollock (Boston bluefish), sole, flounder, anchovy, char, hake, mullet, smelt, Atlantic mackerel, and lake white fish (Health Canada, 2009). Some foods, such as milk and eggs, may have omega-3 and omega-6 fatty acids added to them. Omega-6 fatty acids should not be omitted completely from the diet as linoleic acid and gamma-linolenic acid are essential for maintaining healthy skin and growth in children.

On the basis of their chemical structure, lipids are classified as simple or compound. Glycerides, the simple lipids, are the most common form of lipids. They consist of a glycerol molecule with up to three fatty acids attached. **Triglycerides** (which have three fatty acids) account for more than 90% of the lipids in food and in the body. Triglycerides can contain saturated or unsaturated fatty acids. Saturated triglycerides are found in animal products, such as butter, and are usually solid at room temperature. Unsaturated triglycerides are usually liquid at room temperature and are found in plant products, such as olive oil and corn oil.

Phospholipids contain a glycerol molecule and two fatty acids. They occur naturally in almost all foods. Rich sources include liver, eggs, wheat germ, and peanuts. They work as emulsifiers to keep fats suspended in the blood and other body fluids. They provide structure to the cell membrane and help in the transport of fat-soluble substances across that membrane. Lecithin is the best known phospholipid.

Sterols contain carbon, hydrogen, and oxygen arranged in rings. **Cholesterol**, a sterol, is a fat-like substance that is produced by the body and found in foods of animal origin. Most of the body's cholesterol is synthesized by the liver; however, some is absorbed from the diet.

Cholesterol is needed to create bile acids and to synthesize sex hormones and adrenocortical hormones. Cholesterol is found in all cell membranes. The cholesterol found in food is simply cholesterol—it is neither "good" nor "bad." The terms *good* and *bad* cholesterol are related to the **lipoprotein** (a group of compounds made by the body to move water-insoluble lipids) packages that transport the cholesterol through the blood. Two lipoproteins play a role in cholesterol levels: **low-density lipoproteins (LDLs)** and **high-density lipoproteins (HDLs)**. These endogenous lipoproteins carry fat and cholesterol to the tissues for use in energy production and for exchange with other products in cell metabolism. They are classified according to their ratio of fat to protein, and as their concentration of protein increases, their density increases. Because the LDLs carry cholesterol to the cells and deposit it there, they are considered the so-called *bad* cholesterol. The HDLs carry cholesterol from the tissues to the liver for catabolism and excretion and so are considered the *good* cholesterol.

LIPID DIGESTION Although the chemical digestion of fats begins in the stomach, fats are primarily digested in the small intestine, primarily by bile, pancreatic lipase, and enteric lipase, an intestinal enzyme. The end products of fat digestion are glycerol and fatty acids. Some fat is excreted in the feces.

LIPID METABOLISM Fatty acids and glycerol enter cells where they can be catabolized for energy or rebuilt and stored as triglycerides. Fat catabolism is regulated by adrenocorticotropin, epinephrine, glucagon, and glucocorticoids, whereas fat anabolism is stimulated by insulin.

LIPID STORAGE Lipids are stored in the liver, adipose tissue, and muscle tissue for release when needed for energy. Fat stored in subcutaneous tissue helps to provide insulation to the body. Fat that is stored in fatty tissue acts to protect vital organs by absorbing mechanical forces.

Essential Nutrients: Micronutrients

A **vitamin** is an organic compound that cannot be manufactured by the body and is needed in small quantities to catalyze metabolic processes. Thus, when vitamins are lacking in the diet, metabolic deficits result. Vitamins are generally classified as fat soluble or water soluble. **Water-soluble vitamins** include vitamin C and the B-complex vitamins: B_1 (thiamine), B_2 (riboflavin), B_3 (niacin or nicotinic acid), B_6 (pyridoxine), B_9 (folic acid), B_{12} (cobalamin), pantothenic acid, and biotin. The body cannot store water-soluble vitamins; thus, people must get a daily supply in the diet. Water-soluble vitamins can be affected by food processing, storage, and preparation.

Fat-soluble vitamins include vitamins A, D, E, and K. The body can store these vitamins, although the amounts of vitamins E and K the body can store are limited. Therefore, a daily supply of fat-soluble vitamins is not absolutely necessary. Vitamin content is highest in fresh foods that are consumed as soon as possible after harvest.

Minerals are found in organic compounds as inorganic compounds and as free ions. On oxidation, minerals leave an ash, which can be acidic or alkaline. Calcium and phosphorus make up 80% of all the mineral elements in the body. Minerals come in two categories: (a) macrominerals and (b) microminerals. **Macrominerals** are those that people require in daily amounts of more than 100 mg. They include calcium, phosphorus, sodium, potassium, magnesium, chloride, and sulphur. **Microminerals** are those that people require in daily amounts of less than 100 mg. They include iron, zinc, manganese, iodine, fluoride, copper, cobalt, chromium, and selenium.

Health Canada (2010a) has developed recommendations for the daily intake of these key nutrients. These recommendations are based on sex and age, and whether a woman is pregnant or lactating. **Dietary reference intakes** are four reference values: (a) *recommended dietary allowances,* (b) *adequate intake,* (c) *tolerable upper intake level,* and (d) *estimated average requirement.* These values are used for diet assessment and form the basis of Health Canada's *Eating Well with Canada's Food Guide* (Health Canada, 2007a).

The **recommended dietary allowance** is the amount of a specific vitamin, micromineral, or macromineral that 97% to 98% of healthy individuals should consume based on their age and sex. These recommendations are available online (see the Weblinks section of this chapter for the website). **Adequate intake** is the recommended intake value when a recommended dietary allowance cannot be established; the **tolerable upper intake level** is the maximum amount of a nutrient that should be ingested to avoid any adverse effects (such as with the ingestion of fat-soluble vitamins); and the **estimated average requirement** is the nutrient intake that would meet the needs of 50% of a particular age and sex group.

Common problems associated with the lack of adequate mineral nutrients are iron deficiency resulting in anemia and osteoporosis resulting from loss of bone calcium. Additional information about major minerals associated with the body's fluid and electrolyte balance is found in Chapter 44.

Energy Balance

Energy balance is the relationship between the energy derived from food and the energy used by the body. The body uses energy for voluntary activities, such as walking and talking, and for involuntary activities, such as breathing and secreting enzymes. In theory, a person's energy balance should be determined by comparing his or her energy intake with his or her energy output. It is, however, more complex because each person metabolizes and stores nutrients in a unique way, although the process is the same.

Traditionally, a person's energy balance was determined by considering the caloric value of the nutrients ingested. Recently, the calorie theory has come into question because it does not fully explain the difficulty some individuals have in maintaining a normal weight. An alternative approach to energy balance is related to the glycemic potential of nutrients ingested.

The Caloric Theory Approach

The amount of energy that nutrients or foods supply to the body is their **caloric value**. A **calorie** is a unit of heat energy. A **small calorie** is the amount of heat required to raise the temperature of 1 gram of water by 1°C. This unit of measure is used only in chemistry and physics. A **large calorie (Calorie, kilocalorie [kcal])** is the amount of heat required to raise the temperature of 1 gram of water from 15°C to 16°C and is the unit used in nutrition. It was recommended in 1970 that the unit kilojoule (kJ), a metric measurement, replace the kilocalorie. A **kilojoule** is the amount of energy required when a force of 1 newton (N) moves 1 kilogram of weight to a distance of 1 metre. However, to date, Canada and the United States have not made the change.

One calorie (kcal) equals 4.18 kJ. The energy liberated from the metabolism of food has been determined to be as follows:

- 4 cal/g (about 16 kJ) of carbohydrates
- 4 cal/g (about 16 kJ) of protein
- 7 cal/g (about 28 kJ) of alcohol
- 9 cal/g (about 37 kJ) of fat

The rate of **metabolism,** or metabolic rate, is normally expressed in terms of the rate of heat liberated during the biochemical and physiological processes by which the body grows and maintains itself. The **basal metabolic rate (BMR)** is the baseline number of calories required to support involuntary body functions at rest after a 12-hour fast. The **resting energy expenditure (REE)** is similar to the BMR, but with no 12-hour fasting period. The two terms are often used interchangeably. The REE of healthy persons is generally about 1 cal/kg of body weight/h for men and 0.9 cal/kg of body weight/h for women, although great variation exists among individuals. BMR is calculated by measuring the REE in the early morning, 12 hours after eating. The actual daily expenditure of energy depends on the individual's degree of activity.

Multiple factors influence a person's BMR. Lean body mass (muscle) requires more calories for maintenance than does adipose (fat) tissue. Thus, men and active children, who have a greater proportion of muscle mass, will have a higher BMR than women, who have a greater proportion of adipose tissue. BMR decreases as muscle mass is lost through the aging process, especially if the aging person is sedentary. The thyroid hormones (thyroxine, or T_4, and tri-iodothyronine, or T_3) regulate the BMR. Hyperthyroidism leads to increased BMR; hypothyroidism decreases BMR. Fever and disease states will increase the BMR. Every 0.83°C rise in body temperature will increase the BMR by about 7%. Increased cell activity associated with pathological conditions, such as cancer, head injury, or trauma, will increase the metabolic demand on the body. Pregnancy and lactation increase the metabolic needs of the body. Living in a very hot or very cold environment will increase the metabolic rate because the body uses more energy to regulate its temperature. During a stressful event, the release of stress hormones will raise the BMR. Ingestion of certain drugs can either increase (e.g., amphetamines) or decrease (e.g., opioids, muscle relaxants) the BMR. Some activities require many times the REE. Examples of approximate real caloric expenditures compared with the REE are as follows:

Light housework	210%
Walking steadily	350%
Heavy housework	400%
Labouring	500%
Average jogging/cycling/energetic swimming	700%

Health Canada (2007c) has produced recommendations for the caloric requirements of Canadians that can be retrieved from the Internet.

The Glycemic Index Approach

A food's **glycemic index (GI)** is determined by how quickly blood glucose levels rise after the food, a carbohydrate, is ingested. Understanding the tenets of this approach to energy balance requires understanding the metabolic process and the roles of glucagon and insulin. The primary function of carbohydrates is to provide fuel for energy production. After carbohydrates are ingested, they are broken down into glucose. If the glucose is not used immediately, it can be stored by the liver as glycogen. **Glycemic level** refers to the amount of glucose present in the blood. The glycemic peak, or maximum absorption level, occurs about 30 minutes after ingestion of the food.

If the glycemic level becomes low, a condition called **hypoglycemia**, the body is in need of fuel or glucose. The pancreas then secretes the hormone glucagon, which reestablishes the glycemic level. If the glycemic levels become high, following a glycemic peak, then the pancreas secretes another hormone, insulin. The role of insulin is to eliminate the excess glucose from the blood and facilitate its storage in the liver or muscles or as glycerides in the adipocytes (fat cells). If a carbohydrate has a high GI, then its ingestion will lead to a rapid increase in glucose in the blood—a condition referred to as **hyperglycemia**. The GI of a food can be altered by the way it is processed or prepared. For example, instant potatoes have a GI of 95; baked potatoes have a GI of 90; potatoes boiled without skin have a GI of 70; and potatoes boiled with skin have a GI of 65. Table 40.1 on the next page provides examples of foods with low, medium, and high GIs.

For some people, maintaining a balance between the blood glucose level and the insulin level is problematic. The result can be a state of **hyperinsulinemia**, meaning there is excess insulin present in the blood. If the state of hyperinsulinemia persists, glucose is stored in the adipocytes. In addition, this phenomenon is worsened by the development of **insulin resistance**, in which the sensitivity to insulin by the receptors on the cells is diminished. These two problems are classic hallmarks for the development of type 2 diabetes mellitus and **metabolic syndrome** (a constellation of central obesity, dyslipidemia, hypertension, and insulin resistance, leading to increased risk of type 2 diabetes mellitus and cardiovascular disease).

For people prone to weight gain, watching their caloric intake may not be sufficient. They may need to pay closer attention to the GI of the carbohydrate than to its caloric value. The Canadian Diabetes Association advocates the use of the GI for people with type 1 and type 2 diabetes mellitus.

TABLE 40.1 Glycemic Indices of Selected Foods

Low GI (55 or less)	Medium GI (56–59)	High GI (70 or more)
100% stone ground whole wheat bread	Whole wheat bread	White bread
Heavy mixed grain bread	Rye bread	Kaiser roll
Pumpernickel bread	Pita	Bagel, white
Oat Bran™	Oatmeal	Bran flakes
All-Bran™	Grape Nuts™	Rice Krispies™
Converted or parboiled rice	Basmati rice	Corn Flakes™
Bulgar	Brown rice	Short-grain rice
Pasta/noodles	Couscous	Potato, baking (Russet)
Lentils/kidney/baked beans	Potato, new/white	Rice cakes
Chick peas	Popcorn	Pretzels
Sweet potato/yams	Black bean/green pea soup	French fries

Source: Based on Canadian Diabetes Association. (2008). *Glycemic Index.* Retrieved from http://www.diabetes.ca/files/Diabetes_GL_FINAL2_CPG03.pdf

Factors Affecting Nutrition

Although the nutritional content of food is important to consider in determining an eating plan, other major factors influence the selection and ingestion of food. For many Canadians, patterns of eating are influenced by stage of development, sex, ethnicity and culture, beliefs about food, personal preferences, religious practices, lifestyle, economics, medications or therapy, state of health, alcohol consumption, advertising, and psychological factors.

Stage of Development

People in rapid periods of growth (i.e., infancy and adolescence) have increased need for nutrients. Older people, however, need fewer calories and may need dietary changes in view of the risk of coronary heart disease, osteoporosis, and hypertension. See the section "Nutritional Variations throughout the Lifespan" in this chapter.

Sex

Nutrient requirements are different for men and women because of body composition and reproductive functions. The larger muscle mass of men means a greater need for calories and proteins. Because of menstruation, women require more iron than men do. Pregnant and lactating women have increased caloric and fluid needs.

Ethnicity and Culture

The environment in which an individual is raised plays a major role in that person's food preferences and dietary habits. These dietary traditions have been passed on for generations. However, it is not uncommon for members of different generations of the same family to have different food preferences (e.g. grandparents may eat more traditional fare than their grandchildren). Dietary practices can include the way in which foods are prepared, what to eat or not to eat when a person is ill or pregnant, foods associated with rites of passage, and the variety of foods that are routinely included in the diet.

When a person is unwell or pregnant, it is important that the nurse understands the ramifications that person's culture will have on his or her overall nutritional state. For example, when giving information to a pregnant woman about her need for increased nutrients, the nurse must know whether the information is congruent with the client's ethnic background. If the information is incongruent, then equivalent food sources must be substituted. Teaching this client may also include discussing cultural myths about certain foods. *Eating Well with Canada's Food Guide* takes into account the variety of foods that Canadians enjoy.

Nurses should not use a *good food, bad food* approach but, rather, should realize that variations of intake are acceptable under different circumstances. The only universally accepted guidelines are (a) to eat a wide variety of foods to provide adequate nutrients and (b) to eat moderately to maintain correct body weight. Food preference probably differs as much among individuals of the same cultural background as it does generally between cultures. Not all Italians like pizza, for example, and many undoubtedly enjoy spicy Mexican food.

Beliefs about Food

Beliefs about effects of foods on health and well-being can affect food choices. Many people acquire their beliefs about food from television, magazines, and the Internet.

Food fads that involve nontraditional food practices are relatively common. A **fad** is a widespread but short-lived interest or practice followed with considerable zeal. It may be based either on the belief that certain foods have special powers (e.g., large amounts of yogourt and vitamin E retard the aging process) or on the notion that certain foods are harmful (e.g., eating cabbage and onions sours breast milk). Many fad diets advocate certain eating patterns to stimulate rapid weight loss and are potentially dangerous. Often, such diets do not include the variety of foods necessary for good health. Proponents of the fad may also falsely claim that the body can be tricked into losing weight through the consumption of certain foods. Fad diet gurus often make unrealistic and unscientific claims about the rate of weight loss. It is important for nurses to recognize the popularity of fad diets so that they can promote balanced and nutritious food consumption.

Personal Preferences

People develop likes and dislikes based on associations with a typical food. Parents are key role models in their child's taste preferences. So, if a parent likes or dislikes certain foods, the child will probably have similar preferences. Also, the parents' eating patterns will be mimicked by the child. These preferences and habits are then carried into adulthood.

Individual likes and dislikes can also be related to familiarity. Children often say they dislike a food before they sample it. Some adults are very adventurous and eager to try new foods. Others prefer to eat the same foods over and over again. Preferences in the tastes, smells, flavours (blends of taste and smell), temperatures, colours, shapes, and sizes of food influence a person's food choices. For example, some people may prefer sweet and sour tastes to bitter or salty tastes. Textures play a great role in food preferences. Some people prefer crisp food to limp food, firm to soft, tender to tough, smooth to lumpy, or dry to soggy.

Religious Practices

Religious practice can influence the food selection and preparation. For example, some Protestant faiths prohibit consumption of meat, caffeine, or alcohol. Both Orthodox Judaism and Islam prohibit the consumption of pork or pork products. Some religions have strict guidelines for the preparation of foods or the combinations of foods that cannot be ingested at the same time (such as dairy and meat products in Judaism). The nurse must be sensitive to the client's religious beliefs when issues surrounding nutrition become paramount.

Lifestyle

A person's lifestyle is linked to his or her eating patterns. A less active person requires fewer nutrients than does a person who is engaged in heavy physical activity on a regular basis. For some individuals, meal preparation is either not important or not possible because of busy work schedules. These people often rely on restaurants and convenience foods to meet their nutritional needs. Others place a great deal of importance on what they ingest and how that food is produced and prepared.

Some Canadians may not have access to foods because of their physical state (e.g., cannot walk or drive to buy food). Other Canadians, including some First Nations peoples, may have difficulty accessing fresh fruit and vegetables at certain times of the year. Some people live in institutions and are totally dependent on caregivers to feed and nourish them. Whatever a person's lifestyle, the important consideration is to eat nourishing and well-balanced meals.

Economics

What, how much, and how often a person eats are frequently affected by socioeconomic status. For example, people with limited income may not be able to afford meat, milk, and fresh vegetables. In contrast, people with higher incomes may purchase more proteins and fats and fewer complex carbohydrates. Not all persons have the financial resources for extensive food preparation and storage. The nurse should not assume that clients have their own stove, refrigerator, or freezer. In some low-income areas or in remote villages, food costs at small local grocery stores can be significantly higher than at large chain stores farther away. In 2007–2008, 1.92 million people in Canada aged 12 years or older, including 228 500 children aged 12 to 17 years, lived in food-insecure households. Almost one-third of these people, including 546 100 adults and 60 000 children aged 12 to 17 years, lived in households with severe food insecurity due to quantitative (insufficient intake, household food depletion) or qualitative (nutritional inadequacy, unsuitable food) factors resulting from economic issues. In the case of First Nations peoples living off reserves, 1 in 5 was food insecure (Health Canada, 2011a).

Medications and Therapy

The relationship between drugs and nutrition is a critical consideration for nurses. Some drugs can alter appetite, disturb taste perception, or interfere with nutrient absorption or excretion. Clients should be encouraged to ask their pharmacist if there are known interactions between drugs and foods. For example, the calcium in milk hinders absorption of the antibiotic tetracycline but enhances the absorption of the antibiotic erythromycin. Selected drug and nutrient interactions are shown in Table 40.2.

It is important for the client to know whether the medications should be taken with food or on an empty stomach. Also, it is important for the clients to tell their pharmacist, physician, and nurse if they are taking any herbal remedies or over-the-counter (OTC) medications. These nonprescription remedies and drugs can have a negative interaction with prescribed drugs or with foods they are eating. Older adults are at particular risk for drug–food interactions because of the number of medications they may take, age-related physiological changes affecting medication actions (e.g., a decrease in lean-to-fat ratio, a decrease in renal or hepatic function), and restricted diets. The nurse plays an important role in determining whether the client is knowledgeable about taking medication and in reinforcing correct information. See Chapter 33 for an extensive discussion of medications.

Therapies prescribed for certain diseases can also adversely affect eating patterns and nutrition. Certain antineoplastic agents (drugs that slow down and fight the development of tumours) can give rise to oral ulcers, intestinal bleeding, nausea and vomiting, or diarrhea, resulting in **anorexia** (no appetite or desire to eat) or diminished absorption of nutrients. Radiotherapy of the head and neck can cause decreased salivation, taste distortions, and swallowing difficulties; radiotherapy of the abdomen and pelvis can cause malabsorption, nausea, vomiting, and diarrhea.

Health

An individual's health status greatly affects eating habits and nutritional status. The lack of teeth, ill-fitting dentures, or a sore mouth makes chewing food difficult.

TABLE 40.2 Selected Drug–Nutrient Interactions

Drug	Effect on Nutrition
Acetylsalicylic acid	Decreases serum folate
Antacids containing aluminum or magnesium hydroxide	Increases excretion of vitamin C, thiamine, potassium, amino acids, and glucose
Thiazide diuretics	May cause nausea and gastritis
Potassium chloride	Decrease absorption of phosphate and vitamin A
Laxatives	Inactivate thiamine
Antihypertensives	May cause deficiency of calcium and vitamin D
Anti-inflammatory agents	Increase excretion of sodium, potassium, chloride, calcium, magnesium, zinc, and riboflavin
Antidepressants	May cause anorexia, nausea, vomiting, diarrhea, or constipation
Antineoplastics	Decrease absorption of vitamin B_{12}

Nutrient	Effect on Drugs
Grapefruit	Can cause toxicity when taken with a variety of medications including certain antiarrhythmics (e.g., amiodarone), calcium channel blockers (e.g., nifedipine), statins (e.g., atorvastatin [Lipitor]), erectile dysfunction drugs (e.g., sildenafil), antiseizure agents (e.g., carbamazepine [Tegretol]), and immunosuppressants (e.g., cyclosporine)
Vitamin K	Can decrease the effectiveness of warfarin (Coumadin)
Tyramine (found in aged cheeses, tap beer, dried sausages, fermented soy, sauerkraut)	In combination with monoamine oxidase inhibitor (MAOI) medications, e.g., phenelzine (Nardil), tranylcypromine (Parnate), isocarboxazid (Marplan), isoniazid, and linezolid, creates sudden increase in epinephrine, leading to headaches, increased pulse and blood pressure, and possible death
Milk	Interferes with absorption of tetracycline and ciprofloxacin

Dysphagia (difficulty swallowing) because of a painfully inflamed throat, a cerebrovascular accident (stroke), or a stricture of the esophagus can prevent a person from obtaining adequate nourishment. Disease processes and surgery of the gastrointestinal tract can affect digestion, absorption, metabolism, and excretion of essential nutrients. Gastrointestinal and other diseases also create anorexia, nausea, vomiting, and diarrhea, all of which can adversely affect a person's appetite and nutritional status. Gallstones, which can block the flow of bile, are a common cause of impaired lipid digestion. Metabolic processes can be impaired by diseases of the liver. Diseases of the pancreas can affect glucose metabolism or fat digestion. Allergies to foods are a critical factor to consider.

Lactose intolerance or **lactose maldigestion** occurs when a person has a shortage of the enzyme lactase needed to breakdown lactose, a sugar in dairy products, into glucose and galactose. Symptoms include abdominal pain, bloating, flatulence, cramping, nausea, and diarrhea. Certain people with lactose maldigestion can tolerate small quantities of dairy products, while others require lactase-enzyme supplementation or must avoid dairy products altogether (Dietitians of Canada, 2011a).

Alcohol Consumption

The calories contained in alcoholic drinks include both those of the alcohol itself and of the juices or other beverages added to the drink. In total, these can constitute large numbers of calories, for example, 150 calories for a regular 341 mL beer, 160 calories for a screwdriver (45 mL vodka plus 120 mL orange juice). Drinking alcohol can lead to weight gain through the addition of these calories to the regular diet plus the effect of alcohol on fat metabolism. A small amount of the alcohol is converted directly to fat. However, the greater effect is that the remainder of the alcohol is converted into acetate by the liver. The acetate released to the bloodstream is used for energy instead of fat and the fat is then stored.

Excessive alcohol use contributes to nutritional deficiencies in a number of ways. Alcohol may replace food in a person's diet, and it can also depress the appetite. Excessive alcohol can have a toxic effect on the intestinal mucosa, thereby decreasing the absorption of nutrients. The need for vitamin B increases because it is used in alcohol metabolism. Alcohol can impair the storage of nutrients and increase nutrient catabolism and excretion.

There is some evidence that moderate consumption of alcohol (one to two drinks per day—15 g of any type of alcohol) may reduce the risk of developing cardiovascular disease (Brien, Ronksley, Turner, Mukamal, & Ghali, 2011; Ronksley, Brien, Turner, Mukamal, & Ghali, 2011). Pregnant women should avoid all alcohol consumption to prevent the development of fetal alcohol effects or fetal alcohol syndrome.

Advertising

Food producers try to persuade people to change from the product they currently use to the brand the producer is selling. Often, popular celebrities are used to influence television viewers' or radio listeners' choices. Advertising is thought to influence people's, particularly children's, food choices and eating patterns. Canada and a growing number of countries have adopted regulations prohibiting food advertising on programs targeting young children.

Think about how foods are laid out in a grocery store and what types of food are close at hand at the checkout counter. Such products as alcoholic beverages, cakes and other dessert mixes, soups, tea, coffee, frozen dinners, and soft drinks are more heavily advertised than such products as milk, canned seafood, bread, cheese, poultry, vegetables, and fruits.

Psychological Factors

A person's emotional state is a major factor in his or her eating pattern. The role of various neurotransmitters, such as serotonin, is important to consider in relation to mood and food ingestion. For example, through a complex process, the ingestion of carbohydrates boosts the release of serotonin in the brain. The release of serotonin leads to relaxation and a reduction in anxiety. For some people, being upset or distressed will cause them to eat very little. This reduction of food ingestion could be related to the release of increased amounts of epinephrine, which is a component of stress response. Anorexia and weight loss can indicate severe stress or depression. Anorexia nervosa and bulimia nervosa are severe psychophysiological conditions seen most frequently in female adolescents and are discussed later in this chapter.

Nutritional Variations throughout the Lifespan

Neonates to 1 Year

The neonate's fluid and nutritional needs are met by breast milk or formula. Fluid needs of infants are proportionately greater than those of adults because of a higher metabolic rate, immature kidneys, and greater water losses through the skin and the lungs. The latter is largely due to rapid respirations. Therefore, fluid balance is a critical factor in infants. Under normal environmental conditions, infants do not need additional water; however, neonates in very warm environments may require additional fluids. In these cases, water may be prescribed.

Breast milk should be the sole form of feeding for the first 6 months of life (Canadian Paediatric Society,

Dietitians of Canada, & Health Canada, 2005, reaffirmed in 2009) except in cases where the mother has tested positive for human immunodeficiency virus (HIV) or is taking certain medications (e.g., cyclophosphamide, lithium), when alternatives to breast-feeding are advised (Health Canada, 2005). Breast-feeding can continue until the child is 2 years of age or longer if the mother chooses. Health Canada (2010g) recommends that all breast-fed, healthy, full-term infants in Canada receive a daily vitamin D supplement of 10 mcg (400 IU). Supplementation should begin at birth and continue until the infant's diet includes at least 10 mcg (400 IU) per day of vitamin D from other dietary sources or until the breast-fed infant reaches 1 year of age. If the mother chooses not to or cannot breast-feed, the infant should be fed iron-fortified commercial formulas until 9 to 12 months of age.

Demand feeding (i.e., feeding whenever the child is hungry) tends to decrease the problem of overfeeding or underfeeding the infant. The newborn who is hungry usually cries and exhibits tension in the entire body. The total daily nutritional requirement of the newborn is about 80 mL to 100 mL of breast milk or formula per kilogram of body weight. The newborn infant's stomach capacity is about 90 mL, and feedings are required every 2.5 to 4 hours. During feeding, the infant sucks readily and needs burping after each 30 mL of formula or after 5 minutes of breast-feeding. Burping is done by holding the infant in an upright position while gently patting the back. *Parents should be warned that infant bottles should never be propped up for feeding.* There is a real danger that aspiration or choking could result.

Infants demonstrate satisfaction by slowing their sucking activity or by falling asleep. Once satisfaction has been demonstrated, infants should not be coaxed into finishing the feeding. This could lead to discomfort or overfeeding. When feeding is completed, healthy infants can be placed in a lateral or supine position for sleep during the first 6 months of life to reduce the risk of sudden infant death syndrome (SIDS).

Regurgitation, or spitting up, of digested milk during or after a feeding is a common occurrence during the first year. Although this may be of concern to parents, it does not usually result in nutritional deficiency. Demonstration of adequate weight gain should reassure parents that the infant is receiving adequate nutrition.

The addition of solid food to the diet usually starts at 6 months of age. Six-month-old infants can consume solid food more readily because they can sit up and they have a decreased sucking reflex. Solid foods (strained or pureed) are generally introduced in the following order: iron-fortified cereals (e.g., rice), vegetables (yellow before green), fruits, egg yolks, and strained meats (see Box 40.1). Foods are introduced one at a time, usually with only one new food introduced every 5 days. With the eruption of teeth at about 7 to 9 months, the infant is ready to chew and can begin to experience different textures of food. At this time, the infant enjoys finger

---

BOX 40.1 INFANT AND TODDLER FOOD SAFETY

The following recommendations aim to ensure infant and toddler safety:

- Do not feed honey to infants less than 1 year of age. Honey can be a source of the *Clostridium botulinum* toxin (Health Canada, 2011b).
- To prevent salmonella poisoning, cook all eggs well and do not feed products containing raw eggs to infants and toddlers (Health Canada, 2006).
- Do not feed hard, small and round, smooth, or sticky solid foods (such as candy, hotdogs, popcorn, and peanut butter). They can cause choking and aspiration.
- Always supervise infants and toddlers during feeding.
- Do not allow children to run around with food in their mouths.
- Do not prop up an infant's bottle.
- To prevent the development of food allergies, it is recommended that infants be breast fed until the age of 6 months. Toddlers should not be fed peanuts, nuts, fish or seafood until 3 years of age. Egg whites can be offered after 1 year of age.

---

foods, such as pieces of fruit with skin removed, dry cereal, or toast.

At about 6 months of age, infants require iron supplementation to prevent iron-deficiency anemia. Iron can be obtained in fortified infant cereals. **Iron-deficiency anemia** is a form of anemia caused by inadequate supply of iron for synthesis of hemoglobin. Iron-fortified cereals are usually recommended by 6 months of age and are continued until the child reaches 18 months. Infants should continue to receive a daily 10 mcg (400 IU) vitamin D supplement until the age of 12 months (Health Canada, 2010g).

Whole pasteurized cow's milk can be introduced between 9 and 12 months of age. Before this time, the digestive tract is immature and anemia can result, as cow's milk is a low source of iron and can cause microscopic gastrointestinal bleeding. Weaning from the breast or bottle to the cup takes place gradually and is usually achieved by age 1 year or later. Some infants have difficulty giving up the bottle, particularly at naptime or bedtime. Parents should be warned that having the bottle in bed can lead to **bottle-mouth syndrome** (tooth decay that results from teeth being bathed in liquids containing sugars) as well as aspiration. The term describes decay of the teeth caused by constant contact with sweet liquid from the bottle. Dentists advocate brushing or cleaning the infant's teeth to prevent bottle-mouth syndrome, especially for the infant who requires a bottle only at naptime or bedtime. Weaning from the bottle can be facilitated by increasingly diluting the formula with water until the infant is drinking plain water; most infants do not like to drink plain water. By the age of 1 year, most infants can be completely fed on table food, and milk intake is about 600 mL per day.

Toddlers

Because of a maturing gastrointestinal tract, toddlers can eat most foods and adjust to three meals each day. In addition, by age 3 years, when most of the deciduous teeth have emerged, the toddler is able to bite and chew adult table food. Toddlers' manipulative skills are sufficiently well developed for them to learn how to feed themselves. Before the age of 20 months, most toddlers require help with glasses and cups because their wrist control is limited.

Developing independence may be exhibited through the toddler's refusal of certain foods. Meals should be short because of environmental distractions and the toddler's brief attention span. Often, toddlers display their liking of rituals by eating foods in a certain order, cutting foods a specific way, or accompanying certain foods with a particular drink.

The toddler is less likely to have fluid imbalances than the infant. The toddler's gastrointestinal function is more mature, and the percentage of fluid body weight is lower. A healthy toddler weighing 15 kg needs about 1250 mL of fluid per 24 hours.

During the toddler stage, the caloric requirement decreases to 1200 to 1800 kcal per day because of a decrease in the rate of growth. From 1 to 2 years of age, the toddler may be eating a combination of prepared toddler foods and some table foods. Parents should be instructed to read labels carefully and be aware that the table foods offer more variety, are less expensive, and are more nutritious than prepared toddler foods. Deficiencies of iron, calcium, and vitamins C and A, which are common toddler deficiencies, should also be discussed.

The following suggestions may help parents meet the child's nutritional needs and promote effective parent–child interactions: (a) Make mealtime a pleasant time by avoiding tensions at the table and discussions of bad behaviour; (b) offer a variety of simple, attractive foods in small portions, and avoid meals that combine foods into one dish, such as a stew; (c) do not use food as a reward or punish a child who does not eat; (d) schedule meals, sleep, and snack times that will allow for optimum appetite and behaviour; and (e) avoid the routine use of sweet desserts.

Preschoolers

The preschooler eats adult foods and should have the required amounts from *Eating Well with Canada's Food Guide*. The preschooler requires 1600 kcal per day. Parents should become informed about the diet of their child in daycare or preschool settings so that they can be sure of meeting the child's total nutritional needs. Children at this age are very active and may rush through the meal to return to playing. Parents need to teach the preschooler how to use utensils and should provide them with the opportunity to practise (e.g., spreading margarine on bread). Active children often require snacks between meals. Cheese, fruits, yogourt, raw vegetables, and milk are good choices. Children at this age may enjoy helping in the kitchen, and both girls and boys should be encouraged to do so.

The preschooler is even less susceptible than the toddler to fluid imbalances. The average 5-year-old weighing 20 kg requires at least 75 mL of liquid per kilogram of body weight per day, or 1500 mL every 24 hours.

School-Age Children

Nutrition continues to be a high priority for growing children. School-age children require a balanced diet, including 2400 kcal per day. School-age children eat three meals a day and one or two nutritious snacks. Children need a protein-rich food at breakfast to sustain the prolonged physical and mental effort required at school. Studies have shown that children who skip breakfast become inattentive and restless by late morning and have decreased problem-solving ability.

The average healthy 8-year-old weighing 30 kg requires about 1750 mL of fluid per day. Many school-age children have only one meal a day with their family, at dinner. Mealtime should be a social time enjoyed by all, and families should refrain from watching television or discussing a child's poor eating habits at this time. Parents should be aware that children learn many of their food habits by observing their parents. Eating a balanced diet should be the norm for both parents and children.

The school-age child generally eats lunch at school. The child may bring lunch from home or buy lunch at the school cafeteria. Many dietary problems stem from this independence in food choices. The children may trade their food, not eat lunch at all, or buy sweets or junk food with their lunch money. Parents should discuss with the child the foods that they should eat and continue to provide a balanced diet in the home setting. Strict rules have been enacted in certain provinces and territories to limit unhealthy food choices offered in the school environment (e.g., banning sugary beverages and chocolate bars from vending machines). Many schools now prevent children from bringing foods with common allergens including all forms of peanuts, other nuts, and fish.

Although the rate of childhood obesity is increasing, many Canadian children experience food insecurity and consequently go to school hungry. The Canadian Hunger Count 2010, a survey of food banks conducted by Food Banks Canada, revealed that 867 948 people were assisted by a food bank. Of those individuals, 38% were children under the age of 18 years, and 51% of the assisted families had children (Food Banks Canada, 2010). Undernourished children become fatigued easily and face a greater risk of infection, resulting in frequent absences from school. Children who go to school hungry have difficulty learning and interventions such as school-based breakfast programs improve childhood outcomes, such as academic performance, problem-solving skills, school attendance, and mood (Rampersaud, Pereira, Girard, Adams, & Metzl, 2005).

Despite the prevalence of childhood hunger in Canada, obesity is increasingly a problem that begins in childhood and continues in adolescence and adulthood (see Box 40.2). In the last 30 years, there has been an alarming increase in the prevalence of overweight and obese children in Canada. In 2009, 26% of all boys and girls aged 2 to 18 years were obese (Statistics Canada, 2010a; Shields, 2006). Specifically, from 1978 to 2004, in Canada, the overweight or obesity rate of adolescents aged 12 to 17 years more than doubled from 14% to 29%, and the obesity rate alone tripled from 3% to 9% (Shields, 2006). Among First Nations children, the rates of obesity and overweight are two to three times higher (Public Health Agency of Canada, 2010), likely due, in part, to the high levels of poverty that result in a lack of access to high-quality, nutritious foods. In one recent survey of an Aboriginal Cree community in Northern

Quebec, 98.5% of children in grades 4 to 6 consumed less than five servings of fruits and vegetables per day (Downs, Arnold, Marshall, McCargar, & Willows, 2009).

Poor eating habits and a sedentary lifestyle contribute to obesity. For children, hours of "screen time" result in less physical activity. Obesity in school-age children tends to result in a further decrease in activity, creating a viscious circle. In one study of Cree children in Northern Quebec, 100% of obese children had fitness scores below the 20th percentile for their age and sex (Ng, Marshall, & Willows, 2006). Multifaceted interventions at the level of the family and society as a whole are required to address this wide-reaching public health threat.

Nurses are responsible for identifying individuals at risk and intervening with a family-centred approach. Nurses can work with adults and children to do the following:

- Review the individual's eating habits.
- Alter food choices to better follow *Eating Well with Canada's Food Guide.*

BOX 40.2 THE OBESITY EPIDEMIC

In the last 25 years, there has been an exponential increase in the number of overweight and obese Canadians. Given the clear relationship between excess weight and the development of chronic disease, this trend is very alarming. Nurses play a key role in health promotion and must become proactively involved in addressing this problem at the level of the individual, family, and community. The etiology of obesity is complex. At a basic level, it is caused by a chronic energy imbalance whereby the number of calories consumed exceeds the number of calories expended. For example, over the last century, sedentary employment has replaced physical labour and regular physical activity. However, obesity has many contributing factors, including economics, genetics, culture, media, and education (Public Health Agency of Canada, 2010). It is estimated that in 2006, the direct cost to the Canadian health care system of obesity was $6 billion (Anis, Zhang, Bansback, Guh, Amarsi, & Birmingham, 2010). One in 10 premature deaths of adults between 20 and 64 years of age is attributable to obesity (Lau, Douketis, Morrison, Hramiak, Sharma, & Ur, 2007). The latest data from the 2007 Canadian Health Measures Survey (CHMS) and the 2009 Canadian Community Health Survey (Statistics Canada, 2010b) reveals that 59.2% of Canadian men and 43.9% of women were at increased health risk due to being overweight or obese with a BMI greater than 25 kg/m²; 24.1% are obese with a body mass index greater than 30 kg/m² (Shields, Carroll, & Ogden, 2011).

The health consequences of being overweight or obese are serious. Overweight and obese individuals are at increased risk of type 2 diabetes mellitus, hypertension, dyslipidemia, stroke, coronary artery disease, obstructive sleep apnea, osteoarthritis, and certain cancers (Lau et al., 2007). Obese and overweight surgical patients are at increased risk of atelectasis and urinary retention, poor

wound healing, and wound dehiscence. The psychological ramifications can also be severe. Obese adolescents, for example, are frequently rejected by their peers, badgered by their parents, and ridiculed on television and in the movies. Many feel ugly and socially unacceptable. Depression and low self-esteem are common among obese individuals. Increasingly, the health consequences of excess weight, such as the development of type 2 diabetes mellitus, hypertension, obstructive sleep apnea, polycystic ovary syndrome, and slipped capital femoral epiphysis are being seen in childhood and adolescence (Choudhary, Donnelly, Racadio, & Strife, 2007). Given the health ramifications, obese and overweight children in Nova Scotia had significantly more physician and specialist referrals than their normal-weight peers (Kuhle, Kirk, Ohinmaa, Yasui, Allen, & Veugelers, 2010).

Preventing obesity is key to avoiding lifelong health problems. Convincing evidence suggests that increasing total physical activity decreases the risk of overweight and obesity. Breast-feeding and diets high in whole-grain cereals and dietary fibre, fruit, and vegetables also decrease the risk.

Treatment of obesity includes low-calorie diets in combination with physical activity. In some cases, medication is used. Lifestyle modification and behavioural interventions will work in combination with other approaches. For extreme obesity, bariatric surgery may be indicated. The treatment of excess weight must include education and regular screening and interventions for obesity-related conditions. Regular physical activity is key (Wilding, 2007). Obesity Canada has produced clinical guidelines on the prevention and management of obesity in adults and children. A stepwise algorithm to assist health care professionals in applying the guidelines in clinical practice (Lau et al., 2007) is found in Figure 40.1.

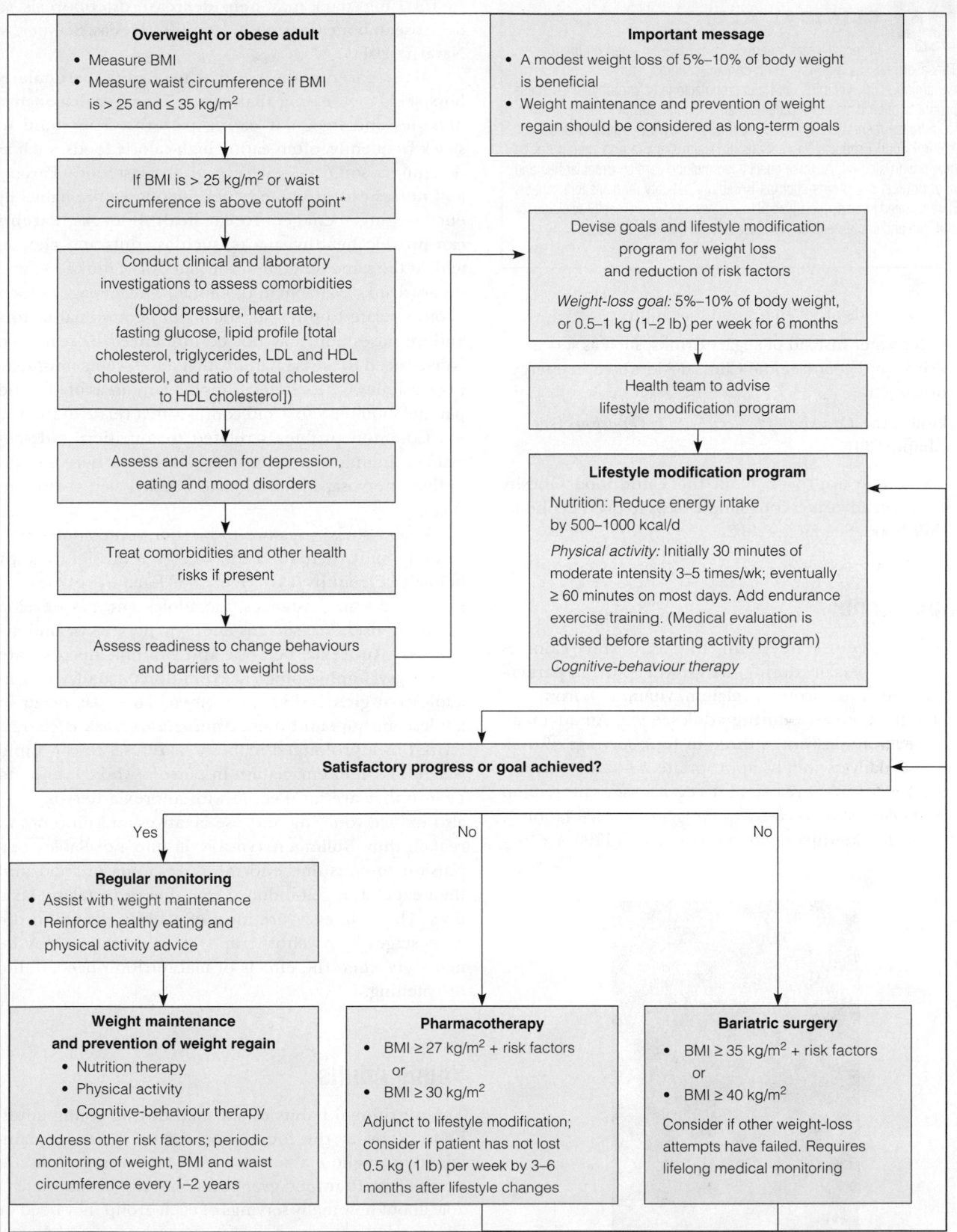

FIGURE 40.1 Algorithm for the assessment and stepwise management of the overweight or obese adult.

*LDL = low-density lipoprotein, HDL = high-density lipoprotein.

Source: Lau, D. C., Douketis, J. D., Morrison, K. M., Hramiak, I. M., Sharma, A. M., & Ur, E. (2007). 2006 Canadian clinical practice guidelines on the management and prevention of obesity in adults and children [summary]. *Canadian Medical Association Journal, 176*(8), s1–s13. This work is protected by copyright and the making of this copy was with the permission of Access Copyright. Any alteration of its content or further copying in any form whatsoever is strictly prohibited unless otherwise permitted by law.

- Use rewards other than food for children.
- Offer water instead of sugary drinks, such as sports drinks and cola (see the Clinical Alert box on energy drinks).
- Follow the *Canadian Physical Activity Guidelines* (see Chapter 39).

A simple approach from the Childhood Obesity Foundation advocates four simple steps to prevent obesity in childhood. See Figure 40.2.

Adolescents

The adolescent's need for nutrients and calories increases, especially during the growth spurt. In particular, the need for protein, calcium, vitamin D, iron, and B vitamins increases during adolescence. An adequate diet for an adolescent is three to four servings of milk products daily as well as appropriate amounts of meat, vegetables, fruits, breads, and cereals (see the section on *Canada's Food Guide* for serving recommendations). Calcium intake during adolescent years (1200 mg/day

to 1500 mg/day) may help decrease osteoporosis (a decrease in bone density) in later life (Mesias, Seiquer, & Navarro, 2011).

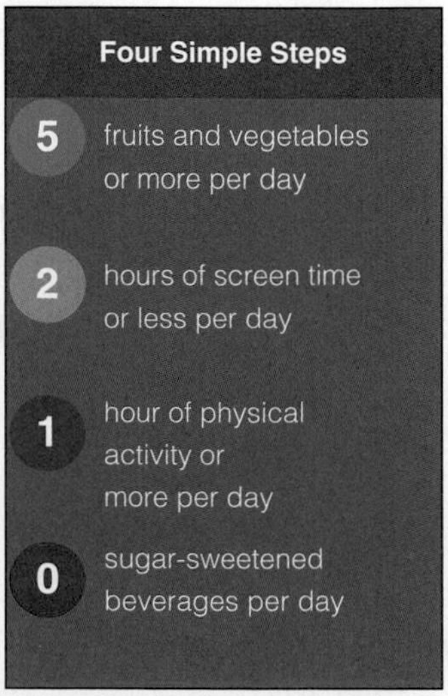

Many parents observe that teenagers, particularly boys, seem to be eating all the time. Teenagers have active lifestyles and irregular eating patterns. They tend to snack frequently, often eating high-calorie foods, such as doughnuts, soft drinks, ice cream, and fast foods. Parents and nurses can promote better lifelong eating habits by encouraging teenagers to eat healthy snacks. Parents can provide healthy snacks, such as fruits and cheese, and, at the same time, limit the amount of junk food and sugary drinks available in the home. The teenager's food choices relate to physical, social, and emotional factors and impulses and may not be influenced by teaching. Nurses need to advise parents that adolescents must take responsibility for their decisions in many areas of life, and parents should try to avoid conflicts that relate to food.

Common problems related to nutrition and self-esteem among adolescents are anorexia nervosa and bulimia nervosa, in addition to obesity, as discussed in Box 40.2.

Under social pressure to be slim, some adolescents severely limit their food intake to a level significantly below that required to meet the demands of normal growth. In some instances, the adolescent may develop an eating disorder, such as anorexia nervosa or bulimia nervosa. Anorexia nervosa and bulimia nervosa are severe psychophysiological conditions usually seen in adolescent girls and young women. They also occur in adolescent boys and men. **Anorexia nervosa** is characterized by a prolonged inability or refusal to eat, rapid weight loss, and emaciation in persons who continue to believe they are fat. People with anorexia nervosa may also induce vomiting and use laxatives and diuretics to remain thin. **Bulimia nervosa** is an uncontrollable compulsion to consume enormous amounts of food and then expel it by self-induced vomiting or by taking laxatives. These illnesses are most effectively treated in the early stages by psychotherapy. Hospitalization may be necessary when the effects of malnutrition become life threatening.

Four Simple Steps

5 fruits and vegetables or more per day

2 hours of screen time or less per day

1 hour of physical activity or more per day

0 sugar-sweetened beverages per day

FIGURE 40.2 Four simple steps to prevent obesity in childhood.

Source: Childhood Obesity Foundation. Vancouver, British Columbia. Retrieved from http://www.childhoodobesityfoundation.ca/ourStory

Young Adults

The nutritional habits established during young adulthood often lay the foundation for the patterns maintained throughout a person's life. Many young adults are aware of the four food groups but may not be knowledgeable about how many servings of each group they need or how much constitutes a serving. The nurse should discuss *Eating Well with Canada's Food Guide* (Figure 40.3) with the young adult client and review serving and portion sizes with them.

Young adult females are at risk for developing iron-deficiency anemia because of blood loss during their

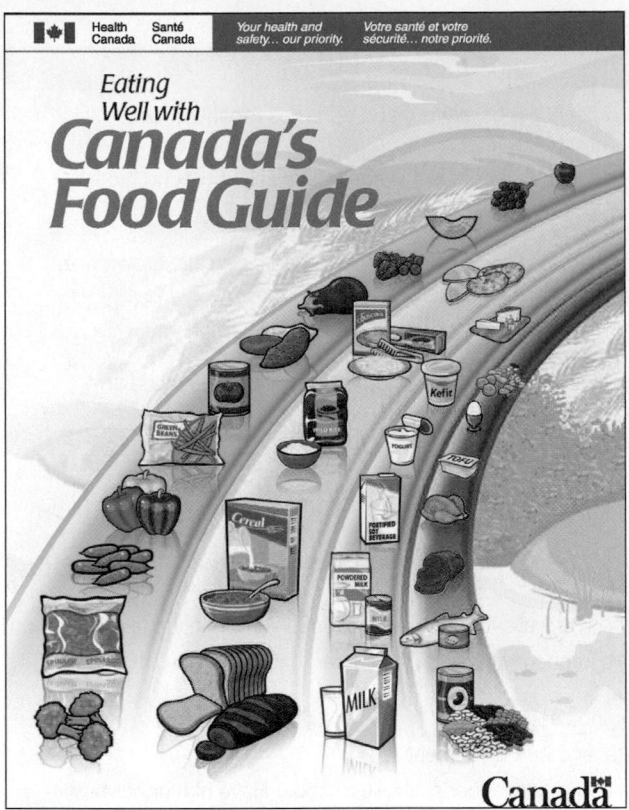

FIGURE 40.3 *Eating Well with Canada's Food Guide.*

Source: Eating Well with Canada's Food Guide. Health Canada, 2011. Reproduced with the permission of the Minister of Health, 2012.

menstrual cycle. Therefore, they need to ensure that they are consuming adequate amounts of iron. Iron-rich foods include red meats, organ meats (liver and kidney), eggs, lentils, sole, cashews, molasses, broccoli, spinach, cooked oatmeal, raisins, and prune juice. Calcium is needed in young adulthood to maintain bones and help decrease the chances of developing osteoporosis in later life. Along with calcium, the person must have adequate vitamin D, which is necessary for the calcium to enter the bloodstream. Vitamin D is made in the skin on exposure to the sun. If the person does not get sufficient sun exposure (15 minutes three times each week), supplements may be indicated. Health Canada (2010g) recommends that supplementation of vitamin D begin at age 50 years, but this may be started earlier if the client does not get adequate sun exposure or have enough dietary intake. See the Clinical Alert box on vitamin supplementation for pregnant women.

> **! CLINICAL ALERT**
>
> Health Canada (2009) recommends that all women who are pregnant or who could become pregnant take a multivitamin with 400 mcg of folic acid (folate). Taking folic acid, a B vitamin, is thought to reduce the likelihood of neural tube defects (such as spina bifida) in the unborn child.

Middle-Aged Adults

Middle-aged adults should follow *Eating Well with Canada's Food Guide* and consume serving sizes and quantities congruent with their activity levels and state of health. This means that they may need to reduce the amount of food eaten on a regular basis. Persons in this group need to be aware of their triglyceride levels and cholesterol (LDLs, HDLs, and total cholesterol) and plan their nutritional intake accordingly. Individuals need to be cognizant of the type of fats they are consuming. In the case of some individuals, it is necessary to monitor the type of carbohydrate and its GI. Osteoporosis Canada (2010) advocates a daily supplement of 400 to 1000 IU of vitamin D for Canadians under age 50 years without osteoporosis. Canadians older than 50 years need up to 2000 IU of vitamin D daily. In the case of calcium, adults under 50 years need 1000 mg per day, and those older than 50 years need 1200 mg. The daily diet should include 2000 mL to 3000 mL of fluid.

Middle-aged adults who gain weight may not be aware of some common facts about this age period. Decreased metabolic activity and decreased physical activity mean a decrease in caloric need. The nurse's role in nutritional health promotion is to counsel clients to prevent obesity by reducing caloric intake and participating in at least 2.5 hours of moderate physical activity (moderate-intensity aerobic activity means you can talk but not sing while participating; it can be broken down into 10 minute intervals) per week (Public Health Agency of Canada, 2011). Referral to dietitians and weight-loss experts may be indicated in some cases.

Older Adults

Older adults should follow a meal plan congruent with their state of health, which may be deteriorating or may include one or more chronic conditions. Portion sizes may need to be reduced if the person is sedentary. Some older adults may need more carbohydrates for fibre and bulk, but most nutrient requirements remain relatively unchanged. Physical changes, such as tooth loss and impaired sense of taste and smell, can affect eating habits. Decreased saliva and gastric juice secretion can also affect a person's nutrition. Psychosocial factors can contribute to nutritional problems. Some older people who live alone may not want to cook for themselves or eat alone. As a result, they may adopt poor dietary habits. Death of the spouse, anxiety, depression, dependence on others, and lowered income all affect eating habits. Table 40.3 on the next page summarizes a range of problems associated with nutrition in the older adult.

Studies have shown that many older adults living in the community are at risk for malnutrition (see the Teaching: Wellness box on the next page for ways that nurses can help), even if they are receiving meals delivered from nutrition support services (Krondl, Lau, Coleman, & Stocker, 2003). Among institutionalized older adults, the risk of

TABLE 40.3 Problems Associated with Nutrition in Older Adults

Problem	Nursing Interventions
Difficulty chewing (may lead to a deficiency in vitamins A and C, minerals, and fibre)	Encourage regular visits to the dentist to have teeth and dentures repaired, refitted, or replaced. Chop fruits and vegetables finely; shred green, leafy vegetables; select ground meat, poultry, or fish.
Lowered glucose tolerance	Have the client eat more carbohydrates (e.g., whole-wheat breads, cereals, brown rice, pasta, potatoes, and legumes) rather than sugar-rich foods.
Decreased social interaction, loneliness	Promote appropriate social interaction at meals, when possible. Encourage the client and significant other to take an interest in food preparation and serving, perhaps as an activity they can do together. If food preparation is not possible, suggest community resources, such as Meals on Wheels. Suggest having picnics in the yard or inviting friends over for meals.
Loss of appetite and senses of smell and taste	Have the client eat essential, nutrient-dense foods first, followed by desserts and low-nutrient-dense foods. Review dietary restrictions, and find ways to make meals appealing within these guidelines. Have the client eat small meals frequently instead of three large meals a day.
Limited income	Suggest the use of generic brands and coupons. Substitute milk, dairy products, and beans for meat. Encourage the client to avoid convenience foods, if able to cook. Have him or her buy foods that are on sale and freeze them for future use. Suggest community resources and nutrition programs.
Difficulty sleeping at night	Have the client eat the major meal at noon and a lighter meal in the evening. Have the client avoid tea, coffee, or other stimulants in the late afternoon or evening.

malnutrition is particularly salient. One study of long-term care facilities in Saskatchewan revealed that the menus did not offer the recommended number of servings of grains and vegetables and fruit identified by *Canada's Food Guide*. Residents were receiving only 88% of the recommended calories for males 50 to 74 years (Lengyel, Zello, Smith, & Whiting, 2003). A small pilot study in a long-term care facility for Canadian veterans revealed that 31% of the mostly male residents were malnourished (Bostrom, Van Soest, Kolewaski, Milke, & Estabrooks, 2011).

TEACHING WELLNESS

Nutrition for Older Adults

Teach clients to include at least the minimal number of servings from each of the following groups from *Eating Well with Canada's Food Guide*:

Vegetables and fruits	7 servings
Grain products	6 servings (female) 7 servings (male)
Milk products	3 servings
Meat and alternatives	2 servings (female) 3 servings (male)

- *Reduce caloric intake.* Caloric needs generally decrease in older people, often because of decreased activity. Older adults need to consume nutrient-dense foods and avoid foods that are high in calories but have few nutrients (empty calorie foods).

- *Reduce fat consumption.* Use leaner cuts of meat, and limit portions to 100 g to 150 g per day. (But be sure that the intake of the meat group is sufficient because older people often consume inadequate amounts of these foods.) Broil, boil, or bake foods instead of frying them. Use low-fat milk and cheese; limit intake of butter, margarine, and salad dressings.

- *Reduce consumption of empty calories.* Substitute fruit or puddings made with low-fat milk in place of pastries, cookies, and rich desserts.

- *Reduce sodium consumption.* Avoid canned soups, ketchup, mustard, and salted, smoked, cured, and pickled meats (e.g., ham and bacon) as they are generally high in sodium. Do not add salt when cooking foods or at the table. Avoid excess use of salt substitutes as they can contain sodium and potassium chloride. Use spices and herbs for seasoning foods.

- *Ensure adequate calcium intake to prevent bone loss.* Older adults need at least 1000 mg of calcium; postmenopausal women need 1200 mg. Milk, cheese, yogourt, cream soups, puddings, and frozen milk products are good sources.
- *Ensure adequate vitamin D intake.* Vitamin D is essential to maintain calcium homeostasis. Include milk because

other dairy products are not usually fortified with vitamin D. Because daily vitamin D intake requirements exceed that which can be provided by following the *Eating Well with Canada's Food Guide*, Health Canada recommends that all Canadians aged over 50 years take a minimum of 400 IU vitamin D supplement.

- *Consume fibre-rich foods and ensure adequate fluid intake to prevent constipation and minimize use of laxatives.* Dietary fibre intake should be from 25 to 30 grams per day.

Standards for a Healthy Diet

Various daily food guides have been developed to help healthy people meet the daily requirements of essential nutrients and to facilitate meal planning. Food group plans emphasize the general types or groups of foods, rather than specific foods, because related foods are similar in composition and often have similar nutrient values. For example, all grains, whether wheat or oats, are significant sources of carbohydrate, iron, and the B vitamin thiamine. *Eating Well with Canada's Food Guide* provides recommendations for healthy nutrition for people aged 2 years and up.

Eating Well with Canada's Food Guide

The goal of *Eating Well with Canada's Food Guide* (see Figure 40.3) is to recommend healthy eating patterns to promote and maintain health. Following the guide allows Canadians to meet their nutrient needs and reduce the risk of obesity, osteoporosis, type 2 diabetes mellitus, coronary artery disease, and some cancers. The *Food Guide* takes into consideration the varied ethnic cultures and cuisines in Canada. Indeed, a specific guide for First Nations, Inuit, and Métis peoples was also developed to account for the consumption of caribou, bannock, and other foods (Health Canada, 2007b). See Figure 40.4. The *Food Guide* is available in English and French as well as in 10 other languages including Farsi, Tagalog, and Urdu; the *First Nations, Inuit, and Métis Food Guide* is available in Inuktitut, Ojibwe, Plains Cree, and Woods Cree.

Eating Well with Canada's Food Guide emphasizes a global pattern of eating over time rather than focusing on any one particular food choice. The *Food Guide* thus represents a total diet approach. Similar to the previous editions of the *Food Guide*, the latest edition depicts foods from all macronutrient groups in a rainbow with four arcs. The smallest arc represents meat and alternative protein sources because this category of foods should have the smallest number of portions per day. Milk

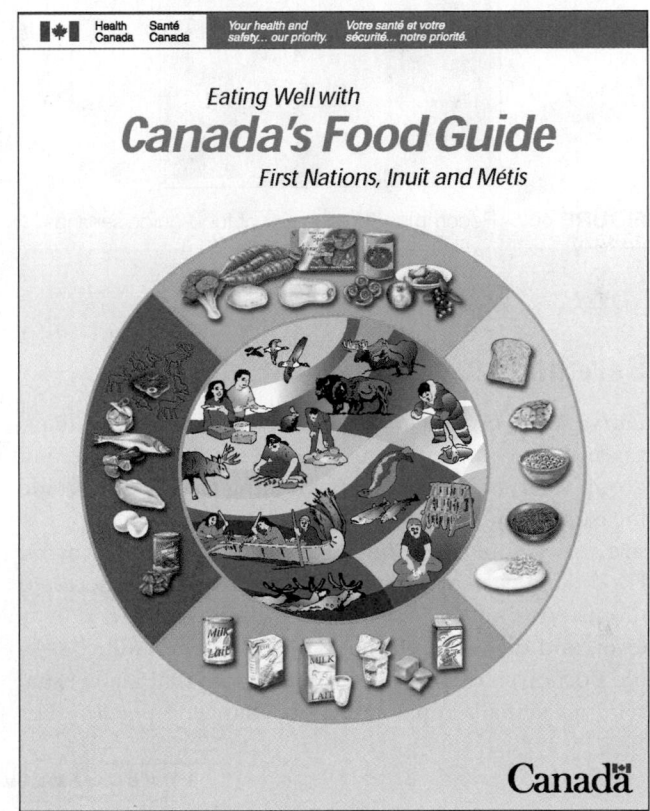

FIGURE 40.4 *Eating Well with Canada's Food Guide: First Nations, Inuit and Métis.*

Source: Eating Well with Canada's Food Guide - First Nations, Inuit and Metis. Health Canada, 2007. Reproduced with the permission of the Minister of Health, 2012.

products appear in the next larger arc, with more servings per day depending on the person's age. Grains are represented in the next larger arc. The largest arc is for fruit and vegetable products because this is the category from which most food intake should be derived. The guidelines stress that people should choose a variety of foods from within each of the four groups. An adult who follows the recommendations of the *Food Guide* will consume between 1800 and 3200 calories. See Figure 40.5 on the next page for the recommended number of daily servings in each of the four food groups. Key directional statements about other nutrition recommendations for Canadians also accompany the guide.

	Recommended Number of Food Guide Servings per day			
	Children 2–3 years old	Children 4–13 years old	Teens and Adults (Females)	(Males)
Vegetables and Fruit Fresh, frozen and canned.	4	5–6	7–8	7–10
Grain Products	3	4–6	6–7	7–8
Milk and Alternatives	2	2–4	Teens 3–4 / Adults (19–50 years) 2 / Adults (50+ years) 3	Teens 3–4 / Adults (19–50 years) 2 / Adults (50+ years) 3
Meat and Alternatives	1	1–2	2	3

FIGURE 40.5 Recommended number of food guide servings per day.

Source: Eating Well with Canada's Food Guide. Health Canada, 2011. Reproduced with the permission of the Minister of Health, 2012.

Serving Sizes

Eating Well with Canada's Food Guide encourages Canadians to eat the recommended number of servings of each food group each day. Rather than counting calories, the guide measures food consumption with portions. The portion size varies depending on the food item in question. My Food Guide is a web-based tool for Canadians interested in customizing the *Food Guide* to their age, sex, activity level, and dietary preferences. Figure 40.6 outlines sample portion sizes. It is important to note that many usual servings actually represent more than one portion. For example, a bagel is actually two servings of grains and 125 mL of juice is one serving of fruit and vegetables.

Food Labels

To be knowledgeable about food, it is helpful to read the food labels on packaged foods. Health Canada stipulates that most food products must have clear labelling indicating *Nutrition Facts*. Each label contains the ingredients in order of proportion and the number of calories supplied for each serving. The caloric content and 13 core nutrients are listed and include proteins, carbohydrates (sugars and fibre), fats (categorized as saturated, monosaturated, or unsaturated and trans), and micronutrients. The **% Daily Value** indicates the percentage of each nutrient in one serving of the product relative to the recommended daily intake. Health Canada's *Using the Nutrition Facts Table* (2010f) is useful in learning how to read *Nutrition Facts* on food labels (see Figure 40.7).

Some of the nomenclature on the label may be unfamiliar to some clients. For example, the salt content of foods is often listed as sodium. Clients with specific health conditions, such as diabetes mellitus, may be more concerned about the carbohydrate content of foods and may need guidance to identify sugars and fibre. As food purchasing is often a shared family responsibility, involving key family members and caregivers in the teaching may be appropriate. Children should be taught from an early age to read labels and to identify fat, sugar, and calorie content to empower them to make healthy food choices. The Teaching: Wellness box describes nutrition recommendations. See also the Clinical Alert box on consumption of fish as part of the diet on page 1224. The Evidence-Informed Practice box on page 1224 discusses sodium intake reduction strategies to improve health.

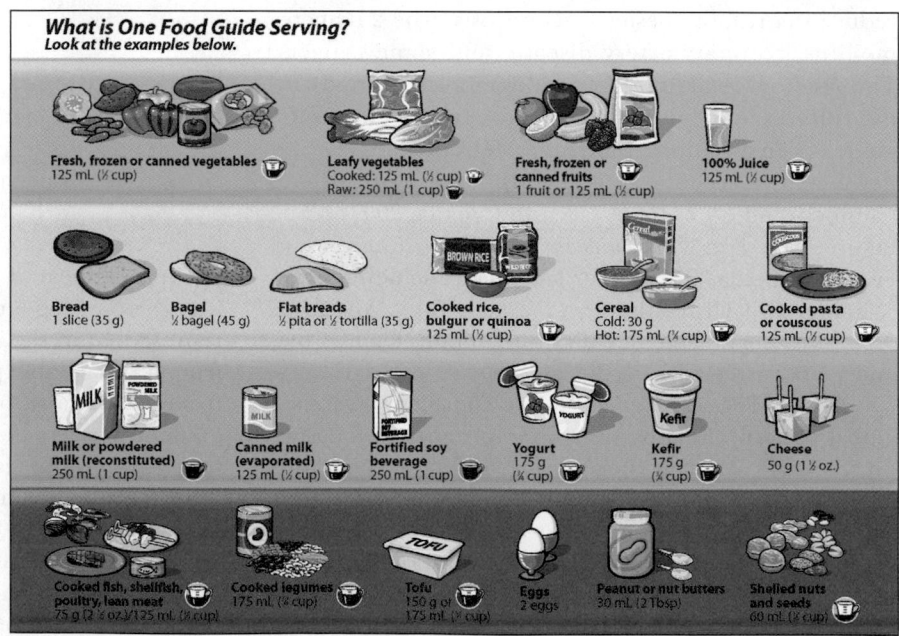

FIGURE 40.6 Portion grid to accompany *Eating Well with Canada's Food Guide.*

Source: Eating Well with Canada's Food Guide. Health Canada, 2011. Reproduced with the permission of the Minister of Health, 2012.

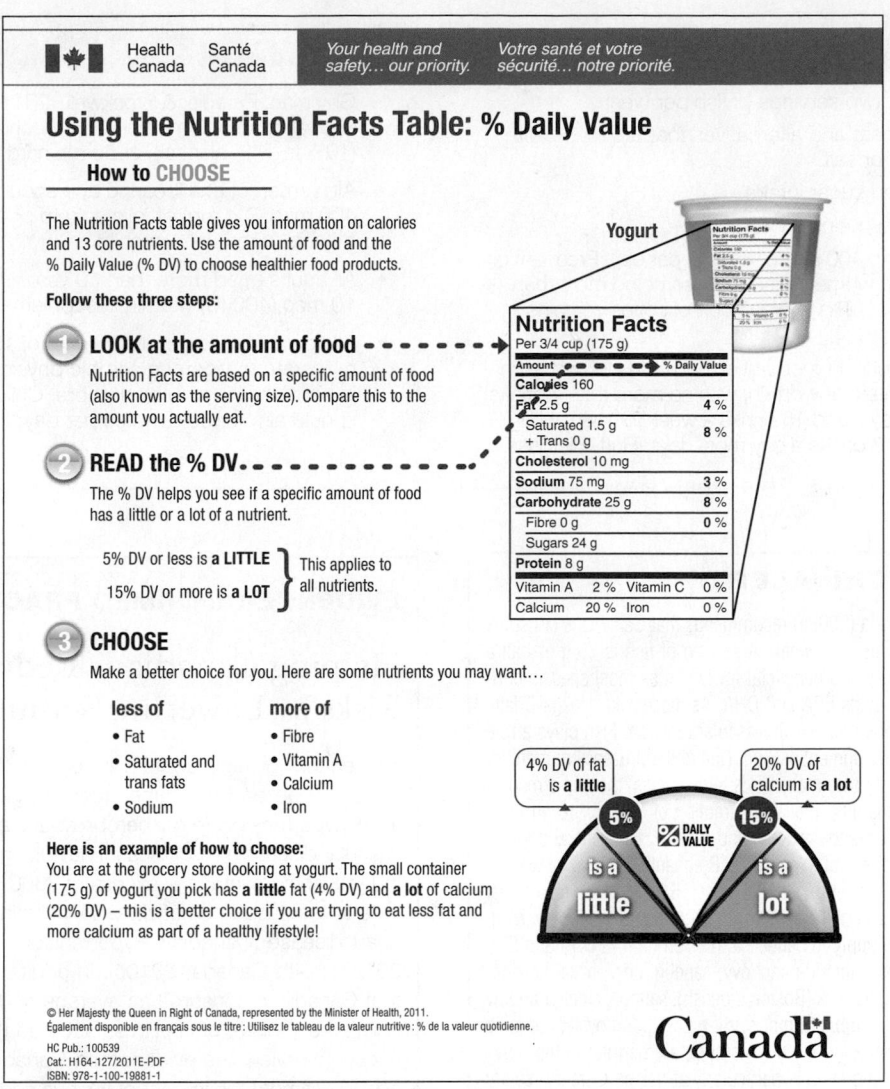

FIGURE 40.7 Using the Nutrition Facts Table: How to Choose.

Source: Eating Well with Canada's Food Guide. Health Canada, 2011. Reproduced with the permission of the Minister of Health, 2012.

Nutrition Recommendations for Canadians

The following recommendations are summarized from *Eating Well with Canada's Food Guide,* Canadian Hypertension Education Program—CHEP (2012), and Health Canada documentation:

- Every day, try to eat at least one orange and one dark green vegetable.
- Eat whole fruits and vegetables rather than drinking juice.
- Prepare vegetables and fruits with little or no added fat or sugar.
- Reduce the average sodium intake per day to *at least* 2300 mg and *ideally* 1500 mg for 19- to 15-year-olds, 1300 mg for 51- to 70-year-olds, and 1200 mg for those over 70 years (CHEP, 2012).

- Prepare foods with little or no added salt. Look for foods that are *salt-free* (<5 mg of sodium per serving), low in sodium (<140 mg of sodium per serving), or reduced in sodium (at least 25% less sodium than the regular product) (Health Canada, 2010c).
- Chose grain products that are lower in fat, sugar, and salt.
- Each day, make sure at least half of your grain products are whole grains.
- Drink lower-fat milk (skim, 1%, or 2%) each day. Children younger than 2 years of age should drink whole milk.
- Select lower-fat dairy products.
- Have meat alternatives, such as tofu, beans, and lentils, more often.

(continued)

TEACHING WELLNESS *(continued)*

- Have at least two servings of fish per week.
- Select lean meat and alternatives that are made with little or no fat or salt.
- Lower salt and sugar intake.
- Drink water to quench thirst.
- Limit caffeine to 400 mg to 450 mg per day. Pregnant or breast-feeding women should consume no more than 300 mg per day. The average cup of coffee contains 200 mg.
- Consume alcohol in moderation, which is defined as 10 drinks a week for women, with no more than 2 drinks a day most days; and 15 drinks a week for men, with no more than 3 drinks a day most days (Butt, Bierness,

Gliksman, Paradis, & Stockwell, 2011). One drink is equivalent to 350 mL beer (5% alcohol), 150 mL wine (10% to 14% alcohol), or 50 mL hard liquor (40% alcohol).

- All women of childbearing age should consume 400 mcg (0.4 mg) of folic acid to prevent neural tube defects in the unborn child.
- All adults aged more than 50 years should take a 10 mcg (400 IU) vitamin D supplement.
- All adults should get a minimum of 150 minutes of moderate to vigorous aerobic physical activity per week in bouts of 10 minutes or more. Children and youth should aim for 60 minutes per day.

CLINICAL ALERT

Health Canada (2008a) recommends that Canadians consume at least two servings of fish per week. A serving of fish is 75 g or half a cup (125 mL). Fish is deemed beneficial for health as most species contain both omega-3 fatty acids EPA and DHA. As discussed, omega-3 fatty acids promote healthy brain and cardiovascular function. Fish plays a role in fetal eye and brain development as well. Due to the presence of mercury that accumulates in the muscle mass of certain species, there is a recommendation that Canadians limit their consumption of fresh or frozen tuna, shark, swordfish, marlin, orange roughy, and escolar. The general population should eat no more than 150 g per week. Pregnant and lactating women should eat only 150 g per month. Children aged 5 to 11 years should eat only 125 g per month, and children 1 to 4 years should have only 75 g. This restriction does not apply to canned tuna. Fish high in DHA and EPA with low levels of mercury include anchovy, capelin, char, hake, herring, Atlantic mackerel, mullet, pollock (Boston bluefish), salmon, smelt, rainbow trout, lake whitefish, blue crab, shrimp, clam, mussel, and oyster. Organic mercury compounds, including methyl mercury, are harmful to the nervous system. The developing fetus is particularly at risk as mercury readily crosses the placental barrier. Mercury exposure, depending on the level, can decrease IQ and cause developmental delays. In an adult, high-level exposure can cause neurological impairment, including tremors, memory loss, intellectual impairment, and loss of muscle coordination and sensation (Health Canada, 2008a).

EVIDENCE-INFORMED PRACTICE

Helping Canadians Reduce Health Risks by Lowering Sodium Intake

The effects of high sodium intake on the development of hypertension and the subsequent complications that arise from hypertension (e.g., cerebrovascular accident, cardiovascular disease, renal disease) have long been documented. Indeed, sodium intake in excess of 2300 mg per day contributes to increased risk of disease including hypertension and heart disease (Canadian Hypertension Education Program, 2012; Health Canada, 2010c). In addition, there is evidence that Canadians consume an average of 3400 mg per day. In 2007, the Minister of Health established the Sodium Working Group to review the evidence on Canadian's sodium intake and to estimate the impact of various sodium reduction strategies on the health of Canadians. The Working Group used the results of public opinion research to understand how Canadians view the health effects of sodium intake. The ultimate goal of the Sodium Reduction Strategy is for as many Canadians as possible to reduce their daily sodium intake to lower than the tolerable upper limit level: 1500 mg per day for 9- to 50-year-olds and less for those younger and older!

NURSING IMPLICATIONS: The nurse plays a key role in health promotion through education and can play a valuable role in helping individuals, families, and communities become aware of the negative effects of high sodium intake on health. While individuals can play a role (e.g., not adding salt to their foods), nurses can advocate using intersectoral collaboration such as encouraging local agencies (e.g., schools cafeterias, soup kitchens) and businesses (e.g., restaurants) to voluntarily reduce the amount of sodium they use in their cooking.

Source: Based on Health Canada. (2010). *Sodium reduction strategy for Canada, Recommendations of the sodium working group.* Ottawa, ON: Author.

Vegetarian Diets

People may become vegetarians for economic, health, religious, ethical, or ecological reasons. Vegetarians generally have lower cholesterol and blood pressure and a reduced occurrence of type 2 diabetes mellitus compared with nonvegetarians (Dietitians of Canada, 2011b). Vegetarian diets come in two basic types: (a) those that consume only plant foods and (b) those that include milk, eggs, and dairy products. Some people eat fish and poultry but not beef, lamb, or pork; others eat only fresh fruit, juices, and nuts; and still others eat plant foods and dairy products but not eggs. See Box 40.3 for a summary of the types of vegetarians.

Vegetarian diets can be nutritionally sound if they include a wide variety of foods and if proper protein complementation and vitamin and mineral supplementation are provided, according to the Dietitians of Canada (2003). Because the proteins found in plant foods are incomplete proteins, vegetarians must eat

BOX 40.3   TYPES OF VEGETARIANS

Type	Description
Vegan	Strict vegetarian; avoids all foods of animal origin
Lacto-ovo vegetarian	Uses dairy products and eggs but avoids eating beef, pork, poultry, fish, shellfish, or animal flesh of any kind
Lacto vegetarian	Uses dairy products but avoids eating eggs and beef, pork, poultry, fish, shellfish, or animal flesh of any kind
Ovo vegetarian	Uses eggs but avoids dairy products and meat products
Pesco vegetarian	Uses dairy products, eggs, and fish but avoids all meat products
Partial vegetarian (semi-vegetarian)	Avoids selected meats (e.g., red meat)
Fruitarian	Uses only fresh (raw) fruits, juices, nuts, honey, and olive oil
Macrobiotic vegetarian	Progresses through 10 dietary stages from a widely inclusive selection to a restrictive selection

BOX 40.4   COMBINATIONS OF PLANT PROTEINS THAT PROVIDE COMPLETE PROTEINS

Grains plus legumes = complete protein
Legumes plus nuts or seeds = complete protein
Grains, legumes, nuts, or seeds plus milk or milk products (e.g., cheese) = complete protein

Grains	Legumes	Nuts and Seeds
Brown rice	Black beans	Almonds
Barley	Kidney beans	Brazil nuts
Corn meal	Lima beans	Cashews
Millet	Soybeans	Pecans
Oats/oatmeal	Lentils	Walnuts
Rye	Tofu	Pumpkin seeds
Whole wheat	Black-eyed peas	Sesame seeds
	Split peas	Sunflower seeds

Examples:

Black-eyed peas and rice

Lentil soup and whole-wheat bread

Beans and tortillas

Lima beans and sesame seeds

Cereal with milk

Macaroni with cheese

complementary protein foods to obtain all the essential amino acids. A plant protein can be *complemented* by combining it with a different plant protein. The combination produces a complete protein (see Box 40.4). Obtaining complete proteins is especially important for growing children and pregnant and lactating women, whose protein needs are high. Generally, legumes (starchy beans, peas, lentils) have complementary relationships with grains, nuts, and seeds. Complementary foods must be eaten in the same meal. Such diets as the fruitarian diet do not provide sufficient amounts of essential nutrients and are not recommended for long-term use.

Foods of animal origin are the best source of vitamin B_{12}. Therefore, vegans (strict vegetarians) need to obtain this vitamin from other sources: brewer's yeast, foods fortified with vitamin B_{12}, or a vitamin supplement. Because iron from plant sources (nonheme iron) is not absorbed as efficiently as is iron from meat (heme iron), vegans should eat iron-rich foods (e.g., green leafy vegetables, whole grains, raisins, and molasses) and iron-enriched foods. They should eat a food rich in vitamin C at each meal to enhance iron absorption. Calcium deficiency is a concern only for strict vegetarians. It can be prevented by including in the diet leafy green vegetables and soymilk and tofu (soybean curd) fortified with calcium. Thus, teaching clients to read food labels is essential to ensure that they consume foods that provide an adequate intake of vitamins and minerals.

Altered Nutrition

Malnutrition is commonly defined as the lack of necessary or appropriate food substances, but in practice, malnutrition includes both undernutrition and overnutrition. In **undernutrition**, the person's caloric intake is less than the daily energy requirements, resulting in weight loss. **Overnutrition** refers to a caloric intake in excess of daily energy requirements, resulting in storage of energy in the form of adipose tissue. As the amount of stored fat increases, the individual becomes overweight or obese. A person is said to be **overweight** when his or her body mass index is between 25 kg/m^2 and 29.9 kg/m^2 and **obese** when the body mass index is more than 30 kg/m^2 (Health Canada, 2008b). **Body mass index (BMI)** is a weight to height ratio, with weight (in kilograms) divided by the height (in metres) squared. (See later in the chapter for a discussion of BMI calculation.) Generally accepted standards for interpreting percentage of ideal body weight (IBW) are shown in Box 40.5.

BOX 40.5   CALCULATING AND INTERPRETING PERCENTAGE OF IDEAL BODY WEIGHT

>120% of ideal body weight (IBW)	Obese
110%–119% of IBW	Overweight
90%–109% of IBW	IBW
80%–89% of IBW	Mildly underweight
70%–79% of IBW	Moderately underweight
<69% of IBW	Severely underweight

To calculate an individual's percentage of IBW use the following formula:

$$\% \text{ IBW} = \frac{\text{Actual body weight (ABW)}}{\text{Ideal body weight (IBW)}} \times 100$$

Excess body weight increases the stress on body organs and predisposes people to chronic health problems, such as hypertension, dyslipidemia, diabetes mellitus, coronary artery disease, obstructive sleep apnea, gall bladder disease, and certain cancers. Obesity that interferes with mobility or breathing is referred to as *morbid obesity*. Obese people may also manifest undernourishment in important nutrients (e.g., essential vitamins or minerals) even though excess calories are ingested.

Adipose tissue located in the visceral area of the abdomen is the most significant in the development of disease conditions. People with visceral fat are more prone to developing metabolic syndrome. In addition, fat located in the abdominal area is highly correlated with obstructive sleep apnea. Men are more likely to develop deposits of visceral fat, especially in midlife. In postmenopausal women, the likelihood of developing abdominal obesity also increases.

Adipose tissue located in the peripheral areas of the body does not place the individual at as high a risk for developing other health problems as does abdominal obesity, but it can lead to problems related to mobility and the development of varicose veins, and it increases the risk of developing osteoarthritis in weight-bearing joints. Peripheral obesity can also contribute to psychological problems associated with a person's attempts to achieve a more perfect body shape because reducing the size of the thighs, upper arms, or hips can be difficult.

Malnutrition occurs when the nutritional reserves are depleted and the nutrients being ingested are insufficient to meet day-to-day demands or the demands placed on the body by added metabolic stress. Malnutrition can occur even though the person is ingesting a large number of calories. For example, a person who primarily eats processed foods high in fats and carbohydrates may have a major deficiency of protein. Improper digestion and absorption of food may lead to malnutrition. An inadequate food intake may be caused by the inability to acquire and prepare food, inadequate knowledge about essential nutrients and a balanced diet, discomfort during or after eating, dysphagia, anorexia (loss of appetite), or nausea or vomiting. Improper digestion and absorption of nutrients can be caused by an inadequate production of hormones or enzymes or by underlying pathological conditions resulting in inflammation or obstruction of the gastrointestinal tract.

A malnourished person may have greater than or less than IBW. **Ideal body weight (IBW)** is the weight recommended for optimal health. To determine an individual's IBW, the nurse can quickly calculate an approximate body weight. See Box 40.6. These approximate weights

---

BOX 40.6 APPROXIMATING IDEAL BODY WEIGHT

Females	Males
45 kg for 1.5 m of height	48 kg for 1.5 m of height
+ 2.3 kg for each 2.5 cm more than 1.5 m	+ 2.8 kg for each 2.5 cm more than 1.5 m
± 10% for body-frame size	± 10% for body-frame size

---

can be increased or decreased by 10%, depending on the person's body frame.

Inadequate nutrition can be associated with weight loss, but not always. It is, however, associated with generalized weakness, altered functional ability, delayed wound healing, increased susceptibility to infection, decreased immunocompetence, and impaired pulmonary function. In the case of the hospitalized patient, malnutrition can prolong the length of time spent in the hospital. When a person is experiencing malnutrition, the stored glycogen is mobilized from the muscle and liver stores. These sources can last for only about 24 hours, and then the body fat stores are mobilized in the form of ketones, an alternative fuel to glucose.

Protein-calorie malnutrition, once associated with starvation in the developing countries, is now recognized as a significant problem for clients with long-term deficiencies in caloric intake (e.g., older adults, fad dieters, those with chronic diseases, those who live in institutions). Characteristics of protein-calorie malnutrition are weakness, apathy, increased risk of infection, poor drug tolerance, and poor wound healing.

Assessing

The purpose of a nutritional assessment is to gather and interpret data to determine the client's nutritional status and to identify issues. Components of a nutritional assessment are shown in Table 40.4 and can be remembered as *ABCD data*:

- Anthropometric
- Biochemical
- Clinical
- Dietary

A nutritional assessment is a collaborative endeavour. The nurse can conduct the initial nutritional assessment and, if necessary, additional in-depth screening can be performed by a nutritionist or dietitian and the physician. Nutritional assessment in children is complicated by the fact that children often eat at home, school, and at their friends' homes. Parents may not always be aware of their children's habits. As discussed, the lunch sent to school may not be the lunch the child actually eats. Including the child in the assessment process may increase the reliably of the report.

TABLE 40.4 Components of a Nutritional Assessment

	Screening Data	Additional In-Depth Data
Anthropometric Data	• Height • Weight • Weight change • Usual or ideal body weight • Body mass index	• Waist circumference • Waist-to-hip ratio • Skinfold thickness (optional)
Biochemical Data	• Hemoglobin, hematocrit • Serum albumin • Total lymphocyte count • Total serum cholesterol • LDL, HDL, Total cholesterol:HDL ratio • Fasting blood glucose	• Serum transferrin level • Urinary urea nitrogen (UUN), blood urea nitrogen (BUN) • Urinary creatinine excretion, serum creatinine • Thyroid stimulating hormone (TSH)
Clinical Data	• Skin • Hair and nails • Mucous membranes • Activity level • History of current and past health issues • Drugs: prescribed and over the counter, herbal remedies, or recreational drugs	• Hair analysis • Neurological testing
Dietary Data	• Diet history • 24-hour food recall • Food frequency record • Food preferences • Ability to prepare food • Food allergies or intolerances	• Selective food frequency record • Food diary • Diet history

Nutritional Screening

Nurses carry out nutritional screening during routine nursing histories and physical examinations. Custom screening tools designed for a particular population (e.g., older adults or pregnant women) and specific disorders (e.g., cardiac disease) are available. Screening tools include the patient-generated subjective global assessment (PG-SGA). The PG-SGA is a method of classifying clients as either well nourished, moderately malnourished, or severely malnourished based on a dietary history and physical examination. It was established primarily for use in people with cancer but has been widely tested and is appropriate for both inpatient and outpatient clients with various diagnoses. Clients who are found to be at moderate or high risk are followed up with a comprehensive assessment by a dietitian. Box 40.7 provides a summary of risk factors for nutritional problems.

BOX 40.7 SUMMARY OF RISK FACTORS FOR NUTRITIONAL PROBLEMS

Some factors can put clients at risk for nutritional problems:

DIET HISTORY

• Chewing or swallowing difficulties (because of ill-fitting dentures, dental caries, missing teeth, or cranial nerve deficits)
• Inadequate food intake
• Restricted or fad diets
• Intravenous fluids (other than total parenteral nutrition for 10 or more days)
• Inadequate food budget
• Inadequate food-preparation facilities
• Inadequate food-storage facilities

• Physical disabilities
• Living and eating alone

MEDICAL HISTORY

• Unintentional weight loss or gain of 10% within 6 months
• Fluid and electrolyte imbalance
• Oral and gastrointestinal surgery
• Dental problems: difficulty chewing, ill-fitting dentures
• Gastrointestinal problems: anorexia, dysphagia, nausea, vomiting, diarrhea, constipation
• Chronic illness: end-stage renal disease, liver disease, human immunodeficiency virus (HIV) infection, chronic obstructive pulmonary disease (COPD), cancer

(continued)

BOX 40.7 *(continued)*

- Alcohol or problematic substance use
- Neurological or cognitive impairment
- Psychiatric conditions: depression, anorexia nervosa, and bulimia nervosa
- Catabolic or hypermetabolic condition: burns, trauma
- Adolescent pregnancy or closely spaced pregnancies

MEDICATION HISTORY*

- Aspirin
- Antacid
- Antidepressants

- Antihypertensives
- Anti-inflammatory agents
- Antineoplastic agents
- Digitalis
- Laxatives
- Diuretics (thiazides)
- Hypoglycemic agents
- Glucocorticosteroids
- Potassium chloride

---

*The potential effects of some medications on nutrition are shown in Table 40.2 on page 1212.

The PG-SGA dietary history consists of five key components:

1. History of weight loss over the preceding 2 weeks and 6 months
2. Current pattern of dietary intake in comparison with the usual pattern
3. Presence of gastrointestinal symptoms that may reduce food intake
4. Functional capacity (ranging from bedridden to fully ambulatory)
5. Primary medical diagnosis and metabolic demands created by the underlying disease

The PG-SGA physical examination emphasizes three features:

1. Loss of subcutaneous fat
2. Muscle wasting
3. Presence of edema and ascites

These physical features are scored as normal (0), mild (1), moderate (2), and severe (3). The PG-SGA is able to provide approximately 80% positive identification of malnutrition when comparing the PG-SGA with traditional assessment methods that included anthropometrics and laboratory tests. Because the PG-SGA is a subjective assessment, the effectiveness of the tool depends largely on the experience of the health care professional collecting and interpreting the data (Green & Watson, 2006).

Dietary Data

A dietary history includes data about the client's usual eating patterns and habits; allergies and food intolerances; frequency, types, and quantities of foods consumed; and social, economic, ethnic, or religious factors influencing nutrition. Specific factors to consider include, but are not limited to, living and eating alone, ability to purchase foods and prepare a meal, and the availability of refrigeration and cooking facilities.

Other information that is important addresses the client's appetite and hunger. These are two different aspects of eating and should not be considered the same. A client may claim to have a good appetite and yet ingest very little food. Others may say they are never hungry, and yet they are observed to be eating frequently. For these reasons, keeping a food diary with associated mood states may help the person realize how much, in fact, is being consumed and why. It is important to know whether the client has eating binges. Does the client eat frequently in restaurants? What does the client know and understand about healthy nutrition and *Eating Well with Canada's Food Guide*?

Four possible methods for collecting dietary data are a 24-hour food recall, a food-frequency record, a food diary, and a diet history.

For a **24-hour food recall**, the nurse asks the client to recall all the food and beverages the client consumes during a typical 24-hour period. The data obtained is then generally evaluated according to *Canada's Food Guide* to judge overall adequacy.

A **food-frequency record** is a checklist that indicates how often general food groups or specific foods are eaten. Frequency may be categorized as times/day, times/week, times/month, or frequently, seldom, never. This record, like the 24-hour food recall, provides information about the types of foods eaten but not the quantities. When specific foods or nutrients are suspected of being deficient or excessive, the health care professional may use a selective food-frequency record that focuses, for example, on fat, fruit, vegetable, and fibre intake.

A **food diary** is a detailed record of measured amounts (portion sizes) of all food and fluids a client consumes during a specified time, usually 3 to 7 days.

A **diet history** is a comprehensive, time-consuming assessment of a client's food intake that involves an extensive interview by a nutritionist or dietitian. It includes characteristics of foods usually eaten, as well as the frequency and amount of food consumed. Thus, it may include a 24-hour recall, a food-frequency record, and a food diary. Medical and psychosocial factors are also assessed to evaluate their impact on nutritional requirements, food habits, and choices. Data obtained are analyzed by computer and translated into caloric and nutrient intake. Results are compared with the recommended dietary allowances that are appropriate for the client's age, sex, and condition.

Health History

Information about the client's current health status and past health status needs to be obtained. This information should include medications, both prescribed and over-the-counter drugs (e.g., vitamins, herbal preparations) that the client is taking. The use and frequency of use of recreational drugs also needs to be addressed. This may be the best time to find out what the client knows about the interactions between food and the drugs being taken. Information about the client's family history needs to be collected. Is there a history of heart disease, obesity, eating disorders, diabetes, and so on? Does the client exercise on a regular basis? Does the client use tobacco? If so, how much, how often, and for how long? Does the client consume alcohol? If so, how much, and how often? Does the client have any disabilities that may limit the ability to prepare food or eat? For example, if a person has advancing multiple sclerosis, he or she may have an intention tremor that causes the hands to shake so much that it is difficult to cook or use a regular fork or spoon. Does the client have difficulty swallowing? Does the client have a problem with choking or aspiration of food when eating?

Some of the health history information may have to be obtained from family members if the client has a cognitive impairment or speech disability. Also, some of this information may be obtained from other health care professionals' histories if the nurse has access to such documentation.

Physical Examination

Physical examination reveals nutritional deficiencies and excesses in addition to obvious weight changes. Assessment focuses on rapidly proliferating tissues, such as skin, hair, nails, eyes, and mucosa, but also includes a systematic review comparable with any routine physical examination. See Box 40.8. The signs of malnutrition must be viewed as *suggestive* of malnutrition because the signs are nonspecific. For example, a red conjunctiva may indicate an infection, rather than a nutritional deficit, and dry, dull hair may be related to excessive exposure to the sun rather than *kwashiorkor* (severe protein depletion). To confirm malnutrition, clinical findings need to be substantiated with laboratory tests and dietary data.

BOX 40.8 CLINICAL SIGNS OF MALNUTRITION

Area of Examination	Signs Associated with Malnutrition
General appearance and vitality	Apathetic, listless, looks tired, easily fatigued
Weight	Overweight or underweight
Skin	Dry, flaky, or scaly; pale or pigmented; presence of petechiae or bruises; lack of subcutaneous fat
Nails	Brittle, pale, ridged, or spoon-shaped (iron)
Hair	Dry, dull, sparse, loss of colour, brittle (see Figure 40.8A on the next page)
Eyes	Pale or red conjunctiva, xerophthalmia (dryness), keratomalacia (soft cornea), dull cornea, night blindness (vitamin A deficiency)
Lips	Swollen, angular stomatitis (red cracks at side of mouth), cheilosis (vertical fissures caused by vitamin B deficiency) (see Figure 40.8B)
Tongue	Swollen; beefy red or magenta coloured (vitamin B deficiency); smooth appearance (vitamin B deficiency); decrease or increase in size (see Figure 40.8C)
Gums	Spongy, swollen, inflamed; bleed easily (vitamin C deficiency) (see Figure 40.8D)
Muscles	Underdeveloped, flaccid, wasted, soft
Gastrointestinal system	Anorexia, indigestion, diarrhea, constipation, enlarged liver, protruding abdomen
Nervous system	Decreased reflexes, sensory loss, paresthesias (burning and tingling of hands and feet caused by vitamin B deficiency), mental confusion or irritability

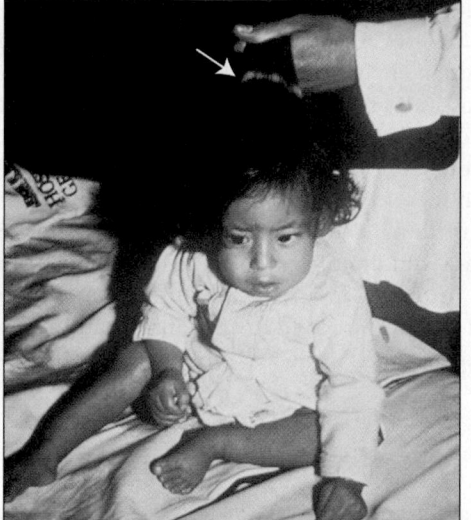
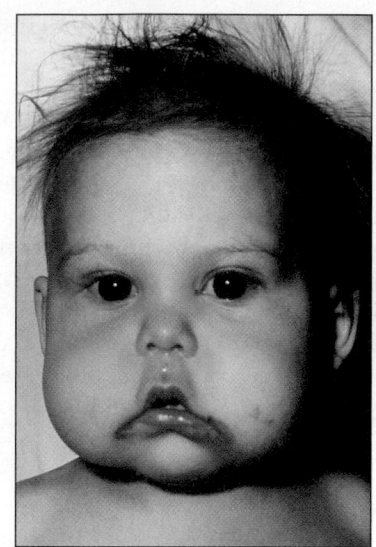
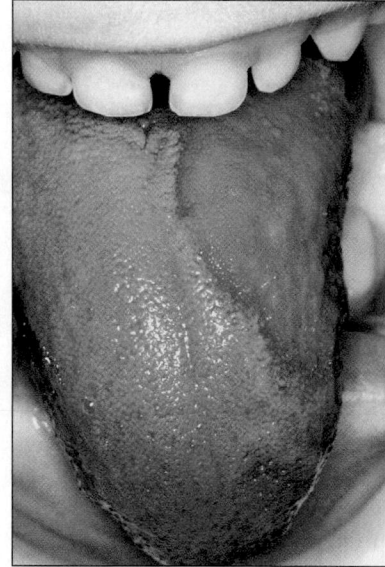
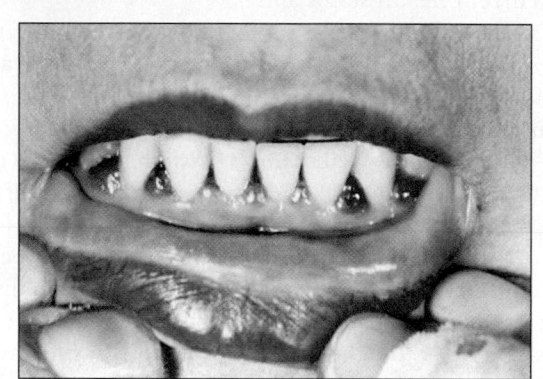

FIGURE 40.8 Examples of nutritional deficiencies: **A:** Dull, sparse hair from protein deficiency; **B:** Inflammation of the corners of the mouth from riboflavin deficiency; **C:** Inflammation of the tongue from niacin, B_6, or riboflavin deficiency; **D:** Spongy, bleeding gums from vitamin C deficiency.

Anthropometric Measurements

Anthropometric measurements are noninvasive techniques that aim to quantify changes in body composition. The client's height and weight should be obtained. Self-reported data are often inaccurate, so accurate equipment and standardized procedures must be used to ensure accurate and precise readings. A beam-balance scale can be used to obtain weight and to measure the person's height. The person should not be wearing shoes and should have on only light clothing when stepping onto the scale. The client should be able to stand on the scale without any support, and should have voided before being weighed. If the patient is bedridden or unable to stand independently, a metabolic scale can be used, if available. A person should be weighed at the same time each day if repeated weight recordings are required. Bathroom scales are not always accurate, so they should only be used to obtain an approximation of the person's weight. The weight obtained should be compared with the client's usual and ideal body weights to determine weight change. Refer to Box 40.9.

BOX 40.9   CALCULATING AND INTERPRETING THE PERCENTAGE OF DEVIATION FROM USUAL BODY WEIGHT AND THE PERCENTAGE OF WEIGHT LOSS

Calculating Percentage of Usual Body Weight

$$\% \text{ usual body weight} = \frac{\text{Current weight}}{\text{Usual body weight}} \times 100$$

Mild malnutrition	85%–90%
Moderate malnutrition	75%–84%
Severe malnutrition	less than 74%

Calculating Percentage of Weight Loss

$$\% \text{ weight loss} = \frac{\text{Usual body weight} - \text{Current weight}}{\text{Usual weight}} \times 100$$

Significant weight loss	**Severe weight loss**
5% over 1 month	>5% over 1 month
7.5% over 3 months	>7.5% over 3 months
10% over 6 months	>10% over 6 months

CALCULATING PERCENTAGE OF WEIGHT GAIN OR LOSS

Accurate assessment of the client's height, current body weight (CBW), and **usual body weight (UBW)** is essential. Although the client's CBW can be compared with an IBW discussed earlier, the IBW is based on healthy people and does not account for changes in the client's body composition that accompany illness or reflect any changes in weight. The client's UBW better reflects weight change and the possibility of malnutrition. Calculation and interpretation of the percentage of deviation from UBW and the percentage of weight loss are shown in Box 40.9. An important aspect of weight assessment, obtained in the nursing history, is a description of **weight change**. The nurse should describe any weight loss or gain, the duration of the change, and whether the weight change was intentional or unintentional.

BMI is an indicator of body composition for individuals over 18 years who are not pregnant nor breast-feeding. The BMI is an indicator of overall adiposity or obesity and can be used to determine whether an individual is at risk for developing serious health problems due to being overweight or underweight. A BMI, however, must be used with caution for certain individuals—for example, those who have a large lean body mass or who have ascites (peritoneal cavity fluid)—because their weight may not be attributable to adipose tissue. To calculate BMI, refer to the following steps or to the nomogram in Table 40.5.

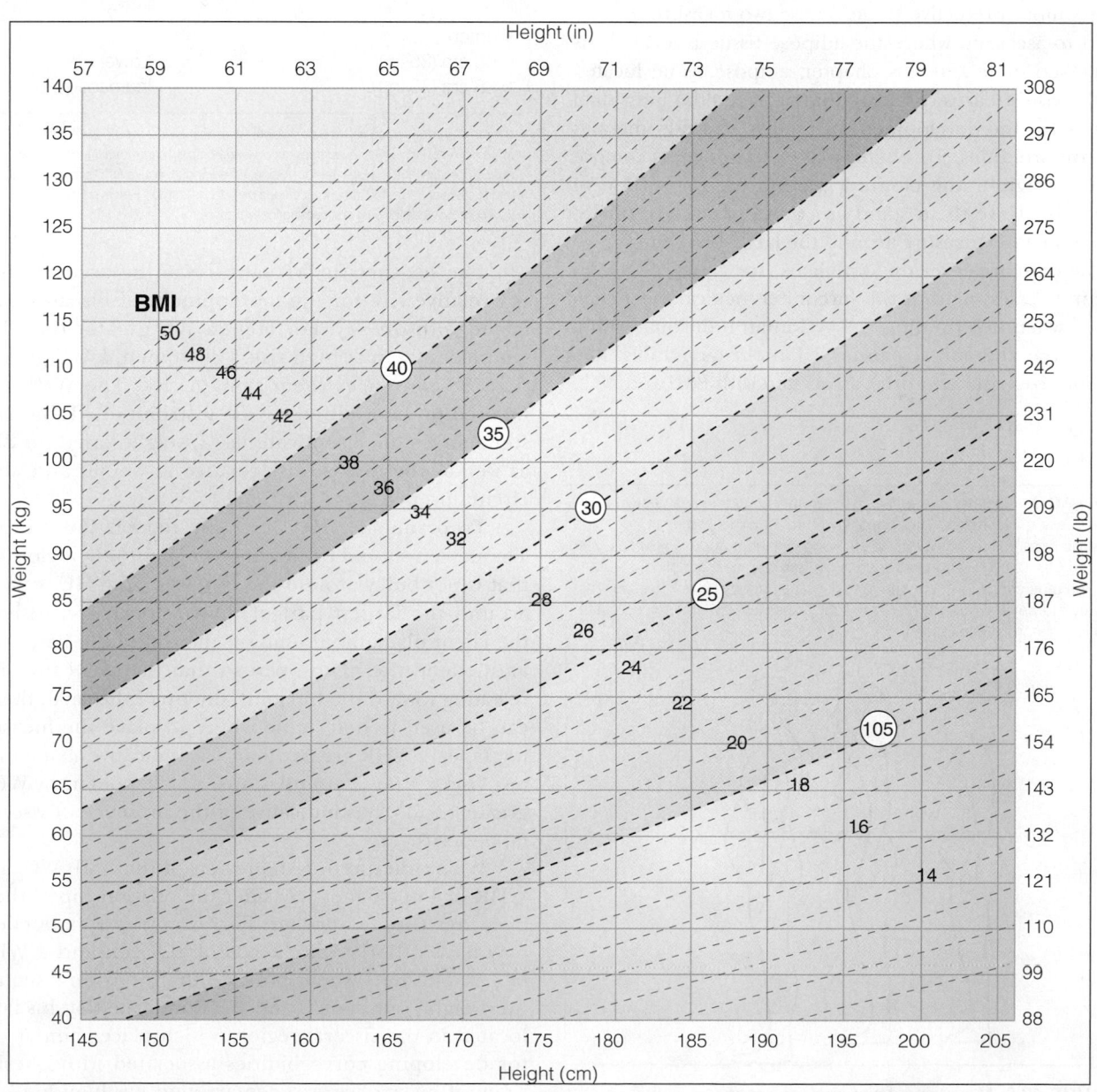

TABLE 40.5 Body Mass Index Nomogram.

Source: Canadian Guidelines for Body Weight Classification in Adults. Health Canada, 2003. Reproduced with the permission of the Minister of Health, 2012.

1. Measure the person's height in metres (e.g., 1.5 m).
2. Measure the weight in kilograms (e.g., 60 kg).
3. Calculate the BMI by using the following formula:

$$\% \, BMI = \frac{Weight \, in \, kilograms}{(Height \, in \, metres)^2}$$

or

$$\frac{60 \, kg}{(1.5 \, m)^2} = 26.6 \, kg/m^2$$

Other important measures to obtain when determining degree of adiposity and location of adipose tissue are the **waist circumference (WC)** and the **hip circumference (HC)**. The ratio of the waist circumference to the hip circumference is called the **waist-to-hip ratio (WHR)**. WC offers more predictive value. These two measures can be used to ascertain where the adipose tissue is located. As discussed earlier in this chapter, adipose tissue located in the visceral area of the abdomen places the individual at risk for the development of metabolic syndrome and its comorbidities. To obtain a WC, have clients remove belts or tight-fitting clothing around the midsection of the body. Have them stand erect and breathe normally. Place the tape measure around the largest circumference of the waist area over the umbilicus (see Figure 40.9). An accurate assessment of this circumference can be a challenge when determining the WC in an individual with a very large abdominal pannus (skinfold fat). Table 40.6 summarizes risk categories associated with BMI and WC.

TABLE 40.6 Body Weight Classification and Risk of Health Problems by Body Mass Index and Waist Circumference

Measure (BMI, kg/m²)	Weight Classification	Risk of Health Problems
< 18.5	Underweight	Increased
18.5–24.9	Normal weight	Least
25.0–29.9	Overweight	Increased
≥ 30.0	Obese:	
30.0–34.9	Class I	High
35.0–39.9	Class II	Very high
≥ 40.0	Class III	Extremely high
Waist circumference		
Men		
< 102 cm (40 in.)		Lower
≥ 102 cm (40 in.)		Increased
Women		
< 88 cm (35 in.)		Lower
≥ 88 cm (35 in.)		Increased

Source: Canadian guideline for Body Weight Classification in Adults - Quick reference tool for professionals. Retrieved from http://www.hc-sc.gc.ca/fn-an/alt_formats/hpfb-dgpsa/pdf/nutrition/cg_quick_ref-ldc_rapide_ref-eng.pdf; Centers for Disease Control and Prevention. "Healthy Weight - it's not a diet, it's a lifestyle!" Retrieved from http://www.cdc.gov/healthyweight/assessing/index.html

The sex-specific WC cutoffs can be used to identify relative risk for the development of diseases associated with obesity. For men, a WC greater than 102 cm places them at high risk. For women, a WC greater than 88 cm places them at high risk. The WHR can be used to determine body fat distribution. Table 40.6 summarizes the classifications of weight based on BMI as well as the disease risk relative to weight and waist circumference.

To obtain the HC, have the person stand erect. The person should be wearing very lightweight clothing that is not bulky around the hip area. The HC is taken around the largest part of the buttocks. If you have the client place the thumb on the top of the iliac crest and extend the hand open so that the small finger is reaching toward the hip joint, the tip of the small finger can be used to determine where to place the measuring tape. A WHR greater than 1 is indicative that a man has visceral fat accumulations. For a woman, a WHR greater than 0.8 is indicative of the presence of visceral fat deposits.

When interpreting the results of the BMI, WC, and WHR, the nurse must consider the relationship of these measures to one another. For example, a male client may have a BMI of 26, a WC of 103 cm, and a WHR of 1.2. The BMI would indicate that he is only slightly overweight, but his WC and WHR indicate that his fat is located in the visceral region, which places him at risk for developing comorbidities associated with obesity. Then, if he smokes, is sedentary, and has high levels of LDL cholesterol and low levels of HDL, his risk factors are increased.

The WC is measured at the part of the trunk located midway between the lower costal margin (bottom of lower rib) and the iliac crest (top of pelvic bone) while the person is standing, with feet about 25-30 cm apart (10-12 in). The measurer should stand beside the individual and fit the tape snugly, without compressing any underlying soft tissues. The circumference should be measured to the nearest 0.5 cm (1/4 in), at the end of a normal expiration.

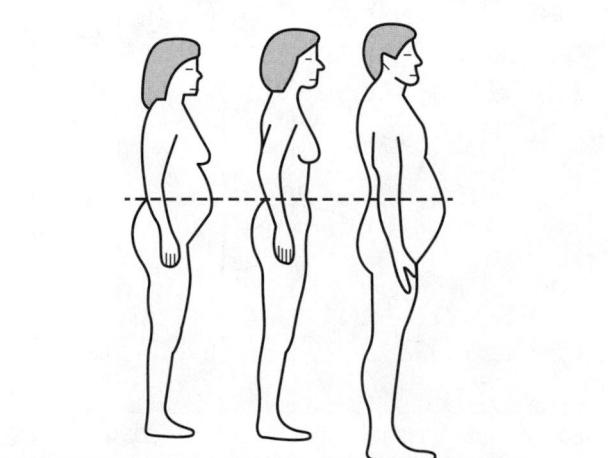

FIGURE 40.9 Measuring waist circumference.

Source: Canadian Guidelines for Body Weight Classification in Adults. Health Canada, 2003. Reproduced with the permission of the Minister of Health, 2012.

Skinfold thicknesses can be obtained to determine fat stores. The fold of skin measured includes subcutaneous tissue but not the underlying muscle. It is measured in millimetres by using special calipers. The most common site for measurement is the triceps skinfold (TSF). To measure the TSF, the nurse locates the midpoint of the upper arm (halfway between the acromion process and the olecranon process), then grasps the skin on the back of the upper arm along the long axis of the humerus (Figure 40.10). The nurse places the calipers 1 cm below his or her fingers and measures the thickness of the fold to the nearest millimetre.

The midarm circumference (MAC) is a measure of fat, muscle, and skeleton. To measure the MAC, ask the client to sit or stand with the arm hanging freely and the forearm flexed to horizontal. Measure the circumference at the midpoint of the arm, recording the measurement in centimetres, to the nearest millimetre (e.g., 24.6 cm) (Figure 40.11).

The midarm muscle circumference (MAMC) is then calculated by using reference tables or by using a formula that incorporates the TSF and the MAC. The MAMC is an estimate of lean body mass, or skeletal muscle reserves. If tables are not available, the nurse uses the following formula to calculate the MAMC from the triceps skinfold and MAC direct measurements:

$$\text{MAMC cm} = \text{MAC (cm)} - \frac{3.143 \; \text{TSF (mm)}}{10}$$

Standard values for anthropometric measurements for adults are shown in Table 40.7.

Changes in anthropometric measurements often occur slowly and reflect chronic, rather than acute, changes in nutritional status. They are, therefore, used to monitor the client's progress over months to years, rather than days to weeks. Ideally, initial and subsequent measurements need to be taken by the same clinician. In addition, measurements obtained need to be interpreted with caution. Fluctuations in hydration status that often occur during illness can influence the accuracy of results. Further, normal standards often do not account for normal changes in body composition, such as those that occur with aging.

Laboratory Tests

Laboratory tests provide objective data to the nutritional assessments, but because many factors can influence these tests, no single test specifically predicts nutritional risk or measures the presence or degree of a nutritional problem. The tests most commonly used are serum proteins (hemoglobin, albumin, transferrin), total lymphocyte count, total serum cholesterol, LDL, HDL, fasting blood glucose, thyroid stimulating hormone, and urinary urea nitrogen and creatinine.

BLOOD TESTS

Serum Proteins Serum protein levels, as mentioned earlier, provide an estimate of visceral protein stores. Tests commonly include hemoglobin, albumin, transferrin, and total iron-binding capacity. A low *hemoglobin* level may be evidence of iron-deficiency anemia. However, abnormal blood loss or a pathological process, such as gastrointestinal cancer, must be ruled out before iron deficiency related to diet is confirmed.

Edema may be present if the client is experiencing malnutrition. When the serum protein is low, edema results because of the loss of colloidal osmotic pressure

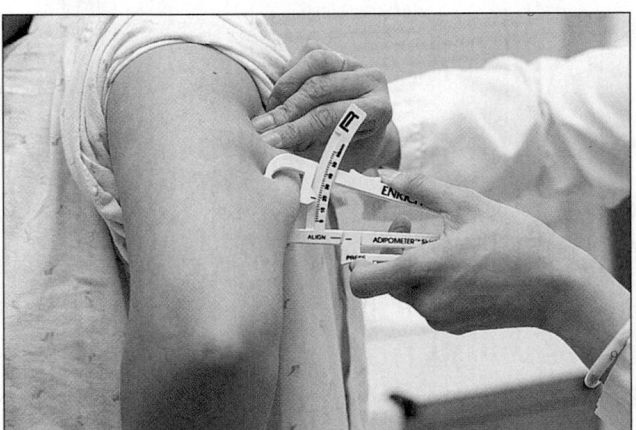

FIGURE 40.10 Measuring the triceps skinfold.

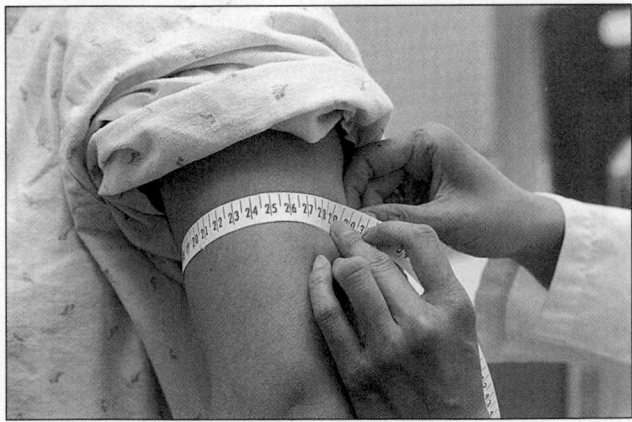

FIGURE 40.11 Measuring midarm circumference.

TABLE 40.7 Standard Values for Anthropometric Measurements for Adults

Measurement	Male	Female
Triceps skinfold (mm)	12	20
Midarm circumference (cm)	32	28
Midarm muscle circumference (cm)	54	30

Source: From *The Merck Manual of Diagnosis and Therapy*, Edition 18, edited by Mark H. Beers. Copyright 2006 by Merck & Co., Inc., Whitehouse Station, NJ. Reprinted with permission.

required to maintain the normal shift of fluid between the capillaries and the surrounding interstitial spaces. The edema may be present around the ankles or hands because of gravitational forces on the extremities, or it may affect the heart and lung actions in severe conditions.

Albumin, which accounts for more than 50% of the total serum proteins, is one of the most common visceral proteins evaluated as part of the nutritional assessment. Because there is so much albumin in the body and because it is not broken down very quickly (i.e., it has a long half-life [18–20 days]), albumin concentrations change slowly. Thus, a low serum albumin level is a useful indicator of prolonged protein depletion rather than acute or short-term changes in nutritional status. However, many conditions besides malnutrition can depress albumin concentration, such as altered liver function, hydration status, and losses from open wounds and burns.

Transferrin is a protein that binds and carries iron from the intestine through the serum. Because it has a shorter half-life compared with albumin (8–9 days), transferrin is likely to respond more quickly to protein depletion than albumin. Serum transferrin can be measured directly or by a *total iron-binding capacity (TIBC) test,* which indicates the amount of iron in the blood to which transferrin can bind. Conversion of the TIBC reading to a transferrin measurement is calculated by a standard mathematical formula. Transferrin levels below normal indicate protein loss, iron-deficiency anemia, pregnancy, hepatitis, and liver dysfunction. An increase in total iron-binding capacity can indicate iron deficiency; a decrease can indicate anemia.

Total Lymphocyte Count Certain nutrient deficiencies and forms of protein-calorie malnutrition can depress the immune system. The total number of lymphocytes decreases as protein depletion occurs.

Cholesterol Tests Total serum cholesterol is a measure of all cholesterol (HDL, LDL, very-low density lipoprotein [VLDL]). It does not separate the HDL and the LDL, so they must be measured separately. High levels of total cholesterol are indicative of being at risk for cardiovascular disease. The levels of LDL and HDL more accurately reflect the risk factor for cardiovascular disease.

Glucose Tests Fasting blood glucose level is conducted to screen for such illnesses as diabetes mellitus as well as monitor control in people diagnosed with diabetes or receiving total parenteral nutrition. An elevated blood glucose level is an indicator of excess glucose in the blood. Skill 40.1 outlines how to obtain a capillary blood specimen to measure blood glucose by using a portable meter.

SKILL 40.1 OBTAINING A CAPILLARY BLOOD SPECIMEN TO MEASURE BLOOD GLUCOSE

PURPOSES

- To determine or monitor blood glucose levels of clients at risk for hyperglycemia or hypoglycemia
- To promote blood glucose regulation by the client
- To evaluate the effectiveness of insulin or oral hypoglycemic medication administration in the case of diabetes mellitus treatment

ASSESSMENT

- Before obtaining a capillary blood specimen, determine the following:
  - The frequency and type of testing
  - The client's understanding of the procedure
  - The client's response to previous testing
- Assess the client's skin at the puncture site to determine that it is intact and the circulation is not compromised. Check colour, warmth, and capillary refill.
- Review the client's record for medications that may prolong bleeding, such as anticoagulants.
- Assess the client's self-care abilities that may affect accuracy of test results, such as visual impairment and finger dexterity.

Equipment

- Blood glucose meter (glucometer)
- Blood glucose reagent strip compatible with the meter

- Gauze
- Warm cloth or other warming device (optional)
- Antiseptic swab
- Disposable gloves
- Sterile lancet and lancet injector

IMPLEMENTATION

Preparation

Review the type of meter and manufacturer's instructions. Assemble the equipment at the bedside.

Performance

1. Before performing the procedure, introduce yourself and verify the client's identity using two identifiers or per agency protocol. Explain to the client what you are going to do, why it is necessary, and how he or she can participate. Discuss how the results will be used in planning further care or treatments.

2. Perform hand hygiene, and follow other appropriate infection prevention and control procedures (e.g., gloves).

3. Provide for client privacy.

4. Prepare the equipment.
   - Calibrate the meter, if necessary, and run a control sample according to the manufacturer's instructions. Many meters are now self-calibrating.

- Place the strip into the meter, according to the manufacturer's instructions.

5. Select and prepare the vascular puncture site.

- Choose a vascular puncture site (e.g., the side of an adult's finger). Avoid sites beside bone. Wrap the finger first in a warm cloth, *or* hold a finger in a dependent position. If the earlobe is used, rub it gently with a small piece of gauze. **Rationale: These actions increase the blood flow to the area, ensure an adequate specimen, and reduce the need for a repeat puncture**.

- Clean the site with the antiseptic swab or soap and water, and allow it to dry completely. **Rationale: Alcohol can affect accuracy and the site burns when punctured when wet with alcohol**.

6. Obtain the blood specimen.

- Put on gloves.

- Place the injector, if used, against the site, and release the needle, thus permitting it to pierce the skin. Make sure the lancet is perpendicular to the site (see ❶). **Rationale: The lancet is designed to pierce the skin at a specific depth when it is in a perpendicular position relative to the skin**.

- *Or* prick the site with a lancet or needle by using a darting motion.

- Gently squeeze (but do not touch) the puncture site until a large drop of blood forms. The size of the drop of blood can vary depending on the meter. Some meters require as little as 0.3 to 1 μL (microlitre) or not much larger than the period at the end of this sentence.

- Hold the reagent strip against the puncture site until adequate blood covers the indicator square. The pad will absorb the blood and a chemical reaction will occur. Do not smear the blood (see ❷). **Rationale: This will cause an inaccurate reading**. When the puncture site is touched with the edge of the strip, some meters will wick the blood onto the strip.

- Ask the client to apply pressure to the skin puncture site with gauze. **Rationale: Pressure will assist hemostasis**.

- Follow the manufacturer's recommendations on the glucose meter and monitor for the amount of time indicated by the manufacturer. **Rationale: The blood must remain in contact with the test pad for a prescribed time to obtain accurate results**.

7. Measure the blood glucose.

- After the designated time, most glucose meters will display the glucose reading automatically. Correct timing ensures accurate results (see ❸).

- Turn off the meter and discard the test strip and gauze in a biohazard container. Discard the lancet into a sharps container.

8. Document the method of testing and results on the client's record. If appropriate, record the client's understanding and ability to demonstrate the technique. The client's record may also include a flowsheet on which capillary blood glucose results and the amount, type, route, and time of insulin or hypoglycemic medication administration are recorded.

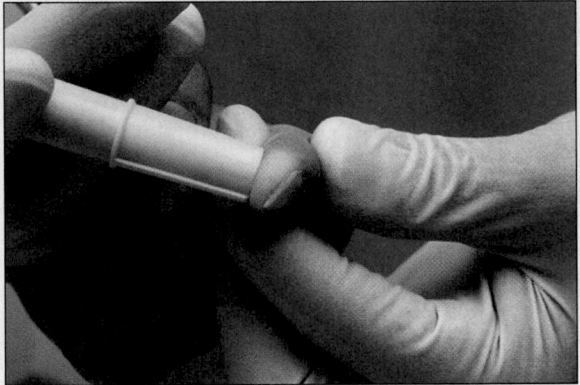

❶ Place the injector against the site.

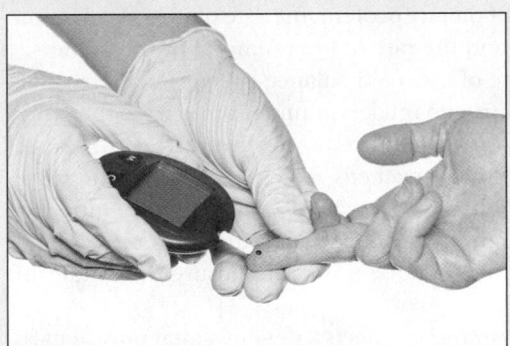

❷ Hold the reagent strip against the puncture site.

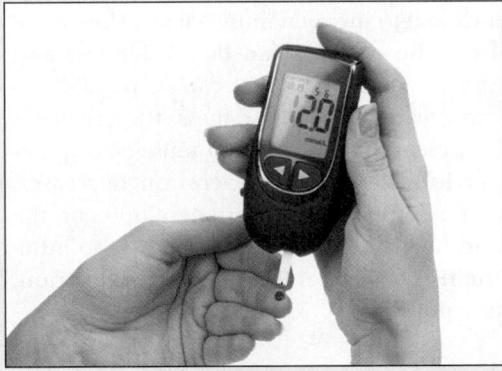

❸ The glucose meter will display the glucose reading.

EVALUATION

- Compare glucose meter reading with normal blood glucose level, status of puncture site, and motivation of the client to perform the test independently.

- Report abnormal results to the appropriate member of the health care team.

THYROID FUNCTION Assessing the function of a client's thyroid is important to determining whether his or her BMR is being regulated normally. If a client's thyroid stimulating hormone (TSH) levels are elevated, it is indicative that the thyroid is not producing adequate amounts of thyroxine (T_4) and triiodothyronine (T_3), and hence the rate of metabolism may be slowed.

URINARY TESTS *Urinary urea nitrogen* (UUN) and *urinary creatinine* are measures of protein catabolism and the state of nitrogen balance. **Urea**, the chief end product of amino acid metabolism, is formed from ammonia detoxified by the liver, circulated in the blood, and transported to the kidneys for excretion. UUN and blood urea nitrogen (BUN), therefore, directly reflect the intake and breakdown of dietary protein, the rate of urea production in the liver, and the rate of urea removal by the kidneys.

The state of nitrogen balance is determined by comparing the nitrogen intake (grams of protein) to the nitrogen output over 24 hours. A positive nitrogen balance exists when intake exceeds nitrogen output; a negative nitrogen balance occurs when output exceeds nitrogen intake. Protein intake must be accurately recorded and kidney function must be normal to ensure the validity of a UUN.

Urinary creatinine reflects a person's total muscle mass because creatinine is the chief end product of the creatine produced when energy is released during skeletal muscle metabolism. The rate of creatinine formation is directly proportional to the total muscle mass. Creatinine is removed from the bloodstream by the kidneys and excreted in the urine at a rate that closely parallels its formation. The greater the muscle mass, the greater is the excretion of creatinine. As skeletal muscle atrophies during malnutrition, creatinine excretion decreases. Standards for creatinine excretion are developed on the basis of sex and height. Urinary creatinine is also influenced by protein intake, exercise, age, renal function, and thyroid function.

Diagnosing

Nursing diagnoses related to nutritional problems are numerous and can include overweight, obesity, underweight, risk for childhood obesity, excess dietary sodium intake, and inadequate nutritional intake relative to *Canada's Food Guide*. Given the many factors that influence healthy nutrition, it is important to identify the factors that contribute to the health issues in diagnoses related to nutrition. For example, the client with *inadequate nutritional intake* as the broad diagnosis will have improved quality of care if it is clear that the inadequate intake is *related to insufficient funds to purchase quality foods, poor appetite related to anosmia and social isolation, and poor dentition*. Other diagnoses may apply to areas of human

functioning that nutritional problems often affect, for example, fatigue related to iron-deficiency anemia; constipation as a result of inadequate fluid intake and fibre intake; anxiety and fear related to bullying from being overweight; poor concentration in school related to hunger.

Planning

Major goals for clients with or at risk for nutritional problems include the following:

- Maintain or restore optimal nutritional status
- Promote healthy nutritional practices
- Prevent complications associated with malnutrition
- Decrease weight
- Regain specified weight

Examples of desired outcomes related to some of these goals, although established in the planning phase, are provided in the Evaluating section of this chapter.

Examples of nursing interventions to enhance an individual's nutrition include the following:

- Nutritional counselling
- Nutrition management
- Nutritional monitoring
- Nutrition therapy
- Assistance with weight reduction
- Assistance with weight gain
- Energy management
- Exercise promotion
- Behaviour modification
- Enteral tube feeding
- Total parenteral nutrition (TPN) administration

Specific nursing activities associated with each of these interventions can be selected to meet the individual needs of the client. A Sample Care Plan that uses nursing interventions and selected activities is provided using the Obesity Canada clinical guidelines as a framework for guiding data collection and interventions.

Planning for Home Care

To provide for continuity of care, the nurse must consider the client's need for assistance with nutrition. Some clients will need help with feeding, purchasing food, and preparing meals; others will need instructions about enteral and total parenteral nutrition (TPN) therapy.

Home care planning incorporates an assessment of the client's and family's abilities for self-care, financial

Sample Care Plan for Nutrition

Assessment Data

Nursing Assessment

Mrs. Rose Santini, a 59-year-old homemaker from New Brunswick, attends a community hospital-sponsored health fair. She approaches the nutrition information booth and discusses with the nurse that she is very upset about her 9-kg weight gain over the last year. She relates that since the death of her husband 12 months ago, she has lost interest in many of her usual physical and social activities. She no longer attends exercise and swimming sessions and has lost contact with her couples' bridge group. Mrs. Santini states she is very unhappy about her appearance as she has always prided herself on her figure. She says her eating habits have changed considerably. She snacks while watching TV and rarely prepares a complete meal.

Physical Examination

Height: 1.62 m

Weight: 77 kg

BMI: 29.34 (up from 26.29 1 year ago)

Temperature: 37°C

Pulse: 76 beats/min

Respirations: 16/min

Blood pressure: 144/84 mm Hg

Diagnostic Data

CBC (complete blood count) normal, urinalysis normal, thyroid profile within normal limits

Nursing Diagnosis

Overweight related to excess caloric intake and reduced physical activity; inadequate quality of nutritional intake related to changes in social situation. Both issues likely related to her emotional reactions to the loss of her husband.

Client Goals

While Mrs. Santini will need help and support related to coping with her loss, the nutrition-related goals that she would like to address are as follows: (a) improve the quality of her nutritional intake; (b) avoid gaining any further weight; and (c) lower her BMI to 27 within 1 year.

Desired Health Outcomes

1. Plans meals and healthy snacks that follow *Eating Well With Canada's Food Guide* recommendations

2. Develops a physical activity plan that engages her in 2.5 hours of moderate physical activity a week

3. Feels more positive about her body image

Nursing Interventions

Improving the quality of nutritional intake:

- Determine current eating patterns by having Mrs. Santini keep a diary of what, when, and where she eats. **Rationale: A diary increases the client's awareness of activities and foods that contribute to excessive intake.**

- Provide Mrs. Santini with a copy of *Eating Well with Canada's Food Guide* and discuss the major recommendations including portion size and number of servings of the various food groups as well as foods to avoid, for example, those containing "empty calories," high sodium, high fat content. **Rationale:** *Canada's Food Guide* **provides evidence-based nutritional guidelines that are clear and comprehensive.**

- Discuss food likes and dislikes and develop a daily meal plan with these in mind. **Rationale: Incorporating food preferences into the dietary plan will promote adherence to the plan.**

- Explore triggers that lead to snacking so as to limit these and/or identify healthy snacks. **Rationale: Awareness of factors that contribute to overeating will assist the individual in planning strategies to avoid situations that prompt excess food consumption; healthy snacks are a way of meeting the recommended number of servings of a particular nutrient in a day.**

- Help her consider the social nature of eating and its impact on the quality of her nutritional intake and develop strategies to cope with this situation. **Rationale: Social and psychological factors play a role in**

healthy nutrition—a major factor in Mrs. Santini's situation is that she has no companionship during meals and may lack both internal motivation (related to loss) and the external motivation (having someone to prepare a meal with/for and share that meal)—in identifying these factors, she may be able to think of ways to help her situation such as inviting friends or family over for a meal.

Avoiding further weight gain and lowering BMI:

- Help Mrs. Santini understand the need to balance a healthy nutritional intake with physical activity.

  Set a realistic weekly goal of gradually increasing physical activity (such as resuming swimming and exercise sessions) with an aim of achieving 2.5 hours of moderate physical activity a week. **Rationale: Weight loss is enhanced when energy expenditure is in excess of energy intake; physical activity promotes a sense of well-being—she previously enjoyed swimming and exercise classes so resuming these activities may also help her feel more like her "usual self" as well as possibly help her reconnect with friends and acquaintances.**

- Encourage use of internal reward systems as she accomplishes increased physical activity while improving the quality of her nutritional intake. **Rationale: Given that she now lives alone, she will need to rely on herself for motivation—focusing on such aspects as feeling fitter, clothes fitting more comfortably, and "doing something for me" may help reinforce her activities.**

- Discuss whether she feels attendance at a support group for weight loss or a community weight control program would motivate her. **Rationale: Support groups can provide companionship, increase motivation, and offer practical solutions to problems associated with dieting.**

(continued)

Sample Care Plan for Nutrition (continued)

- Set and evaluate short-term goals in relation to weight loss.
  Rationale: With Mrs. Santini having gained 9 kg in 1 year, it is reasonable to hypothesize that she could lose the 9 kg in 1 year; although 1 year may be realistic for getting back to her previous weight, achieving short-term goals (e.g., weight loss of 1.5 kg/month) provides for a more "stepwise" way of measuring her success or difficulty in achieving the ultimate goal. While successful weight loss will likely motivate her to continue, no weight loss or weight gain may lead to reduced motivation; strategies may need to be revised if the latter occurs.

Evaluation

Goal partially met at 6 months with a BMI of 27.8. Mrs. Santini kept a dietary log and identified boredom as a major trigger for snacking in excess. She also realized that she was not buying a variety of foods to avoid spoilage—as she noted: "I avoided buying variety so I would not have any waste—it ended up that I would make something and end up eating the same thing 3 or 4 days in a row!" While her weight fluctuated up and down the first 6 weeks, she was motivated to continue in her swimming and exercise classes because she was reconnecting with friends and realized that she needed the structure in her routine

that these outings gave her. She has discovered that she is not alone as she has met several widows and widowers at a local support group—she and a few members of this group have now started a communal kitchen. She notes, "We make four or five batches of different foods, such as lasagna a and meatloaf, and we then split the batches into individual portions so that we each leave with four or five different meals for the week. It sure beats eating the same thing 3 days in a row! We even make sure we get our orange vegetables in per *Canada's Food Guide!*"

---

resources, and the need for referrals and home health services. The Assessment: Home Care box outlines a home care assessment for nutritional problems and needs. A major aspect of discharge planning involves instructional needs of the client and family. See the Teaching: Wellness box on healthy nutrition.

ASSESSMENT | **HOME CARE**

Nutrition

Before discharging clients, nurses need to assess their nutrition needs and any problems:

CLIENT AND ENVIRONMENT

- *Self-care abilities:* Assess the ability to feed self, to purchase food, and to prepare meals.
- *Adaptive feeding aids required:* Determine the need for special drinking cups, plates, or feeding utensils (see "feeding aids" later in this chapter).
- *Instructional needs:* Consider nutritional requirements (e.g., *Eating Well with Canada's Food Guide,* dietary guidelines, special diet); adaptive aids available; recommended lifestyle variations; and management of enteral or parenteral nutrition.
- *Physical environment:* Assess for the adequacy of water, electricity, refrigeration, and telephone facilities and for the presence of a clean, secure area to store and set up enteral or parenteral equipment, as needed.
- *Abilities to manage enteral or parenteral nutrition* (discussed later in this chapter): Assess for the cognitive abilities to manage procedures and follow a prescribed schedule; the adequacy of manual dexterity to open sterile packages and handle equipment; the adequacy of visual acuity to read numbers on syringes and pumps; the ability to prepare formulas; and the ability to evaluate the status of the enteral or parenteral access device and report problems.

FAMILY

- *Caregiver availability, skills, and willingness:* Assess for primary and secondary persons able to assist with food

purchase, meal preparation, and feeding and who are able to comprehend and administer special diets or the enteral or parenteral nutrition required.
- *Family role changes and coping:* Consider the effect on parenting and spousal roles, financial resources, and social roles.
- *Alternative potential primary or respite caregivers:* Assess, for example, other family members, volunteers, church members, paid caregivers, or housekeeping services, available community respite care (adult daycare, senior centres), and so on.

COMMUNITY

- *Current knowledge, use, and experience with community resources:* Determine the familiarity with nutritional counselling services; home health agencies for enteral or parenteral nutrition support; dietitian or nutritionist for planning appropriate meals for prescribed diet, planning ways to include ethnic food preferences into the diet, and providing written meal plans; medical equipment and supply sources; financial assistance services; support and educational services, such as the following:
  - Weight-management programs (e.g., Weight Watchers, Curves, TOPS [Take Off Pounds Successfully])
  - Dietitians of Canada for information on all nutrition topics
  - Health Canada
  - Meals on Wheels

TEACHING WELLNESS

Healthy Nutrition

Discharge planning also includes teaching clients and their families about healthy nutrition:

- Instruct clients about the content of a healthy diet based on *Eating Well with Canada's Food Guide.*
- Encourage clients, particularly older clients, to reduce dietary fat.
- Instruct strict vegetarians, as needed, about complementary proteins and additional vitamin and mineral supplementation.
- Discuss foods high in specific required nutrients, such as protein, iron, calcium, vitamin C, and fibre.
- Discuss the importance of properly fitted dentures and dental care.
- Discuss safe food preparation and preservation techniques, as appropriate.

DIETARY ALTERATIONS

- Explain the purpose of the diet.
- Discuss allowed and excluded foods.
- Explain how to interpret food labels when selecting foods including "% Daily Value."
- Include family or significant others as appropriate.
- Reinforce information provided by the dietitian or nutritionist as appropriate.
- Discuss herbs and spices as alternatives to salt, and discuss substitutes for sugar.

FOR OVERWEIGHT CLIENTS

- Assist client in establishing their own realistic weight-loss goals.
  - Discuss physiological, psychological, and lifestyle factors that predispose people to weight gain.
- Provide information about normal weight range and recommended calorie intake.
- Discuss principles of a well-balanced diet (see *Canada's Food Guide* or other food guidelines) and high-calorie and low-calorie foods.
- Encourage intake of low-calorie, caffeine-free beverages and plenty of water.
- Discuss ways to adapt eating practices by using smaller plates, smaller servings, chewing each bite a specified number of times, and putting the fork down between bites.

- Discuss ways to control the desire to eat by taking a walk, drinking a glass of water, or doing slow deep-breathing exercises.
- Discuss the importance of exercise and help the client plan an exercise program.
- Discuss stress-reduction techniques.
- Provide information about available community resources (e.g., weight-loss groups, dietary counselling, exercise programs, self-help groups).

FOR UNDERWEIGHT CLIENTS

- Discuss factors contributing to inadequate nutrition and weight loss.
- Discuss recommended calorie intake and normal weight range.
- Provide information about the content of a balanced diet based on *Canada's Food Guide.*
- Provide information about ways to increase calorie intake (e.g., high-protein or high-calorie foods and nutritional supplements).
- Discuss ways to manage, minimize, or alter the factors contributing to malnourishment.
- If appropriate, discuss ways to purchase low-cost nutritious foods.
- Provide information about community agencies that can assist in providing food (e.g., Meals on Wheels).

PREVENTING FOOD-BORNE ILLNESS

- Reinforce hygienic handling of food and dishes:
  - Wash hands before preparing foods.
  - Wash hands and all dishes and utensils with hot water and soap after contact with raw meats.
  - Defrost frozen foods in the refrigerator.
  - Cook beef, poultry, and eggs thoroughly. Use a cooking thermometer.
  - Refrigerate leftovers promptly (at 5°C or less) and keep no more than 3 to 5 days.
  - Wash or peel raw fruits and vegetables.
  - Do not use foods from containers that have been damaged or have opened seals.
  - Follow the rules "Keep hot foods hot and cold foods cold" and "When in doubt, throw it out."
- Recommend that the client consider preventive vaccination for hepatitis A.
- Instruct clients to seek medical attention for prolonged vomiting, fever, abdominal pain, or severe diarrhea following a meal.

Implementing

Nursing interventions to promote optimal nutrition for hospitalized patients are often provided in collaboration with the physician, who writes the diet orders, and the dietitian, who works with the interprofessional team and the patient to implement special diets and prepare feeding protocols. The nurse reinforces this instruction and, in addition, creates an atmosphere that encourages eating, provides assistance with eating, monitors the

patient's appetite and food intake, administers enteral and parenteral feedings, and consults with the physician and dietitian about nutritional problems that arise.

In the community setting, the nurse's role is largely educational. For example, nurses promote optimal nutrition at health fairs, in schools, at prenatal classes, and with well or ill clients and support people in their homes. In the home setting, nurses also initiate nutritional screens, refer clients at risk to appropriate resources, instruct clients about enteral and parenteral feedings, and offer nutrition counselling, as needed. Nutrition counselling involves more than simply providing information. The nurse must help clients integrate diet changes into their lifestyles and provide strategies to motivate them to change their eating habits. For children, the school setting is the ideal place to introduce the concepts of healthy nutrition. *Eating Well with Canada's Food Guide* should play an essential part in the curriculum and cafeterias not selling junk food should be encouraged.

Assisting with Special Diets

Alterations in the client's diet are often needed to treat a disease process, such as diabetes mellitus, to prepare for a special examination or surgery, to increase or decrease weight, to restore nutritional deficits, or to allow an organ to rest and promote healing. Diets are modified in one or more of the following aspects: texture, calories, specific nutrients, seasonings, or consistency.

Patients who do not have special needs eat the *regular* (standard or house) *diet,* a balanced diet that supplies the metabolic requirements of a sedentary person (about 2000 kcal). Most agencies offer patients a daily menu from which to select their meals for the next day; others provide standard meals to each patient on the general diet. Certain foods (e.g., cabbage, which tends to produce flatus, and highly seasoned and fried foods, which are difficult for some people to digest) are usually omitted from the regular diet.

TEMPORARY CONSISTENCY MODIFICATIONS Diets that are modified in consistency are often given to patients before and after surgery or to promote healing in patients with gastrointestinal distress. These diets include nothing by mouth (nil per ora), clear fluid, full fluid, soft, and diet as tolerated.

Nothing by Mouth   In **nothing by mouth (nil per ora [NPO])**, food and fluid are prohibited, for example, before anesthesia to prevent aspiration of stomach contents. NPO status should be limited as much as possible to minimize nutritional and dehydration risks. Alternative methods of nutrition and hydration (e.g., parenteral feeding) should be considered if the patient must remain without food or fluid.

Clear Fluid Diet   The **clear fluid diet** is limited to water, tea, coffee, clear broths, ginger ale or other carbonated beverages, strained and clear juices, and plain gelatin. This diet provides the person with fluid and carbohydrate (in the form of sugar) but does not supply adequate protein, fat, vitamins, minerals, or calories. It is a short-term diet (24 to 36 hours) provided for patients after certain surgery or in the acute stages of infection, particularly of the gastrointestinal tract. The major objectives of this diet are to relieve thirst, prevent dehydration, and minimize stimulation of the gastrointestinal tract. Examples of foods allowed in clear diets are shown in Box 40.10.

Full Fluid Diet   The **full fluid diet** contains only liquids or foods that turn to liquid at body temperature, such as ice cream (see Box 40.10). Full fluid diets are often eaten by patients who have gastrointestinal disturbances or are otherwise unable to tolerate solid or semisolid foods. This diet is not recommended for long-term use because it is

---

BOX 40.10   FOODS FOR CLEAR FLUID, FULL FLUID, AND SOFT DIETS

The following are some examples of allowed foods on clear fluid, full fluid, and soft diets:

Clear Fluid	**Full Fluid**	**Soft**
Coffee, regular and decaffeinated	All foods on clear fluid diet, plus the following:	All foods on full and clear fluid diets, plus the following:
Tea (black, green, or white)	Milk and milk drinks	*Meat:* All lean, tender meat, fish, or poultry (chopped, shredded); spaghetti sauce with ground meat over pasta
Carbonated beverages	Puddings, custards	
Bouillon, fat-free broth	Ice cream, sherbet	*Meat alternatives:* Scrambled eggs, omelette, poached eggs; cottage cheese and other mild cheese
Clear fruit juices (apple, cranberry, grape)	Vegetable juices	
Other fruit juices, strained	Refined or strained cereals (e.g., cream of wheat)	*Vegetables:* Mashed potatoes, sweet potatoes, or squash; vegetables in cream or cheese sauce; other cooked vegetables as tolerated (e.g., spinach, cauliflower, asparagus tips), chopped and mashed, as needed; avocado
Popsicles	Cream, butter, margarine	
Gelatin	Eggs (in custard and pudding)	*Fruits:* Cooked or canned fruits; bananas; grapefruit and orange sections without membranes; applesauce
Sugar, honey	Smooth peanut butter	
Hard candy	Yogourt	*Breads and cereals:* Enriched rice, barley, pasta; all breads; cooked cereals (e.g., oatmeal)
		Desserts: Soft cake, bread pudding

low in iron, protein, and calories. In addition, its cholesterol content is high because of the amount of milk offered. Patients who must receive only liquids for long periods are usually given a nutritionally balanced oral supplement, such as Ensure or Boost. The full fluid diet is monotonous and difficult for patients to accept. Planning six or more feedings per day may encourage a more adequate intake.

Soft Diet The **soft diet** is easily chewed and digested. It is often ordered for patients who have difficulty chewing and swallowing. It is a low-residue (low-fibre) diet containing very few uncooked foods; however, restrictions vary among agencies and according to individual tolerance. Examples of foods that can be included in a soft or semisoft diet are shown in Box 40.10. The **pureed diet** is a modification of the soft diet. Liquid can be added to the food, which is then blended to a semisolid consistency.

Diet as Tolerated **Diet as tolerated (DAT)** is ordered when the patient's appetite, ability to eat, and tolerance for certain foods may change. For example, on the first postoperative day, a patient may be given a clear fluid diet. If no nausea occurs, normal intestinal motility has returned, and the patient feels like eating, the diet may be advanced to a full fluid, light, or regular diet.

MODIFICATION FOR DISEASE Many special diets are prescribed to meet the requirements for disease process or altered metabolism. For many medical conditions, specific diets may be prescribed. Patients with diabetes mellitus may be prescribed a diet that follows the glycemic index suggested by the Canadian Diabetes Association. Patients with hypertension will need a sodium-reduced diet. Those with coronary artery disease or those at significant risk (e.g., because of family history of heart attack or cerebrovascular accident) may need a diet low in cholesterol and saturated fats. Patients with celiac disease who are intolerant to wheat gluten must avoid all gluten-containing products and may need to replace all grains with rice-based products. Individuals with renal insufficiency need to limit the number of grams of protein they eat per day to protect their kidneys, and those with renal failure must avoid ingesting too much potassium because they cannot excrete it.

People with severe food allergies must take extreme precaution to avoid exposure to their triggers as well as carry an EpiPen (epinephrine autoinjector) at all times in case of accidental exposure. See the Clinical Alert box on food allergies.

Some patients must adapt their diets because of the medications they take. For example, patients who are taking antineoplastic medications and who have severely depressed immune systems (e.g., neutropenia) may need to eat only well-cooked foods to prevent the risk of infection. Patients who are glucocorticosteroid dependent are encouraged to eat a low-carbohydrate, high-protein diet to prevent weight gain and muscle wasting.

CLINICAL ALERT

In Canada, as many as 3% to 4% of the adult population and 6% of children are affected by food allergies, and the prevalence of such allergies is increasing (Health Canada, 2010b). Common food allergens include peanuts, tree nuts, sesame, soy, fish and seafood, wheat, eggs, and milk. When people are affected by food allergens, exposure to very tiny amounts of the food can trigger a reaction. Symptoms include difficulty breathing, facial swelling, itching, rash, cramps, and diarrhea. Full-blown anaphylaxis can occur. Patients who have food allergies must be taught how to avoid triggers, what to do in the case of accidental exposure, and how to use an EpiPen (epinephrine autoinjector). It is crucial that the nurse reiterate the importance of carrying this life-saving device at all times to increase patient adherence. These patients should wear a medical identification bracelet or necklace. Many schools now restrict certain foods to prevent accidental exposure. In 2011, the Canadian government introduced regulations requiring food producers to use more colloquial language and to declare "hidden" allergens, gluten sources, and sulphites in their products. This will enable Canadians to make more informed and safer food choices (Health Canada, 2011c).

Some clients must follow their special diets (e.g., as for diabetes) for a lifetime. If the diet is for the long term, the client must not only understand the diet but also develop a healthy, positive attitude toward it. Assisting clients and support persons with special diets is a function shared by the dietitian or nutritionist and the nurse. The dietitian informs the client and support persons about the specific foods allowed and not allowed and assists the client with meal planning. The nurse reinforces this instruction, assists the client to make changes, and evaluates the client's responses. All dietary instructions must be individually designed to meet the client's cognitive status, motivation level, lifestyle, culture, and economic status. Both nutritionists and dietitians help to adapt a diet to suit the client. Simple verbal instructions need to be given and reinforced with written material. Family and support persons must be included in the dietary instruction.

Dysphagia Some clients may have no difficulty choosing a healthy diet but may be at risk for nutritional problems because of dysphagia. These clients may have inadequate solid or fluid intake, be unable to swallow their medications, or aspirate food or fluids into the lungs, causing pneumonia. Clients at risk for dysphagia include older adults, those who have experienced a cerebrovascular accident, cancer patients who have had radiation therapy to the head and neck, and others with cranial nerve dysfunction. Nurses may be the first persons to detect dysphagia and are in an excellent position to recommend further evaluation, implement specialized feeding techniques and diets, and work with clients, family members, and other health care professionals to develop a plan to assist the client with difficulties. If the client's condition suggests dysphagia, the nurse should review the history in detail; interview the client or family; assess the mouth, throat, and chest; and observe the client swallowing. The presence of the gag reflex, often thought to indicate that the client can swallow safely, has not been shown to be a reliable indicator. Confirmation of the tendency for food to divert to the trachea is best done with radiography.

The National Dysphagia Diet (American Dietetic Association, 2003) has delineated standards of food textures to help in the treatment of dysphagia. The four levels of liquid foods are (a) thin, (b) nectar-like, (c) honey-like, and (d) spoon-thick liquids. The four levels of semisolid or solid foods are (a) pureed, (b) mechanically altered, (c) advanced or mechanically soft, and (d) regular or general. In consultation with the dietitian, the occupational therapist, the swallowing specialist, the speech-language pathologist, or the physician, these levels can be used to determine a consistent approach to a particular client's dysphagia. For example, a mechanically soft diet may result in lower pneumonia rates than a pureed diet in stroke patients with a history of aspiration pneumonia. Early detection and intervention can prevent the adverse outcomes of dysphagia in most clients.

Stimulating the Appetite

Physical illness, unfamiliar or unpalatable food, environmental and psychological factors, medications or therapies, and physical discomfort or pain may depress the appetites of many patients. A short-term decrease in food intake usually is not a problem for adults; over time, however, it leads to weight loss, decreased strength and stamina, and other nutritional problems. A decreased food intake is often accompanied by a decrease in fluid intake, which may cause fluid and electrolyte problems. Stimulating a person's appetite requires the nurse to determine the reason for the lack of appetite and then to deal with the problem. Some interventions for improving the client's appetite are summarized in Box 40.11.

Assisting Patients with Meals

Because patients in health care agencies are frequently confined to their beds, meals are often brought to the patient. The patient receives a tray that has been assembled in a central kitchen. Nursing personnel may be responsible for giving out and collecting the trays; however, in most settings, this is done by special dietary personnel. Long-term care facilities and some hospitals serve meals to ambulatory patients in a special dining area. Other agencies have a coffee shop for food or machines from which patients can obtain sandwiches and beverages. Guidelines for providing meals to patients and residents are summarized in Box 40.12.

Two groups of people frequently require help with their meals: (a) older adults who are weakened and (b) persons with disabilities, such as those who are visually impaired, those who must remain in a supine position, or those who cannot use their hands. The

---

> **BOX 40.11** IMPROVING APPETITE
>
> Nurses can try the following to help improve a client's appetite:
>
> - Relieve illness symptoms that depress appetite before mealtime; for example, give an analgesic for pain, an antipyretic for fever, or allow rest for fatigue. Treat the patient's nausea well before the meal is presented.
> - Provide familiar food that the person likes. Often, the relatives of patients are pleased to bring food from home but may need some guidance about special diet requirements.
> - Select small portions so as to not discourage the patient with anorexia.
> - Avoid unpleasant or uncomfortable treatments immediately before or after a meal.
> - Provide a tidy, clean environment that is free of unpleasant sights and odours. The sight and smell of a soiled dressing, a used bedpan, an uncovered irrigation set, or even used dishes can negatively affect the appetite.
> - Encourage or provide oral hygiene before mealtime. This improves the patient's ability to taste.
> - Reduce psychological stress. A lack of understanding of therapy, the anticipation of an operation, and fear of the unknown can cause anorexia. Often, the nurse can help by discussing feelings with the patient, giving information and assistance, and allaying fears.
> - Stimulate the patient's appetite by having the patient remember favourite foods and to think about those foods and their tastes. If possible, have family members supply these foods.

---

patient's nursing care plan will indicate that assistance is required with meals.

The nurse must be sensitive to patients' feelings of embarrassment, resentment, and loss of autonomy. Whenever possible, the nurse should help incapacitated patients feed themselves, rather than feed them. Some patients become depressed because they require help and because they believe they are burdensome to busy nursing personnel. Although feeding a patient is time consuming, nurses should try to appear unhurried and convey that they have ample time. Sitting at the bedside is one way to convey this impression.

When feeding a patient, ask in which order the patient would like to eat the food. If the patient cannot see, tell the patient which food is being given. Always allow ample time for the patient to chew and swallow the food before offering more. Also, provide fluids as requested, or if the patient is unable to communicate, offer fluids after every three or four mouthfuls of solid food. It is important to make the time a pleasant one, choosing topics of conversation that are of interest to patients who want to talk.

Although normal utensils should be used whenever possible, special utensils may be needed to help a patient eat. For patients who have difficulty drinking from a cup or glass, a straw often permits them to obtain liquids with less effort and less spillage. Special drinking cups are also

BOX 40.12 PROVIDING MEALS TO PATIENTS

Nurses should observe the following guidelines when providing meals:

- Offer the patient assistance with hand hygiene and oral hygiene before a meal.

- Most people sit up during a meal; if it is permitted, assist the patient to a comfortable position in bed or in a chair, whichever is appropriate.

- Clear the overbed table so that there is space for the tray. If the patient must remain in a lying position in bed, arrange the overbed table close to the bedside so that the patient can see and reach the food.

- Check each tray for the patient's name, the type of diet, and completeness. Do *not* leave a diet that is incorrect for the patient.

- Assist the patient, as required, to remove the food covers, put spreads on the bread, pour the tea, and cut the meat.

- For a person who is visually impaired, identify the placement of the food as you would describe the time on a clock. For instance, the nurse may say, "The potatoes are at 8 o'clock, the chicken at 12 o'clock, and the green beans at 4 o'clock."

- After the patient has completed the meal, observe how much and what the patient has eaten and the amount of fluid taken. Record fluid intake and calorie count, as required.

- If the patient is on a special diet or is having problems eating, record the amount of food eaten and any pain, fatigue, or nausea experienced.

- If the patient is not eating, document this so that changes can be made, such as rescheduling the meals, providing smaller, more frequent meals, or obtaining special self-feeding aids.

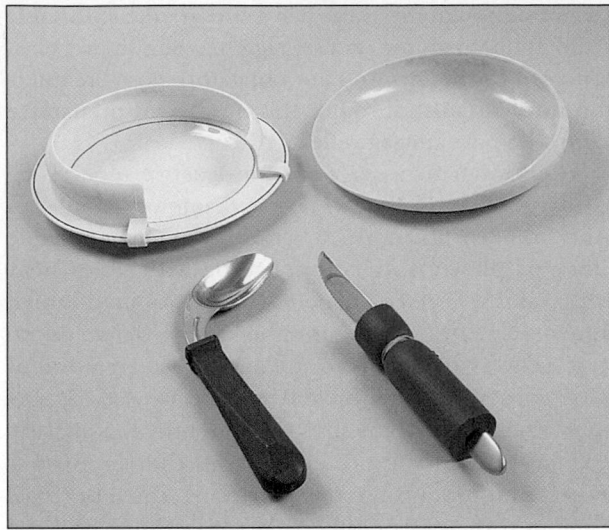

FIGURE 40.12 Dinner plate with guard attached and lip plate facilitate scooping; wide-handled spoon and knife facilitate grip.

Providing Special Community Nutritional Services

In many places, community programs have been developed to help special groups of the population meet their nutritional needs. For older people who cannot prepare meals or leave their homes, ready-to-eat meals or frozen dinners are delivered to the home by local organizations. Online or telephone ordering with home delivery can be an option for people who can prepare meals but are unable to shop for groceries in person.

Providing Enteral Nutrition

Alternative feeding methods to ensure adequate nutrition include both enteral (through the gastrointestinal system) and parenteral (intravenous) methods. **Parenteral nutrition** involves the intravenous infusion of water, protein, carbohydrates, electrolytes, minerals, and vitamins through a central vein. **Enteral nutrition (EN)**, also referred to as **total enteral nutrition (TEN)**, is provided when the client is unable to ingest foods or the upper gastrointestinal tract is impaired and the transport of food to the small intestine is interrupted. EN can also be used to supplement the client's own food intake when it is insufficient to meet daily needs. Enteral feedings are administered through nasogastric and small-bore feeding tubes or through gastrostomy or jejunostomy tubes.

ENTERAL ACCESS DEVICES Enteral access is achieved by means of nasogastric or nasointestinal (nasoenteric) tubes, or gastrostomy or jejunostomy tubes. A **nasogastric tube** is inserted through one of the nostrils, down the nasopharynx, and into the alimentary tract. In some instances, the tube is passed through the mouth and

available. One model has a spout; another is specially designed to permit drinking with less tipping of the cup than is normally required.

Many adaptive feeding aids are available to help patients maintain independence. A standard eating utensil with a built-up or widened handle helps patients who cannot grasp objects easily. Utensils with wide handles can be purchased, or a regular eating utensil can be modified by taping foam around the handle. The foam increases friction and, thus, steadies the patient's grasp. Handles can be bent or angled to compensate for limited motion. Collars or bands that prevent the utensil from being dropped can be attached to the end of the handle and fit over the patient's hand.

Plates with rims and plastic or metal plate guards enable the patient to pick up the food by first pushing it against this raised edge. A suction cup or damp sponge or cloth can be placed under the dish to keep it from moving while the patient is eating. No-spill mugs and two-handled drinking cups are especially useful for persons with impaired hand coordination. Stretch terry cloth and knitted or crocheted glass covers enable the patient to keep a secure grasp on a glass. Lidded tip-proof glasses are also available. Figure 40.12 shows some of these aids.

pharynx, although this route may be more uncomfortable for the adult client and cause gagging. This approach is often used for infants who are obligatory nose breathers (who must breathe through the nose) and premature infants who have no gag reflex.

Traditional firm *large-bore* nasogastric tubes (i.e., those larger than 12 French [Fr] in diameter) are placed in the stomach. Examples are the *Levin tube*, a flexible rubber or plastic single-lumen tube with holes near the tip, and the *Salem sump tube*, with a double lumen (Figure 40.13). The larger tube of the Salem sump allows delivery of liquids to the stomach or removal of gastric contents. When the Salem tube is used for suction of gastric contents, the smaller vent lumen (the proximal port is often referred to as the *blue pigtail*) allows for an inflow of atmospheric air, which prevents a vacuum if the gastric tube adheres to the wall of the stomach. Irritation of the gastric mucosa is thereby avoided. Softer, more flexible, and less irritating *small-bore nasoenteric tubes* (smaller than 12 Fr in diameter) are frequently used (Figure 40.14).

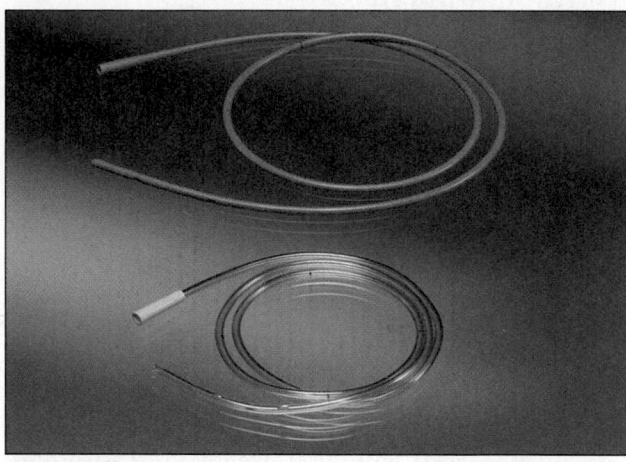

A

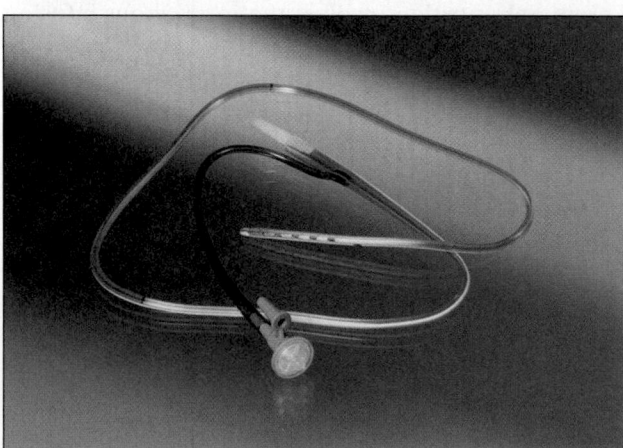

B

FIGURE 40.13 A: Single-lumen Levin tube; **B:** Double-lumen Salem sump tube with filter on air vent port and connector on suction port.

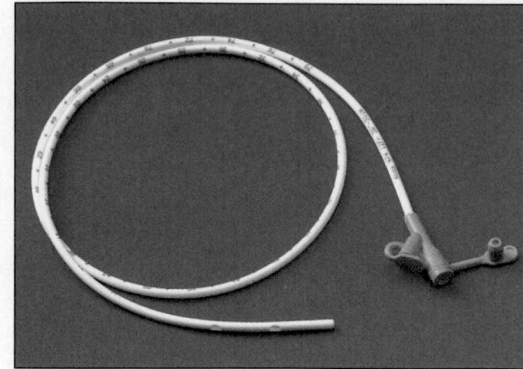

A

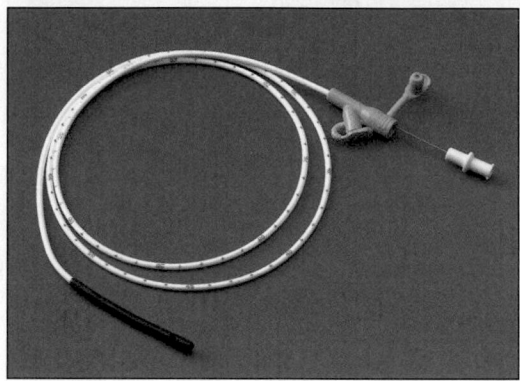

B

FIGURE 40.14 Nasoenteric feeding tubes: **A:** 12 French; **B:** 8 French. Opaque, stylet, weighted tip. Note that both have a Y-port connector to permit irrigation and medication administration without disconnecting feeding device.

Nasogastric tubes are used for patients who have intact gag and cough reflexes, who have adequate gastric emptying, and who require short-term feedings. Skill 40.2 provides guidelines for inserting a nasogastric tube. See also the Lifespan Considerations box on inserting a nasogastric tube on page 1247. Skill 40.3 on page 1248 outlines the steps for removing a nasogastric tube.

A **nasoenteric tube**, a longer tube than the nasogastric tube (at least 16 cm for an adult), is inserted through one nostril down into the upper small intestine. See Figure 40.15A on page 1249. Some agencies may require specially trained nurses or physicians for this procedure. Nasoenteric tubes are used for patients who are at risk for aspiration. Patients at risk for aspiration are those that manifest the following:

- Decreased level of consciousness
- Poor or absent cough or gag reflexes
- Endotracheal intubation
- Recent extubation
- Inability to cooperate with the procedure
- Restlessness or agitation

Gastrostomy and **jejunostomy** devices are used for long-term nutritional support, generally more than 6 to 8 weeks. Tubes are placed surgically or by laparoscopy through the abdominal wall into the stomach

SKILL 40.2 INSERTING A NASOGASTRIC TUBE

PURPOSES

- To administer tube feedings and medications to patients unable to eat by mouth or swallow a sufficient diet without aspirating food or fluids into the lungs

- To establish a means for suctioning stomach contents to prevent gastric distension, nausea, and vomiting

- To remove stomach contents for laboratory analysis

- To lavage (wash) the stomach in case of poisoning or overdose of medications

ASSESSMENT

- Check for a history of nasal surgery or deviated septum. Assess patency of nares.

- Determine presence of gag reflex.

- Assess mental status or ability to cooperate with the procedure.

PLANNING

Before inserting a nasogastric tube, determine the size of tube to be inserted and whether the tube is to be attached to suction.

Equipment

- Large- or small-bore tube (nonlatex preferred)
- Nonallergenic adhesive tape, 2.5 cm wide
- Clean gloves
- Water-soluble lubricant
- Facial tissues
- Glass of water and drinking straw
- 20-mL to 50-mL syringe with an adapter
- Basin
- pH test strip or meter
- Bilirubin dipstick (optional)
- Stethoscope
- Disposable pad or towel
- Clamp or plug (optional)
- Antireflux valve for air vent if Salem sump tube is used
- Suction apparatus
- Safety pin and elastic band

IMPLEMENTATION

Preparation

- Assist the patient to a high-Fowler's position if his or her health condition permits, and support the head on a pillow. **Rationale: It is often easier to swallow in this position, and gravity helps the passage of the tube**.

- Place a towel or disposable pad across the chest.

Performance

1. Before performing the insertion, introduce yourself and verify the patient's identity using two identifiers or per agency protocol. Explain to the patient what you are going to do, why it is necessary, and how he or she can participate.

The passage of a gastric tube is unpleasant because the gag reflex is activated during insertion. Establish a method for the patient to indicate distress and a desire for you to pause the insertion. Raising a finger or hand is often used for this.

2. Perform hand hygiene, and follow other appropriate infection prevention and control procedures (e.g., clean gloves).

3. Provide for patient privacy.

4. Assess the patient's nares.

   - Ask the patient to hyperextend the head, and, using a flashlight, observe the intactness of the tissues of the nostrils, including any irritations or abrasions.

   - Examine the nares for any obstructions or deformities by asking the patient to breathe through one nostril while occluding the other.

   - Select the nostril that has the greater airflow.

5. Prepare the tube.

   - If a small-bore tube is being used, ensure stylet or guide wire, if present, is secured in position. **Rationale: An improperly positioned stylet or guide wire can traumatize the nasopharynx, the esophagus, and the stomach**.

6. Determine how far to insert the tube.

   - Use the tube to mark off the distance from the tip of the patient's nose to the tip of the earlobe and then from the tip of the earlobe to the tip of the xiphoid (see ❶). **Rationale: This length approximates the distance from the nares to the stomach. This distance varies among individuals.**

   - Mark this length with adhesive tape if the tube does not have markings.

7. Insert the tube.

   - Put on gloves.

   - Lubricate the tip of the tube well with water-soluble lubricant or water to ease insertion. **Rationale: A water-soluble lubricant dissolves if the tube accidentally enters the lungs. An oil-based lubricant, such as**

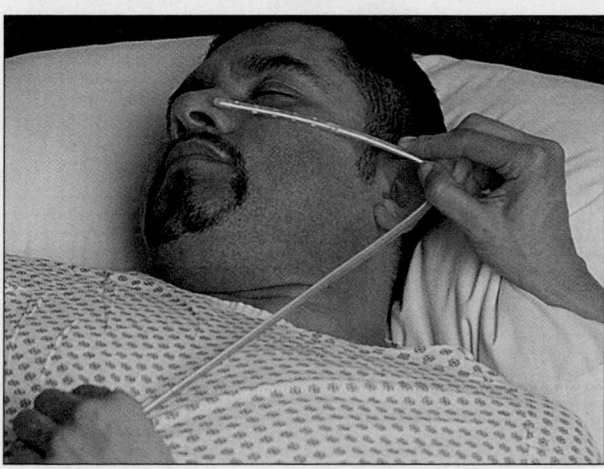

❶ Measuring the appropriate length to insert a nasogastric tube

(continued)

SKILL 40.2 INSERTING A NASOGASTRIC TUBE (continued)

petroleum jelly, will not dissolve and could cause respiratory complications if it enters the lungs.

- Insert the tube, with its natural curve toward the patient, into the selected nostril. Ask the patient to hyperextend the neck, and gently advance the tube toward the nasopharynx. **Rationale: Hyperextension of the neck reduces the curvature of the nasopharyngeal junction.**

- Direct the tube along the floor of the nostril and toward the ear on that side. **Rationale: Directing the tube along the floor avoids the turbinates (projections) along the lateral wall.**

- Slight pressure and a twisting motion are sometimes required to pass the tube into the nasopharynx, and some patient's eyes may water at this point. **Rationale: Tearing is a natural body response.** Provide the patient with tissues as needed.

- If the tube meets resistance, withdraw it, relubricate it, and insert it in the other nostril. **Rationale: The tube should never be forced against resistance because of the danger of injury.**

- Once the tube reaches the oropharynx (throat), the patient will feel the tube in the throat and may gag and retch. Ask the patient to tilt the head forward, and encourage the patient to drink and swallow (see ➋). **Rationale: Tilting the head forward facilitates passage of the tube into the posterior pharynx and esophagus rather than into the larynx; swallowing moves the epiglottis over the opening to the larynx.**

- If the patient gags, stop passing the tube momentarily. Have the patient rest, take a few breaths, and take sips of water to calm the gag reflex.

- In cooperation with the patient, pass the tube 5 cm to 10 cm with each swallow, until the indicated length is inserted.

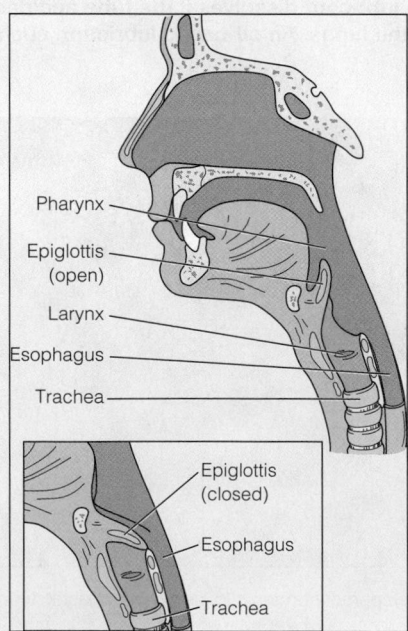

➋ Swallowing closes the epiglottis.

Pharynx
Epiglottis (open)
Larynx
Esophagus
Trachea

Epiglottis (closed)
Esophagus
Trachea

- If the patient continues to gag and the tube does not advance with each swallow, withdraw it slightly, and inspect the throat by looking through the mouth. **Rationale: The tube may be coiled in the throat.** If so, withdraw it until it is straight, and try again to insert it.

8. Ascertain correct placement of the tube. **Rationale: It is imperative that the placement of the tube be verified immediately after installation. Inadvertent placement of the tube in the respiratory track can result in serious morbidity or even death. Instilling feeding solution into a tube placed in a bronchus or the trachea can result in aspiration pneumonia and even death.**

- All nasogastric tubes are radiopaque, and position should be confirmed with radiography. **Rationale: X-ray confirmation of NG tube placement is the gold standard in that it can detect serious mispositioning that otherwise could be missed using the other bedside techniques** (Séguin, Le Bouquin, Aguillon, Maurice, Laviolle, & Mallédant, 2005). If a small-bore tube is used, leave the stylet or guide wire in place until correct position is verified with radiography. If the stylet has been removed, never reinsert it while the tube is in place. **Rationale: The stylet is sharp and could pierce the tube and injure the patient or cut off the tube end.**

- Other methods to ascertain placement in conjunction with, but not replacing, initial radiographic verification:

  - Aspirate stomach contents and check the pH, which should be acidic. **Rationale: Gastric contents are commonly pH 1 to 5; 6 or greater would indicate the contents are from lower in the intestinal tract or in the respiratory tract. A pH greater than 5 should be followed by further confirmation of tube location** (Bankhead, Boullata, Brantley, Corkins, Guenter, Krenitsky . . . & ASPEN Board of Directors, 2009). **It should not replace radiographic confirmation.**

  - Aspirated stomach contents can also be tested for bilirubin. Bilirubin levels in the lungs should be almost zero, while levels in the stomach will be approximately 25.7 mmol/L and in the intestine over 171 mmol/L.

- Place a stethoscope over the patient's epigastrium, and inject 10 mL to 30 mL of air into the tube while listening for a whooshing sound. Although still one of the methods used, do not use this method as the *primary* method for determining placement of the feeding tube *because it does not guarantee tube position*.

- If the signs indicate placement in the lungs, remove the tube and begin again.

- If the signs do not indicate placement in the lung or stomach, advance the tube 5 cm, and repeat the tests.

9. Secure the tube by taping it to the bridge of the patient's nose.

- If the patient has oily skin, wipe the nose first with alcohol to defat the skin.

- Cut 7.5 cm of tape, and split it lengthwise at one end, leaving a 2.5 cm tab at the end.

- Place the tape over the bridge of the patient's nose, and bring the split ends either under and around the tubing, or under the tubing and back up over the nose (see ➌).

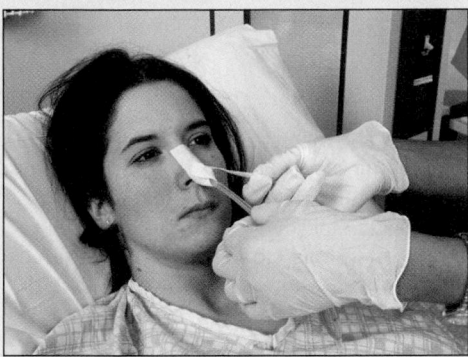

❸ Taping a nasogastric tube to the bridge of the nose

Rationale: Taping in this manner prevents the tube from pressing against and irritating the edge of the nostril.

10. Once correct position has been determined, attach the tube to a suction source or feeding apparatus as ordered, or clamp the end of the tubing.

11. Secure the tube to the patient's gown.
    - Loop an elastic band around the end of the tubing, and attach the elastic band to the gown with a safety pin.
    - *Or* attach a piece of adhesive tape to the tube, and pin the tape to the gown. **Rationale: The tube is attached to prevent it from dangling and pulling.**
    - If a Salem sump tube is used, attach the antireflux valve to the vent port (if used), and position the port above the patient's waist. **Rationale: Doing this ensures that gastric contents do not flow into the vent lumen.**

12. Document relevant information: the insertion of the tube, the means by which correct placement was determined, and patient responses (e.g., discomfort or abdominal distension).

13. Establish a plan for providing daily nasogastric tube care.
    - Inspect the nostril for discharge and irritation.
    - Clean the nostril and tube with moistened, cotton-tipped applicators.
    - Apply water-soluble lubricant to the nostril if it appears dry or encrusted.
    - Change the adhesive tape, as required.
    - Give frequent mouth care. Because of the presence of the tube, the patient may breathe through the mouth.

14. If suction is applied, ensure that the patency of both the nasogastric and suction tubes is maintained.
    - Irrigations of the tube may be required at regular intervals. In some agencies, irrigations must be ordered by the physician or dietitian.
    - If a Salem sump tube is used, follow agency policies for irrigating the vent lumen with air to maintain patency of the suctioning lumen. Often, a sucking sound can be heard from the vent port if it is patent.
    - Keep accurate records of the patient's fluid intake and output, and record the amount and characteristics of the drainage.

15. Document the type of tube inserted, date and time of tube insertion, type of suction used, colour and amount of gastric contents, and the patient's tolerance of the procedure.

EVALUATION

Conduct appropriate follow-up, such as degree of patient comfort, patient tolerance of the nasogastric tube, correct placement of nasogastric tube in stomach, patient understanding of restrictions, colour and amount of gastric contents if attached to suction, or stomach contents aspirated.

LIFESPAN CONSIDERATIONS

Inserting a Nasogastric Tube

INFANTS AND YOUNG CHILDREN

- Restraints may be necessary during tube insertion and throughout therapy. **Rationale: Restraints will prevent accidental dislodging of the tube.**
- Place the infant in an infant seat, or position the infant with a rolled towel or pillow under the head and shoulders.
- When assessing the nares, obstruct one of the infant's nares, and feel for air passage from the other. If the nasal passageway is very small or is obstructed, an orogastric tube may be more appropriate.
- Measure appropriate nasogastric tube length from the nose to the tip of the earlobe and then to the point midway between the umbilicus and the xiphoid process.
- If an orogastric tube is used, measure from the tip of the earlobe to the corner of the mouth to the xiphoid process.
- Do not hyperextend or hyperflex an infant's neck. **Rationale: Hyperextension or hyperflexion of the neck could occlude the airway.**
- Tape the tube to the area between the end of the nares and the upper lip, as well as to the cheek.

Although the focus of this chapter is nutrition, nasogastric tubes are inserted for reasons other than providing a route for feeding the patient. These include the following:

- To prevent nausea, vomiting, and gastric distension following surgery (in this case, the tube is attached to a suction source)
- To remove stomach contents for laboratory analysis
- To lavage (wash) the stomach in cases of poisoning or overdose of medications

SKILL 40.3 **REMOVING A NASOGASTRIC TUBE**

ASSESSMENT

- Assess for the presence of bowel sounds.
- Assess for the absence of nausea or vomiting when tube is clamped.

Equipment

- Disposable pad or towel
- Tissues
- Clean gloves
- 50-mL syringe (optional)
- Plastic trash bag

IMPLEMENTATION

Preparation

- Confirm the physician's order to remove the tube.
- Assist the patient to the sitting position if the patient's health permits.
- Place the disposable pad or towel across the patient's chest to collect any spillage of secretions from the tube.
- Provide tissues to the patient to wipe the nose and mouth after tube removal.

Performance

1. Before performing the removal, introduce yourself and verify the patient's identity using two identifiers or per agency protocol. Explain to the patient what you are going to do, why it is necessary, and how he or she can participate. Discuss how the results will be used in planning further care or treatments.

2. Perform hand hygiene, and follow other appropriate infection prevention and control procedures (e.g., clean gloves).

3. Provide for patient privacy.

4. Detach the tube.
   - Disconnect the nasogastric tube from the suction or feeding apparatus, if present.
   - Unpin the tube from the patient's gown.
   - Remove the adhesive tape securing the tube to the nose.

5. Remove the nasogastric tube.
   - Put on clean gloves.
   - (*Optional*) Instill 50 mL of air into the tube. **Rationale: The instilled air clears the tube of any contents, such as feeding or gastric drainage.**
   - Ask the patient to take a deep breath and to hold it. **Rationale: Doing this closes the glottis, thereby preventing accidental aspiration of any gastric contents.**
   - Pinch the tube with the gloved hand. **Rationale: Pinching the tube prevents any contents inside the tube from draining into the patient's throat.**
   - Withdraw the tube in a smooth motion.
   - Place the tube in the plastic bag. **Rationale: Placing the tube immediately into the bag prevents the transference of microorganisms from the tube to other articles or people.**
   - Observe the intactness of the tube.

6. Ensure patient comfort.
   - Provide oral care, if desired by the patient.
   - Assist the patient as required to blow the nose. **Rationale: Excessive secretions may have accumulated in the nasal passages.**

7. Dispose of the equipment appropriately.
   - Place the pad, bag with tube, and gloves in the receptacle designated by the agency. **Rationale: Correct disposal prevents the transmission of microorganisms.**

8. Document all relevant information.
   - Record the removal of the tube, the amount and appearance of any drainage if connected to suction, and any relevant assessments of the patient.

EVALUATION

- Perform a follow-up examination, such as presence of bowel sounds, absence of nausea or vomiting when tube is removed, and intactness of tissues of the nares.
- Relate findings to previous assessment data, if available.
- Report significant deviations from normal to the appropriate members of the health care team.

(gastrostomy) or into the jejunum (jejunostomy). See Figure 40.15B. A **percutaneous endoscopic gastrostomy (PEG)** (Figure 40.16) or **percutaneous endoscopic jejunostomy (PEJ)** (Figure 40.17) is created by using an endoscope to visualize the inside of the stomach, making a puncture through the skin and subcutaneous tissues of the abdomen into the stomach, and inserting the PEG or PEJ catheter through the puncture.

The surgical opening is sutured tightly around the tube or catheter to prevent leakage. Care of this opening before it heals requires surgical asepsis. The catheter

has an external bumper and an internal inflatable retention balloon to maintain placement. When the tract is established (about 1 month), the tube or catheter can be removed and reinserted for each feeding. Alternatively, a skin-level tube can be used that remains in place (Figure 40.18). A feeding set is attached when needed.

TESTING FEEDING TUBE PLACEMENT Before feedings are introduced, tube placement is confirmed with radiography. After placement is confirmed, the nurse marks the tube with indelible ink or tape at its exit point from

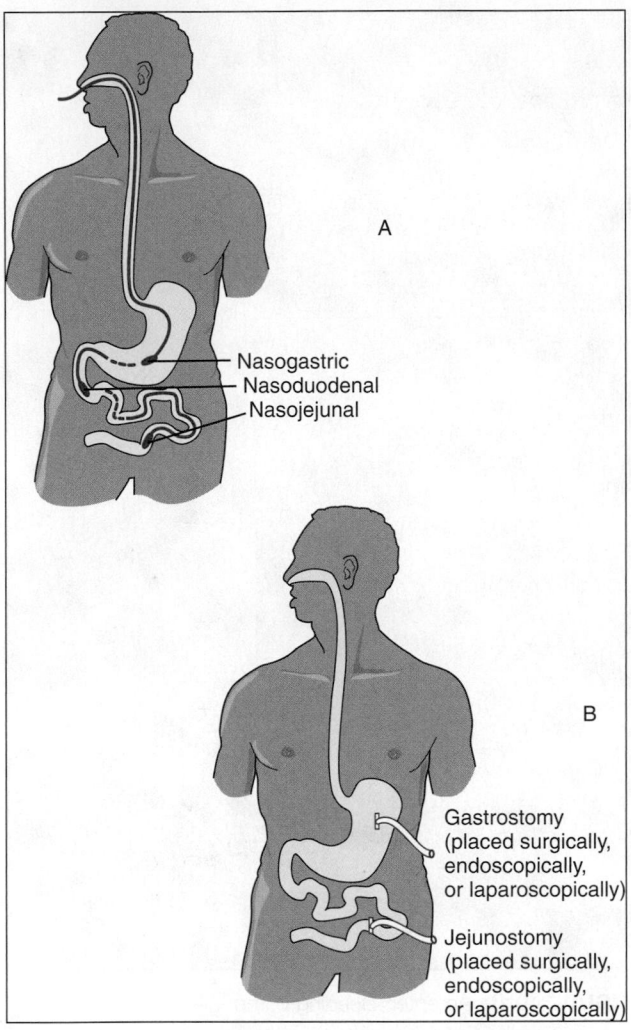

FIGURE 40.15 Placements for enteral access: **A:** For nasoenteric/nasointestinal tubes; **B:** For gastrostomy and jejunostomy tubes.

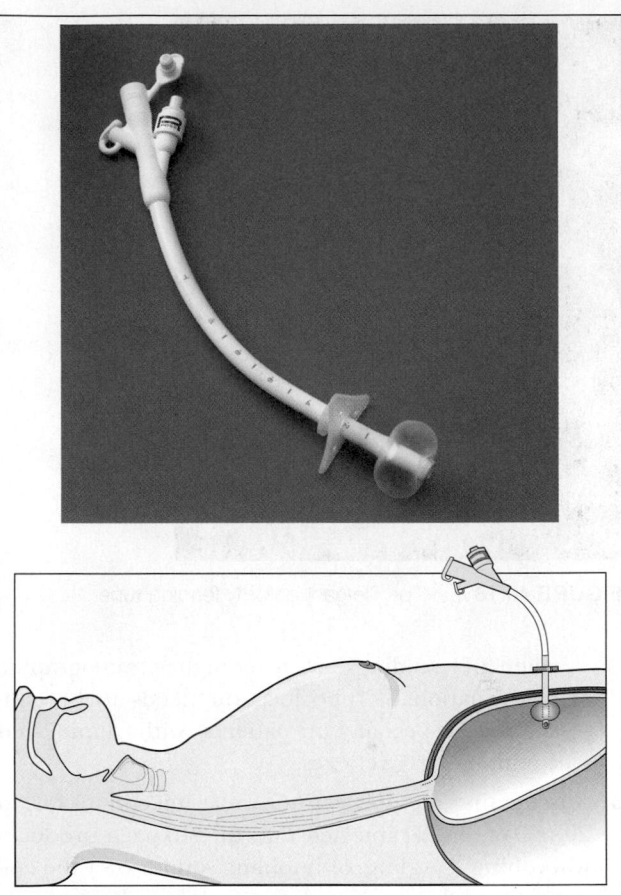

FIGURE 40.16 Percutaneous endoscopic gastrostomy (PEG) tube.

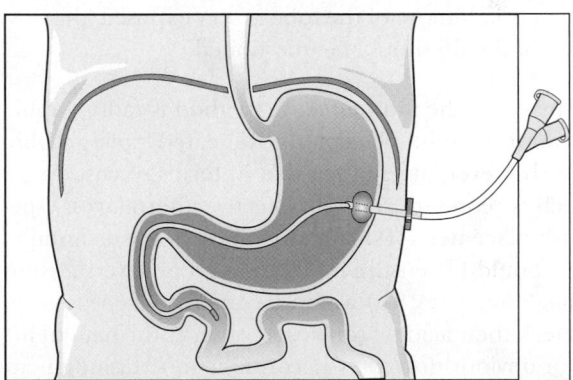

FIGURE 40.17 Percutaneous endoscopic jejunostomy (PEJ) tube.

the nose and documents the length of visible tubing for baseline data. The nurse is responsible for verifying tube placement (i.e., gastrointestinal placement versus respiratory placement) before each intermittent feeding and at regular intervals (e.g., at least once per shift) when continuous feedings are being administered.

Methods nurses use to check tube placement include the following:

1. *Aspirating gastrointestinal secretions.* Small-bore tubes offer more resistance during aspirations than large-bore tubes and are more likely to collapse when negative pressure is applied. Gastric secretions tend to be grassy green, off-white, or tan in colour; intestinal fluid is stained with bile and is golden yellow or brownish green in colour.

2. *Measuring the pH of aspirated fluid.* This is the recommended method to determine tube placement. Testing the pH of aspirates can help distinguish gastric from respiratory and intestinal placement (Bankhead et al., 2009) as follows:

- Gastric aspirates tend to be acidic and have a pH of 1 to 4 but may be as high as 6 if the patient is receiving medications that control gastric acid.
- Small intestine aspirates generally have a pH equal to or higher than 6. Respiratory secretions are more alkaline, with values of 7 or higher. However, a slight possibility exists of respiratory placement when the pH reading is as low as 6. Therefore,

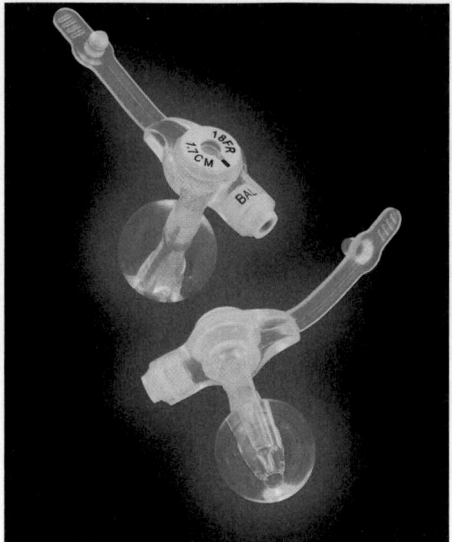

FIGURE 40.18 Low-profile gastrostomy feeding tube.

when pH readings are 6 or higher, radiographic confirmation of tube location needs to be considered, especially in patients with diminished cough and gag reflexes.

3. Auscultating the epigastrium while injecting 5 mL to 20 mL of air. Air injected into the stomach produces whooshing, gurgling, or bubbling sounds over the epigastrium and the upper left quadrant. The accuracy of this method in confirming placement is less reliable than pH testing (American Association of Critical Care Nurses, 2005).

4. Confirming the length of tube insertion with the insertion mark. If more of the tube is now exposed, the position of the tip should be questioned.

Currently, the most effective method is radiographic verification of tube placement. Repeated radiographic studies, however, are not feasible in terms of cost. More research is required to devise effective alternatives, especially for placement of small-bore tubes. In the meantime, nurses should (a) ensure initial radiographic verification of small-bore tubes, (b) aspirate contents when possible and check their acidity, (c) closely observe the patient for signs of obvious distress, (d) consider tube dislodgment after episodes of coughing, sneezing, and vomiting, and (e) measure length of tube extending from patient and compare to length upon insertion.

ENTERAL FEEDINGS The type and frequency of feedings and amounts to be administered are ordered by the physician or the dietitian. Liquid feeding mixtures are available commercially or can be prepared by the dietary department in accordance with the physician's orders. A standard formula provides 1 kcal/mL of solution with protein, fat, carbohydrate, minerals, and vitamins in specified proportions.

Enteral feedings can be given intermittently or continuously. Intermittent feedings are the administration of

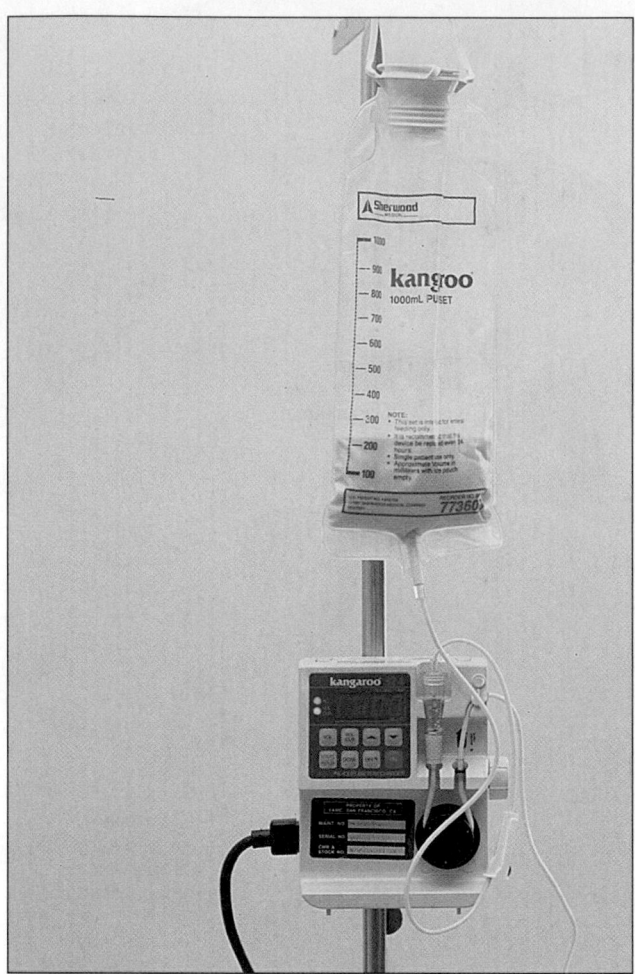

FIGURE 40.19 An enteric feeding pump.

300 mL to 500 mL of enteral formula several times per day. The stomach is the preferred site for these feedings, which are usually administered over at least 30 minutes. Bolus intermittent feedings are those that use a syringe to deliver the formula into the stomach. Because the formula is delivered rapidly by this method, it is not usually recommended but can be used in long-term situations if the patient tolerates it. These feedings must be given only into the stomach; the patient must be monitored closely for distension and aspiration.

Continuous feedings are generally administered over 24 hours by using an infusion pump that guarantees a constant flow rate (Figure 40.19). Continuous feedings are essential when feedings are administered in the small bowel. They are also used when smaller-bore gastric tubes are in place or when gravity flow is insufficient to instill the feeding.

Cyclical feedings are continuous feedings that are administered in less than 24 hours (e.g., 12 to 16 hours). These feedings, often administered at night and referred to as nocturnal feedings, allow the patient to attempt to eat regular meals through the day. Because nocturnal feedings may use higher nutrient densities and faster infusion rates than the standard continuous feeding, particular attention needs to be given to monitoring fluid status and circulating volume overload.

Enteral feedings are administered to patients through open or closed systems. Open systems use an open-top container or a syringe (without plunger) for administration. Enteral feedings for use with open systems are provided in flip-top cans or powdered formulas that are reconstituted with sterile water. Sterile water, rather than tap water, is used to reduce the risk of microbial contamination. Open systems should have no more than 8 hours of formula poured into them (Bankhad et al., 2009). At the end of that time, the remaining formula should be discarded and the container rinsed before new formula is poured. In some institutions, the bag and tubing are discarded after 24 hours. Closed systems consist of a prefilled container that is spiked with enteral tubing and attached to the enteral access device. Prefilled containers generally have 1 L of formula and can hang safely for 24 to 48 hours if sterile technique is used (Bankhead et al., 2009).

Skill 40.4 provides the essential steps involved in administering a tube feeding, and Skill 40.5 indicates the steps involved in administering a gastrostomy or jejunostomy tube feeding. See the Clinical Alert box on adding coloured food dye to tube feedings on page 1255.

SKILL 40.4 ADMINISTERING A TUBE FEEDING

PURPOSES

- To restore or maintain nutritional status
- To administer medications

ASSESSMENT

Assess

- Any clinical signs of malnutrition or dehydration
- Allergies to any ingredient in the feeding; if the patient is lactose intolerant, check the tube feeding formula; notify the physician or dietitian if any incompatibilities exist
- The presence of bowel sounds
- Any problems that suggest lack of tolerance of previous feedings (e.g., delayed gastric emptying, abdominal distension, diarrhea, cramping, or constipation)

PLANNING

Before commencing a tube feeding, determine the type, amount, and frequency of feedings and tolerance of previous feedings.

Equipment

- Correct type and amount of feeding solution
- 60-mL catheter-tip syringe
- Emesis basin
- Clean gloves
- pH test strip or meter
- Large syringe or calibrated plastic feeding bag with label and tubing that can be attached to the feeding tube or prefilled bottle with a drip chamber, tubing, and a flow-regulator clamp
- Measuring container from which to pour the feeding (if using an open system)
- Water (60 mL unless otherwise specified) at room temperature
- Feeding pump as required

IMPLEMENTATION

Preparation

Assist the patient to a Fowler's position (at least 45 degrees elevation) in bed or the sitting position in a chair, the normal position for eating. If the sitting position is contraindicated, a slightly elevated side-lying (right) position is acceptable. **Rationale: These positions enhance the gravitational flow of the solution and prevent aspiration of fluid into the lungs**.

Performance

1. Before performing the feeding, introduce yourself and verify the patient's identity using two identifiers or per agency protocol. Explain to the patient what you are going to do, why it is necessary, and how he or she can participate. Inform the patient that the feeding should not cause any discomfort but may cause a feeling of fullness.

2. Perform hand hygiene, and follow other appropriate infection prevention and control procedures (e.g., clean gloves).

3. Provide privacy for this procedure if the patient desires it. Tube feedings are embarrassing to some people.

4. Assess tube placement.
   - Attach the syringe to the open end of the tube and aspirate. Check the pH.
   - Allow 1 hour to elapse before testing the pH if the patient has received a medication.

5. Assess gastric residual volumes (GRVs). *Clinical note:* There is little standardization with regard to how and when to measure GRVs. There is also no clear definition of an elevated GRV and what it implies for the client (Bankhead et al., 2009).
   - Check gastric residuals every 4 hours during the first 48 hours for patients who receive feedings into the stomach. Do not check gastric residuals for feedings into the small intestine. Once the feeding goal rate is achieved, decrease verifications to q6–8h in a noncritical care setting and q4h in a critical care setting. Aspirate all contents of the stomach with a 60-mL syringe and measure the amount before administering the feeding. **Rationale: This step is done to evaluate absorption of the last feeding, that is, whether undigested formula from a previous feeding remains. If the tube is in the small intestine, residual contents cannot be aspirated**.
   - If the GRV is more than 250 mL, recheck in 3 to 4 hours. If it remains more than 250 mL during the next assessment, a promotility pharmacological should be considered in adult clients. A GRV of more than 500 mL should result in holding EN and reassessing patient tolerance, for example, physical assessment, evaluation of glycemic control, minimization of sedation (Bankhead et al., 2009). Check your agency protocol. **Rationale: At some agencies,**

(continued)

SKILL 40.4 ADMINISTERING A TUBE FEEDING *(continued)*

a feeding is delayed when the specified amount or more of formula remains in the stomach. The feeding rate may need to be adjusted if gastric emptying is delayed.

- *Or* reinstill the gastric contents into the stomach if this is the agency policy or the health care provider's order. **Rationale: Removal of the contents could disturb the patient's electrolyte balance.**

6. Administer the feeding.
   - Before administering the feeding, check the expiration date of the feeding. Warm the feeding to room temperature. **Rationale: An excessively cold feeding can cause abdominal cramps.**
   - When an open system is used, clean the top of the feeding container with alcohol before opening it. **Rationale: This step minimizes the risk of contaminants entering the feeding syringe or feeding bag.**
   - Flush tubing with 30 mL of water before beginning an intermittent feeding.

Feeding Bag (Open System)
- Hang the labelled bag from an infusion pole about 30 cm above the tube's point of insertion into the patient.
- Clamp the tubing and add the formula to the bag.
- Open the clamp, run the formula through the tubing, and reclamp the tube. **Rationale: The formula will displace the air in the tubing, thus preventing the instillation of excess air into the patient's stomach or intestine.**
- Attach the bag to the feeding tube (see ❶) and regulate the drip by adjusting the clamp to the drop factor on the bag (e.g., 20 drops/mL) if not placed on a pump.

Syringe (Open System)
- Remove the plunger from the syringe and connect the syringe to a pinched or clamped nasogastric tube. **Rationale: Pinching or clamping the tube prevents excess air from entering the stomach and causing distension.**
- Add the feeding to the syringe barrel (see ❷).

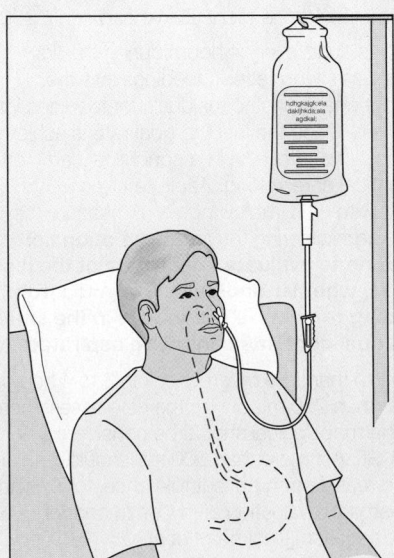
❶ Using a calibrated plastic bag to administer a tube feeding

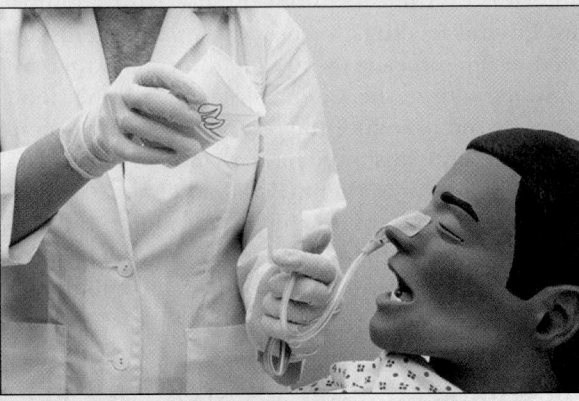
❷ Using the barrel of a syringe to administer a tube feeding

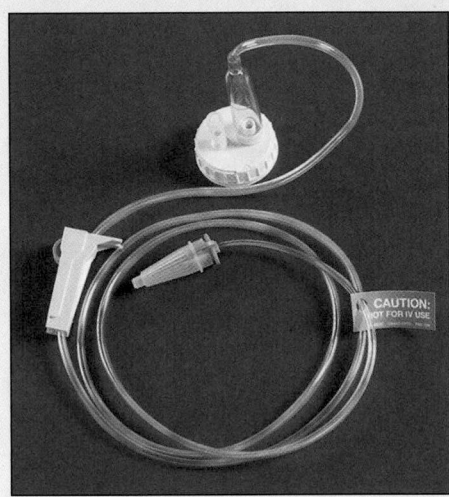
❸ Feeding set tubing with drip chamber

- Permit the feeding to flow in slowly at the prescribed rate. Raise or lower the syringe to adjust the flow as needed. Pinch or clamp the tubing to stop the flow for a minute if the patient experiences discomfort. **Rationale: Rapidly administered feedings can cause flatus, cramps, and/or vomiting.**

Prefilled Bottle with Drip Chamber (Closed System)
- Gently shake the prefilled bottle to ensure the contents have not separated. Remove the screw-on cap from the container, and attach the administration set with the drip chamber and tubing (see ❸).
- Close the clamp on the tubing.
- Hang the container on an intravenous pole about 30 cm above the tube's insertion point into the patient. **Rationale: At this height, the formula should run at a safe rate into the patient's stomach or the intestine.**
- Squeeze the drip chamber to fill it to one-third to one-half of its capacity.
- Open the tubing clamp, run the formula through the tubing, and reclamp the tube. **Rationale: The formula will displace the air in the tubing, thus preventing the instillation of excess air.**
- Attach the feeding set tubing to the feeding tube and regulate the drip rate to deliver the feeding over the desired length of time, or attach to a feeding pump.

7. When the feeding is finished, and if another bottle is not to be immediately hung, flush the feeding tube with 30 mL of water after intermittent feedings in an adult patient and every 4 hours during continuous feeding (Bankhead et al., 2009). **Rationale: Water flushes the lumen of the tube, preventing future blockage by sticky formula.**

   • Be sure to add the water before the feeding solution has drained from the neck of a syringe or from the tubing of an administration set. **Rationale: Adding the water before the syringe or tubing is empty prevents the instillation of air into the stomach or intestine and thus prevents unnecessary distension.**

8. Clamp the feeding tube. Remove the tubing of the administration set between feedings.

   • Clamp the feeding tube before all the water is instilled. **Rationale: Clamping prevents leakage and air from entering the tube if done before water is instilled.**

9. Ensure patient comfort and safety.

   • Secure the tubing to the patient's gown. **Rationale: This minimizes pulling of the tube, thus preventing discomfort and dislodgment.**

   • Ask the patient to remain sitting upright in Fowler's position or in a slightly elevated right lateral position for at least 60 minutes. **Rationale: These positions facilitate digestion and movement of the feeding from the stomach along the gastrointestinal tract and prevent the potential aspiration of the feeding into the lungs.**

   • Check the agency's policy on the frequency of changing the nasogastric tube and the use of smaller lumen tubes if a large-bore tube is in place. **Rationale: These measures prevent irritation and erosion of the pharyngeal and esophageal mucous membranes.**

10. Dispose of equipment appropriately.

    • If the equipment is to be reused, wash it thoroughly with soap and water so that it is ready for reuse.

    • Change the equipment every 24 hours or according to agency policy.

11. Document all relevant information.

    • Document the feeding, including amount and kind of solution taken, duration of the feeding, and assessments of the patient.

    • Record the volume of the feeding and water administered on the patient's intake and output record.

12. Monitor the patient for possible problems.

    • Carefully assess patients receiving tube feedings for problems.

• To prevent dehydration, give the patient supplemental water in addition to the prescribed tube feeding, as ordered. The quantity of water to administer will be determined by physician or dietitian orders in some cases, or by agency policy.

Variation: Continuous-Drip Feeding

• Clamp the tubing at least every 4 to 6 hours, or as indicated by agency protocol or the manufacturer, and aspirate and measure the gastric contents. Then flush the tubing with 30 mL of water. **Rationale: This step determines adequate absorption and verifies correct placement of the tube.** If placement of a small-bore tube is questionable, a repeat radiographic assessment should be done.

• Determine agency protocol regarding withholding a feeding. Many agencies withhold the feeding if more than 75 mL to 100 mL of feeding is aspirated.

• To prevent spoilage or bacterial contamination, do not allow a feeding solution in an open system to hang longer than 8 hours. A closed-bottle feeding may be able to hang for 24 to 48 hours. *Check agency policy or manufacturer's recommendations regarding time limits.*

• Follow agency policy regarding how frequently to change the feeding bag and tubing. Changing the feeding bag and tubing every 24 hours reduces the risk of contamination.

EVALUATION

• Perform a follow-up examination of the following:

  • Tolerance of feeding (e.g., nausea, cramping, gastric residual)
  • Bowel sounds
  • Regurgitation and feelings of fullness after feedings
  • Weight gain or loss
  • Fecal elimination pattern (e.g., diarrhea, flatulence, constipation)
  • Skin turgor
  • Urine output and specific gravity
  • Glucose and acetone in urine
  • Capillary blood glucose
  • Serum electrolytes, including potassium and sodium
  • Relate findings to previous assessment data, if available. Report significant deviations from normal to the appropriate members of the health care team.

SKILL 40.5 | **ADMINISTERING A GASTROSTOMY OR JEJUNOSTOMY FEEDING**

PURPOSES
See Skill 40.4.

ASSESSMENT
See Skill 40.4.

PLANNING
Before commencing a gastrostomy or jejunostomy feeding, determine the type and amount of feeding to be instilled, frequency of feedings, and any pertinent information about previous feedings (e.g., the position in which the patient best tolerates the feeding).

(continued)

SKILL 40.5 ADMINISTERING A GASTROSTOMY OR JEJUNOSTOMY FEEDING (*continued*)

Equipment

- Correct amount of feeding solution
- Graduated container and tubing with clamp to hold the feeding
- 60-mL catheter-tip syringe

For a Tube That Remains in Place

- Mild soap and water
- Clean gloves
- Petrolatum, zinc oxide ointment, or other skin protectant
- Precut 10 cm × 10 cm gauze squares
- Uncut 10 cm × 10 cm gauze squares

For Tube Insertion

- Clean gloves
- Moisture-proof bag
- Water-soluble lubricant
- Feeding tube (if needed)

IMPLEMENTATION

Preparation

See Skill 40.4.

Performance

1. Before performing the feeding, introduce yourself and verify the patient's identity using two identifiers or per agency protocol. Explain to the patient what you are going to do, why it is necessary, and how he or she can participate. Discuss how the results will be used in planning further care or treatments.

2. Perform hand hygiene, and follow other appropriate infection prevention and control procedures (e.g., clean gloves).

3. Provide for patient privacy.

4. Assess and prepare the patient. (See Skill 40.4.)

5. Insert a feeding tube, if one is not already in place.

   - While wearing gloves, remove the dressing. Then discard the dressing and gloves in the moisture-proof bag.
   - Apply new clean gloves.
   - Lubricate the end of the tube, and insert it into the ostomy opening 10 cm to 15 cm.

6. Check the location and patency of a tube that is already in place.

   - Determine correct placement of the tube by aspirating secretions and checking the pH.
   - Follow agency policy for amount of residual formula (do not do this for a patient being fed by jejunostomy). This may include withholding the feeding, rechecking in 3 to 4 hours, or notifying the health care provider if a large residual remains.
   - For continuous feedings, check the residual every 4 to 6 hours and hold feedings, according to agency policy.

- Remove the syringe plunger. Pour 15 mL to 30 mL of water into the syringe, remove the tube clamp, and allow the water to flow into the tube. **Rationale: This step determines the patency of the tube. If water flows freely, the tube is patent.**

- If the water does not flow freely, notify the nurse in charge and the physician.

7. Administer the feeding.

   - Hold the barrel of the syringe 7 cm to 15 cm above the ostomy opening.
   - Slowly pour the solution into the syringe, and allow it to flow through the tube by gravity.
   - Just before all the formula has run through and the syringe is empty, add 30 mL of water. **Rationale: Water flushes the tube and preserves its patency.**
   - If the tube is to remain in place, hold it upright, remove the syringe, and then clamp or plug the tube to prevent leakage.
   - If a catheter was inserted for the feeding, remove it.

8. Ensure patient comfort and safety.

   - After the feeding, ask the patient to remain in the sitting position or a slightly elevated right lateral position for at least 60 minutes. **Rationale: This position minimizes the risk of aspiration.**
   - Assess the status of peristomal skin. **Rationale: Gastric or jejunal drainage contains digestive enzymes that can irritate skin. Document any redness and broken skin areas.**
   - Check orders about cleaning peristomal skin, applying a skin protectant, and applying appropriate dressings. Generally, peristomal skin is washed with mild soap and water at least once daily. The tube may be rotated between thumb and forefinger to release any sticking and promote tract formation. Petrolatum, zinc oxide ointment, or other skin protectant can be applied around the stoma, and precut 10 cm × 10 cm gauze squares can be placed around the tube. The precut squares are then covered with regular 10 cm × 10 cm gauze squares, and the tube is coiled over them.
   - Observe for common complications of enteral feedings: aspiration, hyperglycemia, abdominal distension, diarrhea, and fecal impaction. Report findings to the appropriate members of the health care team. Often, a change in formula or rate of administration can correct problems.
   - When appropriate, teach the patient how to administer feedings and when to notify the health care provider concerning problems.

9. Document all assessments and interventions.

Variation

The feeding can also be administered with a feeding bag or with a prefilled bottle with a drip chamber. (See Skill 40.4.)

EVALUATION

See Skill 40.4.

CLINICAL ALERT

Do not add coloured food dye to tube feedings. Previously, blue dye was often added to assist in recognition of aspiration. However, Health Canada reports cases of adverse reactions to the dye, including toxicity and death.

Before administering a tube feeding, the nurse must determine if the patient has any food allergies and assess tolerance to previous feedings. Table 40.8 lists essential assessments to conduct before administering tube feedings. The nurse must also check the expiration date on a commercially prepared formula or the preparation date and time of agency-prepared solution, discarding any formula that has passed the expiration date or that was prepared more than 24 hours previously. See the Lifespan Considerations box on administering a tube feeding on the next page.

Feedings are usually administered at room temperature unless the order specifies otherwise. The nurse warms the specified amount of solution in a basin of warm water or leaves it to stand until it reaches room temperature. Because a formula that is warmed can grow microorganisms, it should not hang longer than the manufacturer recommends. Continuous feeding should be kept cold; excessive heat coagulates feedings of milk and egg, and hot liquids can irritate the mucous membranes. However, excessively cold feedings can reduce the flow of digestive juices by causing vasoconstriction and may cause cramps.

Enteral feedings may be continued beyond hospital care in the client's home or may be initiated in the home. Guidelines for teaching clients and families about administration of tube feedings in the home are found in the Teaching: Home Care box on the next page.

ADMINISTERING MEDICATION THROUGH A FEEDING TUBE Medication that is normally taken by mouth may be administered via the nasoenteric tube if the patient cannot swallow. In most cases, medication in pill form will be crushed and mixed with a small amount of water and then inserted into the feeding tube. Each medication should be administered separately and liquid dosage forms should be used when available. Do not crush sustained-release capsules or cytotoxic drugs; crushing enteric-coated medications may cause adverse reactions. Do not mix medication into the feeding solutions. In all cases, it is important to flush the feeding tube with at least 30 mL after administration to prevent clogging (Bankhead et al., 2009). When administering medication

TABLE 40.8 Assessing Patients Receiving Tube Feedings

Assessment	Rationale
Allergies to any food in the feeding	Common allergenic foods include milk, eggs, and soy.
Bowel sounds before each feeding or, for continuous feedings, every 4 to 8 hours	Doing this helps determine peristalsis (intestinal activity).
Abdominal distension; at least daily, measure abdominal girth at the umbilicus	Abdominal distension can indicate intolerance to a previous feeding.
Correct placement of tube, before feedings	This step helps prevent aspiration of feedings.
Presence of regurgitation and feelings of fullness after feedings	This finding may indicate delayed gastric emptying, need to decrease quantity or rate of the feeding, or high-fat content of the formula.
"Dumping syndrome": nausea, vomiting, diarrhea, cramps, pallor, sweating, heart palpitations, increased pulse rate, and fainting after a feeding	Jejunostomy clients may experience these symptoms, which result when hypertonic foods and liquids suddenly distend the jejunum. To make the intestinal contents isotonic, body fluids shift rapidly from the client's vascular system.
Diarrhea, constipation, or flatulence	The lack of bulk in liquid feedings may cause constipation. The presence of hypertonic or concentrated ingredients may cause diarrhea and flatulence.
Urine for sugar and acetone	Hyperglycemia may occur if the sugar content is too high.
Hematocrit and urine specific gravity	Both increase as a result of dehydration.
Serum BUN, glucose and sodium levels	Feeding formula may have a high protein content. If a high protein intake is combined with an inadequate fluid intake, the kidneys may not be able to excrete nitrogenous wastes adequately.

Administering a Tube Feeding

INFANTS

- Feeding tubes may be reinserted at each feeding to prevent irritation of the mucous membrane, nasal airway obstruction, and stomach perforation, which can occur if the tube is left in place continuously. Check agency practice.

CHILDREN

- Position a small child or infant in your lap, provide a pacifier, and hold and cuddle the child during feedings. This promotes comfort, supports the normal sucking instinct of the infant, and facilitates digestion.

OLDER ADULTS

- Physiological changes associated with aging may make older adults more vulnerable to complications associated with enteral feedings. Decreased gastric emptying may necessitate checking frequently for gastric residual. Diarrhea from administering the feeding too fast or at too high a concentration can cause dehydration. If the feeding has a high concentration of glucose, assess for hyperglycemia. Because with aging, the body has a decreased ability to handle increased glucose levels.

- Such conditions as a hiatal hernia and diabetes mellitus may cause the stomach to empty more slowly. This delay increases the risk of aspiration in a patient receiving a tube feeding. Checking for gastric residual more frequently can help document this if it is an ongoing problem. Changing the formula or the rate of administration, repositioning the patient, or obtaining a physician's order for a medication to increase stomach emptying may resolve this problem.

TEACHING | **HOME CARE**

Tube Feedings

Clients and caregivers need guidance to manage these feedings in the home:

- *Preparation of the formula.* Include the name of the formula and how much and how often it is to be given; the need to inspect the formula for expiration date and leaks and cracks in bags or cans; how to mix or prepare the formula, if needed; and aseptic techniques, such as swabbing the container's top with alcohol before opening it, and changing the syringe administration set and reservoir every 24 hours. Advise family not to create "home-made" feeding solutions or place liquefied food in the tube as this may cause the tube to clog.

- *Proper storage of the formula.* Include the need to refrigerate diluted or reconstituted formula and formula that contains additives.

- *Administration of the feeding.* Include proper hand hygiene and how to fill and hang the feeding bag. Discuss strategies for hanging formula containers if an IV pole is not available or is inconvenient. Review the operation of an infusion pump, if indicated; the feeding rate; and client positioning during and after the feeding. Plan for optimal timing of feedings to allow for daily activities. Many clients can tolerate having the majority of their feedings run during sleep so they are free from the equipment during the day.

- *Management of the enteral access device.* Teach and explain to the client or caregiver the rationale for how to assess for tube placement by using pH measurement before administering the feeding. Instruct regarding actions to take if the pH is greater than 6. Include site care, aseptic precautions, dressing change, as indicated, how the site should look normally, and flushing protocols (e.g., type of irrigant and schedule).

- *Daily monitoring needs.* Include temperature, weight, and intake and output.

- *Signs and symptoms of complications to report.* Include fever, increased respiratory rate, decrease in urine output, increased or decreased stool frequency, and altered level of consciousness.

- *Whom to contact regarding questions or problems.* Include emergency telephone numbers of home care agency, nursing clinician or physician, or other 24-hour on-call emergency number.

---

via a feeding tube, the nurse must take additional precautions to ensure patient safety:

- Ensure that the medication can be crushed (see Box 33.5, page 900). Consult the physician and pharmacist to determine whether an alternative formulation or administration route is available.

- Verify that the medication is compatible with the feeding solution. For example, Dilantin (phenytoin), an antiseizure medication, cannot be administered when a feeding solution is running, as absorption of the drug will be decreased. If the patient is on continuous feeds, an alternative route must be considered or the feed must be held for 1 to 2 hours before and after drug administration (Dickerson, Tidwell, & Brown, 2003).

- Use a clean mortar and pestle when crushing pills, and ensure that the pills are ground up to a fine powder so that larger pieces will not block the tube. Administer only one crushed pill at a time and flush with water between each one.

- Administer medication mixed only in water. Do not mix medication directly into feeding solution before administration.

MANAGING CLOGGED FEEDING TUBES Even if feeding tubes are flushed with water before and after feedings and medications, they can still become clogged. This blockage can occur when the feeding container runs dry, solid medication is not adequately crushed, or medications are mixed with formula. Even the important practice of aspirating to check residual volume increases the incidence of clogging (Reising & Neal, 2005). To avoid the necessity of removing the tube and reinserting a new tube, both prevention and intervention strategies must be used.

To prevent clogged feeding tubes, flush liberally (at least 30 mL of water) before, between, and after each separate medication is instilled, by using a 60-mL piston syringe. The larger the barrel of the syringe, the less the pressure exerted. Too great a pressure can rupture the tube, especially small-bore feeding tubes. Do not add medications to formula or to each other.

Many strategies have been used to try to unclog feeding tubes. The first strategy that should be tried is to reposition the patient (this may allow a kink to straighten). Alternately flush and aspirate the tube with water. Strategies that have shown inconsistent effectiveness include instilling meat tenderizer, carbonated beverages, or cranberry juice, or flushing with small barrel syringes with or without digestive enzymes, such as papain or chymotrypsin (Bankhead et al., 2009; Reising & Neal, 2005).

Providing Parenteral Nutrition

Parenteral nutrition (PN), also referred to as *total parenteral nutrition* (TPN) or *intravenous hyperalimentation* (IVH), is provided when the gastrointestinal tract is nonfunctional because of an interruption in its continuity or because its absorptive capacity is impaired. Parenteral nutrition is administered intravenously through a central venous catheter into the superior vena cava.

Parenteral feedings are solutions of dextrose, water, fat, proteins, electrolytes, vitamins, and trace elements; it is the provision of all needed calories. Because TPN solutions are *hypertonic* (highly concentrated in comparison to the solute concentration of blood), they are injected only into high-flow central veins, where they are diluted by the patient's blood.

TPN is a means of achieving an anabolic state in patients who are unable to maintain a normal nitrogen balance. Such patients may include those with severe malnutrition, severe burns, bowel disease disorders (e.g., ulcerative colitis or enteric fistula), acute renal failure, hepatic failure, metastatic cancer, or major surgeries in which nothing can be taken by mouth for more than 5 days.

TPN is not risk free. Infection prevention and control is of utmost importance during TPN therapy. The nurse must always observe surgical aseptic technique when changing solutions, tubing, dressings, and filters. Patients are at increased risk of fluid, electrolyte, and glucose imbalances and require frequent evaluation and modification of the TPN mixture.

TPN solutions are a mixture of 10% to 50% dextrose in water, amino acids, and special additives, such as vitamins (e.g., B complex, C, D, K), minerals (e.g.,

potassium, sodium, chloride, calcium, phosphate, magnesium), and trace elements (e.g., cobalt, zinc, manganese). Additives are adapted to each patient's nutritional needs. Fat emulsions may be given to provide essential fatty acids to correct or prevent essential fatty acid deficiency or to supplement the calories for patients who, for example, have high-calorie needs or cannot tolerate glucose as the only calorie source. Note that 1000 mL of 5% glucose or dextrose contains 50 grams of sugar. Thus, a litre of this solution provides fewer than 200 calories!

Because TPN solutions are high in glucose, infusions are started gradually to prevent hyperglycemia. The patient needs to adapt to TPN therapy by increasing insulin output from the pancreas. For example, an adult patient may be given 1 L (40 mL/h) of TPN solution the first day; if the infusion is tolerated, the amount may be increased to 2 L (80 mL/h) for 24 to 48 hours, and then to 3 L (120 mL/h) within 3 to 5 days. Glucose levels are monitored during the infusion.

When TPN therapy is to be discontinued, the TPN infusion rates are decreased slowly to prevent hyperinsulinemia and hypoglycemia. Weaning a patient from TPN can take up to 48 hours but can occur in 6 hours as long as the patient receives adequate carbohydrates either orally or intravenously.

Peripheral parenteral nutrition (PPN) is delivered into the smaller peripheral veins. PPN cannot handle as concentrated a solution as central lines (maximum 10% to 12% dextrose), but can accommodate lipids. PPN is considered a safe and convenient form of therapy. One major disadvantage is the frequent incidence of phlebitis associated with PPN. PPN is generally administered to clients whose needs for intravenous nutrition will last only a short time or in whom placement of a central intravenous catheter is contraindicated. It is a form of therapy used more frequently to prevent nutritional deficits than to correct them.

Evaluating

The goals established in the planning phase are evaluated according to specific desired outcomes also established in that phase. Examples of these are shown in Table 40.9 on the next page.

If the outcomes are *not* achieved, the nurse should explore the reasons why. The nurse might consider the following questions:

- Was the cause of the problem correctly identified?
- Was the family included in the teaching plan? Are they supportive?
- Is the client experiencing symptoms that cause loss of appetite (e.g., pain, nausea, fatigue)?
- Were the outcomes unrealistic for this person?
- Were the client's food preferences considered?
- Is anything interfering with digestion or absorption of nutrients (e.g., vomiting, diarrhea)?

TABLE 40.9 Evaluation Goals and Outcomes

Goal	Examples of Desired Health Outcomes
Maintain or improve nutritional status	• Weight within normal range for height and body frame • Body mass index within expected range • Ingests recommended servings from *Eating Well with Canada's Food Guide* • Uses fats sparingly • Uses salt, sodium, sugars, and alcohol in moderation
Decrease weight	• Identifies factors contributing to excess weight (or risk of excess weight) • Monitors eating habits for specified period (e.g., 1 week) and identifies behaviours that need to be modified to lose weight (or prevent weight gain) • Chooses and ingests a diet that reduces daily caloric intake (e.g., reduces calories by 500 per day for each 0.5 kg of weight loss desired per week) • Establishes a physical activity program of 150 minutes per week of moderate to vigorous intensity aerobic activity • Loses prescribed amount of weight (specify) • Verbalizes improvement in feelings about self and satisfaction with support provided

Regain specified weight	• Identifies factors contributing to inadequate nutritional intake
	• Identifies necessary dietary alterations and foods high in needed nutrients (e.g., calcium, iron, protein, total calories)
	• Consumes a well-balanced diet to restore deficient nutrients
	• Demonstrates decrease (or absence) of signs of malnutrition, as evidenced by:
	  a. Weight gain of specified kilograms per week
	  b. Skinfold measurements reach standard values
	  c. Reports of increased energy (specify)
	  d. Hemoglobin, serum albumin, serum transferrin, and lymphocyte counts within normal ranges

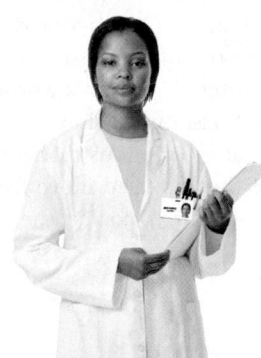

Case Study 40

Mrs. Fai Lee, from Vancouver, is a 75-year-old woman who has recently been diagnosed with chronic lung disease, which has left her very susceptible to pneumonia. As a result, her physician has ordered three different oral medications that have resulted in her losing her appetite and suffering a 10-kilogram weight loss. Once overweight, Mrs. Lee is now within weight standards for her age and height. Mrs. Lee tells her visiting nurse, "Nothing sounds good and nothing tastes good. Meat is particularly distasteful to me right now." Mrs. Lee lives alone and is responsible for her own meal preparation.

CRITICAL THINKING QUESTIONS

1. How do Mrs. Lee's age and health status affect her nutritional needs?

2. What further information do you need regarding Mrs. Lee's present diet?

3. What alternatives can you offer while Mrs. Lee is unable to tolerate meat?

4. Offer suggestions for ways to enhance Mrs. Lee's intake during this period of decreased appetite.

5. Do you think that Mrs. Lee is a good candidate for a feeding tube? Why, or why not?

Check the eText in MyNursingLab for answers and explanations.

KEY TERMS

% Daily Value *p. 1222*

24-hour food
  recall *p. 1228*

adequate intake *p. 1208*

anabolism *p. 1206*

anorexia *p. 1212*

anorexia nervosa *p. 1218*

basal metabolic rate
  (BMR) *p. 1209*

body mass index
  (BMI) *p. 1225*

bottle-mouth
  syndrome *p. 1214*

bulimia nervosa *p. 1218*

caloric value *p. 1208*

calorie *p. 1208*

catabolism *p. 1206*

cholesterol *p. 1207*

clear fluid diet *p. 1240*

complete proteins
  p. 1205

demand feeding *p. 1214*

diet as tolerated
  (DAT) *p. 1241*

diet history *p. 1229*

dietary reference
  intakes *p. 1208*

disaccharides *p. 1204*

dysphagia *p. 1213*

enteral nutrition (EN)
  p. 1243

enzymes *p. 1205*

essential amino acids
  p. 1205

essential fatty acids
  p. 1206

estimated average
  requirement *p. 1208*

fad *p. 1211*

fat-soluble vitamin
  p. 1208

fatty acids *p. 1206*

fibre *p. 1205*

food diary *p. 1228*

food-frequency
  record *p. 1228*

full fluid diet *p. 1240*

gastrostomy *p. 1244*

glucagon *p. 1205*

glycemic index (GI)
  p. 1209

glycemic level *p. 1209*

glycogen *p. 1205*

glycogenesis *p. 1205*

high-density lipoproteins
  (HDLs) *p. 1207*

hip circumference
  p. 1232

hyperglycemia *p. 1209*

hyperinsulinemia *p. 1209*

hypoglycemia *p. 1209*

ideal body weight
  (IBW) *p. 1226*

incomplete proteins
  p. 1205

insoluble fibre *p. 1205*

insulin *p. 1205*

insulin resistance *p. 1209*

iron-deficiency
  anemia *p. 1214*

jejunostomy *p. 1244*

kilojoule *p. 1208*

lactose intolerance
  (lactose
  maldigestion) *p. 1213*

large calorie (Calorie,
  kilocalorie) *p. 1208*

lipids *p. 1206*

lipoprotein *p. 1207*

low-density lipoproteins
  (LDLs) *p. 1207*

macrominerals *p. 1208*

macronutrients *p. 1204*

malnutrition *p. 1225*

metabolic syndrome
  p. 1209

metabolism *p. 1209*

microminerals *p. 1208*

micronutrients *p. 1204*

minerals *p. 1208*

monosaccharides *p. 1204*

monounsaturated fatty
  acids *p. 1206*

nasoenteric tube *p. 1244*

nasogastric tube *p. 1243*

nitrogen balance *p. 1206*

nonessential amino
  acids *p. 1205*

nothing by mouth (nil per
  ora [NPO]) *p. 1240*

nutrients *p. 1204*

nutrition *p. 1204*

nutritive value *p. 1204*

obese *p. 1225*

omega-3 fatty
  acids *p. 1206*

omega-6 fatty
  acids *p. 1206*

overnutrition *p. 1225*

overweight *p. 1225*

parenteral
  nutrition *p. 1243*

partially complete
  proteins *p. 1205*

percutaneous endoscopic
  gastrostomy (PEG)
  p. 1248

percutaneous endoscopic
  jejunostomy (PEJ)
  p. 1248

phospholipids *p. 1207*

polysaccharides *p. 1204*

polyunsaturated fatty
  acids *p. 1206*

protein-calorie
  malnutrition *p. 1226*

pureed diet *p. 1241*

recommended dietary
  allowance *p. 1208*

regurgitation *p. 1214*

resting energy
  expenditure (REE)
  p. 1209

saturated fatty acids
  p. 1206

small calorie *p. 1208*

soft diet *p. 1241*

soluble fibre *p. 1205*

starches *p. 1204*

sterols *p. 1207*

sugars *p. 1204*

tolerable upper intake
  level *p. 1208*

total enteral nutrition
  (TEN) *p. 1243*

trans fats *p. 1206*

triglycerides *p. 1207*

undernutrition *p. 1225*

unsaturated fatty acids
  p. 1206

urea *p. 1236*

usual body weight
  p. 1231

vitamin *p. 1208*

waist circumference
  (WC) *p. 1232*

waist-to-hip ratio
  (WHR) *p. 1232*

water-soluble vitamin
  p. 1208

weight change *p. 1231*

CHAPTER HIGHLIGHTS

- Although people are continually bombarded with information about what to eat and what not to eat, each person is responsible for selecting foods that provide essential nutrients. Nurses can assist people to evaluate the information they receive about nutrients.

- Essential nutrients are grouped into six categories: water, carbohydrates, fats, proteins, vitamins, and minerals.

- Nutrients serve three basic purposes: forming body structures (such as bones and blood), providing energy, and helping to regulate the body's biochemical reactions.

- Energy balance is the relationship between the energy derived from food and the energy used by the body.

- The amount of energy that nutrients or foods supply to the body is their caloric value. The amount of energy required to maintain basic body functions is referred to as the resting energy expenditure (REE). The basal metabolic rate (BMR) is the rate at which the body metabolizes food to maintain the energy and requirements of a person who is awake and at rest.

- A person's state of energy balance can be determined by comparing caloric intake with caloric expenditure.

- Ideal body weight (IBW) is the weight recommended for optimal health.

- Body mass index (BMI) is one indicator of whether a person's weight is appropriate for height, and it may provide a useful estimate of nutrition.

- Factors influencing a person's nutrition include development, sex, ethnicity and culture, beliefs about foods, personal preferences, religious practices, lifestyle, economics, medications and medical therapy, health status, alcohol consumption, advertising, and psychological factors, such as stress, isolation, and depression.

- Nutritional needs vary considerably according to age, growth, and energy requirements. Adolescents have high energy requirements because of their rapid growth; a diet plentiful in milk, meats, green and yellow vegetables, and fresh fruits is required. Older adults often have a reduction in metabolic rate and activity levels. With this being said, older adults living in the community and in long-term care residences have been found to be at increased risk of malnutrition.

- Fats, sugary foods, and sodium must be limited in the diets of Canadians as excess calories are contributing to an epidemic of overweight and obesity. The average diet contains significantly more than the recommended amount of sodium. Excess sodium consumption is related to the development of hypertension and cardiac disease.

- The prevalence of obese and overweight Canadians of all ages has increased dramatically in the past 30 years. The long-term effects of certain nutrient excesses are among the many factors involved in certain diseases, such as coronary artery disease, diabetes mellitus, hypertension, and cancer. Canadian nurses must be proactive in the fight against obesity.

- Various daily food guides have been developed to help healthy people meet the daily requirements of essential nutrients and to facilitate meal planning. This includes *Eating Well with Canada's Food Guide* and *Eating Well with Canada's Food Guide: First Nations, Inuit and Métis*.

- Both inadequate and excessive intakes of nutrients result in malnutrition. The effects of malnutrition can be general or specific, depending on which nutrients and what level of deficiency or excess are involved.

- Assessment of nutritional status may involve all or some of the following: nursing history data, nutritional screening, physical examination, calculation of the percentage of weight loss, a dietary history, anthropometric measurements, and laboratory data.

- Major goals for clients with or at risk for nutritional problems include the following: maintaining or restoring optimal nutritional status, decreasing or regaining specified weight, promoting healthy nutritional practices, and preventing complications associated with malnutrition.

- Assisting patients and support persons with therapeutic diets is a function shared by the nurse and the dietitian. The nurse reinforces the dietitian's instructions, assists the patient to make beneficial changes, and evaluates the patient's response to planned changes.

- Because many hospitalized patients have poor appetites, a major responsibility of the nurse is to provide nursing interventions that stimulate their appetites.

- Whenever possible, the nurse should help incapacitated patients to feed themselves; a number of self-feeding aids can help patients who have difficulty handling regular utensils.

- Enteral feedings, administered through nasogastric, nasoenteric, gastrostomy, or jejunostomy tubes, are provided when the patient is unable to ingest foods or the upper gastrointestinal tract is impaired.

- A nasogastric or nasoenteric tube is used to provide enteral nutrition for short-term use (less than 6 weeks), whereas a gastrostomy or jejunostomy tube can be used to supply nutrients via the enteral route for long-term use.

- The use of feeding tubes for the administration of medication must be done judiciously by the nurse to avoid drug interaction and inappropriate dosing when sustained-release medications are crushed.

- Parenteral nutrition, provided when the gastrointestinal tract is nonfunctional (e.g., absorptive capacity impaired), is given intravenously into a large central vein (e.g., the superior vena cava) or through a peripheral vein, depending on the type of solution.

ASSESS YOUR LEARNING

1. A 36-year-old adult male reports eating the following each day, on average: 2 servings of milk and alternatives, 2 servings of fruit, 3 serving of vegetables, 3 servings of meat and alternatives, and 8 servings of grain products. When following the recommendations of *Eating Well with Canada's Food Guide,* the nurse would counsel the client to do which of the following?

   a. Maintain the diet; the servings are adequate

   b. Increase the number of servings of milk and alternatives

   c. Increase the number of servings of vegetables and fruits

   d. Decrease the number of servings of grain products

2. Which of the following are allowed on a full liquid diet?

   a. Chocolate pudding, tomato juice, hard candy, cream of wheat cereal, and fruit smoothies

   b. Scrambled eggs, tomato juice, mashed potatoes, and fruit smoothies

   c. Scrambled eggs, tomato juice, mashed potatoes, cream of wheat cereal, and oatmeal cereal

   d. Tomato juice, cream of wheat cereal, oatmeal cereal, and fruit smoothies

3. Which of the following is the BEST indication of proper placement of a nasogastric tube in the stomach?

   a. The client is able to speak and is not coughing.

   b. A radiograph confirms placement in the stomach.

   c. The pH of the aspirate is less than 5.

   d. A whooshing noise is heard with a stethoscope when air is injected into the tube.

4. What is the proper technique for gravity tube feeding?

   a. Hanging the feeding bag 30 cm higher than the tube's insertion point into the client

   b. Administering the next feeding only if there is less than 25 mL of residual volume from the previous feeding

   c. Placing the client in the left lateral position while the feeding is being administered

   d. Administering the feeding directly after removing it from the refrigerator to prevent spoilage

5. A 55-year-old female is about 9 kg more than her desired weight. She has been on a low-calorie diet with no improvement. Which of the following statements reflects a healthy approach to the desired weight loss?

   a. "I need to engage in 150 minutes of aerobic physical activity a week."

   b. "I need to switch to a low-carbohydrate, low-fat diet."

   c. "I need to keep a list of my forbidden foods on hand and write down what I eat."

   d. "I need to buy more organic foods and fewer processed foods."

6. A resident of a long-term care facility has mild dysphagia from a recent cerebrovascular accident (stroke). The nurse plans the client's meals based on which of the following?

   a. The need to have at least one serving of thickened milk and alternatives (e.g., pudding, ice cream) per meal

   b. The need to eliminate the beer occasionally ingested on weekends

   c. The results of a complete swallowing assessment

   d. The need to increase the calories from lipids to 40%

7. Two months ago, a client weighed 88.4 kg. The client now weighs 82.5 kg. Calculate the client's percentage weight loss, and determine its significance.

   a. 6.7%, not significant weight loss

   b. 6.7%, significant weight loss

   c. 13.4%, severe weight loss

   d. 3.3%, not significant weight loss

8. A 52-year-old man has a waist circumference of 106 cm. He is 180 cm tall and weighs 98 kg. What is this individual's risk status with respect to the development of cardiovascular disease, type 2 diabetes, and hypertension, given his body mass index (BMI) and waist circumference?

   a. No increased risk

   b. High risk

   c. Very high risk

   d. Extremely high risk

9. A 4-month-old infant should consume which of the following each day?

   a. Breast milk only, or formula in certain circumstances

   b. Breast milk at night and cow's milk in a bottle when the infant is at daycare

   c. Iron-fortified cereal four times a day with breast milk when the infant is hungry between meals

   d. Iron-fortified cereal makes up the bulk of the calories consumed; the infant is breastfed if the mother desires

10. Mrs. Hassan, 38 years old, has been sent home with a gastric feeding tube. Her husband will be administering a bolus feeding every 6 hours. What is the most important consideration the nurse should teach Mr. Hassan when administering gastric feedings?

    a. Flushing the tube with water before and after feedings

   b. Ensuring that Mrs. Hassan is supine with the head of her bed raised

   c. Placing Mrs. Hassan in a side-lying position

   d. Administering Mrs. Hassan's feedings rapidly

Check the eText in MyNursingLab for answers and explanations.

WEBLINKS

Breakfast for Learning

http://www.breakfastforlearning.ca

This national nonprofit organization is dedicated to ensuring child nutrition programs in Canada.

Dietitians of Canada

http://www.dietitians.ca

This site introduces the Dietitians of Canada and the services that it provides to its members and the public.

Health Canada: Food and Nutrition

http://www.hc-sc.gc.ca/fn-an/index_e.html

This site is sponsored by Health Canada and provides an introduction to public information on food and nutrition. The site also has a search tool and permits access to Canadian legislative policy, allergy alerts, and other federal resources.

Healthy Canadians: A Source for a Healthier Lifestyle

http://www.healthycanadians.ca

This site is operated by the Government of Canada and provides information on health-related promotional campaigns supported by Health Canada and the Public Health Agency of Canada.

Canadians can find information about physical activity, healthy eating (e.g., % Daily Value), and smoking cessation here.

Canadian Obesity Network

http://www.obesitynetwork.ca

The Canadian Obesity Network is a registered nonprofit organization dedicated to reducing the burden of obesity in Canada by helping to coordinate obesity funding, research, and prevention and treatment strategies.

Canadian Diabetes Association

http://www.diabetes.ca

Operated by the Canadian Diabetes Association, this site contains valuable information for health care providers and patients. The latest clinical guidelines for diabetes care are contained on this site.

Health Canada: Dietary References Intake Tables and Recommended Dietary Allowances

http://www.hc-sc.gc.ca/fn-an/nutrition/reference/table/index-eng.php

This site lists the daily recommended intakes for vitamins, microminerals, and macrominerals, categorized by sex and age.

MyNursingLab

REFERENCES

American Association of Critical Care Nurses. (2005). *Verification of feeding tube placement. Revised 2009.* Retrieved from http://www.aacn.org/WD/Practice/Docs/PracticeAlerts/Verification_of_Feeding_Tube_Placement_05-2005.pdf

American Dietetic Association. (2003). *National dysphagia diet: Standardization for optimal care.* Chicago, IL: Author.

Anis, A. H., Zhang, W., Bansback, N., Guh, D. P., Amarsi, Z., & Birmingham, C. L. (2010). Obesity and overweight in Canada: An updated cost-of-illness study. *Obesity Reviews, 11,* 31–40.

Bankhead, R., Boullata, J., Brantley, M. S., Corkins, M., Guenter, P., Krenitsky, M. S., . . . & ASPEN Board of Directors. (2009). Enteral nutrition practice recommendations. *Journal of Parenteral and Enteral Nutrition, 33*(2), 122–167.doi: 10.1177/0148607108330314

Bostrom, A.-M., Van Soest, D., Kolewaski, B., Milke, D. L. & Estabrooks, C. A. (2011). Nutrition status among residents living in a veterans long-term care facility in western Canada: A pilot study. *Journal of the American Medical Directors Association, 12*(3), 217–225.

Brien, S. E., Ronksley, P. E., Turner, B. J., Mukamal, K. J., & Ghali, W. A. (2011). Effect of alcohol consumption on biological markers associated with risk of coronary heart disease: Systematic review and meta-analysis of interventional studies. *British Medical Journal, 342,* d636. doi: 10.1136/bmj.d636

Butt, P., Beirness, D., Gliksman, L., Paradis, C., & Stockwell, T. (2011). Alcohol and health in Canada: A summary of evidence and guidelines for low-risk drinking. Ottawa, ON: Canadian Centre on Substance Abuse.

Canadian Diabetes Association. (2008). *The glycemic index.* Retrieved from http://www.diabetes.ca/files/Diabetes_GL_FINAL2_CPG03.pdf

Canadian Hypertension Education Program. (2012). *2012 Canadian hypertension education program recommendations.* Ottawa, ON: Author. Retrieved from http://www.hypertension.ca/chep-recommendations

Canadian Paediatric Society, Dietitians of Canada, & Health Canada. (2005) (Reaffirmed 2009). *Nutrition for healthy term infants.* Ottawa, ON: Minister of Public Works and Government Services. Retrieved from http://www.hc-sc.gc.ca/ fn-an/pubs/infant-nourrisson/nut_infant_nourrisson_term_e.html

Choudhary, A. K., Donnelly, L. F., Racadio, J. M., & Strife, J. L. (2007). Diseases associated with childhood obesity. *American Journal of Roentgenology, 188,* 1118–1130.

Dickerson, R. N., Tidwell, A. C., & Brown, R. O. (2003). Adverse effects from inappropriate medication administration via a jejunostomy feeding tube. *Nutrition in Clinical Practice, 18*(5), 402–405.

Dietitians of Canada. (2003). A new food guide for North American vegetarians. *Canadian Journal of Dietetic Practice, 64*(2), 81–86.

Dietitians of Canada. (2011a). Managing lactose intolerance. Retrieved from http://www.dietitians.ca/Nutrition-Resources-A-Z/Fact-Sheet-Pages%28HTML%29/Lactose/Managing-Lactose-Intolerance.aspx

Dietitians of Canada. (2011b). I recently became a vegetarian. Is it possible to get all the nutrients I need on a vegetarian diet? Retrieved from http://www.dietitians.ca/getattachment/6c6e507c-39ce-4501-b752-0fe241962429/FactSheet—I-recently-became-a-vegetarian.pdf.aspx

Downs, S. M., Arnold, A., Marshall, D., McCargar, L. J., & Willows, N. D. (2009). Associations among the food environment, diet quality and weight status in Cree children in Québec. *Public Health Nutrition, 12*(9), 1504–1511. doi: 10.1017/S1368980008004515

Food Banks Canada. (2010). *HungerCount 2010.* Toronto, ON: Food Banks Canada. Retrieved from http://foodbankscanada.ca/documents/HungerCount2010_web.pdf

Green, S. M., & Watson, R. (2006). Nutritional screening and assessment tools for use by nurses: Literature review. *Journal of Advanced Nursing, 54*(4), 477–490.

Harris, W. S. (2006). The omega-6/omega-3 ratio and cardiovascular disease risk: Uses and abuses. *Current Atherosclerosis Reports, 8,* 453–459.

Harris, W. S., Mozaffarian, D., Rimm, E., Kris-Etherton, P., Rudel, L. L., & Appel, L. J. (2009). Omega-6 fatty acids and risk for cardiovascular disease: A science advisory from the American Heart Association Nutrition Subcommittee of the Council on Nutrition, Physical Activity, and Metabolism; Council on Cardiovascular Nursing; and Council on Epidemiology and Prevention. *Circulation, 119,* 902–907. doi: 10.1161/CIRCULATIONHA.208.191627

Health Canada. (2003). Canadian guideline for body weight classification in adults—Quick reference tool for professionals. Retrieved from http://www.hc-sc.gc.ca/fn-an/alt_formats/hpfb-dgpsa/pdf/nutrition/cg_quick_ref-ldc_rapide_ref-eng.pdf

Health Canada. (2005). *Nutrition for healthy term infants—statement of the joint working group: Canadian Paediatric Society, Dietitians of Canada and Health Canada.* Retrieved from http://www.hc-sc.gc.ca/fn-an/pubs/infant-nourrisson/nut_infant_nourrisson_term_e.html

Health Canada. (2006). It's your health: Salmonella prevention. Retrieved from http://www.hc-sc.gc.ca/hl-vs/iyh-vsv/food-aliment/salmonella-eng.php#mi

Health Canada. (2007a). *Eating well with Canada's food guide.* Ottawa, ON: Author.

Health Canada. (2007b). *Eating well with Canada's food guide: First Nations, Inuit and Métis.* Ottawa, ON: Author.

Health Canada. (2007c). *Estimated energy requirements.* Retrieved from http://www.hc-sc.gc.ca/fn-an/food-guide-aliment/basics-base/1_1_1-eng.php

Health Canada. (2008a). *Mercury in fish.* Retrieved from http://www.hc-sc.gc.ca/fn-an/securit/chem-chim/environ/mercur/cons-adv-etud-eng.php

Health Canada. (2008b). *Canadian guidelines for body weight classification in adults.* Retrieved from http://www.hc-sc.gc.ca/fn-an/nutrition/weights-poids/guide-ld-adult/cg_quick_ref-ldc_rapide_ref-eng.php

Health Canada. (2009). *Prenatal nutrition guidelines for health professionals.* Retrieved from http://www.hc-sc.gc.ca/fn-an/alt_formats/hpfb-dgpsa/pdf/pubs/folate-eng.pdf

Health Canada. (2010a). *Dietary reference intakes.* Retrieved from http://www.hc-sc.gc.ca/fn-an/alt_formats/hpfb-dgpsa/pdf/pubs/omega3-eng.pdf

Health Canada. (2010b). *Food allergies and intolerances.* Retrieved from http://www.hc-sc.gc.ca/fn-an/securit/allerg/index-eng.php

Health Canada. (2010c). *Multi-Stakeholder working group on sodium reduction.* Retrieved from http://www.hc-sc.gc.ca/fn-an/nutrition/sodium/sodium-working-travail-group-eng.php

Health Canada. (2010d). *Safe use of energy drinks.* Retrieved from http://www.hc-sc.gc.ca/hl-vs/alt_formats/pdf/iyh-vsv/food-aliment/boissons-energ-drinks-eng.pdf

Health Canada. (2010e). *Sodium.* Retrieved from http://www.hc-sc.gc.ca/fn-an/nutrition/sodium/index-eng.php

Health Canada. (2010f). *Using the Nutrition Facts Table: How to Choose.* Ottawa, ON: Author. Retrieved from http://www.hc-sc.gc.ca/fn-an/label-etiquet/nutrition/cons/fact-fiche-eng.php

Health Canada. (2010g). *Vitamin D and calcium: Updated dietary reference intakes.* Retrieved from http://www.hc-sc.gc.ca/fn-an/nutrition/vitamin/vita-d-eng.php

Health Canada. (2011a). *Household food insecurity in Canada in 2007-2008: Key statistics and graphics.* Retrieved from http://www.hc-sc.gc.ca/fn-an/surveill/nutrition/commun/insecurit/key-stats-cles-2007-2008-eng.phphttp://www.hc-sc.gc.ca/fn-an/pubs/fnim-pnim/index_e.html

Health Canada. (2011b). It's your health: Infant botulism. Retrieved from http://www.hc-sc.gc.ca/hl-vs/iyh-vsv/diseases-maladies/botu-eng.php

Health Canada. (2011c). *Food allergen labelling.* Retrieved from http://www.hc-sc.gc.ca/fn-an/label-etiquet/allergen/index-eng.php

Krondl, M., Lau, D., Coleman, P., & Stocker, G. (2003). Tailoring of nutritional support for older adults in the community. *Journal of Nutrition for the Elderly, 23,* 17–32.

Kuhle, S., Kirk, S., Ohinmaa, A., Yasui, Y., Allen, A. C., & Veugelers, P. J. (2010). Use and cost of health services among overweight and obese Canadian children. *International Journal of Pediatric Obesity, 6*(2), 142–148.

Lau, D. C., Douketis, J. D., Morrison, K. M., Hramiak, I. M., Sharma, A. M., & Ur, E. (2007). 2006 Canadian clinical practice guidelines on the management and prevention of obesity in adults and children [summary]. *Canadian Medical Association Journal, 176*(8), s1–s13.

Lengyel, C. O., Zello, G. A., Smith, J. T., & Whiting, S. J. (2003). Evaluation of menu and food service practices of long-term care facilities of a health district in Canada. *Journal of Nutrition for the Elderly, 22,* 29–42.

Mesias, M., Seiquer, I., & Navarro, P. (2011). Calcium nutrition in adolescence. *Critical Reviews in Food Science, 51*(3), 195–209.

Ng, C., Marshall, D., & Willows, N. (2006). Obesity, adiposity, physical fitness and activity levels in Cree children. *International Journal of Circumpolar Health, 65*(4), 322–330.

Osteoporosis Canada. (2010). *2010 Clinical Practice guidelines for the diagnosis and management of osteoporosis in Canada. Executive summary.* Retrieved from http://www.osteoporosis.ca/multimedia/pdf/oc_executivesum_0410.pdf

Pischon, T., Hankison, S. E., Hotamisligil, G. S., Rifai, N., Willett, W. C., & Rimm, E. B. (2003). Habitual dietary intake of n-3 and n-6 fatty acids in relation to inflammatory markers among US men and women. *Circulation, 108,* 155–160.

Public Health Agency of Canada. (2010). *Childhood obesity and the role of the government of Canada.* Retrieved from http://www.phac-aspc.gc.ca/ch-se/obesity/obesity-eng.php

Public Health Agency of Canada. (2011). *Physical activity.* Retrieved from http://www.phac-aspc.gc.ca/hp-ps/hl-mvs/pa-ap/07paap-eng.php

Rampersaud, G. C., Pereira, M. A., Girard, B. L., Adams, J., & Metzl, J. D. (2005). Breakfast habits, nutritional status, body weight, and academic performance in children and adolescents. *Journal of the American Dietetic Association, 105,* 743–760.

Reising, D. L., & Neal, R. S. (2005). Enteral tube flushing: What you think are the best practices may not be. *American Journal of Nursing, 105*(3), 58–64.

Ronksley, P. E., Brien, S. E., Turner, B. J., Mukamal, K. J., & Ghali, W. A. (2011). Association of alcohol consumption with selected cardiovascular disease outcomes: A systematic review and meta-analysis. *British Medical Journal, 342,* d671. doi: 10.1136/bmj.d671

Séguin, P., Le Bouquin, V., Aguillon, D., Maurice, A., Laviolle, B., & Mallédant, Y. (2005). Évaluation prospective de trois méthodes de positionnement de la sonde nasogastrique en réanimation. *Annales Françaises d'Anesthésie et de Réanimation, 24*(6), 594–599.

Shields, M. (2006). Overweight and obesity among children and youth. *Health Reports, 17*(27), 42.

Shields, M., Carroll, M. D., & Ogden, C. L. (2011). *Obesity prevalence in Canada and the United States. NCHS Data Reports.* Retrieved from http://www.cdc.gov/nchs/data/databriefs/db56.pdf

Simopoulos, A. P. (2008). The importance of the omega-6/Omega-3 fatty acid ratio in cardiovascular disease and other chronic diseases. *Experimental Biology and Medicine, 233,* 674–688.

Statistics Canada. (2010a). *Canadian health measures survey 2007-2009. Body mass index (BMI) for children and youth 2007 to 2009.* Component of Statistics Canada Catalogue no. 82-625-X no. 2010001. Retrieved from http://www.statcan.gc.ca/pub/82-625-x/2010001/article/11090-eng.pdf

Statistics Canada. (2010b). *Overweight and obese adults (self-reported) 2009.* Retrieved from http://www.statcan.gc.ca/pub/82-625-x/2010002/article/11255-eng.htm

Weicker, M. O., & Pfeiffer, A. F. H. (2008) Metabolic effects of dietary fiber consumption and prevention of diabetes. *Journal of Nutrition, 138,* 439–442.

Wilding, J. P. H. (2007). Treatment strategies for obesity. *Obesity Reviews, 8*(Suppl. 1), 137–144.

Chapter 41

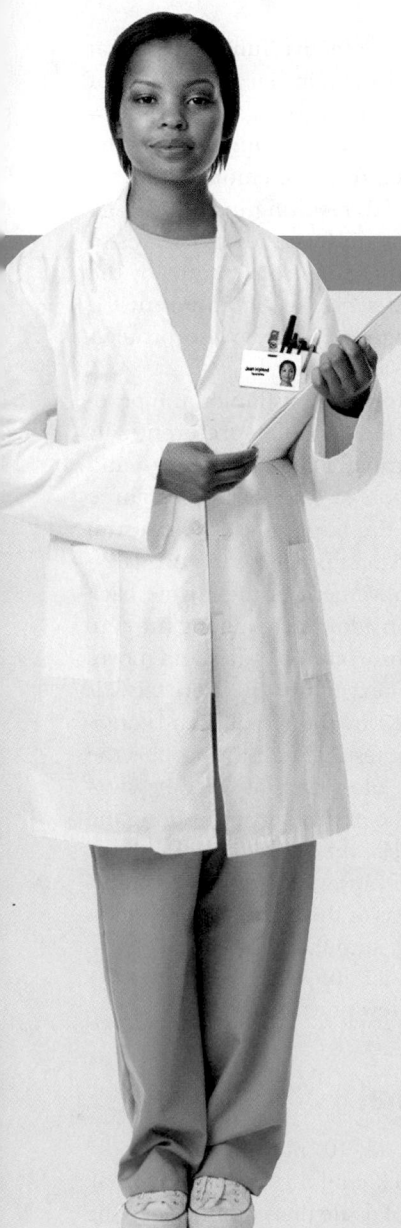

Fecal Elimination

LEARNING OUTCOMES

After studying this chapter, you will be able to:

1. Describe the physiology of defecation.

2. Identify 11 factors that influence fecal elimination and patterns of defecation.

3. Distinguish normal from abnormal characteristics and constituents of feces.

4. Conduct a thorough assessment of fecal elimination.

5. Differentiate five fecal elimination problems.

6. Identify common causes and effects of selected fecal elimination problems.

7. List examples of nursing diagnoses, outcomes, and interventions for clients with elimination problems.

8. Discuss measures that promote regular defecation.

9. Relate common interventions to specific fecal elimination problems.

10. Describe essentials of stoma care for clients with fecal ostomies.

11. Verbalize the steps used in (a) administering an enema and (b) changing a bowel diversion ostomy appliance.

12. State desired health outcomes essential for evaluating the client's progress.

T he elimination of feces is essential to the maintenance of good overall health. Important factors in maintaining normal bowel patterns include such things as exercise, diet, and stress levels. Bowel health is a concern of many people. Generally considered a private and personal matter that is not commonly discussed in public, nurses frequently are consulted or involved in assisting clients with identifying what is healthy about their bowel function as well as understanding and dealing with fecal elimination problems. These problems can be embarrassing to clients and can cause considerable discomfort. With colorectal cancer as the second leading cause of cancer in Canadian men and women (Canadian Cancer Society, 2012), many adults are becoming vigilant about the health of their intestines and nurses are playing an important role in raising awareness of health issues related to bowel health and fecal elimination.

Physiology of Defecation

Elimination of the waste products of digestion from the body is essential to health. These excreted waste products are referred to as **feces** or **stool**.

Large Intestine

The large intestine extends from the ileocecal (ileocolic) valve to the anus. The colon (large intestine) in the adult is generally about 125 cm to 150 cm long. It has seven parts: the cecum; ascending, transverse, and descending colons; sigmoid colon; rectum; and anus or external orifice (Figure 41.1).

The large intestine is a muscular tube lined with mucous membrane. The muscle fibres are both circular and longitudinal, permitting the intestine to enlarge and contract in both width and length. The longitudinal muscles are shorter than the colon and, therefore, cause the large intestine to form pouches, or **haustra**.

The colon's main functions are absorption of water and nutrients, the mucoid protection of the intestinal wall, and fecal elimination. The contents of the colon normally represent foods ingested over the previous 4 days, although most of the waste products are excreted within 48 hours of ingestion (the act of taking food). The digested products leaving the stomach through the small intestine and then passing through the ileocecal valve are called **chyme**. The ileocecal valve, located at the junction of the ileum of the small intestine and the first part of the large intestine, regulates the flow of chyme into the large intestine and prevents backflow into the ileum. The colon absorbs water and significant amounts of sodium and chloride as food passes along it. As much as 1500 mL of chyme passes into the large intestine daily, and all but about 100 mL is absorbed in the proximal half of the colon. The 100 mL of fluid is excreted in feces.

The colon also serves a protective function in that it secretes mucus. This mucus contains large amounts of bicarbonate ions. The mucus secretion is stimulated by excitation of parasympathetic nerves. During extreme stimulation—for example, as a result of emotions—large amounts of mucus are secreted, resulting in the passage of stringy mucus with little or no feces. Mucus serves to protect the wall of the large intestine from trauma by the acids formed in feces, and it serves as an adherent for holding the fecal material together. Mucus also protects the intestinal wall from bacterial activity.

The colon acts to transport along its lumen the products of digestion (flatus and feces), which are eventually eliminated through the anal canal. **Flatus** is largely air and the byproducts of the digestion of carbohydrates. Three types of movement occur in the large intestine: haustral churning, colon peristalsis, and mass peristalsis (Figure 41.2). **Haustral churning** involves movement of the chyme back and forth within the haustra. In addition to mixing the contents, this action aids in the absorption of water and moves the contents forward to the next haustrum. **Peristalsis** is wave-like movement produced by the circular and longitudinal muscle fibres of the intestinal walls; it propels the intestinal contents forward. Colon peristalsis is very sluggish and is thought to move the chyme very little along the large intestine. **Mass peristalsis**, the third type of colonic movement, involves a wave of powerful muscular contraction that moves over large areas of the colon. Usually, mass peristalsis occurs after eating, stimulated by the presence of food in the stomach and small intestine. In adults, mass peristaltic waves occur only a few times a day.

Rectum and Anal Canal

The rectum in the adult is usually 10 cm to 15 cm long; the most distal portion, 2.5 cm to 5 cm long, is the anal canal. In the rectum are three folds of tissue that extend across the rectum and several folds that extend vertically. Each vertical

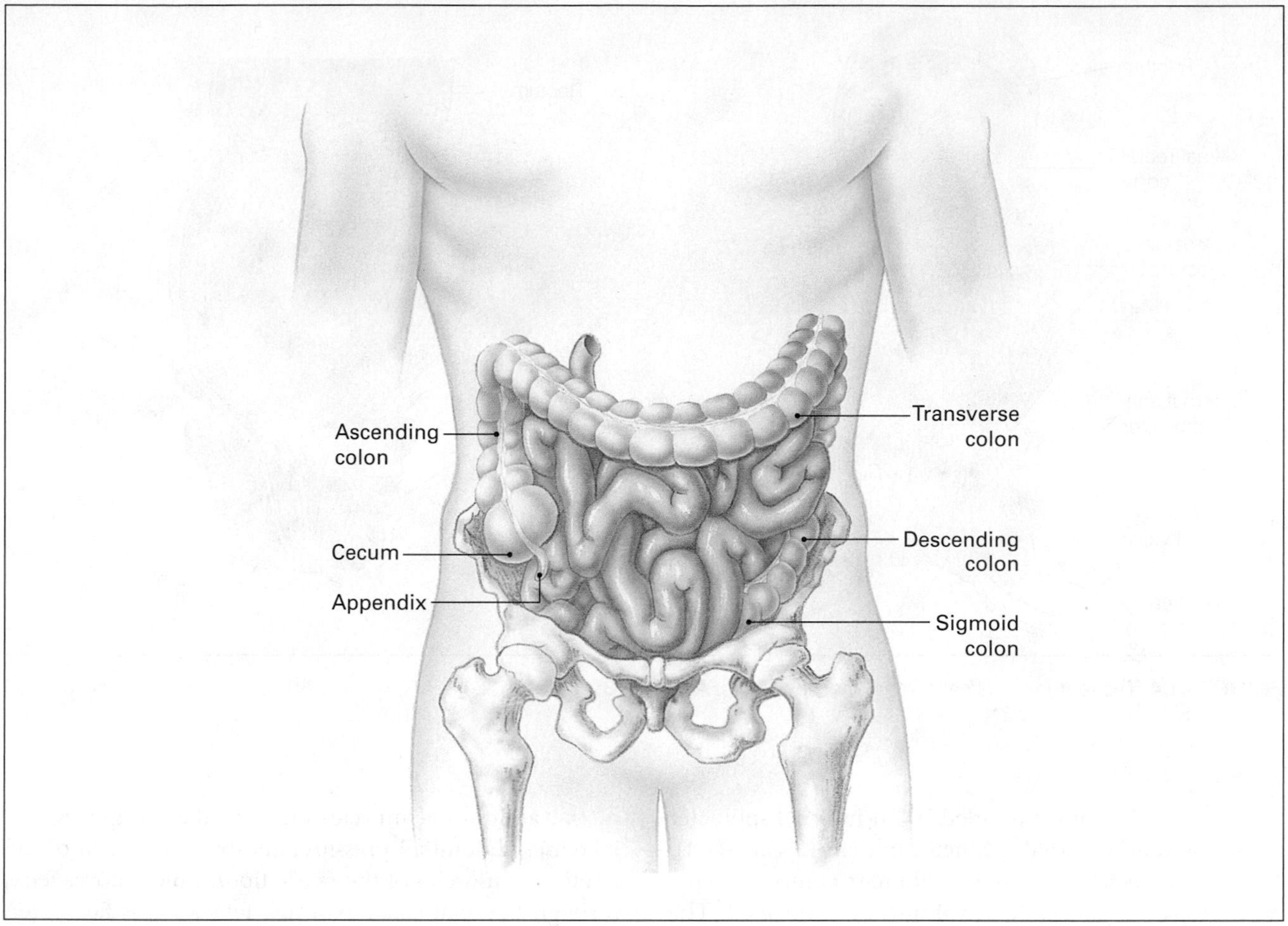

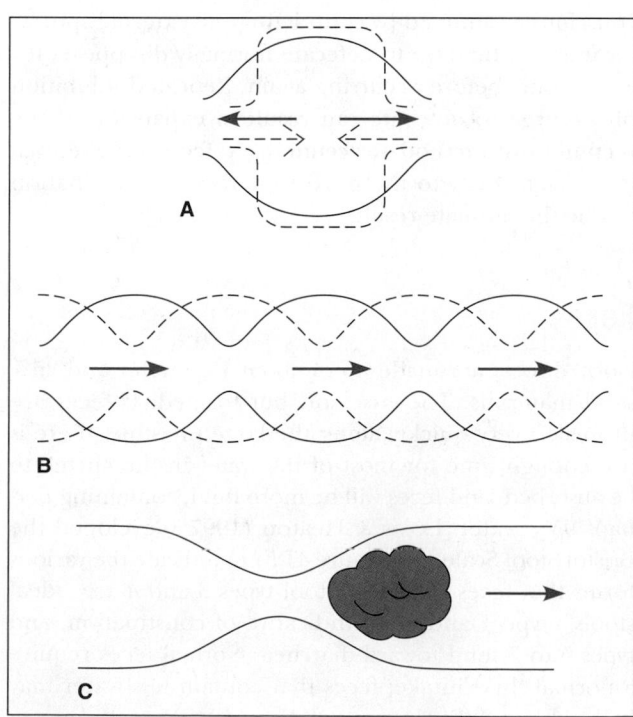

FIGURE 41.1 The large intestine.

Source: Fremgan, B. F., and Frucht, S. S. (2005). *Medical terminology: A living language* (3rd ed.). Upper Saddle River, NJ: Pearson Education Inc. Electronically reproduced with permission of Pearson Education Inc., Upper Saddle River, New Jersey.

fold contains a vein and an artery. It is believed that these folds help retain feces within the rectum. When the veins become distended, as can occur with repeated pressure, a condition known as **hemorrhoids** occurs. Hemorrhoids can present internally or externally (Figure 41.3).

FIGURE 41.2 Three types of intestinal movements: **A:** Haustral churning; **B:** Peristalsis; **C:** Mass peristalsis.

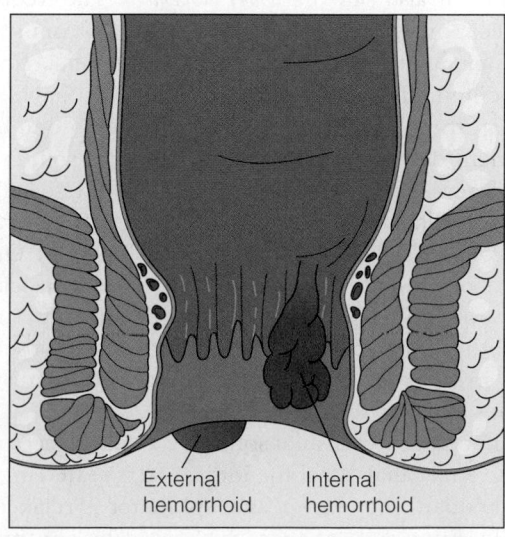

FIGURE 41.3 Internal and external hemorrhoids.

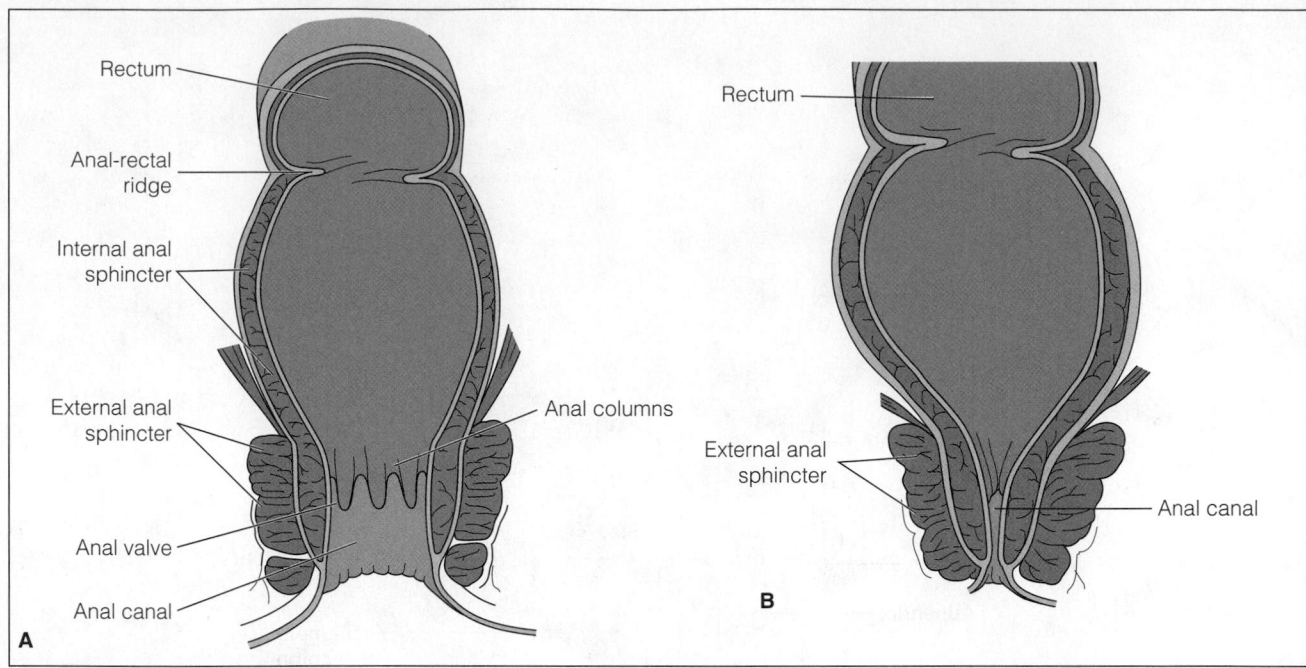

FIGURE 41.4 The rectum, anal canal, and anal sphincters: **A:** Open; **B:** Closed.

The anal canal is bounded by an internal sphincter muscle and an external sphincter muscle (Figure 41.4). The *internal sphincter* is under involuntary control, and the *external sphincter* normally is voluntarily controlled. The external sphincter's action is augmented by the levator ani muscles of the pelvic floor. The internal sphincter muscle is innervated by the autonomic nervous system; the external sphincter is innervated by the somatic nervous system.

Defecation

Defecation is the expulsion of feces from the anus and rectum. It is also called a *bowel movement.* The frequency of defecation is highly individual, varying from several times per day to two or three times per week. Normal bowel elimination in the adult is defined as "equal to or less than three bowel movements per day to one bowel movement daily or at least every other day; soft, brown, formed stool, equal to or greater than 250 mL to 500 mL, with use of laxatives restricted to stool softeners and/or bulk-forming agents" (Sisters of Charity of Ottawa Health Services, cited in Registered Nurses' Association of Ontario [RNAO], 2011). When peristaltic waves move feces into the sigmoid colon and the rectum, the sensory nerves in the rectum are stimulated and the individual becomes aware of the need to defecate.

When the *internal* anal sphincter relaxes, feces move into the anal canal. After the individual is seated on a toilet or bedpan, the *external* anal sphincter is relaxed voluntarily. Expulsion of feces is assisted by contraction of the abdominal muscles and the diaphragm, which increases abdominal pressure, and by contraction of the levator ani muscles of the pelvic floor, which moves feces through the anal canal. Normal defecation is facilitated by (a) thigh flexion, which increases the pressure within the abdomen, and (b) a sitting position, which increases the downward pressure on the rectum.

If the defecation reflex is ignored or if defecation is consciously inhibited by contracting the external sphincter muscle, the urge to defecate normally disappears for a few hours before occurring again. Repeated inhibition of the urge to defecate can result in expansion of the rectum to accommodate accumulated feces and eventual loss of sensitivity to the need to defecate. Constipation can be the ultimate result.

Feces

Normal feces are made up of about 75% water and 25% solid materials. They are soft but formed. If feces are propelled very quickly along the large intestine, there is not enough time for most of the water in the chyme to be absorbed, and feces will be more fluid, containing perhaps 95% water. Lewis & Heaton (1997) developed the Bristol Stool Scale (see Figure 41.5) to indicate the various forms that feces can take. Stool types 3 and 4 are "ideal stools"; type 1 and 2 are indicative of constipation, and types 5 to 7 tend toward diarrhea. Normal feces require a normal fluid intake; feces that contain less water may be hard and difficult to expel. Feces are normally brown, chiefly because of the presence of stercobilin and urobilin,

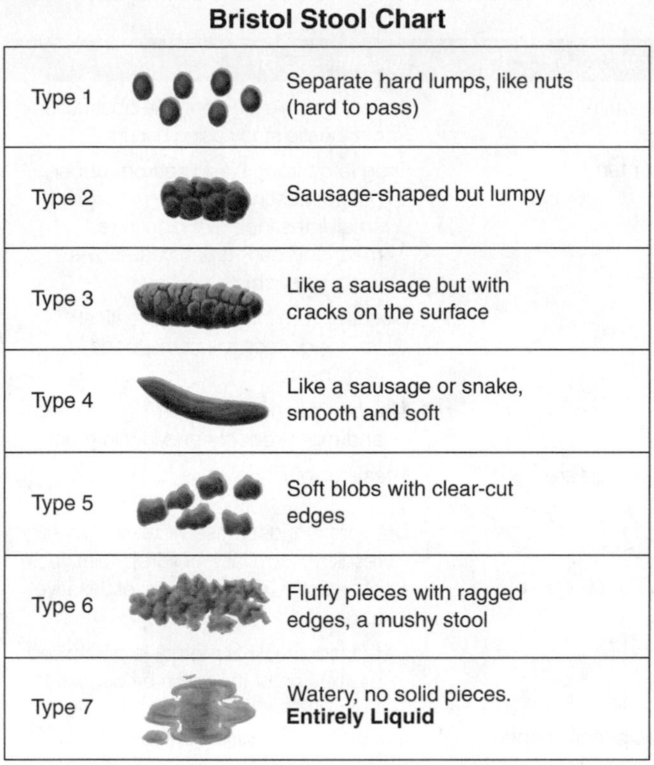

Bristol Stool Chart

Type 1		Separate hard lumps, like nuts (hard to pass)
Type 2		Sausage-shaped but lumpy
Type 3		Like a sausage but with cracks on the surface
Type 4		Like a sausage or snake, smooth and soft
Type 5		Soft blobs with clear-cut edges
Type 6		Fluffy pieces with ragged edges, a mushy stool
Type 7		Watery, no solid pieces. **Entirely Liquid**

FIGURE 41.5 Bristol Stool Chart. Types 1 and 2 indicate constipation. Types 3 and 4 are considered "ideal." Types 5 to 7 progress to diarrhea.

Source: S.J Lewis and K.W Heaton, *Scandinavian Journal of Gastroenterology*, 1997; 32 (9): 920–924, © 1997, Informa Healthcare. Reproduced with permission of Informa Healthcare.

which are derived from bilirubin (a red pigment in bile). Another factor that affects fecal colour is the action of bacteria, such as *Escherichia coli* or staphylococci, which are normally present in the large intestine. The action of microorganisms on the chyme is also responsible for the odour of feces. See Table 41.1 on the next page for characteristics of normal and abnormal feces.

An adult usually forms 7 L to 10 L of flatus (gas) in the large intestine every 24 hours. The gases include carbon dioxide, methane, hydrogen, oxygen, and nitrogen. Some gases are swallowed with food and fluids taken by mouth; some are formed through the action of bacteria on the chyme in the large intestine; and other gas diffuses from the blood into the gastrointestinal tract.

Factors that Affect Defecation

Defecation patterns vary at different stages of life. Circumstances of development, diet, fluid intake and output, activity, psychological factors, habits, medications, diagnostic procedures, anesthesia and surgery, pathological conditions, and pain also affect defecation.

Development

NEWBORNS AND INFANTS **Meconium** is the first fecal material passed by the newborn, normally up to 24 hours after birth. It is black, tarry, odourless, and sticky. Transitional stool, which follows for about a week, is generally greenish yellow; it contains mucus and are loose.

Infants pass stool frequently, often after each feeding. Because the intestine is immature, water is not well absorbed and stool is soft, liquid, and frequent. When the intestine matures, bacterial flora increase. After solid foods are introduced, stool becomes less frequent and firmer. Infants who are breast fed have bright yellow to golden feces, and infants who are taking formula will have dark yellow or tan stool that is more formed.

TODDLERS Some control of defecation starts at 1.5 to 2 years of age. By this time, children have learned to walk, and the nervous and muscular systems are sufficiently well developed to permit bowel control. A desire to control daytime bowel movements and to use the toilet generally starts when the child becomes aware of (a) the discomfort caused by a soiled diaper, and (b) the sensation that indicates the need for a bowel movement. Daytime control is normally attained by age 2.5 years after a process of toilet training.

SCHOOL-AGE CHILDREN AND ADOLESCENTS School-age children and adolescents have bowel habits similar to those of adults. Patterns of defecation vary in frequency, quantity, and consistency. Some school-age children may deliberately delay defecation (functional constipation) because of an activity, such as play. **Encopresis**, the passage or leakage of feces in children who are past the age of toilet training, generally after 4 years of age, can present as a bowel-management problem. Involuntary encopresis is frequently associated with constipation and can indicate fecal impaction. Deliberate soiling can indicate a developmental or emotional problem.

OLDER ADULTS Constipation is a common bowel-management problem in the older adult population. This experience occurs partly because of reduced activity levels, muscle weakness, swallowing or chewing difficulties, and inadequate amounts of fluid and fibre intake. Physiologically, older adults secrete less mucus in the large intestine. Many older people believe that *regularity* means a bowel movement every day. Those who do not meet this criterion often seek over-the-counter (OTC) preparations to relieve what they believe to be constipation. Older clients should be advised that normal patterns of bowel elimination vary considerably. For some, a normal pattern may be every other day; for others, twice a day. Adequate roughage in the diet, adequate exercise, and six to eight glasses of fluid daily are essential preventive measures for constipation. Responding to the **gastrocolic reflex** (increased

TABLE 41.1 Characteristics of Normal and Abnormal Feces

Characteristic	Normal	Abnormal	Possible Cause
Colour	Adult: brown Infant: yellow	Clay or white	Absence of bile pigment (bile obstruction); diagnostic study using barium
		Black or tarry	Drug (e.g., iron); bleeding from upper gastrointestinal tract (e.g., stomach, small intestine); diet high in red meat and dark green vegetables (e.g., spinach)
		Red	Bleeding from lower gastrointestinal tract (e.g., rectum); some foods (e.g., beets)
		Pale	Malabsorption of fats; diet high in milk and milk products and low in meat
		Orange or green	Intestinal infection
Consistency	Formed, soft, semisolid, moist	Hard, dry	Dehydration; decreased intestinal motility resulting from lack of fibre in diet, lack of exercise, emotional upset, laxative abuse
		Diarrhea	Increased intestinal motility (e.g., caused by irritation of the colon by bacteria)
Shape	Cylindrical (contour of rectum), about 2.5 cm in diameter in adults	Narrow, pencil-shaped, or string-like stool	Obstructive condition of the rectum
Amount	Varies with diet (about 100 g to 400 g per day)		
Odour	Aromatic: affected by ingested food and person's own bacterial flora	Pungent	Infection, blood
Constituents	Small amounts of undigested roughage, sloughed dead bacteria and epithelial cells, fat, protein, dried constituents of digestive juices (e.g., bile pigments), inorganic matter (calcium, phosphates)	Pus	Bacterial infection
		Mucus	Inflammatory condition
		Parasites	Pinworms, tapeworms, ascariasis
		Blood	Gastrointestinal bleeding
		Large quantities of fat	Malabsorption
		Foreign objects	Accidental ingestion

peristalsis of the colon after food has entered the stomach) is also an important consideration. For example, toileting is recommended 5 to 15 minutes after meals, especially after breakfast when the gastrocolic reflex is strongest (RNAO, 2011). Older adults with impaired mobility may have difficulty getting to the bathroom before the gastrocolic reflex wanes, making them more prone to constipation.

The older adult should be warned that consistent use of laxatives inhibits natural defecation reflexes and is thought to cause, rather than cure, constipation. The habitual user of laxatives eventually requires larger or stronger doses because the effect is progressively reduced with continual use. Laxatives can also interfere with the body's electrolyte balance and decrease the absorption of certain vitamins. The reasons for constipation can range from lifestyle habits (e.g., lack of exercise) to serious malignant disorders. The nurse should evaluate any complaints of constipation carefully for each individual. A change in bowel habits over several weeks with or without weight loss, pain, or fever should be referred to a physician for a complete medical evaluation.

Diet

Sufficient bulk (cellulose, fibre) in the diet is necessary to provide fecal volume. Dietary fibre in the range of 25 g to 30 g per day is recommended (RNAO, 2011). However, high-fibre diets with insufficient amounts of fluids can cause constipation. Insoluble fibre, such as that in whole wheat flour, wheat bran, nuts, and many vegetables, increases stool bulk and promotes the movement of fecal material through the digestive tracts. Soluble fibre, such as that found in fruits, oats, barley, and psyllium, also add to fecal bulk (see Chapter 39 for a complete discussion on the benefits of fibre). Low-residue foods, such as rice, eggs, and lean meats, move more slowly through the intestinal tract. Increasing fluid intake with such foods increases their rate of movement.

Certain foods are difficult or impossible for some people to digest. This inability results in digestive system upsets and, in some instances, the passage of watery stool. Irregular eating can also impair regular defecation. Individuals who eat at the same times every day usually have a regularly timed, physiological response to the food intake and a regular pattern of peristaltic activity in the colon.

Spicy foods can produce diarrhea and flatus in some individuals. Excessive sugar can also cause diarrhea. Other foods that can influence bowel elimination include the following:

- Gas-producing foods, such as cabbage, onions, cauliflower, bananas, and apples
- Foods with laxative effect, such as bran, prunes, figs, chocolate, and alcohol
- Constipation-producing foods, such as cheese, pasta, eggs, and lean meat

Fluid

When intake is inadequate or output (e.g., urine or vomitus) is excessive for any reason, the body continues to absorb fluid from chyme as it passes along the colon. As a result, chyme becomes drier than normal, resulting in hard feces. In addition, reduced fluid intake slows chyme's passage along the intestines, further increasing the reabsorption of fluid from chyme. Healthy fecal elimination usually requires a minimum daily fluid intake of 1500 mL to 2000 mL. Caffeine and alcoholic beverages should be limited because their diuretic properties result in a loss of fluid (RNAO, 2011). If chyme moves abnormally quickly through the large intestine, however, there is less time for fluid to be absorbed into the blood; as a result, feces are soft or even watery.

Activity

Activity stimulates peristalsis, thus facilitating the movement of chyme along the colon. Weak abdominal and pelvic muscles are often ineffective in increasing the intra-abdominal pressure during defecation or in controlling defecation. Weak muscles can result from lack of exercise, immobility, or impaired neurological functioning. Walking 15 to 20 minutes a day can aid in fecal elimination. Clients confined to bed are often constipated. Bedridden clients can be given exercises to perform, such as pelvic tilts, low trunk rotation, and single leg lift exercises.

Psychological Factors

Some people who are anxious or angry experience increased peristaltic activity and subsequent diarrhea. In contrast, people who are depressed may experience slower intestinal motility, which results in constipation. How a person responds to these emotional states is the result of individual differences in the response of the enteric nervous system to vagal stimulation from the brain.

Defecation Habits

Early bowel training can establish the habit of defecating at a regular time. Many people defecate after breakfast, when the gastrocolic reflex causes mass peristaltic waves in the large intestine. If a person ignores this urge to defecate, water continues to be absorbed, making the feces harder and more difficult to expel. When the normal defecation reflexes are inhibited or ignored, these conditioned reflexes tend to be progressively weakened. When habitually ignored, the urge to defecate is ultimately lost. Adults may ignore these reflexes because of the pressures of time or work. Hospitalized clients may suppress the urge because of embarrassment about using a bedpan, because of a lack of privacy, or because defecation is too uncomfortable. See the Clinical Alert box on warning signs of colorectal cancer.

! CLINICAL ALERT

Any client who complains of general discomfort in the abdomen (gas pains, bloating, fullness, or cramps), a change in bowel habits (e.g., diarrhea or constipation) for no apparent reason, bright red or very dark blood in stool, stool that is narrower than usual, vomiting, feeling very tired, and weight loss must immediately be referred for a complete health assessment, as these are signs and symptoms of colorectal cancer.

Medications

Some drugs have side effects that can interfere with normal elimination. Medications that have an anticholinergic effect (e.g., certain antihypertensive, antidepressant, and analgesic agents), antacids containing aluminum, iron supplements, opioids, antiparkinsonism drugs, and antihistamines are some of the common agents known to cause constipation.

Some medications directly affect elimination. **Laxatives** are medications that stimulate bowel activity and so assist fecal elimination. Other medications soften stool, facilitating defecation. Certain medications, such as dicyclomine hydrochloride, suppress peristaltic activity and sometimes are used to treat diarrhea.

Some medications affect the appearance of feces. Any drug that causes gastrointestinal bleeding (e.g., acetylsalicylic products) can cause stool to be red or black. Iron salts can cause stool to be black because of the oxidation of the iron; antibiotics can cause a grey-green discoloration because of effects on digestion; and antacids can cause a whitish discoloration or white specks in stool.

Diagnostic Procedures

Before certain diagnostic procedures, such as *colonoscopy* (visualization of the colon), the client is often restricted from ingesting food or fluid. The client may also be given a cleansing enema before the examination. In these instances, the client usually will not defecate normally until eating has resumed.

Anesthesia and Surgery

General anesthesia causes normal colonic movements to cease or slow down by blocking parasympathetic stimulation to the muscles of the colon. Clients who have regional or spinal anesthesia are less likely to experience this problem.

Surgery that involves direct handling of the intestines or the effects of general anesthesia can cause a **paralytic ileus**, a temporary paralysis (cessation) of intestinal movement causing obstruction that usually lasts 24 to 48 hours. Listening for bowel sounds that reflect intestinal motility is an important nursing assessment following surgery. See Chapter 28 for assessment of bowel sounds.

Pathological Conditions

Spinal cord injuries and acquired head injuries can decrease the sensory stimulation for defecation. Impaired mobility may limit the client's ability to respond to the urge to defecate when the client is unable to reach a toilet or summon assistance. As a result, the client may experience *constipation* or *fecal incontinence*. Poorly functioning sphincters can also result in *fecal incontinence*.

Pain

Clients who experience discomfort when defecating (e.g., following childbirth or in the presence of a rectal fissure) often suppress the urge to defecate to avoid the pain. Such clients can experience constipation as a result. Clients taking opioid analgesics for pain can also experience constipation as a side effect of the medication.

Fecal Elimination Problems

Five problems related to fecal elimination are (a) constipation, (b) fecal impaction, (c) diarrhea, (d) bowel incontinence, and (e) flatulence.

Constipation

Constipation may be defined as fewer than three bowel movements per week and the passage of small, dry, hard stool that is difficult to eliminate. It occurs when the movement of feces through the large intestine is slow, thus allowing time for additional absorption of fluid from the large intestine. Because of difficult evacuation of stool, there is increased effort or straining of the voluntary muscles of defecation. The person may also have a feeling of incomplete stool evacuation after defecation. It is important to define constipation in relation to the person's regular elimination pattern. Some people normally defecate only a few times a week; if their stool is soft in consistency, they are not considered to be constipated.

The Rome 111 diagnostic criteria (2006) identify that chronic constipation exists when a person experiences two of the following for at least 25% of defecations for at least 3 months, with symptom onset at least 6 months before diagnosis: straining, passage of lumpy or hard stool, sensation of incomplete evacuation, sensation of blockage in the rectum, the need for manual manoeuvres (e.g., digital stimulation) to prompt voiding, and fewer than three defecations a week. In addition, the presence of loose stool only with the use of laxatives would also be classified as constipation. Infants, toddlers, and children who are defecating large-diameter stool so large that it may even block the toilet or who experience painful or hard bowel movements or fecal incontinence or have fewer than two defecations a week need to be assessed for constipation. Careful assessment of the person's habits is necessary before a diagnosis of constipation is made. Box 41.1 lists the frequent defining characteristics of constipation. See the Evidence-Informed Practice box on constipation.

Many causes and factors contribute to constipation. Among them are the following:

- *Lifestyle related:* insufficient fibre intake, insufficient fluid intake, insufficient activity or immobility, irregular defecation habits, changes in daily routine, lack of privacy

- *Emotional disturbances:* for example, depression or mental confusion

---

BOX 41.1   SAMPLE DEFINING CHARACTERISTICS OF CONSTIPATION

Fewer than three defecations a week accompanied by one of the signs or symptoms below:

- Hard, dry, lumpy stool
- Straining or pain during defecation
- Sensation of incomplete bowel evacuation (often described as "fullness" or "pressure" in the rectum)
- Abdominal pain, cramps, or distension
- Anorexia, nausea
- Passage of stool large enough to block the toilet

EVIDENCE-INFORMED PRACTICE

Is Abdominal Massage an Effective Strategy in Relieving Constipation?

Constipation is an uncomfortable experience that can have an impact on someone's quality of life related to feeling "irregular" as well as cause potentially severe physical complications, such as rectal tears and fecal impaction. Canadians spend millions of dollars each year on products, some of them having risky side effects, aimed at relieving the problem. Abdominal massage was used in the 1870s as an intervention to treat constipation; it then fell out of favour but has now had a resurgence, particularly in palliative care, where constipation is a common experience arising from the use of opioids, reduced mobility, and fluid imbalance. It is hypothesized that manual abdominal massage increases intra-abdominal pressure and may elicit rectal waves in some cases, thus contributing to peristalsis and movement of the feces. This systematic review seeks to answer the clinical question: *Does abdominal massage decrease physical or psychological morbidity and symptom distress and improve quality of life in adults with a diagnosis of chronic idiopathic constipation?* The authors will look at all randomized controlled trials and quasi-randomized trials in their review. The review will also look at any adverse effects of this intervention—if the intervention is found to have no or slightly positive outcomes, it will be important to know if there are any negative outcomes that could outweigh the benefits.

NURSING IMPLICATIONS: Nurses spend a lot of time helping clients deal with such basic issues as elimination, and although there are many strategies that can be tried to help people with chronic constipation, having an inexpensive, relatively "easy to perform" strategy that is noninvasive would provide an ideal new option. Families and caregivers could easily learn this strategy if it is found to be effective.

Source: Based on McClurg D., Hagen S., & Dickinson L. (2011). Abdominal massage for the treatment of constipation (Protocol). *Cochrane Database of Systematic Reviews* 2011, *Issue* 4. Art. No.: CD009089. doi: 10.1002/14651858.CD009089

- *Medical conditions:* peripheral neurogenic disorders (e.g., diabetes mellitus); central neurogenic disorders (e.g., multiple sclerosis, Parkinson's disease, spinal cord injury); non-neurogenic disorder (e.g., hypothyroidism, hypokalemia, pregnancy, myotonic dystrophy)
- *Physiological condition:* pelvic floor dysfunction or muscle damage
- *Medications:* such as opioids, iron supplements, antacids, antidepressants, antihistamines, anticholinergics, anesthetics, calcium channel blockers, 5HT3 antagonists, or chronic use of laxatives or enemas

Constipation can cause health problems for some people. Straining associated with constipation often

is accompanied by holding the breath. This is called *Valsalva manoeuvre* and can present serious problems to people with heart disease, brain injuries, or respiratory disease. Holding the breath while bearing down increases intrathoracic and intracranial pressures. In addition, vagal tone is increased, resulting in a slowing of the heart rate (LeMone & Burke, 2008). To some degree, this pressure can be reduced if the person exhales through the mouth while straining. However, avoidance of straining altogether is the best precaution. Hemorrhoids and anal fissures (narrow openings in the anus) are also complications of constipation (Wray, Ijaz, & Lidder, 2008).

Fecal Impaction

Fecal impaction is a mass or collection of hardened feces in the folds of the rectum. Impaction results from prolonged retention and accumulation of fecal material. In severe impactions, the feces accumulate and extend well up into the sigmoid colon and beyond. A person who has fecal impaction can experience the passage of liquid fecal seepage that can be misconstrued as diarrhea. The liquid portion of the feces seeps out around the impacted mass (Figure 41.6). A careful health history and physical examination is necessary to ensure that the liquid seepage is not misdiagnosed as "diarrhea" rather than "seepage" around a hardened mass of fecal matter. Impaction can also be assessed by digital examination of the rectum, during which the hardened mass can often be palpated.

Along with fecal seepage and constipation, symptoms include frequent but nonproductive desire to defecate and rectal pain. A generalized feeling of illness results; the client becomes anorexic, the abdomen becomes distended, and nausea and vomiting may occur.

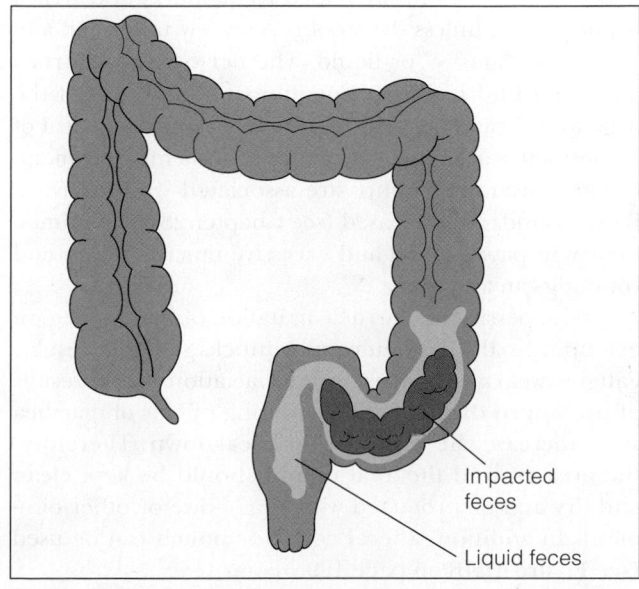

FIGURE 41.6 A fecal impaction with liquid feces passing around the impaction.

The causes of fecal impaction are usually poor defecation habits and constipation. Administration of some medications, such as anticholinergics and antihistamines, increase the risk of fecal impaction. Barium used in radiological examinations of the upper and lower gastrointestinal tracts can also be a causative factor. Therefore, after these examinations, measures are usually taken to ensure removal of the barium.

An impaction can sometimes be palpated through the client's abdomen. Digital examination of the impaction through the rectum should be done gently and carefully because stimulation of the vagus nerve in the rectal wall can slow the client's heart.

Fecal impaction can generally be prevented; however, digital removal of impacted feces is sometimes necessary. Although digital rectal examination is within the scope of nursing practice, some agency policies require a physician's order for digital manipulation and removal of a fecal impaction.

When fecal impaction is suspected, the client is often given an oil retention enema, a cleansing enema 2 to 4 hours later, and daily additional cleansing enemas, suppositories, or stool softeners, as prescribed by an appropriate member of the health care team. If these measures fail, manual removal is often necessary.

Diarrhea

Diarrhea refers to the passage of three or more loose (mushy) or watery feces per day or more frequently than is usual for that person (World Health Organization, 2011). It is the opposite of constipation and results from rapid movement of fecal contents through the large intestine. Rapid passage of chyme reduces the time available for the large intestine to absorb water and electrolytes. Some people pass stool with increased frequency, but diarrhea is not present unless the stool is relatively unformed and excessively "mushy" or liquid. The person with diarrhea may even find it difficult or impossible to control the urge to defecate for very long. Diarrhea and the threat of incontinence are sources of concern and embarrassment. Often, spasmodic cramps are associated with diarrhea. Bowel sounds are increased (see Chapter 28). Sometimes, the client passes blood and excessive mucus; nausea and vomiting can also occur.

With persistent diarrhea, irritation of the anal region extending to the perineum and buttocks generally results. Fatigue, weakness, malaise, and emaciation are the results of prolonged diarrhea. The irritating effects of diarrhea stool increase the risk for skin breakdown. Therefore, the area around the anal region should be kept clean and dry and be protected with zinc oxide or other ointment. In addition, a fecal collector pouch can be used (see Figure 41.18 on page 1294).

When irritants in the intestinal tract are the cause of diarrhea, the diarrhea is thought to be a protective flushing mechanism. It can create serious fluid and electrolyte losses (particularly sodium and potassium) in the body; however, this can develop within an alarmingly short time, particularly in infants and small children. Metabolic acidosis can result from the bicarbonate losses associated with diarrhea. Antibiotic therapy can cause diarrhea because the balance of microbes in the gastrointestinal tract is altered. The development of *Clostridium difficile*-associated diarrhea (CDAD), the most common health care–associated infectious diarrhea, carries a high risk because of the high mortality rate associated with this type of diarrhea (Macleod-Glover & Sadowski, 2010). In fact, over the last decade there has been a marked increase in the incidence and severity of CDAD in North America and Europe (O'Donoghue & Kyne, 2011). Unfortunately the antibiotic treatment used for this diarrhea can lead to an exacerbation of the diarrhea itself (Nelson, 2007). See Chapter 34 for a full discussion on *Clostridium difficile*. Osmotic diarrhea can develop in patients receiving tube feedings or ingesting laxatives that are hyperosmolar (see Chapter 44 for further discussion). Table 41.2 lists some of the major causes of diarrhea and the physiological responses of the body.

TABLE 41.2 Major Causes of Diarrhea

Cause	Physiological Effect
Psychological stress (e.g., anxiety)	Increased intestinal motility and mucus secretion
Medications:	
• Antibiotics	Inflammation and infection of mucosa caused by overgrowth of pathogenic intestinal microorganisms
• Iron	Irritation of intestinal mucosa
• Cathartics	Irritation of intestinal mucosa
Allergy to food, fluid, drugs	Incomplete digestion of food or fluid
Osmotic shifts	Administration of hyperosmolar solutions (e.g., concentrated elemental tube feeding; ingestion of large amounts of sweetened juices by children) into the intestinal tract causes fluid shifts into the gastrointestinal tract
Diseases of the colon:	
• Malabsorption syndrome	Reduced absorption of fluids
• Crohn's disease	Inflammation of the mucosa often leading to ulcer formation

Bowel Incontinence

Bowel incontinence, also called **fecal incontinence**, refers to the loss of voluntary ability to control fecal and gaseous discharges through the anal sphincter. The incontinence may occur at specific times, such as after meals, or it may occur irregularly. Two types of bowel incontinence are described: partial and major. *Partial incontinence* is the inability to control flatus or to prevent minor soiling. *Major incontinence* is the inability to control feces of normal consistency.

Fecal incontinence is generally associated with impaired functioning of the anal sphincter or its nerve supply, such as in some neuromuscular diseases, spinal cord trauma, and tumours of the external anal sphincter muscle.

Fecal incontinence is an emotionally distressing problem that can ultimately lead to social isolation. Affected persons withdraw into their homes or, if in the hospital, the confines of their room to minimize the embarrassment associated with soiling. They may come to prefer easily washable night garments to street clothes. Incontinent feces are acidic and contain digestive enzymes that are highly irritating to skin. Therefore, as with diarrhea, the area around the anal region should be kept clean and dry and be protected with zinc oxide or other ointment. In addition, a rectal pouch can be used. Several surgical procedures are also used for the treatment of fecal incontinence. These include repair of the sphincter and fecal diversion or colostomy.

Flatulence

Flatus, air or gas in the gastrointestinal tract, has three primary causes: (a) action of bacteria on the chyme in the large intestine, (b) swallowed air, and (c) gas that diffuses from the bloodstream into the intestine.

Flatulence is the presence of *excessive* flatus in the intestines and leads to stretching and inflation of the intestines (*intestinal distension*). This condition is also referred to as *abdominal distension*. Large amounts of air and other gases can accumulate in the stomach, resulting in gastric distension.

Most gases that are swallowed are expelled through the mouth by **eructation** (belching). The gases formed in the large intestine are chiefly absorbed through the intestinal capillaries into the circulation. Flatulence can occur in the colon from a variety of causes, such as foods (e.g., cabbage, onions), abdominal surgery, or opioid analgesics. If the gas is propelled by increased colon activity before it can be absorbed, it may be expelled through the anus. If excessive gas cannot be expelled through the anus, it may be necessary to insert a rectal tube or provide a return flow enema to remove it.

Bowel Diversion Ostomies

An **ostomy** is a surgically constructed artificial excretory opening. Bowel ostomies are named relative to their anatomical location in the bowel; for example, an **ileostomy** is an opening into the ileum (small bowel), and a **colostomy** is an opening into the colon (large bowel). Bowel ostomies divert and drain fecal material and are often classified according to (a) their status as permanent or temporary, (b) their anatomical location, and (c) the nature of the construction of the **stoma**, the opening created in the abdominal wall by the ostomy.

Permanence

Colostomies can be either temporary or permanent. Temporary colostomies are generally performed for traumatic injuries or inflammatory conditions of the bowel. They allow the distal diseased portion of the bowel to rest and heal. Permanent colostomies are performed to provide a means of elimination when the rectum or anus is nonfunctional as a result of a birth defect or a disease, such as cancer of the bowel.

Anatomical Location

An ileostomy generally empties from the distal end of the small intestine. A cecostomy empties from the cecum (the first part of the ascending colon). An ascending colostomy empties from the ascending colon. A transverse colostomy empties from the transverse colon. A descending colostomy empties from the descending colon. A sigmoidostomy empties from the sigmoid colon (Figure 41.7).

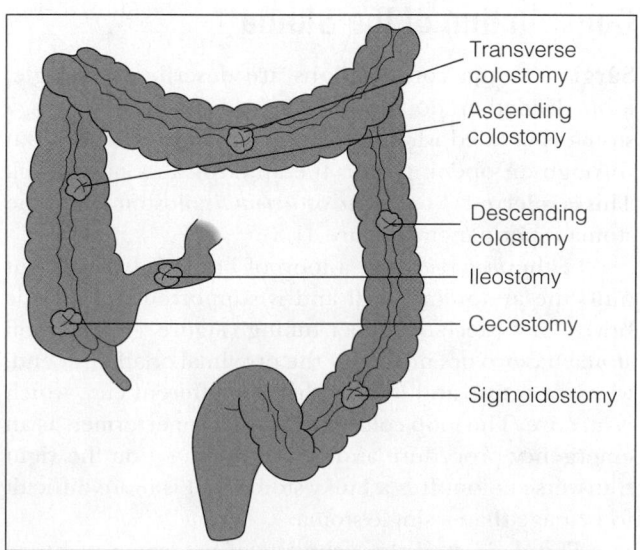

FIGURE 41.7 The locations of bowel diversion ostomies.

The location of the ostomy influences the character and management of the fecal drainage. The farther along the bowel its location, the more formed stool is because the large bowel absorbs water from the fecal mass. In addition, more control over the frequency of stomal discharge can be established:

- An ileostomy produces liquid fecal drainage. Drainage is constant and cannot be regulated. Ileostomy drainage contains some digestive enzymes, which are damaging to the skin. For this reason, ileostomy clients must wear an appliance continuously and take special precautions to prevent skin breakdown. Compared with colostomies, however, odour is minimal because fewer bacteria are present.

- An ascending colostomy is similar to an ileostomy in that the drainage is liquid and cannot be regulated, and digestive enzymes are present. Odour, however, is a problem requiring control (e.g., a deodorant inside the appliance).

- A transverse colostomy produces a malodorous, mushy drainage because some of the liquid has been absorbed. There is usually no control.

- A descending colostomy produces increasingly solid fecal drainage. Stool from a sigmoidostomy is of normal or formed consistency, and the frequency of discharge can be regulated. People with a sigmoidostomy may not have to wear an appliance at all times, and odours can usually be controlled.

The length of time that an ostomy is in place also helps determine the consistency of stool, particularly with transverse and descending colostomies. Over time, stool becomes more formed because the remaining functioning portions of the colon tend to compensate by increasing water absorption.

Construction of the Stoma

Surgical stoma constructions are described as single, loop, divided, or double-barrelled colostomies. The *single* stoma is created when one end of bowel is brought out through an opening onto the anterior abdominal wall. This is referred to as an *end* or *terminal* colostomy, and the stoma is permanent (Figure 41.8).

In the *loop colostomy,* a loop of bowel is brought out onto the abdominal wall and is supported by a plastic bridge or a piece of rubber tubing (Figure 41.9). A loop stoma has two openings: (a) the proximal or afferent end, which is active, and (b) the distal or efferent end, which is inactive. The loop colostomy is usually performed as an emergency procedure and is often situated on the right transverse colon. It is a bulky stoma that is more difficult to manage than a single stoma.

The *divided colostomy* consists of two edges of bowel brought out onto the abdomen but separated from each

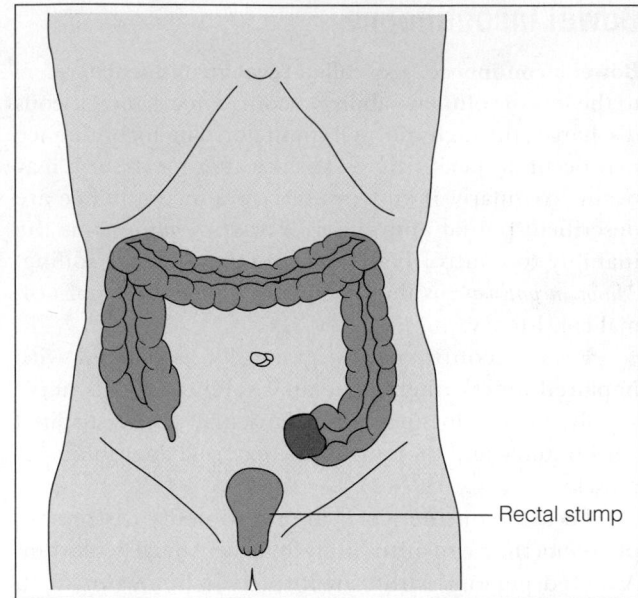

FIGURE 41.8 End colostomy; the diseased portion of bowel is removed and a rectal pouch remains.

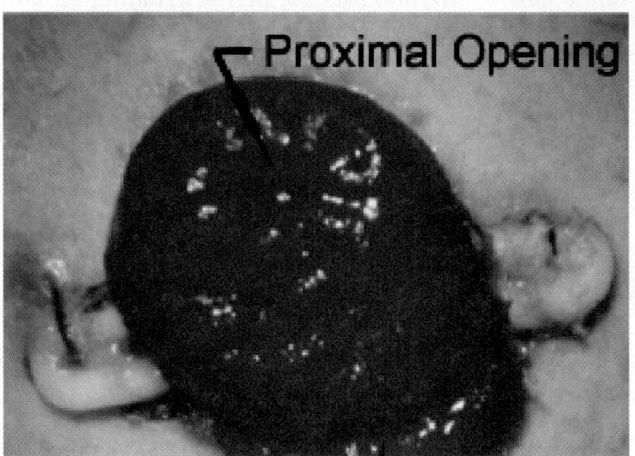

FIGURE 41.9 Loop colostomy.

other (Figure 41.10). The opening from the digestive or proximal end is the colostomy. The distal end in this situation is often referred to as a *mucous fistula,* since this section of bowel continues to secrete mucus. The divided colostomy is often used in situations where spillage of feces into the distal end of the bowel needs to be avoided.

The *double-barrelled colostomy* resembles a double-barrelled shotgun (Figure 41.11). In this type of colostomy, the proximal and distal loops of bowel are sutured together for about 10 cm and both ends are brought up onto the abdominal wall.

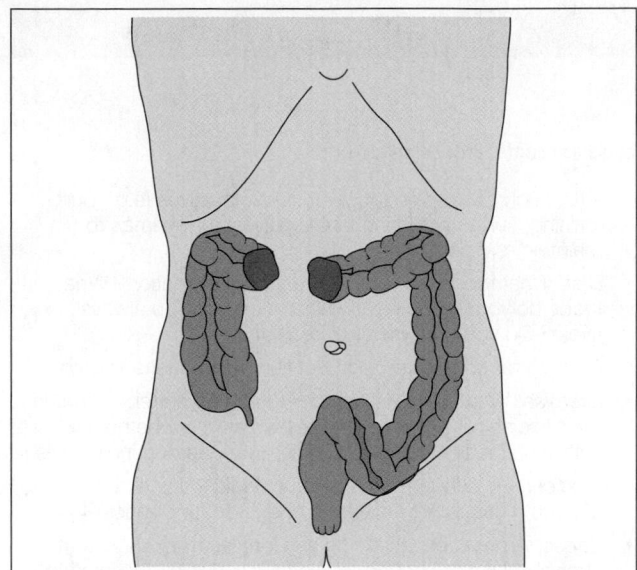

FIGURE 41.10 Divided colostomy with two separated stomas.

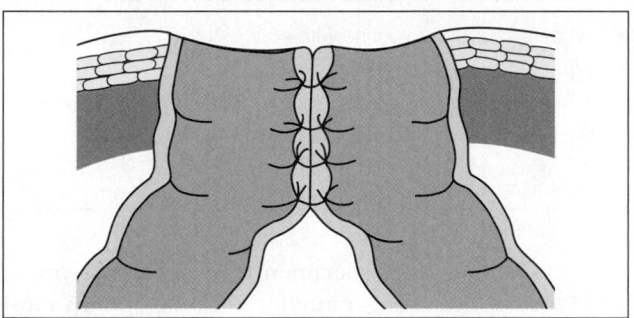

FIGURE 41.11 Double-barrelled colostomy.

Assessing

Assessment of fecal elimination includes taking a nursing history; performing a physical examination of the abdomen, rectum, and anus; and inspecting the feces. The nurse also should review any data obtained from relevant diagnostic tests.

Nursing History

A nursing history for fecal elimination helps the nurse ascertain the client's normal pattern. The nurse elicits a description of usual feces and any recent changes and collects information about any past or current problems with elimination, the presence of an ostomy, and factors influencing the elimination pattern.

Examples of interview questions to elicit this information are shown in the Assessment: Interview box on the next page. The number of questions to ask is adapted to the individual client, according to the client's responses in the first three categories. For example, questions about

factors influencing elimination might be addressed only to clients who are experiencing problems.

When eliciting data about the client's defecation pattern, the nurse needs to understand that the time of defecation and the amount of feces expelled are as individual as the frequency of defecation. Often, the patterns individuals follow depend largely on early training and on convenience.

Physical Examination

Physical examination of the abdomen in relation to fecal elimination problems includes inspection, auscultation, percussion, and palpation with specific reference to the intestinal tract. Auscultation precedes palpation because palpation can alter peristalsis. Examination of the rectum and anus includes inspection and palpation. Physical examination of the abdomen, rectum, and anus is discussed in Chapter 28.

Inspecting Feces

The client's stool is inspected for colour, consistency, shape, amount, odour, and the presence of abnormal constituents. See Table 41.1 (page 1269) for a summary of normal and abnormal characteristics of stool and possible causes.

Diagnostic Studies

Diagnostic studies of the gastrointestinal tract include direct and indirect visualization techniques and laboratory tests for abnormal constituents.

VISUALIZATION TECHNIQUES *Direct visualization techniques* are invasive and include **anoscopy**, the viewing of the anal canal; **proctoscopy**, the viewing of the rectum; **proctosigmoidoscopy**, the viewing of the rectum and sigmoid colon; and **colonoscopy**, the viewing of the large intestine. *Indirect visualization* of the gastrointestinal tract is noninvasive and achieved by radiography. Radiographs of the gastrointestinal tract can detect strictures, obstructions, tumours, ulcers, inflammatory disease, or other structural changes, such as hiatal hernias. Visualization of the tract is enhanced by the introduction of a radiopaque substance, such as barium. For examination of the upper gastrointestinal tract or small bowel, the client drinks barium sulphate. This examination is often referred to as a *barium swallow*. For examination of the lower gastrointestinal tract, the client is given an enema containing barium. This examination is commonly referred to as a *barium enema*. These radiographs usually include *fluoroscopic examination*, that is, projection of the x-ray films onto a screen that permits continuous observation of the flow of barium. Nurses are responsible for preparing clients before these studies and for follow-up care.

Fecal Elimination

The nurse can use these kinds of questions to gather information related to clients' fecal elimination:

DEFECATION PATTERN

- What is the frequency and time of day of defecation?
- Has this pattern changed recently?

DESCRIPTION OF FECES AND ANY CHANGES

- How would you describe your stool in terms of colour, texture (hard, soft, watery), shape, odour?
- Have you noticed any changes in your stool recently?

FECAL ELIMINATION PROBLEMS

- What problems have you had or do you now have with your bowel movements (constipation, diarrhea, excessive flatulence, seepage, or incontinence)?
- When and how often does it occur?
- What do you think causes it (food, fluids, exercise, emotions, medications, disease, surgery)?
- What have you done to try to solve the problem, and how effective was it?

FACTORS INFLUENCING ELIMINATION

- *Use of elimination aids.* What routines do you follow to maintain your usual defecation pattern? Do you use natural aids, such as specific foods or fluids, laxatives (e.g., bulk forming, surfactant, stimulant laxatives), or enemas to maintain elimination?
- *Diet.* What foods do you believe affect defecation? What foods do you typically eat? What foods do you always avoid? Do you take meals at regular times?
- *Fluid.* What amount and kind of fluid do you take each day?
- *Exercise.* What is your usual daily exercise pattern? (Obtain specifics about exercise, rather than asking whether it is sufficient; ideas of what is sufficient vary among individuals.)
- *Medications.* Have you taken any medications that could affect the gastrointestinal tract (e.g., iron, antibiotics)?
- *Stress.* Are you experiencing any long-term or short-term stressors? If so, what are these? Do you think these affect your defecation pattern? How?

PRESENCE AND MANAGEMENT OF BOWEL OSTOMY

- What is your usual routine with your ostomy?
- What type of appliance do you wear?
- What problems, if any, do you have with it?
- How can the nurses help you manage your ostomy?

Laboratory Tests

COLLECTING STOOL SPECIMENS Some of the reasons for testing feces include determining the presence of **occult blood** (hidden blood) that can result from gastrointestinal ulcers, inflammatory disease, or tumours; assessing for **steatorrhea** (fat in stool) that can result from faulty absorption of fat from the small intestine due to reduced bile flow from certain types of liver or gallbladder disease; detecting the presence of ova and parasites, bacteria and viruses. Before obtaining a specimen, the nurse needs to determine the reason for collecting a stool specimen and the correct method of obtaining and handling it (e.g., how much stool to obtain, whether a preservative needs to be added to stool, and whether it needs to be sent immediately to the laboratory). It may be necessary to confirm this information by checking with the agency laboratory. In many situations, only a single specimen is required; in others, timed specimens are necessary, and every stool passed is collected within a designated period.

Nurses need to give clients the following instructions:

- Defecate in a clean bedpan or bedside commode.
- If possible, do not contaminate the specimen with urine or menstrual discharge. Void before the specimen collection.
- Do not place toilet tissue in the bedpan after defecation. Contents of the paper can affect the laboratory analysis.
- Notify the nurse as soon as possible after defecation, particularly for specimens that need to be sent to the laboratory immediately.

To secure a stool specimen from a baby or young child who is not toilet trained, the nurse obtains most recently passed feces from the diaper.

When obtaining stool samples, that is, when handling the client's bedpan, when transferring the stool sample to a specimen container, and when disposing of the bedpan contents, the nurse follows aseptic technique meticulously. Wear disposable gloves to prevent hand contamination, and take care not to contaminate the outside of the specimen container. Use one or two clean tongue blades to transfer the specimen to the container and then wrap them in a paper towel before disposing of them in the waste container. This practice lessens the chance of contact with other articles and the spread of microorganisms. The amount of stool to be sent depends on the purpose for which the specimen is collected. Usually about 2.5 cm of formed stool or 15 mL to 30 mL of liquid stool is adequate. For some timed specimens, however, the entire passed stool may need to be sent. Visible pus, mucus, or blood should be included in sample specimens. For a stool culture, the nurse dips a sterile swab into the specimen, preferably where purulent fecal matter is present and, by using sterile technique, places the swab in a sterile test tube.

Because fresh specimens provide the most accurate results, the nurse sends the specimen to the laboratory immediately. If this is not possible, the nurse follows the directions on the specimen container. In some instances, refrigeration is indicated because bacteriological changes take place in stool specimens left at room temperature.

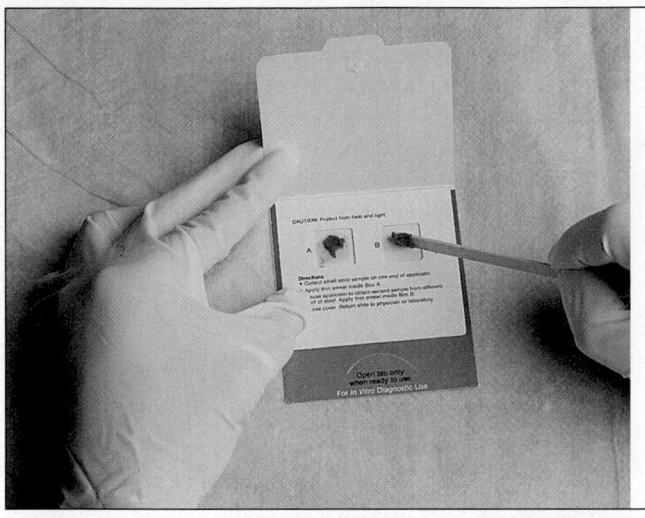
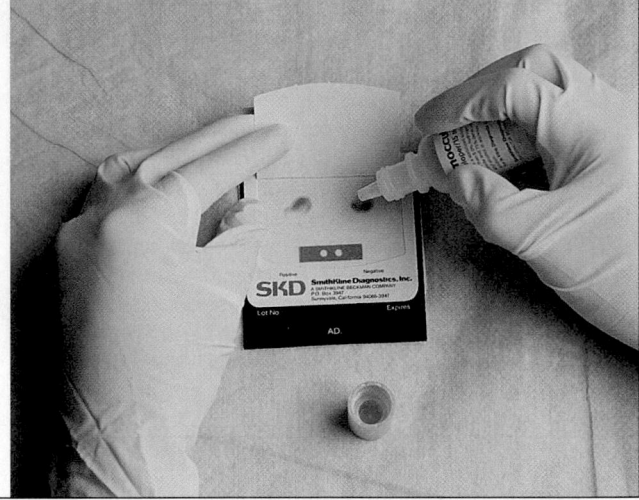

A   **B**

FIGURE 41.12 A: Opening the front cover of a Hemoccult slide and applying a thin smear of feces on the slide; **B:** Opening the flap on the back of the slide and applying two drops of reagent over each smear.

Fecal Occult Blood Testing (FOBT) Stool is tested for occult (hidden) blood to detect gastrointestinal bleeding not visible to the eye. Bleeding can occur as a result of such health problems as ulcers, inflammatory disease, or tumours. Two methods for testing stool for occult blood are the guaiac method (e.g., *Hemoccult test)* and the immunochemical method (e.g., *fecal immunochemical test [FIT]*). The former method involves using a wooden stick to smear a small amount of stool on a card with guaiac paper. The card is turned over and hydrogen peroxide is then applied to the smear on the back of the card to check for the presence of the enzyme peroxidise in the hemoglobin molecule. A blue discoloration indicates a guaiac-positive result—that is, the presence of occult blood. No colour change or any colour other than blue is a negative finding, indicating the absence of blood in stool (Figure 41.12). The guaiac method uses three samples over 3 days; and the client must follow detailed instructions, as the test can yield a false positive in the presence of medications that can cause gastrointestinal bleeding (e.g., acetylsalicylic acid), animal hemoglobin (e.g., beef, lamb, liver), or vitamin C. The Teaching: Clinical box has the instructions that need to be given to the client. The FIT is specific to human hemoglobin and requires a single sample for analysis. There are no dietary or medication restrictions with the FIT. While much easier for clients to use, most Canadian provinces or territories do not cover the cost of the test. Both methods

---

TEACHING | CLINICAL

Assessing Stool for Occult Blood Using Guaiac Method

The following are guidelines for clients to assess their stool for occult blood using the guaiac method:

- Avoid restricted foods, medications, and vitamin C for the period recommended by the manufacturer and during the test. Usually, specified foods and vitamin C are restricted for 3 days before the test and specified medications for 7 days before the test, as recommended by the physician.

- Use a ballpoint pen to label the specimens with your name, address, age, and date of specimen. Usually, three specimens are collected from consecutive and different bowel movements. Each specimen must be dated accurately.

- Avoid collecting specimens during your menstrual period and for 3 days afterward or while you have bleeding hemorrhoids or blood in your urine.

- Remove toilet bowl cleaners from the toilet bowl. Flush the toilet twice before proceeding with the test.

- Avoid contaminating the specimen with urine or toilet tissue. Empty your bladder before the test. To facilitate specimen collection, transfer the stool specimen to a clean, dry container. Wear disposable gloves.

- Use the tongue blade provided to transfer the specimen to the test folder or tape. Only a small amount of stool is required. Take the sample from the centre of a formed stool to ensure a uniform sample.

- Wrap the tongue blade in a paper towel and dispose of it in the waste receptacle. Do not flush the stick.

- Follow the manufacturer's directions explicitly for the test product being used. Test products vary. For example, for the *Hemoccult test,* a thin layer of feces is smeared over the boxes inside the envelope, and when complete the envelope is either directly returned or mailed (using special envelopes); the test centre will then apply a developing solution to the opposite side of the specimen paper. For the *Hematest,* a thin layer of feces is smeared onto guaiac filter paper, sent in for assessment, a tablet is placed in the middle of the specimen, and two or three drops of water are added to the tablet.

- Consult your health care provider if there is any problem understanding the instructions.

- Return completed specimens to your health care provider or laboratory, as instructed.

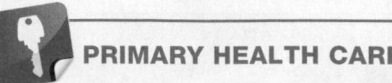

can be used at home and mailed to testing centres for analysis. Chapter 28 discusses FOBT recommendations for colorectal cancer screening guidelines for average-risk Canadians.

See the Reflect on Primary Health Care box on healthy fecal elimination.

Diagnosing

Possible diagnoses related to fecal elimination problems can include: constipation as evidenced by meeting the Rome 111 diagnostic criteria; risk for constipation related to such factors as reduced mobility, inadequate fluid intake, reduced fibre intake, and/or medications affecting peristalsis; bowel incontinence, as evidenced by involuntary passage of stool; diarrhea, as evidenced by the passage of loose, unformed stool.

Because fecal elimination problems can affect many areas of human functioning, other possible nursing

diagnoses include the following: risk for isoosmolar or hyperosmolar fluid volume deficit related to diarrhea; risk for metabolic acidosis related to loss of bicarbonate in diarrhea; risk for impaired skin integrity related to diarrhea or ostomy device; risk for perianal fissure related to passage of hard stool; risk for negative body image related to bowel ostomy or uncontrolled bowel movements. (See Table 41.3.)

Planning

The major goals for clients with fecal elimination problems are to do the following:

- Maintaining or restoring normal bowel elimination pattern
- Maintaining or regaining normal stool consistency
- Preventing associated risks, such as fluid and electrolyte imbalance, skin breakdown, abdominal distension, and pain

Examples of desired outcomes related to each of these goals, although established in the planning phase, are provided in the "Evaluating" section of this chapter.

Appropriate nursing interventions that relate to these broad goals must be identified. Preventive and corrective interventions to maintain or enhance fecal elimination include such strategies as promoting regular defecation, teaching about medications that influence fecal elimination, relieve impaction (such as by digital removal or administering enemas), implementing bowel training programs, and helping clients manage ostomy care, to name a few.

Sample nursing activities related to helping a client with altered bowel elimination are provided in the Sample Care Plan.

TABLE 41.3 Clinical Application: Assessment Data and Exemplar Nursing Diagnoses

Data Cluster	Nursing Diagnosis
Mrs. Amy Ballaster states she feels fullness in her rectum and wants to move her bowels but cannot, even with straining. Her last bowel movement was 4 days ago and was "lumpy." She lives alone and tends to eat only tea, toast, and noodle soup. Because of arthritis, her activities (gardening and walking) have decreased. Bowel sounds are decreased.	Constipation related to inadequate physical activity and insufficient fibre in diet
Marvin Lombardi reports having 4–5 loose, liquid, light brown stool per day for 2 days. Passage of stool is associated with cramping abdominal pain. Bowel sounds are increased; his abdomen is soft and not distended. Temperature is 38°C. He has not taken any medications but reports a feeling of general malaise. He states he "ate at a fast-food restaurant 2 nights ago."	Diarrhea of unknown etiology, possibly related to food contamination; at risk for fluid, electrolyte imbalance
Mary Kuoko has had involuntary leakage of stool. She states her clothing is soiled several times a day. She says she is too embarrassed to go out with her friends because of the fecal odour. Last bowel movement was more than 4 days ago. Digital examination reveals impaction.	Bowel incontinence related to fecal impaction; at risk for skin breakdown and social isolation

Sample Care Plan for Altered Bowel Elimination

ASSESSMENT DATA

Nursing Assessment

Mrs. Anna Margaret Brown is 78 years old. She has been a widow for 9 months. She lives alone in a low-income housing complex for older people. Her two children live with their families in a city approximately 240 km away. She always enjoyed cooking for her family; however, now that she is alone, she does not cook for herself. As a result, she has developed irregular eating patterns and tends to prepare soup-and-toast meals. She gets little exercise and has bouts of insomnia since her husband's death. For the past month, Mrs. Brown has been having a problem with constipation. She states she has a bowel movement about every 3 to 4 days, and her stool is hard and painful to excrete. Mrs. Brown decides to attend the health fair sponsored by the housing complex and seeks assistance from the public health nurse who arranges to meet with Mrs. Brown in her apartment.

Physical Examination

Height: 162 cm

Weight: 65 kg

Temperature: 36.2°C

Pulse: 82 beats/min

Respirations: 20/min

Blood pressure: 128/74 mm Hg

Active bowel sounds in all four quadrants approximately 15/min; LLQ (lower left quadrant) of her abdomen slightly distended; no abdominal mass; hard and mobile feces in rectum on digital examination

Diagnostic Data

Urinalysis: negative

FOBT: negative

Nursing Diagnosis

Constipation related to low-fibre diet and inactivity, as evidenced by infrequent, hard stool; painful defecation; abdominal distension; may be having difficulty coping with the loss of her husband, as evidenced by the change in sleeping and exercise habits; at risk for social isolation;

it is a strength that she is seeking help from the public health nurse.

Client Goals

Mrs. Brown will (a) establish a regular pattern of bowel elimination, (b) develop and maintain an exercise program, and (c) initiate nutritional alterations that will enhance regular bowel elimination. The nurse also identified goals related to coping with loss however these are not discussed at this time.

Desired Health Outcomes

1. Increases daily fluid intake to 1500 mL to 2000 mL unless contraindicated
2. Obtains a daily intake of 25–30 g fibre in her diet
3. Increases physical activity with an aim to takes part in at least 2.5 hours of moderate- to vigorous-intensity aerobic activity each week, potentially spread out into sessions of 10 minutes or more if need be (in accordance with *Canada's Physical Activity Guide* for people >65 years).
4. Verbalizes relief of constipation by the second week

Nursing Interventions	Rationale
Constipation Management	
• Identify factors (e.g., medications, activity level, diet) that can cause or contribute to constipation.	*Assessing causative factors is an essential first step in teaching and planning for improved bowel elimination.*
• Encourage increased fluid intake, unless contraindicated.	*Sufficient fluid intake is necessary for the bowel to absorb sufficient amounts of liquid and promote proper stool consistency.*
• Evaluate her medication profile for gastrointestinal side effects.	*Constipation is a common side effect of many drugs, including opioid analgesics and antacids.*
• Teach Mrs. Brown how to keep a food diary.	*An appraisal of food intake will help identify whether Mrs. Brown is eating a well-balanced diet and consuming adequate amounts of fluid and fibre.*
• Instruct Mrs. Brown on a high-fibre diet.	*Fibre absorbs water, which adds bulk and softness to stool and speeds up passage through the intestines.*
• Instruct her on the relationship of diet, exercise, and fluid intake to constipation.	*Fibre without adequate fluid can aggravate, not facilitate, bowel function.*

Nursing Interventions	Rationale
Promotion of Physical Activity	
• Encourage verbalization of feelings about exercise or the need for exercise.	*Perceptions of the need for exercise can be influenced by misbeliefs, cultural and social beliefs, fears, or age.*
• Teach about *Canada's Physical Activity Guide* for older adults >65 years (see Chapter 39, "Activity and Exercise")	Canada's Physical Activity Guide *for older adults takes into account the health benefits and challenges of performing regular activity for Canadians over age 65 years; spreading out the activity into 10 minute sessions will likely be manageable for Mrs. Brown as she begins to increase her activity.*
• Assist in identifying an exercise "partner" (e.g., neighbour or friend), if desired by the client.	*Exercising with someone else may assist Mrs. Brown by providing incentive and enhancing motivation. Activity influences bowel elimination by improving muscle tone and stimulating peristalsis, including other cardiovascular and general health benefits.*

(continued)

Sample Care Plan for Altered Bowel Elimination (continued)

Nursing Interventions	Rationale

Promotion of Physical Activity

- Inform Mrs. Brown about the health benefits and physiological effects of exercise.

- Assist Mrs. Brown to set short-term and long-term goals for the exercise program.

Mrs. Brown's age and lack of activity should be considered in planning the level of activity.

Realistic goal setting provides direction and motivation.

EVALUATION

Goals partially met. Mrs. Brown has kept a food diary and is able to identify the need for more fluid and fibre but has not consistently included fibre in her diet. Her daily intake of fluid and nutrients is best when she is socializing (e.g., eating with neighbour, friends, family) but inadequate when she is alone. She has started a walking program with a neighbour and has been able to progress to brisk walks lasting for 10 minutes but only four times a week. She has enjoyed these walks but worries about falling—she and her walking partner are exploring a local community centre for an exercise program. She states her last bowel movement was 2 days ago and that it was not hard and therefore easy to pass. She has started taking an OTC bulk-forming laxative.

Planning for Home Care

Clients who have bowel diversion ostomies requiring fecal incontinence pouches, or who have other ongoing elimination problems, will need continuing care in the home setting. In preparation for discharge, the nurse needs to assess the client's and the family's abilities to meet specific care needs. The Assessment: Home Care box on fecal elimination outlines the specific assessment data required before developing a home care plan. By using the assessment data, the nurse designs a teaching plan for the client and family (see the Teaching: Home Care box on fecal elimination).

ASSESSMENT | **HOME CARE**

Fecal Elimination

Assess the following to aid in developing a home care plan:

CLIENT AND ENVIRONMENT

- *Self-care abilities for toileting:* Ability to get to the toilet, to manipulate clothing for toileting, to perform toilet hygiene, and to flush the toilet

- *Mechanical aids required:* Walker, cane, wheelchair, raised toilet seat, grab bars, bedpan, commode

- *Mechanical barriers that limit access to the toilet or are unsafe:* Poor lighting, cluttered pathway to bathroom, narrow doorway for wheelchair, and so on

- *Bowel elimination problem:* Alterations in characteristics of feces, diarrhea, constipation, incontinence, presence of ostomy, and methods of handling these

- *Level of knowledge:* Planned bowel management or training program, prescribed medications, ostomy care, dietary alterations, and fluid and exercise requirements or restrictions

- *Facilities:* Adequacy of bathroom facilities to make possible toilet hygiene and ostomy care, and to contain potentially infectious fecal effluent or stool

FAMILY

- *Caregiver availability and skills:* People able to assist with toileting, medications, ostomy care, or other prescribed therapeutic measures

- *Family role changes and coping:* Effect on financial status, parenting and spousal roles, sexuality, social roles

- *Alternative potential primary or respite caregivers:* For example, other family members, volunteers, church members, paid caregivers or housekeeping services; available community respite care (adult daycare, senior centres)

COMMUNITY

- *Availability of and familiarity with possible sources of assistance:* Equipment and supply companies, financial assistance, home care agencies

TEACHING HOME CARE

Fecal Elimination

The nurse uses the assessment data to create a teaching plan for the client and family:

Facilitating Toileting

- Ensure safe and easy access to the toilet. Make sure lighting is appropriate, scatter rugs are removed or securely fastened, and so on.
- Facilitate instruction, as needed, about transfer techniques. Contact a physical therapist or other appropriate health care professional.
- Suggest ways that garments can be adjusted to make disrobing easier for toileting (e.g., Velcro closing on clothing).

Monitoring Bowel Elimination Pattern

- If appropriate, instruct the client to keep a record of the time and frequency of stool passage, any associated pain, and colour and consistency of stool.

Dietary Alterations

- Provide information about required food and fluid alterations to promote defecation (see the Teaching: Wellness box on healthy defecation and Teaching: Clinical box on managing diarrhea).

Medications

- Discuss problems associated with the overuse of laxatives, if appropriate, and the use of alternatives to laxatives, suppositories, and enemas.

- Discuss the addition of a fibre supplement if the client is taking a constipating medication (e.g., opioid analgesic).

Measures Specific to Elimination Problem

- Provide instructions associated with specific elimination problems and treatment, such as the following:
  - Constipation
  - Diarrhea
  - Ostomy care

Community Agencies and Other Sources of Help

- Make appropriate referrals to home care or community care for assistance with resources, such as installation of grab bars and raised toilet seats, structural alterations for wheelchair access, homemaker or home care aide services to assist with the activities of daily living (ADLs), and an enterostomal therapy nurse for assistance with stoma care and selection of ostomy appliances.
- Provide information about companies from which durable medical equipment (e.g., raised toilet seats, commodes, bedpans, urinals) can be purchased, rented, or obtained free, and where medical supplies, such as incontinence pads or ostomy irrigating supplies and appliances, can be obtained.
- Suggest additional sources of information and help, such as ostomy self-help and support groups or clubs.

TEACHING WELLNESS

Healthy Defecation

Nurses should teach clients how to achieve regular defecation:

- Establish a regular exercise regimen.
- Include high-fibre foods (25 g to 30 g a day), such as vegetables, fruits, and whole grains, in the diet.
- Maintain fluid intake of at least 1500 mL to 2000 mL a day.

- Do not ignore the urge to defecate.
- Allow time to defecate, preferably at the same time each day.
- Avoid over-the-counter medications to treat constipation and diarrhea.

TEACHING CLINICAL

Managing Diarrhea

Ensure the client follows these guidelines in managing diarrhea:

- Ensure oral rehydration with frequent, small amounts of liquids (preferably isotonic) in amounts to meet daily fluid requirements (1.5 L to 2 L per day) to prevent dehydration in adults.
- Avoid alcohol, beverages with caffeine, foods and liquids with a lot of sugar (e.g., carbonated soft drinks,

gelatine desserts), and excessively hot or cold fluids, which aggravate the problem.

- Ingest foods with sodium and potassium. Most foods contain sodium. Potassium is found in dairy products, meats, and many vegetables and fruits, especially tomatoes, potatoes, bananas, cantaloupe, and apricots.

TEACHING CLINICAL (continued)

- Limit foods containing insoluble fibre, such as whole-wheat and whole-grain breads and cereals, and raw fruits and vegetables.
- Increase foods containing soluble fibre, such as rice, oatmeal, and skinless fruits and potatoes.
- Limit fatty foods (e.g., dairy products and packaged processed meats).
- Thoroughly clean and dry the perianal area after passing stool to prevent skin irritation and breakdown. Use soft toilet tissue to clean and dry the area. Apply a moisture-barrier cream or ointment, such as zinc oxide or petrolatum, or an alcohol-free film barrier, as needed.

- Discontinue medications, as recommended by the physician, that cause diarrhea.
- Ingest foods containing probiotics, such as fermented dairy products like yogourt or yogourt drinks.
- Consult a health care provider immediately if weakness, dizziness, change in mental status, or high output of diarrhea, or if diarrhea persists more than 48 hours, or if there are alarming physical assessment findings (e.g., high fever, rigid abdomen, blood in the feces, persistent vomiting, hypotension). Children with diarrhea accompanied with vomiting or who have a fever or who are less than 6 months of age must be referred for complete medical assessment.

Implementing

Promoting Regular Defecation

The nurse can help clients achieve regular defecation by attending to (a) the provision of privacy, (b) timing, (c) nutrition and fluids, (d) exercise, and (e) positioning. See the Teaching: Wellness box on healthy defecation on the previous page.

PRIVACY Privacy during defecation is extremely important to many people. The nurse should, therefore, provide as much privacy as possible to clients but may need to stay with clients who are too weak to be left alone. Some clients also prefer to wipe, wash, and dry themselves after defecating. A nurse may need to provide water and a washcloth and towel for this purpose. Clients should be assisted with hand hygiene following defecation. (See the Clinical Alert box on hand hygiene.)

TIMING A client should be encouraged to defecate when the urge to defecate is recognized. To establish regular bowel elimination, the client and nurse can discuss when mass peristalsis normally occurs and provide time for defecation. Many people have well-established times and routines for defecation that should be part of the client's schedule. Other activities, such as bathing and ambulating, should not interfere with the defecation time. Also, clients should not be hurried and should be given adequate time to defecate.

NUTRITION AND FLUIDS The diet a client needs for regular normal elimination varies, depending on the kind of feces the client currently has, the frequency of defecation, and the types of foods that the client finds assist normal defecation.

For Constipation Have the client increase daily fluid intake, and instruct the client to drink hot liquids and fruit juices, especially prune juice. Encourage the client to include fibre in the diet, that is, such foods as prunes, raw fruit, bran products, and whole-grain cereals and bread.

For Diarrhea Encourage oral intake of isotonic fluids and bland food; have the client avoid foods with a high sugar content as these may contribute to osmotic shifts and exacerbate the diarrhea. Children may require oral rehydration solutions (e.g., Pedialyte) to prevent dehydration. Eating small amounts of bland foods can be helpful because they are more easily absorbed. Diarrhea can lead to potassium loss. See the discussion of hypokalemia in Chapter 44. Excessively hot or cold fluids should be avoided because they stimulate peristalsis. In addition, highly spiced foods and high-fibre foods can aggravate diarrhea. The BRAT (bananas, rice, applesauce, toast) diet was popular at one time, but there is no evidence to support its effectiveness; in fact, the BRAT diet alone does not provide sufficient fluid or electrolytes to meet daily requirements. There is evidence that when used along with rehydration therapy, probiotics (e.g., *Lactobacillus* or *Bifidobacterium*) are safe and have beneficial effects in shortening the duration (by as much as 25 hours) and reducing stool frequency in acute infectious diarrhea (Allen, Martinez, Gregorio, & Dans, 2010). See the Teaching: Clinical box on managing diarrhea (above).

CLINICAL ALERT

Hand hygiene is an essential preventative measure to reduce the spread of antibiotic resistant organisms and to decrease health care–associated infections (HCAIs). Nurses can aid in the reduction of these drug-resistant bacteria by promoting good hand hygiene practices with visitors and staff members. The use of alcohol-based hand rub (ABHR) is considered the gold standard for hand hygiene in most health care facilities; however, concern has been raised about their lack of efficacy against spore-forming organisms like *Clostridium difficile* (Allegranzi & Pittet, 2009). In a clinical review by MacLeod-Glover and Sadowski (2010), it was reported that the use of ABHR is unlikely to negatively or positively influence the rate of CDAD. In another study on ABHR, the conclusion was that overall hand hygiene compliance may be a more significant factor when attempting to control the spread of *C. difficile* infection than the actual hand hygiene product that is used (Knight, Strait, Anthony, Lovell, Norton, Sautter, & Scobey, 2010).

EXERCISE   Regular exercise helps clients develop a regular defecation pattern. A client with weak abdominal and pelvic muscles (which impede normal defecation) may be able to strengthen them with the following isometric exercises:

- In a supine position, the client tightens the abdominal muscles as though pulling them inward, holding them for about 10 seconds, and then relaxing them. This should be repeated 5 to 10 times, four times a day, depending on the client's health.

- Again in a supine position, the client can contract the thigh muscles and hold them contracted for about 10 seconds, repeating the exercise 5 to 10 times, four times a day. This helps the client confined to bed gain strength in the thigh muscles, thereby making it easier to use a bedpan.

POSITIONING   Although the squatting position best facilitates defecation, on a toilet seat the best position for most people seems to be leaning forward.

For clients who have difficulty moving themselves to and from the toilet, an elevated toilet seat can be attached to a regular toilet. Clients then do not have to lower themselves far down onto the seat and do not have to lift themselves as far off the seat. Elevated toilet seats can be purchased for use in the home.

A bedside **commode**, a portable chair with a toilet seat and a receptacle beneath that can be emptied, is often used for the adult client who can get out of bed but is unable to walk to the bathroom. Some commodes can slide over the base of a regular toilet when the waste receptacle is removed, thus providing clients the privacy of a bathroom. Some commodes have a seat and can be used as a chair (Figure 41.13). Potty chairs are available for children.

Clients restricted to bed may need to use a **bedpan**, a receptacle for urine and feces. Female clients use a bedpan for both urine and feces; male clients use a bedpan for feces and a urinal for urine.

There are two main types of bedpans, the regular high-back pan and the slipper, or fracture, pan (Figure 41.14). The slipper pan has a low back and is used for clients unable to raise their buttocks because of physical problems or therapy that contraindicates such movement. Many older adults benefit from the use of a slipper pan. See Practice Guidelines 41.1 on the next page, about giving and removing a bedpan. Many agencies are using biodegradable moulded pulp paper bedpans as an infection control measure. Follow the manufacturer's instructions on how to dispose of the bedpan and its contents. Clients are positioned on to the moulded pulp bedpans in the same manner as the conventional bedpans.

Teaching about Medications

Laxatives are drugs that ease or stimulate defecation. They can act either directly on the fecal matter, such as by reducing the surface tension of stool, or by affecting the intestine, such as inhibiting water absorption in the bowel thus increasing intraluminal electrolytes and water. Most laxatives produce a *laxative effect* that leads

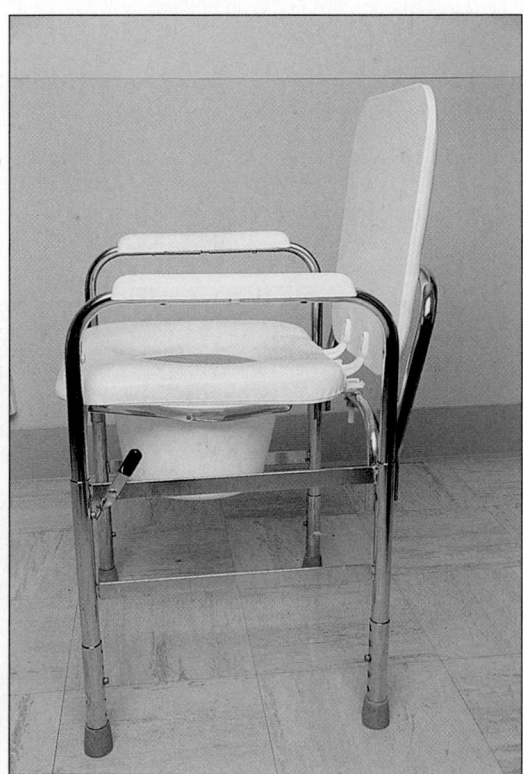

FIGURE 41.13 A commode with overlying seat.

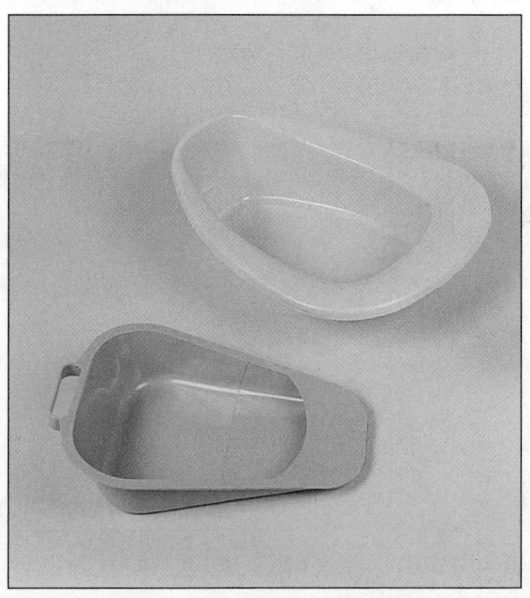

FIGURE 41.14 Top: The high-back or regular bedpan; **Bottom:** The slipper or fracture pan.

PRACTICE GUIDELINES 41.1

Giving and Removing a Bedpan

Guidelines	Rationales
Perform hand hygiene, and follow appropriate infection prevention and control procedures. Put on disposable gloves.	*Routine practices and additional precautions prevent the spread of infection.*
Provide privacy.	*Procedures involving elimination are embarrassing to most clients.*
If the bedpan is metal, warm it by rinsing it with warm water.	*A warmed bedpan will help to promote comfort and sphincter relaxation.*
Elevate the side rail on the opposite side to prevent the client from falling out of bed.	*Raising the side rail will help prevent the client from falling out of bed.*
Adjust the bed to a height appropriate to prevent back strain. Ask the client to assist by flexing the knees, resting the weight on the back and heels, and raising the buttocks, or by using a trapeze bar, if present.	*The use of proper body mechanics decreases the risk of injury to the nurse. Encourage the client to participate in self-care when able.*
Help the client with lifting, as needed, by placing one hand under the lower back, resting your elbow on the mattress, and using your forearm as a lever.	*The use of proper lifting techniques prevents injury to the nurse's back and increases the client's sense of security.*
Place a regular bedpan so that the client's buttocks rest on the smooth, rounded rim. Place a slipper pan with the flat, low end under the client's buttocks (Figure 41.15).	*Proper positioning of the bedpan promotes client comfort and avoids spillage.*
For the client who cannot assist, obtain the assistance of another nurse to help place the client onto the bedpan. Turn the client on his or her side, place the bedpan against the buttocks (Figure 41.16), and roll the client back onto the bedpan.	*Obtaining assistance ensures that the nurse does not sustain a back injury. The client movement to the side and then back ensures proper placement of the bedpan without having to lift the client.*
To provide a more normal position for the client's lower back, elevate the client's bed to a semi-Fowler's position, if permitted. If elevation is contraindicated, support the client's back with pillows, as needed.	*Elevation of the bed or the use of pillows facilitates client comfort and reduces the risk of hyperextension of the back.*
Cover the client with bed linen.	*Being covered maintains client comfort and dignity.*
Provide toilet tissue, place the call light within reach, lower the bed to the low position, elevate the side rails, and leave the client alone, if not contraindicated.	*Many clients find it difficult to have a bowel movement in the presence of another person. Allowing an able client to wipe himself or herself promotes self-care and self-worth.*

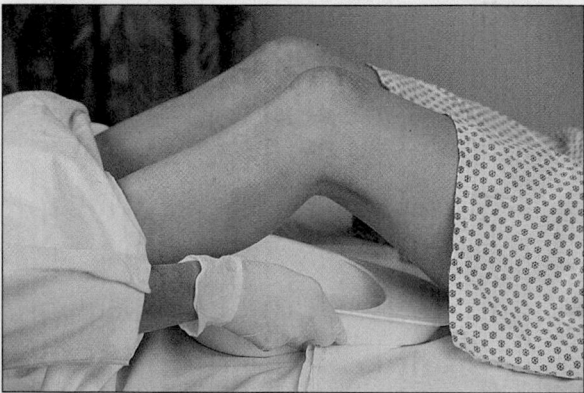

FIGURE 41.15 Placing a slipper pan under the buttocks.

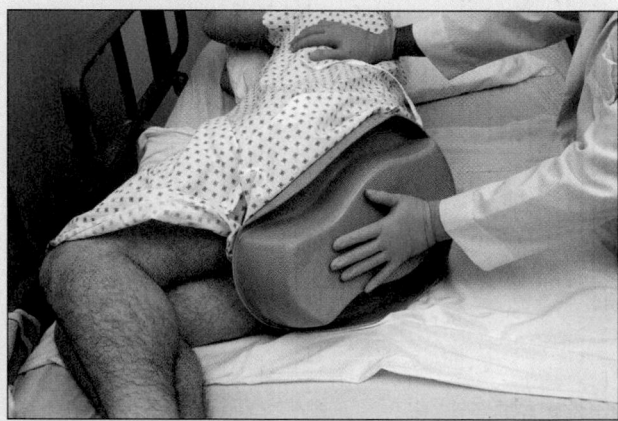

FIGURE 41.16 Placing a regular bedpan against the client's buttocks.

Guidelines	Rationales
Answer the call bell promptly. Do not leave anyone on a bedpan longer than 15 minutes unless he or she is able to remove the pan by himself or herself.	*Lengthy stays on a bedpan can cause pressure ulcers.*
Put on gloves when removing the bedpan, hold the bedpan steady, cover the bedpan, and place it on a disposable pad on an adjacent chair. Return the bed to the position used when giving the bedpan.	*These actions prevent spillage of the bedpan's contents, avoids contamination of client-use surfaces (e.g., the chair), and maintains client dignity and comfort.*
If the client needs assistance, wipe perineal area with several layers of toilet tissue. If specimens are to be collected, discard the soiled tissue into a moisture-proof receptacle other than the bedpan. For female patients, wipe from the urethra toward the anus.	*Wiping "front to back" prevents the transfer of rectal microorganisms into the urinary meatus.*
Wash the perineal area of dependent clients with soap and water as indicated and thoroughly dry the area.	*Cleansing prevents excoriation caused by stool left on the client's skin.*
For all clients, offer warm water, soap, a washcloth, and a towel to wash the hands. Assist the client to a comfortable position, empty and clean the bedpan, and return it to the bedside.	*These steps prevent infection and promote client comfort.*
Remove and discard your gloves and wash your hands.	*Hand hygiene prevents cross-contamination.*
Spray the room with air freshener, as needed, to control odour, unless contraindicated because of respiratory problems, allergies, or institutional policies.	*Clients are often self-conscious about the odour.*
Document colour, odour, amount, and consistency of urine and feces, and the condition of the perineal area.	*Documentation is important to track changes and to prevent complications (e.g., constipation).*

to the production of soft, formed stool over a period of 1 or more days; some laxatives exert a *cathartic effect* that is prompt and purgative leading to evacuation of the bowel—these laxatives are sometimes referred to as *cathartics*. Laxatives that produce a laxative effect include psyllium and docusate sodium; cathartics include castor oil, cascara, and bisacodyl (Dulcolax). Table 41.4 on the next page describes the different types of laxatives.

Laxative abuse is believed to be a common problem. Older adults, in particular, often use laxatives improperly. Persistent self-administration of laxatives can, in fact, result in chronic constipation. The trend now is toward the natural laxative approach, that is, increasing dietary fibre, such as that found in fruits and vegetables, to obtain a laxative effect.

Laxatives are contraindicated in the client who has nausea, cramps, colic, vomiting, or undiagnosed abdominal pain. Clients need to be informed about the dangers of laxative use. Some are known to interfere with absorption of medications or nutrients; for example, medications taken at the same time as a bulk-forming laxative may not be absorbed as they become part of the "mass" created by the agent; oils may interfere with the absorption of water-soluble vitamins and nutrients across the epithelium of the bowel. Continual use of laxatives to encourage bowel evacuation weakens the bowel's natural responses to fecal distension, resulting in chronic constipation. To eliminate chronic laxative use, it is usually necessary to teach the client about dietary fibre, regular

exercise, taking sufficient fluids, and establishing regular defecation habits. In addition, any medication regimen should be examined to see whether it could cause constipation.

Some laxatives (e.g., glycerin, bisacodyl) are given in the form of a **suppository**, a solid, cone-shaped, medicated substance inserted into the rectum. Suppositories act in various ways: by softening the feces; by releasing carbon dioxide to distend the rectum (e.g., potassium bitartrate, sodium bicarbonate); or by stimulating the nerve endings in the rectal mucosa. The best results can be obtained by inserting the suppository 30 minutes before the client's usual defecation time or when the peristaltic action is greatest, such as after breakfast.

ANTIFLATULENT MEDICATIONS Antiflatulent agents, such as simethicone (Gas-X), do not decrease the formation of flatus, but they do coalesce the gas bubbles and facilitate their passage via belching through the mouth or expulsion through the anus. A combination of simethicone and loperamide (Imodium Advanced) is effective in relieving abdominal bloating and gas associated with diarrhea. Suppositories can also be given to relieve flatus by increasing intestinal motility. Alpha-galactosidase (Beano) reduces flatulence caused by eating fermentable carbohydrates (e.g., beans, bran, and fruit).

ANTIDIARRHEAL MEDICATIONS Specific antidiarrheal agents are used to treat the cause of the diarrhea. Nonspecific agents act on or within the bowel to provide

TABLE 41.4 Types of Laxatives

Type	Action	Examples	Pertinent Teaching Information
Bulk-forming	Nonabsorbable; forms large hydrophilic mass increasing bulk in the intestines, thereby stimulating peristalsis	Psyllium hydrophilic mucilloid (Metamucil)	Bulk-forming laxatives help produce soft, formed stool 1 to 3 days after onset of treatment. Sufficient fluid must be taken to facilitate swallowing the product as well as enhance the bulk of stool. Do not take oral medications at the same time, as the medications can become part of the "bulk" matter and may not be absorbed.
Surfactant (stool softener)	Lowers the surface tension of the feces, thus helping water to penetrate; causes secretion of water and electrolytes into the intestine	Docusate sodium (Colace)	Surfactants are available in syrup and liquid formats. Surfactants may take several days to take effect.
Stimulant	Stimulates nerve endings in the wall of the intestine, causing rapid propulsion of the contents; increases water and electrolytes in the intestine	Bisacodyl (Dulcolax), Senna (Senokot), sennoside (Ex-Lax), cascara, castor oil	A semiliquid stool can be produced within 6–12 hours.
Emollient	Nonabsorbable; lubricates feces in the colon	Mineral oil	Use of emollients may cause cramps.
Saline or osmotic	Draws water into the intestine by osmosis, distends bowel, and stimulates peristalsis	Epsom salts, magnesium hydroxide (milk of magnesia), magnesium citrate, sodium phosphate (Fleet enema), glycerin	These laxatives may be rapid acting and can cause fluid and electrolyte imbalance, particularly in older adults and children with cardiac and/or renal disease. These laxatives are not generally recommended, except for such situations as opioid-induced constipation. Prolonged use inhibits the absorption of some fat-soluble vitamins.
		Electrolyte-free polyethylene glycol (Peg3550) (Miralax)	This is a relatively new laxative helpful in the treatment of constipation in children. Tasteless powder is mixed in flavoured liquid, such as juice.

relief. The following are examples of nonspecific antidiarrheal agents: opioids (e.g., Loperamide, Lomotil) are effective in treating diarrhea as they decrease intestinal motility; bismuth subsalicylate (e.g., Pepto-Bismol) is effective for prevention and treatment of mild diarrhea; bulk-forming agents (e.g., methylcellulose) absorb water and cause a formed stool; however, the underlying cause for the diarrhea remains (Lehne, 2010, p. 79).

Administering Enemas

An **enema** is a solution introduced into the rectum and large intestine. An enema works by distending the intestine and sometimes irritating the intestinal mucosa, thereby increasing peristalsis and the excretion of feces and flatus.

TYPES OF ENEMAS Enemas are classified into four groups: (a) cleansing, (b) carminative, (c) retention, and (d) return flow.

Cleansing Enemas Cleansing enemas are intended to remove feces. They are given chiefly to do the following:

- Prevent the escape of feces during surgery
- Prepare the intestine for certain diagnostic tests, such as radiography or visualization tests (e.g., colonoscopy)
- Remove feces in instances of constipation or impaction
- Establish regular bowel function as part of a bowel training program

Cleansing enemas use a variety of solutions. See Table 41.5 for commonly used solutions.

TABLE 41.5 Commonly Used Enema Solutions

Solution	Constituents	Action	Time to Take Effect	Adverse Effects
Hypertonic	90 mL to 120 mL of solution (e.g., sodium phosphate)	Draws water into the colon	5–10 min	Retention of sodium
Hypotonic	500 mL to 1000 mL of tap water	Distends colon, stimulates peristalsis, and softens feces	15–20 min	Fluid and electrolyte imbalance; water intoxication
Isotonic	500 mL to 1000 mL of normal saline	Distends colon, stimulates peristalsis, and softens feces	15–20 min	Possible sodium retention
Soapsuds	500 mL to 1000 mL (3 mL to 5 mL of soap to 1000 mL of water)	Irritates mucosa, distends colon	10–15 min	Irritation and possible damage to mucosa
Oil (mineral, olive, cottonseed)	90 mL to 120 mL	Lubricates feces and colonic mucosa	1–3 hours	Uncommon

Hypertonic solutions (e.g., sodium phosphate, saline) exert osmotic pressure, which draws fluid from the interstitial space into the colon. The increased volume in the colon stimulates peristalsis and hence defecation. A commonly used hypertonic enema is the commercially prepared Fleet enema.

Hypotonic solutions (e.g., tap water) exert a lower osmotic pressure than the surrounding interstitial fluid, causing water to move from the colon into the interstitial space. Before the water moves from the colon, it stimulates peristalsis and defecation. Because the water moves out of the colon, the tap water enema should not be repeated because of the danger of circulatory overload when the water moves from the interstitial space into the circulatory system.

Isotonic solutions (e.g., physiological [normal] saline) are considered the safest enema solutions to use. They exert the same osmotic pressure as the interstitial fluid surrounding the colon. Therefore, there is no fluid movement into or out of the colon. The instilled volume of saline in the colon stimulates peristalsis.

Soapsuds enemas stimulate peristalsis by increasing the volume in the colon and irritating the mucosa. Only pure soap (i.e., soap containing only fatty acids and alkali without other ingredients) (e.g., castile soap) should be used to minimize mucosal irritation.

Some enemas are *large volume* (e.g., 500 mL to 1000 mL) for an adult and others are *small volume,* including hypertonic solutions. The latter, available commercially, act by drawing water into the colon, thus stimulating defecation. The amount of solution administered for a high-volume enema will depend on the age and medical condition of the individual. See Table 41.5 for approximate volumes of solutions.

Cleansing enemas can also be described as *high* or *low.* A *high enema* is given to cleanse as much of the colon as possible. The client changes from the left lateral position to the dorsal recumbent position and then to the right lateral position during administration so that the solution can follow the large intestine (see Figure 41.1 on page 1267). The low enema is used to clean the rectum and sigmoid colon only. The client maintains a left lateral position during administration. A medical prescription should specify when a high-enema technique is to be used.

The force of flow of the solution is governed by (a) the height of the solution container, (b) size of the tubing, (c) viscosity of the fluid, and (d) resistance of the rectum. The higher the solution container is held above the rectum, the faster is the flow and the greater is the force (pressure) in the rectum. During most adult enemas, the solution container should be no higher than 30 cm above the rectum. During a high cleansing enema, the solution container is usually held 30 cm to 45 cm above the rectum because the fluid is instilled farther to clean the entire bowel. For an infant, the solution container is held no more than 7.5 cm above the rectum.

Carminative Enema A *carminative enema* is given primarily to expel flatus. The solution instilled into the rectum releases gas, which, in turn, distends the rectum and the colon, thus stimulating peristalsis. For an adult, 60 mL to 80 mL of fluid is instilled.

Retention Enema A *retention enema* introduces oil or medication into the rectum and sigmoid colon. The oil is retained for a relatively long period (e.g., 1 to 3 hours). It acts to soften the feces and to lubricate the rectum and anal canal, thus facilitating passage of the feces. Antibiotic enemas are used to treat infections locally; anthelminitic enemas kill helminths, such as worms and intestinal parasites.

Return-Flow Enema A *return-flow enema* is used occasionally to expel flatus. Alternating flow of 100 mL to 200 mL of fluid into and out of the rectum and sigmoid colon stimulates peristalsis. This process is repeated five or six times until the flatus is expelled and abdominal distension is relieved.

The nurse must consider that some people may perceive this procedure as a significant violation of personal space and approach the client with utmost sensitivity. Defecation in and of itself is a very private matter, and people are not generally used to having others observing defecation or manipulating the rectal area. In addition, anyone who has a history of sexual abuse may find the procedure extremely traumatic.

Skill 41.1 describes how to administer an enema. See also the Home Care Considerations box and the Lifespan Consideration box on administering an enema on page 1292.

SKILL 41.1 ADMINISTERING AN ENEMA

PURPOSE

- To achieve one or more of the following actions: cleansing, carminative, retention, or return flow

ASSESSMENT

Assess

- When the client last had a bowel movement and the amount, colour, and consistency of the feces
- Presence of abdominal distension (the distended abdomen appears swollen and feels firm, rather than soft, when palpated)
- Whether the client has sphincter control
- Whether the client can use a toilet or commode or must remain in bed and use a bedpan

Clinical Reasoning

As enemas can be embarrassing and unpleasant for clients to receive, consider if all measures have been taken to avoid the need for administering an enema.

PLANNING

Before administering an enema, determine whether a physician's order is required. At some agencies, a physician or other designated health care professional must order the kind of enema and the time to give it, for example, the morning of the examination. When the client has rectal disease, the size of the rectal tube to use may be specified. At other agencies, enemas are given at the nurse's discretion (i.e., as necessary on a prn [as needed] order). In addition, determine the presence of kidney or cardiac disease that contraindicates the use of a hypotonic solution. For people receiving a retention enema, consider that it may be difficult to retain the fluid and the client may need to empty the bowel sooner than desired.

Equipment

- Disposable linen-saver pad
- Bath blanket
- Bedpan or commode
- Disposable gloves
- Water-soluble lubricant, if tubing is not prelubricated
- Paper towel

Large-Volume Enema

- Solution container with tubing of correct size and tubing clamp
- Correct solution, amount, and temperature (solution should be at body temperature for adults)

Small-Volume Enema

- Prepackaged container of enema solution with lubricated tip

IMPLEMENTATION

Preparation

- Lubricate about 5 cm of the rectal tube (some commercially prepared enema sets already have lubricated nozzles). **Rationale: Lubrication facilitates insertion through the sphincters and minimizes trauma**.
- Run some solution through the connecting tubing of a large-volume enema set and the rectal tube to expel any air in the tubing; then close the clamp. **Rationale: Air instilled into the rectum, although not harmful, causes unnecessary distension**.

Performance

1. Before performing the procedure, introduce yourself and verify the client's identity using two identifiers or per agency protocol. Explain to the client what you are going to do, why it is necessary, and how he or she can participate. Indicate that the client may experience a feeling of fullness while the solution is being administered.

2. Perform hand hygiene, put on clean gloves, and follow other appropriate infection prevention and control procedures.

3. Provide for client privacy and be sensitive to client's emotional response to this intrusive procedure.

4. Assist the adult client to the left lateral position, with the right leg as acutely flexed as possible (see ❶) and the linen-saver pad under the buttocks. **Rationale: This position facilitates the flow of solution by gravity into the sigmoid and descending colon, which are on the left side. Having the right leg acutely flexed provides for adequate exposure of the anus**.

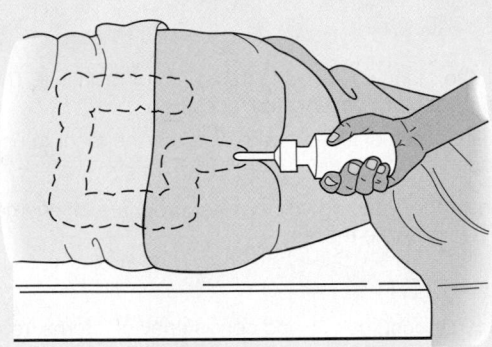

❶ Assuming a left lateral position for an enema. Note the commercially prepared enema.

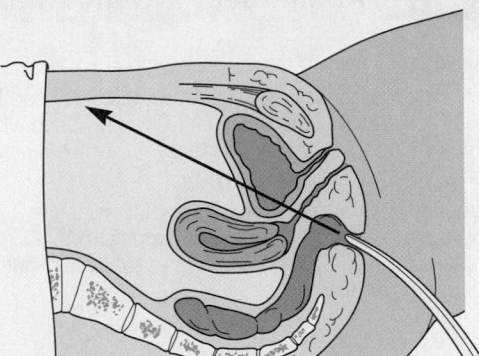

❸ Inserting the rectal tube following the direction of the rectum.

5. Insert the enema tube.

- For clients in the left lateral position, lift the upper buttock (see ❷). **Rationale: This step helps ensure good visualization of the anus**.

- Insert the tube smoothly and slowly into the rectum, directing it toward the umbilicus (see ❸). **Rationale: The angle follows the normal contour of the rectum. Slow insertion prevents spasm of the sphincter**.

- Insert the tube 7 cm to 10 cm. **Rationale: Because the anal canal is about 2.5 cm to 5 cm long in the adult, insertion to this point places the tip of the tube beyond the anal sphincter into the rectum**.

- If resistance is encountered at the internal sphincter, ask the client to take a deep breath, then run a small amount of solution through the tube. **Rationale: This manoeuvre will help relax the internal anal sphincter**.

- Never force tube or solution entry. If instilling a small amount of solution does not permit the tube to be advanced or the solution to freely flow, withdraw the tube. Check for any stool that may have blocked the tube during insertion. If present, flush it and retry the procedure. You may also perform a digital rectal examination to determine if there is an impaction or other mechanical blockage. If resistance persists, end the procedure and report the resistance to the appropriate health care provider and the nurse in charge.

- Raise the solution container, and open the clamp to allow fluid flow.

- *Or* compress a pliable container by hand.

- During most low enemas, hold or hang the solution container no higher than 30 cm above the rectum. **Rationale: The higher the solution container is held above the rectum, the faster is the flow and the greater is the force (pressure) in the rectum.** During a high enema, hang the solution container about 45 cm. **Rationale: The fluid must be instilled farther to clean the entire bowel**. See agency protocol.

- Administer the fluid slowly. If the client complains of fullness or pain, lower the container or use the clamp to stop the flow for 30 seconds, and then restart the flow at a slower rate. **Rationale: Administering the enema slowly and stopping the flow momentarily decreases the likelihood of intestinal spasm and premature ejection of the solution**.

- If using a plastic commercial container, roll it up as the fluid is instilled (see ❹).

- After all the solution has been instilled or when the client cannot hold any more and feels the desire to defecate (the urge to defecate usually indicates that sufficient fluid has been administered), close the clamp, and remove the enema tube from the anus.

- Place the enema tube in a disposable towel as you withdraw it.

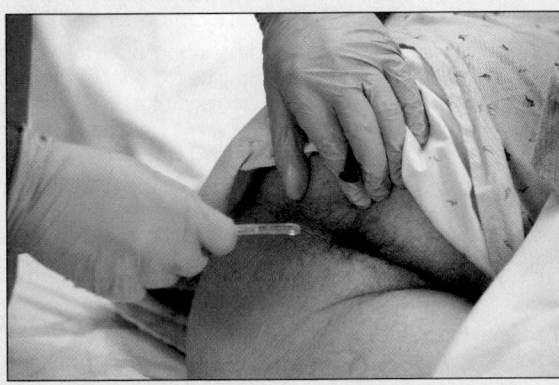

❷ Inserting the enema tube.

6. Slowly administer the enema solution.

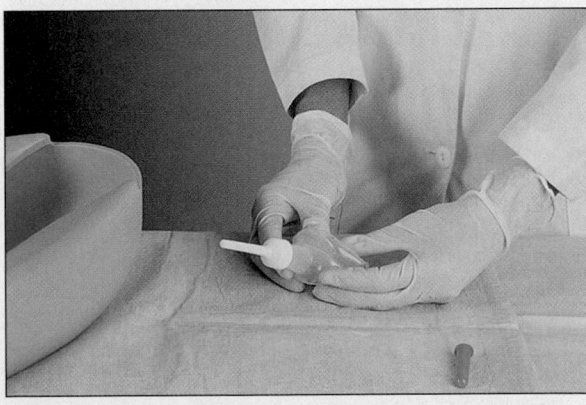

❹ Rolling up a commercial enema container.

(continued)

SKILL 41.1 ADMINISTERING AN ENEMA *(continued)*

7. Encourage the client to retain the enema.
   - Ask the client to remain lying down. It is easier for the client to retain the enema when lying down than when sitting or standing, because gravity promotes drainage and peristalsis.
   - Request that the client retain the solution for the appropriate amount of time, for example, 5 to 10 minutes for a cleansing enema or at least 30 minutes for a retention enema.

8. Assist the client to defecate.
   - Assist the client to a sitting position on the bedpan, commode, or toilet. A sitting position facilitates the act of defecation.

   - Ask the client who is using the toilet not to flush it. The nurse needs to observe the feces.
   - If a specimen of feces is required, ask the client to use a bedpan or commode.

9. Document the type and volume, if appropriate, of enema given. Describe the results.

EVALUATION

Evaluate the amount, colour, and consistency of returns; relief of flatus or abdominal distension; and any problems encountered (e.g., resistance at the external or internal sphincter when inserting the rectal tube).

HOME CARE CONSIDERATIONS

Administering an Enema

Teach the caregiver or the client the following:

- Use enemas only as directed. Do not rely on them for regular bowel evacuation.
- Before administration, make sure a bedpan, commode, or toilet is nearby.

Digital Removal of a Fecal Impaction

Digital removal involves breaking up the fecal mass digitally and removing it in portions. Because the bowel mucosa can be injured during this procedure, some agencies restrict and specify the personnel permitted to conduct digital disimpaction. Rectal stimulation is also contraindicated for some people because it may cause an excessive vagal response resulting in cardiac arrhythmias. Before disimpaction, it may be suggested that an

---

LIFESPAN CONSIDERATIONS

Administering an Enema

INFANTS AND CHILDREN

- Ensure that the reason for which the enema was prescribed is still applicable so as to avoid undue discomfort.
- Provide a careful explanation to the parents and child before the procedure; toddlers and preschool-age children may perceive the enema as a violation of their body space.
- The enema solution should be isotonic (usually saline) to avoid fluid and electrolyte shifts.
- Infants and small children do not exhibit sphincter control and need to be assisted in retaining the enema. The nurse administers the enema while the infant or child is lying with the buttocks over the bedpan, and the nurse firmly presses the buttocks together to prevent the immediate expulsion of the solution. Older children can usually hold the solution if they understand what to do and are not required to hold it for too long.

- Enema temperature should be 37.7°C unless otherwise ordered.
- Large-volume enemas consist of 50 mL to 200 mL in children younger than 18 months old; 200 mL to 300 mL in children age 18 months to 5 years; and 300 mL to 500 mL in children age 5 to 12 years.
- Careful explanation is essential for the preschool-age child as the enema is viewed as intrusive and threatening.
- For infants and small children, the dorsal recumbent position is frequently used. Position them on a small padded bedpan with support for the back and head. Secure the legs by placing a diaper under the bedpan and then over and around the thighs. Place the under pad under the client's buttocks to protect the bed linen, and drape the child with the bath blanket.
- Insert the tube 5 cm to 7.5 cm in the child and only 2.5 cm to 3.75 cm in the infant.

- For children, lower the height of the solution container appropriately for the age of the child. Check your agency protocol.
- To assist a small child in retaining the solution, apply firm pressure over the anus with tissue wipes, or firmly press the child's buttocks together.
- Provide support after the enema; the child may be experiencing embarrassment or discomfort.

OLDER ADULTS

- Monitor the client's tolerance throughout the procedure and during evacuation, watching for vagal episodes, dysrhythmias, and fluid and electrolyte disturbances.
- Avoid overexertion or fatigue for older clients.
- Protect older adults' skin from prolonged exposure to moisture.
- Assist older clients with perineal care, as indicated.

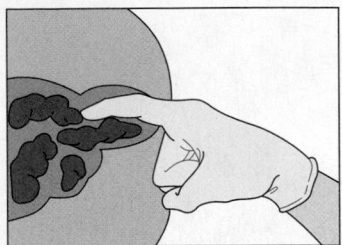

FIGURE 41.17 Digital removal of fecal impaction.

oil retention enema be given and held for 30 minutes. (Check agency policy and physician's order.) After a disimpaction, the nurse can use various interventions to remove remaining feces, such as a cleansing enema or the insertion of a suppository as prescribed by the physician.

For digital removal of a fecal impaction, follow these steps:

1. If indicated, obtain assistance from a second person who can comfort the client during the procedure.
2. Ask the client to assume the left or right side-lying position, with the knees flexed and the back toward the nurse. When the person lies on the right side, the sigmoid colon is uppermost; thus, gravity can aid in removal of the feces. Positioning on the left side allows easier access to the sigmoid colon.
3. Place a disposable absorbent pad under the client's buttocks and a bedpan nearby to receive stool.
4. Drape the client for comfort and to avoid unnecessary exposure of the body.
5. Put on a pair of clean gloves, and liberally lubricate the index finger to be inserted.
6. Gently insert the index finger into the rectum, and move the finger toward the client's umbilicus along the length of the rectum.
7. Loosen and dislodge stool by gently massaging around it. Break up stool by working the finger into the hardened mass, taking care to avoid injury to the mucosa of the rectum (Figure 41.17).
8. Carefully work stool downward to the end of the rectum and remove it in small pieces. Continue to remove as much fecal material as possible. Periodically assess the client for signs of fatigue, such as facial pallor, diaphoresis, or change in pulse rate. Manual stimulation should be minimal.
9. Following disimpaction, assist the client to clean the anal area and buttocks. Then, assist the client onto a bedpan or commode for a short time because digital stimulation of the rectum often induces the urge to defecate.

Decreasing Flatulence

Flatus can be reduced or prevented in a number of ways, including getting exercise, moving in bed, ambulating, and avoiding gas-producing foods. Movement stimulates peristalsis, the escape of flatus, and the reabsorption of gases into the intestinal capillaries. One method of treating flatulence involves the insertion of a rectal tube:

1. Use a rectal tube 22 to 30 French for adults and a smaller size for children.
2. Have the client assume the left side-lying position.
3. Lubricate the rectal tube to reduce mucous membrane irritation.
4. Expose the anus and insert the rectal tube into the rectum 7.5 cm to 10 cm. The rectal tube will stimulate peristalsis. Do not force the tube in if it does not insert easily. Secure the tube in place.
5. Wrap an abdominal or incontinence pad around the end of the rectal tube to catch any liquid that may be expelled. Some nurses suggest inserting the rectal tube and then placing the end into a receptacle filled with water. The passage of flatus will be seen as bubbles are produced.
6. Leave the tube in no longer than 30 minutes to avoid irritation of the rectal mucosa. If abdominal distension is not relieved, the tube can be inserted every 2 to 3 hours.
7. Encourage the client to assume various positions in bed.

If a rectal tube does not relieve flatus, consult with the physician about a suppository, enema, or medication.

Creating Bowel Training Programs

For clients who have chronic constipation, frequent impactions, or fecal incontinence, a *bowel training program* may be helpful. The program is based on factors within the client's control and is designed to help the client establish normal defecation. Such matters as food and fluid intake, exercise, and defecation habits are all considered. Before beginning such a program, clients must understand it and want to be involved. The major phases of the program are as follows:

- Determine the client's usual bowel habits and factors that help and hinder normal defecation.
- Design a plan with the client that includes the following:
  a. Fluid intake of at least 1500 mL to 2000 mL per day, unless contraindicated
  b. Intake of hot drinks, especially just before the usual defecation time
  c. Increase in exercise
- Maintain the following daily routine for 2 to 3 weeks:
  a. Administer a cathartic suppository (e.g., bisacodyl) 30 minutes before the client's defecation time to stimulate peristalsis.

b. When the client experiences the urge to defecate, assist the client to the toilet or commode or onto a bedpan. Note the length of time between the insertion of the suppository and the urge to defecate.

c. Provide the client with privacy for defecation and a time limit; 15 minutes is usually sufficient to allow for defecation while minimizing the risk of skin breakdown.

d. Teach the client to lean forward at the hips, to apply pressure on the abdomen with the hands, and to bear down for defecation. These measures increase pressure on the colon. Straining should be avoided because it can cause hemorrhoids.

• Provide positive feedback when the client successfully defecates. Refrain from negative feedback if the client fails to defecate.

• Offer encouragement to the client, and convey that patience is often required. Many clients require weeks or months of training to achieve success.

Using a Fecal Incontinence Pouch

To collect and contain large volumes of feces, the nurse may place a fecal incontinence collector pouch around the anal area (Figure 41.18). The purpose of the pouch is to prevent progressive perianal skin irritation and breakdown and frequent linen changes necessitated by incontinence.

A fecal collector is secured around the anal opening and may or may not be attached to drainage. Pouches are best applied before the perianal skin becomes excoriated. If perianal skin excoriation is present, the nurse either (a) applies a dimethicone-based moisture-barrier cream or alcohol-free barrier film to the skin to protect it from feces until it heals and then applies the pouch, or (b) applies a skin barrier or hydrocolloid barrier underneath the pouch to achieve the best possible seal.

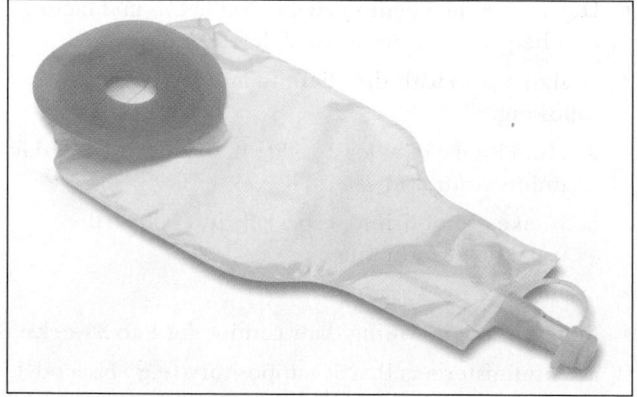

FIGURE 41.18 A drainable fecal collector pouch.

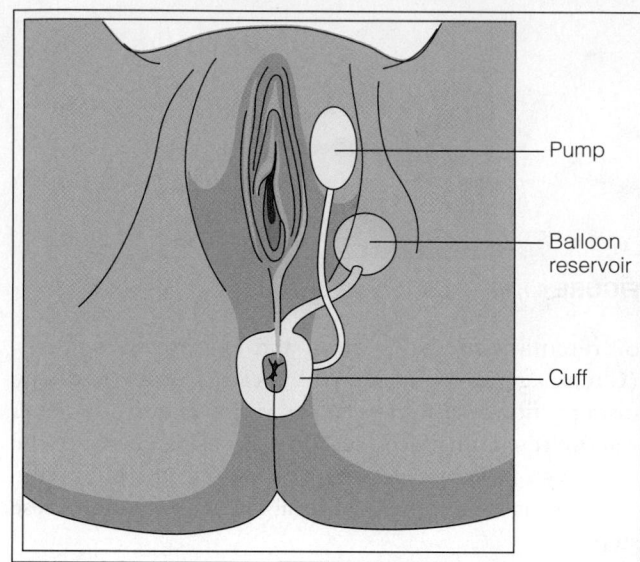

FIGURE 41.19 Inflatable artificial sphincter.

Nursing responsibilities for clients with a rectal pouch include (a) regular assessment and documentation of the perianal skin status, (b) changing the bag every 72 hours or sooner if there is leakage, (c) maintaining the drainage system, and (d) providing explanations and support to the client and family.

Some clients (e.g., post-trauma, quadriplegic, paraplegic, or poststroke) may be treated for fecal incontinence with surgical repair of a damaged sphincter or with an artificial bowel sphincter. The artificial sphincter consists of three parts: (a) a cuff around the anal canal, (b) a pressure-regulating balloon, and (c) a pump that inflates the cuff (Figure 41.19). The cuff is inflated to close the sphincter, maintaining continence. To have a bowel movement, the client deflates the cuff. The cuff automatically reinflates (generally in 10 minutes). Management of this device is usually specific to the device; contact the manufacturing company for details.

Managing an Ostomy

Clients with fecal diversions need considerable psychological support, instruction, and physical care. This section is limited to the nurse's physical interventions of stoma assessment, application of an appliance to collect feces, and promotion of predictable evacuation with colostomy irrigation. Many agencies have enterostomal therapy nurses to assist these clients. National organizations, such as the United Ostomy Association of Canada, aim to improve the quality of life of individuals who have or will require an ostomy.

STOMA AND SKIN CARE Care of the stoma and skin is important for all clients who have ostomies. The fecal material from a colostomy or ileostomy is irritating to the peristomal skin. This is particularly true of stool from an

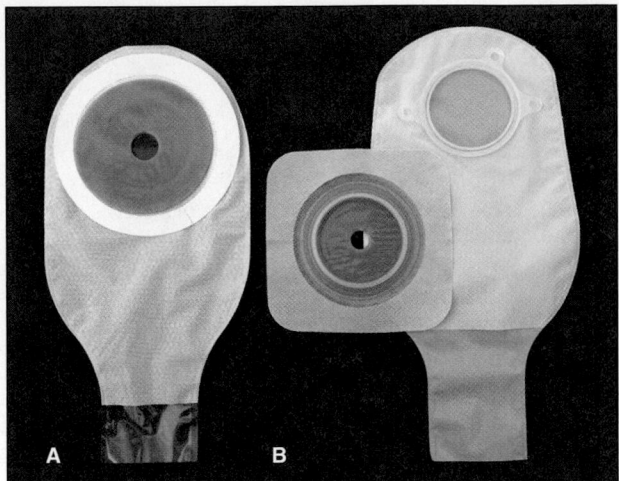

FIGURE 41.20 A: A one-piece ostomy appliance or pouching system; **B:** A two-piece ostomy appliance or pouching system.

ileostomy, which contains digestive enzymes. It is important to assess the peristomal skin for irritation each time the appliance is changed. Any irritation or skin breakdown needs to be treated immediately. The skin is kept clean by washing off any excretion and drying thoroughly.

An ostomy appliance should protect the skin, collect stool, and control odour. The appliance consists of a skin barrier and a pouch. Appliances can be one piece, in which the skin barrier is already attached to the pouch (Figure 41.20A), or an appliance can consist of two pieces: (a) a separate pouch with a flange and (b) a separate skin barrier with a flange where the pouch fastens to the barrier at the flange (Figure 41.20B). The pouch can be removed without removing the skin barrier when using a two-piece appliance.

Pouches can be closed or drainable. A drainable pouch usually has a clip where the end of the pouch is folded over the clamp and clipped (Figure 41.21). Newer drainable pouches have an integrated closure system instead of a clamp. Drainable pouches are generally used by people who need to empty the pouch more than twice a day.

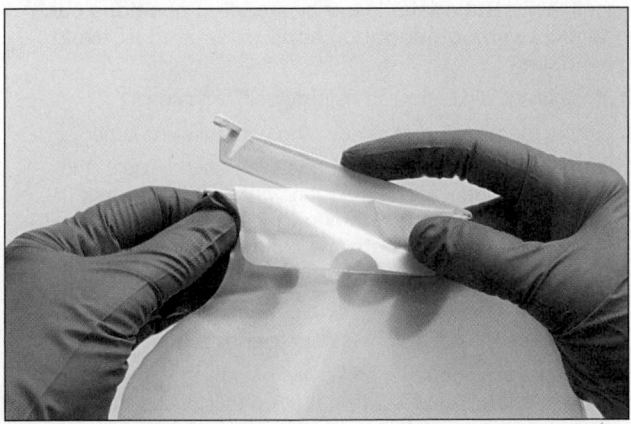

FIGURE 41.21 Applying a clamp to a drainable pouch.

Closed pouches are often used by people who have a regular stoma discharge (e.g., sigmoid colostomy) and have to empty the pouch only one or two times a day. Some people find it easier to change a closed pouch than to empty a drainable pouch, which requires some dexterity.

Odour control is essential to clients' self-esteem. As soon as clients are ambulatory, they can learn to work with the ostomy in the bathroom to avoid odours at the bedside. Selecting the appropriate kind of appliance promotes odour control. An intact appliance contains odours. Most pouches contain odour-barrier material and some have a pouch filter that allows gas out of the pouch but not the odour.

Ostomy appliances can be applied for up to 7 days. The pouch should be changed on a regular basis, before leakage occurs. The most common routine for changing the appliance is twice weekly. It is important that the peristomal skin is cleaned and inspected at this time. If the skin is erythematous, eroded, or ulcerated, the appliance should be changed every 24 to 48 hours to allow appropriate treatment of the skin. More frequent changes are recommended if the client complains of pain or discomfort.

The type of ostomy and amount of output influences how often the pouch is emptied. The pouch is emptied when it is one-third to one-half full. If the pouch overfills, it can cause separation of the skin barrier from the skin and stool comes in contact with the skin. This results in the entire appliance needing to be removed and a new one applied.

Skill 41.2 on the next page explains how to change a bowel diversion ostomy appliance. See also the Home Care Considerations box on changing an ostomy appliance on page 1298.

COLOSTOMY IRRIGATION A colostomy irrigation, similar to an enema, is a form of stoma management used only for clients who have a sigmoid or descending colostomy. It is not done for ileostomies because the feces are usually liquid. The purpose of irrigation is to distend the bowel sufficiently to stimulate peristalsis, which stimulates evacuation. When a regular evacuation pattern is achieved, the wearing of a colostomy pouch is unnecessary. Currently, colostomy irrigations are not routinely taught to most clients. Routine daily irrigations for control of the time of elimination ultimately become the client's decision. Some clients prefer to control the time of elimination through rigid dietary regulation and not be bothered with irrigations, which can take up to an hour to complete. When regulation by irrigation is chosen, it should be done at the same time each day.

For most clients, a relatively small amount of fluid (300 mL to 500 mL) stimulates evacuation. For others, up to 1000 mL may be needed because a colostomy has no sphincter and the fluid tends to return as it is instilled. This problem is reduced by the use of a cone on the irrigating catheter. The cone helps hold the fluid within the bowel during the irrigation. Clients that have used irrigation for several years are more prone

SKILL 41.2 CHANGING A BOWEL DIVERSION OSTOMY APPLIANCE

Before changing a bowel diversion ostomy appliance, determine the kind of ostomy and its placement on the abdomen. It is important to confirm which is the functioning stoma and any orders about the care of the stomas.

PURPOSES

* To assess and care for peristomal skin
* To collect stool for assessment of the amount and type of output
* To minimize odours for the client's comfort and self-esteem

ASSESSMENT

Assess

* *Stoma colour:* The stoma should appear red, similar in colour to the mucosal lining of the inner cheek. Very pale or darker-coloured stomas with a bluish or purplish hue indicate impaired blood circulation to the area. Notify the surgeon immediately.
* *Stoma size and shape:* Most stomas protrude slightly from the abdomen. New stomas normally appear swollen, but swelling generally decreases over 2 or 3 weeks or for as long as 6 weeks. Failure of swelling to recede may indicate a problem, such as blockage.
* *Stomal bleeding:* Slight bleeding initially when the stoma is touched is normal, but other bleeding should be reported.
* *Status of peristomal skin:* Any redness and irritation of peristomal skin—5 cm to 12.5 cm of skin surrounding the stoma—should be noted. Transient redness after removal of adhesive is normal.
* *Amount and type of feces:* Assess the amount, colour, odour, and consistency. Inspect for abnormalities, such as pus or blood.
* *Symptoms:* Statements of burning sensation under the skin barrier may indicate skin breakdown. The presence of abdominal discomfort or distension also needs to be determined.
* The client's and the family members' learning needs regarding the ostomy and self-care.
* The client's emotional status, especially strategies used to cope with the body image changes and the ostomy.

Equipment

* Clean gloves
* Bedpan
* Moisture-proof bag (for disposable pouches)
* Cleaning materials, including tissues, warm water, mild soap (optional), washcloth or cotton balls, towel
* Tissue or gauze pad
* Skin barrier (paste, powder, water, or liquid skin sealant)
* Stoma measuring guide
* Pen or pencil and scissors
* New ostomy appliance
* Tail closure clamp
* Deodorant for pouch (optional)

IMPLEMENTATION

Preparation

1. Determine the need for an appliance change.
   * Assess the used appliance for leakage of stool. **Rationale: Stool can irritate peristomal skin**.
   * Ask the client about any discomfort at or around the stoma. **Rationale: A burning sensation may indicate breakdown beneath the faceplate of the pouch**.
   * Assess the fullness of the pouch. **Rationale: The weight of an overly full bag can loosen the skin barrier and separate it from skin, causing stool to leak and irritate peristomal skin**.

2. If there is pouch leakage or discomfort at or around the stoma, change the appliance.

3. Select an appropriate time to change the appliance.
   * Avoid times close to meal or visiting hours. **Rationale: Ostomy odour and stool may reduce appetite or embarrass the client**.
   * Avoid times immediately after meals or the administration of any medications that may stimulate bowel evacuation. **Rationale: It is best to change the pouch when drainage is least likely to occur**.

Performance

1. Before performing the procedure, introduce yourself and verify the client's identity using two identifiers or per agency protocol. Explain to the client what you are going to do, why it is necessary, and how he or she can participate. Discuss how the results will be used in planning further care or treatments. Changing an ostomy appliance should not cause discomfort, but it may be distasteful to the client. Communicate acceptance and support to the client. It is important to change the appliance competently and quickly. Include support persons, as appropriate.

2. Perform hand hygiene, put on clean gloves, and follow other appropriate infection prevention and control procedures.

3. Provide for client privacy, preferably in the bathroom, where clients can learn to deal with the ostomy as they would at home.

4. Assist the client to a comfortable sitting or lying position in bed or preferably the sitting or standing position in the bathroom. **Rationale: Lying or standing positions can facilitate smoother pouch application, that is, avoid wrinkles**.

5. If the client is wearing an ostomy belt, unfasten it.

6. Empty the pouch and remove the ostomy skin barrier.
   * Empty the contents of a drainable pouch through the bottom opening into a bedpan or toilet. **Rationale: Emptying before removing the pouch prevents spillage of stool onto the client's skin**.
   * If the pouch uses a clamp, do not throw it away as it can be reused.
   * Assess the consistency, colour, and amount of stool.
   * Peel the skin barrier off slowly, beginning at the top and working downward, while holding the client's skin taut.

Rationale: Holding the skin taut minimizes client discomfort and prevents abrasion of the skin.
- Discard the disposable pouch in a moisture-proof bag.

7. Clean and dry the peristomal skin and stoma.
   - Use toilet tissue to remove any excess stool.
   - Use warm water, mild soap (optional), and a washcloth to clean the skin and stoma (see ❶). Check agency practice on the use of soap. **Rationale: Soap is sometimes not advised because it can be irritating to the skin.** If soap is allowed, do not use deodorant or moisturizing soaps. **Rationale: These products may interfere with the adhesives in the skin barrier.**
   - Dry the area thoroughly by patting with a towel. **Rationale: Excess rubbing can abrade the skin.**

8. Assess the stoma and peristomal skin.
   - Inspect the stoma for colour, size, shape, and bleeding.
   - Inspect peristomal skin for any redness, ulceration, or irritation. Transient redness after the removal of adhesive is normal.

9. Place a piece of tissue or gauze over the stoma, and change it, as needed. **Rationale: The material absorbs any seepage from the stoma while the ostomy appliance is being changed.**

10. Prepare and apply the skin barrier (peristomal seal).
    - Use the guide (see ❷) to measure the size of the stoma.
    - On the backing of the skin barrier, trace a circle the same size as the stomal opening.
    - Cut out the traced stoma pattern to make an opening in the skin barrier (see ❸). Make the opening no more than 0.3 cm to 0.4 cm larger than the stoma. **Rationale: This allows space for the stoma to expand slightly when functioning and minimizes the risk of stool contacting peristomal skin.**
    - Remove the backing to expose the sticky adhesive side. The backing can be saved and used as a pattern when making an opening for future skin barriers.

For a One-Piece Pouching System:
- Centre the skin barrier over the stoma (see ❹), and gently press it onto the client's skin for 30 seconds (see ❺). **Rationale: The heat and pressure help activate the adhesives in the skin barrier.**

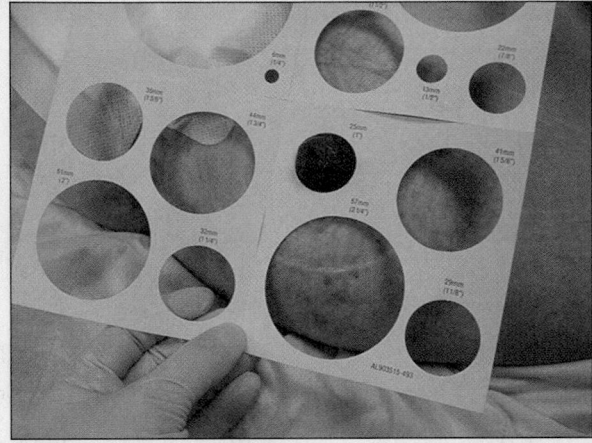

❷ A guide for measuring the stoma.

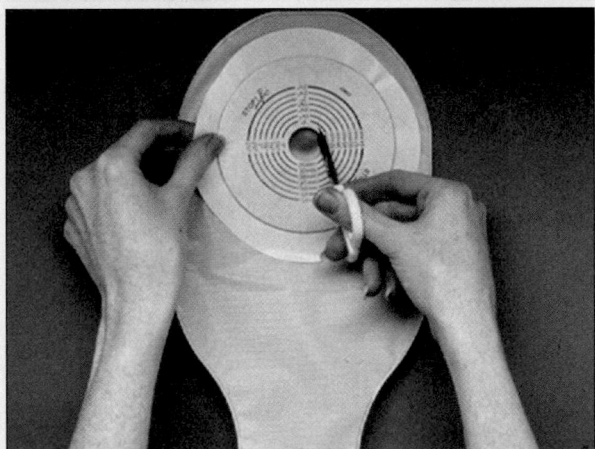

❸ The nurse is making a stoma opening on a disposable one-piece pouch.

For a Two-Piece Pouching System:
- Centre the skin barrier over the stoma, and gently press it onto the client's skin for 30 seconds.

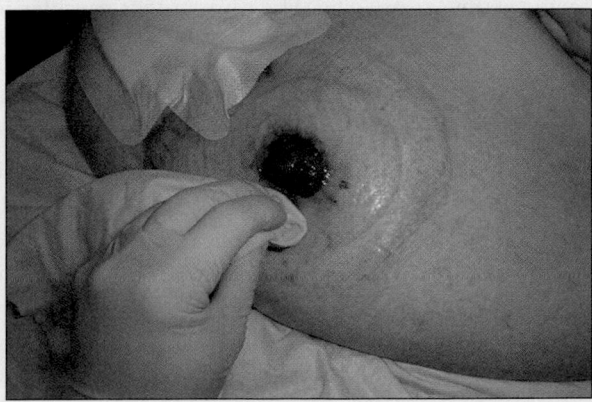

❶ Cleaning the skin.

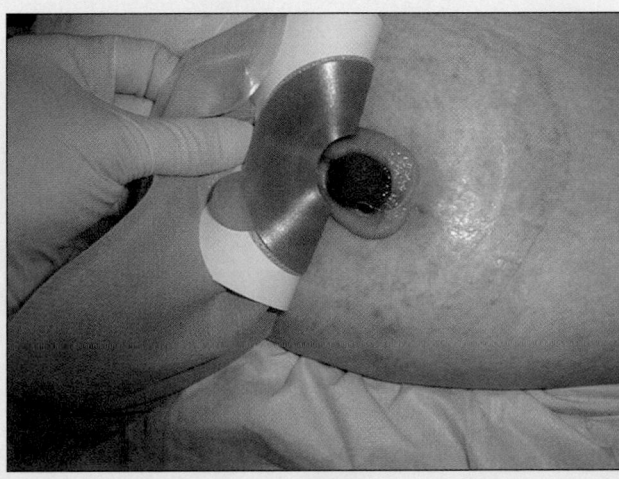

❹ Centring the skin barrier over the stoma.

(continued)

SKILL 41.2 **CHANGING A BOWEL DIVERSION OSTOMY APPLIANCE** *(continued)*

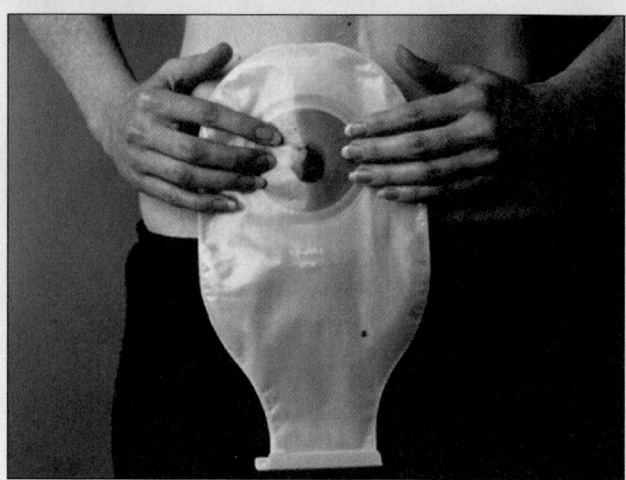

5 Pressing the skin barrier of a disposable one-piece pouch for 30 seconds to activate the adhesives in the skin barrier.

- Remove the tissue over the stoma before applying the pouch.
- Snap the pouch onto the flange or skin barrier wafer.

- For drainable pouches, close the pouch according to the manufacturer's directions.

11. Remove and discard gloves. Perform hand hygiene.

12. Document the procedure in the client record by using forms or checklists supplemented by narrative notes, when appropriate. Report and record pertinent assessments and interventions. Report any increase in stoma size, change in colour indicative of circulatory impairment, and presence of skin irritation or erosion. Record on the client's chart any discoloration of the stoma, the appearance of peristomal skin, the amount and type of drainage, the client's reaction to the procedure, the client's experience with the ostomy, and skills learned by the client.

EVALUATION

- Relate findings to previous data, if available. Adjust the teaching plan and nursing care plan, as needed. Reinforce the teaching each time the care is performed.
- Perform detailed follow-up based on findings that deviated from expected for the client. Report such deviations to the appropriate member of the health care team.

HOME CARE CONSIDERATIONS

Changing an Ostomy Appliance

- Provide the client with the names and phone numbers of an enterostomal therapist and a supply vendor.
- Suggest additional sources of information, such as the Crohn's and Colitis Foundation of Canada and the Canadian Association of Gastroenterology.
- Inform the client of signs to report to the appropriate health care provider (e.g., peristomal redness, skin breakdown, and changes in stomal colour).

to peristomal hernias, bowel perforation, and electrolyte imbalance with large-volume irrigations (500 mL to 1000 mL). Careful observation and assessment of this practice may be required in older, more fragile clients.

Evaluating

The goals established during the planning phase are evaluated according to specific desired outcomes also established in that phase. Examples of desired

outcomes for someone dealing with constipation include the following: The client identifies factors that alter bowel function; ingests adequate amount of fibre; reports (a) bowel movement at least every 3 days, (b) regular time for defecation, and (c) easy passage of stool; verbalizes understanding of need to decrease use of laxatives, enemas, and suppositories. Outcomes for someone dealing with diarrhea might include reduced frequency of bowel evacuation (e.g., no more than two bowel movements per day); maintenance of hydration and serum electrolyte balance (especially sodium and potassium) and acid–base balance; and skin integrity intact.

If outcomes are not achieved, the nurse should explore the reasons why. The nurse might consider some or all of the following questions:

- Were the client's fluid intake and diet appropriate?
- Was the client's activity level appropriate?
- Are prescribed medications or other factors affecting the gastrointestinal function?
- Do the client and family understand the provided instructions well enough to comply with the required therapy?
- Were sufficient physical and emotional supports provided?

Case Study 41

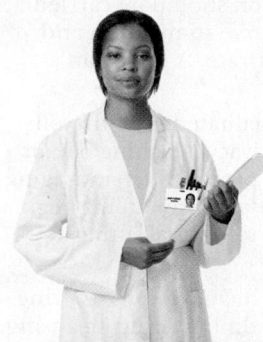

Mr. Dubois is a 62-year-old man who suffered a cerebrovascular accident (stroke) about 3 months ago. He underwent aggressive medical management and extensive physical and occupational therapy, which improved his overall functioning. Currently, Mr. Dubois is able to provide much of his own care but must rely on an assistive device for safe ambulation. He is being followed on an outpatient basis by community health services. During your visit with Mr. Dubois at his home, you learn that he has been experiencing abdominal discomfort, increased flatulence, and intermittent diarrhea for the past several days. He states that he usually has a bowel movement every 1 to 2 days, and his last normal bowel movement was about 6 or 7 days ago. His partner says that he is not eating or drinking well because he feels bloated and uncomfortable much of the time.

CRITICAL THINKING QUESTIONS

1. What conclusions, if any, can be drawn about Mr. Dubois's abdominal distress, diarrhea, and flatulence?

2. You learn that Mr. Dubois's stool has been liquid, in very small amounts, and at infrequent intervals, generally occurring when he feels the urge to defecate. What additional data are important to obtain from him?

3. What nursing intervention is most appropriate before making suggestions to correct the problem he is experiencing?

4. What suggestions can you give him about maintaining a regular bowel pattern?

5. Explain why laxatives are generally contraindicated for people in Mr. Dubois's situation.

Check the eText in MyNursingLab for answers and explanations.

KEY TERMS

anoscopy   *p. 1277*

bedpan   *p. 1285*

bowel incontinence
   p. 1275

chyme   *p. 1266*

colonoscopy   *p. 1277*

colostomy   *p. 1275*

commode   *p. 1285*

constipation   *p. 1272*

defecation   *p. 1268*

diarrhea   *p. 1274*

encopresis   *p. 1269*

enema   *p. 1288*

eructation   *p. 1275*

fecal impaction   *p. 1273*

fecal incontinence
   p. 1275

feces   *p. 1266*

flatulence   *p. 1275*

flatus   *p. 1266*

gastrocolic reflex   *p. 1269*

haustra   *p. 1266*

haustral churning   *p. 1266*

hemorrhoids   *p. 1267*

ileostomy   *p. 1275*

laxatives   *p. 1271*

mass peristalsis   *p. 1266*

meconium   *p. 1269*

occult blood   *p. 1278*

ostomy   *p. 1275*

paralytic ileus   *p. 1272*

peristalsis   *p. 1266*

proctoscopy   *p. 1277*

proctosigmoidoscopy
   p. 1277

steatorrhea   *p. 1278*

stoma   *p. 1275*

stool   *p. 1266*

suppository   *p. 1287*

CHAPTER HIGHLIGHTS

- The primary functions of the large bowel are the absorption of nutrients and water, the mucoid protection of the intestinal wall, and fecal elimination.

- Patterns of fecal elimination vary greatly among people, but a regular pattern of fecal elimination with formed, soft stool is essential to health and a sense of well-being.

- A variety of factors affects defecation: developmental level, diet, fluid intake, activity and exercise, psychological factors, defecation habits, medications, diagnostic procedures, anesthesia, pathological conditions, and pain.

- Fecal elimination problems include constipation, fecal impaction, diarrhea, bowel incontinence, and

flatulence. Each has specific defining characteristics and contributing causes that often relate to or are identical to the factors that affect defecation.

- Assessment relative to fecal elimination includes a nursing history; physical examination of the abdomen, rectum, and anus; and in some situations, visualization studies and inspection and analysis of stool for abnormal constituents, such as blood.

- A nursing history includes data about the client's defecation pattern, description of feces and any changes or problems associated with elimination, and data about possible factors altering bowel elimination.

- Physical examination of the abdomen includes methods of inspection, auscultation, percussion, and palpation. Physical examination of the rectum and anus includes inspection and palpation.

- When inspecting the client's stool, the nurse must observe its colour, consistency, shape, amount, and odour, and the presence of abnormal constituents.

- A function of the nurse is to assist clients with endoscopic and radiographic studies of the large intestine. Client assistance for visualization involves diet and bowel preparation before the study and appropriate follow-up care after the study.

- Clients also often need assistance to obtain stool specimens for laboratory analysis. In many agencies, nurses test stool for occult blood.

- Lack of exercise, irregular defecation habits, stress, bland diets, and overuse of laxatives are all thought to contribute to constipation. Sufficient fluid and fibre intake are required to keep feces soft.

- An adverse effect of constipation is straining during defecation, during which the Valsalva manoeuvre may be used. Cardiac problems may ensue.

- An adverse effect of prolonged diarrhea is fluid and electrolyte imbalance.

- Digital removal of an impaction should be carried out gently because of vagal nerve stimulation and subsequent depressed cardiac rate. A physician's order is often necessary.

- Normal defecation is often facilitated in both well and ill clients by providing privacy, teaching clients to attend to defecation urges promptly, encouraging appropriate food and fluid intake, scheduling regular exercise, and assisting clients to normal sitting positions, whenever possible.

- Additional nursing strategies include administering laxatives and antidiarrheals; administering cleansing, carminative, retention, or return-flow enemas; removing an impaction digitally; inserting rectal tubes to decrease flatulence; applying protective skin agents; monitoring fluid and electrolyte balance; and instructing clients in ways to promote normal defecation.

- Clients who have bowel diversion ostomies require special care, with attention to psychological adjustment, diet, and stoma and skin care.

ASSESS YOUR LEARNING

1. Clients should be taught that repeatedly ignoring the sensation of needing to defecate can result in which of the following?

   a. Constipation

   b. Diarrhea

   c. Incontinence

   d. Hemorrhoids

2. Mrs. Dejardin, a 45-year-old woman who is clinically obese, presents to the emergency department with complaints of right-sided back pain. In removing her bedpan you note white, pasty stool. What would be the MOST appropriate action?

   a. Encouraging Mrs. Dejardin to increase her fluid intake

   b. Encouraging Mrs. Dejardin to increase her fibre intake

   c. Documenting the findings and notifying the appropriate member of the health care team

   d. Obtaining a thorough dietary history for the past 72 hours

3. Jonathon O'Reilly has been ordered a barium swallow before a lower gastrointestinal computed tomography (CT) scan. What action should the nurse take after the procedure?

   a. Maintaining Jonathon NPO (nothing by mouth) until the barium is expelled

   b. Assessing his abdomen for distension

   c. Encouraging fluids and ambulation

   d. Using special precautions with his bodily waste

4. What is a potential complication of a digital removal of a fecal impaction?

   a. Increased vagal tone

   b. Trauma to the rectum

   c. Pain

   d. Bowel perforation

5. In assessing a new colostomy, the nurse notes that the stoma is pale and grey. Which of the following actions is MOST appropriate?

   a. Removing the appliance and examine the skin beneath the adhesive

   b. Notifying the surgeon

   c. Documenting the findings and continuing to monitor

   d. Irrigating the colostomy

6. Mr. John is a 65-year-old man with chronic alcoholism. He is admitted with a peptic ulcer. On emptying Mr. John's bedpan, the nurse notes his stool is black and tarry. What is the MOST probable explanation?

   a. The discoloration is a side effect of iron supplements.

   b. He is experiencing an upper gastrointestinal bleed.

   c. The discoloration is a side effect of taking acetyl-salicylic acid (ASA).

   d. The discoloration is caused by his ingestion of beets.

7. A young client with *neutropenia* (an abnormally low number of neutrophils in the blood), was recently discharged from hospital. She calls complaining of foul-smelling diarrhea occurring 5 to 6 times a day. What instructions should the nurse provide?

a. Increase fluid intake to 8 glasses/day to prevent dehydration.

b. Take an over-the-counter antidiarrheal medication, such as Imodium.

c. Eat a bland diet until the frequency of the diarrhea decreases.

d. Obtain a stool sample and make an appointment with her family physician.

8. Jane is going to the operating room for bowel surgery. She has been prescribed an enema the evening before the procedure. What would the nurse do before administering the enema?

a. Place the client in the left lateral position with the solution container at 25 cm above the rectum and reposition to the right lateral position after 10 minutes

b. Place the client in the right lateral position with the solution container 25 cm above the rectum and reposition to the dorsal recumbent position

c. Place the client in the left lateral position with the solution container 45 cm above the rectum and reposition to the right lateral position after 15 minutes

d. Place the client in the left lateral position with the solution container 45 cm above the rectum

and reposition to the dorsal recumbent and right lateral positions

9. Ann is a 50-year-old client admitted from the operating room following an ileostomy. When the nurse assesses Ann's ostomy, she notes that the adhesive backing has buckled. What is the nurse's immediate concern?

a. Skin breakdown

b. Infection

c. Swelling

d. Discomfort

10. A patient is prescribed morphine for pain associated with bladder cancer. What health teaching must be reinforced on discharge?

a. Morphine is addictive and should only be used when absolutely necessary.

b. Fluid and fibre intake should be increased when taking morphine.

c. Fluid and fibre intake should be decreased when taking morphine.

d. Activity level should be reduced because of the sedation properties of morphine.

Check the eText in MyNursingLab for answers and explanations.

WEBLINKS

The Canadian Celiac Association
http://www.celiac.ca

This organization provides support and education for people who have celiac disease, a medical condition in which the absorptive surface of the small intestine is damaged by gluten.

Colonversation—Cancer View Canada
http://www.colonversation.ca

This website is filled with facts about colon cancer. It is directed at the layperson and uses animations and humour to address this serious topic. The main message is: "Get checked for colon cancer. Spread the word. Have a colonversation."

Crohn's and Colitis Foundation of Canada
http://www.ccfc.ca

This Canadian foundation is a national nonprofit organization committed to finding a cure for inflammatory bowel disease through raising funds for medical research. The website provides

educational resources, including books, FAQs, and downloadable brochures. A lovely section is dedicated to youth—the "gutsy generation."

The United Ostomy Association of Canada
http://www.ostomycanada.ca

The United Ostomy Association of Canada is dedicated to assisting all persons with gastrointestinal or urinary diversions. The website provides information about ostomies and support groups.

The Canadian Association for Enterostomal Therapy
http://www.caet.ca

The Canadian Association for Enterostomal Therapy is a nonprofit association specializing in the nursing care of patients with challenges in wound, ostomy, and continence. The website provides useful information and brochures for patients, families, and professionals dealing with clients who have ostomies.

MyNursingLab

REFERENCES

Allegranzi, B., & Pittet, D. (2009). Role of hand hygiene in healthcare-associated infection prevention. *Journal of Hospital Infection, 73,* 305–315.

Allen, S. J., Martinez, E. G., Gregorio, G. V., & Dans, L. F. (2010). Probiotics for treating acute infectious diarrhoea. *Cochrane Database of Systematic Reviews 2010, Issue 11.* Art. No.: CD003048. doi: 10.1002/14651858.CD003048.pub3

Canadian Cancer Society's Steering Committee on Cancer Statistics. (2012). *Canadian cancer statistics 2012.* Toronto, ON: Canadian Cancer Society.

Knight, N., Strait, T., Anthony, N., Lovell, R., Norton, J., Sautter, R., & Scobey, M. (2010). *Clostridium difficile* colitis: A retrospective study of incidence and severity before and after institution of an alcohol-based hand rub policy. *American Journal of Infection Control, 38,* 523–528.

Lehne, R. (2010). *Pharmacology for nursing care* (7th ed.). St. Louis, MO: Saunders.

LeMone, P., & Burke, K. M. (2008). *Medical surgical nursing: Critical thinking in client care* (4th ed.). Upper Saddle River, NJ: Prentice Hall.

Lewis, S. J, & Heaton, K. W. (1997). Stool form scale as a useful guide to intestinal transit time.

Scandinavian Journal of Gastroenterology, 32(9): 920–924. doi: 10.3109/00365529709011203. PMID 9299672

MacLeod-Glover, N., & Sadowski, C. (2010). Efficacy of cleaning products for *C difficile. Canadian Family Physician, 56,* 417–423.

Nelson, R. (2007). Antibiotic treatment for *Clostridium difficile–*associated diarrhea in adults. *Cochrane Database of Systematic Reviews, 3,* Art. No.: CD004610.

O'Donoghue, C., & Kyne, L. (2011). Update on *Clostridium difficile* infection. *Current Opinion in Gastroenterology, 1,* 38–47.

Registered Nurses' Association of Ontario. (2011). *Best practice guideline supplement: Prevention of constipation in the older adult population.* Toronto, ON: Author.

Rome 111 diagnostic criteria for functional gastrointestinal disorders. Retrieved from http://www.romecriteria.org/assets/pdf/19_RomeIII_apA_885-898.pdf

World Health Organization. (2011). Health topics: Diarrhea. Retrieved from http://www.who.int/topics/diarrhoea/en/

Wray, D., Ijaz, S., & Lidder, S. (2008). Anal fissure: A review. *British Journal of Hospital Medicine, 69*(8), 455–458.

Chapter 42

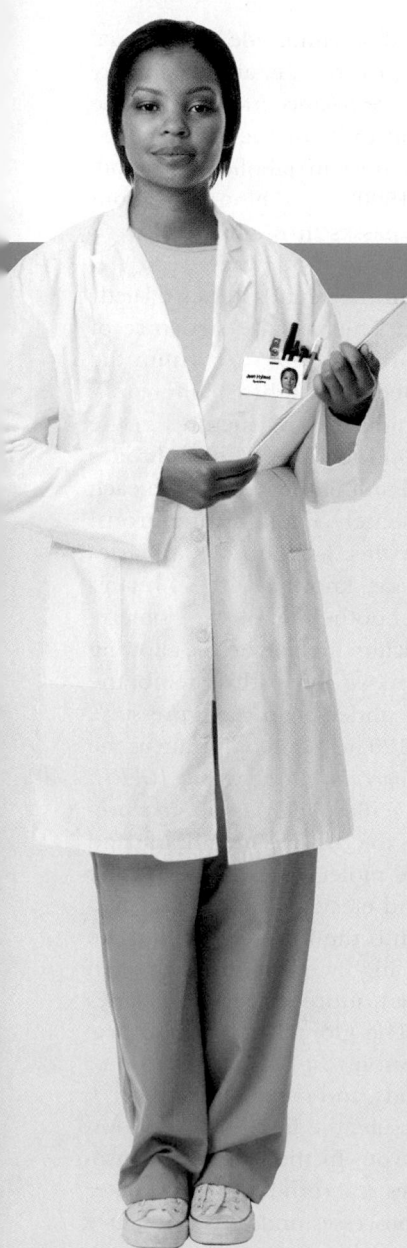

Urinary Elimination

Elimination from the urinary tract is usually taken for granted, although it is the main mechanism for the removal of waste products in the body. Only when a problem arises do most people become aware of their urinary habits and any associated symptoms.

A person's urinary habits depend on physiological processes as well as sociocultural, familial, and personal norms and habits. In Canada, most people are accustomed to privacy and clean (even decorative) surroundings while they urinate. Personal habits regarding urination are affected by the social practices regarding urination, such as privacy, gender, culturally acceptable practices, and physiological processes, such as bladder training. The physiology of the urinary system is complex and is discussed in detail in this chapter.

Physiology of Urinary Elimination

Urinary elimination depends on effective functioning of the renal system, made up of the four urinary tract structures: (a) kidneys, (b) ureters, (c) the bladder, and (d) the urethra (Figure 42.1).

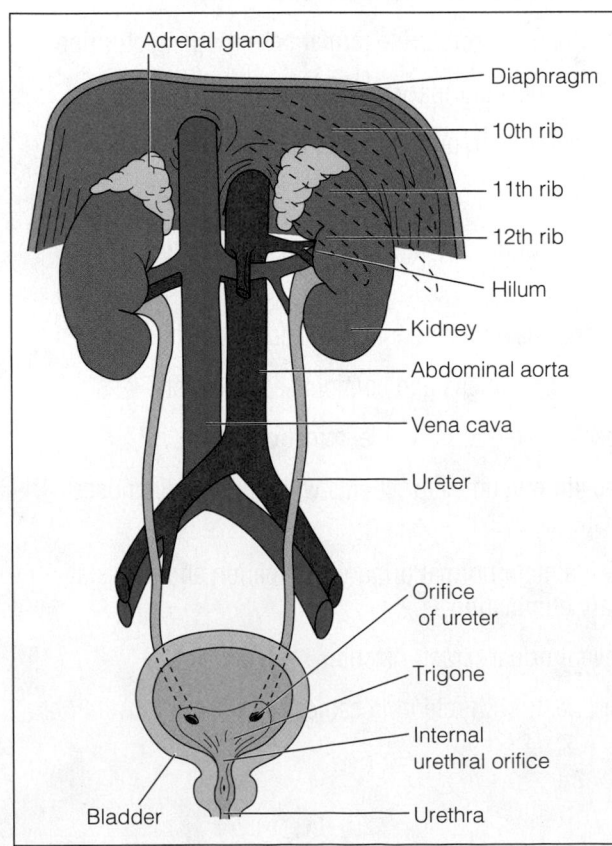

FIGURE 42.1 Anatomical structures of the urinary tract.

Kidneys

The paired kidneys are situated on either side of the spinal column, behind the peritoneal cavity. They are the primary regulators of fluid and acid–base balance in the body (see Chapter 44). The functional units of the kidneys, the nephrons, filter blood and remove metabolic waste products. In the average adult, 1500 mL of blood, or about 25% of the cardiac output, passes through the kidneys every minute. The blood flow to the kidneys is, therefore, excellent, deriving from the renal arteries directly from the descending aorta. The vascular structure of the kidneys also ensures that blood pressure within the renal capillaries is maintained at a slightly higher pressure than generally found in capillary structures in the body, supporting the filtration functions. The **nephron** is the structural and functional unit of the kidney with each kidney containing approximately 1 million nephrons! Each nephron has a **glomerulus**, a group of capillaries surrounded by an enclosing sac, known as the **Bowman's capsule** (Figure 42.2). The endothelium of the glomerular capillaries is one cell thick and highly porous, allowing fluid and solutes to readily move across this membrane into the glomerular capsule under hydrostatic pressure. The kidneys produce about 120 mL/min of filtrate in the glomeruli (known as the *glomerular filtration rate [GFR]*). Blood cells and larger molecules, such as plasma proteins, are normally too large to cross the membrane and so remain in blood. Glucose molecules are close to the threshold size and shape and electrical charge for molecules that will easily pass into the filtrate, so when the glucose concentration rises highly in blood (such as in the case of diabetes mellitus), more glucose molecules also pass into the filtrate. The glomerular filtrate produced is similar in composition to plasma, made up of water, electrolytes, amino acids, and metabolic wastes.

From the Bowman's capsule, the filtrate moves down into the tubule of the nephron. In the proximal convoluted tubule, passive processes reabsorb most of the water and electrolytes, and active processes under the influence

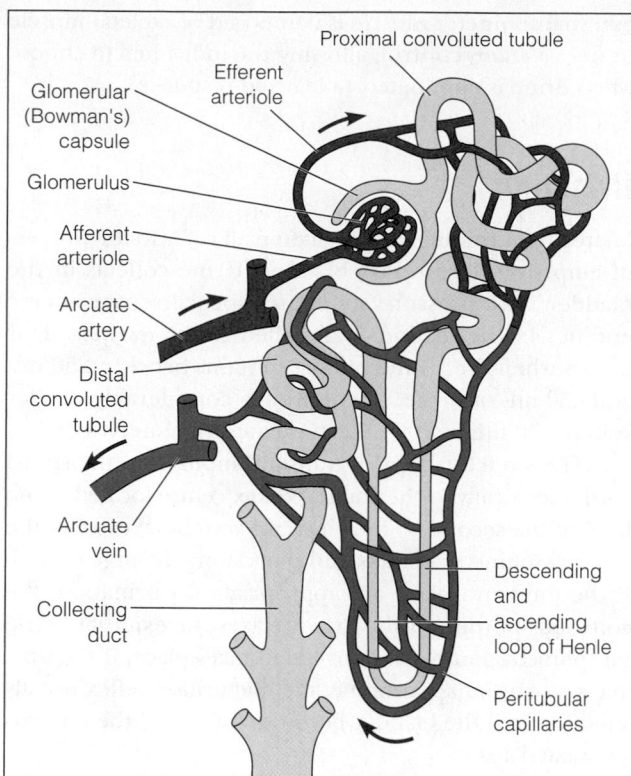

FIGURE 42.2 The nephrons of the kidney have six parts: glomerulus, Bowman's capsule, proximal convoluted tubule, loop of Henle, distal convoluted tubule, and collecting duct.

of atrial natriuretic peptide (ANP) and brain natriuretic peptide (BNP) decrease the reabsorption of sodium ions and water. In the loop of Henle, sodium, potassium, and chloride ions are actively reabsorbed and water is further passively reabsorbed by means of physiological mechanisms that concentrate sodium in the surrounding medulla, further concentrating the filtrate. In the distal convoluted tubule, additional water and sodium are actively reabsorbed under the control of the hormone aldosterone and, to some extent, antidiuretic hormone (ADH) (although this has a more pronounced effect in the collecting ducts). When aldosterone is released from the adrenal cortex, sodium and water are reabsorbed in greater quantities, increasing the blood volume and decreasing urinary output. In the distal tubule, pH is also regulated by the active excretion of hydrogen ions and the regeneration of bicarbonate. In the collecting ducts that drain the nephrons to the renal pelvis and ureters, further water is finally reabsorbed, also under the influence of aldosterone and ADH. When fluid intake is low or the concentration of solutes in the blood is high, ADH is released from the anterior pituitary, more water is reabsorbed in the distal tubule, and less urine is excreted. By contrast, when fluid intake is high or the blood solute concentration is low, ADH is suppressed. Without ADH, the distal tubule and collecting duct becomes impermeable to water, and more urine is excreted. There are other active processes that excrete specific substance into the filtrate,

and many of these remain poorly understood. However, overall this controlled reabsorption in the nephrons and collecting ducts allows fine regulation of fluid and electrolyte balance in the body.

Ureters

Once the urine is formed in the kidneys, it moves through the collecting ducts into the calyces of the renal pelvis and from there into the ureters. The ureters are from 25 cm to 30 cm long in the adult and about 1.25 cm in diameter. The upper end of each ureter is funnel shaped as it enters the kidney. The lower ends of the ureters enter the bladder at the posterior corners of the floor of the bladder (see Figure 42.1). At the junction between the ureter and the bladder, a flap-like fold of mucous membrane acts as a valve to prevent reflux (backflow) of urine up the ureters, closing when the bladder is distended.

Urinary Bladder

The urinary bladder is a hollow, muscular organ that serves as a reservoir for urine and as the organ of excretion. When empty, it lies behind the symphysis pubis. In the male, the bladder lies in front of the rectum and above the prostate gland (see Figure 42.3); in the female, it lies in front of the uterus and vagina (see Figure 42.4 on the next page). The wall of the bladder is made up of four layers: (a) an inner mucous layer; (b) a connective tissue layer; (c) three layers of smooth muscle fibres, some of which extend lengthwise, some obliquely, and some more or less circularly; and (d) an outer serous layer. The smooth muscle layers of the urinary bladder are collectively called the **detrusor muscle**. The detrusor muscle allows the bladder to expand as it fills with urine and to contract to release urine to the outside of the body during voiding. The **trigone** at the base of the bladder is a triangular area marked by the ureter openings at the posterior corners and the opening of the urethra at the anterior inferior corner. Urine exits the bladder through the urethra.

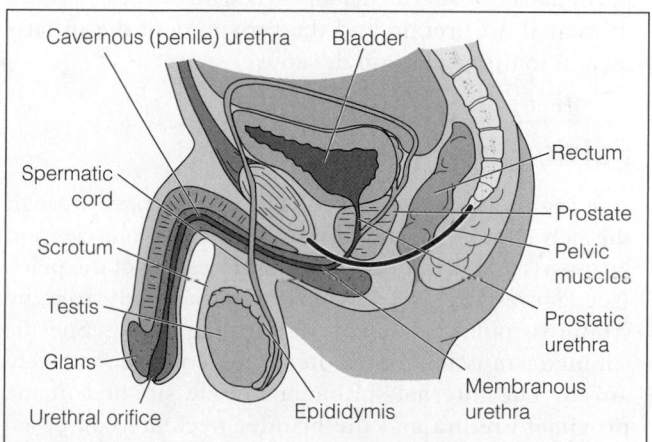

FIGURE 42.3 The male urogenital system.

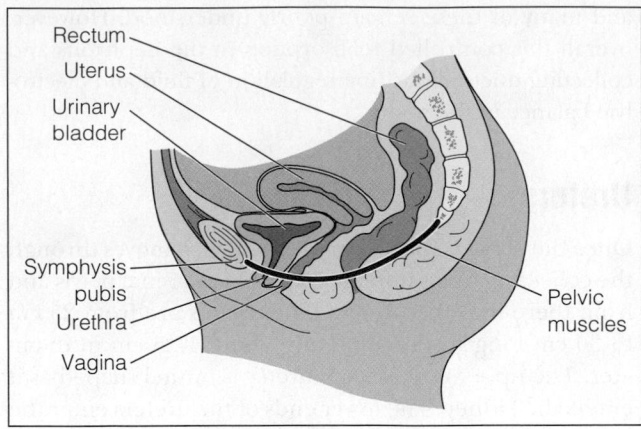

Rectum
Uterus
Urinary bladder
Symphysis pubis
Urethra
Vagina
Pelvic muscles

FIGURE 42.4 The female urogenital system.

The bladder is capable of considerable distension because of rugae (folds) in the mucous membrane lining and because of the elasticity of its walls. When full, the dome of the bladder may extend above the symphysis pubis; in extreme situations, it may extend as high as the umbilicus. Normal bladder capacity is between 300 mL and 600 mL of urine.

Urethra

The urethra extends from the bladder to the urinary **meatus** (opening). In the adult female, the urethra lies directly behind the symphysis pubis, anterior to the vagina, and is about 4.0 cm long (see Figure 42.4). The urethra serves only as a passageway for the elimination of urine. The urinary meatus is located between the labia minora, in front of the vagina and below the clitoris. The male urethra is about 20 cm long and serves as a passageway for semen as well as urine (see Figure 42.3). The meatus is located at the distal end of the penis.

In both males and females, the urethra has a mucous membrane lining that is continuous with the bladder and the ureters. Thus, an infection of the urethra can extend through the urinary tract into the kidneys. Women are particularly prone to urinary tract infections because of their short urethra and the proximity of the urinary meatus to the vagina and the anus.

Pelvic Floor

The vagina, the urethra, and the rectum pass through the pelvic floor, which consists of sheets of muscles and ligaments that provide support to the viscera of the pelvis (see Figures 42.3 and 42.4). The floor extends from the symphysis pubis to the coccyx, forming a sling. Specific sphincter muscles contribute to the continence mechanism. The internal sphincter muscle situated in the proximal urethra and the bladder neck are composed of smooth muscle under *involuntary* control. It provides active tension designed to close the urethral lumen. The

external sphincter muscle is composed of skeletal muscle under *voluntary* control, allowing the individual to choose when urine is eliminated (a learned response).

Urination

Micturition, **voiding**, and **urination** all refer to the process of emptying the urinary bladder. Urine collects in the bladder until pressure stimulates special sensory nerve endings in the bladder wall called *stretch receptors*. This occurs when the adult bladder contains between 250 mL and 450 mL of urine. In children, a considerably smaller volume, 50 mL to 200 mL, stimulates these nerves.

The stretch receptors transmit impulses to the spinal cord, specifically to the voiding reflex centre located at the level of the second to fourth sacral vertebrae, causing the internal sphincter to relax and stimulating the urge to void. If the time and place are appropriate for urination, the conscious portion of the brain relaxes the external urethral sphincter muscle and urination takes place. If the time and place are inappropriate, the micturition reflex usually subsides until the bladder becomes fuller and the reflex is stimulated again.

Voluntary control of urination is possible only if the nerves supplying the bladder and urethra, the neural tracts of the spinal cord and brain, and the motor area of the cerebrum are all intact. The individual must be able to sense that the bladder is full. Injury to any of these parts of the nervous system—for example, from a cerebral hemorrhage or spinal cord injury above the level of the sacral region—results in intermittent involuntary emptying of the bladder. Older people whose cognition is impaired may not be aware of the need to urinate or be able to respond to this urge by seeking toilet facilities.

Factors Affecting Voiding

Numerous factors affect the volume and characteristics of the urine produced and the manner in which it is excreted.

Developmental Factors

INFANTS Urine output varies according to fluid intake but usually is about 15 mL to 60 mL a day after birth, increasing to 250 mL to 500 mL a day during the first year. An infant may urinate as often as 20 times a day owing to a lack of urinary control. The kidney's ability to concentrate urine is minimal in infants (specific gravity of 1.008), and urine appears light yellow in colour.

TODDLERS AND PRESCHOOLERS Kidney function reaches maturity between the first and second years of life, and urine is concentrated effectively and has an amber colour. Between 18 and 24 months, the child starts to recognize bladder fullness and is able to hold urine beyond the urge to void. At approximately 2½ to 3 years of age, the child can perceive bladder fullness, hold urine after the urge to void, and communicate the need to urinate. Full urinary control usually occurs at age 4 or 5 years, with daytime control normally preceding nighttime control.

The preschooler is able to take responsibility for independent toileting. Parents need to realize that accidents do occur, and the child should never be punished or scolded for this. Children often forget to wash their hands or flush the toilet, and they need instruction on wiping themselves.

SCHOOL-AGE CHILDREN The school-age child's elimination system reaches maturity during this period. The kidneys double in size between the ages of 5 and 10 years. During this period, the child urinates six to eight times a day and averages one to two bowel movements per day (see the Lifespan Considerations box). **Enuresis** refers to discrete episodes of urinary incontinence. **Nocturnal enuresis** (synonymous with *intermittent nocturnal incontinence*) refers to urinary incontinence during sleep in children age 5 years or older (Nevéus, von Gontard, Hoebeke, Hjälmås, Bauer, Bower, W., . . . & Djurhuus, 2006). Approximately 15% of 5-year-olds experience enuresis; some 20% of children with nighttime enuresis also have daytime wetting problems, called *complex* or *complicated enuresis.*

Nocturnal enuresis is referred to as primary when the child has never achieved nighttime urinary control and has many causes, including failure to awaken, nocturnal polyuria (overproduction of urine at night), detrusor overactivity, small nocturnal bladder capacity, or a combination of these. The incidence of primary enuresis declines as the child matures. Secondary enuresis appears after the child has achieved dryness for 6 consecutive months and is often ascribed to stressful events such as dealing with parental divorce or the birth of a sibling. However, the exact cause of secondary enuresis remains unknown. Recent research indicates that accurate assessment is important to identify any underlying systemic illness and instigated waking and reward systems can prove very effective in management (Wooton & Norfolk, 2010).

OLDER ADULTS The excretory function of the kidney diminishes with age but usually not significantly below normal levels, unless a disease process intervenes. Blood flow can be reduced by vascular changes and decreases in cardiac output, impairing renal function. With age, the number of functioning nephrons decreases, with an estimated 30% of nephrons lost by age 80 (see the Lifespan Considerations box). Conditions that alter normal fluid intake and output, such as having influenza or having surgery, can compromise the kidney's ability to filter, maintain the acid–base balance, and maintain the electrolyte balance in older adults. The decrease in kidney function also places older adults at

LIFESPAN CONSIDERATIONS

Factors Affecting Voiding

INFANTS AND CHILDREN

- Urinary tract infections (UTIs) are the second most common infection in children, after respiratory infections. They are seen more frequently in newborn and young infant boys than girls and are most often caused by obstructions or malformations of the urinary system in these children (Ball, Bindler, & Cohen, 2010). Among older infants and children, girls experience UTIs more frequently than boys do, usually because of contamination of the urethra with stool.
- Teaching proper perineal hygiene can reduce infection. Girls should learn to wipe from front to back and wear clothing, especially underwear, that is easily permeable to air (e.g., cotton).
- Children should be taught to go to the bathroom as soon as the sensation to void is felt and not try to hold in urine.

OLDER ADULTS

- Many older men have enlarged prostate glands, which can inhibit complete emptying of the bladder. This results in urinary retention and urgency, which sometimes causes incontinence.
- Women past menopause have decreased estrogen, which results in a decrease in perineal tone and support of the bladder, vagina, and supporting tissues. This often results in urgency and stress incontinence and can even increase the incidence of UTI (Delancey, 2010).
- Increased stiffness and pain in joints, previous joint surgery, and neuromuscular problems can impair mobility and make it difficult to get to the bathroom.
- Cognitive impairment, such as in dementia, can prevent the person from understanding the need to urinate and the actions needed to perform the activity. Habit training, such as taking the person to the bathroom at a regular, scheduled time, can be effective in ensuring regular urinary elimination in people with cognitive impairments.
- Safe, easy access to the bathroom or bedside commode, whether at home or in an institution, which includes a well-lit room, safe environment, and proper assistive devices within reach (such as walkers, canes), are important variables in ensuring safety when voiding.

higher risk for toxicity from medications if excretion rates are longer.

The more noticeable changes with age are those related to the bladder. Complaints of urinary urgency and urinary frequency are common. In men, these changes are often caused by an enlarged prostate gland; in women, they are often caused by weakened muscles supporting the bladder or weakness of the urethral sphincter. The capacity of the bladder and its ability to completely empty diminish with age. These factors explain **nocturia** (awakening to urinate at night; some definitions indicate urination more than two times during the night) and urinary retention (the failure to fully empty the bladder of residual urine), predisposing the older adult to bladder infections.

Psychosocial Factors

For many people, a set of conditions helps stimulate the micturition reflex. These conditions include socio-cultural norms regarding privacy, normal position, sufficient time, and occasionally, the sight and sound of running water. Circumstances that counter the client's accustomed conditions can produce anxiety and muscle tension. As a result, the person is unable to relax the abdominal and perineal muscles and the external urethral sphincter, and voiding is inhibited. People may also voluntarily suppress urination because of perceived time pressures; for example, nurses often ignore the urge to void until they are able to take a break. This behaviour can increase the risk of UTIs.

Fluid and Food Intake

The healthy body maintains a balance between the amount of fluid ingested and the amount of fluid eliminated. Therefore, when the amount of fluid intake increases, the output normally increases. Certain fluids, such as alcohol, increase fluid output by inhibiting the production of antidiuretic hormone. Fluids that contain caffeine (e.g., coffee, tea, and cola drinks) also increase urine production. By contrast, food and fluids high in sodium can cause fluid retention as water is retained to maintain the normal concentration of electrolytes.

Some foods and fluids can change the colour of urine. For example, beets can cause urine to appear red; foods containing carotene can cause the urine to appear more yellow than usual.

Medications

Many medications, particularly those affecting the autonomic nervous system, interfere with the normal urination process and may cause retention (see Box 42.1).

Diuretics (e.g., chlorothiazide and furosemide) are drugs that increase urine formation by preventing the reabsorption of water and electrolytes from the tubules of the kidney into the bloodstream. Some medications may alter the colour of the urine (e.g., amitriptyline can discolour urine blue-green; rifampin can cause orange-yellow urine).

Muscle Tone and Activity

Strong muscle tone is important for maintaining the stretch and contractility of the detrusor muscle so the bladder can fill adequately and empty completely. Clients who require a retention catheter for a long period may have poor bladder muscle tone because continuous drainage of urine prevents the bladder from filling and emptying normally. Abdominal and pelvic floor muscle

---

BOX 42.1 SELECTED MEDICATIONS THAT MAY CAUSE URINARY RETENTION*

- Anticholinergics/antispasmodics
  - hyoscyamine (e.g., Levbid, Cystospaz, Anaspaz, Gastrosed)
  - oxybutynin (e.g., Ditropan, Ditropan XL, Oxytrol)
  - tolterodine (e.g., Detrol, Detrol LA)
  - propantheline (e.g., Pro-Banthine)
- Antihistamines
  - fexofenadine (e.g., Allegra)
  - diphenhydramine (e.g., Benadryl)
  - chlorpheniramine (e.g., Chlor-Trimeton)
  - cetirizine (e.g., Zyrtec)
- Antihypertensives
  - hydralazine (e.g., Apresoline)
  - methyldopate (e.g., Aldomet)
- Antiparkinsonism drugs
  - levodopa, trihexyphenidyl (e.g., Artane),
  - benztropine mesylate (e.g., Cogentin)
- Beta-adrenergic blockers
  - propranolol (e.g., Inderal)
- Opioids
  - morphine
  - hydrocodone
- Tricyclic antidepressants
  - imipramine (e.g., Tofranil)
  - amitriptyline (e.g., Elavil, Endep)
  - nortriptyline (e.g., Aventyl, Pamelor)
  - doxepin (e.g., Novo-Doxepin, Sinequan)

*Generic names are given in lower case and trade names in parentheses.

---

tone also contribute to normal emptying: abdominal muscle contraction assists in bladder emptying; pelvic floor muscle tone is a factor in the ability to retain urine voluntarily once the urge to urinate is perceived.

Pathological Conditions

Some diseases and pathologies can affect the formation and excretion of urine. Diseases of the kidneys can affect the ability of the nephrons to produce urine. Abnormal amounts of protein or blood cells can be present in urine, or the kidneys can virtually stop producing urine altogether, a condition known as renal failure. Heart and circulatory disorders, such as heart failure, shock, or hypertension, can affect blood flow to the kidneys, interfering with urine production. If abnormal amounts of fluid are lost through another route (e.g., vomiting or high fever), water is retained by the kidneys and urinary output falls.

Processes that interfere with the flow of urine from the kidneys to the urethra affect urinary excretion. A urinary calculus (stone) can obstruct a ureter, blocking urine flow from the kidney to the bladder. Hypertrophy (enlargement) of the prostate gland, a common condition affecting older men, can partially obstruct the urethra, impairing urination and bladder emptying.

Surgical and Diagnostic Procedures

Some surgical and diagnostic procedures can affect the passage of urine as well as urine itself. The urethra may swell following a cystoscopy, and surgical procedures on any part of the urinary tract can result in some postoperative bleeding; as a result, urine may be red-tinged or pink-tinged for a time.

Spinal anesthetics can affect the passage of urine because they decrease the person's awareness of the need to void. Surgery on structures adjacent to the urinary tract (e.g., the uterus) can also affect voiding because of swelling in the lower abdomen.

Altered Urine Production

Although people's patterns of urination are highly individual, most people void about five to seven times a day. People usually void when they first awaken in the morning, before they go to bed, and around mealtimes. Table 42.1 shows the average urinary output per day at different ages.

TABLE 42.1   Average Daily Urine Output by Age

Age	Amount (mL)
1 to 2 days	15 to 60
3 to 10 days	100 to 300
10 days to 2 months	250 to 450
2 months to 1 year	450 to 500
1 to 3 years	500 to 600
3 to 5 years	600 to 700
5 to 8 years	700 to 1000
8 to 14 years	800 to 1400
14 years through adulthood	1500
Older adulthood	1500 or less

Polyuria

Polyuria refers to the production of abnormally large amounts of urine by the kidneys, often several litres more than the client's usual daily output. Polyuria can follow **polydipsia** (excessive thirst and fluid intake) or can be associated with such diseases as diabetes mellitus, diabetes insipidus, or chronic nephritis. Polyuria can cause excessive fluid loss, leading to intense thirst, dehydration, and weight loss.

Oliguria and Anuria

The terms *oliguria* and *anuria* are used to describe decreased urinary output. **Oliguria** is low urine output, usually less than 500 mL a day or 30 mL an hour for an adult. Although oliguria can occur as a result of abnormal fluid losses or a lack of fluid intake, it often indicates impaired blood flow to the kidneys or impending renal failure and should be promptly reported to the appropriate member of the health care team. Restoring renal blood flow and urinary output promptly can prevent renal failure and its complications. **Anuria** refers to a lack of urine production.

Altered Urinary Elimination

Despite normal urine production, a number of factors or conditions can affect urinary elimination. Frequency, nocturia, urgency, and dysuria often are manifestations of underlying conditions, such as a UTI. Enuresis, incontinence, retention, and neurogenic bladder, conversely, may be either a manifestation or the primary problem affecting urinary elimination. Selected factors associated with altered patterns of urine elimination are identified in Table 42.2 on the next page.

Frequency and Nocturia

Urinary frequency is voiding at frequent intervals, that is, more often than usual—generally, more than six times a day. An increased intake of fluid causes some increase in the frequency of voiding. Some conditions, such as UTIs, stress, and pregnancy, can cause frequent voiding of small quantities (50 mL to 100 mL) of urine. Total fluid intake and output may be normal.

Nocturia, voiding two or more times at night, can be indicative of several health problems, such as heart failure and prostatic hypertrophy. It can be unsettling for clients as their sleep is disturbed. In older adults, or people with health problems, going to the toilet during the night can pose a risk for falls. Similar to frequency, it is usually expressed in terms of the number of times the person gets out of bed to void, for example, "nocturia × 4."

TABLE 42.2 Selected Factors Associated with Altered Urinary Production and Elimination

Altered Production	Selected Associated Factors	Pattern	Selected Associated Factors
Polyuria	Ingestion of fluids containing caffeine or alcohol	Enuresis	Family history of enuresis
	Prescribed diuretic		Difficult access to toilet facilities
	Presence of thirst, dehydration, and weight loss		Home stresses
	History of diabetes mellitus, diabetes insipidus, or kidney disease	Incontinence	Bladder inflammation, cerebrovascular accident, spinal cord injury, or other disease
Oliguria, anuria	Decrease in fluid intake		Difficulties in independent toileting (mobility impairment)
	Signs of dehydration		Leakage when coughing, laughing, sneezing
	Presence of hypotension, shock, or heart failure		Cognitive impairment
	History of kidney disease		Constipation
	Signs of renal failure, such as elevated blood urea nitrogen (BUN) and serum creatinine, edema, hypertension	Retention	Distended bladder on palpation and percussion
Frequency or nocturia	Pregnancy		Associated signs, such as pubic discomfort, restlessness, frequency, and small urine volume
	Increase in fluid intake		Recent anesthesia
	Urinary tract infection		Recent perineal surgery
	Any known contributing or initiating causes, such as stress		Presence of perineal swelling
Urgency	Presence of psychological stress		Medications prescribed
	Urinary tract infection		Lack of privacy or other factors inhibiting micturition
Dysuria	Urinary tract inflammation, infection, or injury		
	Hesitancy, hematuria, pyuria (pus in the urine), frequency		

Urgency

Urinary urgency is feeling the sudden *strong* desire to void. The bladder may or may not have a great deal of urine, but the person feels a need to void immediately. Urgency accompanies psychological stress and irritation of the trigone and urethra. It is also common in young children and people who have poor external sphincter control and unstable bladder, and people with UTIs. This is an abnormal finding.

Dysuria

Dysuria means voiding that is either painful or difficult. It can accompany a stricture (decrease in calibre) of the urethra, urinary infections, and injury to the bladder and urethra. Often, clients will say they have to push to void or that burning accompanies or follows voiding. The burning may be described as severe, like being touched with a hot poker, or more subdued, like a sunburn. Often, **urinary hesitancy** (a delay and difficulty in initiating voiding) is associated with dysuria.

Enuresis

Nocturnal enuresis, the involuntary urination during sleep in children over 5 years of age, and daytime enuresis (sometimes referred to as complicated enuresis) can be a difficult experience for the child and family owing to the many sociocultural values placed on controlling urination.

Urinary Incontinence

Urinary incontinence (UI), or involuntary leakage of urine or loss of bladder control, is a symptom, not a disease. It can have a significant impact on the client's life, creating physical problems, such as skin breakdown, and possibly leading to psychosocial problems, such as embarrassment, isolation, and social withdrawal. Approximately 4% of Canadians experience some sort of urinary incontinence, with women experiencing more UI than men (Irwin, Milsom, Hunskaar, Reilly, Kopp, Herschorn, & . . . Abrams, 2006) and as many as half of women older than 65 years experience UI. This experience is not unique to older clients: 10% of men and 16% of women age 18 to 40 years experience UI. Although incontinence is common in older adults, it is *not* a normal consequence of aging and can often be treated. Common causes of incontinence include UTIs, urethritis, pregnancy, hypercalcemia, volume overload, delirium, restricted mobility, stool impaction, and psychological causes (Wellbery, 2008). Urinary incontinence can be transient (acute) or established (chronic).

Transient UI usually arrives suddenly, lasts 6 months or less, and has reversible causes. The etiology of transient incontinence is generally from nonurinary system causes, such as infection, atrophic urethritis or vaginitis, restricted mobility, use of pharmaceuticals (e.g., diuretics), stool impaction or constipation, and delirium or acute confused state. Some of these factors are readily reversible, with a lessening of symptoms if not complete resolution of urinary incontinence.

Urinary incontinence may be a longstanding or chronic problem. Different types of chronic incontinence, each having a different etiology, include stress, urge, overflow, reflex, functional, and total incontinence (discussed later in the section "Diagnosing").

The preliminary assessment and identification of the symptom of urinary incontinence is truly within the scope of nursing practice (see Clinical Alert box). All clients should be asked about their voiding patterns. Older adults who are incontinent while in their home or who manage to contain or conceal their incontinence from others may not consider themselves incontinent. Therefore, when asked if they are incontinent, they may deny it. However, asking if they lose urine when they do not want to or if they need to use some sort of incontinence product may provide more accurate information. If incontinence is described, a thorough history and assessment is indicated. Treatment can include surgery, medication, or behavioural therapies. Nursing management of incontinence includes implementing individualized bladder programs, containment of urine, and meticulous skin care.

> ### ! CLINICAL ALERT
>
> The new onset of urinary incontinence in any client must be assessed thoroughly. Constipation, trigger medications (muscle relaxants, diuretics), fecal impaction, and infection are possible causes of acute urinary incontinence. The treatment of incontinence can be determined only after the cause is identified.

Urinary Retention

When the emptying of the bladder is impaired, residual urine accumulates and the bladder becomes over-distended, a condition known as **urinary retention**. Overdistension of the bladder causes poor contractility of the detrusor muscle, further impairing urination. Common causes of urinary retention include

prostatic hypertrophy, surgery, and some medications (see Box 42.1 on page 1308).

Clients with urinary retention may experience overflow voiding or incontinence, eliminating 25 mL to 50 mL of urine at frequent intervals. The bladder is firm and distended on palpation and may be displaced to one side of midline.

Neurogenic Bladder

Impaired neurological function can interfere with the normal mechanisms of urine elimination, resulting in a **neurogenic bladder**. The client with a neurogenic bladder does not perceive bladder fullness and is unable to control the urinary sphincters. The bladder may become flaccid and distended or spastic, with frequent involuntary urination.

Assessing

A complete assessment of a client's urinary function includes the following:

- Collecting a nursing history
- Conducting a physical assessment of the genitourinary system, hydration status, and examination of the urine
- Relating the data obtained to the results of any diagnostic tests and procedures

NURSING HISTORY The nurse determines the client's normal voiding pattern and frequency, the appearance of the urine and any recent changes, any past or current problems with urination, the presence of an ostomy, and the factors influencing the elimination pattern.

Examples of questions to elicit this information are shown in the Assessment: Interview box on the next page. The number of questions asked depends on the individual and the responses to the first three categories.

PHYSICAL ASSESSMENT Complete physical assessment of the urinary tract usually includes percussion of the kidneys to detect areas of tenderness. Palpation and percussion of the bladder are also performed. (See Chapter 28.) If the client's history or current problems indicate a need for it, the urethral meatus of both male and female clients is inspected for swelling, discharge, and inflammation.

Because problems with urination can affect the elimination of wastes from the body, it is important that the nurse assess the skin for colour, texture, and tissue turgor as well as the presence of edema. If incontinence, dribbling, or dysuria is noted in the history, the skin of the perineum should be inspected for irritation because contact with urine can excoriate the skin.

Urinary Elimination

The nurse can use the following questions to learn about the client's urinary elimination:

VOIDING PATTERN

- How many times do you urinate during a 24-hour period?
- Has this pattern changed recently?
- Do you need to get out of bed to urinate at night? How often?

DESCRIPTION OF URINE AND ANY CHANGES

- How would you describe your urine in terms of colour, clarity (clear, transparent, or cloudy), and odour (faint or strong)?

URINARY ELIMINATION PROBLEMS

- What problems have you had or do you now have with passing your urine?
- Passage of small amounts of urine?
- Voiding at more frequent intervals?
- Trouble getting to the bathroom in time or feeling an urgent need to void?
- Painful voiding?
- Difficulty starting the urine stream?
- Frequent dribbling of urine or feeling of bladder fullness associated with voiding small amounts of urine?
- Reduced force of stream?
- Accidental leakage of urine?
    If so, when does this occur (e.g., when coughing, laughing, or sneezing; at night; during the day)?
- Past urinary tract illness, such as infection of the kidney, bladder, or urethra; urinary calculi; surgery of kidney, ureters, or bladder?

PRESENCE AND MANAGEMENT OF URINARY DIVERSION OSTOMY

- What is your usual routine with your ostomy?
- What problems, if any, do you have with it?

FACTORS INFLUENCING URINARY ELIMINATION

- *Medications.* Do you take any medications that could increase urinary output (e.g., diuretic) or cause retention of urine (e.g., anticholinergic–antispasmodic, antidepressant–antipsychotic, antiparkinsonism, antihistamines, antihypertensives)? Note specific medication, dosage, and frequency.
- *Fluid intake.* What amount and kind of fluid do you take each day?
- *Environmental factors.* Do you have any problems with toileting (e.g., mobility, removing clothing, toilet seat too low, facility without grab bar)?
- *Presence of long-term catheter.* How do you care for your catheter? Do you have any discomfort with it or other problems? How can the nurse help you manage it?
- *Stress.* Are you experiencing any long-term or short-term stress? If so, what are the stressors? Do you think these affect your urinary pattern?
- *Disease.* Have you had or do you have any illnesses that can affect urinary function, such as hypertension, heart disease, neurological disease, cancer, prostatic enlargement, diabetes mellitus, or diabetes insipidus?
- *Diagnostic procedures.* Have you recently had a cystoscopy or spinal anesthetic?

ASSESSING URINE Normal urine consists of 96% water and 4% solutes. Organic solutes include urea, ammonia, creatinine, and uric acid. Urea is the chief organic solute. Inorganic solutes include sodium, chloride, potassium, sulphate, magnesium, and phosphorus. Sodium chloride is the most abundant inorganic salt. Characteristics of normal and abnormal urine are shown in Table 42.3.

Measuring Urinary Output Normally, the kidneys produce urine at a rate of approximately 60 mL per hour or about 1500 mL per day. Urine output is affected by many factors, including fluid intake, body fluid losses through other routes, such as perspiration and breathing, and the cardiovascular and renal status of the individual.

Urine outputs of less than 30 mL per hour may indicate low blood volume or kidney malfunction and must be reported. In children, normal urine volume is 300 mL to 1500 mL per day (see Table 42.1 on page 1309).

To measure fluid output, the nurse follows these steps:

- Wear clean gloves to prevent contact with microorganisms or blood in the urine.

- Ask the client to void in a clean urinal (see Figure 42.5 on page 1314 for male urinal and Figure 42.6 for female urinal), bedpan, commode, or toilet collection device (*hat*) (see Figure 42.7).
- Instruct the client to keep urine separate from feces and to avoid putting toilet paper in the urine collection container.
- Pour the voided urine into a calibrated container.
- Hold the container at eye level and read the amount in the container. Containers usually have a measuring scale on the inside.
- If a clean specimen is required, pour some urine into the specimen container and discard the remainder, unless all urine is to be saved.
- Record the amount on the fluid intake and output sheet, which may be at the bedside or in the bathroom.
- Rinse the urine collection and measuring containers with cool water and store appropriately.
- Remove gloves and perform hand hygiene.
- Calculate and document the total output on the client's chart at the end of each shift and at the end of 24 hours.

TABLE 42.3 Characteristics of Normal and Abnormal Urine

Characteristic	Normal	Abnormal	Nursing Considerations
Amount in 24 hours (adult)	1200 mL to 1500 mL	Less than 1200 mL More than 1500 mL or a large amount more than intake	Urinary output is generally similar to fluid intake. Output of less than 30 mL/h may indicate decreased blood flow to the kidneys and should be immediately reported. Increased urine production may indicate excess fluid intake, hormonal imbalance such as inadequate antidiuretic hormone, or inability of the kidneys to concentrate urine.
Colour, clarity	Straw, amber Transparent	Dark amber Cloudy Dark orange Red or dark brown Mucous plugs, viscid, thick	Concentrated urine is darker in colour. Diluted urine can appear almost clear or very pale yellow. Some foods and drugs can colour urine (e.g., beets, phenazopyridine, phenytoin). Red blood cells in the urine (hematuria) may be evident as pink, bright red, or rusty brown urine. Menstrual bleeding can also colour urine but should not be confused with hematuria. White blood cells, bacteria, pus, or contaminants, such as prostatic fluid, sperm, or vaginal drainage, can cause cloudy urine.
Odour	Faint aromatic	Offensive	Some foods (e.g., asparagus) cause a musty odour; infected urine can have a fetid odour; urine high in glucose has a sweet odour.
Sterility	No microorganisms present	Microorganisms present	Urine in the bladder is sterile. Urine specimens, however, may be contaminated by bacteria from the perineum during collection.
pH	4.5 to 8	Less than 4.5 More than 8	Freshly voided urine is normally somewhat acidic. More acidic urine (low pH) is found in acidosis, starvation, diarrhea, or with a diet high in protein foods or cranberries. Alkaline urine may indicate a state of alkalosis, urinary tract infection (UTI), or a diet high in fruits and vegetables.
Specific gravity	1.010 to 1.025	Less than 1.010 More than 1.025	Diluted urine has a lower specific gravity; concentrated urine has a higher specific gravity.
Glucose	Not present	Present	Glucose in urine indicates high blood glucose levels and may be indicative of undiagnosed or uncontrolled diabetes mellitus.
Ketone bodies (i.e., beta-hydroxybutyrate, acetone, acetoacetic acid)	Not present	Present	Ketones, the end product of the breakdown of fatty acids, are not normally present in the urine. They may be present in the urine of clients who have uncontrolled diabetes mellitus, are in a state of starvation, or who have ingested excessive amounts of acetylsalicylic acid.
Blood	Not present	Occult (microscopic) Bright red	Blood may be present in the urine of clients who have UTI, kidney disease, or bleeding from the urinary tract.

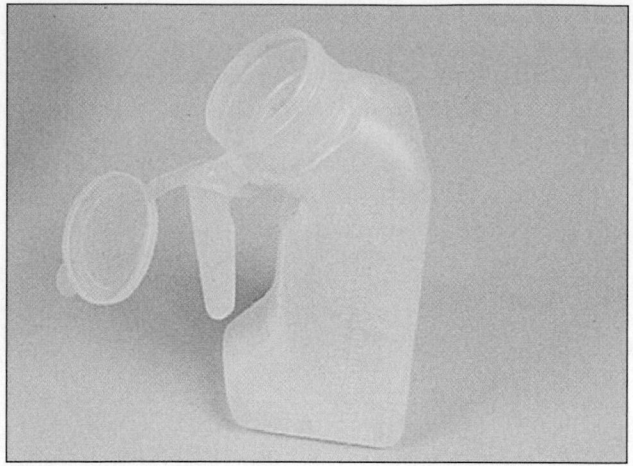

FIGURE 42.5 Male urinal.

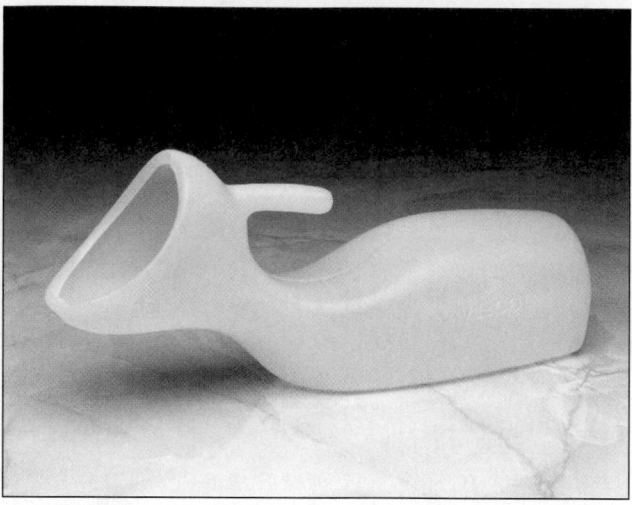

FIGURE 42.6 Female urinal.

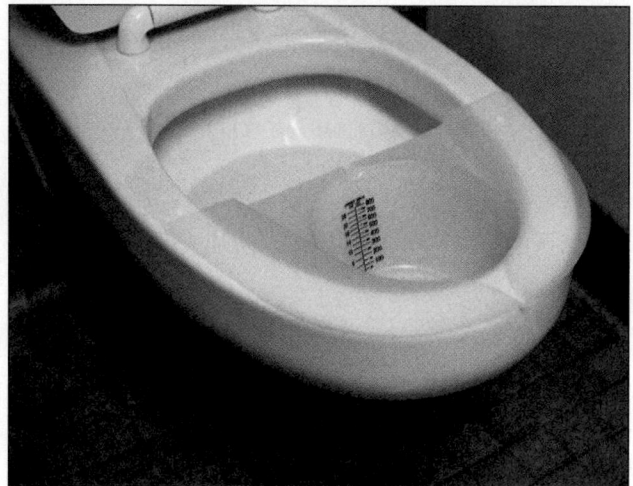

FIGURE 42.7 A urine "hat": a urine collection device for the toilet.

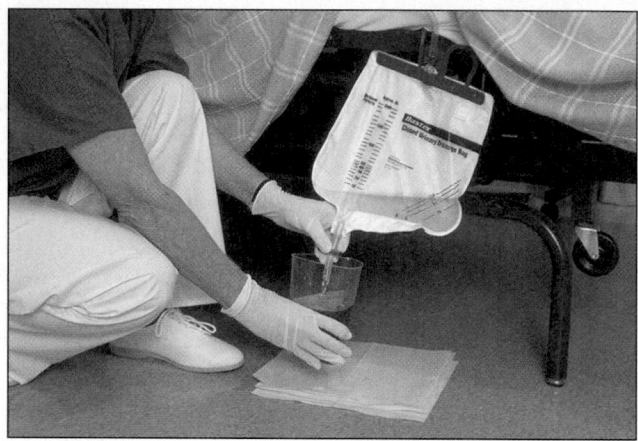

FIGURE 42.8 Urine being measured from a urine collection bag.

Many clients can measure and record their own urine output when the procedure is explained to them.

When measuring urine from a client who has an indwelling catheter, follow these steps:

- Put on clean gloves.
- Take the clean calibrated container to the bedside.
- Place the container under the urine collection bag so that the spout of the bag is above the container but not touching it. The calibrated container is not sterile, but the inside of the collection bag is sterile (Figure 42.8).
- Open the spout and permit the urine to flow into the container.
- Close the spout, and then proceed as described in the previous list.

Measuring Residual Urine **Residual urine** (urine remaining in the bladder following the voiding) is normally 50 mL to 100 mL. However, a bladder outlet obstruction (e.g., enlargement of the prostate gland) or loss of bladder muscle tone can interfere with complete emptying of the bladder during urination. Manifestations of urine retention include frequent voiding of small amounts (e.g., less than 100 mL in an adult). Urinary stasis and UTIs are possible consequences of incomplete bladder emptying. Residual urine is measured to assess the amount of retained urine after voiding and determine the need for interventions (e.g., medications to promote detrusor muscle contraction).

To measure residual urine, the nurse catheterizes or bladder scans (Figure 42.9) the client immediately after voiding. The amount of urine voided and the amount

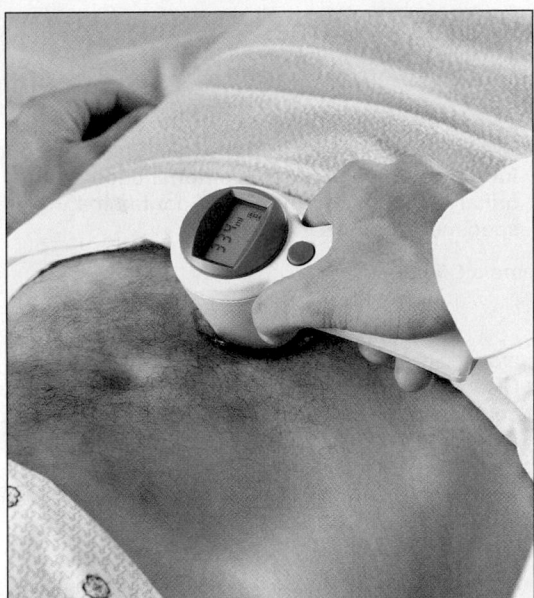

FIGURE 42.9 A handheld, portable bladder ultrasound scanner.

Source: Courtesy of Verathon Medical, USA.

obtained by catheterization or bladder scan are measured and recorded. An indwelling catheter may be inserted if the residual urine exceeds a specified amount.

COLLECTING URINE SPECIMENS   The nurse is responsible for collecting urine specimens for a number of tests: clean voided specimens for routine urinalysis, *clean-catch* or *midstream urine specimens* for urine culture, and timed urine specimens for a variety of tests, depending on the client's specific health problem.

Clean Voided Urine Specimen   A clean voided specimen is usually adequate for routine examination. Many clients are able to collect a clean voided specimen and provide the specimen independently, with minimal instructions. Male clients generally are able to void directly into the specimen container, and female clients usually sit or squat over the toilet, holding the container between their legs during voiding. About 120 mL of urine is generally required. Clients who are seriously ill, physically incapacitated, or disoriented may need to use a bedpan or urinal in bed; others may require supervision or assistance in the bathroom. Whatever the situation, explicit directions are required:

- The specimen must be free of fecal contamination, so urine must be kept separate from feces.
- Any toilet tissue should be discarded in the toilet or in a waste bag, rather than in the bedpan, because tissue in the specimen makes laboratory analysis more difficult.
- The lid must be closed tightly on the container to prevent spillage of the urine and contamination of other objects.

- If the outside of the container has been contaminated by urine, clean it with a disinfectant and place in a clean plastic bag.
- If the outside of the container has been contaminated by urine, it should be cleaned with disinfectant.

The nurse must (a) make sure that the specimen label and the laboratory requisition carry the correct information, and (b) attach them securely to the specimen. Inappropriate identification of the specimen can lead to errors of diagnosis or therapy for the client.

Clean-Catch or Midstream Urine Specimen   Clean-catch or midstream voided specimens are collected when a urine culture is ordered to identify microorganisms causing UTIs. Although some contamination by skin bacteria can occur with a clean-catch specimen, the risk of introducing microorganisms into the urinary tract through catheterization is more significant. Care is taken to ensure that the specimen is as free as possible from contamination by microorganisms around the urinary meatus. Clean-catch specimens are collected into a sterile specimen container with a lid. Disposable clean-catch kits are available (Figure 42.10). Skill 42.1 on the next page explains how to collect a clean-catch urine specimen for culture.

Timed Urine Specimen   Some urine examinations require collection of all urine produced and voided over a specific period, ranging from 1 to 2 hours to 24 hours (see the Home Care Considerations box on page 1317). Timed specimens generally either are refrigerated or contain a preservative to prevent bacterial growth or decomposition of urine components. Each voiding of urine is collected in a small, clean container and then emptied immediately into the large refrigerated bottle or carton.

To collect a timed urine specimen, follow these steps:

- Obtain a specimen container with preservative (if indicated) from the laboratory. Label the container with identifying information for the client, the test to be performed, time started, and time of completion.
- Provide a clean receptacle to collect urine (bedpan, commode, or toilet collection device).

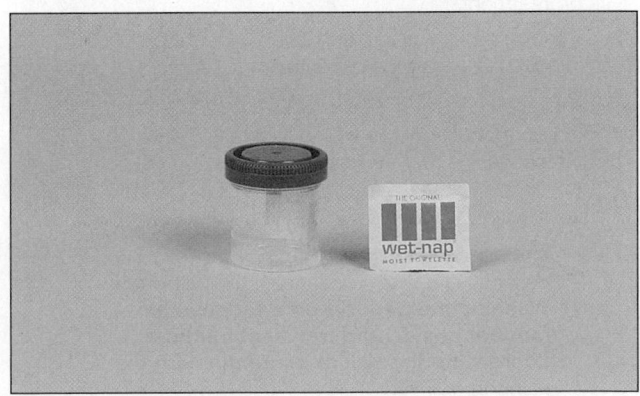

FIGURE 42.10 Disposable clean-catch specimen equipment.

SKILL 42.1 COLLECTING A URINE SPECIMEN FOR CULTURE AND SENSITIVITY BY CLEAN CATCH

PURPOSE

- To determine the presence of microorganisms, the type of organism(s), and the antibiotics to which the organisms are sensitive

ASSESSMENT

- Determine the ability of the client to provide the specimen.
- Assess the colour, odour, and consistency of the urine and the presence of clinical signs of UTI (e.g., frequency, urgency, dysuria, hematuria, flank pain, cloudy urine with foul odour).

Equipment

Equipment used varies from agency to agency. Some agencies use commercially prepared disposable clean-catch kits. Others are agency-prepared sterile trays. Both prepared trays and kits generally contain the following items:

- Clean gloves
- Antiseptic towelettes
- Sterile cotton balls or 5 cm × 5 cm gauze pads
- Sterile specimen container
- Specimen identification label

  In addition the nurse needs to obtain the following:
- Completed laboratory requisition form
- Urine receptacle, if the client is not ambulatory
- Basin of warm water, soap, washcloth, and towel for the nonambulatory client

IMPLEMENTATION

Preparation

Gather the necessary equipment for the collection of the specimen. Use visual aids, if available, to assist the client to understand the midstream collection technique.

Performance

1. Before performing the procedure, introduce yourself and verify the client's identity using two identifiers or per agency protocol. Explain to the client that a urine specimen is required, give the reason, and explain the method to be used to collect it. Discuss how the results will be used in planning further care or treatments.

2. Perform hand hygiene, and follow other appropriate infection prevention and control procedures.

3. Provide for client privacy.

4. For an ambulatory client who is able to follow directions, instruct the client on how to collect the specimen.

   - Direct or assist the client to the bathroom.
   - Ask the client to wash and dry the genitals and perineal area with soap and water. **Rationale: Washing the perineal area reduces the number of skin and transient bacteria, decreasing the risk of contaminating the urine specimen.**

   - Instruct the client on how to clean the urinary meatus with antiseptic towelettes. **Rationale: The antiseptic further reduces bacterial contamination of the urinary meatus and the risk of contaminating the specimen.**

   For Female Clients
   - Use each towelette only once. Clean the perineal area from front to back and discard the towelette. Use all towelettes provided (usually two or three) (see ❶). **Rationale: Cleaning from front to back cleans the area of least contamination to the area of greatest contamination.**

   For Male Clients
   - If the client is uncircumcised, retract the foreskin slightly to expose the urinary meatus.
   - Using a circular motion, clean the urinary meatus and the distal portion of the penis. Use each towelette only once, and then discard it. Clean several centimetres down the shaft of the penis (see ❷). **Rationale: This cleans from the area of least contamination to the area of greatest contamination.**

5. For a client who requires assistance, prepare the client and equipment.
   - Wash the perineal area with soap and water, rinse, and dry.
   - Assist the client onto a clean commode or bedpan. If using a bedpan or urinal, position the client as upright

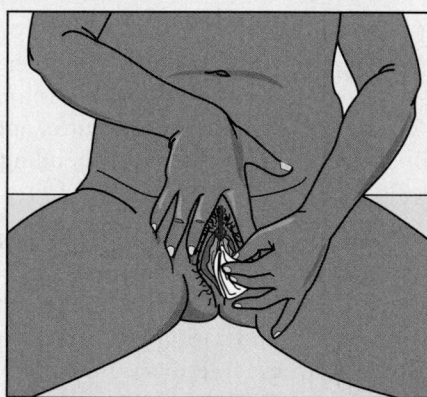

❶ Cleansing the female urinary meatus: spread the labia with one hand, and with the other hand, cleanse the perineal area from front to back.

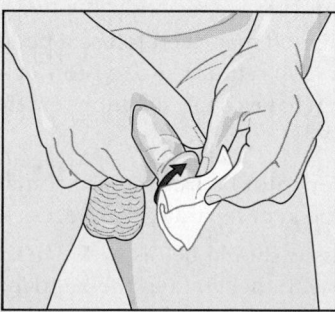

❷ Cleansing the male urinary meatus. Retract the foreskin, if needed. Using a towelette, cleanse the urinary meatus by moving in a circular motion from the centre of the urethral opening, around the glans, and down the distal portion of the shaft of the penis.

as allowed or tolerated. **Rationale: Assuming a normal anatomical position for voiding facilitates urination.**

- Open the clean-catch kit, taking care not to contaminate the inside of the specimen container or lid. **Rationale: It is important to maintain sterility of the specimen container to prevent contamination of the specimen.**
- Put on clean gloves.
- Clean the urinary meatus and perineal area.

6. Collect the specimen from a nonambulatory client or instruct an ambulatory client on how to collect it.

- Instruct the client to start voiding. **Rationale: Bacteria in the distal urethra and at the urinary meatus are cleared by the first few millilitres of urine expelled.**
- Place the specimen container into the midstream of urine and collect the specimen, taking care not to touch the container to the perineum or penis. **Rationale: It is important to avoid contaminating the interior of the specimen container and the specimen itself.**
- Collect urine in the container.
- Cap the container tightly, touching only the outside of the container and the cap. **Rationale: This action prevents contamination or spilling of the specimen.**
- If necessary, clean the outside of the specimen container with disinfectant. **Rationale: This measure prevents transfer of microorganisms to others.**

7. Label the specimen and transport it to the laboratory.
- Ensure that the specimen label is attached to the specimen cup, not the lid, and the laboratory requisition provides the correct information. Place the specimen in a plastic bag that has a biohazard label on it. Attach the requisition securely to the bag. **Rationale: Inaccurate identification or information on the specimen container has the risk of errors in diagnosis or therapy.**
- Arrange for the specimen to be sent to the laboratory immediately. **Rationale: Bacterial cultures must be started immediately before any contaminating organisms can grow, multiply, and produce false results.**

8. Document pertinent data.
- Record collection of the specimen, any pertinent observations of the urine, such as colour, odour, or consistency, and any difficulty in voiding that the client experienced.
- Indicate on the lab slip if the client is taking any current antibiotic therapy or if the client is menstruating.

EVALUATION

- Report and discuss laboratory results with the appropriate members of the health care team.
- Conduct appropriate follow-up nursing interventions, as needed, such as administering ordered medications and client teaching.

HOME CARE CONSIDERATIONS

If the client will have to collect urine at home, consider the following:

- Assess the client's ability and willingness to collect a timed urine specimen. If poor eyesight or hand tremors are a problem, suggest using a clean funnel to pour the urine into the container.
- Always wash hands well with warm, soapy water before and after collecting urine samples.
- Always wear gloves if handling another person's urine.
- The home should have a refrigerator or other method for cooling the urine samples. Tell the client to keep the specimen container in plastic in the refrigerator, separate from other refrigerator contents. The client can also use a cooler with ice.

- Post signs in the client's chart, Kardex, room, and bathroom alerting personnel to save all urine during the specified time.
- At the start of the collection period, have the client void and discard this urine.
- Save all urine produced during the timed collection period in the container, refrigerating or placing the

container on ice, as indicated. Avoid contaminating the urine with toilet paper or feces.

- At the end of the collection period, instruct the client to completely empty the bladder and save this voiding as part of the specimen. Take the entire amount of urine collected to the laboratory with the completed requisition.
- Record collection of the specimen, time started and completed, and any pertinent observations of the urine on appropriate records.

Indwelling Catheter Specimen Sterile urine specimens can be obtained from closed drainage systems, generally through designated ports. Historically, nurses would insert a sterile needle attached to a syringe through the urinary drainage tubing just above where it connected with the collecting tubing (Figure 42.11A on the next page). Newer urinary catheters have access ports that allow urine to be aspirated into a syringe. When urinary catheters with self-sealing rubber ports are used, the needle is inserted into the port and the urine is aspirated (Figure 42.11B). More and more, closed drainage urinary systems now have needleless ports, so a needle does not have to be used to obtain a sample. This protects the nurse from a needle-stick

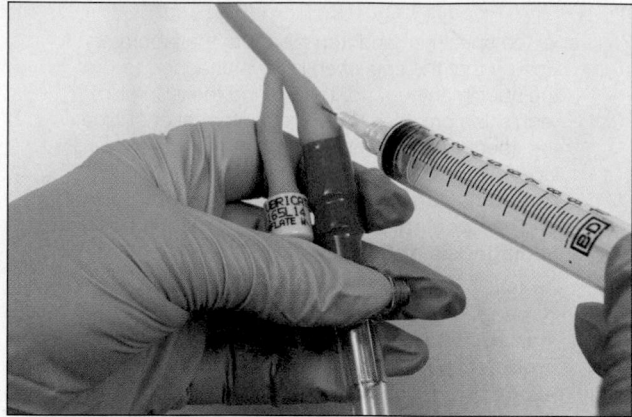

A

B

FIGURE 42.11 Obtaining a urine specimen from a retention catheter: **A:** From a specific area near the end of the catheter; **B:** From an access port in the tubing.

injury and maintains the integrity and sterility of the catheter system by eliminating the need to puncture the tubing. The needleless port accepts a Luer-Lok syringe (Figure 42.12). Position the syringe perpendicular to the centre of the port and insert, twist, and lock into the port. When the specimen is obtained and the syringe removed, the port seals itself.

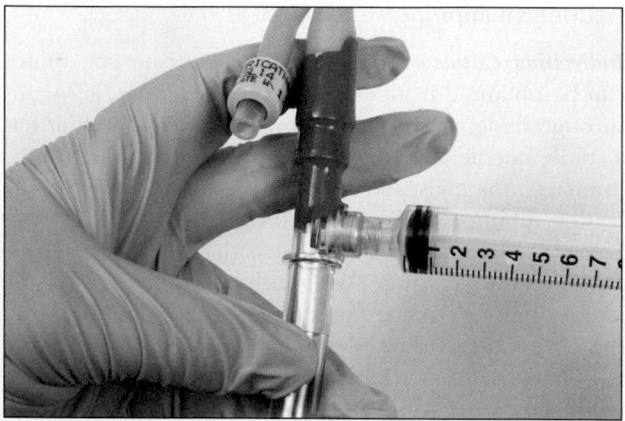

FIGURE 42.12 Obtaining a urine specimen from a retention catheter using a needleless port.

To collect a specimen from a Foley (retention) catheter or a drainage tube, follow these steps:

- Put on disposable gloves.
- If there is no urine in the catheter, clamp the drainage tubing at least 8 cm below the sampling port for about 15 to 20 minutes. This allows fresh urine to collect in the catheter.
- Wipe with a disinfectant swab the area in which the needle or Luer-Lok will be inserted. The site should be distal to the tube leading to the balloon to avoid puncturing this tube. Disinfecting the needle insertion site removes any microorganisms on the surface of the catheter, thereby avoiding contamination of the needle and the entrance of microorganisms into the catheter.
- If using an older urinary catheter without a port, insert the needle at a 30- to 45-degree angle (see Figure 42.11A). This angle of entrance facilitates self-sealing of the rubber. If using a port, insert the needle or needless syringe at a 90-degree angle (see Figures 42.11B and 42.12).
- Withdraw the required amount of urine, for example, 3 mL for a urine culture or 30 mL for a routine urinalysis.
- Transfer the urine to the specimen container. Make sure that neither the needle or needless syringe touches the outside of the container if a sterile culture tube is used.
- If using a needle, do not recap and discard the syringe and needle in an appropriate sharps container.
- Cap the container.
- Unclamp the drainage tubing.
- Remove gloves and discard appropriately.
- Label the container, and send the urine specimen to the laboratory immediately for analysis or refrigeration.
- Record collection of the specimen and any pertinent observations of the urine on the appropriate records.

URINE TESTING Several simple urine tests are often done by nurses on the nursing units. These include tests for specific gravity, pH, and the presence of abnormal constituents, such as glucose, ketones, protein, and occult blood.

Nurses in a health care facility or clients in the home setting can use commercially prepared kits to test abnormal constituents in the urine. These kits contain the required equipment and an appropriate reagent, which may be in the form of a tablet, fluid, or paper test strip or dipstick. When the urine contacts the reagent, a chemical reaction occurs, causing a colour change that is then compared with a chart to interpret the significance of the colour (Figure 42.13). Specific directions for the amount of urine needed, the time required for the chemical reaction, and the meaning of the colours produced vary among manufacturers. Thus, it is essential that nurses and clients read and follow directions supplied by each

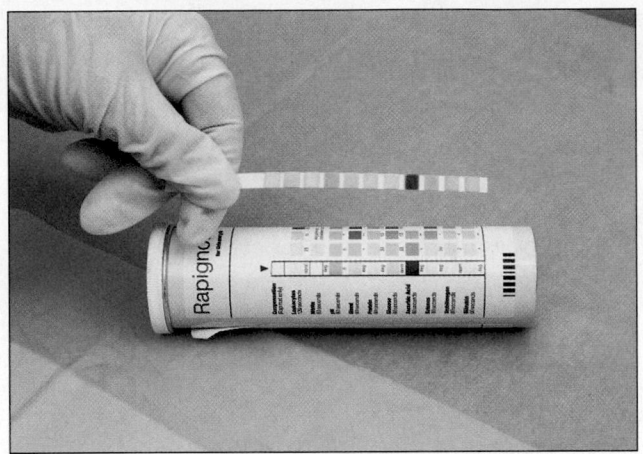

FIGURE 42.13 After dipping the reagent strip (dipstick) into fresh urine, wait the stated time and compare the results to the colour chart.

manufacturer. In addition, testing materials need to be checked to ascertain that they have not expired.

Specific Gravity The urine specific gravity is an indicator of urine concentration, or the amount of solutes (metabolic wastes and electrolytes) present in urine. The specific gravity of distilled water is 1.000; the specific gravity of urine normally ranges from 1.010 to 1.025. As urine becomes more concentrated, its specific gravity increases. Excess fluid intake or diseases affecting the ability of the kidneys to concentrate urine can result in low specific gravity readings. A high specific gravity can indicate fluid deficit or dehydration, or excess solutes, such as glucose, in urine. Specific gravity can be measured with the use of a multiple-test dipstick that has a separate reagent area for specific gravity.

Urinary pH Urinary pH is measured to determine the relative acidity or alkalinity of urine and assess the client's acid–base status. Quantitative measurements of urine pH can be performed in the laboratory, but dipsticks or litmus paper often are used on nursing units or in clinics to obtain less precise pH measurements. Urine normally is slightly acidic, with an average pH of 6 (7 is neutral, less than 7 is acidic, greater than 7 is alkaline). Because the kidneys play a critical role in regulating acid–base balance, assessment of urine pH can be useful in determining whether the kidneys are responding appropriately to acid–base imbalances. In metabolic acidosis, urine pH should decrease as the kidneys excrete hydrogen ions; in metabolic alkalosis, the pH should increase (see Chapter 44).

Glucose Urine is tested for glucose to screen clients for diabetes mellitus and to assess clients during pregnancy for abnormal glucose tolerance. Normally, the amount of glucose in the urine is negligible. Owing to varying glucose thresholds in the kidney, a lack of glucose in the urine does not mean that the person has normal blood glucose levels.

Ketones Ketone bodies, a product of the breakdown of fatty acids, normally are not present in urine. They may, however, be found in the urine of clients with poorly controlled diabetes. Urine ketone testing with reagent tablets or a dipstick also is used to evaluate ketoacidosis in clients with alcoholism and in those who are fasting, starving, or consuming high-protein diets.

Protein Protein molecules normally are too large to escape from glomerular capillaries into the filtrate. If the glomerular membrane has been damaged, however (e.g., because of an inflammatory process, such as glomerulonephritis), it can become *leaky*, allowing proteins to escape. Urine testing for the presence of protein generally is done with a reagent strip, commonly referred to as a *dipstick*.

Occult Blood Normal urine is free of blood. When blood is present, it may be clearly visible or occult (not visible). Commercial reagent strips are used to test for occult blood in urine.

Metabolic Substances Blood levels of two metabolically produced substances, urea and creatinine, are routinely used to evaluate renal function. The kidneys, through filtration and tubular secretion, normally eliminate both. Urea, the end product of protein metabolism, is measured as **blood urea nitrogen (BUN)**. **Creatinine** is produced in relatively constant quantities by the muscles and is excreted by the kidneys. Thus, the amount of creatinine in the blood relates to renal excretory function. The **creatinine clearance** test uses 24-hour urine and serum creatinine levels to determine the glomerular filtration rate (**GFR**), a sensitive indicator of renal function.

VISUALIZATION PROCEDURES Visualization procedures also can be used to evaluate urinary function. A radiograph of the kidneys, ureters, and bladder is commonly referred to as *KUB* (kidney-ureter-bladder). **Intravenous pyelography (IVP)** and **retrograde pyelography** also are radiographic studies used to evaluate the urinary tract. In an intravenous pyelogram, contrast medium is injected intravenously; during retrograde pyelography, the contrast medium is instilled directly into the renal pelvis via the urethra, bladder, and ureters. Following injection or instillation of the contrast medium, radiographs are taken to evaluate urinary tract structures. **Renal ultrasonography** is a noninvasive test that uses reflected sound waves to visualize the kidneys. During a **cystoscopy**, the bladder, ureteral orifices, and urethra can be directly visualized using a **cystoscope**, a lighted instrument inserted through the urethra.

Nurses are responsible for preparing clients before these studies and for follow-up care.

Diagnosing

Possible diagnoses for urinary elimination problems include stress incontinence, as evidenced by sudden leakage of urine with increased abdominal pressure (e.g., sneezing, coughing); urinary retention, as evidenced by residual volume of >100 mL; nocturia, as evidenced by repeated risings during the night to urinate; overflow urinary incontinence, as evidenced by involuntary loss of urine associated with an overdistended bladder.

TABLE 42.4 Assessment Data and Examples of Nursing Diagnoses

Data Cluster	Nursing Diagnosis
Mrs. Amy Brown, 75 years old, reports accidental loss of urine before she is able to reach the toilet. She is aware of the urge to void but states, "Because of my stroke, I sometimes can't get there soon enough."	Functional urinary incontinence related to mobility deficit
Anthony Chou, a teenager with a spinal cord injury, has no awareness of bladder filling, the urge to void, or feelings of bladder fullness. He reports loss of urine at fairly regular intervals.	Reflex urinary incontinence related to neurological impairment (spinal cord lesion)
Tammy Tyndale reports dribbling whenever she laughs, coughs, or sneezes. She is 8 months pregnant.	Stress urinary incontinence related to high intra-abdominal pressure associated with pregnancy
Gail Brady reports urinary urgency, difficulty in getting to the bathroom in time, frequency (more often than every 2 hours), and leakage of urine when unable to reach the toilet in time.	Urge urinary incontinence related to unknown etiology

Clinical examples of assessment data and related nursing diagnoses are shown in Table 42.4.

Problems of urinary elimination can become the etiology for other problems experienced by the client. Examples include the following:

- *Risk for Infection* if the client has urinary retention or undergoes an invasive procedure, such as catheterization.

- *Low Self-Esteem* or *Social Isolation* if the client is incontinent. Incontinence can be physically and emotionally distressing to clients because it is considered socially unacceptable. Often, the client is embarrassed about dribbling or having an accident and may restrict normal activities for this reason.

- *Risk for Impaired Skin Integrity* if the client is incontinent. Bed linens and clothes saturated with urine irritate and excoriate the skin. Prolonged skin dampness leads to dermatitis (inflammation of the skin) and subsequent formation of dermal ulcers.

- *Self-Care Deficit: Toileting* if the client has functional incontinence.

- *Risk for Deficient Fluid Volume* or *Excess Fluid Volume* if the client has impaired urinary function associated with a disease process.

- *Disturbed Body Image* if the client has a urinary diversion ostomy.

- *Risk for Caregiver Role Strain* if the client is incontinent and being cared for by a family member for extended periods.

Planning

The goals established will vary according to the diagnosis and defining characteristics. Examples of overall goals for clients with urinary elimination problems may include the following:

- Maintain or restore a normal voiding pattern

- Regain normal urine output

- Prevent associated risks, such as infection, skin breakdown, fluid and electrolyte imbalance, and lowered self-esteem

- Perform toilet activities independently with or without assistive devices

- Contain urine with the appropriate device, catheter, ostomy appliance, or absorbent product.

Examples of desired outcomes for each of these goals are provided in Table 42.5 in the "Evaluating" section (page 1344).

Selected nursing strategies to achieve the goals for problems of altered urinary elimination are discussed in the "Implementing" section. For example, for *urinary incontinence,* the following strategies may be considered: keeping a voiding record or diary; scheduled toileting; prompted voiding; Kegel (pelvic floor muscle) exercises; dietary and fluid intake alterations; assistive devices, such as a bedside commode, mobility aids, or a raised toilet seat; and incontinence aids, such as a condom drainage device for males, absorbent pads, and protective clothing.

For *urinary retention,* the nurse may consider such strategies as bladder training, positioning and relaxation techniques, Credé's manoeuvre, intermittent self-catheterization, and parasympathomimetic medications, as indicated and prescribed.

Examples of interventions to manage urinary elimination problems include the following:

- Urinary elimination management
- Urinary incontinence care
- Prompted voiding
- Urinary habit training
- Urinary bladder training
- Urinary retention care
- Pelvic floor muscle exercise

Specific nursing activities associated with each of these interventions can be selected to meet the individual needs of the client. A Sample Care Plan for urinary elimination follows.

Sample Care Plan for Urinary Elimination

Assessment Data

Nursing Assessment

John Baker is a 68-year-old shopkeeper who came to the emergency department with acute urinary retention. Mr. Baker states he has noticed urinary frequency during the day for the past 2 weeks and that he does not feel he has emptied his bladder after urinating. He also has to get up two or three times during the night to urinate. Over the past few days, he has had difficulty starting urination, and urine dribbles afterward. He verbalizes the embarrassment his urinary problems cause in his dealings with the public. Mr. Baker is concerned about the cause of this urinary problem. He is diagnosed with benign prostatic hypertrophy and referred to an urologist, who suggests a resection of the prostate in 1 month.

Physical Examination

Height: 185.4 cm

Weight: 85.7 kg

Temperature: 38.1°C

Pulse: 88 beats/min

Respirations: 20/min

Blood pressure: 146/86 mm Hg

In-and-out urinary catheterization for urinary retention yielded 300 mL amber urine.

Diagnostic Data

CBC (complete blood count) normal; urinalysis: amber, clear, pH 6.5, specific gravity 1.025, negative for glucose, protein, ketones, RBCs (red blood cells), and bacteria; IVP (intravenous pyelography): evidence of enlarged prostate gland

Nursing Diagnosis

Urinary retention and overflow incontinence related to bladder neck obstruction by enlarged prostate gland, as evidenced by dysuria, frequency, nocturia, dribbling, hesitancy, and bladder distension; at risk for social isolation related to feeling embarrassed about urinary difficulties; at risk for urinary bladder infection related to stagnant urine and invasive procedure; at risk for uncertainty as he awaits surgery; at risk for falling related to getting up at night to urinate. Strengths include absence of urinary tract infection.

Client Goals

The client will demonstrate an understanding of prostatic hypertrophy and its treatment, and will improve urinary elimination patterns.

Desired Health Outcomes

1. Reports reduction of incontinent episodes (increased dryness; reduction of embarrassment if he has incontinence)

2. Monitors urinary output so as to evaluate for urinary retention

3. Describes how an enlarged prostate gland interferes with urination

4. Describes one or two aspects of treatment

5. Maintains his work and public presence

Nursing Interventions	Rationales
• Monitor urinary elimination, including odour, volume, clarity, and colour, and coach Mr. Baker in when he needs to consult with a health care professional (e.g., hematuria, malodorous and cloudy urine)	*These parameters help determine adequacy of urinary tract function and the need for medical follow-up.*
• Help the client select an appropriate incontinence garment or a pad for short-term management while he awaits surgery.	*Appropriate undergarments can help diminish the embarrassing aspects of urinary incontinence and help ensure that he continues to go to work.*
• Instruct Mr. Baker to limit fluids for 2 to 3 hours before bedtime.	*Decreased fluid intake several hours before bedtime may decrease the incidence of urinary retention and overflow incontinence and promote rest during the night.*
• Instruct him to drink a minimum of 1500 mL per day.	*Increased fluids during the day will increase urinary output and discourage bacterial growth.*
• Limit ingestion of bladder irritants (e.g., alcohol, colas, coffee, tea, and chocolate).	*Alcohol and caffeine have a natural diuretic effect and are bladder irritants.*
Urinary Retention Care	
• Instruct Mr. Baker to record his urinary output and monitor for signs and symptoms of urinary bladder distension	*This serves as an indicator of urinary tract and renal function and of fluid balance. Mr. Baker needs to know how to assess for the need to consult*
• Discuss with the urologist the possible need for home bladder scan monitoring, as Mr. Baker will need to know when he should return to a clinic for intermittent urinary catheterization, if necessary.	*An enlarged prostate compresses the urethra so that urine is retained. Checking for residual urine provides information about bladder emptying so as to monitor for overdistension, which can result in reduced urinary bladder tone. A bladder scan can provide convenient and objective data based on which he can make decisions for seeking appropriate medical intervention (e.g., repeat intermittent catheterization) in the event that his retention worsens.*

(continued)

Sample Care Plan for Urinary Elimination (continued)

Nursing Interventions	Rationales
• Provide enough time for bladder emptying (10 minutes).	*In addition to the effect of an enlarged prostate on the bladder, stress or anxiety can inhibit relaxation of the urinary sphincter. Sufficient time should be allowed for micturition.*
• Instruct the client in ways to avoid constipation or stool impaction.	*Impacted stool can place pressure on the bladder outlet, contributing to urinary retention.*
Teaching: Illness Process	
• Appraise Mr. Baker's current level of knowledge about benign prostatic hypertrophy (BPH).	*Assessing the client's knowledge will provide a foundation for building a teaching plan based on his present understanding of his condition.*
• Explain the pathophysiology of BPH and how it relates to urinary anatomy and function (ideally using photos or teaching resources geared to his education level).	*In this case, urinary retention and overflow incontinence are caused by obstruction of the bladder neck by an enlarged prostate gland.*
• Describe the rationale behind management, therapy, and treatment recommendations (e.g., surgery).	*Adequate information about treatment options is important to diminish anxiety and enhance decision making.*
• Instruct Mr. Baker on which signs and symptoms to report to the appropriate member of the health care team (e.g., burning on urination, hematuria, oliguria).	*In the individual with prostatic hypertrophy, urinary retention and an overdistended bladder reduce blood flow to the bladder wall, making it more susceptible to infection from bacterial growth. Monitoring for these manifestations of urinary tract infection is essential to prevent urosepsis.*

EVALUATION

Outcomes partially met. Mr. Baker reported continued difficulty initiating a urinary stream but experienced less dribbling of urine. He selected an undergarment that was discreet and comfortable and reported that he no longer feared going to work or out to social events as he felt confident. He appreciated the teaching about BPH, as he thought it was only related to prostate cancer. For 2 weeks after the need for an in-and-out urinary catheterization, he managed to empty his bladder sufficiently to feel comfortable and no signs or symptoms of UTI were noted; however, 1 week prior to the planned surgery, his bladder became painfully distended, and he returned to the urologist for insertion of an indwelling catheter that remained in place until he had his surgery, necessitating the need for ongoing teaching and learning related to caring for an indwelling device.

PLANNING FOR HOME CARE To provide for continuity of care, the nurse needs to consider the client's needs for teaching and assistance with care in the home. Discharge planning includes assessment of the client's and family's resources and abilities for self-care, available financial resources, and the need for referrals and home care services. The Assessment: Home Care box outlines an assessment of home care capabilities related to urinary elimination problems and needs. The Teaching: Home Care box addresses the learning needs of the client and family in relation to urinary elimination.

ASSESSMENT HOME CARE

Urinary Elimination

Assess for the following:

CLIENT AND ENVIRONMENT

• *Self-care abilities:* Ability to consume adequate fluids, to perceive bladder fullness, to ambulate and get to the toilet, to manipulate clothing for toileting, and to perform hygiene measures after toileting

• *Assistive devices required:* Ambulatory aids, such as walker, cane, or wheelchair; safety devices, such as grab bars; toileting aids, such as raised toilet seat, urinal, commode, or bedpan; a urinary catheter

• *Home environment for factors that interfere with toileting:* Distance to the bathroom from living areas or bedrooms; barriers, such as stairways, scatter rugs, clutter, or narrow doorways that interfere with bathroom access; lighting (including night lighting that allows gradual transition from dark bedroom to light bathroom)

• *Urinary elimination problems:* Type of incontinence and precipitating factors; manifestations of urinary tract infections (UTIs), such as dysuria, frequency, urgency; evidence of prostatic hypertrophy and effect on urination; ability to perform self-catheterization and care for other urinary elimination devices, such as indwelling catheter, urinary diversion ostomy, or condom drainage

- *Current level of knowledge:* Fluid and dietary intake modifications to promote normal patterns of urinary elimination; bladder training methods and specific techniques to promote voiding; care for indwelling catheter or ostomy (if appropriate)

FAMILY

- *Caregiver availability, skills, and responses:* Ability and willingness to assume responsibilities for care, including assisting with toileting, intermittent catheterization, indwelling catheter care, urinary drainage devices or ostomy care; ready access to laundry facilities; access to and willingness to use respite or relief caregivers

- *Family role changes and coping:* Effect on spousal and family roles, sleep–rest patterns, sexuality, and social interactions

- *Financial resources:* Ability to purchase protective pads and garments, supplies for catheterization or ostomy care

COMMUNITY

- *Environment:* Access to public restrooms and sanitary facilities

- *Current knowledge of and experience with community resources:* Medical and assistive equipment, home care agencies, local pharmacies, available financial assistance, support, and educational organizations

---

Urinary Elimination

Address the learning needs of the client and family in relation to urinary elimination:

Facilitating Urinary Elimination Self-Care

- Teach the client and family to maintain easy access to toilet facilities, including removing scatter rugs and ensuring that halls and doorways are free of clutter.
- Suggest graduated lighting for nighttime voiding: a dim night light in the bedroom and low-wattage hallway lighting.
- Advise the client and family to install grab bars and elevated toilet seats, as needed.
- Provide for instruction in safe transfer techniques. Contact physical therapy to provide training, as needed.
- Suggest clothing that is easily removed for toileting, such as elastic-waist pants or Velcro closures.

Promoting Urinary Elimination

- Instruct the client to respond to the urge to void as soon as possible; avoid voluntary urinary retention.
- Teach the client to empty the bladder completely at each voiding.
- Emphasize the importance of maintaining hydration.
- Teach female clients about pelvic floor muscle exercises (training) to strengthen perineal muscles.
- Inform the client about the relationship between tobacco use and bladder cancer and provide information about smoking cessation programs, as indicated.
- Teach the client to promptly report any of the following to the appropriate member of the health care team: pain or burning on urination, changes in urine colour or clarity (e.g., bright red, rusty, or cloudy urine), malodorous urine, or changes in voiding patterns (e.g., nocturia, frequency, dribbling).

Infection Prevention

- Teach the client to maintain perineal–genital cleanliness, washing with soap and water daily and cleansing the anal and perineal area after defecating.

- Instruct female clients to wipe from front to back (from the urinary meatus toward the anus) after voiding, and to discard toilet paper after each swipe.
- Provide information about products to protect the skin and clothing, and assistive devices for clients who are incontinent. Emphasize the importance of cleaning and drying the perineal area after incontinence episodes. Instruct in the use of protective skin barrier products, as needed.
- Teach clients with an indwelling catheter and their family about care measures, such as cleaning the urinary meatus, managing and emptying the collection device, maintaining a closed system, and bladder irrigation or flushing, if ordered.
- For clients with an incontinent urinary diversion, teach about care of the stoma, drainage devices, and surrounding skin. For continent diversions, teach the client how to catheterize the stoma to drain urine.
- For clients with an indwelling catheter or urinary diversion, emphasize the importance of maintaining fluid intake of 1500 mL/day and of promptly reporting changes in urinary output; signs of urinary retention, such as abdominal pain and a palpable bladder; and manifestations of UTIs, such as malodorous urine, abdominal discomfort, fever, or confusion.

Medications

- Emphasize the importance of taking medications, as prescribed. Instruct the client to take the full course of antibiotics prescribed to treat a UTI, even after symptoms are relieved.
- Inform the client and family about any expected changes in urine colour or odour associated with prescribed medications.
- For clients with urinary retention, emphasize the need to contact the appropriate member of the health

TEACHING	HOME CARE *(continued)*

care team before taking any medication (even over-the-counter medications, such as antihistamines) that may exacerbate symptoms (see Box 42.1 on page 1308).

- For clients taking medications that can damage the kidneys (e.g., aminoglycoside antibiotics), stress the importance of maintaining a generous fluid intake while taking the medication.
- Suggest measures to reduce anticipated side effects of prescribed medications, such as increasing intake of potassium-rich foods when taking a potassium-depleting diuretic, such as furosemide.

Dietary Alterations

- Teach the client about dietary changes to promote urinary function, such as consuming foods that acidify the urine (e.g., eggs, chicken, peanuts, whole grains). It is thought that the fructose and flavanols found in cranberry juice prevent bacteria (particularly *Escherichia coli*) from adhering (sticking) to the wall of the bladder, especially in young women (Jepson & Craig, 2008). The actual amount of daily intake of such foods has not been determined.
- Instruct clients to limit their intake of caffeinated beverages (e.g., tea, coffee, cola drinks) and alcohol as these are bladder irritants that may increase incontinence. Also teach clients to limit their evening fluid intake to reduce the risk of nighttime incontinence episodes.

Measures Specific to Urinary Problems

- Provide instructions for clients with specific urinary problems or treatments, such as the following:
  - Timed urine specimens
  - Urinary incontinence
  - Urinary retention
  - Retention catheters

Referrals

- Make appropriate referrals to home care agencies, community agencies, or social services for assistance with resources, such as grab bars and raised toilet seats; providing wheelchair access to bathrooms; obtaining toileting aids, such as commodes, urinals, or bedpans; and services, such as home care aides, for assistance with activities of daily living.

Community Agencies and Other Resources

- Provide information about resources for durable medical equipment, such as commodes or raised toilet seats; possible financial assistance; and medical supplies, such as drainage bags, incontinence briefs, or protective pads.
- Suggest additional sources of information and help, such as the United Ostomy Association of Canada, Canadian Continence Foundation, or the Kidney Foundation of Canada.

Implementing

MAINTAINING NORMAL URINARY ELIMINATION Most interventions to maintain normal urinary elimination are independent nursing functions. These include promoting adequate fluid intake, maintaining normal voiding habits, and assisting with toileting.

Promoting Fluid Intake Increasing fluid intake increases urine production, which, in turn, stimulates the micturition reflex. A normal daily intake averaging 1500 mL of measurable fluids is adequate for most adult clients.

Many clients have increased fluid requirements, necessitating a higher daily fluid intake. For example, clients who have diaphoresis (are perspiring excessively) or who are experiencing abnormal fluid losses through vomiting, gastric suction, diarrhea, or wound drainage require fluid to replace these losses in addition to their normal daily intake requirements.

Clients who are at risk for UTIs or urinary calculi (stones) should consume 2000 mL to 3000 mL of fluid daily. Evidence suggests that ingesting cranberry juice (or capsules) may prevent UTIs, especially in young women (Jepson & Craig, 2008). Dilute urine and frequent urination reduce the risk of UTIs and stone formation.

Increased fluid intake may be contraindicated for some clients, such as those with kidney failure or heart failure. For these clients, a fluid restriction may be necessary to prevent fluid overload and edema.

Maintaining Normal Voiding Habits Prescribed medical therapies often interfere with a client's normal voiding habits. When a client's urinary elimination pattern is adequate, the nurse helps the client adhere to normal voiding habits as much as possible. See Practice Guidelines 42.1.

Assisting with Toileting Clients who are weakened by a disease process or have a physical impairment may require assistance to toilet. The nurse should assist these clients to the bathroom and remain with them if the client is at risk for falling. The bathroom should contain an easily accessible call signal to summon help, if needed. Clients also need to be encouraged to use handrails placed near the toilet.

For clients unable to use bathroom facilities, the nurse provides urinary equipment close to the bedside (e.g., urinal, bedpan, commode) and provides the necessary assistance to use them.

PREVENTING URINARY TRACT INFECTIONS The rate of UTI is greater in women than in men because of the short urethra and its proximity to the anal and vaginal areas. UTIs are the most common type of health care–associated infection found in long-term care facilities (Nicolle, 2008). Most UTIs are caused by bacteria

PRACTICE GUIDELINES 42.1

Maintaining Normal Voiding Habits

Guidelines	Rationales
Positioning	
Assist the client to a normal position for voiding: standing for males; for females, squatting or leaning slightly forward when sitting. If the client is unable to ambulate to the lavatory, use a bedside commode for females and a urinal for males standing at the bedside, if possible.	*These positions enhance movement of urine through the urinary tract by gravity.*
Relaxation	
Provide privacy for the client, and allow the client sufficient time to void.	*Many people cannot void in the presence of another person or in a rushed environment. Defecation will also be ensured, reducing the risk of constipation, which is a factor in the development of incontinence.*
Suggest that the client read or listen to music. Provide sensory stimuli that may help the client relax.	*These distractions help the client relax and not focus on voiding.*
Pour warm water over the perineum of a female or have the client sit in a warm bath. Apply warmed blankets or towels to the lower abdomen of both men and women.	*The warmth can promote relaxation.*
Turn on running water within hearing distance of the client.	*This aids in stimulating the voiding reflex and masks the sound of voiding for people who find this embarrassing.*
Provide prescribed analgesics and emotional support.	*This helps to relieve physical and emotional discomfort and decrease muscle tension.*
Timing	
Assist clients who have the urge to void immediately. Offer toileting assistance to the client at usual times of voiding, for example, on awakening, before or after meals, and at bedtime.	*Delays only increase the difficulty in starting to void, and the desire to void may pass.*
For clients who are confined to bed	
Warm the bedpan.	*A cold bedpan can prompt contraction of the perineal muscles and inhibit voiding.*
Elevate the head of the client's bed to Fowler's position, place a small pillow or rolled towel at the small of the back, and have the client flex the hips and knees.	*This position simulates the normal voiding position as closely as possible and increases physical support and comfort.*

common to the intestinal environment (e.g., *Escherichia coli*). These gastrointestinal bacteria can colonize the perineal area and move into the urethra, especially when there is urethral trauma, irritation, or manipulation. See the Clinical Alert box on UTIs.

> ### ! CLINICAL ALERT
>
> UTIs are the most common problem associated with urinary catheterization and are the most common health care–associated infection. Nurses should ensure urinary catheters are used only when absolutely necessary and removed as soon as possible. Routine cleaning of the perineal area and use of strict aseptic technique during insertion and manipulation of the catheter is critical in preventing infection.

For women who have experienced a UTI, nurses need to provide instructions about ways to prevent a recurrence. The following guidelines are useful for anyone:

- Drink six to eight 250-mL glasses of water per day to "flush" bacteria out of the urinary system. Avoid fluids that irritate the bladder, such as alcohol and caffeine.

- Practise frequent voiding (every 2 to 4 hours) to flush bacteria out of the urethra and prevent organisms from ascending into the bladder. Void when the urge arises as much as possible rather than inhibiting the urge to void, which would result in an accumulation of stagnant urine in the bladder. Void after sexual intercourse.

- Keep the genital area clean and dry. Avoid the use of harsh soaps, bubble bath, powder, or sprays in the perineal area. These substances can be irritating to the urethra and encourage inflammation and bacterial infection.

- Do not douche or use similar feminine hygiene measures.

- Avoid tight-fitting pants or other clothing that creates irritation to the urethra and prevents ventilation of the perineal area.

- Wear underwear made from breathable fabrics, such as cotton, rather than nylon. Accumulation of perineal moisture facilitates bacterial growth and cotton enhances ventilation of the perineal area.

- Girls and women should always wipe the perineal area from front to back following urination or defecation to prevent introduction of gastrointestinal bacteria into the urethra.

- If recurrent urinary infections are a problem, take showers, rather than baths. Bacteria present in bathwater can readily enter the urethra.

MANAGING URINARY INCONTINENCE Urinary incontinence, the unintentional loss of urine, is *not* a normal part of aging and often is treatable. Independent nursing interventions for clients with urinary incontinence include (a) a behaviour-oriented continence training program that may consist of bladder training, habit training, prompted voiding, pelvic floor muscle exercises, and positive reinforcement; (b) meticulous skin care; and (c) for males, application of an external drainage device (condom-type catheter device).

Continence (Bladder) Training A continence training program requires the involvement of the nurse, the client, and support people. Clients must be alert and physically able to follow a program. Clients who are unable to remain continent for more than 2 hours may have difficulty in adhering to a continence training program. A bladder training program may include the following (Roe, Flanagan, Jack, Barrett, Chung, Shaw, & Williams, 2011):

- **Bladder training** requires that the client postpone voiding, resist or inhibit the sensation of urgency, and void according to a timetable rather than according to the urge to void. The goals are to gradually lengthen the intervals between urination to correct the client's habit of frequent urination, to stabilize the bladder, and to diminish urgency. This form of training can be used for clients who have bladder instability and urge incontinence. Delayed voiding provides larger voided volumes and longer intervals between voiding. Initially, voiding may be encouraged every 2 to 3 hours, except during sleep, and then every 4 to 6 hours. A vital component of bladder training is inhibiting the urge-to-void sensation. To do this, the nurse instructs the client to practise deep, slow breathing until the urge diminishes or disappears. This breathing is performed every time the client has a premature urge to void. See Practice Guidelines 42.2.

- **Habit training**, also referred to as *timed voiding* or *scheduled toileting*, attempts to keep clients dry by identifying their natural voiding pattern and developing

PRACTICE GUIDELINES 42.2

Bladder Training

Guidelines	Rationales
Determine the client's voiding pattern by completing a 3-day voiding record (RNAO, 2011) and encourage voiding at those times, or establish a regular voiding schedule. Help the client to maintain the schedule whether the client feels the urge or not (e.g., on awakening, every 1 or 2 hours during the day and evening, before retiring at night, and every 4 hours at night).	*The stretching-relaxing sequence of such a schedule tends to increase bladder muscle tone and promote more voluntary control.*
Encourage the client to inhibit the urge-to-void sensation when a premature urge to void is experienced. Instruct the client to practise slow, deep breathing until the urge diminishes or disappears.	*Deep breathing aids in distracting the client from the urge to void.*
When the client finds that voiding can be controlled, the intervals between voiding can be lengthened slightly without loss of continence.	*Lengthening the interval will help increase muscle tone and decrease time spent in toileting.*
Regulate fluid intake, particularly during evening hours.	*Regulated fluid intake helps reduce the need to void during the night.*

Guidelines	Rationales
Avoid excessive consumption of citrus juices, carbonated beverages (especially those containing artificial sweeteners), alcohol, and drinks containing caffeine.	*These fluids irritate the bladder and tend to cause detrusor instability, increasing the risk of incontinence.*
Schedule diuretics early in the morning if taken once a day; if diuretics are taken twice a day then recommend that the second dose be taken before or at supper time (unless medically not recommended)	*This step helps reduce the client's need to void during the night.*
Explain to clients that adequate fluid intake is required to ensure adequate urine production, which stimulates the micturition reflex.	*Clients may decrease fluid intake in an attempt to reduce episodes of incontinence.*
Apply protector pads to keep the bed linen dry, and provide specially made waterproof underwear. Avoid using diapers, which are demeaning and also suggest that incontinence is permissible.	*These measures aid in containing urine and decrease the client's embarrassment.*
Assist the client with an exercise program to increase the tone of abdominal and pelvic floor muscles.	*Increasing tone of abdominal and pelvic floor muscles will foster continence through the voluntary control of voiding.*
Provide positive reinforcements to encourage continence. Praise clients for attempting to go to the toilet and for maintaining continence.	*Positive reinforcement will increase clients' self-esteem and promote compliance with the training program.*
Maintain a voiding record to monitor the effectiveness of interventions; for example, a 3-day voiding record should be initiated at least 3 weeks and at most 8 weeks after a prompted voiding intervention is tested (RNAO, 2011).	*Objective evidence provides evaluation feedback as to the effectiveness of the bladder training program.*

an individualized schedule of regular toileting with the aim of avoiding involuntary bladder emptying. With habit training, there is no attempt to motivate the client to delay voiding if the urge occurs. This approach can be effective in children who are experiencing urinary dysfunction. Biofeedback therapy in which the child is taught to relax the pelvic floor can also decrease incidents of wetting.

- **Prompted voiding** supplements habit training by encouraging the client to try to use the toilet (prompting) and reminding the client when to void (Registered Nurses' Association of Ontario [RNAO], 2011). This intervention is used for clients who need timely reminders from caregivers owing to their physical or cognitive deficits. Caregivers using prompted voiding use three primary behaviours:

  1. *Monitoring:* Asking the person with incontinence, at regular intervals, if he or she needs to use the toilet and taking the client to the toilet at regular intervals

  2. *Prompting:* Prompting the client to regularly use the toilet (e.g., "It is time to use the toilet. Do you need any help?") as well as encouraging toilet use between prompted voiding sessions

  3. *Praising:* Giving positive feedback for the maintenance of bladder control

Pelvic Floor Muscle Exercises Pelvic floor muscle exercises (PFME) (sometimes referred to as pelvic floor muscle training), or *Kegel exercises,* help to strengthen pelvic floor muscles and can reduce episodes of urinary incontinence (Dumoulin & Hay-Smith, 2010; Holroyd-Leduc, Straus, Thorpe, Davis, Schmaltz, & Tannenbaum, 2011). The client can identify perineal muscles by stopping urination midstream or by tightening the anal sphincter as if to hold a bowel movement.

Specific client instructions for performing PFME are summarized in the Teaching: Clinical box on pelvic floor muscle exercises (Kegels) on the next page. There is some evidence that biofeedback using vaginal or anal devices to measure the pressure of the pelvic muscles during the PFMEs may provide additional benefit to pelvic floor muscle training in women with urinary incontinence (Herderschee, Hay-Smith, Herbison, Roovers, & Heineman, 2011). See the Evidence-Informed Practice box on the use of mechanical devices in the management of female urinary incontinence on the next page.

Maintaining Skin Integrity Skin that is continually moist becomes macerated. Urine that accumulates on skin is converted to ammonia, which is very irritating to skin. Because both skin irritation and maceration predispose the client to skin breakdown and ulceration, the incontinent person requires meticulous skin care. To maintain skin integrity, the nurse washes the client's

Pelvic Floor Muscle Exercises (Kegels)

Nurses can teach clients how to perform pelvic floor muscle exercises correctly:

- Sit, lie, or stand in a comfortable, relaxed position with legs apart.
- Contract your pelvic floor muscles whereby you pull your rectum, urethra, and vagina up inside, and hold for a count of 3 to 5 seconds. Then relax the same muscles for a count of 3 to 5 seconds.
- Initially perform each contraction 10 times, five times daily. Gradually increase the count to 10 seconds for both contraction and relaxation.
- Develop a schedule that will help remind you to do these exercises, for example, while driving to work, when washing dishes at the kitchen sink, or at scheduled times (e.g., 0700, 1000, 1300, 1600, and 1900 hours).
- Try to start and stop your stream of urine.
- To control episodes of stress incontinence, brace the muscles and use the Kegel manoeuvre when doing any activity that increases intra-abdominal pressure, such as coughing, laughing, sneezing, or lifting.

perineal area with soap and water after episodes of incontinence, rinses it thoroughly, dries it thoroughly, and provides clean, dry clothing or bed linen. If skin is irritated, the nurse applies barrier ointments or creams to protect skin from contact with urine. If it is necessary to pad the client's clothes for protection, the nurse should use products that absorb wetness and leave a dry surface in contact with skin.

Specially designed incontinence drawsheets can be used that provide significant advantages over standard drawsheets for clients with incontinence confined to bed. These sheets are like a drawsheet but are double layered, with a quilted upper nylon or polyester surface and an absorbent viscose rayon layer below. The rayon soaker layer generally has a waterproof backing on its underside. Fluid (i.e., urine) passes through the upper quilted layer and is absorbed and dispersed by the viscose rayon, leaving the quilted surface dry to the touch. This absorbent sheet helps maintain skin integrity; it does not stick to skin when wet, it decreases the risk of bedsores, and it reduces odour.

Applying External Urinary Drainage Devices The application of a condom or external catheter connected to a urinary drainage system is commonly prescribed for male clients with incontinence. Use of a condom appliance is preferable to insertion of a retention catheter because the risk of UTIs is minimal.

Methods of applying condoms vary and the nurse should follow the manufacturer's instructions

EVIDENCE-INFORMED PRACTICE

Are Mechanical Devices Effective in the Management of Adult Female Urinary Incontinence?

The intervention review conducted by Lipp, Shaw, and Glavind set out to determine the effectiveness of mechanical devices (e.g., diaphragms, pessaries, urethral plugs, intravaginal sponge) in the management of adult female urinary incontinence. Although over 500 articles on the topic were found, very few met the stringent criteria for inclusion in this systematic review. In the end, seven randomized or quasi-randomized controlled trials involving 732 women were deemed quality research studies for the review. Two studies compared the use of tampons and pessaries with no treatment and found that use of such mechanical devices may have some helpful benefits but the "evidence for this was inconclusive"; in addition, some women reported discomfort with these devices. Of the trials that compared one mechanical device with another, different outcome measures were used, thus making it difficult to do a true comparison of results. The author's conclusions were that there is little evidence on which to judge whether the use of mechanical devices might be better than no treatment.

NURSING IMPLICATIONS: Women suffering from incontinence may seek out a nurse's opinion on the use of mechanical devices, as some are readily available in pharmacies and online. This intervention review did not provide sufficient evidence that nurses should be recommending mechanical devices with confidence in their effectiveness. The devices may or may not provide any relief from incontinence, and one must also question if they can cause harm. Some of the studies included in the review noted "discomfort," and some others questioned the possibility of urethral trauma or increased urinary tract infection with the use of some mechanical devices. As such, the nurse must question the possible but yet to be conclusive benefits of mechanical devices with any unwanted effects. Many women may opt to try mechanical devices and nurses can help them evaluate their effectiveness at an individual level, including monitoring for any complications. In addition, nurses can help the women learn about other interventions, such as pelvic floor muscle exercises.

Source: Based on Lipp A., Shaw C., & Glavind, K. (2011). Mechanical devices for urinary incontinence in women. *Cochrane Database of Systematic Reviews,* Issue 7. Art. No.: CD001756. doi: 10.1002/14651858.CD001756.pub5 1

accordingly. First, the nurse determines when the client experiences incontinence, as some clients may require a condom appliance at night only, whereas others may need it continuously. Skill 42.2 describes how to apply and remove an external urinary device.

MANAGING URINARY RETENTION Interventions that assist the client to maintain a normal voiding pattern, discussed earlier, also apply when dealing with urinary

SKILL 42.2 APPLYING AN EXTERNAL (CONDOM) URINARY DEVICE

PURPOSES

- To collect urine and control urinary incontinence
- To permit the client to engage in physical activity without fear of embarrassment because of leaking urine
- To prevent skin irritation as a result of urinary incontinence

ASSESSMENT

- Review the client record to determine a pattern of voiding and other pertinent data (e.g., times of urinary incontinence, amount of urine passed).
- Put on clean gloves, and examine the client's penis for swelling or excoriation that would contraindicate the use of the condom catheter.

PLANNING

- Discuss the use of the external urinary device with the client and/or family.
- Determine whether the client has had an external catheter previously and any difficulties with it.
- Perform any procedures that are best completed without the catheter in place, for example, weighing the client would be easier without the tubing and bag.

Equipment

- Leg drainage bag, if ambulatory, or urinary drainage bag with tubing, if confined to bed
- Condom sheath of appropriate size: small, medium, large, extra-large. Use the manufacturer's size guide as indicated. Use latex-free silicone for clients with latex allergies. Use self-adhering condoms or those with Velcro, tape, or other external securing device (see ❶)
- Drape (e.g., sheet or bath blanket)
- Clean gloves
- Basin of warm water and soap
- Washcloth and towel

IMPLEMENTATION

Preparation

- Assemble the leg drainage bag or urinary drainage bag for attachment to the condom sheath.
- Roll the condom outward onto itself to facilitate easier application (see ❷). On some models, an inner flap will be exposed. This flap is applied around the urinary meatus to prevent the reflux of urine.

Performance

1. Before performing the procedure, introduce yourself and verify the client's identity using two identifiers or per agency protocol. Explain to the client what you are going to do, why it is necessary, and how he can participate.
2. Perform hand hygiene, and follow other appropriate infection prevention and control procedures.

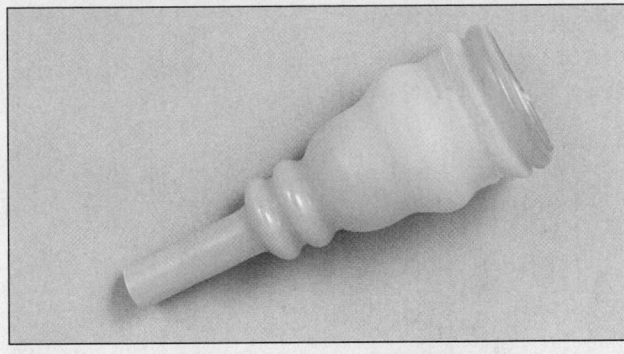

❶ An external or condom catheter.

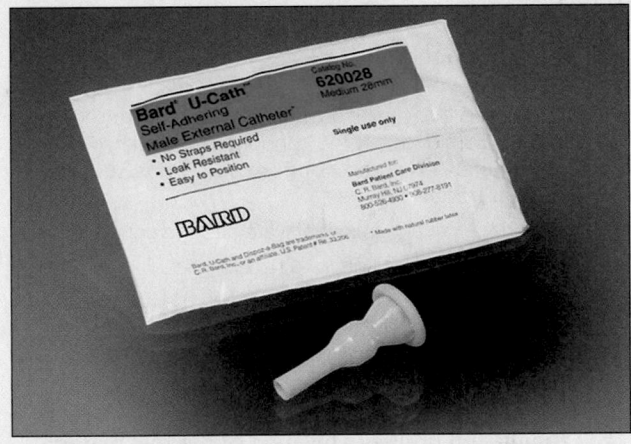

❷ Before application, roll the condom outward onto itself.

3. Position the client in either a supine or a sitting position.
   - Provide for client privacy.
   - Drape the client appropriately with the bath blanket, exposing only the penis.
4. Apply clean gloves.
5. Inspect and clean the penis.
   - Clean the genital area and dry it thoroughly. **Rationale: Doing this minimizes skin irritation and excoriation after the condom is applied.**
6. Apply and secure the condom.
   - Roll the condom smoothly over the penis, leaving 2.5 cm. between the end of the penis and the rubber or plastic connecting tube (see ❸). **Rationale: This space prevents irritation of the tip of the penis and provides for full drainage of urine.**
   - Secure the condom firmly, but not too tightly, to the penis. Some condoms have an adhesive inside the proximal end that adheres to the skin of the base of the penis. Many condoms are packaged with special tape. If neither is present, use a strip of elastic tape or Velcro around the base of the penis over the condom. Ordinary tape is contraindicated because it is not flexible and can stop blood flow.

(continued)

SKILL 42.2 APPLYING AN EXTERNAL (CONDOM) URINARY DEVICE (*continued*)

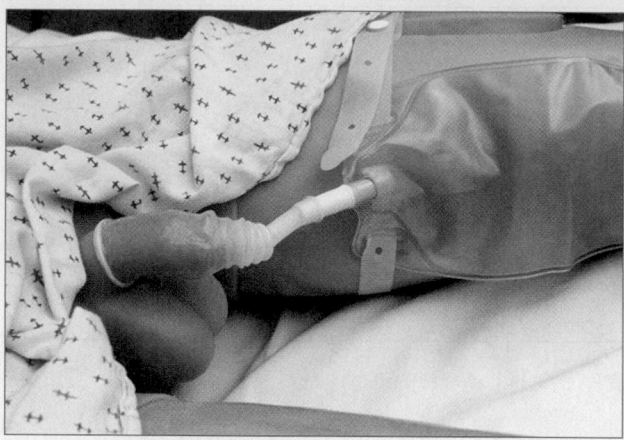

③ The condom rolled over the penis.

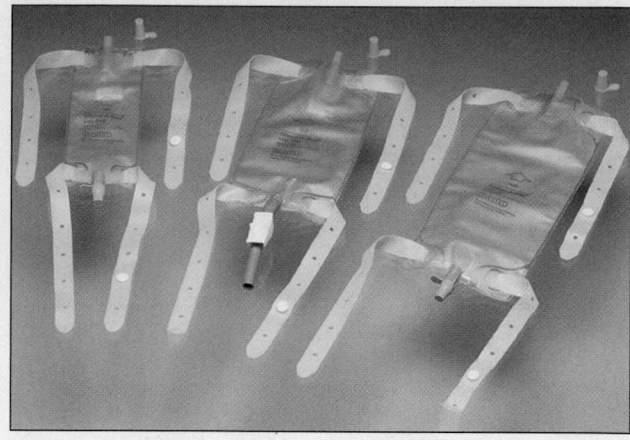

④ Urinary drainage leg bags.

7. Securely attach the urinary drainage system.
   - Make sure that the tip of the penis is not touching the condom and that the condom is not twisted. **Rationale: A twisted condom could obstruct the flow of urine.**
   - Attach the urinary drainage system to the condom.
   - Remove gloves and perform hand hygiene.
   - If the client is to remain in bed, attach the urinary drainage bag to the bed frame.
   - If the client is ambulatory, attach the bag to the client's leg (see **④**). **Rationale: Attaching the drainage bag to the leg helps control the movement of the tubing and prevents twisting of the thin material of the condom appliance at the tip of the penis.**

8. Teach the client about the drainage system.
   - Instruct the client to keep the drainage bag below the level of the condom and to avoid loops or kinks in the tubing.

9. Inspect the penis 30 minutes following the condom application, and check urine flow. Document these findings.
   - Assess the penis for swelling and discoloration, which indicates that the condom is too tight.

- Assess urine flow if the client has voided. Normally, some urine is present in the tube if the flow is not obstructed.

10. Change the condom, as indicated (minimum daily), and provide skin care.
    - Remove the elastic or Velcro strip, apply clean gloves, and roll off the condom.
    - Wash the penis with soapy water, rinse, and dry it thoroughly.
    - Assess the foreskin for signs of irritation, swelling, and discoloration.
    - Reapply a new condom.

11. Document in the client record by using forms or checklists supplemented by narrative notes when appropriate. Record the application of the urinary device, the time, and pertinent observations, such as irritated areas on the penis.

EVALUATION

- Perform a detailed follow-up based on findings that deviated from expected or normal for the client. Relate findings to previous assessment data, if available.
- Report significant deviations from normal to the appropriate member of the health care team.

retention. If these actions are unsuccessful, the appropriate health care provider may order a cholinergic drug, such as bethanechol chloride (Urecholine) to stimulate bladder contraction and facilitate voiding. Clients who have a **flaccid bladder** (weak, soft, and lax bladder muscles) may use **Credé's manoeuvre** (or *Credé's method*) whereby manual pressure is placed on the bladder to promote bladder emptying. This manoeuvre is not advised without a physician's order and is used only for clients who have lost and are not expected to regain voluntary bladder control. When all measures fail to initiate voiding, urinary catheterization may be necessary to empty the bladder completely. An indwelling Foley catheter may be inserted until the underlying cause is treated; alternatively, intermittent straight catheterization (every 3 to 4 hours)

may be performed because the risk of UTIs is believed by some to be less than with an indwelling catheter.

Urinary Catheterization Urinary catheterization is the introduction of a catheter through the urethra into the urinary bladder. This is usually performed only when *absolutely necessary* because the procedure has certain hazards. Because the urinary tract is normally sterile, except at the end of the urethra, the danger exists of introducing microorganisms into the bladder. Clients who have lowered immune resistance are at the greatest risk. Once an infection is introduced into the bladder, it can ascend the ureters and eventually involve the kidneys. The hazard of infection remains after the catheter is in place because normal defence mechanisms, such as intermittent flushing of microorganisms from the urethra through voiding, are bypassed. Thus, strict sterile technique is used for catheterization.

Another hazard is trauma, particularly in the male client, whose urethra is longer and more tortuous. It is important to insert a catheter along the normal contour of the urethra. Damage to the urethra can occur if the catheter is forced through strictures or at an incorrect angle. In males, the urethra is normally curved, but it can be straightened by elevating the penis to a position perpendicular to the body.

Catheters are commonly made of rubber, silicone, plastics or thermoplastics, such as polyvinylchloride (PVC) or latex. Latex catheters are seldom used now because of the risk of allergies. They are sized by the diameter of the lumen by using the French (Fr) scale: the larger the number, the larger is the lumen. Either *straight catheters*, inserted to drain the bladder and then immediately removed, or *indwelling catheters*, which remain in the bladder to drain urine, can be used.

The straight catheter is a single-lumen tube with a small eye or opening about 1.25 cm from the insertion tip (Figure 42.14). The *coudé catheter* is a variation of the straight catheter. It is more rigid than other straight catheters and has a tapered, curved tip (Figure 42.15). This catheter may be used for men with prostatic hypertrophy as it is more easily controlled and less traumatic on insertion.

The *indwelling (retention) catheter*, or *Foley catheter*, is a double-lumen catheter. The larger lumen drains urine from the bladder. A second, smaller lumen is used to inflate a balloon near the tip of the catheter to hold the catheter in place within the bladder (Figures 42.15 and 42.16). Clients who require continuous or intermittent bladder irrigation may have a *three-way Foley catheter* (Figure 42.17). The three-way catheter has a third lumen through which sterile irrigating fluid can flow into the bladder. The fluid then exits the bladder through the drainage lumen along with the urine.

The balloons of indwelling catheters are sized by the volume of fluid used to inflate them. The three commonly used sizes are 5-mL, 10-mL, and 30-mL balloons. The size of the balloon is indicated on the catheter, along with the

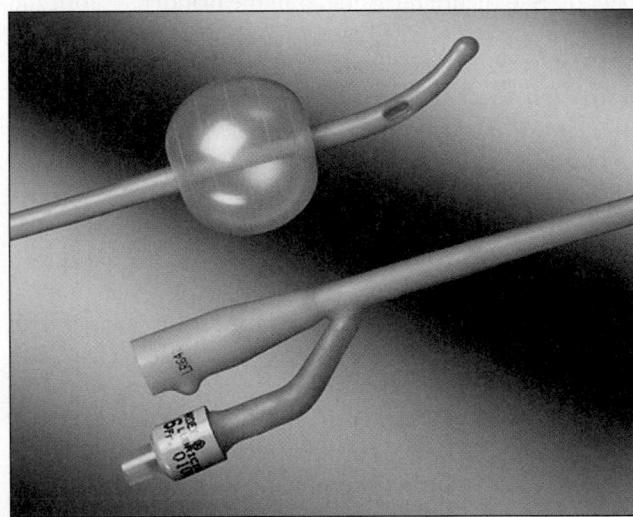

FIGURE 42.15 An indwelling coudé catheter with balloon inflated (note the curved tip).

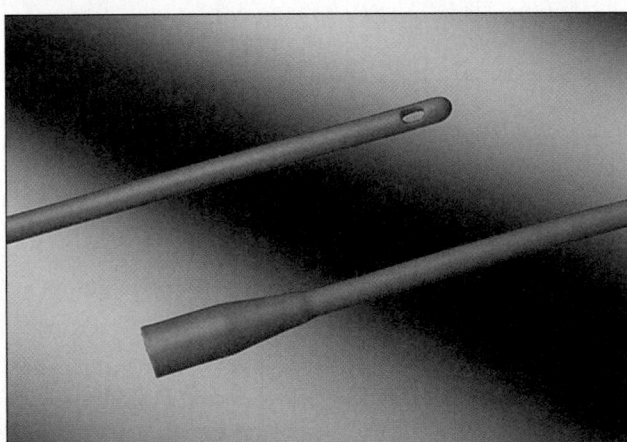

A

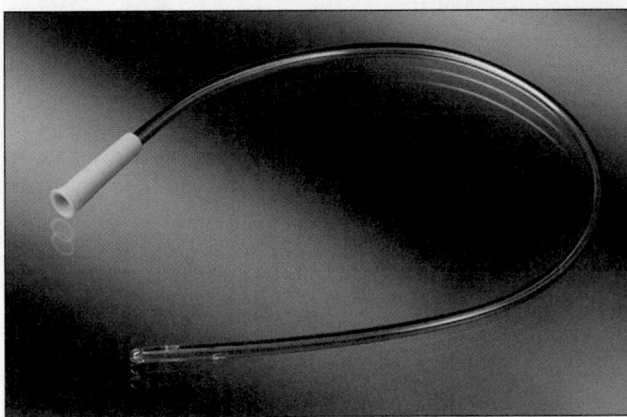

B

FIGURE 42.14 Straight catheters: **A:** Red-rubber; **B:** Robinson.

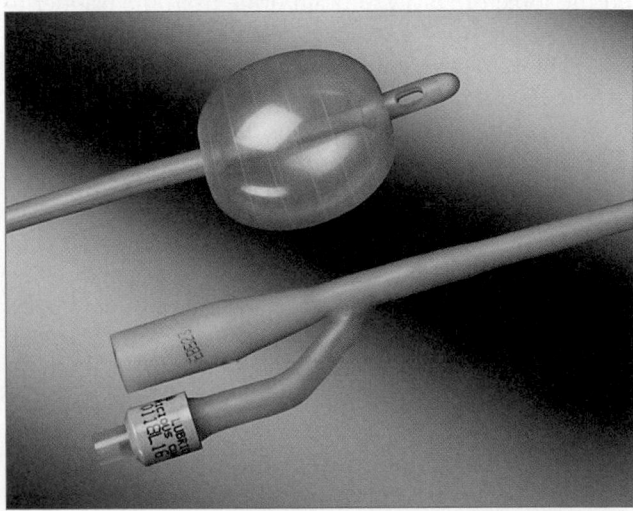

FIGURE 42.16 An indwelling or retention (Foley) catheter with balloon inflated.

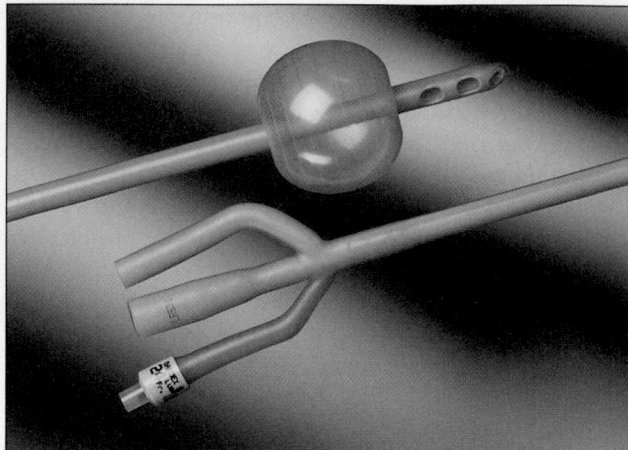

FIGURE 42.17 A three-way Foley catheter (often used for continuous bladder irrigation).

diameter, for example, "18 Fr–5 mL." The purpose of the balloon is to secure the catheter in the bladder. Historically, nurses pretested the catheter balloon to prevent insertion of a defective catheter. Some catheter manufacturers (e.g., Bard) test the balloon as part of their quality assurance process and do *not* recommend pretesting the balloon by the nurse. Pretesting silicone balloons is *not* recommended because the silicone can form a cuff or crease at the balloon area that can cause trauma to the urethra during catheter insertion. It is important to follow the manufacturer's instructions for the proper volume to use for balloon inflation For example, a 5-mL balloon must be inflated with between 9 to 10 mL of sterile water for some devices. Box 42.2 provides guidelines for catheter selection.

Indwelling catheters usually are connected to a *closed gravity drainage system.* This system consists of the catheter, drainage tubing, and a collecting bag for the urine. A closed system should not be opened anywhere along the system from catheter to collecting bag. Closed systems reduce the risk of microorganisms entering the system and infecting the urinary tract. Urinary drainage systems typically depend on the force of gravity to drain urine from the bladder to the collecting bag.

Skill 42.3 describes urethral urinary catheterization of females and males, using straight and indwelling catheters. See the Home Care Considerations box on page 1336 and the Lifespan Considerations box on page 1337 for additional information.

NURSING INTERVENTIONS FOR CLIENTS WITH INDWELLING CATHETERS   Nursing care of the client with an indwelling catheter and continuous drainage is largely directed toward preventing infection of the urinary tract and encouraging urinary flow through the drainage system. It includes encouraging adequate amounts of fluid intake, accurately recording the fluid intake and output, changing the retention catheter and tubing, maintaining the patency of the drainage system, preventing contamination of the drainage system, and teaching these measures to the client.

Fluids   The client with an indwelling catheter should drink up to 3000 mL per day, if permitted. Increased fluid intake ensures an increased urine output, which keeps the bladder flushed out and decreases the likelihood of urinary stasis and subsequent infection. Large volumes of urine also minimize the risk of sediment or other particles obstructing the drainage tubing.

Perineal Care   Generally, no special cleaning other than routine hygienic care is necessary for clients with indwelling catheters, nor is special meatal care recommended. The retention catheter should be cleaned by swabbing down the tubing away from the meatus. Agency practices regarding catheter care vary considerably. The nurse should check agency practice in this regard.

Changing the Catheter and Tubing   Indwelling catheters are used only when absolutely necessary and removed as soon as possible. However, some clients require long-term catheterization. Whenever possible, the closed catheter drainage system should be maintained, and the tubing not disconnected from the catheter for any reason. Routine changing of catheter and tubing is not recommended. Collection of sediment in the catheter or tubing or impaired urine drainage are indicators for changing the catheter and drainage system. When this occurs, the catheter and drainage system are removed and discarded, and a new sterile catheter with a closed drainage system is inserted.

SKILL 42.3 PERFORMING URINARY CATHETERIZATION

PURPOSES

- To relieve discomfort from bladder distension or to provide gradual decompression of a distended bladder
- To assess the amount of residual urine if the bladder empties incompletely
- To obtain a sterile urine specimen
- To empty the bladder completely before surgery
- To facilitate accurate measurement of urinary output for critically ill clients whose output needs to be monitored hourly
- To provide for intermittent or continuous bladder drainage or irrigation
- To prevent urine from contacting an incision after perineal surgery
- To manage incontinence when all other measures have failed

ASSESSMENT

- Determine the most appropriate method of catheterization based on the purpose and any criteria specified in the order, such as total amount of urine to be removed or size of catheter to be used.
- Use a straight catheter if only a one-time urine specimen is needed, if the amount of residual urine is being measured, or if temporary decompression/emptying of the bladder is required.
- Use an indwelling/retention catheter if the bladder must remain empty, intermittent catheterization is contraindicated or continuous urine measurement/collection is needed.
- Assess the client's overall condition. Determine whether the client is able to participate and hold still during the procedure and whether the client can be positioned supine with head relatively flat. For female clients, determine if she can have knees bent and hips externally rotated.
- Determine when the client last voided or was last catheterized.
- Percuss the bladder to check for fullness or distension or perform a bladder scan to assess the amount of urine present in the bladder.

Clinical Reasoning

Prior to performing the urinary catheterization, have all attempts to avoid this invasive procedure been tried? Take some time to anticipate how the client will interpret this procedure—for example, will he or she feel helpless? embarrassed? concerned about issues related to sexuality, such as a man worrying about getting an erection while the catheter is being inserted? Will a female client be concerned about having a male nurse perform the procedure? Will a male client have different concerns about having either a male or a female nurse perform the procedure?

PLANNING

Allow adequate time to perform the catheterization. Although the entire procedure can require as little as 15 minutes, several sources of difficulty could result in a much longer time.

Discuss the need for urinary catheterization with the client and/or family as this procedure can be frightening, embarrassing, and unpleasant for some. Ensure the client that all efforts will be made to ensure dignity.

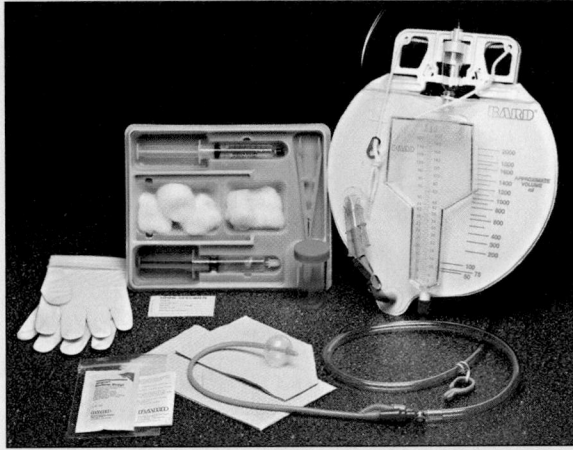

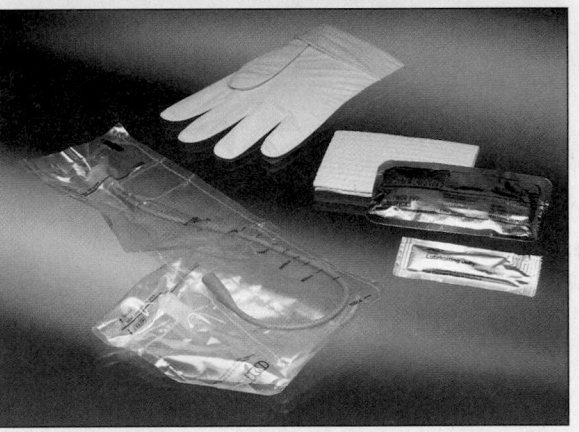

❶ Catheterization insertion kits: **A:** Indwelling; **B:** Straight.

Equipment

- Sterile catheter of appropriate size (an extra catheter should be at hand)
- Catheterization kit (see ❶) or individual sterile items:
  - Sterile gloves
  - Waterproof drapes
  - Antiseptic solution
  - Cleansing balls
  - Forceps
  - Water-soluble lubricant
  - Urine receptacle
  - Specimen container
- For an indwelling catheter:
  - Syringe prefilled with sterile water in amount specified by catheter manufacturer
  - Collection bag and tubing
  - 10 mL–15 mL 2% xylocaine gel for male urethral injection (if agency permits)
  - Clean gloves
  - Supplies for performing perineal cleansing
  - Bath blanket or sheet for draping the client
  - Adequate lighting (use a flashlight or lamp, if necessary)

(continued)

SKILL 42.3 **PERFORMING URINARY CATHETERIZATION** (*continued*)

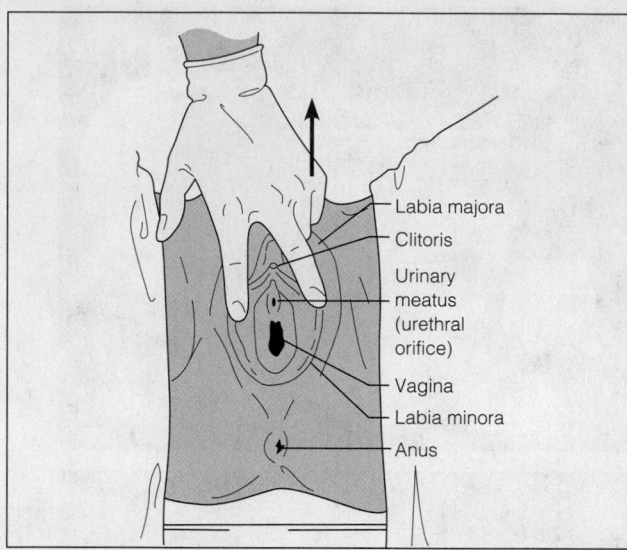

❷ To expose the urinary meatus, separate the labia minora and retract the tissue upward.

Labia majora
Clitoris
Urinary meatus (urethral orifice)
Vagina
Labia minora
Anus

IMPLEMENTATION

Preparation

If using a catheterization kit, read the label carefully to be sure all necessary items are included. Put on clean gloves, and perform routine perineal care to cleanse gross contamination. For women, use this time to locate the urinary meatus relative to surrounding structures (see ❷). Remove and discard gloves. Perform hand hygiene.

Performance

1. Before performing the procedure, introduce yourself and verify the client's identity using two identifiers or per agency protocol. Explain to the client what you are going to do, why it is necessary, and how he or she can participate.

2. Perform hand hygiene, and follow other appropriate infection prevention and control procedures.

3. Provide for client privacy.

4. Place the client in the appropriate position and drape all areas except the perineum
   - *Female:* supine with knees flexed, feet about 50 cm apart, and hips slightly externally rotated, if possible
   - *Male:* supine, thighs slightly abducted or apart

5. Establish adequate lighting. Stand on the client's right if you are right-handed, on the client's left if you are left-handed.

6. If you are using a collecting bag and it is not contained within the catheterization kit, open the drainage package and place the end of the tubing within reach. **Rationale: Since one hand is needed to hold the catheter once it is in place, open the package while two hands are still available.**

7. If agency policy permits, put on clean gloves and inject 10 mL to 15 mL xylocaine gel into the urethra of the male client. Wipe the underside of the shaft to distribute the gel up the urethra. Wait at least 5 minutes for the gel to take effect before inserting the catheter. Remove and discard gloves. Perform hand hygiene.

8. Open the catheterization kit. Place a waterproof drape under the buttocks (female) or penis (male), without contaminating the centre of the drape with your hands.

9. Put on sterile gloves.

10. Organize the remaining supplies:
    - Saturate the cleansing balls with the antiseptic solution.
    - Open the lubricant package.
    - Remove the specimen container and place it nearby, with the lid loosely on top.

11. Attach the prefilled syringe to the indwelling catheter inflation hub. Follow the manufacturer's instructions relative to testing the balloon. **Rationale: Not all manufacturer's recommend pretesting the balloon; for those who do, pretesting is a means of checking for balloon malfunctions, at which time another catheter would need to be used.**

12. Lubricate the catheter (2.5 cm to 5 cm for females; 5 cm to 15 cm for males), and place it with the drainage end inside the collection container.

13. If desired, place the fenestrated drape over the perineum, exposing the urinary meatus.

14. Cleanse the meatus. *Note:* The nondominant hand is considered contaminated once it touches the client's skin.

    a. *For women:* Use your nondominant hand to spread the labia. Ensure that there is enough pressure to keep the labia spread apart without causing discomfort to the client. The antiseptic may make the tissues slippery but the labia must not be allowed to return over the cleaned meatus. Pick up a cleansing ball with the forceps in your dominant hand, and wipe one side of the labia majora in an anteroposterior direction (see ❸). Use great care that wiping the client does not contaminate this sterile hand. Use a new cleansing ball for the opposite side. Repeat for the labia minora. Use the last ball to cleanse directly over the meatus.

    b. *For men:* Use your nondominant hand to grasp the penis just below the glans. If necessary, retract the

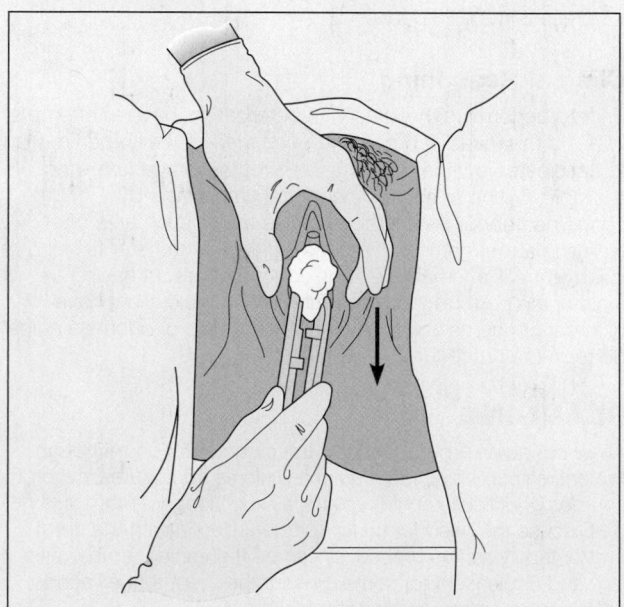

❸ When cleaning the urinary meatus, move the swab downward.

foreskin. Hold the penis firmly upright, with slight tension. **Rationale: Lifting the penis so that it is perpendicular to the body helps straighten the urethra.** Pick up a cleansing ball with the forceps in your dominant hand, and wipe from the centre of the meatus in a circular motion around the glans. Use great care that wiping the client does not contaminate this sterile hand. Use a new cleansing ball and repeat three more times. The antiseptic may make the tissues slippery, but the foreskin must not be allowed to return over the cleaned meatus or the penis be dropped.

15. Insert the catheter.

    • Grasp the catheter firmly 5 cm to 7.5 cm from the tip. Ask the client to take a slow deep breath; insert the catheter as the client exhales. Slight resistance is expected as the catheter passes through the sphincters. If necessary, twist the catheter or hold pressure on the catheter until the sphincter relaxes.

    • Advance the catheter 5 cm farther after the urine begins to flow through it. **Rationale: Doing this ensures that the catheter is fully in the bladder.** For male clients, according to some agency's policies and procedures, the catheter should be advanced to the Y bifurcation of the catheter.

    • If the catheter accidentally contacts the labia or slips into the vagina, it is considered contaminated and a new, sterile catheter must be used. The contaminated catheter can be left in the vagina until the new catheter is inserted to avoid mistaking the vaginal opening for the urethral meatus.

16. Hold the catheter with the nondominant hand. In males, lay the penis down onto the drape, being careful that the catheter does not get pulled out.

17. For an indwelling catheter, inflate the retention balloon with the designated volume.

    • Without releasing the catheter, hold the inflation valve between two fingers of your nondominant hand while you attach the syringe (if not left attached earlier when testing the balloon), and inflate with your dominant hand. If the client complains of discomfort, immediately withdraw the instilled fluid, advance the catheter farther, and attempt to inflate the balloon again.

    • Pull *gently* on the catheter until resistance is felt to ensure that the balloon has inflated and to place it in the trigone of the bladder (see ❹).

18. Collect a urine specimen if needed. Allow 20 mL to 30 mL to flow into the bottle without touching the catheter to the bottle.

19. Allow the straight catheter to continue draining. If necessary, attach the drainage end of an indwelling catheter to the collecting tubing and bag.

20. Examine and measure the urine. In some cases, only 750 mL to 1000 mL of urine are to be drained from the bladder at one time. Check agency policy for further instructions if this should occur.

21. Remove the straight catheter when urine flow stops. For an indwelling catheter, secure the catheter tubing to the inner thigh for female clients (see ❺) or the upper thigh or abdomen for male clients (see ❻) with enough slack to allow usual movement. Tape or a manufactured catheter-securing device (see ❼) should be used to secure the catheter tubing to the client. **Rationale: Securing the catheter prevents unnecessary trauma to the urethra.**

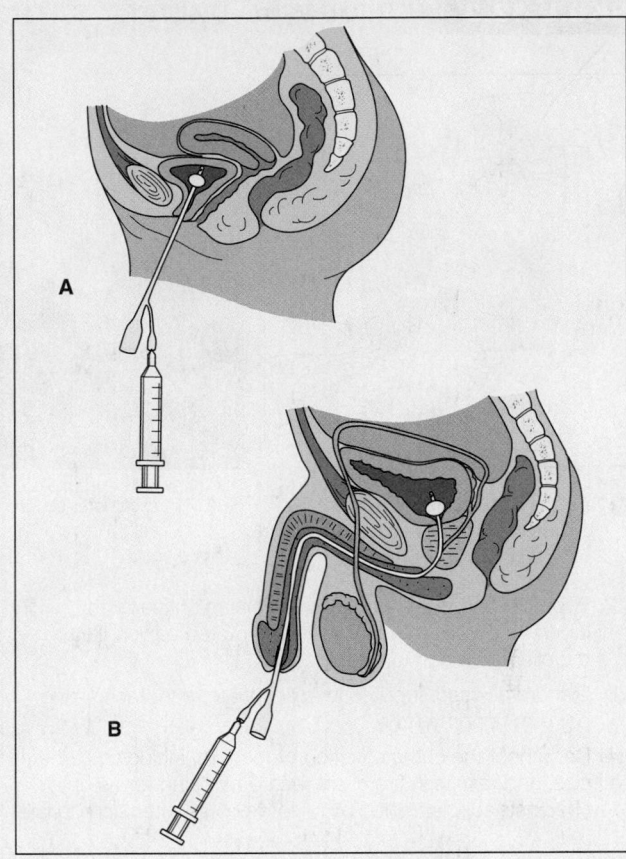

❹ Placement of indwelling catheter and inflated balloon: **A:** Female client; **B:** Male client.

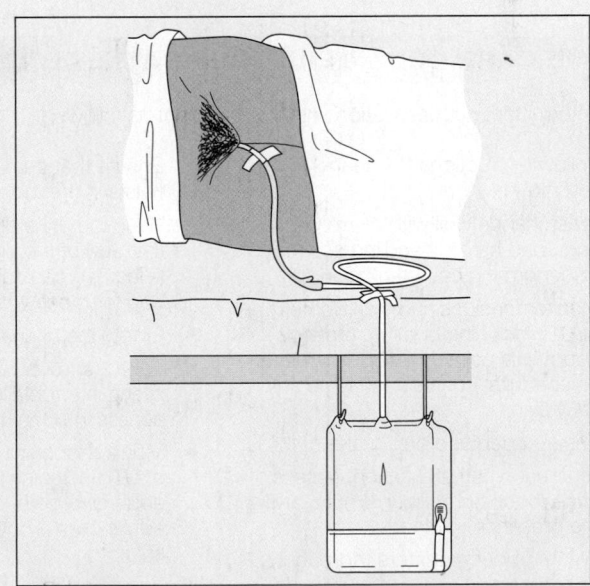

❺ Tape the catheter to the inside of a female's thigh.

Next, hang the collecting bag below the level of the bladder with no tubing falling below the top of the bag (see ❽).

(continued)

SKILL 42.3 PERFORMING URINARY CATHETERIZATION (*continued*)

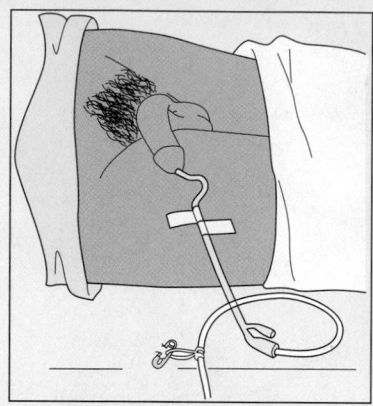

⑥ Tape the catheter to the thigh or abdomen of a male client.

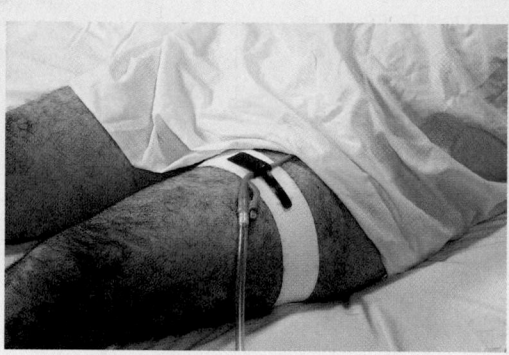

⑦ A Velcro catheter securement device.

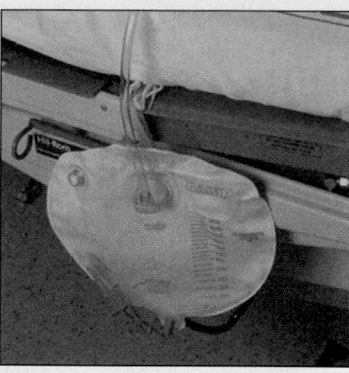

⑧ Correct position for urine drainage bag and tubing.

22. Wipe the perineal area of any remaining antiseptic or lubricant. Replace the foreskin if retracted earlier. Return the client to a comfortable position.

23. Discard all used supplies in appropriate receptacles, and perform hand hygiene.

24. Document the catheterization procedure, including catheter size, and results in the client record by using forms or checklists supplemented by narrative notes when appropriate.

EVALUATION

Conduct appropriate follow-up, such as notifying the appropriate member of the health care team of the catheterization results. Perform a detailed follow-up based on findings that deviated from expected or normal for the client. Relate findings to previous assessment data, if available. Teach the client how to care for the indwelling catheter, advise him or her to drink more fluids, and offer other appropriate instructions.

HOME CARE CONSIDERATIONS CATHETERIZATION

For intermittent catheterization, instruct the client as follows:

- Follow instructions for clean technique.
- Wash hands well with warm water and soap before handling equipment or performing catheterization.
- Monitor for signs and symptoms of UTI, including burning, urgency, abdominal pain, and cloudy urine; in older adults, confusion may be an early sign.
- Ensure adequate oral intake of fluids.
- After each catheterization, assess the urine for colour, odour, clarity, and the presence of blood.
- Wash rubber catheters thoroughly with soap and water after use, dry, and store in a clean place.

  For indwelling catheters, instruct the client as follows:

- Never pull on the catheter.
- Secure the catheter tubing to your leg by using a catheter-securing device.

- Ensure that there are no kinks or twists in the tubing.
- Keep the urine drainage bag below the level of the bladder (Figure 42.18). A leg bag can substitute for a hanging bag for those who are upright.
- Empty the drainage bag regularly.
- Take a shower rather than a tub bath; sitting in a tub allows bacteria easier access into the urinary tract.
- Monitor for signs and symptoms of UTI, including burning, urgency, abdominal pain, cloudy urine; in older adults confusion may be an early sign.
- Ensure adequate oral intake of fluids.
- Clients who have indwelling catheters for lengthy periods need to have the catheter and bag changed at regular intervals. Changing equipment once a month is often the standard, although agency policy may differ.

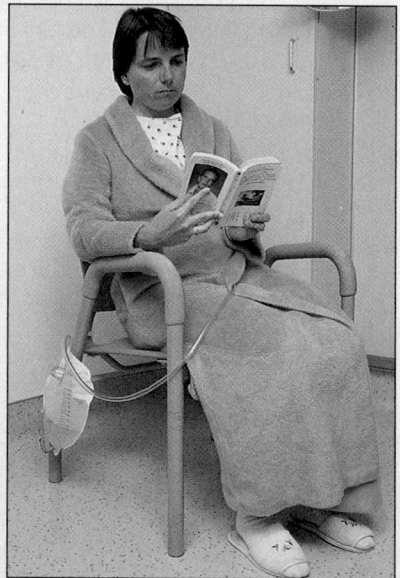

FIGURE 42.18 Positioning the collecting bag and tubing when sitting in a chair.

LIFESPAN CONSIDERATIONS

Catheterization

INFANTS AND CHILDREN

- Adapt the size of the catheter for pediatric clients.
- Ask a family member to assist in holding the child during the catheterization, if appropriate.
- Explain the procedure to the family and the child in terms the child can understand.

OLDER ADULTS

- When catheterizing older adults, be very attentive to problems of limited movement, especially in the hips. Arthritis, or previous hip or knee surgery, can limit movement and cause discomfort. Modify the position (e.g., side-lying) as needed to perform the procedure safely, and comfortably.
- For women, obtain the assistance of another nurse to flex and hold client's knees and hips as necessary or place her in the modified Sims' position.

Guidelines to prevent catheter-associated UTIs are given in Practice Guidelines 42.3. Ongoing assessment of clients with retention catheters is a high priority (see Box 42.3).

Removing Indwelling Catheters   Indwelling catheters are removed after their purpose has been achieved, usually on the order of the physician. If the catheter has been in place for a short time (e.g., a few days), the client usually has little difficulty regaining normal urinary elimination patterns. Swelling of the urethra, however, may initially interfere with voiding, so the nurse should regularly assess the client for urinary retention until normal voiding is reestablished.

BOX 42.3   ONGOING ASSESSMENT OF CLIENTS WITH INDWELLING CATHETERS

It is essential that the nurse regularly assess clients with retention catheters:

- Ensure that there are no obstructions in the drainage tubing. Check that there are no kinks in the tubing, the client is not lying on the tubing, and the tubing is not clogged with mucus or blood.
- Check that there is no tension on the catheter or tubing, that the catheter is securely taped to the thigh or abdomen, and that the tubing is fastened appropriately to the bedclothes.
- Ensure that gravity drainage is maintained. Make sure there are no loops in the tubing below its entry to the drainage receptacle and that the drainage receptacle is below the level of the client's bladder.
- Ensure that the drainage system is well sealed or closed. Check that there are no leaks at the connection sites in open systems.
- Observe the flow of the urine every 2 or 3 hours, and note colour, odour, and any abnormal constituents. If sediment or blood clots are present, check the catheter more frequently to assess patency.

Clients who have had an indwelling catheter for a prolonged period may require bladder retraining to regain bladder muscle tone. With an indwelling catheter in place, the bladder muscle does not stretch and contract regularly as it does when the bladder fills and empties by voiding. A few days before removal, the catheter may be clamped for specified periods (e.g., 2 to 4 hours), and then released to

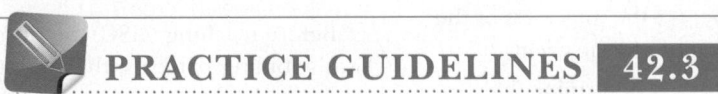

PRACTICE GUIDELINES   42.3

Preventing Catheter-Associated Urinary Tract Infections

Guidelines	Rationales
Have an established infection prevention and control program.	*Evidence-informed standards of practice that are used consistently by health care professionals reduce the risk of infection.*
Catheterize clients only when necessary, using aseptic technique, sterile equipment, and trained personnel.	*Aseptic technique eliminates the risk of introducing bacteria into the bladder.*
Maintain a sterile closed-drainage system. Do not disconnect the catheter and drainage tubing unless absolutely necessary.	*A closed system reduces the risk of bacteria entering the system.*
Remove the catheter as soon as possible.	*The risk of infection increases with the length of time the catheter is in place.*
Follow and reinforce good hand hygiene practices.	*This prevents the introduction of bacteria.*
Provide routine perineal hygiene, including cleansing with soap and water after defecation. Prevent contamination of the catheter with feces in the client with incontinence.	*Keeping the catheter and perineal area clean prevents the migration of fecal bacteria into the bladder.*

allow the bladder to empty. This allows the bladder to distend and stimulates its musculature.

To remove an indwelling catheter, the nurse follows these steps:

- Obtain a receptacle for the catheter (e.g., a disposable basin), a clean towel, disposable gloves, and a sterile syringe to deflate the balloon. The syringe should be large enough to withdraw *all* the solution in the catheter balloon. The size of the balloon is indicated on the label at the end of the catheter.

- Ask the client to assume the supine position as for catheterization.

- *Optional:* Obtain a sterile specimen before removing the catheter. Check agency protocol.

- Remove the tape attaching the catheter to the client, put on gloves, and then place the towel between the legs of the female client or over the thighs of the male.

- Insert the syringe into the injection port of the catheter, and withdraw the fluid from the balloon. If all the fluid cannot be removed, report this fact to the nurse in charge before proceeding.

- Do *not* pull the catheter while the balloon is inflated; doing so may injure the urethra.

- After all the fluid is withdrawn from the balloon, gently withdraw the catheter, and place it in the waste receptacle.

- Dry the perineal area with a towel.

- Remove gloves.

- Measure the urine in the drainage bag, and record the removal of the catheter. Include in the recording (a) the time the catheter was removed; (b) the amount, colour, and clarity of the urine; (c) the intactness of the catheter; and (d) instructions given to the client.

- Following removal of the catheter, determine the time of the first voiding and the amount voided during the first 8 hours. Compare this output with the client's intake.

- Observe for dysfunctional voiding behaviours (e.g., less than 100 mL per void), which might indicate urinary retention. If this occurs, perform an assessment of postvoid residuals by using a bladder scanner, if available. Generally, postvoid residuals greater than 200 mL will require straight catheterization, as needed. Depending on the client's intake, failure to void after 6 to 8 hours may also indicate urinary retention and must be assessed further for possible recatheterization.

CLEAN INTERMITTENT SELF-CATHETERIZATION
Clean intermittent self-catheterization (CISC) is performed by many clients who have some form of chronic neurogenic bladder dysfunction, such as that caused by spinal cord injury. Given the risks of infection with long term self-catheterization, much research has been completed in an attempt to develop best practices; however, very few quality studies exist. The authors of a systematic

review of the evidence related to practices that minimize urinary tract infection in people who use intermittent urinary catheterization found that "there is a lack of evidence to state that incidence of UTI is affected by use of sterile or clean technique, coated or uncoated catheters, single (sterile) or multiple use (clean) catheters, self-catheterisation or catheterisation by others, or by any other strategy" (Moore, Fader, & Getliffe, 2007).

CISC achieves the following:

- Improvement in self-care and independence

- Reduction in incidence of complications of indwelling catheters (e.g., UTI)

- Reduction in the need for equipment (e.g. drainage bags)

- Less interference with intimacy and sexual activities

- Potential reduction in lower urinary tract symptoms (frequency, urgency, incontinence) between catheterizations

- Freedom from embarrassing dribbling

The procedure for CISC is similar to that used by the nurse to catheterize a client. The steps are outlined in the Teaching: Clinical box. Because the procedure requires great motivation and physical and mental preparation, client assessment is important (Newman & Willson, 2011).

The client should have the following:

- Sufficient manual dexterity to manipulate a catheter

- Sufficient mental ability

- Motivation and acceptance of the procedure

- For females, reasonable agility to access the urethra

- Bladder capacity not less than 100 mL

Before teaching CISC, the nurse should establish the client's voiding patterns, the volume voided, fluid intake, and residual amounts. Self-catheterization is easier to learn for males because of the visibility of the urinary meatus. Females need to learn initially with the aid of a mirror but eventually should perform the procedure by using only the sense of touch (see the Teaching: Clinical box on CISC).

URINARY IRRIGATIONS An irrigation is a flushing or washing out with a specified solution. *Bladder irrigation* is carried out on a physician's order, usually to wash out the bladder and sometimes to apply a medication to the bladder lining. *Catheter irrigations* may be performed to maintain or restore the patency of a catheter, for example, to remove pus or blood clots blocking the catheter. Quality studies on the effectiveness of regular irrigation or flushing of long-term indwelling catheter with saline or acidic solutions to prevent catheter blockage are lacking, with preliminary results indicating that there is no benefit to regular flushing (Hagen, Sinclair, & Cross, 2010).

The *closed method* is the preferred technique for catheter or bladder irrigation because it is associated with a lower risk of UTI. Closed catheter irrigations may be either continuous or intermittent. A three-way, or triple

Clean Intermittent Self-Catheterization

It is essential that the client understand how to perform self-catheterization properly:

- Catheterization must be performed as often as needed to maintain an acceptable residual urine volume. At first, catheterization may be necessary every 2 to 3 hours, decreasing to 4 to 6 hours.
- Attempt to void before catheterization; insert the catheter to remove residual urine if unable to void or if amount voided is insufficient (e.g., less than 100 mL).
- Assemble all needed supplies ahead of time. Good lighting is essential, especially for women.
- If female, remove a tampon (if applicable) before carrying out intermittent self-catheterization. A tampon can inhibit catheterization.
- Perform hand hygiene.
- Clean the urinary meatus with either a towelette or soapy washcloth, and then rinse with a wet washcloth. If female, clean the area from front to back.
- Assume a position that is comfortable and that facilitates passage of the catheter, such as a semi-reclining position in bed or sitting on a chair or the toilet. Men may prefer to stand over the toilet; women may prefer to stand with one foot on the side of the bathtub.
- Apply lubricant to the catheter tip (2.5 cm to 5 cm for women; 5 cm to 15 cm for men).
- Insert the catheter until urine flows through.

a. If female, locate the meatus by using a mirror or other aid, or use the touch technique as follows:
  - Place the index finger of your nondominant hand on your clitoris.
  - Place the third and fourth fingers at the vagina.
  - Locate the meatus between the index and third fingers.
  - Separate the labia with your dominant hand.
  - Direct the catheter through the meatus and then upward and forward toward the umbilicus.

b. If male, hold the penis with a slight upward tension at a 60- to 90-degree angle to insert the catheter. Return the penis to its natural position after catheter insertion when urine starts to flow.

- Hold the catheter in place until all urine is drained.
- Withdraw the catheter slowly to ensure complete drainage of urine.
- Wash the catheter with soap and water; store in a clean container. Replace the catheter when it becomes difficult to clean, or too soft or hard to insert easily.
- Contact your health care provider if your urine appears cloudy or contains sediment; if you have bleeding, difficulty, or pain when passing the catheter; or if you have a fever.
- Drink at least 2000 mL to 2500 mL of fluid a day, unless contraindicated, to ensure adequate bladder filling and flushing.

lumen, catheter generally is used for closed irrigations. The irrigating solution flows into the bladder through the irrigation port of the catheter and out through the urinary drainage lumen of the catheter.

Occasionally, an *open irrigation* may be necessary to restore catheter patency. The risk of injecting microorganisms into the urinary tract is greater with open irrigations as the connection between the indwelling catheter and the drainage tubing is broken. Strict precautions to maintain the sterility of the drainage tubing connector and interior of the indwelling catheter must be taken to minimize this risk. The open method of catheter or bladder irrigation is performed with double-lumen indwelling catheters; it may be necessary for clients who develop blood clots and mucous fragments that occlude the catheter and when it is undesirable to change the catheter. Techniques for catheter irrigation are outlined in Skill 42.4.

SKILL 42.4 PERFORMING BLADDER IRRIGATION

PURPOSES

- To maintain the patency of a urinary catheter and tubing (closed continuous irrigation)
- To free a blockage in a urinary catheter or tubing (open intermittent irrigation)

ASSESSMENT

- Determine the client's current urinary drainage system. Review the client record for recent intake and output and any difficulties the client has been experiencing with the system. Review the results of previous irrigations.

- Assess the client for any discomfort, bladder spasms, or distended bladder.

PLANNING

Before irrigating a catheter or bladder, check the following: (a) the reason for the irrigation; (b) the prescription authorizing the continuous or intermittent irrigation (in most agencies, a physician or nurse practitioner's order is required); (c) the type of sterile solution, the amount and strength to be used, and the rate (if continuous); and (d) the type of catheter in place. If these are not specified on the client's chart, check agency protocol.

(continued)

SKILL 42.4 PERFORMING BLADDER IRRIGATION (*continued*)

Equipment

- Clean gloves (2 pairs)
- Retention catheter in place
- Drainage tubing and bag (if not in place)
- Drainage tubing clamp
- Antiseptic swabs
- Sterile receptacle
- Sterile irrigating solution warmed or at room temperature (label the irrigant clearly with the words *Bladder Irrigation*, including the information about any medications that have been added to the original solution, and the date, time, and nurse's initials)
- Infusion tubing
- IV pole

IMPLEMENTATION

Performance

1. Before performing the procedure, introduce yourself and verify the client's identity using two identifiers or per agency protocol. Explain to the client what you are going to do, why it is necessary, and how he or she can participate. The irrigation should not be painful or uncomfortable. Discuss how the results will be used in planning further care or treatments.

2. Perform hand hygiene, and follow other appropriate infection prevention and control procedures.

3. Provide for client privacy.

4. Put on clean gloves.

5. Empty, measure, and record the amount and appearance of urine present in the drainage bag. Discard urine and gloves. **Rationale: Emptying the drainage bag allows more accurate measurement of urinary output after the irrigation is in place or completed. Assessing the character of the urine provides baseline data for later comparison.** Perform hand hygiene.

6. Prepare the equipment.
    - Connect the irrigation infusion tubing to the irrigating solution and flush the tubing with solution, keeping the tip sterile. **Rationale: Flushing the tubing removes air and prevents it from being instilled into the bladder.**
    - Put on clean gloves, and cleanse the port with antiseptic swabs.
    - Connect the irrigation tubing to the input port of the three-way catheter.
    - Connect the drainage bag and tubing to the urinary drainage port if not already in place.
    - Remove gloves, and perform hand hygiene.

7. Irrigate the bladder.
    a) For *closed continuous bladder irrigation*, open the flow clamp on the urinary drainage tubing (if present). See ❶. **Rationale: This allows the irrigating solution to flow out of the bladder continuously.**
    - Open the regulating clamp on the irrigating tubing and adjust the flow rate as prescribed by the appropriate member of the health care team or to 40 to 60 drops per minute, if not specified.

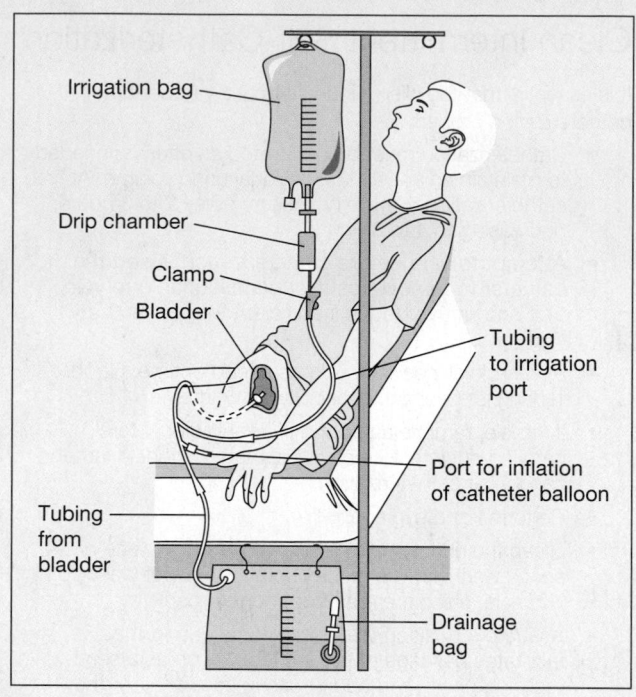

❶ A closed continuous bladder irrigation (CBI) setup.

Irrigation bag
Drip chamber
Clamp
Bladder
Tubing to irrigation port
Port for inflation of catheter balloon
Tubing from bladder
Drainage bag

- Assess the drainage for amount, colour, and clarity. The amount of drainage should equal the amount of irrigant entering the bladder plus expected urine output.

    b) For *closed intermittent bladder irrigation*, determine whether the solution is to remain in the bladder for a specified time.
    - If the solution is to remain in the bladder (a bladder irrigation or instillation), apply the flow clamp to the urinary drainage tubing. **Rationale: Closing the flow clamp allows the solution to be retained in the bladder and in contact with bladder walls.**
    - If the solution is being instilled to irrigate the catheter, open the flow clamp on the urinary drainage tubing. **Rationale: Irrigating solution will flow through the urinary drainage port and tubing, removing mucous shreds or clots.**
    - Open the flow clamp on the irrigating tubing, allowing the specified amount of solution to infuse. Clamp the tubing.
    - After the specified period for which the solution is to be retained, open the drainage tubing flow clamp, and allow the bladder to empty.
    - Assess the drainage for amount, colour, and clarity. The amount of drainage should equal the amount of irrigant entering the bladder plus expected urine output.

8. Assess the client and the urinary output.
    - Assess the client's comfort.
    - Empty the drainage bag and measure the contents. Subtract the amount of irrigant instilled from the total volume of drainage to obtain the volume of urine output.

9. Document the procedure and results in the client record by using forms or checklists supplemented by narrative notes when appropriate.
    - Note any abnormal constituents, such as blood clots, pus, or mucous shreds.

Variation: Open Irrigation by Using a Two-Way Indwelling Catheter

1. Assemble the equipment. Use an irrigation set (see ❷) or assemble individual items, including the following:
   - Clean gloves
   - Sterile gloves
   - Disposable water-resistant towel
   - Sterile irrigating solution
   - Sterile irrigation tray
   - Sterile basin
   - Sterile 30–50-mL irrigating syringe
   - Antiseptic swabs
   - Sterile protective cap (for catheter drainage tubing)

2. Prepare the client (see steps 1 to 5 of main procedure for catheter irrigation).

3. Prepare the equipment.
   - Perform hand hygiene.
   - By using aseptic technique, open supplies and pour the irrigating solution into the sterile basin or receptacle. **Rationale: Aseptic technique is vital to reduce the risk of introducing microorganisms into the urinary tract during the irrigation.**
   - Place the disposable water-resistant towel under the catheter.
   - Put on clean gloves. Disconnect the catheter from the drainage tubing. Place the sterile protective cap over the end of the drainage tubing. **Rationale: The end of the drainage tubing will be considered contaminated if it touches the bed linen or skin surfaces.**
   - Remove clean gloves, and put on sterile gloves.
   - Withdraw the prescribed amount of irrigating solution into the syringe, maintaining the sterility of the syringe and solution.

4. Irrigate the bladder.
   - Insert the tip of the syringe into the catheter opening.
   - Gently and slowly inject the solution. In adults, about 30 mL to 40 mL generally is instilled for catheter irrigations; 100 mL to 200 mL may be instilled for bladder irrigation. **Rationale: Gentle instillation reduces the risks of injury to bladder mucosa and of bladder spasms.**

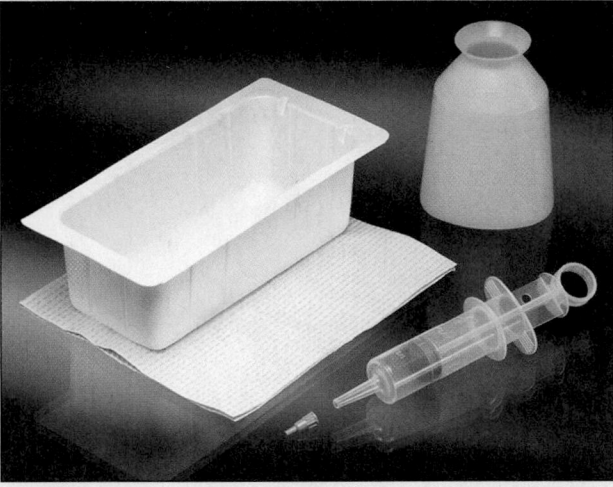

❷ An irrigation set.

   - Remove the syringe and allow solution to drain into the basin.
   - Continue to irrigate client's bladder until fluid returns are clear or clots are removed.
   - Remove the protective cap from the drainage tube and wipe with antiseptic swab or alcohol sponge.
   - Reconnect the catheter to drainage tubing.
   - Assess the drainage for amount, colour, and clarity. The amount of drainage should equal the amount of irrigant entering the bladder. Determine the amount of fluid used for the irrigation and subtract from total output on the client's intake and output (I&O) record.

5. Assess the client and the urinary output and document the procedure as in steps 8 and 9 above.

EVALUATION

- Perform detailed follow-up based on findings that deviated from expected or normal for the client. Relate findings to previous assessment data, if available.
- Report significant deviations from normal to the appropriate member of the health care team.

SUPRAPUBIC CATHETER CARE A **suprapubic catheter** is inserted through the abdominal wall above the symphysis pubis into the urinary bladder (Figure 42.19 on the next page). The catheter is sometimes used for short-term catheterization in pelvic surgical procedures, or urinary tract obstruction. The physician inserts the catheter intraoperatively or by using local anesthesia. The catheter may be secured in place with sutures, with a body seal, or with both sutures and a body seal. The catheter is then attached to a closed drainage system. Some evidence suggests that short-term suprapubic catheterization may present lower risks of bacteriuria, less need for recatheterization, and less discomfort in comparison to indwelling or intermittent catheterization (Niël-Weise

& van den Broek, 2005), although recent work also suggests that intermittent catheterization may support a more rapid return to normal micturition and shorter hospitalization (Dixon, Dolan, Brown, & Hilton, 2010).

Care of clients with a suprapubic catheter includes regular assessments of the client's urine, fluid intake, and comfort; maintenance of a patent drainage system; skin care around the insertion site; periodic clamping of the catheter preparatory to removing it; and measurement of residual urine. Orders generally include leaving the catheter open to drainage for 48 to 72 hours, then clamping the catheter for 3- to 4-hour periods during the day until the client can void satisfactorily amounts. Satisfactory

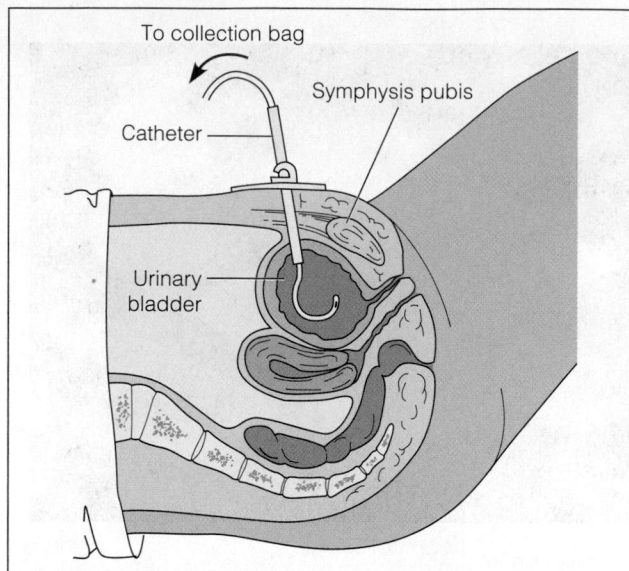

FIGURE 42.19 A suprapubic catheter in place.

voiding is determined by measuring the client's residual urine after voiding.

Care of the catheter insertion site involves sterile technique. Dressings around the suprapubic catheter are changed whenever they are soiled with drainage to prevent bacterial growth around the insertion site and reduce the potential for infection. Procedures for cleaning wounds and changing dressings are discussed in Chapter 35. Any redness and discharge at the skin around the insertion site must be reported.

URINARY DIVERSIONS A **urinary diversion** is the surgical rerouting of urine from the kidneys to a site other than the bladder. Two categories of diversions are available: (a) incontinent and (b) continent.

Incontinent Diversions With incontinent diversions, clients have no control over the passage of urine and require the use of an external ostomy appliance to contain the urine. Urinary diversions may or may not involve

a *cystectomy* (the removal of the urinary bladder). Examples of incontinent diversions include ureterostomy, nephrostomy, vesicostomy, and ileal conduits. In a **ureterostomy**, one or both of the ureters is brought directly to the side of the abdomen to form small stomas. This procedure, however, has some disadvantages in that the stomas provide direct access for microorganisms from skin to the kidneys, the small stomas are difficult to fit with an appliance to collect the urine, and they may narrow, impairing urine drainage. A **nephrostomy** diverts urine from the kidney to a stoma (Figure 42.20). A **vesicostomy** may be formed when the bladder is left intact but voiding through the urethra is not possible (e.g., because of an obstruction or a neurogenic bladder). The ureters remain connected to the bladder, and the bladder wall is surgically attached to an opening in the skin below the navel, forming an incontinent stoma.

The most common urinary diversion is the **ileal conduit** or ileal loop (Figure 42.21). In this procedure, a segment of the ileum is removed and the intestinal ends are reattached. One end of the portion removed is closed with sutures to create a pouch, and the other end is brought out through the abdominal wall to create a stoma. The ureters are implanted into the ileal pouch. The ileal stoma is more readily fitted with an appliance than are ureterostomies because of its larger size. The mucous membrane lining of the ileum also provides some protection from ascending infection. Urine drains continuously from the ileal pouch.

Continent Diversions With continent diversions, a continence mechanism is created, giving clients control over the passage of urine, either by intermittent catheterization of the internal reservoir (e.g., *Indiana pouch*) or by strained voiding (*neobladder*). The Indiana pouch is created by attaching the client's ureters to a portion of the ileum that is shaped into a reservoir (like a pouch) for urine. The client with this type of pouch inserts a catheter through an opening in the abdominal wall to empty the reservoir, generally every 4 hours. A **neobladder** replaces

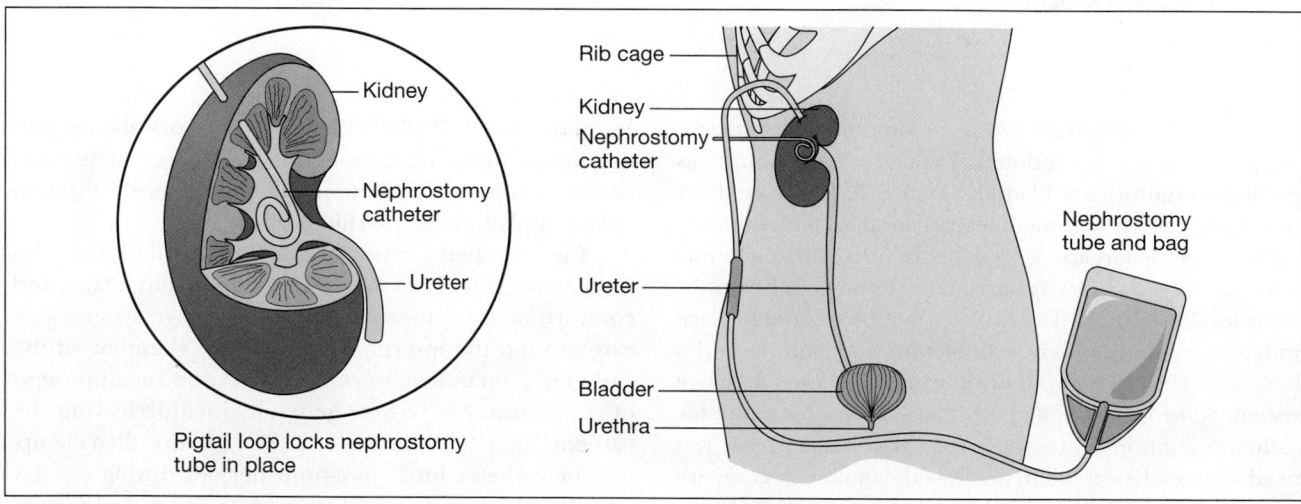

FIGURE 42.20 A nephrostomy.

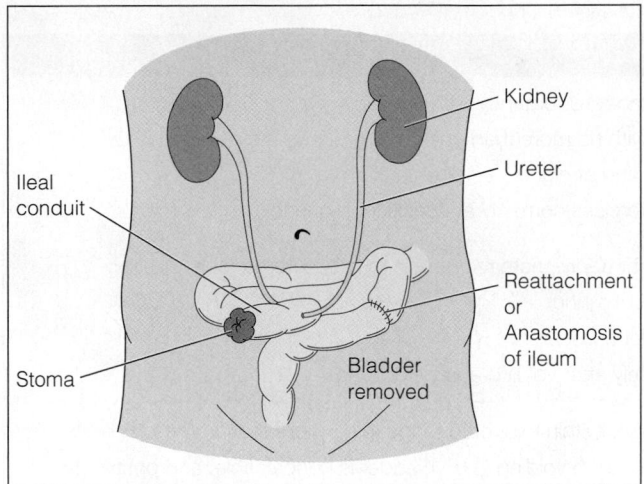

FIGURE 42.21 An incontinent urinary diversion (ileal conduit).

a diseased or damaged bladder with a piece of ileum, thus making a new bladder. This new bladder is then sutured to the functional urethra, allowing the person to urinate normally (Figure 42.22).

When caring for clients with a urinary diversion, the nurse must accurately assess intake and output, note any changes in urine colour, odour, or clarity (mucous shreds are commonly seen in the urine of clients with an ileal diversion), and frequently assess the condition of the stoma and surrounding skin. Clients who must wear a urine collection appliance are at risk for impaired skin integrity because of irritation by urine. Well-fitting appliances are vital. The nurse should consult with the wound ostomy continence nurse to identify strategies for management of stoma and peristomal problems and the most appropriate appliance for the client's needs.

The steps of changing a urostomy appliance are similar to those described in the procedure for changing a

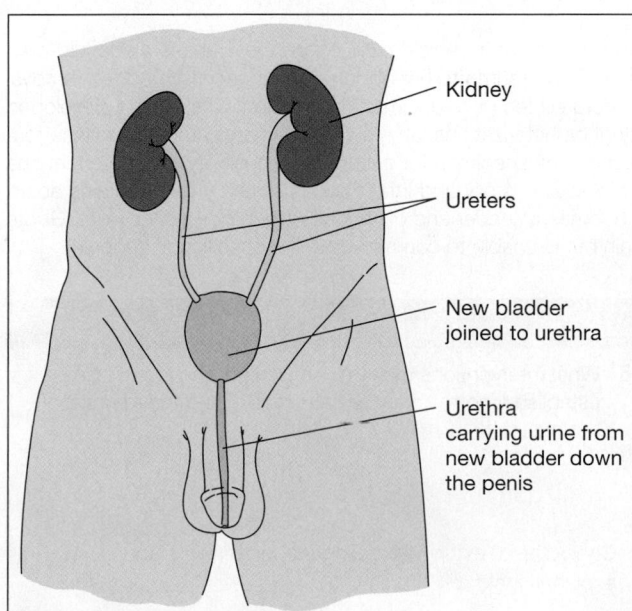

FIGURE 42.22 A neobladder.

bowel diversion appliance (see Chapter 41). However, there are some differences, including the following: incontinent urinary diversions drain continually; as a result, some type of material (e.g., dry gauze) can be placed under the stoma to collect the urine throughout the measurement and change of the ostomy appliance. Immediately following surgery, ureteral stents may be present and protruding from the stoma. They remain in place for 10 to 14 days postop and are removed, depending on institutional protocol, by either the surgeon or the nurse. Ureteral stents are used to maintain the patency of ureters at the anastomotic sites.

Clients with urinary diversions may experience problems with their body image and sexuality and may require assistance in coping with these changes and managing the stoma. Most clients are able to resume their normal activities and lifestyle.

Evaluating

By using the overall goals and desired outcomes identified in the planning stage, the nurse collects data to evaluate the effectiveness of nursing activities. Examples of desired health outcomes for the identified goals are listed in Table 42.5 on the next page.

If the desired outcomes are not achieved, explore the reasons why before modifying the care plan. For example, if the outcome "remains dry between voidings and at night" is not met, examples of questions that need to be considered include the following:

- What is the client's perception of the problem?
- Does the client understand and comply with the health care instructions provided?
- Is access to toilet facilities a problem?
- Can the client manipulate clothing for toileting? Are there adjustments that can be made to allow easier undressing?
- Are scheduled toileting times appropriate?
- Is there adequate transition lighting for nighttime toileting?
- Are mobility aids, such as a walker, elevated toilet seat, or grab bar, needed? If currently used, are they appropriate or adequate?
- Is the client performing pelvic floor muscle exercises appropriately as scheduled?
- Is the client's fluid intake adequate? Does the timing of fluid intake need to be adjusted (e.g., restricted after dinner)?
- Is the client restricting caffeine, citrus juice, carbonated beverages, and artificial sweetener intake?
- Is the client taking a diuretic? If so, when is the medication taken? Do the times need to be adjusted (e.g., taking second dose no later than 4 p.m.)?
- Should continence aids, such as a condom catheter or absorbent pads, be considered or used?

TABLE 42.5 Evaluation Goals and Outcomes: Urinary Elimination

Goal	Examples of Desired Outcomes
Restore normal voiding pattern	Absence of pain, burning, hesitancy, or urgency with urination
	Voids at 3- to 4-hour intervals with no more than one voiding during the night
	Remains dry between voidings and at night
	Performs pelvic floor muscle exercises correctly at specified frequency
Perform toilet activities independently with or without assistive devices	Is able to access toilet facilities or appropriate receptacle (urinal, commode) for voiding
	Is able to manipulate clothing for voiding
	Is able to get on and off the toilet unassisted
	Cleans perineal area appropriately after voiding and defecating
Regain normal urine output	Quantity of urine at each voiding is within expected range (e.g., more than 150 mL)
	Bladder empties completely with each voiding (e.g., bladder is nonpalpable, and postvoid residual is less than 100 mL)
	Urine colour, clarity, and odour are within normal limits
	Urinalysis values are within expected ranges (specific gravity, pH, protein, glucose, and ketones)
Avoid complications associated with altered urinary elimination (urinary tract infection, skin breakdown, fluid and electrolyte imbalance, body image disturbance, social isolation)	Absence of manifestations of urinary tract infections (UTI), such as dysuria, frequency, urgency, hematuria, or pyuria (pus in the urine)
	Identifies symptoms of and measures to prevent UTI
	Drinks at least 2000 mL to 2500 mL of fluid daily
	Serum electrolytes remain within expected values
	Skin of perineal area and over bony prominences (sacrum, hips), or around urinary stoma, if client has one, remains intact
	Cares for urinary stoma and drainage collection devices, as instructed
	Demonstrates appropriate technique in performing intermittent self-catheterization
	States or demonstrates acceptance of urinary diversion and ability to adjust to change in lifestyle
	Maintains or returns to previous social involvement

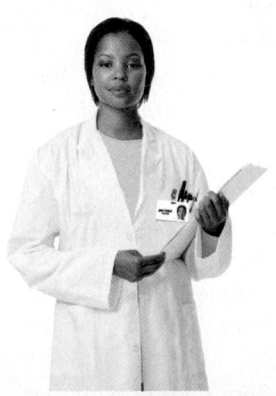

Case Study 42

Mrs. Gupta, 48 years old, is recovering from a motor vehicle collision on the Trans-Canada Highway 4 days ago. In the collision, she sustained blunt trauma to her abdomen that necessitated the removal of her spleen. Additionally, she has a fractured femur and a mild concussion. Mrs. Gupta developed urinary retention and, after four intermittent catheterizations, an indwelling urinary catheter was inserted. On entering Mrs. Gupta's room to collect a urine specimen for culture and sensitivity, you note that she is restless and moaning. Her abdominal dressing is dry and intact and her urinary bag contains about 200 mL of amber coloured urine. Her abdomen is tender and distended. When questioned, Mrs. Gupta is able to communicate that she is in pain but is unable to communicate the specifics of her pain.

CRITICAL THINKING QUESTIONS

1. Is it correct to hypothesize that Mrs. Gupta's pain is caused by her incision? Why, or why not?

2. What actions should be taken before administering analgesia to Mrs. Gupta?

3. What precautions should be taken when collecting a urine sample from a person with an indwelling urinary catheter, and why?

4. What measures can be taken to prevent Mrs. Gupta from developing a urinary tract infection if it is not already present?

5. What interventions may be useful in helping Mrs. Gupta establish a normal urinary pattern following the removal of her catheter?

Check the eText in MyNursingLab for answers and explanations.

KEY TERMS

anuria *p. 1309*

bladder training *p. 1326*

blood urea nitrogen
(BUN) *p. 1319*

Bowman's capsule *p. 1304*

creatinine *p. 1319*

creatinine
clearance *p. 1319*

Credé's
manoeuvre *p. 1330*

cystoscope *p. 1319*

cystoscopy *p. 1319*

detrusor muscle *p. 1305*

dysuria *p. 1310*

enuresis *p. 1307*

flaccid bladder *p. 1330*

glomerulus *p. 1304*

habit training *p. 1326*

ileal conduit *p. 1342*

intravenous pyelography
(IVP) *p. 1319*

meatus *p. 1306*

micturition *p. 1306*

neobladder *p. 1342*

nephron *p. 1304*

nephrostomy *p. 1342*

neurogenic
bladder *p. 1311*

nocturia *p. 1307*

nocturnal enuresis *p. 1307*

oliguria *p. 1309*

pelvic floor muscle
exercises *p. 1327*

polydipsia *p. 1309*

polyuria *p. 1309*

prompted voiding *p. 1327*

renal ultrasonography
p. 1319

residual urine *p. 1314*

retrograde
pyelography *p. 1319*

suprapubic
catheter *p. 1341*

trigone *p. 1305*

ureterostomy *p. 1342*

urinary diversion *p. 1342*

urinary frequency *p. 1309*

urinary hesitancy *p. 1310*

urinary incontinence
(UI) *p. 1310*

urinary retention *p. 1311*

urinary urgency *p. 1310*

urination *p. 1306*

vesicostomy *p. 1342*

voiding *p. 1306*

CHAPTER HIGHLIGHTS

- Urinary elimination depends on normal functioning of the urinary, cardiovascular, and nervous systems.

- Urine is formed in the nephron, the structural and functional unit of the kidney, through a process of filtration, reabsorption, and secretion. Hormones, such as antidiuretic hormone (ADH), aldosterone, and antinatriuretic peptide affect the reabsorption of sodium and water, thus affecting the amount of urine formed.

- The normal process of urination is stimulated when sufficient urine collects in the bladder to stimulate stretch receptors. Impulses from stretch receptors are transmitted to the spinal cord and the brain, causing relaxation of the internal sphincter (unconscious control) and, if appropriate, relaxation of the external sphincter (conscious control).

- In the adult, urination generally occurs after 250 mL to 450 mL of urine has collected in the bladder.

- Many factors influence a person's urinary elimination, including growth and development, psychosocial factors, fluid and food intake, medications, muscle tone and activity, various diseases, and surgical and diagnostic procedures.

- Alterations in urine production and elimination include polyuria, oliguria and anuria, frequency or nocturia, urgency, dysuria, enuresis, incontinence, and retention. Each may have various influencing and associated factors that need to be identified.

- Assessment of a client's urinary function includes (a) a nursing history that identifies normal voiding patterns, usual urine output and recent changes, past and current problems with urination, and factors influencing the elimination pattern; (b) a physical assessment of the genitourinary system; (c) inspection of the urine for amount, colour, clarity, and odour, and if indicated, (d) testing of urine for specific gravity, pH, and the presence of glucose, ketones, protein, and occult blood.

- Incontinence can be physically and emotionally distressing to clients because it is considered socially unacceptable.

- Bladder training can often reduce episodes of incontinence.

- Clients with urinary retention not only experience discomfort but also are at risk of urinary tract infection.

- The most common cause of urinary tract infection is invasive procedures, such as catheterization and cystoscopic examination. Females, in particular, are prone to ascending urinary tract infections because of their short urethras.

- Goals for the client with problems with urinary elimination include maintaining or restoring normal elimination patterns and preventing associated risks, such as skin breakdown.

- In planning for home care, the nurse considers the client's needs for teaching and assistance or assistive devices in the home.

- Nursing interventions related to urinary elimination are generally directed toward facilitating the normal functioning of the urinary system or toward assisting the client with particular problems.

- Interventions include (a) assisting the client to maintain an appropriate fluid intake, (b) assisting the client to maintain normal voiding patterns, (c) monitoring the client's daily fluid intake and output, and (d) maintaining cleanliness of the genital area.

- Urinary catheterization is frequently required for clients with urinary retention but is performed only after all other measures to facilitate voiding fail.

Sterile technique is essential to prevent ascending urinary infections.

- Care of clients with indwelling catheters is directed toward preventing infection of the urinary tract and encouraging urinary flow through the drainage system.
- Clients with urinary retention can be taught to perform intermittent self-catheterization to promote their independence, reduce the risk of infection, and eliminate incontinence.

- Bladder or catheter irrigations can be used to apply medication to bladder walls or maintain catheter patency.
- When the urinary bladder is removed, a urinary diversion is formed to allow urine to be eliminated from the body. The ileal conduit or ileal loop is the most common diversion and requires that the client wear a urine collection device continually over the stoma.

ASSESS YOUR LEARNING

1. Mr. Smith returns from the operating room with a three-way indwelling catheter following a prostatectomy. He suddenly complains of severe lower abdominal pain. What is the nurse's BEST first action?

   a. Assess the client for surgical pain and administer the prescribed analgesic.
   b. Assess the patency of the catheter drainage system.
   c. Palpate Mr. Smith's bladder in the suprapubic region.
   d. Notify the surgeon of the client's pain.

2. Following the irrigation of an indwelling catheter, it is critical for the nurse to do which of the following?

   a. Ensure the drainage tubing is not kinked.
   b. Document findings in the chart.
   c. Send a urine specimen.
   d. Determine urine output.

3. Mrs. Chiu, 80 years old, is admitted to the hospital unit with urinary retention. After inserting an indwelling catheter, the nurse notes a pungent odour and heavily sedimented urine with specks of blood. What is the nurse's MOST appropriate action?

   a. Obtain a specimen for culture and sensitivity and send to the lab.
   b. Notify the appropriate member of the health care team about these findings.
   c. Teach Mrs. Chiu the importance of adequate fluid intake.
   d. Document the results and monitor Mrs. Chiu's vital signs.

4. Mr. Dupree is being discharged to his son's home following a cerebrovascular accident. He is incontinent of urine and feces and requires assistance with mobilization. Mr. Dupree's son is a busy executive and has hired a personal support worker to stay with his father during the day. What is an appropriate nursing diagnosis that may

negatively affect the son's ability to care for his father?

   a. Deficient knowledge related to incontinence
   b. Social isolation related to his father's incontinence
   c. Risk for infection
   d. Risk for caregiver role strain

5. Sanjay Dhara was admitted to the ward following an all-terrain vehicle accident 2 weeks ago in which he suffered a moderate brain injury. Which of the following methods would be MOST appropriate for maintaining Sanjay's continence?

   a. Bladder training
   b. Prompted voiding
   c. Habit training
   d. Pelvic floor muscle exercises

6. Mr. Brown, 65 years old, underwent abdominal surgery 5 days ago. He is eating and drinking well, so his intravenous has been discontinued and his IV analgesic switched to oral morphine. His indwelling catheter was discontinued 24 hours ago. Mr. Brown has been incontinent of large amounts of urine since the beginning of the shift. The MOST appropriate action would be which of the following?

   a. Request a prescription to replace the indwelling catheter so as to prevent skin breakdown
   b. Apply an incontinence brief and provide frequent pericare
   c. Palpate Mr. Brown's bladder in the suprapubic region
   d. Request a prescription for insertion of a straight urinary catheter

7. Which of the following behaviours indicates that the client on a bladder training program has met the expected outcomes?

   a. Voids each time there is an urge
   b. Practises slow, deep breathing until the urge decreases

c. Uses incontinence briefs, just in case

d. Drinks citrus juices and carbonated beverages

8. Melanie Borschnek, 32 years old, underwent surgery for an ileal conduit 4 days ago. She is currently refusing to participate in the care of her device. What is the most appropriate nursing diagnosis?

  a. Deficient knowledge

  b. Social isolation

  c. Low self-esteem

  d. Disturbed body image

9. June Foster, 45 years old, has her left leg in traction. She complains of the inability to void on the bedpan. What actions can the nurse take that may help the client to void?

  a. Closing the bedside curtain

  b. Running warm water over the bedpan before positioning it under June

c. Running water in the sink

d. Placing the bed in high-Fowler's position

10. Elizabeth Newman underwent brain surgery for removal of a tumour 2 days ago. Her urine output for the last 8 hours is 1200 mL (intake 600 mL). What is the accurate description for her output?

  a. Polyuria

  b. Dysuria

  c. Diuresis

  d. Enuresis

Check the eText in MyNursingLab for answers and explanations.

WEBLINKS

Canadian Nurse Continence Advisors

http://www.cnca.ca

This national association, promotes education, research, and clinical practice for the conservative management of incontinence.

The Canadian Continence Foundation

http://www.canadiancontinence.ca

This nonprofit organization has as its focus the support of individuals with continence problems. The site provides fact sheets and information regarding incontinence. Free registration is required.

The Kidney Foundation of Canada

http://www.kidney.ca

The Kidney Foundation of Canada is a volunteer association that provides support to individuals with kidney disease. The site provides comprehensive information pertaining to kidney disease.

The Canadian Association for Enterostomal Therapy

http://www.caet.ca

This nonprofit association specializes in the nursing care of clients with challenges in wound, ostomy, and continence. The website provides some useful information and brochures for clients, families, and professionals dealing with ostomies.

National Kidney and Urologic Diseases Information Clearinghouse

http://kidney.niddk.nih.gov

This excellent website provides information and online publications on all diseases and conditions affecting the kidneys and urological system.

MyNursingLab

REFERENCES

Ball, J. W., Bindler, R. C., & Cowen, K. J. (2010). *Child health nursing: Partnering with children and families.* Upper Saddle River, NJ: Pearson Education.

Delancey, J. (2010). Why do women have stress urinary incontinence? *Neurourology and Urodynamics, 29*(Suppl 1), S13–S17.

Dixon, L., Dolan, L., Brown, K., & Hilton, P. (2010). RCT of urethral versus suprapubic catheterization. *British Journal of Nursing, 19*(18), S7–S13.

Dumoulin, C., & Hay-Smith, J. (2010). Pelvic floor muscle training versus no treatment, or inactive control treatments, for urinary incontinence in women. *Cochrane Database of*

Systematic Reviews 2010, Issue 1. Art. No.: CD005654. doi: 10.1002/14651858.CD005654.pub2

Hagen, S., Sinclair, L., & Cross, S. (2010). Washout policies in long-term indwelling urinary catheterisation in adults. *Cochrane Database of Systematic Reviews 2010*, Issue 3. Art. No.: CD004012. doi: 10.1002/14651858.CD004012.pub4

Herderschee, R., Hay-Smith, E. J. C., Herbison, G. P., Roovers, J. P., & Heineman, M. J. (2011). Feedback or biofeedback to augment pelvic floor muscle training for urinary incontinence in women. *Cochrane Database of Systematic Reviews 2011*, Issue 7. Art. No.: CD009252. doi: 10.1002/14651858.CD009252

Holroyd-Leduc, J. M., Straus, S., Thorpe, K., Davis, D. A., Schmaltz, H., & Tannenbaum, C. (2011). Translation of evidence into a self-management tool for use by women with urinary incontinence. *Age & Ageing, 40*(2), 227–233.

Irwin, D., Milsom, I., Hunskaar, S., Reilly, K., Kopp, Z., Herschorn, S., & . . . Abrams, P. (2006). Population-based survey of urinary incontinence, overactive bladder, and other lower urinary tract symptoms in five countries: Results of the EPIC study. *European Urology, 50*(6), 1306–1314.

Jepson, R. G., & Craig, J. C. (2008). Cranberries for preventing urinary tract infections. *Cochrane Database of Systematic Reviews 2008*, Issue 1. Art. No.: CD001321. doi: 10.1002/14651858.CD001321.pub4

Moore, K. N., Fader, M., & Getliffe, K. (2007). Long-term bladder management by intermittent catheterisation in adults and children. *Cochrane Database of Systematic Reviews 2007*, Issue 4. Art. No.: CD006008. doi: 10.1002/14651858.CD006008.pub2

Nevéus, T., von Gontard, A., Hoebeke, P., Hjälmås, K., Bauer, S., Bower, W., . . . & Djurhuus, J. C. (2006). The standardization of terminology of lower urinary tract function in children and adolescents: Report from the Standardisation Committee of the International Children's Continence Society. *Journal of Urology, 176*(1), 314.

Newman, D. K., & Willson, M. M. (2011). Review of intermittent catheterization and current best practices. *Urologic Nursing*, 31(1), 12–48.

Nicolle, L. (2008). Urinary tract infections in older people. *Reviews in Clinical Gerontology, 18*(2), 103–114.

Niël-Weise, B. S., & van den Broek, P. J. (2005). Urinary catheter policies for short-term bladder drainage in adults. *Cochrane Database of Systematic Reviews 2005*, Issue 3. Art. No.: CD004203. doi: 10.1002/14651858.CD004203.pub2

Registered Nurses' Association of Ontario. (2011). *Promoting continence using prompted voiding: Guideline supplement* (Rev. ed.). Toronto, ON: Author.

Roe, B., Flanagan, L., Jack, B., Barrett, J., Chung, A., Shaw, C., & Williams, K. (2011). Systematic review of the management of incontinence and promotion of continence in older people in care homes: Descriptive studies with urinary incontinence as primary focus. *Journal of Advanced Nursing, 67*(2), 228–250

Wellberg, C. (2008). Distinguishing types of urinary incontinence in women. *American Family Physician, 78*(11), 3–4.

Wootton, J., & Norfolk, S. (2010). Nocturnal enuresis: Assessing and treating children and young people. *Community Practitioner: The Journal of the Community Practitioners' & Health Visitors' Association, 83*(12), 37–39.

Chapter 43

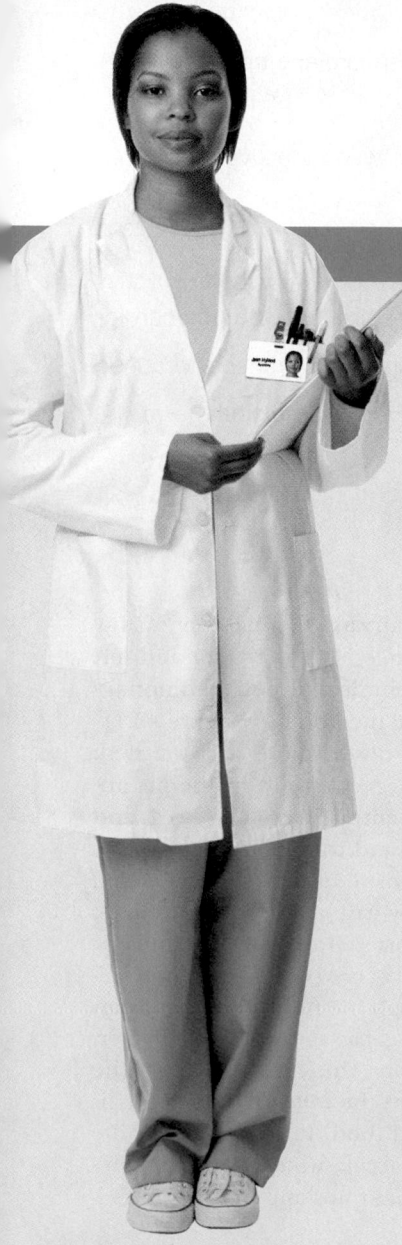

Oxygenation and Circulation

LEARNING OUTCOMES

After studying this chapter, you will be able to:

1. Outline the structure and function of the respiratory and cardiovascular systems.

2. Describe the processes of pulmonary ventilation and respiration.

3. Identify seven factors that influence respiration and circulatory function.

4. List the clinical manifestations of hypoxemia and hypoxia.

5. Identify 10 types of altered breathing patterns.

6. Differentiate among the signs and symptoms of upper, lower, partial, and completely obstructed airways.

7. Identify three major conditions that can alter respiratory function and three major conditions that can alter cardiovascular function.

8. Describe the nurse's role in caring for clients undergoing diagnostic procedures related to cardiorespiratory function.

9. Identify and describe nursing measures to promote cardiorespiratory function and oxygenation.

10. Explain the use of therapeutic measures, such as artificial airways, medications, oxygen therapy, inhalation therapy, pharyngeal and tracheal suctioning, and chest drainage, to promote cardiorespiratory function.

11. Describe the critical nature of cardiopulmonary resuscitation.

12. State outcome criteria for evaluating client responses to measuring and promoting adequate oxygenation and circulation.

Oxygen (O_2) is a clear, odourless gas that constitutes approximately 21% of the air we breathe. Oxygen is necessary for all living cells, and the absence of oxygen can lead to death. The transport of oxygen to body tissues and the removal of carbon dioxide (CO_2) and other byproducts is a complex process. The major systems involved in this process include the lungs, the heart, and blood.

Although all systems in the body are indirectly involved in the oxygenation process, the respiratory system (lungs) and the cardiovascular system (heart and vasculature) are directly and interdependently involved. Impaired function of either system can negatively affect the other system. This impairment can cause significant changes in the ability to breathe, transport gases, and eliminate wastes, and can result in respiratory failure, cardiac dysfunction, and general inability to participate in activities of daily living.

Respiration is the process of gas exchange between the individual and the environment. The process of respiration involves three components:

1. Pulmonary ventilation or breathing, the movement of air between the atmosphere and the alveoli of the lungs as we inhale and exhale

2. Gas exchange, which involves diffusion of oxygen and carbon dioxide between the alveoli and the pulmonary capillaries

3. Transport of oxygen from the lungs to tissues, and carbon dioxide from tissues to the lungs

The respiratory system has a major role in the first two components of respiration, while the cardiovascular system has a major role in the third component. Any impairment in gas transport caused by either a respiratory or a cardiovascular disease will lead to compromised gas exchange at the cellular level.

Physiology of the Respiratory System

The primary function of the respiratory system is gas exchange. Oxygen from inspired air diffuses from alveoli in the lungs into blood in the pulmonary capillaries. Carbon dioxide, a waste product produced during cell metabolism, diffuses from blood into the alveoli and is exhaled. Exchange of oxygen and carbon dioxide occurs at the alveolar–capillary membrane. The organs of the respiratory system facilitate this gas exchange and protect the body from foreign matter, such as particulates and pathogens.

Structure of the Respiratory System

The respiratory system is divided structurally into the *upper* and *lower respiratory tract*. The mouth, nose, and pharynx compose the upper airway. The larynx connects the upper and the lower airways. The lower airway includes the trachea and lungs, with the right and left mainstream bronchi, bronchioles, alveoli, pulmonary capillary network, and pleural membranes (Figure 43.1).

Air enters through the nose, where it is warmed, humidified, and filtered. Large particles in the air are trapped by the hairs at the entrance of the nares, and smaller particles are filtered and trapped as air changes direction on contact with the nasal turbinates and septum. The *sneeze reflex* is initiated by irritants in nasal passages, which stimulate the respiratory centre in the medulla by the trigeminal nerve (cranial nerve [CN] V). A large volume of air rapidly exits through the nose and mouth during a sneeze, helping clear nasal passages of foreign matter.

Inspired air passes from the nose through the pharynx, commonly known as the *throat*. The pharynx is a shared pathway for air and food. It includes both the nasopharynx and the oropharynx, which are richly supplied with lymphoid tissue that traps and destroys pathogens entering with the air.

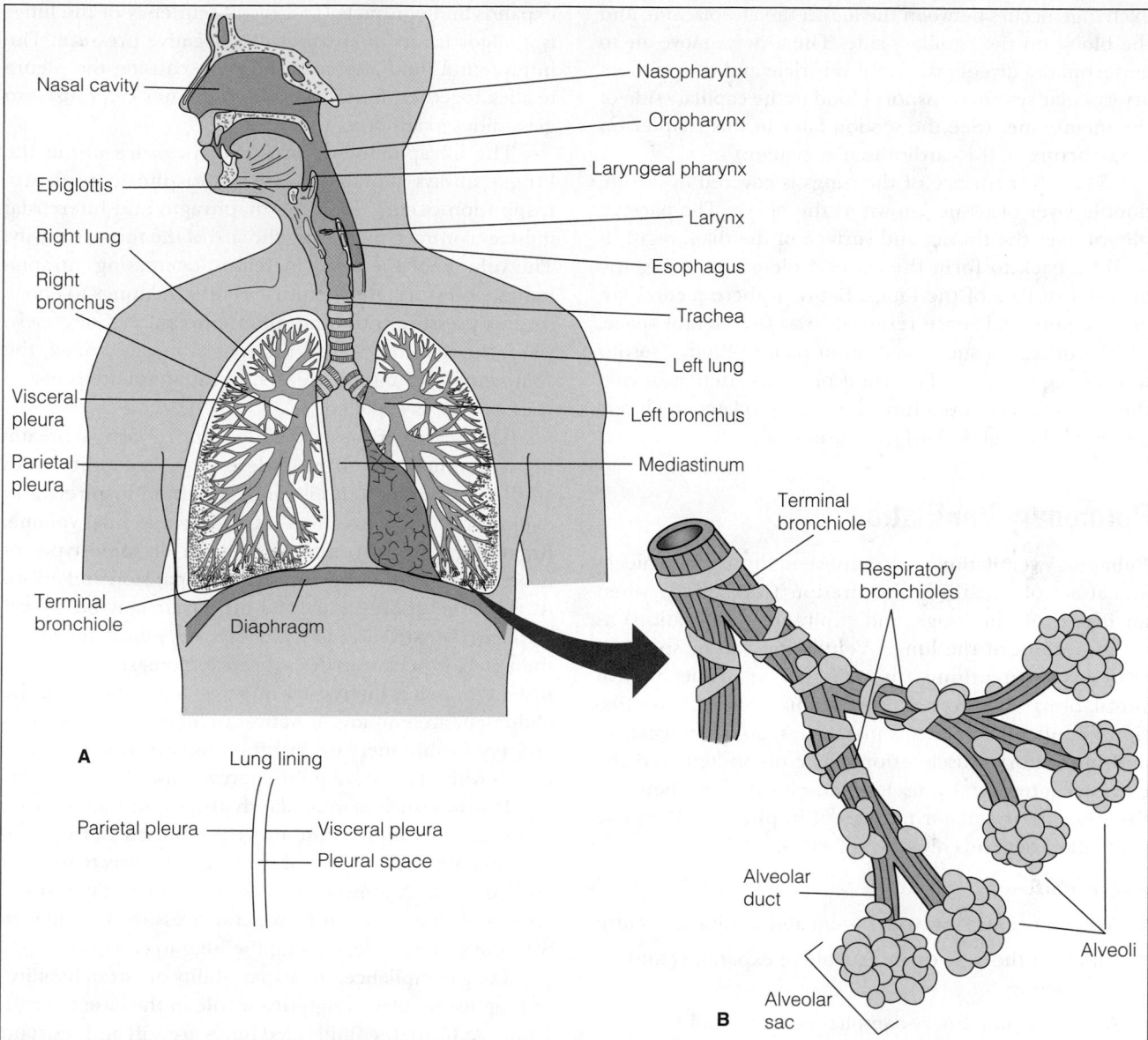

FIGURE 43.1 The lower respiratory tract—the larynx, trachea, bronchi, and lungs with an expanded view showing the structures of an alveolus and the pulmonary blood vessels.

The larynx is a cartilaginous structure that can be identified externally as the "Adam's apple." In addition to its role in providing for speech, the larynx is important for maintaining airway patency and protecting the lower airways from swallowed food and fluids. During swallowing, the inlet to the larynx (the epiglottis) closes, routing food to the esophagus. The epiglottis is open during breathing, allowing air to move freely into the lower airways.

Below the larynx, the trachea leads to the right and left main bronchi (primary bronchi) and the conducting airways of the lungs. Within the lungs, the primary bronchi divide repeatedly into smaller and smaller bronchi, ending with the terminal bronchioles. Together, these airways are known as the *bronchial tree.* The trachea and bronchi are lined with mucosal epithelium. These cells produce a thin layer of mucus, the *mucous blanket,* which

traps pathogens and microscopic particulate matter. These foreign particles are then swept upward toward the larynx, throat, and nasopharynx by cilia (tiny hair-like projections on the epithelial cells), where they are either swallowed or expectorated. The *cough reflex* is triggered by irritants in the larynx, trachea, or bronchi and ensures that mucus and any foreign particles are dislodged from the lower respiratory tract and propelled up and out.

Until air passes through the terminal bronchioles and enters the respiratory bronchioles and alveoli, no gas exchange occurs. The respiratory zone of the lungs includes the respiratory bronchioles (which have scattered air sacs in their walls), the alveolar ducts, and the alveoli (see Figure 43.1). Alveoli have very thin walls composed of a single layer of epithelial cells covered by a thick mesh of pulmonary capillaries. The alveolar and capillary walls form the alveolar–capillary membrane, where gas exchange occurs between the air on the alveolar side and the blood on the capillary side. The airways move air to and from the alveoli; the right ventricle and the pulmonary vascular system transport blood to the capillary side of the membrane. (See the section later in this chapter on the structure of the cardiovascular system.)

The outer surface of the lungs is covered by a thin, double layer of tissue known as the *pleura*. The parietal pleura lines the thorax and surface of the diaphragm. It doubles back to form the visceral pleura, covering the external surface of the lungs. Between these pleural layers is a potential space referred to as the **pleural space**, which contains a small amount of pleural fluid, a serous lubricating solution. This fluid prevents friction during the movements of breathing and serves to keep the layers adherent through its surface tension.

Pulmonary Ventilation

Pulmonary ventilation is accomplished through the mechanical act of breathing: inspiration (inhalation) when air flows into the lungs, and expiration (exhalation) as air moves out of the lungs. Ventilation can be spontaneous (as in breathing) or artificial (as in mechanical ventilation). The forces that are involved with ventilation include elastic recoil properties, airway resistance, and inspiratory muscle efforts. The diaphragm and the external intercostal muscles (muscles that are between the ribs) are the major muscles of inspiration. Adequate ventilation depends on several factors:

- Clear airways
- An intact central nervous system and respiratory centre
- An intact thoracic cavity capable of expanding and contracting
- Adequate pulmonary compliance and recoil

As noted previously, a number of mechanisms, including ciliary action and the cough reflex, work to keep airways open and clear. In some cases, however, these defences can be overwhelmed. The inflammation, edema, and excess mucous production that occur with some types of pneumonia can clog small airways, impairing ventilation of the distal alveoli.

The respiratory centres of the medulla and pons in the brain stem control breathing. Severe head injury or drugs that depress the central nervous system (e.g., opioids, anesthetics, or barbiturates) can affect the respiratory centres, impairing the drive to breathe.

Expansion and recoil of the lungs occurs passively in response to changes in pressures within the thoracic cavity and the lungs themselves. The **intrapleural pressure** (pressure in the pleural cavity surrounding the lungs) is always slightly negative in relation to atmospheric pressure. This negative or subatmospheric pressure is essential because it creates suction that holds the visceral pleura and the parietal pleura together as the chest cage

expands and contracts. The recoil tendency of the lungs is a major factor in creating this negative pressure. The intrapleural fluid also contributes by causing the pleura to stick together, much like a film of water can cause two glass slides to adhere.

The **intrapulmonary pressure** (pressure within the lungs) always equalizes with atmospheric pressure. Inspiration occurs when the diaphragm and intercostal muscles contract, increasing the size of the thoracic cavity. The volume of the lungs increases, decreasing intrapulmonary pressure. Air then rushes into the lungs to equalize this pressure with atmospheric pressure. Conversely, when the diaphragm and intercostal muscles relax, the volume of the lungs decreases, intrapulmonary pressure rises, and air is expelled.

The degree of chest expansion during normal breathing is minimal, requiring little energy expenditure. In adults, approximately 500 mL of air is inspired and expired with each breath. This is known as **tidal volume**. Breathing during strenuous exercise or some types of heart disease requires greater chest expansion and effort. At this time, more than 1500 mL of air may be moved with each breath. *Accessory muscles of inspiration,* including the anterior neck muscles, sternocleidomastoid muscles, scalene muscles, intercostal muscles, and muscles of the abdomen, are employed. Active use of accessory muscles and noticeable increase in breathing effort are seen in clients with obstructive pulmonary disease.

Diseases, such as muscular dystrophy, or trauma, such as spinal cord injury, can affect the muscles of respiration, impairing the ability of the thoracic cavity to expand and contract. A gunshot wound or other trauma to the chest wall may allow intrapleural pressure to equalize with the atmosphere, causing the lung to collapse.

Lung compliance, the expansibility or "stretchability" of lung tissue, plays a significant role in the ease of ventilation. At birth, the fluid-filled lungs are stiff and resistant to expansion, similar to that of a new balloon that is difficult to inflate. With each subsequent breath, the alveoli become more compliant and easier to inflate, just as a balloon becomes easier to inflate after several tries. Lung compliance tends to decrease with aging, making it more difficult to expand the alveoli and increasing the risk of **atelectasis**, or collapse of a portion of the lung. The decreased compliance in older adults may be the result of chest wall rigidity from calcification of intercostal cartilage, decreased mobility of the ribs, or loss of elastic fibres in the lungs.

In contrast to lung compliance is **lung recoil** (elasticity), the continual tendency of the lungs to collapse away from the chest wall. Just as lung compliance is necessary for normal inspiration, lung recoil is necessary for normal expiration. Although elastic fibres in lung tissue contribute to lung recoil, the *surface tension* of fluid lining the alveoli has the greatest effect on recoil. Fluid molecules tend to draw together, reducing the size of the alveoli. **Surfactant**, a lipoprotein produced by specialized alveolar cells, acts like a detergent, reducing the surface tension of alveolar fluid. Without surfactant, lung expansion is exceedingly difficult and the lungs collapse. Premature infants whose lungs are not yet capable of producing adequate surfactant develop *respiratory distress syndrome (RDS)*; adults can develop *adult respiratory distress syndrome (ARDS)*, usually as a complication of serious illness or trauma.

Respiration

Respiration is the process of delivering O_2 to the cells for utilization and the removal of CO_2; it involves (a) alveolar gas exchange by diffusion in the lungs; (b) the transport of O_2 and CO_2 through the circulatory system; and (c) systemic diffusion of these gases between the capillaries and the tissues and cells.

ALVEOLAR GAS EXCHANGE This exchange involves the diffusion of O_2 from the alveoli into the pulmonary blood vessels. **Diffusion** is the movement of gases or other particles from an area of greater pressure or concentration to an area of lower pressure or concentration. Pressure differences in the gases on each side of the respiratory membrane obviously affect diffusion. When the pressure of O_2 is greater in the alveoli than in blood, O_2 diffuses into blood. The **partial pressure** (the pressure exerted by each individual gas in a mixture according to its concentration in the mixture) of O_2 (PO_2) in the alveoli is about 100 mm Hg, whereas the PO_2 in the venous blood of the pulmonary arteries is about 60 mm Hg. These pressures rapidly equalize, however, so that the arterial O_2 pressure also reaches about 100 mm Hg. By contrast, CO_2 in venous blood entering the pulmonary capillaries has a partial pressure of about 45 mm Hg (PCO_2), whereas that in the alveoli has a partial pressure of about 40 mm Hg. Therefore, CO_2 diffuses from blood into the alveoli where it can be eliminated with expired air. When referring to the pressure of gas in arterial blood, the abbreviation is PaO_2. When referring to partial pressure in venous blood, the abbreviation is PvO_2.

TRANSPORT OF OXYGEN AND CARBON DIOXIDE The transport of O_2 and CO_2 to and from the cells is complex and requires a *transport mechanism*—the circulatory system. Several factors affect the transport of oxygen from the lungs to the tissues, including cardiac output, the quantity and quality of **erythrocytes** (red blood cells [RBCs]), and exercise.

Normal *cardiac output* (the amount of blood pumped by the ventricles in 1 minute) is approximately 5 L per minute (see page 1356 for full discussion on cardiac output). Any pathological condition that decreases cardiac output (e.g., damage to the heart muscle, blood loss, or pooling of blood in the peripheral blood vessels) diminishes the amount of oxygenated blood delivered to tissues. The heart attempts to compensate for inadequate output by increasing its pumping rate (heart rate), but with severe damage or blood loss, this compensatory mechanism may not restore adequate blood flow and O_2 to the tissues.

Effective transportation of O_2 also requires an adequate quantity (e.g., number, proportion relative to plasma) and quality (e.g., shape, hemoglobin content) of erythrocytes. Normally, most of the O_2 (97%) combines loosely with hemoglobin in the erythrocytes and is carried to the tissues as **oxyhemoglobin** (the compound of O_2 and hemoglobin). The remaining oxygen is dissolved and transported in the fluid of the plasma and cells. The actual number of circulating erythrocytes is measured as cells per litre of blood: normal ranges are 4.5×10^{12}/L to 5.3×10^{12}/L in men and 4.1×10^{12}/L to 5.1×10^{12}/L in women. The proportion of erythrocytes to plasma is reflected in the **hematocrit**—a normal hematocrit is 0.37 to 0.49 in men and 0.36 to 0.46 in women. Increasing the RBCs (such as in polycythemia) or decreasing the plasma component (such as in dehydration) of blood will result in an increased hematocrit (blood will be more viscous) which results in more resistance and a slower blood flow, reducing the cardiac output and, therefore, reducing oxygen transport. While people may have an adequate number of RBCs, their quality is also important. The healthy shape of the RBC is a flexible biconcave disc enabling efficient gas exchange and passage through even the smallest of capillaries. The amount of **hemoglobin** (Hgb), a protein molecule in erythrocytes, reflects the O_2-carrying capacity of the RBC as O_2 binds to the heme on the hemoglobin molecule. Normal hemoglobin levels are 138 g/L to 180 g/L in men and 120 g/L to 160 g/L in women. Variations in the transport of gases can be affected by an alteration in either of the quantity and/or quality of the RBCs. For example, a client can have an adequate number of erythrocytes but have an abnormal shape, such as in sickle cell anemia, or have inadequate hemoglobin within the erythrocyte, such as in microcytic anemia. Clients can have normal "quality" of RBCs but lack sufficient numbers, such as in hemorrhage.

Exercise also has a direct influence on O_2 transport. In well-trained athletes, O_2 transport can be increased up to 20 times the normal rate, in part because of an increased cardiac output and in part because of increased use of O_2 by the cells (utilization coefficient).

CO_2, continually produced in the processes of cell metabolism, is transported from the cells to the lungs in three ways: (a) the majority (about 65%) is carried inside the RBCs as bicarbonate (HCO_3^-) and is an important component of the bicarbonate buffer system (see Chapter 44); (b) a moderate amount of CO_2 (30%) combines with hemoglobin as *carbaminohemoglobin* for transport; and (c) smaller amounts (5%) are transported in solution in the plasma and as *carbonic acid* (H_2CO_3) (the compound formed when CO_2 combines with water).

SYSTEMIC DIFFUSION Systemic diffusion involves diffusion of O_2 and CO_2 between the capillaries and the tissues and cells down to a concentration gradient similar to diffusion at the alveolar capillary level. As cells consume oxygen, the PO_2 in the tissues decreases, causing the O_2 at the arterial end of the capillary to diffuse into the cells. When the cells consume more O_2, such as during exercise or stress, the pressure gradient increases and diffusion is enhanced, allowing the cells to regulate their own flow of O_2. CO_2 from metabolic processes accumulates in the tissues and diffuses into the capillaries where the PCO_2 is lower. In reduced blood flow states, such as shock, capillary blood flow may decrease, interfering with tissue O_2 delivery.

Respiratory Regulation

Respiratory regulation includes both neural and chemical controls to maintain the correct concentrations of O_2, CO_2, and hydrogen ions in body fluids. The nervous system adjusts the rate of alveolar ventilations to meet the needs of the body so that PO_2 and PCO_2 remain relatively constant. The body's respiratory centre consists of two groups of neurons located in the medulla oblongata and pons of the brain (dorsal respiratory group, pneumotaxic centre of upper and lower pons).

A chemosensitive centre in the medulla oblongata is highly responsive to increases in blood CO_2 and hydrogen ion concentration. By influencing other respiratory centres, this centre can increase the activity of the inspiratory centre and the rate and depth of respirations. In addition to this direct chemical stimulation of the respiratory centre in the brain, special neural receptors sensitive to decreases in O_2 concentration are located outside the central nervous system in the carotid bodies (just above the bifurcation of the common carotid arteries) and aortic bodies. Decreases in arterial O_2 concentrations stimulate these *chemoreceptors*, and they, in turn, stimulate the respiratory centre to increase ventilation. Of the three blood gases (hydrogen, O_2, and CO_2) that can trigger chemoreceptors, increased CO_2 concentration is the strongest stimulator of respiration.

However, in clients with certain lung ailments, such as emphysema, O_2 concentrations, *not carbon dioxide concentrations*, play a major role in regulating respiration. For such clients, decreased O_2 concentrations are the main stimuli for respiration. This is sometimes called the *hypoxic drive*. Increasing the concentration of O_2 can depress the respiratory rate, and, therefore, it is important that only low concentrations of supplemental O_2 be administered to these clients.

Physiology of the Cardiovascular System

The cardiovascular system consists of the heart and blood vessels. Together with blood, the cardiovascular system is the main transport system of the body, delivering O_2 and nutrients to cells and organs as well as facilitating gas exchange. The heart serves as the system pump, moving blood through the vessels to the cells and tissues and then back to the heart.

The Heart

The heart (Figure 43.2) is a hollow, cone-shaped organ about the size of a fist. It is located in the mediastinum, between the lungs and behind the sternum. It is surrounded by a double-layered fibroserous membrane known as the **pericardium**. The outer parietal layer of the pericardium protects the heart and anchors it to surrounding structures. The inner visceral pericardium adheres to the heart's outermost layer, the **epicardium**. A thin layer of serous fluid separates the parietal pericardium from the visceral pericardium and allows the heart to beat in the chest without any friction between the two layers of membrane. The heart wall contains two additional layers: the **myocardium**, cardiac muscle cells that form the bulk of the heart and contract with each beat, and the **endocardium** lining the inside of the heart's chambers and great vessels.

The heart consists of four chambers—two upper **atria** and two lower **ventricles**, which are separated longitudinally by the *interventricular septum*. The atria and ventricles are separated from each other by the *atrioventricular valves*, the *tricuspid valve* on the right and the *bicuspid* or *mitral valve* on the left. The ventricles, in turn, are separated from the great vessels (the pulmonary arteries and aorta) by the *semilunar valves*: the *pulmonic valve* on the right and the *aortic valve* on the left. The valves serve to direct the flow of blood, allowing it to move from the atria to the ventricles and from the ventricles to the great vessels, but preventing backflow.

Deoxygenated blood from the venous system enters the right atrium of the heart via the superior and inferior venae cavae. Blood then flows into the right ventricle, which pumps this blood through the pulmonary artery into the lungs for gas exchange. Freshly oxygenated blood returns to the left atrium via the pulmonary veins. From the left atrium, blood enters the left ventricle to be pumped out to the systemic circulation through the aorta.

Cardiac Cycle

With each heartbeat, the myocardium goes through a cycle of systole and diastole. In **systole**, the heart contracts and ejects blood into the pulmonary and systemic circulation. In **diastole**, the ventricles relax and fill with blood. The diastolic phase of the cardiac cycle is twice as long as the systolic phase. This is important because diastole (or ventricular filling) is largely a passive process. The longer diastolic phase allows this filling to occur; at the end of the diastolic phase, the atria contract, adding additional volume to the ventricles. This volume is sometimes called the *atrial kick*.

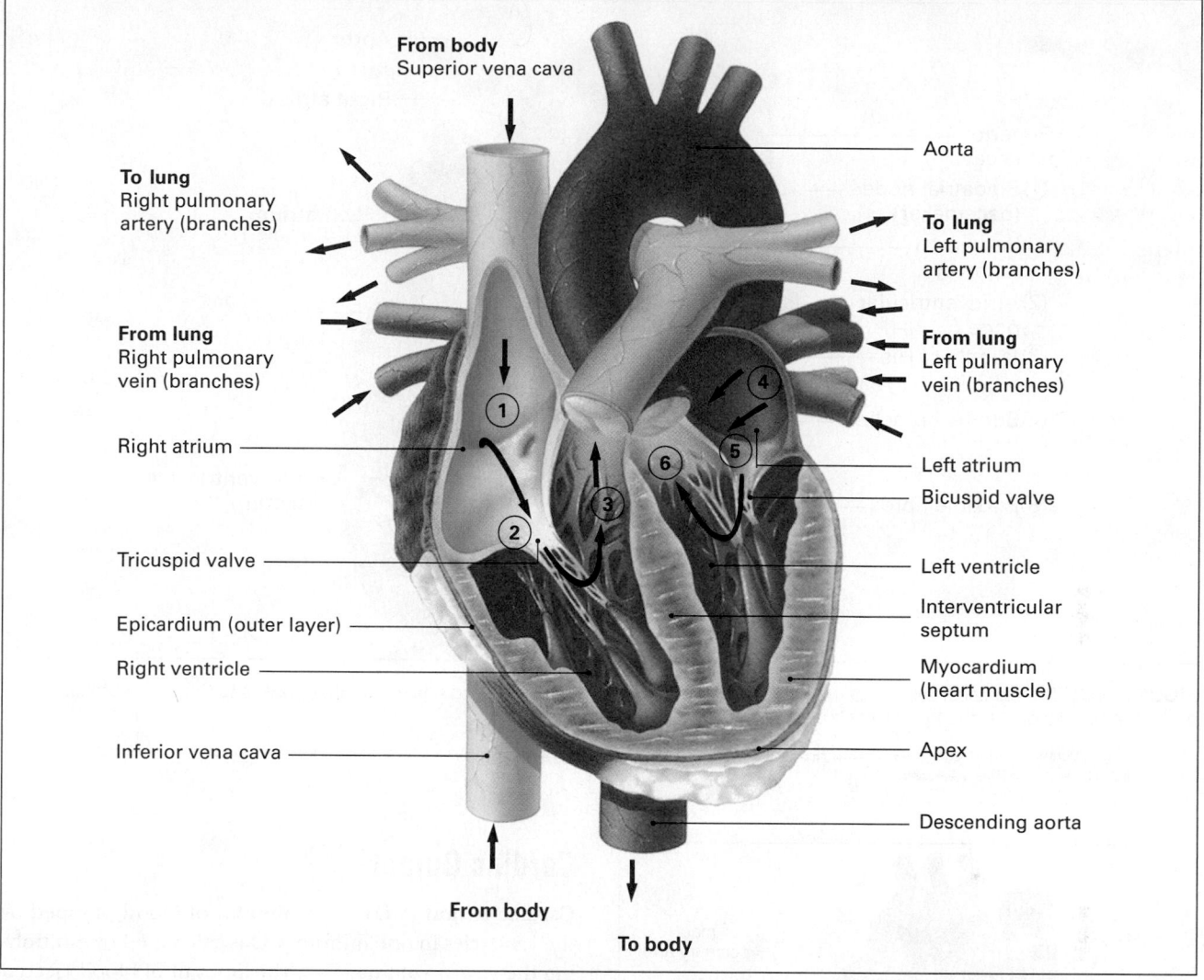

From body
Superior vena cava

To lung
Right pulmonary
artery (branches)

From lung
Right pulmonary
vein (branches)

Right atrium

Tricuspid valve

Epicardium (outer layer)

Right ventricle

Inferior vena cava

Aorta

To lung
Left pulmonary
artery (branches)

From lung
Left pulmonary
vein (branches)

Left atrium

Bicuspid valve

Left ventricle

Interventricular
septum

Myocardium
(heart muscle)

Apex

Descending aorta

From body

To body

FIGURE 43.2 The heart: The diagram shows blood flow through the heart from the vena cava, right atrium (1), tricuspid valve (2), right ventricle (3), pulmonic valve, pulmonary arteries, pulmonary veins, left atrium (4), mitral valve (5), left ventricle (6), aortic valve, and the aorta.

Source: Fremgan, Bonnie F.; Frucht, Suzanne S., *Medical Terminology: A Living Language*, 3rd Ed., © 2005. Reprinted and Electronically reproduced with permission of Pearson Education Inc., Upper Saddle River, New Jersey.

Cardiac Conduction System

Cardiac muscle contraction is a mechanical event that occurs in response to electrical stimulation. Cardiac muscle is unique in that, unlike skeletal muscle, it can generate electrical impulses and contractions independently of the nervous system. A network of specialized cells and pathways known as the *cardiac conduction system* normally controls the electrical activity and contraction of the heart.

The primary pacemaker of the heart is the **sinoatrial (SA or sinus) node**, located at the junction of the right atrium and superior vena cava. The SA node normally initiates electrical impulses that are conducted throughout the atria and result in atrial contraction. In adults, it usually fires at a regular rate of 60 to 100 times per minute, the "normal" heart rate. The impulse then spreads throughout the atria via the *interatrial pathways*. These conduction pathways converge and narrow through the **atrioventricular (AV) node**, slightly

delaying transmission of the impulse to the ventricles. This delay allows the atria to contract slightly before ventricular contraction occurs. From the AV node, the impulse then spreads through the ventricular conduction pathways: the *bundle of His,* the right and left *bundle branches,* and the *Purkinje fibres.* These fibres terminate in ventricular muscle, stimulating contraction (Figure 43.3 on the next page).

CORONARY CIRCULATION The heart muscle moves blood to the lungs and peripheral tissues but receives no O_2 or nourishment from blood within its chambers. Instead, blood is supplied to the heart by its own vascular system known as the *coronary circulation.* The **coronary arteries** originate at the base of the aorta, branching out to encircle and penetrate the myocardium. The two main coronary arteries are (a) the right coronary artery and (b) the left main coronary artery. Each further divides into branches (Figure 43.4 on the next page). The

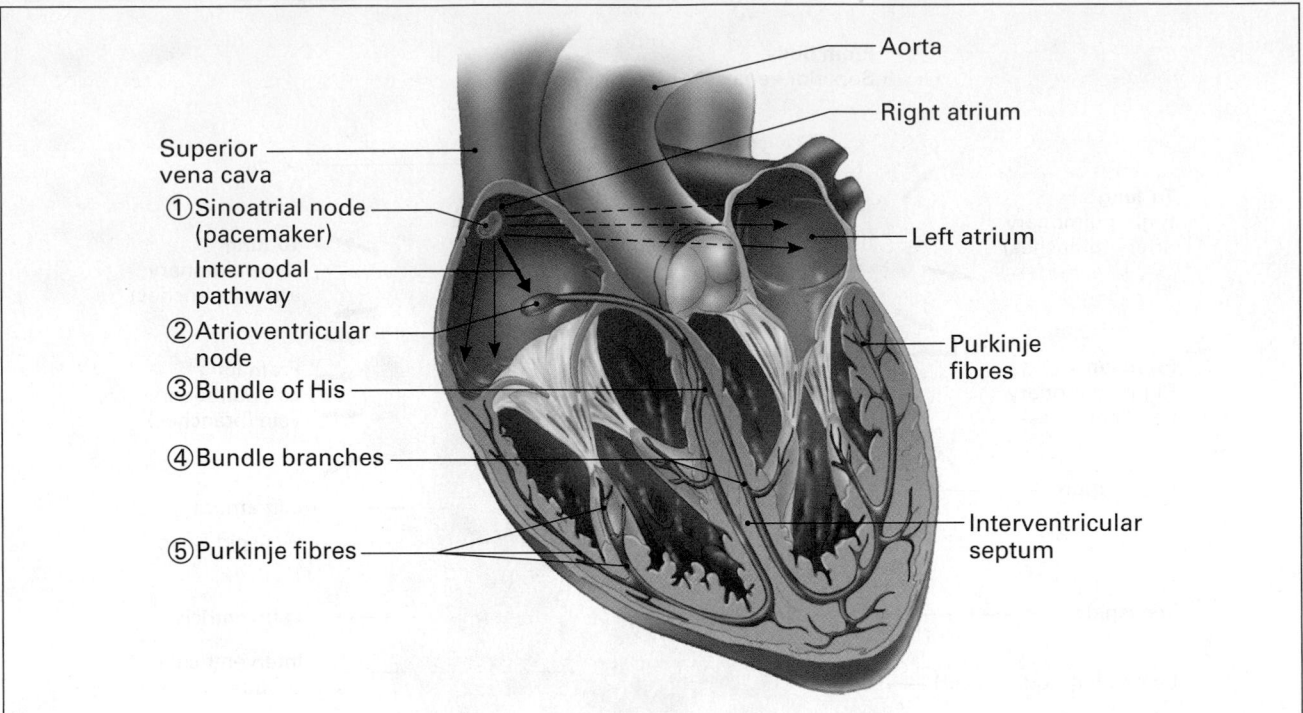

FIGURE 43.3 The electrical system of the heart. The impulse is initiated by the sinoatrial node, then travels to the atrioventricular node, the bundle of His, the bundle branches, and finally to the Purkinje fibres.

Source: Fremgan, Bonnie F.; Frucht, Suzanne S., *Medical Terminology: A Living Language*, 3rd Ed., © 2005. Reprinted and Electronically reproduced with permission of Pearson Education Inc., Upper Saddle River, New Jersey.

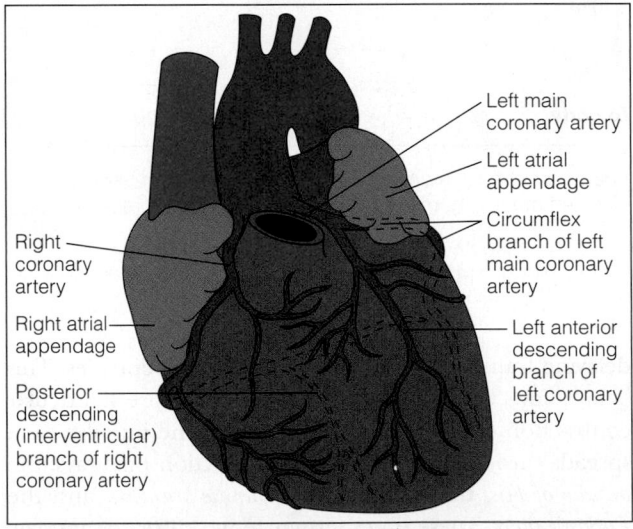

FIGURE 43.4 The coronary arteries supply the heart muscle with oxygenated blood.

coronary arteries fill during diastole, bringing oxygen-rich blood to the myocardium. If these arteries become clogged with atherosclerotic plaque or are obstructed by a blood clot, the myocardium area that is being supplied is deprived of O_2, and the client may develop angina (chest pain) or experience a myocardial infarction (MI, heart attack). The *cardiac veins* drain the deoxygenated blood from the myocardium into the *coronary sinus,* which empties into the right atrium.

Cardiac Output

Cardiac output (CO) is the amount of blood pumped by the ventricles in one minute. CO is calculated by multiplying the **stroke volume (SV)** (the amount of blood ejected with each contraction) by the heart rate ($CO = SV \times HR$). The stroke volume is determined by the preload, cardiac contractility, and afterload. In adults, the average SV is about 70 mL per beat. The CO is an important indicator of how well the heart is functioning as a pump. If the cardiac output is poor, tissue perfusion is decreased, and as a result, less O_2 and fewer nutrients reach the cells.

Cardiac output is affected by several factors:

- *Heart rate* is determined by the SA node and is influenced by the autonomic nervous system, blood pressure, hormones, some medications, and physical activity. Tachycardia (heart rate [HR] above 100 in adults) increases CO even if the SV does not change. However, heart rates that are very high (e.g., more than 150 beats/min) may not allow adequate time for the ventricles to fill, causing cardiac output to drop. CO decreases when the heart rate falls, if the stroke volume remains constant.

- **Preload** reflects the amount of stretching of the cardiac myocytes prior to contraction—given that this "stretch" cannot be measured clinically, other indices of preload are used such as ventricular end-diastolic volume or pressure (Klabunde, 2011). Preload largely depends on the amount of blood returning to the heart from the venous circulation. Increased ventricular end-diastolic volume causes increased stretch, leading to a more forceful contraction of cardiac muscle fibres. For example, exercise increases venous return and the amount of blood in the ventricle before contraction; therefore, the heart contracts more forcefully, and SV and CO increase during exercise. During hemorrhage, there is reduced venous return, which results in a decrease in preload, leading to weaker contraction of cardiac muscle fibres.

- **Contractility** is the inherent ability of cardiac muscle fibres to contract. Stroke volume decreases if contractility is poor, reducing CO. Contractility also is affected by the autonomic nervous system and certain drugs. Positive inotropic drugs (e.g., digoxin, catecholamines [epinephrine, dopamine]) increase contractility, and negative inotropic drugs (e.g., calcium channel blockers, beta-blockers) decrease the contractile strength.

- **Afterload** is the resistance against which the heart must pump to eject blood into the circulation. To move blood into the circulatory system, the ventricles must generate sufficient pressure to overcome the *systemic vascular resistance* or the pressure within the arteries. Systemic vasoconstriction and aortic valve stenosis (narrowing) lead to an increased afterload, which also increases cardiac workload. In contrast, vasodilation, such as with angiotensin-converting enzyme (ACE) inhibitor therapy, reduces afterload and the workload of the heart.

Blood Vessels

With each cardiac contraction, blood is ejected into a closed system of blood vessels that transports blood to the tissues and returns it to the heart. The heart supports two circulatory systems: (a) the low-pressure pulmonary system, and (b) the higher-pressure systemic circulatory system.

Deoxygenated blood from the right ventricle enters the pulmonary vascular system through the pulmonary arteries. The pulmonary arteries subdivide into lobar arteries. These lobar arteries follow the main bronchi into the lungs and then branch out to form arterioles and the dense capillary networks that encompass the alveoli. O_2 diffuses into blood from the alveoli, and CO_2 diffuses into the alveoli from blood. Blood then returns to the left side of the heart via the venules and the *pulmonary veins*. Note that the pulmonary vascular system is the only part of the circulatory system in which *arteries* (which transport blood away from the heart) carry deoxygenated blood and *veins* (which transport blood toward the heart) contain oxygenated blood.

The muscular left ventricle of the heart pumps oxygenated blood into the *aorta*. The blood then moves into major arteries that branch from the aorta into successively smaller arteries, *arterioles,* and, finally, the thin-walled

capillary beds of organs and tissues. It is in the capillary beds that O_2 and nutrients are exchanged for metabolic waste products. The deoxygenated blood then returns to the heart through a series of *venules* and veins that become progressively larger until they empty into the right atrium via the superior and inferior venae cavae.

With the exception of capillaries, blood vessel walls have three distinct layers, or *tunics*. The innermost layer, the *tunica intima,* is smooth endothelium that facilitates blood flow. The *tunica media* is made up of elastic fibres and smooth muscle cells innervated by the autonomic nervous system. This allows vessels to constrict or dilate depending on the needs of the body. The tunica media is thicker and more muscular in arteries than in veins, a feature that helps maintain blood pressure and continuous circulation to the tissues. As individuals age, the tunica media wall lining becomes less elastic and thicker and begins to degenerate and calcify. The outermost layer of blood vessels is the *tunica adventitia,* a layer of connective tissue that supports, protects, and anchors the vessel to surrounding tissues. Capillaries contain only one thin layer of tunica intima, allowing gases and molecules to diffuse between blood and the tissues.

ARTERIAL CIRCULATION The arterial circulation moves blood pumped by the heart to the tissues by maintaining a constant flow to the capillary beds.

Blood flow—the volume of blood flowing through a given vessel, an organ, or the entire circulation over a specific time—is determined by *pressure differences* and *resistance*. Blood always moves from an area of higher pressure to an area of lower pressure. The greater the difference between pressures, the greater is the blood flow. The **blood pressure** is the force exerted on arterial walls by the blood flowing within the vessel (see Chapter 29). The *mean arterial pressure* (*MAP*) is the average pressure over one cardiac cycle. The MAP is thought to be a very good estimate of the perfusion seen by the organs. In many situations, the MAP is a better indicator of overall perfusion than the systolic pressure. A MAP of greater than 60 mm Hg indicates adequate perfusion. Most patient monitoring systems (noninvasive and invasive) automatically calculate the MAP. The formula for calculating the MAP reflects (at normal heart rates) the extended time the heart is in diastole during the cardiac cycle. The formula: MAP = [(systolic pressure) + (diastolic pressure × 2)]/3 *or* CO (cardiac output) × PVR (peripheral vascular resistance) = MAP. Resistance is the opposition to blood flow. An inverse relationship exists between the movement of blood through the vascular system and resistance (e.g., as blood flow decreases, resistance increases). **Systemic vascular resistance (SVR)** impedes or opposes blood flow to the tissues and is determined by the viscosity, or thickness, of the blood, blood vessel length, and blood vessel diameter.

VENOUS RETURN In contrast to the high-pressure arterial system, venous pressure is too low to adequately return blood from peripheral tissues to the heart without assistance. The fall in intrathoracic pressure that occurs with inspiration and expiration draws blood upward toward the heart, is an adaptation known as the *respiratory pump*. Skeletal muscle activity contributes to the *muscular pump*, as muscle contractions push blood toward the heart. Venous valves are vital in making these pumps work by counteracting the force of gravity; once blood passes a valve, it cannot flow backward away from the heart. Figure 43.5 depicts the relationship between arteries and veins and the entire circulatory system.

Blood

Blood is transported within the cardiovascular system, bringing oxygen and nutrients from the lungs and gastrointestinal system to the body's cells. Blood is a complex

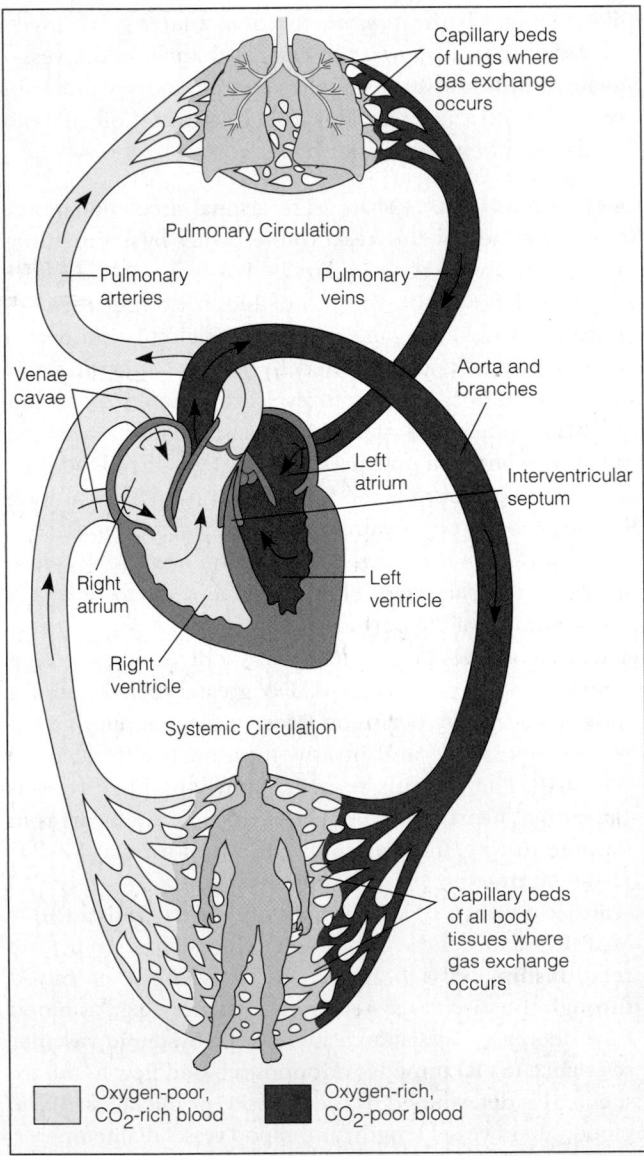

FIGURE 43.5 The heart and blood vessels: The left side of the heart pumps oxygenated blood into the arteries. Deoxygenated blood returns via the venous system into the right side of the heart.

mixture of living formed elements (blood cells) and proteins suspended in plasma (fluid). Its primary functions are as follows:

- Supplies oxygen, nutrients, and hormones needed for cell metabolism to the cells, and transports metabolic wastes away from the tissues for elimination
- Regulates acid–base balance, body temperature, pH, and fluid volume
- Prevents infection and blood loss

Most oxygen is transported bound to hemoglobin. Hemoglobin is a major component of erythrocytes, whose predominant responsibility is tissue oxygenation. Hemoglobin binds easily with oxygen, releasing it in the body tissues. When all four heme groups of the hemoglobin molecule are bound to oxygen, it is said to be *fully saturated*. Oxygen binding is affected by several factors, including the PO_2, temperature, pH, and PCO_2. Up to a certain point (about 70 mm Hg), the higher the PO_2, the greater the affinity of hemoglobin for oxygen and the more saturated the hemoglobin molecules. The relationship to temperature, pH, and PCO_2 is the opposite: At higher temperatures, lower pH (greater hydrogen ion concentration), and higher PCO_2 levels, the affinity for oxygen decreases, and hemoglobin releases its oxygen molecules. *Anemia* (too few RBCs that contain too little or abnormal hemoglobin) interferes with oxygen delivery to the tissues, which often leads to fatigue and activity intolerance. See previous discussion in this chapter (p. 1353) related to the blood's role in transporting O_2 and CO_2.

Factors Affecting Respiratory and Cardiovascular Function

Factors that influence oxygenation affect the cardiovascular system as well as the respiratory system. These factors include age and development, environment, lifestyle, health status, pharmacological agents, stress and coping, and gender.

Lifespan Considerations

At birth, profound changes occur in the respiratory and cardiovascular systems. The fluid-filled lungs drain, the PCO_2 rises, and the neonate takes the first breath. The lungs gradually expand with each subsequent breath, reaching full inflation by 2 weeks of age. As the lungs expand, pressures in the pulmonary vascular system fall, changing pressure relationships within the heart. The *foramen ovale* between the atria closes as pressures on the right side of the heart fall and pressures on the left side increase. Arterial PaO_2 rises and arterial $PaCO_2$ falls, prompting closure of the *ductus arteriosus* between the pulmonary artery and aorta.

Respiratory and pulse rates are highest and most variable in newborns. The respiratory rate of a neonate is 40 to 80 breaths per minute; in infancy, it averages about 30 per minute. The rate gradually decreases, averaging around 25 per minute in the preschooler and reaching the adult rate of 12 to 18 per minute by late adolescence. Because of their rib cage structure, infants rely almost exclusively on diaphragmatic movement for breathing. An infant's breathing pattern is primarily abdominal breathing, with the abdomen rising and falling with each breath.

The resting heart rate for a neonate ranges from 80 to 200 beats per minute, decreasing to 80 to 150 in infancy and early childhood, and reaching the adult rate of 60 to 100 by about age 10 years. Irregular heart rates are common in infants and young children, often increasing and decreasing with each breath. This pattern of irregularity is known as *sinus arrhythmia,* a normal variation of the heart rate.

As the conversion from fetal circulation takes place and pressures in the left side of the heart rise, the arterial blood pressure increases. Immediately after birth (1 to 3 days of age) the blood pressure averages about 65/40 mm Hg. By 1 month, the arterial pressure is about 90/55 mm Hg. It rises gradually to the adult norm of 120/80 mm Hg.

Congenital heart defects may affect infants and children; however, acquired heart diseases are rare in childhood. *Rheumatic fever* is a group A beta-hemolytic streptococcal infection (e.g., strep throat) that can go on to damage the heart valves. For most people, the heart continues to function effectively well into older adulthood unless the blood supply to the heart muscle is impaired by blood vessel disease.

During infancy and childhood, upper respiratory infections are common and, fortunately, usually not serious. Infants and preschoolers also are at risk for airway obstruction by foreign objects, such as coins, peanuts, and small toys. *Cystic fibrosis* is a congenital disorder that affects the lungs, causing them to become congested with thick, tenacious (sticky) mucus. *Asthma* is another chronic disease often identified in childhood. The airways of the asthmatic child respond to such stimuli as allergens, exercise, or cold air by constricting, becoming edematous and producing excessive mucus. Airflow is impaired, and the child may wheeze as air moves through narrowed air passages.

As individuals age, the chest wall becomes more rigid and the lungs less elastic. More air is retained in the lungs at the end of each breath, and the **vital capacity**, or maximum amount of air that can be exchanged with each breath, decreases. The client with severe elasticity problems may have a *barrel chest,* with an anteroposterior (AP) diameter approximately equal to the lateral diameter (normally, the AP diameter is about half the lateral diameter in adults). The older client is at increased risk

for acute respiratory diseases, such as pneumonia, and chronic diseases, such as emphysema and chronic bronchitis. *Chronic obstructive pulmonary disease (COPD)* is seen more frequently in older adults, particularly after years of exposure to cigarette smoke or industrial pollutants.

During middle adulthood, the incidence of *hypertension,* or an elevated blood pressure, increases significantly. Hypertension, also known as "the silent killer" because of its lack of symptoms, is a major risk factor for cardiovascular disease. (See Chapter 29 for more discussion on hypertension.) *Cardiovascular disease (CVD)* is the second leading cause of death in Canada (Statistics Canada, 2008, modified 2011). *Atherosclerosis,* the buildup of fatty plaque within the arteries, is the major contributor. With aging, blood pressure continues to rise as arteriosclerosis affects the blood vessels, narrowing their lumen and decreasing their ability to dilate.

Environment

Altitude, heat, cold, and air pollution affect oxygenation. The higher the *altitude,* the lower is the PO_2 an individual breathes. As a result, the person at high altitudes has increased respiratory and cardiac rates and increased respiratory depth, which usually become most apparent when the individual exercises.

The peripheral blood vessels dilate in response to *heat,* consequently, blood flows to skin, increasing the amount of heat lost from the body surface. With vasodilation, the lumens of the blood vessels enlarge, thus decreasing the resistance to blood flow. In response, the heart rate and CO increase to maintain blood pressure. The increased cardiac output requires additional oxygen, which causes increased rate and depth of breathing. In contrast, in a *cold* environment, the peripheral blood vessels constrict, raising the blood pressure, which, in turn, decreases cardiac action, thereby reducing the need for O_2.

Healthy people exposed to *air pollution,* such as smog, may experience stinging of the eyes, headache, dizziness, coughing, and choking. Second-hand smoke or environmental tobacco smoke contains more than 40 chemical compounds known to cause cancer. People who have existing lung conditions or disease and altered respiratory function experience varying degrees of respiratory difficulty in a polluted environment. Some individuals are unable to maintain the activities of daily living in such an environment and require health care assistance.

Lifestyle

Physical exercise or activity increases the rate and depth of respirations and the heart rate and hence the supply of oxygen in the body. With regular vigorous exercise, the heart muscle becomes more powerful and efficient.

Aerobic exercise reduces the risk of cardiovascular disease by slowing the atherosclerotic process. People who lead sedentary lives, by contrast, have a higher risk of cardiovascular disease. They also lack the alveolar expansion and deep breathing patterns of people who participate in regular activity, and they are less able to respond effectively to respiratory stressors. Chapter 39 provides a detailed discussion of the role of activity and exercise in contributing to cardiac and respiratory health.

Diet and other lifestyle factors also affect both cardiac and respiratory functions. A healthy diet with adequate calories, protein, and other nutrients is important to maintaining good immune function and increasing resistance to disease. Along with certain vitamins and minerals, dietary protein is important in preventing anemia. Similarly, a strong link exists between elevated serum lipid levels and the development of coronary heart disease. Lipoproteins circulate in the blood and are made up of cholesterol, triglycerides, and phospholipids. A high dietary intake of saturated fats is the most critical factor for the development of elevated serum lipids. In Canada, more than 40% of men and women have elevated total plasma cholesterol levels. The Heart and Stroke Foundation of Canada (2011a) recommends that no more than 20% to 35% of total calories (about 45 g/day to 75 g/day for a woman; about 60 g/day to 105 g/day for a man) come from fats. See Chapter 40 for a detailed discussion on fats.

High sodium intake (greater than 2300 mg/day) can affect blood pressure and contribute to the development of hypertension (Canadian Hypertension Education Program, 2012). The Heart and Stroke Foundation of Canada and the members of a national sodium working group have issued guidelines that recommend reducing the daily sodium consumption of adult Canadians to 2300 mg (no more than 5 mL or 1 teaspoon of salt per day) to lower the rates of hypertension, the number one risk factor for stroke and a major risk factor for MI. Once this goal is achieved (by 2016, it is hoped), the next goal would be to lower the sodium intake to 1200 to 1500 mg by 2020. Presently, most Canadians consume on average 3100 mg/day of sodium, excluding the salt added at the dinner table and in cooking (cited in Joffres, Campbell, Manns, & Tu, 2007; Heart and Stroke Foundation of Canada, 2011a). High intake of sodium can contribute to hypertension in two ways. First, it can increase the release of natriuretic hormone, which indirectly contributes to hypertension. Additionally, sodium stimulates vasopressor mechanisms, which cause vasoconstriction. Evidence suggests that other factors, such as low potassium, calcium, and magnesium intake, can contribute to vasoconstriction and the development of hypertension. High consumption of dairy products and dietary calcium has been found to reduce blood pressure levels (Ruidavets et al., 2006). (Chapter 29 and Chapter 40 discuss hypertension and the role of sodium in more detail.)

Recent studies suggest that moderate *alcohol use*, in particular, red wine, may reduce the risk of heart disease; however, excessive alcohol intake negatively affects the body in several other ways (Saremi & Arora, 2008). Alcohol is a respiratory depressant, slowing respirations. Alcohol abusers often are malnourished, thereby increasing their risk of anemia and infections. Excess alcohol intake also increases the risk of hypertension, liver disease, and coagulation problems. The current recommendations suggest that if you drink alcohol, you should limit yourself to one or two standard drinks per day, to a weekly maximum of 9 for women and 14 for men (Heart and Stroke Foundation, 2011a). Keep in mind that one drink equals:

- 341 mL/12 oz (1 bottle) of regular strength beer (5% alcohol)
- 143 mL/5 oz wine (12% alcohol)
- 43 mL/1 1/2 oz spirits (40% alcohol)

The cardiovascular and respiratory systems are affected by *cigarette smoking*. Nicotine causes an increase in heart rate, blood pressure, and systemic vascular resistance, which, in turn, increases the heart's workload. Smoking causes vasoconstriction of vessels, increased viscosity of the blood, and platelet adherence. Smoking can also potentiate further damage to the intimal wall lining of vessels, particularly if those vessels are already affected by athelerosclerosis, causing impairment of tissue oxygenation. Indeed, tobacco use is the leading preventable cause of premature death, disease, and disability, as it increases the risk of cardiovascular and respiratory diseases, including cancers. Smoking is also linked to adverse effects in pregnancy, gastrointestinal problems, and tooth and gum problems. It is responsible for about one-third of potential years of life lost due to cancer, about one-fourth of potential years of life lost due to cardiac diseases, and about one-half of potential years of life lost due to respiratory disease. With a Canadian national smoking rate of 19% (TobaccoFreeRNAO, 2011), the annual rate of death as a direct result of smoking is estimated to be more than 47 000 among Canadians age 35 years or older. See the Evidence-Informed Practice box on nursing interventions that promote smoking cessation.

Health Status

In the healthy person, the cardiovascular and respiratory systems can provide sufficient O_2 to meet the body's needs. Diseases of the cardiovascular system often affect the delivery of O_2 to the cells of the body, whereas diseases of the respiratory system can adversely affect the oxygenation of the blood.

Numerous respiratory and cardiovascular diseases affect oxygenation. One cardiovascular condition that affects oxygenation but is often overlooked is anemia (described in the section "Cardiovascular Alterations" later in this chapter). Obesity, dyslipidemia, and metabolic syndrome (Met-S) are major factors in the development of cardiac disease—these are discussed in Chapter 40.

EVIDENCE-INFORMED PRACTICE

Transforming Evidence into Reality: Nursing Interventions That Promote Smoking Cessation

The Registered Nurses' Association of Ontario (RNAO) has developed a series of best practice guidelines (BPGs) based on a broad review and rigorous analysis of evidence related to several nurse sensitive issues. The original series of BPGs, released in the early 2000s, have subsequently undergone further review and revision in light of new evidence. The RNAO has done a commendable job in addressing common nursing issues, succinctly summarizing recommendations, and translating the evidence-based recommendations in very *practical* ways (such as video clips, one-pagers for nurses, tools for patients). The RNAO has now gone one step further in bridging the gap between evidence and practice with its TobaccoFreeRNAO initiative, emphasizing the leadership role that nurses can take relative to smoking cessation. The following are a sample of some of the 11 summary practice recommendations for nurses: implement minimal tobacco use intervention using the "Ask, Advise, Assist, Arrange" protocol with all clients; introduce intensive smoking cessation intervention (more than 10 minutes duration) when their knowledge and time enables them to engage in more intensive counselling; recognize that tobacco users may relapse several times before achieving abstinence and need to re-engage clients in the smoking cessation process; be knowledgeable about community smoking cessation resources, for referral and follow-up; implement, wherever possible, intensive intervention with women during pregnancy and in the postpartum period; and encourage persons who smoke, as well as those who do not, to make their homes smoke-free and to protect children, families, and themselves from exposure to second-hand smoke. The RNAO provides web-based resources for nurses to help them integrate these BPGs, including acknowledging nurses who themselves smoke and the need for nurses to connect with each other as a "community" of practice.

NURSING IMPLICATIONS: Nurses play an important role in prompting clients to quite smoking. Having access to a full range of resources is important so that nurses can tailor the recommended smoke cessation strategies to the particular needs of their clients.

Source: Based on Registered Nurses' Association of Ontario (RNAO). (2011). *RNAO best practice guideline: Integrating smoking cessation into daily nursing practice, TobaccoFreeRNAO National Initiative.* Retrieved from http://tobaccofreernao.ca/en/resources/best-practices-guidelines/nurses-practice-recommendations

Pharmacological Agents

A variety of medications can decrease the rate and depth of respiration. The most common medications with this effect are the benzodiazepine sedative–hypnotics and antianxiety drugs, such as diazepam (Valium), lorazepam (Ativan), and midazolam (Versed); barbiturates, such as phenobarbital; and opioids, such as morphine. Other pharmacological agents that can affect respiratory and cardiac function include bronchodilators and beta-blockers. Bronchodilators, although given to improve oxygenation by dilating the bronchial tree, can also cause increased cardiac workload by increasing heart rate and blood pressure. Caution must be used when giving beta-blockers to individuals with a history of bronchospastic respiratory conditions because these medications can cause an increase in bronchoconstriction, thereby further compromising respiratory status. When administering bronchodilators, beta-blockers, and opioids, the nurse must monitor the client's respiratory status on an ongoing basis.

Stress and Coping

When stress and stressors are encountered, both psychological and physiological responses can affect oxygenation. Some people may hyperventilate in response to stress. When this occurs, PaO_2 rises, and $PaCO_2$ falls. The person may experience lightheadedness and numbness and tingling of the fingers, toes, and around the mouth as a result.

Physiologically, when an individual experiences stress, the sympathetic nervous system is stimulated and epinephrine and norepinephrine are released. Epinephrine causes the heart to contract more forcefully and the bronchioles to dilate, increasing blood flow and O_2 delivery to active muscles. Norepinephrine increases blood pressure by causing vasoconstriction. Although these responses are adaptive in the short term, when stress continues, they can be destructive, increasing the risk of cardiovascular disease by increasing heart rate and blood pressure. See Chapter 48 for further discussion of stress and coping.

Sex

Cardiovascular disease (heart disease and stroke) is a leading cause of death in Canadian women. Women tend to be safeguarded from heart disease prior to menopause because of the protective effect of estrogen. However, this is not always the case. For example, premenopausal women with diabetes have risk similar to that of men of the same age because diabetes cancels out the protective effect of estrogen. It is important for every woman to know about their risk factors and recognize the warning signs for heart disease and stroke so that they can prevent and manage them (Heart and Stroke Foundation of Canada, 2011b).

Alterations in Function

Respiratory Alterations

Respiratory function can be altered by conditions that affect the following:

- The movement of air into or out of the lungs

- The diffusion of O_2 and CO_2 between the alveoli and the pulmonary capillaries
- The transport of O_2 and CO_2 via blood to and from the tissue's cells

Conditions Affecting Movement of Air

Having a patent (open) airway is essential for ventilation. A completely or partially obstructed airway can occur anywhere along the upper or lower respiratory passageways. An upper airway obstruction—that is, in the nose, pharynx, or larynx—can be caused by a foreign object, such as food; by the tongue falling back into the oropharynx when a person is unconscious; or by secretions collecting in the passageways. *Obstructive sleep apnea* is repeated obstruction of the upper airway by the tongue or relaxed muscles of the pharynx for several seconds during sleep. Lower airway obstruction involves partial or complete occlusion of the passageways in the bronchi and lungs, most often caused by increased accumulation of mucus or inflammatory exudate.

Assessing for and maintaining a patent airway is a nursing responsibility, one that often requires immediate action. Partial obstruction of the upper airway passages is indicated by a low-pitched snoring sound during inhalation. Complete obstruction is indicated by extreme inspiratory effort that produces no chest movement. Such a client, in an effort to obtain air, may also exhibit marked sternal and intercostal retractions. Lower airway obstruction is not always as easy to observe. **Stridor**, a harsh, high-pitched sound, may be heard during inspiration. The client may have altered arterial blood gas levels, restlessness, anxiety, dyspnea, and **adventitious breath sounds** (abnormal breath sounds). See Table 28.8 (page 641) for details on adventitious breath sounds.

The movement of air is also affected by breathing patterns, which include the rate, volume, rhythm, and relative ease or effort of respiration. Normal respiration (**eupnea**) is quiet, rhythmic, and effortless. **Tachypnea** (rapid respiratory rate) is seen with fevers, metabolic acidosis, pain, and hypoxemia. **Bradypnea** is an abnormally slow respiratory rate, which may be seen in clients who have metabolic alkalosis (an increased intracranial pressure [e.g. from a brain injury]), who have been given anesthetic gases (a respiratory depressant), or who have taken drugs such as morphine or sedatives. **Apnea** is the cessation of breathing; *sleep apnea* is the cessation of breathing during sleep.

Hyperventilation, often called *alveolar hyperventilation*, is an increased movement of air into and out of the lungs. During hyperventilation, the rate and depth of respirations increase, and more CO_2 is eliminated than is produced. One particular type of hyperventilation that accompanies metabolic acidosis is **Kussmaul's respiration**, by which the body attempts to achieve a return to normal pH by blowing off the CO_2 through deep and rapid breathing. Hyperventilation can also occur in response to stress, as mentioned earlier.

Hypoventilation is inadequate alveolar ventilation and may be caused by either slow or shallow breathing or both, such as can happen with diseases of the respiratory muscles (e.g., amyotrophic lateral sclerosis) or certain medications (e.g., anesthetic agents). Hypoventilation can also occur as a result of collapse of the alveoli, leaving too few functioning alveoli to meet the body's ventilation needs, or it can result from airway obstruction. Hypoventilation may lead to **hypercapnia** (increased levels of CO_2) or hypoxemia (low levels of O_2 in the blood).

Other abnormal breathing patterns may create breathing irregularity. Irregular respiratory rhythms include the following:

- **Cheyne-Stokes respiration.** Marked rhythmic waxing and waning of respirations from very deep to very shallow breathing and temporary apnea. Common causes include heart failure, increased intracranial pressure, and drug overdose.
- **Biot's (cluster) respiration.** Shallow breaths interrupted by apnea; may be seen in clients with central nervous system disorders.

The sensation of difficult breathing or breathlessness is called **dyspnea**. Because this experience is the most common disabling symptom of chronic obstructive pulmonary disease (COPD), dyspnea is often considered the sixth vital sign in the assessment of people with COPD (RNAO, 2010). The dyspneic person often appears anxious and may describe his or her experience as being short of breath (SOB) or having a feeling of being unable to "get enough air." Often, the nostrils are flared because of the increased effort of inspiration. The skin and mucous membranes may appear dusky and the heart rate is usually increased. **Orthopnea** is the inability to breathe except in an upright or a standing position.

Conditions Affecting Diffusion

Impaired diffusion may affect levels of gases in the blood, particularly O_2, which does not diffuse as readily as CO_2. **Hypoxemia**, or reduced O_2 levels in the blood (e.g., O_2 saturation <90%, PO_2 <norms), may be caused by conditions that impair diffusion at the alveolar–capillary level, such as pulmonary edema or atelectasis (collapsed alveoli) or by low hemoglobin levels. The cardiovascular system compensates for hypoxemia by increasing heart rate and cardiac output, in an attempt to transport adequate O_2 to the tissues. If the cardiovascular system is unable to compensate or hypoxemia is severe, tissue **hypoxia** (insufficient O_2 anywhere in the body) results, potentially causing cellular injury or death. Although the terms *hypoxemia* and *hypoxia* are often used interchangeably, they are different concepts. The following examples may help. Despite no hypoxemia (i.e., the person has normal O_2 saturation and PO_2), he or she may experience tissue hypoxia, such as when a blocked coronary artery leads to hypoxia in the heart tissue and causes

Box 43.1 Oxygenation and Circulation **1363**

BOX 43.1

Hypoxemia	Hypoxia
Signs and symptoms related to systemic lack of oxygen and compensatory mechanisms as well as end-organ effects of reduced oxygen in the circulatory system:	Signs and symptoms related to local effects of inadequate oxygen in the tissue. Site-specific symptoms depend on the area not receiving oxygen:

- Tachycardia and tachypnea (sympathetic nervous system response to hypoxemia)
- Restlessness or lightheadedness; agitation, confusion (because of lack of oxygen circulating in arterial blood to the brain)
- Flaring of the nares and/or intercostal retractions or indrawing (trying to increase ventilation)
- Chest pain if the hypoxemia is severe enough to provide inadequate oxygen to the heart
- Generalized cyanosis

- Angina, if the coronary arteries are occluded
- Restlessness or lightheadedness, agitation, confusion if a cerebral artery is occluded
- Necrotic bowel, if the mesenteric artery is occluded
- Cool, pale arm; prolonged capillary refill time with an obstruction in the brachial artery
- Localized cyanosis (e.g., left leg cyanosis in the case of an occluded left femoral artery)

angina or when a clot embolizes from an artery in the neck and occludes a cerebral artery leading to hypoxia in the brain tissue and subsequent "brain attack." A patient who develops compartment syndrome in a limb following a severe trauma will have normal circulating levels of O_2 in the bloodstream (no hypoxemia) but can experience severe tissue hypoxia as a result of edema compressing arterial circulation to the limb. Hypoxia to vital organs, such as the heart or lungs, will ultimately lead to hypoxemia, as complications of hypoxia in these organs will directly affect their ability to meet the oxygenation needs within the circulatory system. Although a person can have hypoxia without hypoxemia, people with hypoxemia are at great risk for hypoxia. Box 43.1 summarizes signs and symptoms of hypoxemia and hypoxia.

Cyanosis a bluish discoloration of the skin, nail beds, and mucous membranes caused by reduced hemoglobin–oxygen saturation, may be present with hypoxemia or hypoxia. Cyanosis requires two conditions: (a) the blood must contain about 5 g or more of unoxygenated hemoglobin per 100 mL of blood and (b) the surface blood capillaries must be dilated. Factors that interfere with either of these conditions (e.g., severe anemia or the administration of epinephrine) will eliminate cyanosis as a sign, even if the client is experiencing hypoxia.

Adequate oxygenation is essential for cerebral functioning. The cerebral cortex can tolerate hypoxia for only 3 to 5 minutes before permanent damage occurs. The face of the acutely hypoxic person usually appears anxious, tired, and drawn. The person usually assumes a sitting position, often leaning forward slightly to permit greater expansion of the thoracic cavity.

With *chronic* hypoxemia, the client often appears fatigued and is lethargic. The client's fingers and toes may be clubbed as a result of long-term lack of oxygen in the arterial blood supply. With clubbing, the base of the nail becomes swollen and the ends of the fingers and toes increase in size. The angle between the nail and the base of the nail increases to more than 180 degrees (see Figure 28.10, page 612).

Conditions Affecting Transport

Once O_2 moves into the lungs and diffuses into the capillaries, the cardiovascular system transports the O_2 to all body tissues and transports CO_2 from the cells back to the lungs where it can be exhaled. Conditions that decrease cardiac output, such as heart failure or hypovolemia, affect tissue oxygenation and also the body's ability to compensate for hypoxemia.

Cardiovascular Alterations

Cardiovascular function can be altered by conditions that affect the following:

1. The function of the heart as a pump (cardiac output)
2. Blood flow to organs and to peripheral tissues (tissue perfusion)
3. The composition of the blood and its ability to transport O_2 and CO_2 (blood alterations)
4. Cardiac dysrhythmias

DECREASED CARDIAC OUTPUT Alterations in the structure of the heart can affect cardiac output. For example, congenital heart defects result in abnormal blood flow and may even allow venous and arterial blood to mix. The oxygen supply to the tissues is affected in this case. An illness, such as rheumatic fever, can damage the heart valves, affecting the flow of blood within the heart and to the great vessels. For example, if the mitral (bicuspid) valve becomes scarred and *stenotic* (constricted), it may not open fully, impairing filling of the left ventricle. Or if the mitral valve does not fully close (*mitral insufficiency*), blood may escape back or *regurgitate* into the left atrium instead of entering the aorta each time the ventricle contracts. Cardiac muscle damage, especially damage to the left ventricle, such as can occur with an MI, can lead to a reduction in cardiac output as the affected muscle no longer contracts.

HEART FAILURE Approximately 500 000 Canadians live with heart failure (Ross et al., 2006). **Heart failure** is a clinical syndrome in which the ventricle is unable to fill or eject blood. This abnormality of cardiac function results in the heart's inability to deliver adequate volumes of blood to tissues at rest or during normal activity.

Heart failure can occur as a result of MI, cardiomyopathy (disease of the myocardium—the heart muscle), uncontrolled hypertension, or extensive arteriosclerosis. In *congestive heart failure* (CHF), the vessels of the pulmonary system become congested or engorged with blood. This may cause fluid to escape into the alveoli and interfere with gas exchange, a condition known as *pulmonary edema.* Signs of heart failure include SOB, tachycardia, tachypnea, peripheral edema, and distended jugular veins. Other diseases, such as myocarditis (inflammation of the myocardium) and cardiomyopathy, also can affect the heart muscle, impairing its ability to contract and pump.

IMPAIRED TISSUE PERFUSION Within the arterial circulation, atherosclerosis is the most common cause of impaired blood flow to organs and tissues. Any artery in the body can be affected by atherosclerosis, although the effects are often related to coronary arteries, vessels supplying blood to the brain, and arteries in peripheral tissues.

The major modifiable risk factors for atherosclerosis include the following:

- Cigarette smoking
- High alcohol consumption
- High fat intake (dyslipidemia)
- Obesity
- Sedentary lifestyle
- Hypertension
- Stress
- Diabetes

Risk factors that cannot be modified include the following:

- Age
- Sex
- Race
- Family history

Some of these risk factors can be modified, treated, or controlled, and others cannot. The more risk factors a person has, the greater is the chance of developing atherosclerosis some time in that person's life (Perrin, 2009, p. 154).

The coronary arteries supply blood and oxygen to the myocardium. Because of plaque buildup and atherosclerosis, the myocardium can become deprived of blood and O_2. Thrombus formation and further plaque formation eventually narrow the coronary arteries, causing ischemia and death of myocardial tissue. **Ischemia** occurs if the demand for O_2 exceeds its supply. Demand for myocardial O_2 increases with exercise, stress, and sympathetic nervous system stimulation. A **myocardial infarction (MI)** occurs when the heart muscle is abruptly deprived of O_2. When the heart is deprived of O_2, it proceeds through several phases of tissue injury. The first phase is the area of ischemia. If treatment is not immediate, the tissue damage will continue on to injury and then on to necrosis (Perrin, 2009, p. 157).

The classic sign or symptom a patient experiences during the cardiac event is pain. It is important for the nurse to differentiate the pain of an MI or angina attack from a multitude of other pain syndromes that can mimic a coronary event. In the past, it was believed that women and men had different warning signs of heart attack. This may not be the case. Both women and men may experience typical or nontypical symptoms, such as nausea; sweating; pain in the arm, throat, and jaw; or pain that is unusual. However, the pain experienced and described by women may be different from that of men. Nevertheless, the most common symptom in women and men is still chest pain (Heart and Stroke Foundation of Canada, 2011b).

The immediate treatment goals for the patient with MI are to restore coronary artery blood flow, limit the infarction size, and balance myocardial O_2 supply and demand (Perrin, 2009, p. 163). Following an MI, most patients are started on standard pharmacological therapy that includes Aspirin, a cholesterol-lowering agent, an ACE inhibitor, a beta-blocker, an antiplatelet agent, and nitrates.

On the venous side of the circulatory system, incompetent valves may allow blood to pool in the veins, causing edema and decreasing venous return to the heart (Figure 43.6). Veins also can become inflamed, reducing blood flow and increasing the risk of thrombus (clot) formation. A thrombus can then break loose, becoming an embolus (note, plural of *thrombus* is *thrombi*; that of *embolus* is *emboli*). Emboli can travel as far as the pulmonary circulation, where they become trapped in pulmonary vessels, occluding blood supply to the capillary side of the alveolar–capillary membrane (*pulmonary embolism*). Although alveolar ventilation to the affected area often remains adequate if the clots are relatively small, no gas exchange occurs because of impaired blood flow. Signs

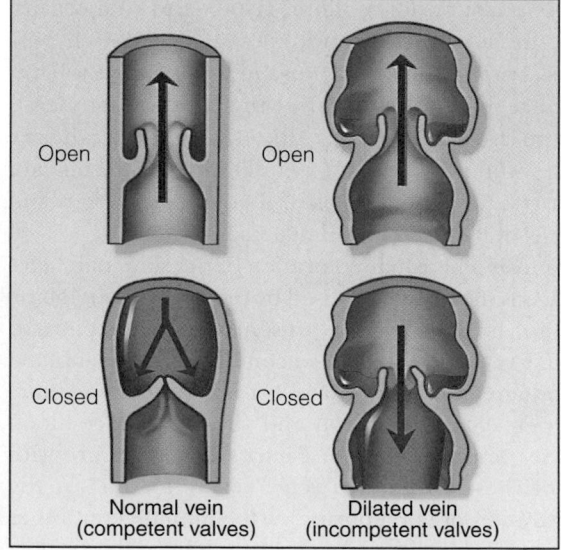

FIGURE 43.6 Vein with competent valve and vein with incompetent valve that allows blood to pool in the veins.

Source: Fremgan, Bonnie F.; Frucht, Suzanne S., *Medical Terminology: A Living Language*, 3rd Ed., © 2005. Reprinted and Electronically reproduced with permission of Pearson Education Inc., Upper Saddle River, New Jersey.

of acute pulmonary embolism (PE) include sudden onset of SOB and pleuritic pain (sharp pain in the chest that worsens with coughing and deep breathing).

BLOOD ALTERATIONS Because most O_2 is transported to tissues in combination with hemoglobin, the problems of inadequate red blood cells (RBCs), low hemoglobin levels, or abnormal hemoglobin structure can affect tissue oxygenation. Anemia has several different causes: RBCs are lost along with other components because of acute or chronic bleeding; if the diet is deficient in iron or folic acid, hemoglobin and RBCs are not formed adequately; lack of the hormone erythropoietin (such as in severe renal disease) leads to reduced production of RBCs; and some disorders cause RBCs to break down excessively. People with sickle-cell anemia produce an abnormal form of hemoglobin and can experience tissue ischemia during exacerbations of the disease. People experiencing moderate to severe anemia may experience chronic fatigue, pallor, SOB, and hypotension.

Blood volume also affects tissue oxygenation. If blood volume is inadequate, as in hemorrhage or severe dehydration, then blood pressure and CO fall, and tissues may become ischemic. Conversely, clients with *hypervolemia* (excess blood volume), which can result from fluid retention or kidney failure, may develop heart failure and peripheral edema, also leading to tissue ischemia.

Cardiac Dysrhythmias

Cardiac dysrhythmias may be life threatening, markedly altering CO and causing deterioration in vital signs, or they may be benign, or somewhere in between. Some pathological causes of cardiac dysrhythmias include degenerative diseases (coronary artery disease), ischemia (post-MI), fluid and electrolyte imbalances, and effects of certain medications. Examples of common dysrhythmias include the following:

- Sinus dysrhythmias (sinus tachycardia, sinus bradycardia, sinus arrhythmia, sinus arrest, sinus pause)
- Atrial dysrhythmias (atrial fibrillation, atrial flutter, premature atrial contractions [PACs], supraventricular tachycardia)
- Junctional dysrhythmias
- Atrial ventricular blocks
- Ventricular dysrhythmias (premature ventricular contractions [PVCs], ventricular tachycardia, ventricular fibrillation)

Although many of these dysrhythmias are generally not considered life threatening or lethal, careful and deliberate assessment of the patient must be a continuous process, as with all dysrhythmias.

Atrial fibrillation is the most commonly sustained dysrhythmia in older adults because the incidence of atrial fibrillation increases with age and heart disease. This dysrhythmia results in approximately 24% of cerebrovascular accidents in clients age 80 to 89 years (Fang, Chen, & Rich, 2007). These clients are frequently prescribed anticoagulants (e.g., warfarin) because of the high risk of these embolic events.

Assessing

Nursing assessment of oxygenation and circulation status includes a history, physical examination, and review of relevant diagnostic data.

NURSING HISTORY A comprehensive nursing history status should include data about current and past respiratory and cardiovascular problems; lifestyle; the presence of pain; medications for heart, blood pressure, circulation, or breathing; and the presence of risk factors for impaired oxygenation or circulatory status. Examples of interview questions to elicit this information are shown in the Assessment: Interview box.

PHYSICAL EXAMINATION In assessing a client's oxygenation status, the nurse uses all four physical examination techniques: (a) inspection, (b) palpation, (c) percussion, and (d) auscultation. The nurse first observes the rate, depth, rhythm, and quality of respirations, noting the position the client assumes for breathing. Some clients with chronic respiratory problems prefer to bend forward at the waist to ease breathing or to sit leaning over a table because these positions permit greater lung expansion. Lying on the back or on either side restricts expansion of part of the thorax (the underlying portion). This relatively small increase in expansion may be important to a dyspneic client. Variations in the shape of the thorax may indicate adaptation to chronic respiratory conditions. For example, clients with emphysema frequently develop a barrel chest (see Figure 28.26 on page 640).

To examine the cardiovascular system, the nurse evaluates the blood pressure in both arms (the results should be within 10 mm Hg of each other) and palpates peripheral pulses for their strength and equality. Auscultation is done to determine the apical pulse rate, rhythm, and the quality of heart sounds, and carotid arteries are auscultated for bruits (the abnormal sound blood makes as it rushes past an obstruction). Information about the cardiovascular system is obtained by assessing the skin for colour, temperature, hair distribution, lesions, and peripheral edema. Clients with extensive peripheral vascular disease may have cool feet with weak pulses and shiny, nearly hairless shins. Pitting edema of the feet and ankles may be noted in clients with heart failure. The **ankle-brachial index (ABI)** is a calculated number that indicates the amount of arterial blood flow to the extremity; it compares the ratio of the ankle systolic pressure with the higher of the two brachial systolic pressures (British Columbia Provincial Nursing Skin and Wound Committee, 2011) (see Box 43.2 on page 1367). Chapter 28 provides detailed information on assessing the respiratory and cardiac systems.

Oxygenation and Circulation

The following selected questions can help the nurse obtain information about a client's respiratory and cardiovascular systems:

CURRENT RESPIRATORY PROBLEMS

- Have you noticed any changes in your breathing pattern (e.g., shortness of breath, difficulty breathing, need to be in upright position to breathe, or rapid and shallow breathing)?
- If so, what activities might cause these symptoms to occur? What helps, if anything, to alleviate these symptoms?
- How many pillows do you use to sleep at night?

HISTORY OF RESPIRATORY DISEASE

- Have you had colds, allergies, asthma, tuberculosis, bronchitis, pneumonia, or emphysema?
- How frequently have these occurred? How long did they last? And how were they treated?

CURRENT OR PAST CARDIOVASCULAR PROBLEMS

- Do you have hypertension (high blood pressure)?
- Do you have any history of heart disease, such as angina, heart attack, or heart failure? Have you ever had a cardiac catheterization, angiography, or angioplasty?
- Have you ever been diagnosed with rheumatic fever, endocarditis, pericarditis, or other diseases of the heart? If so, when?
- Have you ever been told that you have peripheral vascular disease? Do you ever develop pain in the calves of your legs when walking? How far can you walk before it occurs? What do you do to relieve it?
- Do you have pain in your lower limbs when resting? Does changing your position make the symptoms better or worse? Do you have pain, redness, or swelling in your calves?
- Do your feet and ankles ever swell or feel very cold, numb, or tingling?
- Do you become extremely fatigued with activity? Have you ever been told that you are anemic?

LIFESTYLE

- Do you smoke? If so, how much? Do you want to stop? If you don't smoke, did you smoke previously, and when did you stop?
- Are you exposed to cigarette smoke or other pollutants (e.g., fumes, dust, coal, asbestos) in your environment?
- Do you use alcohol? If so, how many drinks (mixed drinks, glasses of wine, or beers) do you usually have per day or per week?

- Describe your exercise patterns. What exercise (types) do you participate in? How often do you exercise, and for how long?
- Describe your diet relative to sodium (salt) intake and fat content. Do you follow the *Canada Food Guide*?

PRESENCE OF COUGH

- How often and how much do you cough?
- Does the cough occur during certain activities or at certain times of the day?
- Is it *productive,* that is, accompanied by sputum, or *nonproductive,* that is, dry?
- If the cough is productive, what is the amount, colour, thickness, and odour? Is it ever tinged with blood?

PRESENCE OF CHEST PAIN

- Do you experience any pain with breathing or activity?
- If there is pain, describe the pain (e.g., where it is located, how it feels, what makes it worse or better, how long it lasts, how it affects your breathing, what precipitates the pain, what relieves the pain).
- Do you experience any other symptoms when the pain occurs (e.g., nausea, shortness of breath or difficulty breathing, lightheadedness, palpitations)?

PRESENCE OF RISK FACTORS

- Do you have a family history of lung cancer, asthma, other respiratory diseases, cardiovascular disease (including cerebrovascular accidents), or tuberculosis?

    The nurse should also note the client's height, weight, body mass index, activity pattern, and dietary assessment. In addition to smoking, risk factors include obesity, sedentary lifestyle, and a diet high in saturated fats.

MEDICATION HISTORY

- Have you taken or do you take any medications for heart disease, blood pressure, or breathing (e.g., bronchodilator, inhalant, opioid), including any over-the-counter medications (e.g., cough remedies)?
- If so, which ones? And what are the dosages, times taken, and results, including side effects?
- Do you use any herbal supplements? If so, which?

DIAGNOSTIC STUDIES   A range of diagnostic tests are available to assess respiratory and cardiac status, function, and level of oxygenation. Included are sputum samples, throat cultures, pulmonary function tests, venous and arterial blood specimens, cardiac monitoring, and visualization procedures.

Specimens   **Sputum** is the mucous secretion from the lungs, bronchi, and trachea. It is important to differentiate it from *saliva,* the clear liquid secreted by the salivary glands in the mouth, sometimes referred to as *spit.*

Healthy individuals do not produce sputum. Clients need to cough to *expectorate* (bring up) sputum from the lungs, bronchi, and trachea into the mouth in order to expectorate it into a collecting container. Sputum specimens are usually collected for one or more of the following reasons:

- For *culture and sensitivity,* to identify a specific microorganism and its drug sensitivities.
- For *cytology,* to identify the origin, structure, function, and pathology of cells. Specimens for cytology often require serial collection of three early-morning

BOX 43.2   MEASUREMENT OF AN ANKLE-BRACHIAL INDEX (ABI)

The ABI measurement compares the systolic blood pressure of the lower extremity with the higher of the two systolic blood pressures of the brachial artery. The ABI is calculated by dividing either the posterior tibial or dorsalis pedis (whichever is higher) systolic pressure by the higher brachial systolic pressure. For example, if a client has a left brachial systolic pressure of 130 and a right brachial systolic pressure of 126 and a dorsalis pedis systolic pressure of 130 then the ABI is 1 (130 divided by 130); a client with a left brachial systolic pressure of 120 and a right brachial systolic pressure of 116 and a dorsalis pedis systolic pressure of 80 has an ABI is 0.66 (80 divided by 120)—this value warrants further investigation.

Measurement of ABI between 0.91 to 1.3 indicate absence of significant arterial disease; an ABI between 0.41 and 0.9 indicates mild to severe arterial compromise requiring referral; an ABI ≤0.4 indicates critical limb ischemia and requires immediate referral; an ABI >1.31 indicates calcified arteries (common in people with diabetes mellitus).

Source: Based on British Columbia Provincial Nursing Skin and Wound Committee. (2011). *Procedure: Ankle brachial index (ABI) in adults.* Retrieved from http://www.clwk.ca/cop/skin-wound-care/clinical-dsts

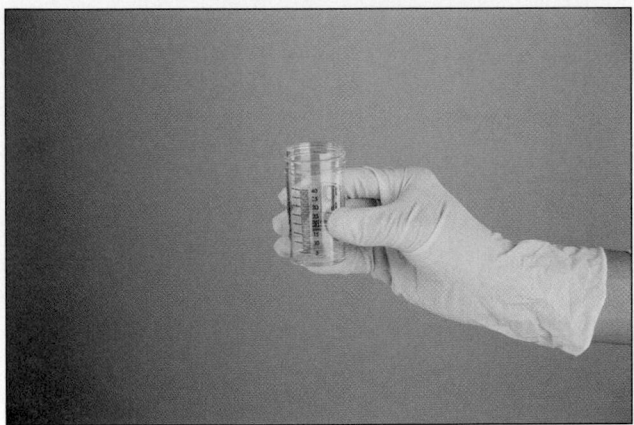

FIGURE 43.7 Sputum specimen container.

specimens that are tested to identify cancer in the lung and its specific cell type.

- For *acid-fast bacillus* (AFB), which also requires serial collection, often for 3 consecutive days, to identify the presence of tuberculosis (TB). Some agencies use a special glass container when the presence of AFB is suspected.

- To assess the *effectiveness of therapy.*

Sputum specimens are often collected in the morning. On awakening, the client can cough up the secretions that have accumulated during the night. Sometimes, specimens are collected during postural drainage, when the client can more readily produce sputum. When a client cannot cough, the nurse must sometimes use pharyngeal suctioning to obtain a specimen. To collect a sputum specimen, follow these steps:

- Offer mouth care so that the specimen will not be contaminated with microorganisms from the mouth. Do not use mouthwash.

- Ask the client to breathe deeply and to cough up 15 mL to 30 mL of sputum.

- Wear gloves to avoid direct contact with the sputum. Follow special precautions if tuberculosis is suspected, obtaining the specimen in a room equipped with a special airflow system or ultraviolet light. If these options are not available, wear a mask capable of filtering droplet nuclei.

- Ask the client to expectorate the sputum into the specimen container. Make sure the sputum does not contact the outside of the container (Figure 43.7). If the

outside of the container does become contaminated, wash it with a disinfectant. Place the container in a plastic bag for transport to the lab.

- Label and arrange transport of the specimen to the laboratory. If transport cannot occur immediately, refrigerate the specimen. Bacterial cultures must be started immediately before any contaminating microorganisms can grow, multiply, and produce false results.

- Following sputum collection, offer mouthwash to remove any unpleasant taste.

- Document the amount of sputum collected, colour, odour, consistency (thick, tenacious, watery), and presence of **hemoptysis** (blood in the sputum).

Skill 43.4 (see page 1393) describes how to obtain a sputum specimen during oropharyngeal, nasopharyngeal and nasotracheal suctioning.

A **throat culture** sample is collected from the mucosa of the oropharynx and tonsillar regions by using a culture swab. The sample is then cultured and examined for the presence of disease-producing microorganisms. To obtain a throat culture specimen, the nurse inserts the swab into the oropharynx and runs the swab along the tonsils and areas on the pharynx that are reddened or contain exudate. The gag reflex, active in some clients, may be decreased by having the client sit upright if health permits, open the mouth, extend the tongue, and say "ah," and by taking the specimen quickly. The sitting position and extension of the tongue help expose the pharynx; saying "ah" relaxes the throat muscles and helps minimize contraction of the constrictor muscle of the pharynx (the gag reflex). If the posterior pharynx cannot be seen, use a light and depress the tongue with a tongue blade (Figure 43.8 on the next page). See the Lifespan Considerations box for additional guidelines on taking specimens from infants, children, and older adults.

Pulmonary Function Tests   Pulmonary function tests measure lung volume and capacity. Clients undergoing pulmonary function tests, which are usually carried out by a respiratory therapist, do not require an anesthetic. The

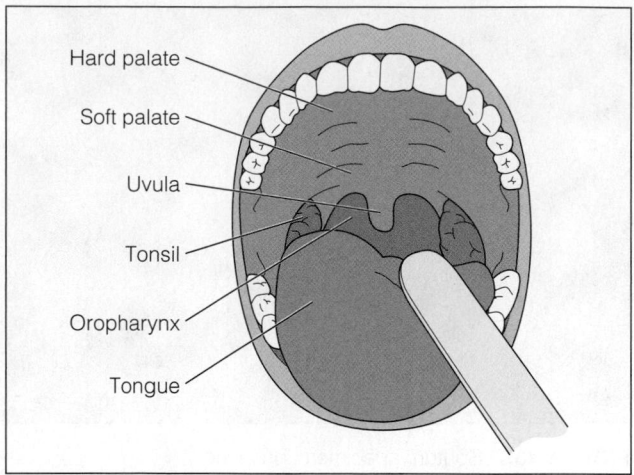

FIGURE 43.8 Depressing the tongue to view the pharynx.

tests are painless, but the client's cooperation is essential. Clients breathe into a machine and forcefully exhale all their breath and then inhale again. Pulmonary readings are recorded throughout the procedure and compared with any previous readings and with the baseline normal according to age, sex, height, and weight. Nurses need to explain the tests to people beforehand and help clients rest afterward because the tests are often tiring. Table 43.1 describes the measurements taken and Figure 43.9 shows their relationships and normal adult values.

BLOOD TESTS Specimens of venous blood are taken for a *complete blood count* (CBC), which includes hemoglobin and hematocrit measurements, erythrocyte (red blood cell [RBC]) count, leukocyte (white blood cell [WBC]) count, RBC indices, and a differential WBC count.

The *hemoglobin* is a measure of the total amount of hemoglobin in the blood. The normal reference range

for hemoglobin is 138 g/L to 180 g/L in men and 120 g/L to 160 g/L in women. The *hematocrit* measures the portion of erythrocytes (RBCs) in the plasma. The normal reference range for hematocrit is 0.37 to 0.49 of plasma in men and 0.36 to 0.46 of plasma in women. Hemoglobin and hematocrit increase with dehydration, as the blood becomes more concentrated, and decrease with hypervolemia and resulting hemodilution. Both the hemoglobin and the hematocrit counts are related to the erythrocyte count, the number of RBCs in whole blood. The normal reference range for RBCs is 4.5×10^{12}/L to 5.3×10^{12}/L

TABLE 43.1 Pulmonary Volumes and Capacities

Measurement	Description
Tidal volume (V_T)	Volume inhaled and exhaled during normal, quiet breathing
Inspiratory reserve volume (IRV)	Maximum amount of air that can be inhaled over and above a normal breath
Expiratory reserve volume (ERV)	Maximum amount of air that can be exhaled following a normal exhalation
Residual volume (RV)	The amount of air remaining in the lungs after maximal exhalation
Total lung capacity (TLC)	The total volume of the lungs at maximum inflation; calculated by adding the V_T, IRV, ERV, and RV
Vital capacity (VC)	Total amount of air that can be exhaled after a maximal inspiration; calculated by adding the V_T, IRV, and ERV
Inspiratory capacity (IC)	Total amount of air that can be inhaled following normal quiet exhalation; calculated by adding the V_T and IRV
Functional residual capacity (FRC)	The volume left in the lungs after normal exhalation; calculated by adding the ERV and RV
Minute volume (MV)	The total volume or amount of air breathed in 1 minute

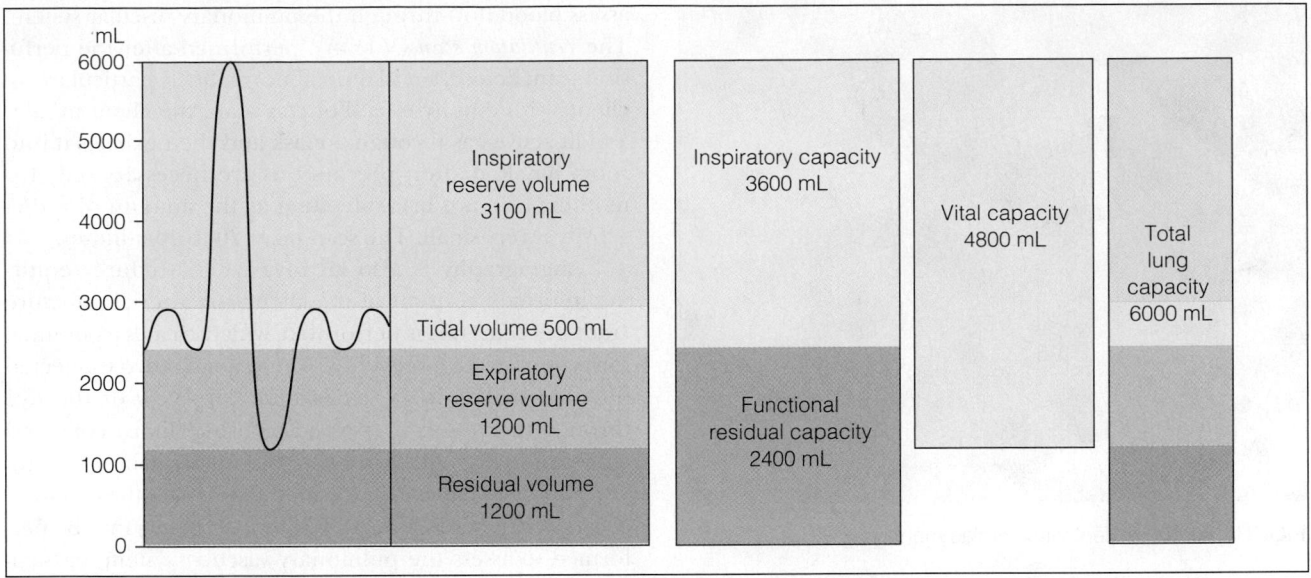

FIGURE 43.9 The relationship of lung volumes and capacities: volumes (mL) shown are for an average adult male; female volumes are 20% to 25% smaller.

in men and 4.1×10^{12}/L to 5.1×10^{12}/L in women. It also varies by age. Low RBC counts are indicative of anemia; clients with chronic hypoxia may develop higher than normal counts, a condition known as *polycythemia*. *RBC indices* may be performed as part of the CBC to evaluate the size, weight, and hemoglobin concentration of RBCs.

The *leukocyte* or *white blood cell* count determines the number of circulating WBCs in whole blood. The normal reference range for WBCs is 4.5×10^9/L to 11.0×10^9/L. High WBC counts are often seen in the presence of a bacterial infection; by contrast, WBC counts may be low if a viral infection is present. In the WBC differential, leukocytes are identified by type (e.g., neutrophil), and the percentage of each type is determined. This information is useful in diagnosing certain disorders that have characteristic patterns of distribution.

A number of other tests may be performed on blood plasma. These often are referred to as *blood chemistries*. Common chemistry examinations include determining serum electrolytes (sodium, potassium, chloride, calcium, and bicarbonate); certain enzymes, including lactic dehydrogenase (LDH), creatine phosphokinase (CPK) (also referred to as creatine kinase [CK, not to be confused with creatinine kinase]), troponin, aspartate aminotransferase (AST), and alanine aminotransferase (ALT); serum glucose; hormones, such as thyroid hormone, erythropoietin; metabolic waste products, such as creatinine and blood urea nitrogen (BUN); and other substances, such as cholesterol and triglycerides. These tests provide valuable diagnostic cues. For example, **creatine phosphokinase** and **troponin** are cardiac enzymes that are released into the blood when there is acute myocardial injury and damage. Both these tests are very useful in the diagnosis of an acute MI. Troponin I is the most accurate marker of myocardial injury. This marker

appears in the blood stream 4 to 12 hours after the onset of injury and will peak within 12 hours, and often remains elevated for 4 to 12 days. In addition, elevated levels of these enzymes can help differentiate between an MI and chest pain from a different cause, such as angina or pleuritic pain. **B-type natriuretic peptide (BNP)** is released in response to increased ventricular filling pressures and is a routine blood test for diagnosing heart failure.

Measurement of *arterial blood gases* is another important diagnostic procedure (see Chapter 44). Specimens of arterial blood are normally taken by respiratory or specialty nurses or medical technicians. Blood for these tests is taken from the radial, brachial, or femoral arteries. Because of the relatively great pressure of the blood in these arteries, it is important to prevent hemorrhaging by applying pressure to the puncture site for at least 5 minutes after removing the needle. Pulse oximetry is a noninvasive means of assessing the O_2 saturation (SpO_2) level and is especially useful when invasive ABG sampling is not feasible to assess arterial oxygen saturation (SaO_2). Pulse oximetry is detailed in Skill 29.7 on page 731.

CARDIAC MONITORING **Cardiac monitoring** allows for continuous observation of the client's heart rhythm. It is used for clients who have known or suspected cardiovascular disease, during and after surgery, to monitor responses to drug therapy, and to monitor clients at risk for serious complications, such as shock. Electrodes placed on the client's chest can be attached to a bedside monitor (Figure 43.10 on the next page); these electrodes transmit the electrical impulses of the heart to an oscilloscope or graphic recorder. The monitor is equipped with alarms used to warn of potential problems, such as very fast or very slow heart rates and lethal arrhythmias. The alarm limits are set for 20 beats more and fewer than the client's baseline rate, often at 100 to 110 and 50 to 55,

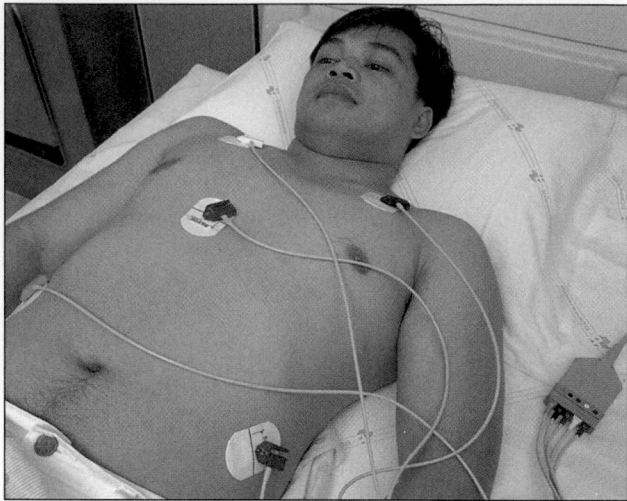

FIGURE 43.10 A client with cardiac monitoring.

respectively, for adults. The wave forms produced by the **electrocardiography (ECG)**, can then be examined to detect dysrhythmias and alterations in conduction indicative of myocardial ischemia or damage, enlargement of the heart, or drug effects.

For ambulatory clients (in the hospital or at home), the electrodes connect to a transmitter unit. This unit electronically sends the signal to a central monitor for display or may store the information to be retrieved later in the physician's office. The Holter monitor is a type of ambulatory monitoring. Electrodes are attached and the client wears the monitor for 24 hours. Continuous ECG is performed and the recordings later analyzed for irregularities. ECG is most commonly a recording of 12 leads or 12 different views of the heart. In contrast, cardiac monitoring uses only one or two leads at a time. Some clients may undergo *stress electrocardiography* to assess the response to an increased cardiac workload during exercise. As the body's demand for O_2 increases with exercise, the cardiac workload increases, as does the O_2 demand of the heart muscle itself. Clients with coronary artery disease may develop chest pain and characteristic ECG changes during exercise.

Visualization Procedures A number of visualization procedures can be done to examine the respiratory tract and the cardiovascular system. As these procedures are invasive, they require written informed consent. Radiography (x-ray), lung scan, coronary or pulmonary angiography, echocardiography, and endoscopy (bronchoscopy and laryngoscopy) are a few.

Radiographic examination of the chest is done both to diagnose disease and to assess the progress of a disease. For a radiographic examination, the nurse needs to inform the client that jewellery and clothing from the waist up must be removed.

A **lung scan**, also known as a V/Q (ventilation/perfusion) scan, records the emissions from radioisotope-tagged albumin injected intravenously as it circulates through the lung. The *perfusion scan* (Q scan) is used to assess blood flow through the pulmonary vascular system. The *ventilation scan* (V scan), performed after the perfusion scan, detects ventilation abnormalities, particularly in clients with emphysema. For this scan, the client inhales a radioactive gas through a mask and then exhales it into room air. Radiation precautions are necessary only for mothers who are breast-feeding as the amount of radioactivity is very small. The scan takes 20 to 40 minutes.

Angiography is also an invasive procedure requiring informed consent of the client. An arterial puncture (radial or femoral) is performed, which creates a potential for postprocedure bleeding. A radiopaque dye is injected into the vessels to be examined. The flow of the dye through the vessels is assessed by using fluoroscopy and x-rays, and areas of narrowing or blockage can be observed. *Coronary angiography* is performed to evaluate the extent of coronary artery disease; *pulmonary angiography* may be performed to assess the pulmonary vascular system, particularly if pulmonary emboli are suspected. Other vessels that can be studied include the carotid and cerebral arteries, the renal arteries, and the vessels of the lower extremities.

Echocardiography is a test that uses ultrasound to visualize structures of the heart and evaluate left ventricular function. Images are produced as ultrasound waves reflect back to a transducer after striking cardiac structures. Transthoracic echocardiography is noninvasive, and the client needs to be informed that this test causes no discomfort, although the conductive gel used may be cold. In cases where there is a desire to increase visualization of heart chambers and/or valves, transesophageal echocardiography may be done, which involves sedation and local anesthesia in the throat, creating a need for the client to be NPO (nil per ora, nothing by mouth) before the procedure and until the gag reflex returns after the procedure.

Laryngoscopy and **bronchoscopy** are sterile procedures that use a laryngoscope and bronchoscope, respectively. During the procedure, tissue samples may be taken for biopsy. A local anesthetic (e.g., xylocaine) and muscle relaxant (e.g., midazolam) are usually given before the examination. The local anesthetic is sprayed on the client's pharynx to prevent gagging; alternatively, the client gargles with the anesthetic to anesthetize the throat. The bronchoscope is then inserted to visualize the larynx or bronchi (Figure 43.11). Informed consent is required for these procedures. Food and fluids are withheld after the procedure until the gag reflex returns.

Diagnosing

Multiple nursing diagnoses can relate to oxygenation and circulation problems, such as impaired gas exchange (O_2 and/or CO_2), impaired pumping action of the heart, impaired ventilation, impaired arterial and/or venous circulation, unhealthy lifestyle, increasing risk for cardiac and/or respiratory compromise, and many more. These diagnoses may also be the etiology of several other diagnoses, for example, inability to fulfill work- and family-related

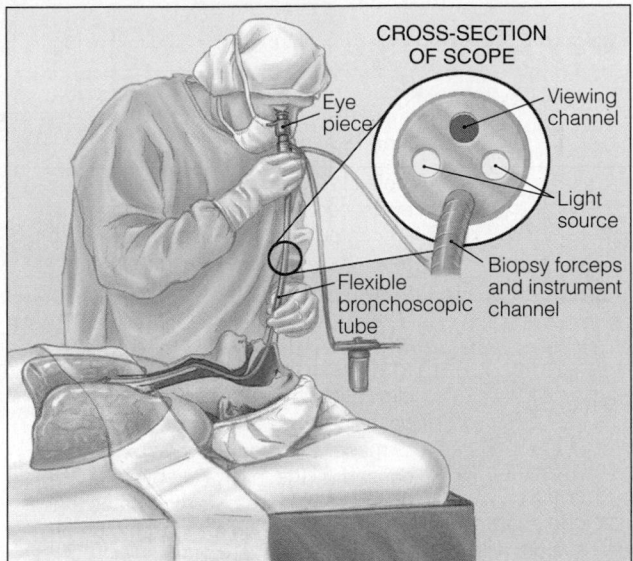

FIGURE 43.11 Bronchoscopy.

Source: Fremgan, Bonnie F.; Frucht, Suzanne S., *Medical Terminology: A Living Language*, 3rd Ed., © 2005. Reprinted and Electronically reproduced with permission of Pearson Education Inc., Upper Saddle River, New Jersey.

roles related to cardiac and respiratory compromise, anxiety related to dyspnea, insomnia related to orthopnea, fear related to chronic disabling respiratory and/or cardiac illness, social isolation related to activity intolerance and inability to travel to usual social activities.

Planning

The overall goals for a client with oxygenation and circulation problems are as follows:

- Maintaining a patent airway
- Improving comfort and ease of breathing
- Maintaining or improving pulmonary ventilation and oxygenation
- Maintaining or improving tissue perfusion
- Maintaining or restoring an adequate cardiac output
- Improving ability to participate in physical activities
- Preventing risks associated with oxygenation problems, such as skin and tissue breakdown, syncope, acid–base imbalances; feelings of hopelessness and social isolation

These desired health outcomes provide direction for planning interventions and as criteria for evaluating client progress. A clinical example of desired health outcomes, interventions, and activities is provided in the Sample Care Plan on the next page.

PLANNING FOR HOME CARE To provide for continuity of care, the nurse needs to consider the client's learning needs and needs for assistance with care in the home. Planning incorporates an assessment of the client's and family's knowledge and abilities for self-care, financial

resources, and evaluation of the need for referrals and for home care services. The Assessment: Home Care box on page 1373 outlines issues related to the client's oxygenation problems and needs at home.

Implementing

PROMOTING OXYGENATION Most people in normal health give little thought to their respiratory and cardiovascular functions. Changing position frequently, ambulating, and exercising usually maintain adequate ventilation, gas exchange, and cardiovascular function. The Teaching: Wellness boxes on page 1374 list other ways to promote healthy breathing and maintain a healthy heart.

When people become ill, their respiratory and cardiovascular functions may be inhibited for such reasons as pain and immobility. Shallow respirations inhibit both diaphragmatic excursion and lung distension. The result of inadequate chest expansion is stasis and pooling of respiratory secretions, which ultimately harbour microorganisms and promote infection.

Interventions by the nurse to maintain the normal respirations of clients include the following:

- Positioning the client to allow for maximum chest expansion
- Encouraging or providing frequent changes in position
- Encouraging ambulation
- Implementing measures that promote comfort, such as giving analgesia
- Providing fluids and humidification
- Encouraging deep breathing and coughing

The semi-Fowler's or high-Fowler's position (see Chapter 39) allows for maximum chest expansion in clients confined to beds, particularly dyspneic clients. Dyspneic persons often sit in bed and lean over their over-bed tables (which are raised to a suitable height), usually with a pillow for support. This *orthopneic position* is an adaptation of the high-Fowler's position. It has a further advantage in that, unlike in high-Fowler's, the abdominal organs are not pressing on the diaphragm. Also, a client in the orthopneic position can press the lower part of the chest against the table to facilitate exhaling (Figure 43.12 on page 1374).

PROMOTING CIRCULATION Immobility is detrimental to cardiovascular function. Without exercise of the calf and leg muscles, blood pools in the veins of the lower extremities. This stagnant blood flow may allow clots to develop (*venous thrombosis*). With time, these clots can break loose and become emboli, eventually lodging in the small vessels of the pulmonary vascular system. Blood flow and gas exchange in the lungs are then impaired.

Many nursing interventions can help maintain cardiovascular function. They can be classified as vascular or cardiac.

Sample Care Plan for Ineffective Airway Clearance

ASSESSMENT DATA

Nursing Assessment

Johti Singh is a 39-year-old secretary who was admitted to the hospital with an elevated temperature, fatigue, tachypnea with laboured respirations, and mild dehydration. The nursing history reveals that Ms. Singh has had a "bad cold that would not go away" for several weeks. She has been dieting for several months and skipping meals. Ms. Singh mentions that in addition to her full-time job as a secretary, she is attending university classes two evenings a week. She has smoked one package of cigarettes per day since she was 18 years old. Chest radiography confirms pneumonia.

Physical Examination

Height: 167.6 cm

Weight: 54.4 kg

Temperature: 39.4°C orally

Pulse: 116 beats/min, regular, 2+ amplitude

Respirations: 26/min

Blood Pressure: 118/70 mm Hg

Skin pale; cheeks flushed; chills; nasal flaring; inspiratory crackles with diminished air entry to right middle lobe (RML) and right lower lobe (RLL); expectorating thick, yellow sputum with no odour

Diagnostic Data

Chest x-ray: RML and RLL infiltration
WBC: 14.0×10^9/L
pH: 7.34
(normal 7.35–7.45)
$PaCO_2$: 46 mm Hg
(normal 35–45 mm Hg)
HCO_3^-: 23 mmol/L
(normal 22–26 mmol/L)
PaO_2: 76 mm Hg
(normal 80–100 mm Hg)
SaO_2: 92% (normal 95%–100%)

Nursing Diagnosis

Ineffective gas exchange, as evidenced by hypercapnia causing respiratory acidosis (uncompensated) and hypoxemia likely secondary to pneumonia and presence of thick sputum. Tachypnea and tachycardia are likely compensatory mechanisms to increase the availability of O_2 in the circulation in response to the impaired gas exchange in the lungs as well as to meet the increased metabolic needs caused by the fever. Retention of CO_2 despite tachypnea likely indicates that that the surface area for exchange of CO_2 is greatly affected.

Client Goals

One of the goals for this client is as follows: The client will demonstrate effective coughing and increased gas exchange.

Desired Health Outcomes

1. Coughs and deep breathes q1h within first 24 hours
2. Expectorates secretions from airway, whenever necessary
3. Increases fluid intake to 3000 mL
4. Exhibits normal breath sounds throughout all lung fields

Nursing Interventions	Rationales
Enhance Coughing	
• Assist Ms. Singh to a sitting position with head slightly flexed, shoulders relaxed, and knees flexed.	*Lying flat causes the abdominal organs to shift toward the chest, crowding the lungs and making it more difficult to breathe.*
• Encourage her to take several deep breaths.	*Deep breathing promotes oxygenation before controlled coughing.*
• Encourage her to take a deep breath, hold for 2 seconds, and cough two or three times in succession.	*Controlled coughing is accomplished by the closure of the glottis and the explosive expulsion of air from the lungs by the work of abdominal and chest muscles.*
• Encourage the use of incentive spirometry, as appropriate.	*Breathing exercises help maximize ventilation.*
• Promote systemic fluid hydration, as appropriate.	*Adequate fluid intake enhances liquefaction of pulmonary secretions and facilitates expectoration of mucus.*

Nursing Interventions	Rationales
Respiratory Monitoring	
• Monitor rate, rhythm, depth, and effort of respirations.	*Monitoring these measurements provides a basis for evaluating adequacy of ventilation.*
• Note chest movement, watching for symmetry, use of accessory muscles.	*The presence of nasal flaring and the use of accessory muscles of respiration can occur in response to ineffective ventilation.*
• Auscultate breath sounds, noting areas of decreased or absent ventilation and presence of adventitious sounds.	*As fluid and mucus accumulate, abnormal breath sounds can be heard, including crackles and diminished breath sounds, owing to fluid-filled air spaces and diminished lung volume.*

Nursing Interventions	Rationales
Respiratory Monitoring	
• Auscultate lung sounds after treatments to note results.	*Performing these actions assists in evaluating prescribed treatments and client outcomes.*
• Monitor the client's ability to cough effectively.	
• Monitor client's respiratory secretions.	*Respiratory tract infections alter the amount and character of secretions. An ineffective cough compromises airway clearance and prevents mucus from being expelled.*
• Institute respiratory therapy treatments (e.g., nebulizer), as needed.	*People with pneumonia commonly produce rust-coloured, purulent sputum.*
• Monitor for increased restlessness, anxiety, and air hunger.	*A variety of respiratory therapy treatments can be used to open constricted airways and liquefy secretions.*
• Note changes in O_2 saturation, tidal CO_2, and changes in arterial blood gas values, as appropriate.	*These clinical manifestations are indicators of hypoxemia.*

Nursing Interventions	Rationales
Oxygen Therapy	
• Instruct Ms. Singh about the importance of leaving the oxygen delivery device on.	*Oxygen demand is greater during febrile illness and physical activity.*
• Periodically check the oxygen delivery device to ensure that the prescribed concentration is being delivered.	*Too much or too little oxygen can be detrimental, especially in the client with a history of smoking.*

EVALUATION

Goal partially met. Ms. Singh coughs and deep breathes purposefully q1–2h during the day. Her fluid intake is approximately 1500 mL each day. Cough continues to be productive, but sputum is clearer. Inspiratory crackles continue to be present in RLL but less than before; good air entry to RML. Her PaO_2 is 85 mm Hg, and her SaO_2 is 95% on nasal prongs 2 L/minute.

Note: Other aspects of care in this situation would include antibiotic therapy for the pneumonia.

ASSESSMENT HOME CARE

Oxygenation

Assess the following areas related to the client's oxygenation problems and needs at home:

CLIENT

- *Self-care abilities:* Ability to ambulate and perform activities of daily living (ADLs) independently
- *Exercise and activity pattern:* Type and regularity of usual exercise, perceived and actual energy for desired and required leisure activities
- *Assistive devices required:* Supplemental oxygen, humidifier, nebulizer treatments or inhalers; walker, cane, or wheelchair; grab bars, shower chair, and other devices to promote safety and minimize energy expenditure; scale to monitor weight on a regular basis
- *Home environment:* Assessment for factors that impair airway clearance, gas exchange, or activity tolerance; indoor pollutants, such as cigarette smoke and dust; allergens, such as pets; dry air; and barriers, such as stairs
- *Current level of knowledge:* Importance of avoiding smoking and other pollutants; dietary salt and other restrictions (if appropriate); recommended activities; medications; need to limit exposure to respiratory infections; use of prescribed nebulizer, multidose inhaler, powdered dose inhaler, home oxygen; activity level

FAMILY

- *Caregiver availability, skills, and responses:* Ability and willingness to provide care, as needed (helping with ADLs, providing meals, assisting with transportation and shopping, caring for dependants; performing treatments, such as percussion and postural drainage)
- *Family role changes and coping:* Effect on financial status, parenting and spousal roles, sexuality, social roles
- *Alternative potential primary or respite caregivers:* For example, other family members, volunteers, church members, paid caregivers or housekeeping services; available community respite care (e.g., adult daycare, senior centres)

COMMUNITY

- *Environment:* Usual temperature and humidity; presence of air pollutants, such as automobile exhaust, industrial smoke and pollutants, smoke from field burning
- *Current knowledge of and experience with community resources:* Medical and assistive equipment and supply companies, respiratory and physical therapy services, home care agencies, local pharmacies, available financial assistance, support and educational organizations, such as the local lung association, COPD support groups

Promoting Healthy Breathing

The nurse can the following instructions to clients to promote healthy breathing:

- Sit straight and stand erect to permit full lung expansion.
- Exercise regularly.
- Breathe through the nose.
- Breathe in so as to expand the chest fully.
- Do not smoke cigarettes, cigars, or pipes; do not use chewing tobacco.
- Eliminate or reduce the use of household pesticides and irritating chemical substances.
- Avoid exposure to second-hand smoke.
- Use building materials that do not emit vapours.
- Make sure furnaces, ovens, wood stoves, and fireplaces are correctly ventilated.
- Support a pollution-free environment.

Promoting a Healthy Heart

The nurse can provide the following instructions to clients to promote heart health:

- Exercise regularly, according to Canadian fitness guidelines (e.g., adults should participate in at least 150 minutes of moderate- to vigorous-intensity aerobic physical activity per week in bouts of 10 minutes or more).
- Follow *Eating Well with Canada's Food Guide*, which takes into consideration energy and nutrient needs, including fibre and limiting sodium and fat intake in the diet.
- Do not smoke.
- Maintain your body mass index within healthy norms (see Chapter 40).
- Drink alcohol in moderation, if at all, consuming no more than 30 mL of alcohol a day (one cocktail, one to one-and-a-half glasses of wine or beer).
- Reduce stress, and manage anger.
- Effectively manage diabetes and hypertension, maintaining blood glucose and blood pressure levels within normal limits.
- Consult your health care provider about the advisability of low-dose Aspirin therapy to further reduce the risk of cardiovascular disease.

Vascular Vascular nursing interventions to maintain cardiovascular function include the following:

- Positioning the client with the legs elevated to promote venous return to the heart; although this intervention is important for people with venous dysfunction, care should be taken to avoid this position

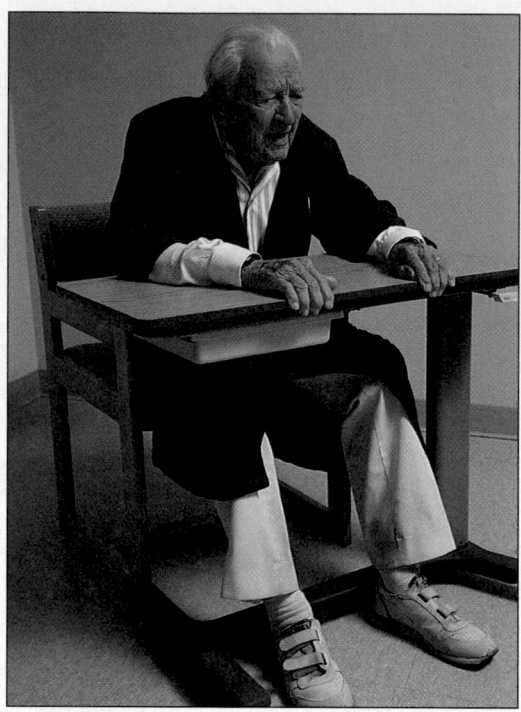

FIGURE 43.12 A patient using the overbed table to assist with breathing.

in clients with cardiac dysfunction because it will increase preload and may stress a dysfunctional heart

- Avoiding placing pillows under the client's knees or more than 15 degrees of knee flexion, to improve blood flow to the lower extremities and reduce venous stagnation
- Avoiding crossing the client's legs or ankles
- Encouraging leg exercises, such as flexion and extension of the feet and active contraction and relaxation of calf muscles, for a client on bed rest, and promoting ambulation as soon as possible
- Encouraging or providing frequent position changes

Cardiac Cardiac nursing interventions to maintain cardiovascular function include the following:

- Positioning the client in high-Fowler's position to decrease preload and reduce pulmonary congestion
- Monitoring intake and output; fluid restriction is not usually required for clients with mild to moderate cardiac dysfunction; with severe heart failure, fluid restriction may be required

DEEP BREATHING AND COUGHING The nurse can facilitate respiratory functioning by encouraging deep-breathing exercises and coughing to remove secretions. Breathing exercises are frequently indicated for clients with restricted chest expansion, such as those with COPD or clients recovering from thoracic surgery and pneumonia.

A commonly employed breathing exercise is abdominal (diaphragmatic) and pursed-lip breathing. *Abdominal* (*diaphragmatic*) *breathing* permits deep full breaths with little effort. *Pursed-lip breathing* helps the client develop control over breathing. The pursed lips create a resistance to the air flowing out of the lungs, thereby prolonging exhalation and preventing airway collapse by maintaining positive airway pressure. The client purses the lips as if about to whistle and breathes out slowly and gently, tightening the abdominal muscles to exhale more effectively. The client usually inhales to a count of three and exhales to a count of seven.

Forceful coughing is highly effective, but some clients may lack the strength or ability to cough normally. Normal forceful coughing involves the client inhaling deeply and then coughing twice while exhaling. Alternative cough techniques, such as forced expiratory technique or huff coughing, may be taught as alternatives for those clients who are unable to perform a normal forceful cough. A client with COPD is instructed to exhale through pursed lips and to exhale with a "huff" sound in midexhalation. The huff cough helps prevent the high expiratory pressures that collapse diseased airways.

The Teaching: Clinical boxes address (a) abdominal (diaphragmatic) and pursed-lip breathing; and (b) forced expiratory technique (huff coughing).

HYDRATION Adequate hydration maintains the moisture of the respiratory mucous membranes. Normally, respiratory tract secretions are thin and, therefore, are moved readily by ciliary action. However, when the client is dehydrated or when the environment has a low humidity, the respiratory secretions can become thick and tenacious. Fluid intake should be individually determined on the basis of respiratory and cardiovascular status. See Chapter 44 for normal daily fluid intake.

HUMIDIFIERS **Humidifiers** are devices that add water vapour to inspired air. Room humidifiers provide cool mist to room air. Nebulizers are used to deliver humidity and medications. They may be used with oxygen delivery systems to provide moistened air directly to the client. Their purposes are to prevent mucous membranes from drying and becoming irritated and to loosen secretions for easier expectoration. It is important to follow the manufacturer's directions for cleaning and maintaining humidifiers to reduce potential sources of bacterial growth.

MEDICATIONS A number of types of medications can be used for clients with oxygenation problems. Bronchodilators, anti-inflammatory drugs, expectorants, and cough suppressants are some medications that are used to treat respiratory problems.

Bronchodilators, including sympathomimetic drugs and xanthines, reduce bronchospasm, opening tight or congested airways and facilitating ventilation. These drugs can be administered orally or intravenously, but the preferred route is through inhalation to prevent many systemic side effects. Since drugs used to dilate the bronchioles and improve breathing are usually drugs that enhance the sympathetic nervous system, clients must be monitored for

---

TEACHING | CLINICAL

Abdominal (Diaphragmatic) and Pursed-Lip Breathing

The following are instructions for abdominal (diaphragmatic) and pursed-lip breathing:

- Assume a comfortable semi-sitting position in bed or a chair *or* the lying position in bed with one pillow.
- Flex your knees to relax the muscles of the abdomen.
- Place one or both hands on your abdomen, just below the ribs.
- Breathe in deeply through your nose, keeping your mouth closed.
- Concentrate on feeling your abdomen rise (expand) as far as possible; stay relaxed, and avoid arching your back. If you have difficulty raising your abdomen, take a quick, forceful breath through the nose.
- Then, purse your lips as if about to whistle, and breathe out slowly and gently, making a slow "whooshing" sound without puffing out the cheeks. This *pursed-lip breathing* creates a resistance to air flowing out of the lungs, increases pressure within the bronchi (main air passages), and minimizes collapse of smaller airways, a common problem for people with COPD.
- Concentrate on feeling the abdomen fall or sink, and tighten (contract) the abdominal muscles while breathing out to enhance effective exhalation. Count to seven during exhalation.
- Use this exercise every 2 hours and whenever you are feeling short of breath. Increase gradually to 5 to 10 minutes 4 times a day. Regular practice will help you do this type of breathing without conscious effort. The exercise, once learned, can be performed when sitting upright, standing, and walking.

TEACHING | CLINICAL

Forced Expiratory Technique (Huff Coughing)

- After using a bronchodilator treatment (if prescribed), inhale deeply, and hold your breath for a few seconds.
- Cough twice. The first cough loosens the mucus; the second expels secretions.
- For huff coughing, lean forward and exhale sharply with a "huff" sound. This technique helps keep your airways open while moving secretions up and out of the lungs.
- Inhale by taking rapid short breaths in succession ("sniffing") to prevent mucus from moving back into smaller airways.
- Rest and breathe slowly between coughs.
- Try to avoid prolonged episodes of coughing as these may cause fatigue and/or hypoxemia.

TEACHING CLINICAL

Using Cough Medications

Provide the following instructions to clients to be used as guidelines before starting a cough medication:

- Do not take cough medications in excessive amounts because of adverse side effects. Consult your nurse, pharmacist, or physician, as needed.
- If you have diabetes mellitus, avoid cough syrups that contain sugar or alcohol; these can disturb glucose metabolism.
- Be aware of side effects (e.g., drowsiness) that can make driving or operating machinery dangerous.
- Be aware of interactions of cough medications with prescription and other nonprescription medications.

side effects of increased heart rate, blood pressure, anxiety, and restlessness. This is especially important in older adults, who may also have cardiac problems.

Another class of drugs used are the *anti-inflammatory drugs,* such as glucocorticoids. They can be given orally, intravenously, or via inhalers. They work by decreasing the edema and inflammation in the airways (as in asthma) and allowing a better air exchange. If both bronchodilators and anti-inflammatory drugs are ordered to be administered via inhalers, the client should be instructed to use the bronchodilator inhaler first and then the antiinflammatory inhaler. If the bronchioles are dilated first, more tissue is exposed for the anti-inflammatory drugs to act on. (Chapter 33 discusses administration of medications through inhalation.)

The *leukotriene modifiers* are relatively new medications that suppress the effects of leukotrienes on the smooth muscle of the respiratory tract. Leukotrienes cause bronchoconstriction, mucus production, and edema of the respiratory tract.

Expectorants liquefy mucus and make it easier to expectorate. Guaifenesin is a common expectorant found in many prescription and nonprescription cough syrups. When frequent or prolonged coughing interrupts sleep, a *cough suppressant,* such as codeine, may be prescribed. See the Teaching: Clinical box on using cough medications.

Other medications can be used to improve oxygenation by improving cardiovascular function. The *cardiac glycosides* (e.g., digoxin) act directly on the heart to improve the strength of contraction and slow the heart. The *beta-adrenergic agonists,* such as metoprolol (Lopressor), affect the sympathetic nervous system to reduce the workload of the heart. These drugs can negatively affect people with asthma or COPD, as they can constrict airways.

Some medications, such as *nitrates, calcium channel blockers,* and *ACE inhibitors,* reduce the workload of the heart and prevent vasoconstriction. In addition, various drugs, such as amiodarone (e.g., Cordarone), beta-blockers (e.g., metoprolol), calcium channel blockers (e.g., diltiazem), and digoxin (e.g., Lanoxin), are used to treat cardiac dysrhythmias. *Direct vasodilators* may be used for clients with peripheral vascular disease.

INCENTIVE SPIROMETRY Incentive spirometers (Figure 43.13), also referred to as *sustained maximal inspiration devices* (SMIs), measure the flow of air inhaled through a mouthpiece and are used to do the following:

- Maintain or improve pulmonary ventilation
- Counteract the effects of anesthesia or hypoventilation
- Loosen respiratory secretions

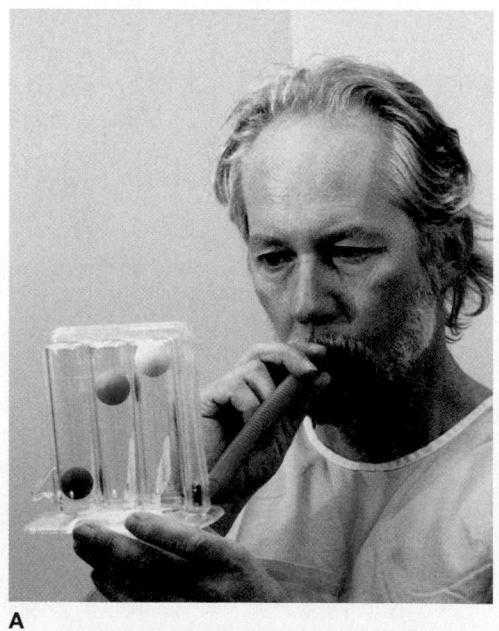
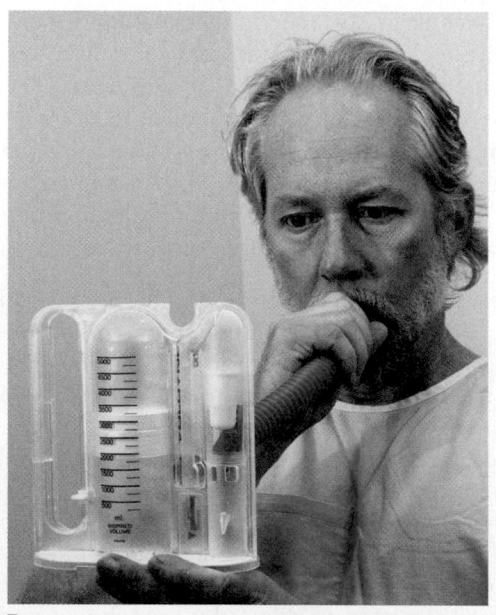

FIGURE 43.13 A: Flow-oriented sustained maximal inspiration (SMI) device; **B**: Volume-oriented SMI device.

- Facilitate respiratory gaseous exchange
- Expand collapsed alveoli

SMI devices offer an incentive to improve *inhalation* and are designed to mimic natural sighing or yawning by encouraging the client to take long, slow, deep breaths. Flow-oriented spirometers consist of one or more clear plastic chambers containing feely movable coloured balls or discs. The client inhales and elevates the ball—the longer the client keeps the ball "up," the larger is the volume of inhaled air, so the client is encouraged to take slow deep breaths. Volume-oriented spirometers measure the inhalation volume maintained by the client with a cylinder rising to mark the volume of inspiration. When using an SMI device, the client should be assisted into position, preferably an upright sitting position in bed or a chair, that facilitates maximum ventilation. The Teaching: Clinical box on using an incentive spirometer provides specific instructions for clients.

PERCUSSION, VIBRATION, AND POSTURAL DRAINAGE

Percussion, vibration, and postural drainage (PVD) are performed according to a physician's order and agency policy. While generally performed by respiratory or physical therapists, nurses may perform this procedure in some agencies. Percussion, sometimes called *clapping*, is forceful striking of the skin with cupped hands. Mechanical percussion cups and vibrators are also available. When the hands are used, the fingers and thumb are held together and flexed slightly to form a cup, as if scooping up water. Percussion over congested lung areas can mechanically dislodge tenacious secretions from the bronchial walls. Cupped hands trap the air against the chest. The trapped air sets up vibrations through the chest wall. PVD is contraindicated in some conditions (e.g., rib fractures and bleeding disorders).

To percuss a client's chest, follow these steps:

- Position the client (the lateral position is recommended if tolerated by client).
- Cover the area with a towel or gown to reduce discomfort.
- Ask the client to breathe slowly and deeply to promote relaxation.
- Alternately flex and extend the wrists rapidly to strike the chest (Figure 43.14).

TEACHING | **CLINICAL**

Using an Incentive Spirometer

The following are guidelines for clients to use an incentive spirometer:

- Hold or place the spirometer in an upright position. A tilted *flow-oriented* device requires less effort to raise the balls or cylinder; a *volume-oriented* device will not function correctly unless upright.
- Exhale normally.
- Seal your lips tightly around the mouthpiece.
- Take in a *slow, deep breath* to elevate the balls or cylinder, and then hold the breath for 2 seconds initially, increasing to 6 seconds (optimum), to keep the balls or cylinder elevated, if possible.
- For a *flow-oriented* device, avoid brisk, low-volume breaths that snap the balls to the top of the chamber. Greater lung expansion is achieved with a very slow inspiration than with a brisk, shallow breath, even though it may not elevate the balls or keep them elevated while you hold your breath. Sustained elevation of the balls or cylinder ensures adequate ventilation of the alveoli (lung air sacs).
- If you have difficulty breathing only through your mouth, a nose clip can be used.
- Remove the mouthpiece, and exhale normally.
- Cough after the incentive effort. Deep ventilation can loosen secretions, and coughing can facilitate their removal.
- Relax, and take several normal breaths before using the spirometer again.
- Repeat the procedure several times and then four or five times hourly. Practice increases inspiratory volume, maintains alveolar ventilation, and prevents atelectasis (collapse of the air sacs).
- Clean the mouthpiece with water, and shake it dry.

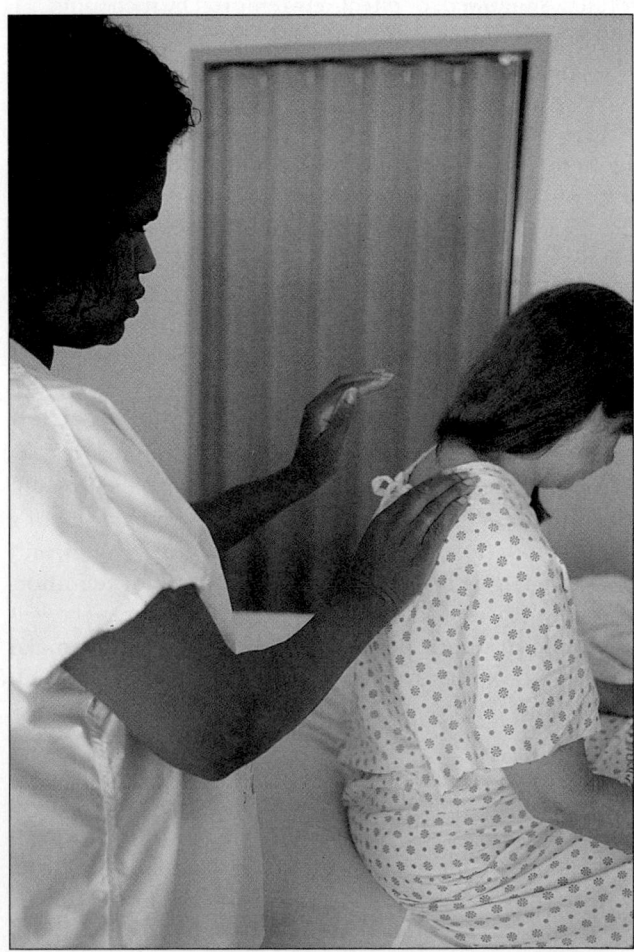

FIGURE 43.14 Percussing the upper posterior chest.

• Percuss each affected lung segment for 1 to 2 minutes or according to agency policy.

When done correctly, the percussion action should produce a hollow, popping sound. Percussion is avoided over certain easily injured structures, such as the breasts, sternum, spinal column, and kidneys.

Vibration is a series of vigorous quiverings produced by hands that are placed flat against the client's chest wall. Vibration is used after percussion to increase the turbulence of the exhaled air and, thus, loosen thick secretions. It is often done alternately with percussion. The client takes a deep breath in and then exhales; during the exhalation, the nurse tenses all hand and arm muscles, and using most of the heel of the hand, vibrates the hands, moving them downward. The vibration stops when the client has completed exhalation. Vibration is usually done for five exhalations over one affected lung segment. The client is encouraged to cough after each vibration.

Postural drainage is the drainage by gravity of secretions from various lung segments. Secretions that remain in the lungs or respiratory airways promote bacterial growth and subsequent infection. They also can obstruct the smaller airways and cause atelectasis. Secretions in the major airways, such as the trachea and the right and left main bronchi, are usually coughed into the pharynx, where they can be expectorated, swallowed, or effectively removed by suctioning.

A wide variety of positions is necessary to drain all segments of the lungs, but not all positions are required for every client. Only those positions that drain specific affected areas are used. The lower lobes require drainage most frequently because the upper lobes drain during normal daily activities. Before postural drainage, the client may be given a bronchodilator medication or nebulization therapy to loosen secretions, as ordered by a physician. Frequently, postural drainage treatments are scheduled two or three times daily, as ordered, depending on the degree of lung congestion. Be aware of the client's exercise tolerance, as postural drainage can be tiring. Postural drainage should also be avoided after meals as it puts the client at risk for vomiting and aspiration.

The nurse needs to evaluate the client's tolerance of postural drainage by assessing the stability of the client's vital signs, particularly the pulse and respiratory rates, and by noting signs of intolerance, such as pallor, diaphoresis, dyspnea, and fatigue. Some clients do not react well to certain drainage positions, and the nurse must make appropriate adjustments. For example, some become dyspneic in the Trendelenburg position and require only a moderate tilt or a shorter time in that position.

The sequence for PVD is usually as follows: positioning, percussion, vibration, and removal of secretions by coughing or suction. Each position is usually assumed for 10 to 15 minutes, although beginning treatments may start with shorter times that are gradually increased. Usually, the entire treatment, including preparatory nebulization, deep breathing, and all postures, takes 30 minutes.

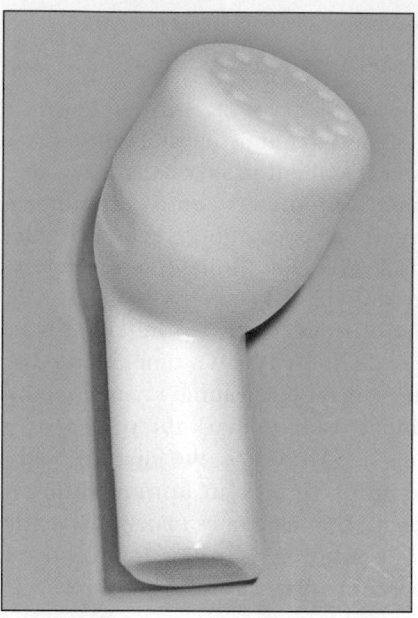

FIGURE 43.15 Flutter mucus clearance device.

Before and immediately after PVD, the nurse should auscultate the client's lungs and compare the findings with baseline data. Following PVD, document the amount, colour, and character of expectorated secretions, and note how well the client tolerated the procedure.

MUCUS CLEARANCE DEVICES A **mucus clearing device (MCD)** is used for clients with excessive secretions, such as in COPD and cystic fibrosis. The Flutter™ MCD is a small, handheld device with a hard mouthpiece at the end and a perforated cover at the other end. Inside the device is a steel ball that sits in a circular cone shape (Figure 43.15). The client inhales slowly and then, keeping the cheeks firm, exhales fast through the device, causing the steel ball to move up and down. This movement causes vibrations that loosen mucus from the airways and assist its movement up the airway to be expectorated (Ignatavicius & Workman, 2010).

OXYGEN THERAPY Clients who have difficulty ventilating all areas of their lungs, those whose gas exchange is impaired, or people with heart failure may require O_2 therapy to prevent hypoxia. The concentration, method of delivery, and number of litres per minute of O_2 should be prescribed by a physician or nurse practitioner. In certain circumstances (e.g., sudden onset of chest pain or shortness of breath), registered nurses may initiate O_2 therapy, according to agency policy.

Safety precautions are essential during O_2 therapy (see Box 43.3). Although O_2 by itself will not burn or explode, it does facilitate combustion. For example, a bed sheet ordinarily burns slowly when ignited in the atmosphere; however, if saturated with free-flowing O_2 and ignited by a spark, it will burn rapidly and explosively. Because O_2 is colourless, odourless, and tasteless, people are often unaware of its presence.

BOX 43.3 OXYGEN THERAPY SAFETY PRECAUTIONS

Follow these guidelines when using oxygen therapy with clients:

- Place cautionary signs reading "No smoking: Oxygen in use" on the client's door, at the foot or head of the bed, and on the oxygen equipment.
- Instruct the client and visitors about the hazard of smoking with oxygen in use.
- For home oxygen use, teach family members and roommates to smoke only outside or in rooms well away from the client.
- Make sure that electric devices (such as razors, hearing aids, radios, televisions, and heating pads) are in good working order to prevent the occurrence of short-circuit sparks.
- Avoid materials that generate static electricity, such as woollen blankets and synthetic fabrics. Cotton blankets should be used, and clients and caregivers are advised to wear cotton fabrics.
- Avoid the use of volatile, flammable materials, such as oils, greases, alcohol, ether, and acetone (e.g., nail polish remover) near clients receiving oxygen.
- Ground electric monitoring equipment, suction machines, and portable diagnostic machines.
- Make known the location of fire extinguishers, and make sure personnel are trained in their use and in protocols associated with fire safety.

REFLECT ON PRIMARY HEALTH CARE

The *appropriate use of technology* is evident when home oxygen therapy lets clients with severe cardiac or respiratory disease achieve their developmental and life goals. Consider how the legislation that requires nicotine products to be behind closed cabinets serves as a *health-promotion* strategy to ensure cardiac and respiratory health.

Low O_2 concentrations are essential for clients with COPD. A high CO_2 level in the blood is the normal stimulus to breathe. However, people with COPD may chronically have a high CO_2 level, and their stimulus to breathe is hypoxemia (low blood O_2 level). High concentrations of O_2 can potentially relieve this hypoxemia, removing the stimulus to breathe; low concentrations, by contrast, maintain a slightly hypoxemia state, maintaining the respiratory drive.

Oxygen is supplied in several different ways. In hospitals and long-term care facilities, it is usually piped into wall outlets at the client's bedside, making it readily available for use at all times. Tanks or cylinders of O_2 under pressure are also frequently available for use when wall O_2 either is unavailable or is impractical (e.g., for transporting clients who are dependent on O_2 between treatment areas).

Clients who require O_2 therapy in the home can use small cylinders of O_2, O_2 in liquid form, or an O_2 concentrator (see the Reflect on Primary Health Care box). Portable O_2 delivery systems are available to increase the client's independence. Home O_2 therapy services are available in most communities. These services generally supply the O_2 and delivery devices, training for the client and family, equipment maintenance, and emergency services should a problem occur.

Oxygen administered from a cylinder or wall-outlet system is dry. Dry gases dehydrate the respiratory mucous membranes. Humidifying devices that add water vapour to inspired air are thus an essential adjunct of O_2 therapy, particularly for litre flows of more than 2 L per minute

(Figure 43.16). These devices provide 20% to 40% humidity. The O_2 passes through sterile distilled water or tap water and then along a line to the device through which the moistened O_2 is inhaled (e.g., a cannula, nasal catheter, or oxygen mask).

Humidifiers prevent mucous membranes from drying and becoming irritated, and they loosen secretions for easier expectoration. Oxygen passing through water picks up water vapour before it reaches the client. The more bubbles created during this process, the more water vapour is produced. Very low litre flows (e.g., 1 L to 2 L/min by nasal cannula) do not require humidification.

Oxygen cylinders need to be handled and stored with caution and strapped securely in wheeled transport devices

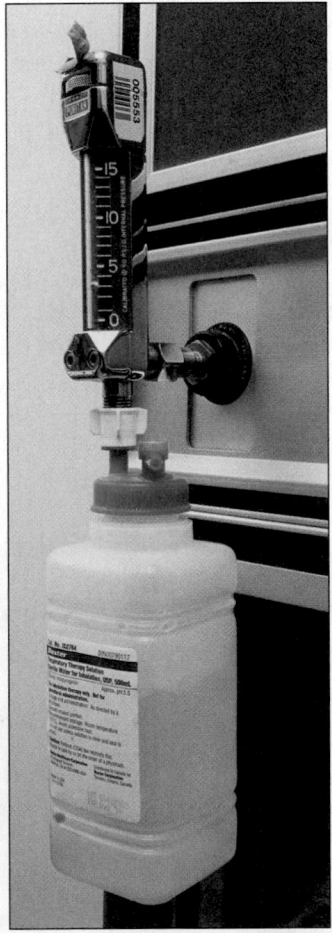

FIGURE 43.16 An oxygen humidifier attached to a wall outlet oxygen flow meter set at 3 L/min.

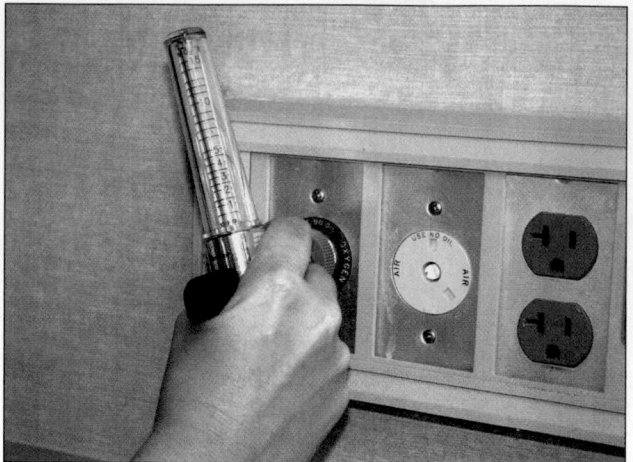

FIGURE 43.17 Insert the flow meter into the wall unit.

or stands to prevent possible falls and outlet breakages. They should be placed away from traffic areas and heaters.

To use an O_2 wall outlet, carry out these steps:

- Attach the flow meter (Figure 43.17) to the wall outlet, exerting firm pressure. The flow meter should be in the off position.
- Fill the humidifier bottle with sterile distilled water in accordance with agency protocol. (This can be done before coming to the bedside.) The sterile distilled water should be changed every 24 hours or according to agency policy.
- Attach the humidifier bottle to the base of the flow meter.
- Attach the prescribed O_2 tubing and delivery device to the humidifier.
- Regulate the flow meter to the prescribed level. The line for the prescribed flow rate (e.g., 3 L/min) should be in the middle of the ball of the flow meter (see Figure 43.16).

OXYGEN DELIVERY SYSTEMS Low-flow and high-flow systems are available to deliver O_2 to the client. The choice of system depends on the client's O_2 needs, comfort, and developmental considerations. Low-flow systems deliver O_2 via small-bore tubing. Low-flow administration devices include nasal cannulas, facemasks, O_2 tents, and transtracheal catheters. Because with these types of devices, room air is also inhaled along with the supplemental O_2, the fraction of inspired O_2 (FiO_2) will vary, depending on the respiratory rate, tidal volume, and litre flow. High-flow systems supply all the O_2 required during ventilation in precise amounts, regardless of the client's respirations. The high-flow system used to deliver a precise and consistent FiO_2 is the Venturi mask with large-bore tubing.

Cannula The nasal cannula (nasal prongs) is the most common and inexpensive device used to administer O_2 (Figure 43.18). The nasal cannula is easy to apply and does not interfere with the client's ability to eat or talk. It is relatively comfortable, permits some freedom of movement, and is usually well tolerated by the client. It delivers a relatively low concentration of O_2 (24% to 45%) at flow rates of 2 L to 6 L per minute. At more than 6 L per minute, the client tends to swallow air, and the FiO_2 is *not* increased. Limitations to the cannula include its inability to deliver higher concentrations of O_2 and the fact that it can be drying and irritating to the mucous membranes. Reservoir nasal cannulas store O_2 in a reservoir while the client breathes out and then delivers a 100% O_2 bolus when the client breathes in. As a result, it delivers a higher O_2 concentration at a lower flow rate than the plain nasal cannula because it conserves O_2. The moustache and pendant reservoirs are two styles of reservoir nasal cannula (see Figure 43.18). Humidification is not necessary with the reservoir cannula, because it collects water vapour while the client breathes out and returns it when the client breathes in.

Administering O_2 by cannula is detailed in Skill 43.1.

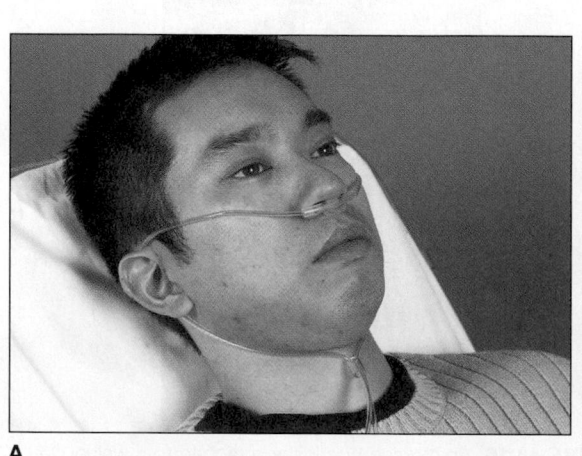
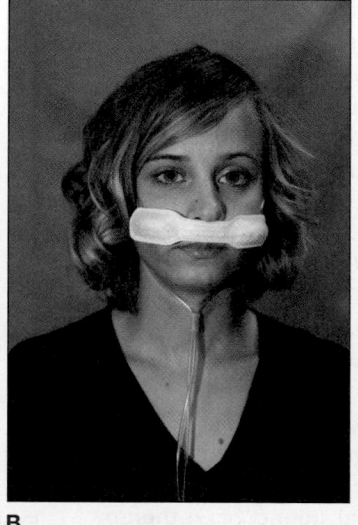
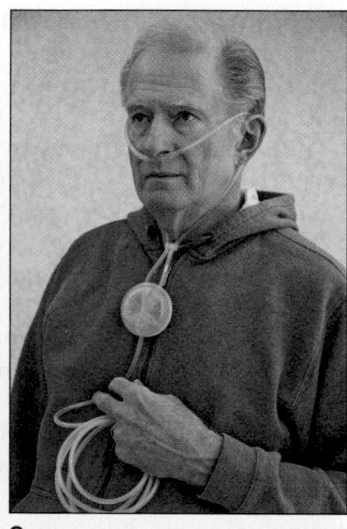

A   B   C

FIGURE 43.18 A: Nasal cannula; **B:** Moustache reservoir nasal cannula; **C:** Pendant reservoir nasal cannula.

SKILL 43.1 ADMINISTERING OXYGEN BY CANNULA, FACEMASK, OR FACE TENT

Before administering O_2, check (a) the prescription for O_2, including the administering device and the litre flow rate (L/min) or the percentage of O_2; (b) the PO_2 and PCO_2 levels in the client's blood (normal arterial values are PaO_2 80 mm Hg to 100 mm Hg; $PaCO_2$ 35 mm Hg to 45 mm Hg); (c) whether the client chronically retains CO_2, such as in COPD; (d) the SaO_2; and (e) the hemoglobin.

PURPOSES

Cannula
- To deliver a relatively low concentration of O_2 when only minimal O_2 support is required
- To allow uninterrupted delivery of O_2 while the client ingests food or fluids

Facemask
- To provide moderate O_2 support and a higher concentration of O_2 or humidity than is provided by cannula

Face Tent
- To provide high humidity
- To provide O_2 when a mask is poorly tolerated
- To provide a high flow of O_2 when attached to a Venturi system

ASSESSMENT

See Chapter 28 for complete details on respiratory and cardiac assessments.

Assess vital signs, with emphasis on pulse rate and quality, and respiratory rate, rhythm, and depth; arterial blood gas levels if available or SpO_2 by pulse oximetry (see Skill 29.7 on page 731); lung sounds; signs of hypoxemia (e.g., tachycardia, tachypnea, restlessness, dyspnea, pallor of mucous membranes, confusion); signs of hypercapnia (e.g., restlessness, headache, lethargy, tremor); patency of nares (if nasal cannula is to be used); signs of O_2 toxicity (e.g., tracheal irritation, cough, decreased pulmonary ventilation).

Equipment

Cannula
- O_2 supply with a flow meter and adapter
- Humidifier with distilled water or tap water, according to agency protocol
- Nasal cannula and tubing
- Padding for the elastic band

Facemask
- O_2 supply with a flow meter and adapter
- Humidifier with sterile distilled or tap water, according to agency policy
- Prescribed facemask of the appropriate size
- Padding for the elastic band

Face Tent
- O_2 supply with a flow meter and adapter
- Humidifier with sterile distilled or tap water, according to agency policy
- Face tent of the appropriate size

IMPLEMENTATION

Preparation

1. Determine the need for O_2 therapy, and verify the prescription for the therapy.
   - In an emergency situation, provide the client with O_2 first before commencing a complete respiratory assessment.
   - Perform a respiratory assessment to determine the need for O_2 therapy and to develop baseline data, if not already available.

2. Prepare the client and the support people.
   - Assist the client to the semi-Fowler's position, if possible. **Rationale: The semi-Fowler's position permits easier chest expansion and, hence, easier breathing**.
   - Explain that O_2 is not dangerous when safety precautions are observed and that it will ease the discomfort of dyspnea. Inform the client and the support people about the safety precautions regarding O_2 use.

Performance

1. Before performing the procedure, introduce yourself and verify the client's identity using two identifiers or per agency protocol. Explain to the client what you are going to do, why it is necessary, and how he or she can participate. Discuss how the effects of the O_2 therapy will be used in planning further care or treatments.

2. Perform hand hygiene, and follow other appropriate infection prevention and control procedures.

3. Provide for client privacy, if appropriate.

4. Set up the O_2 equipment and the humidifier.
   - Attach the flow meter to the wall outlet or tank. The flow meter should be in the "off" position.
   - If needed, fill the humidifier bottle. (This can be done before coming to the bedside.)
   - Attach the humidifier bottle to the base of the flow meter.
   - Attach the prescribed O_2 tubing and delivery device to the humidifier.

5. Turn on the O_2 at the prescribed rate, and ensure proper functioning.
   - Check that the O_2 is flowing freely through the tubing. There should be no kinks in the tubing, and the connections should be airtight. Bubbles should be seen in the humidifier as the O_2 flows through the water and O_2 flow should be felt at the outlets of the cannula, mask, or tent.
   - Set the O_2 at the flow rate prescribed.

6. Apply the appropriate O_2 delivery device.

Cannula
- Put the cannula over the client's face, with the outlet prongs fitting into the nares and the elastic band around the head (see Figure 43.18). Some models have a strap to adjust under the chin.
- If the cannula will not stay in place, tape it at the sides of the face.

(continued)

SKILL 43.1 ADMINISTERING OXYGEN BY CANNULA, FACEMASK, OR FACE TENT (continued)

- Pad the tubing and band over the ears and cheekbones, as needed.

Facemask

- Guide the mask toward the client's face, and apply it from the nose downward.
- Fit the mask to the contours of the client's face (Figure 43.19). **Rationale: The mask should mould to the face so that very little O_2 escapes into the eyes or around the cheeks and chin**.
- Secure the elastic band around the client's head so that the mask is snug but comfortable.
- Pad the band behind the ears and over bony prominences. **Rationale: Padding will prevent irritation from the mask**.

Face Tent

- Place the tent over the client's face, and secure the ties around the head (see Figure 43.23).

7. Assess the client regularly.

- Assess vital signs, level of anxiety, colour, and ease of respirations and provide support while the client adjusts to the therapy.
- Assess the client in 15 to 30 minutes, depending on the client's condition, and regularly thereafter.
- Assess the client regularly for clinical signs of hypoxia (e.g., tachycardia, confusion, dyspnea, restlessness, anxiety). Review O_2 saturation or ABGs, if they are available.

Nasal Cannula

- Assess the client's nares for encrustations and irritation. Apply a water-soluble lubricant, as required, to soothe the mucous membranes.
- Assess the top of the client's ears for any signs of irritation from the cannula strap. If present, padding with a gauze pad may relieve the discomfort.

Facemask or Tent

- Inspect the facial skin frequently for dampness or chafing, and dry and treat it, as needed.

8. Inspect the equipment on a regular basis.

- Check the litre flow and the level of water in the humidifier in 30 minutes and whenever providing care to the client.
- Empty any water that collects in dependent loops of tubing.
- Make sure that safety precautions are being followed.

9. Document relevant data, including when the therapy commenced and the client's response.

EVALUATION

- Perform follow-up based on findings that deviated from expected or normal for the client. Relate findings to previous data, if available (e.g., check SaO_2 or SpO_2 to evaluate adequate oxygenation).
- Report significant deviations from normal to the appropriate members of the health care team.

Facemask Facemasks that cover the client's nose and mouth can be used for O_2 inhalation. Exhalation ports on the sides of the mask allow exhaled CO_2 to escape. A variety of O_2 masks are marketed:

- The *simple facemask* delivers O_2 concentrations from 40% to 60% at litre flows of 5 L/min and 8 L/min, respectively (see Figure 43.19).

- The *partial rebreather mask* delivers oxygen concentrations of 60% to 90% at litre flows of 6 L/min to 10 L/min, depending on client respiratory rate and depth. The O_2 reservoir bag that is attached allows the client to rebreathe about the first third of the exhaled air in conjunction with O_2 (Figure 43.20). Thus, it increases the FiO_2 by recycling expired O_2. The partial rebreather bag must not totally deflate

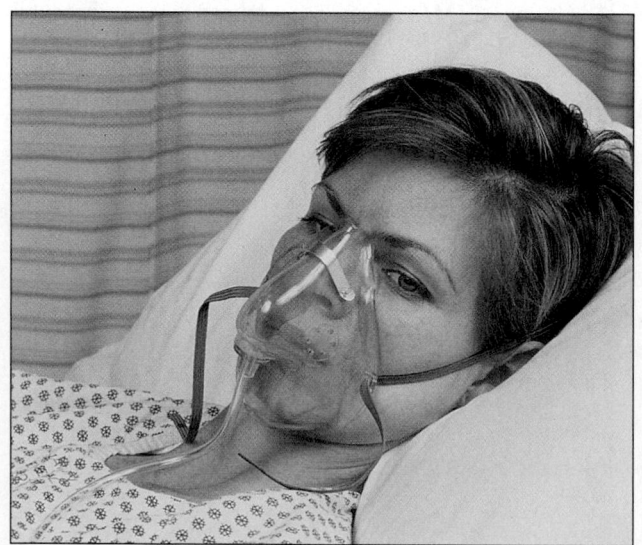

FIGURE 43.19 A simple facemask.

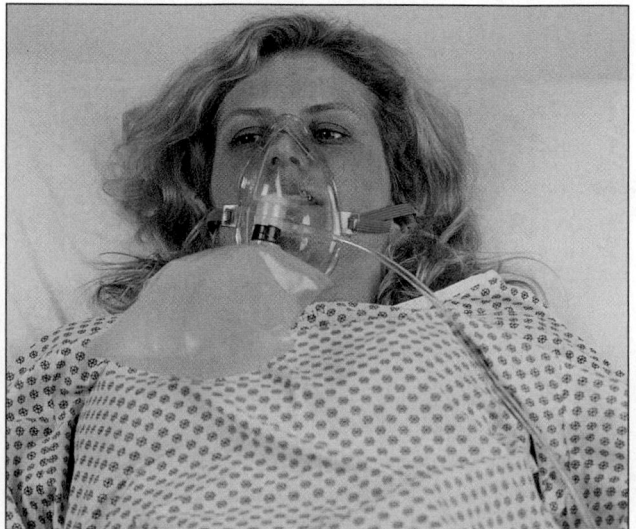

FIGURE 43.20 A partial rebreather mask.

during inspiration to avoid CO_2 buildup. If this problem occurs, the nurse increases the litre flow of O_2.

- The *nonrebreather mask* delivers the highest O_2 concentration possible—that is, 95% to 100%—by means other than intubation or mechanical ventilation, depending on client respiratory rate and depth. One-way valves on the mask and between the reservoir bag and the mask prevent the room air and the client's exhaled air from entering the bag so that only the O_2 in the bag is inspired (Figure 43.21). To prevent CO_2 buildup, the nonrebreather bag must not totally deflate during inspiration. If it does, the nurse can correct this problem by increasing the litre flow of O_2.

- The *Venturi mask* delivers O_2 concentrations varying from 24% to 50% at litre flows of 4 L/min to 10 L/min (Figure 43.22). The Venturi mask has wide-bore tubing and colour-coded jet adapters that correspond to a precise O_2 concentration and litre

flow. For example, one colour-coded adapter delivers a 24% concentration of O_2 at 4 L/min, and another colour-coded adapter delivers a 35% concentration of O_2 at 8 L/min. The Venturi mask can be humidified through room air or additional humidification may be necessary. Follow the manufacturer's directions and agency policy for use of the Venturi mask.

Initiating O_2 by mask is much the same as initiating O_2 by cannula except that the nurse must find a mask of appropriate size. Smaller sizes are available for children. Administering O_2 by mask or face tent is detailed in Skill 43.1 on page 1381. Limitations of masks include difficulty in achieving a proper fit and poor tolerance by some clients who may complain of feeling hot or "smothering."

Face Tent Face tents (Figure 43.23) can replace O_2 masks when masks are poorly tolerated by clients. Face tents provide varying concentrations of O_2, for example, 30% to 50% concentration of O_2 at 4 L/min to 8 L/ min. Frequently inspect the client's facial skin for dampness or chafing, and dry and treat, as needed. As with facemasks, the client's facial skin must be kept dry.

When the client is an infant or a child, an O_2 hood or an O_2 tent (see Figure 43.24 on the next page) can be used. See the Lifespan Considerations box on the next page. The Home Care Considerations box on page 1385 outlines three major oxygen systems for home care use.

Transtracheal Catheter A transtracheal catheter (Figure 43.25) is placed through a surgically created tract in the lower neck directly into the trachea. Once the tract has matured (healed), the client removes and cleans the catheter two to four times per day. Oxygen applied to the catheter at greater than 1 L/min should be humidified. Maximum oxygen flow through a transtracheal catheter is generally limited to 12 L/min and heated humidification is required at flow rates above 5–6 L/min.

Noninvasive Positive Airway Pressure Ventilation (NPPV) In certain circumstances clients require mechanical assistance to maintain adequate breathing. This assistance may

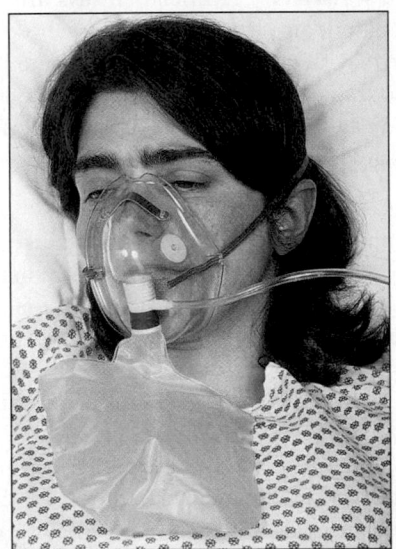

FIGURE 43.21 A nonrebreather mask.

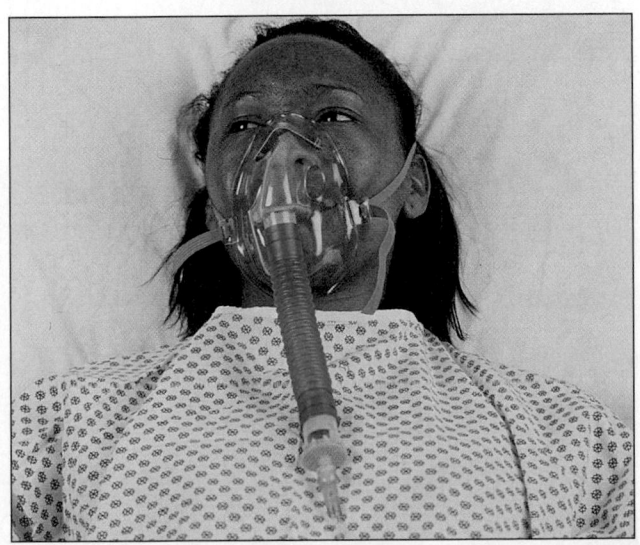

FIGURE 43.22 A venturi mask.

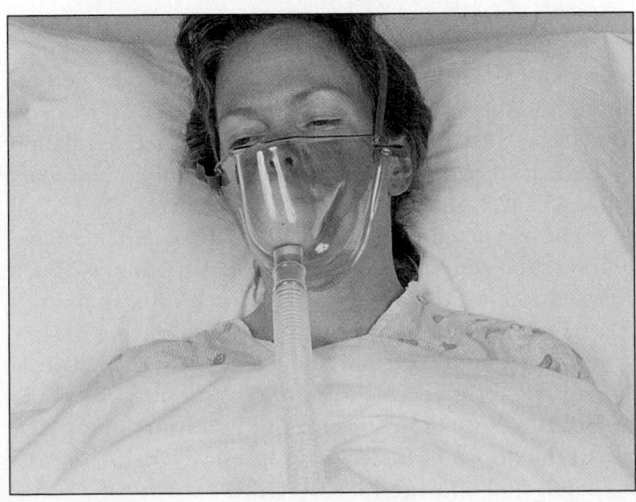

FIGURE 43.23 An oxygen face tent

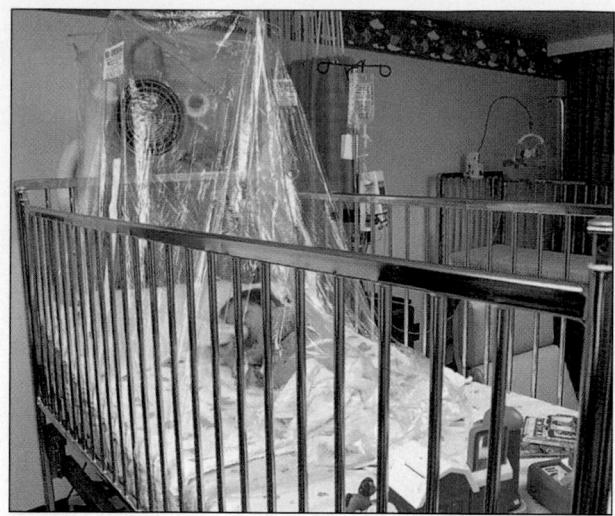

FIGURE 43.24 Pediatric oxygen tent.

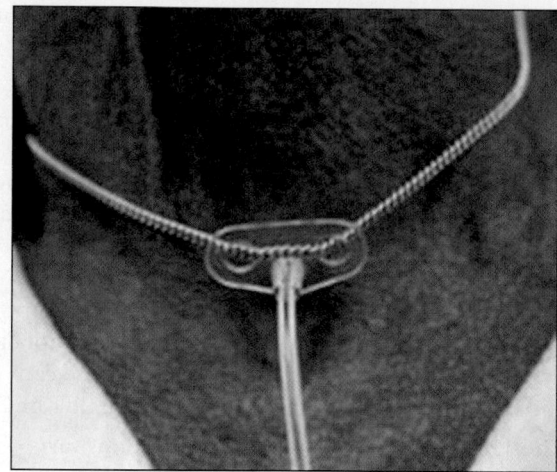

FIGURE 43.25 Transtracheal catheter.

Source: Courtesy of Transtracheal Systems.

ARTIFICIAL AIRWAYS Artificial airways are inserted to maintain a patent air passage for clients whose airway has become or may become obstructed. A patent airway is necessary so that air can flow to and from the lungs. Four of the more common types of airways are oropharyngeal, nasopharyngeal, endotracheal, and tracheostomy.

Oropharyngeal and Nasopharyngeal Airways Oropharyngeal and nasopharyngeal airways are used to keep the upper air passages open when they may become obstructed by secretions or the tongue. These airways are easy to insert and have a low risk of complications. Sizes vary and should be appropriate to the size and age of the client. The airway should be well lubricated with water or water-soluble gel before inserting.

Oropharyngeal airways (Figure 43.29 on page 1386) stimulate the gag reflex and are used only for clients with altered levels of consciousness (e.g., because of general

be accomplished by the use of noninvasive ventilation, the delivery of air or O_2 under pressure without the need for an invasive tube, such as an endotracheal tube or tracheostomy tube. Conditions requiring noninvasive ventilation include acute and chronic respiratory failure, pulmonary edema, COPD, and obstructive sleep apnea (Figure 43.26).

The most common type of NPPV mask and pump system is called **continuous positive airway pressure (CPAP)**. A variation of CPAP is *bilevel positive airway pressure (BiPAP)*, in which the pressure delivered during exhalation is less than the pressure delivered during inhalation. The nurse's primary role in caring for clients using CPAP or BiPAP devices is to ensure optimal functioning and use of the device by the client, as prescribed.

Skill 43.2 on page 1386 describes how to use a CPAP machine.

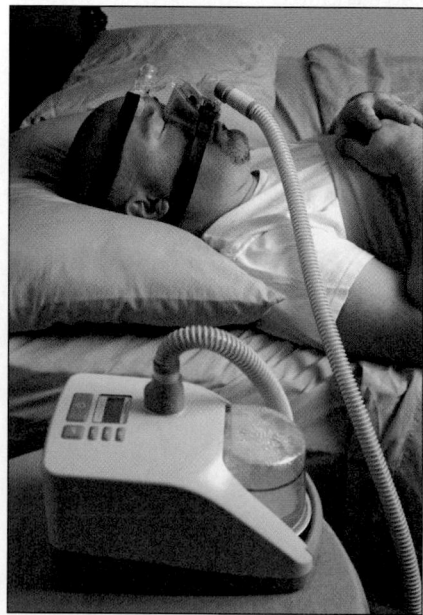

FIGURE 43.26
A continuous positive airway pressure (CPAP) mask is held in place by a headgear, and tubing goes from the mask to the CPAP unit. The CPAP unit is plugged into an electrical outlet and provides a constant flow of air or oxygen to the mask.

HOME CARE CONSIDERATIONS

Oxygen Equipment

Three major oxygen systems for home care use are available in most communities: (a) cylinders or tanks of compressed gas, (b) liquid (cryogenic) oxygen, and (c) oxygen concentrators.

1. *Cylinders ("green tanks"):* Cylinders are the system of choice for clients who need oxygen episodically. Advantages are that cylinders deliver all litre flows (1 L/min to 15 L/min), and O_2 evaporation does not occur during storage. Disadvantages are that the cylinders are heavy and awkward to move, the supply company must be notified when a refill is needed, and they are costly for the high-use client. A size D tank weighs about 3.5 kg and stores 425 L of oxygen; a size E tank holds 680 L and is transported on wheels (Figure 43.27). The gauge on a full tank reads a pressure of at least 2000 pounds per square inch (psi), and a tank is considered empty when it reads less than 500 psi.

2. *Liquid oxygen:* Liquid systems have two parts: (a) a large stationary container and (b) a portable unit with a small lightweight tank that is refilled from the stationary unit. Liquid reservoirs store oxygen at –212°C in a smaller amount of space than for compressed gas. The advantages are that these reservoirs are lighter and cleaner than cylinders, and they are easier to operate. The disadvantages of liquid O_2 are that many home care medical supply and service companies are not able to handle it, O_2 evaporation occurs when the unit is not used, only low flows (1 L/min to 4 L/min) can be used or freezing will occur, and the portable unit designed to be carried over the shoulder weighs 3.5 kg to 4 kg, a possible burden to the typical COPD client (Figure 43.28). A wheeled cart can be used to carry the unit but may be awkward.

3. *Oxygen concentrators:* Concentrators are electrically powered systems that manufacture O_2 from room air. The advantages are that they look better, resembling

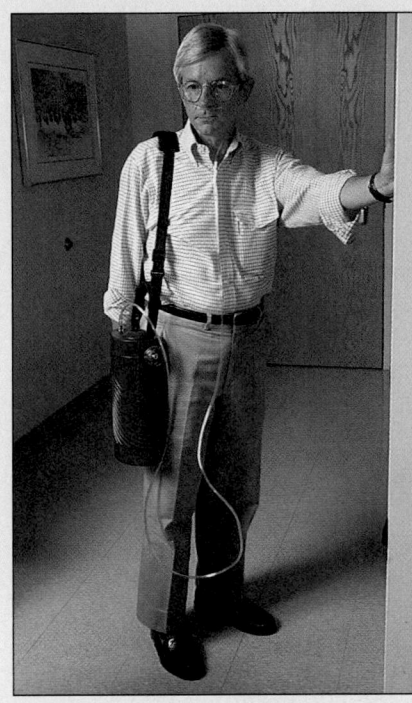

FIGURE 43.28
A portable liquid oxygen supply.

furniture rather than medical equipment; they eliminate the need for regular delivery of O_2 or refilling of cylinders; they alleviate the client's anxiety about running out of O_2 because the supply of O_2 is constant; and they are the most economical system when continuous use is required. The major disadvantages of a concentrator are that it is expensive; lacks real portability (small units weigh 12 kg to 15 kg); tends to be noisy; and is powered by electricity (an emergency backup O_2 tank must be provided for clients for whom a power failure could be life threatening). Further, heat produced by the concentrator motor is a problem for those who live in trailers, small houses, or warm climates where air conditioners are required. The O_2 concentrator must also be checked periodically with an O_2 analyzer to ensure that it is providing an adequate delivery of O_2.

It is important that the client has appropriate help in choosing a reputable home O_2 vendor. Services furnished should include the following:

- Twenty-four-hour emergency service
- Trained personnel to make the initial delivery and instruct the client in safe and appropriate use of the O_2 and maintenance of the equipment
- At least monthly follow-up visits to check the equipment and reinstruct the client, as necessary
- A regular cost review to ensure that the system is the most cost-effective one for that client, with routine notification of the physician or home care professional if it seems that another system is more appropriate

The nurse needs to also ensure that the client knows about the financial reimbursements available from insurance agencies.

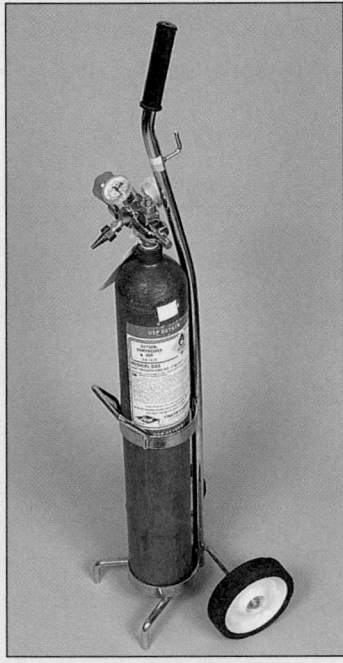

FIGURE 43.27 An E cylinder oxygen tank on a wheeled stand.

SKILL 43.2 ADMINISTERING CONTINUOUS POSITIVE AIRWAY PRESSURE (CPAP)

PURPOSES

- To deliver constant positive pressure air or O_2 in a continuous flow to the upper respiratory airway to keep it open during sleep
- To maintain ventilation during sleep

ASSESSMENT

Assess respiratory status, including ease of breathing, rate, rhythm, depth, and SpO_2 (see Skill 29.7 on page 731) before and during sleep; dry nose, mouth, or throat; nasal congestion; epistaxis (nosebleed); and dry, irritated, or swollen eyes.

PLANNING

- Check the manufacturer's instructions for maintaining the CPAP machine.

Equipment

- Continuous positive airway pressure machine
- Corrugated tubing
- Prescribed face, nasal, or mouth mask of the appropriate size
- Headgear

IMPLEMENTATION

Preparation

1. Before performing the procedure, introduce yourself and verify the client's identity using two identifiers or per agency protocol.
2. Prepare the client.
   - Inform the client of the prescription of CPAP and the

benefits of the intervention.

3. Choose an appropriate secure location close to where the client sleeps to install the CPAP machine. **Rationale: The equipment requires a physical location in proximity to the client and needs to be in a location where it will not fall**.

Performance

1. Perform hand hygiene, and follow other appropriate infection prevention and control procedures.
2. Provide for client privacy, if appropriate.
3. Assess the client's nares for encrustations and irritation. Apply a water-soluble lubricant, as required, to soothe the mucous membranes.
4. Attach the corrugated tubing to the machine.
5. Attach the mask (nasal, mouth, or face) to the corrugated tubing.
6. Connect the headgear to the mask (follow the manufacturer's instructions).
7. Turn on the CPAP machine at the prescribed pressure.
8. Position the headgear and mask on the client.
9. Document the initiation and duration of the therapy and all nursing assessments.

EVALUATION

Perform follow-up based on the client's response to the use of CPAP. For example, was the client comfortable during the night? Did the client experience any adverse outcomes, such as disrupted sleep?

anesthesia, overdose, or head injury). To insert the airway, follow these steps:

- Place the client in the supine or semi-Fowler's position.
- Perform hand hygiene, and follow other appropriate infection prevention and control procedures.

- Put on clean gloves.
- Hold the lubricated airway by the outer flange, with the distal end pointing up.
- Open the client's mouth, and insert the airway along the top of the tongue.

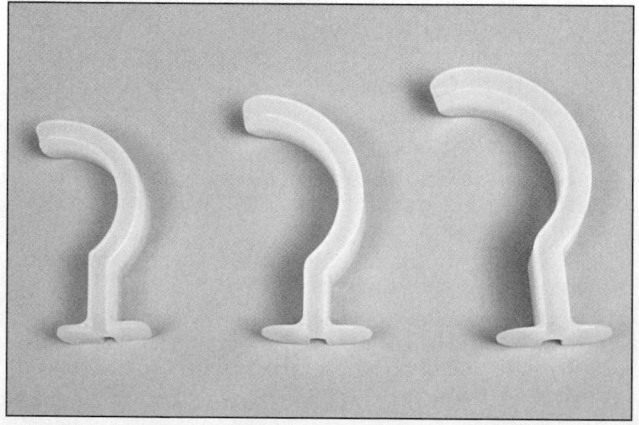
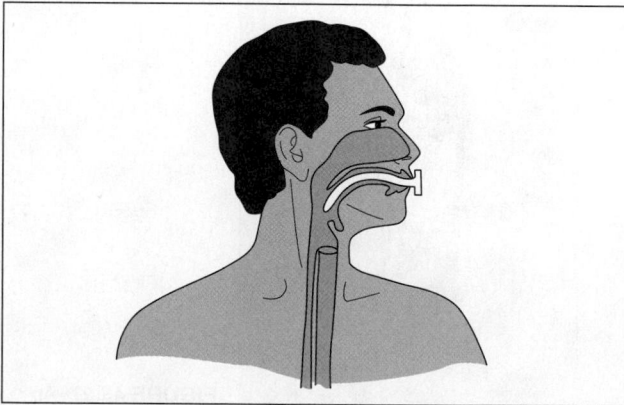

FIGURE 43.29 A: Oropharyngeal airways; **B:** An oropharyngeal airway in place.

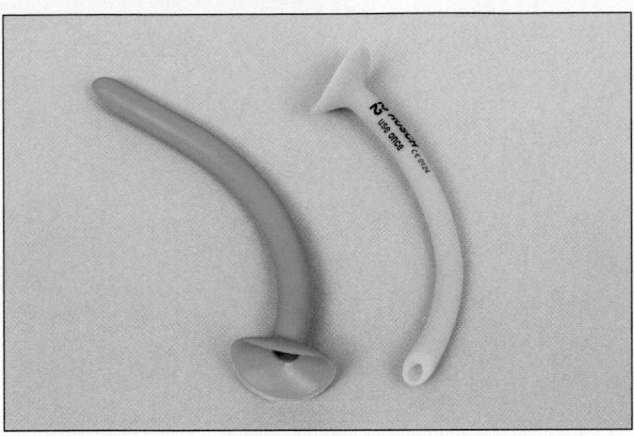

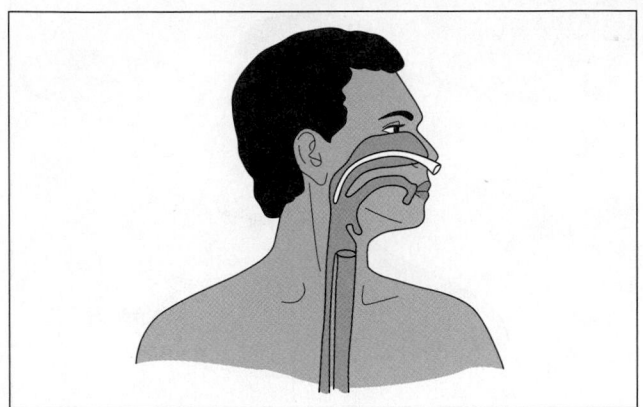

FIGURE 43.30 A: Nasopharyngeal airways; **B:** A nasopharyngeal airway in place.

Source: Berman, Audrey J.; Snyder, Shirlee, *Skills in Clinical Nursing*, 7th Ed., © 2012. Reprinted and Electronically reproduced by permission of Pearson Education, Inc., Upper Saddle River, New Jersey.

- When the distal end of the airway reaches the soft palate at the back of the mouth, rotate the airway 180 degrees downward, and slip it past the uvula into the oral pharynx.
- If not contraindicated, place the client in the side-lying position to allow secretions to drain out of the mouth.
- The oropharynx may be suctioned as needed by inserting the suction catheter alongside the airway.
- Do not tape the airway in place; remove it when the client begins to cough or gag.
- Provide mouth care at least every 2 hours, keeping suction available at the bedside.

As appropriate for the client's condition, remove the airway every 8 hours to assess the mouth and provide oral care. Reinsert the airway immediately.

Nasopharyngeal airways are tolerated better by alert clients. They are inserted through the nares, terminating in the oropharynx (Figure 43.30). When caring for a client with a nasopharyngeal airway, provide frequent oral and nares care, repositioning the airway in the other nare every 8 hours or as ordered to prevent necrosis of the mucosa.

Endotracheal Tubes Endotracheal tubes (Figure 43.31) are most commonly inserted for clients who have had general anesthesia or for those in emergency situations where mechanical ventilation is required. An endotracheal tube can be inserted through either the mouth or the nose and into the trachea with the guide of a laryngoscope by the physician or nurse with specialized education. The tube terminates just superior to the bifurcation of the trachea into the bronchi. The tube may have an air-filled cuff to prevent air leakage around it. Because an endotracheal tube passes through the epiglottis and glottis, the client

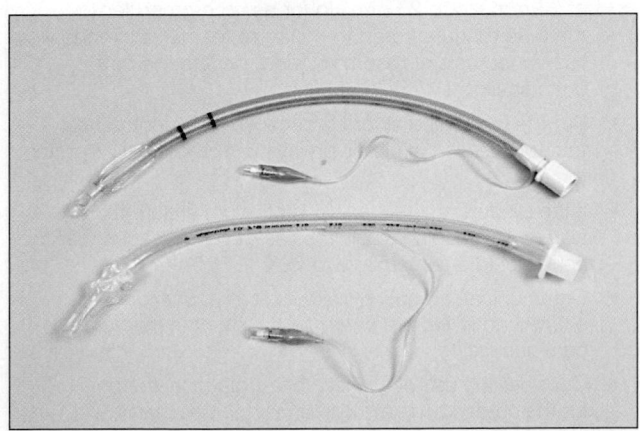

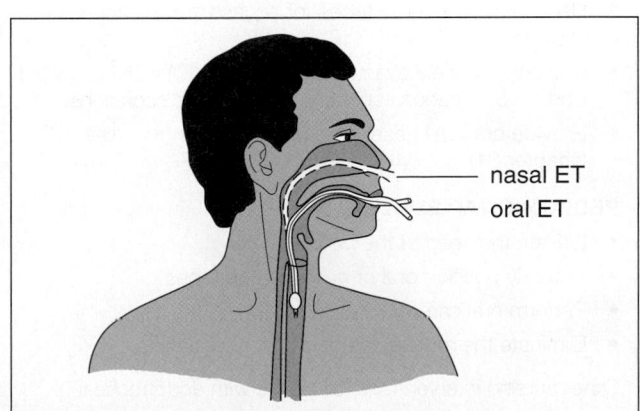

FIGURE 43.31 A: Endotracheal tubes; **B:** An endotracheal tube in place.

Source: Berman, Audrey J.; Snyder, Shirlee, *Skills in Clinical Nursing*, 7th Ed., © 2012. Reprinted and Electronically reproduced by permission of Pearson Education, Inc., Upper Saddle River, New Jersey.

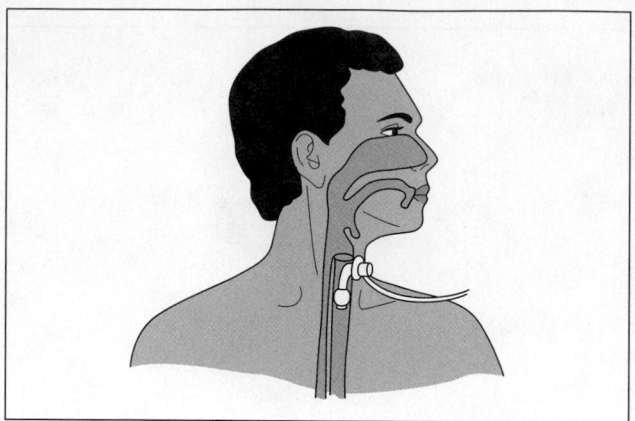

FIGURE 43.32 A tracheostomy tube in place.

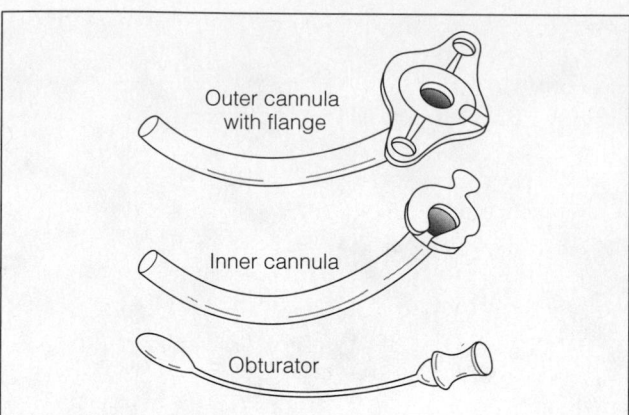

FIGURE 43.33 Components of a tracheostomy tube.

is unable to speak while it is in place. Nursing interventions for clients with endotracheal tubes are shown in Box 43.4.

Tracheostomy   Clients who need long-term airway support may have a **tracheotomy**, a surgical incision in the trachea just below the larynx. A **tracheostomy** is the opening made for the tube itself. A curved tracheostomy tube is inserted to extend through the stoma into the trachea (Figure

43.32). Tracheostomy tubes may be either plastic or metal and are available in different sizes.

Tracheostomy tubes (Figure 43.33) have an outer cannula that is inserted into the trachea and a flange that rests against the neck and allows the tube to be secured in place with tape or ties. All tubes also have an obturator, used to insert the outer cannula and then removed. The obturator is kept at the client's bedside in case the tube becomes dislodged and needs to be reinserted. Some

---

BOX 43.4   NURSING INTERVENTIONS FOR CLIENTS WITH ENDOTRACHEAL TUBES

Ventilator-associated pneumonia (VAP) is the leading cause of death among hospital-acquired infections and substantially increases the likelihood of mortality for ventilated patients. To prevent VAP, Safer Healthcare Now! (2009) makes the following recommendations:

ADULT VAP BUNDLE:
- Elevate the head of the bed between 30 and 45 degrees.
- Temporarily interrupt sedation and conduct a spontaneous breathing trial each day to assess readiness to extubate.
- Use oral versus nasal tubes for access to the trachea or stomach.
- Use endotracheal evacuation tubes (EVAC) with integrated port for continuous aspiration of subglottic secretions.
- Provide oral and nasal care every 2 to 4 hours (see Chapter 31).

PEDIATRIC VAP BUNDLE:
- Elevate the head of the bed.
- Properly position oral or nasal gastric tubes.
- Perform oral care.
- Eliminate the routine use of instil for suctioning.

Other nursing interventions for clients with endotracheal tubes are as follows:
- Assess the client's respiratory status at least every 1 to 2 hours, or more frequently, if indicated. Include respiratory

rate, rhythm, depth, equality of chest excursion, and lung sounds; level of consciousness; and colour of skin and mucous membranes in the assessment.
- Secure the endotracheal tube with tape to prevent accidental movement of the tube further into or out of the trachea. Assess the position of the tube frequently. Notify the physician immediately if the tube is dislodged out of the airway. If the tube advances into a main bronchus, it may need to be slightly withdrawn to ensure ventilation of both lungs.
- Closely monitor cuff pressure, maintaining a pressure of 20 mm Hg to 25 mm Hg (or as recommended by the tube manufacturer) to minimize the risk of tracheal tissue necrosis. If recommended, deflate the cuff periodically.
- Provide humidified air or O_2 because the endotracheal tube bypasses the upper airways, which normally moisten the air.
- If the client is on mechanical ventilation, ensure that all alarms are enabled at all times as the client cannot call for help should an emergency occur.
- Communicate frequently with the client, providing a note pad or picture board for the client to use for communicating.
- Consider the use of a kinetic bed (rotational therapy) for the client who is at highest risk for atelectasis and pneumonia, such as someone who is sedated and requires a resuscitator for more than 3 to 4 days and for whom manual turning and positioning is difficult.

tracheostomy tubes have an inner cannula that can be removed for periodic cleaning.

Cuffed tracheostomy tubes are surrounded by an inflatable cuff that produces an airtight seal between the tube and the trachea. This seal prevents aspiration of oropharyngeal secretions and air leakage between the tube and the trachea. Cuffed tubes are often used immediately after a tracheostomy and are essential when ventilating a tracheostomy client with a mechanical ventilator. Children do not require cuffed tubes because their tracheas are small enough to seal the air space around the tube.

Low-pressure cuffs (Figure 43.34) are commonly used to distribute a low, even pressure against the trachea, thus decreasing the risk of tracheal tissue necrosis. They do not need to be deflated periodically to reduce pressure on the tracheal wall. Foam cuffed tracheostomy tubes do not require injected air; instead, when the port is opened, ambient air enters the balloon, which then conforms to the client's trachea. Air is removed from the cuff before insertion or removal of the tube.

The nurse provides tracheostomy care for the client with a new or recent tracheostomy to maintain patency of the tube and reduce the risk of infection. Initially, a tracheostomy may need to be suctioned (see the section on suctioning that follows) and cleaned as often as

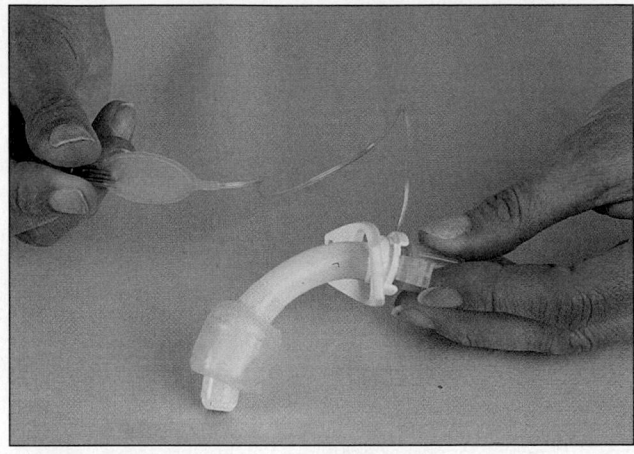

FIGURE 43.34 A tracheostomy tube with a low-pressure cuff.

every 1 to 2 hours. After the initial inflammatory response subsides, tracheostomy care may need to be done only once or twice a day, depending on the client. Skill 43.3 describes tracheostomy care.

When the client breathes through a tracheostomy, air is no longer filtered and humidified as it is when passing through the upper airways; therefore, special precautions are necessary. Humidity can be provided with a

---

SKILL 43.3 PROVIDING TRACHEOSTOMY CARE

PURPOSES
- To maintain airway patency
- To maintain cleanliness and prevent infection at the tracheostomy site
- To facilitate healing and prevent skin excoriation around the tracheostomy incision
- To promote comfort

ASSESSMENT

Assess
- Respiratory status, including ease of breathing, rate, rhythm, depth, lung sounds, and O_2 saturation levels
- Pulse rate, rhythm, and amplitude
- Character and amount of secretions from tracheostomy site
- Presence of drainage on tracheostomy dressing or ties
- Appearance of incision (note any redness, swelling, purulent discharge, or odour)

Equipment
- Sterile disposable tracheostomy cleaning kit or supplies, including sterile containers, sterile nylon brush or pipe cleaners, sterile applicators, gauze squares
- Towel or drape to protect bed linens
- Sterile suction catheter kit (suction catheter and sterile container for solution)

- Sterile normal saline and soaking solution, per agency policy (solutions include normal saline, mixture of equal parts hydrogen peroxide and 0.9% sodium chloride, mixture of equal parts hydrogen peroxide and sterile water)
- Sterile gloves (two pairs—one is for suctioning, if needed)
- Mask and goggles, if required
- Recommended cleaning solution for cannula
- Clean gloves
- Moisture-proof bag
- Sterile tracheostomy dressing
- Cotton twill ties or Velcro collar
- Clean scissors

IMPLEMENTATION

Performance
1. Before performing the procedure, introduce yourself and verify the client's identity using two identifiers or per agency protocol. Explain to the client what you are going to do, why it is necessary, and how he or she can participate. Provide for a means of communication, such as eye blinking or raising a finger, to indicate pain or distress. Follow through by carefully observing the client throughout the procedure, offering periodic eye contact, caring touch, and verbal assurance.
2. Perform hand hygiene, and follow other appropriate infection prevention and control procedures.
3. Provide for client privacy.

(continued)

SKILL 43.3 PROVIDING TRACHEOSTOMY CARE (continued)

4. Prepare the client and the equipment.
   - Assist the client to the semi-Fowler's or Fowler's position. **Rationale: These positions promote lung expansion.**
   - Suction the tracheostomy tube, if necessary (see Skill 43.5 on page 1396). If required, allow the client to rest and restore O₂.
   - Open the tracheostomy kit or sterile basins.
   - Establish a sterile field.
   - Open other sterile supplies, as needed, including sterile applicators, suction kit, tracheostomy dressing, and disposable inner cannula, if applicable. Pour the recommended cleaning solution into containers.
   - Put on clean gloves.
   - Remove the O₂ source (if applicable).
   - Using the gloved hand, unlock the inner cannula (if present) and remove it by gently pulling it out toward you in line with its curvature. Place the inner cannula in the soaking solution. **Rationale: The solution moistens and loosens dried secretions.**
   - Remove the soiled tracheostomy dressing. Place the soiled dressing in your gloved hand and peel the glove off so that it turns inside out over the dressing. Discard the glove and the dressing.
   - Put on sterile gloves. Keep your dominant hand sterile during the procedure.

5. Clean the inner cannula (see Variation for using a disposable cannula).
   - Remove the inner cannula from the soaking solution.
   - Clean the lumen and entire inner cannula thoroughly by using the brush or pipe cleaners moistened with sterile normal saline (some agencies use hydrogen peroxide) (see ❶). Inspect the cannula for cleanliness by holding it at eye level and looking through it into the light.
   - Rinse the inner cannula thoroughly in sterile normal saline—some agencies soak the cannula in alcohol for 30 minutes prior to rinsing; proceed per agency protocol. **Rationale: Thorough rinsing is important to remove the soaking or cleaning solution from the inner cannula.**

   - After rinsing, gently tap the cannula against the inside edge of the sterile saline container. Use a pipe cleaner folded in half to dry only the inside of the cannula; do not dry the outside. **Rationale: Drying removes excess liquid from the cannula and prevents possible aspiration by the client while leaving a film of moisture on the outer surface to lubricate the cannula for reinsertion.**

6. Replace the inner cannula, securing it in place.
   - Insert the inner cannula by grasping the outer flange and inserting the cannula in the direction of its curvature.
   - Lock the cannula in place by turning the lock (if present) into position to secure the flange of the inner cannula to the outer cannula.

7. Clean the incision site and tube flange.
   - Using sterile applicators or premanufactured specific tracheostomy-sponge dressings moistened with a normal saline, clean the incision site (see ❷). Use each applicator or gauze dressing only once and then discard it. **Rationale: This measure avoids contaminating a clean area with a soiled gauze dressing or applicator.**
   - Thoroughly rinse the cleaned area by using gauze squares moistened with sterile normal saline (check agency policy, as some may use different solutions; half-strength hydrogen peroxide has been used in the past, however, it can be irritating to the skin if not thoroughly removed).
   - Clean the flange of the tube in the same manner.
   - Thoroughly dry the client's skin and tube flanges with dry gauze squares.

8. Apply a sterile tracheostomy dressing.
   - Place the dressing under the flange of the tracheostomy tube as shown in ❸.
   - While applying the dressing, ensure that the tracheostomy tube is securely supported. **Rationale: Excessive movement of the tracheostomy tube irritates the trachea.**

9. Change the tracheostomy ties or Velcro collar.
   - Change, as needed, to keep the skin clean and dry.

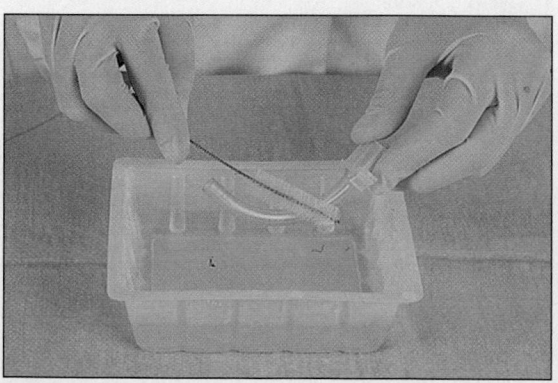

❶ Cleaning the inner cannula with a brush.

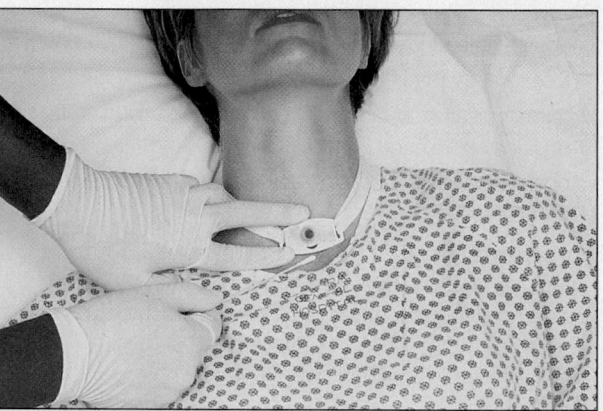

❷ Using an applicator stick to clean the tracheostomy site.

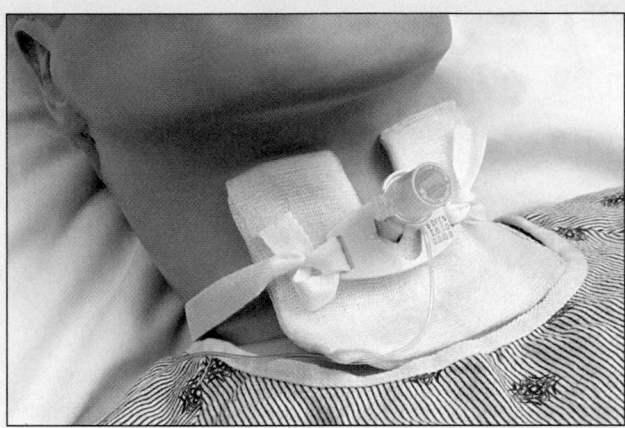

❸ A tracheostomy dressing placed under the flange of the tracheostomy tube.

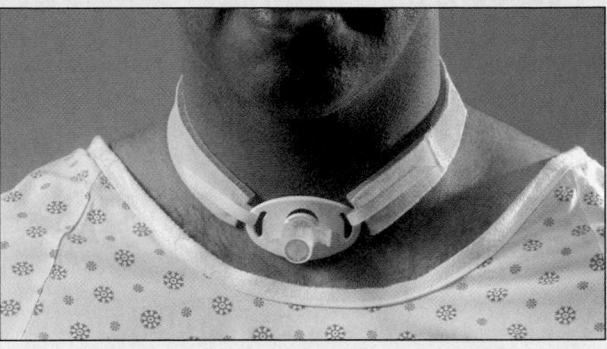

❹ A Velcro tracheostomy tie.

- Twill tape and specially manufactured Velcro ties are available. Twill tape is inexpensive and readily available, however, it is easily soiled and can trap moisture that leads to irritation of the skin of the neck. Velcro ties are becoming more commonly used (see ❹). They are wider and more comfortable and cause less skin abrasion.

Two-Strip Method

- Cut two unequal strips of twill tape, one approximately 25 cm long and the other about 50 cm long. **Rationale: Cutting one tape longer than the other allows them to be fastened at the side of the neck for easy access and to avoid the pressure of a knot on the skin at the back of the neck**.

- Cut a 1-cm lengthwise slit approximately 2.5 cm from one end of each strip. To do this, fold the end of the tape back onto itself about 2.5 cm, and then cut a slit in the middle of the tape from its folded edge.

- Leaving the old ties in place, thread the slit end of one clean tape through the eye of the tracheostomy flange from the bottom side; then thread the long end of the tape through the slit, pulling it taut until it is securely fastened to the flange. **Rationale: Leaving the old ties in place while securing the clean ties prevents inadvertent dislodging of the tracheostomy tube. Securing tapes in this manner avoids the use of knots, which can come untied or cause pressure and irritation**.

- If the old ties are very soiled or if it is difficult to thread new ties onto the tracheostomy flange with old ties in place, have an assistant don a sterile glove and hold the tracheostomy in place while you replace the ties. This is very important because movement of the tube during this procedure can cause irritation and stimulate coughing. Coughing can dislodge the tube if the ties are undone.

- Repeat the process for the second tie.

- Ask the client to flex the neck. Slip the longer tape under the client's neck, place a finger between the tape and the client's neck (see ❺), and tie the tapes together at the side of the neck. **Rationale: Flexing the neck increases its circumference the way coughing does. Placing a finger under the ties prevents making the ties too tight, which could interfere with coughing or place pressure on the jugular veins**.

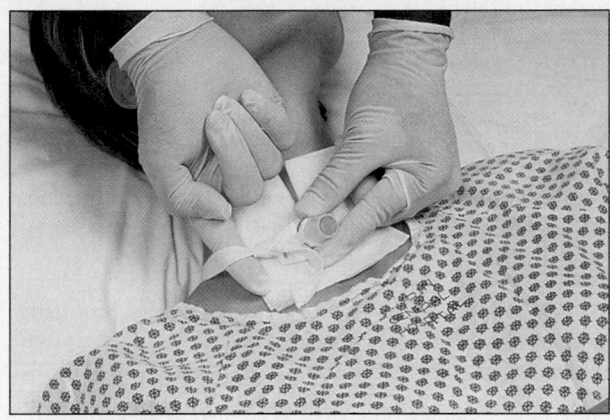

❺ Placing a finger underneath the tie tape before tying it.

- Tie the ends of the tapes by using square knots. Cut off any long ends, leaving approximately 1 cm to 2 cm. **Rationale: Square knots prevent slippage and loosening. Adequate ends beyond the knot prevent the knot from inadvertently untying**.

- Once the clean ties are secured, remove the soiled ties and discard.

Velcro Collar Method

- Thread one piece of the collar with the Velcro end into the slot on one side of the flange.

- Take the collar around the back of the client's neck, keeping it flat.

- Thread the other piece of the collar with the Velcro end into the slot on the other side of the flange.

- Take the second piece of the collar around the back of the client's neck, keeping it flat.

- Have the client flex the neck and secure the two pieces of the collar together with the Velcro, allowing space for two fingers between the collar and the client's neck.

- Check the tightness of the collar as with the tie method.

10. Remove and discard sterile gloves. Perform hand hygiene.

11. Document all relevant information.
    - Record suctioning, tracheostomy care, and the dressing change, noting your assessments.

(continued)

SKILL 43.3 PROVIDING TRACHEOSTOMY CARE (*continued*)

Variation: Using a Disposable Inner Cannula

- Check policy for frequency of changing inner cannula, because standards vary among institutions.
- Open a new cannula package.
- Using a gloved hand, unlock the current inner cannula (if present) and remove it by gently pulling it out toward you in line with its curvature.

- Check the cannula for amount and type of secretions, and discard properly.
- Pick up the new inner cannula, touching only the outer locking portion.
- Insert the new inner cannula into the tracheostomy.
- Lock the cannula in place by turning the lock (if present) or clipping in place.

EVALUATION

- Perform appropriate follow-up, such as determining character and amount of secretions, drainage from the tracheostomy, appearance of the tracheostomy incision, pulse rate, respiratory status compared with baseline data, and complaints of pain or discomfort at the tracheostomy site.

- Relate findings to previous assessment data, if available.
- Report significant deviations from normal to the appropriate members of the health care team.

---

mist collar (Figure 43.35). Clients with long-term tracheostomies can wear a light scarf or a gauze held in place with a cotton tie over the stoma to filter air as it enters the tracheostomy.

SUCTIONING When clients have difficulty handling their secretions or an airway is in place, suctioning may be necessary to clear air passages. **Suctioning** refers to the aspiration of secretions through a catheter connected to a suction machine or wall suction outlet. Even though the oropharynx and nasopharynx are not sterile, sterile technique is recommended for all suctioning to avoid introducing pathogens.

Suction catheters are either open tipped or whistle tipped (Figure 43.36). The whistle-tipped catheter is less irritating to respiratory tissues, although the open-tipped catheter may be more effective for removing thick mucous plugs. An oral suction tube, or Yankauer device,

is used to suction the oral cavity (Figure 43.37). Most suction catheters have a thumb port on the side to control the suction. The catheter is connected to suction tubing, which, in turn, is connected to a collection chamber and suction control gauge (Figure 43.38).

The nurse decides when suctioning is needed by assessing the client for signs of respiratory distress or

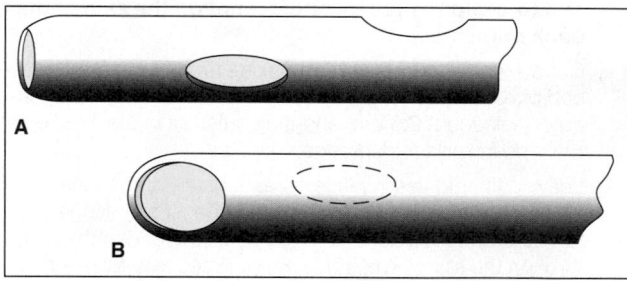

FIGURE 43.36 Types of suction catheters: **A:** Open tipped; **B:** Whistle tipped.

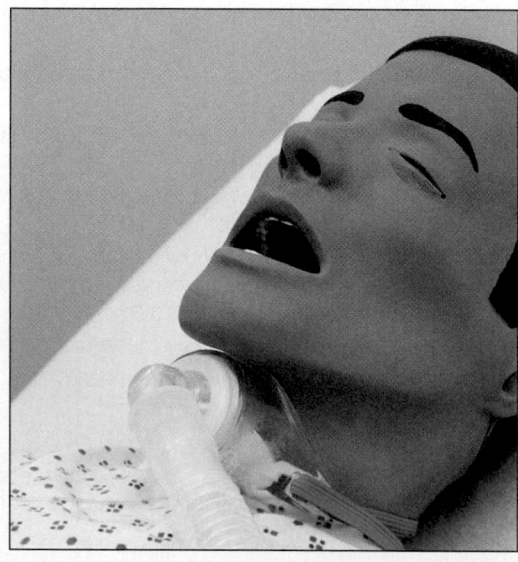

FIGURE 43.35 A tracheostomy mist collar.

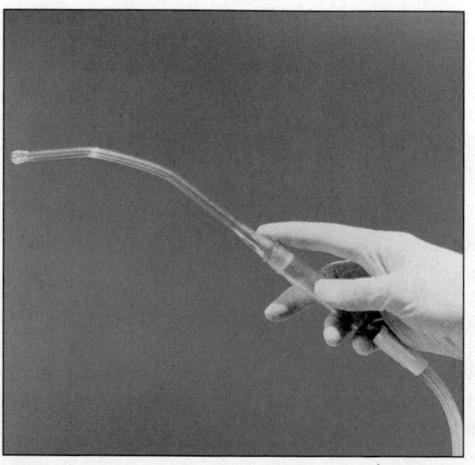

FIGURE 43.37 Oral (Yankauer) suction tube.

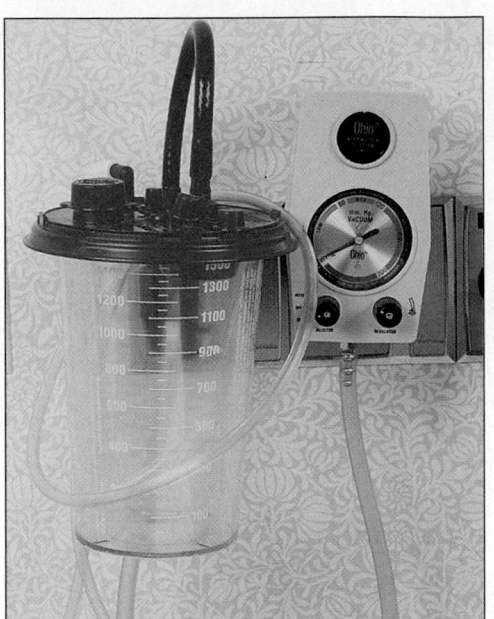

FIGURE 43.38 A wall suction unit.

evidence that the client is unable to cough up and expectorate secretions. Dyspnea, bubbling or rattling breath sounds, poor skin colour or cyanosis, or decreased SaO_2 may indicate the need for suctioning. Accurate nursing judgment is necessary, because suctioning irritates mucous membranes and can increase secretions if performed too frequently. In other words, suctioning is based on clinical need, not a fixed schedule.

Oral and nasopharyngeal suctioning removes secretions from the upper respiratory tract. Nasopharyngeal and nasotracheal suctioning provide closer access to the trachea and require sterile technique. Skill 43.4 outlines oropharyngeal and nasopharyngeal suctioning.

Following endotracheal intubation or a tracheotomy, the trachea and surrounding respiratory tissues are irritated and react by producing excessive secretions. Sterile suctioning is necessary to remove these secretions and maintain a patent airway. The frequency of suctioning depends on the client's assessment data and how recently the intubation was done. Additionally, suctioning may be necessary in clients who have increased secretions

SKILL 43.4   OROPHARYNGEAL, NASOPHARYNGEAL, AND NASOTRACHEAL SUCTIONING

PURPOSES

- To remove secretions that obstruct the airway
- To facilitate ventilation
- To obtain secretions for diagnostic purposes
- To prevent infection that may result from accumulated secretions

ASSESSMENT

Assess for clinical signs indicating the need for suctioning:

- Restlessness
- Gurgling sounds during respiration
- Adventitious breath sounds when the chest is auscultated
- Change in mental status
- Colour of skin and mucous membranes
- Rate and pattern of respirations
- Pulse rate and rhythm
- Decreased oxygen saturation

Equipment

Oral and Nasopharyngeal or Nasotracheal Suctioning

- Towel or moisture-resistant pad
- Portable or wall suction machine with tubing and collection receptacle
- Sterile disposable container for fluids
- Sterile normal saline or water
- Goggles or face shield, if appropriate
- Moisture-resistant disposal bag
- Sputum trap, if specimen is to be collected

Oral and Oropharyngeal Suctioning

- Yankauer suction catheter or suction catheter kit
- Clean gloves

Nasopharyngeal or Nasotracheal Suctioning

- Sterile gloves and clean gloves
- Sterile suction catheter kit (12–18 Fr for adults; 8–10 Fr for children, and 5–8 Fr for infants)
- Water-soluble lubricant
- Y-connector

IMPLEMENTATION

Performance

1. Before performing the procedure, introduce yourself and verify the client's identity using two identifiers or per agency protocol. Explain to the client what you are going to do, why it is necessary, and how he or she can participate. Inform the client that suctioning will relieve breathing difficulty and that the procedure is painless but may be uncomfortable and stimulate the cough, gag, or sneeze reflex. **Rationale: Knowing that the procedure will relieve breathing problems is often reassuring and enlists the client's cooperation**.

2. Perform hand hygiene, and follow other appropriate infection prevention and control procedures.

3. Provide for client privacy.

4. Prepare the client.

   - Position a *conscious* person who has a functional gag reflex in the semi-Fowler's position with the head turned to one side for oral suctioning or with the neck hyperextended for nasal suctioning. **Rationale: The semi-Fowler's position facilitates the insertion of the catheter and helps prevent aspiration of secretions**.

(continued)

SKILL 43.4 OROPHARYNGEAL, NASOPHARYNGEAL, AND NASOTRACHEAL SUCTIONING (*continued*)

- Position an *unconscious* client in the lateral position, facing you. **Rationale: The lateral position allows the tongue to fall forward so that it will not obstruct the catheter on insertion. This position also facilitates drainage of secretions from the pharynx and prevents the possibility of aspiration**.
- Place the towel or moisture-resistant pad over the pillow or under the chin.

5. Prepare the equipment.
   - Turn the suction device on and set to appropriate negative pressure on the suction gauge. The amount of pressure should be high enough to clear secretions but not too high. **Rationale: Too high a pressure can cause the catheter to adhere to the tracheal wall and cause irritation or trauma.** Use the lowest amount of suction pressure needed to clear the secretions. The following are generally accepted ranges: adult: 80 mm Hg to 120 mm Hg; child: 95 mm Hg to 110 mm Hg; infant: 50 mm Hg to 95 mm Hg.

Oral and Oropharyngeal Suctioning

- Put on clean gloves.
- Moisten the tip of the Yankauer or suction catheter with sterile water or saline. **Rationale: This measure reduces friction and eases insertion**.
- Pull the client's tongue forward, if necessary, using gauze.
- Do not apply suction (that is, leave your finger off the port) during insertion. **Rationale: Applying suction during insertion causes trauma to the mucous membrane**.
- Advance the catheter about 10 cm to 15 cm along one side of the mouth into the oropharynx. **Rationale: Directing the catheter along the side prevents gagging**.
- It may be necessary during oropharyngeal suctioning to apply suction to secretions that collect in the vestibule of the mouth and beneath the tongue.

Nasopharyngeal and Nasotracheal Suctioning

- Open the lubricant if performing nasopharyngeal or nasotracheal suctioning.
- Open the sterile suction package.
   a. Set up the cup or container, touching only the outside.
   b. Pour sterile water or saline into the container.
   c. Put on the sterile gloves, or put a clean glove on the nondominant hand and then a sterile glove on the dominant hand. **Rationale: The sterile gloved hand maintains the sterility of the suction catheter, and the clean glove prevents the transmission of microorganisms to the nurse**.
- With your sterile gloved hand, pick up the catheter and attach it to the suction unit (see ❶). If needed, apply or increase supplemental oxygen.

6. Test the pressure of the suction and the patency of the catheter by applying your sterile gloved finger or thumb to the port or open branch of the Y-connector (the suction control) to create suction.

7. Lubricate and introduce the catheter.
   - Lubricate the catheter tip with sterile water, saline, or water-soluble lubricant. **Rationale: This measure reduces friction and eases insertion**.

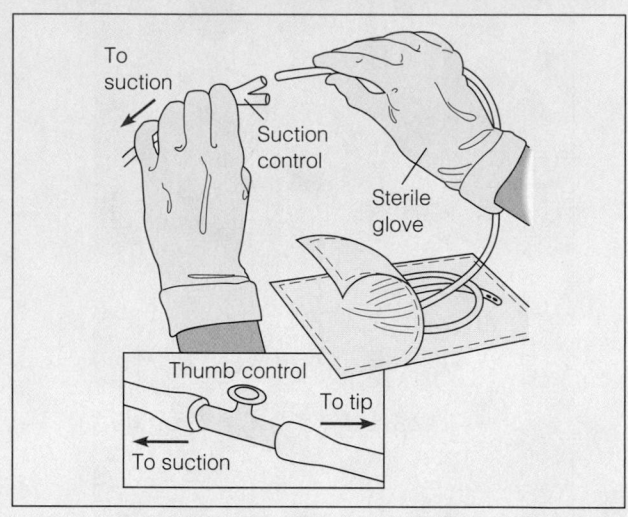

❶ Attaching the catheter to the suction unit.

- Remove the O_2 device with nondominant hand, if appropriate.
- *Without applying suction,* insert the catheter the premeasured or recommended distance into either nares, and advance it along the floor of the nasal cavity. **Rationale: Doing this avoids the nasal turbinates**.
- Never force the catheter against an obstruction. If one nostril is obstructed, try the other.

8. Perform suctioning.
   - Apply your finger to the suction control port to start suction, and gently rotate the catheter. **Rationale: Gentle rotation of the catheter ensures that all surfaces are reached and prevents trauma to any one area of the respiratory mucosa because of prolonged suction**.
   - Apply intermittent suction for 5 to 10 seconds while slowly withdrawing the catheter, then remove your finger from the control, and remove the catheter.
   - A suction attempt should last only 10 to 15 seconds. During this time, the catheter is inserted, the suction applied and discontinued, and the catheter removed.

9. Rinse the catheter, and repeat suctioning as above.
   - Rinse and flush the catheter with sterile water or saline.
   - Relubricate the catheter, and repeat suctioning until the air passage is clear.
   - Allow 30-second to 1-minute intervals between each suction, and limit suction attempts to two or three times. Assess cardiopulmonary status between each suctioning attempt. **Rationale: Applying suction for too long may cause secretions to increase or may decrease the client's oxygen supply**.
   - Encourage the client to breathe deeply and to cough between suctions. Use supplemental O_2, if appropriate. **Rationale: Coughing and deep breathing help carry secretions from the trachea and bronchi into the pharynx, where they can be reached with the suction catheter. Deep**

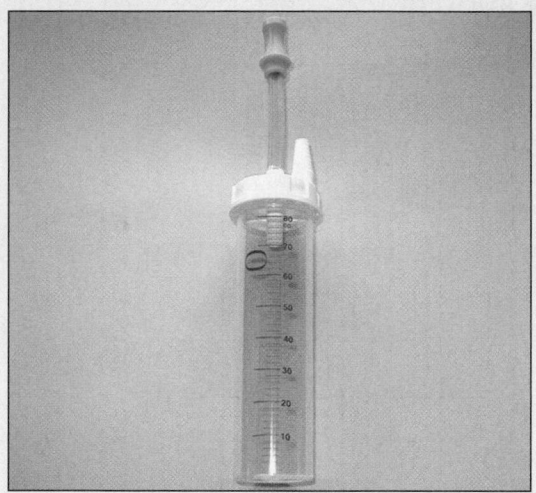

❷ A sputum collection trap.

breathing and supplemental O₂ provide O₂ to the alveoli.

10. Obtain a specimen, if required. Use a sputum trap (see ❷) as follows:
    - Attach the suction catheter to the rubber tubing of the sputum trap.
    - Attach the suction tubing to the sputum trap air vent.
    - Suction the client's nasopharynx or oropharynx. The sputum trap will collect the mucus during suctioning.
    - Remove the catheter from the client. Disconnect the sputum trap rubber tubing from the suction catheter.
    - Remove the suction tubing from the trap air vent.
    - Connect the rubber tubing of the sputum trap to the air vent. **Rationale: This helps retain any microorganisms in the sputum trap**.
    - Connect the suction catheter to the tubing.
    - Flush the catheter to remove secretions from the tubing.

11. Promote client comfort.
    - Offer to assist the client with oral or nasal hygiene.
    - Assist the client to a position that facilitates breathing.

12. Dispose of equipment and ensure availability for the next suction.
    - Dispose of the catheter, gloves, water, and waste container. Wrap the catheter around your sterile gloved hand, holding it as the glove is removed over it for disposal.
    - Rinse the suction tubing, as needed, by inserting the end of the tubing into the water container. Empty and rinse the suction collection container, as needed or indicated by protocol. Change the suction tubing and container at least daily.
    - Ensure that supplies are available for the next suctioning (suction kit, gloves, water or normal saline).

13. Assess the effectiveness of suctioning.
    - Auscultate the client's breath sounds to ensure they are clear of secretions. Observe the client's skin colour and mucous membranes, dyspnea, level of anxiety, vital signs, and O₂ saturation level.

14. Document relevant data.
    - Record the procedure: the amount, consistency, colour, and odour of sputum; the number of suctioning attempts; and the client's breathing status before, during, and after the procedure. This may include lung sounds, rate and character of breathing, and O₂ saturation.

EVALUATION

- Conduct appropriate follow-up, such as appearance of secretions suctioned; breath sounds; respiratory rate, rhythm, and depth; pulse rate and rhythm; and skin colour.
- Compare findings with previous assessment data, if available.
- Report significant deviations from normal to the appropriate members of the health care team.

because of pneumonia or an inability to clear secretions because of an altered level of consciousness.

Suctioning is associated with several complications: hypoxemia, trauma to the airway, health care–associated infection, and cardiac dysrhythmias, which are related to the hypoxemia. Techniques to minimize or decrease these complications include the following (according to agency policy):

- *Hyperinflation*. This involves giving the client breaths that are 1 to 1.5 times the tidal volume set on the ventilator through the ventilator circuit or via a manual resuscitation bag. Three to five breaths are delivered before and after each pass of the suction catheter.

- *Hyperoxygenation*. This can be done with a manual resuscitation bag or through the ventilator and is performed by increasing the oxygen flow (usually

to 100%) before suctioning and between suction attempts.

For tracheostomy and endotracheal suctioning, the diameter of the suction catheter should be about half the inside diameter of the tracheostomy or endotracheal tube so that hypoxia can be prevented. The nurse uses sterile techniques to prevent infection of the respiratory tract (see Skill 43.5 on the next page). The traditional method of suctioning an endotracheal tube or tracheostomy is sometimes referred to as the *open method*. If a client is connected to a ventilator, the nurse disconnects the client from the ventilator, suctions the airway, reconnects the client to the ventilator, and discards the suction catheter. Drawbacks to the open airway suction system include the nurse needing to wear personal protective equipment (e.g., goggles or face shield, gown) to avoid exposure to the client's sputum

SKILL 43.5 SUCTIONING A TRACHEOSTOMY OR ENDOTRACHEAL TUBE

PURPOSES

- To maintain a patent airway and prevent airway obstructions
- To promote respiratory function (optimal exchange of O_2 and CO_2 into and out of the lungs)
- To prevent pneumonia that may result from accumulated secretions

ASSESSMENT

Assess the client for the presence of congestion on auscultation of the thorax. Note if the client is unable to remove the secretions through coughing.

Equipment

- Resuscitation bag (Ambu bag) connected to 100% O_2
- Sterile towel (optional)
- Equipment for suctioning the oropharyngeal cavity (see Skill 43.4 on page 1393)
- Goggles and mask, if necessary
- Gown, if necessary
- Sterile gloves
- Moisture-resistant bag

IMPLEMENTATION

Performance

1. Before performing the procedure, introduce yourself and verify the client's identity using two identifiers or per agency protocol. Explain to the client what you are going to do, why it is necessary, and how he or she can participate. Inform the client that suctioning usually causes some intermittent coughing and that this assists in removing secretions.

2. Perform hand hygiene, and follow other appropriate infection prevention and control procedures.

3. Provide for client privacy.

4. Prepare the client.
   - If not contraindicated, place the client in the semi-Fowler's position to promote deep breathing, maximum lung expansion, and productive coughing. **Rationale: Deep breathing oxygenates the lungs, counteracts the hypoxic effects of suctioning, and may induce coughing. Coughing helps loosen and move secretions**.
   - If necessary, provide analgesia as ordered by the physician before suctioning. **Rationale: Premedication can increase the client's comfort during the suctioning procedure**.

5. Prepare the equipment. Attach the resuscitation apparatus to the O_2 source (see ❶). Adjust the O_2 flow to 100%.
   - Open the sterile supplies in readiness for use.
   - Place the sterile towel, if used, across the client's chest below the tracheostomy.
   - Turn on the suction, and set the pressure in accordance with agency policy. For a wall unit, a pressure setting between 80 and 120 mm Hg is normally used for adults, 60 to 100 mm Hg for children.
   - Put on goggles, mask, and gown, if necessary.
   - Put on sterile gloves.

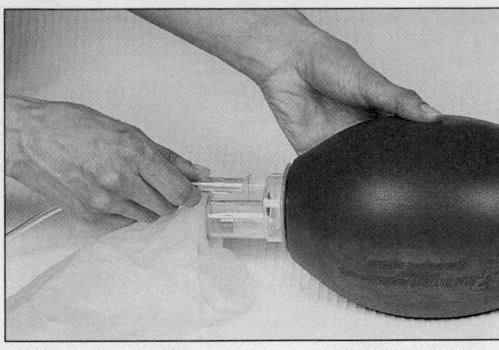

❶ Attaching the resuscitation apparatus to the oxygen source.

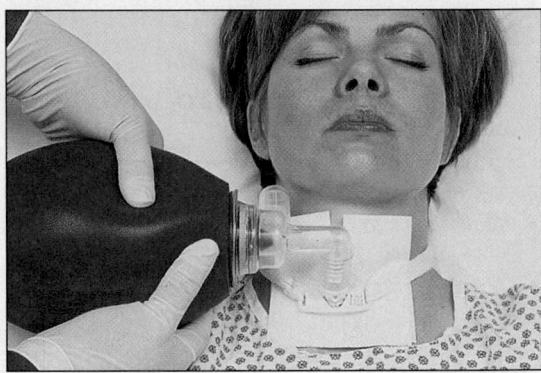

❷ Attaching the resuscitator to the tracheostomy.

   - Holding the catheter in the dominant hand and the connector in the nondominant hand, attach the suction catheter to the suction tubing (see Skill 43.4, ❶).

6. Flush and lubricate the catheter.
   - Using the dominant hand, place the catheter tip in the sterile saline solution.
   - Using the thumb of the nondominant hand, occlude the thumb control and suction a small amount of the sterile solution through the catheter. **Rationale: This determines that the suction equipment is working properly and lubricates the outside and the lumen of the catheter. Lubrication eases insertion and reduces tissue trauma during insertion. Lubricating the lumen also helps prevent secretions from sticking to the inside of the catheter**.

7. If the client does not have copious secretions, hyperventilate the lungs with a resuscitation bag before suctioning, as ordered by a physician and according to agency policy.
   - Summon an assistant, if one is available, for this step.
   - Using your nondominant hand, turn on the O_2 to 12 L/min to 15 L/min.
   - If the client is receiving O_2, disconnect the oxygen source from the tracheostomy tube by using your nondominant hand.
   - Attach the resuscitator to the tracheostomy or endotracheal tube (see ❷).
   - Compress the Ambu bag three to five times as the client *inhales*. This is best done by a second person

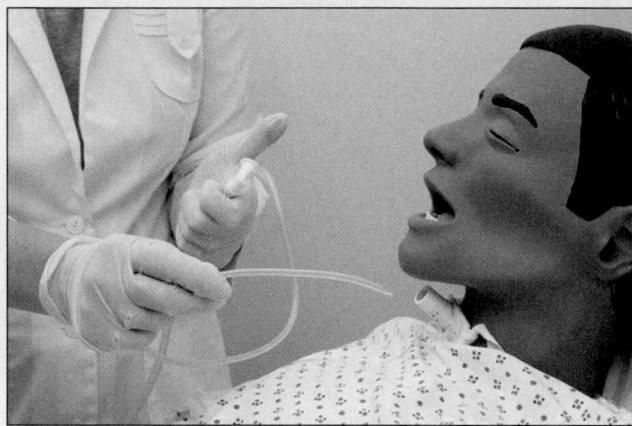

③ Inserting the catheter into the trachea through the tracheostomy tube. *Note:* Suction is not applied *while* inserting the catheter.

who can use both hands to compress the bag, providing a greater inflation volume.

- Observe the rise and fall of the client's chest to assess the adequacy of each ventilation.

- Remove the resuscitation device, and place it on the bed or the client's chest with the connector facing up.

8. If the client has copious secretions, keep the regular O_2 delivery device on, and increase the litre flow or adjust the FiO_2 to 100% for several breaths before suctioning, according to agency policy. **Rationale: Hyperventilating a client who has copious secretions can force the secretions deeper into the respiratory tract**.

9. Quickly but gently insert the catheter *without* applying any suction.

- With your nondominant thumb off the suction port, quickly but gently insert the catheter into the trachea through the tracheostomy tube (see **③**). **Rationale: To prevent tissue trauma and oxygen loss, suction is not applied during insertion of the catheter**.

- Insert the catheter about 12.5 cm for adults, less for children, or less if the client coughs or you feel resistance. **Rationale: Resistance usually means that the catheter tip has reached the bifurcation of the trachea**. To prevent damaging the mucous membranes at the bifurcation, withdraw the catheter about 1 cm to 2 cm before applying suction.

10. Perform suctioning.

- Apply intermittent suction for 5 to 10 seconds by placing and removing the nondominant thumb over the thumb port. **Rationale: Suction time is restricted to 10 seconds or less to minimize oxygen loss**.

- Rotate the catheter by rolling it between your thumb and forefinger while slowly withdrawing it. **Rationale: This prevents tissue trauma by minimizing the suction time against any one part of the trachea**.

- Withdraw the catheter completely, and release the suction.

- Hyperventilate the client.

- Suction again, if needed.

11. Reassess the client's oxygenation status, and repeat suctioning.

- Observe the client's respirations and skin colour. Check the client's pulse, if necessary, by using your nondominant hand.

- Encourage the client to breathe deeply and to cough between suctions.

- Allow 2 to 3 minutes between suctions, when possible. **Rationale: This provides an opportunity for reoxygenation of the lungs**.

- Flush the catheter, and repeat suctioning two or three times until the air passage is clear and the breathing is relatively effortless and quiet.

- After each suction, pick up the resuscitation bag with your nondominant hand and ventilate the client with no more than three breaths.

12. Dispose of the catheter, and ensure that the suction tubing is available for the next suction.

- Flush the catheter and suction tubing.

- Turn off the suction, and disconnect the catheter from the suction tubing.

- Wrap the catheter around your sterile hand, and peel off the glove so that it turns inside out over the catheter.

- Discard the glove and the catheter in the moisture-resistant bag.

- Secure the suction tubing so that it is ready for the next suction (many units have a clip on the wall where the suction tubing is attached; the tubing may be coiled and stored in a package).

- Be sure that the ventilator and oxygen settings are returned to presuctioning settings. **Rationale: On some ventilators, this is automatic, but always check**.

13. Provide for client comfort and safety.

- Assist the client to a comfortable, safe position that aids breathing. If the person is conscious, the semi-Fowler's position is frequently indicated. If the person is unconscious, Sims' position aids in the drainage of secretions from the mouth.

14. Document relevant data.

- Record the suctioning procedure, including the amount and description of suction returns, cardiopulmonary assessment before and after suctioning, and client response.

Variation: Closed Airway or Tracheal Suction System (Inline Catheter)

- If a catheter is not attached, put on clean gloves, aseptically open a new closed catheter set, and attach the ventilator connection on the T piece to the ventilator tubing. Attach the client connection to the endotracheal tube or tracheostomy.

- Attach one end of the suction connecting tubing to the suction connection port of the closed system and the other end of the connecting tubing to the suction device.

- Turn on the suction, occlude or kink tubing, and depress the suction control valve (on the closed catheter system) to set suction to the appropriate level. Release the suction control valve.

(continued)

SKILL 43.5 SUCTIONING A TRACHEOSTOMY OR ENDOTRACHEAL TUBE *(continued)*

- Use the ventilator to hyperoxygenate, and hyperinflate the client's lungs.

- Unlock the suction control mechanism, if required by the manufacturer.

- Advance the suction catheter enclosed in its plastic sheath with the dominant hand. Steady the T piece with the nondominant hand.

- Depress the suction control valve, and apply suction for no more than 10 seconds. Gently withdraw the catheter.

- Repeat, as needed, remembering to provide hyperoxygenation and hyperinflation, as needed.

- When completed suctioning, withdraw the catheter into its sleeve and close the access valve, if appropriate. **Rationale: If the system does not have an access valve on the client connector, you need to observe for the**

potential of the catheter migrating into the airway and partially obstructing the artificial airway.

- Flush the catheter by instilling normal saline into the irrigation port and applying suction. Repeat until the catheter is clear.

- Close the irrigation port and close the suction valve.

EVALUATION

- Perform a follow-up examination of the client to determine the effectiveness of the suctioning (e.g., respiratory rate, depth, and character; breath sounds; colour of skin and nail beds; character and amount of secretions suctioned; changes in vital signs).

- Relate findings to previous assessment data, if available.

- Report significant deviations from normal to the appropriate members of the health care team.

and the potential cost of one-time catheter use, especially if the client requires frequent suctioning.

With the *closed airway/tracheal suction system* (*inline suctioning*) (Figure 43.39), the suction catheter attaches to the ventilator tubing and the client does not need to be disconnected from the ventilator. The nurse is not exposed to any secretions because the suction catheter is enclosed in a plastic sheath. The catheter can be reused as many times as necessary until the system is changed. The nurse needs to inquire about the agency's policy for changing the closed suction system.

CHEST TUBES AND DRAINAGE SYSTEMS If the thin, double-layered pleural membrane is disrupted by lung disease, surgery, or trauma, the negative pressure between the

pleural layers can be lost. The lung then collapses because it is no longer drawn outward as the diaphragm and intercostal muscles contract during inhalation. When air collects in the pleural space, it is known as a **pneumothorax**. A collection of blood in the pleural space, a **hemothorax**, or fluid, a pleural effusion, places pressure on lung tissue and interferes with lung expansion. Chest tubes can be inserted into the pleural cavity to restore negative pressure and drain collected fluid or blood. Because air rises, chest tubes for pneumothorax often are placed in the upper anterior thorax, whereas chest tubes used to drain fluid are generally placed in the lower lateral chest wall.

When chest tubes are inserted, they must be connected to a sealed drainage system or a one-way valve that allows air and fluid to be removed from the chest cavity

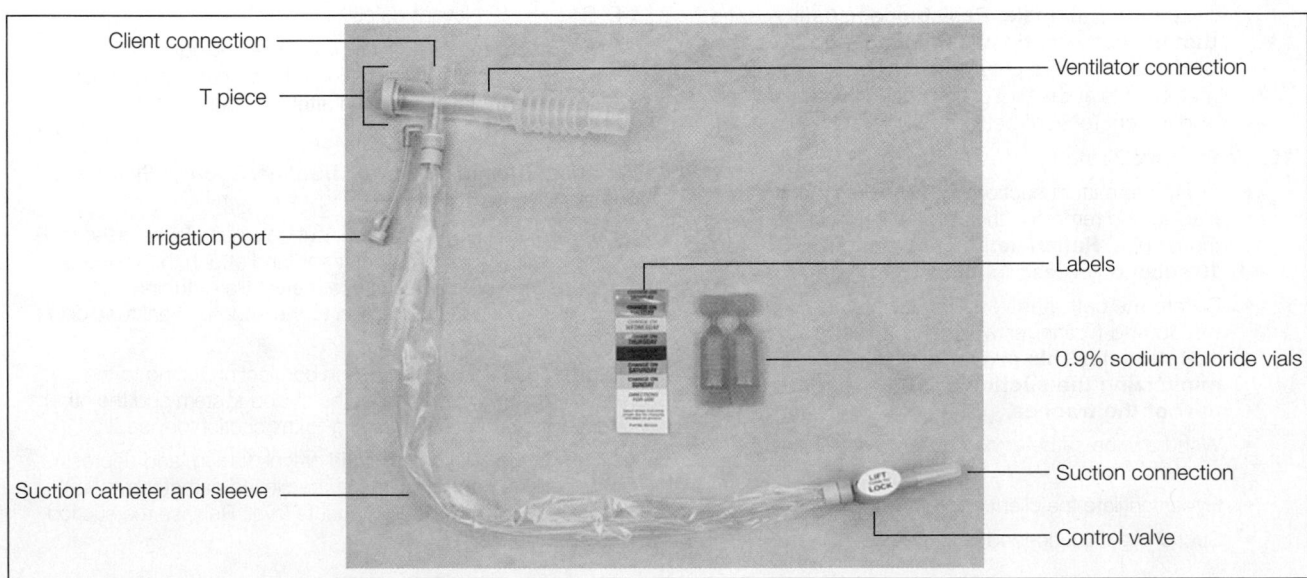

FIGURE 43.39 A closed airway suction (inline) system.

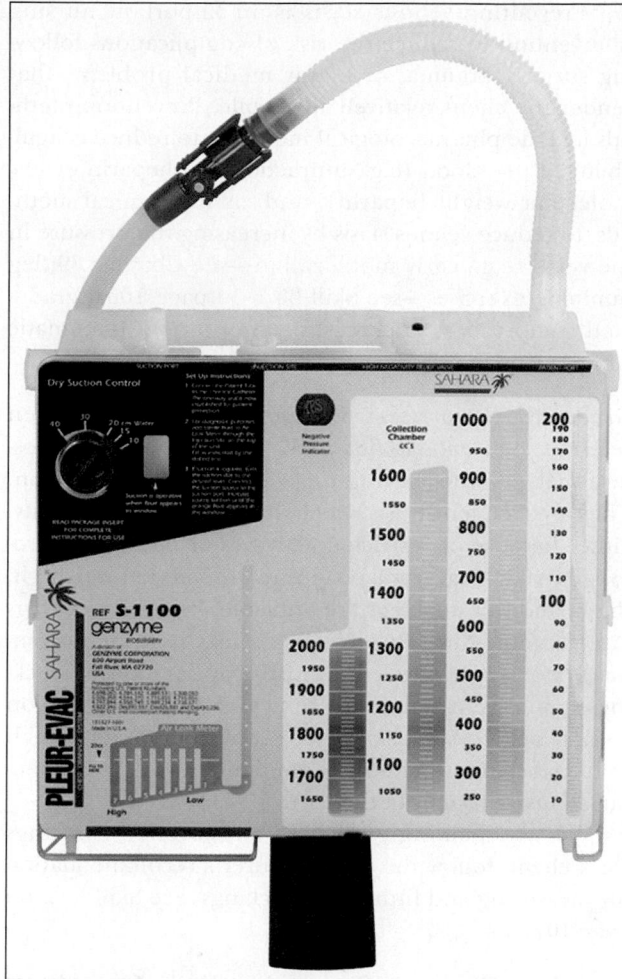

FIGURE 43.40 A disposable chest drainage system.

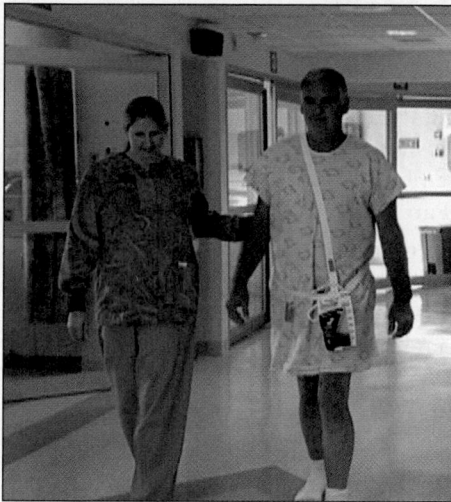

FIGURE 43.41 A mobile chest drain system allows the client freedom of movement.

but prevents air from entering from the outside. Water-seal drainage systems are used to prevent outside air from entering the chest tube. Sterile disposable systems commonly are used. These systems typically have a suction control chamber, a water seal chamber, and a closed collection chamber for drainage (Figure 43.40). With the water-seal system, when the client inhales, the water prevents air from entering the system from the atmosphere. During exhalation, however, air can exit the chest cavity, bubbling up through the water. Suction can be added to the system to facilitate removing air and secretions from the chest cavity. The drainage system should always be kept below the level of the client's chest to prevent fluid and drainage from being drawn back into the chest cavity.

Newer light-weight and compact chest drainage systems are available that allow clients to be ambulatory (Figure 43.41).

Nursing responsibilities regarding drainage systems include the following:

- Monitor and maintain the patency and integrity of the drainage system.
- Assess the client's vital signs, O$_2$ saturation, cardiovascular status, and respiratory status. Check the breath sounds bilaterally, and check for symmetry of breath sounds.
- Observe the dressing site at least every 4 hours. Inspect the dressing for excessive and abnormal drainage, such as bleeding or foul-smelling discharge. Palpate around the dressing site, and listen for a crackling sound indicative of subcutaneous emphysema. *Subcutaneous emphysema is air in the subcutaneous tissues and can result from a poor seal at the chest tube insertion site.* If subcutaneous emphysema is present, inform the physician.
- Determine the client's level of discomfort with and without activity, and medicate for pain, if indicated.
- Encourage deep-breathing and coughing exercises every 2 hours (this may be contraindicated in clients who have had a lung removed). Have the client sit upright to perform the exercises, and splint the chest around the tube insertion site with a pillow or with a hand to minimize discomfort.
- Assist the client with range-of-motion exercises of the affected shoulder three times per day to maintain joint mobility.
- Ensure that the chest tube is secured to the client's chest wall and that connections are securely taped to avoid disconnection.
- Keep the collection devices below the client's chest level.
- Frequently check the water seal and suction control chambers. The water can evaporate, and sterile water may need to be added to either chamber. The water seal level should fluctuate with respiratory effort.
- Assess the drainage in the tubing and collection chamber. The drainage is measured at regularly scheduled times (per agency policy). Mark the date and time at the fluid level on the drainage chamber. If drainage suddenly increases or if there is more than

100 mL/h of blood drainage, inform the appropriate member of the health care team.

- Avoid aggressive chest tube manipulation (e.g., milking or stripping the tube) to remove clots, as milking can create excessive negative pressure that can harm the pleural membranes and/or surrounding tissues (Coughlin & Parchinsky, 2006, p. 40).

- Avoid clamping the chest tube, unless ordered, as this increases the risk of a **tension pneumothorax**. Some agencies allow clamping of a chest tube in the following critical circumstances: (a) when disconnecting the chest drainage system to change the unit, (b) when the chest drainage system breaks or the integrity is disrupted for any reason, or (c) when removing the chest tube.

- If the tube becomes disconnected from the collecting system, submerge the end in 2 cm of sterile saline or water to maintain the seal. If the chest tube is inadvertently pulled out, the wound should be immediately covered with a dry sterile dressing. If you can hear air leaking out the site, ensure that the dressing is not occlusive. *If the air cannot escape, this would lead to a tension pneumothorax.*

- When transporting and ambulating the client, do the following:
  - Keep the water-seal unit below chest level and upright.
  - Disconnect the drainage system from the suction apparatus before moving the client and make sure the air vent is open.

Chest tube insertion and removal require sterile technique and must be done without introducing air or microorganisms into the pleural cavity. Removal of a chest tube is a brief but quite painful procedure. Medicate the client before the removal. Remove the dressing around the tube, and prepare the dressing that will cover the insertion site. This will be an occlusive dressing if there is no purse-string suture around the insertion site to prevent air from entering the chest. Generally, the physician performs the removal but, in some areas, specially trained nurses may be permitted to do so.

PREVENTING VENOUS STASIS When clients have limited mobility or are confined to bed, venous return to the heart is impaired and the risk of venous stasis increases. Immobility is a problem not only for ill or debilitated clients but also for some travellers who sit with their legs dependent for long periods in a motor vehicle or on an airplane. Venous stasis can lead to thrombus formation, often in the deep veins of the lower limbs—referred to as *deep vein thrombosis (DVT)*. With DVT, the thrombus can embolize and travel to the pulmonary circulation and cause a pulmonary embolism (PE), which can be fatal. The term *venous thromboembolism (VTE)* incorporates DVT and PE. VTE is one of the most common preventable causes of hospital-related death (Safer Healthcare Now! 2011).

Preventing venous stasis is an important nursing intervention to reduce the risk of complications following surgery, trauma, or major medical problems that render the client relatively immobile. Prevention methods include pharmacological methods, to reduce coagulability of the blood (e.g., unfractionated heparin or low molecular weight heparin), and/or mechanical methods, to reduce venous stasis by increasing the pressure in the veins (e.g., early mobilization—see Chapter 39; leg pumping exercises—see Skill 36.1 on page 1064; graduated compression stockings; or intermittent pneumatic compression devices).

Graduated Compression Stockings (GCS) GCS (often referred to as *antiembolism stockings*) are firm elastic hosiery that provide varying degrees of leg compression. They are frequently used in clients with limited mobility, either because of restricted activities or because of prolonged standing (e.g., restaurant servers). Knee-high, thigh, and full stockings are available. Presized stockings are commonly used; some clients may require custom-made stockings. The length of the antiembolism stockings should be based on the individual client's condition (e.g., if a client has a history of popliteal clots, thigh-high or full stockings would be recommended to facilitate venous return throughout the leg).

When obtaining graduated compression stockings for a client, follow the manufacturer's recommendation for measuring and fitting the stockings. See Skill 36.2 on page 1071.

Intermittent Pneumatic Compression (IPC) **Intermittent pneumatic compression** (sometimes referred to as *sequential compression*) involves the use of pneumatic pressure devices to promote venous return from the legs (see ❶ in Skill 43.6). IPC devices alternately inflate and deflate different portions of plastic sleeves wrapped around the legs or feet (as in the venous foot pump) to promote venous flow. For the knee or thigh length IPC, the ankle area inflates first, followed by the calf region, and then the thigh area.

The IPC is removed for ambulation and is usually discontinued when the client resumes activities. IPCs are useful in *preventing* thrombi and edema from venous stasis, but they are not used for clients who have arterial insufficiency, cellulitis, infection of the extremity, or existing venous thrombosis. Pressure devices are available for rent or purchase for home use.

Skill 43.6 outlines how to apply intermittent pneumatic compression.

CARDIOPULMONARY RESUSCITATION **Cardiopulmonary resuscitation (CPR)** is a combination of oral resuscitation (mouth-to-mouth breathing or use of a mask), which supplies oxygen to the lungs, and external cardiac massage (chest compression), which is intended to re-establish cardiac function and blood circulation. CPR is also referred to as *basic life support (BLS)*.

SKILL 43.6 APPLYING INTERMITTENT PNEUMATIC COMPRESSION

PURPOSES

- To promote venous return from the legs
- To decrease the risk of venous thromboembolism (VTE), including deep vein thrombosis (DVT) and pulmonary embolism (PE)

ASSESSMENT

Assess for baseline data:

- Cardiovascular status, including heart rate and rhythm, peripheral pulses, and capillary refill
- Colour and temperature of extremities
- Movement and sensation of feet and lower extremities

Equipment

- Measuring tape
- Intermittent pneumatic compression (IPC) device, including disposable sleeves, air pump, and tubing

IMPLEMENTATION

Performance

1. Before performing the procedure, introduce yourself and verify the client's identity using two identifiers or per agency protocol. Explain to the client what you are going to do, why it is necessary, and the procedure for applying the sequential compression device. **Rationale: The client's understanding and comfort will be increased by understanding the rationale for applying the IPC**.

2. Perform hand hygiene, and follow other appropriate infection prevention and control procedures.

3. Provide for client privacy.

4. Prepare the client.
   - Place the client in the dorsal recumbent or semi-Fowler's position.
   - Measure the client's legs as recommended by the manufacturer if a thigh-length sleeve is required. **Rationale: Foot and knee-length sleeves come in just one size; the thigh circumference determines the size needed for a thigh-length sleeve**.

5. Apply the IPC sleeves.
   - Place a sleeve under each leg with the opening at the knee.
   - Wrap the sleeve securely around the leg, securing the Velcro tabs (see ❶). Allow two fingers to fit between the leg and the sleeve. **Rationale: This amount of space ensures that the sleeve does not impair circulation when inflated**.

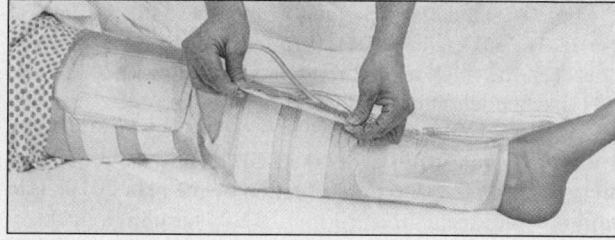

❶ Applying a sequential compression device to the leg.

6. Connect the sleeves to the control unit and adjust the pressure, as recommended.
   - Connect the tubing to the sleeves and control unit, ensuring that arrows on the plug and the connector are in alignment and that the tubing is not kinked or twisted. **Rationale: Improper alignment or obstruction of the tubing by kinks or twists will interfere with operation of the IPC**.
   - Turn on the control unit, and adjust the alarms and pressures, as needed. The sleeve cooling control and alarm should be on; ankle pressure should be set as recommended by the manufacturer, generally 35 mm Hg to 55 mm Hg. **Rationale: It is important to have the sleeve cooling control on for comfort and to reduce the risk of skin irritation from moisture under the sleeve. Alarms warn of possible control unit malfunctions**.

7. Document the procedure.
   - Record baseline assessment data and application of the IPC. Note control unit settings.
   - Assess and document skin integrity and neurovascular status regularly according to agency policy while the IPC is in place. Remove the unit and notify the physician if the client complains of numbness, tingling, or leg pain. **Rationale: These complaints can be symptoms of nerve compression**.

EVALUATION

- Perform appropriate follow-up assessments, such as cardiovascular status, including pedal pulses, skin colour and temperature, skin integrity, and neurovascular status, including movement and sensation.
- Compare with baseline data, if available.
- Report significant deviations from normal to the appropriate members of the health care team.

A **respiratory arrest** (pulmonary arrest) is the cessation of breathing. It often occurs as a result of a blocked airway, but it can occur following a cardiac arrest and for other reasons. A respiratory arrest may occur abruptly or be preceded by short, shallow breathing that becomes increasingly laboured. A **cardiac arrest** is the cessation of cardiac function; the heart stops beating. Often, a cardiac arrest is unexpected and sudden. When it occurs, the heart no longer pumps blood to any of the organs of the body. Breathing then stops, and the person becomes unconscious and limp. Within 20 to 40 seconds of a cardiac arrest, the victim is clinically dead. After 4 to 6 minutes, the lack of O_2 supply to the brain causes permanent and extensive damage.

The three cardinal signs of a cardiac arrest are apnea, absence of a carotid or femoral pulse, and dilated pupils. The person's skin and mucous membranes appear pale or greyish and the skin feels cool. The pupils may be dilated. Cyanosis is evident when respiratory function fails before heart failure.

The latest American Heart Association recommendations for cardiopulmonary resuscitation (CPR) and emergency cardiac care (ECC) (Travers et al., 2010) is a change in the basic life support (BLS) sequence of steps from "A-B-C" (airway, breathing, chest compressions) to "C-A-B" (chest compressions, airway, breathing) for adults and pediatric patients (children and infants, excluding newborns). Although the experts agreed that it is important to reduce time to first chest compressions, they were aware that a change in something as established as the A-B-C sequence would require re-education of everyone who has ever learned CPR. The *2010 AHA Guidelines for CPR and ECC* recommend this change for the following reasons: The vast majority of cardiac arrests occur in adults, and the highest survival rates from cardiac arrest are reported among patients of all ages with witnessed arrest and a rhythm of ventricular fibrillation or pulseless ventricular tachycardia (VT). In these patients, the critical initial elements of CPR are chest compressions and early defibrillation. In the A-B-C sequence, chest compressions are often delayed while the responder opens the airway to give mouth-to-mouth breaths or retrieves a barrier device or other ventilation equipment. By changing the sequence to C-A-B, chest compressions will be initiated sooner and ventilation only minimally delayed until completion of the first cycle of chest compressions (30 compressions should be accomplished in approximately 18 seconds).

It is vital that all nurses be trained to perform CPR so that resuscitation measures can be initiated immediately when a cardiac or respiratory arrest occurs. Nurses also can be instrumental in increasing community awareness of the need for CPR training and ensuring its availability. Most health care agencies have established practices and policies regarding CPR.

Evaluating

By using the goals and desired health outcomes identified in the planning stage of the nursing process, the nurse collects data to evaluate the effectiveness of interventions. Examples of desired health outcomes for the goals identified for clients with oxygenation problems are found in Table 43.2.

If outcomes are *not* achieved, the nurse, client, and support person, if appropriate, need to explore the reasons why before modifying the care plan.

TABLE 43.2 Evaluation Goals and Outcomes: Oxygenation and Circulation

Goal	Examples of Desired Health Outcomes
Maintain a patent airway	• Unlaboured respirations and rate within expected range • Clear lung sounds • No stridor or wheezing • Expels secretions effectively with coughing
Improve comfort and ease of breathing	• Quiet, rhythmic, and effortless breathing pattern • Respiratory rate, depth, and rhythm within expected range • No dyspnea, shortness of breath (SOB), or orthopnea • No restlessness or agitation • Uses pursed-lip breathing, as needed
Maintain or improve pulmonary ventilation and oxygenation	• Arterial blood gases within normal range • SaO_2 is greater than 90% • Respiratory rate, rhythm, and depth within expected range • Symmetrical chest expansion • No auscultated adventitious breath sounds • No restlessness, agitation, cyanosis, or confusion
Maintain (or promote) cardiac function and output	• Blood pressure (systolic and diastolic) within expected range • Apical–radial heart rate and rhythm within expected range • Heart and lung sounds normal • Urinary output of 30 mL/h to 50 mL/h or greater • No lethargy or extreme fatigue
Maintain or improve tissue perfusion	• Capillary refill is brisk • Strong and equal peripheral pulses • Skin pink and warm, mucous membranes moist and pink; sensation intact • No peripheral edema noted • No localized extremity pain or pain with activity

Goal	Examples of Desired Health Outcomes
Maintain (or improve) ability to participate in physical activities	• Performs usual personal care activities (e.g., bathing, dressing, grooming, toileting) without shortness of breath or fatigue • Food and fluid intake adequate to maintain energy level • Blood tests within normal range (e.g., hemoglobin, blood gases) • Balances rest and activity • Adapts lifestyle to energy limitations
Avoid risks associated with oxygenation problems (acid–base imbalances, skin and tissue breakdown, syncope, hopelessness, social isolation)	• Skin intact and adequate perfusion • Serum electrolytes and blood gases within normal limits • Neurological status within normal limits • Cognitive status satisfactory (e.g., alert and oriented) • Maintains participation in usual social activities • Expresses positive future outlook and sense of inner peace

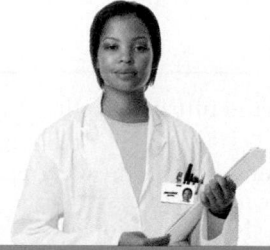

Case Study 43

Jerry Markert, 21 years old, was admitted to the hospital following a biking accident in which he received multiple injuries, including a hemothorax. He is receiving 6 L of O_2, as ordered, by a nasal cannula, has a chest tube connected to a closed drainage system, and is attached to a pulse oximeter that indicates an O_2 saturation level of 98%. He is alert, stable, and progressing well.

CRITICAL THINKING SKILLS

1. If Mr. Markert is stable and progressing well, why is his O_2 saturation being monitored?

2. Speculate about why Mr. Markert is receiving O_2 by a nasal cannula as opposed to a facemask.

3. Compare and contrast a hemothorax and a pneumothorax.

4. What precautions need to be taken when caring for Mr. Markert while his chest tube is in place?

5. Offer suggestions that would help Mr. Markert, or any person with a respiratory problem, to establish healthy breathing after his chest tube is removed.

Check the eText in MyNursingLab for answers and explanations.

KEY TERMS

adventitious breath sounds *p. 1362*

afterload *p. 1357*

angiography *p. 1370*

ankle-brachial index (ABI) *p. 1365*

apnea *p. 1362*

atelectasis *p. 1352*

atria *p. 1354*

atrioventricular (AV) node *p. 1355*

B-type natriuretic peptide (BNP) *p. 1369*

Biot's (cluster) respiration *p. 1362*

blood pressure *p. 1357*

bradypnea *p. 1362*

bronchoscopy *p. 1370*

cardiac arrest *p. 1401*

cardiac monitoring *p. 1369*

cardiac output (CO) *p. 1356*

cardiopulmonary resuscitation (CPR) *p. 1400*

Cheyne-Stokes respiration *p. 1362*

continuous positive airway pressure (CPAP) *p. 1384*

contractility *p. 1357*

coronary arteries *p. 1355*

creatine phosphokinase *p. 1369*

cyanosis *p. 1363*

diastole *p. 1354*

diffusion *p. 1353*

dyspnea *p. 1362*

echocardiography *p. 1370*

electrocardiography (ECG) *p. 1370*

endocardium *p. 1354*

epicardium *p. 1354*

erythrocytes *p. 1353*

eupnea *p. 1362*

heart failure *p. 1363*

hematocrit *p. 1353*

hemoglobin *p. 1353*

hemoptysis *p. 1367*

hemothorax *p. 1398*

humidifiers *p. 1375*

hypercapnia *p. 1362*

hyperventilation *p. 1362*

hypoventilation *p. 1362*

hypoxemia *p. 1362*

hypoxia *p. 1362*

incentive spirometers *p. 1376*

intermittent pneumatic compression *p. 1400*

intrapleural pressure *p. 1352*

CHAPTER HIGHLIGHTS

- Respiration is the process of gas exchange between the individual and the environment.

- The respiratory system contributes to effective respiration through pulmonary ventilation (the movement of air between the atmosphere and the lungs) and the diffusion of oxygen (O_2) and carbon dioxide (CO_2) across the pulmonary membrane.

- The cardiovascular system transports these gases in the blood to and from the tissues and facilitates the diffusion of gases between the capillaries and body tissues.

- Alveoli and the capillaries that surround them form the respiratory membrane where gas exchange between the lungs and blood occurs.

- Effective pulmonary ventilation, or breathing, requires clear airways, an intact central nervous system and respiratory centre, an intact thoracic cavity and musculature, and adequate pulmonary compliance (stretch) and recoil.

- Gas exchange occurs by diffusion as gas molecules move from an area of higher concentration to an area of lower concentration. At the respiratory membrane, O_2 moves from the alveolus into blood, while CO_2 moves from blood into the alveolus.

- Most O_2 (97%) is carried to the tissues loosely combined with hemoglobin in erythrocytes (red blood cells [RBCs]). Anemia, which is too few RBCs or low hemoglobin levels, impairs O_2 transportation.

- CO_2 is transported within RBCs as bicarbonate or combined with hemoglobin, and in blood plasma as carbonic acid.

- The heart and blood vessels make up the cardiovascular system, which, together with blood, is the major system for transporting O_2 and nutrients to the tissues and waste products away from the tissues for elimination.

- The right side of the heart receives deoxygenated blood from the body and pumps it to the lungs via the pulmonary arteries; the left side receives oxygenated blood from the lungs and pumps it out to the body via the aorta.

- Coronary arteries supply O_2 and nutrients to the heart muscle.

- The cardiac conduction system controls the electrical activity of the heart and the cardiac cycle: systole, contraction of the heart muscle and ejection of blood; and diastole, the relaxation period during which the heart fills with blood.

- Cardiac output depends on stroke volume, or amount of blood ejected during systole, and heart rate.

- The systemic blood vessels carry blood to the tissues through a system of arteries, arterioles, and capillaries and return it to the heart through the venules, veins, and venae cavae.

- Heart and respiratory rates normally are highest in neonates and infants, gradually slowing to adult ranges; the blood pressure rises gradually from birth to reach the adult range in adolescence.

- Aging affects both the respiratory and the cardiovascular systems: the chest wall becomes more rigid and lungs less elastic; atherosclerosis causes fatty plaque to develop within arteries.

- Other factors affecting oxygenation include the environment, lifestyle, health status, opioid analgesics, stress and coping, and sex.

- Hypoxia, insufficient O_2 in the tissues, can result from impaired ventilation (hypoventilation) or diffusion, or from impaired O_2 transportation to the tissues because of anemia or decreased cardiac output.

- Normal respirations are quiet and effortless; altered respiratory patterns include tachypnea, bradypnea, hyperventilation, hypoventilation, and dyspnea. Shortness of breath is a subjective sensation of not getting enough air.

- Airway obstruction interferes with ventilation. A low-pitched snoring sound, stridor, and abnormal breath sounds may accompany partial airway obstruction. Extreme inspiratory effort with no chest movement indicates complete upper airway obstruction.

- Decreased cardiac output, impaired tissue perfusion, and disorders affecting the blood are the major cardiovascular problems that can affect oxygenation.

- Cardiac output may fall with a myocardial infarction, heart failure, dysrhythmias, and structural alterations of the heart (e.g., valve deformities).

- The most common cause of impaired blood flow to tissues is atherosclerosis; this can lead to tissue ischemia and pain.

- To assess oxygenation, the nurse conducts a nursing history, performs a complete physical assessment of the client, and reviews relevant diagnostic data.

- The nursing history includes questions about current or past respiratory and cardiovascular problems, including hypertension; about lifestyle; presence of symptoms, such as cough or shortness of breath; smoking and other risk factors; and medications.

- Physical assessment should include a general assessment, as well as specific examination of the respiratory and cardiovascular systems.

- Cardiac monitoring is used for continuous observation of the heart rate and rhythm.

- Diagnostic tests that may be performed to assess oxygenation include sputum and throat culture specimens; blood tests, such as the complete blood count (CBC), hemoglobin, and hematocrit, blood chemistries, and arterial blood gases; electrocardiography (ECG) and stress ECG; pulmonary function tests; visualization procedures, such as radiography, lung scans, angiography, echocardiography, laryngoscopy, and bronchoscopy.

- The nurse is responsible for obtaining specimens for diagnostic tests, preparing the client and the support people for diagnostic procedures, monitoring the client's response to certain procedures, and reviewing records and reports of diagnostic tests.

- Multiple nursing diagnoses can relate to oxygenation and circulation problems, such as impaired gas exchange; impaired pumping action of the heart; impaired ventilation; impaired arterial and/or venous circulation; unhealthy lifestyle increasing risk for cardiac and/or respiratory compromise; and many more.

- In planning care for clients with problems of oxygenation, the nurse establishes goals such as maintaining a patent airway; improving ease and comfort of breathing; maintaining ventilation and oxygenation; ensuring tissue perfusion; maintaining cardiac output; improving the client's activity tolerance; and preventing risks, such as tissue breakdown and infection.

- In discharge and home care planning, the nurse assesses the client's self-care abilities and need for assistive devices, home environment, compliance with medical regimen, and knowledge level. The ability of the family or support people to provide assistance and financial support and to cope with the changes are also assessed, as are community factors, such as the environment and resources.

- The nurse teaches the client about home care activities to maintain a patent airway and gas exchange, to promote healthy breathing, and to maintain cardiac output and tissue perfusion. Dietary modifications, prescribed medications, and specific procedures also are taught, and the nurse makes referrals to community agencies, as needed.

- Nursing interventions to promote oxygenation include promoting healthy breathing and a healthy heart, deep breathing and coughing, and hydration; administering medications; implementing measures to clear secretions (e.g., incentive spirometry, percussion, vibration, and postural drainage); initiating and monitoring O_2 therapy; initiating or assisting with procedures to maintain the airway (e.g., artificial airways, suctioning, and continuous positive airway pressure therapy); providing tracheostomy care; monitoring chest drainage systems; using antiembolic stockings and intermittent pneumatic compression to prevent venous stasis; and administering cardiopulmonary resuscitation.

- The effectiveness of nursing interventions is evaluated by using the goals and desired health outcomes identified in the planning stage of the nursing process. If a goal is not met, the nurse asks pertinent questions to assess the reason for not meeting the goal.

ASSESS YOUR LEARNING

1. A client with chronic pulmonary disease has a bluish tinge around the lips. This would MOST accurately be documented as which of the following?

   a. Hypoxia

   b. Hypoxemia

   c. Dyspnea

   d. Cyanosis

2. A client with a chronic lung disorder requires some supplemental oxygen (O_2). Which of the following should the nurse consider as safe delivery?

   a. O_2 at 2 L/min per nasal cannula

   b. O_2 at 6 L/min per facemask

   c. O_2 at 8 L/min per partial rebreather mask

   d. O_2 at 10 L/min per nonrebreather mask

3. Which of the following represents proper naso-pharyngeal or nasotracheal suction technique?

   a. Lubricating the suction catheter with petroleum jelly (e.g., Vaseline) before and between insertions

   b. Applying suction intermittently while inserting the suction catheter

   c. Rotating the catheter and applying suction while slowly withdrawing the catheter

   d. Hyperoxygenating the client with 100% oxygen for 30 minutes before and after suctioning

4. Which of the following statements by the client indicates successful teaching regarding the proper use of an incentive spirometer?

 a. "I should breathe out as fast and hard as possible into the device."

 b. "I should inhale slowly and steadily to keep the balls up."

 c. "I should use the device three times a day, after meals."

 d. "The entire device should be washed thoroughly in sudsy water once a week."

5. The nurse is caring for a client with chest tubes. During ambulation, the connection between the tube and the water seal comes apart. Which of the following actions is MOST appropriate?

 a. Assisting the client with ambulation back to bed

 b. Reconnecting the tube to the water seal

 c. Assessing the client's lung sounds with a stethoscope

 d. Having the client cough forcibly several times

6. Which of the following clients should be watched MOST closely for a problem with the transport of O_2 from the lungs to tissues?

 a. A client who has anemia

 b. A client who has an infection

 c. A client who has a fractured rib

 d. A client who has a tumour of the medulla

7. The nurse is planning to perform percussion and postural drainage with a client. Which of the following is an important aspect of the planning?

 a. Percussion and postural drainage should be done before lunch on an empty stomach.

 b. The order should be coughing, percussion, positioning, and then suctioning.

 c. Percussion and postural drainage should be done in the morning after breakfast when the client is well rested.

 d. Percussion and postural drainage should always be preceded by 3 minutes of 100% oxygen.

8. Which of the following would MOST likely be included in the evaluation of the client goal of "demonstrate adequate tissue perfusion"?

 a. Symmetrical chest expansion

 b. Pursed-lip breathing

 c. Brisk capillary refill

 d. Appetite

9. To prevent postoperative complications, the nurse assists the client with coughing and deep-breathing exercises. Which of the following would the nurse recommend to the client?

 a. Performing coughing exercises 1 hour before meals and deep breathing 1 hour after meals

 b. Coughing forcefully as many times as tolerated throughout the day

 c. Performing huff coughing every 2 hours or as needed

 d. Using diaphragmatic and pursed-lip breathing 5 to 10 times, four times a day

10. Mr. Jacobs, 53 years old, was admitted to the hospital because of chest pain. His condition has deteriorated, and he develops crackles in his lower lobes of the lungs. He is feeling short of breath and anxious. The physician prescribes morphine sulphate (morphine) 4 mg IV and furosemide (Lasix) 40 mg IV. Which of the following changes in condition BEST indicates that Mr. Jacobs is responding favourably to the medications?

 a. Decreased respiratory rate, decreased crackles

 b. Decreased crackles, large diuresis

 c. Increased pulse, increased respiratory rate

 d. Decreased respiratory rate, decreased blood pressure

Check the eText in MyNursingLab for answers and explanations.

WEBLINKS

Canadian Lung Association
http://www.lung.ca
This is the umbrella association for the provincial and territorial groups; the website provides a variety of educational material for the public and health care professionals. The Canadian Respiratory Health Professionals network offers a forum for dialogue at this site.

Heart and Stroke Foundation of Canada
http://www.heartandstroke.ca
This national association provides information and support to the public and health care professionals.

TobaccoFreeRNAO
http://tobaccofreernao.ca/en
This is an excellent resource for nurses, and it includes links to an immense array of resources to help clients—and nurses themselves—quit smoking.

MyNursingLab

REFERENCES

Ball, J. W., & Bindler, R. C. (2008). *Pediatric nursing: Caring for children* (4th ed.). Upper Saddle River, NJ: Pearson/Prentice Hall.

British Columbia Provincial Nursing Skin and Wound Committee. (2011). *Procedure: Ankle brachial index (ABI) in adults.* Retrieved from http://www.clwk.ca/cop/skin-wound-care/clinical-dsts

Canadian Hypertension Education Program. (2012). *2012 CHEP recommendations for the management of hypertension.* Ottawa, ON: Author. Retrieved from http://www.hypertension.ca/chep-recommendations

Coughlin, A. M., & Parchinsky, C. (2006). Go with the flow of chest tube therapy. *Nursing, 36*(3), 36–41.

Fang, M. C., Chen, J., & Rich, M. W. (2007). Atrial fibrillation in the elderly. *American Journal of Medicine, 120*(6), 481–487.

Heart and Stroke Foundation of Canada. (2011a). *Excessive alcohol consumption.* Retrieved from http://www.heartandstroke.com/site/c.ikIQLcMWJtE/b.3484033/k.2811/Heart_disease__Excessive_alcohol_consumption.htm

Heart and Stroke Foundation of Canada. (2011b). *Women and heart disease and stroke.* Retrieved from http://www.heartandstroke.com/site/c.ikIQLcMWJtE/b.3484041/k.D80A/Heart_disease__Women_and_heart_disease_and_stroke.htm

Ignatavius, D., & Workman, M. L. (2010). *Medical-surgical nursing* (6th ed.). St. Louis, MO: Mosby.

Joffres, M. R., Campbell, N. R. C., Manns, B., & Tu, K. (2007). Estimate of the benefits of a population-based reduction in dietary sodium additives on hypertension and its related health care costs in Canada. *Canadian Journal of Cardiology, 23*(6), 437–443.

Klabunde, R. E. (2011). *Cardiovascular physiology concepts* (2nd ed.). Philadelphia, PA: Lippincott Williams & Wilkins.

Perrin, K. (2009). *Understanding the essentials of critical care nursing.* Upper Saddle River, NJ: Pearson/Prentice Hall.

Registered Nurses' Association of Ontario. (2010). *Nursing care of dyspnea: The 6th vital sign in individuals with chronic obstructive pulmonary disease (COPD)—Guideline Supplement.* Toronto, ON: Author.

Ross, H., Howlett, J., Arnold, J. M., Lu, P., O'Neill, B. J., Simpson, C. S., ... & Glasgow, K.; Canadian Cardiovascular Society Access to Care Working Group. Treating the right patient at the right time: Access to heart failure care. *Canadian Journal of Cardiology, 22*(9), 749–754.

Ruidavets, J., Bongard, V., Simon, C., Dallongeville, J., Ducimetiere, P., Arveiler, D., ... & Ferrieres, J. (2006). Independent contribution of dairy products and calcium intake to blood pressure variations at a population level. *Journal of Hypertension, 24,* 671–681.

Safer Healthcare Now! (2009). *Getting started kit: Prevention of ventilator-associated pneumonia in adults and children.* Retrieved from http://www.saferhealthcarenow.ca/EN/Interventions/VAP/Documents/VAP%20Getting%20Started%20Kit.pdf

Safer Healthcare Now! (2011). Venous thromboembolism (VTE). Retrieved from http://www.saferhealthcarenow.ca/en/interventions/vte/pages/default.aspx

Saremi, A., & Arora, R. (2008). The cardiovascular implications of alcohol and red wine. *American Journal of Therapeutics, 15,* 265–277.

Statistics Canada. (2008, modified 2011). Leading causes of death in Canada. Retrieved from http://www.statcan.gc.ca/pub/84-215-x/2011001/hl-fs-eng.htm

TobaccoFreeRNAO; Registered Nurses' of Ontario. (2011). *Nurses: Practice recommendations.* Retrieved from http://tobaccofreernao.ca/en/resources/best-practices-guidelines/nurses-practice-recommendations

Travers, A. H., Rea, T. D., Bobrow, B. J., Edelson, D. P., Berg, R. A., Sayre, M. R., ... & Swor, R. (2010). CPR overview: 2010 American Heart Association guidelines for cardiopulmonary resuscitation and emergency cardiovascular care. *Circulation, 122*(Suppl 3), S676–S684.

Chapter **44**

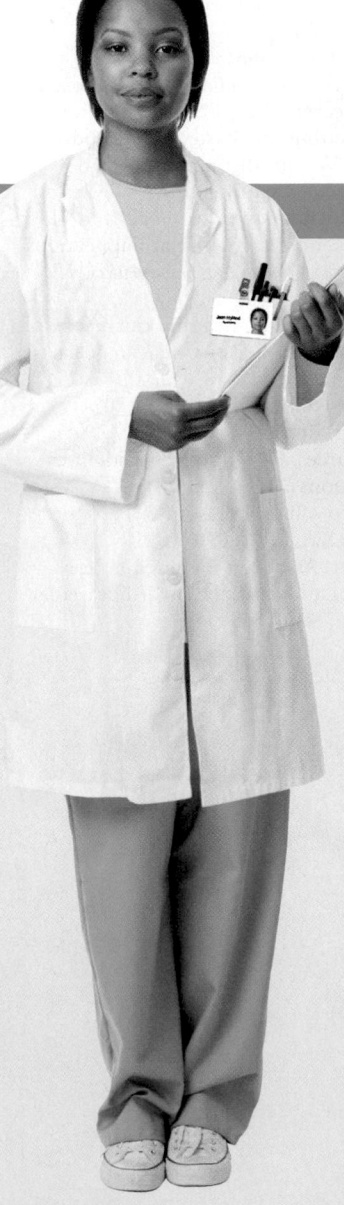

Fluid, Electrolyte, and Acid–Base Balance

LEARNING OBJECTIVES

After studying this chapter, you will be able to:

1. Discuss the function, distribution, movement, and regulation of fluids and electrolytes in the body.

2. Describe the regulation of acid–base balance in the body, including the roles of buffers, the lungs, and the kidneys.

3. Identify factors affecting normal body fluid, electrolyte, and acid–base balance

4. Outline the risk factors for and the causes and effects of fluid, electrolyte, and acid–base imbalance.

5. Collect assessment data related to the client's fluid, electrolyte, and acid–base balance.

6. Select appropriate nursing diagnoses for clients with altered fluid, electrolyte, or acid–base balance.

7. Teach clients ways to maintain fluid and electrolyte balance.

8. Implement measures to correct imbalances of fluids and electrolytes or acids and bases, such as enteral or parenteral replacements and blood transfusions.

9. Evaluate the effect of nursing and collaborative interventions on the client's fluid, electrolyte, or acid–base balance.

n good health, a delicate balance of fluid, electrolytes, acids, and bases maintains the body. This balance depends on multiple physiological processes that regulate fluid intake and output, as well as the movement of water and the substances dissolved in it between the body compartments.

Almost every illness has the potential to threaten this balance. Even in daily living, factors such as excessive temperatures or vigorous activity can disturb homeostasis if adequate water and salt intake are not maintained. Therapeutic measures, such as the use of diuretics or nasogastric suction, can also disturb the body's homeostasis unless water and electrolytes are replaced.

Body Fluids and Electrolytes

The proportion of the human body composed of fluid is surprisingly large. Approximately 60% of the average healthy adult's weight is water, the primary body fluid. In good health, this volume remains relatively constant, and a person's weight varies by less than 0.2 kg in 24 hours, regardless of the amount of fluid ingested.

Water is vital to health and normal cellular function, serving as the following:

- A medium for metabolic reactions within cells
- A transporter for nutrients, waste products, and other substances
- A lubricant
- An insulator and a shock absorber
- A means of regulating and maintaining body temperature

Age, sex, and body fat affect total body water. Infants have the highest proportion of water, accounting for 70% to 80% of their body weight. The proportion of body water decreases with age. In people older than 60 years of age, it represents only about 50% of total body weight. Women generally have a lower percentage of body water than men. In both women and older adults, this is due to lower levels of muscle mass and a greater percentage of fat tissue. Fat tissue is essentially free of water, whereas lean tissue contains a significant amount of water. Therefore, water makes up a greater percentage of a lean person's body weight than that of a person who is obese.

Distribution of Body Fluids

The body's fluid is divided into two major components: (a) intracellular fluid and (b) extracellular fluid (see Figure 44.1). **Intracellular fluid (ICF)** is found within the cells of the body. It constitutes approximately two-thirds

of the total body fluid in adults. **Extracellular fluid (ECF)** is found outside the cells and accounts for about one-third of total body fluid. Extracellular fluid is further subdivided in two compartments. The two main compartments of ECF are intravascular and interstitial. **Intravascular fluid (IVF)**, or **plasma**, accounts for approximately 20% of ECF and is found within the vascular system. **Interstitial fluid (ISF)**, accounting for approximately 75% of ECF, surrounds the cells. The other compartments of ECF include the lymph and transcellular fluids. Examples of **transcellular fluid** include cerebrospinal, pericardial, pancreatic, pleural, intraocular, biliary, peritoneal, and synovial fluids.

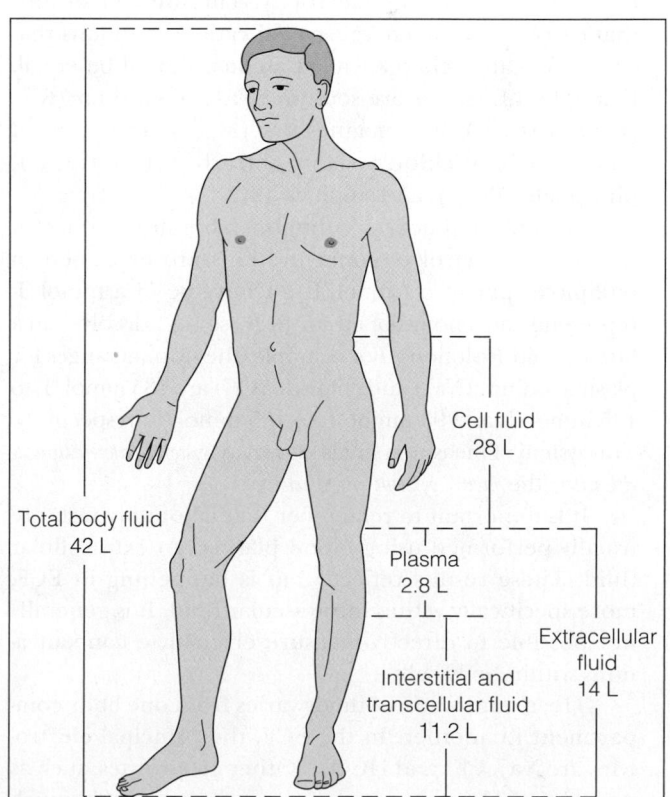

Total body fluid
42 L

Cell fluid
28 L

Plasma
2.8 L

Interstitial and transcellular fluid
11.2 L

Extracellular fluid
14 L

FIGURE 44.1 Total body fluid amounts to about 42 L in an adult male weighing 70 kg.

Intracellular fluid is vital to normal cell functioning. It contains solutes, such as oxygen (O_2), electrolytes, and glucose, and it provides a medium in which metabolic processes of the cell take place.

Although ECF is in the smaller of the two compartments, it is the transport system that carries O_2 and nutrients to, and waste products from, body cells. For example, plasma carries O_2 from the lungs and glucose from the gastrointestinal tract to the capillaries of the vascular system. From there, the O_2 and glucose move across the capillary membranes into the interstitial spaces and then across the cellular membranes into the cells. The opposite route is taken for waste products, such as carbon dioxide (CO_2) going from the cells to the lungs, and metabolic wastes going to the kidneys. Interstitial fluid transports wastes from cells by way of the lymph system, as well as directly into the blood plasma through capillaries.

Composition of Body Fluids

Extracellular and intracellular fluids contain O_2 from the lungs, dissolved nutrients from the gastrointestinal tract, excretory products of metabolism, such as carbon dioxide, and charged particles called **ions**.

Many salts dissociate in water into electrically charged ions. The salt called sodium chloride breaks up into one ion of sodium (Na^+) and one ion of chloride (Cl^-). These charged particles are called **electrolytes** because they are capable of conducting electricity. The number of ions that carry a positive charge, called **cations**, and ions that carry a negative charge, called **anions**, should be equal. Examples of cations are sodium (Na^+), potassium (K^+), calcium (Ca^{2+}), and magnesium (Mg^{2+}). Examples of anions include chloride (Cl^-), bicarbonate (HCO_3^-), phosphate (PO_4^-), and sulphate (SO_4^{2-}).

In clinical practice, common laboratory values of the body's electrolyte concentrations are expressed in millimoles per litre (mmol/L). The value of a mmol/L represents the amount of electrolytes (solute) dissolved in a litre of fluid (solution). For example, the normal ranges for plasma sodium (Na^+) and chloride (Cl^-) are 135 mmol/L to 145 mmol/L and 95 mmol/L to 105 mmol/L, respectively. This system of measurement is known as *Système Internationale d'Unités* (the *metric system*) or *SI units*.

It is important to remember that laboratory tests are usually performed using blood plasma, an extracellular fluid. These results reflect what is happening in ECF, more specifically within intravascular fluid. It is generally not possible to directly measure electrolyte concentrations within body cells.

The composition of fluids varies from one body compartment to another. In the ECF, the principal electrolytes are Na^+, Cl^-, and HCO_3^-. Other electrolytes, such as potassium, calcium, and magnesium, are present in much smaller quantities. Plasma and interstitial fluid, the two primary components of ECF, contain similar electrolytes and solutes, with the exception of protein. Plasma is a protein-rich fluid containing large amounts of albumin; in contrast, interstitial fluid contains very little protein.

The composition of ICF differs significantly from that of ECF. Potassium and magnesium are the primary cations present in ICF, with phosphate and sulphate being the major anions. As in ECF, other electrolytes are present within the cell but in much smaller concentrations (Figure 44.2).

Maintaining a balance of fluid volumes and electrolyte compositions in the fluid compartments of the body is essential to health. Normal and unusual fluid and electrolyte losses must be replaced if homeostasis is to be maintained.

Other body fluids, such as gastric and intestinal secretions, also contain electrolytes. This is of particular concern when these fluids are lost from the body, such as in severe vomiting or diarrhea, or when gastric suctioning removes gastric secretions.

Movement of Body Fluids and Electrolytes

The body fluid compartments are separated from one another by cell membranes. Although these membranes are completely permeable to water, they are selectively permeable to solutes as substances move across them with varying degrees of ease. Small particles, such as ions, O_2, and carbon dioxide, easily move across these membranes, but larger molecules, such as glucose and proteins, have more difficulty moving between fluid compartments.

Solutes are substances dissolved in a liquid. For example, when sugar is added to coffee, the sugar is the solute. Solutes can be **crystalloids** (salts that dissolve readily into true solutions) or **colloids** (substances, such as large protein molecules, that do not readily dissolve into true solutions). A **solvent** is the component of a solution that can dissolve a solute. In the previous example, coffee is the solvent for the sugar. The concentration of solutes in body fluids is usually expressed as the **osmolality**. Osmolality is determined by the total solute concentration within a fluid compartment and is measured as parts of solute per kilogram of water. Osmolality is determined by the total solute concentration within a fluid compartment and is measured as part of solute per kilogram of water.

Osmolality is reported as milliosmoles per kilogram (mOsm/kg). Sodium is, by far, the greatest determinant of the osmolality of plasma, or *serum osmolality*, although glucose and urea also contribute. Potassium, glucose, and urea are the primary contributors to the osmolality of intracellular fluid. The term *tonicity* can be used to refer to the osmolality of one solution in relation to another solution. Solutions may be termed *isotonic, hypertonic,* or *hypotonic.* In relation to body fluid, an **isotonic** solution has the same osmolality as ECF. Normal saline, 0.9% sodium chloride, is an example of an isotonic solution.

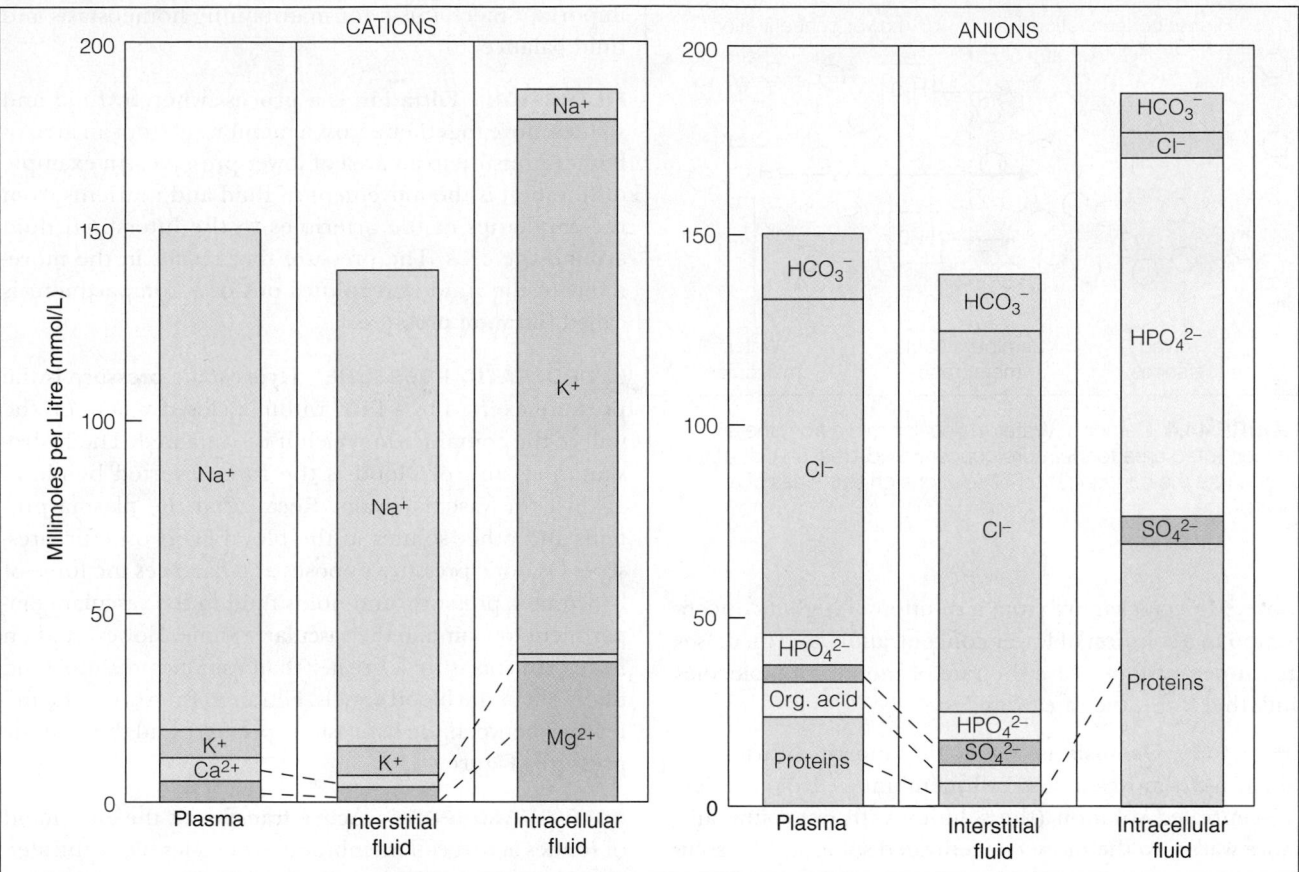

FIGURE 44.2 Electrolyte composition (cations and anions) of body fluid compartments.

Source: From Martini, F. H., & Halyard, R. H., (2006). *Fundamentals of anatomy and physiology interactive* [Media ed.] (7th ed.). Upper Saddle River, NJ: Pearson Education, Inc. Reproduced with permission of Pearson Education, Inc., Upper Saddle River, New Jersey.

Hypertonic solutions, such as 3% sodium chloride, have a higher osmolality than ECF. **Hypotonic** solutions, such as 0.45% sodium chloride, have a lower osmolality compared with ECF.

Osmotic pressure is the power of a solution to pull water across a semipermeable membrane. When two solutions of different concentrations are separated by a semipermeable membrane, the solution with the higher solute concentration exerts a higher osmotic pressure, pulling water across the membrane to equalize the concentrations of the solutions. For example, infusing a hypertonic intravenous solution, such as 3% sodium chloride, will pull fluid out of erythrocytes (red blood cells [RBCs]), causing the cells to shrink. In contrast, a hypotonic solution administered intravenously will cause the RBCs to swell as water is pulled into the cells by their higher osmotic pressure. In the body, plasma proteins exert an osmotic pull called **colloid osmotic pressure (COP)** or **colloid oncotic pressure**, holding water in plasma, and when necessary, pulling water from the interstitial spaces into the vascular compartment. This is an important mechanism in maintaining vascular volume.

The methods by which water and solutes move in the body are called *diffusion, osmosis, filtration,* and *active transport.*

DIFFUSION **Diffusion** occurs when two solutes of different concentrations are separated by a semipermeable membrane (Figure 44.3). The rate of diffusion of a solute varies according to the size of the molecules, the concentration of the solution, and the temperature of the solution. Larger molecules move less quickly than smaller ones because large molecules require more energy to

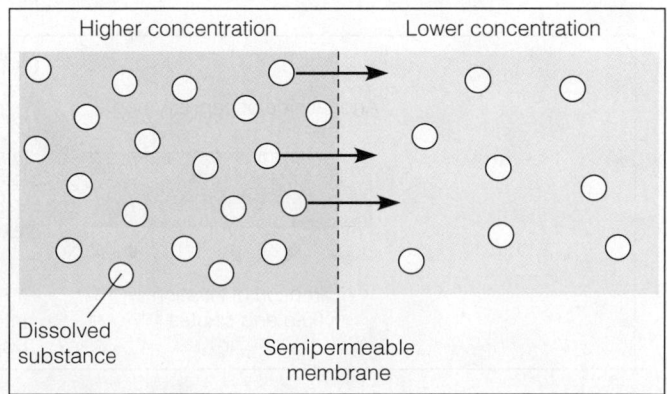

FIGURE 44.3 Diffusion: The movement of molecules through a semipermeable membrane from an area of higher concentration to an area of lower concentration.

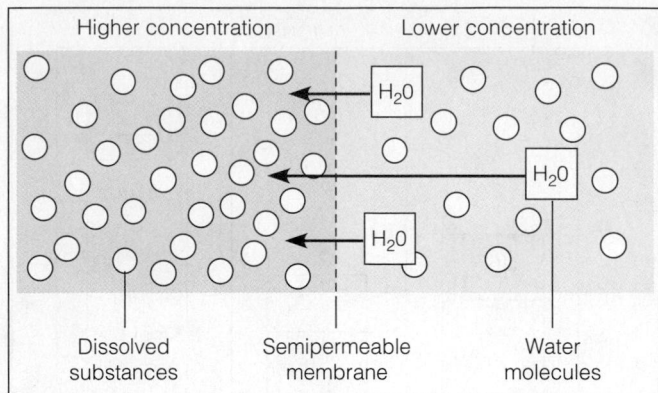

Higher concentration   Lower concentration

Dissolved substances

Semipermeable membrane

Water molecules

FIGURE 44.4 Osmosis: Water molecules move from the less concentrated area to the more concentrated area in an attempt to equalize the concentration of solutions on two sides of a membrane.

move. Molecules move from a solution of higher concentration to a solution of lower concentration, and increases in temperature increase the rate of motion of molecules and, therefore, the rate of diffusion.

OSMOSIS **Osmosis** is a specific kind of diffusion in which *water* moves across cell membranes, from the less concentrated solution (the solution with less solute and more water) to the more concentrated solution (the solution with more solute and less water) (Figure 44.4). In other words, water moves toward the higher concentration of solute in an attempt to equalize the concentrations of both water and solute.

Osmosis occurs in the body when the concentration of solutes is higher on one side of a selectively permeable membrane, such as the capillary membrane, than on the other side. For example, a marathon runner loses a significant amount of body water through perspiration, increasing the concentration of solutes in the plasma. This higher solute concentration draws water from the interstitial spaces and cells into the vascular compartment to equalize the concentration of solutes in all fluid compartments. Osmosis is an

important mechanism for maintaining homeostasis and fluid balance.

FILTRATION **Filtration** is a process whereby fluid and solutes move together across a membrane from an area of higher pressure to an area of lower pressure. An example of filtration is the movement of fluid and nutrients from the capillaries of the arterioles to the interstitial fluid around the cells. The pressure that results in the movement of the fluid and solutes out of a compartment is called **filtration pressure**.

HYDROSTATIC PRESSURE **Hydrostatic pressure** is the pressure exerted by a fluid within a closed system on the wall of the container in which it is contained. The hydrostatic pressure of blood is the force exerted by blood against the vascular walls. Recall that the plasma proteins and other solutes in the blood exert osmotic pressure. Osmotic pressure opposes and balances the force of hydrostatic pressure, and holds fluid in the vascular compartment to maintain the vascular volume. However, when hydrostatic pressure is greater than osmotic pressure, fluid filters out of the blood vessels. Filtration pressure is the difference between the hydrostatic pressure and the osmotic pressure (Figure 44.5).

ACTIVE TRANSPORT **Active transport** is the movement of solutes across cell membranes from a less concentrated solution to a more concentrated one (Figure 44.6). This process differs from diffusion and osmosis in that metabolic energy is expended. In active transport, a substance combines with a carrier on the outside surface of the cell membrane, and they move to the inside surface of the cell membrane. Once inside, they separate, and the substance is released to the inside of the cell. A specific carrier is required for each substance.

The process of active transport is of particular importance in maintaining the differences in sodium and potassium ion concentrations of ECF and ICF. Under normal conditions, sodium concentrations are higher in the ECF, and potassium concentrations are higher inside the cells. To maintain these proportions, the active transport

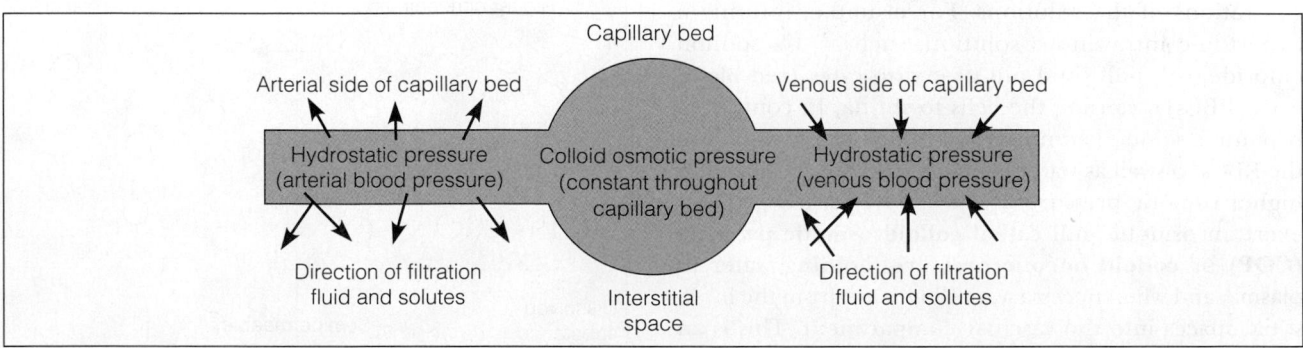

Capillary bed

Arterial side of capillary bed

Venous side of capillary bed

Hydrostatic pressure (arterial blood pressure)

Colloid osmotic pressure (constant throughout capillary bed)

Hydrostatic pressure (venous blood pressure)

Direction of filtration fluid and solutes

Interstitial space

Direction of filtration fluid and solutes

FIGURE 44.5 Schematic of filtration pressure changes within a capillary bed. On the arterial side, arterial blood pressure exceeds colloid osmotic pressure so that water and dissolved substances move out of the capillary and into the interstitial space. On the venous side, venous blood pressure is less than colloid osmotic pressure so that water and dissolved substances move into the capillary.

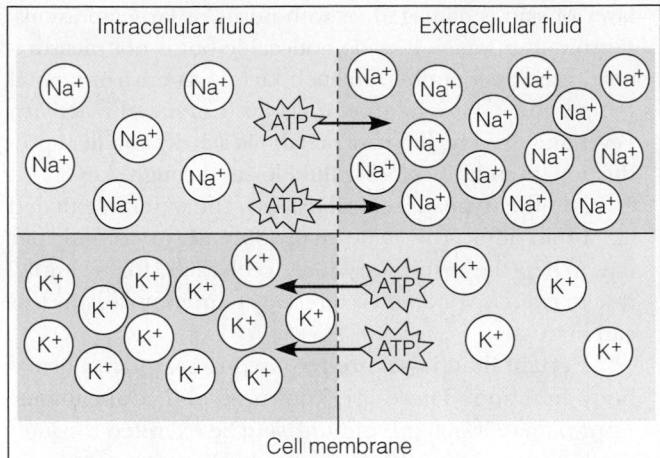

Intracellular fluid   Extracellular fluid

Cell membrane

FIGURE 44.6 An example of active transport. Energy (adenosine triphosphate [ATP]) is used to move sodium molecules and potassium molecules across a semipermeable membrane against sodium's and potassium's concentration gradients (i.e., from areas of lesser concentration to areas of greater concentration).

mechanism (the sodium–potassium pump) is activated, moving sodium from the cells and potassium into the cells. Active transport moves and holds sodium and potassium against their diffusion gradients.

Regulating Body Fluids

In a healthy person the volumes and chemical composition of the fluid compartments stay within narrow limits. Normally, fluid intake and fluid loss are balanced. Illness can upset this balance, causing the body to have too little or too much fluid.

FLUID INTAKE During periods of moderate activity at moderate temperature, the average adult requires a fluid intake of 30 mL/kg/day to 40 mL/kg/day (on average, 2500 mL/day). Fluid intake comes from oral fluids as well as from solid foods that contain water. The oxidation of foods during metabolic processes produces approximately 200 mL per day. The water content of food is relatively high: Fresh vegetables are approximately 90% water, fresh fruits, about 80%, and lean meats, around 60%. See Table 44.1.

TABLE 44.1 Average Daily Fluid Intake for an Adult

Source	Amount (mL)
Oral fluids	1200 to 1500
Water in foods	1000 to 1100
Water as byproduct of food metabolism	200
Total	2400 to 2800

Minimum daily fluid intake requirements for children are higher per kilogram of body weight owing to the greater proportion of body fluid, especially in newborns and infants. The following are formulae for minimum daily fluid requirements in children:

- Body weight 1 kg to 10 kg: requirement = 100 mL/kg (e.g., a baby weighing 5.5 kg requires a minimum of 550 mL fluid intake a day)
- Body weight 10 kg to 20 kg: requirement = 1000 mL + 50 mL/kg above 10 kg (e.g., a 15 kg child requires 1000 + 5 (50) = 1250 mL minimum fluid intake per day)
- Body weight more than 20 kg: requirement = 1500 mL + 20 mL/kg above 20 kg (e.g., a child weighing 22 kg requires 1500 + 2 (20) = 1540 mL minimum fluid intake per day)

The thirst mechanism is the primary regulator of fluid intake. The thirst centre is located in the hypothalamus of the brain. A number of stimuli trigger this centre, including the osmotic pressure of body fluids, vascular volume, and *angiotensin II* (a hormone released in response to decreased blood flow to the kidneys, causing the sensation of thirst and the desire to drink fluids).

Thirst is normally relieved immediately after drinking a small amount of fluid, even before it is absorbed from the gastrointestinal tract. However, this relief is only temporary, and the thirst returns in about 15 minutes. The thirst is again temporarily relieved by drinking a small amount of fluid. This mechanism protects the individual from drinking too much, because it takes between 30 minutes to 1 hour for the fluid to be absorbed and distributed throughout the body (Figure 44.7 on the next page).

FLUID OUTPUT Fluid losses from the body counterbalance the intake of fluid, as shown in Table 44.2 on the next page. The routes of fluid output include the following:

- Urine
- Feces
- Insensible losses (through the skin as perspiration and through the lungs as water vapour in the expired air)

Urine Urine is formed by the kidneys and excreted from the urinary bladder, and is the major route of fluid output. Normal urine output for an adult is 1400 mL to 1500 mL per 24 hours, or at least 30 mL to 50 mL per hour. In healthy people, urine output may vary noticeably from day to day. Urine volume automatically increases as fluid intake increases. If fluid loss through perspiration is large, however, urine volume decreases to maintain fluid balance in the body.

Feces The chyme that passes from the small intestine into the large intestine contains both water and electrolytes. The volume of chyme entering the large intestine in an adult is normally about 1500 mL per day. Of this amount, all but about 100 mL to 200 mL is reabsorbed in

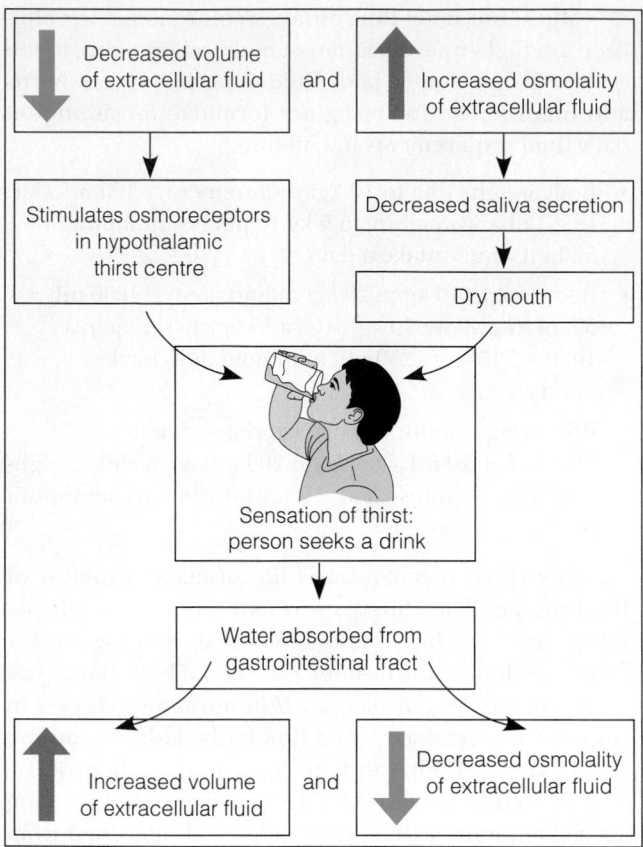

FIGURE 44.7 Factors stimulating water intake through the thirst mechanism.

Source: LeMone, Priscilla; Burke, Kkaren M., *Medical Surgical Nursing: Critical Thinking in Client Care, Single Volume*, 4th Ed., © 2008. Reprinted and reproduced with the permission of Pearson Education, Inc., Upper Saddle River, New Jersey.

TABLE 44.2 Average daily fluid output for an adult

Route	Amount (mL)
Urine	1400 to 1500
Insensible losses: • Lungs • Skin	 350 to 400 350 to 400
Sweat	100
Feces	100 to 200
Total	2200 to 2600

the proximal half of the large intestine. The reabsorbed volume contains primarily water and electrolytes.

Insensible Losses **Insensible water losses** occur through skin and the lungs. They are called *insensible* because it is usually not noticeable and cannot be measured. Insensible fluid loss through skin occurs in two ways: (a) diffusion and (b) perspiration. Water losses through diffusion are not noticeable but normally account for 300 mL to 400 mL per day. This loss can be significantly increased if the protective

layer of skin is damaged, as with burns or large abrasions. Perspiration, which may be noticeable but is not measureable, varies depending on such factors as environmental temperature, body temperature, and metabolic activity. Fever and exercise increase metabolic activity and heat production, thereby increasing fluid losses through skin.

Another type of insensible loss is the water in exhaled air. In an adult, this is normally 350 mL to 400 mL per day. When the respiratory rate accelerates, for example, due to exercise or an elevated body temperature, this loss can increase.

Certain fluid losses are required to maintain normal body function. These are known as **obligatory losses**. Approximately 500 mL of fluid *must* be excreted through the kidneys of an adult each day to eliminate metabolic waste products. Water lost through respirations, through skin, and in feces also are obligatory losses, necessary for temperature regulation and elimination of waste products. The total of all these losses is approximately 1300 mL per day.

MAINTAINING HOMEOSTASIS The volume and composition of body fluids are regulated through several homeostatic mechanisms. A number of organs and systems contribute to this regulation, including the kidneys, lungs, and the cardiovascular and gastrointestinal systems. Hormones, such as antidiuretic hormone (ADH), also known as arginine vasopressin (AVP), the renin–angiotensin–aldosterone system, and the atrial natriuretic factor are also involved, as are mechanisms to monitor and maintain vascular volume.

Kidneys The kidneys are the primary regulator of body fluids and electrolyte balance. They regulate the volume and osmolality of ECF by regulating water and electrolyte excretion. The kidneys control the reabsorption of water from plasma filtrate and, ultimately, the amount excreted as urine. Although 135 L to 180 L of plasma per day is normally filtered in an adult, only about 1.5 L of urine is excreted. Electrolyte balance is maintained by selective retention and excretion by the kidneys. The kidneys also play a significant role in acid–base regulation, excreting hydrogen ions (H^+) and retaining HCO_3^-.

Hormones Several neuroendocrine control mechanisms help control fluid and electrolyte balance.

Antidiuretic Hormone (ADH) ADH, which regulates water excretion from the kidneys, is synthesized in the anterior portion of the hypothalamus and stored in the posterior pituitary gland. ADH acts on the collecting ducts of the nephrons. When serum osmolality rises, ADH is produced, causing the collecting ducts to become more permeable to water. This increased permeability allows more water to be reabsorbed into blood. As more water is reabsorbed, urine output falls and serum osmolality decreases because the water dilutes body fluids. Conversely, if serum osmolality decreases, ADH is suppressed, the collecting ducts become less permeable to water, and urine output increases. Excess water is excreted, and serum osmolality returns to normal. Other factors also affect the production and release of ADH, including blood volume, temperature, pain, stress, and some drugs, such as opiates, barbiturates, caffeine, alcohol, and nicotine. See Figure 44.8.

Renin–Angiotensin–Aldosterone System The renin–angiotensin–aldosterone system is another neuroendocrine control mechanism that contributes to maintaining fluid balance. Specialized receptors in the kidneys respond to changes in renal perfusion, stimulating the renin–angiotensin–aldosterone system. If blood flow or pressure to the kidneys decreases, renin is released. Renin causes the conversion of angiotensinogen to angiotensin I, which is then converted to angiotensin II by angiotensin-converting enzyme (ACE). Angiotensin II acts directly on the nephrons to promote sodium and water retention. In addition, it stimulates the release of aldosterone from the adrenal cortex. Aldosterone also promotes sodium retention in the distal nephron. The net effect of the renin–angiotensin–aldosterone system is to increase blood volume (and renal perfusion) through sodium and water retention.

Atrial Natriuretic Factor Atrial natriuretic factor (ANF) is released from cells in the atrium of the heart in response to excess blood volume and stretching of the atrial walls. Acting on the nephrons, ANF promotes sodium wasting and acts as a potent diuretic, thus decreasing blood volume. ANF also inhibits thirst, reducing fluid intake.

Regulating Electrolytes

Electrolytes, which are charged ions capable of conducting electricity, are present in all body fluids and fluid compartments. Just as maintaining the fluid balance is vital to

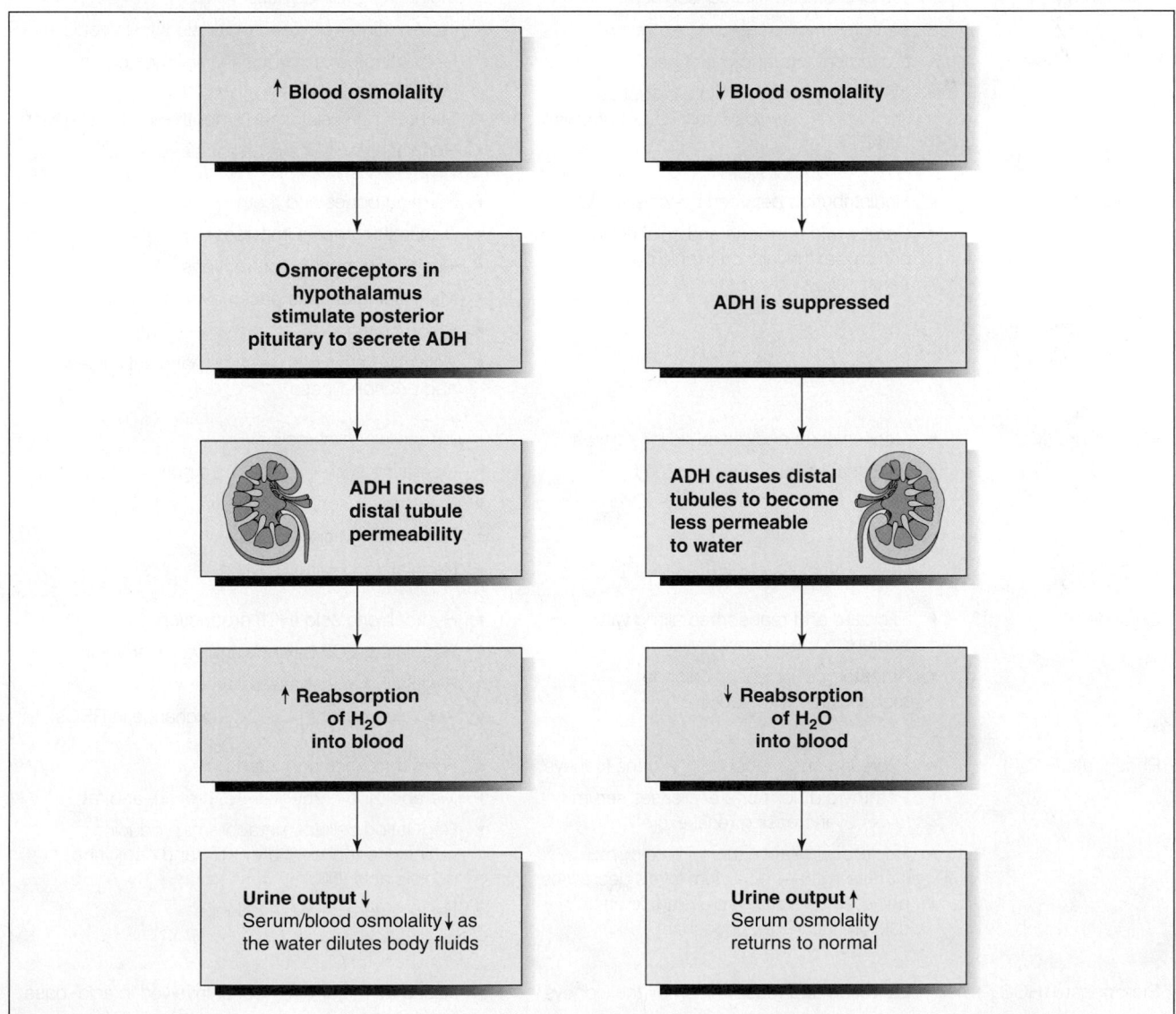

FIGURE 44.8 Antidiuretic hormone (ADH) regulates water excretion from the kidneys.

normal body functions, so is maintaining electrolyte balance. Although the concentration of specific electrolytes differs between fluid compartments, a balance of cations (positively charged ions) and anions (negatively charged ions) always exists. Electrolytes are important for the following:

* Maintaining fluid balance
* Contributing to acid–base regulation
* Facilitating enzyme reactions
* Transmitting neuromuscular reactions

Most electrolytes enter the body through dietary intake and are excreted in the urine. Some electrolytes, such as sodium, are not stored by the body and must be consumed daily to maintain normal levels. Other electrolytes, such as calcium, are stored in the body; when serum levels drop, ions can shift out of storage into the blood to maintain adequate serum levels for normal functioning, at least in the short term. The regulatory mechanisms and functions of the major electrolytes are summarized in Table 44.3.

TABLE 44.3 Regulation and Functions of Electrolytes

Electrolyte	Regulation	Function
Sodium (Na^+)	• Renal reabsorption or excretion • Aldosterone increases Na^+ reabsorption in collecting duct of nephrons	• Regulating ECF volume and distribution • Maintaining blood volume • Transmitting nerve impulses and contracting muscles
Potassium (K^+)	• Renal excretion and conservation • Aldosterone increases K^+ excretion • Movement into and out of cells • Insulin helps move K^+ into cells; tissue damage and acidosis shift K^+ out of cells into ECF	• Maintaining ICF osmolality • Transmitting nerve and other electrical impulses • Regulating cardiac impulse transmission and muscle contraction • Maintaining skeletal and smooth muscle function • Regulating acid–base balance
Calcium (Ca^{2+})	• Redistribution between bones and ECF • Parathyroid hormone and calcitriol increase serum Ca^{2+} levels; calcitonin decreases serum levels	• Forming bones and teeth • Transmitting nerve impulses • Regulating muscle contractions • Maintaining cardiac pacemaker (automaticity) • Blood clotting • Activating enzymes, such as pancreatic lipase and phospholipase
Magnesium (Mg^{2+})	• Conservation and excretion by kidneys • Intestinal absorption increased by vitamin D and parathyroid hormone	• Intracellular metabolism • Operating sodium–potassium pump • Relaxing muscle contractions • Transmitting nerve impulses • Regulating cardiac function
Chloride (Cl^-)	• Excreted and reabsorbed along with sodium in the kidneys • Aldosterone increases chloride reabsorption with sodium	• Hydrochloric acid (HCl) production • Regulating ECF balance and vascular volume • Regulating acid–base balance • Acting as buffer in O_2–CO_2 exchange in RBCs
Phosphate (PO_4^-)	• Excretion and reabsorption by the kidneys • Parathyroid hormone decreases serum levels by increasing renal excretion • Reciprocal relationship with calcium: increasing serum calcium levels decreases phosphate levels; decreasing serum calcium increases phosphate	• Forming bones and teeth • Metabolizing carbohydrate, protein, and fat • Regulating cellular metabolism; producing adenosine triphosphate (ATP) and deoxyribonucleic acid (DNA) • Regulating acid–base balance • Regulating calcium levels
Bicarbonate (HCO_3^-)	• Excretion and reabsorption by the kidneys • Regeneration by kidneys	• Acting as major body buffer involved in acid–base regulation

SODIUM Sodium (Na^+) is the most abundant cation in ECF and a major contributor to serum osmolality. Normal serum sodium levels are 135 mmol/L to 145 mmol/L. Sodium functions mainly in controlling and regulating water balance. When sodium is reabsorbed from the kidney tubules, chloride and water are reabsorbed with it, thus maintaining ECF volume. Sodium is found in many foods, and in especially high levels in foods such as bacon, ham, processed cheese, and table salt.

POTASSIUM Potassium (K^+) is the major cation in ICF, with only a small amount found in plasma and interstitial fluid. ICF levels of potassium are usually 125 mmol/L to 140 mmol/L, while normal serum potassium levels are 3.5 mmol/L to 5.0 mmol/L. The ratio of intracellular to extracellular potassium must be maintained for neuromuscular response to stimuli. Potassium is a vital electrolyte for skeletal, cardiac, and smooth muscle activity. It is involved in maintaining acid–base balance, and it contributes to intracellular enzyme reactions. Potassium must be ingested daily because the body cannot conserve it. Many fruits and vegetables, meat, fish, and other foods contain potassium (see Box 44.1).

CALCIUM The vast majority (99%) of calcium (Ca^{2+}) in the body is in the skeletal system, with a relatively small amount in extracellular fluid. Although the calcium outside the bones and teeth amounts to only about 1% of the total calcium in the body, it is vital in regulating neuromuscular function, including muscle contraction and relaxation, as well as cardiac function. ECF calcium is regulated by a complex interaction of parathyroid hormone, calcitonin (a hormone produced by the thyroid), and calcitriol (a metabolite of vitamin D). When calcium levels in ECF fall, parathyroid hormone and calcitriol cause calcium to be released from bone into ECF and increase the absorption of calcium in the intestines, thus raising serum calcium levels. Conversely, calcitonin stimulates the deposition of calcium in bone, reducing the concentration of calcium ions in the blood.

BOX 44.1 POTASSIUM-RICH FOODS

VEGETABLES	FRUITS
Avocado	Dried fruits (e.g., raisins
Raw carrot	and dates)
Baked potato	Banana
Raw tomato	Apricot
Spinach	Cantaloupe
	Orange
MEATS AND FISH	
Beef	**BEVERAGES**
Cod	Milk
Pork	Orange juice
Veal	Apricot nectar

With increasing age, the intestines absorb calcium less effectively, and more calcium is excreted via the kidneys. Calcium shifts out of bone to replace these ECF losses, increasing the risk of osteoporosis and fractures of the wrists, vertebrae, and hips. Lack of weight-bearing exercise (which helps keep calcium in the bones) and a vitamin D deficiency contribute to this risk, as do genetics and lifestyle factors.

Milk and milk products are the richest sources of calcium, with other foods, such as dark green leafy vegetables and canned salmon, containing smaller amounts. Osteoporosis Canada (2011) recommends the following daily calcium intake: 1000 mg for children age 4 to 8 years; 1300 mg for those age 9 to 18 years; 1000 mg for adults age to 50 years. Postmenopausal women should ingest 1200 mg of calcium per day; however, the consumption of calcium supplements above 2000 mg/day can lead to adverse effects (Health Canada, 2010).

Serum calcium levels are often reported in two ways based on the way it is circulating in the plasma. Approximately 50% of serum calcium circulates in a free or unbound form. The other 50% circulates in the plasma, bound to either plasma proteins or other non-protein ions. The normal total serum calcium level, which ranges from 2.2 mmol/L to 2.58 mmol/L, represents both bound and unbound calcium. The ionized serum calcium level, which ranges from 1.0 mmol/L to 1.15 mmol/L, represents calcium circulating in the plasma in free, or unbound, form.

MAGNESIUM Magnesium (Mg^{2+}) is primarily found in the skeleton and in ICF, where it is the second most abundant intracellular cation. It is important for intracellular metabolism, particularly in the production and use of ATP. Magnesium is also necessary for protein and DNA synthesis within the cells. Only about 1% of the body's magnesium is in ECF, and it has a normal serum level of 0.65 mmol/L to 1.05 mmol/L. In ECF, it is involved in regulating neuromuscular and cardiac function. Maintaining and ensuring adequate magnesium levels is an important part of care of clients with cardiac disorders. Cereal grains, nuts, dried fruit, legumes, and green leafy vegetables are good sources of magnesium in the diet, as well as dairy products, meat, and fish.

CHLORIDE Chloride (Cl^-) is the major anion of ECF, and normal serum levels are 95 mmol/L to 105 mmol/L. Chloride functions with sodium to regulate serum osmolality and blood volume. The concentration of Cl^- in ECF is regulated secondarily to Na^+; when Na^+ is reabsorbed in the kidneys, Cl^- usually follows. Chloride is a major component of gastric juice as HCl and is involved in regulating acid–base balance. It also acts as a buffer in the exchange of O_2 and CO_2 in RBCs. Chloride is found in the same foods as sodium.

PHOSPHATE Phosphate (PO_4^-) is the major anion of ICF. It is also found in ECF, bone, skeletal muscle, and nerve tissue. Normal serum levels of PO_4^- in adults range from 0.97 mmol/L to 1.45 mmol/L. Children have much higher PO_4^- levels compared with adults, with that of a newborn being nearly twice that of an adult. Higher levels of growth hormone and a faster rate of skeletal growth probably account for this difference. Phosphate is involved in many chemical actions of cells, and is essential for functioning of muscles, nerves, and red blood cells. It is also involved in the metabolism of protein, fat, and carbohydrate. Phosphate is absorbed from the intestine and is found in many foods, such as meat, fish, poultry, milk products, and legumes.

BICARBONATE Bicarbonate (HCO_3^-) is present in both ICF and ECF. The normal serum HCO_3^- level in adults is 22 mmol/L to 26 mmol/L. Its primary function is regulating acid–base balance as an essential component of the body's buffering system. Extracellular HCO_3^- levels are regulated by the kidneys. HCO_3^- is excreted when too much is present; if more is needed, the kidneys both regenerate and reabsorb HCO_3^- ions. Unlike other electrolytes that must be consumed in the diet, adequate amounts of HCO_3^- are produced through metabolic processes.

Acid–Base Balance

An important part of body fluid homeostasis is regulating acidity or alkalinity. An **acid** is a substance that releases hydrogen ions (H^+) in solution. Strong acids, such as HCl, release all or nearly all their hydrogen ions; weak acids, such as carbonic acid (H_2CO_3), release some hydrogen ions. **Bases**, or *alkalis*, have a low hydrogen ion concentration and can accept hydrogen ions in solution. The relative acidity or alkalinity of a solution is measured by its **pH**. The pH reflects the hydrogen ion concentration of the solution: The higher the hydrogen ion concentration, the lower is the pH; the lower the hydrogen ion concentration, the higher is the pH. Water has a pH of 7 and is neutral. Solutions with a pH lower than 7 are acidic; those with a pH higher than 7 are alkaline. The pH scale is logarithmic: a solution with a pH of 5 is 10 times as acidic as one with a pH of 6.

Regulation of Acid–Base Balance

Body fluids are normally maintained within a narrow range that is slightly alkaline. The normal pH of arterial blood is between 7.35 and 7.45 (Figure 44.9). Acids are continually produced during metabolism. Several body systems, including the respiratory and renal systems and buffers, are actively involved in maintaining the narrow pH range necessary for optimal function. Buffers help maintain acid–base balance by neutralizing excess acids or bases. The lungs and the kidneys help maintain a normal pH by either excreting or retaining acids and bases, as needed.

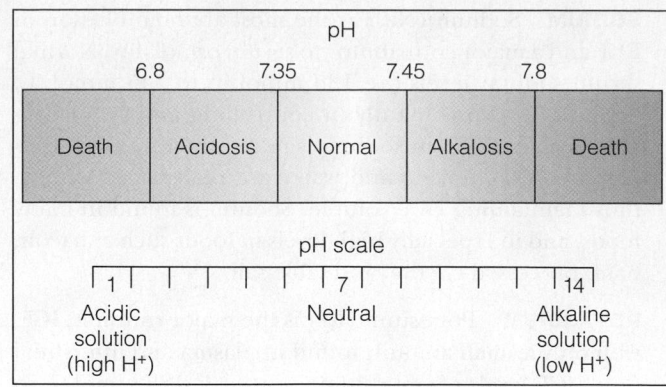

FIGURE 44.9 Body fluids are normally slightly alkaline, between a pH of 7.35 and 7.45.

BUFFERS **Buffers** prevent excessive changes in pH by binding with or releasing hydrogen ions. If body fluids become acidic, meaning excess hydrogen ions are present in body fluids, buffers bind with the hydrogen ions. If body fluids become too alkaline, meaning not enough hydrogen ions are present in body fluids, buffers can release hydrogen ions. The action of a buffer is immediate but limited in its capacity to maintain or restore normal acid–base balance.

The major buffer system in ECF is the bicarbonate (HCO_3^-) and carbonic acid (H_2CO_3) system. The amount of HCO_3^- and H_2CO_3 in the body varies; however, as long as a ratio of 20 parts of HCO_3^- to 1 part of H_2CO_3 is maintained, the pH remains in its normal range of 7.35 to 7.454. However, adding a strong acid to ECF can change this ratio, as HCO_3^- is depleted in neutralizing the acid. When this happens, the pH drops, a condition called **acidosis**. The ratio can also be upset by adding a strong base to ECF, depleting H_2CO_3 as it combines with the base. In this case, the pH rises, and the client has **alkalosis**.

In addition to the HCO_3^-–H_2CO_3 buffer system, plasma proteins, hemoglobin, and phosphates also function as buffers in body fluids.

RESPIRATORY REGULATION The lungs help regulate acid–base balance by eliminating or retaining carbon dioxide (CO_2), a potential acid. When combined with water, CO_2 forms carbonic acid ($CO_2 + H_2O = H_2CO_3$). This chemical reaction is reversible; H_2CO_3 breaks down into CO_2 and H_2O. The lungs help regulate acid–base balance by altering the rate and depth of respirations. The response of the respiratory system to changes in pH is rapid, occurring within minutes. CO_2 is a powerful stimulator of the respiratory centre in the brain. When blood levels of H_2CO_3 and CO_2 rise, the respiratory centre is stimulated, and the rate and depth of respirations increase. This causes an increased amount of CO_2 to be exhaled, and H_2CO_3 levels fall. By contrast, when blood levels of H_2CO_3 and CO_2 fall, the rate and depth of respirations decrease. This causes an increased level of CO_2 to be retained, H_2CO_3 levels rise, and the excess HCO_3^- is neutralized.

BOX 44.2 PHYSIOLOGICAL REGULATION OF ACID–BASE BALANCE

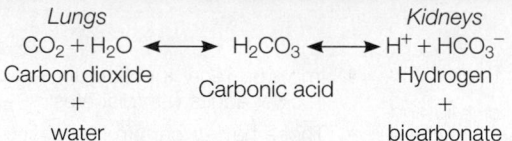

Lungs   *Kidneys*

$$CO_2 + H_2O \longleftrightarrow H_2CO_3 \longleftrightarrow H^+ + HCO_3^-$$

Carbon dioxide   Carbonic acid   Hydrogen
+   +
water   bicarbonate

The lungs and kidneys are the two major systems that are working on a continuous basis to help regulate the acid–base balance in the body. In the biochemical reactions above, the processes are all reversible and go back and forth as the body needs change. The lungs can work very quickly and do their part by either retaining or getting rid of carbon dioxide by changing the rate and depth of respirations. The kidneys work much more slowly; they may take hours to days to regulate the balance by either excreting or conserving hydrogen and bicarbonate ions. Under normal conditions, the two systems work together to maintain homeostasis.

CO_2 levels in the blood are measured as PCO_2, the partial pressure of the dissolved gas in venous blood, and $PaCO_2$, the partial pressure of the dissolved CO_2 in arterial blood. The normal $PaCO_2$ is 35 mm Hg to 45 mm Hg.

RENAL REGULATION Although buffers and the respiratory system can compensate for changes in pH, the kidneys are the ultimate long-term regulators of acid–base balance. They are slower to respond to changes, requiring hours to days to correct imbalances, but their response is more permanent and selective than those of the other systems.

The kidneys maintain acid–base balance by selectively excreting or conserving bicarbonate and hydrogen ions. When excess hydrogen ions are present and the pH falls (acidosis), the kidneys reabsorb and regenerate bicarbonate and excrete hydrogen ions. When insufficient hydrogen ions are present and pH rises (alkalosis), excess bicarbonate is excreted, and hydrogen ions are retained. Normal arterial serum bicarbonate is 22 mmol/L to 26 mmol/L. The relationship of the respiratory and renal regulation of acid–base balance is further explained in Box 44.2.

Factors Affecting Body Fluid, Electrolytes, and the Acid–Base Balance

The ability of the body to adjust fluids, electrolytes, and acid–base balance is influenced by age, sex, body size, environmental temperature, and lifestyle.

Age

Infants and growing children have much greater fluid turnover than have adults because their higher metabolic rate increases fluid loss. Infants lose more fluid through the kidneys because immature kidneys are less able to conserve water than adult kidneys. In addition, infants' respiratory rate is much higher than that of adults, and their body surface area is proportionately greater than that of adults, both of which increase insensible fluid losses. This higher turnover of fluid, combined with the losses produced by disease, can create critical fluid imbalances in children much more rapidly than in adults.

In older adults, the normal aging process may affect fluid balance (see the Lifespan Considerations box on the next page), increasing the risk of dehydration. The thirst response is often diminished. ADH levels remain normal or may even be elevated, but the nephrons become less able to conserve water in response to ADH. Higher levels of ANF may also contribute to this impaired ability to conserve water. These normal changes of aging increase the risk of dehydration. When combined with the increased likelihood of heart disease and impaired renal function, the older adult's risk for fluid and electrolyte imbalance is significant. Additionally, it is important to consider that the older adult has thinner, more fragile skin and veins, which can make an intravenous insertion more difficult.

Sex and Body Size

Total body water also is affected by sex and body size. Fat cells contain little or no water, but lean tissue has a high water content; therefore, people with a higher percentage of body fat have less body water than people with a higher percentage of lean muscle. Women generally have proportionately more body fat and, therefore, less body water than men. Water accounts for approximately 80% of a newborn's weight, 60% of an adult male's weight, but only 52% of an adult female's weight. In an obese individual, this percentage may be even smaller, with water accounting for only 30% to 40% of the person's weight.

Environmental Temperature

People with an illness and those participating in strenuous activity are at increased risk for fluid and electrolyte imbalances when the environmental temperature is high. Fluid losses through sweating are increased in hot environments as the body attempts to dissipate heat. These losses are even greater in people who are not accustomed to a hot environment.

Both electrolytes and water are lost through sweating. When only water is replaced, electrolyte depletion is a risk. A person who is electrolyte depleted may experience fatigue, weakness, headache, and gastrointestinal symptoms, such as anorexia and nausea. The risk

Fluid and Electrolyte Balance

INFANTS AND CHILDREN

Infants are at high risk for fluid and electrolyte imbalance because of the following:

- Their immature kidneys cannot concentrate urine.
- They have a rapid respiratory rate and proportionately larger body surface area than adults, leading to greater insensible fluid loss through skin and respirations.
- They cannot express thirst, nor can they actively seek fluids.

Vomiting and/or diarrhea in infants and young children can lead quickly to electrolyte imbalance. Oral rehydration therapy (ORT) with electrolyte solutions (such as Pedialyte) should be used to restore fluid and electrolyte balance in mild to moderate dehydration. Prompt treatment with ORT can prevent the need for intravenous therapy and hospitalization. Even if the child is vomiting, small sips of ORT can be helpful.

OLDER ADULTS

Older adults are at high risk for fluid and electrolyte imbalance because of the decreases in the following:

- Thirst sensation
- Ability of the kidneys to concentrate urine
- Intracellular fluid and in total body water
- Response to body hormones that help regulate fluid and electrolytes

Other factors that may influence fluid and electrolyte balance in older adults are as follows:

- Use of diuretics for hypertension and heart disease
- Decreased intake of food and water, especially in older adults with dementia or who are dependent on others to feed them and offer them fluids
- Preparations for diagnostic tests that include being NPO (nil per os; nothing by mouth) for long periods, laxatives, or contrast dyes

- Impaired renal function, for example, in older adults with diabetes
- Those having certain diagnostic procedures (dyes used for some procedures, such as arteriograms and cardiac catheterizations, can cause further renal problems; ensure the client is well hydrated before, during, and after the procedure to help in diluting and excreting the dye; if the client is NPO for the procedure, the nurse should check with the appropriate health care provider to see whether IV fluids are needed)

All these factors increase older adults' risk for fluid and electrolyte imbalance, particularly under conditions that tax the normal compensatory mechanisms, such as a fever, influenza, surgery, or heat exposure. The change can happen quickly and become serious in a short time. A change in mental status may be the first symptom of impairment and must be further evaluated to determine the cause.

---

of adverse effects is even greater if loss of water is not replaced. Body temperature rises, and the person is at risk for heat exhaustion or heatstroke; this happens when a person's heat production exceeds the body's ability to dissipate heat. Consuming adequate amounts of cool liquids, particularly during strenuous activity, reduces the risk of adverse effects from heat.

Lifestyle

Lifestyle factors, such as diet, exercise, stress, and alcohol consumption, affect fluid, electrolyte, and acid–base balance. The intake of fluids and electrolytes is affected by diet. People with eating disorders are at risk for severe fluid and electrolyte imbalances because of inadequate intake or purging regimens (e.g., inducing vomiting, using diuretics and laxatives). Seriously malnourished people have decreased serum albumin levels and may develop edema because the osmotic draw of fluid into the vascular compartment is reduced. When calorie intake is not adequate to meet the body's needs, fat stores are broken down and fatty acids are released, increasing the risk of acidosis.

Regular weight-bearing exercise, such as walking, running, or bicycling, has a beneficial effect on calcium balance. The rate of bone loss that occurs in postmenopausal women and older men is slowed with weight-bearing exercise, reducing the risk of osteoporosis.

Stress can increase cellular metabolism, blood glucose concentration, and catecholamine levels. In addition, stress can increase production of ADH, which, in turn, decreases urine production. The overall response of the body to stress is to increase the blood volume.

Heavy alcohol consumption affects electrolyte balance, increasing the risk of low calcium, magnesium, and phosphate levels. In addition, the risk of acidosis associated with breakdown of fat tissue is greater in people who drink large amounts of alcohol.

Disturbances in Fluid, Electrolyte, and Acid–Base Balance

A number of factors, such as illness, trauma, surgery, and medications, can affect the body's ability to maintain fluid, electrolyte, and acid–base balance. The kidneys play a major role in maintaining fluid, electrolyte, and acid–base balance. Renal disease is a significant cause of fluid, electrolyte and acid–base imbalance. In addition, decreased blood flow to the kidneys, due to impaired cardiac function, stimulates the renin–angiotensin–aldosterone system, causing sodium and water retention. Medications, such as diuretics or corticosteroids, can result in abnormal losses of electrolytes and fluid loss or retention. Diseases, such as diabetes mellitus or chronic obstructive pulmonary disease (COPD) and cancer, can affect acid–base balance. Clients who are confused or unable to communicate their needs are at risk for inadequate fluid intake. Vomiting, diarrhea, or nasogastric suction can cause significant fluid and electrolyte losses. Tissue trauma, such as burns, causes fluid and electrolytes to be lost from damaged cells. Medications, such as diuretics or corticosteroids, can result in abnormal losses of electrolytes and fluid loss or retention.

Fluid Imbalances

Fluid imbalances are of two basic types: (a) isotonic and (b) osmolar. **Isotonic imbalance** occurs when water and electrolytes are lost or gained in equal proportions so that the osmolality of body fluids remains constant. **Osmolar imbalance** involves the loss or gain of *only* water, so that the osmolality of the serum is altered. Thus, four categories of fluid imbalances may occur: (a) an isotonic loss of water and electrolytes, (b) an isotonic gain of water and electrolytes, (c) a hyperosmolar loss of only water, and (d) a hypoosmolar gain of only water. These are referred to, respectively, as *fluid volume deficit, fluid volume excess, dehydration* (hyperosmolar imbalance), and *overhydration* (hypoosmolar imbalance).

FLUID VOLUME DEFICIT Isotonic **fluid volume deficit (FVD)** occurs when the body loses both water and electrolytes from the ECF in similar proportions. Thus, the decreased volume of fluid remains isotonic. In FVD, fluid is initially lost from the intravascular compartment, so it often is called **hypovolemia.**

FVD generally occurs as a result of (a) abnormal losses through the skin, gastrointestinal tract, or kidneys; (b) decreased intake of fluid; (c) bleeding; or (d) movement of fluid into a third space. See the section on "third space syndrome" that follows.

For the risk factors, clinical manifestations, and nursing interventions related to fluid volume deficit, see Table 44.4.

Third Space Syndrome In **third space syndrome**, fluid shifts from the vascular space into an area where it is not readily accessible. This fluid remains in the body but is essentially unavailable for use, causing an isotonic fluid volume deficit. Fluid may be sequestered in the bowel, in the interstitial space as edema, in inflamed tissue, or in potential spaces, such as the peritoneal or pleural cavities.

TABLE 44.4 Isotonic Fluid Volume Deficit

Risk Factors	Clinical Manifestations	Nursing Interventions
Loss of water and electrolytes from the following: • Vomiting • Diarrhea • Excessive sweating • Polyuria • Fever • Nasogastric suction • Abnormal drainage or wound losses • Bleeding Insufficient intake caused by the following: • Anorexia • Nausea • Inability to access fluids • Impaired swallowing • Confusion, depression	Complaints of weakness and thirst Weight loss • 2% loss = mild FVD • 5% loss = moderate FVD • 8% loss = severe FVD Fluid intake less than output Decreased tissue turgor Dry mucous membranes, sunken eyeballs, decreased tearing Subnormal temperature Weak pulse, tachycardia Decreased blood pressure Postural (orthostatic) hypotension Flat neck veins, decreased capillary refill Decreased central venous pressure (CVP) Decreased urine volume (<30 mL/h) Increased specific gravity of urine (>1.030) Increased hematocrit (HCT) Increased blood urea nitrogen (BUN)	Assess for clinical manifestations of fluid volume deficit (FVD). Monitor weight and vital signs, including temperature. Assess capillary refill time. Assess tissue turgor. Assess breath sounds. Monitor fluid intake and output. Monitor laboratory findings. Administer oral and intravenous fluids, as indicated. Provide frequent mouth care so as to decrease unpleasant taste in the mouth and stimulate thirst. Implement measures to prevent skin breakdown. Provide for safety, for example, provide assistance to a client rising from bed.

The client with third space syndrome has an isotonic fluid deficit but may not manifest apparent fluid loss or weight loss. Careful nursing assessment is vital to effectively identify and intervene for clients experiencing third spacing. Because the fluid shifts back into the vascular compartment after time, assessment for manifestations of fluid volume excess or hypervolemia is also vital.

FLUID VOLUME EXCESS **Fluid volume excess (FVE)** occurs when the body retains both water and sodium in similar proportions to normal ECF. This is commonly referred to as **hypervolemia** (increased blood volume). FVE is always secondary to an increase in the total body sodium content, which leads to an increase in total body water. Because both water and sodium are retained, the serum sodium concentration remains essentially normal and the excess volume of fluid is isotonic. Specific causes of FVE include (a) excessive intake of sodium chloride; (b) the administration of sodium-containing infusions too rapidly, particularly to clients with impaired regulatory mechanisms; and (c) disease processes that alter regulatory mechanisms, such as heart failure, renal failure, cirrhosis of the liver, and Cushing's syndrome.

The risk factors, clinical manifestations, and nursing interventions for FVE are summarized in Table 44.5.

Edema In fluid volume excess, both intravascular and interstitial spaces have an increased water and sodium content. Excess ISF is known as **edema**. Edema typically is most apparent in areas where the tissue pressure is low, such as around the eyes, and in dependent tissues (known as *dependent edema*) where hydrostatic capillary pressure is high.

Edema can be caused by several different mechanisms. The three main mechanisms are (a) increased capillary hydrostatic pressure, (b) decreased plasma oncotic pressure, and (c) increased capillary permeability. Edema may be due to FVE that increases capillary hydrostatic pressure, pushing fluid into the interstitial tissues. This type of edema is often seen in dependent tissues, such as the feet, hands, ankles, and sacrum, because of the effects of gravity. Low levels of plasma proteins from malnutrition or liver or kidney diseases can reduce the plasma oncotic pressure so that fluid is not drawn into the capillaries from interstitial tissues, causing edema. With tissue trauma and some disorders, such as allergic reactions, capillaries become more permeable, allowing fluid to escape from the capillaries into interstitial tissues. Obstructed lymph flow also impairs the movement of fluid from interstitial tissues back into the vascular compartment, resulting in edema.

Pitting edema is edema that leaves a small depression or pit after finger pressure is applied to the swollen area. The pit is caused by movement of fluid to adjacent tissue, away from the point of pressure (Figure 44.10). The pit normally disappears within 10 to 30 seconds, as fluid returns to the area.

DEHYDRATION **Dehydration**, or hyperosmolar imbalance, occurs when water is lost from the body, leaving the client with excess sodium. Because water is lost while electrolytes, particularly sodium, are retained, the serum osmolality and serum sodium levels increase. Water is drawn into the vascular compartment from the interstitial spaces and cells, resulting in cellular dehydration. Older adults are at particular risk for dehydration because of decreased thirst sensation. Dehydration can also affect clients who are hyperventilating, have a prolonged fever, are in diabetic ketoacidosis, or are receiving enteral feedings with insufficient water intake.

TABLE 44.5 Isotonic Fluid Volume Excess

Risk Factors	Clinical Manifestations	Nursing Interventions
Excess intake of sodium-containing intravenous fluids	Weight gain	Assess for clinical manifestations of FVE.
Excess ingestion of sodium in diet or medications (e.g., sodium bicarbonate antacids, such as Alka-Seltzer; or hypertonic enema solutions, such as Fleet)	• 2% gain = mild FVE • 5% gain = moderate FVE • 8% gain = severe FVE	Monitor weight and vital signs.
	Fluid intake greater than output	Assess for edema.
	Moist mucous membranes	Assess breath sounds, dyspnea.
Impaired fluid balance regulation related to heart failure, renal failure, and/or cirrhosis of the liver	Full, bounding pulse; tachycardia	Monitor fluid intake and output.
	Increased blood pressure and central venous pressure (CVP)	Monitor laboratory findings.
	Distended neck and peripheral veins; slow vein emptying	Place client in Fowler's position.
	Moist crackles in lungs; dyspnea, shortness of breath	Administer diuretics, as ordered.
	Mental confusion	Restrict fluid intake, as ordered.
	Peripheral edema	Restrict dietary sodium, as ordered.
		Implement measures to prevent skin breakdown.

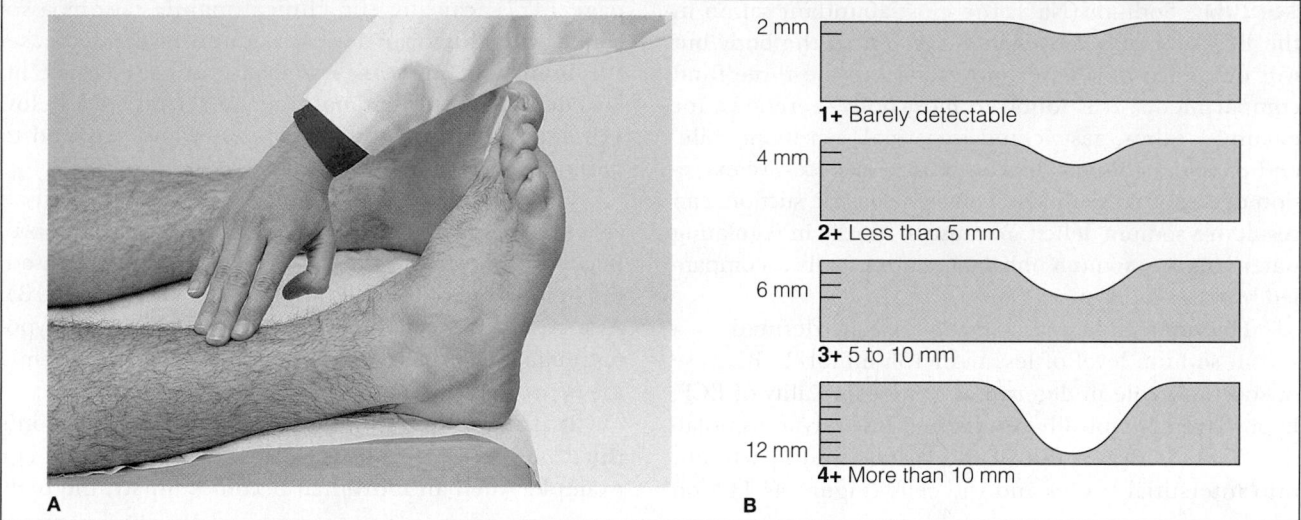

FIGURE 44.10 Evaluation of edema: **A:** Palpating for edema over the tibia, as shown here, and behind the medial malleolus and over the dorsum of each foot; **B:** Four-point scale for grading edema.

OVERHYDRATION **Overhydration**, also known as *hypoosmolar fluid imbalance*, occurs when water is gained in excess of electrolytes, resulting in low serum osmolality and low serum sodium levels. Water is drawn into the cells, causing them to swell. In the brain, this can lead to cerebral edema and impaired neurological function. Overhydration, sometimes called water intoxication, often occurs when both fluid and electrolytes are lost, for example, through excessive sweating, but only water is replaced. It can also result from the syndrome of inappropriate antidiuretic hormone (SIADH), acquired immunodeficiency syndrome

(AIDS), head injury, or administration of certain drugs, such as barbiturates or anesthetics. The characteristics of fluid volume gains and losses are noted in Table 44.6.

Electrolyte Imbalances

The most common and clinically significant electrolyte imbalances involve sodium, potassium, calcium, magnesium, chloride, and phosphate. Table 44.7 on the next page lists risk factors, clinical manifestations, and nursing interventions for several electrolyte imbalances.

TABLE 44.6 Comparison of Fluid Volume Gains and Fluid Volume Losses

Fluid Volume Gains	Etiology
Isotonic fluid volume excess (FVE) (hypovolemia)	Excessive intake of sodium chloride
	Administration of sodium-containing infusions too rapidly
	Disease processes that alter regulatory mechanisms, such as heart failure, renal failure, cirrhosis of the liver, and Cushing's syndrome
Overhydration (hypoosmolar imbalance or water excess)	Increased water, not sodium, as can occur with excess ADH, head injury, human immunodeficiency virus (HIV), some drugs, water-only replacement
Fluid Volume Losses	**Etiology**
Isotonic fluid volume deficit (FVD) (hypovolemia)	Increased losses through the skin, gastrointestinal tract, or kidney
	Decreased intake of fluid
	Bleeding
	Movement of fluid into a third space
Dehydration (hyperosmolar imbalance)	Older adults with decreased thirst sensation
	Athletes with excessive sweating or hyperventilating
	Prolonged fever
	Diabetic ketoacidosis
	Enteral feedings with insufficient water intake

SODIUM   Sodium (Na^+), the most abundant cation in the ECF, not only moves into and out of the body but will influence how water moves among the three fluid compartments. It is found in most body secretions, for example, saliva, gastric and intestinal secretions, bile, and pancreatic fluid. The continuous or excessive excretion of any of these fluids, such as via gastric suction, can result in a sodium deficit. Because of its role in regulating water balance, sodium imbalances are usually accompanied by water imbalances.

Hyponatremia is a sodium deficit, defined as a serum sodium level of less than 135 mmol/L. Because of sodium's role in determining the osmolality of ECF, hyponatremia typically results in a low serum osmolality. Water is drawn out of the vascular compartment into interstitial tissues and the cells (Figure 44.11A on page 1427), causing the clinical manifestations associated with this disorder. As sodium levels decrease, the brain and nervous system are affected by cellular edema. Severe hyponatremia, a serum level below 110 mmol/L, is a medical emergency and can lead to permanent neurological damage.

Hypernatremia is a sodium excess in ECF, defined as a serum sodium level of greater than 145 mmol/L. Because the osmotic pressure of the ECF is increased, fluid moves out of the cells into the ECF (Figure 44.11B). As a result, the cells become dehydrated. As in hyponatremia, the primary manifestations of hypernatremia are neurological in nature.

It is important to note that, normally, a person's thirst mechanism protects against hypernatremia. For example, when an individual becomes thirsty, the body

TABLE 44.7   Electrolyte Imbalances

Risk Factors	Clinical Manifestations	Nursing Interventions
Hyponatremia		
Loss of sodium:	Lethargy, confusion, apprehension	Assess clinical manifestations.
• Gastrointestinal fluid loss	Muscle twitching	Monitor fluid intake and output.
• Sweating	Abdominal cramps	Monitor laboratory data
• Use of diuretics	Anorexia, nausea, vomiting	(e.g., serum Na^+).
	Headache	Assess client closely if administering
Gain of water:	Seizures, coma	hypertonic saline solutions.
• Hypotonic tube feedings		Encourage food and fluid high in Na^+,
• Excessive drinking of water	*Laboratory findings:*	if permitted (e.g., processed foods,
• Excess hypotonic IV solution administration (e.g., D_5W [5% dextrose in water])	Serum sodium below 135 mmol/L	table salt).
	Serum osmolality below 280 mOsm/kg	Limit water intake, as indicated.
Syndrome of inappropriate ADH (SIADH):		
• Head injury		
• Acquired immunodeficiency syndrome (AIDS)		
• Malignant tumours		
• Brain surgery		
Hypernatremia		
Loss of water:	Thirst	Monitor fluid intake and output.
• Insensible water loss (hyperventilation, fever)	Dry, sticky mucous membranes	Monitor behaviour changes (e.g., restlessness, disorientation).
• Diarrhea	Tongue red, dry, swollen	Monitor laboratory findings
• Water deprivation	Weakness	(e.g., serum Na^+).
	Postural hypotension, dyspnea	Encourage fluids, as ordered.
Gain of sodium:	Severe hypernatremia:	Monitor diet, as ordered (e.g., restrict
• Parenteral administration of saline solutions		intake of salt and foods high in sodium).
• Hypertonic tube feedings without adequate water	• Fatigue, restlessness	
• Excessive use of table salt (1 tsp or 5 mL contains 2300 mg of sodium)	• Decreasing level of consciousness	
	• Disorientation	
Conditions, such as the following:	• Convulsions	
• Diabetes insipidus	*Laboratory findings:*	
• Heatstroke	Serum sodium above 145 mmol/L	
	Serum osmolality above 300 mOsm/kg	

TABLE 44.7 Electrolyte Imbalances (*continued*)

Risk Factors	Clinical Manifestations	Nursing Interventions
Hypokalemia		
Loss of potassium: • Vomiting and gastric suction • Diarrhea • Heavy perspiration Use of potassium-wasting drugs (e.g., diuretics) Poor intake of potassium (as with debilitated clients, clients with alcoholism or anorexia nervosa) Hyperaldosteronism	Muscle weakness, leg cramps Fatigue, lethargy Anorexia, nausea, vomiting Decreased bowel sounds, decreased bowel motility Cardiac dysrhythmias Depressed deep-tendon reflexes *Laboratory findings:* Serum potassium below 3.5 mmol/L Arterial blood gases (ABGs) may show alkalosis T wave flattening and ST segment depression on electrocardiography (ECG)	Monitor heart rate and rhythm and ECG. Monitor clients receiving digitalis closely because hypokalemia increases risk of digitalis toxicity. Administer oral K^+, as ordered, with food or fluid to prevent gastric irritation. Administer diluted intravenous K^+ solutions at a rate no faster than 10–20 mmol/h; never administer undiluted potassium intravenously. For clients receiving IV potassium, monitor for pain and inflammation at the injection site. Teach client about potassium-rich foods. Teach clients how to prevent excessive loss of K^+ (e.g., through avoiding abuse of diuretics and laxatives).
Hyperkalemia		
Decreased potassium excretion: • Renal failure • Hypoaldosteronism • Potassium-conserving diuretics High potassium intake: • Excessive use of potassium-containing salt substitutes • Excessive or rapid IV infusion of potassium Potassium shift out of the tissue cells into the plasma (e.g., infections, burns, acidosis)	Gastrointestinal hyperactivity, diarrhea Irritability, apathy, confusion Cardiac dysrhythmias or arrest Muscle weakness, absence of reflexes Paresthesias and numbness in extremities *Laboratory findings:* Serum potassium above 5.0 mmol/L Peaked T wave, widened QRS on ECG	Closely monitor cardiac status and ECG. Administer diuretics and other medications, such as glucose and insulin, as ordered. Hold K^+ supplements and potassium-conserving diuretics as ordered. Monitor serum K^+ levels carefully; a rapid drop can occur as potassium shifts into the cells. Teach clients to avoid foods high in K^+ and salt substitutes.
Hypocalcemia		
Surgical removal of the parathyroid glands Conditions, such as the following: • Hypoparathyroidism • Acute pancreatitis • Hyperphosphatemia • Thyroid carcinoma Inadequate vitamin D intake Malabsorption Hypomagnesemia Alkalosis Sepsis Alcohol abuse	Numbness, tingling of the extremities and around the mouth Muscle tremors, cramps; if severe, can progress to tetany and convulsions Cardiac dysrhythmias; decreased cardiac output Positive Trousseau's and Chvostek's signs Confusion, anxiety, possible psychoses Blood clots Bone fractures *Laboratory findings:* Serum calcium less than 2.2 mmol/L (total) or 1.0 mmol/L (ionized)	Closely monitor respiratory and cardiovascular status. Take precautions to protect a confused client. Administer oral or parenteral calcium supplements, as ordered. When administering intravenously, closely monitor cardiac status and ECG during infusion. Teach clients at high risk for osteoporosis about the following: • Dietary sources rich in calcium • Recommendation for 1200 mg of calcium per day for adults >50 years • Calcium supplements, as ordered • Regular exercise • Estrogen replacement therapy for postmenopausal women, as ordered Monitor respiratory and cardiovascular status.

(continued)

TABLE 44.7 Electrolyte Imbalances (*continued*)

Risk Factors	Clinical Manifestations	Nursing Interventions
Hypercalcemia		
Prolonged immobilization	Lethargy, weakness	Increase client movement and exercise.
Conditions such as the following:	Depressed deep-tendon reflexes	Encourage oral fluids, as permitted, to maintain a dilute urine.
• Hyperparathyroidism	Anorexia, nausea, vomiting	Teach clients to limit intake of food and fluid high in calcium.
• Malignancy of the bone	Constipation	Encourage ingestion of fibre to prevent constipation.
• Paget's disease	Polyuria, hypercalciuria	Protect a confused client; monitor for pathological fractures in clients with long-term hypercalcemia.
	Flank pain secondary to urinary calculi	
	Dysrhythmias, possible heart block	Encourage intake of acid-ash fluids (e.g., prune or cranberry juice) to counteract deposits of calcium salts in the urine.
	Bone pain, fractures	
	Laboratory findings:	Increase client movement and exercise.
	Serum calcium greater than 2.58 mmol/L (total) or 1.15 mmol/L (ionized)	Encourage oral fluids, as permitted, to maintain dilute urine.
	Shortened QT intervals	
	Shortened ST segments	
Hypomagnesemia		
Excessive loss from the gastrointestinal tract (e.g., from nasogastric suction, diarrhea, fistula drainage)	Neuromuscular irritability with tremors	Monitor respiratory and cardiovascular status.
	Increased reflexes, tremors, convulsions	Assess clients receiving digitalis for digitalis toxicity. Hypomagnesemia increases the risk of toxicity.
Long-term use of certain drugs (e.g., diuretics, aminoglycoside antibiotics)	Positive Chvostek's and Trousseau's signs	Take protective measures when there is a possibility of seizures.
Conditions such as the following:	Tachycardia, elevated blood pressure, dysrhythmias	• Assess the client's ability to swallow water before initiating oral feeding.
• Chronic alcoholism	Disorientation, confusion, vertigo	• Initiate safety measures to prevent injury during seizure activity.
• Pancreatitis	Anorexia, dysphagia	• Carefully administer magnesium salts as ordered.
• Burns	*Laboratory findings:*	Encourage clients to eat magnesium-rich foods, if permitted (e.g., whole grains, meat, seafood, and green leafy vegetables).
	Serum magnesium below 0.65 mmol/L	
	Prolonged PR and QT intervals, widened QRS, flat T wave; ST depression	Refer clients to alcohol treatment programs, as indicated.
Hypermagnesemia		
Abnormal retention of magnesium, as in the following:	Peripheral vasodilation, flushing	Monitor respiratory and cardiovascular status.
• Renal failure	Nausea, vomiting	Monitor vital signs and level of consciousness when clients are at risk.
• Adrenal insufficiency	Muscle weakness, paralysis	
• Treatment with magnesium salts	Hypotension, bradycardia	If patellar reflexes are absent, notify the physician.
	Depressed deep-tendon reflexes	Advise clients who have renal disease to contact their care provider before taking over-the-counter drugs.
	Lethargy, drowsiness	
	Respiratory depression, coma	
	Respiratory and cardiac arrest, if hypermagnesemia is severe	
	Laboratory findings:	
	Serum magnesium above 1.05 mmol/L	
	Prolonged PR and QT interval; widened QRS complexes	

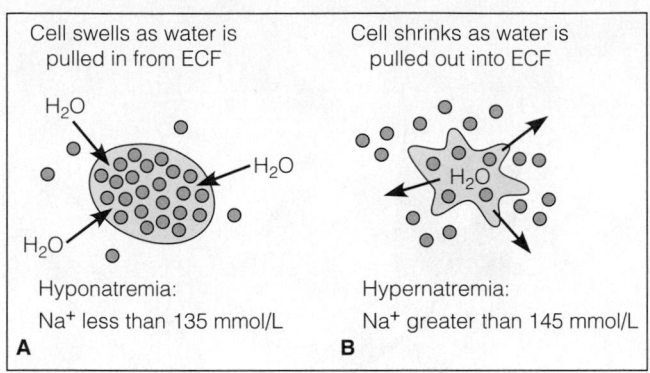

Cell swells as water is pulled in from ECF

H_2O
H_2O
H_2O

Hyponatremia: Na^+ less than 135 mmol/L

A

Cell shrinks as water is pulled out into ECF

H_2O

Hypernatremia: Na^+ greater than 145 mmol/L

B

FIGURE 44.11 The extracellular sodium level affects cell size: **A:** In hyponatremia, cells swell; **B:** In hypernatremia, cells shrink.

is stimulated to drink water, which helps correct the hypernatremia. Clients at risk for hypernatremia are those who are unable to access water (e.g., unconscious; unable to request fluids, such as infants or older adults with dementia; or ill clients with an impaired thirst mechanism).

POTASSIUM   Although the amount of potassium (K^+) in ECF is small, it is vital to normal neuromuscular and cardiac function. Normal renal function is important for maintenance of potassium balance as 80% of potassium is excreted by the kidneys. Potassium must be replaced daily to maintain its balance, which normally happens through food intake. See Box 44.1 on page 1417 to review foods high in potassium. Abnormalities in potassium balance represent the most common electrolyte imbalance in hospitalized patients.

Hypokalemia is a potassium deficit, defined as a serum potassium level of less than 3.5 mmol/L. Gastrointestinal losses of potassium through vomiting and gastric suction are common causes of hypokalemia, as is the use of potassium-wasting diuretics, such as thiazides or loop diuretics (e.g., furosemide). Symptoms of hypokalemia are usually mild until the level drops below 3 mmol/L, unless the decrease in potassium is rapid. When the decrease is gradual, the body compensates by shifting potassium from the intracellular environment into the serum.

Hyperkalemia is a potassium excess, defined as a serum K^+ level greater than 5.0 mmol/L. Hyperkalemia is less common than hypokalemia and rarely occurs in clients with normal renal function. It is, however, more dangerous than hypokalemia and can lead to cardiac arrest. As with hypokalemia, symptoms are more severe and occur at lower levels when the increase in potassium is rapid. See the Clinical Alert box on intravenous administration of potassium.

CALCIUM   Levels of calcium (Ca^{2+}) in the body can be affected by many factors. **Hypocalcemia** is a calcium deficit, defined as a total serum Ca^{2+} level of less than 2.2 mmol/L (total) or an ionized Ca^{2+} level of less

⚠ CLINICAL ALERT

Potassium may be given intravenously for severe hypokalemia. It must always be diluted appropriately and never be given as an intravenous (IV) push. Potassium that is to be given intravenously should be mixed in the pharmacy and double-checked by two nurses before administration. The usual concentration of IV K^+ is 20 to 40 mmol/L.

than 1.0 mmol/L. Severe depletion of Ca^{2+} can cause tetany (muscle spasms) and paresthesias (numbness and tingling around the mouth or in the hands or feet) and can lead to convulsions. Two signs indicate hypocalcemia: (a) Chvostek's sign is contraction of the facial muscles that is produced by tapping the facial nerve in front of the ear (Figure 44.12A on the next page); and (b) Trousseau's sign is a carpal spasm that occurs by inflating a blood pressure cuff on the upper arm to 20 mm Hg greater than the systolic pressure for 2 to 5 minutes (Figure 44.12B). Clients at greatest risk for hypocalcemia are those whose parathyroid glands have been removed. This is frequently associated with total thyroidectomy or other neck surgeries, which can result in unintentional removal or damage to the parathyroid glands. Low serum magnesium levels (hypomagnesemia) and chronic alcoholism also increase the risk of hypocalcemia.

Hypercalcemia is a calcium excess, defined as a total serum Ca^{2+} level greater than 2.58 mmol/L (total) or an ionized Ca^{2+} level greater than 1.15 mmol/L, which most often occurs when Ca^{2+} is released in excess from the bony skeleton. This is usually caused by malignancy or prolonged immobilization.

MAGNESIUM   The majority of magnesium (Mg^{2+}) is found intracellularly. Many organs, including nerves and muscles, depend on magnesium. Imbalances may go unrecognized in hospitalized clients.

Hypomagnesemia is a magnesium deficiency defined as a serum Mg^{2+} level of less than 0.65 mmol/L. It occurs more frequently than hypermagnesemia. Chronic alcoholism is the most common cause of hypomagnesemia. Magnesium deficiency may also aggravate the manifestations of alcohol withdrawal, such as delirium tremens (DTs). **Hypermagnesemia** is a magnesium excess, defined as a serum Mg^{2+} level above 1.05 mmol/L. It is often iatrogenic, that is, caused by medical treatment; usually the cause is oversupplementation of magnesium.

CHLORIDE   Because of the relationship between sodium ions and chloride ions (Cl^-), imbalances of chloride commonly occur in conjunction with sodium imbalances. **Hypochloremia** is a chloride deficit, defined as a serum Cl^- level below 95 mmol/L, and is usually related to excess losses of Cl^- through the gastrointestinal (GI) tract, kidneys, or sweating. Hypochloremic clients are at risk for alkalosis and may experience muscle twitching,

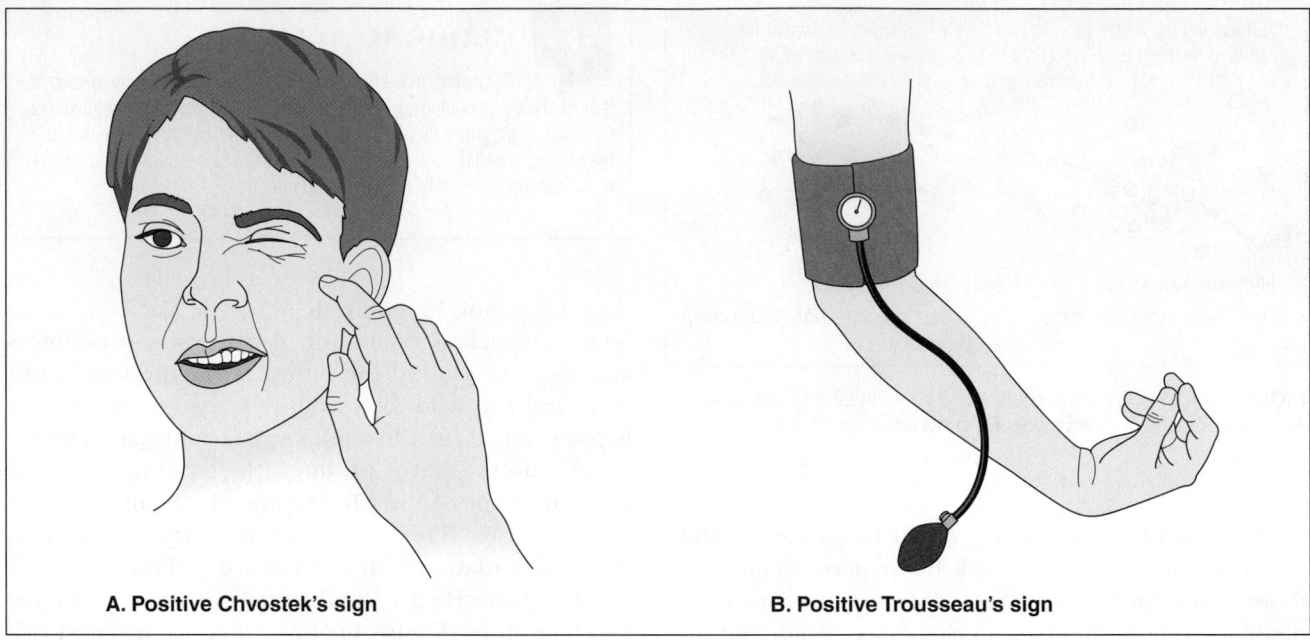

A. Positive Chvostek's sign

B. Positive Trousseau's sign

FIGURE 44.12 A: Positive Chvostek's sign; **B:** Positive Trousseau's sign.

Source: From LeMone, P., & Burke, K. (2008). *Medical surgical nursing: Critical thinking in client care* (4th ed.). Upper Saddle River, NJ: Pearson Education, Inc. Reproduced with the permission of Pearson Education, Inc., Upper Saddle River, New Jersey.

tremors, or tetany. **Hyperchloremia** is a chloride excess, defined as a serum Cl⁻ level above 108 mmol/L. Excess replacement of sodium chloride or potassium chloride is a risk factor for high serum Cl⁻ levels, as are conditions that lead to hypernatremia. The manifestations of hyperchloremia include acidosis, weakness, and lethargy, with a risk of dysrhythmias and coma.

PHOSPHATE The phosphate anion (PO_4^-) is found in ICF and ECF. Most of the phosphorus (P^+) in the body exists as PO_4^-. Phosphate is critical for cellular metabolism because it is a major component of adenosine triphosphate (ATP). Phosphate imbalances frequently are related to therapeutic interventions for other disorders.

Hypophosphatemia is a phosphate deficit defined as a serum PO_4^- level of less than 0.9 mmol/L. Glucose and insulin administration and total parenteral nutrition can cause PO_4^- to shift into the cells from extracellular fluid compartments, leading to hypophosphatemia. Alcohol withdrawal, acid–base imbalances, and the use of antacids that bind with phosphate in the GI tract are other possible causes. Manifestations of hypophosphatemia include paresthesias, muscle weakness and pain, mental changes, and possible seizures.

Hyperphosphatemia occurs when PO_4^- shifts out of the cells into ECF (e.g., due to tissue trauma, cancer chemotherapy, etc.), in renal failure, or when excess phosphate is administered or ingested. Infants who are fed cow's milk and clients who use phosphate-containing enemas or laxatives are at risk for hyperphosphatemia. Manifestations of hyperphosphatemia include numbness and tingling around the mouth and in the fingertips, muscle spasms, and tetany.

Acid–Base Imbalances

Acid–base imbalances are usually classified as respiratory or metabolic according to the underlying cause of the disorder. H_2CO_3 levels are normally regulated by the lungs through the retention or excretion of CO_2, and problems lead to respiratory acidosis or alkalosis. HCO_3^- and hydrogen ion levels are regulated by the kidneys, and problems lead to metabolic acidosis or alkalosis. Healthy regulatory systems will attempt to correct acid–base imbalances, a process called **compensation**.

RESPIRATORY ACIDOSIS Any condition that causes carbon dioxide retention, either due to hypoventilation or impaired lung or respiratory muscle function, causes H_2CO_3 levels to increase and the pH to fall below 7.35, a condition known as **respiratory acidosis**. Asthma and chronic obstructive pulmonary disease (COPD) are common causes of respiratory acidosis. Central nervous system depression due to anesthesia or opioid overdose can slow the respiratory rate enough to cause CO_2 retention. When respiratory acidosis occurs, the kidneys retain bicarbonate to restore the normal H_2CO_3 to HCO_3^- ratio. Recall, however, that the kidneys are relatively slow to respond to changes in acid–base balance, so this compensatory response may require hours to days to restore the normal pH.

RESPIRATORY ALKALOSIS When a person hyperventilates, more CO_2 than normal is exhaled, H_2CO_3 levels fall, and the pH rises to greater than 7.45. This condition is called **respiratory alkalosis**. Anxiety-related hyperventilation is a common cause of respiratory alkalosis. Other causes include fever and respiratory infections. In respiratory alkalosis, the kidneys will excrete bicarbonate to return the pH to within the normal range. Often, however, if the cause of the hyperventilation is eliminated, the pH returns to normal before renal compensation occurs.

METABOLIC ACIDOSIS When bicarbonate levels are low in relation to the amount of H_2CO_3 in the body, the pH falls and **metabolic acidosis** develops. One cause of metabolic acidosis is renal failure and the inability of the kidneys to excrete hydrogen ions and produce HCO_3^-. It can also occur when too much acid is produced in the body, for example, in diabetic ketoacidosis or starvation when fat tissue is broken down for energy. Metabolic acidosis stimulates the respiratory centre, and the rate and depth of respirations increase. CO_2 is then eliminated and H_2CO_3 levels fall, minimizing the change in pH. This respiratory compensation occurs within minutes of onset of the pH imbalance.

METABOLIC ALKALOSIS In **metabolic alkalosis**, the amount of HCO_3^- in the body exceeds the normal 20 to 1 ratio. Ingestion of bicarbonate of soda as an antacid is one cause of metabolic alkalosis. Another cause is prolonged vomiting with loss of hydrochloric acid from the stomach. The respiratory centre is depressed in metabolic alkalosis, and respirations slow and become shallower. CO_2 is then retained, and H_2CO_3 levels increase, helping balance the excess HCO_3^-. The risk factors, manifestations, and nursing interventions for acid–base imbalances are listed in Table 44.8.

Assessing

Assessing clients for fluid, electrolyte, and acid–base imbalances is an important nursing responsibility. Components of the assessment include (a) the nursing history, (b) physical assessment of the client, (c) clinical measurements, and (d) review of laboratory test results.

NURSING HISTORY The nursing history is particularly important for identifying clients who are at risk for fluid, electrolyte, and acid–base imbalances. A client's

TABLE 44.8 Acid–Base Imbalances

Risk Factors	Clinical Manifestations	Nursing Interventions
Respiratory Acidosis	**Acute:**	
Acute lung conditions that impair alveolar gas exchange (e.g., pneumonia, acute pulmonary edema, aspiration of foreign body, pneumothorax)	Increased pulse and respiratory rates	Frequently assess respiratory status and lung sounds.
	Headache, dizziness	Monitor airway and ventilation; insert artificial airway and prepare for mechanical ventilation, as necessary.
	Confusion, decreased level of consciousness (LOC)	
Chronic lung disease (e.g., asthma, cystic fibrosis, or emphysema)	Convulsions	Administer pulmonary therapy measures, such as inhalation therapy, percussion and postural drainage, bronchodilators, and antibiotics, as ordered.
	Warm, flushed skin	
	Chronic:	
Overdose of opioids or sedatives that depress respiratory rate and depth	Weakness	Monitor fluid intake and output, vital signs, and arterial blood gases (ABGs). Administer opioid antagonists, as indicated.
	Headache	
Brain injury that affects the respiratory centre	*Laboratory findings:*	
Airway obstruction	Arterial blood pH less than 7.35	Maintain adequate hydration (2–3 L of fluid per day), unless contraindicated.
	$PaCO_2$ above 45 mm Hg	
	HCO_3^- normal or slightly elevated in acute; above 26 mmol/L in chronic	
Respiratory Alkalosis		
Hyperventilation due to the following:	Complaints of shortness of breath, chest tightness	Monitor vital signs and ABGs.
• Extreme anxiety	Lightheadedness with circumoral paresthesias and numbness and tingling of the extremities	Assist client to breathe more slowly.
• Elevated body temperature		Help client breathe into a paper bag or apply a rebreather mask (to inhale CO_2).
• Overventilation with a mechanical ventilator	Difficulty concentrating	Treat underlying problem, as ordered.
• Hypoxia	Tremulousness, blurred vision	
• Salicylate overdose	*Laboratory findings (in uncompensated respiratory alkalosis):*	
Brain stem injury	Arterial blood pH above 7.45	
Increased basal metabolic rate (such as in fever)	$PaCO_2$ less than 35 mm Hg	

(continued)

TABLE 44.8 Acid–Base Imbalances (*continued*)

Risk Factors	Clinical Manifestations	Nursing Interventions
Metabolic Acidosis		
Conditions that increase nonvolatile acids in the blood (e.g., renal impairment, diabetes mellitus, starvation)	Kussmaul's respirations (deep, rapid respirations)	Monitor ABG values, intake and output, LOC, and respiratory status.
Conditions that decrease bicarbonate (e.g., prolonged diarrhea)	Lethargy, confusion	Administer IV sodium bicarbonate carefully, if ordered.
Excessive infusion of chloride-containing IV fluids (e.g., sodium chloride [NaCl])	Headache	Treat underlying problem, as ordered.
	Weakness	Assess cardiovascular status.
Excessive ingestion of acids, such as salicylates	Nausea and vomiting	
Cardiac arrest	*Laboratory findings:*	
	Arterial blood pH below 7.35	
	Serum bicarbonate less than 22 mmol/L	
	$PaCO_2$ less than 35 mm Hg with respiratory compensation	
Metabolic Alkalosis		
Excessive acid losses due to the following:	Decreased respiratory rate and depth	Monitor intake and output closely.
• Vomiting	Dizziness	Monitor vital signs, especially respirations, LOC, and intake and output.
• Gastric suction	Circumoral paresthesias, numbness and tingling of the extremities	Administer ordered IV fluids carefully.
Excessive use of potassium-losing diuretics	Hypertonic muscles, tetany	Treat underlying problem, as ordered.
Excessive adrenal corticoid hormones due to the following:	*Laboratory findings:*	Assess cardiovascular status.
• Cushing's syndrome	Arterial blood pH above 7.45	Monitor intake and output closely.
• Hyperaldosteronism	Serum bicarbonate greater than 26 mmol/L	
Excessive bicarbonate intake from the following:	$PaCO_2$ higher than 45 mm Hg with respiratory compensation	
• Antacids		
• Parenteral $NaHCO_3^-$		

current and past medical history reveals such conditions as chronic lung disease or diabetes mellitus, which can disrupt normal balances. Medications prescribed to treat acute or chronic conditions (e.g., diuretic therapy for hypertension) also may place the client at risk for altered homeostasis. Functional, developmental, and socio-economic factors must also be considered in assessing a client's risk. Older people and very young children, clients who must depend on others to meet their nutrition and hydration needs, and people who cannot afford or do not have the means to cook food for a balanced diet are at greater risk for fluid and electrolyte imbalances.

When obtaining a nursing history, the nurse also needs to elicit data about the client's food and fluid intake, fluid output, and the presence of signs or symptoms suggestive of altered fluid and electrolyte balance. The Assessment: Interview box provides examples of questions to elicit information regarding fluid, electrolyte, and acid–base balance.

PHYSICAL ASSESSMENT Physical assessment to evaluate a client's fluid, electrolyte, and acid–base status focuses on skin, the oral cavity and mucous membranes, eyes, and the cardiovascular, respiratory, urinary, gastrointestinal, neurological, and musculoskeletal systems. Data from this physical assessment are used to expand and verify information obtained in the nursing history. The focused physical assessment is summarized in Table 44.9; refer to Tables 44.4 through 44.8 for possible abnormal findings related to specific imbalances discussed in this chapter.

CLINICAL MEASUREMENTS Three simple clinical measurements that the nurse can initiate are daily weights, vital signs, and fluid intake and output (I&O).

Daily Weights Daily weight measurements provide a relatively accurate assessment of a client's fluid status. Significant changes in weight over a short time (e.g., more than 2 kg in a week or more than 1 kg in 24 hours) are indicative of acute fluid changes. Each kilogram of weight gained or lost corresponds to 1 L of fluid gained or lost. Such fluid gains or losses indicate changes in total body fluid volume, rather than in any specific compartment, such as the intravascular

ASSESSMENT **INTERVIEW**

Fluid, Electrolyte, and Acid–Base Balance

These questions can help the nurse elicit data about the client during the nursing history:

CURRENT AND PAST MEDICAL HISTORY

- Are you currently receiving treatment of any chronic diseases, such as kidney disease, heart disease, hypertension, diabetes insipidus, or thyroid or parathyroid disorders?
- Have you recently experienced any acute conditions, such as gastroenteritis, severe trauma, head injury, or surgery? If so, describe them.

MEDICATIONS AND TREATMENTS

- Are you currently taking any medications on a regular basis, such as diuretics, steroids, potassium supplements, calcium supplements, hormones, salt substitutes, or antacids?
- Have you recently undergone any treatments, such as dialysis, parenteral nutrition, tube feedings, or been on a ventilator? If so, when, and why?

FOOD AND FLUID INTAKE

- How much and what type of fluids do you drink each day?
- Describe your diet for a typical day. (Pay particular attention to intake of foods high in sodium content, of protein, and of whole grains, fruits, and vegetables.)
- Have there been any recent changes in your food or fluid intake?
- Are you on any type of restricted diet?

- Has your food or fluid intake recently been affected by changes in appetite, nausea, or other factors, such as pain or difficulty breathing?

FLUID OUTPUT

- Have you noticed any recent changes in the frequency or amount of urine output?
- Have you recently experienced any problems with vomiting, diarrhea, or constipation? If so, when, and for how long?
- Have you noticed any other unusual fluid losses, such as excessive sweating?

FLUID, ELECTROLYTE, AND ACID–BASE IMBALANCES

- Have you gained or lost weight in recent weeks?
- Have you recently experienced any symptoms, such as excessive thirst, dry skin or mucous membranes, dark or concentrated urine, or low urine output?
- Do you have problems with swelling of your fingers, hands, feet, or ankles? Do you ever have difficulty breathing, especially when lying down or at night? How many pillows do you use to sleep?
- Have you recently experienced any of the following symptoms: difficulty concentrating or confusion; dizziness or feeling faint; muscle weakness, twitching, cramping, or spasm; excessive fatigue; abnormal sensations, such as numbness, tingling, burning, or prickling; abdominal cramping or distension; heart palpitations?

TABLE 44.9 Focused Physical Assessment for Fluid, Electrolyte, or Acid–Base Imbalance

System	Assessment Focus	Technique	Possible Abnormal Findings
Skin	Colour, temperature, moisture	Inspection, palpation	Flushed, warm, very dry
			Moist or diaphoretic
			Cool and pale
	Turgor	Gently pinch up a fold of skin over sternum or inner aspect of thigh for adults, on the abdomen or medial thigh for children	Poor turgor: Skin remains tented for several seconds instead of immediately returning to normal position
	Edema	Inspect for visible swelling around eyes, in fingers, and in lower extremities	Skin around eyes is puffy, lids appear swollen; rings are tight; shoes leave impressions on feet
		Compress the skin over the dorsum of the foot, around the ankles, over the tibia, in the sacral area	Depression remains (pitting): see scale for describing edema in Figure 44.10
Mucous membranes	Colour, moisture	Inspection	Mucous membranes dry, dull, pale in appearance; tongue dry and cracked; edema
Eyes	Firmness	Gently palpate eyeball with lid closed	Mucous membranes dry, dull, pale in appearance; tongue dry and cracked; edema

(continued)

TABLE 44.9 Focused Physical Assessment for Fluid, Electrolyte, or Acid–Base Imbalance (*continued*)

System	Assessment Focus	Technique	Possible Abnormal Findings
Fontanelles (infant)	Firmness, level	Inspect and gently palpate anterior fontanelle	Fontanelle bulging, firm Fontanelle sunken, soft
Cardiovascular system	Heart rate	Auscultation, cardiac monitor	Tachycardia, bradycardia; ECG changes; dysrhythmias
	Peripheral pulses	Palpation	Weak and thready; bounding; absent
	Blood pressure	Auscultation of Korotkoff sounds	Hypotension; hypertension
		BP assessment lying and standing	Postural hypotension
	Capillary refill	Palpation	Slowed capillary refill
	Venous filling	Inspection of jugular veins and hand veins	Jugular venous distension; flat jugular veins; poor venous refill
Respiratory system	Respiratory rate and pattern	Inspection	Increased or decreased rate and depth of respirations; use of accessory muscles
	Lung sounds	Auscultation	Crackles
Neurological system	Level of consciousness (LOC)	Observation, stimulation Glasgow coma scale (GCS)	Decreased LOC, lethargy, stupor, or coma, change in GCS score
	Orientation, cognition	Questioning	Disoriented, confused; difficulty concentrating
	Motor function	Strength testing	Weakness, decreased motor strength
	Reflexes	Deep tendon reflex (DTR) testing	Hyperactive or depressed DTRs
	Abnormal reflexes	*Chvostek's sign:* Tap over facial nerve about 2 cm anterior to tragus of ear (see Figure 44.12A)	Facial muscle twitching including eyelids and lips on side of stimulus
		Trousseau's sign: Inflate a blood pressure cuff on the upper arm to 20 mm Hg greater than the systolic pressure, leave in place for 2 to 5 minutes (see Figure 44.12B)	Carpal spasm: contraction of hand and fingers on affected side
Urinary and gastrointestinal systems	Intake/output	Measurement of intake of oral or parenteral fluids	Fluid intake or urinary output less than normal
		Output: urine, liquid stool, vomit, drainage from a wound or operative site, drainage from a nasogastric tube	Excess losses from a surgical drain or vomiting
		Auscultate bowel sounds	High-pitched bowel sounds or absent bowel sounds
		Palpate bladder and abdomen	Firm bladder indicating possible distension

compartment. Rapid losses or gains of 5% to 8% of total body weight indicate moderate to severe fluid volume deficits or excesses.

To obtain accurate weight measurements, the scale should be balanced before each use and the client should be weighed (a) at the same time each day (e.g., before breakfast and after the first void), (b) wearing the same or similar clothing, and (c) on the same scale. The type of scale (i.e., standing, bed, or chair) should be documented.

Regular assessment of weight is particularly important for clients in the community and extended care facilities who are at risk for fluid imbalance. For these clients, measuring intake and output may be impractical because of lifestyle or problems with incontinence. Regular weight measurement, either daily, every other day, or weekly, provides valuable information about the client's fluid volume status.

Vital Signs   Changes in the vital signs may indicate, or in some cases precede, fluid, electrolyte, and acid–base imbalances. For example, elevated body temperature may be a result of dehydration or a cause of increased body fluid losses.

Tachycardia is an early sign of hypovolemia. Pulse volume will decrease in FVD and increase in FVE. Irregular pulse rates may occur with electrolyte imbalances. Changes in respiratory rate and depth may cause respiratory acid–base imbalances or indicate a compensatory mechanism in metabolic acidosis or alkalosis.

Blood pressure, a sensitive measure for detecting blood volume changes, may fall significantly with FVD and hypovolemia or increase with FVE and overhydration. Postural, or orthostatic, hypotension may also occur with FVD and hypovolemia.

To assess for orthostatic hypotension, measure the client's baseline blood pressure and pulse in a supine position. Allow the client to remain in that position for 3 to 5 minutes, leaving the blood pressure cuff on the arm. Ask the client to stand up, and immediately reassess the blood pressure and pulse. For a client who is too dizzy or weak to stand, assess supine and then sitting with legs dangling. A drop of 10 to 15 mm Hg in the systolic blood pressure with a corresponding drop in diastolic pressure and an increased pulse rate (by 10 or more beats per minute) is indicative of orthostatic or postural hypotension.

Fluid Intake and Output   The measurement and recording of all fluid I&O during a 24-hour period provides important data about the client's fluid and electrolyte balance. Generally, I&O are measured for hospitalized at-risk clients. Most agencies have a form for recording I&O, usually a bedside record on which the nurse lists all items measured and their quantities per shift. Recording the specifics of IV fluids, such as the type of solution, additives, time started, and amounts absorbed are often noted on the I&O record.

It is important to inform clients, family members, and all caregivers that accurate measurements of the client's fluid I&O are required, explaining why and emphasizing the need to use a bedpan, urinal, commode, or in-toilet collection device (unless a urinary drainage system is in place). Instruct the client not to put toilet tissue into the container with urine. Clients who wish to be involved in recording fluid intake measurements need to be taught how to compute the values and what foods are considered fluids.

To measure fluid intake, each item of fluid consumed or administered is recorded, specifying the time and type of fluid. All the following fluids need to be recorded:

- *Oral fluids.* Water, milk, juice, soft drinks, coffee, tea, cream, soup, and any other beverages. Include water taken with medications. To assess the amount of water consumed from a water pitcher, measure what remains and subtract this amount from the volume of the full pitcher (generally 1 L). Then, refill the pitcher.

- *Ice chips.* Record these as fluids at approximately one-half the volume of the ice chips. For example, if the ice chips fill a cup holding 200 mL and all the ice chips have been consumed, the volume consumed would be recorded as 100 mL.

- *Foods that are or become liquid at room temperature.* These include ice cream, sherbet, custard, and gelatin (Jell-O). Do *not* measure foods that are pureed because purees are simply solid foods prepared in a different form.

- *Tube feedings.* Remember to include the volume of water instilled before and after medication administration, intermittent or continuous feedings, residual checks, or any other water given via a feeding tube.

- *Parenteral fluids.* The exact amount of IV fluid administered is to be recorded, since some fluid containers may be overfilled. Blood transfusions are included.

- *Intravenous medications.* IV medications that are administered as an intermittent or continuous infusion must also be included (e.g., ceftazidime 1 g in 50 mL of NS).

- *Catheter or tube irrigants.* Fluid used to irrigate nasogastric tubes or intestinal tubes must be recorded, if not immediately withdrawn as part of the irrigation.

To measure *fluid output*, measure the following fluids (remember to use appropriate infection prevention and control precautions):

- *Urinary output.* Following each voiding, pour the urine into a measuring container, note and record the amount and time on the I&O form. For clients with retention catheters, empty the drainage bag into a measuring container at the end of the shift (or at prescribed times, if output is to be measured more often). Note and record the amount of urine output. In intensive care areas, urine output is often measured hourly. If the client is incontinent of urine, estimate and record these outputs. For example, for an incontinent client, the nurse might record "Incontinent 3 times" or "Drawsheet soaked in 30 cm diameter." A more accurate estimate of the urine output of infants and incontinent clients may be obtained by first weighing diapers or incontinence pads that are dry, and then subtracting this weight from the weight of the soiled items. Each gram of weight left after subtracting is equal to 1 mL of urine. If urine is frequently soiled with feces, the number of voidings can be recorded, rather than the volume of urine.

- *Vomitus and liquid feces.* The amount and type of fluid and the time need to be specified.

- *Tube drainage,* such as gastric or intestinal drainage. The amount and type of fluid and time need to be recorded.

- *Wound and fistula drainage.* Drainage may be recorded by documenting the type and number of dressings or linen saturated with drainage or by measuring the exact amount of drainage collected in a vacuum drainage (e.g., Hemovac) or gravity drainage system.

Fluid I&O measurements are totalled at the end of the shift, and the totals are recorded in the client's permanent record. In intensive care areas, nurses may record I&O more frequently. Usually, the nurses on night shift total the amounts of I&O recorded for each shift and record the 24-hour total.

To determine whether fluid output is proportional to fluid intake or whether there are any changes in the client's fluid status, the nurse compares (a) the total 24-hour fluid output measurement with the total 24-hour fluid intake measurement, and (b) both with previous measurements. Urinary output is normally equivalent to the amount of fluids ingested; the usual range is 1500 to 2000 mL in 24 hours, or 40 to 80 mL in 1 hour (0.5 mL/kg per hour). Clients whose output substantially exceeds intake are at risk for fluid volume deficit. By contrast, clients whose intake substantially exceeds output are at risk for fluid volume excess. In assessing the client's fluid balance, it is important to consider additional factors that may affect I&O. For example, a client who is extremely diaphoretic or who has rapid, deep respirations has fluid losses that cannot be measured but must still be considered in evaluating fluid status.

When a significant discrepancy exists between intake and output or when fluid intake or output is inadequate (e.g., urine output of less than 500 mL in 24 hours for an adult), this information should be reported to the appropriate member of the health care team.

LABORATORY TESTS   Many laboratory studies are conducted to determine the client's fluid, electrolyte, and acid–base status. Some of the more common tests are discussed here.

Serum Electrolytes   Serum electrolyte levels are often routinely ordered for any client admitted to hospital as a screening test for electrolyte and acid–base imbalances. Serum electrolytes also are routinely assessed for clients at risk in the community, for example, clients who are being treated with diuretics for hypertension or heart failure. The most commonly ordered serum tests are for sodium, potassium, chloride, magnesium, and bicarbonate ions. Normal values of commonly measured electrolytes are summarized in Box 44.3.

Some agencies use a diagram format for keeping track of the client's sodium (Na^+), potassium (K^+), chloride (Cl^-), bicarbonate (HCO_3^-), blood urea nitrogen (BUN), and creatinine (CR) when documenting in the client's progress notes. See Figure 44.13.

Complete Blood Count (CBC)   The CBC, another basic screening test, includes information about

BOX 44.3 NORMAL ELECTROLYTE VALUES FOR ADULTS*	
Venous blood	
Sodium	135–145 mmol/L
Potassium	3.5–5.0 mmol/L
Chloride	95–105 mmol/L
Calcium (total)	2.2–2.58 mmol/L
Calcium (ionized)	1.0–1.15 mmol/L
Magnesium	0.65–1.05 mmol/L
Phosphate (phosphorus)	0.97–1.45 mmol/L
Serum osmolality	280–300 mmol/kg water

*Normal laboratory values vary from agency to agency.

hematocrit (Hct). **Hematocrit** is the portion of blood plasma that is composed of erythrocytes (red blood cells [RBCs]). Because Hct is measured in relation to plasma, it is directly affected by changes in plasma volume. Thus, hematocrit increases with dehydration and decreases with overhydration. Normal Hct values are 0.37 to 0.49 (males) and 0.36 to 0.46 (females).

Osmolality   Serum osmolality is a measure of the solute concentration of the blood. The solutes included are sodium ions, glucose, and blood urine nitrogen (BUN). Serum osmolality can be estimated by doubling the serum sodium value because sodium and its associated chloride ions are the major determinants of serum osmolality. Serum osmolality values are used primarily to evaluate fluid balance. Normal values are 280 to 300 mmol/kg. An increase in serum osmolality indicates a fluid volume deficit; a decrease reflects a fluid volume excess.

Urine osmolality is a measure of the solute concentration of urine. The particles included are nitrogenous wastes, such as creatinine, urea, and uric acid. Normal values are 500 to 800 mmol/kg. An increased urine osmolality indicates a fluid volume deficit; a decreased urine osmolality reflects a fluid volume excess.

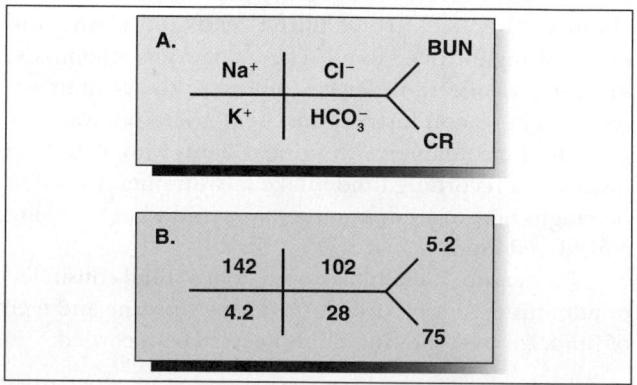

FIGURE 44.13   A: Format for a diagram of serum electrolyte, blood urea nitrogen, and creatinine results; **B:** Example that may be seen in documentation notes.

Urine Specific Gravity   **Specific gravity** is an indicator of urine concentration that correlates with urine osmolality, and it can be measured quickly and easily. Normal specific gravity ranges from 1.010 to 1.025. When the concentration of solutes in the urine is high (FVD), the specific gravity rises; when the concentration of solutes in the urine is low (FVE), the specific gravity is low.

Urine pH   Measurement of urine pH can be obtained by laboratory analysis or by using a dipstick on a freshly voided specimen. Because the kidneys play a critical role in regulating acid–base balance, assessment of urine pH can be useful in determining whether the kidneys are responding appropriately to acid–base imbalances. Normally, the pH of the urine is relatively acidic, averaging about 6, but a range of 4.5 to 8 is considered normal. In metabolic acidosis, urine pH should decrease as the kidneys retain HCO_3^- and excrete hydrogen ions; in metabolic alkalosis, the pH should increase as the kidneys retain hydrogen ions and excrete HCO_3^-.

Arterial Blood Gases   **Arterial blood gases (ABGs)** are performed to evaluate the client's acid–base balance and oxygenation. Arterial blood is used because it provides a more accurate reflection of gas exchange in the pulmonary system than venous blood. Blood gases may be drawn by laboratory technicians, respiratory therapy personnel, or nurses with specialized skills. Because a high-pressure artery is used to obtain blood, it is important to apply pressure to the puncture site for at least 5 minutes after the procedure to reduce the risk of bleeding or bruising.

Six measurements are commonly used to interpret arterial blood gases:

1. pH is a measure of the relative acidity or alkalinity of the blood and is an inverse measure of the number of hydrogen ions in a solution. An acidic solution has more hydrogen ions, and this is reflected in a lower pH. An alkaline solution has fewer hydrogen ions, and this is reflected in a higher pH. The normal range for arterial pH is narrow, and death may ensue with pH values below 6.8 or above 7.8.

2. PaO_2 is the partial pressure exerted by O_2 dissolved in arterial plasma, and is an indirect measure of blood O_2 content. PaO_2 represents one of the two forms in which O_2 is transported in the blood, and accounts for only about 3% of O_2 content in blood.

3. $PaCO_2$ is the partial pressure of CO_2 in arterial plasma and is the respiratory component of acid–base determination. Because carbon dioxide is regulated by the lungs, $PaCO_2$ is used to determine if an acid–base imbalance is respiratory in origin.

4. HCO_3^- is a measure of the bicarbonate dissolved in arterial plasma and represents the metabolic component of acid–base balance.

5. Base excess (BE) is a calculated value of HCO_3^- levels, also reflective of the metabolic component of acid–base

balance. If the number is preceded by a plus sign, it represents a base excess and indicates alkalosis; if preceded by a minus sign, it is a base deficit and indicates acidosis.

6. O_2 saturation (SaO_2) is the percentage of hemoglobin saturated (combined) with O_2. This represents the other form in which O_2 is transported in the blood and accounts for about 97% of the O_2 in the blood. Pulse oximetry can also be used to measure O_2 saturation. This noninvasive procedure measures SpO_2. Measuring O_2 saturation by using pulse oximetry is detailed in Skill 29.7 on page 731.

Table 44.10 lists normal ABG values and also summarizes changes seen in common acid–base imbalances. Note that although the PaO_2 and SaO_2 are important for

TABLE 44.10   Arterial Blood Gas Values

Normal Values of Arterial Blood Gases (ABGs)*	
pH	7.35–7.45
PaO_2	80–100 mm Hg
$PaCO_2$	35–45 mm Hg
HCO_3^-	22–26 mmol/L
Base excess	–2 to +2 mmol/L
O_2 saturation	95%–100%

Arterial Blood Gas Values in Common Acid–Base Disorders		
Disorder		**ABG Values**
Respiratory acidosis	pH	<7.35
	$PaCO_2$	>45 mm Hg (excess CO_2 and H_2CO_3)
	HCO_3^-	Normal; or >26 mmol/L with renal compensation
Respiratory alkalosis	pH	>7.45
	$PaCO_2$	<35 mm Hg (inadequate CO_2 and H_2CO_3)
	HCO_3^-	Normal; or <22 mmol/L with renal compensation
Metabolic acidosis	pH	<7.35
	$PaCO_2$	Normal; or <35 mm Hg with respiratory compensation
	HCO_3^-	<22 mmol/L (inadequate HCO_3^-)
Metabolic alkalosis	pH	>7.45
	$PaCO_2$	Normal; or >45 mm Hg with respiratory compensation
	HCO_3^-	>26 mmol/L (excess HCO_3^-)

*Normal laboratory values will vary from agency to agency. Nurses are advised to use the normal values issued by the agency when interpreting laboratory results.

BOX 44.4 INTERPRETING ABGS: A FOUR-STEP GUIDE

Nurses must use a systematic approach when evaluating ABG results:

1. Look at each number separately.
   - Label the pH:
     - If the pH is less than 7.35, the problem is acidosis.
     - If the pH is greater than 7.45, the problem is alkalosis.
     - If the pH is normal but either $PaCO_2$ or HCO_3^- is abnormal, then there has been "full compensation."
   - Label the $PaCO_2$:
     - If the $PaCO_2$ is less than 35 mm Hg, more CO_2 is being exhaled than normal and indicates respiratory alkalosis or compensation for a metabolic imbalance.
     - If the $PaCO_2$ is greater than 45 mm Hg, less CO_2 is being exhaled than normal and indicates respiratory acidosis or compensation for a metabolic imbalance.
   - Label the HCO_3^-:
     - If the HCO_3^- is less than 22 mmol/L, HCO_3^- levels are lower than normal, indicating metabolic acidosis or compensation for a respiratory imbalance.
     - If the HCO_3^- is greater than 26 mmol/L, HCO_3^- levels are higher than normal, indicating metabolic alkalosis or compensation for a respiratory imbalance.

2. Determine the cause of the acid–base imbalance.
   - Look at the pH: Is it acidosis, alkalosis, or within the normal range?

3. Determine whether the origin of the imbalance is respiratory or metabolic.
   - Check the $PaCO_2$ and HCO_3^-: Which one corresponds with the same acid–base status as the pH?

4. Look for evidence of compensation.
   - Look at the value that does *not* match the pH.

- If it (e.g., $PaCO_2$ or HCO_3^-) is within normal range, there is no compensation.
- If it (e.g., $PaCO_2$ or HCO_3^-) is above or below normal range, the body is compensating.

EXAMPLES

a. In respiratory acidosis (pH < 7.35, $PaCO_2$ > 45 mm Hg), if the HCO_3^- is greater than 26 mmol/L, the kidneys are retaining HCO_3^- to minimize the acidosis: renal compensation.

b. In respiratory alkalosis (pH > 7.45, $PaCO_2$ < 35 mm Hg), if the HCO_3^- is less than 22 mmol/L, the kidneys are excreting HCO_3^- to minimize the alkalosis: again, renal compensation.

c. In metabolic acidosis (pH < 7.35, HCO_3^- < 22 mmol/L), if the $PaCO_2$ is less than 35 mm Hg, CO_2 is being eliminated to minimize the acidosis: respiratory compensation.

d. In metabolic alkalosis (pH > 7.45, HCO_3^- > 26 mmol/L), if the $PaCO_2$ is greater than 45 mm Hg, CO_2 is being retained to compensate for excess base: again, respiratory compensation.

e. Analyze the following ABG:

   pH = 7.33 (acidosis); $PaCO_2$ = 55 (acidosis); HCO_3^- = 29 (alkalosis)

   Cause of imbalance = acidosis as pH < 7.35

   $PaCO_2$ (acidosis) *matches* the pH (acidosis) = respiratory problem

   HCO_3^- is high so renal compensation is occurring; however, insufficient to render pH within normal range

Conclusion: Client has respiratory acidosis with partial compensation.

Note: If the value that does not match (e.g., $PaCO_2$ or HCO_3^-) is above or below normal and the pH is within normal range, the body has completely compensated. Complete compensation takes time to develop and is the result of a chronic condition (e.g., chronic respiratory acidosis with COPD).

---

assessing respiratory status, they generally do not provide useful information for assessing acid–base balance and so are not included in this table.

When evaluating ABG results to determine acid–base balance, it is important to use a systematic approach such as the one outlined in Box 44.4.

Diagnosing

There are numerous diagnoses that can relate to fluid, electrolyte, and acid–base imbalances such as actual or at risk for fluid volume deficit; actual or at risk for fluid volume excess; electrolyte imbalance (e.g., hypokalemia, hypernatremia, hypocalcemia); respiratory and/or metabolic alkalosis and/or acidosis. Each of these diagnoses can be related to multiple factors, for example, hypokalemia related to inadequate intake and excess loss in vomiting; respiratory acidosis related to presence of pulmonary edema, hypoventilation, and partial airway obstruction.

Fluid, electrolyte, and acid–base imbalances affect many other body areas, and, as a consequence, may be the etiology of many other nursing diagnoses, such as the following: acute confusion related to electrolyte imbalance; impaired skin integrity related to dehydration or edema; at risk for fall related to muscle weakness caused by hypokalemia; reduced tissue perfusion related to decreased cardiac output secondary to deficient fluid volume or edema; at risk for injury related to calcium shift out of bones into extracellular fluids.

Planning

When planning care, the nurse identifies nursing interventions that will assist the client to achieve these broad goals:

- Maintain or restore normal fluid balance
- Maintain or restore normal balance of electrolytes in the intracellular and extracellular compartments

- Maintain or restore gas exchange and oxygenation
- Prevent associated risks (tissue breakdown, decreased cardiac output, confusion, other neurological signs)
- Maintain or repair renal function

Nursing activities to meet goals and outcomes related to fluid, electrolyte, and acid–base imbalances are discussed in the next section. These include (a) monitoring fluid I&O, cardiovascular and respiratory status, and results of laboratory tests; (b) assessing the client's weight; the location and extent of edema, if present; skin turgor and skin status; specific gravity of urine; and level of consciousness and mental status; (c) fluid intake modifications; (d) dietary changes; (e) parenteral fluid, electrolyte, and blood replacement; and (f) other appropriate measures, such as administering prescribed medications and O_2, providing skin care and oral hygiene, positioning the client appropriately, and scheduling rest periods.

PLANNING FOR HOME CARE   Home care planning includes assessment of the client's and family's needs, strengths, and resources, as well as their readiness for home care. The Assessment: Home Care box describes the specific assessment data required to establish a home care plan. On the basis of the data gathered in assessment of the home situation, the nurse individualizes the teaching plan for the client and family (see the Teaching: Home Care box on the next page).

Implementing

PROMOTING WELLNESS   Most people rarely think about their fluid, electrolyte, or acid–base balance. They know it is important to drink adequate fluids and consume a balanced diet, but they may not understand the potential effects when this is not done. Nurses can promote clients' health by providing wellness teaching that will help them maintain fluid and electrolyte balance. See the Teaching: Wellness box on fluid and electrolyte balance on page 1441.

ENTERAL FLUID AND ELECTROLYTE REPLACEMENT   Fluids and electrolytes can be provided orally in the home and hospital if the client's health permits, that is, if the client is not vomiting, has not experienced an excessive fluid loss, and has an intact GI tract and gag and swallow reflexes. Clients who are unable to ingest solid foods may be able to ingest fluids.

FLUID INTAKE MODIFICATIONS   Increased fluids (ordered as "push fluids") are often prescribed for clients with actual or potential fluid volume deficits arising, for example, from mild diarrhea or mild to moderate fevers. Guidelines for helping clients increase fluid intake are shown in the Practice Guidelines boxes. Restricted fluids may be necessary for clients who have fluid volume excess as a result of renal failure, heart failure, SIADH, or other disease processes.

Fluid restrictions vary from NPO (nil per os, or "nothing by mouth") to a precise amount ordered by a

---

ASSESSMENT   HOME CARE

Fluid, Electrolyte, and Acid–Base Balance

Assess for the following:

CLIENT

- *Risk factors for imbalances:* The client's age, medications such as diuretic therapy or corticosteroids, and presence of chronic diseases, such as diabetes mellitus, heart disease, lung disease, or dementia
- *Self-care abilities for maintaining food and fluid intake:* Mobility; ability to chew and swallow, ability to access fluids and respond to thirst, to purchase food and prepare a balanced diet
- *Current level of knowledge (as appropriate):* Prescribed diet, any fluid restrictions, activity restrictions, actions and side effects of prescribed medications, regular weight monitoring, gastric tube care and enteral feedings, central line or peripherally inserted central catheter (PICC) care, and parenteral fluids and nutrition

FAMILY

- *Caregiver availability, skills, and responses:* Availability and willingness to assume responsibility for care, knowledge

and ability to provide assistance with preparing food and maintaining adequate intake of food and fluids, knowledge of risk factors and early warning signs of problems
- *Family role changes and coping:* Effect on financial status, parenting and spousal roles, social roles
- *Alternative potential primary or respite caregivers:* For example, other family members, friends, volunteers, church members, paid caregivers or housekeeping services; available community care (e.g., adult daycare), senior centres

COMMUNITY

- *Current knowledge of and experience with community resources:* Home care agencies, organizations that offer financial assistance or assistance with food preparation, meal services, pharmacies, home intravenous services, respiratory care services

TEACHING HOME CARE

Fluid, Electrolyte, and Acid–Base Balance

After the assessment of the home situation, the nurse individualizes the teaching plan:

MONITORING FLUID INTAKE AND OUTPUT

- Teach and provide the rationale for monitoring fluid I&O to the client and family, as appropriate. Include instructions for using a commode or collection device (urine hat) in the toilet, emptying and measuring urinary catheter drainage, or counting or weighing diapers.
- Instruct and provide rationale for regular weight monitoring to the client and family. Weigh at the same time of day, after the client has voided, using the same scale, and with the client wearing the same amount of clothing.
- Educate and provide rationale to the client and family regarding when to contact a health care professional, such as in the cases of a significant change in urine output; any change of 2.5 kg or more in a 1- to 2-week period or 1 kg in a 24-hour period; prolonged episodes of vomiting, diarrhea, or inability to eat or drink; dry, sticky mucous membranes; extreme thirst; swollen fingers, feet, ankles, or legs; difficulty breathing, shortness of breath, need for an increased number of pillows to sleep on, or rapid heartbeat; and changes in behaviour or mental status.

MAINTAINING FOOD AND FLUID INTAKE

- Instruct the client and family about any diet or fluid restrictions, such as a low-sodium diet. Contact a dietitian to provide appropriate teaching.
- Teach family members the rationale for offering fluids regularly to clients who are unable to meet their own needs because of age, impaired mobility or cognition, or other conditions, such as impaired swallowing because of a cerebrovascular accident.
- If the client is receiving enteral fluids or IV (parenteral) fluids at home, teach and provide rationales to caregivers about proper administration and care. Contact a home health or home IV service to provide services and teaching.

SAFETY

- Instruct and provide the rationale to the client regarding the need to change positions slowly, if appropriate, especially when moving from a supine to the sitting or standing position.
- Inform and provide the rationale to the client and family about the importance of good mouth and skin care.
- Teach the client to change positions frequently and to elevate the feet on a stool when sitting for a long period.

- Teach the client and family how to care for IV access sites or gastric tubes. Include instructions about what to do if tubes become dislodged.

MEDICATIONS

- Emphasize the importance and rationale of taking medications as prescribed.
- Instruct clients taking diuretics to take the medication in the morning. If a second daily dose is prescribed, they should take it in the late afternoon to avoid disrupting sleep for urinating.
- Inform clients about any expected side effects of prescribed medications and how to handle them (e.g., if a potassium-depleting diuretic is prescribed, increase intake of potassium-rich foods).
- Teach clients when to contact their health care provider, for example, if they are unable to take a prescribed medication or have signs of an allergic or a toxic reaction to a medication.

MEASURES SPECIFIC TO CLIENT'S PROBLEM

- Provide instructions and rationale specific to the client's fluid, electrolyte, or acid–base imbalance, such as the following:
  a. Deficient fluid volume
  b. Impaired exchange of carbon dioxide
  c. Fluid volume excess

REFERRALS

- Make appropriate referrals to home care or community services for assistance with resources, such as meal preparation and food delivery, IV infusions and access, enteral feedings, and homemaker or home care aide services to help with activities of daily living (ADLs).

COMMUNITY AGENCIES AND OTHER SOURCES OF HELP

- Provide information about companies or agencies that can provide medical equipment, such as commodes, lift chairs, or hospital beds for purchase, for rental, or free.
- Provide a list of sources for supplies, such as catheters and drainage bags, measuring devices, tube feeding formulas, and electrolyte replacement drinks.
- Suggest additional sources of information and help, such as a dietitian, wellness centre, or public health office.

physician. The restriction of fluids can be difficult for some clients, particularly if they are experiencing thirst. Guidelines for helping clients to increase fluid intake are shown in Practice Guidelines 44.1 and to restrict fluid intake are shown in Practice Guidelines 44.2.

DIETARY CHANGES Specific fluid and electrolyte imbalances may require simple dietary changes. For

example, clients receiving potassium-depleting diuretics need to be informed about foods with high potassium content (e.g., bananas, oranges, and leafy greens). Some clients with fluid retention need to avoid foods high in sodium.

ORAL ELECTROLYTE SUPPLEMENTS Some clients can benefit from oral supplements of electrolytes,

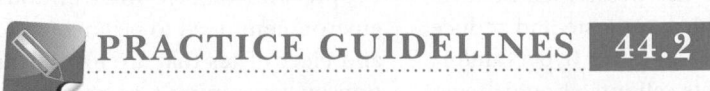

PRACTICE GUIDELINES 44.1

Facilitating Fluid Intake

Guidelines	Rationales
Explain to the client the reason for the required intake and the specific amount needed.	*This explanation promotes understanding and may enhance adherence.*
Establish a 24-hour plan for ingesting the fluids. For the hospitalized or long-term care client, half the total volume is generally given during the day shift, and the other half is divided between the evening and night shifts, with most of that ingested during the evening shift. For example, if 2500 mL is to be ingested in 24 hours, the plan may specify 7–3 (1500 mL); 3–11 (700 mL); and 11–7 (300 mL).	*Distributing fluid intake throughout waking hours and in conjunction with usual mealtimes helps to ensure the required fluids are ingested.*
Set short-term outcomes that the client can realistically meet. Examples include ingesting a glass of fluid every hour while awake.	*The client can be positively reinforced for achieving the desired outcome; if the outcome is not achieved, then alternative strategies can be tested to ensure the 24-hour fluid intake goal is achieved.*
Identify fluids the client likes, and make available a variety of those items, including fruit juices and milk (if allowed). Coffee and tea consumption should be limited.	*Fluids that are palatable to the client will enhance motivation; caffeinated beverages can have a diuretic effect.*
Help clients to select foods that tend to become liquid at room temperature (e.g., gelatin, custard, sherbet), if these are allowed.	*These foods contribute significantly to daily fluid intake.*
For clients who are confined to bed, supply appropriate cups, glasses, and straws, and keep fluids within easy reach.	*Fluid intake for these clients requires additional functional and safety requirements.*
Make sure fluids are served at the appropriate temperature (i.e., hot and cold fluids) and according to client's preference.	*The appropriate temperature ensures the palatability of the fluids.*
Encourage clients to participate in maintaining the fluid intake record, when possible.	*Maintaining the intake record assists the client in evaluating the achievement of desired health outcomes.*
Be alert to any cultural implications of food and fluids.	*Some cultures restrict certain foods and fluids and view others as having healing properties.*

PRACTICE GUIDELINES 44.2

Helping Clients Restrict Fluid Intake

Guidelines	Rationales
Explain the reason for the restricted intake and how much and what types of fluids are permitted orally. Many clients need to be informed that ice chips, gelatin, and ice cream, for example, are considered fluid.	*This explanation promotes understanding and may enhance adherence.*
Help the client decide the amount of fluid to be taken with each meal, between meals, before bedtime, and with medications. For the client in a hospital or long-term care facility, half the total volume is generally scheduled during the day shift when the client is most active, receives two meals, and takes most oral medications. A large part of the remainder is scheduled for the evening shift.	*Dividing the intake throughout the day will permit fluids with meals and evening visitors and avoid periods of thirst.*

(continued)

PRACTICE GUIDELINES 44.2

Helping Clients Restrict Fluid Intake (continued)

Guidelines	Rationales
Identify fluids or fluid-like substances the client likes, and make sure that these are provided, unless contraindicated. A client who is allowed only 200 mL of fluid for breakfast, for example, should receive the type of fluid the client prefers.	*Having something the client likes will help ensure quality of life despite fluid restrictions.*
Set short-term goals that make the fluid restriction more tolerable, that is, schedule a specified amount of fluid at 1- or 2-hour intervals between meals. Some clients may prefer fluids between meals only if the food provided at mealtime helps relieve thirst.	*Scheduling may help make the fluid restriction more tolerable.*
Place allowed fluids in small containers, such as a 120 mL juice glass, to allow the perception of a full container; periodically offer the client ice chips as an alternative.	*Doing so can help make the fluid restriction seem less restrictive (e.g., ice chips are approximately half of the frozen volume after they melt).*
Provide frequent mouth care and rinses.	*These care measures reduce the thirst sensation.*
Instruct the client to avoid ingesting or chewing salty or sweet foods (e.g., hard candy or gum).	*These foods tend to produce thirst. Sugarless gum may be an alternative for some clients.*
Encourage the client to participate in maintaining the fluid intake record, if possible.	*Maintaining the record assists the client in evaluating the achievement of desired health outcomes.*

---

particularly when a medication that affects electrolyte balance is prescribed. Supplements may also be used when dietary intake is inadequate for a specific electrolyte or when fluid and electrolyte losses are extreme as a result of excessive perspiration.

Corticosteroids and many diuretics can cause too much potassium to be eliminated through the kidneys. For clients taking these medications, potassium supplements may be prescribed. Instruct clients taking oral potassium supplements to take the prescribed medication with juice to mask the unpleasant taste and reduce the possibility of gastric distress. Because hyperkalemia can have serious cardiac effects, clients should never increase the amount of potassium being taken without a physician's order to do so. In addition, inform clients that most salt substitutes contain potassium, so it is important to consult with their health care providers before using salt substitutes.

People who ingest insufficient milk products benefit from calcium supplements. The recommended daily allowance for calcium is 1000 to 1300 mg depending on age. It is generally recommended that postmenopausal women take 1200 mg of calcium per day to reduce the risk of osteoporosis. Long-term use of corticosteroid drugs can also cause calcium loss from the bones, and calcium supplements may help reduce this loss. Clients who are predisposed to developing renal calculi and who take supplemental calcium need to maintain a fluid intake

of at least 2500 mL per day (unless contraindicated) to reduce the risk of kidney stones, which are commonly composed of calcium salts.

Although routine supplements for other electrolytes generally are not recommended, clients who have poor dietary habits, who are malnourished, or who have difficulty accessing or eating fresh fruits and vegetables may benefit from electrolyte supplements. A daily multiple vitamin with minerals may achieve the desired goal. People who engage in strenuous activities in a warm environment need to be encouraged to replace the water and electrolytes that are lost through excessive perspiration by consuming a sports drink or other commercial fluid and electrolyte solution.

Liquid nutritional supplements are often given to clients who are malnourished or have poor eating habits. They are used with frequency in older adults to bolster nutritional status and caloric intake. It is very important for clients to read the product labels and to be aware of the contents of the supplement. Some of them are very high in protein and high in potassium, which may be contraindicated in an individual with impaired renal function.

PARENTERAL FLUID AND ELECTROLYTE REPLACEMENT

Intravenous (IV) fluid therapy is essential when clients are unable to take food and fluids orally. It is an efficient and effective method of supplying fluids directly into the intravascular fluid compartment and replacing electrolyte losses. IV fluid therapy is usually ordered by the physician or nurse practitioner. The nurse is responsible for administering and maintaining the therapy and for teaching the client and significant others how to continue the therapy at home, if necessary. See the Teaching: Wellness box on promoting healthy fluid and electrolyte balance.

Intravenous Solutions IV solutions can be classified as *isotonic*, *hypotonic*, or *hypertonic*. Isotonic solutions are often used to restore and maintain vascular volume. Hypertonic solutions have a greater concentration of solutes than plasma; hypotonic solutions have a lesser concentration of solutes. Table 44.11 provides examples of IV solutions and nursing implications.

IV solutions can also be categorized according to their purpose. Nutrient solutions contain some form of carbohydrate, such as dextrose or glucose, and water. Water is supplied for fluid requirements and carbohydrate for calories and energy. For example, 1 L of 5% dextrose provides 170 calories. Nutrient solutions are useful in preventing dehydration and ketosis but do not provide sufficient calories to promote wound healing, weight gain, or normal growth in children. Common nutrient solutions are 5% dextrose in water (D_5W) and 5% dextrose in 0.45% sodium chloride ($D_5 \frac{1}{2}$ NS).

Electrolyte solutions contain varying amounts of cations and anions. Commonly used solutions are normal saline (0.9% sodium chloride), Ringer's solution (which contains sodium, chloride, potassium, and calcium),

TEACHING WELLNESS

Promoting Healthy Fluid and Electrolyte Balance

Nurses should provide the following instructions to clients on how to maintain homeostasis:

- Consume 2000 mL to 2500 mL water daily, unless contraindicated.
- Avoid excess amounts of foods or fluids high in salt, sugar, and caffeine.
- Eat a well-balanced diet according to *Eating Well with Canada's Food Guide* (see Chapter 40).
- Limit alcohol intake because it has a diuretic effect.
- Increase fluid intake before, during, and after strenuous exercise, particularly when the environmental temperature is high, and replace lost electrolytes from excessive perspiration as needed with commercial electrolyte solutions.
- Maintain a normal body weight and body mass index for age and sex.
- Learn about and monitor side effects of medications that affect fluid and electrolyte balance (e.g., diuretics) and ways to handle side effects.
- Recognize possible risk factors for fluid and electrolyte imbalance, such as prolonged or repeated vomiting, frequent watery stools, or inability to consume fluids because of illness.
- Seek prompt professional health care for notable signs of fluid imbalance, such as sudden weight gain or loss, decreased urine volume, swollen ankles, shortness of breath, dizziness, or confusion.

TABLE 44.11 Selected Intravenous Solutions

Type/Examples	Comments/Nursing Implications
Isotonic Solutions 0.9% sodium chloride (NaCl; normal saline [NS]) Lactated Ringer's, or Ringer's solution	Isotonic solutions, such as NS and Ringer's solution, initially remain in the vascular compartment, expanding vascular volume. Ringer's is considered a physiologic (balanced electrolyte) solution. Assess clients carefully for signs of hypervolemia, such as bounding pulse and shortness of breath.
5% dextrose in water (D_5W)	D_5W is defined as isotonic, but becomes a hypotonic solution in the plasma. Upon administration, dextrose is rapidly metabolized, providing only free water, and therefore expanding intracellular and extracellular fluid volumes. D_5W is avoided in clients at risk for increased intracranial pressure (IICP) because it can increase cerebral edema.
Hypotonic Solutions 0.45% NaCl (half normal saline–½ NS) 0.33% NaCl (one-third normal saline–⅓ NS)	Hypotonic solutions are used to provide free water and treat cellular dehydration. These solutions promote waste elimination by the kidneys. Do not administer to clients at risk for IICP or third-space fluid shift.
Hypertonic Solutions 5% dextrose in normal saline (D_5NS) 5% dextrose in 0.45% NaCl ($D_5 \frac{1}{2}$ NS)* 5% dextrose in Lactated Ringer's (D_5LR)	Hypertonic solutions draw fluid out of the intracellular and interstitial compartments into the vascular compartment, expanding vascular volume. Do not administer to clients with kidney or heart disease or clients who are dehydrated. Watch for signs of hypervolemia. * Defined as hypertonic but becomes a hypotonic solution in the plasma as dextrose is rapidly metabolized on infusion providing NS

and lactated Ringer's (which contains sodium, chloride, potassium, calcium, and lactate). Lactate is metabolized in the liver to form HCO_3^-. Saline and balanced electrolyte solutions are commonly used to restore vascular volume, particularly after trauma or surgery. They also may be used to replace fluid and electrolytes for clients with continuing losses, for example, those experiencing gastric suction or wound drainage.

Lactated Ringer's solution is an alkalinizing solution that may be given to treat metabolic acidosis. Acidifying solutions, in contrast, are administered to counteract metabolic alkalosis. Examples of acidifying solutions are 5% dextrose in 0.45% sodium chloride and 0.9% sodium chloride solution.

Volume expanders are solutions used to increase the blood volume following severe loss of blood (e.g., from hemorrhage) or loss of plasma (e.g., from severe burns, which draw large amounts of plasma from the bloodstream to the burn site). Examples of volume expanders are plasma and human serum albumin.

Venipuncture Sites   The site chosen for venipuncture varies with the client's age, the length of time the infusion is to run, the type of solution used (e.g., vesicant or irritant), condition of veins, physical and functional assessment, and patient preference (Registered Nurses' Association of Ontario [RNAO], 2008). For adults, veins in the hand and arm are commonly used; for infants, veins in the scalp and dorsal foot are often used. The larger veins of the adult forearms are preferred over the metacarpal veins of the hands for infusions that need to be given rapidly and for solutions that are hypertonic, or highly acidic or alkaline, or could be irritating (e.g., certain medications).

The loss of subcutaneous tissues, thinning of the skin, and fragile veins in the older adult can be a challenge for the nurse when performing a venipuncture. It is common practice for the initial venipuncture to be in the most distal portion of the arm because this allows for subsequent venipunctures to move upward. The veins of the hands of the older adults, however, are not the best initial sites for venipunctures because of loss of subcutaneous tissue and thinning of the skin (Rosenthal, 2006).

The metacarpal, basilic, and cephalic veins are commonly used for intermittent or continuous infusions (Figure 44.14B). The ulna and the radius act as natural splints at these sites, and the client has greater freedom of arm movements for activities, such as eating. Although the basilic and median cubital are convenient sites for venipuncture, they are usually kept for blood samples, bolus injections of medication, and insertion sites for a peripherally inserted central catheter (PICC) line (see Figure 44.14A). See Practice Guidelines 44.3 for vein selection and general tips for easier IV starts. See the Evidence-Informed Practice box on the best practice guidelines for maintaining vascular access devices.

Historically, nurses have used their eyes and hands to locate a suitable vein for a venipuncture. This could be especially challenging in some clients, such as older adults, clients who are obese, infants and children, as well as dark-skinned clients because their veins may not be visible or palpable. Transillumination (ultrasound) devices using lights to allow for the location and identification of blood vessels are becoming increasingly available in clinical settings. Focusing bright, visible light onto and under the skin is promising to assist the nurse in locating superficial veins, regardless of skin colour.

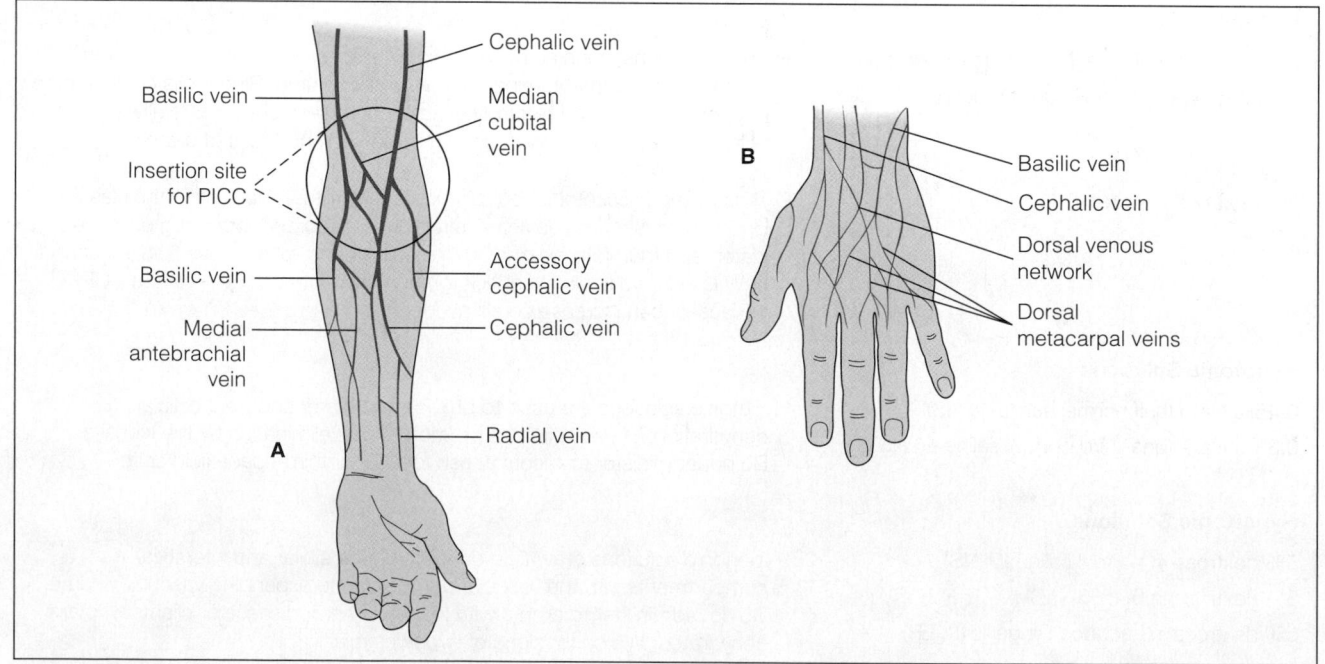

FIGURE 44.14 Commonly used venipuncture sites: **A:** Arm; **B:** Hand; **A** also shows the site used for a peripherally inserted central catheter (PICC).

EVIDENCE-INFORMED PRACTICE

What Are Best Practice Guidelines for Maintaining Vascular Access Devices?

The Registered Nurses' Association of Ontario (RNAO, 2008) produced a document that outlines the best practices in caring for and maintaining vascular access devices. The guidelines are the result of a significant review of literature, critique of studies, and synthesis of material on the topic. The document gives detailed and concise recommendations for a range of venous access device issues, from cleaning solutions through taping procedures to frequency of tubing change. The RNAO builds in a regular review process to ensure that any literature is incorporated into the original guidelines in the form of a supplement.

NURSING IMPLICATIONS: This document provides an excellent resource for nurses. The concise and specific recommendations will ensure that knowledge transfer of research findings occurs in the clinical world.

Source: Based on Registered Nurses' Association of Ontario. (2008). *Care and maintenance to reduce vascular access complications—guideline supplement.* Toronto, ON: Author.

Physical assessments that reveal lymphedema, tissue damage, or deformity can help determine site selection with efforts made to avoid any area that is already compromised. A client who requires crutches to function must, if at all possible, have a venipuncture site chosen that does not further impede mobility. Collaborating with the client and family in site selection not only enhances the client's self-efficacy but also ensures that any additional and relevant information is factored into the venipuncture site decision-making process (RNAO, 2008).

When long-term IV therapy is anticipated, or the client is receiving IV medications that are damaging to vessels (e.g., chemotherapy, fluids with an osmolarity >600 mOsm/L, such as parenteral nutrition), a **central venous catheter** may be inserted. Central venous catheters usually are inserted into the subclavian or jugular vein, with the distal tip of the catheter resting in the superior vena cava just above the right atrium (Figure 44.15 on the next page). They may be inserted at the client's bedside, or for longer-term access, surgically inserted. Subclavian central venous catheters permit freedom of movement for ambulation; however, there is greater risk of complications, including hemothorax or pneumothorax, cardiac perforation, thrombosis, and infection. Assess the client closely for manifestations, such as shortness of breath, chest pain, cough, hypotension, tachycardia, and anxiety, after the insertion procedure.

A **peripherally inserted central catheter (PICC)** is inserted in the basilic or cephalic vein just above or below the antecubital space of the right arm. The tip of the catheter rests in the lower portion of the superior vena cava. The risk of pneumothorax is eliminated with PICC. These catheters are frequently used for long-term

---

PRACTICE GUIDELINES 44.3

Vein Selection

Guidelines	Rationales
Use distal veins of the arm first.	*Distal vein selection provides for more proximal alternatives if subsequent venipuncture is required; if proximal veins are used first and they become sclerosed, all access to distal veins will be blocked.*
Use the client's nondominant arm, whenever possible.	*Using this arm helps to ensure that the client can continue to perform the activities of daily living.*
Select a vein that is (a) easily palpated and feels soft and full; (b) naturally splinted by bone; and (c) large enough to allow adequate circulation around the catheter.	*These factors ensure ease of insertion and patency once the catheter is in the vein.*
Avoid using veins that are in areas of flexion (e.g., the antecubital fossa) and in the ventral surface of the wrist; are damaged by previous use, inflammation or infiltration; are sclerosed, knotted, or tortuous; that are continually distended with blood; or are in a compromised or injured extremity (e.g., avoid veins in the limb with dialysis access or paralysis or paresis; or same side as a mastectomy).	*These situations can involve impaired circulation and cause discomfort for the client.*
Consider client preference.	*Having a choice helps to ensure client self-efficacy and nurse–client partnership; the client can provide helpful input to ensure quality of life and care issues are addressed.*

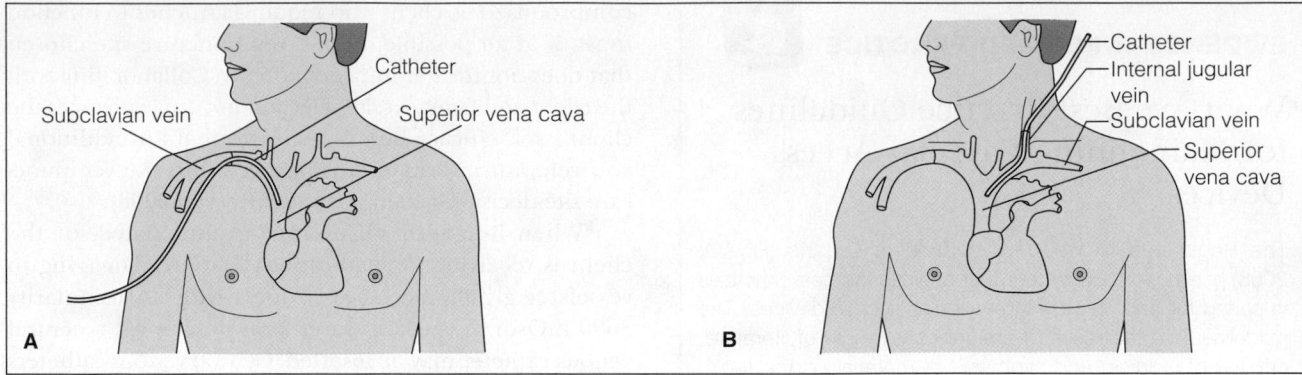

FIGURE 44.15 Central venous lines: **A:** Subclavian vein insertion; **B:** Left jugular insertion.

intravenous access when the client is receiving IV therapy at home.

Implantable venous access devices or ports (Figures 44.16 and 44.17) are used for clients with chronic illness who require long-term IV therapy (e.g., intermittent medications, vesicants such as certain chemotherapy, total parenteral nutrition, and frequent blood samples).

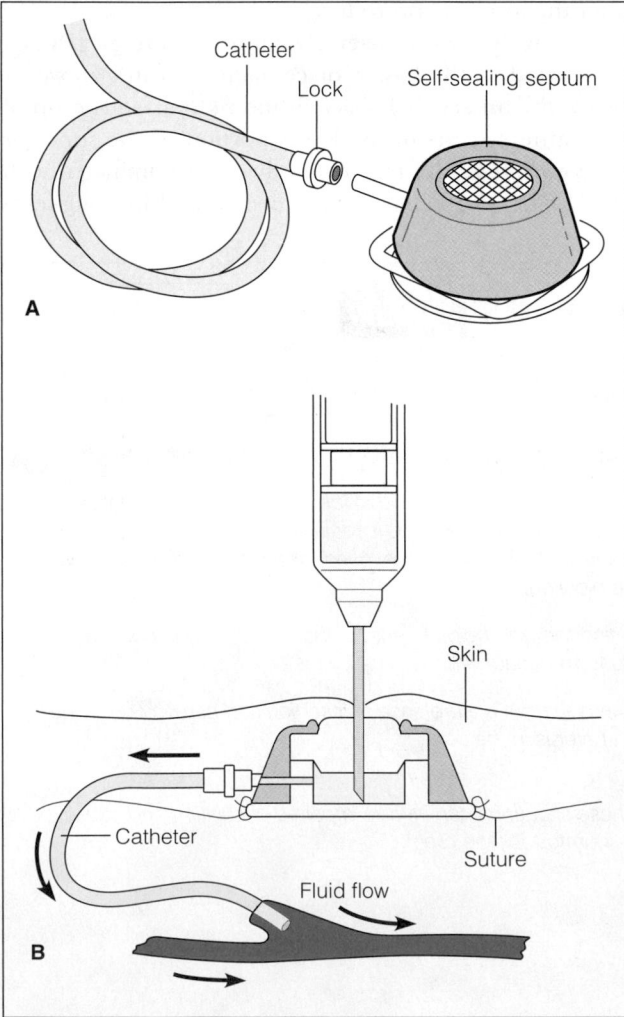

FIGURE 44.16 An implantable venous access device:
A: Components; **B:** The device in place.

This type of device is designed to provide repeated access to the central venous system, avoiding the trauma and complications of multiple venipunctures. Using local anesthesia, implantable ports are surgically placed into a small subcutaneous pocket under the skin, usually on the upper anterior chest near the clavicle, and no part of the port is exposed. The distal end of the catheter is placed in the subclavian or jugular vein. Different kinds of implantable venous access devices are available and they may be tunnelled or nontunnelled. Special precautions need to be taken with all central lines and venous access ports to ensure asepsis and catheter patency. Nursing care of clients with these devices is outlined in the Practice Guidelines 44.4.

An alternative form of therapy, hypodermoclysis is sometimes used to treat adults with dehydration. **Hypodermoclysis** is the subcutaneous infusion of fluid, generally isotonic. This procedure does not require venous access and has been shown to be effective for the treatment of mild to moderate dehydration in adults, in particular those receiving home palliative care, and it can be performed at home by family members (Slesak, Schnurle, Jakob, Dietz, 2003). The fine-gauge device is inserted under the skin in such locations as the upper arm, chest wall, abdomen, or thigh. Site rotation is recommended every 3 to 7 days (Infusion Nurses Society, 2011).

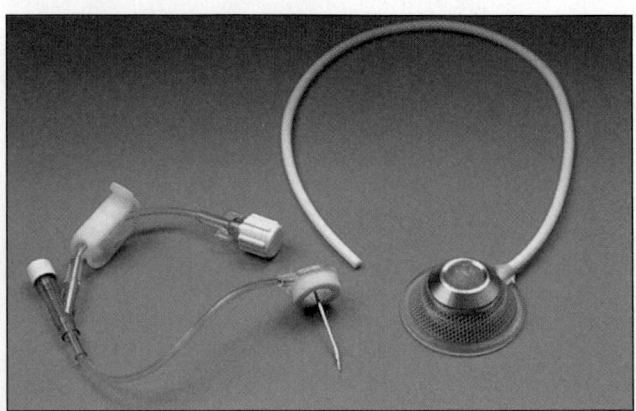

FIGURE 44.17 An implantable venous access device (*right*) and a Huber needle with extension tubing.

PRACTICE GUIDELINES 44.4

Caring for Clients with a Venous Access Device (VAD)

Guidelines	Rationales
After insertion, document the date; the insertion site; the brand, gauge, and catheter length; the location of the catheter tip (verified by radiography); the length of the external segment; and client teaching.	*Appropriate documentation is required and correct placement of the device must be ensured via radiography before commencing infusion therapy.*

Site Care

Use strict aseptic technique (including the use of sterile gloves and mask) when caring for central lines and long-term VADs.	*Venous access devices provide a portal of entry for microorganisms.*
The frequency of dressing changes is dependent on the dressing material. Transparent semipermeable membrane (TSM) dressing or tape and gauze are acceptable, though TSM dressing is preferable. Dressings also should be changed when loose or soiled.	*Gauze dressings do not allow for visualization of the insertion site and need to be changed every 48 hours; in contrast, TSM dressings allow for visualization and can be left in place for a maximum of 7 days if it remains clean, dry, and intact.*
Assess the site for any redness, swelling, tenderness, or drainage. Compare the length of the external portion of the catheter with its documented length. Obtain a chest radiograph to determine the catheter tip's position if in doubt. Report and document any position changes or sign of infection.	*Infection and displacement are possible complications of venous access devices.*
Follow agency protocol for cleaning solutions and types of dressings; chlorhexidine gluconate is the preferred agent to clean the insertion site.	*Following these protocols ensures infection prevention and control.*
Clean the skin around the site with chlorhexidine (or per agency policy) using a back-and-forth or side-to-side motion. Allow the site to air dry.	*Taking this precaution minimizes the risk of infection.*
Secure the catheter with a new stabilization device, and cover the entry site and external portion of the catheter with a sterile occlusive dressing.	*Taking this measure minimizes risk of infection and helps to prevent catheter displacement.*
Provide routine care of the incision site for the implant device until it is healed. Once it heals, no care is necessary when the port is idle.	*Ongoing care will minimize risk of infection.*

Catheter Care and Flushing

Change the catheter cap as indicated by agency protocol. Adding a 15-second scrub of the connection surface of the needleless connector before the removal of the cap has been shown to prohibit microorganism entry on the surface (Moureau & Dawson, 2010).	*Taking this precaution minimizes risk of infection.*
The solution used and frequency of flushing are determined by agency protocol for the specific type of port being used. If heparin is used as part of the flushing protocol, the concentration should not be in amounts that cause systemic anticoagulation, but in the lowest possible concentration to maintain patency. Many agencies are switching to needleless IV connectors that can be flushed with normal saline solution only.	*Flushing ensures patency and prevents contact between incompatible medications or fluids. Heparin-induced thrombocytopenia has been reported with the use of heparin flush solution and saline flushes have been effective in maintaining patency.*
Flush the catheter before and after each dose of medication. The frequency of flushes between uses may vary from every 12 hours to once a week or less, depending on the type of catheter.	*The initial flush is to assess patency of the catheter, and the flush after administration of the medication is to ensure that the complete dose has entered the bloodstream. The frequency of flushing varies with the size of the catheter gauge, the concentration of the flush fluid, and the nature of the catheter product.*

(continued)

PRACTICE GUIDELINES 44.4

Caring for Clients with a Venous Access Device (VAD) (continued)

Guidelines	Rationales
Use a 10-mL syringe to flush the catheter. Never apply force if you feel resistance.	*The syringe size ensures adequate pressure to deliver the flush without damaging the catheter. Note that the smaller the syringe, the greater the amount of pressure.*
Remember to flush all lumens for multiple-lumen catheters.	*Flushing helps maintain patency.*
A needle with a 90-degree angle is generally used to access an implanted port for infusions. Stabilizing the port between the thumb and index finger of the nondominant hand, insert the needle through the centre of the port until the resistance of the platform is felt.	*Specially designed needles are easier to stabilize and are more comfortable for the client.*
To remove the needle after a treatment, again stabilize the port and use even pressure to withdraw the needle.	*Stabilizing the port to promote client comfort. Positive pressure ensures catheter patency.*
Maintain positive pressure by withdrawing the needle as the last millilitre of flush solution is being instilled.	
Flush idle implanted ports in accordance with agency protocol or at least every 8 weeks.	*Flushing ensures patency.*

Teaching

Provide clients with the following instructions:

- Do not allow anyone to take a blood pressure on the arm in which a PICC line is inserted.

- Wear a Medic Alert tag or bracelet if the device is to be in place for a long period.

- For a PICC line, you do not need to restrict activities, except that the arm should not be immersed in water. Showering is allowed if the site and catheter are covered by a TSM dressing.

- For an implanted central venous port, there are no activity restrictions, but the port or catheter tip can become dislodged. Signs of a dislodged catheter tip include pain in the neck or ear on the affected side, swishing or gurgling sounds, or palpitations; signs of a dislodged port include free movement of the port, swelling, or difficulty accessing the port. Notify the physician should any of these occur or if symptoms of infection develop.

Clients must learn many details related to the care of their catheter to ensure patency and minimize risk of displacement and infection.

Source: Hadaway, L. C. (2008) Targeting therapy with central venous access devices. *Nursing, 36*(6), 34–40. Guidelines adapted with permission.

Intravenous Equipment Because equipment varies according to the manufacturer, the nurse must become familiar with the equipment used in each particular agency.

Intravenous (IV) equipment consists of IV catheter, catheter stabilization devices, solutions containers, infusion and administration sets, IV filters, and IV poles.

Intravenous Catheters The type of IV catheters to be used depends on the kinds of vascular needs, which are based

on the prescribed therapy and length of treatment. The catheter size used should be the smallest size and shortest length that will accommodate the prescribed therapy (RNAO, 2008). Furthermore, all catheters must be radiopaque (RNAO, 2008). A peripheral-short catheter is less than or equal to 7.6 cm (3 in.) in length. Over-the-needle catheters, also known as *angiocaths*, are commonly used for adult clients. The plastic catheter fits over a

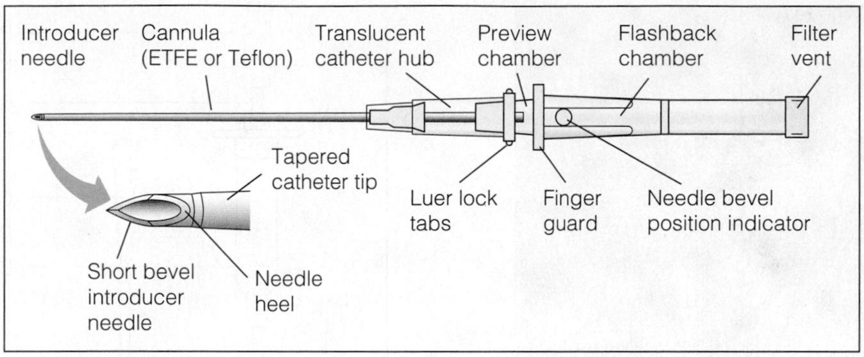

Introducer needle | Cannula (ETFE or Teflon) | Translucent catheter hub | Preview chamber | Flashback chamber | Filter vent

Tapered catheter tip

Short bevel introducer needle | Needle heel | Luer lock tabs | Finger guard | Needle bevel position indicator

FIGURE 44.18 Schematic of an over-the-needle catheter.

needle used to pierce the skin and vein wall (Figure 44.18). Once inserted into the vein, the needle is withdrawn and discarded, leaving the catheter in place. With the original over-the-needle catheters, the sharp stylet remained exposed until placed in a sharps container. This resulted in needlestick injuries to nurses. A variety of safety devices on IV catheters are now available and their use is becoming a recommended standard of care (Infusion Nurses Society, 2011). The safety devices can be either an active safety device that requires activation by the nurse or a passive safety device in which the safety feature is automatically activated after the stylet is removed from the catheter.

Butterfly, or wing-tipped, needles with plastic flaps attached to the shaft are sometimes used (Figure 44.19). The flaps are held tightly together to hold the needle securely during insertion; after insertion, they are flattened against the skin and secured with tape. The butterfly needle is most frequently used for short-term therapy (e.g., less than 24 hours), such as for IV push medication.

Catheter Stabilization Devices Securing or stabilizing an IV catheter helps decrease movement of the catheter in and out of the insertion site, and the catheter is less likely

to be dislodged. Historically, nonsterile tape was used to secure peripheral IV catheters. The RNAO (2008) standards now recommend the use of manufactured catheter stabilization devices (Figure 44.20).

Solution containers are available in various sizes (50, 100, 250, 500, or 1000 mL); the smaller containers are often used to administer medications. Most solutions are dispensed in plastic bags (Figure 44.21 on the next page). However, glass bottles may need to be used if the administered medications are incompatible with plastic. Glass bottles require an air vent so that air can enter the bottle and replace the fluid that enters the client's vein. Some bottles contain a tube that serves as a vent; other containers require a vent on the administration set. Air vents usually have filters to prevent contamination from the air that enters the container. Air vents are not required for plastic solution bags because the bags collapse under atmospheric pressure when the solution enters the vein. It is essential that the solution be sterile and clear. Cloudiness, evidence that the container has been opened previously, or leaks indicate possible contamination. Always check the expiration date on the label. Return any questionable or contaminated solutions to the pharmacy.

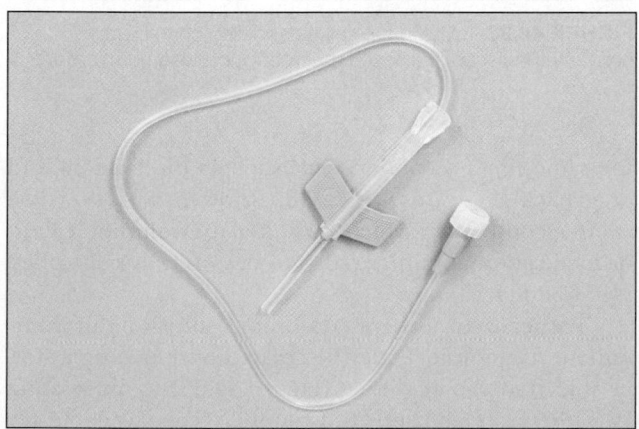

FIGURE 44.19 A butterfly IV needle.

Source: Berman, A., & Snyder, S. (2012). *Skills in clinical nursing* (7th ed) (Fig 18-3, p. 488). Upper Saddle River, NJ: Pearson Education Inc.

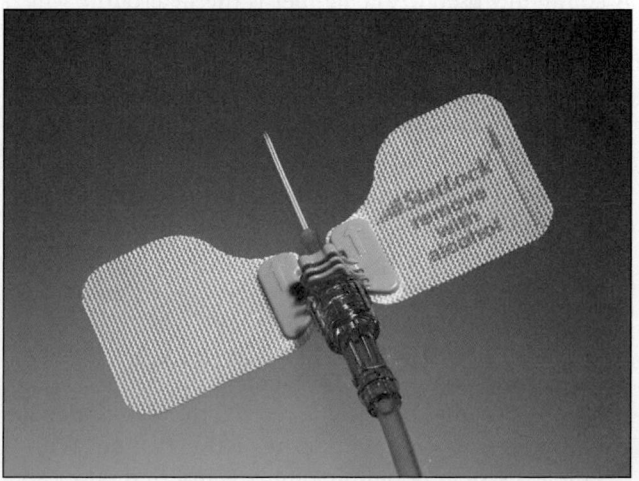

FIGURE 44.20 Manufactured catheter stabilization device.

Photo courtesy of C.R. Bard, Inc.

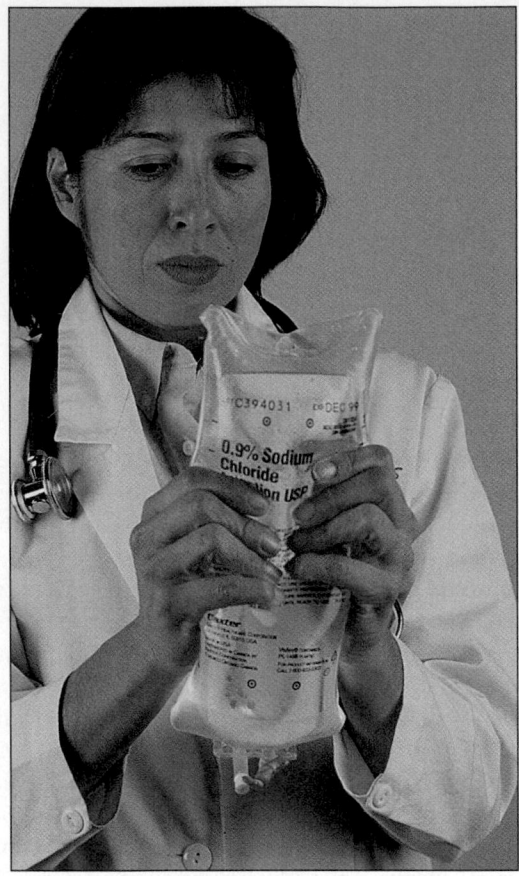

FIGURE 44.21 A plastic intravenous fluid container.

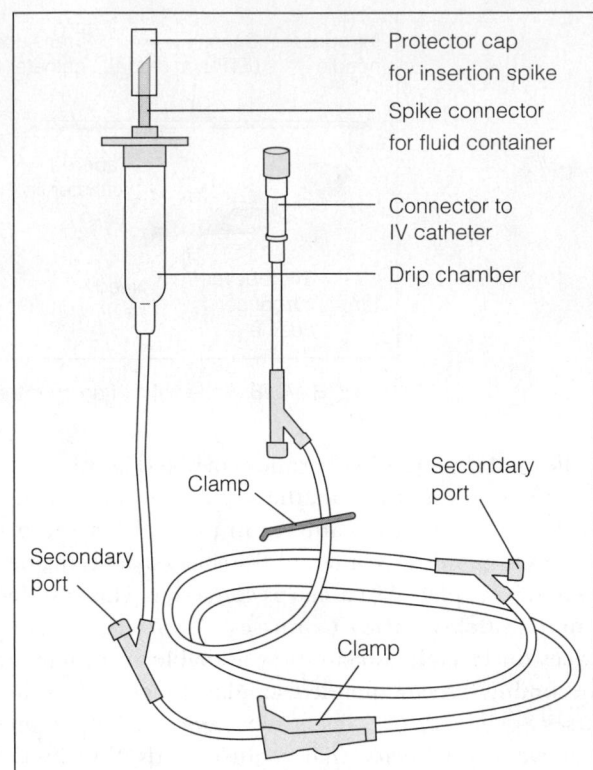

FIGURE 44.22 A standard IV administration set.

Labels on figure: Protector cap for insertion spike; Spike connector for fluid container; Connector to IV catheter; Drip chamber; Secondary port; Clamp; Secondary port; Clamp

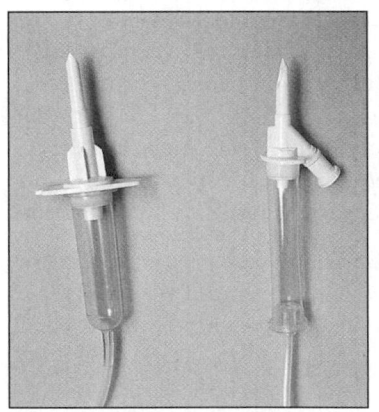
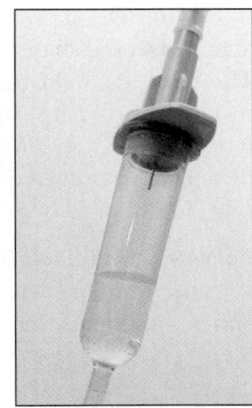

FIGURE 44.23 Infusion set spikes and drip chambers: nonvented macrodrip, vented macrodrip, nonvented microdrip.

Infusion administration sets consist of an insertion spike, a drip chamber, a roller valve or screw clamp, tubing with secondary ports, and a protective cap over the IV catheter adapter (Figure 44.22). The insertion spike is kept sterile and inserted into the solution container when the equipment is set up and ready to start. The drip chamber permits a predictable amount of fluid to be delivered. A commonly used drip chamber is the macrodrip, which delivers 10 to 20 drops/mL of solution. This information is found on the package. There are also microdrip sets, which deliver 60 drops/mL of solution (see Figure 44.23). The roller valve or clamp, which compresses the lumen of the tubing, controls the rate of the flow. The protective cap over the needle adapter maintains the sterility of the end of the tubing so that it can be attached to a sterile needle or catheter inserted in the client's vein. A special infusion set may be required if the IV flow rate will be regulated by an infusion pump.

Most infusion sets include one or more injection ports for administering IV medications or secondary infusions. Needleless systems reduce the risk of needlestick injury and contamination of the IV line. With a needleless system, a blunt cannula is inserted into a special injection port or adapter on the IV tubing to administer medications or secondary infusions (Figure 44.24). When more than one solution needs to be infused at the same time, secondary sets, such as the tandem and piggyback IV setups, are used. Another variation is a volume-control set, which is used if the volume of fluid or medication administered is to be carefully controlled (see Chapter 33).

Rather than using a continuous infusion, an intermittent infusion lock may be created by attaching a sterile injection cap or device (Figure 44.25) to an existing IV catheter. This keeps the venous access available for the administration of intermittent or emergency medications. The device is commonly referred to as a saline lock because periodic injection with saline is used to keep blood from coagulating within the tubing.

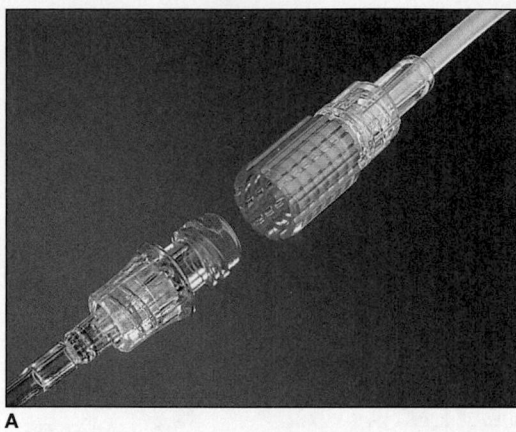

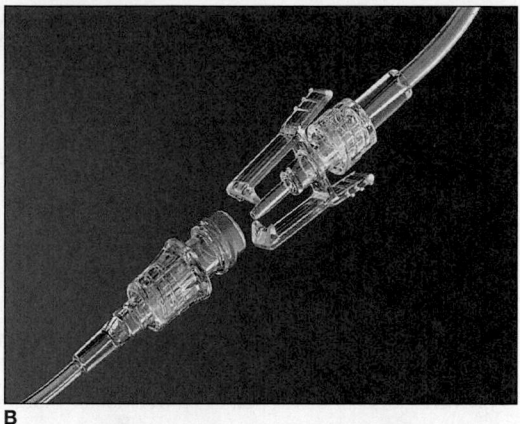

A **B**

FIGURE 44.24 Cannulae used to connect the tubing of additive sets to primary infusions: **A:** Threaded-lock cannula; **B:** Lever-lock cannula.

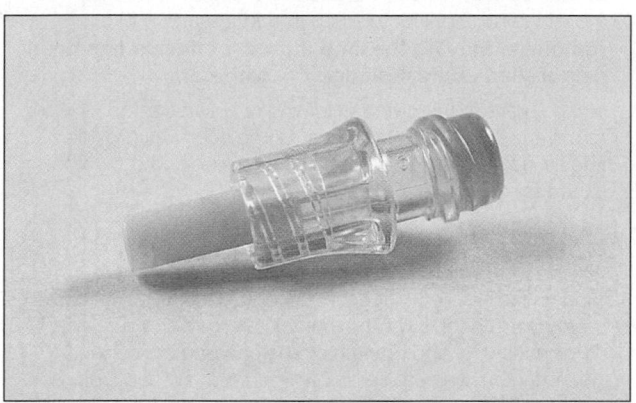

FIGURE 44.25 Intermittent infusion device with injection port.

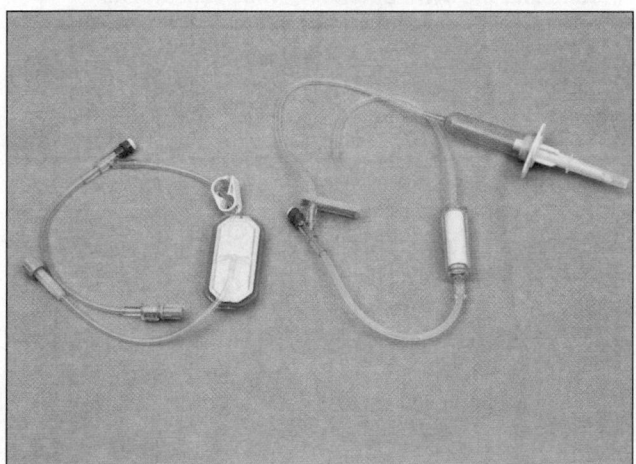

FIGURE 44.26 Two types of IV filters.

Intravenous Filters IV filters are used to remove air and particulate matter from IV infusions and to reduce the risk of complications (e.g., infusion-related phlebitis) associated with routine IV therapies (Figure 44.26). Most IV filters consist of a membrane (pore size of 0.22 micron, although sizes vary). Some problems associated with filters include (a) clogging of the filter surface, which may stop or slow the flow rate when debris accumulates; and (b) binding of some drugs (e.g., insulin and amphotericin B) to the surface of the filter.

Intravenous poles are used to hang the solution container. Some poles are attached to hospital beds or hang from the ceiling; others are floor models with casters that can be pushed along when the client is up and walking. The height of most poles is adjustable. In the home, robe hooks, kitchen cabinet knobs, or an S-hook over the top of a door can be used to hang solution containers. The higher the solution container, the greater is the force of the solution as it enters the client's vein and the faster the rate of flow.

Starting an Intravenous Infusion Although the physician is generally responsible for prescribing IV therapy for clients, nurses initiate, monitor, and maintain the infusion. This is true not only in hospitals and long-term care facilities but also increasingly in community-based settings, such as clinics and clients' homes. Nurses may be required to be certified for initiation of intravenous therapy by their employing agencies.

Before preparing an infusion, the nurse determines the following:

- The type and amount of solution to be infused
- The exact amount (dose) of any medications to be added to a compatible solution
- The rate of flow or the time over which the infusion is to be completed

If solutions are prepared by the pharmacy or another department, the nurse must verify that the solution supplied exactly matches what the physician prescribed.

Understanding the purpose for the infusion is as important as assessing the client. For example, the nurse should question an order for 5% dextrose in water (D_5W) at 150 mL/h if the client has peripheral edema and other signs of fluid overload.

To perform venipuncture and start an IV infusion, see Skill 44.1 on the next page.

SKILL 44.1   STARTING AN INTRAVENOUS INFUSION

Before preparing the infusion, first verify the prescription indicating the type of solution, the amount to be administered, the rate of flow of the infusion, and any client allergies (e.g., to tape or latex). Check agency policy.

PURPOSES

- To supply fluid when clients are unable to take in an adequate volume of fluids by mouth
- To provide salts and other electrolytes needed to maintain electrolyte balance
- To provide glucose (dextrose), the main fuel for metabolism
- To provide water-soluble vitamins and medications
- To establish a lifeline for rapidly needed medications

ASSESSMENT

Assess

- Vital signs (pulse, respiratory rate, and BP) for baseline data
- Skin turgor
- Allergy to latex (e.g., tourniquet), tape, iodine
- Bleeding tendencies
- Disease or injury to extremities
- Status of veins to determine appropriate venipuncture site. Avoid sites that have been used recently. **Rationale: Recently used sites will be more prone to complications and discomfort.**
- Whether patient is right-handed or left-handed. **Rationale: The dominant hand should be left free, if possible.**
- The agency policy about clipping hair in the area before a venipuncture. Shaving is not recommended because of the possibility of nicking the skin and subsequent infection.

PLANNING

- Before initiating the IV infusion, consider how long the client is likely to have the IV, what kinds of fluids will be infused, and what medications the client will be receiving or is likely to receive. These factors may affect the choice of vein and catheter size. Review the client record regarding previous infusions. Note any complications and how they were managed.

Equipment

Substitute appropriate supplies if the client has tape, antiseptic, or latex allergies.

- Infusion set
- Sterile parenteral solution
- IV pole
- Nonallergenic tape
- Moisture-permeable transparent dressing
- Tourniquet
- Antiseptic swabs (preferably 2% chlorhexidine gluconate with alcohol)
- IV catheter (choose an IV catheter of the appropriate type and size based on the size of the vein and the purpose of the IV. A 20- to 22-gauge catheter is indicated for most

adults. Always have an extra catheter and ones of different sizes available.)

- Clean gloves
- Sterile gauze dressing or transparent semipermeable membrane (TSM) dressing
- Arm splint, if required
- Towel or pad
- Electronic infusion device or pump, as necessary
- Local anesthetic (optional, and per agency policy)

IMPLEMENTATION

Preparation

- Unless initiating IV therapy is urgent, provide any scheduled care before establishing the infusion to minimize movement of the affected limb during the procedure. **Rationale: Moving the limb after the infusion has been established could dislodge the catheter.**
- Make sure that the client's clothing or gown can be removed over the IV apparatus. Some agencies provide special gowns that open over the shoulder and down the sleeve for easy removal.

Performance

1. Before performing the procedure, introduce yourself and verify the client's identity using two identifiers or per agency protocol. Explain what you are going to do, why it is necessary, and how he or she can participate. A venipuncture can cause discomfort for a few seconds, but there should be no discomfort while the solution is flowing. Use a doll to demonstrate for children, and explain the procedure to the parents. **Rationale: Pain and anxiety stimulate the sympathetic nervous system and trigger vasoconstriction and vasovagal reactions.**

2. Perform hand hygiene, and follow other appropriate infection prevention and control procedures.

3. Position the client appropriately.
   - Assist the client into a comfortable position, either sitting or lying. Expose the limb to be used, but provide for client privacy.

4. Apply a timing label on the solution container (Figure 44.27 on page 1455).

5. Open and prepare the infusion set.
   - Remove tubing from the container and straighten it out.
   - Slide the tubing clamp along the tubing until it is just below the drip chamber to facilitate its access.
   - Close the clamp.
   - Leave the ends of the tubing covered with the plastic caps until the infusion is started. **Rationale: This will maintain the sterility of the ends of the tubing.**

6. Spike the solution container.
   - Remove the protective cover from the entry site of the bag.
   - Remove the cap from the spike, and insert the spike into the insertion site of the bag or bottle (see ❶), following the manufacturer's instructions.

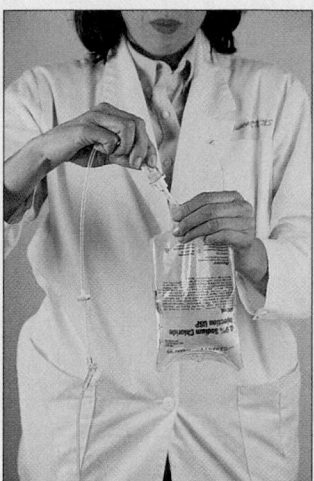

❶ Inserting the spike.

7. Hang the solution container on the pole.

   • Adjust the pole so that the container is suspended about 1 m above the client's head. **Rationale: This height is needed to enable gravity to overcome venous pressure and facilitate flow of the solution into the vein.**

8. Partially fill the drip chamber with solution.

   • Squeeze the chamber gently until it is half full of solution (see ❷). **Rationale: The drip chamber is partly filled with solution to prevent air from moving down the tubing.**

9. Prime the tubing, as described below. The term prime means "to make ready," but in common use refers to flushing the tube to remove air.

   • Remove the protective cap and hold the tubing over a container. Maintain the sterility of the end of the tubing and the cap.

   • Release the clamp and let the fluid run through the tubing until all bubbles are removed. Tap the tubing, if necessary, with your fingers to help the bubbles move. **Rationale: The tubing is primed to prevent the introduction of air into the client.**

   • Air bubbles smaller than 0.5 mL usually do not cause problems in peripheral lines.

   • Reclamp the tubing and replace the tubing cap, maintaining sterile technique.

   • For caps with air vents, do not remove the cap when priming this tubing. **Rationale: The flow of solution through the tubing will cease when the cap is moist with one drop of solution.**

   • If an infusion control pump, electronic device, or controller is being used, follow the manufacturer's directions for inserting the tubing and setting the infusion rate.

10. Perform hand hygiene again just before client contact.

11. Select the venipuncture site as per Practice Guidelines 44.3 (page 1443).

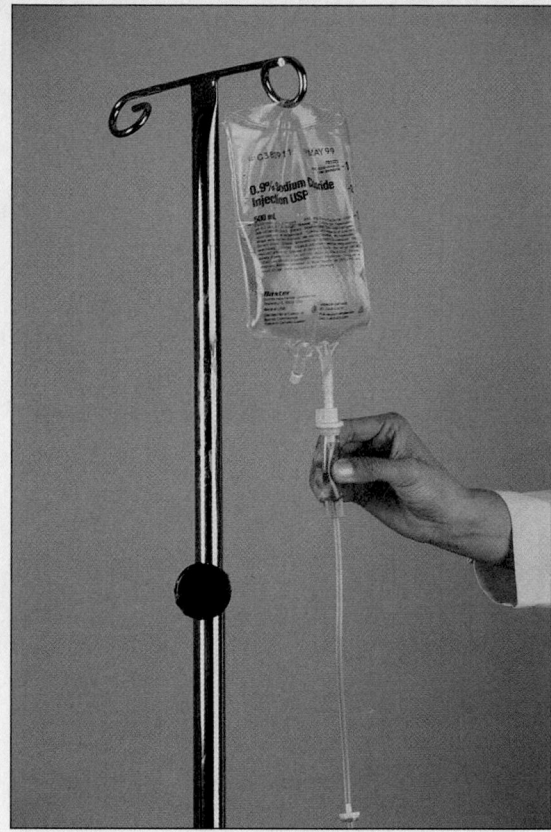

❷ Squeezing the drip chamber.

   • If the site is very hairy, remove hair by clipping with scissors. **Rationale: Shaving increases the risk of microabrasions, which can lead to infection.**

   • Place a towel or bed protector under the extremity to protect linens (or furniture if in the home).

12. Dilate the vein.

   • Place the extremity in a dependent position (at a level lower than the client's heart). **Rationale: Gravity slows venous return and distends the veins. Distending the veins makes it easier to insert the needle properly.**

   • Apply a tourniquet firmly 15 to 20 cm above the venipuncture site (see ❸). Explain that the tourniquet will feel tight. **Rationale: The tourniquet must be tight enough to obstruct venous flow but not so tight that it occludes arterial flow. Obstructing arterial flow inhibits venous filling. If a radial pulse can be palpated, the arterial flow is not obstructed. Use the tourniquet on only one client. This avoids cross-contamination to other clients.**

   • For older adults with fragile skin, instead of applying a tourniquet, place the arm in a dependent position to allow the vein to engorge. **Rationale: The tourniquet can cause tissue damage and may not be needed to allow the vein to dilate.**

(continued)

SKILL 44.1 **STARTING AN INTRAVENOUS INFUSION (continued)**

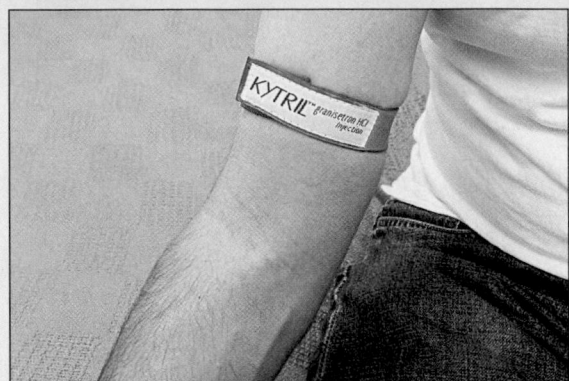

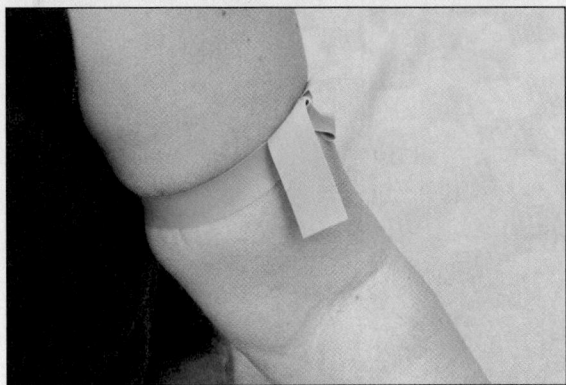

❸ Two types of tourniquets.

- If the vein is not sufficiently dilated, do the following:

  a. Massage or stroke the vein distal to the site and in the direction of venous flow toward the heart. **Rationale: This action helps fill the vein.**

  b. Encourage the client to clench and unclench the fist. **Rationale: Contracting the muscles compresses the distal veins, forcing blood along the veins and distending them.**

  c. Lightly tap the vein with your fingertips. **Rationale: Tapping may distend the vein.**

- If the preceding steps fail to distend the vein so that it is palpable, remove the tourniquet, and apply a warm towel to the entire extremity for 10 to 15 minutes. **Rationale: Heat dilates superficial blood vessels, causing them to fill.** Then, repeat steps to dilate the vein.

13. Minimize insertion pain as much as possible. Although the pain of insertion should be brief, prevention can and should be offered. Transdermal analgesic creams (e.g., eutectic mixture of local anesthetics [EMLA]) may also be used, depending on policy. Allow at least 30 minutes for the topical analgesic to take effect (Phillips, 2010).

14. Apply clean gloves and clean the venipuncture site. **Rationale: Gloves protect the nurse from contamination by the client's blood.**

- Clean the skin at the site of entry with a topical antiseptic swab (e.g., 2% chlorhexidine). Some institutions may use 70% isopropyl alcohol or 10% povidone-iodine swabs (check agency policy). Check for allergies to iodine before cleansing skin with Betadine or iodine products.

- Use a circular motion, moving from the centre outward for several centimetres. **Rationale: This motion carries microorganisms away from the site of entry.**

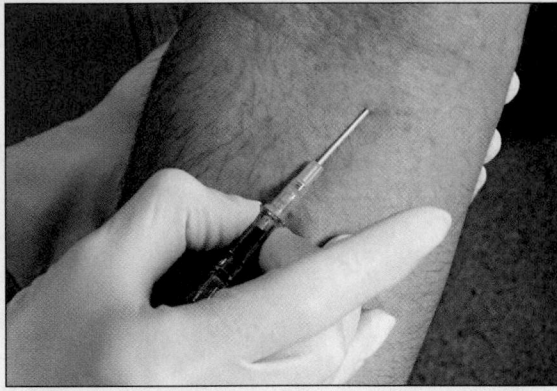

❹ Blood is noted in the flashback chamber once the stylet has entered the vein.

- Permit the solution to dry on the skin (2% chlorhexidine gluconate and povidone-iodine require 2 minutes to dry). **Rationale: Allowing the solution to air dry will increase effectiveness.**

15. Insert the catheter, and initiate the infusion.

- Remove the catheter assembly from its sterile packaging. Review instructions for using the catheter because a variety of needle-safety devices are manufactured. Remove the cover of the needle.

- Use the nondominant hand to pull the skin taut below the entry site. **Rationale: Doing this stabilizes the vein and makes the skin taut for needle entry. It can also make initial tissue penetration less painful.**

- Holding the over-the-needle catheter at a 15- to 30-degree angle with needle (stylet) bevel up, insert the catheter through the skin and into the vein in one movement. A sudden lack of resistance is felt as the needle enters the vein. Jabbing, stabbing, or quick thrusting should be avoided because it may cause rupture of delicate veins.

- Once blood appears in the lumen of the needle or you feel the lack of resistance, lower the angle of the catheter until it is almost parallel with the skin, and advance the needle and catheter approximately 0.5 cm to 1 cm farther. See ❹. Holding the needle portion steady, advance the catheter until the hub is at the venipuncture site. **Rationale: The catheter is advanced to ensure that it, and not just the metal needle, is in the vein.** The exact technique depends on the type of catheter used.

- If there is no blood return, try redirecting the catheter assembly toward the vein. If the stylet has been withdrawn from the catheter even a small distance, or the catheter tip has been pulled out of the skin, the catheter must be discarded and a new one used. **Rationale: Reinserting the stylet into the catheter can result in damage or slicing of the catheter. A catheter that has been removed from the skin is considered contaminated and cannot be reused.**

- If blood begins to flow out of the vein into the tissues as the catheter is inserted, creating a hematoma, the insertion has not been successful. This is sometimes referred to as a *blown vein*. Immediately release the tourniquet and remove the catheter, applying pressure over the insertion site with dry gauze. Attempt the

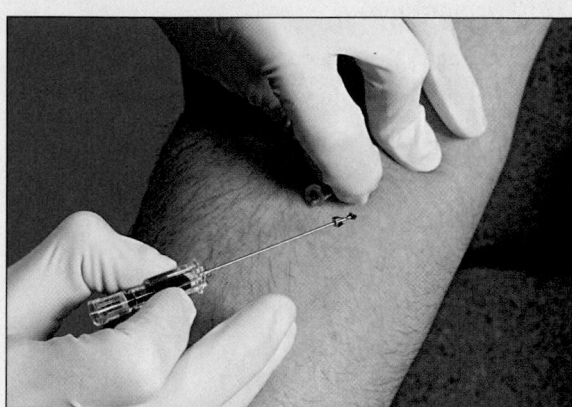

❺ Occlude the vein with one finger while removing the stylet.

venipuncture with another site, and the opposite arm, if possible. **Rationale: Placing the tourniquet back on the same arm above the unsuccessful site may cause it to bleed. Placing the IV below the unsuccessful site could result in infusing fluid into the already punctured vein, causing it to bleed.**

- Release the tourniquet.

- Put pressure on the vein proximal to the catheter to eliminate or reduce blood oozing out of the catheter. Stabilize the hub with thumb and index finger of the nondominant hand.

- Remove the protective cap from the distal end of the tubing, and hold it ready to attach to the catheter, maintaining sterility of the end.

- Stabilize the catheter hub (unless using newer closed IV catheter systems), and apply pressure distal to the catheter with your fingers. See ❺. **Rationale: This prevents excess blood flow through the catheter.**

- Carefully remove the needle, engage the needle safety device, and attach the end of the infusion tubing to the catheter hub. Place the stylet directly into a sharps container.

- Initiate the infusion or flush the catheter with sterile normal saline. **Rationale: Blood must be removed from the catheter lumen and tubing immediately. Otherwise, the blood will clot inside the lumen.**

- Watch closely for any signs that the catheter is infiltrated. Infiltration occurs when the tip of the IV is outside the vein and the fluid is entering the tissues instead. It is manifested by localized swelling, coolness, pallor, and discomfort at the IV site. **Rationale: Inflammation or infiltration necessitates removal of the IV needle or catheter to avoid further trauma to the tissues.**

Note: If you miss the venipuncture, offer an honest explanation in a matter-of-fact and friendly manner. Think about what you can do to improve the next attempt, and explain what you will do differently (if anything). It is generally recommended to limit your attempts to two; if unsuccessful after two tries, ask another member of the health care team to try again a little later.

16. Dress, stabilize, and label the catheter and tubing, according to agency policy.

- Secure the catheter using a sterile TSM dressing (see ❻) or according to agency policy. Newer catheters have built in stabilizing devices (see ❼) and should be considered the preferred alternative to tape (Infusion

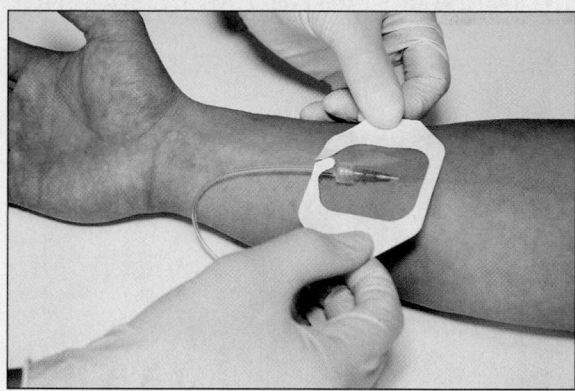

❻ Cover insertion site with transparent dressing.

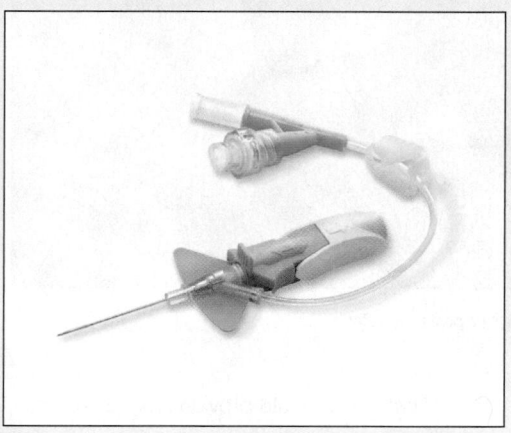

❼ A closed IV catheter system with built in stabilizing device.

Source: BD; Becton, Dickinson and Company. Copyright © 2012 BD. BD Nexia Closed IV Catheter System. Retrieved from *http://www.bd.com/ infusion/products/ivcatheters/nexiva/*. Reprinted with permission.

Nurses Society, 2011, p. S46). **Rationale: Transparent semipermeable membrane dressing secures the cannula while allowing for visual inspection of the insertion site. This type of dressing can be left on for 48 to 72 hours** (RNAO, 2008).

- Label the dressing with the date and time of insertion, type and gauge of needle or catheter used, and your initials (see ❽).

- Apply an IV site protector, if available. See ❾. Protecting devices are available that help prevent dislodgment of

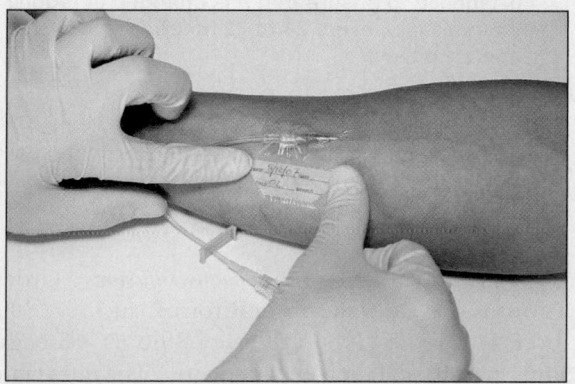

❽ Label IV site with date, time, size of catheter, and initials.

(continued)

SKILL 44.1 STARTING AN INTRAVENOUS INFUSION (*continued*)

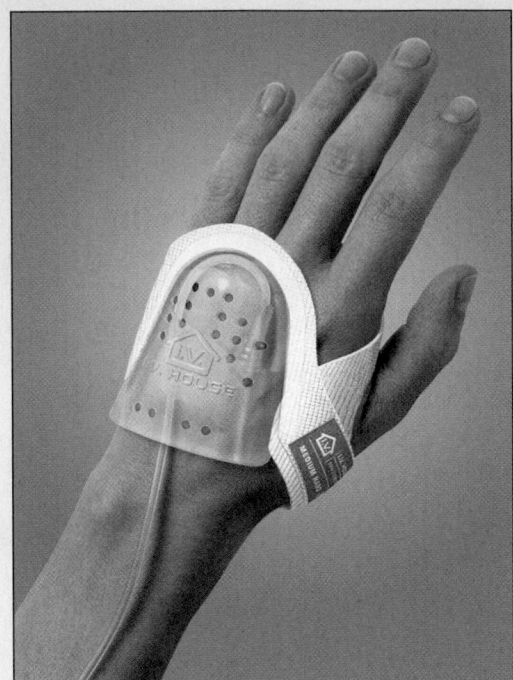

9 IV protective device.

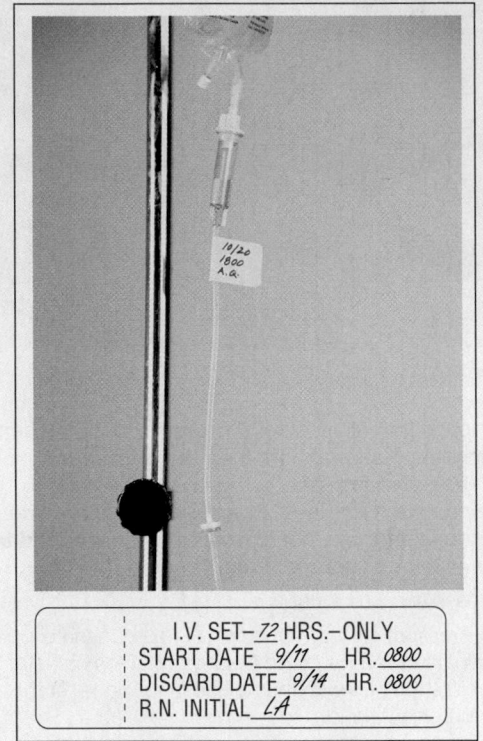

| I.V. SET– *72* HRS.–ONLY |
| START DATE *9/11* HR. *0800* |
| DISCARD DATE *9/14* HR. *0800* |
| R.N. INITIAL *LA* |

10 Tubing labelled with date, time of attachment, and nurse's initials; also shown is a preprinted label.

the IV catheter and still provide easy assessment of the IV site.

- Loop the tubing, and secure it with tape. **Rationale: Looping and securing the tubing prevent the weight of the tubing or any movement from pulling on the needle or catheter**.

- Discard the tourniquet. Remove soiled gloves, and discard appropriately. Perform hand hygiene.

17. Ensure appropriate infusion flow.

- Apply a padded arm board to splint the joint, as needed.

- Adjust the infusion rate of flow according to the prescription.

18. Label the IV tubing.

- Label the tubing with the date and time of attachment and your initials (see **10**). This labelling can also be done when the infusion is started. **Rationale: The tubing is labelled to ensure that it is changed at regular intervals (i.e., every 24 to 72 hours, according to agency policy)**.

19. Document all assessments and interventions.

- Record the start of the infusion on the client's chart. Some agencies provide a special form for this purpose. Include the date and time of the venipuncture; amount

and type of solution used, including any additives (e.g., kind and amount of medications); container number; flow rate; type, length, and gauge of the needle or catheter; venipuncture site; how many attempts were made and location of each attempt; the type of dressing applied; and the client's general response.

EVALUATION

- Regularly assess the client for intended and adverse effects of the infusion.

- At least every 4 hours, assess the skin status at IV site (warm temperature and absence of pain, redness, swelling, and draining), status of the dressing, IV flow rate consistent with prescription, the client's ability to perform self-care activities, and the client's understanding of any mobility limitations.

- Perform follow-up based on findings or outcomes that deviated from what is expected or normal for the client. Relate findings to previous data, if available.

- Report significant deviations from normal to the appropriate member of the health care team.

Regulating and Monitoring Intravenous Infusions Orders for IV infusions can take several forms, such as "3000 mL over 24 hours"; "1000 mL every 8 hours × 3 bags"; "125 mL/h until oral intake is adequate." The nurse initiating the IV calculates the correct flow rate, regulates the infusion, and monitors the client's response. Unless an

infusion control device is used, the nurse manually regulates the drops per minute of flow by using the roller clamp to ensure that the prescribed amount of solution will be infused in the correct span. If the flow is incorrect, such problems as hypervolemia, hypovolemia, electrolyte imbalances, or inadequate medication administration can result. It is recommended that an infusion control device be used whenever possible, particularly with administration of medications.

The number of drops delivered per millilitre of solution varies with different brands and types of infusion sets. This rate, called the **drop factor** or **drip factor**, is printed on the package of the infusion set. Macrodrops commonly have drop factors of 10, 15, or 20 drops/mL; the drop factor for microdrip sets are always 60 drops/mL (see Figure 44.23 on page 1448).

To calculate flow rates, the nurse must know the volume of fluid to be infused and the specific time for the infusion. Two commonly used methods of indicating flow rates are (a) designating the number of millilitres to be administered in 1 hour (mL/h); or (b) designating the number of drops to be given in 1 minute (gtt/min). Because 1 mL of fluid displaces 1 cc (cubic centimetre) of space, the volume to be infused in the first method can also be designated as cubic centimetres per hour (cc/h). *Note:* However, the abbreviation "cc" can be mistaken for other meanings and should not be used; "mL" is the preferred abbreviation.

Occasionally, the IV rate order will read "keep vein open" (KVO). This order does not provide adequate direction for the nurse unless agency policy specifies the millilitres per hour equivalent for this order. Generally, the KVO rate is less than 50 mL per hour. Some IV pumps have a keep open rate choice built in. If the IV is not on this type of pump and no policy exists, contact the primary care provider for clarification.

Millilitres per Hour Hourly rates of infusion can be calculated by dividing the total infusion volume by the total infusion time in hours. For example, if 1000 mL is to be infused in 8 hours, the number of millilitres per hour is as follows:

$$\frac{1000 \text{ mL (total infusion volume)}}{8 \text{ h (total infusion time)}} = 125 \text{ mL/h}$$

Nurses need to check infusions at least every hour to ensure that the indicated millilitres per hour have infused and that IV patency is maintained. A strip of adhesive marking the exact time or amount to be infused can be taped to the solution container. Some agencies make premarked labels available (Figure 44.27).

Drops per Minute The nurse initiating and monitoring an infusion must regulate the drops per minute to ensure that the prescribed amount of solution will infuse. Drops per minute are calculated by the following formula:

$$\text{Drops per minute} = \frac{\text{Total infusion volume} \times \text{Drop factor}}{\text{Total time of infusion in } \textit{minutes}}$$

In our previous example, if the requirements are 1000 mL in 8 hours and the drip factor is 20 drops/mL, the drops per minute should be as follows:

$$\frac{1000 \text{ mL} \times 20 \text{ gtt/mL}}{8 \text{ h} \times 60 \text{ min/h}} = 41.66 \text{ gtt/min}$$

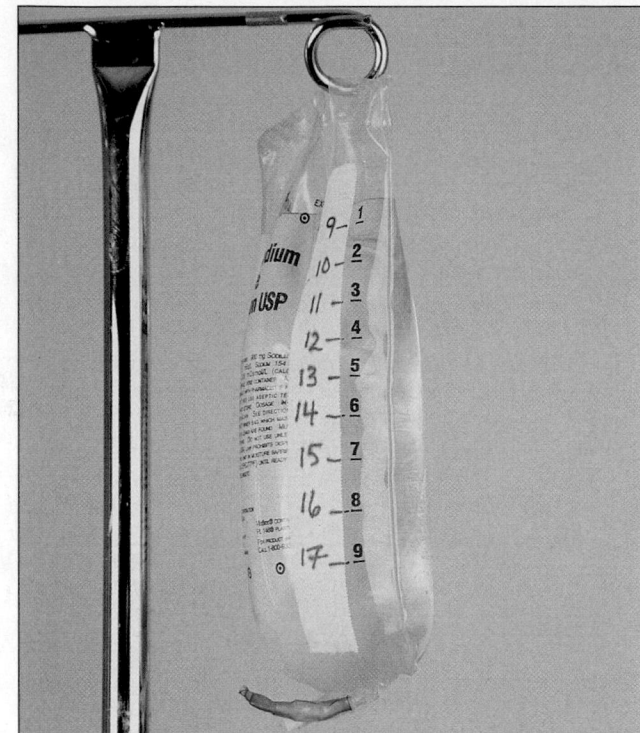

FIGURE 44.27 Timing label on an intravenous container. The first time marked (0900 hours) would be correct for a bag hung at 0800 hours with a rate of 100 mL per hour.

Approximating this rate as 42 drops/min, the nurse regulates the drops per minute by tightening or releasing the IV tubing clamp and counting the drops for 15 seconds, then multiplying that number by 4 (e.g., 10 to 11 drops/15 sec). A number of factors influence flow rate (see Box 44.5 on the next page).

Devices to Control Infusions A number of devices are used to control the rate of an infusion. Electronic infusion devices (EIDs) regulate the infusion rate at preset limits. They also have an alarm that is triggered when the solution in the IV bag is low, when there is air in the tubing, or when flow is impeded by an occlusion. The *Dial-A-Flo* inline device (Figure 44.28 on the next page) is a manual regulator that controls the amount of fluid to be administered. The Dial-A-Flo may be used in situations where a pump is not available or required, but prevention of fluid overload is important. The nurse presets the volume to be infused by rotating the dial to the desired rate. Another variation is a volume-control set, or *Volutrol*, which is used if the volume of fluid administered is to be carefully controlled. The set, which holds a maximum of 100 mL of solution, is attached below the solution container, and the drip chamber is placed below the set. Volume-control sets are frequently used in pediatric settings, where the volume administered is critical.

Devices such as battery-operated controllers and infusion pumps with alarm systems facilitate a regulated flow. Newer systems are programmable and include

BOX 44.5 FACTORS INFLUENCING FLOW RATES

Flow rates can be affected by a number of factors:

- *The position of the forearm.* Sometimes, a change in the position of the client's arm decreases flow. Pronation, supination, extension, or elevation of the forearm on a pillow can increase flow.
- *The position and patency of the tubing.* Tubing can be obstructed by the client's weight, a kink, or a clamp closed too tightly. The flow rate also diminishes when part of the tubing dangles below the puncture site.
- *The height of the infusion bottle.* Elevating the height of the infusion bottle a few centimetres can speed the flow by creating more pressure.
- *Possible infiltration or fluid leakage.* Swelling, a feeling of coldness, and tenderness at the venipuncture site may indicate infiltration.

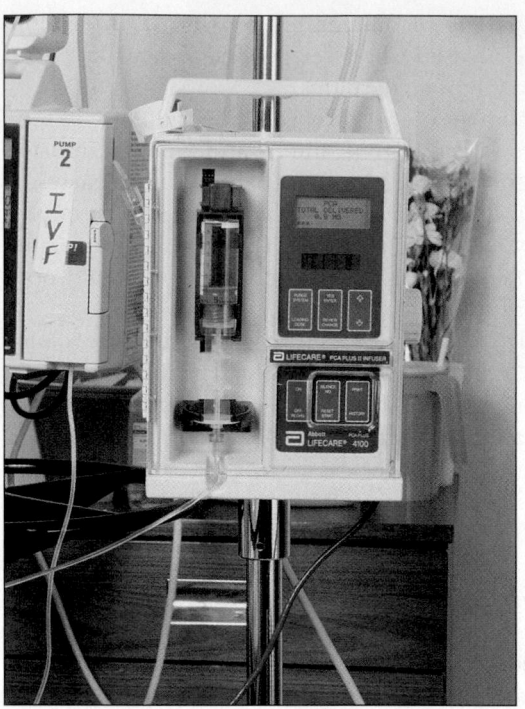

FIGURE 44.29 An intravenous infusion pump.

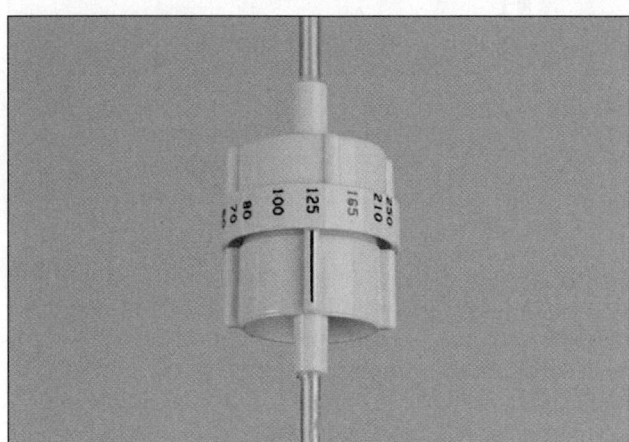

FIGURE 44.28 The Dial-A-Flo inline device.

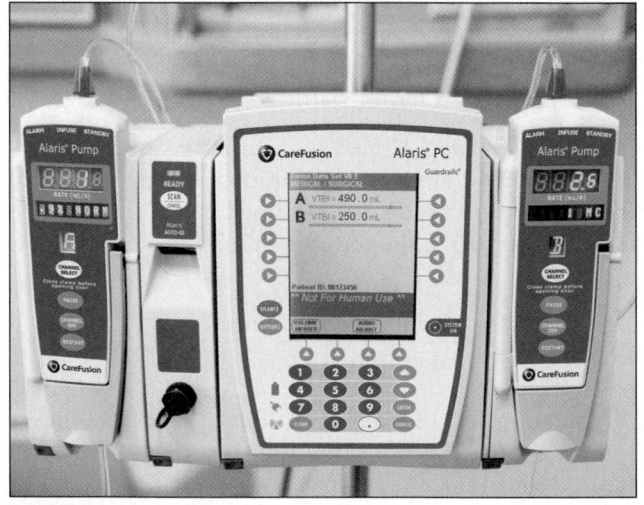

FIGURE 44.30 Programmable infusion pump.

drug libraries with dose rate calculators, automatic flushing between medication, dual or triple simultaneous line control, memory, multiple alarm settings, air inline, pressure/resistance, battery, schedule reminders, volume settings down to 0.1 mL, panel locks, and digital displays. An infusion pump (Figures 44.29 and 44.30) delivers fluids intravenously by exerting positive pressure on the tubing or on the fluid. In situations where the fluid flow is unrestricted, the pump pressure is comparable with that of gravity flow. However, if restrictions develop (increased venous resistance), the pump can maintain the fluid flow by increasing the pressure applied to the fluid.

A volumetric infusion controller, by contrast, operates solely by gravitational force. The delivery pressure depends on the height of the container in relation to the venipuncture site. The container must be at least 76 cm above the venipuncture site for a controller to work. A controller does not have the ability to add pressure to the line and to overcome resistance to fluid flow. See the Clinical Alert box on flow rate control devices.

Skill 44.2 outlines the steps involved in monitoring an intravenous infusion.

⚠ CLINICAL ALERT

A flow rate control device should be used when administering IV fluid to older adult or pediatric clients. Both of these age groups are especially at risk for complications of fluid overload, which can occur with rapid infusion of IV fluids.

SKILL 44.2 MONITORING AN INTRAVENOUS INFUSION

PURPOSES

- To maintain the prescribed flow rate
- To prevent complications associated with IV therapy

ASSESSMENT

Assess

- Appearance of infusion site and the patency of system
- Type of fluid being infused and rate of flow
- Response of the client

IMPLEMENTATION

Preparation

1. Prepare the client.
   - Before performing the procedure, introduce yourself and verify the client's identity using two identifiers or per agency protocol. Explain the procedure to the client.

2. Gather pertinent data.
   - From the physician's order, determine the type and sequence of solutions to be infused, and determine the rate of flow and infusion schedule.

Performance

1. Perform hand hygiene, and follow other appropriate infection prevention and control procedures.

2. Ensure that the correct solution is being infused.
   - If the solution in incorrect, slow the rate of flow to a minimum to maintain the patency of the catheter. (If client is at risk for developing an adverse reaction, infusion must be stopped and the catheter saline-locked.) **Rationale: Stopping the infusion completely will allow a thrombus to form in the IV catheter. If this occurs, the catheter must be removed and another venipuncture performed before the infusion can be resumed.**
   - Change the solution to the correct one. Document and report the error, according to agency protocol.

3. Observe the rate of flow every hour.
   - Compare the rate of flow regularly, for example, at least every hour, against the infusion schedule. **Rationale: Infusions that are off schedule can be harmful to a client.**
   - If the rate is *too fast,* check agency policy. **Rationale: Solution administered too quickly may cause a significant increase in circulating blood volume.**
   - Assess the client for manifestations of hypervolemia and its complications, including dyspnea; rapid, laboured breathing; cough; crackles in the lung bases; tachycardia; and bounding pulses.
   - If the rate is *too slow,* check agency policy. Some agencies permit nursing personnel to adjust a rate of flow by a specified amount. Adjustments above this rate may require a physician's order. **Rationale: Solution that is administered too slowly can supply insufficient fluid, electrolytes, or medication for a client's needs.**
   - If the rate of flow is 150 mL/h or more, check the rate of flow more frequently, for example, every 15 to 30 minutes.

4. Inspect the patency of the IV tubing and catheter.
   - Observe the position of the solution container. If it is less than 1 m above the IV site, readjust it to the correct height (unless the infusion is on a pump). Recheck the rate of flow any time the height of the solution container is changed. **Rationale: If the container is too low, the solution may not flow into the vein because there is insufficient gravitational pressure to overcome the pressure of the blood within the vein.**
   - Observe the drip chamber. If it is less than half full, squeeze the chamber to allow the correct amount of fluid to flow in.
   - Inspect the tubing for pinches or kinks or obstructions to flow. Arrange the tubing so that it is lightly coiled and under no pressure.
   - Observe the position of the tubing. If it is dangling below the venipuncture, coil it carefully on the surface of the bed. **Rationale: The solution cannot flow upward into the vein against the force of gravity.**
   - Determine catheter position, such as by lowering the solution container below the level of the infusion site, and observe for a return flow of blood from the vein. **Rationale: A return flow of blood indicates that the needle is patent and in the vein. Absence of blood return may indicate that the catheter is no longer in the vein or that the tip of the catheter is partially obstructed by a thrombus, the vein wall, or a valve in the vein.** *Note:* With some catheters, no blood may appear even with patency because the soft catheter walls collapse during siphoning.
   - If leakage occurs, locate the source. If the leak is at the catheter connection, tighten the tubing into the catheter. If the leak cannot be stopped, slow the infusion as much as possible without stopping it, and replace the tubing with a new sterile set. Estimate the amount of solution lost.

5. Inspect the insertion site for fluid infiltration at least every hour.
   - When an IV catheter becomes dislodged from the vein, fluid flows into interstitial tissues, causing swelling. This is known as *infiltration* and is manifested by localized swelling, coolness, pallor, and discomfort at the IV site.
   - If an infiltration is present, stop the infusion and remove the catheter. Restart the infusion at another site.
   - Apply a warm compress to the site of the infiltration. **Rationale: Warmth promotes comfort and vasodilation, facilitating absorption of the fluid from interstitial tissues.**

6. If the infiltration involves a *vesicant drug* (a drug that can cause tissue necrosis), it is called *extravasation,* and other measures may be indicated. Extravasated vesicant drugs can cause severe tissue injury or destruction. The extravasation of a vesicant drug should be considered an emergency (Hadaway, 2009).
   - Stop the infusion immediately. Disconnect the tubing as close to the catheter hub as possible, and attempt to aspirate any drug remaining in the hub. If an injectable antidote is available, the catheter should remain in place.
   - The appropriate member of the health care team should be notified and, if ordered, the antidote administered.

(continued)

SKILL 44.2 MONITORING AN INTRAVENOUS INFUSION (*continued*)

- The affected arm should be elevated and, depending on the drug, heat or cold therapy should be implemented.

7. Inspect the insertion site for phlebitis (inflammation of a vein).

- Inspect and palpate the site at least every 8 hours. Phlebitis can occur as a result of injury to a vein, for example, because of mechanical trauma or chemical irritation. Chemical injury to a vein can occur from IV (especially potassium and magnesium) and some medications.

    The signs and symptoms of phlebitis include pain, tenderness, erythema (redness), warmth, swelling at the intravenous site, and/or palpable venous cord (Infusion Nurses Society, 2011).

- If phlebitis is detected, discontinue the infusion, and apply warm compresses to the venipuncture site as ordered and according to agency policy. Do not use this injured vein for further infusions.

8. Inspect the intravenous site for bleeding.

- Oozing or bleeding into the surrounding tissues can occur while the infusion is freely flowing but is more likely to occur after the catheter has been removed from the vein.

- Observation of the venipuncture site is extremely important for clients who bleed readily, such as those receiving anticoagulants.

9. Provide instructions, such as the following, to the client to maintain the infusion system:

- Avoid sudden twisting or turning movements of the arm with the catheter.

- Avoid stretching or placing tension on the tubing.

- Try to keep the tubing from dangling below the level of the catheter.

- Notify a nurse, if any of the following occurs:
    - **a.** The flow rate suddenly changes or the solution stops dripping.
    - **b.** The solution container is nearly empty.
    - **c.** There is blood in the IV tubing.
    - **d.** Discomfort or swelling is experienced at the IV site.

10. Document all relevant information.

EVALUATION

Evaluate the following:

- Amount of fluid infused according to the schedule
- Intactness of IV system
- Appearance of IV site (e.g., dry, tissue infiltration, discomfort)
- Urinary output compared with intake
- Tissue turgor; specific gravity of urine
- Vital signs and lung sounds compared with baseline data

Changing Intravenous Containers, Tubing, and Dressings for Peripheral Intravenous Sites IV solution containers are changed when only a small amount of fluid remains in the neck of the container and fluid still remains in the drip chamber. However, all IV bags should be changed every 24 hours, regardless of how much solution remains, to minimize the risk of contamination. Change primary administration sets and secondary tubing that remains continuously attached to them every 72 hours. Change intermittent infusion sets without a primary infusion every 24 hours or whenever their sterility is in question (Gillies, O'Riordan, Wallen, Morrison, Rankin, & Nagy, 2005). Add-on devices (e.g., extension sets, filters, stopcocks) should be changed at the same time the administration set is changed. Agency policy and manufacturer's recommendations must also be considered in the decision-making process. Skill 44.3 provides guidelines for changing an IV solution container, tubing, and the IV site dressing.

SKILL 44.3 CHANGING AN INTRAVENOUS CONTAINER, TUBING, AND DRESSING

PURPOSES

- To maintain the flow of required fluids
- To maintain sterility of the IV system and decrease the incidence of phlebitis and infection
- To maintain patency of the IV tubing
- To prevent infection at the IV site and the introduction of microorganisms into the bloodstream

ASSESSMENT

Assess

- Presence of fluid infiltration, bleeding, or phlebitis at IV site
- Allergy to tape or iodine

- Infusion rate and amount absorbed
- Blockages in IV system
- Appearance of the dressing for integrity, moisture, and need for change
- The date and time of the previous dressing change

PLANNING

Review the physician's orders for changes in fluid administration.

Equipment

- Container with the correct kind and amount of sterile solution, according to physician's orders
- Administration set, including sterile tubing and drip chamber

- Timing label
- Receptacle (e.g., a basin) for discarded fluid

For the Dressing

- Clean gloves
- Sterile gauze or transparent dressing
- Adhesive remover
- Antiseptic swab (preferably 2% chlorhexidine gluconate)
- Catheter stabilization device
- Tape
- Towel

IMPLEMENTATION

Preparation

1. Prepare the client.
   - Before performing the procedure, introduce yourself and verify the client's identity using two identifiers or per agency protocol. Explain the procedure to the client.
2. Obtain the correct solution container.
   - Read the label of the new container.
   - Verify that you have the correct solution, correct client, correct additives (if any), and correct dose (number of bags or total volume ordered).
   - Check clarity of solution and expiry date.

Performance

1. Perform hand hygiene, and follow other appropriate infection prevention and control procedures.
2. Set up the intravenous equipment with the new container, and label them.
   - See Skill 44.1, steps 2 to 9, on page 1450.
   - Apply a timing label to the container.
   - Prime the tubing.
   - Label the tubing as described in Skill 44.1.
3. Prepare the dressing equipment near the client.
   - Open all equipment: solution or swabs, dressing and adhesive bandage. **Rationale: Doing this facilitates access to supplies.**
   - Place a towel under the extremity. **Rationale: The towel prevents soiling of bed linens.**
   - Apply clean gloves.
4. Remove the soiled dressing and stabilization device.
   - Remove the old dressing carefully. **Rationale: Taking this precaution prevents dislodgement of the catheter or needle in case tubing becomes entangled between layers of dressing.**
   - Discard the used dressing materials in the appropriate container.
5. Assess the IV site.
   - Inspect the IV site for the presence of infiltration or inflammation. **Rationale: Inflammation or infiltration necessitates removal of the IV needle or catheter to avoid further trauma to the tissues.**

- Go to step 6, or discontinue and relocate the IV site, if indicated. See Skills 44.1 and 44.4.
6. Disconnect the used tubing or remove the cap on an intermittent device.
   - Apply clean gloves. Place a sterile swab under the hub of the catheter. **Rationale: The swab absorbs any leakage that might occur when the tubing is disconnected.**
   - Clamp the tubing. With the fourth or fifth finger of the nondominant hand, apply pressure to the vein above the end of the catheter. **Rationale: The pressure helps prevent blood from coming out of the needle during the change of tubing.**
   - Holding the hub of the catheter with the thumb and index finger of the nondominant hand, loosen the tubing with the dominant hand, using a twisting, pulling motion. **Rationale: Holding the catheter firmly but gently maintains its position in the vein.**
   - Remove the used IV tubing.
   - Place the end of the tubing in the basin or other receptacle.
7. Connect the new tubing, and re-establish the infusion.
   - Continue to hold the catheter, and grasp the new tubing with the dominant hand.
   - Remove the protective tubing cap, maintaining sterility, and insert the tubing end securely into the needle hub. Twist it to secure it.
   - Open the clamp to start the solution flowing.
8. Clean the IV site.
   - Using chlorhexidine, or solution recommended by agency policy, clean the site, beginning at the catheter and cleaning outward in a 5-cm diameter. **Rationale: Cleaning in this manner prevents contamination of the IV site from bacteria on peripheral skin areas. Antiseptics reduce the number of microorganisms present at the site, thus reducing the risk of infection.**
9. Resecure the catheter. See Skill 44.1.
   - Remove gloves. Perform hand hygiene.
10. Label the dressing, and secure the IV tubing.
    - Place the date and time of the dressing change and your initials either on the label provided or directly over the top of the dressing but where it will not obstruct the assessment of the venipuncture site.
    - Secure IV tubing with additional tape, as required.
11. Regulate the rate of flow of the solution according to the order on the chart.
12. Document all relevant information.
    - Record the change of the solution container, tubing, and dressing in the appropriate place on the client's chart. Also record the fluid intake, according to agency practice. Also record your assessments.

EVALUATION

Evaluate the following:

- Status of IV site
- Patency of IV system
- Accuracy of flow

When an IV infusion is no longer necessary to maintain the client's fluid intake or to provide a route for medication administration, the infusion is either discontinued and the catheter removed, or the catheter is left in place and converted to a saline lock. Guidelines for discontinuing an IV infusion or converting the catheter to a lock are outlined in Skills 44.4 and 44.5, respectively.

CHANGING PERIPHERAL INTRAVENOUS SITES The Centers for Disease Control and Prevention (CDC, 2011) guidelines established 3 days (72 hours) as the maximum time for a catheter to dwell in the same peripheral vein. When a vein is prone to phlebitis, the length of dwell should be even shorter (e.g., 48 to 72 hours). Clinical assessment of the site is ongoing and the intravenous site should be changed earlier than

---

SKILL 44.4   DISCONTINUING A PERIPHERAL INTRAVENOUS INFUSION

PURPOSE

- To discontinue an IV infusion when the therapy is complete or when the IV site needs to be changed

ASSESSMENT

Assess

- Appearance of the venipuncture site
- Any bleeding from the infusion site
- Amount of fluid infused
- Appearance of IV catheter

Equipment

- Clean gloves
- Small sterile dressing and tape
- Linen-saver pad

Planning

Review the physician's orders, and check agency policy.

IMPLEMENTATION

Preparation

- Before performing the procedure, introduce yourself and verify the client's identity using two identifiers or per agency policy. Explain to the client what you are going to do, why it is necessary, and how he or she can participate. Explain the reason for discontinuing the IV and that the procedure should cause no discomfort, other than that associated with removing the tape.

Performance

1. Perform hand hygiene, and follow other appropriate infection prevention and control procedures.

2. Assist the client into a comfortable position, either sitting or lying. Expose the IV site, but provide for client privacy. Place a linen-saver pad under the extremity that has the IV.

3. Prepare the equipment.
   - Clamp the infusion tubing. **Rationale: Clamping the tubing prevents the fluid from flowing out of the needle onto the client or bed.**
   - Put on clean gloves.

- Remove the dressing, stabilization device, and tape at the venipuncture site while holding the catheter firmly and applying countertraction to the skin. **Rationale: Movement of the catheter can injure the vein and cause discomfort to the client. Countertraction prevents pulling the skin and causing discomfort.**

- Apply the sterile gauze above the venipuncture site. Only touch the upper portion of the gauze pad and maintain sterility of the lower portion that is in contact with the venipuncture site.

4. Withdraw the catheter from the vein.
   - Withdraw the catheter by pulling it out along the line of the vein. **Rationale: Pulling it out in line with the vein avoids injury to the vein.**
   - Immediately apply firm pressure to the site by using the sterile gauze for 2 to 3 minutes. **Rationale: Pressure helps stop the bleeding and prevents hematoma formation.**
   - Hold the client's arm above the body if any bleeding persists. **Rationale: Raising the limb decreases blood flow to the area.**
   - Teach the client to inform the nurse if the site begins to bleed at any time or the client notes any abnormalities in the area.

5. Examine the catheter removed from the client
   - Examine the catheter to make sure it is intact. **Rationale: If a piece of tubing remains in the client's vein, it could move centrally (toward the heart or lungs).**
   - Report a broken catheter to the nurse in charge or physician immediately.
   - If the broken piece can be palpated, apply a tourniquet above the insertion site. Application of a tourniquet decreases the possibility of the piece moving until a physician is notified.

6. Cover the venipuncture site.
   - Apply a new sterile dressing. **Rationale: The dressing continues the pressure and covers the open area in the skin, preventing infection.**
   - Discard used supplies appropriately.
   - Remove and discard gloves. Perform hand hygiene.

7. Note the amount of solution remaining in the IV solution container prior to discarding the IV solution.

8. Document all relevant information.
   - Record the amount of fluid infused on the intake and output record and in the chart, according to agency practice. Include the container number, type of solution used, time of discontinuing the infusion, and the client's response.

EVALUATION

Perform follow-up based on findings or outcomes that deviated from expected or normal for the client. Relate findings to previous data, if available. Report significant deviations from normal to the appropriate member of the health care team.

SKILL 44.5 CHANGING A PERIPHERAL INTRAVENOUS CATHETER TO AN INTERMITTENT INFUSION LOCK

PURPOSE

- To permit IV administration of medications or fluids on an intermittent basis

ASSESSMENT

Assess

- Patency of the IV catheter
- Appearance of the site (evidence of inflammation or infiltration)

PLANNING

Review the physician's order.

- A specific order may be written to convert an IV access to a saline lock. The order also may be implied, for example, IV fluids are to be discontinued but the client has orders for an IV antibiotic every 6 hours or is receiving analgesics intravenously.
- From the physician's order, determine the type and sequence of intermittent infusion.

Equipment

- Intermittent infusion cap or device
- Clean gloves
- Sterile 2 × 2 or 4 × 4 gauze
- Sterile saline for injection (without preservative) using a 3-mL syringe with a 25-gauge needle, or a needleless infusion device
- Isopropyl alcohol wipe
- Tape
- Clean emesis basin

IMPLEMENTATION

Preparation

- Before performing the procedure, introduce yourself and verify the client's identity using two identifiers or per agency policy. Explain to the client what you are going to do, why it is necessary, and how he or she can participate. Explain the reason for the intermittent device and that changing an IV

to a saline lock should cause no discomfort other than that associated with removing tape from the IV tubing.

- Obtain the needed equipment, and take it to the client's bedside.

Performance

1. Perform hand hygiene, and follow other appropriate infection prevention and control procedures.

2. Assist the client to a comfortable position, either sitting or lying. Expose the IV site, but provide for client privacy.

3. Assess the IV site and determine the patency of the catheter (see Skill 44.2, page 1457). If the catheter is not fully patent or there is evidence of phlebitis or infiltration, discontinue the catheter and establish a new IV site.

   - Expose the IV catheter hub, and loosen any tape that is holding the IV tubing in place, or it will interfere with insertion of the intermittent infusion plug into the catheter.

   - Clamp the IV tubing to stop the flow of IV fluid.

   - Open the gauze pad, and place it under the IV catheter hub. **Rationale: This absorbs any leakage that might occur when the tubing is disconnected.**

   - Open the alcohol wipe and intermittent infusion plug, leaving the plug in its sterile package.

4. Remove the IV tubing and insert the intermittent infusion plug into the IV catheter.

   - Put on clean gloves.

   - Stabilize the IV catheter with your nondominant hand, and use the little finger to place slight pressure on the vein *above* the end of the catheter. Twist the IV tubing adapter to loosen it from the IV catheter and remove it, placing the end of the tubing in a clean emesis basin. See ❶.

   - Pick up the intermittent infusion plug from its package, and remove the protective sleeve from the male adapter (blue in Figure 44.25), maintaining its sterility. Insert the plug into the IV catheter, twisting it to seat it firmly, or engage the Luer lock.

5. Instill saline per agency policy. **Rationale: Saline is used to maintain patency of the IV catheter when fluids are not infusing through the catheter. The intermittent lock will need to be flushed with a prescribed**

(continued)

| SKILL 44.5 | CHANGING A PERIPHERAL INTRAVENOUS CATHETER TO AN INTERMITTENT INFUSION LOCK (*continued*) |

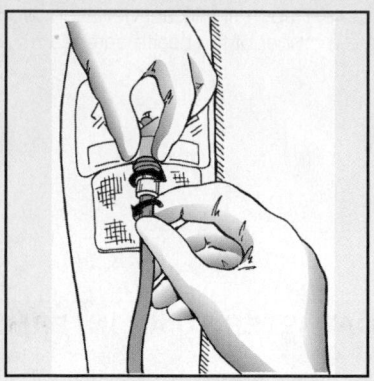

❶ Separating the IV catheter from the infusion tubing.

Source: Berman, Audrey J.; Snyder, Shirlee, *Skills in Clinical Nursing*, 7th Ed., © 2012. Reprinted and Electronically reproduced by permission of Pearson Education, Inc., Upper Saddle River, New Jersey.

solution after each use or every 8 to 12 hours if not in use, or according to agency policy.

6. Cover the site with a transparent dressing. **Rationale: The transparent dressing provides protection from infection, allows for ease of assessment of**

venipuncture site, and also promotes comfort, preventing the plug from catching on clothing or bedding.

7. Remove and discard gloves. Perform hand hygiene.
8. Teach the client how to maintain the lock.
   - Notify the appropriate member of the health care team if the plug or catheter comes out, if the site becomes red, inflamed, or painful, or if any drainage or bleeding occurs at the site.
9. Document all relevant information.
   - Record the dates and time when the infusion device was converted, the status of the IV insertion site, and any adverse responses of the client.

EVALUATION

Perform follow-up based on findings or outcomes that deviated from expected or normal for the client. Relate findings to previous data, if available. Evaluate the patency of the catheter, the appearance of the site, and the ease of flushing. Report significant deviations from normal to the appropriate member of the health care team.

these guidelines in cases of infiltration, signs of infection, or severe discomfort.

BLOOD TRANSFUSIONS IV fluids can be effective in restoring intravascular (blood) volume; however, they do not affect the O_2-carrying capacity of blood. When red and white blood cells, platelets, or blood proteins are lost because of hemorrhage or disease, it may be necessary to replace these components to restore blood's ability to transport O_2 and CO_2, to clot, to fight infection, and to keep ECF within the intravascular compartment. A blood transfusion is the introduction of whole blood or blood components into the venous circulation.

Blood Groups Human blood is commonly classified into four main groups (A, B, AB, and O). The surface of an individual's RBCs contains a number of proteins known as **antigens** (substances capable of inducing the formation of antibodies) that are unique for each person. Many blood antigens have been identified, but the A, B, and Rh antigens are the most important in determining blood group or type. Because antigens promote *agglutination* or clumping of blood cells, they are also known as **agglutinogens**. The A antigen or agglutinogen is present on the RBCs of people with blood group A, the B antigen is present in people with blood group B, and both A and B antigens are found on the RBC surface in people with group AB blood. Neither antigen is present on the RBCs of people with group O blood.

Preformed **antibodies** to RBC antigens are present in the plasma; these antibodies are often called **agglutinins**. People with blood group A have B antibodies (agglutinins); A antibodies are present in people with blood group B; and people with blood group O have antibodies to both A and B antigens. People with group AB blood do not have antibodies to either A or B antigens. When blood is transfused, the blood group of the donor and recipient must match to avoid an antigen–antibody reaction and hemolysis (destruction) of RBCs.

Rhesus (Rh) Factor The Rh factor antigen is present on the RBCs of approximately 85% of people. Blood that contains the Rh factor is known as *Rh-positive* (Rh^+); blood that does not contain the Rh factor is known as *Rh negative* (Rh^-). In contrast to the ABO blood groups, Rh^- blood does not naturally contain Rh antibodies. However, after exposure to blood containing Rh factor (e.g., an Rh^- mother carrying a fetus with Rh^+ blood, or transfusion of Rh^+ blood into a client who is Rh^-), Rh antibodies develop. Subsequent exposure to Rh^+ blood places the client at risk for an antigen–antibody reaction and hemolysis of RBCs.

Blood Typing and Cross-matching To avoid transfusing incompatible RBCs, both blood donor and recipient are typed, and their blood is cross-matched. Blood typing is done to determine the ABO blood group and Rh factor status. This test is also performed on pregnant women and neonates to assess for possible intrauterine exposure

TABLE 44.12 ABO Compatibility and Rh Compatibility of RBC

Recipient	Donor
ABO Compatibility of RBC	
A	A, O
B	B, O
AB	AB, A, B, O
O	O
Rh Compatibility of RBC	
Rh-positive	Rh-positive or Rh-negative
Rh-negative	Rh-negative

Source: Based on Canadian Blood Services. (2007). *Clinical guide to transfusion* (p. 79). Retrieved from http://www.transfusionmedicine.ca/resources/clinical-guide-transfusion

TABLE 44.13 Blood Products for Transfusion

Product	Use
Whole blood	Not commonly used except for extreme cases of acute hemorrhage. Replaces blood volume and all blood products: RBCs, plasma, plasma proteins, platelets, and other clotting factors.
Packed red blood cells (PRBCs)	Used to increase the oxygen-carrying capacity of blood in anemias, surgery, disorders with slow bleeding. One unit of PRBCs has the same amount of oxygen-carrying RBCs as a unit of whole blood.
Autologous red blood cells	Used for blood replacement following planned elective surgery. Clients donate their own blood 4 to 5 weeks before surgery for autologous transfusion.
Platelets	Replaces platelets in clients with bleeding disorders or platelet deficiency. Fresh platelets are most effective.
Fresh frozen plasma	Expands blood volume and provides clotting factors. Does not need to be cross-matched (contains no RBCs). ABO compatibility must be confirmed.
Albumin and plasma protein fraction	Blood volume expander. Provides plasma proteins.
Clotting factors and cryoprecipitate	Used for clients with clotting factor deficiencies. Each provides different factors involved in the clotting pathway. Cryoprecipitate also contains fibrinogen.

of the mother or baby to an incompatible blood type (particularly Rh factor incompatibilities).

Because blood typing only determines the presence of the major ABO and Rh antigens, cross-matching is also necessary prior to transfusion to identify possible interactions of minor antigens with their corresponding antibodies. RBCs from the donor blood are mixed with serum from the recipient; a reagent (Coombs' serum) is added, and the mixture is examined for visible agglutination. If the recipient's serum does not contain antibodies to the donor's RBCs, agglutination does not occur, and the risk of a transfusion reaction is small.

Table 44.12 provides a summary of what types of donated blood a recipient can receive based on their ABO and Rh designations.

Selection of Blood Donors Screening of blood donors is rigorous. Criteria have been established to protect the donor from possible ill effects of donation and to protect the recipient from exposure to diseases transmitted through blood. Blood donors are unpaid volunteers. Potential donors are eliminated by a history of hepatitis, HIV infection (or risk factors for HIV infection), heart disease, most cancers, severe asthma, bleeding disorders, or exposure to malaria. Donation may be deferred for people in situations of pregnancy, surgery, anemia, or high or low blood pressure, and if the donor is taking certain drugs.

Blood and Blood Products for Transfusion Not all clients require transfusion of whole blood; many times, transfusion of a particular blood component is more appropriate. Table 44.13 lists some of the common blood products that can be transfused.

Transfusion Adverse Reactions Transfusion of ABO or Rh incompatible blood can result in a **hemolytic transfusion reaction**, which causes destruction of the transfused RBCs

and subsequent risk of kidney damage or failure. To avoid hemolytic transfusion reaction, blood from the donor and the recipient is tested for compatibility. This is referred to as "*type and cross-match.*" Other forms of transfusion adverse reactions may also occur, including febrile or allergic reactions, circulatory overload, and sepsis. Because the risk of an adverse reaction is high when blood is transfused, clients must be frequently and carefully assessed before and during transfusion. Many reactions become evident within 5 to 15 minutes of initiating the transfusion, but reactions can develop any time during a transfusion; for this reason, clients are most closely monitored during the initial period of the transfusion. Stop the transfusion immediately if signs of a reaction develop. Some of the possible transfusion adverse reactions, their clinical signs, and nursing implications are listed in Table 44.14.

Administering Blood Special precautions are necessary when administering blood. When a transfusion is ordered, obtain blood from the blood bank just before starting the transfusion. Do not store blood in the refrigerator on the nursing unit; lack of temperature control can damage blood. Once blood or a blood product is removed from the refrigerator, it must be administered within a limited amount of time (e.g., packed RBCs should not be left hanging for more than 4 hours after being removed from the blood bank refrigerator). Agencies following

TABLE 44.14 Transfusion Adverse Reactions

Reaction: Cause	Clinical Signs	Nursing Interventions*
Hemolytic reaction: ABO-incompatibility (such as can result from improper labelling, testing errors, or error in patient identification)	Chills, fever, hemoglobinuria (dark coloured urine) nausea/vomiting, dyspnea, chest pain, hypotension	1. Discontinue the transfusion immediately. *Note:* When the transfusion is discontinued, the blood tubing must be removed as well. Use new tubing for the normal saline infusion. 2. Maintain vascular access with normal saline, or according to agency protocol. 3. Notify the physician immediately. 4. Monitor vital signs. 5. Monitor fluid intake and output. 6. Send the remaining blood, bag, filter, tubing, a sample of the client's blood, and a urine sample to the hospital transfusion service (blood bank).
Febrile non-hemolytic reaction: sensitivity of the client's blood to cytokines in the plasma of the transfused blood component	Fever during or up to several hours after transfusion; chills, rigors, nausea, vomiting, hypotension	1. Discontinue the transfusion immediately. *Note:* When the transfusion is discontinued, the blood tubing must be removed as well. Use **new** tubing for the normal saline infusion. 2. Notify the appropriate member of the health care team immediately. 3. Keep the vein open with normal saline solution. 4. Give antipyretics, as ordered; meperidine may be used for severe rigors, as prescribed.
Allergic reaction (mild): sensitivity to infused plasma proteins	Flushing, urticaria with or without itching	1. Stop or slow the transfusion, depending on agency protocol. 2. Notify the appropriate member of the health care team. 3. Administer medication (antihistamines, steroids), as ordered.
Allergic reaction (severe): antibody–antigen reaction; transfusing an allergen (e.g., penicillin) consumed by the donor to a sensitized patient	Hypotension, dyspnea/cough, tachycardia, facial edema, laryngeal edema (stridor), shock (circulatory collapse)	1. Stop the transfusion immediately. *Note:* When the transfusion is discontinued, the blood tubing must be removed as well. Use **new** tubing for the normal saline infusion. 2. Keep the vein open with normal saline solution. 3. Notify the appropriate member of the health care team immediately. 4. Monitor vital signs. 5. Administer medications (e.g., antihistamines, epinephrine) and oxygen, as ordered. 6. Provide supportive care; administer cardiopulmonary resuscitation (CPR), if needed.
Circulatory overload: impaired cardiac function and/or blood administered faster than the circulatory system can accommodate	Dyspnea, orthopnea, cyanosis, tachycardia, hypertension	1. Interrupt the transfusion. 2. Place the client upright with feet dependent. 3. Notify the appropriate member of the health care team immediately. 4. Administer diuretics and oxygen, as ordered.

*Nurses should follow agency protocol regarding interventions. This may vary among agencies.

Canadian Blood Services (CBS, 2007, p. 79) recommendations will require the following:

- Verifying ABO and Rh compatibility of the product and recipient (see Table 44.12 on page 1463)

- Verifying that the unique patient identifiers on the product match those of the intended recipient

- Verifying that the unique product identifiers on the product label match those on the accompanying transfusion service form/tag.

Most agencies require an independent double-check of the above completed by two registered nurses. See the Clinical Alert box on administering normal saline during blood transfusions.

Blood is preferably administered through a #19-gauge or larger IV catheter (CBS, 2007); a smaller gauge may be necessary for small children or clients with small, fragile veins. An unvented Y-type blood transfusion set with an inline or add-on filter is used when administering blood to remove debris in the form of blood clots and aggregates of cells (CBS, 2007) (Figure 44.31). One arm of the administration set connects to the blood, and normal saline (0.9% NaCl) is attached to the other arm of the Y-type set. Saline is used to completely wet the filter

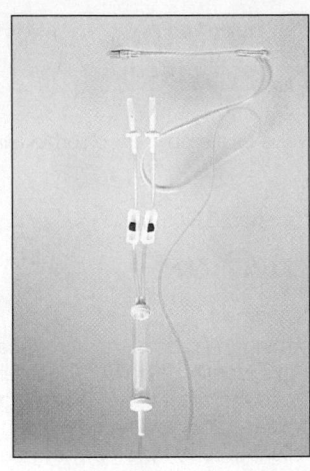

FIGURE 44.31 Y-type blood transfusion tubing.

Source: Berman, Audrey J.; Snyder, Shirlee, *Skills in Clinical Nursing*, 7th Ed., © 2012. Reprinted and Electronically reproduced by permission of Pearson Education, Inc., Upper Saddle River, New Jersey.

and prime the set before administering blood. No other IV solution or medication should be added to the blood bag or tubing (CBS, 2007). One unit of RBCs usually takes 1.5 to 2 hours to infuse; the transfusion should be completed within 4 hours of initiation. The risk of sepsis increases if blood is left hanging for a longer period. The CBS (2007) indicates that "various standards indicate that blood administration sets should be changed within four hours, eight hours, or up to 24 hours following initiation of the transfusion. Four to eight hours is a reasonable time frame with up to four units being transfused in this interval prior to filter change" (p. 74).

For the correct steps for initiating, maintaining, and terminating a blood transfusion, see Skill 44.6.

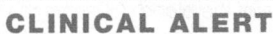

CLINICAL ALERT

Normal saline should always be used when giving a blood transfusion. Solutions other than saline can cause damage to the blood components.

SKILL 44.6 INITIATING, MAINTAINING, AND TERMINATING A BLOOD TRANSFUSION

PURPOSES

- To restore blood volume after hemorrhage
- To restore the O_2-carrying capacity of the blood
- To provide plasma factors, such as antihemophilic factor (AHF) or factor VIII, or platelet concentrates to prevent or treat bleeding

ASSESSMENT

Assess for clinical signs of transfusion adverse reaction (see Table 44.14); manifestations of hypovolemia or hypervolemia; status of infusion site; vital signs; blood test results, such as hemoglobin values or platelet count; or any unusual symptoms.

PLANNING

- Review the client's record regarding previous transfusion. Note any complications and how they were managed (allergies or previous transfusion adverse reactions).
- Check the physician's order for the number and type of units and the desired speed of infusion.

- Confirm client consent, and obtain baseline data before transfusion.
- Assess blood pressure, pulse, respiratory rate and depth, and temperature.
- Note specific signs related to the client's pathology and the reason for the transfusion. For example, for a client with anemia, note the hemoglobin and hematocrit levels.
- Note any premedication ordered (e.g., acetaminophen or diphenhydramine). Schedule their administration (usually 30 minutes prior to transfusion).

Equipment

- Blood product
- Blood administration set
- IV pump, if needed
- 250 mL normal saline for infusion
- IV pole
- Venipuncture set containing a 19-gauge or larger-gauge needle or catheter (if one is not already in place) or, if blood is to be administered quickly, a larger catheter (e.g., 14 gauge), per agency policy

(continued)

SKILL 44.6   **INITIATING, MAINTAINING, AND TERMINATING A BLOOD TRANSFUSION** (*continued*)

- Antiseptic swabs (preferably 2% chlorhexidine gluconate)
- Tape
- Clean gloves

IMPLEMENTATION

Preparation

1. Before performing the procedure, introduce yourself and verify the client's identity using two identifiers or per agency policy. Explain to the client what you are going to do, why it is necessary, and how he or she can participate. Instruct the client to report promptly any sudden chills, nausea, itching, rash, dyspnea, back pain, or other unusual symptoms.

2. Provide for client privacy, and prepare the client.
   - Assist the client into a comfortable position, either the sitting or lying position. Provide for client privacy, and expose only the IV site.
   - If the client has an intravenous solution infusing, check whether the catheter and solution are appropriate to administer blood. The preferred catheter is a 19 gauge or larger, and the solution must be normal saline. Dextrose (which causes lysis of RBCs), Ringer's solution, medications and other additives, and hyperalimentation solutions are incompatible. See step 5 below if the infusing solution is not compatible.
   - If the client does not have an IV solution infusing, check agency policy. In some agencies, an infusion must be running before the blood is obtained from the blood bank. In this case, you will need to perform a venipuncture on a suitable vein (see Skill 44.1 on page 1450) and start an IV infusion of normal saline.

Performance

1. Perform hand hygiene, and follow other appropriate infection prevention and control procedures.

2. Prepare the infusion equipment.
   - Ensure that the blood filter inside the drip chamber is suitable for the blood product to be transfused. Attach the blood tubing to the blood filter, if necessary. **Rationale: Blood filters have a surface area large enough to allow the blood components through easily but are designed to trap clots and cellular debris.**
   - Put on gloves.
   - Close all the clamps on the Y-set: the main flow rate clamp and both Y-line clamps.
   - Hang the container on the IV pole about 1 m above the planned venipuncture site.
   - Insert the spike into the 0.9% saline solution.
   - Hang the container on the IV pole about 1 m above the venipuncture site.

3. Prime the tubing.
   - Open the upper clamp on the normal saline tubing, and squeeze the drip chamber until it covers the filter and one-third of the drip chamber above the filter.
   - Tap the filter chamber to expel any residual air in the filter.
   - Open the main flow rate clamp, and prime the tubing with saline.
   - Close both clamps.

4. Start the saline solution.
   - If an IV solution incompatible with blood is infusing, stop the infusion and discard the solution and tubing, according to agency policy.
   - Attach the blood tubing primed with normal saline to the IV catheter.
   - Open the saline and main flow rate clamps, and adjust the flow rate. Use only the main flow rate clamp to adjust the rate.
   - Allow a small amount of solution to infuse to make sure there are no problems with the flow or with the venipuncture site. **Rationale: Infusing normal saline before initiating the transfusion also clears the IV catheter of incompatible solutions or medications.**

5. Obtain the correct blood component for the client.
   - Check the physician's order with the requisition.
   - Check the requisition form and the blood bag label with a laboratory technician or according to agency policy. Specifically, check the client's name, unit identification number, blood type (A, B, AB, or O) and Rh group (see Table 44.12 on page 1463), the blood donor number, and the expiry date of the blood. Observe the blood for abnormal colour, RBC clumping, gas bubbles, and extraneous material. Return outdated or abnormal blood to the blood bank.
   - With another nurse (most agencies require an RN), compare the laboratory blood record (or according to agency policy) for the following:
     - *Order:* Check the blood or component against the physician's written order.
     - *Client identification:* The name and identification number on the client's identification band must be *identical* to the name and number attached to the unit of blood.
     - *Unit identification:* The unit identification number on the blood container, the transfusion form, and the tag attached to the unit must *all* agree.
     - *ABO group and Rh type:* The ABO group and Rh type on the primary label of the donor unit must agree with those recorded on the transfusion form.
     - *Expiration:* The expiration date and time of the donor unit should be verified as acceptable.
     - *Compatibility:* The interpretation of compatibility testing must be recorded on the transfusion form and on the tag attached to the unit.
   - If any of the information does not match *exactly*, notify the charge nurse and the blood bank. Do not administer blood until discrepancies are corrected or clarified.
   - Sign the appropriate form and complete documentation with the other nurse.
   - Make sure that the blood is left at room temperature for no more than 30 minutes before starting the transfusion (check agency policy). **Rationale: As blood**

components get warm, the risk of bacterial growth also increases. Agencies may designate different times at which the blood must be returned to the blood bank if it has not been used. If the start of the transfusion is unexpectedly delayed, return the blood to the blood bank. Do not store blood in the unit refrigerator. **Rationale: The temperature of unit refrigerators is not precisely regulated, and the blood may be damaged.**

6. Prepare the blood bag.
   - Invert the blood bag gently several times to mix the cells with the plasma. **Rationale: Rough handling can damage the cells.**
   - Expose the port on the blood bag by pulling back the tabs (see ❶).
   - Insert the remaining Y-set spike into the blood bag.
   - Suspend the blood bag.

7. Establish the blood transfusion.
   - Close the upper clamp below the IV saline solution container.
   - Open the upper clamp below the blood bag. The blood will run into the saline-filled drip chamber. If necessary, squeeze the drip chamber to re-establish the liquid level with drip chamber one-third full. (Tap the filter to expel any residual air within the filter.)
   - Readjust the flow rate with the main clamp.
   - Remove and discard gloves. Perform hand hygiene.

8. Observe the client closely for the first 15 minutes, remaining with the client. Assess frequently for the next 30 minutes after that.
   - Run the blood slowly for the first 15 minutes, at 5 mL per minute. **Rationale: This small amount is enough to produce a severe reaction but small enough that the reaction could be treated successfully** (Phillips, 2010, p. 749).
   - Note adverse reactions, such as chilling, nausea, vomiting, skin rash, urticaria, dyspnea, facial edema, or change in vital signs. **Rationale: The earlier a transfusion reaction occurs, the more severe it tends to be. Identifying such reactions promptly helps minimize the consequences.**
   - Remind the client to tell a nurse *immediately* if any unusual symptoms are felt during the transfusion.
   - If any of these reactions occur, report these to the nurse in charge, and take appropriate nursing action (see Table 44.14 on page 1464).

9. Document all the relevant data.
   - Record initiation of the blood transfusion, including vital signs, type of blood, blood unit number, sequence number (e.g., no. 1 of 3 ordered units), site of the venipuncture, size of the needle, and drip rate.

10. Monitor the client.
    - Fifteen minutes after initiating the transfusion, check the client's vital signs. If there are no signs of a reaction, establish the required flow rate. Follow physician's orders and agency policy with regard to length of time for transfusion. Most adults can tolerate receiving one unit of blood in 1.5 to 2 hours (CBS, 2007). Do not transfuse a unit of blood for longer than 4 hours.

- Assess the client, including vital signs, every 30 minutes or more often, depending on the client's health status, until 1 hour after transfusion. If the client has a reaction and the blood is discontinued, send the blood bag and tubing to the laboratory for investigation of the blood.

11. Terminate the transfusion.
    - Perform hand hygiene, and follow other appropriate infection prevention and control precautions.
    - Put on clean gloves.
    - If no infusion is to follow, clamp the blood tubing. Follow agency protocol related to disposal of the blood bag and tubing, such as in a biohazard container. The IV line can be discontinued or capped with an adaptor or a new infusion line and solution container may be added. If another transfusion is to follow, clamp the blood tubing and open the saline infusion arm. Blood administration sets are changed within 8 to 24 hours or after 4 units of blood, per agency protocol.
    - If the primary IV is to be continued, flush the maintenance line with saline solution. Disconnect the blood tubing system, and re-establish the intravenous infusion by using new tubing. Adjust the drip to the desired rate. **Rationale: Often, a normal saline or other solution is kept running in case of delayed reaction to the blood.**
    - Remove gloves.

12. Follow agency protocol for appropriate disposal of the blood bag.
    - On the requisition attached to the blood unit, fill in the time the transfusion was completed and the amount transfused.
    - Generally, agency policy involves returning the bag to the blood bank in the event of subsequent or delayed adverse reaction.

13. Document relevant data.
    - Record completion of the transfusion, the amount of blood transfused, the blood unit number, and the vital signs and any signs and symptoms noted. If the primary intravenous infusion was continued, record connecting it. Also record the transfusion on the IV flowsheet and I&O record.

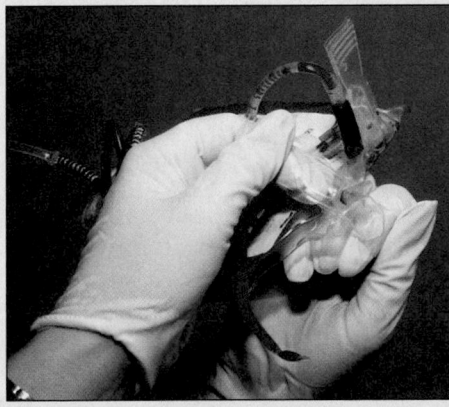

❶ Exposing the port on the blood bag by pulling back the tabs.

(continued)

SKILL 44.6	INITIATING, MAINTAINING, AND TERMINATING A BLOOD TRANSFUSION (continued)

EVALUATION

Evaluate the following:

• Perform follow-up based on findings and outcomes that deviated from expected or normal for the client. Relate

findings to previous data and the reason why the client required a transfusion.

• Report any significant deviations from normal to the appropriate member of the health care team.

Evaluating

The nurse collects data to evaluate the effectiveness of interventions by using the overall goals identified in the planning stage of maintaining or restoring fluid balance; maintaining or restoring pulmonary gas exchange and oxygenation; maintaining or restoring normal balance of electrolytes; and preventing associated risks of fluid, electrolyte, and acid–base imbalances. Examples of desired health outcomes for the identified goals are found in Table 44.15.

If desired outcomes are not achieved, the nurse, client, and support person, if appropriate, need to explore the reasons before modifying the care plan. For example, if the outcome "fluid intake of 2.3 L per day" is not achieved, questions to be considered might include the following: Does the client understand the need for the fluid? Is the client motivated to achieve this objective? Are the types of fluid provided palatable to the client? Is there a problem with access to the fluid?

TABLE 44.15 Evaluation Goals and Outcomes: Fluid, Electrolyte, and Acid–Base Balances

Goal	Examples of Expected Health Outcomes
Maintain or restore normal fluid balance	Vital signs and central venous pressure are within expected ranges. Lung sounds are clear. Urine output is greater than 1300 mL per day and within 500 mL of intake. Skin turgor is elastic; tongue and mucous membranes are moist. No edema is evident. Thirst is absent. Weight is within normal range for client. Laboratory values within normal range (serum osmolality, serum sodium, hematocrit, urine specific gravity). Client explains measures to prevent or treat fluid volume deficit or excess and symptoms that need to be reported to a health care provider
Maintain or restore normal balance of electrolytes in the ICF and ECF compartments	Vital signs are stable and within expected ranges. Client is alert; is oriented to person, place, and time; and speech is clear. Muscle strength is normal. Abnormal sensations, such as numbness, tingling around mouth or distal extremities, are absent. Laboratory values are within normal range (serum sodium, potassium, calcium, chloride, magnesium). Client verbalizes measures to prevent future imbalances, including diet and medications.
Maintain or restore pulmonary gas exchange and oxygenation	Respiratory rate is within normal range; there is no dyspnea or shortness of breath. Client demonstrates effective cough. Lung sounds are clear. Client identifies specific factors leading to impaired airway clearance.
Prevent associated risks (tissue breakdown, decreased cardiac output, confusion, other neurological signs)	Skin and mucous membranes are intact. Skin is warm and pink. Capillary refill is less than 3 seconds. Lung sounds are clear. Client is alert and oriented; no confusion is evident.

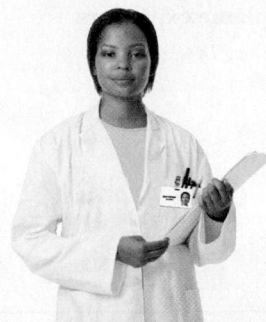

Case Study 44

Mr. Nelson, 74 years old, was admitted to the hospital with a diagnosis of acute gastroenteritis following a 3-day episode of fever and severe diarrhea. He is 1.78 m tall and weighs 78 kg. His oral temperature is 38.7°C; pulse 98 and regular; respirations 32; and blood pressure (BP) 106/86. His skin is flushed and diaphoretic. His lungs are clear on auscultation. His abdomen is tender throughout, and bowel sounds are hyperactive in all quadrants. His urine output is scanty and concentrated. He has an intravenous infusion of Ringer's solution infusing at 125 mL/h via an infusion pump.

CRITICAL THINKING QUESTIONS

1. Predict the possible consequences of Mr. Nelson's fever, diarrhea, and diaphoresis on his fluid, electrolyte, and acid–base status.

2. Why do you think Ringer's solution was prescribed for Mr. Nelson rather than another type of fluid replacement, such as 5% dextrose in water?

3. Why is it important to monitor Mr. Nelson's intake and output?

4. Is it correct to assume that Mr. Nelson's intravenous infusion does not need to be monitored, since it is being administered by an infusion pump? Why, or why not?

5. How would you know if Mr. Nelson was developing an acid–base imbalance related to his severe diarrhea?

Check the eText in MyNursingLab for answers and explanations.

KEY TERMS

CHAPTER HIGHLIGHTS

- A balance of fluids, electrolytes, acids, and bases in the body is necessary for health and life.

- The body fluid is divided into two major compartments: the intracellular fluid (ICF) inside the cells and extracellular fluid (ECF) outside the cells.

- Extracellular fluid is subdivided into three compartments: intravascular (plasma), interstitial, and transcellular. ECF constitutes about one-third of total body fluid.

- ECF is in constant motion throughout the body. It is the transport system that carries nutrients to, and waste products from, cells.

- The percentage of total body fluids varies according to the individual's age, body fat, and sex. The younger the person, the higher is the proportion of water in the body. The less body fat present, the greater is the proportion of body fluid. Postadolescent females have a smaller percentage of fluid in relation to total body weight than do men.

- There are two types of electrolytes (ions): cations (positively charged ions) and anions (negatively charged ions).

- The principal ions of ECF are sodium and chloride; the principal ions of ICF are potassium and phosphate.

- Fluids and electrolytes move among the body compartments by osmosis, diffusion, filtration, and active transport.

- The major fluid pressures exerted as part of the movement of fluid and electrolytes from one compartment to another are osmotic pressure, oncotic pressure, and hydrostatic pressure.

- The three sources of body fluid are fluids taken orally, food ingested, and the oxidation of food. Fluid intake is regulated by the thirst mechanism.

- Fluid output occurs chiefly through excretion of urine, although body fluid is also lost through sweat, feces, and insensible water loss.

- In healthy adults, measurable fluid intake and output should balance. The output of urine normally approximates the oral intake of fluids. Water from food and oxidation is balanced by fluid loss through skin, the respiratory process, and feces.

- A number of body systems and organs are involved in regulating the volume and composition of body fluids: the kidneys, the endocrine system, the cardiovascular system, the lungs, and the gastrointestinal system. The kidneys are the primary regulator of fluid and electrolyte balance.

- Hormones, such as antidiuretic hormone, the renin–angiotensin–aldosterone system, and the atrial natriuretic factor, are also involved in maintaining fluid balance.

- Fluid imbalances include (a) fluid volume deficit, also referred to as hypovolemia; (b) fluid volume excess, also referred to as hypervolemia; (c) dehydration, a deficit in water and increase in serum sodium level; and (d) overhydration, an excess of water and decrease in serum sodium level.

- The most common electrolyte imbalances are deficits or excesses in sodium, potassium, and calcium.

- The acid–base balance (pH) of body fluids is maintained within a precise range of 7.35 to 7.45.

- Acid–base balance is regulated by buffers that neutralize excess acids or bases; the lungs, which eliminate or retain carbon dioxide, a potential acid; and the kidneys, which excrete or conserve bicarbonate and hydrogen ions.

- Acid–base imbalance occurs when the normal 20-to-1 ratio of bicarbonate to carbonic acid is upset. Imbalances can be either respiratory or metabolic in origin; either can result in acidosis or alkalosis.

- Factors that influence an individual's fluid, electrolyte, and acid–base balance include age, sex, body size, environmental temperature, and lifestyle. Illness, trauma, surgery, and certain medications can place individuals at risk for fluid, electrolyte, and acid–base imbalances.

- Fluid, electrolyte, and acid–base imbalance is most accurately determined through laboratory examination of blood plasma.

- Assessment relative to fluid, electrolyte, and acid–base balances includes (a) a nursing history; (b) physical examination; (c) measurement of body weight, vital signs, and fluid intake and output; and (d) various diagnostic studies of blood and urine.

- A nursing history includes data about the client's fluid and food intake; fluid output; signs of fluid, electrolyte, and acid–base imbalances; and medications, therapies, or disease processes that can disrupt these balances.

- Several nursing diagnoses relate specifically to fluid, electrolyte, and acid–base imbalances' including actual or at risk for fluid volume excess; electrolyte imbalance (e.g., hypokalemia, hypernatremia, hypocalcemia); respiratory and/or metabolic alkalosis and/or acidosis.

- In many instances, fluids and electrolytes are provided orally to clients who are experiencing or at risk of developing fluid deficits. The nurse needs to establish with the client a 24-hour plan for ingesting the necessary fluids and to respect the client's fluid preferences.

- For clients with fluid retention, fluids may need to be restricted; a schedule and short-term goals that make the fluid restriction more tolerable need to be developed.

- For clients experiencing excessive fluid losses, the administration of fluids and electrolytes intravenously

is necessary. Meticulous aseptic technique is required when caring for clients with intravenous infusions.

- Preventing complications, such as infiltration, phlebitis, hypervolemia (circulatory overload), and infection, is an important aspect of intravenous therapy.

- The administration of blood transfusions involves accurately matching and identifying the blood for the individual, correctly identifying the recipient, and monitoring the client throughout the procedure for transfusion reactions.

ASSESS YOUR LEARNING

1. A nursing home resident has refused to eat or drink for several days and is admitted to the hospital. The nurse should expect which of the following findings?
   a. Increased blood pressure
   b. Weak, rapid pulse
   c. Moist mucous membranes
   d. Jugular vein distension

2. An older adult man brings his wife to the emergency department. He states that she has been vomiting and has had diarrhea for the past 2 days. She appears lethargic and is complaining of leg cramps. What should the nurse do first?
   a. Start an IV with 10 mmol of potassium/litre
   b. Review the results of serum electrolytes
   c. Offer the woman foods that are high in sodium and potassium content
   d. Administer an antiemetic

3. During a blood transfusion, the client becomes anxious and complains of a headache and dyspnea. The nurse notes that the client is flushed. What should the nurse do first?
   a. Administer antihistamines, as ordered
   b. Discontinue the transfusion
   c. Establish a second IV for emergency drugs
   d. Start oxygen at 100% by mask

4. Which of the following arterial blood gas (ABG) results indicates respiratory acidosis?
   a. pH 7.54; $PaCO_2$ 28 mm Hg; HCO_3^- 22 mmol/L
   b. pH 7.32; $PaCO_2$ 48 mm Hg; HCO_3^- 24 mmol/L
   c. pH 7.31; $PaCO_2$ 35 mm Hg; HCO_3^- 20 mmol/L
   d. pH 7.50; $PaCO_2$ 37 mm Hg; HCO_3^- 28 mmol/L

5. Mr. Blanchard, 42 years old, has been diagnosed with cancer and is being discharged with a peripherally inserted central catheter (PICC) for medication administration. Which of the following instructions would the nurse provide to Mr. Blanchard's family about working with a PICC?

   a. Inspect the area for redness and swelling on a daily basis.
   b. Flush the catheter daily.
   c. Use hydrogen peroxide to cleanse the site.
   d. Change the tubing every 72 hours.

6. Which of the following client statements indicates a need for further teaching regarding treatment for hypokalemia?
   a. "I will use avocado in my salads."
   b. "I will be sure to check my heart rate before I take my digoxin."
   c. "I will take my potassium in the morning after eating breakfast."
   d. "I can continue using my salt substitute."

7. An older adult man is admitted to the medical unit with a diagnosis of severe dehydration with severe hypernatremia. Which of the following signs or symptoms are MOST representative of this type of sodium imbalance?
   a. Hyperreflexia
   b. Disorientation
   c. Irregular pulse
   d. Muscle weakness

8. The client's arterial blood gas results are pH 7.31; $PaCO_2$ 35; HCO_3^- 19. Which type of acid–base imbalance do these results indicate?
   a. Metabolic acidosis
   b. Respiratory acidosis
   c. Metabolic alkalosis
   d. Respiratory alkalosis

9. A client is admitted to the hospital for hypocalcemia. Nursing interventions relating to which system would have the HIGHEST priority?
   a. Renal
   b. Cardiac
   c. Gastrointestinal
   d. Neuromuscular

10. The nurse would assess for signs of hypomagnesemia in which of the following clients?

    a. A client taking digoxin

    b. A client with adrenal insufficiency

    c. A client with bone cancer

    d. A client with chronic alcoholism

Check the eText in MyNursingLab for answers and explanations.

WEBLINKS

The Kidney Foundation of Canada

http://www.kidney.ca

This foundation is a national volunteer organization dedicated to improving the health and quality of life of people living with kidney disease. The organization funds research and related clinical education, provides services for special needs of individuals, and actively promotes the awareness of organ donation.

Canadian Vascular Access Association (CVAA)

http://www.cvaa.info

This is a professional nursing organization dedicated to promoting standards for IV therapy and educational programs to enhance the care of patients requiring IV therapy. Note: This organization was previously named the Canadian Intravenous Nurses Association.

MyNursingLab

REFERENCES

Canadian Blood Services. (2007). *Clinical guide to transfusion.* Retrieved from http://www.transfusionmedicine.ca/resources/clinical-guide-transfusion

Centres for Disease Control and Prevention. (2011). *Guidelines for the prevention of intravascular catheter-related infections, 2011.* Retrieved from http://www.cdc.gov/hicpac/pdf/guidelines/bsi-guidelines-2011.pdf

Gillies, D., O'Riordan, L., Wallen, M., Morrison, A., Rankin, K., & Nagy, S. (2005). Optimal timing for intravenous administration set replacement. *Cochrane Database of Systematic Reviews, 4,* Art. No.: CD003588.

Hadaway, L. (2009). Protect patients from IV infiltration. *American Nurse Today, 4*(7), 10–11.

Health Canada. (2010). Vitamin D and calcium. Retrieved from http://www.hc-sc.gc.ca/fn-an/nutrition/vitamin/vita-d-eng.php

Infusion Nurses Society. (2011). Infusion nursing: Standards of practice. *Journal of Intravenous Nursing, 34*(1S).

Moureau, N. L., & Dawson, R. B. (2010). Keeping needleless connectors clean, part 2. *Nursing, 40*(6), 61–63.

Osteoporosis Canada. (2011). How much calcium do we need? Retrieved from http://www.osteoporosis.ca/index.php/ci_id/5535/la_id/1.htm

Phillips, L. D. (2010). *Manual of I.V. therapeutics. Evidence-based practice for infusion therapy* (5th ed.). Philadelphia, PA: F.A. Davis.

Registered Nurses' Association of Ontario. (2008). *Assessment and device selection for vascular access–guideline supplement.* Toronto, ON: Author.

Registered Nurses' Association of Ontario. (2008). *Care and maintenance to reduce vascular access complications–guideline supplement.* Toronto, ON: Author.

Rosenthal, K. (2006). Intravenous fluids: The whys and wherefores. *Nursing, 36*(7), 26–27.

Slesak, G., Schnurle, J. W., Jakob, J., & Dietz, P. K. (2003). Comparison of subcutaneous and intravenous rehydration in geriatric patients: A randomized trial. *Journal of American Geriatric Society, 51,* 155–60.

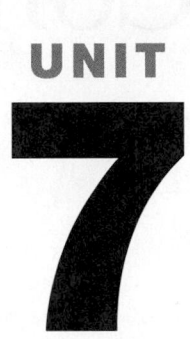

UNIT 7

Promoting Psychosocial Health

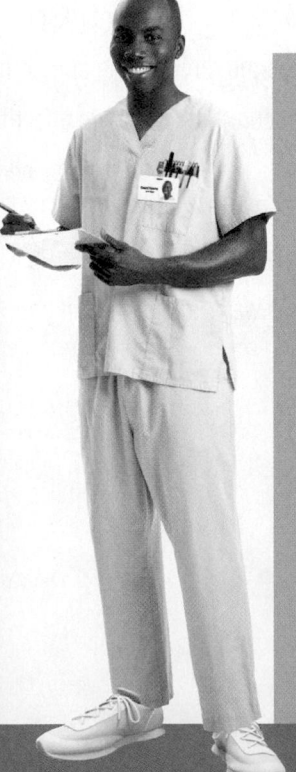

Chapter 45

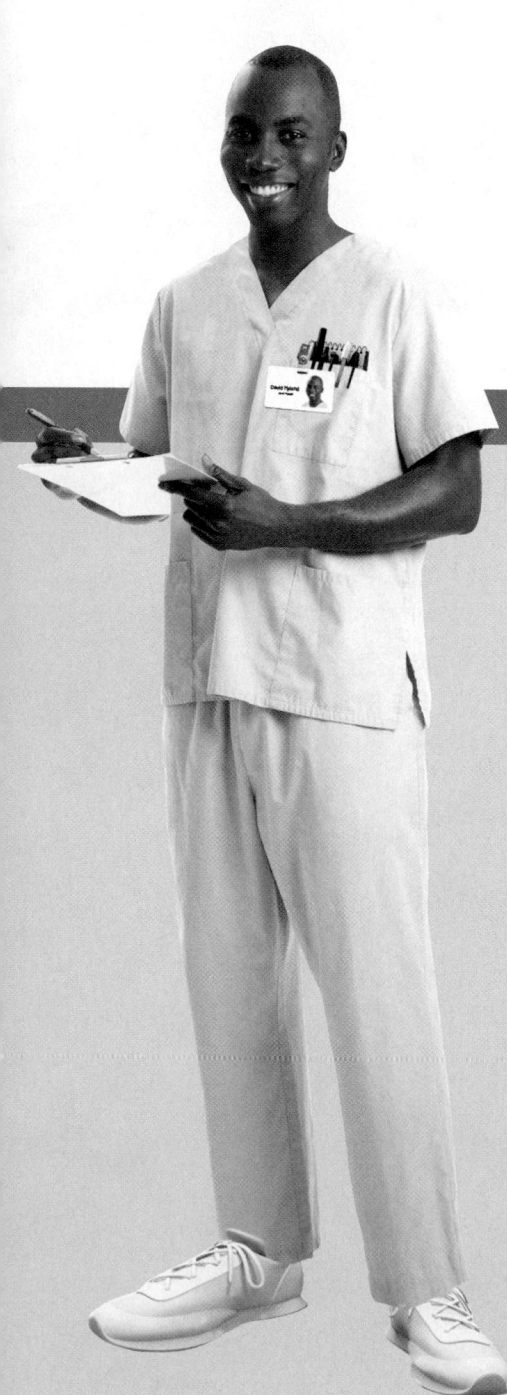

Self-Concept

After studying this chapter, you will be able to:

1. Summarize the development of self-concept and self-esteem, including the framework described by Erikson.

2. Describe the dimensions and components of self-concept.

3. Identify common stressors affecting self-concept and coping strategies.

4. Perform a self-concept assessment using communication and the nurse–client relationship related theory.

5. Design a care plan for a person with a nursing diagnosis of altered self-concept.

6. Describe ways to enhance client self-esteem.

Self-concept is one's mental image of oneself. A positive self-concept is essential to a person's mental and physical health. Individuals with a positive self-concept are better able to develop and maintain interpersonal relationships and resist psychological and physical illness. They have greater control of their environments and are better able to accept or adapt to changes over the lifespan. Individuals who have a poor self-concept may express feelings of worthlessness, self-dislike, or even self-hatred. They may feel sad or hopeless and may lack energy to perform the simplest of tasks (Kraus, Chen, & Keltner, 2011). Nurses have a responsibility to assess clients who have a negative self-concept and to identify the possible causes to help them develop a more positive view of themselves.

Self-Concept

Self-concept involves all the self-perceptions—appearance, values, and beliefs—that influence behaviour and are referred to when using the words *I* or *me*. Self-concept influences the following:

- How one thinks, talks, and acts
- How one sees and treats another person
- Choices one makes
- Ability to give and receive love
- Ability to take action and to change things

Self-concept has four dimensions:

1. *Self-knowledge:* insight into one's own abilities, nature, and limitations
2. *Self-expectation:* what one expects of oneself; may be realistic or unrealistic expectations
3. *Social self:* how a person is perceived by others and society
4. *Social evaluation:* the appraisal of oneself in relationship to others, events, or situations

People who value "how I perceive me" above "how others perceive me" can be termed *me-centred.* They try to live up to their own expectations and compete only with themselves. In contrast, strongly *other-centred* people have a need to live up to the expectations of others, comparing, competing, and evaluating themselves in relation to others. They tend to have difficulty asserting themselves, and fear disapproval. The positive self-concept, therefore, is me-centred and is formed with limited reference to others' opinions.

The nurse's awareness of one's own self-concept helps in the accurate assessment and promotion of positive self-concept with clients. Nurses who possess a positive self-concept are better able to understand the needs, desires, feelings, and conflicts of their clients and are more likely to help clients meet their needs (Eckroth-Bucher, 2010).

Self-awareness is the relationship between a person's own perception of self in comparison with others' perceptions of him or her. Self-awareness in a nurse is crucial for the development of therapeutic nurse–client relationships. A nurse needs to look inward at personal beliefs, attitudes, motivations, strengths, and limitations (Richards, Campenni, & Muse-Burke, 2010). A nurse gains self-awareness through working with others and accepting constructive feedback. While in the caregiver role, the self-aware nurse is able to suspend judgment and focus on the needs of the client, even if they differ from those of the nurse. When conflicts arise, the nurse can analyze his or her reactions through **introspection** and by asking questions such as the following:

- Why do I react this way (fear, anger, anxiety, annoyance, worry)?
- Can I change the way I respond to this situation to affect the client's reaction in a helpful way?

Formation of Self-Concept

A person is not born with a self-concept; rather, it develops as a result of social interactions with others. See Chapter 17 for a discussion on the development of self-concept, including Erikson's stages of development, Piaget's cognitive developmental stages, and Havighurst's developmental tasks.

According to Erikson (1963), throughout life people face developmental tasks associated with eight psychosocial stages. The development of a healthy self-concept is dependent on the success of accomplishing these developmental tasks. Inability to complete developmental tasks may lead to a poor self-concept. Table 45.1 on the next page lists behaviours that indicate successful or unsuccessful accomplishment of developmental tasks.

TABLE 45.1 Examples of Behaviours Associated with Erikson's Stages of Psychosocial Development

Stage: Developmental Tasks	Behaviours Indicating Positive Resolution	Behaviours Indicating Negative Resolution
Infancy: trust versus mistrust	Requesting assistance and expecting to receive it Expressing belief of another person Sharing time, opinions, and experiences	Being unable to accept assistance Refusing to provide a person with personal information Restricting conversation to superficialities
Toddlerhood: autonomy versus shame and doubt	Accepting the rules of a group but also expressing disagreement when it is felt Expressing one's own opinion Easily accepting deferment of a wish fulfillment	Failing to express needs Not expressing one's own opinion when opposed Overly concerned about being clean
Early childhood: initiative versus guilt	Starting projects eagerly Expressing curiosity about many things Demonstrating original thought	Verbalizing fear about starting a new project Apologizing and being very embarrassed over small mistakes Imitating others rather than developing independent ideas
Early school years: industry versus inferiority	Completing a task once it has been started Working well with others Using time effectively	Not completing tasks started Not assisting with the work of others Not organizing work
Adolescence: identity versus role confusion	Asserting independence Planning realistically for future roles Establishing close interpersonal relationships	Failing to assume responsibility for directing one's own behaviour Failing to set goals in life Accepting the values of others without question
Early adulthood: intimacy versus isolation	Establishing a close, intimate relationship with another person Making a commitment to that relationship, even in times of stress and sacrifice Accepting sexual behaviour as desirable	Remaining alone Avoiding close interpersonal relationships Withdrawing from sexual relationships
Middle-aged adults: generativity versus stagnation	Being willing to share with another person Guiding others Establishing a priority of needs, recognizing both self and others	Talking about oneself instead of listening to others Showing concern for oneself in spite of the needs of others Being unable to accept interdependence
Older adults: integrity versus despair	Using past experience to assist others Maintaining productivity in some areas Accepting limitations	Demanding unnecessary assistance and attention from others Procrastinating and being apathetic Not accepting changes

Self-concept development comprises three broad steps:

1. The infant learns that the physical self is separate and different from the environment.
2. The child internalizes others' attitudes toward self.
3. The child and adult internalize the standards of society.

The term **global self** refers to the collective beliefs and images a person holds about the self (Bosson & Swann, 2009). It is also a person's frame of reference for experiencing and viewing the world. Some of these beliefs and images represent statements of fact, for example, "I am a woman"; "I am a father"; "I am short." Others refer to less tangible aspects of self, for instance, "I am competent"; "I am shy."

Each separate image and belief has a bearing on self-concept. The various images and beliefs people hold about themselves are not equal in weight and prominence, but they constitute the **core self-concept** to the person's identity. For example, "I am very smart"; "I am female." Images and beliefs that are less important to the person are on the periphery. For example, "I am left-handed"; "I am not athletic."

People are thought to base their self-concept on how they perceive and evaluate themselves in these areas:

- Vocational performance
- Intellectual functioning
- Personal appearance and physical attractiveness
- Sexual attractiveness and performance
- Being liked by others
- Ability to cope with and resolve problems
- Independence
- Particular talents

Self-concept in these areas influences the choices people make and perceptions they have about their health. Persons with a strong positive self-concept about appearance are likely to value healthy behaviours and take action to maintain the health of their skin, hair, and body tone. Persons with negative self-concepts may be less proactive about health-promotion and illness-prevention activities.

Maintaining and evaluating a self-concept is an ongoing process. Events or situations may change the level of self-concept over time. As one ages, engaging in social activity is key to maintaining self-concept and possibly enhancing one's identity (Lodi-Smith & Roberts, 2010). Having a basic self-concept includes how we see ourselves and how we are seen by others. The **ideal self** is how we should be or would prefer to be. The ideal self is the individual's perception of how one should behave based on certain personal standards, aspirations, goals, and values. Adults usually hold some thoughts about their **perceived self**, how they see themselves versus how they are seen by others. A discrepancy between the ideal self and the perceived self can be an incentive to self-improvement. However, when the discrepancy is great, low self-esteem can result.

The increased use of Internet, e-mail, instant messaging, video gaming, and cell phones by today's generation can impact on the development of self-concept and self-esteem. Digital technology and cyberspace interactions tend to create social isolation without actual face-to-face contacts, and may exert a negative influence on the development of self-concept and self-esteem (Jackson, vonEye, Fitzgerald, Zhao, & Witt, 2010).

Nurses, like other adults, view themselves based on both internal and external inputs acquired during their educational and subsequent work experience. The ability to appraise one's own strengths, the desire to follow in the steps of role models, and the feedback received from colleagues and clients are some of the influences on the nurse's self-concept.

Components of Self-Concept

Self-concept has four components: (a) personal identity, (b) body image, (c) role performance, and (d) self-esteem.

Personal Identity

Personal identity is the conscious sense of individuality and uniqueness that is continually evolving throughout life. People often view their identity in terms of name, gender, age, race, ethnic origin or culture, occupation or roles, talents, and other situational characteristics (e.g., marital status and education).

Personal identity also includes beliefs and values, personality, and character. For instance, is the person outgoing, friendly, reserved, generous, or selfish? Personal identity thus encompasses both the tangible and factual, such as name and gender, and the intangible, such as values and beliefs. Identity is what distinguishes the self from others.

A person with a strong sense of identity has integrated body image, role performance, and self-esteem into a complete self-concept. This sense of identity provides a person with a feeling of continuity and a unity of personality. Furthermore, the individual sees himself or herself as a unique person. For example, as Canadian adolescents are becoming more open and are disclosing their sexual orientation, their sense of self is negatively impacted when exposed to homophobic terms such as *faggot*, *queer*, *lezbo*, and *dyke*. To build a sense of school community where diversity is celebrated, schools need to establish and enforce antihomophobia policies (Taylor & Peter, 2011).

Body Image

The image of physical self, or **body image**, is how a person perceives the size, appearance, and functioning of the body and its parts. Body image has both cognitive and affective aspects. The cognitive aspect is the knowledge of the physical body; the affective aspect includes the sensations of the body, such as pain, pleasure, fatigue, and physical movement. Body image is the sum of these attitudes, conscious and subconscious, that a person has toward his or her body.

Body image includes clothing, makeup, hairstyle, jewellery, tattooing, body piercing, and other things intimately connected to the person (Figure 45.1 on the next page). It also includes body prostheses, such as artificial limbs, dentures, and hairpieces, as well as devices required for functioning, such as wheelchairs, canes, and eyeglasses. Past and present perceptions and how the body has evolved over time are part of body image.

A person's body image develops partly from others' attitudes and responses and partly from the individual's own exploration of the body. Body image develops in infancy in response to how the parents or caregivers respond to the child with smiles, holding, and touching. The child's exploration of his or her own body sensations during breast-feeding, thumb sucking, and the bath are equally as important on attitude development. In addition, cultural and societal values also influence a person's body image.

All sources of media influence how individuals view themselves and others. The "ideal" body image frequently portrayed influences women's and men's perceptions of what constitutes a healthy, normal appearance.

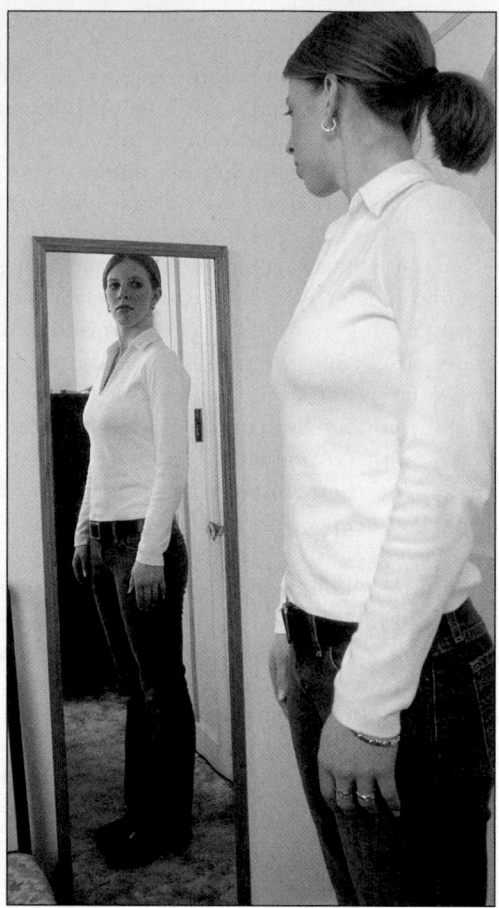

FIGURE 45.1 Body image is the sum of a person's conscious and unconscious attitudes about his or her body. Persons do not always appear to themselves as they appear to others.

Overweight women in particular are more at risk to experience depression, engage in negative self-talk, and develop an eating disorder in response to body image dissatisfaction (Sides-Moore & Tochkov, 2011).

During adolescence, concerns related to body image are of paramount concern (see the Reflect on Primary Health Care box).

If a person's body image closely resembles that person's body ideal, the individual is more likely to think positively about the physical and nonphysical components of the self. The body ideal is greatly influenced by

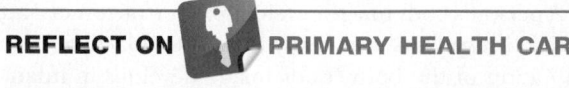

REFLECT ON **PRIMARY HEALTH CARE**

Public health nurses work collaboratively with teachers in school settings to develop sexual health education programs for preadolescent students. One of the activity components is to guide these students to develop a positive self-concept that will enable them to explore relationships and assertiveness, including ways to negotiate safe sex. This activity illustrates the principles of *health promotion* and *intersectoral collaboration*. Consider how nurses can implement the principle of *public participation* by engaging students to determine how best to deliver such sexual health education.

cultural standards. For example, in North America, the fit, well-toned body is admired.

Different parts of the body have different values for different people. Some parts of the body have greater significance for different people than other parts. For example, some women desire to have larger breasts, some may be upset with greying hair or hair loss, and some others do not place a high importance on these physical attributes.

A person with a healthy body image will engage in activities that make them look and feel better. This person will take responsibility to improve health at times of illness and institute health-promoting activities. In contrast, a person with an unhealthy body image may neglect such activities as sleep and a healthy diet that are important to health.

The individual who has a body image disturbance may ignore a body part that is significantly changed in structure by illness or trauma. Some individuals may express feelings of helplessness, hopelessness, powerlessness, and depression in relation to the body image changes that occur over time. These feelings can be so intense that they contribute to self-destructive behaviour, such as overeating, undereating, or suicide attempts. But in today's society the option of cosmetic surgery is readily available. It has given female breast cancer survivors the option of breast reconstruction following mastectomy and has contributed positively to reducing aging anxiety in middle-aged women (Slevec & Tiggemann, 2010). On the other hand, one may also argue that women needing plastic surgery to "reduce aging anxiety" may reflect their inability to accept their aging body and therefore embrace a positive self concept of healthy aging.

Role Performance

People undergo numerous role changes throughout life. A **role** is a set of expectations about how a person in a certain role should behave. **Role performance** is how an individual fulfills the expected duties of a particular role. **Role mastery** means that the individual is successful in meeting the expectations of that assigned role. Expectations or standards of behaviour of a role are set by society, a cultural group, or a smaller group to which a person belongs. Each person usually has several roles, such as husband, parent, brother, son, employee, friend, nurse, and church member. Some roles are only temporary. With the introduction of each new role, there needs to be a period of **role development,** which involves socialization into that particular role. For example, nursing students are socialized into nursing through exposure to their professors, practice experience, classes, laboratory simulations, and seminars.

To act appropriately, people need to know who they are in relation to others and what are the societal expectations for certain roles. Nolan and Harold (2010) used the tenets of image congruity theory to study what attracted participants to certain job opportunities. Results showed that prospective job seekers are attracted to organizations with personalities they perceive as similar to their own actual and ideal self-concepts. **Role ambiguity** occurs when people are unclear of role responsibilities and do not know what to do or how to do it and are unable to predict the reactions of others to their behaviour. Ambiguity causes feelings of frustration and inadequacy leading to role failure, often causing lowered self-esteem.

Self-concept is also affected by role strain and role conflicts. **Role strain** occurs when people feel or are made to feel inadequate or unsuited to a role. Role strain is often associated with gender-role stereotypes. For example, women in occupations traditionally held by men might be treated as having less knowledge and competence than men in the same roles.

Role conflicts arise from opposing or incompatible expectations of a role or position. In an *interpersonal conflict*, people have different expectations about a particular role. For example, a grandparent may have different expectations from those of the mother about how she should care for her children. In an *interrole conflict*, one person's or group's role expectations differ from the expectations of another person or group. For example, a woman working full time in a job may have a role conflict if her husband expects her to handle all childcare problems. In a *person–role conflict*, role expectations violate the beliefs or values of the individual fulfilling the role. For example, a nurse in a family planning clinic may be expected to advise couples about birth control methods that are inconsistent with the nurse's belief system regarding prevention or management of unwanted pregnancy. Role conflict can lead to tension, a decrease in self-esteem, and embarrassment. See the Clinical Alert box on Maslow's category of love and belonging needs.

> **! CLINICAL ALERT**
>
> According to Maslow, if an individual's love and belonging needs are met, they are more likely to achieve the need for self-esteem. Achieving this need is an important element in striving for self-actualization.

Self-Esteem

Self-esteem is a person's judgment of his or her own worth, that is, how that person's standards and performances compare with those of others and with his or her ideal self. If a person's self-esteem does not match the ideal self, then low self-concept results.

Self-esteem comes in two types: (a) global and (b) specific. **Global self-esteem** is how much a person likes himself or herself as a whole. **Specific self-esteem** is how much a person approves of a certain part of himself or herself. Global self-esteem is influenced by specific self-esteem. For example, if a man places little value on his cooking skills, then how well or badly he cooks will have little influence on his global self-esteem.

Self-esteem is derived from the self and others. In infancy, self-esteem is related to the caregiver's evaluations and acceptances. Later, the child's self-esteem is affected by competition with others. As an adult, a person who has high self-esteem has feelings of significance, feelings of competence, the ability to cope with life, and control over his or her destiny.

The foundation for self-esteem is established during early life experiences, usually within the family structure. However, an adult's level of overall self-esteem is affected by what is happening in one's life at any given time. Severe stress related to prolonged illness or unemployment can substantially lower a person's self-esteem. Individuals who experience a disability or illness that is viewed negatively by society may have lower self-esteem. Also, females, with the exception of the 11- to 12-year-olds, had consistently higher levels of social physique anxiety and lower levels of physical self-esteem compared with males (Hagger & Stevenson, 2010). People frequently focus more on their negative aspects and less on their positive aspects. It is important for them to recognize both their strengths and weaknesses. See the Evidence-Informed Practice box

EVIDENCE-INFORMED PRACTICE

What Is the Relationship between Adolescents' Self-Esteem and Body Image?

Seventh-grade students (*N* = 1553) from five Montreal-area schools were asked to participate in a research project to determine if self-esteem and body image affect adolescents' success in coping with developmental challenges. This study asked three questions: (a) Are the intraindividual developmental trajectories of self-esteem and body image stable across adolescence? (b) What is the direction of the relations between body image and self-esteem over time? (c) What is the role of gender, ethnicity, and pubertal development on those trajectories?

The results showed that levels of self-esteem were positively influenced by levels of body image. The effects of the onset of puberty on body image and self-esteem levels indicated non-Caucasian females adjusted better to a more advanced pubertal development. Caucasian females presented the lowest self-esteem and body image levels, but with maturity, they experienced a slight rise in body image. Girls, in general, experienced lower levels of body image and self-esteem compared with their male counterparts. The majority of adolescents adapt well to the physical, emotional, and social changes associated with this stage.

NURSING IMPLICATIONS: The majority of youth successfully cope with normal adolescent developmental changes with proper support and resources. However, nurses caring for adolescents need to be sensitive to the normal developmental challenges facing this age group, in particular Caucasian girls, who, in this study, were found to display the lowest levels of self-esteem and body image. Nursing interventions that focus on creating a positive body image would also result in an increased self-esteem for this age category.

Source: Based on Morin, A. J. S., Maïano, C., Marsh, H. W., Janosz, M., & Nagengast, B. (2011). The longitudinal interplay of adolescents' self-esteem and body image: A conditional autoregressive latent trajectory analysis. *Multivariate Behavioral Research, 46,* 157–201.

on the relationship between adolescents' self-esteem and body image.

Factors That Affect Self-Concept

Major factors such as stage of development, family and culture, stressors, resources, history of success and failure, and illness can impact an individual's self-concept.

Stage of Development

During the various stages of development, conditions affecting the development of self-concept change. For example, an infant requires a supportive, caring environment, while a child requires freedom to explore and learn. An older adult's self-concept is based on experiences and accomplishments in progressing through life's stages.

Family and Culture

A young child's values are largely influenced by the family and culture. In later years, peers have a greater influence on the child and the sense of self. When the child is confronted with conflicting expectations from family, culture, and peers, the child's sense of self is often confused (Figure 45.2). For example, an underage adolescent is instructed by parents not to consume alcohol, but some of their peers may drink alcohol regardless of parental restrictions.

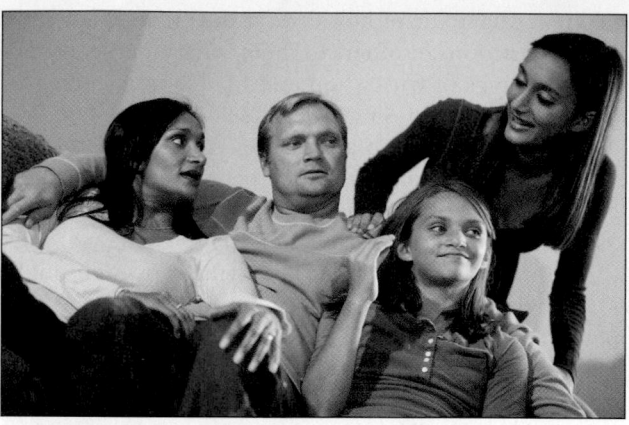

FIGURE 45.2 A child is often pulled in opposite directions by family and peer expectations.

Stressors

Stressors can strengthen the self-concept as an individual copes successfully with problems. Conversely, overwhelming stressors can cause maladaptive responses, including problematic substance use, withdrawal, and anxiety if coping strategies fail. A person's ability to handle stressors will largely depend on personal resources. See Box 45.1 for examples of stressors that may place a client at risk for problems with self-concept.

Resources

An individual's resources are internal and external. Examples of internal resources include confidence and values; external resources include a support network, sufficient finances, and organizations. Generally, the greater

---

BOX 45.1 STRESSORS AFFECTING SELF-CONCEPT

Many different stressors can interfere with a positive self-concept:

IDENTITY STRESSORS
- Change in physical appearance (e.g., facial wrinkles)
- Decline in physical, mental, or sensory abilities
- Inability to achieve goals
- Relationship concerns
- Sexuality concerns
- Unrealistic ideal self

BODY IMAGE STRESSORS
- Loss of body parts (e.g., amputation, mastectomy, hysterectomy)
- Loss of body functions (e.g., from stroke, spinal cord injury, neuromuscular disease, arthritis, declining mental or sensory abilities)
- Disfigurement (e.g., resulting from pregnancy, severe burns, facial blemishes, colostomy, tracheotomy)

- Unrealistic body ideal (e.g., a muscular configuration that cannot be achieved)

SELF-ESTEEM STRESSORS
- Lack of positive feedback from significant others
- Repeated failures
- Unrealistic expectations
- Abusive relationship
- Loss of financial security

ROLE STRESSORS
- Loss of parent, spouse, child, or close friend
- Change in or loss of job or other significant role
- Divorce
- Illness
- Ambiguous or conflicting role expectations
- Inability to meet role expectations

the number of resources a person has and uses, the more positive is the effect on the self-concept.

History of Success and Failure

People who have a history of failure often see themselves as failures. Those who have a history of success are more likely to have a positive self-concept. Likewise, people with a positive self-concept tend to find contentment in their level of success, while having a negative self-concept can lead people to view their life situation as negative.

Illness

Illness and trauma can also affect the self-concept. A woman with a mastectomy may see herself as less attractive, and the loss of a breast may affect how she acts and values herself. People respond to stressors, such as illness and alterations in function related to aging, in a variety of ways. Acceptance, denial, withdrawal, and depression are common reactions.

Nursing Management

Assessing

A comprehensive health assessment includes a psychosocial assessment of the client and the family or support person, because this provides clues to actual or potential problems. The nurse assessing self-concept focuses on the four components: (a) personal identity, (b) body image, (c) role performance, and (d) self-esteem.

Before conducting a psychosocial assessment, the nurse must establish trust and a working relationship with the client. Guidelines for conducting a psychosocial assessment include the following:

- Create a quiet, private environment.
- Minimize interruptions, if possible.
- Maintain appropriate eye contact.
- Sit at eye level with the client.
- Listen and attend to the client's concerns.
- Remain nonjudgmental in your body language and verbal responses.
- Ask open-ended and relevant questions to encourage the client to share information.
- Obtain the client's permission to record pertinent data during the interview.
- Ask permission prior to seeking additional information from others, if indicated.
- Maintain confidentiality.

BOX 45.2 CULTURALLY COMPETENT CARE: ASSESSING SELF-CONCEPT

It is the nurse's responsibility to use therapeutic communication and to remain sensitive to the effect that cultural influences will have on the client's behaviours and needs. Cultural background is not only assessed directly but also considered as a factor in the areas of self-perception, role relationships, major stressors, and coping strategies. In the area of behaviours that may suggest low self-esteem, nurses need to ask themselves the following questions: Is this really a behaviour that would suggest a low self-esteem, or is it part of the cultural behaviour of the client? Might the client be experiencing cultural dissonance, a situation in which there are conflicting beliefs and attitudes between the client's culture and the one in which the client is living?

- Be aware of your own biases and discomforts that could influence the assessment.
- Be culturally sensitive (see Box 45.2).

A nurse needs to assess how a client will react to a stressor. A positive, growth-oriented perception of stressful events reinforces self-worth. A negative, hopeless, defeatist perception leads to decreased self-esteem. A true indication of how someone will handle a stressor is to note how they reacted to previous stressors. The nurse should examine the client's usual response to stress by asking the client questions, such as the following:

- When you have a problem or face a stressful situation, how do you usually deal with it?
- Do these methods work?

PERSONAL IDENTITY When assessing self-concept, the information the nurse first needs is about the client's personal identity. This involves who the client believes he or she is. See the Assessment: Interview Personal Identity box for examples of questions to ask the client.

ASSESSMENT   INTERVIEW

Personal Identity

The nurse can use the following questions to assess self-concept:
- How would you describe your personal characteristics? or How do you see yourself as a person?
- How do others describe you as a person?
- What do you like about yourself?
- What do you do well?
- What are your personal strengths, talents, and abilities?
- What would you change about yourself if you could?
- Does it bother you a great deal if you think someone does not like you?

ASSESSMENT | INTERVIEW

Body Image

Assessing body image is very important.

- Is there any part of your body you would like to change?
- Are you comfortable discussing your surgery?
- Do you feel different or inferior to others?
- How do you feel about your appearance?
- What changes in your body do you expect following your surgery?
- How have significant others in your life reacted to changes in your body?

BODY IMAGE If a client displays signs of a body image disturbance, the nurse should assess the client carefully for possible functional or physical problems. The disturbance may be a result of a present deformity or malfunction or an anticipated one. In addition to the stated responses about the problem, it is important to assess related behaviour. See the Assessment: Interview: Body Image box above for examples of questions to ask about body image.

ROLE PERFORMANCE The nurse assesses the client's satisfactions and dissatisfactions associated with family roles, work roles, student roles, and social roles. Family roles are especially important to people because of the closeness of family relationships. Relationships can be supportive and growth producing or, at the opposite extreme, highly stressful if they contain violence or abuse. Assessment of family role relationships may begin with structural aspects, such as the number in the family group, ages, and residence locations. To obtain data

related to the client's family relationships and satisfaction or dissatisfaction with work roles and social roles, the nurse might ask some of the questions shown in the Assessment: Interview: Role Performance box below. Remember to keep questions relevant to the individuals and their culture, age, and situation.

SELF-ESTEEM A nurse can ask the following questions to assess a client's self-esteem:

- Are you satisfied with your life?
- How do you feel about yourself?
- Are you accomplishing what you want?
- What goals in life are important to you?

It is important for the nurse to assess the client's cultural background first to avoid misinterpreting specific behaviours. The following behaviours can indicate low self-esteem, but they can also be part of the client's cultural background:

- Avoids eye contact
- Stoops in posture and moves slowly
- Is poorly groomed and has an unkempt appearance
- Is hesitant or halting in speech
- Is overly critical of self (e.g., "I'm no good"; "I'm ugly"; or "People don't like me.")
- May be overly critical of others
- Is unable to accept positive remarks about self
- Apologizes frequently
- Verbalizes feelings of hopelessness, helplessness, and powerlessness, such as "I really don't care what happens"; "I'll do whatever anyone wants"; "Whatever is destined will happen."

ASSESSMENT | INTERVIEW

Role Performance

Use these questions as a base to construct questions to learn about the client's roles:

FAMILY RELATIONSHIPS

- Tell me about your family.
- What is your home like?
- How is your relationship with your spouse/partner/significant other? [if appropriate]
- What are your relationships like with your other relatives?
- How are important decisions made in your family?
- What are your responsibilities in the family?
- How well do you feel you accomplish what is expected of you?
- What about your role or responsibilities would you like changed?
- Are you proud of your family members?
- Do you feel as if your family members are proud of you?

WORK ROLES AND SOCIAL ROLES

- Do you like your work?
- How do you get along at work?
- What about your work would you like to change if you could?
- How do you spend your free time?
- Are you involved in any community groups?
- Are you most comfortable alone, with one other person, or in a group?
- Who is most important to you?
- Whom do you seek out for help?

Diagnosing

Three nursing diagnoses relating specifically to the domain of self-perception and the classes of self-concept, self-esteem, and body image include the following:

- *Disturbed Body Image*
- *Ineffective Role Performance*
- *Chronic Low Self-Esteem*

Additional nursing diagnoses that may apply to clients with problems of self-concept include the following:

- *Disturbed Personal Identity*
- *Anxiety Related to Changed Physical Appearance* (e.g., amputation, mastectomy)
- *Ineffective Coping*, with role change related to death of spouse
- *Grieving* or *Complicated Grieving*, related to change in physical appearance
- *Hopelessness*
- *Powerlessness*
- *Parental Role Conflict*
- *Readiness for Enhanced Self-Concept*

- *Disturbed Sleep Pattern*
- *Social Isolation*
- *Spiritual Distress*
- *Disturbed Thought Processes*

Planning

The nurse develops plans in collaboration with the client and his or her support system, when possible, according to the client's state of health, level of anxiety, resources, coping mechanisms, and sociocultural and religious affiliations. The nurse who has little experience in intervening with clients with altered self-concept may want to consult with a more experienced nurse to develop effective plans. The nurse and client set goals together to enhance the client's self-concept.

The goals established will vary according to the diagnoses and defining characteristics related to each individual. Examples of desired outcomes, interventions, and activities are shown in the Sample Care Plan box. Specific nursing orders associated with each of these activities can be selected to meet the individual needs of the client.

Sample Care Plan for Clients with Self-Concept and Role Problems

DATA CLUSTER: Frank Sawyers had a permanent colostomy 7 days ago for cancer of the sigmoid colon. When the nurse was changing the colostomy appliance, Frank said, "I am really repulsed by this." He avoided looking at the stoma and put his arm over his eyes.

Nursing Diagnosis	Desired Health Outcomes	Nursing Activities
Disturbed Body Image/ Confusion in mental picture of one's physical self	Positive body image • Attitude toward touching affected body part • Adjustment to changes in body function	To enhance client's body image and self-care, do the following: • Assist client to discuss changes caused by illness/surgery. • Assist client in identifying parts of his body that have positive perceptions associated with them. • Facilitate contact with individuals with similar changes in body image. • Encourage independence but intervene when client is unable to perform.

DATA CLUSTER: George Kawazi, a first-year university student, is studying liberal arts and the sciences. George states that even though he attends all his classes and studies every day and on weekends, his grades do not please his father, who expects straight A's. "I've always had trouble measuring up to Father's expectations. He never thought I was as good as my older brother."

*Chronic Low Self-Esteem/*Long-standing negative self-evaluation/feelings about self or self-capabilities	Positive self-esteem and self-worth • Acceptance of self-limitations • Willingness to confront others • Description of success in school	To enhance client's self-esteem and self-worth, do the following: • Determine client's confidence in own judgment • Reinforce strengths the client identifies • Assist in setting realistic goals • Explore previous experiences of success

Implementing

Nursing interventions to promote a positive self-concept include helping a client to identify areas of strength. In addition, for clients who have an altered self-concept, nurses should establish a therapeutic relationship and help clients evaluate themselves and make behavioural changes.

IDENTIFYING AREAS OF STRENGTH Healthy people often perceive their problems and weaknesses more easily than their assets and strengths. People with low self-esteem tend to focus more on their limitations, be less aware of their strengths, and perceive themselves as having many more problems. When a client has difficulty identifying personality strengths and assets, the nurse provides the client with a set of guidelines or a framework for identifying those personality strengths (Box 45.3).

Nurses can employ the following specific strategies to reinforce strengths:

- Stressing positive thinking
- Identifying and reinforcing client strengths
- Encouraging clients to set realistic goals
- Acknowledging goals that have been met
- Providing honest, positive feedback

ENHANCING SELF-ESTEEM Nurses must establish a therapeutic relationship with clients who have an altered self-concept. To do this, the nurse must have self-awareness and effective communication skills. The following nursing strategies may help clients identify their problems and enhance their self-concept:

- Encouraging clients to appraise the situation and express their feelings
- Encouraging clients to ask questions
- Providing accurate information
- Becoming aware of distortions, inappropriate or unrealistic standards, and faulty labels in clients' speech

- Exploring clients' positive qualities and strengths
- Encouraging clients to examine more on positive self-evaluation than negative self-evaluation
- Avoiding criticism
- Teaching clients to substitute negative self-talk ("I can't walk to the store anymore") with positive self-talk ("I can walk half a block each morning"). Negative self-talk reinforces a negative self-concept.

Certain strategies vary depending on the age of the client (see the Lifespan Considerations box).

Evaluating

The nurse uses data collected during interactions with the client and significant others to determine whether client outcomes have been met. If outcomes are not achieved, the nurse should explore the reasons and consider asking the following questions:

- Have old situations recurred, triggering feelings or behaviours associated with low self-esteem?
- Have new stressful situations occurred with which the client feels unable to cope, resulting in continuing or recurrent low self-esteem?
- Are new or additional roles causing increased stress in adapting?
- Are significant others supporting the client adequately in attempts to improve self-esteem?
- Did the client follow through on referrals to appropriate agencies? Did the agencies provide the expected services?
- Were the client's expectations realistic in relation to the time needed for successful resolution of self-esteem problems?

BOX 45.3 FRAMEWORK FOR IDENTIFYING PERSONALITY STRENGTHS

Note past, present, and anticipated future participation in the following:

- Hobbies and crafts
- Expressive arts, such as writing, painting, sketching, or music appreciation
- Sports and outdoor activities, including spectator sports
- Education, training, and related areas (including self-education)
- Work, vocation, job, or position

In addition, determine the following:

- Sense of humour and the ability to laugh at self and take "kidding"
- Health status, including healthy aspects of body function and good health maintenance practices

- Special aptitudes, such as sales or mechanical ability; having "a green thumb"; the ability to recognize and enjoy beauty; the ability to solve problems; a liking for adventure or pioneering; perseverance and the drive needed to get things done
- Relationship strengths, including the ability to make people feel comfortable, the capacity to enjoy being with people, the ability to be aware of people's needs and feelings, and the ability to listen
- Emotional strengths, including the capacity to give and receive warmth, affection, and love; the ability to control anger and to feel and express a wide range of emotions; and the capacity for empathy
- Spiritual strengths, such as faith, love of God, and hope.

LIFESPAN CONSIDERATIONS

Enhancing Self-Esteem

CHILDREN

Children build strong self-esteem if they develop five basic attitudes: (a) security and trust, (b) identity, (c) belonging, (d) purpose, and (e) personal competence.

- Security and trust are developed early in life; for example, infants should not be left "to cry it out," but they should learn that they can rely on their parents to meet their needs promptly and consistently. With older children, trust and security are strengthened when adults spend time with them, listening, playing, reading, or just being there. Both emotional and physical contacts, such as a hug, convey warmth and caring.

- Identity is developed when children are allowed to explore and experiment with the world around them and to express themselves as unique individuals in that world. They should be given opportunities to practise who they are. Preschoolers, for example, love to dress themselves and should be allowed to wear outlandish outfits (within limits of weather and safety) if they choose to. Teenagers who try new hair colours and styles, some of which may upset their parents, are engaging in a crucial developmental step.

- Belonging is essential for all humans, and having a sense that others in your social network care about you, want you there, and benefit by your contribution is important to healthy self-esteem. Children gain this sense of belonging by being included in activities, by being praised for their efforts and achievements, and by being valued by parents, siblings, caregivers, and other adults. Parents should make an effort to catch their children doing well and praise them for it (e.g., "I like the way you share with your brother"). Children should also hear that they are valued just for being themselves (e.g., "I like doing things with you. Remember when we went to the park? Wasn't that fun?").

- Purpose and belonging are closely related. Children need opportunities to participate in the family and their community to discover what they can best contribute based on their strengths and skills. For example, a mother might say, "Leo (age 4) is our actor. He is wonderful with costumes and can make any of us smile when he starts his routine." Leo may never become an actor, but he knows he makes a significant contribution to his family's well-being. He brings them joy.

- Personal competence grows as children identify and refine their skill sets. Children develop competence as they confront and solve problems, face challenges, expand their thinking, and are asked to do more than they think they can do. Adults must, however, provide children with support, guidance, appropriate assistance, and constructive feedback (including praise) to prevent the child from being overwhelmed. Too much frustration or uncertainty can lead to giving up, avoidance, lying, bullying, and other antisocial behaviours. If adults help children to accomplish goals that are important to them, children are more likely to develop a sense of personal competence and independence.

- Key ingredients for helping children develop high self-esteem are love, acceptance, firmness, consistency, and the establishment of expectations. Such qualities provide children with a safe, loving, supportive, and predictable world to live in.

ADOLESCENTS

- Provide increasing levels of responsibility. Adolescents need to experience successes and failures and the consequences of their own behaviour.

- Encourage discussion about issues, including problems and mistakes.

- Show appreciation for effort and contributions. Emphasize the process, not just the result.

- Ask for their opinions and suggestions.

- Encourage participation in decision making in areas that affect the adolescent. Show confidence in the teen's judgments.

- Avoid comparison with others, and avoid ridicule or punishment in front of others.

- Assist in the creation of realistic goals and standards.

- Adolescents often engage in volunteer activities in their schools or communities, helping them to identify their strengths and find meaning in their activities. Knowing that they have a purpose and make a difference gives them strong self-esteem.

ADULTS

- Explore the meaning of self-esteem and how the client's self-esteem has influenced past behaviours and actions (and can influence present and future plans and decisions).

- Assist the client in assessing the internal and external forces contributing to or weakening his or her self-esteem.

- Act in ways that demonstrate belief that the person can cope with the realities and demands of life and is worthy of experiencing joy and happiness.

- Avoid comparisons with other people.

- Discourage statements about the self that are negative.

- Encourage the use of affirmations to enhance self-esteem with such statements as "I like myself" or "I am a valuable person."

- Encourage associations with positive, supportive people.

- Make positive statements about the person's past successes (major or minor).

- Help the person to make a list of his or her positive qualities and to review this list often.

- Suggest the person do things for others. Making a positive contribution enhances positive feelings of self-worth.

OLDER ADULTS

The older adult who becomes increasingly dependent can develop low self-esteem. Old age is frequently accompanied by changes, such as reduced income, decline in physical health, loss of friends and family, and retirement. In addition to those actions listed above, nurses can use the following strategies to help older adults enhance their self-esteem:

- Encourage clients to participate in planning their own care.

- Listen carefully to their concerns.

- Assist clients to identify and use their own strengths.

- Encourage them to participate in activities in which they can be successful.

- Be respectful and address the client by name. Focus on the client's strengths and knowledge.

- Encourage clients to stay connected with their memories through reminiscing by writing or recording an autobiography and story telling.

- Promote privacy and respect.

- Encourage creative activities to tap their resources. Examples are music, art, storytelling, quilting, and photography.

- Work with clients to establish achievable goals to bolster self-esteem.

The nurse, client, and significant others need to understand that to change beliefs, feelings, and behaviours affecting self-esteem requires time and ongoing effort. Unlike many physical problems (e.g., wounds) where healing can be quickly observed, improvement in the self-concept can be difficult to evaluate. New crises can cause clients to doubt themselves and revert to former feelings of inadequacy. People can learn from each new situation and gain new strategies for feeling satisfied with themselves.

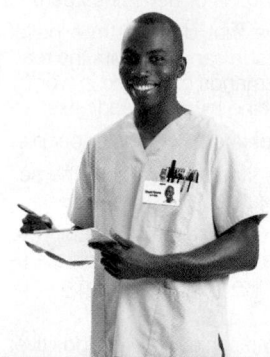

Case Study 45

Craig is a 20-year-old male university student. He was involved in an automobile accident 3 days ago and had to have his left lower leg amputated. Craig's mother has stayed in hospital with him since the accident and is very supportive. His father is grief stricken and is having difficulty dealing with Craig's condition; Craig was captain of his university basketball team and had aspirations of becoming a professional athlete. Craig's condition is stable and he will be transferred to a rehabilitation facility as soon as possible, where he will be fitted for a leg prosthesis. Craig's personality has changed from outgoing to sombre and uncommunicative. He refuses to look at his stump during dressing changes and he will not discuss his rehabilitation program.

CRITICAL THINKING QUESTIONS

1. Given Craig's age, discuss if Craig's self-concept is at risk because of his disability.

2. What data suggest that Craig's self-esteem is negatively affected by his amputation?

3. What factors will have an impact on Craig's ability to adapt to his amputation and to actively engage in the rehabilitation program?

4. How would your nursing interventions differ for a 70-year-old client suffering the loss of a leg in a traumatic incident?

5. How would your approach to this client change if he were from a different culture?

6. What other groups of clients, in addition to those with amputations, are at risk for the development of altered self-esteem or body image?

Check the eText in MyNursingLab for answers and explanations.

KEY TERMS

body image *p. 1477*	introspection *p. 1475*	role conflicts *p. 1479*	self-awareness *p. 1475*
core self-concept *p. 1476*	perceived self *p. 1477*	role development *p. 1478*	self-concept *p. 1475*
global self *p. 1476*	personal identity *p. 1477*	role mastery *p. 1478*	self-esteem *p. 1479*
global self-esteem *p. 1479*	role *p. 1478*	role performance *p. 1478*	specific
ideal self *p. 1477*	role ambiguity *p. 1478*	role strain *p. 1479*	self-esteem *p. 1479*

CHAPTER HIGHLIGHTS

- A positive self-concept is essential to a person's physical and psychological well-being.

- A person's self-perception can differ from the person's perception of how others see him or her and from the ideal self, that is, how the person would like to be.

- Interactions with significant others create the conditions that influence self-concept throughout life.

- When individuals are able to conceptualize the self, they begin a lifelong process of deciding whether and to what extent they are valuable and worthy.

- Individuals who grow up in families whose members value one another are likely to feel good about themselves.

- Factors affecting self-concept include development, family and culture, stressors, resources, history of success and failure, and illness.

- The nurse assesses four areas of self-concept: personal identity, body image, self-esteem, and role performance.

- Because a positive self-concept is basic to health, one of the nurse's major responsibilities is to help clients whose self-concept is disturbed to develop a more positive and realistic image of themselves.

- A trusting client–nurse relationship is essential for the effective assessment of a client's self-concept, for providing help and support, and for motivating client behaviour change.

ASSESS YOUR LEARNING

1. Julie, 10 years old, is newly diagnosed with type 1 diabetes mellitus. The nurse is assisting Julie and her family to understand this new diagnosis. Julie's parents are unsure if she should resume playing soccer. Julie cries and states, "I will never be normal again." What is the nurse's MOST appropriate response?

   a. "That's not true. Crying will only make you feel worse."

   b. "You are normal, Julie, even with diabetes."

   c. "Even with diabetes, you can still lead a normal life."

   d. "Other children have been diagnosed with diabetes."

2. Students who are juggling the responsibilities of work, school, and family are MOST likely to experience which of the following?

   a. Role ambiguity

   b. Role strain

   c. Role conflict

   d. Role enhancement

3. Which of the following is an appropriate desired health outcome for clients with situational low self-esteem?

   a. The client will demonstrate restored self-esteem.

   b. The client will consistently verbalize self-acceptance.

   c. The client will teach adaptive skills.

   d. The client will describe preoccupation with altered self.

4. An 89-year-old client states, "I'm a lost cause. I can't even stand long enough to cook my own meals anymore." Which of the following is the MOST appropriate response?

   a. "That must be difficult. What things are you still able to do?"

   b. "Well, that is to be expected at your age."

   c. "Do you have someone else who can cook for you?"

   d. "Do you consider yourself a good cook?"

5. An adult who has failed to satisfactorily resolve the developmental task of adolescence—identity versus confusion—is MOST likely to show which of the following behaviours?

   a. Is able to assert independence

   b. Is unable to express personal desires

   c. Has difficulty working as a member of a team

   d. Goes along with the crowd in all activities

6. When asked to describe herself, a client newly diagnosed with a chronic illness describes only those roles involving others (e.g., wife, mother, medical assistant) and no personal hobbies or interests. Which of the following would be a priority nursing intervention for this client?

   a. The nurse should encourage the client to identify how her treatment will affect her ability to perform those roles.

   b. The nurse should encourage the client to explore the importance of and need for personal hobbies or interests.

   c. The nurse should encourage the client to insist that her family be present while the treatment plan is being developed.

   d. The nurse should encourage the client to go for psychological counselling for role performance in addition to her medical treatment.

7. You are caring for a client who has a nursing diagnosis of *Chronic Low Self-Esteem*. Which of the following behaviours is consistent with this diagnosis?

   a. The client is assertive with authority figures.

   b. The client consistently performs his family role of father.

   c. The client works hard to achieve personal goals.

   d. The client has difficulty making positive observations about himself.

8. Which of the following interventions are appropriate for a client with low or poor self-concept?

   a. Encourage the client to compare herself with others.

   b. Encourage the client to say positive things about herself.

   c. Recommend the client avoid situations of having to care for others.

   d. Communicate very low expectations of the client.

9. You are caring for a client with a diagnosis of *Low Self-Esteem* who is from a different cultural background. Which of the following nursing interventions BEST demonstrates awareness of the need to be sensitive to cultural differences?

   a. Use therapeutic silence appropriately for the client's culture.

   b. Avoid discussing issues of noncompliance with the client.

   c. Frequently use therapeutic touch to communicate with the client.

   d. Have the client validate your perceptions of what he is saying or doing.

10. You are caring for Mrs. Johnston, a 65-year-old client with a history of demanding and aggressive behaviour. She reminds you of your grandmother. When you find yourself avoiding this client, you become concerned and seek out a colleague with

whom to share your feelings about this situation. What does this behaviour BEST indicate?

a. An ineffective coping strategy

b. Insufficient knowledge about the client

c. Your lack of self-confidence in handling difficult clients

d. An appropriate response based on your awareness of your own behaviour

Check the eText in MyNursingLab for answers and explanations.

WEBLINKS

Growing Healthy Canadians

http://www.growinghealthykids.com/english/home/index.html

This site contains a guide for positive child development developed around six perspectives, what is known about the factors that promote the healthy development of all children and youth, and the concept of developmental transitions; and four areas of focus: positive outcomes, important influences, multiple contributors, and effective strategies.

Public Health Agency of Canada

http://www.phac-aspc.gc.ca

This site provides access to a number of publications relevant to self-concept and self-esteem issues of Canadians across the lifespan. A search engine allows for easy access to articles and links.

MyNursingLab

MyNursingLab's guided learning path makes reviewing and test preparation straightforward.

– Content summaries, animations, and videos reinforce key concepts and skills

– Practice questions help with test prep by showing gaps in knowledge

– An eText, available online and via the iPad, makes searching, highlighting, and note-taking easy

---

This QR code appears at the end of every chapter and provides learning resources that you can access with your smartphone to study on the go. Access self-review quizzes, flashcards, and more!

REFERENCES

Bosson, J. K., & Swann, W. B., Jr. (2009). Self-esteem: Nature, origins, and consequences. In R. Hoyle & M. Leary (Eds.), *Handbook of individual differences in social behavior* (pp. 527–546). New York, NY: Guilford.

Eckroth-Bucher, M. (2010). Self-awareness: A review and analysis of a basic nursing concept. *Advances in Nursing Science, 33*(4), 297–309.

Erikson, E. H. (1963). *Childhood and society* (2nd ed.). New York, NY: Norton.

Hagger, M. S., & Stevenson, A. (2010). Social physique anxiety and physical self-esteem: Gender and age effects. *Psychology & Health, 25*(1), 89–110. doi: 10.1080/08870440903160990

Jackson, L., vonEye, A., Fitzgerald, H., Zhao, Y., & Witt, E. (2010). Self-concept, self-esteem, gender, race and information technology use. *Computers in Human Behavior, 26*(3), 323–328. doi: 10.1016/j.chb.2009.11.001

Kraus, M., Chen, S., & Keltner, D. (2011). The power to be me: Power elevates self-concept, consistency and authenticity. *Journal of Experimental Social Psychology, 47*(5), 974–980. doi: 10.1016/j.jesp.2011.03.017

Lodi-Smith, J., & Roberts, B. W. (2010). Getting to know me: Social role experiences and age differences in self-concept clarity during adulthood. *Journal of Personality, 78*(5), 1383–1410. doi:10.1111/j.1467-6494.2010.00655.x

Nolan, K. P., & Harold, C. M. (2010). Fit with what? The influence of multiple self-concept images on organizational attraction. *Journal of Occupational & Organizational Psychology, 83*(3), 645–662. doi: 10.1348/096317909X465452

Richards, K. C., Campenni, C., & Muse-Burke, J. L. (2010). Self-care and well-being in mental health professionals: The mediating effects of self-awareness and mindfulness. *Journal of Mental Health Counseling, 32*(3), 247–264.

Sides-Moore, L., & Tochkov, K. (2011). The thinner the better? Competitiveness, depression and body image among college student women. *College Student Journal, 45*(2), 439–448. Retrieved from http://www.readperiodicals .com/201106/2384154341.html

Slevec, J., & Tiggemann, M. (2010). Attitudes toward cosmetic surgery in middle-aged women: Body image, aging anxiety, and the media. *Psychology of Women Quarterly, 34*(1), 65–74. doi:10.1111/j.1471-6402.2009.01542.x

Taylor, C., & Peter, T. (2011). We are not aliens, we're people, and we have rights. *Canadian Review of Sociology, 48*(3), 275–312. doi:10.1111/j.1755-618X.2011.01266.x

Chapter 46

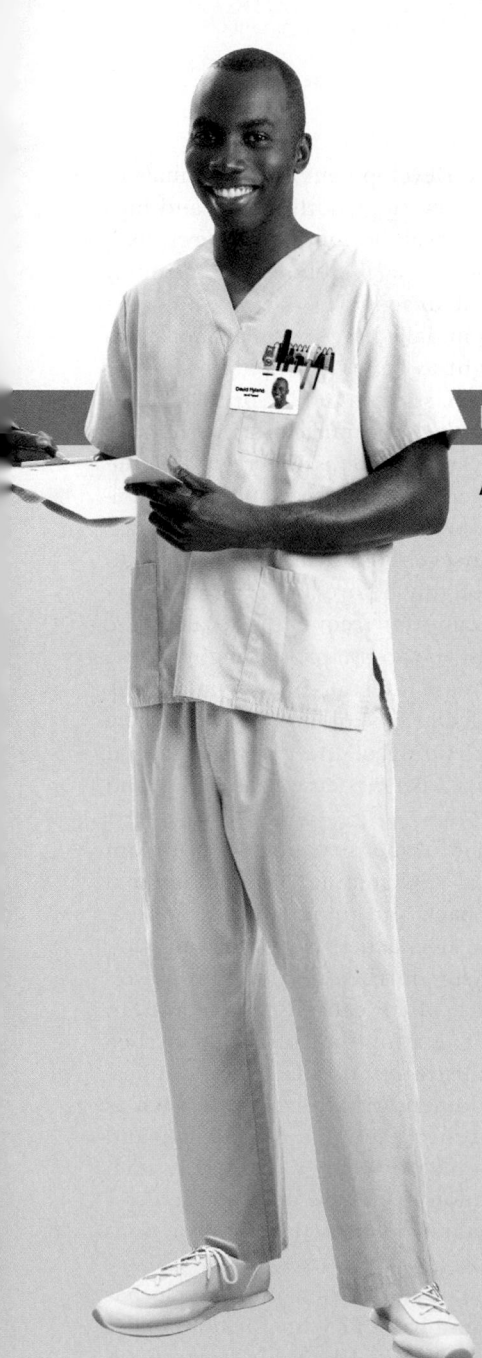

Sexuality

LEARNING OUTCOMES

After completing this chapter, you will be able to:

1. Describe sexual development and concerns across the lifespan.

2. Define sexual health.

3. Discuss the varieties of sexuality.

4. Give examples of how the family, culture, religion, and personal expectations and ethics influence one's sexuality.

5. Describe physiological changes in males and females during the sexual response cycle.

6. Identify the forms of male and female altered sexual function.

7. Prepare basic sexual questions the nurse should ask during client assessment.

8. Formulate nursing diagnoses and interventions for the client experiencing sexual problems.

9. Recognize health-promotion teaching related to reproductive structures.

H umans are sexual beings. Regardless of gender, age, race, socioeconomic status, religious beliefs, physical and mental health, cultural practices, or other demographic factors, sexuality is individually expressed in a variety of ways throughout people's lives. **Sexuality** is "a central aspect of being human throughout life . . . and can be expressed in thoughts, fantasies, desires, beliefs, attitudes, values, behaviours, practices, roles, and relationships. . . . Sexuality is influenced by the interaction of biological, psychological, social, economic, political, cultural, ethical, legal, historical, religious and spiritual factors" (Public Health Agency of Canada, 2008, p. 5). Satisfying or "normal" sexual expression can generally be described as whatever behaviours give pleasure and satisfaction to those adults involved, without threat of coercion or injury to self or others. What constitutes normal sexual expression, however, varies among religions and cultures.

Development of Sexuality

The development of sexuality begins with conception and continues throughout the lifespan. Table 46.1 outlines characteristics of sexual development through the lifespan, with nursing interventions and teaching guidelines for each developmental stage.

Birth to 12 Years

The ability of the human body to experience a sexual response is present even before birth. When babies find their fingers and toes, they also find their genitals. They seem to experience a pleasurable sensation from the touch, but one would not call this a *sexual experience*. By the age of 3 years, more purposeful **masturbation** (excitation of one's own or another's genital organs by means other than sexual intercourse) begins, and the orgasmic response is quite common, although males do not ejaculate until after puberty. By age 2½ or 3 years, children know their gender and have a beginning awareness of genital differences between males and females.

Around age 9 or 10 years, the first physical changes of puberty begin: the development of breast buds in girls and the growth of pubic hair in both males and females. As the adrenal glands mature, they produce more testosterone and estradiol, which contribute to the first experiences of sexual attraction to another person. Girls need to be taught about **menstruation** (monthly uterine bleeding) and related self-care.

Adolescence

During early adolescence (12 to 13 years), primary and secondary sex characteristics continue to develop. In boys, the testes and scrotum increase in size, the skin over the scrotum becomes darker, pubic hair grows, and

axillary sweating begins. Development of the genitals to adult size takes 5 to 6 years. In girls, the pelvis and hips broaden, breast tissues develop, pubic hair grows, axillary sweating begins, and vaginal secretions become milky and change from alkaline to acid pH.

Teenage girls may initially have irregular menstruation. They can be taught to be aware of subtle signs of impending menstruation, such as tender breasts, water retention or bloating, or the appearance of skin eruptions or pimples. Girls should also be counselled regarding the variety of feminine hygiene products available (e.g., sanitary pads and tampons) so that they can make appropriate choices. Parents and nurses should advise teenage girls to wash their hands thoroughly before and after inserting a tampon, to change tampons frequently, to alternate them with sanitary pads, and to use pads at night. These measures will help decrease infection, including the risk of "toxic shock," a particular type of *Staphylococcus aureus* infection. Thorough cleaning of the genital area and wiping from front to back will also decrease infection and prevent odours.

Dysmenorrhea (painful menstruation) is prevalent among adolescent females. Cramping, lower abdominal pain radiating to the back and upper thighs, nausea, vomiting, diarrhea, and headaches may occur for a few hours up to 3 days. Dysmenorrhea results from powerful uterine contractions, which cause ischemia and, in turn, cramping pain. The symptoms of dysmenorrhea are treated with administration of analgesics; application of heat to the abdomen; certain exercises, such as abdominal muscle strengthening; biofeedback; and nonsteroidal anti-inflammatory drugs (NSAIDs), such as ibuprofen. Masturbation to achieve orgasm also eases cramping through the associated uterine contractions and increased blood flow (Levin, 2007).

In Canada, the mean age of first intercourse has gradually been decreasing from 17 years for both males and females since the 1960s to 16.5 years (Roterman, 2005). Compared with young men in other countries,

TABLE 46.1 Sexual Development throughout Life

Stage	Characteristics	Nursing Interventions and Teaching Guidelines
Infancy		
Birth to 18 months	Given gender assignment of male or female Differentiates self from others gradually External genitals sensitive to touch Penile erections in male infants; vaginal lubrication in female infants	Self-manipulation of genitals is normal. Caregivers need to recognize these behaviours as common in children.
Toddler		
1–3 years	Continues to develop gender identity Able to identify own gender	Body exploration and genital fondling are normal. Children use names for body parts. Children from single-parent homes should have contact with adults of both sexes.
Preschooler		
4–5 years	Becomes increasingly aware of self Explores own and playmates' body parts Learns correct names for body parts Learns to control feelings and behaviour Focuses love on parent of the opposite sex	Answer questions about "where babies come from" honestly and simply. Parental overreaction to exploration of genitals and masturbation can lead to feelings that sex is "bad."
School Age		
6–12 years	Has strong identification with parent of same gender Tends to have friends of the same gender Has increasing awareness of self Increased modesty; desire for privacy Continues self-stimulating behaviour Learns the role and concepts of own gender as part of the total self-concept At about 8 or 9 years becomes concerned about specific sexual behaviours and often approaches parents with explicit concerns about sexuality and reproduction	Provide parents and children with opportunities to express their concerns and ask questions regarding sex. Answer all questions with factual data and perhaps follow up with appropriate books and other material. Advise parents to discuss basic information about sexual intercourse, menstruation, and reproduction with children at about 10 years of age. Give children reading material, and then discuss it with them.
Adolescence		
12–18 years	Development of primary and secondary sex characteristics Occurrence of menarche Development of relationships with interested partners Masturbation a common occurrence May participate in sexual activity May experiment with homosexual relationships At risk for pregnancy and sexually transmitted infections (STIs)	Adolescents require information about body changes. Peer groups have great importance at this time and assist in forming gender roles. Dating helps adolescents prepare for adult roles. Parents influence values and beliefs regarding behaviour. Teenagers require information about contraceptive measures and precautions to STIs.
Young Adulthood		
18–40 years	Sexual activity common Establishes own lifestyle and values Homosexual identity usually established by mid-20s Couples sharing financial obligations and household tasks	Young adults often require information about measures to prevent unwanted pregnancies (i.e., abstinence or contraceptive devices). They require information to prevent STIs. Regular communication is required to understand partner's sexual needs and to work through problems and stresses.

(continued)

TABLE 46.1   *(continued)*

Stage	Characteristics	Nursing Interventions and Teaching Guidelines
Middle Adulthood		
40–65 years	Men and women experience decreased hormone production. Menopause occurs in women, usually any time between 40 and 55 years. The climacteric occurs gradually in men. The quality, rather than the number, of sexual experiences becomes important. Individuals establish independent moral and ethical standards.	Women and men may need help adjusting to new roles. People may require counselling to help them re-evaluate and direct their energies. Encourage couples to look at the positive aspects of this time of life.
Late Adulthood		
65 years and over	Interest in sexual activity often continues. Sexual activity may be less frequent. Women's vaginal secretions diminish, and breasts atrophy. Men produce fewer sperm and need more time to achieve an erection and to ejaculate.	Older adults often continue to be sexually active. Couples may require counselling about adapting their affection and sexual needs to physical limitations.

those under the age of 16 years are less likely to have had their first intercourse. Canadian adolescents who are having intercourse at a younger age are likely to be Canadian-born youth who are from lower-income households and those who drop out of school. These groups tend to form a particular subset of youth, who are marginalized in a number of ways, which may contribute to early sexual activity (Smylie, Medaglia, & Maticka-Tyndale, 2006). However, according to the Toronto Teen Survey, Asian or East Asian youth were less likely to engage in higher levels of sexual behaviour. Those who were Muslim and those not born in Canada were also less likely to report these behaviours (Pole & Flicker, 2010).

Adolescence is a time for sexual experimentation. According to the Canadian report *Sexual Health in Canada–Baseline 2007* (Canadian Federation for Sexual Health, 2007), adolescent pregnancy, abortion, and birth rates are declining, which suggests that young Canadian women are exercising greater control over their fertility. The number of sexually active youth who report having only one lifetime partner is increasing, and the number who report having six or more partners is decreasing. The greater majority report using some form of contraception during their last intercourse, and yet many are not choosing safer sex practices, such as condom use. The STI rates among youth continue to rise. In another report (Rothermann, 2008) in 2005, 58% of Quebec teens reported having had sexual intercourse compared with 37% in Ontario and 40% in British Columbia. Teen pregnancy is still widely prevalent in Canada (Health Nexus Santé, 2007, 2008, 2009).

Human immunodeficiency virus (HIV) and acquired immunodeficiency syndrome (AIDS) are spread mainly through intravenous drug use, and the rates are rising among Aboriginals and Canadian women between the ages of 15 and 29 years. Although the highest number of new HIV and hepatitis C virus infections continues to be among gay men (45%), 27% of new infections are among women, who now make up more than 20% of the 58 000 Canadians living with HIV or AIDS, and many are unaware of their infections (Miller, Strathdee, Kerr, Li, & Wood, 2006). Human papilloma virus (HPV) infection is now a well-established cause of cervical cancer. Canada has a population of 13.53 million women ages 15 years and older who are at risk of developing cervical cancer. Cervical cancer ranks as the twelfth most frequent cancer among women in Canada, and the third most frequent cancer among women between 15 and 44 years of age. The HPV vaccine is currently recommended for females in the 9-to-26–year age group. STIs are the most common bacterial infections among adolescents (see Table 46.2). Teens need education about these diseases, preventive measures, and early treatment.

Adolescents want to know about sexual behaviours but are often uneasy about discussing these concerns with their parents. Nurses, the schools, and the family need to provide accurate information. During the nursing assessment, teenagers should be asked directly what they know about sex, contraception, and reproduction.

Often, a lot of the teenager's information is based on popular myths and little, if any, on fact. The nurse should discuss factual information about sex, sexual activities and their consequences, the individual's right to make a decision regarding ways to express oneself sexually, and the

TABLE 46.2 Sexually Transmitted Infections

Infection	Male	Female
Gonorrhea	Painful urination; urethritis with watery white discharge, which may become purulent	May be asymptomatic; or vaginal discharge, pain, and urinary frequency may be present
Syphilis	Chancre, usually on glans penis, which is painless and heals in 4–6 weeks; secondary symptoms—skin eruptions, low-grade fever, inflammation of lymph glands—in 6 weeks to 6 months after chancre heals	Chancre on cervix or other genital areas, which heals in 4–6 weeks; symptoms same as for male
Genital warts (*Condyloma acuminatum*)	Caused by human papilloma virus (HPV); single lesions or clusters of lesions growing beneath or on the foreskin, at external meatus, or on the glans penis; on dry skin areas, lesions are hard and yellow-grey; on moist areas, lesions are pink or red and soft with a cauliflower-like appearance	Certain strains of HPV linked to cervical cancer; lesions may be found on vulva, urethra, vagina, cervix, and anus
Chlamydial urethritis	Urinary frequency; watery, mucoid urethral discharge	Commonly carriers; vaginal discharge, dysuria, urinary frequency
Trichomoniasis	Slight itching; moisture on top of penis; slight, early morning urethral discharge; many males asymptomatic	Itching and redness of vulva and skin inside thighs; copious watery, frothy vaginal discharge
Candidiasis	Itching, irritation, discharge, plaque of cheesy material under foreskin	Red and excoriated vulva; intense itching of vaginal and vulvar tissues; thick, white, cheesy or curd-like discharge
Acquired immunodeficiency syndrome (AIDS)	HIV attacks the person's immune system, diminishing the number of CD4 cells and lowering the person's resistance to opportunistic infections. A person is diagnosed with AIDS by the presence of 1 of the 21 opportunistic infections or a CD4 level of <200. Symptoms can appear anytime from several months to several years after acquiring the virus; reduced immunity to other diseases; symptoms include any of the following for which there is no other explanation: persistent heavy night sweats; extreme fatigue; severe weight loss; enlarged lymph glands in neck, axillae, or groin; persistent diarrhea; skin rashes; blurred vision or chronic headache; harsh, dry cough; thick grey-white coating on tongue or throat	
Herpes genitalis (herpes simplex of the genitals)	Primary herpes involves the presence of painful sores or large, discrete vesicles that last for weeks; vesicles rupture; recurrent herpes itchy rather than painful; lasts for a few hours to 10 days	
Hepatitis B	No symptoms in 30% of infected people; symptoms, if present, include jaundice (yellowing of the skin and eyes), fatigue, loss of appetite, joint pain, abdominal pain, and general feelings of malaise	
Human papilloma virus (HPV)	More than 100 known types of HPV, which are sexually transmitted; can cause anal-genital warts in men and women, although infections are often asymptomatic; the high-risk type HPV is linked to cervical cancer in women and penile cancer in men; no tests available for the detection of HPV, but Papanicolaou (Pap) test can increase chances of early detection of abnormalities or precancerous cells in the cervix	

responsibilities of each person with respect to sexual activity. (See Table 46.3 on the next page).

Adulthood

During early adulthood, many people form emotional and sexual relationships and cohabitate with partners. Individuals establish their own value systems and develop lifestyles that reflect these personal values. Although some young adults partner in marriage and start to raise children, others cohabitate with sexual partners, live alone, or live with persons with whom they are not sexually involved.

Sexual activity is common throughout adulthood and includes not only sexual intercourse but also touching, masturbation, oral sex, sexual fantasies, and other sources of pleasure. Difficulties can arise in heterosexual relationships because of differences in sexual desire and sexual response between individuals. Gay and lesbian couples often fare better in this respect. Couples need to

TABLE 46.3 Common Sexual Misconceptions

Misconception	Fact
Nearly all men over 70 years old have erectile dysfunction.	Sexual ability is not lost due to aging. Changes are commonly due to disease or medication.
Masturbation causes certain mental instabilities.	Masturbation is a common and healthy behaviour.
Sexual activity weakens a person.	There is no evidence that sexual activity weakens a person.
Women who have experienced orgasm are more likely to become pregnant.	Conceiving is not related to experiencing orgasm.
"Nice" girls should not feel entitled to sexual satisfaction.	As women become more comfortable with their own sexuality, they advocate for their own sexual fulfillment.
A large penis provides greater sexual satisfaction to women than does a small penis.	There is no evidence that a large penis provides greater satisfaction.
Alcohol is a sexual stimulant.	Alcohol is a relaxant and central nervous system depressant. Chronic alcoholism is associated with erectile dysfunction.
Intercourse during menstruation is dangerous (i.e., it will cause vaginal tissue damage).	There is no physiological basis for abstinence during menses.
The face-to-face coital position is the moral or proper one.	The position that offers the most pleasure and is acceptable to both partners is the correct one.

communicate their sexual needs to each other to support the growth and development of a successful intimate relationship. Young adults should also be aware that because sexual needs and responses may change, each partner should listen and respond to the needs of the other.

Sexual desire and response are affected by social, religious, and cultural circumstances and biological changes throughout adulthood. During pregnancy, for example, some women and men express concerns about sexual intercourse. Intercourse is generally safe in a healthy pregnancy up to the last month before delivery. The sexual lives of young adults are also affected by the demands of raising young children and the fatigue and stress of busy schedules (Polomeno & Dubeau, 2009).

During middle adulthood, both men and women experience decreased hormone production, causing the climacteric, usually called **menopause** in women. **Andropause** is the phase in men's lives in which they experience a gradual reduction in the production of testosterone and sperm by the testes (see Chapter 19).

Older adults may define sexuality far more broadly and include in their definition such things as touching, hugging, romantic gestures (e.g., giving or receiving roses), comfort, warmth, dressing up, joy, spirituality, and beauty. Interest in sexual activity is not lost as people age. For men, however, more time is needed to achieve an erection and to ejaculate (the erection may last longer than at a younger age); more direct genital stimulation is required to achieve an erection; the volume of ejaculated fluid decreases; and the intensity of contractions with orgasm may decrease. The refractory period after orgasm

is longer. Older women remain capable of multiple orgasms and may, in fact, experience an increase in sexual desire after menopause. Vaginal lubrication and elasticity decrease with menopause and decreased estrogen, and phases of the sexual response cycle may take longer to occur. There is a possibility of pain during sexual activity and intercourse (dyspareunia) related to vaginal dryness or chronic health conditions (e.g., diabetes or arthritis). Lack of privacy may be a concern for older adults who live with family or in a rehabilitation or nursing home facility. Many products are available to assist older adults with enhancing their sexual experiences. These range from simple lubricants (Andelloux, 2010) to medications and surgically implanted devices that enable penile erections. The nurse should never assume that they are less interested or motivated to have an active sex life.

Sexual Health

Sexual health is an individual and constantly changing phenomenon falling within the wide range of human sexual thoughts, feelings, needs, and desires. For most people, sexual health is not a concern until its absence or impairment is noticed. **Sexual health** is defined as "a state of physical, emotional, mental and social well-being in relation to sexuality: it is not merely the absence of disease, dysfunction or infirmity. Sexual health requires a positive and respectful approach to sexuality and sexual relationships, as well as the possibility of having

BOX 46.1 CHARACTERISTICS OF SEXUAL HEALTH

- Knowledge about sexuality and sexual behaviour
- Ability to express one's full sexual potential, excluding all forms of sexual coercion, exploitation, and abuse
- Ability to make autonomous decisions about one's sexual life within a context of personal and social ethics
- Experience of sexual pleasure as a source of physical, psychological, cognitive, and spiritual well-being
- Capability to express sexuality through communication, touch, emotional expression, and love
- Right to make free and responsible reproductive choices
- Ability to access sexual health care for the prevention and treatment of all sexual concerns, problems, and disorders

Source: From World Association of Sexology. (1999). *Declaration of sexual rights.* Adopted at the 14th World Congress of Sexology, Hong Kong and People's Republic of China.

EVIDENCE INFORMED PRACTICE

What Motivates Women to Remove Their Pubic Hair?

In this exploratory, descriptive study on women's motivations and practices regarding pubic hair removal, 660 Canadian women, ages 15 to 50 years, were asked about their reasons for, methods of, and side effects associated with this practice. Appearance in a bathing suit and the desire to feel more attractive and cleaner were the most common reasons. The three most common methods were shaving, salon waxing, and trimming with scissors. Side effects included razor bumps, ingrown hairs, rash, pimples, and cuts.

NURSING IMPLICATIONS: The practice of pubic hair removal is becoming more common among women, especially those in the younger age group. Microabrasions, contact dermatitis, and skin disruption pose the risk for the transmission of viruses, including HIV, hepatitis virus, herpes simplex virus, and human papilloma virus. Little is known about hygienic practices in salons and other aesthetics services that remain unregulated. Best practice guidelines for nurses in relation to this practice need to be developed to prevent the transmission of infection.

Source: Based on Riddell, L., Varto, H., & Hodgson, Z. G. (2010). Smooth talking: The phenomenon of pubic hair removal in women. *Canadian Journal of Human Sexuality, 19*(3), 121–130.

pleasurable and safe sexual experiences, free of coercion, discrimination and violence. For sexual health to be attained and maintained, the sexual rights of all persons must be respected, protected and fulfilled" (Public Health Agency of Canada, 2008). The characteristics of sexual health are listed in Box 46.1.

Components of Sexual Health

Five critical components of sexual health are (a) sexual self-concept, (b) body image, (c) gender identity, (d) gender-role behaviour, and (e) freedoms and responsibilities.

One's **sexual self-concept** (how one values oneself as a sexual being) determines with whom one will have sex, the gender and kinds of people a person is attracted to, and the values about when, where, with whom, and how one expresses sexuality. A positive sexual self-concept enables people to form intimate relationships throughout life. A negative sexual self-concept may impede the formation of relationships.

Body image is how a person feels about his or her body. Pregnancy, aging, trauma, disease, and therapies can alter an individual's appearance and function, which can affect body image. People who feel good about their bodies are likely to be comfortable with and enjoy sexual activity. People who have a poor body image may respond negatively to sexual arousal. A major influence on body image for women is the media focus on physical attractiveness and breast size. Likewise, many men worry about penis size. The myth that "larger is better," particularly if the penis is erect and has staying power, is pervasive in North America. A person's body image can suffer when unable to achieve these expectations. (See the Evidence-Informed Practice box.)

Gender identity is one's self-image as a female or male. More than just the biological component, it also includes social and cultural norms. Gender identity is the result of a long series of developmental events that may or may not conform to one's apparent biological sex. Once gender identity is established, it cannot be easily changed.

Gender-role behaviour is an expression of a person's sense of maleness or femaleness as well as what is perceived as gender-appropriate behaviour. Each society defines its roles for males and females; boys are expected to behave in a "masculine" way, and girls are reinforced for "feminine" behaviours (see Figure 46.1).

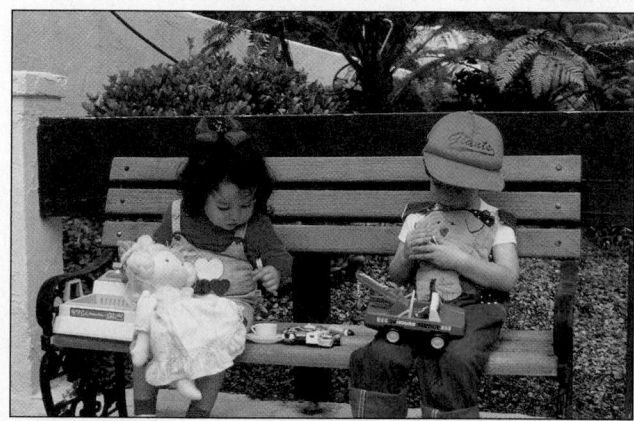

FIGURE 46.1 Children express gender role behaviour at an early age.

In North America, expected adult male roles include breadwinner, lover, father, and athlete. Expected male behaviours include wearing trousers, demonstrating physical strength, and expressing feelings in a controlled fashion. Women are expected to express their emotions more freely and to be gentler in their physical responses; they also have a broader choice of clothing than men do.

Androgyny, or flexibility in gender roles, is the belief that most characteristics and behaviours are human qualities that should not be limited to one specific gender or the other. Androgynous describes the degree of flexibility a person has regarding gender-stereotypic behaviours. Adults who can behave flexibly regarding their sexual roles may be able to adapt better than those who adopt rigid stereotyped gender roles.

Sexual health includes both freedoms and responsibilities. Sexually healthy people engage in activities that are freely chosen, including both self-pleasuring and shared-pleasuring activities. Individuals also have freedom of their sexual thoughts, feelings, and fantasies. Sexually healthy people are ethically motivated to exercise behavioural, emotional, economic, and social responsibility for themselves (Kleinplatz, 2012).

Variations in Sexuality

People differ in the way they prioritize sexuality in their lives. Variations in how people experience and express their sexuality include sexual orientation, gender identity, and erotic preferences.

Sexual Orientation

One's attraction to people of the same sex, to people of the opposite sex, or to both sexes is referred to as **sexual orientation**. Sexual orientation lies along a continuum, with a wide range between the two extremes of exclusively heterosexual attraction and exclusively homosexual attraction. Individuals who are attracted to people of both genders are referred to as *bisexuals*.

The origins of sexual orientation are still not well understood. Some biological theories describe sexual orientation in terms of the genetic composition of the individual. Psychological theories stress the role of early learning experiences and cognitive processes. Other theories acknowledge the confluence of genetics and the environment in the development of sexual orientation.

Estimates of the percentage of the population with a homosexual orientation vary, although the usual figure is 5% to 10% of men and 2% to 4% of women (Rayside, 2008). Because these individuals are aware of the discrimination they face, many do not disclose their sexual orientation; thus, actual figures are not available. In 2009, the first Canadian Health Survey (Statistics Canada,

2010) included a question on sexual orientation, and found that 1% of Canadians ages 18 to 59 years reported that they considered themselves homosexual (gay or lesbian), and 0.7% in the same age group reported that they considered themselves bisexual.

Gay, lesbian, bisexual, transgendered, and queer (LGBTQ) youth often remain closeted (not disclosing their sexual orientation) in their interactions with friends, family, and in school throughout adolescence. In the first Canadian study on gay, lesbian, and bisexual youth in high schools (Taylor et al., 2011), 74% of transgendered students, 55% of sexual minority students, and 26% of non-LGBTQ students reported having been verbally harassed about their gender expression, and 37% of transgendered students, 32% of female sexual minority students, and 20% of male sexual minority students reported being verbally harassed daily or weekly about their sexual orientation. More than 1 in 5 (21%) LGBTQ students reported being physically harassed or assaulted because of their sexual orientation. During adolescence, many young people deal with issues related to self-esteem, belonging, and identity. For lesbian, gay, and bisexual youth, these struggles are increased with the tensions of living in a heteronormative society and few visible role models for their development. For immigrant youth from other countries, this situation becomes more critical, as LGBTQ people may be shunned in their former countries. Homosexuality is considered illegal in certain countries.

Gender Identity

Western culture is deeply committed to the idea that there are only two genders. In some cases, sex is clear; in other cases, such as in transsexuals, cross-dressers, or a blending of both sexes within the same individual, it is unclear.

INTERSEX About 1 in every 2000 babies is born with an **intersex** condition, in which contradictions exist among chromosomal sex, gonadal sex, internal organs, and external genital appearance. The sex of an intersexed person is ambiguous; some parts usually associated with males and some parts usually associated with females. Intersex anatomy may not be apparent at birth. Sometimes, it is undetected until puberty, until the person is identified as an infertile adult, or until the person dies and an autopsy is performed.

TRANSGENDERISM The medical profession considers **transgender individuals** to have a condition called *gender dysphoria* (strong and persistent feelings of discomfort with the assigned gender) or *gender identity disorder*. For the transgendered person, sexual anatomy is not consistent with gender identity. Those who are born physically male but are emotionally and psychologically female are called male-to-female (MTF) transgenders. Those who are born female but are emotionally and psychologically male are called female-to-male (FTM) transgenders (Beemyn, Rankin, & Beemyn, 2011).

Most transgendered people have felt gender dysphoria since early childhood. They often suffer for many years and try to hide the situation from family and friends for fear of being considered mentally unstable. Being transgendered puts women and men at extreme risk of the following:

- Being ridiculed and humiliated
- Being in constant jeopardy in getting and keeping a job
- Being evicted without cause from restaurants and stores
- Being denied housing
- Being refused medical treatment, even to save their lives (Girshick & Green, 2009)

As self-understanding and acceptance increase, many transgendered individuals live partly or fully as members of the opposite sex. Their sexual orientation may be heterosexual, homosexual, or bisexual.

CROSS-DRESSERS **Cross-dressing** (dressing in the clothing of the opposite sex) makes one's outward appearance consistent with their inner identity and gender role and increases their comfort with themselves. Cross-dressers are typically males who cross-dress to express the feminine side of their personality. Cross-dressers usually are not interested in permanently altering their bodies through surgical means. The majority of them are comfortable with their original birth gender identity and behaviour in their public and professional lives.

Cross-dressing is a conscious choice and may occur at home or in public settings. It occurs more frequently in cultures where males are expected to be strong, independent, and unemotional protectors. Some men may need to express their gentleness and dependence by creating a separate world and female persona within that rigid social climate.

Erotic Preferences

Sexual fantasies and single-partner sex are the most common sexual outlets for women and men, single and coupled persons, and heterosexual, gay/lesbian, and bisexual persons. Masturbation is the way erotic feelings are discovered and sexual response is learned. Mutual masturbation can provide sexual pleasuring and intimacy without hurrying to genital interaction before both partners are ready.

The technical term for male-to-female or female-to-female **oral–genital sex** is *cunnilingus*. This involves kissing, licking, or sucking of the female genitals, including the mons pubis, vulva, clitoris, labia, and vagina. Fellatio is oral stimulation of the penis by licking and sucking.

The term "sixty-nine" refers to simultaneous oral–genital stimulation by two persons. Preconceptions and myths are a major deterrent for those who have not tried oral sex. However, like most sexual practices, oral–genital sex is not completely free of the risk for transmission of STIs, and safe sex practices must be used.

Anal stimulation can be a source of sexual pleasure because the anus has a rich supply of nerves. Stimulation may be applied with fingers, mouth, or sex toys, such as vibrators. The anus is surrounded by strong muscles, and the rectum contains no natural lubrication. Thus, inserting a finger or penis in the rectum requires relaxation and a water-soluble lubricant.

A common form of sexual activity for heterosexual couples is **genital intercourse**. Penile–vaginal intercourse (coitus) can be both physically and emotionally satisfying. Various positions are assumed for this kind of intercourse; the most common is lying face to face (with female or male on top). Side-lying, standing, sitting, and rear-entry positions are also used. Side-lying, female-on-top, and rear-entry positions facilitate clitoral stimulation, either by penile or manual contact. The choice of intercourse positions and activities depends on physical comfort and beliefs, values, and attitudes about different practices.

During intercourse, the man moves the penis back and forth along the vaginal walls by rhythmic thrusting movements of his hips. At the same time, the woman may move her own body to match the partner's hip movements. Movements continue until orgasm is achieved by one or both partners. Simultaneous orgasm may be difficult to achieve. After coitus, caressing, hugging, and kissing can increase the shared intimacy and should be encouraged.

The other form of genital intercourse is anal intercourse, during which the penis is inserted into the anus and rectum of the partner. Anal intercourse is commonly practised by gay men, but a number of heterosexual couples engage in it as well.

Current practice dictates the use of a condom in both genital and anal forms of intercourse to prevent the transmission of infections. Because anorectal tissue is not self-lubricating, a lubricant must be used on the condom. Also, because normal bacterial flora from the bowel can produce infection in other parts of the body, the used condom should be removed and another applied before inserting the penis into other body orifices.

There are many other varieties of sexuality that are beyond the scope of this chapter. These include several or many partners, nudism, swinging, group sex, fetishism, sexual sadism, and sexual masochism. A particular sexual practice that is slowly becoming common in Canada originates from Africa and is called **Kunyaza**. In this sexual practice, the man taps the internal area of his partner's vagina with the tip of his penis. He does this either with vertical or horizontal movements. The clitoris can also be "tapped" from left to right. Using a lubricant can help during the tapping. The woman may have an orgasm within 5 minutes if this is done well by the male partner.

Factors Influencing Sexuality

The following section discusses how family, culture, religion, personal expectations and ethics, and health and illness influence a person's sexuality.

Family

Families are the fabric of our day-to-day lives. Through family interactions, we learn about our gender roles and identity, body image, sexual self-concept, capacity for intimacy, social relationships, gender roles, and our expectations of others and ourselves (see Figure 46.2). From earliest beginnings, children observe their parents and model themselves after these role models. If parents are able to share affection with each other and other family members, children will most likely become adults who are able to give and receive affection. If parents seldom hug, hold hands, or kiss each other, their children may become adults who are very uncomfortable with romantic touch.

Family messages about sex range from "sex is so shameful it should not be talked about" to "sex is a joyful part of adult relationships." Some common sexual messages children learn from their families are as follows:

- Sex is dirty.
- Premarital sex is sinful.
- Good girls do not do it.
- Masturbation is disgusting.
- Men should be the sexual experts.
- Sex is mainly for procreation.
- Bodies, including genitals, are beautiful.
- Sex should be fun for both women and men.
- Sexual thoughts and feelings are natural.
- Masturbation is a common, pleasurable activity.
- There is great variety in sexual behaviours.

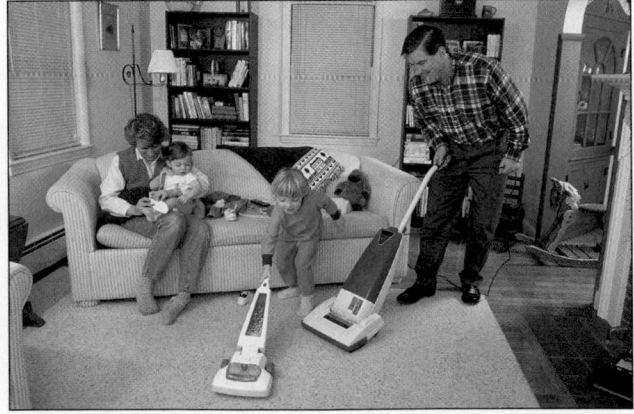

FIGURE 46.2 Children often imitate their parents' roles.

Culture

Sexuality is governed by the individual's culture and societal attitudes. For example, culture influences the sexual nature of dressing, rules about marriage, expectations of role behaviour and social responsibilities, and specific sexual practices. Attitudes about childhood sexual play with the self or other children may be restrictive or permissive. Premarital and extramarital sexual relationships may be considered unacceptable or tolerated. Polygamy (several partners) or monogamy (one partner) may be the norm.

Cultures differ with regard to which body parts they find to be erotic. In some cultures, legs are erotic, and breasts are not. Body weight may also be a determinant of sexual attractiveness. There is a great deal of pressure in North American culture to be very thin. Women who would be considered obese in North America are found highly attractive in other countries. The degree of public nudity ranges from women's entire bodies and faces being covered in Islamic societies to complete nudity in some cultures in New Guinea and Australia.

Female circumcision, also known as *female genital mutilation, female ritual cutting (FRC),* or *female genital cutting (FGC),* is a dangerous practice found in parts of Africa. Some of the cultural beliefs behind the practice include the following: Female genitals are offensive to men; if not removed, the clitoris will become the size of a penis; the labia get in the way of intercourse; and the cutting enhances fertility and prepares the woman for childbirth. Removal of the clitoris may or may not be accompanied by removal of the labia and closure of the vaginal entrance except for a small opening. Long-term medical complications include urinary incontinence, chronic urinary tract infections, vaginal scarring, pain syndromes, infertility, and sexual dysfunctions. FGC is illegal in several African and European countries and in Canada and the United States (Shah, Susan, & Furcroy, 2009).

Male circumcision is one of the oldest recorded operative procedures and one of the most controversial issues. Some professional groups support newborn circumcision, believing that it will prevent the spread of HIV and other infections (Siegfried, Muller, Deeks, & Volmink, 2009). In 2009, the Public Health Agency of Canada reported a circumcision rate of 31.9% among male babies for Canada overall for 2006–2007, with the rate lowest in Nova Scotia (6.8%) and highest in Alberta (44.3%) (Sauvé & Royle, 2009). The data for Nunavut, Yukon, and Newfoundland and Labrador were not available.

Religion

Religion influences sexual expression. It provides guidelines for sexual behaviour and acceptable circumstances for the behaviour, as well as prohibited sexual behaviour and the consequences of breaking the sexual rules. For example, some religions view that forms of sexual expression other than heterosexual intercourse are unnatural and hold virginity before marriage to be the rule. Some religious values conflict with the more liberal values of Canadian society. (See Chapter 47.)

Personal Expectations and Ethics

Cultures reflect the written or unwritten codes of conduct based on ethical principles. Personal expectations concerning sexual behaviour come from these cultural norms. What one person views as bizarre, perverted, or wrong may be completely natural and right for another person. Examples include values regarding masturbation, oral or anal intercourse, and cross-dressing. Many people accept a variety of sexual expressions if they are performed by consenting adults, are practised in private,

and are not harmful. Couples need to explore and communicate clearly about various types of acceptable sexual expression to prevent domination of sexual decision making by one member of the couple. To assess a few of your personal values, complete the statements in Box 46.2.

Health and Illness

SEXUALLY TRANSMITTED INFECTIONS The presence of an STI in one partner induces fear of transmission in the other, resulting in abstinence of sexual contact. In some situations, the presence of an STI is unknown, and transmission occurs without the knowledge of one or both persons involved. See Table 46.2 on page 1493.

BOX 46.2 ASSESSING PERSONAL SEXUAL VALUES

- I believe sexual satisfaction is . . .
- When I think of my parents having sex, I . . .
- If I were to care for a transgendered client, I would . . .
- When I think about lesbians, gays, and bisexuals, I . . .
- Masturbation is . . .
- My beliefs about oral sex are . . .

Sexual Response Cycle

Commonly occurring phases of the human sexual response follow a similar sequence in both females and males regardless of sexual orientation. Table 46.4 provides a summary of the physiological changes associated with each of the phases of the cycle.

TABLE 46.4 Physiological Changes Associated with the Sexual Response Cycle

Phase of the Sexual Response Cycle	Signs Present in Both Sexes	Signs Present in Males Only	Signs Present in Females Only
Excitement/Plateau	Muscle tension increases as excitement increases Sex flush, usually on chest Nipple erection	Penile erection; glans size increases as excitement increases Appearance of a few drops of lubricant, which may contain sperm	Erection of the clitoris Vaginal lubrication Labia may increase 2 to 3 times in size Breasts enlarge Inner two-thirds of vagina widens and lengthens; outer third swells and narrows Uterus elevates
Orgasmic	Respirations may increase to 40 breaths per minute Involuntary spasms of muscle groups throughout the body Diminished sensory awareness Involuntary contractions of the anal sphincter Peak heart rate (110 to 180 beats/min), respiratory rate (40/min or greater), and blood pressure (systolic 30 to 80 mm Hg and diastolic 20 to 50 mm Hg above normal)	Rhythmic, expulsive contractions of the penis at 0.8-sec intervals Emission of seminal fluid into the prostatic urethra from contraction of the vas deferens and accessory organs (stage 1 of the expulsive process) Closing of the internal bladder sphincter just before ejaculation to prevent retrograde ejaculation into bladder Orgasm can occur without ejaculation Ejaculation of semen through the penile urethra and expulsion from the urethral meatus The force of ejaculation varies from man to man and at different times but diminishes after the first two to three contractions (stage 2 of the expulsive process)	Approximately 5 to 12 contractions in the orgasmic platform at 0.8-sec intervals Contraction of the muscles of the pelvic floor and the uterine muscles Varied pattern of orgasms, including minor surges and contractions, multiple orgasms, or a simple intense orgasm similar to that of the male

(continued)

TABLE 46.4 *(continued)*

Phase of the Sexual Response Cycle	Signs Present in Both Sexes	Signs Present in Males Only	Signs Present in Females Only
Resolution	Reversal of vasocongestion in 10 to 30 min; disappearance of all signs of myotonia within 5 min Genitals and breasts return to their pre-excitement states Sex flush disappears in reverse order of appearance Heart rate, respiratory rate, and blood pressure return to normal Other reactions include sleepiness, relaxation, and emotional outbursts such as crying or laughing	A refractory period during which the body will not respond to sexual stimulation; varies, depending on age and other factors, from a few moments to hours or days	Some women experience multiple successive orgasms followed by a longer period of resolution.

The response cycle starts in the brain, with conscious sexual desires called the **desire phase**. Sexually arousing stimuli, often called *erotic stimuli,* may be real or symbolic. Sight, hearing, smell, touch, and imagination (sexual fantasy) can all invoke sexual arousal. Sexual desire fluctuates within each person and varies from person to person. If people suppress or block out conscious sexual desires, they may not experience any physiological response. Although psychological issues are the more common causes of lack of sexual desire, medications, drugs, and hormone imbalances can also interfere.

The **excitement phase** involves two primary physiological changes (see Figure 46.3). Vasocongestion is an increase in the blood flow to various body parts resulting in erection of the penis and clitoris and swelling of the labia, testes, and breasts. Vasocongestion stimulates sensory receptors within these body parts that, in turn, transmit messages to the conscious brain where they are usually interpreted as pleasurable sensations. When stimulation is continued, vasocongestion increases until it either is released by orgasm or fades away. Likewise, myotonia, an increase of tension in muscles, may increase until released by orgasm, or it may also simply fade away.

The **orgasmic phase** is the involuntary climax of sexual tension, accompanied by physiological and psychological release. This phase is considered the measurable peak of the sexual experience. Although the entire body is involved, the major focus of the orgasm is felt in the pelvic region. Male orgasms usually last 10 to 30 seconds while female orgasms last 10 to 50 seconds. Men usually have an ejaculation and expel semen as part of their orgasm. Before puberty and in later years, males experience orgasms without ejaculation.

The **resolution phase**, the period of return to the unaroused state, may last 10 to 15 minutes after orgasm, or longer if there is no orgasm. This phase in females is quite varied as some women experience multiple

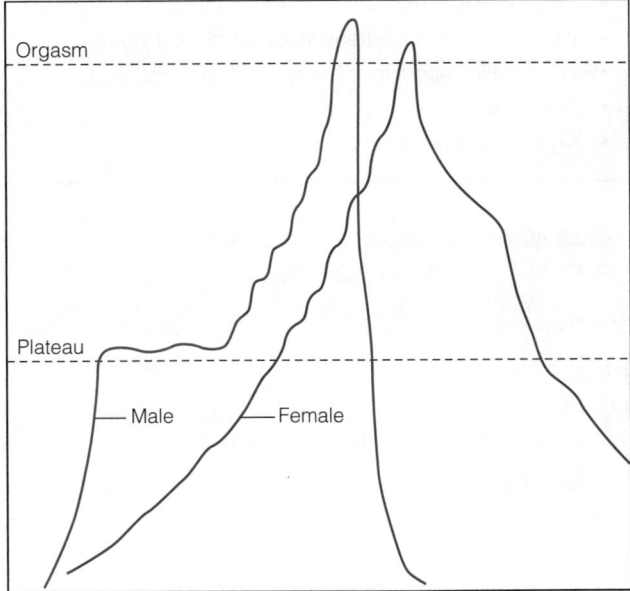

FIGURE 46.3 Phases of the sexual response cycle.

successive orgasms followed by a longer period of resolution. See MyNursingLab for sections in R. Basson's *Model of Sexual Response and Emotional Intimacy for Women and Problems with Sexual Satisfaction* (Basson, 2005).

Alternative Sexual Function

Some individuals experience transient or lifelong problems with their ability to respond to sexual stimulation or to maintain the response. The problems may be generalized to all sexual interactions and settings, or they may be situational, occurring in a specific setting or with specific types of sexual activity. It is often difficult to sort out the multiple factors contributing to an individual's or a couple's sexual problems. Generally, a number of past and current factors are involved.

Past and Current Factors

Sociocultural factors interfering in sexual function include a very strict upbringing accompanied by inadequate sex education. Rigid gender-role socialization may inhibit exploration of sexual activities, positions, toys, and other lovemaking behaviours. If people's religious affiliations believe that sex is only for procreation, there may be great difficulty in celebrating the pleasure and fun of a loving sexual relationship. Another factor may be parental punishment for normally exploring one's genitals or for normal childhood sex play. The pressures of family and work often leave couples with too little time and not enough energy to enjoy sex.

Psychological factors may include negative feelings, such as guilt, anxiety, or fear that interfere with the ability to experience pleasure and joy. Some people experience guilt when they simply enjoy sex or when they participate in what they label "unusual" sexual activities, or guilt regarding the choice of the partner. Adults who have been sexually abused at any time of their lives may experience overwhelming anxiety when faced with the decision to engage in sex. Fears may include pregnancy, STIs, or pain. Because vulnerability and intimacy are inherent in most sexual relationships, fear of these may lead to an avoidance of sex. Fear of failure in sexual performance often becomes a vicious cycle. Individuals may worry excessively if they will lose their erection, if they will have an orgasm, or if their abdomen is too flabby. Depressed people lose interest in sexual activity and often experience a complete loss of sexual desire and fulfillment.

Cognitive factors include the internalization of negative expectations and beliefs. Those with low self-esteem may not understand how another person could value and love them and also find them sexually attractive. For those who have not yet accepted their sexual orientation or gender identity, this cognitive conflict may interfere with sexual relationships.

Sexual problems may also be symptomatic of relationship problems. Conflict and anger with one's partner are not conducive to positive sexual interaction. Some individuals lose the physical attraction to another or feel more attracted to someone else. Failure to communicate may result in one or both partners not knowing how to please the other. Disagreements in sexual frequency and/or sexual activities may lead to further relationship conflict.

Sexual Desire Disorders

Most people's sexual desire varies from day to day as well as over the years. Some people, however, report a persistently low interest or a total lack of interest in sexual activity; these clients suffer from **hypoactive sexual desire disorder**. Typically, there is a disparity of sexual needs, and the person with the greater desire becomes dissatisfied with the sexual relationship. The key issue in the relationship is not frequency but rather the dovetailing of partners' needs.

Sexual aversion disorder is a severe distaste for sexual activity or the thought of sexual activity, which then leads to a phobic avoidance of sex. It occurs in both women and men. Intense emotional dread of an impending sexual interaction also can trigger the physiological symptoms of anxiety: sweating, increased heart rate, and extreme muscle tension. The person then stops the sexual interaction or prevents it from even beginning. The most common cause of sexual aversion disorder is childhood sexual abuse or adult rape. The severe trauma can lead to a phobic response to sexual activity (Hertlein, Weeks, & Gambescia, 2008).

Sexual Arousal Disorders

Sexual arousal refers to the physiological responses and subjective sense of excitement experienced during sexual activity. Lack of lubrication and failure to attain or maintain an erection are the major disorders of the arousal phase. In **female sexual arousal disorder**, the lack of vaginal lubrication causes discomfort or pain during sexual intercourse. The diagnosis of **male erectile disorder** is usually made when the man has erection problems during 25% or more of his sexual interactions. Some men cannot attain a full erection, and others lose their erection prior to orgasm. The condition used to be called *impotency,* which implied that the man is feeble, inadequate, and incompetent, but the correct term is *erectile dysfunction* (ED), which is objectively descriptive and not judgmental. Arousal disorder may occur in individuals with persistent or recurring lack of subjective sexual excitement or pleasure (see the Teaching: Wellness box on erectile dysfunction on the next page).

Orgasmic Disorders

Female orgasmic disorder refers to women who are incapable of responding sexually or do not experience orgasm. Studies indicate that 10% to 15% of women are preorgasmic (never experienced an orgasm), and another 20% to 22% report irregular orgasms. Compounding the orgasmic difficulty is the associated anxiety. In the preoccupation with orgasm, the real goal of being sexual—mutual pleasuring and intimacy—is lost, and the interchange becomes one of anxiety, frustration, and anger (Hertlein, Weeks, & Sendak, 2009).

Men with **male orgasmic disorder** can maintain an erection for long periods (an hour or more) but have extreme difficulty ejaculating (referred to as *retarded ejaculation*). In heterosexual intercourse, the difficulty may be limited to ejaculation in the vagina. Some men ejaculate after self-stimulation or manual or oral stimulation by the

Phosphodiesterase Type 5 (PDE5) Inhibitor (sildenafil citrate [Viagra]; tadalafil [Cialis]; vardenafil [Levitra])

The Client Taking Medication for Erectile Dysfunction

In erectile dysfunction (ED), the sexually stimulated penis does not achieve or maintain an erection, often due to restricted blood flow to the penis. These medications inhibit the breakdown of the enzymes and products that allow the muscle relaxation which, in turn, facilitates adequate blood flow to the penis. Thus, the medications do not enhance sexual desire or cure the ED but allow the stimulated penis to obtain and sustain an erection.

Nursing Responsibilities

- ED medications are contraindicated for men with cardiovascular risk factors, uncontrolled high or low blood pressure, cerebrovascular accident, renal or liver problems, vision loss, or bleeding disorders.
- Men with an anatomically deformed penis should consult with the primary care provider prior to taking these medications.
- Medications come in different dose strengths and may require adjustment.

Client and Family Teaching

- General safety in using these medications is the same as for engaging in sexual activity overall. The risk of adverse outcomes of sexual activity after taking these medications is not increased.
- Explain that men who take medications that are nitrates—those that are prescribed (e.g., nitroglycerin) or those that are recreational (e.g., amyl nitrate–"poppers")—should not take these medications.
- The client should take the medication about 1 hour prior to sexual activity (up to 4 hours prior) and not more than once per day.
- Teach side effects to immediately report to the primary care provider: loss of vision, or an erection that lasts more than 4 hours.
- Other common side effects may include headache, muscle pain, flushing, or stuffy nose.
- These medications do not prevent pregnancy or STIs.

Note: Prior to administering any medication, review all aspects with a current drug handbook or other reliable source.

partner, whereas others have great difficulty ejaculating with any type of stimulation.

Rapid ejaculation is one of the most common sexual dysfunctions among men. This condition is the involuntary control of ejaculation, which ranges from ejaculating before being touched, ejaculating before penetration, ejaculating with one internal thrust, to ejaculating within a minute or two of penetration. A more helpful description is *absence of voluntary control of ejaculation.*

Sexual Pain Disorders

Both women and men can experience **dyspareunia**, pain during or immediately after intercourse. It is associated with many physiological causes, especially those that inhibit lubrication. Thus, skin irritations, vaginal infections, estrogen deficiencies, and use of medications that dry vaginal secretions can cause women to experience discomfort with intercourse.

Pelvic disorders, such as infections, lesions, endometriosis, scar tissue, or tumours, can result in painful intercourse. Similarly, in males, infection or inflammation of the glans penis or other genitourinary organs can cause pain with intercourse. Also, some contraceptive foams, creams, sponges, or latex products can irritate either the vagina or penis.

Vaginismus is the involuntary spasm of the outer one-third of the vaginal muscles, making penetration of the vagina painful and sometimes impossible. The woman often experiences desire, excitement, and orgasm with stimulation of the external sexual structures. Attempts at intercourse, however, elicit the involuntary spasm. She may have similar difficulty undergoing pelvic exams and inserting tampons or a diaphragm.

Vulvodynia is constant, unremitting burning that is localized to the vulva with an acute onset. The girl or woman has problems in sitting, standing, and sleeping related to the intensity of pain. **Vestibulitis** causes severe pain only on touch or attempted vaginal penetration. Half of the women with vestibulitis report lifelong dyspareunia. Women with either of these disorders report a negative impact on their sexual functioning and partner relationship, as well as their self-esteem and mental health (Jodoin, 2008; Kingdon, 2009; Ponte, Klemperer, Sahay, & Chren, 2009).

Effects of Medications on Sexual Function

Many prescription medications and social drugs can affect sexual desire and response (see Table 46.5). These include central nervous system depressants, such as opiates; antianxiety agents, such as barbiturates and benzodiazepines; anticholinergic agents, such as atropine; cardiovascular agents, such as antiarrhythmics, antihypertensives, diuretics, and beta-blocking agents;

TABLE 46.5   Effects of Medications on Sexual Function

Medication	Possible Effects*
Alcohol	Moderate amounts: increased sexual functioning; chronic use: decreased sexual desire, orgasmic dysfunction, and erectile dysfunction
Alpha-blockers	Inability to ejaculate
Amphetamines	Increased sex drive, delayed orgasm
Amyl nitrate	Reported enhanced orgasm; vasodilation, fainting
Anabolic steroids	Decreased sex drive, shrinking of testicles and infertility in men
Antianxiety agents	Decreased sexual desire; orgasmic dysfunction in women; delayed ejaculation
Anticonvulsants	Decreased sexual desire; reduced sexual response
Antidepressants	Decreased sexual desire; orgasmic delay or dysfunction in women; delayed or failed ejaculation; painful erection
Antihistamines	Decreased vaginal lubrication; decreased desire
Antihypertensives	Decreased sexual desire; erectile failure; ejaculation dysfunction
Antipsychotics	Decreased sexual desire; orgasmic dysfunction in women; delayed ejaculation; ejaculatory failure
Barbiturates	In low doses, increased sexual pleasure; in large doses, decreased sexual desire, orgasmic dysfunction, and erectile dysfunction
Beta-blockers	Decreased sexual desire
Cardiotonics	Decreased sexual desire
Cocaine	Increased intensity of sexual experience; with chronic use, decreased sexual desire and sexual dysfunction
Diuretics	Decreased vaginal lubrication; decreased sexual desire; erectile dysfunction
Marijuana	As above for cocaine, but prolonged use reduces testosterone levels and reduces sperm production
Narcotics	Inhibited sexual desire and response; erectile and ejaculatory dysfunctions

*Nurses and clients must familiarize themselves with the specific medication prescribed or used, as effects vary in each category of drug.

antidepressants and antipsychotics; and social drugs, such as alcohol and marijuana.

Nursing Management

Assessing

Sexuality is a normal, healthy part of life and part of holistic nursing care. Clients are often hesitant and may be too embarrassed to discuss the topic of sex with their primary health care providers. Information about a client's sexual health status should always be an integral part of a nursing assessment. The amount and kind of data collected depend on the client's reason for seeking health care and how the client's sexuality interacts with other problems Generally, the nurse conducts a sexual history on the following categories of clients:

- Those receiving care for pregnancy, infertility, contraception, or an STI
- Those whose illness or therapy will affect sexual functioning (e.g., clients with diabetes, gynecological problems, heart disease)
- Those currently experiencing a sexual problem (e.g., erectile dysfunction)

NURSING HISTORY   To introduce the topic of sexuality to all clients, all nursing histories should at least include a question, such as "Have there been any changes in your sexual functioning that might be related to your illness or the medications you take?" Nurses might also facilitate communication by saying, "I'm concerned about all aspects of your health, both when they are well and when they are ill. When I take your history, sexual concerns are included to help plan a comprehensive treatment approach."

Interviewing a client regarding sexual health may be uncomfortable for some nurses (and for the client). Nurses must be aware of their own feelings and beliefs so that they can prepare approaches for gathering data and creating the nursing care plan. The nurse sets aside personal values about sexual practices and uses a culturally sensitive, nonjudgmental, nonthreatening, and reassuring approach. It is extremely important to create an atmosphere that facilitates open communication and comfort for the client. Remind the client that all personal health information is handled in a confidential manner. Also see Chapter 5 for a review of values clarification and Chapter 12 for more information on the health history.

The Assessment: Interview box provides questions that nurses may ask as part of the health history after a rapport has been established.

PHYSICAL EXAMINATION   Physical examination of the female genitals and reproductive tract and the male genitals is part of a routine physical examination in some agencies. See Chapter 31 for details of the examination. Nursing history data indicating the need for a physical examination include the following:

- Suspicion of infertility, pregnancy, or an STI
- Reports of discharge, presence of a lump or sore, or change in colour, size, and shape of a genital organ
- Changes in urinary function
- Need for Papanicolaou test
- Request for birth control

IDENTIFYING CLIENTS AT RISK   Clients at risk for altered sexual patterns include those experiencing the following:

- Altered body structure or function caused by trauma, pregnancy, recent childbirth, anatomic abnormalities of the genitals, or a variety of diseases

- Physical, psychosocial, emotional, or sexual abuse; sexual assault
- Disfiguring conditions, such as burns, skin conditions, birthmarks, scars (e.g., mastectomy), and ostomies
- Specific medication therapy that cause sexual problems such as decreases sexual drive or causes erectile or ejaculatory dysfunction (see Table 46.5).
- Temporary or long-term impaired physical ability to perform and maintain sexual attractiveness
- Value conflicts between personal beliefs and religious doctrine
- Loss of a partner
- Lack of knowledge or misinformation about sexual functioning and expression

Diagnosing

Nursing diagnoses relating specifically to sexuality include the following (NANDA International, 2012):

- *Ineffective Sexuality Pattern:* the state in which an individual experiences a change in sexual function during the sexual response phases of desire, excitation, and/or orgasm, which is viewed as unsatisfying, unrewarding, or inadequate
- *Sexual Dysfunction:* expression of concern regarding own sexuality

Sexual problems can also be the etiology of other diagnoses, including the following:

- *Deficient Knowledge* (e.g., about conception, STIs, contraception, or normal sexual changes over the lifespan) related to misinformation and sexual myths
- *Pain* related to inadequate vaginal lubrication or effects of genital surgery
- *Anxiety* related to loss of sexual desire or functioning
- *Fear* related to history of sexual abuse or dyspareunia

ASSESSMENT   INTERVIEW

Sexual Health History

- Are you currently sexually active? with men, women, or both?
- Are you sexually active with one or more than one partner?
- Describe the positive and negative aspects of your sexual functioning.
- Do you have difficulty with sexual desire? arousal? orgasm? satisfaction?
- Do you experience any pain during sexual interaction?

- If there are problems, how have they influenced how you feel about yourself? How have they affected your partner? How have they affected the relationship?
- Do you expect your sexual functioning to be altered because of your illness?
- What are your partner's concerns about your future sexual functioning?
- Do you have any other sexual questions or concerns that I have not addressed?

- *Disturbed Body Image* (e.g., mastectomy) related to perceived sexual rejection by partner

See Box 46.3 for examples of application of nursing diagnoses and their related desired outcomes and nursing interventions in the Nursing Care Plan.

Planning

Overall goals to meet clients' sexual needs include the following:

- Maintaining, restoring, or improving sexual health
- Increasing knowledge of sexuality and sexual health
- Preventing the occurrence or spread of sexually transmitted infections
- Preventing unwanted pregnancy
- Increasing satisfaction with the level of sexual functioning
- Improving sexual self-concept

The nurse needs to communicate with both clients and family members in a culturally sensitive manner. Nursing interventions to promote sexual health and function focus largely on the nurse's teaching role. For example, clients need to be taught about normal sexual function, the effects of medications on sexual function, the prevention of STIs, how to perform testicular self-examination, and how to gain an awareness of what is

normal for their breasts. Additionally, nurses can help clients maintain a healthy sexual self-concept by doing the following:

- Providing privacy during intimate body care
- Giving attention to the client's appearance and dress
- Giving clients privacy to meet their sexual needs alone or with a partner within physically safe limits

Implementing

On the basis of the data obtained and the identified nursing diagnoses, interventions are directed at preventing problems the client is at risk for, providing information about sexual health, and counselling for altered sexual function. Nurses require six basic skills to help clients in the area of sexuality:

1. Self-knowledge of and comfort with their own sexuality
2. Acceptance of sexuality as an important area for nursing intervention and a willingness to work with clients who express their sexuality in a variety of ways
3. Knowledge of sexual growth and development throughout the life cycle
4. Knowledge of basic sexuality, including how certain health problems and treatments may affect sexuality and sexual function and which interventions facilitate sexual expression and functioning

---

BOX 46.3 IDENTIFYING NURSING DIAGNOSES, OUTCOMES, AND INTERVENTIONS FOR CLIENTS WITH SEXUALITY PROBLEMS

DATA CLUSTER Marsha Ogilvy, 55 years old, reports vaginal burning and pain whenever she and her husband have intercourse. Her last menses was 14 months ago. She says her husband is concerned about the lack of her usual response to lovemaking.

Nursing Diagnosis	Desired Outcome	Intervention
Sexual Dysfunction/the state in which an individual experiences a change in sexual function during the sexual response phases of desire, excitation, and/or orgasm, which is viewed as unsatisfying, unrewarding, or inadequate	No deviation from sexual functioning	• Determine current health knowledge and lifestyle behaviours of individual and family. • Incorporate strategies to enhance the client's self-esteem. • Teach strategies that can be used to minimize client's discomfort and enhance sexual pleasure.

DATA CLUSTER Larry Stogyn, 52 years old, has a history of hypertension for which he has been taking an antihypertension. He says he has lost interest in sex in the past few months, and when he does have sex, he has trouble keeping an erection.

Ineffective Sexuality Patterns	Often demonstrated • sustained penile erection • uses assistive device as needed • adapts sexual techniques as needed	• Discuss the effect of medication on sexuality. • Discuss any alternative forms of sexual expressive medication that might be acceptable to the client. • Provide referral to other members of the health care team as appropriate to explore other medical interventions (e.g., use of prosthesis or Viagra, etc.).

5. Therapeutic communication skills

6. Ability to recognize the need for all clients and family members to have the topic of sexuality introduced not only in written or audiovisual materials but also in a verbal discussion.

Providing Sexual Health Teaching

Providing education for sexual health is an important component of nursing implementation (see the Reflect on Primary Health Care box). Many sexual problems exist as a result of sexual ignorance; many others can be prevented with effective sexual health teaching. Examples of important areas of teaching include (a) sex education, (b) self-examination and (c) responsible sexual behaviour.

REFLECT ON **PRIMARY HEALTH CARE**

Sexual health education applies the principle of *health promotion* by aiming at preventing STIs and unplanned pregnancies. Through *intersectoral cooperation,* sexual health information is integrated in the school curriculum, with public health nurses working closely with the teachers and the school board. Together, they design the best approaches, such as small groups, games, drama education, and use of the Internet (appropriate technology) to meet the learning needs of adolescents about sex, sexuality, and sexual health. Consider how the application of these primary health care principles can transform the schools into caring communities for these young people.

SEX EDUCATION Nurses can help clients understand their anatomy and how their bodies function. For example, understanding the anatomy of the genitals may help women learn how their bodies respond to sexual stimulation. Both men and women need to learn the kind of stimulation that is pleasing and causes arousal. The importance of open communication between partners should also be encouraged. Women may also benefit from learning *Kegel exercises.* These exercises involve contraction and relaxation of the pubococcygeal muscle, the muscle that contracts when a person prevents urine flow. The benefits of Kegel exercises include increased pelvic floor muscle tone, increased vaginal lubrication during sexual arousal, increased sensation during intercourse, increased genital sensitivity, stronger gripping of the base of the penis, earlier postpartum recovery of the pelvic floor muscle, and increased flexibility of episiotomy scars (Katz, 2009). (See Chapter 42.)

Details about physiological changes that occur during major developmental crises should be provided as part of general health care. For example, the nurse needs to discuss the effects of puberty, pregnancy, menopause,

and the male climacteric on sexual function. When clients experience illness or surgery that alters sexual function, the nurse needs to discuss effects of treatment (e.g., medications) and any changes that need to be undertaken to ensure safe sex (e.g., position changes or a safe time to resume sexual intercourse after a myocardial infarction).

Parents often need assistance to learn ways to answer questions and what information to provide for their children starting in the preschool years. Parents need to be the primary educators of children at an early age; however, peers, teachers, media, and toys also teach about sexual issues. It is important that nurses learn about the beliefs clients hold and provide up-to-date information.

AWARENESS AND SELF-EXAMINATION

Breast Cancer Awareness Although the overall breast cancer death rates have declined in all ages since the mid 1990s, the incidence of breast cancer is on the rise. Breast cancer is the most common cancer among Canadian women and some men. In 2010, about 22 700 new Canadian women were diagnosed with breast cancer. One in nine women is expected to develop breast cancer during her lifetime, and 1 in 29 will die from it. According to estimates, 200 men will be diagnosed with breast cancer (Canadian Cancer Society's Steering Committee on Cancer Statistics, 2012).

In November 2011, the Canadian Task Force on Preventive Health Care announced new breast cancer screening guidelines for women at *average risk* of breast cancer aged 40 to 74 years. Women aged 40 to 49 should not undergo routine mammography screening and the mammography screening interval is now extended from every 2 years to every 2 to 3 years for women aged 50 to 74 years. Women at average risk should not have routine magnetic resonance imaging (MRI) screening, mammography, clinical breast exams, and breast self-examinations. These recommendations do not apply to women at higher risk due to personal history of breast cancer, history of breast cancer in a first-degree relative, known *BRCA1/BRCA2* mutation, or prior chest wall radiation (Canadian Task Force on Preventive Health Care, 2011). All women should be breast aware (i.e., know how their breasts normally look and feel). (See the Teaching: Wellness box on breast awareness and mammography.)

Testicular Cancer Awareness The incidence of testicular cancer has remained the same since 2009. Testicular cancer tends to be a young male's cancer, as it is the most common type of cancer among Canadian men aged 15 to 29 years, peaks around age 30 years, and declines by age 60 years. All men, from the time they are 15 years old, should learn how to perform testicular self-examination (TSE) and should be doing it on a regular basis (Canadian Testicular Cancer Association, 2011).

Breast Awareness and Mammography

Breast Awareness

Women should become breast aware by following these five steps:

1. Know how your breasts normally look and feel.
2. Know what changes to look for.
3. Look and feel for changes.
4. Report any changes to a doctor or nurse.
5. Have regular mammograms, if age appropriate or if recommended by a doctor.

Look and feel for the following changes by using the finger pads (tips) of the three middle fingers, moving in small circles, from the outside of the breast to the nipple, covering the surface (above and below) of each breast, including the armpit:

- Changes to the size or shape of one or both breasts
- Thickenings, dimples, or puckered skin of one or both breasts
- Unusual, persistent pain in the breast or armpit area
- Swelling under the armpit or below the collarbone

- Changes in the nipples, such as the shape or position of a nipple, a nipple turning inward, or crusting or scaling on a nipple

Mammography

Mammography is a type of radiography that can reveal changes inside your breasts that are too small to feel. Mammography also gives you and your doctor information about changes in your breasts that you find or that a health care professional finds during a physical examination of the breasts.

All women should discuss the risks and benefits of mammography with their doctor. Women between 50 and 74 years should have a mammogram every 2 to 3 years. If you are under age 50 or over 74 years and are at a higher risk for breast cancer, you should discuss with your doctor when mammography may be appropriate for you.

Breast screening programs vary. All provinces and territories have breast cancer screening programs for women ages 50 to 74 years. They can make an appointment at a screening centre without a doctor's referral. Women outside that age range may need a referral.

Sources: Information adapted from Canadian Cancer Society. (2010). *What is breast cancer?* Retrieved from http://www.cancer.ca/Canada-wide/About%20cancer/Types%20of%20cancer/What%20is%20breast%20cancer.aspx?sc_lang=en; and Canadian Task Force on Preventive Health Care. (2011). *Screening for breast cancer: Summary of recommendations for clinicians and policy-makers.* Retrieved from http://www.canadiantaskforce.ca/recommendations/2011_01_eng.html

According to a Cochrane review on testicular cancer screening (Ilic & Misso, 2011), male patients with an increased risk of developing testicular cancer, such as a family history of testicular cancer, undescended testis (cryptorchidism), or testicular atrophy, should be informed of the potential benefits and harms associated with screening. (See the Teaching: Wellness box on testicular self-examination and Figure 46.4 on the next page for specific techniques of self-examination techniques.)

RESPONSIBLE SEXUAL BEHAVIOUR Responsible sexual behaviour involves the prevention of STIs, the prevention of unwanted pregnancy, and the avoidance of sexual harassment or abuse.

STI Prevention The prevention of STIs is an essential part of sexual health teaching. Increases in STIs are caused by two factors: (a) changing sexual morality that has permitted increased sexual activity and (b) an increase in the number of sexual partners. Because the term *STIs* elicits feelings of guilt, shame, and fear, people frequently do not seek medical help as early as they should. Clients need education about these infections, preventive measures, and early treatment (see the Nursing and Canadian Society box on the next page and the Teaching: Wellness

box on page 1509). Many STIs can be treated quickly and effectively. Others may have serious consequences. For example, women may develop pelvic inflammatory disease (PID) resulting in damage to the reproductive structures and possible infertility. Currently, AIDS has no cure. The anxiety about AIDS transmission has caused many individuals to alter their sexual behaviour, such as using a condom during genital or anal sex.

Box 46.4 on page 1509 lists the common signs of STIs for which people should seek medical care.

Prevention of Unplanned Pregnancies Prevention of unplanned pregnancies must be addressed not only with adolescents but also with couples who are timing their first birth and want to space children and limit family size (see Figure 46.5 on page 1509). Nurses need to be familiar with various contraceptive methods and their advantages, disadvantages, contraindications, effectiveness, safety, and cost. It is beyond the scope of this text to discuss contraceptives in detail. See Box 46.5 on page 1509 for the various methods of contraception.

Avoiding Sexual Harassment and Abuse Sexual harassment exists when someone in a position of power threatens another person's job or status in exchange for unwanted sexual acts. Such harassment can be severe enough to be

Testicular Self-Examination

Testicular self-examination (TSE) can help detect testicular cancer early. All men should perform a TSE once each month from the time they are 15 years old. Ideally, you should examine your testicles during or after a hot bath or shower because the warmth will cause your testicles to descend and the skin of your scrotum to relax, making it easier to feel any lumps, growths, or tenderness.

- Choose one day of each month (e.g., the first or last day of each month) to examine yourself.
- Examine yourself when you are taking a warm shower or bath.
- Support the testicle underneath with one hand. Place the fingers of the other hand under the testicle and the thumb on top (this may be easier to do if the leg on that side is raised).
- Roll each testicle between the thumb and fingers of your hand, feeling for lumps, thickening, or any hardening (Figure 46.4). The testes should feel smooth.
- Palpate the epididymis, a cord-like structure on the top and back of the testicle. The epididymis should feel soft and not as smooth as a testicle.

- Locate the spermatic cord, or vas deferens, which extends upward from the scrotum toward the base of the penis. It should feel firm and smooth.
- By using a mirror, inspect your testicles for swelling, any enlargement, or lumps in the skin of the testicle.
- Report any lumps or other changes to your health care provider promptly.

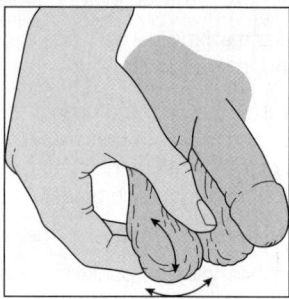

FIGURE 46.4 Rolling the testicle between the thumb and fingers.

 Nursing and Canadian Society

Facts	Implications for Nursing Practice
Chlamydia is the most common form of STI. The national number of reported cases for Chlamydiasis increased from 43 709 in 2009 to 45 460 in 2010. Ontario had the highest number of reported cases for both years, followed by Quebec and Alberta. However, the rate for Alberta decreased significantly from 2009 to 2010 (PHAC, 2010c).	Nurses need to be aware of the trends and significance of STIs and to educate clients about safe sexual practices.
For the same period (2009–2010), the national rates for gonorrhea and infectious syphilis decreased, but these rates continued to rise in Ontario and Quebec. Alberta showed a drastic decrease in these infections using provincial-wide STI campaigns (gonorrhoea: 821 cases in 2009, 541 cases in 2010; syphilis: 158 cases in 2009, 97 cases in 2010) (PHAC, 2010c).	Nurses need to promote public awareness to reduce STIs via sexual health teaching in school and community centres and to educate expectant parents about the importance of prenatal screening programs for selected communicable diseases.
Some forms of human papilloma virus (HPV) are sexually transmitted, and particular strains of the virus have been linked to cervical cancer. Canada has a population of 13.53 million women aged 15 years and older who are at risk of developing cervical cancer. About 9.9% of women in the general population are estimated to harbour cervical HPV infection at a given time, and 74.3% of invasive cervical cancers are attributed to HPVs (WHO/ICO, 2010).	The HPV vaccine is available to immunize young girls and women against contracting HPV infection. Nurses can teach parents about the vaccine and the prevention of HPV.
HIV is the virus that causes AIDS. At the end of 2008, there were an estimated 65 000 people in Canada living with HIV, up from 57 000 in 2005. Of these, around 26% were unaware of their infection. It is estimated that between 2300 and 4300 new HIV infections occur in Canada each year. Gay, bisexual, and other men who have sex with men (MSM) continued to comprise the greatest proportion (44%) of new HIV infections in 2009. By the end of 2009, of 21 681 AIDS diagnoses in Canada, at least 13 449 people with AIDS have died (PHAC, 2010d).	Nurses must continue to educate the public about HIV and AIDS. Sexual health teaching in different types of settings for gay, bisexual, and MSM must continue. Teaching of First Nations peoples needs to continue as the rates are increasing at an alarming rate.

BOX 46.4 SEXUALLY TRANSMITTED INFECTIONS AMONG CANADIANS

The following are some facts about STIs among Canadians:

- Human papilloma virus (HPV) is a virus that can manifest in different parts of the body that are vulnerable to infection; some forms of HPV are sexually transmitted. Particular strains of the virus have been linked to cervical cancer. It is estimated that more than 70% of sexually active Canadians will have a sexually transmitted HPV infection in their lifetimes (PHAC, 2010a).
- HIV is the virus that causes AIDS. By the end of 2008, an estimated 65 000 Canadians were living with HIV infection and AIDS, an increase of 14% since from 2005 (PHAC, 2011).
- Hepatitis B is approximately 100 times more infective than HIV and carries with it a 15% to 25% risk of death from liver disease and damage. The prevalence in Canada is estimated at 0.7% to 0.9%; people who have unprotected sex with multiple partners are at high risk for contracting the infection (PHAC, 2010b).

TEACHING   WELLNESS

Preventing Transmission of Sexually Transmitted Infections

Clients need to know how to prevent STIs:

- Talk openly with partners about how to have safe sex, and honestly discuss any history of an STI.
- Use condoms in all sexual relationships.
- Abstain from sexual activity with a partner *known* to have or *suspected* of having an STI.
- Report to a health care facility for examination whenever in doubt about possible exposure or when signs of an STI are evident.
- When an STI is diagnosed, notify all partners, and encourage them to seek treatment.
- Consider the use of vaccinations now available for hepatitis B and human papilloma virus (HPV).
- Women should have regular Pap tests for the early detection of STI-related cervical cell changes.

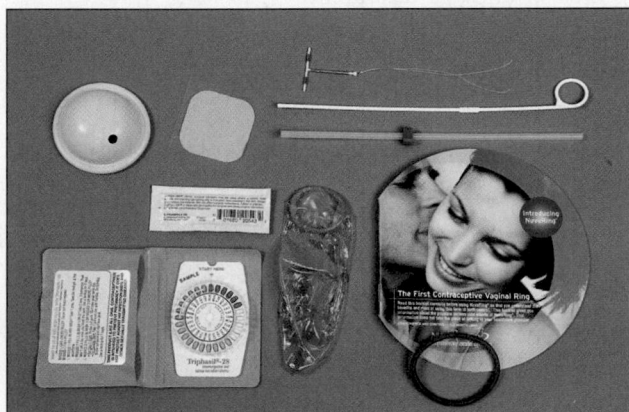

FIGURE 46.5 Methods of contraception.

BOX 46.5 METHODS OF CONTRACEPTION

- Abstinence
- Withdrawal of the penis before ejaculation (coitus interruptus)
- Fertility awareness (identification of the days of the month when conception is most likely to occur and abstaining during that time)
- Mechanical barriers: vaginal diaphragm, cervical cap, condom (*Note:* There are three types of condom materials: latex, lambskin, and polyurethane. All are equally effective at preventing pregnancy. Latex condoms are the least expensive. Lambskin pore size does not protect against STIs as well as the others. Polyurethane condoms are recommended if contact with latex should be avoided. Polyurethane is the material used in female condoms.)
- Chemical barriers: insertion of spermicidal foams, creams, jellies, or suppositories into the vagina before intercourse
- Intrauterine devices (IUDs)
- Hormonal: oral contraceptives (birth control pills), subdermal implants of synthetic progestin, transdermal patches (*Note:* Certain antibiotics decrease the effectiveness of oral contraceptives and patches. Women on these antibiotics must use an alternative method of contraception until their antibiotic treatment is completed. Other drug interactions can occur with implants.)
- Surgical sterilization: tubal ligation and vasectomy
- Abortion

considered abuse, but sexual abuse (also called *molestation*) is forced, unwanted sexual activity of any kind. Prevention is the most important role of the nurse, and this can best be accomplished through educating adult clients and families of children about their rights and support services available if they believe there is sexual harassment or abuse. Assessing for, diagnosing, and intervening in possible situations of sexual harassment or abuse is a significant undertaking, and not every nurse will be skilled in these roles (Donohoe, 2010). However, every nurse must be aware of the proper methods of reporting suspected abuse. See MyNursingLab for "Warning Signs of Abuse."

Counselling for Altered Sexual Function

One technique nurses can use to help clients with altered sexual function is the PLISSIT model, developed by Annon (1974) for this purpose. The model involves four progressive levels represented by the acronym PLISSIT:

P   Permission giving
LI Limited information
SS Specific suggestions
IT Intensive therapy

At each level, the nurse provides additional guidance and information to the client and, therefore, requires more specialized and specific knowledge and skill. All professional nurses should be able to function at the first three levels, described below.

Permission Giving Clients may feel that they need permission to be sexual beings, to ask questions, to show affection, and to express themselves sexually. Giving permission means that the nurse, by attitude or word, lets the client know that sexual thoughts, fantasies, and behaviours between informed, consenting adults are allowed. Giving permission begins when the nurse acknowledges the client's spoken and unspoken sexual concerns and conveys the attitude that sexual concerns and needs are important to health and recovery.

For example, the nurse might ask a client recuperating from a heart attack the following questions:

- "Now that you're recuperating and you've had some time to sort out your feelings, have you thought about how your heart attack might alter your sex life?"

- "Have you and your partner discussed how you both feel about it?"

Limited Information Clients need accurate but concise information. The nurse might explain what is normal; how some medical conditions, treatments, injuries, or surgeries can affect sexuality and functioning; or how aging can affect sexuality and functioning.

Continuing with the preceding example, the nurse shares information and informs the client about how the heart attack might affect the client's sex life, including the following:

- "Your heart attack will not alter your capacity for sexual responsiveness. Most people can resume intercourse in 4 to 6 weeks, but this should be confirmed by your doctor. If you can climb a flight of stairs without having chest pain you should be able to resume having sex, since it takes about the same amount of energy."

- "Many clients who have suffered a heart attack fear sexual intercourse because of increased heart and respiratory rates associated with it. However, your prescribed program of progressive physical activity will also increase your tolerance for sexual activity."

Many clients recuperating from childbirth, for example, or a specific illness or disease (e.g., heart attack) need instructions about safe sexual activities and the effects that therapy can have on sexual functioning. The following topics need to be considered:

- When sexual activity is safe
- Specific sexual activities that are unsafe and why
- Adaptations needed for resuming a satisfactory sexual life
- The side effects of prescribed medications on sexual functioning and the need to notify the primary care provider for possible dose or medication adjustment should problems develop.

Specific Suggestions At the level of specific suggestions, the nurse requires specialized knowledge and skill about how sexuality and functioning can be affected by a disease process or therapy and what interventions might be effective. The nurse offers suggestions to help the client adapt sexual activity to promote optimal functioning, such as what measures might be used to alleviate vaginal dryness, safe positions for intercourse following a total hip replacement, safe and unsafe sexual practices following a heart attack, and ways to handle ostomy appliances, urinary catheters, casts, or other devices (e.g., prostheses) during sexual activity. Similarly, nurses on a cardiac unit need specialized knowledge about sexual readjustment during cardiac rehabilitation, and nurses working with clients with spinal cord injuries need information about the sexual consequences of spinal injuries at various levels.

Using the example of the client recuperating from a heart attack, the nurse may offer the following suggestion: "Many people express concern about the stress of certain positions for intercourse, but you may use whatever position is comfortable for you and your partner, or try side-lying or partner-on-top positions."

Intensive Therapy At this level of intervention, nurses must have specialized preparation and knowledge of sexual and gender identity disorders. Sex counselling helps clients incorporate their sexual knowledge into satisfying lifestyles and socially responsible behaviour. Sex therapy is a highly specialized, in-depth treatment to help clients resolve serious sexual problems.

DEALING WITH INAPPROPRIATE SEXUAL BEHAVIOUR
Nurses, both male and female, may encounter a variety of sexually inappropriate behaviours for a variety of reasons. The behaviour may be either aggressive or nonaggressive. Clients may act out sexually in the following ways:

- Exposing themselves
- Asking the nurse to provide intimate physical care, such as bathing genital areas, when they are capable of doing this themselves
- Touching or grabbing the nurse's genitals or buttocks
- Making blatant sexual statements to the nurse
- Offering sex to the nurse
- Whistling; making comments about the nurse's attractiveness or desirability
- Making sexual comments to another client in the same room or to visitors about the "hot" nurse or what they would like to do sexually with the nurse

Possible reasons for this inappropriate behaviour are as follows:

- Fear or anxiety over future ability to function sexually
- Unmet needs for intimacy and sexual closeness because of hospitalization, injury, illness, treatment, lack of a partner, or lack of privacy
- Misinterpretation of the nurse's behaviour as sexual or provocative

- Need for reassurance that they are still sexual beings and still sexually attractive
- Need for attention
- Confusion: Neurological impairment or trauma can lead clients to use profane sexual language, engage in masturbation, expose themselves, or inappropriately touch or grab at the nurse
- Need to control: Clients may be experiencing loss of control over their lives because of hospitalization, injury, or illness
- Need for power
- Belief that flirtatious behaviour is expected because of media portrayal of nurses as sexy, available, and experienced

Before implementing any nursing interventions, the nurse should first ensure that the behaviour is inappropriate and not an attempt to communicate a physical need. For example, clients may expose themselves if they are febrile, pull at the penis if a catheter is uncomfortable or irritating, or reach for the nurse if unable to communicate verbally. Nursing strategies to deal with inappropriate sexual behaviour are shown in Box 46.6.

Evaluating

The goals established during the planning phase are evaluated according to specific desired health outcomes also established during that phase. If any outcomes have *not* been achieved, the nurse should explore the reasons why with such questions as the following:

- Were risk factors correctly identified?
- Did the client convey all significant fears and concerns about sexuality?

BOX 46.6   NURSING STRATEGIES FOR INAPPROPRIATE SEXUAL BEHAVIOUR

- Communicate that the behaviour is not acceptable by saying, for example, "I really do not like the things you are saying," or "I see you are not dressed. I will be back in 10 minutes and will help you with breakfast when you get your clothes on."
- Tell the client how the behaviour makes you feel: "I am very uncomfortable. It makes it hard for me to give you the kind of nursing care you need."
- Identify the behaviour you expect: "Please call me by my name, not 'Honey'"; or "I expect you to keep yourself covered when I am in the room."
- Set firm limits: Take the client's hand and move it away, use direct eye contact, and say, "Don't do that!"
- Try to refocus clients from the inappropriate behaviour to their real concerns and fears; offer to discuss sexuality concerns: "You have been making very personal sexual comments about yourself. Sometimes people talk like that when they are concerned about the sexual part of their life and how their illness will affect them. Are there things that you have questions about or would like to talk about?"
- Report the incident to the nurse in charge and, if appropriate, the primary care provider. Discuss the incident, your feelings, and possible interventions.
- Clarify the consequences of continued inappropriate behaviour (avoidance, withdrawal of services, no chance to help resolve underlying concerns of client).

- Was the client more comfortable following discussions about sexual matters?
- Did the client understand the nurse's teaching?
- Was the health teaching compatible with the client's culture and religious values?
- Was the client ready to deal with sexuality problems?

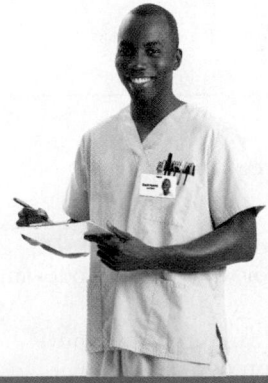

Case Study 46

Mr. Curry, a 50-year-old Canadian male of African origin, has diabetes and suffered a heart attack 3 weeks ago. He is doing well and is in a cardiac rehabilitation program. His diabetes is controlled with diet, and his only medications consist of a daily Aspirin and an antihypertensive medication. During a routine checkup, you inquire how he is feeling and whether he is doing well on his medications. Reluctantly, he admits that he is having some sexual problems. You encourage further discussion of the matter by displaying interest and explaining that it is okay for him to share his concerns with you. Mr. Curry states that he is having some difficulty achieving erections, but is more concerned that he will have another heart attack if he engages in sexual activities.

CRITICAL THINKING QUESTIONS

1. Speculate about Mr. Curry's reluctance to discuss his sexual concerns.
2. What factors influence nurses' abilities to discuss sexual concerns with their clients?
3. What is the relationship between health and sexual function?

4. How can you best intervene to help Mr. Curry?

Check the eText in MyNursingLab for answers and explanations.

KEY TERMS

anal stimulation *p. 1497*	female sexual arousal	male erectile disorder	sexual aversion disorder
androgyny *p. 1496*	disorder *p. 1501*	*p. 1501*	*p. 1501*
andropause *p. 1494*	gender identity *p. 1495*	male orgasmic disorder	sexual health *p. 1494*
body image *p. 1495*	gender-role behaviour	*p. 1501*	sexuality *p. 1490*
cross-dressing *p. 1497*	*p. 1495*	masturbation *p. 1490*	sexual orientation *p. 1496*
desire phase *p. 1500*	genital intercourse	menopause *p. 1494*	sexual self-concept *p. 1495*
dysmenorrhea *p. 1490*	*p. 1497*	menstruation *p. 1490*	transgender individuals
dyspareunia *p. 1502*	hypoactive sexual desire	oral–genital sex *p. 1497*	*p. 1496*
excitement phase *p. 1500*	disorder *p. 1501*	orgasmic phase *p. 1500*	vaginismus *p. 1502*
female orgasmic	intersex *p. 1496*	resolution phase	vestibulitis *p. 1502*
disorder *p. 1501*	Kunyaza *p. 1497*	*p. 1500*	vulvodynia *p. 1502*

CHAPTER HIGHLIGHTS

- Sexuality is important in developing self-identity, interpersonal relationships, intimacy, and love.

- There is a tremendous range of variation in how people express their sexuality, including sexual orientation, gender identity, and erotic preferences.

- Factors that affect sexuality include family, culture, religion, personal expectations and ethics, disease processes, medications, and relationship problems.

- Sexual problems include desire disorders, arousal disorders, orgasmic disorders, sexual pain disorders, and problems with satisfaction.

- Assessing risk for or actual sexual problems is part of the initial nursing assessment.

- Nurses assess attitudes toward sexuality, including factors that affect attitudes and behaviours.

- Before assisting clients with sexual problems, nurses must be aware of their own feelings and beliefs so that they can objectively prepare approaches for

gathering data and creating the nursing care plan. The nurse uses a culturally sensitive, nonjudgmental, nonthreatening, and reassuring approach.

- Nursing diagnoses for clients with sexual problems are related to altered body structure or function, lack of knowledge or misinformation about sexual matters, physical or psychological abuse, value conflicts, and loss or lack of a partner. Common nursing diagnoses include ineffective sexuality pattern and sexual dysfunction.

- Nursing interventions focus largely on teaching clients about sexual health and function, responsible sexual behaviour that includes the prevention of STIs and unwanted pregnancies, breast awareness and breast screening, and self-examination of the testicles.

- Counselling clients with altered sexual functions can be facilitated by using the PLISSIT model: permission giving (P), limited information (LI), and specific suggestions (SS). Intensive therapy (IT) requires intervention by clinical nurse specialists or sex therapists.

ASSESS YOUR LEARNING

1. Breast cancer is one of the leading causes of death for Canadian women. Which of the following is the BEST method to routinely detect breast cancer for women age 50 years and older?

   a. They should be aware of what their breasts look and feel like normally.

   b. They should have a clinical breast examination monthly.

   c. They should have a mammography every 2 to 3 years.

   d. They should ask for blood tests for breast cancer genetic screening.

2. What is the BEST way for the nurse to promote safe sexual practices in a group of adolescents?

   a. Provide condoms

   b. Encourage abstinence

   c. Teach ways to prevent pregnancy

   d. Teach safe sex practices

3. Clients are unlikely to introduce the topic of sex with health care providers for which of the following reasons?

   a. They assume that health care providers know little about sexual functioning.

   b. Most clients have few, if any, questions or problems.

   c. Female clients prefer to discuss problems with female health care providers.

   d. They are too embarrassed to introduce the topic of sex.

4. A client informs the nurse that he is a transsexual. Which of the following is MOST representative of this client?

   a. Gonadal gender, internal organs, and external genitals are contradictory.

   b. Sexual anatomy is not consistent with gender identity.

   c. Sexual attraction is to individuals of both genders.

   d. Gender identity is altered by acute psychosis.

5. A nurse informs a client who is 8½ months pregnant that it is best to abstain from intercourse until after the birth of the baby. This communication is MOST representative of which component of the PLISSIT model?

   a. Permission giving (P)

   b. Limited information (LI)

   c. Specific suggestions (SS)

   d. Intensive therapy (IT)

6. A male client is starting on an antidepressant medication. Which of the following should be included in the teaching?

   a. "Your partner will be pleased because your sexual functioning is going to improve."

   b. "You may find that your desire for sex will decrease while on this medication."

   c. "Retrograde ejaculation is a common problem when taking antidepressants."

   d. "Your skin will probably become supersensitive to touch, so you may need to change your activity during sex."

7. A 75-year-old male client reports decreased frequency of sexual intercourse, but he does not express any dissatisfaction or difficulty. He seems a little embarrassed by the discussion but is engaged and asks some questions. An appropriate nursing diagnosis would be which of the following?

   a. Sexual dysfunction

   b. Disturbed body image

   c. Sedentary lifestyle

   d. Readiness for enhanced knowledge

8. Which of the following outcomes may indicate the need for referral to a more highly skilled therapist?

   a. The client verbalizes methods of modifying sexual activity according to physical limitations.

   b. The client requests the phone number of a sex education support group.

   c. Suggestions given by the nurse are ineffective in reaching the desired goals.

   d. The client reports experimenting with new sexual activities.

9. A client reports having dyspareunia. Which of the following questions is the MOST appropriate for the nurse to ask?

   a. "Have you talked with your partner about this discomfort?"

   b. "Have you had these spasms since you became sexually active?"

   c. "Do you have pain before your period begins?"

   d. "Do your breasts swell large enough to need a larger bra?"

10. Including at least some sexual health history questions would be most relevant for clients taking which of the following classification of drugs?

   a. Anti-inflammatories (such as ibuprofen)

   b. Hypnotics (sleeping pills)

   c. Antihypertensives (blood pressure medications)

   d. Antihistamines (cold medications)

Check the eText in MyNursingLab for answers and explanations.

WEBLINKS

Public Health Agency of Canada
http://www.phac-aspc.gc.ca/std-mts/sti-its/guide-lignesdir-eng.php
This site provides the publication Canadian Guidelines on Sexually Transmitted Infections.

The Society of Obstetricians and Gynaecologists of Canada
http://www.sexualityandu.ca (English)
http://www.masexualite.ca (en français)
An initiative of Obstetricians and Gynaecologists of Canada, this website provides accurate and up-to-date information on sexual health and healthy sexuality.

Sex Information and Education Council of Canada
http://www.sieccan.org
This nonprofit association was established to promote education about human sexuality.

VIDEO

TSE – Self Exam – How to

http://www.tctca.org/index.php?option=com_content&view=article&id=49&Itemid=67

For specific techniques of self-examination.

MyNursingLab

REFERENCES

Andelloux, M. (2010). Products for sexual lubrication: Understanding and addressing options with your patients. *Nursing for Women's Health, 15*(3), 253–257.

Annon, J. (1974). The behavioural treatment of sexual problems. Vol. 1. *Brief Therapy*. New York, NY: Harper & Row.

Basson, R. (2005). Women's sexual dysfunction: Revised and expanded definitions. *Canadian Medical Association Journal, 172*(10), 1327–1333.

Beemyn, B. G., Rankin, S. R., & Beemyn, G. (2011). *The lives of transgender people*. New York, NY: Columbia University Press.

Canadian Cancer Society's Steering Committee on Cancer Statistics. (2012, May). *Canadian cancer statistics 2012.* Toronto, ON: Canadian Cancer Society.

Canadian Federation for Sexual Health. (2007). *Sexual health in Canada—Baseline 2007.* Ottawa, ON: Author.

Canadian Task Force on Preventive Health Care. (2011). *Screening for breast cancer: Summary of recommendations for clinicians and policy-makers*. Retrieved from http://www.canadiantaskforce.ca/recommendations/2011_01_eng.html

Canadian Testicular Cancer Society. (2011). *What is testicular cancer?* Retrieved from http://www.tctca.org/index.php?option=com_content&view=article&id=47&Itemid=37

Donohoe, J. (2010). Uncovering sexual abuse: Evaluation of the effectiveness of the victims of violence and abuse prevention program. *Journal of Psychiatric & Mental Health Nursing, 17,* 9–18. doi: 10.1111/j.1365-2850.2009.01479.x

Girshick, L. B., & Green, J. (2009). *Transgender voices: Beyond women and men.* Lebanon, NH: University Press of New England.

Health Nexus Santé. (2007). Update report on teen pregnancy prevention. Toronto, ON: Best Start: Ontario's Maternal Newborn and Early Child Development Resource Centre. Retrieved from http://www.beststart.org/resources/rep_health/pdf/teen_pregnancy.pdf

Health Nexus Santé. (2008). Teen pregnancy prevention: Exploring out-of-school approaches. Toronto, ON. Best Start. Ontario's Maternal Newborn and Early Child Development Resource Centre. Retrieved from http://www.nfhs-pg.org/media/1_Prevention/teen_pregnancy.pdf

Health Nexus Santé. (2009). Subsequent teen pregnancies: Exploring the issues, impact and effectiveness of prevention strategies. Toronto, ON: Best Start: Ontario's Maternal Newborn and Early Child Development Resource Centre. Retrieved from http://www.beststart.org/resources/preconception/subsequent_teen_preg.pdf

Hertlein, K. M., Weeks, G., & Gambescia, N. (2008). *Systemic sex therapy.* New York, NY: Routledge.

Hertlein, K. M., Weeks, G., & Sendak, S. (2009). *A clinician's guide to systemic sex therapy.* New York, NY: Routledge.

Ilic, D., & Misso, M. L. (2011). *Screening for testicular cancer* (review). The Cochrane Collaboration, Issue 2. Retrieved from http://www.update-software.com/BCP/WileyPDF/EN/CD007853.pdf

Jodoin, M., Bergeron, S., Khalife, S., Dupuis, M. J., Desrochers, G., & Leclerc, B. (2008). Male partners of women with provoked vestibulodynia. *Journal of Sexual Medicine, 5,* 2862–2870. doi: 10.1111/j.1743-6109.2008.00950.x

Katz, A. (2009). When worlds collide: Urinary incontinence and female sexuality. *American Journal of Nursing, 109*(3), 59–63.

Kingdon, J. (2009). Vulvodynia: A comprehensive review. *Nursing for Women's Health. 13*(1), 48–57. doi: 10.1111/j.1751-486X.2009.01373.x

Kleinplatz, P. (2012). *New directions in sex therapy: Innovations and alternatives.* New York, NY: Routledge.

Levin, R. J. (2007). Sexual activity, health and well-being: The beneficial roles of coitus and masturbation. *Sexual and Relationship Therapy, 22,* 135–148. doi: 10.1080/14681990601149197

Miller, C. L., Strathdee, M., Kerr, T., Li, K., & Wood, E. (2006). Factors associated with early adolescent initiation into injection drug use: Implication for intervention programs. *Journal of Adolescent Health, 38*(4), 462–464.

NANDA International. (2012). *Nursing diagnoses: Definitions and classification 2012–2014.* Oxford, United Kingdom: Wiley-Blackwell.

Pole, J., & Flicker, S. (2010). Sexual behaviour profile of a diverse group of urban youth: An analysis of the Toronto Teen Survey. *The Canadian Journal of Human Sexuality, 19*(4), 145–156.

Polomeno, V., & Dubeau, D. (2009). La sexopérinatalité: Où en sommes-nous? *L'Infirmière clinicienne, 6*(2), 20–24.

Ponte, M., Klemperer, E., Sahay, A., & Chren, M.-M. (2009). Effects of vulvodynia on quality of life. *Journal of the American Academy of Dermatology, 60*(1), 70–76.

Public Health Agency of Canada (2008). *Canadian guidelines for sexual health education.* Retrieved from http://www.phac-aspc.gc.ca/publicat/cgshe-ldnemss/pdf/guidelines-eng.pdf

Public Health Agency of Canada. (2010a). *Human papillomavirus (HPV)*. Retrieved from http://www.phac-aspc.gc.ca/std-mts/hpv-vph/fact-faits-eng.php

Public Health Agency of Canada. (2010b). *Hepatitis B—Get the facts*. Retrieved from http://www.phac-aspc.gc.ca/hcai-iamss/bbp-pts/hepatitis/hep_b-eng.php

Public Health Agency of Canada. (2010c). *Reported cases of notifiable STI from January to June 30, 2009 and January 1 to June 30, 2010 and corresponding annual rates for the years 2009 and 2010*. Retrieved from http://www.phac-aspc.gc.ca/std-mts/stdcases-casmts/index-eng.php

Public Health Agency of Canada. (2010d). *HIV and AIDS in Canada. Surveillance Report to December 31, 2009*. Retrieved from http://www.phac-aspc.gc.ca/aids-sida/publication/survreport/2009/dec/pdf/2009-Report-Rapport.pdf

Public Health Agency of Canada. (2011). *HIV/AIDS Epi Updates—July 2010*. Retrieved from http://www.phac-aspc.gc.ca/aids-sida/publication/epi/2010/1-eng.php

Rayside, D. (2008). *Queer inclusions, continental divisions.* Toronto, ON: University of Toronto Press.

Rotermann, M. (2005). Sex, condoms, and sexually transmitted infections among young people. *Statistics Canada Report, 16*(3), 39–49.

Rothermann, M. (2008). Trends in teen sexual behaviour and condom use. *Statistics Canada Report, 19*(3), 1–5.

Sauvé, R., & Royle, C. (2009). Male circumcision. In Public Health Agency of Canada. *What mothers say: The Canadian Maternity Experiences Survey* (pp. 222–225). Retrieved from http://www.phac-aspc.gc.ca/rhs-ssg/pdf/survey-eng.pdf

Shah, G., Susan, L., & Furcroy, J. (2009). Female circumcision: History, medical and psychological complications and initiatives to eradicate this practice. *Canadian Journal of Urology, 16*, 4576–4579.

Siegfried, N., Muller, M., Deeks, J. J., & Volmink, J. (2009). Male circumcision for prevention of heterosexual acquisition of HIV in men. *Cochrane Database of Systematic Reviews 2009, 2*(CD003362). doi: 10.1002/14651858.CD003362.pub2

Smylie, L., Medaglia, S., & Maticka-Tyndale, E. (2006). The effect of social capital and socio-demographics on adolescent risk and sexual health behaviours. *Canadian Journal of Sexuality, 15*(2), 95–112.

Statistics Canada. (2010, updated July 8, 2011). *Gay pride . . . by the numbers.* Retrieved from http://www42.statcan.gc.ca/smr08/2011/smr08_158_2011-eng.htm

Taylor, C. & Peter, T., with McMinn, T. L., Elliott, T., Beldom, S., Ferry, A., Gross, Z., Paquin, S., & Schachter, K. (2011). *Every class in every school: The first national climate survey on homophobia, biphobia, and transphobia in Canadian schools.* Final report. Toronto, ON: Egale Canada Human Rights Trust.

WHO/ICO (2010). Human papillovirus and related cancers—summary report update, September 15, 2010–Canada. Barcelona, Spain: WHO/ICO Information Centre on HPV and Cervical Cancer (HPV Information Centre. Retrieved from http://apps.who.int/hpvcentre/statistics/dynamic/ico/country_pdf/CAN.pdf?CFID=4005139&CFTOKEN=50211239

Chapter 47

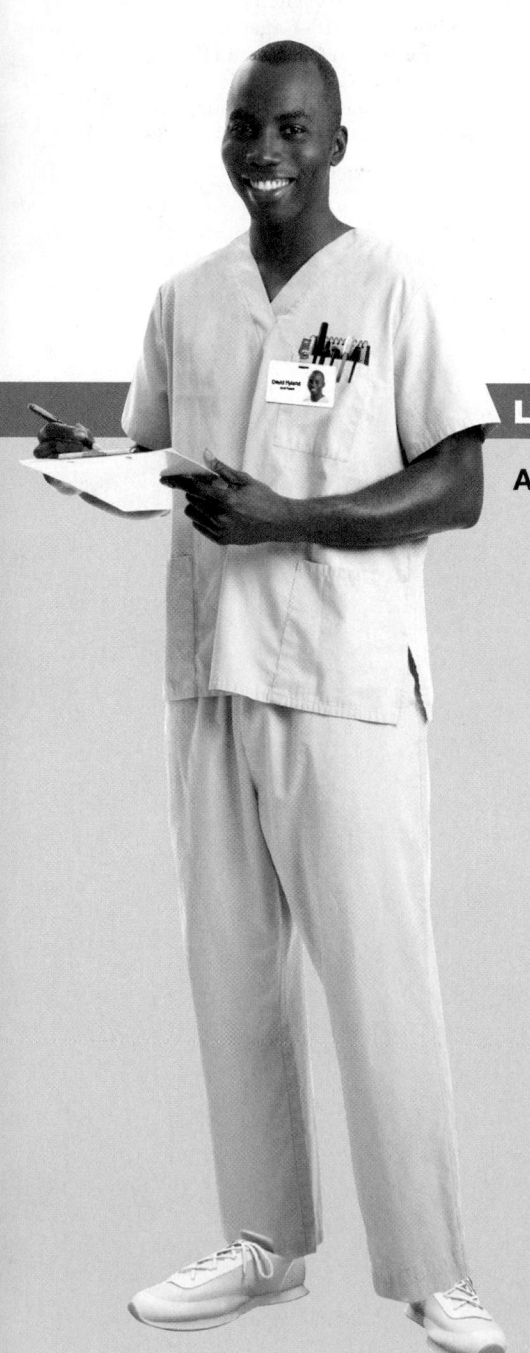

Spirituality

The nurse provides care not only for the physical body and mind but also for the client's spirit, soul, or inner essence. Assessing and responding to the client's spiritual needs can decrease suffering and aid in physical and mental healing (see the Nursing and Canadian Society box).

Nursing and Canadian Society

Fact	Implications for Nursing Practice
About 75% of Canadians say they have spiritual needs. A further breakdown appears below: • 38% say spirituality is very important to them. • 82% believe in God. • 65% say they believe that "God or a higher power cares for them personally." • 72% of Canadians pray (daily, 27%; rarely, 19%) • 84% of Canadians identify with a specific religion (Bibby, 2006).	Nurses should engage clients with basic assessment questions that include recognition of spirituality, and intervention should include interdisciplinary teamwork with spiritual care professionals to address clients' spiritual and religious issues or needs.

To provide holistic care, nurses need to not only care for the physical body and mind but also be attentive to the client's spirit (Carpenter, Girvin, Kitner, & Ruth-Sahd, 2008). To assess for spiritual care needs and offer interventions, nurses require multidimensional listening skills and an ability to establish trusting nurse–client relationships that are attentive to caring for the human spirit. A client's spirituality is complex and individual. Each person or family unit inevitably approaches their health challenges, decisions, suffering, and life implications with a world view that reflects what are typically considered spiritual or religious beliefs (Pesut, Fowler, Reimer-Kirkham, Taylor, & Sawatzky, 2009; Van Leeuwen, Tiesinga, Jochemsen, & Post, 2007). Because involvement in spiritual care is personal for both the nurse and the client, nurses need to communicate with sensitivity and empathy, have a good understanding of their own world view as well as spiritual and religious beliefs, and understand how this can affect their ability to provide spiritual care (Chung, Wong, & Chan, 2007). They need to familiarize themselves with the concept of spirituality as something that is broad and diversely understood but also meaningful and integral for whole-person, or holistic, care.

Nurses cannot rely solely on their own spiritual and religious beliefs, learning, or practices when providing spiritual care as a dimension of holistic care. They need to be knowledgeable about various religious traditions and spiritual practices that express clients' spirituality. Furthermore, nurses need to know when they have reached limitations of their understanding about spirituality and how to access specially educated spiritual care providers. Optimal spiritual care recognizes that clients benefit most when approached collaboratively and in light of their unique needs (Baldacchino, 2006). Many clients have spiritual strengths that the nurse can nurture to help the client attain or maintain a feeling of spiritual health, recover from illness, or face death peacefully. Likewise, many clients have had traumatic experiences that have wounded their spirits and will need interdisciplinary teamwork to facilitate spiritual health.

Spirituality and Related Concepts

Spirituality, religion, and faith are distinct entities, yet the words are often used interchangeably by clients and professionals alike. The word *spiritual* derives from the Hebrew *ruah* (wind) and the Latin *spiritus,* meaning "to blow" or "to breathe," and has come to mean something that gives life or essence to being human. A recent nursing concept analysis defined **spirituality** as "that most human of experiences that seeks to transcend self and find meaning and purpose through connection with others, nature, and/or a Supreme Being, which may or may not involve religious structures or traditions" (Buck, 2006, p. 288). Although numerous nurses have analyzed the concept of spirituality, they still often complain that there is a lack of consensus among nurses as to what it is, and that definitions are too vague and "elastic" to be helpful (Paley, 2008). Other nurse scholars suggest that this elasticity is essential so that persons from diverse viewpoints can use the concept (Pesut, 2008).

Spirituality involves the following essential elements (Chiu, Emblen, Van Hofwegen, Sawatzky, & Meyerhoff, 2004):

- Experiencing life with existential awareness—including hope, meaning-making, and purposeful living

- Being in relationship and connectedness—including relating to self, others, Other

- Opening to that which transcends or goes beyond current situations and circumstances

- Being motivated through energizing, unifying, and life-giving forces—including inspiration, guidance, striving for wholeness

Although spirituality is a broad concept, **religion** is more practical and acts as a container or holding environment that offers ways to express spirituality. World religions serve as formal, socially recognized communities within which people share common values, beliefs, and practices (Clark & Olson, 2000). Diverse religious traditions provide guidance for believers in responding to life's questions and challenges. According to a classic study by Vardey (1996), organized religions offer (a) a sense of community bound by common beliefs, (b) the collective study of sacred texts (Torah, Bible, Koran, or others), (c) the performance of ritual, (d) the use of disciplines and practices, commandments, and sacraments, and (e) ways of taking care of the person's soul (such as fasting, prayer, and meditation). Many traditional religious practices and rituals are related to such life events as birth, transition from childhood to adulthood, marriage, illness, and death. Religious principles can also apply to matters of daily life, such as dress, food, social interaction, menstruation, and sexual relationships (Marks, 2004). It is important to be aware, however, that a client can follow certain religious practices and yet not internalize the symbolic meaning behind the practices.

Just as a rich language surrounds the concept of spirituality, a complex composition of terms and cautions are frequently associated with religiosity. Kendler, Liu, Gardner, McCullough, Larson, and Prescott (2003) identify seven dimensions of religiosity (see Box 47.1). These diverse descriptions can exist in nurse and client alike. There is reason, therefore, to hold diversity of both spirituality and religions in balance. Religious beliefs, influences, traditions, and structures form part of the client's total capacity for mindfulness, coping, and meaning-making. In this light, an **agnostic** will question the existence of God or a supreme being, whereas an **atheist** will not acknowledge belief in the existence of God. At the same time both agnostics and atheists, while wanting to be respected for their nonbelief, still desire to find meaning in life and to remain connected to close persons and the natural world at the end of life (Smith-Stoner, 2007). In a different vein, some religions describe themselves as **theistic** (e.g., Baha'i, Christianity, Hinduism, Islam, Judaism) based on belief in a higher

BOX 47.1	DIMENSIONS OF RELIGIOSITY
General Religiosity	A person's concern and involvement with spiritual issues; active involvement with God on a day-to-day basis and at times of crisis
Social Religiosity	Interaction with other religious individuals and frequency of attendance at a church or other places of worship
Involved-God Religiosity	Belief in a deity who is actively and positively involved in human affairs
Forgiveness Religiosity	A caring, loving, and forgiving approach to the world
God-as-Judge Religiosity	Belief in a deity who is judgmental and punitive
Unvengefulness Religiosity	An attitude toward the world that emphasizes personal retaliation rather than forgiveness
Thankfulness Religiosity	Feelings of thankfulness versus anger toward life and God

Source: Adapted from Kendler, K., Liu, X., Gardner, C., McCullough, M., Larson, D., & Prescott, C. (2003). Dimensions of religiosity and their relationship to lifetime psychiatric and substance use disorders. *American Journal of Psychiatry, 160,* 496–503.

power or God. Other religions focus attention on noble **truths** (Buddhism), principles of **consciousness** (Hare Krishna), or Earth's **seasons** and cycles (Aboriginal peoples, Wiccan traditions). Being aware of diversity and of complexity are important nursing skills when seeking to care for the human spirit.

A third related concept is *faith.* This term is often used to describe the relational essence of spirituality and religion as these are experienced in everyday life. Faith points to the human need to connect with nature, family, various communities, and realities that transcend normal activities. **Faith** has been described as "being in relationship with" the various others that make life meaningful, such as God, loved ones, and social contacts (Clark, 2000, p. 19). Over time, meaning attached to the concept of *faith* has included that it is a "constitutive dimension" of human existence (Panikkar, 1971), a "universal" feature of living, acting, and self-understanding (Fowler & Keen, 1985), an allegiance, commitment, trust, or loyalty innately human and present in both religious and nonreligious people (Bowker, 1997), and an aspect of ongoing human development (Fowler & Dell, 2006).

Spiritual, Religious, and Faith Development

A number of authors have contributed to understanding the concepts of spirituality, religion, and faith as **developmental**. Some have highlighted "stages" (Fowler, 1981; Fowler & Dell, 2006) through which people move over the course of their lifetime. Others have emphasized faith development as a "journey" that can be "mapped" (Fowler & Keen, 1985). This image is helpful in assisting clients to see their lives in time (chronological dates) and space (geographical places), and to reflect on events that have occurred as they would reflect on various aspects of travelling.

Ford (1988) used the metaphor of "life spirals" by combining the faith development theory of James Fowler (1981) and the psychosocial theory of Erik Erikson (1963) to describe multidimensional processes that occur as life transitions (see Table 47.1). The spiral is an ancient transcultural and multifaith image that is used all over the world to communicate connections that exist in

TABLE 47.1 Faith Development Models: Highlighting the Spiral Faith Model in Connection to James Fowler's and Erik Erikson's Development Theories

J. Fowler (1981) Stages of Faith	I. Ford (1988) Spiral Faith Model	E. Erikson (1963) [With I. Ford (1988) added] Psychosocial Task
Undifferentiated (Birth to 2 years)	**INCARNATING FAITH** "Ahh…" (Birth to circa 6 months) Faith Gift: Trust [embedded in the family]	INFANCY (birth to 18 months) Conflict: Basic Trust vs. Mistrust
	EXPLORING FAITH "Yes, Yes . . . No, No" (Circa 6 months to 2 years) Faith Gift: Joy [embedded in feelings]	EARLY CHILDHOOD (18 months to 3 years) Conflict: Autonomy vs. Shame
Intuitive–projective (4 to 6 years)	**SELFING FAITH** "That's mine!" (Circa 2 to 5 years) Faith Gift: OK-ness [embedded in needs]	LATE CHILDHOOD (3 to 6 years) Conflict: Initiative vs. Guild
Mythic–literal (7 to 12 years)	**SCHOOLING FAITH** "Can I?" (Circa 6 to 11 years) Faith Gift: Life Stories [embedded in skills]	SCHOOL AGE (6 to 12 years) Conflict: Industry vs. Inferiority
Synthetic–conventional (Adolescent to adult)	**INTER-PERSONAL FAITH** "Why should I?" (Circa 12 to 14 years) Faith Gift: Forgiveness [embedded in the peer group]	[I. Ford added] Conflict: Affiliation vs. Abandonment
Individuating–reflective (After 18 years)	**INTRA-INDIVIDUAL FAITH** "Why did I?" (Circa 15 to 21 years) Faith Gift: Acceptance of Difference [embedded in cultural systems]	ADOLESCENT (12 to 18 years) Conflict: Identity vs. Role Confusion
	INTRO-VOCATIONAL FAITH "Show me how." (Circa 22 to 29 years) Faith Gift: Love [embedded in discipleship/roles]	YOUNG ADULT (18 to 25 years) [I. Ford added] Conflict: Intimacy vs. Isolation
Paradoxical–consolidative (After 30 years)	**INTRO-WORLD FAITH** "I care." (Circa 30 to 39 years) Faith Gift: Caring [embedded in stewardship]	ADULTHOOD (25 to 65 years) Conflict: Generativity vs. Stagnation
Universalizing (Maybe never)	**EXTRA-SELF FAITH** "It's too much!" (Circa 40 to 55 years) Faith Gift: Acceptance of Limits [embedded in experience]	MATURITY (65 years to death) Conflict: Integrity vs. Despair
	SPIRITUAL FAITH "Hanging loose." (Circa 55 to 65 years) Faith Gift: Letting Go [embedded in perspective]	[I. Ford added] Conflict: Interiorizing vs. Separating
	TRANSITIONAL FAITH "Now what?" (Circa 65 to 75 years) Faith Gift: Hope [embedded in change]	[I. Ford added] Conflict: Expanding vs. Constricting
	TRANSCENDING FAITH "My life is held." (Circa 75 plus years) Faith Gift: Peace [embedded in faith]	[I. Ford added] Conflict: Trust vs. Fear

Source: From Ford, I. M. (1988). *Life spirals: The faith journey* (pp. 19–20). Burlington, ON: Welch Publishing Company. Used by permission of the author.

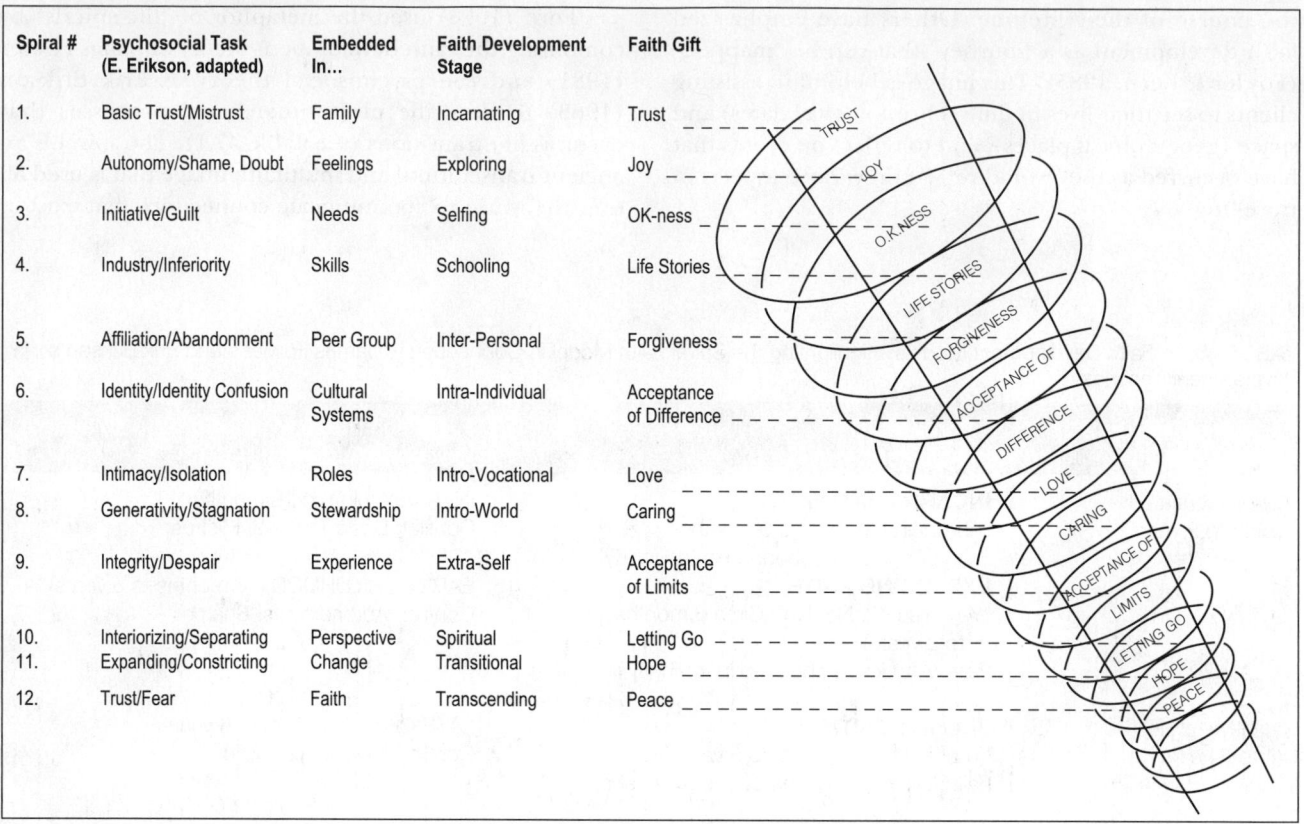

Spiral #	Psychosocial Task (E. Erikson, adapted)	Embedded In...	Faith Development Stage	Faith Gift
1.	Basic Trust/Mistrust	Family	Incarnating	Trust
2.	Autonomy/Shame, Doubt	Feelings	Exploring	Joy
3.	Initiative/Guilt	Needs	Selfing	OK-ness
4.	Industry/Inferiority	Skills	Schooling	Life Stories
5.	Affiliation/Abandonment	Peer Group	Inter-Personal	Forgiveness
6.	Identity/Identity Confusion	Cultural Systems	Intra-Individual	Acceptance of Difference
7.	Intimacy/Isolation	Roles	Intro-Vocational	Love
8.	Generativity/Stagnation	Stewardship	Intro-World	Caring
9.	Integrity/Despair	Experience	Extra-Self	Acceptance of Limits
10.	Interiorizing/Separating	Perspective Change	Spiritual Transitional	Letting Go
11.	Expanding/Constricting			Hope
12.	Trust/Fear	Faith	Transcending	Peace

FIGURE 47.1 Spiral Faith Model: Spiral by Spiral Description.

Source: From Ford, I. M. (1988). *Life spirals: The faith journey* (pp. 19–20). Burlington, ON: Welch Publishing Company. Used by permission of the author.

chronological and situational spiritual experiences. In her spiral faith model (see Figure 47.1), Iris Ford (1988) depicted each spiral as a "cluster of opportunities" fashioned by "maturation, experience, and previous opportunities" (p. 15). One by one, and taken together, the 12 faith development spirals invite individuals and groups to face what life offers, both the positive and negative, with an attitude of hope.

The other key concept associated with depicting spiritual, religious, and faith development is **world view**. This concept derives from the German word *Weltanschauung* and aligns with various approaches to the term *environment* found in the nursing metaparadigm. World view focuses attention on the context within which people move toward health. An individual's or a group's geographical location, psychosocial–spiritual circumstances and resources, and socioeconomic position contribute to their world view. These variables influence how people see and interpret the world insofar as they filter perceptions based on a person's or group's set of **beliefs**, **values**, and **assumptions** about life and the universe. Nurses need to notice and empathically engage the belief statements expressed by their clients to more fully understand the world view out of which they are operating (Dy-Liacco, Piedmont, Murray-Swank, Rodgerson, & Sherman, 2009).

Spiritual and Religious Care in Contemporary Context

Global events of the late twentieth century and the early twenty-first century changed health care professionals' approaches to spiritual and religious care. With both the decade of buildup to a new millennium and the impact of terrorist attacks in the United States on September 11, 2001, came a great deal of reflection on historical, theological, and sociopolitical themes. Of particular note has been literature on millennialism, religious fundamentalism, and globalization (Salzman, 2008), and the United Nations Millennium Declaration (United Nations General Assembly, 2000). Ongoing uncertainty and unpredictability related to terrorism, hotspots of military conflict, climate change, and pandemic threats, continue to bring to the fore awareness of the interfaces among world religions, politics, and economics. Consequently, one health implication for spiritual and religious care today is the prominence of **generalized anxiety**—a state of mental uneasiness, apprehension, or dread that produces an increased level of arousal—and its potential to evoke spiritual distress in individuals as well as groups.

The practical implications of these developments on spiritual and religious care by nurses include the need to do the following:

- Thinking globally while acting locally
- Realizing that diverse subgroups or denominations exist within many world religions
- Engaging differing spiritual and religious perspectives with respectful inquiry
- Recognizing the health implications that flow out of clients' spiritual and religious views and practices, and gaining greater skill in assessing spiritual health and spiritual needs through interdisciplinary education and professional collaboration

Spiritual Health and Spiritual Distress

Several concepts used in the literature speak about healthy spirituality. These include the ancient idea of *holiness,* as well as the more contemporary terms *wholeness, spiritual well-being, spiritual wellness,* and *spiritual health.* **Spiritual well-being** refers to the "ability to experience and integrate meaning and purpose in life through connectedness with self, others, art, music, literature, nature, and/or a power greater than oneself that can be strengthened (NANDA International, 2009, p. 292). **Spiritual wellness** is "a way of living, a lifestyle that views and lives life as purposeful and pleasurable, that seeks out life-sustaining and life-enriching options to be chosen freely at every opportunity, and that sinks its roots deeply into spiritual values and/or specific religious beliefs" (Pilch, 1988, p. 31). **Spiritual health** is a feeling of being "generally alive, purposeful, and fulfilled" (Ellison, 1983, p. 332).

People enhance or nurture their spirituality in many ways. Some of these focus on development of the inner self or world; others focus on the expression of their inner essence to others or the outer world. Relating to the inner self or soul can be achieved through having an inner dialogue with a higher power or with the self; praying or meditating; analyzing dreams; communing with nature; listening quietly to music; or experiencing the inspiration of art, drama, or dance. The expression of a person's inner essence to others is manifested in loving relationships with and service to others, joy and laughter, and participation in spiritual or religious rituals.

Spiritual distress refers to a disturbance in or a challenge to the core value system that provides strength, hope, and meaning to a person's life. Many factors are associated with spiritual distress: physiological problems, treatment-related concerns, or situational concerns. A fourth factor associated with spiritual distress is that of developmental transitions (Clark & Olson, 2000). Physiological problems include having a medical diagnosis of a terminal or debilitating disease or experiencing pain, the loss of bodily function, or a miscarriage or stillbirth.

Treatment-related factors include the recommendation for blood transfusions, surgery, dietary restrictions, amputation of a body part, or isolation. Situational factors can involve the death or illness of a significant other, barriers to or embarrassment at practising rituals (Carpenito-Moyet, 2008). NANDA International (2007) offered the following as defining characteristics of spiritual distress:

- Experiencing a disturbance in a personal belief system
- Questioning the meaning of life, death, or suffering
- Questioning the credibility of a personal belief system
- Demonstrating discouragement or despair
- Choosing not to practise usual religious rituals
- Having ambivalent feelings (doubts) about beliefs
- Not having a reason for living
- Feeling a sense of spiritual emptiness
- Showing emotional detachment from self and others
- Expressing concern (e.g., anger, resentment, fear) over the meaning of life, suffering, or death
- Requesting spiritual assistance for a disturbance in a belief system

Interdisciplinary Spiritual Care Planning and Intervention

With the benefits of increased awareness and interest in the topics of spirituality, religion, and faith, nurses, together with their interdisciplinary colleagues in chaplaincy, social work, psychology, rehabilitation sciences, and medicine, are in a position to examine the spiritual and religious values and assumptions embedded in health care language and treatment paradigms. Helpful in this regard are the insights of Gottlieb and Ezer (1997) in their writing about the McGill model of nursing. They emphasized that understandings of health are learned within diverse family configurations, and these understandings can be engaged through professional activities that recognize clients' potential and resources for taking greater ownership of their health.

Foundational to the McGill model is the promotion of inquiry and an exploratory approach to data collection. This approach is conducive to interdisciplinary dialogue and can result in obtaining an overall profile of health. According to Olson (2000), health or wholeness can become "the goal toward which we strive during times of transition" including "health risks and health potentials as these exist in transitional times" (p. 224). A complete assessment of health risks and potentials requires the knowledge and skill of diverse health care professionals. Each profession that includes spiritual care as central to its reason for being (i.e., chaplaincy) or associative to its optimal provision of care (i.e., nursing, social work, psychology, rehabilitation sciences, and medicine) needs to be included in assessing, planning, implementing, and evaluating processes. Learning skills of interdisciplinary assessment, dialogue, collaboration, and referral in the spiritual and religious care of clients is a developing topic in the literature.

According to Puchalski, Lunsford, Harris, and Miller (2006), for example, interdisciplinary spiritual care means that all health care professionals on the team, including the chaplain, interact with one another to develop and implement the spiritual care plan for the patient in a fully collaborative model. In their book *Making Health Care Whole*, Puchalski and Ferrell (2010) distinguish three approaches to spiritual planning and intervention:

> Spiritual screening *or triage is a quick determination of whether a person is experiencing a serious spiritual crisis and therefore needs immediate referral to a professional chaplain. . . .* Spiritual history-taking *is the process of interviewing a patient and asking him or her questions about his or her life to come to a better understanding of the patient's spiritual needs and resources . . . .* Spiritual assessment *refers to an extensive, in-depth, ongoing process of actively listening to a patient's story as it unfolds in a relationship with a professional chaplain and summarizing the needs and resources that emerge. The summary includes a spiritual care plan with expected outcomes that should be communicated to the rest of the treatment team.* (pp. 94–95)

Puchalski and Ferrell believe that spiritual screening and history taking are built on sets of questions that can be employed in either quick conversations or extended interviews. By contrast, they see spiritual assessment being built on interpretive frameworks that require specialized knowledge and clinical training insofar as it is focused on in-depth relational listening to the client's story as it unfolds in the clinical relationship. Taylor (2003a) as well as Fitchett and Risk (2009) provide helpful resources for screening and history taking. In professional chaplaincy, a type of learning called *Clinical Pastoral Education* (CPE) has become the standard of specialized training for developing in-depth relational listening skills (VandeCreek, 2003). Courses in CPE are sometimes taken by nurses and have been especially valued by parish nurses (Derrickson, 2002).

Nurses are consistently at the frontlines of patient and client care across the continuum of health services. They are in an ideal position to screen, take history, assess, and refer for optimal interdisciplinary responsiveness to spiritual needs and resources. According to Taylor (2003b), it is imperative that nurses consider how they can address patient preconceptions and requisites for spiritual caregiving, and educate the public regarding their role as holistic and spiritual care providers.

Spiritual and Religious Practices Affecting Nursing Care

Spiritual holy days, sacred writings, spiritual symbols, prayer and meditation practices, rituals, and religious guidelines associated with diet, nutrition, dress, birth, and death are among the factors to consider when giving nursing care. Whenever these factors become obvious in their work with clients, nurses need to be aware that it is possible to impose personal spiritual beliefs on clients without intending to do so. Observing the following guidelines for ethical conduct in spiritual caregiving is essential. These guidelines for nurses were offered by Winslow and Wehtje-Winslow (2007):

- Seek a basic understanding of clients' spiritual needs, resources, and preferences (i.e., assess).

- Follow the client's expressed wishes regarding spiritual care.

- Do not prescribe or urge clients to adopt certain spiritual beliefs or practices, and do not pressure them to relinquish such beliefs or practices.

- Strive to understand personal spirituality and how it influences caregiving.

- Provide spiritual care in a way that is in harmony with personal beliefs.

HOLY DAYS A **holy day** is a day set aside for special religious observance. Most Christians observe Sunday as the Sabbath, while Jews and some Christians observe Saturday as the day of the week devoted to rest and worship. Muslims hold their congregational prayer on Fridays. These observances are in response to religious directives. Holy days can also be special days of celebration and feasting that occur once a year, such as Christmas and Easter (Christian), Eid al-Fitr and Eid al-Adha (Islam), and Sukkoth or the Feast of Tabernacles (Jewish).

Solemn religious observances throughout the year may be referred to as *high holy days* and may include fasting, reflection, and prayer. Examples of such holy days are Rosh Hashanah and Yom Kippur (Jewish), Good Friday (Christian), and the month-long observance of Ramadan (Islam). Many religions require fasting, extended prayer, and reflection or ritual observances on sacred days; however, believers who are seriously ill are often exempt from such requirements. Many hospitals and health care organizations facilitate ritual observances for clients and staff on holy days. For example, a hospital may provide nonmeat entrees on Ash Wednesday and Good Friday for Catholic clients, or equip separate kitchens to prepare halal dietary options for Muslim clients or kosher foods for Jewish clients. Finally, as many religions follow calendars that are different from the Gregorian calendar, a multifaith calendar can be used to identify the holy days of various faith traditions and religious groups (Griffith, 1996).

SACRED TEXTS Each religion has its sacred writings or scriptures, believed to be the thoughts or words of the Supreme Being as written by appointed prophets or disciples. Christians rely on the *Bible*; Jews on the *Torah* and *Talmud*; Muslims on the *Koran*; Hindus on several holy texts called *Vedas*; and Buddhists on the canons or teachings found in *Tripitakas* (see Box 47.2). Sacred writings frequently impart religious laws or commandments, and these are often used as the basis for secular law, such as laws regarding committing murder or stealing. Religious law can affect a client's willingness to accept treatment suggestions. For example, blood transfusion is in conflict with the religious law of Jehovah's Witnesses.

People often gain strength and hope from reading religious writings when they are ill or in crisis. See Box 47.2 for a list of sacred texts. A religion's sacred texts frequently tell the stories of religious leaders, heroes, and heroines (Boehm, 2004). Some examples include stories of Abraham, Miriam, and Samuel (Jewish); Jesus, Mary Magdalene, and Paul (Christian); Hagar or the Prophet Muhammad (Islam); Rama and Sita (Hindu); or revered Monks and their disciples (Buddhist).

SPIRITUAL SYMBOLS Spiritual symbols include jewellery, medals, amulets, icons, totems, or body ornamentation (e.g., tattoos) that carry religious or spiritual significance. They may be worn to proclaim a person's faith, to provide spiritual protection, or to be a source of comfort or strength. People may wear religious medals at all times, and they may want to wear them when they are undergoing diagnostic studies, medical treatment, or surgery. Roman Catholics may carry a *rosary* for prayer, Buddhists and Hindus carry *mala* prayer beads, and Muslims carry *subhah* prayer beads.

People may have religious icons or statues in their homes, cars, or places of work as personal reminders of their faith or as part of personal places of worship or meditation. Hospitalized clients or long-term care residents may want to have their spiritual icons or statues with them as a source of comfort.

PRAYER AND MEDITATION Most faith traditions describe practices of prayer and meditation. According to Ameling (2000) **prayer** is "the simple act of turning our mind and our heart to the sacred" (p. 42) and **meditation** is a form of spiritual practice that seeks to "still the active mind" (p. 43) so that one's attention can focus on a fixed point, word, or image. For centuries, faith traditions have differentiated active forms of prayer into the following categories: petition, intercession, confession, lamentation, adoration, invocation, and thanksgiving (Ameling, 2000). Forms of meditation may be active (guided imagery, mindfulness, repeating a mantra) or passive (detachment, self-emptying, centring). The diversity of prayerful and meditative expression is helpful to those who are experiencing illness or healing and is seen as a health promoting means through which to cope (Banziger, Van Uden, & Janssen, 2008; Levine, 2008). Some religions prescribe daily prayers or dictate specific times for prayer and worship, such as the five daily prayers (*Salat*) of the Muslims or the daily *Kaddish* of the Jews. Some religions have prescribed prayers that are printed in a prayer book, such as the *Anglican Book of Common Prayer* or the *Catholic Missal*. People who are ill may want to continue or increase their prayer practices (Narayanasamy & Narayanasamy, 2008). They may need uninterrupted quiet time during which they have their prayer books, rosaries, malas, or other icons available to them.

BELIEFS AFFECTING DIET Many religions have proscriptions regarding diet, including rules about which foods and beverages are allowed and which are prohibited. For example, Orthodox Jews may not eat shellfish or pork, and Muslims may not drink alcoholic beverages or eat pork. Mormons, who are members of the Church of Jesus Christ of Latter-day Saints, may not drink caffeinated or alcoholic beverages. Some older Catholics may choose not to eat meat on Fridays because of early Catholic religious doctrine. Religious law may also dictate how food is prepared. For example, many Jewish people require **kosher** food, that is, food prepared according to Jewish law.

Some solemn religious observances are marked by fasting, or not eating food, for a specified time. Some religions also restrict beverages; others allow drinking of water or other sustaining beverages on fast days. Examples of religions that observe fasting include Islam, Judaism, and Christianity. During the month of Ramadan, devout Muslims eat no food and avoid beverages during daylight

BOX 47.2 SACRED TEXTS	
Christianity	Bible
Judaism	Torah
	Talmud
Islam: Muslim	Koran
Hindu	Ramayana
	Mahabharata
	Vedas
	Upanishads
Sikh	Granth
Buddhism	Sutras
	Tripitakas
Zoroastrianism	Avesta
	Gathas

hours; the fast can be broken after sunset. Members of Jewish synagogues fast on Yom Kippur, the Day of Atonement; and devout Christians may fast on Good Friday. Most religions lift the fasting requirements for seriously ill clients and believers for whom fasting may be a detriment to health, such as clients with diabetes. Some religions may exempt nursing mothers or menstruating women from fasting requirements.

It is important for health care providers to prescribe diet plans with an awareness of the client's beliefs related to foods and fasting.

BELIEFS RELATED TO DRESS Many religions have laws or traditions that dictate dress. For example, Orthodox and Conservative Jewish men believe that it is important to have their head covered at all times and, therefore, wear a *yarmulke*. Orthodox Jewish women may wear a wig or scarf to cover their hair as a sign of respect. As well, Muslim women may cover their hair with a *hijab* (headscarf) in compliance with religious law and in accordance with their particular ethnic or national background. Mormons may wear temple undergarments in compliance with religious law.

Some religions require that women dress in a conservative manner, which may include not wearing sleeveless or low-cut tops and skirts that are above the knees. Some religions, Islam for example, require that the body (torso, arms, and legs) be covered. Hindu women accustomed to wearing saris prefer to cover all of the body except arms and feet. Hospital gowns may make women who want to comply with religious dress codes uneasy and uncomfortable. Clients may be especially disconcerted when undergoing diagnostic tests or treatments, such as mammography, that require body parts to be bared.

BELIEFS RELATED TO BIRTH For all faith traditions the birth of a child is an important event giving cause for celebration. Many religions have specific ritual ceremonies that consecrate the new child to God.

When a Muslim child is born, it is customary for the father, or a respected member of the local community, to whisper the *Adhan* into the baby's right ear. These words include the name of Allah the Creator and are followed by the Declaration of Faith. On the seventh day after birth, the child is named, and a tuft of hair is shaved from the head (Gatrad & Sheikh, 2001).

In the Christian faith, meaningful birth rituals include baptism, christening, and naming. Not all Christian denominations believe in the baptism of infants; therefore, it is important to inquire about a family's preference for their child. Christian parents of seriously ill infants may want a ceremony performed at birth. Whenever possible, it is beneficial to have a professional chaplain involved, since they are trained to celebrate baptisms and other meaningful rituals. In an emergency, however, any health care professional may provide baptism (Campbell & Campbell, 2005).

In the Jewish religion, the ritual circumcision conducted on male children on the eighth day after birth is an expression of the religious bond between the prophet Abraham, his descendants, and their God. Following the circumcision by the ritually trained surgeon, called a *mohel,* the child is named. Girls are named in the synagogue on the Sabbath after the birth (Fishbane, 1993).

When nurses are aware of the religious needs of families and their infants, they can assist families in fulfilling their religious hopes and obligations. This help is especially important when the newborn is seriously ill or in danger of dying because some people believe that if religious obligations are not fulfilled, the infant will not be accepted into the community of the faithful after death.

BELIEFS RELATED TO DEATH Spiritual and religious beliefs play a significant role in the believer's approach to death, just as they do in other major life events. Many believe that the person who dies transcends this life for a better place or state of being.

Some spiritual traditions have special rituals surrounding dying and death that must be observed by the faithful. Observance of these rituals provides comfort to the dying person and their loved ones. Rituals may be carried out while the person is still alive as a way of preparing for death, warding off evil, or even seeking to prevent or defer the death. These rituals may include placing a sacred book or object on or near the person, saying special prayers, such as the "Anointing of the Sick" (previously referred to as "Last Rites"), singing or chanting, and reading sacred writings. Following a person's death is another time when rituals are performed. These may include offerings of reminiscence, respect, and remembering, and may find expression through formal prayers, wailing or lamentation, and memorial or funeral services (Lobar, Youngblut, & Brooten, 2006).

Several faith traditions have specific practices that require the awareness of health care professionals. Many Muslims who are dying will want their body or head turned toward Mecca. Jews have a tradition of burial within 24 hours following death, except on the Sabbath, and they "sit Shiva" (gather to pay respects), draping any mirrors with black cloth to ensure that guests are focused on the memory of the deceased rather than on themselves. Tibetan Buddhists read the *Tibetan Book of the Dead* within 7 days of the death to release the soul of the deceased from the *Bardos,* or nether worlds. Hindus cremate the body within 24 hours to release the soul from any earthly attachment.

Some religions require that the body of the deceased be touched only by members of that faith. In both the Muslim (Denny, 1993) and the Jewish (Fishbane, 1993) religions, devout believers require that a ritual bath be given after death either by a family member or by a ritual burial society. Many religions require that a family member or other believer stay with the body at all times until it is buried or cremated. Religious symbols or objects should be treated with respect and kept with the body (Griffith, 1996). The nurse can support the family of the deceased by providing an environment conducive to the performance of death rituals.

Spiritual Health and the Nursing Process

The nursing process, which includes assessing, diagnosing, planning, implementing, and evaluation, has often been applied to spiritual care. Although this can be a helpful approach, it is now thought to misguide spiritually sensitive nursing care (Sawatzky & Pesut, 2006). Spiritual care is not a linear process in that it is not about measuring a level of spirituality, trying to fix spiritual pain, prescribing spiritual therapy, or solving spiritual problems. Rather, nursing care of the human spirit involves conversation and observation about what gives meaning and purpose through diverse relational connections and how these resources are experienced in times of changing health.

Nurses can play a pivotal role in supporting clients' spirituality. At times, offering spiritual support may include drawing on personal beliefs and practices. When considering accessing personal beliefs in the care of others, a nurse must consider the following questions:

- For what purpose am I sharing my beliefs or practices? By doing so, am I meeting my needs or my client's?
- Is my spiritual care reflecting a spiritual assessment?
- Am I imposing my beliefs on a vulnerable client?
- Am I offering my beliefs and practices in a manner that allows my client to refuse comfortably?
- Does my spiritual care hurt or contribute to a therapeutic relationship with the client?

In their professional practice, nurses need to know when they have reached the limits of their understanding about spirituality and how to access specially educated spiritual care providers. Spiritual care experts include chaplains, clergy, and other spiritual mentors that clients may identify. Likewise, although many clients view nurses as important sources of spiritual support, they often view their family and friends as primary spiritual caregivers (Hanson, Dobbs, Usher, Williams, Rawlings, & Daaleman, 2008). There may be times when nurses experience moral distress (Jameton, 1944; Pauly, Varcoe, Storch, & Newton, 2009) related to the spiritual or religious beliefs of a client conflicting with the nurse's own personal, spiritual, religious, or professional values and beliefs. It is important to acknowledge and reflect on this conflict whenever it arises. In that

process, the nurse can differentiate elements of the conflict that might impact optimal client care. For example, one's conflicting feelings may emanate from personal values (what would I do in this situation?), religious values (what does my religion have to say about the right or wrong of this situation?), and professional values (how can I respect every person's right and need for nursing care?). Often, the spiritual care experts available to clients within health care settings are also available to nursing staff in situations of moral distress. If the conflict cannot be resolved and moral distress continues, the nurse may want to explore other options available, such as removing oneself from the situation and drawing on the assistance of a nursing colleague to ensure optimal nursing care.

Assessing

Data about a client's spiritual needs, spiritual and religious practices, and spiritual resources are obtained from the client's general history; through a nursing history; and by clinical observations of the client's behaviour, verbalizations, mood, and so on. Even when a particular religion is identified, nurses should never assume that a client follows all the practices of the stated religion. Individual assessment is required to determine the nature of spiritual needs, usual spiritual and religious practices, and available spiritual resources. Clients' spiritual needs can be as important to them as their health care needs (see the Reflect on Primary Health Care box).

NURSING HISTORY The spiritual assessment is best integrated into nursing care once the nurse has developed a good relationship with the client or support person. The questions provided in the Assessment: Interview box on the next page can help begin the spiritual assessment process. In general, the nurse obtains data about the client's concept of a divine being, deity, or creative force; sources of hope and strength; religious and spiritual beliefs and practices; rituals; and any relationship perceived between spiritual beliefs and state of health.

A multitude of spiritual assessment tools have been developed from various disciplines and theoretical perspectives (Fitchett, 1993; O'Connor, Meakes, O'Neill,

REFLECT ON   PRIMARY HEALTH CARE

When examining the principles of primary health care, look at spiritual care as contributing to the principle of health promotion. Promoting health can be enhanced through the inclusion of spiritual elements in nursing care of the individual or family. This incorporation can be accomplished wherever the patient or client is encountered by the nurse and whatever the client's physical or mental health status.

ASSESSMENT	INTERVIEW

Spirituality

Asking the following questions can help the nurse assess a client's spiritual needs:

- Are any particular religious or spiritual practices important to you? If so, could you please tell me about them?
- Will being in this health care setting interfere with or complicate your religious or spiritual practices?
- In what ways is your faith important to you right now?
- In what ways can I help you connect with your faith? For example, would you like me to read your sacred writings to you or assist you with prayer or meditation?
- Would you like a visit from your spiritual counsellor, faith group leader, or a chaplain?
- What are your hopes and your sources of strength right now?
- What spiritual or religious beliefs influence you the most as you make health care decisions?

Prenner, VanStaalduinen, & Davis, 2005). These can be used as guides to assist practitioners with integrating spiritual assessment into overall health assessment. Spiritual assessment is also important when conducting family assessment and in planning family interventions. Specific guidelines have been developed for family spiritual assessments (Tanyi, 2006).

CLINICAL ASSESSMENT Cues to spiritual and religious preferences, strengths, concerns, or distress may be revealed by one or more of the following (Taylor, 2002):

1. *Environment.* Does the client have a Bible, Torah, Koran, other prayer book, devotional literature, religious symbols (i.e., prayer beads, cross, Star of David), or religious get-well cards in the room? Does a faith community send flowers or worship service bulletins?

2. *Behaviour.* Does the client appear to pray before meals or at other times or read religious literature? Does the client have nightmares and sleep disturbances, or express anger at religious representatives or a deity?

3. *Verbalization.* Does the client mention a divine being, deity, or creative force, prayer, faith, the church, synagogue, mosque, temple, spiritual or religious leader, or religious topics? Does the client ask about a visit from a spiritual mentor or faith leader? Does the client express fear of death, concern about the meaning of life, inner conflict about religious beliefs, concern about a relationship with the deity, questions about the meaning of existence, the meaning of suffering, or the moral or ethical implications of treatment options?

4. *Affect and attitude.* Does the client appear lonely, depressed, angry, anxious, agitated, apathetic, or preoccupied?

5. *Interpersonal relationships.* Who visits? How does the client respond to visitors? Do faith leaders or chaplains visit? How does the client relate to other clients and nursing personnel?

Diagnosing

Nursing diagnoses related to spirituality may be specifically related to spiritual issues themselves or may impact other areas of functioning, where the distress of the spirit becomes the etiology. The following are some sample diagnoses:

- Spiritual distress is the challenge to the individual's ability to connect with those elements that are important to life—for example, values; fine arts, such as music and art; significant others; the world of nature; or a higher power within his or her life. An individual can also be at risk for spiritual distress. Clinical examples of assessment data and related nursing diagnoses are shown in Table 47.2.

TABLE 47.2 Clinical Application: Assessment Data and Related Nursing Diagnoses for Clients with Spiritual Distress

Data	Nursing Analysis
Marilyn Eckhardt, 72 years old, is crying, fingering her rosary, and voicing concern that she has not seen her priest for confession since being admitted to the hospital. She states that she is afraid to die without confessing her sins. She also states that she does not want to see the hospital chaplain but would prefer to see her own priest, whose parish is about 18 kilometres away. The hospital record indicates that Ms. Eckhardt is Roman Catholic.	Spiritual distress related to demonstrating discouragement and requesting spiritual assistance (confession with parish priest)
John Ames, 42 years old, is in a terminal state with an acquired immunodeficiency syndrome (AIDS)–related condition. He has become withdrawn but states to the nurse, "What have I done that God has punished me so?" The nurse observes religious literature on his bedside cabinet.	Spiritual distress related to questioning the meaning of life and the credibility of a personal belief

- Conversely, the client can demonstrate a willingness to expand his or her spiritual well-being through increased or enhanced connectedness to those same elements. Some people will respond to adversity with increased spiritual strength that provides hope and comfort.

- Any anxiety or *fear* as the individual contemplates the soul's future after death and his or her level of preparedness for death

- A poor self-assessment of the patient's ability to follow the rituals of the chosen faith

- Difficulty in sleeping or coping with the health challenges because of spiritual distress, feelings of abandonment by God, loss of religious faith

- Any inability to consider a treatment plan in light of religious or spiritual beliefs

Planning

In the planning phase, the nurse identifies interventions to help the client achieve the overall goal of maintaining or restoring spiritual health so that spiritual strength, serenity, and satisfaction are realized. For example, goals may include the following:

- Maintaining a meaningful personal relationship with a deity

- Maintaining harmonious supportive relationships with others

Examples of desired outcomes to achieve each of these goals, developed in the planning phase, are provided in Table 47.3.

Planning in relation to spiritual needs should be designed to do one or more of the following:

- Help the client fulfill spiritual and religious obligations

- Help the client draw on and use inner resources more effectively to meet the present situation

- Help the client maintain or establish a dynamic, personal relationship with self, others, and a divine being in the face of unpleasant circumstances

- Help the client find meaning in existence and the present situation

- Promote a sense of hope

- Provide new spiritual resources

Implementing

Spiritual interventions promote health and healing and may include noting clients' coping mechanisms, capacity for humour, self-determination, and optimism. It can also include assisting the client to leave a legacy by recording life stories for family and friends, and encouraging creative expression through art, music, and writing. Fostering ways for clients to keep in touch with nature and maintain a sense of wonder are also forms of spiritual care. Nursing actions most desired by clients to meet their spiritual needs include (a) providing presence, (b) supporting spiritual and religious practices, (c) assisting clients with prayer and meditation, (d) referring clients to spiritual care professionals and faith group leaders, and (e) maintaining connections with others (Taylor & Mamier, 2005).

PROVIDING PRESENCE "Probably the greatest tool available to nurses for meeting spiritual needs is their own presence and an ability to touch another, both physically and spiritually" (Carson, 1989, p. 164). Empathic presence means being willing to suffer with another, to offer and share oneself, and to gain insight into the client's meaning and purpose in life, sickness, and health. The nurse provides presence through the development of a professional caring relationship with the client, a relationship that enables the nurse to experience the client's uniqueness. The client, in turn, experiences the nurse as a genuine human person. The nurse that becomes fully present to a client will be confident, comfortable, and wholly focused on the client. In providing presence, the nurse communicates a willingness to care, to listen, and to be available to the client. "Presence itself touches the client's spirit, just as a cool hand might soothe a fevered brow" (Carson, 1989, p. 165).

The act of being present for clients involves qualities considered to be humanistic: compassion, kindness,

TABLE 47.3 Evaluation Goals and Outcomes: Spiritual Well-Being

Goal	Examples of Desired Outcomes
Maintains meaningful personal relationships with deity	Verbalizes satisfaction with relationship with deity
	Carries out usual religious practices using resources available
	Expresses feelings of inner peace and spiritual fulfillment
	States faith provides strength to understand and endure suffering
Maintains harmonious, supportive relationships with others	Conveys warmth and compassion to family, friends, and others
	Shares thoughts, feelings, and faith with others

BOX 47.3 SUPPORTING SPIRITUALITY AND RELIGIOUS PRACTICES

In Hospital or Other Care Centre

Being able to continue their spiritual practices is important to many clients:

- Inform the client about religious services provided in the agency. Many agencies provide nondenominational religious services or several services for different denominations.

- Ensure opportunities for privacy for the client and family for prayer, meditation, or counsel. Many agencies have quiet areas for these purposes.

- Support the client's desire to have spiritual icons, statues, jewellery, or other religious items with him or her and protect them from damage or loss.

- With the client's permission, facilitate arrangements for the client's minister, priest, rabbi, or other spiritual adviser or healer to visit. Many hospitals also provide the services of an agency chaplain or a list of clergy to call when needed. Hospital chaplains can also be used as a resource for finding representatives for various religious groups.

- If sacraments or other rituals are to be performed by spiritual leaders or healers, prepare the client's room appropriately. For example, clear the bedside table, draw the bed curtains, and make sure there is a seat near the bedside for the religious counsellor.

- Make arrangements with the dietitian for dietary practices to be met. If the agency cannot accommodate the client's needs, ask the family to bring in their own food.

- Consult with the client, family, or spiritual adviser before removing special amulets, garments, or body hair for tests, treatments, or surgery. For example, Sikhism requires that men wear a turban 24 hours a day and have uncut hair. Some Sikhs, therefore, may refuse to have any body hair cut (e.g., for electrodes or an intravenous infusion).

In the Home

- Explore resources available, such as audiotapes of weekly religious services, taped meditations or inspirational music, televised religious services, and clergy who routinely make home visits.

- Consult with family members to consider ways to help the client, such as reading scriptures on a regular basis, having prayer sessions, providing inspirational literature, and so on.

---

honesty, love, gentleness, and patience. Being present to clients asks nurses to engage with others in times of uncertainty, not so much to fix or answer but to be in mystery with another. "Spiritual care-giving calls us to be with another in openness and love, creating a safe and sacred place in which to explore the questions, delve into the mystery, and seek meaning" (Burkhardt & Nagai-Jacobson, 2002, p. 50).

SUPPORTING SPIRITUAL AND RELIGIOUS PRACTICES During the assessment of the client, the nurse obtains specific information about the client's spiritual and religious preference and practices. These will be considered when planning nursing care, especially when it is affected by client preferences and practices about birth, death, dress, diet, prayer, spiritual symbols, sacred texts, and holy days. As highlighted in Box 47.3, when nurses intentionally support spirituality and facilitate religious practices for their clients, they are also teaching wellness.

ASSISTING CLIENTS WITH PRAYER AND MEDITATION In a health care context, prayer is often associated with coping. It involves a sense of love, connection, and a reaching out. It is recognized as an ancient human practice that has many health benefits and healing properties.

Clients may choose to participate in personal prayer or want community prayer with family, friends, or representatives of their faith. Likewise, meditation practices may be integral to a person's faith tradition. In such situations, the nurse's major responsibility is to ensure a quiet environment and privacy. Nursing care may need to be adjusted to accommodate periods for prayer and meditation.

Illness can interfere with some clients' ability to pray. Feelings of anxiety, fear, guilt, grief, despair, and isolation can produce barriers to relationships in general and in the relationship the person has with his or her deity. In these instances, clients may ask the nurse to pray with them. Prayers with clients should only be done when there is mutual agreement between the clients and those praying with them. Because prayer can take various forms, Carson (1989) offered the following guidelines:

- Ask the client to whom they pray and whether there is a special prayer that has personal significance. The client may be comforted by reciting such a prayer with the nurse.

- Use a conversational type of prayer that reflects the client's concerns and needs. For example, "Please comfort Mrs. Wilson as she enters surgery. Lift her fear and in its place give her peace and strength. Let her know you are with her. . . ."

- Tell the client that you will say a private prayer if you are not comfortable praying out loud or if the client is uncomfortable with the spoken prayer.

- Offer to be with clients during private prayer or personal meditation.

Nurses who are unaccustomed to praying aloud or in public may find it helpful to have a formal prayer or a religious passage readily available. Because prayer can evoke deep feelings, the nurse needs to spend time with the client following a prayer to enable the client to express these feelings.

REFERRING CLIENTS TO SPIRITUAL CARE PROFESSIONALS AND FAITH GROUP LEADERS There are times when spiritual care is best referred to other members of the health care team. Referrals can be made for hospitalized clients and their families through the hospital chaplain's office if one is available. Nurses in home and community health settings can identify spiritual resources by checking directories of community service agencies, telephone directories, or religious directories that describe available spiritual care professionals and the services provided through the religious community. See the Evidence-Informed Practice box on when nurses refer patients to professional chaplains.

Many faith group leaders will provide assistance to members of their faith who are not members of their specific religious community. For example, a priest, a rabbi, an imam, or a minister may all attend on a client in the hospital or at home, even if the person is not a member of the faith leader's local faith community.

Referrals may be necessary when the nurse makes a diagnosis of spiritual distress. In this situation, the nurse and spiritual care professional or faith group leader can work together to meet the client's needs. One situation the nurse may encounter is client refusal of necessary medical intervention because of religious tenets. In this case, the nurse encourages the client, the physician, and the spiritual adviser to discuss the conflict and consider alternative methods of treatment. The nurse's major role is to provide the information the client needs to make an informed decision and then to support the client's decision.

Referrals can also be made to parish nurses, registered nurses who function as members of a congregation's ministry team, combining nursing and health expertise in the context of a faith community's mission. They believe that spiritual health is the core of an individual's wellness and that it influences all aspects of well-being. Parish nurses build on the strengths of individuals, families, and the community, assisting and empowering them to become more active in their own health. They work in partnership with faith group leaders and congregational members to enable the faith community to become a place of health and healing (Clark & Olson, 2000; Solari-Twadell & McDermott, 1999).

MAINTAINING CONNECTIONS WITH OTHERS As human beings, our belonging needs are strong and our very survival depends on our connection with others (Burkhardt & Nagai-Jacobson, 2002). At times of stress and during illness, these connections are even more important than when life flows along smoothly. The nurse can carry out important spiritual care interventions when facilitating clients' connections with loved ones in times of stress and illness. Being aware of the client's most significant relationships enables the nurse to seek ways to encourage these connections to promote health and healing. When actual connections with significant others are not possible, access to photos, phone calls, and electronic communication can be facilitated. It is also important to be aware of relationships that cause stress for the client. Nurses may need to offer support at times when these interactions are inevitable. Finally, assisting family members and friends with their questions and concerns about interacting with clients during times of illness and treatment can be an important nursing role. See the Sample Care Plan for spiritual distress on the next page.

EVIDENCE-INFORMED PRACTICE

When Do Nurses Refer Patients to Professional Chaplains?

Weinberger-Litman, Muncie, Flannelly, & Flannelly (2010) examined the types of issues around which nurses make referrals to chaplains. A questionnaire was distributed to 133 hospital staff who were mainly registered nurses. Data analysis of variance (ANOVA) indicated that issues most referred to chaplains involved complex family dynamics, end-of-life rituals, or need for emotional support in challenging health situations rather than treatment related concerns.

NURSING IMPLICATIONS: "Nurses desire to meet patients' spiritual needs" (p. 44). Therefore, nurses need to be able to engage in collaborative spiritual assessment and formulate interdisciplinary spiritual care plans.

Source: Based on Weinberger-Litman, S., Muncie, M., Flannelly, L., & Flannelly, K. (2010). When do nurses refer patients to professional chaplains? *Holistic Nursing Practice*, 24(1), 44–48.

Evaluating

Typically, the effectiveness of delivering spiritual care to clients is evaluated as a final step of the nursing process. However, there is need for caution when discussing the evaluation of spiritual care. Does spiritually sensitive nursing care lead to observable and measurable client outcomes? If it does not, then is it unsuccessful or unimportant? And what outcomes indicating movement toward improved spiritual health are appropriate for nurses to consider? Taylor (2007) suggested that clinicians' spiritually healing responses often move a client *incrementally* toward spiritual healthiness. Nurses with theistic religious beliefs might add that a client's movement toward spiritual health is evidence of God's grace, and ultimately something that is not within the purview of any clinician or person. Given that many health care institutions require spiritual care be documented in nursing care plans, an example of how this can be done is provided in Tables 47.2 (page 1526) and 47.3 (page 1527).

Sample Care Plan for Spiritual Distress

Assessment Data

Nursing Assessment

Sally Horton, 60 years old, is hospitalized at Vancouver General Hospital and is recovering from a right radical mastectomy. Yesterday, she was told by her physician that because of metastases of the cancer, her prognosis is poor. This morning her primary nurse finds her tearful, stating she slept poorly and has no appetite. She asks the nurse, "Why is this happening to me? Perhaps it's because I have sinned in my life. I've not gone to church or spoken to a minister in several years. Is there a chapel in the hospital where I could go and pray? I'm terribly afraid of dying and what awaits me."

Physical Examination

Height: 165.1 cm

Weight: 54.0 kg

Temperature: 36.6°C

Pulse: 88 beats/min

Respirations: 22/min

Blood Pressure: 146/86 mm Hg

Large surgical dressing right chest wall and axillary region, dry and intact. Slight edema right hand and arm.

Nursing Diagnosis

Spiritual distress related to separation from religious rituals (as evidenced by questioning credibility of personal beliefs, depression, expressions of resentment and fear of death, requests for chapel visits).

Client Goals

The client will regain a sense of spiritual satisfaction.

Desired Health Outcomes

1. Expresses desire to perform religious or spiritual practices
2. Visits with chaplain by day 2
3. Displays absence of feelings of anger and resentment by day 5
4. Verbalizes increase in psychological and spiritual comfort with illness, prognosis, and death

Diagnostic Data		Normal
RBC: 3.5×10^{12}/L	Female: $4.1–5.1 \times 10^{12}$/L	Male: $4.5–5.3 \times 10^{12}$/L
Hgb: 105 g/L	Female: 120–160 g/L	Male: 130–180 g/L
Hct: 0.35	Female: 0.36–0.46	Male 0.37–0.49

Selected Nursing Interventions with Rationales [in bold]

Spiritual Support

- Allow Mrs. Horton to express her feelings regarding her illness and death.
  Rationale: Being open to those expressions encourages her to reveal inner concerns and fears and allows her to see the worth of tackling issues.

- Encourage her to voice and alleviate her anger in a constructive manner.
  Rationale: Constructive expressions of anger can be an excellent source of energy and produce a sense of freedom for the client.

- Help Mrs. Horton to identify and clarify her beliefs and values through exercises such as values clarification.
  Rationale: Indecision and conflicts can arise when values and beliefs are not clear. Clarification will assist clients to make decisions that are congruent with their values and beliefs, including their spiritual beliefs.

- Use active listening to ascertain desire for prayer or important spiritual rituals.
  Rationale: The speed and quality of recovery or the redefinition of hope and finding meaning in death is often affected by the spiritual care offered and received.

- When these desires are expressed, facilitate Mrs. Horton's participation in meditation, prayer or other religious rituals.
  Rationale: Health professionals sometimes overlook spiritual needs. Giving recognition and respect to these needs is an important nursing advocacy role.

- Give assurance of nursing and other support in times of suffering.
  Rationale: One fear is that of dying alone—expressions of presence and support will assist in alleviating this.

Coping Enhancement

- Create an environment that is nonjudgmental and accepting.
  Rationale: This is an essential step in creating a therapeutic relationship—this can promote communication and freedom of expression.

- Be open to positive and negative expressions of perceptions, feelings and fears. Ensure Mrs. Horton has time for grieving.
  Rationale: These expressions and the nurse's acceptance of them helps the client to give meaning to her experience.

- Encourage Mrs. Horton to link her values to behaviours in previous situations and settings.
  Rationale: This will assist her in using past experience to further develop her values, and to engage in behaviours in this situation that are congruent with past and present values.

EVALUATION

Goal met. Mrs. Horton has been visited on several occasions by the chaplain. She reads scripture each day and has found consolation in reading the Book of Psalms. She states, "God is merciful and will help me bear my suffering."

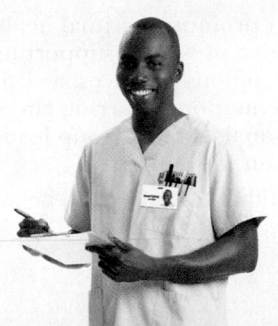

Case Study 47

Linh Van, a 32-year-old woman from Edmonton, Alberta, received several units of blood following an automobile accident in the late 1990s. Five years ago she was diagnosed with AIDS and is now in the hospital. She is very ill, and you sense she is discouraged by the seriousness of her illness but know from both your own experience and routine reports at change of staff that she does not speak about such matters. Ms. Van is a devout Buddhist, and you have noticed her daily practices of meditation and ritual. In light of her grave prognosis, including the probability of severe pain, you wonder about discussing the topic of spiritual care with her.

CRITICAL THINKING QUESTIONS

1. On what basis are you sensing that Ms. Van is discouraged by the seriousness of her illness? Explain.

2. What does Ms. Van's silence in the face of her illness tell you about her spiritual beliefs?

3. How might Ms. Van's behaviour in the face of her illness and suffering be affected by her spiritual beliefs? by her religious beliefs?

4. How might a spiritual assessment be of benefit to both you and the client?

5. If you were to discuss the topic of spirituality and spiritual care with Ms. Van, what is the first question you might ask?

Check the eText in MyNursingLab for answers and explanations.

KEY TERMS

agnostic   *p. 1518*

assumptions   *p. 1520*

atheist   *p. 1518*

beliefs   *p. 1520*

consciousness   *p. 1518*

developmental   *p. 1518*

faith   *p. 1518*

generalized anxiety   *p. 1520*

holy day   *p. 1522*

kosher   *p. 1523*

meditation   *p. 1523*

prayer   *p. 1523*

religion   *p. 1518*

seasons   *p. 1518*

spiritual distress   *p. 1521*

spiritual health   *p. 1521*

spiritual well-being
   p. 1521

spiritual wellness   *p. 1521*

spirituality   *p. 1517*

theistic   *p. 1518*

truths   *p. 1518*

values   *p. 1520*

world view   *p. 1520*

CHAPTER HIGHLIGHTS

- Clients have a right to receive care that respects their individual spiritual and religious beliefs, values, and practices.

- The spiritual needs of clients and support persons often come into focus at a time of illness. Spiritual beliefs and religious practices often help people accept illness and plan for the future.

- Spirituality and religion are distinct concepts. Spirituality is a broad concept that encompasses relationships with a divine being, deity, or creative force; with the self; with nature; and with others.

- Religion is more practical and acts as a container or holding environment that offers ways to express spirituality. Both spiritual and religious beliefs influence lifestyle, attitudes, and feelings about health, illness, and death.

- Spiritual health is described as a feeling of being generally alive, purposeful, and fulfilled. It is manifested by a person's communication that reveals meaning and purpose to existence, inner peace, trusting relationships, and inner strength that is directed toward ultimate values of love, meaning, hope, beauty, and truth.

- Spiritual distress refers to a disturbance in or a challenge to a person's core value system that provides strength, hope, and meaning to life. Possible factors in spiritual distress include physiological problems, treatment-related concerns, situational and developmental concerns. Spiritual distress can be reflected in a number of behaviours, including depression, anxiety, verbalizations of unworthiness, and fear of death.

- Spiritual screening, spiritual history taking, and spiritual assessment are best carried out after the nurse has developed a good relationship with the client. Information may be elicited about the client's concept of the deity or creative force, the client's source of hope and strength, the significance of spiritual or religious practices and rituals, and the relationship the client perceives between health and spiritual or religious beliefs.

- Home health nurses can observe cues in the home that may indicate client spiritual beliefs and practices. Nurses in community settings should be aware of spiritual and religious resources in the community and what services they provide.

- To implement spiritual care, nurses need to be skilled in establishing a trusting nurse–client relationship.
- Nurses can support clients' spiritual and religious practices if they understand needs related to holy days, sacred texts, spiritual symbols, prayer and meditation, diet practices, dress requirements, birth rituals, and death rituals.

- Nursing interventions that promote spiritual health include offering a supportive presence, supporting the client's spiritual and religious practices, assisting clients with prayer and meditation, referring clients to a spiritual care professional or faith group leader, and maintaining connection with others.
- Nurses need to be aware of their own spiritual beliefs in order to be comfortable assisting others.

ASSESS YOUR LEARNING

1. Mr. Marshall tells the nurse that his friend was killed in the all-terrain vehicle mishap. When the nurse is talking to Mr. Marshall about his feelings, he states, "I can't believe God can be so cruel. I am so angry and frustrated!" What should be the nurse's initial response?

    a. Acknowledge Mr. Marshall's spiritual concerns.

    b. Reassure Mr. Marshall that accidents are unavoidable.

    c. Refer Mr. Marshall to a grief counsellor.

    d. Ask whether Mr. Marshall would like to talk to a chaplain.

2. Mrs. Smith is an older adult residing in your skilled nursing facility. She is searching for a way to make life meaningful. When planning care for Mrs. Smith, which of the following nursing actions would be MOST beneficial?

    a. Assessing the client for depression

    b. Diagnosing and documenting that the client has spiritual distress

    c. Keeping the client busy with social activities

    d. Engaging the client in a spiritual assessment

3. Mr. Hussein, a Muslim patient, is given a grave prognosis. His wife asks the nurse for prayer support. Which of the following is the nurse's BEST initial response in determining further nursing interventions?

    a. "May I call the chaplain for you to discuss your concerns?"

    b. "I know your faith is important to you. My faith is important to me, too."

    c. "How may I best help you in getting prayer support?"

    d. "Isn't it wonderful that we have Jesus with whom we can share our concerns?"

4. A client reports, "Cancer is the best thing that has happened to me! It is making me appreciate life so much more." Based on this statement, which nursing diagnosis might be appropriate?

    a. Spiritual distress related to denial of illness

    b. Risk for ignoring treatment while engaging in new activities

    c. Effective coping with life-threatening illness

    d. Denial related to diagnosis of life-threatening illness

5. A dying client states, "Part of what makes dying hard is that I don't know for sure where I'm going. Nurse, what do you believe happens in the hereafter?" Which ethical guideline should guide your response?

    a. Never share personal spiritual beliefs.

    b. Share all spiritual beliefs, favouring none.

    c. Share only your beliefs.

    d. First, assess client beliefs.

6. A client in the emergency department needs red blood cells. She is a Jehovah's Witness, whose religious beliefs make it impossible for her to accept the prescribed blood transfusion. Which of the following statements would MOST likely lead to a resolution of this conflict?

    a. "You must accept the transfusion or else leave the emergency department so others can receive care."

    b. "Please accept the transfusion; you can ask for pardon after taking the blood."

    c. "May I call a representative of your religion to facilitate discussion about alternative methods of treatment?"

    d. "I understand your position. Without the transfusion you will die, but I'll be here to support you."

7. An 88-year-old Buddhist woman has just been admitted to a skilled nursing facility. She tells the nurse that she has been a spiritual practitioner for many years and hopes to continue her daily meditations. How should the nurse initially respond to this request?

    a. "Tell me more about your daily meditation practice."

    b. "I think there is a Buddhist temple listed in the phone book."

    c. "I studied Buddhism in my world religions class in university."

    d. "Unfortunately, you are our only Buddhist client."

8. Which of the following is an appropriate spiritual screening or assessment question?

    a. "Tell me more about your religion and religious practices."

    b. "How can we support your spiritual and religious beliefs and practices?"

    c. "How has your prayer experience been affected by your illness?"

    d. "What do you see as the purpose or mission for your life?"

9. The mother of a pediatric client states, "I can't understand why God would allow this to happen to my innocent child!" Based on this statement, which nursing diagnosis might the nurse consider?

    a. Spiritual distress related to the search for meaning in a child's illness

    b. Altered religiosity related to anger at God

    c. Ineffective coping related to anger

    d. Hopelessness related to seriousness of child's diagnosis

10. A client's spirituality is complex and individual. What is the main reason for assessing and responding to spiritual needs and resources in providing nursing care?

    a. To uncover needs that could be referred to spiritual care professionals

    b. To decrease suffering and aid in physical and mental healing

    c. To fulfill nursing's obligation to do no harm

    d. To be able to help clients observe their unique practices

Check the eText in MyNursingLab for answers and explanations.

WEBLINKS

Canadian Association for Parish Nursing Ministry

http://www.capnm.ca

Parish nursing is recognized as an essential dimension in the integration of faith and health within diverse faith communities throughout Canada. The Canadian Association for Parish Nursing Ministry is committed to the development of parish nursing as a health and ministry resource within Canada.

Canadian Association for Spiritual Care

http://www.spiritualcare.ca

The Canadian Association for Spiritual Care (CASC) is a national multifaith organization that is committed to the professional education, certification, and support of people involved in spiritual care and pastoral counselling. CASC is concerned with a holistic approach to health care and personal development, with a special focus on spiritual and religious care.

Canadian Research Institute of Spirituality and Healing

http://www.crish.org

The Canadian Research Institute of Spirituality and Healing is a Canadian professional organization that promotes multidisciplinary research and education in spirituality, culture, healing, and health care. It was initiated in 2006 and is associated with regular international multidisciplinary conferences focusing on spirituality and health.

Multifaith Calendar

http://www.multifaithcalendar.org

The multifaith calendar stimulates dialogue and discussion for people of many cultures and faiths.

North American Interfaith Network

http://www.nain.org

The North American Interfaith Network (NAIN) is a nonprofit association of interfaith organizations and agencies in Canada, Mexico, and the United States. NAIN offers networking opportunities to persons of many religious traditions and numerous interfaith organizations.

Ontario Multifaith Council

http://www.omc.ca

The Ontario Multifaith Council on Spiritual and Religious Care is a nonprofit charitable organization representing a wide range of faith groups in Ontario. It is recognized as one of North America's largest organizations dedicated to advocacy of spiritual care and the protection of religious rights. This site includes a searchable multifaith library feature.

MyNursingLab

REFERENCES

Ameling, A. (2000). Prayer: An ancient healing practice becomes new again. *Holistic Nursing Practice, 14*(3), 40–48.

Baldacchino, D. L. (2006). Nursing competencies for spiritual care. *Journal of Clinical Nursing, 15*(7), 885–896.

Banziger, S., Van Uden, M., & Janssen, J. (2008). Praying and coping: The relation between varieties of praying and religious coping styles. *Mental Health, Religion & Culture, 11(1),* 101–118.

Bibby, R. W. (2006). *The boomer factor: What Canada's most famous generation is leaving behind.* Toronto, ON: Bastian Books.

Boehm, R. (Ed.) (2004). *Images of women in spiritual traditions: Role models for global understanding.* Edmonton, AB: Intercultural Action Committee for the Advancement of Women.

Bowker, J. (Ed.). (1997). *The Oxford dictionary of world religions.* New York, NY: Oxford University Press.

Buck, H. G. (2006). Spirituality: Concept analysis and model development. *Holistic Nursing Practice, 20,* 288–292.

Burkhardt, M., & Nagai-Jacobson, M. (2002). *Spirituality: Living our connectedness.* Albany, NY: Delmar.

Campbell, A., & Campbell, D. (2005). Emergency baptism by health professionals. *Paediatric Nursing, 17*(2), 39–42.

Carpenito-Moyet, L. J. (2008). *Nursing diagnosis: Application to clinical practice* (12th ed.). Philadelphia, PA: Lippincott.

Carpenter, K., Girvin. L., Kitner, W., & Ruth-Sahd, L. A. (2008). Spirituality: A dimension of holistic critical care nursing. *Dimensions of Critical Care Nursing, 27*(1), 16–20.

Carson, V. B. (1989). *Spiritual dimensions of nursing practice.* Philadelphia, PA: Saunders.

Chiu, L., Emblen, J., Van Hofwegen, L., Sawatzky, R., & Meyerhoff, H. (2004). An integrative review of the concept of spirituality in the health sciences. *Western Journal of Nursing Research, 26*(4), 405–428.

Chung, L. Y. F., Wong, F. K. Y., & Chan, M. F. (2007). Relationship of nurses' spirituality to their understanding and practice of spiritual care. *Journal of Advanced Nursing, 58*(2), 158–170.

Clark, M. (2000). Characteristics of faith communities. In M. Clark & J. Olson (Eds.), *Nursing within a faith community: Promoting health in times of transition* (pp. 17–29). Thousand Oaks, CA: Sage.

Clark, M. & Olson, J. (2000). *Nursing within a faith community: Promoting health in times of transition.* Thousand Oaks, CA: Sage.

Denny, F. M. (1993). Islam and the Muslim community. In H. Byron Earhart (ed.), *Religious traditions of the world* (pp. 603–712). New York, NY: HarperSanFrancisco.

Derrickson, P. (2002). Parish nursing and clinical pastoral education. *Journal of Health Care Chaplaincy 11*(2), 15–25.

Dy-Liacco, G., Piedmont, R., Murray-Swank, N., Rodgerson, T., & Sherman, M. (2009). Spirituality and religiosity as cross-cultural aspects of human experience. *Psychology of Religion and Spirituality 1*(1), 35–52.

Ellison, C. W. (1983). Spiritual well-being: Conceptualization and measurement. *Journal of Psychology and Theology, 11,* 330–340.

Erikson, E. (1963). *Childhood and society.* New York, NY: Norton.

Fishbane, M. (1993). Judaism: Revelation and traditions. In H. Byron Earhart (Ed.), *Religious traditions of the world* (pp. 373–484). New York, NY: HarperSanFrancisco.

Fitchett, G. (1993). *Assessing spiritual needs.* Minneapolis, MN: Augsburg.

Fitchett, G., & Risk, J. (2009). Screening for spiritual struggle. *Journal of Pastoral Care and Counseling 63*(1,2), 4.1–4.12.

Ford, I. M. (1988). *Life spirals: The faith journey.* Burlington, ON: Welch.

Fowler, J. W. (1981). *Stages in faith.* New York, NY: Harper & Row.

Fowler, J., & Dell, M. (2006). Stages of faith from infancy through adolescence: Reflections on three decades of faith development theory. In E. Roehlkepartain, P. Ebstyne King, L. Wagener, & P. Benson (Eds.), *Handbook of spiritual development in childhood and adolescence* (pp. 35–45). Thousand Oaks, CA: Sage.

Fowler, J., & Keen, S. (1985). *Life maps: Conversations in the journey of faith.* Waco, TX: Word Books.

Gatrad, A., & Sheikh, A. (2001). Muslim birth customs. *ADC Fetal Neonatal Ed, 84,* F6–F8.

Gottlieb, L. & Ezer H. (Eds.). (1997). *A perspective on health, family, learning and collaborative nursing: A collection of writing on the McGill model of nursing.* Montreal, PQ: McGill University School of Nursing.

Griffith, J. K. (1996). *The religious aspects of nursing care.* Vancouver, BC: Author.

Hanson, L. C., Dobbs, D. , Usher, B., Williams, S., Rawlings, J., & Daaleman, T. P. (2008). Providers and types of spiritual care during illness. *Journal of Palliative Medicine, 11,* 907–914.

Jameton, A. (1984). *Nursing practice: The ethical issues.* Englewood Cliffs, NJ: Prentice Hall.

Kendler, K., Liu, X., Gardner, C., McCullough, M., Larson, D., & Prescott, C. (2003). Dimensions of religiosity and their relationship to lifetime psychiatric and substance use disorders. *American Journal of Psychiatry, 160*(3), 496–503.

Levine, M. (2008). Prayer as coping: A psychological analysis. *Journal of Health Care Chaplaincy, 15,* 80–98.

Lobar, S., Youngblut, J., & Brooten, D. (2006). Cross-cultural beliefs, ceremonies, and rituals surrounding death of a loved one. *Pediatric Nursing, 32*(1), 44–50.

Marks, L. (2004). Sacred practices in highly religious families: Christian, Jewish, Mormon, and Muslim perspectives. *Family Process, 43*(2), 217–231.

NANDA International. (2007). *Nursing diagnoses: Definitions and classification, 2007–2008.* Philadelphia, PA: Author.

NANDA International. (2009). *Nursing diagnoses: Definitions and classification, 2009-2011.* Oxford, United Kingdom: Wiley-Blackwell.

Narayanasamy, A., & Narayanasamy, N., (2008). The healing power of prayer and its implications for nursing. *British Journal of Nursing, 17,* 394–398.

O'Connor, T., Meakes, E., O'Neill, K., Prenner, C., VanStaalduinen, G., & Davis, K. (2005). Not well known, used little and needed: Canadian chaplains' experiences of published spiritual assessment tools. *Journal of Pastoral Care and Counselling, 59,* 97–107.

Olson, J. (2000). Health promotion during times of transition. In *Nursing within a faith community: Promoting health in times of transition* (pp. 223–232). Thousand Oaks, CA: Sage.

Paley, J. (2008). Spirituality and nursing: A reductionistic approach. *Nursing Philosophy 9*(1), 3–18.

Panikkar, R. (1971). Faith, a constitutive dimension of man. *Journal of Ecumenical Studies, 8*(2), 223–254.

Pauly, B., Varcoe, C., Storch, J., & Newton, L. (2009). Registered nurses' perceptions of moral distress and ethical climate. *Nursing Ethics 16*(5), 561–573.

Pesut, B. (2008). A conversation on diverse perspectives of spirituality in nursing literature. *Nursing Philosophy, 9*(2), 98–109.

Pesut, B., Fowler, M., Reimer-Kirkham, S., Taylor, E.J., & Sawatzky, R. (2009). Particularizing spirituality in points of tension: Enriching the discourse. *Nursing Inquiry, 16,* 1–10.

Pilch, J. J. (1988). Wellness spirituality. *Health Values, 12*(May/June), 28–31.

Puchalski, C. & Ferrell, F. (2010). *Making health care whole: Integrating spirituality into patient care.* West Conshohocken, PA: Templeton Press.

Puchalski, C., Lunsford, B., Harris, M., & Miller, T. (2006). Interdisciplinary spiritual care for seriously ill and dying patients: A collaborative model. *Cancer Journal, 12*(5), 398–416.

Salzman, M. (2008). Globalization, religious fundamentalism and the need for meaning. *International Journal of Intercultural Relations, 32*(4), 318–327.

Sawatsky, R. & Pesut, B. (2006). Attributes of spiritual care in nursing practice. *Journal of Holistic Nursing, 23,* 19–33.

Smith-Stoner, M. (2007). End-of-life preferences for atheists. *Journal of Palliative Medicine, 10,* 923–928.

Solari-Twadell, P., & McDermott, M. A. (Eds.). (1999). *Parish nursing: Promoting whole person health within faith communities.* Thousand Oaks, CA: Sage.

Tanyi, R. A. (2006). Spirituality and family nursing: Spiritual assessment and intervention for families. *Journal of Advanced Nursing 53*(3), 287–294.

Taylor, E. J. (2002). *Spiritual care: Nursing theory, research, and practice.* Upper Saddle River, NJ: Pearson.

Taylor, E. J. (2003a). Spiritual needs of patients with cancer and family caregivers. *Cancer Nursing 26*(4), 260–266.

Taylor, E. J. (2003b). Nurses caring for the spirit: Patients with cancer and family caregiver expectations. *Oncology Nursing Forum, 30*(4), 585–590.

Taylor, E. J. (2007). Spiritual pain. *Advance for Nurses, 9*(21), 15–16.

Taylor, E. J. & Mamier, I. (2005). Spiritual care nursing: What cancer patients and family caregivers want. *Journal of Advanced Nursing, 49,* 260–267.

United Nations General Assembly. (2000). *United Nations millennium declaration.* New York, NY: United Nations. Retrieved from www.un.org/millennium/declaration/ares552e.htm

VandeCreek, L. (Ed.). (2003). *Professional chaplaincy and clinical pastoral education should become more scientific: Yes and no.* New York, NY: Routledge.

Van Leeuwen, R., Tiesinga, L. J., Jochemsen, H., & Post, D. (2007). Aspects of spirituality concerning illness. *Scandinavian Journal of Caring Science, 21,* 482–489.

Vardey, L. (Ed.). (1996). *God in all worlds: An anthology of contemporary spiritual writings.* Toronto, ON: Vintage Canada.

Winslow, G. R. & Wehtje-Winslow, B. W. (2007). Ethical boundaries of spiritual care. *Medical Journal of Australia, 186*(10 Suppl), S63–S66.

Chapter 48

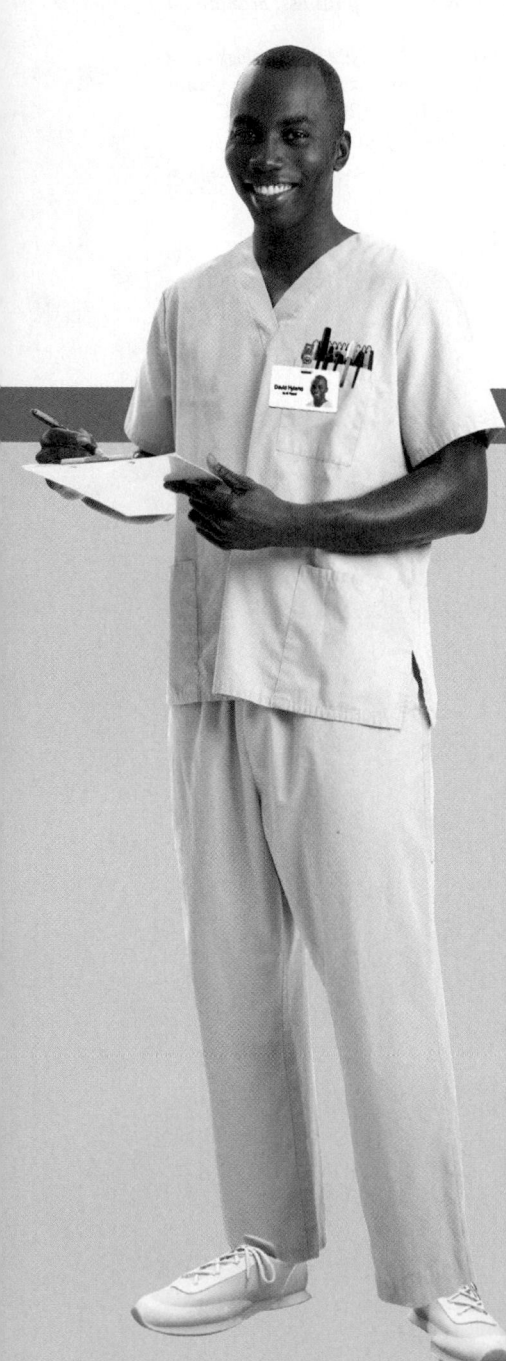

Stress and Coping

After studying this chapter, you will be able to:

1. Differentiate the concepts of stress as a stimulus, as a response, and as a transaction.

2. Describe the three stages of Selye's general adaptation syndrome.

3. Identify physiological, psychological, and cognitive indicators of stress.

4. Explain the role of the hypothalamic–pituitary–adrenal (HPA) axis in regulating the stress response.

5. Differentiate four levels of anxiety.

6. Discuss types of coping and coping strategies.

7. Identify essential aspects of assessing a client's stress and coping patterns.

8. Explain nursing diagnoses related to stress.

9. Describe interventions to help clients minimize and manage stress.

Stress is a universal phenomenon. All people experience it. Parents refer to the stress of raising children, working people talk of the stress of their jobs, and students at all levels talk of the stress of school. Stress can result from both positive and negative experiences. For example, a bride preparing for her wedding or a graduate preparing to start a new job may have stress reactions to these positive experiences, and a husband concerned about caring for his wife and family following a diagnosis of cancer may experience similar stress reactions.

The concept of stress is important because it provides a way of understanding the person as a unified being who responds in totality (mind, body, and spirit) to a variety of changes that take place in daily life.

Concept of Stress

Stress is a condition in which the person experiences changes in the normal balanced state. A **stressor** is any event or stimulus that causes an individual to experience a biological or psychological reaction to it. When a person faces stressors, responses are referred to as *coping strategies, coping responses,* or *coping mechanisms.*

Sources of Stress

Stress has many sources. They can be broadly classified as internal or external stressors, or developmental or situational stressors. *Internal stressors* originate within a person, for example, an infection or feelings of depression. *External stressors* originate outside the individual, for example, a move to another city, a death in the family, or pressure from peers. *Developmental stressors* occur at predictable times throughout an individual's life (Table 48.1). *Situational stressors* are unpredictable and can occur at any time during life. Examples of situational stressors include the death of a significant other, getting or losing a job, or an acute illness.

The degree to which any of these sources of stress has positive or negative effects may depend, to some degree, on an individual's developmental stage. For example, the death of a parent may be more stressful for a 12-year-old than for a 40-year-old. See the Lifespan Considerations box on the next page.

Effects of Stress

Stress can have physical, emotional, intellectual, social, and spiritual consequences. Usually the effects are mixed because stress affects the whole person. Physically, stress can threaten a person's physiological homeostasis. Emotionally, stress can produce negative or

TABLE 48.1 Selected Stressors Associated with Developmental Stages

Developmental Stage	Stressors
Child	Resolving conflict between independence and dependence
	Beginning school
	Establishing peer relationships and adjustments
	Coping with peer competition
Adolescent	Accepting changing physique
	Developing relationships involving sexual attraction
	Achieving independence
	Choosing a career
Young adult	Getting married
	Leaving home
	Managing a home
	Getting started in an occupation
	Continuing education
	Rearing children
Middle-aged adult	Accepting physical changes of aging
	Maintaining social status and standard of living
	Helping teenage children to become independent
	Helping aging parents
Older adult	Accepting decreasing physical abilities and health
	Accepting changes in residence
	Adjusting to retirement and reduced income
	Coping with death of spouse or partner and friends

Stress and Coping

People experience stress at all stages of life, as described below:

INFANTS AND CHILDREN

- Children's perceptions of and responses to stress are dependent on their developmental stage. Infants sense stressors in their environment and respond in a diffuse way, often crying and clinging. Toddlers and preschool-age children may be frightened and react by withdrawing or losing control. School-age children and adolescents are more capable of thinking about incidents that cause stress (e.g., a catastrophic accident) and talking about them with adults.

- Temperament is a factor that influences how children respond to stress. An outgoing, low-sensitivity child, for example, is less likely than a timid, intense child to be upset by a family move to a different province.

- Anxiety disorders are the most common psychiatric disorders in children and adolescents but are frequently unrecognized (Kodish, Rockhill, Ryan, & Varley, 2011).

- As children grow, they are able to develop more coping skills to manage stressful situations. Nurses have an important role in teaching parents to recognize stress in their children and to help their children cope.

YOUNG ADULTS

- Young adults are increasingly experiencing stress related to the transition to adulthood. Many university and college students juggle school demands with employment necessary to support their studies. The increasing cost of tuition and the need to achieve high grades are serious sources of stress for students. School-based counselling and mental health services are seeing an increase in demand for their services as a result.

MIDDLE-AGED ADULTS

- Middle-aged adults are often called the *sandwich generation*. They find themselves caring for children or grandchildren and often caring for aging parents at the same time. When these activities become time and energy consuming, there is often not enough time left for attention to the self. A 2009 poll of working Canadians reported that 13% assist their parents in carrying out domestic activities and that 78% of those find the situation very or somewhat stressful (Desjardins Financial Security, 2011). Nurses need to be aware of this and assist in suggesting resources and effective planning to ease the strain.

OLDER ADULTS

- Older adults experience many losses and changes in their lives. The losses may be incremental and, over time, become stressful and possibly overwhelming. Changes in health, decreased functional ability and independence, need for relocation, loss of family and friends, and becoming a caregiver for a spouse or friend are a few of the stresses often experienced by older adults. Many of them have survived significant challenges in their earlier lives and have learned effective coping skills. Nurses can help them plan, evaluate their strategies, and learn new strategies, if needed. Informal and formal social supports are very important in learning to successfully live with these changes and stress.

- Some effective coping methods for older adults are exercise, learning different relaxation techniques, participating in activities, getting adequate nutrition and rest, and engaging in expressive creative activities, such as art, music, and journalling. Referral to community resources and supports should be done when appropriate. It is most important to see older adults as unique individuals, with unique past experiences and very specific needs as they age.

---

unconstructive feelings about the self. Intellectually, stress can influence a person's perceptual and problem-solving abilities. Socially, stress can alter a person's relationships with others. Spiritually, stress can challenge one's beliefs and values. Many medical conditions have been linked to stress. The field of **psychoneuroimmunology** examines the links between stress, the concomitant endocrine and immunological responses and the development or exacerbation of illness (Figure 48.1).

Models of Stress

Models of stress help nurses to identify the stressor operating in a particular situation and to predict the individual's responses. Nurses can use the knowledge of these models to assist clients in strengthening healthy coping responses and in adjusting less healthy or unproductive responses. Three main models of stress are stimulus-based, response-based, and transaction-based.

Stimulus-Based Models

In **stimulus-based stress models**, stress is defined as a stimulus, a life event, or a set of circumstances that arouses physiological or psychosocial reactions that may increase the individual's vulnerability to illness. In their classic work, Holmes and Rahe (1967) assigned a numerical value to 43 life changes or events. The most recent version of that scale includes 77 items (Miller & Rahe, 1997), and a shortened version (54 items, full stress and coping inventory completed in 15 minutes) was created more recently (Rahe & Tolles, 2002). The scale of stressful life events is used to document a person's relatively recent experiences, such as divorce, pregnancy, and retirement. In this view, both positive and negative events are considered stressful.

Other similar scales have been developed, but all such scales require caution because the degree of stress an event presents can be highly individual. For example, a divorce may be highly traumatic to one person and cause relatively little anxiety to another. In addition,

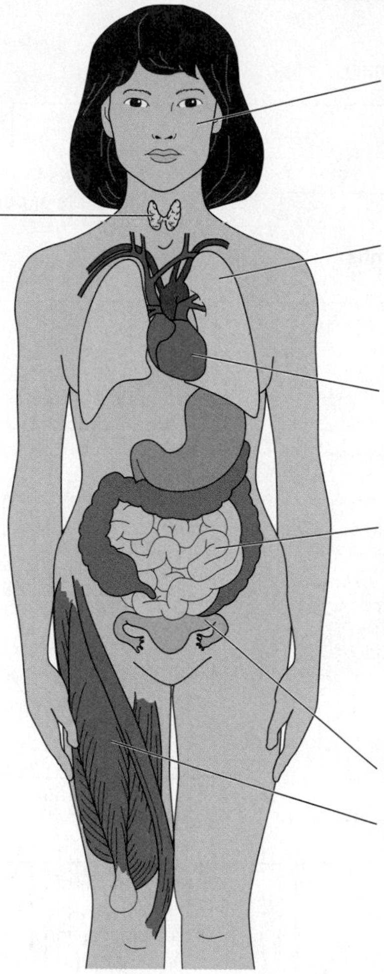

FIGURE 48.1 Some disorders can be caused or aggravated by stress.

Source: From Edin, G., & Golanty, E. (2007). *Health and wellness: A holistic approach* (9th ed.) (p. 40). Boston, MA: Jones & Bartlett. Adapted with permission of the authors.

many scales have not been tested for age, socioeconomic status, or cultural sensitivity.

Response-Based Models

Stress can also be considered as a response. This definition was developed and described by Selye (1956, 1976) as "the nonspecific response of the body to any kind of demand made upon it" (1976, p. 1). Schafer (1992, p. 9) defined stress as the "arousal of mind and body in response to demands made upon them." Regardless of the cause, circumstances, or psychological interpretation of a demanding situation, Selye's stress response is characterized by the same chain or pattern of physiological events. This nonspecific response is called the **general adaptation syndrome (GAS)** or *stress syndrome.*

To differentiate the cause of stress from the response to stress, Selye created the term *stressor* (1976) to denote any factor that produces stress and disturbs the body's equilibrium. Because stress is a state of the body, it can be observed only by the changes it produces in the body. This

response of the body, the stress syndrome (GAS) occurs with the release of certain adaptive hormones and subsequent changes in the structure and chemical composition of the body. Parts of the body particularly affected by stress are the gastrointestinal tract, the adrenal glands, and the lymphatic structures. With prolonged stress, the adrenal glands enlarge considerably; the lymphatic structures, such as the thymus, spleen, and lymph nodes, atrophy (shrink); and deep ulcers appear in the lining of the stomach.

In addition to adapting globally, the body can also react locally; that is, one organ or a part of the body reacts alone. This is referred to as the **local adaptation syndrome (LAS)**. One example of the LAS is inflammation. Selye (1976) proposed that both the GAS and the LAS have three stages: (a) alarm reaction, (b) resistance, and (c) exhaustion.

ALARM REACTION   The initial reaction of the body is the **alarm reaction (AR)**, which alerts the body's defences against the stressor, whether the stressor is heat, bacteria, or a verbal or physical attack from someone. Selye divided

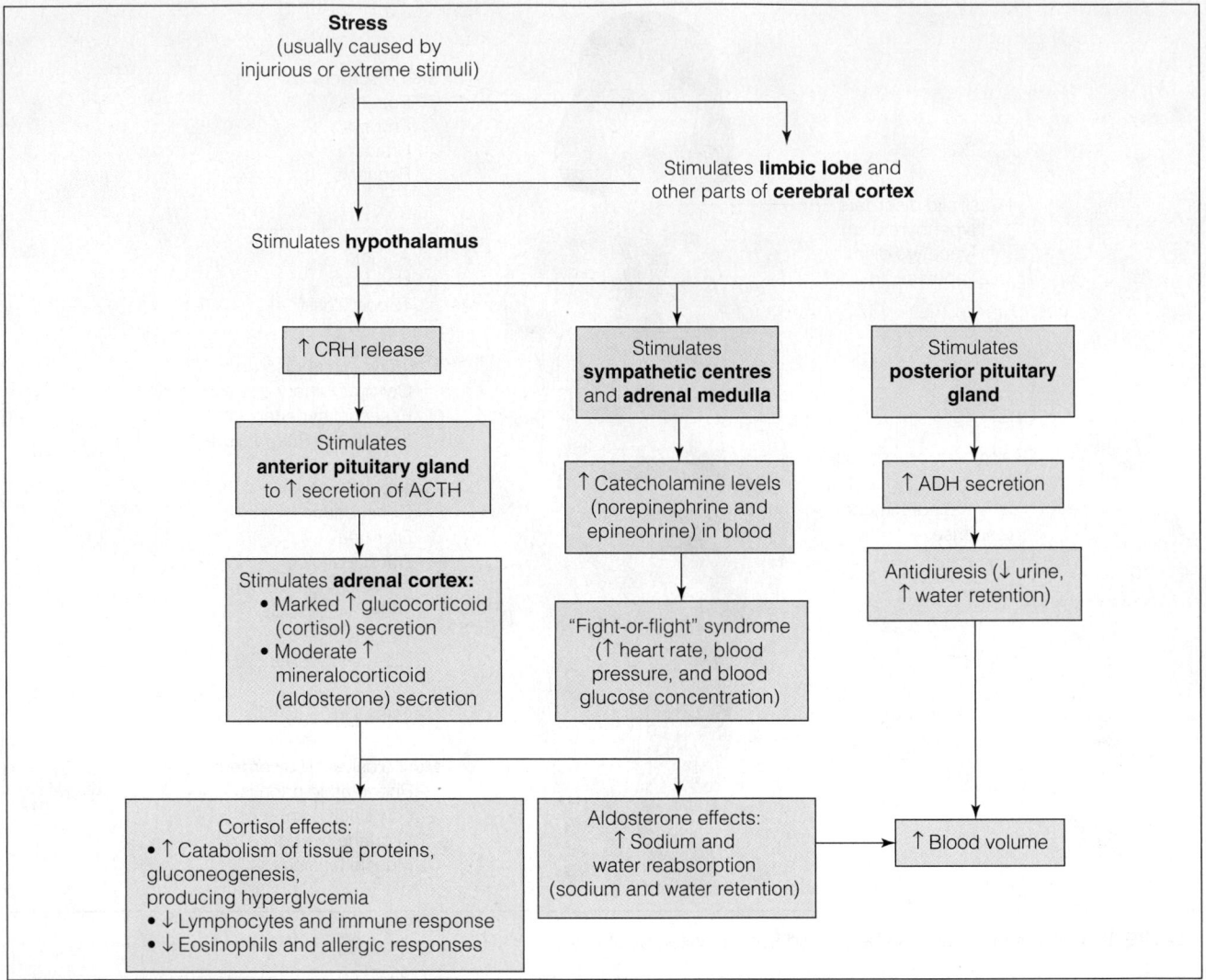

FIGURE 48.2 Effects of stress hormones. *ACTH,* adrenocorticotropic hormone; *ADH,* antidiuretic hormone; *CRH,* corticotropin-releasing hormone.

Source: Adapted from *Medical-Surgical Nursing in Canada*, 2nd Edition, Sharon L. Lewis et al., p. 138, Copyright © Elsevier (2010).

this stage into two parts: (a) the shock phase and (b) the countershock phase.

During the **shock phase**, as named by Selye, the stressor is perceived consciously or unconsciously by the individual via the cortex. The event is evaluated in light of previous experiences and the limbic system mediates the emotional response. The limbic system then stimulates the hypothalamic–pituitary–adrenal (HPA) axis. The stress response has both a nervous and an endocrine component. Once stimulated, a cascade of hormones prepares the body to cope with the stressor, in what is called the "fight-or-flight response," originally named by Cannon in 1929.

The hypothalamus also stimulates the sympathetic nervous system to directly release norepinephrine into the bloodstream. The principal effect of norepinephrine is decreased blood flow to the kidneys and increased secretion of renin. Renin is an enzyme that hydrolyzes

angiotensinogen to produce angiotensin. Angiotensin increases the blood pressure by constricting arterioles. The increase in blood pressure then allows for better perfusion of muscles and key organs.

The endocrine response is mediated by the release of corticotropin-releasing hormone (CRH) from hypothalamus, which stimulates the anterior pituitary gland to release adrenocorticotropic hormone (ACTH). ACTH acts on the adrenal cortex to release aldosterone (to retain fluid) and cortisol to increase the availability of energy and modulate the immunological and inflammatory responses of the body. At the same time, the posterior pituitary is stimulated by CRH and releases antidiuretic hormone (ADH), to retain body fluid to support blood pressure while combating the stressor. The initial stressor also stimulates the adrenal medulla to release epinephrine, a catecholamine (Johnson & Renn, 2006).

Significant body responses to epinephrine include the following:

1. Increased myocardial contractility, which increases cardiac output and blood flow to active muscles
2. Bronchial dilation, which allows increased oxygen intake
3. Increased blood clotting
4. Increased cellular metabolism
5. Increased fat mobilization to make energy available and to synthesize other compounds needed by the body

The sum of all of these adrenal hormonal effects permits the person to perform far more strenuous physical activity than would otherwise be possible. The person is then ready for "fight or flight." This primary response is short lived, lasting from 1 minute to 24 hours (Figure 48.2).

The second part of the AR is called the **countershock phase**. During this time, the changes produced in the body during the shock phase are reversed. Thus, a person is best mobilized to react during the shock phase of the AR.

STAGE OF RESISTANCE The second stage in the GAS and LAS syndromes, the **stage of resistance (SR)**, is when the body's adaptation takes place. In other words, the body attempts to cope with the stressor and to limit the stressor to the smallest area of the body that can deal with it.

STAGE OF EXHAUSTION During the third stage, the **stage of exhaustion**, the adaptation that the body made during the second stage cannot be maintained. This means that the ways used to cope with the stressor have been exhausted. If adaptation has not overcome the stressor, the stress effects may spread to the entire body. At the end of this stage, the body may either rest and return to normal, or death may be the ultimate consequence. The end of this stage depends largely on the adaptive energy resources of the individual, the severity of the stressor, and the external adaptive resources that are provided, such as oxygen.

Transaction-Based Models

Transactional theories of stress are based on the work of Lazarus (1966), who stated that the stimulus theory and the response theory do not consider individual differences. Neither theory explains which factors lead some people and not others to respond effectively, nor interprets why some people are able to adapt for longer periods than others.

Although Lazarus (2006) recognized that certain environmental demands and pressures produce stress in substantial numbers of people, he emphasized that people and groups differ in their sensitivity and vulnerability to certain types of events, as well as in their interpretations and reactions. For example, in terms of illness, one person may respond with denial, another with anxiety, and still another with depression. To explain variations among individuals under comparable conditions, the Lazarus model takes into account cognitive processes that intervene between the encounter and the reaction, and the factors that affect the nature of this process. In contrast to Selye, who focused on physiological responses, Lazarus included mental and psychological components or responses as part of his concept of stress.

The Lazarus **transactional stress theory** encompasses a set of cognitive, affective, and adaptive (coping) responses that arise out of person–environment transactions. The person and the environment are inseparable; each affects and is affected by the other. Stress refers to "any event in which environmental demands, internal demands, or both tax or exceed the adaptive resources of an individual, social system, or tissue system" (Monat & Lazarus, 1991, p. 3). The individual responds to perceived environmental changes by adaptive or coping responses. See the section "Coping" later in this chapter.

Psychoneuroimmunology

The field of *psychoneuroimmunology* emerged in the 1950s in an attempt to understand the links between the brain, behaviour, and the endocrine and immune systems. Recent epidemiological studies at the time had shown there was a relationship between stress and increased risk of morbidity and mortality (Irwin, 2008). A clear link was shown in patients who had experienced the recent death of a spouse. These patients had significantly decreased T cell function, rendering them susceptible to illness (Bartrop, Lazarus, Luckhurst, Kiloh, & Penny, 1977). Researchers are now exploring the links between stress and the development of cancer and autoimmune and cardiovascular diseases. Nurses need to be aware of the role that psychosocial stress can play in the development and exacerbation of illness.

Indicators of Stress

Indicators of an individual's stress can be physiological, psychological, and cognitive.

Physiological Indicators

Responses to stress vary depending on the individual's perception of events. The physiological signs and symptoms of stress result from the activation of the sympathetic and neuroendocrine systems of the body. The Clinical Manifestations box on the next page lists physiological indicators of stress.

Physiological Indicators of Stress

When a person is experiencing stress, he or she can also experience the following physiological changes:

- Pupils dilate to increase visual perception when serious threats to the body arise.
- Diaphoresis (sweat production) increases to control elevated body heat caused by increased metabolism.
- Heart rate and cardiac output increase to transport nutrients and byproducts of metabolism more efficiently.
- Skin is pallid because of constriction of peripheral blood vessels, an effect of norepinephrine.
- Sodium and water retention increase because of the release of mineralocorticoids, which increase blood volume.
- Rate and depth of respiration increases because of dilation of the bronchioles, promoting hyperventilation.
- Urinary output decreases.
- Mouth may be dry.
- Peristalsis of the intestines decreases, resulting in possible constipation and flatulence. In some cases, people experience increased peristalsis resulting in diarrhea.
- For serious threats, mental alertness improves.
- Muscle tension increases to prepare for rapid motor activity or defence.
- Blood sugar increases because of release of glucocorticoids and gluconeogenesis.

Psychological Indicators

Psychological manifestations of stress include anxiety, fear, anger, and depression. Some of these coping patterns are helpful; others are a hindrance, depending on the situation and the length of time they are used or experienced.

ANXIETY AND FEAR   A common reaction to stress is **anxiety**, a state of mental uneasiness, apprehension, dread, or foreboding or a feeling of helplessness related to an impending or anticipated unidentified threat to the self or significant relationships. Anxiety can be experienced at the conscious, subconscious, or unconscious levels. The incidence of anxiety has been increasing in Canada in recent years and 12% of Canadians have been diagnosed with an anxiety disorder (Anxiety Disorders Association of Canada, 2007).

Anxiety can manifest at four levels:

1. *Mild anxiety* produces a slight arousal state that enhances perception, learning, and productive abilities. Most healthy people experience mild anxiety, perhaps as a feeling of mild restlessness that prompts a person to seek information and ask questions.
2. *Moderate anxiety* increases the arousal state to a point where the person expresses feelings of tension, nervousness, or concern. Perceptual abilities are narrowed.

Attention is focused more on a particular aspect of a situation than on peripheral activities.

3. *Severe anxiety* consumes most of the person's energies and requires intervention. Perception is further decreased. The person, unable to focus on what is really happening, focuses on only one specific detail of the situation generating the anxiety.
4. *Panic* is an overpowering, frightening level of anxiety causing the person to lose control. It is less frequently experienced than other levels of anxiety. The perception of a panicked person can be altered to the point where the person distorts events.

See Table 48.2 for indicators of these levels of anxiety.

Fear is an emotion or a feeling of apprehension aroused by impending or seeming danger, pain, or other perceived threat. The fear may be in response to something that has already occurred, in response to an immediate or current threat, or of something the person believes will happen. The object of fear may or may not be based in reality. For example, the beginning nursing student may be fearful in anticipation of the first experience in a client care setting. The student may fear that the client will not want to be cared for by the student or that the client might inadvertently harm the client.

Anxiety and fear differ in four ways:

1. The source of anxiety may not be identifiable; the source of fear is identifiable.
2. Anxiety is related to the future, that is, to an anticipated event. Fear is related to the present.
3. Anxiety is vague, whereas fear is definite.
4. Anxiety is the result of psychological or emotional conflict; fear is the result of a discrete physical or psychological entity.

See the Clinical Alert box on anxiety.

ANGER   **Anger** is an emotional state consisting of a subjective feeling of animosity or strong displeasure. People feel guilty when they feel anger because they have learned that to feel angry is wrong. However, anger can be expressed in a nonalienating verbal manner; it is then considered a positive emotion and a sign of emotional maturity because growth and beneficial interactions result from it.

A person's verbal expression of anger can be considered a signal to others of internal psychological

TABLE 48.2 Indicators of Levels of Anxiety

| | Level of Anxiety | | | |
Category	Mild	Moderate	Severe	Panic
Verbalization changes	Increased questioning	Voice tremors and pitch changes	Communication difficult to understand	Communication may not be understandable
Motor activity changes	Mild restlessness Sleeplessness	Tremors, facial twitches, and shakiness Increased muscle tension	Increased motor activity, inability to relax Fearful facial expression	Increased motor activity, agitation Unpredictable responses Trembling, poor motor coordination
Perception and attention changes	Feelings of increased arousal and alertness Uses learning to adapt	Narrowed focus of attention Able to focus but selectively inattentive Learning slightly impaired	Inability to focus or concentrate Easily distracted Learning severely impaired	Perception distorted or exaggerated Unable to learn or function
Respiratory and circulatory changes	None	Slightly increased respiratory and heart rates	Tachycardia	Dyspnea, palpitations, choking, chest pain or pressure
Other changes	None	Mild gastric symptoms, e.g., "butterflies in the stomach"	Headache	Feeling of impending doom Paresthesia, sweating

Sources: Carpenito-Moyet, L. J. (2010). *Nursing diagnosis: Application to clinical practice* (13th ed.) (pp. 75–76). Philadelphia, PA: Lippincott; and Fontaine, K. L., & Fletcher, J. S. (2009). *Mental health nursing* (6th ed.) (p. 227). Upper Saddle River, NJ: Prentice Hall.

discomfort and a call for assistance to deal with perceived stress. In contrast, *hostility* is usually marked by overt antagonism and harmful or destructive behaviour; *aggression* is an unprovoked attack or a hostile, injurious, or destructive action or outlook; and *violence* is the exertion of physical force to injure or abuse. Verbally expressed anger differs from hostility, aggression, and violence, but it can lead to destructiveness and violence if the anger persists unabated.

A clearly expressed verbal communication of anger, when the angry person tells the other person about the anger and carefully identifies the source, is constructive. This clarity of communication gets the anger out into the open so that the other person can deal with it and help alleviate it. The angry person gets it off his or her chest and prevents an emotional buildup.

DEPRESSION Depression is a common reaction to events that seem overwhelming or negative. **Depression,** an extreme feeling of sadness, despair, dejection, lack of worth, or emptiness, affects thousands of Canadians a year. The prevalence of depression in Canadians has increased because of the recent economic downturn. Before September 2008, the prevalence was 5.1% in an adult Albertan sample and between March 1, 2009, and October 1, 2009, there was a significant increase to 7.6%

(Wang, Smailes, Sareen, Fick, Schmitz, & Patten, 2010). The signs and symptoms of depression and the severity of the problem vary with the client and the significance of the precipitating event. Emotional symptoms can include feelings of tiredness, sadness, emptiness, or numbness. Behavioural signs of depression include irritability, inability to concentrate, difficulty making decisions, loss of sexual desire, crying, sleep disturbance, and social withdrawal. Physical signs of depression may include loss of appetite, weight loss, constipation, headache, and dizziness. Many people may experience short periods of depression in response to overwhelming stressful events, such as the death of a loved one or loss of a job; prolonged depression, however, is a cause for concern and may require treatment.

Cognitive Indicators

Cognitive indicators of stress are thinking responses that include problem solving, structuring, self-control or self-discipline, suppression, and fantasy. *Problem solving* involves thinking through the threatening situation by using specific steps similar to those of the nursing process to arrive at a solution. The person assesses the situation or problem, analyzes or defines it, chooses alternatives, carries out the selected alternative, and evaluates whether the solution was successful.

Structuring is the arrangement or manipulation of a situation so that threatening events do not occur. For example, a nurse can structure or control an interview with a client by asking only direct, closed questions. This strategy avoids information or questions that may be threatening to the nurse's knowledge or values. Structuring, however, can be productive in certain situations. A person who schedules a dental examination semiannually to prevent severe dental disease is using productive structuring.

Self-control (discipline) is assuming a manner and facial expression that convey a sense of being in control or in charge, no matter what the situation is. When self-control prevents panic and harmful or unproductive actions in a threatening situation, it is a helpful response that conveys strength. Self-control carried to an extreme, however, can delay problem solving and prevent a person from receiving the support of others, who may perceive the person as handling the situation well, as cold, or as unconcerned.

Suppression is consciously and willfully putting a thought or feeling out of mind: "I won't deal with that today. I'll do it tomorrow." This response relieves stress temporarily but does not solve the problem. A person who keeps ignoring a toothache, pushing it out of mind fearing the pain of having a filling, will not relieve symptoms or find the solution.

Fantasy or *daydreaming* is likened to make-believe. Unfulfilled wishes and desires are imagined as fulfilled, or a threatening experience is reworked or replayed so that it ends differently from reality. Experiences can be relived, everyday problems solved, and plans for the future made. The outcome of current problems can also be fantasized. For example, a client who is awaiting the results of a breast biopsy may fantasize the surgeon saying, "You do not have cancer." Fantasy responses can be helpful if they lead to problem solving. For example, the client awaiting breast biopsy results might say to herself, "Even if the doctor says, 'You have cancer,' as long as the doctor also says it can be treated, I can accept that." Fantasies can be destructive and unproductive if a person uses them to excess and retreats from reality.

Coping

Coping can be described as dealing with change, successfully or unsuccessfully. A **coping strategy (coping mechanism)** is an innate or acquired way of responding to a changing environment or specific problem or situation. According to Folkman and Lazarus (1991), coping is "the cognitive and behavioural effort to manage specific external and/or internal demands that are appraised as taxing or exceeding the resources of the person" (p. 210).

Two types of coping strategies have been described: (a) problem-focused coping and (b) emotion-focused coping. *Problem-focused coping* refers to efforts to improve a situation by making changes or taking some action. *Emotion-focused coping* includes thoughts and actions that relieve emotional distress. Emotion-focused coping does not improve the situation, but the person often feels better. Both types of strategies usually occur together (Lazarus, 2006).

Coping strategies are also viewed as short-term or long-term strategies. *Short-term coping strategies* can reduce stress to a tolerable limit temporarily but are ineffective ways to permanently deal with reality. They may even have a destructive or detrimental effect on the person. Examples of short-term strategies are using alcoholic beverages or drugs, daydreaming and fantasizing, relying on the belief that everything will work out, and giving in to others to avoid anger.

Long-term coping strategies can be constructive and realistic. For example, in certain situations, talking with others and trying to find out more about the situation are long-term strategies. Other long-term strategies include a change in lifestyle patterns, such as eating a healthy diet, exercising regularly, balancing leisure time with working, or using problem solving in decision making instead of anger or other unconstructive responses.

Coping strategies vary among individuals (see the Nursing and Canadian Society box) and are often related to the individual's perception of the stressful event. Three approaches to coping with stress are to alter the stressor, adapt to the stressor, or avoid the stressor. A person's coping strategies often change with a reappraisal of a situation. There is always more than one way to cope. Some people choose avoidance; others confront a situation as a means of coping. Still others seek information or rely on religious beliefs as a means of coping.

See Table 48.3 for some examples of the effects of stress on basic human needs.

Coping can be adaptive or maladaptive. *Adaptive coping* helps the person to deal effectively with stressful events and minimizes the distress associated with them. *Maladaptive coping* can result in unnecessary distress for the person and others associated with the person or stressful event. In the nursing literature, effective and ineffective coping are often differentiated. *Effective coping* results in adaptation; *ineffective coping* results in maladaptation. Nurses may be able to teach clients coping skills.

Although coping behaviour may not always seem appropriate, the nurse needs to remember that coping is always purposeful. The effectiveness of an individual's coping is influenced by a number of factors, including the following:

• The number, duration, and intensity of the stressors
• Past experiences of the individual

Nursing and Canadian Society

Fact	Implications for Nursing Practice
According to a 2009 Desjardins Financial Security National Health Survey, about of 30% of surveyed working Canadians said their stress levels had increased in the last year. They reported insomnia, headaches, and muscle tension. Working longer hours, they reported that their job was the biggest stressor in their lives with worries centred around money, workload, and job security. Canadians feel that they have limited control over their stress levels, especially when it comes to work and finances. Exercise and use of distraction, such as reading, could be helpful strategies.	Nurses can help people develop strategies for stress relief in areas over which they do have control. Something as prevalent as feeling out of control over stress levels indicates that nurses must assess this area when monitoring and intervening in client situations.
It is estimated that upward of 10% of Canada's peacekeepers returning from recent war efforts will experience some form of post-traumatic stress disorder (PTSD) or war-related stress (Veterans Affairs Canada, 2008). The number of veterans with PTSD have tripled since the onset of military deployment in Afghanistan in 2005 (Canadian Press, 2008). Individuals who experience highly traumatic events, such as acts of war, life-threatening diseases, and crimes, are at risk of developing PTSD in the months and years that follow such an event. Symptoms include dreams or images "flashbacks" of the event, the perception of reliving the event, and significant anxiety, including hypervigilance, insomnia, irritability, and an exaggerated startle response (Varcarolis, 2011) are also common.	Assessing for PTSD in returning service people is relevant in determining the long-term effects of military service during wartime. Appropriate referral to Veterans Affairs Canada for a range of services will benefit those who suffer from PTSD.
The Canadian Mental Health Association (2005) offers tips on dealing with holiday stress. Although generally a time to celebrate, the holiday season can be particularly stressful for people who lack finances or social support. It can be a difficult time for people who are isolated or who have trouble coping with even minor changes in routine. The Canadian Mental Health Association notes an increased incidence of depression around the holidays in December.	Although many Canadians enjoy holiday festivities, nurses must be sensitive to the adverse effects of holiday seasons on people. Exacerbation of depression or suicidal ideation may be present in people who are overwhelmed with the demands and pressures of a holiday season.

TABLE 48.3 Examples of the Effects of Stress on Basic Human Needs

Need	Example
Physiological	Has altered elimination pattern Experiences changes in appetite Has altered sleep pattern
Safety and security	Expresses nervousness and feelings of being threatened Focuses on stressors and inattention to safety measures
Love and belonging	Isolated and withdrawn Becomes overly dependent Blames others for own problems
Self-esteem	Fails to socialize with others Becomes a workaholic Draws attention to self
Self-actualization	Is preoccupied with own problems Shows lack of control Is unable to accept reality

- Support systems available to the individual
- Personal qualities of the person

If the duration of the stressors is extended beyond the coping powers of the individual, that person becomes exhausted and may develop increased susceptibility to health problems. Reaction to long-term stress is seen in family members who undertake the care of a person at home for a long period. This stress is called **caregiver burden** and produces such responses as chronic fatigue, sleeping difficulties, and high blood pressure. In the case of caregiver burden, the caregiver also becomes the nurse's client and a plan to intervene should be created (Nguyen, 2009). Prolonged stress can also result in mental illness. As coping strategies or **defence mechanisms** become ineffective, the individual may have interpersonal problems, work difficulties, and a significant decrease in abilities to meet basic human needs. See Table 48.4, the Reflect on Primary Health Care, and the Clinical Alert box on the next page.

TABLE 48.4 Clinical Application: Assessment Data and Related Nursing Diagnoses: Stress and Coping Abilities

Data	Nursing Analysis
Darryl Johnson, a 48-year-old accountant, was admitted to the emergency department with a myocardial infarction. He says, "I'm scared about this. My dad died of a heart attack when he was 48 years old." He appears restless, questions everything that is going on, and is hyperventilating.	Anxiety related to change in health status and threat of dying
Sonia Park, a 33-year-old mother of three, returned to nursing after taking a refresher course. She says, "I'm so tired since I started work. I'm not keeping up with housekeeping the way I should, and I'm not spending as much time with the kids. I'm too tired to shop and go to my son's baseball game. Everyone is helping out and not complaining, but I just keep thinking the children wish I still baked cookies for them and played more with them. I'm sure not sleeping well, and I'm having awful headaches."	Decisional Conflict related to work versus home responsibilities causing emotional and physical stress; possible uncertainty about course of action when the choice among competing actions involves risk, loss, or challenge to personal life values

REFLECT ON PRIMARY HEALTH CARE

Reducing stressors in people's lives as well as helping them to cope with stress when it does occur is an excellent opportunity for *intersectoral coordination*. Individuals and families in crisis rely on the coordination of services across sectors so that their needs can be met in a timely and effective manner. An example of a coordinated approach in some communities occurs after police have been called to a home because of a domestic dispute. The police immediately file a report with the health and social services department of their community health centre so that follow-up can be made and underlying conflicts addressed.

CLINICAL ALERT

Informal caregivers of seriously ill patients with cancer have been found to suffer from significant dysregulation of inflammation control due to a disturbance in the HPA axis. Caregivers of patients with glioblastoma multiforme (an aggressive brain tumour) were followed for a year while their loved one underwent radiotherapy. It was noted that the caregivers (average age 50.4 +/− 3.5 years) exhibited significant increases in C-reactive protein compared with controls. C-reactive protein is a marker of systemic inflammation, associated with the stress response. At the same time, there was a decrease in the levels of messenger ribonucleic acid (mRNA) for anti-inflammatory signalling molecules. This finding is significant in that is occurred in relatively young caregivers. It indicated that these individuals, in addition to the psychological and financial burdens they faced, were also at risk for developing pathologies that stem from increased systemic inflammation, such as worsening autoimmune disease and coronary artery disease (CAD) (Rohleder, Marin, Ma, & Miller, 2009).

Assessing

Nursing assessment of a client's stress and coping patterns includes (a) nursing history, and (b) physical examination of the client for indicators of stress (e.g., nail biting, nervousness, weight changes) or stress-related health problems (e.g., hypertension, dyspnea). When obtaining the nursing history of any client, the nurse poses questions about client-perceived stressors or stressful incidents, manifestations of stress, and past and present coping strategies. The nurse can also assess the effect of stress on others in the client's life (see the Evidence-Informed Practice box). During the physical examination, the nurse observes for verbal, motor, cognitive, or other physical manifestations of stress. Remember, however, that clinical signs and symptoms may not occur when cognitive coping is effective.

In addition, the nurse should be aware of expected developmental transitions (predictable tasks that must be accomplished if the person is to grow psychologically as well as physically; see Chapters 17 to 19). This knowledge

EVIDENCE-INFORMED PRACTICE

What Are the Effects of Postnatal Maternal Anxiety on Children?

Although many studies have examined the effects of maternal depression on children, few have examined the effects of postnatal maternal anxiety. The prevalence of postnatal maternal anxiety is unclear, with some estimating that it is as high as 43%. This systematic review identified 14 studies employing various measures of maternal anxiety and different childhood outcomes in the somatic, psychological, and developmental domains. The authors concluded that there is insufficient evidence to make concrete conclusions about the effects of maternal anxiety due to the dearth of well-constructed studies. While some studies link maternal anxiety to infant colic or temperament at 6 months, there is a need for longitudinal examination of mother–child dyads with consistent measures and control of confounding variables.

NURSING IMPLICATIONS: Nurses working with women during the perinatal and postnatal periods should assess their clients' anxiety levels. While some level of apprehension is normal during this life-changing period, nurses can help women develop their coping skills and refer them for further assessment when appropriate.

Source: Based on Glasheen, C., Richardson, G. A., & Fabio, A. (2010). A systematic review of the effects of postnatal maternal anxiety on children. *Archives of Women's Mental Health, 13,* 61–74. doi: 10.1007/s00737-009-0109-y

ASSESSMENT INTERVIEW

Stress and Coping Patterns

The nurse can use the following questions to learn about a client's stress and coping pattern:

- On a scale of 0 to 10, how would you rate the stress you are experiencing in the following areas?
  a. Home
  b. Work or school
  c. Finance
  d. Recent illness or loss of loved one
  e. Your health
  f. Family responsibilities
  g. Relationships with friends
  h. Relationship with parents or children
  i. Relationship with partner
  j. Recent hospitalization
  k. Other (specify)
- How long have you been dealing with these stressors?

- How do you usually handle stressful situations? If the client does not adequately describe, prompt with the following:
  a. Cry
  b. Get angry
  c. Talk to someone (Who?)
  d. Withdraw from the situation
  e. Control others or situation
  f. Go for a walk or perform physical exercise
  g. Try to arrive at a solution
  h. Pray
  i. Laugh, joke, or use some other expression of humour
  j. Meditate or use some other relaxation technique, such as yoga or guided imagery
- How well does your usual coping strategy work?

helps the nurse identify additional stressors that are present and the client's response to them. Table 48.1 provided an overview of developmental stressors. Questions to elicit data about the client's stress and coping patterns are shown in the Assessment: Interview box.

Diagnosing

There are many possible nursing diagnoses related to stress, adaptation, and coping. Some might include the following:

- Mild, moderate, severe, or panic levels of anxiety related to any number of causes (e.g. uncertainty, impending danger, threat)
- Fear and/or anger related to any number of causes (e.g. uncertainty, impending danger, threat)
- Reduced problem-solving abilities related to anxiety or threat or reduced coping options
- Effective coping related to use of effective problem-solving skills and/or effective emotion-focused coping and/or viewing situation as manageable and a challenge
- Ineffective coping related to use of ineffective problem solving skills and/or ineffective emotion-focused coping and/or viewing situation as not manageable and a threat

Planning

The nurse develops plans in collaboration with the client and significant support people, when possible, according to the client's state of health (e.g., ability

to return to work), level of anxiety, support resources, coping mechanisms, and sociocultural and religious affiliation. The nurse who has little experience intervening with clients undergoing stress may want to consult with a clinical specialist or a more experienced nurse to develop effective plans. The nurse and client set goals to change the existing client responses to the stressor or stressors.

The overall client goals for persons experiencing stress-related responses are as follows:

- Decrease or resolve anxiety
- Increase ability to manage or cope with stressful events or circumstances
- Improve role performance

Examples of specific desired outcomes, although established in this phase, are provided in Table 48.5 in the "Evaluating" section of this chapter (page 1553).

Examples of interventions include the following:

- Promoting anxiety reduction
- Body image enhancement
- Caregiver support
- Coping enhancement
- Crisis intervention
- Decision-making support
- Role enhancement

Specific nursing activities related to each of these interventions can be selected to individualize client care. The Sample Care Plan provides selected interventions and activities.

Sample Care Plan to Promote Coping

Assessment Data

Nursing Assessment

Amanda Crosby, a 55-year-old mother of four children from the Gaspésie, Quebec, is hospitalized because of breast cancer. She is scheduled for a simple mastectomy the following day. This procedure will be followed by daily external beam radiation. Amanda was relatively healthy until she found a lump in her right breast 2 weeks ago. She and her husband are extremely anxious about the surgery. Amanda confides to the admitting nurse, "I can't stand the idea of having one of my breasts cut off; I don't know how I'm going to be able to even look at myself. I will be scarred from the radiation, too." Mr. Crosby informs the nurse that Amanda has been abusing alcohol since her diagnosis and neglecting her responsibilities as a mother. She is tearful and does not see how she will be able to continue her work as a dress designer.

Physical Examination

Height: 164 cm
Weight: 58 kg
Temperature: 37°C
Pulse: 88 beats/min
Respirations: 16/min
Blood Pressure: 142/88 mm Hg

Diagnostic Data

Chest radiography negative, CBC (complete blood count) and urinalysis within normal limits

Nursing Diagnosis

Ineffective coping related to personal vulnerability secondary to mastectomy (as evidenced by verbalization of inability to cope, substance abuse, inability to meet role expectations)

Client Goal

The client will demonstrate effective coping strategies.

Desired Health Outcomes

Coping, as evidenced by often demonstrating the ability to do the following:

1. Identify effective and ineffective coping patterns, including a reduction in the ineffective patterns
2. Report decrease in negative feelings
3. Verbalize a sense of control
4. Participate in activities of daily living postoperatively

Social support is evidenced by substantial reports of the following:

1. Willingness to call on others for help
2. Emotional assistance provided by others

Selected Nursing Interventions and Activities with Rationales [in bold]

Coping Enhancement

- Ensure an accepting environment.
  Rationale: A first step in therapeutic communication is establishing rapport. An atmosphere of trust and warmth encourages recognizing problems and sharing feelings through client self-reflection.

- Provide or ensure accurate knowledge of client diagnosis, treatment and prognosis.
  Rationale: A solid foundation for exploring feelings and coping strategies is factual information. Persons under stress often misunderstand information and need repetition of facts to promote understanding, which will also help to relieve stress.

- Assess Amanda's perception of changes to her body image.
  Rationale: Body image may be a big issue for Amanda. A thorough and accurate appraisal can facilitate therapeutic intervention, assisting her to reappraise her situation and ensure successful coping strategies.

- Facilitate autonomous decision-making.
  Rationale: This increases self-esteem, personal achievement and a sense of control.

- Investigate her previous ways of coping with life issues.
  Rationale: Exploring present and past can build on previous success, avoid ineffective methods and ensure new skill development when required for the present situation. It also helps determine the risk for self-harm.

- Encourage expression of fears, feelings and perceptions.
  Rationale: Nonthreatening discussion can assist in identifying influential factors and confronting issues.

- Assist Amanda in identifying her personal strengths and abilities.
  Rationale: She can use these attributes to build effective coping strategies for the present situation. This improves self-concept and stress management abilities.

- Encourage realistic appraisal of Amanda's change in role.
  Rationale: Persons under stress may not have realistic perceptions. A description of her present and future roles assists her in being realistic in her personal goal-setting.

- Encourage constructive expressions of anger and hostility.
  Rationale: Anger can be a positive energy and prevent potential harm to self and others.

Support System Enhancement

- Watch family interactions.
  Rationale: This helps to identify Amanda's sources of support or lack of that support.

- Identify barriers to available support.
  Rationale: Support may be available, but Amanda may not accept it or know how to use it.

- Involve her significant others in planning and care.
  Rationale: If Amanda allows, significant others can assist her in coping with and accepting changes in her appearance. They may also assist in identifying strengths and coping behaviours.

- Discuss with concerned others how they can help.
  Rationale: Within the bounds of confidentiality, support from others will provide a foundation for her own acceptance and adjustment.

(continued)

- Discuss referral to a community-based breast cancer support group.
  Rationale: Individuals who have experienced some of her issues may be able to be more supportive than family and friends who are unsure how to help. Sharing with others in her situation may encourage acceptance of her personal situation.

EVALUATION

The coping outcome was minimally met. Following surgery, Amanda was withdrawn. During bathing, she would not assist and turned her head away when the dressing was removed. She refused to learn how to manage the wound drain, discuss her feelings, or plan for the future. She did identify that alcohol was not an effective coping strategy. Because patients having a mastectomy are often only hospitalized for a few days, it may be that she requires more time to reach the desired outcome.

Social support outcome partly met. Amanda allows her husband to provide direct care and emotional support for her. She was discharged to the care of her family, and a community nurse was consulted to care for and help her to cope with her ongoing issues. Amanda expressed an interest in receiving a call from the breast cancer support group member before deciding if she would attend an actual face-to-face meeting.

Planning for Home Care

Clients who are experiencing stress may require ongoing nursing support or referral to community agencies that can provide support to meet client needs and enhance client coping. The determination of how much and what type of planning and home care follow-up is based in great part on the nurse's knowledge of how the client and family have coped with previous stressors and the nature of the present stressor. The Assessment: Home Care box describes data to be gathered for home care or follow-up assessment.

Implementing

Although stress is part of daily life, it is also highly individual; a situation that to one person is a major stressor may not affect another. Some methods to help reduce stress will be effective for one person; other methods will be appropriate for a different person. A nurse who is sensitive to clients' needs and reactions can choose those methods of intervention that will be most effective for each individual.

Encouraging Health-Promotion Strategies

Several health-promotion strategies are often appropriate as interventions for clients with stress-related nursing diagnoses. Among these are physical exercise, optimal nutrition, adequate rest and sleep, and time management.

EXERCISE Regular exercise promotes both physical and emotional health. Physiological benefits include improved muscle tone, increased cardiopulmonary function, and weight control. Psychological benefits include

---

ASSESSMENT | **HOME CARE**

Stress and Coping

Nurses must assess clients and their families and whether they will need follow-up care after discharge:

CLIENT

- *Knowledge:* Client's understanding of the nature of the stressors
- *Current coping strategies:* Effectiveness of current coping strategies and willingness to learn new stress management techniques
- *Self-care abilities:* Physical, emotional, social, and financial ability to minimize associated stressors
- *Role expectations:* Client's perception of the need to return to prior roles and possible stressors associated with these roles

FAMILY

- *Knowledge:* Family members' and significant others' understanding of the nature of the client's stressors and their own relationship with client stressors

- *Family coping strategies:* Effectiveness of family members' and significant others' coping strategies and willingness to learn new stress management techniques
- *Role expectations:* Family members' and significant others' perception of the need for the client to return to family and work roles
- *Support people's availability and skills:* Family and significant others' sensitivity to the client's emotional and physical needs and ability to provide a supportive environment

COMMUNITY

- *Resources:* Availability of and familiarity with possible sources of assistance for stress management, such as massage therapists, religious or spiritual centres, physical care providers, support groups, and so on

relief of tension, a feeling of well-being, and relaxation. Canadian health guidelines recommend adults accumulate 2.5 hours of moderate to vigorous physical activity per week, which can be broken into 10 minute sessions (Canadian Society for Exercise Physiology, 2011). See Chapter 39 for more detailed information.

NUTRITION Optimal nutrition is essential for health and for increasing the body's resistance to stress. To minimize the effects of a stress response (e.g., irritability, hyperactivity, anxiety), people need to avoid excesses of caffeine, salt, sugar, and fat, and deficiencies in vitamins and minerals. Guidelines for a well-balanced, healthy diet are detailed in Chapter 40. See the Clinical Alert box on comfort foods.

CLINICAL ALERT

Many persons have "comfort foods"—foods they like to eat that actually make them feel better emotionally. These should be allowed in moderation whenever they are not contraindicated by the person's health condition. Often these foods are high in carbohydrates and calories and can contribute to increasing body mass index (BMI) over the long term.

REST AND SLEEP Rest and sleep restore the body's energy levels and are an essential aspect of stress management. To ensure adequate rest and sleep, clients may need help to attain comfort (such as pain management) and to learn techniques that promote peace of mind and relaxation. (See "Using Relaxation Techniques" later in this chapter.)

TIME MANAGEMENT People who manage their time effectively usually experience less stress because they feel more in control of their circumstances. Clients who feel overwhelmed often need help to prioritize tasks and to consider whether modifications can be made to decrease role demands. Some working mothers, for example, may need to consider delegating more tasks to family members or hiring part-time help. Controlling the demands of others is also an important aspect of effective time management because all requests made by others cannot always be met. Clients may need to learn to develop an awareness of which requests they can meet without undue stress, which ones can be negotiated, and which ones need to be declined. Feelings of control can also be enhanced when clients schedule a daily or weekly time to deal with specific tasks.

Time management must address both what is important to the client and what can realistically be achieved. For example, clients may need to consider whether a clean house and time spent with the children can both be accomplished satisfactorily and, if not, which is more important. Often, clients who are feeling overwhelmed need to re-examine the "should, ought, and must" approach to their actions and develop more realistic self-expectations.

Reducing Anxiety

Nurses carry out measures to minimize clients' anxiety and stress. For example, nurses encourage clients to take deep breaths before an injection, explain procedures before they are implemented, including sensations likely to be experienced during the procedure, administer a back or neck rub to help the client relax, and offer support to clients and families during times of illness. General guidelines for helping clients who are stressed and feeling anxious are outlined in Box 48.1.

BOX 48.1 MINIMIZING STRESS AND ANXIETY

The nurse can use these methods to help clients who are experiencing stress or anxiety:

- Listen attentively; try to understand the client's perspective of the situation.
- Provide an atmosphere of warmth and trust; convey a sense of caring and empathy.
- Provide factual information, as needed, to prepare clients for tests, treatments, and so on.
- Encourage clients to participate in the plan of care; give them choices about appropriate aspects of care without overwhelming them with the need to make decisions.
- Stay with clients, as needed, to promote safety and feelings of security and to reduce fear.
- Control the environment to minimize additional stressors, such as by reducing noise, limiting the number of persons in the room, and providing care by the same nurse as much as possible.
- Help clients to do the following:
  a. Determine situations that precipitate anxiety and identify signs of anxiety.
  b. Verbalize feelings, perceptions, and fears as appropriate. Some cultures discourage the expression of feelings.
  c. Identify personal strengths.
  d. Recognize usual coping patterns and differentiate positive from negative coping mechanisms.
  e. Identify new strategies for managing stress (e.g., exercise, massage, progressive relaxation).
  f. Identify available support systems.
- Teach clients about the following:
  a. The importance of adequate exercise, a balanced diet, and rest and sleep to energize the body and enhance coping abilities.
  b. The support groups that are available, such as Alcoholics Anonymous, Weight Watchers, or Overeaters Anonymous, and parenting and child abuse support groups.
  c. The educational programs that are available, such as time management, assertiveness training, and meditation groups.

Mediating Anger

Often, nurses find clients' anger difficult to handle. Caring for the client who is angry is difficult for two reasons:

- Clients seldom state, "I feel angry or frustrated," or indicate the reason for their anger. Instead, they may refuse treatment, become verbally abusive or demanding, threaten violence, or become overly critical. Their complaints rarely reflect the cause of their anger.

- Anger from clients can elicit fear and anger in the nurse, who may respond in a manner that intensifies the client's anger, even to the point of violence. The majority of nurses respond in a way that reduces their own stress, rather than the client's stress.

Fontaine (2009) recommends the following strategies for dealing with clients' anger:

- Know and understand your own response to the feelings and expressions of anger.
- Accept the client's right to be angry; feelings are real and cannot be discounted or ignored.
- Try to understand the meaning of the client's anger.
- Ask the client what contributed to the anger.
- Help clients "own" the anger—do not assume responsibility for their feelings.
- Let clients talk about their anger.
- Listen to the client, and act as calmly as possible.
- After the interaction is completed, take time to process your feelings and your responses to the client with your colleagues.

Always ensure the safety of the client and others. Know the agency procedures to call for assistance from other staff or security personnel if you believe someone (including you) is in danger. See the Clinical Alert box on working with an angry client.

CLINICAL ALERT

A nurse who is concerned for his or her own safety while working with an angry client should withdraw immediately from the situation and obtain support from another individual.

Using Relaxation Techniques

Several relaxation techniques can be used to quiet the mind, release tension, and counteract the fight-or-flight responses of GAS discussed earlier in this chapter. Nurses can teach these techniques to clients and then encourage clients to use them to control stress throughout life. Nurses can also encourage clients admitted to hospitals to use these techniques when they encounter stressful situations in a hospital setting. Examples of these situations are (a) during childbirth, (b) postoperatively to cope with pain, and (c) before and during a painful procedure. Many agencies now have relaxation recordings available. Some clients make their own recordings for use on their personal mobile devices, for example. Specific relaxation techniques are discussed in Chapter 30 and include the following:

- Breathing exercises
- Massage
- Progressive relaxation
- Imagery
- Biofeedback
- Yoga
- Meditation
- Therapeutic touch
- Music therapy
- Humour and laughter

Performing Crisis Intervention

A **crisis** is an acute, time-limited state of disequilibrium resulting from situational, developmental, or societal sources of stress. A person in crisis is temporarily unable to cope with or adapt to the stressor by using previous methods of problem solving. People in crisis generally have a distorted perception of the event, do not have adequate situational support, and do not have adequate coping mechanisms. Common characteristics of crises are shown in Box 48.2.

Crisis intervention is a short-term helping process of assisting clients to (a) work through a crisis to its resolution, and (b) restore their pre-crisis level of functioning. It is a process that includes not only the client in crisis but also various members of the client's

---

BOX 48.2 COMMON CHARACTERISTICS OF CRISES

Crises typically have the following characteristics:

- All crises are experienced as sudden. The person is usually not aware of a warning signal, even if others could "see it coming." The individual or family may feel that they have little or no preparation for the event or trauma.
- The crisis is often experienced as ultimately life threatening, whether this perception is realistic or not.
- Communication with significant others is often decreased or cut off.
- Perceived or real displacement from familiar surroundings or loved ones can occur.
- All crises have an aspect of loss, whether actual or perceived. The losses can include an object, a person, a hope, a dream, or any significant factor for that individual.

support network. Crisis intervention is not the domain of any one professional group. People who intervene in crises come from the fields of nursing, medicine, psychology, social work, and theology. Police officers, teachers, school guidance counsellors, and rescue workers, among others, are often on the spot in moments of crisis.

Because a state of disequilibrium is so uncomfortable, a crisis is self-limiting. However, a person experiencing a crisis alone is more vulnerable to unsuccessful resolution than a person working through a crisis with help. Working with another person increases the likelihood that the person in crisis will resolve it in a positive way. Often, a state of crisis offers the individual or family great potential for growth and change.

The traditional steps of the nursing process correspond closely to the steps of crisis intervention. *Assessment* is the first phase of crisis intervention. The nurse or helper must focus on the person and the problem, collecting data about the client, the client's coping style, the precipitating event, the situational supports, the client's perception of the crisis, and the client's ability to handle the problem. Assessment is an essential and critical step of crisis intervention. This information is the basis for later decisions about how and when to intervene and whom to call. An individual's perception of the event and personal response will determine the nursing diagnoses. The most common nursing diagnoses for people in crisis are similar to those cited earlier in this chapter. Effective *planning* for crisis intervention must be based on careful assessment and developed in active collaboration with the person in crisis and the significant people in that person's life.

Implementation involves crisis counselling and home crisis visits. **Crisis counselling** focuses on solving immediate problems and it involves individuals, groups, or families. Crisis intervention centres rely heavily on telephone counselling by volunteers who have professional consultation available to them. Also known as *hotlines* and often available around the clock, they allow callers to remain anonymous and test what it feels like to ask for assistance. The volunteers usually work within a protocol that indicates what information they need from the client to assess the crisis. Their goal is to plan steps to provide immediate relief and then long-term follow-up, if necessary.

Crisis home visits are made when telephone counselling does not suffice or when the crisis workers need to obtain additional information by direct observation or to reach a client who is unobtainable by telephone. Home visits are appropriate when crisis workers need to initiate contacts rather than waiting for clients to come to them, such as when a telephone caller is assessed to be highly suicidal or when a concerned neighbour, physician, or clergy member informs the agency of clients in potential crisis.

Stress Management for Nurses

Nurses, like clients, are susceptible to experiencing anxiety and stress. Nursing practice involves many stressors related to both clients and the work environment: understaffing and increasing client care assignments, adjusting to various work shifts, being expected to assume responsibilities for which the nurse does not feel prepared, receiving inadequate support from supervisors and peers, visiting homes that are depressing, caring for dying clients, and so on.

The Registered Nurses' Association of Ontario has developed best practice guidelines to promote healthy work environments for nurses throughout Canada in an attempt to alleviate work-related stress. These can be accessed at http://rnao.ca.

Although most nurses cope effectively with the physical and emotional demands of nursing, in some situations, nurses become overwhelmed and develop **burnout**, a complex syndrome of behaviours that can be likened to the exhaustion stage of GAS. The nurse with burnout manifests physical and emotional depletion, a negative attitude and self-concept, and feelings of helplessness and hopelessness.

Nurses can prevent burnout by using the techniques to manage stress discussed for clients. Nurses must first recognize their stress and become attuned to such responses as feelings of being overwhelmed, fatigue, angry outbursts, physical illness, and increases in coffee drinking, smoking, or other substance use. Once attuned to stress and personal reactions, it is necessary to identify which situations produce the most pronounced reactions so that steps can be taken to reduce the stress:

- Plan a daily relaxation program with meaningful quiet times to reduce tension (e.g., read a novel, listen to music, soak in a hot bath, or meditate).

- Establish a regular exercise program to direct energy outward (e.g., jog, play badminton, or join a yoga class).

- Develop assertiveness techniques to overcome feelings of powerlessness in relationships with others. Learn to say no.

- Learn to accept failures—your own and others'—and make it a constructive learning experience. Recognize that most people do the best they can. Learn to ask for help, to show your feelings with colleagues, and to support your colleagues in times of need.

- Accept what cannot be changed. Every situation has certain limitations. Get involved in constructive change efforts if organizational policies and procedures cause stress.

- Develop collegial peer support groups to deal with feelings and anxieties generated in the work setting.

- Participate in professional organizations to address workplace issues.

- Seek counselling, if indicated, to get clarifications for concerns.

Evaluating

Using the desired outcomes developed during the planning stage as a guide, the nurse collects data needed to determine whether client goals and outcomes have been achieved. Examples of client goals and related outcomes are shown in Table 48.5.

If outcomes are not achieved, the nurse, client, and support people, if appropriate, need to explore the reasons why before modifying the care plan. Such questions as the following need to be considered:

- How does the client perceive the problem?
- Is there an underlying problem that has not been identified?
- Have new stressors occurred that interfere with successful coping?
- Were existing coping strategies sufficient to meet intended outcomes?
- How does the client perceive the effectiveness of the new coping strategies?
- Did the client implement the new coping strategies properly?
- Did the client access and use available resources?
- Have family members and significant others provided effective support?

TABLE 48.5 Evaluation Goals and Health Outcomes: Stress and Coping

Goal	Examples of Desired Outcomes
Decrease or resolve anxiety	Describes causes and level of anxiety Eliminates causes of anxiety, as appropriate Verbalizes feelings related to anxiety Decreases external stimuli when experiencing anxiety Verbalizes an increase in emotional and physical comfort
Improve ability to manage or cope with stressful events	Describes usual coping patterns Identifies personal strengths Develops new coping strategies for managing stress Plans coping strategies for stressful situations Uses effective coping strategies in managing anxiety Verbalizes a sense of control Reports decreased stress
Improve role performance	Describes realistic personal role expectations Reports strategies for role change, as appropriate Maintains role performance Performs family roles Performs effective work or school role Maintains social relationships

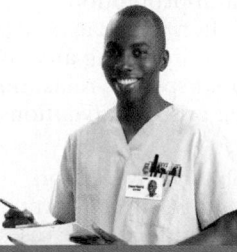

Case Study 48

Refer to the "Sample Care Plan to Promote Coping" on page 1548 and answer the following questions.

CRITICAL THINKING QUESTIONS

1. If Amanda had been able to choose a lumpectomy rather than a mastectomy (less visible, smaller, potentially less "meaningful" tissue removal), would the nursing diagnosis and expected outcomes remain the same? Why, or why not?

2. Does Amanda's situation reflect more of a stimulus-based or a response-based model of stress? Why?

3. While you are working with Amanda, she becomes very angry and says to you, "You don't understand. You've never had to go through this." How would you respond?

4. On the basis of the evaluation above, do you believe that Amanda is in crisis? What factors led to your decision? How does your view change the modifications indicated in her care plan?

Check the eText in MyNursingLab for answers and explanations.

KEY TERMS

alarm reaction (AR)
 p. 1539

anger *p. 1542*

anxiety *p. 1542*

burnout *p. 1552*

caregiver burden
 p. 1545

coping *p. 1544*

coping strategy (coping mechanism) *p. 1544*

countershock phase
 p. 1541

crisis *p. 1551*

crisis counselling
 p. 1552

CHAPTER HIGHLIGHTS

- Stress is a state of physiological and psychological tension that affects the whole person, physically, emotionally, intellectually, socially, and spiritually.

- Models view stress as a stimulus, stress as a response, and stress as a transaction.

- Psychoneuroimmunology is the study of the interactions between stress, the brain, and the endocrine and immune systems.

- Physiological responses to stress are described by the general adaptation syndrome (GAS) and the local adaptation syndrome (LAS).

- General adaptation syndrome (GAS) is a multisystem response to stress and involves three stages: alarm reaction, resistance, and exhaustion.

- Local adaptation syndrome (LAS) is a localized physiological response that also expresses the three stages of GAS. An example of LAS is the inflammatory response.

- Stress has physiological, psychological, and cognitive indicators. Physiological indicators are the result of increased activity of the sympathetic and neuroendocrine systems.

- Common psychological indicators are anxiety, fear, anger, and depression. Anxiety, the most common response, has four levels: mild, moderate, severe, and panic.

- Cognitive indicators or thinking responses to stress include problem solving, structuring, self-control (discipline), suppression, and fantasy.

- Coping strategies to deal with stress vary significantly among individuals. Strategies can be problem-focused or emotion-focused, long-term or short-term, and effective or ineffective.

- The effectiveness of individual coping depends on the number, duration, and intensity of the stressors; past experience; support systems available; and the personal qualities of the person.

- Prolonged stress and ineffective coping interfere with the meeting of basic needs and can affect physical and mental health.

- Nursing assessment of a client experiencing stress involves a nursing history to identify perceptions of and duration of stressors and coping strategies, and a physical examination for physical indicators of stress.

- Nursing interventions for clients who are stressed are aimed at encouraging health-promotion strategies (exercise, balanced diet, adequate rest and sleep, and time management), minimizing anxiety, mediating anger, teaching about specific relaxation techniques, and implementing crisis interventions, as needed.

- Because nursing practice involves many stressors related to both clients and the work environment, nurses are susceptible to anxiety and, in some cases, burnout. Like clients, they need to implement stress-reduction measures.

ASSESS YOUR LEARNING

1. After the death of several long-term clients, which of the following actions indicates that the nurse is demonstrating ineffective coping?

   a. The nurse talks at length to her partner about the deaths.

   b. The nurse keeps busy with other actions and does not think about the deaths for several days.

   c. The nurse offers to work extra shifts for several weeks.

   d. Several nurses schedule a group session with the agency clergy to discuss the deaths.

2. A 50-year-old client, newly diagnosed with diabetes mellitus, is to begin giving insulin injections. The nurse helps identify previously successful coping strategies that may be useful in the current situation. Which of the following stressors is closely related to the new stressor?

   a. An interview for a new job

   b. The death of a pet when the person was a teenager

   c. The person's partner filing for divorce

   d. Starting to wear eyeglasses at age 30 years

3. Two people have been in a car accident and have similar injuries. According to the transaction-based model, their degree of stress from the accident would be which of the following?

   a. Based on previous experience and personal characteristics

   b. Very similar since they had the same stimulus

   c. The identical physiological alarm reaction

   d. Different depending on their external resources and support levels

4. A client who was informed of a cancer diagnosis assures the nurse he is fine. Which of the following is MOST indicative physical evidence to the nurse of the client's stress?

   a. Constricted pupils

   b. Dilated peripheral blood vessels

   c. Hyperventilation

   d. Decreased heart rate

5. Immediately after the parents of a hospitalized child are informed that the child has leukemia, the father responds by continuing his usual work schedule, rarely visiting, and asking when the child can return to school. Of the following, which would be an appropriate nursing diagnosis at this time?

   a. Ineffective denial

   b. Caregiver role strain

   c. Readiness for enhanced coping

   d. Decisional conflict

6. A nurse has begun working with young adults. Which of the following would the nurse recognize as sources of stress common to that population?

   a. Coping with aging parents

   b. Starting a new job

   c. Accepting decreased physical abilities

   d. Accepting a changing body structure

7. Which of the following would be the most important health-promotion strategy for a middle-aged male client who is experiencing stress because fear of a job layoff has led him to accept projects that require a great deal of international travel?

   a. Exercise

   b. Sleep

   c. Nutrition

   d. Time management

8. On entering the client's room for the first time, the nurse finds the client on the phone. Within the next few seconds, the client slams down the phone, sweeps everything off the overbed table, and demands that the nurse perform several duties "this very minute." Which of the following would be the MOST appropriate response for the nurse?

   a. Tell the client, "I will return," and then leave the room.

   b. Tell the client no care will be given until the screaming ends.

   c. Begin providing needed care calmly and quietly.

   d. Allow the client to complete venting and then respond calmly.

9. Mr. Jonas, 67 years old, will soon be discharged home from the cardiac unit. He indicates that he is concerned about his discharge because his home situation can be stressful. What strategy should the nurse employ to help him cope with stressful situations?

   a. Encourage him to plan his daily activities.

   b. Inform him that a nurse will visit him at home.

   c. Reassure him that stress is normal and that he should just rest.

   d. Have him practise a stress-reduction method that he has found effective.

10. Which of the following interventions best facilitates successful stress management with clients?

   a. Teaching relaxation techniques

   b. Suggesting talking with others

   c. Encouraging problem solving

   d. Promoting self-awareness

Check the eText in MyNursingLab for answers and explanations.

WEBLINKS

Canadian Mental Health Association (CMHA)

http://www.cmha.ca

This website contains educational information, links to multiple Canadian and international mental health sites, information regarding CMHA provincial and territorial locations (except Nunavut), and a discussion site.

Health Canada—Healthy Living

http://www.hc-sc.gc.ca/hl-vs/iyh-vsv/life-vie/stress-eng.php

This website is funded by Health Canada and contains information on many health issues, including stress and stress management for Canadians.

Centre for Addiction and Mental Health

http://www.camh.net

The Centre for Addiction and Mental Health site contains information on addiction, community health and education, mental health, and research at the centre.

Canadian Nurses Association

http://www.cna-nurses.ca

The Canadian Nurses Association (CNA) is a federation of 11 provincial and territorial registered nurses associations and colleges representing all Canadian nurses and nurse practitioners. Includes documents describing the code of ethics and clinical best practices.

Registered Nurses' Association of Ontario (RNAO)

http://www.rnao.org

The RNAO has produced numerous guidelines to assist nurses in dealing with clients in crisis and promoting well-being and healthy work environments.

MyNursingLab

REFERENCES

Anxiety Disorders Association of Canada. (2007). *About anxiety disorders.* Retrieved from http://www.anxietycanada.ca/english/index.php

Bartrop, R. W., Lazarus, L., Luckhurst, E., Kiloh, L. G., & Penny, R. (1977). Depressed lymphocyte function after bereavement. *Lancet, 16,* 834–836.

Canadian Mental Health Association. (2005). *Holiday angst hits everyone.* Retrieved from http://www.cmha.bc.ca/files/5-12-05.pdf

Canadian Press. (2008, February 28). *Post-traumatic stress disorder surges among Canadian veterans.* Retrieved from http://www.cbc.ca/news/health/story/2008/02/29/ptad-report.html

Canadian Society for Exercise Physiology. (2011). *Canadian physical activity guidelines.* Retrieved from http://www.csep.ca/english/view.asp?x=804

Cannon, W. B. (1929). *Bodily changes in pain, hunger, fear, and rage.* New York, NY: Appleton-Century-Crofts.

Desjardins Financial Security. (2011). *National health surveys.* Retrieved from http://www.desjardinslifeinsurance.com/en/life-events/thinking-health/Pages/national-health-surveys.aspx

Desjardins Financial Security. (2009). *Health is cool 2009: Employee Survey Summary–regional results.* Retrieved from http://www.desjardinslifeinsurance.com/en/life-events/Documents/Health%20survey%202009%20Highlights%20employees.pdf

Folkman, S., & Lazarus, R. S. (1991). Coping and emotion. In A. Monat & R. S. Lazarus (Eds.). *Stress and coping* (pp. 207–227). New York, NY: Columbia University Press.

Fontaine, K. L.(2009). *Mental health nursing* (6th ed.). Upper Saddle River, NJ: Prentice Hall.

Holmes, T. H., & Rahe, R. H. (1967). The social re-adjustment rating scale. *Journal of Psychomatic Research, 11*(August), 213–218.

Irwin, M. R. (2008). Human psychoneuroimmunology: 20 Years of discovery. *Brain, Behavior and Immunity, 22*(2), 129–139. doi: 10.1016/j.bbi.2007.07.013

Kodish, I., Rockhill, C., Ryan, S., & Varley, C. (2011). Pharmacotherapy for anxiety disorders in children and adolescents. *Pediatric Clinics of North America, 58(1),* 55–72. doi: 10.1016/j.pcl.2010.10.002

Johnson, K. L., & Renn, C. (2006). The hypothalamic-pituitary-adrenal axis in critical illness. *AACN Clinical Issues, 17(1),* 39–49.

Lazarus, R. S. (1966). *Psychological stress and the coping process.* New York, NY: McGraw-Hill.

Lazarus, R. S. (2006). *Stress and emotion: A new synthesis.* New York, NY: McGraw-Hill.

Miller, M. A., & Rahe, R. H. (1997). Life changes scaling for the 1990s. *Journal of Psychosomatic Research, 43,* 279–292. doi: 10.1016/S0022-3999(97)00118-9

Monat, A., & Lazarus, R. S. (Eds.) (1991). *Stress and coping* (3rd ed.). New York, NY: Columbia University Press.

Nguyen, M. (2009). Nurse's assessment of caregiver burden. *MEDSURG Nursing, 18,* 148–152.

Rahe, R. H., & Tolles, R. L. (2002). The brief stress and coping inventory: A useful stress management instrument. *International Journal of Stress Management, 9,* 61–70. doi: 10.1023/A:1014950618756

Rohleder, N., Marin, T. J., Ma, R., & Miller, G. E. (2009). Biologic cost of caring for a cancer patient: Dysregulation of pro- and anti-inflammatory signaling pathways. *Journal of Clinical Oncology, 27,* 2909–2915.doi: 10.1200/JCO.2008.18.7435

Schafer, W. (1992). *Stress management for wellness* (2nd ed.). Fort Worth, TX: Harcourt Brace Janovich.

Selye, H. (1956). *The stress of life.* New York, NY: McGraw-Hill.

Selye, H. (1976). *The stress of life* (Rev. ed.). New York, NY: McGraw-Hill.

Varcarolis, E. (2011). *Manual of psychiatric nursing care planning* (4th ed.), St. Louis, MO: Saunders.

Veterans Affairs Canada. (2008). *Post-traumatic stress disorder (PTSD) and war-related stress.* Ottawa, ON: Minister of Veterans Affairs.

Wang, J., Smailes, E., Sareen, J., Fick, G. H., Schmitz, N., & Patten, S. B. (2011). The prevalence of mental disorders in the working population over the period of global economic crisis. *Canadian Journal of Psychiatry, 55(9),* 598–605.

Chapter 49

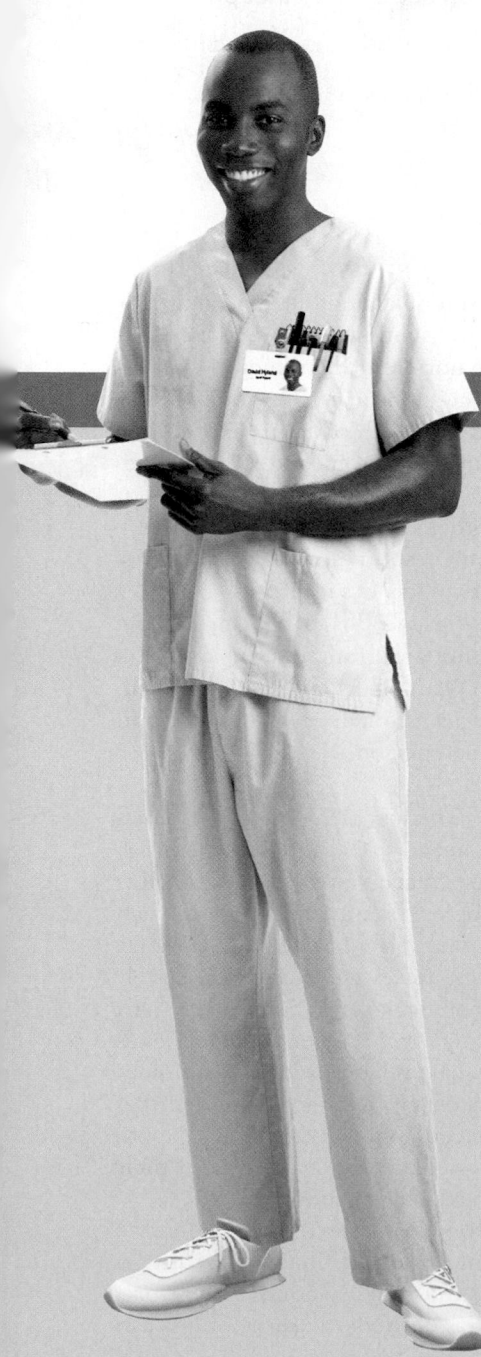

Loss, Grieving, and Death

LEARNING OUTCOMES

After studying this chapter, you will be able to:

1. Describe types and sources of losses.

2. Describe the experience of grief as a response to loss that is individually experienced and expressed.

3. Outline eight factors affecting grief responses.

4. Identify measures that facilitate the journey of grief.

5. List clinical signs of impending and of actual death.

6. Describe the nurse's legal and moral responsibilities regarding end-of-life care and such issues as advance directives, artificial nutrition, and do-not-resuscitate (DNR) orders.

7. Describe relational communication as authentic presence of the nurse.

8. Describe six strategies for helping clients die with dignity.

9. Identify nursing measures for care of the body after death.

10. Describe the role of the nurse in working with families or caregivers of dying clients.

Loss, grieving, and death are experienced by everyone at some time during their life. People may suffer the loss of valued relationships through life changes, such as moving from one city to another, separation, divorce, or the death of a parent, spouse, or friend. People may grieve changing life roles as they watch grown children leave home or when they retire from their life-long work. *Loss* is a generic term that signifies absence of an object, position, ability, or attribute. The term is often applied to the death of an individual, and it is the bereaved person who is considered to have experienced a loss. In the clinical setting, the nurse encounters clients who are experiencing grief related to declining health, loss of a body part, terminal illness, or their impending death or that of a significant other. Nurses interact with dying clients and their families or caregivers in a variety of settings, from the demise of a fetus, to that of an adolescent victim of an accident, to that of an older adult client who finally succumbs to a chronic illness. Nurses must recognize the various influences on the dying process—legal, ethical, religious and spiritual, biological, and personal—and be prepared to provide sensitive, skilled, and supportive care to all those affected.

Loss and Grief

Loss is an actual or a potential situation in which something that is valued is changed, no longer available, or gone. People can experience the loss of body image, a significant other, a sense of well-being, a job, personal possessions, beliefs, or a sense of self. Illness and hospitalization often produce losses.

Death is a fundamental loss, both for the dying person and for those who survive. Death is inevitable, and it is an experience that each person ultimately faces alone. Yet death, like loss, can stimulate people to grow in their understanding of themselves and others. Death can be viewed not simply as loss of life but also as the dying person's final opportunity to experience life in ways that bring meaning and fulfillment.

Types and Sources of Loss

The two general types of loss are actual loss and perceived loss. Both losses can be anticipatory. An **actual loss** can be identified by others and can arise either in response to or in anticipation of a situation. For example, a woman whose husband is dying may experience actual loss in anticipation of his death. A **perceived loss** is experienced by one person but cannot be verified by others. Psychological losses are often perceived losses in that they are not directly verifiable. For example, a woman who leaves her employment to care for her children at home may perceive a loss of independence and freedom. An **anticipatory loss** is experienced before the loss actually occurs.

Loss can be viewed as situational or developmental. The loss of a job, the death of a child, and the loss of functional ability as a result of acute illness or injury, for example, are unexpected situational losses. Losses that occur in the process of normal development—such as the departure of grown children from the home, retirement from a career, and the death of aged parents—are developmental losses that can, to some extent, be anticipated and prepared for. How individuals work through loss is closely related to their life stages and past experiences, personal and family resources, social support systems, and their beliefs about the loss itself.

Many sources of loss exist: (a) loss of an aspect of the self: a body part, a physiological function, or a psychological attribute, (b) loss of an object external to the self, (c) separation from an accustomed environment, and (d) loss of a loved or valued person.

ASPECT OF THE SELF   The loss of an aspect of the self changes a person's body image, even though the loss may not be obvious to others. A face scarred from a burn is generally obvious to people; loss of part of the stomach or loss of ability to feel emotion may not be as obvious. The degree to which these losses affect a person largely depends on the integrity of the person's body image (part of self-concept). Any change that the person perceives as negative in the way he or she relates to the environment can be considered a loss of self. It should be noted that *self* is a culturally influenced concept; therefore, experiences of self-loss are particular to individuals and their particular cultural and personal influences.

Such losses as divorce can have a considerable impact. A divorce may mean loss of financial security, a home, daily routines, and a role as spouse. Therefore, even when the divorce was desired, the sense of loss can be substantial.

During old age, changes can occur in physical and mental capabilities. Again the self-image is vulnerable. Old age is the time when people usually experience many losses: of employment, of usual activities, of independence, of health, of friends, and of family.

EXTERNAL OBJECTS   Loss of external objects includes (a) loss of inanimate objects that have importance to the person, such as the loss of money or the burning down of a family's house, and (b) loss of animate objects, such as pets that provide love and companionship.

FAMILIAR ENVIRONMENT   Separation from an environment and people who provide security can result in a sense of loss. The 6-year-old is likely to feel loss when first leaving the usual environment to attend school. The university student who moves away from home for the first time also experiences a sense of loss.

LOVED ONES   The loss of a loved one or valued person through illness, separation, or death can, among other experiences, create suffering. In some illnesses, a person may undergo personality changes that make friends and family feel they have lost that person.

Significant current research on grief indicates that the death of a loved one initiates a change in family relationships that constantly changes and evolves over time to bring new meanings to family members left behind (Moules, Simonson, Prins, Angus, & Bell, 2004). Making room for grief and death is not a popular concept (Moules et al., 2004). In past societies, death was considered a normal, natural event, and life was seldom long. In contemporary North American society, death is often denied. People may be uncomfortable talking about death and being around people who are dying. Sometimes, in an effort to escape the finality of death, people resort to extraordinary measures to prolong and preserve life.

Historical and Shifting Ways of Conceptualizing Grief

It is generally agreed that there are no single "correct" or "true" theories that explain the experience of **grief**. Individuals vary markedly in the type of grief they experience, its intensity, its duration and the way they express, live, and accept the reality of loss. From a historical lens, grief has been explained in many of the early theorists' works as a process involving progression through a series of stages or phases requiring work or particular tasks that result in a final resolution of grief feelings. Out of this explanation, stage model theories, some of which are based on Kubler-Ross's (1969) work on death and dying, have provided one template for understanding the experience of grief. One criticism of stage model theories is that although they may provide some understanding, recognition, and language for the experience of grief, they may also serve to obscure unique and individual experiences of grief (Moules, 1998; Moules, Simonson, Fleiszer, Prins, & Glasgow, 2007; Moules et al., 2004). They can narrowly focus on psychological responses while overlooking social, spiritual, familial, and physical domains of the experience of grief. To understand grief as a staged experience can mistakenly invite the belief that grief occurs passively in expected sequences that disregard individual experiences and that fail to resonate with the experiences people actually undergo in grieving.

Martocchio (1985) discussed five clusters of grief, which exemplify common experiences in the grief response. These include (a) shock and disbelief; (b) yearning and protest; (c) anguish, disorganization, and despair; (d) identification in bereavement; and (e) reorganization and restitution. This way of seeing grief boxes people in to a single correct way or timetable. Grief that does not follow a predictable or an expected course is often described as abnormal, complicated, pathological, unresolved, chronic, morbid, prolonged, dysfunctional, exaggerated, or disenfranchised. This pathologizing view of any divergence of expected and typical responses to loss can serve to intensify the suffering of grief, and add, in addition to the experience of loss, a sense of personal failure and incompetence (Moules, 1998; Moules et al., 2004; Moules et al., 2007).

Furthermore, socially sanctioned notions about grief invite the idea that the work of grief resolution is to find a way to let go of the person who is lost and to say goodbye. Alternatively, White (1989) and Moules (1998; Moules et al., 2004; Moules et al., 2007) suggested that when people lose a loved one, they continue to feel in relationship to the person, and although the relationship is necessarily changed and altered through physical absence, it continues in their emotional and spiritual life. Grief then becomes the process of learning how to live with this new and changed relationship in such a way that it offers aspects of connection and comfort, rather than pain and suffering. In describing grief, Moules has used the metaphor of an unwanted visitor that arrives within the context of the experience of loss. It sweeps into every domain of a person's life: biological, psychological, social, emotional, and spiritual. Grief endures in a way that shifts over time, eventually creating a mutable or changing and evolving but, most often, a lifetime relationship with the loss. Unwanted or not, this visitor, grief, takes up residence in lives. Moules offers that nurses have an opportunity in therapeutic listening and being with individuals to open space other than suffering and in inviting them to remember their lost other and say hello to a new and changed relationship (Moules, 1998; Moules et al., 2004; Moules et al., 2007).

Grief, however, is not without its complications. Researchers have identified the diagnostic criteria for complicated grief disorder (Horowitz, Siegel, Holen, Bonanno, Milbrath, & Stinson, 1997). These criteria include "the current experience (>1 year after a loss) of intensive intrusive thoughts, pangs of severe emotion, distressing yearnings, feeling excessively alone and empty, excessively avoiding tasks reminiscent of the deceased, unusual sleep disturbances, and maladaptive levels of loss of interest in personal activities" (p. 904). Other researchers have underscored the need for specification of complicated grief as a unique disorder and have developed *The Inventory of Complicated Grief,* to measure maladaptive symptoms of loss (Prigerson, Maciejewski, & Reynolds, 1995). This inventory has been said to be helpful to practitioners because it has been useful in differentiating between depression and complicated grief. Finally, it is the severity of symptomatology and the duration of the severe symptoms that distinguishes complicated from normal grief.

Factors Influencing Loss and Grief

A number of factors affect a person's response to a loss or death. These factors include age, significance of the loss, culture, spiritual beliefs, gender, socioeconomic status, support systems, and the cause of the loss or death. Nurses can learn general concepts about the influence of these factors on the grieving experience, but the constellation of these factors and their significance will vary from individual to individual.

AGE Age affects a person's understanding of and reaction to loss. With experience, people usually increase their understanding and acceptance of life, loss, and death.

People do not usually experience the loss of loved ones at regular intervals. As a result, preparation for these experiences is difficult. Coping with other losses in life, such as the loss of a pet, the loss of a friend, the loss of a job, and the loss of youth, can prepare people for the more severe loss of death.

Childhood Children differ from adults not only in their understanding of loss and death but also in how they are affected by the loss of others. The child's patterns progress rapidly; adult patterns of growth and development are generally stable. The loss of a parent or other significant person can threaten the child's ability to develop, and regression sometimes results. Assisting the child with the grief experience includes helping the child regain the normal continuity and pace of emotional development.

The hesitancy of children to exhibit their own sadness so as not to upset their parents requires that professionals encourage parents to give their children permission to be sad when that is how they feel. By taking care of their parents, children may not receive the attention they require. Careful work with bereaved children is especially necessary because experiencing a loss in childhood can have serious effects later in life.

Early and Middle Adulthood As people grow, they come to experience loss as part of normal development. By middle age, for example, the loss of a parent through death seems a normal occurrence compared with the death of a younger person. Coping with the death of an aged parent has even been viewed as a necessary developmental task of the middle-aged adult.

The middle-aged adult can experience losses other than death. For example, losses resulting from impaired health or body function and losses of various role functions can be difficult for the middle-aged adult. How the middle-aged adult responds to such losses is influenced by previous experiences with loss, the person's sense of self-esteem, and the strength and availability of support.

Late Adulthood Losses experienced by older adults include loss of health, loss of mobility, loss of independence, and loss of work role. Limited income and the need to change living accommodations can also lead to feelings of loss and grieving.

For older adults, the loss through death of a longtime mate is profound. Although individuals differ in their ability to deal with such a loss, research originally suggested that health problems for widows and widowers increase during the first year following the death of the spouse (Richter, 1984). It has recently been suggested that psychological reactions to loss may reflect a broader array of cultural contexts. Other cultural factors including patterns of household structure and filial piety, and attitudes toward life and death, may condition the experience of older bereaved persons (Carr, 2008). However, because the majority of deaths occur among older adults and because the number of older people is increasing in North America, nurses will need to be especially alert to the potential problems of older adults who are grieving.

SIGNIFICANCE OF THE LOSS The significance of a loss depends on the perceptions of the individual experiencing the loss. One person may experience a great sense of loss over a divorce; another may find it only mildly disrupting. A number of factors affect the significance of the loss:

- The value placed on the lost person, object, or function
- The degree of change required because of the loss
- The person's beliefs and values

For older people who have already encountered many losses, an anticipated loss, such as their own death, may not be viewed as a highly negative loss, and they may be apathetic about it instead of reactive. More than fearing death, some may fear loss of control or becoming a burden.

CULTURE Culture influences an individual's reaction to loss. How grief is expressed is often determined by the customs of the culture. In the United States and Canada, unless an extended family structure exists, grief is handled by the nuclear family. The death of a family member in a typical nuclear North American family leaves a great void because the same few individuals fill most of the roles. In cultures in which several generations and extended family members either reside in the same household or are physically close, the impact of a family member's death may be softened because the roles of the deceased are quickly filled by other relatives.

Many North Americans appear to have adopted the belief that grief is a private matter to be endured internally. Therefore, feelings tend to be repressed and may remain unidentified. People who have been socialized to "be strong" and "make the best of the situation" may not express deep feelings or personal concerns when they experience a serious loss.

Some cultural groups value social support and the expression of loss. In some groups, the expression of grief through wailing, crying, physical prostration, and other outward demonstrations are acceptable and encouraged. Other groups may frown on demonstration as a loss of control, favouring a quieter and more stoic expression of grief. In cultural groups in which strong kinship ties are maintained, physical and emotional support and assistance are provided by family members.

SPIRITUAL BELIEFS Spiritual beliefs and practices greatly influence both a person's reaction to loss, the way they make sense of their lives, and a person's subsequent meaning and behaviour. When this meaning extends beyond a materialistic account and includes a transcendent reality (God), then we are dealing with faith or religion. Most religious groups have practices related to dying, and these are often important to the client and support people. For additional information, see Chapter 47. To provide support at a time of death, nurses need to understand the client's particular beliefs and practices. A part of a person's spirituality is represented in, and influences, the way that person makes meaning of the experience of loss. Asking questions of a spiritual nature is within the domain of nursing practice (Moules, 1999; Wright, 1999, 2008).

GENDER Men and women do grieve differently, however the context, age, social class, generation and culture all impact their response (Martin & Dolka, 2000). For example, widows are more likely to seek emotional support from others; widowers more often turn to work, religion, creative expression, or alcohol. Differences between genders narrow as people age, perhaps because they become more androgynous in coping. Research results are inconclusive. Results from some studies have shown men to have better outcomes, others have shown women to do better, and still others show no significant difference or mixed results (Martin & Dolka, 2000).

SOCIOECONOMIC STATUS The socioeconomic status of an individual often affects the support system available at the time of a loss. Financial concerns resulting from the need to decrease work hours or quit their jobs because of caregiving responsibilities have been shown to increase stress levels in families who care for their loved ones (Ferrario, Cardillo, & Vicario, 2004). In Canada,

only 35% of households with caregivers report income over $45 000. Twenty-five percent of caregivers report their employment situation has been affected because of their caregiving responsibilities. Caregivers can be young or old, but most are women (77%). Family caregivers are often forced to give up their paid work. While often unavoidable, this sacrifice represents more than a loss of wages. It has long-term effects, such as reducing eligibility for the Canada Pension Plan (CPP) and other retirement pension plans (Senate of Canada, 2010).

SUPPORT SYSTEMS The people closest to the grieving individual are often the first to recognize and provide needed emotional, physical, and functional assistance. However, because many people are uncomfortable or inexperienced in dealing with losses, the usual support people may instead withdraw from the grieving individual. Also, support may be available when the loss is first recognized, but as the support people return to their usual activities, the need for ongoing support may be unmet. Sometimes, the grieving individual is unable or unready to accept support when it is offered.

CAUSE OF LOSS OR DEATH Individual and societal views on the cause of a loss or death can significantly influence the grief response. Some diseases are considered clean, such as cardiovascular disorders, and engender compassion; others may be viewed as repulsive and less unfortunate. A loss or death that is beyond the control of those involved may be more acceptable than one that is preventable, such as a drunk driving accident. Injuries or deaths occurring during respected activities, such as in the line of duty, are considered honourable, whereas those occurring during illicit activities may be considered the individual's just rewards.

Assessing

Nursing assessment of the client and family experiencing a loss includes three major components: (a) nursing history, (b) assessment of personal coping resources, and (c) physical assessment. During the routine health assessment of every client, the nurse poses questions regarding previous and current losses. The nature of the loss and the meaning of such losses to the client must be explored.

If the client has experienced a current or recent loss, greater detail is needed in the assessment. Because clients do not always associate physical ailments with emotional responses, such as grief, the nurse may need to probe to identify possible loss-related stresses. If the client reports significant losses, it is important to examine how the client usually copes with loss and what resources are available to assist the client in coping. Data regarding general health status; other personal stressors; cultural and spiritual traditions, rituals, and beliefs related to loss and grieving; and the person's support network will be needed in order to determine a plan of care (see the Assessment: Interview box on the next page).

ASSESSMENT	INTERVIEW

Loss and Grieving

The following questions can help the nurse determine a client's ability to cope with loss:

PREVIOUS LOSSES

- Have you ever lost someone or something very important to you?
- Have you or your family ever moved your home?
- What was it like for you when you first started school? moved away from home? got a job? retired?
- Are you physically able to do all the things you like to do? used to do?
- Has anyone important or close to you died?
- Do you think there will be any losses in your life in the near future?

PREVIOUS GRIEVING

- Tell me about (the loss). What was losing _____ like for you?
- Did you have trouble sleeping? eating? concentrating?
- What kinds of things did you do to make yourself feel better when something like that happened?
- Are there spiritual or cultural practices you observed when you had a loss like that?
- Whom did you turn to if you were very upset about (the loss)?
- How long did it take you to feel more like yourself again and go back to your usual activities?

CURRENT LOSS

- What have you been told about (the loss)? Is there anything else you would like to know or do not understand?
- What changes do you think this (illness, surgery, problem) will cause in your life? What do you think it will be like without (the lost object)?
- Have you ever experienced a loss like this before?
- Can you think of anything good that might come out of this?
- What kind of help do you think you will need? Who is going to be helping you with this loss?
- Are there any people or organizations in your community that might be able to help?

CURRENT GRIEVING

- Are you having trouble sleeping? eating? concentrating? breathing?
- Do you have any pain or other new physical problems?
- Are you taking any drugs or medications to help you cope with this loss?
- What are you doing to help you deal with this loss?

In assessing the client's response to a current loss, the nurse may identify complications of grief that may be best treated by a health care professional who is expert in assisting such clients. If the nursing assessment reveals severe physical or psychological signs and symptoms, the client should be referred to an appropriate care provider. Such complications include clinical depression, extensive social isolation and withdrawal, severe physiological symptoms, suicidal thoughts or urges, or unrelenting and oppressive sorrow that persists for prolonged periods and is not balanced by any relief or joy-filled experiences.

Implementing

The skills most relevant to situations of loss and grief are attentive listening, silence, open and closed questioning, paraphrasing, clarifying and reflecting feelings, and summarizing. Less helpful to clients are responses that give advice and evaluation, those that interpret and analyze, and those that give unwarranted reassurance. The offering of platitudes is often a temptation to those trying to comfort someone who is suffering a loss. Though well intended and often arising out of a loss for words, such platitudes as "It must have happened for a reason; you need to accept it," "Time heals all wounds," "Try not to think about it," "You'll get over it in time," or "Now you've got a little angel in heaven" serve only to contribute to

messages that a visible grief is unhealthy and that grief is time limited (Moules & Amundson, 1997). These messages deny the right and need of the bereaved to fully experience, acknowledge, and express grief as a part of incorporating loss into their lives. What the nurse says or does is always best guided by the client and in response to the client's needs. Sometimes, a simple statement of "I am sorry for your loss," or a silent presence is what is most needed. To ensure effective communication, the nurse must make an accurate assessment of what is appropriate for the client.

Communication with grieving clients needs to be relevant to meeting clients at the point of *their* needs, not the nurse's needs. To determine the point of a client's need, the nurse has to be willing to listen to the client's pain and suffering and not be tempted to try to take the pain away or heal it, even if such a thing were possible.

In addition to effective communication skills, a nurse can support and care in specific ways for a client experiencing loss. Of these, probably the most important is that the nurse "make room for grief" (Moules, 1998, p. 100). This means that the nurse accepts, facilitates, and normalizes the experience and expression of grief, which can be done through actions and attitudes:

- Be present, be comfortable with silence, and offer touch if the person indicates that would be comforting.

- Acknowledge pain and suffering.
- Encourage talk about the loss and the loved one, but accept it if clients cannot or do not want to do so.
- Explore and respect clients' racial, cultural, religious, personal, and family values in their expression of grief.
- Explore their support system and personal resources. Who is available to be with them? Who would be most helpful right now? Who can help them take care of practical arrangements and details?
- Assist clients and families in understanding that grief is expressed differently by different people and individuals cannot be expected to adhere to others' expectations of appropriate responses to grief.
- If children are involved, encourage family members to be truthful and to allow the children to participate in the grieving activities of others.
- Though maybe not at the time of the immediate loss, support clients in exploring the meaning they have made of their loss, how they have come to understand it or live with it, and how they have come to make room for a relationship with grief in their lives.
- Provide resource and support information, such as local grief support groups or counselling.

Dying and Death

The concept of death is developed over time, as the person grows, experiences various losses, and reflects on concrete and abstract concepts. In general, humans move from a childhood belief in death as a temporary state, to adulthood in which death is accepted as very real but also very frightening, and to older adulthood in which death may be viewed as more desirable than living with a poor quality of life. Table 49.1 describes some of the specific beliefs common to different age groups. The nurse's knowledge of these developmental stages helps in understanding some of the client's responses to a life-threatening situation.

End-of-Life Care for Older Adults

Canada's population is aging. As a result, the Canadian Hospice Palliative Care Association (CHPCA) estimates that the next 40 years demand for hospice palliative care services will continue to increase (CHPCA, 2010). By 2031 the number of older adults will account for between 6.1% and 6.5% of the total population (Statistics Canada, 2010). In 2004, Statistics Canada projected that the rate of deaths in Canada will increase by 33% by the year 2020 to more than 330 000 deaths per year.

Older adults may have comorbid medical conditions that contribute an added symptom burden to the

TABLE 49.1 Development of the Concept of Death

Age	Beliefs and Attitudes
Infancy to 5 years	Does not understand concept of death Infant's sense of separation forms basis for later understanding of loss and death Believes death is reversible, a temporary departure, or sleep Emphasizes immobility and inactivity as attributes of death
5 to 9 years	Understands that death is final Believes own death can be avoided Associates death with aggression or violence Believes wishes or unrelated actions can be responsible for death
9 to 12 years	Understands death as the inevitable end of life Begins to understand own mortality, expressed as interest in afterlife or as fear of death
12 to 18 years	Fears a lingering death May fantasize that death can be defied, acting out defiance through reckless behaviours (e.g., dangerous driving, problematic substance use) Seldom thinks about death, but views it in religious and philosophic terms May seem to reach adult perception of death but be emotionally unable to accept it May still hold concepts from previous developmental stages
18 to 45 years	Has attitude toward death influenced by religious and cultural beliefs
45 to 65 years	Accepts own mortality Encounters death of parents and some peers Experiences peaks of death anxiety Death anxiety diminishes with emotional well-being
65+ years	Fears prolonged illness Encounters death of family members and peers Sees death as having multiple meanings (e.g., freedom from pain, reunion with already deceased family members)

palliative care population. The presence of chronic medical conditions is associated with disability and increased health care use, including institutionalization and hospitalization. Given the multisystemic nature of illness at the end of life, the pattern of symptoms is usually diverse and can include pain as well as dyspnea, dysphagia, edema,

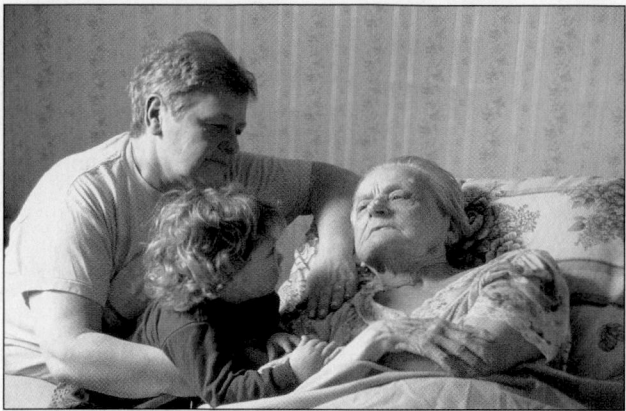

FIGURE 49.1 Family members may be closely involved in both physical and psychological support of the dying.

shortness of breath, and delirium. These will be discussed later in the chapter. Furthermore, the presence of existing comorbidities and disabilities renders older adults more susceptible to the complications of new illnesses and their treatments. The trajectory of death in older adults is also less predictable, encompassing many acute episodic illnesses that eventually result in a slow decline of functional and cognitive abilities.

Typically, family members meet care needs of older individuals and, more often than not, these individuals are women (see Figure 49.1). Caregiver burden is well documented in the literature and includes a great number of depressive symptoms, anxiety, diminished physical health, financial problems, and disruption from work (Stajduhar, Martin, & Cairns, 2010). Older adult patients requiring symptom care are more likely than younger patients to have an increased dependence on others for basic activities of daily living, such as bathing, meal preparation, eating, and ambulating. If the patient is confused or agitated, the burden is even greater, often requiring 24-hour care. For older adults with chronic illnesses, the duration of caregiving can be several years. When people have no family caregivers, or care needs become too great (as with Alzheimer's disease), patients are often placed in a long-term care facility. Seventy percent of deaths today still take place in hospitals and long-term care facilities (Statistics Canada, 2010).

Responses to Dying and Death

Understanding responses to death and dying begins with the recognition that dying individuals exist within a family system. The nurse considers the impact of the dying individual's illness on the whole family and the family's responses that affect the patient. Caring for the dying individual's family involves understanding family in the broadest sense. The family is a group of individuals who are inextricably linked in ways that are constantly interactive and mutually reinforcing. Family may include direct blood relatives, relationships through an emotional commitment, or the group or person unrelated by blood or marriage may function as family.

Both the client who is dying and the family members grieve as they recognize the loss. The literature on family factors thought to influence end-of-life decision making, including ways in which the acuity of onset or phase of the illness can intersect with family adaptation is emerging (Rolland, 2003, 2004). As well, families are thought to move into and out of periods of relative closeness versus distance based on their characteristic style of adaptation and the phase of illness (Winchester Nadeau, 2008). Clinical literature (King, Shields, & Wynne, 2005; Qualls, 2000; Walsh & McGoldrick, 2004) and research (Kissane, Bloch, Onghena, McKenzie, Synde, & Dowe, 1996; Kissane, 2003; Weihs & Reiss, 1996) suggest that families have different levels of relational ability based on their history of shared experiences, as well as the strengths and vulnerabilities of individual family members.

Nurses and other health care professionals must strive to understand the meaning of the grief experience to the dying individual and the family. Grieving can include feelings of fear, inability to focus, hopelessness without a sense of moving beyond the death, powerlessness, losing control over emotions, and despair and depression. People may also have many physical symptoms, including increased pulse and respirations, dry mouth, anorexia, difficulty sleeping, and nightmares. If meaningful care is to be provided to the dying individuals and their families, the nurse must understand their beliefs and values related to the experience, how the relationships fit together, and the many factors that affect the experience of dying and illness. See the Evidence-Informed Practice box on what makes grief difficult for families and health care professionals.

Caregivers, both professionals and support people, also are affected by the impending death. The ongoing responsibilities for providing physical, ethical, and emotional support to a dying person can create extreme stress for all providers in whatever setting care is provided (Simon, Ramsenthaler, Bausewein, Krischke, & Geiss, 2009). Often, the length of time between a terminal diagnosis and when death will occur is unknown and the people supporting the dying person become fatigued and depressed and feel empty. They may feel anger because of lost time and resources for personal activities or attention for other people. The impending death can pose a challenge to family roles and day-to-day functioning. In this situation, the family may be unable to meet the physical, emotional, or spiritual needs of the members and may have difficulty communicating and problem solving.

Nurses who have developed a close relationship with the dying individual and family may themselves experience a sense of loss and suffer with them as they care for them in the journey of dying (Raffin, 2002; Raffin Bouchal, 2007). Nurses who spend many hours, even days, with the dying individual and family "do not simply

EVIDENCE-INFORMED PRACTICE

What Makes Grief Difficult for Families and Health Care Professionals?

Family members who assume care giving roles for their loved one who is dying start the bereavement process having experienced taxing emotional and physical ups and downs throughout the illness journey. The bereavement experience is impacted by a number of factors, including health problems, financial concerns, social support, and family relationships. Stajduhar, Martin, and Cairns (2010) reported on findings from a secondary analysis of qualitative data from a study examining the experiences of family caregiver coping in end-of-life care for patients with cancer, to describe, from the perspectives of bereaved family caregivers, their perspectives on what made their grief difficult. Three focus groups with family caregivers ($n = 19$) and two focus groups with health care professionals ($n = 14$) were analyzed using interpretive analysis. The findings of this study suggest three broad areas that make family caregivers' grief difficult: (a) dealing with occurrences in everyday life (dual care giving responsibilities, relationships with others, being employed); (b) dealing with challenges specific to the care giving situation (missing the death, health problems, decision making responsibilities); and (c) dealing with the health care system (lack of knowledge about the patient's health status, timely access to information, provision of services).

NURSING IMPLICATIONS: The findings provide an important beginning point in understanding the types of issues that seem to make grief difficult for family caregivers of patients with cancer at the end of life and can help nurses and other health care professionals to understand what is needed by family caregivers in terms of support and delivery of services. The following are a few selected examples. This study suggests that missing the death of their relative results in considerable feelings of guilt that influence caregiver's grief in a negative way. Although this is not important for all family caregivers, many reported intense guilt feelings. Given the potential impact, nurses should discuss this with family and make an effort to ensure that family members who desire to be present are able to. This study and other research has shown family members who have roles outside of caregiving, such as being a parent or being employed, have little time to focus on their own health and well-being. Thus, dual care giving makes grief difficult and nurses should raise awareness within the health care team and advocate for additional support for these families in order to prevent possible complications in bereavement.

Sources: Based on Stajduhar, K., Martin, W., & Cairns, M. (2010). What makes grief difficult? Perspectives from bereaved family caregivers and healthcare providers of advanced cancer patients. *Palliative and Supportive Care, 8,* 277–289. doi: 10.1017/S14789551510000076

care for the dying individual's physical bodies, they also tend to their spirit, gently, respectfully, and knowingly" (Moules, 2000, p. 4). The very nature of palliative care nursing is such that, every day, practitioners face some of the most fundamental and poignant issues confronting humanity (Perry, 2008). Nurses are invited to share in the intimate journey of living and dying where suffering is present. This sharing often entails a commitment of developing a meaningful relationship as a way to know and understand the dying experience. The relationship, although rewarding, often places the nurse in a vulnerable position. Nurses are affected by this position (Raffin, 2002; Raffin Bouchal, 2007).

Caring for the dying and the bereaved is one of the nurse's most complex and challenging responsibilities, bringing into play all the skills needed for care of the whole person—mind, body, and spirit. To care for the whole person, nurses must be aware of and comfortable with their own values and beliefs about death, dying, and suffering, as these will surely affect the care they are able to give others.

Legal and Moral Issues Related to End-of-Life Care

Many legal issues surround the event of death, including a legal definition as to when a person is considered clinically dead. Few jurisdictions in Canada provide a legislative definition of the moment of death. Physicians, until well into the twentieth century, concurred that a person was dead when all vital signs (pulse, respiration) had ceased. Since the last half of the twentieth century, medical technology has allowed physicians to sustain the lives of seriously ill individuals by means of artificial support that maintains blood circulation. As well, the advances of medical transplant technology have made possible transplantation of viable organs from deceased individuals to living recipients.

It has become apparent that the traditional medical criteria for determining the fact of death have become inadequate. In 1975, Manitoba became the first (and, so far, the only) province to enact a legal definition of death. The Manitoba Vital Statistics Act suggests that "the death of a person takes place at the time at which irreversible cessation of all that person's brain function occurs" (cited by Lazar, Shemie, Webster, & Dickens, 2001, p. 834). This definition conforms to the accepted medical practice. With this definition, the client still may be able to breathe but is irreversibly unconscious. People who support this definition of death believe that the cerebral cortex—which holds the capacity for thought, voluntary action, and movement—*is* the individual.

ADVANCE CARE PLANNING AND ADVANCE DIRECTIVES (LIVING WILLS) Individuals receiving health care sometimes worry that if they become incapacitated and unable to express their wishes, they will be hooked up to machines and receive treatment that they do not want. The Terry Schiavo case in the United States uncovered the complexity and possible issues people may face at the end of life. Advance directives have been suggested as one way to address this problem. The Canadian Nurses Association (CNA, 1998) and other sponsors produced a joint statement on advance directives for nurses' use in practice. **Advance directives** are "the means used to document and communicate a person's preferences regarding life-sustaining treatment in the event that they become incapable of expressing those wishes for themselves" (CNA, 1998, p. 1). Advance directives are commonly expressed in two ways: (a) an instruction directive, or **living will**, which identifies what life-sustaining treatment a person wants in certain situations; or (b) a **proxy directive**, which explains who is to make health care decisions if the person becomes incompetent. A proxy directive is often referred to as a power of attorney for personal care (CNA, 1998). The CNA encourages nurses and other health care professionals to communicate with clients regarding their health care and treatment to ensure that clients have informed choices and identify how clients want end-of-life issues to be addressed (CNA, 2008). Making and documenting decisions about future treatment options, including cardiopulmonary resuscitation (CPR), is often referred to as *Advance Care Planning* (CNA, 2008) Nurses' roles in advance care planning include encouraging clients to discuss and document their wishes should they become incapable with their family.

The legal right of each individual to decide future health care has been recognized by Canadian courts for some time and is also reflected in the Canadian Constitution. If the construction and the execution of the directive complies with the legal requirements set out by the province or territory in the individual's jurisdiction, then it will be legally binding (Tapp, 2006). It is necessary for nurses to be aware of the legal status of all types of advance directives in their province or territory. As outlined by the CNA (2008), some provinces and territories recognize only proxy directives as legally binding, whereas others recognize both proxy and instructional directives (Tapp, 2006). In addition, nurses need to become familiar with laws and documents regarding a person's competence to consent, issues regarding CPR, and issues at the end of life, as these are closely related to advance directives (Figure 49.2).

Health care professionals, including nurses, are responsible for ensuring that advance directives are addressed, not only as an admission duty but also as a part of the ongoing communication among all members providing and receiving care. A significant part of this process is to discuss and obtain a statement of the individual's personal values. This inquiry highlights the person's value system and beliefs about health, well-being, choice, and dignity. Identification of the person's values will enable the nurse to approach the client's hospital experience in a more holistic manner.

ARTIFICIAL NUTRITION AND HYDRATION Artificial nutrition and hydration (ANH) (non-oral means of administering nutrition to a patient) are common but controversial issues at the end of life. Although regularly used in certain populations, strong scientific evidence regarding the benefits of these therapies is lacking, making care decisions even more complex. Provision of food and fluids is a fundamental caregiving activity; issues arise when patients with progressive, life-limiting illness refuse or cannot take oral nourishment and fluids. Deciding whether or not to initiate ANH is an important conversation to have with patients and their families.

Artificial nutrition is an emotionally charged issue for many caregivers. Maintaining nutrition is a natural life-sustaining measure and a common part of the nursing role. Families often believe that their loved ones will suffer without nutrition. It is important for nurses and other health care professionals to help family members understand that loss of appetite is an integral part of the dying process. Studies of terminally ill cognitively intact patients with anorexia have shown that they do not suffer hunger and that symptoms of thirst can be relieved with good oral hygiene, artificial saliva, and sips of water (Heuberger, 2010).

Current literature suggests fluids should not be routinely administered to dying individuals or automatically withheld from them, but rather given based on the goals of care and a careful assessment of the client's comfort. A position statement by the CNA (2008) on end-of-life care stresses the importance of the health care team working together to determine whether food and fluid are beneficial or harmful to a client. The following questions may help health care professionals in thinking about the goals of care (Bennett Jacobs & Taylor, 2005; Ganzini, 2006): Will the client's well-being be enhanced by artificial nutrition? Are there symptoms that could be relieved or aggravated? Could hydration enhance the client's mental status or level of consciousness? Will it temporarily prolong the client's life? Is that what the client and family want? When food and hydration are administered for a prolonged period to a client who is not expected to improve, some nurses will view this care as extraordinary or heroic, whereas others will see it as humane. It is important to stress to families that dying individuals who are not receiving artificial nutrition or hydration will still be provided with adequate care.

EUTHANASIA The act of **euthanasia** can mean different things to different people. The word *euthanasia* comes from Greek words meaning "good death." The term is often used synonymously with the term **mercy killing**, a concept that has drawn much controversy over the years. The most widely accepted definition of euthanasia in Western health care is considered "deliberate, rapid, and painless termination of a life of a person afflicted with incurable and progressive disease" (Roy, Williams, & Dickens, 1994, p. 411). Euthanasia has two forms: *active* and *passive*. These terms are meant to convey the difference between committing an act that causes death and omitting to take a life-sustaining act, allowing death to ensue.

Sample Directive: Stating Instructions

Personal Directive

I, _____, of _____, Alberta, do hereby
declare that if I am unable to participate in decisions about my own future care, this Directive
should be interpreted as a carefully considered expression of my wishes and directions.

If at such a time the situation arises in which there is no reasonable expectation of my
recovery from severe physical or mental disability to a state of meaningful interaction with
loved ones, family or friends, I direct that I be allowed to die and note be kept alive by
medications or artificial means. In particular, I would like the following directions to be followed:

1.   Measures of artificial life-support, in the above stated situation, that I refuse are:

      o Cardiopulmonary resuscitation and admittance into an intensive care unit.
      o Mechanical respiration when I cannot breathe by myself.
      o Prolonged gastric tube or intravenous feeding when I am indefinitely unable to eat
         through my mouth.
      o Antibiotic medication to treat or prevent infection.
      o Other: _____

2.   I request to live my last days at home rather than a hospital, if my family agrees.

3.   If any of my tissues or organs are healthy and useful for other people I give permission for
      all such donation, or as specified, *during* my *life*:

      _____

      _____

4.   I do wish to have medication mercifully administered to me in order to avoid suffering even
      though this may shorten my remaining life.

Dated at _____ in the Province of Alberta, this _____ day of

_____, 20_____.

_____   _____

        Witness Signature   Maker's Signature

*The appearance of this sample personal directive does not imply endorsement by the
Provincial Health Ethics Network; it is provided for information purpose only. PHEN assumes
no liability for any loss or damage suffered by any person by reason of their reliance on the
information contained herein.*

FIGURE 49.2 Sample advance directive appointing an agent and stating instructions.

Source: Provincial Health Ethics Network. (2010). *Sample directive: Stating instructions*. Alberta: Author. Retrieved from
http://www.phen.ab.ca/perdir/sample-instruct.asp

The issue is an ethical one that remains unsettled. It revolves around two fundamental beliefs: the right of the individual to decide his or her own time and means of dying, and the equally strong argument that all measures must be tried before death is accepted. Often, it becomes a matter of to treat or not to treat.

Euthanasia and physician-assisted suicide are illegal in Canada. The Criminal Code of Canada prohibits culpable homicide (sections 222 and 229), which includes helping to end another's life through voluntary euthanasia, and makes counselling a person to commit suicide or aiding a suicide punishable offences (section 241). Section 14 of the Code makes it clear that having the consent of the person does not alter the criminal nature of the act. Although there has been significant debate about voluntary euthanasia and assisted suicide (physician or other) over the past few years, there has been no change in the law.

The withholding or withdrawing of treatments and the provision of compassionate palliative care, even when life is shortened, is considered to be good and ethical medical practice (Lowy, Sawyer, & Williams, 1993). A discussion between the physician and family members to determine when treatment should be stopped or withdrawn is ethical and common practice. Patients and family members may request that a dying individual not be subjected to resuscitative measures in the event of death, in which case the physician should write "do-not-resuscitate (DNR) order" in the patient's chart.

Individuals who argue against euthanasia base their reasoning on the principle of the sanctity of life and on the traditional rules and laws prohibiting the taking of life except in situations of self-defence or war. Many are also concerned about the potential for abuse if euthanasia were to become legal. They see a law like this slipping (the slippery slope argument) to extend to such others as the chronically ill, the very old, and the person with dementia.

Those individuals who support euthanasia believe that in some situations, life is not worth living. They believe that competent individuals should be given the right to end their life when it is burdened with physical, emotional, and psychological pain that it is no longer possible to eliminate. These individuals believe that sanctity of life is not an absolute principle and can be overridden out of respect for individual autonomy and for the dignity of human life.

DO NOT RESUSCITATE ORDERS Cardiopulmonary resuscitation (CPR) has become a standard intervention because of its potential benefits if implemented immediately. This standard, coupled with the lack of advance care planning, creates the routine use of CPR (Gilbert, Counsell, & Guin, 2001; Golin, Wegner, & Liu, 2000). The question of whether this intervention should be used for all patients at all times has been the topic of several research studies. The results indicate that CPR can do harm to certain patients (those of advanced age and with comorbidities), bringing about a lesser quality of life (Brindley, Markland, Mayers, & Kutsogiannis, 2002; Robinson, 2002). Inappropriate use of CPR and inappropriate prolongation of life in general are among the most troubling issues for registered nurses (Storch, 2006). Nurses and others involved in resuscitative interventions with little perceived benefit may experience moral distress. Nurses and physicians in direct care roles often perform CPR on patients who might not have had the opportunity to articulate a preference for or against it. Alternatively, many times, the patient's age, history, and even personal directives are ignored to accommodate our "never give up attitude" (Lazaruk, 2006, p. 22).

When a client or surrogate has requested no CPR in the event of a respiratory or cardiac arrest, or if no medical benefit is apparent, a do not resuscitate (DNR) order can be written. Health care institutions commonly have a policy for obtaining a DNR order. Approaching treatment decisions in palliative care, especially DNR orders, can be particularly troublesome for the team if advance directives are not available or are not followed. An ethical approach includes clarifying patient and family goals of care, balancing the potential burden and benefit of the proposed treatment, and, to some extent, considering the availability of resources for providing treatment. Health care professionals need to consider the following question in their deliberations: Should resuscitation be presented as a treatment option when it almost certainly will not be successful? Advance care planning provides an opportunity for thoughtful consideration of CPR as an intervention.

The CNA (1995) issued a joint policy statement to provide guidance for developing policies on the appropriate use of CPR. The following principles are integral to the development of the CPR policy (pp. 2–3):

1. *Good health care requires open communication, discussion and sensitivity to cultural and religious differences among caregivers, potential recipients of care, their family members and significant others.*

2. *A person must be given sufficient information about the benefits, risks and likely outcomes of all treatment options to enable him or her to make informed decisions.*

3. *A competent person has the right to refuse, or withdraw consent to, any clinically indicated treatment, including life-saving or life-sustaining treatment. Competence can be difficult to assess because it is not always a constant state. A person may be competent to make decisions regarding some aspects of life but not others; as well, competence can be intermittent—a person may be lucid and oriented at certain times of the day and not at others. The legal definition and assessment of competence are governed by the provinces or territories. Facilities should be aware of the laws (e.g., capacity to consent and age of consent) regarding the assessment and documentation of incompetence.*

4. *When a person is incompetent, treatment decisions must be based on his or her wishes, if these are known. The person's decision may be found in an advance directive or may have been communicated to the physician, other members of the health care team or other relevant people. In some jurisdictions, legislation specifically addresses the issue of decision-making concerning medical treatment for incompetent people; the legislative requirements should be followed.*

5. *When an incompetent person's wishes are not known, treatment decisions must be based on the person's best interests, taking into account:*
   i *the person's known values and preferences;*
   ii *information received from those who are significant in the person's life and who could help in determining his or her best interests;*
   iii *aspects of the person's culture and religion that would influence a treatment decision; and,*
   iv *the person's diagnosis and prognosis.*

   In some jurisdictions legislation specifies who should be recognized as designated decision-makers (proxies) for incompetent people; this legislation should be followed. The term "proxy" is used broadly to identify those people who make a treatment decision based on the decision a person would have made for himself or herself (substitute decision-maker), people who help in determining what decision would be in the person's best interest and people whose appropriateness to make treatment decisions for the person is recognized under provincial legislation.

6. *There is no obligation to offer a person futile or nonbeneficial treatment. Futile and nonbeneficial treatments are controversial concepts when applied to CPR. Policymakers should determine how these concepts should be interpreted in the policy on resuscitation, in light of the facility's mission, the values of the community it serves, and ethical and legal developments. For the purposes of this document and in the context of resuscitation, "futile" and "nonbeneficial" are understood as follows. In some situations a physician can determine that a treatment is "medically" futile or nonbeneficial because it offers no reasonable hope of recovery or improvement or because the person is permanently unable to experience any benefit. In other cases the utility and benefit of a treatment can only be determined with reference to the person's subjective judgement about his or her overall well-being. As a general rule a person should be involved in determining futility in his or her case. In exceptional circumstances such discussions may not be in the person's best interests. If the person is incompetent the principles for decision making for incompetent people should be applied.*

Families often need time to absorb information presented, seek additional information, discuss it among themselves, and observe that the client is not recovering before being able to accept a DNR decision. In ethical nursing practice, as in all areas of practice, respect for persons is a prime concern. The CNA believes that nurses have an important role in encouraging all individuals, whether healthy or ill to express their goals and wishes related to end-of life care, and whether they would like life-sustaining treatments, such as CPR (CNA, 2008). For further guidance, nurses should refer to the guidelines set out by the Canadian Nurses Protective Society (CNPS, 2006).

Death-Related Religious and Cultural Practices

Various cultural and religious traditions and practices associated with death, dying, and the grieving process help people cope with these experiences. Nurses are often present through the dying process and at the moment of death. Knowledge of the client's religious and cultural heritage helps nurses provide individualized care to clients and their families, even though they may not participate in the rituals associated with death.

Dying in solitude is generally unacceptable in most cultures. In many cultures, people prefer a peaceful death at home rather than in the hospital. Members of some ethnic groups may request that health care professionals not reveal the prognosis to dying clients. They believe the person's last days should be free of worry and pain. People in other cultures prefer that a family member (preferably a male in some cultures) be told the diagnosis so that the client can be tactfully informed by a family member in gradual stages or not be told at all. Nurses also need to determine whom to call and when as the impending death draws near.

Beliefs and attitudes about death, its cause, and the soul also vary among cultures. Unnatural deaths, or bad deaths, are sometimes distinguished from good deaths. The death of a person who has behaved well in life may be considered less threatening based on the belief that the person will be reincarnated into a good life.

Beliefs about preparation of the body, autopsy, organ donation, cremation, and prolonging life are closely allied to the person's religion. *Autopsy,* for example, may be prohibited, opposed, or discouraged by Eastern Orthodox religions, Muslims, Jehovah's Witnesses, and Orthodox Jews. Some religions prohibit the removal of body parts and dictate that all body parts be given appropriate burial. The practice of *organ donation* varies among faiths. *Cremation* is discouraged, opposed, or prohibited by the Mormon, Eastern Orthodox, Islamic, and Jewish Orthodox faiths. Hindus, in contrast, prefer cremation and cast the ashes in a holy river. *Prolongation of life* is generally encouraged; however, some religions, such as Christian Science, are unlikely to use medical means to prolong life, and the Jewish faith generally opposes prolonging life after irreversible brain damage. In hopeless illness, Buddhists may permit euthanasia.

Nurses also need to be knowledgeable about the client's death-related rituals, such as last rites (see Figure 49.3 on the next page) and administration of Holy Communion, chanting at the bedside, and special procedures for washing, dressing, positioning, and shrouding the dead. For example, in some cultures family members of the same sex wash and prepare the body for burial and cremation. Muslims customarily turn the body toward Mecca. Nurses need to ask family members about their preference and verify who will carry out these activities. Burial clothes and other cultural or religious items are often important symbols for the funeral. For example, faithful Mormons are often dressed in their temple clothes. Some Aboriginals may be dressed in elaborate apparel and jewellery and wrapped in new blankets with money. The nurse must ensure that any ritual items present in the health care agency be given to the family or to the funeral home.

Relational Communication: Authentic Presence in Opening Conversations

The nurse gets to know the dying individual's and family's beliefs, desires, and needs in the journey of dying. Through continued assessment the nurse also collects a complete patient and family history, which includes

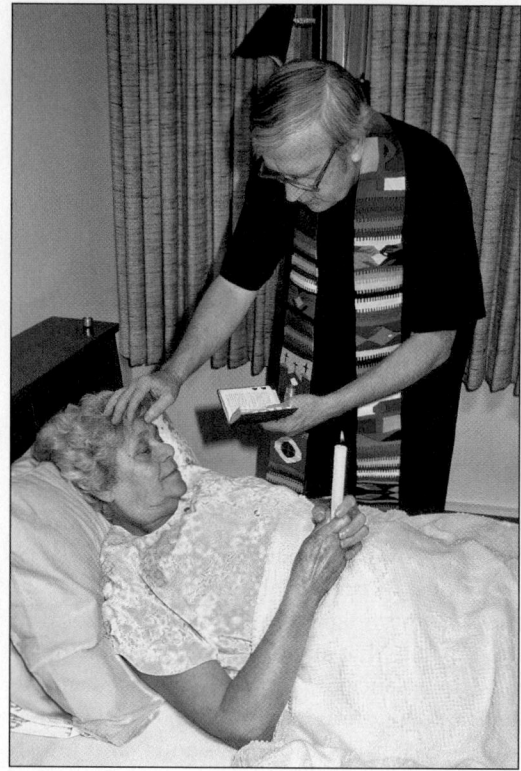

FIGURE 49.3 Catholic clients may request last rites or the sacrament of the sick.

physical, emotional, social, and spiritual dimensions. In this relationship, the nurse becomes aware of the living and dying transitions that the dying individual and family experience. Knowing the dying individual and family allows the nurse to respond in a way that best supports the patient and family. When approaching end-of-life discussions the ethics of being in relation to the patient and family is an obligation to supportive and quality palliative care. **Relational communication** is not about knowing the right thing to say or do, or about having the appropriate communication skills to effectively deal with patients and family members. Hartwick Doane and Varcoe (2005) stated that the most important resource each nurse brings to practice is the person he or she is. "Although you might learn communication skills and techniques that can improve your ability to be in-relation, the best way to be effective relationally is to be yourself" (p. 190). Dr. David Kuhl (2002) offered the belief that whatever questions you ask of others, you must ask of yourself. Personal awareness involves insight into how one's sensations, emotional life, past experiences, thoughts, beliefs, attitudes and values influence our life experience, including our interactions with patients, families, and other professionals. Personal awareness includes awareness of self, others, and the environment.

There is an important difference between natural relational capacity and a behavioural process of relating. The CASN (2009) Palliative Care Competencies states that nurses "engage in relational practice, which is characterized by: skill with listening; the ability to engage in difficult conversations; the ability to be present with

patients; responsiveness; respect for lived experience and meanings arising; appreciating patient and family choices and strengths; collaborative care; and fostering dignity" (p. 5). Nurses find courage to open themselves in their own vulnerability to hear these difficult conversations. Effective communication relating to the patients experience, including many issues that are a part of terminal illness, will assist the nurse to alleviate the persons' and families distress and total pain and suffering.

Assessment during the Transition of Active Dying

Nursing care and support for the dying individual and family includes making an accurate assessment of the physiological signs of approaching death. In addition to signs related to the individual's specific disease, certain other physical signs are indicative of impending death. The four main characteristic changes are loss of muscle tone, slowing of the circulation, changes in respirations, and sensory impairment. See Box 49.1 for indications of impending clinical death.

BOX 49.1 SIGNS OF IMPENDING CLINICAL DEATH

Nurses must be able to recognize the signs of impending clinical death:

LOSS OF MUSCLE TONE
- Relaxation of the facial muscles (e.g., the jaw may sag)
- Difficulty speaking
- Difficulty swallowing and gradual loss of the gag reflex
- Decreased activity of the gastrointestinal tract, with subsequent nausea, accumulation of flatus, abdominal distension, and retention of feces, especially if opioids or tranquilizers are being administered
- Possible urinary and rectal incontinence because of decreased sphincter control
- Diminished body movement

SLOWING OF THE CIRCULATION
- Diminished sensation
- Mottling and cyanosis of the extremities
- Cold skin, first in the feet and later in the hands, ears, and nose (the client, however, may feel warm because of elevated body temperature)
- Decelerated and weaker pulse
- Decreased blood pressure

CHANGES IN RESPIRATIONS
- Rapid, shallow, irregular, or abnormally slow respirations; Cheyne-Stokes respirations (periodic breathing); noisy breathing, referred to as the *death rattle,* caused by the collection of mucus in the throat; mouth breathing, which leads to dry oral mucous membranes

SENSORY IMPAIRMENT
- Blurred vision
- Impaired sense of taste and smell

Various consciousness levels occur just before death. Some individuals are alert, whereas others are drowsy, stuporous, or comatose. Hearing is thought to be the last sense that is lost. As death approaches, the nurse assists the family and other significant people to prepare themselves. Depending, in part, on knowledge of the dying individual's state of awareness, the nurse asks questions that help identify ways to provide support before and after death. In particular, the nurse needs to know what the family expects to happen when the person dies so accurate information can be given. See the Assessment: Interview box for sample interview questions. When the family members know what to expect, they are better able to support the dying person and others who are grieving. In addition, they may be able to make certain decisions about events surrounding the death, such as whether they will want to view the body after death.

Planning a Peaceful Death

Major desires of dying individuals are (a) maintaining physiological and psychological comfort, and (b) achieving a dignified and peaceful death, which includes maintaining personal control and accepting declining health status. When planning care with these individuals, the dying person's bill of rights can be a useful guide (see Box 49.2).

Examples of specific desired outcomes, although established in the planning phase, are provided in Table 49.4 later in this chapter (page 1578).

Examples of nursing interventions for the dying individual include the following:

- Helping individuals die with dignity
- Meeting physiological needs
- Providing spiritual support
- Supporting the family
- Providing postmortem care

ASSESSMENT | INTERVIEW

The Dying Individual

Ask the spouse, partner, or significant others the following questions:

- Have you ever been close to someone who was dying?
- What have you been told about what may happen when death occurs?
- Do you have questions about what may happen at the time of death?
- Do you have questions about how we are caring for [the person] during these last days?
- How do you think you would like to say goodbye?
- How are you taking care of yourself during these times?
- Who can you turn to for help at this time?
- Is there anyone you would like us to contact now or when death occurs?

BOX 49.2 THE DYING PERSON'S BILL OF RIGHTS

I have the right to be treated as a living human being until I die.

I have the right to maintain a sense of hopefulness, however changing its focus may be.

I have the right to be cared for by those who can maintain a sense of hopefulness, however changing this might be.

I have the right to express my feelings and emotions about my approaching death in my own way.

I have the right to participate in decisions concerning my care.

I have the right to expect continuing medical and nursing attention even though "cure" goals must be changed to "comfort" goals.

I have the right not to die alone.

I have the right to be free from pain.

I have the right to have my questions answered honestly.

I have the right not to be deceived.

I have the right to have help from and for my family in accepting my death.

I have the right to die in peace and dignity.

I have the right to retain my individuality and not be judged for my decisions, which may be contrary to beliefs of others.

I have the right to discuss and enlarge my religious and/or spiritual experiences, whatever these may mean to others.

I have the right to expect that the sanctity of the human body will be respected after death.

I have the right to be cared for by caring, sensitive, knowledgeable people who will attempt to understand my needs and will be able to gain some satisfaction in helping me face my death.

Source: Based on Barbus, A. J. (1975). The dying person's bill of rights. *American Journal of Nursing, 75,* 99. Copyright © 1975, American Journal of Nursing Company. Reprinted with permission from the *American Journal of Nursing.*

Planning for Home Care

Dying clients have been cared for in the home by nurses since early in the development of the profession. In Canada, the development of palliative care programs began in hospitals. This trend continued late into the 1990s, with up to 80% of deaths occurring in hospital (Wilson et al., 2001). Recently, a shift toward community care and more home deaths has occurred for various reasons, including increasing costs in hospital care, changing environments in hospitals that do not meet the needs of all patients, the growing expertise of health care providers, and advancing technology that allows even complex care to be given at home. Growing numbers of patients and families are advocating for increased community care, and society has begun to value care for the dying and to embrace the expansion of a palliative care philosophy as paramount to quality end-of-life care.

A major factor in determining whether a person will die in a health care facility or at home is the availability of willing and able caregivers. If the dying person wants to be at home, and the family or others can provide care to maintain symptom control and meet other basic needs of the dying individual, the nurse should facilitate a referral to home care services. Home care nurses and other interdisciplinary team members will then conduct a full assessment of the home and the care provider's skills.

The issue of transfer of funds from hospital to homes, however, is not adequately addressed in all areas of Canada. Most home care programs do not fund 24-hour care over the long term, expecting that family members will provide most of the care. Unless families are able to privately fund home care, including the cost of medications, home medical equipment and supplies, transportation, and respite services, the probability of staying at home until death is not always a reality.

Home care providers are typically characterized as formal or informal caregivers. As mentioned, family and friends (informal caregivers) provide the majority of the care, especially for older adults with multiple comorbidities requiring care for many years. Formal caregivers consist of all disciplines, the majority being registered nurses and personal care attendants or licensed practical nurses. Registered nurses are considered to be the coordinators of care, providing skilled assessments in pain and symptom management and providing direction for other nurses and paraprofessionals. Nurses provide the client and family with bereavement care. The goal and related nursing responsibilities for dying individuals is to assist them to a peaceful death. More specific responsibilities are the following:

- To provide relief from loneliness, fear, and depression
- To maintain the client's sense of security, self-confidence, dignity, and self-worth
- To maintain hope
- To help the client accept losses
- To provide physical comfort

Not all clients can manage or choose to remain at home. Individuals facing death need help accepting that they will have to depend on others. Some dying individuals require only minimal care and can be cared for at home; others need continuous care and attention and require the services of a hospital and palliative care interdisciplinary team. Families and dying individuals need support and guidance, well in advance of death, to plan for the transition to death. They need to consider what might happen and how and where they would like to die.

Helping Individuals Die with Dignity

Perhaps one of the most interesting and applicable ways for nurses to think about dignity when caring for dying individuals comes from the writings of Arthur Frank (2004). Frank's discussion of dignity is relational and places emphasis on the local nature of dignity, which conceptualizes it as "an event happening between persons, rather than a fixed quality" (p. 207). This postmodern understanding of dignity as *relational* places the value of dignity as a human experience in a different light. It serves to remind us that "caring is not a unidirectional administration of a standardized treatment. Care that takes dignity seriously is a dialogue" (p. 207).

Frank (2004) emphasized that caring requires the caregiver to reflect on his or her own values of care. Dignity is sustained in nurses' acts of caring; dignity can be enacted in silence. Dignity is inherent in the context of the nurse–client relationship. Nurses can facilitate care that allows for dying individuals to retain some control by making their own choices about the location of care (e.g., hospital, home, or hospice), times of appointments with health care professionals, activity schedule, use of health care resources, and times of visits from relatives and friends.

Many dying individuals want to be able to manage the events preceding death so they can die peacefully. Nurses can facilitate dialogue that opens possibilities for individuals to find meaning and completeness and to determine their own physical, psychological, and social priorities. Dying individuals often strive for self-fulfillment more than for self-preservation, and they need to find meaning in dying while continuing to live. Part of the nurses' challenge is to help facilitate day-to-day comfort and care so that the individual's transition to death is peaceful.

Sometimes, nurses have difficulty discussing death with clients who are dying. Although it is natural for people to be uncomfortable discussing death, steps can be taken to make such discussions easier for both the nurse and the client. Callanan (1994) proposed the following strategies:

- Identify personal feelings about death and how they can influence interactions with clients. Acknowledge personal fears about death, and discuss them with a friend or colleague.
- Focus on the client's needs. The client's fears and beliefs may be different from the nurse's. It is important that the nurse avoid imposing personal fears and beliefs on the client or family.
- Understand the client and how the client copes. Talk to the client or the family about how the client usually copes with stress. Clients will use their usual coping strategies for dealing with impending death. For example, if they are usually quiet and reflective, they will become quieter and more withdrawn when facing terminal illness.

- Establish a communication relationship that shows concern for and commitment to the client. Communication strategies that let the client know you are available to talk about death include the following:

    a. Describe what you see: for example, "You seem sad. Would you like to talk about what's happening to you?"

    b. Clarify your concern: for example, "I'd like to know better how you feel and how I can help you."

    c. Acknowledge the client's struggle: for example, "It must be difficult to feel so uncomfortable. I care about you and would like to help you be more comfortable."

    d. Provide a caring touch. Holding the client's hand or offering a comforting massage can encourage the client to verbalize feelings.

- Determine what the client knows about the illness and prognosis.

- Respond with honesty and directness to the client's questions about death.

- Make time to be available to the client to provide support, listen, and respond.

HOSPICE PALLIATIVE CARE Hospice or palliative care has emerged as a specialized field only within the past 30 years (Billings, 1998). The **hospice care** model was developed to address the specific needs of the dying and their families, so neglected by the medical system of care (see Figure 49.4). The modern hospice movement started in England in 1967 through the work of Dame Cicely Saunders and colleagues at St. Christopher's Hospice in London. The hospice movement came to North America in the mid-1970s, when Dr. Florence Wald, a nursing pioneer, led an interdisciplinary team to create the first American hospice (Wald, 1999). Typically, hospice care is for those individuals with a life expectancy of 6 months or less.

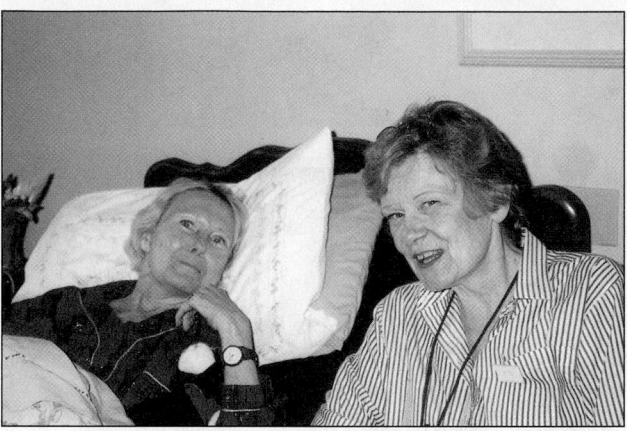

FIGURE 49.4 The patient and family are the "unit of care" in hospice palliative care.

In the United Kingdom, a hospice is the building in which dying persons are cared for. In the United States, the term refers to a specific model for delivering palliative care. The **palliative care** model evolved from the traditional hospice perspective to address quality-of-life concerns for those patients living for prolonged periods with a progressive debilitating disease.

Historically, the terms *hospice* and *palliative care* in Canada were used in a variety of ways. The term *hospice* included a philosophy of care, often community-based, volunteer-driven programs providing care in the home, in a long-term care facility, or in a freestanding hospice (Brenneis & Brown, 2006). New terminology in Canada was proposed in 2002. The words *hospice* and *palliative care* were combined to recognize the convergence of hospice and palliative care into one movement. The national organization for palliative care, which at that time was called the Canadian Palliative Care Association, adjusted its name to include the term **hospice palliative care**, becoming the Canadian Hospice Palliative Care Association (CHPCA) (Brenneis & Brown, 2006). See the Nursing and Canadian Society box.

 Nursing and Canadian Society

Fact	Implications for Nursing Practice
The Canadian Hospice Palliative Care Association (CHPCA) is the recognized national organization for leadership in palliative care. The mission of the CHPCA is to promote palliative care awareness, education, and research, advocating at a national level for policy development, resource allocation, and support for caregivers.	Nurses need to be aware of the policy papers on nursing care of the dying that have been accepted by each professional association, in accordance with the CHPCA standards.
The principles and practice of palliative care nursing and palliative care competencies for Canadian nurses was established in September 2009	Educational institutions should consider these standards when developing curricula in palliative care.
The CNA board of directors has designated palliative care as a specialty, making it the twelfth discipline to gain that status. The first hospice palliative care nursing certification examination was offered in 2004.	In achieving hospice palliative care nursing certification in Canada, nurses share in the enhancement of hospice palliative care for all Canadians.

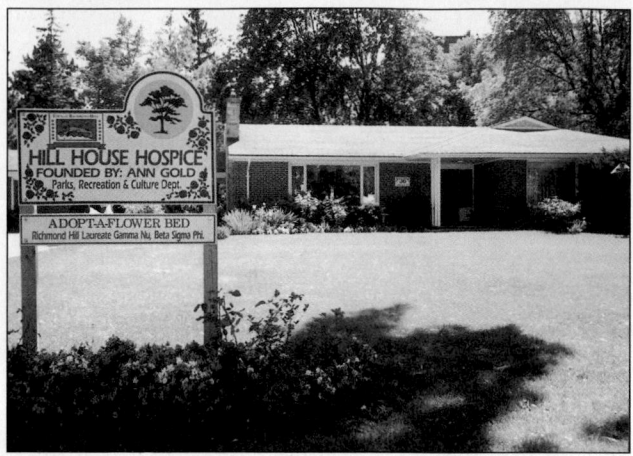

FIGURE 49.5 Hospice care is based on the principles of providing care to improve the dying individual's quality of life.

Regardless of location or type of program, hospice palliative care is based on the principles of providing care to improve the dying individual's quality of life, rather than aiming for cure (Figure 49.5). The care is patient and family centred, focusing on needs and concerns that are most important to them. A hallmark of hospice palliative care since Cicely Saunders founded the modern hospice movement has been the combination of scientific rigour and personal concern. At St. Christopher's Hospice, Saunders developed an education program for palliative care that embraced three broad areas: (a) the science and techniques of pain management and symptom control; (b) the knowledge of psychosocial, social, and spiritual aspects of dying and grieving; and (c) self-knowledge on the part of caregivers, especially related to personal beliefs about death and loss (Barnard, Towers, Boston, & Lambrinidou, 2000). Hospice palliative care is always provided by a multidisciplinary team of primarily physicians, nurses, social workers, and chaplains.

MEETING THE PHYSIOLOGICAL NEEDS OF THE DYING INDIVIDUAL The physiological needs of people who are dying are related to a slowing of body processes and to homeostatic imbalances. Interventions include providing personal hygiene measures; controlling pain; relieving respiratory difficulties; assisting with movement, nutrition, hydration, and elimination; and providing measures related to sensory changes. See also Table 49.2.

SENSORY PERCEPTUAL NEEDS Changes in the level of consciousness may be the first symptom of dying, occurring over weeks or days. Changes may include **clouding of consciousness** or thought, drowsiness, **delirium**, **stupor** or unresponsiveness, **coma**, and, in some individuals, confusion or agitation. Consciousness is an integral aspect of being human; the ability to relate to others and the environment allows the individual an important sense

TABLE 49.2 Physiological Needs of Dying Persons

Problem	Nursing Interventions
Ineffective airway clearance	30° Fowler's position: conscious clients Lateral, throat suctioning: conscious clients Sims', 30° lateral, and lateral position: unconscious clients
Self-care deficit: bathing or hygiene	Frequent baths and linen changes Mouth care
Impaired physical mobility	Assist client out of bed periodically, if client is able Regularly change bedridden client's position Support client's position with pillows, blanket rolls, or towels, as needed Elevate client's legs when sitting up to prevent pooling of blood
Imbalanced nutrition: less than body requirements	Antiemetics or small amount of alcoholic beverage to stimulate appetite Encourage liquid foods, as tolerated
Constipation	Dietary fibre Laxatives
Impaired urinary elimination	Skin care in response to incontinence of urine or feces Bedpan, urinal, or commode chair within easy reach Call light within reach for assistance onto bedpan or commode Absorbent pads placed under incontinent client; linen changed as often as needed Catheterization, if necessary Keep room as clean and odour free as possible
Disturbed sensory perception: visual, tactile	Clients prefer a well-lit room Hearing is not diminished; speak clearly and do not whisper Touch is diminished, but client will feel pressure of touch

of control. Even though individuals may have mentally accepted the fact that they are dying, the actual process of losing consciousness and the awareness of death may be a frightening experience. The fatigue and exhaustion of illness may prompt a wish of "falling asleep and not waking up." Others may struggle to continue to live and, thus, be very restless and unsettled until death. As the client's body slows down, the nurse must use the knowledge of normal physiological changes to prepare the client for death and lessen anxiety (see Table 49.3).

PAIN MANAGEMENT One of the greatest fears of dying individuals is that they will experience intense, unbearable pain. However, this fear is largely unfounded because the majority of patients with terminal illness can obtain pain relief. Nurses are critical members of the palliative care team, particularly when it comes to pain management (Paice & Fine, 2006). The prevalence of pain in the terminally ill varies by diagnosis and other factors. Approximately one-third of individuals actively receiving treatment for cancer and two-thirds of those with advanced malignant disease experience pain (Chang, Hwang, Feuerman, & Kasimis, 2000; Meuser et al., 2001; Morita, Ichiki, Tsunoda, Inoue, & Chihaa, 1998; Wells, 2000).

In studies of patients admitted to palliative care units, pain is often the dominant symptom, along with fatigue and dyspnea (Jenkins, Taube, Ken, Hanson, & Bruera, 1998; Ng & von Gunten, 1998). Pain control is essential because pain alters sleep, appetite, mobility, energy levels, and psychological functioning. Barriers to good pain relief are numerous and pervasive. Often, because of lack

---

TABLE 49.3 State of Consciousness in Dying Patients

A. Consciousness: To be fully conscious is to be aware of one's self and the surrounding environment. There are two aspects:

1. *Content.* The sum of mental processes, including the ability to discriminate among both the sensory inputs and the internal cognitive aspects.

2. *Arousal.* A state of wakefulness or alertness to external and internal processes.

B. Clouding of Consciousness: Defined as a reduced state of wakefulness or awareness.

1. *Mild Clouding.* For the terminal patient, fatigue and periods of drowsiness are not uncommon. After a period of rest, the patient remains fully conscious. Several other features may not be observed or appreciated by caregivers in the early part of this phase. These features include the following:

   - Excitability and irritability, which alternate with drowsiness
   - Startled by minor stimuli
   - Easily distracted
   - Misjudges sensory perception, especially visual
   - Cannot think clearly or quickly

   These features may be intermittent and mistaken for anxiety.

2. *Advanced or subacute confusional state.* In this phase, the intensity and persistence of the symptoms is increased. The patient is "confused."

   - Stimuli are more consistently misinterpreted.
   - Attention span is shortened.
   - The patient is bewildered and has difficulty following commands.
   - There is some disorientation to time and sometimes to place and person.
   - Memory is faulty.
   - Drowsiness is often prominent (may alternate with nighttime agitation).

3. *Delirium.* The next "lower" level of consciousness is delirium. Although defined and used here in the classic sense, the term "delirium" is not consistently used in all practice settings where care of the dying is provided. The word has a connotation of being "crazy" and is inappropriate in working with dying patients. The next phases are referred to as lower levels of consciousness. Symptoms at this level include the following:

   - Intensified disorientation
   - Misinterpretation of stimuli; often visual hallucinations
   - Lucid periods that often alternate with delirium
   - Delusions
   - Loud, talkative, offensive, suspicious, or agitated behaviour

4. *Stupor.* "Stupor" is defined as a state in which the patient is unresponsive but briefly arousable, only during vigorous and repeated stimuli, and then immediately drifts back to unresponsiveness. In this stage, the patient may moan or be briefly restless when being turned or when given skin care. Staff need to ascertain whether this "moaning" is due to insufficient pain control or simply being partially roused from a deeper level. This is not a "withdrawn" state in which the patient, lying in a fetal position, is conscious but does not respond to people. In this type of case, the patient will initially appear to be in a stupor but is, in fact, conscious and just not responding to family or caregivers. Management (and prognosis) of this state is very different from that for the truly stuporous patient.

5. *Coma.* This is the true comatose state, defined as complete unarousable unresponsiveness or "the absence of any psychologically understandable response to external stimuli or inner need." This is exemplified in a patient who is breathing on his or her own but is totally unarousable by any physical stimulus, such as pinching, heat or cold, and yelling or sudden noise. There is no intake by the patient.

Source: Based on Victoria Hospice Society. (1998). *Hospice resource manual. Volume 1: Medical care of the dying* (3rd ed.) Victoria, BC: Author.

of education, misbeliefs, and attitudinal issues, these barriers prevent many individuals from receiving adequate pain relief (Parageon & Hailey, 1999).

Most nurses are educated in the observation and assessment of acute pain, which is very different from chronic pain. The dramatic signs and symptoms of acute pain warrant fast and immediate action. Outward signs of chronic pain are not as obvious and, therefore, may go untreated. Lack of expression does not mean lack of pain. Comprehensive assessment of pain is imperative. This must be conducted initially, regularly throughout treatment, and during any changes in the patient's experience of pain. Performing an individualized pain assessment is the first step to ensuring baseline data and continued treatment resulting in an improved quality of life for the dying individual.

Treatment of pain in older adults generally follows the same guidelines as in younger adults, with opioid therapy remaining the cornerstone of pain management. There is conflicting evidence on changes that occur in the nociceptive system with aging (Helme, Meliala, & Gibson, 2004). Even if nociceptive perception is decreased in older adults, diseases likely to cause chronic pain have a higher prevalence in older adults. These diseases include arthritis, polymyalgia rheumatica, atherosclerotic disease, zoster (shingles), and peripheral neuropathy. Pain assessment in older adults is often complicated by the existence of cognitive impairment. The cognitively impaired patient is often unable to express pain adequately or request analgesics; this increases the risk of undertreatment. The fear of precipitating or exacerbating a delirious episode by employing opioids in the management of pain may also lead to inadequate pain management.

Once the individual's pain has been assessed, an analgesic medication to control the pain is selected (opioid or nonopioid analgesic). The World Health Organization (1996) recommended the use of an analgesic ladder to assist with analgesic selection. With chronic pain, analgesics are generally most effective if administered regularly (or around the clock) rather than on an as-needed basis. Frequently, when patients receive a regular dose of medication, pain can break through and require additional doses to keep it under control. Opioid or controlled substances are used for managing moderate to severe pain. For primarily historical reasons, morphine is the strong opioid of choice. Nonopioid medications are commonly used to ease pain, lower fever, and manage mild to moderate pain.

Medications for pain management are not limited to analgesics; they can include corticosteroids, antidepressants, anticonvulsants, and anxiolytics, determined by the type of pain assessed. Other than medications for the control of pain, the nurse can offer therapeutic comfort measures, such as helping the patient relax, providing music, giving warm and soothing baths or a massage, and providing distraction. The presence of the nurse to ensure support, conversation, and genuine concern is most important and assists in the process of reducing pain and promoting comfort.

BREATHING NEEDS **Dyspnea** (shortness of breath) is an uncomfortable awareness of breathing. Like pain, dyspnea is a subjective sensation involving both the perception of breathlessness and the individual's reaction to it. The prevalence of dyspnea varies according to the disease. Approximately 50% of the general outpatient cancer population experiences some breathlessness, with this number rising to 55% to 70% in the terminal phase of the disease (Dudgeon, Kristjanson, Sloan, & Lertzman, 2001; Fainsinger, MacEachern, Hanson, Miller, & Bruera, 1991). In older adults, shortness of breath can be a symptom associated with chronic disease, such as emphysema and heart failure, or acute bronchopulmonary pneumonia.

Dyspnea, like pain, is multidimensional in nature, with physical symptoms and affective components, which are shaped by an individual's past experience with dyspnea (Dudgeon, 2006). Dyspnea, like pain, is not always evident to the observer. The nurse should inquire specifically about shortness of breath. Occasionally, dying individuals have physical signs of tachypnea and appear to be in distress; however, they may not feel dyspneic or distressed. The opposite can also occur, with individuals who are not tachypneic or in apparent respiratory distress describing feeling very short of breath. The extent of breathlessness experienced by a patient may or may not be related to the oxygen saturation level. Therefore, the patient's own assessment of the level of dyspnea may be a more reliable indicator than the oxygen saturation level. Dyspnea is, thus, a symptom that needs to be reported by the dying individual. A complete clinical assessment of dyspnea includes symptom history, including its temporal onset (acute or chronic), whether it is affected by positioning, its qualities, its associated symptoms, its precipitating and relieving events and activities, and its responses to medications. A past history of smoking, underlying lung or cardiac disease, concurrent medical condition, allergies, and details of previous medications or treatment should be elicited (Dudgeon, 2006).

The nurse provides many comfort measures to help relieve, decrease the perception of, and comfort the experience of dyspnea, including (a) administering medications, such as opioids, bronchodilators, and diuretics; (b) creating a therapeutic environment in which the individual engages in distraction therapy and relaxation exercises, is allowed to rest, or is allowed to be with family; (c) assisting the individual to a position that makes breathing easier (usually a high sitting position is best) and offering a fan to reduce the perception of breathlessness; (d) offering fluids and using a humidifier to loosen mucus so that coughing is easier; and (e) administering oxygen therapy by mask or nasal cannula. If the client is hypoxic, maintain oxygen saturation around 88% to 90%. The nurse has to be cautious in offering oxygen to a patient with chronic obstructive pulmonary disease (COPD); in these individuals, oxygen saturation should be kept around 90% or as ordered by the physician (Pereira & Bruera, 2001). Oxygen therapy relieves symptoms, improves exercise tolerance, and is the only therapy proven to prolong life in patients with COPD. It is important that the nurse offer these interventions early in the experience of dyspnea to reduce anxiety and improve quality of life.

The importance of teaching the dying individual and family cannot be overlooked. Strategies to relieve the acute experience of dyspnea include (a) using positioning and structured relaxation techniques, (b) knowing the signs and symptoms of an impending exacerbation, (c) using techniques to conserve energy and prioritize activities, and (d) understanding ways to maximize the effectiveness of medications, such as by using a spacer with inhaled drugs and taking an additional dose of the medications before activity, as ordered.

ACKNOWLEDGING AND STRENGTHENING SPIRITUALITY Spirituality is an inherent, integrating, and, often, extremely valued dimension of the journey of dying for individuals and their families. Spirituality is immensely personal, abstract, and illusive in nature (Sinclair, 2011; Sinclair, Raffin, Pereria, & Guebert, 2006). Spiritual distress, or *soul pain,* is a common experience in those who are dying and, sometimes, an experience that is not addressed or understood. The experiences are complex, varied, and individual, and if left unaddressed, they may stifle the opportunity for growth, heighten the loss of a sense of meaning and purpose, and contribute to poorly controlled symptoms (Raffin, 2002).

The relationship between spirituality and religion is important for the nurse to understand, as each client and family will embrace a unique interconnection. A common understanding of the relationship presents spirituality as the overarching umbrella, with religion being only one of the many forms of spiritual expression. A review of the literature from many disciplines discusses religion as being correlated with an organized faith system, beliefs, worship, religious rituals, and relationship with a divine being (Sinclair, Pereira, & Raffin, 2006). Often, the experience of suffering prompts people, whether or not they see themselves as religious, to ask deeply spiritual questions and turn to God or a spiritual guide for solace. Even in the case of those who are avowedly religious, suffering can lead to questioning of fundamental beliefs (Anderson, 1989). To appreciate individual responses to suffering, it is imperative that the nurse attempt to understand the religious and spiritual views of the sufferer.

Spirituality delves into the nature of humanity and the deep mysteries of life (Sinclair, 2011; Sinclair et al., 2006). Nurses caring for dying individuals need to embrace values, meaning, and purpose; turn inward to the human traits of honesty, love, caring, wisdom, and compassion; help others to search for a higher authority, guiding spirit, or transcendence that is mystical; and help create healing of body, mind, and spirit that may or may not involve organized religion (Raffin, 2002). Nurses, in helping others find their expression of spirituality, need to allow for an open interpretation of what the individual considers to be divine or a transcendent Other.

Nurses have a responsibility not to impose their own religious or spiritual beliefs on a client but to respond to the client in relation to the client's own background and needs. Openness and honesty are most important in helping the client articulate needs and in developing a sense of caring and trust.

Specific interventions may include facilitating expressions of feeling, prayer, meditation, reading, and discussion with appropriate clergy or a spiritual adviser. It is important for nurses to establish an effective interdisciplinary relationship with other health care professionals for quality patient and family care. Spirituality is inherently relational and shapes the care provided by palliative care professionals. Palliative care can also serve as a catalyst for interdisciplinary team members' own spiritual journeys (Sinclair et al., 2006). For a further discussion of spiritual issues, see Chapter 47. Death-related beliefs and practices of selected groups are discussed earlier in this chapter.

Evaluating the Process of Care

To evaluate the achievement of client goals, the nurse collects data in accordance with the desired outcomes established in the planning phase. Evaluation activities may include the following:

- Listening to the client's reports of feeling in control of the environment surrounding death, such as control over pain relief, visitation of family and support people, or treatment plans
- Observing the client's relationship with significant others
- Listening to the client's thoughts and feelings related to hopelessness or powerlessness

Finally, examples of goals and desired outcomes in fostering a peaceful death are shown in Table 49.4 on the next page.

Caring for the Family

At no time is the family more important than during the times of death and dying. Nurses have an obligation not only to include the family in the care of the client but also to honour their wisdom, their beliefs, their wishes, and their needs. In this act of honouring, it is important to meet families at the point of their needs, rather than have set and unbending expectations of how family members will react to and involve themselves during the profound and difficult experience of watching a loved one die.

TABLE 49.4 Goals in Fostering a Peaceful Death

Goal	Examples of Desired Outcomes
Maintain personal control over present situation	Identifies areas of personal control
	Participates in self-care activities in accordance with health status
	Makes choices related to care and treatment
	Expresses sense of control over the present situation
Maintain comfort	Maintains physiological comfort
	Maintains psychological comfort
	Skin and oral tissues hydrated
	Absence of constipation or urinary retention
	Absence of restlessness
Accept declining health status	Shares values and personal meaning of life
	Verbalizes acceptance of situation
	Accepts limitations and seeks help, as needed

The most important thing a nurse can do to care for family members is to acknowledge them and include them. If the nurse shifts her or his thinking from considering the dying individual as the client to accepting the entire family as the client, then care becomes focused on the very significant event that is happening not just to the person but also to the entire family system.

Acknowledging family members includes consulting the family in terms of care of client and honouring their knowledge of the dying individual. It involves a collaborative evolution of ways in which the family needs to be involved and ways in which they prefer the nurse to assume care. For example, some family members want to be involved in physical care, whereas other family members are more comfortable with the nurse assuming these caring practices. It is important, in asking the family members' preferences, not to imply that the nurse has an expectation that they assume these acts, but rather that the nurse respects the family members' level of comfort. One way to approach this delicate establishment of roles and involvement would be to say to the family, "Sometimes family members like to be involved in the physical care of their ill members, and others prefer the nurse to assume these things. What would be most comfortable for you in this area?" Family members may want other kinds of involvement, rather than physical care, but be unsure of how to offer this. The nurse can help guide family members in knowing that it may be soothing to dying individuals to speak to them, read to them, hold their hands, or simply be present.

A part of what a nurse offers a family is a caring and compassionate presence. *Compassion* is defined as "suffering with." Though the nurse is not suffering as the family is, the nurse has in some ways entered the world of the family's suffering. "In entering the world of the one who is suffering, we do have to open space to where we listen to the pain, where we see, touch, and feel the pain" (Moules, 1999, p. 255). Nurses create a context in which family members feel as though they can be open about their pain, suffering, and grief. Nurses can offer information about the process of what is occurring and thereby walk alongside the family in understanding this experience (Raffin Bouchal, 2007).

When the individual dies, family members should be invited to spend time with the body (if they so desire) as this important ritual can serve as a significant event in making room for grief and grieving. Some people ask for mementos, such as locks of hair. Children should not be discouraged from being involved in this important ritual of viewing the body, and, at times, nurses can offer encouragement or even permission to families that it is appropriate to include children. Family members may have specific desires to participate in some care of the body, as in the case of a mother who asked to bathe her child one last time and dress him in special clothes. The nurse, in this instance, helped prepare clean towels and a basin for the mother, showing sensitivity in commenting that the water needed to be warmer, and then returning with warm water. The mother later reported that this simple act of kindness was of great comfort to her. In a health care system that is often short of beds, the nurse may, at times, need to act as an advocate for families to ensure that they have all the time they need to spend with the body to begin saying goodbye to the physical presence of this person in their lives.

Postmortem Care

Rigor mortis is the stiffening of the body that occurs about 2 to 4 hours after death. It results from a lack of adenosine triphosphate (ATP), which is not synthesized because of a lack of glycogen in the body. ATP is necessary for muscle fibre relaxation. Its lack causes the muscles to contract, which, in turn, immobilizes the joints. Rigor mortis starts in the involuntary muscles (heart, bladder, and so on), then progresses to the head, neck, and trunk, and finally reaches the extremities.

Because the deceased person's family often wants to view the body and because it is important that the deceased appear natural and comfortable, nurses need to position the body, place dentures in the mouth, as needed, and close the eyes and mouth *before* rigor mortis sets in. Rigor mortis usually leaves the body about 96 hours after death.

Algor mortis is the gradual decrease of the body's temperature after death. When blood circulation terminates and the hypothalamus ceases to function, body temperature falls about 1°C per hour until it reaches room temperature. Simultaneously, the skin loses its elasticity and can easily be broken when removing dressings and adhesive tape.

After blood circulation has ceased, the red blood cells break down, releasing hemoglobin, which discolours surrounding tissues. This discoloration, referred to as **livor mortis**, appears in the lowermost or dependent areas of the body.

Nursing personnel may be responsible for care of a body after death. Postmortem care should be carried out according to the policy of the hospital or agency. Because care of the body may be influenced by religious beliefs, the nurse should check the client's religion and make every attempt to comply. If the deceased's family or friends want to view the body, it is important to make the environment as clean and pleasant as possible and to make the body appear natural and comfortable. All equipment, soiled linen, and supplies should be removed from the bedside. Some agencies require that all tubes in the body remain in place; in other agencies, tubes may be cut to within 2.5 cm of the skin and taped in place; in others, all tubes are removed. Legal issues surrounding the death (e.g., coroner's case) may necessitate that all tubes remain in place.

Normally, the body is placed in a supine position with the arms either at the sides, palms down, or across the abdomen. One pillow is placed under the head and shoulders to prevent blood from discolouring the face by settling in it. The eyelids are closed and held in place for a few seconds so they remain closed. Dentures are usually inserted, as needed, to help give the face a natural appearance. The mouth is then closed.

Soiled areas of the body are washed; however, a complete bath is not necessary because the body will be washed by the **mortician** (also referred to as an *undertaker*), a person trained in care of the body after death.

Absorbent pads are placed under the buttocks to take up any feces and urine released because of relaxation of the sphincter muscles. A clean gown is placed on the client, and the hair is brushed and combed. The top bed linens are adjusted neatly to cover the client to the shoulders. Soft lighting and chairs are provided for the family.

In the hospital, after the body has been viewed by the family, additional identification tags are applied. The body is wrapped in a **shroud**, a large piece of plastic or cotton material used to enclose a body after death. Identification is then applied to the outside of the shroud. The body is taken to the morgue if arrangements have not been made to have a mortician pick it up from the client's room.

Educating Nurses in Palliative Care

Recently, in Canada, there have been numerous important developments in education and training for new health care professionals, including nurses. Since 2004, the CNA has offered Hospice Palliative Care Certification. A new educational resource by the CASN Task Force on palliative and end-of-life care was developed for educators to consult in curriculum development in palliative care nursing. The Task Force has identified core competencies specific to this particular field of care as well as general competencies nurses need when providing palliative and end-of-life care (CASN, 2009). Research indicates that palliative end-of-life education positively influences student nurses attitudes toward death and caring for dying persons (Mallory, 2003; Mok, Lee & Wong, 2002) and that early introduction and exploration with death issues with practice integration helps to better prepare nurses to care for dying individuals. The CASN (2009) guidelines are informed and developed by nurses to ensure and maintain relevant and comprehensive care. See the Weblinks section below for detailed information.

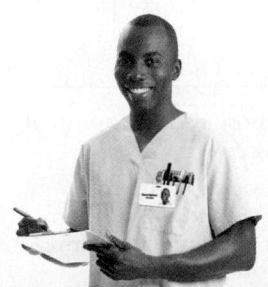

Case Study 49

Jacob Frank, a 40-year-old father of two, lives in a small town in rural Alberta. Jacob, who has advanced prostate cancer, has decided not to pursue further active chemotherapy. Jacob shares with the palliative home care nurse that his father died when he was only 8 years old. He recalls not being told that his father was very ill and that he was not permitted to attend the funeral service.

CRITICAL THINKING QUESTIONS

1. How should the nurse respond to this information? In her conversation with Jacob, what should she explore further?

2. How can the nurse help Jacob clarify his beliefs and values about living and dying now that he is dealing with his own terminal illness?

3. What therapeutic interventions would be important for the nurse to explore with Jacob's family?

Check the eText in MyNursingLab for answers and explanations.

KEY TERMS

actual loss *p. 1558*	**delirium** *p. 1574*	**livor mortis** *p. 1579*	**relational**
advance directives	**dyspnea** *p. 1576*	**loss** *p. 1558*	**communication**
p. 1566	**euthanasia** *p. 1566*	**mercy killing** *p. 1566*	*p. 1570*
algor mortis *p. 1578*	**grief** *p. 1559*	**mortician** *p. 1579*	**rigor mortis** *p. 1578*
anticipatory loss *p. 1558*	**hospice care** *p. 1573*	**palliative care** *p. 1573*	**shroud** *p. 1579*
clouding of	**hospice palliative care**	**perceived loss** *p. 1558*	**stupor** *p. 1574*
consciousness *p. 1574*	*p. 1573*	**proxy directive** *p. 1566*	
coma *p. 1574*	**living will** *p. 1566*		

CHAPTER HIGHLIGHTS

- Nurses help clients deal with all kinds of losses, including loss of body image, loss of a loved one, loss of a sense of well-being, and loss of a job.

- Loss, especially loss of a loved one or a valued body part, can be viewed as either a situational or a developmental loss and as either an actual or a perceived loss (both of which can be anticipatory).

- Grieving is a normal, subjective emotional response to loss; it is essential for mental and physical and spiritual health. Grieving allows the bereaved person to cope with loss gradually and to accept it as part of reality.

- Knowledge of different stages or phases of grieving and factors that influence the loss reaction can help the nurse understand the responses and needs of clients, but recent research studies suggest that grief is an experience that is ongoing and changes over time, and involves a continuing relationship with the deceased.

- How an individual deals with loss is closely related to the individual's stage of development, personal resources, and social support system.

- Caring for the dying and the bereaved is one of the nurse's most complex and challenging responsibilities.

- Nurses' beliefs, values, and attitudes about death and dying directly affect their ability to provide care.

- Nurses must consider the entire family as requiring care in situations involving loss, especially death.

- Nurses must be knowledgeable about their responsibilities in regard to ethical and legal issues surrounding death: advance directives, withdrawing food and fluid, euthanasia, and do not resuscitate orders.

- Nurses need to consider palliative care educational competencies developed for the delivery of safe and quality palliative care.

- Dying clients require open communication, physical help, and emotional and spiritual support to ensure a peaceful and dignified death. They need to maintain a sense of control in managing the events preceding death.

ASSESS YOUR LEARNING

1. The hospice palliative care nurse educator is presenting a session to student nurses about the beliefs, attitudes, and practices essential to hospice palliative care. Which of the following BEST describes these practices?

   a. Palliative care is best provided by an interdisciplinary team working collaboratively with the person and family to address physical, psychological, social, and spiritual concerns.

   b. Palliative care is best provided by an interdisciplinary team working collaboratively with the person to address physical, emotional, and practical concerns.

   c. Palliative care is best provided by the nurse and physician working with the person and family

   to address physical, psychosocial, and spiritual concerns related to dying.

   d. Palliative care is best provided by an interdisciplinary team in a specialized setting working with the person and family to address identified social and emotional needs.

2. Which of the following is the best statement about do not resuscitate (DNR) orders in advanced terminal illness?

   a. DNR orders are seldom appropriate. The principle of nursing is that all life is valuable and should be preserved at all costs.

   b. When the disease progresses to the point that the heart stops beating or the person stops breathing, efforts to resuscitate will always fail and are an inappropriate use of resources.

   c. Palliative care units do not have the capabilities to provide advanced life support. Therefore, people need to agree to a DNR on admission to the palliative care unit.

   d. The goal of palliative care is to alleviate suffering and enhance quality of life. Resuscitation may prolong suffering and impede a peaceful death.

3. What is the BEST strategy the hospice nurse can use to support a person and family in making decisions and coping with advanced illness and the dying experience?

   a. Assist the family to begin detaching from the dying person to help with the grieving process, allowing the team to provide appropriate care.

   b. Facilitate the expression and understanding of the emotions of both the dying person and the family, allowing the person or family as much control as possible.

   c. Facilitate discussions with the family about the dying person's roles within the family so that the family can make decisions about the dying experience.

   d. Assess the person's or family's communication style and teach them the best communication strategies.

4. Which of the following is characteristic of stupor in the dying person?

   a. Drowsiness is prominent

   b. Cannot think quickly or clearly

   c. Unresponsive but briefly arousable

   d. Does not react to physical stimuli

5. The hospice palliative care nurse has been following a client who is in bereavement. Which of the signs and symptoms might suggest grief that needs to be medically assessed?

   a. Crying at any time of the day or night without warning

   b. Continuing to experience sadness, loss, and depression not relieved over time or offset by periods of pleasure and joy

   c. Feeling pain and loss that reoccur with various memories and significant dates

   d. Experiencing grief that interrupts daily life activities and at certain times causes the bereaved person to withdraw

6. Which of the following is a characteristic of an advance directive?

   a. Writing one should occur only when the client is facing a life-threatening situation.

   b. Writing one involves exploring the client's goals and values if he or she should face a life-threatening event.

   c. Writing one typically does not involve family members.

   d. After one is written, it is signed by the client and never reviewed again.

7. Which of the following is an experience of suffering at the end of life?

   a. It is often linked to an individual's search for meaning.

   b. It is alleviated with good symptom control.

   c. It is always understood when the sufferer searches for religious beliefs.

   d. It can always be alleviated by the nurse.

8. Dyspnea is defined as which of the following?

   a. A subjective sensation that appears only in certain diseases, such as COPD

   b. The medical term for hyperinflation of the chest

   c. A state that is always related to the client's oxygen saturation level

   d. A subjective sensation involving both the individual's perception of breathlessness and his or her reaction to it

9. Which of the following is the truest statement about chronic pain at the end of life?

   a. It can be managed like acute pain, with opioid analgesics given as needed.

   b. Analgesics are most effective if administered regularly (around the clock), with breakthrough medication, if needed.

   c. Once pain is stabilized, the routine of how analgesics are administered should not be altered.

   d. Chronic pain usually is treated with one type of medication that works best for the client.

10. Mr. Hume, 64 years old, is a retired university professor. He has insulin-dependent diabetes and has required hemodialysis three times per week for the past year (for renal failure). He has been admitted for an exacerbation of his condition. After working with his nephrologist and social worker, Mr. Hume decides he no longer wishes to continue with dialysis and is ready to die. What is the MOST appropriate action for the nurse to take?

   a. Tell Mr. Hume that this must have been a difficult decision and that she will continue to care for him.

   b. Notify Mr. Hume's son that his father has decided to discontinue dialysis.

   c. Try to convince Mr. Hume to continue with dialysis for another week.

   d. Share with Mr. Hume that her own father made the same choice a few years ago so she understands his decision.

Check the eText in MyNursingLab for answers and explanations.

WEBLINKS

Canadian Association Schools of Nursing (CASN) (Palliative Care Competencies for Canadian Nurses)

http://www.casn.ca/en/Palliative_Care_122/items/3.html

The CASN is pleased to post a new educational resource developed by the CASN Task Force on palliative and end-of-life care that educators may consult in curriculum development in this area of nursing care. The Task Force has identified core competencies specific to this particular field of care as well as general competencies nurses need when providing palliative and end-of-life care.

Caregiver Network Inc.

http://caregiver.ca/content_main.html

Caregiver Network Inc. (CNI), the first of its kind in Canada, is a resource centre created to help caregivers of older adults and people who are ill. The goal of the network is to make caregivers' lives easier by providing information on the internet and in a newsletter (see CNI Services); education through the 13-part TV/video series "Caregiving with June Callwood"; the Canadian Aging and Caregiving Resource Guide; and personal assistance and support through seminar series, care management consulting service, the Caregiver Club, and Care Across the Border.

Canadian Hospice Palliative Care Association

http://www.chpca.net/about_us/mission_statement.htm

The Canadian Hospice Palliative Care Association (CHPCA) is the national association that provides leadership in hospice palliative care in Canada. The CHPCA uses collaboration and representation, increased awareness, knowledge, and skills related to hospice palliative care of the public, health care providers, and volunteers; development of national standards of practice for hospice palliative care in Canada; support of research on hospice palliative care; advocacy for improved hospice palliative care policy; resource allocation; and supports for caregivers to pursue excellence in care for persons approaching death so that the burdens of suffering, loneliness, and grief are lessened.

Hospice Association of Ontario

http://www.hospicelifeline.com

The Hospice Association of Ontario provides information about a wide range of hospice palliative care services and such resources as hospice palliative care programs, hospice palliative care units, community-based services, pain and symptom management, bereavement support services, and palliative care education.

Canadian Virtual Hospice

http://www.virtualhospice.ca

The virtual hospice is a network of information and support for people dealing with life-threatening illness and loss. The website does not offer direct medical advice or clinical care but does offer information and resources that may help people to better understand the physical, emotional, and spiritual aspects of their experiences. The Canadian Virtual Hospice is an interactive network designed to facilitate information exchange, communication, and mutual support among patients, their friends and family, health care providers, and palliative care volunteers.

MyNursingLab

REFERENCES

Anderson, H. (1989). After the diagnosis: An operational theology for the terminally ill. *Journal of Pastoral Care, 43,* 141–150.

Barnard, D., Towers, A., Boston, P., & Lambrinidou, Y. (2000). *Crossing over: Narratives of palliative care.* New York, NY: Oxford University Press.

Bennett Jacobs, B., & Taylor, C. (2005). Seeing artificial hydration and nutrition through an ethical lens. *Home Healthcare Nurse, 23*(11), 749–743.

Billings, J. (1998). What is palliative care? *Journal of Palliative Medicine, 1*(1), 73–81.

Brenneis, C., & Brown, P. (2006). International models of excellence: Palliative care in Canada. In B. Ferrell & N. Coyle (Eds.). *Textbook of palliative nursing* (2nd ed.) (pp. 1147–1159). New York, NY: Oxford University Press.

Brindley, P., Markland, D., Mayers, I., & Kutsogiannis, D. (2002). Predictors of survival following in-hospital adult cardiopulmonary resuscitation. *Canadian Medical Association Journal, 167*(4), 343–348.

Callanan, M. (1994). Dealing with death: Breaking the silence. *American Journal of Nursing, 94,* 22–23.

Canadian Association Schools of Nursing. (2009). *The principles and practice of palliative care nursing and palliative care competencies for Canadian Nurses.* Ottawa, ON: Author.

Canadian Hospice Palliative Care Association. (2010). *Fact Sheet: Hospice palliative care in Canada.* Ottawa, ON: Author.

Canadian Nurses Association. (1995). *Policy Statement: Joint statement on resuscitative interventions.* Ottawa, ON: Author.

Canadian Nurses Association. (1998). *Advance directives: The nurse's role.* Ottawa, ON: Author.

Canadian Nurses Association. (2008). *Providing care at the end of life.* Ottawa, ON: Author.

Canadian Nurses Protective Society. (2006). *Consent for CPR, Infolaw, 15*(2), Ottawa, ON: Author.

Carr, D. (2008). Factors that influence late-life bereavement: Considering data from the changing lives of older couples study. In M. Strobe, R., Hannsson, H., Schut, & W. Strobe (Eds.). *Handbook of bereavement research and practice,* (pp. 417–440). Washington, DC: American Psychological Association.

Chang, V., Hwang, S., Feuerman, M., & Kasimis, B. (2000). Symptom and quality of life survey of medical oncology patients at a veterans' affairs medical center: A role for symptom assessment. *Cancer, 88,* 1175–1183.

Dudgeon, D. (2006). Dyspnea, death rattle and cough. In B. Ferrell & N. Coyle (Eds.). *Textbook of palliative nursing* (2nd ed.) (pp. 249–264). New York, NY: Oxford University Press.

Dudgeon, D., Kristjanson, L., Sloan, J., & Lertzman, M. (2001). Dyspnea in cancer patients: Prevalence and associated factors. *Journal of Pain and Symptom Management, 21*(2), 95–102.

Fainsinger, R., MacEachern, T., Hanson, J., Miller, M., & Bruera, E. (1991). Symptom control during the last week of life on a palliative care unit. *Journal of Palliative Care, 7,* 5–11.

Ferrario, R., Cardillo, V., & Vicario, F. (2004). Advanced cancer at home: Caregiving and bereavement. *Palliative Medicine, 18,* 129–136.

Frank, A. (2004). Dignity, dialogue and care. *Journal of Palliative Care, 20*(3), 207–211.

Ganzini, L. (2006). Artificial nutrition and hydration at the end of life: Ethics and evidence. *Palliative and Supportive Care, 4,* 135–143.

Gilbert, M., Counsell, C., & Guin, P. (2001). Determining the relationship between end-of-life decisions expressed in advance directives and resuscitation efforts during cardiopulmonary resuscitation. *Outcomes Management for Nursing Practice, 5*(2), 87–92.

Golin, C., Wegner, N., & Liu, H. (2000). A prospective study of patient-physician communication about resuscitation. *Journal of American Geriatric Society, 48,* 52–60.

Hartwick Doane, G., & Varcoe, C. (2005). *Family nursing as relational inquiry: Developing heath promoting practice.* Philadelphia, PA: Lippincott Williams & Wilkin.

Helme, R., Meliala, A., & Gibson, S. (2004). Methodologic factors which contribute to variations in experimental pain threshold reported for older people. *Neuroscience Letters, 361*(1–3), 144–146.

Heuberger, R. (2010). Artificial nutrition and hydration at the end-of life. *Journal of Nutrition in Gerontology and Geriatrics, 29*(4), 347–385.

Horowitz, M., Siegel, B., Holen, A., Bonanno, G., Milbrath, C., & Stinson, C. (1997). Diagnostic criteria for complicated grief disorder. *American Journal of Psychiatry, 154,* 904–910.

Jenkins, C., Taube, A., Ken, T., Hanson, J., & Bruera, E. (1998). Initial demographic, symptom, and medication profiles in patients admitted to palliative care units. *Journal of Pain and Symptom Management, 16,* 163–170.

King, D. A., Shields, C. G., & Wynne, L. C. (2005). Family intervention and therapy with older adults. In B. J. Sadock & V. A. Sadock (Eds.). *Comprehensive textbook of psychiatry* (8th ed.) (pp. 3763–3769). Philadelphia, PA: Lippincott, Williams &Wilkins.

Kissane, D. W. (2003). Psychosocial morbidity associated with patterns of family functioning in palliative care: Baseline data from the family focused grief therapy controlled trial. *Palliative Medicine, 17,* 527–537.

Kissane, D. W., Bloch, S., Onghena, P., McKenzie, D., Synde, R., & Dowe, D. (1996). The Melbourne family grief study, II: Psychosocial morbidity and grief in bereaved families. *American Journal of Psychiatry, 13,* 659–666.

Kubler-Ross, E. (1969). *On death and dying.* New York, NY: Macmillan.

Kuhl, D. (2002). *What dying patients want: Practical wisdom for the end of life.* Doubleday Canada

Lazar, N., Shemie, S., Webster, G., & Dickens, B. (2001). Bioethics for clinicians: Brain death. *Canadian Medical Association Journal, 164*(6), 833–836.

Lazaruk, T. (2006). The CPR question. *Canadian Nurse, 102*(2), 22–24.

Lowy, F., Sawyer, D., & Williams, J. (1993). *Canadian physicians and euthanasia.* Ottawa, ON: Canadian Medical Association.

Mallory, J., (2003). The impact of a palliative care educational component on attitudes toward care of the dying in undergraduate nursing students. *Journal of Professional Nursing, 19*(5), 305–312.

Martin, T., & Dolka, K. (2000). *Men don't cry, women do: Transcending gender stereotypes of grief.* Philadelphia, PA: Brunner/Mazel.

Martocchio, B. C. (1985). Grief and bereavement: Healing through hurt. *Nursing Clinics of North America, 20,* 327–341.

Meuser, T., Pietruck, C., Radbruch, L., Stute, P., Lehmann, K., & Grond, S. (2001). Symptoms during cancer pain treatment following WHO guidelines: A longitudinal follow-up study of symptom prevalence, severity, and etiology. *Pain, 93,* 247–257.

Mok, E., Lee, W., & Wong, F. (2002). The issue of death and dying: Employing problem based learning in nursing education. *Nurse Education Today, 22*(4), 319–329.

Morita, T., Ichiki, T., Tsunoda, J., Inoue, S., & Chihaa, S. (1998). A prospective study on the dying process in terminally ill cancer patients. *American Journal of Hospice and Palliative Care, 15,* 217–222.

Moules, N. J. (1998). Legitimizing grief: Challenging beliefs that constrain. *Journal of Family Nursing, 4*(2), 142–166.

Moules, N. J. (1999). Suffering together: Whose words were they? *Journal of Family Nursing, 5*(3), 251–258.

Moules, N. J. (2000). Funerals, families and family nursing: Lessons of love and practice. *Journal of Family Nursing, 6*(1), 3–8.

Moules, N. J., & Amundson, J. K. (1997). Grief—An invitation to inertia: A narrative approach to working with grief. *Journal of Family Nursing, 3*(4), 378–393.

Moules, N., Simonson, K., Fleiszer, A., Prins, M., & Glasgow, B. (2007). The soul of sorrow work: Grief and therapeutic interventions with families. *Journal of Family Nursing, 13*(1), 1–25.

Moules, N., Simonson, K., Prins, M., Angus, P., & Bell, J. (2004). Making room for grief: Walking backwards and living forward. *Nursing Inquiry, 11*(2), 99–107.

Ng, K., & von Gunten, C. (1998). Symptoms and attitudes of 100 consecutive patients admitted to an acute hospice/palliative care unit. *Journal of Pain and Symptom Management, 16,* 307–316.

Paice, J., & Fine, P. (2006). Pain at the end of life. In B. Ferrell & N. Coyle (Eds.), *Textbook of palliative nursing* (2nd ed.) (pp. 131–153). New York, NY: Oxford University Press.

Parageon, K., & Hailey, B. (1999). Barriers to effective cancer pain management: A review of the literature. *Journal of Pain and Symptom Management, 18,* 358–368.

Perry, B. (2008). Why exemplary oncology nurses seem to avoid compassion fatigue. *Canadian Oncology Nursing Journal, 18*(2), 87–99.

Pereira, J., & Bruera, E. (2001). *Alberta palliative care resource book.* Edmonton, AB: Alberta Cancer Board.

Prigerson, H., Maciejewski, P., & Reynolds, C. (1995). Inventory of complicated grief: A scale to measure maladaptive symptoms of loss. *Psychiatry Research, 59,* 65–79.

Qualls, S. (2000). Therapy with aging families: Rationale, opportunities and challenges. *Aging Mental Health, 4,* 191–199.

Raffin, S. (2002). *Accompanying the dying: Nurses create a moral space for suffering.* Unpublished doctoral dissertation, University of Alberta, Edmonton, Canada.

Raffin Bouchal, S. (2007). Moral meanings in caring for the dying. In N. E. Johnston & A. Scholler-Jaquish (Eds.). *Meaning in suffering: Caring practices in the health professions. Vol. VI of interpretive studies in healthcare and the human sciences* (pp. 232–275). Chicago, IL: University of Wisconsin Press.

Richter, J. M. (1984). Crisis of mate loss in the elderly. *American Nursing Society, 6*(4), 45–54.

Robinson, E. M. (2002). An ethical analysis of cardiopulmonary resuscitation for elders in acute care. *AACN Clinical Issues, 13*(1), 132–144.

Rolland, J. S. (2003). Mastering family challenges in illness and disability. In F. Walsh (Ed.). *Normal family process* (3rd ed.) (pp. 460–489). New York, NY: Guilford.

Rolland, J. S. (2004). Helping families with anticipatory loss and terminal illness. In F. Walsh & M. McGoldrick (Eds.). *Living beyond loss: Death in the family* (2nd ed.) (pp. 213–236). New York: WW Norton.

Roy, D., Williams, J., Dickens, B. (1994). *Bioethics in Canada.* Scarborough, ON: Prentice-Hall.

Senate of Canada, (2010). *Raising the bar: A roadmap for the future of palliative care in Canada.* Ottawa, ON: Author

Simon, S., Ramsenthaler, C., Bausewein, C., Krischke, N., & Geiss, G. (2009). Core attitudes of professionals in palliative care: A qualitative study. *International Journal of Palliative Nursing, 14*(8), 405–411.

Sinclair, S. (2011). Impact of death on the personal lives and practices of palliative care professionals. *Canadian Medical Association Journal, 183*(2), 180–187.

Sinclair, S., Pereira, J., & Raffin, S. (2006). A thematic review of the spirituality literature within palliative care. *Journal of Palliative Medicine, 9*(2), 464–479.

Sinclair, S., Raffin, S., Pereira, J., & Guebert, N. (2006). Collective soul: The spirituality of an interdisciplinary palliative care team. *Palliative and Supportive Care, 4,* 13–24.

Statistics Canada. (2010). *Projections for Canada, provinces and territories*—2005–2031. Statistics Canada, Catalogue #91-520. p. 50.

Statistics Canada. (2010). *Deaths in hospital and elsewhere, Canada, provinces and territories,* annual CANSIM (database) Statistics Canada, Table 102-0509. Retrieved from http://cansim2.stancan.gc.ca/cgi-win/cnsmcgi.pgm

Stajduhar, K., Martin, W., & Cairns, M. (2010). What makes grief difficult? Perspectives from bereaved family caregivers and healthcare providers of advanced cancer patients. *Palliative and Supportive Care, 8,* 277–289. doi: 10.1017/S1478951510000076

Storch, J. (2006). The CPR question: Commentary. *Canadian Nurse, 102*(2), 23–24.

Tapp, A. (2006). Advance directives. *Canadian Nurse, 102*(2), 26.

Wald, L. (1999). Hospice care in the United States: A conversation with Florence S. Wald. *Journal of the American Medical Association, 281,* 1683–1685.

Walsh, F., & McGoldrick, M. (Eds.). (2004). *Living beyond loss: Death in the family* (2nd ed.). New York, NY: WW Norton.

Weihs, K., & Reiss, D. (1996). Family re-organization in response to cancer: A developmental perspective. In L. Baider & C. Cooper (Eds.). *Cancer and the family* (pp. 3–29). Oxford, UK: John Wiley & Sons.

Wells, N. (2000). Pain intensity and pain interference in hospitalized patients with cancer. *Oncology Nursing Forum, 27,* 985–991.

White, M. (1989). Saying hello again: The incorporation of the lost relationship in the resolution of grief. In M. White (Ed.). *Selected papers* (pp. 29–36). Adelaide, Australia: Dulwich Centre.

Wilson, D., Northcott, H., Truman, C., Smith, S., Anderson, M., Fainsinger, R., & Stingl, M. J. (2001). Location of death in Canada: A comparison of 20th century hospital and non-hospital locations of death and corresponding population trends. *Evaluation and the Health Professions, 24*(4), 385–403.

Winchester Nadeau, J. (2008). Meaning making in bereaved families: Assessment, intervention, and future research. In M. Stroebe, R. Hansson, W. Stroebe, & H. Schut (Eds.). *Handbook of bereavement research: Consequences, coping and care* (pp. 511–530). Washington, DC: American Psychological Association.

World Health Organization. (1996). *Cancer pain relief and palliative care. Report of a WHO expert committee* (2nd ed.). Geneva, Switzerland: Author. WHO Technical Series #804.

Wright, L. M. (1999). Spirituality, suffering, and beliefs: The soul of healing with families. In F. Walsh (Ed.). *Spiritual resources in families and family therapy* (pp. 61–75). New York, NY: Guilford Press.

Wright, L. M. (2008). Softening suffering through spiritual care practices: One possibility for healing families. *Journal of Family Nursing, 14,* 394. doi: 10.1177/1074840708326493

Glossary

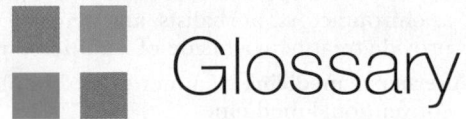

% Daily Value the percentage of each nutrient in one serving of a product relative to the recommended daily intake

24-hour food recall a record of food and fluid intake for a 24-hour period

Aboriginal population people who can trace their origins to First Nations, Inuit, or Métis in Canada

Absorption the process by which a drug passes into the bloodstream

Accessibility residents of a province or territory must have reasonable access to insured services

Accidents unexpected or unplanned events that cause harm and are neither foreseeable nor preventable

Accommodation a process of change whereby cognitive processes mature sufficiently to allow a person to solve problems that were previously unsolvable

Accountability responsibility for one's own actions and acceptance of the consequences of one's own behaviour

Acid a substance which yields hydrogen ions in solution and from which hydrogen may be displaced by a metal to form a salt

Acidosis a condition that occurs with increases in blood carbonic acid or with decreases in blood bicarbonate; blood pH lower than 7.35

Active-assistive range-of-motion (ROM) exercise the client, with the nurse's assistance, uses a stronger, opposite arm or leg to move each of the joints of a limb incapable of active motion

Active immunity a resistance of the body to infection in which the host produces its own antibodies in response to natural or artificial antigens

Active living adding physical activity to the time spent at home, at work, at school, at play

Active range-of-motion (ROM) exercise isotonic exercises in which the client moves each joint in the body through its complete range of movement, maximally stretching all muscle groups within each plane, over the joint

Active transport movement of substances across cell membranes against the concentration gradient

Activity-exercise pattern refers to a person's pattern of exercise, activity, leisure, and recreation

Activity theory describes the best way to age as staying physically active during these years

Activity tolerance the type and amount of exercise or daily activities an individual is able to perform

Actual loss can be identified by others and can arise either in response to or in anticipation of a situation

Actual nursing diagnosis a client problem that is present at the time of the nursing assessment

Acupressure form of massage in which firm, gentle pressure is applied to the acupuncture points of the body

Acupuncture a Chinese practice of piercing specific superficial nerves with needles, often to treat pain

Acute confusion a mental state in which a person appears bewildered and may make inappropriate statements and answers to questions

Acute illness rapidly occurring illness that runs its course and the individual then returns to previous level of functioning

Acute pain pain that lasts only through the expected recovery period and is purposeful, informing the person that something is wrong

Acute wound a wound that heals within an expected time frame

Adaptation the process of modifying to meet new, changing, or different conditions

Adaptive mechanisms (defence mechanisms) learned behaviours that assist an individual to adjust to the environment

Addiction a psychological dependence characterized by craving for and compulsive use of opioids for an effect other than pain relief

Additional precautions measures used in addition to routine practices for clients with *known* or *suspected* infections that are spread by airborne transmission, by droplet transmission, or by contact to prevent the spread of infection

Additive effect when two of the same types of drug increase the action of each other

Adequate intake the recommended intake value of a specific vitamin, micromineral, or macromineral when a recommended dietary allowance cannot be established

Adherence a client's willingness to follow a treatment regimen

Adolescence the period during which a person becomes physically and psychologically mature and acquires a personal identity; usually from 12 to 18 or 20 years of age in North America

Advance directive a statement the client makes prior to receiving health care specifying the client's desires regarding health care decisions

Adventitious breath sounds abnormal or acquired breath sounds

Adverse effect (secondary effect) an unintended and undesired effect of a drug; they are usually predictable

Adverse event unintended injuries or complications that result in death, disability, or prolonged hospital stays as a result of health care management

Adverse event reporting reporting of injuries related to health care management rather than disease process; the event is an unplanned, undesired harmful outcome directly associated with care service

Advocacy pleading and supporting clients' rights by respecting client decisions and enhancing client autonomy

Aerobic exercise any activity during which the body takes in more or an equal amount of oxygen than it expends

Aesthetic knowing the art of nursing; expressed by the individual nurse through his or her creativity and style in meeting the needs of clients

Afebrile absence of a fever

Affective domain feelings, emotions, interests, attitudes, and appreciations, and five major learning categories

Afterload (peripheral resistance) the resistance against which the heart must pump to eject the blood into the circulation

Ageism the stereotypes that promote negative views of older adults as frail, dependent, and in need of long-term care

Agglutinins specific antibodies formed in the blood

Agglutinogens substances that act as antigens and stimulate the production of agglutinins

Aging in place a process that enables older adults to age within the comfort and familiarity of their own homes

Agnostic a person who doubts the existence of God or a supreme being or believes the existence of God has not been proved

Agonist a drug that interacts with a receptor to produce a response

Agonist–antagonist analgesic drugs that can act like opioids and relieve pain when given to a client who has not taken any pure opioids but can block or inactivate other opioid analgesics when given to a client who has been taking pure opioids

Agriculture assets that come from cultivating soil, producing crops, and raising livestock to create wealth

Airborne precautions practices initiated to prevent the spread of airborne microorganisms

Airborne transmission when air currents transport the microorganism

Alarm reaction (AR) the initial stage of the adaptation syndrome described by Selye

Albinism the complete or partial lack of melanin in the skin, hair, and eyes

Alcohol-based hand rub (ABHR) a hand sanitizer that kills microorganisms and is more effective than soap and water in reducing hand contamination

Algor mortis the gradual decrease of the body's temperature after death

Alkalosis a condition that occurs with increases in blood bicarbonate or decreases in blood carbonic acid; blood pH above 7.45

Allodynia the sensation of pain from a stimulus that normally does not produce pain

Alopecia the loss of scalp hair (baldness) or body hair

Alternative care providers health care workers, such as chiropractors, herbalists, and acupuncturists, who provide treatment outside of traditional medicine

Alternative medicine treatments used in place of conventional medicine

Alzheimer's disease the most common type of dementia; characterized by plaques (numerous tiny dense and toxic deposits scattered throughout the brain) and tangles, both of which interefere with vital process, eventually choking off living cells

Amblyopia reduced visual acuity in one eye

Ambulation the act of walking

Ampule a small glass container for individual doses of liquid medications

Anabolism a process in which simple substances are converted by the body cells into more complex substances (e.g., building tissue, positive nitrogen balance)

Anaerobic exercise exercise that involves activity in which the muscles cannot draw out enough oxygen from the bloodstream; used in endurance training

Anal stimulation sexual stimulation of the anus, applied with fingers, mouth, or sex toys

Anaphylactic reaction a severe allergic reaction

Andragogy the art and science of helping adults learn

Androgyny the belief that most characteristics and behaviours are human qualities that should not be limited to one specific gender or the other

Andropause the phase in men's lives in which they experience a gradual reduction in the production of testosterone and sperm by the testes

Anesthesia loss of sensation or feeling; induced loss of the sense of pain

Anger a subjective emotional state of strong displeasure

Angiography a diagnostic procedure enabling radiographic visual examination of the vascular system after injection of a radiopaque dye

Angle of Louis the junction between the body of the sternum and the manubrium; the starting point for locating the ribs anteriorly

Animal-assisted therapy the use of specifically selected animals as a treatment modality in health and human service settings

Anions ions that carry a negative charge: chloride, bicarbonate, phosphate, sulphate

Anisocoria unequal pupils

Ankle flare an ulcer near or on the ankle associated with venous hypertension or varicose veins

Ankle-brachial index (ABI) a calculated number that indicates the amount of arterial blood flow to the extremity

Anorexia lack of appetite

Anorexia nervosa a disease characterized by a prolonged inability or refusal to eat, rapid weight loss, and emaciation in persons who continue to believe they are fat

Anoscopy visual examination of the anal canal using an anoscope (a lighted instrument)

Antagonist a drug that interferes with a cell receptor without stimulating it and blocks the action of an agonist

Antibodies (immunoglobulin) protective protein substances produced in the body to counteract antigens

Anticipatory loss the state in which an individual or group experiences reactions in response to an expected significant loss

Antigens substances capable of inducing the formation of antibodies

Antihelix the semicircular ridge on the anterior of the ear and parallel to the helix

Antimicrobial agents materials that kill or slow the growth of infectious agents

Antiseptic an agent that inhibits the growth of some microorganisms

Anuria the failure of the kidneys to produce urine, resulting in a total lack of urination or output of less than 100 mL per day in an adult

Anxiety a state of mental uneasiness, apprehension, or dread producing an increased level of arousal caused by an impending or anticipated threat to self or significant relationships

Apex the pointed end of a cone-shaped part

Apgar scores a scoring system to assess newborn babies

Aphasia inability to communicate through speech, writing, or signs, caused by dysfunction of the brain centre

Apical pulse a central pulse located at the apex of the heart

Apical–radial pulse measurement of the apical beat and the radial pulse at the same time

Apnea a complete absence of respirations

Apocrine glands glands that increase secretions and become fully functioning during puberty; release sweat in response to emotional stimuli

Application software computer programs that allow someone using a computer to perform functions or work tasks

Applied research research that uses knowledge to solve immediate problems

Appreciative inquiry (AI) an approach to organization change that focuses on what is positive by asking participants to share their experiences and successes, examine the challenges, and explore what is working well

Arcus senilis partial or complete glossy, white circle around the periphery of the cornea; appears later in life

Aromatherapy the therapeutic use of essential oils of plants in which the odour or fragrance plays an important part

Arrhythmia (dysrhythmia) a pulse with an abnormal rhythm

Arterial blood gases (ABGs) oxygen and carbon dioxide concentrations (PO_2, PCO_2), hydrogen ion concentration (pH), and oxygen saturation of the hemoglobin in arterial blood; also describe the laboratory tests that measure these levels

Asepsis freedom from infection or infectious material

Aseptic technique (clean technique) the absence of almost all but not all microorganisms

Asphyxiation (suffocation) a lack of oxygen intake that can ultimately lead to unconsciousness and death

Assault an attempt or threat to touch another person unjustifiably

Assessing the process of collecting, organizing, validating, and recording data (information) about a client's health status

Assimilation (of a group) the blending of attitudes and beliefs; the process by which members of a foreign culture learn the values and behaviours of a culture to which they have immigrated

Assumptions statements of fact or suppositions that people accept as the underlying theoretical foundation for conceptualizations about a phenomenon

Astigmatism an uneven curvature of the cornea that prevents horizontal and vertical rays from focusing on the retina

Atelectasis a condition that occurs when ventilation is decreased and pooled secretions accumulate in a dependent area of a bronchiole and block it

Atheist a person who denies the existence of God

Atria (of the heart) two upper hollow chambers within the heart

Atrioventricular (AV) node in place in the heart where the conduction pathways converge and narrow, slightly delaying transmission of the impulse to the ventricles

At-risk aggregate a subgroup within the community or population that is at greater risk of illness or poor recovery

Atrophie blanche white atrophic lesions often associated with venous disease

Atrophy wasting away; decrease in size of organ or tissue (e.g., muscle)

Attachment lasting, strong emotional bonds

Attentive listening using all the senses and body positioning to listen to the client

Attitudes mental stances that are composed of many different beliefs; usually involving positive or negative judgments toward a person, object, or idea

Audit (nursing) a process in which the nursing interventions are monitored and measured against established standards

Auricle (pinna) flap of the ear

Auscultation the process of listening to sounds produced within the body

Auscultatory gap the temporary disappearance of sounds normally heard over the brachial artery when the sphygmomanometer cuff pressure is high and the sounds reappear at a lower level

Authority the power given by an organization to direct the work of others; the right to act

Autoantigen an antigen that despite being a constituent of normal tissue is the target of a cell-mediated response

Autocratic (authoritarian, directive) leaders have an authoritarian style of leadership in which the leader makes decisions for the group

Autonomy (respect for persons) the state of being independent and self-directed without outside control to make one's own decisions

Awareness the ability to perceive environmental stimuli and body reactions and to respond appropriately through thought and action

Axillary tail of Spence a projection of breast tissue into the axilla

Ayurveda the Indian system of medicine that views illness as a state of imbalance among the body's systems

Baby boomers the generation of people born between 1945 and 1964, who are characterized as being extremely hard working

Baccalaureate nursing degrees programs offered by universities, university colleges, and polytechnical institutes that lead to an undergraduate degree in nursing

Bacteremia bacteria in blood

Bacteria infection-causing agents

Bactericidal capable of killing some microorganisms (bacteria)

Balance consists of mental, physical, emotional, spiritual, and environmental components and is attained when each component reaches a state of equilibrium

Bandage a strip of cloth used to wrap some part of the body

Bandwidth the speed of information transmission online

Basal metabolic rate (BMR) the rate of energy utilization in the body required to maintain essential activities, such as breathing

Basal metabolism the minimal energy expended for the maintenance of all physical and chemical processes

Base (heart) sometimes used to refer to the upper portion of the heart (both atria)

Base (alkali) the nonacid part of a salt; a substance that combines with acids to form salts

Base of support the area on which an object rests

Basic research research that generates knowledge; sometimes called *pure research*

Battery the willful or negligent touching of a person (or the person's clothes or even something the person is carrying), which may or may not cause harm

Bed rest restriction of a client's activities, either partially or completely

Bedpan a receptacle for urine and feces used by people confined to bed

Behavioural domain the cultural skill that enables the health care provider to learn about client's cultural values, beliefs, and practices to determine the most appropriate goals and interventions

Behavioural effect questions explores the effect of one family member's behaviour on another

Beliefs interpretations or conclusions that a person accepts as true

Beneficence the moral obligation to do good or to implement actions that benefit clients and their support persons

Bevel the slanted part at the tip of a needle

Bicultural used to describe a person who crosses two cultures, lifestyles, and sets of values

Bioelectromagnetic therapy treatment that involves the use of electromagnetic fields, such as pulsed fields, magnetic fields, or alternating current or direct current fields, in people with diseases ranging from asthma and arthritis, poisoning and tubal pregnancy, to wrinkles

Biofeedback a stress management technique that brings under conscious control bodily processes normally thought to be beyond voluntary command

Biot's (cluster) respiration shallow breaths interrupted by apnea

Bioterrorism the use of a microorganism with the deliberate intent of causing infection to achieve certain goals

Biotransformation (detoxification, metabolism) the process by which a drug is converted to a less active form

Bladder training a program designed to assist clients experiencing difficulty in controlling the flow of urine

Blanch test a test during which the client's fingernail is temporarily pinched to assess capillary refill and peripheral circulation

Blindness visual acuity of 20/200 with the best correction possible

Blood-borne pathogens infectious microorganisms in human blood that can cause disease, such as HIV, hepatitis B, and hepatitis C

Blood pressure the pressure of blood against the walls of blood vessels

Blood urea nitrogen (BUN) a measure of blood level of urea, the end product of protein metabolism

Body image how a person perceives the size, appearance, and functioning of their body and its parts

Body mass index (BMI) indicates whether weight is appropriate for height

Body mechanics the efficient and coordinated use of the body to produce motion and maintain balance during activity

Body temperature the balance between the heat produced by the body and the heat lost from the body

Boomerang kids young adults who move back into their parents' homes after an initial period of independent living

Borborgymi hyperactive or increased bowel sounds

Bottle-mouth syndrome the decay of an infant's teeth caused by constant contact with the sweet liquid in a bottle

Boundaries limits in which a person may act or refrain from acting within a designated time or place

Boundary a real or imaginary line that differentiates one system from another system or a system from its environment

Bowel incontinence (fecal incontinence) refers to the loss of voluntary ability to control fecal and gaseous discharges through the anal sphincter

Bowman's capsule the central capsule of each nephron

Bradycardia abnormally slow pulse rate, fewer than 60 per minute

Bradypnea abnormally slow respiratory rate, usually fewer than 10 respirations per minute

Brand name (trade name) the name given by the drug manufacturer

Bromhidrosis foul-smelling perspiration

Bronchoscopy visual examination of the bronchi using a bronchoscope

Bruit a blowing or swishing sound created by turbulence of blood flow

B-type natriuretic peptide (BNP) a peptide released in response to increased ventricular filling pressures and is a routine blood test for diagnosing heart failure

Buccal pertaining to the cheek

Buffers agents or systems that tend to maintain constancy or that prevent changes in the chemical concentration of a substance

Bulimia nervosa an uncontrollable compulsion to eat large amounts of food and then expel it by self-induced vomiting or by taking laxatives

Bullying an abusive, intimidating treatment of someone who is in a vulnerable position or a position with less power

Bureaucratic leader has a style of leadership in which the leader is impersonal and inflexible; policies, procedures, and rules serve as the bases for decision making

Burn injury to tissue caused by contact with dry or moist heat

Burnout a complex syndrome of behaviours that can be likened to the exhaustion stage of the general adaptation syndrome; an overwhelming feeling that can lead to physical and emotional depletion, a negative attitude and self-concept, and feelings of helplessness and hopelessness

Callus a thickened portion of skin

Caloric value the amount of energy that nutrients or foods supply to the body

Calorie (large calorie, C, Cal, kilocalorie, kcal) a unit of heat energy equivalent to the amount of heat required to raise the temperature of 1 kg of water 1°C

Cannula (shaft) a tube with a lumen (channel) that is inserted into a cavity or duct and is often fitted with a trocar during insertion

Capacity the client's ability to understand the relevant information and appreciate the consequences of his or her decision that might reasonably be foreseen

Capacity building a long-term, continual process of development that involves all stakeholders in a population and uses a country's human, scientific, technological, and organizational resources and capabilities

Carbon monoxide a colourless, odourless, toxic gas that is a product of incomplete combustion; exposure can cause symptoms of headaches, dizziness, weakness, nausea, vomiting, or loss of muscle control, leading to unconsciousness, brain damage, or death

Cardiac arrest the cessation of heart function

Cardiac monitoring continuous observation of the client's cardiac rhythm

Cardiac output (CO) the amount of blood ejected by the heart with each ventricular contraction

Cardiopulmonary resuscitation (CPR) artificial stimulation of the heart and lungs; also referred to as *basic life support (BLS)*

Caregiver burden strain placed on informal care providers, usually family members, because of the care required by an individual

Caries (dental) tooth cavities

Caring the feeling and expressing of empathy for other; it is an essential aspect of nursing but varies among cultures in its expressions, processes, and patterns

Caring practice nursing practice that involves connection, mutual recognition, and involvement between the nurse and the client

Carrier a person or animal that harbours a specific infectious agent and serves as a potential source of infection, yet does not manifest any clinical signs of disease

Case management a method for delivering nursing care in which the nurse is responsible for a case load of clients across the health care continuum

Case managers health care professionals who coordinate care for a specific client population and collaborate with other health care professionals and clients to achieve established outcomes

Case method a method in which one nurse is assigned to and is responsible for the comprehensive care of a group of clients over a shift

Catabolism a process in which complex substances are broken down into simpler substances (e.g., breakdown of tissue)

Cataracts opacity of the lens or capsule of the eye

Cations ions that carry a positive charge: sodium, potassium, calcium, magnesium

Ceiling dose the level at which increasing the dose results in no further increase in analgesia

Ceiling effect larger doses of a medication have progressively smaller incremental effects

Cell-mediated defences (cellular immunity) occurs through the T cell system

Cellular immunity (cell-mediated defence) occurs through the T cell system

Cementum bony tissue covering the root of the tooth that is embedded in the jaw

Central disinhibition causes hyperexcitability of the central pain neurons because of the loss of control mechanisms that usually inhibit the conduction of a pain signal

Central neuropathic pain pain that results from malfunctioning nerves in the central nervous system, such as spinal cord injury pain, poststroke pain, and multiple sclerosis pain

Central sensitization prolonged firing of nociceptors with severe and persistent injury, such as surgery, causes dorsal horn spinal cord neurons to become more responsive to all inputs

Central venous catheter a venous access device commonly introduced into the subclavian or internal jugular veins and passed to the superior vena cava just above the right atrium

Centre of gravity the point at which the mass (weight) of the body is centred

Certification the voluntary practice of validating that an individual nurse has met minimum standards of nursing competence in a specialty area

Cerumen the wax-like substance secreted by glands in the external ear canal

Change the process of modifying or altering something

Change agent a person (or group) who initiates changes or who assists others in making modifications in themselves or in the system

Change-of-shift report report usually given to nurses starting the next shift

Charismatic leader is able to evoke strong feelings of commitment to the leader and the leader's cause and beliefs

Chart (client record) the clinical record

Charting (recording) keeping a clinical record of the facts about a client and the progression of an illness

Charting by exception a documentation system in which only significant findings or exceptions to norms are recorded

Chemical name the name by which a chemist knows the drug; describes the constituents of the drug precisely

Chemical restraints medications used to control socially disruptive behaviour

Chemical thermogenesis the stimulation of heat production in the body through increased cellular metabolism caused by increases in thyroxine output

Chemotaxis the action by which leukocytes are attracted to injured cells

Cheyne-Stokes respirations rhythmic waxing and waning of respirations from very deep breathing to very shallow breathing with periods of temporary apnea, often associated with cardiac failure, increased intracranial pressure, or brain damage

Chiropractic therapy treatment that focuses on the spine and its relation to the component bone structures, muscles, and nerves and treats a variety of symptoms thorough spinal manipulation or adjustment

Choking a person's trachea being obstructed by either a foreign body, such as a chunk of food, or a liquid, such as vomitus; can lead to suffocation

Cholesterol a lipid that does not contain fatty acid but possesses many of the chemical and physical properties of other lipids

Chronic illness sickness that lasts for an extended period, usually longer than 6 months

Chronic pain pain that lasts beyond the usual course for recovery and has no purpose

Chronic wound any break or alteration in the skin that remains for 3 months or more or recurs frequently

Chyme digested products that leave the stomach through the small intestine and then pass through the ileocecal valve

Cicatrix scar

Circadian rhythm the roughly 24-hour cycle in the sleep–wake processes that are regulated in all mammals by the suprachiasmatic nuclei of the hypothalamus

Circulating nurse during operations, the nurse who coordinates activities and manages client care by continually assessing client safety, aseptic practice, and the environment

Circulatory diseases diseases that affect the circulatory system, which is the system that moves blood throughout the body, comprising the heart, arteries, capillaries, and veins

Civil law legislative rules that regulate relationships among people

Claudication reduced arterial elasticity, which may result in diminished blood circulation to such areas as the legs, resulting in calf muscle pain on exertion

Clean technique (aseptic technique) the absence of almost all but not all microorganisms

Clean-contaminated wounds surgical wounds in which the respiratory, alimentary, genital, or urinary tract has been entered under controlled conditions and without unusual contamination

Clean wounds uninfected operative wounds without inflammation

Cleansing baths bathing done for hygiene purposes

Clear fluid diet a diet consisting of water, tea, coffee, clear broths, ginger ale or other carbonated beverages, strained and clear juices, and plain gelatin

Client a person who engages the advice or services of another person who is qualified to provide this service

Client education a major aspect of nursing practice; providing information and teaching on issues for which clients have expressed needs and in a manner that is meaningful and relevant to them to promote, protect, maintain, and restore health, and cope with illness or altered health status

Client health outcomes the anticipated, predetermined outcomes that the client selects in collaboration with the nurse to guide and inform nursing practice

Client record (chart) the clinical record

Clients' rights self-determination and control over clients' own bodies when they were ill through informed consent, confidentiality, and the right of the client to accept or refuse treatment are all aspects of this self-determination

Climacteric the point in development when reproduction capacity in the female terminates (menopause) and the sexual activity of the male decreases (andropause)

Climate change occurs when long-term weather patterns change

Clinical judgment the interpretation or conclusion about a client's needs, concerns, or health problems, or the decision to take action (or not), use or modify standard approaches, or improvise new ones as deemed appropriate by the client's response

Clinical Judgment Model a model that includes four aspects that can be used within continuously evolving practice environments: noticing, interpreting, responding, and reflection

Clinical reasoning a thought process used to assess a client's evolving situation and health care concerns, gather data, and make decisions to solve problems within a particular clinical context to achieve better client outcomes

Closed questions restrictive questions requiring only a short answer

Closed system a system that does not exchange energy, matter, or information with its environment

Closed-wound drainage system a drain connected to either an electric suction or a portable drainage suction

Clouding of consciousness a reduced state of wakefulness or awareness

Clubbing (of a nail) elevation of the proximal aspect of the nail and softening of the nail bed

Coanalgesic (formerly known as an *adjuvant*) a medication that is not classified as a pain medication but has properties that may reduce pain alone or in combination with other analgesics, relieve other discomforts, potentiate the effect of pain medications, or reduce the pain medication's side effects

Cochlea a seashell-shaped structure found in the inner ear; essential for sound transmission and hearing

Code of ethics a formal statement of a group's ideals and values; a set of ethical principles shared by members of a group, reflecting their moral judgments and serving as a standard for professional actions

Cognitive the act of knowing or the development of knowledge

Cognitive development the manner in which people learn to think, reason, and use language; it involves a person's intelligence, perceptual ability, and ability to process information, and represents a progression of mental abilities from illogical to logical thinking, from simple to complex problem solving, and from understanding concrete ideas to understanding abstract concepts

Cognitive domain six intellectual skills from the simple to the complex, beginning with knowing, comprehending, and applying

Cognitive skills referring to intellectual processes, such as remembering, thinking, perceiving, abstracting, and generalizing

Cognitive theory depicts learning as a complex cognitive activity, that is, largely a mental or intellectual or thinking process

Colic acute abdominal pain caused by periodic contractions of the intestines during the first 3 months of life

Collaborative care plan a standardized plan that outlines the care required for clients with common, predictable (usually medical) conditions

Collaborative interventions actions the nurse carries out in collaboration with other health care team members

Collaborative relational stance a position that values the multiple ideas and perspectives that are encountered within a family

Collagen a protein found in connective tissue; a whitish protein substance that adds tensile strength to a wound

Collective prescription (protocol order) a set of criteria and orders under which a medication is to be administered

Colloid osmotic pressure (oncotic pressure) a pulling force exerted by colloids that help maintain the water content of blood

Colloids substances, such as large plasma protein molecules, that do not readily dissolve in true solution

Colonialism the ruling of one country or people by another through policies that keep the colony dependent on the rulers

Colonization the presence of organisms in body secretions or excretions in which strains of bacteria become resident flora but do not cause illness

Colonoscopy visual examination of the interior of the colon with a colonoscope

Colostomy an opening into the colon (large bowel)

Coma a state of unconsciousness in which the person shows no response to maximum painful stimuli, absence of reflexes, and absence of muscle tone in the extremities

Commendations statements of praise or support

Commode a portable chair with a toilet seat and a receptacle beneath that can be emptied that is used for the adult client who can get out of bed but is unable to walk to the bathroom

Common law the body of principles that evolves from court decisions

Communicability the ability of a disease to be spread from one person to another

Communicable disease a disease that can spread from one person to another

Communication a two-way process involving the sending and receiving of messages

Community-based health care (CBHC) a system that provides health-related services within the context of people's daily lives; that is, in places where people spend their time in the community

Community health assessment a holistic assessment that involves many areas, including community members, physical environments, socioeconomic environments, health and social services, culture and religion, communication, transportation, government and politics, law and safety, and education and healthy childhood development.

Community health nurses (CHNs) registered nurses whose practice specialty promotes the health of individuals, families, communities, and populations, and an environment that supports health

Compensation (acid–base imbalance) a process whereby healthy regulatory systems attempt to correct acid–base imbalances

Compensatory counterbalancing

Competent care the ability to make sound or rational informed decisions regarding health care, demonstrating understanding and ability to see consequences of care

Complementary medicine treatment that is used together with conventional or Western medicine

Complete proteins proteins that contain all of the essential amino acids as well as many nonessential ones

Complex regional pain syndrome a term used for a number of pain conditions whose etiology is poorly understood

Compliance (client) the extent to which an individual's behaviour coincides with medical or health advice

Compliance (of arteries) the distensibility of the arteries (i.e., their ability to contract and expand)

Comprehensiveness the health services provided by hospitals and medical practitioners are insured in all health care insurance plans of each province and territory

Compress a moist gauze dressing applied frequently to an open wound, sometimes medicated

Compromised hosts any person at increased risk for an infection

Computer provider order entry (CPOE) a computer system that allows a clinician or provider to enter treatment and medication orders electronically

Concept an abstract idea or mental image of phenomena or reality

Concept map pieces of information or ideas presented in a visual scheme with links or relationships among them

Concept mapping a technique that uses a graphic depiction of nonlinear and linear relationships to represent critical thinking

Conceptual framework a group of related concepts

Conceptual model a graphic illustration of the relationships between concepts

Concurrent audit the evaluation of practices as they occur or while the client is still in the institution

Conduction the transfer of heat from one molecule to another in direct contact

Conduction hearing loss a form of hearing loss in which sound is inadequately conducted through the external or middle ear to the sensorineural apparatus of the inner ear

Confidential information intimate or private knowledge protected under a duty of confidentiality of a health care professional

Confidentiality the right of a client or research subject that any information revealed by that individual will not be made public or available to others

Congruent communication when words and behaviour coincide or are unified

Conjunctivitis inflammation of the bulbar and palpebral conjunctiva

Conscious sedation a minimal depression of level of consciousness during which the client retains the ability to consciously maintain a patent airway and respond appropriately to verbal and physical stimuli

Consciousness (spirituality) the focus of the Hare Krishnas

Consequence-based (teleological) theories examine the outcome of an action in judging whether that action is right or wrong

Constant data information that does not change over time

Constant fever a state in which the body temperature fluctuates minimally but always remains above normal

Constipation passage of small, dry, hard stool or passage of no stool for an abnormally long time

Consumer an individual, a group of people, or a community that uses a service or commodity

Contact precautions precautions taken to prevent the possibility of illnesses easily transmitted by direct contact

Contaminated wound an open, fresh, accidental wound; or a surgical wound involving a major break in sterile technique or gross spillage from the gastrointestinal tract and incisions in which acute, nonpurulent inflammation is visible

Contamination bacteria are present but are neither attached to a wound surface nor replicating

Continuing nursing education lifelong learning or the continuous enhancement of knowledge, skills, and critical thinking required to meet client needs in a changing health care system; planned learning experiences undertaken following a basic nursing education

Continuity of care coordination of services provided to individuals before, during, and after entry into a health care facility

Continuity theory a belief that people maintain their values, habits, and behaviours in old age

Continuous positive airway pressure (CPAP) a therapy that provides a continuous flow of pressurized air to keep upper airway passages open during sleep; often prescribed for the client experiencing obstructive sleep apnea

Continuum of care care given in a variety of settings from the onset of the health challenge to the point at which the recipient of care no longer requires it

Contract a written or verbal agreement between two or more people to do or not do some lawful act

Contractility the inherent ability of cardiac muscle fibres to shorten or contract

Contractual obligations the duty of care established by the presence of an expressed or implied contract

Contractual relationships a legal agreement between two or more parties

Contracture permanent shortening of a muscle and subsequent shortening of tendons and ligaments

Convection the dispersion of heat by air currents

Coordinating the process of ensuring that plans are carried out and evaluating outcomes

Coping the process through which the individual manages the demands of the person–environment relationship that are appraised as stressful

Coping strategy (coping mechanism) any mechanism directed toward stress management

Core self-concept the beliefs and images that are most central to the person's identity

Core temperature the temperature of the deep tissues of the body (e.g., thorax, abdominal cavity); relatively constant at 37°C

Corn a conical, circular, painful, raised area on the toe or foot

Coronary arteries arteries that originate at the base of the aorta, branching out to encircle and penetrate the myocardium; they fill during ventricular relaxation, bringing oxygen-rich blood to the myocardium

Costal breathing (thoracic breathing) breathing involving the external intercostal muscles and other accessory muscles, such as the sternocleidomastoid muscles

Countershock phase part of the alarm phase described by Selye

Creatine phosphokinase an enzyme released into the blood during a myocardial infarction

Creatinine a nitrogenous waste that is excreted in urine

Creatinine clearance a test that uses 24-hour urine and serum creatinine levels to identify the glomerular filtration rate

Creativity the ability to develop and implement new and better solutions or ideas

Credé's manoeuvre manual exertion of pressure on the bladder to force urine out

Crepitation a crackling, grating sound produced by bone rubbing against bone

Crisis an acute, time-limited state of disequilibrium resulting from situational, developmental, or societal sources of stress

Crisis counselling solving immediate problems involving individuals, groups, or families

Crisis intervention a problem-solving technique to promote adaptation and improve future coping

Critical analysis a set of questions a person can apply to a particular situation or idea to determine essential information and ideas and discard superfluous information and ideas

Critical incident an error made in practice that may or may not lead to an adverse event

Critical pathways multidisciplinary guidelines for client care based on specific medical diagnoses designed to achieve predetermined outcomes

Critical thinking a cognitive process that includes creativity, problem solving, and decision making

Critiquing intensive scrutiny of a study, including its strengths and weaknesses, its statistical and clinical significance, and the generalizability of the results

Cross-dressing people who dress in the clothing of the opposite sex

Crown the exposed part of the tooth that is outside the gum

Crystalloids salts that dissolve readily in true solutions

Cues any pieces of information or data that influence decisions

Cultural awareness conscious and informed recognition of the differences and similarities between different cultural or ethnic groups

Cultural competence possessing the required knowledge, skill, and ability to provide safe and effective health care regardless of population or setting

Cultural identity the characteristics of the group which gives the person a sense of identity

Cultural safety considers power relations and the uniqueness of human beings and avoids stereotyping to provide quality nursing care for people from all cultures within their cultural values and norms

Cultural sensitivity respect and appreciation for cultural behaviours based upon an understanding of the other person's perspective

Culturally competent care nursing care that preserves the client's familiar lifeways, makes accommodations in care that are satisfying to clients, and repatterns nursing care to help the client move toward wellness

Culture a world view and set of traditions used and transmitted from generation to generation by a particular group, includes related attitudes and institutions

Culture-specifics those values, beliefs, and patterns of behaviour that tend to be unique to a designated culture

Culture-universals commonalities of values, norms of behaviour, and life patterns among different cultures

Cumulative effect occurs when the body cannot metabolize a drug before additional dosages are administered

Cyanosis bluish discoloration of skin and mucous membranes caused by reduced oxygen in blood

Cystoscope a lighted instrument used to visualize the interior of the urinary bladder

Cystoscopy visual examination of the urinary bladder with a cystoscope

Cytokines chemical mediators produced by leukocytes

Dacryocystitis inflammation of the lacrimal sac

Data information

Database all information about a client, including nursing health history and physical assessment, physician's history and physical examination, and laboratory and diagnostic test results

Data collection the process of gathering information about a client's health status

Deafness when a person has little of no functional hearing and depends on visual rather than auditory communication

Debridement removal of necrotic or devitalized tissue that interferes with wound healing

Decision making the process of establishing criteria by which alternative courses of action are developed and selected

Decision-support systems computer systems that analyze raw data and nursing assessments to suggest nursing diagnoses and recommended interventions

Decode relate the communication message to the receiver's storehouse of information and experiences

Deductive reasoning making specific observations from a generalization

Defecation expulsion of feces from the rectum and anus

Defence mechanisms (adaptive mechanisms) any reaction that serves to protect against something physically or psychologically harmful

Defining characteristics client signs and symptoms that must be present to validate a nursing diagnosis

Dehiscence the partial or total rupturing of a sutured wound; usually involves an abdominal wound in which the layers below skin also separate

Dehydration insufficient fluid in the body

Delayed primary intention healing (tertiary intention healing) healing that occurs when a wound is left open for 3 to 5 days to allow edema or infection to resolve or exudate to drain and are then closed with sutures, staples, or adhesive skin closures

Delegating care directs the practice of care to another health care professional

Delegation assigning responsibility and authority for performing specific tasks to another person

Delirium mental confusion, restlessness, and incoherence

Demand feeding the infant is fed when hungry

Dementia a global impairment of cognitive function that usually is progressive and may be permanent; interferes with normal social and occupational activities

Democratic (participative, consultative) leaders have a participative style of leadership in which the leader encourages group discussion and decision making

Demography the study of population, including statistics about distribution by age and place of residence, mortality, and morbidity

Dental caries tooth decay

Dentin the chief substance of the teeth

Dentist a health care professional who diagnoses, prevents, and treats diseases, conditions, and disorders of the teeth, mouth, and surrounding tissues and structures

Denver Developmental Screening Test (DDST-II) a screening test used to assess children from birth to 6 years of age

Dependent functions nurses are obligated to carry out physician-prescribed therapies and treatments

Dependent interventions activities carried out under the physician's orders or supervision, or according to specified routines

Dependent variable the behaviour, characteristic, or outcome that the researcher wants to explain or predict

Depression feelings of sadness and dejection, often accompanied by physiological change, such as a decreased functional activity

Descriptive statistics procedures that summarize large volumes of data; used to describe and synthesize data, showing patterns and trends

Desire phase the first phase of the sexual response cycle, which starts in the brain with conscious sexual desires

Desired effect (of drug) the primary effect intended of a drug; reason the drug is prescribed

Desired health outcomes (goals) the end results that the client and the nurse are working toward through the care plan; often identified in relation to nursing diagnosis

Detoxification (biotransformation, metabolism) process by which a drug is converted to a less active form

Detrusor muscle the collective smooth muscle layers of the bladder

Development an individuals increasing capacity and skill in functioning, related to growth

Developmental (spiritual) people move through spiritual, religious, and faith stages in their lifetime

Developmental milestones the developmental sequences and patterns that are predictable in a child's growth

Developmental task skills and behaviour patterns learned during stages of development

Diabetes a group of metabolic diseases characterized by high blood glucose levels, which result from defects in insulin secretion, action, or both

Diagnosis a statement or conclusion concerning the nature of some phenomenon

Diagnostic labels titles used in writing a nursing diagnoses

Diapedesis the movement of blood corpuscles through a blood vessel wall

Diaphragmatic breathing (abdominal breathing) breathing that involves the contraction and relaxation of the diaphragm

Diarrhea defecation of liquid feces and increased frequency of defecation

Diastole the period during which the ventricles relax

Diastolic pressure the pressure of blood against the arterial walls when the ventricles of the heart are at rest

Diet as tolerated (DAT) foods are added back slowly to ensure that each is tolerated

Diet history a comprehensive assessment of a client's food intake, usually by a dietitian or nutritionist

Dietary reference intakes a set of four reference values produced by Health Canada: recommended dietary allowances, adequate intake, tolerable upper intake level, and estimated average requirement; used for diet assessment and form the basis of *Eating Well with Canada's Food Guide*

Dietary therapy the consumption of specific types of diets or supplements, including vitamins, minerals, amino acids, herbs and other botanicals, and miscellaneous substances, such as enzymes and fish oils, for the purpose of preventing or treating illness

Dietitian a health care professional who has specialized knowledge about the diets required to maintain health and to treat disease

Difference questions explore differences among people, relationships, or ideas

Diffusion the mixing of molecules or ions of two or more substances as a result of random motion; the movement of gases or other particles from an area of greater pressure or concentration to an area of lower pressure or concentration

Digital transition the movement of significant professional and scholarly information from paper to digital form

Dignity ability to function as a significant and integrated person

Diploma programs programs offered by community colleges in partnership with universities that lead to a diploma in nursing

Direct contact transmission immediate and direct transfer of microorganisms from person to person through touching, biting, kissing, or sexual intercourse, that is, body surface to body surface

Directing a management function that involves communicating the task to be completed and providing guidance and supervision

Directive interview a highly structured interview that uses closed questions to elicit specific information

Dirty (infected) wounds old traumatic wounds with retained dead tissue and wounds that involve existing clinical infection or perforated viscera

Disaccharides sugars that are composed of double molecules

Discharge planning the process of anticipating and planning for client needs after discharge

Disclosure the provision of information needed for the parties to make an informed decision

Discrimination the differential treatment of individuals or groups based on such categories as race, ethnicity, gender, social class, age, or exceptionality

Discussion specific dialogue or interaction between people

Disease an alteration in body function resulting in a reduction of capacities or shortening of the normal lifespan

Disease prevention measures to prevent and control common risk factors for diseases

Disengagement theory aging involves mutual withdrawal between an older adult and others within that person's environment

Disinfectant an agent that destroys all microorganisms

Disinfection cleaning that reduces the number of microorganisms but does not eliminate them all or kill most spores

Distribution the transportation of a drug from its site of absorption to its site of action

Diversity differences, often used in reference to cultural groups and people

Documenting written recording of pertinent information related to the client

Dorsal recumbent (supine) position a back-lying position with the head and shoulders slightly elevated

Drip factor (drop factor) the number of drops per millilitre of solution delivered for a particular drip chamber

Droplet nuclei residue of evaporated droplets that remains in the air for long periods

Droplet precautions practices initiated to prevent the spread of large particle microorganisms

Droplet transmission respiratory secretions larger than 5 microns in diameter that are generated by sneezing, coughing, spitting, singing, or talking, or procedures, such as suctioning; they are projected a short distance

Drug (medication) a chemical compound taken for disease prevention, diagnosis, cure, or relief or to affect the structure or function of the body

Drug abuse (problematic substance use) inappropriate intake of a substance, either continually or periodically

Drug allergy an immunological reaction to a drug

Drug dependence the inability to keep the intake of a drug or substance under control

Drug–drug interaction when one drug interacts with another drug and has an effect on the body; can take the following forms: one drug altering the absorption of another drug; one drug altering the distribution of another drug; some drugs can either enhance or delay metabolism or excretion of other drugs

Drug–food interaction when food interacts with a drug and has an effect on the body; food can enhance or diminish the absorption of certain medications

Drug habituation a mild form of psychological dependence, where the individual develops the habit of taking the substance and feels better after taking it

Drug interaction the beneficial or harmful interaction of one drug with another drug

Drug misuse improper use of common medications in ways that can lead to acute and chronic toxicity

Drug tolerance a condition in which successive increases in the dosage of a drug are required to maintain a given therapeutic effect

Drug toxicity the quality of a drug that exerts a deleterious effect on an organism or tissue

Dullness (of sound) a thud-like sound produced during percussion by dense tissue of body organs, such as the liver, spleen, or heart

Duration (of sound) the length of time that a sound is heard

Dynamics of difference understanding the rituals, customs, and practices of cultural groups that give rise to cultural differences

Dysmenorrhea painful menstruation

Dyspareunia pain experienced by a woman during intercourse

Dysphagia difficulty or inability to swallow

Dyspnea difficult or laboured breathing

Dysrhythmia (arrhythmia) a pulse with an irregular rhythm

Dysuria painful or difficult voiding

Eccrine glands glands that produce sweat; found over most of the body

Echocardiography (ECG) a graph of the electrical activity of the heart

Ecomap an assessment tool identifying the family's relationship to the environment

Edema the presence of excess interstitial fluid in the body

Effectiveness the ability to produce a specific result

Efficiency a measurement of competency

Ego includes consciousness and memory, which serves to mediate between primitive instinctual drives (id), internal social prohibitions (superego), and reality

eHealth electronic health

Ejaculation expulsion of seminal fluid and sperm

Elasticity of the arterial wall the ability of the arterial wall to expand and contract

Elective surgery performed when surgical intervention is the preferred treatment for a condition that is not imminently life-threatening or to improve the client's life

Electrocardiography (ECG, EKG) a graph of the electrical activity of the heart

Electrolytes chemical substances that develop an electric charge and are able to conduct an electric current when placed in water; ions

Electronic communication communication conducted electronically, most commonly through e-mail

Electronic documentation the capturing, transcribing, and adding of information to a client's electronic health record

Electronic health record (EHR) a health record of an individual that is accessible online from many separate, interoperable automated systems within an electronic network and that can be retrieved by caregivers, administrators, accreditors, and other persons authorized to access it; includes an electronic medical record and an electronic patient record for that individual; it links institutions

Electronic medical record (EMR) the part of a person's electronic health record that is kept in a clinic, by a family health team, or in a health practitioner's office

Electronic patient record (EPR) the part of a person's electronic health record that includes a record of a patient's demographic data, such as name and date of birth, the patient's diagnosis, and details about assessments and interventions provided by health professionals during an episode of care from one health organization

E-mail the most common form of electronic communication

Embolus a blood clot (or a substance, such as air) that has moved from its place of origin and is causing obstruction to circulation elsewhere (plural: emboli)

Emergency surgery an operation that is performed immediately to preserve function or the life of the client

Emigration movement of leukocytes through the blood vessel wall into affected tissue

Emmetropic normal refraction so that the eyes focus images on the retina

Emotional intelligence the ability to form work relationships with colleagues, display maturity in a variety of situations, manage emotions, consider the emotions of others, and resolve conflicts by interacting with colleagues constructively to achieve a positive outcome

Empathy the ability to discriminate what the other person's world is like and to communicate to the other this understanding in a way that shows that the helper understands the client's feelings and the behaviour and experience underlying these feelings

Empirical knowing knowledge that is systematically organized into laws and theories for the purpose of describing, explaining, and predicting phenomena or special concern to the discipline of nursing

Empiricist tradition suggests that there is a single reality that exists independent of our knowledge of it

Empowerment an assertion of personal power to mastery over something

Enamel the white, compact, hard substance covering the crown of a tooth

Encoding involves the selection of specific signs or symbols to transmit message during communication

Encopresis the passage or leakage of feces in children who are past the age of toilet training

Endocardium the lining inside the heart's chambers and great vessels

End-of-life care humane, compassionate care of the dying, often provided by nurses and others, such as family members, who are not hospice palliative care specialists

Enema a solution introduced into the rectum and sigmoid colon to remove feces or flatus

Energy the force that integrates and connects the body, mind, and spirit

Enteral through the gastrointestinal system

Enteral nutrition (EN) feedings administered through nasogastric or small-bore feeding tubes or through gastrostomy or jejunostomy tubes

Entry-to-practice the minimum educational requirement for entry into the practice of nursing; it is a baccalaureate degree in nursing

Enuresis bedwetting; involuntary passing of urine in children after bladder control is achieved

Environment the practice setting

Environmental control programs programs that address contaminants in the air, food, and water that will affect the health of future generations

Environmental health/factors the factors of the environment (climate change, access to safe water, sanitation, and indoor and outdoor pollution) that exert significant influence on human health in all countries

Environmental restraints things that control or limit a person's mobility (e.g., a secured unit or raised bed rails)

Enzymes a biological catalyst that speeds up chemical reactions

Epicardium the outermost layer of the heart

Epidemiological transition occurs as a country undergoes the process of modernization from third-world status to first-world status

Epidural into the epidural space

Epidural (peridural) anesthesia the injection of an anesthetic agent into the epidural space (the area inside the spinal column but outside the dura mater)

Epistemology investigates the nature of knowledge

Equianalgesia the relative potency of various opioid analgesics compared with a standard dose of parenteral morphine

Equianalgesic dose the dose of one analgesic that has the same pain-relieving effect as another drug

Equilibrium a state of balance

Equitable health care residents of a province or territory should all have access to the same or similar health care

Equity focuses on equality of outcomes, meaning that people with unequal need require different of differential treatment to achieve identical results

Eructation belching; the expulsion of swallowed gases through the mouth

Erythema redness associated with a variety of skin rashes

Erythrocytes red blood cells

Eschar thick necrotic tissue produced by burning, by a corrosive application, or by death of tissue associated with loss of vascular supply, bacterial invasion, and putrefaction

Essential amino acids amino acids that cannot be manufactured in the body and must be supplied as part of the protein ingested in the diet

Essential fatty acids lipids that are required for normal growth and development but that cannot be synthesized by the body

Estimated average requirement the nutrient intake that would meet the needs of 50% of a particular age and gender group

Ethical knowing knowledge that focuses on matters of obligation or what ought to be done and goes beyond following the ethical codes of discipline

Ethical obligations responsibilities imposed as a result of ethical imperatives

Ethics the rules or principles that govern right conduct

Ethics of care suggest that individuals have a moral obligation to each other

Ethnic belonging to a specific group of individuals who share a common social and cultural heritage

Ethnocentrism the belief that the person's own culture is superior to all others

Ethnographic research a qualitative design used to describe social behaviours with a particular group or setting; the goal is to understand the culture and norms from the participant's viewpoint

Ethnopharmacology the study of the effect of ethnicity on responses to prescribed mediation

Ethnorelativity the ability to appreciate and respect the viewpoints of other cultures

Etiology the causal relationship between a problem and its related or risk factors

Eupnea normal, quiet breathing

Eustachian tube the part of the middle ear that connects the middle ear to the nasopharynx; stabilizes air pressure between the external atmosphere and the middle ear

Euthanasia (mercy killing) the act of painlessly putting to death persons suffering from incurable or distressing disease

Evaluation a planned, ongoing, purposeful activity in which client and health care professionals determine the client's progress toward goal achievement and the effectiveness of the nursing care plan

Evaluative statement a statement that has a conclusion (a statement on whether the goal or desired health outcome was met) and supporting data (the list of

client responses that support the conclusion) and is written on the care plan or in the nurse's notes

Evaporation continuous vaporization of moisture from the respiratory tract, from the mucosa of the mouth, and from skin

Evidence-based practice (evidence-informed practice) nursing practice that includes the use of clinical evidence in patient-care decisions

Evidence-informed nursing practice nursing practice that includes the use of clinical evidence in client care decisions

Evisceration extrusion of the internal organs

Exacerbation the period during a chronic illness when symptoms reappear after remission

Excitement phase the second phase of the sexual response cycle that involves two primary physiological changes: vasocongestion (increase in the blood flow to various body parts) and myotonia (increase in tension in muscles)

Excretion elimination of a waste product produced by the body cells from the body

Exercise a type of physical activity; a planned, structured, and repetitive bodily movement done to improve or maintain one or more components of physical fitness

Exhalation (expiration) the movement of gases from the lungs to the atmosphere

Exophthalmos protrusion of the eyeballs with elevation of the upper eyelids, resulting in a startled or staring expression

Expanded practice nursing that goes beyond the traditional roles of registered nurses

Experimental design a research method in which the investigator manipulates the independent variable by administering a treatment to some subjects while withholding it from others

Expert power power that is based on the person's expertise or knowledge

Expiration (exhalation) the outflow of air from the lungs to the atmosphere

Express consent an oral or written agreement

External auditory meatus the entrance to the ear canal

External respiration the interchange of oxygen and carbon dioxide between the alveoli of the lungs and the pulmonary blood

External stimuli things that are visual (sight), auditory (hearing), olfactory (smell), tactile (touch), and gustatory (taste)

Extinction the failure to perceive touch on one side of the body when two symmetric areas of the body are touched simultaneously

Extracellular fluid (ECF) fluid found outside the body cells

Exudate material, such as fluid and cells, that has escaped from blood vessels during the inflammatory process and is deposited in tissue or on tissue surfaces

Fad a widespread but short-lived interest, or a practice followed with considerable zeal

Failure to thrive delayed infant development without any physical cause; the infant is often malnourished and fails to gain weight and grow normally

Faith an active "mode of being-in-relation" to another or others in which we invest commitment, belief, love, and hope

Fall an unexpected even in which a person comes to rest on the ground, floor, or lower level

False imprisonment the unlawful restraint or detention of another person against his or her wishes

Family any combination of two or more persons bound together over time by ties of mutual consent, birth or adoption, or placement, and who assume responsibilities for any combination of physical maintenance and care of group members, addition of new members through procreation or adoption, socialization of children, social control of members, production, consumption, distribution of goods and services, or affective nurturance

Family nursing refers to those relational practices that involve family members in care

Family support a form of social support that helps to buffer stress

Family unit as the client of care attention is simultaneously directed toward the individual and the family, with the family in the foreground

Fasciculation an abnormal contraction or shortening of a bundle of muscle fibres

Fat-soluble vitamins A, D, E, and K vitamins that the body can store

Fatty acid the basic structural unit of most lipids; made up of carbon chains and hydrogen

Fear an emotional response to an actual, present danger

Febrile pertaining to a fever; feverish

Fecal impaction a mass or collection of hardened, putty-like feces in the folds of the rectum

Fecal incontinence (bowel incontinence) the loss of voluntary ability to control fecal and gaseous discharges through the anal sphincter

Fecal–oral route the transfer or microoganisms from fecal particles from a carrier through food or water to a another person

Feces (stool) body wastes and undigested food eliminated from the rectum

Feedback (communication) the response or message that the receiver returns to the sender during communication

Feedback (homeostasis) the mechanism by which some output of a system is returned to the system as input

Female orgasmic disorder refers to women who are incapable of responding sexually or do not experience orgasm

Female sexual arousal disorder the lack of vaginal lubrication causes discomfort or pain during sexual intercourse

Fetal alcohol spectrum disorder impaired mitochondrial development in the fetus, which leads to microcephaly, intellectual disorders, learning disorders, and other central nervous system defects; results from alcohol use by pregnant women

Fever elevated body temperature

Fever spike a temperature that rises to fever level rapidly following a normal temperature and then returns to normal within a few hours

Fibre an indigestible carbohydrate derived from plants

Fibrin an insoluble protein formed from fibrinogen during the clotting of blood

Fibrinogen a plasma protein that is converted to fibrin when it is released into the tissues and, together with thromboplastin and platelets, forms an interlacing network making a barrier to wall off an area

Fibrous (scar) tissue common connective tissue composed of elastic and collagen fibres

Fidelity a moral principle that obligates the individual to be faithful to agreements and responsibilities the person has undertaken

Filtration passage through a material that restricts or prevents passage of certain molecules

Filtration pressure the stress or strain exerted during the passage through a filter

First-level manager a manager responsible for the work of nonmanagerial personnel and the day-to-day activities of a specific work group or groups

First-pass effect oral drugs first pass through the liver and are partially metabolized before reaching the target organ

Fissures clefts or grooves

Fit checking assessing the adequacy of the seal when donning a respirator; should be done each time a respirator is worn

Fit testing fitting a respirator mask to an individual based on size and style to ensure and adequate seal of a mask around the mouth and nose

Fixation immobilization or the inability of the personality to proceed to the next developmental stage because of anxiety

Flaccid weak or lax or soft, especially in relation to muscles

Flaccid bladder weak, soft, and lax bladder muscles

Flatness (of sound) an extremely dull sound produced, during percussion, by very dense tissue, such as muscle or bone

Flatulence the presence of excessive amounts of gas in the stomach or intestines

Flatus gas or air normally present in the stomach or intestines

Flowsheets records of the progress of specific or specialized data, such as vital signs, fluid balance, or routine medications; often charted in graph form

Fluid volume deficit (FVD) an abnormal reduction in blood volume

Fluid volume excess (FVE) an abnormal increase in the body's blood volume; circulatory overload

Foam swabs equipment used to clean mouths of dependent clients

Focus charting a method of charting that uses key words or foci to describe what is happening to the client

Focused assessment an examination that focuses on a specific problem area noted from the nursing assessment

Food diary a detailed record of measured amounts of all food and fluid consumed during a specific period

Food security a state that exists when all people at all times have access to sufficient, safe, and nutritious food to maintain a healthy and active life

Food-frequency record a checklist that indicates how often general food groups or specific foods are eaten

Formal care plan usually a written guide to direct the efforts of nurses as they work with patients to achieve goals that are mutually agreed upon

Formal leader an appointed leader selected by an organization and given official authority to make decisions and act

Four-point alternate gait a crutch gait in which the client moves the right crutch ahead a suitable distance; moves the left front foot forward, preferably to the level of the left crutch; moves the left crutch forward; and moves the right foot forward; the client must be able to bear weight on both legs to use this gait

Fowler's position a bed sitting position with the head of the bed raised to 45 degrees

Frailty a general decline in an older adult's physical functioning that can result in increased vulnerability to illness

Fremitus the faintly perceptible vibration of the vocal cords felt through the chest wall when the client speaks

Friction rubbing; the force that opposes motion

Full agonist a painkiller that binds to opioid receptors, mimicking the effects of endogenous opioids, or endorphins

Full disclosure all information required by the client will be provided prior to participation in a research study

Full fluid diet a diet consisting of only liquids or foods that turn to liquid at body temperature

Full-thickness wound wounds that involve the dermis, epidermis, subcutaneous tissue, and possibly muscle and bone; require connective tissue repair

Functional age age based on the fact that aging is a multi-faceted, diverse process in which individuals at a specific chronological age are either older or younger than their peers in terms of some relevant skill or experience

Functional method a model for delivering nursing care which focuses on the tasks to be completed

Functional strength the ability of the body to perform work

Fungi infection-causing microorganisms that include yeasts and moulds

Gait the way a person walks

Gait belt an assistive device used to help a client during ambulation; it enhances safety and prevents back injury to the nurse

Gaiter area the area from 2.5 cm below the malleolus to the lower third of the calf

Gastrocolic reflex increased peristalsis of the colon after food has entered the stomach

Gastrostomy an opening through the abdominal wall into the stomach

Gastrostomy tube a tube inserted through the abdominal wall into the stomach

Gauge the size of the shaft of the needle; varies from 18 gauge to 28 gauge; the larger the gauge number, the smaller is the diameter of the shaft

Gender identity indicates biological male or female status

Gender-role behaviour the expression of a person's sense of maleness or femaleness as well as what is perceived as gender-appropriate behaviour

General adaptation syndrome (GAS) a general arousal response of the body to a stressor that is characterized by certain physiological events and that is dominated by the sympathetic nervous system

General anesthesia sedative drugs that produce relaxation of skeletal muscles and reduced or absent reflex action

Generalized anxiety a state of mental uneasiness, apprehension, or dread that produces an increased level of arousal

Generation X the generation of people born between 1965 and 1978, who are characterized as being independent, resilient, confident, and loyal and committed to colleagues and clients over the employer; willing to share their expertise with colleagues and clients; and letting care be guided more by their client's desire than by rules and policies in the organization

Generation Y the generation of people born between 1979 and 2000

Generativity (Erikson) concern for establishing and guiding the next generation

Generic name (of drug) a drug name not protected by trademark and usually describing the chemical structure of the drug

Genital intercourse penile–vaginal intercourse (coitus)

Genogram a concise visual depiction of the family structure and relevant situational information

Geragogy the process involved in stimulating and helping older adults to learn

Geriatrics the medical care (e.g., diseases and disabilities) of older adults

Gerontology the study of all aspects of the aging process, including biological, psychological, and sociological

Gingiva the gum tissue

Gingivitis red, swollen gingiva (gums)

Glaucoma a disturbance in the circulation of aqueous fluid; causes an increase in intraocular pressure

Global health health issues and concerns that transcend national borders, race, ethnicity, and culture

Global self the collective beliefs and images a person holds about himself or herself; the most complete description that individuals can give of themselves at any one time

Global self-esteem how much a person likes his or her perceived self as a whole

Glomerulus a collection of capillary vessels within the kidney involved in the initial formation of urine

Glossitis inflammation of the tongue

Glucagon a hormone released by the pancreas that causes the liver to release glycogen

Glycemic Index (GI) an index that measures how much the blood glucose increases in the 2 or 3 hours after a person eats

Glycemic level the amount of glucose present in blood

Glycogen the chief carbohydrate stored in the body, particularly in the liver and muscles

Glycogenesis the process of glycogen formation

Goals (desired health outcomes) the end results that the client and the nurse are working toward through the care plan; often identified in relation to nursing diagnoses

Good Samaritan a health care practitioner or layperson who provides aid to a person in an emergency

Goodness of fit whether parents' expectations of their child's behaviour are consistent with the child's temperament type

Granulation tissue young connective tissue with new capillaries formed in the wound healing process

Grief emotional suffering often caused by bereavement

Grounded theory a qualitative design used to develop nursing theory from collected data; theory may be generated for relatively new areas where very little is known, or for more familiar areas where a fresh viewpoint is sought

Group two or more people with shared purposes and goals

Group dynamics forces that determine the behaviour of the group and the relationships among the group members

Growth physical change and increase in size

Guided imagery a relaxation technique using self-chosen positive images to achieve specific health-related goals (i.e., stress reduction, pain control)

Habit training (schedule toileting) the attempt to keep clients dry by having them void at regular intervals

Half-life (of a drug) the time interval required for the body's elimination processes to reduce the concentration of the drug in the body by one half

Hand hygiene both hand washing and use of hand sanitizers

Hardware the physical elements of a computer

Harm reduction a health-promotion approach that aims to minimize harm or reduce the negative consequences of risk behaviour by keeping people as safe and healthy as possible in their current lifestyle realities

Haustra pouches within the large intestine

Haustral churning the movement of the chyme back and forth within the haustra, in the large intestine

Healing touch a group of noninvasive energy-based techniques that incorporate therapeutic touch and can be helpful in promoting relaxation, reducing pain, and managing stress

Health a state of being physically fit, mentally stable, and socially comfortable; it encompasses more than the state of being free of disease

Health care system the totality of services offered by all health disciplines

Health education a strategy of health promotion concerned with the communication of information and the fostering of motivation, skills, and confidence to take action to improve health

Health field concept the theory that biology, lifestyles, environment, and health care organizations are the four elements that determine health

Health literacy the ability to read, understand, and act on health information, including such tasks as comprehending prescription labels, interpreting appointment slips, completing health insurance form, and following instructions for diagnostic tests

Health promotion any activity undertaken for the purpose of achieving a higher level of health and well-being

Health protection activities focused on preventing, avoiding, or minimizing preventable illnesses and injuries that individuals have little or no control over

Health restoration a process of restoring ill or injured people to more optimal levels of health and functioning, emphasizing the importance of helping clients to function adequately in the physical, mental, social, economic, and vocational areas of their lives

Health risk appraisal a tool that indicates a client's risk of diseases or injury over time by comparing the client with a large national sample with similar demographic data

Health care–associated infections infections associated with the delivery of health care services in a health care facility, including hospitals, long-term or continuing care facilities, community care, home care, health care professionals' offices, or test centres

Heart failure the inability of the heart to maintain a circulation sufficient to meet the body's needs

Heat balance the state a person is in when the amount of heat produced by the body exactly equals the amount of heat lost

Heat exhaustion the result of excessive heat and dehydration; signs include pallor, dizziness, nausea, vomiting, fainting, and a moderately increased temperature (38.5°C to 39°C)

Heat stroke can result from exercising in hot weather; signs include warm, flushed skin, a lack of sweating, and a temperature of 41°C or higher; can cause the person to be delirious, lose consciousness, or have seizures

Heave an abnormal lateral movement of the chest related to enlargement of the left ventricle

Helix the posterior curve of the flap of the ear

Helminths (worms) multicelled parasites

Hematocrit the proportion of red blood cells (erythrocytes) to the total blood volume

Hematoma a collection of blood in a tissue, organ, or space due to a break in the wall of a blood vessel

Hemoglobin the red pigment in red blood cells that carries oxygen

Hemolytic transfusion reaction a response that occurs when incompatible blood is transfused into a patient that should have been given blood of a different type

Hemoptysis the presence of blood in the sputum

Hemorrhage excessive loss of blood from the vascular system

Hemorrhoids distended veins in the rectum

Hemostasis cessation of bleeding

Hemothorax a collection of blood in the pleural cavity

Herbal medicine using herbs to treat disease or supplement other treatments

Herbal therapy treatment in which the routine use of herbs helps to prevent disease or promote health

Hernia a protrusion of the intestine through the inguinal canal

High-density lipoproteins (HDLs) lipoproteins that carry cholesterol from the tissues to the liver for catabolism and excretion

High-Fowler's position a bed-sitting position in which the head of the bed is elevated 90 degrees

Hip circumference the measurement around the largest part of the buttocks and hips

Hirsutism abnormal hairiness, particularly in women

Holism all living organisms are seen as interacting, unified wholes that are more than the sums of their parts

Holistic being concerned with the individual as a whole, not as an assembly of parts and processes

Holistic health a model of health based on the belief that the whole is more than the sum of its parts

Holistic health belief holds that forces of nature must be maintained in balance or harmony

Holistic health care a system that considers all the components of health: health promotion, health maintenance, health education and illness prevention, and restorative–rehabilitative care

Holy day a day set aside for special religious observance

Home health nurse (HHN) community health nurses who provide, in a client's home, school, or workplace, clinical care and treatment that is directed toward health restoration, maintenance, or palliation

Homeopathy an alternative therapy based on the theory that the cure for the disease lies in the disease itself; thus, treatment is with highly diluted amounts of substances that at a higher concentration would produce the same symptoms as the disease

Homeostasis (balance) the tendency of the body to maintain a state of balance or equilibrium while continually changing; a mechanism in which deviations from normal are sensed and counteracted

Homeostasis (feedback) the mechanism by which some output of a system is returned to the system as input

Homeostatic drive (of sleep) restores normal levels of activity and normal balance among parts of the nervous system, including the autonomic nervous system

Hordeolum (sty) redness, swelling, and tenderness of the hair follicle and glands that empty at the edge of the eyelids

Horticultural therapy an adjunct therapy to occupational and physical therapy that has people view nature, visit a healing garden or a wander garden, or actually participate in gardening to decrease social isolation, foster interactions with others, stimulate the five senses, provide leisure activities, improve motor function, provide a sense of achievement, and improve self-esteem

Hospice care care that addresses the specific needs of the dying and their families

Hospice–palliative care end-of-life care based on holistic concepts that emphasize care to improve the quality of life, rather than cure; nurse can specialize in hospice–palliative care, with that care often limited to persons experiencing difficult dying processes

Hub the part of the needle that fits onto the syringe

Humanism learning that focuses on the feelings and attitudes of learners, the importance of the individual in identifying learning needs and taking responsibility for them, and the self-motivation of the learners to work toward self-reliance and independence

Humanist the view that the mind and body are indivisible, people have the power to solve their own problems, people are responsible for the patterns of their lives, and well-being is a combination of personal satisfaction and contributions to the larger community

Humidifiers devices that add water vapour to inspired air

Humoral (circulating) immunity antibody-mediated defence; resides ultimately in the B lymphocytes and is mediated by the antibodies produced by B cells

Humour the ability to discover, express, or appreciate the comical or absurdly incongruous, to be amused by our own imperfections or the whimsical aspects of life, and to see the funny side of an otherwise serious situation

Hydrostatic pressure the pressure a liquid exerts on the sides of the container that holds it; also called *filtration force*

Hygiene the science of health and its maintenance

Hyperalgesia extreme sensitivity to pain

Hypercalcemia an excess of calcium in the blood plasma

Hypercapnia accumulation of carbon dioxide in the blood

Hyperchloremia an excess of chloride in the blood plasma

Hyperemia increased blood flow to an area

Hyperesthesia greater than normal sensation

Hyperexcitability an increase in dorsal horn neuron sensitivity

Hyperglycemia an excessive concentration of sugar in blood

Hyperhidrosis excessive perspiration

Hyperinsulinemia the state that exists when excess insulin is present in blood

Hyperkalemia an excess of potassium in blood plasma

Hypermagnesemia an excess of magnesium in blood plasma

Hypernatremia an excess of sodium in blood plasma

Hyperopia abnormal refraction in which light rays focus behind the retina; farsightedness

Hyperopic farsighted

Hyperphosphatemia an excess of phosphate in blood plasma

Hyperpyrexia (hyperthermia, pyrexia) an extremely high body temperature (e.g., 41°C)

Hyperresonance an abnormal booming sound produced during percussion of the lungs

Hypersomnia excessive sleep

Hypertension an abnormally high blood pressure: more than 140 mm Hg systolic or 90 mm Hg diastolic

Hyperthermia (hyperpyrexia, pyrexia) an extremely high body temperature (e.g., 41°C)

Hypertonic describes solutions that have a higher osmolality than body fluids

Hypertrophy enlargement of a muscle or organ

Hyperventilation very deep, rapid respirations

Hypervolemia an abnormal increase in the body's blood volume; circulatory overload

Hypnosis a trance state or an altered state of consciousness in which an individual's concentration is focused and distraction is minimized

Hypoactive sexual desire disorder people who report a persistently low interest or a total lack of interest in sexual activity

Hypocalcemia deficiency of calcium in blood plasma

Hypochloremia deficiency of chloride in blood plasma

Hypodermoclysis the introduction of fluid in subcutaneous tissues

Hypoesthesia less than normal sensation

Hypoglycemia a reduced amount of glucose in blood

Hypokalemia deficiency of potassium in blood plasma

Hypomagnesemia deficiency of magnesium in blood plasma

Hyponatremia deficiency of sodium in blood plasma

Hypophosphatemia deficiency in phosphate in blood plasma

Hypotension an abnormally low blood pressure: less than 100 mm Hg systolic in an adult

Hypothalmic integrator the centre in the brain that controls the core temperature; located in the preoptic area of the hypothalamus

Hypothermia a core body temperature lower than the lower limit of normal

Hypothesis in an experiment, a prediction of the relationship between two or more concepts (plural: hypotheses)

Hypothetical or future-oriented questions explore family options and alternative actions or implications in the future

Hypotonic describes solutions that have a lower osmolality than body fluids

Hypoventilation very shallow respirations

Hypovolemia an abnormal reduction in blood volume

Hypoxemia a condition in which the level of oxygen in the blood is less than normal; characterized by a low partial pressure of oxygen in arterial blood or low hemoglobin saturation

Hypoxia insufficient oxygen anywhere in the body

Iatrogenic disease usually an infection that is acquired as a result of treatment or diagnostic procedure

Id the source of instinctive and unconscious psychological urges

Ideal body weight the weight recommended for optimal health

Ideal self how a person would prefer to be; the individual's perception of how he or she should behave based on certain personal standards, aspirations, goals, or values

Identification perceiving the self as similar to and behaving like another person

Idiosyncratic effect a different, unexpected, or individual effect from the normal one usually expected from a medication; the occurrence of unpredictable and unexplainable symptoms

Ileal conduit most commonly used urinary diversion procedure

Ileostomy an opening into the ileum (small bowel)

Illicit drug a drug that is sold illegally; a street drug

Illness a highly personal state in which the person feels unhealthy or ill, may or may not be related to disease

Illness and injury prevention such practices as providing immunizations, identifying risk factors for illnesses, and helping people take measures to prevent both acute and chronic illnesses from occurring

Illness narratives seek understanding of the person's or family's experience of illness in experiences of daily life

Imagination ability to fantasize

Imitation copying the behaviours and attitudes of another person

Immunization the process of becoming immune or rendering someone immune

Immunoglobulins (antibodies) a part of the body's plasma proteins

Implications suggestions for ways of thinking about the phenomenon in the future

Implied consent permission that is assumed in an emergency when consent cannot be obtained from the client or a relative

Impulse conduction the movement of an impulse along nerve pathways to the spinal cord or directly to the brain; vibrations received in the inner ear are translated into electric impulses that travel along the acoustic nerve to the brain

Incentive spirometers devices that measure the flow of air through a mouthpiece

Incident reports a report completed by the nurse when the care provided is not consistent with standard practice, causing injury, harm, or loss to the client, and negatively affecting the quality of client care; also known as event or occurrence reports

Incivility rude, discourteous, or disrespectful behaviour that reflects a lack of regard for others

Incomplete proteins proteins that lack one or more essential amino acids; usually derived from vegetables

Incus middle of the three ossicles of the ear

Independent functions those areas of health care that are unique to nursing

Independent interventions those activities that nurses are licensed to initiate on the basis of their knowledge and skills

Independent variable the behaviour, characteristic, or outcome that a researcher wants to explain

Indigenous peoples people who live in geographically distinct traditional habitats, who identify themselves as being part of a distinct cultural group, and who are descended from groups present in the area before colonists arrived

Indirect contact transmission passive transfer of microorganisms from the reservoir to an intermediate inanimate object in the client's immediate environment and then to the recipient, for example, hands touch a contaminated doorknob, pick up microorganisms, and transfer them to the recipient's mucous membrane

Individualized care plans tailored to meet the needs of a specific client

Inductive reasoning making generalizations from specific data

Infection the disease process produced by microorganisms

Infection control practitioners health care practitioners whose role includes monitoring rates and trends of infections; identifying and managing outbreaks; educating and consulting with staff; developing, implementing, and evaluating policies and procedures surrounding infection prevention and control; and acting as consultants to a variety of committees on issues related to infection prevention and control

Infectious agent a microorganism that invades body tissue and proliferates, with damage to host tissue

Inferences interpretation or conclusions made based on cues or observed data

Inflammation the local and nonspecific defensive tissue response to injury or destruction of cells

Influence an informal strategy used to gain the cooperation of others without exercising formal authority

Informal care plan an unwritten plan of action to address a client health problem

Informal leader an individual selected by the group as its leader because of seniority, age, special abilities, or charisma

Information the result when data are interpreted, organized, or structured in a meaningful way

Information and computer technology (ICT) a term used to describe various informatics devices, software, hardware, or systems

Information (digital) literacy the proficiencies of knowing, identifying, finding and organizing, evaluating, and using information (e.g., critical evaluation of and production of new knowledge) that advance research skills and critical thinking

Information dissemination the use of a variety of media to educate the public and raise awareness about the risks of particular lifestyle choices and personal behaviours, as well as the benefits of changing those behaviours and improving the quality of life

Informed consent a client's agreement to accept a course of treatment or a procedure after receiving complete information, including the risks of treatment and facts relating to it, from the physician

Infusion administration sets consist of an insertion spike, a drip chamber, a roller valve or screw clamp, tubing with secondary ports, and a protective cap over the IV catheter adapter

Inhalation (inspiration) the act of breathing in; the intake of air or other substances into the lungs

Inhibiting effect the administration of one drug before, at the same time as, or after another drug decreases the effects of the drug

Injury physical harm, hurt, trauma, or damage to the body caused by an exchange of energies that exceeds the body's tolerance; typically predictable and preventable

Input consists of information, material, or energy that enters a system

Insensible heat loss heat loss that occurs from evaporation (vaporization) of moisture from the respiratory tract, mucosa of the mouth, and skin

Insensible water loss fluid loss that is not perceptible to the individual

In-service education a program administered by an employer that is designed to upgrade the knowledge or skills of employees, such as informing nurses about a new piece of equipment, about specific isolation practices, or about methods of implementing a nurse theorist's conceptual framework for nursing

Insoluble fibre fibre that acts as roughage and draws water into the colon, preventing constipation; sources include wheat bran and the skins of some fruits and vegetables

Insomnia inability to obtain a sufficient quality or quantity of sleep

Inspection visual examination

Inspiration (inhalation) the act of breathing in; the intake of air or other substances into the lungs

Institutional discrimination uneven access by various groups or group members to resources, status, and power resulting from policies and practices of organizations and institutions

Insulin a hormone secreted by the pancreas that enhances the transport of glucose into the cells

Insulin resistance the sensitivity to insulin by the cell's receptors is decreased

Insulin syringe a type of syringe used to administer insulin; it has a "unit" scale specially designed for insulin and is the only syringe that should be used to administer insulin

Integrative medicine treatment that combines Western medicine and complementary and alternative medicine (CAM) to achieve maximum safety and effectiveness of care

Intensity (amplitude) the loudness or softness of a sound

Intention tremor an involuntary trembling when a person attempts voluntary movement

Intentional injuries damage to the body that results from purposeful harm, such as child abuse, assault, or homicide

Intentional torts a tort where the person intends to do the action that causes harm to victims

Interdisciplinary or interprofessional approaches ways to increase the effectiveness of health care delivery by interrelating with many other health care professionals from all areas

Interferons molecules produced by virus-infected cells that move to and enter neighbouring cells where they prevent binding of the virus to the uninfected cell or interfere with viral replication in the cell

Intermittent fever a body temperature that alternates at regular intervals between periods of fever and periods of normal temperature

Intermittent pneumatic compression the use of pneumatic pressure devices to promote venous return from the legs; sometimes referred to as sequential compression

Internal respiration the interchange of oxygen and carbon dioxide between the circulating blood and the cells of the body tissues

Internal stimuli things that are kinesthetic or visceral

International health the health status among nations; emphasizes differences among countries rather than their commonalities

International nursing nursing that focuses on health and wellness issues in all nations

Internationally educated nurses nurses who have been educated in other countries and apply to have their credentials assessed

Interpersonal skills all the verbal and nonverbal activities people use when communicating directly with one another

Interpretive tradition suggests that there is no single fixed reality against which knowledge can be measured

Interprofessional collaboration or interprofessional cooperation health care professionals from all areas working together to further client care

Interprofessional education (IPE) health professionals being educated together to provide a greater understanding of the roles each of them play, and help them work together more effectively after graduation

Intersex a condition in which contradictions exist among chromosomal sex, gonadal sex, internal organs, and external genital appearance; the sex of an intersexed person is ambiguous

Interstitial fluid (ISF) liquid that surrounds the cells, includes lymph

Interview a planned communication; a conversation with a purpose

Intimacy (Erikson) the development of affectionate relationships and lengthy attachments and the making of personal commitments to another that may include marriage or sexual relations

Intimate partner violence (IPV) dating and cohabiting violence, same-sex violence, and violence by heterosexual women; can include physical violence and nonphysical abuses, including emotional, psychological, economic, and social abuse

Intra-arterial into an artery

Intra-articular into a joint

Intracardiac into the heart muscle

Intracellular fluid (ICF) fluid found within the body cells, also called *cellular fluid*

Intradermal under the epidermis; into the dermis

Intramuscular into the muscle

Intraoperative phase the phase during surgery that begins when the client is transferred to the operating room and ends when the client is admitted to the recovery room

Intraosseous into bone

Intrapleural within the pleural cavity

Intrapleural pressure pressure within the pleural cavity

Intrapulmonary pressure pressure within the lungs

Intraspinal (intrathecal) into the spinal canal

Intrathecal (intraspinal) into the spinal canal

Intravascular fluid (IVF) plasma

Intravenous within a vein

Intravenous block (Bier block) an anesthesia procedure used for the arm, wrist, and hand

Intravenous poles used to hand the solution container for an IV set

Intravenous pyelography (IVP) radiographic filming of the kidney and ureters after injection of a radiopaque material into the vein

Introjection the assimilation of the attributes of others

Introspection a person's consideration of his or her own beliefs, attitudes, motivations, strengths, and limitations

Intuition the understanding or learning of things without the conscious use of reasoning

Invasion of privacy release of personal information without the individual's consent

Invasive (open) surgery surgery that involves large incisions made to visualize and provide direct access to the area requiring surgery

Ions atoms or a group of atoms that carry a positive or negative electric charge; electrolytes

Iritis inflammation of the iris

Iron-deficiency anemia a form of anemia caused by inadequate supply of iron for synthesis of hemoglobin

Irrigation (lavage) a flushing or washing-out of a body cavity, organ, or wound with a specified solution

Ischemia deficiency of blood supply caused by obstruction of circulation to the body part

Isokinetic (resistive) exercise exercise that involves muscle contraction or tension against resistance

Isolation (geographical) a state of physical separation from others

Isolation precautions measures designed to prevent the spread of infections or potentially infectious micro-organisms to health care personnel, clients, and visitors

Isometric (static or setting) exercise tensing of a muscle against an immovable outer resistance, which does not change muscle length or produce joint motion

Isotonic describes solutions that have the same osmolality as body fluids

Isotonic (dynamic) exercise exercise in which muscle tension is constant and the muscle shortens to produce muscle contraction and active movement

Isotonic imbalance a state that occurs when water and electrolytes are lost or gained in equal proportions so that the osmolality of body fluids remains constant

Jaundice a yellowish colour of the sclera, mucous membranes, or skin

Jejunostomy an opening through the abdominal wall into the jejunum

Justice the process that distributes fairly risks, benefits, and costs

Kardex the trade name for a charting method that makes use of a series of cards to concisely organize and record client data and instructions for daily nursing care, especially care that changes frequently and must be kept up to date

Keloid a hypertrophic scar containing an abnormal amount of collagen

Kilojoule (kJ) a metric measurement referring to the amount of energy required when a force of 1 newton (N) moves 1 kilogram of weight 1 metre distance

Kinesthetic refers to awareness of the position and movement of body parts

Knowledge synthesizes information to identify relationships that provide fuller understanding of an issue or subject

Koilonychia the condition in which the nail curves upward from the nail bed

Korotkoff's sounds a series of five sounds produced by blood within the artery with each ventricular contraction

Kosher food that is acceptable or prepared according to Jewish law

Kunyaza a sexual practice originating in Africa in which the man taps the internal area of his partner's vagina with the tip of his penis

Kussmaul's respiration deep rapid breathing; a dyspnea occurring in paroxysms often preceding diabetic coma; air hunger

Kyphosis excessive convex curvature of the thoracic spine

Laboratory/radiologic technologist health care workers who assist or complete diagnostic tests—often laboratory or radiology tests

Lactose intolerance (lactose maldigestion) a shortage of the enzyme lactase, which is needed to breakdown lactose, a sugar in dairy products; symptoms include abdominal pain, bloating, flatulence, cramping, nausea, and diarrhea

Laissez-faire (nondirective, permissive, ultraliberal) leader has a nondirective style of leadership in which the leader assumes a "hands-off" approach, allowing group members to perform tasks in their area of expertise while the leader acts as a resource person

Lanugo the fine, woolly hair or down on the shoulders, back, sacrum, and earlobes of the unborn child that may remain for a few weeks after birth

Large calorie (**Calorie**, kilocalorie, kcal, C, Cal) a unit of heat energy equivalent to the amount of heat required to raise the temperature of 1 kg of water 1°C

Laryngoscopy visual examination of the larynx with a laryngoscope

Lateral (side-lying) position a side-lying position

Lateral violence physical, verbal, or emotional abuse or aggression directed at coworkers at the same organizational level; also known as horizontal violence or horizontal hostility

Lavage (irrigation) a flushing or washing-out of a body cavity, organ, or wound with a specified solution

Law rules made by humans that regulate social conduct in a formally prescribed and binding manner

Laxatives medications that stimulate bowel activity

Leader a person who influences others to work together to accomplish a specific goal

Leadership style the traits, behaviours, motivations, and choices used by individuals to effectively influence others

Leading question a question that influences the client to give a particular answer

Learning a change in human disposition or capability that persists over a period and cannot be solely accounted for by growth

Learning need a desire or requirement to know something that is presently unknown

Least restraint the policy of using the minimum amount of restraint needed to ensure safety

Leukocyte white blood cell

Leukocytosis an increase in the number of white blood cells

Leukoplakia white patches or spots on the mucous membrane of the tongue or cheek

Libido urge or desire for sexual activity

Lice parasitic insects that infest mammals

Licensing examination a test for the specific nursing group (e.g., registered nurse [RN], licensed practical nurse [LPN], registered practical nurse [RPN]) provided by the appropriate provincial or territorial regulatory authorities; successful candidates become licensed in that province or territory

Licensure the granting by a nursing regulatory body, such as a college or provincial or territorial nursing association, to a qualified nurse the right to practise within a province or territory, according to standards of care and ethics and scope of practice specified in the licence

Lifestyle and behaviour change programs programs that require the active participation of the individuals and are geared toward enhancing their quality of life and extending their lifespan

Lifestyle assessment appraisal of the personal lifestyle and habits of the client as they affect health

Lift an abnormal anterior movement of the chest related to enlargement of the right ventricle

Line of gravity an imaginary vertical line running through the centre of gravity

Lipids organic substances that are greasy and insoluble in water

Lipodermatosclerosis ulcers in the gaiter area caused by areas of connective tissue in the deep dermis and fat, producing a woody hardening of tissue

Lipoproteins water-soluble substances that are the form in which lipids are transported in blood

Living will a document that states medical treatments the client chooses to omit or refuse in the event that the client is unable to make these decisions

Livor mortis discoloration of skin caused by breakdown of the red blood cells; occurs after blood circulation has ceased; appears in the dependent areas of the body

Lobule small segment or lobe

Local adaptation syndrome (LAS) the reaction of one organ or body part to stress

Local anesthesia a process in which an anesthetic agent interrupts the transmission of nerve impulses to that area; used for minor surgical procedures

Local infection an infection that is limited to the specific part of the body where the microorganisms remain

Local infiltration a process in which an anesthetic agent is injected into a specific area

Locus of control a concept about whether clients believe their health status is under their own or other's control

Logical positivism a philosophical doctrine that asserts that scientific knowledge is the only kind of factual knowledge

Logrolling a technique used to turn a client whose body must at all times be kept in straight alignment (like a log), such as a client with a spinal injury

Long-term memory the repository for information stored for very long periods

Lordosis an exaggerated concavity in the lumbar region of the vertebral column

Loss an actual or potential situation in which a valued ability, object, or person is inaccessible or changed so that it is perceived as no longer valuable

Low-density lipoproteins (LDLs) lipoproteins that carry cholesterol to the cells and deposit it there

Low-Fowler's position a bed-sitting position in which the head of the bed is elevated between 15 and 45 degrees, with or without knee flexion

Lung compliance expansibility of the lung

Lung recoil the tendency of lungs to collapse away from the chest wall

Lung scan an image of the lung produced using a detector or a moving beam of radiation

Maceration the wasting away or softening of a solid as if by the action of soaking; often used to describe degenerative changes and eventual disintegration

Macrominerals the minerals that people require daily in amounts of more than 100 mg

Macronutrients energy-producing nutrients (carbohydrates, fats, and proteins)

Macrophages large phagocytic cells that destroy microorganisms or harmful cells

Major surgery an operation that involves a high degree of risk for a variety of reasons; it may be complicated or prolonged; large losses of blood may occur; vital organs may be involved; postoperative complications may occur

Male erectile disorder when a man experiences erection problems during 25% or more of his sexual interactions

Male orgasmic disorder when a man can maintain an erection for long periods (an hour or more) but has extreme difficulty ejaculating

Malignant hyperthermia a pharmacogenetics disease that can be triggered by exposure to certain anesthetic agents; signs include elevated carbon dioxide production, profuse sweating, tachycardia, and skeletal muscle rigidity, prior to developing a life-threatening rapid increase in core body temperature

Malleus largest of the three ossicles of the ear

Malnutrition a disorder of nutrition; insufficient nourishment of the body cells

Manager a person who is appointed to a position in an organization which gives the power to guide and direct the work of others

Manubrium uppermost portion of the sternum

Margination the aggregating or lining up of substances along a surface or edge (e.g., the lining up of white blood cells against the wall of a blood vessel during the inflammatory process)

Mass peristalsis involves a wave of powerful muscular contraction that moves over large areas of the colon; usually occurs after eating

Massage healing done through touch to stimulate the production of certain chemicals in the immune system that promote healing

Master's programs graduate study programs offered by universities that lead to a master's degree in nursing or a master's degree in science; they provide specialized knowledge and skills that enable nurses to assume advanced roles in practice, education, administration, and research

Mastoid a bony prominence behind the ear

Masturbation manual self-stimulation of the genital organs or other erogenous areas

Maturity the state of maximal function and integration; the state of being fully developed

Mean a measure of central tendency, computed by summing all scores and dividing by the number of subjects; commonly symbolized as X or M

Measures of central tendency measures that describe the centre of a distribution of data, denoting where most of the subjects lie; include mean, median, and mode

Measures of variability measures that indicate the degree of dispersion or spread of the data; include range, variance, and standard deviation

Meatus an opening, passage, or channel

Mechanical loads extrinsic forces, such as pressure, friction, and shear, that cause soft tissue damage and potentially lead to blood flow impedance, tissue necrosis, and pressure ulcer development

Meconium the first fecal material passed by the newborn, normally up to 24 hours after birth

Media literacy the application of critical thinking in assessing information grains from the mass media

Median a measure of central tendency, representing the exact middle score or value in a distribution of scores; the median is the value above and below which 50% of the scores lie

Medical diagnosis a diagnosis that refer to disease processes—specific pathophysiological responses that are fairly uniform from one client to another

Medical futility an effort to achieve a result that is possible but that experience suggests is highly improbable and cannot systematically be reproduced

Medical narratives provide information related to the nature and onset of physical symptoms, diagnosis, and treatment of a disease process

Medication (drug) a substance administered for the diagnosis, cure, treatment, mitigation, or prevention of disease

Medication history includes information about the drugs the client is taking currently or has taken recently

Medication reconciliation a formal process that aims to prevent potential medication errors and adverse drug events

Medicine wheel a way to describe the holistic world view of health and wellness held by Aboriginal people; it has many variations, but all emphasize "the way of good life" or "everyday good living" in the context of human behaviour and interaction

Meditation a mental exercise that directs the mind to think inwardly by closing the sense organs to external stimulation

Menarche onset of menstruation

Menopause cessation of menstruation

Menstruation the monthly discharge of blood through the vagina occurring in women who are not pregnant, from puberty to menopause

Mentors persons who serve as experienced guides, advisers, or advocates and assume responsibility for promoting the growth and professional advancement of less experienced individuals

Mercy killing (euthanasia) the act of painlessly putting to death persons suffering from incurable or distressing diseases

Message an expression of thoughts or feelings with verbal or nonverbal communication

Metabolic acidosis a condition characterized by a deficiency of bicarbonate ions in the body in relation to the amount of carbonic acid in the body, in which the pH falls to lower than 7.35

Metabolic alkalosis a condition characterized by an excess of bicarbonate ions in the body in relation to the amount of carbonic acid in the body; the pH rises to greater than 7.45

Metabolic syndrome a constellation of central obesity, dyslipidemia, hypertension, and insulin resistance leading to increased risk of type 2 diabetes mellitus and cardiovascular disease

Metabolism the sum of all the physical and chemical processes by which living substance is formed and maintained and by which energy is made available for use by the organism

Metabolism (of a drug; **detoxification, biotransformation**) the process by which a drug is converted to a less active form

Metabolites end products or enzymes

Metaparadigm a specific relationship among the four major abstract concepts related to nursing

Metered-dose inhaler (MDI) a handheld nebulizer that can be used by clients to self-administer an aerosol medication

mHealth mobile health; health care applications for smartphones and tablets

Microbial load the number of infectious agents present

Microminerals the minerals that people require daily in amounts less than 100 mg

Micronutrients vitamins and minerals

Micturition (urination, voiding) the process of emptying the bladder

Middle-level managers managers who supervise a number of first-level managers and are responsible for the activities in the departments supervised

Migration the movement of people, usually from one country to another

Millennial generation or **Generation Y** nurses born from 1979 to 2000 who are characterized as being at ease with computers, video games, and cell phones; and being able to multitask and easily establish rapport with team members, clients, and families

Millennium Development Goals (MDGs) eight goals identified in the United Nations Millennium Declaration to significantly reduce poverty and promote development by developing economic and social conditions in the world's poorest countries

Minerals substances found in organic compounds as inorganic compounds and as free ions

Minimally invasive surgery surgery that involves multiple small incisions through which specialized telescopic equipment is inserted to provide indirect visualization and manipulation of a specific body site or organ; sometimes referred to as *laparoscopic* or *keyhole surgery*

Minor surgery an operation that involves little risk, produces few complications, and is often performed in a day surgery facility

Miosis constricted pupils

Mixed hearing loss a combination of conduction and sensorineural loss

Mobile technology the use of smartphones, tablets, personal digital assistants, etc. by nurses to support health care delivery

Mobility the ability to move about freely, easily, and purposefully in the environment

Mode the score or value that occurs most frequently in a distribution of scores

Modelling observing the behaviour of people who have successfully achieved a goal that the person has set and, through observing, acquiring ideas for behaviour and coping strategies

Modulation a pain mechanism in which noxious impulses stimulate regions of the midbrain and then descending spinal fibres, from the thalamus through the midbrain and medulla to the dorsal horn, conduct nociceptive inhibitory impulses, and release endogenous opioids

Monosaccharides sugars that are composed of single molecules

Monounsaturated fatty acids fatty acids with one double bond

Moral aspect of ethics; concerned with what constitutes right action

Moral agents beings that are capable of actions that have a moral quality

Moral behaviour the way an individual perceives and responds to the requirements of people living together within a society

Moral development the pattern of change in moral behaviour with age

Moral dilemmas situations involving conflicting ethical claims

Moral distress occurs when the individual knows the ethically correct action to take but is unable to take the action because of internal or external barriers

Moral integrity the quality of one's character and integrated virtues, including honesty and truthfulness

Moral theories a set of abstract moral principles

Morality a doctrine or system denoting what is right and wrong in conduct, character, or attitude

Mortician a person trained in the care of the dead; also called an *undertaker*

Motivation the desire to learn

Mucus clearing device (MCD) a device used to help clients clear excessive secretions

Multidisciplinary care plan a standardized plan that outlines the care required for clients with common, predictable (usually medical) conditions

Musculoskeletal disorders (MSDs) a painful group of disorders affecting muscles, joints, tendons, ligaments, and nerves and typically affect the back, neck, shoulders, upper limbs, and knees

Music therapy treatment that consist of listening, rhythm, body movement, and singing to alter ordinary levels of consciousness and achieve the mind's fullest potential, induce relaxation, or promote self-expression

Mutual a quality of social support where individuals attempt to be supportive of each other

Mydriasis enlarged pupils

Myocardial infarction (MI) cardiac tissue necrosis owing to obstruction of blood flow to the heart

Myocardium cardiac muscle cells that form the bulk of the heart and contract with each beat

Myopia abnormal refraction in which light rays focus in front of the retina; nearsightedness

Myopic nearsighted

Narcolepsy a condition in which an individual experiences an uncontrollable desire for sleep or attacks of sleep during the day

Narrative charting a descriptive record of client data and nursing interventions, written in sentences and paragraphs

Nasoenteric tube a long tube that is inserted through one nostril and down into the upper small intestine

Nasogastric tube a plastic or rubber tube inserted through the nose into the stomach for the purpose of feeding or irrigating the stomach

Natural disasters events that disrupt the normal infrastructure of a country or region on a large scale that are usually climate related

Natural health products (NHPs) vitamins and minerals, herbal remedies, homeopathic medicines, traditional medicines, probiotics, and other products like amino acids and essential fatty acid

Natural resources assets that come from extracting resources supplied by nature, such as oil, coal, water, and timber, that can be used to create wealth

Naturalistic paradigm the assumption that there are multiple perspectives of reality, each existing within a context

Naturopathic medicine treatment that involves botanical medicine, homeopathy, clinical nutrition, hydrotherapy, naturopathic manipulation, traditional Chinese medicine, acupuncture, or prevention and lifestyle counselling

Negative feedback feedback that inhibits change

Negligence failure to behave in a reasonable and prudent manner; an unintentional tort

Neobladder a piece of ileum that replaces a diseased or damaged bladder, thus making a new bladder that is sutured to the functional urethra

Nephron the structural and functional unit of the kidney with each kidney containing approximately 1 million nephrons

Nephrostomy a surgical procedure that diverts urine from the kidney to a stoma

Nerve block chemical interruption of a nerve pathway by injecting a local anesthetic

Nervous system plasticity the fact that pain mechanisms in the peripheral and central nervous systems can change in response to continued noxious stimulation

Networking a process by which people develop linkages throughout the profession to communicate, share ideas and information, and offer support and direction to each other

Neurogenic bladder interference with the normal mechanisms of urine elimination in which the client does not perceive bladder fullness and is unable to control the urinary sphincters; the result of impaired neurological function

Neuropathic pain the result of a disturbance of the peripheral or central nervous system that results in pain that may or may not be associated with an ongoing tissue-damaging process

Neuroplasticity the ability of the brain to recognize its signalling and the processing of stimuli in accordance with the input from the environment

Neutral question a query that does not direct or pressure a client to answer in a certain way

Nitrogen balance when nitrogen output equals nitrogen intake

Nociception the physiological processes related to pain perception

Nociceptors receptors that transmit noxious information

Nocturia increased frequency of urination at night that is not a result of increased fluid intake

Nocturnal emissions orgasm and emission of semen during sleep

Nocturnal enuresis involuntary urination at night

Nondirective interview an interview using open-ended questions and empathetic responses to build rapport and learn client concerns

Nonessential amino acids amino acids that the body can manufacture

Nonexperimental design a research method in which the investigator does not manipulate the independent variable; used to measure characteristics and determine relationships or correlations among these variables

Nonmaleficence the duty to do no harm

Nonspecific defences bodily defences that protect a person against all microorganisms, regardless of prior exposure

Nonsteroidal anti-inflammatory drugs (NSAIDs) drugs that relieve pain by acting on the peripheral nerve endings to inhibit the formation of the prostaglandins that tend to sensitize nerves to painful stimuli; have analgesic, antipyretic, and anti-inflammatory effects; include acetyl salicylic acid (ASA) and ibuprofen

Nonverbal communication communication other than words, including gestures, posture, and facial expressions

Norm (standard) an ideal or fixed standard; an expected standard of behaviour of group members

Normal flora (resident flora) microorganisms that normally reside on the skin, mucous membranes, and inside the respiratory and gastrointestinal tracts

Normocephalic normal head size

Normocephaly normal head circumference at birth; usually 35 cm

Nosocomial infections infections that originate in a hospital or similar institution; this term is no longer used and has been replaced by *health care–associated infections*

Nothing by mouth (nil per ora [NPO]) all foods and fluids are prohibited

NREM sleep (non–rapid eye movement sleep) a deep restful sleep state; also called *slow-wave sleep*

Nurse informaticians nurses who have specialized knowledge and skills within the informatics discipline

Nurse practitioner health care professionals who diagnose and treat human illness and assist in rehabilitation, with their role also expected to be holistic and health promotive

NurseONE portal a website developed by the CAN to provide nurses with timely, easily accessible information on all aspects of health care

Nursing care conference a meeting of a group of nurses to discuss possible solutions to certain problems of a client

Nursing diagnosis the nurse's clinical judgment about individual, family, or community responses to actual and potential health problems or life processes to provide the basis for selecting nursing interventions to achieve outcomes for which the nurse is accountable

Nursing informatics the science of using computer information systems in the practice of nursing

Nursing Interventions Classification (NIC) a taxonomy of standardized nursing interventions

Nursing Outcomes Classification (NOC) a taxonomy of standardized nurse-sensitive client outcomes

Nursing practice standards provide guidelines for determining the quality of nursing care that a patient or client receives

Nursing process a systematic, rational method of planning and providing nursing care

Nursing research the systematic, objective investigation of phenomena (experiences, events, or circumstances) of importance to nursing, with the goal of improving practice

Nursing rounds procedures in which a group of nurses visits selected clients at each client's bedside to obtain information that will help plan nursing care, provide clients the opportunity to discuss their care, evaluate the nursing care the client has received, and identify alternative nursing possibilities from research and experienced nurses

Nutrients organic or inorganic substances found in food; nutrients are digested and absorbed in the gastrointestinal tract and then used in the body's metabolic processes

Nutrition the sum of the process of taking in, assimilating, and using nutrients

Nutritionist a person who has specialized knowledge about nutrition and food

Nutritive value the nutrient content of a specified amount of food

Nystagmus involuntary rapid movement of the eyeball

Obese having a body mass index of more than 30 kg/m^2

Objective data information (data) that is detectable by an observer or can be tested against an accepted standard; can be seen, heard, felt, or smelled

Obligatory losses the essential fluid losses required to maintain body functioning

Occult blood presence of blood that is undetectable to the naked eye

Occupational exposure reasonably anticipated skin, eye, mucous membrane, or parenteral contact with blood or other potentially infectious materials that may result from the performance of an employee's duties

Occupational therapist a health care professional who assists clients with impaired function to gain the skills required to perform activities of daily living

Official name (of drug) the name under which a drug is listed in one of the official publications (e.g., the *Canadian Formulary*)

Oliguria production of abnormally small amounts of urine by the kidney

Omega-3 fatty acids essential fatty acids and polyunsaturated fats that have been shown to lower serum triglyceride levels, reduce blood pressure, and decrease factors contributing to blood clotting and strokes; found primarily in cold-water fish, walnuts, flax, hemp, and canola oil

Omega-6 fatty acids essential fatty acids and polyunsaturated fats that have anti-inflammatory, vasodilator, and antithrombotic properties; arachidonic acid, found in meat, poultry, and eggs, is associated with an increased risk of coronary artery disease, diabetes mellitus, osteoporosis, and some autoimmune disorders; linoleic acid and gamma-linolenic acid can be found in cooking oils, including sunflower, safflower, corn, cottonseed, and soybean oils

Oncotic pressure (colloid osmotic pressure) a pulling force exerted by colloids that help maintain the water content of blood

One-point discrimination the ability to sense whether one area of the skin is being stimulated by pressure

Onset of action the time after administration until the body initially responds to the drug

Ontology investigates the nature of being

Onychocryptosis the inward growing of the nail into the soft tissue around it

Open system a system in which energy, matter, and information move into and out of the system through the system boundary

Open-ended questions queries that specify only the broad topic to be discussed and invite clients to discover and explore their thoughts and feelings about the topic

Ophthalmic related to the eye

Opportunistic pathogen a microorganism causing disease only in a susceptible individual

Oral related to the mouth

Oral–genital sex sexual stimulation of the genitals using the lips, tongue, and mouth; called cunnilingus when performed on a female and fellatio when performed on a male

Organizing to systematize or to provide structure

Orgasmic phase the involuntary climax of sexual tension, accompanied by physiological and psychological release

Orthopnea the ability to breathe only when in an upright position (sitting or standing)

Orthopneic position a sitting position to relieve respiratory difficulty in which the client leans over and is supported by an overbed table across the lap

Orthostatic hypotension decrease in blood pressure related to positional or postural changes from lying to sitting or standing positions

Osmolality the concentration of solutes in solution; the osmolar concentration of a solution expressed in osmols per litre of solution

Osmolar imbalance a state that involves the loss or gain of *only* water, so that the osmolality of the serum is altered

Osmosis passage of a solvent through a semipermeable membrane from an area of lesser solute concentration to one of greater solute concentration

Osmotic pressure pressure exerted by the number of nondiffusable particles in a solution; the amount of pressure needed to stop the flow of water across a membrane

Ossicles bones of sound transmission

Osteoporosis demineralization of the bone

Ostomy a suffix denoting the formation of an opening or outlet, such as an opening on the abdominal wall, for the elimination of feces or urine

Otic instillations instillations or irrigations of the external auditory canal; generally carried out for cleaning purposes

Otoscope an instrument used to examine the ears

Outcome evaluation focuses on demonstrable changes in clients' health status as a result of nursing care

Output energy, matter, or information from a system given out by the system as a result of its processes

Overhydration excess water in the extracellular fluid

Overnutrition a caloric intake in excess of daily energy requirements, resulting in storage of energy in the form of adipose tissue

Overweight body mass index between 25 kg/m^2 and 29.9 kg/m^2

Oxyhemoglobin hemoglobin combined with molecular oxygen for transportation in blood

Pace the number of steps taken per minute or the distance taken in one step when walking

Pain the unpleasant sensory and emotional experience associated with actual or potential damage, or described in terms of such damage

Pain management the alleviation of pain or a reduction to a level of comfort

Pain threshold the amount of pain stimulation a person requires before feeling pain

Pain tolerance the maximum amount and duration of pain that an individual is willing to endure

Palliative care care provided to reduce or alleviate uncomfortable symptoms but not to produce a cure; care that addresses quality of life concerns for those patients living for prolonged periods with a progressive debilitating disease

Pallor the absence of underlying red tones in the skin and may be most readily seen in the buccal mucosa

Palpation the examination of the body using the sense of touch

Pap (Papanicolaou) test a method of taking a sample of cervical cells for microscopic examination to detect malignancy

Paradigm (world view) is a particular way of thinking based on a specific set of beliefs, values, and assumptions

Paralytic ileus temporary (24 to 48 hours) cessation of intestinal movement caused by surgery that involves direct handling of the intestines

Paramedical technologist workers who assist or complete diagnostic tests, such as in radiology, laboratory, or nuclear medicine

Parasites microorganisms that live in or on another from which they obtain nourishment

Parasomnia a kind of sleep disorder in which abnormal events occur during sleep, such as sleepwalking or talking

Parenteral drug administration occurring outside the alimentary tract; injected into the body through some route other than the alimentary canal (e.g., intramuscularly)

Parenteral nutrition the intravenous infusion of water, protein, carbohydrates, electrolytes, minerals, and vitamins through a central vein

Paresis paralysis

Paresthesia an abnormal sensation of burning or prickling

Paronychia infection of the tissue surrounding the nail

Parotitis inflammation of the parotid salivary gland

Partial agonists drugs that block the mu receptors or are neutral at that receptor but bind at a kappa-receptor site; have good analgesic potency

Partial pressure the pressure exerted by each individual gas in a mixture according to its percentage concentration in the mixture

Partially complete proteins proteins that contain less than the required amount of one or more essential amino acids; cannot alone support continued growth

Partial-thickness wound a wound confined to the dermis and epidermis; heal by regeneration

Passive immunity a resistance of the body to infection in which the host receives natural or artificial antibodies produced by another source

Passive range-of-motion (ROM) exercise exercise in which another person moves each of the client's joints through their complete range of movement, maximally stretching all muscle groups within each plane over each joint

Paternalism an action that is based on what a parent would do

Pathogen a microorganism with the potential to cause disease

Pathogenicity the ability to produce pathological changes or disease

Pathological fractures a break resulting from weakened bone tissue; often caused by neoplasms or osteoporosis

Patient a person who is waiting for or undergoing medical treatment and care

Patient safety the reduction and mitigation of unsafe acts within the health care system

Patient-controlled analgesia (PCA) a pain management technique that allows the client to take an active role in managing pain

Patient-focused care a delivery model that brings all services and care providers to the client

Peak plasma level (of drug) the concentration of a drug in the blood plasma that occurs when the elimination rate equals the rate of absorption

Pedagogy the discipline concerned with helping children learn

Pediculosis infestation by head lice

Peer groups collection of individuals of equal status

Peer review when nurses functioning in the same capacity appraise the quality of care or practice performed by other equally qualified nurses

PERRLA an acronym used to record normal assessment of the pupils: pupils equally round and react to light and accommodation

Pelvic floor muscle exercises exercises that help to strengthen pelvic floor muscles and can reduce episodes of urinary incontinence; also called Kegel exercises

Perceived loss the loss experienced by a person that cannot be verified by others

Perceived self how a person sees himself or herself and how he or she is seen by others

Perception the ability to interpret the environment through the senses

Percussion (in assessment) a method in which the body surface is struck to elicit sounds that can be heard or vibrations that can be felt

Percutaneous the route of absorption of topical medications through skin

Percutaneous endoscopic gastrostomy (PEG) a procedure in which a PEG catheter is inserted into the stomach through the skin and subcutaneous tissues of the abdomen; used as a feeding tube

Percutaneous endoscopic jejunostomy (PEJ) see percutaneous endoscopic gastrostomy; inserted into the jejunum

Perfusion passage of blood constituents through the vessels of the circulatory system

Pericardium the double layer of fibroserous membrane that surrounds the heart, protects it, and anchors it to surrounding structures

Periodontal disease (pyorrhea) disorder of the supporting structures of teeth

Perioperative period refers to the three phases of surgery: preoperative, intraoperative, and postoperative

Peripheral neuropathic pain pain that follows damage or sensitization of peripheral nerves, such as phantom limb pain, postherpetic neuralgia, and carpal tunnel syndrome

Peripheral pulse a pulse located in the periphery of the body (e.g., foot, wrist)

Peripheral sensitization after injury, surgery, or inflammation, damaged cells release chemicals, such as bradykinin, histamine, and prostaglandins, which can change nociceptors so that they transmit spontaneous discharges, and respond at a lowered threshold to both nociceptive and non-nociceptive stimuli

Peripherally inserted central catheter (PICC) a catheter is inserted in the basilic or cephalic vein just above or below the antecubital space of the right arm

Peristalsis wave-like movements produced by circular and longitudinal muscle fibres of the intestinal walls; it propels the intestinal contents onward

Person in the context of the family the individual is viewed as the primary focus of nursing care and the family is viewed as a contextual influence

Personal digital assistant (PDA) a handheld device that allows nurses to access mobile health technologies

Personal hygiene the self-care that includes bathing, toileting, general body cleaning, and grooming

Personal identity the conscious sense of individuality and uniqueness that is continually evolving throughout life

Personal knowing knowledge that is concerned with the knowing, encountering, and actualizing of the concrete, individual self

Personal power power that is associated with admiration by others, which comes from such attributes as strength of character, passion, inspiration, or wisdom

Personal protective equipment (PPE) equipment that acts as a barrier to reduce a health care worker's exposure to microorganisms and reduce carriage of microorganisms by the health care worker on hands and clothes; includes gloves, gowns, facial protection, and respirators

Personal space the distance people prefer in interactions with others

Personal values standards internalized from the society or culture in which a person lives

Personality the outward expression of the inner self

pH a measure of the relative alkalinity or acidity of a solution; a measure of the concentration of hydrogen ions

Phagocytes white blood cells; they ingest microorganisms, other cells, and foreign particles

Pharmacist a person licensed to prepare and dispense drugs and prescriptions

Pharmacodynamics study of the actions of drugs

Pharmacogenetics how genetic variations, such as gender, size, and body composition, influence clients' responses to a drug

Pharmacokinetics the study of the absorption, distribution, biotransformation, and excretion of drugs

Pharmacology the scientific study of the actions of drugs on living animals and humans

Pharmacy the art of preparing, compounding, and dispensing drugs

Phenomenology a qualitative design that regards each human as having a unique experience; the researcher attempts to derive meaning from individuals' descriptions of their experiences through in-depth conversations

Phospholipids a glycerol molecule and two fatty acids together; work as emulsifiers to keep fats suspended in the blood and other body fluids; rich sources include liver, eggs, wheat germ, and peanuts

Photophobia sensitivity to light

Physical activity bodily movement produced by skeletal muscles that requires energy expenditure and can produce progressive health benefits

Physical dependence (on a drug) a physiological process in which the body adapts to the presence of an opioid such that its abrupt withdrawal or cessation results in physical symptoms

Physical restraints any manual method or physical or mechanical device, material, or equipment attached to the client's body that restrict the client's movement

Physician a health care professional who prevents, diagnoses, and treats human illness and assists in rehabilitation after the onset of disease or injury

Physiological dependence a type of drug dependence that is caused by biochemical changes in body tissues, especially in the nervous system

Physiotherapist primary health care professionals who analyze the impact of injury, disease, and disorders of movement and function

Picture and archiving communication systems (PACS) an application software system that allows digital images to be securely transferred and accessed by multiple health care providers

PIE an acronym for a charting model that follows a recording sequence of *p*roblems, *i*nterventions, and *e*valuation of the effectiveness of the interventions

Piggyback (additive setup or alignment) when an intermittent infusion is used to administer, at regular intervals, a medication mixed in a small amount of intravenous (IV) solution, a secondary set connects the second container to the tubing of the primary container at the upper port

Pilates a method of physical movement and exercise designed to stretch, strengthen, and balance the body, in particular the core or centre, including the abdominal region

Pilot study a small-scale trial run done before an actual quantitative study begins, to determine the feasibility of the data collection plan, identify flaws, and refine the research methodology

Pinna (auricle) flap of the ear

Pitch the frequency or number of the vibrations heard during auscultation

Pitting edema edema that leaves a small depression or pit after finger pressure is applied to the swollen area

Placebo response the experience of pain relief from an intervention that may not be directly related to the actual pain relief method employed

Planned change an intended, purposive attempt to make something different

Planning an ongoing process that includes assessment of the client and establishment of a plan of care

Plantar warts warts on the sole of the foot

Plaque an invisible soft film consisting of bacteria, molecules of saliva, and remnants of epithelial cells and leukocytes that adheres to the enamel surface of teeth

Plasma the fluid portion of the blood in which blood cells are suspended

Plateau a maintained concentration of a drug in the plasma during a series of scheduled doses

Pleural space the potential space between the pleural layers of the lungs

Pleximeter in percussion, the middle finger of the dominant hand placed firmly on the client's skin

Plexor in percussion, the middle finger of the nondominant hand or a percussion hammer used to strike the pleximeter

Pneumothorax accumulation of gas or fluid in the pleural cavity

Point of care (POC) technology and devices that can assist nurses in collecting and documenting data at or near the location of care

Point of care risk assessment a risk assessment prior to each individual encounter with a client to identify the most appropriate strategies to implement to reduce transmission of infectious agents

Point of maximal impulse (PMI) the point where the apex of the heart touches the anterior chest wall

Policy principles or rules that set standards of behaviour; plans or course of action

Pollution noxious or toxic substances that are in the air we breathe; can be both indoor or outdoor in nature

Polydipsia excessive thirst

Polysaccharides branched chains of dozens, sometimes hundreds, of glucose molecules; starches

Polysomnography electroencephalographic recording of activity (movements, struggling, noisy respirations) during sleep

Polyunsaturated fatty acids fatty acids with more than one double bond (or many carbons not bonded to a hydrogen atom)

Polyuria the production of abnormally large amounts of urine by the kidneys without an increased fluid intake

Population used in research to describe all possible members of the group who meet the inclusion criteria for the study

Portability the health care insurance plan of a province or territory can set only a limited waiting period for eligibility and pay the cost of insured health services provided while temporarily absent from the province or territory but within Canada

Portal of entry the entry point a microorganism uses to enter another person or host

Portal of exit the route by which a microorganism leaves a reservoir before establishing an infection in another host

Portals websites that allow a user to view information that is personalized and/or relevant to their role

Position power power that is related to the authority associated with a role or title and includes the power to manage people or command resources

Positive feedback feedback that stimulates change

Positive reinforcement giving rewards, such as praise for a learner's achievements

Possible nursing diagnosis a diagnosis in which evidence about a health problem is incomplete or unclear; requires more data either to support or to refute it

Postexposure prophylaxis any prophylactic treatment started immediately after exposure to a pathogen to prevent infection by the pathogen and the development of disease

Postformal thought a period following Piaget's formal operational stage that includes creativity, intuition, and the ability to consider information related to other ideas; postformal thinkers can comprehend and balance arguments created by both logic and emotion

Postoperative phase begins with the admission of the client to the postanesthesia area and ends when healing is complete

Postural drainage the drainage, by gravity, of secretions from various lung segments

Postural tonus sustained contraction of the muscles supporting the body's upright position

Potentiating effect the administration of one drug before, at the same time as, or after another drug increases the effects of the drug

Poverty a complex concept that includes low income as well as the limited choices and opportunities associated with low income

Power the capacity to influence another person in some way or to produce change

Prayer an appeal to a higher power; spiritual or religious context

Preceptor an experienced nurse who assists the novice nurse in improving nursing skill and judgment

Precordium an area of the chest overlying the heart

Preemptive analgesia the administration of analgesics before an invasive or operative procedure to treat pain before it occurs

Prefilled unit-dose system a prefilled syringe ready for use or a prefilled sterile cartridge and needle that require the attachment of a reusable holder (injection system) before use

Prejudice a strongly held option about some topic or group of people

Preload the degree to which muscle fibres in the ventricle are stretched at the end of the relaxation period (diastole)

Preoperative phase the period before an operation; begins when the decision for surgery has been made and ends when the client is transferred to the operating room bed

Presbycusis loss of hearing related to aging

Presbyopia loss of elasticity of the lens and thus loss of ability to see close objects as a result of the aging process

Prescription the written direction for the preparation and administration of a drug

Pressure ulcer an area of localized damage to skin and underlying tissue, usually as a result of external forces, such as pressure, friction, and shear

Primary health care (PHC) the point of entry into the health care system at which initial health care is given

Primary intention healing healing that occurs in a wound in which the tissue surfaces are or have been approximated and there is minimal or no tissue loss; it is characterized by the formation of minimal granulation tissue and scarring

Primary nursing one nurse is responsible for the total care of clients 24 hours a day, 7 days a week, and associates provide care when the primary nurse is not available

Primary port the port farthest from the client

Primary sexual characteristics relate to the organs necessary for reproduction

Primary skin lesions lesions that appear in response to some change in the external or internal environment of skin

Primary sleep disorders the person's main problem is a sleep disorder

Principle of utility the view that a good act is one that brings the most good and the least harm for the greatest number of people

Principles-based (deontological) theories ethical approaches or frameworks that emphasize duties, obligations, principles, and rationality in judging whether an action is right or wrong

Priority setting the process of establishing a preferential order of nursing diagnoses, client health outcomes, and interventions

Privacy a deserved degree of social retreat that provides a comfortable feeling

Prn order an "as needed" order, which permits the nurse to give a medication when, in the nurse's judgment, the patient requires it

Problematic substance use (drug abuse) a disruption in any area of an individual's life (medical, physical, financial, occupational, family, interpersonal, social, legal, or academic) caused by excessive intake of a substance either continually or periodically

Problem-oriented medical record (POMR) or problem-oriented record (POR) data about the client are recorded and arranged according to the client's problems, rather than according to the source of the information

Problem solving the process of recognizing, defining, and solving a problem

Procedures methods developed to govern the handling of frequently occurring situations

Process evaluation focuses on how care is given

Process recording the verbatim (word-for-word) account of a conversation

Proctoscopy visual examination of the interior of the rectum with a lighted instrument (proctoscope)

Proctosigmoidoscopy visual examination of the rectum and the sigmoid colon with a lighted instrument (proctosigmoidoscope)

Productivity a measure of performance

Profession an occupation that requires extensive education or a calling that requires special knowledge, skill, and preparation

Professional values beliefs that are acquired during socialization into nursing

Progress notes chart entries made by a variety of methods and by all health care professionals involved in a client's care for the purpose of describing a client's problems, treatments, and progress toward desired outcomes

Progressive relaxation a formalized relaxation technique designed to reduce stress and chronic pain

Prompted voiding clues provided to a client to support urination

Prone position face-down lying position, with or without a small pillow

Proprioception awareness of posture, movement, and changes in equilibrium and the knowledge of position, weight, and resistance of objects in relation to the body

Proprioceptors sensory receptors that are sensitive to movement and the position of the body

Protein-calorie malnutrition a serious nutritional deficiency; associated with starvation

Protocol order (collective prescription) a set of criteria and orders under which a medication is to be administered

Protocols preprinted and preplanned plans specifying the procedure to be followed in a particular situation

Protozoa single-celled parasites

Proxy directive a legal statement that appoints a proxy to make medical decisions for the client in the event the client is unable to do so

Psychological dependence emotional reliance on a drug to maintain a sense of well-being, accompanied by feelings of need or cravings for that drug

Psychomotor domain motor skills, such as giving an injection

Psychoneuroimmunology a field of study that examines the links between stress, the concomitant endocrine and immunological responses, and the development or exacerbation of illness

Puberty the first stage of adolescence, in which sexual organs begin to grow and mature

Public administration the nonprofit operation of health care insurance plans in each province and territory by a public authority appointed or designated by the government

Public health nurse (PHN) community health nurses whose practice focuses on the health promotion of populations and work in such settings as community health centres, schools, street clinics, youth centres, and nursing outposts

Pulmonary ventilation the movement of air between the atmosphere and the lungs

Pulp cavity the centre of the tooth, which contains the blood vessels and nerves

Pulse the wave of blood within an artery that is created by contraction of the left ventricle of the heart

Pulse deficit the difference between the apical pulse and the radial pulse

Pulse oximeter a noninvasive device that measures the arterial blood oxygen saturation by means of a sensor attached to the finger

Pulse pressure the difference between the systolic blood pressure and the diastolic blood pressure

Pulse rhythm the pattern of beats and intervals between beats

Pulse volume the strength or amplitude of the pulse; the force of blood exerted with each heart beat

Pureed diet a modification of the soft diet, which includes foods that are easily chewed and digested; liquid may be added to the food, which is then blended to a semisolid consistency

Purulent exudate an exudate consisting of leukocytes, liquefied dead tissue debris, and dead and living bacteria

Pus a thick liquid associated with inflammation and composed of cells, liquid, microorganisms, and tissue debris

Pyogenic bacteria bacteria that produce pus

Pyorrhea purulent periodontal disease

Pyrexia (hyperthermia, hyperpyrexia) a body temperature above the normal range; fever

Pyrogens chemicals that stimulate the production of fever

Qigong a Chinese discipline consisting of breathing and mental exercises combined with body movements

Qualifiers words that have been added to some NANDA labels to give additional meaning to the diagnostic statement, such as *deficient, impaired, decreased, ineffective, or compromised*

Qualitative designs a research method through which the researcher seeks to derive meaning and understanding from human experiences

Qualitative research an inductive approach to analysis; no formal instruments are used and instead, loosely structured narrative data are collected; data are analyzed by identifying themes and patterns that emerge

Quality (of sound) a subjective description of a sound (e.g., whistling, gurgling)

Quality assurance the evaluation of nursing services provided and the results achieved against an established standard

Quality improvement (QI) an organizational commitment and approach used to continuously improve all processes in the organization with the goal of meeting and exceeding customer expectations and outcomes; also known as *total quality management (TQM)* and *continuous quality improvement (CQI)*

Quality practice environments practice environments that have the organizational and human support allocations necessary for safe, competent, and ethical nursing care

Quantitative research a systematic, logical approach to studying phenomena that lend themselves to precise measurement by using quantification and statistical analysis

Quasi-experimental design a research method in which the investigator manipulates the independent variable but either the randomization or the control that characterizes true experiments is lacking

Race classification of people according to shared biological characteristics and physical features

Racism the assumption of inherent racial superiority or inferiority and the consequent discrimination against certain races

Radiation the transfer of heat from the surface of one object to the surface of another without contact between the two objects

Radiographic examination an examination done to diagnose a disease or assess the progress of a disease

Range the difference between the lower and upper ranges of a variable

Range of motion (ROM) the degree of movement possible for each joint

Rapport a relationship between two or more people that facilitates effective communication

Rationale the scientific reason for selecting a specific action

Reactive hyperemia a bright red flush on skin occurring after pressure is relieved

Readiness to learn behaviours or cues that reflect a learner's motivation to learn at a specific time

Receiver the listener, who must listen, observe, and attend

Recent memory information held in the brain for a few hours

Receptor the terminal of a sensory nerve that is sensitive to specific stimuli

Reciprocal mutual; to each other

Recommended dietary allowance is the amount of a specific vitamin, micromineral, or macromineral that 97% to 98% of healthy individuals should consume based on their age and sex

Reconstitution the technique of adding a solvent to a powdered drug to prepare it for injection

Record a written communication providing formal, legal documentation of a client's progress

Recording (charting) the process of making written entries about a client on the medical record

Referred pain discomfort perceived to be in one area but whose source is another area

Reflection thinking from a critical point of view

Reflective practice a nurse's ability to take information about experience, knowledge, or skills levels based on assessments, analyze this information, and determine how to act upon this information in the future

Reflective questions invite family members to think differently about themselves, health and illness concerns, and options for addressing concerns; they are nursing interventions because they can facilitate change

Reflective thinking thinking that focuses on the critique and evaluation of actions taken and lessons learned

Reflex an automatic response of the body to a stimulus

Reflexology a treatment based on massage of the feet to relieve symptoms in other parts of the body

Regeneration (tissue) renewal, regrowth, or the replacement of destroyed tissue cells by cells that are identical or similar in structure and function

Regional anesthesia the temporary interruption of the transmission of nerve impulses to and from a specific area or region of the body; the client loses sensation in an area of the body but remains conscious

Registration the listing of an individual's name and other information on the official roster of a governmental or nongovernmental agency

Regression a defence mechanism in which the person adapts behaviour that was comforting earlier in life to overcome the discomfort and insecurity of the present situation

Regulatory bodies nursing organizations that, through provincial or territorial laws, are delegated authority to monitor and discipline their own membership

Regurgitation the spitting up or backward flow of undigested food

Rehabilitation the process of restoring clients to useful function in physical, mental, social, economic, and vocational areas of their lives

Reiki a healing technique that channels life energy to someone through the hands to reduce stress and aid in relaxation

Relapsing fever the occurrence of short febrile periods of a few days interspersed with periods of 1 or 2 days of normal temperature

Related factors one or more probable causes of the health problem

Relational communication a style of communication used in palliative care that conveys being in relation to the patient and family; it is not about knowing the right thing to say or do or about having the appropriate communication skills—it is simply being yourself

Relational ethics theories suggest that individuals have a moral obligation to each other

Relational stance the thoughtful and purposeful choices that nurses make in clinical practice about the ways that they will interact with families

Relationship power the respect others have for someone's personal abilities, knowledge, or skills

Relationships-based (caring) theories an approach to ethics that, in judging the rightness or wrongness of an action, focuses on individual care and responsibility in promoting and maintaining relationships

Relaxation response (RR) a healthful physiological state that can be elicited through deep relaxation breathing with emphasis on a prolonged exhalation phase

Reliability the degree to which an instrument produces consistent results on repeated use

Religion an organized system of worship

REM sleep (rapid eye movement sleep) sleep during which the person experiences rapid eye movements

Remission a period during a chronic illness when there is a lessening of severity or cessation of symptoms

Remittent fever the occurrence of a wide range of temperature fluctuations (more than 2°C) over the 24-hour period, all of which are above normal

Remote (geographical) located far away from urban and even rural centres

Renal ultrasonography a noninvasive test that uses reflected sound waves to visualize the kidneys

Report a prepared account of an event for formal presentation

Repositioning changing the client's body position on the same surface

Repression a defence mechanism in which painful thoughts, experiences, and impulses are removed from awareness

Research a methodical investigation to discover facts, prove or revise a theory, or create a plan of action

Research-based nursing practice nursing practice that is informed by valid and reliable research findings obtained from scientific investigations

Research design the method that will be used in the study or investigation to answer the research question

Research problem the situation that needs to be described, explained, or predicted

Research process a formalized, logical, systematic approach to problem solving

Research question the statement, question, or hypothesis that a researcher will be addressing

Reservoirs sources of microorganisms

Resident flora (normal flora) microorganisms that normally reside on skin, mucous membranes, and inside the respiratory and gastrointestinal tracts

Residual urine the amount of urine remaining in the bladder after a person has voided

Resolution phase the period of return to an unaroused state after sexual stimulation or orgasm

Resonance a low-pitched, hollow sound produced over normal lung tissue when the chest is percussed

Respiration the act of breathing; transport of oxygen from the atmosphere to the body cells and transport of carbon dioxide from the cells to the atmosphere

Respirators masks made of a high-filtration material that are designed to create a tight seal around the mouth and nose

Respiratory acidosis a state of excessive carbon dioxide in the body

Respiratory alkalosis a state of excessive loss of carbon dioxide from the body

Respiratory arrest the sudden cessation of breathing

Respiratory diseases disease that affect the respiratory system, which are the organs involved in breathing (the nose, throat, larynx, trachea, bronchi, and lungs)

Respiratory hygiene coughing or sneezing into tissues or cloth rather than the hands to reduce transmission of infectious agents through respiratory secretions

Respiratory quality or respiratory character those aspects of breathing that are different from normal, effortless breathing; includes the amount of effort exerted to breathe and the sounds produced by breathing

Respiratory rhythm or pattern the regularity of the expirations and the inspirations, which are normally evenly spaced

Respiratory therapist health care professionals who assist physicians with the diagnosis and treatment of lung disorders

Respite care temporary relief services for the primary care provider of a dependent adult

Responsibility an obligation to complete a task

Resting energy expenditure (REE) the baseline number of calories required to support involuntary body functions without a previous 12-hour fasting period

Resting tremor a tremor that is apparent when the client is at rest and diminishes with activity

Restorative justice an approach to criminal justice that involves righting the wrong, as much as possible, through reconciliation, healing, and building peace within communities

Restraints protective devices used to limit physical activity of the client or a part of the client's body

Reticular activating system (RAS) part of the brain stem; mediates the arousal mechanism through two components: the reticular excitatory area (REA) and the reticular inhibitory area (RIA)

Retrograde pyelography radiography performed after a contrast medium is injected through ureteral catheters into the kidneys

Retrospective audit the evaluation of client outcomes and nursing care after the client has been discharged from the agency; frequently uses chart review and client interviews

Review of the literature a determination of what is known and what is not known about a problem based on published research results

Right of self-determination subjects in research studies should feel free of undue influence to participate in a study

Rigor mortis the stiffening of the body that occurs after death

Rinne test a test to compare air conduction to bone conduction

Risk factors features that cause a client to be vulnerable to developing a health problem

Risk nursing diagnosis a clinical judgment that a problem does not yet exist, but the presence of risk factors indicates that a problem is likely to develop unless the nurse intervenes

Role the set of expectations about how a person occupying a specific position behaves

Role ambiguity unclear role expectations; people do not know what to do or how to do it and are unable to predict the reactions of others to their behaviour

Role conflicts clashes between the beliefs or behaviours imposed by two or more roles fulfilled by one person

Role development socialization into a specific role

Role mastery performance of role behaviours that meet social expectations

Role of the nurse in health promotion the role can involve advocacy, consultation, teaching, facilitation, or coordination of health care services

Role performance what a person does in a particular role in relation to the behaviours expected of that role

Role strain a generalized state of frustration or anxiety experienced with the stress of role conflict and ambiguity

Routine practices measures used in the care of all clients regardless of their diagnosis or possible infection status that are used to prevent infections

Rural a word to describe places, such as the countryside, towns, and small cities outside urban centres

S_1 the first heart sound, which occurs when the atrioventricular valves (mitral and tricuspid) close

S_2 the second heart sound, which occurs when the semilunar valves (aortic and pulmonic) close

Safe water water that is safe for human consumption; it is considered a basic human right that is essential to the full enjoyment of life and all other human rights

Sample portion of a larger group of subjects in a research study

Sandwich generation individuals who are providing for the needs of both their children and their aging parents

Sanguineous exudate an exudate containing large amounts of red blood cells

Sanitation the treatment and disposal of waste products making them safe for public health

Sarcopenia a steady decrease in muscle fibres that occurs with aging

Saturated fatty acids fats whose molecular structures are saturated with hydrogen, such as fats in meat, butter, and eggs

SBAR situation-background-assessment recommendation; a communication tool commonly used during change-of-shift reports to promote and maintain effective communication between the health care team when discussing a client's condition and progress

Scabies a contagious skin infestation caused by an arachnid, the itch mite

Scald a burn caused by hot liquid or vapour

Scientific method a logical, systematic approach to solving problems

Scientific or biomedical health belief the belief that life and life processes are controlled by physical and biochemical processes that can be manipulated by humans

Screening examination a brief review of essential functioning of various body parts or systems

Scrub nurse during operations, the nurse who assists the surgeon

Seasons (spirituality) the focus of some religions (Aboriginal peoples, Wiccan traditions) on Earth's seasons

Sebaceous glands minute glands in the skin that secrete fluid through hair follicles

Sebum the oily, lubricating secretion of glands in the skin called sebaceous glands

Secondary (side) effect (adverse effect) an unintended and undesired effect of a drug; they are usually predictable

Secondary intention healing healing that occurs in a wound in which the tissue surfaces are not approximated and there is extensive tissue loss; it is characterized by the formation of excessive granulation tissue and scarring

Secondary port the port closes to the client

Secondary sexual characteristics physical characteristics that differentiate the male from the female but do not relate directly to reproduction

Secondary skin lesions a lesion that does not appear initially but results from modifications, such as chronicity, trauma, or infection of the primary lesion

Secondary sleep disorders sleep disturbances caused by another clinical disorder

Seizure a sudden onset of excessive electrical discharges in one or more areas of the brain

Seizure precautions safety measures taken by the nurse to protect clients from injury in the event of a seizure

Self-awareness the relationship between a person's perception of himself or herself and others' perceptions of him or her

Self-concept the collection of ideas, feelings, and beliefs a person has about himself or herself

Self-esteem the value a person has for himself or herself; self-confidence

Self-regulation the homeostatic mechanisms that come into play automatically in a healthy person

Semicircular canals the passages in the inner ear

Semi-Fowler's position a bed-sitting position in which the head of the bed is elevated 15 to 45 degrees, with or without knee flexion

Sender a person or group who wants to convey a message to another

Sensitization pain mechanisms in the PNS and CNS changing in response to continued noxious stimulation

Sensorineural hearing loss is the result of damage to the inner ear, the auditory nerve, or the hearing centre in the brain

Sensoristasis the need for sensory stimulation

Sensory deficit partial or complete impairment of any sensory organ

Sensory deprivation insufficient sensory stimulation for a person to function

Sensory memory momentary perception of stimuli by the senses

Sensory overload an overabundance of sensory stimulation

Sensory perception the organization and translation of stimuli into meaningful information

Sensory reception the process of receiving environmental stimuli

Separation anxiety the fear and frustration experienced by young children that comes with parental absences

Septicemia a systemic disease associated with presence of pathogenic microorganisms or their toxins in blood

Serosanguineous exudate an exudate composed of serum and blood

Serous exudate inflammatory material composed of serum (clear portion of blood) derived from blood and serous membranes, such as the peritoneum, pleura, pericardium, and meninges; is watery in appearance and has few cells

Servant leaders a subtype of the transformational leader based on the concept that leaders serve their followers

Sexual aversion disorder a severe distaste for sexual activity or the thought of sexual activity, which then leads to a phobic avoidance of sex

Sexual health the integration of the somatic, emotional, intellectual, and social aspects of sexuality in ways that are positively enriching and that enhance personality, communication, and love

Sexuality the collective characteristics that mark the differences between the male and female, the constitution and life of the individual as related to sex

Sexual orientation a person's attraction to people of the same sex, to people of the opposite sex, or to both sexes

Sexual self-concept how a person views him or herself as a sexual being

Shaft (cannula) a tube with a lumen (channel) that is inserted into a cavity or duct and is often fitted with a trocar during insertion

Shaken baby syndrome (SBS) a constellation of severe injuries, such as cerebral damage, neurological defects, blindness, and intellectual disorders, caused by deliberate whiplash shaking of an infant; injuries often occur without external evidence of head injury; should be suspected in infants younger than 1 year old who have apnea, seizures, lethargy or drowsiness, bradycardia, or respiratory difficulty, who are in coma, or who die

Shared governance a method that aims to distribute decision making among a group of people

Shared leadership a contemporary theory of leadership that recognizes the leadership capabilities of each member in a professional group and assumes that appropriate leadership will emerge in relation to the challenges that confront the group

Shearing a combination of friction and pressure that when applied to the skin results in damage to blood vessels and tissues

Shock phase the second stage of the general adaptation syndrome described by Selye

Short-term memory information held in the brain for a few minutes

Shroud a large piece of plastic or cotton material that wraps a body after death

Silent Generation nurses born from 1933 to 1944 who are characterized as having a traditional work ethic and good critical thinking skills, being disciplined and loyal team players, and sharing knowledge and expertise readily with their colleagues

Sims' (semi-prone) position a side-lying position with the lowermost arm behind the body and uppermost leg flexed

Single order a one-time order (e.g., of medication)

Sinoatrial (SA or sinus) node the primary pacemaker of the heart

Situational leaders leaders who adopt their style of leadership on the basis of the readiness and willingness of the group

Sitz bath a hip bath used to soak a client's pelvic area by using a special tub or chair that immerses the client from the midthighs to the iliac crests or umbilicus

Sleep a period of rest for the body and mind in which bodily functions are partially suspended

Sleep apnea periodic cessation of breathing during sleep

Sleep architecture the basic organization of normal sleep

Slow-wave sleep (SWS) deep sleep in which the sleeper's heart and respiratory rates drop 20% to 30% lower than those exhibited during waking hours, the sleeper is difficult to arouse, the person is not disturbed by sensory stimuli, the skeletal muscles are very relaxed, the reflexes are diminished, and snoring is most likely to occur

Small calorie (c, cal, calorie) the amount of heat required to raise the temperature of 1 g of water 1°C

SOAPIER an acronym for a charting method that follows a recording sequence of *s*ubjective data, *o*bjective data, *a*ssessment, *p*lanning, *i*nterventions, *e*valuation, and *r*evision

Social determinants of health differences in the health status of populations based on the unequal distribution of power, income, goods, and services, both globally and nationally

Social justice a concept based on the principles of equity, equality, and respect for human rights; broadly concerned with the equitable bearing of burdens and reaping of benefits in society

Social media websites that allow users to generate and share content with others

Social support help that fosters successful coping and promotes satisfying and effective living

Social support systems others outside the immediate family unit who provide strength, encouragement, and assistance to the family, especially during a crisis

Social worker a professional who promotes social change aimed at improving conditions that affect the health and well-being of individuals, families, groups, and communities

Socialization a process by which a person learns the ways of a group or society to become a functioning participant

Socratic questioning questions that let nurses look beneath the surface, recognize and examine assumptions, search for inconsistencies, examine multiple points of view, and differentiate what they know from what they merely believe

Soft diet foods that are easily chewed and digested

Software applications or programs that control computer hardware and, in essence, are instructions that direct a computer's hardware to function

Soluble fibre fibre that, as it passes through the digestive tract, breaks down and forms a gel that is thought to reduce the amount of cholesterol that is absorbed; sources include oats, legumes, some seeds, brown rice, barley, oats, fruits, some green vegetables, and potatoes

Solutes substances dissolved in a liquid

Solution containers IV containers that are available in various sizes

Solvent the liquid in which solutes are dissolved

Somatic pain discomfort that arises from ligaments, tendons, bones, blood vessels, and nerves

Sordes accumulation of foul matter (food, microorganisms, and epithelial elements) on teeth and gums

Source-oriented record a record in which each person or department makes notations in a separate section or sections of the client's chart

Spastic the sudden, prolonged involuntary muscle contractions of clients with damage to the central nervous system

Specific defences ways the body defends itself from microorganisms, mostly involving the immune system, which responds to foreign proteins in the body

Specific gravity the weight or degree of concentration of a substance compared with that of an equal volume of another, such as distilled water, taken as a standard

Specific self-esteem how much an individual approves of a certain part of himself or herself

Spinal anesthesia anesthesia produced by injecting an anesthetic agent into the subarachnoid space surrounding the spinal cord

Spiritual distress a disturbance in or a challenge to a person's belief or value system that provides strength, hope, and meaning to life

Spiritual health a feeling of inner peace and of being generally alive, purposeful, and fulfilled; the feeling is rooted in spiritual values or specific religious beliefs

Spiritual well-being harmonious interconnectedness, creative energy, and faith in a power greater than oneself

Spiritual wellness a way of life that is rooted in spiritual values or beliefs and views life as purposeful and pleasurable

Spirituality belief in or relationship with some higher power, creative force, driving being, or infinite source of energy

Sputum the mucus secretion from the lungs, bronchi, and trachea

Stage of exhaustion the third phase of Selye's general adaptation syndrome

Stage of resistance (SR) the second phase of Selye's general adaptation syndrome

Stagnation (Erikson) a sense of boredom and impoverishment experienced by middle-age adults who are unable to expand their interests and who do not assume the responsibilities of middle age

Standard a generally accepted rule, model, pattern, or measure

Standard deviation the most frequently used measure of variability, indicating the average to which scores deviate from the mean; commonly symbolized as *SD* or *S*

Standardized care plans preprinted guides for giving nursing care of clients with common needs (e.g., a nursing diagnosis)

Standardized language the use of a body of terms that has been agreed upon by an overarching authority or by general consent

Standards of care detailed guidelines describing the minimal nursing care that can reasonably be expected to ensure high quality care in a defined situation (e.g., a medical diagnosis or a diagnostic test)

Standing order a written and approved document containing rules, policies, procedures, regulations, and orders for the conduct of client care in various identified clinical settings

Stapes one of the three ossicles of the ear

Starches insoluble, nonsweet forms of carbohydrate

Stat order a single order of medication that is to be administered immediately

Steatorrhea fat in stool

Stereognosis the ability to recognize objects by touching and manipulating them

Stereotyping assuming that all members of a culture or ethnic group are alike

Sterile field a specified area that is considered free from microorganisms

Sterile technique those practices that keep an area or object free of all microorganisms

Sterilization a process that destroys all microorganisms, including spores

Sternum breastbone

Sterols carbon, hydrogen, and oxygen arranged in rings

Stimulus an agent or act that stimulates a nerve receptor

Stimulus-based stress models frameworks in which stress is perceived as a stimulus that may trigger an individual's vulnerability to illness

Stoma an artificial opening in the abdominal wall; it may be permanent or temporary

Stomatitis inflammation of the oral mucosa

Stool (feces) waste products excreted from the large intestine

Strabismus squinting or crossing of the eyes; uncoordinated eye movements

Stress (as a stimulus) an event or set of circumstances causing a disrupted response; the disruption caused by a noxious stimulus or stressor

Stressor any factor that produces stress or alters the body's equilibrium

Stridor a harsh, crowing sound made on inhalation caused by constriction of the upper airway

Stroke volume (SV) the amount of blood ejected from the heart with each ventricular contraction

Structure evaluation focuses on the setting in which care is given

Study purpose what the researcher intends to do with the research problem identified; includes *what* the researcher will do, *who* the subjects will be, and *where* the data will be collected

Stupor a state in which the client is unresponsive but briefly arousable only during vigorous and repeated stimuli, and then immediately drifts back to unresponsiveness

Sty (hordeolum) redness, swelling, and tenderness of the hair follicle and glands that empty at the edge of the eyelids

Subarachnoid block anesthesia produced by injecting an anesthetic agent into the subarachnoid space surrounding the spinal cord

Subculture a group whose members share characteristics not common to the larger cultural group

Subcutaneous beneath the layers of skin

Subjective data data that are apparent only to the person affected; can be described or verified only by that person

Sublingual under the tongue

Substitute decision makers decision makers who know the client and can represent his or her best interests (speak on behalf of the client)

Subsyndromal delirium a person with one or more of the signs or symptoms of delirium, but he or she does not progress to delirium

Suctioning the aspiration of secretions by a catheter connected to a suction machine or wall outlet

Sudden infant death syndrome (SIDS) the sudden and unexpected death of an infant, in which a postmortem examination usually fails to reveal a cause

Sudoriferous (sweat) glands a gland of the dermis that secretes sweat

Suffocation (asphyxiation) lack of oxygen intake that can ultimately lead to unconsciousness and death

Sugars water-soluble carbohydrates that are produced naturally by both plants and animals

Suicide the act of a person deliberately causing his or her own death

Sulcular technique a technique of brushing teeth under the gingival margins

Superego the conscience of personality; the source of feelings of guilt, shame, and inhibition

Supine (dorsal) position a back-lying position; lying on the back with the face upward without support for the head and shoulders

Suppository a solid, cone-shaped, medicated substance inserted into the rectum, vagina, or urethra

Suppuration the formation of pus

Suprapubic catheter a catheter inserted above the pubic arch

Surface temperature the temperature of skin, the subcutaneous tissue, and fat; variable in response to environmental temperature changes

Surfactant a surface-active agent (e.g., soap or a synthetic detergent); in pulmonary physiology, a mixture of phospholipids secreted by alveolar cells into the alveoli and respiratory air passages that reduces the surface tension of pulmonary fluids and, thus, contributes to the elastic properties of pulmonary tissue

Surveillance monitoring disease outbreaks and threats to public health

Susceptible host any person who is at risk for infection

Sustainability in terms of global health, refers to the long-term maintenance of developed programs in a society

Sustainable happiness happiness that contributes to individual, community, or global well-being and does not exploit other people, the environment, or future generations

Suture (wound) a surgical stitch used to close accidental or surgical wounds; can also refer to the material used to sew the wound

Swing-through gait a crutch gait in which the client moves both crutches forward together and then lifts his or her body weight by the arms and *swings through and beyond* the crutch

Swing-to gait a crutch gait in which the client moves both crutches ahead together and then lifts his or her body weight by the arms and swings to the crutches

Synergistic effect the effect when one agent enhances the actions of another

System a set of interacting identifiable parts or components

System software computer programs that include instructions for the initiation, input, output, and storage mechanisms of a computer

Systemic infection an infection that affects the body as a whole

Systemic vascular resistance (SVR) impedes or opposes blood flow to the tissues and is determined by the viscosity, or thickness of blood, blood vessel length, and blood vessel diameter

Systole the period during which the ventricles contract

Systolic pressure the pressure of the blood against the arterial walls when the ventricles of the heart contract

Tachycardia an abnormally rapid pulse rate, greater than 100 beats per minute

Tachypnea abnormally fast respirations, usually more than 24 respirations per minute

Tacit knowledge knowledge that is learned from experience and once known often occurs without conscious thought

Tai Chi a discipline that combines physical fitness, meditation, and self-defence through soft, slow, continuous movements that are circular in nature

Tandem (additive setup or alignment) when an intermittent infusion is used to administer at regular intervals a medication mixed in a small amount of IV solution, the second container is attached to the line of the first container at the lower, secondary port

Tartar a visible, hard deposit of plaque and dead bacteria that forms at the gum lines

Task group a common type of work-related group in which the completion of a specific task if the main focus

Task power the ability to influence who is able to help with a process or task

Teaching planned method of instruction to an individual or group

Team nursing a group of nurses organized to do a task together

Technical skills "hands-on" skills, such as those required to manipulate equipment, administer injections, and move or reposition patients

Technological determinism a perspective that identifies technology as the primary actor in social changes

Telehealth the sharing of nursing information using electronic means, such as a telephone or the Internet, to answer consumers' questions

Telemedicine the use of technology to transmit electronic medical data about clients to persons at distant locations

Temperament the way individuals respond to their external and internal environments

Tension pneumothorax occurs when there is buildup of air in the pleural space that cannot escape, causing increased pressure, which can eventually compromise cardiovascular function

Teratogen anything that adversely affects normal cellular development in the embryo or fetus

Territoriality a concept of the space and things that individuals consider their own

Tertiary intention healing (delayed primary intention healing) healing that occurs when a wound is left open for 3 to 5 days to allow edema or infection to resolve or exudate to drain and are then closed with sutures, staples, or adhesive skin closures

Testicular self-examination a means of early identification of testicular cancer done by a man himself

Theistic based on a belief in a higher power or God

Theory a system of ideas that is proposed to explain a given phenomenon (e.g., theory of gravity)

Therapeutic baths bathing done for physical effects, such as to soothe irritated skin or to treat an area

Therapeutic communication an interactive process between nurse and client that helps the client overcome temporary stress, to get along with other people, to adjust to the unalterable, and to overcome psychological blocks which stand in the way of self-realization

Therapeutic effect (desired effect) (of drug) the primary effect intended of a drug; reason the drug is prescribed

Therapeutic touch (TT) a process by which practitioners believe they can transmit energy to a person who is ill or injured to potentiate the healing process without making contact

Third space syndrome a shift of body fluid into a space from which it is not easily obtained

Three-point gait a crutch gait in which the client moves both crutches and the weaker leg forward, and then moves the stronger leg forward; the client must be able to bear the entire body weight on the unaffected leg

Thrill a vibrating sensation over a blood vessel which indicates turbulent blood flow

Throat culture a specimen collected from the mucosa of the oropharynx and tonsillar regions using a culture swab

Thrombophlebitis inflammation of a vein followed by formation of a blood clot

Thrombus a solid mass of blood constituents in the circulatory system; a clot (plural: thrombi)

Throughput the process of moving from input to output within an open system

Ticks small grey-brown parasites that bite into tissue and suck blood, and can transmit several diseases to people, in particular Rocky Mountain spotted fever, Lyme disease, and tularemia

Tidal volume the volume of air that is normally inhaled and exhaled

Tinea pedis a fungal infection of the foot (athlete's foot)

Tolerable upper intake level the maximum amount of a nutrient that should be ingested to avoid any adverse effects

Tolerance (of drugs) a physiological process resulting in a larger dose of medication being required to obtain the same effect

Topical applied externally (e.g., to the skin or mucous membranes)

Topical (surface) anesthesia temporary interruption of the transmission of nerve impulses to and from a specific area of the body; applied directly to skin and mucous membranes

Tort a civil wrong committed against a person or a person's property

Tort law law that defines and enforces duties and rights among private individuals that are not based on contractual agreements

Total enteral nutrition (TEN) feedings administered through nasogastric or small-bore feeding tubes or through gastrostomy or jejunostomy tubes

Tracheostomy creation of an opening into the trachea through the neck

Tracheotomy incision of the trachea through the skin and muscles of the neck

Trade name (brand name) the name given by the drug manufacturer

Traditional Chinese medicine (TCM) the Chinese system of medicine that sees the body as a delicate balance of *yin* and *yang*: two opposing and inseparable forces

Traditional medicine refers to ways of protecting and restoring health that existed before the arrival of Western health care practices

Tragus the cartilaginous protrusion at the entrance to the ear canal

Transactional leader a leader who practises a contemporary theory of leadership in which resources are exchanged as an incentive for loyalty and performance

Transactional stress theory a theory that encompasses a set of cognitive, affective, and adaptive (coping) responses that arise out of persons–environment transactions; the person and the environment are inseparable and affect each other

Transcellular fluid a set of fluids that are outside of the normal compartments

Transcutaneous electric nerve stimulation (TENS) a noninvasive, nonanalgesic pain control technique that allows the client to assist in the management of acute as well as chronic pain

Transdermal patch a type of topical or dermatologic medication delivery system that administers sustained-action medications via multilayered films containing the drug and an adhesive layer

Transduction a pain mechanism in which the excited nociceptor converts the surrounding noxious stimulus into an electrochemical impulse that is then carried to the central nervous system

Trans fats fats that are made during partial hydrogenation of vegetable oils; also known as *trans fatty acids*

Transfer the movement of a client from one surface to another

Transfer belt an assistive device used when moving or transferring a client; it enhances safety and helps prevent back injury to the nurse

Transformational leader a leader who practises a contemporary theory of leadership in which the leader inspires and empowers others to share in a goal

Transgender individuals people who do not feel there is consistency between their sexual anatomy and their gender identity

Transmission a pain mechanism in which noxious information is conducted along two types of nociceptive fibres, A-delta and C fibres

Treatment nursing care intended to relieve illness or injury

Tremor an involuntary trembling of a limb or body part

Trial and error a type of problem solving where a number of approaches are tried until a solution is found

Triangular fossa a depression of the antihelix

Triglycerides substances that have three fatty acids; they account for more than 90% of the lipids in food and in the body

Trigone a triangular area at the base of the bladder marked by the ureter openings at the posterior corners and the opening of urethra at the anterior corner

Trimesters 3-month periods during pregnancy marking certain landmarks for developmental changes in mother and the fetus; three trimesters occur during pregnancy

Tripod (triangle) position the proper standing position with crutches; the crutches are 15 cm in front of the feet and 15 cm out laterally

Troponin an enzyme released into the blood during a myocardial infarction

Truths (spirituality) the focus of some religions (Buddhism) on noble truths

Tuberculin syringe a narrow gauge syringe calibrated in tenths and hundredths of a millilitre (up to 1 mL)

Tui Na a body massage treatment that uses acupressure, the purpose of which is to bring the body into balance; it is accomplished through a series of pressing, tapping, and kneading with palms, fingertips, knuckles, or implements that help the body to remove blockages along the meridians of the body and stimulates the flow of qi and blood to promote healing

Turgor normal fullness and elasticity

Two-point alternate gait a crutch gait in which the client moves the left crutch and the right foot forward together and then moves the right crutch and the left foot ahead together; the client must be able to bear at least partial weight on each foot

Two-point discrimination the ability to sense whether two areas of the skin are being stimulated by pressure

Tympanic membrane the eardrum

Tympany a musical or drum-like sound produced during percussion over an air-filled stomach and abdomen

Unconscious mind the mental life of a person of which the person is unaware

Undernutrition a caloric intake of less than the daily energy requirements, resulting in weight loss

Unintentional injuries harm that results from unplanned events, such as motor vehicle collisions, falls, drowning, fire, or ingestion of foreign objects

Universality all people in a province or territory must have access to the insured health services in the health care insurance plan of that province or territory

Unplanned change haphazard change that occurs without control by any person or group

Unregulated care providers (UCP) a health care provider who RNs can delegate certain components of nursing care to; the types of tasks that can be delegated vary nationally

Unsaturated fatty acids fatty acids that could accommodate more hydrogen atoms than they currently do

Upper-level managers organizational executives who are primarily responsible for establishing goals and developing strategic plans

Urea a substance found in urine, blood, and lymph; the main nitrogenous substance in blood

Ureterostomy a surgical procedure that brings one or both of the ureters to the side of the abdomen to form small stomas

Urgent surgery surgical intervention that is required within 24 to 48 hours

Urinary diversion the surgical rerouting of urine from the kidneys to a site other than the bladder

Urinary frequency the need to urinate often

Urinary hesitancy a delay and difficulty in initiating voiding; often associated with dysuria

Urinary incontinence (UI) a temporary or permanent inability of the external sphincter muscles to control the flow of urine from the bladder

Urinary reflux backward flow of urine

Urinary retention the accumulation of urine in the bladder and the inability of the bladder to empty itself

Urinary stasis stagnation of urinary flow

Urinary urgency the need to urinate with urgency

Urination (micturition, voiding) the process of emptying the bladder

Usual body weight the amount that an individual usually weighs

Utilitarianism a specific, consequence-based, ethical theory that judges as right the action that does the most good and least amount of harm for the greatest number of persons

Vacuum-assisted closure an adjunctive therapy that employs negative pressure (a vacuum) to remove fluid from difficult-to-heal wounds

Vaginismus the irregular and involuntary contraction of the muscles around the outer third of the vagina when sexual intercourse is attempted

Validation the determination that the diagnosis accurately reflects the problem of the client, that the methods used for data gathering were appropriate, and that the conclusion or diagnosis is justified by the data

Validity the degree to which an instrument measures what it is intended to measure

Valsalva manoeuvre forceful exhalation against a closed glottis, which increases intrathoracic pressure and, thus, interferes with venous blood return to the heart

Values personal beliefs about the worth of a given idea or behaviour

Values clarification a process by which individuals define their own values

Value set all the values (e.g., personal, professional, religious) that a person holds

Value system the organization of a person's values along a continuum of relative importance

Variable data information that can change quickly, frequently, or rarely, including such data as blood pressure, level of pain, and age

Variance a variation or deviation from a critical pathway; goals not met or interventions not performed according to the time frame

Variances nursing goals that are not met

Vector-borne transmission an animal or insect that serves as an intermediate means to transport an infectious agent into a susceptible host

Vectors of disease animals such as rats, ticks, flies, and mosquitoes that migrate and bring old diseases to new areas or give rise to new diseases

Vehicle-borne transmission a substance that serves as an intermediate means to transport an infectious agent into a susceptible host

Ventilation the movement of air in and out of the lungs; the process of inhalation and exhalation

Ventricles (of the heart) two lower hollow chambers within the heart

Veracity a moral principle that holds that people should tell the truth and not lie

Verbal communication use of verbal language to send and receive messages

Vernix caseosa a protective covering that develops over the fetus' skin; a white, cheese-like substance that adheres to the skin and can become 3 mm thick by birth

Vesicostomy a surgical procedure that attaches the bladder wall to an opening in the skin below the navel, forming an incontinent stoma

Vestibule contains the organs of equilibrium; found in the inner ear

Vestibulitis severe pain that occurs only when the woman's vagina is touched or vaginal penetration is attempted

Vial a glass medication container with a sealed rubber cap, for single or multiple doses

Vibration a series of vigorous quiverings produced by hands that are placed flat against the chest wall to loosen thick secretions

Vicarious liability the liability of an employer for the negligent acts of an employee done within the scope of the employee's authority or employment

Virions new virus particles

Virtue of good character

Virulence the power of a microorganism to overcome host defences and produce disease

Virulence factors evasion mechanisms of microorganisms

Viruses minute infectious agents smaller than bacteria

Visceral referring to the viscera

Visceral pain results from stimulation of pain receptors in the abdominal cavity, cranium, and thorax

Vision the mental image of a possible and desirable future state

Visual acuity the degree of detail the eye can discern in an image

Visual fields the area an individual can see when looking straight ahead

Vital capacity the maximum amount of air that can be exhaled after a maximum inhalation

Vital signs measurements of physiological functioning, specifically temperature, pulse, respiration, and blood pressure

Vitamin an organic compound that cannot be manufactured by the body and is needed in small quantities to catalyze metabolic processes

Vitiligo patches of hypopigmented skin, caused by the destruction of melanocytes in the area

Voiding (urination, micturition) the process of emptying the bladder

Volume expanders solutions given to replace volume when a client has lost a lot of body fluids but does not need red blood cells

Volume-control infusion set a small fluid container attached below the primary infusion container used to administer intermittent intravenous medications

Voluntariness the client's right to come to a decision without force, coercion, or manipulation from others

Vulvodynia constant, unremitting burning that is localized to the vulva with an acute onset

Waist circumference (WC) the measurement of the waist

Waist-to-hip ratio (WHR) the ratio of the waist and the hip measurements

Water-soluble vitamins vitamins that the body cannot store, so people must get a daily supply in the diet; include C and B-complex vitamins

Weber's test a test to assess bone conduction

Weight change comparison of usual and ideal body weight

Well-being a subjective perception of balance, harmony, and vitality

Wellness a state of well-being; engaging in attitudes and behaviours that enhance quality of life and maximize personal potential

Wellness assessment programs the use of positive methods of enhancement to apprise individuals of the risk factors that are inherent in their lives to motivate them to reduce specific risks and develop positive health habits

Wellness nursing diagnoses clinical judgments that identify transition toward a higher state of wellness; they may relate to an individual, family, or group and relate to health processes; form the basics of nursing interventions

Whistle-blowers people who report a perceived wrongdoing

Wind-up a condition where the spinal cord neurons become hyperresponsive and their receptive fields in the corresponding organs expand

Workflow a process of interconnected steps that depict an action or behaviour

World view a particular way of thinking based on a specific set of beliefs, values, and assumptions

World Wide Web (WWW) a collection of Internet software applications that allows the transfer of text, images, audio, and video

Xerostomia dry mouth

Yoga a type of meditation that is a system of exercises for attaining bodily or mental control and well-being

Zoomers older adults who tend to be informed consumers of health care

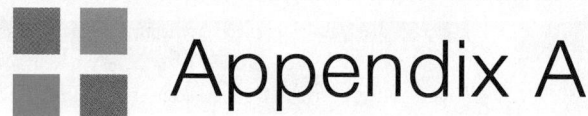

Appendix A

Laboratory Values

Abbreviations and symbols:

$<$ = less than

$>$ = greater than

fL = femtolitre (10^{-15} L)

IU = international unit

g = gram

mg = milligram (10^{-3} g)

µg = microgram (10^{-6} g)

ng = nanogram (10^{-9} g)

pg = picogram (10^{-12} g)

TABLE A.1 Hematology: Complete Blood Count with Clinical Implications

Component	Description	Normal Findings* (Adult)	Possible Causes of Abnormal Findings	
			Increased	Decreased
Erythrocyte (red blood cell [RBC]) count	The number of RBCs per litre of blood	M: 4.5×10^{12}/L to 5.3×10^{12}/L F: 4.1×10^{12}/L to 5.1×10^{12}/L	Primary polycythemia (e.g., polycythemia vera) Secondary polycythemia or erythrocytosis, usually caused by oxygen need (e.g., chronic lung disease, congenital heart defects)	Abnormal loss of erythrocytes Abnormal destruction of erythrocytes Lack of needed elements or hormones for erythrocyte production Bone marrow suppression
Hemoglobin (Hgb)	Composed of a pigment (heme), which contains iron, and globin (a protein)	M: 138 g/L to 180 g/L F: 120 g/L to 160 g/L	Polycythemia	Blood loss Hemolytic anemia Bone marrow suppression Sickle cell disease
Hematocrit (Hct)	The hematocrit represents the proportion of RBCs to the plasma	M: 0.37 to 0.49 F: 0.36 to 0.46	Polycythemia Dehydration Burns	Blood loss Overhydration Dietary deficiency Anemia

(continued)

TABLE A.1 Hematology: Complete Blood Count with Clinical Implications *(continued)*

Component	Description	Normal Findings* (Adult)	Possible Causes of Abnormal Findings	
			Increased	Decreased
Red blood cell indices (RBC indices)				
Mean corpuscular volume (MCV)	The mean or average size of the individual RBC	M: 78 fL to 100 fL F: 78 fL to 102 fL	Liver disease Alcoholism Pernicious anemia	Iron-deficiency anemia Lead poisoning
Mean corpuscular hemoglobin (MCH)	Amount of Hgb present in one cell	25 pg to 35 pg	Rarely seen	Iron-deficiency anemia
Mean corpuscular hemoglobin concentration (MCHC)	The proportion of each cell occupied by Hgb	0.31 to 0.37	Rarely seen	Iron-deficiency anemia
White blood cell (WBC) count	Count of the total number of WBCs in a litre of blood	4.5×10^9/L to 11×10^9/L	(Leukocytosis) Infection	(Leukopenia) Autoimmune disease
Differential count	The proportion of each of the five types of WBCs in a sample of 100 WBCs			
Neutrophils		55% to 70%	Stress Acute infection	Viral diseases Some drugs (e.g., chemotherapy, antibiotics such as nafcillin, penicillin, and cephalosporins) Radiation therapy
Lymphocytes		20% to 40%	Viral infection Mononucleosis Tuberculosis Chronic bacterial infections Lymphocytic leukemia	Adrenal corticosteroids and other immuno-suppressive drugs Autoimmune diseases (e.g., lupus erythematosus) Severe malnutrition
Monocytes		2% to 8%	Chronic inflammatory disorders Tuberculosis Protozoan infections (e.g., malaria) Chronic ulcerative colitis	Drug therapy: Prednisone
Eosinophils		1% to 4%	Allergic reactions (e.g., hay fever, medication) Parasitic infestations (e.g., round worms)	Corticosteroid therapy
Basophils		0% to 2%	Leukemia	Acute allergic reaction Corticosteroids Acute infections

(continued)

TABLE A.1   Hematology: Complete Blood Count with Clinical Implications *(continued)*

Component	Description	Normal Findings* (Adult)	Possible Causes of Abnormal Findings	
			Increased	Decreased
Platelet count	Platelets are fragments of cytoplasm that function in blood coagulation	150×10^9/L to 350×10^9/L	Malignant tumours Polycythemia vera	Idiopathic (unknown cause) Thrombocytopenic purpura Viral infections, including AIDS Systemic lupus erythematosus Chemotherapy drugs Some types of anemia

Normal laboratory values vary from agency to agency.

TABLE A.2   Hematology: Coagulation

Component	Normal Findings* (Adult)
Bleeding time	180 to 570 seconds
APTT (activated partial thromboplastin time)	24 to 36 seconds
PTT (partial thromboplastin time)	25 to 35 seconds
PT (prothrombin time)	11 to 13 seconds
INR (international normalized ratio)	0.81 to 1.2
Thrombin time	8 to 12 seconds
Fibrinogen	2 g/L to 4 g/L

Normal laboratory values vary from agency to agency.

TABLE A.3   Serum Electrolytes

Component	Normal Findings* (Adult)
Sodium (Na^+)	135 mmol/L to 145 mmol/L
Potassium (K^+)	3.5 mmol/L to 5.0 mmol/L
Calcium (Ca^{2+}) (total)	2.2 mmol/L to 2.58 mmol/L
Calcium (ionized)	1.0 mmol/L to 1.15 mmol/L
Magnesium (Mg^{2+})	0.65 mmol/L to 1.05 mmol/L
Chloride (Cl^-)	95 mmol/L to 105 mmol/L
Phosphate (PO_4^-)	0.97 mmol/L to 1.45 mmol/L
Serum osmolality	280 mmol/kg water to 300 mmol/kg water

Normal laboratory values vary from agency to agency.

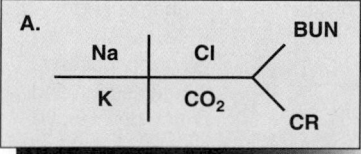

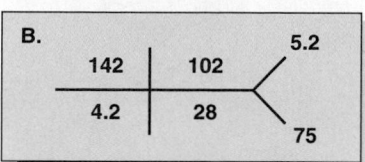

A: Format for a diagram of serum electrolyte results.
B: Example that may be seen in documentation notes.

TABLE A.4 Blood Chemistry Tests with Clinical Implications

Test	Normal Findings* (Adult)	Significance	Possible Causes of Increased	Possible Causes of Decreased
Glucose Regulation				
Random blood glucose (casual plasma glucose)	4 mmol/L to 6 mmol/L	Glucose provides body with energy; insulin produced by pancreas controls plasma glucose levels	Diabetes mellitus; stress response	Pancreatic disorders; liver disease; insulin overdose
Fasting plasma glucose (FPG)	3.6 mmol/L to 5.6 mmol/L	No oral intake for 8 hours		
Oral glucose tolerance (OGT)	< 7.8 mmol/L	Blood glucose measured 2 hours after ingestion of 75 g glucose solution	7.8 mmol/L to 11.0 mmol/L: impaired glucose tolerance (IGT); ≥11.1 mmol/L: diabetes mellitus	Not applicable
Hemoglobin A_{1c} (HbA$_{1c}$) (also referred to as glycosylated hemoglobin)	4% to 6%	A measure of the blood glucose bound to hemoglobin; reflects the blood glucose levels during the prior 3 to 4 months	Diabetes mellitus	Hemoglobinopathy; invalid test in people with beta-thalassemia
Liver Function Tests				
ALT (alanine aminotransferase)	M: 10 U/L to 55 U/L F: 7 U/L to 30 U/L	Marker of hepatic injury	Hepatitis; infectious mononucleosis; acute pancreatitis; acute myocardial infarction; heart failure	Not clinically significant
AST (aspartate aminotransferase)	M: 10 U/L to 40 U/L F: 9 U/L to 25 U/L	Found in heart, liver, and skeletal muscle; marker of hepatic injury	Liver damage (e.g., hepatitis, alcoholism, drug toxicity); acute myocardial infarction anemias, skeletal muscle diseases	Chronic renal dialysis; vitamin B6 deficiency
Albumin	35 g/L to 48 g/L; panic value: < 15 g/L	A protein produced by the liver	No pathology causes the liver to produce more albumin; an increased level may reflect dehydration	Chronic liver dysfunction; AIDS; severe burns; malnutrition; renal disease; acute and chronic infections
Alkaline phosphatase	25 U/L to 100 U/L	Found in the tissues of the liver, bone, intestine, and kidney. Used as an index of liver and bone disease when correlated with other clinical findings	Liver disease; bone disease; hyperparathyroidism; myocardial infarction; chronic renal failure; heart failure	Malnutrition; pernicious anemia and severe anemias; hypothyroidism; magnesium and zinc deficiency
Ammonia	35 µmol/L to 65 µmol/L	A byproduct of protein metabolism (converted by the liver into urea, which is excreted by the kidneys)	Liver disease; gastrointestinal hemorrhage	Renal failure

(continued)

TABLE A.4 Blood Chemistry Tests with Clinical Implications *(continued)*

Test	Normal Findings* (Adult)	Significance	Possible Causes of Increased	Possible Causes of Decreased
Amylase	< 125 U/L	An enzyme that catalyzes the hydrolysis of carbohydrates	Hepatitis (acute and chronic)	Liver disease (cirrhosis, acute alcoholism)
Bilirubin	Total: 5.1 mmol/L to 17 mmol/L Direct: 0.0 mmol/L to 3.4 mmol/L Indirect: 1.7 mmol/L to 17 mmol/L Panic value: > 20 mmol/L	A product of the catabolism of heme in red blood cells; excreted from the body in bile and urine	Total: Hepatitis; obstruction of the common bile or hepatic ducts; pernicious anemia; sickle-cell disease Direct: Cancer of the head of the pancreas; choledocholithiasis Indirect: Hemolytic anemias; drug toxicity; transfusion reaction	Not clinically significant
GGT (gamma-glutamyl transferase or gamma-glutamyl transpeptidase)	M: 1 U/L to 94 U/L F: 1 U/L to 70 U/L	Found primarily in the liver; also found in kidney, prostate, and spleen	Liver disease; alcohol abuse	Not clinically significant
Prothrombin	11 to 13 seconds Critical value: > 20 seconds for persons not on anticoagulants	A protein produced by the liver for clotting of blood	Liver disease, damage; vitamin K deficiency; obstruction of common bile duct; deficiency of factors II, V, VII, or X	Thrombophlebitis; malignant tumour
Cardiac Markers				
CPK (creatine phosphokinase) (also known as creatine kinase [CK])	Total: M: 38 U/L to 174 U/L F: 26 U/L to 140 U/L Isoenzymes: MM (CK_3): 96% to 100% MB (CK_2): 0% to 6% BB (CK_1): 0%	An enzyme found in the heart and skeletal muscles; has three isoenzymes: BB or CK_1, MB or CK_2, and MM or CK_3	Total: Acute myocardial infarction (MI); myocarditis; after open heart surgery; acute cerebrovascular disease, muscular dystrophy; chronic alcoholism CK Isoenzymes: MB (CK_2): Myocardial infarction; myocardial ischemia, angina pectoris	Not clinically significant
Troponin I (cTnI)	Troponin I: > 0.35 µg/L Critical value: > 1.5 µg/L	Cardiac troponin is highly concentrated in the heart muscle; this test is used in the early diagnosis of MI; after an MI, troponin I begins to increase within 4 hours, peaks at 12 hours, and remains elevated for 4 to 12 days	Troponin I: small infarct; myocardial injury	Not clinically significant

(continued)

TABLE A.4 Blood Chemistry Tests with Clinical Implications *(continued)*

Test	Normal Findings* (Adult)	Significance	Possible Causes of Increased	Possible Causes of Decreased
Lipoprotein Profile				
Cholesterol	Desirable: < 5.2 mmol/L	This test is an important screening test for heart disease	Type II familial hypercholesterolemia; biliary cirrhosis; chronic renal failure; poorly controlled diabetes mellitus; alcoholism	Severe hepatocellular disease; hyperthyroidism; malnutrition, chronic anemias, severe burns
HDL-C (high-density lipoprotein cholesterol)	Desirable: > 1.5 mmol/L	A class of lipoproteins produced by the liver; higher levels are beneficial.	HDL excess; chronic liver disease; long-term aerobic or vigorous exercise	Familial hypo-lipoproteinemia; familial hyper-triglyceridemia, poorly controlled diabetes mellitus, chronic renal failure
LDL (low-density lipoprotein)	Ideal: < 3.5 mmol/L; < 2.0 mmol/L = target level for people at moderate or high risk of heart disease	Up to 70% of the total serum cholesterol is present in the LDL. Lower levels are beneficial.	Familial type 2 hyperlipidemia Secondary causes can include a diet high in cholesterol and saturated fat, nephritic syndrome, multiple myeloma, diabetes mellitus, chronic renal failure	Hypolipoproteinemia; hyperthyroidism, chronic anemias, severe hepatocellular disease
Triglycerides	Desirable: 0.45 mmol/L to 1.69 mmol/L	This test evaluates suspected atherosclerosis and measures the body's ability to metabolize fat	Hyperlipoproteinemia; liver disease; renal disease; hypothyroidism; pancreatitis; myocardial infarction	Malnutrition; hyperthyroidism; brain infarction; chronic obstructive lung disease
Renal Function				
Creatinine	44 μmol/L to 133 μmol/L	Produced as the result of protein metabolism (especially from muscles) and is excreted solely by the kidneys	Renal disease; rhabdomyolysis; heart failure; shock; severe dehydration	Low muscle mass (e.g., muscular dystrophy, debilitation); severe liver disease
Blood urea nitrogen (BUN)	3.6 mmol/L to 7.1 mmol/L	End product of protein metabolism	Renal disease; severe dehydration; heart failure; gastrointestinal bleed	Severe liver disease; celiac disease; severe malnutrition; overhydration

*Normal laboratory values vary from agency to agency.

TABLE A.5 Arterial Blood Gas

Component	Normal Findings (Adult)
pH	7.35 to 7.45
Bicarbonate (HCO_3^-)	22 mmol/L to 26 mmol/L
$PaCO_2$	35 mm Hg to 45 mm Hg
PaO_2	80 mm Hg to 100 mm Hg
SaO_2 (oxygen saturation)	95% to 100%

TABLE A.6 Urine Analysis

Component	Normal Findings (Adult)
Colour, clarity	Straw, amber, transparent
Odour	Faint aromatic
Sterility	No microorganisms present
pH	4.5 to 8
Specific gravity	1.010 to 1.025
Glucose	None
Ketone bodies	None
Protein	None
Blood	None
Osmolality	500 mmol/kg to 800 mmol/kg

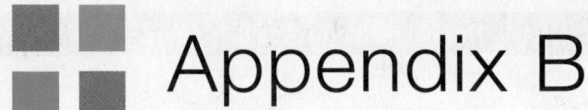 # Appendix B

Formulae

This appendix summarizes formulae that have been presented within the text.

Body Weight (see Chapter 40)

Body Mass Index (BMI)	BMI = weight (in kg/m^2) Normal: 18.5 to 24.9 (see Chapter 40, Table 40.6)
Waist-to-hip ratio (WHR)	WHR = WC ÷ HC (WC = waist circumference; HC = Hip circumference) Normal: F: < 0.8 M: < 1.0

Circulatory Indices (see Chapter 43)

Cardiac output (CO)	CO = HR × SV (HR = heart rate; SV = stroke volume)
Mean arterial pressure (MAP)	MAP = CO × SVR OR MAP = [(systolic pressure) + (diastolic pressure x 2)] / 3 (CO = cardiac output; SRV = systemic vascular resistance)
Ankle-brachial index (ABI)	ABI = posterior tibial *or* dorsalis pedis (whichever is higher) systolic pressure ÷ brachial artery systolic pressure Normal: 0.91 to 1.3 (absence of significant arterial disease)

Fluid Requirements (see Chapter 44)

Children Body weight 1 kg to 10 kg	100 mL/kg
Body weight 10 kg to 20 kg	1000 mL + 50 ml/kg for each kg above 10 kg
Body weight >20 kg	1500 mL + 20 ml/kg for each kg above 20 kg
Adults	30 mL/kg/day to 40 mL/kg/day

Intravenous infusion (see Chapter 44)

Millilitres per hour (mL/h)	mL/h = Total infusion volume ÷ Number of hours for infusion
Drops per minute (DPM; gtt/min)	DPM = (Total infusion volume × Drop factor) ÷ Total time of infusion in minutes

Medication dosage (see Chapter 33)

D = desired dose (i.e., dose ordered)

H = dose on hand (i.e., dose on label of bottle, vial, ampule)

V = vehicle (i.e., form in which the drug comes, such as tablet or liquid)

Basic formula $= \dfrac{D \times V}{H} =$ amount to administer

Ratio and proportion method: H : V :: D : x

Fractional equation method: $\dfrac{H}{V} = \dfrac{D}{x}$

Child dosages by using body surface area

$$\text{Child's dose} = \frac{\text{surface area of child (m}^2)}{1.7 \text{ m}^2} \times \text{Normal adult dose}$$

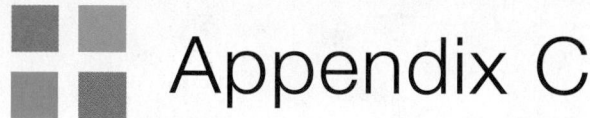

Appendix C

Vital Signs

Oral Temperature (see Chapter 29)

Hypothermia	$< 36°C$
Normal range	$36°C$ to $\leq 38°C$
Pyrexia	$> 38°C$ to $\leq 41°C$
Hyperpyrexia	$> 41°C$

Pulse and Respirations (see Chapter 29)

Age	Pulse (Average and Ranges)	Respirations (Average and Ranges)
Newborns (0–4 weeks)	130 (80–180)	35 (30–80)
< 1 year	120 (80–140)	30 (20–40)
1–4 years	110 (80–120)	25 (20–30)
5–8 years	100 (75–120)	20 (15–25)
9–10 years	70 (50–90)	19 (15–25)
11–19 years	75 (50–90)	18 (15–20)
20–64 years	80 (60–100)	16 (12–20)
≥ 65 years	70 (60–100)	16 (15–20)

Pulse Volume

Three Point Scale	Description of Pulse
0	Absent, not discernible
+1	Thready or weak, difficult to feel
+2	Normal, detected readily, obliterated by strong pressure
+3	Bounding, difficult to obliterate

Four Point Scale	Description of Pulse
0	Absent, not discernible
+1	Thready or weak, difficult to feel
+2	Normal, detected readily, obliterated by strong pressure
+3	Increased
+4	Bounding

Blood Pressure (Adults) (see Chapter 29, Table 29.6)

Category	Systolic (mm Hg)	Diastolic (mm Hg)
Normal	<130	and/or <85
High–Normal	130–139	and/or 85–89
Grade 1 HTN	140–159	and/or 90–99
Grade 2 HTN	160–179	and/or 100–109
Grade 3 HTN	≥180	and/or ≥110
Isolated Systolic HTN (ISH)	>140	and/or >90

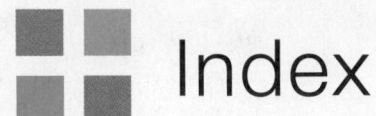

Index

Photo Credits

Chapter 1 1.1 – Hôtel Dieu, Quebec. From Gibbon, J., Mathewson, M. (1947). Three Centuries of Canadian Nursing. Toronto: McMillian; 1.2 – Library and Archives Canada/C-022763; 1.3 – Library and Archives Canada/Canadian Nurses Association fonds/e00241489; 1.4 – Library and Archives Canada/Health Canada fonds/e002504605. © Government of Canada. Reproduced with the permission of the Minister of Public Works and Government Services Canada (2012); 1.5 – Courtesy of the Victorian Order of Nurses Canada; 1.6, 1.7 – From Gibbon, J., Mathewson, M. (1947). Three Centuries of Canadian Nursing. Toronto: McMillian; 1.8 – Courtesy of the Wilberforce Heritage Guild Collection.; 1.9, 1.10, 1.11 – Courtesy of Cynthia Toman and Jayne Elliot, held by the AMS Nursing History Research Unit, University of Ottawa; 1.12 – © Elena Dorfman/Addison Wesley

Chapter 5 5.1 – Courtesy of the Faculty of Nursing, University of Calgary; 5.2 – Lynette Stamler; 5.3 – American Association of Critical Care Nurses (AACN) from AACN Ethics Work Group. (2004). The 4 A's to Rise above moral distress. Aliso Viejo, CA: AACN.

Chapter 10 Intro Box – Shutterstock/ Joachim Wendler.

Chapter 11 11.1 – Courtesy of Holly Graham-Marrs, Celia B. E. Clennell, and Aiyana Graham; 11.2 – Photo courtesy of the Aboriginal Healing Foundation, www.ahf.ca.

Chapter 12 12.2a – © Anne W. Krause/ CORBIS; 12.2b – Shutterstock/ fotorobs; 12.2c – Shutterstock/ Huntstock.com.

Chapter 14 14.1 – Courtesy of Kristen Knibbs; 14.2 – © Tetra Images / Alamy.

Chapter 16 16.2 – © Yuri Arcurs/ Fotolia.

Chapter 18 18.2, 18.7, 18.8 – © Elena Dorfman/Addison Wesley; 18.4 – © Jane Wattenburg/Addison Wesley.

Chapter 19 19.1, 19.2 – © Elena Dorfman/Addison Wesley.

Chapter 20 20.1 – © Yuri Arcurs / Fotolia, LLC; 20.2, 20.3 – Elena Dorfman/Addison Wesley.

Chapter 22 22.3 – © Alain McLaughlin/Addison Wesley; 22.5, 22.6 – © Elena Dorfman/Addison Wesley.

Chapter 24 24.5 – Neehr Perfect® networked educational EHR featuring WorldVistA. Courtesy of Archetype Innovations, LLC 2010.; 24.6 – © Blend Images / Alamy; 24.7 – © uwimages / Fotolia, LLC.

Chapter 25 25.2 – Courtesy of Royal Victoria Regional Health Centre, Barrie, Ontario.

Chapter 26 26.1 – © Alain McLaughlin/Addison Wesley; 26.3 – © Elena Dorfman/Addison Wesley.

Chapter 27 27.1a – c – © Alain McLaughlin/Addison Wesley.

Chapter 28 28.1 – © Richard Tauber/Addison Wesley; Table 28.3 – © Elena Dorfman/Addison Wesley; 28.2, 28.3 – © Richard Tauber/Addison Wesley;

28.4 – © Elena Dorfman/Addison Wesley; 28.5 – © Richard Tauber/Addison Wesley; 28.8 (1)–(7) DERMATOLOGY SECRETS IN COLOR 2/E. Fitzpatrick et al. Copyright © Elsevier (2001), (8) Reproduced with permission from the American Academy of Dermatology, Copyright © 2012. All rights reserved.; Skill 28.6 – (1)–(5) Richard Tauber/ Addison Wesley, (6), (8)–(10) – Patrick Watson, Pearson Education/PH; Skill 28.7 – (3), (5)–(7) Patrick Watson, Pearson Education/PH; Skill 28.8 – (1) © Elena Dorfman/Addison Wesley; Skill 28.9 – (1)–(4) © Elena Dorfman/Addison Wesley; Skill 28.10 – (1)–(3) © Elena Dorfman/Addison Wesley; Skill 28.11 – (1), (5) © Elena Dorfman/Addison Wesley; Skill 28.14 – (2)–(3) Patrick Watson/ Pearson Education/PH; Skill 28.15 – (1)–(9) © Elena Dorfman/Addison Wesley; Skill 28.16 – (1) © Elena Dorfman/Addison Wesley; Skill 28.17 – (1)–(6), (8), (10)–(16) © Elena Dorfman/Addison Wesley, (7), (9) Al Dodge, Pearson Education/PH, (1), (7) Patrick Watson, Pearson Education/PH; 28.36 – Patrick Watson.

Chapter 29 29.4a – Photo courtesy of Welch Allyn, Inc.; 29.4b – © doomu / Fotolia; 29.7 – Steve Gorton © Dorling Kindersley; 29.8 – © mihai romeo bogdan/ Shutterstock; Skill 29.1 – (1), (4) Madeleine Buck, (2)–(3) Patrick Watson; (5)a, (5)b Copyright © Exergen Corporation. All rights reserved; 29.9 – Patrick Watson; 29.10, 29.11 – From D'Amico, D., Barbarito, C., Twomey, C., & Harder, N. (2012). Health & Physical Assessment in Nursing, Canadian Edition, Pearson Education Canada. Reprinted with permission by Pearson Canada Inc.; 29.12 – © Elena Dorfman/Addison Wesley; Skill 29.2 – (1) c © Richard Tauber/Addison Wesley; Skill 29.3 – (1)–(3) Patrick Watson, (4)–(5) © Elena Dorfman/Addison Wesley; 29.15 – Madeleine Buck; 29.17 and Skill 29.6 – From D'Amico, D., Barbarito, C., Twomey, C., & Harder, N. (2012). Health & Physical Assessment in Nursing, Canadian Edition, Pearson Education Canada. Reprinted with permission by Pearson Canada Inc.; 29.20 – © Elena Dorfman/Addison Wesley; 29.21 – Courtesy of Nonin Medical, Inc.

Chapter 31 31.1, 31.2 – © Jenny Thomas Photography/ Addison Wesley; 31.4, 31.5 – Courtesy of Sara Daniels RN, MN; Skill 31.1 – (1), (2)a – c, (3), (4), (6), (8) Al Dodge/Pearson Education/PH College, (5) Patrick Watson, (7) © Jenny Thomas Photography/Addison Wesley; Skill 31.2 – (1), (2) From Berman, A. and Snyder, S. Skills in Clinical Nursing, 7th edition. Pearson: New Jersey, p. 192; Skill 31.4 – Al Dodge/Pearson Education/PH College; Skill 31.5 – © Elena Dorfman/Addison Wesley; Skill 31.7 – © Jenny Thomas Photography/Addison Wesley; 31.11 – © DAVID PARKER/SCIENCE PHOTO LIBRARY; 31.12 – © Sean Justice/Corbis; 31.13 – Courtesy of Sonic Innovations; 31.14a, 31.15 – © JANE SHEMILT/SCIENCE PHOTO LIBRARY; 31.14b – © rolafoto/ Fotolia; 31.16 – Courtesy of Starkey Hearing Technologies; Skill 31.9 – (1) Al Dodge/ Pearson Education/PH College, (2), (3), (6) Patrick Watson, (7) © Alain McLauglin/Addison Wesley; Skill 31.10 – Al Dodge/Pearson Education/PH College.

Chapter 32 32.1 – Left: © Tony Freeman/ PhotoEdit Inc., Right: © Peter Hudeck / Fotolia; 32.2 – © Michael Pettigrew/ Fotolia; 32.3 – © mocker_bat/ Fotolia; 32.4 – © dimedrol68 / Fotolia; 32.5 – © bst2012 / Fotolia; 32.6 – Advanta ™ Bed is a trademark of Hill-Rom Services, Inc. © 2010 Hill-Rom Services, Inc. REPRINTED WITH PERMISSION – ALL RIGHTS RESERVED.; Skill 32.1 – ① Courtesy of AlertCare, ② Image provided by Posey Company, Arcadia, California.; 32.7 – Image courtesy of Labelsource Ltd; 32.8, 32.10 – © Jenny Thomas Photography/Addison Wesley; Skill 32.3 – ②: Al Dodge/Pearson Education/PH College; 32.11 – Roy Ramsey/Pearson Education/PH College.

Chapter 33 Skill 33.1 – ③ Patrick Watson; 33.11 – Shirlee Snyder; 33.13, 33.15 – Patrick Watson; 33.20 – Elena Dorfman; 33.24a,b – © Richard Tauber/Addison Wesley; 33.25a – c – Patrick Watson; Skill 33.3 – ①–③ Patrick Watson; Skill 33.4 – ①–④ Patrick Watson; Skill 33.6 – ② Elena Dorfman; 33.29 – Copyright © 2012 Custom Medical Stock Photo – Custom Medical Stock Photo, All Rights Reserved.; 33.30 – Jenny Thomas; 33.31 – Courtesy of Logical Images, Inc.; 33.32 – Copyright © 2012 Eric Nelson – Custom Medical Stock Photo, All Rights Reserved.; 33.34 – Copyright © 2012 Custom Medical Stock Photo. – Custom Medical Stock Photo, All Rights Reserved; 33.37a and 33.38 – Courtesy and © Becton, Dickinson and Company.; Skill 33.9 – ①–④, ⑥ Berman, A. & Snyder, S. (2012), ⑤ Madeleine Buck. Skills in Clinical Nursing. (7th ed). Upper Saddle River, NJ: Pearson (Photos 1 – 6, Ch 17, p. 477).; Skill 33.10 – ① Jenny Thomas, ③ Courtesy and © Becton, Dickinson and Company.; 33.40 – Madeleine Buck; 33.41 – Adams, Michael; Josephson, Dianne L.; Holland, Leland N., Pharmacology in Nursing: A Pathophysiologic Approach, 1st Ed., © 2005. Reprinted and Electronically reproduced by permission of Pearson Education, Inc., Upper Saddle River, New Jersey.; Skill 33.11 – ②–③ Jenny Thomas; Skill 33.12 – ① Jenny Thomas, ② Patrick Watson; 33.47 – Courtesy of Briggs Healthcare; 33.49, 33.51 – Jenny Thomas.

Chapter 34 34.2 – Copyright © 2012 – Custom Medical Stock Photo, All Rights Reserved.; Skill 34.1 – © Queen's Printer for Ontario, 2008. Reproduced with permission.; Skill 34.2 – ①, ③–⑤ Al Dodge/Pearson Education/PH College, ② © Alain McLaughlin/Addison Wesley; Skill 34.3 – ①–④, ⑬ Al Dodge/Pearson Education/PH College, ⑤–⑥ Elena Dorfman, ⑦–⑩ Patrick Watson, ⑪–⑫ Alexandra Truitt & Terry Marshall; Skill 34.4 – ①–④ Al Dodge/Pearson Education/PH College; Skill 34.5 – ①, ④–⑦ Alain McLaughlin/Addison Wesley.

Chapter 35 35.1 – Photographs: Courtesy of Cory Patrick Hartley RN, Nurse consulting service, Dublin CA.; 35.2 – Copyright © 2012 Educational Images Ltd. – Custom Medical Stock Photo, All Rights Reserved.; 35.6 – Courtesy of Cory Patrick Hartley RN, Nurse consulting service, Dublin CA.; 35.8 – R.A. Penne-Casanova / Science Source; 35.9 – Clinitron ® Rite Hite® bed image is a registered trademark of Hill-Rom Services; Inc; © 2013 Hill-Rom Services, Inc. REPRINTED WITH PERMISSION – ALL RIGHTS RESERVED.; 35.10 – Image provided by Posey Company, Arcadia, California.; 35.12 – © Jenny Thomas/Addison Wesley; 35.13 – Berman, Audrey J.; Snyder, Shirlee, Skills in Clinical Nursing, 7th Ed., © 2012. Reprinted and Electronically reproduced by permission of Pearson Education, Inc., Upper Saddle River, New Jersey; Skill 35.4 – Courtesy of Cory Patrick Hartley RN, Nurse consulting service, Dublin CA.; 35.17a – c – Courtesy of Cory Patrick Hartley RN, Nurse consulting service, Dublin CA.; 35.18 – R.A. Penne-Casanova / Science Source; 35.19, 35.20 – Elena Dorfman/Addison Wesley; 35.27 – Patrick Watson; 35.29, 35.30 – Richard Tauber/Addison Wesley.

Chapter 36 Skill 36.1, Skill 36.4 – Elena Dorfman / Addison Wesley; 36.8 – Jenny Thomas; 36.9 – Richard Tauber/Addison Wesley.

Chapter 37 37.3 – Richard Tauber/Addison Wesley.

Chapter 39 39.1 – Patrick Watson; 39.31 – Patrick Watson; 39.43 – Courtesy of Wright Products, Inc.; Box 39.2 – ②–③ Provided courtesy of Posey Company, Arcadia, California; Skill 39.1 – ①–② Reprinted with permission of Glenys Moran and participants in the photo; Skill 39.2 – ①b Reprinted with permission of Glenys Moran and participants in the photo.; 39.51, 39.52 – Image provided by Posey Company, Arcadia, California.; Skill 39.6 – ② Reprinted with permission of Glenys Moran and participants in the photo., ③ Jenny Thomas Photography/ Addison Wesley; Skill 39.7 ①–③ Reprinted with permission of Glenys Moran and participants in the photo.; 39.56 – Jenny Thomas Photography/ Addison Wesley; 39.68 – 39.70 – Richard Tauber/Addison Wesley.

Chapter 40 40.8a, b – Centers for Disease Control and Prevention (CDC), retrieved from http://phil.cdc.gov/ phil/home.asp; 40.8c © 2012 Edward H. Gill – Custom Medical Stock Photo, All Rights Reserved.; 40.10, 40.11 – Elena Dorfman/Addison Wesley; Skill 40.1 – ② © karamysh / Shutterstock, ③ © Dmitry Lobanov/ Fotolia; 40.13a, b – Courtesy of C. R. Bard, Inc.; 40.14a, b – Courtesy of Abbott Laboratories.; Skill 40.2 – ① Elena Dorfman/ Addison Wesley; 40.16a – Courtesy of Abbott Laboratories.; 40.18 – © Kimberly-Clark Worldwide, Inc; Skill 40.4 – ③ Courtesy of Abbott Laboratories.

Chapter 41 41.12a, b – © Elena Dorfman/Addison Wesley; 41.14 – © Jenny Thomas Photography/Addison Wesley; 41.15 – © Elena Dorfman/Addison Wesley; Skill 41.1 – ④ © Elena Dorfman/Addison Wesley; 41.18 – Permission to use these copyrighted images has been granted by the owner, Hollister Incorporated.; Skill 41.2 – ①–②, ④ Courtesy of Cory Patrick Hartley RN, Nurse consulting service, Dublin CA., ③, ⑤ Courtesy of ConvaTec Inc.

Chapter 42 42.10 – © Jenny Thomas Photography/ Addison Wesley; Skill 42.2 – ②, ④ Courtesy of C. R. Bard, Inc. U-Cath is a trademark of C. R. Bard, Inc.; 42.14 – 42.17 – Courtesy of C. R. Bard, Inc.; Skill 42.3 – ①, ⑦ Courtesy of C. R. Bard, Inc.; Skill 42.4 – ①, ② – Courtesy of C. R. Bard, Inc.

Chapter 43 43.7 – © Elena Dorfman/Addison Wesley; 43.14 – © Richard Tauber/Addison Wesley; 43.17 – Shirlee Snyder; 43.19 – © Jenny Thomas Photography/ Addison Wesley; 43.20, 43.21 – © Elena Dorfman/ Addison Wesley; 43.22 – © Richard Tauber/Addison Wesley; 43.23 – © Jenny Thomas Photography/Addison